THE INTERNATIONAL TEXTBOOK OF CARDIOLOGY

Pergamon Titles of Related Interest

Verstraete/Vermylen THROMBOSIS
Duncan/Weston-Smith THE ENCYCLOPEDIA OF MEDICAL IGNORANCE

Related Journals

(Free sample copies available on request)

JOURNAL OF APPLIED CARDIOLOGY
THROMBOSIS RESEARCH
CLINICAL HEMORHEOLOGY

THE INTERNATIONAL TEXTBOOK OF CARDIOLOGY

Edited by
Tsung O. Cheng, M.D.
Professor of Medicine
The George Washington University School of Medicine and Health Sciences
Washington, D.C.
and
Visiting Professor of Medicine
Shanghai Second Medical University
Shanghai, China

PERGAMON PRESS
New York Oxford Beijing Frankfurt São Paulo Sydney Tokyo Toronto

Pergamon Press Offices:

U.S.A.	Pergamon Press, Maxwell House, Fairview Park, Elmsford, New York 10523, U.S.A.
U.K.	Pergamon Press, Headington Hill Hall, Oxford OX3, 0BW, England
PEOPLE'S REPUBLIC OF CHINA	Pergamon Press, Qianmen Hotel, Beijing, People's Republic of China
FEDERAL REPUBLIC OF GERMANY	Pergamon Press, Hammerweg 6, D-6242 Kronberg, Federal Republic of Germany
BRAZIL	Pergamon Editora, Rua Eça de Queiros, 346, CEP 04011, São Paulo, Brazil
AUSTRALIA	Pergamon Press (Aust.) Pty. P.O. Box 544, Potts Point, N.S.W. 2011, Australia
JAPAN	Pergamon Press, 8th Floor, Matsuoka Central Building, 1-7-1 Nishishinjuku, Shinjuku-ku, Tokyo 160, Japan
CANADA	Pergamon Press Canada, Suite 104, 150 Consumers Road, Willowdale, Ontario, M2J 1P9, Canada

---

First Printing 1986
Reprinted 1989

Library of Congress Cataloging-in-Publication Data

The International Textbook of Cardiology.

Includes index.
1. Cardiology. 2. Cardiology—International cooperation. I. Cheng, Tsung O. [DNLM: 1. Cardiology. 2. Cardiovascular Diseases. WG 100 I615]
RC667.158 1986 616.1'2 86-5094
ISBN 0-08-034310-4
ISBN 0-02-946026-3 (International Edition)

IE Printing: 1 2 3 4 5 Year: 9 0 1 2 3

Printed in the Republic of Singapore

ISBN 0-02-946026-3

To

My Loving Family,

My Inspiring Teachers, and

My Supportive Friends Throughout the World

Who All Made the Writing of This Text Possible

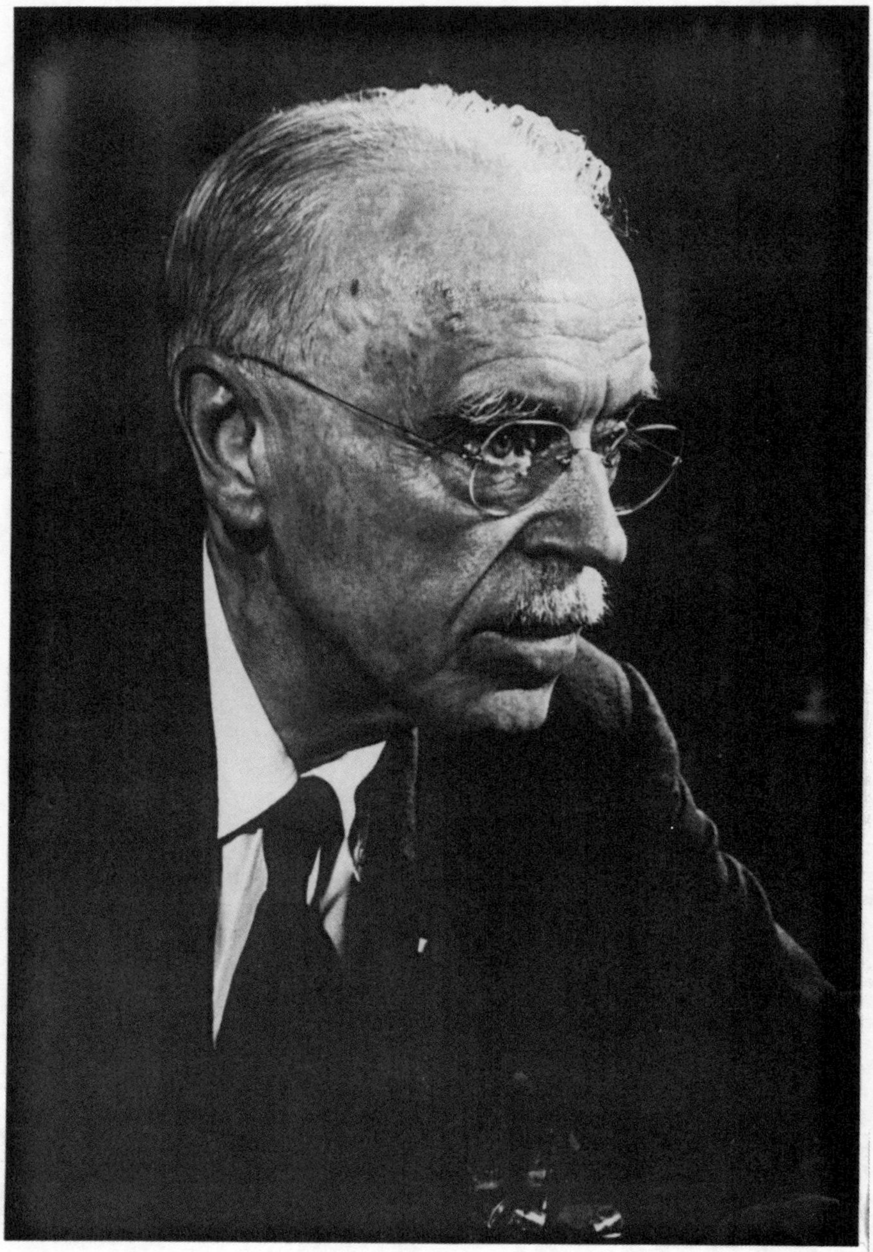

To Tsung O. and Mark Dudley Cheng
with kindest regards and best wishes
from Paul Dudley White

June 11,
1969

Foreword

When Dr. Cheng asked me if I would write a short foreword for his book *The International Textbook of Cardiology*, memories came flooding back to me of our wonderful early trips to China and the Soviet Union, to the many other countries we visited, and to the many friends we made there. A whole portrait gallery of those who came here to Boston to study and work and visit is imprinted on my mind. What a rich inheritance!

I am well aware of the distinguished position Dr. Cheng holds among his colleagues, of the tremendous number of outstanding contributions he has made in the field of cardiology. It is indeed an honor to write a short foreword to his book. There is another reason that is more personal and that delights me. Dr. Cheng has a son, Mark Dudley Cheng, named after Paul, born in 1957 in Boston when Dr. Cheng was at the Massachusetts General Hospital working with Dr. White. In 1972 Dr. Cheng visited the People's Republic of China, the first China-born physician from the United States to have that privilege. In 1973 he went again to China, this time taking his son, Mark Dudley.

For many years Dr. White thought, as most physicians do now, that the science and practice of medicine have a special role to play in bringing the people of the world together. Physicians have "no axe to grind," their sole purpose being to work and study together to help solve the multiplicity of problems that face them for the betterment of all people.

This book, edited by Dr. Cheng, would have been of enormous interest to Dr. White because it draws from the scientific studies done by Dr. Cheng and by other men and women from all parts of the world.

I thank Dr. Cheng for giving me the opportunity to feel again the excitement and value of this great work.

Mrs. Paul D. White

Ina Reid White
(Mrs. Paul Dudley White)

Foreword

[illegible]

Contents

VII. INTERRELATIONSHIP BETWEEN THE HEART AND OTHER BODY SYSTEMS

VIII. CARDIOVASCULAR PHARMACOLOGY

IX. ANTIBODIES IN CARDIOLOGY

X. CARDIOPULMONARY REHABILITATION

XI. NONCARDIAC SURGERY IN CARDIAC PATIENTS

XII. ANESTHESIA IN HEART SURGERY

XIII. RECENT DEVELOPMENTS IN CARDIOVASCULAR SURGERY

XIV. GERIATRIC CARDIOLOGY

XV. ENVIRONMENTAL FACTORS AFFECTING THE HEART

XVI. COMPUTERS AND CARDIOVASCULAR PRACTICE

XVII. PREVENTIVE CARDIOLOGY

XVIII. CARDIOVASCULAR NURSING

XIX. NEW CARDIOVASCULAR DRUG DEVELOPMENT

XX. MEDICAL COMMUNICATIONS IN CARDIOLOGY

Contributors

WILBERT S. ARONOW, M.D.
Medical Director, Hebrew Hospital for Chronic Sick, Inc., Bronx, New York, U.S.A.

JOHN C. BALDWIN, M.D.
Assistant Professor of Cardiovascular Surgery, Stanford University School of Medicine, Stanford, California, U.S.A.

JOHN B. BARLOW, M.D., F.R.C.P.
Professor of Cardiology, Department of Cardiology, University of the Witwatersrand Medical School; Chief Physician, Cardiac Unit, Johannesburg Hospital, Johannesburg, South Africa

NEIL D. BERMAN, M.D., F.R.C.P.(C), F.A.C.P., F.A.C.C.
Associate Professor of Medicine, University of Toronto; Director, Pacemaker Clinic, Toronto Western Hospital, Toronto, Ontario, Canada

RICHARD J. BING, M.D.
Professor of Medicine Emeritus, University of Southern California; Director of Experimental Cardiology and Scientific Development, Huntington Medical Research Institutes, Huntington Memorial Hospital, Pasadena, California, U.S.A.

VIKING O. BJÖRK, M.D.
Professor Emeritus, Karolinska Institute, Stockholm, Sweden; Director of Research, Heart Institute of the Desert, Rancho Mirage, California, U.S.A.

PETER C. BLOCK, M.D.
Director, Cardiac Catheterization Laboratory, Massachusetts General Hospital; Associate Professor of Medicine, Harvard Medical School, Boston, Massachusetts, U.S.A.

DAVID BREGMAN, M.D.
Chairman, Department of Surgery, St. Joseph's Hospital and Medical Center, Paterson, New Jersey; Associate Clinical Professor of Surgery, Columbia University College of Physicians & Surgeons, New York, New York, U.S.A.

GRACE E. BROWN, M.A., R.N., F.A.A.N.
Associate Director, Inpatient and Acute Services, University of Wisconsin Hospital and Clinics, Madison, Wisconsin, U.S.A.

EWALD W. BUSSE, M.D.
Associate Provost and Dean Emeritus, J.P. Gibbons Professor of Psychiatry, Duke University Medical Center, Durham, North Carolina, U.S.A.

SUPHACHAI CHAITHIRAPHAN, M.D., F.A.C.P., F.A.C.C., F.C.C.P.
Associate Professor of Medicine and Chief, Division of Cardiology, Department of Medicine, Siriraj Hospital and Faculty of Medicine, Mahidol University, Bangkok, Thailand

THOMAS C. CHALMERS, M.D.
Distinguished Service Professor, The Clinical Trials Unit, Mount Sinai School of Medicine, New York, New York, U.S.A.

MING C. CHAN, M.D.
Vice Chairman, Department of Medicine, Third Teaching Hospital, Beijing Medical College, Beijing, China; Research Fellow, Western Heart Institute, St. Mary's Hospital and Medical Center, San Francisco, California, U.S.A.

ALTAGRACIA M. CHAVEZ, M.D.
Department of Thoracic and Cardiovascular Surgery, The Cleveland Clinic Foundation, Cleveland, Ohio, U.S.A.

EUGENE I. CHAZOV, M.D., Ph.D.
Director General, U.S.S.R. Cardiology Research Centre, Moscow, U.S.S.R.

SHU-XIA CHEN, M.D.
Lecturer of Medicine and Vice Chief, Department of Teaching and Research in Medicine, Shanghai Second Medical University, Shanghai, China

TSUNG O. CHENG, M.D., M.S. (Med.), F.A.C.P., F.A.C.C., F.C.C.P., F.A.C.A., F.I.C.A.
Professor of Medicine, The George Washington University School of Medicine and Health Sciences, Washington, D.C., U.S.A.; Visiting Professor of Medicine, Shanghai Second Medical University, Shanghai, China

TE-CHUAN CHOU, M.D.
Professor of Medicine, University of Cincinnati College of Medicine, Cincinnati, Ohio, U.S.A.

DANIEL S. J. CHOY, M.D., F.A.C.P.
Director, Laser Laboratory, and Research Scientist, Investigative Cardiology Laboratory, St. Luke's-Roosevelt Hospital Center and Columbia University College of Physicians & Surgeons, New York, New York, U.S.A.

DOUGLAS C. CONAWAY, M.D.
Assistant Professor of Medicine, Temple University School of Medicine, Philadelphia, Pennsylvania, U.S.A.

DENTON A. COOLEY, M.D.
Surgeon-in-Chief, Texas Heart Institute; Clinical Professor of Surgery, University of Texas Medical School at Houston, Houston, Texas, U.S.A.

RICHARD A. CRASS, M.D.
Associate Professor of Surgery, University of California at San Francisco School of Medicine, San Francisco, California, U.S.A.

MARK A. CREAGER, M.D.
Assistant Professor of Medicine, Harvard Medical School; Director, Noninvasive Vascular Laboratory, Division of Vascular Medicine and Atherosclerosis, Brigham and Women's Hospital, Boston, Massachusetts, U.S.A.

J. MICHAEL CRILEY, M.D.
Professor of Medicine and Radiologic Sciences, UCLA School of Medicine; Chief, Division of Cardiology, Harbor-UCLA Medical Center, Torrance, California, U.S.A.

T. S. DANOWSKI, B.A., M.D.
Clinical Professor of Medicine, University of Pittsburgh; Chief of Endocrinology and Metabolism, Shadyside Hospital, Pittsburgh, Pennsylvania, U.S.A.

B. N. DATTA, M.D.
Professor, Department of Pathology, Postgraduate Institute of Medical Education and Research, Chandigarh, India

MICHAEL E. DeBAKEY, M.D.
Olga Keith Weiss Professor of Surgery, Chairman, Department of Surgery, and Chancellor, Baylor College of Medicine, Houston, Texas, U.S.A.

ROBERT F. DeBUSK, M.D.
Professor of Medicine and Director, Cardiac Rehabilitation Program, Stanford University School of Medicine, Stanford, California, U.S.A.

ANTONIO C. de LEON, Jr., M.D.
Medical Director, Cardiovascular Institute, St. John Medical Center; Clinical Professor of Medicine and Chief of Cardiology, University of Oklahoma Tulsa Medical College, Tulsa, Oklahoma, U.S.A.

MIGUEL del RIO, M.D.
Attending Cardiologist, Service of Hemodynamics, Italian Hospital, Buenos Aires, Argentina

PEDRO del RIO, M.D.
Chief, Intensive Care Unit, San Camilo Clinic, Buenos Aires, Argentina

LEONARD S. DREIFUS, M.D.
Professor of Medicine, Jefferson Medical College, Thomas Jefferson University; Chief of Cardiovascular Division, Lankenau Hospital, Philadelphia, Pennsylvania, U.S.A.

VICTOR J. DZAU, M.D.
Associate Professor of Medicine, Harvard Medical School; Chief, Division of Vascular Medicine and Atherosclerosis, Brigham and Women's Hospital, Boston, Massachusetts, U.S.A.

MYRVIN H. ELLESTAD, M.D.
Chief, Division of Cardiology, Memorial Medical Center of Long Beach, Long Beach, California; Clinical Professor of Medicine, University of California, Irvine, California U.S.A.

MARY ALLEN ENGLE, M.D.
Stavros S. Niarchos Professor of Pediatric Cardiology, Professor of Pediatrics, and Director of Pediatric Cardiology, The New York Hospital-Cornell Medical Center, New York, New York, U.S.A.

TOMMY N. EVANS, M.D.
Professor of Obstetrics and Gynecology, University of Colorado Health Sciences Center, Denver, Colorado, U.S.A.; Past President, American College of Obstetrics and Gynecology.

GREGORY K. FELD, M.D.
Assistant Professor of Medicine, UCLA; Research Associate (Cardiology), Wadsworth Veterans Administration Hospital, Los Angeles, California, U.S.A.

ZHUO-RONG FENG, B.S., M.D.
Professor of Surgery, Chief Cardiothoracic Surgeon, and Vice Chairman of Surgical Faculty, The Ren Ji Hospital, Shanghai Second Medical University, Shanghai, China

O. H. FRAZIER, M.D.
Director, Cardiac Transplant Program and Cardiovascular Surgical Research Laboratories, Texas Heart Institute; Associate Professor of Surgery, University of Texas Medical School at Houston, Houston, Texas, U.S.A.

ALLAN GIBOFSKY, M.D.
Hospital for Special Surgery, Cornell University Medical College, New York, New York, U.S.A.

ANTHONY P. GOLDMAN, M.D.
Research Associate, Division of Cardiovascular Disease, Albert Einstein Medical Center, Philadelphia, Pennsylvania, U.S.A.

LEE GOLDMAN, M.D.
Associate Professor of Medicine, Harvard Medical School; Assistant Physician-in-Chief, Brigham and Women's Hospital, Boston, Massachusetts, U.S.A.

JOHN F. GOODWIN, M.D., F.R.C.P., F.A.C.C., F.A.C.P.
Emeritus Professor of Clinical Cardiology, Royal Postgraduate Medical School, University of London; Consultant Physician, Hammersmith Hospital, London, England

BO-QI GU, M.D.
Associate Professor of Pathology, Department of Pathology, Shanghai Medical University, Shanghai, China

RICHARD S. GUBNER, M.D., F.A.C.P.
Clinical Professor of Medicine, State University of New York Downstate College of Medicine; Editorial Board, Medical Tribune and Circulation, New York, New York, U.S.A.

EDGAR HABER, M.D.
Chief, Cardiac Unit, Massachusetts General Hospital; Higgins Professor of Medicine, Harvard Medical School, Boston, Massachusetts, U.S.A.

CHARLES HAHN, M.D.
Professor of Cardiovascular Surgery, Faculty of Médicine, University of Geneva; Head, Cardiovascular Research Center, Arzier, Switzerland; Honorary Professor of Cardiovascular Surgery, Beijing Heart, Lung and Blood Vessel Medical Center and Anzhen Hospital, Beijing, China

ROBERT J. HALL, M.D., F.A.C.C.
Director of Cardiology, St. Luke's Episcopal Hospital; Medical Director, Texas Heart Institute; Clinical Professor of Medicine, Baylor College of Medicine; Clinical Professor, Department of Internal Medicine, The University of Texas Medical School at Houston, Houston, Texas, U.S.A.

JI-SHENG HAN, M.D.
Professor and Chairman, Department of Physiology, Beijing Medical College, Beijing, China

E. WILLIAM HANCOCK, M.D.
Professor of Medicine (Cardiology), Stanford University Medical Center, Stanford, California, U.S.A.

W. CLARK HARGROVE, III, M.D.
Assistant Professor of Surgery (Cardiovascular Surgery), University of Pennsylvania, Philadelphia, Pennsylvania, U.S.A.

ALDEN H. HARKEN, M.D.
Professor and Chairman, Department of Surgery, University of Colorado Health Sciences Center, Denver, Colorado, U.S.A.

J. WARREN HARTHORNE, M.D.
Associate Professor of Medicine, Harvard Medical School; Director, Pacemaker Laboratory, Massachusetts General Hospital, Boston, Massachusetts, U.S.A.

MING-XIN HUANG, M.D., D.Sc.
Professor of Medicine, Shanghai Second Medical University, Shanghai, China

HENRI A. JAHN, M.D.
Professor and Chief, Department of Nephrology, Université Louis Pasteur, Strasbourg, France

THOMAS N. JAMES, M.D., M.A.C.P.
The Mary Gertrude Waters Professor of Cardiology and Distinguished Professor of the University, University of Alabama in Birmingham, Birmingham, Alabama, U.S.A.

STUART W. JAMIESON, M.B., F.R.C.S.
Associate Professor of Cardiovascular Surgery, Stanford University School of Medicine, Stanford, California, U.S.A.

HARRY S. JONAS, M.D.
Dean, University of Missouri-Kansas City, Kansas City, Missouri, U.S.A.

JORGE JORDANA
Director, Bioimplant Canada Inc. Laboratory, Saint Hyacynthe, Quebec, Canada

PETER S. KASKEL
Department of Surgery, Columbia University College of Physicians & Surgeons, New York, New York, U.S.A.

EVA KEMENY, M.D.
The Rockefeller University, New York, New York, U.S.A.

HUGO KESTELOOT, M.D.
Professor of Cardiology, and Head of Department of Epidemiology, St. Rafaël University Hospital, Leuven, Belgium

ASHWANI K. KHANNA, Ph.D.
The Rockefeller University, New York, New York, U.S.A.

E. GREG KOSKI, M.D.
Assistant in Anesthesia, Department of Anesthesia, Massachusetts General Hospital; Assistant Professor of Anesthesia, Harvard Medical School, Boston, Massachusetts, U.S.A.

MORRIS N. KOTLER, M.D.
Chief of Cardiology, Albert Einstein Medical Center; Professor of Medicine, Temple University, Philadelphia, Pennsylvania, U.S.A.

JAY H. KOZLOWSKI, M.D.
Clinical Assistant Professor of Medicine, Wayne State University School of Medicine, Detroit, Michigan, U.S.A.

PETER T. KUO, M.D.
John G. Detwiler Professor of Cardiology and Director of Atherosclerosis Research, University of Medicine and Dentistry of New Jersey, Rutgers Medical School, New Brunswick, New Jersey, U.S.A.

CHARLES S. LaMONTE, M.D.
Chief, Cardiopulmonary Service, Memorial Sloan-Kettering Cancer Center, New York, New York, U.S.A.

XI-CH'UN LAN, M.D.
Professor of Surgery and Advisor to the President, Shanghai Second Medical University; Director of Shanghai Institute of Biomedical Engineering, Shanghai, China

ROBERT LEACHMAN, M.D.
Clinical Professor of Medicine, Baylor College of Medicine; Senior Cardiologist, Texas Heart Institute, Houston, Texas, U.S.A.

GARRETT LEE, M.D.
Director of Research, Western Heart Institute, St. Mary's Hospital and Medical Center, San Francisco, California, U.S.A.

CLAUDE LENFANT, M.D.
Director, National Heart, Lung and Blood Institute, National Institutes of Health, Bethesda, Maryland, U.S.A.

DOMINGO LIOTTA, M.D.
Chief of Cardiovascular Surgery, Italian Hospital, Buenos Aires; Clinical Professor of Surgery, National University of Cordoba, Cordoba, Argentina

XIUJIE LIU, M.D.
Assosciate Professor and Chief of Nuclear Medicine, Fu Wai Hospital and Cardiovascular Institute, Chinese Academy of Medical Sciences, Beijing, China

YU-QING LIU, M.D.
Director, Department of Radiology, Fu Wai Hospital & Cardiovascular Institute, Chinese Academy of Medical Sciences, Beijing, China; Consulting Editor, *Cardiovascular and Interventional Radiology.*

FLOYD D. LOOP, M.D.
Chairman, Department of Thoracic and Cardiovascular Surgery, The Cleveland Clinic Foundation, Cleveland, Ohio, U.S.A.

EDWARD LOWENSTEIN, M.D.
Anesthetist, Massachusetts General Hospital; Professor of Anesthesia, Harvard Medical School, Boston, Massachusetts, U.S.A.

VALERIE S. MANDELL, M.D.
Assistant Professor of Radiology, Harvard Medical School; Associate Radiologist, Department of Radiology, Beth Israel Hospital, Boston, Massachusetts, U.S.A.

VLADIR MARANHAO, M.D.
Chief, Department of Cardiology and Head, Hemodynamic Laboratories, Deborah Heart and Lung Center, Browns Mills, New Jersey, U.S.A.

PAUL A. MARKS, M.D.
President and Chief Executive Officer, Memorial Sloan-Kettering Cancer Center, New York, New York, U.S.A.

DEAN T. MASON, M.D.
Physician-in-Chief, Western Heart Institute, St. Mary's Hospital and Medical Center, San Francisco, California, U.S.A; Editor-in-Chief, *American Heart Journal.*

HUGH A. McALLISTER, Jr., M.D., F.A.C.C.
Chief of Cardiovascular Pathology, St. Luke's Episcopal Hospital & Texas Heart Institute; Clinical Professor of Pathology, Baylor College of Medicine, Houston, Texas, U.S.A.

CHARLES H. McCOLLUM, M.D.
Associate Professor of Surgery, Department of Surgery, Baylor College of Medicine, Houston, Texas, U.S.A.

DAN G. McNAMARA, M.D.
Professor of Pediatrics, Baylor College of Medicine; Chief of Pediatric Cardiology, Texas Children's Hospital, Houston, Texas, U.S.A.

ALLEN R. MYERS, M.D.
Professor of Medicine, Temple University School of Medicine, Philadelphia, Pennsylvania, U.S.A.

KOONLAWEE NADEMANEE, M.D.
Assistant Professor, UCLA; Director, Clinical Electrophysiology Laboratory, Wadsworth Veterans Administration Hospital, Los Angeles, California, U.S.A.

K. G. NAIR, M.D. Ph.D.
Honorary Senior Cardiologist, Jaslok Hospital and Research Center, Bombay, India; President, Association of Physicians of India.

JOSE A. NAVIA, M.D.
Deputy Chief, Cardiovascular Surgery, Italian Hospital, Buenos Aires, Argentina

HAROLD C. NEU, M.D.
Professor of Medicine and Pharmacology, and Chief, Division of Infectious Diseases, College of Physicians & Surgeons of Columbia University, New York, New York, U.S.A.

HENRY N. NEUFELD, M.D.
Professor of Cardiology, Sackler School of Medicine, Tel-Aviv University; Director, The Heart Institute, Chaim Sheba Medical Center, Tel Hashomer, Israel

JAMES T. NIEMANN, M.D.
Assistant Professor of Medicine, UCLA School of Medicine; Associate Chairman, Department of Emergency Medicine, Harbor-UCLA Medical Center, Torrance, California, U.S.A.

MICHAEL R. NIHILL, M.D.
Associate Professor of Pediatrics, Baylor College of Medicine; Associate in Pediatric Cardiology, Texas Children's Hospital, Houston, Texas, U.S.A.

JAMES J. NORA, M.D., M.P.H.
Professor of Genetics, Preventive Medicine and Pediatrics, and Director of Preventive Cardiology, University of Colorado School of Medicine; Director of Genetics, Rose Medical Center, Denver, Colorado, U.S.A.

JAMES D. O'TOOLE, M.D., F.A.C.C.
Clinical Associate Professor of Medicine, University of Pittsburgh; Director of Cardiology, Shadyside Hospital, Pittsburgh, Pennsylvania, U.S.A.

PHILIP E. OYER, M.D., Ph.D.
Associate Professor of Cardiovascular Surgery, Stanford University School of Medicine, Stanford, California, U.S.A.

WILLIAM C. PAGANELLI, M.D., Ph.D.
Department of Physiology, Harvard Medical School, Boston, Massachusetts, U.S.A.

WAYNE R. PARRY
Chief Research Technician, Division of Cardiovascular Disease, Albert Einstein Medical Center, Philadelphia, Pennsylvania, U.S.A.

SVEN PAULIN, M.D.
Professor of Radiology, Harvard Medical School; Chief of Radiology, Beth Israel Hospital, Boston, Massachusetts, U.S.A.

DWIGHT I. PERETZ, M.D.
Clinical Professor of Medicine/Cardiology, University of British Columbia; Director, Coronary Care Unit, St. Paul's Hospital, Vancouver, British Columbia, Canada

OMAR LIMA QUINTANA, M.D.
Attending Cardiologist, Assistance Circulation Unit, Italian Hosptial, Buenos Aires, Argentina

ERIC L. RITMAN, M.D., Ph.D.
Head, Biodynamic Research Unit, Department of Physiology and Biophysics, Mayo Foundation; Professor of Physiology and Medicine, Mayo Medical School, Rochester, Minnesota, U.S.A.

ARTHUR M. SACKLER, M.D.
International Publisher, *Medical Tribune*; Chairman, International Task Force on World Health Manpower for the World Health Organization.

RENEE L. SCHMITT, M.D.
Senior Associate Physician in Nephrology, University Hospital Center, Strasbourg, France

DOMINIQUE C. SCHOHN, M.D.
Senior Associate Physician in Nephrology, Cardiac Catheterization Laboratory, Department of Nephrology, Université Louis Pasteur, Strasbourg, France

PREDIMAN K. SHAH, M.D., F.A.C.C.
Director, Inpatient Cardiology and Cardiac Care Unit, Cedars-Sinai Medical Center; Associate Professor of Medicine, UCLA School of Medicine, Los Angeles, California, U.S.A.

S. SHARMA, M.D.
Associate Professor of Cardiology, T. N. Medical College and B. Y. L. Nair Hospital, Bombay, India

WILLIAM C. SHELDON, M.D.
Chairman, Department of Cardiology, The Cleveland Clinic Foundation, Cleveland, Ohio, U.S.A.

NORMAN E. SHUMWAY, M.D., Ph.D.
Professor and Chairman, Department of Cardiovascular Surgery, Stanford University School of Medicine, Stanford, California, U.S.A.

BRAMAH N. SINGH, M.D., Ph.D., F.R.C.P. (London)
Professor of Medicine, UCLA; Assistant Chief of Cardiology and Director of Cardiovascular Research, Wadsworth Veterans Administration Hospital, Los Angeles, California, U.S.A.

HOWARD M. SPIRO, M.D.
Professor of Medicine, Yale University School of Medicine, New Haven, Connecticut, U.S.A.

JOHN A. SPITTELL, Jr., M.D., F.A.C.P., F.A.C.C.
Mary Lowell Leary Professor of Medicine, Mayo Medical School; Consultant, Division of Cardiovascular Diseases and Internal Medicine, Mayo Clinic and Mayo Foundation, Rochester, Minnesota, U.S.A.

JEREMIAH STAMLER, M.D.
Professor and Chairman, Department of Community Health and Preventive Medicine, Northwestern University Medical School, Chicago, Illinois, U.S.A.

EUGENE A. STEAD, Jr., M.D.
Professor and Chairman Emeritus, Department of Medicine; Distinguished Professor of the Veterans Administration, Duke University, Durham, North Carolina, U.S.A.

EDWARD B. STINSON, M.D.
Professor of Cardiovascular Surgery, Stanford University School of Medicine, Stanford, California, U.S.A.

JAY M. SULLIVAN, M.D.
Professor of Medicine and Chief of Cardiology, The University of Tennessee Center for the Health Sciences, Memphis, Tennessee, U.S.A.

H. J. C. SWAN, M.D., Ph.D., M.A.C.P.
Director, Division of Cardiology, Cedars-Sinai Medical Center; Professor of Medicine, UCLA School of Medicine, Los Angeles, California, U.S.A.

VICHAI TANPHAICHITR, M.D., Ph.D., F.A.C.P., F.A.C.N.
Professor of Medicine and Chief, Division of Nutrition and Biochemical Medicine, Department of Medicine, Ramathibodi Hospital, Mahidol University, Bangkok, Thailand

MORRIS TRAUBE, M.D.
Assistant Professor of Medicine, Gastroenterology Unit, Department of Medicine, Yale University School of Medicine, New Haven, Connecticut, U.S.A.

DONALD D. TRUNKEY, M.D.
Chief of Surgery, San Francisco General Hospital; Professor and Vice Chairman, Department of Surgery, University of California School of Medicine, San Francisco, California, U.S.A.

CHENG LANG TUNG, M.D.
Consultant in Medicine, Shanghai Sixth People's Hospital; Editor-in-Chief, Shanghai Medical Journal; Editor-in-Chief, Excerpta Medica (Cardiology) in Chinese; Honorary Advisor, Chinese Medical Association, Beijing, China

FRANS VAN DE WERF, M.D.
Associate Professor of Medicine, Division of Cardiology, University of Leuven, Campus Gasthuisberg, Leuven, Belgium

NAGAMMAL VENKATESH, M.D.
Assistant Professor of Medicine, UCLA School of Medicine, Los Angeles, California, U.S.A.

ZVI VERED, M.D.
Head, Echocardiography Laboratory, The Heart Institute, Chaim Sheba Medical Center, Tel-Hashomer, Israel

HENRY N. WAGNER, Jr., M.D.
Professor of Medicine, Radiology and Environmental Health Sciences; Director, Division of Nuclear Medicine and Radiation Health Sciences, The Johns Hopkins Medical Institutions, Baltimore, Maryland, U.S.A.

JOHN I. WALKER, M.D.
Assistant Professor of Psychiatry, Psychiatric Director of Combined Medical Specialty Unit, Duke University Medical Center, Durham, North Carolina, U.S.A.

YI-SHAN WANG, B.S., M.D.
Professor of Surgery, Shanghai Second Medical University; Director, First Division of Cardiovascular Research, Department of Thoracic-Cardiovascular Surgery, The Ren Ji Hospital, Shanghai, China

KARLMAN WASSERMAN, M.D., Ph.D.
Professor of Medicine, UCLA School of Medicine; Chief, Division of Respiratory Physiology and Medicine, Harbor-UCLA Medical Center, Torrance, California, U.S.A.

YOSHIO WATANABE, M.D.
Professor of Medicine and Director, Cardiovascular Institute, Fujita-Gakuen University School of Medicine, Toyoake, Aichi, Japan

ARNOLD M. WEISSLER, M.D.
Chairman, Department of Medicine, Rose Medical Center; Professor of Medicine, University of Colorado, Denver, Colorado, U.S.A.

LARS WERKÖ, M.D., F.R.C.P.
Former Vice President for Research, AB ASTRA; Professor of Medicine Emeritus, University of Gothenburg, Stockholm, Sweden

DELON WU, M.D., F.A.C.C.
Professor of Medicine, Chang Gung Medical College; Chairman, Department of Medicine, Chang Gung Memorial Hospital, Taipei, Taiwan, China

SING SAN YANG, M.D.
Head, Cardiac Non-Invasive Laboratory, Deborah Heart and Lung Center, Browns Mills, New Jersey, U.S.A.

HIROFUMI YASUE, M.D.
Professor of Medicine and Chief, Division of Cardiology, Kumamoto University, School of Medicine, Kumamoto City, Japan

CHUN-XIU YE, B.S., M.D., M.A.O. (Hon.)
Associate Professor of Surgery, Shanghai Second Medical University; Vice Director, First Division of Cardiovascular Research, The Ren Ji Hospital, Shanghai, China

JOHN B. ZABRISKIE, M.D.
The Rockefeller University, New York, New York, U.S.A.

CHI-SUNG ZEE-CHENG, M.D.
Assistant Professor of Medicine (Cardiology), Department of Medicine, University of Missouri-Kansas City; Director, Cardiac Catheterization Laboratory, Truman Medical Center, Kansas City, Missouri, U.S.A.

Preface

As Dr Paul D. White said, cardiology knows no international boundary and is the world's best ambassador. The science of medicine—and, for that matter, of cardiology—is universal in its relevance. Cardiovascular disease is the greatest killer and crippler throughout the world, be it in Beijing, China or Washington, DC.

However, biological variations and socio-economo-ethno-racial differences exist among different parts of the world. For example, coronary artery disease is significantly less prevalent in China than in the United States, although hypertension is almost equally common in both countries. The damage from hypertension to the target organs varies in different countries: in China, Japan, and India, stroke leads the list of complications of hypertension, whereas cardiovascular and renal complications are more frequent than cerebrovascular accidents in the United States. Another example is Keshan disease, an endemic cardiomyopathy in China, which has a different etiology from cardiomyopathy in the Western world. Gene pools have been modified by natural selection; for example, balanced polymorphism seems to have given rise to a high incidence of sickle cell disease with its usual cardiovascular complications only where the associated hyperresistance to falciparum malaria constitutes a significant biological advantage. Pulmonary embolism is rather rare among the Chinese. Such examples of differing gene pools in ethnic groups abound.

On the other hand, much more impressive is the constancy of human biology among the world population. Out of infinite possibilities, the same heart pumps blood around every human body, extracts oxygen from the same coronary blood supply, and maintains well-being 24 hours a day in all human beings without regard for national borders, ethnic background, or cultural differences. Thus, the basic principles that underlie the functioning of the cardiovascular system, and consequently the practice of cardiology throughout the world, remain the same.

On the basis of these observations, I undertook the preparation of this comprehensive textbook on the international practice of cardiology. This book tries to do three things that have not been done before. First, it presents a full coverage of up-to-date information on all aspects of modern cardiology, including the prevalence of heart disease, herbal pharmacology in cardiovascular therapeutics, acupuncture anesthesia in open heart surgery and its neurochemical and physiological basis, computers in cardiovascular practice, collaborative trials in cardiology, the pharmaceutical industry and cardiology, medical communication in cardiology, cardiovascular nursing, tropical heart disease including parasitic heart disease, antibodies in cardiology, geriatric cardiology, and preventive cardiology.

Second, it takes advantage of the expertise of many authorities around the world by presenting contributions from nearly every continent. About one third of the contributing authors in the book are from outside the United States, including contributors from Argentina, Belgium, Canada, England, France, India, Israel, Japan, The Soviet Union, South Africa, Sweden, Switzerland, and Thailand; twenty are Chinese.

Third, the authors attempt, wherever possible, to point out international differences, for example, cardiac manifestations in anemias between sickle cell disease in black Americans and the thalassemia and hemoglobinopathy syndromes in Thailand and the

Far East, as well as the similarities. Thus, the book gives every serious student of international cardiology a source of reference in one single textbook.

According to Sir William Osler, medicine is the only worldwide profession following the same methods everywhere, activated by the same ambition, and pursuing the same ends. An international approach is important, however, because the actual practice of medicine varies greatly in different parts of the world. Environmental factors, incidence, ethno-racial background, clinical manifestations, diagnostic approaches, and therapeutic options of different cardiovascular diseases differ from one part of the world to another. In fact, it is difficult to find any disorder with equal geographical prevalence. Such authorities as Dr Barlow from South Africa for whom Barlow's syndrome is named, Dr Yasue from Japan where variant angina seems to be very prevalent, and Dr Gu from China, who was the first to discover a connection between white muscle disease in domestic animals due to selenium deficiency and Keshan disease in humans, are my coauthors of the chapters on mitral valve prolapse, coronary artery spasm, and Keshan disease, respectively. Dr Chazov from Moscow, who administered the world's first intracoronary thrombolytic treatment in acute myocardial infarction in 1976, presents a Russian viewpoint of the current status of thrombolytic therapy in cardiology, a very important contemporary subject of worldwide interest. Thus, this textbook attempts to bring together authoritative coverage of all the cardiological subjects by an international group of specialists with a vast firsthand knowledge of the disease entities, providing cardiologists, internists, pediatricians, surgeons, epidemiologists, and other specialists throughout the world with reliable information on diseases either indigenous to, or relatively abundant in, the regions of the authors, or furnished by the most authoritative data sources in the world today. Nowadays, with increasing international travel and massive migration of refugees, diseases which used to be native to one region may frequently be encountered in other parts of the world.

The practice of medicine, to which cardiology is no exception, requires a frame of reference which, for this book, is the Western world with its ready availability of sophisticated diagnostic technology and innovative therapeutic modalities. We combine the best of both worlds: the excellence of hardware in the West with the abundance of software in the East. By working together, we may reach a better understanding; the prospect for more successful management of heart disease and, ultimately, improved health of all the people in the entire world seems brighter. All the authors in this book, to whom I owe heartfelt gratitude for their time and effort, cherish the hope that each and every one of us contribute to the achievement of these goals.

THE INTERNATIONAL TEXTBOOK OF CARDIOLOGY

1 Prevalence and Incidence of Heart Disease

Tsung O. Cheng, MD

Cardiovascular disease is the main cause of death in developed countries and is of increasing importance in developing countries. In the developed countries where infectious diseases and malnutrition have largely been controlled, a steady, progressive increase in cardiovascular disease has been recorded, so that it now accounts for nearly 50% of deaths from all causes.[1] Even in developing countries, heart disease takes its steady toll. However, the prevalence* of various forms of heart disease varies from country to country and from race to race (Table 1.1). Furthermore, the trend has shown a tendency to change in recent years (Table 1.2). Although epidemiologic studies offer a scientific explanation for most of the changes, there is still no unequivocal reason for some of the trends.[2] This discussion will be limited to the world's five major etiologic types of heart disease, namely, coronary heart disease, hypertension and its cerebrovascular complications, rheumatic fever and rheumatic heart disease, congenital heart disease, and cardiomyopathies.

CORONARY HEART DISEASE

Until the mid-1970s coronary heart disease was recognized as the major killer of the century. However, it came as a surprise when first reports ten years ago indicated that a decline in mortality from coronary heart disease had begun in the United States.[3] In 1978 a major conference was convened by the National Heart, Lung, and Blood Institute, National Institutes of Health, Bethesda, Maryland,[4] to examine in detail the trend in the United States and to make international comparisons. It was concluded at the Bethesda Conference that primary prevention must play a role in explaining the decreased mortality from coronary heart disease in the United States. Furthermore, recent developments in the medical care of patients with clinical coronary artery disease provide evidence that both primary and secondary prevention have been at work.[5] (See chapter 80 on Preventive Cardiology.)

In a recent forum on the changing trends in mortality from coronary heart disease, among the 11 countries selected, seven countries including the United States, Australia, New Zealand, Finland, Norway, Belgium, and Israel showed a declining mortality from coronary heart disease during the 1970s, whereas four countries including Sweden, Poland, Italy, and Spain showed an increase.[6] It was suggested that poor dietary habits, as reflected in the elevated mean serum cholesterol levels of the population, and smoking were contributing factors. (See Table 12 in chapter 80 on Preventive Cardiology.) In those countries where total mortality from coronary heart disease has decreased during the past decade, not only have the women participated in this favorable trend, but also the decline in mortality was often greater among women.[7] Coronary deaths decreased 20% in US women between 1968 and 1976, with a more prominent decline in mortality among young women.[4] However, a recent study from Göteborg, Sweden, showed little or no change in the incidence of myocardial infarction in women younger than 65 years of age between 1968 and 1977.[8] Equally distressing is the recent report from Scotland that mortality rates for coronary heart disease among Scottish men have become among the highest in the world: 11% of Scotsmen currently die of coronary heart disease by the age of 65.[9]

It may be true that with the control of infectious disease and a decrease in infant mortality, more persons reach old age and therefore are more prone to the development of atherosclerosis. The increasing incidence cannot, however, be attributed to an increasing aged population alone[10] (Figure 1.1), nor can it be attributed to modern civilization or more accurate diagnosis, as coronary artery

* "Prevalence" refers to the number of cases existing in a population at the time of a survey; "incidence" refers to the number of cases developing per year per unit population. Many clinicians use "incidence" rather loosely to apply to both prevalence and incidence; I prefer to hold to strict epidemiologic usage.

Table 1.1. Age-Standardized Mortality (in descending order) from Heart Disease in 1980*

Country	Male	Female	Country
United Kingdom (Northern Ireland)	689†	244	United Kingdom (Scotland)
Finland	648	238	United Kingdom (Northern Ireland)
United Kingdom (Scotland)	634	212	Romania
Ireland	563	204	New Zealand
Czechoslovakia (1981)	537	202	Ireland
United Kingdom (England and Wales)	524	201	Hungary
New Zealand	511	194	Israel
Hungary	509	194	Yugoslavia
United States of America	498	190	Czechoslovakia (most recent 10 yr)
Poland	478	180	United States of America
Australia	465	169	United Kingdom (England and Wales)
Canada	437	156	Poland
Denmark	426	155	Australia
Norway	424	149	Bulgaria
Sweden	416	145	Austria
Germany (Federal Republic)	409	145	Canada
Austria	405	142	Finland
Israel	383	129	Denmark
Netherlands	380	125	Germany (Federal Republic)
Romania	380	115	Belgium
Yugoslavia	375	106	Netherlands
Belgium (1979)	361	106	Sweden
Bulgaria	324	105	Norway
Switzerland	296	104	Italy
Italy	295	80	Switzerland
France	213	66	Japan
Japan	137	64	France

* Adapted from Uemara and Pisa.[1]

† Rates per 100,000 population aged 40 to 69 years.

Table 1.2. Percentage Change in Age-Standardized Death Rates From Heart Disease*

Country	Period	Males	Females
Canada	1972–1982	−24.1%	−21.3%
United States of America	1970–1980	−25.9%	−26.1%
Israel	1975–1980	−7.2%	−17.6%
Japan	1972–1982	−1.1%	−19.5%
Austria	1972–1982	1.0%	−12.9%
Belgium	1971–1981	−22.9%	−30.9%
Bulgaria	1972–1982	42.5%	4.7%
Czechoslovakia	1972–1982	19.1%	10.9%
Denmark	1972–1982	−8.0%	−12.2%
Finland	1970–1980	−16.3%	−33.9%
France	1971–1981	−14.2%	−28.0%
Germany (Fed. Rep.)	1972–1982	−4.6%	−12.0%
Hungary	1972–1982	29.9%	−1.2%
Ireland	1970–1980	9.4%	−0.5%
Italy	1970–1980	−4.9%	−28.6%
Netherlands	1972–1982	−14.4%	−18.5%
Norway	1972–1982	−6.7%	−18.6%
Poland	1970–1980	37.5%	10.1%
Romania	1972–1982	10.9%	−9.2%
Sweden	1972–1982	0.7%	−21.9%
Switzerland	1971–1981	−4.1%	−22.7%
United Kingdom			
England and Wales	1972–1982	−12.0%	−11.9%
Northern Ireland	1971–1981	−1.1%	4.6%
Scotland	1973–1983	−9.9%	−13.8%
Yugoslavia	1971–1981	26.4%	15.3%
Australia	1971–1981	−30.9%	−35.0%
New Zealand	1971–1981	−21.1%	−15.0%

* Modified from Uemara and Pisa.[1]

disease was found in a 50-year-old Chinese woman who died of acute myocardial infarction 2,100 years ago[11] (Figure 1.2).

HYPERTENSION AND CEREBROVASCULAR DISEASE

Hypertension and its cerebrovascular complications appear to be common in all races throughout the world. However, large differences exist among blood pressure levels in people from different parts of the world.[12] Nations with an Islamic culture (the Arabic-speaking countries, Turkey, and Iran) and the nations of the Far East and Latin America have the lowest blood pressure levels, whereas the nationals of countries in black Africa have the highest; the prevalence of hypertension in the former is almost a quarter that of the latter[13] (Table 1.3). In the United States, hypertension is more prevalent among the black population.[14]

Although genetic predisposition may account for part of the differences, the dietary factor with interplay of sodium, potassium, calcium, and other electrolytes plays an important role. Although increased sodium intake[15] is a major factor in the development of hypertension, deficiencies of potassium[16] and calcium[17] may be contributing factors. Several electrolytes including magnesium seem to exert independent influences on blood pressure.[18]

Although obesity favors the development of hypertension,[19] it does not seem to have a decisive influence on the differences in arterial pressure among the people of various nations[14] (Figure 1.3). Despite this interesting observation and the recent report that blood pressure is less predictive of mortality from coronary heart disease

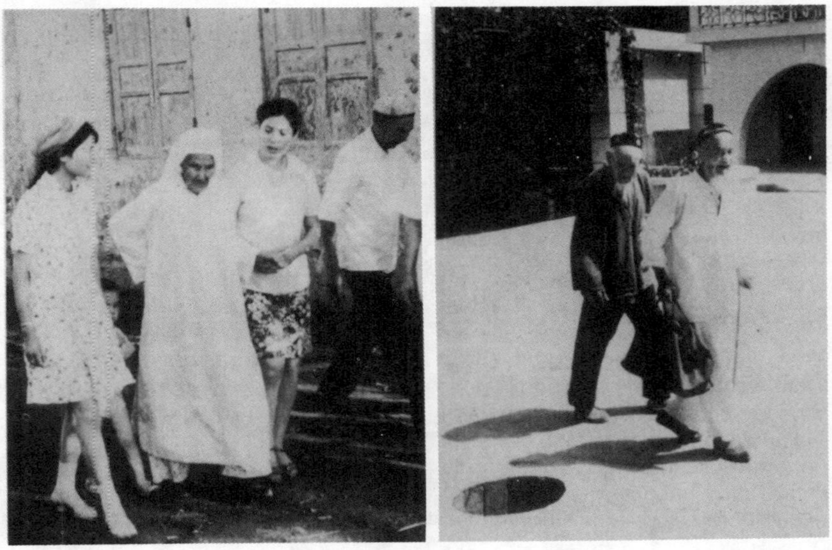

Figure 1.1A. A 108-year-old woman (*left*) strolling with her family and (*right*) a man of 99 walking behind a man of 95 years of age in Turpan, Xinjiang (Sinkiang), China.

in obese than in nonobese subjects,[20] there is undeniable evidence that obesity increases the risk of hypertension.[20]

Hypertension is the major risk factor in coronary heart disease as well as in cerebrovascular accidents.[21-23] Mortality from cerebrovascular disease has decreased in the last 15 to 20 years in many countries.[1] However, this disease remains a major cause of death in most developing countries, and hypertension has been shown to be the primary risk factor. This certainly is true in Japan where the mortality rate for stroke is still the highest in the world.[24] It is of note that in Japan cerebrovascular diseases have a higher incidence than does coronary artery disease which, by contrast, occurs more frequently in Europe and America.[25] A local factor in addition to hypertension must be incriminated, and cerebral arteriosclerosis is considered a major contributing factor.[26]

RHEUMATIC FEVER AND RHEUMATIC HEART DISEASE

The incidence of rheumatic fever and rheumatic heart disease, prevalent throughout the world in the late 19th and early 20th centuries, has been declining rapidly in many western countries in the past two decades.[27,28] There is little doubt that chronic rheumatic heart disease occurring in 40- to 50-year-old persons in the western world reflects an acute attack of rheumatic fever that had occurred 30 years previously. The changing incidence is due to worldwide recognition of the importance of the group A hemolytic streptococcus as the offending etiologic agent, the prompt use of penicillin in the eradication of streptococcal throat infections, and possible mutation of the epidemic strain into a more attenuated group A streptococcus.

In Sweden the incidence of acute rheumatic fever declined from 2.6 cases per 10,000 inhabitants in 1930 to 1934 to 0.2 in 1970 to 1974.[29] In New Zealand the incidence of rheumatic fever declined markedly from 1971 to 1981 except among the Maoris.[30] In New York it is only found in black, Puerto Rican, and Haitian population groups in which poverty, overcrowding and suboptimal medical conditions exist.[28] Acute rheumatic fever has virtually disappeared from the relatively affluent population of North America and Europe. The incidence should continue to decline and with it the incidence of rheumatic heart disease. However, in many underdeveloped countries of the world, in the Middle East and in the developing countries of Southeast Asia and Africa with their fast growing populations, and in the poverty-stricken Central and South Americas, rheumatic heart disease is still prevalent and continues to have its impact on the health of the population.[28,31]

Carditis was the dominant feature of rheumatic fever in the 1960s and 1970s, but joint involvement has become more common in recent years.[31-33] Rheumatic subcutaneous nodules, chorea, or erythema marginatum are rarely encountered nowadays. Therefore, it is a fallacy to use the revised Jones criteria[34] which may lead to underdiagnosing rheumatic fever in the underdeveloped countries where the disease is still prevalent. The classic picture of acute rheumatic fever with carditis and severe mitral regurgitation so often seen in the third world countries is almost unknown to most physicians trained in western medical schools. We must not miss the diagnosis of rheumatic fever which is now a preventable disease.

Sequelae are essentially limited to the heart and depend on the presence and severity of carditis during the acute attack. This is true in both developed[35] and developing[36] countries where the major risk factors adversely affecting the outcome are the severity of carditis, inadequacy of medical service, noncompliance of chemoprophylaxis, rheumatic fever recurrence, poor socioeconomic status, and high prevalence of group A streptococci. There is no uniform "Oriental type" natural history of rheumatic fever and rheumatic heart disease; the natural history varies greatly among countries.[36]

CONGENITAL HEART DISEASE

According to a recent world survey by Taussig,[37] although the incidence of specific malformations may vary from country to country, continent to continent, or race to race, the common congenital heart diseases are prevalent throughout the world. Thus, ventricular septal defect, patent ductus arteriosus, atrial septal defect, tetralogy of Fallot, and pulmonic stenosis were among the

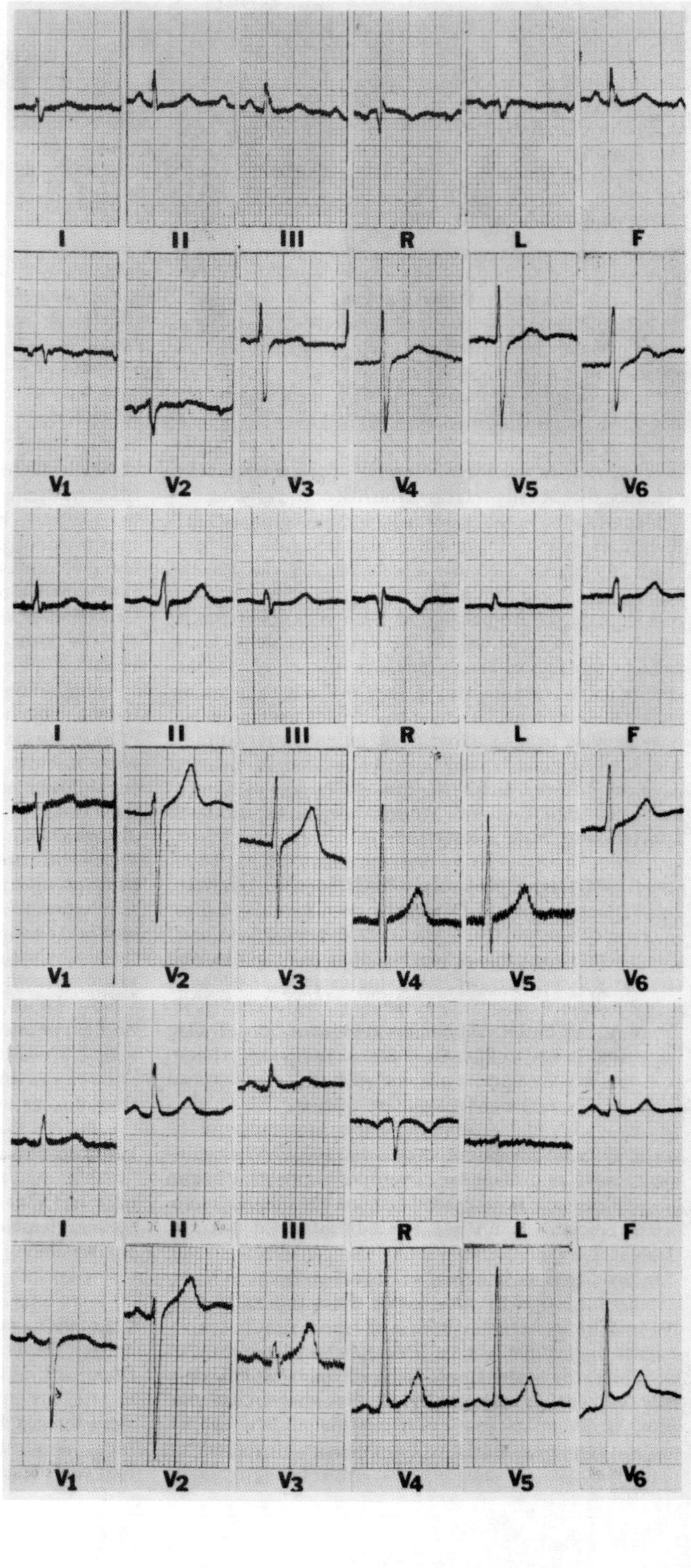

Figure 1.1B. Normal electrocardiograms of the 108-year-old (*top*), 99-year-old (*middle*), and 95-year-old (*bottom*) persons in Figure 1.1A. (From Cheng,[10] with permission.)

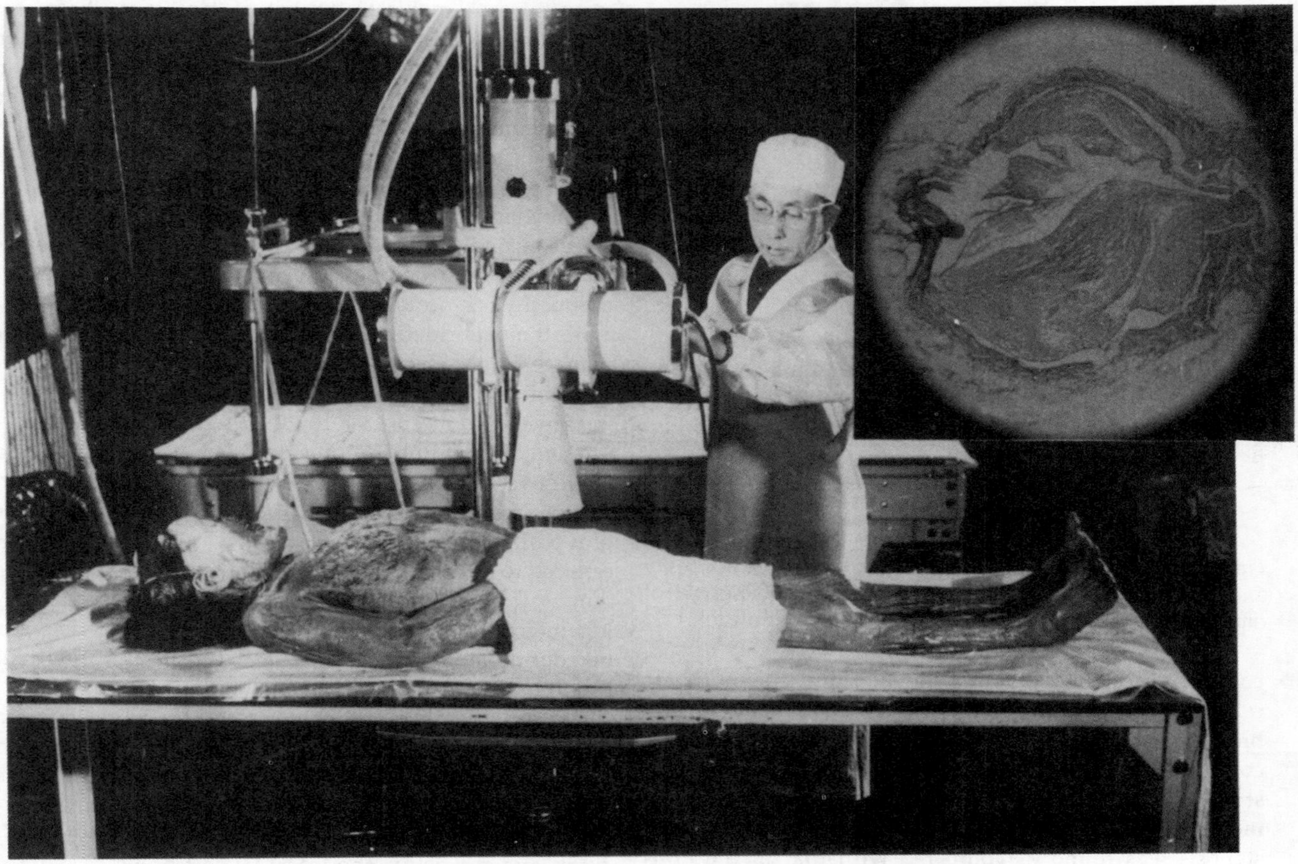

Figure 1.2. Severe atherosclerotic occlusive disease in the proximal left coronary artery (*inset*) of a 50-year-old Chinese woman who died of acute myocardial infarction over 2,100 years ago.

commonest congenital heart malformations found in her surveys of countries including North and South Africa, Singapore, Australia, Greenlandic Eskimos, and India. In Africa, congenital heart disease was as common in blacks as whites.[38–40] Congenital heart disease was as prevalent in the tropics and subtropics as in the temperate zone,[41,42] and among the aborigines of Australia[43] and Greenlandic Eskimos[44] as in the general population.

However, ethnic differences in the incidence of various congenital heart malformations do exist. For example,

Table 1.3. Prevalence of Diastolic Arterial Hypertension (%) in Men of Different National Groups*

Geographic Areas	n	Mean† (20–59)	Age (yr) 20–29	30–39	40–49	50–59
Nations of Islamic culture	222	8.0	4	6	4	16
Far East	114	9.5	0	5	5	23
Latin America	183	10.3	0	2	11	22
United States and Canada	365	13.7	0	6	13	26
Italy, Spain, and Portugal	401	13.7	8	6	16	20
Soviet Union	249	14.0	6	9	16	21
Australia and New Zealand	69	14.1	0	7	12	30
Germanic-speaking nations	380	15.0	0	8	15	27
Switzerland	469	15.1	5	12	12	25
United Kingdom	374	17.3	0	7	17	32
Nations speaking Slavic languages (except USSR)	124	19.6	0	15	17	33
India and Sri Lanka	138	20.3	0	14	22	31
France	959	20.3	5	13	20	34
Nations of black Africa	123	35.2	0	17	28	73

* Adapted from Fabre et al.[13]

† Adjusted for age ($P < 0.001$).

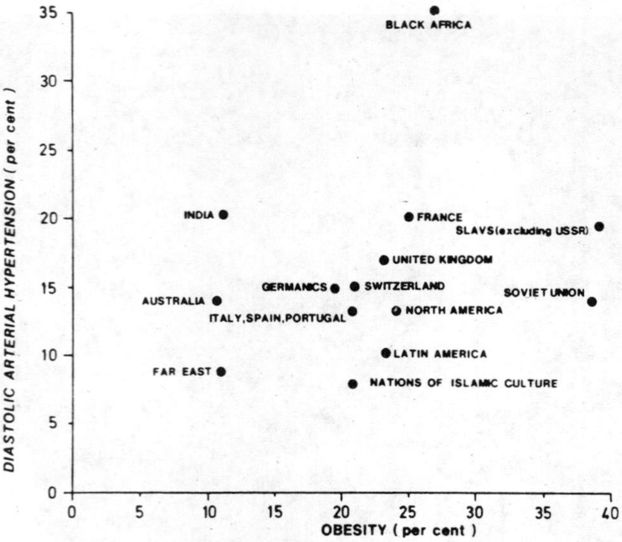

Figure 1.3. Lack of correlation between the degree of obesity and severity of arterial hypertension among the people of different countries. (From Fabre et al,[13] with permission.)

coarctation of the aorta and valvular aortic stenosis are relatively uncommon in various Asian countries[45-46] (Table 1.4), whereas ruptured sinus of Valsalva is relatively common in China.[47] It is interesting to note that in a study of North American Indian children a similar low incidence of coarctation of the aorta and valvular aortic stenosis was found as compared with that in the non-Indian population in the same geographic area.[48] Because no environmental factor, dietary or otherwise, was clinically evident, Anderson[48] postulated that this similarity was related to the ancestral origin of the North American Indians from the Asiatic mainland.

Conversely, environmental factors do play some role. For example, in a recent citation by Cheng[46] of a Chinese epidemiologic study of the increased prevalence of congenital heart disease among children born on the Qinghai plateau, only 7% were born at sea level, 25% at an altitude 2,261 m above sea level, 34% at 2,500 to 3,050 m above sea level, and 35% at 3,200 to 5,157 m above sea level.[46]

A study of congenital heart disease based on data collected by a central registry may underestimate the true incidence of some lesions, because symptom-free patients

Table 1.4. Rarity of Coarctation of the Aorta and Aortic Stenosis Reported in Asian Countries

Country	Patients (no.)	Coarctation of Aorta	Aortic Stenosis
Japan[45]	322	1	1
Korea[45a]	132	0	6
Taiwan[45b]	356	4	0
Thailand[45c]	1800*	1	0
China[45d]	35†	1	0
China[46]	118‡	1	0

* Based on author's estimate of 10-20 pediatric cardiac patients seen per day over a 4-month period.

† In an epidemiologic survey of 11,230 children in Chengdu, China.

‡ In an epidemiologic survey of 13,446 children born on the Qinghai plateau.

may not seek medical attention.[49] However, the recent Czechoslovakian report of an autopsied child population seemed to confirm the clinical impression that ventricular septal defect and patent ductus arteriosus are indeed the two commonest congenital cardiac defects.[50]

CARDIOMYOPATHIES

Knowledge about the cardiomyopathies, "heart muscle disease of unknown cause,"[51] has advanced enormously in the last two decades. Nowadays, the term "cardiomyopathy" is no longer adequate; classification and diagnosis must be defined with precision so that appropriate management can be instituted. The World Health Organization Expert Committee on Cardiomyopathies met in Geneva from April 18 to 20, 1983, and classified cardiomyopathy into three types: dilated, hypertrophic, and restrictive.[52] The terms "primary" and "secondary" cardiomyopathy used in the past have been withdrawn. The group of diseases previously known as "primary" is now referred to as cardiomyopathy and the "secondary" group is now known as specific heart muscle disease, including infective, metabolic, and general systemic diseases, heredofamilial abnormalities, and sensitivity and toxic reactions.[52]

Cardiomyopathies occur throughout the world. Certain types of cardiomyopathy show geographic, racial, and cultural differences, and areas of relatively high incidence exist in various parts of the world. Dilated cardiomyopathy appears to be the most widely distributed condition and restrictive the least. Hypertrophic cardiomyopathy appears to lie somewhere between the two, and for this condition racial differences have been reported. Dilated and hypertrophic cardiomyopathies are found throughout the Asian and Pacific areas. Endomyocardial fibrosis is most frequent in Africa and Central and South America; however, except for certain parts of India,[53] it is rare in other Asian countries. Keshan disease, a specific form of cardiomyopathy, is found only in China.[54] (See chapter 44 on Keshan Disease.)

Dilated cardiomyopathy is found in all parts of the world. Although several large studies were reported from centers in Germany, Japan, the United Kingdom, and the United States of America, accurate data on disease prevalence and incidence have not been obtained because these studies were based on selected patients.[52] Nevertheless, five studies from different parts of the world were noteworthy. In Chandigarb, North India, where the autopsy rate is 90%, 3.3% of cardiovascular deaths were due to cardiomyopathy; of the 38 cases autopsied, dilated cardiomyopathy was found in 28, endomyocardial fibrosis in nine, and hypertrophic cardiomyopathy in one.[55] Two Swedish studies, both from the same center in Malmö, a city of 250,000 inhabitants, over an eight-year and a subsequent extended period, found an incidence of five and ten patients, respectively, per 100,000 persons per year.[56,57] In another study from China involving 66,000 factory workers, school teachers, and government employees in Nanning district, Guant-Xi province, 56 persons were found to have cardiomyopathies, and of these, 52 had the dilated and four the hypertrophic form of the disease.[58] In western Denmark with a population of 2,798,000, a two-year study from 1980 through 1981 yielded 41 patients with dilated cardiomyopathy, an overall incidence of 7.3/10^6 population per year and 20 patients with hypertrophic cardiomyopathy; in men aged 40 to 59 years the incidence of dilated cardiomyopathy was 23.4/10^6 population per year.[59] In England the prevalence of dilated cardiomyopathy was 8.317 per 100,000 population in areas covering a total sample of 913,836 inhabitants.[60] Because most of these studies were retrospective and diagnosis was made only on well-established cases, the prevalence most likely will even be higher, especially with recent reports of a causal relation between myocarditis and dilated cardiomyopathy.[61–64]

Hypertrophic cardiomyopathy also has a worldwide distribution, although it seems to be rare in Negroes.[65] Hypertensive heart disease, which is common in Negroes, may interfere with the correct diagnosis of hypertrophic cardiomyopathy, especially in the elderly.[66,67] In a recent autopsy study from Iceland,[68] 11 patients with hypertrophic cardiomyopathy were found in a series of 5,780 autopsies from 1966 to 1977, an incidence of 0.19%. By using the autopsy rate in Iceland, which was 34% in this period, and the aforementioned incidence, it can be estimated that an average of 2.5 patients per year died of hypertrophic cardiomyopathy, corresponding to 0.17% of the deaths in the population. Nine of the 11 Icelandic patients died under the age of 50 and eight were male. Hypertrophic cardiomyopathy therefore accounts for a considerable proportion of cardiac deaths among young males.[68] However, this is only the "inconspicuous rump of the iceberg."[69] When all accessible close relatives of these 11 patients were studied by echocardiography, 41% of the first degree relatives had hypertrophic cardiomyopathy as compared with none of an age-matched control group.[70] In Japan, hypertrophic cardiomyopathy is common; there were 84 confirmed cases of congestive (or dilated) cardiomyopathy, 57 cases of hypertrophic nonobstructive cardiomyopathy, and 52 cases of hypertrophic obstructive cardiomyopathy collected from 15 cardiology divisions of university or national hospitals in Japan.[71] It is worth noting that cases of hypertrophic cardiomyopathy exceeded those of congestive cardiomyopathy and cases of hypertrophic nonobstructive cardiomyopathy exceeded those of hypertrophic obstructive cardiomyopathy. The reason most likely is that annual physical examinations are so popular in schools or factories in Japan and that patients with asymptomatic hypertrophic cardiomyopathy showing abnormal electrocardiograms are frequently referred for echocardiographic examination. Another noteworthy finding in the Japanese report is that the ten-year survival rate after diagnosis was 34.2% for congestive cardiomyopathy, 81.7% for hypertrophic nonobstructive cardiomyopathy, and 84.4% for hypertrophic obstructive cardiomyopathy.[71]

Japanese investigators[72,73] recently described a variety of hypertrophic cardiomyopathy characterized by giant precordial negative T waves and angiographic or echocardiographic evidence of apical hypertrophy, the so-called "ace-of-spades" configuration at end-diastole on a left ventricular with the tip of the spade directed

Table 1.5. Level of Cardiovascular Mortality in 1980 and Recent Trends in 27 Countries*

Recent Trends†		
Improving	**Stable**	**Deteriorating**
High Mortality		
Finland	Czechoslovakia	Bulgaria
United Kingdom (Scotland)	Ireland	Hungary
	Romania	Poland
	United Kingdom (Northern Ireland)	
Medium Mortality		
Canada		Yugoslavia
Israel		
Austria		
Germany (Federal Republic)		
United Kingdom (England and Wales)		
United States of America		
Australia		
New Zealand		
Low Mortality		
Japan		
Belgium		
Denmark		
France		
Italy		
Netherlands		
Norway		
Sweden		
Switzerland		

* Adapted from Uemara and Pisa.[1]

†Trends: improving = decrease of +10%; stable = change within ±10%; deteriorating = increase of +10%.

toward the apex. For years, apical hypertrophic cardiomyopathy was reported only from Japan, and the cardiologic world began to wonder whether this was a specific Japanese entity. In recent years, however, there have been reports from other parts of the world including United States,[74-76] Singapore,[77] India,[78] South Africa,[79] Israel,[80] and Canada.[81]

Restrictive cardiomyopathy includes endomyocardial disease, believed to be confined to tropical areas, and Löffler's endocarditis parietalis fibroplastica, believed to occur mainly in temperate zones. Evidence continues to indicate a close connection between the two. There is now strong evidence that endomyocardial disease represents a single disease entity irrespective of its geographic distribution.[82] Since the original descriptions, cases have been reported from many parts of the world including Africa, South and Central America, Southeast Asia, especially southern India, as well as the United States and several European countries. The prevalence of the disease is greater in tropical regions. In Uganda, 14% of patients dying of heart failure have been diagnosed as having endomyocardial fibrosis, whereas in Nigeria the figure is 10% of all cases.[52] On the Ivory Coast, endomyocardial fibrosis accounts for 20% of deaths from heart failure in persons less than 40 years of age.[52] In Africa, the disease is prevalent in the forest regions where certain population groups are more affected (eg, the group on the Ivory Coast), probably because of conducive ecologic rather than genetic factors.[52]

CONCLUSIONS

Despite recent advances in medical technology in developed countries and improved medical conditions in developing countries, considerable differential still exists in the morbidity and mortality from cardiovascular disease among various countries (Table 1.5). Whereas recent trends in many countries are encouraging, the situation in a few others seems to be worsening. Therefore, there is room for improvement. The reduction in cardiovascular and stroke mortality in Japan has been remarkable.[83] The same favorable trend in China is discussed in the next chapter.

The great difference between the high and low mortality rates for cardiovascular disease in different countries has serious public health implications. Despite progress in the identification of the risk factors involved and continuous efforts to identify the reasons for the different trends, there is still no unequivocal explanation for the trends.

To answer this question, the World Health Organization recently launched a multinational collaborative research project, known as MONICA[84] (Monitoring the Trends and Determinants in Cardiovascular Disease). It attempts to measure, over a ten-year period, both mortality and morbidity due to cardiovascular disease as well as changes in risk factors, life-styles, and medical care in defined study populations in close to 30 participating countries. The MONICA methodology also could be used as an information tool for countries that are not involved in the project itself. This World Health Organization project therefore represents a true international cooperative effort in an attempt on an unprecedented scale to monitor, prevent, control, and treat cardiovascular diseases in the world population.

Acknowledgment: Figure 1.2 is reproduced through the courtesy of China Pictorial, Beijing, China, and Dr. L. X. Peng, Hunan Medical College, Changsha, China.

REFERENCES

1. Uemura K, Pisa Z: Recent trends in cardiovascular disease mortality in 27 industrialized countries. *World Health Stat Q* 1985; 38:142–162.
2. Smith WC, Tunstall-Pedoe H: European regional variation in cardiovascular mortality. *Br Med Bull* 1984; 40:374–379.
3. Gordon T, Thom T: The recent decrease in CHD mortality. *Prev Med* 1975; 4:115–125.
4. Havlik R, Feinleib M: Proceedings of the Conference on the Decline in Coronary Heart Disease Mortality. US Department of Health, Education and Welfare. Public Health Service, NIH Publ No. 79–1610, National Institutes of Health, Washington, DC, 1979.
5. Stamler J: The marked decline in coronary heart disease mortality rates in the United States, 1968-1981: summary of findings and possible explanations. *Cardiology* 1985; 72:11–22.
6. Pyorala K, Epstein FH, Kornitzer M: Changing trends in coronary heart disease mortality: possible explanations. *Cardiology* 1985; 72:5–10.
7. Wenger NK: Coronary disease in women. *Ann Rev Med* 1985; 36:285–294.
8. Johansson S, Vedin A, Wilhelmsson C, Wedel H, Wilhelmsen L: Myocardial infarction among women in Gothenburg, Sweden: a community study of mortality and incidence, 1968-1977. *Am J Epidemiol* 1984; 119:603–609.
9. Tunstall-Pedoe H, Smith WCS, Symmers W, Watt G, Kenicer M, Crombie IK, Irving M: Coronary heart disease in Scotland and the programme of the cardiovascular epidemiology unit in Dundee (abstr). *Eur Heart J* 1985; 6(suppl 1):7.
10. Cheng TO: Medicine and health care along the silk road in China. *Am J Med* 1985; 78:3–8.
11. Cheng TO: Glimpses of the past from the recently unearthed ancient corpse in China. *Ann Intern Med* 1984; 101:714–715.
12. Epstein FH, Eckoff RD: The epidemiology of high blood pressure. Geographic distributions and etiological factors, in Stamler J, Stamler R, Pullman TN (eds): *The Epidemiology of Hypertension.* New York, Grune & Stratton, 1967, pp 155–166.
13. Fabre J, Baczko A, Laravoire P, Dayer P, Fox H: Arterial hypertension and ethnic factors. *Adv Nephrol* 1983; 12:19–39.
14. Hall WD, Saunders E, Shulman NB: *Hypertension in Blacks: Epidemiology, Pathophysiology and Treatment.* Chicago, YearBook Medical Publishers, 1985.
15. Fregly MJ, Kare MR: *The Role of Salt in Cardiovascular Hypertension.* New York, Academic Press, 1982.
16. Grim CE, Luft FC, Miller JZ, Meneely GR, Battarbee HD, Hames CD, Dahl LK: Racial differences in blood pressure in Evans County, Georgia: relationship to sodium and potassium intake and plasma renin activity. *J Chronic Dis* 1980; 33:87–94.
17. McCarron DA, Morris CD, Cole C: Dietary calcium in human hypertension. *Science* 1982; 217:267–269.
18. Kesteloot H, Huang DX, Geboers J: Blood pressure and urinary electrolytes in the People's Republic of China (abstr). *Eur Heart J* 1985; 6(suppl I):104.
19. Health Implications of Obesity. National Institutes of Health Consensus Development Conference (Feb 11-13, 1985) Statement. Vol 5, Number 9.
20. Barrett-Connor E, Khaw KT: Is hypertension more benign when associated with obesity? *Circulation* 1985; 72:53–60.
21. McMahon SW, Leeder SR: Blood pressure levels and mortality from cerebrovascular disease in Australia and the United States. *Am J Epidemiol* 1984; 120:865-875.
22. Shimizu Y, Kato H, Lin CH, Kodama K, Peterson AV, Prentice RL: Relationship between longitudinal changes in blood pressure and stroke incidence. *Stroke* 1984; 15:839–846.
23. Lindholm L, Ejlertsson G, Schersten B: High risk of cerebrocardiovascular mortality in well treated male hypertensives. A retrospective study of 40–59-year-old hypertensives in a Swedish primary care district. *Acta Med Scand* 1984; 216:251–259.
24. Kannel WB: Current status of the epidemiology of brain infarction associated with occlusive arterial disease. *Stroke* 1971; 2:295–318.
25. Worth RM, Kato H, Rhoads GG, Kagan A, Syne SL: Epidemiologic study of coronary heart disease and stroke in Japanese men living in Japan, Hawaii and California: mortality. *Am J Epidemiol* 1975; 102:481–490.

26. Konishi M: Epidemiological studies on cerebrovascular diseases with the special references to the pathological findings on stroke in Akita district. *Jpn J Public Health* 1974; 21:485–500.
27. Strasser T: Rheumatic fever and rheumatic heart disease in the 1970s. *WHO Chron* 1978; 32:18–25.
28. Gotsman MS: Rheumatic fever in the 80s. Part II. *Cardiovasc Rev Rep* 1985; 6:935–957.
29. Persson B: The natural history of rheumatic fever and rheumatic heart disease in Malmö. *Acta Med Scand* 1982; 666(suppl):11–172.
30. Wabitsch KR, Prior IAM, Stanley DG, Pearce N: New Zealand trends in acute rheumatic fever and chronic rheumatic heart disease 1971-1981. *NZ Med J* 1984; 97:594–597.
31. Padmavati S: Rheumatic fever and rheumatic heart disease in developing countries. *Bull WHO* 1978; 56:543–550.
32. Woo KS, Kong SM, Wai KH: The changing prevalence and pattern of acute rheumatic fever and rheumatic heart disease in Hong Kong (1968-1978). *Aust NZ J Med* 1983; 13:151–156.
33. Majeed HA, Yousof AM, Shaltout A, Khuffash FA: Acute rheumatic fever below the age of five years: a prospective study of the clinical profile. *Ann Trop Paediatr* 1984; 4:37–40.
34. American Heart Association Committee on Rheumatic Fever and Bacterial Endocarditis: Jones criteria (revised) for guidance in the diagnosis of rheumatic fever. *Circulation* 1984; 69:204A–208A.
35. United Kingdom and United States Joint Report: The evolution of rheumatic heart disease in children. Five-year report of a cooperative clinical trial of ACTH, cortisone, and aspirin. *Circulation* 1960; 22:503–515.
36. Lue HC, Chen CL, Wei HY, Okuni M, Mabilangan LM, Dharmasakti D, Hanafiah A: The natural history of rheumatic fever and rheumatic heart disease in the Orient. *Jpn Heart J* 1979; 20:237–252.
37. Taussig HB: World survey of the common cardiac malformations: developmental error or genetic variant? In Engle MA, Perloff JK (eds): *Congenital Heart Disease After Surgery: Benefits, Residua, Sequelae.* New York, Yorke Medical Books, 1983, pp 1-42.
38. Schrire V: Experience with congenital heart disease at Groote Schuur Hospital, Capetown. An analysis of 1439 patients over an 11-year period. *S Afr Med J* 1963; 37:1175–1180.
39. Schrire V: The racial incidence of the less common forms of heart disease at Groote Schuur Hospital, Capetown 1952-1961. *S Afr Med J* 1964; 38:598–601.
40. McLaren MJ, Lachman AS, Barlow JB: Prevalence of congenital heart disease in black school children of Soweto, Johannesburg. *Br Heart J* 1979; 41:554–558.
41. Caddell JL, Conner DH: Congenital heart disease in Ugandan children. *Br Heart J* 1966; 28:766–767.
42. Caddell JL, Morton P: The pattern of congenital heart disease in Yoruba children of Western Nigeria. *Am Heart J* 1967; 73:431–432.
43. Tofler OB: Congenital heart disease in aboriginals. *Med J Aust* 1979; 1:620.
44. Harvald B, Hels J: Incidence of cardiac malformations in Greenlandic Eskimos. *Humangenetik* 1972; 15:257–260.
45. Wada J: Congenital heart disease. *Jpn Circ J* 1963; 27:251–253.
45a. Cho KY, Nahm CC, Such CS, Lee DY, Cho CB: Heart disease in Korea. *Proceedings Third Asian-Pacific Congress of Cardiology.* Kyoto, Kawakita Printing Co, 1964, p 190.
45b. Shann MKM: Congenital heart disease in Taiwan, Republic of China. *Circulation* 1969; 39:251–258.
45c. Ongley PA: Pediatric cardiology in Thailand. *Circulation* 1966; 34:1–3.
45d. Qian YQ, Zheng DY, Zeng FY, Li MJ, Sun ZQ: Epidemiological study of children under 6 years of age in Chengdu for congenital heart disease. *Chin J Cardiol* 1984; 12:4.
46. Cheng TO: Prevalence of cardiovascular diseases among the national minorities of China. *Ann Intern Med* 1984; 101:562–563.
47. Cheng TO: Cardiology in People's Republic of China, in Russek HI (ed): *New Horizons in Cardiovascular Practice.* Baltimore, University Park Press, 1975, pp 1-29.
48. Anderson RC: Congenital heart malformations in North American Indian children. *Pediatrics* 1977; 59:121–123.
49. Hoffman JIE: Natural history of congenital heart disease. Problems in its assessment with special reference to ventricular septal defects. *Circulation* 1968; 37:97–125.
50. Samanek M, Goetzova J, Benesova D: Distribution of congenital heart malformations in an autopsied child population. *Int J Cardiol* 1985; 8:235–248.
51. Report of the WHO/ISFC task force on the definition and classification of cardiomyopathies. *Br Heart J* 1980; 44:672–673.
52. WHO Report on Cardiomyopathies. WHO Technical Report Series 697. Geneva, WHO, 1984, pp 7-68.
53. Vijayaraghavan G, Cherian G, Krishnaswami S, Sukumar IP: Left ventricular endomyocardial fibrosis in India. *Br Heart J* 1977; 39:563–568.
54. Yang DY: Keshan disease (endemic cardiomyopathy). *Chin J Intern Med* 1984; 23:445–447.
55. Babu SK, Khatri HN, Datta BN, Bidwai PS, Sapru RP, Wahi PL: Cardiomyopathy in Northern India: a clinicopathological study. *Indian Heart J* 1977; 29:35–42.
56. Torp A: Incidence of congestive cardiomyopathy. *Postgrad Med J* 1978; 54:435–437.
57. Torp A: Incidence of congestive cardiomyopathy, in Goodwin JF, Hjalmarson A, Olsen EGJ (eds): *Congestive Cardiomyopathy.* Moelndal, Sweden; AB Hassle, 1981, pp 18–22.
58. Prevalence of cardiomyopathy in a survey study of 66,632 subjects in Nanning district, Guang-Xi province. *Bull Guang-Xi Med Coll* 1979; 1:57–70.
59. Bagger JP, Baandrup U, Rasmussen K, Moller M, Vasterlund T: Cardiomyopathy in western Denmark. *Br Heart J* 1984; 52:327–331.
60. Williams DG, Olsen EGJ: Prevalence of overt dilated cardiomyopathy in two regions of England. *Br Heart J* 1985; 54:153–155.
61. Zeo-Cheng CS, Tsai CC, Palmer D, Codd JE, Penoington DG, Williams GA: High incidence of myocarditis by endomyocardial biopsy in patients with idiopathic congestive cardiomyopathy. *J Am Coll Cardiol* 1984; 3:63–70.
62. O'Connell JB, Fowles RE, Robinson JA, Subramanian R, Henkin RE, Gunnar RM: Clinical and pathologic findings of myocarditis in two families with dilated cardiomyopathy. *Am Heart J* 1984; 107:127–135.
63. Yang LD, Chen HZ, Pu SY, Zhu JR, Shi OS, Yang YZ: Possible etiological association of Coxsackie B viruses with idiopathic dilated cardiomyopathy. *Chin J Cardiol* 1984; 12:86–89.
64. Dec GW, Palacios IF, Fallon JT, Aretz HT, Mills J, Lee DCS, Johnson RA: Active myocarditis in the spectrum of acute dilated cardiomyopathies. Clinical features, histologic correlates and clinical outcome. *N Engl J Med* 1985; 312:885–890.
65. Beck W: Cardiomyopathies in South Africa: a brief survey of the problems and current therapeutic approaches. *Postgrad Med J* 1978; 54:469–474.
66. Topol EJ, Traill TA, Fortuin NJ: Hypertensive hypertrophic cardiomyopathy of the elderly. *N Engl J Med* 1985; 312:277–283.
67. Soloff LA: Hypertensive hypertrophic cardiomyopathy. *N Engl J Med* 1985; 312:1455–1456.
68. Bjarnason I, Hallgrimsson J: Hypertrophic cardiomyopathy: an autopsy study of the years 1966-78. *Icelandic Med J* 1980; 66:205–209.
69. Hardarson T: Subclinical hypertrophic cardiomyopathy: the inconspicuous rump of the iceberg. *Acta Med Scand* 1984; 216:1–2.
70. Bjarnason I, Jonsson S, Hardarson T: Mode of inheritance of hypertrophic cardiomyopathy in Iceland. Echocardiographic study. *Br Heart J* 1982; 47:122–129.
71. Kawai C, Sakurai T, Fujiwara H, Matsumori A, Yui Y: Hypertrophic obstructive and non-obstructive cardiomyopathy in Japan. Diagnosis of the disease with special reference to endomyocardial catheter biopsy. *Eur Heart J* 1983; 4(suppl F):121–125.
72. Yamaguchi H, Nakanishi S, Nishijo T, Nagasaki F, Matsumoto S, Ishimura T: Hypertrophic cardiomyopathy with giant negative T waves. *Jpn Circ J* 1976; 40(suppl l):110–111.
73. Yamaguchi H, Ishimura T, Nishiyama S, Nagasaki F, Nakanishi S, Takatsu F, Nishijo T, Umeda T, Machii K: Hypertrophic nonobstructive cardiomyopathy with giant negative T-waves (apical hypertrophy): ventriculographic and echocardiographic features in 30 patients. *Am J Cardiol* 1979; 44:401–412.
74. Maron BJ, Bonow RO, Seshagiri TNR, Roberts WC, Epstein SE: Hypertrophic cardiomyopathy with ventricular septal hypertrophy localized to the apical region of the left ventricle (apical hypertrophic cardiomyopathy). *Am J Cardiol* 1982; 49:1838–1848.
75. Kereiakes DJ, Anderson DJ, Crouse L, Chatterjee K: Apical hypertrophic cardiomyopathy. *Am Heart J* 1983; 105:855–856.
76. Vacek JL, Davis WR, Bellinger RL, McKiernan TL: Apical hypertrophic cardiomyopathy in American patients. *Am Heart J* 1984; 108:1501–1506.
77. Lock CB, Ng R, Oh V, Ee B, Tan L: Apical hypertrophic cardiomyopathy in an Indian male. *Singapore Med J* 1981; 22:298–301.
78. Krishnaraj N, Rajan S, Jayakrishnan TK, Raghuram AR, Moorthy JS, Abraham KA, Subramanyam R: Apical hypertrophic cardiomyopathy. *Indian Heart J* 1982; 34:133–137.
79. Przybojewski JZ, Blake RS: Hypertrophic non-obstructive apical cardiomyopathy. A case presentation and review of the literature. *S Afr Med J* 1984; 66:492–496.
80. Keren G, Belhassen B, Sherez J, Miller H, Megidish R, Berenfeld D, Laniado S: Apical hypertrophic cardiomyopathy: evaluation by noninvasive and invasive techniques in 23 patients. *Circulation* 1985; 71:45–56.
81. Wigle ED, Sasson Z, Henderson MA, Ruddy TD, Fulop J, Rakowski H, Williams WG: Hypertrophic cardiomyopathy. The importance of the site and the extent of hypertrophy. A review. *Progr Cardiovasc Dis* 1985; 28:1–83.
82. Olsen EGJ, Spry CJF: Relation between eosinophilia and endomyocardial disease. *Progr Cardiovasc Dis* 1985; 27:241–254.
83. Ohno Y: Health development in Japan: determinants, implications and perspectives. *World Health Stat Q* 1985; 38:176–192.
84. Pisa Z: The MONICA project for cardiovascular disease. *World Health Forum* 1982; 3:336–337.

2 The Changing Incidence of Heart Disease in Modern China

Cheng Lang Tung, MD and Tsung O. Cheng, MD

Changes in the average life expectancy in modern China bear a close relation to the incidence of heart disease in the population at large. The average life span has nearly doubled in the last 30 years. In old China the average life span was 35 to 40 years according to various estimates, whereas in 1981 it was 67.88 years (66.43 years for males and 69.35 years for females) for the country as a whole.[1] For urban Shanghai, it was 42.6 years for males and 45.7 years for females in 1951; the corresponding figures were 72.78 and 75.37 years in 1980.[1] Similar lengthening of life span was observed in other parts of China.[2] With this prolongation of life and its associated decrease in mortality due to infectious diseases and malnutrition, both the morbidity and mortality rates of heart disease registered a marked increase. Whether this increase in the number of deaths from heart disease is relative or absolute will be discussed subsequently.

AVAILABLE CRUDE AND CAUSE-SPECIFIC MORTALITY DATA

According to the *World Health Statistics Quarterly*[3] and *Annual*[4] in 1981, the crude death rate each year per 1,000 persons in urban and rural areas of China was about 25.0 before 1949, 18.0 in 1950, 10.80 in 1957, 9.55 in 1965, 7.34 in 1971, 7.36 in 1975, and 6.29 in 1978. The latest population census from China showed that the mortality rate was 6.36 per 1,000 persons in 1982.[5] These data show that during the past 30-year period, the health of the Chinese people has greatly improved. At the same time, the cause-specific mortality rate from heart disease per 100,000 persons had risen from fourth place (44.65 to 68.58 in urban and rural areas) in the period 1954 to 1959 to first place in 1974 to 1978 (113.13 to 130.67 in urban and 111.14 to 151.79 in rural areas), the latter figures accounting for over 17% of all causes of death, a remarkable increase in the mortality rate from heart disease of about 90%. However, an investigation conducted in certain Chinese cities for a more recent period apparently disclosed cerebrovascular disease as the number two killer, second only to heart disease.[5]

AVAILABLE HOSPITAL ADMISSION DATA

Although the ratio of cardiac patients to total number of admissions to the medical services of large, metropolitan hospitals and the proportion of various etiologic types of heart disease among these cardiac patients do not necessarily mirror the prevalence of heart disease in general and of its etiologic types in particular in the population at large of the area or areas studied, hospital data still possess certain intrinsic value, such as close study and often prolonged observation periods coupled with necessary laboratory facilities, so that the diagnoses are comparatively reliable. Moreover, in a socialist country like China, practically all patients that need hospitalization are admitted to the various types of hospitals. Therefore, it appears to us that hospital practice data from large general hospitals have at least supportive value in our survey of the prevalence of heart disease in China.

That there has been a definite increase in the proportion of cardiac patients among all patients admitted to the general medical services of the hospitals in Shanghai may be seen from the following statistics. In the 32-year period from 1948 through 1979, a total of 25,597 cardiac patients were studied in the three general hospitals of Shanghai (Shanghai Sixth People's Hospital and Zhongshan and Huashan Hospitals of the Shanghai First Medical College). The proportion of cardiac patients among all admissions to the general medical services of these hospitals registered an increase from 10.17% from 1948 to 1958 to 22.03% from 1959 to 1971 and 23.16% from 1972 to 1978.[6]

CHANGING PROPORTION OF VARIOUS ETIOLOGIC TYPES

Of greater significance, however, is the magnitude as well as the nature of the changing proportion of various etiologic types of heart disease in Shanghai during the last 32-year period (Table 2.1). Analysis of these 25,597 cardiac inpatients in this period[6] indicates that aside from the dramatic decline in syphilitic heart disease and the less noticeable decline in hypertensive heart disease, the most impressive changes in the proportion of various types of heart disease involve those of rheumatic heart disease (RHD) and coronary or ischemic heart disease (IHD). Rheumatic heart disease decreased by 50% in proportion in the 32-year period, whereas IHD registered a spectacular increase of nearly 500% in this period. Doubtlessly, this remarkable increase in the hospital incidence of IHD is partly relative in nature, but we have reason to believe that it also represents a true increase in the incidence of this disease in China, as evidenced by a similar trend reported in another recent survey from Shanghai of 15,696 patients during the same period.[7]

There are at least two reasons for the relative increase in IHD. First, because of improved living conditions and nationwide health care programs, more persons live to the age of 50 and over, when coronary atherosclerosis becomes more prevalent than in the young. Second, as already mentioned, the virtual elimination of syphilitic aortitis and the significant decrease in rheumatic and hypertensive heart disease increase the relative proportion of IHD. The availability of portable electrocardiographs may also be partly responsible for the apparent increase in morbidity of IHD, but this cannot be an important factor. It is our conviction that there has been an absolute increase in the incidence of this disease in modern China. First, its spectacular increase in proportion from 6% to 29% in our hospital practice is too great to be accounted for simply by the modest decline in the proportion of RHD in this period. Second, our experience in clinical cardiology of over half a century, when one of us (CLT) was in charge of the cardiology service at the Peiping Union Medical College* Hospital (PUMC of Rockefeller Foundation) from 1931 to 1941, where electrocardiographic examinations were readily available without charge in the outpatient and emergency clinics and in all wards of this 500-bed then modern hospital, a case of acute myocardial infarction (AMI), so eagerly looked for at that time, would be a topic of the weekly medical grand rounds. In the three-year period from April 1938 to March 31, 1941, only nine patients with AMI were observed in the PUMC, averaging only three Chinese patients per year (Caucasian patients not included).[8] Similar conclusions concerning the rarity of coronary artery disease were drawn by Snapper,[9] then Professor of Medicine at PUMC. Snapper made a remark to one of us (CLT) that the aortic intima of some elderly Chinese patients at autopsy was so smooth and soft in texture, with so little atherosclerotic change, that it resembled that of young European patients. This clinical experience was fully supported by Professor of Pathology, Dr. C.H. Hu, who concluded that aortic and coronary atherosclerosis of the same degree appeared an average of 15 to 20 years later in Chinese than in Caucasian patients (based on 885 autopsies at PUMC, 816 Chinese and 69 Caucasian cases).[10] This rarity of AMI in the 1920s, 1930s, and 1940s was in sharp contrast to the commonplace observation of several such patients in a present-day small medical ward.

VARIOUS ETIOLOGIC TYPES IN OTHER PARTS OF CHINA

Similar findings on the changing proportion of various types of heart disease were reported from other medical centers, such as Shenyang in the Northeast and Guangdong province in the South. In Shenyang, among admissions to the cardiac medical service of its teaching hospital, RHD declined in proportion from 80% in 1949 to 1958, to 54% in 1959 to 1968, and then to 37% in 1969 to 1978, whereas the proportion of IHD increased from 8% in the first decade to 16% in the second decade and 32% in the third decade.[11] In Guangdong province in south China, RHD declined in proportion from 43.9% in the period 1954 to 1958, to 34.1% from 1962 to 1966, and then to 24.3% from 1975 to 1979, whereas the proportion of IHD increased from 11.2% in the first period

*Called Peking Union Medical College as of June 5, 1985.

Table 2.1. Changing Proportion of Various Types of Heart Disease in Shanghai, 1948 to 1979

Etiologic Types	1948–1958 (%)	1959–1971 (%)	1972–1979 (%)
Ischemic heart disease	6	13	29
Rheumatic heart disease	50	40	26
Congenital heart disease	4	9	15
Myocarditis	1	2	8
Chronic cor pulmonale	8	11	6
Hypertensive heart disease	16	12	5
Cardiomyopathies	1	1	3
Pericarditis	2	2	1
Syphilitic heart disease	7	2	1
Thyroid heart disease	2	1	1
Others	3	2	5

to 20.8% in the second and then to 34.6% in the third period.[11]

REGIONAL DIFFERENCES

A study of AMI by a collaborating group of 16 hospitals in Beijing (Peking) showed that total admissions of new cases steadily increased from 604 in 1972 to 1,264 in 1979, with no significant change in age composition.[12] The mortality rate declined from 25% in 1972 to 1973 to 12% after 1977.[12] Tao[13] concluded that the number of patients with AMI admitted to a relatively large general hospital in the northern cities like Beijing and Tianjin (Tientsin) has approximated 100 per year, but it was only 20 or even less in southern cities like Shanghai, Zhongqing (Chungking), and Guangzhou (Canton). In a recent clinical analysis of 1,544 cases of AMI studied during the ten-year period 1970 through 1979 in ten general hospitals in Shanghai, there was a tendency toward a gradual increase in the incidence of AMI relative to total admissions to the general medical services from 0.80% to 2.09% (mean for the ten-year period being 1.54%) per year. Total admissions for AMI were 78 in 1970 and 249 in 1979. The latter figure yielded 25 cases per hospital, the highest in the ten-year period, but still well below those of Beijing and Tianjin.[14] Such a striking discrepancy in the regional incidence of AMI, which agrees with our general experience, defies any rational explanation at present but could be due to differences in diet.

Other reports concerning differences in the prevalence of IHD should also be noted. In a general survey of 52,298 people over 40 years of age in 22 different parts of China in the early 1970s, the average incidence of coronary heart disease was 6.46%, but marked differences existed in various parts of China.[15] The lowest incidences were those of 0.6% among 1,625 fishermen in Choushan Archipelago, Zhejian, reported by Cheng[16] in 1973, and 1.92% in Zhonggang,[15] and the highest were those of 19.75% among 81 male nomads in Sinkiang (where the cadres had an incidence of 2.46%)[16] and 14.29% in people living in Inner Mongolia.[15] The reasons advanced were that the nomads eat predominantly animal fat, whereas the fishermen's diet of shellfish, crabs, and lobsters is rich in cholesterol but has a high polyunsaturated to saturated fatty acid ratio.

Clinical evidence of an increase in the incidence of IHD in modern China appears to be corroborated by a recent survey of data on coronary atherosclerosis from autopsies collected from various pathology laboratories in China.[17] In comparison with Wang and Hu's figures published in 1957,[10] the prevalence of atherosclerosis is higher in the present pathologic study, although definite conclusions cannot yet be drawn owing to possible differences in the nature and scope of the two pathologic studies. Another feature of interest is that the prevalence of coronary atherosclerosis is higher in Beijing and Tianjin than in the other regions of China.[13]

CHANGES IN CERTAIN ENVIRONMENTAL FACTORS

Any attempts to explain this increasing incidence of IHD in modern China must consider the effects of certain changes of risk or environmental factors in operation, although it is difficult to prove these effects. Many factors such as stress and strain in modern society, hypertension, cigarette smoking, diet, and associated hyperlipoproteinemia may play a causative role in coronary atherosclerosis. Indeed, certain segments of the Chinese people are more intense today than before in both their life and work, but judging from Western standards they are by no means at full stress. The increase in cigarette smoking, particularly among the younger generation, may be related more to the increase in the incidence of hypertension and certain cardiac arrhythmias than to the increased prevalence of IHD, because the widespread use of antihypertensive drugs has reduced greatly the incidence of hypertensive heart disease. Therefore, it appears to us that hypertension is not a factor that could account for the recent increase in IHD. Next come the recent changes in the quality of diet with its attendant increase in blood lipid levels, at least in the large cities. The consumption of dietary pork and eggs has increased sharply among the population. Investigation of 1,200 workers' households by the Beijing Municipal Statistics Department[18] showed that in Beijing people are consuming more pork and eggs and less grain; pork consumption per capita per year increased from 12.2 kilos in 1978 to 19.6 kilos in 1981, and that of eggs from 4.3 to 6.6 kilos. These figures did not include food consumed at restaurants, where meat and eggs are served ad libitum, or prepared foods. A similar increase was observed in the consumption of beef, mutton, fish, shrimp, and poultry. Investigation showed that for the city residents the ratio of meat and poultry, on the one hand, and vegetables and fruits, on the other, by weight in kilograms was 28:72 in 1978 and 34:66 in 1981.[18] In another recent dietary survey in Beijing the proportion of saturated fat to polyunsaturated fat was 2.6:1, the ideal proportion being 1:1.[18a]

The uniform increase in serum cholesterol levels at the different age levels in 728 subjects examined in 1981 was significant when compared with a similar group of 509 subjects in 1958 (Table 2.2). The mean increase in serum

Table 2.2. Comparative Mean Serum Cholesterol Levels of Free Living Chinese in 1958 and 1981

	1958		1981	
Age Group (yr)	No.	Mean (mg%)	No.	Mean (mg%)
Males				
20–29	43	142.7	59	168.41
30–39	68	154.9	39	180.80
40–49	97	154.4	50	205.64
50–59	54	168.9	42	205.11
Over 60	23	155.4	21	212.48
Total	285	155.3	211	191.21
Females				
20–29	56	151.5	199	173.87
30–39	52	149.1	109	176.98
40–49	55	160.1	152	197.73
50–59	45	173.3	57	213.40
Over 60	16	168.4	...	...
Total	224	158.64	517	185.9

cholesterol was 30 mg% in 1981 in both males and females. The techniques used in the quantitative determination of serum cholesterol were the same in 1958 and 1981. Similar findings of higher serum cholesterol levels were reported from three medical centers in north and central China. In 789 healthy subjects, the figure averaged 185 mg% in those under 40 and 213 mg% in those over 40.[19] If this modest increase in total serum levels can be confirmed for the population samples at large, then changes in the diet with its attendant changes in blood lipid levels may largely be responsible for alterations in the proportion of IHD cases among hospital admissions in the last 32 years.[6]

RHEUMATIC HEART DISEASE

Rheumatic heart disease was the most common form of heart disease in China before 1949 and for about 25 years since. It currently ranks only second to coronary artery disease, and it is particularly prevalent in northern and northeastern provinces. During a period of about 50 years (1920 to 1970), rheumatic fever and RHD dominated the cardiac service in our general hospitals, with many fulminating cases of rheumatic pancarditis; rheumatic pleurisy and pneumonitis, subcutaneous nodules, and chorea were also not uncommon. According to necropsy data in 107 cases of RHD at PUMC reported in 1955,[20] the mitral valve was affected in 100%, with isolated mitral valve disease in 46.7% and combined mitral and aortic valvular disease in 34.5%, whereas the aortic valve was affected in 48.5%, tricuspid valve in 12.2%, and pulmonary valve in only 6.5% of cases. Clinically, pure or predominant mitral stenosis is undoubtedly the most commonly encountered form of RHD.

As a result of improvement in the socioeconomic status of the people and the widespread use of penicillin therapy for beta-hemolytic streptococcal infections, there has been a significant nationwide decline in the prevalence of rheumatic fever and RHD in China.[11]

OTHER ETIOLOGIC FORMS OF HEART DISEASE

Heart disease due to malnutrition such as beriberi heart disease and anemic heart disease, so common in the past,[21] have now practically disappeared. So have diphtheric myocarditis and syphilitic aortitis, the latter being a common cause of angina pectoris in the 1930s and 1940s.[22] However, chronic cor pulmonale is an important form of heart disease, especially in cold plateau areas. A special form of primary myocardial disease, Keshan disease, named after the county in Heilungkiang province in northeastern China where it was first discovered, afflicts almost exclusively the rural population in certain regions in northeast and southwest China. It may be acute or chronic. The pathologic changes consist of scattered focal myocardial necrosis located beneath the endocardium along the distribution of the coronary vessels. Its etiology is unknown. Hypotheses advanced are that (1) the disease is related to selenium deficiency in the soil and water supply,[23] (2) people who had long been living on a "single type of food" harvested from the fields in endemic areas with a particular background of water/soil conditions may suffer from Keshan disease,[24] and (3) it is caused by Coxsackie B virus infection of the myocardium.[25] Other forms of primary cardiomyopathies are also encountered in our hospital practice, particularly the dilated (congestive) and the obstructive (subaortic) hypertrophic types. Viral myocarditis is a probable precursor of dilated cardiomyopathy in most instances, because alcoholic cardiomyopathy is uncommon in China.[26] In a recently completed national survey, the highest incidence of viral myocarditis was found in Harbin in northeast China and the lowest in Fuzhou in south China (41.86 and 8.03 per 100,000 persons, $P < 0.001$).[27]

REFERENCES

1. Seminar opens on China's census. *China Daily,* March 27, 1984.
2. Cheng TO: Medicine and health care along the Silk Road in China. *Am J Med* 1985; 78:3–8.
3. Ling RZ: A brief account of 30 years' mortality of Chinese population. *W H Stat Q* 1981; 31:127–134.
4. *World Health Statistics Annual,* Annex 4, Geneva, WHO, 1981.
5. Anonymous: China conducts nationwide mortality survey. *Chin Med J* 1984; 97:605.
6. Tung CL, Chen WC, Liang SP, Pan SR, Xue W: A reappraisal of the changing proportion of the various types of heart diseases in Shanghai and its relationship to serum cholesterol levels. *Chin Med J* 1984; 97:171–174.
7. Chen H, Lin Y, Dai R, He W, Yuan J, Li J, Wu S, Yang Y: Changes in etiologic types of heart disease in Shanghai during the past 32 years. An analysis of 15,696 patients. *Chin Med J* 1985; 98:151–156.
8. Tung CL: Coronary thrombosis among the Chinese. *Chin Med J* 1948; 66:587–592.
9. Snapper I: *Chinese Lessons to Western Medicine.* New York, Interscience Publishers, 1941, p 160.
10. Wang TX, Hu CH: A study of arteriosclerosis in 885 autopsies in Peking. *Natl Med J China* 1957; 43:411–421.
11. Cooperative Research Group of Guangdong Cardiovascular Institute: Clinical analysis of rheumatic heart disease in the past 30 years in Guangdong Province. *Chin J Intern Med* 1981; 20:3–5.
12. Tao SQ, Chen ZJ, Cui JJ, Xu YS, Kou WR: Trends in incidence, fatality and mortality of acute myocardial infarction in Beijing. A study on hospitalized patients. *Chin Med J* 1982; 95:239–244.
13. Tao SQ: Epidemiologic study of cardiovascular disease in the People's Republic of China. Lecture at WHO Study Group, Beijing, 1980.
14. Shanghai Myocardial Infarction Research Cooperative Group: Clinical analysis of 1544 cases of acute myocardial infarction in Shanghai between 1970 and 1979. *Chin J Int Med* 1984; 23:273–280.
15. Chen HZ: Cardiovascular diseases in China. *Nature J* 1983; 6:586–592.
16. Cheng TO: Cardiology in the People's Republic of China, in Russek HI (ed): *New Horizons in Cardiovascular Practice.* Baltimore, University Park Press, 1975, p 4.
17. Wu YK, Wu ZS, Yao CH: Epidemiologic studies of cardiovascular diseases in China. *Chin Med J* 1983; 96:201–205.
18. Xinhua News Agency: Beijing people are eating more meat. *China Daily*, July 9, 1982.
18a. Yao CH, Hao EH, Wu YY: Dietary survey in Beijing in 1983. *Chin Med J* 1985; 98:439–441.
19. Tao SQ: Coronary atherosclerosis and arteriosclerotic heart disease, in Tung CL, Tao SQ (eds): *Practical Cardiology.* Shanghai, Shanghai Science and Technology Publishers, 1978, p 695.
20. Liu Y: Pathologic changes in rheumatic heart disease. *Chin J Pathol* 1955; 1:104–110.
21. Tung CL, Bien WN, Chiu YC: The heart in severe anemia. *Chin Med J* 1937; 52:479–500.
22. Tung CL, Mu JW: Immediate effects of the intravenous administration of neoarsphenamine on the electrocardiogram in cases of syphilitic aortitis. *Am Heart J* 1940; 19:529–540.
23. Keshan Disease Research Group of the Chinese Academy of Medical Sciences, Beijing: Epidemiologic studies on the etiologic relationship of selenium and Keshan disease. *Chin Med J* 1979; 92:477–482.
24. Yang SY: An endemic cardiomyopathy in China-Keshan disease, in Doyle EF, Engle MA, Gersony WM, Rashkind WJ, Talner NS (eds): *Pediatric Cardiology*. New York, Springer-Verlag, 1986, pp 975–977.

25. Gu BQ: Pathology of Keshan disease. A comprehensive review. *Chin Med J* 1983; 96:251–261.
26. Cheng TO: Prevalence of cardiovascular diseases among the national minorities of China. *Ann Intern Med* 1984; 101:562–563.
27. Li CY, Li J, Chen GF, Guo XP, Yang SY, Han RC: Investigation on incidence of virus myocarditis in children, in Doyle EF, Engle MA, Gersony WM, Rashkind WJ, Talner NS (eds): *Pediatric Cardiology*. New York, Springer-Verlag, 1986.

3 Cardiovascular Risk Factors Distribution: A Comparison Between East and West

Hugo Kesteloot, MD

Significant differences in the distribution of cardiovascular risk factors and in the prevalence and incidence of cardiovascular disease, together with important variations in diet exist in different parts of the world. The purpose of the study presented in this chapter was to evaluate the significance of these differences in the distribution of cardiovascular risk factors measured in a standardized way between Korea, with a typically Oriental diet, and Belgium, with a typically Western diet, and to try to identify the factors responsible for these differences. The study mainly focused on the distribution of arterial blood pressure and serum lipid levels between the two populations. Moreover, our findings will be put into a historical perspective.

METHODOLOGY

Great attention was given to standardization of the methods of measuring various biologic parameters. No standardization was necessary for height and weight, although in Korea one is always weighed naked whereas in Belgium light clothing (such as underwear or trousers) is usual when weight is determined.

For age, however, some problems exist in Korea because calendar age is frequently used. This means that anyone born on December 31 is considered one year old on January 1. Moreover, age is often expressed according to a Buddhist habit which starts counting age from a date approximately nine months before the actual birth. Therefore, age determination in older people is often difficult. However, in all cases birth date was used for the determination of age.

BLOOD PRESSURE MEASUREMENT

Standardization of blood pressure measurement is extremely difficult when measurements are made in different parts of the world. We have followed the recommendations of two working groups instituted by the medical research council of the European Communities and dedicated to this problem.[1,2] In summary, to minimize the methodologic, biologic, and circadian factors influencing blood pressure measurement, home reading of blood pressure by the participants themselves was performed in Belgium and Korea, using the same blood pressure measurement devices (Auto-test SK, Pressostabil, Germany). Measurements were taken at the same biologically important moments, namely, on arising from bed in the morning and on retiring to bed at night, both in the standing and in the supine positions. Measurements were carried out on three consecutive days and the results of the measurements were pooled per individual to obtain mean systolic and diastolic blood pressure. Phase 5 (disappearance of Korotkoff sounds) was used to determine diastolic blood pressure.[1,2] In Belgium, home reading was taught to the participants by physicians; and in Korea by trained nurses. Blood pressure was expressed in millimeters of mercury and measured to the nearest even number.

TWENTY-FOUR-HOUR URINE COLLECTION

Strict instructions were given to avoid urine over- or undercollection. Bladder emptying before defecation was ordered. The urine was slightly acidified by the addition of 20 ml of pure glacial acetic acid. Volume was measured to the nearest 40 ml. In Korea, the 24-hour urine collection was performed on three consecutive days, whereas in Belgium, collection was performed on ten nonconsecutive days. For uniformity, the three first days of the Belgian collection only were used in this analysis. Aliquots of urine from Korean subjects were put in deep-freezers and sent to Belgium by airmail for analysis. Measurements of calcium, sodium, potassium, and creatinine were performed on the 24-hour urine samples in the laboratory of the St. Rafaël University Hospital. Creatinine was measured according to the colorimetric method of Jaffé.[3]

SERUM LIPID STUDY

In Belgium as well as in Korea, different population groups were examined for the blood pressure study and for the serum lipid study.[4–8] Therefore, these populations will be studied separately. The nutritional status of the Korean population was excellent.

POPULATION CHARACTERISTICS

Blood Pressure Study

The examined population group in Belgium consisted of a suburban population from the city of Leuven which generally can be considered middle class. Measurements were performed during the years 1972 and 1973. In Korea the participants were partly farmers from the southwest (about 150 km southwest of Seoul) and partly inhabitants of the city of Seoul.[9,10] The city inhabitants generally lived in the neighborhood or were acquaintances of student nurses who introduced the participants to the method of home blood pressure measurement, as indicated herein.

In Korea, examinations were performed between September and December when the climate is generally moderate and becoming progressively colder. This was done to minimize electrolyte loss through sweating, as summers are hot and humid in Korea. The study was performed in Korea in the period 1976 to 1978.

Serum Lipid Study

Koreans, for philosophical reasons, are reluctant to let blood samples be taken for biologic determination. The investigated subjects consisted partly of volunteer workers for work in the Middle East who were obligatorily submitted to serum analysis for the Bordet-Wasserman test to detect syphilis. On this occasion, blood samples were collected for serum lipid determinations. The female participants were nurses and other hospital personnel including cleaning women. Some of the participants came from Taegu, 300 km south of Seoul, a city of 1.5 million inhabitants, and the participants were mainly soldiers, students, nurses, and farmers. The Belgian participants were clerical and manual workers of a chemical plant in the neighborhood of Antwerpen. In the Belgian plant the participation rate was 99%. Both the Korean and the Belgian studies were performed in the period 1978 to 1979.

STATISTICAL ANALYSIS

To study the independent influence of factors considered to be dependent variables, multiple regression analysis was performed in a step-up fashion. In the first analysis, all factors are included, of which a possible effect on the dependent variable is expected. At each step the least significant factor is eliminated until only factors significant at the $P<0.05$ level remain. Whenever combinations of several groups were made, interaction variables, taking into account the interrelation between these groups and the independent variables, were included in the multiple regression analysis which corresponds to the use of multiple covariance analysis.

RESULTS

BLOOD PRESSURE STUDY

Anthropometric characteristics, blood pressure data, and mean sodium and potassium excretion in the population studied are given in Table 3.1 for Korea and in Table 3.2 for Belgium. For both sexes, sodium excretion is significantly higher and potassium excretion lower in Korea compared with Belgium. Both male and female subjects are more obese in Belgium than in Korea, as appears from the height-to-weight ratio.

When blood pressure was calculated from the equation between blood pressure and age, height and weight as independent variables, both systolic and diastolic blood pressure were markedly higher in Korea than in Belgium.[11] The crude data also showed systolic and diastolic blood pressure to be higher in Korea than in Belgium, notwithstanding the marked obesity of the Belgian population. From multiple regression analysis it appears that the overall influence of sodium on blood pressure was positive in Korea, but not significant in Belgian men, and of only borderline significance in Belgian women. Only in Korean men did potassium levels significantly correlate with blood pressure. The t value of the independent relation of sodium and potassium is given in Table 3.3. Results of the complete analysis, using multiple regression analysis with inclusion of the interaction terms for group (Belgian and Korean) and sex, is given in Table 3.4. As can be seen from the regression coefficients for sodium and potassium, their overall influence on blood pressure remains small: about 2 mm Hg per 100 mmol of 24-hour sodium excretion for systolic and 1 mm Hg for diastolic. An increase in 24-hour potassium intake of 100 mmol causes a decrease in systolic blood pressure of 5 mm Hg. However, total mean 24-hour potassium intake (men and women) is only 56 mmol in Korea and 70 mmol in Belgium (Tables 3.1 and 3.2).

This analysis also indicates that men have a higher blood pressure than women and that systolic blood pressure is 6 mm Hg higher in Korea compared with Belgium.

Recently we also became interested in the relation be-

Table 3.1. Anthropometric Data, Urinary Electrolyte Excretion, and Blood Pressure (Mean Values ± SD; Men and Women/Belgium)

	Men (No. = 133)		Women (No. = 167)	
	Mean	**SD**	**Mean**	**SD**
Age (yr)	39.3	± 11.0	40.0	± 12.2
Height (cm)	174.0	± 6.4	161.3	± 6.4
Weight (kg)	75.4	± 10.8	60.7	± 8.2
Weight/height² (× 100)	0.25	± 0.003	0.23	± 0.031
Sodium (mmol/24 h)	183.9	± 44.6	152.6	± 43.8
Potassium (mmol/24 h)	76.7	± 15.4	65.3	+ 12.5
Systolic blood pressure (mm Hg)	121.4	± 12.6	114.6	± 13.9
Diastolic blood pressure (mm Hg)	78.5	± 8.6	73.0	± 8.4

SD = standard deviation.

Table 3.2. Anthropometric Data, Urinary Electrolyte Excretion, and Blood Pressure (Mean Values ± SD; Men and Women/Korea)

	Men (No. = 200)	Women (No. = 258)	Men + Women (No. = 458)
Age (yr)	37.5 ± 14.3	39.7 ± 13.7	38.8 ± 14
Height (cm)	166.6 ± 6.6	155.4 ± 5.2	160.3 ± 8
Weight (kg)	60.2 ± 8.2	50.4 ± 7.3	54.7 ± 9.1
Weight/height² (× 100)	0.22 ± 0.024	0.21 ± 0.029	0.21 ± 0.027
Sodium (mmol/24 h)	294.2 ± 133.4	266.5 ± 107.6	278.6 ± 120.2
Potassium (mmol/24 h)	57.1 ± 43.8	54.7 ± 27.5	55.8 ± 35.6
Systolic blood pressure (mm Hg)	125.2 ± 14.2	120.5 ± 18.6	122.6 ± 16.9
Diastolic blood pressure (mm Hg)	81.2 ± 10.6	77.9 ± 12.0	79.4 ± 11.5

SD = standard deviation.

tween calcium and blood pressure. This resulted from the finding that in a large epidemiologic study in Belgian male subjects, a highly significant relation was found (by both uni- and multivariate analysis) between serum calcium and blood pressure.

A positive and significant relation was also found in the same Belgian study, the preliminary data of which have been published,[12] and in the Korean study between 24-hour urinary calcium and blood pressure (Table 3.5). It should be noted that 24-hour urinary calcium excretion was somewhat higher in Koreans than in Belgians, being 5.1 ± 2.9 mmol in Belgian men compared with 5.3 ± 3.3 mmol in Korean men and 4.1 ± 2.7 mmol in Korean women.

SERUM LIPID STUDY

Anthropometric data for the studied populations, which have previously been published, are similar to the values given in Tables 3.1 and 2. These data again demonstrate the increased obesity of the Belgian population. The total cholesterol values obtained in the Korean and Belgian populations for men are given in Table 3.6 and for women in Table 3.7. The values of HDL-cholesterol in men are presented in Table 3.8 and in women in Table 3.9. It is clear from the tables that total serum cholesterol is higher in Belgium than in Korea and that the difference increases with age. In contrast, the HDL-cholesterol level is about the same in Belgian and Korean men but markedly lower in Korean women. The difference in HDL-cholesterol levels between male and female subjects is much higher in Belgium than in Korea.

DISCUSSION

Studies of differences in life-styles and diet between populations can be considered as natural experiments that cannot be duplicated in the laboratory. For example, it would be impossible to reproduce in the laboratory the effect of eating a high-salt diet for 50 years, but this effect can be studied in populations having such a diet.

Much evidence points to diet as a causal factor in several important and extremely common cardiovascular diseases such as ischemic heart disease and hypertensive cardiovascular disease. However, dietary habits within populations are rather uniform, and it is extremely difficult, if not impossible, to change them radically in a short time. Even then, the biologic and metabolic consequences of the former diet might well influence the results obtained by the dietary change. It therefore is interesting to look at populations with markedly different life-styles to study their influence on the distribution of some important cardiovascular risk factors. Already more than 60 years ago, working in Indonesia, de Langen found

Table 3.3. Independent *t* Values of Sodium (Na) and Potassium (K)

			SBP		DBP		R	
		No.	Na	K	Na	K	SBP	DBP
Belgium	M	133	...	...	...	...	0.51	0.53
	F	167	...	...	+2.01*	...	0.55	0.59
	M+F	300	...	...	...	...	0.55	0.61
Korea	M	200	+3.0*	−3.1†	...	...	0.37	0.34
	F	258	...	...	+2.1*	...	0.32	0.28
	M+F	458	+2.8†	−2.2*	...	...	0.37	0.33
Korea (+HR)	M	200	+3.4‡	−2.6†	...	...	0.46	0.46
	F	258	+2.4†	...	+2.9†	...	0.41	0.44
	M+F	458	+4.1‡	...	+2.6†	...	0.45	0.45
Belgium + Korea	M	333	+2.9†	−2.7†	...	...	0.44	0.42
	F	425	...	...	+2.0*	...	0.41	0.42
	M+F	758	+3.0†	−2.0*	+2.1*	...	0.45	0.47

* $P < 0.05$; † $P < 0.01$; ‡ $P < 0.001$.

DBP = diastolic blood pressure; F = females; HR = heart rate; M = males; R = value of the multiple correlation coefficient obtained with all significant factors included (age, Quetelet index, 24-h urinary excretion of Na, K, and creatinine and HR when specified); SBP = systolic blood pressure.

Table 3.4. Multivariate Analysis of Blood Pressure (Men and Women; Belgium and Korea) (No. = 758)

	Blood Pressure		t Value
SBP = (mm Hg)	82.52		
	+0.3845	A	9.18
	+7214.06	W/H^2	3.94
	+0.01908	Na	3.02
	−0.04758	K	−1.90
	+0.004184	Creatinine	2.79
	−3.08	G	−3.75
	+4.99	S	2.97
	−0.0836	S × A	−2.05
R = 0.45; R^2 = 0.20; SEy = 14.32 mm Hg			
DBP = (mm Hg)	55.78		
	+0.2985	A	10.42
	+4107.89	W/H^2	3.31
	+0.0082	Na	2.13
	+0.04273	G × A	2.14
	+465.27	G × S × W/H^2	2.78
	−0.002776	Creatinine	−4.53
	+2.186	S	5.91
R = 0.47; R^2 = 0.22; SEy = 9.75 mm Hg			

A = age (yr); G = group: BE+1, KO−1; H = height (cm); S = sex: M+1, F−1; Na, K (mmol/24 h); creatinine (mg/24 h); W = weight (kg).

a difference in serum cholesterol levels between Dutch and Indonesian subjects.[13] However, the numbers were small, standardization of methods was nonexistent, and his interest was mainly centered on the difference in the prevalence of gallstones between the two populations, although he also included some side remarks on the possible bearing of this finding on the distribution of ischemic heart disease. Subsequently, however, de Langen[14] paid special attention to the importance of a cholesterol-free diet in the prevention of atherosclerosis and embolism in the Javanese population. This finding was confirmed by Snapper[15,16] in a Northern Chinese population, who also found that the diet of the Chinese was richer in polyunsaturated fat and poorer in saturated fat than the Western diet. In the first edition of his book, *Chinese Lessons to Western Medicine* in 1941, he was rather skeptical about the relation between the Chinese diet and the absence of atherosclerosis, but he changed his view in commentaries to the second edition of his book in 1965 where he adopted de Langen's view on the relation between diet and atherosclerosis. Although Snapper devoted a chapter of his book to hypertensive cardiovascular disease, he did not find Chinese blood pressure particularly high nor did he mention the high salt intake of the Northern Chinese population. However, comparative blood pressure studies are difficult to perform, as mentioned in the methodologic section, and standardization of blood pressure was nonexistent at that time. Moreover, salt intake was probably also high in Europe in the 1930s. Another important contribution made by de Langen was the observation that Javanese stewards working on Dutch passenger ships, whose diet was similar to the European diet, also had serum cholesterol levels similar to those found in Europeans.[14] This again stressed the importance of diet as the major determinant of serum cholesterol levels, and it also demonstrated the minor importance of racial differences. It is a well-known fact that ischemic heart disease is rare and cerebrovascular disease more common in Korea and Japan than in Western countries. During a stay in Korea as visiting professor in cardiology at the Kyung Hee University in Seoul, I was prompted by this finding to initiate some comparative studies on the distribution of cardiovascular risk factors in Belgium and Korea. The Korean diet is a typically Oriental diet which derives most of its calories from rice. Its major distinction from a Western diet, however, is the nearly complete absence of saturated fat, fat delivering only about 10% of the total calories.[17,18] In the Western diet, most fat is saturated and it delivers about 40% of the total calories. However, the Korean diet contains much more sodium and less potassium than the Western diet and contains less protein from animal origin. Our findings confirm the much lower serum cholesterol levels of Oriental populations compared with Western populations. Our studies also demonstrate the significant difference of the HDL-cholesterol to total cholesterol ratio between Belgium and Korea, the values being much higher in Korea. This ratio has been linked to the genesis of atherosclerosis, and a high HDL-cholesterol to total cholesterol ratio has been described as protective against the development of atherosclerosis. Our findings are strengthened by the fact that the serum lipid determinations were performed in the same laboratory, by the same technician, using the same methods.[4-8]

Table 3.5. Slope of Urinary Calcium (mmol/24 h) on Blood Pressure

Blood Pressure (mm Hg)	Analysis	Belgium (1979–1980) M (No. = 3541)	Korea (1976–1978) M (No. = 200)	Korea (1976–1978) F (No. = 258)
Systolic	Univariate	0.394*	1.267*	1.350†
	Multivariate‡	0.316§	0.912§	1.064†
Diastolic	Univariate	0.327*	0.676†	0.995§
	Multivariate‡	0.222§	0.475‖	0.807†

* $P < 0.0001$.

† $P < 0.01$.

‡ With the inclusion of age, height, weight, heart rate (Korea only), social class (Korea only), region (urban or rural, Korea only), and 24-h urinary sodium, potassium, and creatinine levels.

§ $P < 0.001$.

‖ $P < 0.05$.

Table 3.6. Comparative Serum Cholesterol Values Between Belgian and Korean Men*

Age (yr)	Belgium No.	Belgium Cholesterol (mg%)	Korea No.	Korea Cholesterol (mg%)
<20	48	172.6 ± 33.7	23	137.4 ± 15.4
20+	193	173.2 ± 29.4	131	149.0 ± 29.1
25+	335	187.2 ± 33.7	166	156.6 ± 30.6
30+	431	201.4 ± 36.6	145	165.4 ± 32.4
35+	325	215.8 ± 41.2	112	156.9 ± 25.0
40+	239	224.2 ± 40.5	58	170.1 ± 37.5
45+	189	229.1 ± 45.4	...	...
50+	144	224.5 ± 43.1	...	...
55+	50	238.3 ± 43.1	...	...

* All differences are significant to the $P<10^{-5}$ level.

Of special interest is our finding that the difference in HDL-cholesterol levels between Belgian and Korean men is relatively small, the Korean values being slightly lower.

Our data are in agreement with recent findings showing that in 13 countries, of which two were Asian (the Philippines and Pakistan), the HDL-cholesterol levels are rather similar, the European values being moderately higher.[19] This shows that the important differences between populations in the level of physical exercise, alcohol intake, total caloric intake, obesity, saturated and polyunsaturated fat intake, and intake of contraceptive hormones result in only small differences in HDL-cholesterol levels. Therefore, it will be extremely difficult to change the HDL-cholesterol level in populations. However, as LDL-cholesterol can be manipulated by dietary means, it makes decreasing the LDL-cholesterol levels all the more important.

One unexplained finding is the much higher HDL-cholesterol level in Belgian compared with Korean women, resulting in much smaller male-female difference in HDL-cholesterol in Korea. Korean women smoke less, use fewer contraceptive pills, are less obese, and are more active than Belgian women. As smoking decreases the HDL-cholesterol level, whereas the effect of contraceptive pills is variable,[20] these differences cannot explain the lower HDL-cholesterol level in Korean women. Whether this is due to a genetic factor remains to be established. This absence of a marked difference in HDL-cholesterol levels between men and women was also found in other Oriental populations in Polynesia[21] and in the People's Republic of China (H. Kesteloot et al, unpublished data).

Our studies also confirmed the higher blood pressure levels in the Korean compared with the Belgian population. In Korea we were able to demonstrate by multiple regression analysis that sodium correlated positively with blood pressure and potassium correlated negatively. This was much less evident in the Belgian population. Many reasons can be invoked to explain the absence of a relation between salt intake and blood pressure in our Belgian population:

1. In Belgium, salt intake has been decreasing with time.[22] People consumed more sodium 10 and 20 years ago than now. The influence of this previously high salt intake could still exist now. Such important changes presumably did not occur in Korea.
2. The standard deviation of the population's salt intake is about twice as high in Korea as in Belgium.
3. In Belgium, people with high blood pressure will probably decrease their salt intake more than will people with normal blood pressure, who might even increase their salt intake in the belief that they are immune to hypertension.
4. Alcohol plays a confounding factor in the Belgian population: high beer intake reduces other food intake and thus presumably also salt intake, but alcohol increases blood pressure levels.
5. Interrelations exist among the effects of sodium, potassium, and calcium on blood pressure.[23,24] We have shown that a positive correlation exists between urinary calcium and blood pressure. In Korea a negative correlation was found between potassium and blood pressure levels. Urinary calcium excretion was actually higher in Korea than in Belgium. Of great theoretic importance is that a negative correlation exists between the amount of urinary-excreted sodium and a positive one with the urinary-excreted potassium and with serum calcium.[24] Serum calcium correlates positively with blood pressure[23] and the interactions among sodium, potassium and calcium make the study of the effect of those ions on blood pressure more complex.
6. Three 24-hour urine samples are insufficient to characterize the mean salt intake of an individual.[25]
7. Methodologic problems in collecting exact 24-hour urine samples and in measuring blood pressure also act as a confounding factor.

The foregoing make the study of the relation between sodium intake and blood pressure difficult. Moreover, genetic factors undoubtedly also play a role in the pathogenesis of hypertension.

Ten years ago butter and cheese were virtually nonexistent in Korea, but this is gradually changing. Also, more refrigerators are being sold, and therefore salt for food preservation is no longer needed. These dietary changes, coupled with dietary changes occurring in the Belgian population, will be interesting to follow in the future to determine their effects on mortality and morbidity.

Our findings agree with recent theories on the pathogenesis of hypertension.[26-28] In sensitive subjects, possibly because of a deficiency in the handling of sodium by the kidney, a high salt intake increases intracellular and blood volume. As a result, a natriuretic hormone is produced which influences sodium-potassium exchange

Table 3.7. Comparative Serum Cholesterol Values Between Belgian and Korean Women*

Age (yr)	Belgium No.	Belgium Cholesterol (mg%)	Korea No.	Korea Cholesterol (mg%)
15+	84	185.7 ± 29.0	440	164.5 ± 28.4
25+	48	203.6 ± 39.1	106	157.9 ± 28.5
35+	55	204.5 ± 31.2	43	161.6 ± 31.2
45+	54	231.3 ± 41.4	33	170.9 ± 37.2
55+	13	255.8 ± 56.4	16	179.8 ± 42.8

* All differences are significant to the $P<10^{-5}$ level.

Table 3.8. Comparative Serum HDL-Cholesterol Values Between Belgian and Korean Men

	Belgium		Korea	
Age (yr)	No.	HDL-Cholesterol (mg%)	No.	HDL-Cholesterol (mg%)
< 20	48	51.3 ± 10.2	23	45.6 ± 8.5*
20+	193	49.2 ± 10.6	131	44.3 ± 8.2†
25+	335	47.8 ± 9.5	166	43.9 ± 9.9†
30+	431	46.2 ± 10.3	145	43.1 ± 10.9‡
35+	325	45.5 ± 10.4	112	42.0 ± 9.6†
40+	239	45.1 ± 10.1	58	45.1 ± 13.2 (NS)
45+	189	45.5 ± 10.4	...	...
50+	144	45.5 ± 9.6	...	...
55+	50	46.1 ± 9.6	...	...

* $P < 0.05$.

† $P < 0.001$.

‡ $P < 0.01$.

NS = not significant.

through the cell membrane, leading to an accumulation of sodium in the vascular smooth muscle cell. This, in turn, through the inhibition of transmembrane sodium-potassium exchange, leads to an accumulation of calcium in the cell. It increases vascular tone and vascular contractility and consequently increases peripheral resistance leading to hypertension. This theory combines the effects of sodium, potassium, and calcium and agrees with our findings of a blood pressure increasing effect of serum calcium (in a separate Belgian study) and of urinary 24-hour calcium and sodium, as indicators of sodium and calcium intake, and a blood pressure lowering effect of 24-hour urinary potassium.

It should be realized, however, that the 24-hour urinary excretion of calcium is only an imperfect indicator of calcium intake, as vitamin D concentration in food, saturated fat intake,[29] and protein intake[30] influence the proportion of calcium absorbed from the intestine. At the population level, however, there can be little doubt that in adults urinary calcium excretion is a function of calcium intake.

Mortality and morbidity due to ischemic heart disease or peripheral arterial disease are low in Korea, whereas cerebrovascular disease and hypertensive heart disease are common. Although reliable morbidity data are unavailable in Korea because of the widespread practice of Oriental medicine as well as Western medicine, several stays in Korea and discussions with clinicians and pathologists have convinced me of the reality of this fact. This is confirmed by autopsy findings in Korea and in Japan in which only 75 cases of myocardial infarction were found among 10,000 autopsies; they also confirm the low prevalence of high-grade coronary sclerosis in Japan.[31]

It should be mentioned that notwithstanding the fact that cigarette smoking is common in Korean and Japanese men, atherosclerosis is rare. Diabetes is also common in China but is rarely accompanied by gangrene of the legs, a fact already mentioned by Snapper[15] in 1941. In Western countries, cigarette smoking and diabetes are invariably associated with an increased risk of ischemic heart disease. This apparent contradiction has been explained by the fact that smoking and diabetes accelerate the atherosclerotic process but only in the presence of a causal factor, in this case a diet rich in saturated fat.[32]

A high salt intake has also been described in Japan, particularly in Northern Honshu,[33,34] together with a high morbidity and mortality due to cerebrovascular disease and a high prevalence of hypertension. Comparative studies of serum lipid levels among Japanese living in Japan, Hawaii, and California have demonstrated how the serum lipid levels in Japanese approached those of Westerners according to the westernization of their diet.[35,36] Their mortality and morbidity patterns in relation to atherosclerotic disease changed accordingly. This once again demonstrates that possible genetic differences between populations are largely overruled by environmental or, in this case, dietary factors.

No doubt much can be learned from comparative studies of different populations. This is particularly true in studies that imply dietary components, as it is difficult

Table 3.9. Comparative Serum HDL-Cholesterol Values Between Belgian and Korean Women*

	Belgium		Korea	
Age (yr)	No.	HDL-Cholesterol (mg%)	No.	HDL-Cholesterol (mg%)
15+	84	60.3 ± 13.1	440	47.9 ± 11.3
25+	48	58.8 ± 13.0	106	47.9 ± 9.8
35+	55	62.6 ± 16.4	43	42.1 ± 8.9
45+	54	64.6 ± 13.2	33	43.8 ± 12.1
55+	13	58.7 ± 16.1	16	40.7 ± 7.5

* All differences are significant at the $P < 10^{-3}$ level.

to change the dietary habits of populations within a reasonable time. In this endeavor the way was undoubtedly shown by de Langen[13] who entitled his lecture before the Dutch Society for the Advancement of Medicine in Batavia (Djakarta) in 1915: "Cholesterin metabolism and the pathology within (different) races."

REFERENCES

1. Kesteloot H (ed): Methodology and standardization of noninvasive blood pressure measurement in epidemiological studies. Eur 5544e, Commission of the Eur. Comm., 1976.
2. Kesteloot H, Joossens JV: Methodology of blood pressure measurement and epidemiology of hypertension. *Acta Cardiol (Brux)* 1978; 33:67–70.
3. Jaffé M: Über den Niederschlag welche Pikrinsaure in normalem Harn erzeugt und über eine Reaktion des Kreatinins. *Z Phys Chem* 1886; 10:391–400.
4. Abell LL, Levy BB, Brodie BB, Kendall FE: Simplified method for the estimation of total cholesterol in serum and demonstration of its specificity. *J Biol Chem* 1952; 195:357–366.
5. Bachorik PS, Wood PD, Albers JJ, Steiner P, Dempsey M, Kuba K, Warnik R, Karlsson L: Plasma high-density lipoprotein cholesterol concentrations determined after removal of other lipoproteins by heparin-manganese precipitation or by ultracentrifugation. *Clin Chem* 1976; 22:1828–1834.
6. Lambert D, Mejean L, Drouin P, Debry G: Stability of lipid and protein composition of very low-density lipoproteins during the storage after freezing of whole serum and isolated lipoproteins (French). *Clin Chem Acta* 1978; 88:135–142.
7. Assmann G, Schriewer H: Möglichkeiten und Grenzen der Analytik des HDL-Cholesterins. *J Clin Chem Biochem* 1981; 19:1–6.
8. Kesteloot H, Lee CS, Park HM, Kegels C, Geboers J, Claes JH, Joossens JV: A comparative study of serum lipids between Belgium and Korea. *Circulation* 1982; 65:795–799.
9. Kesteloot H, Park BC, Lee CS, Brems-Heyns E, Claessens J, Joossens JV: A comparative study of blood pressure and sodium intake in Belgium and Korea. *Eur J Cardiol* 1980; 11:169–182.
10. Kesteloot H, Song CS, Song JS, Brems-Heyns E, Joossens JV: An epidemiological survey of arterial blood pressure in Korea using home reading, in Rorive E, Van Cauwenberge H (eds): *The Arterial Hypertensive Disease.* New York, Masson, 1976, pp 141–148.
11. Kesteloot H: Epidemiology of arterial blood pressure. *Arch Mal Coeur* 1975; 68(suppl):149–151.
12. Kesteloot H, Vuylsteke M, Costenoble A: Relationship between blood pressure and sodium and potassium intake in a Belgian male population group, in Kesteloot H, Joossens JV (eds): *Epidemiology of Arterial Blood Pressure.* The Hague, Martinus-Nijhoff Publishers, 1980, pp 345–352.
13. de Langen CD: Significance of geographic pathology in race problems in medicine (Dutch). *Geneesk Tijdschr Ned Indië* 1933; 73:1026–1044.
14. de Langen CD: Cholesterol metabolism and racial pathology (Dutch). *Geneesk Tijdschr Ned Indië* 1916; 56:1–34.
15. Snapper I: *Chinese Lessons to Western Medicine.* ed 1. New York, Interscience Publishers Inc, 1941; ed 2 with commentaries. New York and London, Grüne & Stratton, 1965.
16. Snapper I: Diet and atherosclerosis: truth and fiction. *Am J Cardiol* 1963; 11:283–289.
17. Park Y, Chun SK: Food consumption and nutrition survey in Korean rural areas. *Korean J Nutr* 1976; 9:87–93.
18. Ahn BH, Ryoo UH, Chung SK, Kim ES, Hong SA, Suh DK: A nationwide food consumption survey in Korea. *Human Sci (Korea)* 1977; 1:13–20.
19. Knuiman JT, West CE: HDL-cholesterol in men from thirteen countries. *Lancet* 1981; 2:367–368.
20. Criqui MH, Wallace RB, Heiss G, Mischkel M, Schonfeld G, Jones GTL: Cigarette smoking and plasma high density cholesterol levels. The Lipid Research Clinics Program Prevalence Study. *Circulation* 1980; 62(suppl IV):70–76.
21. Egusa G, Bennett PH, Aleck K, Taylor R, Howard BV: Hyperlipemia and arteriosclerotic cardiovascular disease in the Polynesian population of Rarotonga. *Atherosclerosis* 1984; 53:241–254.
22. Joossens JV: Stroke, stomach cancer and salt. A possible clue to the prevention of hypertension, in Kesteloot H, Joossens JV (eds): *Epidemiology of Arterial Blood Pressure.* The Hague, Boston, London, Martinus Nijhoff Publishers, 1980, pp 489–508.
23. Kesteloot H, Geboers J: Calcium and blood pressure. *Lancet* 1982; 1:813–815.
24. Kesteloot H, Geboers J, Van Hoof R: Epidemiological study of the relationship between calcium and blood pressure. *Hypertension* 1983; 5(suppl II):52–56.
25. Liu K, Cooper R, McKeever J, Byington R, Soltero I, Stamler R, Gosch F, Stevens E, Stamler J: Assessment of the association between habitual salt intake and high blood pressure: methodological problems. *Am J Epidemiol* 1979; 110:219–226.
26. De Wardener HE: Natriuretic hormone. *Clin Sci Mol Med* 1977; 53:1–8.
27. Haddy FJ, Pamnani MB, Clough DL: Humoral factors in the sodium-potassium pump in volume expanded hypertension. *Life Sci* 1979; 24:2105–2118.
28. Blaustein MP: Sodium ions, calcium ions, blood pressure regulation and hypertension: a reassessment and a hypothesis. *Am J Physiol* 1977; 232:C165–C173.
29. Southgate DAT, Widdowson EM, Smits BJ, Cooke WT, Walker CHM, Mathers NP: Absorption and excretion of calcium and fat by young infants. *Lancet* 1969; 1:487–489.
30. Margen S, Chu JY, Kaufmann NA, Calloway DH: Studies in calcium metabolism. The calciuretic effect of dietary protein. *Am J Clin Nutr* 1974; 27:584–589.
31. Kimura N: Analysis of 10,000 post-mortem examinations in Japan, in Keys A, White PD (eds): *World Trends in Cardiology. I. Cardiovascular Epidemiology.* New York, Hoeber-Hayer, 1956, pp 22–33.
32. Kesteloot H, Vuylsteke M, Wulleman G, Vertenten E, Van Houte O: Causes of cardiovascular mortality and morbidity in a longitudinal epidemiological study. *Rheinisch-Westfälische Akad Wiss* 1978; 63:514–521.
33. Sasaki N: Epidemiological studies on hypertension in the North-Eastern part of Japan. *Japan Circ J* 1977; 41:1139–1142.
34. Shigiya R, Kimura N, Komachi Y, Isomura K, Kojima S, Watanabe T: Nutritional status of Japanese with special reference to cerebrovascular and coronary heart disease, in Shigiya R, Asahima K (eds): *Physiological Adaptability and Nutritional Status of the Japanese.* Tokyo, University Press, 1975, pp 123–165.
35. Kato H, Tillotson J, Nichaman MZ, Rhoads GG, Hamilton HB: Epidemiologic studies of coronary heart disease and stroke in Japanese living in Japan, Hawaii and California: serum lipids and diet. *Am J Epidemiol* 1973; 97:372–385.
36. Kagan A, Harris BR, Winkelstein W Jr, Johnson KG, Kato H, Syme SL, Rhoads GG, Gay ML, Nichaman MZ, Hamilton HB, Tillotson J: Epidemiologic studies of coronary heart disease and stroke in Japanese men living in Japan, Hawaii, and California: demographic, physical, dietary and biochemical characteristics. *J Chron Dis* 1974; 27:345–364.

4 History and Physical Examination

Antonio C. de Leon, Jr, MD and Tsung O. Cheng, MD

Current technology available in medicine has led many to increased reliance on these helpful tools. It is unfortunate that as a result of these, there has been less emphasis and interest in the basic clinical skills. Actually, our enhanced understanding of clinical disease entities has made the clinical history and the various aspects of the physical examination more powerful tools than ever before.

SYMPTOMS

CHEST PAIN ASSOCIATED WITH CORONARY ARTERY DISEASE

The clinical history of chest pain raises a host of diagnostic possibilities. Careful refinement of that symptom in terms of location, mode of onset, duration, areas of radiation, sex, and age of the patient are but some of the factors that allow for reduction of the diagnostic possibilities to a few or even a single clinical entity.

Angina Pectoris

Chest discomfort of myocardial ischemia has variously been described by patients as pain, ache, pressure, or even an ill-defined discomfort or sensation. At the moment of the symptom, myocardial ischemia is present and represents a disparity between oxygen supply and demand. Although in most the initial area of discomfort is substernal, occasionally it may be precordial, interscapular, shoulder, arm, neck, jaw, or epigastric in location. Radiation of pain is usually to the left arm along the ulnar surface, but it may also be to the right arm, neck, or jaw. In each patient, the discomfort is usually predictably reproduced by a given level of physical effort or by emotional stress. Factors that further increase stress, such as a large meal, cold weather, or walking against a wind, may precipitate the symptoms. The discomfort usually lasts for two to five minutes, is relieved by rest or discontinuance of activity, and is also promptly relieved by sublingual nitrates. The frequency of these episodes is variable from patient to patient. However, in any one patient, the frequency is usually predictable, hence the term "stable angina." In trying to identify angina from all the other causes of chest pain, its predictable reproduction with physical effort or emotional stress is the most useful characteristic.

Unstable Angina

Progression of coronary atherosclerosis, development of associated coronary vasospasm, anemia, significant arrhythmia, and hyperthyroidism are elements that can alter stable angina. The chest pain episodes progressively increase in severity, frequency, and duration. In some, the magnitude of increase in severity and duration is such that an acute myocardial infarction becomes clinically difficult to exclude. Some patients with new-onset angina can present with a progressively increasing frequency of angina rather than the more typical stable angina.

Variant Angina

Chest pain at rest or in the early morning hours suggests coronary artery spasm as an important factor in the symptom genesis. Originally described by Prinzmetal as being associated with ST-segment elevation,[1] current knowledge suggests that ST-segment depression may also occur, and that the state of coronary arteries can vary from normal to fixed, high-grade obstructive lesions.[2] The character, radiation, and duration of the pain are not dissimilar to those in stable angina. Rather, it is the lack of a relation between the occurrence of pain and a demonstrable reason for increased oxygen demand (ie, at rest or on minimal effort) that makes this form of angina "variant." (See also chapter 36 on Coronary Artery Spasm.)

Myocardial Infarction

Acute myocardial infarction occurs when there is sufficient deprivation of myocardial blood flow for a long enough time to result in necrosis. Thrombosis, embolism, coronary vasospasm, and high-grade fixed obstructive lesions usually represent the underlying disease. The clinical presentation of chest pain differs from angina pectoris mainly in that it is long and sustained (30 minutes or more), and it is more likely to be associated with other symptoms such as nausea, diaphoresis, giddiness, or lightheadedness. The severity of pain may also be greater than that experienced with previous anginal episodes. In some, the sensation described is one of heavy pressure rather than pain. In the elderly, it may present as shortness of breath, or alteration in sensorium.[3]

CHEST PAIN ASSOCIATED WITH OTHER CARDIOVASCULAR ENTITIES

Chest pain is a common symptom of patients with mitral valve prolapse.[4] It is usually atypical of angina pectoris in that the pain is brief but recurrent for long periods, occurring at rest or exercise without any demonstrable consistency, and variable in chest wall location and radiation. Response to nitrates is unpredictable.

Chest pain also occurs with pericarditis.[5] It may be sharp, stabbing, dull, or described as an ache; may wax and wane in intensity, but is usually present for hours. Aggravation of the discomfort by lying down or by the act of swallowing and relief on sitting up or leaning forward are helpful historical clues to recognition.

Chest pain from aortic dissection is usually of sudden onset, severe and excruciating, sometimes described as a "tearing" sensation, and may radiate prominently or appear to localize to the interscapular area of the back. It may be exceedingly difficult to relieve even with the use of opiates. Other areas of radiation may closely mimic that of angina pectoris or acute myocardial infarction.[6]

Chest pain may occur with pulmonary embolism, either as the result of associated pulmonary infarction or because of the development of pulmonary hypertension. When due to pulmonary infarction, the increased severity of pain with respiration (pleuritic pain) serves as a helpful clue.[7] When the pain is noted in portions of the chest wall other than the substernal region, it is easier to differentiate from angina or acute myocardial infarction.

Chest pain from pulmonary hypertension of any cause, including that from pulmonary embolism, is presumably an ischemic (right ventricular) form of chest discomfort. Its recognition primarily rests on the demonstration by physical examination (or other ancillary diagnostic procedures) of pulmonary hypertension.[8]

In all the foregoing cardiovascular entities that may cause chest pain of noncoronary etiology, usually the physical examination (or other ancillary diagnostic procedures, or both) enables recognition of the clinical entity.

CHEST PAIN DUE TO NONCARDIOVASCULAR ENTITIES

Chest pain from noncardiovascular causes constitutes a constant differential diagnostic problem for anyone presenting with this symptom. For the clinician, there is no getting away from a careful, detailed history and physical examination if cardiovascular causes are to be eliminated as possibilities.

Chest pain from reflux esophagitis or esophageal spasm, or both, might be recognized from a description of substernal burning or pain brought on by the recumbent position, large meals or spicy foods, associated dysphagia, relief from antacids or bland food, and a history of previously documented sliding hiatus hernia. In esophageal spasm, both relief from the administration of nitrates and provocation by ergonovine[9] can occur. Clearly, the absence of any stigmas of cardiovascular disease on physical examination is a useful aid in the recognition of this noncardiac cause of chest pain.

Chest wall pain constitutes another frequent differential diagnostic point for angina pectoris. A description of diffuse pain, ache, or tightness over the anterior chest, especially the precordium, without a consistent, dependable relation to physical effort and especially when reproducible by chest wall palpation are useful clues. In some, the symptom complex is described as a fleeting or momentary, sharp or stabbing inframammary pain. Again, there usually is no reproducible relation with effort and the event, although recurrent over time, is exceedingly brief. As a rule, such patients are able to continue what they are doing despite the discomfort. Other chest wall syndromes, such as those arising from cervical nerve root compression or stimulation, and costochrondritis (Tietze's syndrome), can be appropriately identified by careful physical examination, particularly when the pain can be reproduced by the examiner.

Gastrointestinal entities such as peptic ulcer, gall bladder disease, or irritable bowel syndrome may result in epigastric pain or discomfort with substernal or precordial radiation. Other aspects of the clinical history such as a relation to the intake of fatty foods, relief from bland foods or antacids, gaseous distension, and relief from belching or flatulence are helpful in their recognition.

DYSPNEA

Dyspnea or shortness of breath is a sensation experienced by patients and is not specific for cardiac failure. It may be seen in the absence of demonstrable organic disease such as anxiety, hyperventilation, and neurocirculatory asthenia. Pulmonary parenchymal or vascular disease, as well as thoracic cage or thoracic muscle abnormalities, may also cause the symptom. When due to cardiac disease, the severity of effort needed to bring about the dyspnea is useful clinical information for assessment of the severity of the cardiac problem as well as the modality and intensity of therapeutic management. The New York Heart Association classification of functional cardiac status[10] has gained general acceptance and use (Table 4.1).

In a few instances, dyspnea with effort or emotion (without anginal pain) describes the presentation of ischemic heart disease. It lasts the same length as angina and is relieved by rest or nitrates. It can therefore be viewed as an anginal equivalent (blockpnea[11]).

PAROXYSMAL NOCTURNAL DYSPNEA

Typical paroxysmal nocturnal dyspnea is a breathless sensation that awakens a patient two to four hours after having fallen asleep. Relief is usually obtained by sitting up with the legs dangling over the side of the bed or actually getting up to stand or walk around. Some feel a compulsion to open a window to get more fresh air. When present, it usually indicates left heart failure. The presumed pathophysiologic mechanism for this symptom is the gradual resorption of interstitial fluid, resulting in increased intravascular volume sufficient to increase the mean left atrial pressure to a point of pulmonary venous congestion, interstitial edema, or even alveolar edema, which then results in the dyspnea that awakens the patient.

ORTHOPNEA

Orthopnea is breathlessness shortly upon assuming the recumbent position and results from recruitment of blood from the lower extremities and abdomen, causing the mean left atrial pressure to increase further, worsening the degree of pulmonary venous congestion, thus increasing the work of breathing. It represents a more advanced state of left heart failure than that of the patient who only experiences paroxysmal nocturnal dyspnea. When true orthopnea is present, it usually indicates overt left heart failure. Typically, the patient needs two to three pillows to elevate the head and upper trunk, or instead elevates the head of the bed for relief. In its milder form, the patient may only note cough on recumbency, and in its more severe form, there is relief only when sitting fully upright. One should always make certain that the use of two or three pillows to sleep is not the result of habit before concluding that orthopnea due to left heart failure is present.

Table 4.1. Functional Cardiac Status

Class	Symptoms
1	Symptoms only with unusual exertion
2	Symptoms with ordinary exertion
3	Symptoms with minimal exertion
4	Symptoms at rest

ACUTE PULMONARY EDEMA

Alveolar edema represents the extreme end of pulmonary venous hypertension. Such patients are overtly dyspneic even sitting fully upright and dyspnea is often associated with cough productive of pink frothy sputum.

Unlike orthopnea and paroxysmal nocturnal dyspnea, there are noncardiac causes of acute pulmonary edema. Thus, high altitude and abnormal capillary permeability can also produce alveolar edema, even with normal pulmonary venous pressure. Again, careful physical examination in which left heart disease is eliminated, together with other clinical information (high altitude location, vasculitis, toxin exposure, allergic reaction, etc), should identify its noncardiac origin.

PERIPHERAL EDEMA

Edema of the lower extremities, ascites, or both are not symptoms specific for cardiac disease. However, when they occur with evidence of an elevated mean right atrial pressure (see discussion under Physical Examination), right heart failure would be a reasonable presumption. The presence of symptoms of left heart failure, as discussed previously, also makes peripheral edema likely to be due to right heart failure.

Clinical onset is usually gradual: weight gain, tightness of clothing (secondary to hepatic congestion or ascites) or of shoes (pedal edema), increasing dyspnea (pleural effusion), urinary frequency, especially nocturia, and subsequently, overt pitting edema observed by the patient are common modes of presentation.

SYNCOPE

Syncope is the transient loss of consciousness resulting from inadequate cerebral blood flow. Its milder version (near syncope) may present as light-headedness, faintness, or dizziness. This symptom is not specific and there are several noncardiac or vascular causes.

Among the cardiac causes are the various disturbances in rhythm, as well as the various forms of obstruction to right and left ventricular outflow (Table 4.2). The clinical triad of symptoms of left heart failure, angina, and syncope during, or shortly after, effort is a common presentation of obstruction to left ventricular outflow.[12] Exertional syncope, especially in a young female without cardiac murmur, is a clinical presentation seen in primary pulmonary hypertension.[13] Syncope associated with cyanosis should prompt a consideration of Fallot's tetralogy.[14]

HEMOPTYSIS

Hemoptysis, or coughing up blood, can have cardiac as well as noncardiac causes. A more detailed history that elicits the character and circumstances of the hemoptysis can be most helpful in elucidating some of the causes. Some cardiac entities such as mitral stenosis may even present with various forms of hemoptysis:

In acute pulmonary edema, the fairly intimate admixture of red blood cells, air, and alveolar edema fluid results in the characteristic "pink, frothy" sputum produced during coughing spells.

Table 4.2. Cardiac Causes of Syncope

I. Alteration in cardiac rhythm:
  A. Bradycardia: sinus, atrial, or ventricular asystole and second or third degree heart block
  B. Tachycardia: very rapid supraventricular tachycardia, ventricular tachycardia, and ventricular fibrillation
II. Obstruction to left ventricular outflow:
  A. Hypertrophic cardiomyopathy with obstruction
  B. Subvalvular aortic stenosis
  C. Valvular aortic stenosis
  D. Supravalvular aortic stenosis(?)
III. Obstruction to right ventricular outflow:
  A. Infundibular pulmonic stenosis
  B. Valvular pulmonic stenosis
  C. Pulmonary embolism
  D. Severe pulmonary vascular obstructive disease
IV. Intracardiac mass lesions, particularly left or right atrial myxoma
V. Carotid sinus hypersensitivity
VI. Orthostatic hypotension including vasodepressor syncope

Bronchial mucosal bleeding that can result from severe coughing spells in bronchitis which may accompany mitral stenosis results in blood-streaked sputum.

Rupture of submucosal bronchial veins because of pulmonary venous hypertension results in the spontaneous welling up of bright red (oxygenated) blood of considerable volume (teaspoon to a cup) and is usually self-limited.

Pulmonary embolism with resulting pulmonary infarction can result in a rusty colored or frankly bloody sputum.

Other cardiovascular entities to consider include Eisenmenger's physiology, pulmonary arteriovenous fistula, collagen vascular disease, necrotizing pulmonary arterial lesions, and even aortic aneurysm eroding into or rupturing into a portion of the tracheobronchial tree.

FATIGUE

Fatigue or general weakness is also not a specific symptom that identifies a cardiovascular cause. However, in the context of a patient with heart disease, it suggests low or inadequate cardiac output, particularly when the symptom is present not only with effort but also at rest. Severe regurgitant valvular lesions may present with this symptom. It can also be the result of massive diuresis as a side effect of drug therapy.

PALPITATION

This is a term that many patients use to refer to their awareness of the heart beat. Thus, it does not necessarily imply tachycardia, but it may be an awareness of forceful heart beat. A "fluttering," "jumping," "skipping," or "flip-flop" sensation may be descriptive terms that a patient may use. It is, therefore, helpful to have the patient elaborate further. Is it rapid, regular, irregular, slow, or simply forceful? When it is tachycardia, is the onset and offset sudden? Has the patient learned how to terminate the episode? With extrasystoles, it is often the cardiac cycle following the pause that the patient is most aware of, because it represents a more forceful contraction following a larger end-diastolic volume.

CYANOSIS

Central cyanosis is noted as a bluish discoloration of the nail beds and mucous membranes. In certain races, the nail beds appear naturally dark, and cyanosis is best appreciated in the conjuctivae and oral mucous membrane. Usually, it requires 5 g/100 ml or more of reduced hemoglobin for cyanosis to be clinically apparent. Arterial oxygen saturation is usually 85% or less. It is of considerable value to inquire whether cyanosis was present since birth or noted later in life, occurs only with effort, or is asymmetrical.

Differential cyanosis is a useful clue to two types of congenital heart disease. In patent ductus arteriosus with pulmonary hypertension and reversed shunt, only the toes and sometimes also the fingers of the left hand are cyanotic. Differential cyanosis in which the toes are less cyanotic than the fingers is a rare but distinctive sign of complete transposition of the great vessels with patent ductus arteriosus. Differential cyanosis can be brought out or exaggerated by exercise or by having the patient put the hands and feet in warm water.

Peripheral cyanosis secondary to a low cardiac output or exposure to cold is associated with a normal arterial oxyhemoglobin saturation but a widened arteriovenous oxygen difference due to peripheral stasis of blood flow. Peripheral cyanosis can be distinguished from central cyanosis by warming the hands and feet. Warming abolishes peripheral cyanosis but exaggerates central cyanosis. Furthermore, peripheral cyanosis is neither associated with clubbing of the fingers and toes nor accompanied by polycythemia.

PHYSICAL EXAMINATION

GENERAL APPEARANCE

Facial and general appearance are readily evident to the clinician in the course of obtaining the clinical history. Awareness of the common cardiovascular abnormalities that can be associated with specific appearance and habitus can be a valuable additional aid during history taking and can especially alert the physician to potential findings on the subsequent physical examination.

Marfan's syndrome can be suspected in a tall person who has inappropriately long limbs compared to the trunk. Arachnodactyly and joint hyperextensibility are other features readily recognized. During physical examination, pectus excavatum is common and ectopia lentis may be demonstrable. The cardiovascular conditions that may be present are aortic regurgitation, aneurysm of the ascending aorta, or mitral valve prolapse.[15] Other less common connective tissue disorders are associated with cardiovascular disease. Pseudoxanthoma elasticum, recognized by a "plucked chicken" appearance resulting from skin laxity, is associated with the occurrence of premature atherosclerosis, hypertension, angina, and congestive failure.[16]

The Ehlers-Danlos syndrome presents with hyperextensible skin and joints, skin nodules, and easy bruisability. It can be associated with mitral valve prolapse or dilatation of the aortic root or sinus of Valsalva.[17]

Supravalvular aortic stenosis syndrome is recognized by "elfin facies," characterized by protruding lips, low-set eyes, epicanthic folds, and strabismus. It is associated with supravalvular narrowing of the aorta above the sinus of Valsalva. Associated pulmonary artery stenosis may also occur.[18]

Down's syndrome (trisomy 21) is recognized from the "mongoloid"appearance characterized by widely set eyes, upward slanting palpebral fissures, epicanthal folds, and a large tongue with or without transverse fissuring (see section on Mouth, Tongue, Teeth, and Gums). The most common associated cardiovascular abnormalities are persistent common atrioventricular canal, isolated ventricular septal defect, or, less frequently, tetralogy of Fallot.[19]

Turner's syndrome results from an XO chromosomal anomaly in a female. Females with this syndrome are recognized by their short stature, neck webbing, cubitus valgus, and a facies characterized by a small mandible, prominent ears, low posterior hairline, ptosis, and epicanthic folds. Coarctation of the aorta is the most common cardiovascular anomaly.[20]

Ullrich-Noonan syndrome occurs in patients with XX or XY chromosomes who have the physical characteristics of Turner's syndrome. The most common associated cardiovascular anomaly is pulmonary stenosis with a dysplastic valve.[21]

Acromegaly, caused by abnormally high levels of growth hormone, results in enlargement of the cartilaginous and bony structures of the head, face, hands, and feet. Systemic hypertension is the most common cardiovascular problem noted in these patients.[22]

Holt-Oram syndrome is recognized from the characteristic appearance of the hands. There is usually hypoplasia or aplasia of the radial aspect of the hand. In some instances, the thumb is absent or rudimentary (Figure 4.1). Secundum atrial septal defect and ventricular septal defect are the most common associated cardiac lesions.[23]

Subcutaneous nodules (Figure 4.2) represent one of the pathognomonic features of acute rheumatic fever. Their seriousness lies in their association with active carditis. It is important to recognize these nodules not only because they are occasionally evanescent but also because in some of the recurrent attacks of rheumatic fever they may represent the only local manifestation of rheumatic fever recrudescence.

There are many other clinical entities, such as scleroderma, ankylosing spondylitis, osteogenesis imperfecta, rheumatoid arthritis, and Duchenne muscular dystrophy that may be recognizable from the physical appearance and have known associated cardiovascular abnormalities.[24-27]

EARLOBE CREASE

The diagonal earlobe crease (Figure 4.3) has significantly been associated with coronary artery disease throughout the world, including the United States,[28] China,[29] Russia,[30] Poland,[31] Israel,[32] Finland,[33] Denmark,[34] and Canada.[35] Although the first report suggesting a connection between the earlobe crease and coronary artery disease was made in 1973,[36] such an association existed even in ancient Rome, whose Emperor Hadrian had coronary artery disease and bilateral earlobe creases.[37] Although not a diagnostic criterion, it is a risk factor and may contribute to early detection of coronary artery disease, particularly during mass screening of the population.[30]

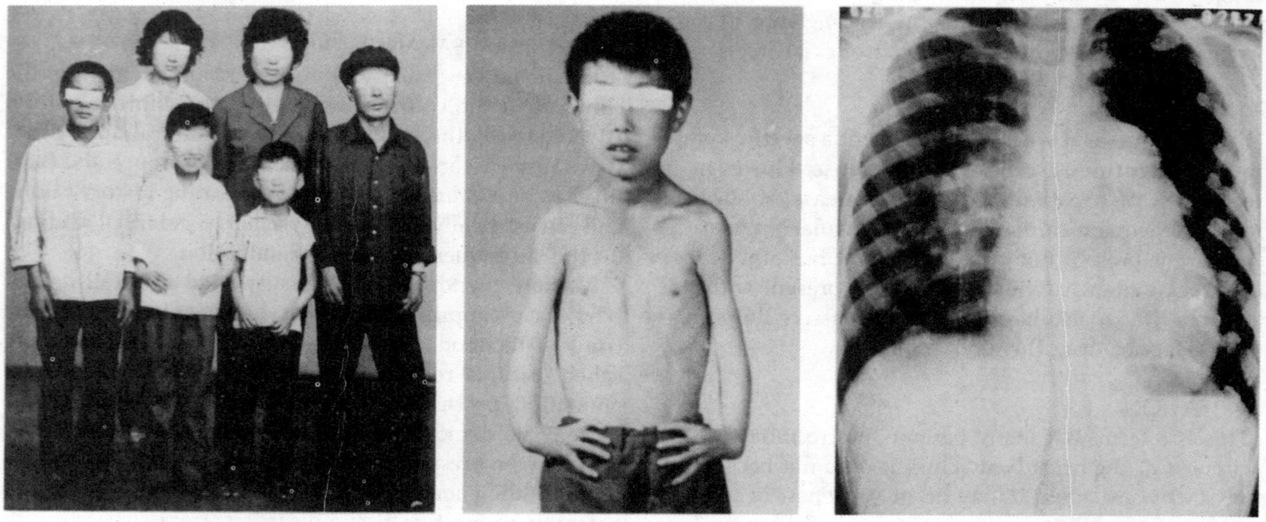

Figure 4.1. Holt-Oram syndrome in a Chinese family. *Left,* All of its male members are affected: father (right) with a ventricular septal defect and two younger sons (middle) with a secundum atrial septal defect in each. *Middle,* The middle son has bilateral absence of thumbs and short forearms. *Right,* Chest roentgenogram of the middle son with a secundum atrial septal defect. (From Zhang KZ, Sun QB, Cheng TO: Holt-Oram syndrome in China: a collective review of 18 cases. *Am Heart J* 1986; 111:572–577. With permission.)

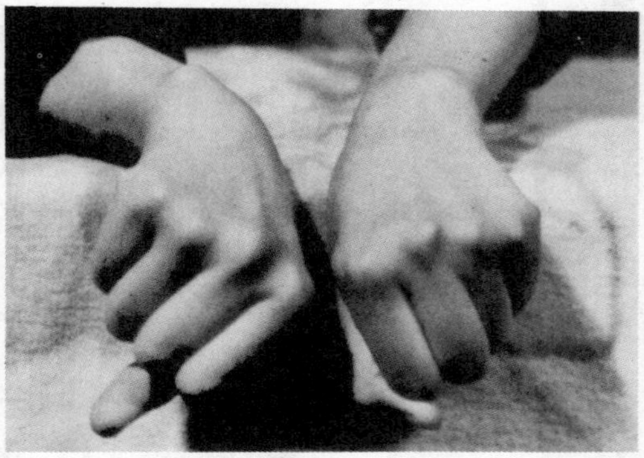

Figure 4.2. Subcutaneous nodules in a 16-year-old Chinese girl with acute rheumatic carditis. (Courtesy of Dr CL Tung, Shanghai, China.)

MOUTH, TONGUE, TEETH, AND GUMS

Examination of the mouth, especially the tongue (Figure 4.4), teeth (Figure 4.5), and gums (Figure 4.6), is often very informative.

Tongue

Visual examination of the tongue is a useful aid in cardiovascular diagnosis. The Chinese physicians, especially those trained in traditional medicine, made astute diagnoses from careful inspection of the tongue along with palpation of the pulse. The latter will be discussed in the section on Arterial Pulse.

A normal tongue is soft, pink, and moist, with a thin and clear fur coating that is neither too dry nor too moist. The tongue coating becomes thick when disease sets in. However, attention should be paid to false impressions often created on the tongue coating by staining from food, drink, or cigarettes (Figure 4.4, top left). Tongue fissures, when vertical (scrotal tongue) (Figure 4.4, top middle), are a normal variant. However, transverse fissuring of the tongue (Figure 4.4, top right) is abnormal and occurs in a high percentage of patients with Down's syndrome. Combined horizontal, vertical, and diagonal fissuring (Figure 4.4, bottom left) is often seen in patients with cardiac arrhythmias. Geographic tongue or erythema migrans is due to loss of papillae with subsequent regeneration, giving the appearance of migration, hence the term *geographic tongue.* Although it can be a normal finding, it is a frequent occurrence in patients with coronary artery spasm and cerebral vasospasm (Figure 4.4, bottom middle). "Chicken heart" tongue (Figure 4.4, bottom right), due to repeated central denudation, is often seen in patients with coronary artery disease.

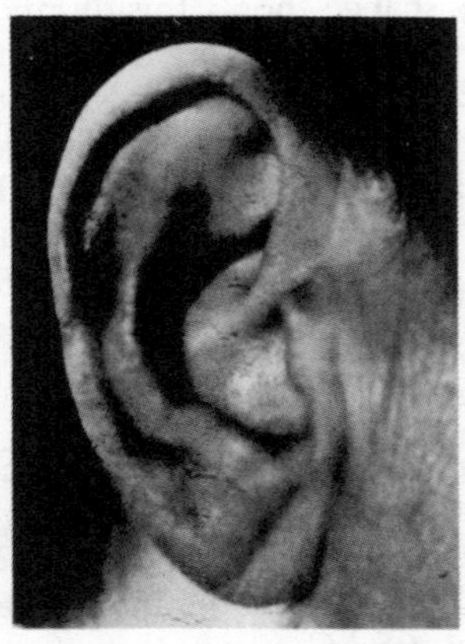

Figure 4.3. Earlobe crease in a Chinese patient. (From Chen et al,[29] with permission.)

An enlarged tongue is seen in Down's syndrome, amyloidosis, hypothyroidism, glycogen storage disease, and the mucopolysaccharidoses, particularly Hurler's syndrome and Morquio's syndrome.

Teeth

In congenital syphilis the upper central incisors are widely spaced, centrally notched, and tapered in the manner of a screwdriver (Hutchinson's teeth).

In the Ellis-van Creveld syndrome the teeth may be either absent or peg-shaped, and there are multiple frenula binding the upper lip to the gingiva[38] (Figure 4.5).

Gums

Hyperplasia of gingivae of epileptic patients treated with phenytoin (Dilantin®) is well known. Phenytoin being also an antiarrhythmic agent, it may result in some degree of gingival hyperplasia in about 10% to 30% of all patients treated regularly with this drug.[39]

Recently gingival hyperplasia has also been reported following the administration of nifedipine[39] (Figure 4.6) and cyclosporine.[40] Because these drugs are being increasingly used in cardiac patients, nifedipine as a calcium channel blocker in patients with coronary artery spasm and cyclosporine as an immunosuppressive drug in heart transplantation, physicians should be aware of this side effect.

JUGULAR VENOUS PULSE

"The neck veins were flat" or "the neck veins were distended" are fairly common statements seen in a physical examination report if one is fortunate enough to find any reference at all to the jugular veins. Careful and critical examination of the jugular veins can be far more informative than the foregoing statements imply.

In the same manner that we currently use balloon-tipped catheters placed in the pulmonary artery to obtain a pulmonary capillary wedge pressure as a reflection of left atrial events, the jugular veins are naturally occurring extensions of the superior vena cava and therefore can provide us with valuable information of right atrial events. The internal jugular vein is larger than the external jugular and hence more likely to reflect right atrial events more accurately. Because of its location beneath the sternocleidomastoid muscle, it is not readily visible except when venous pulsations are larger than normal. Thus, the degree of distension and the waveform assessment of modest amplitude are often carried out using the smaller external jugular vein which is superficial and crosses in front of the sternocleidomastoid muscle. Although the right jugular veins are most often used, it is always worthwhile to observe both sides to ensure that they are iden-

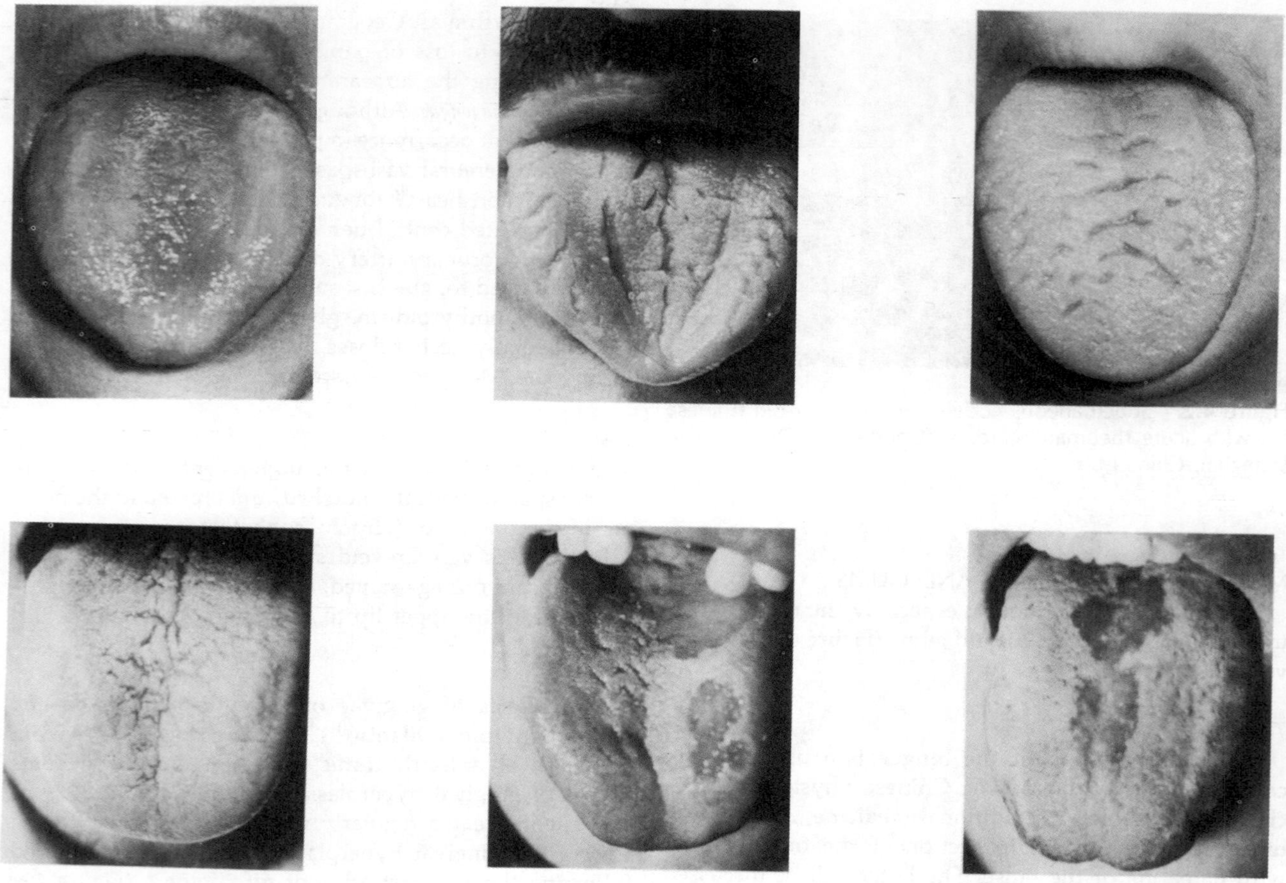

Figure 4.4. Tongue appearances in different cardiovascular diseases. *Top left,* Normal coated tongue of a cigarette smoker with nicotine staining. *Top middle,* Normal or fissured tongue (scrotal tongue). *Top right,* Transverse fissuring of the tongue in Down's syndrome. (From Zatouroff's *Color Atlas of Physical Signs in General Medicine.* Year Book Medical Publishers, 1976, reproduced with permission.) *Bottom left,* Combined horizontal, vertical, and diagonal fissuring of the tongue in a patient with cardiac arrhythmias. *Bottom middle,* Geographic tongue in a patient with coronary artery disease and cerebral artery spasm. *Bottom right,* "Chicken heart" tongue in a patient with coronary artery disease. (Courtesy of Dr TB Song, Chinese Traditional Medical College, Peking, China.)

tical, and in some cases the waveforms are better seen on the left.

Mean right atrial pressure is reflected in the height of the column of blood in the superior vena cava and jugular veins. Thus, the level of distension of jugular veins or the midpoint of venous excursion relative to the mid-right atrium represents mean venous pressure. In most clinical circumstances, the vertical distance from the mid-right atrium to the sternal angle of Louis (transverse sternal ridge at the insertion level of the second rib) is 5 cm. For the normally shaped thorax this distance is the same whether the patient is supine or sitting upright. An imaginary horizontal line should be drawn from the highest point of jugular vein distension to the area above the sternal angle and this distance measured.[41] Normal mean venous pressure is 8 cm H_2O or less from the mid-right atrium. This value in millimeters of water/13.6 translates the measurements into millimeters of mercury.

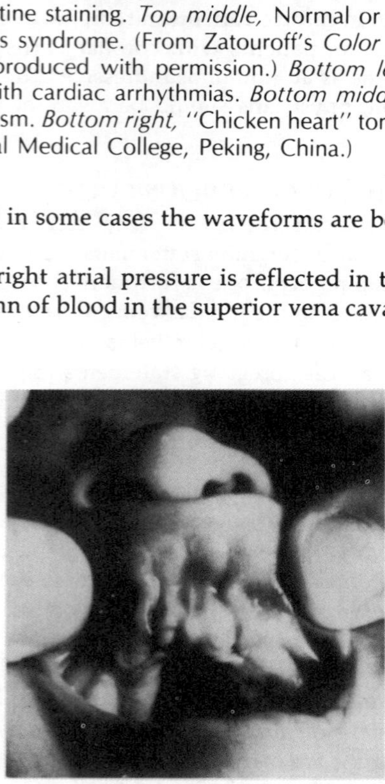

Figure 4.5. Infant with Ellis-van Creveld syndrome demonstrating multiple frenula binding the upper lip to the gingiva and no teeth. (From Lynch et al,[38] with permission.)

NORMAL WAVEFORMS

When recordings of the jugular venous pulse are obtained, there are two major upward deflections, the A and V waves, and two major downward deflections, the X and Y descents. The X descent is interrupted by a small upward deflection (the C wave), then continues downward as the X′ descent (Figure 4.7, top tracing).

The A wave represents the increase in right atrial pres-

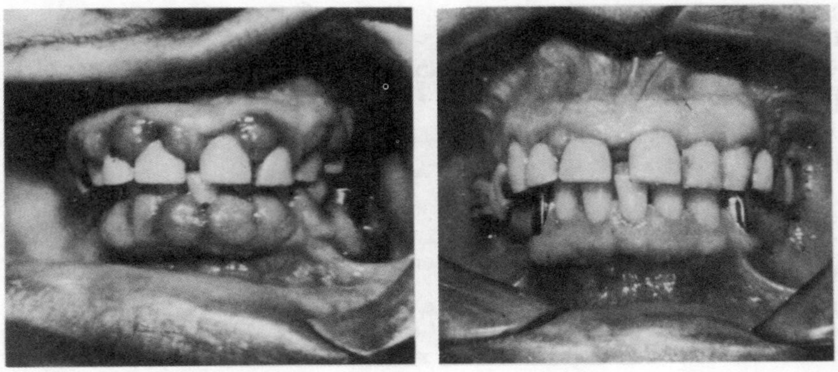

Figure 4.6. Gingival hyperplasia in a patient on nifedipine (*left*) and its disappearance following discontinuation of the drug (*right*). (From Ramon et al,[39] with permission.)

sure with right atrial systole. This is followed by the X descent as atrial relaxation occurs.[42] With the onset of ventricular systole and closure of the tricuspid valve, the C wave occurs and the following X′ descent results from the increase in right atrial cavity dimension as the contracting ventricle pulls down the atrioventricular anulus.[43]

The V wave represents the passive increase in atrial pressure as the right atrium fills during ventricular systole. The V wave is therefore a systolic (ventricular) event, with the peak of the V wave occurring close to the second heart sound. The following Y descent results from the decrease in right atrial pressure as passive right ventricular filling occurs (Figure 4.8).

ABNORMAL WAVEFORMS

Giant A waves result from abnormally forceful right atrial contraction. In the patient with normal sinus rhythm, these giant A waves occur with the same regularity as the arterial pulse (Figure 4.7, middle panel). Their presence indicates either significant obstruction of the tricuspid orifice (eg, tricuspid stenosis), or significant right ventricular hypertrophy (eg, pulmonic stenosis or pulmonary hypertension).[44,45] Correlation of this clinical finding with precordial palpation (ie, presence or absence of a right ventricular or pulmonary artery lift, or both) allows the examiner to attribute a specific clinical inference from the presence of the giant A wave.

Cannon A waves are the result of atrial contraction while the tricuspid valve is closed.[46] The force of right atrial contraction is thus transmitted to the neck veins and indicates the occurrence of atrioventricular dissociation. Thus, they are seen in complete heart block or ventricular tachycardia, in patients who have a ventricular pacemaker, and with ventricular extrasystoles. Because cannon A waves require the fortuitous presence of a P wave (atrial contraction) at the time of ventricular systole, they occur intermittently as opposed to the regularity of giant A waves. Cannon A waves also tend to have a more brisk rate of rise as well as a higher peak than that noted with giant A waves. In junctional tachycardia with retrograde atrial capture, cannon A waves occurring with each ventricular systole may be present and mistaken for giant A waves unless the examiner appreciates that these A waves are in timing with ventricular systole (carotid pulse) rather than preceding it, as is the case with giant A waves.

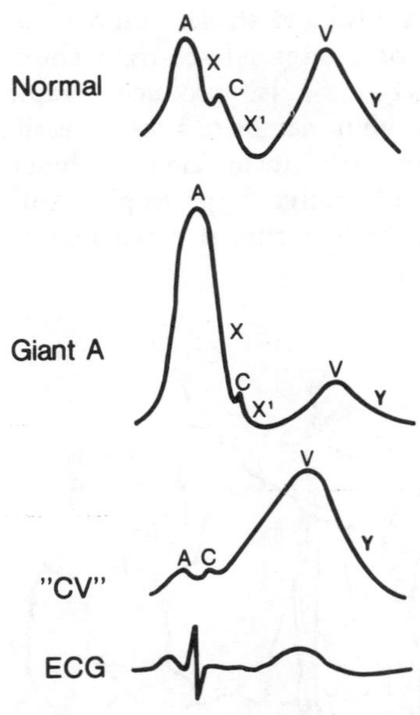

Figure 4.7. Top tracing demonstrates a normal jugular venous pulse. Second tracing demonstrates a giant A wave. Third tracing demonstrates the CV wave of tricuspid regurgitation. Fourth tracing is from an electrocardiogram (ECG).

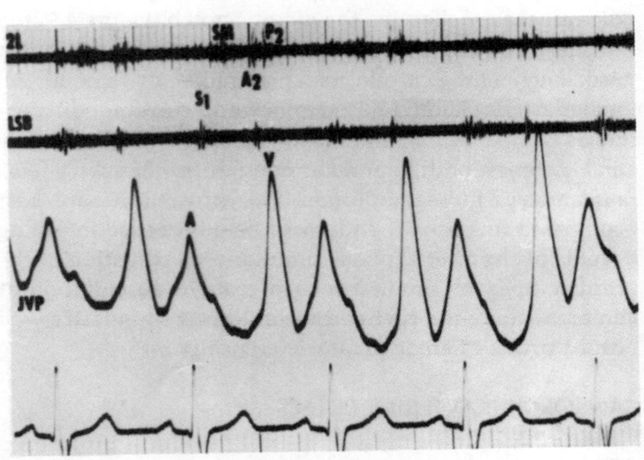

Figure 4.8. A jugular venous pulse recording in a normal person with a dominant V wave.

Abnormal V waves result from tricuspid valve regurgitation. The V wave is abnormal in that it is tall (ie, taller than the A wave) and begins sooner, thus encroaching or even obliterating the X′ descent.[47] With pulse recording, the C wave may be seen to continue on upwards to blend with the following V so that the term *CV wave* is also used to refer to an abnormal V wave (Figure 4.7, lower panel). Mild tricuspid regurgitation does not usually alter the V wave, but as the severity of tricuspid regurgitation increases, encroachment on the X′ descent occurs until one has a CV wave. The clinical finding, therefore, not only identifies the hemodynamic problem but also quantifies the severity.

The Y descent reflects the rate of passive right atrial emptying during early right ventricular diastole. Thus, when there is significant impediment to passive right atrial blood flow into the right ventricle (as in tricuspid stenosis), the rate of Y descent may be slow, especially in the context of the height of the V wave.

Restriction to right ventricular filling such as that encountered in constrictive pericarditis and restrictive cardiomyopathy results in an elevated mean venous pressure and prominent X and Y descents which produce the M- or W-shaped venous pulse.[48] Furthermore, because of the restriction to filling, the increase in venous return from inspiration results in elevation of venous pressure with inspiration (Kussmaul's sign).[49]

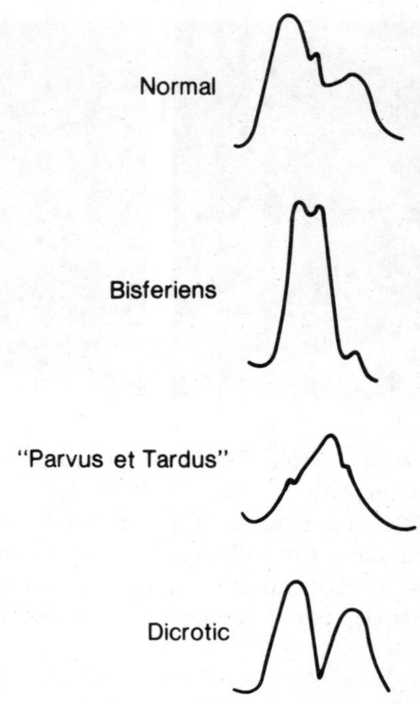

Figure 4.9. Top tracing demonstrates a normal arterial pulse. Second tracing demonstrates a rapid-rising bifid (bisferiens) arterial pulse. Third tracing demonstrates a slow-rising late-peaking pulse (parvus et tardus) of aortic stenosis. Fourth tracing demonstrates a dicrotic pulse.

THE ARTERIAL PULSE

The arterial pulse has been used in clinical diagnosis by the earliest Chinese, Greek, Hindu, and Roman physicians.[50,51] In present day medicine, the arterial pulse is most commonly used to determine heart rate or to recognize the presence of cardiac arrhythmia. However, this need not be the case. Important clinical and diagnostic information can be obtained from careful assessment of the character and contour of the arterial pulse.

Proper examination of the arterial pulses requires that the examiner be comfortable and all fingers, especially the middle three, be relaxed so that varying pressure can be applied on the arterial wall. In this manner, the examiner can assess the rate of increase, amplitude of the pulse, timing and character of the peak or peaks, and the dicrotic wave following the dicrotic notch (Figure 4.9, top tracing). For this purpose, a relatively large artery is best used such as the carotid, brachial, radial, or femoral. All major arteries should be examined and corresponding arteries compared by simultaneous palpation, ie, both brachial arteries, both femoral arteries, or brachial with femoral artery. Pulse amplitude and arrival time are best compared this way. If additional help is needed in timing events of the arterial pulse, simultaneous palpation of the cardiac apex or simultaneous precordial auscultation at an area where the first and second heart sounds are well heard provides an adequate reference point.

ABNORMAL ARTERIAL PULSES

Rapid-Rising Arterial Pulse

Individuals under conditions of excitement, exercise, fever, anemia, and hyperthyroidism may have a brisk, rapid-rising, large-amplitude pulse with a brief peak.[52] In some, a double systolic peak may be present (pulsus bisferiens) and is most commonly seen in pure aortic insufficiency or combined aortic stenosis and insufficiency (Figure 4.9, second panel). The collapsing or water-hammer pulse of aortic insufficiency may be appreciated by firmly grasping the patient's wrist with the arm held above the head (Figure 4.10). Conditions that divert part of the left ventricular stroke volume, such as mitral regurgitation or a large left-to-right shunting ventricular septal defect, may also produce a rapid-rising arterial pulse, although it may be of lesser overall amplitude than that seen in aortic insufficiency. Hypertrophic cardiomyopathy (idiopathic hypertrophic subaortic stenosis) may also exhibit a similar rapid-rising arterial pulse[53] (Figure 4.11).

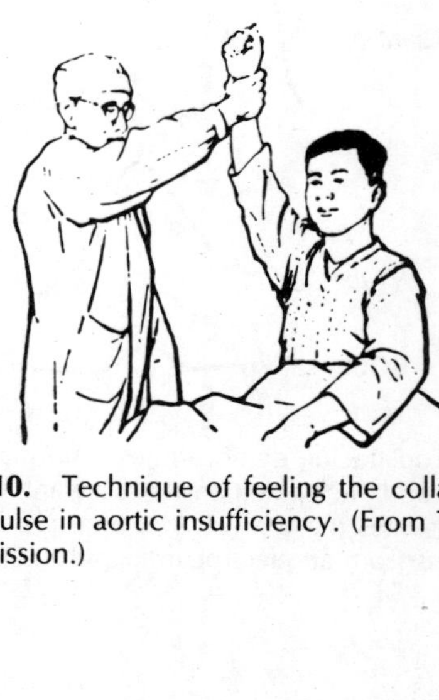

Figure 4.10. Technique of feeling the collapsing or water-hammer pulse in aortic insufficiency. (From Tung and Tao,[63] with permission.)

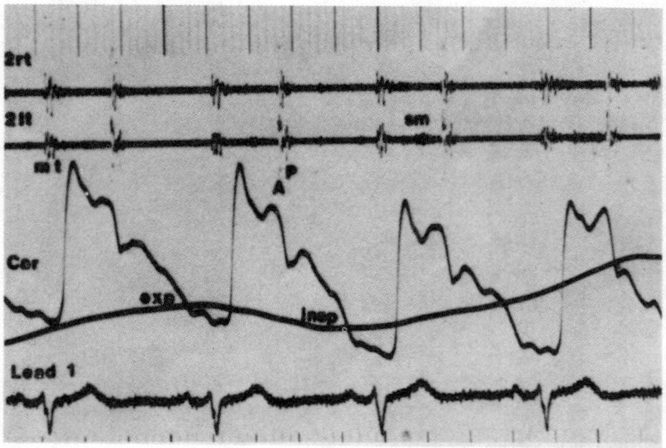

Figure 4.11. A patient with obstructive hypertrophic cardiomyopathy. The carotid pulse (Car) shows the typical rapid-rising pulse in this entity. The phonocardiograms are obtained at the right second (2 rt) and left second (2 lt) interspaces.

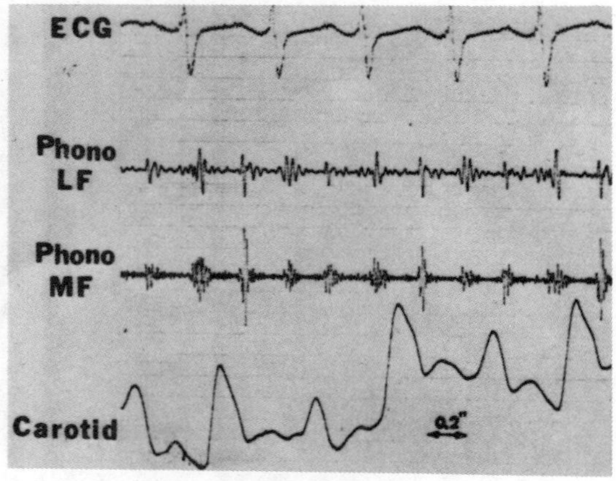

Figure 4.12. Alternating intensities of first and second heart sounds in pulsus alternans. (Modified from Cheng and Leet.[60])

Slow-Rising Arterial Pulse

Left ventricular failure with a resulting decrease in stroke volume results in a small arterial pulse. The peak of the pulse is usually not appreciably delayed.

In contrast, with moderate to severe fixed-orifice aortic stenosis, the arterial pulse is a slow-rising pulse that may have an anacrotic notch, shudder or thrill, a small overall amplitude, and a late peak (parvus et tardus)[54] (Figure 4.9, third tracing). In infants and children and in the elderly, moderate to severe aortic stenosis may be seen with apparently normal carotid arterial pulse.[50]

Dicrotic Pulse

The dicrotic pulse is a twin-peaked arterial pulse that differs from all other twin-peaked arterial pulses in that the second peak is diastolic and is the result of a large, palpable dicrotic wave (Figure 4.9, fourth tracing). Earlier descriptions of this pulse noted its presence in typhoid fever and attributed it to low systemic vascular resistance.[55] Subsequent studies suggest that a high peripheral vascular resistance, low cardiac output because of left ventricular failure, and relative youth for arterial resiliency are necessary ingredients for genesis of the pulse.[56]

Pulsus Alternans

Alternating strong and weak arterial pulses serve as a useful clinical clue to left ventricular failure.[57,58] In its most subtle form, the tactile sensation of alternation can be the result of alternation of arterial rate of rise rather than a difference in peak pressure.[50] Careful employment of the technique of varying the pressure of the examining thumb or finger against the arterial wall is needed to elicit this finding. Palpating the radial pulse when the arm is elevated or the patient is in an upright position enhances the recognition of this physical finding. Patients with pulsus alternans may also have alternation in intensity of heart sounds and murmurs[59,60] (Figure 4.12).

Paradoxical Pulse

Kussmaul originally described the decrease in amplitude or disappearance of the arterial pulse on inspiration in adhesive pericarditis.[61] In the normal individual, inspiration results in a decrease in systolic pressure of 10 mm Hg or less. An inspiratory decrease exceeding 10 mm Hg is considered abnormal and this decrease in strength of the pulse can be appreciated. Kussmaul pointed out the disparity between cardiac action and the arterial pulse, hence the term *paradoxic.*[50] In current practice, the most common cause of an exaggerated decrease in systolic arterial pressure on inspiration is chronic obstructive lung disease. Pericardial effusion with cardiac tamponade and, less frequently, constrictive pericarditis are the other two common cardiac considerations.[62]

Unequal Pulses

Occlusive arterial abnormalities, aberrant arterial origin and course, cervical rib, scalenus anticus syndrome, and aortic dissection are among the many considerations when a specific arterial pulse is absent or diminished (compared to its opposite counterpart). Coarctation of the aorta is, of course, clinically recognized when femoral pulses are bilaterally absent. When the femoral pulse is present, the amplitude may be less or the arrival time is later compared to the brachial pulses, or both.

CHINESE PULSE-LORE

The Chinese pulse-lore (Figure 4.13) appears to have developed even before the dawn of Hippocratic medicine.[51] The skillful physician often can make a determination of the diagnosis, prognosis, and treatment from the pulse alone. During pulse palpation the physician should banish all other thoughts from his mind to concentrate on the pulse. This is important because the pulse is being timed by the respiration of the physician, four pulsations to each respiration being the natural rate. The pulse should be palpated at three separate places (寸關尺 in Figure 4.13) by the physician's ring, middle, and index fingers, respectively (Figure 4.14). At each place, light, moderate, and firm pressure is applied in turn so as to elicit the superficial and deep pulses. The pulse should be examined at both wrists (Figure 4.13), the physician using his right hand for the patient's left pulse and vice versa (Figure 4.14).

In Chinese traditional medicine each body organ has its proper pulse (Figure 4.13), and 28 kinds of pulses are

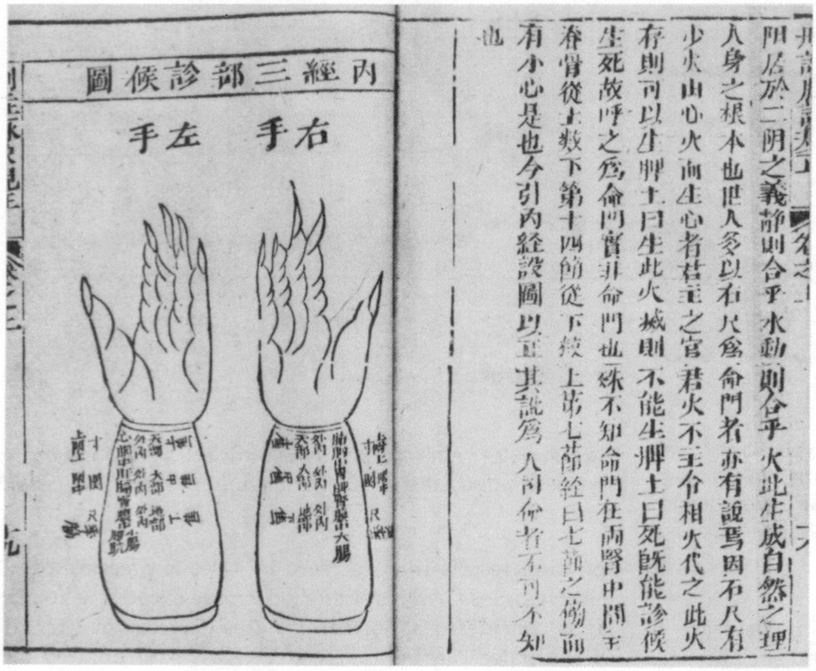

Figure 4.13. Chinese pulse lore published in 1693. 寸 corresponds to upper part of the body, including the heart on the left and lungs on the right, palpated by the ring finger; 関 , middle part of body, by middle finger; 尺 , lower part of body by index finger. (Courtesy of Wellcome Institute Library, London, England.)

described.[63] Among those that are of importance in the evaluation and management of cardiovascular diseases are:

1. 细脉,微脉,伏脉 (fine pulse, filiform pulse, and hidden pulse). Fine pulse is felt as a thin thread and seen in severe mitral stenosis, tricuspid stenosis, constrictive pericarditis, and pericardial effusion. Filiform pulse is felt as almost imperceptible below the fingers and found in cardiogenic shock. Hidden pulse is hidden (or sunken) and is seen in aortitis.
2. 洪脉 (flooding pulse). This corresponds to the bounding pulse in Western medicine.
3. 芤脉,革脉 (hollow pulse and leather pulse). Hollow pulse, "like the stalk of a spring onion," is seen in conditions associated with peripheral vasodilation and decreased peripheral vascular resistance. Leather pulse, "like tapping the skin of a drum," corresponds to the water-hammer pulse in aortic valve incompetence.

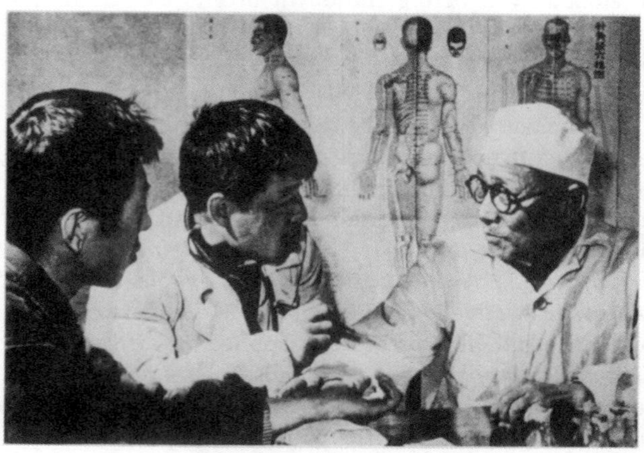

Figure 4.14. Chinese traditional medical doctor palpating the patient's pulse.

4. 迟脉 (slow pulse). Slow pulse means three pulsations per each respiration, normal being four. It is seen in sinus bradycardia and various degrees of heart block.
5. 促脉,结脉,代脉 (hasty pulse, knotted pulse, and intermittent pulse with long pauses). They represent various tachyarrhythmias and bradyarrhythmias.

BLOOD PRESSURE MEASUREMENT

When control of hypertension and prevention of its dreaded complications became an accepted worldwide practice, routine blood pressure measurement became a standard medical practice. Although it is a simple office procedure which is often delegated to a nurse or other paramedical personnel, there are several factors that often may lead to erroneous readings, misdiagnoses, and consequent mismanagement. The following points need special emphasis:

1. Palpate the radial pulse during inflation of the sphygmomanometric cuff. Defer auscultation over the brachial artery until the radial pulse has disappeared, thus avoiding the "auscultatory gap" that may result in a falsely low reading, especially in hypertensive subjects. Because the "auscultatory gap" tends to occur when there is venous distension or reduced velocity of arterial flow into the forearm, have the patient clench the fist 10 to 20 times beforehand. Palpating the pulseless radial or brachial artery distal to the point of occlusion by the cuff (Osler's maneuver[64]) is also useful in differentiating true hypertension from pseudohypertension, a condition in which the cuff pressure is inappropriately higher than the intraarterial pressure because of excessive arteriosclerosis common in the elderly, and the Osler maneuver is therefore positive.[64]
2. Use the lightest possible pressure on the head of the

stethoscope. Although excessive pressure on the stethoscopic head does not affect the systolic blood pressure value, it does erroneously lower diastolic reading and frequently causes the sounds to persist to zero.[65]

3. Record both the fourth (muffling) and fifth (disappearance of sound) phases of Korotkoff sounds to measure "true" diastolic pressure. In a recent survey of hospital personnel, it was found that although most of the faculty and nursing staff recorded phase 5, almost half of the housestaff and medical students used phase 4.[66] Since the Hypertension Detection and Follow-up Program (HDFP),[67] which suggested that mild hypertension (diastolic pressure 90 to 104 mm Hg) be treated, used phase 5 as diastolic, physicians using phase 4 diastolic blood pressure readings, which may be 5 to 10 mm Hg higher than those of phase 5, may be inappropriately treating some patients.
4. Indicate whether blood pressure was measured in the right or left arm. The American Heart Association stated that on the initial examination blood pressure should be determined in both arms and thereafter pressure should be taken on the side that initially had the highest pressure.[68] Recently, however, in large-population blood pressure studies, either the arm that was tested was not specified[69] or the pressure was taken only on the right side.[67] Although the pressure difference between the arms is small in most people[70] it is often unpredictable. Therefore, arm or other aspects should always be considered when taking comparative blood pressure measurements.
5. Take the blood pressure with the patient seated and with the arm supported in a horizontal position at heart level. A recent British survey showed that blood pressure measurements made with the arm dependent at the side were consistently higher than those made with the arm horizontal at heart level and that blood pressures recorded in the sitting position were lower than the supine pressure provided that the arm was at heart level.[71] Therefore, it is advisable to specify not only the arm, whether right or left, but also the body position of the patient, whether supine or sitting, in which the blood pressure was taken and also to record both phase 4 and phase 5 of the Korotkoff sounds, eg, blood pressure equals 130/90/80 mm Hg, right arm, sitting.
6. Be aware of seasonal and population variations and iatrogenic factors in blood pressure measurement. Blood pressures are usually lower in summer than in winter and spring, as documented in both a Belgian[72] and an American[73] study. Population differences arising from ethnicity, socioeconomic background, or environment certainly account for the discrepancies in blood pressure distribution among high school students in a recent Canadian survey.[74] It has long been recognized that even during relatively stable and nonstressful situations blood pressure can vary considerably during a 24-hour period. This was recently confirmed by studies from Greece[75] and Italy[76] using 24-hour continuous intraarterial catheter monitoring of blood pressure in both normotensive and hypertensive free-living patients. The best assessment of resting blood pressure is probably made by the patient at home to avoid the pitfalls of the so-called "white coat hypertension." Blood pressure measurements should always be taken at the end rather than at the beginning of the visit.[77] Because blood pressure measurements frequently are used to determine the course of treatment for mild or borderline hypertension and for modifying therapeutic regimens in poorly controlled hypertension, these seasonal and iatrogenic variations could affect the decision on how to treat millions of patients. They further demonstrate the necessity of maintaining appropriate controls whenever drug, diet, behavioral changes, or other therapeutic manipulations are implicated in reducing blood pressure levels.

PRECORDIAL PALPATION

Inspection and palpation of the thorax are an expertise that more and more physicians appear to use less often, particularly with the readily available array of present day noninvasive diagnostic tools. It is still worth the physician's time and can provide useful information which can be used in the context of the other clinical findings from the venous and arterial pulse as well as auscultation.[78,79]

Search for thrills! Their location and direction of radiation can provide important clues to the diagnostic possibilities. When present, a corresponding murmur of grade 4/6 or greater is certain to be present. With very loud murmurs which transmit widely, it may be difficult to judge by auscultation the area of maximal intensity; the location of the thrill can help in this localization. A second right interspace systolic thrill, especially with radiation superiorly toward the right side of the neck, suggests valvular aortic stenosis. A second left interspace systolic thrill which may radiate toward the left side of the neck suggests pulmonary stenosis. A continuous thrill at the left second interspace suggests an aortopulmonary communication, usually a patent ductus arteriosus. A left parasternal systolic thrill, especially if it radiates across the sternum toward the right parasternal area, suggests a ventricular septal defect. A systolic thrill at the cardiac apex (occupied by left ventricle) suggests mitral regurgitation and a diastolic apical thrill may be due to mitral stenosis. Thrills over intercostal arteries (usually best noted in the posterior or lateral thorax, or both) suggest enlarged intercostal arteries with large flow, a tip-off of abnormal collateral circulation, such as that seen in aortic coarctation.

Palpate for sounds! When palpable, and not readily explainable by a thin chest, the implication is that the sound is of abnormal intensity. Therefore, a loud first heart sound (S_1 mitral closure component) and mitral opening snap may be palpable at the cardiac apex, a loud pulmonic closure sound (P_2) at the second left interspace, and a loud aortic closure sound (A_2) at the second right interspace. Ejection sounds, especially the aortic ejection sound, may be palpable (and mistaken for a palpable S_1). The systolic clicks of mitral valve prolapse are not usually palpable.

Observe for visible precordial motion. Areas of retraction are better seen than felt. Right ventricular volume load abnormality such as in atrial septal defect can result in hyperdynamic parasternal motion which is more impressive visually than is the brief, nonsustained lift noted by the palpating fingers or hand. At the very least, areas of visualized movement can be correspondingly palpated.

Palpation of precordial movements is best carried out using the palmar surface of the hand, the fingertips, and interphalangeal or metacarpophalangeal junction depending on whether one is palpating a diffuse or localized event, or is looking for a high frequency event (thrill) as well. For the latter, the interphalangeal or metacarpophalangeal joints are usually better because bone is a better conductor of vibration than is soft tissue.

The apical impulse should be assessed in the supine as well as left lateral decubitus position. In the supine position, an abnormal location of this impulse may indicate dextrocardia, or with a normal cardiac position it may be a useful gross index of whether or not cardiomegaly is present. Thus, with left ventricular dilatation the usual left ventricular apex is displaced lateral to the left midclavicular line or downward below the fifth interspace, or both, provided the heart itself is not abnormally shifted for other reasons. The character of the apex impulse should also be assessed. The normal impulse is a brief tap, whereas that of left ventricular hypertrophy is sustained and usually well localized (Figure 4.15). The apex impulse of a volume-loaded left ventricle tends to occupy a larger area, and when visible, it is more diffuse (Figure 4.16). Hyperkinetic states result in a more vigorous but brief apex impulse. In the left lateral decubitus position, the apex is brought close to the chest wall and its character can even be better assessed. Pre-systolic and mid-diastolic distension may be both visible and palpable and is equivalent to the S_4 (Figure 4.15) and S_3 noted on auscultation. The double systolic outward thrust noted in some patients with hypertrophic cardiomyopathy (IHSS) may also be felt (Figure 4.17). With careful observation, an area of retraction can usually be observed. Its location relative to the apex impulse provides the clinical clue on which ven-

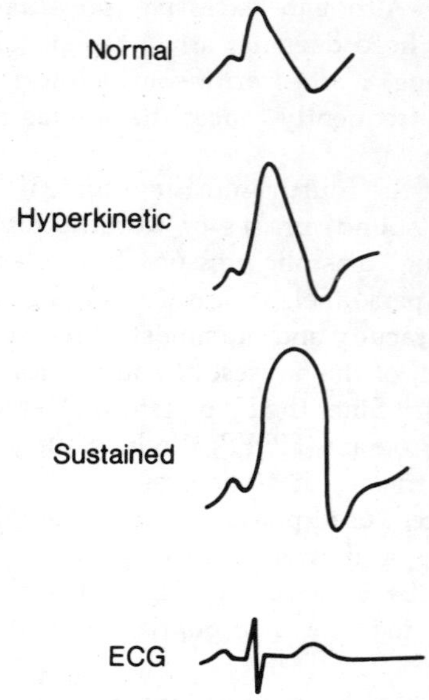

Figure 4.16. Top tracing demonstrates the brief tap of a normal apex impulse. Second tracing demonstrates the vigorous but brief tap of the cardiac apex in hyperkinetic states. Third tracing demonstrates the sustained outward thrust of left ventricular hypertrophy. Fourth tracing is the electrocardiogram. The initial small upward deflection preceding the apex impulse represents atrial presystolic distension (atrial kick).

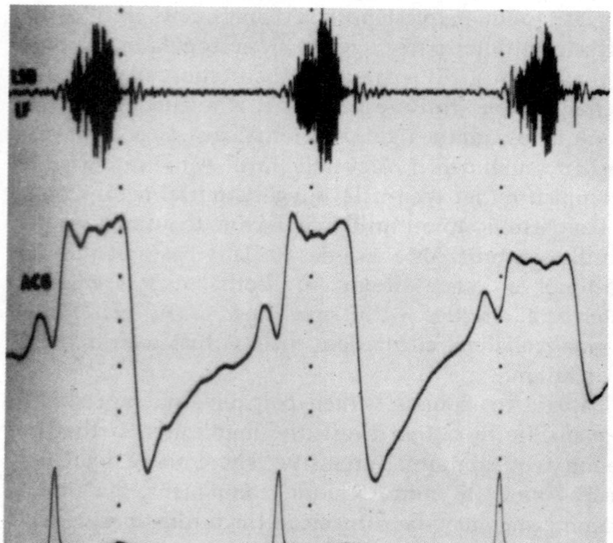

Figure 4.15. A patient with aortic stenosis and left ventricular hypertrophy. The apex cardiogram (ACG) shows presystolic distension and a sustained outward thrust. A phonocardiogram at the lower left sternal border (LSB) demonstrates the systolic ejection murmur.

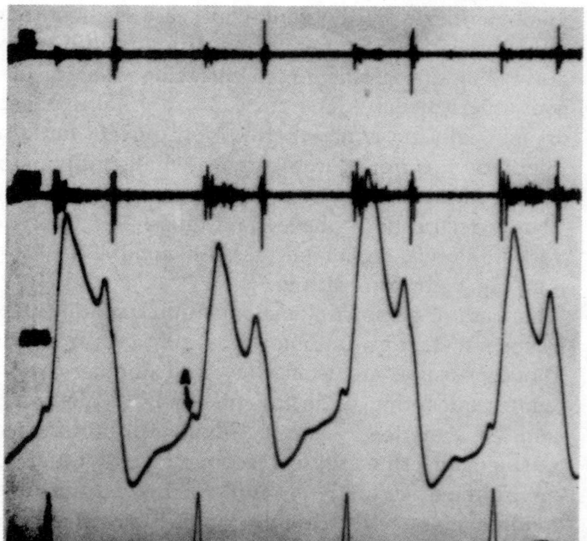

Figure 4.17. A patient with obstructive hypertrophic cardiomyopathy. The apex cardiogram (ACG) demonstrates the presystolic distension (A), and a double systolic apical thrust. The phonocardiogram along the lower left sternal border (LSB) demonstrates the systolic murmur.

tricle occupies the apex impulse. When the left ventricle occupies the apex, the area of retraction is medial, and when the right ventricle occupies the apex, retraction is lateral to it. In the latter, the apex impulse and the parasternal systolic lift are contiguous.

The left parasternal area should be assessed. Normally, there is little or no detectable motion. However, with right ventricular hypertrophy, a sustained left parasternal systolic impulse may be appreciated and, just as indicated, the right ventricle may also occupy the apex impulse. With hyperkinetic and volume-loaded states such as atrial septal defect, the systolic parasternal lift is exaggerated over normal but is brief. Timing of the systolic lift is important, because left atrial expansion from mitral regurgitation results in forward displacement of the overlying right ventricle. In this instance, the left parasternal lift has a late systolic onset with peak motion in time with the peak of the left atrial V wave.[80] The abnormal right ventricular impulse can also be appreciated in the subxiphoid area and is felt as systolic pulsation against the tips of the examiner's fingers. This is especially useful when the anteroposterior diameter of the chest is increased.[79]

The area of the precordium above and medial to the apex (lateral to the left parasternal area) is commonly referred to as the area for "ectopic" impulses. Systolic expansion of the left ventricular wall during systole can be appreciated in this area.[81] The systolic expansion may be the result of a physiologic or anatomic ventricular aneurysm.[82]

Other areas of the precordium should be examined, because aneurysms of the aorta may produce a second right interspace systolic impulse, and pulmonary hypertension a left second interspace systolic impulse.

AUSCULTATION

Auscultation is most rewarding when all the important ingredients are carefully and deliberately incorporated. The room should be quiet and all possible sources of extraneous noise excluded. The patient should be comfortable and the possibility of extraneous friction noise caused by clothing eliminated. The stethoscope used should have a bell and a diaphragm. The examiner should be comfortable and also aware that the bell applied lightly on the skin just to secure a good seal is best for low frequency events and that the diaphragm applied firmly is best for high frequency events. The patient should be examined in positions that best enhance the particular auscultatory events (supine, left lateral decubitus, sitting, standing, and leaning forward). The examiner should develop the ability to "tune in" to each auscultatory event one at a time while simultaneously "tuning out" other sound events.[83] Developing the habit of drawing a diagram of the sounds and murmurs heard in one complete cardiac cycle is a good way to ensure that each event has been carefully heard and considered.

All of the foregoing details serve only as a prelude to what makes auscultation one of the most powerful tools of the cardiac examination. It is the mental translation of events heard into pathophysiologic correlates that ultimately enables the examiner to infer the absence or presence of heart disease, determine the abnormality present, and assess the resulting severity of hemodynamic disturbance. The mental exercise of carefully weighing the diagnostic possibilities from the previously obtained clinical history, inspection, the jugular venous and arterial pulses, and precordial examination allows the examiner to especially "tune in" and search for particular auscultatory events.

SOUNDS

First Heart Sound

The first heart sound serves as the auscultatory landmark for the onset of ventricular systole. It normally consists of two audible components: mitral valve closure (M_1) and tricuspid valve closure (T_1). Although there is a temporal relation between atrioventricular (AV) valve closure and occurrence of the first heart sound, the sound does not occur at the moment of leaflet coaptation. Rather, it occurs at the moment of abrupt deceleration of the valve structures as they reach the point of maximal bulge into the respective atrial cavity.[84,85] The intensity of the sound generated is primarily a function of the force of deceleration of the valve leaflet structures. Because the force of deceleration is a function of the force of acceleration immediately preceding it, the major determinants of the intensity of sound generated are the leaflet positions immediately preceding ventricular systole and the rate of pressure development in the ventricle. Because the rate of pressure development in the ventricle progressively increases as systole begins, the later the AV valve closes, the greater the closing force and, hence, the intensity of sound produced.[86,87] Thus, the first heart sound (M_1) is loud with a short PR interval in mitral stenosis and hyperkinetic states. Conversely, it is softer than normal in first degree AV block, acute myocardial infarction, congestive cardiomyopathy, and aortic valve regurgitation severe enough to result in mitral valve closure before ventricular systole. Loss of valve mobility and elasticity, such as occurs with calcification or dense fibrotic changes or both, also results in a soft or even absent sound (both closure and opening). The tricuspid component of the first heart sound is loud in atrial septal defects[88] and in Ebstein's anomaly.[89] Complete heart block, AV dissociation, and atrial fibrillation result in changing intensity of the first heart sound.[83] Variation in the position of the AV valves or changes in the rate of ventricular pressure development caused by the change in left ventricular end-diastolic volume (changing RR intervals), or both, explain the change in intensity of the first heart sound.

Second Heart Sound

The second heart sound represents the end of ventricular systole and normally has two distinct components. The sound results from the abrupt checking of the closing motion of the aortic and pulmonary semilunar valves. Clinically, it is recognized that elevated diastolic pressure in the aorta or pulmonary arteries with resulting increased pressure gradient across the semilunar valve results in increased intensity of the second heart sound. More recent physiologic data suggest that the intensity of the semilunar valve closure sound is related to the rate of decline in ventricular pressure, which in turn affects the rate of change in pressure gradient across the valve.[90]

Normally, aortic closure (A_2) precedes pulmonic closure (P_2). With respiration there is a normal increase in separation between A_2 and P_2 on inspiration (inspiratory splitting), and these components come together to form a single second heart sound on expiration. This normal sequence is termed *physiologic splitting* (Figure 4.18, top tracing). An earlier A_2 (from decreased pulmonary venous return to the left heart) accounts for a small portion of this inspiratory splitting. The major contribution to the inspiratory splitting is the delay in P_2. Increased venous return to the right heart is a partial explanation. The major contributor to delay in P_2 appears to be continued forward flow of blood into the pulmonary arterial bed while the right ventricle has already begun to relax and right ventricular pressure is declining. This delayed occurrence of the dicrotic notch in the pulmonary arterial pressure has been termed "hang-out"[91] and is caused by the inspiratory decrease in pulmonary vascular impedance.[92]

It is especially important to pay critical attention to the movement of the two components of the second heart sound because they can directly provide clues to the presence of some specific clinical entities and are also important in the assessment of some cardiac murmurs. An increase in the degree of inspiratory splitting can occur from earlier aortic valve closure (A_2) or from a delay in pulmonary valve closure (P_2). Earlier A_2 occurs with significant mitral regurgitation or a large left-to-right shunting ventricular septal defect, both of which unload the left ventricle and shorten left ventricular ejection time. Despite the wider splitting, normal movement toward expiratory fusion of the two components would be expected. Delay in P_2 occurs with complete right bundle branch block, because the conduction abnormality delays the onset of right ventricular systole. Movement of the two components closer together or even normal fusion occurs on expiration. In idiopathic dilatation of the pulmonary artery and in mild pulmonic stenosis, the increased inspiratory splitting due to delay in P_2 is due to "hang-out" resulting from increased capacitance of the pulmonary vascular bed.[91] Expiratory movement closer together or even fusion into a single second sound is expected on expiration. With severe pulmonic stenosis, prolongation of right ventricular systole contributes to the delay in P_2, and although the second sound splitting is less on expiration, it does not usually become single. Additionally, the intensity of P_2 is usually decreased. Left-to-right shunt at atrial level, particularly atrial septal defect, results in wide splitting of the second heart sound which shows little or no variation with expiration (fixed splitting) and is a diagnostic feature of this cardiac abnormality (Figure 4.18, middle tracing; Figure 4.19). It is important that the lack of movement of the two components of the second sound on expiration be also demonstrated in the sitting position before concluding that fixed splitting is present.[93]

Reversal of the normal A_2-P_2 relation so that P_2 precedes A_2 results in paradoxic splitting of the second heart sound (Figure 4.18, third tracing). This auscultatory finding is commonly noted in complete left bundle branch block (delay in onset of left ventricular systole, hence delay in the end of systole (A_2) (Figure 4.20). The normal inspiratory delay in P_2 and earlier A_2 brings the two components closer together or they even fuse as a single second heart sound on inspiration, and conversely on expiration wider splitting is present. Individuals with a transvenous right ventricular pacemaker also have paradoxic splitting of S_2 because of delayed activation of the left ventricle. Conditions that prolong the duration of left ventricular systole such as obstruction to left ventricular outflow (aortic stenosis) can also delay A_2 and result in paradoxic splitting of the second heart sound.[83] When present in a patient with aortic stenosis, significant obstruction can be assumed. In calcific aortic stenosis, mobility and compliance of the aortic leaflets are likely to be impaired, so the sound of valve closure (A_2) may be soft or even absent and a single second heart sound thus results. Paradoxic splitting may also occur in coronary heart disease due to prolongation of left ventricular systole resulting from myocardial ischemia.[94] In patent ductus arteriosus the increased left ventricular diastolic volume may also prolong the left ventricular systole and result in paradoxic splitting, although the accentuation of

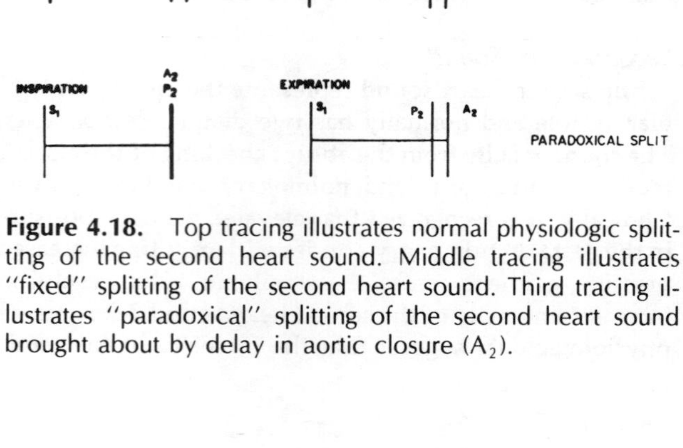

Figure 4.18. Top tracing illustrates normal physiologic splitting of the second heart sound. Middle tracing illustrates "fixed" splitting of the second heart sound. Third tracing illustrates "paradoxical" splitting of the second heart sound brought about by delay in aortic closure (A_2).

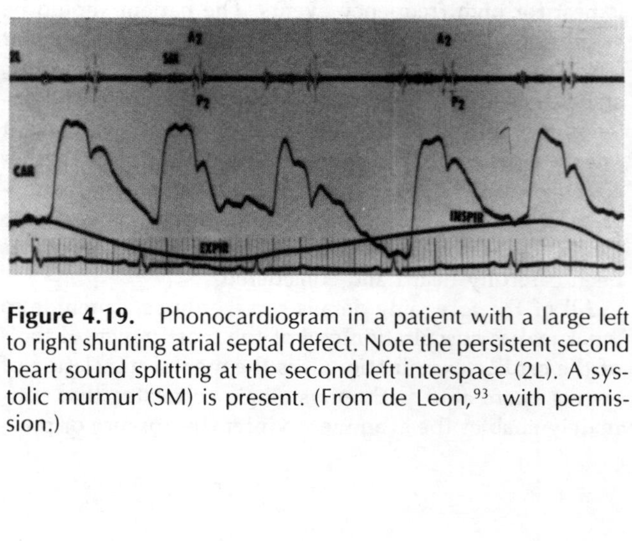

Figure 4.19. Phonocardiogram in a patient with a large left to right shunting atrial septal defect. Note the persistent second heart sound splitting at the second left interspace (2L). A systolic murmur (SM) is present. (From de Leon,[93] with permission.)

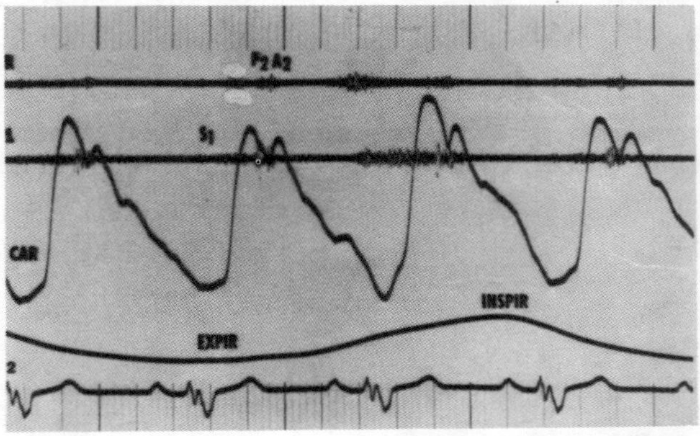

Figure 4.20. Phonocardiogram of a patient with dilated cardiomyopathy and complete left bundle branch block. Note the wide second sound splitting on expiration (EXPIR) caused by delay in aortic closure (A_2) which follows rather than precedes pulmonary closure (P_2).

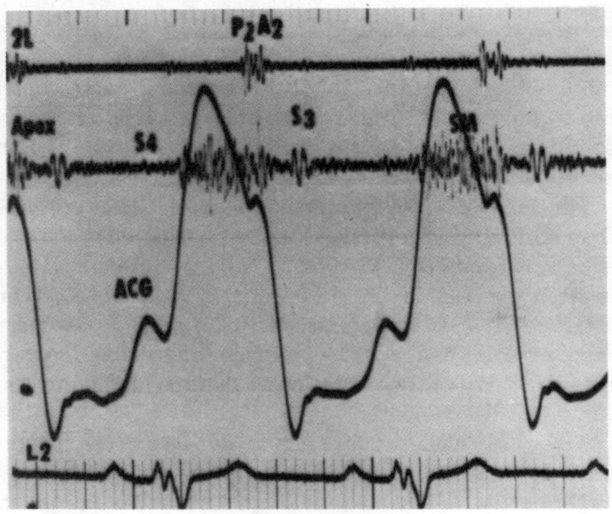

Figure 4.21. The same patient with dilated cardiomyopathy as in Figure 4.20 demonstrating a systolic murmur of mitral regurgitation (SM), and both an atrial (S_4) as well as a ventricular diastolic gallop (S_3). The apex cardiogram (ACG) demonstrates the presystolic outward thrust, which corresponds to S_4, and the early diastolic rapid-filling wave, which corresponds to S_3.

the continuous murmur at the time of the second sound makes its recognition difficult. A false impression of paradoxic splitting can occur in patients with an increased anteroposterior diameter, because a soft P_2 may become inaudible on inspiration, and if close expiratory splitting is present, the single second sound (A_2) heard on inspiration leads to misdiagnosis.

Third Heart Sound

The third heart sound (S_3) occurs in early diastole during the period of early passive diastolic filling of the ventricle. It is usually 0.14 to 0.16 second after the second heart sound and is of low frequency and hence best heard using the bell of the stethoscope over the cardiac apex. It is frequently present in normal children and young adults, and in the absence of heart disease, it is also referred to as a physiologic third heart sound. In the context of cardiac disease it is referred to as a ventricular gallop or S_3 gallop (Figure 4.21).

The precise genesis of the third heart sound remains unsettled. The sudden tension on the mitral valve structures and traction on the apical myocardium have been proposed[95] and other recent studies suggest that the sound occurs with the sudden intrinsic limitation of longitudinal expansion of the left ventricular wall.[96–98] Others propose that the sound results from the physical impact of the heart on the chest wall.[99] Still others believe that deceleration of inflow by the left ventricular wall in diastole is responsible for the sound.[100,101]

Clinically, the sound is present when there is left ventricular myocardial failure from many causes (eg, ischemic heart disease and cardiomyopathy) and it decreases in intensity as cardiac compensation is restored with therapy. Conditions that result in ventricular diastolic volume overloading also produce the sound. Thus, the third heart sound appears when mitral regurgitation progresses from mild to moderate or severe. Conversely, a left ventricular third heart sound would not be the usual finding in tight mitral stenosis. A left ventricular third heart sound would be a feature of a large left-to-right shunting ventricular septal defect and patent ductus arteriosus, because both result in increased left ventricular diastolic volume load.

Right ventricular failure can also result in a third heart sound of right-sided origin. It can be recognized by the inspiratory augmentation of intensity of the sound and is best heard along the left sternal border, xiphoid area, or even the cardiac apex when the right ventricle occupies it.

The pericardial knock sound is a term especially given to the early diastolic sound heard in constrictive pericarditis.[83] It occurs earlier (0.10 to 0.12 second) and tends to have a higher frequency than the usual third heart sound. Because the encasing pericardium restricts ventricular filling, diastolic ventricular dimensions reach their limits sooner and provide a tempting explanation for the earlier occurrence of the sound. The frequency characteristic of the sound and its closeness to the second heart sound may lead to its being mistaken for an opening snap. The absence of diastolic rumble, elevated jugular venous pressure, and positive Kussmaul sign should help in its proper identification.

Fourth Heart Sound

The fourth heart sound (S_4) is a low frequency event that occurs after the P wave on the electrocardiogram and is therefore heard immediately preceding the first heart sound. Like the third heart sound, it is best heard with the bell of the stethoscope applied lightly over the cardiac apex. Because the sound is not present in atrial fibrillation, atrial contraction is a necessary ingredient for its presence. The precise genesis of the sound is likely to be similar to that of the third heart sound.[100]

An audible fourth heart sound is not a common normal finding in children and young adults. In persons above age 50, the sound can be recorded in the phonocardiogram in 73% of those without cardiovascular disease.[102] The yield of audible S_4 is likely to be lower but nevertheless sufficiently frequent to make the sole presence of the sound an inadequate indicator of heart disease. Furthermore, prolongation of the PR interval (first degree heart block) can unmask the atrial component of the first heart sound complex[103] and cause a distinct, audible S_4. In certain specific clinical entities, the presence of S_4 can be of clinical value. In valvular aortic stenosis in patients less than 40 years of age, presence of an S_4 suggests the presence of a significant gradient.[104] An S_4 is a frequent finding in hypertrophic cardiomyopathy,[105] acute myocardial infarction,[106,107] during episodes of angina,[108] primary myocardial disease[109] (Figure 4.21), and systemic hypertension.[110] All of these conditions share in common a less compliant left ventricle.

Right ventricular origin of an S_4 can also occur. Therefore, it may be encountered in severe pulmonary hypertension[111] and in pulmonic stenosis. In the latter, its presence can be a useful clinical index of severity.[112]

Summation Gallop

Sinus tachycardia results in a decrease in the diastolic period of the cardiac cycle. Hence, in patients with both a third and fourth heart sound, the two events may occur simultaneously resulting in a loud sound, a summation gallop. On occasion, this sound can be louder than either the first or second heart sound and thus be misinterpreted as the first sound resulting in the mistiming of associated murmurs present. It is usually encountered in the setting of severe congestive heart failure. As therapy succeeds and heart rate decreases, the presence of both the third and fourth heart sounds becomes evident.

Ejection Sound

Normally, the opening of the aortic or pulmonary semilunar valves and the onset of ventricular ejection does not produce a clinically audible sound. In certain cardiac abnormalities, a sharp, high-frequency sound is heard shortly after the first heart sound and because its genesis is related to the start of ventricular ejection, it has been termed *ejection sound* (or ejection click). Congenital aortic or pulmonary valvular abnormality (bicuspid and unicuspid) produces the sound as the opening motion of the valve is abruptly halted. The sound also occurs in the absence of valve stenosis in patients with a dilated ascending aorta or main pulmonary artery. In these cases, the initial movement of the column of blood above the valve as it opens distends the great vessel wall and may be an explanation for the sound that is slightly earlier than the ejection sound of valvular origin.[113]

The aortic ejection sound noted in aortic stenosis implies the presence of a congenitally biscupid or unicuspid valve (Figure 4.22). It may be an isolated finding (bicuspid valve) or, as is usually the case, may introduce a systolic ejection murmur. The presence of the sound requires mobility and compliance of the valve and therefore may disappear when heavy calcification of the leaflets supervenes. The ejection sound is heard at the second right interspace, but it may be equally or better heard over the left ventricular cardiac apex. When present in the apex, the sound may be mistaken for the first heart sound.

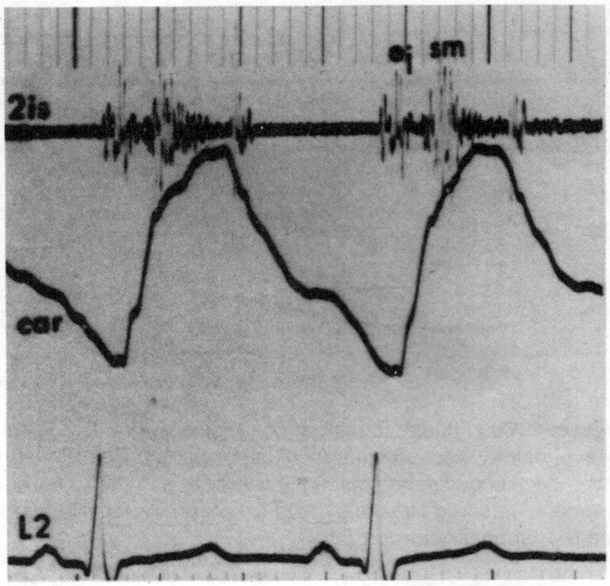

Figure 4.22. Phonocardiogram at the right second interspace (2is) of a patient with coarctation of the aorta and a bicuspid aortic valve. The carotid arterial pulse (car) used for timing shows some "shudder" of the upstroke. ej = ejection click; sm = systolic murmur. (From de Leon,[93] with permission.)

There is no discernible intensity variation in the sound with respiration. Dilatation of the ascending aorta from various causes such as aneurysm or hypertension may also be associated with an ejection sound (Figure 4.23). In coarctation of the aorta, the frequently associated presence of a bicuspid aortic valve is the more likely cause of the sound. The clinical recognition of the sound is important, because it may be the only clue to the presence of an abnormal valve (bicuspid) for which prophylaxis against bacterial endocarditis should be instituted.

The pulmonary ejection sound of valvular pulmonic stenosis[114] is likewise the result of the abrupt halt in the opening motion of the valve. It is of relatively high frequency and exhibits selective respiratory variation (Figure 4.24). Therefore, on inspiration, the sound is soft or absent, and on expiration, the sound gets louder. It is usually best heard at the second left interspace and lower left sternal border and would be heard at the cardiac apex only when the sound is very loud or when the right ventricle occupies the apex. The presence of an ejection sound also serves to differentiate pulmonic valvular stenosis from infundibular stenosis. However, a pulmonic ejection sound may be heard in supravalvular pulmonary stenosis due to associated pulmonary artery dilatation.[115] Idiopathic dilatation of the pulmonary artery with a normal pulmonary valve may also be associated with a pulmonary ejection sound.[116] Selective respiratory variation in intensity, when present, also serves to identify its right-sided origin.

Systolic Clicks

Sounds in systole of intracardiac origin, not related to semilunar valve stenosis or great vessel dilatation, are referred to as nonejection systolic clicks. Most are prob-

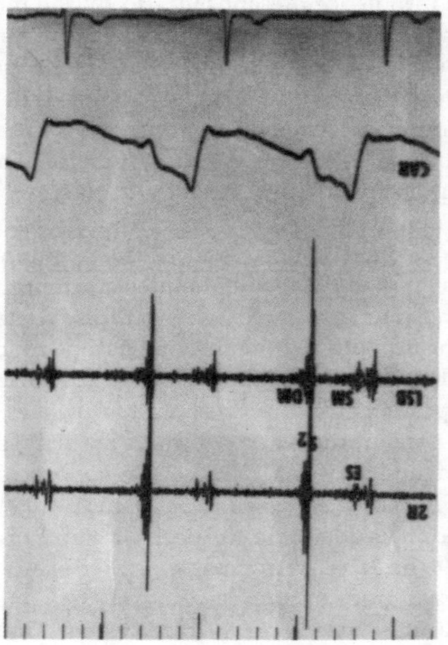

Figure 4.23. A patient with ascending aortic aneurysm. Phonocardiographic recording at the second right interspace (2R) and lower left sternal border (LSB). An aortic ejection sound (ES) is present, followed by a short systolic ejection murmur (SM). Aortic insufficiency is manifest in the diastolic murmur (DM) which is decrescendo from the second heart sound (S_2). A carotid arterial pulse (CAR) is simultaneously recorded.

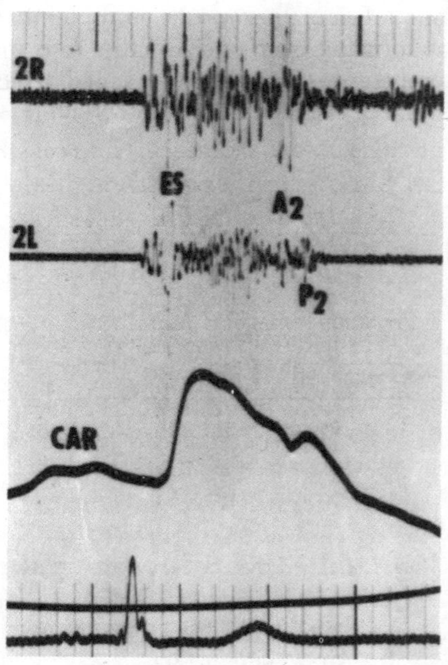

Figure 4.24. A patient with valvular pulmonary stenosis. The recordings at the second right (2R) and left (2L) interspaces demonstrate the pulmonary ejection sound (ES) which precedes the systolic ejection murmur. Note as well the delay of pulmonary closure sound (P_2). A carotid arterial pulse (CAR) is also simultaneously recorded.

ably due to the abrupt halt and tensing that occurs as a prolapsing mitral leaflet reaches maximum travel into the left atrium.[117] It is entirely possible that prolapse of the tricuspid leaflets may also produce clicks. However, in most cases in which tricuspid prolapse is demonstrated, mitral valve prolapse is also present.

Single or multiple clicks may be present and variation in the number of clicks occurs in the same patient with different cardiac cycles. In some, the numerous, multiple clicks occur in such close succession that they are misinterpreted for a systolic murmur. The clicks are usually best heard at the apex and lower left sternal border. When a single click is present and is in early systole, it may be mistaken for an ejection sound. The latter, however, preserves its location in early systole despite maneuvers that alter the ventricular volume. In systolic clicks of mitral valve prolapse, changes in ventricular volume alter their location in systole. Therefore, in the recumbent position it may be in mid- to late systole and move into early systole on assuming the sitting or standing position. This very mobility of the clicks with the various bedside maneuvers also identifies their intracardiac origin and helps to separate them from extracardiac clicks of pleuropericardial origin. The systolic click of mitral valve prolapse will be discussed in greater detail in chapter 31 on Mitral Valve Billowing and Prolapse.

Opening Snap

Mitral or tricuspid valve opening does not normally produce an audible sound. Pathologic changes that result in mitral or tricuspid stenosis, or both, make the valve opening audible. It is an early diastolic event. The point of maximal opening travel and abrupt checking of valve motion results in the sound called the opening snap (OS). The OS of the mitral valve is most frequently encountered in, and usually is the result of, rheumatic mitral stenosis. It is a relatively high-frequency sound, heard best at the cardiac apex and along the lower left sternal border. On occasion, the sound is loud enough to be heard at the second interspace and can therefore be confused as a component of the second heart sound. It is therefore important to observe that there actually are three separate sounds on inspiration (A_2-P_2-OS) and only two on expiration (S_2-OS). Thus, the opening snap does not manifest detectable respiratory movement.

Because the OS is related to mitral valve opening, factors that make the valve open earlier (or later) influence the timing of the opening snap relative to aortic valve closure (A_2). The more elevated the left atrial pressure, the earlier is pressure cross-over with left ventricular pressure and hence an earlier opening snap. For this reason, the interval between A_2 and OS can range from 0.04 to 0.12 second. The shorter interval (earlier OS) indicates more severe stenosis, and the long interval (0.12 second), mild stenosis. This sound is present in both sinus rhythm and atrial fibrillation.

The stenotic tricuspid valve may also produce a tricuspid opening snap. Because rheumatic tricuspid stenosis usually coexists with rheumatic mitral stenosis, it is not always possible to clearly identify the tricuspid opening snap.

A diastolic click may sometimes be heard in mitral valve prolapse[118] and mistaken for an opening snap. The differential diagnosis may at times be very difficult, especially because mitral valve prolapse may coexist with mitral stenosis.[119]

Artificial Valve Sounds

The most common therapy for valvular heart disease is prosthetic valve replacement. It, therefore, is essential to learn both normal and abnormal auscultatory findings.[120,121] This task is compounded by the variety of valves as well as the various models of each valve type in current use. Furthermore, the position of the valve (mitral, aortic, or tricuspid) also determines the sound it produces. In general, the homo- and heterograft valves produce a closing sound that most closely mimics normal heart sounds. They produce either a soft or an absent opening sound. Conversely, the various mechanical prosthetic valves generally produce a prominent or readily heard closing sound. The valve opening sound may be soft or absent (bileaflet or tilting valve) or readily heard and even prominent (caged disk or caged ball).

Prosthetic ball or disk valves produce an audible closing sound in the mitral position and would correspond to the M_1 component of S_1. The opening sound produced would correspond to the OS of the mitral valve.

In the aortic position, these same valves produce an audible opening sound that would correspond to an "ejection sound" in timing. Valve closure, which is also audible, would correspond to A_2.

Alteration, therefore, in sound intensity, presence and timing of the sound, intermittent presence, and the features of associated murmurs become important factors in assessment of the state of valve function.

Other Sounds

Pacemaker stimulation of skeletal muscle can produce a loud sound at the time of the pacemaker stimulus. This so-called "pacemaker heart sound" precedes the normally produced S_1 and is therefore a diastolic or presystolic event.[122–124]

Mobile intracardiac tumors, such as left atrial myxoma, may produce a sound as they reach the apex of the travel allowed by their attached pedicle. It is usually diastolic, of low-frequency, and times as a mitral opening snap.[125] It has been referred to as a "tumor plop." Less frequently, tumor travel back into the atrium with ventricular systole will also produce a systolic sound.[126]

MURMURS

Murmurs represent noise created by turbulence of blood flow.[127] Therefore, they have an opportunity to occur only when there is movement of blood from one chamber (or site) to another. Sufficient velocity or volume, or both, must be present for the turbulence created to be of a magnitude that produces audible sound. The murmur is usually loudest over the site of genesis and radiation is toward the direction of blood flow. Hence, on clinical auscultation, an effort is made to establish where the murmur is loudest and where it radiates. The intensity of the murmur is determined not only by the degree of turbulence present but also by the intervening structures between the site of genesis and the surface of the chest wall. For example, obesity and emphysema tend to muffle intensity, and an asthenic build or narrow anteroposterior chest diameter makes relatively faint events easier to hear. The currently used system for categorizing murmur intensity is that of Levine and Harvey[83] and consists of six grades: grade 1, faint murmur heard only after a period of concentration; grade 2, faint murmur heard immediately; grade 3, moderate intensity murmur; grade 4, loud murmur associated with a thrill; grade 5, loud murmur heard with part of the stethoscope touching the chest wall; and grade 6, loud murmur heard without the stethoscope touching the chest wall. However, because in certain parts of the world a 4-grade system (soft, moderate, loud, and very loud), which was advocated by Paul Wood (*British Medical Journal* 1954; 1:1051–1063), is still being used, it is advisable to specify a murmur as grade 3/6 or 3/4 for ease of comparison. A grade 3 murmur based on a 6-grade system is obviously less loud than a grade 3 murmur based on a 4-grade system. On the basis of the portion of the cardiac cycle occupied, murmurs are usually classified as systolic, diastolic, or continuous. This simple categorization of a murmur in itself limits the number of possible pathophysiologic mechanisms, and efforts to achieve further subcategories help refine and reduce diagnostic possibilities.

Systolic Murmurs

Murmurs that occur only in systole fall into this broad category. They can be further subdivided according to their site of genesis. Thus, the systolic murmur that occurs in the process of ventricular ejection into a corresponding great vessel is a systolic ejection murmur (Figure 4.25). The systolic murmur that results from ventricular blood flowing abnormally from one structure into another (AV valve incompetence or a ventricular septal defect) is called a holosystolic or regurgitant murmur (Figure 4.26).

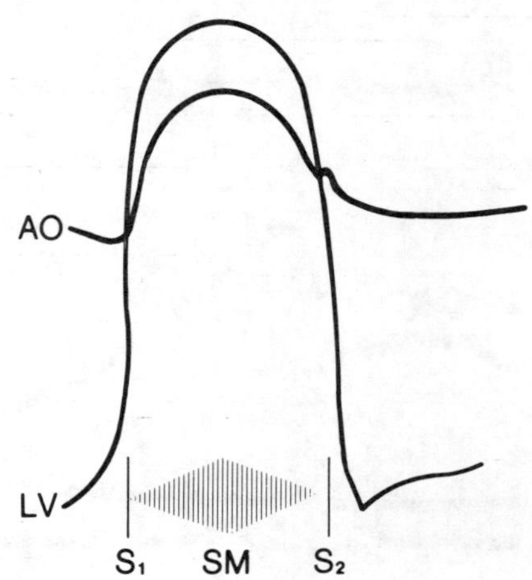

Figure 4.25. Diagrammatic illustration of a systolic ejection murmur (SM). Note its onset is after isometric contraction of the ventricle (LV), and ends with semilunar valve closure (S_2). The murmur has a crescendo-decrescendo (diamond-shaped) configuration.

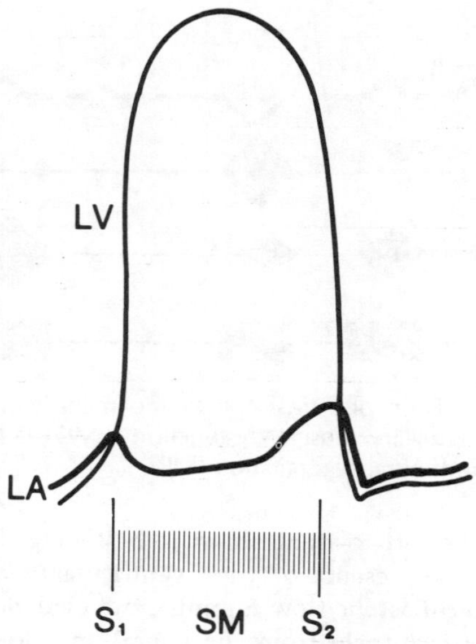

Figure 4.26. Diagrammatic illustration of the typical holosystolic murmur (SM). Onset of murmur is with the first heart sound (S_1) and continues past semilunar valve closure (S_2) into the period of isometric relaxation of the ventricle. The murmur is even in frequency throughout systole.

Innocent Systolic Murmur

The systolic ejection murmur, commonly heard in normal children and young adults, results from turbulent blood flow of right ventricular ejection into the pulmonary artery or left ventricular ejection into the aorta[128] and may therefore be heard best at the left or right second interspace. The murmur is short, occurs in early systole, has a crescendo-decrescendo configuration, and is usually grade 3/6 or less in intensity. It is characterized also by normal, physiologic splitting of the second sound; the absence of any abnormal heart sounds such as an ejection sound, systolic clicks, or opening snap; and the frequent presence of a physiologic third heart sound. In some, the systolic murmur is best heard along the left sternal border, and is recognized as innocent by its musical or groaning character (Still's murmur).[83]

The presence of a narrow anteroposterior diameter resulting from pectus excavatum or a straight thoracic spine, or both, makes turbulence from right ventricular ejection into the pulmonary artery more easily audible as an early systolic murmur.[129] Conditions that result in a large stroke volume (eg, slow heart rate) or hyperkinetic states causing more vigorous ventricular contraction (fever, thyrotoxicosis, and anemia) also produce a short, early systolic murmur in the absence of cardiac structural abnormality.

There are also innocent systolic murmurs of vascular origin such as the supraclavicular bruit,[130] a vascular thyroid gland, lactating breast, and over the placenta in pregnancy.[83] Supraclavicular bruit, which may sometimes be mistaken for a murmur of aortic stenosis, can be made to disappear by hyperextension of the shoulder.[130]

Abnormal Systolic Murmur

Ejection Murmurs. The early systolic ejection murmur in the second left interspace, resulting from turbulence of blood flow with right ventricular ejection into the pulmonary artery, occurs in atrial septal defect and with mild pulmonic stenosis. Recognition that cardiac abnormality is present comes from the fixed splitting of the second heart sound (atrial septal defect) or the presence of a pulmonic ejection sound (valvular pulmonic stenosis). A similar murmur occurs in the right second interspace with mild aortic stenosis, and its recognition comes from the presence of an aortic ejection sound (mild valvular aortic stenosis). In the elderly, degenerative changes (sclerosis) of the aortic leaflets result in a short, early systolic ejection murmur in the second right interspace and may be heard at the cardiac apex as well, sometimes with a musical quality.

In the context of obstruction to ventricular outflow, especially in the right heart, the length of the systolic ejection murmur serves as a clinical index of severity of obstruction. As obstruction becomes more severe, the peak of murmur intensity also occurs in later systole.[131] Because the murmur relates to ventricular ejection, the longest murmur always ends when the appropriate semilunar valve closes. Thus, in pulmonic stenosis, it ends just before pulmonary valve closure (P_2), but in so doing, it may extend beyond aortic closure (A_2). In aortic stenosis, the murmur ends before aortic valve closure (A_2). In the right heart, the obstructive lesions to consider are infundibular, valvular, and supravalvular pulmonary stenosis. In the left heart, the levels of obstruction can be supravalvular, valvular, subvalvular (congenital membrane), and muscular (hypertrophic cardiomyopathy) (Figures 4.27 and 4.28).

Short, systolic ejection murmurs also occur because of dilatation of the great vessels (ascending aortic aneurysm and idiopathic dilatation of the aorta) or because of a large ventricular stroke volume (significant aortic insufficiency and complete heart block).

Vascular stenotic lesions may also give rise to systolic crescendo-decrescendo murmurs. Some examples are carotid artery stenosis, pulmonary artery branch stenosis, and coarctation of the aorta. In these instances, the location of maximal murmur intensity provides the appro-

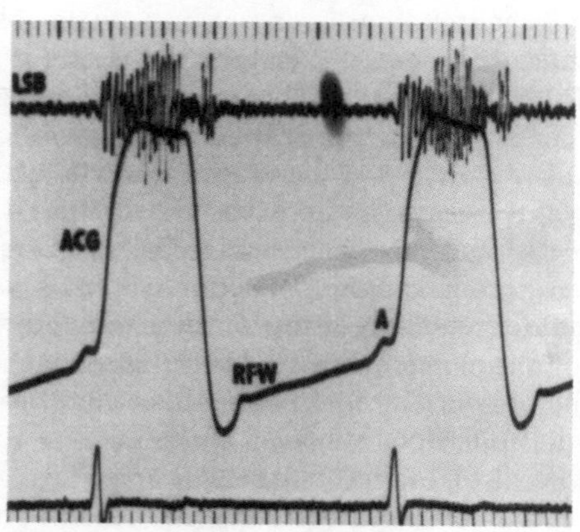

Figure 4.27. A patient with congenital subvalvular aortic stenosis. Phonocardiographic recording at the lower left sternal border (LSB) shows the systolic ejection murmur. The apex cardiogram (ACG) shows presystolic distension (A) and a sustained systolic outward thrust. After systole, a rapid-filling wave (RFW) is recorded.

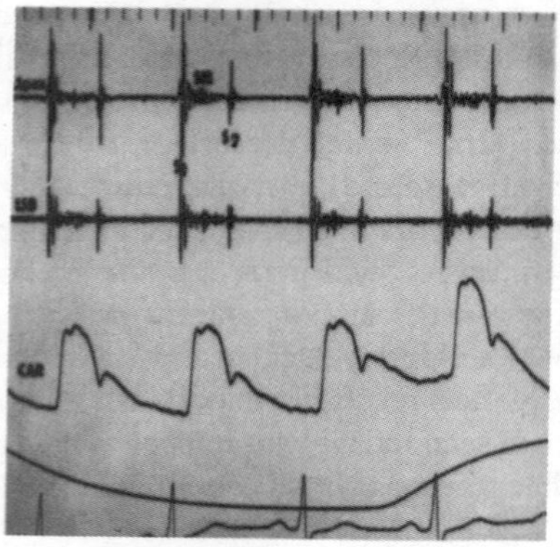

Figure 4.28. A patient with obstructive hypertrophic cardiomyopathy. Recordings at the cardiac apex (Apex) and lower left sternal border (LSB) demonstrate the systolic ejection murmur (SM). A simultaneous carotid pulse tracing (CAR) shows a rapid rate of rise and a double peak.

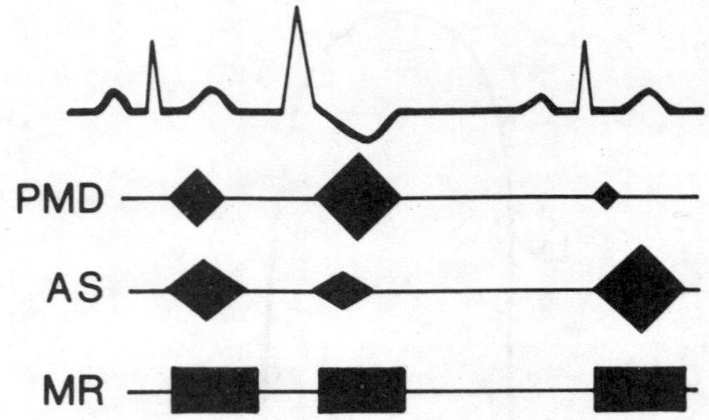

Figure 4.29. Effect of extrasystole on the intensity of systolic murmurs of papillary muscle dysfunction (PMD), aortic stenosis (AS), and mitral regurgitation (MR).

priate clue, ie, over the carotid artery for carotid artery stenosis, the posterior and lateral thorax for pulmonary artery branch stenosis, and the interscapular area for aortic coarctation.

Holosystolic Murmurs. The typical holosystolic murmur starts with the first heart sound and extends beyond its corresponding second heart sound into part of the period of ventricular isometric relaxation (Figure 4.26). They are, therefore, encountered in mitral regurgitation, tricuspid regurgitation, and ventricular septal defect. The murmur is usually of even frequency and intensity, blowing in character, and best heard over the appropriate area of genesis.

The holosystolic murmur of mitral regurgitation is best heard over the left ventricular apex and radiates to the mid-axilla or posterior thorax, or both. It may also radiate toward the left sternal border and second interspace if the incompetent posterior mitral leaflet deflects the regurgitant jet toward the interatrial septum. When the systolic murmur of mitral regurgitation radiates to the base, it may be mistaken at times as aortic stenosis. However, in addition to its holosystolic character, the murmur of mitral regurgitation does not accentuate following a postextrasystolic pause, whereas the murmur of aortic stenosis becomes louder. This response to extrasystole is of further diagnostic importance, as the systolic murmur of papillary muscle dysfunction decreases in intensity following a postextrasystolic pause[132,133] (Figure 4.29). Anterior leaflet incompetence tends to deflect the regurgitant jet toward the lateral and posterior left atrial wall, hence the posterior radiation of the murmur. Hemodynamic severity of mitral regurgitation is best judged at the bedside from the presence of a left ventricular third heart sound, a mid-diastolic flow murmur, a late systolic parasternal lift, and a displaced left ventricular apex, suggesting enlargement of left ventricular internal dimensions.

The holosystolic murmur of a left-to-right shunting ventricular septal defect is best heard along the lower left sternal border. The murmur radiates across the sternum to the right sternal border and superiorly toward the left second interspace. In some patients, the murmur may also have a crescendo-decrescendo configuration. The magnitude of the left-to-right shunt is best judged at the bedside by the presence of a left ventricular third heart sound, a mid-diastolic flow murmur, and evidence of an enlarged left ventricle from the lateral and downward displacement of the left ventricular apex.

The holosystolic murmur of tricuspid valve regurgitation is best heard along the lower left sternal border or xiphoid area and is best recognized by the increase in murmur intensity during inspiration (Rivero-Carvallo sign) or hepatojugular reflux.[134] The severity of tricuspid regurgitation can be judged by the presence of a right ventricular third heart sound, a parasternal mid-diastolic murmur that may also increase in intensity and duration with inspiration, the abnormal CV wave of the jugular venous pulse, and hepatic systolic expansion.

Variant Presentation of Mitral Regurgitation. Acute severe mitral regurgitation results in an exceptionally large left atrial V wave, which in turn results in a substantially diminished transvalvular gradient between the left ventricle and left atrium in late systole. The systolic murmur, if holosystolic, therefore decreases in intensity in the latter part of systole.[135] In most severe cases, the murmur not only attenuates in late systole, but it may in fact end well before the second heart sound (A_2) and is therefore less than holosystolic (Figure 4.30).

Mitral valve prolapse may present only with a late systolic murmur which either is crescendo-decrescendo or is crescendo to the second heart sound.[136] In some, the murmur is holosystolic, starts with the first heart sound but increases in intensity in late systole.[137] In addition, systolic clicks may be present. The reader is referred to chapter 31 on Mitral Valve Billowing and Prolapse for illustrations.

Papillary muscle dysfunction presents in a variable manner. It may be early or midsystolic, late systolic, or holosystolic and may also have a late systolic increase in intensity.[132,138,139]

In all the foregoing variations of murmur presentations of mitral regurgitation, the systolic murmur is best heard over the left ventricular apex. As previously mentioned, the incompetent leaflet, which serves as a baffle, determines the direction of major murmur radiation. In mitral regurgitation resulting from a mitral prosthetic paravalvular leak, the severe regurgitation may be silent or, if a murmur is present, be less than holosystolic.

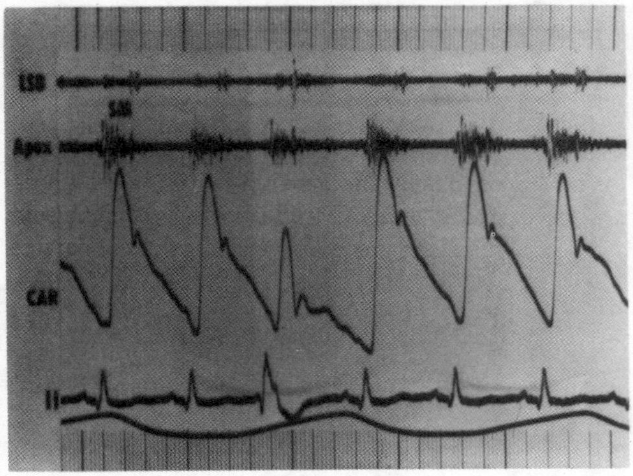

Figure 4.30. A patient with acute severe mitral regurgitation. Phonocardiographic recording at the cardiac apex (Apex) demonstrates a systolic murmur (SM) which is decrescendo toward late systole. The carotid pulse tracing (CAR) demonstrates a rapid-rising arterial pulse. Note the lack of effect of a premature ventricular contraction on the intensity of the mitral regurgitant murmur.

Variant Presentation of Ventricular Septal Defect. The small muscular ventricular septal defect may become physiologically closed as contraction of the interventricular septum occurs. In these cases, the loud parasternal murmur, which begins with the first heart sound, may abruptly cease in midsystole and hence is less than holosystolic.[140]

The patient with ventricular septal defect and severe pulmonary hypertension may only have a brief left-to-right shunt in early systole and hence only an early systolic murmur along the lower left sternal border.[111] However, there would be other clinical evidence of pulmonary hypertension, such as a sustained right ventricular lift, palpable pulmonary artery systolic impulse, and loud pulmonary valve closure (P_2).

Variant Presentation of Tricuspid Regurgitation. Severe tricuspid regurgitation occurring with normal or only moderately elevated right ventricular pressure (eg, tricuspid valve endocarditis) can result in right atrial CV waves which are almost identical to right ventricular pressure. Because the transvalvular gradient may be nil or occur only in early systole, the resulting murmur may either be inaudible or only be early systolic.[141,142]

Diastolic Murmurs

Diastolic murmurs occur from turbulent blood flow across the mitral and aortic valves, from incompetence of the aortic and pulmonary semilunar valves, or from coronary artery stenosis. The diastolic murmurs resulting from flow across the AV valves are normally of low frequency and hence are rumbling in character. They are best heard using the bell of the stethoscope applied lightly to the skin for an air seal. Firm pressure with the bell or using the stethoscope diaphragm will usually attenuate or abolish the murmur. They are usually heard in a small area and have limited radiation. The diastolic murmur of aortic valve incompetence is usually of high frequency, blowing in character, and best heard using the diaphragm of the stethoscope. The pulmonary valve insufficiency murmur is of high frequency when pulmonary hypertension is present, and medium or low frequency when pulmonary artery pressure is normal. The mid-diastolic murmur caused by coronary artery stenosis may mimic mitral stenosis, although it is higher in pitch and shows decrease in intensity instead of increase, as in mitral stenosis after amyl nitrite inhalation.[143]

Mitral Diastolic Murmur. In the absence of any obstructive valvular disease, increased blood flow across the valve can result in sufficient turbulence to produce a murmur. Therefore, large left-to-right shunting ventricular septal defect or patent ductus arteriosus (or aortopulmonary communication), and moderate to severe mitral regurgitation all may produce the murmur. They are usually introduced by a third heart sound and occur in mid-diastole during the period of rapid, passive ventricular filling.

With mitral valve stenosis, the narrowed orifice results in turbulent diastolic blood flow which is heard as a diastolic murmur.[144] It is usually introduced by an opening snap and the murmur continues as long as a diastolic pressure gradient is present across the mitral valve. In patients in normal sinus rhythm, the presystolic increase in gradient induced by atrial contraction results in an increase in the intensity of the diastolic murmur (presystolic murmur). With patients in atrial fibrillation, the wide variation in cycle length provides the examiner with longer diastolic filling periods. Therefore, the length of the diastolic rumble gives an estimate of the diastolic time period needed to achieve equalization of left atrial and ventricular pressures. This, of course, can be an index of the severity of obstruction, ie, the longer diastolic murmur represents more severe mitral stenosis. The auscultatory spectrum of severe mitral stenosis consists of a loud first heart sound (M_1), a loud second heart sound (P_2 if pulmonary hypertension is present), an opening snap, a mid-diastolic murmur, and a presystolic crescendo murmur (when in normal sinus rhythm).

Severe aortic valve insufficiency may also result in a rumbling or "blubbery" diastolic murmur (mid-diastolic and presystolic). This murmur is called an Austin Flint murmur.[83] Turbulent diastolic flow across the mitral valve occurs because the regurgitant jet coming from the aorta strikes the ventricular surface of the anterior mitral leaflet and moves it toward a closed position with a resulting decrease in the effective mitral orifice.

All mitral diastolic murmurs are best heard over the left ventricular cardiac apex. Auditory appreciation of the murmur is usually further enhanced when auscultation at the cardiac apex is carried out with the patient in the left lateral decubitus position or following amyl nitrite inhalation.

Tricuspid Diastolic Murmur. Conditions that increase blood flow across the tricuspid valve also can produce a diastolic murmur. A large left-to-right shunt at the atrial level (usually atrial septal defect) or severe tricuspid regurgitation often produces a mid-diastolic, low-frequency murmur (Figure 4.31). Tricuspid valve stenosis also produces a mid-diastolic murmur and, when in normal sinus rhythm, a crescendo-decrescendo late diastolic (presystolic) murmur.[145] Demonstration of increased intensity of the diastolic murmur with inspiration is a helpful clue to its tricuspid valve origin. The murmur is best heard along the lower left sternal border or in the xiphoid region.

Aortic Diastolic Murmur. Aortic valve insufficiency results in a regurgitant jet into the left ventricle when the aortic leaflets close. The resulting murmur therefore starts from aortic valve closure (A_2), and the large transvalvular pressure gradient between aorta and left ventricle produces a high velocity jet, hence a high-frequency, blowing, decrescendo murmur (Figure 4.32). The murmur may be best heard along the left sternal border (Erb's area), but it may also be well heard at the cardiac apex and second right interspace. When the diastolic murmur is louder on the right second, third, and fourth interspaces compared to the left, dilatation or aneurysm of the ascending aorta should be considered as a possible etiology for the insufficiency.[146]

Acute severe aortic insufficiency results in severe regurgitation into a normal or only slightly enlarged left ventricular cavity. The resulting rapid and substantial increase in left ventricular end-diastolic pressure causes premature mitral valve closure and rapid equilibration between aortic diastolic and left ventricular end-diastolic pressures. The resulting early diastolic murmur is relatively short and soft. Tachycardia is usually present, and with the shortened diastolic filling period caused by premature mitral valve closure, systole and diastole can be interchanged and the murmurs mistimed.[147]

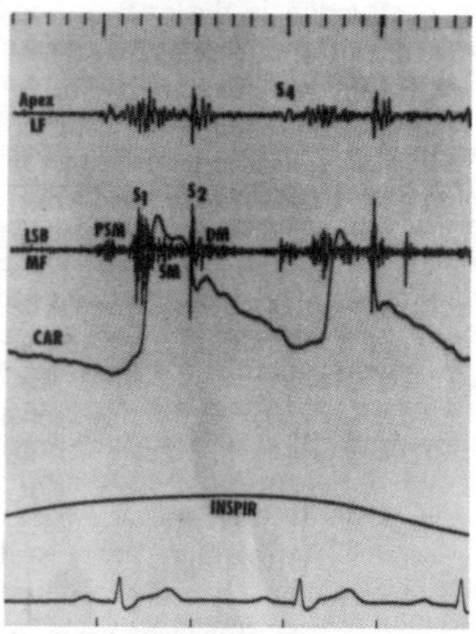

Figure 4.31. A patient with Ebstein's anomaly and tricuspid regurgitation. Note at the lower left sternal border (LSB) a presystolic murmur (PSM), the systolic murmur (SM) of tricuspid regurgitation, and a diastolic flow murmur (DM) across the tricuspid valve. A carotid pulse tracing (CAR) is recorded simultaneously. The murmurs were best heard and recorded on inspiration (INSPIR).

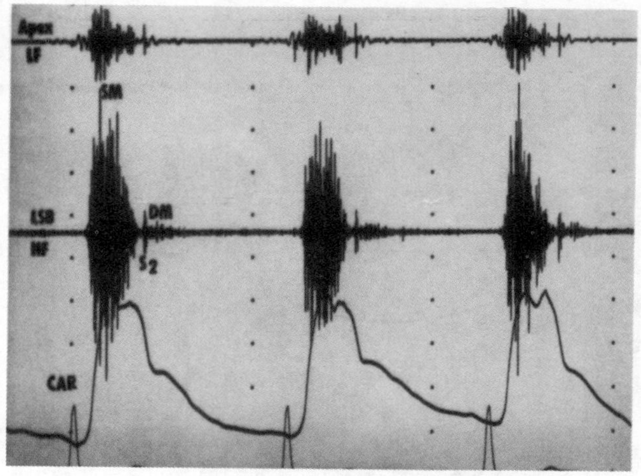

Figure 4.32. A patient with aortic stenosis and insufficiency. The systolic murmur is recorded well both at the apex (Apex) and lower left sternal border (LSB). Note the decrescendo diastolic murmur (DM) after the second heart sound (S_2) at the left sternal border. A high frequency recording (HF) was utilized to emphasize the diastolic murmur. Simultaneous carotid tracing (CAR) is also recorded.

An early systolic ejection murmur is usually present in moderate to severe aortic regurgitation because of the large left ventricular stroke volume. Its presence should not always elicit associated aortic stenosis as a diagnostic consideration. As previously noted under mitral diastolic murmurs, an apical mid-diastolic murmur (Austin-Flint) may also be heard and need not represent associated mitral stenosis.

Pulmonary Diastolic Murmurs. When pulmonary hypertension is present, the diastolic murmur of pulmonary valve insufficiency occurs right after valve closure (P_2) and has the same high-frequency decrescendo characteristics and configuration as chronic aortic insufficiency (Graham Steell murmur).[111] It is best heard at the second and third left sternal border using the diaphragm of the stethoscope. In some, inspiratory increase in murmur intensity may be demonstrated. Presence of a giant A in .e jugular venous pulse, a sustained right ventricular lift, and a loud pulmonary valve closure sound (P_2) serve to alert the examiner to the right-sided origin of the murmur.

When pulmonary artery pressure is normal, the diastolic murmur of pulmonary valve insufficiency may start at some interval after the second sound (P_2), thus being more mid-diastolic (Figure 4.33).[147a] It is usually of low or medium frequency, with a crescendo-decrescendo configuration, and is best heard at the second and third left interspaces.[148] Demonstrable increase in murmur intensity with inspiration or assumption of a supine position is usually a feature, in contrast to the diastolic murmur of aortic valve insufficiency which is better heard in held expiration and in the sitting position.

Continuous Murmurs

Cardiac abnormalities that result in a holosystolic (or long ejection systolic) and an early diastolic murmur are sometimes mistaken for a continuous murmur. The com-

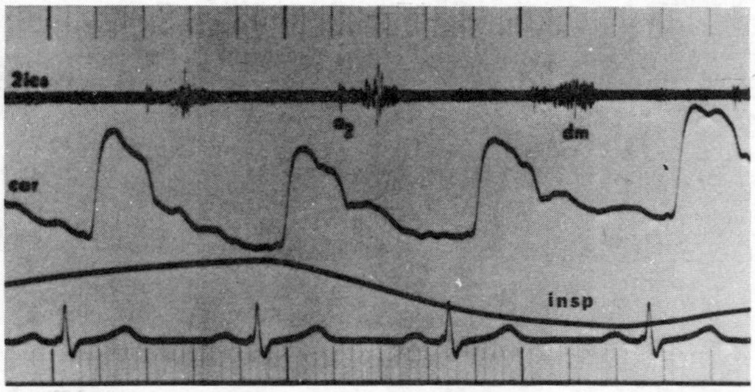

Figure 4.33. A patient with congenital pulmonary valve insufficiency. Recording at the second left interspace (2ics) documents the crescendo-decrescendo mid-diastolic murmur (dm) of pulmonary valve insufficiency which increases with inspiration (insp). (From de Leon,[147a] with permission.)

bination of a ventricular septal defect and aortic insufficiency, mitral and aortic insufficiency, or aortic stenosis and insufficiency are examples (Figure 4.34).[147a] They can be recognized as two separate murmurs by the difference in the frequency and quality between the systolic and diastolic murmur. Careful attention to the second heart sound should also reveal that the systolic murmur ends before or with it, whereas the diastolic murmur begins thereafter.

Continuous murmurs extend from systole into diastole through the second heart sound.[149] The "innocent" continuous murmurs result from rapid blood flow through a blood vessel. Examples are the venous hum generated through the internal jugular vein and the mammary soufflé heard over a lactating breast. The venous hum is common in children and young adults, and also occurs in thyrotoxicosis and anemia. The venous hum is loudest in diastole and can be abolished by transient compression of the internal jugular vein. Because some venous hums are loud enough to radiate below the clavicles, they can be mistaken for organic causes of a continuous murmur such as a patent ductus arteriosus. The mammary soufflé is loudest in systole and can be obliterated by pressure immediately adjacent and lateral to the breast.

Continuous murmurs, which represent disease, occur in conditions in which blood can flow from a high pressure to a low pressure structure throughout systole and diastole despite closed semilunar valves. The continuous murmur of a patent ductus arteriosus peaks at the second heart sound (Figure 4.35). Other forms of aortopulmonary communication (ie, aortopulmonary window, Blalock-Taussig shunt, and Waterston shunt) have similar features. Development of pulmonary hypertension progressively shortens the diastolic component of the continuous murmurs, so that when pulmonary arterial pressure equals systemic pressure, only a short systolic murmur may remain.

Arteriovenous fistulas also produce a continuous murmur. At present, those most commonly encountered come from the arteriovenous shunt surgically created for hemodialysis. Aortic communication with the right heart (ruptured aneurysm of the sinus of Valsalva) and coronary arteriovenous communication are other examples. High grade arterial stenosis also produces a continuous murmur. Usually the murmur achieves maximal intensity in systole.

PERICARDIAL FRICTION RUB

The pericardial rub results from friction between inflamed visceral and parietal pericardium. It typically has three components: a presystolic component related to atrial systole, a loud systolic component related to ventricular systole, and a mid-diastolic component related to ventricular filling. It usually has a rough, leathery character, sounds superficial, and waxes and wanes with respiration.[83] It is usually heard along the lower left sternal border or xiphoid region. When all three components are present, it is easily recognized. Even two components

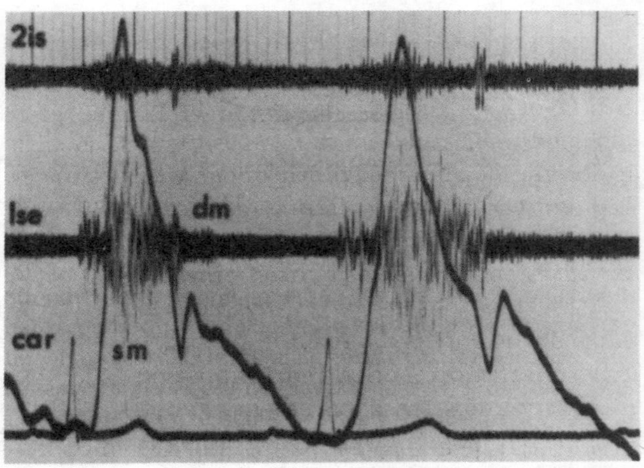

Figure 4.34. A patient with ventricular septal defect and aortic insufficiency. Phonocardiogram at the right second interspace (2is) and especially the lower left sternal edge (lse) demonstrates the systolic (sm) and diastolic (dm) murmurs. (From de Leon,[147a] with permission.)

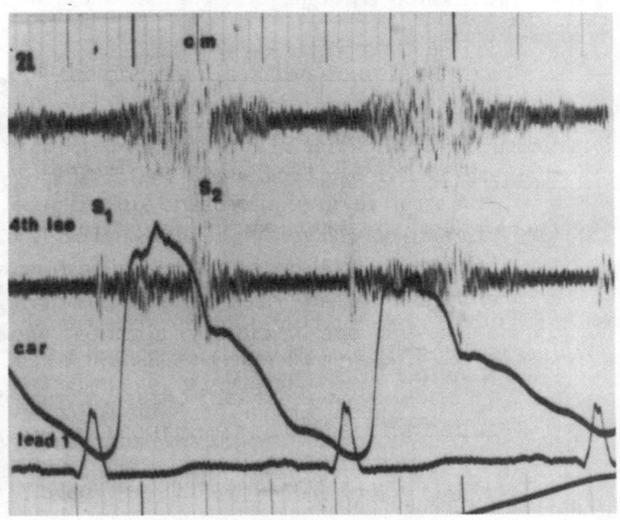

Figure 4.35. A patient with a left-to-right shunting patent ductus arteriosus. The phonocardiogram at the second left interspace (2L) demonstrates the continuous murmur (cm) which peaks at the second heart sound (S_2). A carotid tracing (car) is simultaneously recorded.

(systolic and mid-diastolic) may be recognized because of the character of the rub. However, when only the systolic component is present, it may be mistaken for a systolic murmur.

BEDSIDE MANEUVERS AND PHARMACOLOGIC AGENTS

Throughout the discussion of the various heart sounds and murmurs, the hemodynamic changes induced by respiration were of great value in their assessment. Of value also are changes in the diastolic filling period caused by changing cycle length, as in atrial fibrillation, and the long diastolic period of the compensatory pause following a ventricular premature beat. The latter, as described earlier, is very useful in distinguishing an ejection systolic murmur of aortic stenosis from the holosystolic murmur of mitral regurgitation, irrespective of the site where the murmur is best heard (Figure 4.29).

Other bedside maneuvers serve to exaggerate or diminish venous return as well as alter systemic resistance and hence central aortic pressure. They therefore serve to accentuate or decrease[150] murmurs, depending on their mechanism.

The Valsalva maneuver, by reducing ventricular volume, causes the murmur of obstructive hypertrophic cardiomyopathy to intensify (Figure 4.36). In mitral valve prolapse, the maneuver may bring out a late systolic murmur or transform into a holosystolic murmur.

Prompt squatting increases the murmur of aortic insufficiency by increasing central aortic diastolic pressure. This maneuver softens or abolishes the murmur of obstructive hypertrophic cardiomyopathy and intensifies the systolic ejection murmur of valvular aortic stenosis or discrete subaortic stenosis, the systolic murmur of pulmonary stenosis or Fallot's tetralogy, the systolic murmur of ventricular septal defect, and the mitral regurgitant murmur.[151]

Isometric handgrip also elevates systemic arterial pressure and, when properly done, produces the same changes as prompt squatting.

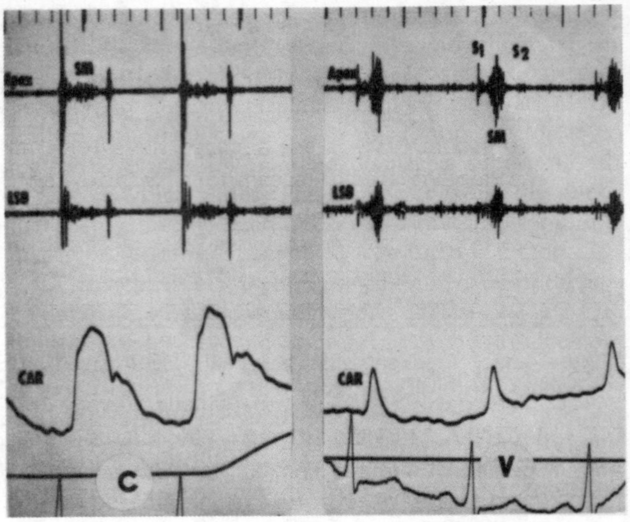

Figure 4.36. A patient with obstructive hypertrophic cardiomyopathy. Phonocardiographic recordings are at the cardiac apex (Apex) and lower left sternal border (LSB). Note the change in intensity of the systolic murmur (SM) from control (C, *left panel*) to that following a sustained Valsalva maneuver (V, *right panel*). A substantial increase in murmur intensity is demonstrated.

Amyl nitrite, a vasodilator, causes a decrease in systemic resistance and pressure. Hence, the murmurs of ventricular septal defect, mitral regurgitation, and aortic insufficiency decrease in intensity, whereas the murmur of obstruction to left ventricular outflow at all levels increases in intensity.[152] The mid-diastolic murmur in mitral stenosis increases in intensity, whereas the mid-diastolic murmurs in coronary artery stenosis[143] and aortic insufficiency (Austin-Flint murmur)[153] decrease. Vasopressors influence murmurs in a manner opposite to that of amyl nitrite and produce physiologic changes similar to those of isometric handgrip and prompt squatting. All of these relatively simple maneuvers should be a routine and integral part of a cardiac examination.

REFERENCES

1. Prinzmetal M: Angina pectoris. I. A variant form of angina pectoris. Preliminary report. *Am J Med* 1959; 27:375–388.
2. Groves B: Variant angina, an electrocardiographic and arteriographic spectrum produced by coronary artery spasm. *Curr Probl Cardiol* 1977; 2:1–71.
3. Pathy MS: Clinical presentation of myocardial infarction in the elderly. *Br Heart J* 1967; 29:190–199.
4. O'Rourke RA, Crawford MH: The systolic click-murmur syndrome: Clinical recognition and management. *Curr Probl Cardiol* 1976; 1:1–60.
5. Fowler NO: Diseases of the pericardium. *Curr Probl Cardiol* 1978; 2:6–38.
6. Hirst AE Jr, Johns VJ Jr, Kime SW Jr: Dissecting aneurysm of the aorta: review of 505 cases. *Medicine* 1958; 37:217–279.
7. Bell WR, Simon TL, DeMets DL: The clinical features of submassive and massive pulmonary emboli. *Am J Med* 1977; 62:355–360.
8. Sleeper JC, Orgain ES, McIntosh HD: Primary pulmonary hypertension. Review of clinical features and pathologic physiology with a report of pulmonary hemodynamics derived from repeated catheterization. *Circulation* 1962; 26:1358–1369.
9. Cheng TO: Esophageal function in patients with angina and normal coronary arteriograms. *Ann Surg* 1984; 199:123.
10. Criteria Committee, New York Heart Association, Inc: *Diseases of the Heart and Blood Vessels. Nomenclature and Criteria for Diagnosis,* ed 6. Boston, Little Brown & Co, 1964.
11. Chevalier H: Blockpnea on effort in emphysematous patients, a diagnostic challenge. *Am Heart J* 1967; 73:579–581.
12. Chizer MA, Pearle DL, de Leon AC Jr: The natural history of aortic stenosis in adults. *Am Heart J* 1980; 99:419–424.
13. Howarth S, Lowe JB: The mechanism of effort syncope in primary pulmonary hypertension and cyanotic congenital heart disease. *Br Heart J* 1953; 15:47–54.
14. Wood P: Attacks of deeper cyanosis and loss of consciousness (syncope) in Fallot's tetralogy. *Br Heart J* 1958; 20:282–286.
15. Pyeritz RE, McKusick VA: The Marfan syndrome: diagnosis and management. *N Engl J Med* 1979; 300:772–777.
16. Przybojewski JZ, Maritz F, Tiedt FAC, van der Walt JJ: Pseudoxanthoma elasticum with cardiac involvement. A case report and review of the literature. *S Afr Med J* 1981; 59:268–275.
17. Leier CV, Call TD, Fulkerson PK, Wooley CF: The spectrum of cardiac defects in the Ehlers-Danlos syndrome, types I and III. *Ann Intern Med* 1980; 92:171–178.
18. Beuren AJ, Schulze C, Eberle P, Harmjanz D, Apitz J: The syndrome of supravalvular aortic stenosis, peripheral pulmonary stenosis, mental retardation and similar facial appearance. *Am J Cardiol* 1964; 13:471–483.
19. Tandon R, Edwards JE: Cardiac malformations associated with Down's syndrome. *Circulation* 1973; 47:1349–1355.
20. Nora JJ, Torres FG, Sinha AK, McNamara DG: Characteristic cardiovascular anomalies of XO Turner syndrome, XX and XY phenotype and XO/XX Turner mosaic. *Am J Cardiol* 1970; 25:639–641.
21. Nora JJ, Nora AH, Sinha AK, Spangler RD, Lubs HA: The Ullrich-Noonan syndrome (Turner phenotype). *Am J Dis Child* 1974; 127:48–55.

22. McGuffin WL Jr, Sherman BM, Roth J, Gordon P, Kahn CR, Roberts WC, Frommer PL: Acromegaly and cardiovascular disorders. A prospective study. *Ann Intern Med* 1974; 81:11–18.
23. de Leon AC Jr: Musculoskeletal abnormalities and heart disease, in Horwitz LD, Groves BM (eds): *Signs and Symptoms in Cardiology*. Philadelphia, JB Lippincott, 1985, pp 106–107.
24. Gottdiener JS, Moutsopoulos HM, Decker JL: Echocardiographic identification of cardiac abnormality in scleroderma related disorders. *Am J Med* 1979; 66:391–398.
25. Stein D, Kloster FE: Valvular heart disease in osteogenesis imperfecta. *Am Heart J* 1977; 94:637–641.
26. Nomeir AM, Turner R, Watts E, Smith D, West G, Edmonds J: Cardiac involvement in rheumatoid arthritis. *Ann Intern Med* 1973; 79:800–806.
27. Perloff JK, de Leon AC Jr, O'Doherty D: The cardiomyopathy of progressive muscular dystrophy. *Circulation* 1966; 33:625–648.
28. Elliott WJ: Ear lobe crease and coronary artery disease. 1000 patients and review of the literature. *Am J Med* 1983; 75:1024–1032.
29. Chen WC, Xue W, Lu WZ, Zhao TM, Liu DZ, Zheng SQ: Ear lobe sign, hypercholesterolemia and HLA. *Shanghai Med J* 1982; 5:204–206.
30. Khalfen ES, Alekaeva LD, Veselov VV, Alekseev IG: The diagonal fold of the ear lobe in coronary heart disease. *Kardiologiia* 1984; 24:43–46.
31. Wermut W, Jaszczenko S, Ruszel A: Earlobe crease as a risk factor in coronary arterial disease. *Wiad Lek* 1980; 33:435–438.
32. Shoenfeld Y, Mor R, Weinberger A, Avidor I, Pinkhas J: Diagonal earlobe crease and coronary risk factors. *J Am Geriatr Soc* 1980; 27:184–187.
33. Kaukola S: The diagonal ear-lobe crease, a physical sign associated with coronary heart disease. *Acta Med Scand* 1978; 619:1–49.
34. Christiansen JS, Mathiesen B, Anderson AR, Calberg H: Diagonal ear-lobe crease in coronary heart disease. *N Engl J Med* 1975; 293:308–309.
35. Pasternac A, Sami M: Predictive value of the ear lobe crease sign in coronary artery disease. *Can Med Assoc J* 1982; 126:645–649.
36. Frank ST: Aural sign of coronary artery disease. *N Engl J Med* 1973; 289:327–328.
37. Petrakis NL: Diagonal earlobe creases, type A behavior, and the death of Emperor Hadrian. *West J Med* 1980; 132:87–91.
38. Lynch JI, Perry LW, Takakuwa T, Scott LP III: Congenital heart disease and chondroectodermal dysplasia. Report of two cases, one in a Negro. *Am J Dis Child* 1968; 115:80–87.
39. Ramon Y, Behar S, Kishon Y, Engelberg IS: Gingival hyperplasia caused by nifedipine, a preliminary report. *Int J Cardiol* 1984; 5:195–204.
40. Rateitschak-Pluss EM, Hefti A, Lortscher R, Thiel G: Initial observation that cyclosporin-A induces gingival enlargement in man. *J Clin Periodontol* 1983; 10:237–246.
41. Ewy GA, Marcus FI: Bedside estimation of venous pressure. *Heart Bull* 1968; 17:41–44.
42. Cheng TO: Mechanism of x descent in atrial pressure pulse. *Arch Intern Med* 1973; 132:114–115.
43. Constant J: The X prime descent in jugular contour nomenclature and recognition. *Am Heart J* 1974; 88:372–379.
44. Wood P: *Diseases of the Heart and Circulation*, ed 3. Philadelphia, JB Lippincott Co, 1968, p 52.
45. Kitchin A, Turner R: Diagnosis and treatment of tricuspid stenosis. *Br Heart J* 1964; 26:354–379.
46. Colman AL: *Clinical Examination of the Jugular Venous Pulse*. Springfield, Illinois, Charles C Thomas Publisher, 1966.
47. Hartman H: The jugular venous tracing. *Am Heart J* 1960; 59:698–717.
48. Lisa CP, Hood G, Tavel ME: The jugular pulse in pericardial constriction: its differentiation from that of cardiomyopathy. *Am Heart J* 1972; 84:409–414.
49. Hancock EW: On the elastic and rigid forms of constrictive pericarditis. *Am Heart J* 1980; 100:917–923.
50. Schlant RC, Felner JM: The arterial pulse, clinical manifestations. *Curr Probl Cardiol* 1977; 2:1–50.
51. Bedford DE: The ancient art of feeling the pulse. *Br Heart J* 1951; 13:423–437.
52. Marx HJ, Yu PN: Clinical examination of the arterial pulse. *Progr Cardiovasc Dis* 1967; 10:207–235.
53. Wigle ED: The arterial pressure pulse in muscular subaortic stenosis. *Br Heart J* 1963; 25:97–105.
54. Epstein EJ, Coulshed N: Assessment of aortic stenosis from the external carotid pulse wave. *Br Heart J* 1964; 26:84–96.
55. MacKenzie J: *The Study of the Pulse, Arterial, Venous and Hepatic and of the Movement of the Heart.* London, Young J Pentland, 1902, p. 25.
56. Ewy GA, Rios JC, Marcus FI: The dicrotic arterial pulse. *Circulation* 1969; 39:655–661.
57. Ryan JM, Schieve JF, Hull HB, Oser BM: Experiences with pulsus alternans. Ventricular alternation of the stage of heart failure. *Circulation* 1956; 14:1099–1103.
58. Gleason WL, Braunwald E: Studies on Starling's law of the heart. VI. Relationships between left ventricular end-diastolic volume and stroke volume in man with observations on the mechanism of pulsus alternans. *Circulation* 1962; 25:841–848.
59. Cooper T, Braunwald E, Morrow AG: Pulsus alternans in aortic stenosis. Hemodynamic observations in 50 patients studied by left heart catheterization. *Circulation* 1958; 18:64–70.
60. Cheng TO, Leet CJ: Pulsus alternans. Its response to amyl nitrite inhalation. *Angiology* 1984; 35:115–121.
61. Shapiro E, Salick AI: A clarification of the paradoxic pulse. Adolf Kussmaul's original description. *Am J Cardiol* 1965; 16:426–31.
62. Shabetai R, Fowler NO, Guntheroth WG: The hemodynamics of cardiac tamponade and constrictive pericarditis. *Am J Cardiol* 1970; 26:480–489.
63. Tung CL, Tao SC: *Practical Cardiology*. Shanghai, Science Technology Publishers, 1978, pp 44–46.
64. Messerli FH, Ventura HO, Amodeo C: Osler's maneuver and pseudohypertension. *N Engl J Med* 1985; 312:1548–1551.
65. Londe S, Klitzner TS: Auscultatory blood pressure measurement, effect of pressure on the head of the stethoscope. *West J Med* 1984; 141:193–195.
66. Levine SR: "True" diastolic blood pressure. *N Engl J Med* 1981; 304:362–363.
67. Hypertension Detection and Follow-up Program Cooperative Group: Five-year findings of the hypertension detection and follow-up program. I. Reduction in mortality of persons with high blood pressure including mild hypertension. *JAMA* 1979; 242:2562–2571.
68. Kirkendall WM, Feinleib M, Freis EA, Mark AL: Recommendations for human blood pressure determination by sphygmomanometers. *Circulation* 1980; 62:1146A–1155A.
69. Australian National Blood Pressure Study Management Committee: The Australian therapeutic trial in mild hypertension. *Lancet* 1980; 1:1261–1267.
70. Hashimoto F, Hunt W, Hardy L: Differences between right and left arm blood pressures in the elderly. *West J Med* 1984; 141:189–192.
71. Webster J, Newnham D, Petrie JC, Lovell HG: Influence of arm position on measurement of blood pressure. *Br Med J* 1984; 288:1574–1575.
72. Kesteloot H, Van Houte O: An epidemiologic survey of arterial blood pressure in a large male population. *Am J Epidemiol* 1974; 99:14–29.
73. Khaw KT, Barrett-Connor E, Suarez L: Seasonal and secular variation in blood pressure in man. *J Cardiol Rehab* 1984; 4:440–444.
74. Handa SP, Wolfe HK: Blood pressure distribution in students of junior and senior high school in Saint John, NB. *Can Med Assoc J* 1985; 132:29–32.
75. Stamatelopoulos S, Petrou P, Georgilis K, Mouskos C, Papamichael C, Moulopoulos S: 24-hour blood pressure monitoring during basic conditions, abstracted. *Eur Heart J* 1984; 5: (suppl 1)152.
76. Mancia G, Bertinieri G, Grassi G, Parati G, Pomidossi G, Ferrari A, Gregorini L, Zanchetti A: Effects of blood pressure measurement by the doctor on patient's blood pressure and heart rate. *Lancet* 1983; II: 695–698.
77. O'Brien E, Fitzgerald D, O'Malley K: Blood pressure measurement: current practice and future trends. *Br Med J* 1985; 290:729–734.
78. Abrams J: Precordial motion in health and disease. *Mod Concepts Cardiovasc Dis* 1980; 49:55–60.
79. Ewy GA: Bedside evaluation of precordial pulsations. *Cardiology in Practice* 1984; 1:127–133.
80. Ewy GA, Gomez L, Marcus FI: Left parasternal pulsations in patients with mitral insufficiency. *Circulation* 1965; 32 (suppl II): II-83.
81. Eddleman EE Jr, Langley JO: Paradoxical pulsation of the precordium in myocardial infarction and angina pectoris. *Am Heart J* 1962; 63:579–581.
82. Cheng TO: Incidence of ventricular aneurysm in coronary artery disease. An angiographic appraisal. *Am J Med* 1971; 50:340–355.
83. Levine SH, Harvey WP: *Clinical Auscultation of the Heart*, ed 2. Philadelphia, WB Saunders Co, 1959.
84. Laniado S, Yellin EL, Miller H, Frater RWM: Temporal relation of the first heart sound to closure of the mitral valve. *Circulation* 1973; 47:1006–1014.
85. O'Toole JD, Reddy SP, Curtiss EI, Griff FW, Shaver JA: The contribution of tricuspid valve closure to the first heart sound. An intracardiac micromanometer study. *Circulation* 1976; 53:752–758.
86. Leech G, Brooks N, Green-Wilkinson A, Leatham A: Mechanism of influence of PR interval on loudness of first heart sound. *Br Heart J* 1980; 43:138–142.
87. Thompson ME, Shaver JA, Heidenreich FP, Leon DF, Leonard JJ: Sound, pressure and motion correlates in mitral stenosis. *Am J Med* 1970; 49:436–450.
88. Schrire V, Vogelpoel L: Atrial septal defect. *Am Heart J* 1964; 68:263–277.
89. Pocock WA, Tucker RBK, Barlow JB: Mild Ebstein's anomaly. *Br Heart J* 1969; 31:327–336.
90. Stein PD, Sabbah HN, Anbe DT, Khaja F: Hemodynamic and anatomic determinants of relative differences in amplitude of the aortic and pulmonary components of the second heart sound. *Am J Cardiol* 1978; 42:539–544.
91. Shaver JA, Nadolny RA, O'Toole JD, Thompson ME, Reddy PS, Leon

DF, Curtiss EI: Sound pressure correlates of the second heart sound: an intracardiac sound study. *Circulation* 1974; 49:316–325.

92. Curtiss EI, Matthews RG, Shaver JA: Mechanism of normal splitting of the second heart sound. *Circulation* 1975; 51:157–164.
93. de Leon AC Jr: Atrial septal defect in the adult, in Harvey WP et al (Eds): *Current Problems in Cardiology*. Chicago, Year Book Medical Publishers, Inc, 1976.
94. Yurchak PM, Gorlin R: Paradoxical splitting of the second heart sound in coronary heart disease. *N Engl J Med* 1963; 269:741–743.
95. Fleming JS: Evidence for a mitral valve origin of the left ventricular third heart sound. *Br Heart J* 1969; 31:192–199.
96. Ozawa Y, Smith D, Craige E: Origin of the third heart sound. I. Studies in dogs. *Circulation* 1983; 67:393–398.
97. Ozawa Y, Smith D, Craige E: Origin of the third heart sound. II. Studies in humans. *Circulation* 1983; 67:399–404.
98. Ishimitsu T, Smith D, Berko B, Craige E: Origin of the third heart sound: comparison of ventricular wall dynamics in hyperdynamic and hypodynamic types. *J Am Coll Cardiol* 1985; 5:268–272.
99. Reddy PS, Meno F, Curtiss EI, O'Toole JD: The genesis of gallops sounds: investigation by quantitative phono- and apexcardiography. *Circulation* 1981; 63:922–933.
100. Van de Werf F, Minten J, Carmeliet P, DeGeest H, Kestleloot H: The genesis of the third and fourth heart sounds. A pressure-flow study in dogs. *J Clin Invest* 1984; 73:1400–1407.
101. Van de Werf F, Bobel A, Geboers J, Minten J, Willems J, DeGeest H, Kestleloot H: Diastolic properties of the left ventricle in normal adults and in patients with third heart sound. *Circulation* 1984; 69:1070–1078.
102. Spodick DH, Quarry VM: Prevalence of the fourth heart sound by phonocardiography in the absence of cardiac disease. *Am Heart J* 1974; 87:11–14.
103. Kincaid-Smith P, Barlow J: The atrial sound and the atrial component of the first heart sound. *Br Heart J* 1959; 21:470–478.
104. Caulfield WH, de Leon AC Jr, Perloff JK, Steelman RB: The clinical significance of the fourth heart sound in aortic stenosis. *Am J Cardiol* 1971; 28:179–182.
105. Harris A, Donmoyer T, Leatham A: Physical signs in differential diagnosis of left ventricular obstructive cardiomyopathy. *Br Heart J* 1969; 31:501–510.
106. Hill JC, O'Rourke RA, Lewis RP, McGranahan GM: The diagnostic value of the atrial gallop in acute myocardial infarction. *Am Heart J* 1969; 78:194–201.
107. Turner P, Hunter J: The atrial sound in ischemic heart disease. *Br Heart J* 1973; 35:657–662.
108. Proudfit WL, Hodgman JR: Physical signs during angina pectoris. *Prog Cardiovasc Dis* 1968; 10:283–286.
109. Harvey WP, Segal JP, Gurel T: The clinical spectrum of primary myocardial disease. *Prog Cardiovasc Dis* 1964; 7:17–42.
110. Kontos HA, Shapiro W, Kemp VE: Observations on the atrial sound in hypertension. *Circulation* 1963; 28:877–884.
111. Perloff JK: Auscultatory and phonocardiographic manifestations of pulmonary hypertension. *Prog Cardiovasc Dis* 1967; 9:303–340.
112. Yahini JH, Dulfano MJ, Toor M: Pulmonic stenosis. A clinical assessment of severity. *Am J Cardiol* 1960; 5:744–757.
113. Whittaker AV, Shaver JA, Gray S, Leonard JJ: Sound pressure correlates of the aortic ejection sound. An intracardiac sound study. *Circulation* 1969; 39:475–486.
114. Hultgren HN, Reeve R, Cohn K, McLeod R: The ejection click of valvular pulmonic stenosis. *Circulation* 1969; 40:631–640.
115. Cheng TO: Early systolic ejection click associated with supravalvular pulmonary stenosis. *Am J Cardiol* 1966; 18:292–296.
116. Leatham A, Vogelpoel L: The early systolic sound in dilatation of the pulmonary artery. *Br Heart J* 1954; 16:21–33.
117. Ronan JA, Perloff JK, Harvey WP: Systolic clicks and the late systolic murmur. Intracardiac phonocardiographic evidence of their mitral valve origin. *Am Heart J* 1965; 70:319–325.
118. Cheng TO: Diastolic click in mitral valve prolapse. *Arch Intern Med* 1977; 137:696.
119. Cheng TO: Coexistent mitral valve prolapse and mitral stenosis. *Chest* 1982; 81:526–527.
120. Smith ND, Raizada V, Abrams J: Auscultation of the normally functioning prosthetic valve. *Ann Intern Med* 1981; 95:594–598.
121. de Leon AC Jr: How to recognize prosthetic valve dysfunction. *Cardiovasc Med* 1984; 9:631–646.
122. Harris A: Pacemaker 'heart sound'. *Br Heart J* 1967; 29:608–615.
123. Kramer DH, Moss AJ, Shah PM: Mechanisms and significance of pacemaker-induced extracardiac sound. *Am J Cardiol* 1970; 25:367–371.
124. Cheng TO, Ertem G, Vera Z: Heart sounds in patients with cardiac pacemakers. *Chest* 1972; 62:66–70.
125. Pitt A, Pitt B, Schaefer J, Criley JM: Myxoma of the left atrium: hemodynamic and phonocardiographic consequences of sudden tumor movement. *Circulation* 1967; 36:408–416.
126. Martin CE, Hufnagel CA, de Leon AC Jr: Calcified atrial myxoma: diagnostic significance of the "systolic tumor sound" in a case presenting as tricuspid insufficiency. *Am Heart J* 1969; 78:245–250.
127. Sabbah HN, Stein PD: Turbulent blood flow in humans: its primary role in the production of ejection murmurs. *Circ Res* 1976; 38:513–525.
128. Stein PD, Sabbah HN: Aortic origin of innocent murmurs. *Am J Cardiol* 1977; 39:665–671.
129. de Leon AC, Perloff JK, Twigg H, Majd M: The straight back syndrome. Clinical cardiovascular manifestations. *Circulation* 1965; 32:193–203.
130. Nelson W, Hall R: The innocent supraclavicular arterial bruit: utility of shoulder maneuvers in its recognition. *N Engl J Med* 1968; 278: 778.
131. Gamboa R, Hugenholtz PG, Nadas AS: Accuracy of the phonocardiogram in assessing severity of aortic and pulmonic stenosis. *Circulation* 1964; 30:35–46.
132. Cheng TO: Some new observations on the syndrome of papillary muscle dysfunction. *Am J Med* 1969; 47:924–945.
133. Cheng TO: Non-invasive techniques in the evaluation of the patient with coronary heart disease. *Angiology* 1975; 26:820–836.
134. Maisel AS, Atwood JE, Goldberger AL. Hepatojugular reflux: useful in the bedside diagnosis of tricuspid regurgitation. *Ann Intern Med* 1984; 101:781–782.
135. Ronan JA Jr, Steelman RB, de Leon AC Jr, Waters TJ, Perloff JK, Harvey WP: The clinical diagnosis of acute severe mitral insufficiency. *Am J Cardiol* 1971; 27:284–290.
136. Barlow JB, Bosman CK, Pocock WA, Marchand P: Late systolic murmurs and non-ejection ("mid-late") systolic clicks. *Br Heart J* 1968; 30:203–218.
137. de Leon AC Jr: Mitral valve prolapse: etiology, diagnosis and management. *Postgrad Med* 1980; 67:66–77.
138. Burch GE, DePasquale NP, Phillips JH: The syndrome of papillary muscle dysfunction. *Am Heart J* 1968; 75:399–415.
139. Cheng TO: Late systolic murmur in coronary artery disease. *Chest* 1972; 61:346–356.
140. Nadas AS, Scott LP, Hauck AJ, Rudolph AM: Spontaneous functional closure of ventricular septal defects. *N Engl J Med* 1961; 264:309–316.
141. Rios JC, Massumi RA, Breesman WT, Sarin RK: Auscultatory features of acute tricuspid regurgitation. *Am J Cardiol* 1969; 23:4–11.
142. Cheng TO: Hydrogen and ascorbate dilution curves. A simplified method for routine use in detection of intracardiac shunt and valvular regurgitation. *Chest* 1972; 62:304–310.
143. Cheng TO: Diastolic murmur caused by coronary artery stenosis. *Ann Intern Med* 1970; 72:543–546.
144. Wood P: An appreciation of mitral stenosis. Part I. Clinical features. *Br Med J* 1954; 1:1051–1063.
145. Perloff JK, Harvey WP: Clinical recognition of tricuspid stenosis. *Circulation* 1960; 22:346–364.
146. Harvey WP, Corrado MA, Perloff JK: "Right-sided" murmurs of aortic insufficiency (diastolic murmurs better heard to the right of the sternum rather than to the left). *Am J Med Sci* 1963; 245:533–542.
147. Reddy PS, Leon DF, Krisnaswami V, O'Toole JD, Salerni R, Shaver JA: Syndrome of acute aortic regurgitation. *Am Heart Assoc Monogr* 1975; 46:166–174.

147a. de Leon AC: Non-invasive diagnosis of congenital heart disease, in *Non-invasive Methods in Cardiology*. Springfield, Illinois, Charles C Thomas, 1974.

148. Criscitiello MG, Harvey WP: Clinical recognition of congenital pulmonary valve insufficiency. *Am J Cardiol* 1967; 20:765–771.
149. Myers JD: The mechanisms and significances of continuous murmurs. *Am Heart Assoc Monogr* 1975; 46:201–208.
150. Dohan MC, Criscitiello MG: Physiological and pharmacologic manipulations of heart sounds and murmurs. *Mod Concepts Cardiovasc Dis* 1970; 39:121–127.
151. Cheng TO: Prompt squatting and systolic murmurs. *Am Heart J* 1969; 77:433.
152. de Leon AC Jr, Harvey WP: Pharmacologic agents and auscultation. *Mod Concepts Cardiovasc Dis* 1975; 44:23–28.
153. Nasser W, Tavel ME, Feigenbaum H, Fisch C: Austin-Flint murmur versus murmur of organic mitral stenosis. *N Engl J Med* 1966; 275:1007–1009.

5 Electrocardiography and Vectorcardiography

Te-Chuan Chou, MD

The electrical activity of the heart may be recorded from the body surface in the form of the conventional scalar electrocardiogram or the vectorcardiogram. The major difference between the two is the method of display. The conventional electrocardiogram depicts the variation in the magnitude of the cardiac potential in relation to time in the 12 or more leads routinely obtained (Figure 5.1). In vectorcardiography all the cardiac electrical forces are assumed to originate from one point (E point) and the vectorcardiogram displays the vectorial sum of the electrical forces generated at each instantaneous moment of a cardiac cycle. The changing magnitude and direction of the vectors during each cardiac cycle inscribe a certain course (Figure 5.2). To simplify the graphic presentation of the forces, the termini of the successive vectors are joined and vector loops are formed. The vector loops are usually interrupted at a certain time interval to facilitate identification of the vectors at a given moment.

To observe the spatial characteristics of the cardiac forces, the vectorcardiogram is recorded in three mutually perpendicular planes: transverse, sagittal, and frontal (Figure 5.3). The sagittal plane may be viewed from left or right. The latter is the one used in this text. The transverse plane projection of the vectorcardiogram is produced by the interaction of the potential variation of the horizontal (X) and posteroanterior (Z) leads. The sagittal plane projection is formed by the interaction of the posteroanterior (Z) and superoinferior (Y) leads, and the frontal plane, X and Y leads. The transverse plane vectorcardiogram has its counterpart in the precordial leads of the conventional electrocardiogram and the frontal plane vectorcardiogram, the limb leads. The scalar electrocardiogram may be derived from the projection of the vectors on the axis of the lead in question (Figure 5.4). Various systems of electrode placement have been suggested to record the X, Y, and Z leads.[1–4] The Frank system is simple to use and has been widely accepted (Figure 5.5).

Although the vectorcardiogram clearly demonstrates the phasic changes of the action potential, it usually records only the event of one cardiac cycle. The scalar electrocardiogram is needed to study cardiac arrhythmias. The vector concept is helpful in correlating electrophysiologic changes with electrocardiographic findings. On most subjects in this chapter the vectorcardiographic findings will be presented first, but their electrocardiographic changes will be dealt with in more detail because of the more extensive use of the conventional electrocardiogram in clinical practice.

SEQUENCE OF CARDIAC ACTIVATION AND THE NORMAL VECTORCARDIOGRAM AND ELECTROCARDIOGRAM

ATRIAL VECTOR AND ELECTROCARDIOGRAM

Atrial activation begins in the sinoatrial (SA) node and spreads in a radial fashion to depolarize the right atrium,

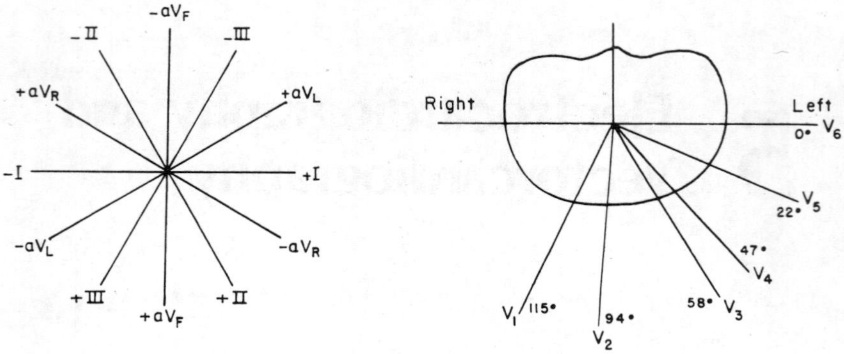

Figure 5.1. Lead axes of the 12-lead conventional electrocardiogram.

the interatrial septum, and then the left atrium.[5,6] Although specialized pathways connecting the SA node to the atrioventricular (AV) node and the two atria have been identified,[7] their role in human atrial impulse conduction under normal circumstances is still not clear. For practical purposes the early atrial forces may be considered to be generated by the right atrium, the late forces by the left atrium, and the mid forces by both atria and the interatrial septum. Anatomically, the right atrium is located anteriorly and the left atrium posteriorly. Because the SA node is located at the right upper posterior portion of the right atrium, the direction of spread of the activation impulse is essentially from above downward, from the right toward the left, and at first anteriorly (when the right atrium is activated) and then posteriorly (when the left atrium is activated). If the initial right atrial forces are represented by mean spatial vector P1 (Figure 5.6), the vector will be directed inferiorly, slightly toward the left, and anteriorly. If the combined right and left atrial forces that follow are represented by vector P2, the vector will be pointed inferiorly, more to the left, and either slightly anteriorly or slightly posteriorly. The late left atrial forces may be represented by vector P3, which is directed inferiorly, further to the left, and posteriorly.

On the vectorcardiogram, the normal spatial P loop is

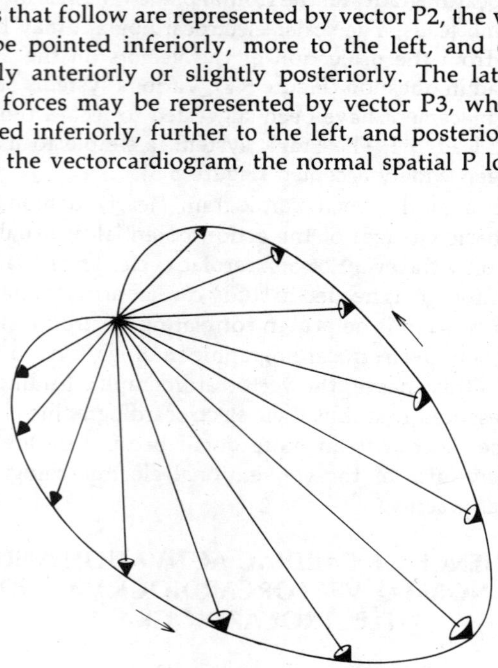

Figure 5.2. Diagram depicting the magnitude and direction of 12 representative instantaneous spatial vectors. A spatial vector loop is formed by joining the terminals of the vectors.

small and elongated, requiring great magnification to study its characteristics in detail[8-10] (Figure 5.7). The loop is often marked by one or more small notches. Because of the atrial repolarization potential, the loop does not close. It terminates at a point (O point) superior and slightly posterior and to the right of its origin (E point). Therefore, the direction of the spatial atrial T vector (Ta vector) is usually opposite the direction of the spatial P loop itself. In the transverse plane projection the antero-posterior and right-left components of the spatial P loop are viewed. Because all vectors are directed to the left and the early forces are anterior and the late forces posterior, the course of the vectors inscribed a counterclockwise loop, although a figure eight contour is also seen. The average direction of the maximum P vector in the transverse plane is −5° with a normal range of −50° to +60°. Its magnitude is less than 0.1 mV. In the right sagittal plane the anteroposterior and superoinferior components of the vectors are recorded. The early anteroinferior and late inferoposterior directions of the vectors inscribe a clockwise loop. The maximum P vector in this projection has an average direction of 85° with a normal range of 50° to 110°. The magnitude of the maximum vector is less than 0.2 mV. In the frontal plane the superoinferior and right-left components of the P vectors are viewed. Because all the vectors are directed inferiorly, the increasing leftward orientation of the successive vectors inscribes a counterclockwise loop. The average direction of the maximum P vector in this projection is 65°, and the normal range is 15° to 90°. The magnitude of the maximum vector does not exceed 0.2 mV.

On the scalar electrocardiogram the duration of the normal adult P wave varies from 0.08 to 0.11 second.[11,12] The P wave axis in the frontal plane ranges from 0° to 75° with the majority falling between 45° and 60°.[13] Therefore, the P wave is always upright in leads I and II and inverted in lead aVR. In lead III it may be upright, diphasic, or inverted. The P wave in lead aVL is also variable in polarity. A negative P wave is quite common in this lead. In lead aVF the P wave is usually upright, but a diphasic or flat P wave may also be seen. In the precordial leads the P wave is upright except in leads V_1 and V_2, where it may be diphasic. Because the early right atrial forces are directed anteriorly and the late atrial forces posteriorly, the diphasic P wave, if seen in these leads,

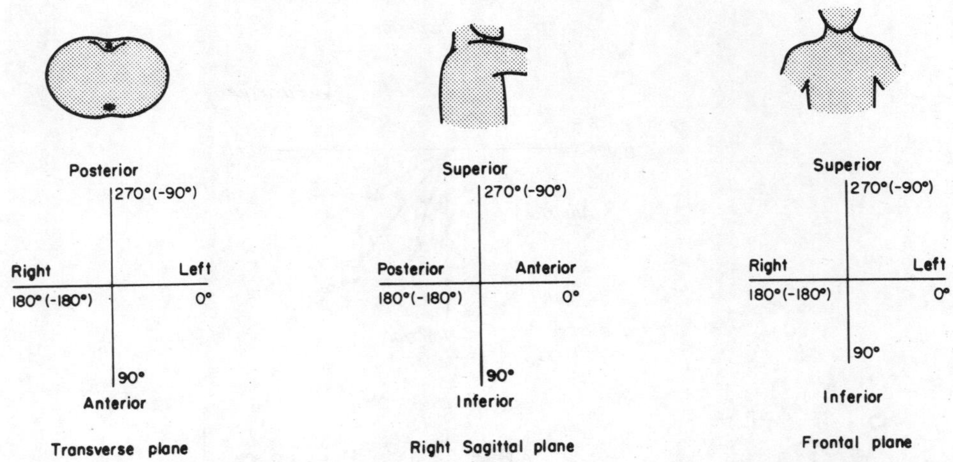

Figure 5.3. Planes of projection and reference frames used for display and analysis of the vectorcardiogram.

has positive-negative morphologic characteristics. An entirely negative deflection may also be recorded in lead V_1, but normally the P wave in lead V_2 is seldom entirely negative. The amplitude of the normal P waves in the limb leads seldom exceeds 0.25 mV. In the precordial leads the positive component of the P wave is less than 0.15 mV. In lead V_1 the negative deflection, if present, is usually less than 0.1 mV. The total area of the negative component in lead V_1 as represented by the product of the maximum negative amplitude in millivolts and the duration of the negative deflection in seconds should not exceed 0.003 mV.[14]

PR INTERVAL

The PR interval represents the interval between the onset of atrial depolarization and the onset of ventricular depolarization. In normal AV conduction it involves the time required for the activation impulse to advance from the atria through the AV node, bundle of His, bundle branches, and the Purkinje fibers until the ventricular myocardium begins to depolarize. As the depolarization process involving the AV node and the His-Purkinje system generates low potential, no significant electrical forces can be detected from the body surface. The duration of AV conduction is difficult to measure on the vectorcardiogram. The scalar leads are needed. In adults the normal PR interval is between 0.12 and 0.20 second, with the most common value being 0.16 second. The PR interval is generally shorter in children and longer in older persons. The PR segment, which is the horizontal line

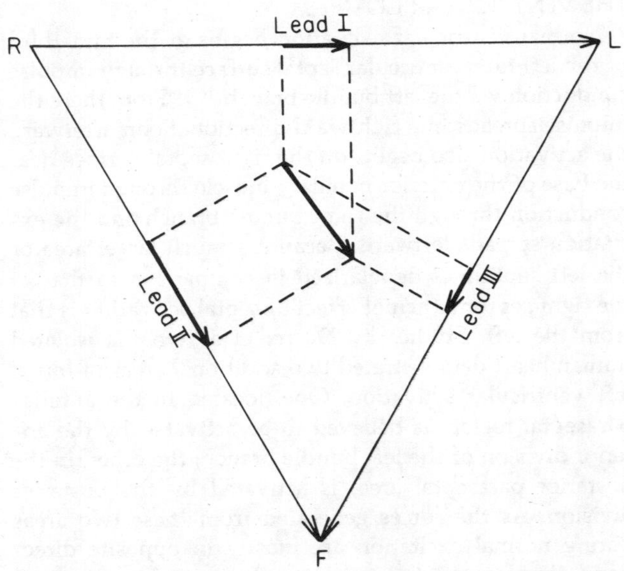

Figure 5.4. Derivation of the magnitude and polarity of the deflections in the three limb leads from a vector. Similarly, the projection of a vector on each of the 12 leads may be obtained by using the lead axes depicted in Figure 5.1.

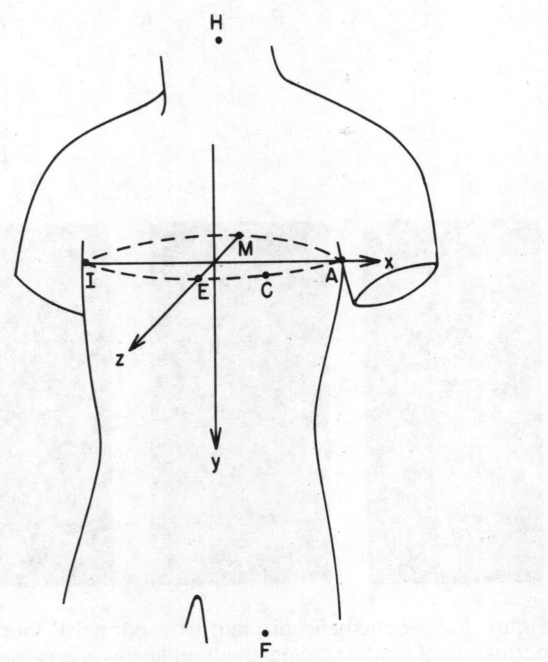

Figure 5.5. Frank system of lead placement. Seven electrodes are used. Leads X, Y, and Z are formed by connecting the electrodes in various combinations. (See Frank[1] for the specific locations of the electrodes and lead connections.)

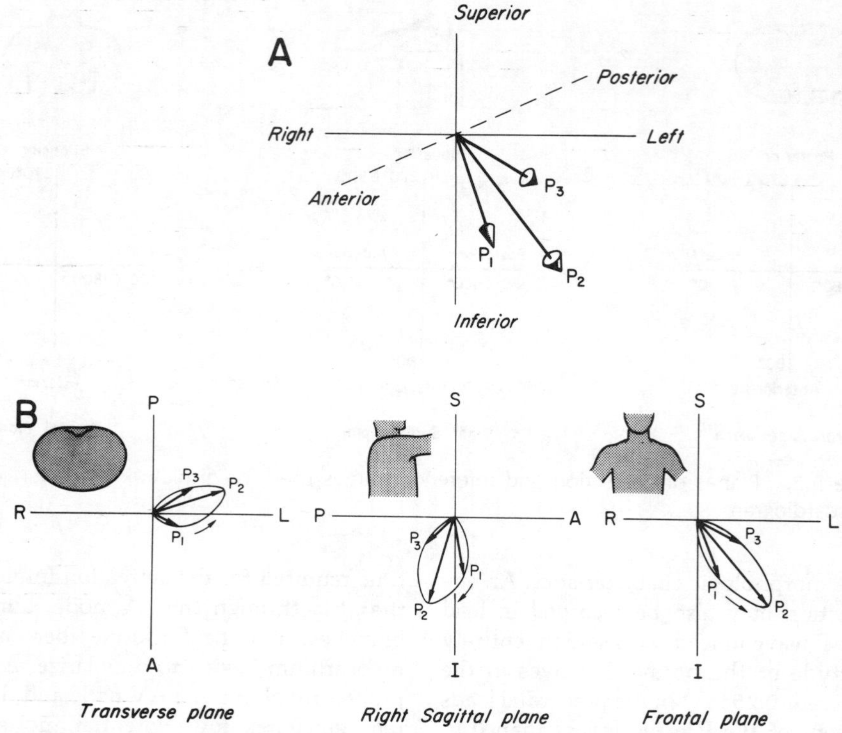

Figure 5.6. Three representative spatial P vectors are illustrated in *A*. P_1 represents the initial, P_2 the middle, and P_3 the late P vectors. Their projections on the three planes and the corresponding P loops are illustrated in *B*. See text. (From Chou et al,[54] with permission.)

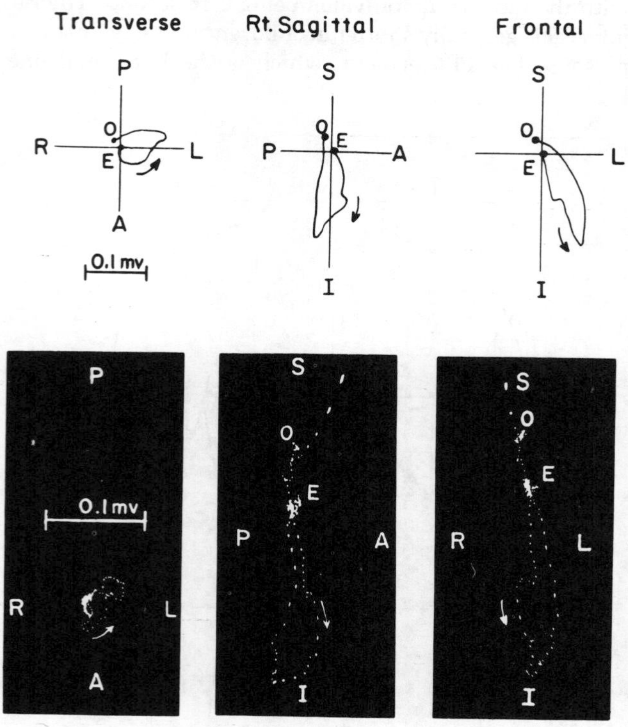

Figure 5.7. Schematic diagram of a normal P loop and a normal atrial vectorcardiogram. E indicates the beginning of the P loop and corresponds to the point on the isoelectric line at the beginning of the P wave on the scalar electrocardiogram. O indicates the beginning of the QRS loop, which is omitted in this illustration. In the vectorcardiographic recording the loops are interrupted every 2 ms. The blunt end of the teardrop represents the front end.

between the end of the P wave and the beginning of the QRS complex, is usually displaced in a direction opposite to the polarity of the P wave. This displacement is mainly due to atrial repolarization (atrial T wave). In normal subjects the amount of PR-segment depression is usually less than 0.8 mm.[15]

THE VENTRICULAR COMPLEX

Normal ventricular excitation begins at the mid-third of the left interventricular septal surface through impulse conduction via the left bundle branch.[16–19] From there the impulse spreads in a rightward direction. Soon afterward the activation also begins on the right septal surface near the base of the anterior papillary muscle through impulse conduction through the right bundle branch and the excitation spreads leftward. Because a much larger area of the left septum is depolarized in comparison to that of the right septum, the net effect of septal activation is that from the left. Studies by Durrer et al[17] in the isolated human heart demonstrated two additional areas of initial left ventricular activation. One, located in the anterior paraseptal region, is believed to be activated by the anterior division of the left bundle branch; the other, in the posterior paraseptal area, is activated by the posterior division. As the forces generated from these two areas during normal excitation are mostly in opposite directions, they are neutralized by each other. The direction of the initial left ventricular forces is, therefore, determined mainly by the forces generated from the midseptum.

Soon after the beginning of septal and paraseptal activation, the excitation impulse arrives at most of the endocardial layers of the myocardium of the apical and lateral free wall of both ventricles through the Purkinje network. Within the inner layers of the ventricular wall, due to deep penetration of the Purkinje fibers into the myocardium, the activation waves spread in all directions. As a result, their effects cancel each other and little electrical activity is detected outside the area. The thickness of the layers to be activated in this manner is estimated to be one third to two thirds of the entire wall. In the outer layers of the ventricles the impulse spreads more uniformly in the endocardial-to-epicardial direction. Because of its greater muscle mass, the left ventricle generates more electrical forces than does the right. Consequently, the resultant vectors are oriented in the direction of the left ventricular free wall, ie, leftward, inferiorly, and posteriorly.

In the last phase of ventricular activation the posterobasal region of the septum and ventricles is depolarized. The late arrival of the activation front has been explained by the rarity of the Purkinje fibers in these areas. The electrical forces generated from these areas are directed posteriorly.

In summary, because of its larger muscle mass, the left ventricle contributes most of the resultant QRS forces. As illustrated in Figure 5.8, the initial left septal activation generates vectors directed rightward and anteriorly. Most of the ventricular forces from the free wall are oriented leftward and inferiorly. The late excitation of the posterobasal portion of the ventricles is accompanied by terminal QRS forces directed posteriorly.

On the vectorcardiogram the normal QRS loop has a smooth contour without notches or irregularities. In the transverse plane, projection is always inscribed counterclockwise (Figures 5.9 and 5.10). The majority of the loop area is located in the left posterior quadrant. The initial forces are usually directed to the right and anteriorly, but occasionally they may be directed anteriorly and to the left. The duration of the initial anterior forces is more than 0.02 but less than 0.05 second. The terminal vectors are directed posteriorly and slightly to the right or left. The maximum QRS vector has an average direction of −10°, with a normal range of −80° to 20°. The magnitude of the maximum vector varies from 0.85 to 1.95 mV (Figure 5.10).

In the right sagittal plane the QRS loop is inscribed clockwise. Most of the loop area is located inferiorly and posteriorly. The initial forces are directed anteriorly and usually superiorly. The terminal forces are oriented posteriorly and either superiorly or inferiorly. The maximum QRS vector has an average direction of 100°, but it may vary from 50° to 165°. Its magnitude ranges from 0.3 to 1.9 mV.

In the frontal plane projection the normal QRS loop appears narrow. In contrast to the other two planar projections the direction of inscription of the QRS loop is quite variable in this plane. It may be inscribed clockwise or counterclockwise or display a figure eight pattern. The direction of inscription of the loop is somewhat related to the orientation of its maximum vector. When the maximum QRS vector is more vertical than 40°, the loop is

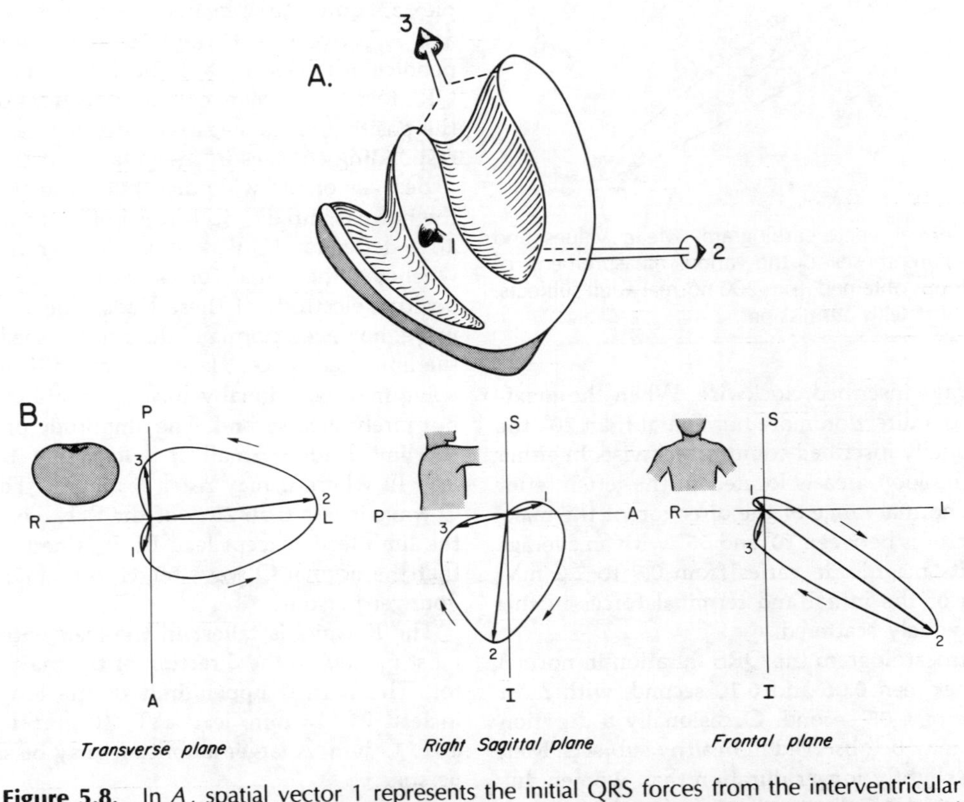

Figure 5.8. In *A*, spatial vector 1 represents the initial QRS forces from the interventricular septum. Vector 2 represents the resultant QRS forces from the free wall of the ventricles and vector 3 from the posterobasal part of the septum and ventricles. In *B*, the planar projections of the three representative spatial QRS vectors and the QRS loop are shown. (From Chou et al,[54] with permission.)

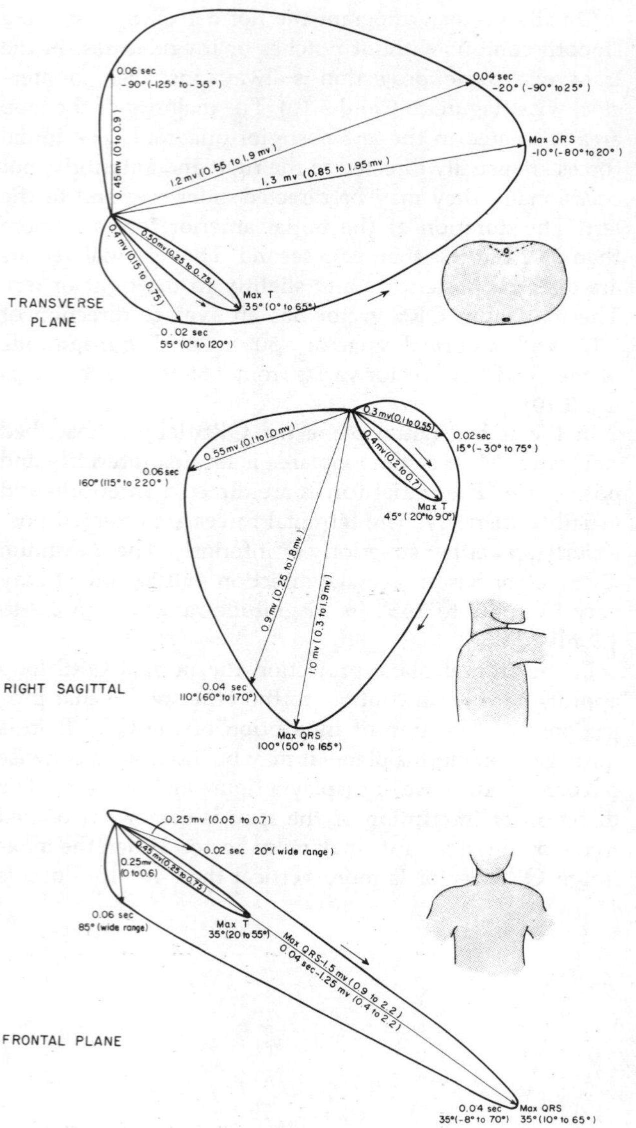

Figure 5.9. Normal vectorcardiogram. Mean values and 95% ranges (in parentheses) of the various measurements of the QRS and T loops obtained from 200 normal adult subjects. (From Chou et al,[54] with permission.)

practically always inscribed clockwise. When the maximum vector has a direction more horizontal than 20°, the QRS loop is usually inscribed counterclockwise. In either case most of the loop area is located in the left inferior quadrant. The normal range of the direction of the maximum QRS vector is between 10° and 65°, with an average value of 35°. Its magnitude varies from 0.9 to 2.2 mV. The directions of the initial and terminal forces in this projection are widely scattered.

On the electrocardiogram the QRS duration in normal adults varies between 0.06 and 0.10 second, with most having a value of 0.08 second. Occasionally a duration of 0.11 second may be observed in healthy subjects. Men tend to have a slightly longer duration than women. Infants and young children may have a duration of less than 0.06 second. The QRS axis calculated from the limb leads has a normal range between −30° and +105°.[12,20] Most people have a value between −30° and +75°. There is a tendency toward a leftward shift of the axis in older persons. In subjects under the age of 30 years the axis is seldom superior to 0°. After the age of 40 years the axis is seldom to the right of 90°. A thin person is likely to have a more vertical axis and overweight subjects tend to have a more leftward axis.

The amplitude of the QRS complex is also affected by constitutional variables. With advancing age the QRS complex generally becomes smaller. Men usually have a larger QRS amplitude than do women. The black population has a higher voltage than does the white population. With increasing body weight the QRS decreases in amplitude. The normal values of the amplitudes of the Q, R, and S waves in men and women of different ages have been compiled by Lepeschkin.[21]

The morphologic characteristics of the QRS complex in the limb leads depend on the orientation and amplitude of the QRS vectors in the frontal plane. As most of the QRS forces are directed leftward and inferiorly, lead I usually records a dominant R wave except in younger subjects with a rightward shift of the QRS forces resulting in an R/S ratio of less than 1. This is especially true in lead aVL where the entire QRS complex may be negative if the QRS axis is greater than 60°. Normally, lead II always has a prominent R wave as the projection of the major QRS forces on its lead axis is invariably on the positive side. In contrast, lead aVR always records a negative deflection. An essentiallly upright complex is more common in lead aVF, especially in younger subjects. In lead III the morphologic characteristics of the QRS complex are quite variable. Because in most subjects the QRS axis is between +30° and 75° and is more or less perpendicular to lead III, a slight shift in the direction of the QRS forces may change their projections on the lead from the positive to the negative side, or vice versa, with corresponding changes in the polarity of the complex.

Because of the wide distribution in the orientation of the normal initial QRS forces in the frontal plane, a negative deflection (Q wave) may be seen in any limb leads whenever the initial forces are directed away from the positive electrode of these leads. The duration of the Q wave, however, normally does not exceed 0.03 second in the limb leads except leads III and aVR. In lead III the Q wave may occasionally have a duration of 0.04 second but rarely 0.05 second. The amplitude of the Q wave in the limb leads is small. It is less than 4 mm, except in lead III where it may reach 5 mm.[13,20] The depth of the Q wave is less than 25% of the R-wave amplitude in all the limb leads except lead III. It is pertinent to mention that the normal Q wave tends to be more prominent in younger persons.

The R wave is tallest in the lead with its axis being most parallel to the direction of the maximum QRS vector. The normal upper limit of the R-wave amplitude in lead I is 15 mm; lead aVL, 10 mm; leads II, III, and aVF, 19 mm. A larger amplitude may be seen in younger persons.[22]

The S wave is most prominent in lead aVR, as this lead has a polarity opposite to the direction of the major QRS forces. A relatively large S wave may sometimes be seen

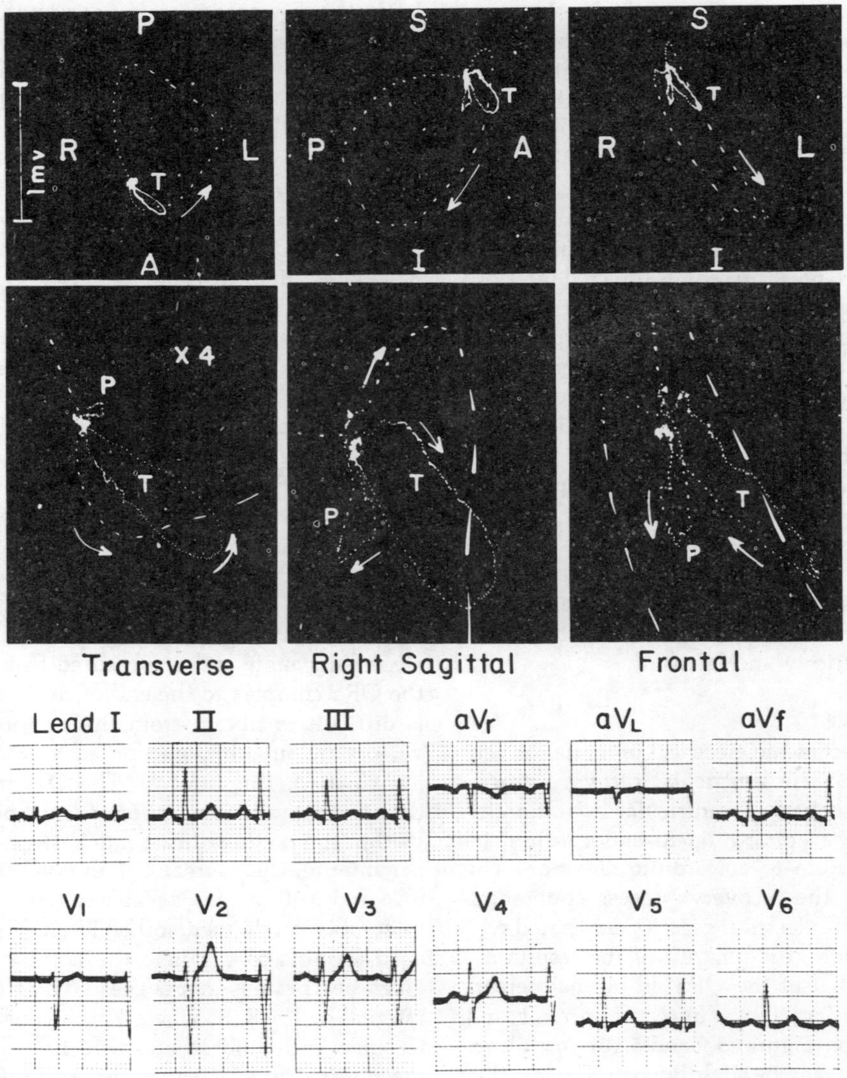

Figure 5.10. Normal vectorcardiogram and electrocardiogram of a 39-year-old man. (From Chou et al,[54] with permission.)

in leads III and aVL depending on the QRS axis, but its magnitude seldom exceeds 9 mm. In leads I, II, and aVF the S waves are less than 5 mm.[20]

In the precordial leads the predominantly negative deflections (S waves) are recorded in leads V_1 and V_2 and upright deflections (R waves) are recorded in leads V_5 and V_6. The location of the lead having a positive and a negative deflection of the same magnitude represents the transitional zone which is normally located at or between leads V_3 and V_4. Small Q waves are present in the left precordial leads (V_5 and V_6) in most normal subjects. They are often referred to as "septal" Q waves, implying that they are generated from the left-to-right septal activation. A Q wave may also be seen in lead V_4 but is rare in lead V_3. The normal duration of the Q waves in the left precordial leads is 0.03 second or less. Their amplitude is usually 3 mm or less.

R-wave amplitude increases from the right toward the left precordium. In lead V_1 it may be absent and a QS deflection is recorded. However, a QS complex is rare in lead V_2 in healthy subjects. The height of the R wave in lead V_1 seldom exceeds 6 mm, except in younger adults.[20,21] The tallest R wave in the precordial leads is most commonly seen in leads V_4 and V_5. The upper normal limit of the R-wave amplitude in leads V_5 and V_6 is generally considered to be 25 mm, although it is often higher in younger subjects.[23,24]

In the right precordial leads (V_1 and V_2) the S waves are normally less than 30 mm.[20] In lead V_1 an S wave of less than 3 mm is considered abnormally small. In the left precordial leads the S wave is often absent.

ST VECTOR AND ST SEGMENT

On the vectorcardiogram, the ST vector is obtained by joining the origin of the QRS loop (O point) to the beginning of the T loop, with the latter being the terminus of the vector. It represents the electrical potential existing during the interval between the end of ventricular depolarization and the beginning of its repolarization. It is small in normal subjects and usually does not exceed 0.1

mV in any of the planar projections. It is directed anteriorly, inferiorly, and to the left. The corresponding ST segment on the electrocardiogram is the segment between the end of the QRS complex (J point) and the beginning of the T wave. In the limb leads the ST segment is isoelectric in about 75% of normal adults.[12] ST-segment elevation or depression up to 1 mm is generally considered within normal limits.[22] However, ST-segment depression is seldom present in leads I, II, and aVF because the ST vector in the frontal plane, if present, is directed inferiorly and leftward. For the same reason, ST-segment elevation is more common in the inferior leads. In the precordial leads, ST-segment elevation is present in over 90% of normal subjects. The elevation is most common and prominent in leads V_2 and V_3 where the amplitude may reach 2 to 3 mm. In the left precordial leads the elevation usually does not exceed 1 mm. The upward displacement of the ST segment is generally more pronounced in younger persons. It may be higher in persons with the "early repolarization" pattern, which is a normal variant.[25] Any ST-segment depression in the precordial leads is abnormal because the normal ST vector in the horizontal plane is directed anteriorly and leftward.

T LOOP AND T WAVE

The T vectors represent the electrical potential of ventricular repolarization. The ventricular recovery process generally follows the course of ventricular excitation except it proceeds in the epicardium-to-endocardium instead of the endocardium-to-epicardium direction. This opposite direction of the recovery process counterbalances the reversal of the electrical polarity associated with repolarization. Therefore, the polarity of the resultant T vectors is similar to that of the QRS. In normal persons the orientation of the T vectors is leftward, inferior, and, in most adults, anterior (Figures 5.9 and 5.10). In children and young adults they may be slightly posterior, but they become increasingly anterior with advancing age. The normal T loop is elliptical and elongated with a smooth contour. The efferent limb of the T loop is always inscribed slower than the afferent limb. In the transverse plane projection the T loop is inscribed counterclockwise. The maximum T vector has a normal range of 0° to 65°. Its magnitude varies from 0.25 to 0.75 mV. In the right sagittal plane the T loop is inscribed clockwise. The direction of the maximum T vector has a normal range of 20° to 90°. Its magnitude varies from 0.2 to 0.7 mV. In the frontal plane the T loop may be inscribed either clockwise or counterclockwise. Furthermore, the rotation may not necessarily be the same as that of the QRS loop, as is the case in the transverse and right sagittal planes. The direction of the maximum T vector has a normal range of 20° to 55° and its magnitude varies from 0.25 to 0.75 mV.

On the electrocardiogram the normal T waves are always upright in leads I and II and inverted in lead aVR as the T vectors are directed leftward and inferiorly. They may be upright or inverted in leads III and aVL depending on whether the T vectors are more vertical or horizontal. In lead aVF the T wave is usually upright, but it may occasionally be flat or slightly inverted. In the precordial leads the T waves are always upright in leads V_4, V_5, and V_6. T-wave inversion is quite common in lead V_1, especially in women.[12] It is much less common in lead V_2 and is only occasionally seen in lead V_3, mostly in the younger age group. T-wave inversion in leads V_1 and V_2 or V_1 to V_3 in healthy adults is called the "persistent juvenile pattern."

T-wave amplitude is normally less than 6 mm in all the limb leads.[21] In leads I and II the amplitude should not be less than 0.5 mm. The T waves in the precordial leads are tallest in leads V_2 and V_3. The amplitude is higher in males than females, its average value being 6 mm in males, and 3 to 4 mm in females. It may reach 12 mm or more in younger men.

The normal T wave is asymmetrical. The slope of the first half of the T wave is more gradual than that of the second half. The first portion has an upward concavity if the T wave is upright and a downward concavity if the T wave is inverted.

QT INTERVAL

The QT interval represents the duration of ventricular electrical systole and is measured from the beginning of the QRS complex to the end of the T wave. The interval is difficult to obtain from the vectorcardiogram as the vectors are superimposed on each other during a significant part of this interval. The QT interval varies with the heart rate and is lengthened as the heart rate decreases. Within the range of heart rate between 45 and 115 beats per minute, the normal QT interval may vary between 0.46 and 0.30 second.[26] Women have slightly longer QT intervals than do men and children. The most commonly used formula to calculate the normal QT interval for a given heart rate is that suggested by Bazett[27]: normal QT interval $= K\sqrt{\text{R-R}}$, where K is a constant, equal to 0.37 for men and children and 0.40 for women, and R-R is the interval between two successive R waves. The QT interval corrected for heart rate, or QTc, may be obtained by dividing the measured QT interval by the square root of R-R. The upper limit of the corrected QT interval for men is 0.39 second and for women 0.41 second.[21]

U LOOP AND U WAVE

The genesis of this low level potential is still a subject of controversy.[28] One of the proposed mechanisms is that it represents the afterpotentials of the ventricular myocardium. The repolarization of the muscle at the end of the action potential proper is incomplete. The potential follows the action potential proper and is called the afterpotential. Another theory suggests that the U wave is the result of repolarization of the Purkinje fibers.[29]

On the vectorcardiogram the normal U loop is difficult to recognize. It requires much magnification of the area around the null (E) point to be viewed. The U loop of normal subjects has a configuration resembling a small slightly curved "club." Its direction and rotation are similar to those of the T loop.[30]

On the electrocardiogram the normal U wave is upright in the limb leads and precordial leads except in lead aVR. The amplitude of the U waves is usually proportional to that of the T wave, being about 5% to 20% of the latter's voltage. It is tallest in leads V_2 and V_3, where it may reach 2.0 mm, but it has an average amplitude of 0.33 mm.[31] It generally becomes more prominent during slower heart rate.

ATRIAL ABNORMALITIES

An abnormal P loop in patients with sinus rhythm may be due to atrial enlargement or an intraatrial conduction defect. The term "atrial enlargement" is generally used to imply the presence of atrial hypertrophy or dilatation, or both. The electrovectorcardiographic diagnosis of right and left atrial enlargement is based mainly on the fact that the right atrium contributes mostly to the early anterior forces and the left atrium to the late posterior forces.[8–10] Right atrial enlargement is present if there is an abnormal increase in the magnitude of the maximum P vector and the P loop is displaced anteriorly. Left atrial enlargement is present if the magnitude of the maximum P vector is increased and the P loop is displaced posteriorly. These changes are best seen in the transverse and sagittal projections (Figure 5.11). In the frontal plane the direction of the maximum P vector is more vertical in right atrial enlargement and often approaches 90°. The P loop tends to be narrow in configuration. In left atrial enlargement the maximum P vector is more horizontal. The P loop may be quite irregular and in some cases bifid in appearance. The duration of the P loop is often increased. In biatrial enlargement there is an increase in both the early anterior and the late posterior components of the atrial forces. In the sagittal plane the enlarged P loop is often triangular in shape.

The P loop in intraatrial conduction defects often displays many bites. Some portions of the P loop often are slowly inscribed. The duration of the P loop is increased. Some or all of these changes may be seen in patients with left atrial enlargement in which an intraatrial conduction defect frequently coexists.

On the electrocardiogram the more vertical orientation of the increased maximum P vector in right atrial enlargement is manifested as tall and peaked P waves in the inferior leads (Figure 5.11). The increased early anterior atrial forces are associated with an increase in the positive initial deflection of the P wave in the precordial leads V_1 and V_2. The commonly used criteria in the diagnosis of right atrial enlargement include: (1) a tall and peaked P wave with a height of 2.5 mm or more in leads II, III, or aVF, with a normal duration, the P pulmonale, (2) a P-wave axis in the frontal plane of 75° or greater, or (3) a positive deflection of the P wave in leads V_1 or V_2 greater than 1.5 mm (Figure 5.11). It is important to note that many other conditions may present similar P-wave changes in the limb leads. The P pulmonale pattern may be seen in patients with chronic obstructive lung disease without cor pulmonale,[32,33] and in patients with hypertensive heart disease without left or right ventricular failure.[8] The P-wave amplitude often increases with the standing position and simulates P pulmonale.[34] Tall P waves may occur during tachycardia and exercise. In my experience an abnormally tall P wave in the right precordial leads is a more specific finding for right atrial enlargement. Conversely, many patients with right atrial enlargement fail to reveal any electrocardiographic signs, especially when right atrial enlargement is due to acquired heart disease.

In the electrocardiographic diagnosis of left atrial enlargement, the following criteria are most frequently used: (1) The P terminal force in lead V_1 is equal to or more negative than −0.04 mm second. This measurement is the product of the depth of the terminal negative deflection (in millimeters) and its duration (in seconds).[14] (2) The P wave is notched with a duration of 0.12 second or more, the P mitrale pattern.[35] (3) The presence of leftward shift of the P-wave axis in the frontal plane to 15° or beyond, or a leftward shift of the terminal P forces in the frontal plane. A prominent negative deflection of the P wave in lead V_1 was seen in about one third of the patients with definite left atrial enlargement proven at surgery.[36] However, it is also seen in patients with chronic obstructive lung disease, pectus excavatum[37] and straight back syndrome.[38] The P mitrale pattern, as the name implies, is commonly seen in patients with mitral valve disease, especially mitral stenosis. The pattern is most often observed in leads I and II and in the left precordial leads. It was observed in one third of the patients with isolated mitral stenosis proven at surgery.[36] As previously stated, notching of the P wave with an increase in its duration may be due to an intraatrial conduction defect secondary to atrial myocardial damage.[39] Abnormal bifid P waves are also seen in patients with constrictive pericarditis.[40,41]

The presence of biatrial enlargement may be suspected on the electrocardiogram when signs of both left and right atrial enlargement coexist. The most useful combination of signs to suggest the diagnosis is a large diphasic P wave in lead V_1 with the initial positive component greater than 1.5 mm and the terminal negative component reaching 1 mm in amplitude and 0.04 second in duration.

VENTRICULAR HYPERTROPHY

LEFT VENTRICULAR HYPERTROPHY

In left ventricular hypertrophy an increase in left ventricular muscle mass is associated with accentuation of the left ventricular potential. The normally preponderant leftward and posterior QRS forces further increase in magnitude. This increase in QRS voltage is the most characteristic finding in left ventricular hypertrophy. The increase in thickness of the left ventricular wall prolongs ventricular activation time and may result in lengthening of the QRS duration. Secondary changes in the ST segment and T wave often occur. Because of the delay in completion of the endocardium-to-epicardium depolarization process, repolarization may now begin in the subendocardial instead of subepicardial layer of the myocardium. This reversal in the direction of repolarization is associated with a change in the direction of the ST and T vectors.

On the vectorcardiogram the significant changes are best seen in the transverse plane[42–44] (Figures 5.12 and 5.13). The QRS loop in this projection is usually elongated, it is inscribed counterclockwise in most cases, but a figure eight pattern may be seen especially when the hypertrophy is severe. The maximum QRS vector is di-

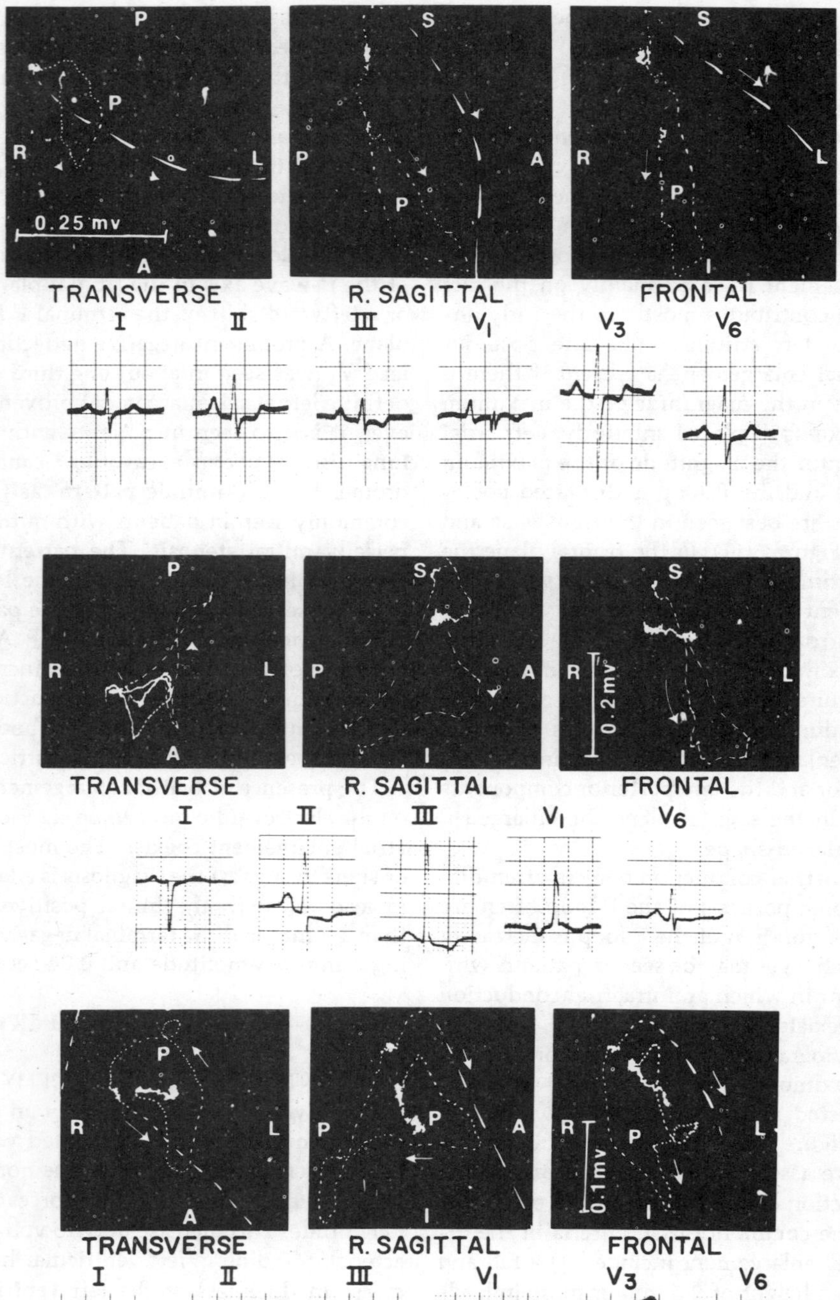

Figure 5.11. Atrial enlargement. *Top panel*, an example of right atrial enlargement. The vectorcardiogram shows an increase in the maximum P vector in all three planes and the P loop is displaced anteriorly. The electrocardiogram demonstrates tall P waves in leads II, V_1, and V_3. *Middle panel*, a case of left atrial enlargement. The vectorcardiogram shows an abnormally large P loop which is displaced posteriorly. The electrocardiogram demonstrates a prominent negative component in the P wave in lead V_1. *Bottom panel*, a case of biatrial enlargement. The P loop has prominent anterior forces to suggest right atrial enlargement. Lead II of the electrocardiogram reveals a broad and notched P wave consistent with P mitrale.

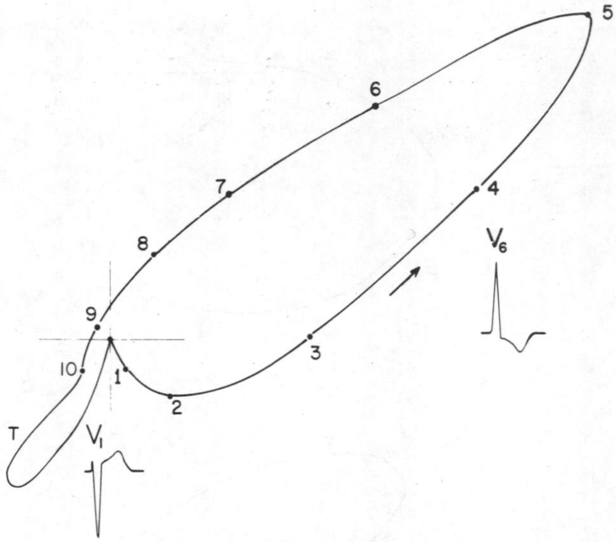

Figure 5.12. Schematic diagram of the transverse plane QRS and T loops in left ventricular hypertrophy. The numerals in this and subsequent similar diagrams indicate the time in hundredths of a second after the beginning of the QRS loop. The corresponding QRS-T complex in scalar leads V_1 and V_6 is also illustrated.

rected to the left and more posteriorly than normal. Its magnitude is increased and often exceeds 2.0 mV. There also is a tendency for the initial and terminal forces to be displaced leftward.[45] The magnitude of the ST vector is often increased. Both the ST vector and the T loop tend to be displaced anteriorly and to the right. In the other two planar projections, an increase in magnitude of the maximum QRS vector and displacement of the ST and T vectors in the opposite direction of the QRS loop are also seen.

On the electrocardiogram the presence of left ventricular hypertrophy is suggested if one or more of the following criteria are met[46–48]: (1) an R wave in lead I + S wave in lead III greater than 25 mm; (2) an R wave in lead aVL greater than 11 mm; (3) an R wave in lead aVF greater than 20 mm; (4) an R wave in lead V_5 or V_6 greater than 26 mm; (5) an R wave in lead V_5 or V_6 + S wave in lead V_1 greater than 35 mm; (6) largest R wave + S wave in the precordial leads greater than 45 mm.

The diagnosis of left ventricular hypertrophy by these voltage criteria is further supported by the presence of ST-segment depression and T-wave inversion in the left precordial leads and in those limb leads whose major QRS deflection is upright. A point score system using a combination of the various findings was proposed by Romhilt and Estes.[49] In addition to the increase in QRS voltage and ST- and T-wave changes, the presence of left atrial

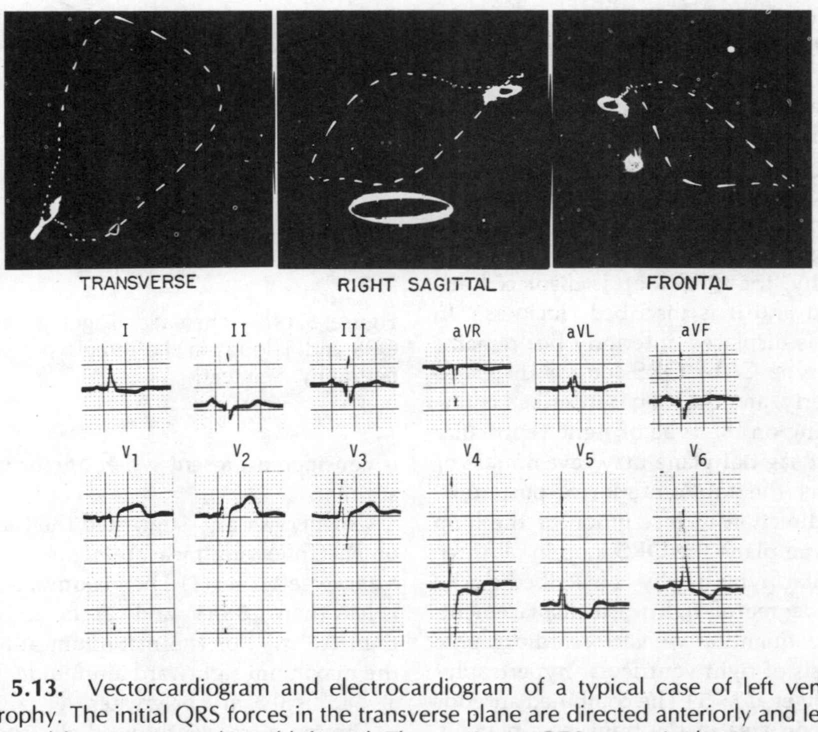

Figure 5.13. Vectorcardiogram and electrocardiogram of a typical case of left ventricular hypertrophy. The initial QRS forces in the transverse plane are directed anteriorly and leftward, the terminal forces posteriorly and leftward. The maximum QRS vector in the transverse plane exceeds 2mV. The QRS loop is inscribed counterclockwise. The T loop is discordant to the QRS. In the right sagittal and frontal planes the QRS loop is inscribed clockwise and the T loop is also discordant to the QRS. The electrocardiogram shows increased QRS voltage in the precordial leads with secondary ST-segment and T-wave changes due to left ventricular hypertrophy.

enlargement, left axis deviation, and increased QRS duration is also taken into consideration in the diagnosis of left ventricular hypertrophy in their point score system.

The sensitivity of the electrocardiogram in the diagnosis of left ventricular hypertrophy has been reported to be between 54% and 85%.[49–52] A false-positive diagnosis may be made in 11% to 15% of cases.[52,53] Generally speaking, high voltage in the precordial leads is the most sensitive criterion in the diagnosis of left ventricular hypertrophy. However, it is also less specific, especially in young adults. The additional presence of ST- and T-wave changes of the so-called "strain" pattern increases the specificity of the diagnosis. Inverted U waves in leads I, V_5, and V_6 are also helpful supporting signs of the diagnosis.[31]

The vectorcardiogram is usually less sensitive than the electrocardiogram in the diagnosis of left ventricular hypertrophy.[54] However, changes in the configuration of the QRS loop supply additional information that may improve diagnostic reliability.

RIGHT VENTRICULAR HYPERTROPHY

Normally, right ventricular forces are mostly masked by the dominant left ventricular potential. In right ventricular hypertrophy the increased anterior and rightward forces will modify the resultant QRS vectors to a degree in proportion to the severity of the hypertrophy. In mild cases no apparent changes may be detected. In severe right ventricular hypertrophy, however, the normally dominant left posterior QRS forces may be replaced by prominent right anterior forces. Intermediate degrees of abnormality may be observed when the hypertrophy is moderate. Secondary changes in the ST and T vectors often occur. They may be displaced leftward and posteriorly, opposite to the major QRS forces.

The vectorcardiographic findings in right ventricular hypertrophy may be classified into three types based on the morphologic characteristics of the QRS loop in the transverse plane[55] (Figures 5.14 and 5.15). In type A right ventricular hypertrophy, the QRS loop is displaced anteriorly and rightward and it is inscribed clockwise. In type B the QRS loop is displaced anteriorly but remains counterclockwise. In type C the QRS loop is displaced rightward but posteriorly, and the loop is inscribed counterclockwise. Depending on the type of right ventricular hypertrophy, the right sagittal plane may reveal most of the QRS loop in either the anteroinferior or posteroinferior quadrant. The direction of inscription of the loop is variable. In the frontal plane the QRS loop in all three types of right ventricular hypertrophy is inscribed clockwise with a variable degree of rightward displacement. The following simple quantitative vectorcardiographic criteria for the diagnosis of right ventricular hypertrophy were proposed by Chou et al[56]: (1) The combined anterior and rightward QRS loop area in the transverse plane is greater than 70% of the total. (2) The QRS loop area in the right posterior quadrant in the transverse plane is greater than 20% of the total. (3) The QRS loop area in the right inferior quadrant in the frontal plane is greater than 20% of the total. Right ventricular hypertrophy

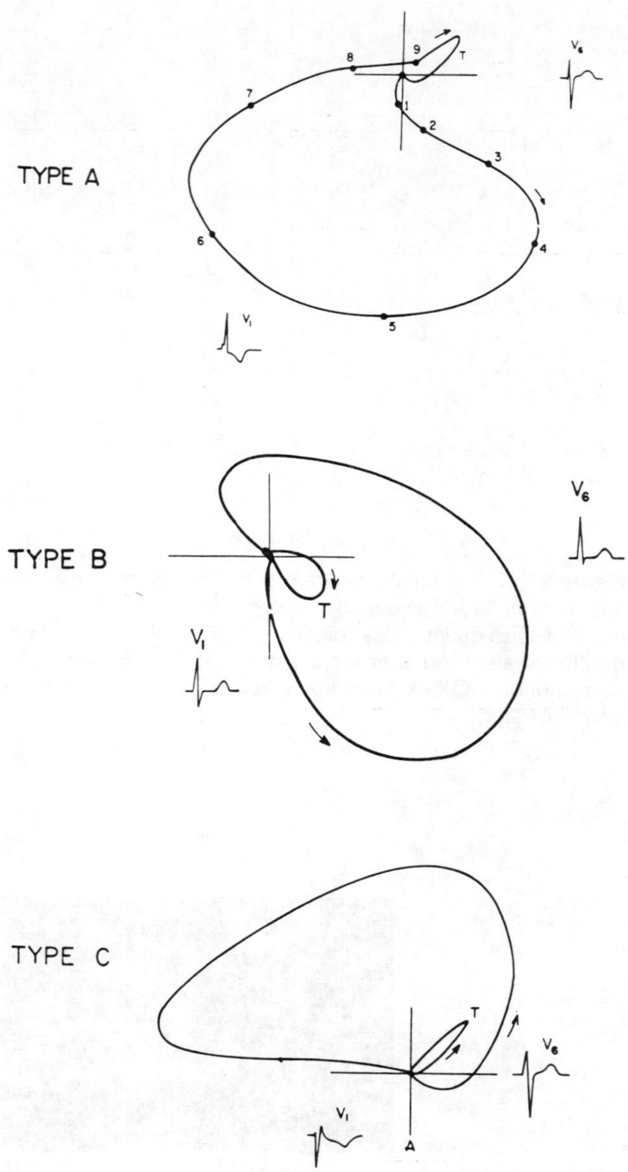

Figure 5.14. Schematic diagrams of the transverse plane QRS and T loops in the three types of right ventricular hypertrophy. See text.

is considered present when one or more of these criteria are met.

Cowdery et al[57] suggested the following criteria based on the following measurements of the QRS loop in the transverse plane: (1) The maximum transverse magnitude is less than 1.8 mV, and (2) the amplitude at −45° is less than 0.3 mV, or the maximum anterior amplitude plus the maximum rightward amplitude minus the magnitude at −45° is 0.5 mV or greater.

The more frequently used electrocardiographic criteria for the diagnosis of right ventricular hypertrophy are as follows[58–60]: (1) right axis deviation of +110° or more; (2) R/S ratio in lead V_1 (or V_{3R}) greater than 1; (3) R wave in lead V_1 7 mm or greater; (4) S wave in lead V_1 less than 2 mm; (5) qR pattern in lead V_1 (or V_{3R}); (6)

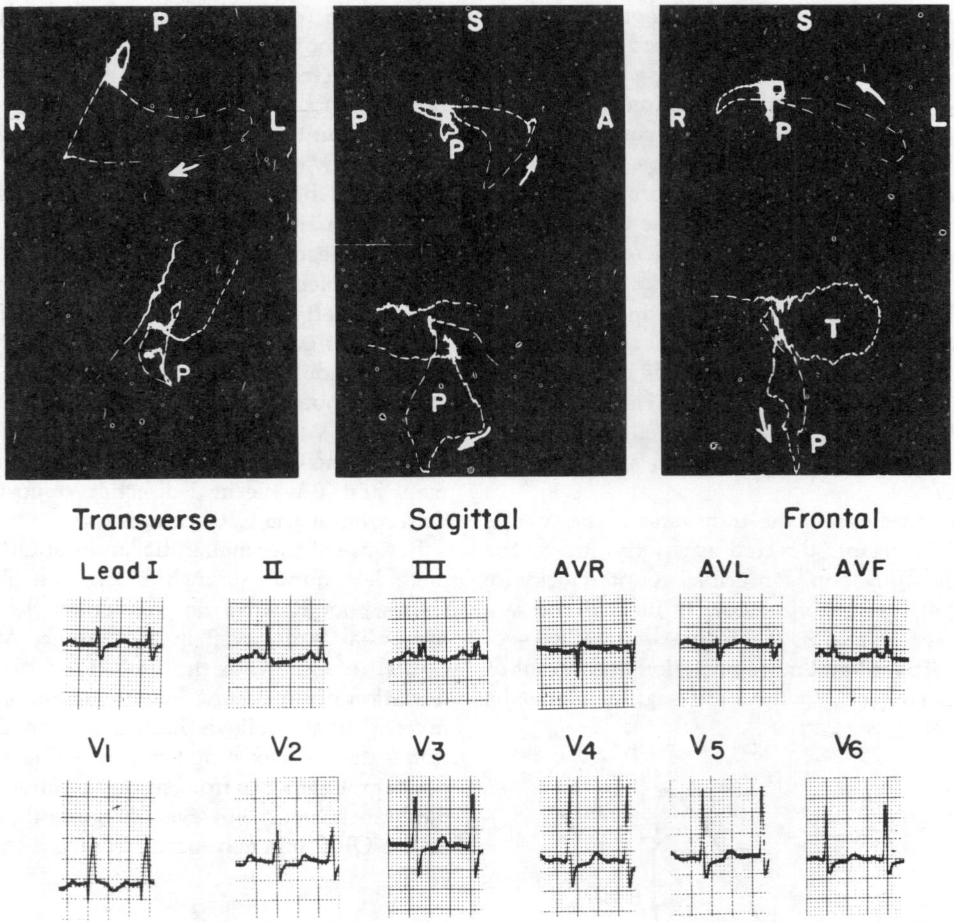

Figure 5.15. Right ventricular hypertrophy in a patient with severe mitral stenosis. The vectorcardiogram shows type A right ventricular hypertrophy with clockwise inscription of the QRS loop in the transverse plane and counterclockwise inscription in the right sagittal plane. In the frontal plane it is inscribed counterclockwise, which is atypical of right ventricular hypertrophy. The T loop is discordant to the QRS in all three planar projections. The electrocardiogram indicates borderline right axis deviation. A QR pattern is present in lead V_1. T-wave inversion is present in the right precordial and inferior leads. (From Chou et al,[54] with permission.)

R wave in lead V_1 + S wave in lead V_5 or V_6 greater than 10.5 mm; (7) R/S ratio in lead V_5 or V_6 of 1 or less; (8) rSR′ in lead V_1 with R′ 10 mm or greater.

The electrocardiogram is not a sensitive tool for the diagnosis of right ventricular hypertrophy unless the hypertrophy is severe. Using one or more of the criteria just listed, 32% to 66% of proven cases of right ventricular hypertrophy may be recognized.[56,61] The sensitivity of the individual criterion is generally less than 20%.[62] Criteria that depend on the increase in depth of the S waves in the left precordial leads are generally more sensitive but less specific, whereas the reverse is true if the diagnosis is based on an increased R-wave amplitude and especially a QR pattern in lead V_1. Several studies have indicated that the vectorcardiogram is more sensitive than the electrocardiogram in the diagnosis of right ventricular hypertrophy.[56,57,60,63–65] Of the proven cases of right ventricular hypertrophy, 60% to 83% were recognized by the vectorcardiogram compared with 27% to 66% by the electrocardiogram.[56,57] The specificity of the vectorcardiographic criteria was found to be greater than 90%.[57,66]

VENTRICULAR CONDUCTION ABNORMALITIES

LEFT BUNDLE BRANCH BLOCK

Interruption of impulse conduction through the left bundle branch results in the initiation of ventricular activation in the right, instead of the left, septum and free wall of the right ventricle through the right bundle branch. Because electrical forces from the right septum and the free wall of the right ventricle are opposite in direction, they are mostly cancelled by each other. The manifested initial QRS forces originate mostly from endocardium-to-epicardium activation of the right ventricular apex. Therefore, they are directed leftward, anteriorly, and inferiorly. As right-to-left septal depolarization continues and involves the left septum, the QRS forces generated will be oriented leftward, posteriorly, and inferiorly. After the excitation impulse arrives at the free wall of the left ventricle, the activation continues in the leftward direction through muscle conduction, although the Purkinje system may also be involved.[35,67] Because the conduction pathway is abnormal and often does not follow the Purkinje network, the time required for the completion of depolarization is increased and the QRS duration is prolonged to 0.12 second or more.

The abnormal ventricular activation in left bundle branch block is associated with secondary changes in the repolarization process. The latter proceeds in a generally right-to-left direction, and the resulting electrical forces are opposite in polarity to those generated by depolarization. Therefore, the ST and T vectors are discordant with the QRS.

On the vectorcardiogram the transverse plane reveals small initial QRS vectors directed anteriorly and to the left. Most of the QRS loop is inscribed counterclockwise and the speed of inscription is slow in its mid and late portions (Figures 5.16 and 5.17). The maximum QRS vector is directed leftward and more posteriorly than that of average normal subjects. In the right sagittal plane the initial QRS forces are directed anteriorly and inferiorly. The QRS loop is inscribed clockwise with the maximum vector directed posteriorly, either inferiorly or partly superiorly. In the frontal plane the loop is invariably inscribed counterclockwise. The maximum vector is directed leftward and may be displaced superiorly, the degree of which varies. The ST vector is usually abnormally large and directed opposite to the QRS loop in all of the projections. This is also true for the T loop.

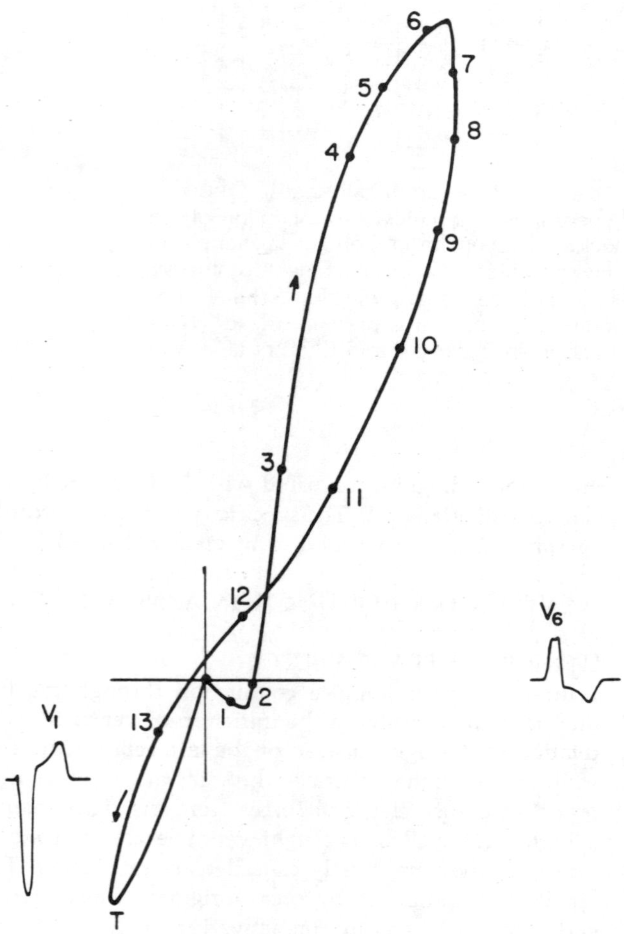

Figure 5.16. Schematic diagram of the transverse plane QRS and T loops and leads V_1 and V_6 in complete left bundle branch block.

On the electrocardiogram the characteristic findings in complete left bundle branch block consist of (1) a QRS duration of 0.12 second or greater; (2) the presence of a broad monophasic R wave in leads I, V_5, and V_6, which is usually notched or slurred; (3) the absence of a Q wave in leads I, V_5, and V_6 due to the initial leftward orientation of the QRS forces; (4) displacement of the ST segment and T wave in a direction opposite to the major deflection of the QRS complex.

Because of the small initial anterior QRS forces in complete left bundle branch block, the electrocardiogram shows poor R-wave progression in the right and midprecordial leads, even in the absence of anterior myocardial infarction. In the limb leads, abnormal left axis deviation often occurs, but its genesis is debated. Some investigators[68] believe that the abnormal left axis deviation is due to coexisting left anterior hemiblock. The preponderant evidence from studies of intermittent left bundle branch block, however, suggests that a marked shift of the QRS axis may occur from the conduction defect alone.[69,70]

LEFT ANTERIOR AND LEFT POSTERIOR HEMIBLOCK

The left bundle branch divides into the anterior and posterior divisions shortly after its departure from the His bundle. The anterior division supplies Purkinje fibers to the anterior and lateral wall of the left ventricle and the posterior division, the inferior and posterior wall.[71,72] In left anterior hemiblock the activation impulse from the main stem of the left bundle branch is conducted through the posterior division first and arrives at the anterior division retrograde. Early activation of the inferior wall of the left ventricle results in displacement of the initial QRS forces inferiorly. The delayed depolarization of the anterolateral wall of the left ventricle supplied by the anterior division results in superior displacement of the late QRS forces (Figure 5.18). In left posterior hemiblock the sequence of left ventricular activation is reversed. The early activation of the anterolateral wall is associated with initial QRS forces directed leftward and superiorly. The delayed depolarization of the posterior and inferior wall results in inferior and rightward displacement of the late QRS vectors.

On the vectorcardiogram the most characteristic findings are displayed in the frontal plane.[73–76] In left anterior hemiblock the initial QRS vectors are directed inferiorly and mostly to the right. Occasionally they may be oriented inferiorly and slightly leftward. The QRS loop is always inscribed counterclockwise with most of the loop area located in the left superior quadrant. The loop is usually wide. In left posterior hemiblock the initial leftward and superior forces and late inferior and rightward

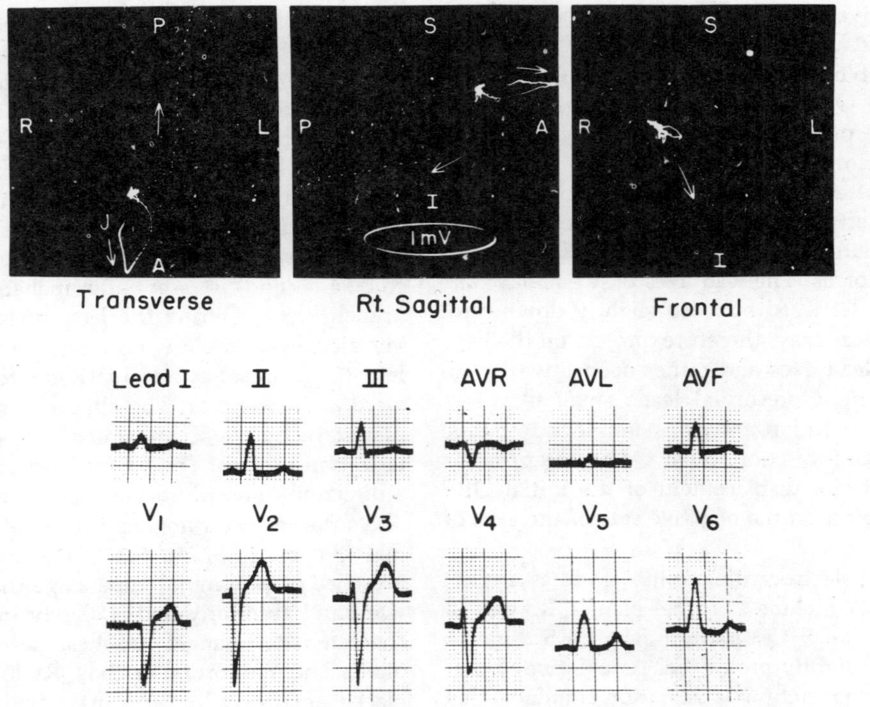

Figure 5.17. Complete left bundle branch block. On the transverse plane vectorcardiogram, the initial QRS forces are small and directed anteriorly and leftward. The QRS loop has a figure eight pattern with clockwise inscription of most of the loop. Its midportion is slowly inscribed. The ST vector and T loop are discordant to the QRS. In the frontal plane the QRS loop is inscribed counterclockwise even though the maximum QRS vector in this projection is directed at about 55°. On the electrocardiogram the QRS complex is abnormally wide and Q waves are absent in leads I, V_5, and V_6. Slurring of the R wave is best seen in leads I and V_5. The repolarization changes are not as clearly demonstrated as on the vectorcardiogram.

forces inscribed a QRS loop which is clockwise.[74,77] Most of the loop area is located inferiorly with an abnormally large portion rightward. These findings in left posterior hemiblock are similar to those seen in patients with right ventricular hypertrophy. In both left anterior and left posterior hemiblock the duration of the QRS loop may be slightly prolonged, but it usually does not exceed 0.10 second. The ST vector and T loop do not show significant abnormalities in either type of hemiblock.

The diagnostic electrocardiographic findings in left anterior hemiblock consist of (1) displacement of the mean QRS axis in the frontal plane to between −30° and −90° (abnormal left axis deviation); (2) a qR deflection (or an R wave) in leads I and aVL and an rS deflection in leads II, III, and aVF; and (3) a slightly prolonged or normal QRS duration.

There are considerable controversies in regard to the degree of left axis deviation required for the diagnosis of left anterior hemiblock.[70,71,78] Currently most electrocardiographic interpreters consider a QRS axis of, or superior

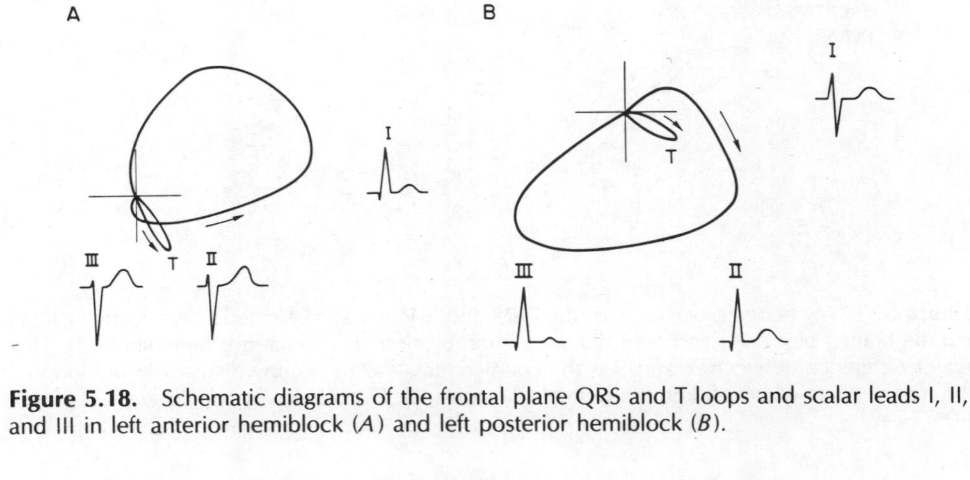

Figure 5.18. Schematic diagrams of the frontal plane QRS and T loops and scalar leads I, II, and III in left anterior hemiblock (*A*) and left posterior hemiblock (*B*).

to, −30° as indicative of left anterior hemiblock. Although a small Q wave is usually present in leads I and aVL in left anterior hemiblock, its absence does not exclude the diagnosis.[79] Such Q waves often remain absent or unchanged from the previous tracings in newly developed cases of left anterior hemiblock.[80,81]

Deep S waves often develop in the left precordial leads in patients with left anterior hemiblock. These negative deflections are related to marked superior displacement of the late QRS forces. The lead axes of V_5 and V_6 are directed not only leftward but also slightly downward. The late QRS vectors may, therefore, project on the negative side of the lead axes and rather deep S waves are recorded. In the right precordial leads small Q waves occasionally develop in left anterior hemiblock to mimic anterior myocardial infarction. Such Q waves appear as a result of the inferior displacement of the initial QRS vectors, which project on the negative side of the axes of these leads.[71,82]

The significant electrocardiographic findings in left posterior hemiblock include a frontal plane QRS axis of +90° to 180° with an S_1Q_3 pattern. The QRS duration may be normal or slightly prolonged. As mentioned previously, the abnormal right axis deviation simulates that of right ventricular hypertrophy and additional information is needed to separate these two entities. Because of the rightward shift of the late QRS forces, prominent S waves are recorded in the left precordial leads.[70,71,83,84]

RIGHT BUNDLE BRANCH BLOCK

Activation of the right ventricular septum and the free wall of the right ventricle is delayed in right bundle branch block. The left ventricular septum and free wall are depolarized in the normal fashion through the intact left bundle branch system. The activation impulse spreads from the left to the right ventricle and the two ventricles are depolarized sequentially rather than simultaneously.[85] The time required for completion of ventricular excitation, and therefore the QRS duration, is prolonged. Because normally the morphology of the QRS complex is determined mainly by the dominant left ventricular potential, the early part of the QRS complex (usually 0.03 to 0.04 second) is essentially unchanged in right bundle branch block. During the later phase the delayed right ventricular potential is no longer masked by that of the left. It manifests as terminal QRS forces directed rightward and anteriorly. The abnormal sequence of ventricular activation is accompanied by a change in the repolarization process. The ST and T vectors are displaced in a direction opposite to that of the terminal QRS forces.

On the vectorcardiogram the initial QRS forces are normal (Figures 5.19 and 5.20). The typical finding is the presence of a terminal appendage that is directed rightward and anteriorly and is slowly inscribed.[86–88] These characteristic changes are best seen in the transverse plane. The midportion of the QRS loop may also be displaced anteriorly and the main body of the QRS loop may be inscribed counterclockwise or clockwise depending on the degree of anterior displacement of its midportion.

On the electrocardiogram complete right bundle branch block is diagnosed when (1) the QRS duration is prolonged to 0.12 second or longer, and (2) a secondary R wave (R′) is present in the right precordial leads (especially in lead V_1), resulting in an RSR′ or RR′ pattern. This secondary R wave is the equivalent of the terminal

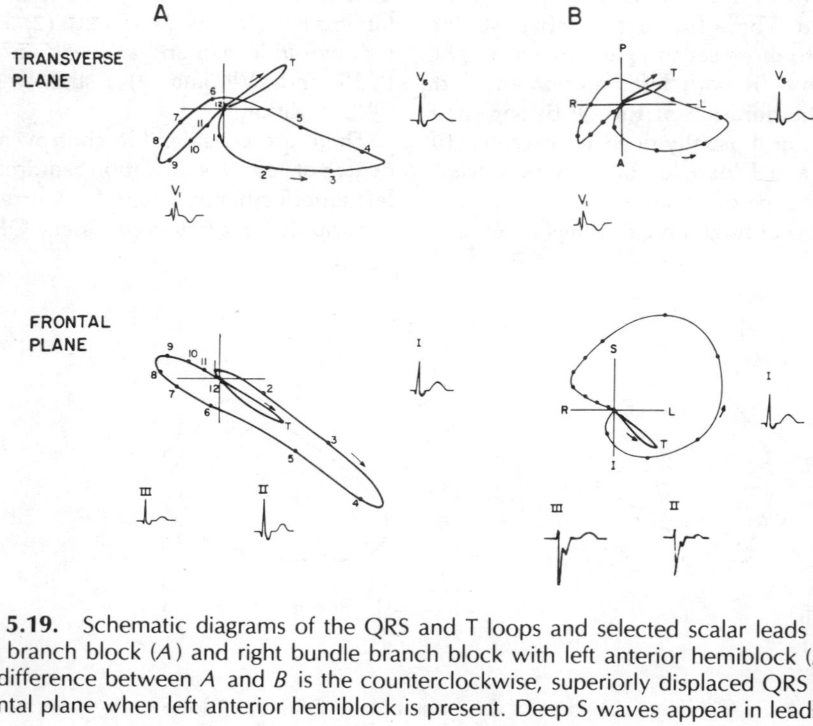

Figure 5.19. Schematic diagrams of the QRS and T loops and selected scalar leads in right bundle branch block (*A*) and right bundle branch block with left anterior hemiblock (*B*). The major difference between *A* and *B* is the counterclockwise, superiorly displaced QRS loop in the frontal plane when left anterior hemiblock is present. Deep S waves appear in leads II and III.

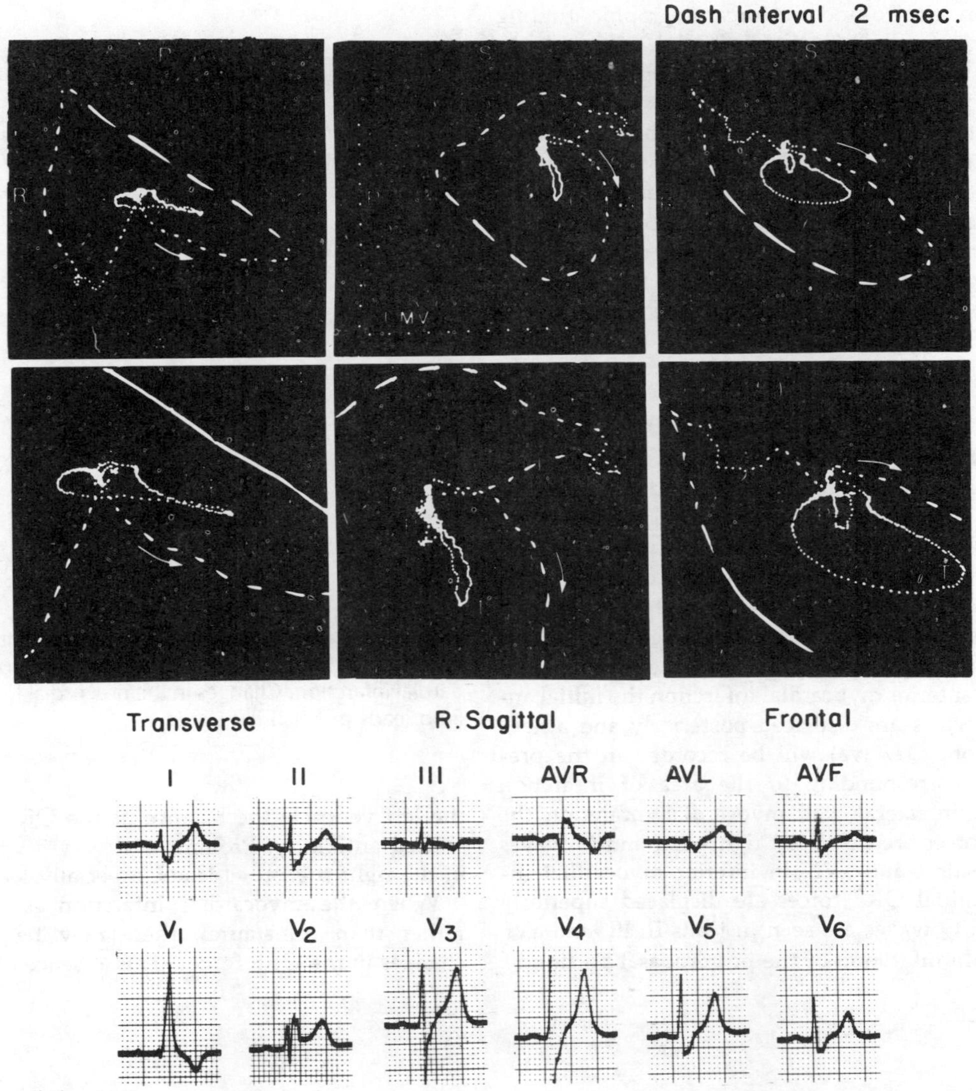

Figure 5.20. Complete right bundle branch block. Note the slowly inscribed terminal appendage which is directed anteriorly and rightward in the transverse plane. This terminal appendage is the equivalent of R′ in lead V_1 and the wide and slurred S waves in leads V_5 and V_6. (From Chou et al,[54] with permission.)

appendage in the vectorcardiogram and is manifested in the left precordial leads and lead I as wide and deep S waves. In right bundle branch block there is no significant displacement of the ST segment, and the T waves are inverted in the right precordial leads where prominent R′ waves are recorded. The T waves are upright in lead I and left precordial leads in the absence of other abnormalities.

Right bundle branch block is called incomplete if the morphology of the QRS complex is similar to that of the complete variety but the QRS duration is less than 0.12 second. The essential finding is the wide, slowly inscribed R′ in lead V_1 with a duration of 0.04 second or more.

Although right bundle branch block, either complete or incomplete, is usually due to lesions in the main bundle itself, recent observations during cardiac surgery and electrophysiologic studies suggest that similar electrocardiographic findings may occur when the damage occurs in its more distal branches.[89,90] This is also true when the injury involves the more peripheral right ventricular Purkinje network.[91]

BIFASCICULAR BLOCKS

The intraventricular conduction system may be considered as a trifascicular system consisting of the right bundle branch and the left anterior and posterior divisions of the left bundle branch. The three types of bifascicular blocks are: (1) right bundle branch block with left anterior hemiblock, (2) right bundle branch block with left posterior hemiblock, and (3) combined left anterior and left posterior hemiblocks causing electrocardiographic changes similar to those of block at the main branch of the left bundle.

Right bundle branch block with left anterior hemiblock

is a common electro-and vectorcardiographic finding, whereas right bundle branch block with left posterior hemiblock is not.[71,92–96] These bifascicular blocks may be recognized by dividing the QRS complex or QRS loop into two portions. The first half (usually 0.06 second) of the QRS forces shows leftward and superior displacement (abnormal left axis deviation) with counterclockwise inscription in left anterior hemiblock (Figure 5.19B). In left posterior hemiblock, it shows inferior and rightward displacement with clockwise inscription of the loop. The second half of the QRS forces displays the typical slowly inscribed terminal appendage seen in right bundle branch block.

MYOCARDIAL INFARCTION, MYOCARDIAL INJURY, AND MYOCARDIAL ISCHEMIA

The QRS vectors recorded from the body surface represent the resultants of the electrical forces generated from various areas of the myocardium during ventricular activation. In myocardial infarction the area of necrosis becomes electrically silent. The balance of the forces tends to be displaced away from this area as the opposing potentials from other regions become more dominant. Therefore, in anterior myocardial infarction the initial anterior QRS vectors are displaced posteriorly and a negative deflection (Q wave) will be recorded in the precordial leads corresponding to the area of infarction (Figure 5.21). In lateral wall myocardial infarction the initial QRS forces are displaced rightward and Q waves develop in leads I and aVL. In inferior myocardial infarction the initial QRS forces are displaced superiorly and abnormal Q waves are seen in leads II, III, and aVF (Figure 5.22). In infarction of the posterobasal portion of the left ventricle the balance of the QRS forces will be shifted anteriorly. Prominent R waves will be recorded in the right precordial leads, especially lead V_1.

When the myocardial infarction is subendocardial rather than transmural, there may be no significant changes in the QRS forces. This absence of QRS changes

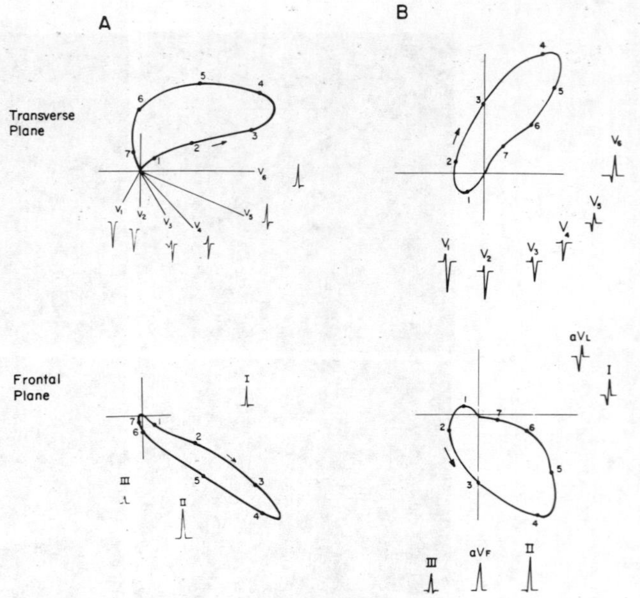

Figure 5.21. Schematic diagrams of the transverse and frontal plane QRS loop in anterior (*A*) and anterolateral (*B*) myocardial infarction. Changes in the precordial leads and selected limb leads are also illustrated.

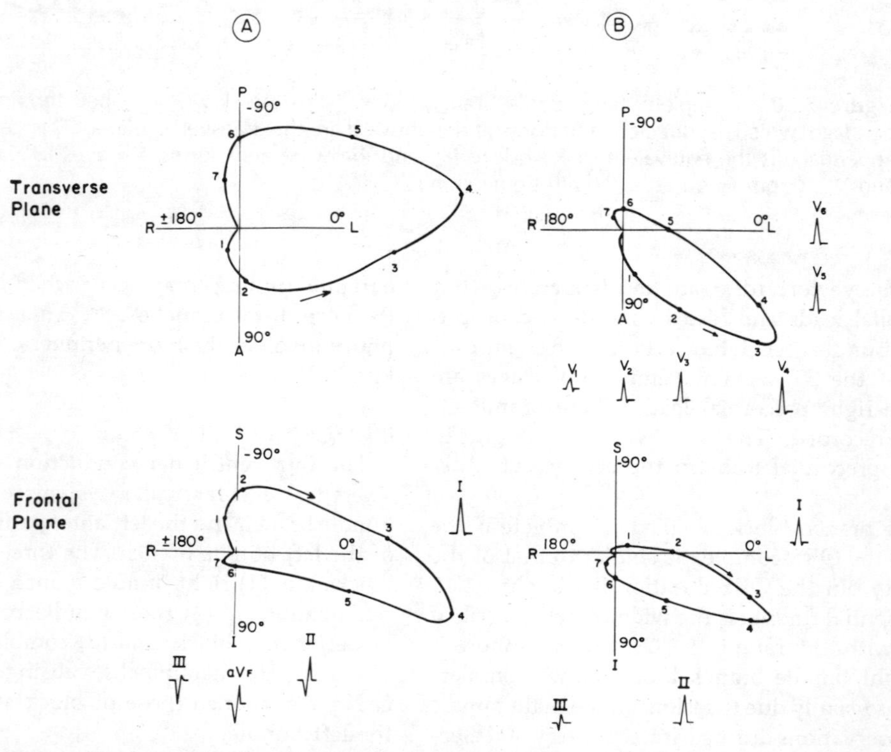

Figure 5.22. Schematic diagrams of the QRS loop and scalar lead QRS complexes in inferior (*A*) and true posterior (*B*) myocardial infarction.

is explained by the deep penetration of the Purkinje fibers into the myocardium.[97] Within the inner layers of the ventricular wall the activation impulse spreads in all directions and the forces generated are cancelled by each other. Therefore, there is little change in the QRS voltage if the myocardial infarction is limited to the subendocardium.

Many theories have been proposed to explain the ST-segment displacement in acute myocardial injury.[98] For the sake of simplicity the theory of incomplete depolarization is chosen in this chapter. At the end of depolarization the area of injury remains electrically more positive than the rest of the myocardium. Therefore, the ST vector will be directed toward the zone of injury. If an exploring electrode is placed in this region, the relatively positive potential will cause an elevation in the ST segment. Conversely, if the electrode is placed over the myocardium opposite to the injured area, it will face the negative end of the ST vector and ST-segment depression will be recorded. Similarly, if the injury is limited to the subendocardial layer of the ventricular wall, the exploring electrode will be separated from the area by a layer of normal myocardium. At the end of depolarization the persistent positivity of the injured endocardium will result in an ST vector pointing away from the exploring electrode. ST-segment depression will appear.

In myocardial ischemia the repolarization process is delayed in the involved area.[99] Consequently, the ischemic zone is electrically more negative than the unaffected area during the recovery phase and the resultant T vectors are pointing away from it. If an exploring electrode is placed over the area of ischemia, it will record a negative T wave. If the ischemia is subendocardial rather than transmural, the normal epicardium-to-endocardium direction of the recovery process is not altered. The additional delay in repolarization in the subendocardium, however, allows its electrical potential to be unopposed. The resulting T vectors increase in amplitude. A recording electrode facing the epicardium of that area of the ventricle will record an abnormally tall T wave.

In acute transmural myocardial infarction the area of necrosis is surrounded by a zone of injury and a zone of ischemia. Therefore, ST-segment elevation and T-wave abnormalities are recorded in the lead displaying the abnormal Q waves as well as in the leads adjacent to the infarcted area.

MYOCARDIAL INFARCTION

Vectorcardiographic criteria for the diagnosis of myocardial infarction[100–110] are as follows (Figures 5.23 to 5.26):

A. Anterior myocardial infarction (1 or 2)*:
   1. Absent initial anterior QRS forces
   2. 0.02-second QRS vector directed posteriorly
B. Anterolateral myocardial infarction (1, 2, and 3):
   1. Normal initial anterior septal forces
   2. Initial rightward QRS forces greater than 0.022 second

* The numbers in parentheses after each infarction location indicate the minimum requirements for the diagnosis.

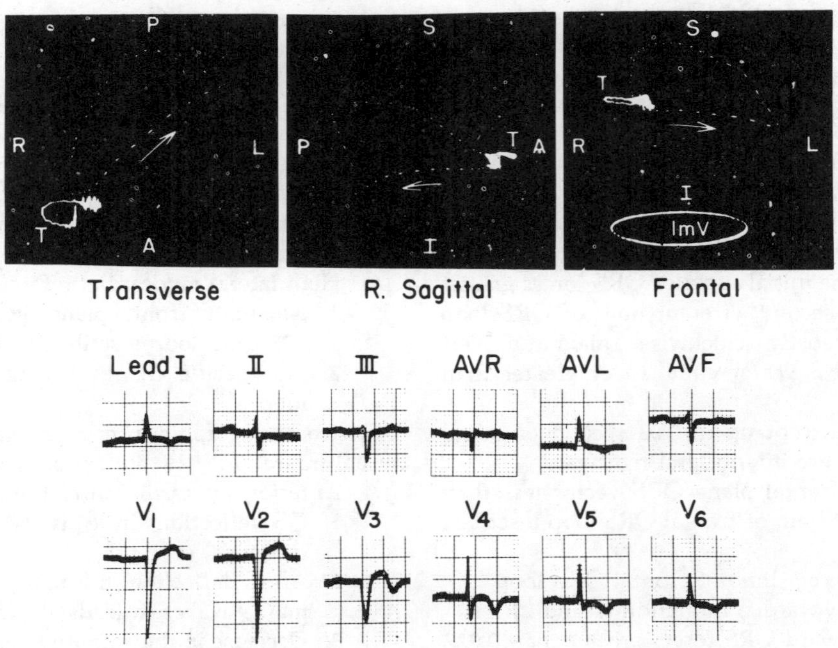

Figure 5.23. Anterior myocardial infarction. On the vectorcardiogram the initial anterior QRS forces are absent. The QRS loop is displaced superiorly and inscribed counterclockwise in the frontal plane, consistent with left anterior hemiblock. The T loop is displaced rightward, consistent with lateral wall myocardial ischemia. The electrocardiogram indicates first degree AV block. The QRS changes are consistent with left anterior hemiblock and anterior myocardial infarction. The T-wave inversion in leads I, aVL, and V_3 to V_6 are suggestive of anterolateral myocardial ischemia.

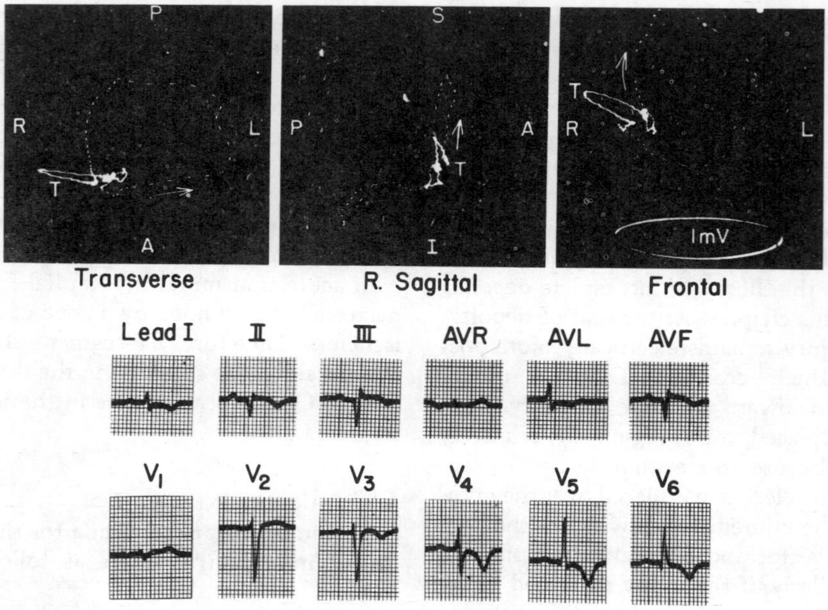

Figure 5.24. Inferior myocardial infarction. On the vectorcardiogram there is superior displacement of the initial and mid-QRS forces, as shown in the sagittal and frontal planes. The T loop is displaced rightward, posteriorly and superiorly. The rightward and posterior displacement is consistent with anterolateral myocardial ischemia and the superior displacement is related to inferior myocardial infarction. On the electrocardiogram, QR deflections are present in leads II, III, and aVF. There is slight ST-segment elevation with T-wave inversion in these leads. Symmetrical T-wave inversion is seen in the anterolateral leads. Although the S wave in lead V_1 is small and suggests posterior myocardial infarction, there is no reduction in the amplitude of the posterior QRS forces in the vectorcardiogram.

3. Clockwise inscription of the efferent limb of the transverse plane QRS loop
4. Initial rightward QRS forces greater than 0.16 mV
5. Maximum frontal plane QRS vector greater than 40°, QRS loop inscribed counterclockwise

C. Extensive anterior myocardial infarction (1 and 2):
1. Absent initial anterior QRS forces
2. Transverse plane QRS loop inscribed clockwise

D. Inferior myocardial infarction (1 or more):
1. Frontal plane initial superior QRS forces greater than 0.025 second, efferent limb of QRS loop inscribed mostly clockwise, maximum left superior QRS vector equal to or greater than 0.3 mV
2. Same as 1 except up to 0.01 second of initial QRS forces are inferior and rightward
3. Maximum frontal plane QRS vector less than 10°, efferent limb of frontal QRS loop inscribed clockwise
4. Bites in afferent limb of frontal QRS loop

E. Inferolateral myocardial infarction (1 and 2):
1. Initial rightward QRS forces greater than 0.022 second
2. Initial superior QRS forces greater than 0.025 second
3. Efferent limb of frontal plane QRS loop inscribed clockwise
4. Initial rightward QRS forces greater than 0.16 mV

F. True posterior myocardial infarction (1 or more) in the transverse plane:
1. Anterior loop area greater than 70% of total QRS area
2. Maximum QRS vector anterior to 20°
3. Duration of anterior QRS forces greater than 0.05 second
4. Half-area QRS vector anterior to 10°
5. Maximum anterior QRS voltage 0.6 mV or greater

G. High lateral myocardial infarction (1 and 2):
1. Maximum frontal plane QRS vector greater than 40°, QRS loop inscribed counterclockwise
2. No specific changes in transverse plane QRS loop

Electrocardiographic criteria for the diagnosis of myocardial infarction[111-121] are as follows:

A. Anterior myocardial infarction:
1. QS deflections in leads V_1, V_2, V_3, and sometimes V_4, or
2. An rS deflection in lead V_1 followed by abnormal Q waves in leads V_2 to V_4; or
3. Decrease in the amplitude of the initial R waves from leads V_1 to V_4

B. Anterolateral myocardial infarction:
1. Abnormal Q waves in leads V_4 to V_6, I, and aVL

C. Extensive anterior myocardial infarction:
1. QS deflections in all or nearly all the precordial leads

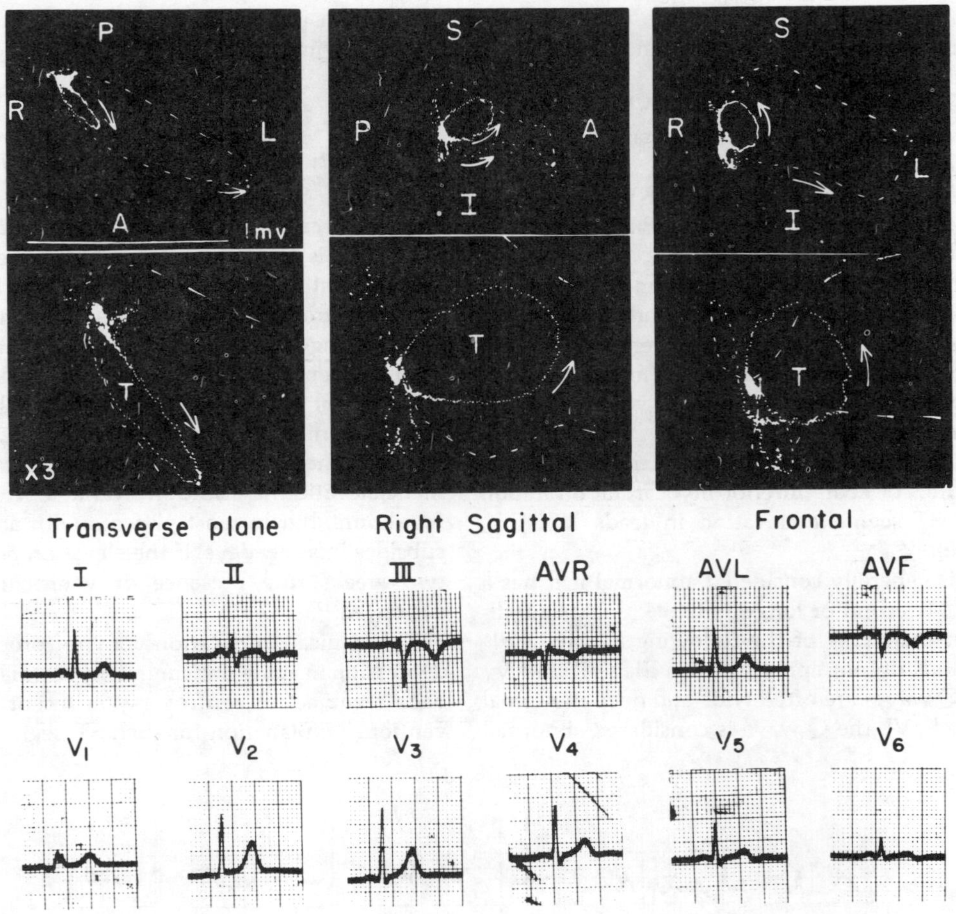

Figure 5.25. True posterior myocardial infarction. On the vectorcardiogram there is anterior displacement of the QRS and T loops, with the latter being inscribed clockwise. There is also superior displacement of the QRS and T loops as shown in the frontal and sagittal planes. The T loop is abnormally wide. The electrocardiogram shows the absence of an S wave in the right precordial leads with the T waves being upright in these leads. The T waves are inverted in the inferior leads and are consistent with inferior myocardial ischemia. (From Chou et al,[54] with permission.)

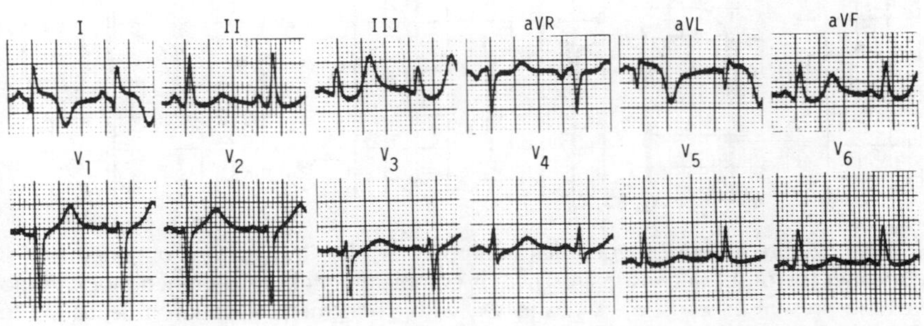

Figure 5.26. Acute high lateral myocardial infarction. Abnormal Q waves with ST-segment elevation and T-wave inversion are present in leads I and aVL. The QT interval is prolonged. These abnormalities developed two days after the onset of chest pain and were associated with elevated cardiac enzyme levels.

D. High lateral myocardial infarction:
   1. Abnormal Q waves in leads I and aVL
E. Inferior myocardial infarction:
   1. Q waves in leads II, III, and aVF, with the Q wave in lead aVF being abnormal
F. Inferolateral myocardial infarction:
   1. Q waves in leads II, III, and aVF which met the criteria for inferior infarction, plus abnormal Q waves in leads V_5 and V_6
G. True posterior myocardial infarction:
   1. Initial R waves in leads V_1 and V_2 having a duration of 0.04 second or longer, with an R/S ratio equal to or greater than 1 (in patients over 30 years of age without right ventricular hypertrophy)
H. Right ventricular myocardial infarction:
   1. Findings of acute inferior myocardial infarction plus ST-segment elevation in leads V_1, V_{3R}, and/or V_{4R}

A Q wave is generally considered abnormal if it has a duration of 0.04 second or longer[111,116,118,119] or its amplitude is greater than 25% of the following R wave.[111,116] These definitions do not apply to leads III, aVR and V_1 in which the Q waves are often wide and deep in normal persons. In lead aVL the Q wave is considered abnormal only when it has an amplitude of greater than 50% of the following R wave in the presence of an upright P wave.[116]

Evolutionary Changes in Acute Transmural Myocardial Infarction

In most cases the first indication of acute myocardial infarction is the appearance of an abnormally large ST vector pointing at the area of infarction (Figure 5.27). The scalar electrocardiogram reveals ST-segment elevation in leads facing the area of infarction with reciprocal ST-segment depression in the opposite leads. The degree of ST-segment elevation varies greatly. The elevation decreases significantly in the first 7 to 12 hours after the onset of chest pain.[122,123] The total duration of ST-segment elevation is also quite variable. It may last only a few hours, but in most patients with acute infarction it subsides in a few days. If the elevation persists more than two weeks, the presence of ventricular aneurysm is suggested.[124]

The clinical implications of "reciprocal" ST-segment depression in acute transmural myocardial infarction have been a subject of controversy in recent years. The conventional explanation for such ST-segment depression is

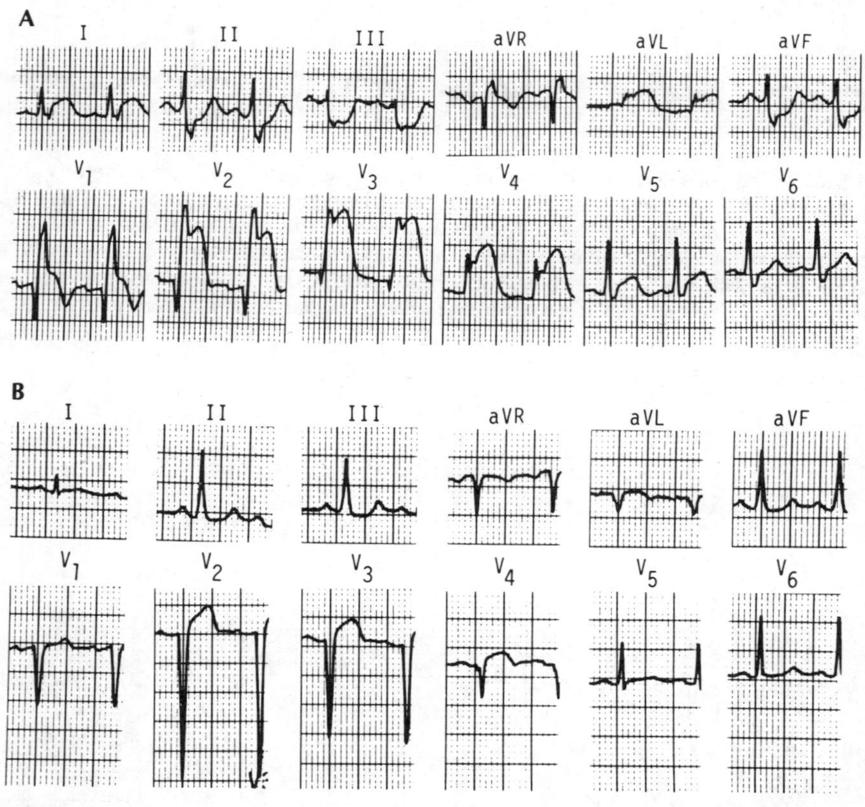

Figure 5.27. Acute anterior myocardial infarction. *A*, The tracing was obtained one and a half hours after the onset of chest pain. There is complete right bundle branch block. Abnormal Q waves are present in leads V_1, V_2, and V_3, with ST-segment elevation in leads V_1 to V_5, I, and aVL. *B*, Five hours and 25 minutes later, the tracing no longer shows changes of right bundle branch block. QS deflection has developed in leads V_1 to V_4. ST-segment elevation is less pronounced and is confined to leads V_1 through V_4. A coronary arteriogram revealed a critical obstructive lesion in the proximal portion of the left anterior descending artery. No other significant lesions were found.

that it represents a simple electrical phenomenon. The negative potential is recorded by the electrodes facing the negative end of the ST vector which points in the direction of the area of acute injury. However, some recent angiographic and radionuclide studies suggest that this reciprocal ST-segment depression may be due to a more extensive area of ischemia or coexistence of disease of other coronary vessels.[125–129] Other studies did not substantiate these relations and reciprocal ST-segment depression was also observed in patients with acute myocardial infarction due to single vessel disease.[130,131]

Tall and peaked T waves occasionally may be the earliest sign of acute myocardial infarction and are believed to be due to subendocardial ischemia.[132,133] They are transient and most tracings fail to record such changes.

Loss of QRS forces or the appearance of abnormal Q waves in the leads corresponding to the area of acute infarction usually occurs within several hours or days after the onset of chest pain. Most commonly they develop while the ST segment is still elevated. Although they usually persist indefinitely, in 12% to 30% of the patients with transmural myocardial infarction the Q waves may become either nondiagnostic or absent.[134–137]

During the evolution of acute myocardial infarction, symmetrical inversion of the T waves appears as the ST-segment elevation begins to subside. The inverted T waves become progressively deeper as the ST segment returns to the isoelectric line. Both ST-segment elevation and T-wave changes are seen in more leads than are the abnormal Q waves. The symmetrical T-wave inversion may disappear within months or years, but it also may persist indefinitely.

Various terms such as *acute, subacute, recent, remote, previous*, or *old* have been used to describe the various stages of myocardial infarction. The precise definitions of these terms have not been generally agreed upon. It is important to note that staging of the infarction is difficult when previous electrocardiograms or clinical information is not available. It is my practice to define the infarction as old if it was known to exist at least two months.

Subendocardial Infarction

Pathologically the term *subendocardial infarction* (Figure 5.28) refers to infarction involving no more than the inner half of the ventricular wall.[138,139] Subendocardial infarction is estimated to occur in about 25% of all infarctions.[140–142] The most consistent electrocardiographic changes in acute subendocardial infarction are ST-segment depression and T-wave inversion in the leads facing the epicardial surface of the infarcted area. In typical cases no appreciable abnormalities are seen in the QRS complex.[139] However, abnormal Q waves are recorded in some patients.[138,143–148] Therefore, the differentiation of transmural and subendocardial infarction based on the presence or absence of abnormal Q waves alone may not be justifiable.

Right Ventricular Infarction

Myocardial infarction involving the free wall of the right ventricle (Figure 5.29) rarely occurs in isolated form, but it is present in 14% to 36% of the patients with transmural left ventricular inferior wall infarction.[149–152] On the electrocardiogram the presence of right ventricular infarction is suggested when there is ST-segment elevation in one or more of the rightsided chest leads (V_1, V_{3R}, and V_{4R}) associated with signs of acute inferior myocardial infarction.[112–115,153] ST-segment elevation is usually short-lived and subsides within ten hours after the onset of chest pain in half the patients.[112] Although changes in the QRS complex have been observed in experimental right ventricular infarction, whether they occur in humans is still to be determined.[154,155]

Reliability of the Electrocardiogram and Vectorcardiogram in the Diagnosis of Myocardial Infarction

Many factors influence the accuracy of the electrocardiographic and vectorcardiographic diagnosis of myocardial infarction. The accuracy is affected by the size, age, location of the infarct, the presence or absence of multiple infarcts, and the presence or absence of ventricular hy-

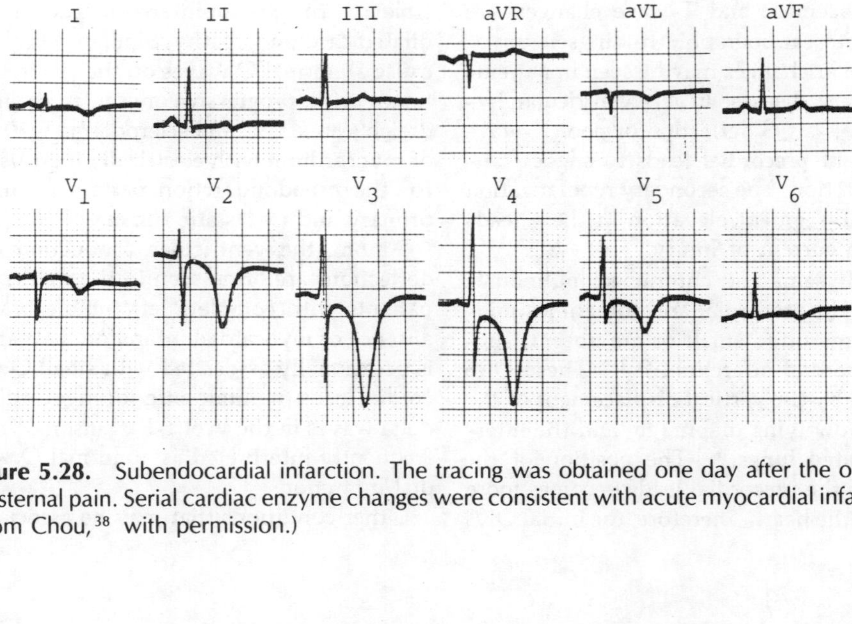

Figure 5.28. Subendocardial infarction. The tracing was obtained one day after the onset of substernal pain. Serial cardiac enzyme changes were consistent with acute myocardial infarction. (From Chou,[38] with permission.)

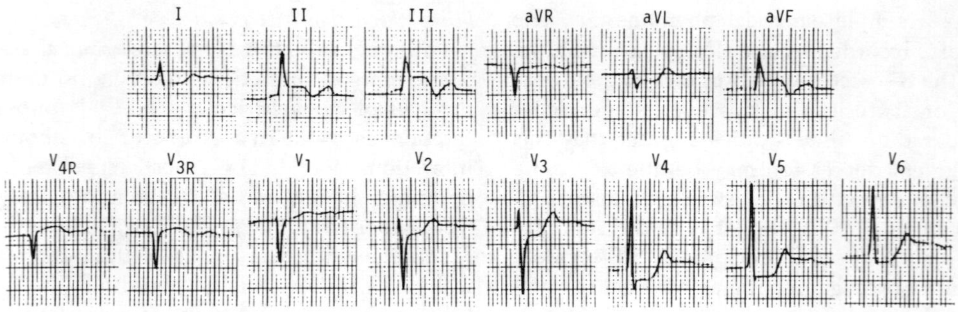

Figure 5.29. Acute inferior myocardial infarction with right ventricular infarction. The electrocardiogram was obtained a few hours after the onset of chest pain. A rhythm strip shows complete AV block. There is ST-segment elevation in leads II, III, and aVF with ST-segment depression in leads I, aVL, and V_2 to V_6. ST-segment elevation is present in lead V_{4R}. Serial tracings and cardiac enzyme levels were consistent with acute inferior myocardial infarction. Hemodynamic data and radionuclide studies were indicative of right ventricular infarction, which is suggested on the electrocardiogram by the ST-segment elevation in lead V_{4R}.

pertrophy and ventricular conduction abnormality. The availability of adequate number of records, especially those before infarction occurs, greatly improves the ability to recognize it. In the absence of an intraventricular conduction defect the reported sensitivity of the electrocardiogram in the recognition of myocardial infarction proven at autopsy varies from 48% to 82%.[102,147,156–159] Acute infarction is less likely to be missed. Anterior infarction generally is more easily recognized than inferior or true posterior infarction. Subendocardial infarction is less likely to be diagnosed than is transmural infarction. Furthermore, electrocardiographic prediction of the exact location of the infarct is often inaccurate.[102]

Studies comparing the reliability of electrocardiographic and vectorcardiographic diagnosis of myocardial infarction suggest that the vectorcardiogram is more sensitive but not more specific than the electrocardiogram.[103,160–163] The increased sensitivity of the vectorcardiogram is more apparent in patients with inferior myocardial infarction.

The Pseudoinfarctions

Although abnormal Q waves, especially accompanied by ST-segment displacement and T-wave changes, are the characteristic electrocardiographic findings in myocardial infarction, similar changes may be seen in patients without coronary artery disease. In left ventricular hypertrophy there often is a QS deflection or poor R-wave progression in the right precordial leads to suggest anterior myocardial infarction. The secondary repolarization abnormalities with ST-segment elevation in these leads may be mistaken as a current of injury.

In pulmonary emphysema and chronic cor pulmonale the R waves in the right precordial and sometimes mid-precordial leads become quite small or are absent, suggesting anterior myocardial infarction.[164–167] These QRS changes are explained by the vertical displacement of the heart secondary to a low lying diaphragm and the intervention of hyperinflated lungs.[166] The position of the exploring electrode of the precordial leads becomes more superior in relation to the heart. Therefore, the initial QRS forces are likely to be perpendicular or directed toward the negative side of the electrical axes of these leads and small R or Q waves may be recorded to mimic anterior myocardial infarction. The pseudoinfarction pattern may also be seen in patients with either spontaneous or artificial pneumothorax.[168,169] The voltage of the QRS complex may be reduced. QS deflection may appear in the right precordial leads.[170] The T waves are often inverted and symmetrical to resemble "ischemic" T waves in coronary artery disease. In pulmonary embolism the appearance of Q waves in lead III (as part of the S_1Q_3 pattern) and sometimes in lead aVF accompanied by ST-segment and T-wave changes is often interpreted as inferior myocardial infarction.[171–173] In addition to T-wave inversion with or without an rSr′ pattern in the right precordial leads due to acute right heart strain, QS complexes with ST-segment elevation may occasionally develop in these leads and mimic acute anterior myocardial infarction.[174]

In hypertrophic cardiomyopathy abnormal Q waves are often seen especially in the left precordial leads and lead I.[175–177] These Q waves have been attributed to ventricular septal hypertrophy. Myocardial fibrosis is often responsible for the pseudoinfarction pattern in patients with dilated cardiomyopathy. Similar pathologic changes may cause abnormal Q waves on the electrocardiogram of patients with progressive muscular dystrophy,[178,179] Friedreich's ataxia,[180] and scleroderma.[181,182] The replacement of myocardium with electrically inert tissue is responsible for the pseudoinfarction pattern in amyloidosis[183] and primary and metastatic tumors of the heart.[184,185]

Among the ventricular conduction disturbances, QS deflections are often seen in the right precordial leads in patients with complete left bundle branch block in the absence of myocardial infarction. Left anterior hemiblock is occasionally associated with small Q waves in the precordial leads to mimic anterior myocardial infarction. The delta waves in the Wolff-Parkinson-White syndrome are frequently interpreted as abnormal Q waves of myocardial infarction.

Other conditions that may be associated with electrocardiographic changes simulating myocardial infarction include intracranial hemorrhage,[186,187] hyperkalemia,[188] and acute pericarditis. The electrocardiographic changes in hyperkalemia and pericarditis will be discussed subsequently in this chapter.

Diagnosis of Myocardial Infarction in the Presence of Ventricular Conduction Defects

In uncomplicated right bundle branch block, activation of the left ventricle is not disturbed. Initial QRS forces are not altered. Because most myocardial infarctions cause abnormalities of the initial QRS forces, the presence of right bundle branch block does not interfere with recognition of the infarction.[157] However, when left bundle branch block is present, the diagnosis of myocardial infarction is difficult. Changes in the sequence of ventricular excitation in left bundle branch block produce marked alterations in both the initial and late QRS forces. Many conventional criteria in the diagnosis of myocardial infarction are no longer applicable.[189] A useful sign of myocardial infarction in the presence of left bundle branch block is the appearance of Q waves with a duration of 0.04 second or greater in leads I, V_5, and V_6.[190] The presence of myocardial injury or infarction is also suggested if there is ST-segment elevation in leads that normally display ST-segment depression. For example, the development of ST-segment elevation in the anterolateral leads in patients suspected of having acute myocardial infarction would be highly suggestive of the diagnosis. Similarly, such ST-segment changes can be used in the diagnosis of myocardial infarction in the presence of the Wolff-Parkinson-White syndrome.[191,192]

MYOCARDIAL INJURY AND ISCHEMIA

Acute ST-segment elevation suggestive of myocardial injury often may be seen without QRS changes. Acute myocardial infarction may or may not have occurred. Not infrequently, ST-segment elevation is the result of coronary artery spasm and is associated with reciprocal ST-segment depression. ST-segment elevation also may occur in many noncoronary events. In acute pericarditis the ST segment is diffuse, and reciprocal ST-segment depression is not observed. ST-segment elevation is often seen in normal persons as a normal variant due to early repolarization.[133] It is more common in younger subjects, especially men. Such elevation generally remains unchanged over a long period. Other entities often associated with ST-segment elevation were discussed under the topic of pseudoinfarction.

Myocardial ischemia may be manifested on the electrocardiogram as one of the following findings: (1) abnormally tall T waves, (2) symmetrically or deeply inverted T waves (Figure 5.30A), (3) horizontal ST-segment depression with or without T-wave inversion, (4) normalization of abnormal T waves (Figure 5.30B), and (5) nonspecific ST- and T-wave changes. As many other conditions may cause such changes, clinical correlation is needed to support the electrocardiographic interpretation.

On the vectorcardiogram the repolarization abnormalities associated with myocardial ischemia include changes

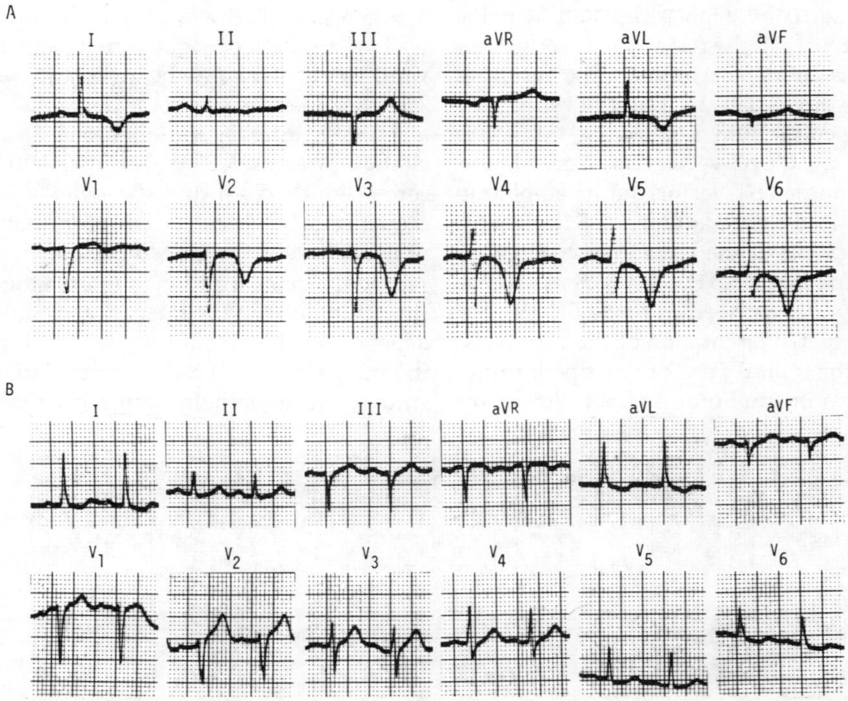

Figure 5.30. Anterior and lateral myocardial ischemia. *A*, T-wave inversion is shown in leads I, II, aVL, and all of the precordial leads. The patient is known to have angina and these T-wave changes have been present for over a year. During an episode of angina, pseudonormalization of the inverted T waves is demonstrated (*B*). The deeply inverted T waves in the anterior and lateral leads on the baseline electrocardiogram are replaced by upright or biphasic T waves.

in the orientation or amplitude of the T vectors and sometimes reversal in the direction of inscription of the T loop. The T loop may be inscribed at a uniform speed and does not show the normal slower inscription of its efferent limb. It may be abnormally wide, with its length-to-width ratio being less than the normal value of 2.6 to 1[101] (Figure 5.25).

Coronary Artery Spasm

Angina pectoris and myocardial infarction occasionally may be caused by coronary artery spasm.[193–199] The spasm may involve vessels with or without organic obstructive lesions, and the typical symptom is angina at rest. During the anginal episodes the electrocardiogram may reveal ST-segment elevation, ST-segment depression, increased T-wave amplitude, or pseudonormalization of inverted T waves. Among the various presentations of vasospastic angina, variant (Prinzmetal) angina is the most widely recognized. This variant form of angina is characterized by the development of chest pain when the patient is at rest. The pain is recurrent and is accompanied by transient ST-segment elevation. Cardiac arrhythmias, most often ventricular in origin, occur in about 50% of the cases during pain. An AV conduction defect also may be observed.[200,201]

PERICARDITIS

Electrocardiographic findings in acute pericarditis are generally attributed to associated subepicardial myocarditis.[202] The inflammatory process induces a zone of injury in the superficial layer of the myocardium. The injured zone is only partially depolarized and remains electrically more positive than the rest of the myocardium at the end of ventricular depolarization. The resulting abnormal ST vector is directed away from the ventricular cavity and toward the epicardium, ie, leftward, inferiorly, and anteriorly. Therefore, the ST vector has an orientation similar to that of the normal ST vector, but its amplitude is increased. In the 12-lead electrocardiogram ST-segment elevation is present in most of the leads except lead aVR in which it is depressed (Figure 5.31). ST-segment depression occasionally may also be seen in leads III, aVL, or V_1, depending of the spatial orientation of the ventricles. During the course of the typical cases of acute pericarditis the ST vector decreases in amplitude and is followed by displacement of T vectors to the right, posteriorly, and superiorly. The electrocardiogram records T-wave inversion in leads that normally display upright T waves. Such T-wave changes are probably due to delay in recovery of the injured subepicardial layer of the myocardium. In some patients the PR segment (STa) is depressed because of atrial subepicardial injury. PR-segment depression is seen in leads that display ST-segment elevation.[203–205]

In patients in whom significant pericardial effusion develops, the short-circuiting effect of the pericardial fluid may reduce the amplitude of the QRS forces. Occasionally there is a regular alternation in the configuration or magnitude of the electrocardiographic complexes, called electrical alternans. The alternation may involve the P, QRS, or T waves, or all three. Electrical alternans may occur in the absence of pericardial effusion, and the incidence of this phenomenon in pericardial effusion is quite low. When the electrical alternans involves all three waves (P, QRS, and T), however, pericardial effusion with tamponade is almost invariably present.[206] The genesis of electrical alternans in the presence of pericardial effusion is most likely anatomic alternation of the cardiac position. When pericardial effusion is absent, the probable mechanism is an alternation in the pathway of depolarization.

WOLFF-PARKINSON-WHITE SYNDROME

The Wolff-Parkinson-White syndrome is also called the ventricular preexcitation syndrome. In its classical form there is an accessory AV pathway, namely, the bundle of Kent, which allows the atrial impulse to bypass the AV node and depolarize the ventricle prematurely.[207] The accessory pathway may be located between the free wall of the left or right atrium and the corresponding ventricle, or between the atrial and ventricular septa.[208] The characteristic electrocardiographic findings consist of a short PR interval and abnormal QRS complex. Preexcitation of an area of the ventricle alters the initial QRS forces which constitute the delta wave. The abnormal sequence of ventricular activation that follows results in prolongation of the QRS duration and is associated with secondary repolarization abnormalities. The degree of shortening of the PR interval and widening of the QRS depends on the prematurity of atrial impulse arriving at the ventricle. The ventricular depolarization may depend entirely on the impulse transmitted through the bypass,

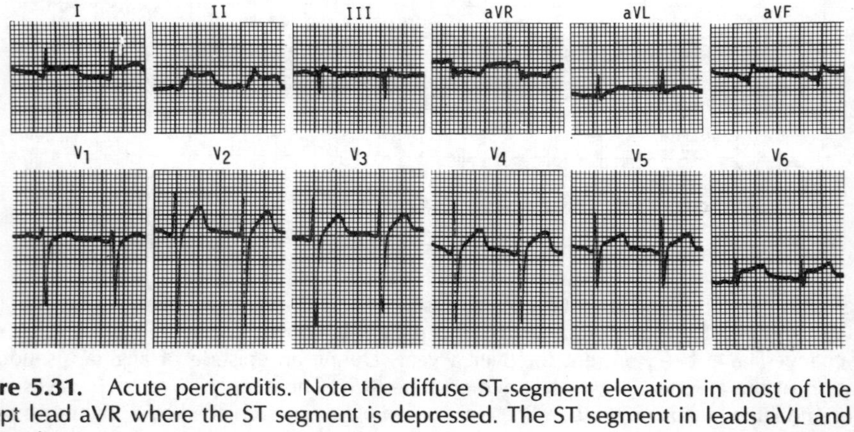

Figure 5.31. Acute pericarditis. Note the diffuse ST-segment elevation in most of the leads except lead aVR where the ST segment is depressed. The ST segment in leads aVL and V_1 is isoelectric.

or is accomplished partially by impulse conducted through the accessory bundle and partly through the normal AV conduction system. In the latter case the QRS complex represents a fusion beat.

There are several variant forms of the preexcitation syndrome. In the Lown-Ganong-Levine syndrome the PR interval is shortened, but the QRS complex is normal.[209] The accelerated AV conduction is due to the presence of a paranodal pathway, described by James, which bypasses the upper and central AV node to connect with the lower third of the node, or directly with the bundle of His.[210] Most of the normal AV conduction delay is, therefore, avoided. Another form of ventricular preexcitation is due to the presence of the bypass fibers described by Mahaim and Winston.[211] The Mahaim fibers serve as a short direct connection between the lower AV node or His bundle and the ventricular septum. The PR interval is normal, but there is a delta wave that is due to preexcitation of the ventricular septum. There are other patients who have concealed bypass between the atrium and the ventricle.[212–214] The accessory pathway is able to conduct impulse only in the retrograde (ventriculoatrial) direction. During sinus rhythm the electrocardiogram shows a normal PR interval and QRS complex.

In the Wolff-Parkinson-White syndrome and its variants the presence of an accessory pathway establishes a reentry circuit. Therefore, paroxysmal tachycardia frequently occurs in patients with this syndrome. In most cases the normal AV bundle is used for antegrade conduction during tachycardia, and the QRS complex is normal. Tachycardias using such a mechanism are called orthodromic reentrant tachycardias. If the antegrade conduction uses the accessory bundle during reentrant tachycardia, wide QRS complexes will be recorded and the tachycardia is called antidromic tachycardia.[215]

On the vectorcardiogram the most characteristic finding in the Wolff-Parkinson-White syndrome is the presence of a slowly inscribed initial portion of the QRS loop, representing the delta deflection (Figures 5.32 and 5.33). The duration of the delta deflection usually ranges from 0.02 to 0.07 second. Depending on the direction of the delta deflection (vectors) in the transverse plane, the Wolff-Parkinson-White syndrome may be classified into three types. In type A Wolff-Parkinson-White syndrome the delta vectors are directed anteriorly, either to the left or slightly to the right. They are anterior to 25°. There is also anterior displacement of the rest of the QRS loop with the maximum QRS vector located in the left anterior quadrant. The direction of inscription of the QRS loop is usually counterclockwise, although a figure eight pattern is occasionally seen. Type A Wolff-Parkinson-White syndrome is generally associated with left-sided accessory pathway.[216] Ventricular preexcitation begins at the epicardium of the posterior basal region of the left ventricle and spreads anteriorly. This direction of impulse conduction probably accounts for the anterior direction of the delta vectors. In type B Wolff-Parkinson-White syndrome the ventricular preexcitation probably begins at the epicardium of the basal portion of the right ventricle at its lateral border. The impulse spreads in a right-to-left direction. Therefore, the delta vectors are oriented to

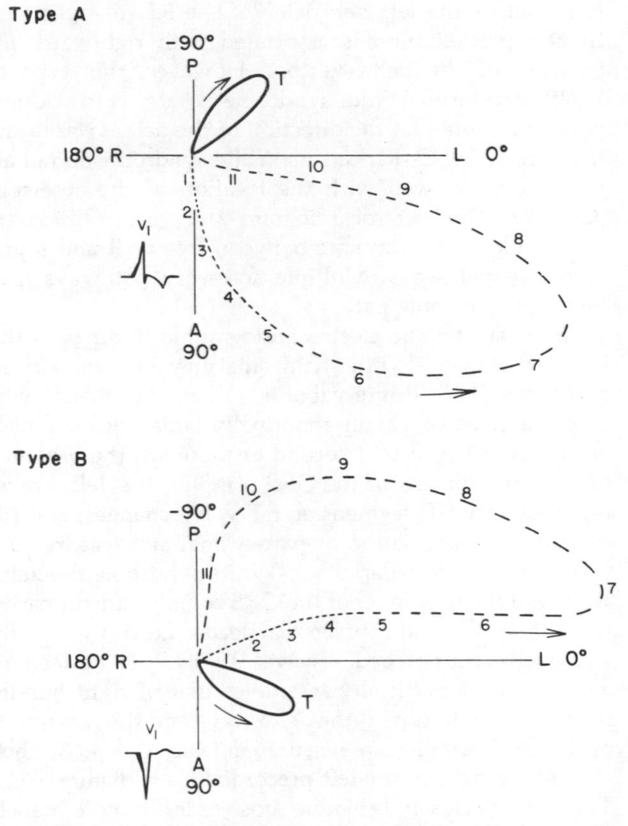

Figure 5.32. Schematic diagrams of the transverse plane QRS and T loops in type A and type B Wolff-Parkinson-White syndrome. In type A the slowly inscribed initial deflection is directed anteriorly, and lead V_1 shows an upright delta wave. In type B the initial deflection of the QRS loop is directed leftward and posteriorly, and the delta wave in lead V_1 is downward.

the left, usually superiorly but sometimes slightly inferiorly. Most of the delta vectors are posterior to 25° in the transverse plane. Most of the QRS loop area is located in the left posterior quadrant. The direction of inscription of the loop is quite variable. In type C Wolff-Parkinson-White syndrome the area of preexcitation is in the lateral

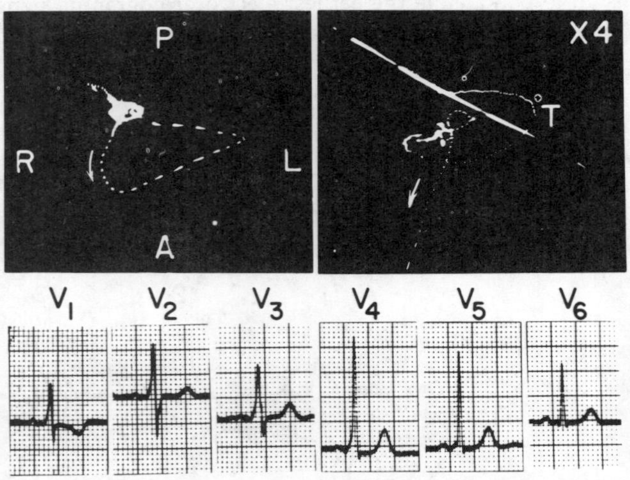

Figure 5.33. Type A Wolff-Parkinson-White syndrome; transverse plane vectocardiogram and the precordial leads of the electrocardiogram are shown.

free wall of the left ventricle.[217] The left-to-right ventricular preexcitation is associated with rightward orientation of the delta vectors. However, this type of Wolff-Parkinson-White syndrome is rare. It is also important to note that the direction of the delta vectors and the type of Wolff-Parkinson-White syndrome do not always correlate well with the location of the accessory pathway. The electrocardiogram and vectorcardiogram are unable to discriminate between free wall and septal accessory pathways. Multiple accessory pathways may be present in some patients.

The characteristic electrocardiographic findings in the Wolff-Parkinson-White syndrome may be summarized as follows: (1) a PR interval of less than 0.12 second, with a normal P wave; (2) an abnormally wide QRS complex with a duration of 0.11 second or more; (3) the presence of an initial slurring of the QRS complex, the delta wave; (4) secondary ST-segment and T-wave changes; and (5) the frequent association of paroxysmal tachycardia.

In type A Wolff-Parkinson-White syndrome the delta wave and the remainder of the QRS complex are primarily upright in all of the precordial leads. Lead V_1 usually shows either a notched R wave, RS, or RSR' deflection. The pattern superficially resembles that of right bundle branch block. In type B the delta wave and the remainder of the QRS complex are negative in leads V_1 and V_2, but they are upright in the left precordial leads (Figure 5.34). The changes closely resemble those of left bundle branch block. In type C the delta wave is negative in leads V_5 and V_6 but positive in leads V_1 to V_4.[218,219]

ELECTROLYTE IMBALANCE

The electrocardiogram is useful in the recognition of electrolyte imbalance, especially relating to potassium and calcium. Abnormalities of these electrolytes alter the normal ionic concentration gradient across the cellular membrane and the movement of the ions. The configuration, duration, and amplitude of the action potential may be changed. On the electrocardiogram, evidence of repolarization, depolarization, or conduction abnormalities is often seen.

In hyperkalemia the earliest electrocardiographic signs of an elevated serum potassium level are tall, narrow, and peaked "tent-shaped" T waves[220] (Figure 5.35). The corrected QT (QTc) interval is either normal or decreased.[221] As the degree of hyperkalemia becomes more severe and the serum potassium concentration exceeds 6.5 mEq/L, the QRS complex often becomes prolonged.[221] As a rule, widening of the QRS complex is diffuse. In extreme cases of hyperkalemia they may appear as sine waves. The P-wave amplitude may also decrease and its duration increase when the serum potassium concentration exceeds 7.0 mEq/L. The P waves become invisible as the concentration increases further.[221] Occasionally, ST-segment elevation suggesting myocardial infarction may occur in advanced hyperkalemia.[222] Atrioventricular block of various degrees including complete AV block may also occur.[223,224] Death in patients with hyperkalemia, however, is usually due to ventricular tachycardia and fibrillation.

The typical electrocardiographic changes in hypokalemia consist of ST-segment depression, lowering of the T-wave amplitude, and prominent U waves (Figure 5.36). These changes are found in more than three-fourths of the patients with a serum potassium level below 2.7 mEq/L.[221] The prominent U waves give a common impression that the QTc interval is prolonged in hypokalemia. When the U wave is excluded, the QT interval is actually not prolonged. There are many other conditions that could increase the amplitude of the U wave. Prominent U waves are seen in patients receiving class I antiarrhythmic drugs such as quinidine and procainamide, and psychotropic drugs such as the phenothiazines. They may be prominent in patients with cerebrovascular accidents. The U-wave amplitude is also increased in bradycardia and left ventricular hypertrophy.

Hypokalemia may cause many types of cardiac arrhythmia such as paroxysmal atrial tachycardia with block, AV dissociation, first and second degree AV block, and ventricular arrhythmias including premature ventricular beats, ventricular tachycardia, and fibrillation.

The effects of abnormal serum concentration of calcium on the electrocardiogram involve mainly the QT interval. Hypercalcemia causes shortening and hypocalcemia lengthening of the QT interval. The changes are mainly at the expense of the ST-segment portion of the QT interval.[221,225–228]

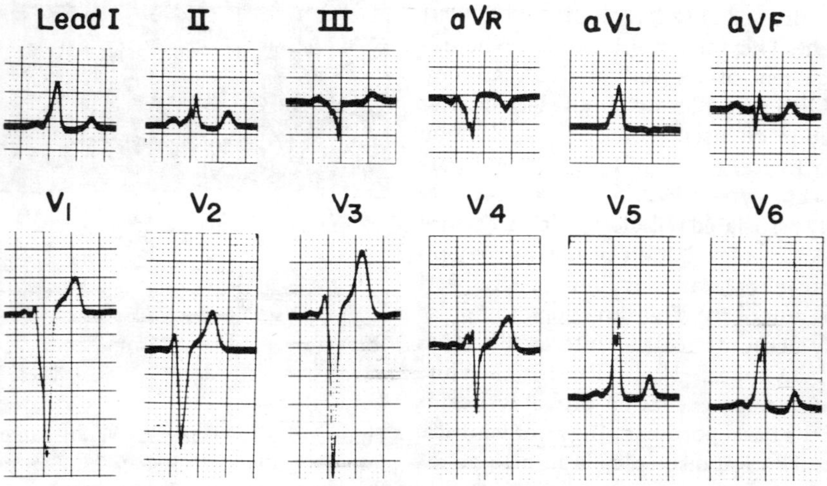

Figure 5.34. Type B Wolff-Parkinson-White syndrome.

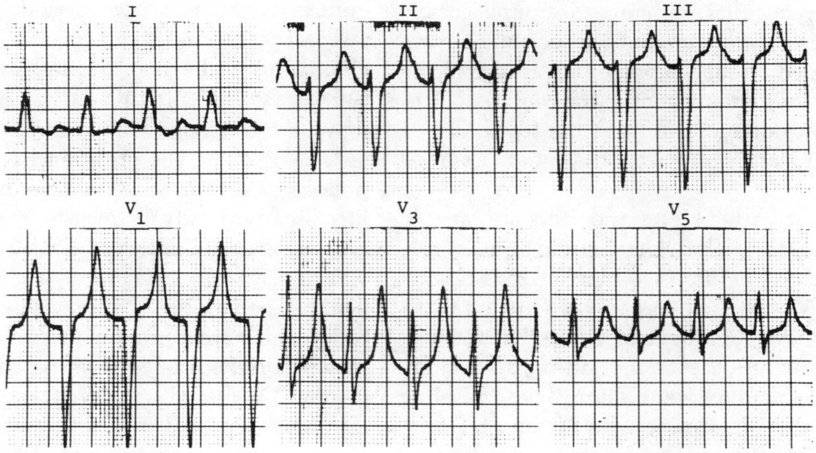

Figure 5.35. Hyperkalemia. The electrocardiogram shows first degree AV block and the P waves are small. The QRS duration is prolonged to 0.14 second. The T waves are tall and peaked. The serum potassium was 8.3 mEq/L shortly before this tracing was obtained. The abnormal left axis deviation was present before hyperkalemia developed. (From Chou,[38] with permission.)

PROLONGED QT INTERVAL

Prolongation of the QT interval has attracted much attention in recent years because of its relation to serious ventricular arrhythmias, syncope, and sudden cardiac death. The association is particularly evident in patients receiving antiarrhythmic agents such as quinidine and procainamide, and in patients with an idiopathic long QT syndrome. Marked asynchrony of ventricular repolarization is probably the underlying mechanism responsible for the development of life-threatening ventricular arrhythmias.[229] Conditions that may be associated with a prolonged QT interval are as follows[99,229,230]:

I. Idiopathic long QT interval syndrome
   A. The Jervell-Lange-Nielson syndrome
   B. The Romano-Ward syndrome
   C. Sporadic long QT syndrome
II. Secondary (acquired) types of QT prolongation
   A. Coronary artery disease: myocardial ischemia and myocardial infarction
   B. Mitral valve prolapse and cardiomyopathy
   C. Central nervous system disease, especially intracranial hemorrhage
   D. Autonomic nervous system dysfunction secondary to radical neck dissection, carotid endarterectomy, and transabdominal truncal vagotomy
   E. Metabolic disturbances: electrolyte imbalance (such as hypocalcemia), liquid protein diet, and intracoronary injection of contrast agents
   F. Cardiac drugs: quinidine, procainamide, disopyramide, and amiodarone
   G. Psychotropic drugs: phenothiazines, tricyclic antidepressants, and lithium
   H. Miscellaneous conditions: severe bradycardia, high-degree AV block, post-Stokes–Adams seizures, hypothyroidism, hypothermia, pheochromocytoma, and organophosphorus poisoning.

AMBULATORY ELECTROCARDIOGRAM

Ambulatory electrocardiogram, also called a Holter electrocardiogram, is recorded with a portable tape recorder while the patient continues usual physical activities.[231] The recording is commonly used to detect cardiac

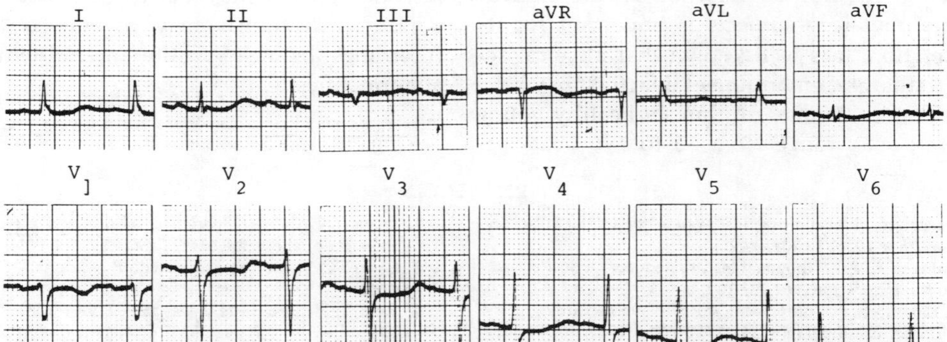

Figure 5.36. Hypokalemia. The serum potassium was 2.7 mEq/L. The electrocardiogram shows diffuse ST-segment depression, T-wave flattening, and prominent U waves. (From Chou,[38] with permission.)

arrhythmias and myocardial ischemia. Scanning equipment is used to select and print out the pertinent parts of the tracing recorded on tape. A major advantage of the ambulatory electrocardiogram over the conventional electrocardiogram or bedside monitoring is the feasibility of correlating the electrocardiogram with the patient's symptoms and activities.

Most of the currently used Holter monitors are capable of recording two leads of the electrocardiogram simultaneously for at least 24 hours. Two bipolar leads resembling leads V_1 and V_5 are used. In patients who are monitored because of chest pain a set of controlled tracings is taken with the patient in the supine, sitting, and standing positions and during hyperventilation. These baseline tracings are essential to determine whether any ST-segment changes are significant. The recorder usually provides a clock and an event marker to be activated when symptoms occur.

Most of the commercially available playback equipment is capable of scanning the tape recording at several different speeds, up to 240 times real time. They differ in their features of computerized recognition, classification, and quantification of ectopic beats. Certain playback systems print out the electrocardiogram from the entire Holter tape in a condensed form, and selected portions of the tracing may then be reproduced at slower paper speed. Others automatically print out a segment of the tape whenever the event marker has been activated. Some provide a 24-hour trend sheet or digital printout to display the heart rate and ST-segment changes in relation to the time of day as well as the number and characteristics of ectopic beats on an hourly basis. With any system the technician scanning the Holter tape plays an important role in obtaining accurate results. The computer interpretation may not always be reliable and artifacts are frequently the cause of error. The technician should also be able to select the pertinent parts of the recording to print out for the physician to analyze and interpret. Therefore, it is essential that the technician is experienced in electrocardiographic interpretation and knows the clinical significance of the common cardiac arrhythmias.

AMBULATORY ELECTROCARDIOGRAM IN NORMAL SUBJECTS

A knowledge of the normal variation on the electrocardiogram of ambulatory subjects is important for its proper interpretation. It is well known that physical activity, mental status, and environmental factors may have a significant effect on cardiac rhythm. In healthy young adults, heart rate may range from 35 to 190 beats per minute during a 24-hour period.[232–234] The slowest heart rate occurs during sleep, usually between 3 and 5 AM. Fluctuation in heart rate is less evident in the elderly.[235] Isolated supraventricular and ventricular ectopic beats may be seen in one half to three fourths of healthy subjects.[232–234,236,237] The prevalence is low and the number of premature ectopic beats is few in young subjects, but it increases with advancing age.[237,238] Complex ventricular ectopic beats are observed occasionally, and short runs of ventricular tachycardia rarely are detected in an otherwise healthy person.[232,234] Short episodes of "benign" atrial tachycardia are common in persons without heart disease.[239] Brief episodes of sinus pauses and first and second degree AV block with Wenckebach phenomenon have also been reported in normal subjects,[232,234,236] mostly in younger persons and during sleep.

INDICATIONS FOR AMBULATORY ELECTROCARDIOGRAM

The common indications for Holter monitoring[239–241] are: (1) evaluation of symptoms such as palpitations, dizziness, and syncope that may be caused by cardiac arrhythmias; (2) evaluation of symptoms that may be due to myocardial ischemia by analysis of the ST-segment changes; (3) detection of arrhythmias that may be of prognostic or therapeutic importance in specific heart disease such as coronary artery disease and cardiomyopathy; (4) evaluation of the therapeutic effects of antiarrhythmic agents; and (5) assessment of cardiac response, such as rhythm and ST-segment changes, to specific physical and emotional stresses that cannot be duplicated readily in the hospital or office.

For optimal utilization of the information supplied by the ambulatory electrocardiogram, the reason for the monitoring should be known to the interpreter. A 12-lead electrocardiogram and a list of medications that the patient is receiving should also be available. The importance of the patient's diary in regard to activities and symptoms cannot be overemphasized. Both positive and negative correlations of electrocardiographic changes and symptoms are equally useful information to be included in the report. Because certain arrhythmias are often observed in otherwise healthy subjects, their clinical significance has to be determined on an individual basis in conjunction with other clinical data. Conversely, important arrhythmias may be missed despite repeated recordings because of the intermittent nature of the abnormalities.

Acknowledgment: I thank Jean Johnson for typing the manuscript and Zenia Frantz for checking the references.

REFERENCES

1. Frank E: An accurate, clinically practical system for spatial vectorcardiography. *Circulation* 1956; 13:737–749.
2. McFee R, Parungao A: An orthogonal lead system for clinical electrocardiography. *Am Heart J* 1961; 62:93–100.
3. Schmitt OH, Simonson E: The present status of vectorcardiography: symposium on electrocardiography. *Arch Intern Med* 1955; 96:574–590.
4. Helm RA: An accurate lead system for spatial vectorcardiography. *Am Heart J* 1957; 53:415–424.
5. Lewis T, Meakins J, White PD: The excitatory process in the dog's heart. Part I. The auricles. *Philos Trans R Soc* 1914; 205B:375.
6. Puech P, Esclavissat M, Sodi-Pallares D, Cisneros F: Normal auricular activation in the dog's heart. *Am Heart J* 1954; 47:174–191.
7. James TN, Sherf L: Specialized tissues and preferential conduction in the atria of the heart. *Am J Cardiol* 1971; 28:414–427.
8. Chou TC, Helm RA: The pseudo P pulmonale. *Circulation* 1965; 32:96–105.
9. Sano T, Hellerstein HK, Vayda E: P vector loop in health and disease as studied by the technique of electrical dissection of the vectorcardiogram (differential vectorcardiography). *Am Heart J* 1957; 53:854–879.
10. Scheuer J, Kahn M, Bleifer S, Donoso E, Grishman A: The atrial vectorcardiogram in health and disease. *Am Heart J* 1960; 60:33–50.
11. Caceres CA, Kelser GA: Duration of the normal P wave. *Am J Cardiol* 1959; 3:449–452.

12. Hiss RG, Lamb LE, Allen MF: Electrocardiographic findings in 67,375 asymptomatic patients. *Am J Cardiol* 1960; 6:200–231.
13. Lamb LE: *Electrocardiography and Vectorcardiography*. Philadelphia, WB Saunders, 1965.
14. Morris JJ Jr, Estes EH Jr, Whalen RE, Thompson HK, McIntosh HD: P-wave analysis in valvular heart disease. *Circulation* 1964; 29:242–252.
15. Charles MA, Benzinger TA, Glasser SP: Atrial injury current in pericarditis. *Arch Intern Med* 1973; 131:657–662.
16. Amer NS, Stuckey JH, Hoffman BF, Cappelletti RR, Domingo RT: Activation of the interventricular septal myocardium studied during cardiopulmonary bypass. *Am Heart J* 1960; 59:224–237.
17. Durrer D, vanDam RT, Freud GE, Janse MJ, Meijler FL, Arzbaecher RC: Total excitation of the isolated human heart. *Circulation* 1970; 41:899–912.
18. Lewis T, Rothschild MA: The excitatory process in the dog's heart. II. The ventricles. *Phil Trans R Soc Lond* 1915; 206B:181–226.
19. Scher AM: The sequence of ventricular excitation. *Am J Cardiol* 1964; 14:287–293.
20. Simonson E: *Differentiation Between Normal and Abnormal in Electrocardiography*. St. Louis, CV Mosby, 1961.
21. Lepeschkin E: Duration of electrocardiographic deflections and intervals: Man. In Altman PL, Dittmer DS (eds): *Respiration and Circulation*. Bethesda, MD, Federation of American Societies for Experimental Biology, 1971, pp 277–278.
22. Kossman CE: The normal electrocardiogram. *Circulation* 1953; 8:920–936.
23. Leatham A: The chest lead electrocardiogram in health. *Br Heart J* 1950; 12:213–231.
24. Manning GW, Smiley JR: QRS-voltage criteria for left ventricular hypertrophy in a normal male population. *Circulation* 1964; 29:224–230.
25. Wasserburger RH, Alt WJ, Lloyd CJ: The normal RS-T segment elevation variant. *Am J Cardiol* 1961; 8:184–192.
26. Simonson E, Cady LD, Woodbury M: The normal Q-T interval. *Am Heart J* 1962; 63:747–753.
27. Bazett HC: An analysis of the time-relations of electrocardiograms. *Heart* 1920; 7:353–370.
28. Lepeschkin E: Physiologic basis of the U wave, in Schlant RC, Hurst JW (eds): *Advances in Electrocardiography*. New York, Grune & Stratton, 1976, Vol 2, pp 353–375.
29. Watanabe Y: Purkinje repolarization as a possible cause of the U wave in the electrocardiogram. *Circulation* 1975; 51:1030–1037.
30. Sano T, Tsuchihashi H, Takigawa S, Shimamoto T: U vector loop or arc in normal subjects and in those with left ventricular hypertrophy. *Am Heart J* 1961; 61:802–810.
31. Lepeschkin E: The U wave of the electrocardiogram. *Mod Conc Cardiovasc Dis* 1969; 38:39–45.
32. Calatayud JB, Abad JM, Khoi NB, Stanbro WW, Silver HM: P-wave changes in chronic obstructive pulmonary disease. *Am Heart J* 1970; 79:444–453.
33. Spodick DH, Hauger-Klevene JH, Tyler JM, Muench H, Dorr CA: The electrocardiogram in pulmonary emphysema: relationship of characteristic electrocardiographic findings to severity of disease as measured by degree of airway obstruction. *Am Rev Respir Dis* 1963; 88:14–19.
34. Shleser IH, Langendorf R: The significance of the so-called P-pulmonale pattern in the electrocardiogram. *Am J Med Sci* 1942; 204:725–734.
35. Sodi-Pallares D, Calder RM: *New Bases of Electrocardiography*. St. Louis, CV Mosby Co, 1956.
36. Saunders JL, Calatayud JB, Schulz KJ, Maranhao V, Gooch AS, Goldberg H: Evaluation of ECG criteria for P-wave abnormalities. *Am Heart J* 1967; 74:757–765.
37. DeOliveira JM, Sambhi MP, Zimmerman HA: The electrocardiogram in pectus excavatum. *Br Heart J* 1958; 20:495–501.
38. Chou TC: *Electrocardiography in Clinical Practice*. New York, Grune & Stratton, 1986, pp 30–31.
39. Abildskov JA: The atrial complex of the electrocardiogram. *Am Heart J* 1959; 57:930–941.
40. Dalton JC, Pearson RJ Jr, White PD: Constrictive pericarditis: a review and long-term follow-up of 78 cases. *Ann Intern Med* 1956; 45:445–458.
41. Thomas P, DeJong D: The P wave in the electrocardiogram in the diagnosis of heart disease. *Br Heart J* 1954; 16:241–254.
42. Romhilt DW, Greenfield JC Jr, Estes EH Jr: Vectorcardiographic diagnosis of left ventricular hypertrophy. *Circulation* 1968; 37:15–19.
43. Varriale P, Alfenito JC, Kennedy RJ: The vectorcardiogram of left ventricular hypertrophy: analysis and criteria (Frank lead system). *Circulation* 1966; 33:569–576.
44. Wallace AG, McCall BW, Estes EH Jr: The vectorcardiogram in left ventricular hypertrophy: a study using the Frank lead system. *Am Heart J* 1962; 63:466–476.
45. Abbott-Smith CW, Chou TC: Vectorcardiographic criteria for the diagnosis of left ventricular hypertrophy. *Am Heart J* 1970; 79:361–369.
46. Gubner R, Ungerleider HE: Electrocardiographic criteria of left ventricular hypertrophy. *Arch Intern Med* 1943; 72:196–209.
47. Sokolow M, Lyon TP: The ventricular complex in left ventricular hypertrophy as obtained by unipolar precordial and limb leads. *Am Heart J* 1949; 37:161–186.
48. McPhie J: Left ventricular hypertrophy: electrocardiographic diagnosis. *Aust Ann Med* 1958; 7:317–327.
49. Romhilt DW, Estes EH: Point-score system for the ECG diagnosis of left ventricular hypertrophy. *Am Heart J* 1968; 75:752–758.
50. Rosenfeld I, Goodrich C, Kassebaum G, Winston AL, Reader G: The electrocardiographic recognition of left ventricular hypertrophy. *Am Heart J* 1962; 63:731–742.
51. Scott RC, Seiwert VJ, Simon DL, McQuire J: Left ventricular hypertrophy: study of accuracy of current electrocardiographic criteria when compared with autopsy findings in one hundred cases. *Circulation* 1955; 11:89–96.
52. Selzer A, Ebnother CL, Packard P, Stone AO, Quinn JE: Reliability of electrocardiographic diagnosis of left ventricular hypertrophy. *Circulation* 1958; 17:255–265.
53. Chou TC, Scott RC, Booth RW, McWhorter HB: Specificity of the current electrocardiographic criteria in the diagnosis of left ventricular hypertrophy. *Am Heart J* 1960; 60:371–377.
54. Chou TC, Helm RA, Kaplan S: *Clinical Vectorcardiography*. New York, Grune & Stratton, 1974, pp 71–84.
55. Chou TC, Helm RA, Kaplan S: *Clinical Vectorcardiography*. New York, Grune & Stratton, 1974, pp 85–114.
56. Chou TC, Masangkay MP, Young P, Conway GF, Helm RA: Simple quantitative vectorcardiographic criteria for the diagnosis of right ventricular hypertrophy. *Circulation* 1973; 48:1262–1267.
57. Cowdery CD, Wagner GS, Starr JW, Rogers G, Greenfield JC Jr: New vectorcardiographic criteria for diagnosing right ventricular hypertrophy in mitral stenosis: comparison with electrocardiographic criteria. *Circulation* 1980; 62:1026–1032.
58. Barker JM, Valencia F: The precordial electrocardiogram in incomplete right bundle branch block. *Am Heart J* 1949; 38:376–406.
59. Myers GB, Klein HA, Stofer BE: The electrocardiographic diagnosis of right ventricular hypertrophy. *Am Heart J* 1948; 35:1–40.
60. Sokolow M, Lyon TP: The ventricular complex in right ventricular hypertrophy as obtained by unipolar precordial and limb leads. *Am Heart J* 1949; 38:273–294.
61. Scott RC: The electrocardiographic diagnosis of right ventricular hypertrophy in the adult. *Heart Bull* 1967; 16:65–67.
62. Flowers NC, Horan LG: Subtle signs of right ventricular enlargement and their relative importance, in Schlant RC, Hurst JW (eds): *Advances in Electrocardiography*. New York, Grune & Stratton, 1972, pp 297–308.
63. Cueto J, Toshima H, Armijo G, Tuna N, Lillehei W: Vectorcardiographic studies in acquired valvular disease with reference to the diagnosis of right ventricular hypertrophy. *Circulation* 1966; 33:588–598.
64. Gamboa R, Hugenholtz PG, Nadas AS: Corrected (Frank), uncorrected (Cube), and standard electrocardiographic lead systems in recording augmented right ventricular forces in right ventricular hypertension. *Br Heart J* 1966; 28:62–74.
65. McCaughan D, Koroxenidis GT, Hopff LG, Williams C: New vector cardiographic criteria for the diagnosis of acquired right ventricular hypertrophy: comparison with standard electrocardiographic criteria (abstr). *Circulation* 1963; 28:766.
66. Curtiss EI, Cecchetti AA: QRS loop areas in selective right ventricular overload: relation to hemodynamic status. *J Electrocardiol* 1983; 16:53–58.
67. Becker RA, Scher AM, Erickson RV: Ventricular excitation in experimental left bundle branch block. *Am Heart J* 1958; 55:547–556.
68. Grant RP: Left axis deviation. An electrocardiographic-pathologic correlation study. *Circulation* 1956; 14:233–249.
69. Lepeschkin E: The electrocardiographic diagnosis of bilateral bundle branch block in relation to heart block. *Prog Cardiovasc Dis* 1964; 6:445–471.
70. Pryor R, Blount SG Jr: The clinical significance of true left axis deviation. *Am Heart J* 1966; 72:391–413.
71. Rosenbaum MB, Elizari MV, Lazzari JO: *The Hemiblocks*. Oldsmar, Fla, Tampa Tracings, 1970.
72. Rosenbaum MB: The hemiblocks: diagnostic criteria and clinical significance. *Mod Conc Cardiovasc Dis* 1970; 39:141–146.
73. Benchimol A, Barreto EC, Pedraza A: The Frank vectorcardiogram in left anterior hemiblock. *J Electrocardiol* 1971; 4:116–128.
74. Chou TC, Helm RA, Kaplan S: *Clinical Vectorcardiography*. New York, Grune & Stratton, 1974, pp 147–185.
75. Kulbertus H, Collignon P, Humblet L: Vectorcardiographic study of the QRS loop in patients with left anterior focal block. *Am Heart J* 1970; 79:293–304.
76. Medrano GA, Brenes C, DeMicheli A, Sodi-Pallares D: Clinical electrocardiographic and vectorcardiographic diagnosis of left anterior subdivision block isolated or associated with RBBB. *Am Heart J* 1972; 83:447–458.
77. Benchimol A, Desser KB: The Frank vectorcardiogram in left posterior hemiblock. *J Electrocardiol* 1971; 4:129–136.

78. Grant RP: Left axis deviation. *Mod Conc Cardiovasc Dis* 1958; 27:437–440.
79. Burchell HB, Tuna N: The interpretation of gross left axis deviation in the electrocardiogram. *Eur J Cardiol* 1979; 10:259–277.
80. Fernandez F, Scebat L, Lenegre J: Electrocardiographic study of left intraventricular hemiblock in man during selective coronary arteriography. *Am J Cardiol* 1970; 26:1–5.
81. Rabkin SW, Mathewson FAL, Tate RB: Natural history of marked left axis deviation (left anterior hemiblock). *Am J Cardiol* 1979; 43:605–610.
82. McHenry PL, Phillips JF, Fisch C, Corya BR: Right precordial qrS pattern due to left anterior hemiblock. *Am Heart J* 1971; 81:498–502.
83. Pryor R: Fascicular blocks and the bilateral bundle branch block syndrome. *Am Heart J* 1972; 83:441–446.
84. Rizzon R, Rossi L, Baissus C, Demoulin C, DiBiase M: Left posterior hemiblock in acute myocardial infarction. *Br Heart J* 1975; 37:711–720.
85. Erickson RV, Scher AM, Becker RA: Ventricular excitation in experimental bundle-branch block. *Circ Res* 1957; 5:5–10.
86. Chou TC, Helm RA, Kaplan S: *Clinical Vectorcardiography*. New York, Grune & Stratton, 1974, pp 131–146.
87. Penaloza D, Gamboa R, Sime F: Experimental right bundle branch block in the normal human heart: electrocardiographic, vectorcardiographic and hemodynamic observations. *Am J Cardiol* 1961; 8:767–779.
88. Scherlis L, Lee Y-C: Right bundle branch block following open heart surgery: electrocardiographic and vectorcardiographic study. *Am J Cardiol* 1961; 8: 780–791.
89. Krongard E, Hefler SE, Bowman FO, Malm JR, Hoffman BF: Further observations on the etiology of the right bundle branch block pattern following right ventriculotomy. *Circulation* 1974; 50:1105–1113.
90. Okoroma EO, Guller B, Maloney JD, Weidman WH: Etiology of right bundle-branch block pattern after surgical closure of ventricular septal defects. *Am Heart J* 1975; 90:14–18.
91. Horowitz LN, Alexander JA, Edmunds LH: Postoperative right bundle branch block: identification of three levels of block. *Circulation* 1980; 62:319–328.
92. Rosenbaum MB, Elizari MV, Lazzari JO, Nau GS, Levi RJ, Halpern MS: Intraventricular trifascicular blocks. Review of the literature and classification. *Am Heart J* 1969; 78:450–459.
93. Kulbertus H, Collignon P, Humblet L: Vectorcardiographic study of QRS loop patients with left superior axis deviation and right bundle-branch block. *Br Heart J* 1970; 32:386–392.
94. Medrano GA, Brenes C, DeMicheli A, Sodi-Pallares D: Clinical electrocardiographic and vectorcardiographic diagnosis of the left anterior subdivision block isolated or associated with RBBB. *Am Heart J* 1972; 83:447–458.
95. Pryor R: Fascicular blocks and the bilateral bundle branch block syndrome. *Am Heart J* 1972; 83:441–446.
96. Varriale P, Kennedy RJ: Right bundle branch block and left posterior fascicular block. Vectorcardiographic and clinical features. *Am J Cardiol* 1972; 29:459–465.
97. Prinzmetal M, Shaw C McK Jr, Maxwell MH, Flamm EJ, Goldman A, Kimura N, Rakita L, Borduas JL, Rothman S, Kennamer R: Studies of the mechanism of ventricular activity. VI. The depolarization complex in pure subendocardial infarction; role of the subendocardial region in the normal electrocardiogram. *Am J Med* 1954; 16:469–489.
98. Samson WE, Scher AM: Mechanism of S-T segment alteration during acute myocardial injury. *Circ Res* 1960; 8:780–787.
99. Surawicz B: The pathogenesis and clinical significance of primary T-wave abnormalities, in Schlant RC, Hurst JW (eds): *Advances in Electrocardiography*. New York, Grune & Stratton, 1972, pp 377–421.
100. Chou TC, Helm RA, Kaplan S: *Clinical Vectorcardiography*. New York, Grune & Stratton, 1974, pp 187–254.
101. Chou TC, Helm RA, Lach R: The significance of a wide TsE loop. *Circulation* 1964; 30:400–410.
102. Gunnar RM, Pietras RJ, Blackaller J, Dadmun SE, Szanto PB, Tobin JR Jr: Correlation of vectorcardiographic criteria for myocardial infarction with autopsy findings. *Circulation* 1967; 35:158–171.
103. Gunnar RM, Winslow EBJ, Cabin G, Pietras R, Rosewall J, Szanto R: Autopsy correlation of vectorcardiographic criteria for the diagnosis of myocardial infarction, in Hoffman I, Hamby RI, Glassman E (eds): *Vectorcardiography 2*. Amsterdam, North Holland Pub Co, 1971, pp 333–342.
104. Hoffman I, Taymor RC, Gootnick A: Vectorcardiographic residua of inferior infarction. Seventy-eight cases studied with the Frank system. *Circulation* 1964; 29:562–576.
105. Hoffman I, Taymor RC, Morris MH, Kittell I: Quantitative criteria for the diagnosis of dorsal infarction using the Frank vectorcardiogram. *Am Heart J* 1965; 70:295–304.
106. Hugenholtz PG, Whipple GH, Levine HD: A clinical appraisal of the vectorcardiogram in myocardial infarction. I. The cube system. *Circulation* 1961; 24:808–824.
107. Mathur VS, Levine HD: Vectorcardiographic differentiation between right ventricular hypertrophy and posterobasal myocardial infarctions (abstr). *Am J Cardiol* 1966; 17:131.
108. McConahay DR, McCallister BD, Hallermann FJ, Smith RE: Comparative quantitative analysis of the electrocardiogram and the vectorcardiogram. Correlations with the coronary arteriogram. *Circulation* 1970; 42:245–259.
109. Young E, Williams C: The frontal plane vectorcardiogram in old inferior myocardial infarction. Criteria for diagnosis and electrocardiographic correlation. *Circulation* 1968; 37:604–623.
110. Young E, Levine HD, Vokonas PS, Kemp HG, Williams RA, Gorlin R: The frontal plane vectorcardiogram in old inferior myocardial infarction. II. Mid-to-late QRS changes. *Circulation* 1970; 42:1143–1162.
111. Barker JM: *The Unipolar Electrocardiogram: A Clinical Interpretation*. New York, Appleton-Century-Crofts, 1952.
112. Braat S, Brugada P, DeZwaan C, Coenegracht JM, Wellens HJJ: Value of electrocardiogram in diagnosing right ventricular involvement in patients with an acute inferior wall myocardial infarction. *Br Heart J* 1983; 49:368–372.
113. Candell-Riera J, Figueras J, Valle V, Alvarex A, Gutierrez L, Cortadellas J, Cinca J, Salas A, Rius J: Right ventricular infarction: Relationships between ST segment elevation in V_{4R} and hemodynamic, scintigraphic, and echocardiographic findings in patients with acute inferior myocardial infarction. *Am Heart J* 1981; 101:281–287.
114. Chou TC, van der Bel-Kahn J, Allen J, Brockmeier L, Fowler NO: Electrocardiographic diagnosis of right ventricular infarction. *Am J Med* 1981; 70:1175–1180.
115. Croft CH, Nicod P, Corbett JR, Lewis SE, Huxley R, Mukharji J, Willerson JT, Rude RE: Detection of acute right ventricular infarction by right precordial electrocardiography. *Am J Cardiol* 1982; 50:421–427.
116. Goldberger E: *Unipolar Lead Electrocardiography and Vectorcardiography* ed 3. Philadelphia, Lea & Febiger, 1953.
117. Myers GB, Klein HA, Hiratzka T: II. Correlation of electrocardiographic and pathologic findings in large anterolateral infarcts. *Am Heart J* 1948; 36:838–881.
118. Myers GB, Klein HA, Hiratzka T: V. Correlation of electrocardiographic and pathologic findings in posterior infarction. *Am Heart J* 1949; 38:547–592.
119. Myers GB, Klein HA, Hiratzka T: VI. Correlation of electrocardiographic and pathologic findings in posterolateral infarction. *Am Heart J* 1949; 38:837–862.
120. Myers GB, Klein HA, Stofer BE: VII. Correlation of electrocardiographic and pathologic findings in lateral infarction. *Am Heart J* 1949; 37:374–417.
121. Perloff JK: The recognition of strictly posterior myocardial infarction by conventional scalar electrocardiography. *Circulation* 1964; 30:706–718.
122. Essen RV, Merx W, Effert S: Spontaneous course of ST-segment elevation in acute anterior myocardial infarction. *Circulation* 1979; 59:105–112.
123. Zmyslinski RW, Akiyama T, Biddle TL, Shah PM: Natural course of the S-T segment and QRS complex in patients with acute anterior myocardial infarction. *Am J Cardiol* 1979; 43:29–34.
124. Mills RM, Young E, Gorlin R, Lesch M: Natural history of S-T segment elevation after acute myocardial infarction. *Am J Cardiol* 1975; 35:609–614.
125. Gibson RS, Crampton RS, Watson DD, Taylor GJ, Carabello BA, Holt ND, Beller GA: Precordial ST-segment depression during acute inferior myocardial infarction: clinical, scintigraphic and angiographic correlations. *Circulation* 1982; 66:732–741.
126. Goldberg HL, Borer JS, Jacobstein JG, Kluger J, Scheidt SS, Alonso DR: Anterior S-T segment depression in acute inferior myocardial infarction: indicator of posterolateral infarction. *Am J Cardiol* 1981; 48:1009–1015.
127. Haraphongse M, Tanomsup S, Jugdutt BI: Inferior ST segment depression during acute anterior myocardial infarction: clinical and angiographic correlations. *J Am Coll Cardiol* 1984; 4:467–476.
128. Salcedo JR, Baird MG, Chambers RJ, Beanlands DS: Significance of reciprocal S-T segment depression in anterior precordial leads in acute inferior myocardial infarction: concomitant left anterior descending coronary artery disease? *Am J Cardiol* 1981; 48:1003–1008.
129. Shah PK, Pichler M, Berman DS, Maddahi J, Peter T, Singh BH, Swan HJC: Non-invasive identification of a high-risk subset of patients with acute inferior myocardial infarction. *Am J Cardiol* 1980; 46:915–921.
130. Croft CH, Woodward W, Nicod P, Corbett JR, Lewis SE, Willerson JT, Rude RE: Clinical implications of anterior S-T segment depression in patients with acute inferior myocardial infarction. *Am J Cardiol* 1982; 50:428–436.
131. Fuchs RM, Achuff SC, Grunwald L, Yin FCP, Griffith LSC: Electrocardiographic localization of coronary artery narrowings: studies during myocardial ischemia and infarction in patients with one-vessel disease. *Circulation* 1982; 66:1168–1176.
132. Dressler W, Roesler H: High T waves in the earliest stage of infarction. *Am Heart J* 1947; 34:627–645.
133. Wasserburger RH, Alt WJ: The normal RS-T segment elevation variant. *Am J Cardiol* 1961; 8:184–192.

134. Anderssen N, Skjaeggestad O: The electrocardiogram in patients with previous myocardial infarction. *Acta Med Scand* 1964; 176:123–126.
135. Cox CJB: Return to normal of the electrocardiogram after myocardial infarction. *Lancet* 1967; 1:1194–1197.
136. Kalbfleisch JM, Shadaksharappa KS, Conrad LL, Sarkar NK: Disappearance of the Q-deflection following myocardial infarction. *Am Heart J* 1968; 76:193–198.
137. Kaplan BM, Berkson DM: Serial electrocardiogram after myocardial infarction. *Ann Intern Med* 1964; 60:430–435.
138. Cook RW, Edwards JE, Pruitt RD: Electrocardiographic changes in acute subendocardial infarction. I. Large subendocardial and large nontransmural infarcts. *Circulation* 1958; 18:603–612.
139. Georas CS, Dahlquist E, Cutts FB: Subendocardial infarction. Correlation of clinical, electrocardiographic, and pathologic data in 17 cases. *Arch Intern Med* 1963; 111:146–155.
140. Lown B, Vassaux C, Hood WB, Fakhro AM, Kaplinsky E, Roberge G: Unresolved problems in coronary care. *Am J Cardiol* 1967; 20:494–508.
141. Rosenberg BA, Malach M: Acute myocardial infarction in a city hospital: follow-up study of 131 survivors. *Am J Cardiol* 196l; 8:799–806.
142. Stimmel B, Katz AM, Donoso E: Q-wave development in acute subendocardial infarction. *Arch Intern Med* 1973; 131:676–678.
143. Freifeld AG, Schuster EH, Bulkley BH: Nontransmural versus transmural myocardial infarction. *Am J Med* 1983; 75:423–432.
144. Myers GB, Sears CH, Hiratzka T: Correlation of electrocardiographic and pathologic findings in ringlike subendocardial infarction of the left ventricle. *Am J Med Sci* 1951; 222:417–426.
145. Raunio H, Rossanen V, Romppanen T, Jokinen Y, Rehnberg S, Helin M, Pyorala K: Changes in the QRS complex and ST segment in transmural and subendocardial myocardial infarctions. A clinicopathologic study. *Am Heart J* 1979; 98:176–184.
146. Savage RM, Wagner GS, Ideker RE, Podolsky SA, Hackel DB: Correlation of postmortem anatomic findings with electrocardiographic changes in patients with myocardial infarction. *Circulation* 1977; 55:279–285.
147. Sullivan W, Vlodaver Z, Tuna N, Long L, Edwards JE: Correlation of electrocardiographic and pathologic findings in healed myocardial infarction. *Am J Cardiol* 1978; 42:724–732.
148. Yu PN, Stewart JM: Subendocardial myocardial infarction with special reference to the electrocardiographic changes. *Am Heart J* 1950; 39:862–880.
149. Forman MB, Goodin J, Phelan B, Kopelman H, Virmani R: Electrocardiographic changes associated with isolated right ventricular infarction. *J Am Coll Cardiol* 1984; 4:640–643.
150. Isner JM, Roberts WC: Right ventricular infarction complicating left ventricular infarction secondary to coronary heart disease. Frequency, location, associated findings and significance from analysis of 236 necropsy patients with acute or healed myocardial infarction. *Am J Cardiol* 1978; 42:885–894.
151. Ratliff NB, Hackel DB: Combined right and left ventricular infarction: pathogenesis and clinicopathologic correlations. *Am J Cardiol* 1980; 45:217–221.
152. Wartman WB, Hellerstein HK: The incidence of heart disease in 2,000 consecutive autopsies. *Ann Intern Med* 1948; 28:41–65.
153. Erhardt LR, Sjogren A, Wahlberg I: Single right-sided precordial lead in the diagnosis of right ventricular involvement in inferior myocardial infarction. *Am Heart J* 1976; 91:571–576.
154. Cardenas M, Diaz del Rio A, Gonzalez-Hemosillo JA, deLeon O, Renteria V, Verdejo J: El infarto agudo del miocardio del ventriculo derecho. *Arch Inst Cardiol Mex* 1980; 50:295–312.
155. Chou TC, Fowler NO, Gabel M, van der Bel-Kahn J, Feltner EJ: Electrocardiographic and hemodynamic changes in experimental right ventricular infarction. *Circulation* 1983; 67:1258–1267.
156. Burch GE, Horan LG, Ziskind J, Cronvich JA: A correlative study of postmortem electrocardiographic and spatial vectorcardiographic data in myocardial infarction. *Circulation* 1958; 18:325–340.
157. Horan LG, Flowers NC, Johnson JC: Significance of the diagnostic Q wave of myocardial infarction. *Circulation* 1971; 43:428–436.
158. Weiss MM, Weiss MM Jr: The electrocardiogram in myocardial infarction *Arch Intern Med* 1958; 101:1126–1128.
159. Woods JD, Laurie W, Smith WG: The reliability of the electrocardiogram in myocardial infarction. *Lancet* 1963; 2:265–269.
160. Wolff L, Wolff R, Samartzis MD, Mazzoleni A, Soffe AM, Reiner L, Matsuoka S: Vectorcardiographic diagnosis: a correlation with autopsy findings in 167 cases. *Circulation* 1961; 23:861–880.
161. Hugenholtz PG, Forkner CE Jr, Levine HD: A clinical appraisal of the vectorcardiogram in myocardial infarction. II. The Frank system. *Circulation* 1961; 24:825–850.
162. Starr JW, Wagner GS, Behar VS, Walston A, Greenfield JC: vectorcardiographic criteria for the diagnosis of inferior myocardial infarction. *Circulation* 1974; 49:829–836.
163. Starr JW, Wagner GS, Draffin RM, Reed JB, Walston A, Behar VS: Vectorcardiographic criteria for the diagnosis of anterior myocardial infarction. *Circulation* 1976; 53:229–234.
164. Littman D: The electrocardiographic findings in pulmonary emphysema. *Am J Cardiol* 1960; 5:339–348.
165. Murata K, Hashiba K, Ikeda M, Seki M: QS- and QR-pattern in leads V_3 and V_4: electrocardiographic and pathologic correlation of 41 cases, including 25 cases without myocardial infarction. *Jpn Cir J* 1963; 27:359–366.
166. Phillips JH, Burch GE: Problems in the diagnosis of cor pulmonale. *Am Heart J* 1963; 66:818–832.
167. Surawicz B, VanHorne RG, Urbach JR, Bellet S: QS- and QR-pattern in leads V_3 and V_4 in absence of myocardial infarction. Electrocardiographic and vectorcardiographic study. *Circulation* 1955; 12:391–405.
168. Armen RN, Frank TV: Electrocardiographic patterns in pneumothorax. *Dis Chest* 1949; 15:709–719.
169. Copeland RB, Omenn GS: Electrocardiogram changes suggestive of coronary artery disease in pneumothorax. Their reversibility with upright posture. *Arch Intern Med* 1970; 125:151–153.
170. Chou TC: Pseudo-infarction (noninfarction Q waves). *Cardiovasc Clin* 1973; 5:199–218.
171. Cutforth RH, Oram S: The electrocardiogram in pulmonary embolism. *Br Heart J* 1958; 20:41–60.
172. McGinn S, White PD: Acute cor pulmonale resulting from pulmonary embolism. *JAMA* 1935; 104:1473–1480.
173. Phillips E, Levine HD: A critical evaluation of extremity and precordial electrocardiography in acute cor pulmonale. *Am Heart J* 1950; 39:205–216.
174. Romhilt D, Susilavorn B, Chou TC: Unusual electrocardiographic manifestation of pulmonary embolism. *Am Heart J* 1970; 80:237–241.
175. Braudo M, Wigle ED, Keith JD: A distinctive electrocardiogram in muscular subaortic stenosis due to ventricular septal hypertrophy. *Am J Cardiol* 1964; 14:599–607.
176. Frank S, Braunwald E: Idiopathic hypertrophic subaortic stenosis. *Circulation* 1968; 37:759–788.
177. Marriott HJL: Electrocardiographic abnormalities, conduction disorders and arrhythmias in primary myocardial disease. *Prog Cardiovasc Dis* 1964; 7:99–114.
178. Perloff JK, Roberts WC, DeLeon AC, O'Doherty D: The distinctive electrocardiogram of Duchenne's progressive muscular dystrophy. *Am J Med* 1967; 42:179–188.
179. Slucka C: The electrocardiogram in Duchenne progressive muscular dystrophy. *Circulation* 1968; 38:933–940.
180. Hejtmancik MR, Bradfield JY, Miller GV: Myocarditis and Friedreich's ataxia. *Am Heart J* 1949; 38:757–765.
181. Sackner MA, Heinz ER, Steinberg AJ: The heart in scleroderma. *Am J Cardiol* 1966; 17:542–559.
182. Windesheim JH, Parkin TW: Electrocardiograms of ninety patients with acrosclerosis and progressive diffuse sclerosis (scleroderma). *Circulation* 1959; 17:874–881.
183. Buja LM, Khoi NB, Roberts WC: Clinically significant cardiac amyloidosis. *Am J Cardiol* 1970; 26:394–405.
184. Geha AS, Weidman WH, Soule EH, McGoon DC: Intramural ventricular cardiac fibroma. Successful removal in two cases and review of the literature. *Circulation* 1967; 36:427–440.
185. Harris TR, Copeland GD, Brody DA: Progressive injury current with metastatic tumor of the heart. Case report and review of the literature. *Am Heart J* 1965; 69:392–400.
186. Chou TC, Susilavorn B: Electrocardiographic-pathological conference. Electrocardiographic changes in intracranial hemorrhage. *J Electrocardiol* 1969; 2:193–196.
187. Cropp GJ, Manning GW: Electrocardiographic changes simulating myocardial ischemia and infarction associated with spontaneous intracranial hemorrhage. *Circulation* 1960; 22:25–38.
188. Levine HD, Wanzer SH, Merrill JP: Dialyzable currents of injury in potassium intoxication resembling acute myocardial infarction or pericarditis. *Circulation* 1956; 13:29–36.
189. Horan LG, Flowers NC, Tolleson WJ, Thomas JR: The significance of diagnostic Q waves in the presence of bundle branch block. *Chest* 1970; 58:214–221.
190. Scott RC: Left bundle branch block: a clinical assessment. Part II. *Am Heart J* 1965; 70:691–712.
191. Sodi-Pallares D, Cisneros F, Medrano GA, Bisteni A, Testelli MR, deMicheli A: Electrocardiographic diagnosis of myocardial infarction in the presence of bundle branch block (right and left), ventricular premature beats and Wolff-Parkinson-White syndrome. *Prog Cardiovasc Dis* 1963; 6:107–136.
192. Wolff L, Richman JL: The diagnosis of myocardial infarction in patients with anomalous atrioventricular excitation (Wolff-Parkinson-White syndrome). *Am Heart J* 1953; 45:545–570.
193. Cheng TO, Bashour T, Kelser GA, Weiss L, Bacos J: Variant angina of Prinzmetal with normal coronary arteriograms: a variant of the variant. *Circulation* 1973; 47:476–485.
194. Cheng TO, Bashour T, Singh BK, Kelser GA: Myocardial infarction in the absence of coronary arteriosclerosis. Result of spasm? *Am J. Cardiol* 1972; 30:680–682.

195. Hart NJ, Silverman ME, King SB: Variant angina caused by coronary artery spasm. *Am J Med* 1974; 56:269–274.
196. Maseri A, L'Abbate A, Chierchia S, Parodi O, Severi S, Biagini A, Distante A, Marzilli M, Ballestra AM: Significance of spasm in the pathogenesis of ischemic heart disease. *Am J Cardiol* 1979; 44:788–792.
197. Maseri A, L'Abbate A, Baroldi G, Chierchia S, Marzilli M, Ballestra AM, Severi S, Parodi O, Biagini A, Distante A, Pesola A: Coronary vasospasm as a possible cause of myocardial infarction. A conclusion derived from the study of "preinfarction" angina. *N Engl J Med* 1978; 299:1271–1277.
198. Oliva PB, Breckinridge JC: Arteriographic evidence of coronary arterial spasm in acute myocardial infarction. *Circulation* 1977; 56:366–374.
199. Oliva PB, Potts DE, Pluss RG: Coronary arterial spasm in Prinzmetal angina. Documentation by coronary arteriography. *N Engl J Med* 1973; 288:745–751.
200. Prinzmetal M, Ekmekci A, Kennamer R, Kwoczynski JK, Shubin H, Toyoshima H: Variant form of angina pectoris. Previously undelineated syndrome. *JAMA* 1960; 174:1794–1800.
201. Prinzmetal M, Kennamer R, Merliss R, Wada T, Bor N: Angina pectoris. I. A variant form of angina pectoris; preliminary report. *Am J Med* 1959; 27:375–388.
202. Bellet S, McMillan TM: Electrocardiographic patterns in acute pericarditis. Evolution, causes and diagnostic significance of patterns in limb and chest leads; a study of 57 cases. *Arch Intern Med* 1938; 61:381–400.
203. Spodick DH: The electrocardiogram in acute pericarditis: distributions of morphologic and axial changes in stages. *Am J Cardiol* 1974; 33:470–474.
204. Spodick DH: Diagnostic electrocardiographic sequences in acute pericarditis. Significance of PR segment and PR vector changes. *Circulation* 1973; 48:575–580.
205. Spodick DH: Differential diagnosis of acute pericarditis. *Prog Cardiovasc Dis* 1971; 14:192–209.
206. Littman D, Spodick DH: Total electrical alternation in pericardial disease. *Circulation* 1958; 17:912–917.
207. Wolferth CC, Wood FC: The mechanism of production of short P-R intervals and prolonged QRS complexes in patients with presumably undamaged hearts: hypothesis of an accessory pathway of auriculoventricular conduction (bundle of Kent). *Am Heart J* 1933; 8:297–311.
208. Sealy WC, Gallagher JJ, Pritchett ELC: The surgical anatomy of Kent bundles based on electrophysiological mapping and surgical exploration. *J Thorac Cardiovasc Surg* 1978; 76:804–815.
209. Lown B, Ganong WF, Levine SA: The syndrome of short P-R interval, normal QRS complex and paroxysmal rapid heart action. *Circulation* 1952; 5:693–706.
210. James TN: Morphology of the human atrioventricular node, with remarks pertinent to its electrophysiology. *Am Heart J* 1961; 62:756–771.
211. Mahaim I, Winston MR: Recherches d'anatomie comparée et de pathologie experimentale sur les connexions hautes du faisceau de His-Taware. *Cardiologie* 1941; 5:189–260.
212. Gillette PC: Concealed anomalous cardiac conduction pathways: a frequent cause of supraventricular tachycardia. *Am J Cardiol* 1977; 40:848–852.
213. Sung RJ, Gelband H, Castellanos A, Aranda JM, Myerburg RJ: Clinical and electrophysiologic observations in patients with concealed accessory atrioventricular bypass tracts. *Am J Cardiol* 1977; 40:839–847.
214. Wellens HJJ, Durrer D: The role of an accessory atrioventricular pathway in reciprocal tachycardia. Observations in patients with and without the Wolff-Parkinson-White syndrome. *Circulation* 1975; 52:58–72.
215. Wellens HJJ: Wolff-Parkinson-White syndrome. I. Diagnosis, arrhythmias, and identification of the high risk patient. *Mod Conc Cardiovasc Dis* 1983; 52:53–56.
216. Tonkin AM, Wagner GS, Gallagher JJ, Cope GD, Kasell J, Wallace AG: Initial forces of ventricular depolarization in the Wolff-Parkinson-White syndrome. *Circulation* 1975; 52:1030–1036.
217. Gallagher JJ, Pritchett ELC, Sealy WC, Kosell J, Wallace AG: The preexcitation syndromes. *Prog Cardiovasc Dis* 1978; 20:285–327.
218. Ferrer MI: *Pre-Excitation, Including the Wolff-Parkinson-White and Other Related Syndromes*. Mount Kisco, NY, Futura Publ Co, 1976.
219. Lev M, Fox SM, Bharati S, Greenfield JC Jr, Rosen KM, Pick A: Mahaim and James fibers as a basis for a unique variety of ventricular preexcitation. *Am J Cardiol* 1975; 36:880–888.
220. Levine HD, Vazifdar JP, Lown B, Merrill JP: "Tent-shaped" T waves of normal amplitude in potassium intoxication. *Am Heart J* 1952; 43:437–450.
221. Surawicz B: Relationship between electrocardiogram and electrolytes. *Am Heart J* 1967; 73:814–834.
222. Levine HD, Wanzer SH, Merrill JP: Dialyzable currents of injury in potassium intoxication resembling acute myocardial infarction of pericarditis. *Circulation* 1956; 13:29–36.
223. Surawicz B: Role of electrolytes in etiology and management of cardiac arrhythmias. *Prog Cardiovasc Dis* 1966; 8:364–386.
224. Levine HD, Merrill JP, Somerville W: Advanced disturbances in cardiac mechanisms in potassium poisoning. *Circulation* 1951; 3:889–905.
225. Bronsky D, Dubin A, Waldstein SS, Kushner DS: Calcium and the electrocardiogram. I. The electrocardiographic manifestations of hyperparathyroidism. *Am J Cardiol* 1961; 7:823–832.
226. Bronsky D, Dubin A. Waldstein SS, Kushner DS: Calcium and the electrocardiogram. II. The electrocardiographic manifestations of hyperparathyroidism and of marked hypercalcemia from various other etiologies. *Am J Cardiol* 1961; 7:833–839.
227. Bronsky D, Dubin S, Kushner DS, Waldstein SS: Calcium and the electrocardiogram. III. The relationship of the intervals of the electrocardiogram to the level of serum calcium. *Am J Cardiol* 1961; 7:840–843.
228. Nierenberg DW, Ransil BJ: Q-aTc interval as a clinical indicator of hypercalcemia. *Am J Cardiol* 1979; 44:243–248.
229. Surawicz B, Knoebel SB, Long QT: Good, bad or indifferent? *J Am Coll Cardiol* 1984; 4:398–413.
230. Moss AJ, Schwartz PJ: Delayed repolarization (QT or QTU prolongation) and malignant ventricular arrhythmias. *Mod Conc Cardiovasc Dis* 1982; 51:85–90.
231. Holter, NJ: New method for heart studies. Continuous electrocardiography of active subjects over long periods is now practical. *Science* 1961; 134:1213–1220.
232. Brodsky M, Wu D, Denes P, Kanakis C, Rosen KM: Arrhythmias documented by 24 hour continuous electrocardiographic monitoring in 50 male medical students without apparent heart disease. *Am J Cardiol* 1977; 39:390–395.
233. Kostis JB, Moreyra AE, Amendo MI, Pietro JD, Cosgrove N, Kuo PT: The effect of age on heart rate in subjects free of heart disease. Studies by ambulatory electrocardiography and maximal exercise stress test. *Circulation* 1982; 65:141–145.
234. Sobotka PA, Mayer JH, Bauernfeind RA, Kanakis C, Rosen KM: Arrhythmias documented by 24-hour continuous ambulatory electrocardiographic monitoring in young women without apparent heart disease. *Am Heart J* 1981; 101:753–759.
235. Camm AJ, Evans KE, Ward DE, Martin A: The rhythm of the heart in active elderly subjects. *Am Heart J* 1980; 99:598–603.
236. Clarke JM, Shelton JR, Hamer J, Taylor S, Venning GR: The rhythm of the normal human heart. *Lancet* 1976; 2:508–512.
237. Glasser SP, Clark PI, Appelbaum HJ: Occurrence of frequent complex arrhythmias detected by ambulatory monitoring. Findings in an apparently healthy asymptomatic elderly population. *Chest* 1979; 75:565–568.
238. Raftery EB, Cashman PMM: Long-term recording of the electrocardiogram in normal population. *Postgrad Med J* 1976; 52 (suppl 7):32–38.
239. Chou TC, Caeser JH: Ambulatory electrocardiogram: clinical applications, in Fowler NO (ed): *Noninvasive Diagnostic Methods in Cardiology. Cardiovascular Clinics*. Philadelphia, FA Davis Co, 1983, pp 321–334.
240. Sheffield LT, Berson A, Bragg-Remschel D, Gillette PC, Hermes RE, Hinkle L, Kennedy H, Mirvis DM, Oliver C: Recommendations for standards of instrumentation and practice in the use of ambulatory electrocardiography. The Task Force of the Committee on Electrocardiography and Cardiac Electrophysiology of the Council on Clinical Cardiology. *Circulation* 1985; 71:626A–636A.
241. Morganroth J: Ambulatory Holter electrocardiography: choice of technologies and clinical uses. *Ann Intern Med* 1985; 102:73–81.

6 Echocardiography and Doppler Echocardiography

Morris N. Kotler, MD, Wayne R. Parry, and Anthony P. Goldman, MD

Clinical echocardiography developed as a result of the application of sonar which was used during World War II for submarine detection. Edler and Hertz[1] in 1954 recorded motion of the anterior mitral leaflet and thought they were looking at the left atrial wall. Their initial studies recorded mitral valve motion and were predominantly employed in the evaluation of mitral stenosis.[2] Subsequent investigators, including Joyner et al[3] and Feigenbaum et al[4] in the United States, expanded the application to include pericardial effusion, tricuspid valve disease, and clinical disorders affecting the mitral valve. Gramiak and Shah[5] in 1968 used intracardiac contrast injections for the validation of cardiac anatomy in man. In 1973, Bom et al[6] described multiscan echocardiography as a potential new tool for evaluating cardiac anatomy. This was followed up in 1974 by Griffith and Henry[7] who developed a sector scanner for real-time two-dimensional (2-D) echocardiography. Shortly thereafter, Eggleton and Feigenbaum[8] provided cross-sectional cardiac anatomic images using real-time B-mode ultrasonic scanners. Von Ramn et al[9] in 1976 described a phased-array ultrasound system. With the advent of combining instrumentation that uses the Doppler principle with standard pulse ultrasound imaging, it is now possible to image the heart and obtain a Doppler signal from areas within it. The principles and applications of pulsed Doppler echocardiography were described in 1977 by Baker et al.[10] By means of gating the Doppler sample in an anatomic portion of the heart as seen on M-mode or 2-D echocardiography, the Doppler signal can be received from that precise area of the heart. Holen et al[11] in 1976 used continuous wave Doppler echocardiography to quantitate the pressure decrease in mitral stenosis. Brubakk et al[12] in 1977 described the clinical application of a Doppler instrument that provides both pulsed and continuous wave Doppler echocardiography. The routine use of pulsed and continuous wave Doppler echocardiography has currently become an acceptable tool in evaluating valvular and congenital heart lesions. As a result of combined M-mode, 2-D, and Doppler echocardiography, clinical applications have been expanded considerably over the past 30 years. All three techniques are now regarded as an essential diagnostic tool in the evaluation of patients with cardiac disorders.

The major disadvantage of M-mode echocardiography is that a limited "ice pick" one-dimensional view of the heart is obtained. The entire left ventricular cavity, apex of the left ventricle, right atrium, and three leaflets of the tricuspid valve cannot always be evaluated by M-mode echocardiography. In addition, intracardiac structures are displayed in an unfamiliar format that bears little resemblance to cardiac anatomy. Spatial orientation of cardiac structures cannot always be readily appreciated by M-mode techniques. However, M-mode echocardiography, by providing good axial resolution, is able to measure dimensions accurately to within 1 mm. In addition, with combining phonocardiography, the timing of intracardiac events, such as valve motion, as well as opening and closing sounds can be matched with the motion of the valve being interrogated. This has led us to a better understanding of normal and abnormal heart sounds as well as normal and abnormal prosthetic valve sounds. In contrast, 2-D echocardiography, by providing spatial orientation, allows appreciation of lateral as well as axial distances between structures. The resulting images obtained by the various 2-D systems resemble heart structures in motion. The newer real-time 2-D imaging devices are capable of extraordinary rapid image formation times, offering the viewer a remarkable appreciation of the heart in motion. With the sophisticated phased-array systems or the new mechanical sector scanners, an 80° to 90° sector scan of the heart can be obtained. This scan allows complete visualization of the entire left ventricular cavity, cardiac apex, right ventricle, right and left atrium, and interatrial septum as well as the tricuspid and pulmonary valves and great vessels. As with M-mode echocardiography, suboptimal 2-D images may be obtained in obese and emphysematous patients or in persons with chest deformities.

Pulsed and continuous wave Doppler techniques share similar complementary roles. Although pulsed Doppler echocardiography provides a precise sample volume for localization of flow abnormalities, blood velocity from even moderately stenotic lesions exceeds the limits of this technique. Conversely, continuous wave Doppler echocardiography can accurately measure extremely high velocities and hence quantitate stenotic lesions, but it has no range resolution at all. Combining these two in one instrument allows both location of a flow disturbance and quantitation of the pressure difference.[12,13]

PHYSICAL PRINCIPLES

ECHOCARDIOGRAPHY

M-mode echocardiography depends on sound waves of high frequency that are generated by a piezoelectric crystal incorporated into a transducer that converts electrical to vibratory or sound-wave energy. As the name implies, ultrasound represents vibrations above 20,000 c/s (20 kHz), which is the upper limit of audible sound. In echocardiography, the sonic frequency ranges from 1 to 7 million c/s (1 to 7 MHz). In adults, the frequencies that are commonly employed are 2 to 3.5 MHz, whereas in children they are usually higher, ranging from 3.5 to 7 MHz. The piezoelectric crystal is used as both a signal transmitter and a receiver and generates high frequency vibrations generally in the range of 2.5 to 5 MHz. The resolution of the system, which is the ability to distinguish two objects that are spatially close together, varies directly with the frequency and inversely with the wavelength. Therefore, high frequency (short wavelengths) ultrasound can identify separate objects that are less than 1 mm apart. In contrast, systems that have lower frequencies and longer wavelengths have poorer resolution. The degree of penetration, which is the ability to transmit sufficient ultrasonic energy into the chest, is inversely proportional to the frequency of the signal. Therefore, high frequency systems operating at 3 or 5 MHz may be unable to penetrate a thick chest wall, so low frequency ultrasonic beams are used in adults. All transmitted sound from a single pulse travels through the thorax and returns before the next pulse so that there is no interference between sequential pulses. High frequency sound waves are reflected best from the interface of tissues of a different acoustic impedance (density). Subsequent returning sound energies are converted to an electrical impulse that can be displayed on a strip chart recorder coupled with other parameters for timing of cardiac events such as the electrocardiogram or phonocardiogram. Velocity of sound in soft tissues of the body is approximately 1,540 m/s. As a sound pulse travels through soft tissue, it loses some energy by reflection, some by refraction, and some by absorption; therefore, sound returning from distant structures in relation to the transducer has lower energy than sound reflected from surfaces nearer the transducer. For this reason, a depth compensation circuit is used in most commercial instruments so that the intensity of echoes near the transducer is attenuated whereas more distant echoes are relatively enhanced. Most M-mode systems employ focused transducers that collimate, ie, focus, the emitted sound beam and thus reduce the lateral spread. In effect, M-mode recordings are a continuous plot of the depth of structures with respect to time.

The original 2-D system consisted of a multielement transducer.[6] Twenty separate crystals were arranged linearly. Each crystal was pulsed sequentially and the resultant image was displayed as a series of single line reflections. However, significant image dropout resulted because of the position of the ribs and lungs. Subsequently, a mechanical sector scanner was introduced consisting of a single transducer that was allowed to oscillate rapidly by means of an electronic motor through a 30° to 60° arc.[7] This relatively inexpensive system provided good quality images. However, because of the narrow angle, noise, and vibrating sensation, the more popular phased-array systems were developed.[9] More recently, wide-angle 80° to 90° mechanical sector scanners using multiple rotating or single oscillating crystals have been developed.

Phased-array systems provide a distinct advantage in 2-D echocardiography. A 90° sector scan of the heart is obtained at a scan rate of 30 frames/s. Some commercial systems may use up to 48 piezoelectric crystals. The ultrasound beam is steered through an arc of 90° by excitation of the crystals almost simultaneously but slightly out of phase, so that a crystal at one end of the transducer is excited slightly before the next one. In this manner, the resultant beam is transmitted at a constant angle to the face of the transducer. In addition, by rapidly changing the sequence of pulsations, the beam can be electronically steered in various directions, thus creating the sector image. In a "dynamically focused" phased-array system, the pulse sequence is further manipulated to provide uniform focusing throughout the sector. The phased-array system can time share the firing of the transducer to create simultaneous M-mode, 2-D, and, more recently, Doppler recordings. Images are represented in real time and the sector images are recorded on 1/2" to 3/4" videotapes at 30 frames/s. Generally, individual frames can be photographed by a Polaroid® camera attachment or can be directly obtained in a printout by other freeze frame recorders. Because each video frame consists of two interlacing fields and the still frame consists of only a single field, there is half the information and, therefore, significant degradation of image quality occurs. In addition, still frame images lack the visual integration apparent in successive frames of real-time imaging. For this reason, some illustrations in this presentation that suffer from image degradation may be accompanied by an idealized diagram. Although current mechanical sector transducer technology has approximated the size of phased-array transducers, they still share the disadvantage of not providing simultaneous 2-D and M-mode or Doppler imaging, or both.

DOPPLER ECHOCARDIOGRAPHY

A comprehensive description of the physical principles of Doppler echocardiography is beyond the scope of this chapter, and an excellent review of the subject is provided by Hatle and Angelsen.[14] With regard to Doppler echocardiography, the Doppler principle states that the velocity of an object can be determined if one knows (1) the frequency of transmitted sound waves (F_t), (2) the frequency of returning sound waves (F_r), (3) the speed of ultrasound in blood (c), and (4) the angle of incidence (o) of the sound beam with respect to the motion of the reflecting object (Figure 6.1). The reflectors of interest in Doppler echocardiography are red blood cells and, to a lesser degree, cardiac valves. The former provide valuable hemodynamic parameters and the latter are useful for timing cardiac events.

In some instruments, the Doppler signal is displayed as a plot of frequency shifts over time. Newer systems solve the Doppler equation in real time by either digital or analog techniques, and they provide a spectral display of the distribution of velocities with respect to time. By convention, flow toward the transducer is shown above the baseline and that away from the transducer, below the baseline. The density of the spectral display is proportional to the intensity of returning signals. In normal laminar flow, most red blood cells are traveling at similar speeds in approximately the same direction, and the spectral flow profile shows a relatively narrow distribution of velocities. In disturbed or turbulent flow, rapid fluctuation in both the speed and the direction of flow causes "spectral broadening" commonly seen in flow distal to stenotic valves (Figure 6.1). Although flow within a stenotic jet is usually laminar, turbulent flow adjacent to and downstream from the jet frequently is recorded as well.

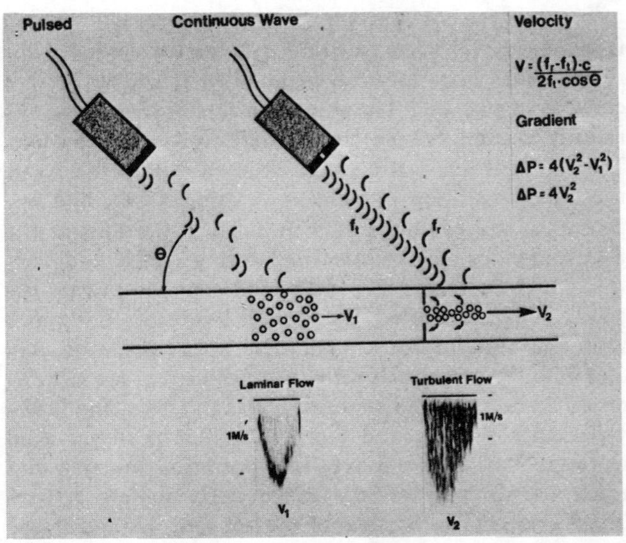

Figure 6.1. Schematic representation of the principles of pulsed and continuous wave Doppler echocardiography with representative spectral recordings of laminar and turbulent blood flow. See text for details. The Bernoulli equation, which measures the pressure drop (ΔP) across a valve or structure, is simplified to equal four times the maximum velocity (V_2) squared.

There are three principal types of Doppler modes currently in clinical use: (1) pulsed Doppler, (2) continuous wave Doppler, and (3) color flow imaging. Each modality has advantages and limitations (Table 6.1), and together they provide a comprehensive approach to the noninvasive assessment of cardiovascular flow abnormalities (Table 6.2).

Pulsed Doppler Imaging

Pulsed Doppler imaging is functionally similar to imaging echocardiography in that short bursts of sound waves are rapidly transmitted, with the transducer acting as a receiver between transmissions. By using a time gate in the receive mode, signals from a localized region along the sound beam (sample volume) can be selectively recorded. To determine the location of a sample volume with certainty (range resolution), each pulse must be sampled before another one returns. The pulse repetition frequency (PRF) is generally much higher than that used in imaging echocardiography and is directly proportional to the maximum measurable velocity. When examining a shallow structure, a relatively high PRF can be used to detect high flow velocities. As the sample volume is positioned deeper in the thorax, the PRF must be reduced to avoid the phenomenon of range ambiguity, ie, more than one sample volume in the field of interest at one time. When the maximum velocity is excessive, frequency aliasing or the inability to determine the velocity or direction of flow, or both, occurs (Figure 6.2).

A variation of pulsed Doppler imaging, high PRF, uses a rapid pulse sequence at greater depths to increase the maximum measurable blood flow velocity. In high PRF Doppler imaging, several sample volumes are present in the field of view at one time, and range ambiguity or the inability to determine the precise source of the flow signal is introduced. Although high PRF is a useful adjunct to pulsed Doppler imaging, it is more cumbersome to use than continuous wave Doppler imaging.

Continuous Wave Doppler Imaging

Two ultrasound crystals are simultaneously used in continuous wave Doppler imaging; one continuously

Table 6.1. Comparison of Different Doppler Techniques

	Advantage	Disadvantage
Pulsed	Range resolution	Velocity limit/aliasing
Continuous wave	No velocity limit	No range resolution
High pulse repetition frequency	Measure high velocity	Range ambiguity
Color flow imaging	Direct visualization of flow patterns	Velocity limit/aliasing Unable to precisely determine flow velocity

Table 6.2. Clinical Applications of Doppler Echocardiography

(1) Differentiation of innocent and pathologic murmurs
(2) Detection and quantification of stenotic valvular and vascular lesions
(3) Detection and estimation of severity of regurgitant lesions
(4) Detection and quantification of intra- and extracardiac shunts
(5) Estimation of intracardiac pressures
(6) Evaluation of prosthetic valve function
(7) Estimation of cardiac output

transmits sound waves, whereas the other continuously receives reflected sound waves. Velocities well in excess of physiologic limits can be measured without aliasing. However, continuous wave Doppler imaging records all velocities along the entire length of the ultrasound beam and hence has no range resolution. In high flow states, pulsed Doppler imaging can be used to locate the site of disturbed flow and continuous wave Doppler imaging can be used to detect maximum velocities for the calculation of pressure gradients using the Bernoulli equation (Figure 6.1).[4]

Color Flow Imaging (Two-Dimensional Doppler Flow Imaging)

Systems recently have been developed that sample Doppler shifts throughout the imaging plane and provide a composite image of blood flow and two dimensional anatomy in real time.[15,16] Blood flow is color coded to indicate the direction and extent of flow, with brightness of the signal indicating the relative velocity of flow. Although the clinical significance of simultaneous blood flow and anatomic imaging has yet to be determined, preliminary reports indicate that color flow imaging has significant advantages over conventional Doppler and contrast angiography in the evaluation of valvular heart disease,[17–21] congenital heart disease,[16,19–22] and dissecting aortic aneurysms.[23] The potential application of the technique in congenital heart disease is enormous.

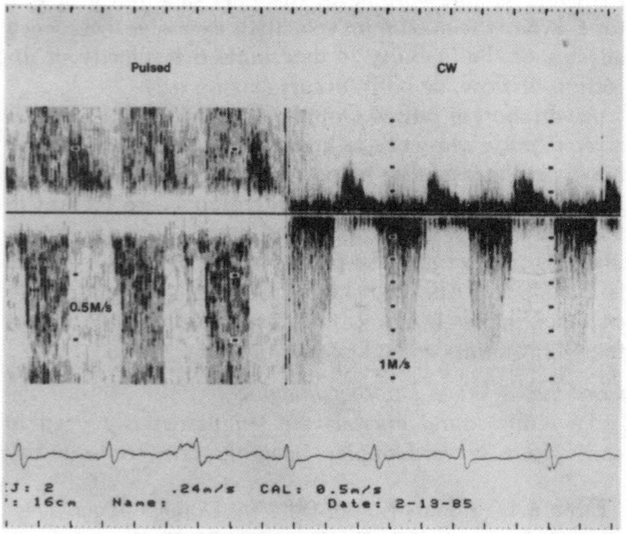

Figure 6.2. Pulsed (*left panel*) and continuous wave (CW) Doppler (*right panel*) recording from the apical position in a patient with mitral regurgitation. With the pulsed Doppler sample volume placed in the left atrium, the velocity of regurgitant flow exceeds the maximum measurable velocity at this sample depth, and frequency aliasing occurs. Both the direction of flow and peak velocity during systole cannot be discerned. During diastole, antegrade mitral valve flow is displayed above the baseline. With CW Doppler recording, a peak regurgitant flow velocity of approximately 6 m/s is directed away from the transducer and is displayed below the baseline.

TECHNIQUE

ECHOCARDIOGRAPHY

With the patient in a supine or semirecumbent position and with the trunk elevated between 15° and 45°, an M-mode transducer is applied to the chest wall in the third or fourth interspace 1 to 5 cm lateral to the left sternal border. A water-soluble gel is used to ensure contact between the transducer and the skin. The transducer is directed slightly medially from a true anteroposterior direction until the mitral valve is located. The mitral valve is usually found at a depth of 5 to 8.5 cm from the chest wall. Maximum amplitude of mitral valve motion is obtained by directing the ultrasound beam to the tip of the mitral valve. Once the mitral valve has been identified, the septum and left ventricular posterior wall can also be recognized by angulating the transducer inferolaterally away from the tip of the mitral valve. As the transducer is rotated toward the apex, the posterior mitral leaflet merges into posterior chordal structures and papillary muscles (Figure 6.3). The two mitral leaflets (anterior and posterior) move in diastole in an M-shaped, mirror-image pattern. At the onset of systole, the leaflets merge at the C point. During systole the two leaflets move slightly anterior to the D point. With the onset of diastole the anterior leaflet opens to the E point. The early diastolic velocity of the leaflet (E-F slope) is dependent on the rate of filling of the left ventricle. If the transducer is angulated from the mitral valve position in a medial-cephalad direction, the aortic root can be identified. The aortic root consists of two undulating intense echoes that move anteriorly during systole and posteriorly during diastole. Two aortic valve leaflets may be seen within the aortic root; they separate in systole, creating a box-like appearance, and come together in diastole. Portions of the tricuspid valve may be identified during systole and diastole when the transducer is directed medially toward the spine. When identified, the tricuspid valve is contiguous with the anterior aortic wall. The posterior aortic wall and anterior mitral valve are in continuity as are the anterior aortic wall and septum. During systole, the interventricular septum and left ventricular posterior wall thicken. The septum moves in a posterior direction and the left ventricular wall moves anteriorly; therefore, there is reduction in the diameter of the left ventricle and shortening of the minor axis is usually greater than 25%. The right ventricle is usually seen anterior to the septum and the left atrium is posterior to the aortic root. The normal M-mode echocardiographic measurements[24] are listed in Table 6.3.

With regard to 2-D echocardiography, a committee of the American Society of Echocardiography has estab-

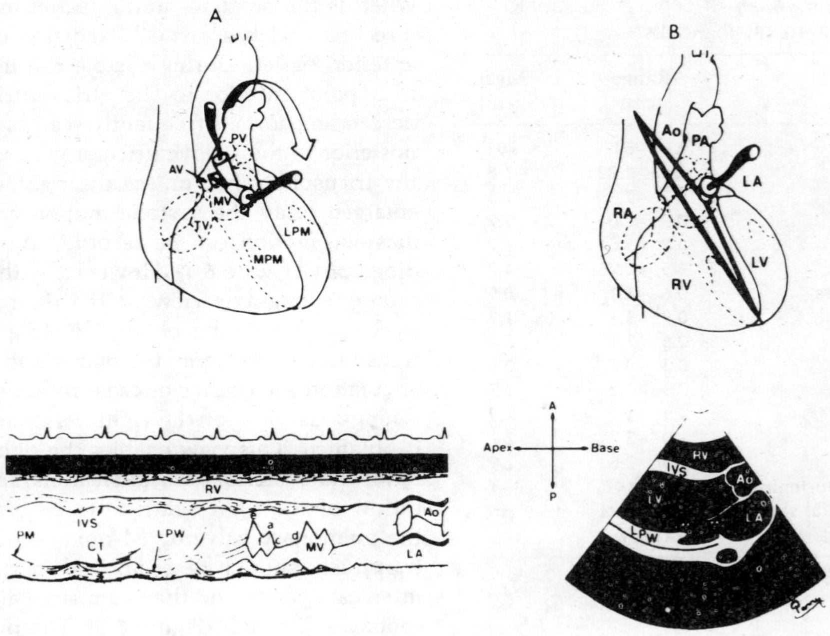

Figure 6.3. *A*, The M-mode transducer is in the third interspace pointing toward the mitral as well as the aortic valve. An M-mode echocardiographic sweep from the aortic root to the left ventricular cavity is shown diagrammatically below this. The electrocardiogram is demonstrated for timing events. Anteriorly, the right ventricular wall, cavity, and septum are demonstrated. Posteriorly, the left ventricular cavity and posterior wall structures are identified. *B*, A two-dimensional transducer placed in the long axis of the left ventricle. Anterior and to the right is the aorta, and posterior is the left atrium. The right ventricular cavity is separated from the left ventricular cavity by the interventricular septum. The circular structure posterior to the atrioventricular junction is the descending aorta. Ao = aorta; AV = aortic valve; CT = chordal structures; IVS = interventricular septum; LA = left atrium; LPM = lateral papillary muscle; LPW = left ventricular posterior wall; MPM = medial papillary muscle; MV = mitral valve; LV = left ventricle; PA = pulmonary artery; PM = papillary muscle; PV = pulmonary valve; RA = right atrium; RV = right ventricle; TV = tricuspid valve. (From Kotler et al,[261] with permission.)

lished guidelines for nomenclature and standards for image orientation.[25] The location on the body from which the echocardiographic studies can be obtained are suprasternal, parasternal (either left or right), subcostal, or apical (which is assumed to be left-sided unless otherwise stated). When the transducer is placed in the suprasternal notch, the suprasternal location is the term used. When the transducer is placed beneath the lowest ribs near the midline of the body, this is referred to as the subcostal location. The apical location is a position used when the transducer is located over the apex impulse. The area bounded superiorly by the left clavicle and inferiorly by the apical region is referred to as the parasternal location. Three basic orthogonal, ie, mutually perpendicular planes, are used to describe 2-D imaging planes that transect the heart. The imaging plane that transects the heart perpendicular to the dorsal and ventral surface of the body and parallel to the long axis of the heart is the long-axis plane. The plane that transects the heart perpendicular to the dorsal and ventral surfaces of the body but perpendicular to the long axis of the heart is the short-axis plane. The plane that transects the heart approximately parallel to the dorsal and ventral surfaces of the body is the four-chamber plane.

The committee has also recommended that 2-D images be identified by referring to the transducer position as well as the imaging plane. For example, if the transducer is placed in the parasternal location and oriented so that the imaging plane transects the heart parallel to the long axis of the heart, the resulting image should be called a parasternal long-axis view. The long-axis view of the left ventricle as obtained by 2-D echocardiography is shown in Figure 6.3. The transducer is positioned in the third or fourth interspace and the ultrasound beam is directed parallel to a line joining the right shoulder and the left flank. The image obtained represents a section through the long axis of the left ventricle. The image is oriented so that the aorta is displayed to the right, the cardiac apex to the left, the chest wall and right ventricle anteriorly, and the left ventricular posterior wall and left atrium posteriorly. In this view, practically the entire left ventricular cavity except for a small portion of the apex can be visualized. During diastole, the anterior mitral leaflet opens and approximates the left ventricular septal surface,

Table 6.3. Normal Values of Echocardiographic Measurements in Adults*

Measurement	Range (cm)	Mean (cm)
Age (yr)	13 –54	26
Body surface area	1.45–2.22	1.8
RVD supine flat	0.7 –2.3	1.5
RVD left lateral	0.9 –2.6	1.7
LVIDd supine flat	3.7 –5.6	4.7
LVIDd left lateral	3.5 –5.7	4.7
Posterior LV wall thickness	0.6 –1.1	0.9
Posterior LV wall amplitude	0.9 –1.4	1.2
IVS wall thickness	0.6 –1.1	0.9
Mid IVS amplitude	0.3 –0.8	0.5
Apical IVS amplitude	0.5 –1.2	0.7
Left atrial dimension	1.9 –4.0	2.9
Aortic root dimension	2.0 –3.7	2.7
Aortic cusps' separation	1.5 –2.6	1.9
Percentage of fractional shortening†	34%–44%	36%
Mean rate of circumferential shortening‡	1.02–1.94 circ/s	1.3 circ/s

* Adapted from Feigenbaum[24], with permission.

† $EF = \frac{LVIDd - LVIDs}{LVIDd}$

‡ VCF or mean normalized shortening velocity $= \frac{LVIDd - LVIDs}{LVIDd \times \text{Ejection Time}}$

d = end-diastole; IVS = interventricular septum; LV = left ventricle; LVID = left ventricular internal dimension; RVD = right ventricular dimension; s = end-systole.

whereas the posterior mitral leaflet moves in a posterior direction and has a small excursion compared with the anterior leaflet. During systole the mitral leaflets coapt to a point inferior to the atrioventricular groove. The descending aorta is frequently seen as a circular structure posterior to the atrioventricular groove.[26] With regard to the tricuspid valve, unless the right ventricle is grossly enlarged, only the systolic motion and portions of the diastolic motion can be recorded by M-mode echocardiography (Figure 6.4). However, with 2-D echocardiography, a long-axis view of the right ventricular inflow tract can readily be obtained[27] (Figure 6.4). With the transducer in the same interspace and with inferomedial angulation and slight clockwise rotation of the transducer, a long-axis view of the right ventricle and right atrium is obtained. This view enables the right atrial cavity, anterior and posterior tricuspid leaflets, and right ventricular inflow of the right ventricle to be visualized. To locate the pulmonary valve by M-mode echocardiography, the transducer should be positioned in the second or third intercostal space and the beam angulated in a lateral and cephalad direction (Figure 6.5). The pulmonary artery is identified as a sonolucent space 1 to 2 cm from the anterior chest wall and is anterior and to the right of the aorta. Generally, the posterior cusp of the pulmonary valve can be recognized in most subjects. It opens during systole and has a fairly prominent "a" wave. The "a"

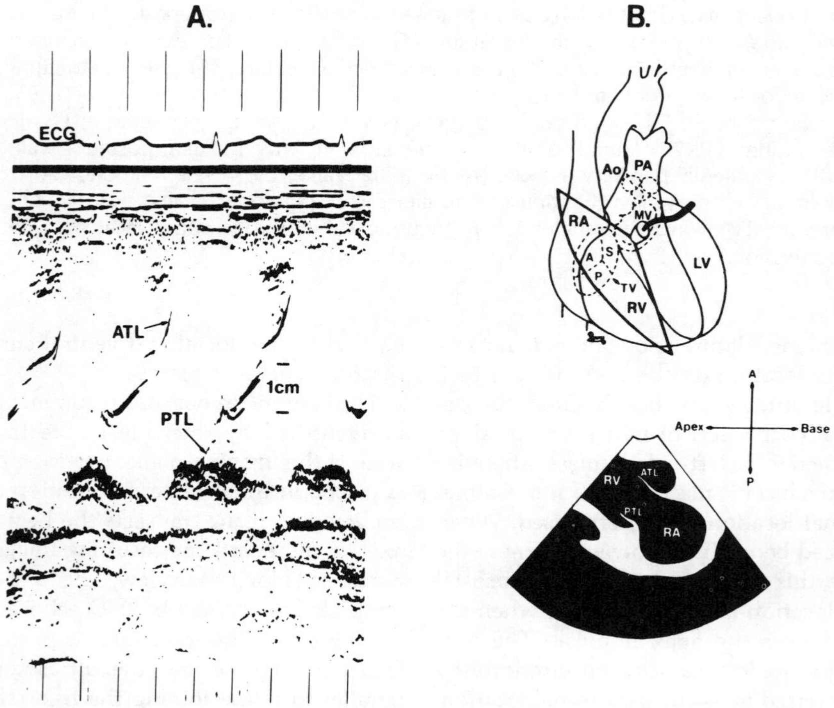

Figure 6.4. *A*, An M-mode echocardiogram with the transducer pointed medially and toward the spine, showing portions of the tricuspid valve. *B*, Two-dimensional view of the right ventricular inflow tract with a transducer placed in the third intercostal space and angulated slightly medially. In the idealized diagram, the right ventricle is anterior, the right atrium is posterior, and two leaflets of the tricuspid valve are clearly visualized. Ao = aorta; ATL = anterior tricuspid leaflet; ECG = electrocardiogram; LV = left ventricle; MV = mitral valve; PA = pulmonary artery; PTL = posterior tricuspid leaflet; RA = right atrium; RV = right ventricle; TV = tricuspid valve. (From Kotler et al,[261] with permission.)

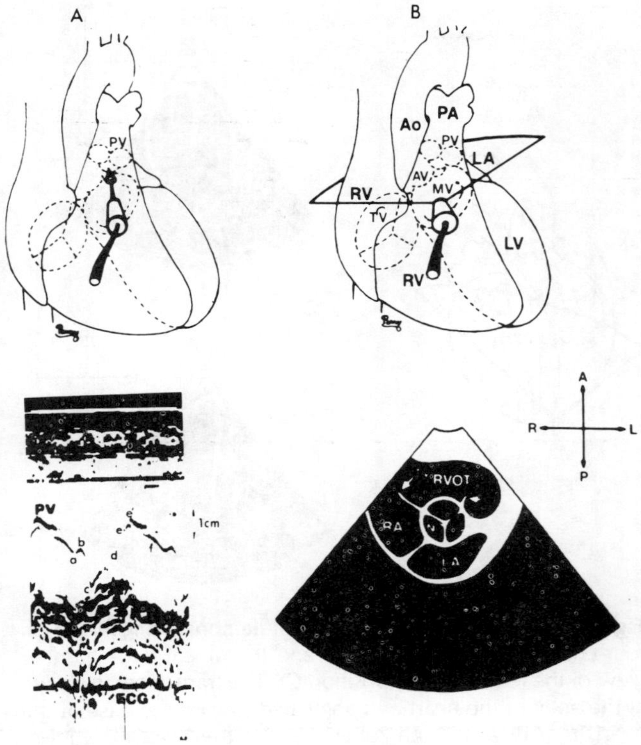

Figure 6.5. *A*, M-mode transducer in the second interspace pointing laterally toward the left shoulder. The pulmonary valve is superior, anterior, and lateral to the aortic valve. The recording of the posterior pulmonic leaflet is depicted below. *B*, Cross-sectional view at the level of the great vessels. The aorta appears as a circle with a tri-leaflet aortic valve. Anteriorly, the outflow tract of the right ventricle (RVOT) is sausage-shaped in appearance, and the pulmonic valve (PV) can be seen. The tricuspid valve is medial, and the interatrial septum separates the left and right atrium. Ao = aorta; AV = aortic valve; LA = left atrium; LC = left coronary cusp; LV = left ventricle; MV = mitral valve; NC = noncoronary cusp; PA = pulmonary artery; PV = pulmonary valve; RA = right atrium; RC = right coronary cusp; RV = right ventricle; TV = tricuspid valve. (From Kotler et al,[261] with permission.)

wave represents the effect of atrial contraction on the pulmonic leaflet. To visualize the pulmonic valve with 2-D techniques the transducer is placed in the parasternal position in the third or fourth intercostal space and the short-axis view of the heart is obtained by rotating the transducer so that the plane of the ultrasound beam is perpendicular to the plane of the long axis of the left ventricle (Figure 6.5). The transducer is pointed cephalad and the great arteries are sectioned in a transverse plane. The aorta appears as a circle with a tri-leaflet aortic valve, which during diastole has the appearance of the letter Y. The right ventricular outflow tract crosses anterior to the aorta and has a sausage-like appearance. The pulmonary valve is visualized anterior and to the right of the aorta. During systole, the pulmonic valve leaflets are open and approximate the anterior and posterior walls of the pulmonary artery. The anterior leaflet of the tricuspid valve can also be seen on the left of the image. Other structures recorded in this view include the left atrium, interatrial septum, and right atrium to the left of the image. To visualize the main pulmonary artery and its bifurcation, the transducer can be rotated slightly clockwise and tilted beyond the pulmonary valve.

Additional cross-sectional views of the left ventricle can be obtained with 2-D techniques by inferior movement of the transducer. At the level of the body of the left ventricle, the transducer beam transects the mitral valve and the anterior and posterior mitral leaflets are widely separated, creating a fish-mouth appearance during diastole (Figure 6.6). During systole, the leaflets are in a closed position and can appear as a single line. The circular left ventricular myocardium can be seen contracting during systole and relaxing during diastole. Anterior and to the left, the right ventricle is visualized. With further tilting or motion of the transducer beam inferiorly, a cross section at the level of the papillary muscle is obtained. The left ventricular myocardium represents a circular structure and the anterolateral and posteromedial papillary muscles project into the left ventricular cavity and are visualized approximately at the 4 and 8 o'clock positions, respectively (Figure 6.6). The left and right ventricular walls can be divided into separate segments (Figure 6.7). Further transducer motion in an inferior direction displays a cross-sectional view at the ventricular apex. In this view, the ventricular cavity is small and surrounded by thickened, circular myocardium. Two of the most important views are the apical four-chamber and apical two-

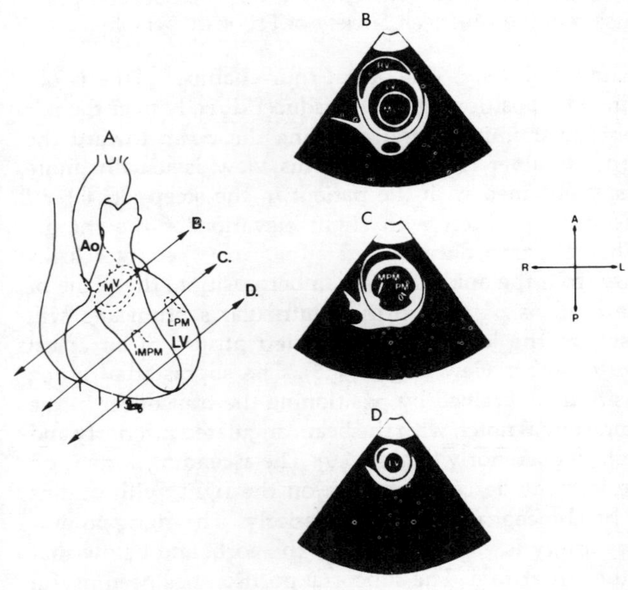

Figure 6.6. Cross-sectional view of the left ventricle. *A*, Diagrammatic view of the heart showing various cross-sectional planes taken from the level of the mitral valve (MV) toward the apex of the left ventricle (LV). *B*, Cross-sectional view of the LV at the level of the MV. The right ventricle (RV) is anterior and to the left of the LV. The LV appears as a circular structure. The mitral valve orifice (MVO) has a fish-mouth appearance during diastole. *C*, Cross-sectional view of the LV at the level of the papillary muscles (LPM, MPM) which project in the left ventricular cavity at approximately the 4 and 8 o'clock positions. *D*, Cross-sectional view of the LV at its apex. It is small and surrounded by thick circular muscle. Ao = aorta; R = right; A = anterior; L = left; P = posterior. (From Kotler et al,[261] with permission.)

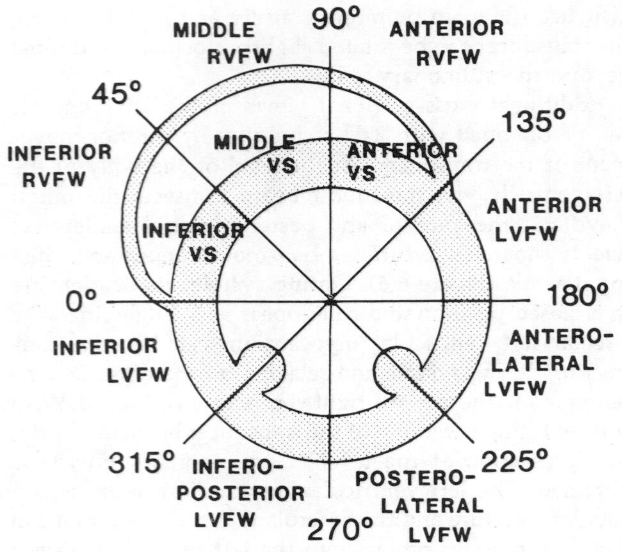

Figure 6.7. Short-axis view of the midventricular region, demonstrating the method of subdividing the myocardial wall into segments. A coordinate system consisting of eight lines that are 45° apart is used. With this system the left ventricular wall (LVFW) is divided into five segments, whereas the ventricular septum (VS) and right ventricular wall (RVFW) are subdivided into three segments each. (From *Report of the American Society of Echocardiography Committee on Nomenclature and Standards: Identification of myocardial wall segments.* Raleigh, NC, November 1982. Reproduced by permission of the American Society of Echocardiography.)

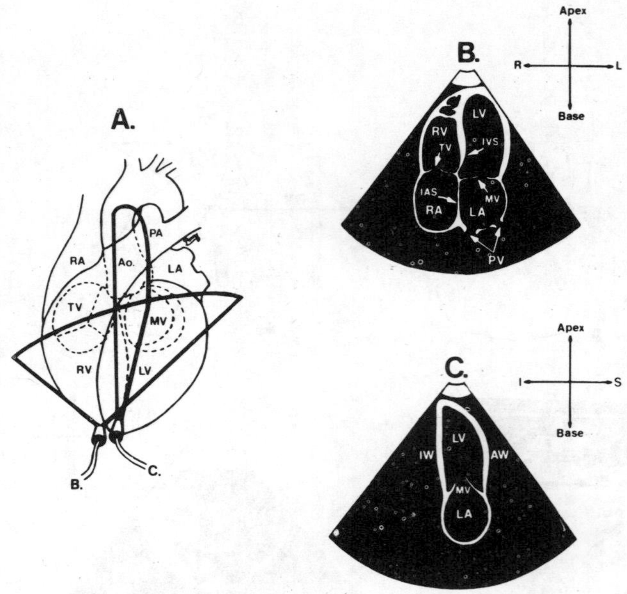

Figure 6.8. *A*, Drawing of the heart demonstrating the apical four-chamber view (position B) and the apical two-chamber view of the left ventricle (position C). The transducer is placed at the apex of the heart and angulated toward the base of the heart. *B*, Apical four-chamber view of the heart. The interventricular septum (IVS) separates the right and left ventricles (RV and LV). The interatrial septum (IAS) separates the right and left atrium (RA and LA). The attachments of the tricuspid valve (TV, inferiorly situated) and mitral valve (MV) are seen. Pulmonary veins (PV) may be seen entering the left atrium. The apices of both ventricles are situated anteriorly, and the base of the heart is situated posteriorly. *C*, Apical two-chamber view of the heart. The apex of the left ventricle is anterior. The left atrium (LA) is posterior. The inferior wall (IW) and anterior wall (AW) of the left ventricle are seen. Ao = aorta.

chamber views.[28] The apical four-chamber plane is obtained by positioning the transducer directly over the left ventricular impulse and directing the beam toward the right shoulder (Figure 6.8). This view is usually more easily obtained with the patient in the steep left lateral decubitus position with slight elevation of the thorax. When the transducer is rotated 60° to 90° counterclockwise from the apical four-chamber position, the plane of the beam is parallel to the ventricular septum and will visualize the left ventricle and left atrium in an apical two-chamber view (Figure 6.8). The suprasternal notch position is obtained by positioning the transducer in the suprasternal notch with the beam angulated inferiorly and slightly posteriorly (Figure 6.9). The ascending aorta is on the left, the descending aorta on the right, with origins of brachiocephalic vessels superiorly. The right pulmonary artery is visualized below the aorta and below that is the left atrium. The subcostal position has been useful in patients with chronic obstructive lung disease and chest wall deformities when the parasternal ultrasonic window is obliterated because of hyperinflated lungs. It is also useful in evaluating infants and children with congenital cardiac disorders as the beam is usually directed perpendicular to the interatrial and interventricular septa. Atrial and ventricular septal defects can frequently be visualized with this approach. Subcostal examination is performed by placing the transducer in the midline or slightly to the patient's right with the transducer pointed toward the spine. In this position, the liver, hepatic veins, inferior vena cava, and right atrium are identified (Figure 6.9). To obtain a four-chamber view of the heart, the transducer should be placed along the coronal plane parallel to a line between the patient's shoulders with a scan plane tilted about 20° downward from the plane of the anterior chest wall. This view allows visualization of both atrial cavities, the atrial and ventricular septa, left and right ventricular cavities, and the atrioventricular valves (Figure 6.10).

DOPPLER TECHNIQUE AND IMAGE ORIENTATION

In imaging echocardiography, the best results are obtained when structures are perpendicular to the ultrasound beam. In contrast, the best Doppler signals are obtained when the beam is aligned in the direction of blood flow, ie, parallel to cardiac and vascular walls. Hence, the "usual" acoustic windows for these techniques are frequently different. The apical views are useful in assessing mitral and tricuspid inflow, both atria, right ventricle, left ventricular outflow tract, and proximal ascending aorta. The subcostal approach is particularly useful in evaluating the inferior vena cava, hepatic vein, right ventricular outflow tract, and pulmonary artery as well as in detecting atrial and ventricular septal defects. The left parasternal approach provides access to the right ventricular outflow tract, pulmonary artery, right ventricle, and right atrium. The high right sternal border and suprasternal notch usually provide the maximum velocity of flow in aortic stenosis and coarctation of the aorta.

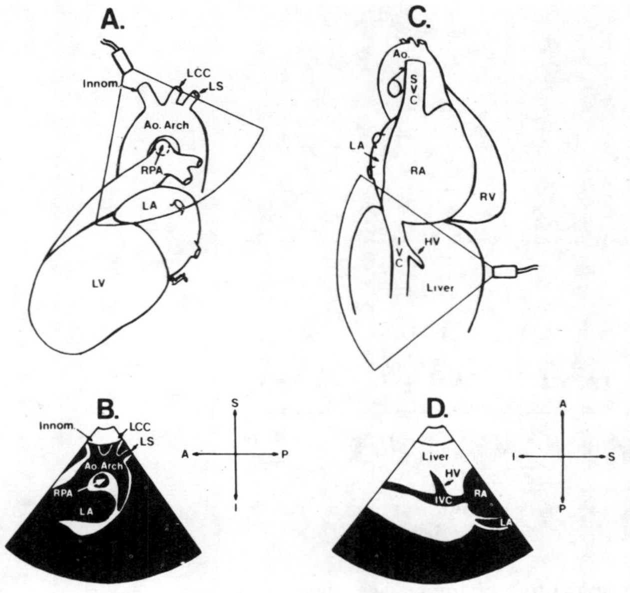

Figure 6.9. *A*, Drawing of the heart and great vessels with the transducer in the suprasternal notch position and directed inferiorly and slightly posteriorly and to the left. *B*, Diagrammatic representation of the sector scan. The ascending aorta (Ao) is on the left, the aortic arch is anterior, and the descending aorta is on the right. The origins of the brachiocephalic vessels can be seen, as can a cross-section of the right pulmonary artery (RPA). Posteriorly, the left atrium can be seen. *C,* Drawing of the heart with the transducer in the subcostal position and angulated toward the patient's spine. *D,* Diagrammatic representation of sector scan. Anteriorly, the liver and junction of the inferior vena cava, hepatic vein, and right atrium (RA) are also demonstrated. The interatrial septum and left atrium (LA) may also be seen. A = anterior; HV = hepatic vein; I = inferior; Innom = innominate artery; LCC = left common carotid artery; LS = left subclavian artery; P = posterior; S = superior; SVC = superior vena cava. (From Kotler et al,[262] with permission.)

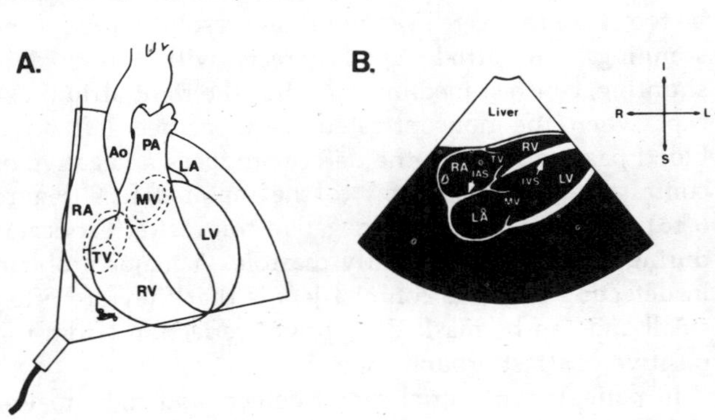

Figure 6.10. *A*, Subxiphoid view of a two-dimensional echocardiogram with the transducer placed in the subxiphoid position and angulated toward the base of the heart. *B*, Diagrammatic representation of sector scan. The right atrium and right ventricle are anteriorly situated, and the left atrium and left ventricle are posteriorly situated. The interatrial and interventricular septa and the tricuspid and mitral valves are also demonstrated. Ao = aorta; IAS = interatrial septum; IVS = interventricular septum; LA = left atrium; LV = left ventricle; MV = mitral valve; PA = pulmonary artery; RA = right atrium; RV = right ventricle; TV = tricuspid valve. (From Kotler et al,[261] with permission.)

Mitral Valve Flow

Using the standard apical four-chamber view, the sample volume is placed in the left ventricle, just distal to the tips of the mitral valve leaflets (Figure 6.11). Normal diastolic flow velocity in sinus rhythm is biphasic and resembles an M-mode recording of the anterior mitral leaflet. The early diastolic peak represents rapid filling and usually has a velocity of 0.9 to 1.0 m/s (Table 6.4). The second, smaller peak occurs with atrial systole and is absent in atrial fibrillation as well as rapid heart rates. During ventricular systole, left ventricular outflow velocity is frequently seen below the baseline.

Tricuspid Valve Flow

Tricuspid valve flow velocity is best recorded by positioning the sample in the right ventricle, inferior to the tips of the anterior and septal tricuspid valve leaflets (Figure 6.12). The ratio of maximum tricuspid to mitral valve flow velocity is usually 0.6 (Table 6.4).[5] Aside from the reduced maximum flow velocity, tricuspid flow also differs from mitral flow in that two distinct diastolic peaks are frequently inapparent and flow velocity increases with inspiration.

Left Ventricular Outflow

The left ventricular outflow tract and proximal ascending aorta can be assessed with slight caudal angulation of the imaging plane from the apical four-chamber view. From this position (the apical five-chamber view), left ventricular outflow is displayed as a spectral waveform below the baseline during systole (Figure 6.13). Peak systolic velocity is approximately 1 m/s (Figure 6.4) and increases slightly when the sample volume is placed in the proximal ascending aorta. Acceleration of velocity is rapid and reaches its peak in early systole.

Aortic Flow

Blood flow velocity in both the ascending and descending aorta can be obtained with the transducer oriented in the suprasternal long-axis view of the aortic arch (Figure 6.14). Blood flow in the ascending aorta is easier to assess using a small, nonimaging Doppler transducer. The spectral display is similar to that obtained from the proximal ascending aorta from the apical approach except that flow from this position is toward the transducer and is displayed above the baseline. A brief period of negative flow is commonly seen in protodiastole and probably reflects reversal of flow associated with aortic valve closure. With the sample in the aortic arch, bidirectional flow can be seen, and in the descending aorta, flow is displayed below the baseline.

Right Ventricular Outflow

Blood flow in the right ventricular outflow tract and pulmonary artery is obtained from either the parasternal or the subcostal short-axis view at the level of the great vessels. From both positions, flow is away from the transducer and is displayed below the baseline (Figure 6.15). The spectral display is similar to that seen in the aorta except that acceleration of flow is slower, and a lower peak velocity occurs later in systole (Table 6.4). In the

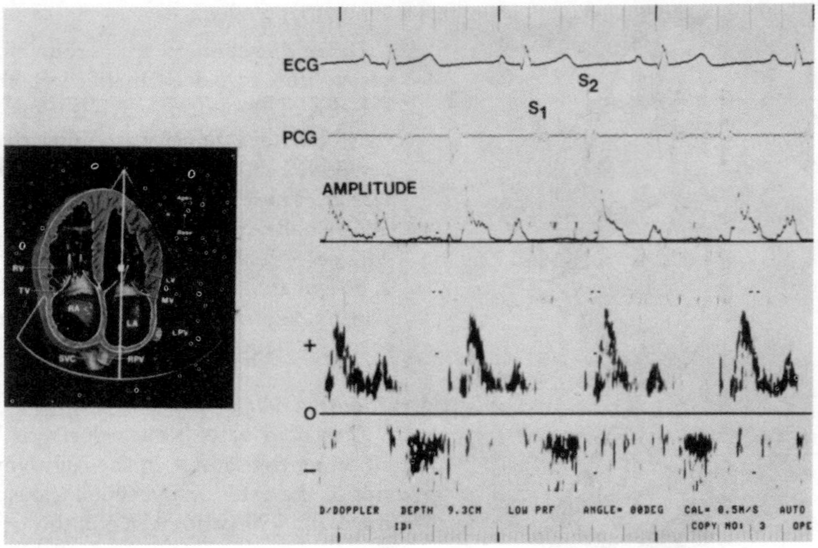

Figure 6.11. *Left*, Artist's rendition of an apical four-chamber view illustrating the technique used to record mitral valve flow. The sample volume is positioned in the left ventricle (LV) just distal to the tips of the mitral valve (MV) leaflets. *Right*, Pulsed Doppler recording in a normal subject with simultaneously recorded electrocardiogram (ECG), phonocardiogram (PCG), and Doppler amplitude. During diastole, flow is directed toward the transducer and is displayed above the baseline. Normal mitral valve flow has a characteristic 'M' shaped pattern similar to an M-mode recording of the anterior mitral valve. Early diastolic flow commences shortly after the second heart sound (S_2) and reaches a peak velocity of approximately 1 m/s in early diastole. Mitral flow velocity decreases rapidly until a second, smaller peak is inscribed after left atrial (LA) contraction. During systole, flow in the left ventricular outflow tract is displayed below the baseline. LPV = left pulmonary vein; RA = right atrium; RPV = right pulmonary vein; RV = right ventricle; S_1 = first heart sound; SVC = superior vena cava; TV = tricuspid valve.

right ventricular outflow tract, negative presystolic flow from atrial contraction is usually seen, especially during inspiration.

CONTRAST ECHOCARDIOGRAPHY

Injection of an agitated solution into the intravascular space will produce many microbubbles that appear as a cloud of echoes on the echocardiogram. A variety of contrast agents have been used[29] (Table 6.5), most commonly hand-agitated saline solution and indocyanine green dye. Recently, agents that liberate oxygen and carbon dioxide such as hydrogen peroxide[30] and combined sodium bicarbonate and vitamin C[31] have been employed. Since it was first described in 1968,[5] the clinical application of contrast echocardiography has steadily increased (Table 6.6).

Table 6.4. Maximal Velocities Recorded Noninvasively With Doppler Ultrasound in Normal Persons*

	Children (m/s)	Adults (m/s)
Mitral flow	1.00 (0.8–1.3)	0.90 (0.6–1.3)
Tricuspid flow	0.60 (0.5–0.8)	0.50 (0.3–0.7)
Pulmonary artery	0.90 (0.7–1.1)	0.75 (0.7–0.9)
Left ventricle	1.00 (0.7–1.2)	1.90 (0.7–1.1)
Aorta	1.50 (1.2–1.8)	1.35 (1.0–1.7)

* From Hatle and Angelsen,[14] with permission.

Contrast echocardiography has widely been used in the detection of right-to-left and left-to-right shunts. The technique provides information about flow patterns and may identify communications within the heart that may be too small to image even with high resolution real-time scanning.[32] In atrial septal defects with left-to-right shunting, contrast medium opacifies the right atrium except when the noncontrasted, nonopacified left atrial blood passing through the defect produces a negative or contrast-free area adjacent to the septal defect (Figure 6.16).[33] The timing of the negative contrast effect occurs during end-systole and early diastole. A major problem in detecting negative contrast jets is that they are often small and can be masked by bright reflections from the positive contrast around them.[32]

In patients with atrial septal defects and right-to-left shunts, the contrast microbubbles can be detected in the left side of the heart within a few cardiac cycles after injection of the contrast medium (Figure 6.17).

In patients with right-to-left shunts and ventricular septal defects, contrast echoes may be visualized in the left ventricle during peripheral contrast injection. The negative contrast effect is seldom present in patients with ventricular septal defects and left-to-right shunts. Similarly, shunting can be detected through a patent ductus arteriosus with the aid of 2-D echocardiography from the suprasternal and parasternal short-axis views.[32]

Additional uses of contrast echocardiography include

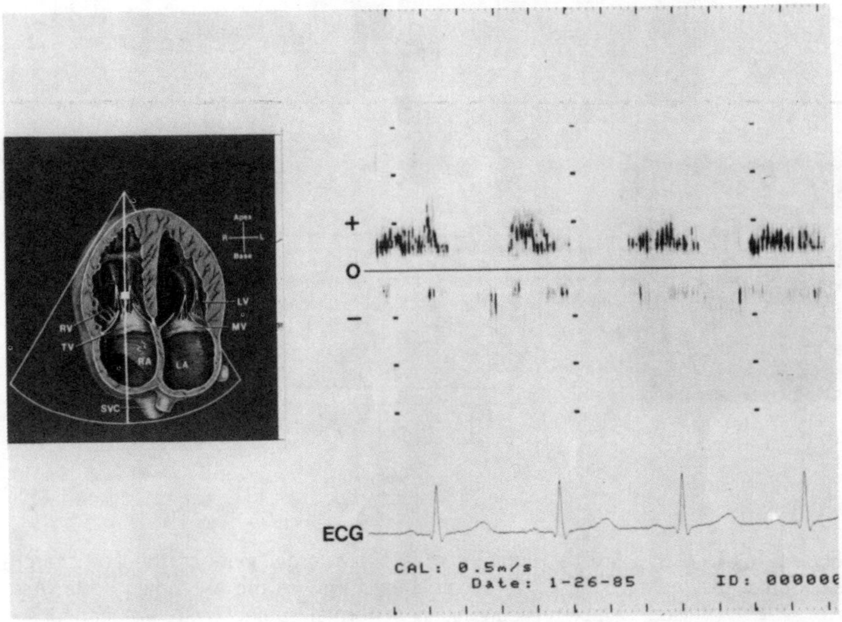

Figure 6.12. *Left*, Artist's rendition of an apical four-chamber view illustrating the technique used to record tricuspid valve flow. The sample volume is placed in the right ventricle (RV) just distal to the tips of the tricuspid valve (TV) leaflets. *Right*, Pulsed Doppler recording in a normal subject shows inspiratory augmentation of tricuspid flow velocity (beats 1 and 2). Peak diastolic velocity is approximately 60% of mitral valve flow and the characteristic 'M' pattern is often missing in normal subjects. ECG = electrocardiogram; LA = left atrium; LV = left ventricle; MV = mitral valve; RA = right atrium; SVC = superior vena cava.

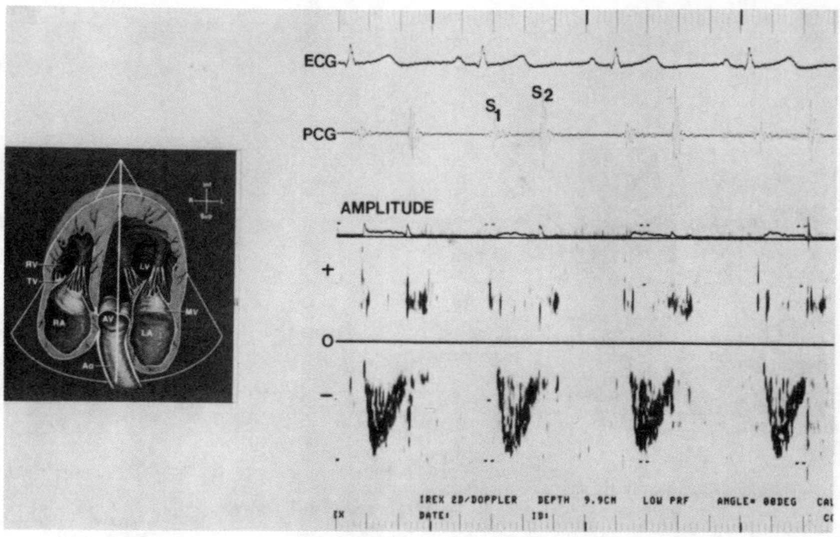

Figure 6.13. *Left*, Artist's rendition of an apical five-chamber view illustrating the technique used to record flow in the left ventricular outflow tract and proximal ascending aorta (Ao). *Right*, Pulsed Doppler recording of the proximal ascending aorta of a normal subject with simultaneously recorded electrocardiogram (ECG), phonocardiogram (PCG), and Doppler amplitude. With the sample placed just above the aortic valve (AV) (not shown), flow during systole is directed away from the transducer and displayed below the baseline. Flow begins shortly after the first heart sound (S_1), reaching a peak velocity in early systole, and it ends with the second heart sound (S_2). A brief period of reversed flow is commonly recorded in protodiastole and probably represents reversal of blood flow associated with aortic valve closure. LA = left atrium; LV = left ventricle; MV = mitral valve; RA = right atrium; RV = right ventricle, TV = tricuspid valve.

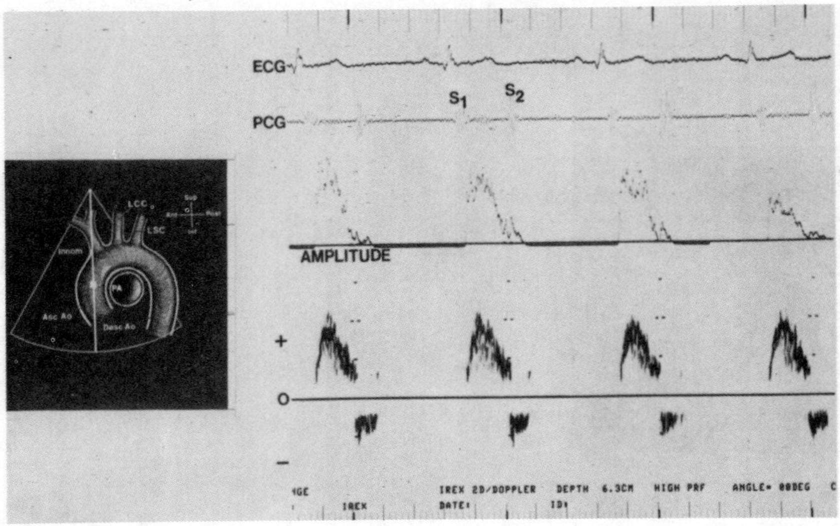

Figure 6.14. *Left*, Artist's rendition of a suprasternal view of the aortic arch illustrating the technique used to record blood flow in the ascending aorta (Asc Ao). *Right*, Pulsed Doppler recording in a normal subject with simultaneously recorded electrocardiogram (ECG), phonocardiogram (PCG), and Doppler amplitude. From this position, systolic flow is toward the transducer and displayed above the baseline. Protodiastolic reversal of flow is noted below the baseline. Desc Ao = descending aorta; Innom = innominate artery; LCC = left common carotid artery; LSC = left subclavian artery; PA = right pulmonary artery.

detection of paradoxic embolism with the aid of the Valsalva maneuver,[34] determination of cardiac output using video densitometric indicator-dilution curves,[35] and determination of area of risk for necrosis after acute coronary occlusion,[36] a useful technique for evaluating myocardial blood flow distribution in patients with coronary heart disease. The severity of coronary stenosis can be assessed by measuring the echo intensity disappearance

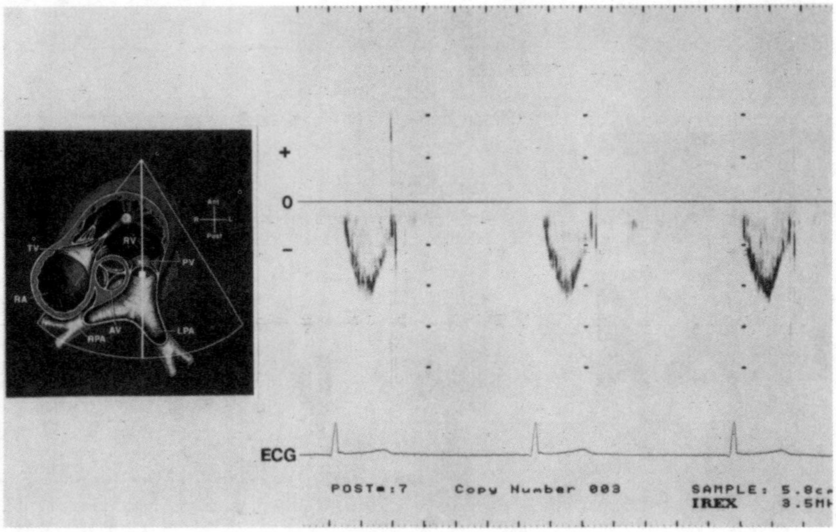

Figure 6.15. *Left*, Artist's rendition of a parasternal short-axis view at the level of the great vessels, illustrating the technique used to record flow in the main pulmonary artery. *Right*, Pulsed Doppler recording of the main pulmonary artery in a normal subject. Flow is away from the transducer and displayed below the baseline. The velocity profile is similar to that recorded in the proximal ascending aorta from the apical position. In general, peak flow velocity in the pulmonary artery occurs later and its magnitude is slightly less than that seen in the aorta. Pulmonic valve closure is seen at end-systole in this example. AV = aortic valve; ECG = electrocardiogram; LPA = left pulmonary artery; PV = pulmonic valve; RA = right atrium; RV = right ventricle; RPA = right pulmonary artery; TV = tricuspid valve.

Table 6.5. Contrast Agents

(1) Degassed tap water
(2) 5% dextrose in water
(3) 0.9% sodium chloride
(4) Indocyanine green
(5) Carbonated saline solution
(6) 70% sorbitol
(7) 50% or 70% dextrose in water*
(8) Renografin-76*
(9) Hydrogen peroxide
(10) Sodium bicarbonate solution + vitamin C
(11) Mixture 1:1 ratio 25% mannitol and 0.9% saline solution
(12) Mixture 1:1 ratio of Renografin-76 and 0.9% saline solution*
(13) Mixture 1:1 ratio of 70% sorbitol and 5% dextrose in water

* Liquids that have also undergone sonication produce contrast agents consisting of relatively uniform, stable and small (< 10μ diameter) gaseous microbubbles suspended in liquid solutions.

rate (T½) of the myocardium.[37,38] Intraoperative cardioplegic contrast echocardiography is useful in assessing myocardial perfusion during open heart surgery.[39] The latter technique has the potential of identifying segments at greatest ischemic risk and guiding the surgeon in determining the sequence of coronary artery bypass grafting and in providing improved intraoperative myocardial protection. Intraoperative contrast echocardiography has also been used to evaluate mitral valve operations.[40] A second operative procedure can be undertaken before chest closure in some patients with persistent mitral regurgitation detected by intraoperative 2-D contrast echocardiography.

The risk of side effects has been carefully studied and the results reported by the American Society of Echocardiography.[41] Fortunately, the risk is low (about 0.062%) and no residual side effects or long-term complications were observed. The most distressing side effect is a transient neurologic disturbance, probably as a result of gas embolization of microbubbles of various sizes. In a recent report, a transient cerebrovascular defect was noted after contrast echocardiography, which improved after 24 hours.[42] Other side effects reported include auditory hallucinations, paresthesias, and abdominal pain. These symptoms resemble paraben toxicity and were en-

Table 6.6. Clinical and Potential Research Applications of Contrast Echocardiography

(1) Identification or verification of anatomic structures, or both
(2) Detection of cardiac shunts
  (a) Left-to-right–negative contrast effect
  (b) Right-to-left and bidirectional shunts at the atrial, ventricular, and great vessel level
(3) Detection of regurgitation
  (a) Right-sided lesions with peripheral venous injections
  (b) Left-sided lesions with catheter injections
(4) Estimation of cardiac output
(5) Evaluating myocardial perfusion in relation to varying degrees of coronary stenosis
  (a) Direct catheter injection
  (b) Venous injections of small contrast agents that cross pulmonary circulation
(6) Intraoperative contrast echocardiography
  (a) Assessing myocardial perfusion during open heart surgery
  (b) Evaluation of success of mitral valve surgical procedures

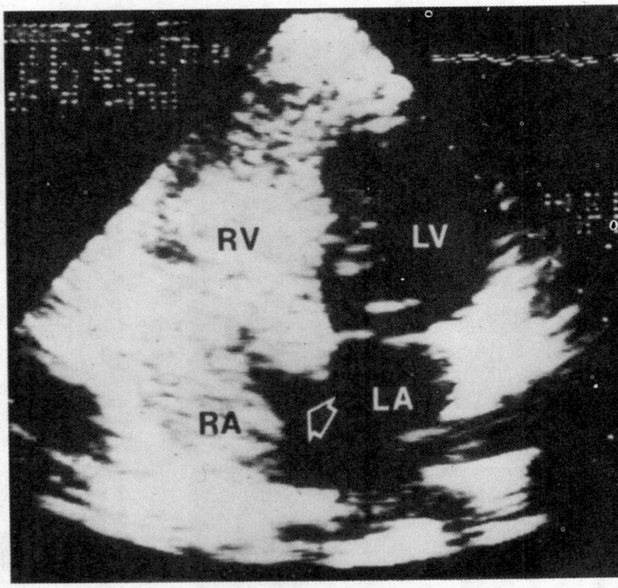

Figure 6.16. Apical four-chamber view in a patient with atrial septal defect. After opacification of the right atrium (RA) and right ventricle (RV) with a peripheral contrast injection, the negative contrast effect (*large arrow*) is seen. LA = left atrium; LV = left ventricle.

countered only during injections of bacteriostatic saline solution and not after injections of pure saline solution. Paraben-related substances have been used as preservative agents for injectable saline. Idiosyncratic reactions have been reported when green dye was used as a contrast agent. Other reported reactions include vagovagal effects and anxiety reactions that may be related to the injection itself or to venipuncture. Great precaution should be taken not to inject visible amounts of air especially in patients with right-to-left shunts or during arterial catheter injections. More recently, sonicated solutions have been used that provide small bubbles that cross the pulmonary circulation and visualize the left ventricular cavities as well as the myocardium during the coronary perfusion phase.[43] Because Doppler echocardiography inherently has a better signal-to-noise ratio than do conventional echocardiographic imaging systems, detection of abnormal contrast flow is significantly improved with this technique.[44]

CLINICAL APPLICATIONS

VALVULAR HEART DISEASE

Mitral Stenosis

Although M-mode echocardiography was originally thought to be precise in diagnosing the presence of mitral stenosis, it is not accurate in determining the severity of the lesion. Several studies have correlated the size of the mitral valve orifice as obtained on 2-D echocardiography with the size of the valve measured at surgery or calculated from cardiac catheterization data.[45–47] The results show a good correlation. However, there are limitations and pitfalls when evaluating mitral valve areas with 2-D techniques. In some patients, adequate examination can-

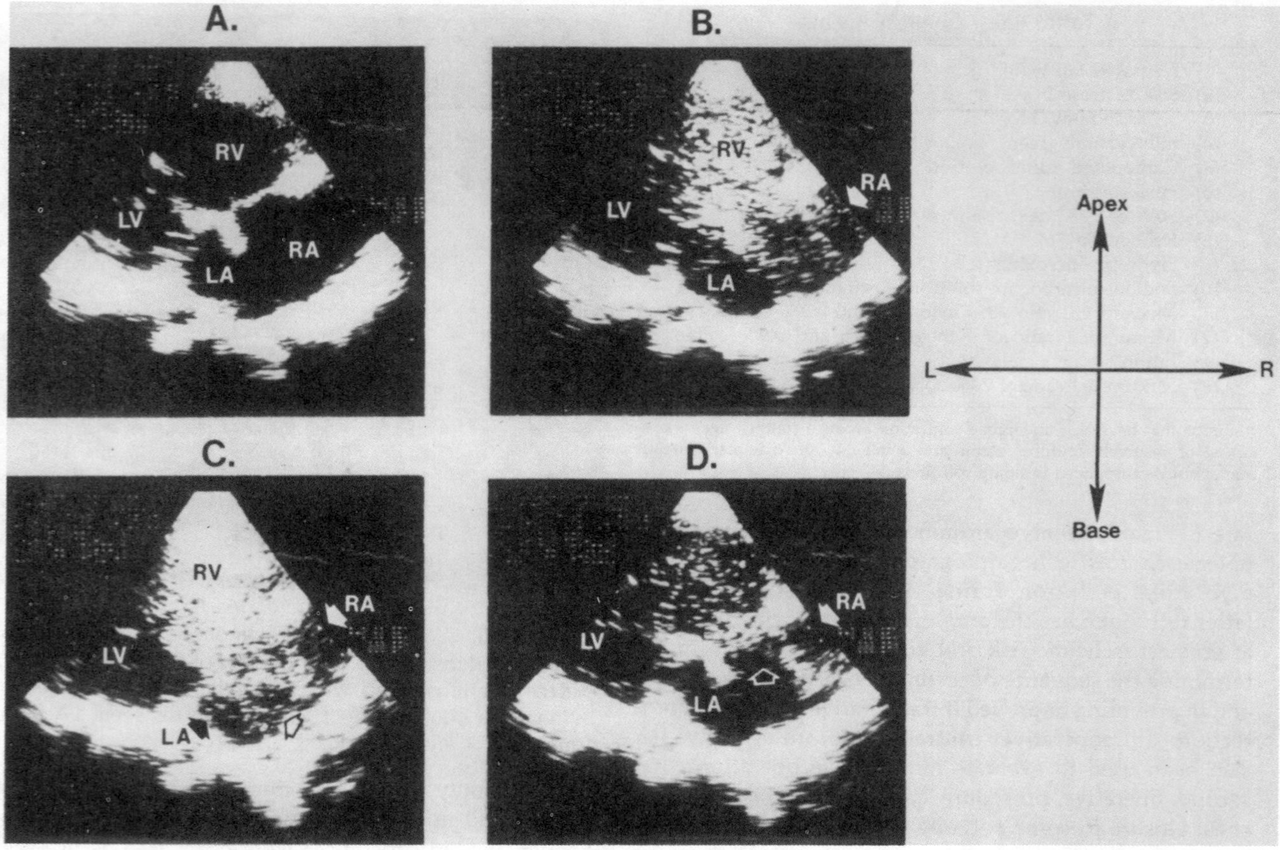

Figure 6.17. Modified off-axis parasternal view of the right and left ventricular chambers in a patient with atrial septal defect and bidirectional shunting. Contrast bubbles are seen to cross over from the right atrium (RA) to left atrium (LA) best seen in frame C, *dark arrow*. The negative contrast effect (*light arrows*) is also evident in frame D. RA = right atrium; RV = right ventricle.

not always be obtained because of the association of chest wall deformities or emphysema or both. In addition, careful attention should be paid to technique, and the transducer must be aligned superiorly and inferiorly to locate the smallest area separating the atrium and ventricle (Figure 6.18). The stenotic mitral valve assumes the shape of a funnel, and if the leaflets are imaged and cross-sectioned at the level of the body or at the base of the leaflets, a spuriously enlarged mitral valve orifice can be obtained. In addition, oblique angulation of the beam may produce a spuriously enlarged mitral valve orifice as a result of imaging the large anterior mitral leaflet, especially when it assumes an obtuse angle bend during diastole. The area determined by planimetry may also be inaccurate because of an irregularity in the margin of the orifice or an increased line of thickness from persistence of the video imaging system. Of utmost importance, in patients with heavy calcification or dense fibrosis of the valve tips, a spuriously small valve area may be obtained especially if the gain is improperly adjusted (Figure 6.18). In severely calcified leaflets, excess echo reflections from the calcium deposit may cause a leaflet to appear thicker and the mitral valve orifice to appear smaller than its actual size (Figure 6.18). Problems with lateral beam resolution and image dropout, particularly in the region of the commissures, may contribute to errors in measurement. Another 2-D echocardiographic feature of rheumatic mitral stenosis is diastolic doming of the anterior mitral leaflet with an obtuse angular bend during diastole, best appreciated in the parasternal long-axis view. Generally, the tips of the leaflets are restricted by chordae tendineae that are thickened, shortened and/or fused. The left atrium is enlarged in all views and should be examined carefully for thrombi[48] (Figure 6.19), especially in the area of the left atrial appendage.[49] Two-dimensional echocardiography is useful in detecting restenosis after mitral valve commissurotomy.[50]

Mitral stenosis is one of the more readily assessable lesions by Doppler echocardiography. Using continuous wave Doppler imaging from an apical window, maximum velocities are readily obtained and correlate well with simultaneously recorded gradients at cardiac catheterization.[51,52] In addition, the mitral valve area can be calculated using the pressure half-time technique reported by Hatle et al.[53] Pressure half-time is obtained by dividing the early, peak diastolic velocity by $\sqrt{2}$ (= 1.4) and measuring the time it takes for the velocity to decrease from its peak to this value. In general, pressure half-time measurements in excess of 220 ms indicate a mitral valve area of 1 cm^2 or less.[53,54] The mitral valve area (MVA) can be estimated by the formula: MVA (cm^2) = 220/pressure half-time (ms). Pressure half-time appears to be inde-

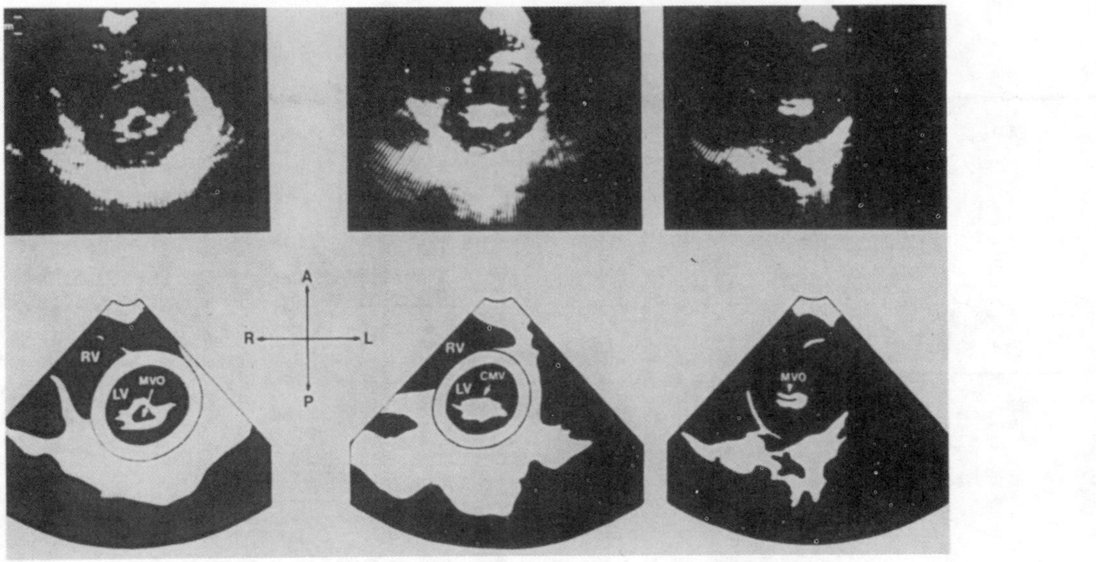

Figure 6.18. Parasternal short-axis images in patients with mitral stenosis. *Left*, the mitral valve orifice is considerably reduced in size and the mitral valve area measures 0.5 cm^2. *Middle*, Cross-sectional two-dimensional echocardiogram at the level of the mitral tips in a patient with severe mitral stenosis and calcified mitral valve (CMV). With normal gain setting, no mitral valve is demonstrated. *Right*, Same patient as in B with the gain setting decreased. The mitral valve orifice (MVO) can barely be appreciated, but the mitral valve area could not be calculated. LV = left ventricle; RV = right ventricle. (From Kotler et al,[262] with permission.)

pendent of cardiac output whether associated mitral regurgitation is present or not (Figure 6.20). In patients with atrial fibrillation and aortic regurgitation, care must be taken to differentiate transmitral flow from regurgitant aortic flow (Figure 6.21).

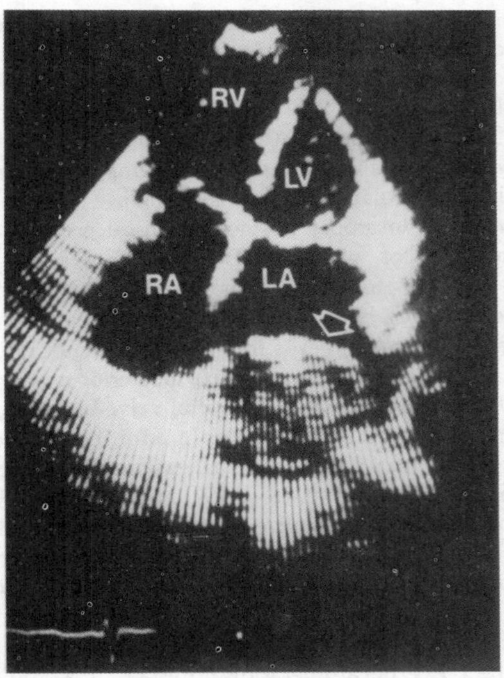

Figure 6.19. Apical four-chamber view in a patient with rheumatic mitral valve disease, demonstating an enlarged left atrium and a large thrombus adjacent to the posterolateral wall of the left atrium (*arrow*). LA = left atrium; LV = left ventricle; RA = right atrium; RV = right ventricle.

Assessment of pulmonary artery pressure is important in patients with mitral stenosis. Doppler recordings of pulmonary artery flow recently were shown to correlate well with pulmonary artery pressure measured at cardiac catheterization. Several groups have found a strong negative correlation between pulmonary activation times and systolic[55] and mean[56,57] pulmonary artery pressure. Activation time is measured as the time interval from the onset of flow to peak flow, and patients with activation time less than 100 m/s usually have mean pulmonary artery pressure in excess of 20 mm Hg.[55,56] Hatle et al[58] have used Doppler echocardiography to measure right ventricular isovolumic relaxation time. Using a nomogram previously described by Burstin,[59] they demonstrated a good positive correlation of this parameter with systolic pulmonary artery pressure. Figure 6.20 illustrates transmitral and pulmonary artery flow in a patient with severe mitral stenosis and pulmonary hypertension. Mitral valve area is calculated by the pressure half-time technique and mean pulmonary artery pressure (PAP) by the formula: mean PAP = 90 − 0.62 (activation time).[56]

Mitral Regurgitation

Mitral regurgitation may occur as a result of abnormal function of the mitral anulus, mitral valve leaflets, chordae tendineae, papillary muscles, and left ventricular myocardium. Although the severity of mitral regurgitation may not always be reliably detected by 2-D echocardiography, it is useful in evaluating the cause of mitral regurgitant murmurs.[60–62] The most common causes of mitral regurgitation today are mitral valve prolapse and rheumatic heart disease. Less common causes include ruptured chordae tendineae, papillary muscle dysfunction, anular calcification, hypertrophic obstructive cardiomyopathy, cleft mitral valve, and atrial myxoma. In a

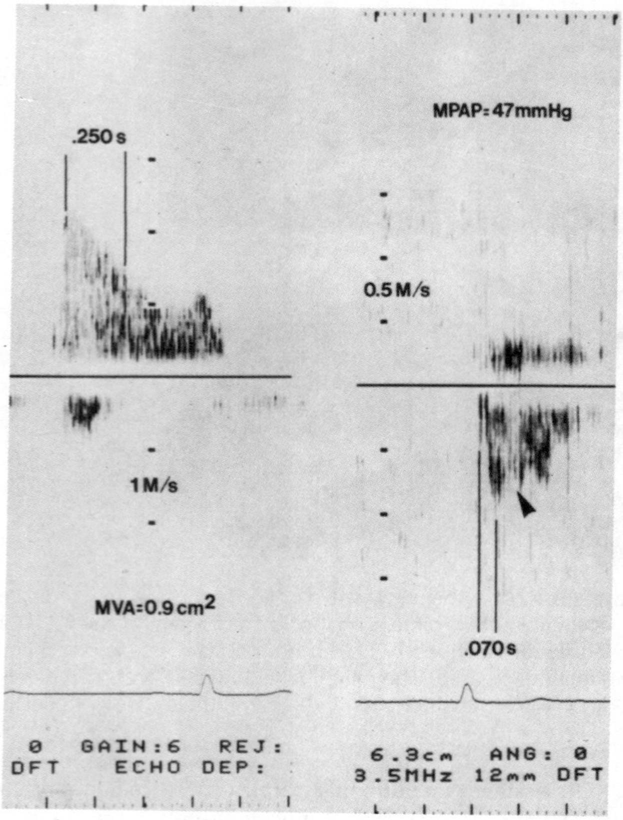

Figure 6.20. *Left*, continuous wave Doppler recording from the apical position in a patient with severe mitral stenosis. The early diastolic velocity measures 2.3 m/s for a peak diastolic gradient of 21 mm Hg. With the pressure half-time technique, the mitral valve area (MVA) is estimated to be 0.9 cm^2. See text for details. *Right*, Parasternal pulsed Doppler recording of the main pulmonary artery in the same patient. The time interval from the onset of flow to peak systolic velocity (ACT) is markedly shortened and measures 0.07 s. Using the formula of Mahan et al,[56] the mean pulmonary artery pressure (MPAP) is estimated to be 47 mm Hg. Midsystolic "notching" of the velocity spectrum (arrowhead) is commonly seen in severe pulmonary hypertension. See text for details.

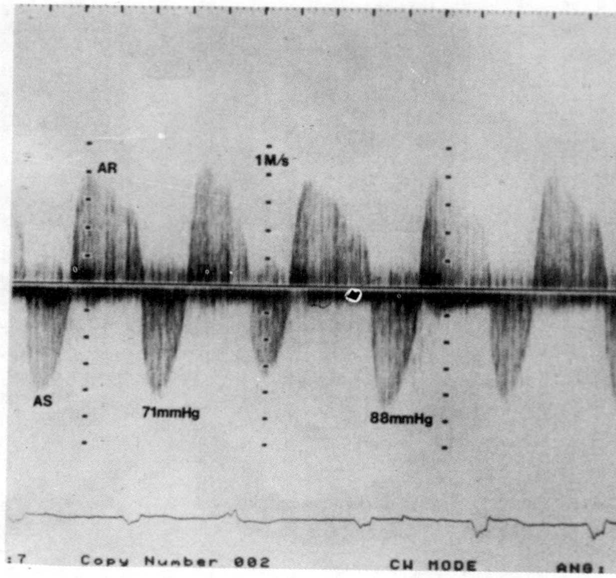

Figure 6.21. Continuous wave Doppler recording from the apical position in a patient with aortic stenosis (AS) and aortic regurgitation (AR). During systole, flow in the proximal ascending aorta is directed away from the transducer and is displayed below the baseline. A peak systolic velocity of 4.2 m/s indicates a peak systolic gradient of 71 mm Hg. On the beat following the premature contraction, the aortic valve gradient increases to 88 mm Hg. During diastole, flow of aortic regurgitation is directed toward the transducer and is displayed above the baseline. Regurgitant flow begins immediately after aortic valve closure, and this feature can be used to differentiate flow due to mitral stenosis. (This occurs irrespective of whether the patient is in sinus rhythm or atrial fibrillation.)

small percentage of cases only has 2-D echocardiography been unable to provide accurate diagnosis with regard to etiology. The echocardiographic features of rheumatic mitral regurgitation appear identical to those of stenosis in the parasternal long-axis view. However, in the parasternal short-axis view the mitral valve area is not as significantly reduced as in mitral stenosis or it may be only mildly reduced. In the parasternal short-axis view during systole, failure of coaptation leaflets of small areas of either the medial or lateral aspect of the valve leaflets has been associated with minimal regurgitation.[63] In patients with significant mitral regurgitation, failure of both sides to close has been noted.

A recent report on mitral valve prolapse by Albert et al.[64] demonstrated that a combination of arching of one or both mitral leaflets in the parasternal long-axis view (Figure 6.22C) and bowing of one or both leaflets in an apical four-chamber view in association with posterior coaptation of the leaflets in relation to the mitral anulus in both views resulted in a sensitivity of 87% and a specificity of 97%.

Echocardiographic diagnosis of mitral valve prolapse may occur more frequently as compared with clinical or phonocardiographic findings.[65] In a recent study, only 2% of 100 patients had 2-D echocardiographic evidence of mitral valve prolapse.[66] An additional four patients had midsystolic clicks without echocardiographic evidence of mitral valve prolapse. A "pseudoprolapse" pattern was produced by improper M-mode transducer angulation. The question of whether 2-D echocardiography is the "gold standard" for the diagnosis of mitral valve prolapse has been argued by some investigators.[67]

There are some patients in whom 2-D echocardiography fails to demonstrate the rapid posterior motion of a relatively small portion of the mitral valve because of the low frame rate of 2-D imaging. In addition, 2-D echocardiography may not allow visualization of all three scallops of the posterior mitral leaflet, and "off-axis" views may be required to visualize a localized area of prolapse. Some investigators have argued that the M-mode criteria of prolapse, ie, a fairly abrupt posterior motion of the mitral valve apparatus in late systole or holosystolic prolapse throughout systole, or both,[68] may be better defined than the 2-D echocardiographic criteria.[67] In a study employing M-mode, 2-D echocardiography and Doppler echocardiography, Abbasi et al[69] improved the sensitivity of diagnosis of mitral valve prolapse with all three techniques. With M-mode alone, the sensitivity was 50%, with 2-D echocardiography 68%, with combined M-mode and 2-D echocardiography 77%, whereas with

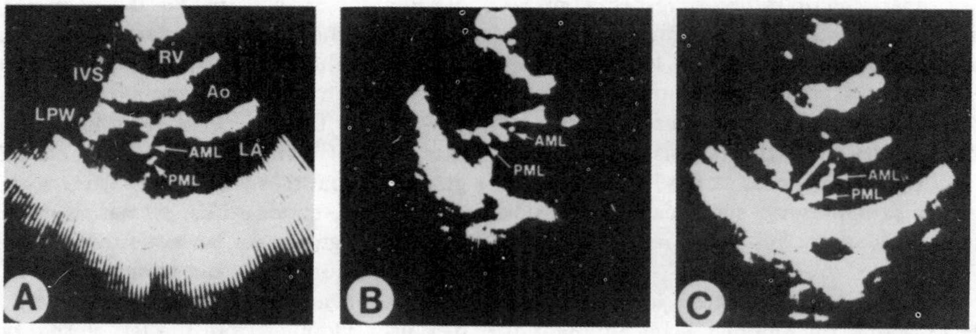

Figure 6.22. Two-dimensional images all obtained in the parasternal long-axis view during systole. *A*, Flail posterior leaflet. The tip of the posterior mitral leaflet (PML) has moved beyond the line of mitral closure into the left atrium (LA). *B*, Flail anterior leaflet. The tip of the anterior mitral leaflet (AML) was bent perpendicular to the body of the AML and has moved beyond the line of mitral closure into the left atrium. *C*, Anterior and posterior mitral leaflet prolapse. The AML and PML have prolapsed beyond the mitral annulus (*large white arrow*) and both leaflets are arched superiorly into the left atrium. Note that the coaptation point, although posteriorly situated, is preserved in prolapse, in contrast to flail leaflets. Ao = aorta; IVS = interventricular septum; LPW = left ventricular posterior wall; RV = right ventricle. (From Kotler et al,[263] with permission. Copyright © 1980 by Year Book Medical Publishers, Inc , Chicago.)

all three techniques combined, the sensitivity increased to 93%.

Ruptured chordae tendineae with a flail mitral leaflet is easily detected by 2-D echocardiography. Findings include rapid systolic motion of the involved leaflet beyond the line of valve closure into the left atrium best appreciated in the parasternal long-axis view.[70] The maximum abnormal systolic motion is greatest at the tip of the leaflet with loss of normal coaptation point (Figure 6.22A and B). The 2-D echocardiographic criteria for the detection of a flail mitral leaflet are clearly superior to the M-mode criteria.[71] Not all patients with flail mitral leaflets require surgery, and 2-D echocardiography is a useful technique in following such patients.[72] In patients who remained asymptomatic, left ventricular ejection fraction and left atrial volumes by 2-D echocardiography were stable, whereas patients who became more symptomatic and required surgery showed progressive increases in both left ventricular and left atrial volumes.

Mitral anular calcification can readily be diagnosed by echocardiography and is generally best appreciated in the parasternal long- and short-axis views. In the parasternal short-axis view, mitral anular calcification appears as a crescent mass of echoes visualized beneath the posterior mitral leaflet and anterior to the left ventricular posterior wall. When the calcification was close to the conduction system, 53% of patients had conduction abnormalities versus 26% of patients with posterior mitral anular calcification only that was remote from the conduction system.[73] In patients with mitral anular calcification, atrial fibrillation was 12 times more frequent than in those without it.[74] Other recognizable complications of mitral anular calcification on 2-D echocardiography include rapidly progressive mitral stenosis[75] and cerebral emboli.[76]

The severity of mitral regurgitation has been calculated by computing the left atrial emptying volume and subtracting the diastolic from the systolic atrial volume.[77] Patients with significant mitral regurgitation had left atrial volumes greater than 40 ml.[77,78]

Mitral regurgitation is best detected using pulsed Doppler echocardiography from either the apical or left parasternal approach. With the sample volume placed immediately superior to the mitral valve, regurgitant systolic flow is detected.[79,80] Because the regurgitant flow velocity usually exceeds the limit of the pulsed mode, aliasing occurs and the signal is seen on both sides of the baseline (Figure 6.2). If continuous wave Doppler is used from the apex, the signal is seen below the baseline, indicating flow away from the transducer. Mitral regurgitation is easily differentiated from aortic outflow and tricuspid regurgitation by the timing of flow and respiratory variation. Several techniques for quantitating the severity of mitral regurgitation have been reported. With the flow mapping technique, pulsed Doppler recording is used to map the extent of flow disturbance within the left atrium. Generally, the greater the distance from the mitral valve and the greater the area occupied by disturbed flow, the greater will be the severity of regurgitation as assessed by contrast angiography.[81,82] The new technique of color flow imaging has proved particularly useful in the semiquantitative assessment of all regurgitant lesions.[16,17,20] Another quantitative approach is to measure the regurgitant fraction. This is accomplished by measuring flow across the mitral valve (forward and regurgitant flow) and comparing it to the stroke volume through the aortic valve, or an average of aortic and pulmonary stroke volume (forward flow).[83] Finally, the spectral recording itself can give clues to the severity of regurgitation. In severe regurgitation, the intensity of the spectral tracing will be increased, the maximum velocity will decrease toward end-systole, and the velocity of antegrade diastolic flow will greatly be increased[14] (Figure 6.21).

Aortic Stenosis

The echocardiographic features of aortic stenosis include thickening of the leaflets with reduction of valve excursion. Attempts have been made to separate maximal aortic valve opening in normal subjects and patients with aortic stenosis.[84,85] However, there is individual overlap between groups of patients with varying degrees of maximal aortic opening measurements. As a general rule of thumb, most patients with critical aortic stenosis (aortic valve areas of 0.75 cm^2 or less) have demonstrated maximal aortic cusp separation of 11 mm or less. In contrast, a normal patient will usually have separation of 20 mm or more. Leaflet separation greater than 13 mm usually has been associated with mild lesions and aortic valve areas of 1 cm^2 or greater. Additional indirect criteria for determining the severity of aortic stenosis can be ascertained by measuring the thickness of the left ventricular wall. However, in patients with systemic hypertension or left ventricular dilatation this measurement may be unreliable.

In an adult population, aortic stenosis is considerably more difficult to assess by Doppler echocardiography than is mitral stenosis. Peak systolic velocities are usually best recorded with continuous wave Doppler echocardiography from a high right parasternal position, the suprasternal notch, or the apical position. It is important to interrogate the aortic valve from a variety of ultrasonic windows as it cannot be predicted which window will produce the highest velocity in a given patient. In a recent reported study, high velocity jets were best recorded from the cardiac apex and less frequently from the right parasternal and suprasternal areas.[86] Pulsed Doppler echocardiography is useful in detecting the level of obstruction and assessing associated aortic regurgitation.[13] The audio signal is a useful guide in obtaining peak velocities. A high-pitched, whistling sound is heard when the Doppler beam is in the stenotic jet. A good correlation has been found between the peak systolic gradient on Doppler echocardiography and the peak instantaneous gradient at cardiac catheterization.[54,87–89] The peak systolic gradient on Doppler echocardiography overestimates the peak-to-peak and mean gradients commonly reported at catheterization. Mean systolic gradients by both techniques show excellent agreement.[90]

Doppler-derived peak systolic gradients are influenced by cardiac output. Therefore, patients with critical aortic stenosis and low cardiac output may only show modest increases in velocity. Conversely, patients with significant aortic regurgitation and only moderate aortic stenosis may be classified as having severe aortic stenosis. Assessment of velocity of flow in the left ventricular outflow tract can be useful in making the distinction. A new Doppler technique involves calculation of aortic valve area using cardiac output determined either noninvasively[91] or by thermodilution.[92] Shown in Figure 6.21 is a tracing of a patient with moderately severe aortic stenosis with associated aortic regurgitation.

Aortic Regurgitation

Recently, it was demonstrated that 2-D echocardiography is of value in determining the cause of aortic regurgitation, being able to differentiate valvular from aortic root causes.[93] Rheumatic aortic regurgitation and that due to endocarditis were the most common causes. In patients with infective endocarditis and aortic regurgitation, echoes from a vegetation or portion of the disrupted aortic valve frequently prolapse into the left ventricular outflow tract during diastole. The most useful echocardiographic finding in aortic regurgitation is fine fluttering of the anterior leaflet of the mitral valve during diastole and, rarely, that of the posterior leaflet or the left side of the interventricular septum. These movements are presumably caused by the regurgitant jet flowing into the left ventricle. When the aortic valve is disrupted or flail, it may flutter during diastole and is a reliable, but insensitive, finding in patients with chronic aortic regurgitation. In patients with acute aortic regurgitation usually secondary to endocarditis, premature mitral valve closure can be recognized by M-mode techniques.

Aortic regurgitation can be detected with pulsed or continuous wave Doppler echocardiography from the apex or pulsed Doppler from the left sternal border with the sample volume placed just inferior to the aortic valve (Figure 6.21). Moderate to severe aortic regurgitation can also be detected in the aorta itself.[94,95] Doppler echocardiography is highly sensitive and specific for the detection of aortic regurgitation and estimation of its severity.[96–98] Mapping the extent of regurgitant flow into the left ventricle gives a good estimate of its severity as compared with contrast angiography.[96,97] Although there was overlap between groups with mild and those with moderate aortic regurgitation, severe regurgitation was clearly differentiated. A comparison of forward and reverse flow in the aorta is also useful in assessing the degree of regurgitation.[94,95,98] In patients with severe (3+ to 4+) aortic regurgitation, the diastolic blood pressure measured by cuff sphygmomanometer, and end-diastolic aortic-left ventricular pressure gradient, measured by Doppler echocardiography, can be used to predict left ventricular end-diastolic pressure.[99]

Interest in defining the optimum time of valve replacement in patients with aortic regurgitation and the predictors of outcome after valve replacement have led investigators to use noninvasive techniques pre- and postoperatively.[100] The end-diastolic dimension and fractional shortening measured by echocardiography have been proposed as prognostic predictors. However, the results have been controversial.[100–102] In a series of 50 consecutive patients undergoing aortic valve replacement, Henry et al[100] reported a high risk group of patients who died either at operation or subsequently from congestive heart failure. In the patients who died, 9 of 13 patients had a preoperative left ventricular systolic dimension 55 mm or greater; only one patient died late of congestive heart failure.

In another study reported by Fioretti et al,[101] 47 consecutive patients underwent aortic valve replacement for isolated, asymptomatic aortic regurgitation. Of the 27 patients with a preoperative end-systolic dimension 55 mm or greater and 20 patients with a preoperative end-systolic dimension less than 55 mm, there were no pre- or postoperative deaths in a late follow-up period averaging 41 months. In both groups, the left ventricular end-diastolic dimension decreased considerably. Despite the controversy of recommending aortic valve replacement for asymptomatic patients with a large end-systolic dimension, limitations with regard to M-mode echocardiography occur.[102] In patients with grossly enlarged left ventricles, the dimensions may vary as much as 20%, depending on angulation of the transducer and position of the patient.

Tricuspid Stenosis and Regurgitation

Disorders of the tricuspid valve can readily be assessed with 2-D echocardiography, because all three leaflets of the tricuspid valve can be identified. Tricuspid regurgitation can be demonstrated by contrast echocardiography and imaging the inferior vena cava. Contrast bubbles that appear only during systole are diagnostic of tricuspid regurgitation.[103] In a recent study of 372 patients with rheumatic mitral valve disease, 23 (6%) had tricuspid valve involvement.[104] The 2-D echocardiographic criteria of rheumatic tricuspid valve disease include thickened leaflets with restricted motion, diastolic doming, and encroachment of the leaflet tips on the ventricular inlet. By combining contrast echocardiography, Doppler echocardiography, and the anatomic features of the tricuspid valve, differentiation between organic and functional tricuspid valve disease can readily be made. Although the 2-D features of rheumatic tricuspid stenosis are identical to those of mitral stenosis, it is usually not possible to image the tricuspid valve area on cross-section, and therefore the severity of tricuspid stenosis should be determined using Doppler techniques. Other disorders that affect the tricuspid valve such as carcinoid heart disease,[105] Ebstein's anomaly of the tricuspid valve,[106] tricuspid valve prolapse,[107] and endocarditis[108] can readily be diagnosed by 2-D echocardiography.

Doppler echocardiographic detection and quantification of tricuspid regurgitation is similar to the technique used for mitral regurgitation (Figure 6.23). Mapping the right atrium can readily be performed from the apex or left sternal border to provide a rough approximation of severity.[109] In addition, the subcostal position can be used to assess antegrade diastolic and retrograde systolic flow in the inferior vena cava[110] and hepatic vein (Figure 6.24).[111,112] Similar results have been obtained by examining the superior vena cava from the suprasternal notch.[113] Although considerable overlap exists in the derived indexes of mild and moderate tricuspid regurgitation, severe regurgitation is clearly separated with these techniques.[110–113] The incidence of Doppler-detected tricuspid regurgitation has been reported to be from 47% to 96% in normal subjects as well as in patients with various forms of heart disease.[114,115] Although often not clinically significant, the presence of tricuspid regurgitation can provide valuable information about right heart hemodynamics. By adding right atrial pressure, as estimated from the jugular venous pulse, to the Doppler-derived peak right ventricular–right atrial systolic gradient, a noninvasive estimate of right ventricular systolic pressure is obtained.[116,117] In the absence of right ventricular outflow obstruction, this value will also represent systolic pulmonary artery pressure.

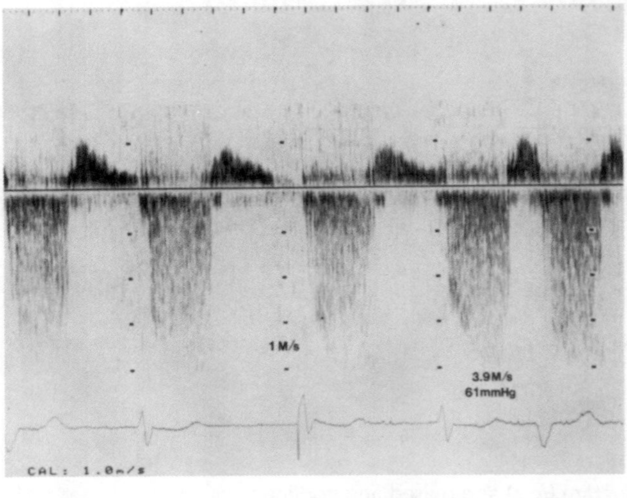

Figure 6.23. Continuous wave Doppler recording from the apical position in a patient with severe tricuspid regurgitation. During diastole, antegrade tricuspid flow velocity is increased to approximately 1.1 m/s. During systole, peak regurgitant flow velocity is 3.9 m/s, indicating a right ventricular-to-right atrial pressure decrease of 61 mm Hg. The right atrial pressure was estimated to be 10 mm Hg from the jugular venous pulse, indicating right ventricular peak systolic pressure of 71 mm Hg.

Spectral recording of tricuspid stenosis is similar to that of mitral stenosis. However, peak diastolic velocity is usually not as high as that in mitral stenosis, and exaggerated inspiratory augmentation of flow velocity is frequently present.[14,118]

Pulmonic Stenosis

M-mode echocardiography has been useful in evaluating valvular pulmonic stenosis. An increase in posterior deflection of the posterior pulmonary leaflet after atrial contraction has been demonstrated.[119] Doming of the pulmonic valves with restricted motion can also be seen with 2-D techniques[120] (Figure 6.25).

Pulmonic stenosis is easily evaluated in both adults and children because of the favorable orientation of the pulmonary artery. Using continuous wave Doppler echocardiography, the pulmonary artery is sampled from either a parasternal or subcostal short-axis view at the level of the great vessels. Doppler echocardiographic gradients show excellent correlation with those obtained at cardiac catheterization.[14,121,122] Infundibular and valvular pulmonic stenosis can be differentiated with pulsed Doppler sampling.[14,122]

Pulmonic Regurgitation

Pulmonic regurgitation can be recognized predominantly by Doppler techniques and should be suspected in all patients with enlarged pulmonary arteries as seen on 2-D echocardiography. The same ultrasonic window is used for pulmonic regurgitation and stenosis. The pulsed Doppler sample volume is placed beneath the pulmonic valve in the right ventricular outflow tract. With normal diastolic pulmonary artery pressure, the early diastolic regurgitant velocity is much less than that seen in aortic regurgitation and the diastolic slope of the velocity recording is steep.[123] In pulmonary hypertension, early diastolic regurgitant velocities are high, showing little diminution throughout diastole.[123] With significant pulmonic regurgitation, regurgitant flow can also be recorded in the pulmonary artery. Pulmonic regurgitation is frequently found by Doppler echocardiography in patients with congenital (Figure 6.25) and acquired heart disease[114,115] as well as in apparently normal persons.[114,115]

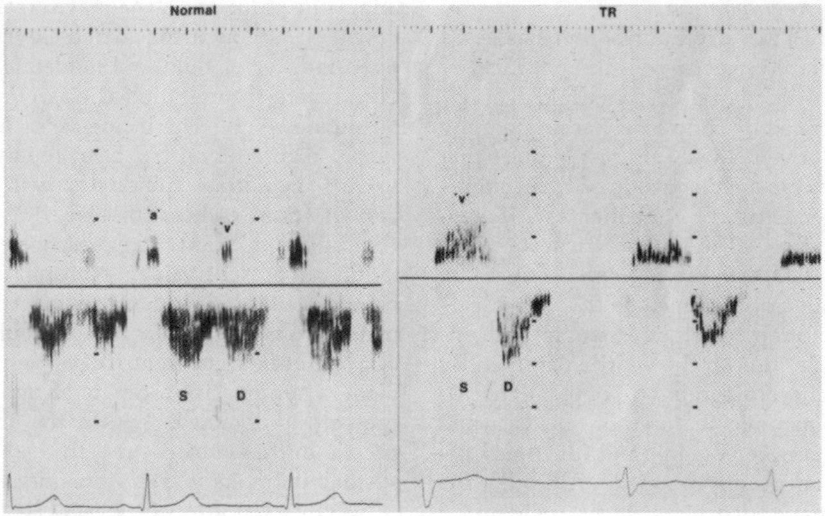

Figure 6.24. Pulsed Doppler recordings of hepatic vein flow in a normal subject (*left*) and in a patient with moderately severe tricuspid regurgitation (*right*) obtained from a subcostal approach. In the normal subject, flow away from the transducer is noted during systole (S) and diastole (D). Brief periods of reversed flow occur during atrial contraction and in early diastole and correspond to the 'a' and 'v' waves seen in right atrial pressure recordings. On the right, tricuspid regurgitation (TR) is seen as systolic flow above the baseline.

PROSTHETIC VALVES

Combining phonocardiography and M-mode echocardiography is a useful noninvasive technique in differentiating normal from abnormal metallic prosthetic valve function. The A_2-mitral valve opening interval is a valuable measurement.[124] This interval can be recorded in patients in whom the opening click is not well heard by measuring the interval from the aortic valve closure sound on phonocardiography to the maximal opening of the mitral prosthesis recorded on echocardiography. A short-

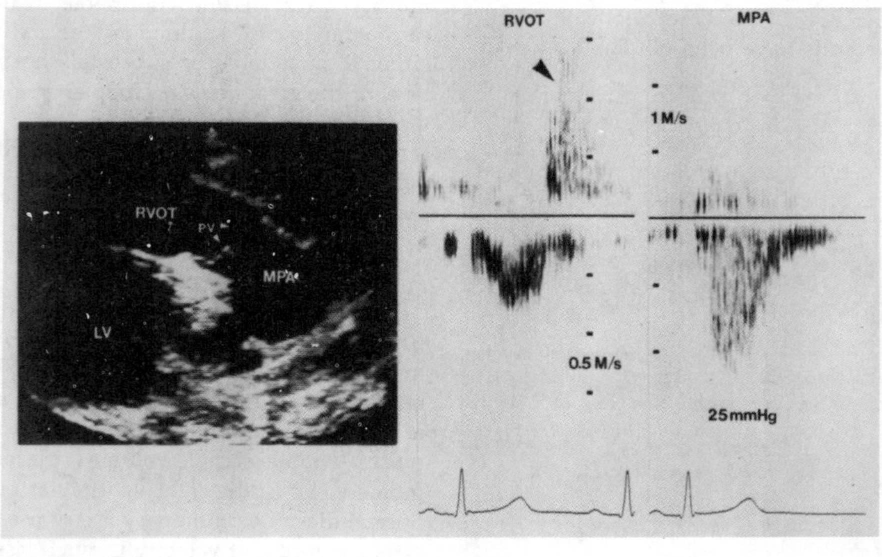

Figure 6.25. Two-dimensional echocardiogram (*left*) and pulsed and continuous wave Doppler recordings (*middle* and *right*) from the parasternal position in a patient with mild valvular pulmonic stenosis and regurgitation. During systole, classic doming of the pulmonic valve leaflets (PV) is noted (*left*). With the sample volume positioned in the right ventricular outflow tract (RVOT), diastolic flow from pulmonic regurgitation is displayed above the baseline (*middle*). Using continuous wave Doppler recording, a peak systolic velocity of 2.5 m/s is recorded in the main pulmonary artery (MPA), indicating a peak systolic gradient of 25 mm Hg across the pulmonic valve (*right*). The mean pulmonic valve gradient was 13 mm Hg. LV = left ventricle.

ened A_2-mitral valve opening interval may indicate mitral obstruction or severe regurgitation. However, it may also occur in the presence of severe left ventricular dysfunction. A prolonged A_2-mitral valve opening interval may indicate a sticking valve with clot or tissue ingrowth as well as left ventricular dysfunction. The intensity of opening and closing clicks and associated functional murmurs will depend on the type of prosthetic valve, heart rate, rhythm, and underlying hemodynamic status.[125] Arrhythmias or conduction disturbances, or both, may produce motion patterns that mimic the echocardiographic signs of malfunctioning prosthetic valves. With regard to mechanical valves, 2-D echocardiography is of limited help in assessing patients with metallic prosthetic valves because of reverberating artifacts and sidelobe echoes.[126] However, 2-D echocardiography is useful in excluding underlying left ventricular dysfunction. It also allows precise determination of the alignment of the prosthetic valve for optimal M-mode and Doppler evaluation.[127] Two-dimensional echocardiography can also allow a diagnosis of pericardial effusion and exclusion of other valvular abnormalities. With regard to bioprosthetic valves, 2-D echocardiography appears to be superior to M-mode in detecting primary valve failure.[126,128] In addition, detection of vegetations, valve alignment, ring, and individual leaflet motion can readily be accomplished with 2-D echocardiography. When considering the value of noninvasive techniques in assessing prosthetic valve function, it is most important to recognize that the patient must serve as his or her own control in the follow-up.

Doppler echocardiography has been of considerable value in evaluating prosthetic valve stenosis and regurgitation. Although moderate and severe valve dysfunction is easily detected by Doppler techniques, minimal information is available for precisely defining velocities in a wide variety of prostheses. The ability of Doppler echocardiography to diagnose mild forms of valve dysfunction with confidence has not adequately been shown. Holen et al[129] in a study of 19 patients with Björk-Shiley, Hancock, and Lillehei-Kaster mitral prostheses in the immediate post-operative period found that obstruction to flow was often quite significant. In another study of nine patients with Björk-Shiley mitral valves, the mean diastolic gradients ranged from 2 to 12.5 mm Hg.[130] Hatle and Angelsen[14] reported 76 cases of various mitral tilting disk and tissue prostheses. The mean diastolic gradients in the tilting disk valves were between 2 and 5 mm Hg and the pressure half-time ranged from 60 to 130 ms. Twelve patients with perivalvular leaks had mean diastolic gradients in the 4- to 8-mm Hg range. Patients with mitral tissue prostheses had higher gradients. There was no apparent correlation between valve size and gradient. These same investigators reported a large series of various aortic valve prostheses. The mean pressure gradient ranged from approximately 5 to 35 mm Hg.[14] Of 87 patients, 54 (62%) had some degree of aortic regurgitation. In 81% of these patients, regurgitant signals extended less than 2 cm below the aortic valve and were considered mild or insignificant. In five patients, regurgitant signals were recorded at the mid-ventricular level, and in another five, the signals extended through more than two thirds of the ventricle. These were considered moderate and severe, respectively. Doppler assessment of the severity of aortic regurgitation correlated well with contrast angiography.[14] In a more recent study, Williams and Labovitz[131] reported similar results. Seventy patients had either Björk-Shiley, porcine, or Starr-Edwards aortic valve prostheses and 64 patients had one of the same types of mitral valve prostheses. There was a wide range of "normal" transvalvular gradients, and valvular regurgitation was not uncommon.[131] Whether or not Doppler echocardiography is too sensitive to differentiate benign, "physiologic" regurgitation from true, pathologic regurgitation will require further study. Furthermore, many types of metallic prosthetic valves have complex, eccentric flow profiles and the maximum measured velocity may not represent the average pressure decrease across the entire orifice of the valve. Figure 6.26 is from a patient with Björk-Shiley aortic and mitral prostheses. Continuous wave Doppler echocardiography is used from the apical position to record maximum aortic outflow velocity. A peak systolic gradient of 25 mm Hg is recorded and during diastole, the flow toward the transducer suggests aortic regurgitation. However, on careful examination of the tracing, an 0.08-second hiatus between aortic valve closure and onset of diastolic flow is noted. Hence, this is normal transmitral and not regurgitant aortic flow.

BACTERIAL ENDOCARDITIS

The reported prevalence of vegetations detected on echocardiography in patients with infective endocarditis ranges from 13% to 78% with a mean of 30% to

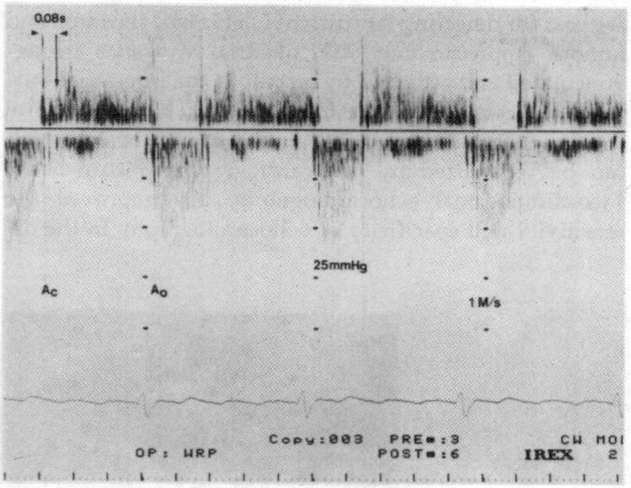

Figure 6.26. Continuous wave Doppler recording from the apical position in a patient with Björk-Shiley mitral and aortic prostheses. During systole, the aortic valve opening (Ao) and closing (Ac) clicks are well recorded. A peak systolic velocity of 2.5 m/s in the ascending aorta indicates a peak instantaneous aortic valve gradient of 25 mm Hg. During diastole, flow towards the transducer suggests prosthetic aortic valve regurgitation. On close examination of beat 1, an 0.08 s hiatus is noted from the aortic valve closure to the onset of diastolic flow, indicating that this is normal flow through the prosthetic mitral valve and not aortic regurgitation.

50%.[132–136] Both M-mode and 2-D echocardiography play a complementary role in the diagnosis of endocarditis as well as in providing pathophysiologic information. The 2-D echocardiographic features of vegetations appear as rapidly oscillating masses that either attach to or replace normal valve tissue (Figure 6.27).[135] Vegetations are generally localized to individual leaflets and the size and mobility of the vegetation can readily be assessed. The complications of bacterial endocarditis such as aortic root abscess, annular or myocardial abscess, aneurysms of the sinus of Valsalva, and flail leaflets can be detected more readily by 2-D than by M-mode echocardiography.[133] There are limitations with regard to echocardiography in diagnosing vegetations. These include size of vegetation, stage of development of vegetation, preexisting valvular disease such as myxomatous mitral valve leaflets, rheumatic mitral valve disease, and calcified bicuspid aortic valves, and evaluation of patients with a previous episode of endocarditis. Detection of right-sided endocarditis by echocardiography in intravenous drug addicts and in those with recurrent septic emboli provides a basis for rational therapy.[108] In our reported series,[136] patients with echocardiographically demonstrated vegetations have a higher incidence of congestive heart failure and major embolic events, but the precise treatment of such an individual remains controversial.

INTRACARDIAC MASSES

A significant advance in 2-D echocardiography has been to accurately localize and recognize intracardiac masses. The technique allows more precise appreciation of the size, shape, mobility, and origin of the lesion, features that are not always recognized by M-mode techniques. The apical four-chamber and two-chamber views are best for detecting left thrombi, left atrial thrombi, and tumors. Approximately 90% of atrial myxomas are pedunculated and attached by a stalk to the interatrial septum in the region of the fossa ovalis. The stalk allows the tumor to move in relation to the cardiac cycle, which can be recognized by echocardiography (Figure 6.28). Two-dimensional echocardiography has improved the sensitivity and specificity of echocardiography in the diagnosis of myxomas and provides information regarding size, shape, location, and mobility of the tumors.[137–140] If the myxoma is sessile and does not prolapse through the mitral orifice, 2-D echocardiography may still offer accurate diagnostic information (Figure 6.29).[141]

Left atrial thrombus usually occurs in a setting of reduced flow, as in mitral stenosis or an enlarged left atrium, or both. Although most thrombi are situated in the left atrial appendage, an area that is difficult to assess by 2-D echocardiography, some may be situated adjacent to the posterior and lateral wall of the left atrium (Figure 6.19). To improve the sensitivity of identifying thrombi of the left atrial appendage, Herzog et al[49] have suggested a modified short-axis parasternal view which visualizes the aorta and pulmonary artery. From this standard view and with slight lateral tilting, the left atrial appendage below the pulmonary artery can be visualized.

Two-dimensional echocardiography is the technique of choice in the detection of right atrial masses and can differentiate abnormal masses from normal intracardiac structures such as a eustachian valve, catheters, pacemaker electrodes, and artifacts.[141] The most common right atrial lesions are right atrial thrombi and myxomas. Right atrial thrombi may occur in the presence of cardiomyopathy; after insertion of intracardiac catheters, postoperatively, in patients with idiopathic right atrial dilatation; and in some patients with tricuspid stenosis.[141] Mobile thrombi in the right atrium and inferior vena cava (Figure 6.30) during transition from the leg veins have recently been reported.[142,143] The detection of these transitional thrombi may be ominous because most patients have massive pulmonary emboli. Two-dimensional echocardiography can define tumor thrombus in the right atrium that has extended from the inferior vena cava in patients with hypernephroma of the kidney.[144] Detection of such a lesion is of major importance, because such lesions can be considered for resection and surgical curative results can be obtained without necessarily implying inoperability and distant metastatic disease. Continuous wave and pulsed Doppler are sensitive techniques in the assessment of associated valvular obstruction and regurgitation.[14]

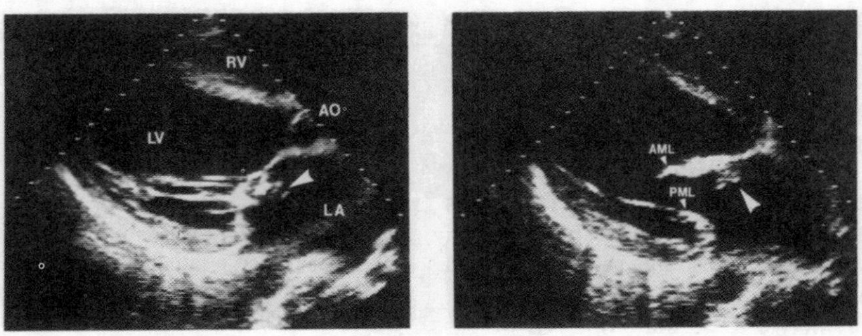

Figure 6.27. Parasternal long-axis views (*left*, systole; *right*, diastole) in a patient with bacterial endocarditis of the anterior mitral leaflet (AML). The large shaggy vegetation (*white arrow*) is attached to the AML on the atrial surface. The entire anterior mitral leaflet is thickened. The left ventricle (LV) and left atrium (LA) are enlarged because of significant mitral regurgitation. Ao = aorta; PML = posterior mitral leaflet; RV = right ventricle.

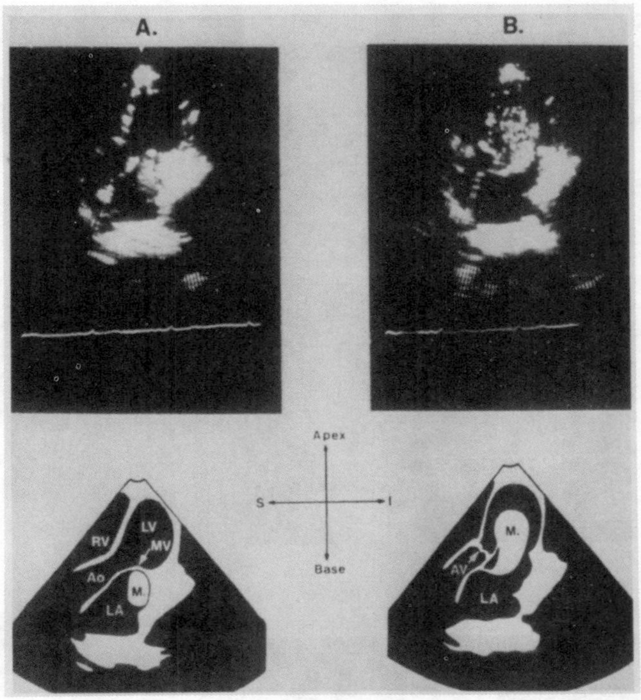

Figure 6.28. Apical right anterior oblique equivalent view of the left ventricle (LV) and left atrium (LA) in a patient with left atrial myxoma. During systole (*left*) a large echogenic mass (M) is seen posterior to the mitral valve (MV) and located in the left atrium. During diastole (*right*) the mass prolapses through the mitral valve into the left ventricle. The stalk of the mass is clearly defined. Ao = aorta; AV = aortic valve; RV = right ventricle. (From DePace et al,[48] with permission.)

CORONARY ARTERY DISEASE

Two-dimensional echocardiography is ideally suited for the determination of both global and regional left ventricular function, because it allows direct visualization of the entire left ventricle and identification of zones of abnormal myocardial thickening or thinning, or both. Abnormal regional wall motion is a sensitive and early indicator of myocardial ischemia and fibrosis.[145] It should be noted that temporal heterogeneity and regional variability of contractions per se may not necessarily indicate the presence of ischemia or infarction, as it has been reported in normal subjects.[146,147] However, dyskinesia, or aneurysmal bulging of part of the ventricle during systole that results in an increased segment area has not been observed in normal subjects.[148] It is therefore a specific indicator of regional transmural ischemia or acute infarction. Infarct size may be overestimated by two-dimensional echocardiography when the circumferential extent of dyskinesia is compared with the circumferential extent of the infarction found at pathologic examination.[149,150] The cause of the contraction abnormality in the normal segments has been attributed to mechanical tethering of normal myocardium by the adjacent infarcted myocardium. Several studies have compared regional wall motion abnormalities as assessed by 2-D echocardiography with angiography.[145,151] In a double blind study, Kisslo et al[145] found good agreement between the two techniques, with 2-D echocardiography correctly identifying wall motion characteristics in 87% of segments examined. Discrepancies between the two techniques were related to limitations of both techniques. Some echocardiographic limitations include inadequate target visualization due to endocardial echocardiographic dropout and tangential angulation of the transducer resulting in distortion of wall motion. Other investigators have used a more quantitative approach,[151] using echocardiographic short-axis images that were divided into segments and segmental area shrinkage during systole calculated for each segment. Localization of infarction by 2-D echocardiography was then compared with electrocardiographic and angiographic localization. The sensitivity and specificity in the detection of abnormally moving segments by 2-D echocardiography were 95% and 89%, respectively. Another group of investigators found that dyskinesia or akinesia correlated well with transmural infarction.[152] Only 8% of the akinetic or dyskinetic segments were not transmurally infarcted. Hypokinesia, conversely, was associated with both subendocardial infarcted myocardium and normal myocardium; therefore, the difficulty of interpreting hypokinesia on 2-D echocardiographic studies poses clinical and prognostic problems. Quantitative measurements of wall motion indexes from 2-D echocardiography show good correlation with clinical parameters of left ventricular function and therefore may be useful in predicting in-hospital prog-

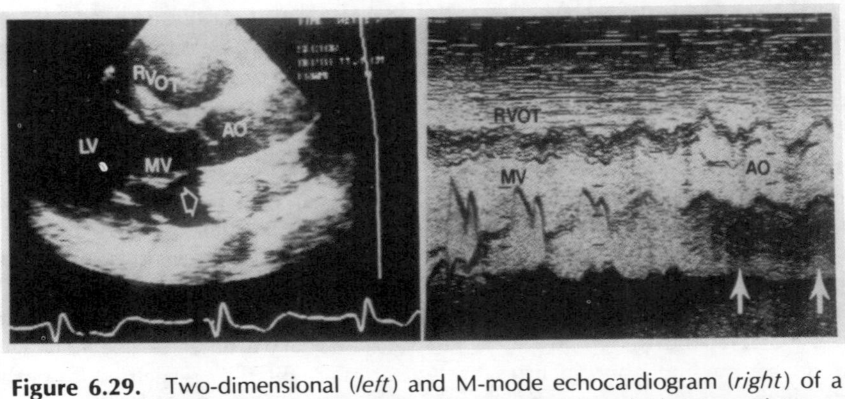

Figure 6.29. Two-dimensional (*left*) and M-mode echocardiogram (*right*) of a nonmobile nonprolapsing atrial myxoma (proven at surgery). Arrows point to a dense echogenic mass. Ao = aorta; MV = mitral valve; RVOT = right ventricular outflow tract; LV = left ventricle.

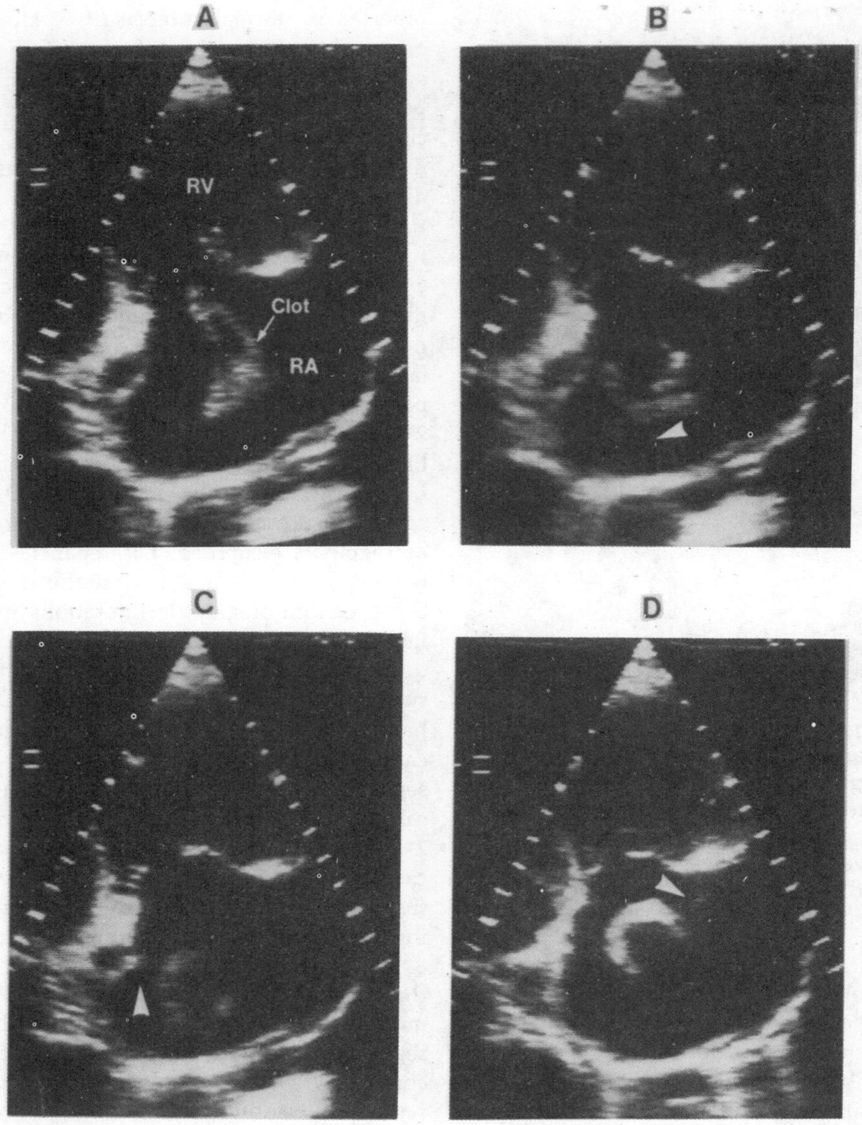

Figure 6.30. Sequential frames obtained from apical two-chamber right ventricular view in a patient with a migratory thrombus that had become entrapped in the eustachian valve. The thrombus has a serpentine motion and changes position and direction throughout the various phases of the cardiac cycle (*white arrows*). RA = right atrium; RV = right ventricle.

nosis.[153,154] Some investigators believe that the degree of wall motion abnormality has more prognostic predictive value than overall global left ventricular function in patients with acute myocardial infarction.[153,155] In single-vessel disease, regional asynergy could be correlated with infarction in the distribution of the narrow vessel, and areas of remote asynergy were not present.[153] However, in multivessel disease, Stamm et al[154] showed that asynergy may be present both in the distribution of the occluded vessel and in remote areas served by the vessels with severe stenosis.

During the ischemic phase in patients having unstable angina, transient and persistent wall motion abnormalities have been identified by 2-D echocardiography.[156] The effect of reperfusion on contraction abnormalities has generated considerable interest since the advent of streptokinase and percutaneous transluminal angioplasty. Experimental studies have shown that regional contractile function may remain depressed up to several weeks following transient ischemia and reperfusion.[157,158] Segmental contractile function can slowly improve after several weeks. Significant tissue salvage by reperfusion generally is not detected in the early stages by 2-D echocardiography;[159] however, this is not to say that it may not improve in the latter period. Further studies are necessary to determine the clinical implications of these findings.

IMAGING OF THE CORONARY ARTERIES

Normally, the dimensions of the coronary arteries are at or below the resolving limits of 2-D echocardiography and only the most proximal portions of the left main or right coronary arteries can be visualized. When coronary arteries are dilated or calcified, or both, these arteries can be identified more readily. Kawasaki's syndrome is an acute systemic inflammatory disorder of unknown etiology primarily seen in infants and children and it may be associated with necrotizing vasculitis of the epicardial coronary arteries. During the healing phase, coronary artery aneurysms can develop. Several investigators have described the 2-D echocardiographic features of Kawasaki's disease.[160–162] Generally, the coronary artery aneurysms are localized bulges in the proximal coronary vessels best seen in the parasternal short-axis views at the level of the aortic valve. Occasionally, a subcostal 2-D echocardiographic approach can detect aneurysmal dilatations of the peripheral left and right coronary arteries.[162] Miyatake et al[163] reported the complementary roles of 2-D and Doppler echocardiography in the detection of coronary arteriovenous fistula.

EXERCISE ECHOCARDIOGRAPHY

Exercise echocardiography has been reported by several investigators.[164–167] In most series reported, an adequate echocardiogram during exercise can be obtained in 70% to 85% of cases. However, with newer techniques such as image averaging and increased endocardial resolution capabilities, the success rate may be increased. Exercise-induced regional wall motion abnormalities have been detected and correlate with the presence of significant coronary disease by angiography.[165] In addition, global left ventricular performance can also be accurately assessed.[166] Assessment of asynergic segments by echocardiography during exercise has been correlated with reversible thallium perfusion defects.[164]

COMPLICATIONS OF MYOCARDIAL INFARCTION

Right Ventricular Infarction

The incidence of anatomic right ventricular infarction at autopsy is about 14% in all patients with acute myocardial infarction and 24% among those with inferior wall infarction.[168] Right ventricular infarction generally is associated with left ventricular infarction and significant obstruction of the right coronary artery. Two-dimensional echocardiography has demonstrated right ventricular dilatation and regional wall motion abnormalities of the diaphragmatic or free right ventricular wall (Figure 6.31).[169,170] Generally, right ventricular wall motion is best studied in the apical four-chamber view, subcostal views, and an apical two-chamber right ventricular view. The apical two-chamber right ventricular view can be obtained by rotating the transducer approximately 90° counterclockwise from the apical four-chamber plane, angulating anteriorly and medially until the right heart chambers and portions of the tricuspid valve are visualized. Right ventricular apical aneurysms are visualized and the presence of tricuspid regurgitation can be recognized by contrast and Doppler echocardiography.

Left Ventricular Aneurysm

A frequent complication of myocardial infarction that can be visualized by 2-D echocardiography is left ventricular aneurysm. Most aneurysms occur at the left ventricular apex and therefore are best visualized from the apical and subcostal positions. The characteristic 2-D echocardiographic finding in an aneurysm is a well-demarcated apical segment that shows systolic expansion or bulging during the period of inward contraction of the left ventricle.[171,172] Generally, a "hinge point" separates the normal myocardium from the dyskinetic portion (Figure 6.32). Often, however, akinesia rather than actual systolic expansion may be observed and such aneurysms may be less well demarcated pathologically. Echocardiographically, true aneurysms distort the shape of the left ventricle during diastole and systole, whereas dyskinetic segments, which have to be differentiated from aneurysms, distort the geometry only during systole. Two-dimensional echocardiography has also been useful in describing inferior and posterior aneurysms that can occur but are less common than apical aneurysms. Inferior aneurysms are generally identified in the parasternal long-axis view, but they are also seen in the apical four- and two-chamber views. Two-dimensional echocardiography is extremely useful in differentiating true aneurysms from pseudoaneurysms.[173] The latter frequently develop after rupture of a recently infarcted segment of the myocardial wall with perforations through the endocardium and myocardium, with resultant localized hemopericardium that is confined by an adherent, parietal pericardium. Two-dimensional echocardiographic characteristics of a pseudoaneurysm (Figure 6.33) include (1) sharp discontinuity of the endocardial image at the site of the pseudoaneurysm communication with the left ventricular cavity; (2) a saccular or globular contour of the false aneurysm chamber; (3) the presence of a narrow orifice compared with the diameter of the pseudoaneurysm; and (4) occasional displacement of other cardiac

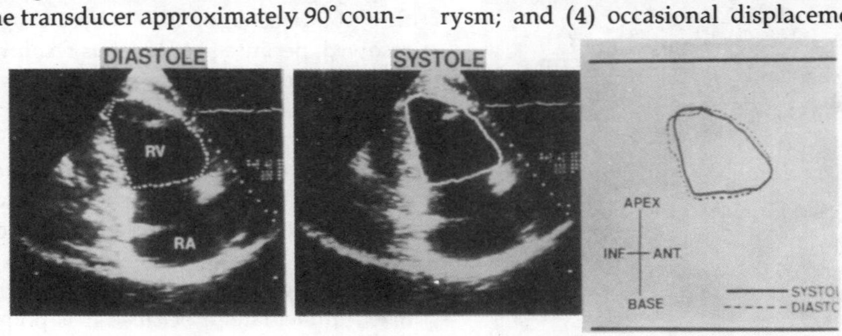

Figure 6.31. Apical right ventricular (RV) two-chamber view in a patient with right ventricular infarction. Akinesia to dyskinesia of the distal RV free wall (right wall of RV) and severe hypokinesia of the diaphragmatic wall (left wall of RV) are present. RA = right atrium. (From Panidis IP, Ron JS, Ross J, Kotler MJ, Mintz GS, Kane S, Iskandrian AS: Two-dimensional echocardiographic estimation of right ventricular ejection fraction in patients with coronary artery disease. *J Am Coll Cardiol* 1983; 2:911–918, with permission.)

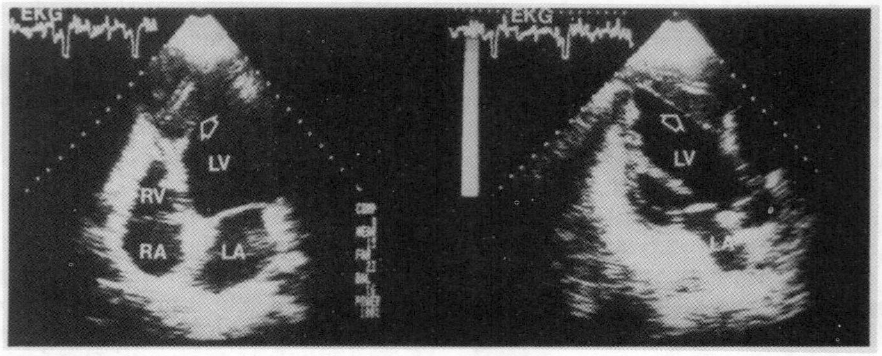

Figure 6.32. Apical four- (*left*) and two-chamber (*right*) views in a patient with a large anteroapical aneurysm of the left ventricle (LV). A well-demarcated apical thrombus is present (*large arrow*). LA = left atrium; RA = right atrium; RV = right ventricle.

chambers such as compression of the right ventricle. In contrast, true aneurysms are characterized by a wide neck, with the diameter of the neck comparable to the maximum diameter of the aneurysm (Figure 6.32).

Left Ventricular Thrombus

Left ventricular thrombus classically occurs in the setting of an existing aneurysm and in patients with a dilated or ischemic cardiomyopathy.[174–176] Patients with acute anterior wall or transmural myocardial infarction complicated by significant areas of asynergy are particularly prone to the development of thrombus.[175] Thrombi may be detected by 2-D echocardiography as early as 72 hours after infarction. The characteristic echocardiographic features include a mass of discrete echoes that are present in systole and diastole and that project into the ventricular cavity and are contiguous with the endocardium (Figure 6.32). Small apical thrombi may frequently be overlooked on echocardiography. Artifacts have to be differentiated from thrombi, because most thrombi usually are seen at the apex.[176,177] The problem of machine artifact or near-field noise may often produce confusion. Generally, near-field noise is ill-defined and occurs immediately posterior to a bright reflector. Thrombi generally protrude discretely in the left ventricular cavity, are usually seen in multiple views, and are associated with wall motion abnormalities (Figure 6.32). Recently, the ability of 2-D echocardiography to differentiate thrombi that may have potential embolic complications has been described.[178] These echocardiographic features include (1) mobile thrombus, (2) thrombus that clearly protrudes well into the left ventricular cavity and is not laminated against the wall, and (3) those that occur early during the course of anterior wall infarction. The question of whether to employ anticoagulation in all patients with myocardial thrombi detected on 2-D echocardiography has not been resolved, because spontaneous resolution may or may not occur without subsequent embolic events.[179]

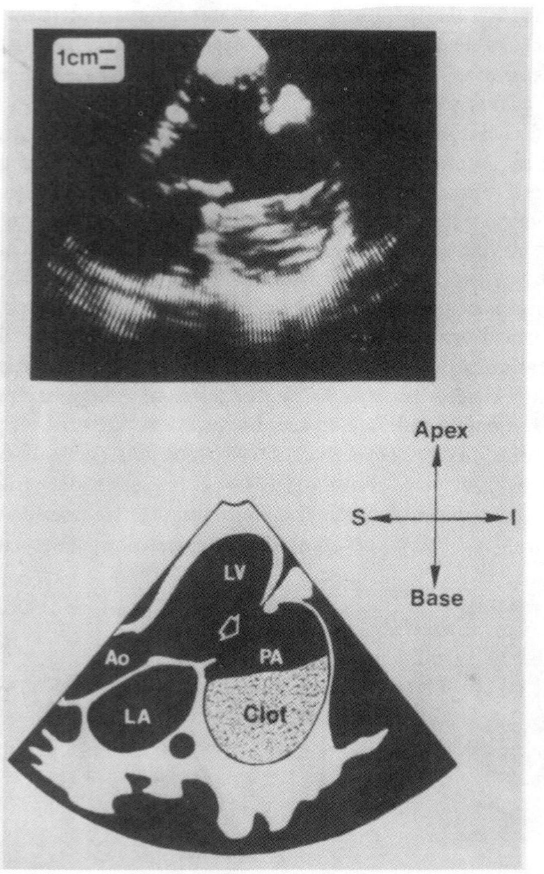

Figure 6.33. Apical two-chamber view in a patient with a large pseudoaneurysm (PA) involving the inferior wall (*arrow*). The aneurysm is filled with clot and the mouth of the aneurysm is narrowed in relation to the total diameter of the false chamber. Ao = aorta; LA = left atrium; LV = left ventricle. (From Catherwood et al,[173] with permission.)

Papillary Muscle Rupture

Although papillary muscle rupture is rare, being reported in about 0.9% of patients after acute myocardial infarction, the clinical presentation is often dramatic, with progressive pulmonary edema and shock not infrequently encountered. Papillary muscle rupture has to be recognized immediately, because it is potentially treatable by surgery. As shown in Figure 6.34 during systole, the tip of the anterior leaflet moves beyond the posterior leaflet in the left atrium, resulting in a lack of coaptation. In addition, a portion of the papillary muscle can be visualized as a mass attached to the flail leaflet.[180] Most patients with isolated papillary muscle or partial papillary

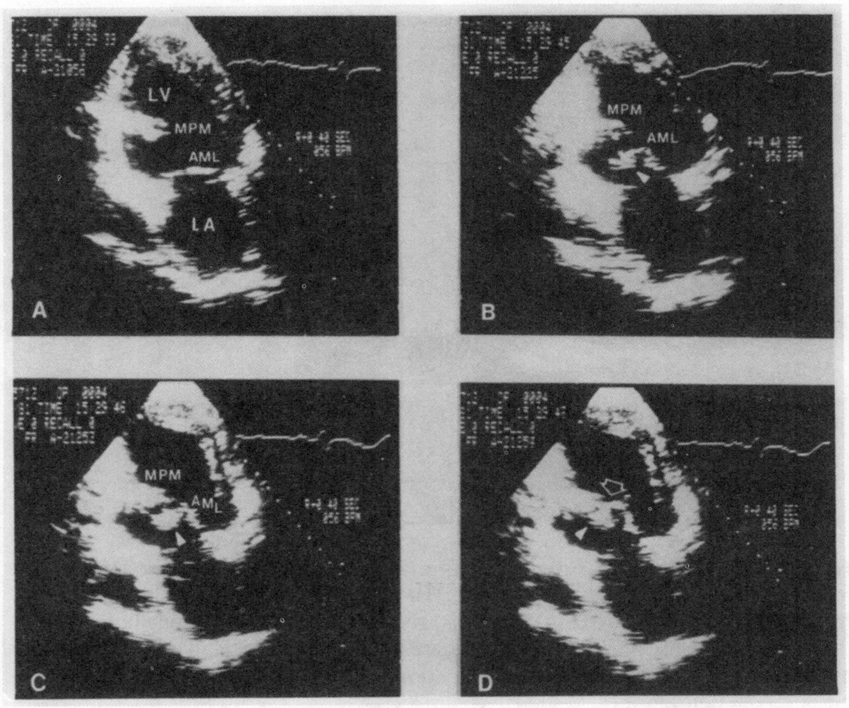

Figure 6.34. Papillary muscle rupture. These apical sequential stop-frame images are from a patient with partial papillary muscle rupture. Normal mitral valve closure is seen in frame A. The actual disruption of the heads of the papillary muscle from the body of the papillary muscle is shown in frames B and C and represented by the large arrow in frame D. AML = anterolateral papillary muscle; LA = left atrium; LV = left ventricle; MPM = posteromedial papillary muscle. (From Kotler et al,[180] with permission.)

muscle rupture have limited areas of asynergy, usually confined to the inferior wall. In addition, motion of the interventricular septum may be hyperdynamic. Papillary muscle rupture or partial rupture has to be differentiated from papillary muscle dysfunction which is frequently encountered after inferior wall infarction.[181] In papillary muscle dysfunction, the posterior mitral leaflet appears apically retracted and held in a rigid position. The motion of the leaflet may be reduced during systole and in diastole in contrast to the normal motion of the anterior leaflet. In the parasternal short-axis view, the posteromedial papillary muscle frequently appears more echogenic and dense than the anterolateral papillary muscle. Color-coding systems of echocardiographic intensity may enhance the ability to detect localized areas of myocardial fibrosis.[182] Mitral regurgitation is easily detected and can be differentiated from ventricular septal defect by Doppler echocardiography.[14,183] The finding of a decreasing peak regurgitant velocity throughout systole may indicate near-equilibration of left ventricular and left atrial pressure, especially if the left atrium is normal in size.

Ventricular Septal Rupture

Ventricular septal rupture also is an uncommon complication of infarction, occurring in less than 1% of patients with coronary artery disease and infarction. The high prevalence of first infarct, single-vessel coronary artery disease and the absence of septal collateral vessels suggest an abrupt reduction in blood flow which may be responsible for the rupture. Ventricular septal rupture occurs equally in anterior as well as inferior wall infarction. Generally, ventricular septal rupture occurs at the center of the septal aneurysm. Septal tissue adjacent to the defect may be thin, dense, and fibrotic. During systole the septal aneurysm bulges and the defect widens.[181] The site of the defect and the characteristic left-to-right shunt can classically be evaluated by combined 2-D echocardiographic and Doppler echocardiography (Figure 6.35). In contrast to traumatic ventricular septal rupture, which is easily seen because of the clear-cut nature of the trauma, acquired ventricular septal rupture may not always be visualized directly by 2-D echocardiography. It may be necessary to angulate the transducer in off-axis views to locate the defect. In addition, the anatomy of the defect may make it difficult to detect by echocardiography. Pathologically, the defects, when acute, have ragged edges, may have a serpentine course through the septum, and consist of multiple small defects, all contributing to nonvisualization. In addition, defects may be obscured by right ventricular trabeculations. With contrast echocardiography, positive contrast microbubbles entering the left ventricle through the ventricular septal defect have been seen.[184] The so-called negative contrast effect (washout of right ventricular bubbles by left ventricular blood crossing the ventricular septal defect) was less frequently encountered.

Doppler echocardiography has been highly sensitive and specific in the detection of both congenital[185,186] and

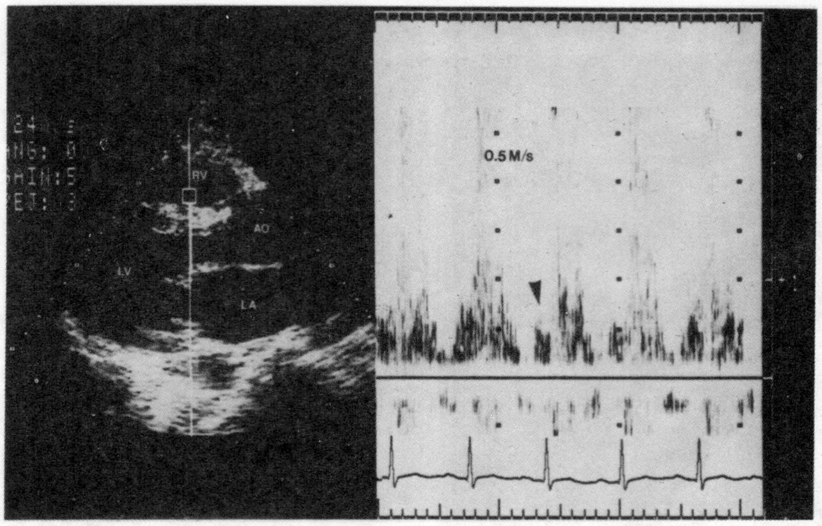

Figure 6.35. Simultaneous two-dimensional and pulsed Doppler echocardiogram from the parasternal long-axis position. The sample volume is positioned in the right ventricle (RV) close to the ventricular septum (*left*). *Right*, systolic flow toward the transducer indicates left-to-right shunting at the ventricular level. Following atrial contraction, diastolic left-to-right shunting is also noted (arrow head). AO = aorta, LA = left atrium; LV = left ventricle.

acquired[14,187] ventricular septal defects. Differentiation of ventricular septal defect and mitral regurgitation is easily accomplished with this technique.[14,183] Using pulsed Doppler echocardiography, an apical, parasternal, or subcostal ultrasonic window is used, depending on the site of the defect. In a recent series of 11 patients with ventricular septal rupture, 2-D echocardiography visualized the defect in seven patients and Doppler echocardiography detected the presence of a left-to-right shunt in all 11 patients.[187] Several groups of investigators have demonstrated the reliability of the Doppler-derived ratio of pulmonic-to-systemic blood flow in a variety of intra- and extracardiac shunts.[188–190] In ventricular septal defect, flow across the tricuspid and aortic valves represents systemic blood flow and that across the pulmonic and mitral valves, pulmonary blood flow. Using continuous wave Doppler recording, right ventricular and pulmonary artery systolic pressure can be estimated by subtracting the peak left ventricular–right ventricular pressure gradient from the systolic blood pressure measured by cuff sphygmomanometer.[14] Doppler echocardiography is also useful postoperatively for assessing the integrity of ventricular septal patches.[191]

LEFT VENTRICULAR FUNCTION

Although M-mode echocardiography is useful in evaluating left ventricular function in normal subjects and in those with global left ventricular dysfunction, it is unreliable in evaluating left ventricular function in patients with regional left ventricular dysfunction.

Several studies have attested to the feasibility of using standard geometric formulas for calculating left ventricular volume and ejection fraction.[192–195] Most studies report that 2-D echocardiography tends to underestimate ventricular volumes as compared with ventriculography, but it appears more reliable when ejection fraction is used.

Some of the reasons for these discrepancies[196] are: (1) Because of lateral beam width resolution problems, the endocardium appears falsely thickened. (2) Two-dimensional echocardiography uses the tips of the erect columnae carneae to delineate the left ventricular perimeter. By overlooking the interstices of these endocardial projections, it underestimates chamber size as compared with ventriculography which includes the interstices of the endocardium. The two imaging techniques agree more closely during systole, when the bunching of these columns squeezes blood out of the trabecular space. (3) Frequently, if the transducer is incorrectly applied to the apex of the left ventricle, foreshortening of the left ventricle will occur.

Quantitative assessment of left ventricular function has been advanced significantly with the aid of off-line computer-assisted analysis systems.[197] Portions of the analog video display can be digitized and stored in computer memory or other media such as floppy disks. Once in digital format, a variety of complex manipulations, such as image averaging, digital subtraction, and contrast equalization, can be employed to improve image quality. Using a joystick or light pen, the end-diastolic and end-systolic endocardial border can be traced from two orthogonal views, and biplane volumes and ejection fractions are rapidly obtained using algorithms such as Simpson's rule, bullet formula, and area-length method. Endocardial and epicardial borders can be divided into a number of radial chords or areas to analyze regional wall motion and wall thickening, frame by frame. Many systems allow the operator to translate or rotate the end-systolic image, or both, with respect to the long axis and center of mass of the end-diastolic image. Of particular interest is the ability to play back two different studies simultaneously in a split screen format.

Intraoperative 2-D echocardiography can be used to

determine left ventricular function before and after coronary bypass grafting and valve replacement.[198] In patients with a significant decrease in left ventricular ejection fraction after open heart surgery, inotropic support or intraaortic balloon counterpulsation, or both, should be instituted to afford maximal survival in this high-risk group.

Left ventricular mass can also be calculated by 2-D echocardiographic techniques:[199] left ventricular mass = epicardial enclosed volume − endocardial enclosed volume × 1.05.

Biplane area length formula and Simpson's rule can be used to calculate epicardial and endocardial volume. The calculation of left ventricular mass in patients with hypertension and aortic valve disease allows an accurate means of assessing response to therapy and whether regression indeed does occur.[200] In a recent study from our laboratory, left ventricular mass correlated better with exercise systolic blood pressure than with blood pressure at rest in a group of hypertensive patients.[201]

Noninvasive cardiac output has been validated in studies using both pulsed[202–204] and continuous wave Doppler echocardiography.[205–207] To determine stroke volume (SV), three parameters must be obtained: (1) The mean spatial velocity of blood flow (V), (2) the period of flow, or ejection time (ET), and (3) the cross-sectional area of flow (CSA). Stroke volume is calculated by the formula: SV = V × ET × CSA. Blood flow velocity can be obtained in the aorta[205–207] or, more recently, across any of the cardiac valves.[205,208,209] The velocity curve is either manually planimetered or automatically integrated by computer technique to produce the so-called time-velocity integral, expressed as a distance in centimeters. The cross-sectional area of flow is obtained directly from 2-D echocardiography or derived from A-mode or M-mode diameter measurements. The product of these two parameters yields the stroke volume in milliliters. Cardiac output is obtained when stroke volume is multiplied by heart rate.

The major source of error to date has been in determining the cross-sectional area of flow. Indeed, an error in diameter of only a few millimeters can lead to serious under- or overestimation of cardiac output. If a patient is used as his or her own control, percent change in cardiac output can be obtained without knowledge of the cross-sectional area of flow. This approach has been useful in assessing drug intervention[210,211] and mode of physiologic pacing.[212,213]

RIGHT VENTRICULAR FUNCTION

Quantitative 2-D evaluation of right ventricular function appears to be useful. The right ventricle is more difficult to image than the left ventricle because its trabeculated muscle, three papillary muscles, and separate infundibulum tend to obscure the endocardial border. Whereas the left ventricle is conveniently ellipsoidal, the right ventricle is a complex triangular or crescent shape that does not lend itself to conventional geometric formulas for volume calculation. The right ventricular shape varies with loading conditions. Several studies have demonstrated the feasibility and reliability of 2-D echocardiography in evaluating ventricular function in normal subjects and in those with right ventricular overload.[214–216] Most studies use the apical or subcostal and four- and two-chamber views and the standard algorithms (biplane area-length method or Simpson's rule using two paired orthogonal views) to calculate right ventricular volume and ejection fraction. A simplified formula has been employed using the apical four-chamber view and subcostal right ventricular outflow tract views to obtain right ventricular volume and ejection fraction.[215] Thus, right ventricular volume = 2/3 × area of right ventricle (apical four-chamber view) × long-axis measurement of right ventricular outflow tract.

Another method recently described is relatively simple and fast, and eliminates the need for tracing endocardial borders and imperfect geometric formulas.[217] The approach involves obtaining an apical four-chamber view and drawing a straight line from the midpoint of the origin of the echocardiographic fan to the junction of the right ventricular free wall and tricuspid valve in end-diastole. Next, the plane where the tricuspid anulus dissects this line in end-systole is marked, and excursion of the tricuspid valve plane from end-diastole to end-systole is measured. The tricuspid valve moves towards the right ventricular apex during ventricular systole because of longitudinal shortening of the interventricular septum and right ventricular free wall and reflects wall motion and integrity of both walls. In patients with right ventricular ejection fractions less than 25%, tricuspid anular plane systolic excursion (TAPSE) had scores below 8 to 15 mm, whereas TAPSE scores greater than 15 mm were indicative of normal ejection fraction.

PERICARDIAL DISORDERS

Pericardial Effusion

Echocardiography is ideally suited to the diagnosis of pericardial effusion. The echocardiographic features of pericardial effusion include the presence of an echo-free space posterior to the heart with a tendency for disappearance of the space at the edge of the atrioventricular junction. The echo-free space separates the visceral, or epicardial, and parietal pericardial surfaces which are imaged as two reflected interfaces.[218] As the effusion enlarges, absence of motion of the parietal pericardium may be noted. The volume of fluid can be roughly estimated and semiquantification of mild-to-moderate and significant pericardial effusion can readily be made by 2-D echocardiography. Large effusions, those greater than 500 ml, usually accumulate posteriorly, but they are also seen laterally, apically, and anteriorly[219] (Figure 6.36). Dramatic swings of the heart may occur within the pericardial space. Abnormal swings over several cardiac cycles may be associated with electrical alternans.[220] In some patients with significant pericardial effusion, the echo-free space may extend behind the posterior wall of the left atrium to the point of insertion of the pulmonary veins. False-positive echocardiographic studies can occur in a variety of disorders, particularly left pleural effusion, pericardial tumors, fat pads, large hernias of the foramen of Morgagni, pericardial cysts, and gigantic left atria or pseu-

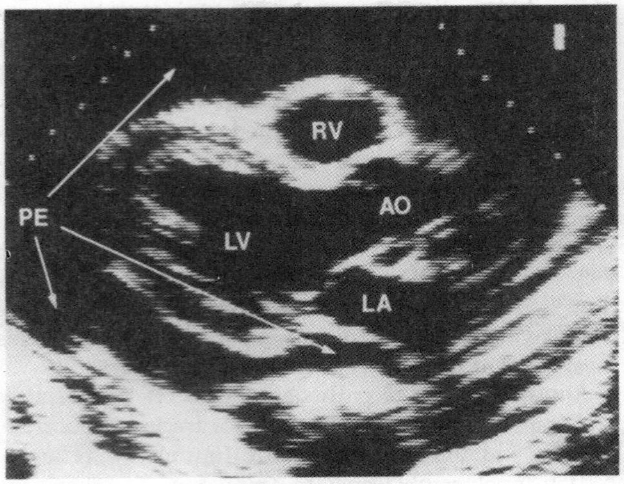

Figure 6.36. A two-dimensional echocardiogram obtained in a patient with large pericardial effusion (PE), showing accumulation of fluid toward the apex. Although this image was obtained from the parasternal long-axis view, the apical accumulation of fluid could be seen in a variety of image planes. In this example, fluid extends posterior to the left atrium (LA) as well, and the right ventricle (RV) is compressed at the apex. AO = aorta; LV = left ventricle; RV = right ventricle.

doaneurysms.[221] The descending aorta is a reliable landmark in differentiating pericardial from pleural effusion.[222] In pericardial effusion, the descending aorta is displaced from the left ventricular posterior wall, whereas in pleural effusion, intimate contact is maintained between the descending aorta and left ventricular posterior wall. Malignant effusions are frequently large and tumors have been identified (Figure 6.37).[223,224] Although the diagnosis of cardiac tamponade is a clinical one, certain echocardiographic features may support the diagnosis of tamponade.[225-228] Right ventricular compression appears to be a reliable sign and occurs early after mitral valve opening (Figure 6.36). Late diastolic and early systolic indentation of the right atrium has also been described as a reliable sign with tamponade (Figure 6.38); however, in a recent reported series it appears to be less sensitive than the right ventricular collapse sign.[228] On the basis of animal experiments, right ventricular diastolic collapse is a pressure-related phenomenon that occurs late in the course of tamponade and is immediately relieved on reducing intrapericardial pressure. It appears to be caused by right ventricular pressure decreasing below the pericardial pressure in early diastole. In patients who have right ventricular dysfunction secondary to pulmonary hypertension and increased right ventricular pressure, the right ventricular diastolic collapsing sign may be absent.[229] Pericardial effusion can be loculated after open heart surgery, and tamponade can occur even in the presence of isolated loculated effusion.[230,231] Several centers have reported that echocardiography can be a useful guide in pericardiocentesis.[221,232] Patients with loculated pericardial effusion, little or no fluid inferiorly, or extensive pericardial adhesions were more prone to complications such as inadvertent cardiac puncture during pericardiocentesis.[221] In a recent report, Doppler-detected flow velocity paradoxus was found in the pulmonary artery and aorta. This finding appeared to be a sensitive sign of cardiac tamponade.[233]

Constrictive Pericarditis

The echocardiographic diagnosis of constrictive pericarditis has been disappointing. The finding of a dilated

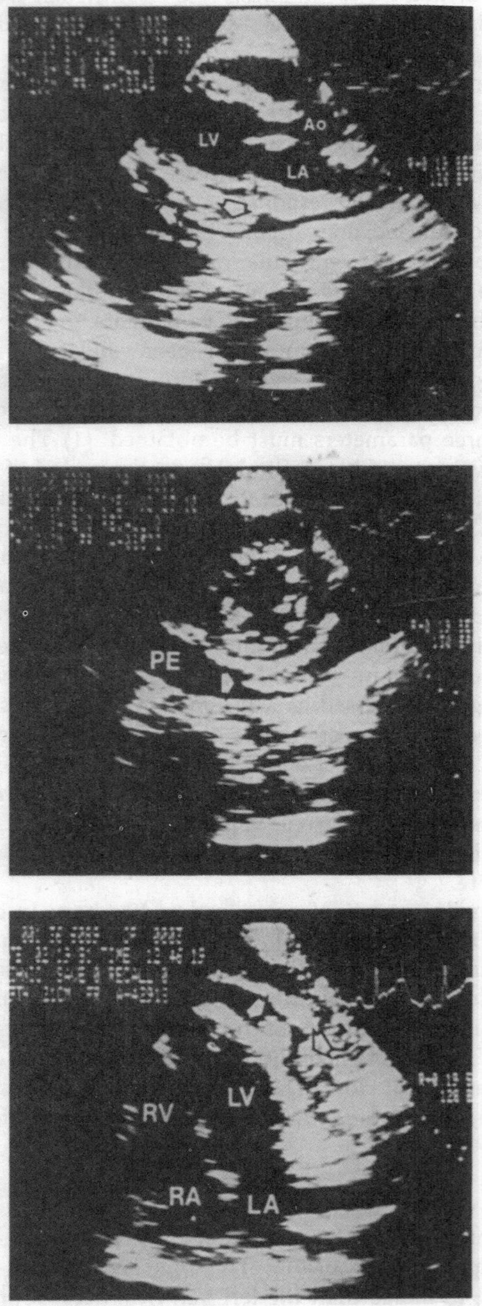

Figure 6.37. Two-dimensional echocardiogram of a patient with cytologic confirmation of metastatic pericardial disease. Discrete masses (*arrows*) attached to the visceral and parietal pericardium are noted. *Top*, parasternal long-axis view; *middle*, parasternal short-axis view, *bottom*, apical four-chamber view. Ao = aorta; LA = left atrium; LV = left ventricle; RA = right atrium; RV = right ventricle. (From Friedman et al,[224] with permission.)

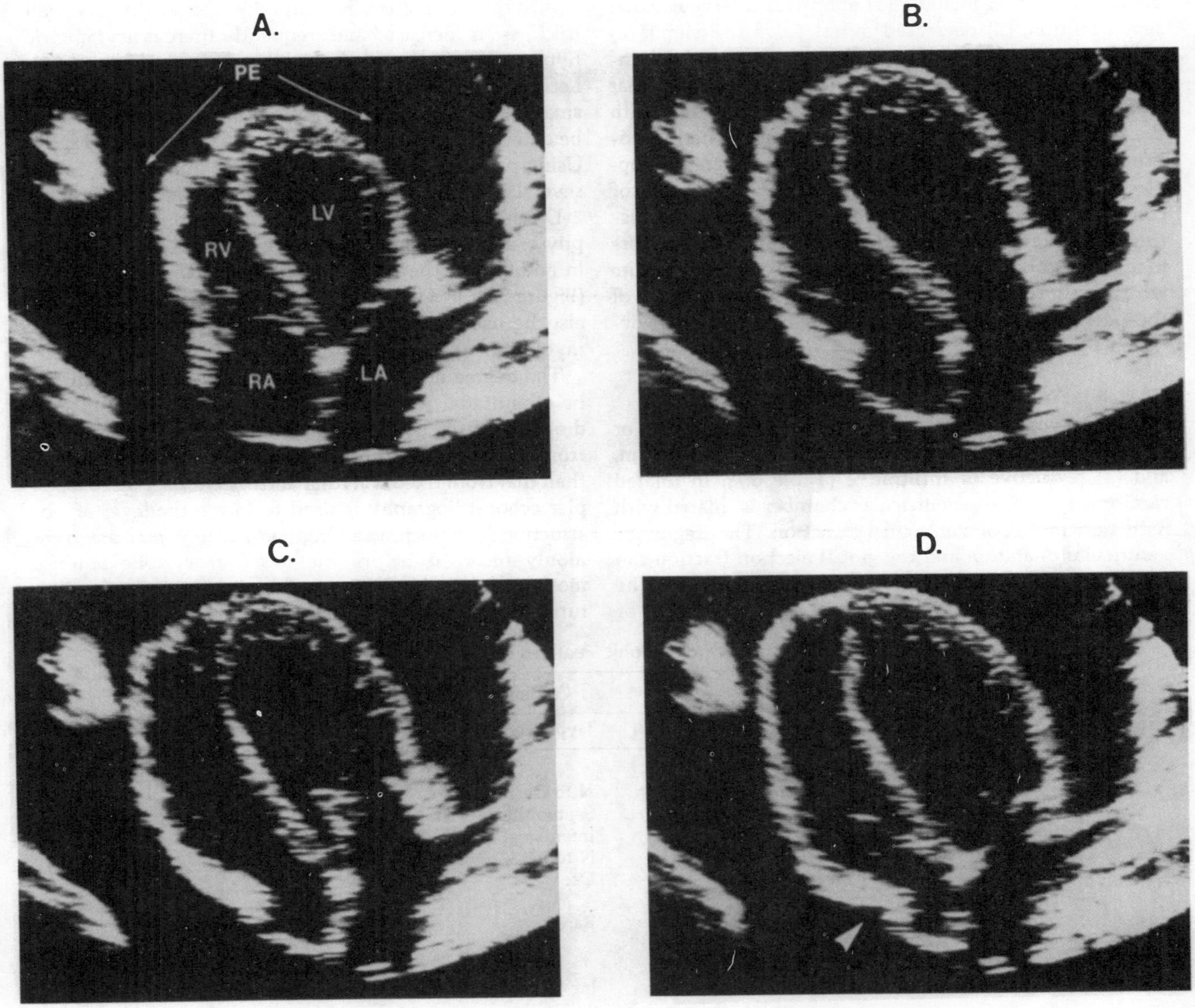

Figure 6.38. An apical four-chamber view obtained throughout multiple periods of the cardiac cycle in a patient with a large malignant pericardial effusion (PE). The right atrium (RA) begins to invaginate in mid-diastole (*B, C*) and invaginates more (*white arrows*) during late diastole and early systole (*D*). During early diastole, the right atrium is not compressed (*A*) and appears normal. The apical localization of pericardial effusion is present. LA = left atrium; LV = left ventricle; RV = right ventricle.

inferior vena cava with little or no respiratory variation in size, the presence of normal left and right ventricular function, and normal wall thickness should alert the clinician to the diagnosis of constrictive pericarditis.[234] Thickening or calcification of the pericardium, or both, may be more reliably accomplished by computerized tomographic scanning and magnetic resonance imaging.[235] Several M-mode findings have been reported in constrictive pericarditis which include: (1) abnormal interventricular septal motion, (2) decreased mitral valve E-F slope, (3) premature opening of the pulmonic valve, and (4) increased slope of the diastolic motion of the left ventricular wall with abrupt cessation occurring and coinciding with the pericardial knock followed by minimal posterior motion during the remainder of diastole.[236] Recently, Doppler echocardiography was useful in the diagnosis of constrictive pericarditis. Altered filling patterns did distinguish patients with constrictive pericarditis from normal subjects.[237] Other abnormalities of the pericardium which include pneumopericardium,[238] partial absence of the pericardium, and pericardial cysts[239] have been detected by echocardiography.

CARDIOMYOPATHY

Cardiomyopathies can be classified as (1) congestive or dilated, (2) hypertrophic with and without obstruction, and (3) restrictive or infiltrative (Table 6.7). In dilated cardiomyopathy, the ventricular chamber is dilated with reduction in global ventricular function. The degree of ventricular dilatation and the global ejection fraction can readily be determined and mural thrombi identified. The ratio of cavity size to wall thickness and the percent of systolic thickening of the left ventricular wall are two M-mode echocardiographic measurements that provide prognostic information.[240,241] Two-dimensional echocardiography and Doppler cardiac output determination may be helpful in following patients with dilated cardiomyopathy with regard to assessment of prognosis or treatment, or both, especially in patients who have viral myocarditis.

In hypertrophic cardiomyopathy, the ventricular wall thickness is increased and frequently there is asymmetric hypertrophy of the interventricular septum (Figure 6.39). Left ventricular cavity dimensions are either normal or small.[240] Systolic anterior motion of the mitral valve may be detected on both M-mode and 2-D echocardiography. Using parasternal short-axis views, Maron et al[242] found several patterns of hypertrophy of the left ventricle by 2-D echocardiography. The commonest type is hypertrophy of the anterior and posterior portions of the septum in addition to the anterolateral wall of the left ventricle (Figure 6.40). Two-dimensional echocardiography may also be useful in evaluating patients undergoing septal myotomy-myectomy.[243]

The degree of left ventricular outflow obstruction can be quantitated with continuous wave Doppler echocardiography from the apical position. Peak systolic velocity from dynamic subaortic stenosis occurs later in systole than that from fixed, valvular aortic stenosis. Pulsed Doppler echocardiography is used to locate the level of obstruction.[14] Velocities as high as 2.5 to 3 m/s are commonly recorded before the onset of systolic anterior motion of the mitral valve and tends to support the venturi effect as the mechanism of systolic anterior motion

Table 6.7. Echocardiographic Features of Cardiomyopathies

	Cardiomyopathies		
	Congestive	**Hypertrophic**	**Restrictive**
Left ventricle			
(a) Size	Inc +++	N to Dec	N to Inc +
(b) Wall thickness	N to Dec Rarely Inc	Septum Inc +++ Inferobasal Wall N	Inc ++ Inc ++
(c) Systolic function	Dec	N to Inc	N to Dec
(d) Diastolic function	N	Dec	Dec
(e) Mural thrombi	Common	Rare	Rare except in hypereosinophilic syndrome
Left atrial size	Inc	Inc with mitral regurgitation	Inc
Mitral valve	Inc E-point septal separation AC shoulder	SAM (with obstruction) Dec E-F slope	Normal to thickened valve Normal to Dec E-F slope
Aortic valve	Gradual systolic closure	Mid-systolic closure (with obstruction)	N
Right ventricle			
Size	Inc	N	N
Wall thickness	N	N to Inc	Inc
Right atrium			
Size	N to Inc	N	N to Inc
Thickness, especially	N	N	N to Inc

Dec = decreased; Inc = increased; N = normal; SAM = systolic anterior motion.

Pluses indicate the magnitude, "+" being mild; "++" being moderate; "+++" being marked.

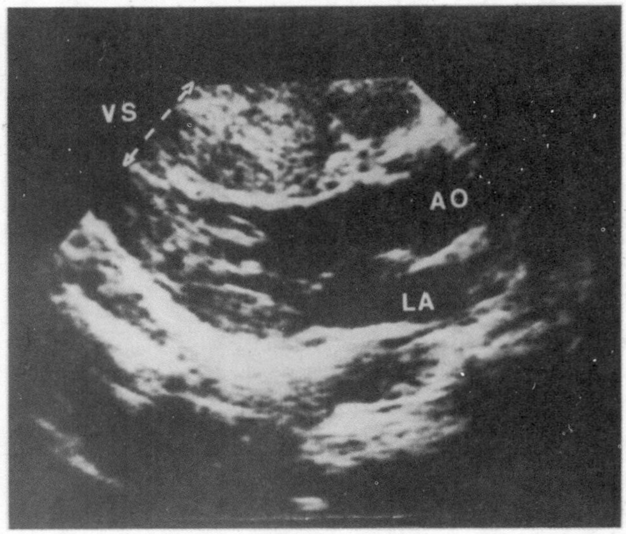

Figure 6.39. Parasternal long-axis view in a patient with hypertrophic cardiomyopathy. The markedly thickened septum (VS) in relation to the posterior wall is apparent. AO = aorta; LA = left atrium.

in this disorder.[14] In a recent study of 28 patients, Doppler echocardiography detected mitral regurgitation in all patients with outflow obstruction and in 50% of those without obstruction, the latter being assessed as mild.[244]

In restrictive cardiomyopathy, the ventricular cavities are normal in size and the ventricular walls are thickened. Systolic contraction may be normal initially, but it becomes reduced as the disease progresses. In amyloid heart disease, the right ventricle and interatrial septum are also thickened.[245] Additional findings in amyloid heart disease include thickening of the cardiac valves and the presence of pericardial effusion. A sparkling appearance of the myocardium has been described in patients with infiltrative cardiomyopathy[245] as well as in the interventricular septum in patients with hypertrophic cardiomyopathy.[246]

AORTA AND DISORDERS AFFECTING THE AORTA

The entire thoracic and abdominal aorta can be evaluated by 2-D echocardiography using a variety of views which include: the left parasternal long- and short-axis view, the long and short-axis view of the second right intercostal space, a suprasternal notch view, and a subcostal long- and short-axis view of the distal descending thoracic and abdominal aorta.[247–249] In addition, a modified apical approach has been recommended to visualize the descending thoracic aorta.[250] The main value of 2-D echocardiography is its ability to identify the type, location, and extent of aortic aneurysms and dissection.[251,252] Saccular and fusiform aneurysms can be differentiated from dissecting aneurysms. In dissecting aneurysms, visualization of the intimal flap by 2-D echocardiography has been described (Figure 6.41). To increase the sensitivity and specificity of 2-D echocardiography in the diagnosis of aortic dissection, optimal visualization of the entire aorta is required and multiple on- and off-axis views should be obtained. False-positive echocardiographic studies may result from extension of reverberation from other cardiac structures or spurious echoes within the aortic lumen. Atherosclerotic plaques in the aortic wall and those projecting within the aortic lumen can also simulate an intimal flap by echocardiography.[253] Although intimal flaps may oscillate, suggesting differential rates of filling of false and true lumens, blood flow patterns can more reliably be assessed by Doppler techniques.[254] Color flow imaging Doppler echocardiography is particularly useful in assessing blood flow in the lumina as well as in defining the sites of exit and reentry.[23] Patients with Marfan's syndrome and anuloaortic ectasia may have aneurysmal dilatation of the ascending thoracic aorta beginning at the aortic valve anulus and terminating proximally at the innominate artery.[255] The importance of recognizing such patients is that they are at greater risk of developing acute aortic dissections and hemodynamically significant aortic regurgitation.

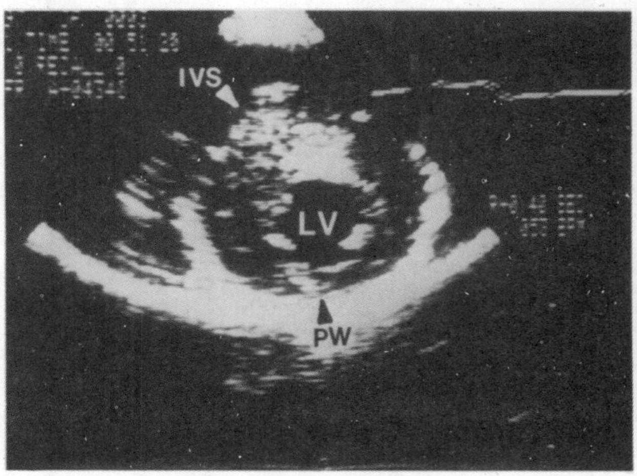

Figure 6.40. Parasternal short-axis view in a patient with hypertrophic cardiomyopathy. The markedly thickened septum (IVS) (anterior and posterior portion) and anterolateral wall of the left ventricle (LV) in relation to the posterior wall (PW) are evident.

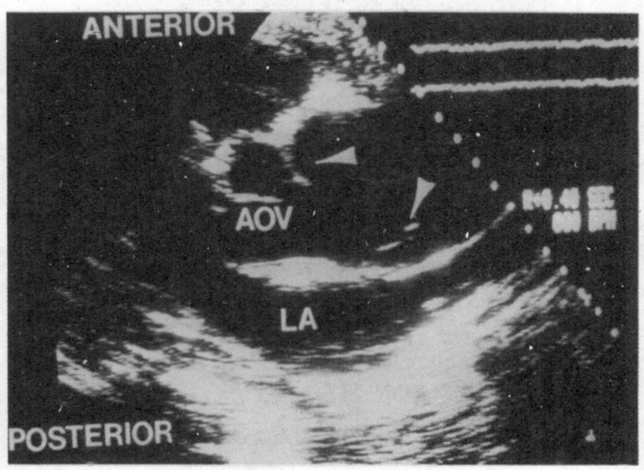

Figure 6.41. Parasternal long-axis view of the ascending aorta in a patient with Marfan's syndrome and dissecting aneurysm. The ascending aorta is markedly dilated and measures 6.0 cm. *White arrows* point to the intimal flaps. AOV = aortic valve; LA = left atrium. (From Mattleman et al,[247] with permission.)

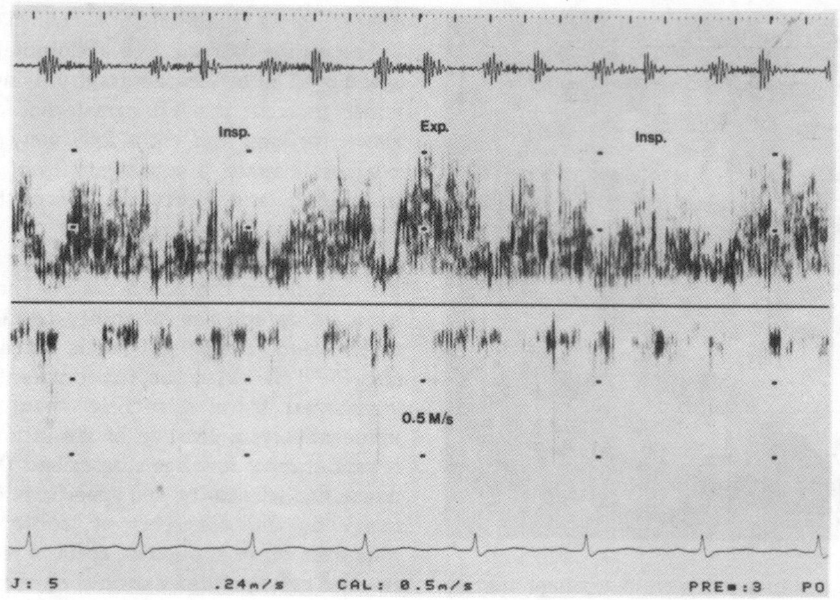

Figure 6.42. Pulsed Doppler recording from the subcostal position with the sample volume placed in the right atrium close to the interatrial septum. Flow toward the transducer during late systole and early to mid-diastole indicates left-to-right shunting at the atrial level. During inspiration (insp), the amount of left-to-right shunting decreases with increased venous return to the right atrium. Exp. = expiration.

CONGENITAL HEART DISEASE

In congenital heart disease, 2-D echocardiography provides extremely useful anatomic information with regard to identification of ventricles, atria, valves, and outflow vessels.[218,256,257] The approach directed toward the patient with complex congenital heart lesions should include: (1) identification of the atrial situs, (2) identification of the ventricular situs, (3) great vessel orientation, (4) the pattern in which great vessels are connected to ventricular chambers, (5) the presence and direction of intracardiac shunts, especially determined by Doppler echocardiography, and (6) the presence, location, and severity of aortic

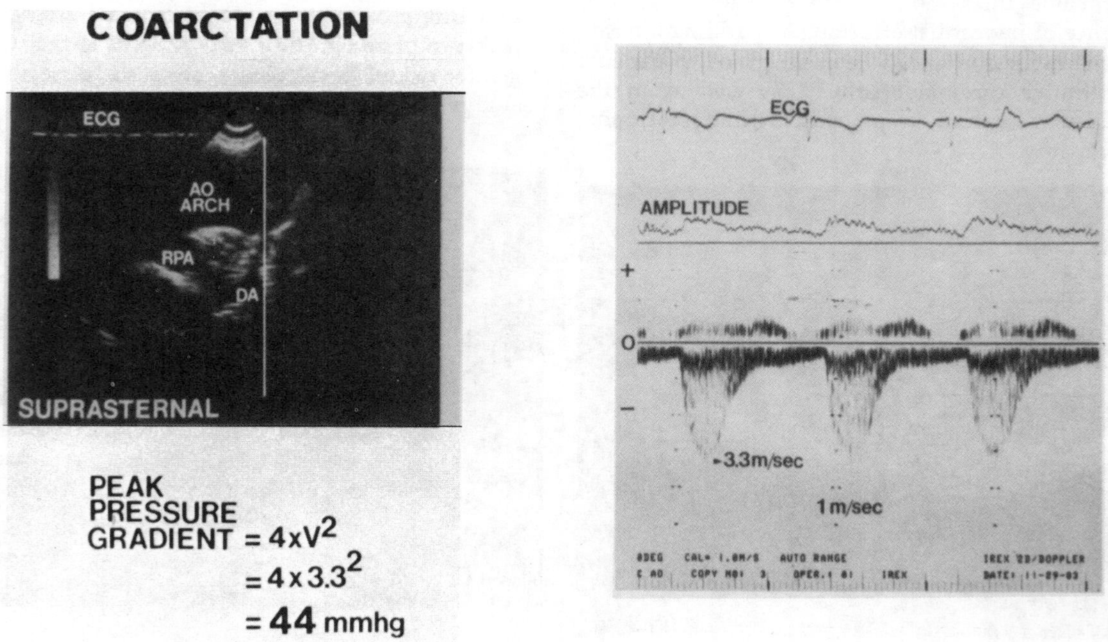

Figure 6.43. Two-dimensional echocardiogram (*left*) and continuous wave Doppler recording (*right*) from the suprasternal notch in a patient with coarctation of the aorta. On the left, the aortic (Ao) arch is dilated and the descending aorta (DA) is narrowed just distal to the origin of the left subclavian artery. The *white line* indicates the position of the Doppler beam. On the right, a peak systolic velocity of 3.3 m/s is recorded from the descending aorta, indicating a peak systolic pressure gradient of 44 mm Hg across the coarctation. ECG = electrocardiogram; RPA = right pulmonary artery.

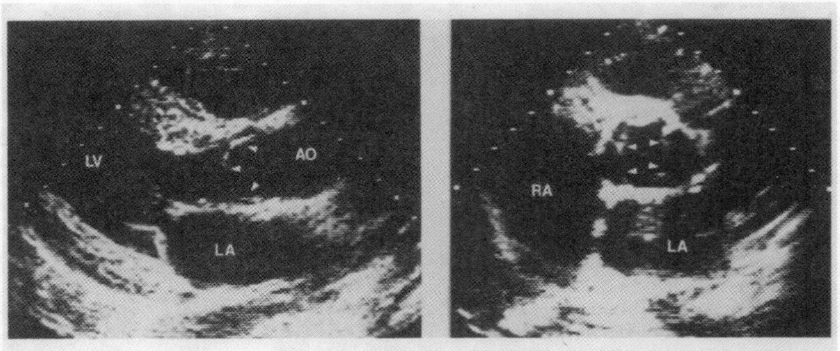

Figure 6.44. Parasternal long- (*left*) and short-axis (*right*) views of the aortic valve in a patient with a bicuspid aortic valve. In the parasternal long-axis view in diastole, the leaflets are bowing into the left ventricular outflow tract (*white arrows*). In the parasternal short-axis view in systole, the commissures are situated at the 1 and 6 o'clock positions and the leaflets assume a fish-mouth appearance (*white arrows*). Normally during systole the open leaflets have an inverted triangular appearance. AO = aorta; LA = left atrium; LV = left ventricle; RA = right atrium.

or pulmonary outflow obstruction with both 2-D and Doppler echocardiography.

Combined 2-D and Doppler echocardiography is particularly useful in diagnosing intracardiac shunts, especially atrial septal defects (Figure 6.42), and in assessing flow across the tricuspid valve.[258] Ventricular septal defects and patent ductus arteriosus are also readily assessed by Doppler echocardiography. In addition, coarctation of the aorta can readily be diagnosed by 2-D echocardiography and the severity of the constricting lesion can also be reliably assessed by Doppler echocardiography (Figure 6.43).

Bicuspid aortic valve is a common congenital cardiac anomaly occurring in 0.4% to 2.0% of the adult population. Although stenosis due to calcification commonly ensues, the real importance of recognizing a patient with a biscuspid aortic valve is to attempt prophylaxis with antibiotics in such a person to prevent endocarditis.

Bicuspid valves may have three unequal aortic sinuses and a tall raphe along the conjoined cusp or only two aortic sinuses and a shallow raphe.[259] Two-dimensional echocardiography is useful in identifying these anatomic variations. Although asymmetric closure of cusps is frequent in patients with bicuspid aortic valves with M-mode echocardiography, it can also occur normally, depending on transducer angulation. The parasternal short-axis view of the aortic valve is ideally suited to determine the number of cusps and location of the commissures.[259] In a bicuspid aortic valve, the commissures are usually located at the 4 and 10 o'clock or 1 and 6 o'clock positions (Figure 6.44) instead of the normal 2, 6, and 10 o'clock positions.[259] In addition, the cusps assume a fish-mouth appearance during systole (Figure 6.44). On the basis of comparative 2-D echocardiographic studies with surgical and pathologic inspection, Brandenburg et al[259] found that echocardiography is a sensitive and highly specific technique for diagnosing bicuspid aortic valve. In the parasternal long-axis view, aortic valve prolapse can frequently occur during diastole (Figure 6.44). It appears that the greater the degree of prolapse, the more the likelihood of aortic regurgitation.[260]

Acknowledgment: Figures 11 to 15 were supplied through the courtesy of John Ross, RCPT, Hahnemann University, and Johnson & Johnson Ultrasound, Inc.

REFERENCES

1. Edler I, Hertz CH: Use of ultrasonic reflectoscope for continuous recording of movements of heart walls. *Kurgl Fysiogr, Sallad i Lund Forhandl* 1954; 24:5–19.
2. Edler I: Diagnostic use of ultrasound in heart disease. *Acta Med Scand* 1955; 308:32–41.
3. Joyner CR, Hey BE, Johnson J, Reid JM: Reflected ultrasound in the diagnosis of tricuspid stenosis. *Am J Cardiol* 1967; 19:66–73.
4. Feigenbaum H, Zaky A, Grabhorn L: Cardiac motion in patient with pericardial effusion: a study using ultrasound cardiography. *Circulation* 1966; 34:611–619.
5. Gramiak R, Shah P: Echocardiography of the aortic root. *Invest Radiol* 1968; 3:356–388.
6. Bom N, Lancee C, van Zweiten G, Kloster FE, Roelandt J: Multiscan echocardiography. I. Technical description. *Circulation* 1973; 48:1066–1074.
7. Griffith JM, Henry WL: A sector scanner for real-time, two-dimensional echocardiography. *Circulation* 1974; 49:1147–1152.
8. Eggleton RC, Feigenbaum H, Johnston KW, Weyman AE, Dillon JC, Chang S: Visualization of cardiac dynamics with real-time B-mode ultrasonic scanner, in White D (ed): *Ultrasound in Medicine.* New York, Plenum Press, 1975; vol 1, pp 385–393.
9. von Ramm OT, Thurstone FL: Cardiac imaging using a phased array ultrasound system. 1. System design. *Circulation* 1976; 53:258–262.
10. Baker DW, Rubenstein SA, Lorch GS: Pulsed Doppler echocardiography: principles and applications. *Am J Med* 1977; 63:69–80.
11. Holen J, Aaslid R, Landmark K, Simonsen S: Determination of pressure gradient in mitral stenosis with a non-invasive ultrasound Doppler technique. *Acta Med Scand* 1976; 199:455–460.
12. Brubakk AO, Angelsen BAJ, Hatle L: Diagnosis of valvular heart disease using transcutaneous Doppler ultrasound. *Cardiovasc Res* 1977; 11:461–469.
13. Hatle L: Noninvasive assessment and differentiation of left ventricular outflow obstruction with Doppler ultrasound. *Circulation* 1981; 64:381–387.
14. Hatle L, Angelsen B: Doppler ultrasound in cardiology: physical principles and clinical applications. 2nd ed. Philadelphia, Lea & Febiger, 1985.
15. Bommer WJ, Miller L: Real-time two-dimensional color-flow Doppler: enhanced Doppler flow imaging in the diagnosis of cardiovascular disease (abstr). *Am J Cardiol* 1982; 49:944.
16. Miyatake K, Okamoto M, Kinoshita N, Kyo S, Tsumi S, Owa M, Takao S, Sakakibar H, Nimura Y: Clinical applications of a new type

of real-time two-dimensional Doppler flow imaging system. *Am J Cardiol* 1984; 54:857–868.

17. Omoto R, Yokote Y, Takamoto S, Ueda K, Asano H, Namekawa K, Kasai C, Kondo Y, Koyano A, et al: The development of real-time two-dimensional Doppler echocardiography and its clinical significance in acquired valvular diseases with special reference to the evaluation of valvular regurgitation. *Jpn Heart J* 1984; 25:325–340.
18. Sakakibara H, Miyatake K, Izumi S, Kinoshita N, Asonuma H, Nimura Y: Assessment of mitral and aortic regurgitation by real-time two-dimensional and Doppler flow imaging system (abstr). *Circulation* 1984; 70 (suppl II): II–406.
19. Stevenson JG, Brandestein MA: Real time imaging of directional blood flow: value of detection of blood flow in an abnormal direction, location or time in the cardiac cycle (abstr). *Circulation* 1984; 70 (suppl II):II–39.
20. Asaka T, Yoshikawa K, Yoshida K, Okumachi F, Yangihara K, Kato H, Shiratori K: Sensitivity and specificity of real-time two-dimensional Doppler flow imaging system in the detection of valvular regurgitation (abstr). *Circulation* 1984; 70 (suppl II): II–38.
21. Omoto R (ed): *Color Atlas of Real-Time Two-Dimensional Doppler Echocardiography*. Tokyo, Shindan-to-Chiryo Co, 1984.
22. Kyo S, Omoto R, Takamato S, Takanawa E: Clinical significance of color flow mapping real-time two-dimensional Doppler echocardiography (2-D Doppler) in congenital heart disease (abstr). *Circulation* 1984; 70 (suppl II): II–37.
23. Takamoto S: Aortic disease, in Omoto R (ed): *Color Atlas of Real-Time Two-Dimensional Doppler Echocardiography*. Tokyo, Shindan-to-Chiryo Co, 1984, pp 135–160.
24. Feigenbaum H: Echocardiography, in Braunwald E (ed): *Heart Disease*. Philadelphia, W.B. Saunders Co, 1984, pp 88–145.
25. Henry WL, DeMaria A, Gramiak R, King DL, Kisslo JA, Popp RL, Sahn DJ, Schiller NB, Tajik A, Teicholz LE, Weyman AE: Report of the American Society of Echocardiography Committee on Nomenclature and Standards in Two-Dimensional Echocardiography. *Circulation* 1980; 62:212–217.
26. Mintz GS, Kotler MN, Segal BL, Parry W. The two-dimensional echocardiographic recognition of the descending thoracic aorta. *Am J Cardiol* 1979; 44:232–238.
27. Tajik AJ, Seward JB, Hagler DJ, Mair DD, Lie JT: Two-dimensional real-time ultrasonic imaging of the heart and great vessels. Technique, image orientation, structure, identification and validation. *Mayo Clin Proc* 1978; 53:271–303.
28. Silverman NH, Schiller NB: Apex cardiography. A two-dimensional technique for evaluating congenital heart disease. *Circulation* 1978; 57:503–511.
29. Feinstein SB, Folkert J, Ten Cate J, Zwehl W, Ong K, Maurer G, Tei C, Shah PM, Meerbaum S, Corday E: Two-dimensional contrast echocardiography. I. In vitro development and quantitative analysis of echo contrast agents. *J Am Coll Cardiol* 1984; 3:14–20.
30. Wang XF, Wang JE, Chen HR, Lu CF: Contrast echocardiography with hydrogen peroxide. II. Clinical application. *Chin Med J* 1979; 92:693–702.
31. Jiang L, Pu SY, Yang MZ, Lu YZ, Chen HZ: Left heart contrast echocardiography using a carbon dioxide producing agent. *Circulation* 1984; 70 (suppl II): II–5.
32. Valdes-Cruz LM, Sahn DJ: Ultrasonic contrast studies for the detection of cardiac shunts. *J Am Coll Cardiol* 1984; 3:978–985.
33. Weyman AE, Wann LS, Caldwell RL, Hurwitz RA, Dillon JC, Feigenbaum H: Negative contrast echocardiography: a new method for detecting left to right shunts. *Circulation* 1979; 59:498–505.
34. Cheng TO: Echocardiography and paradoxical embolism. *Ann Intern Med* 1981; 95:515.
35. DeMaria AN, Bommer W, Kwan OL, Riggs K, Smith M, Waters J: In vivo correlation of thermodilution cardiac and videodensitometric indicator - dilution curves obtained from contrast two-dimensional echocardiograms. *J Am Coll Cardiol* 1984; 3:999–1004.
36. Kaul S, Pandian NG, Okada RD, Pohost GM, Weyman AE: Contrast echocardiography in acute myocardial ischemia. I. In vivo determination of total left ventricular "area at risk." *J Am Coll Cardiol* 1984; 4:1272–82.
37. Matsumoto M, Yasui K, Shimazu T, Maeda T, Matsuyama T, Nishioka H, Ozaki H, Fujiwara M, Tada M, Minamino T: Evaluation of severity of coronary stenosis by contrast echomyocardiography in clinical cases. *Circulation* 1984; 70 (suppl II):II–393.
38. Matsumoto M, Yasui K, Inoue M: Contrast echomyocardiography: contrast enhanced echography of the myocardium. *Echocardiography* 1985; 2:57–66.
39. Goldman ME, Mindich BP: Intraoperative cardioplegic contrast echocardiography for assessing myocardial perfusion during open heart surgery. *J Am Coll Cardiol* 1984; 5:1029–1034.
40. Goldman ME, Mindich BP, Teichholz LE, Burgess N, Staville K, Fuster V: Intraoperative contrast echocardiography to evaluate mitral valve operations. *J Am Coll Cardiol* 1984; 5:1035–1040.
41. Bommer WJ, Shah PM, Allen H, Meltzer R, Kisslo J: The safety of contrast echocardiography: report of the committee on contrast echocardiography for the American Society of Echocardiography. *J Am Coll Cardiol* 1984; 3:6–13.
42. Lee F, Ginzton L: A central nervous sytem complication of contrast echocardiography. *J Clin Ultrasound* 1983; 11:292–294.
43. Ten Cate FJ, Feinstein S, Zwehl W, Meerbaum S, Fishbein M, Shah P, Corday E: Two-dimensional contrast echocardiography. II. Transpulmonary studies. *J Am Coll Cardiol* 1984; 3:21–27.
44. Goldberg SJ, Valdes-Cruz LM, Feldman L, Sahn DJ, Allen HD: Range gated doppler ultrasound detection of contrast echographic microbubbles for cardiac and great vessel blood flow patterns. *Am Heart J* 1981; 101:793–796.
45. Henry WL, Griffith JM, Michaelis LL, McIntosh CL, Morrow AG, Epstein SE: Measurement of mitral orifice area in patients with mitral valve disease by real-time two-dimensional echocardiography. *Circulation* 1975; 52:827–831.
46. Nichol PM, Gilbert BW, Kisslo JA: Two-dimensional echocardiographic assessment of mitral stenosis. *Circulation* 1977; 55:120–128.
47. Wann LS, Weyman AE, Feigenbaum H, Dillon JC, Johnston KW, Eggleton RC: Determination of mitral valve area by cross-sectional echocardiography. *Ann Intern Med* 1978; 88:337–341.
48. DePace NL, Soulen RL, Kotler MN, Mintz GS: Two-dimensional echocardiographic detection of intraatrial masses. *Am J Cardiol* 1981; 48:954–966.
49. Herzog CA, Bass D, Kane M, Asinger R: Two-dimensional echocardiographic imaging of left atrial appendage thrombi. *J Am Coll Cardiol* 1984; 3:1340–1344.
50. Heger JJ, Wann LS, Weyman AE, Dillon JC, Feigenbaum H: Long-term changes in mitral valve area after successful mitral commissurotomy. *Circulation* 1979; 59:443–448.
51. Holen J, Simonsen S: Determination of pressure gradient in mitral stenosis with Doppler echocardiography. *Br Heart J* 1979; 41:529–535.
52. Hatle L, Brubakk A, Tromsdal A, Angelsen B: Noninvasive assessment of pressure drop in mitral stenosis by Doppler ultrasound. *Br Heart J* 1978; 40:131–140.
53. Hatle L, Angelsen B, Tromsdal A: Noninvasive assessment of atrioventricular pressure half-time by Doppler ultrasound. *Circulation* 1979; 60:1096–1104.
54. Stamm RB, Martin RP: Quantification of pressure gradients across stenotic valves by Doppler ultrasound. *J Am Coll Cardiol* 1983; 2:707–718.
55. Kosturakis D, Goldberg SJ, Allen HD, Loeber C: Doppler echocardiographic prediction of pulmonary arterial hypertension in congenital heart disease. *Am J Cardiol* 1984; 53:1110–1115.
56. Mahan G, Dabestani A, Gardin J, Allfie A, Burn C, Henry W: Estimation of pulmonary artery pressure by pulsed Doppler echocardiography (abstr). *Circulation* 1983; 68 (suppl III):III–367.
57. Kitabataki A, Inoue M, Asao M, Masuyama T, Tanouchi J, Morita T, Mishima M, Uematsu M, Shimazu T, Hori M, Abe H: Noninvasive evaluation of pulmonary hypertension by a pulsed Doppler technique. *Circulation* 1983; 68:302–309.
58. Hatle L, Angelsen BAJ, Thomsdal A: Noninvasive estimation of pulmonary artery systolic pressure with Doppler ultrasound. *Br Heart J* 1981; 45:157–165.
59. Burstin L: Determination of pressure in the pulmonary artery by external graphic recordings. *Br Heart J* 1967; 29:396–404.
60. Mintz GS, Kotler MN, Segal BL, Parry WR: Two-dimensional echocardiographic evaluation of patients with mitral insufficiency. *Am J Cardiol* 1979; 44:670–678.
61. Kotler MN, Mintz GS, Parry WR, Segal BL: M-mode and two-dimensional echocardiography in mitral and aortic regurgitation. Pre and post operative evaluation of volume overload of the left ventricle. *Am J Cardiol* 1980; 46:1144–1152.
62. Delaye J, Beaune J, Gayet JL, Fatayri W, Silvestre A: Current etiology of organic mitral insufficiency in adults. *Arch Mal Coeur* 1983; 76:1072–1076.
63. Waun LS, Feigenbaum H, Weyman AE, Dillon JC: Cross-sectional echocardiographic detection of rheumatic mitral regurgitation. *Am J Cardiol* 1978; 41:1258–1263.
64. Alpert MA, Carney RJ, Flaker GC, Sanfelippo JF, Webel RR, Kelly DL: Sensitivity and specificity of two-dimensional echocardiographic signs of mitral valve prolapse. *Am J Cardiol* 1984; 54:792–796.
65. Perloff JK: Evolving concepts of mitral valve prolapse. *N Engl J Med* 1982; 307:369–370.
66. Wann LS, Grove JR, Hess TR, Glisch L, Pfacin MJ, Hughes CV, Gross CM: Prevalence of mitral prolapse by two-dimensional echocardiography in healthy young women. *Br Heart J* 1983; 49:334–340.
67. Popp RL, Rubenson DS, Tucker CR, French JW: Echocardiography: M-mode and two-dimensional method. *Ann Intern Med* 1980; 93:844–856.
68. Markiewicz W, Stoner J, London E, Hunt SA, Popp RL: Mitral valve

prolapse in one hundred presumably healthy young females. *Circulation* 1976; 53:464–473.
69. Abbasi AS, DeCristofaro D, Anabtawi J, Irwin L: Mitral valve prolapse: comparative value of M-mode, two-dimensional and Doppler echocardiography. *J Am Coll Cardiol* 1983; 2:1219–1223.
70. Mintz GS, Kotler MN, Segal BL, Parry WR: Two-dimensional echocardiographic recognition of ruptured chordae tendineae. *Circulation* 1978; 57:244–250.
71. Mintz GS, Kotler MN, Segal BL, Parry WR: A statistical comparison of the M-mode and two-dimensional echocardiographic diagnosis of flail mitral leaflets. *Am J Cardiol* 1980; 45:253–259.
72. DePace NL, Mintz GS, Ren JF, Kotler MN, Mattleman S, Victor MF, Ross J, Mintz PS: The natural history of the flail mitral leaflet syndrome. A serial two-dimensional echocardiographic study. *Am J Cardiol* 1983; 52:789–795.
73. Takamoto T, Popp RL: Conduction disturbances related to the site and severity of mitral annular calcification: a two-dimensional echocardiographic and electrocardiographic correlative study. *Am J Cardiol* 1983; 51:1644–1649.
74. Savage DD, Garrision RJ, Castelli WP, McNamara P, Anderson SJ, Kannel WB, Feinleib M: Prevalence of submitral (annular) calcium and its correlates in a general population-based sample (The Framingham Study). *Am J Cardiol* 1983; 51:1375–1378.
75. DePace NL, Rohrer AH, Kotler MN, Brezin JH, Parry WR: Rapidly progressive massive mitral annular calcification in a patient with chronic renal failure. *Arch Intern Med* 1981; 141:1663–1665.
76. Kalman P, DePace NL, Kotler MN, Mintz GS, Levites R, Ren JF: Mitral annular calcification and echogenic densities in the left ventricular outflow tract in association with cerebral ischemic events. *J Cardiovasc Ultrasonogr* 1982; 1:155–159.
77. Ren JF, Kotler MN, DePace NL, Mintz GS, Kimbiris D, Kalman P, Ross J: Two-dimensional echocardiographic determination of left atrial emptying volume: a non-invasive index in quantifying the degree of non-rheumatic mitral regurgitation. *J Am Coll Cardiol* 1983; 2:729–736.
78. Kotler MN, Ren JF, Mintz GS: Severity of nonrheumatic mitral regurgitation. *Primary Cardiol* 1985; 11:66–76.
79. Blanchard D, Diebold B, Peronneau P, Foult JM, Nee M, Guermonprez JL, Maurke P: Non-invasive diagnosis of mitral regurgitation by Doppler echocardiography. *Br Heart J* 1981; 45:589–593.
80. Knutsen KM, Bac EA, Sivertssen E, Hoiseth A: Detection mitral regurgitation by Doppler ultrasound. *Acta Med Scand* 1981; 210:349–351.
81. Abbasi AS, Allen MW, Decristofaro D, Ungar I: Detection and estimation of the degree of mitral regurgitation by range-gated pulsed Doppler echocardiography. *Circulation* 1980; 61:143–147.
82. Veyrat C, Ameur A, Bas S, Lessana A, Arbitbol G, Kalmanson D: Pulsed Doppler echocardiographic indices for assessing mitral regurgitation. *Br Heart J* 1984; 51:130–138.
83. Stewart WJ, Palacios I, Jiang L, Dinsmore RE, Weyman AE: Doppler measurement of regurgitant fraction in patients with mitral regurgitation: a new quantitative technique (abstr). *Circulation* 1983; 68 (suppl III):III–111.
84. Weyman AE, Feigenbaum H, Dillon JC, Chang S: Cross-sectional echocardiography in assessing the severity of valvular aortic stenosis. *Circulation* 1975; 52:828–834.
85. DeMaria AN, Bommer W, Jaye J, Lee G, Bouteller J, Mason DT: Value and limitations of cross-sectional echocardiography of the aortic valves in the diagnosis and quantification of valvular aortic stenosis. *Circulation* 1980; 62:304–312.
86. Williams GA, Labovitz AJ, Nelson JG, Kennedy HL: Value of multiple echocardiographic views in the evaluation of aortic stenosis in adults by continuous-wave Doppler. *Am J Cardiol* 1985; 55:445–449.
87. Hatle L, Angelsen BA, Tromsdal A: Non-invasive assessment of aortic stenosis by Doppler ultrasound. *Br Heart J* 1980; 43:284–292.
88. Berger M, Berdoff R, Gallerstein PE, Goldberg E: Evaluation of aortic stenosis by continuous wave Doppler ultrasound. *J Am Coll Cardiol* 1984; 3:150–156.
89. Oliveira Lima C, Sahn DJ, Valdes-Cruz LM, Allen HD, Goldberg SJ, Grenadier E, Barron JV: Prediction of the severity of left ventricular outflow tract obstruction by quantitation two-dimensional echocardiographic Doppler studies. *Circulation* 1983; 68:348–354.
90. Smith MD, Dawson P, Elion J, Wisenbaugh T, Handshoe S, Kwan OL, Demaria AN: Comparative correlation of continuous wave Doppler spectral measurements with hemodynamic parameters in patients with aortic stenosis (abstr). *Circulation* 1984; 70 (suppl II):II–116.
91. Kosturakis D, Allen HD, Goldberg SJ, Sahn DJ, Valdez-Cruz LM: Noninvasive quantification of stenotic semilunar valve areas by Doppler echocardiography. *J Am Coll Cardiol* 1984; 3:1256–1262.
92. Warth DC, Stewart WJ, Block PC, Weyman AE: A new method to calculate aortic valve area without left heart catheterization. *Circulation* 1984; 70:978–983.
93. DePace NL, Nestico PF, Kotler MN, Mintz GS, Kimbiris D, Goel IP, Glazier-Laskey E, Ross J: Comparison of echocardiography and angiography in the evaluation of the etiology of severe aortic regurgitation. *Br Heart J* 1984; 52:36–45.
94. Sequeira RF, Watt J: Assessment of aortic regurgitation by transcutaneous aortovelography. *Br Heart J* 1977; 39:929–930.
95. Boughner DR: Assessment of aortic insufficiency by transcutaneous Doppler ultrasound. *Circulation* 1975; 52:874–879.
96. Ciobana M, Abbasi AS, Allen M, Hermer A, Spellberg R: Pulsed Doppler echocardiography in the diagnosis and estimation of severity of aortic insufficiency. *Am J Cardiol* 1982; 49:339–343.
97. Veyrat C, Ameur A, Gourtchiglouion C, Lessana A, Arbitbol G, Kalmonson D: Calculation of pulsed Doppler left ventricular outflow tract regurgitant index for grading the severity of aortic regurgitation. *Am Heart J* 1984; 108:507–515.
98. Diebold B, Peronnau P, Blanchard D, Colonna G, Guermonprez JL, Forman J, Sellier P, Maurice P: Non-invasive quantification of aortic regurgitation by Doppler echocardiography. *Br Heart J* 1983; 49:167–173.
99. Handshoe R, Handshoe S, Kwan OL, Smith MD, DeMaria AN: Value and limitations of Doppler measurements in the estimation of left ventricular end diastolic pressure in patients with aortic regurgitation. *Circulation* 1984; 70 (suppl II): II–117.
100. Henry WL, Bonow RO, Borer JS, Ware JH, Kent KM, Redwood DR, McIntosh CL, Morrow AG, Epstein SE: Observations on the optimum time for aortic regurgitation. I. Evaluation of the results of aortic valve replacement in symptomatic patients. *Circulation* 1980; 61:471–483.
101. Fioretti P, Roelandt J, Bos RJ, Meltzer RS, van Hoogenhuyze D, Serruys PW, Nauta J, Hugenholtz PG: Echocardiography in chronic aortic insufficiency. Is valve replacement too late when left ventricular end systolic dimension reaches 55 mm? *Circulation* 1983; 67:216–221.
102. O'Rourke RA, Crawford MH: Timing of valve replacement in patients with chronic aortic regurgitation. *Circulation* 1980; 61:493–495.
103. Meltzer RS, Hoogenhuyze DV, Serruys PW, Haalebos MMP, Hugenholtz PG, Roelandt J: Diagnosis of tricuspid regurgitation by contrast echocardiography. *Circulation* 1981; 63:1093–1099.
104. Daniels SJ, Mintz GS, Kotler MN: Rheumatic tricuspid valve disease. Two-dimensional echocardiographic, hemodynamic and angiographic correlations. *Am J Cardiol* 1983; 51:492–496.
105. Callahan JA, Wroblewski EM, Reeder GS, Edwards WD, Seward JB, Tajik AJ: Echocardiographic features of carcinoid heart disease. *Am J Cardiol* 1982; 50:762–768.
106. Shiina A, Seward JB, Edwards WD, Hagler J, Tajik AJ: Two-dimensional echocardiographic spectrum of Ebstein's anomaly: detailed anatomic assessment. *J Am Coll Cardiol* 1984; 3:356–370.
107. DePace NL, Ross J, Iskandrian AS, Nestico PF, Kotler MN, Mintz GS, Segal BL, Hakki AH, Morganroth J: Tricuspid regurgitation: non-invasive techniques for determining causes and severity. *J Am Coll Cardiol* 1984; 3:1540–1550.
108. Panidis IP, Kotler MN, Mintz GS, Weber J, Levites R, Ren JF, Ross J: Clinical echocardiographic correlations in patients with right heart endocarditis. *Int J Cardiol* 1984; 6:17–31.
109. Miyatake K, Okamoto M, Kinoshita N, Ohta M, Kozuka T, Sakakibari H, Nimura Y: Evaluation of tricuspid regurgitation by pulsed Doppler and two-dimensional echocardiography. *Circulation* 1982; 66:777–784.
110. Diebold B, Tonati R, Blanchard D, Colonna G, Guermonprez JL, Peronneau P, Forman J, Maurice P: Quantitative assessment of tricuspid regurgitation using pulsed Doppler echocardiography. *Br Heart J* 1983; 50:443–449.
111. Sakai K, Nakamara K, Satomi G, Kondo M, Hirosawa K: Evaluation of tricuspid regurgitation by blood flow pattern in the hepatic vein using pulsed Doppler technique. *Am Heart J* 1984; 108:516–522.
112. Pennestri F, Loperfido F, Salvatori MP, Mongiardo R, Ferrazza A, Guccione P, Manzoli U: Assessment of tricuspid regurgitation by pulsed Doppler ultrasonography of the hepatic veins. *Am J Cardiol* 1984; 54:363–368.
113. Garcia-Dorado D, Falzgraf S, Almazan A, Delcan JL, Lopez-Besco L, Menarguez L: Diagnosis of functional tricuspid insufficiency by pulsed-wave Doppler ultrasound. *Circulation* 1982; 66:1315–1321.
114. Waggoner AD, Quinones MA, Young JB, Brandon TA, Shah AA, Verani MS, Miller RR: Pulsed Doppler echocardiography detection of right-sided valve regurgitation. *Am J Cardiol* 1981; 47:279–286.
115. Yock PG, Naasz C, Schnittger I, Popp RL: Doppler tricuspid and pulmonic regurgitation in normals: Is it real? (abstr). *Circulation* 1984; 70 (suppl II): II–40.
116. Skjaerpe T, Hatle L: Diagnosis and assessment of tricuspid regurgitation with Doppler ultrasound, in Spencer M (ed): *Cardiac Doppler Diagnosis.* The Hague, Martinus Niijhoff, 1983, pp 247–254.
117. Yock PG, Popp RL: Noninvasive estimation of right ventricular systolic pressure by Doppler ultrasound in patients with tricuspid regurgitation. *Circulation* 1984; 70:657–662.
118. Nakamura K, Satomi G, Ogasawara S, Oteki H, Hirosawa K: Noninvasive evaluation of tricuspid stenosis with Doppler echocardiography (abstr). *Circulation* 1984; 70 (suppl II):II–394.

119. Weyman AE: Pulmonary valve echo motion in clinical practice. *Am J Med* 1977; 62:843–855.
120. Weyman AE, Hurwitz RA, Girod DA, Dillon JC, Feigenbaum H, Green D: Cross-sectional echocardiographic visualization of the stenotic pulmonary valve. *Circulation* 1977; 56:769–774.
121. Oliveira-Lima C, Sahn DJ, Valdes-Cruz LM, Goldberg SJ, Barron JV, Allen HD, Grenadier E: Noninvasive prediction of transvalvular pressure gradient in patients with pulmonary stenosis by quantitative two-dimensional echocardiographic Doppler studies. *Circulation* 1983; 67:866–871.
122. Johnson GL, Kivan OL, Handshoe S, Noonan JA, DeMaria AN: Accuracy of combined two-dimensional echocardiography and continuous wave Doppler recordings in the estimation of pressure gradient in right ventricular outlet obstruction. *J Am Coll Cardiol* 1984; 3:1013–1018.
123. Miyatake K, Okamoto M, Kinoshita N, Matsuhisa M, Negata S, Beppu S, Park Y-D, Sakakibara H, Nimura Y: Pulmonary regurgitation studied with the ultrasonic pulsed Doppler technique. *Circulation* 1982; 65:969–976.
124. Brodie BR, Grossman W, McClaurin L, Starek PJK, Craige E: Diagnosis of prosthetic valve malfunction with combined echo-phonocardiography. *Circulation* 1976; 53:93–100.
125. Smith ND, Raijzada V, Abrams J: Auscultation of normally functioning prosthetic valve. *Ann Intern Med* 1981; 95:594–598.
126. Kotler MN, Mintz GS, Panidis I: Non-invasive evaluation of normal and abnormal prosthetic valve function. *J Am Coll Cardiol* 1983; 2:151–173.
127. Felner J, Miller D: Echocardiographic characteristics of mechanical prosthetic heart valves. *Echocardiography* 1984; 1:261–310.
128. Usher BW: Echocardiographic assessment of patients with bioprosthetic valves. *Echocardiography* 1984; 1:311–332.
129. Holen J, Hoie J, Semb B: Obstructive characteristics of Björk-Shiley, Hancock and Lillehei-Kaster prosthetic mitral valves in the immediate postoperative period. *Acta Med Scand* 1978; 204:5–10.
130. Halen J, Simonsen S, Froysaker T: An ultrasound Doppler technique for the noninvasive determination of the pressure gradient in the Björk-Shiley mitral valve. *Circulation* 1979; 59:436–442.
131. Williams GA, Labovitz AJ: Doppler hemodynamic evaluation of prosthetic (Starr-Edwards and Björk-Shiley) and bioprosthetic (Hancock and Carpentier-Edwards) cardiac valves. *Am J Cardiol* 1985; 56:325–332.
132. Dillon JC: Echocardiography in valvular vegetations. *Am J Med* 1977; 62:856–862.
133. Mintz GS, Kotler MN, Segal BL, Parry W: Comparison of two-dimensional and M-mode echocardiography in the evaluation of patients with infective endocarditis. *Am J Cardiol* 1979; 43:738–744.
134. Wann LS, Hallam CC, Dillon JC: Comparison of M-mode and cross-sectional echocardiography in infective endocarditis. *Circulation* 1979; 60:728–733.
135. Gilbert BW, Haney RS, Crawford F, McClellan J, Gallis HA, Johnson ML, Kisslo JA: Two-dimensional echocardiographic assessment of vegetative endocarditis. *Circulation* 1977; 55:346–353.
136. Mintz GS, Kotler MN: Clinical value and limitations of echocardiography. Its use in the study of patients with infectious endocarditis. *Arch Intern Med* 1980; 140:1023–1027.
137. Lappe DL, Bulkley BH, Weiss JL: Two-dimensional echocardiographic diagnosis of left atrial myxoma. *Chest* 1978; 74:55–58.
138. Perry LS, King JF, Zeft HJ, Manley JC, Gross CM, Wann LS: Two-dimensional echocardiography in the diagnosis of left atrial myxoma. *Br Heart J* 1981; 45:667–671.
139. Sutton MG St J, Mercier LA, Giuliani ER, Lie JT: Atrial myxomas. A review of clinical experience in 40 patients. *Mayo Clin Proc* 1980; 55:371–376.
140. Felner JM, Knopf WD: Echocardiographic recognition of intracardiac and extracardiac masses. *Echocardiography* 1985; 2:3–55.
141. Panidis IP, Kotler MN, Mintz GS, Ross J: Clinical and echocardiographic features of right atrial masses. *Am Heart J* 1984; 107:745–758.
142. Nestico IP, Panidis IP, Kotler MN, Mintz GS, Ross J: Surgical removal of right atrial thromboembolus detected by two-dimensional echocardiography in pulmonary embolism. *Am Heart J* 1984; 107:1278–1280.
143. Felner JM, Churchwell AL, Murphy DA: Right atrial thromboemboli: clinical, echocardiographic and pathophysiologic manifestations. *J Am Coll Cardiol* 1984; 4:1041–1051.
144. Goldman A, Parameswaran R, Kotler MN, Hartman J, Parry W: Renal cell carcinoma and right atrial tumor diagnosed by echocardiography. *Am Heart J* 1985; 110:183–186.
145. Kisslo JA, Robertson D, Gilbert BW, von Romm O, Behar VS: A comparison of real-time, two-dimensional echocardiography and cine-angiography in detecting left ventricular asynergy. *Circulation* 1977; 55:134–141.
146. Haendchen RW, Wyatt HL, Maurer G, Zwehl W, Bear M, Meerbaum S, Corday E: Quantitation of regional cardiac function by two-dimensional echocardiography. I. Patterns of contraction in the normal left ventricle. *Circulation* 1983; 67:1234–1245.
147. Pandian NG, Skorton DJ, Collins SM, Falsetti HL, Burke ER, Kerber RE: Heterogeneity of left ventricular segmental wall thickening and excursion in two-dimensional echocardiograms of normal humans. *Am J Cardiol* 1983; 51:1667–1673.
148. Pandian NG, Kerber RE: Two-dimensional echocardiography experimental coronary stenosis. I. Sensitivity and specificity in detecting transient myocardial dyskinesis. Comparison with sonomicrometers. *Circulation* 1982; 66:597–602.
149. Wyatt HL, Meerbaum S, Heng MK, Rit J, Gueret P, Corday E: Experimental evaluation of the extent of myocardial dyssynergy and infarct size by two-dimensional echocardiography. *Circulation* 1981; 63:607–614.
150. Pandian NG, Koyanagi S, Skorton DJ, Collins SM, Eastham LL, Kieso RA, Marcus ML, Kerber RE: Relations between two-dimensional echocardiographic wall thickening abnormalities, myocardial infarct size and coronary risk area in normal and hypertrophied myocardium in dogs. *Am J Cardiol* 1983; 52:1318–1325.
151. Parisi AF, Moynihan PF, Folland ED, Feldman CL: Quantitative detection of regional left ventricular contraction abnormalities by two-dimensional echocardiography. II. Accuracy in coronary artery disease. *Circulation* 1981; 63:761–767.
152. Weiss JL, Bulkley BH, Hutchins GM, Mason SJ: Two-dimensional echocardiographic recognition of myocardial injury in man. Comparison with post-mortem studies. *Circulation* 1981; 63:401–408.
153. Gibson RS, Bishop HL, Stamm HB, Crampton RS, Beller GA, Martin RP: Value of two-dimensional echocardiography in patients with acute myocardial infarction. *Am J Cardiol* 1982; 49:1110–1119.
154. Stamm RB, Gibson RS, Bishop HL, Carabello BA, Beller GA, Martin RP: Echocardiographic detection of infarct-localized asynergy and remote asynergy during acute myocardial infarction: correlation with the extent of angiographic coronary disease. *Circulation* 1983; 67:233–244.
155. Horowitz RS, Morganroth J, Parotto C: Immediate diagnosis of acute myocardial infarction by two-dimensional echocardiography. *Circulation* 1982; 65:323–329.
156. Nixon JV, Brown CN, Smitherman TC: Identification of transient and persistent segmental wall motion abnormalities in patients with unstable angina by two-dimensional echocardiography. *Circulation* 1982; 65:1497–1503.
157. Theroux P, Ross J Jr, Franklin D, Kemper WS, Sasayama S: Coronary arterial reperfusion. III. Early and late effects on regional myocardial function and dimensions in conscious dogs. *Am J Cardiol* 1976; 53:302–314.
158. Lavelle M, Cox D, Patrick TA, Vatner SF: Salvage of myocardial function by coronary artery reperfusion 1, 2, and 3 hours after occlusion in conscious dogs. *Circ Res* 1983; 53:235.
159. Hammerman H, O'Boyle JE, Cohen C, Kloner A, Parisi AF: Dissociation between two-dimensional echocardiographic left ventricular wall motion and myocardial salvage in early experimental acute myocardial infarction in dogs. *Am J Cardiol* 1984; 54:875–879.
160. Yoshikawa J, Yanagihara K, Owaki T, Kato H, Tagaki Y, Okumachi F, Fukaya T, Tomita Y, Baba K: Cross-sectional echocardiographic diagnosis of coronary artery aneurysms in patients with mucocutaneous lymph node syndrome. *Circulation* 1979; 59:133–139.
161. Hiraishi S, Yashiro K, Kusano S: Non-invasive visualization of coronary arterial aneurysm in infants and young children with mucocutaneous lymph node syndrome with two-dimensional echocardiography. *Am J Cardiol* 1979; 43:1225–1233.
162. Maeda T, Yoshida H, Fundabashi T, Nakaya S, Takabatake S, Ohno T, Taniguchi N: Subcostal two-dimensional echocardiographic imaging of peripheral left coronary artery aneurysms in Kawasaki's disease. *Am J Cardiol* 1983; 52:48–52.
163. Miyatake K, Okamoto M, Kinoshita N, Fusejima K, Sakakibara H, Nimura Y: Doppler echocardiographic features of coronary arteriovenous fistula: complementary roles of cross sectional echocardiography and the Doppler technique. *Br Heart J* 1984; 51:508–518.
164. Mawer G, Nanda NC: Two-dimensional echocardiographic evaluation of exercise induced left and right ventricular asynergy. Correlation with thallium scanning. *Am J Cardiol* 1981; 48:720–727.
165. Morganroth J, Chen CC, David D, Sawin HS, Naito M, Parotto C, Meixell L: Exercise cross-sectional echocardiographic diagnosis of coronary artery disease. *Am J Cardiol* 1981; 47:20–26.
166. Crawford MH, Amon KW, Vance WS: Exercise two-dimensional echocardiographic quantification of left ventricular performance in patients with severe angina pectoris. *Am J Cardiol* 1983; 51:1–6.
167. Quinones M: Exercise two-dimensional echocardiography. *Echocardiography* 1984; 1:151–163.
168. Isner JB, Roberts WC: Right ventricular infarction complicating left ventricular infarction secondary to coronary heart disease. *Am J Cardiol* 1978; 42:885–894.
169. Darcy B, Nanda NC: Two-dimensional echocardiographic features of right ventricular infarction. *Circulation* 1982; 65:167–173.
170. Panidis IP, Kotler MN, Mintz GS: Right ventricular function in cor-

onary artery disease as assessed by two-dimensional echocardiography. *Am Heart J* 1984; 107:1187–1194.

171. Weyman AE, Peskoe SM, Williams ES, Dillon JC, Feigenbaum H: Detection of left ventricular aneurysms by cross-sectional echocardiography. *Circulation* 1976; 54:936–944.
172. Visser CA, Kan G, David GK, Lie KI, Durer D: Echocardiographic-cineangiographic correlation in detecting left ventricular aneurysm. A prospective study of 422 patients. *Am J Cardiol* 1982; 50:337–341.
173. Catherwood E, Mintz GS, Kotler MN, Parry WR, Segal BL: Two-dimensional echocardiographic recognition of left ventricular pseudoaneurysm. *Circulation* 1980; 62:294–303.
174. Reeder GS, Tajik AJ, Seward JB: Left ventricular mural thrombus, two-dimensional echocardiographic diagnosis. *Mayo Clin Proc* 1981; 56:77–81.
175. Asinger RW, Mikell FL, Elsperger J, Hodges M: Incidence of left ventricular thrombus after acute transmural myocardial infarction. *N Engl J Med* 1981; 305:297–302.
176. Stratton JR, Lighty GW, Pearlman AS, Ritchie JL: Detection of left ventricular thrombus by two-dimensional echocardiography: sensitivity, specificity and causes of uncertainty. *Circulation* 1982; 66:156–166.
177. Asinger RW, Mikell FL, Sharme B, Hodges M: Observations on detecting left ventricular thrombus with two-dimensional echocardiography. Emphasis on avoidance of false positive diagnoses. *Am J Cardiol* 1981; 47:145–156.
178. Haughland JM, Asinger RW, Mikell FL, Elsperger J, Hodges M: Embolic potential of left ventricular thrombi detected by two-dimensional echocardiography. *Circulation* 1984; 70:588–598.
179. Weinrich DJ, Burke JF, Pauletto FJ: Left ventricular mural thrombi: complicating acute myocardial infarction. *Ann Intern Med* 1984; 100:789–794.
180. Kotler MN, Mintz GS, Segal BL: Operable complications of myocardial infarction: noninvasive diagnosis. *Cardiovasc Med* 1982; 7:1070–1074.
181. Mintz GS, Victor MF, Kotler MN, Parry WR, Segal BL: Two-dimensional echocardiographic identification of surgically correctable complications of acute myocardial infarction. *Circulation* 1981; 64:91–96.
182. Parisi AF, Nieminen M, O'Boyle JE, Moynihan PF, Khuri SF, Kloner RA, Folland ED, Schoen FJ: Enhanced detection of the evolution of tissue changes after acute myocardial infarction using color-encoded two-dimensional echocardiography. *Circulation* 1982; 66:764–770.
183. Stevenson JG, Kawabori I, Dooley T: Differentiation of ventricular septal defects from mitral regurgitation by pulsed Doppler echocardiography. *Circulation* 1977; 56:14–18.
184. Drobac M, Gilbert B, Howard R, Baigne R, Rakowski H: Ventricular septal defect after myocardial infarction. Diagnosis by two-dimensional contrast echocardiography. *Circulation* 1983; 67:335–341.
185. Hatle L, Rokseth R: Noninvasive diagnosis and assessment of ventricular septal defect by Doppler ultrasound. *Acta Med Scand Suppl* 1981; 645 (suppl):47–56.
186. Stevenson JG, Kawabori I, Dooley T, Guntheroth WG: Diagnosis of ventricular septal defect by pulsed Doppler echocardiography. Sensitivity, specificity and limitations. *Circulation* 1978; 58:322–326.
187. Recusani F, Raisaro A, Sgalambro A, Tronconi L, Venco A, Salerno J, Ardissino D: Ventricular septal rupture after myocardial infarction: diagnoses by two-dimensional and pulsed Doppler echocardiography. *Am J Cardiol* 1984; 54:277–281.
188. Sanders SP, Yeager S, Williams RG: Measurement of systemic and pulmonary blood flow and QP/QS ratio using Doppler and two-dimensional echocardiography. *Am J Cardiol* 1983; 51:952–956.
189. Kitabatake A, Inoue M, Asao M, Ito H, Masuyama T, Tanouchi J, Morita T, Hori M, Yoshima H, Ohnishi K, Abe H: Noninvasive evaluation of the ratio of pulmonary to systemic flow in atrial septal defect by duplex Doppler echocardiography. *Circulation* 1984; 69:73–79.
190. Baron JV, Sahn DJ, Valdes-Cruz LM, Lima CO, Goldberg SJ, Grenadier E, Allen HD: Clinical utility of two-dimensional Doppler echocardiographic techniques for estimating pulmonary to systemic blood flow ratios in children with left to right shunting atrial septal defect, ventricular septal defect or patent ductus arteriosus. *J Am Coll Cardiol* 1984; 3:169–178.
191. Stevenson JG, Kawabori I, Stamm SJ, Bailey WW, Hall DG, Mansfield PB, Rittenhouse EA: Pulsed Doppler echocardiographic evaluation of ventricular septal defect patches. *Circulation* 1974; 70 (suppl I):I-38–I-46.
192. Folland ED, Parisi AF, Moynihan PF, Jones DR, Feldman CL, Tow DE: Assessment of left ventricular ejection fraction and volume by real-time two-dimensional echocardiography. A comparison of cineangiographic and radionuclide techniques. *Circulation* 1979; 60:760–766.
193. Schiller NB, Acquatella H, Ports TA, Drew D, Goerke J, Ringertz H, Silverman NH, Brundage B, Botvinik EH, Boswell R, Carlsson E, Parmley WW: Left ventricular volume from paired biplane two-dimensional echocardiography. *Circulation* 1979; 60:547–555.
194. Starling MR, Crawford MH, Sorenson SG, Levi B, Richards KL, O'-Rourke RA: Comparative accuracy of apical biplane cross-sectional echocardiography and gated equilibrium radionuclide angiography for estimating left ventricular size and performance. *Circulation* 1981; 63:1075–1084.
195. Ren JF, Kotler MN, DePace NL, Mintz GS, Iskandrian AS, Hakki AH, Panidis IP, Kimbiris D, Segal BL: Comparison of left ventricular ejection fraction and volumes by two-dimensional echocardiography, radionuclide angiography and cineangiography. *J Cardiovasc Ultrasonogr* 1983; 2:213–222.
196. Schnittger I, Fitzgerald PJ, Daughters GT, Ingels NB, Kantrowitz NE, Schwartzkopf A, Mead CW, Popp RL: Limitations of comparing left ventricular volumes by two-dimensional echocardiography, myocardial markers and cineangiography. *Am J Cardiol* 1982; 50:512–519.
197. Ren JF, Kotler MN, Hakki AH, Panidis IP, Mintz GS, Ross J: Quantitation of regional left ventricular function by two-dimensional echocardiography in normals and patients with coronory artery disease. *Am Heart J* 1985; 110:552–560.
198. Ren JF, Panidis IP, Kotler MN, Mintz GS, Goel I, Ross J: Effect of coronary bypass surgery and valve replacement on left ventricular function: assessment by intraoperative two-dimensional echocardiography. *Am Heart J* 1985; 109:281–289.
199. Reichek N, Helak J, Plappert T, Sutton MSJ, Weber KT: Anatomic validation of left ventricular mass estimates from clinical two-dimensional echocardiography: initial results. *Circulation* 1983; 67:348–352.
200. Panidis IP, Kotler MN, Ren JF, Mintz GS, Ross J, Kalman P: Development and regression of left ventricular hypertrophy. *J Am Coll Cardiol* 1984; 3:1309–1320.
201. Ren JF, Hakki AH, Kotler MN, Iskandrian AS: Exercise systolic blood pressure: a powerful determinant of increased left ventricular mass in patients with hypertension. *J Am Coll Cardiol* 1985; 5:1224–1231.
202. Ihlen H, Ambie PJ, Dale J, Forfang K, Nitter-Hauge S, Otterstad JE, Simonsen S, Myhre E: Determination of cardiac output by Doppler echocardiography. *Br Heart J* 1984; 51:54–60.
203. Loeber CP, Goldberg SJ, Allen HD: Doppler echocardiographic comparison of flows distal to the four cardiac valves. *J Am Coll Cardiol* 1984; 4:268–272.
204. Loeppky JA, Hoekenga DE, Greene ER, Luft UC: Comparison of noninvasive pulsed Doppler and fick measurements of stroke volume in cardiac patients. *Am Heart J* 1984; 107:339–346.
205. Huntsman LL, Stewart DK, Barnes SR, Franklin SB, Colocousis JS, Hessel EA: Noninvasive Doppler determination of cardiac output in man: clinical validation. *Circulation* 1983; 67:593–602.
206. Chandraratna PA, Nanna M, McKay C, Nimalasuriya A, Swinney R, Elkayam U, Rahimtoola SH: Determination of cardiac output by transcutaneous continuous-wave ultrasonic Doppler computer. *Am J Cardiol* 1984; 53:234–237.
207. Nishimura RA, Callahan MJ, Schaff HV, Ilstrup DM, Miller FA, Tajik AJ: Noninvasive measurement of cardiac output by continuous-wave Doppler echocardiography: inital experience and review of the literature. *Mayo Clin Proc* 1984; 59:484–489.
208. Fischer DC, Sahn DJ, Friedman MJ, Larson D, Valdez-Cruz LM, Horowitz S, Goldberg SJ, Allen HD: The mitral valve orifice method for noninvasive two-dimensional echo Doppler determinations of cardiac output. *Circulation* 1983; 67:872–877.
209. Labovitz AJ, Buckingham TA, Habemehl K, Nelson J, Kennedy HL, Williams GA: The effects of sampling site on the two-dimensional echo - Doppler determination of cardiac output. *Am Heart J* 1985; 109:327–332.
210. Elkayam U, Gardin JM, Berkley R, Hughes CA, Henry WL: The use of Doppler flow velocity measurement to assess the hemodynamic response to vasodilators in patients with heart failure. *Circulation* 1983; 67:337–383.
211. Rose JS, Nanna M, Rahimtoola H, Elkayam U, McKay C, Chandraratna PAN: Accuracy of determination of changes in cardiac output by transcutaneous continuous-wave Doppler computer. *Am J Cardiol* 1984; 54:1099–1101.
212. Nanda NC, Bhandari A, Barold SS, Falkoff M: Doppler echocardiographic studies in sequential atrioventricular pacing. *PACE* 1983; 6:811–814.
213. Stewart NJ, Dicola VC, Harthorne WJ, Gillam LD, Weyman AE: Doppler ultrasound measurement of cardiac output in patients with physiologic pacemakers: effects of left ventricular function and retrograde ventriculoatrial conduction. *Am J Cardiol* 1984; 54:308–312.
214. Bommer W, Weinert BS, Neumann A, Neef J, Mason DT, DeMaria A: Determination of right atrial and right ventricular size by two-dimensional echocardiography. *Circulation* 1979; 60:91–100.
215. Levin RA, Gibson TC, Aretz T, Gillam LD, Guyer DE, King ME, Weyman AE: Echocardiographic measurement of right ventricular volume. *Circulation* 1984; 64:497–505.
216. Panidis IP, Ren JF, Kotler MN, Mintz GS, Iskandrian A, Ross J, Kane S: Two-dimensional echocardiographic estimation of right ventricular ejection fraction in patients with coronary artery disease. *J Am Coll Cardiol* 1983; 2:911–918.

217. Kaul S, Tei C, Hopkins JM, Shah PM: Assessment of right ventricular function using two-dimensional echocardiography. *Am Heart J* 1984; 107:526–531.
218. Weyman AE: *Cross-sectional echocardiography*. 1st ed. Philadelphia, Lea & Febiger, 1982.
219. Martin RP, Rakowski H, French JW, Popp RL: Localization of pericardial effusion with wide-angle phased array echocardiography. *Am J Cardiol* 1978; 42:904–912.
220. Feigenbaum N: *Echocardiography*. 3rd ed. Philadelphia, Lea & Febiger, 1981.
221. Chandraratna PAN: Uses and limitations of echocardiography in the evaluation of pericardial disease. *Echocardiography* 1984; 1:55–74.
222. Haaz WS, Mintz GS, Kotler MN, Parry WR, Segal BL: Two-dimensional echocardiographic recognition of the descending thoracic aorta. Value in differentiating pericardial from pleural effusions. *Am J Cardiol* 1980; 46:739–743.
223. Martin RP, Bowden R, Filly K, Popp RL: Intrapericardial abnormalities in patients with pericardial effusions. Findings by two-dimensional echocardiography. *Circulation* 1980; 61:568–572.
224. Friedman T, Mintz GS, Kotler MN, Victor M: Value of two-dimensional echocardiography in the detection of pericardial and pleural metastases. *J Cardiovasc Ultrasonogr* 1982; 1:205–209.
225. Schiller NB, Botvinick EH: Right ventricular compression as a sign of cardiac tamponade. An analysis of echocardiographic ventricular dimensions and their clinical implications. *Circulation* 1977; 56:774–779.
226. Gillam LD, Guyer DE, Gibson TC, King ME, Marshall JE, Weyman AE: Hydrodynamic compression of the right atrium; a new echocardiographic sign of cardiac tamponade. *Circulation* 1983; 68:294–301.
227. Leimgruber PP, Kloffenstein SH, Wann SL, Brooks HL: The hemodynamic derangement associated with right ventricular diastolic collapses in cardiac tamponade: an experimental echocardiographic study. *Circulation* 1983; 68:612–620.
228. Singh S, Wann S, Schuchard GH, Klopfenstein HS, Leimgruber PP, Keelan MH, Brooks HL: Right ventricular and right atrial collapse in patients with cardiac tamponade: a combined echocardiographic and hemodynamic study. *Circulation* 1984; 70:966–971.
229. Wann S: Echocardiography in pericardial disease. *Echocardiography* 1984; 1:111–113.
230. Weitzman LB, Tinker P, Kronzon I, Cohen ML, Glassman E, Spencer FC: The incidence and natural history of pericardial effusion after cardiac surgery. An echocardiographic study. *Circulation* 1984; 69:506–511.
231. Stevenson LW, Child JS, Laks H, Kern L: Incidence and significance of early pericardial effusion after cardiac surgery. *Am J Cardiol* 1984; 54:848–851.
232. Callahan JA, Seward JB, Nishimura RA, Miller FA, Reeder GS, Shub C, Callahan MJ, Schattenberg TT, Tajik AJ: Two dimensional echocardiographically guided pericardiocentesis: experience in 117 consecutive patients. *Am J Cardiol* 1985; 55:476–479.
233. Pandian NG, Rifkin RD, Wang SS: Flow velocity paradoxus: a Doppler echocardiographic sign of cardiac tamponade: exaggerated respiratory variation in pulmonary and aortic blood flow velocities (abstr). *Circulation* 1984; 70 (suppl II):II–381.
234. Mintz GS, Kotler MN, Parry W, Iskandrian A, Kane SA: Real-time inferior vena caval ultrasonography: normal and abnormal findings and its use in assessing right-heart function. *Circulation* 1981; 64:1018–1025.
235. Soulen RL, Stark DD, Higgins CB: Magnetic resonance imaging of constrictive pericardial disease. *Am J Cardiol* 1985; 55:480–484.
236. Voelkel AG, Pietro DA, Folland ED, Fisher ML, Parisi AF: Echocardiographic features of constrictive pericarditis. *Circulation* 1978; 58:871–875.
237. Agatson AS, Rao A, Price RJ, Kinney EL: Diagnosis of constrictive pericarditis by pulsed Doppler echocardiography. *Am J Cardiol* 1984; 54:929–930.
238. Reid CL, Chandraratna PAN, Kawanishi D, Bezdek WD, Schatz R, Nanna M, Rahimtoola SH: Echocardiographic detection of pneumomediastinum and pneumopericardium: the air gap sign. *J Am Coll Cardiol* 1983; 1:916–921.
239. Payvandi MN, Kerber RE: Echocardiography in congenital and acquired absence of pericardium. *Circulation* 1976; 53:86–91.
240. Mintz GS, Kotler MN, Segal BL, Parry WR: Echocardiographic features of cardiomyopathy. *Cardiovasc Clin* 1978; 9:123–137.
241. Ghafour S, Gutgesell HP: Echocardiographic evaluation of left ventricular function in children with congestive cardiomyopathy. *Am J Cardiol* 1979; 44:1332–1338.
242. Maron B, Gottdiener JS, Epstein SE: Patterns and significance of distribution of left ventricular hypertrophy in hypertrophic cardiomyopathy. A wide angle two-dimensional echocardiographic study of 1254 patients. *Am J Cardiol* 1981; 48:418–428.
243. Schapira JN, Stemple DR, Martin RP, Rakowski H, Stinson EB, Popp RL: Single and two-dimensional echocardiographic visualization of the effects of septal myomectomy in idiopathic hypertrophic subaortic stenosis. *Circulation* 1978; 58:850–860.
244. Kinoshita N, Nimura N, Okamato M, Miyatake K, Nagata S, Sakakibara H: Mitral regurgitation in hypertrophic cardiomyopathy. Noninvasive study by two-dimensional Doppler echocardiography. *Br Heart J* 1983; 49:574–583.
245. Siqueira-Filho SG, Cunha CLP, Tajik AJ: M-mode and two-dimensional echocardiographic features in cardiac amyloidosis. *Circulation* 1981; 63:188–196.
246. Martin RP, Rakowski H, French J, Popp RL: Idiopathic hypertrophic subaortic stenosis viewed by wide-angle, phased array echocardiography. *Circulation* 1979; 59:1206–1217.
247. Mattleman S, Panidis I, Kotler MN, Mintz GS, Victor M, Ross J: Dissecting aneurysm in a patient with Marfan's syndrome: recognition of extensive involvement of the aorta by two-dimensional echocardiography. *J Clin Ultrasound* 1984; 12:219–221.
248. Mathew T, Nanda NC: Two-dimensional and Doppler echocardiographic evaluation of aortic aneurysms and dissection. *Am J Cardiol* 1984; 54:379–385.
249. Iliceto S, Antonelli G, Biasco G, Rizzon P: Two-dimensional echocardiographic evaluation of aneurysms of the descending thoracic aorta. *Circulation* 1982; 66:1045–1049.
250. Come PC: Improved cross-sectional echocardiographic technique for visualization of the retrocardiac descending aorta in its long axis. *Am J Cardiol* 1983; 51:1029–1032.
251. DeMaria AN, Bommer W, Neumann A, Weinert L, Bogren H, Mason DT: Identification and localization of aneurysms of the ascending aorta by cross-sectional echocardiography. *Circulation* 1979; 59:755–779.
252. Victor MF, Mintz GS, Kotler MN, Wilson AR, Segal BL: Two-dimensional echocardiographic diagnosis of aortic dissection. *Am J Cardiol* 1981; 48:1155–1159.
253. Nestico P, Panidis IP, Kotler MN, Mintz GS, Mattleman S, Ross J: Atherosclerotic plaque simulating aortic dissection by echocardiography and angiography. *Am Heart J* 1985; 109:607–609.
254. Dany F, Bensaid J, Blanc P, Virot P, Christides C, Kim M: Contribution of continuous wave Doppler ultrasound to the diagnosis of aortic dissection (abstr). *Circulation* 1984; 70 (suppl II):II–395.
255. Fox R, Ren JF, Panidis IP, Kotler MN, Mintz GS, Ross J: Annulo-aortic ectasia. A clinical and echocardiographic study. *Am J Cardiol* 1984; 54:177–181.
256. Kotler MN, Mintz GS, Parry WR, Segal BL: Two-dimensional echocardiography in congenital heart disease. *Am J Cardiol* 1980; 46:1237–1246.
257. Silverman NH, Snider AR (ed): *Two-Dimensional Echocardiography in Congenital Heart Disease*. Norwalk, Appleton-Century-Crofts, 1982.
258. Meijboom EJ, Horowitz S, Valdez-Cruz LM, Sahn DJ, Larson DF, Oliveira Lima C: A Doppler echocardiographic method for calculating volume flow across the tricuspid valve: correlative laboratory and clinical studies. *Circulation* 1985; 71:551–556.
259. Brandenburg RO Jr, Tajik AJ, Edwards WD, Reeder GS, Shub C, Seward JB: Accuracy of 2-dimensional echocardiographic diagnosis of congenitally bicuspid aortic valve: echocardiographic-anatomic correlation in 115 patients. *Am J Cardiol* 1983; 51:1469–1473.
260. Stewart WJ, King ME, Gillam LD, Guyer DE, Weyman AE: Prevalence of aortic valve prolapse with bicuspid aortic valve and its relation to aortic regurgitation. A cross-sectional echocardiographic study. *Am J Cardiol* 1984; 54:1277–1282.
261. Kotler MN, Mintz GS, Segal BL, Parry WR: Clinical echocardiography, in Teplick JG, Haskin ME (ed): *Surgical Radiology*. Philadelphia, W. B. Saunders Co, 1981.
262. Kotler MN, Mintz GS, Segal BL, Parry WR: Clinical use of two-dimensional echocardiography. *Am J Cardiol* 1980; 45:1061–1082.
263. Kotler MN, Mintz GS, Segal BL, Parry WR: Echocardiography, in Rosen K (ed): *Current Cardiol*. Boston, Houghton & Mifflin, 1980, vol 2.

7 Cardiovascular Radiography

Yu-qing Liu, MD

Conventional radiologic study of the cardiovascular system includes two major methods: radiography and fluoroscopy. Considering the relative merits and reduction of unnecessary radiation exposure, the principal procedure should be radiography, the so-called cardiac series. It includes teleoradiograms in the posteroanterior and lateral or the two anterior (left and right) oblique projections, or both. On certain occasions cardiac fluoroscopy, cineradiographic recordings, and roentgenkymography should be performed. Cardiac fluoroscopy with an image intensifier of high resolution is of great advantage in the detection and localization of intracardiac calcification and in studying pulsation of the heart, aorta, and central pulmonary arteries as well as motility of other thoracic structures.

The method generally selected is directly related to the diagnostic yield. Therefore, it is of vital importance to the clinician to be familiar with the value and limitations of each radiologic procedure. It is advisable for the clinician in this respect to consult with a radiologist, especially in certain special situations.

CARDIAC MEASUREMENT

TRANSVERSE DIAMETER AND CARDIOTHORACIC RATIO

The mean value of the transverse diameter ($T = T_1 + T_2$) in healthy Chinese subjects, based on our statistical study of 100 subjects aged 19 to 40 years, is 11.75 ± 0.93 cm; among male subjects it is 12.14 ± 0.83 cm, among female subjects 11.35 ± 0.86 cm[1] (Figure 7.1). The ratio between the transverse diameter of the heart and the maximum width of the thorax is expressed as the cardiothoracic ratio (T/Th). The mean value of the ratio in normal subjects, according to the aforementioned study, is 0.44 ± 0.03 (males 0.43 ± 0.04, females 0.45 ± 0.03). The upper limit of normal generally is 0.5 or 50%. Cardiac enlargement in our practice, as measured and assessed by this ratio, is divided into three grades: mild, 0.51 to 0.55; moderate, 0.56 to 0.60; and gross, 0.61 and larger.

The cardiothoracic ratio, a simple and convenient method, is one of the most commonly used cardiac measurements. However, it cannot reflect enlargement of the anteroposterior diameter of the heart. Therefore, in mitral stenosis or cor pulmonale with enlargement of the left atrium or right ventricle, or both, the cardiothoracic ratio may produce a false-negative result, and in cases of a "transverse heart" due to elevation of the diaphragm and obesity, it may produce a false-positive result.

FRONTAL AREA AND VOLUME

Measurement of the cardiac frontal area developed by Wang and Xie[2] is widely used in China. In a statistical study of 120 healthy adults, they calculated the normal values of the cardiac frontal area among Chinese, using body height and weight as correlation coefficients:

$$\text{Predicted frontal area (cm}^2) = 0.6207 \times \text{height (cm)} + 0.6654 \times \text{weight (kg)} - 42.7646 \text{ (constant)}$$

The frontal area can be measured with a planimeter, and also can be calculated by the following formula (Figure 7.2):

$$\text{Calculated frontal area (cm}^2) = 0.702 \times L \text{ (cm)} \times B \text{ (cm)} + 2.096 \text{ (constant)}$$

where L represents the longitudinal diameter taken between the junction of the right heart border with the

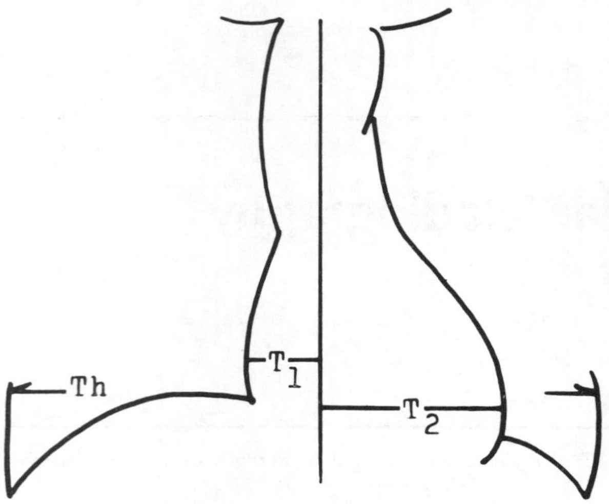

Figure 7.1. Cardiac transverse diameter ($T_1 + T_2 = T$), maximum width of the thorax (Th), and cardiothoracic ratio (T/Th).

superior vena cava and the intersection of the left heart border with the diaphragm, and B is the sum of B_1 and B_2, the perpendicular distances to L from the junction of left heart border with the pulmonary segment and the intersection of the right heart border with the diaphragm, respectively. This method is more accurate than the cardiothoracic ratio, and the frontal area enlargement can also be divided into three grades: mild, 15% to 35%; moderate, 36% to 60%; and gross, greater than or equal to 61%. The foregoing formulas can only be used in adults.

Using length, width, and depth diameters measured on the posteroanterior and lateral plain films, the cardiac volume can be calculated (Figure 7.3). We carried out a statistical study of 200 healthy Chinese subjects (100 males and 100 females aged 20 to 60 years)[3] and derived the normal values for total cardiac volume (V_T) and cardiac volume index (V_I) using the formula:

$$V_T(\text{ml}) = K \times L \times B \times D$$

$$V_I = \frac{V_T}{\text{Body surface area}(\text{m}^2)\ (\text{DuBois})}$$

where L represents the longitudinal diameter between the junction of the right heart border with the superior vena cava and the intersection of the left heart border with the diaphragm; B, the broad diameter between intersection of right heart border with the diaphragm and intersection of left heart border with the pulmonary artery segment; and D, the depth diameter, the maximum horizontal distance between the anterior and posterior heart borders. K value normogram (Figure 7.4), developed by us, is used for correction of individual radiographic projection magnification.[3]

The mean value for total cardiac volume (V_T) in male subjects is 669.43 ± 86.24 ml, in female subjects 567.51 ± 110.74 ml; cardiac volume index (V_I) in male subjects is 390.20 ± 48.22 ml/m^2, in female subjects 365.48 ± 50.38 ml/m^2. The upper limits of normal for cardiac volume index (V_I) are useful clinically and tend to be 460 ml/m^2 for male subjects and 430 ml/m^2 for female subjects.

Cardiac volume determination is the most accurate method of assessing cardiac enlargement. However, it is too complicated and time-consuming to be used as a daily procedure in a busy department.

VISUAL ASSESSMENT AND MEASUREMENT

The visual assessment of cardiac enlargement has the great advantages of speed and simplicity; in the hands of an experienced observer it is reasonably reliable. For the beginner it would be better to check the assessment with one of the aforementioned measurements.[4]

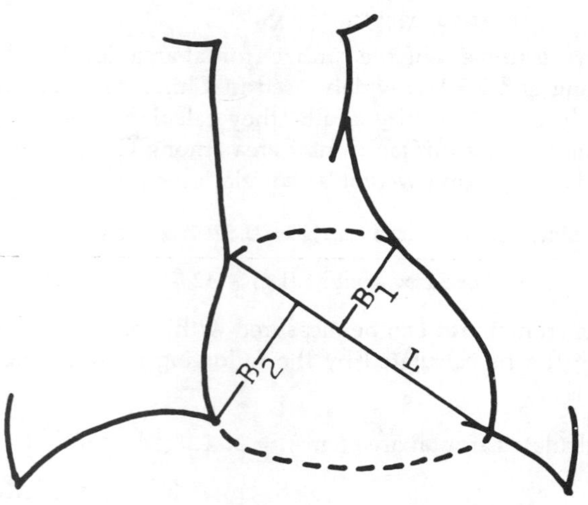

Figure 7.2. Measurement of cardiac frontal area. L = longitudinal diameter; $B_1 + B_2$, broad diameter. (See text.)

ENLARGEMENT OF THE HEART AND ITS CHAMBERS

ENLARGEMENT OF THE HEART

Enlargement of the heart and its change in configuration is one of the most important signs of heart disease. Cardiac enlargement may be generalized or may affect individual chambers, with one or two predominantly involved. The former should be differentiated from massive pericardial effusion; the latter may give rise to some specific configurations of the heart.

ENLARGEMENT OF THE CARDIAC CHAMBERS

Left Atrium

The left atrium occupies the posterosuperior aspect of the heart and does not ordinarily participate in the formation of left and right heart borders. Enlargement of the left atrium may occur first posteriorly, then superiorly, to the left and to the right, or in any combination of the four directions.

1. Localized indentation or displacement of the barium-

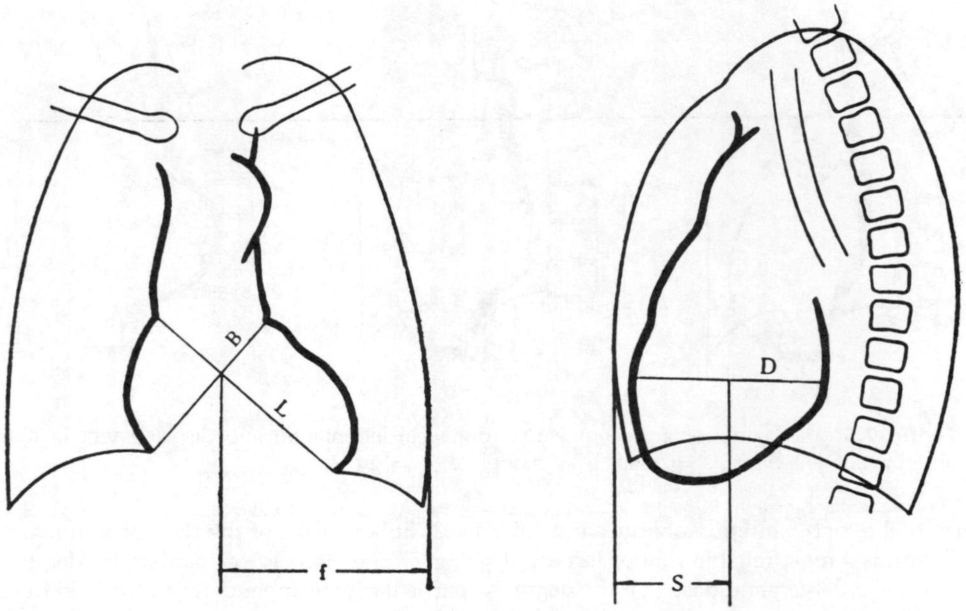

Figure 7.3. Measurement of cardiac volume. B = broad diameter; D = depth diameter; L = longitudinal diameter. f = distance from the heart mid-point to the external costal border (posteroanterior view); S = distance from the heart mid-point to the external sternal border (left lateral view). (See text.)

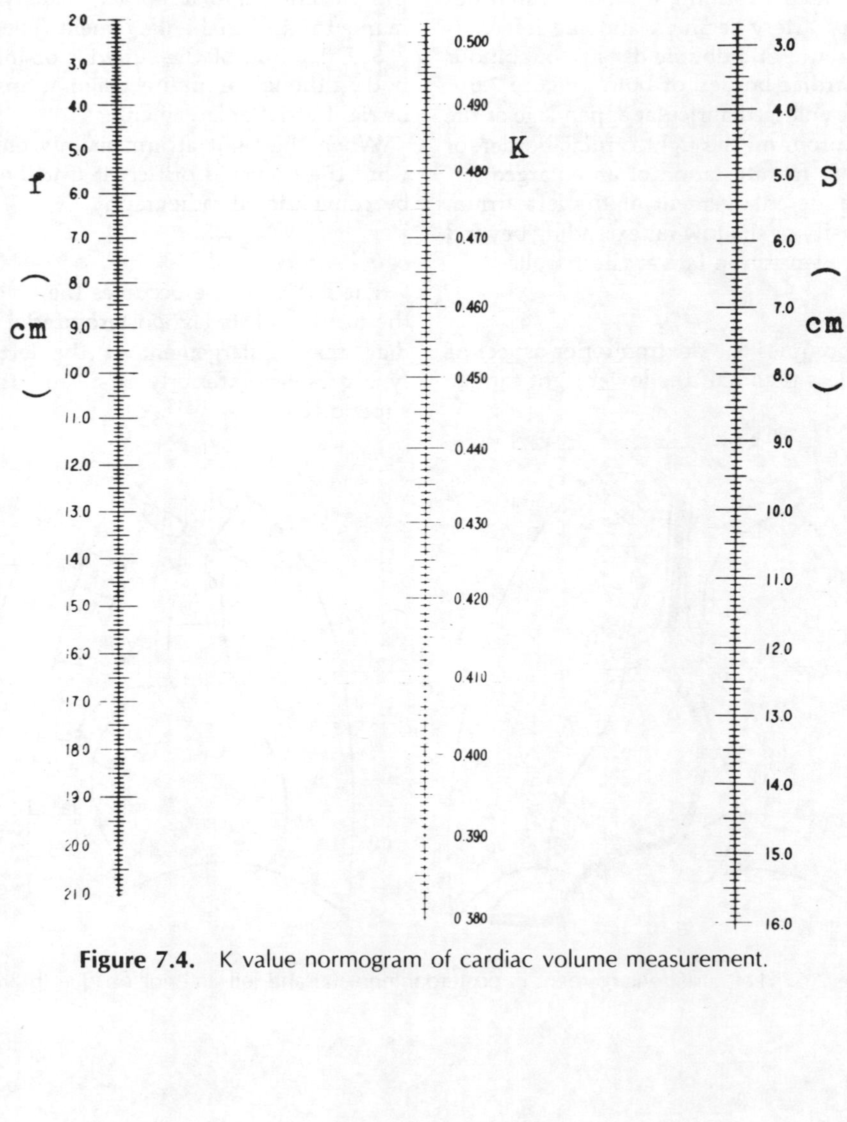

Figure 7.4. K value normogram of cardiac volume measurement.

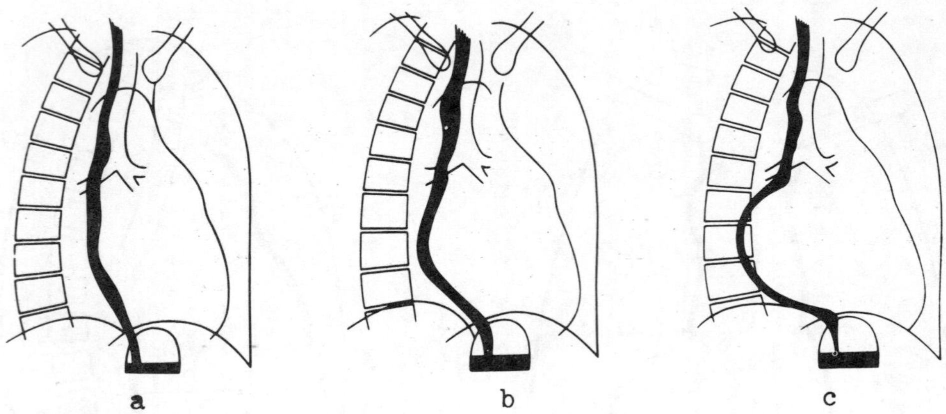

Figure 7.5. Left atrial enlargement with esophageal indentation and displacement in right anterior oblique views. a = mild; b = moderate; c = gross.

filled esophagus in the right anterior oblique and left lateral views, or both, is a most reliable sign of left atrial enlargement. Left atrial enlargement, based on the degree of indentation or displacement of the opacified esophagus, or both, can be graded as mild, moderate, and gross (Figure 7.5).

2. Left atrial enlargement may also manifest in different views as an upward displacement of the left main bronchus, sometimes with widening of the carina, enlargement of the auricular appendage forming a separate arch between the pulmonary artery segment and the left ventricle, and the appearance of a double density or contour on the right lower cardiac border, or both, (Figure 7.6).

3. Occasionally the enlarged auricular appendage or the double density or contour on the right cardiac border, or both, may be the only manifestation of an enlarged left atrium, and the gigantic enlargement of the left atrium may form a huge density or shadow far extending beyond the cardiac contour, even to the lateral chest walls.

Right Atrium

The right atrium occupies the dextroinferior aspect of the heart and forms less than half the lower right cardiac border.

1. Enlargement of the right atrium manifests as a bulging of the right lower cardiac border to the right side, particularly its upper part upwardly in the posteroanterior view (Figure 7.7a).

2. In the left anterior oblique view, right atrial enlargement manifests as an anterior or inferior bulging of the upper part of the anterior border of the cardiac silhouette, or both (Figure 7.7b). In the right anterior oblique view it is indicated by posterior bulging of the lower third of the posterior cardiac border, usually a manifestation of marked right atrial enlargement (Figure 7.7c).

3. Dilatation of the superior or inferior vena cava, or both, although an indirect sign, is an integral component of right atrial enlargement.

When the right atrium mainly enlarges inwardly toward the tricuspid orifice, it usually cannot be detected by conventional radiography.

Left Ventricle

The left ventricle occupies the levoposterior aspect of the heart, and its levoposteroinferior end forms the cardiac apex. Enlargement of the left ventricle generally occurs levoinferiorly first, and then posteriorly and superiorly.

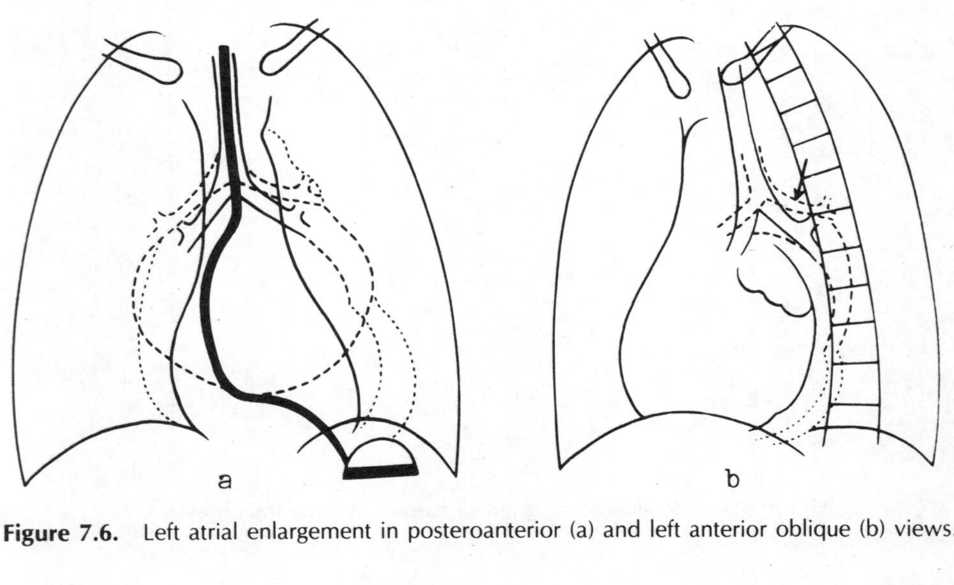

Figure 7.6. Left atrial enlargement in posteroanterior (a) and left anterior oblique (b) views.

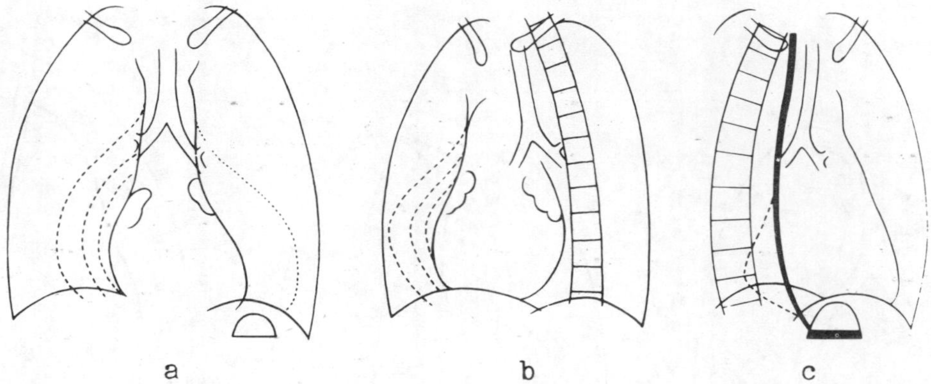

Figure 7.7. Right atrial enlargement in posteroanterior (a), left anterior oblique (b), and right anterior oblique (c) views.

1. Enlargement of the left ventricle is indicated by increased length and convexity of the left ventricular segment, usually associated with downward displacement of the cardiac apex extending below the level of the diaphragm on the posteroanterior view (Figure 7.8a).

2. In the left anterior oblique and left lateral views, progressive enlargement of the left ventricle may be demonstrated as posterior and inferior bulging of the lower segment of the posterior cardiac border, extending posteriorly beyond the anterior border of the thoracic spine in a 60° left anterior oblique view (Figure 7.8b) and more than 1.5 cm beyond the upper segment of the inferior vena cava on lateral view (Figure 7.8c).

3. The marked enlargement of the left ventricle results in leftward rotation of the heart. The left ventricle rotates to the right and anteriorly, with widening of the aortic arch and concavity of the cardiac waist, producing an "aortic configuration" of the cardiac shadow on the posteroanterior view.

Right Ventricle

The right ventricle occupies about three fourths of the anterior aspect of the heart. Enlargement of the right ventricle generally may occur first anteriorly and levosuperiorly and then inferiorly.

1. Enlargement of the right ventricle is indicated by elevation of the cardiac apex, which is usually associated with prominence of the upper part of the left heart border on the posteroanterior view (Figure 7.9a).

2. On left anterior oblique and lateral views, progressive enlargement of the right ventricle may be demonstrated as anterior bulging of the lower segment of the anterior heart border, with increased contact of the sternum in the lateral view (Figure 7.9b and c).

Prominence of the pulmonary artery segment, ie, dilatation of the pulmonary trunk, is an indirect sign of right ventricular enlargement.

3. The marked enlargement of the right ventricle results in rightward rotation of the heart. The right ventricle

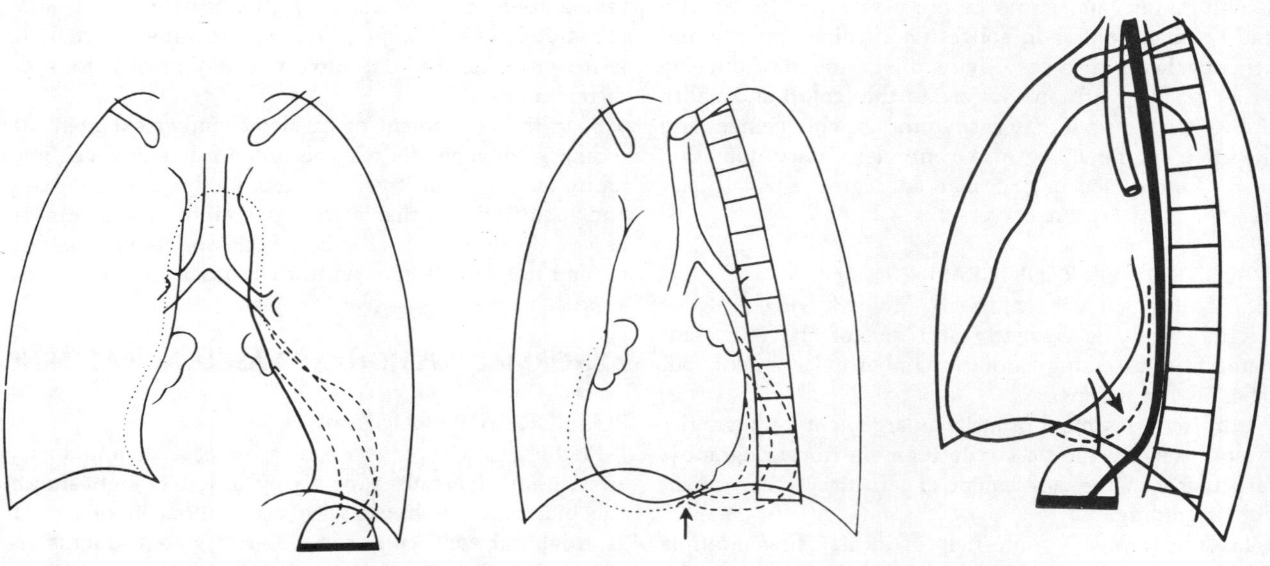

Figure 7.8. Left ventricular enlargement in posteroanterior (a), left anterior oblique (b), and left lateral (c) views.

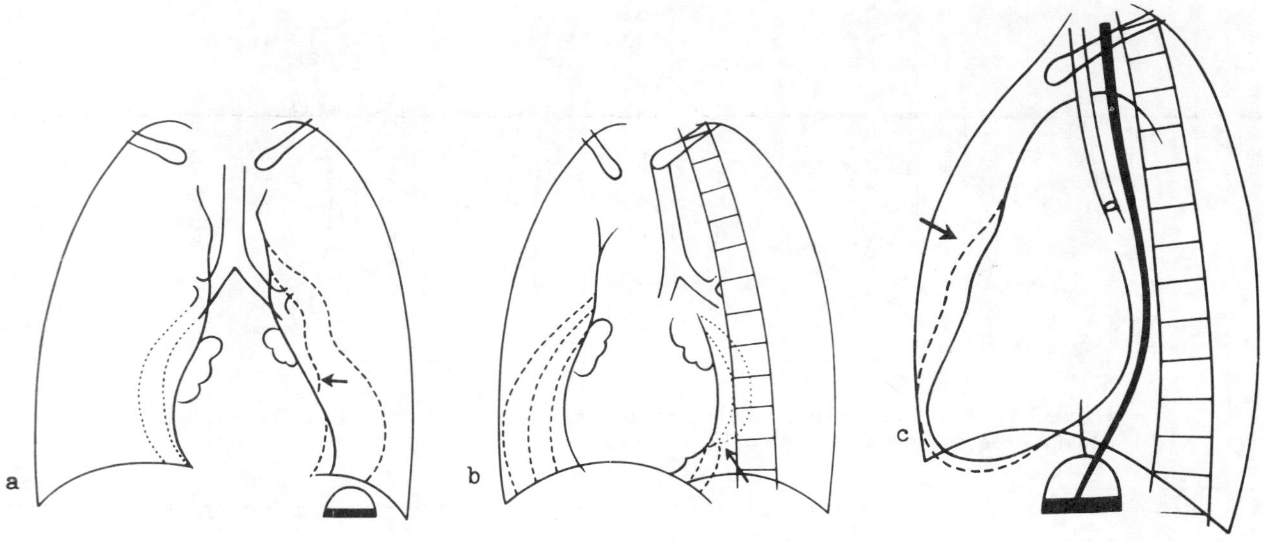

Figure 7.9. Right ventricular enlargement in posteroanterior (a), left anterior oblique (b), and left lateral (c) views.

rotates to the right with prominence of the pulmonary artery segment, which overshadows the aortic arch, producing a "mitral configuration" of the cardiac shadow on the posteroanterior view.

HYPERTROPHY AND DILATATION OF THE VENTRICLES

Radiologic enlargement of the ventricles is caused by dilatation or hypertrophy, or both. Ventricular wall hypertrophy is a response to pressure and resistance overload such as hypertension, valve stenosis, and hypertrophic cardiomyopathy. Pure hypertrophy generally may not give rise to ventricular enlargement until a marked degree is reached. It manifests as rounding and elongation, particularly the outflow portion, of the ventricular segment of the cardiac border. Cavity dilatation is the result of volume overload, such as valve regurgitation and left-to-right shunt, and pump failure of a ventricle can also lead to dilatation, as in congestive cardiomyopathy and ischemic heart disease. Cavity dilatation may develop rather rapidly with an increase in the length and width of a ventricle, and it may easily produce enlargement and alteration in the shape of a ventricle. Cavity dilatation over a long period or of a marked degree is usually accompanied by hypertrophy.

EVALUATION OF RADIOGRAPHY IN THE ASSESSMENT OF CHAMBER ENLARGEMENT

Radiography is currently still one of the important methods of assessing cardiac chamber enlargement, but it has its limitations.

1. In the assessment of atrial enlargement, radiography is more sensitive and accurate than electrocardiography, particularly in the assessment of left atrial enlargement and its grading.

2. Radiography is more helpful in assessing multiple chamber enlargement than single chamber enlargement. The latter is usually an early manifestation of heart disease. For multiple chamber enlargement, it is superior to other methods in demonstrating the number of chambers involved and the severity as well as their spatial relations within the thorax.

3. In some cases of mild left ventricular enlargement of concentric hypertrophy, radiography may have no abnormal findings, but electrocardiography may show definite left ventricular hypertrophy. The same situation may occur in early cor pulmonale with mild right ventricular enlargement.

4. Electrocardiography may reveal no abnormal findings in some cases of biventricular enlargement; radiography may play an important role in their assessment. In biventricular enlargement with one ventricle greater and the other lesser, the latter can easily be missed by either radiography or electrocardiography.

In some cases of cyanotic congenital heart disease, such as tetralogy of Fallot and tricuspid atresia, the radiographic configuration of the heart may be similar, but electrocardiographic demonstration of right or left ventricular hypertrophy may aid greatly in their differentiation.

5. In the assessment of cardiac chamber enlargement, radiography generally may be superior to electrocardiography and less sensitive and accurate, both qualitatively and quantitatively, than echocardiography. The combined use of the various methods, which are complementary to, and not competitive with, each other, may be a wise approach.

ABNORMAL PULMONARY VASCULAR PATTERNS

PLETHORA AND OLIGEMIA

Plethora is a synonym for an increase in pulmonary arterial flow. It is caused mainly by (1) left-to-right shunts and bidirectional shunts with venoarterial mixing, such as atrial and ventricular septal defect, patent ductus arteriosus, transposition of the great arteries, single ventricle, and persistent truncus arteriosus, and (2) increased output of the right ventricle, such as systemic arteriovenous fistula, thyrotoxicosis, anemia, and cor pulmonale with a high cardiac output state.

Radiographically it manifests as (1) an increase in width and in the number of pulmonary arterial markings, the pulmonary veins being correspondingly enlarged, (2) dilatation of the arterial component of the hilar shadow, ie, dilatation of the descending branch of the right pulmonary artery (greater than 1.5 cm in diameter for adults), usually combined with a prominent pulmonary artery segment, and (3) the margins of the dilated vessels being clearly defined and the radiolucency of the lung field remaining in the normal range (Figure 7.10).

Oligemia indicates a decrease in pulmonary arterial flow. It is caused mainly by (1) conditions that obstruct right heart output, with or without right-to-left shunts, such as pulmonic valve stenosis, trilogy of Fallot, tetralogy of Fallot, tricuspid atresia, and pulmonary atresia, and (2) pulmonary embolism, generalized obstructive emphysema, unilateral pulmonary artery agenesis and hypoplasia, unilateral hyperlucent lung, and emphysematous bullae. The latter three may cause unilateral, regional or uneven pulmonary oligemia.

Radiographically it manifests as (1) narrowing and sparsity of pulmonary arterial markings with the pulmonary veins also narrowed correspondingly, (2) reduction in the width of the arterial component of the hilar shadow, ie, narrowing of the descending branch of the right pulmonary artery, usually combined with flatness or concavity of the pulmonary artery segment except in cases of pulmonic valve stenosis with an intact ventricular septum in which the pulmonary artery segment is prominent because of poststenotic dilatation of the main pulmonary artery, and (3) increased radiolucency of the lung field (Figure 7.11a and b).

When the hilar arteries are markedly narrowed or even invisible, and instead the comma-like shadow appears at a higher level of the hilum, usually with numerous tortuous and even mildly dilated reticular vascularities in the lung fields, particularly in the mid-lower zones, we are dealing with manifestations of collateral circulation originating from bronchial or systemic arteries, or both (Figure 7.11c).

The fundamental radiographic signs of plethora and oligemia have a fair correlation with the severity of in-

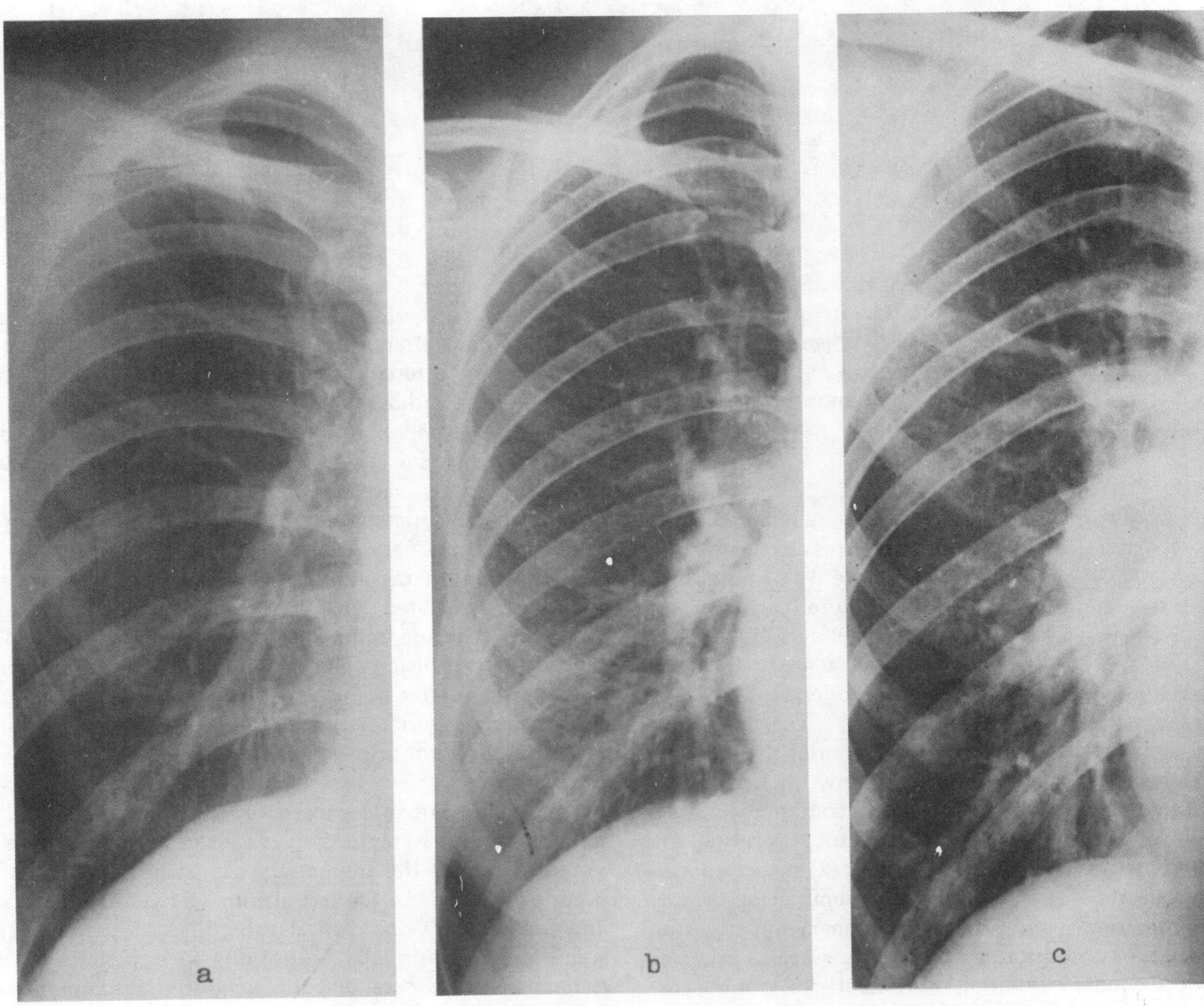

Figure 7.10. Radiographic sign of plethora. a = normal (without heart disease); b = plethora (atrial septal defect proved by operation); c = plethora, marked degree (atrial septal defect proved by operation).

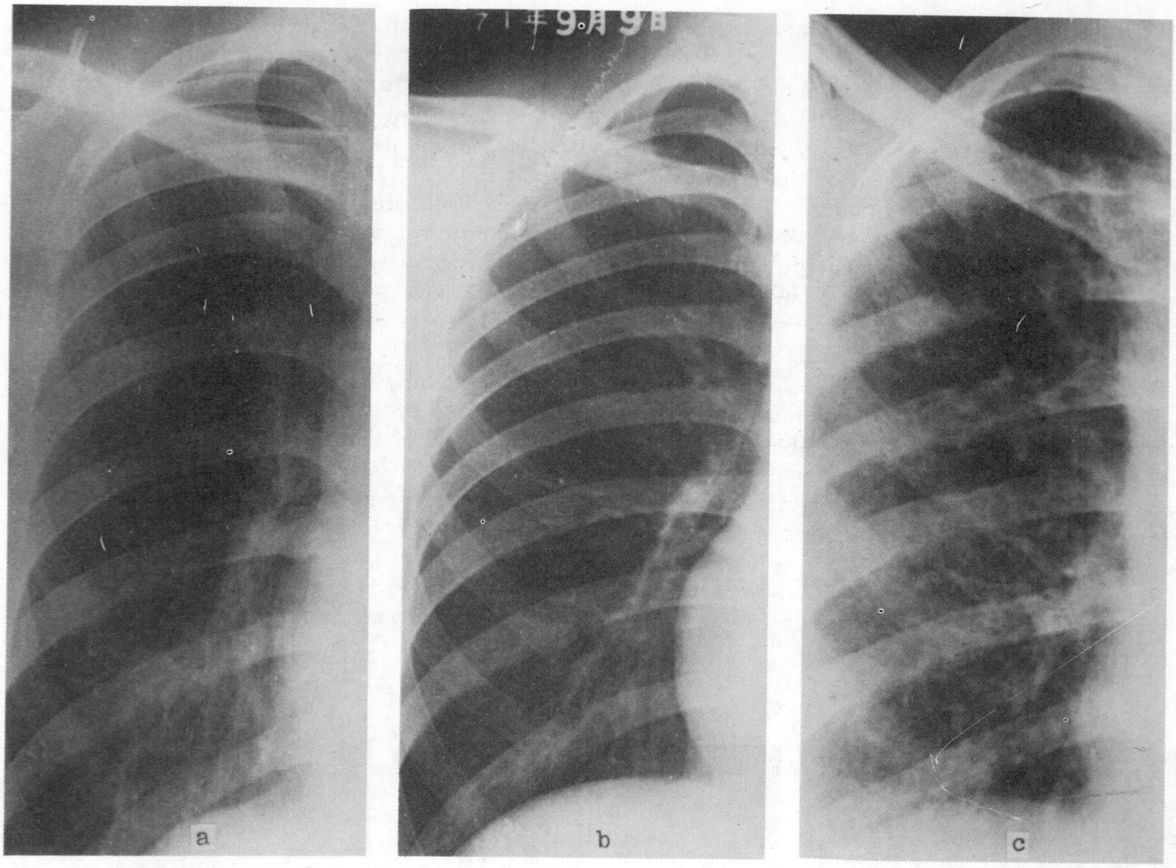

Figure 7.11. Radiographic sign of oligemia. a = mild pulmonic valve stenosis proved by operation; b = marked pulmonic valve stenosis proved by operation; c = oligemia with collateral circulation in tetralogy of Fallot diagnosed by cardiac angiography.

crease and decrease of pulmonary flow. Sometimes mild plethora due to a normal variation in pulmonary vascularity may be difficult to assess. Oligemia with signs of collateral circulation always means a severe reduction in pulmonary flow usually seen in pulmonary atresia with or without ventricular septal defect.

PULMONARY HYPERTENSION

Pulmonary arterial hypertension is present when the pulmonary arterial systolic and mean pressures exceed 30 and 20 mm Hg, respectively. The severity of pulmonary arterial hypertension can be graded more feasibly by the ratio of pulmonary to systemic arterial systolic pressure, ie, PASP/SASP equals 0.25 to 0.45, 0.46 to 0.75, and greater than 0.75, indicating mild, moderate, and severe hypertension, respectively.

The major causes of pulmonary arterial hypertension are (1) increased pulmonary arterial flow, such as left-to-right shunts with massive amounts commonly seen in ventricular septal defect, patent ductus arteriosus, and single ventricle with mixed shunting, (2) increased arteriolar resistance, such as pulmonary embolism, arteritis of various origins, and primary pulmonary hypertension, and (3) thoracorespiratory disorders, such as cor pulmonale secondary to chronic bronchitis or emphysema, or both, pulmonary fibrosis of various causes, and thoracospinal deformities.

The fundamental radiographic signs are (1) a prominent pulmonary artery segment and dilatation of central hilar arteries, (2) narrowing and sparsity of peripheral arterial branches, and (3) an enlarged right ventricle.

Pulmonary arterial hypertension generally does not manifest itself radiographically until the pressure reaches a moderate degree. Pulmonary arterial hypertension secondary to a massive left-to-right shunt is radiographically characterized by narrowing and tortuosity of the peripheral arterial branches on the basis of an increased flow pattern of pulmonary vascularity (Figure 7.12).

Diffuse narrowing and sparsity of pulmonary arterial markings associated with marked enlargement of the heart are common radiographic signs of primary pulmonary hypertension (Figure 7.13a and b), and uneven vascularity, infarct scars, and pleural thickening aid in differentiating pulmonary thromboembolic hypertension (Figure 7.14) from primary pulmonary hypertension.

Pulmonary venous hypertension exists when pulmonary capillary venous pressure exceeds 10 to 15 mm Hg. Pulmonary venous hypertension is caused by increased resistance beyond the pulmonary capillaries, and it may occur at the level of the left atrium, left ventricle, aorta, and pulmonary veins. Mitral valve disease, particularly stenosis, left ventricular failure due to hypertensive or ischemic heart disease, or both, congestive cardiomyopathy, aortic valve disease, and total anomalous pulmonary venous drainage are common etiologic disorders.

The fundamental radiographic signs are (1) dilatation

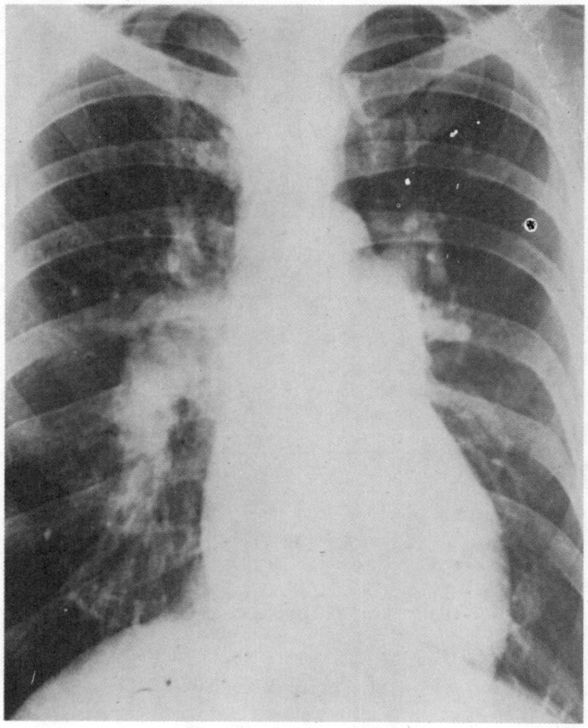

Figure 7.12. Pulmonary arterial hypertension secondary to a massive left-to-right shunt (atrial septal defect proved by operation, pulmonary arterial pressure 98/40 mm Hg).

of the upper pulmonary veins while the lower veins remain normal or constricted, ie, signs of redistribution of pulmonary flow (Figure 7.15a and b), (2) a generalized increase in pulmonary vascular markings with blurred margins, particularly in the mid-lower lung fields (Figure 7.15c); and (3) signs of pulmonary edema, usually mild pleural effusion, and hemosiderosis and ossific nodules (Figure 7.16).

Pulmonary venous and arterial hypertension can cause an increase in pulmonary arteriolar resistance, resulting in coexistent venous and arterial hypertension. The mixed type of pulmonary hypertension is typically seen in chronic mitral stenosis. According to our observations the development and course of pulmonary hypertension in chronic mitral stenosis are as follows: pulmonary venous hypertension usually mild in its early stage and then sustained venous and arterial hypertension; both may rise proportionately and reach moderate and severe degrees. In only a few cases the arterial pressure may increase disproportionately compared with venous pressure. Radiographically it manifests as coexistent signs of both venous and arterial hypertension, ie, upper vessel dilation and interstitial edema combined with a prominent pulmonary artery segment and enlarged hilar arteries associated with constriction of the lower vessels (Figure 7.17).

PULMONARY EDEMA

When pulmonary capillary pressure exceeds plasma osmotic pressure of 25 to 30 mm Hg, fluid may transudate from the capillaries into the interstices and alveoli of the lung, resulting in interstitial and alveolar edema. Any condition that can cause pulmonary venous hypertension may lead to pulmonary edema. Interstitial edema is common in chronic left-sided heart failure and in increased resistance of pulmonary veins, such as mitral stenosis. Alveolar edema is usually an indicator of acute left-sided heart failure. Some extracardiac conditions, such as uremia, excessive parenteral fluid, allergic reactions and cerebral disorders, may also result in acute pulmonary edema.

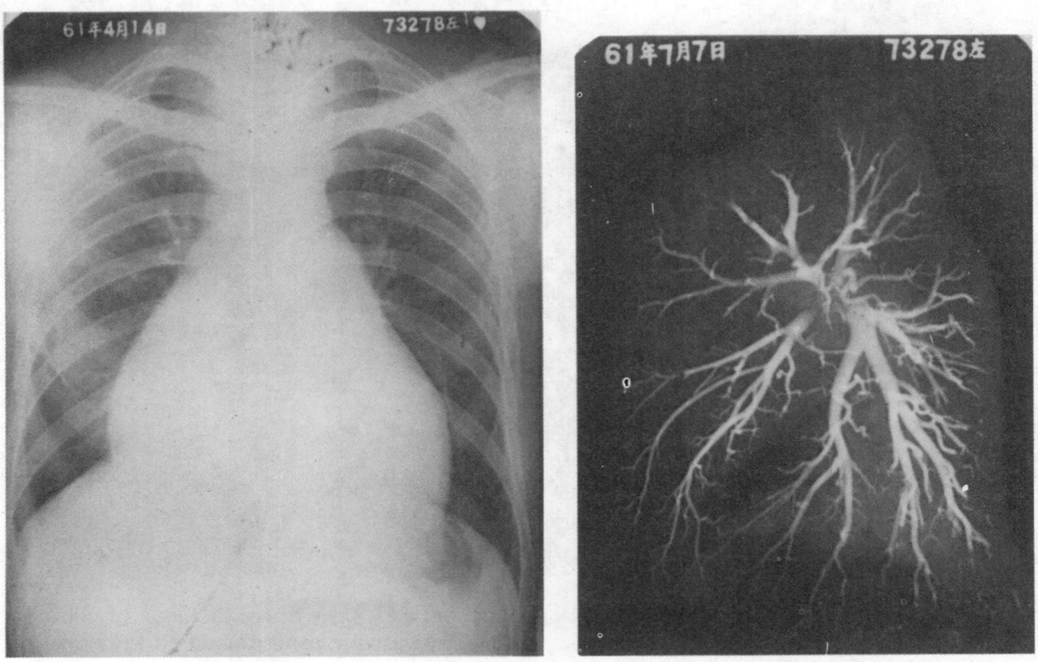

A B

Figure 7.13. Primary pulmonary arterial hypertension proved by autopsy. *A,* posteroanterior plain film; *B,* postmortem pulmonary arteriogram. Pulmonary arterial pressure was 100/80 mm Hg measured at cardiac catheterization before death.

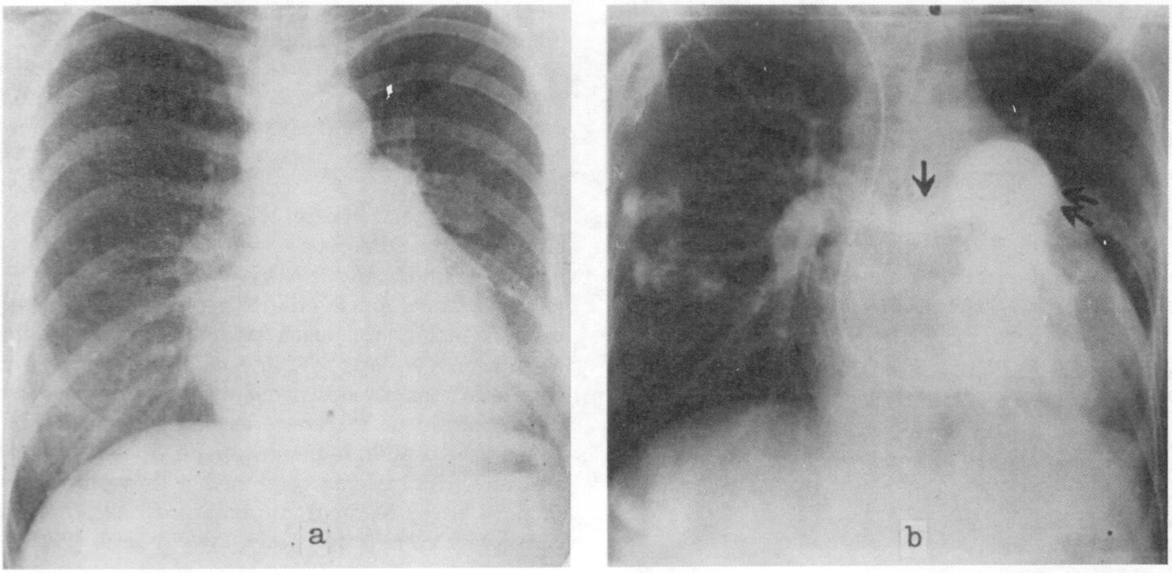

Figure 7.14. Pulmonary thromboembolic hypertension. *a,* posteroanterior plain film; *b,* pulmonary arteriogram showing intraluminal embolus (↓) and occlusion of left pulmonary artery (⇇).

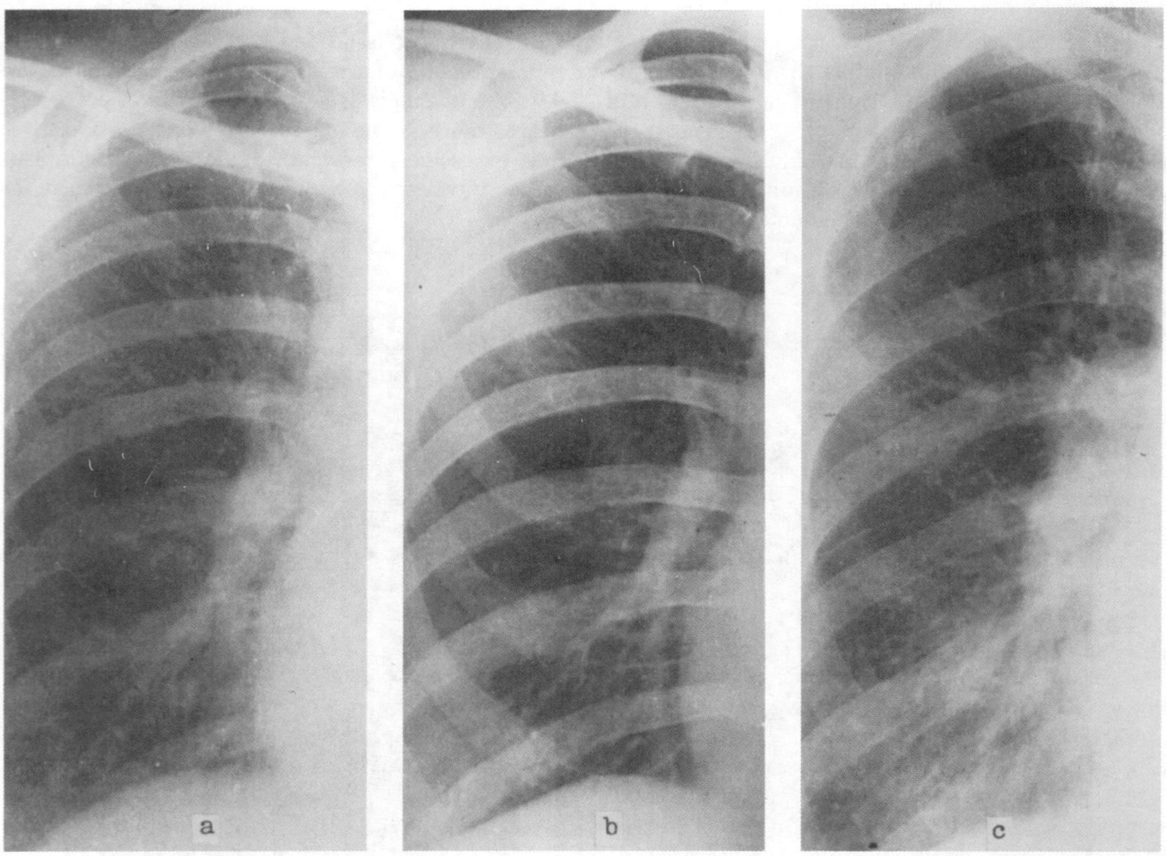

Figure 7.15. Radiographic signs of pulmonary venous hypertension. a = signs of redistribution of pulmonary blood flow with upper pulmonary vein dilatation; b = same patient, pulmonary vascular pattern returned to normal due to effective control of heart failure; c = redistribution of pulmonary flow associated with an increase in generalized pulmonary vascular markings.

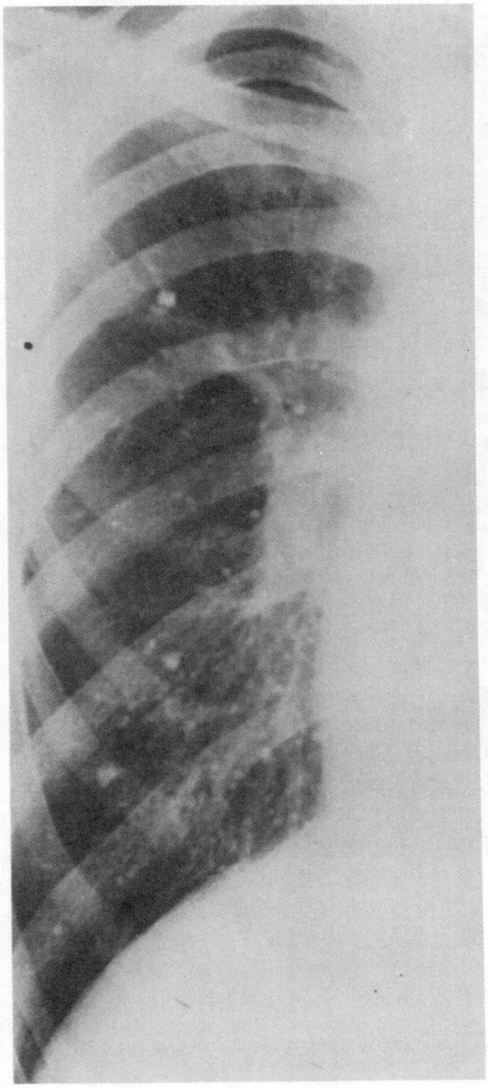

Figure 7.16. Pulmonary hypertension associated with ossific nodules in a case of longstanding rheumatic valvular disease.

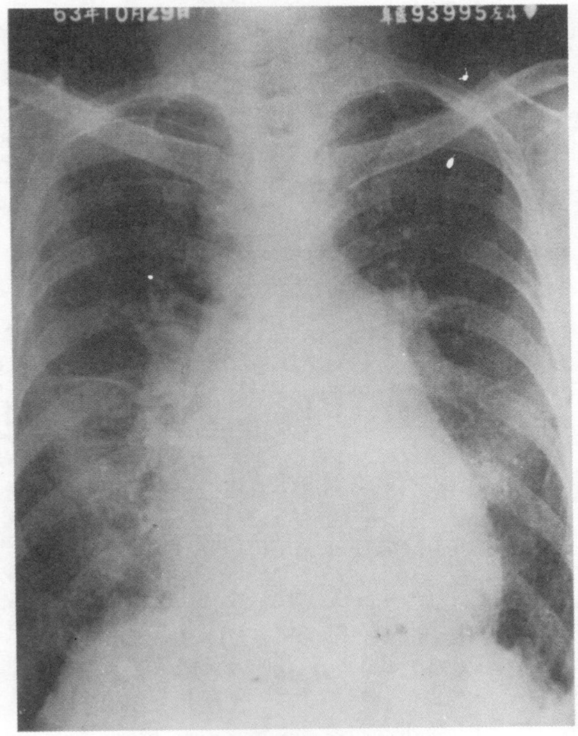

Figure 7.17. Pulmonary venous and arterial hypertension of a severe degree in a case of rheumatic mitral lesion, predominantly stenosis. Cardiac catheterization showed a pulmonary arterial pressure of 96/44 mm Hg, and left atrial pressure of 35 mm Hg.

Interstitial Edema

Radiographically it manifests as follows:

1. There appear septal lines, the most common being sharply defined, horizontal linear densities in the lung base of the costophrenic angle (Kerley B-lines). They are usually 2 to 3 cm in length and 1 to 4 mm in width and may extend into the midportion of the lung fields (Figure 7.18a). Longer straight lines, usually 3 to 6 cm in length, may be seen in any part, more in the mid- to upper portion of the lung fields and pointing towards the hilum (Kerley A-lines) (Figure 7.18b). The septal lines are produced by thickening of the interlobular septa mainly caused by the accumulation of edematous fluid, and partly by the dilated lymphatics.

2. The interlacing and reticular vascular pattern also known as Kerley C-lines (Figure 7.18a) is seen in the mid-lower lung fields with poorly defined borders.

3. Hilar haze, usually mildly enlarged (Figure 7.18c), is caused by a collection of edematous fluid in connective tissue around the hilum, sometimes with edematous enlargement of lymph nodes. Perivascular edema blurs the borders of the vascular markings, and peribronchial edema results in thickening of the bronchial wall appearing as the so-called "cuff sign" when a larger bronchus is seen end-on.

4. Subpleural and small pleural effusions present as thickening and increased density of interlobar fissure (Figure 7.18c) or obliteration of costophrenic angles, or both.

Alveolar Edema

Radiographically it manifests as follows:

1. Widespread macular patchy shadows with ill-defined and fluffy margins of both lung fields, and the shadows tend to be coalescent (Figure 7.19).

2. The "butterfly or bat's wing" shadow, a perihilar and bilateral shadow consisting of massive infiltration or coalescent patchy densities, or both, is the most characteristic appearance of alveolar edema (Figure 7.20). The apices, lung bases, and lateral margins of both lung fields are usually spared, and the air bronchogram sign can always be visualized.

3. Disseminated miliary densities and parenchymal consolidation confined to one lung or even one lobe are rare atypical manifestations of alveolar edema.

4. The shadows appear and disappear rapidly, and change their distribution and density from day to day,

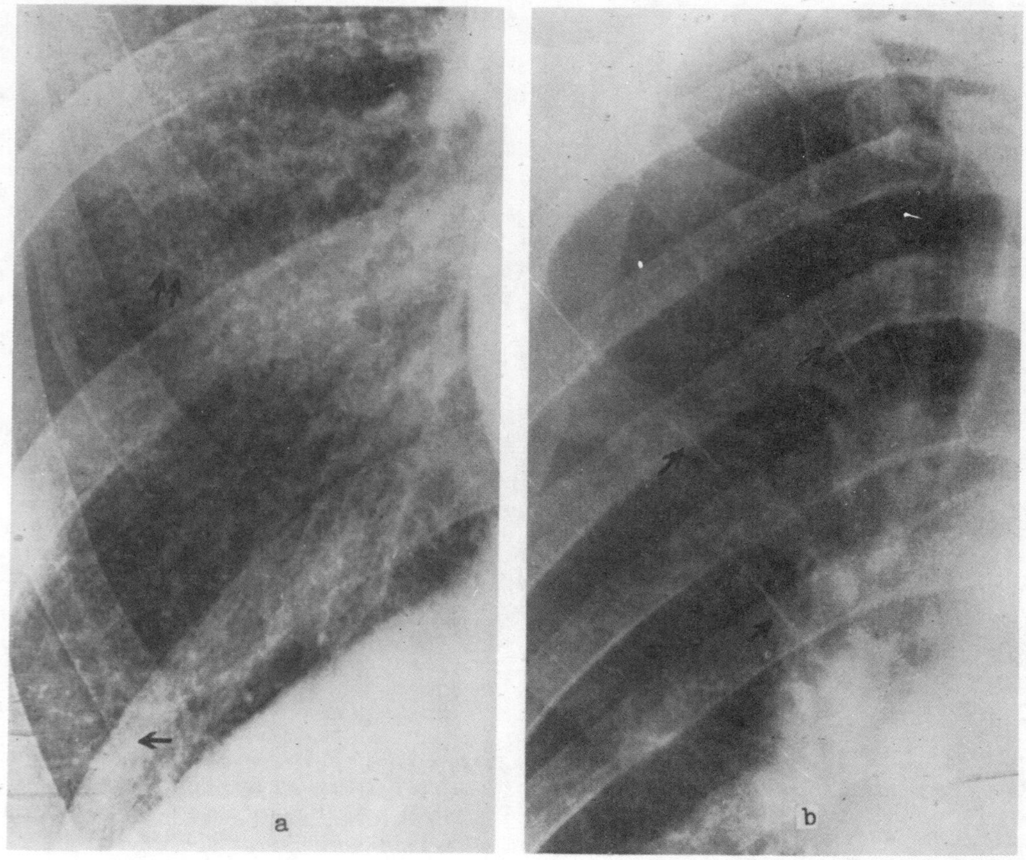

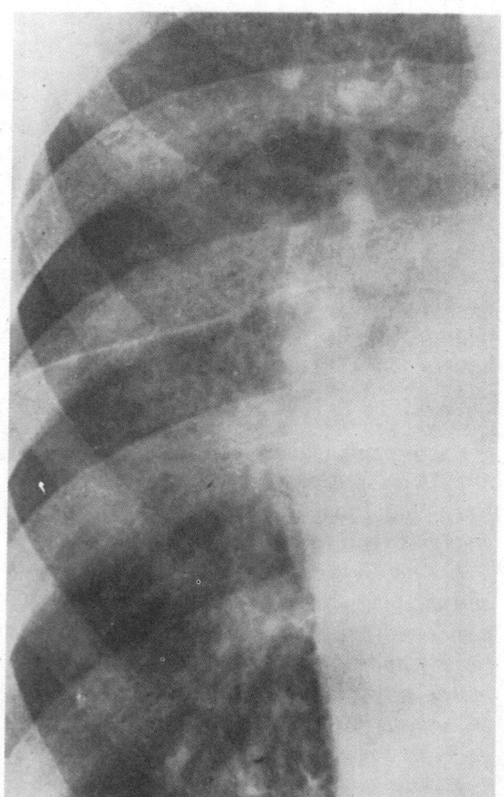

Figure 7.18. Radiographic signs of interstitial edema of the lung. a = Kerley B-lines (←) and the interlacing and reticular vascular pattern (↑↑), the so-called Kerley C-lines; b = Kerley A-lines (↑); c = hilar haze and interlobar thickening (subpleural fluid).

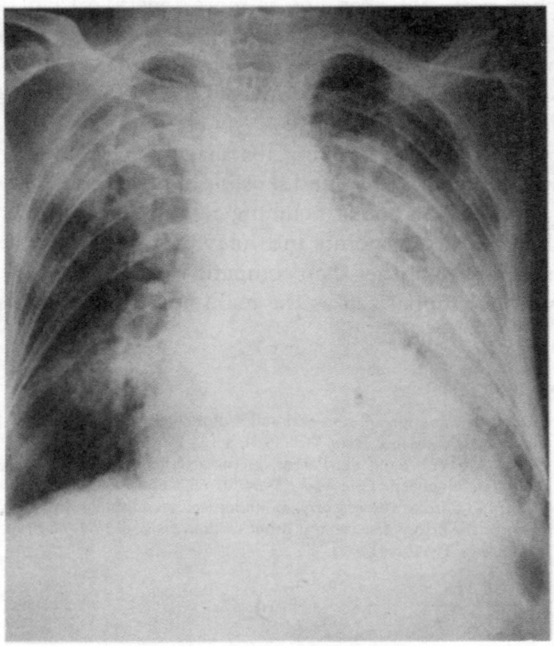

Figure 7.19. Alveolar edema of the lung. Macular patchy shadows with coalescence, particularly on the left side of the lung.

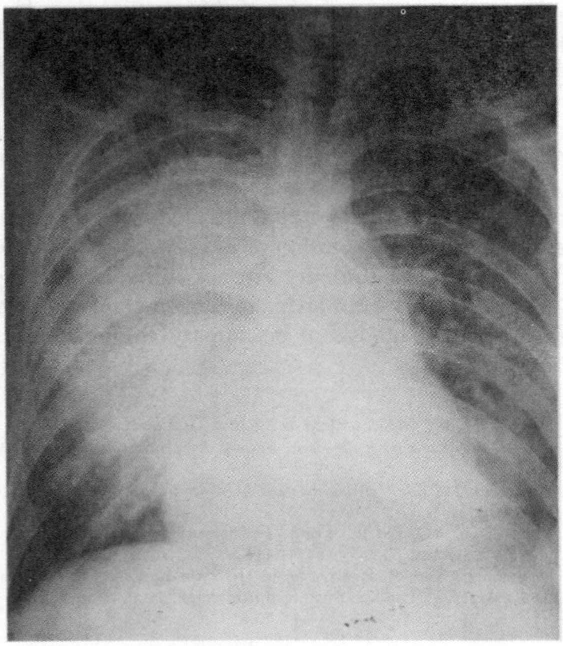

Figure 7.20. Alveolar edema of the lung. Perihilar massive infiltration on the right side, and multiple macular patchy shadows on the left side of the lung.

all important indicators of alveolar edema. Signs of interstitial edema and pleural effusion are often associated.

EVALUATION OF RADIOGRAPHY IN THE DIAGNOSIS OF HEART DISEASE

Conventional radiography has a long history. However, in the era of modern medical imaging technology with the rapid development and refinement of echocardiography, nuclear medicine, computed tomography, and magnetic resonance imaging, it is by no means easy to adequately evaluate the role of conventional radiography in the diagnosis of heart disease. Up to now, based on our practice in China, radiography is still one of the most important and widely used noninvasive methods in the study of heart disease.

The value and limitations of radiography may be concisely summarized as follows[5]:

1. Radiography can provide information on both heart and lung concurrently, particularly in assessing abnormalities of pulmonary circulation on the basis of modern physiology and pathophysiology, such as plethora, oligemia, pulmonary venous and arterial hypertension, and pulmonary edema. It is also quite valuable in correlating thoracorespiratory alterations and the cardiovascular disorder, as in the diagnosis of cor pulmonale. In some cases, a plain film in a posteroanterior view can offer sufficient diagnostic information.

In cardiovascular disorders secondary to systemic diseases, such as Marfan's syndrome, systemic sclerosis, and some skeletal dystrophies, radiography can be used to study both the heart and other organ systems.

2. Radiography currently is the most useful method for demonstrating the shape, size, and position of the heart and its relation to thoracic and abdominal viscera.

In assessing chamber enlargement including cavity dilatation and wall hypertrophy, however, echocardiography is more sensitive and accurate than radiographic examination.

3. Radiography is ideal for obtaining a complete picture of the thoracic aorta and as a basic method in demonstrating tortuosity and elongation, aneurysm, and coarctation of the thoracic aorta. To study aortic root dilatation, echocardiographic examination should mainly be relied on. Integrated application of radiography and radionuclide cardiac pool scanning may improve the accuracy of differential diagnosis between an aneurysm of the thoracic aorta and a mediastinal mass.

4. Radiography is almost useless in "qualitative" diagnosis of some heart diseases, such as ischemic heart disease, myocarditis, cardiomyopathy, and intracardiac tumor. However, it is useful in assessing the degree of cardiovascular impairment. For example, in acute myocardial infarction, radiographic findings, such as cardiac size and alteration in pulmonary vascularity, proved to be important parameters in assessing the severity of disease and in predicting the patient's prognosis. In the early detection and diagnosis of left-sided heart failure, radiography is usually superior to clinical and other parameters.

In the diagnosis and quantitative estimation of pericardial effusion, however, echocardiography is more sensitive and accurate than radiography, particularly in the early detection of a small amount of effusion.

5. In some congenital heart diseases, such as atrial and ventricular septal defect, patent ductus arteriosus, a supracardiac type of total anomalous pulmonary venous drainage, tetralogy of Fallot, and Ebstein's anomaly associated with typical radiographic manifestations, radio-

graphic examination may be of diagnostic value. However, the more complicated the deformity, including multiple deformities, and the younger the age group or the smaller the defect,[6] the more limited is the radiographic method of diagnosis.

6. Cardiac fluoroscopy with a high resolution image intensifier alone or combined with cineradiographic recordings is more sensitive than ultrasonic examination in the detection and localization of intracardiac calcification, such as calcium in coronary arteries and valve leaflets.[7]

7. To assess the pulmonary perfusion state, as for example, in the diagnosis of pulmonary embolism, radionuclide perfusion scanning is more sensitive than radiographic examination, but the latter can concisely demonstrate pulmonary emphysema, bullae, and mass, thus complementing the drawback of less specificity of radionuclide examination.

In conclusion, improving the diagnostic accuracy and ensuring the intelligent and sensible application of various noninvasive methods, including radiography, can bring each one's strong points into play. That they are complementary to, rather than competitive with, one another should be emphasized as the main approach.

REFERENCES

1. Dai YP, Liu YQ: Measurement of the heart and great vessels, in Liu YQ (ed): *Clinical Radiology of the Heart.* Beijing, Beijing Publishing Co, 1981, pp 41–51.
2. Wang SH, Xie ZK: Cardiac measurement among Chinese. *Chin J Radiol* 1956; 4:5–11.
3. Dai RP, Liu YQ, Du JH, Rong ZP: Measurement of Chinese cardiac volume. *Chin Med J* 1983; 96:411–414.
4. Jefferson K, Rees R: Heart size, in Jefferson K, Rees R (eds): *Clinical Cardiac Radiology.* London/Boston, Butterworth, 1980, chap 1, pp 6–8.
5. Liu YQ: Evaluation of conventional radiology in the diagnosi: diovascular disease. *J Practi Med* 1984; 4:13–14.
6. Li YQ, Liu YQ, Jiang SL: Patent ductus arteriosus. Some pro' radiologic diagnosis. *Chin Med J* 1984; 97:657–662.
7. Elliott LP: Cardiac fluoroscopy: an underused technique in the of coronary artery disease and other cardiac diseases. *IM–Inter the Specialist* 1984; 5:61–71.

8 Nuclear Cardiology

Henry N. Wagner, Jr, MD and Xiujie Liu, MD

In 1956 radioactive isotopes began to be used in China for the diagnosis and treatment of patients and for biomedical research. By 1979 all of China's provinces, municipalities, and autonomous regions, except Tibet, ere using nuclear technology in medicine. In the autumn of 1979 a group of American physicians and medical scientists visited China to foster exchange of data and ideas. Nuclear cardiology was an area of science and technology that was part of the modernization program and a topic of considerable interest. The Chinese wanted to know what cardiologists and nuclear medicine physicians were doing with radioactive tracers to learn more about their patients and problems. Because of historical relations in the past, such as that of the Peking Union Medical College and the Rockefeller Foundation, warm feelings were encountered as old friends met and new friendships were made. "Friendship first" was a frequently expressed feeling throughout the visit.

Cooperative efforts during the visit made possible the carrying out of the first studies in China with the Nuclear Stethoscope®*, a device for monitoring cardiac function. A technetium-99m generator was shipped by Mallinckrodt Nuclear Corporation from St. Louis, Missouri, to Peking, China, via Japan's Narita airport. To meet the strict time requirements of radioactive decay, several phases of preparation had to be carried out simultaneously. Production of the Mallinckrodt Ultra-Technekow in St. Louis, Missouri, was more complicated than usual because a special generator had to be built with extra lead shielding. The generator had to be labeled in Chinese and the decay schedule calculated to take into consideration the differences in time between the United States and China. The generator arrived in Japan on Monday, September 24, 1979, a national holiday in Japan, so that the Mallinckrodt staff in Japan had to give up part of their holiday to meet the plane and ensure the transfer of the technetium generator to the flight going to the People's Republic of China. The generator from Mallinckrodt Nuclear made it possible for the first Nuclear Stethoscope study of the heart to be performed by Drs Liu and Wagner in China on September 25, 1979 at Fu Wai Hospital in Beijing (Figure 8.1). Simultaneously with the shipment of the technetium-99m generator was the shipment of the "Nuclear Stethoscope" cardiac probe from Valhalla, New York, to China. This first study was the forerunner of a continuing friendship between nuclear medicine physicians in the People's Republic of China and in the United States of America. For example, between July 1, 1980 and July 31, 1982, Dr Xiujie Liu worked in the Johns Hopkins Hospital in the Division of Nuclear Medicine, and between March 16, 1981 and September 10, 1982, Dr Jiang Mao-Song of Shanghai was at Johns Hopkins as a Fellow in Nuclear Medicine. Since that time, several publications

* Nuclear Stethoscope is a trademark of Bios Inc, 503 Grasslands Road, Valhalla, New York.

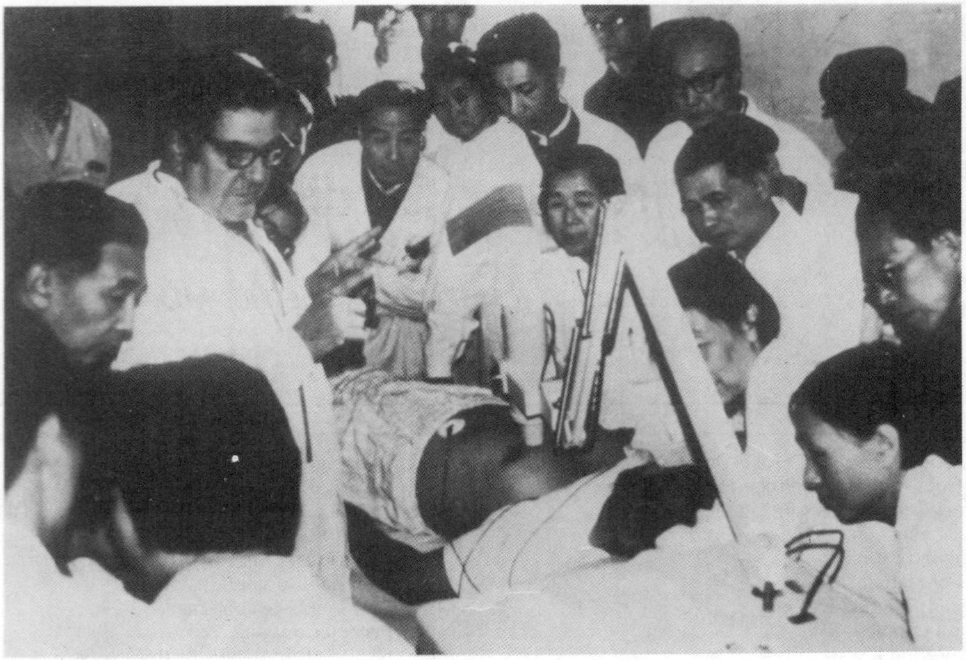

Figure 8.1. Doctors Liu and Wagner performing the first study in China with the Nuclear Stethoscope at the Fu Wai Hospital, September 25, 1979.

have appeared that represent the joint work of Johns Hopkins and Chinese nuclear physicians.[1-6]

Many of these publications involve the use of the cardiac probe, called a "Nuclear Stethoscope," a new tool that provides noninvasive measurement of ventricular function by monitoring the radioactivity within the heart from a radiotracer tagged to the patient's blood pool. Clinical applications focus on two major areas: screening for cardiac disease and acute care monitoring.

THE CARDIAC PROBE

The cardiac probe (Figure 8.2) is a radiation detector that is positioned by hand over the chest and monitors the radioactively labeled red blood cells or albumin within the heart during one or multiple heart beats. Blood volume changes within the heart are detected by changes in radioactivity. The probe allows assessment of the function of the heart by providing information on changes in volumes, rates of filling and emptying, and the times at which hemodynamic events occur within the ventricles.[7,8]

The concept of measuring the function of the heart with radioactive tracers has evolved over the past 60 years from the pioneering work of Blumgart in 1927 to the microprocessor-based Nuclear Stethoscope of today.

WHAT DOES THE CARDIAC PROBE DO?

The probe provides a wide range of information on cardiac function. Results are obtained both from the first pass of an intravenously injected bolus of radioactivity through the heart and from equilibrium studies of individual or composite heartbeats. Figure 8.3 shows typical displays of data from each of the modes of operation. The position/monitor mode is used both for positioning the detector and for measuring changes that occur over a few heartbeats as in the case of arrhythmias, anesthesia, or fast-acting drugs. The highest temporal resolution (10 ms) is used in the ventricular function mode which displays the sum of all beats collected over a selected time interval (30 seconds to 4 minutes). This mode is used, for example, when accurate information on diastolic filling is desired, as in screening for heart disease or in measuring the effects of drug therapy. Peak filling rate (PFR) and time to peak filling (TPFR), measured from high temporal resolution curves, are helpful in the detection of heart disease or assessment of drug effects.[9]

HOW DOES THE CARDIAC PROBE HELP?

When the physician needs to assess cardiac function, he now relies chiefly on clinical signs and symptoms, the electrocardiographic monitor, gamma camera/computer imaging, ultrasound, or cardiac catheterization. Because of the ability of the cardiac probe to provide data on cardiac function rapidly and directly, the major applications of the probe have been in the diagnosis of coronary disease and monitoring the effects of drug therapy.

Examples of usefulness in coronary disease include:

—Assessing ventricular function at the time of initial diagnosis

—Monitoring the effects of exercise on ventricular function[10]

—Evaluating the severity of disease, determining baseline cardiac function, and monitoring the possible development of cardiomyopathy with increasing doses of cardiotoxic drugs, such as doxorubicin.[11,12]

Examples of the usefulness in acute care monitoring/intervention include:

—Assessment of the effects of drug therapies (calcium channel blockers, beta blockers, antiarrhythmics, antihypertensives, and digitalis) for individual or com-

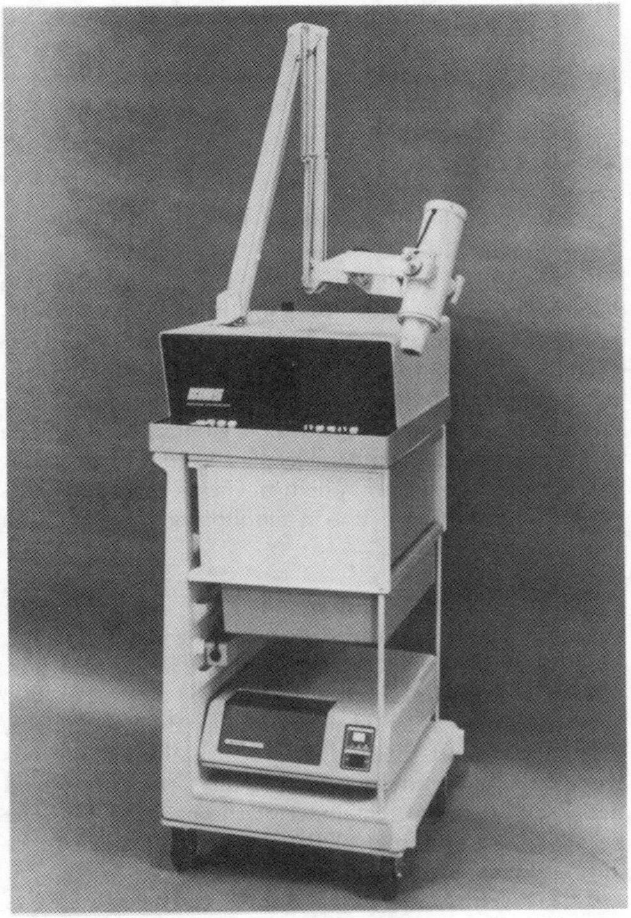

Figure 8.2. The Nuclear Stethoscope™ Cardiac Probe. This cardiac probe is an electrocardiogram gated scintillation detector and computer system developed for the noninvasive real time monitoring of left ventricular function at bedside.

posite beats or both. Individualization of drug and other therapy.

—Assessment of ventricular function in myocardial infarction

—Assessment of ventricular function before and after coronary artery bypass surgery

—Regulation of pacers to provide optimal left ventricular function

—Quantitation of performance of individual beats in patients with arrhythmias

—Management of acute and chronic congestive heart failure

—Assessment of ventricular function of patients with trauma and burn injuries, eg, when large volumes of intravenous fluids are being given.

INDIUM-113M AND THE CARDIAC PROBE

One of the main challenges in the world is to translate technologic advances from highly developed to less highly developed countries. Most in vivo núclear medicine studies involve the use of technetium-99m as a tracer label. Because of its short (six-hour) half-life, it must be obtained from a molybdenum-99 generator that has a half-life of 67 hours. In practice, such a generator must be obtained by a hospital at weekly intervals, which presents problems if the production site is far removed from the hospital. To extend the ability to perform such studies, indium-113m, which has a half-life of 99 minutes, affords several advantages: (1) It can readily be obtained from a parent radionuclide, tin-113, that has a half-life of 115 days and therefore need only be obtained at about 5-month intervals, the indium-113m being obtained by chemical elution several times a day. (2) Indium-113m, because of its short half-life, gives a low radiation dose to the patient. (3) Indium-113m can be used after technetium-99m in dual-isotope studies. (4) It is especially useful in locations where technetium-99m is not available on a regular basis.

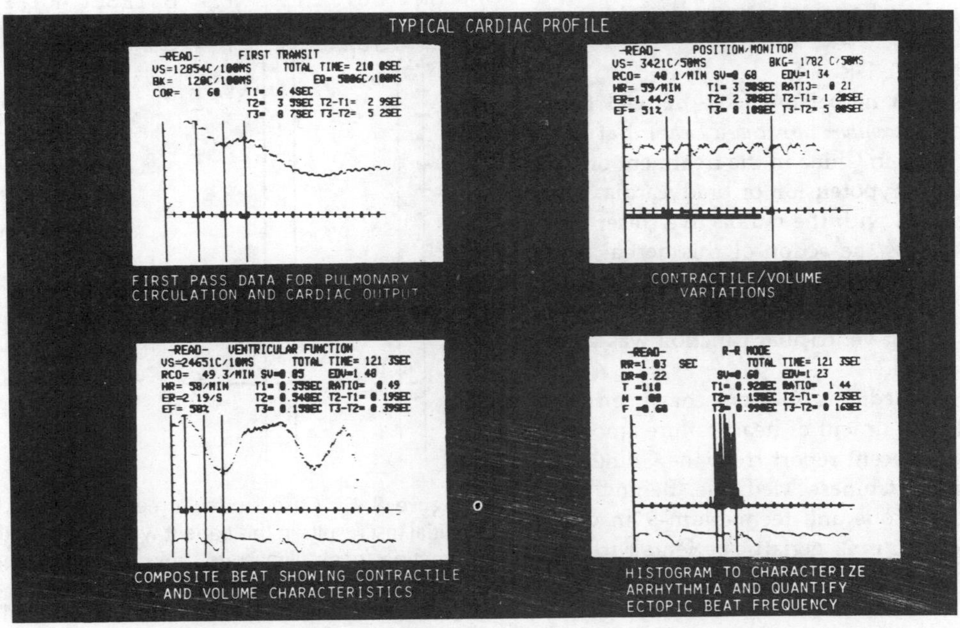

Figure 8.3. Typical cardiac profile—data displays.

Left ventricular ejection fraction can be measured with indium-113m injected intravenously because of its binding to the plasma protein transferrin. We found a close correlation between the results of the cardiac probe and those obtained with a gamma camera in 25 patients with coronary artery disease and 10 patients with regional left ventricular wall motion abnormalities.[1]

DIASTOLIC FUNCTION

Left ventricular peak filling rate and other diastolic parameters can be assessed using the Nuclear Stethoscope. Although measurements of ejection fraction and regional wall motion have been widely used in nuclear cardiology, only recently has attention been paid to diastolic parameters despite the fact that reduction in ejection fraction is a relatively insensitive means of detecting ventricular function, particularly when patients are examined at rest. Because of its greater temporal resolution, the rates of emptying and filling can be assessed with accuracy using the cardiac probe and they provide important indexes of ventricular function.[13]

The cardiac probe can be used in combination with pressure monitoring to generate pressure-volume loops, that is, the relation between intraventricular pressure and left ventricular volume.[14]

BACKGROUND CORRECTION

A major cause of interobserver variability in the use of the Nuclear Stethoscope has been the measurement of background activity, that is, the activity measured from red blood cells not restricted to the intraventricular cavity. We have found that a constant percentage of the measured end-diastolic count rate can be used as the background in calculating ejection fraction. In 17 patients, the background averaged 0.73 ± 0.05 of the end-diastolic count rate. Using this background, the correlation of measurement of ejection fraction with the cardiac probe to that measured by contrast angiography was 0.91.[4] Therefore, it is not necessary for most studies with the cardiac probe to measure background activity.

EFFECTS OF HERBAL DRUGS

Higenamine is an herbal medicine derived from the plant Mankshoot (*Aconitum carmichaeli Debx*) that has been used for many years in China in the treatment of patients with symptoms of hypotension or bradycardia. The cardiac probe was used with the radioactive tracer ionic indium-113m to assess the action of this herbal medicine on left ventricular function. The results of the study in 15 patients with different forms of heart disease indicated that the effect on left ventricular function was similar to that of isoproterenol.[5]

Another herbal medicine, Ginseng, has been used for ages in China for treatment of heart failure among many other disorders. A recent report from the Chinese Academy of Traditional Chinese Medicine, Beijing, China[14a] using the cardiac probe and technetium-99m described its therapeutic effects in 24 geriatric patients with congestive heart failure (coronary heart disease, 14; rheumatic heart disease, 5; hypertensive cardiovascular disease, 3; dilated cardiomyopathy, 1; syphilitic heart disease, 1). Thirty minutes after intravenous injection of Ginseng Co, which contains 2 g of the crude Ginseng, the ejection fraction increased from 0.35 ± 0.02 to 0.42 ± 0.02 ($p < .001$). The Ginseng Co injection also increased the diastolic fast filling rate from 1.15 ± 0.11 to 1.50 ± 0.13 ($p < .001$).

CADMIUM TELLURIDE DETECTOR

To simplify the attachment of the cardiac probe to the chest wall over the left ventricle, a miniature cadmium telluride probe was substituted for the sodium iodide detector of the cardiac probe. In the 25 patients who were examined, left ventricular ejection measured with the cadmium telluride probe agreed well with the left ventricular ejection fraction obtained with a gamma camera. The probe can provide comparable data to that of a scintillation camera-computer system and being small and lightweight is suitable for use in monitoring patients in an intensive care facility.[6]

CLINICAL EXAMPLES

In many patients, heart disease is progressive. There is often an initial period without symptoms during which disease is slowly developing, followed by a phase of mild symptoms over a period of approximately 1 to 2 years, a relatively short phase during which the diagnosis is made by intensive testing, and finally a therapy period which may last the remainder of the patient's life. The following are examples of the use of the cardiac probe during the different phases.

Case 1 is an example of a resting study performed as a screening test during the early phases of the disease (Figure 8.4). The patient, a 60-year-old man, was experiencing chest pain and shortness of breath during mild

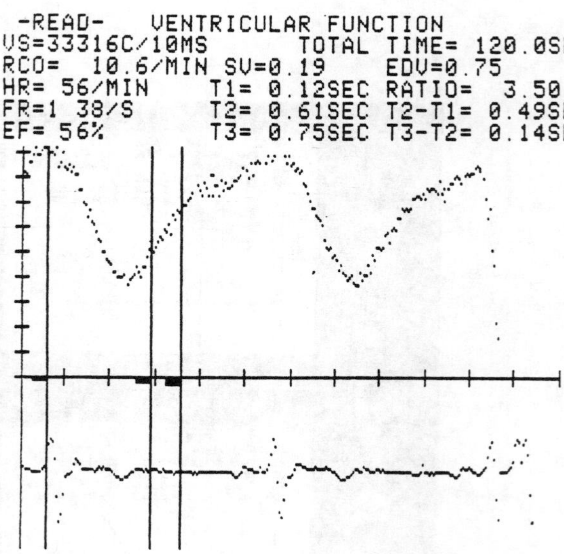

Figure 8.4. Case study: screening for cardiac disease. All initial test results in this patient were normal except for diastolic function (peak filling rate, time to peak filling rate). Diastolic function has been reported to be sensitive and specific for coronary disease. Case contributed by Paul J. Rosch, MD, New York Medical College.

exertion. Physical examination and laboratory tests gave normal results. The cardiac probe study showed normal systolic function with an ejection fraction of 56%. Diastolic function, however, was depressed (PFR = 1.35 EDV/S, normal = 2.5 to 5.0 EDV/S; TPFR = 196 ms, normal ≤ 180 ms), suggesting early left ventricular dysfunction.

Case 2 (Figure 8.5) illustrates an exercise study. The ejection fraction in this patient increased 35% during and immediately after exercise (bicycle). The disappearance of the diastolic plateau (diastasis) during exercise and its early reappearance after exercise can be seen, as well as the increase in ejection rate and ejection fraction. This is the normal response to exercise; in patients with cardiac disease, a decrease or no change in ejection fraction is the usual response.

Therapy monitoring is illustrated by the third and fourth patients. In case 3, the effects of drug selection and dose regulation were monitored in a patient with congestive heart failure. The patient had had a long history of angina and recurrent myocardial infarction and was admitted to the hospital with severe congestive heart failure. His therapy before admission included digoxin, diuretics, and long-acting nitrates, but these were no longer effective. Initial hospital treatment included dobutamine and nitroprusside infusion without apparent benefit. Prazosin and hydralazine were then used in an effort to improve cardiac function. The immediate effectiveness of the drug interventions was monitored using the cardiac probe. The response of various cardiac parameters to two of the drugs, prazosin and hydralazine, is shown in Figure 8.6, *top*. The marked improvement in left ventricular systolic and diastolic function was clearly demonstrated by the probe studies. The patient's function and symptoms continued to respond favorably to the larger dose of hydralazine (Figure 8.6, *bottom*). With the vast number of different types of drugs available today, it would have been difficult to judge their effects alone or in combination in this patient without direct measurement of the response.

Pre- and postoperative studies to evaluate the results of coronary bypass surgery are illustrated in case 4 (Figure 8.7). The patient had had an anteroseptal myocardial infarction, with extremely elevated creatine phosphokinase values, severe anterior and anteroapical akinesia and mild inferior hypokinesia in a gated blood pool scintillation camera study, and a global ejection fraction of 19%. Cardiac catheterization confirmed anteroapical hypokinesia and revealed high-grade stenosis of a dominant right coronary artery with total occlusion of the main left coronary artery. Quadruple bypass grafts to the left anterior descending, diagonal, posterior descending, and circumflex obtuse marginal branches of the coronary arteries were performed. The patient was treated with nifedipine and diuretics. By the ninth postoperative day, the ejection fraction, ejection rate, and peak filling rate had improved to normal or near normal values (EF = 62%). Pre- and postoperative cardiac studies are shown in Figure 8.7.

WHAT ARE THE RISKS?

It is reasonable to ask what risk is associated with the 150 to 300 mrads of radiation received by a patient having a study with the cardiac probe. The most authoritative studies of the biologic effects of ionizing radiation for the United Nations and the US National Academy of Sciences indicate that the risk to a patient of getting cancer from this dose is one in one million. This risk is the same as the risk of dying from traveling 700 miles by plane, working 3 weeks in a coal mine, or living for 2 months in a stone building. The routinely performed gated blood pool study done by a gamma camera/computer requires the same radiopharmaceutical and gives the same dose. The radiopharmaceutical, technetium-99m, has a short (6-hour) half-life, which means the radioactivity is virtually undetectable less than 48 hours after the test. The radioactive tracer studies give significantly less radiation exposure than does cardiac catheterization.

HOW THE STUDIES ARE PERFORMED

The patient's red blood cells are prepared by intravenous injection of stannous pyrophosphate approximately 30 minutes before an injection of 3 to 25 mCi of sodium pertechnetate Tc-99m.[15] If first transit procedures are to be performed, the bolus of sodium pertechnetate must be discrete for a satisfactory study, because the first pass of radioactivity through the heart is to be measured. Posi-

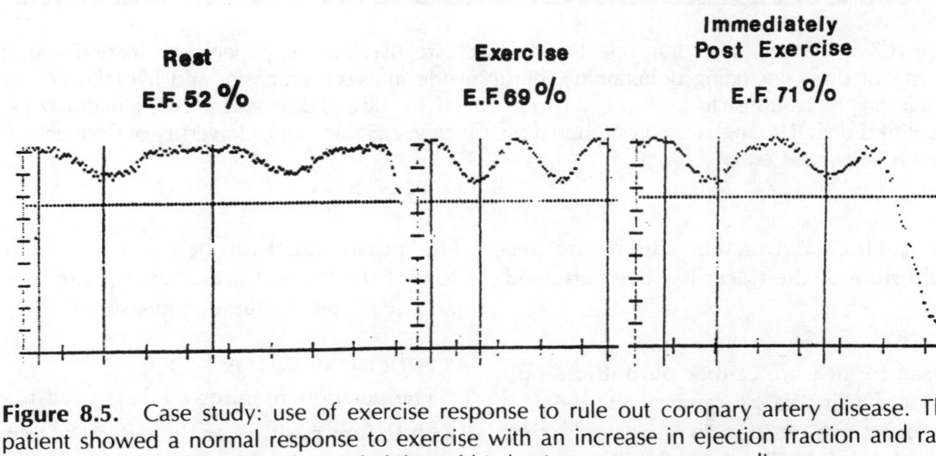

Figure 8.5. Case study: use of exercise response to rule out coronary artery disease. This patient showed a normal response to exercise with an increase in ejection fraction and rate. This significantly decreases the probability of his having coronary artery disease.

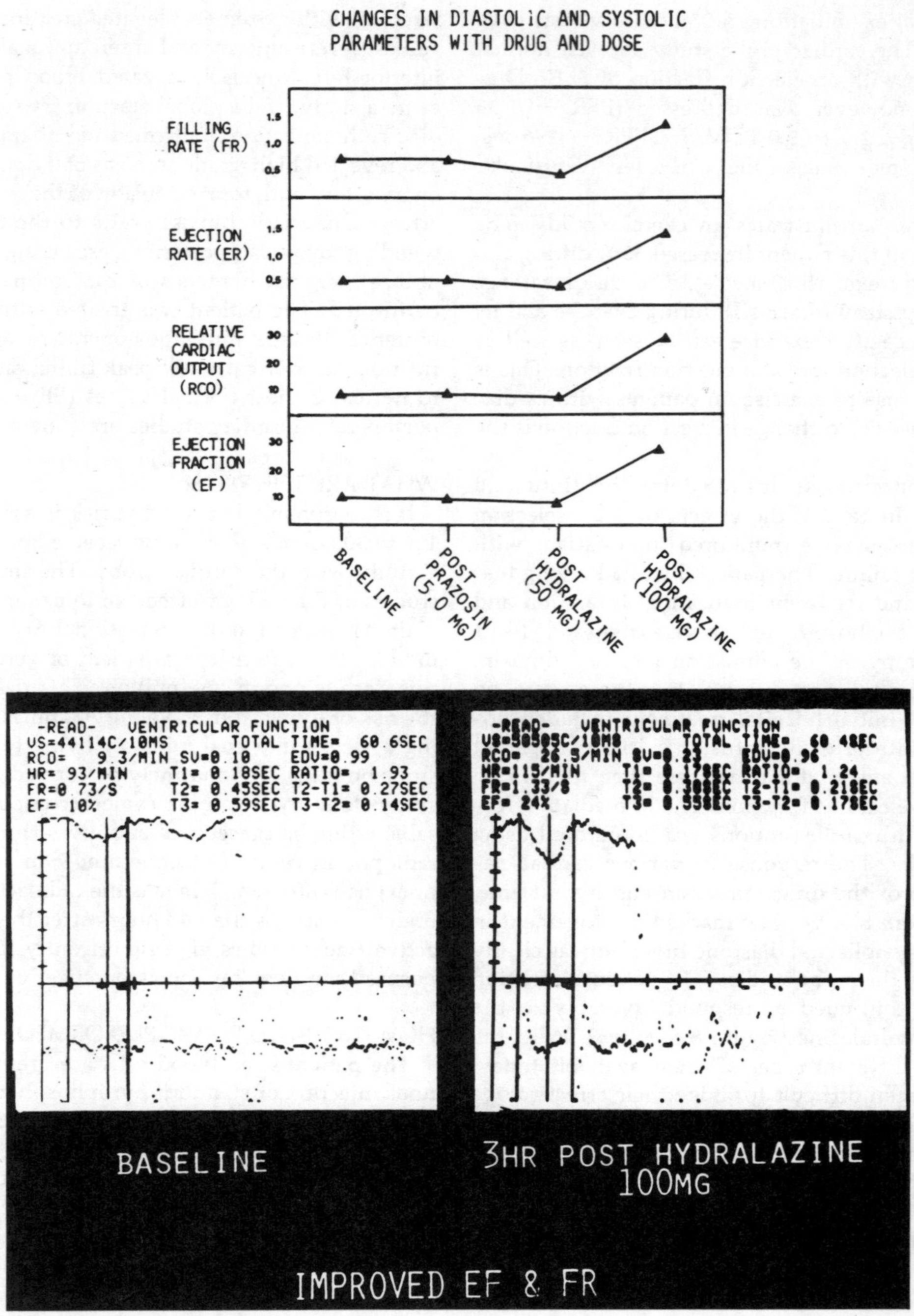

Figure 8.6. Case study: drug selection and dose regulation. The patient was treated with a variety of drugs including dobutamine, nitroprusside infusion, prazosin, and hydralazine. By monitoring his response to each one, the most effective drug and dose was selected (hydralazine, four times daily 100 mg). Case contributed by Vivienne E. Smith, MD, University of Connecticut Health Sciences Center.

tion/monitor and ventricular function studies are performed after equilibrium of the tracer has been attained.

FIRST TRANSIT MODE

This mode is used to measure cardiac output and pulmonary transit time. During measurement, the detector is located over the chest in a position to measure the time course of the tracer through both right and left ventricles. The measurement can be repeated by injecting a second dose of the tracer. Cardiac output can be calculated if the patient's blood volume is measured.

POSITION/MONITOR MODE

The position/monitor mode is used to determine:

—Optimum position of the detector for measurement of left ventricular function

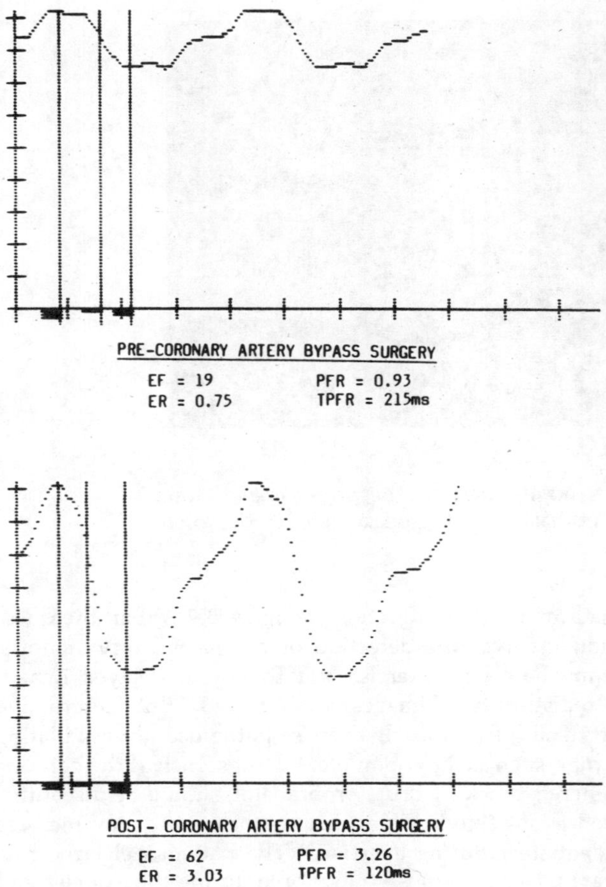

Figure 8.7. Case study: before (*top*) and after (*bottom*) coronary artery bypass surgery. Preoperative values for all parameters of cardiac function were extremely depressed. After the four-vessel bypass, there was a marked improvement in values demonstrated by the results of the follow-up probe study. Case contributed by Kenneth R. Rice, MD, and Ernest V. Gervino, ScD, Harvard Medical School, Beth Israel Hospital.

—Optimum position for measurement of background activity
—Beat to beat left ventricular function and its changes during arrhythmia, ectopy, and drug response.

Continuous activity/time curves are displayed while the operator locates the optimum position for ventricular measurement and monitors the screen to identify the beats of interest. Up to 20 beats may be displayed at any one time, depending on the heart rate of the patient.

POSITIONING

Correct positioning is essential for proper use of the Nuclear Stethoscope. To assist in locating the correct positions, the system uses an indicator bar located just below the horizontal axis on the CRT. The bar responds in real time to changes in the activity/time curves which are sensed as the detector moves over the patient's chest. The microprocessor automatically calculates the value of

$$\frac{\text{stroke counts}}{\text{average counts}}$$

and displays its magnitude as the length of the bar. The bar is updated with each heartbeat. The region of greatest stroke volume and correspondingly longest bar length is normally found over the left ventricle (highest stroke counts, lowest mean counts).

Background activity contributed by surrounding tissue raises the average volume or count level. This activity must be subtracted to determine activity due to the left ventricle for use in heart function calculations. The optimum position for measuring background is at the location where bar length is one to one and a half major scale divisions. This corresponds to a location where there are minimum stroke counts at the highest mean counts.

Proper positioning requires three steps that must be practiced until proficiency is achieved. This usually requires the study of at least 10 to 20 patients. The three steps are:

—Definition of the general size and position of the heart and approximate location of the ventricle
— Definition of the precise location of optimal left ventricle activity
—Definition of background location.

VENTRICULAR FUNCTION

The ventricular function mode provides a high temporal resolution image (10 ms) of a composite beat for measurement of left ventricular parameters. The time interval over which beats are collected can be selected by the operator. The volume/time curve is synchronized with the R wave of the electrocardiogram and updated every two beats. The CRT display shows the composite curve for successive pairs of beats. After data collection is complete, the operator chooses the area of interest, and the system automatically calculates the results. Measurements in the ventricular function mode are made with the probe in the left ventricular position which was found in the P/M mode.

RR HISTOGRAM

When using the ventricular function mode, the operator can display a histogram of the RR intervals of the beats collected during the measurement period. This is used to assess the severity of the arrhythmias.

THE FUTURE

Monitoring a patient's response to drugs will continue to be one of the most important areas for the use of cardiac probes. Evaluating the effects of specific drug therapies will become more critical because of increases in the number and types of drugs available to the physician. Mobility of the current system permits studies to be performed routinely at the patient's bedside.

MYOCARDIAL PERFUSION SCINTIGRAPHY

REGIONAL MYOCARDIAL BLOOD FLOW

The major uses of thallium-201 myocardial imaging are: (1) to aid in the differential diagnosis of patients with chest pain; (2) to assess the degree of myocardial damage in patients with myocardial infarction; (3) to help dis-

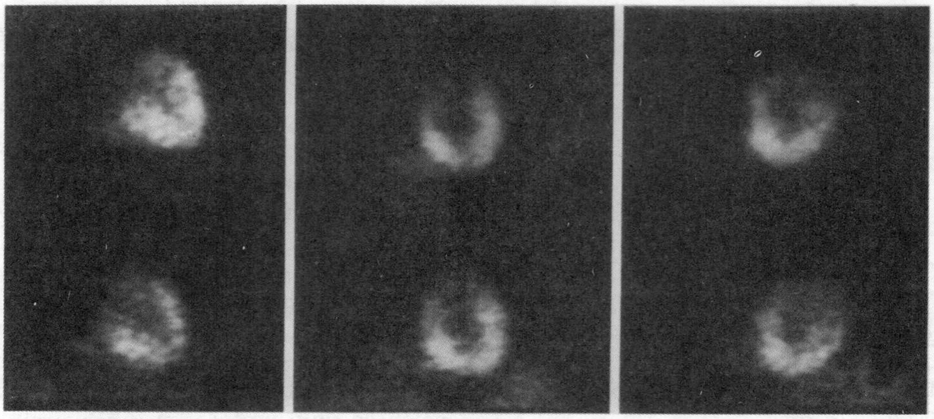

Figure 8.8. An exercise thallium-201 study in a normal person. The *upper images* were obtained immediately after the injection of 2 mCi of thallium-201 at peak exercise. The *lower images* were obtained four hours later.

criminate myocardial infarction from myocardial ischemia after myocardial infarction, ie, the so-called "jeopardized" myocardium; and (4) to assess the state of regional myocardial blood flow after coronary artery bypass surgery.

Thallium-201 imaging may also help determine the hemodynamic significance of small (50%) reductions in coronary artery diameter seen by coronary angiography. Other uses include estimating prognosis after myocardial infarction, detection of noncoronary cardiomyopathy, left ventricular hypertrophy, and left ventricular aneurysm. In many patients with angina pectoris or acute myocardial infarction, thallium-201 imaging is not necessary to establish the diagnosis, but can be helpful when other diagnostic procedures are not completely satisfactory and uncertainty persists, ie, with an a priori probability of between 30% and 70%.[16–18]

In performing a thallium-201 study, the patient is usually fasted to decrease splanchnic accumulation of the tracer.[19] It is also helpful to inject the patient while he is standing. A 1.5 mCi dose is injected intravenously and imaging with an Anger type scintillation camera or single photon emission tomography (SPECT) system. Multiple views are usually obtained: anterior, left anterior oblique (LAO) 30°, LAO 45°, LAO 60°, and left lateral. A thallium-201 study in a normal person is shown in Figure 8.8 and a study in a patient with coronary artery disease who had had myocardial infarction in Figure 8.9. When the question involves the detection of coronary artery stenosis, immediate post-exercise and four-hour delayed images ("redistribution" images) are obtained.[20,21] An alternative to treadmill or bicycle exercise is the use of vasodilating drugs, such as dipyridamole.[21a] Drugs, such as the beta adrenergic blocking drug, propranalol, should be discontinued if possible in order that the heart rate may increase adequately during exercise.[22] The patient's electrocardiogram is continuously monitored during the exercise and the thallium-201 dose injected one minute before the patient stops exercising. The exercise is terminated if: the heart rate reaches 90% of predicted values; 1 mm or more of ST-segment depression is observed; systolic arterial pressure decreases; serious arrhythmias develop; the patient is unable to continue or becomes ataxic. In any case 1.5 to 2.0 mCi of thallium-201 thallous ion is injected one minute before termination of the exercise. An experienced physician will be able to predict successfully when the patient is within one minute of having to stop exercising.

Many techniques have been proposed for processing the images before interpretation. Complete automation of interpretation has not yet been achieved, although this is an important goal of many investigators. Background subtraction and various other types of contrast enhance-

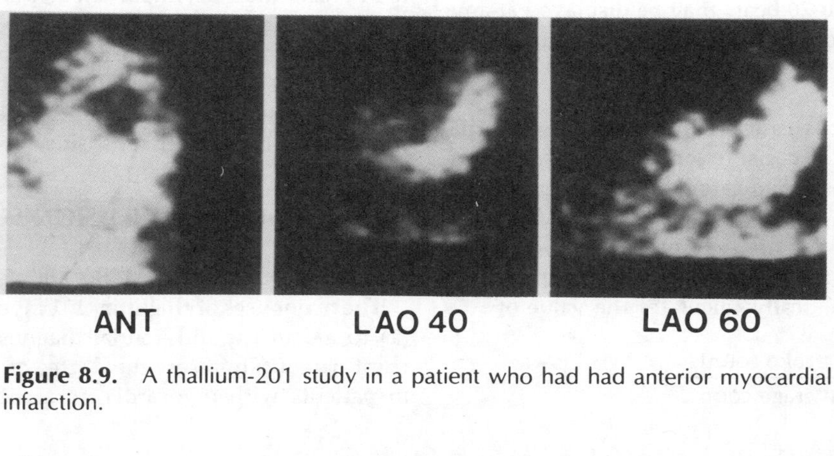

Figure 8.9. A thallium-201 study in a patient who had had anterior myocardial infarction.

ment are usually employed.[23] Quantification of the quantity of the tracer in various parts of the heart is an aid to subjective interpretation of the images.[19,24–26,26a,26b,26c] One of the major advances has been the use of single photon emission computed tomography (SPECT). Several studies have shown the value of SPECT in improving the accuracy of detecting coronary stenoses.[27,28,28a] A particular advantage is the ability to view the distribution of the tracer after the images have been rotated by computer along the longitudinal axis of the heart extending from the apex to the base. Viewing the heart in this way makes it possible to detect abnormal inhomogeneities more easily.

In addition to detecting regional decreases in tracer activity, it is helpful to examine the rate of wash-out of the thallium-201 from the myocardium over the four-hour period after injection.[29] In normal persons, the wash-out half-time is about four hours. To compare the immediate postexercise and delayed images, it is important to position the patient carefully for both studies. Superimposition of the images is also facilitated by the ability to translocate the images of the thallium-201 distribution by means of the computer. Contour images are helpful for this purpose. Delayed wash-out in a particular region increases the likelihood that the segment of myocardium is abnormal.

It is well established that the initial accumulation of thallium-201 is a function of regional myocardial blood flow because extraction of the tracer from the blood is high. Damage such as hypoxia does not significantly reduce the accumulation of thallium-201, whereas ischemia does. When injection is given with the patient in the resting state, right ventricular blood flow is usually too low to permit visualization of the right ventricle in the thallium-201 images. With exercise, right ventricular blood flow is increased and the right ventricle becomes visible. If the right ventricle is visualized in a rest study, the patient probably has right ventricular hypertrophy.[30]

An area of ischemia is differentiated from an area of infarction by the fact that the ischemic region becomes more nearly normal in appearance in the delayed images. In infarction the initial defects remain unchanged. In the case of myocardial scarring the initial and the four-hour delayed images usually are similar in appearance.[31]

In patients with acute myocardial infarction, thallium-201 images obtained at rest should be obtained as soon as possible after the acute episode because the sensitivity decreases from nearly 100% to about 75% if the study is not performed within the first 24 hours. An important use of thallium-201 imaging is in prognosis. If greater than 40% of the left ventricular muscle is impaired, the prognosis is much worse than in the case of small infarcts.[32] In patients with coronary stenosis without infarction, a normal thallium-201 exercise test is a good predictor that the patient has less than a 1% chance of having a major event, such as a myocardial infarction or sudden death or angina, within a period of 5 years.

Rubidium-82 chloride has been proposed for use in positron emission tomography (PET) for measuring regional myocardial blood flow, because it is available from a commercially available generator and therefore does not require a cyclotron for its production at the site of use. Its 75-second half-life makes it possible to make frequent measurements and to assess perturbations. It has been used chiefly in the assessment of relative regional myocardial blood flow in patients with ischemic heart disease.[33–35] Whether its use will become widespread remains questionable.

If a cyclotron is available, other tracers that can be used to measure regional myocardial blood flow include ^{13}N ammonia and oxygen-15 water. Because of its 2.5-minute physical half-life, studies can be repeated frequently after perturbation of flow. Regional oxygen consumption as well as regional blood flow can be measured.

Recently, several Tc-99m isonitrile analogues, eg, Tc-99m t-butylisonitrile (TBI) and Tc-99m carbomethoxyisopropyl isonitrile (CPI), have been developed with promising characteristics. Unlike thallium-201, they redistribute very slowly. Furthermore, because Tc-99m isonitrile analogues are generator, not cyclotron, produced, they can be prepared on site. The characteristics of this new family of Tc-99m–labeled racers suggest that it may not be very long before it rep aces thallium-201 for myocardial scintigraphy.[35a]

MYOCARDIAL INFARCTIOI IMAGING

Since the early 1960s, radioactive tracers that accumulate in myocardial infarction have been used chiefly to establish the diagnosis or to estimate the size of infarcted areas. The most widely used agent for this purpose is technetium-99m phosphates and phosphonates introduced by Bonte et al in 1974.[36] More recently radioiodinated and indium-111 labeled monoclonal antibodies against myocardial myosin have been proposed.[37]

Factors that influence the uptake of infarct-localizing radiotracers include the degree of myocardial damage, the residual blood flow to the infarcted area, and the stage of injury. For both technetium-99m pyrophosphate and indium-111 antimyosin monoclonal antibodies, the accumulation of the tracer is less when blood flow is reduced to less than 10% to 15% of normal myocardial blood flow compared with the accumulation of the tracer in regions where the deficit in flow is between 15% and 85% of normal. Infarct sizing is usually based on the size of the area of abnormal uptake of the tracer rather than on the intensity of uptake.[38] Figure 8.10 shows a ^{99m}Tc-pyrophosphate study in a patient with myocardial infarction.

Large infarcts are at times characterized by a zone of diminished tracer uptake within a ring of increased tracer concentration. This is a sign of serious injury with a poor prognosis.[39,40] For maximum sensitivity in the detection of acute myocardial infarction, imaging should be performed 30 to 48 hours after admission of the patient to the intensive care unit. Two normal studies within 48 hours of admission greatly decrease the likelihood of acute myocardial infarction. One of the most important uses of infarct imaging is the study of a patient known to have had myocardial infarction in the past and in whom the question is whether an acute process has been superimposed.

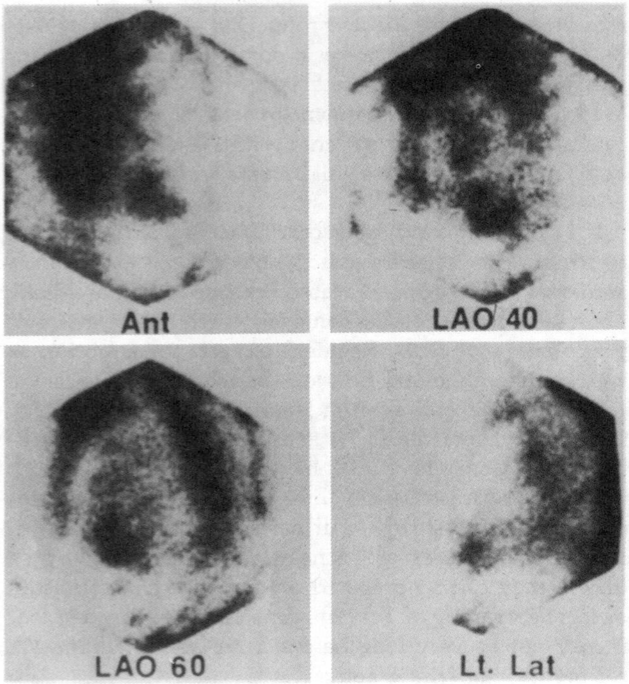

Figure 8.10. An 81-year-old woman with hypertension and a history of previous myocardial infarction was admitted to the hospital with chest pain and inconclusive evidence of acute myocardial infarction. The ^{99m}Tc-pyrophosphate study reveals increased concentration of the tracer in the inferior wall and apex and confirms the occurrence of acute infarction.

BLOOD POOL IMAGING (RADIONUCLIDE VENTRICULOGRAPHY)

Ventricular function can be assessed in several ways using techniques of nuclear cardiology. One is the use of the cardiac probe that we have described previously. The other methods are the use of the large field of view Anger scintillation camera or the multicrystal camera. Two approaches are used: (1) monitoring the first pass of the bolus of injected radioactivity as it passes through the heart and great vessels or (2) gating the radiation-detection device using the patient's electrocardiogram to examine individual phases of the cardiac cycle. The first-pass study in the right anterior oblique position is often used to examine the function of the right ventricle to solve the problem of the overlap of the right and left ventricles. The 30° RAO position is well suited to separate the right atrium from the right ventricle.[41–43]

To image the chambers of the heart, a radiotracer such as technetium-99m labeled red blood cells, which remains in the vascular compartment, is used. The cardiac cycle is divided into 16 to 64 time intervals and images obtained to reflect the chamber volumes and contours throughout the different stages of the cardiac cycle. Because of the limited number of photon emissions coming from the labeled cells within the chambers, usually 100 to 200 cardiac cycles are examined and a composite image is obtained to represent an average cardiac cycle. In patients with severe arrhythmias, computer programs are used to select only those beats that are regular enough to represent the most common cardiac cycle. The individual images are usually displayed in cinematic fashion to portray a motion picture of the filling and emptying of the chambers and the degree of ventricular wall motion. Multiple views, including the anterior and 45° left anterior oblique, are usually obtained routinely.[44] The left anterior oblique view permits separation of the right from the left ventricle. The number of counts coming from within a region of interest such as the left ventricle is proportional to volume, so that end-diastolic and end-systolic count rates can be used to calculate ejection fraction, according to the formula:

$$\text{Ejection fraction} = \frac{\text{EDC-ESC}}{\text{EDC}}$$

where EDC equals end-diastolic counts and ESC equals end-systolic counts.

A gated blood pool study in a normal person, the time activity curve, and calculated ejection fraction are shown in Figure 8.11. The study shown in Figure 8.12 was performed in a 5-year-old boy who had a severe carnitine deficiency which resulted in heart failure. Before treatment the left ventricular ejection fraction was 23%. After treatment it improved to normal, 56%.

Ejection fraction can be abnormally low as the result of either a decreased stroke volume (EDC–ESC) or an increase in end-diastolic volume or both. An abnormally low ejection fraction at rest is a relatively late sign of ventricular disease compared with other measurements such as the rate of diastolic filling.[45] Often abnormalities in the degree of contraction of a particular part of the left ventricular wall can be observed before the overall ejection fraction has decreased below normal levels. Regions of hypokinesia, akinesia, or dyskinesia are often seen in patients with acute myocardial infarction or left ventricular aneurysm.

To increase the sensitivity of measurements of left ventricular overall or global function or the detection of regional left ventricular wall motion abnormalities, it is helpful to examine the patient during various stages of exercise usually performed by means of a bicycle ergometer. When focal ischemia occurs during exercise, a wall motion abnormality may be observed or the ejection fraction will decrease from resting levels or at least fail to increase to the normal degree.[46]

While subjective interpretation of gated blood pool scintigrams remains the most widely used method of analysis, there is also a need for quantification of the various abnormalities, especially of regional wall motion and in the evaluation of therapeutic interventions. Functional imaging by such methods as Fourier phase and amplitude analysis has been recently applied to the evaluation of regional ventricular function in patients with coronary artery disease.[46a]

POSITRON EMISSION TOMOGRAPHY

The concept of tomography has revolutionized medical imaging, including imaging of the heart. Positron emission tomography combines the chemical capabilities of positron-emitting radionuclides and the ability of tomography to quantify regional concentrations of radioactive tracers that decay by the process of positron emission. It

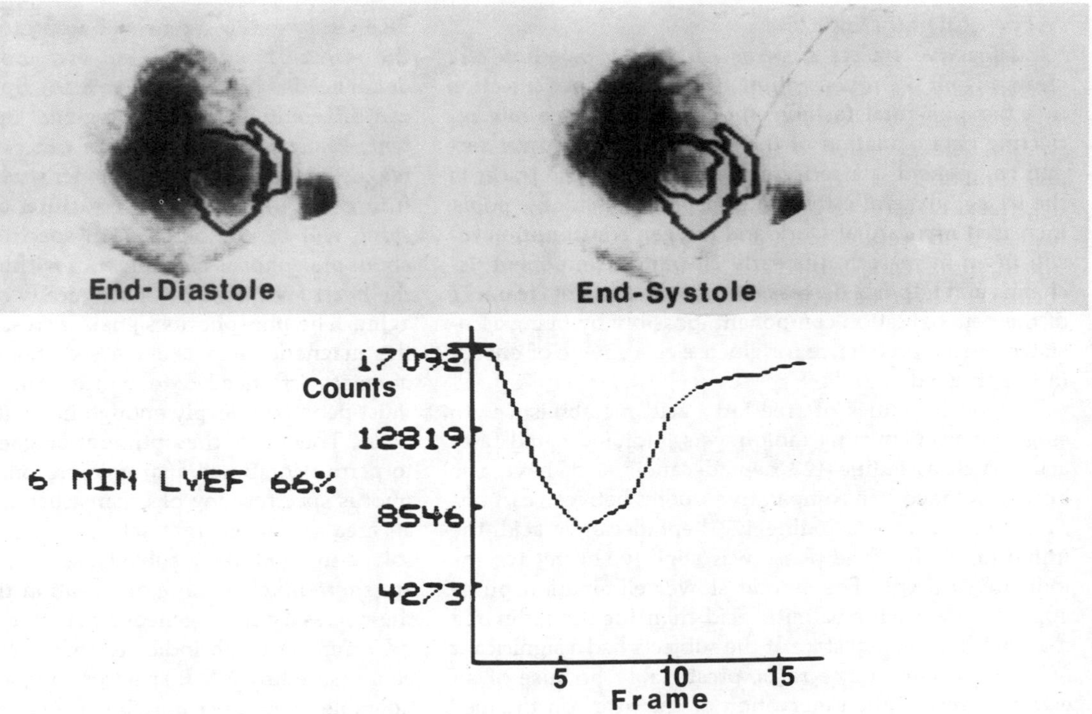

Figure 8.11. End-diastolic and end-systolic images, with left ventricular regions of interest and a background region indicated, obtained in a normal person. The left ventricular ejection fraction, 66%, was obtained from the time activity curve, shown in the lower portion of the figure.

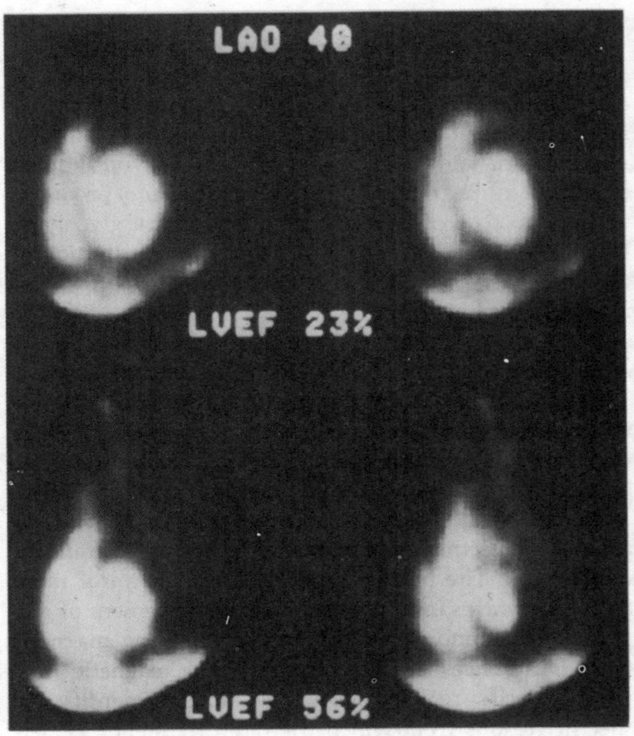

Figure 8.12. A 5-year-old boy with severe carnitine deficiency was admitted to the hospital because of increasing heart failure. A study performed before treatment (*upper images*) revealed a left ventricular ejection fraction of 23%. After treatment with carnitine the ejection fraction increased to 56% (*lower images*).

makes possible measurement of regional myocardial blood flow, substrate utilization, and neuroreceptor activities within the myocardium of living human beings.

REGIONAL GLUCOSE METABOLISM

In the fasting state, the heart relies chiefly on free fatty acids for its energy. Other substrates include lactate and pyruvate, depending on diet, physical activity, and other factors. An increase in blood glucose and secretion of insulin results in an increased utilization of glucose. Physical exercise increases lactate production which becomes the principal source of energy.

Fluorine-18 deoxyglucose is a widely used positron-emitting tracer for the study of myocardial metabolism. The tracer is actively transported into heart muscle cells and then phosphorylated by the enzyme hexokinase to glucose-6-phosphate.[47] Thereafter, the metabolism stops except for small amounts of dephosphorylation. By means of a mathematical model and measurement of arterial blood levels of the tracer, regional exogenous glucose metabolism can be calculated. A major finding to date has been that injured or "stunned" myocardium may be reflected in a preference for glucose rather than other metabolites that are less efficiently metabolized.[48] One hypothesis is that matched decreases in regional blood flow and glucose metabolism are a sign of necrotic or scarred myocardium, whereas reduced flow but increased glucose metabolism reflects injured but living myocardium.[49] Such studies have been proposed as a means of selecting patients who would benefit from coronary artery bypass grafting.

FATTY ACID METABOLISM

Radioactive tracers such as carbon-11 palmitate are cleared from the myocardium after intravenous injection in a biexponential fashion, the initial clearance rate reflecting beta oxidation of the fatty acid. The slower second component is a reflection of storage of the tracer in the triacyl glycerol ester and phospholipid storage pools. Increased myocardial work and oxygen consumption result in an increase in the early clearance component. Ischemia and hypoxia decrease the size and rate of clearance of the beta oxidation component, possibly by being associated with a preference for glucose as a source of energy in the stressed state.[50-53]

To permit studies of free fatty acid metabolism with single-photon emitting radiotracers, radioiodinated fatty acids, such as iodine-123 heptadecanoic acid, have also been developed.[54] In comparative studies between carbon-11 palmitic acid and iodine-123 heptadecanoic acid, the initial rapid clearance phase was slightly shorter for the iodinated tracer.[55] The second slower elimination phase appeared longer for palmitic acid than for the iodinated material. The mental state of the subjects had a significant effect on the clearance rates, presumably because of an effect of autonomic innervation of the heart on the metabolism of fatty acids.[56]

RECEPTOR IMAGING

In 1628 William Harvey stated that, "Every affection of the mind that is attended with either pain or pleasure, hope or fear, is the cause of an agitation whose influence extends to the heart." In his Lumleian lecture in 1910 Sir William Osler described worry as being a constant feature in patients with angina pectoris. Because over half the patients with coronary heart disease are identified only by the occurrence of sudden death, it behooves modern cardiology to make every effort to understand the neurologic and psychiatric factors related to coronary heart disease. One approach is the study of the nervous control of the heart. Of great interest are the alpha- and beta-adrenergic systems and the muscarinic acetylcholine systems. Quinuclidinyl benzilate (QNB) and its methylated analogue have both been investigated. Practolol and propranolol have also been examined, but they present problems of nonspecific binding or low affinity, respectively. Maziere et al (personal communication, 1981) showed that atropine could quantitatively displace bound C-11–labeled N–methyl QNB. The French group was also able to show the relation of the binding of methyl QNB and resting heart rate. Images of the dog heart have also been obtained using iodine-123 iodoQNB. The use of a radiolabeled derivative for quantitative imaging of beta adrenoreceptors and muscarinic cholinergic receptors in the heart now seems feasible.

NUCLEAR MAGNETIC RESONANCE

IMAGING AND SPECTROSCOPY

Nuclear magnetic resonance (NMR) provides both anatomic (NMRI)[56a] and biochemical (NMRS) information of potential value in the care of patients with cardiovascular disease.[57-59] Both cardiac (electrocardiographic) and respiratory gating are needed in proton NMRI to remove the effect of organ motion and provide the structural detail needed (Figures 8.13 to 8.16). Spectroscopic analysis can differentiate between regional lipid and water content. Phosphorus metabolism can be assessed at larger magnet strengths currently under study. In the immediate future it is likely that the structural detail of proton imaging will be combined with spectroscopic information about phosphorus bioenergetics within specific regions of the heart identified by anatomically oriented proton imaging. The phosphorus signals increase as the strength of the magnetic field is increased, but the high radiofrequencies (rf) needed to perturb the phosphorus nuclei must penetrate deeply enough into the body to study the heart. Therefore, the optimum magnet strength required to permit combined anatomic proton imaging and phosphorus spectroscopy of organs such as the heart remains an area of current research. Problems that remain to be solved in "spatially resolved chemical shift spectroscopy" are shortening the long observation times and achieving the necessary homogeneous magnetic fields.

Current research indicates that myocardial lactate can be measured by NMR spectroscopy, an approach of considerable importance in ischemic heart disease. It may also be possible to examine carbon-13–labeled substrates that are metabolized by the heart, although up to now, most NMR spectroscopy of the heart has been directed toward phosphorus bioenergetics, in particular toward measuring the derangements of cardiac energy metabolism during extremes of cardiac work during exercise and under ischemic conditions.

The heart consumes energy to carry out the process of excitation, contraction, relaxation, and repair of wear and tear damage. Adenosine triphosphate provides this energy in two principal ways: (1) oxidative phosphorylation in mitochondria and (2) glycolysis, the anerobic breakdown of glucose into lactate. About 10% of the energy produced under normal conditions comes from anaerobic glycolysis. Under conditions of anoxia, the relative contribution of the latter increases more than the rate of increase of oxidative phosphorylation.

ANATOMICALLY ORIENTED PROTON IMAGING

Proton imaging is used primarily to provide anatomic information, although visualization of the movement of the ventricular walls at various stages of the cardiac cycle by electrocardiographic gating provides functional information as well.[60] As in all diagnostic imaging, NMR imaging uses electromagnetic energy (photons) to transmit information. The NMR signals are in the form of radio frequency waves in resonance with the movement of nuclear protons under the influence of a strong magnetic field. Differences in the strength of the magnetic field within specific regions make it possible to identify the specific regions from which the radio frequency signals arise. The density of the protons within regions as small as 1 mm^3 can be determined, as well as the rate of change of the effects induced by the external radio frequency waves. Several types of signals—hydrogen (proton) density, relaxation times, T_1 and T_2—are measured depending on the time sequence of radio frequency pulses

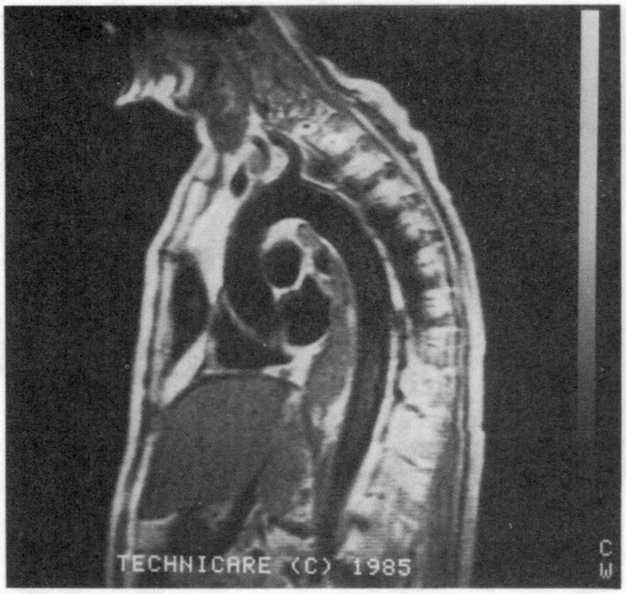

A

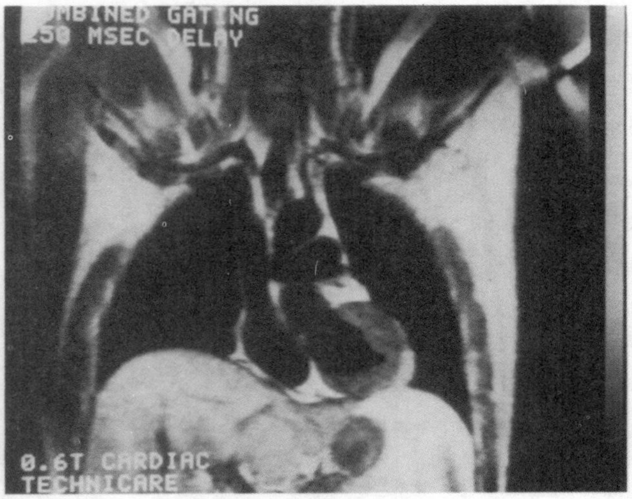

B

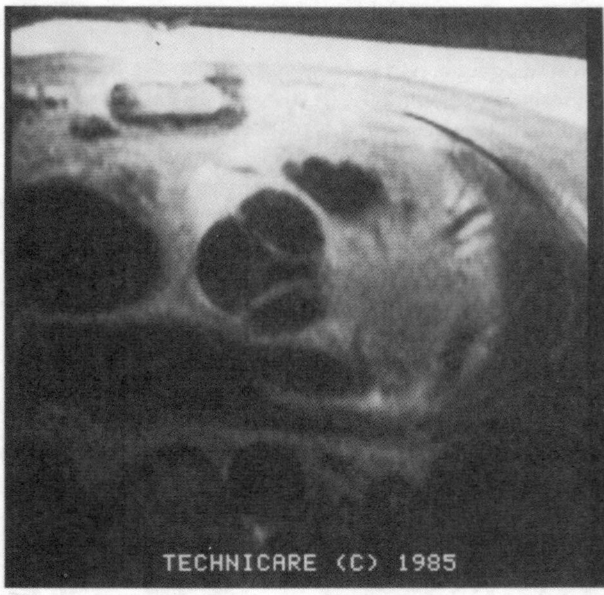

C

Figure 8.13. Nuclear magnetic resonance images of the chest of a normal person in sagittal (A), coronal (B), and transverse (C) planes. The images have been gated to decrease the effects of both cardiac and respiratory motion. The magnet strength was 0.6 tesla. C was taken with a surface coil resulting in a high-resolution image. Images in this and in figures 8.14 and 8.15 were provided courtesy of Technicare, Cleveland, Ohio.

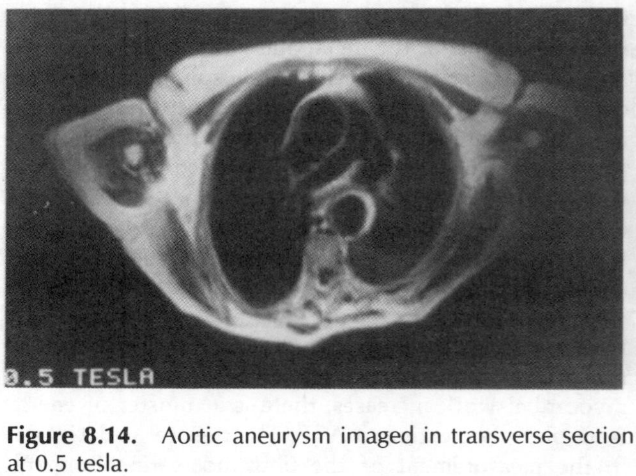

Figure 8.14. Aortic aneurysm imaged in transverse section at 0.5 tesla.

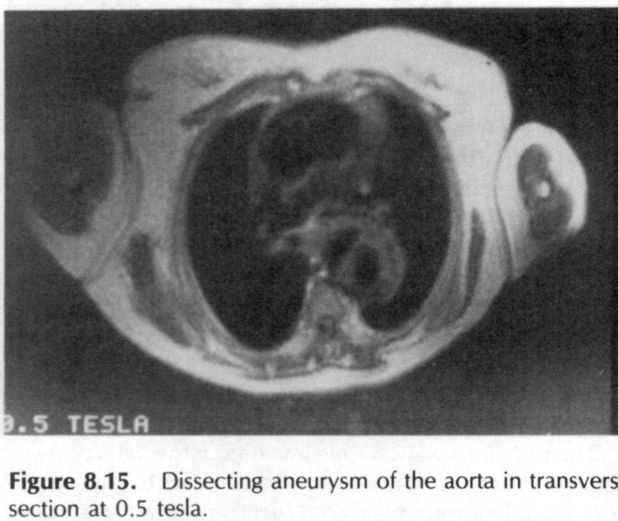

Figure 8.15. Dissecting aneurysm of the aorta in transverse section at 0.5 tesla.

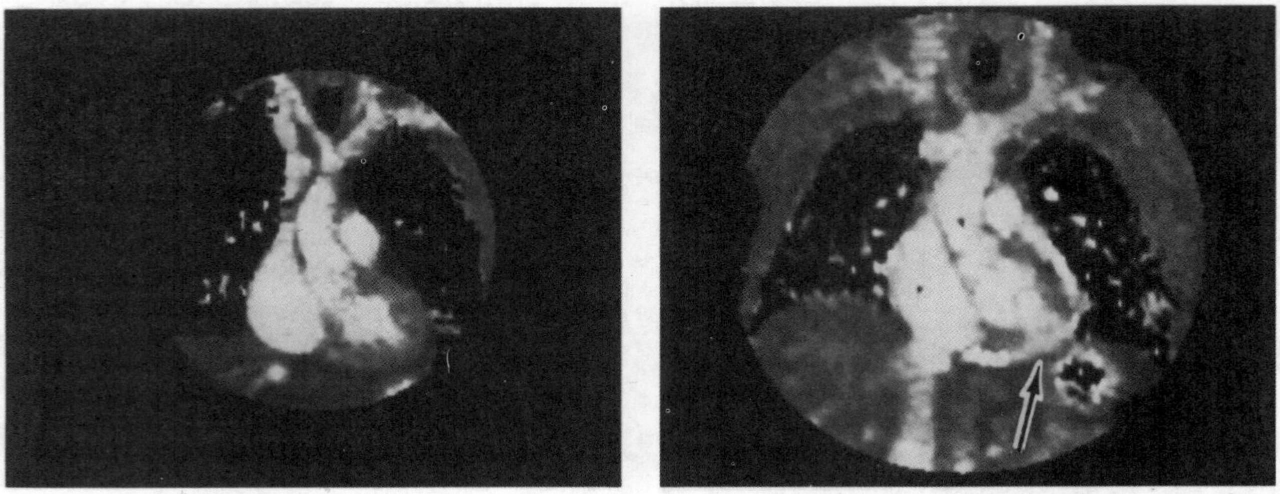

Figure 8.16. Gated magnetic resonance images of a normal subject (*left*) and a man eight days after inferior myocardial infarction (*right*). The infarcted heart shows an area of high spin-lattice relaxation time in the inferoapical region of the left ventricle above the *arrow*. There is also a small amount of pericardial fluid seen as a rim around the heart. (From Been M, Smith MA, Ridgeway JP, Brydon JWE, Douglas RHB, Kean DM, Best JJK, Muir AL: Characterization of acute myocardial infarction by gated magnetic resonance imaging. *Lancet* 1985; 2:348–350. Reproduced by permission.)

and the manner in which the resonant signals are recorded as the return from the regions of interest within the heart. The pulse sequences determine the contrast that is obtained from the various components of the different types of tissue. In addition to proton density and T_1 and T_2 relaxation, signals are affected by the movement of blood and thus it is possible to assess regional blood flow.

CHEMICAL SHIFT

The resonant signals depend not only on the number of protons within a region, but also on the chemical form of the protons. Measurement of the number of pulses of each of the emitted radio frequencies produces an energy spectrum called "chemical shift." This type of spectroscopy can differentiate the various states of phosphorus, such as phosphocreatine, inorganic phosphorus, ATP, and ADP. For "chemical shift imaging," the stronger the magnet the better, although adequate structural information from proton imaging can be obtained with lower magnet strengths, an important consideration because cost and complexity of NMR increase with increasing magnet strength.

APPLICATIONS

In most cases it is not necessary to administer contrast material to differentiate blood pools from structures, because movement of blood itself affects the NMR signals. Pericardium, valves, and interventricular septa can be visualized in addition to the movement of the ventricular walls. The acquisition time for cardiac imaging by NMR is on the order of five minutes, during which the electrocardiogram is used to examine specific parts of the cardiac cycle. Using dimensions obtained from the images, it is possible to calculate ventricular volume, stroke volume, and ejection fraction.

The use of relaxation time imaging in the detection and quantification of the size of areas of acute myocardial infarction looks promising.[60a] Nuclear magnetic resonance proton imaging is particularly suitable for the differential diagnosis of congenital heart disease.[61,62] Valvular lesions, septal defects, atresia, and transposition of the great vessels have all been identified.[63] The clinical role of NMR imaging relative to echocardiography in the identification of such conditions remains to be determined.[63a]

In essence, the great appeal of proton NMR imaging lies in: (1) the lack of ionizing radiation; (2) the high quality images of structure; and (3) the ability to image in any desired plane. Nevertheless, because of the existence of other imaging techniques, such as echocardiography and nuclear cardiology, the structurally oriented proton imaging methods do not create as great excitement as does the examination of other nuclei, particularly phosphorus.

BIOENERGETICS

Phosphorus is a major constituent of the high energy molecules, ATP and phosphocreatine, which provide energy to the cells of the heart. By measuring the relative concentrations of these compounds and their metabolites in different regions of the heart, it is possible to assess their metabolic status. Intracellular lactic acid, another important signal of the metabolic status of the heart, can also be measured. Adenosine triphosphate is an immediate source of energy, whereas phosphocreatine provides an intermediate storage mechanism. Adenosine triphosphate is produced in the heart by glycolysis and mitochondrial oxidative phosphorylation, the former not requiring oxygen. Under normal conditions, when oxygen supply is adequate, anaerobic glycolysis accounts for only about 10% of ATP production. During extreme cardiac work, glycolysis can almost triple. Under conditions of ischemia, glycolysis provides an increasing percentage of the energy needed for contraction and types of work. As myocardial work increases, there is a transfer of energy from phosphocreatine to ATP. The transfer is detectable in the measurement of the phosphocreatine inorganic phosphorus ratio.[64,65] Impairment of energy production is believed to be an important feature of myocardial injury associated with myocardial infarction. In applying mechanical reperfusion techniques or pharmacologic interventions after myocardial infarction, it may soon be possible to assess myocardial bioenergetics to supplement functional information such as regional wall motion and global ventricular ejection fraction.

An optimistic projection for the future is metabolic imaging where images are produced that reflect the distribution and concentration of metabolically important nuclei, such as ^{31}P, within the myocardium.[60a] At present, the time required to generate such images raises concern regarding the clinical feasibility of this technique. Another possibility may be the tandem use of hydrogen magnetic resonance imaging along with ^{31}P spectroscopy sampled from a region of interest within the gated hydrogen MRI of the ventricle. However, although such a combination of imaging and spectroscopy has been shown to be feasible for the human brain, its use in the evaluation of regional myocardial metabolism in patients will require considerable technological advances.

REFERENCES

1. Liu XJ, Harrison KS, Wagner HN Jr: Measurement of left ventricular ejection fraction with ionic indium-113m and a cardiac probe. *Eur J Nucl Med* 1982; 7:410–412.
2. Liu XJ, Liu Y, Wu Q, Zhou B, Zhang W, Kou W, Gao R, Chen Z, Wagner HN Jr: Evaluation of left ventricular diastolic function in patients with coronary artery disease. *Chin J Nucl Med* 1984; 4:200–202.
3. Liu XJ, Wagner HN Jr, Ehrlich W, Harrison KS: Measurement of left ventricular function using a cardiac probe in experimental and clinical studies. *Chin J Nucl Med* 1983; 3:151–154.
4. Liu XJ, Wagner HN Jr, Harrison KS, Douglass KH, Camargo EE: A simplified method for background correction in the measurement of left ventricular ejection fraction. *Chin J Nucl Med* 1983; 3:155–158.
5. Liu XJ, Wagner HN Jr, Tao S: Measurement of effects of the Chinese herbal medicine higenamine on left ventricular function using a cardiac probe. *Eur J Nucl Med* 1983; 8:233–236.
6. Harrison KS, Liu XJ, Han ST, Camargo EE, Wagner HN Jr: Evaluation of a miniature CdTe detector for monitoring left ventricular function. *Eur J Nucl Med* 1982; 7:204–206.
7. Wagner HN Jr, Wake R, Nickoloff E, Natarajan TK: The nuclear stethoscope: a simple device for generation of left ventricular volume curves. *Am J Cardiol* 1976; 38:747–750.
8. Berger HJ, Davies RA, Batsford WP, Hoffer PB, Gottschalk A, Zaret BL: Beat-to-beat left ventricular performance assessed from the equilibrium cardiac blood pool using a computerized nuclear probe. *Circulation* 1981; 63:133–142.
9. Wagner HN Jr: The nuclear cardiac probe. *Hosp Pract* 1982; 17(4):163–177.
10. Wagner HN Jr, Rigo P, Baxter RH, Alderson PO, Douglass KH, Housholder DR: Monitoring ventricular function at rest and during exercise with nonimaging nuclear detector. *Am J Cardiol* 1979; 43:975–979.
11. Strashun A, Horowitz SF, Goldsmith SJ, Teichholz LE, Dicker A, Miceli K, Gorlin R: Noninvasive detection of left ventricular dysfunction with a portable electrocardiographic gated scintillation probe device. *Am J Cardiol* 1981; 47:610–617.
12. Strashun A, Goldsmith SJ, Horowitz SF: Serial Assessment of Doxorubicin Cardiomyopathy With the Computerized Scintillation Probe (abstr). Third World Congress of Nuclear Medicine, Paris, France, 1982.
13. Camargo EE, Harrison KS, Wagner HN Jr, Bourguignon MH, Reid PR, Alderson PO, Baxter RH: Noninvasive beat-to-beat monitoring of left ventricular function by a nonimaging nuclear detector during premature ventricular contractions. *Am J Cardiol* 1980; 45:1219–1224.
14. Berger HJ, Byrd W, Giles R, Orphanoudakis S, Zaret BL: Beat-to-beat left ventricular pressure-volume relationships assessed from the equilibrium cardiac blood pool using a computerized nonimaging nuclear probe. *IEEE Computers in Cardiology* 1981; 55–60.

14a. Liang H, Chen K, Zhou Q, Wang Z, Zhou Z: Clinical effects of Ginseng injection and Ginseng Co injection on the aged patients with heart failure using computerized nuclear stethoscope. *Chin J Integrated Traditional & Western Med* 1986; 6:13–16.

15. Pavel DG, Zimmer AM, Patterson VN: *In vivo* labeling of red blood cells with ^{99m}Tc: a new approach to blood pool visualization. *J Nucl Med* 1977; 18:305–308.
16. Ritchie JL, Zaret BL, Strauss HW, Pitt B, Berman DS, Schelbert HR, Ashburn WL, Berger HJ, Hamilton GW: Myocardial imaging with thallium-201: a multicenter study in patients with angina or acute myocardial infarction. *Am J Cardiol* 1978; 42:345–350.
17. Botvinick EH, Taradash MR, Shames DM, Parmley WW: Thallium-201 myocardial perfusion scintigraphy for the clinical clarification of normal, abnormal and equivocal electrocardiographic stress tests. *Am J Cardiol* 1978; 41:43–51.
18. Hamilton GW, Trobaugh GB, Ritchie JL, Gould KL, DeRouen TA, William DL: Myocardial imaging with ^{201}thallium: an analysis of clinical usefulness based on Bayes theorem. *Seminars Nucl Med* 1978; 8:358–364.
19. Berman DS, Garcia EV, Maddahi J, Rozanski A: Thallium-201 myocardial perfusion scintigraphy, in Freeman LM (ed): *Freeman and Johnson's Clinical Radionuclide Imaging*, ed 3. New York, Grune & Stratton, 1984, vol 1, pp 479–537.
20. Beller GA, Pohost GM: Mechanism for T1-201 redistribution after transient myocardial ischemia (abstr). *Circulation* 1977; 56(suppl III):III–141.
21. Grunwald AM, Watson DD, Holzgrefe HH Jr, Irving JF, Beller GA: Myocardial thallium-201 kinetics in normal and ischemic myocardium. *Circulation* 1981; 64:610–618.

21a. Hurst JW: *The Heart*, ed 6. New York, McGraw-Hill, 1986, pp 1838–1839.

22. Marshall RC, Wisenberg G, Schelbert HR, Henze E: Effect of oral propranolol on rest, exercise and postexercise left ventricular performance in normal subjects and patients with coronary artery disease. *Circulation* 1981; 63:572–583.
23. Goris ML, Daspit SG, McLaughlin P, Kriss JP: Interpolative background subtraction. *J Nucl Med* 1976; 17:744–747.
24. Burow RD, Pond M, Schafer AW, Becker L: "Circumferential profiles": a new method for computer analysis of thallium-201 myocardial perfusion images. *J Nucl Med* 1979; 20:771–777.
25. Garcia E, Maddahi J, Berman D, Waxman A: Space/time quantitation of thallium-201 myocardial scintigraphy. *J Nucl Med* 1981; 22:309–317.
26. Wackers FJ Th, Fetterman RC, Mattera JA, Clements JP: Quantitative planar thallium-201 stress scintigraphy: a critical evaluation of the method. *Sem Nucl Med* 1985; 15:46–66.

26a. Kaul S, Newell JB, Chesler DA, Pohost GM, Okada RD, Guiney TE, Boucher CA: Value of computer analysis of exercise thallium images in the noninvasive detection of coronary artery disease. *JAMA* 1986; 255:508–511.

26b. Van Train KF, Berman DS, Garcia EV, Berger HJ, Sands MJ, Friedman JD, Freeman MR, Pryzlak M, Ashburn WL, Norris SL, Green AM, Maddahi J: Quantitative analysis of stress thallium-201 myocardial scintigrams: a multicenter trial. *J Nucl Med* 1986; 27:17–25.

26c. Kaul S, Boucher CA, Newell JB, Chesler DA, Greenberg JM, Okada RD, Strauss HW, Dinsmore RE, Pohost GM: Determination of the quantitative thallium imaging variables that optimize detection of coronary artery disease. *J Am Coll Cardiol* 1986; 7:527–537.

27. Ritchie JL, Olson DO, Williams DL, Harp G, Caldwell JH, Hamillon GW: Transaxial computer tomography with ^{201}TL in patients with prior myocardial infarction (abstr). *J Nucl Med* 1981; 22:11.
28. Tamaki N, Yonekura Y, Mukai T, Fujita T, Nohara R, Kadota K, Kambara H, Kawai C, Torizuka K, Ishii Y: Segmental analysis of stress thallium myocardial emission tomography for localization of coronary artery disease. *Eur J Nucl Med* 1984; 9:99–105.

28a. Coleman RE, Blinder RA, Jaszczak RJ: Single photon emission computed tomography (SPECT). Part II: clinical applications. *Invest Radiol* 1986; 21:1–11.

29. Maddahi J, Garcia EV, Berman DS, Waxman A, Swan HJC, Forrester J: Improved noninvasive assessment of coronary artery disease by quantitative analysis of regional stress myocardial distribution and washout of thallium-201. *Circulation* 1981; 64:924–935.
30. Wackers FJ, Klay JW, Laks H, Schnitzer J, Zaret BL, Geha AS: Pathophysiologic correlates of right ventricular thallium-201 uptake in a canine model. *Circulation* 1981; 64:1256–1264.
31. Pohost GM, Zir LM, Moore RH, McKusick KA, Guiney TE, Beller GA: Differentiation of transiently ischemic from infarcted myocardium by serial imaging after a single dose of thallium-201. *Circulation* 1977; 55: 294–302.
32. Silverman KJ, Becker LC, Bulkley BH, Burow RD, Mellits ED, Kallman CH, Weisfeldt ML: Value of early thallium-201 scintigraphy for predicting mortality in patients with acute myocardial infarction. *Circulation* 1980; 61:996–1003.
33. Mullani NA, Goldstein RA, Gould KL, Marani SK, Fisher DJ, O'Brien HA Jr, Loberg MD: Myocardial perfusion with rubidium-82. I. Measurement of extraction fraction and flow with external detectors. *J Nucl Med* 1983; 24:898–906.
34. Goldstein RA, Mullani NA, Marani SK, Fisher DJ, Gould KL, O'Brien

HA Jr: Myocardial perfusion with rubidium-82: II. Effects of metabolic and pharmacologic interventions. *J Nucl Med* 1983: 24:907–915.

35. Mullani NA: Myocardial perfusion with rubidium-82: III. Theory relating severity of coronary stenosis to perfusion deficit. *J Nucl Med* 1984; 25:1190–1196.

35a. Holman BL: Replacing thallium 201. *Applied Cardiol* 1986; 14:7.

36. Bonte FJ, Parkey RW, Graham KD, Moore J, Stokely EM: A new method for radionuclide imaging of myocardial infarcts. *Radiology* 1974; 110:473–474.

37. LaFrance ND, Becker L, Takeda K, Gato N, Links JM, Ravert H, Wong D, Wagner HN Jr: Indium-111 antimyosin antibody (Ab) for assessing myocardial damage (abstr). *J Nucl Med* 1985; 26(5):33.

38. Lyons KP, Olson HG, Aronow WS: Pyrophosphate myocardial imaging. *Semin Nucl Med* 1980; 10:168–177.

39. Olson HG, Lyons KP, Aronow WS, Kuperus J, Orlando J, Hughes D: Prognostic value of a persistently positive technetium-99m stannous pyrophosphate myocardial scintigram after myocardial infarction. *Am J Cardiol* 1979: 43:889–898.

40. Rude RE, Parkey RW, Bonte FJ, Lewis SE, Twieg D, Buja LM, Willerson JT: Clinical implications of the technetium-99m stannous pyrophosphate myocardial scintigraphic "doughnut" pattern in patients with acute myocardial infarcts. *Circulation* 1979; 59:721–730.

41. Berger HJ, Gottschalk A, Zaret BL: Radionuclide assessment of left and right ventricular performance. *Radiol Clin North Am* 1980; 18:441–466.

42. Berger HJ, Matthay RA, Pytlik LM, Gottschalk A, Zaret BL: First-pass radionuclide assessment of right and left ventricular performance in patients with cardiac and pulmonary disease. *Semin Nucl Med* 1979; 9: 275–295.

43. Berger HJ, Zaret BL: Nuclear cardiology. *N Engl J Med* 1981; 305:799–807, 855–865.

44. Berger HG, Zaret BL: Radionuclide assessment of cardiovascular performance, in Freeman LM (ed): *Freeman and Johnson's Clinical Radionuclide Imaging*, ed 3. New York, Grune & Stratton, Inc, 1984, pp 364–478.

45. Bonow RO, Bacharach SL, Green MV, Kent KM, Rosing DR, Lipson LC, Leon MB, Epstein SE: Impaired left ventricular diastolic filling in patients with coronary artery disease: assessment with radionuclide angiography. *Circulation* 1981; 64:315–323.

46. Jones RH, McEwan P, Newman GE, Port S, Rerych SK, Scholz PM, Upton MT, Peter CA, Austin EH, Leong KH, Gibbons RJ, Cobb FR, Coleman RE, Sabiston DC Jr: Accuracy of diagnosis of coronary artery disease by radionuclide measurement of left ventricular function during rest and exercise. *Circulation* 1981; 64:586–601.

46a. Green MV, Bacharach SL: Functional imaging of the heart: methods, limitations and examples from gated blood pool scintigraphy. *Progr Cardiovasc Dis* 1986; 28:319–348.

47. Schelbert HR, Phelps ME, Hoffman E, Huang S-C, Kuhl DE: Regional myocardial blood flow, metabolism and function assessed noninvasively with positron emission tomography. *Am J Cardiol* 1980; 46:1269–1277.

48. Schelbert HR, Henze E, Phelps ME, Kuhl DE: Assessment of regional myocardial ischemia by positron-emission computed tomography. *Am Heart J* 1982; 103:588–597.

49. Schelbert HR: Radionuclide assessment of myocardial metabolism, in Freeman LM (ed): *Freeman and Johnson's Clinical Radionuclide Imaging*, ed 3. New York, Grune & Stratton, 1984, vol 1, pp 563–610.

50. Schon HR, Schelbert HR, Robinson G, Najafi A, Huang SC, Hanson H, Barrio J, Kuhl DE, Phelps ME: C-11 labeled palmitic acid for the noninvasive evaluation of regional myocardial fatty acid metabolism with positron-computed tomography. I. Kinetics of C-11 palmitic acid in normal myocardium. *Am Heart J* 1982; 103:532–547.

51. Schelbert HR, Henze E, Keen R, Schon HR, Hansen H, Selin C, Huang SC, Barrio JR, Phelps ME: C-11 palmitate for the noninvasive evaluation of regional myocardial fatty acid metabolism with positron-computed tomography. IV. *In vivo* evaluation of acute demand-induced ischemia in dogs. *Am Heart J* 1983; 106:736–750.

52. Lerch RA, Ambos HD, Bergmann SR, Welch MJ, Ter-Pogossian MM, Sobel BE: Localization of viable, ischemic myocardium by positron-emission tomography with ^{11}C palmitate. *Circulation* 1981; 64:689–699.

53. Schelbert HR, Henze E, Schon HR, Keen R, Hansen HW, Selin C, Huang SC, Barrio JR, Phelps ME: C-11 palmitate for the noninvasive evaluation of regional myocardial fatty acid metabolism with positron computed tomography. III. In vivo demonstration of the effects of substrate availability on myocardial metabolism. *Am Heart J* 1983; 105: 492–504.

54. Freundlieb C, Hock A, Vysha K, Freinendegen LE, Machulla HJ, Stöcklin G: Myocardial imaging and metabolic studies with [17-^{123}I] iodoheptadecanoic acid. *J Nucl Med* 1980; 21:1043–1050.

55. Machulla HJ, Stöcklin G, Kupfernagel Ch, Freundlieb Ch, Höck A, Vyska K, Feinendegen LE: Comparative evaluation of fatty acids labeled with C–11, Cl-34m, Br–77, and I–123 for metabolic studies of the myocardium: *J Nucl Med* 1978; 19:298–302.

56. Deanfield JE, Maseri A, Selwyn AP, Ribeiro P, Chierchia S, Krikler S, Morgan M: Myocardial ischemia during daily life in patients with stable angina. Its relation to symptoms and heart rate changes. *Lancet* 1983: 2:753–758.

56a. Pohost GM, Elgavish GA, Evanochko WT: Nuclear magnetic resonance imaging: with or without nuclear? *J Am Coll Cardiol* 1986; 7:709–710.

57. Pohost GM, Ratner AV: Nuclear magnetic resonance: potential applications in clinical cardiology. *JAMA* 1984; 251:1304–1309.

58. Byrd BF III, Higgins CB, Lanzer P, Botvinick EH, Lipton MJ, Schiller NB: Clinical cardiac magnetic resonance imaging, in Collins SM, Skorton DJ (eds): *Cardiac Imaging and Image Processing*. New York, McGraw-Hill, 1986, pp 407–418.

59. Higgins CB, McNamera MT: Magnetic resonance imaging of ischemic heart disease. *Progr Cardiovasc Dis* 1986; 28:257–266.

60. Wesby G, Higgins CB, Lanzer P, Botvinick E, Lipton MJ: Imaging and characterization of acute myocardial infarction *in vivo* by gated nuclear magnetic resonance. *Circulation* 1984; 69:124–130.

60a. Higgins CB, McNamara MT: Magnetic resonance imaging of ischemic heart disease. *Progr Cardiovasc Dis* 1986; 28:257–266.

61. Fletcher BD, Jacobstein MD, Nelson AD, Riemenschneider TA, Alfidi RJ: Gated magnetic resonance imaging of congenital cardiac malformations. *Radiology* 1984; 150:137–140.

62. Higgins CB, Byrd BF III, Farmer DW, Osaki L, Silverman NH, Cheitlin MD: Magnetic resonance imaging in patients with congenital heart disease. *Circulation* 1984; 70:851–860.

63. Higgins CB, Byrd BF II, McNamara MT, Lanzer P, Lipton MJ, Botvinick E, Schiller NB, Crooks LE, Kaufman L: Magnetic resonance imaging of the heart: a review of the experience in 172 subjects. *Radiology* 1985; 155:671–679.

63a. Lanzier PA, Ortendahl DA, Botvinick EH, Higgins CB: Cardiac imaging by magnetic resonance, in Collins SM, Skorton DJ (eds): *Cardiac Imaging and Image Processing*. New York, McGraw-Hill, 1986, pp 88–104.

64. Neely JR, Morgan HE: Relationship between carbohydrate and lipid metabolism and the energy balance of heart muscle. *Ann Rev Physiol* 1974; 36:413–459.

65. Jacobus WE: General introduction. Myocardial energy transport: current concepts of the problem, in Jacobus WE, Ingwall JS (eds): *Heart Creatine Kinase: The Integration of Isozymes for Energy Transport*. Baltimore, Williams & Wilkins, 1980, pp 1–5.

9 High Speed Computed X-Ray Tomography in Cardiac Imaging

Erik L. Ritman, MD, PhD

The techniques and clinical usefulness of computerized axial tomography (CAT) are well established for head and body imaging. Extending this technique to the cardiovascular system has required the development of new machines. The fundamental problem in imaging the beating heart with CAT is that the time required to complete a scan is lengthy in comparison with the duration of a single cardiac cycle. Although the most serious problem is the motion blurring artifact that results from the scan duration, there is also the problem that a single slice image of the heart (even if scanned at high speed) generally cannot adequately convey the heart's entire three-dimensional shape.

One of the first attempts at cardiac CAT scanning used commercially available whole-body scanners (with a 4- to 5-second scan time) following intravenous injection of a contrast agent. Although the resulting images often appeared good, this was partly due to the so-called "dwell" effect, ie, the heart wall is fairly stationary during its diastolic phase, which at resting heart rates is the predominant fraction of the cardiac cycle. Therefore, the brief, fast-moving systolic phase of the cycle is blurred, leaving the diastolic phase imaged fairly sharply. In hearts with regional hypokinesia, this dwell effect is reinforced in the hypokinetic region. It is unlikely, however, that these images are quantitatively accurate despite their good appearance. For this reason, and for imaging the systolic phase, gated CAT scanning was used.

Gated CAT scanning also used commercial CAT scanners which were modified to reorder the scan data before image reconstruction. A continuous sequence of scans is performed (usually for 10 to 20 seconds), and an electrocardiogram is simultaneously recorded. The time period of one heart cycle is divided into a number of equal time segments (usually 7 to 12 segments per cycle). The recorded projection data corresponding to equivalent cycle segments of sequential cardiac cycles are pooled to give the necessary scan data for each segment of a single representative electrocardiographic cycle. Then image reconstruction for each cycle segment is performed. Many heart cycles are thus used to reconstruct a single, presumably representative, "average" cycle. Reports have appeared in the literature using this method for imaging myocardial infarction,[1] establishing patency of coronary artery bypass grafts,[2] measuring regional contraction[3] and systolic wall thickening,[4] and estimating regional blood flow.[5]

These methods all have the basic limitation that only one slice is scanned at any one time. Even if only one localized structure within the heart is of interest, accurate measurements cannot be made if this slice is not in the right location and orientation relative to the structure of interest.

One solution to the problem of collecting many angles of view and scanning a number of contiguous slices in a short time is provided by the CardioVascular Computed Tomography scanner presently marketed by the Imatron Company of San Francisco.[6] In this system, there is no mechanically moving gantry. Instead, the x-ray source consists of four parallel pairs of semicircular tungsten target rings spanning 210 degrees about the patient. A high intensity electron beam is electromagnetically swept along one target ring at a time, thereby creating a rotating fan beam of x-ray. Opposite each x-ray source target, multiple side-by-side scintillation crystal detectors record incident x-ray intensity. Eight transaxial slices (8 mm thick and at 1-cm intervals) are scanned by sweeping the beam sequentially over the target rings and recording x-ray intensity after passing through the body. Scan speeds of 50 ms per slice (plus an 8-ms reset interval) are being obtained; hence, eight near parallel slices (scanned two per sweep) require approximately 240 ms to complete. The high-speed/multiple slice capability offers significant advantage over the gated conventional CT method, and images over much of the entire apex-to-base extent of the heart can be obtained.[7] The main disadvantage of this system is that it is not fully three-dimensional because its spatial resolution in the cephalocaudal direction is much less than that in the transverse direction. In addition, several sequential eight-slice scans will need to be repeated at different phases of the cardiac cycle (during sequential heart cycles) so that an image is provided for each of the eight slices for each selected phase of the cardiac cycle. This would therefore involve prolonged, intravenous infusion or multiple injections of roentgen contrast agent if the whole cardiac chamber needs to be imaged throughout the cardiac cycle.[7]

DYNAMIC SPATIAL RECONSTRUCTION SCANNER

Another method of rapid cardiac CT scanning is the Dynamic Spatial Reconstructor (DSR) designed and installed at the Mayo Clinic.[8] It is a system capable of dynamic, synchronous *volume** imaging. The scanner has a multisource/multidetector arrangement of 14 x-ray tubes producing overlapping x-ray images on curved fluorescent screens. In turn, the images produced by the fluorescent screens are imaged by 14 video cameras. The x-ray tubes, screens, and cameras are all mounted on a rotating gantry (Figure 9.1). Each tube is pulsed in sequence, creating an image on the fluorescent screen, read by a television camera and recorded on stop-action video disks. The video disk images are later converted to digital values and used for computing up to 120, sequential transverse slices, each 0.9 mm thick and at either 0.9- or 1.8-mm intervals, depending on the scan mode selected. Figure 9.2 depicts a "stack" of transverse images making a volume image. When combined, this image stack describes a cylindrical volume 22 to 39 cm in transaxial diameter and 22 cm in axial height. Once such volume can be scanned every 1/60 second.

A tradeoff exists between time resolution and image quality. Images from sequential scans can be added to improve spatial resolution at the expense of temporal resolution (eg, when four sequential volume images are added, temporal resolution is reduced from 1/60 second to 4/60 second). If this addition is performed during the end-diastolic phase of the cardiac cycle, little blurring results. This ability to perform retrospective digital image manipulation is a powerful advantage.

Dynamic Spatial Reconstructor images may be either qualitative (for showing three-dimensional anatomic shapes, relations, etc), quantitative (for measuring physiologic parameters in space and time), or both. Several display methods in current use were developed to facilitate these two forms of data analysis.

PROJECTION–DISSOLUTION DISPLAY METHOD

This method of display was developed to provide a rapid overview of an entire volume image primarily to facilitate detection of a lesion or of an anatomic feature for measurement. Let us suppose an investigator wishes to view the three-dimensional course of a contrast-filled coronary artery contained within a volume image reconstructed from a DSR scan. An example of a canine coronary artery projection dissolution image is shown in Figure 9.3. The processing computer is instructed to detect only those "voxels" (picture elements in the volume image) that have intensity (CT numbers) corresponding to the concentration of contrast medium in the desired vessel. In effect, by ignoring all other voxels, the computer has "dissolved" unwanted, potentially obscuring or camouflaging structures. The computer then projects the detected voxels onto a television screen, showing the two-dimensional projection of the artery without the surrounding, potentially obscuring, less radiopaque structures. The computer program may now be instructed to project the artery from different angles of view, and when each angle is viewed sequentially in rapid succession, the artery appears to rotate. The computer-generated rotation eliminates the need for repeat injection and angiographic imaging at a new angle of view, commonly necessary in conventional coronary angiography. Another method developed to provide a similar image analysis function in-

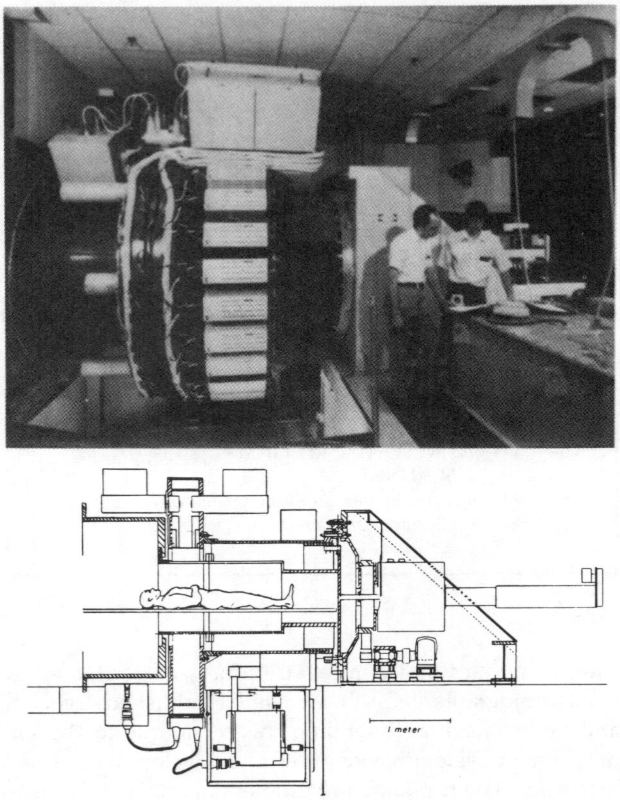

Figure 9.1. *Top,* Dynamic Spatial Reconstructor scanner assembly. The entire structure to the left of the men is cantilevered from the triangular base. Multiple image isocon TV cameras and corresponding x-ray sources are arranged along a vertical plane. Rotation of the cantilevered section increases the number of angles of view per scan in proportion to the programmed duration of the scan. *Bottom,* Midline longitudinal section of the scanner shows relation of human subject lying on table and the surrounding gantry. (From Behrenbeck T, Sinak LJ, Robb RA, Kinsey JH, Ritman EL: Some imaging characteristics of the Dynamic Spatial Reconstructor x-ray scanner system, in Reba RC, Goodenough DJ, Davidson HF [eds]: *Diagnostic Imaging in Medicine.* Boston, Martinus Nijhoff, 1983, pp 254–271, used with permission.)

* A volume image is an image of a three-dimensional object with spatial resolution comparable in all three orthogonal directions.

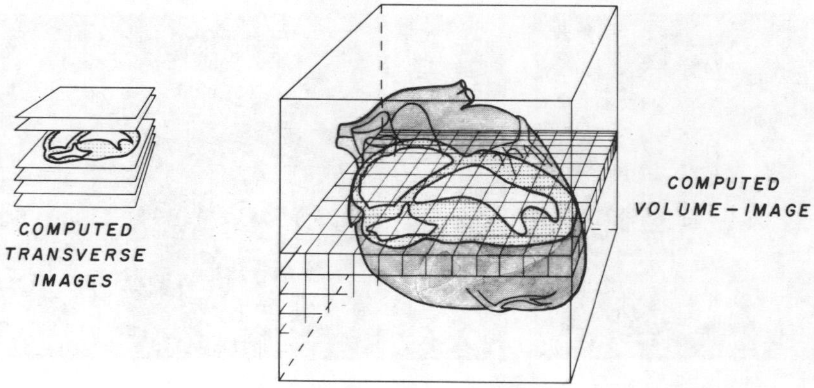

Figure 9.2. Creation of a three-dimensional image from multiple parallel images scanned synchronously within 11 ms. This volume is rescanned every 16.7 ms. This cubic array of volume picture elements (voxels) can be used to compute images of slices in any location, orientation, or thickness within the volume without loss of spatial resolution. (From Ritman EL, Harris LD, Padiyar HR, Chevalier PA, Robb RA: Non-invasive visualization and quantitation of cardiovascular structure and function. *Physiologist* 1979; 22(6):39–43. Used with permission.)

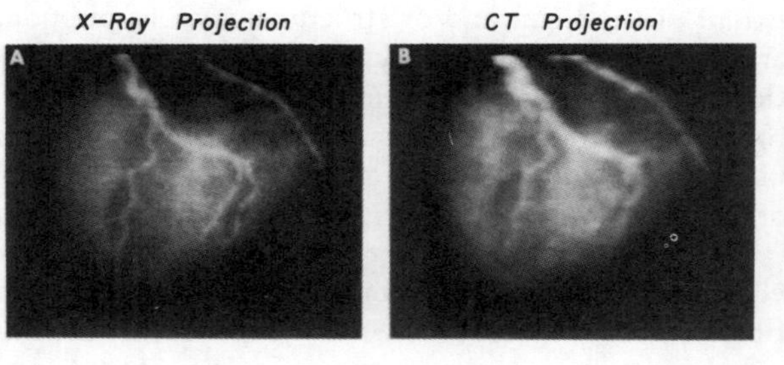

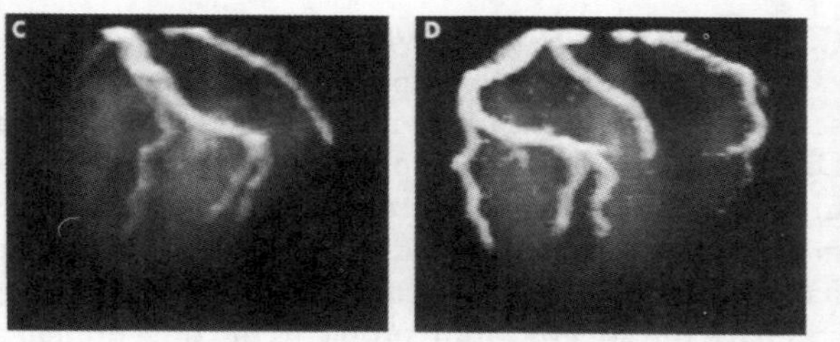

Figure 9.3. Projection images for conveying three-dimensional anatomy of coronary arterial tree. Base of the heart is at the top, apex at the bottom in each panel. *A,* Digital display of radiograph of isolated canine heart with x-ray contrast medium in coronary arteries. *B,* Computer-generated projection of volume reconstruction of the same canine heart. This two-dimensional image, generated from three-dimensional image data obtained by the transaxial reconstruction process, is slightly blurred but otherwise identical to the radiographs. *C,* Before projection, the intensity of the heart wall was selectively reduced, leaving the coronary arteries relatively brighter and more visible. This technique cannot be applied to the radiographs. *D,* Same partially dissolved image data as in *C,* but projected from a different angle of view. This image clearly shows the septal (central) coronary artery, which was obscured by the circumflex (left) coronary artery in *C.* In *C* and *D,* the dissolution was 83.5%; the angle of rotation was 0° and 45°, respectively. (From Ritman EL, Kinsey JH, Robb RA, Gilbert BK, Harris LD, Wood EH: Three-dimensional imaging of heart, lungs, and circulation. *Science* 1980; 210:273–280. Copyright 1980 by the AAAS, used with permission.)

volves the use of a three-dimensional display (analogous to a hologram) which is generated with a varifocal mirror system.[9]

SHADED SURFACE DISPLAYS

If an investigator wishes to view the myocardium itself, the computer may be programmed to select only voxels with image densities (brightness) of muscle. It can assemble these voxels, make each voxel nontransparent, and shade the resulting solid muscle as if illuminated by a light positioned at the observer's eye. Again, because this information is three-dimensional, images from all angles of view may be made, and the object can be rotated. An example is provided in Figure 9.4. Anatomic relations and shapes are easily conveyed with this kind of display.

An additional advantage of the shaded surface display is that because the volume of each voxel is known, counting individual voxels within the displayed anatomic structure permits calculation of the volume of the chambers[10] or the muscle itself.[11]

CROSS-SECTIONAL DISPLAY

Single sections in two-dimensional display are especially useful for measurement, provided the slice is in the right plane relative to the anatomic structure being measured. An interactive computer program used to manipulate the angle and location of an oblique section is demonstrated in Figure 9.5. Three thin orientation sections (from left to right they are sagittal, coronal, and transverse) are displayed across the top of the illustration. Brightened white lines overlaid on these orientation sections convey the intersection of the selected oblique plane with the orientation slice. An image of the selected oblique plane is shown en face in the lower panel of the figure. The computer is given interactive directions for changing the orientation and location of the plane as though the observer himself is moving through the volume image. These images from oblique planes are used to make length, area, and local image density measure-

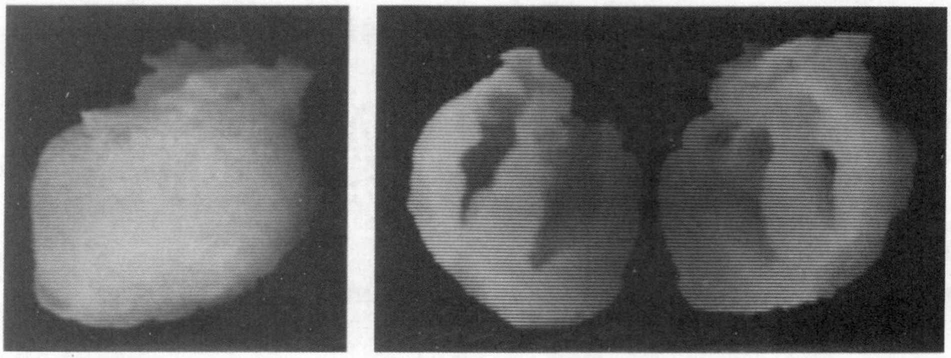

Figure 9.4. Computer-generated three-dimensional shaded surface display of heart determined from reconstructed heart: one after mathematical opening into halves to permit viewing of internal structures is shown. (Reprinted with permission from Robb RA: X-ray computed tomography: an engineering synthesis of multi-scientific principles. *Crit Rev Biomed Eng* 1982; 7:265–333. Copyright CRC Press, inc, Boca Raton, FL).

ments such as those needed for estimating vessel cross-sectional area, cardiac muscle volume, or tissue perfusion.

PARAMETERS FOR MEASUREMENT

Using the retrospective computer manipulation aspect of DSR images, three advances in noninvasive measurement result. First, multiple measurements can be made synchronously; second, measurements can be made with greatly increased accuracy relative to conventional imaging methods, and third, some measurements that were not previously possible using relatively noninvasive techniques can be made. Examples of these advances include measuring time-varying cardiac chamber volumes, cardiac muscle mass, and regional wall thickness[12] over the entire extent of the heart and of structures such as pulmonary arteries,[13] stenosed coronary arteries,[14] or ventricular outflow tracts.[15] Blood flow and tissue perfusion can be estimated by injecting a bolus of contrast medium into the bloodstream and observing changes in the image density of structures versus time.[16,17] Results in experimental animals to date indicate that cardiac chamber and muscle volumes can be estimated correctly to within 95%, blood flow in arteries to within 90% of independently measured values, and coronary artery stenoses down to 0.6 mm in luminal diameter.

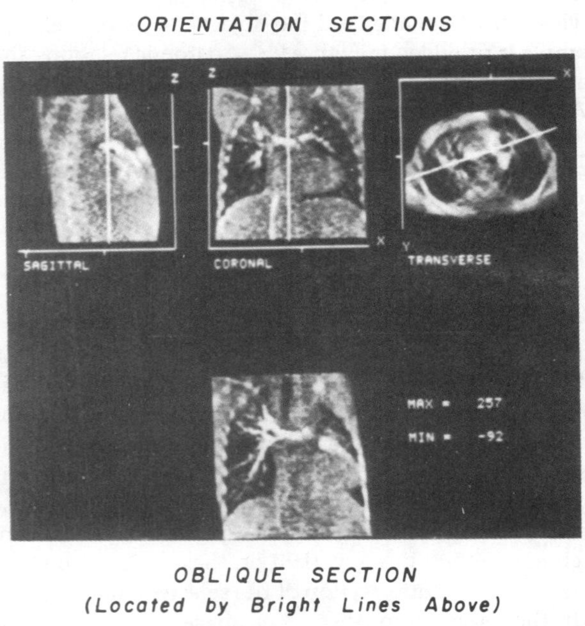

Figure 9.5. Visual feedback used by the operator to identify the orientation of an oblique section through the volume scanned by the Dynamic Spatial Reconstructor. In this case, the selected oblique section (*lower middle panel*) passes along the right pulmonary artery. (From Schwartz RS: Computed tomography in cardiac imaging. *Practical Cardiology* 1983; 9:224–238. Used with permission.)

COMPARATIVE PERSPECTIVE

A brief comment of comparative perspective on CAT scanning with other cardiac imaging methods is in order. Digital subtraction angiography is becoming very popular in recent years. Venous contrast injection is adequate for many important clinical studies because this method enhances angiographic image contrast. However, the images still have the superposition problems of conventional angiography, so that multiple angles of view and repeat angiograms are sometimes necessary. Volume scanning computed tomography overcomes these superposition limitations.

Nuclear magnetic resonance imaging (NMRI) is a new technique currently being tried for imaging cardiovascular structures. It has three-dimensional tomographic capabilities, but it has limited time resolution and hence may be unsuitable for many needs in quantitative cardiologic measurements.

Gated nuclear pooled blood studies are useful clinically for assessing ventricular function, but they have comparatively poor spatial and temporal resolution. Like cineangiographic techniques, this method is also limited by the superposition problem. For example, the left atrium superimposes partially on the left ventricle so that the volume of the ventricle cannot be defined with certainty.

Sector echocardiography is a comparatively inexpensive, noninvasive tomographic imaging technique with adequate spatial and good temporal resolution. However, it is of limited utility in visualizing coronary arteries or in accurately quantitating cardiac chamber or muscle volumes.

It is important to realize that the future of cardiac imaging is by no means decided. There are continual tradeoffs among spatial resolution, temporal resolution, cost, and complexity. It seems medicine has begun a new course in attempting to comprehend the beating heart. Where that course will lead should prove interesting indeed.

Acknowledgment: This work was supported in part by Research Grants HL-04664 and R-02540 from the National Institutes of Health, Bethesda, Maryland.

I thank my colleagues for the use of their image data, Delories C. Darling for typing this manuscript, and James L. Hanson for illustrating the DSR.

REFERENCES

1. Doherty PW, Lipton MJ, Berninger WH, Skioldebrand CG, Carlsson E, Redington RW: Detection and quantitation of myocardial infarction *in vivo* using transmission computed tomography. *Circulation* 1981; 63:597–606.
2. Brundage BH, Lipton MH, Herfkens RJ, Berninger WH, Redingon RW, Chatterjee K, Carlsson E: Detection of patent coronary bypass grafts by computed tomography: a preliminary report. *Circulation* 1980; 61:826–831.
3. Mattrey RF, Higgins CB: Detection of regional myocardial dysfunction during ischemia with computerized tomography. Documentation and physiologic basis. *Invest Radiol* 1982; 17:329–335.
4. Skioldebrand CG, Ovenfors CO, Mavroudis C, Lipton MJ: Assessment of ventricular wall thickness *in vivo* by computed transmission tomography. *Circulation* 1980; 61:960–965.
5. Nassi M, Brody WR: Regional myocardial flow estimation using computed tomography. *Med Phys* 1981; 8:302–307.
6. Boyd DP, Lipton MJ: Cardiac computed tomography. *Proc IEEE* 1983; 71:298–307.
7. Feiring AJ, Rumberger JA, Reiter SJ, Skorton DJ, Collins SM, Lipton MJ, Higgins CB, Ell S, Marcus ML: Determination of left ventricular mass in dogs with rapid-acquisition cardiac computed tomographic scanning. *Circulation* 1985; 72:1355–1364.
8. Ritman EL, Robb RA, Harris LD: *Imaging Physiological Functions: Experience with the DSR.* New York, Praeger, 1985.
9. Harris LD, Camp JJ: Display and analysis of tomographic volumetric images utilizing a varifocal mirror. *Society of Photo-Optical Instrumentation Engineers—Processing and Display of Three-Dimensional Data II* 1984; 507:38–45.
10. Hoffman EA, Ritman EL: Shape and dimensions of cardiac chambers: importance of CT section thickness and orientation. *Radiology* 1985; 155:739–744.
11. Iwasaki T, Sinak LJ, Hoffman EA, Robb RA, Harris LD, Bahn RC, Ritman EL: Mass of left ventricular myocardium estimated with the dynamic spatial reconstructor. *Am J Physiol:* 1984; 246 (*Heart Circ Physiol* 15:H138–142).
12. Schwartz RS, Bove AA, Bahn RC, Ritman EL: A method for quantitative display of three-dimensional regional myocardial function. *IEEE Trans Med Imaging* 1985; MI4:208–214.
13. Sinak LJ, Liu YH, Block M, Mair DD, Julsrud PR, Hoffman EA, Hagler DJ, Seward JB, Ritman EL: Anatomy and function of the heart and intrathoracic vessels in congenital heart disease: evaluation with the Dynamic Spatial Reconstructor. *J Am Coll Cardiol* 1985; 5(suppl): 70S–76S.
14. Block M, Bove AA, Ritman EL: Coronary angiographic examination with the Dynamic Spatial Reconstructor. *Circulation* 1984; 70:209–216.
15. Sinak LJ, Hoffman EA, Schwartz RS, Smith HC, Holmes DR, Bove AA, Robb RA, Harris LD, Ritman EL: Three-dimensional cardiac anatomy and function in heart disease in adults: initial results with the Dynamic Spatial Reconstructor. *Mayo Clin Proc* 1985; 60:383–392.
16. Iwasaki T, Ritman EL, Fiksen-Olsen MH, Romero JC, Knox FG: Renal cortical perfusion—preliminary experience with the Dynamic Spatial Reconstructor (DSR). *Ann Biomed Eng* 1985; 13:259–271.
17. Robb RA, Ritman EL, Harris LD: Digital image processing in x-ray computed tomography: high-speed volume imaging with the DSR, in Collins SM, Skorton DJ (eds), *Cardiac Imaging and Image Processing.* New York, McGraw-Hill, 1986, pp 361–406.

10 The Exercise Test As a Guide to Diagnosis, Management, and Prognosis

Myrvin H. Ellestad, MD and Jay H. Kozlowski, MD

Exercise stress testing has become one of the most commonly used noninvasive methods to evaluate ischemic heart disease. It has been useful in establishing a diagnosis, assessing the prognosis, and helping to formulate activity or exercise guidelines in the field of coronary disease.

HISTORY

In the late 1920s, Fiel and Seigel[1] reported on electrocardiographic changes that occurred during spontaneous episodes of angina pectoris. In the early 1940s, Master et al[2] studied the heart's response to exertion by recording electrocardiograms after a two-step exercise protocol. In the mid-1940s, Master began recording electrocardiographic tracings during his two-step test. From these early attempts at gaining an early assessment came the modern day treadmill stress test and a number of attendant protocols.

PROTOCOLS

Among the protocols commonly used in treadmill stress testing are those of Bruce, Balke, Balke-Ware, Naughton, Sheffield, and Ellestad. These are all designed to provide a graded stress with time for physiologic equilibration within particular stages. In Scandinavia and other parts of Europe, the cycle ergometer is a more popular mode of exercise stress testing. Herein, however, we will concentrate on the treadmill because of its almost universal acceptance in the United States (Figure 10.1).

ISOMETRIC STRESS

Isometric exercise (usually a sustained handgrip) increases cardiac work.[3] An isometric stress test using the handgrip dynamometer has been used in a number of centers. It increases blood pressure more than heart rate, and it is much less sensitive than the treadmill exercise test in diagnosing cardiovascular disease. The double product (heart rate × systolic blood pressure) does not become nearly as great with this type of "exercise." Somewhat surprisingly, when added to an isotonic or dynamic exercise, it may actually decrease the incidence of a positive or abnormal electrocardiographic response, ie, decreasing sensitivity.[4] DeBusk et al[5] showed that ischemic electrocardiographic responses and symptoms were delayed in combined stresses, possibly because of increased myocardial perfusion secondary to an increase in the aortic diastolic blood pressure.

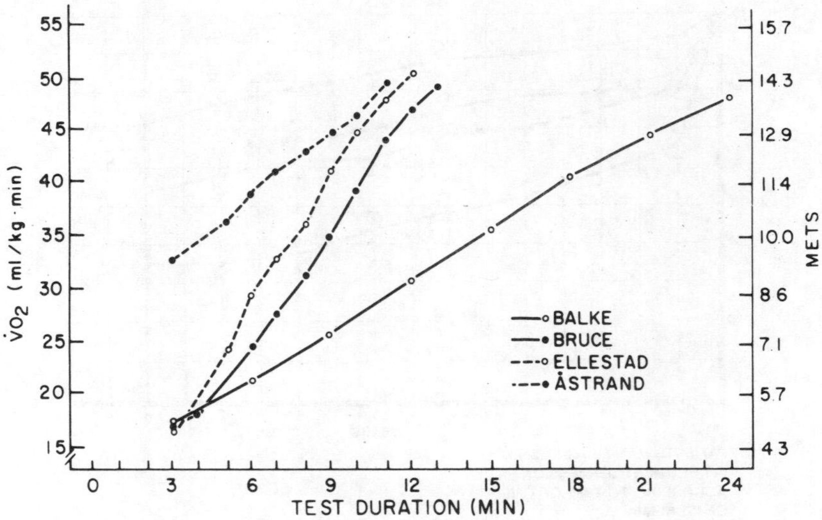

Figure 10.1. Comparison of maximal oxygen consumption and metabolic equivalent of four commonly used stress test protocols. All essentially have the same end point. (From Pollock ML, Bohannon RL, Cooper KH, Ayres JJ, Ward A, White SR, Linnerud AC: A comparative analysis of four protocols for maximal treadmill stress testing. *Am Heart J* 1976; 92:39–46. Used with permission.)

DIURNAL EFFECT

Although much stress testing is performed in the morning, this practice has recently been questioned. Joy et al[6] reported that a test performed in the morning is less likely to be positive or abnormal than one done later in the day. The investigators speculated that the discrepancy might be due to a diurnal variation in vagal tone.

DURATION OF EXERCISE

A stress test is negative or normal (with regard to ischemia) if there are no significant abnormalities (electrocardiographic or otherwise) and if the subject has achieved a satisfactory workload. This decision should be a clinical one and not based entirely on an arbitrary percentage of predicted maximum heart rate. The symptom-limited end point is more commonly used than the heart-rate–limited end point. Considerable information can be gleaned from a suboptimal performance.

ST-SEGMENT MAGNITUDE AND TIMING

Although the relation is not absolute,[7] generally the more pronounced the exercise-induced ST-segment depression, the greater the likelihood of significant coronary artery disease.[8–14] In addition to the configuration of the ST segment and the magnitude of its displacement, the time to onset and the persistence of significant ST-segment depression in recovery give further diagnostic and prognostic information. The significant ST-segment changes that occur early in a stress test at relatively low heart rates (less than 130 beats per minute) or that persist several minutes into recovery, or both, are suggestive of severe disease and an unfavorable prognosis[15,16] (Figure 10.2). The Coronary Artery Surgery Study has shown that exercise duration is an independent and important predictor of survival in patients with significant coronary disease. Perhaps most importantly, this relation held true in patients with severe, triple-vessel disease.[17]

LEAD SYSTEMS

The evaluation of ST-segment shifts during exercise has been the cornerstone of noninvasive assessment for coronary artery disease ever since Master's pioneering work.[2] Detection of exercise-induced ST-segment displacement depends on monitoring an appropriate number of electrocardiographic leads.[18] The use of 12 to 16 leads or more will increase sensitivity but may reduce specificity.[19,20] Most investigators have found that recording three leads is adequate in most clinical situations, and we favor leads V_1 or V_2; leads V_5, V_6, or CM_5; and lead aVF—a slightly altered orthogonal lead system. It has been shown that a single lead (V_5 or CM_5) will reveal about 80% of the ST-segment changes that would have been detected with a multiple lead system.[19,20] Many of the newer recorders now make 12-lead recording convenient, so that almost any lead system can be used.

LOCALIZATION OF DISEASE

Recently, Fox et al[21] found the sensitivity of treadmill stress testing in patients with documented single-vessel coronary artery disease to be similar in 12-lead, 3-lead (V_3, V_5, and aVF), and single-lead (V_5) systems. They further showed that the location of ST-segment depression did not allow prediction of the site of single-vessel obstruction. Other investigators employing thallium scintigraphy demonstrated that coronary artery disease cannot be accurately localized from the leads in which stress-induced ST-segment depression occurred. There was an overall poor correlation between thallium defects and an area of ischemia by electrocardiography.[21–23]

EXERCISE TESTING—INDICATIONS AND CONTRAINDICATIONS

Although indications for exercise stress testing are numerous (Table 10.1), the supervising physician must observe the contraindications, both relative and absolute[24]

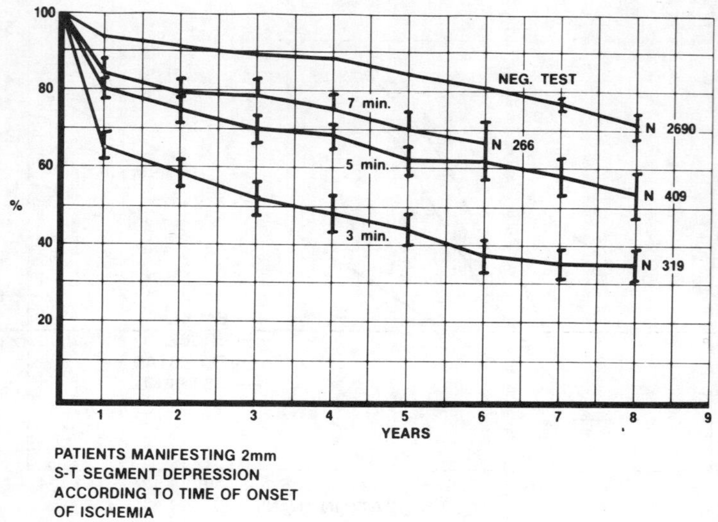

Figure 10.2. Life table data illustrate the prevalence of coronary events according to the time of appearance of ST-segment depression on our protocol. Magnitude of work can be compared by referring to Figure 10.1. (From Ellestad MH, Allen WH, Stuart RJ: Diagnostic and prognostic information derived from exercise testing, in Wenger NK (ed): *Exercise and the Heart*. Philadelphia, FA Davis, 1979. Used with permission.)

(see Table 10.2). Tests performed in persons with potential heart disease should be attended by a physician familiar with exercise testing who is able to handle any resultant complication and is familiar with the principles of exercise physiology. Such a person should know when to postpone or stop a test.

SAFETY

The incidence of fatality resulting from treadmill stress testing is less than 1 per 10,000 persons. The likelihood of either serious arrhythmias or myocardial infarction is less than 1 per 1,000 persons. Therefore, the relative safety of stress testing is well established,[25,26] especially in light of the fact that many patients with severe cardiac disease undergo such testing. Young et al[27] recently evaluated the risk of serious complications from treadmill testing in a group of patients with a history of ventricular fibrillation or tachycardia. They found a 2.3% incidence of sustained arrhythmias requiring prompt intervention. Most of these patients had coronary artery disease. The stated risk of similar complications in a group of test patients without a history of malignant ventricular arrhythmias, however, was much less (0.05%).[27] The relative safety of the procedure was extended by Butman et al[28] who demonstrated that submaximal exercise testing could be safely performed three days after stabilization of unstable angina previously believed to be an absolute contraindication to exercise testing. They went on to suggest that those with abnormal test results should be considered for early angiography.

BAYES' THEOREM

Fundamental to an understanding of the applicability of stress testing and the diagnosis of ischemic heart disease is a familiarity with Bayes' theorem. These concepts have been discussed in depth elsewhere, but they may be summarized by stating that the sensitivity and specificity (and therefore the predictive accuracy) of a test are intimately related to the prevalence of disease in a given population.[29-32] Taking historical and risk factors into account, the pre-test likelihood of disease in an individual can be determined.

Exercise testing is often performed to broaden the data base from which diagnostic decisions are made. The pretest probability of disease, assessed by the patient's history, clinical findings, and evaluation of risk factors in

Table 10.1. Indications for Exercise Testing

1. To help diagnose chest pain etiology
2. To help determine the prognosis and severity of disease
3. To help evaluate functional capacity
4. To help evaluate treatment, both surgical and medical
5. To evaluate dysrhythmias
6. To determine an exercise prescription
7. To help evaluate peripheral vascular disease and lung disease
8. To help screen for asymptomatic coronary artery disease

Table 10.2. *Absolute* Contraindications to Exercise Testing

1. Any recent change in the resting electrocardiogram suggesting the possibility of acute myocardial infarction or ischemia
2. Unstable angina
3. Serious cardiac dysrhythmias, eg, ventricular tachycardia, third-degree atrioventricular block, or uncontrolled atrial fibrillation or tachycardia
4. Acute pericarditis or myocarditis
5. Endocarditis
6. Severe aortic or mitral stenosis
7. Severe left ventricular dysfunction
8. Acute pulmonary embolism or pulmonary infarction
9. Any acute or serious noncardiac disorder
10. Severe physical handicap

large part, determines the diagnostic value of an exercise test. It appears that exercise testing is particularly valuable in individuals with approximately a 50% pre-test probability of disease. Such a patient might be a 45- to 55-year-old man with atypical chest pain and a 20-year history of smoking.

A normal exercise test response in a person with a low pre-test probability of disease will not significantly alter the likelihood of disease.[32,33] Conversely, an abnormal test result in this individual will still suggest a relatively low post-test risk of disease. An abnormal exercise test result in a person with a high pre-test probability of disease will not significantly increase the likelihood of disease. Furthermore, a normal test result in a high-risk individual will not significantly reduce the likelihood of disease. Probability analysis may also be helpful in deciding what further testing (after initial treadmill stress testing) might prove useful in the workup of coronary artery disease.

Sensitivity can be defined as the percentage of subjects with disease or with abnormal test results. Such subjects represent true-positive test results. Those with disease who have normal stress tests are said to have false-negative results.

$$\text{Sensitivity} = \frac{\text{true-positive results}}{\text{true-positive} + \text{false-negative results}}$$

Specificity reflects the ability of a negative test result to give normal results in a patient without disease. Such subjects without disease and normal stress test results are said to have true-negative results. Those without disease who have abnormal test results are said to have false-positive results.

$$\text{Specificity} = \frac{\text{true-negative results}}{\text{true-negative} + \text{false-positive results}}$$

The predictive value of an abnormal test result is the percentage of subjects with abnormal tests that are, in fact, diseased.

$$\text{Predictive value} = \frac{\text{true-positive results}}{\text{true-positive} + \text{false-positive results}}$$

Clearly, this variable, like sensitivity and specificity, is influenced by the prevalence of disease in a given population.

ST-SEGMENT DEPRESSION

ISCHEMIC ST-SEGMENT DEPRESSION

An abnormal electrocardiographic response to exercise is generally defined as 1 mm of ST-segment depression at 80 ms past the J point (junction between the end of the QRS complex and the beginning of the ST segment) in one or more leads.[34,35] Horizontal or downsloping ST-segment depression is regarded as abnormal, whereas the significance of upsloping ST-segment depression is less clear.[36] Most investigators regard the upsloping pattern as a weaker predictor of coronary artery disease.[37-39] Conversely, classifying upsloping patterns as normal reduces the sensitivity of the test. Multivessel coronary artery disease is uncommon with less than 2 mm of upsloping ST-segment depression (Figure 10.3).

Hamby et al[40] found that of 120 patients referred to their center for cardiac catheterization because of ST-segment depression exceeding 2 mm, 57% had three-vessel disease and 16% had left main coronary artery disease. A markedly abnormal electrocardiographic response is therefore a strong predictor of severe coronary artery disease.[40] Interestingly, Hakki et al[41] recently found that patients with low amplitude R waves (less than 11 mm in lead V_5) are less likely to have ST-segment deflections during exercise, given similar degrees of coronary artery disease. These negative results were shown to be falsely negative by nuclear imaging and coronary arteriography.[41]

McHenry et al[42] showed that exercise-induced ST-segment depression in apparently healthy, asymptomatic young and middle-aged men predicted subsequent onset of angina pectoris. These changes were not predictive of myocardial infarction or sudden death as an initial manifestation of coronary artery disease, however.[42] ST-segment analysis, in conjunction with risk factor assessment, can make the treadmill stress test an important screening test for coronary artery disease, but the evaluation of ST-segment shifts alone weaken the predictive power.[43]

FALSE-POSITIVE TEST RESULTS

Factors that may contribute to a false-positive test result are anemia, hypertension, left ventricular hypertrophy, hypokalemia, alkalosis, autonomic disturbances, mitral valve prolapse, and certain other valvular and congenital heart diseases.[44] Diuretics, in part by their potassium-depleting properties,[45,46] digitalis preparations,[47,48] and estrogens[49] may all cause abnormal test results in the absence of significant coronary artery disease. These factors should not, however, alter the accuracy of a negative study. Sketch et al[47] postulated that digoxin may increase the sensitivity of stress testing and unmask subclinical disease. When a test result is suspected of being falsely positive, it might be worthwhile to correct the metabolic disturbance, discontinue the offending medication, or perform additional studies such as an exercise thallium study or a nuclear ventriculographic study. In certain instances, after careful clinical evaluation, coronary arteriography might be needed to adequately define the cardiac status.

FALSE-NEGATIVE TEST RESULTS

More harmful perhaps than mislabeling a person as having disease is classifying someone with significant disease as normal (false-negative test results). Therefore, if a significant suspicion of coronary artery disease exists and the stress test gives normal results, a nuclear study or coronary arteriography should be performed. Medications that have been reported to contribute to false-negative results are nitrates,[50] beta blockers,[51] calcium antagonists,[52] and possibly androgens, quinidine, and diazepam, although there are few data to determine how often this occurs.[53] We are all aware that certain medications (such as beta blockers and calcium antagonists) may effectively lower myocardial oxygen consumption. Whether this effect contributes to false-negative results or whether it just delays the onset of ischemia has been

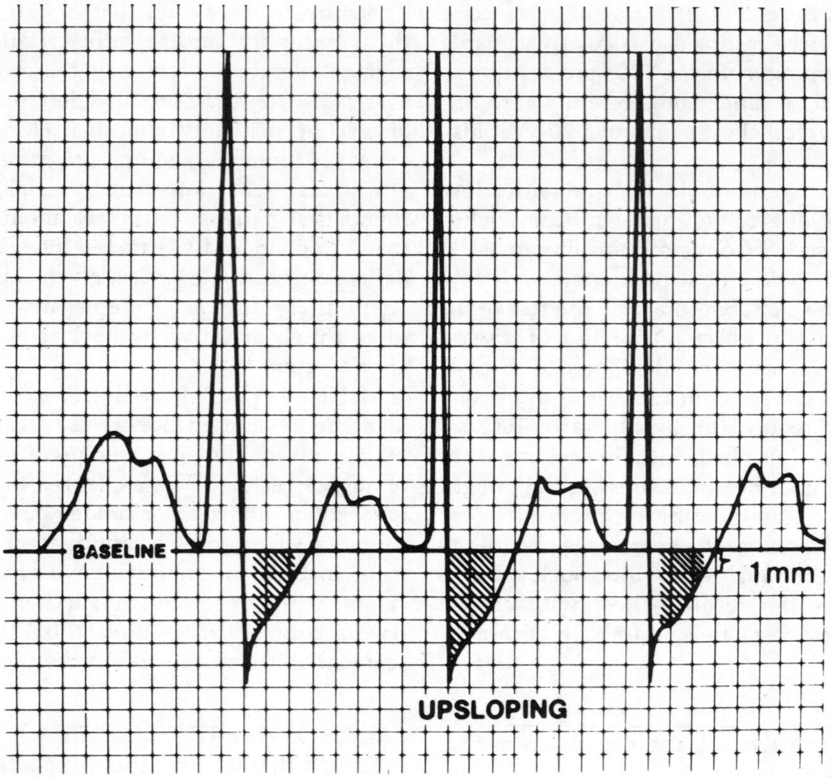

Figure 10.3. Upsloping ST pattern. This pattern is usually associated with ischemia, although it is usually found with lesser degrees of coronary narrowing than horizontal or downsloping ST-segment depression. (From Ellestad MH, Allen WH, Stuart RJ: Diagnostic and prognostic information derived from exercise testing, in Wenger NK (ed): *Exercise and the Heart*. Philadelphia, FA Davis Co, 1979. Used with permission.)

debated. In most cases, the patient becomes ischemic at a certain double product (regardless of which medications he or she is receiving). Zohman and Kattus[35] and later Marcomichelakis et al[54] report that beta blockage fails to normalize the electrocardiogram in patients with true ischemia.

HYPERVENTILATION

Hyperventilation may induce ST-segment depression, probably through a reduction in vagal tone.[55–57] Such responders are often female and a significant percentage might have mitral valve prolapse.[58] This response was shown to be a negative predictor of coronary artery disease, as is other evidence of an overreactive autonomic system.

EFFECTS OF INTERVENTIONS ON STRESS TESTING RESULTS

The heart rate response to exercise may be blunted by beta blockers, and the degree of ST-segment depression at peak exercise may therefore be reduced.[59] The usual effect of beta blockade is to delay the onset of ischemia. This is due, at least in part, to a reduction in double product for comparable workloads. Timolol was shown to increase exercise capacity and decrease the ST-segment abnormalities seen in patients with ischemic heart disease.[59a] Again, much or all of the beta blocker's effect may have been related to attendant decreases in heart rate and blood pressure response to exercise.

Calcium antagonists also increase treadmill time, decrease symptoms, and lessen ST-segment abnormalities.[52] These changes may be due to redistribution of flow to ischemic areas. Nifedipine, a calcium antagonist, may enhance exercise capacity and increase the time to onset of significant ST-segment depression in patients with chronic stable angina pectoris.[59b] These benefits were present in a 6-month follow-up. A recent study showed that diltiazem significantly improved exercise tolerance in patients with coronary artery disease but failed to alter maximal ST-segment depression.[60]

Training may contribute to the improvement but rarely to the normalization of the ischemic response to exercise. Meyers et al[61] showed that there is a tendency toward improvement in ST-segment depression during exercise in patients with coronary artery disease after 1 year of training. They explained the changes by the increase in maximal oxygen uptake and the decreased heart rate at identical workloads.

CONVERSION OF A TEST RESULT FROM NEGATIVE TO POSITIVE

Logic would suggest that when a negative treadmill stress test converts to a positive one, the probability of disease would be high. McHenry et al,[34] however, noted that such a conversion was no more predictive of coronary artery disease than was one that was abnormal initially. In other words, false-positive results occur even in asymptomatic subjects.

SEX DIFFERENCES

Given male and female populations with a similar pretest likelihood of disease, the stress test is a less specific (but probably more sensitive) test in women than in men.[62,63] The higher incidence of ST-segment depression in women with normal coronary arteries has been attributed by some to the vasoconstrictor effect of estrogens. Estrogens are structurally related to digoxin, which is a well-known cause of false-positive test results. It is not known for certain if the digoxin-induced changes are due to vasoconstriction, however.[64]

Hung et al[65] demonstrated that the standard exercise electrocardiogram is a less than ideal diagnostic test in women suspected of having coronary artery disease if they have anything other than typical angina pectoris. In other situations, such as premenopausal patients, the specificity is so low it makes the results very difficult to interpret.[65] It is of interest that exercise-induced ST-segment depression is more common in young women than in those who are postmenopausal in whom the prevalence of coronary artery disease is greater.[66]

ELECTROCARDIOGRAPHIC PATTERNS AND THEIR SIGNIFICANCE

ST-SEGMENT ELEVATION

ST-segment elevation, especially in lead V_1, may be associated with severe proximal left anterior descending coronary artery disease. In patients with a previous infarction, however, it almost always reflects a ventricular aneurysm or a wall motion abnormality.[34,67] As will be discussed, ST-segment elevation may also be seen with vasospastic angina.[67–69,69a]

R-WAVE AMPLITUDE

One of the most controversial electrocardiographic data points used in exercise stress testing is R-wave analysis.[70] Brody[71] in the mid-1950s described a relation between intraventricular volumes and R-wave amplitude. It has since been conclusively shown that increases in the R wave in patients with ischemia are not dependent on changes in ventricular volume.[72] The usefulness of R-wave changes during exercise has been disputed,[73,74] but data to support its value are also available.[75–78] The "normal" R-wave response to exercise is a decrease in amplitude[79]; an "ischemic" response is an increase in amplitude with exercise, which is thought to be due to ischemia-related intraventricular conduction disturbances[80] (see Figure 10.4). A recent commentary on the subject subtitled "Still Controversial" summarizes findings of various studies.[70] There is some evidence that changes in R-wave amplitude can be used to diagnose ischemia in the presence of left bundle branch block.[81,82] Also, a recent report suggests the particular usefulness of R-wave analysis in diagnosing coronary artery disease in women.[83] A note of caution should, however, be made regarding the use of R-wave amplitude change in populations following exercise training, because it has been shown that endurance training in young females may produce an increase in R-wave amplitude during high-intensity exercise.[83a] But this recent finding should not deter from the use of R-wave amplitude in evaluation of patients with coronary artery disease. According to Poyatos et al,[84] persons with increases in R-wave amplitude who have known coronary artery disease are twice as likely to have myocardial infarction or death from cardiovascular origin than are those

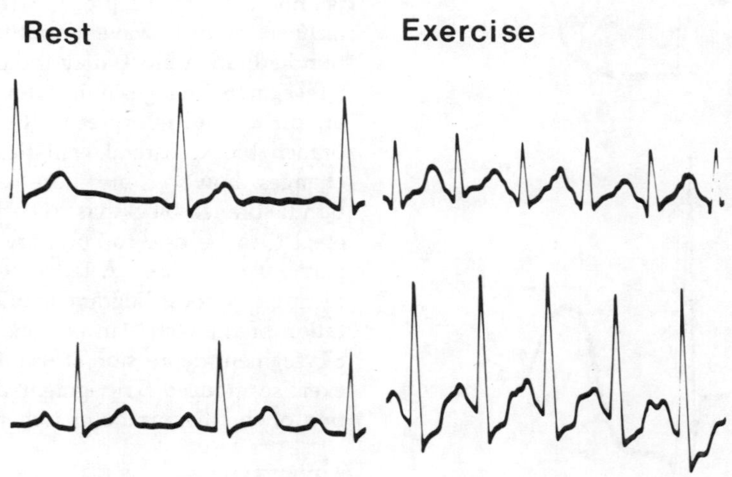

Figure 10.4. R-wave amplitude. The pair of complexes in the lower line were taken from a patient with severe myocardial ischemia. Note that exercise causes an increase in the R wave of the CM_5 lead. This is probably due to changes in intraventricular conduction brought on by ischemia. The upper pair is a normal response with a decrease in R wave immediately after exercise.

who had a normal R-wave response (reduction in amplitude with exercise). Thus, the predictive value suggests it may be most useful in patients with more severe degrees of coronary heart disease.

SEPTAL Q WAVE

It has recently been suggested that analysis of the septal Q wave may prove helpful diagnostically, especially in the case of left anterior descending coronary artery disease.[85] Famularo et al[86] demonstrated that low septal Q-wave amplitude and its failure to increase with exercise (thought to be a normal response) suggest abnormal septal activation and are believed to be due to septal ischemia from left anterior descending stenosis (Figure 10.5).

QT INTERVAL

The QT interval provides an estimate of ventricular systole, and its measurement has been used to evaluate ischemia for years. Some investigators[87,88] have described a prolongation of the QT_c with exercise-induced ischemia. When used independently, it fails to improve sensitivity, specificity, or the predictive value of a stress test. It may prove useful when used in conjunction with other electrocardiographic data points. Vasilomanolakis et al[89] showed that the Q to peaked T interval was likewise often prolonged in an ischemic setting and that its analysis increased sensitivity of the exercise test.

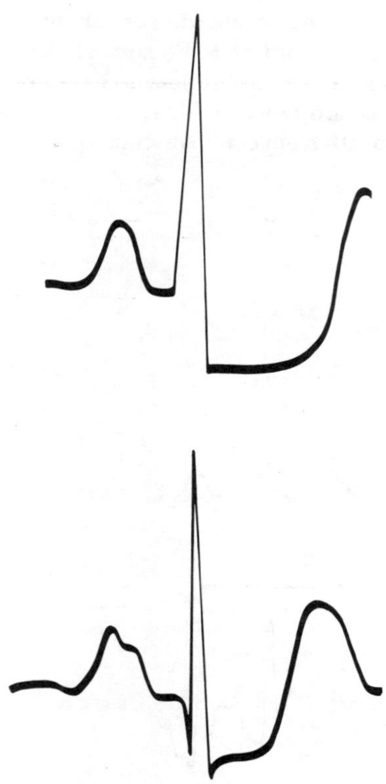

Figure 10.5. Septal Q wave. The septal Q wave is absent in the top complex, indicating true ischemia. The lower complex has a deep septal Q in association with ST-segment depression. This usually denotes a "false-positive" ST-segment depression.

U WAVE

An important, albeit unusual, finding on the exercise electrocardiogram is that of U-wave inversion. This phenomenon is an insensitive but quite specific marker for left anterior descending coronary artery disease.[90,91]

CONDUCTION AND RHYTHM DISTURBANCES

INTRAVENTRICULAR CONDUCTION DEFECTS

Intraventricular conduction defects are another group of electrocardiographic abnormalities that may develop with exercise. However, the incidence of the phenomena is low, probably less than 1%. Boran et al[92] showed that left anterior fascicular block is the most common variety of intraventricular conduction delay, although left posterior fascicular block and complete left or right bundle branch block may also be seen. They also reported on ten patients with intraventricular conduction defects and ischemic ST-segment responses who underwent coronary arteriography and were found to have significant left anterior descending stenosis proximal to the first septal perforator. All patients were treated (eight of ten surgically), and on retesting, nine of the ten no longer showed either an ischemic electrocardiographic response or an exercise-induced conduction defect. Similarly, exercise-induced left bundle branch block was seen in a patient with severe proximal left anterior descending coronary artery disease who later underwent successful coronary angioplasty. On subsequent retesting the exercise-induced left bundle branch block was not elicited.[92a] Stress-related conduction disturbances may be seen in conditions other than coronary artery disease as well.

A person with the Wolff–Parkinson–White syndrome or other forms of preexcitation may develop an exercise-induced intraventricular conduction delay or may have exercise-induced ST-segment depression in the absence of coronary artery disease, or both.[93,94]

It is generally believed that exercise-induced ST-segment deviation in the presence of left bundle branch block is impossible to interpret.[95,96] There is some evidence that an increase in R-wave amplitude in the presence of left bundle branch block may indicate ischemia.[81] Similarly, ST-segment changes in inferior and right precordial leads are difficult to interpret in the presence of right bundle branch block. Lateral wall (ie, leads V_5, V_6, or CM_5) changes, however, are more reliable.[97] The rate-related bundle branch block has recently been shown by Wayne et al[98] to be due to coronary artery disease in a high percentage of cases. A left anterior fascicular block on a resting electrocardiogram should not affect the interpretation of the test.[99] In persons with normal conduction, ST-segment depression at rest should be subtracted from exercise-induced ST-segment depression in the estimation of the magnitude of ischemic changes.[100,101]

ARRHYTHMIAS

Premature atrial beats and short runs of supraventricular tachycardia are not unusual during exercise testing and do not have any diagnostic or prognostic significance for coronary artery disease. Exercise-induced atrial flutter or fibrillation, although rare, may or may not signify ischemic heart disease.[102] Similarly, premature ventricular beats commonly occur during exertion, even in normal subjects. Isolated premature ventricular contractions, therefore, do not seem to provide any diagnostic or prognostic information. A recent report showed that asymptomatic and apparently healthy persons who had nonsustained ventricular tachycardia during stress testing apparently do not have a significant increased risk of cardiac events within 2 years of the test.[103] Further follow-up would be of interest. Malignant forms of ventricular ectopy, however, are more likely to be associated with significant coronary artery disease. This is especially true if other signs of coronary artery disease are present.[104,105] Exercise-induced ventricular tachycardia is usually associated with heart disease, most commonly ischemic heart disease. It occasionally is seen with a prolonged baseline QT interval. Ischemia-related ventricular tachycardia may be abolished by successful coronary artery bypass grafting.[106] Ventricular arrhythmias associated with superior frontal axis shift (−30° to −120°) have been said to be more suggestive of coronary artery disease.[107]

Several studies have shown that ventricular arrhythmias, in the presence of ischemic ST-segment changes, are predictive of significant coronary artery disease and wall motion abnormalities. Frequent premature ventricular contractions (PVCs) in patients with left ventricular dysfunction are predictors of a poor prognosis.[108] Also, in patients with known coronary artery disease, PVCs during treadmill stress testing are indicative of more severe disease.[108] Similarly, in persons clinically suspected of having coronary artery disease, even simple PVCs place them at increased risk of having significant coronary artery disease.[108,109]

BLOOD PRESSURE AND HEART RATE RESPONSES

HYPOTENSION

The normal blood pressure response to exercise is a progressive increase in systolic blood pressure with a possible plateau at peak exercise and a steady or slightly diminishing diastolic pressure. Patients with clinical or subclinical hypertension may have a hypertensive blood pressure response to exercise.[110] According to Sheps et al,[111] an increase in diastolic blood pressure of at least 15 mm Hg is a sign of coronary artery disease and may be seen in the absence of ischemic ST-segment changes. Thus, accurate blood pressure measurements are important during exercise. Ideally, measurements should be made at least once during every two- or three-minute stage. More frequent monitoring should be instituted with the appearance of significant symptoms or electrocardiographic changes. The stress test should be terminated in the event of exertional hypotension.

Characteristic changes in blood pressure may aid in the diagnosis, prognostication, and management of patients with coronary artery disease.[112,113] Hypotension with exertion, defined as a decrease in systolic blood pressure of more than 10 mm Hg or failure of systolic blood pressure to increase above 130 mm Hg, is often seen in conjunction with severe ischemic heart disease and left ventricular dysfunction. Weiner et al[114] recently showed that patients with exertional hypotension were more likely to be men with a history of angina pectoris or previous myocardial infarction, or both. Post-stress test management was randomized and repeat testing after therapy was performed. In most medically managed patients (17 of 20), exertional hypotension persisted, but repeat testing in all who had undergone bypass surgery (22 of 22) revealed a normal blood pressure response.[115] As with exertional angina, the predictive value of an exercise-induced decrease in systolic blood pressure is increased when it is seen with ischemic ST-segment depression.[14] Other causes of exertional hypotension should also be considered, however. Nonischemic causes of hypotension include hypovolemia, left ventricular outflow obstruction, left ventricular failure, and sustained arrhythmias. It should also be noted that stress-induced hypotension is a less specific sign of coronary artery disease in women.[116]

Exertional hypotension may also occur if an individual exercises to and beyond his or her anaerobic threshold. In this circumstance, blood pH decreases as a result of lactic acid accumulation. These changes may cause a decrease in cardiac output, peripheral resistance, and systolic pressure. Clinical differentiation between hypotension of this etiology and that which occurs in severe coronary artery disease is not usually difficult because it comes on late in the exercise test.

Amon et al[117] evaluated a subgroup of patients in whom systolic blood pressure in recovery exceeded that seen at peak exercise. When such a phenomenon was witnessed, they reported a high likelihood of coronary artery disease. Their data need to be confirmed before much confidence can be placed in this finding, however.

HEART RATE RESPONSE

The expected heart rate response to exercise is a progressive and relatively smooth increase. Conditioning of the subject is an important factor in determining the heart rate at a given level of activity. A conditioned individual will respond to a given physical stress with a lower heart rate than will a deconditioned person.[118] A rather precipitous increase in heart rate may also be seen in an individual whose cardiovascular system is marginally compensated. Such a person lacks adequate ventricular reserve to increase stroke volume appropriately, so he responds with a disproportionate increase in heart rate with an attempt to maintain cardiac output[119] (Figure 10.6).

CHRONOTROPIC INCOMPETENCE

A patient who is not a well-trained athlete and has a blunted heart rate response to exercise is said to have chronotropic incompetence.[120] This phenomenon has also been called "sustained relative bradycardia" and can occasionally be seen in patients with ischemic heart disease.[121] It is identified by failure of the heart rate to increase to within two standard deviations of the age-predicted response during exercise. This finding during exercise testing suggests significant coronary artery disease or left ventricular impairment and may be seen in the absence of ST-segment displacement.[53] Wiener et al[122] showed that chronotropic incompetence is a specific but insensitive sign of coronary artery disease. In-

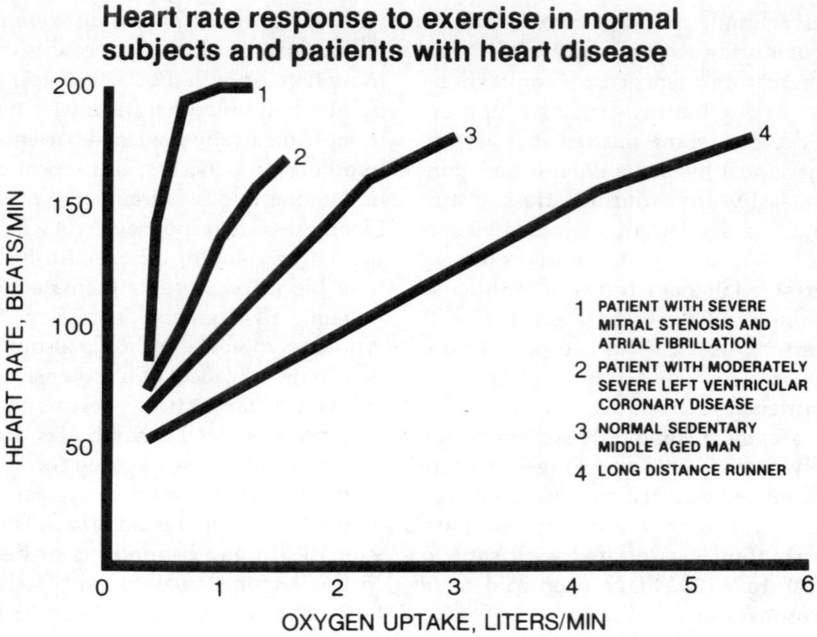

Figure 10.6. The heart rate response to exercise in patients with different functional status. Note that the better the stroke volume, the slower the heart rate in relation to increased work. (From Ellestad MH, Allen WH, Stuart RJ: Diagnostic and prognostic information derived from exercise testing, in Wenger NK (ed): *Exercise and the Heart*. Philadelphia, FA Davis Co, 1979. Used with permission.)

teresting examples of this phenomenon have been published.[53] One case involved a middle-aged man who initially had a normal heart rate response to exercise. He subsequently sustained myocardial infarction and developed chronotropic incompetence on retesting. Another patient was found on initial testing to have an attenuated heart rate response to exertion in addition to ischemic ST-segment depression. He underwent successful bypass surgery and on repeat testing was found to have a normal heart rate response to exercise with no ischemic changes (Figure 10.7).

SYMPTOM AND RISK FACTOR EVALUATION

SYMPTOMS

It is important for the clinician to consider all symptoms that occur during and after the exercise test. Symptoms are often absent in the presence of an ischemic ST-segment response to exercise. In fact, patients with marked ST-segment abnormalities may be asymptomatic. When angina pectoris occurs in association with ST-segment changes, however, the likelihood that these changes are due to coronary artery disease is greater, according to Weiner et al.[122] In other words, the predictive value of the test is enhanced. Interestingly, angina pectoris without ischemic changes may be as predictive of coronary artery disease as are ST-segment changes alone. Patients with angina during exercise are at increased risk of subsequent coronary events[123] (Figure 10.8).

RISK FACTOR EVALUATION

Eliciting a good clinical history is an extremely important step in the evaluation of coronary artery disease. A history suggesting angina is important when present, but a negative history certainly does not exclude significant disease. Hossack and Bruce,[124] in the Seattle Heart Watch Study, found that graded treadmill testing of a population of asymptomatic persons with major risk factors helped identify a high-risk group in which new cardiovascular events were likely to occur. A loud S_4 gallop or a sustained apical impulse on physical examination provides additional information. After history taking, physical examination, and risk factor analysis, the pretest likelihood of disease in an individual can at least be semiquantitatively determined. The factors most important in estimating coronary risk are age, sex, family history, cholesterol level, symptoms, history of smoking, alcohol use or abuse, hypertension, and diabetes. When combined with information from exercise stress testing, these factors form a basis on which a multivariate analysis of risk may be made and the post-test likelihood of disease can be determined.[125,126] Such indexes and guidelines incorporate all available data to make an informed decision on the probability and severity of disease.

Risk analysis helps remind us that although ST-segment depression may be an important indicator of ischemic heart disease, other signs, symptoms, and historical information must be taken into account in evaluating the significance of ST-segment depression.[127]

VASOSPASTIC ANGINA

Vasospastic angina is typically spontaneous, is not exertion related, and is due to alteration of epicardial or intramyocardial coronary vascular tone. This phenomenon may occur in a structurally normal vessel but is probably more likely in one in which atherosclerotic disease is present. The stress electrocardiogram is an insensitive tool in establishing the diagnosis; however, ST-segment

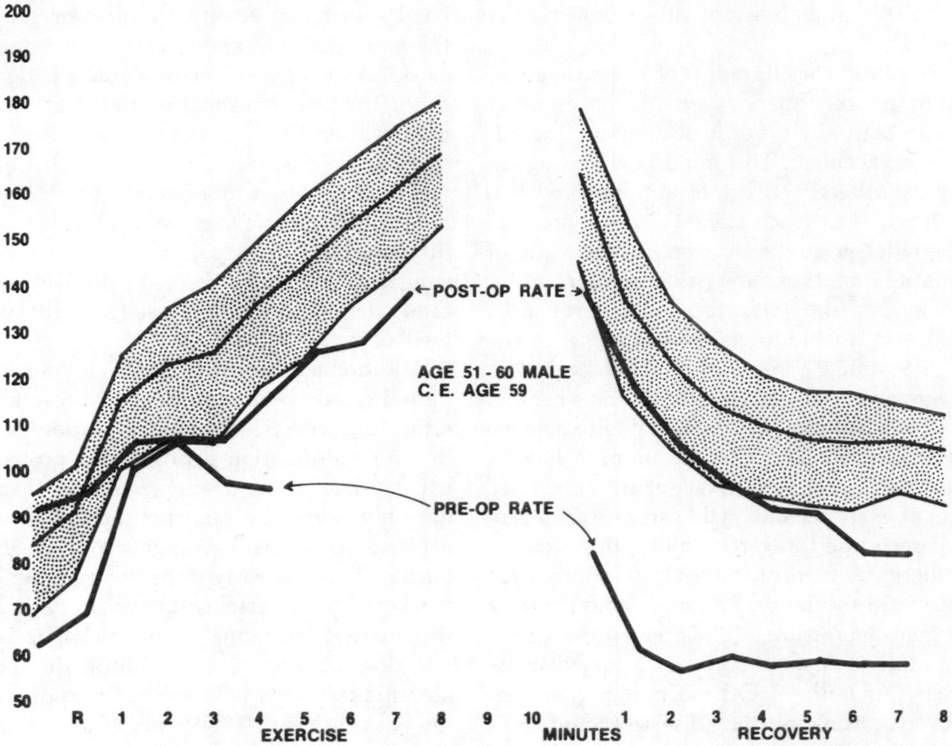

Figure 10.7. Heart rate response before and after bypass surgery as compared with the expected response for age and sex. The "chronotropic incompetence" is an autonomic response that protects the ischemic heart by maintaining a longer diastolic time period.

elevation, depression, or both may occur.[128,129] A patient with vasospastic disease who demonstrates exercise-induced ST-segment depression is likely to have fixed, obstructive coronary artery disease as well.[130] An abnormal exercise electrocardiographic response may normalize with successful treatment, usually with a calcium channel antagonist.

PROGNOSTICATION

Most of the discussion thus far has concentrated on the diagnostic capabilities of treadmill stress testing. Exercise testing also provides invaluable information with regard to the patient's prognosis.[10,11] Although making a diagnosis is not the goal of testing in patients with documented coronary artery disease, a functional assessment

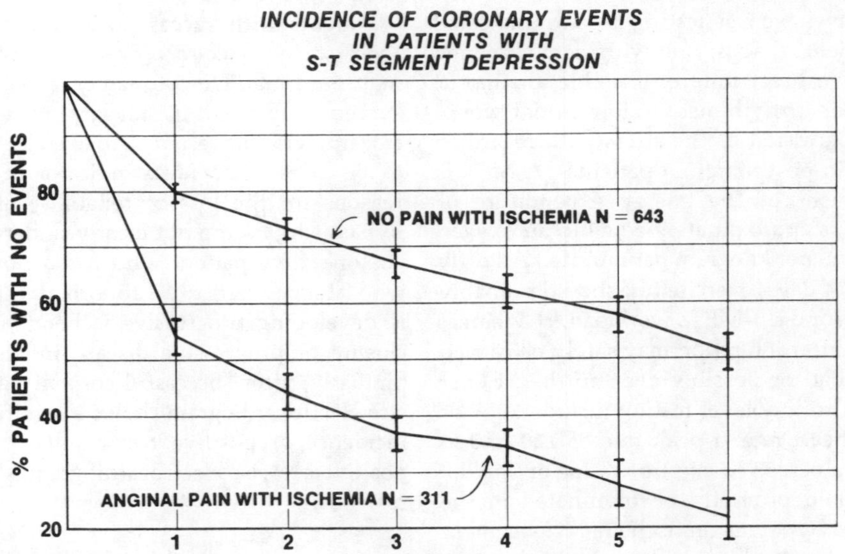

Figure 10.8. Life table of coronary events in patients who had typical anginal pain during the treadmill test as compared with those with ST-segment depression but who were asymptomatic.

and an estimate of the probability of subsequent cardiac events can be made.

McNeer et al[15] found that duration of exercise, a correlate of fitness or aerobic capacity, provided more prognostic information than any other measurement, including ST-segment displacement. This important finding has been confirmed by others.[16] Bruce et al[131] showed that a "healthy" man who can reach stage IV of his protocol (4.2 mph, 16% grade) or attain an exercise heart rate of 160 beats per minute is in a very low risk group for cardiac death—99% one-year and 95% four-year survival.[131] Conversely, a subject unable to complete stage II of the Bruce protocol (2.5 mph, 12% grade) or one who has an abnormal ST-segment response has an 85% one-year and a 63% four-year survival rate. Patients unable to achieve an exercise heart rate of 120 beats per minute have a similarly high mortality rate.[131] McNeer et al[15] concluded that the duration of exercise, maximal heart rate achieved, and ST-segment response to exercise allow the clinician to categorize patients as high or low risk for subsequent cardiac morbidity and mortality. Patients demonstrating marked ST-segment depression at a relatively low workload are likely to have left main coronary artery disease, multivessel disease, or both.[132] Other findings that suggest possible severe coronary artery disease include ST-segment elevation, malignant ventricular arrhythmias, exertional hypotension, chronotropic incompetence, and inverted U waves. Unfortunately, these findings are not 100% specific and they may also be seen in the absence of coronary artery disease.[133,134]

PROGNOSTICATION IN PATIENTS AFTER INFARCTION

Routine low grade exercise testing after myocardial infarction is now performed by many physicians involved in the care of coronary patients.[135,136] Historical and clinical characteristics, in addition to the results of early postinfarction exercise testing, help discriminate patients at high risk of having a coronary event in the subsequent year.[137] Even low level exercise testing is contraindicated in the unstable patient, that is, one with hemodynamic instability, congestive heart failure, unstable angina, or malignant ventricular arrhythmias. A low initial workload and a slow progression of the stress with regard to METs is employed in postinfarction patients. (A MET is a metabolic equivalent of the energy expenditure of standing at rest and is approximately equal to an oxygen consumption of 3.5 ml per kilogram per minute.) An early postinfarction (7 to 14 days) exercise test should probably not be continued beyond a 5-METs workload,[138] whereas a test taken 21 days after infarction may safely be carried to a 7-METs workload or possibly even further. Other arbitrary end points to low level testing include 70% of predicted maximal heart rate, a peak rate of 120 to 130 beats per minute, or a perceived exertion rating of "hard."

Stress testing should promptly be terminated in the event that exertional hypotension, ischemic ST-segment changes, or malignant arrhythmias occur. A test does not necessarily need to be terminated for ST-segment elevation or even mild angina pectoris, assuming that none of the other signs dictating termination is present.

Exercise duration, ischemic response, and exercise-related ventricular ectopy are of some prognostic value in the early postinfarction period. Any degree of exercise-associated ventricular ectopy puts a patient at about eight times the risk for posthospital death. Conversely, if a patient exercises to a target heart rate, is asymptomatic, and has no evidence of residual ischemia, the prognosis has been reported to be good.[139,139a,139b] A seemingly adequate performance on a low grade stress test after infarction allows a patient to expect performances on similarly stressful tasks once discharged. This can certainly help with a patient's self-confidence and emotional well-being.[139b,140]

Additional diagnostic and therapeutic intervention may be indicated when abnormal test results are found. Exertion-induced ST-segment elevation occurs frequently in the postinfarction period and is probably due to ventricular wall motion abnormalities. In and of itself, it does not portend a poor prognosis. Unlike conventional exercise stress testing, angina[138,141] or exertional hypotension[142] in the early postinfarction period is not a good marker of multivessel coronary artery disease. It has been shown that exertional hypotension is often absent on retesting. Angina pectoris during this period, however, identifies patients who are likely to develop angina over the ensuing year.[143] Theroux et al[138] found that significant (greater than 1 mm) ST-segment depression in patients tested soon after having had myocardial infarction imparted a 25% one-year mortality in contrast to a 2% mortality in those without such changes. In patients with normal results on postinfarction treadmill stress tests, a follow-up symptom-limited treadmill should be performed at 6 weeks (or slightly later) after infarction. Such testing can provide further prognostic information and subsequently aid in the management of the patient.[142]

TESTING AFTER CORONARY BYPASS SURGERY AND ANGIOPLASTY

Patients with successful bypass surgery may convert their exercise electrocardiographic response from abnormal to normal. Unfortunately, even unsuccessful bypass surgery may result in this type of response.[144] The electrocardiographic response to exercise is therefore believed to be a less than ideal indicator of graft patency. The reasons for the loss of reliability after coronary artery bypass surgery are not clearly understood. Conversely, a postoperative patient who has a normal stress test and who later converts to an abnormal response almost always is developing progressive ischemia, due to either graft closure or progressive disease in his native circulation. Similarly, after successful coronary angioplasty an exercise electrocardiogram shows a significant decrease in the incidence of positive test results,[145] and a return of a positive exercise electrocardiogram is highly predictive of restenosis.[146]

CONCLUSION

We have emphasized the importance of the exercise stress test in patients with ischemic heart disease. A good deal of information, in addition to ST-segment changes, is available for interpretation. The test can never be interpreted in a vacuum, but only in relation to the patient as a whole. Informed analysis, however, allows more accurate diagnosis and estimation of the severity of disease, management of patients, and establishment of prognosis. When the advantages and limitations of exercise testing are fully understood, it remains one of the most useful procedures available in the management of ischemic heart disease.

REFERENCES

1. Feil H, Siegel ML: Electrocardiographic changes during attacks of angina pectoris. *Am J Med Sci* 1928; 175:255–260.
2. Master AM, Friedman R, Dack S: The electrocardiogram after standard exercise as a functional test of the heart. *Am Heart J* 1942; 24:777–793.
3. Nutter DO, Schlant RC, Hurst JW: Isometric exercise and the cardiovascular system. *Mod Concepts Cardiovasc Dis* 1972; 41:11–15.
4. Kerber RE, Miller RA, Najjar SM: Myocardial ischemic effects of isometric, dynamic, and combined exercise in coronary artery disease. *Chest* 1975; 67:388–394.
5. DeBusk R, Pitts W, Haskell W, Houston N: Comparison of cardiovascular responses to static–dynamic effort and dynamic effort alone in patients with chronic ischemic heart disease. *Circulation* 1979; 59:977–984.
6. Joy M, Pollard CM, Nunan TO: Diurnal variation in exercise responses in angina pectoris. *Br Heart J* 1982; 48:156–160.
7. Levites R, Anderson GJ: Detection of critical coronary lesions with treadmill exercise testing: fact or fiction? *Am J Cardiol* 1978; 42:533–538.
8. Selzer A, Cohn K, Goldschlager N: On the interpretation of the exercise test. *Circulation* 1978; 58:193–195.
9. Cohn PF: Severe asymptomatic coronary artery disease. A diagnostic, prognostic and therapeutic puzzle. *Am J Med* 1978; 62:565–568.
10. Dagenais GR, Rouleau JR, Christen A, Fabia J: Survival of patients with a strongly positive exercise electrocardiogram. *Circulation* 1982; 65:452–456.
11. Ellestad MH: Can stress testing predict the severity of coronary disease? *Chest* 1976; 69:708–710.
12. Goldman S, Tselos S, Cohn K: Marked depth of ST-segment depression during treadmill exercise testing. Indicator of severe coronary artery disease. *Chest* 1976; 69:729–733.
13. Podrid PJ, Graboys TB, Lown B: Prognosis of medically treated patients with coronary-artery disease with profound ST-segment depression during exercise testing. *N Engl J Med* 1981; 305:1111–1116.
14. Sanmarco ME, Pontius S, Selvester RH: Abnormal blood pressure response and marked ischemic ST segment depression as predictors of severe coronary artery disease. *Circulation* 1980; 61:572–578.
15. McNeer JM, Margolis JR, Lee KL, Kisslo JA, Peter RH, Kong Y, Behar VS, Wallace AG, McCants CB, Rosati RA: The role of the exercise test in the evaluation of patients for ischemic heart disease. *Circulation* 1978; 57:64–70.
16. Schneider RM, Seaworth JF, Dohrmann MJ, Lester RM, Phillips HR Jr, Bashore TM, Baker JT: Anatomic and prognostic implications of an early positive treadmill exercise test. *Am J Cardiol* 1982; 50:682–688.
17. Weiner DA, Ryan TJ, McCabe CH, Chaitman BR, Sheffield LT, Ferguson JC, Fisher LD, Tristani F: Prognostic importance of a clinical profile and exercise test in medically treated patients with coronary artery disease. *J Am Coll Cardiol* 1984; 3:772–779.
18. Sketch MH, Nair CK, Esterbrooks DJ, Mohiuddin SM: Reliability of single-lead and multiple-lead electrocardiography during and after exercise. *Chest* 1978; 74:394–401.
19. Chaitman BR, Bourassa MG, Wagniart P, Corbara F, Ferguson RJ: Improved efficiency of treadmill exercise testing using a multiple lead ECG system and basic hemodynamic exercise response. *Circulation* 1978; 57:71–79.
20. Chaitman BR, Waters DD, Bourassa MG, Tubau JF, Wagniart P, Ferguson RJ: The importance of clinical subsets in interpreting maximal treadmill exercise test results: The role of multiple-lead ECG systems. *Circulation* 1979; 59:560–570.
21. Fox KM, Hakki A-H, Iskandrian AS: Relation between electrocardiographic and scintigraphic location of myocardial ischemia during exercise in one-vessel coronary artery disease. *Am J Cardiol* 1984; 53:1529–1531.
22. Abouantoun S, Ahnve S, Savvides M, Witztum K, Jensen D, Froelicher V: Can areas of myocardial ischemia be localized by the exercise electrocardiogram? A correlative study with thallium-201 scintigraphy. *Am Heart J* 1984; 108:933–941.
23. Dunn RF, Freedman B, Bailey IK, Uren RF, Kelly DT: Localization of coronary artery disease with exercise electrocardiography: correlation with thallium-201 myocardial perfusion scanning. *Am J Cardiol* 1981; 48:837–843.
24. Council on Scientific Affairs: Indications and contraindications for exercise testing. *JAMA* 1981; 246:1015–1018.
25. Atterhog JH, Jonsoon B, Samuelsson R: Exercise testing: a prospective study of complication rates. *Am Heart J* 1979; 98:572–579.
26. Stuart RJ, Ellestad MH: National survey of exercise stress testing facilities. *Chest* 1980; 77:94–97.
27. Young DZ, Lampert S, Graboys TB, Lown B: Safety of maximal exercise testing in patients at high risk for ventricular arrhythmia. *Circulation* 1984; 70:184–191.
28. Butman SM, Olson HG, Gardin JM, Piters KM, Hullett M, Butman LK: Submaximal exercise testing after stabilization of unstable angina pectoris. *JACC* 1984; 4:667–673.
29. Wagner HN Jr: Bayes' theorem: an idea whose time has come? *Am J Cardiol* 1982; 49:875–877.
30. Diamond GA, Forrester JS: Analysis of probability as an aid in the clinical diagnosis of coronary artery disease. *N Engl J Med* 1979; 300:1350–1358.
31. Epstein SE: Implications of probability analysis on the strategy used for noninvasive detection of coronary artery disease. Role of single or combined use of exercise electrocardiographic testing, radionuclide cineangiography and myocardial perfusion imaging. *Am J Cardiol* 1980; 46:491–499.
32. Detrano R, Yiannikas J, Salcedo EE, Rincon G, Go RT, Williams G, Leatherman J: Bayesian probability analysis: a prospective demonstration of its clinical utility in diagnosing coronary disease. *Circulation* 1984; 69:541–547.
33. Patterson RE, Eng C, Horowitz SF: Practical diagnosis of coronary artery disease: a Bayes' Theorem nomogram to correlate clinical data with noninvasive exercise tests. *Am J Cardiol* 1984; 53:252–256.
34. McHenry PL, Richmond HW, Weisenberger BL, Rodnay JS, Perry GF, Jordan JW: Evaluation of abnormal exercise electrocardiogram in apparently healthy subjects: labile repolarization (ST-T) abnormalities as a cause of false-positive responses. *Am J Cardiol* 1981; 47:1152–1160.
35. Zohman LR, Kattus AA: Exercise testing in the diagnosis of coronary heart disease: a perspective. *Am J Cardiol* 1977; 40:243–250.
36. Goldschlager N, Selzer A, Cohn K: Treadmill stress tests as indicators of presence and severity of coronary artery disease. *Ann Intern Med* 1976; 85:277–286.
37. Kurita A, Chaitman BR, Bourassa MG: Significance of exercise-induced junctional ST depression in evaluation of coronary artery disease. *Am J Cardiol* 1977; 40:492–497.
38. Rijneke RD, Ascoop CA, Talman JL: Clinical significance of upsloping ST segments in exercise electrocardiography. *Circulation* 1980; 61:671–678.
39. Stuart RJ, Ellestad MH: Upsloping ST segments in exercise stress testing. Six year follow up study of 438 patients and correlation with 248 angiograms. *Am J Cardiol* 1976; 37:19–22.
40. Hamby RI, Davison ET, Hilsenrath J, Shanies S, Young M, Murphy DH, Hoffman I: Functional and anatomic correlates of markedly abnormal stress tests. *J Am Coll Cardiol* 1984; 3:1375–1381.
41. Hakki AH, Iskandrian AS, Kutalek S, Hare TW, Sokoloff NM: R wave amplitude: a new determinant of failure of patients with coronary heart disease to manifest ST segment depresssion during exercise. *J Am Coll Cardiol* 1984; 3:1155–1160.
42. McHenry PL, O'Donnell J, Morris SN, Jordan J: The abnormal exercise electrocardiogram in apparently healthy men: a predictor of angina pectoris as an initial coronary event during long-term follow-up. *Circulation* 1984; 70:547–551.
43. Hopkirk JAC, Uhl GS, Hickman JR, Fischer J, Medina A: Discriminant value of clinical and exercise variables in detecting significant coronary artery disease in asymptomatic men. *J Am Coll Cardiol* 1984; 3:887–894.
44. Bruce RA: Values and limitations of exercise electrocardiography. *Circulation* 1974; 50:1–3.
45. Georgopoulos AJ, Proudfit WL, Page IH: Effect of exercise on electrocardiograms of patients with low serum potassium. *Circulation* 1961; 23:567–572.
46. Soloff LA, Fewell JW: Abnormal electrocardiographic responses to exercise in subjects with hypokalemia. *Am J Med Sci* 1961; 242:724.
47. Sketch MH, Mooss AN, Butler ML, Nair CK, Mohiuddin SM: Digoxin-induced positive exercise tests: their clinical and prognostic significance. *Am J Cardiol* 1981; 48:655–659.
48. Tonkon MJ, Lee G, DeMaria AN, Miller RR, Mason DT: Effects of digitalis on the exercise electrocardiogram in normal adult subjects. *Chest* 1977; 72:714–718.
49. Jaffe MD: Effect of oestrogens on postexercise electrocardiogram. *Br Heart J* 1977; 38:1299–1303.
50. Russek HI, Funk EH Jr: Comparative responses to various nitrates in the treatment of angina pectoris. *Postgrad Med* 1962; 31:150–155.
51. Gianelly RE, Treister BL, Harrison DC: The effect of propranolol on exercise-induced ischemic S-T segment depression. *Am J Cardiol* 1969; 24:161–165.
52. Subramanian B, Bowles M, Lahiri A, Davies AB, Raftery EB: Long-

term antianginal action of verapamil assessed with quantitated serial treadmill stress testing. *Am J Cardiol* 1981; 48:529–535.
53. Ellestad MH: *Stress Testing: Principles and Practice,* ed 3. Philadelphia, FA Davis Co, 1986, pp 441–442.
54. Marcomichelakis J, Donaldson R, Green J, Joseph S, Kelly HB, Taggart P, Somerville W: Exercise testing after beta-blockade: improved specificity and predictive value in detecting coronary heart disease. *Br Heart J* 1980; 43:252–261.
55. Furberg C, Linderholm H: Effects of hyperventilation on ECG in patients with circulatory disturbances. *Acta Med Scand* 1969; 185:167–174.
56. Greenberg PS, Cooke BM Jr, Bible M, Ellestad MH: Use of heart rate responses to standing and hyperventilation at rest to detect coronary artery disease: correlation with the ST response to exercise. *J Electrocardiol* 1980; 13:373–378.
57. Jacobs WF, Battle WE, Ronan JA Jr: False-positive ST-T wave changes secondary to hyperventilation and exercise. A cineangiographic correlation. *Ann Intern Med* 1974; 81:479–482.
58. Gardin JM, Isner JM, Ronan JA Jr, Fox SM: Pseudoischemic "false-positive" ST segment changes induced by hyperventilation in patients with mitral valve prolapse. *Am J Cardiol* 1980; 45:952–958.
59. LeWinter MM, Crawford MH, O'Rourke RA, Karliner JS: The effects of oral propranolol, digoxin and combination therapy on the resting and exercise electrocardiogram. *Am Heart J* 1977; 93:202–209.
59a. Aronow WS, Turbow M, Van Camp S: The effect of timolol versus placebo in angina pectoris. *Circulation* 1980; 61:66–69.
59b. Khurmi NS, Bowles MJ, Subramanian VB: Short- and long-term efficacy of nicardipine, assessed by placebo-controlled single- and double-blind crossover trials in patients with chronic stable angina. *J Am Coll Cardiol* 1984; 4:908–917.
60. Khurmi NS, Bowles MJ, O'Hara MJ: Long-term efficacy of diltiazem assessed with multistage graded exercise tests in patients with chronic stable angina pectoris. *Am J Cardiol* 1984; 54:738–743.
61. Meyers J, Ahnve S, Froelicher V: A randomized trial of the effects of 1 year of exercise training on computer measured ST segment displacement in patients with coronary artery disease. *J Am Coll Cardiol* 1984; 4:1094–1102.
62. Cumming GR, Dufresne C, Kich L, Samm J: Exercise electrocardiogram patterns in normal women. *Br Heart J* 1973; 35:1055–1061.
63. Val PG, Chaitman BR, Waters DD, Bourassa MG, School JM, Ferguson RJ, Wagniart P: Diagnostic accuracy of exercise ECG lead systems in clinical subsets of women. *Circulation* 1982; 65:1465–1474.
64. Sketch MH, Mohiuddin SM, Lynch JD, Zencha AE, Runco V: Significant sex differences in the correlation of electrocardiographic exercise testing and coronary arteriograms. *Am J Cardiol* 1975; 36:169–173.
65. Hung J, Chaitman BR, Lam J: Noninvasive diagnostic test choices for the evaluation of coronary artery disease in women: a multivariate comparison of cardiac fluoroscopy, exercise electrocardiography and exercise thallium myocardial perfusion scintigraphy. *J Am Coll Cardiol* 1984; 4:8–16.
66. Wu SC, Secchi MB, Radice M: Sex differences in the prevalence of ischemic heart disease and in the response to a stress test in a working population. *Eur Heart J* 1981; 2:461–465.
67. Dunn RF, Bailey IK, Uren R, Kelly DT: Exercise-induced ST segment elevation. Correlation of thallium-201 myocardial perfusion scanning and coronary arteriography. *Circulation* 1980; 61:989–995.
68. Dunn RF, Freedman B, Kelly DT, Bailey IK, McLaughlin A: Exercise-induced ST-segment elevation in leads V_1 or aV_L. A predictor of anterior myocardial ischemia and left anterior descending coronary artery disease. *Circulation* 1981; 63:1357–1363.
69. Fortuin NJ, Friesinger GC: Exercise-induced S-T segment elevation: clinical, electrocardiographic and arteriographic studies in twelve patients. *Am J Med* 1970; 49:459–464.
69a. DeServi S, Ardissino D, Mussini A, Angoli L, Bramucci E, Falcone C, Specchia G: Exercise-induced coronary artery spasm. A regional coronary blood flow study. *Jpn Heart J* 1985; 26:1029–1037.
70. Ellestad MH: The mechanism of exercise-induced R wave amplitude changes in coronary heart disease—still controversial. *Arch Intern Med* 1982; 142:963–965.
71. Brody DA: A theoretical analysis of intracavitary blood mass influence on the heart-lead relationship. *Circ Res* 1956; 4:731–738.
72. Battler A, Froelicher V, Slutsky R, Ashburn W: Relationship of QRS amplitude changes during exercise to left ventricular function and volumes and the diagnosis of coronary artery disease. *Circulation* 1979; 60:1004–1013.
73. Fox K, England D, Jonathan A, Selwin A: Inability of exercise-induced R wave changes to predict coronary artery disease. *Am J Cardiol* 1982; 49:674–679.
74. Wagner S, Cohn K, Selzer A: Unreliability of exercise-induced R wave changes as indexes of coronary artery disease. *Am J Cardiol* 1979; 44:1241–1246.
75. Baron DW, Ilsley C, Sheiben I, Poole-Wilson PA, Rickards AF: R wave amplitude during exercise. Relation to left ventricular function and coronary artery disease. *Br Heart J* 1980; 44:512–517.
76. Bonoris PE, Greenberg PS, Castellanet MJ, Ellestad MH: Significance of changes in R wave amplitude during treadmill stress testing: angiographic correlation. *Am J Cardiol* 1978; 41:846–851.
77. Bonoris PE, Greenberg PS, Christison GW, Castellanet MJ, Ellestad MH: Evaluation of R wave amplitude changes versus ST segment depression in stress testing. *Circulation* 1978; 57:904–910.
78. deCaprio L, Cuomo S, Belloti P, Adamo B, Postiglione M, Vigorito C, Rengo F: R wave amplitude changes during stress testing. Comparison with ST segment depression and angiographic correlation. *Am Heart J* 1980; 99:413–418.
79. Wolthuis RA, Froelicher VF, Hopkirk A, Fischer JR, Keiser N: Normal electrocardiographic waveform characteristics during treadmill exercise testing. *Circulation* 1979; 60:1028–1035.
80. David D, Naito M, Michelson E, Watanabe J, Chen CC, Morganroth J, Shaffenburg M, Blenko T: Intramyocardial conduction: a major determinant of R wave amplitude during acute myocardial ischemia. *Circulation* 1982; 65:161–167.
81. Greenberg PS, Ellestad MH: Ability of the R wave change during stress testing to accurately detect coronary disease in the presence of left bundle branch block at rest. *Angiology* 1980; 31:230–237.
82. Uhl GS, Hopkirk JAC: Analysis of exercise-induced R wave amplitude changes in detection of coronary artery disease in asymptomatic men with left bundle branch block. *Am J Cardiol* 1979; 44:1247–1250.
83. Ilsley C, Canepa-Anson R, Westgate C, Webb S, Richards A, Poole-Wilson P: Influence of R wave analysis upon diagnostic accuracy of exercise testing in women. *Br Heart J* 1982; 48:161–168.
83a. Fernhall B, Burkett LN, Walters SC: The effect of training on exercise-induced R-wave amplitude changes in young females. *Med Sci Sports Exerc* 1986; 18:128–133.
84. Poyatos ME, Lerman J, Estrada A, Chiozza M, Perosio A: Predictive value of changes in R-wave amplitude after exercise in coronary heart disease. *Am J Cardiol* 1984; 54:1212–1215.
85. Morales-Ballejo H, Greenberg PS, Ellestad MH, Bible M: Septal Q wave in exercise testing: angiographic correlation. *Am J Cardiol* 1981; 48:247–251.
86. Famularo MA, Paliwal Y, Redd R, Ellestad MH: Identification of septal ischemia during exercise by Q wave analysis: correlation with coronary angiography. *Am J Cardiol* 1983; 51:440–443.
87. Greenberg PS, Friscia DA, Ellestad MH: Predictive accuracy of Q-X/Q-T ratio, Q-T_c interval, ST depression and R wave amplitude during stress testing. *Am J Cardiol* 1979; 44:18–23.
88. O'Donnell J, Knoebel SM, Lovelace DE, McHenry PL: Computer quantitation of Q-T and terminal T wave (aT-eT) intervals during exercise: methodology and results in normal men. *Am J Cardiol* 1981; 47:1168–1172.
89. Vasilomanolakis E, Damian A, Mahan G, Baron D, Ellestad M: Treadmill stress testing in geriatric patients (abstr). *J Am Coll Cardiol* 1984; 3:520.
90. Kishida H, Cole JS, Surawicz B: Negative U wave: a highly specific but poorly understood sign of heart disease. *Am J Cardiol* 1982; 49:2030–2036.
91. Gerson MC, Phillips JF, Morris SN, McHenry PL: Exercise-induced U wave inversion as a marker of stenosis of the left anterior descending coronary artery. *Circulation* 1979; 60:1014–1020.
92. Boran KJ, Oliveros RA, Boucher CA, Beckman CH, Seaworthy JF: Ischemia associated intraventricular conduction disturbances during exercise testing as a predictor of proximal left anterior descending coronary artery disease. *Am J Cardiol* 1983; 51:1098–1102.
92a. Puleo P, Verani MS, Wyndham CR, Hixson J, Raizner AE: Exercise-induced left bundle branch block: resolution after coronary angioplasty. *Am Heart J* 1984; 108:1373–1374.
93. Astrand I, Blomqvist G, Orinius E: ST changes at exercise in patients with short P-R interval. *Acta Med Scand* 1969; 185:205–208.
94. Gazes PG: False-positive exercise test in the presence of the Wolff-Parkinson-White syndrome. *Am Heart J* 1969; 78:13–15.
95. Orzan F, Garcia E, Mathur VS, Hall RJ: Is the treadmill exercise test useful for evaluating coronary artery disease in patients with complete left bundle branch block? *Am J Cardiol* 1978; 42:36–40.
96. Whinnery JE, Froelicher VF Jr, Stewart AJ, Longo MR, Triebwasser JH, Lancaster MC: The electrocardiographic response to maximal treadmill exercise of asymptomatic men with left bundle branch block. *Am Heart J* 1977; 94:316–324.
97. Tanaka T, Friedman MJ, Okada RD, Buckels LJ, Marcus FI: Diagnostic value of exercise-induced ST segment depression in patients with right bundle block. *Am J Cardiol* 1978; 41:670–673.
98. Wayne VS, Bishop RL, Cook L, Spodick DH: Exercise-induced bundle branch block. *Am J Cardiol* 1983; 52:283–286.
99. Mooss AN, Andreadis N, Mohiuddin SM, Sketch MH: Effect of left anterior hemiblock on exercise-induced ST-T segment changes. *Am Heart J* 1979; 98:725–726.
100. Cohn PF, Vokonas PS, Herman MV, Gorlin R: Postexercise electrocardiogram in patients with abnormal resting electrocardiograms. *Circulation* 1971; 43:648–654.
101. Kansal S, Roitman D, Sheffield LT: Stress testing with ST segment depression at rest. *Circulation* 1976; 54:636–639.

102. Jelinek MV, Lown B: Exercise stress testing for exposure of cardiac arrhythmia. *Prog Cardiovasc Dis* 1974; 16:497–522.
103. Fleg JL, Lakatta EG: Prevalence and prognosis of exercise-induced nonsustained ventricular tachycardia in apparently healthy volunteers. *Am J Cardiol* 1984; 54:762–764.
104. Goldschlager N, Cake D, Cohn K: Exercise-induced ventricular arrhythmias in patients with coronary artery disease. Their relation to angiographic findings. *Am J Cardiol* 1973; 31:434–440.
105. Morris SN, McHenry PL: Role of exercise stress testing in healthy subjects and patients with coronary heart disease. *Am J Cardiol* 1978; 42:659–666.
106. Codini MA, Sommerfeldt L, Eybel CE, DeLaria GA, Messer JV: Efficacy of coronary bypass grafting in exercise-induced ventricular tachycardia: *J Thorac Cardiovasc Surg* 1981; 81:502–506.
107. Mardelli TJ, Morganroth J, Dreifus LS: Superior QRS axis of ventricular premature complexes: an additional criterion to enhance the sensitivity of exercise stress testing. *Am J Cardiol* 1980; 45:236–243.
108. Udall JA, Ellestad MH: Predictive implications of ventricular premature contractions associated with treadmill stress testing. *Circulation* 1977; 56:985–989.
109. Califf RM, McKinnis RA, McNeer JF, Harrell FE, Lee KL, Pryor DB, Waugh RA, Harris PJ, Rosati RA, Wagner GS: Prognostic value of ventricular arrhythmias associated with treadmill exercise testing in patients studied with cardiac catheterization for suspected ischemic heart disease. *J Am Coll Cardiol* 1983; 2:1060–1067.
110. Schrager BR, Ellestad MH: The importance of blood pressure measurement during exercise testing. *Cardiovasc Rev & Reports* 1983; 4:381–394.
111. Sheps D, Ernst JC, Briese FW, Myerburg RJ: Exercise-induced increase in diastolic pressure: indicator of severe coronary artery disease. *Am J Cardiol* 1979; 43:708–712.
112. Baker T, Levites R, Anderson GJ: The significance of hypotension during treadmill exercise testing (abstr). *Circulation* 1976; 54(suppl II):II-11.
113. Irving JB, Bruce RA: Exertional hypotension and postexertional ventricular fibrillation in stress testing. *Am J Cardiol* 1977; 39:849–851.
114. Weiner DA, McCabe CH, Cutler SS, Ryan TJ: Decrease in systolic blood pressure during exercise testing: reproducibility, response to coronary bypass surgery and prognostic significance. *Am J Cardiol* 1982; 49:1627–1631.
115. Li W, Riggins RCK, Anderson RP: Reversal of exertional hypotension after coronary bypass grafting. *Am J Cardiol* 1979; 44:607–611.
116. Levites R, Baker T, Anderson GJ: The significance of hypotension developing during treadmill exercise testing. *Am Heart J* 1978; 95:747–753.
117. Amon KW, Richards KL, Crawford MH: Usefulness of the postexercise response of systolic blood pressure in the diagnosis of coronary artery disease. *Circulation* 1984; 70:951–956.
118. Bruce RA, Blackman JR, Jones JW, Strait G: Exercise testing in adult normal subjects and cardiac patients. *Pediatrics* 1963; 32:742–756.
119. Glagov S, Rowley DA, Cramer DB, Page RG: Heart rate during 24 hours of usual activity of 100 normal men. *J Appl Physiol* 1970; 29:799–805.
120. Chin CF, Messenger JC, Greenberg PS, Ellestad MH: Chronotropic incompetence in exercise testing. *Clin Cardiol* 1979; 2:12–18.
121. Hinkle LE, Carver ST, Plakum A: Slow heart rates and increased risk of cardiac death in middle-aged men. *Arch Intern Med* 1972; 129:732–748.
122. Weiner DA, McCabe C, Hueter D: The predictive value of chest pain as an indicator of coronary disease during exercise testing (abstr). *Circulation* 1976; 54(suppl II):II-10.
123. Cole JP, Ellestad MH: Significance of chest pain during treadmill exercise: correlation with coronary events. *Am J Cardiol* 1978; 41:227–232.
124. Hossack KF, Bruce RA: Prognostic value of exercise testing: the Seattle Heart Watch Experience. *J Cardiac Rehab* 1985; 5:9–19.
125. Berman JL, Wynne J, Cohn PF: Value of a multivariate approach for interpreting treadmill exercise tests in coronary artery disease (abstr). *Am J Cardiol* 1978; 41:375.
126. Ellestad MH, Greenberg PS: Multivariate approach to the treadmill stress test: prospective study. *Cardiology* 1981; 68(suppl 2):27–34.
127. Fisher LD, Kennedy JW, Chaitman BR, Ryan TJ, McCabe C, Weiner D, Tristani F, Schloss M, Warner HR Jr: Diagnostic quantification of CASS (Coronary Artery Surgery Study) clinical and exercise test results in determining presence and extent of coronary artery disease. A multivariate approach. *Circulation* 1981; 63:987–1000.
128. Lahiri A, Subramanian B, Millar-Craig M, Crawley J, Raftery EB: Exercise-induced ST segment elevation in variant angina. *Am J Cardiol* 1980; 45:887–894.
129. Waters DD, Szlachcic J, Bourassa MG, School J, Theroux P: Exercise testing in patients with variant angina: results, correlations with clinical and angiographic features and prognostic significance. *Circulation* 1982; 65:265–274.
130. Boden WE, Bough EW, Korr KS, Benham I, Gheorghiade M, Caputi A, Shulman RS: Exercise-induced coronary spasm with ST segment depression and normal coronary arteriography. *Am J Cardiol* 1981; 48:193–197.
131. Bruce RA, DeRouen TA, Hossack KF, Blake B, Hofer V: Value of maximal exercise tests in risk assessment of primary coronary heart disease events in healthy men. Five years' experience of the Seattle Heart Watch Study. *Am J Cardiol* 1980; 46:371–378.
132. Dagenais GR, Rouleau JR, Christen A, Fabia J: Survival of patients with a strongly positive exercise electrocardiogram. *Circulation* 1982; 65:452–456.
133. Doyle JT, Kinch S: The prognosis of an abnormal electrocardiographic stress test. *Circulation* 1970; 41:545–553.
134. Ellestad MH, Wan MKC: Predictive implications of stress testing. *Circulation* 1975; 51:363–369.
135. Miller DH, Borer JS: Exercise testing early after myocardial infarction, risks and benefits. *Am J Med* 1982; 72:427–438.
136. DeBusk RF, Davidson DM, Houston N, Fitzgerald J: Serial ambulatory electrocardiography and treadmill exercise testing after uncomplicated myocardial infarction. *Am J Cardiol* 1980; 45:547–554.
137. DeBusk RF, Kraemer HC, Nash E: Stepwise risk stratification soon after acute myocardial infarction. *Am J Cardiol* 1983; 52:1161–1166.
138. Theroux P, Waters DD, Halphen C, Debaisieux JC, Mizgala HF: Prognostic value of exercise testing soon after myocardial infarction. *N Engl J Med* 1979; 301:341–345.
139. Theroux P, Marpole DF, Bourassa MG: Exercise stress testing in the post-myocardial infarction patient. *Am J Cardiol* 1983; 52:664–667.
139a. Weld FM: Exercise testing early after myocardial infarction. *J Cardiac Rehabil* 1985; 5:20–27.
139b. DeBusk RF: Techniques of exercise testing, in Hurst JW (ed): *The Heart*, ed 6. New York, McGraw-Hill, 1986, pp 1704–1716.
140. Ewart CK, Taylor CB, Reese LB, DeBusk RF: Effects of early post-myocardial infarction exercise testing on self-perception and subsequent physical activity. *Am J Cardiol* 1983; 51:1076–1080.
141. DeBusk RF, Haskell W: Symptom-limited versus heart rate-limited exercise testing soon after myocardial infarction. *Circulation* 1980; 61:738–743.
142. Starling MR, Crawford MH, Kennedy GT. O'Rourke RA: Exercise testing early after myocardial infarction. *Am J Cardiol* 1980; 46:909–914.
143. Davidson DM, DeBusk RF: The prognostic value of a single exercising test three weeks after uncomplicated myocardial infarction. *Circulation* 1980; 61:236–242.
144. McConahay DR, Valdes M, McCallister BD, Crockett JE, Conn RD, Reed WA, Killen DA: Accuracy of treadmill testing in assessment of direct myocardial revascularization. *Circulation* 1977; 56:548–552.
145. Rosing DR, Van Raden J, Mincemoyer RM, Bonow RO, David PR, Ewels CJ, Detie KM, Kent KM: Exercise electrocardiographic and functional responses after percutaneous transluminal coronary angioplasty. *Am J Cardiol* 1984; 53:36C–41C.
146. Val PG, David PR, Bourassa MG, Bosch X, Rapold HJ: Clinical symptom and treadmill exercise testing can detect restenosis ≧ 70% after successful coronary angioplasty (PTCA) (abstr). *J Am Coll Cardiol* 1985; 5:502.

11 Phonocardiography and External Pulse Recording

Frans Van de Werf, MD

Even in a period of increasing use of sophisticated imaging systems (two-dimensional echocardiography, digital subtraction angiography, and nuclear magnetic resonance) the graphic recording of externally registered low-frequency pulsations and high-frequency sounds and murmurs due to the mechanical action of the heart, also called phonomechanocardiography, remains an important noninvasive tool in clinical cardiology. As this method is noninvasive, inexpensive, and bedside applicable, it can be used by cardiologists throughout the world to obtain clinically relevant information regarding the functional state of the heart.

Essentially, the necessary equipment encompasses a microphone (converting the vibrations into electric pulses), an amplifier (to magnify the electrical pulses of small energy originating in the microphone), filters (to pass a given band of frequencies and to attenuate all others), and a graphic recording system (usually a galvanometer or cathode ray tube). Given the characteristics of human perception and because low-frequency vibrations have a much higher energy content, attenuation of the low-frequency components is required to record phonocardiograms that correlate with auscultation. On the contrary, for external pulse recording high frequencies (above 50 Hz) should be filtered out to obtain high quality tracings. An important characteristic of the whole system is its time constant (that is, the time interval necessary for the output level to drop to 37% of its initial maximum value). To reproduce long plateaus without appreciable decay, a time constant of more than 1 second is necessary.

The simultaneous use of multiple channels greatly enhances the diagnostic power of the method. One channel is always used for recording the electrocardiogram; two or more channels can be used for sound recording from a single microphone with different filters or from different microphones with an identical filter over different areas of the chest. If external pulses are to be studied, an additional channel or one of the channels used for sound recording will be required to record the pulse wave. The recording paper speed should be fast enough to allow accurate study of the tracings (at least 100 mm per second).

The advantages of phonomechanocardiographic registrations are numerous. The graphic registration objectifies auscultation or palpation, or both, and hence it may play an important role in the teaching of auscultation and clinical examination; it allows the recording of sounds that are difficult to perceive (eg, gallop sounds) or to differentiate from other sounds or murmurs (eg, ejection click); it permits sequential observations and simultaneous recordings of the electrocardiogram, pulse wave, and phonocardiogram and therefore measurement of multiple time intervals.

PHONOCARDIOGRAPHY

SOUNDS

First and Second Heart Sounds

The exact genesis of heart sounds remains a matter of controversy. According to the "valvular theory," the first and second heart sounds are causally related to the coaptation of the atrioventricular and semilunar valves, respectively.[1,2] Other investigators have claimed that the first and second heart sounds originate from vibrations of the "cardiohemic system" caused by acceleration or deceleration of blood flow when the valves are already closed by the action of the ventricles (contraction and relaxation). According to this theory, coaptation of the valvular cusps (due to small transvalvular pressure gradients) times the onset of the subsequent rapid processes of acceleration and deceleration as valvular closure permits the development of larger pressure gradients and hence more vigorous acceleration or deceleration.[3–5] These theories are not mutually exclusive as both recognize the importance of valvular closure and the generation of transvalvular pressure gradients.

The loudness of the first heart sound depends on the speed of pressure increase during contraction, the completeness of presystolic deceleration of ventricular inflow, and the ability of the atrioventricular valves to close. Therefore, the increased loudness associated with mitral stenosis, a short PR interval, or vigorous contraction, and the decreased intensity associated with a long PR interval, left ventricular failure, or mitral regurgitation can easily be explained.

The aortic and pulmonic components of the second heart sound normally fuse with full expiration and are separated (from 0.02 to 0.06 second) with inspiration. The increased right ventricular and decreased left ventricular ejection time associated with increased filling of the right heart and pooling of blood in the lungs during inspiration explains this "physiologic splitting." Prolonged right ventricular systole (pulmonary stenosis and right bundle branch block) or shortening of left ventricular ejection (mitral regurgitation) may produce wide splitting with respiratory variation. In atrial septal defect, respiration has little or no effect and splitting is called "fixed" even during expiration. As a rule, splitting of more than 0.04 second during held expiration must be considered pathologic. The aortic component normally is louder than the pulmonic component. Hypertension or dilatation of the aorta and pulmonary artery, or both, will increase the intensity of aortic and pulmonic components, respectively. However, valvular stenosis, particularly when the valve is calcified, will reduce the intensity of the sounds.

Ejection Sounds, Midsystolic Clicks, and Opening Snaps

Ejection sounds are of high frequency and occur early in systole (0.02 to 0.09 second after the beginning of the first heart sound). They are probably generated by stenotic (but not calcified) semilunar valves or by the wall of the (dilated) great vessels, or both. Congenital aortic and pulmonic stenosis with rapid acceleration of blood in early systole is the most common condition associated with an ejection sound. The ejection sound is usually followed by a systolic ejection murmur. Midsystolic clicks are associated with prolapse of the mitral valve cusps and may be accompanied by a late systolic murmur due to mitral regurgitation (click-murmur syndrome).

The opening snap is an early diastolic high-frequency sound observed in patients with mitral or tricuspid stenosis. The sound is best recorded between the left sternal border and the apex. The opening snap coincides with the maximum opening of the valve and may be due to tension of the altered valve leaflets or to increased sudden acceleration of blood to the ventricle following opening of the stenotic valve. The time interval from the aortic component of the second heart sound to the opening snap ranges from 0.03 to 0.13 second and is not influenced by respiration. In general, the shorter this time interval, the more severe the stenosis.[6] An opening snap may be absent when valvular movement is severely impaired and cardiac output is low.

Third and Fourth Heart Sounds

The third and fourth heart sounds are of low frequency and occur in early and late diastole, respectively. These sounds are commonly found in normal young individuals (under 40 years) and in athletes in whom they are considered physiologic.

Conditions associated with a pathologic third heart sound or protodiastolic gallop are: an increased early diastolic filling rate (high cardiac output states and mitral regurgitation), congestive heart failure, and restrictive cardiomyopathy. The pathologic third heart sound follows the second heart sound at approximately 0.150 to 0.180 second. Two other early diastolic sounds, the pericardial "knock" of constrictive pericarditis and the "tumor plop" associated with a left atrial myxoma, tend to be of higher frequency and occur earlier after the second heart sound than the third.

A pathologic fourth heart sound or presystolic gallop is associated with altered compliance of the left or right ventricular wall (eg, arterial or pulmonary hypertension, hypertrophic cardiomyopathy, and aortic or pulmonic stenosis). A prolonged PR interval usually enhances the audibility of the fourth heart sound.

Both physiologic and pathologic third and fourth heart sounds nearly have the same timing and frequency characteristics, suggesting an identical production mechanism. Recently, it was shown that the vibrations of these sounds occur during rapid deceleration of left ventricular inflow caused by a reversed (backward) transmitral pressure gradient.[7] These negative pressure gradients are generated by a rapid left ventricular pressure increase in the beginning and at the end of diastole: the so-called rapid filling wave and the A wave, respectively. Ventricular inflow rate, the completeness of ventricular relaxation, the viscoelastic properties of the ventricular wall, and atrial contractility determine the height and steepness of these pressure increases and hence the amount of deceleration of ventricular inflow and the loudness of these sounds.[8–10] This uniform concept for the genesis of both physiologic and pathologic third and fourth heart sounds offers a reasonable explanation for the presence of these sounds under different normal and abnormal hemodynamic conditions. It is also consistent with the recently proposed mechanism for disappearance of the physiologic third heart sound with age, ie, the development of relative left ventricular hypertrophy during adulthood as compared with childhood.[10a]

Other investigators, however, have suggested alternative mechanisms: impact of the heart against the chest wall, sudden intrinsic limitation of longitudinal expansion of the ventricular wall, or valvulvar contributions.[11–15]

Prosthetic Valve Sounds

The sounds generated by artificial valves have different characteristics depending on the type and location of the valve. The caged ball or disk valves produce the loudest sounds (opening and closing), whereas biologic valves produce sounds nearly comparable to those of a normal valve.

Combined M-mode echophonocardiography is a very

sensitive method for detecting malfunction of prosthetic valves.[16,17] For example, a time interval from the beginning of the second heart sound to the mitral valve opening of less than 0.075 second is highly suspicious of paravalvular regurgitation of the Björk–Shiley prosthetic mitral valve.

MURMURS

Murmurs are a series of vibrations of relatively long duration caused by turbulence of blood flow. Turbulence occurs when blood velocity becomes critically high (Reynolds number) in the presence of an obstruction to flow. Narrowing of the blood flow trajectory is usually formed by the valve orifices and hence these sites are the most common areas of murmur production, even in the absence of organic stenosis (eg, so-called functional murmurs).

The frequency of the vibrations caused by turbulence is directly related to flow velocity. The frequency content of a murmur can be estimated from its selective appearance in one or more channels on the phonocardiogram depending on the frequency bands of the filters used in these channels. For clinical purposes, murmurs are best categorized according to their location in the cardiac cycle.

Systolic Murmurs

Ejection murmurs are often diamond shaped, are of medium frequency, and reach their maximum intensity in midsystole. They begin after the first heart sound and end before closure of the semilunar valve on one side of the heart, but they may eventually continue through closure of the semilunar valve of the other side. Aortic and pulmonic stenoses are classic causes of such murmurs. A purely midsystolic ejection murmur is typical for idiopathic hypertrophic subaortic stenosis. Physiologic ejection murmurs often occur in young individuals especially during an increased rate of ejection of blood (fever and exercise). These murmurs occur in protosystole and are always of short duration (usually less than half the systole).

Holosystolic murmurs occur whenever a holosystolic gradient is present as in mitral regurgitation, tricuspid regurgitation, or ventricular septal defect. These murmurs are usually of high frequency and have a blowing quality. Telesystolic murmurs are a sign of mitral valve prolapse and often begin with a click.

Diastolic Murmurs

Diastolic murmurs due to insufficiency of the semilunar valves are of high frequency (blowing and decrescendo). Diastolic murmurs due to mitral and tricuspid stenosis are of low frequency and are called rumbles. They usually begin in early diastole immediately after an opening snap and may intensify during atrial contraction.

Continuous Murmurs

Continuous murmurs occur whenever systolic–diastolic pressure gradients are present as in cases of patent ductus arteriosus, rupture of a sinus of Valsalva into the right heart, arteriovenous fistulas, or stenotic peripheral arteries (eg, coarctation of the aortas and constriction of a peripheral pulmonary artery).

EXTERNAL PULSE RECORDING

The clinical importance of noninvasive recording of external pulses is based on the demonstration that the intracardiac or intravascular pressure is the major determinant of the time course and morphologic aspects of these tracings. A remarkable similarity has been demonstrated between the right and left apexcardiogram and right and left ventricular pressure tracing,[18–22] between the external carotid pulse and the central intraaortic pressure curve,[23] and between the jugular venous pulse and the right atrial pressure.[24]

The method most widely used for the recording of all different kinds of tracings is the displacement method. With this technique the displacement of the skin over the point of maximum impulse, caused by the action of the heart, is recorded by measuring the pressure changes in the air chamber of the pickup device (air-coupled crystal microphone). If required, the resulting signal can be calibrated (in relation to a known displacement volume) and differentiated (in function of an electrical ramp signal with a constant slope).[25,26]

JUGULAR VENOUS PULSE

The jugular venous pulse is best recorded in the supraclavicular region lateral to the medial attachment of the sternocleidomastoid muscle. Although the morphologic aspects of the jugular venous pulse are similar to those of the right atrial pressure, an important time delay exists between both tracings as a result of the transmission of the pressure wave to the superior caval vein.[27] A normal jugular venous pulse consists of two major peaks (a and v) and two major descents (x and y). In addition, a c wave and an h peak can be recorded (Figure 11.1a).

The a wave and the x descent are due to right atrial contraction and relaxation, respectively. The v wave is the result of filling of the right atrium when the atrioventricular waves are closed. The y descent reflects the decrease in right atrial pressure during diastolic emptying. The h wave, following the nadir of the y descent, indicates the end of passive filling of the right ventricle. It can be recorded in normal subjects only when the heart rate is sufficiently low.

The c wave is due to a bulging of the tricuspid valve into the right atrium during isovolumic contraction. In the normal jugular venous pulse the a wave is always the highest, whereas the x depression is always deeper than the y depression. The time interval between the pulmonic component of the second heart sound and the summit of the v wave is an indirect measure of right ventricular relaxation and is normally 0.06 to 0.08 second.

In constrictive pericarditis the y descent is steep, narrow, and nearly symmetrical (Figure 11.1b). The Qh interval is less than 0.07 second. It should be noted that in constrictive epicarditis or constrictive pericarditis complicated by pericardial effusion, the morphologic aspects of the jugular venous pulse closely resemble those of reduced right ventricular compliance, as will be discussed.

The jugular venous pulse in tricuspid regurgitation is characterized by a reduced or obliterated x depression. In severe cases the x depression is replaced by a systolic

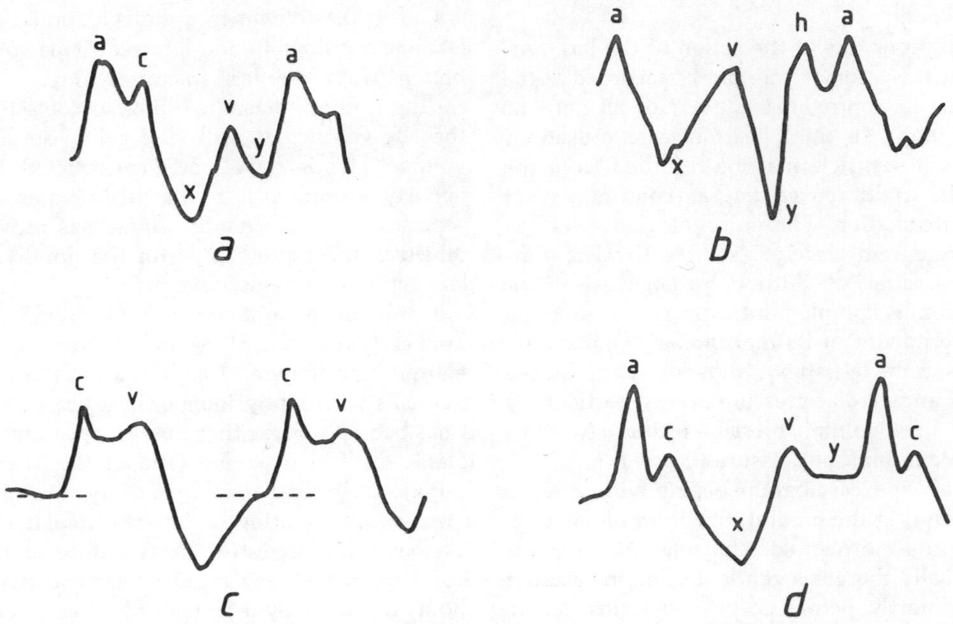

Figure 11.1. Contour of the jugular venous pulse. (*a*) Normal, (*b*) constrictive pericarditis, (*c*) tricuspid regurgitation, and (*d*) reduced right ventricular compliance.

square wave. Even if atrial fibrillation is present, the diagnosis can be made when the systolic wave exceeds the telediastolic level (Figure 11.1c). In these cases a systolic wave can often be recorded over the liver (liver pulse).

A prominent a wave, a marked x descent, and a shallow y depression are present in cases of reduced right ventricular compliance: right ventricular hypertrophy of any origin or reduction of right ventricular dimensions as a consequence of left ventricular hypertrophy (the Bernheim effect) (Figure 11.1d). The jugular venous pulse in tricuspid stenosis with sinus rhythm is similar to the one found in right ventricular hypertrophy, as already described. When atrial fibrillation is present, the morphologic characteristics are less typical. Due to the slow emptying of the right atrium a prolonged Qh interval can be found (if the heart rate is sufficiently low).

EXTERNAL CAROTID PULSE

The indirect carotid pulse is recorded in the mid-neck region (trigonum caroticum) directly over the point of maximum pulsations. Apart from the measurements of systolic time intervals (see chapter 12) contour analysis of the external carotid pulse may provide useful information. The normal carotid pulse shows several waves: the rapid upstroke and its initial peak (the percussion wave), the secondary wave or tidal wave late in systole, the dicrotic notch or incisura due to closure of the aortic valve, and the dicrotic wave (Figure 11.2a). Because of the transmission time of the pulse wave necessary to reach the neck, the mean delay between the incisura of the central aortic pressure and the carotid pulse averages 0.03 second.[23] The carotid pulse in valvular aortic stenosis has a typical contour: slow upstroke, anacrotic notching, superimposed vibrations ("shudder"), and flattening of the dicrotic notch (Figure 11.2b and c).

In aortic regurgitation the dicrotic wave will progressively disappear depending on the degree of insufficiency (Figure 11.2c and d). In severe cases this can lead to a "ventricularized" morphology. In idiopathic hypertrophic subaortic stenosis the carotid pulse is also typical: a rapid initial upstroke followed by an early systolic dip and a small tidal wave (Figure 11.2e). In left ventricular failure (eg, ischemic or idiopathic dilated cardiomyopathy) both upstroke and downstroke of the systolic part are slow and the dicrotic wave is pronounced (Figure 11.2f).

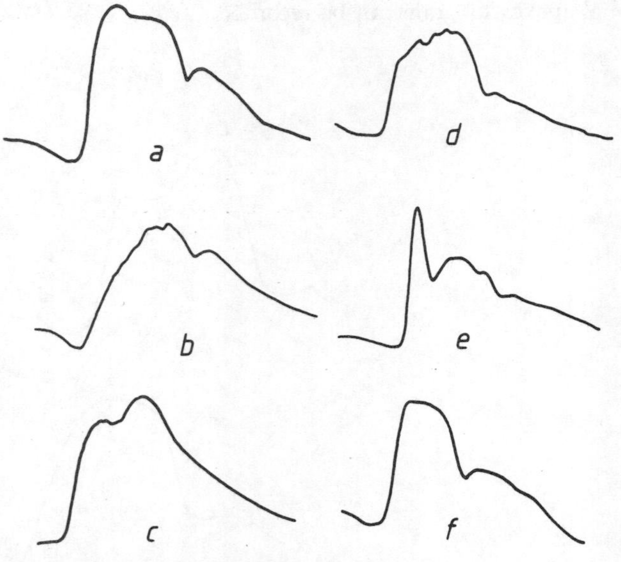

Figure 11.2. Contour of the external carotid pulse. (*a*) Normal, (*b*) valvular aortic stenosis, (*c*) aortic regurgitation, (*d*) combined aortic stenosis and regurgitation, (*e*) idiopathic hypertrophic subaortic stenosis, and (*f*) left ventricular failure.

APEXCARDIOGRAM

Precordial pulsations due to the action of the left ventricle throughout the cardiac cycle can be recorded at the apex of the heart in approximately 90% of all patients (left apexcardiogram). In right heart disease pulsations overlying the right ventricle may be recorded from the left sternal border (right apexcardiogram) and may offer useful clinical information. The morphologic aspects on the left apexcardiogram closely resemble the left ventricular pressure tracing.[18–22] Although the genesis of the left apexcardiogram is complex, intraventricular pressure is the major determinant of its morphologic characteristics. For this reason the left apexcardiogram is well suited for the timing of intracardiac pressure events, particularly the beginning of an isovolumic pressure increase (c point) and protodiastolic minimum pressure (0 point).[20,28]

The normal left apexcardiogram begins with a rapid upstroke which ends at the E point, the onset of ejection. During ejection, the morphologic characteristics are less constant, but usually there is a gentle decline toward the end of systole. Shortly before aortic valve closure the curve shows a sharp decline (onset of isovolumic relaxation) terminated by the protodiastolic nadir. Early diastolic filling produces a rapid filling wave which is followed by slow filling (diastasis) and an A wave as a consequence of left atrial contraction (Figure 11.3a).

During ejection the systolic part of the left apexcardiogram is variable. In pressure-load hypertrophy, a sustained systolic wave plateau after the E point can be recorded (Figure 11.3b). An aneurysm or severely reduced left ventricular function may produce pansystolic "bulging" of the left apexcardiogram with a slowly rising upstroke and an ill-defined E point (Figure 11.3c). In these cases the descending limb is also less steep, indicating delayed relaxation. Late systolic bulging can be seen in patients with ischemic heart disease (Figure 11.3d). In constrictive pericarditis no apex tracing at all or a systolic precordial retraction resembling a mirror image of a normal apexcardiogram can be recorded.

During diastole the morphologic similarity between the left apexcardiogram and left ventricular pressure is even better. Therefore, left apexcardiography has been used for the study of diastolic filling, viscoelastic properties of the left ventricular wall, and gallop sounds. "Pressure-volume" loops have been constructed from simultaneously recorded left apexcardiograms and M-mode echocardiograms. This technique has proven to be very sensitive and reproducible for the noninvasive study of left ventricular hemodynamics.[29]

A pronounced and peaked rapid filling wave indicates rapid early diastolic filling and is often recorded in mitral regurgitation (Figure 11.4a) but also in young normal individuals with a physiologic third heart sound. Recently it has been proposed that the disappearance of the physiologic third heart sound (and of the pronounced rapid filling) may be explained by a delayed relaxation rate and a less sudden halting of left ventricular filling in early diastole.[10] In congestive heart failure or restrictive cardiomyopathy a steep rapid filling wave (without overshoot) followed by a plateau (diastasis) can be recorded (Figure 11.4b). In these cases a pathologic third heart sound is nearly always perceived.

In pure mitral stenosis the rapid filling wave is faded out or completely absent. This, together with absence of an A wave (due to either atrial fibrillation or the stenosis itself), results in a typical gentle ascent of the curve throughout the total duration of diastole (Figure 11.4c).

An increased A wave (greater than 15% of the total height of the left apexcardiogram) excludes the diagnosis of significant mitral stenosis in the presence of sinus rhythm and indicates a diminished compliance of the left ventricular wall (eg, hypertrophy and fibrosis) (Figures 11.3b and 11.4d). As for the rapid filling wave, it has been shown that the speed of rise of the A wave (and not its total height) is the major determinant of the presence of a fourth heart sound.[9]

The introduction of calibrated apexcardiography has been of great help in further understanding the genesis

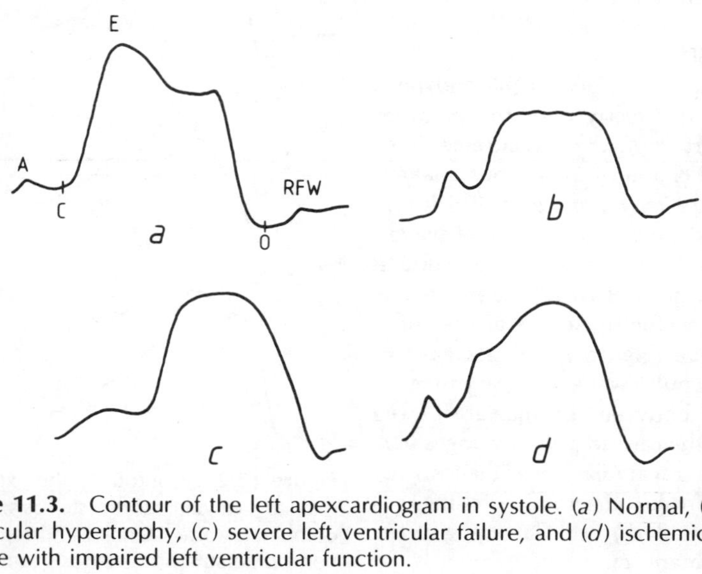

Figure 11.3. Contour of the left apexcardiogram in systole. (*a*) Normal, (*b*) left ventricular hypertrophy, (*c*) severe left ventricular failure, and (*d*) ischemic heart disease with impaired left ventricular function.

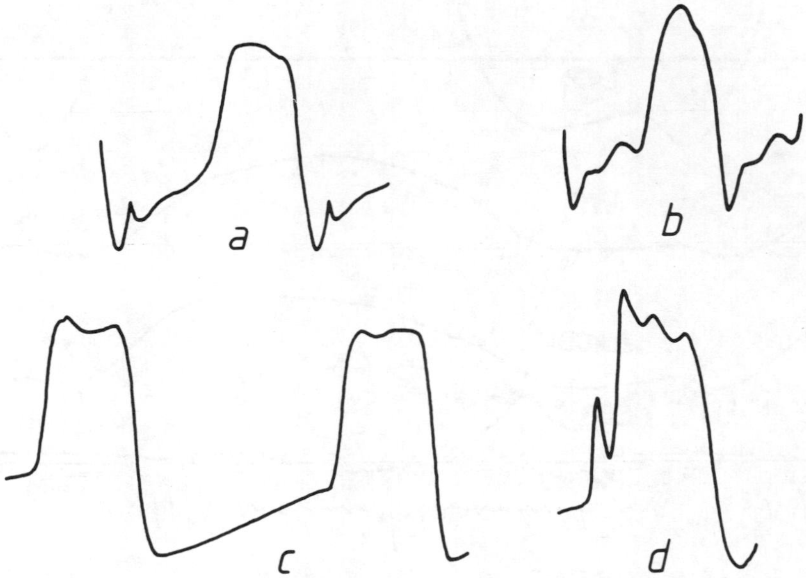

Figure 11.4. Contour of the left apexcardiogram in diastole. (*a*) Severe mitral regurgitation with preserved left ventricular function, (*b*) severe congestive heart failure, (*c*) mitral stenosis, and (*d*) idiopathic hypertrophic subaortic stenosis.

and clinical value of apexcardiography. A great similarity in slope exists between the left apexcardiogram and the left ventricular pressure tracing recorded with a tip-micromanometer (Figure 11.5). The identity in slope is especially prominent in isovolumic beats during which ballistic forces are supposedly nonexistent or minimal.[18] Furthermore, it should be remembered that the major parts of both the upstroke and the descent of the apexcardiogram occur during isovolumic contraction and relaxation. Moreover, as already mentioned, the apexcardiogram is well suited for the timing of intracardiac pressure events, such as the beginning of the systolic upstroke and the protodiastolic nadir.[20,28] From these observations it is apparent that intraventricular pressure plays a dominant role in the genesis of the apexcardiogram.

In the experimental animal significant correlations exist between the magnitudes and the peak first derivatives of left ventricular pressure waves and corresponding calibrated deflections of the apexcardiogram during both systole and diastole.[21,26,30] The higher degree of correlation that exists for diastolic events is probably due to the smaller wall tension in the myocardium during diastole, thus allowing more direct transmission of the intracavitary pressure wave. The greater heart volume during diastole also permits a better coupling of the heart to the thoracic wall.

On the basis of these experimental findings, indexes of contractility have been obtained from the left ventricular pressure tracing and the simultaneously recorded left apexcardiogram in patients with cardiac disease. The "normalized first derivatives" of the calibrated left apexcardiogram ($dD/dt/D$) and the left ventricular pressure ($dP/dt/P$) are similar in magnitude, standard deviation, and variation coefficient.[19] Highly significant linear correlations exist between the normalized first derivative of the apexcardiogram and other indexes of left ventricular function.[19] Moreover, this apexcardiographic index is superior to systolic time intervals for differentiation between normal and abnormal left ventricular function in patients with ischemic heart disease.[31]

Taking into account these results and the easy applicability and high reproducibility of the technique,[25,32–34] quantitative apexcardiography is very useful for repeated assessment of both systolic and diastolic left ventricular function in man. Recording devices for calibrated apexcardiography have been developed and are commercially available; they permit the immediate electronic calculation and recording of the magnitude, first derivative, and normalized first derivative of the different parts of the apical impulse.

HEMODYNAMIC INTERVENTIONS DURING PHONOMECHANOCARDIOGRAPHY

A number of pharmacologic agents can be used to alter the hemodynamic conditions of the recording. Inhalation of amyl nitrite causes arterial vasodilation and an increase in forward flow. Systolic ejection murmurs (aortic stenosis, pulmonic stenosis, and idiopathic hypertrophic subaortic stenosis) increase, whereas the holosystolic murmurs of mitral insufficiency and ventricular septal defect and the diastolic murmur of aortic insufficiency decrease. In idiopathic hypertrophic subaortic stenosis this test also provokes or accentuates the typical morphologic aspects of the carotid pulse (rapid upstroke followed by a pseudoincisura)(Figure 11.2e). Vasopressors such as phenylephrine or methoxamine generally exert opposite effects.

Isometric handgrip exercises increase the systemic blood pressure. As a result, the systolic murmurs of valvular aortic stenosis and idiopathic hypertrophic subaortic

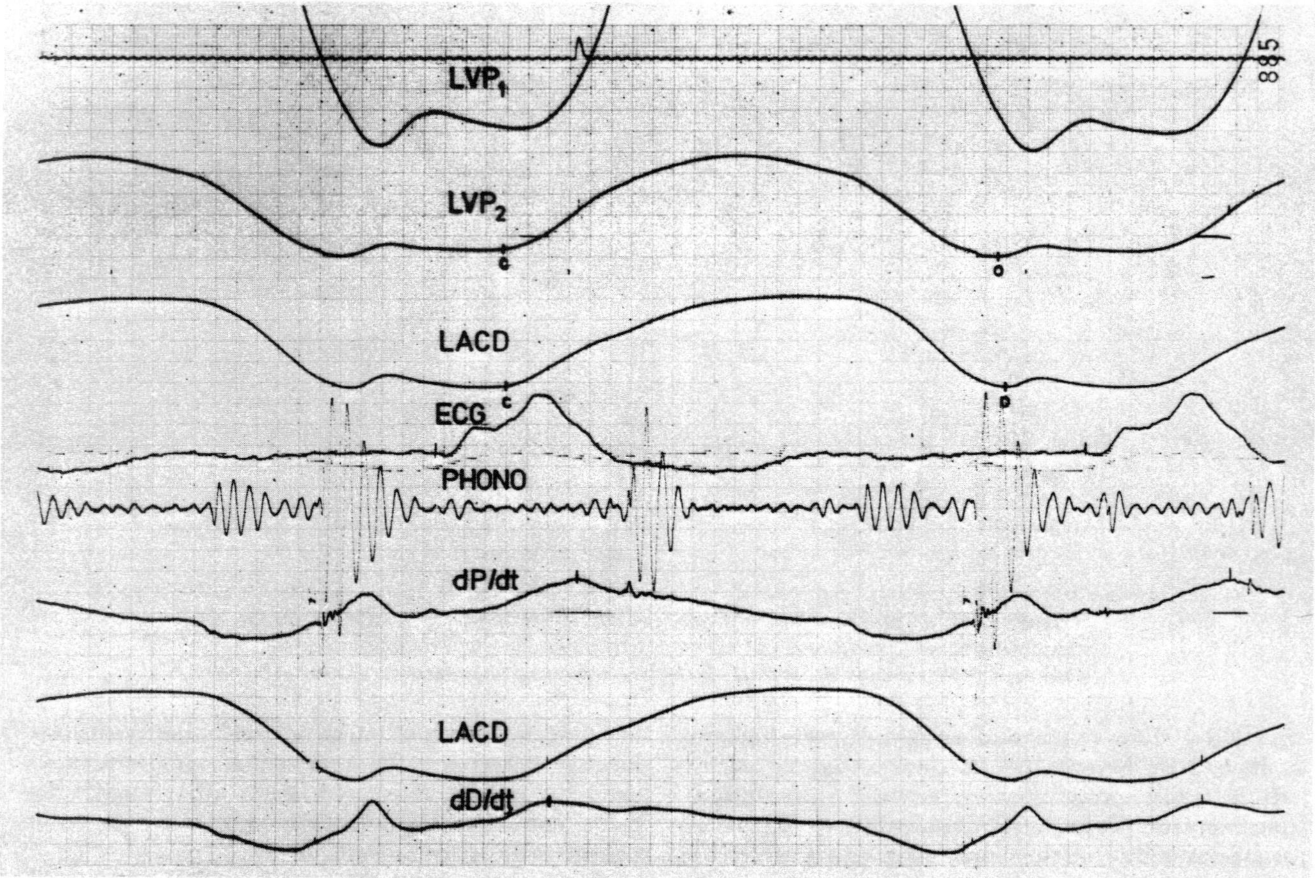

Figure 11.5. Simultaneous, high-speed (250 mm/s) recording of the calibrated displacement left apexcardiogram (LACD) and the left ventricular pressure tracing (LVP_1 = fluid-filled system; LVP_2 = micromanometer) and their corresponding first derivatives (dD/dt and dP/dt) in a patient with severe congestive heart failure. c = beginning of systolic upstroke; ECG = electrocardiogram; o = protodiastolic nadir; PHONO = external phonocardiogram.

stenosis decrease, whereas the diastolic murmur of aortic regurgitation increases. This test should not be used in patients with coronary insufficiency.

Because of technical problems, the Valsalva maneuver and prompt squatting (both influencing the venous return to the heart) are not suitable for graphic registration. These tests are better applied at the bedside during clinical examination.[35]

REFERENCES

1. Mills P, Craige E: Echophonocardiography. *Progr Cardiovasc Dis* 1978; 20:337–358.
2. Craige E: On the genesis of heart sounds: contributions made by echocardiographic studies. *Circulation* 1976; 53:207–209.
3. Rushmer RF: *Cardiovascular Dynamics.* Philadelphia, WB Saunders, 1976, p 241.
4. Luisada AA, Mac Canon DM, Kumar S, Feigen LP: Changing views on the mechanism of the first and second heart sounds. *Am Heart J* 1974; 88:503–514.
5. Piemme TE, Barnett GO, Dexter L: Relationship of heart sounds to acceleration of blood flow. *Circ Res* 1966; 18:303–315.
6. Oriol A, Palmer WH, Nakhajavan F, McGregor M: Prediction of left atrial pressure from the second sound, opening snap interval. *Am J Cardiol* 1965; 16:184–188.
7. Van de Werf F, Minten J, Carmeliet P, De Geest H, Kesteloot H: The genesis of the third and fourth heart sounds. A pressure-flow study in dogs. *J Clin Invest* 1984; 69:1400–1407.
8. Van de Werf F, Boel A, Geboers J, Minten J, Willems J, De Geest H, Kesteloot H: Diastolic properties of the left ventricle in normal adults and in patients with third heart sounds. *Circulation* 1984; 69:1070–1078.
9. Denef B, De Geest H, Kesteloot H: The clinical value of the calibrated A wave and its relationship to the fourth heart sound. *Circulation* 1979; 60:1412–1421.
10. Barrios L, Aubert A, Geboers J, De Geest H, Kesteloot H, Van de Werf F: The disappearance of the physiological third heart sound with age. (abstr) *Circulation* 1984; 70(suppl II):II-262.

10a. Van de Werf F, Geboer S, Kesteloot H, De Geest H, Barrios L: The mechanism of disappearance of the physiologic third heart sound with age. *Circulation* 1986; 73:877–884.

11. Aubert AE, Denys BG, Meno F, Reddy PS: Investigation of genesis of gallop sounds in dogs by quantitative phonocardiography and digital frequency analysis. *Circulation* 1985; 71:989–993.
12. Ozawa Y, Smith D, Craige E: Origin of the third heart sounds. I. Studies in dogs. *Circulation* 1983; 67:393–398.
13. Ozawa Y, Smith D, Craige E: Origin of the third heart sound. II. Studies in human subjects. *Circulation* 1983; 67:399–404.
14. Nixon PGF: The third heart sound in mitral regurgitation. *Br Heart J* 1961; 23:677–689.
15. Fleming JS: Evidence for a mitral valve origin of the left ventricular third heart sound. *Br Heart J* 1969; 31:192–199.
16. Tavel ME: Phonocardiography: clinical use with and without combined echocardiography. *Progr Cardiovasc Dis* 1983; 26:145–175.
17. Brodie BK, Grossman W, McLawin L, Starek P, Craige E: Diagnosis of prosthetic mitral valve malfunction with combined echo-phonocardiography. *Circulation* 1976; 53:93–100.
18. Kesteloot H, Willems J: Relation between the right apexcardiogram and the right ventricular dynamics. *Acta Cardiol* 1967; 22:64–89.
19. Van de Werf F, Piessens J, De Geest H, Kesteloot H: The normalized first derivative of the left apexcardiogram in the assessment of left ventricular function. *Am J Cardiol* 1976; 37:1059–1064.
20. Willems J, De Geest H, Kesteloot H: On the value of apexcardiography for timing intracardiac events. *Am J Cardiol* 1971; 28:59–66.

21. Willems J, Kesteloot H, De Geest H: Influence of acute hemodynamic changes on the apexcardiogram in dogs. *Am J Cardiol* 1972; 29:504–513.
22. Reddy PS, Meno F, Griff FW, O'Toole JD, Shaver JA: Calibrated apexcardiography. *Circulation* 1976; 54(suppl II):II-98.
23. Van de Werf F, Piessens J, Kesteloot H, De Geest H: A comparison of systolic time intervals derived from the central aortic pressure and from the external carotid pulse tracing. *Circulation* 1975; 51:310–316.
24. Hartman H: The jugular venous tracing. *Am Heart J* 1960; 59:698–703.
25. Denef B, Popeye R, De Geest H, Kesteloot H: On the clinical value of calibrated apexcardiography. *Circulation* 1975; 51:541–551.
26. Denef B, Van de Werf F, De Geest H, Kesteloot H: Calibrated apexcardiography and assessment of left ventricular dynamics in man. *Eur J Cardiol* 1976; 4(suppl):143–152.
27. Minten J, Van de Werf F, Aubert A, Kesteloot H, De Geest H: Apparent pulse wave velocity in the canine superior vena cava. *Cardiovasc Res* 1983; 17:627–632.
28. Van de Werf F, Piessens J, Kesteloot H, De Geest H: Value of apexcardiography for the timing of left ventricular events in man. *Acta Cardiol* 1978; 32:295–303.
29. Venco A, Gibson DG, Brown DJ: Relation between apexcardiogram and changes in left ventricular pressure and dimension. *Br Heart J* 1977; 39:117–125.
30. Denef B, De Geest H, Kesteloot H: Influence of change in myocardial contractility on the height and slope of the calibrated apex cardiogram. *Am J Cardiol* 1973; 32:662–669.
31. Van de Werf F, Piessens J, De Geest H, Kesteloot H: Mechanocardiographic assessment of left ventricular function in coronary artery disease. *Br Heart J* 1980; 43:184–190.
32. Bernardi L, Farilla C, Garavani E, Marni E, Trivi M, Zambelli A, Finardi G: Reproducibility of apexcardiographic indices. *Acta Cardiol* 1985; 40:29–32.
33. Linss G, Eisenberg BM, Purfurst WD, Witte J: Reproducibility of apexcardiographic data. *Acta Cardiol* 1985; 40:33–35.
34. Alvares RF: Value of phonomechanocardiography. *Acta Cardiol* 1986; 41:1–8.
35. Nishimura RA, Tajik AJ: The Valsalva maneuver and response revisited. *Mayo Clinic Proc* 1986; 61:211–217.

12 Systolic Time Intervals

Arnold M. Weissler, MD

Among the measures currently employed for assessing the functional state of the ventricular chambers in man by either invasive or noninvasive technique, the systolic time intervals are unique in several aspects. Their determination was the first quantitative measure designed to evaluate the contractile function of the heart in man[1] and the first for which the term noninvasive was designated.[2] Of physiologic significance is that the systolic time intervals represent a dimension of cardiac performance, namely time, that is distinct from other functional measures of the extent and force of ventricular wall contraction, ie, stroke volume, ejection fraction, intraventricular pressure, and wall tension. The ease with which the systolic time intervals can be measured repeatedly with safety and without discomfort to the patient has prompted a host of studies designed to perfect their measurement and to better understand their clinical significance. This chapter, based on these studies, summarizes current concepts pertinent to the measurement and clinical interpretation of the systolic time intervals (STI).

HISTORICAL BACKGROUND

The impetus for measuring the timing of the cardiac contraction cycle in humans probably derived from the invention of the physiologic kymograph by Ludwig[3] in 1847. Employing an adaptation of the Ludwig kymograph and the use of a sensitive transducer, Marey[4] first recorded the arterial and venous pulse in normal individuals and patients with various cardiac afflictions. In 1874, Garrod[1] employed such sphygmographic tracings to determine the duration of the length of systole (in fact, the duration of left ventricular ejection) and its relation to heart rate in humans. From limited observations he inferred that measurement of the duration of systole in this manner might prove useful in uncovering the presence of altered left ventricular contractile function in disorders of the heart. Thurston[5] in 1876 and Chapman[6] in 1894 elaborated on the observations of Garrod. It is of interest that the introduction of the measurement of the duration of systole preceded the invention of such time-honored clinical methods as the chest roentgenogram, the sphygmomanometer, and the electrocardiogram. In 1904, Bowen[7] graphically recorded the changes in the duration of ejection accompanying increasing heart rate during exercise, and in so doing he was the first to introduce exercise testing as a method for assessing cardiac function in man. The first experimental studies of the physiologic significance of the duration of the phases of the cardiac cycle were conducted by Frank[8] and Wiggers.[9,10] The studies of Lombard and Cope[11] in human subjects established the presence of slight but significant differences between males and females and demonstrated the critical influence of changes in posture on the duration of ejection. Katz and Feil,[12,13] who first applied modern electronic recording and photographic technique in the determination of the phases of systole, studied changes in the STI in atrial fibrillation and hypertension. Blumberger,[14] in a classical series of studies on a wide variety of patients, demonstrated their potential clinical usefulness in valvular heart disease and in disorders of left ventricular muscle contraction.

Despite their early introduction, clinical application of the STI has received relatively less attention than have other noninvasive methods for assessing ventricular performance such as echocardiography and radioisotopic imaging. In part this reflects the different nature of the STI, which denotes the timing of events of the cardiac cycle rather than the extent of wall and chamber motion. The fact that time is a more abstract dimension of cardiac function than is the anatomic movement that other methods depict probably adds to this phenomenon. In addition, the fact that the STI is subject to transient circulatory influences, such as changes in diastolic wall stress (preload), systolic outflow impedance (afterload), and intrinsic contractile state (physiologic factors that influence virtually all other measures of ventricular global performance as well), has deterred some from accepting these measures as valid expressions of cardiac performance in man. With better understanding that the temporal events of the cardiac cycle can be delineated accurately and that their measurement and interpretation can uncover the presence of significant alterations in left ventricular performance, the STI have gained wider clinical application in recent years.

METHODOLOGIC BACKGROUND

The STI, which constitutes the sequential phases of left ventricular systole, is precisely and inexpensively determined from simultaneous high-speed recordings of the electrocardiogram, phonocardiogram, and carotid arterial pulse tracing.[2,15,16] In practice, three primary measurements of the phases of systole are determined: duration of electromechanical systole (QS_2), pre-ejection period (PEP) and, left ventricular ejection time (LVET) (Figure 12.1). The QS_2, which is measured directly, is the interval that encompasses the entire systolic period from the onset of the QRS complex on the electrocardiogram to the closure of the aortic valve as denoted in the aortic component of the second heart sound on the phonocardiogram. The

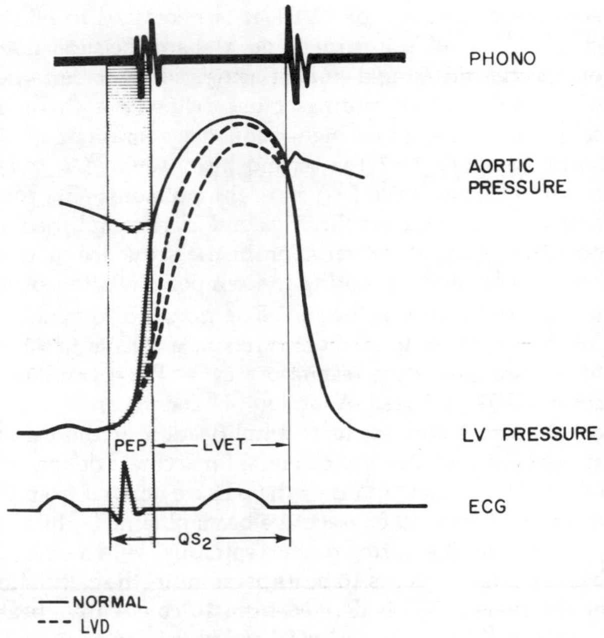

Figure 12.2. Relation of measured systolic time intervals to the normal cardiac cycle (*solid line*). *Dashed lines* illustrate the changes induced in left ventricular decompensation (LVD). ECG = electrocardiogram; phono = phonocardiogram. For other abbreviations, see Figure 12.1.

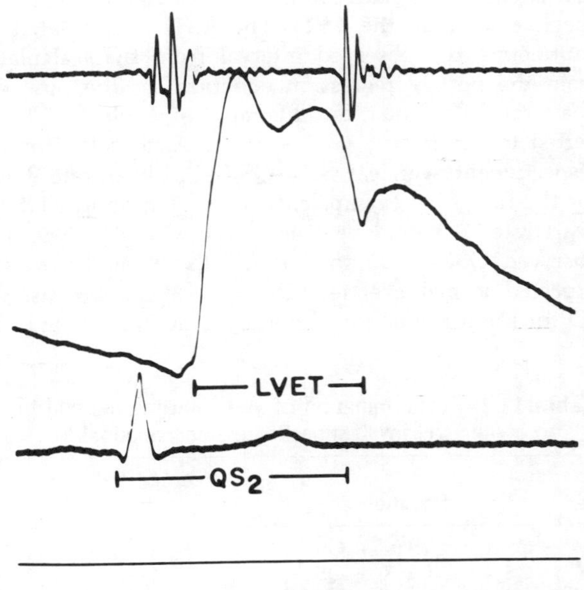

Figure 12.1. Measurement of systolic time intervals from simultaneous recordings at 100 mm/sec paper speed of the electrocardiogram, phonocardiogram, and carotid arterial pulse tracing. LVET = left ventricular ejection time; PEP = preejection period; QS_2 = interval from onset of QRS on electrocardiogram to the aortic component of second heart sound on phonocardiogram. (From Lewis et al,[16] with permission.)

LVET, which is measured directly as well, is the interval from the beginning upstroke to the trough of the incisura on the carotid arterial tracing. It is the phase of systole during which the left ventricle ejects into the arterial system. The PEP, the interval from the onset of ventricular depolarization to the beginning of ejection, is derived by subtracting the LVET from the QS_2 interval. Calculation of the PEP in this manner discounts the error resulting from the delay in transmission of the arterial pulse from the proximal aorta to the point of its detection over the carotid artery. The PEP can be derived alternatively by measuring the interval from the onset of ventricular depolarization to the beginning of the upstroke of the carotid arterial pulse, from which the arterial pulse transmission time (the A_2-incisural interval) is subtracted. The relation of the measured STI to the cardiac cycle is illustrated in Figure 12.2.

To make these measurements accurately, meticulous methodologic detail must be followed. In modern practice the standard or precordial lead that elicits the earliest onset of electrical depolarization is selected. This lead is best determined from simultaneous recordings of electrocardiographic leads that encompass three planes of depolarization force (ie, leads I, aVF, and V_1). The phonocardiogram should be recorded over the upper precordium in the frequency range 100 to 500 Hz. The carotid arterial pulse must be recorded with high-fidelity instrumentation. In our laboratory a strain gauge transducer, which permits a flat frequency and phase response between 0.1 and 30.0 Hz and an infinite time constant, is preferred. An arterial or venous pressure strain gauge transducer used at near maximum gain suffices for this purpose. For accurate delineation of LVET it is necessary to elicit a clearly discernible upstroke and a sharp incisural notch on the carotid arterial pulse tracing. For best definition of the QS_2, the recordings must delineate a sharp inscription of the initial high-frequency vibrations of the aortic component of the second heart sound (A_2). Segregation of the aortic (A_2) from the pulmonic (P_2) component of the second heart sound is accomplished by observing respiratory variation in the sequence of these components and by noting the temporal relation of A_2 to the carotid arterial incisura. The trough of the incisura follows A_2 by 20 to 30 ms and retains a constant relation to A_2 throughout the respiratory cycle. Photographic recordings are preferred. A minimum paper recording speed of 100 mm/s and adequate amplification of the carotid arterial pulse are deemed essential for accurate delineation of the STI.[17] Calculations of the STI are derived from the mean of at least 10 consecutive beats obtained while the patient is supine during quiet respiration. When beat-to-beat variation exceeds 10 beats per minute, the calculation of the average STI is derived from 20 consecutive beats. Studies validating the technical and physiologic principles underlying the measurement of the STI have been summarized by Lewis et al.[17]

The STI can be determined from simultaneous recordings of the M-mode echocardiogram, measuring the interval from the onset of ventricular depolarization to the opening of the aortic valve (PEP) and that between the opening and closing of the aortic valve (LVET).[18–21] This method is most useful in children in whom the temporal landmarks are best delineated by the echocardiogram. Recent studies suggest that the impedance cardiogram[22,23] and ultrasonic Doppler methods[24–26] may be a useful alternative for determining the STI. The consistency of the temporal landmarks with these latter methods needs verification and the relative value of impedance cardiography and Doppler techniques in measuring the STI requires additional clinical study. With respect to the echocardiographic measurement of STI, our preference remains with the method employing simultaneous recordings of the electrocardiogram, phonocardiogram, and carotid arterial pulse because it is less costly and because the echocardiogram does not permit visualization of the onset and termination of ejection as consistently as does the carotid arterial pulse. The two approaches are complementary, however, so that when the temporal landmarks for the STI are not well delineated from graphic recordings of the electrocardiogram, phonocardiogram, and carotid arterial pulse, they may be detected by the echocardiographic approach. The echocardiogram can also be applied to verify observations on the STI when their clinical evaluation from the graphic recordings is in question.

In simplest terms, the STI delineates the duration of the major components of the systolic cycle of the left ventricle, namely, the pre-ejection period (PEP), left ventricular ejection time (LVET), and the duration of total electromechanical systole (QS_2). Measurement of the STI by the noninvasive approach affords an accurate determination of the same intervals measured from high fidelity catheter tip micrometers placed in the left ventricle and aorta.[27,28]

Clinical application of the STI is rooted in the fact that the STI in the normal population falls within narrow physiologic limits that are well defined by linear regression equations[2,15,16] relating the intervals to heart rate.

In practice, each interval (QS_2, PEP, and LVET) can be corrected for heart rate and sex employing the normal regression equations.[2,15,16] In one method, the regression equations are transposed from the slope-intercept form $y = -mx + b$ to the form $b = y + mx$ (where y equals the measured interval, m the regression slope, x the measured heart rate, and b the intercept at 0 heart rate) (Table 12.1). The b value is termed the STI index (QS_2I, LVETI, and PEPI). The STI index so calculated is the intercept of the regression equation at 0 heart rate when the measured interval and heart rate are entered into the regression equation. The calculation assumes that the normal regression slope relating heart rate and interval remains constant. The latter assumption has held for normal individuals as well as patients with heart failure. Deviation from the normal mean interval index is a measure of deviation in the measured interval from the respective normal regression equation at the observed heart rate.

For example, if a male patient is observed to have a QS_2 of 360 at heart rate 70, the QS_2I would be calculated as $360 + (2.1 \times 70) = 507$. The difference between this value and the expected normal index of 546 (546 − 507) is 39 ms. This difference is equivalent to 2.8 standard deviations (SDs) below the normal index; hence, it would be considered abnormally low (greater than 2 SDs below normal).

An alternative means for expressing variation from normal is the direct calculation of the deviation in the respective interval, the ΔSTI. The ΔSTI is calculated by subtracting the observed interval from that calculated from the normal regression equation for the observed heart rate. The equation illustrated in Table 12.1 is inverted to the form $y = b - mx$ so as to solve for the respective interval, ie, $QS_2 = QS_2I - 2.1$ heart rate. Thus, for the foregoing examp-le, the expected normal QS_2 at heart rate 70 would be $(546 - 2.1 \times 70)$ or 399. The observed QS_2 is 360 so that it falls 39 ms below the expected normal level, ie, $\Delta QS_2 = -.39$ ms. Because the SD for the regression equation is 14 ms this value is 2.8

Table 12.1. Determination of Systolic Time Interval Index Values From Resting Regression Equations*

Sex	Equation	Normal Index (ms)	SD
M	$QS_2I = 2.1\ HR + QS_2$	546	14
F	$QS_2I = 2.0\ HR + QS_2$	549	14
M	LVETI = 1.7 HR + LVET	413	10
F	LVETI = 1.6 HR + LVET	418	11
M	PEPI = 0.4 HR + PEP	131	10
F	PEPI = 0.4 HR + PEP	133	10

*The measured heart rate (HR) and systolic interval are entered into the appropriate equation. The difference between observed and normal index is the deviation from normal in the systolic interval for the observed heart rate. The two standard deviation (SD) limit is considered normal. QS_2I, LVETI, and PEPI refer to the respective interval index.

LVETI = left ventricular ejection time index; PEPI = pre-ejection period index; QS_2I = duration of electromechanical systolic index.

SDs below the norm. Note that the deviation in the respective interval from the normal regression line as calculated by either of the foregoing methods constitutes the absolute deviation from the expected normal value.

Determination of the STI and appropriate corrections for heart rate may be processed by computer. Two approaches to computer measurements are applicable. In the first, a technician-assisted method, a light pen is used to delineate the relevant temporal landmarks on the primary recording from which the intervals, their indexes, and the PEP/LVET are computed. In the second, the intervals and their indexes are determined entirely by automated computerized techniques.[29,30] For the purpose of discussion in this chapter the designation of PEPI, LVETI, and QS_2I will refer to the respective intervals corrected for heart rate and expressed as the respective STI index.

In clinical application the PEP/LVET determination is a useful overall expression of the changes induced by left ventricular dysfunction (see next section). The normal PEP/LVET is .34 (1 SD = .04). The PEP/LVET is only slightly influenced by heart rate and sex and for practical purposes requires no correction in the range of heart rate from 50 to 110 beats per minute.

PHYSIOLOGIC DETERMINANTS AND THE INTERPRETATION OF THE SYSTOLIC TIME INTERVALS

Early laboratory studies on the determinants of the duration of the phases of systole in the isolated dog heart employing modern physiologic recording techniques demonstrated that when heart rate was controlled, the duration of the phases of systole related closely to the magnitude of the left ventricular stroke volume.[31] With extreme elevations in arterial pressure and constant heart rate and stroke volume, LVET was increased. Later observations established that the duration of the phases of systole were influenced by sudden alterations in preload, afterload, and the intrinsic contractile state of the myocardium.[32] In a contemporary reevaluation of these physiologic relations, Nakamura et al[33] employed an elegant isolated rat papillary or trabecular left ventricular muscle segment preparation with computer-assisted technology to study the determinants of the duration of the phases of systole. They labeled the intervals the preshortening period (PSP, an analog of the PEP), the isotonic contraction time (ICTC, an analog of LVET), and the duration of electromechanical systole (EMS, an analog of QS_2). These studies confirmed, in the isolated myocardial segment, the independent contributions of loading and intrinsic myocardial function to the duration of the sequential phases of ventricular systole. Thus, increased preload caused an abbreviation in the PSP and an increase in the ICTC with lengthening of the EMS. The ratio of PSP to ICTC (an analog of PEP/LVET) decreased with increased preload. Increases in total load induced opposite changes (lengthening of PSP, abbreviation of ICTC, and an increase in PSP/ICTC) with little influence on the duration of EMS. In these experiments the responses in systolic intervals to the positive inotropic effects of isoproterenol and calcium differed somewhat, suggesting that differences in the mechanisms of inotropic stimulation may yield varying responses in the STI. Isoproterenol induced a shortening of all phases of systole with little change in PSP/ICTC. Calcium induced shortening of PSP and lengthening of ICTC and EMS, while PSP/ICTC decreased.

The responses to loading and inotropic intervention observed in the isolated myocardial strip experiments are reminiscent of, although not identical to, those observed in man as summarized in previous publications[16,34,35] and in Figure 12.3. Thus, increased preload in man induces a decrease in PEPI, a lengthening of LVETI, and a slight prolongation of QS_2I, while PEP/LVET decreases. Decreased preload induces opposite effects. Increases in total load (afterload) induce increased PEPI, decreased LVETI, and increased PEP/LVET with only a slight increase or no effect on QS_2I. Reduced afterload induces opposite effects. It is of importance to note that the effect of afterload on the STI may be influenced by concomitant changes in preload. Thus, pharmacologically induced increases in afterload, when accompanied by concomitant increases in preload (combined preload and afterload increase), may prolong both PEPI and LVETI.[36] The changes induced by positive inotropic agents in man consist of an abbreviation in PEPI and a variable response in LVETI. The latter is dependent upon the magnitude of the inotropic response. Left ventricular ejection time index is reduced or remains unchanged at lower levels of stimulation, whereas it increases with maximum positive inotropic stimulation. Positive inotropic influences induce a consistent decrease in QS_2I usually accompanied by a decrease in PEP/LVET.[16] It is to be emphasized that altered preload and afterload influence QS_2I only minimally (usually no greater than 1 SD change), whereas positive and negative inotropic agents exert major decreases and increases, respectively, in QS_2I (in the range of 2 to 8 SD ms). Because of these characteristics of the QS_2I, useful insight can be gained into the presence of positive (shortened QS_2I) and negative (lengthened QS_2I) inotropic influences when STI alterations are analyzed. The finding of a QS_2I less than 518 in the male (521 in the female) lends evidence for a positive inotropic influence. In supine normal individuals and patients, changes in PEPI, LVETI, and PEP/LVET induced by loading generally do not exceed three normal SD units, whereas positive and negative inotropic influences commonly induce changes in the range of 3 to 8 SD units. Major deviations from normal in PEPI, LVETI, or PEP/LVET (greater than 3 SD units) in the supine subject should not be attributed to the effect of loading alone.

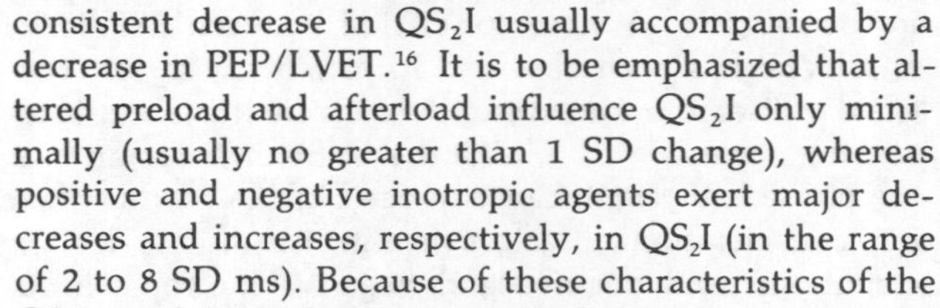

Figure 12.3. Acute interventions that influence the systolic time intervals. See text for details and Figure 12.1 for abbreviations.

Clearly, the duration of the phases of the cardiac cycle is governed by the same factors (baseline ventricular performance, heart rate, changes in systolic preload and afterload, and altered myocardial contractility) that have been demonstrated in the past to control left ventricular stroke volume, stroke work, ejection fraction, and the rate of increase in systolic pressure in the normal and abnormal ventricle. The fact that the responses in the STI are easily discernible and that the intervals can be measured repetitively with no intrusion of the vascular system allows sequential testing of the influence of pharmacologic agents and other therapeutic maneuvers in normal individuals as well as patients with left ventricular dysfunction.

The clinical interpretation of the STI in cardiac disease is founded on the now well-established observation that as left ventricular chamber performance deteriorates in patients with left ventricular disease, a distinct pattern of change in the STI evolves: PEPI lengthens, LVETI shortens, and PEP/LVET increases, whereas QS_2 remains virtually unchanged[2,15,16] (Figure 12.2). The increase in PEP/LVET is closely correlated with the reduction in stroke volume, cardiac output, left ventricular ejection fraction, and an index of left ventricular contractile performance derived from the first derivative of isovolumic left ventricular pressure[2,15,16,37–39] in patients with coronary artery, primary myocardial, and hypertensive disease. Identical directional changes in the STI have been described recently in laboratory-induced Adriamycin® cardiotoxicity in the rabbit.[40] A close correlation between PEP/LVET and LVEF has been observed in patients with left ventricular disease in the presence of cardioactive and load-altering agents.[37–39,41–43] Like the LVEF, interpretation of the physiologic significance of the PEP/LVET must take into consideration all factors (ie, intrinsic disease, loading conditions, and positive and negative inotropic influences) that may influence global left ventricular function. In this regard, changes due to ventricular loading alone rarely alter baseline levels of PEP/LVET beyond 3 normal SD units in the supine subject, whereas left ventricular decompensation generally induces changes in the range of 3 to 12 SD units above normal.

Alterations in ventricular conduction may of themselves induce changes in STI.[16,44–49] Characteristically, the presence of left bundle branch block tends to prolong the PEPI and QS_2I selectively (usually in proportion to the lengthening in QRS), whereas LVETI remains within levels expected for the stroke volume and ejection fraction. The PEP/LVET is therefore increased because of the selective increase in PEP. Prolongation of the PEPI accounts almost completely for the change in QS_2I. Patients with isolated left axis deviation have changes similar in direction but of lesser magnitude in PEPI, QS_2I, and PEP/LVET. Right bundle branch block per se has little influence on the left-sided STI. Patients with combined bundle branch block may demonstrate a disproportionate lengthening of the PEPI and QS_2I similar to that for left bundle branch block. The left bundle branch block type conduction disturbance that is produced by right ventricular pacing is also associated with selective lengthening of the PEPI and QS_2I. The latter effect is particularly well seen in patients in whom atrial pacing alone is alternated with synchronized right atrial and right ventricular pacing. At the same ventricular rate as observed with atrial pacing alone, synchronized ventricular pacing induces prolonged QRS of the left bundle branch block type associated with prolonged PEP and QS_2, whereas LVET is unchanged.[16] In interpreting changes in STI in patients with intraventricular conduction blocks, the influence of left ventricular dysfunction in addition to the conduction delay must be taken into account. In view of their significant influence on the duration of the PEPI, QS_2I, and the PEP/LVET, the possibility of left intraventricular conduction delay must always be considered in interpreting the STI.

The lengthening of the PEPI in left bundle branch block is caused primarily by a delay in the onset of left ventricular mechanical activity and by a diminished rate of pressure increase due to an asynergic contractile pattern during isovolumic systole. A diminution in the rate of pressure increase due to left ventricular contractile dysfunction per se may add to prolongation of the PEPI. The prolongation of PEPI in left bundle branch block is associated with lengthening in its measured subintervals, the Q to onset of left ventricular systole on the apex cardiogram, the Q to onset of the mitral component of the first heart sound on the phonocardiogram, and the Q to opening of the mitral valve on the echocardiogram.

CLINICAL APPLICATIONS OF THE SYSTOLIC TIME INTERVALS

CHRONIC CORONARY ARTERY DISEASE

Studies of the STI in coronary artery disease in recent years have focused on its potential for following the course of left ventricular function and its prognostic implications. The accuracy of PEP/LVET in detecting and quantitating left ventricular dysfunction in chronic coronary artery disease has been studied in patients who survived previous myocardial infarction as well as in those with angina pectoris and no clinical evidence of previous myocardial infarction.[50] In these studies, coronary artery disease was confirmed by diagnostic coronary arteriography and left ventricular function was evaluated by ventriculographic estimates of left ventricular ejection fraction (LVEF). The STI in patients with coronary artery disease was compared with that in a third (control) group of patients who were evaluated for atypical chest pain by cardiac and coronary catheterization and found to have normal coronary arteries and ventricular function. Multiple methods of statistical analysis were applied in testing the accuracy of the STI. Analysis of variance and cumulative distribution plots revealed that the patients with previous myocardial infarction were significantly different in all measures (PEPI, LVETI, PEP/LVET, and LVEF) from normal subjects and patients with coronary artery disease without previous myocardial infarction. The latter two groups did not differ from each other in either LVEF or STI. The discriminating power of the PEP/LVET was virtually identical to that of the LVEF in separating the group with previous myocardial infarction from the normal subjects and patients with angina pectoris without previous myocardial infarction. The PEPI and the LVETI alone were less discriminating than the PEP/LVET in separating the groups. Employing 2 SDs as the lower limit of normal for LVEF (0.52), the presence of an abnormal PEP/LVET (greater than .42) permitted separation of normal and abnormal LVEF with an overall accuracy exceeding 90%. The close parallelism between PEP/LVET and LVEF in defining the presence of normal and abnormal left ventricular global function in patients with established coronary artery disease was thus confirmed.

The close relation between PEP/LVET and LVEF among patients with coronary artery disease occurs in the presence of antianginal drugs, beta blockade therapy, digitalis, and diuretics. The two measures of global left ventricular performance hence are equivalent in their capacity to define and quantitate the level of ventricular dysfunction among treated patients with coronary artery disease.

Additional studies have focused on the relation of left ventribular dysfunction, as detected by PEP/LVET, to the extend of coronary artery disease in patients with and without previous myocardialinfarction.[51] Among patients with angina pectoris in the absence of previous myocardial infarction the relative incidence of abnormal left ventricular global function as measured by PEP/LVET is minimal (4%) at all levels of angiographically defined coronary artery disease. In contrast, among patients with angina pectoris and previous myocardial infarction there is a high incidence of persistent left ventricular global dysfunction (58%) at all levels of coronary artery occlusive disease. Measurements of LVEF by contrast ventriculography among the same groups of patients confirm the high frequency of global dysfunction in patients with previous myocardial infarction and the low frequency of global dysfunction in the absence of previous myocardial infarction.[51] Of special clinical interest is the finding among patients with chronic angina pectoris that an abnormal PEP/LVET is associated with a 95% probability of previous myocardial infarction. The clinical value of STI in assessing left ventricular function in chronic coronary artery disease has been supported by several additional recent studies.[52–56]

A criticism of the clinical value of the STI maintains that these measures offer little beyond conventional clinical findings in detecting the presence of left ventricular dysfunction. We have challenged the validity of this view in a study of 136 patients with established coronary artery disease, among whom the accuracy of STI and clinical indicators was compared employing the LVEF as the independent measure of left ventricular function. The clinical indicators tested included the presence of dyspnea (New York Heart Association class 3 or 4), the presence of S_4 and S_3 gallop on cardiac auscultation, and the measurement of the cardiothoracic ratio on chest roentgenogram. The sensitivity, specificity, positive and negative predictive value, and overall accuracy of the PEP/LVET and the clinical descriptors are summarized in Table 12.2. It is clear from this analysis that none of the clinical descriptors could approach the discriminating power of the PEP/LVET in establishing the presence of left ventricular dysfunction among patients with coronary artery disease.

Other studies have supported the view that STI measurements may provide useful prognostic indicators in patients with established coronary artery disease. Recent studies show a high level of stratification of mortality risk by the level of abnormality in PEP/LVET among patients who have recovered from remote myocardial infarction[57–60] (Figure 12.4). When the relative prognostic potency of the PEP/LVET and the extent of coronary arteriographic disease were compared, the dominant risk determinant was the state of left ventricular performance.[60] Of interest was the finding that irrespective of the extent of arterial occlusive disease, patients with a normal PEP/LVET retain a relatively low mortality risk. Thus, five-year survival in patients with one-, two-, or three-vessel disease and a normal PEP/LVET following recovery from acute myocardial infarction was, respectively, 97%, 92%, and 87%. Among patients with abnormal left ventricular performance (PEP/LVET greater than 0.42), the respective five-year survival was 82%, 51%, and 41%. These studies demonstrate that the determination of left ventricular performance by the STI offers an accurate means for detecting the patient with a high mortality risk following previous myocardial infarction. Of various clinical descriptors applied in the past to detect the high risk patient (severity of angina, dyspnea, S_3 or S_4 gallop, hypertension, hypercholesterolemia, previous myocardial infarction, history of smoking, and cardiomegaly on x-ray), no single or combined grouping proved to be as potent as the noninvasive assessment of left ventricular function.[60]

Table 12.2. Accuracy of Clinical Indicators of Left Ventricular Dysfunction in Patients With Previous Myocardial Infarction*

	Sensitivity (%)	Specificity (%)	Positive Predictive Value (%)	Negative Predictive Value (%)	Accuracy (%)
S_4 gallop	49	46	48	47	48
S_3 gallop	24	95	83	56	60
Dyspnea class III–IV	32	95	86	58	64
CTR > 0.5	37	91	80	59	64
PEP/LVET	88	96	96	89	92

* Data derived from 136 patients with previous myocardial infarction. Accuracy is the percentage of accurate predictions per total predictions. Standard of reference for left ventricular dysfunction is left ventricular ejection fraction < 0.52, PEP/LVET > 0.42.

CTR = cardiothoracic ratio.

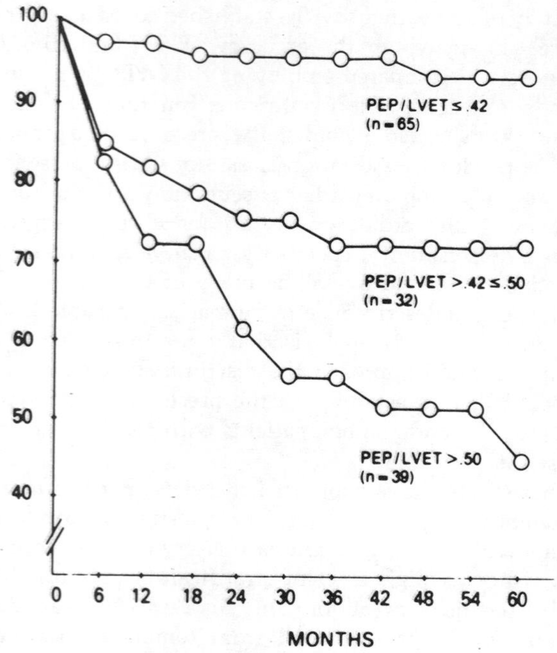

Figure 12.4. Cumulative five-year survival in patients subgrouped according to the presence of a normal ratio of preejection period to left ventricular ejection time (PEP/LVET) (0.42 or less), a moderately abnormal PEP/LVET (0.43 to 0.50), or a severely abnormal PEP/LVET (greater than 0.50). The trend for diminishing survival with increasing left ventricular dysfunction is significant ($P < 0.05$). (From Weissler et al,[60] with permission.)

The PEP/LVET has been valuable in segregating patients with angina pectoris and previous myocardial infarction who are appropriate candidates for coronary bypass surgery.[61] Patients with an abnormal PEP/LVET and two- or three-vessel disease exhibit improved longevity following coronary bypass surgery when compared with medically treated patients. Patients with a normal PEP/LVET and equivalent coronary artery occlusive disease exhibit no improvement in longevity following coronary bypass surgery. Other studies have demonstrated that the STI is of additional value in assessing the influence of coronary bypass surgery on left ventricular function.[62-65] A recent study demonstrated that patients on long-term propranolol therapy following previous myocardial infarction have major improvement in the five-year mortality rate if left ventricular performance indicated by PEP/LVET is below normal (PEP/LVET greater than 0.42), whereas those with a normal PEP/LVET exhibit no significant reduction in mortality.[66] These observations, based on STI data, suggest that the improved longevity in patients on beta-blockade therapy following acute myocardial infarction may be directly related to the enhanced survival of the high risk subgroup with left ventricular dysfunction.

A dominant cause of death among patients with stable coronary artery disease following recovery from acute myocardial infarction is sudden death. In the prognostic studies just outlined, sudden death accounted for two thirds of the deaths. To better define patients at high risk of fatal cardiac arrhythmia, we reinvestigated the value of the duration of the QT interval as a mortality risk indicator. These studies demonstrated that the QT interval corrected for the duration of electromechanical systole was a more sensitive risk indicator than the QT interval corrected for heart rate.[67] Prolongation of the QT interval relative to the duration of electromechanical systole (QT greater than QS_2) appears to be a potent adjunctive indicator for the risk of sudden death among patients with chronic coronary artery disease (Figure 12.5).

The most recent studies have tested the potential prognostic usefulness of the PEP/LVET in combination with the QT interval relative to QS_2. In these studies on 100 patients with previous myocardial infarction followed prospectively for an average of 43 months, all 16 patients who died suddenly had either abnormal left ventricular resting performance (PEP/LVET greater than 0.42) or prolongation of the QT interval relative to QS_2 (QT greater than QS_2) (Figure 12.6).[68] Of 16 patients with an abnormal PEP/LVET and a QT greater than QS_2, 12 died during the follow-up period; 11 of the deaths occurred suddenly. Over the same study period, only one of 43 patients with a normal PEP/LVET and a normal QT interval relative to QS_2 died. These data lend evidence favoring the application of combined noninvasive methods in stratifying mortality risk in patients with coronary artery disease.

ACUTE MYOCARDIAL INFARCTION

The STI changes accompanying an episode of acute myocardial infarction (AMI) have been studied widely.[69-103] The typical pattern of prolonged PEPI, abbreviated LVETI, and normal QS_2I characteristic of left ventricular dysfunction in chronic heart disease is modified in AMI. In large part this reflects the fact that during the initial days following AMI there is a striking increase in adrenergic cardiostimulatory activity as evidenced by in-

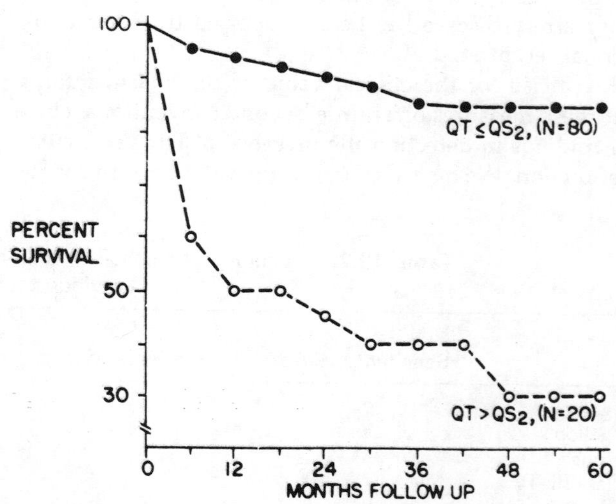

Figure 12.5. Cumulative five-year survival in patients with and without QT > QS_2. The difference in survival curves is significant ($P < 0.001$). See Figure 12.1 for abbreviations. (From Boudoulas et al,[67] with permission.)

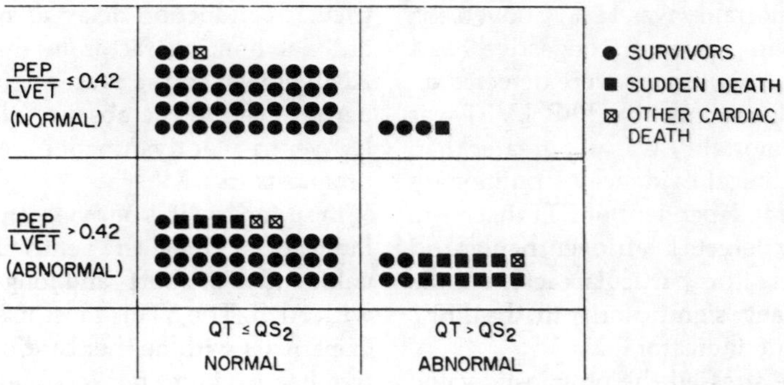

Figure 12.6. Distribution of 100 patients with previous myocardial infarction for the presence of normal and abnormal PEP/LVET and for QT≤QS_2 and QT>QS_2. See Figure 12.1 for abbreviations. (From Weissler and Boudoulas[68] with permission.)

creases in plasma catecholamines and 24-hour urinary epinephrine and norepinephrine excretion.[84] As a consequence, during the initial 24 hours following a first episode of AMI, the QS_2I is generally abbreviated (and remains so for several—five to seven—days thereafter). The abbreviation in QS_2I is accompanied by a variable abbreviation in PEPI and a more consistent decrease in LVETI, whereas the PEP/LVET generally remains within normal limits. Two to three days following an initial episode of AMI, the PEP/LVET increases above its initial level, reaching a maximum on the third or fourth day. Despite the increasing levels during days one through four, the PEP/LVET often remains below 0.42. During days 7 to 21 after AMI the PEP/LVET generally falls toward baseline levels as left ventricular function recovers. In patients with AMI with antecedent left ventricular dysfunction on the basis of previous myocardial infarction or hypertensive heart disease, the PEP/LVET tends to remain increased beyond that for patients with a first uncomplicated episode of myocardial infarction and no previous disease. The abnormal PEP/LVET in this group tends to persist three to six months after the acute episode (Figure 12.7).

Northover[102] reported a comprehensive study on the prognostic value of STI during 601 episodes of AMI in 578 patients admitted to the Leicester Royal Infirmary. Overall survival was 84% and average duration of hospital stay of survivors was 13 days. Serial changes in the STI were followed during the first week after AMI. Of special note was the finding that the magnitude of the first recorded value of PEP/LVET was closely related to subsequent mortality in the hospital. Therefore, among patients whose PEP/LVET was below 0.33 on the first day after AMI (64% of patients), the overall mortality was 5%. By contrast, among patients with a PEP/LVET in the range of 0.34 to 0.37, 0.38 to 0.41, and greater than 0.41 (none of whom had left bundle branch block), in-hospital mortality was, respectively, 17%, 33%, and 60%. The PEP/LVET proved more potent than clinical indicators in predicting early mortality risk. Of note in this regard was the finding that among 11% of patients having no clinical evidence of cardiac failure in whom PEP/LVET

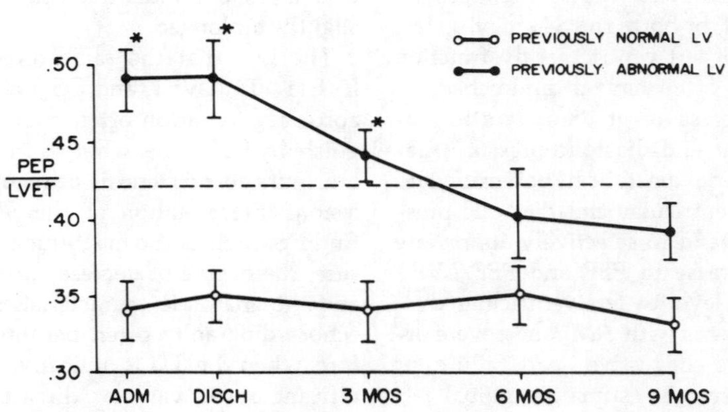

Figure 12.7. Long-term changes in PEP/LVET after acute myocardial infarction; serial mean values for 12 patients with a previously normal left ventricle (LV) (*open circles*) and 13 patients with a previously abnormal left ventricle (*closed circles*). The *horizontal bars* indicate ranges for ± 1 standard error of the mean and the *dashed line* the upper limits of normal for the PEP/LVET (0.42). The dissimilarity between the two groups is striking; *asterisks* indicate significant differences between the two groups ($P < 0.05$). ADM = first three days after admission; DISCH = day before discharge (usually two to three weeks after admission study). (From Lewis et al,[56] with permission.)

was greater than 0.33, the mortality was 14%. Conversely, among 21% of patients with apparent congestive heart failure in whom basal lung crepitations were detected on the first day following AMI and in whom PEP/LVET was less than 0.30, in-hospital mortality was not greater than that of patients with no clinical evidence of pulmonary congestion. Among factors independent of STI that were evaluated statistically, only defects in atrioventricular and intraventricular conduction (in particular left bundle branch block) proved to add significantly to the PEP/LVET as an early prognostic indicator.

Other investigators have stressed the prognostic value of serial STI measurements.[73,76,81,93] In general, failure of abnormal STI to normalize during the first weeks after the acute episode portends a poor prognosis, whereas persistence of an abnormal PEP/LVET beyond 3 weeks presages persistence of postinfarctional left ventricular dysfunction.

Not all investigators agree on the usefulness of the STI in AMI. Some state that the frequency with which the STI falls within normal limits and the variability among individual patients reflect the inadequacy of the method in detecting abnormal function. It is our view that the frequency with which STI falls within normal limits in AMI is not caused by methodologic inadequacy but rather by the magnitude of the left ventricular compensation that normalizes the STI after AMI. In addition, as Northover[102] noted, the variability among studies reflects, at least in part, a failure to adhere to methodologic detail in making the STI measurements, particularly in several older studies. The varying extent of left ventricular necrosis and ischemia, the variable contribution of antecedent myocardial damage, and the variable normalizing effect of increased sympathetic cardiostimulatory activity all affect global left ventricular function and hence the STI changes that follow AMI. The consistency with which the STI has detected patients with good and poor prognoses suggests that their most useful application may be in the stratification of mortality risk following AMI.

In the presence of cardiogenic shock or florid congestive heart failure following AMI, or both, the STI may be less applicable as an indicator of left ventricular dysfunction or mortality. Such patients often have a diminished intraventricular isovolumic pressure gradient (aortic diastolic minus left ventricular end-diastolic pressure) because of the presence of arterial diastolic hypotension and a markedly elevated left ventricular end-diastolic pressure. These factors, which tend to selectively abbreviate the PEP, result in less increase in PEP and PEP/LVET than that expected for the level of left ventricular dysfunction. Therefore, in patients with AMI and severe arterial hypotension or severe congestive heart failure, or both, the STI is less sensitive in estimating global left ventricular performance and prognosis. The poor prognosis in such patients can usually be established on clinical grounds alone. Indeed, rarely are noninvasive methods required to determine the deficiency in left ventricular performance when marked hypotension and overt congestive heart failure are present.

The presence of left bundle branch block, which selectively prolongs the PEP on the basis of the intraventricular conduction delay as noted previously, is an additional limiting factor in the interpretation of STI in AMI. However, the presence of left bundle branch block per se, even in the absence of other clinical evidence of left ventricular dysfunction, remains an indicator of poor prognosis in AMI.

In summary, it is our view that the STI provides a useful indicator of global left ventricular performance and a valuable index of short- and long-term prognosis in patients with AMI. The STI is most useful in the large population of patients with neither cardiogenic shock, florid congestive heart failure, nor left bundle branch block.

VALVULAR HEART DISEASE

In considering patients with valvular heart disease, it is pertinent to recognize that alterations in the STI are caused by the hemodynamic changes induced by the valvular defect or defects, as well as the associated changes in myocardial function secondary to volume or pressure overload, or both. For this reason, interpretation of the STI in patients with valvular heart disease often necessitates the application of other noninvasive measures of left ventricular performance such as echocardiography and nuclear imaging of global left ventricular performance.

Aortic Valvular Disease

In patients with hemodynamically significant aortic stenosis, aortic insufficiency, or combined aortic stenosis and insufficiency, in whom left ventricular function is well compensated, there is an abbreviation in PEPI and prolongation of LVETI associated with a lengthening of QS_2I and a decrease in PEP/LVET.[16,104–109] The lengthening in LVETI per se has proven particularly useful in estimating the severity of aortic overflow obstruction. As left ventricular decompensation supervenes in the course of aortic valvular disease, the PEPI lengthens and the LVETI is shortened while the PEP/LVET increases, thus reversing the primary effects of aortic valvular dysfunction. The QS_2I under these circumstances tends to remain slightly prolonged.

The fact that the same directional changes in PEPI, LVETI, PEP/LVET, and QS_2I occur in aortic stenosis and aortic regurgitation often makes it impossible to distinguish, by STI alone, whether in the presence of combined murmurs aortic stenosis or regurgitation is the dominant lesion. Interpretation of the STI in light of associated findings such as the magnitude of the arterial pulse pressure, the degree of decrease in arterial diastolic pressure, and the anatomic characteristics of the left ventricle on echocardiography often permits this distinction. Therefore, when the STI is indicative of hemodynamically significant aortic valvular disease (short PEPI, prolonged LVETI, increased QS_2I, and decreased PEP/LVET) in the presence of a wide arterial pulse pressure and low diastolic arterial pressure, while the echocardiogram reveals increased left ventricular diastolic volume with only mild diastolic thickening of the left ventricular wall, the diagnosis of dominant aortic regurgitation is almost certain. When the STI is indicative of hemodynamically significant aortic valvular disease in the presence of low arterial pulse pressure and normal diastolic arterial pressure, and echocardiography discloses a normal or decreased left ventricular volume and diameter and a markedly increased left ventricular diastolic wall thickness, the diagnosis of dominant aortic stenosis is highly probable.

In the patient with auscultatory signs of aortic valvular disease, the finding of an abbreviated PEPI, prolonged LVETI, and diminished PEP/LVET should always suggest hemodynamically significant aortic valvular disease. Conversely, in the presence of clinical signs suggesting aortic valvular disease, the finding of unexpectedly prolonged PEPI, abbreviated LVETI, and increased PEP/LVET should strongly suggest a superimposed disorder in left ventricular function. In elderly patients in whom a systolic ejection murmur is often detected in the absence of other evidence of left ventricular dysfunction, the STI is of value in determining whether hemodynamically significant aortic stenosis is the basis for the murmur.

Recent studies in our laboratory have employed combined STI and echocardiography in quantitating the severity of aortic stenosis.[110] Employing the measurement of the LVETI (in msec) in combination with echocardiographic measures of aortic valve leaflet opening (AVO in millimeters) and the thickness (in millimeters) of the interventricular septum (IVSth) and the left ventricular posterior wall (LVPth), an index of severity of aortic stenosis (ASI) has been devised as follows: $ASI = LVETI \times (IVSth + LVPth)/AVO$. The presence of hemodynamically significant aortic stenosis could be detected with 90% accuracy in the presence of an ASI greater than 1,000 even when combined aortic regurgitation and stenosis are clinically evident.

The mechanisms underlying the changes in STI in patients with aortic valvular disease in the absence of left ventricular decompensation are not fully understood. Present evidence favors the explanation that in aortic stenosis abbreviation in PEPI relates to the rapid rate of increase in left ventricular pressure during isovolumic systole in the presence of a high end-diastolic ventricular pressure and a low pressure gradient from left ventricular end-diastole to aortic diastolic pressure, resulting in early opening of the aortic valve. These changes are coupled with late closure of the aortic valve because of its rigidity, so that the LVETI is prolonged. In aortic regurgitation the high rate of isovolumic systolic pressure development together with the low arterial diastolic pressure induces a short PEPI. The large stroke volume and low arterial pressure at the aortic incisura combine to prolong the LVETI. Recent studies[111] have confirmed the presence of a prolonged LVETI and decreased PEP/LVET in experimentally induced aortic outflow obstruction in the rabbit.

It is important that several characteristic landmarks employed in delineation of the STI are often obscured in patients with aortic stenosis and regurgitation. This pertains in particular to the delineation of the aortic closure sound (A_2) and the carotid incisural notch. When these aortic valvular closure events are obscured, it is best to defer to other noninvasive methods for the diagnosis and quantitation of aortic valvular disease.

Note that aortic valve replacement usually normalizes the characteristic abbreviation of PEPI and prolongation of LVETI of aortic valve disease.[105,112–114] The presence of an antecedent abnormality in left ventricular function is uncovered, after prosthetic aortic valve replacement, through the finding of a persistently abnormal prolongation of PEPI and shortening of LVET.

Mitral Valvular Disease

In patients with mitral stenosis, mitral regurgitation, or both, the presence of left ventricular dysfunction is denoted by prolongation of the PEPI, abbreviation of the LVETI, and an increase in PEP/LVET. Our early studies indicated that the same relation between the LVEF and PEP/LVET observed in patients with primary myocardial disease pertained in mitral valvular disease as well.[37] The increased PEP/LVET associated with decreased left ventricular global function has been observed in patients with acute and chronic mitral regurgitation.[115,116] In acute mitral regurgitation, however, the changes are associated with marked abbreviation in QS_2I. The QS_2I generally remains within normal limits in chronic mitral regurgitation. An interesting observation is that the PEP/LVET is increased relative to the echocardiographically measured percentage of change in left ventricular diameter (% ΔD) in patients with hemodynamically severe mitral regurgitation.[115] When left ventricular function is well preserved in mitral regurgitation due to mitral valvular prolapse, the STI remains within normal limits.[117]

HYPERTENSIVE CARDIOVASCULAR DISEASE

Several studies indicate that patients with hypertensive cardiovascular disease frequently exhibit abnormal STI (prolonged PEPI, abbreviated LVETI, and increased PEP/LVET) whereas the QS_2I remains normal in the absence of clinical signs of left ventricular dysfunction.[2,15,16,118–123] More recently, the relation of PEP/LVET to the extent of left ventricular hypertrophy among patients with a broad range of left ventricular mass, estimated by echocardiography, has been studied by our group.[124] Among patients classified according to the presence of mild, moderate, and severe left ventricular hypertrophy (as reflected in left ventricular mass in the range 0 to 2, 2 to 4, and greater than 4 SDs above the normal mean), an increasing abnormality in PEP/LVET was noted to accompany increasing left ventricular hypertrophy. In each category of left ventricular hypertrophy, changes in PEP/LVET exceeded the frequency of abnormality in echocardiographic measures of left ventricular performance (systolic fractional shortening of internal diameter, % ΔD and circumferential shortening rate, Vcf). These changes in PEP/LVET in patients with hypertension were not dependent on the level of arterial diastolic pressure per se. Other studies indicate that although short-term treatment (up to 15 days) may induce a minor abnormality in STI through reduction in preload and adrenergic blockade,[125,126] long-term antihypertensive therapy with a significant decrease in arterial pressure yields evidence of improved left ventricular function by STI measurements.[127–131] Serial measurements of the STI in chronic hypertensive disease, therefore, offer a useful index of the progress of left ventricular function and the influence of antihypertensive therapy.

PRIMARY MYOCARDIAL AND PERICARDIAL DISEASES

The distinctive pattern of changes in STI observed in left ventricular failure consisting of prolongation of the PEPI, abbreviation of LVETI, and an increase in PEP/LVET, while QS_2I remains within normal limits, was early detected as a hallmark of left ventricular dysfunction in patients with congestive cardiomyopathy.[2,15,16] This pattern of change has been demonstrated repeatedly in patients with primary myocardial disease (congestive cardiomyopathy)[39,41,132–138] and has been observed in patients with restrictive cardiomyopathy as well.[41,136–137] In patients with chronic constrictive pericarditis and pericardial effusion in whom left ventricular function is commonly normal, the STI remains within normal limits.[41,136,138] Restrictive myocardial disease and constrictive pericarditis, which often present with similar clinical findings, can readily be differentiated by measurement of the STI.[136] The frequency of congestive cardiomyopathy among chronic alcoholic patients has prompted several studies on the influence of acute alcohol ingestion on the STI.[139–146] Although mild alterations suggesting left ventricular dysfunction have been observed after acute ingestion of alcohol[140–142] and in one study following alcohol ingestion and autonomic blockade,[139] it is not clear whether these changes reflect altered myocardial function or reduced preload. It is of interest that among oriental subjects who experience postalcoholic facial flush with elevated blood acetaldehyde levels, there is a marked decrease in PEP/LVET associated with a decrease in peripheral resistance and ventricular afterload.[143] The STI has been studied in patients with chronic alcoholism.[144–146] There is a suggestion that patients progressing to alcoholic cardiomyopathy may be detected by STI measurements.[144]

Similar changes in STI to those observed in patients with congestive cardiomyopathy have been observed in cardiac amyloidosis,[137] Duchenne's muscular dystrophy,[147,148] systemic lupus erythematosus,[149] and Adriamycin cardiotoxicity.[150–155] Serial monitoring of STI has been suggested as a means of detecting early myocardial toxicity in patients on Adriamycin therapy.

Studies on beat-to-beat changes in STI in patients with congestive cardiomyopathy have proven to be clinically useful in detecting the presence of left ventricular pulsus alternans and pulsus paradoxus[156–158] when other clinical methods do not reveal their presence.

Studies in patients with hypertrophic cardiomyopathy have revealed variable lengthening in LVETI and inconsistent changes in PEPI and PEP/LVET.[159–161] Recent studies from our laboratory have clarified the spectrum of changes in STI in hypertrophic cardiomyopathy.[162] Among patients with echocardiographically diagnosed hypertrophic cardiomyopathy and no resting left ventricular outflow gradient, the LVETI is significantly abbreviated relative to normal, whereas the PEPI and PEP/LVET remain within normal limits. Among patients with a left ventricular outflow gradient greater than 50 mm Hg, the LVETI is significantly prolonged whereas the PEPI and PEP/LVET are distinctly diminished. The STI among patients with hypertrophic cardiomyopathy and a left ventricular outflow gradient between 0 and 50 mm Hg is generally within normal limits. When the LVETI is plotted against the left ventricular outflow gradient, a clear spectrum of variation from an abbreviated LVETI in the absence of an left ventricular outflow gradient to a distinctly prolonged LVETI in patients with a gradient greater than 50 mm Hg is apparent. The presence of an LVETI greater than 423 ms in patients with echocardiographically diagnosed hypertrophic cardiomyopathy is strong evidence for a left ventricular outflow gradient greater than 50 mm Hg (greater than 90% accuracy). Postextrasystolic changes in STI are valuable diagnostic adjuncts in demonstrating the presence of a left ventricular outlfow gradient in patients with hypertrophic cardiomyopathy.[163,164]

MISCELLANEOUS APPLICATIONS

The STI has been widely studied in children with cardiovascular disease. It has been applied as a sensitive means for studying the effects of cardioactive pharmacologic influences on the left ventricle. The STI has proven useful in studying the artificially-paced heart, hypothyroidism, acromegaly, the influence of chronic anemia, high altitude exposure, hemodialysis, febrile states, space travel, chronic pulmonary heart disease, cigarette smoking, and congenital heart disease. For detailed review of these applications of the STI, the reader is referred to the key references on STI[165] as well as the recent literature.[166]

SUMMARY

Measurement of the systolic time intervals (STI) offers a unique reflection of left ventricular global performance which can be reproduced with a high level of accuracy and at low cost. Knowledge of the variables that influence the STI permits their ready interpretation, particularly when they are determined in concert with other noninvasive measures. Their sensitivity permits detection of abnormal ventricular function before it is apparent clinically. As quantitative knowledge of the changes in STI in health and disease and of various pharmacologic perturbations becomes better appreciated, their application as clinically useful measures should become more widespread.

REFERENCES

1. Garrod AH: On some points connected with the circulation of the blood arrived at from a study of the sphygmograph-trace. *Proc Roy Soc London* 1874; 23:351–354.
2. Weissler AM, Harris WS, Schoenfeld CD: Bedside techniques for the evaluation of ventricular function in man. *Am J Cardiol* 1969; 23:577–583.
3. Ludwig C: The influence of respiratory movements on blood flow in the aorta. *Arch Anat Physiol Wiss Med* 1847; 242–302.

4. Marey EJ: De l'emploi du sphygmographe dans le diagnostic des affections valvulaires du coeur et des aneuismes des arteres; extrait d'une note de M. Marey. *C R Acad Sci (D) Paris* 1860; 51:813–817.
5. Thurston E: The length of the systole of the heart, as estimated from sphygmographic tracings. *J Anat Physiol* 1876; 10:494–501.
6. Chapman PM: Abstract of the Goulstonian Lectures on the physics of the circulation. *Br Med J* 1894; 1:511–515.
7. Bowen WP: Changes in heart rate, blood pressure and duration of systole resulting from bicycling. *Am J Physiol* 1904; 11:59–77.
8. Frank O: On the dynamics of cardiac muscle (Chapman CB, Wasserman F, trans). *Am Heart J* 1959; 58:282–317.
9. Wiggers CJ: Studies on the consecutive phases of the cardiac cycle. I. The duration of the consecutive phases of the cardiac cycle and the criteria for their precise determination. *Am J Physiol* 1921; 56:415–438.
10. Wiggers CJ: Studies on the consecutive phases of the cardiac cycle. II. The laws governing the relative durations of ventricular systole and diastole. *Am J Physiol* 1921; 56:439–459.
11. Lombard WP, Cope OM: The duration of the systole of the left ventricle of man. *Am J Physiol* 1926; 77:263–294.
12. Katz LN, Feil HS: Clinical observations on the dynamics of ventricular systole. I. Auricular fibrillation. *Arch Intern Med* 1923; 32:672–692.
13. Feil HS, Katz LN: Clinical observation on the dynamics of ventricular systole. II. Hypertension. *Arch Intern Med* 1924; 33:321–329.
14. Blumberger K: VI. Die Untersuchung der Dynamik des Herzens beim Menschen. *Ergeb Inn Med Kinderheilkd* 1942; 62:424–531.
15. Weissler AM, Harris WS, Schoenfeld CD: Systolic time intervals in heart failure in man. *Circulation* 1968; 37:149–159.
16. Lewis RP, Leighton RF, Forester WF, Weissler AM: Systolic time intervals, in Weissler AM (ed): *Non-Invasive Cardiology*. New York, Grune & Stratton, 1974, pp 301–368.
17. Lewis RP, Rittgers SE, Forester WF, Boudoulas H: A critical review of systolic time intervals. *Circulation* 1977; 56:146–158.
18. Hirschfeld S, Meyer R, Schwartz DC, Korfhagen J, Kaplan S: Measurement of right and left ventricular systolic time intervals by echocardiography. *Circulation* 1975; 51:304–309.
19. Stefadouros MA, Witham C: Systolic time intervals by echocardiography. *Circulation* 1975; 51:114–117.
20. Griebenow R, Meier CH, Saborowski F: Vergleichende Bestimmung der systolischen. (Measurement of systolic time intervals by echocardiographic and conventional methods.) *Zeitintervalle Z Kardiol* 1981; 70:687–692.
21. Vredevoe LA, Creekmore SP, Schiller NB: The measurement of systolic time intervals by echocardiography. *J Clin Ultrasound* 1974; 2:99–105.
22. Bassett Frey MA, Doerr BM: Correlations between ejection times measured from the carotid pulse contour and the impedance cardiogram. *Aviat Space Environ Med* 1983; 54:894–897.
23. Colin J, Carre R, Amoretti R: Mesure des intervalles de temps systoliques par pléthysmographie électrique. *Anesth Analg* 1979; 36:435–438.
24. Lang-Jensen T: Ultrasonic Doppler. A non-invasive method of measuring the rate of circulation and the systolic time intervals. *Ugeskr Laeger* 1981; 143:666–670.
25. Bartolin R, Bouvenot G, Jouve R, Fieschi M, Sellam E, Delboy C: Nouvelle approche de la fonction ventriculaire gauche par mésure d'intervalles de temps systoliques au Doppler carotidien. *Sem Hop Paris* 1981; 57:1206–1208.
26. Hegrenaes L: Left ventricular systolic time intervals. A comparison between conventional carotid pulse curve method and the doppler ultrasound method. *Eur Heart J* 1983; 4:313–319.
27. Metzger CC, Chough CB, Kroetz FW, Leonard JJ: True isovolumic contraction time: its correlation with two external indexes of ventricular performance. *Am J Cardiol* 1970; 25:434–442.
28. Martin CE, Shaver JA, Thompson ME, Reddy PS, Leonard JJ: Direct correlation of external systolic time intervals with internal indices of ventricular function in man. *Circulation* 1971; 44:419–431.
29. Kyle MC, Freis ED: Computer identification of systolic time intervals. *Comput Biomed Res* 1970; 3:637–651.
30. Zecchi P, Iannarelli M, Ardanese F, Loperfido F, Bellocci F, Fenici R, Ansalone G: L'analisi automatica dell'esame poligrafico. *Minerva Med* 1980; 71:3345–3352.
31. Braunwald E, Sarnoff SJ, Stainsby WN: Determinants of duration and mean rate of ventricular ejection. *Circ Res* 1958; 6:319–325.
32. Wallace AG, Mitchell JH, Skinner NS, Sarnoff SJ: Duration of the phases of left ventricular systole. *Circ Res* 1963; 12:611–619.
33. Nakamura Y, Wiegner AW, Gaasch WH, Bing OHL: Systolic time intervals: assessment by isolated cardiac muscle studies. *J Am Coll Cardiol* 1983; 2:973–978.
34. Weissler AM, Garrand CL Jr: Systolic time intervals in cardiac disease. *Mod Concepts Cardiovasc Dis* 1971; 40:1–4.
35. Weissler AM: Current concepts in cardiology. Systolic time intervals. *N Engl J Med* 1977; 296:321–324.
36. Shaver JA, Kroetz FW, Leonard JJ, Paley HW: The effect of steady state increases in systemic arterial pressure on the duration of left ventricular ejection time. *J Clin Invest* 1968; 47:217–230.
37. Garrard CL Jr, Weissler AM, Dodge HT: The relationship of alterations in systolic time intervals to ejection fraction in patients with cardiac disease. *Circulation* 1970; 42:455–462.
38. Ahmed SS, Levinson GE, Schwartz CJ, Ettinger PO: Systolic time intervals as measures of the contractile state of the left ventricular myocardium in man. *Circulation* 1972; 46:559–571.
39. Lewis BS, Armstrong TG, Everson RC, Gotsman MS: Predictive value of the systolic time intervals in primary myocardial disease. *Chest* 1973; 64:431–438.
40. Long HJ, Diamond SS, Barningham RA, Raflo CP: Systolic time interval recordings in rabbits with congestive cardiomyopathy induced by chronic anthracycline administration. *Am J Vet Res* 1983; 44:1375–1377.
41. Armstrong TG, Lewis BS, Gotsman MS: Systolic time intervals in constrictive pericarditis and severe primary myocardial disease. *Am Heart J* 1973; 85:6–12.
42. Adenle B, Weir EK, Chesler E: Advantages of systolic time intervals over echocardiography in the measurement of left ventricular ejection fraction. *Minnesota Med* 1981; 64:479–483.
43. Ambrosi C, Chabrillat Y, Duport G, Valeix B, Berthet-BondetM, Gerard R: Le calcul de la fraction d'éjection d'après les intervalles systoliques et l'angiographie simultanément enregistrés. Etude comparative. *Arch Mal Coeur* 1981; 73:321–328.
44. Bourassa MG, Borteau GM, Allenstein BJ: Hemodynamic studies during intermittent left bundle branch block. *Am J Cardiol* 1962; 10:792–799.
45. Baragan J, Fernandez-Caamano F, Sozutek Y, Coblence B, Lenegre J: Chronic complete bundle-branch block. Phonocardiographic and mechanocardiographic study of 30 cases. *Br Heart J* 1968; 30:196–202.
46. Adolph RJ, Fowler NO, Tanaka K: Prolongation of isovolumic contraction time in left bundle branch block. *Am Heart J* 1969; 78:585–591.
47. Silei M: *Etude Phonomecanocardiographique des Blocs de Branche: á propos de 106 Observations* (thesis). Lyons, Imprimerie Bosc Frères, 1969.
48. Baragan J, Fernandez F, Coblence B, Saad Y, Lenegre J: Left ventricular dynamics in complete right bundle block with left axis deviation of QRS. *Circulation* 1970; 42:797–804.
49. Hultgren HN, Craige E, Fujii J, Nakamura T, Bilisoly J: Left bundle branch block and mechanical events of the cardiac cycle. *Am J Cardiol* 1983; 52:755–762.
50. Stack RS, Sohn YH, Weissler AM: Accuracy of systolic time intervals in detecting abnormal left ventricular performance in coronary artery disease. *Am J Cardiol* 1981; 47:603–609.
51. Weissler AM, Stack RS, Sohn YH: Global left ventricular performance in chronic stable angina pectoris. The critical role of myocardial infarction. *Coeur Med Interne* 1980; 19:143–152.
52. Meng R, Liebson PR, Hollander C, Teran JC, Barresi V, LurieM: The use of noninvasive methods in the evaluation of left ventricular performance in coronary artery disease, in Ciethrich EB (ed): *Noninvasive Cardiovascular Diagnosis, Current Concepts.* Baltimore, University Park Press, 1978, pp 249–265.
53. Oilinki OI, Takkunen JT: The predictive value of mechanocardiographic measurements with respect to myocardial infarction. *Ann Clin Res* 1980; 12:160–167.
54. Venco A, Rampulla C, Mandelli V, Saviotti M, Regalia F, Finardi G: Relation of kinetocardiogram to systolic time intervals in patients with old myocardial infarction. *Cardiology* 1982; 69:11–21.
55. Randazzo A, Sardella F, Martinotti R, Daffara G, Parziale M, Cremonesi G: Evaluation of systolic time intervals in patients with angina pectoris. *Am Heart J* 1983; 105:756–762.
56. Lewis RP, Boudoulas H, Welch TG, Forester WF: Usefulness of systolic time intervals in coronary artery disease. *Am J Cardiol* 1976; 37:787–797.
57. Sharratt GP, Carson P: The prognostic implications of systolic time intervals after acute myocardial infarction. *Acta Cardiol* 1975; 30:279–292.
58. Weissler AM, Stack RS, Sohn YH, Schaffer D: Systolic time intervals, in Fishman AP (ed): *Heart Failure.* Washington, DC, Hemisphere Publishing Corp, 1978, pp 203–214.
59. Gillilan RE, Parnes WP, Khan MA, Bouchard RJ, Warbasse JR: The prognostic value of systolic time intervals in angina pectoris patients. *Circulation* 1979; 60:268–274.
60. Weissler AM, O'Neill WW, Sohn YH, Stack RS, Chew PC, Reed AH: The prognostic significance of systolic time intervals after recovery from myocardial infarction. *Am J Cardiol* 1981; 48:995–1002.
61. Boudoulas H, Sohn YH, O'Neill W, Brown R, Weissler AM: Identification of patients with improved survival following coronary bypass surgery. *Cardiology* 1984; 71:247–254.
62. Johnson AD, O'Rourke RA, Karliner JS, Burian C: Effect of myocardial revascularization on systolic time intervals in patients with left ventricular dysfunction. *Circulation* 1972; 45/46 (suppl 1):91–96.
63. Matlof H, Hultgren HN, Pfeifer JF, Harrison DC: Cardiac function assessed by systolic time intervals after aortocoronary saphenous vein bypass surgery. *Br Heart J* 1973; 35:714–719.
64. Boudoulas H, Lewis RP, Vasko JS, Karayannacos PE, Beaver BM: Left

ventricular function and adrenergic hyperactivity before and after saphenous vein bypass. *Circulation* 1976; 53:802–806.

65. DeCaprio L, Rengo F, Spampinato N, Carlomagno A, Chiariello L, Spinelli L, Romano M: Left ventricular function after coronary artery bypass: non-invasive study by systolic time intervals. *Acta Cardiol* 1980; 35:93–105.
66. Boudoulas H, Sohn Y, Brown R, Weissler AM: Left ventricular dysfunction is a determinant of improved survival with beta-blockade therapy following myocardial infarction. *IRCS Med Sci* 1985; 13:271–272.
67. Boudoulas H, Sohn YH, O'Neill WW, Brown R, Weissler AM: The QT > QS_2 syndrome. A new mortality risk indicator in coronary artery disease. *Am J Cardiol* 1982; 50(6):1229–1235.
68. Weissler AM, Boudoulas H: Prognosis in coronary artery disease: a noninvasive approach. *J Cardiography* 1984; 14(suppl V):52–56.
69. Jezek V: Clinical value of the polygraphic tracing in the study of sequence of events during cardiac contraction. *Cardiologia* 1963; 43:298–316.
70. Schoenfeld CD, Robinson JL, Weissler AM, Warren JV: The left ventricular systolic time intervals in myocardial infarction. *Clin Res* 1967; 15:411.
71. Halpern BL, Hodges M, Dagenais A, Friesinger GC: Left ventricular pre-ejection period and ejection time in patients with acute myocardial infarction. *Circulation* 1969; 40 (suppl III):III–100.
72. Samson R: Changes in systolic time intervals in acute myocardial infarction. *Br Heart J* 1970; 32:839–846.
73. Diamant B, Killip T: Indirect assessment of left ventricular performance in acute myocardial infarction. *Circulation* 1970; 42:579–592.
74. Rufty AJ, Ramo BW, Wallace AG, Whalen RE, McIntosh HD, Clark DO: Correlation of left ventricular ejection time with stroke index in patients with acute myocardial infarction. *Ann Intern Med* 1970; 72:780.
75. Inoue K, Young GM, Grierson AL, Smulyan H, Eich RH: Isometric contraction period of the left ventricle in acute myocardial infarction. *Circulation* 1970; 42:79–90.
76. Heikkila J, Luomanmaki K, Pyorala K: Serial observations on left ventricular dysfunction in acute myocardial infarction. II. Systolic time intervals in power failure. *Circulation* 1971; 44:343–354.
77. Gould L, Michael AH, Gomprecht RF: The systolic time intervals in myocardial infarction. *Angiology* 1971; 22:568–574.
78. Dowling JT, Sloman G, Urquart C: Systolic time interval fluctuations produced by acute myocardial infarction. *Br Heart J* 1971; 33:765–772.
79. Jain SR, Lindahl J: Apexcardiogram and systolic time intervals in acute myocardial infarction. *Br Heart J* 1971; 33:578–584.
80. Perloff JK, Reichek N: Value and limitations of systolic time intervals (pre-ejection period and ejection time) in patients with acute myocardial infarction. *Circulation* 1972; 45:929–932.
81. Fabian J, Epstein EJ, Coulshed N, McKendrick CS: Duration of phases of left ventricular systole using indirect methods. II. Acute myocardial infarction. *Br Heart J* 1972; 34:882–889.
82. Hamosh P, Cohn JN, Engelman K, Broder M, Freis ED: Systolic time intervals and left ventricular function in acute myocardial infarction. *Circulation* 1972; 45:375–381.
83. Hodges M, Halpern BL, Friesinger GC, Dagenais GR: Left ventricular pre-ejection period and ejection time in patients with acute myocardial infarction. *Circulation* 1972; 45:933–942.
84. Lewis RP, Boudoulas H, Forester WF, Weissler AM: Shortening of electromechanical systole as a manifestation of excessive, adrenergic stimulation in acute myocardial infarction. *Circulation* 1972; 46:856–862.
85. Agress CM, Wegner S, Forrester JS, Chatterjee K, Parmley WW, Swan HJC: An indirect method for evaluation of left ventricular function in acute myocardial infarction. *Circulation* 1972; 46:291–297.
86. Loeb HS, Rahimtoola SH, Rosen KM, Sinno MZ, Chuquimia R, Gunnar RM: Assessment of ventricular function after acute myocardial infarction by plasma volume expansion. *Circulation* 1973; 47:720–728.
87. Toutouzas P, Corcondilas A, Papadopoulos P, Avgoustákis D: La systole mécanique du ventricule gauche dans l'infarctus du myocarde. *Arch Mal Coeur* 1974; 8:939–947.
88. Waagstein F, Hjalmarson AC, Wasir HS: Apexcardiogram and systolic time intervals in acute myocardial infarction and effects of practolol. *Br Heart J* 1974; 36:1109–1121.
89. Gunnar RM, Loeb HS, Rahimtoola SH: Left ventricular function in patients with acute myocardial infarction, in Gunnar RM, Loeb HS, Rahimtoola SH (eds): *Shock in Myocardial Infarction*. New York, Grune & Stratton, 1974, pp 65–84.
90. Delahaye JP, Chulliat JC, Bons JP, Beaune J, Touboul P, Porte J, Biron A: Valeur pronostique de l'étude des intervalles systoliques dans l'infarctus myocardique récent. *Arch Mal Coeur* 1974; 67:421–429.
91. DeLuca I, Cristallo E, Valenti P, Fino E, Palma B, Losignore M, Castellaneta G, Bacca F: Valutazione dei tempi sistolici nella fase acuta dell'infarto micocardico. *Boll Soc Ital Cardiol* 1974; 19:557–569.
92. Naqui SZ, Chisholm AM, Shane SJ: Left ventricular function in ischemic heart disease: assessment by noninvasive techniques. *Am Heart J* 1975; 90:312–316.
93. Robijns H, Clement D, Verstreken G, DeGeest H, Kesteloot H, Joossens JV: Left ventricular systolic time intervals during acute myocardial infarction. *Eur J Cardiol* 1975; 2/4:431–441.
94. Sharratt GP, Carson P: The prognostic implication of systolic time intervals after acute myocardial infarction. *Acta Cardiol* 1975; 30:279–292.
95. Wertheimer L: Le tecniche incruente nella diagnosi e nel trattamento delle sindromi cardiache acute. *Clin Med Am*, Padova, Piccin Ed, 1975.
96. Brubakk O, Overskeid K: Systolic time intervals in acute myocardial infarction. *Acta Med Scand* 1976; 199:33–40.
97. Cazor JL, Thiron JM, Letac B: Etude des temps systoliques par phonomeccanocardiographie externe dana l'infarctus du myocarde. *Arch Mal Coeur* 1976; 4:377.
98. Kesteloot H: On the clinical value of mechanocardiography. *Eur J Cardiol* 1976; 4/3:393–397.
99. Letac B, Cazor JL, Thiron JM: Etude des temps systoliques par phonomeccanocardiographie externe dana l'infarctus du myocarde *Arch Mal Coeur* 1976; 4:367–376.
100. Nishi K: Evaluation of left ventricular function in acute and old myocardial infarction by noninvasive method with special reference to systolic time intervals. *Jpn Circ J* 1976; 40:403–405.
101. Sharratt GP, Carson P: The electromechanical interval in normal subjects and after myocardial infarction. *Acta Cardiol* 1976; 31:307–312.
102. Northover BJ: Left ventricular systolic time intervals in patients with acute myocardial infarction. *Br Heart J* 1980; 43:506–513.
103. Sardella F, Martinotti R, Porro F, Monzani V, Randazzo A, Pieri R: A polygraph study of ischemic heart disease: behavior of systolic times in acute myocardial infarction. *Acta Cardiol* 1983; 38:209–225.
104. Moskowitz RL, Wechsler BM: Left ventricular ejection time in aortic and mitral valve disease. *Am J Cardiol* 1965; 15:809–814.
105. Parisi AF, Salzman SH, Schechter E: Systolic time intervals in severe aortic valve disease. Changes in surgery and hemodynamic correlations. *Circulation* 1971; 44:539–547.
106. Bache RJ, Wang Y, Greenfield JC Jr: Left ventricular ejection time in valvular aortic stenosis. *Circulation* 1973; 44:527–533.
107. Bonner AJ Jr, Sacks HN, Tavel ME: Assessing the severity of aortic stenosis by phonocardiography and external carotid pulse recordings. *Circulation* 1973; 48:247–252.
108. Manchanda SC, Kasturi TE: Systolic time intervals in aortic valve disease. *Indian Heart J* 1980; 32:309–312.
109. Nakamura T, Hultgren HN, Shettigar UR, Fowles RE: Noninvasive evaluation of the severity of aortic stenosis in adult patients. *Am Heart J* 1984; 107:959–966.
110. Jawad I, Boudoulas H, Stark G, Brown R, Sohn Y, Weissler AM: A noninvasive index of severity of valvular aortic stenosis (to be published).
111. Murphy ML, Doherty JE, De Soya N, Kane JJ, Straub KD: Systolic time intervals in the experimental animal with aortic outflow obstruction. *Cardiology* 1981; 68:19–29.
112. Benchimol A, Matsuo S: Ejection time before and after aortic valve replacement. *Am J Cardiol* 1971; 27:244–249.
113. Haerten K, Erbel FM, Kuhn H, Leuner C, Loogen F: Die Anwendung der systolischen Zeitintervalle in der Verlaufskontrolle operierter aortenvitien. *Z Kardiol* 1979; 68:469–476.
114. Vardan S, Warner R, Mookherjee S, Mead M, Obeid AI: Echo- and phonocardiographic studies in patients with Lillehei-Kaster aortic valve prostheses. *Jpn Heart J* 1979; 20:277–288.
115. Wanderman KL, Goldberg MJ, Stack RS, Weissler AM: Left ventricular performance in mitral regurgitation assessed with systolic time intervals and echocardiography. *Am J Cardiol* 1976; 38:831–835.
116. Boudoulas H, Lewis RP Dervenagas S, Fontana ME, Vasko JS: Abbreviation of systolic time intervals in acute mitral regurgitation: effect of prosthetic mitral valve replacement. *Am J Cardiol* 1979; 44:595–600.
117. Ramirez J, Flowers NC: Echocardiographic determinations of systolic time intervals in mitral valvular prolapse. *Chest* 1979; 76:493–494.
118. Rossi A, Ziacchi V, Lomanto B: Les intervalles de temps systoliques dans l'hypertension essentielle. *Arch Mal Coeur* 1972; 11:1232–1239.
119. Kolv N, Dencev K: Assessment of left-ventricular function in hypertension disease via phase analysis. *Vutr Boles* 1978; 17:55–62.
120. Srivastava SC, Siwach SB, Singh N, Popli HC: Left ventricular performance in hypertension. A study of systolic time intervals. *Indian Heart J* 1979; 31:358–362.
121. Adesanya CO, Sanderson JE, Verheijen PJT, Brinkman AW: Echocardiographic assessment and systolic time interval measurements in the evaluation of severe hypertension in Nigerian Africans. *Aust NZ J Med* 1981; 11:364–369.
122. Schirripa V, Attisano N, Sarcia G, Grenci G, Martelli G: Studio della funzione ventricolare sinistra con metodo poligrafico in soggetti affetti da ipertensione arteriosa sistemica. *Minerva Med* 1982; 73:77–80.
123. Guadalajara JF, Torres GS, Brizuela F, Leanez A, Casanova JM, Olvera

S: Cardiopatia hipertensiva. Estudio fonomecanocardiografico y revision de sus mecanismos fisiopatologicos. *Arch Inst Cardiol Mex* 1983; 53:39–44.

124. Boudoulas H, Mantzouratos D, Sohn YH, Weissler AM: Left ventricular mass and systolic performance in chronic systemic hypertension. *Am J Cardiol* 57:232–237.

125. Lehner JP, Simon A, Kehder A, Weiss Y, Tzincoca CH, Safar M: Evaluation de la performance cardiaque chez l'hypertendu. Effet d'un bétabloquant: l'atenolol. *Arch Mal Coeur* 1971; 10:1107–1112.

126. Gomez AG, Capestany FG, Hernandez-Canero A, Garcia-Barreto D: Modification of blood pressure and systolic time intervals by diuretics and beta-blockers in essential hypertension. *Cor Vasa* 1983; 25:233–240.

127. Dodek A, Burg JR, Kloster FE: Systolic time intervals in chronic hypertension: alterations and response to treatment. *Chest* 1975; 68:51–55.

128. Rossi A, Ziacchi V, Lomanto B: Les intervalles de temps systoliques dans l'hypertension essentielle. 2. Variations produites par le traitement avec labetalol. *Arch Mal Coeur* 1972; 11:1240–1246.

129. Kyle MC, Freis ED: Serial measurements of systolic time intervals: effects of propranolol alone and combined with other agents in hypertensive patients. *Hypertension* 1980; 2:111–117.

130. Hammond JJ, Kirkendall WM, Jacks-Nagle VL, Plotnick GD, Fisher ML, Hamilton JH, Robinson M, Carliner NH, Janoski AH, Hamilton BP: Pindolol and systolic time intervals in patients with hypertension. *Am Heart J* 1982; 104:456–464.

131. Buch J, Rasmussen S: The use of systolic time intervals in the evaluation of antihypertensive treatment with metoprolol, labetalol and prazosin. *Cor Vasa* 1983; 5:358–366.

132. McDonald IG, Hobson ER: A comparison of the relative value of noninvasive techniques—echocardiography, systolic time intervals, and apexcardiography—in the diagnosis of primary myocardial disease. *Am Heart J* 1974; 88:454–462.

133. Ferro G, Chiariello M, Trimarco B, Perticone F, Laccarino V, Ricciardelli B, Rengo F: Correlation between systolic time intervals and roentgen findings in normal subjects and cardiopathic patients. *Jpn Heart J* 1978; 19:732–740.

134. Fincker JL, Brandt CM, Michel JM, Drui S: Evaluation de la fonction ventriculaire gauche dans les cardiomyopathies. *Cardiology* 1981; 68:86–90.

135. Ferro G, Chiariello M, Trimarco B, Perticone F, Ricciardelli B, Rengo F, Condorelli M: Utilita' dei parametri radiologici nella valutazione funzionale di pazienti cardiopatici non valvolari. *G Ital Cardiol* 1978; 8:962–967.

136. Khullar S, Lewis RP: Usefulness of systolic time intervals in differential diagnosis of constrictive pericarditis and restrictive cardiomyopathy. *Br Heart J* 1976; 38:43–46.

137. Wizenberg TA, Muz J, Sohn YH, Samlowski W, Weissler AM: Value of positive myocardial technetium-99m-pyrophosphate scintigraphy in noninvasive diagnosis of cardiac amyloidosis. *Am Heart J* 1982; 103:468–473.

138. Ghose JC, Ganguli A, Bagchi D, Mukherjee AB: Systolic time intervals in pericardial effusion and congestive cardiomyopathy. *Indian Heart J* 1978; 30:231–232.

139. Child JS, Kovick RB, Levisman JA, Pearce ML: Cardiac effects of acute ethanol ingestion unmasked by autonomic blockade. *Circulation* 1979; 59:120–125.

140. Kupari M, Heikkila J, Ylikahri R: Acute effects of alcohol on left ventricular dynamics during isometric exercise in normal subjects. *Clin Cardiol* 1983; 6:103–108.

141. Gould L, Reddy CVR, Singh BK, Zen B: Cardiac effects of alcohol. *Angiology* 1980; 31:753–759.

142. Kupari M: Acute cardiovascular effects of ethanol. A controlled noninvasive study. *Br Heart J* 1983; 49:174–182.

143. Kupari M, Eriksson CJP, Heikkila J, Ylikahri R: Alcohol and the heart. Intense hemodynamic changes associated with alcohol flush in orientals. *Acta Med Scand* 1983; 213:91–98.

144. Morvai V, Folly G, Kardos G: Changes in cardiac function in the "preclinical" stage of alcoholic heart disease. *Acta Med Acad Sci Hungaricae* 1980; 37:229–237.

145. Askanass A, Udoshi M, Sadjadi SA: The heart in chronic alcoholism: a noninvasive study. *Am Heart J* 1980; 99:9–16.

146. Kupari M, Eriksson CJP, Heikkila J, Ylikahri R: Alcohol and the heart. *Acta Med Scand* 1983; 213:91–98.

147. Matsuo S, Oku Y, Oshibuchi R, Hashiba K: Systolic time intervals in progressive muscular dystrophy. *Jpn Heart J* 1979; 20:23–32.

148. Secchi MB, Wu SC, Obbiassi, Oltrona L, Folli G: Evaluation des intervalles systoliques dans la cardiomyopathie de Duchenne. *Arch Mal Coeur* 1982; 75:1291–1296.

149. Del Rio A, Vazquez JJ, Sobrino JA, Gil A, Bardado J, Mate I, Ortiz-Vazquez J: Myocardial involvement in systemic lupus erythematosus. A noninvasive study of left ventricular function. *Chest* 1978; 74:414–417.

150. Rinehart JJ, Lewis RP, Balcerzak SP: Adriamycin cardiotoxicity in man. *Ann Intern Med* 1974; 81:475–478.

151. Villani F, Beretta G, Guindani A: Evaluation of early doxorubicin-induced cardiotoxicity by means of systolic time intervals. *Cancer Chemother Pharmacol* 1979; 3:249–251.

152. Al-Ismail SAD, Whittaker JA: Systolic time interval as index of schedule-dependent doxorubicin cardiotoxicity in patients with acute myelogenous leukaemia. *Br Med J* 1979; 1:1392–1395.

153. Friedman MJ, Ewy GA, Jones SE, Cruze D, Moon TE: 1-year followup of cardiac status after adriamycin therapy. *Cancer Treatment Rep* 1979; 63:1810–1816.

154. Chaudron JM, Beauduin M, Delwiche JP, Delannoy A, Luwaert R, Majois F, Lebacq EG, Pluygers E: Adriamycin cardiotoxicity. Prognostic value of the systolic time intervals. *Acta Cardiol* 1982; 37:105–115.

155. Lenzhofer R, Dudczak R, Dittrich C, Gumhold G, Moser K, Spitzy KH: Uberwachung der Herzfunktion bei Doxorubicintherapie des metastasierten Mammakarzinoms. *Dtsch Med Wenschr* 1983; 108:771–775.

156. Hada Y, Wolfe C, Craige E: Pulsus alternans determined by biventricular simultaneous systolic time intervals. *Circulation* 1982; 65:617–626.

157. Spodick DH, Paladino D, Flessas AP: Respiratory effects on systolic time intervals during pericardial effusion. *Am J Cardiol* 1983; 51:1033–1035.

158. Cheng TO, Leet CJ: Pulsus alternans. Its response to amyl nitrite inhalation. *Angiology* 1984; 35:115–121.

159. Wigle ED, Auger P, Marquis Y: Muscular subaortic stenosis. The direct relation between the intraventricular pressure difference and the left ventricular ejection time. *Circulation* 1967; 36:36–44.

160. Ibrahim M, Silie M, Delahaye JP, Froment R: Systolic time intervals in valvular aortic stenosis and idiopathic hypertrophic subaortic stenosis. *Br Heart J* 1973; 35:276–283.

161. Stefadouros MA, Canedo MI, Karayannis E, Abdulla A, Frank MJ: Internally recorded systolic time intervals in hypertrophic subaortic stenosis. *Am J Cardiol* 1977; 40:700–706.

162. Boudoulas H, Mantzouratos D, Sohn YH, Lewis RL, Weissler AM: Asymmetric septal hypertrophy: identification of patients with significant obstruction by noninvasive methods, abstr. *Am J Cardiol* 1982; 49:949.

163. White CW, Zimmerman TJ: Prolonged left ventricular ejection time in the post-premature beat. A sensitive sign of idiopathic hypertrophic subaortic stenosis. *Circulation* 1975; 51:306–312.

164. Stefadouros MA, Canedo MI, Abdulla AM, Karayannis E, Baute A, Frank MJ: Postextrasystolic changes in systolic time intervals in the assessment of hypertrophic cardiomyopathy. *Br Heart J* 1982; 47:261–269.

165. Weissler AM, Lewis RP, Boudoulas H: Systolic time intervals—key references. *Circulation* 1981; 64:862–867.

166. Jiang ZD, Xie BC: Left ventricular performance in children with congential heart diseases evaluated with systolic time intervals changes before and after surgery, in Doyl EF, Engle MA, Gersony WM, Rashkind WJ, Talner NS (eds): *Abstracts of Second World Congress of Pediatric Cardiology, June 2–6, 1985, New York.* New York, Springer-Verlag, 1985, p. 170.

13 Cardiac Catheterization

Sing San Yang, MD and Vladir Maranhao, MD

Cardiac catheterization involves several processes. First, a catheter or catheters are introduced into cardiac chambers and great vessels. Second, blood samples and signals (eg, pressure) carrying hemodynamically relevant information are collected. Third, the raw data thus collected are processed, yielding hemodynamic parameters. Fourth, hemodynamic interpretation is applied to these data.

INDICATIONS

In general, cardiac catheterization is indicated when the need for cardiac surgery in a patient with a clinically suspected condition is considered to confirm its presence (anatomic and functional diagnosis), to assess its severity (quantitation) and hemodynamic consequences (eg, pulmonary hypertension and right ventricular failure in severe mitral stenosis), and to exclude, unmask, and/or evaluate the associated cardiac conditions. Usually, angiocardiographic examination is added to complete the overall evaluation, and the resultant information may help to define the feasibility of surgery as well as its potential benefit and risks.

Coronary arteriography is currently probably the most frequently performed cardiac catheterization procedure in this country. It is recommended when coronary revascularization surgery is contemplated in a patient with coronary artery disease, when a patient undergoing valvular or other cardiac surgery for acquired or congenital heart disease is over 40 years of age or suspected of having coronary artery disease, or when the cause of chest pain is unknown and coronary artery disease cannot be ruled out on clinical grounds.

Although recent advances in the diagnostic capability of noninvasive techniques, notably echocardiography, have made it possible to provide a considerable amount of information, anatomic as well as functional, in valvular disease and prompted some[1-3] to advocate surgery without cardiac catheterization in these patients, most cardiologists and cardiac surgeons still consider it mandatory to have invasive hemodynamic evaluation preoperatively to obtain information that is as accurate and complete as possible, leaving little room for error or incompleteness in diagnosis. The establishment of a precise diagnosis is particularly crucial in congenital heart disease where mimics are not uncommon (eg, double outlet right ventricle simulating ventricular septal defect and a single ventricle with pulmonic stenosis mimicking tetralogy of Fallot) and multiple defects are not unusual. To avoid unnecessary surgery as well as unexpected findings on the operating table, which may necessitate alteration in the operative plan, prolong the procedure, and possibly jeopardize the patient's outcome, it is absolutely necessary to have an accurate diagnosis preoperatively.

Cardiac catheterization may be indicated in some symptomatic patients to evaluate the results of surgery (eg, relief of valvular stenosis, residual shunt or regurgitation, coronary bypass graft patency, prosthetic valve function, and right or left ventricular function).

In symptomatic patients with suspected cardiomyopathy, cardiac catheterization may be carried out to rule out potentially correctable conditions such as coronary artery, valvular, and pericardial disease.

Cardiac catheterization employing a balloon-tipped, flow-directed catheter (Swan-Ganz catheter) is now widely undertaken in the intensive care or coronary care unit for continuous monitoring of pulmonary artery and wedge pressures and repeated measurement of the cardiac output in post-operative patients and in those whose condition is clinically unstable following myocardial infarction. These data are of utmost importance in assessing the patient's response to therapy.

Other diagnostic indications include intracardiac phonocardiography,[4] His bundle electrocardiography,[5] and endomyocardial biopsy.[6] Therapeutic uses of cardiac catheterization include transcatheter His bundle ablation,[7] endocavitary cardioversion,[8] percutaneous transluminal coronary angioplasty,[9] intracoronary thrombolysis,[10] percutaneous balloon dilation of pulmonic valvular stenosis,[11] aortic valvular stenosis,[12] and coarctation of aorta,[13] percutaneous intraaortic balloon counterpulsation,[14] balloon atrial septostomy,[15] transcatheter closure of atrial septal defect[16] and patent ductus arteriosus,[17] percutaneous catheter commissurotomy of mitral stenosis,[18,18a] intracardiac catheter retrieval of foreign bodies,[19] catheter embolotherapy for A-V fistula,[19a] and percutaneous arterial embolectomy.[19b]

Table 13.1 lists the preferred cardiac catheterization procedures for the diagnosis of various cardiac conditions.

TECHNIQUES

RIGHT HEART CATHETERIZATION

The first cardiac catheterization in man was performed by Forssmann[20] on himself in 1929. He inserted a ureteral catheter into a left antecubital vein and, under fluoroscopic guidance, advanced it into the right atrium. In 1930, Klein[21] performed right heart catheterization in 11 patients, with passage of a catheter into the right ventricle and measurement of cardiac output by the Fick method. The following decade saw only sporadic application of right heart catheterization to evaluate circulatory function in normal and diseased hearts. In 1941, Cournand and Richards began a series of studies on right heart physiology and paved the way for its clinical application.[22-24] Dexter et al[25] reported their work on congenital heart disease and commented on "the oxygen saturation and source of pulmonary capillary blood" sampled from the catheter in the pulmonary artery wedge position. Their subsequent work[26] and that of Lagerlof and Werko[27] established the basis for the widespread use of "wedge" pressure as an accurate estimate of left atrial pressure. Other pioneers in those early years included McMichael[28] in England, Lenegre[29,30] in France, and Stead and Warren,[31,32] Bing[33-36] Burchell,[37] Wood[38] and others in the United States.

Right heart catheterization is performed with the patient under local anesthesia, using either an open or percutaneous approach. In the open approach, usually an antecubital or saphenous vein is selected for catheter entry, the former being more common. Of the antecubital veins, the cephalic vein is avoided in favor of the basilic or brachial vein because it joins the subclavian vein at a right angle, making it difficult to pass a catheter from the cephalic vein to the right atrium. A 6F or 7F Cournand or Goodale-Lubin catheter is commonly used. (One French unit refers to 0.33 mm in outside diameter of the catheter.) In the antecubital approach, the catheter, having reached the axilla (blindly), is further advanced under fluoroscopic guidance. Manipulation of the catheter from the right atrium to the pulmonary artery is usually accomplished by the J-loop technique. A J loop is formed within the right atrium with the catheter tip against the lateral right atrial wall. Subsequent counterclockwise rotation and slight advancement of the catheter place the catheter tip into the right ventricle through the tricuspid orifice. Usually a few ventricular premature beats are noted on right ventricular entry. As the J loop is still maintained, with its tip pointing toward the right ventricular outflow tract, the catheter can be readily advanced into the pulmonary artery. Further advancement into the "wedged" position can be facilitated by deep inspiration or coughing. This position must be confirmed by the left atrial pressure waveform and the oxygenated blood sample (greater than 95% O_2 saturation).[39] In severe tricuspid regurgitation with a large right atrium, coiling of the catheter within the right atrium can be avoided by introducing

Table 13.1. Approaches to the Diagnosis of Cardiac Disease by Cardiac Catheterization*

Condition Evaluated	Preferred Procedures
Valve stenosis	Pressure gradient, Valve area
	Angiocardiography
Valve regurgitation	Angiocardiography
	Indicator dilution curves
	Pressure pulses
Coronary artery disease	Angiocardiography
	Selective coronary arteriography
	Left ventriculography
Shunts	
Detection	Indicator dilution curves
	Angiocardiography
	Oximetry
Localization	Angiocardiography
	Indicator dilution curves
	Oximetry
Quantitation	Oximetry
	Indicator dilution curves
	Angiocardiography
Complex congenital defect	Angiocardiography
Intracardiac mass	Angiocardiography
Cardiomyopathy	Cardiac output, pressures, and derived parameters
	Angiocardiography
Constrictive pericarditis	Pressures

*The preferred procedures are listed in the order of preference. The relative priority assigned here is that of the authors. Different and possibly better approaches may exist and are subject to the catheterizer's preference.

a straight 0.35 or 0.38 guidewire through the catheter to stiffen its body so that it can be maneuvered into the wedged position.

The percutaneous technique of Seldinger[40] originally used in arteriography is now widely applied in right as well as left heart catheterization. A needle is percutaneously inserted in a vein (eg, femoral vein) at about a 45° angle and the stylet is removed. A flexible metal guidewire is passed through the needle into the vein, and the needle is withdrawn over the guidewire. A catheter is threaded over the guidewire into the vein and the guidewire is removed. In the modified Seldinger technique, instead of advancing the catheter over the guidewire, a vein dilator-sheath assembly is advanced with rotary motion over the guidewire into the vein. The guidewire and the vein dilator are then removed, leaving only the sheath, which remains there throughout the procedure, serving as a conduit through which different types of open or closed tip catheters (eg, Cournand, Swan-Ganz, and Eppendorf) may be introduced.

The Swan-Ganz catheter[41] has been increasingly used in right heart catheterization for bedside monitoring of hemodynamics in the coronary care unit (usually antecubital, internal jugular, or subclavian approach) and for the diagnosis of congenital and acquired heart disease (femoral or antecubital approach). It can be introduced into the vein through a cutdown or percutaneously. It does not require fluoroscopy because its tip can be flow directed to reach the right atrium, right ventricle, and pulmonary artery and its branches, on inflation of the balloon mounted near its tip, after it has been blindly advanced to near the right atrium. With the catheter tip wedged and the balloon inflated, pulmonary artery wedge pressure is recorded, whereas on deflation pulmonary arterial pressure is obtained. A specially designed Swan-Ganz catheter* with a triple lumen (one of which is used for injection of cold indicator) is available for serial cardiac output measurement by thermodilution. It is also possible to record the intracavitary electrogram using a Swan-Ganz catheter with platinum electrodes mounted at specified distances from the tip.

LEFT HEART CATHETERIZATION

The first left heart catheterization in man was reported by Zimmerman et al[42] in 1950. They introduced a 6F Cournand catheter into the ulnar artery and retrogradely advanced it into the left ventricle. In the same year, Limon-Lason and Bouchard[43] also performed retrograde left heart catheterization. The percutaneous technique first introduced by Seldinger[40] has since been widely applied in left as well as right heart catheterization. Transseptal left heart catheterization was developed independently by Ross[44] and Cope[45] in 1959. Selective coronary arteriography, which was developed by Sones et al[46] in 1959, employed an open brachial approach. Subsequently, a percutaneous approach was advocated by Ricketts and Abrams[47] in 1962 and Judkins[48] in 1967.

Of the various methods of left heart catheterization, the retrograde percutaneous femoral arterial approach is probably used most extensively. Alternately, the open brachial approach is used if femoral entry is not feasible because of a severe scar or other skin conditions, or if marked tortuosity or blockage of the arterial passage prevents advancement of the catheter even with the aid of a J guidewire introduced ahead of the catheter. A 6F to 8F Sones catheter is frequently used for this purpose. The retrograde arterial approach permits localization of the level of left ventricular outflow obstruction, assessment of aortic and mitral regurgitation, and selective coronary arteriography. In addition, the specially made Shirey catheter† can be further retrogradely passed into the left atrium, allowing assessment of mitral stenosis.[49]

When the studies of the left heart require that the left atrium be entered (eg, to obtain mitral valve gradient and derive the mitral valve area in mitral stenosis), transseptal left heart catheterization is the method of choice. A Brockenbrough catheter† is percutaneously introduced into the right femoral vein and advanced into the right atrium to its junction with the superior vena cava. A long, curved needle (eg, Brockenbrough needle†) is inserted into the catheter and advanced slightly beyond the tip to puncture the atrial septum in the region of the fossa ovalis. The catheter is advanced over the needle into the left atrium and the needle is withdrawn. The catheter may be further advanced into the left ventricle. The increased demand for coronary arteriography in recent years and wide acceptance of the pulmonary artery wedge pressure as an accurate estimate of left atrial pressure have lessened the need for transseptal left heart catheterization; consequently, many practitioners are inexperienced with this technique. Recent modifications of the technique including the use of right anterior oblique cinefluoroscopy to define septal boundaries during interatrial septal puncture and a preshaped guidewire to catheterize the left ventricle[50] should make it safer and easier to perform. Transseptal left heart catheterization is required to estimate the aortic valve gradient; when crossing the severely stenotic aortic valve or the orifice of a tilting-disk aortic valve prosthesis is not successful by the retrograde arterial approach.

In percutaneous anterior left ventricular puncture, a long, 20- to 23-gauge needle attached to a pressure transducer is inserted directly into the left ventricle in the region of the apical impulse. Because of the relatively high morbidity and mortality of this approach in comparison with those of the transseptal and retrograde approaches, it is used only when all other methods of left heart catheterization fail. It is the only method that can evaluate postoperative double mitral and aortic prosthetic valve function.

Other currently unused techniques, namely, suprasternal left atrial puncture, posterior percutaneous left atrial puncture, and transbronchial left heart catheterization are only of historic interest.

* Swan-Ganz flow-directed thermodilution catheter, Edwards Laboratories, Santa Ana, California.

† United States Catheter and Instruments Corporation, Billerica, Massachusetts.

CARDIAC CATHETERIZATION DATA

PRESSURE MEASUREMENTS

Measurement of pressures in the cardiovascular system is an integral part of cardiac catheterization inasmuch as (1) the pressure pulse visualized on the oscilloscope serves to identify the position of the catheter tip; (2) an abnormality in pressure pulse can be related to the pathologic anatomy and functional pathology of the lesion (eg, ventricularization of the left atrial pressure pulse in severe mitral regurgitation); (3) changes in pressure between chambers or within the same chamber can be related to the pathologic anatomy of the regions traversed by the catheter tip (eg, characteristic intracavitary pressure-electrogram dissociation in Ebstein's anomaly); (4) the pressure gradient across the stenotic valve and the derived estimate of the orifice area permit quantitation of the severity of valvular stenosis; (5) systemic and pulmonary vascular resistance can be obtained from the pressure-flow data; and (6) assessment of ventricular performance can be made from the ventricular end-diastolic pressure, the rate of increase of ventricular pressure (dP/dt) and its derived parameters, and other derived parameters such as wall stress, stroke work, and the end-systolic pressure-volume relation.

Pressure within the cardiac chambers and great vessels can be recorded by a pressure transducer connected to a fluid-filled catheter or attached to the tip of a catheter without an intervening fluid column (catheter-tip micromanometer), the former being more commonly used. A modern fluid-filled transducer is generally an electrical strain gauge with a Wheatstone bridge circuit coupled to a membrane. A pressure change is transmitted through the catheter to the membrane by the blood column within, deforming the membrane and in turn, causing the change in electrical resistance of strain-sensitive wires coupled to the membrane, producing electrical output proportional to the pressure applied. To obtain an accurate recording of the pressure pulses, it is necessary to use a catheter-transducer system with a high natural resonant frequency and optimal damping. The catheter must be relatively short and wide and damping of the system optimal. In addition, meticulous care must be taken to ensure an air-free system because air bubbles in the system decrease the resonant frequency and increase the damping. The number of stopcocks should be kept at a minimum to avoid potential airtrapping and leaking. The connecting tubings between the transducer and the catheter should be stiff, short, and of large diameter to minimize damping. The zero level for pressure measurement must be established by placing the transducer at the estimated heart level; the mid-chest level and 10 cm above the back are probably most widely used. Calibration of the catheter-transducer system must be periodically carried out.

The catheter-tip micromanometers, having high natural frequency and low damping, produce pressure recordings that are practically free of amplitude distortion and delay of pressure waveform and are insensitive to catheter whip and catheter impact.

Table 13.2 lists normal resting pressures in the heart and great vessels.[51] Figures 13.1, 13.3 and 13.4 show the representative normal pressure pulses recorded from various cardiac chambers and the great arteries.

Table 13.2. Normal Pressures in Heart and Great Vessels*

Pressure (mm Hg)	Average	Range
Right atrium		
Mean	2.8	1–5
a wave	5.6	2.5–7
z point	2.9	1–5.5
c wave	3.8	1.5–6
x′ wave	1.7	0–5
v wave	4.6	2–7.5
y wave	2.4	0–6
Right ventricle		
Peak systolic	25	17–32
End-diastolic	4	1–7
Pulmonary artery		
Mean	15	9–19
Peak systolic	25	17–32
End-diastolic	9	4–13
Pulmonary artery wedge		
Mean	9	4.5–13
Left atrium		
Mean	7.9	2–12
a wave	10.4	4–16
z point	7.6	1–13
v wave	12.8	6–21
Left ventricle		
Peak systolic	130	90–140
End-diastolic	8.7	5–12
Brachial artery		
Mean	85	70–105
Peak systolic	130	90–140
End-diastolic	70	60–90

* From Fowler,[51] with permission.

A typical atrial pressure pulse (Figure 13.1) consists of three positive waves, a, c, and v, each followed by negative x, x′ and y descents. The a wave is due to atrial contraction and occurs after the P wave of the electrocardiogram. It is absent in atrial fibrillation. The x descent results from atrial relaxation. The c wave is produced by the bulging of the atrioventricular valve into the atrium during the isovolumic phase of ventricular systole. The z point marks the sudden increase in atrial pressure with the onset of ventricular contraction and is approximately at the peak or nadir of the QRS complex. The x′ descent results from the descent of the atrioventricular valve ring during ventricular ejection and continued atrial relaxation. The v wave is due to atrial filling while the atrioventricular valve is closed. Rapid ventricular filling following atrioventricular valve opening causes a steep decline in atrial pressure, the y descent. This is followed by slow ventricular filling, a slightly upward segment termed diastasis, representing equilibration between atrial and ventricular pressures. Left and right atrial pressure pulses are similar but not equal. The v wave is usually higher than the a wave in the left atrium and vice versa in the right atrium. The mean left atrial pressure is higher than the mean right atrial pressure. The pulmonary artery wedge pressure pulse (Figure 13.1) is obtained by wedging an end-hole catheter into a branch of the pulmonary artery, thus obstructing it. It reflects closely the left atrial pressure pulse but is damped and delayed (0.02 to 0.08 second).[52] The mean pulmonary artery wedge pressure is about 2 mm Hg higher than the mean left atrial pressure.

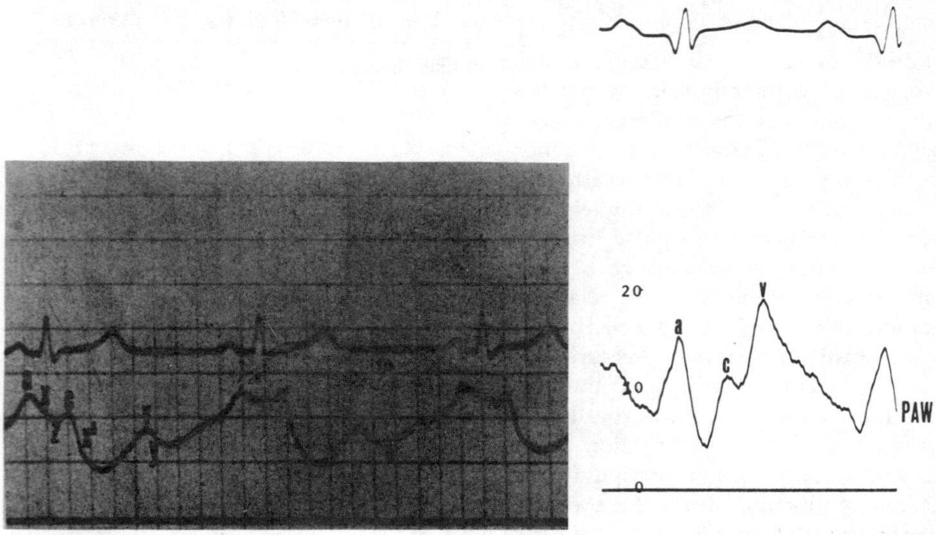

Figure 13.1. Normal right atrial and pulmonary artery wedge pressure pulses. *Left,* Right atrium. A Miller catheter-tip transducer was employed for recording. *Right,* Pulmonary artery wedge.

The left atrial a wave becomes prominent in patients with enhanced left atrial contraction due to mitral valve obstruction (mitral stenosis), decreased left ventricular compliance (eg, aortic stenosis), or left ventricular failure. Increased left atrial pressure with a prominent v wave is seen in patients with increased left atrial filling, as in those with mitral regurgitation, a ventricular septal defect, and patent ductus arteriosus. A prominent right atrial v wave may be due to tricuspid regurgitation, left ventricular–right atrial communication, or Ebstein's anomaly. Increased right atrial pressure with a prominent a wave may be associated with tricuspid stenosis, tricuspid atresia, pulmonic stenosis, total anomalous pulmonary venous drainage, or primary pulmonary hypertension. The appearance of a prominent a wave in ventricular systole suggests second or third degree atrioventricular block. A prolonged diastolic gradient across the atrioventricular valve (between atrium and ventricle) is diagnostic of atrioventricular valve stenosis. In severe mitral or tricuspid regurgitation, there may be an early diastolic gradient across the respective valve. In Ebstein's anomaly, as an electrode catheter with a lumen is withdrawn from the right ventricle to right atrium, dissociation of intracavitary electrogram and pressure (Figure 13.2) is observed as it passes the atrialized right ventricle where the right ventricular electrogram and right atrial pressure are recorded.

The ventricular pressure pulse (Figure 13.3) is divided into two phases, systole and diastole. At the onset of ventricular systole, the atrioventricular valve closes. This point, termed end-diastole, occurs near the peak or nadir of the QRS complex. The systole comprises isovolumic contraction, ejection, and protodiastole. Isovolumic contraction begins with atrioventricular valve closure and ends with semilunar valve opening. Ejection takes place between the semilunar valve opening and the beginning of protodiastole when the slow downslope of the ventricular pressure pulse gives way to a rapid downslope. As the rapidly declining ventricular pressure reaches that of the corresponding great artery, the semilunar valve closes and protodiastole ends. The diastolic phase is divided into isovolumic relaxation, rapid ventricular filling, slow ventricular filling (diastasis), and atrial systole (atrial kick). Isovolumic relaxation occurs between the semilunar valve closure and the atrioventricular valve opening. The decrease in ventricular pressure continues into the rapid ventricular filling period during which the pressure finally begins to increase. The ventricular pressure gradually increases during diastasis. The atrial kick corresponds to the a wave of the atrial pressure pulse.

Increased ventricular end-diastolic pressure may be observed in patients with myocardial failure, decreased ventricular compliance, increased volume overload (eg, aortic and mitral regurgitation), cardiac tamponade, and constrictive pericarditis. A systolic gradient across the semilunar valve (between the ventricle and corresponding great artery) is diagnostic of semilunar valve stenosis. In subaortic stenosis and infundibular pulmonic stenosis, there is a systolic gradient between the body and the outflow tract of the ventricle.

The arterial pressure pulse (Figure 13.4) may increase slightly near the end of the QRS complex as the semilunar valve bulges into the corresponding great artery, caused by isovolumic contraction of the ventricle. Ejection begins with the opening of the semilunar valve, and the arterial pressure pulse increases abruptly. This initial steep increase is followed by a gradual increase to a rounded peak, a subsequent slow decline to the dicrotic notch, which corresponds to the semilunar valve closure, and finally a slow descent to end-diastole. In the central aortic pressure pulse, an anacrotic notch is often present during early ejection. More peripheral arterial pressure pulse shows a higher peak pressure and a steeper ascending limb while the diastolic and mean pressures are lower.

The characteristics of the arterial pressure pulse vary depending on the type of aortic stenosis (Figure 13.5). The aortic pressure pulse in valvular aortic stenosis and

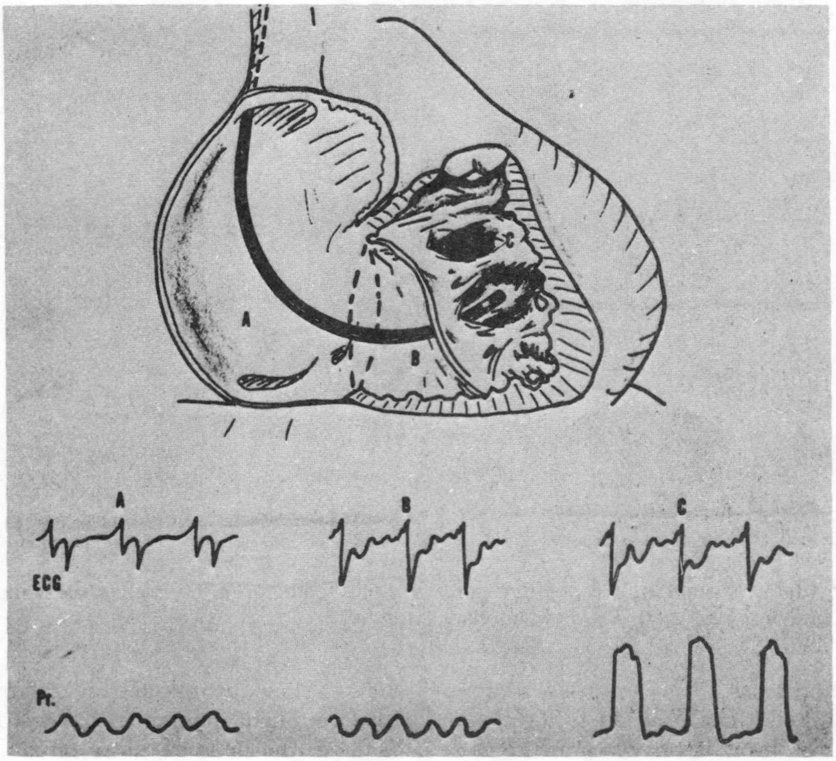

Figure 13.2. Simultaneous recording of intracavitary electrogram and pressure pulse in Ebstein's anomaly. On pullback from right ventricle (C) to right atrium (A), ventricular electrogram and atrial pressure pulse are recorded in the atrialized right ventricle (B). (From Gooch AS, Maranhao V, Goldberg H: *Clues to Diagnosis in Congenital Heart Disease.* Philadelphia, FA Davis, 1969, case 8. Reproduced with permission.)

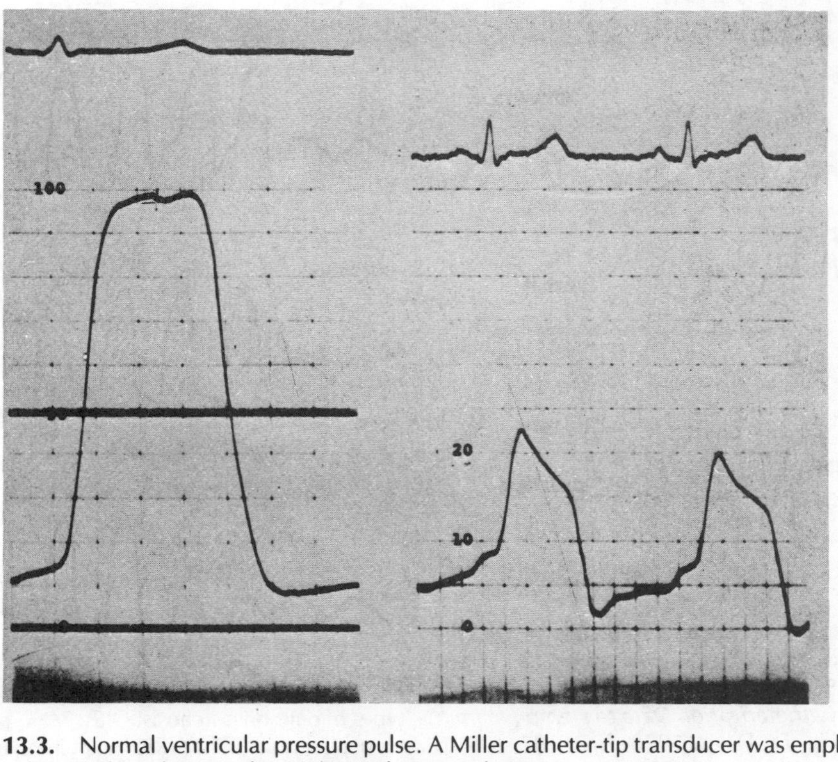

Figure 13.3. Normal ventricular pressure pulse. A Miller catheter-tip transducer was employed for recording. *Left*, Left ventricle. *Right*, Right ventricle.

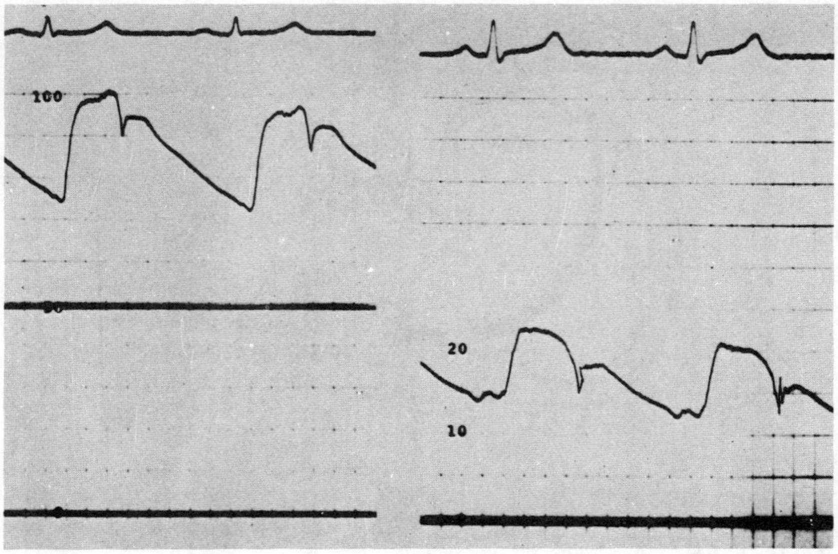

Figure 13.4. Normal arterial pressure pulse. A Miller catheter-tip transducer was employed for recording. *Left*, Aorta. *Right*, Pulmonary artery.

discrete subaortic stenosis has a slow upstroke, a prominent anacrotic notch, and a late peak. In supravalvular aortic stenosis, there may be a disparity in pressure pulse in the right and left carotid and radial arteries, resulting from the forceful jet of blood directed toward the innominate artery. The aortic and peripheral arterial pressure pulse in hypertrophic subaortic stenosis is notable for a rapid upstroke, absence of anacrotic notch, early systolic dip, and a second peak in late systole. In valvular pulmonic stenosis, the pulmonary arterial pressure pulse shows a slow upstroke and an anacrotic notch. In patients with peripheral pulmonic stenosis or pulmonary artery banding, the pressure pulse proximal to obstruction is ventricularized, the peak systolic and end-diastolic pressures being the same as those of the right ventricular pressure (Figure 13.6). A low diastolic pressure with a wide pulse pressure is characteristic of the pressure pulse in aortic regurgitation or other conditions associated with aortic run-off such as patent ductus arteriosus, coronary arteriovenous fistula, and rupture of the sinus of Valsalva

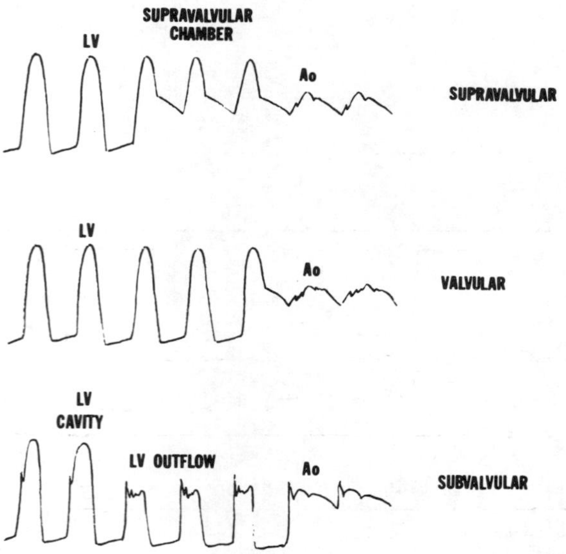

Figure 13.5. Continuous withdrawal pressure in various types of aortic stenosis. Ao = ascending aorta; LV = left ventricle. (From Yang SS, Bentivoglio LG, Maranhao V, Goldberg H: *From Cardiac Catheterization Data to Hemodynamic Parameters.* Philadelphia, FA Davis, 1978, Figure 87, p 180. Reproduced with permission.)

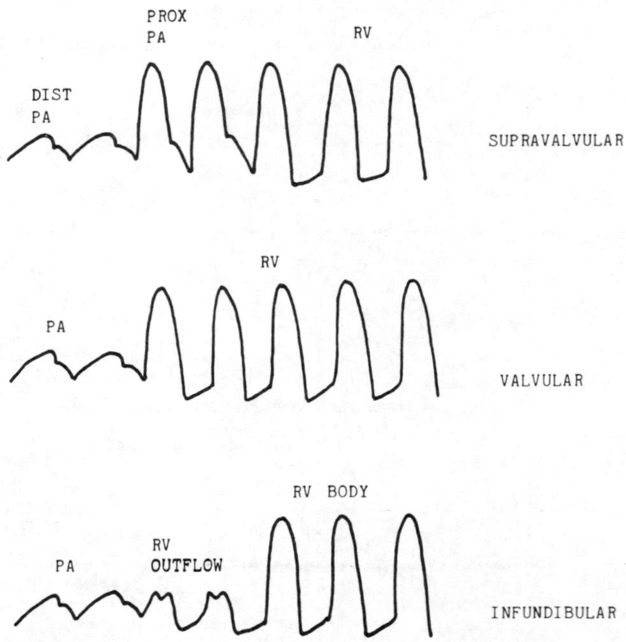

Figure 13.6. Continuous withdrawal pressure in various types of pulmonic stenosis. DIST PA = pulmonary artery distal to obstruction; PROX PA = pulmonary artery proximal to obstruction; RV = right ventricle.

into a right or left heart chamber. Similarly, in pulmonic regurgitation, the pulmonary arterial diastolic pressure is low and the pulse pressure wide.

MEASUREMENT OF CARDIAC OUTPUT

Cardiac output (CO) is the amount of blood ejected from the heart per unit of time, usually expressed in liters per minute. Customarily, it is normalized for body surface area (BSA) on the premise that the CO is proportional to the BSA. Thus the cardiac index (CI) equals CO/BSA, where the BSA is obtained from the Dubois and Dubois[53] height-weight equations:

$$BSA = \frac{71.84}{10{,}000} W^{0.425} H^{0.725}$$

in which BSA, W (weight), and H (height) are in square meters, kilograms, and centimeters respectively.

The direct Fick and indicator dilution methods are the standard techniques for measurement of the cardiac output and are both based on the Fick principle.[54] The Fick principle states that the amount of substance taken up or released by an organ is the product of its blood flow rate and the arteriovenous difference in the concentration of the substance.

Direct Fick Method

In this method, systemic blood flow is assumed to be equal to pulmonary blood flow. Applying the Fick principle, the oxygen taken up by the lungs (O_2 consumption) is calculated as the product of the flow rate and the arteriovenous difference in O_2 content (AV O_2 difference). Thus,

$$O_2 \text{ consumption} = CO \times AV\ O_2 \text{ difference}$$

where the units for O_2 consumption, CO, and AV O_2 difference are milliliters per minute, liters per minute, and milliliters per liter, respectively. Cardiac output is therefore calculated as

$$CO = \frac{O_2 \text{ consumption}}{AV\ O_2 \text{ difference}}.$$

The patient must be in steady-state during the three-minute period when the expired air is collected for measurement of O_2 consumption and the representative systemic arterial and mixed venous blood samples are obtained for measurement of the AV O_2 difference. The difference between the O_2 content of the ambient air (milliliters of O_2/liters of air) and the O_2 content of the expired air is taken as the O_2 consumption per liter of expired air and this, when multiplied by the minute volume (liters per minute), yields the O_2 consumption in milliliters per minute. In determining the AV O_2 difference, any systemic artery can be used for arterial blood sampling, because the O_2 content of arterial blood is uniform throughout the body. The mixed venous blood is sampled from the pulmonary artery where the mixing is adequate. The O_2 content in the arterial and venous samples is ideally measured by the Van Slyke[55] manometric apparatus. This method, although very accurate, is time consuming even for a skilled technician. This has practically been replaced by other methods; the O_2 saturation of hemoglobin is measured by reflectance oximetry, and the O_2 content is calculated by multiplying the O_2 saturation (%) by the O_2 capacity.* These methods must be periodically calibrated against the Van Slyke method.

Indicator Dilution Method

The indicator dilution method was originally proposed by Stewart[56] to calculate CO, but it has since found other applications such as estimation of pulmonary blood volume,[57] cardiac volume,[58,59] cardiovascular shunts,[60,61] and valvular regurgitation.[62,63] The method involves injecting an indicator (eg, indocyanine green) into a systemic vein or right side of the heart, followed by sampling from a systemic artery at a constant rate through a densitometer, with recording of the time-concentration curve (Figure 13.7). The curve consists of an initial rapid ascending limb followed by a slower downslope and a recirculation curve,

* O_2 capacity = blood hemoglobin content (g%) × 1.36 (ml/g) + 0.00326 (vol%/mm Hg) × pO_2 (mm Hg). One gram of hemoglobin binds 1.36 ml of O_2 at saturation and the coefficient of solubility of O_2 in plasma is 0.00326 ml O_2/100 ml per millimeter of mercury pO_2.

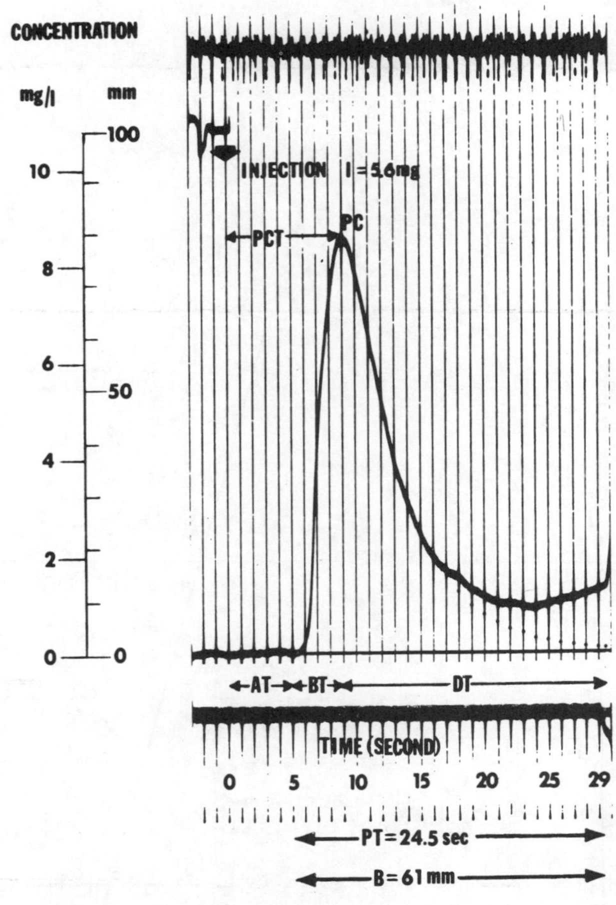

Figure 13.7. Time-concentration curve. AT = appearance time (s); BT = Build-up time (s); DT = Disappearance time (s); PC = peak concentration (mg/L); PCT = Peak concentration time (s). (From Yang SS, Bentivoglio LG, Maranhao V, Goldberg H: *From Cardiac Catheterization Data to Hemodynamic Parameters.* Philadelphia, FA Davis, 1978, Figure 36, p 63. Reproduced with permission.)

the latter beginning before the end of the first circulation. The downslope of the curve has been shown to be exponential until the onset of the recirculation curve. When replotted on semilogarithmic paper, with the indicator concentration on the logarithmic axis, the downslope of the new curve is noted to be a straight line, followed by a recirculation curve (Figure 13.8). Conventionally, a point at which the indicator concentration is 1% of the peak concentration may be arbitrarily chosen as the end of the disappearance time, and the straight line portion of the downslope is therefore extrapolated to this point.

The concentration values on this extrapolated portion are transferred to the original time-concentration curve to construct a complete curve without recirculation (Figure 13.8). Cardiac output is then calculated as follows:

$$CO = \frac{I \times 60}{C_m \times t}$$

where CO equals cardiac output in liters per minute, I equals the amount of indicator injected in milligrams, 60 equals 60 seconds per minute, C_m equals mean indicator concentration in milligrams per liter, and t equals total curve duration.

It is obvious in the foregoing Hamilton equation[64,65] that the denominator is the area under the complete curve. Besides simple planimetry, other methods are available for calculating the curve area and ultimately the CO. The ability of the computer to calculate the time constant of the exponential downslope, reconstruct the complete curve without recirculation, and integrate the curve up to and calculate the curve area beyond a point on the exponential downslope greatly facilitates calculation of CO.

For patients with a distorted disappearance slope, empirical formulas have been used to predict the total area from information derived from the initial ascending limb (ie, peak concentration, peak concentration time, and appearance time) with favorable results in comparison to the Hamilton method.[66,67]

Distortion in indicator dilution curve may arise from

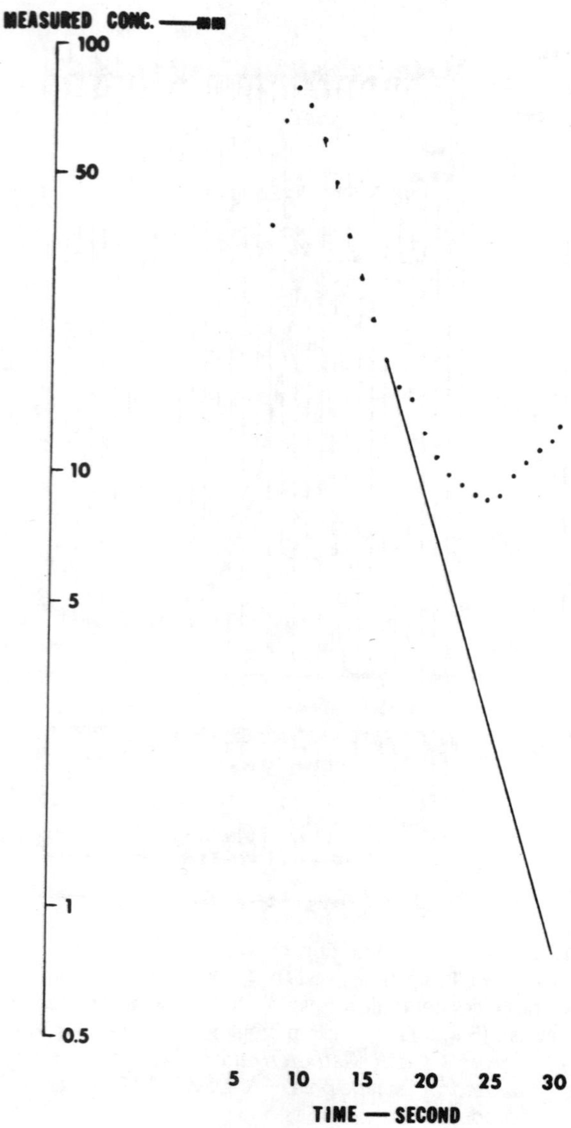

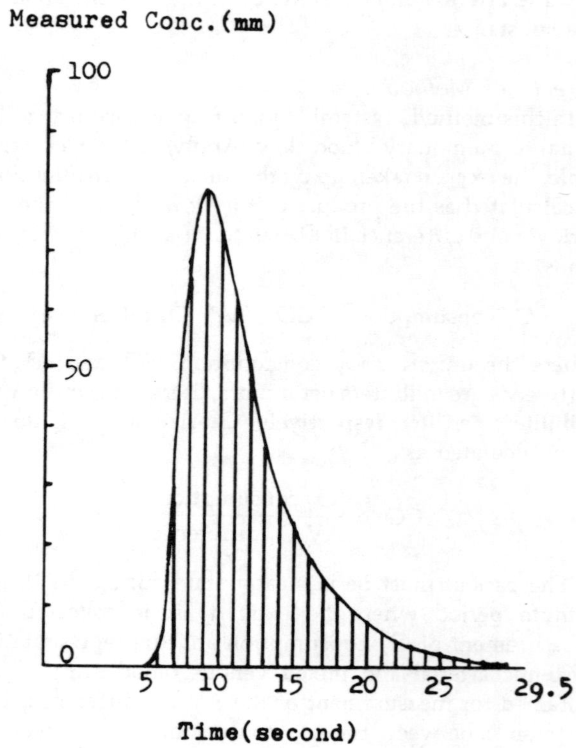

Figure 13.8. Semilogarithmic plot of the time-concentration curve and construction of a complete curve. *Left,* Semilogarithmic plot of the time-concentration curve with extrapolation of the straight segment of the downslope. *Right,* A complete curve without recirculation. (From Yang SS, Bentivoglio LG, Maranhao V, Goldberg H: *From Cardiac Catheterization Data to Hemodynamic Parameters.* Philadelphia, FA Davis, 1978, Figure 37, p 64, and Figure 40, p 71. Reproduced with permission.)

intracardiac shunts, valvular regurgitation, and changes in CO and blood volume between injection and sampling sites during the procedure. Cardiac output may be underestimated if recirculation is undetected, and overestimated if indicator is lost.

The thermodilution technique[68,69] is a unique indicator dilution technique which employs cold liquid (eg, saline solution, 5% dextrose in water, or autologous blood) as indicator. Its advantages over those of the conventional indicator dilution technique are: (1) the indicator is inexpensive; (2) no blood is lost during calibration and curve inscription; (3) rapid mixing and negligible recirculation make possible multiple determinations in a short time; (4) the thermal dilution curve, because of virtual absence of recirculation, lends itself to rapid calculation of the CO by an analog computer; (5) only right-sided catheterization is required for the procedure and systemic arterial entry is unnecessary. A small amount of thermal indicator is injected into the right atrium or vena cava and the resultant change in blood temperature is continuously recorded by a thermistor mounted 2 to 5 cm from the tip of a catheter at the pulmonary artery. Cardiac output is calculated as follows:

$$CO = \frac{V_i S_i C_i (T_b - T_i) \times 0.82 \times 60}{S_b C_b \int_0^{\infty} \Delta D_b(t)dt \times K}$$

where V_i equals volume of injectate in milliliters, S_i equals specific gravity of injectate, S_b equals specific gravity of blood, C_i equals specific heat of injectate, C_b equals specific heat of blood, T_b equals initial temperature of blood (°C), T_i equals initial temperature of injectate (°C), 0.82 equals empirical correction factor for indicator loss between end and tip of the catheter, 60 equals 60 seconds per minute, K equals the calibration factor for the curve (°C per millimeters of deflection), and $\int_0^{\infty} \Delta D_b(t)dt$ equals the area under the deflections-time curve registered following injection of the thermal indicator (°C × second).

Table 13.3 presents the mean values for the Fick CO and related measurements in normal individuals. Comparison of the results of CO measured by the Fick and the indicator dilution methods, respectively, indicates no systematic difference between the values obtained.[70,71] The thermodilution CO correlates well with that obtained by Fick and the standard indicator dilution method.[72,73]

Table 13.3. Normal Values for Cardiac Output and Related Measurements by the Fick Method*

Measurements	Units	±SD
O_2 uptake	143 ml/min/m²	14.3
Arteriovenous O_2 difference	4.1 vol%	0.6
Cardiac index	3.5 L/min/m²	0.7
Stroke index	46 ml/beat/m²	8.1

*Modified from Barratt-Boyes BG, Wood EH: Cardiac output and related measurements and pressure values in the right heart and associated vessels, together with an analysis of the hemodynamic response to the inhalation of high oxygen mixtures in healthy subjects. *J Lab Clin Med* 1958; 51:72–90.

CALCULATION OF ORIFICE AREA IN STENOTIC VALVE

Obstruction to ventricular inflow and outflow produces increased pressure proximal to the obstruction, resulting in a diastolic and a systolic gradient, respectively, across the narrowed atrioventricular (mitral or tricuspid) and semilunar (aortic or pulmonic) valves. These gradients, however, depend not only on the narrowed orifice area but also on the CO as well as the heart rate, the latter especially in inflow obstruction. In the hemodynamic assessment of valvular stenosis, therefore, the valve orifice area is ultimately the single, most important value to be obtained. It can be calculated using Gorlin and Gorlin's[74] hydraulic formula which states that the stenotic orifice area is directly proportional to the blood flow rate across the orifice and inversely proportional to the square root of the pressure gradient. Thus,

$$VA = \frac{VF}{44.5 \times C \sqrt{VG}}$$

where VA equals valve area in square centimeters, VF equals valve flow (milliliters per diastolic filling second or milliliters per systolic ejection second), VG equals valve gradient in millimeters of mecury, and C equals empirical constant, being 1 for the tricuspid and semilunar valves and 0.85 for the mitral valve (44.5 × 0.85 = 38).[75] Valve flow in the foregoing formula is calculated as follows:

$$VF = \frac{CO\ (ml/min)}{DFP\ (s/min)\ or\ SEP\ (s/min)}$$

where DFP equals diastolic filling period per minute = diastolic filling period per beat × heart rate (Figure 13.9) and SEP equals systolic ejection period per minute = systolic ejection period per beat × heart rate (Figure 13.9).

The formula underestimates valve area in the presence of regurgitation, for only the forward flow is incorporated in the formula; the amount of regurgitant flow that on subsequent diastole or systole recrosses the valve is not taken into consideration. Even in the absence of regurgitation, the formula does not always give an accurate estimate of the valve area. This is understandable considering the assumption on which the formula is based, namely, fixed valve area and steady blood flow. It has been shown that the valve orifice area is not constant and is flow and pressure dependent, especially at low flow rates.[76–79] In practice, therefore, to minimize possible error in estimating the valve area when the valve gradient is small, exercise is recommended to increase valve flow and valve gradient. In the estimation of mitral valve gradient, frequently the pulmonary artery wedge pressure is substituted for the left atrial pressure which is more difficult to obtain. Occasionally, what appears to be a technically adequate pulmonary artery wedge pressure pulse may turn out to be damped and may have a significantly higher mean pressure than the corresponding left atrial pressure, accounting for a misleadingly high mitral valve gradient. Therefore, to avoid underestimating the mitral valve area especially in patients being considered for re-

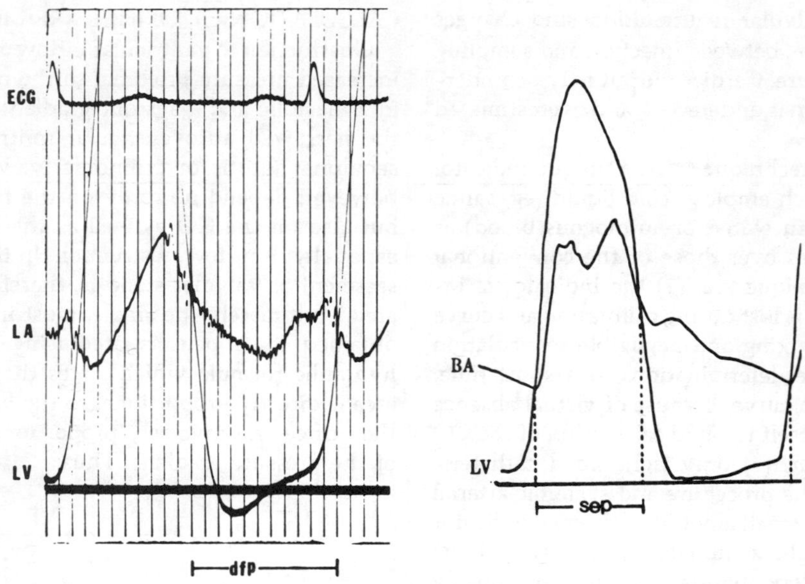

Figure 13.9. Measurement of diastolic filling period and systolic ejection period. dfp = diastolic filling period per beat; sep = systolic ejection period per beat.

peat mitral valve surgery because of possible prosthetic valve stenosis, transseptal catheterization, which allows for more accurate determination of prosthetic valve area, should be performed.[80]

CALCULATION OF VASCULAR RESISTANCE

Vascular resistance is defined, by analogy to Ohm's law, as the ratio of the mean pressure decrease (gradient) across a vascular segment to the flow through it:

$$\text{resistance} = \frac{\text{mean pressure drop}}{\text{flow}}$$

According to Poiseuille, flow (F) in a rigid, cylindrical tube is directly proportional to the mean pressure gradient (P) and the fourth power of the radius (R) of the tube and is inversely proportional to the viscosity (ρ) of the fluid and the length (L) of the tube:

$$F = \frac{\pi P R^4}{8 \rho L}$$

Therefore,

$$\frac{P}{F} = \text{resistance} = \frac{8 \rho L}{\pi R^4}$$

Idealized as it may be, the relation points to the fact that the resistance is highly dependent on the caliber of the vessels. The vascular resistance, as defined, measures the opposition of the vascular bed to the steady component of flow, the pulsatile components of the flow being ignored. Therefore, vascular resistance underestimates the total opposition to flow by an unknown amount. Because the resistance represents a large portion of the total opposition to flow, it remains a useful approximation of the true resistance in the vascular bed.

In hemodynamic laboratories, resistance is expressed in hybrid resistance units* or absolute resistance units. The hybrid resistance unit is the ratio of a driving pressure equal to that produced by a column of mercury, 1 mm high, to a resultant flow of 1 L/min. It has units of millimeters of mercury per liter per minute.

The absolute resistance unit is defined as the ratio of a driving pressure of 1 dyne/cm^2 to a resultant flow of 1 cm^3/s. It has units of dynes·s·cm^{-5}. The resistance expressed in both units is interconvertible:

$$\text{absolute resistance units} = \text{hybrid resistance units} \times 80$$

The following are formulas for vascular resistance commonly used in hemodynamic laboratories:

$$\text{PVR} = \frac{(\text{PA}_m - \text{LA}_m)}{\text{CO}}$$

$$\text{TPR} = \frac{\text{PA}_m}{\text{CO}}$$

$$\text{SVR} = \frac{(\text{SA}_m - \text{RA}_m)}{\text{CO}}$$

where PVR, TPR, and SVR are pulmonary vascular, total pulmonary, and systemic vascular resistance, respectively; PA_m, LA_m, and SA_m are mean pulmonary arterial, mean left atrial, and mean systemic arterial pressures, respectively.

Normal values for resistances are presented in Table 13.4.

ASSESSMENT OF CARDIOVASCULAR SHUNTS

In the hemodynamic assessment of cardiovascular shunts, the indicator dilution method is most sensitive for their detection, whereas quantitation of shunts is best

* Sometimes also referred to as Wood units (Wood P: *Diseases of the Heart and Circulation,* ed 3. Philadelphia, JB Lippincott, 1968, pp 188–189).

Table 13.4. Normal Values for Resistances*

Measurements	Units ± Standard Deviation
Systemic vascular resistance	1,130 ± 178 $dynes{\cdot}s{\cdot}cm^{-5}$
Total pulmonary resistance	205 ± 51 $dynes{\cdot}s{\cdot}cm^{-5}$
Pulmonary vascular resistance	67 ± 23 $dynes{\cdot}s{\cdot}cm^{-5}$

*Modified from Barratt-Boyes BG, Wood EH: Cardiac output and related measurements and pressure values in the right heart and associated vessels, together with an analysis of the hemodynamic response to the inhalation of high oxygen mixtures in healthy subjects. *J Lab Clin Med* 1958; 51:72–90.

accomplished by oximetry. However, angiocardiography during cardiac catheterization has acquired a preeminent diagnostic role because of its ability to visualize and semiquantitate shunts (even a small one) and to outline the location and size of the abnormal communication. Therefore, in most pediatric hemodynamic laboratories, angiocardiography takes precedence over the foregoing techniques. It should be recognized that an abnormal course taken by the catheter during its passage through the cardiovascular chambers and vessels may help detect the abnormal communication. For example, a catheter that is in the left pulmonary artery may suddenly course inferiorly as it enters the descending aorta through a patent ductus arteriosus.

Oximetry

Under steady-state, blood samplings are carried out in rapid sequence from the right, left, and main pulmonary arteries; the right ventricular outflow tract, body, and inflow tract; the low, mid, and high right atrium; the low and high superior vena cava; and the low and high inferior vena cava. Because of incomplete mixing, particularly in the more proximal chambers, allowance is made for variability in the O_2 content and saturation from chamber to chamber, in trying to detect a significant O_2 step-up for the diagnosis of left-to-right shunt.[81] The O_2 step-up required to detect left-to-right shunt in our laboratory is as follows: superior vena cava to right atrium, 1.9 vol% (7%)*; right atrium to right ventricle, 0.9 vol% (5%); and right ventricle to pulmonary artery, 0.5 vol% (3%). Therefore, if there is an O_2 step-up of, for example, 2.2 vol% (O_2 content) and 9% (O_2 saturation) from the superior vena cava to right atrium, a left-to-right shunt into the right atrium is indicated. This may be an atrial septal defect, anomalous pulmonary venous drainage, left ventricular–right atrial communication, coronary-right atrial communication, ruptured sinus of Valsalva into the right atrium, or a ventricular septal defect with tricuspid regurgitation. For a significant O_2 step-up at the ventricular level, ventricular septal defect, ostium primum atrial septal defect, patent ductus arteriosus with pulmonic regurgitation, coronary-right ventricular communication, or a ruptured sinus of Valsalva into the right ventricle is suspected. Possible causes of a significant O_2 step-up at the pulmonary artery level include patent ductus arteriosus, aortico-pulmonary window, and an aberrant coronary artery originating from the pulmonary artery.

*O_2 content (O_2 saturation).

Desaturation of arterialized blood sampled from the left heart chambers and the systemic arteries suggests a right-to-left shunt. If sequential samplings can be made from the left atrium, left ventricle, and aorta, the site of entry of a right-to-left shunt is identified as the first chamber to yield desaturated blood (less than 94%). Technically, however, it is difficult to enter the pulmonary veins and left atrium, especially in the adult.

To quantitate the shunt, the Fick method is used to calculate systemic blood flow (SBF), pulmonary blood flow (PBF), and effective pulmonary blood flow (EPBF) as follows:

$$\text{SBF} = \frac{O_2 \text{ consumption (ml/min)}}{(\text{SA}O_2 - \text{mixed V}O_2) \times 10}$$

$$\text{PBF} = \frac{O_2 \text{ consumption (ml/min)}}{(\text{PV}O_2 - \text{PA}O_2) \times 10}$$

$$\text{EPBF} = \frac{\dot{O}_2 \text{ consumption (ml/min)}}{(\text{PV}O_2 - \text{mixed V}O_2) \times 10}$$

where SAO_2, mixed VO_2, PVO_2, and PAO_2 represent the O_2 content (in vol%) of blood obtained from the systemic artery, mixed venous return, pulmonary vein, and pulmonary artery, respectively. The mixed venous blood is sampled from the chamber immediately proximal to the recipient site of the left-to-right shunt, and in a right-to-left shunt, from the pulmonary artery. In using vena caval blood as mixed venous blood in atrial septal defect, it has been suggested[82] that the following rather than the average of both superior (VC_s) and inferior (VC_i) vena caval blood samples be used:

$$VO_2 = \frac{3VC_sO_2 + VC_iO_2}{4}$$

If the pulmonary vein cannot be entered, an O_2 content based on its assumed O_2 saturation of 95% is used as PVO_2. Thus,

$$PVO_2 = O_2 \text{ capacity} \times \frac{95}{100}$$

where O_2 capacity = blood hemoglobin content (g%) × 1.36 (ml/g) + 0.00326 (vol%/mm Hg) × pO_2(mm Hg). The EPBF is defined as the fraction of mixed venous return that is conveyed to the lungs to be oxygenated.

The left-to-right ($S_{l\text{-}r}$) and right-to-left ($S_{r\text{-}l}$) shunts are calculated as follows[36]:

$$S_{l\text{-}r} = \text{PBF} - \text{EPBF}$$
$$S_{r\text{-}l} = \text{SBF} - \text{EPBF}$$

It should be noted that these formulas apply also to bidirectional shunts. In the left-to-right shunt alone, EPBF equals SBF because SAO_2 and PVO_2 are identical. In the right-to-left shunt alone, EPBF equals PBF because mixed VO_2 equals PAO_2.

The pulmonary-to-systemic flow ratio is calculated as follows:

$$\frac{\text{PBF}}{\text{SBF}} = \frac{\text{SA}O_2 - \text{mixed V}O_2}{\text{PV}O_2 - \text{PA}O_2}$$

Indicator Dilution Method

A left-to-right shunt as small as 5% of the pulmonary blood flow can be detected by sampling from the main pulmonary artery following injection of an indicator into a distal lobar pulmonary artery.[83] The recorded indicator dilution curve will show an early appearance of the indicator. Also sensitive is a method in which hydrogen gas is inhaled and a left-to-right shunt is detected and localized by a platinum electrode placed first in the pulmonary artery and then in the right ventricle and right atrium[84,85] (Figure 13.10). Another method to localize the shunt is serial injections of the indicator into the aorta and left heart chambers with samplings in a systemic artery.[60] An abnormal curve (Figure 13.11) with a low peak and distorted disappearance slope results from injection into or proximal to the compartment from which the shunt originates. In a right-to-left shunt, an abnormal indicator dilution curve will be recorded from a systemic

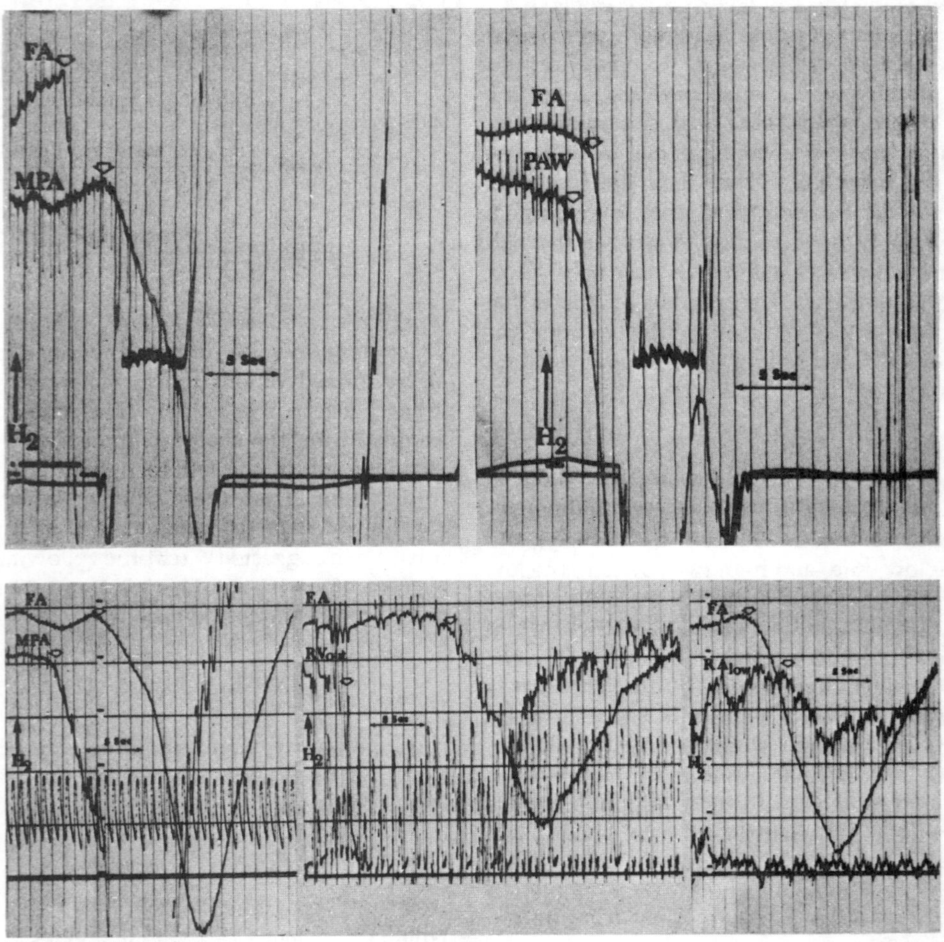

Figure 13.10. *Top,* Negative hydrogen test for a left-to-right shunt. *Left panel* represents simultaneous hydrogen dilution curves from two platinum electrodes, one in the femoral artery (FA) and the other in the main pulmonary artery (MPA), hydrogen (H_2) reaching the former before the latter. *Right panel* shows the venous electrode in the pulmonary artery wedge position (PAW) where hydrogen (H_2) is detected earlier than in the femoral artery (FA). It is advisable to always do a 'control' H_2 test at the PAW position to ensure the sensitivity of the venous electrode. *Bottom,* Positive hydrogen test for a left-to-right shunt through a ventricular septal defect. Hydrogen (H_2) arrives at the main pulmonary artery (MPA, *left panel*) and right ventricular outflow tract (RV_{out}, *middle panel*) earlier, and at the low right atrial level (RA_{low}, *right panel*) later, than the femoral artery (FA). The *solid arrows* indicate the instant of hydrogen inhalation, and the *hollow arrows* the appearance times. The location of the electrode in the right side of the heart is indicated not only by the intracavitary electrocardiogram but by the pressure curves, calibrated 10 mm Hg for each horizontal line starting from zero at the baseline. Note the different appearance times of hydrogen in the femoral artery in each instance, due partly to different depths of inhalation of hydrogen by the sedated patient and partly to the occurrence of multiple ventricular extrasystoles induced by the venous electrode in the outflow tract of the right ventricle. (Figures 13.10 and 13.12 are from Cheng TO: Hydrogen and ascorbate dilution curves. A simplified method for routine use in detection of intracardiac shunt and valvular regurgitation. *Chest* 62:304–310, 1972. Reproduced with permission.)

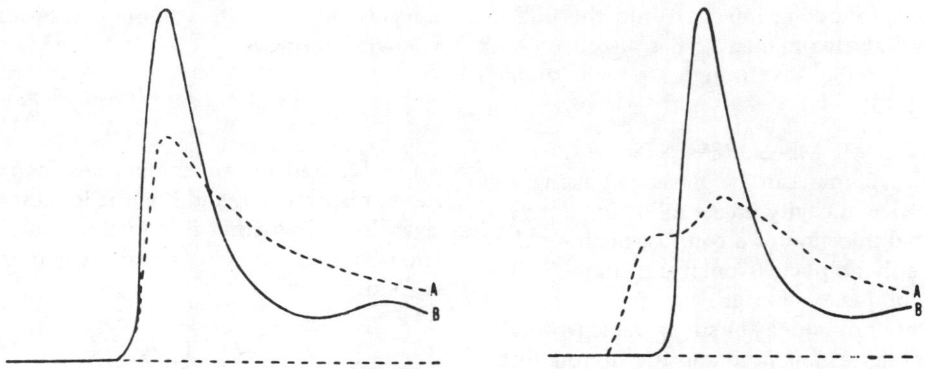

Figure 13.11. Abnormal indicator dilution curve recorded from a systemic artery following injection into or proximal to the compartment from which the shunt originates. *Left,* Left-to-right shunt. *Right,* Right-to-left shunt. A normal curve (*bold line*) results from distal injection. (From Yang SS, Bentivoglio LG, Maranhao V, Goldberg H: *From Cardiac Catheterization Data to Hemodynamic Parameters.* Philadelphia, FA Davis, 1978, Figure 104, p 219, and Figure 107, p 224. Reproduced with permission.)

artery following injection into or proximal to the chamber from which the shunt originates.[61] The abnormality is either early appearance of the indicator, eg, dye[86] (Figure 13.11) and ascorbate solution[85,87] (Figure 13.12), or its unexpected appearance, eg, solution of hydrogen in saline[88] and solution of krypton-85 in saline,[89] when the indicator used is normally cleared by the lungs. The curve is normal when the injection is made distal to the site of origin of the shunt. This technique can detect a right-to-left shunt as small as 2% to 3% of the systemic blood flow.[86] Therefore, the origin of the shunt is located within the chamber immediately proximal to the one showing a normal curve. When a right-to-left shunt associated with an atrial septal defect is very small, its detection can be enhanced by the

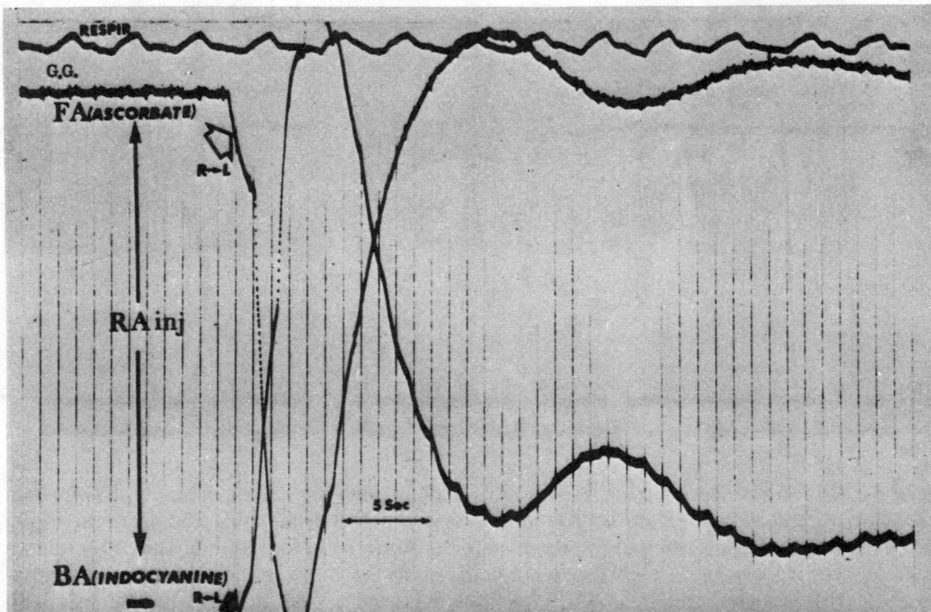

Figure 13.12. Small right-to-left (R → L) shunt at the right atrial (RA) level in a patient with severe pulmonic stenosis and patent foramen ovale, more clearly shown on the ascorbate dilution curve (*hollow arrow*) from the femoral artery (FA) than on the simultaneously recorded indocyanine dilution curve (*solid arrow*) from the brachial artery (BA). Normal curves were recorded following ascorbate injections into right ventricle and pulmonary artery (not shown).

Valsalva maneuver following injection into the inferior vena cava.[90] The Valsalva maneuver has also been used to detect paradoxic embolism through a patent foramen ovale[91] (Figure 13.13).

VENTRICULAR VOLUME MEASUREMENTS

Left ventricular volume can be measured using the opacified left ventricular cavity image following left ventricular or left atrial injection of a contrast medium. Angiocardiography, either biplane (frontal and lateral,[92] right and left anterior oblique,[93] and right anterior oblique and half-axial left anterior oblique[94]) or single plane (frontal[95] or right anterior oblique[96]), is used and the filming technique is either seriography or cinefluorography. The classic biplane, area-length method of Dodge et al[92] assumes that the left ventricular cavity can be represented by an ellipsoid and that its volume can be calculated by the following formula:

$$V = \frac{4}{3}\pi \frac{D_a}{2}\frac{D_l}{2}\frac{L}{2} = \frac{\pi}{6} D_a D_l L$$

where D_a and D_l are minor axes in frontal and lateral views, respectively, and L is the longest measured length regardless of whether it is in the frontal or lateral view. The two minor axes are not measured and are calculated as follows:

$$D_a = \frac{4A_a}{\pi L_a}$$

$$D_l = \frac{4A_l}{\pi L_l}$$

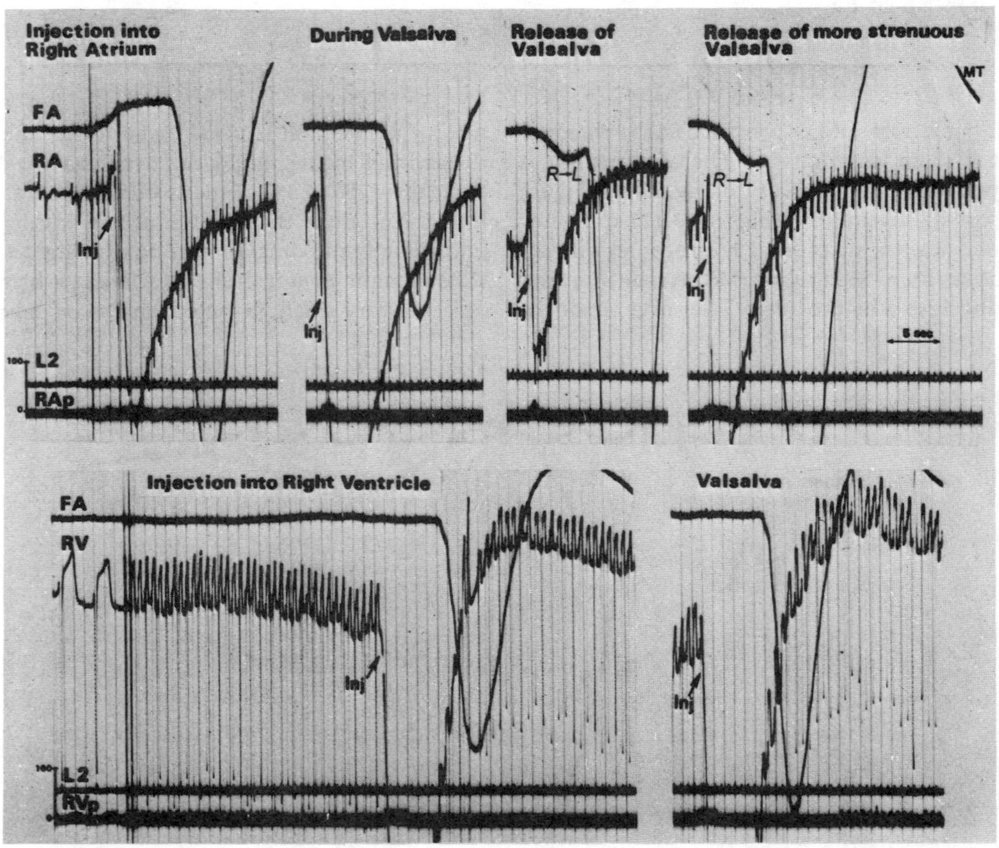

Figure 13.13. Ascorbate dilution curves in a patient with paradoxical cerebral embolism accompanying pulmonary embolism. The study was performed by injecting 300 mg of ascorbate into the right atrium (*top*) and into the right ventricle (*bottom*) before, during, and after release of the Valsalva maneuver. In each the femoral artery (FA) was the sensing site following either right atrial (RA) or right ventricular (RV) injections; recordings were made simultaneously with ECG lead II (L2) and right atrial (RA_p on top) and right ventricular (RV_p on bottom) pressures except in the second and fourth panels on top and parts of the bottom panels where connection to the strain gauge was turned off. There was no evidence of a right-to-left interatrial shunt both before and during the Valsalva maneuver. However, following release of the Valsalva maneuver, there was a small right-to-left (R → L) interatrial shunt which became larger following release of a more strenuous Valsalva maneuver. No right-to-left shunt was demonstrated at the ventricular level with or without a Valsavla maneuver. (From Cheng TO: Paradoxical embolism. A diagnostic challenge and its detection during life. *Circulation* 53:565–568,1976. Reproduced with permission of the American Heart Association.)

where A_a and A_l are areas of the projected images in the frontal and lateral views, respectively, and L_a and L_l are the longest measured lengths in the frontal and lateral views, respectively (Figure 13.14). Each length in both views must first be corrected for nonparallel x-ray distortion as described elsewhere.[97,98]

In the single plane methods, only the long-axis and one short-axis are obtained; the nonvisualized short axis is assumed to be the same as the visualized one. Therefore,

$$V = \frac{\pi}{6} D^2 L \,.$$

Single plane methods are usually combined with cine technique. A calibrated grid is filmed at the assumed level of the left ventricle and is used in deriving a correction factor to correct for the nonparallel x-ray distortion as well as pincushion effect (more magnification at the periphery).[99]

Biplane or single plane, the calculated volume tends to overestimate the actual volume probably because of the inclusion of the papillary muscles and trabeculae carneae in the opacified image and to the inherent overestimation by the formula itself. To correct for this overestimation, regression equations have been derived from in vitro studies using casts or radiopaque paste.[92,93,96,99–103]

The normal left ventricular end-diastolic volume is 70 $\pm$ 20 ml/m^2 (mean $\pm$standard deviation), the end-systolic volume is 24 $\pm$ 10 ml/m^2, and the ejection fraction is 0.67 $\pm$ 0.08.[104]

In aortic and mitral regurgitation, the regurgitant stroke volume is obtained as the total stroke volume minus the forward stroke volume. The total stroke volume is the difference between the end-diastolic and end-systolic volume. The regurgitant fraction is regurgitant stroke volume divided by total stroke volume. A regurgitant fraction of over 60% suggests severe valvular regurgitation.

Despite the irregularity and complexity of the right ventricular internal geometry, several angiocardiographic methods have been proposed to determine right ventricular volume, including modifications of the area-length method.[105–109] Normal right ventricular end-diastolic volume is 76 $\pm$ 11 ml/m^2, end-systolic volume is 26 $\pm$ 6 ml/m^2, and the ejection fraction is 0.66 $\pm$ 0.06.[109]

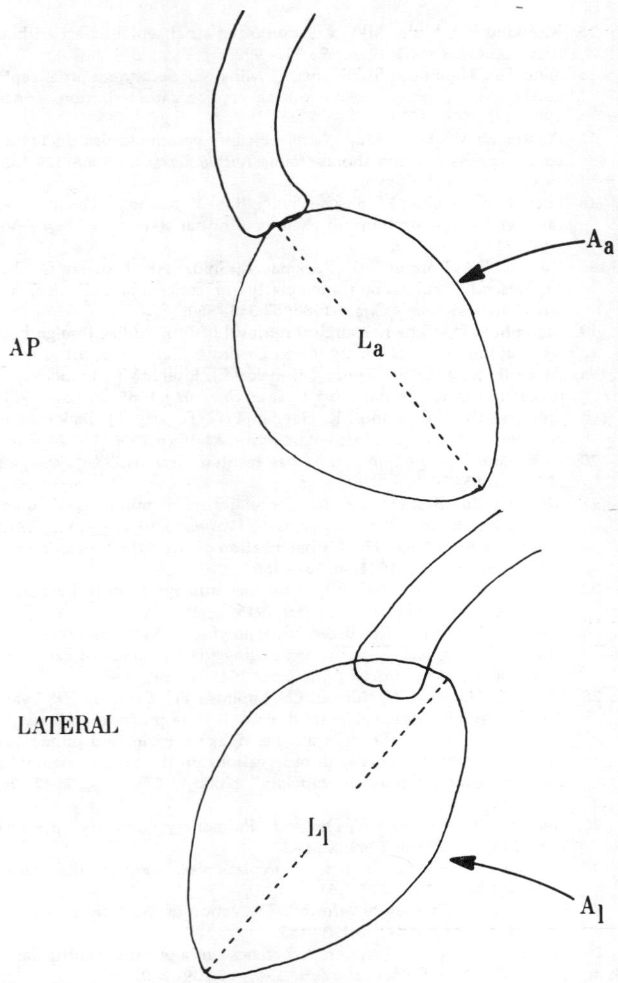

Figure 13.14. Area-length method of Dodge and associates. Diagram depicting the measurement of the longest measured axis and the area of the projected image in anteroposterior (AP) and lateral projections. A_a = area of the projected image in AP view; A_l = area of the projected image in lateral view; L_a = longest measured axis in AP view; L_l = longest measured axis in lateral view. (From Yang SS, Bentivoglio LG, Maranhao V, Goldberg H: *From Cardiac Catheterization Data to Hemodynamic Parameters.* Philadelphia, FA Davis, 1978, Figure 52, p 106. Reproduced with permission.)

REFERENCES

1. St. John Sutton MG, St. John Sutton M, Oldershaw P, Sacchetti R, Paneth M, Lennox SC, Gibson RV, Gibson DG: Valve replacement without preoperative cardiac catheterization. *N Engl J Med* 1981; 305:1233–1238.
2. Borow KM, Wynne J, Sloss LJ, Cohn LH, Collins JJ: Noninvasive assessment of valvular heart disease: surgery without catheterization. *Am Heart J* 1983; 106:443–449.
3. Hall RJC, Kadushi OA, Evemy K: Need for cardiac catheterization in assessment of patients for valve surgery. *Br Heart J* 1983; 49:268–275.
4. Lewis DH, Deitz GW, Wallace JD, Brown JR: Intracardiac phonocardiography in man. *Circulation* 1957; 16:764–775.
5. Scherlag BJ, Lau SH, Helfant RA, Berkowitz WD, Stein E, Damato AN: Catheter technique for recording His bundle activity in man. *Circulation* 1969; 39:13–18.
6. Sakakibara S, Konno S: Endomyocardial biopsy. *Jpn Heart J* 1962; 3:537–543.
7. Scheinman MM, Davis JC: Catheter ablation for treatment of tachyarrhythmias: present role and potential promise. *Circulation* 1986; 73:10–13.
8. Zipes DP, Heger JJ, Miles WM: Synchronous intracardiac cardioversion. *PACE* 1984; 7:522–533.
9. Grüntzig A: Transluminal dilatation of coronary-artery stenosis. *Lancet* 1978; 1:263.
10. Rentrop P, Blanke H, Karsch KR, Daiser H, Kostering H, Leitz K: Selective intracoronary thrombolysis in acute myocardial infarction and unstable angina pectoris. *Circulation* 1981; 63:307–317.
11. Kan JS: Balloon angioplasty-pulmonic stenosis, in Doyle EF, Engle MA, Gersony WM, Rashkind WJ, Talner NS (eds): *Pediatric Cardiology.* New York, Springer-Verlag, 1986, pp 352–354.
12. Lababidi Z, Walls J, Stoeckle H: Percutaneous balloon aortic valvuloplasty, in Doyle EF, Engle MA, Gersony WM, Rashkind WJ, Talner NS (eds): *Pediatric Cardiology.* New York, Springer-Verlag, 1986, pp 334–335.
13. Lock JE, Bass JL, Amplatz K, Fuhrman BP, Castaneda-Zuniga W: Balloon dilation angioplasty of aortic coarctations in infants and children. *Circulation* 1983; 68:109–116.
14. Bregman D, Casarella WJ: Percutaneous intra-aortic balloon pumping: Initial clinical experience. *Ann Thorac Surg* 1979; 29:153–155.

15. Rashkind WJ, Miller MW: Creation of an atrial septal defect without thoracotomy. *JAMA* 1966; 196:991–992.
16. King TD, Thompson SL, Steiner C, Mills NL: Secundum atrial septal defect. Nonoperative closure during cardiac catheterization. *JAMA* 1976; 235:2506–2509.
17. Porstmann W, Wierny L, Warnke H: Der verschluss des ductus arteriosus persistens ohne thorakotomie. *Fortschr Roentgenstr* 1968; 109:133–148.
18. Lock JE, Khalilullah M, Shrivastava S, Bahl V, Keane JF: Percutaneous catheter commissurotomy in rheumatic mitral stenosis. *N Engl J Med* 1985; 313:1515–1518.
18a. Kveselis DA, Rocchini AP, Beekman R, Snider AR, Crowley D, Dick M, Rosenthal A: Balloon angioplasty for congenital and rheumatic mitral stenosis. *Am J Cardiol* 1986; 57:348–350.
19. Bloomfield DA: The nonsurgical retrieval of intracardiac foreign bodies—an international survey. *Cathet Cardiovasc Diagn* 1978; 4:1–14.
19a. Reidy JF, Jones ODH, Tynan MJ, Baker EJ, Joseph MC: Embolisation procedures in congenital heart disease. *Br Heart J* 1985; 54:184–192.
19b. Zimmerman JJ, Cipriano PR, Hayden WG, Fogarty TJ: Balloon embolectomy catheter used percutaneously. *Radiology* 1986; 158:260–262.
20. Forssmann W: Die Sondierung des rechten Herzens. *Klin Wochenschr* 1929; 8:2085–2087.
21. Klein O: Zur Bestimmung des Zerkulatorischen minutens Volumen nach dem Fickschen Prinzip. *Munch Med Wochenschr* 1930; 77:1311–1312.
22. Cournand AF, Ranges HS: Catheterization of the right auricle in man. *Proc Soc Exp Biol Med* 1941; 46:462–466.
23. Richards DW Jr: Cardiac output by the catheterization technique, in various clinical conditions. *Fed Proc* 1945; 4:215–220.
24. Cournand AF, Riley RL, Breed ES, Baldwin EF, Richards DW: Measurement of cardiac output in man using the technique of catheterization of the right auricle. *J Clin Invest* 1945; 24:106–116.
25. Dexter L, Haynes FW, Burwell CS, Eppinger EC, Sagerson RP, Evans JM: Studies of congenital heart disease. II. The pressure and oxygen content of blood in the right auricle, right ventricle, and pulmonary artery in control patients with observations on the oxygen saturation and source of pulmonary "capillary" blood. *J Clin Invest* 1947; 26: 554–560.
26. Hellems HK, Haynes FW, Dexter L: Pulmonary "capillary" pressure in man. *J Appl Physiol* 1949; 2:24–29.
27. Lagerlof H, Werko L: Studies on circulation of blood in man. *Scand J Clin Lab Invest* 1949; 1:147–161.
28. McMichael J, Sharpey-Schafer EP: The action of intravenous digoxin in man. *Q J Med* 1944; 13:123–135.
29. Lenegre J, Maurice P: Premiers recherches sur la pression ventricularire droite. *Bull Mem Soc Med Hop Paris* 1944; 80:239–240.
30. Lenegre J, Maurice P: De quelques resultats obtenus par la derivation directe intracavitaire des courants electriques de l'oreillette et du ventricule droits. *Arch Mal Coeur* 1945; 38:298–302.
31. Stead EA Jr, Warren JV: Cardiac output in man: analysis of mechanisms varying cardiac output based on recent clinical studies. *Arch Intern Med* 1947; 80:237–248.
32. Stead EA Jr, Warren JV, Brannon ES: Cardiac output in congestive heart failure: analysis of reasons for lack of close correlation between symptoms of heart failure and resting cardiac output. *Am Heart J* 1948; 35:529–541.
33. Bing RJ, Hammond MM, Handelsman JC, Powers SR, Spencer FC, Eckenhoff JE, Goodale WT, Italkenschiel JH, Kety SS: Catheterization of coronary sinus and middle cardiac vein in man. *Proc Soc Exp Biol Med* 1947; 66:239–240.
34. Bing RJ, Vandam LD, Gregire F, Handelsman JC, Goodale WT, Eckenhoff JE: Measurement of coronary blood flow, oxygen consumption and efficiency of the left ventricle in man. *Am Heart J* 1949; 38:1–24.
35. Vandam LD, Bing RJ, Gray FD Jr: Physiological studies in congenital heart disease. IV. Measurements of circulation in 5 selected cases. *Bull Johns Hopkins Hosp* 1947; 81:192–215.
36. Bing RJ, Vandam LD, Gray FD Jr: Physiological studies in congenital heart disease. I. Procedures. *Bull Johns Hopkins Hosp* 1947; 80:107–120.
37. Burchell HB: Cardiac catheterization in diagnosis of various cardiac malformations and diseases. *Proc Mayo Clin* 1948; 23:481–487.
38. Wood EH, Geraci JE, Pollack AA, Groom D, Taylor BD, Pender JW, Puch DG: General and special techniques in cardiac catheterization. *Proc Mayo Clin* 1948; 23:494–500.
39. Rapaport E, Dexter L: Pulmonary "capillary" pressure, in Warren JV (ed): *Methods in Medical Research.* Chicago, Year Book Publishers, 1958; vol 7, pp 85–93.
40. Seldinger SI: Catheter replacement of the needle in percutaneous arteriography: a new technique. *Acta Radiol* 1953; 39:368–376.
41. Swan HJC, Ganz W, Forrester J, Marcus H, Diamond G, Chonette D: Catheterization of the heart in man with the use of a flow-directed balloon-tipped catheter. *N Engl J Med* 1970; 283:447–451.
42. Zimmerman HA, Scott RW, Becker ND: Catheterization of the left side of the heart in man. *Circulation* 1950; 1:357–359.
43. Limon-Lason R, Bouchard A: El cateterismo Intracardico: cateterizacion de las cavidades izquierdas en el hombre. Registro simultaneo de presion y electrocardiograma intracavetarios. *Arch Inst Cardiol Mexico* 1950; 21:271–285.
44. Ross J Jr: Transseptal left heart catheterization: a new method of left atrial puncture. *Ann Surg* 1959; 149:395–401.
45. Cope C: Technique for transseptal catheterization of the left atrium: preliminary report. *J Thoracic Surg* 1959; 37:482–486.
46. Sones FM Jr, Shirey EK, Proudfit WL, Westcott RN: Cinecoronary arteriography, abstr. *Circulation* 1959; 20:773.
47. Ricketts JH, Abrams HL: Percutaneous selective coronary cine arteriography. *JAMA* 1962; 181:620–624.
48. Judkins MP: Selective coronary arteriography: a percutaneous transfemoral technique. *Radiology* 1967; 89:815–824.
49. Shirey EK: Retrograde transaortic and mitral valve catheterization for physiological and morphological evaluation of the left side of the heart. *Circulation* 1966; 34 (Suppl III): III-216–III-217.
50. Croft CH, Lipscomb K: Modified technique of transseptal left heart catheterization. *J Am Coll Cardiol* 1985; 5:904–910.
51. Fowler NO: *Cardiac Diagnosis and Treatment,* ed 2. Hagerstown, Harper & Row, 1976, p 12.
52. Connolly DC, Lev R, Kirklin JW, Wood EH: Pulmonary artery wedge pressures in mitral valve disease: relationship to left atrial pressure (abstr). *Fed Proc* 1953; 12:28.
53. Dubois D, Dubois EF: A height–weight formula to estimate the surface area of man. *Proc Soc Exp Biol (NY)* 1916; 13:77–78.
54. Fick A: Uber die Messung des Blutquantums in den Herzventrikeln. *Sitzung Phys med Gesell Würzburg* 1870; July, p 16.
55. Van Slyke DD, Neill JM: The determination of gases in blood and other solutions by vacuum extraction and manometric measurements. *J Biol Chem* 1924; 61:523–573.
56. Stewart GN: Researches on the circulation time and on the influences which affect it. IV. The output of the heart. *J Physiol* 1897; 22:159–183.
57. Kunieda R: Evaluation of pulmonary blood volume in mitral valve disease by T-1824 method (application of direct left atrial puncture). *Respiration and Circulation (Kokyu To Junkan)* 1955; 3:510–518.
58. Holt JP: Estimation of the residual volume of the ventricle of the dog's heart by two indicator-dilution techniques. *Circ Res* 1956; 4:187–195.
59. Thorpe CR, Grodins FS: Estimation of left ventricular volumes from thermodilution curves (abstr). *Fed Proc* 1960; 19:117.
60. Swan HJC, Wood EH: Localization of cardiac defects by dye-dilution curves recorded after injection of T-1824 at multiple sites in the heart and great vessels during cardiac catheterization. *Proc Mayo Clin* 1953; 28:95–100.
61. Swan HJC, Zapata-Diaz J, Wood EH: Dye dilution curves in cyanotic congenital heart disease. *Circulation* 1953; 8:70–81.
62. Korner PI, Shillingford JP: Quantitative estimation of valvular incompetence by dye dilution curves. *Clin Sci* 1955; 14:553–573.
63. Warner HR: Analysis of the role of indicator technics in quantitation of valvular regurgitation. *Circ Res* 1962; 10:519–529.
64. Kinsman JM, Moore JW, Hamilton WF: Studies on the circulation. I. Injection method: physical and mathematical considerations. *Am J Physiol* 1929; 89:322–330.
65. Hamilton WF, Moore JW, Kinsman JM, Spurling RG: Studies on the circulation. IV. Further analysis of the injection method and of changes in hemodynamics under physiological and pathological conditions. *Am J Physiol* 1932; 99:534–551.
66. Dow P: Dimensional relationships in dye-dilution curves from humans and dogs, with an empirical formula for certain troublesome curves. *J Appl Physiol* 1955; 7:399–408.
67. Hetzel PS, Swan HJC, Ramirez DeArellano A, Wood EH: Estimation of cardiac output from first part of the arterial dye dilution curves. *J Appl Physiol* 1958; 13:92–96.
68. Fegler G: Measurement of cardiac output in anesthetized animals by a thermodilution method. *Q J Exp Physiol* 1954; 39:153–164.
69. Ganz W, Donoso R, Marcus HS, Forrester JS, Swan HJC: A new technique for measurement of cardiac output by thermodilution in man. *Am J Cardiol* 1971; 27:392–396.
70. Hamilton WF, Riley RL, Attyah AM, Cournand A, Fowell DM, Himmelstein A, Noble RP, Remington JW, Richards DW, Wheller NC, Witham AC: Comparison of Fick and dye injection methods of measuring cardiac output in man. *Am J Physiol* 1948; 153:309–321.
71. Wade OL, Bishop JM: *Cardiac Output And Regional Blood Flow.* Philadelphia, FA Davis (Blackwell Scientific), 1962, p 23.
72. Goodyer AVN, Huvos A, Eckhardt WF, Ostberg RH: Thermal dilution curves in the intact animal. *Circ Res* 1959; 7:432–441.
73. Fegler G: The reliability of the thermodilution method for determination of the cardiac output and the blood flow in central veins. *Q J Exp Physiol* 1957; 42:254–266.
74. Gorlin R, Gorlin SG: Hydraulic formula for calculation of the area of the stenotic mitral valve, other cardiac valves and central circulatory shunts. *Am Heart J* 1951; 42:1–29.

75. Cohen MV, Gorlin R: Modified orifice equation for the calculation of mitral valve area. *Am Heart J* 1972; 84:839–840.
76. Ubago JL, Figueroa A, Colman T, Ochoteco A, Duran CG: Hemodynamic factors that affect calculated orifice areas in the mitral Hancock xenograft valve. *Circulation* 1980; 61:388–394.
77. Rodrigo FA, Snellen HA: Estimation of valve area and valvular resistance. *Am Heart J* 1953; 45:1–12.
78. Wright JTM: Hydrodynamic evaluation of tissue valves, in Ionescu MI (ed): *Tissue Heart Valves.* London, Butterworth, 1979, p 29–87.
79. Cannon SR, Richards KL, Crawford M: Hydraulic estimation of stenotic orifice area: a correction of the Gorlin formula. *Circulation* 1985; 71:1170–1178.
80. Schoenfeld MH, Palacios IF, Hutter AM Jr, Jacoby SS, Block PC: Underestimation of prosthetic mitral valve areas: role of transseptal catheterization in avoiding unnecessary repeat mitral valve surgery. *J Am Coll Cardiol* 1985; 5:1387–1392.
81. Gorlin R: Normal variations in venous oxygen content, in Warren JV (ed): *Methods in Medical Research.* Chicago, Year Book Publishers, 1958, vol. 7, p 69.
82. Flamm MD, Cohn KE, Hancock EW: Measurement of systemic cardiac output at rest and exercise in patients with atrial septal defect. *Am J Cardiol* 1969; 23:258–265.
83. Wood EH, Swan HJC, Marshall HW: Technic and diagnostic applications of dilution curves recorded simultaneously from the right side of the heart and from the arterial circulation. *Proc Staff Meet Mayo Clin* 1958; 33:536–553.
84. Clark LC Jr, Bargeron LM Jr: Left-to-right shunt detection by an intravascular electrode with hydrogen as an indicator. *Science* 1959; 130:709–710.
85. Cheng TO: Hydrogen and ascorbate dilution curves. A simplified method for routine use in detection of intracardiac shunt and valvular regurgitation. *Chest* 1972; 62:304–310.
86. Castillo CA, Kyle JC, Gilson WE, Rowe GG: Simulated shunt curves. *Am J Cardiol* 1966; 17:691–694.
87. Levy AM, Monroe RG, Hugenholtz PG, Nadas AS: Clinical use of ascorbic acid as an indicator of right-to-left shunt. *Br Heart J* 1967; 29:22–29.
88. Clark LC Jr, Bargeron LM Jr, Lyons C, Bradley MN, MacArthur KT: Detection of right-to-left shunts with an arterial potentiometric electrode. *Circulation* 1960; 22:949–955.
89. Long RTL, Braunwald E, Morrow AG: Intracardiac injection of radioactive krypton: clinical applications of new methods for characterization of circulatory shunts. *Circulation* 1960; 21:1126–1133.
90. Banas JS, Meister SG, Gazzaniga AB, O'Connor NE, Haynes FW, Dalen JE: A simple technique for detecting small defects of the atrial septum. *Am J Cardiol* 1971; 28:467–471.
91. Cheng TO: Paradoxical embolism. A diagnostic challenge and its detection during life. *Circulation* 1976; 33:565–568.
92. Dodge HT, Sandler H, Ballew DW, Lord JD Jr: The use of biplane angiocardiography for the measurement of left ventricular volume in man. *Am Heart J* 1960; 60:762–776.
93. Wynne J, Green LH, Mann T, Levin D, Grossman W: Estimation of left ventricular volumes in man from biplane cineangiograms filmed in oblique projections. *Am J Cardiol* 1978; 41:726–732.
94. Als AV, Paulin S, Aroesty JM: Biplane angiographic volumetry using the right anterior oblique and half-axial left anterior oblique technique. *Radiology* 1978; 126:511–514.
95. Sandler H, Dodge HT: The use of single plane angiocardiograms for the calculation of left ventricular volume in man. *Am Heart J* 1968; 75:325–334.
96. Kennedy JW, Trenholme SE, Kasser IS: Left ventricular volume and mass from single plane cineangiocardiograms. *Am Heart J* 1970; 80:343–352.
97. Yang SS, Bentivoglio LG, Maranhao V, Goldberg H: *From Cardiac Catheterization Data to Hemodynamic Parameters*, ed 2. Philadelphia, FA Davis, 1978, pp 105–109.
98. Rackley CE, Hood WP Jr: Quantitative angiographic evaluation and pathophysiologic mechanism in valvular heart disease. *Prog Cardiovasc Dis* 1973; 15:427–447.
99. Dodge HT: Determination of left ventricular volume and mass. *Radiol Clin North Am* 1971; 9:459–467.
100. Rackley CE, Behar VS, Whalen RE, McIntosh HD: Biplane cineangiographic determination of left ventricular function: pressure–volume relationships. *Am Heart J* 1967; 74:766–779.
101. Greene DG, Carlisle R, Grant C, Bunnell IL: Estimation of left ventricular volume by one-plane cineangiography. *Circulation* 1967; 35:61–69.
102. Rackley CE: Quantitative evaluation of left ventricular function by radiographic techniques. *Circulation* 1976; 54:862–879.
103. Graham TP Jr, Jarmakani JM, Canent RV Jr, Morrow MN: Left heart volume estimations in infancy and childhood: reevaluation of methodology and normal values. *Circulation* 1971; 43:895–904.
104. Kennedy JW, Baxley WA, Figley MM, Dodge HT, Blackmon JR: Quantitative angiocardiography. I. The normal left ventricle in man. *Circulation* 1966; 34:272–278.
105. Arcilla RA, Tsai P, Thilenius O, Ranniger K: Angiographic method for volume estimation of right and left ventricles. *Chest* 1971; 60:446–454.
106. Graham TP Jr, Jarmakani JM, Atwood GF, Canent RV Jr: Right ventricular volume determinations in children. Normal values and observations with volume or pressure overload. *Circulation* 1973; 47:144–153.
107. Gentzler RD, Briselli MF, Gault JH: Angiographic estimation of right ventricular volume in man. *Circulation* 1974; 50:324–330.
108. Fisher EA, DuBrow IW, Hastreiter AR: Right ventricular volume in congenital heart disease. *Am J Cardiol* 1975; 36:67–75.
109. Ferlinz J, Gorlin R, Cohn PF, Herman MV: Right ventricular performance in patients with coronary artery disease. *Circulation* 1975; 52:608–615.

14 Cardiac Angiography

Valerie S. Mandell, MD and Sven Paulin, MD

RADIOGRAPHIC EQUIPMENT AND QUALITY CONTROL

Familiarity with the basic concepts underlying image production as it pertains to the cardiovascular system is important. Although a thorough discussion on x-ray physics would be beyond the scope of this chapter, a brief description will be given on available equipment that is specifically designed for radiologic demonstration of cardiovascular anatomy and function. Because the most widely used format is 35 mm cinematography, this will be dealt with in more detail, particularly with regard to radiographic technique and quality control. Other useful recording modalities such as spot film devices, rapid film changers, and digital subtraction will be briefly reviewed.

Presently along with the great strides being made in the field of medical imaging and computer science, improvement and refinement of angiographic equipment have also taken place. As welcome as such development may be, it has confronted the health care system with escalating costs, which are particularly burdensome to developing countries with limited financial resources. Even in affluent countries, the medical profession may encounter restrictions on expenditures due to governmental concerns about excessive health care costs. Cardiovascular radiologists and cardiologists, therefore, may have to use less sophisticated equipment, not representing the latest medical developments, but capable of delivering studies of high diagnostic quality, provided that they adhere to the basic principles of x-ray physics, and pay attention to cardiovascular anatomy and physiology.

GENERATOR

An x-ray generator consists of a step-up transformer to provide high voltage potentials across the x-ray tube, a step-down transformer to provide low voltage currents for the filament, and a rectifier to convert alternating current into direct current necessary for tube operation.

A control panel on the generator contains settings for three variables: kilovoltage (kV), which determines the energy spectrum of the x-rays; milliamperes (mA), the tube current that controls the number of x-ray photons emitted by the tube per unit time; and milliseconds (ms), the time of exposure, or pulse width in cinematography.[1] To avoid voltage fluctuations during pulsing, the power output of the generator should be at least one and a half to two times the cine pulse output. Thus, modern generators designed for cine angiography have an output of 100 kW at 100 kV or greater. Incoming power should be 440 to 480 V, three-phase, alternating current.[2]

X-RAY TUBE

The cathode, a fine tungsten filament, is the source of electrons, the number of which is controlled by the current applied (mA). When a high voltage (kV) is applied between the cathode and anode target, electrons are accelerated across the vacuum tube and strike the anode, causing an emission of x-ray photons (Figure 14.1). The focal spot size (or x-ray source size) is determined in part by the angle of the anode. A small angle, and hence a small focal spot size, is desirable in cine angiography for production of a sharp image. Focal spot size may be controlled electronically to produce a microfocal spot as small as 0.1 to 0.3 mm.[1]

In an angiographic tube, the anode consists of a rotating disk with a beveled edge corresponding to the anode angle. The rotation of the anode allows the heat produced by the electrons striking the target to be dissipated across a larger surface. The heat produced is expressed in heat units, which are defined as the product of peak tube potential (kVp), and x-ray tube current and exposure time (mAs). Sufficient heat load capacity of the tube is important, particularly when examining dense objects such as large patients or organs, as it permits greater flexibility in the choice of optimal exposure settings.[1] A desirable tube for cine angiography should be able to provide at least 300 mA at 65 to 95 kV with pulse widths (time of exposure) of 4 ms using a 0.6 mm focal spot.[3]

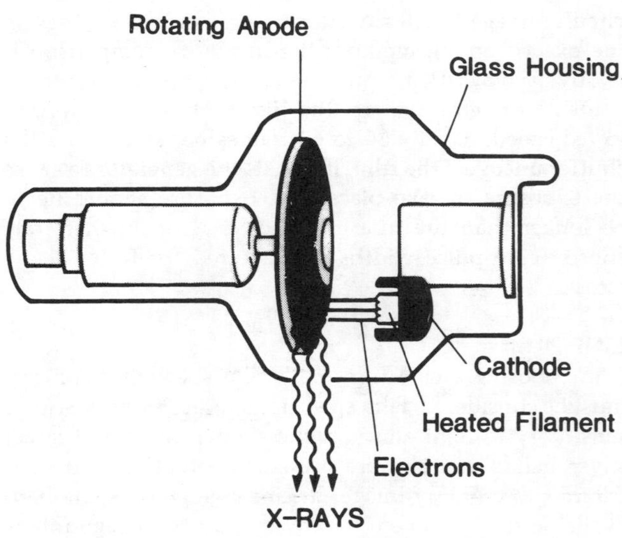

Figure 14.1. Line drawing of an x-ray tube. The heated filament in the cathode liberates electrons that are accelerated by the kilovoltage tube potential and strike the slanted surface of the rotating anode, generating x-ray photons. (Figures 14.1, 14.2, and 14.3 are reproduced from Marco and Paulin.[4] Copyright 1986 by Lea & Febiger. Reproduced with permission.)

PULSING

In contrast to the earliest cine systems in which radiation was delivered without interruption whether the cine camera shutter was open or not, modern systems synchronize the x-ray emission with the open time of the camera shutter. Obviously this reduces radiation to patient and operators by eliminating the unproductive intervals. After the film is advanced, and the camera shutter is opened, the generator is signaled to deliver a short, intense pulse of radiation. The length of each pulse, or the pulse width, determines the time for each individual frame exposure. The exposure time must be sufficient to provide an adequate number of photons (x-ray quanta) to provide a good image. Insufficient photons will result in a grainy image due to quantum mottle. A good balance for cine angiography is a 4 to 6 ms pulse width.[1,2] This pulse width is short enough to eliminate motion blurring.

The kV should be as close to 70 kV as is practical, approximating the K-edge of iodine, to provide optimal attenuation by the radiographic contrast agent. Because such relatively low kV may require, in a given patient, an unattainably high mA, a higher kV may have to be accepted as a compromise, even though some contrast may be lost.[4]

IMAGE INTENSIFIER

The image intensifier's input phosphor screen, usually composed of cesium iodide crystals, is analogous to the light producing screen in the x-ray film cassette. The light produced in response to x-ray photons is detected by a photocathode, which is separated from the input phosphor by a thin transparent membrane. Light absorbed by the photocathode generates low energy electrons in a distribution that corresponds to the light on the input phosphor, representing the spatial relation of x-ray photons that have passed through the patient. These low energy electrons are accelerated within the tube by a separate cathode potential and focused by magnetic lenses to produce an inverted and accurate but minified image on the output phosphor screen. The electrons arriving at the output end of the tube are reconverted into light photons in the output phosphor (Figure 14.2).

The intensification of light from the input phosphor to the output phosphor is achieved not only with electronic gain within the tube, but also by the concentration of available light into a smaller, hence brighter area. A single electron from the input phosphor photocathode can generate on the output phosphor thousands of light photons. The overall gain, both minification and electronic, is 2,400 to 6,000 fold.[1]

An input phosphor of 5 to 7 inches in diameter is preferred for examinations of coronary and congenital heart disease because of its superior resolving power. Larger input phosphors of 9 to 10 inches in diameter are

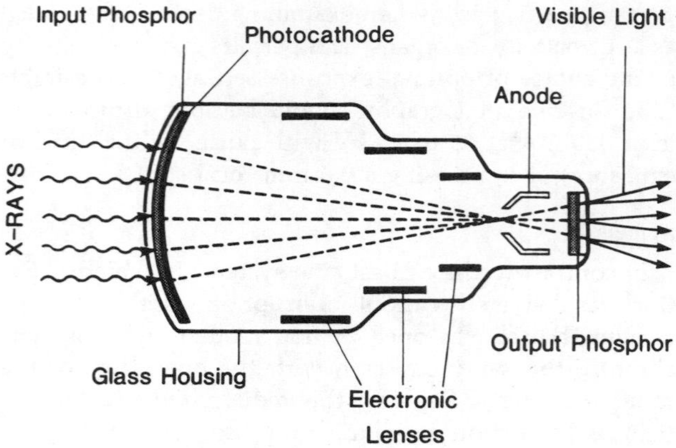

Figure 14.2. Line drawing of image intensifier. X-rays, having passed through the patient, strike the input phosphor and are multiplied electronically. The visible light produced by the output phosphor is viewed by the video and cine cameras.

useful for studies that delineate chambers of the adult heart, particularly in the presence of cardiomegaly where the somewhat lesser resolving power has little consequence on the perception of the object's size, wall dynamics, or contrast filling patterns. To serve both purposes, dual mode intensifiers, with rapidly interchangeable field size are available and provide more versatility than a single mode intensifier.[2]

AUTOMATIC BRIGHTNESS CONTROL

Because of the inherently large differences in density within the chest (heart, lungs, bone, and diaphragm) the movement of the patient under the fluoroscope during panning causes large variations in luminescence in the image intensifier screen. To maintain even, stable brightness for cine filming and video display, brightness control is necessary. Manual control, even by an experienced technologist, is bound to fail and automatic feedback systems are routinely incorporated. These function either by sensing the current flowing through the image intensifier or measuring the brightness of the output phosphor. Based on these measurements, a signal to increase or decrease the x-ray factors is supplied to the generator. Methods for brightness stabilization include variable kV, variable mA, and variable pulse width or some combination of these. A controlled system might begin with setting an optimal mA and kV, brightness being controlled by variation in the exposure time. When the upper limit of the exposure time is reached, however, kV is automatically raised. Conversely, another system might choose an optimal mA with kV varying automatically to regulate brightness.[1,4]

CINE CAMERA

Cameras for diagnostic radiography are essentially commercial movie cameras. Unfortunately, the frame size of cine film is rectangular (18 by 24 mm for 35 mm cameras) whereas the image from the image intensifier is circular. Framing refers to the sizing and placement of the circular image within the rectangular film frame (Figure 14.3). Recording the entire circle on the film (exact framing) wastes film, whereas the opposite extreme (total overframing), in which the circular image spills over the frame in all dimensions, reduces the effective field size. One satisfactory method of framing (maximum horizontal overframing) exactly fills the horizontal dimension of the film with the circular image, losing only the upper and lower parts of the image. Because this method causes the circular image to fill the frame more completely than in the exact framing method, the image by comparison is relatively magnified.[2,4]

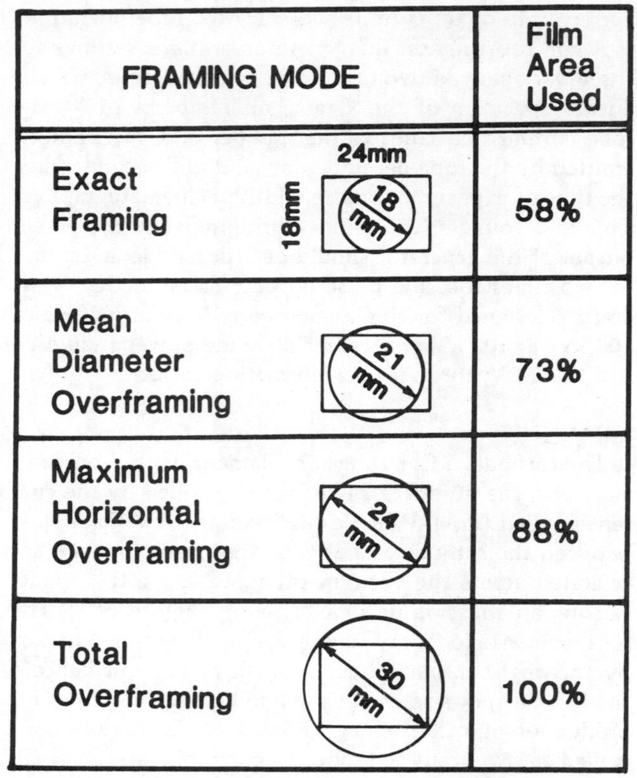

Figure 14.3. Relation of framing method to field size reduction in cinefluoroscopy. (Modified from Friesinger et al.[2])

Inside the cine camera, the film is moved at a preselected speed, usually 30 to 60 frames per second. As the shutter uncovers the film, it signals the generator to cause the exposure to take place. The exposure should never be longer than the time the shutter is open; therefore, shorter cine pulse widths are required for faster frame rates.

CINE FILM

In choosing a cine film, both film speed and contrast must be considered. Film speed is an indicator of the film's sensitivity to light and is highest when more and larger silver halide granules are present, a situation that contributes to a grainy image. In cineangiography, the light available to the camera is provided by the image intensifier, which is monitored by the automatic brightness control and is ultimately a function of x-ray exposure. The use of a high speed film would require either a decrease in the camera aperture or a decrease in the radiation exposure (to decrease light from the image intensifier) to avoid overexposing the film. Although it may seem theoretically ideal to use a high speed film to lower the necessary radiation dose, such a decrease in the number of photons presented to the image intensifier may lead to degradation of the image due to insufficient photons or quantum mottle. Consequently, it is most desirable to choose the optimal radiographic settings based on the size of the patient and then to choose the lowest compatible speed film to minimize the film graininess.

The second important characteristic is film latitude, which is a measure of the range of film contrast. Although high gray scale contrast would seem to be desirable, in cineangiography we are faced with the problem of imaging the coronary arteries superimposed on areas of differing density, such as the lungs, diaphragm, and liver. Although a film of high contrast will be superior in recording objects that have little inherent difference in contrast, its useful range of densities is narrow. In cineangiography, it is advisable to use a film with somewhat lower contrast, but with wider latitude, that is, a wider range of useful densities so that coronary arteries may be imaged even when viewed in areas of highly differing x-ray absorption.[3,4]

FILM PROCESSING

Improper or careless film processing is a major cause of poor cineangiographic image quality. A problem in any of a number of separate aspects of cine film processing may adversely affect the image. Although dedicated automatic cine film processors are usually included in the angiographic facilities, the complexity of the photographic film processing requires continuous and meticulous attention by skilled and knowledgeable technicians. Because the temperature inside the tank controls the rate of chemical reaction, an increase in temperature speeds up the deposition of silver halide crystals on the film and makes it overly dark. Temperature regulation should insure a maximum variation from day to day of no more than 0.3°C (0.5°F). The speed of film travel through the developing solution should not vary more than ±5% because larger variations in contact time with the developer may cause over- or underdeveloping. Fluid agitation must be even to avoid streaks, artifacts, and nonuniform processing. As the developer becomes exhausted, its replenishment is necessary to restore both developer and fixer, to prevent build-up of reaction products, and to maintain the volume of the solution at the proper level. The volume of replenisher required is determined by the number of feet of film processed. A filtration system is necessary to remove particles that might cling to the film and mar the final appearance. Maintenance of a proper drying temperature (about 125°F) is important to avoid overly dried, brittle films or underdried films that would be soft and tacky.[3]

QUALITY CONTROL

Quality control of the radiographic equipment in the catheterization or angiographic laboratory should be performed daily. Both the exposure aspects (x-ray source, image intensifier, brightness control, cine camera) and the developing aspects should be evaluated. A general problem or possible component malfunction may be identified using two strips of film: one to record the cine of a standard test object exposed under identical standardized conditions and one exposed with a standard light sensitometer. When compared with records of previous test strips, a daily variation in the cine strip could indicate a problem in either the cine system or the developing process. A variation in the sensitometric strip, however, is specific to the developing process, whereas a normal sensitrometric strip points to a problem in the exposure-generating components of the equipment chain.[2]

For daily film testing a sensitometer is used which consists of a calibrated light source that delivers constant exposures in the form of a step pattern. After film exposure and processing, densitometric readings are made at different steps. The daily checks include measurement of the inherent blackening of the film after processing and determination of the film's speed and contrast indexes.

DIGITAL IMAGING

Because digital equipment for radiographic use is complex and presently undergoing rapid changes in design, a complete description of its capabilities is beyond the scope of this chapter and the reader is referred to the literature.[5–7] The following, however, may serve as a brief introduction.

A digital x-ray is a computerized image composed of pixels or "picture elements" arranged in rows and columns called the matrix. The size of the matrix is expressed by the number of horizontal and vertical pixels, for example, 256 by 256 or 512 by 512. Each pixel is set up to represent a certain number of shades of gray, in medical imaging, at least 256. To express this many possible numbers using the binary system, each pixel must have eight bits of computer memory, or in digital terminology, each pixel must be eight bits deep. For more shades of gray, more bits are required; for example, for 1,024 shades, a bit depth of ten is necessary.

The larger the matrix size and the greater the bit depth, the greater is the requirement for computer memory. It can be seen mathematically that as one doubles the matrix size, the total number of pixels in the image and hence the need for computer storage are quadrupled. It follows then that for a fixed computer system memory, the greater the matrix size, the fewer the number of images that can be handled.

The equipment chain of a digital system consists of the radiographic components, ie, the tube and the image intensifier to which a television camera coupled with the analog to digital (A/D) converter and the computer itself is added. The output phosphor image of the intensifier is viewed by a video camera and the analog video signal generated is converted to a digital signal by the A/D converter. Once in digital form, an image may be processed by the computer for subtraction, image enhancement, or other densitometric or contourographic measurements. Based on this information and using prepared software programs, translations into physiologic parameters can be made almost instantaneously. Such programs exist for determination of ventricular volumes and ejection fractions, cardiac output and left to right shunts.[8–12]

Radiographic subtraction technique is performed by obtaining a digitized image of the object before the arrival of contrast material. This image, the mask, is stored in the computer's memory (memory A). Another image is then obtained after the arrival of contrast, digitized, and stored in another part of the computer's memory (memory B). Digitization of the images makes it possible to subtract the mask image from the contrasted image, leaving only the contrast itself behind. The computer may be instructed to perform this subtraction in "real time" simply by subtracting the mask from each subsequent frame obtained during the contrast passage. In this way, the images are displayed in subtracted form instantaneously. If the result is imperfect, different masks can be applied retrospectively until the best fit is obtained. The need for the latter procedure occurs frequently in cardiac examinations because of the considerable spatial displacements related to cardiac motion.

Because the mask and the contrasted image are separated from each other in time, this technique is referred to as temporal subtraction. A variation of this technique, specially designed for cardiac contrast imaging, is the subtraction of two contrast-containing images taken sequentially at short time intervals. This technique is referred to as time interval difference subtraction (TID) and has been proposed for analysis of ventricular changes during portions of the cardiac cycle.[13,14]

Once a subtracted image has been obtained, it may be enhanced in one of several different ways. Images may be smoothed by averaging several frames together to minimize quantum mottle, or contrast enhanced using varying window settings similar to computed tomography. If the subtraction is suboptimal due to motion, the mask and contrast frames may be reregistered to obtain a better fit. Digital images may be obtained either serially, with pulsed x-ray exposures at rates typically of one or more frames per second (fps), or dynamically, at rapid frame rates such as 30 fps, using either a continuous or pulsed mode fluoroscopy.

To eliminate the problems of subtraction misregistration due to motion, another technique called dual energy subtraction has been explored.[15] In this case two images are obtained in rapid sequence using significantly different kilovoltages for each exposure. As attenuation differences for iodine in the contrast medium at the two different radiation energy levels are unequal to those of bone or soft tissue, appropriately performed digital subtraction can enhance and isolate the contrast medium. Because the two images are taken only milliseconds apart, motion as a cause of misregistration is eliminated. For details of various subtraction and filtration techniques, the reader is referred to the literature.[16–18]

Data storage is a significant problem because of the exponential increase in storage space needed as matrix size and gray scale depth increase. For example, although eighty 512 by 512 images can be stored on a 20-megabyte Winchester disk, only four such images can be stored on an 8-inch floppy disk. If the matrix size were increased to 1,024 by 1,024, twenty such images could be stored on the hard disk, but only one on the 8-inch disk. In practical terms, the performance of a coronary angiogram at the relatively slow rate of 7.5 fps for a total of 50 seconds of acquisition time (or 400 images), using a 1,024 by 1,024 matrix, would require a 400-megabyte capacity. The problem of storage may be solved in the future with the arrival of high capacity laser disks capable of storing up to 13 billion bytes each.[19]

RADIATION RISKS

EXPOSURE TO PATIENTS

Radiation exposure to the patient during fluoroscopy occurs at a skin dose rate of 0.5 to 1.0 R/mA per minute* and at a dose of 20 to 30 μR per frame during 35 mm cineangiography.[3] Total patient dose for a particular examination, then, is dependent on fluoroscopy time, cine frame rate, and duration of cine. As a general approximation, 1 second of cine filming generates a patient exposure similar to 20 seconds of fluoroscopy. In cardiac angiography, filming rather than fluoroscopy delivers the major portion of the dose to both patient and personnel.[20,21] Patient skin dose during a typical cardiac catheterization with angiography ranges from 20 to 47 R per study. The relative magnitude of this dose can be better appreciated when compared with that received with other common clinical radiologic examinations: lumbar spine series, 3.46 R; barium enema, 2 to 5 R; intravenous pyelogram, 3.3 R; posteroanterior and lateral chest film, 95 to 150 mR.[22] Naturally occurring background radiation is about 50 to 100 mR per year.

EXPOSURE TO PERSONNEL

Of equal concern is the radiation risk to the angiographer and other personnel whose careers may last 20 years or more under occupational exposure. Controllable variables such as length of fluoroscopy time, and length and frame rate of cine, affect the dosage ranges reported from different institutions.[20,23,24] Reuter's review[21] revealed a range of 6.4 to 30 mR to the eye, 3.5 to 33 mR to the thyroid, and 4.6 to 154 mR to the hand of the angiographer during a typical cardiac catheterization and angiographic procedure. Guidelines for permissible yearly exposure have been set up in the United States by the National Council on Radiation Protection and Measurement (NCRP) and the International Commission on Radiological Protection (ICRP). NCRP recommendations in rems per year are as follows: whole body, 5 rems; hands, 75 rems; thyroid, 15 rems; limbs, 5 rems.

If, for example, an average dose per study of 20 mR is considered, an angiographer would have to perform only five studies per week (100 mR) to reach a yearly maximal permissible dose of 5 R; however, if he were in a slightly more distant position from the patient, as in an assistant's position, he could perform nearly three times the studies and still receive less than the recommended upper dose limit.[21]

Because there is no known safe amount of radiation, every effort must be made to minimize exposure to both patient and operator. Useful measures include careful

*Radiation units: The Roentgen (R) is a unit of radiation exposure; the rad is the unit of absorbed dose; the rem is the unit of dose equivalent or rads multiplied by a quality factor, essentially a measure of biologic effectiveness of radiation. For all practical purposes, these three units can be thought of as equal.[1]

beam collimation, avoidance of prolonged fluoroscopy, use of at least 0.5-mm lead aprons, eyeglasses, and thyroid shields for personnel, as well as shielding devices around the table when practical. No operator or assistant should be nearer the patient than absolutely necessary for safe performance of the study. Placement of television monitors, physiologic recorders, and equipment control panels behind lead glass enclosures in a separate control room is recommended.

RADIOGRAPHIC CONTRAST AGENTS

The conventional intravascular contrast agents, complex organic molecules with iodine atoms bound to them, are ionic compounds, dissociating in solution into a cation (+) and an anion (−). The two most widely employed cations are sodium and the organic ion methylglucamine. The three most commonly employed anions are diatrizoate, iothalamate, and metrizoate.

PHYSIOLOGIC EFFECTS

Many adverse effects of ionic contrast agents are felt to be related to their hypertonicity. When compared with the osmolarity of blood (300 mOsm/L), the ionic contrast agents are hypertonic with osmolarities as high as 2,000 mOsm/L. These hypertonic solutions, particularly when administered in large quantity, cause a rapid transport of water from the interstitial and intracellular spaces into the intravascular compartment with a resultant significant expansion of plasma volume as shown experimentally.[25] In a normal individual with prompt renal clearance and good cardiac reserve, this volume challenge can be handled. In the presence of an already compromised cardiac state, eg, reduced myocardial function or an abnormal valve, such a sudden volume increase may precipitate decompensation. Fluid and electrolyte changes caused by this contrast-related osmotic effect are particularly dangerous in infants.

The well-known hypotensive effect of radiographic contrast media is probably the result of both a direct effect on the vasculature itself, causing dilatation of the arterioles that govern peripheral vascular resistance, and a direct effect on the myocardium, depressing contractility.[26] It is likely that the extent to which one dominates is determined by the site of contrast injection. Thus, a thoracic aortogram, followed by temporary hypotension, tachycardia, and increased cardiac output, is an example of the former mechanism, whereas a selective injection into a coronary artery, causing a temporary blood pressure decrease because of reduced myocardial contraction, smaller stroke volume, and increased diastolic filling pressure in the left ventricle, is an example of the latter. Left ventriculography, exposing both the coronary and systemic circulation to the agent, involves both mechanisms.

Often elevation of the left ventricular end-diastolic and left atrial pressures is seen after contrast administration, an effect that is more pronounced in patients with ventricular dysfunction.[27,28] The frequently encountered increase in heart rate, however, is the response to peripheral vasodilatation. Injection in the right side of the heart may cause an elevation in pulmonary arterial pressure, thought to be related in part to sludging of red cells in the pulmonary capillary bed and in part to elevation of left atrial pressure as a consequence of the agent's circulation through the left heart and subsequently the systemic circulation.[28]

The ionic media have also been studied extensively as to their propensity to cause ventricular fibrillation. Injection of contrast medium into the coronary arterty decreases the ventricular fibrillation threshold for nearly one minute and increases the vulnerability of the canine heart to developing a serious arrhythmia to experimentally delivered electrical stimulation.[29] Selective injections into the coronary arteries may cause bradycardia or even asystole, probably due to a toxic effect on the sinoatrial or the atrioventricular node, or both.[30] Optimal ionic contrast agents for coronary arteriography contain a small percentage of sodium ion to achieve near physiologic serum levels, because sodium-free agents as well as agents with an overabundance of sodium were found to result in a high incidence of ventricular fibrillation.[31,32]

Contrast is handled by the kidney primarily by glomerular filtration, and its administration induces osmotic diuresis in the normal individual. Renal failure following contrast administration is dose related, exacerbated by dehydration, and seen more frequently in patients with multiple myeloma, renal insufficiency, and diabetes mellitus.[33,33a] Contrast dose reduction in patients with limited renal function may be facilitated by arterial digital subtraction angiography, a technique that can be performed using contrast diluted to one quarter of the usual strength. This technique can allow adequate angiographic studies in patients who would otherwise be at risk for excessive contrast burden.

Subjectively experienced side effects are common and include sensation of warmth or pain, metallic taste, and nausea. The frequent development of a few hives or itching is considered to warrant treatment with an antihistamine, although the true allergic nature of these manifestations is in question. True anaphylaxis, leading to cardiovascular collapse and fatality, fortunately is rare and occurs in 1 in 10,000 to 1 in 40,000 patients.[34] If angiography is unavoidable in patients with a history of previous anaphylaxis, pretreatment with steroids and antihistamines is generally advised, in spite of inconclusive evidence for its effectiveness. Recent evidence indicates that anaphylactoid reactions may occur less often with non-ionic agents.[35]

NEW CONTRAST AGENTS

The fact that many of the adverse effects of ionic contrast agents have been shown experimentally to be related to their hyperosmolarity has stimulated research for the development of new contrast agents that are either nonionic or dimer molecules and therefore of much lower osmolarity.[36] Many of these agents have been widely used in Europe for more than 10 years and have proven to be better tolerated but have not been approved for use in the United States by the Food and Drug Administration (FDA). Metrizamide, the first nonionic agent available, was initially approved for myelography. More recently, it as well as ioxaglate, a dimeric molecule, are now authorized for clinical intravascular use in the United States.

A substantial amount of experimental evidence exists to support the clinically favorable results gained in other countries with these compounds. With regard to cardiac examinations, they cause fewer ventricular arrhythmias, cause less significant changes in blood pressure and heart rate,[37] and less depression of myocardial contractility.[38,39] Clinical trials authorized by the FDA in this country have included a great variety of the most common angiographic examinations such as pulmonary angiography, aortography, left ventriculography, and coronary arteriography, with most favorable results in all instances.[40]

COMPLICATIONS

The risks for complications of cardiac catheterization and angiography are related to the invasive procedure, application of the contrast agent, and clinical status of the patient. Placement of the catheter through a vein or artery is associated with a small but real risk of injury to the vessel. Whereas venous injury is usually of fairly little consequence, arterial damage may be serious. Various large studies have reported local vascular complication rates of 0.6% to 1.4%.[41–45] These include local thrombosis, intimal dissection, arteriovenous fistula, hematoma, or rarely pseudoaneurysm. Adams' retrospectively performed survey reported a 1.7% incidence of thrombosis following brachial cutdown catheterization, and a 1.2% incidence of thrombosis with the femoral percutaneous technique. The difference is probably related to the different calibers of the artery at the site of catheter introduction, but other factors, not controlled by the study, such as the use of prophylactic heparin, catheter dimension and shape, and experience of the operator, may play an important role. Attempts have been made to compare the brachial and femoral techniques also with regard to mortality and morbidity, but they have failed to demonstrate a significant difference.[41,42,45] The important revelation was that the incidence of complications from either method is lowest in those hospitals in which a large number of procedures are performed annually.

Maneuvering the catheter within the heart may cause transient arrhythmias, usually premature contractions. Induction of a permanent right bundle branch block related to catheterization is rare but has been reported.[46] Perforation of the heart, although uncommon, especially with the use of pigtail catheters, may cause cardiac tamponade, necessitating pericardiocentesis and open heart repair. A severe cardiac complication consists of myocardial infarction, occurring in association with coronary arteriography in 0.07% to 0.6%.[41,42]

Because the catheter advancement for cardiac angiography occurs in close proximity to the cerebral vessels, there exists the danger of severe, permanent brain damage if cerebral embolism occurs. The reported incidence of neurologic complications was 0.03% to 14% in the same reports previously cited. There has been a reduction in the incidence of catheterization-related coronary and cerebral transient or permanent ischemia since the institution of systemic heparinization for the duration of the study,[43,45,47] suggesting that these complications were the result of catheter-induced thromboembolism. Reversal of temporary heparinization by protamine is widely used to minimize bleeding complications.

The most significant risk of catheterization is death, usually due to acute myocardial infarction, arrhythmia, or cardiac failure. In some instances fatalities may be the result of cerebrovascular accident. The mortality in various series ranges from 0.1% to 0.5%.[41,42,44,48] The report of the Inter-Society Commission for Heart Disease Resources has stated that a mortality rate of over 0.3% is unacceptable and that mortality rates of 0.1% or less are to be strived for.[2] Patients at high risk for death related to cardiac catheterization have been identified.[42,48] The mortality rate for patients under the age of 1 year is particularly high, probably reflecting to some degree the seriousness of conditions leading to catheterization. In the adult population, there is a significant correlation in procedure-related mortality with age, functional class, and left ventricular performance. Thus, patients over the age of 60 have a reported mortality of 0.25% compared with 0.07% for those under the age of 60. The corresponding results for clinical functional classes I and II were 0.02% versus 0.67% for class IV. Significantly reduced ejection fraction in the left ventricular angiogram (less than 30%) appears particularly ominous as the mortality rate in these patients was 0.8% to 1.2%. Another significant variable is the presence of left main coronary artery stenosis, which has been reported to have an examination mortality rate of 0.8% to 0.9%.[42,48]

TECHNIQUE

VASCULAR APPROACH

Access to the vascular system for angiographic purposes may be obtained by either surgical cutdown or percutaneous puncture technique. Details of both femoral and brachial arterial and venous cutdown techniques are described elsewhere.[49]

The percutaneous technique was developed in the early 1950s by Seldinger.[50] The ingenious concept of needle replacement by a guidewire for subsequent catheter introduction revolutionized diagnostic angiography and paved the way for the development of the many interventional procedures used today. More easily mastered than the technically demanding cutdown approach, this technique may be used for either venous or arterial entrance from brachial, axillary, or femoral sites.

The procedure is performed under local anesthesia following which percutaneous puncture of the vessel is performed with a thin-walled 18 gauge needle. Following successful entry, a guidewire is passed through the needle into the lumen of the vessel and advanced into the aorta or vena cava under fluoroscopic control. Gentle manual pressure on the puncture site achieves hemostasis over the guidewire as the needle is removed. After establishing guidewire access, the angiographer is free to insert over the wire an end-hole catheter or may choose to place a sheath to facilitate multiple catheter exchanges, allow use of a nonend-hole catheter, or permit continuous pressure monitoring by a side-arm pressure port.

The technical ease of this procedure should not invoke an unjustified feeling of safety for this invasive approach. Meticulous technique and gentle catheter manipulations are necessary to avoid intimal injury, air embolism, and other potential complications. Because both catheters and guidewires are thrombogenic, systemic heparinization and heparinized saline for flush are used to avoid thrombotic and embolic complications.[47] A single dose of 3,000 to 5,000 units of heparin (depending on the patient's size) is administered immediately following arterial catheter introduction. Reversal with 30 to 50 mg of protamine at the end of the procedure will help to prevent local hemorrhagic complications at the puncture site.

VASCULAR ACCESS IN INFANTS AND CHILDREN

In the neonate with a congenital heart condition, vascular access may be obtained by catheterizing either the umbilical vein, which will allow passage through the ductus venosus into the inferior vena cava and into the right heart, or one of the umbilical arteries, which offers direct access to the aorta. After the first few days of life these convenient avenues can no longer be used and catheterization usually requires a cutdown of the femoral artery or vein, but in some instances it can be performed percutaneously. Obviously, the older and larger the child, the easier it is to perform the percutaneous technique. When the use of balloon catheters without end-holes is desired, it will be necessary to use a sheath. The advantage of balloon catheters is that they are less likely to cause arrhythmias or myocardial staining during the injection than conventional catheters. Pigtail end-hole catheters of size 5F or 6F are also very atraumatic and permit rapid flow rates. Catheterization of the left side of the heart in an infant or young child is often possible by passing the right heart catheter across a patent foramen ovale. Similarly, the presence of a large ventricular septal defect may permit entry into the aorta from the right ventricle, particularly if aortic override is present as it is in many common cyanotic abnormalities. Thus, frequently, the more traumatic arterial catherization may be avoided in this young age group.

CATHETERS

A wide range of catheter materials is available including woven Dacron®, polyethylene, polyurethane, and Teflon®. By making use of different physical properties of elasticity, viscosity, melting point, rigidity, memory, and surface characteristics, manufacturers working with physicians have produced a wide variety of catheters designed for many specific uses.

Basically, there are two different approaches to selective catheterization. The first and the oldest requires the use of a relatively soft catheter, or one that softens at body temperature (often Dacron), which is introduced via cutdown and advanced to the site of interest. This pliable catheter, when meeting resistance at various anatomic sites, is gently curved by careful advancement, forming loops of varying sizes and configuration. Appropriate rotation of the catheter combined with advancement or retraction is required to direct the catheter tip to the desired location. Typical examples include the catheters for right heart and pulmonary artery catheterization and the Sones catheters for selective coronary arteriography. A popular modification of this principle is the Swan–Ganz pulmonary catherization technique in which a soft catheter is floated into the pulmonary circulation carried by an inflatable balloon at the catheter tip.

The second catheterization approach makes use of stiffer catheter materials that are preshaped in accordance with the expected vascular anatomy. During the catheterization procedure these preshaped catheters are inserted over guidewires and hence straightened temporarily. Their selective shape usually returns after removal of the guide- wire, but sometimes requires reforming by manipulation in the aorta. Such catheters, notably the Judkins coronary catheters, are very effective in achieving stable selective positions, but because their shape is so specific, they may require multiple exchanges if several different arteries or chambers are to be injected, as in right and left coronary angiography and left ventriculography.

Contrast injection into large vascular compartments such as the aorta, pulmonary artery, vena cava, or right atrium requires high flow rates and therefore thin-walled catheters of relatively large internal diameter. To insure adequate contrast and blood mixing, to minimize catheter recoil, and to prevent damage to intima or endocardium, or both, multiple sideholes are required. For example, closed tip catheters with multiple side holes at the distal end, such as the Eppendorf or National Institutes of Health type, are used for rapid right and left heart injections. Their introduction, however, requires vascular cutdown or percutaneous sheath placement. The popular pigtail, with its multiple sideholes and tight distal curl with an open end-hole, is the preferred catheter for use with the percutaneous puncture approach. High flow injections in the adult patient usually require a catheter caliber of 7F or 8F, whereas in pediatric patients, smaller catheters of 5F or 6F are preferred.

Catheters designed for selective arterial injections such as are performed in coronary angiography do not require high flow rates, but they do need good shape memory and torque control. Such catheters therefore have thicker walls often reinforced by braiding and are usually 7F or 8F shaft size, although the distal tip end is tapered to 5F for safe entry into the coronary ostium.

Certain standard approaches have emerged over time. Presently, right heart and pulmonary artery catheterization for angiography is performed using a percutaneously introduced pigtail catheter, the rounded leading end of which is considered to be safe for atraumatic passage through the right heart. Retrograde left ventriculography, which requires passage through the aortic valve apparatus, also makes use of similar pigtail-end shaped catheters, which avoids inadvertent entrance into a coronary artery and separates gently the delicate valve cusps during end-systole without causing damage.

A stenotic aortic valve makes this approach more difficult, as the narrowed opening will not permit the pigtail end to be advanced through it. In such situations, the end of the catheter may be straightened out over a straight, floppy tipped guidewire, which, once negotiated through the stenosis, allows subsequent advancement of the catheter into the ventricle. Straight catheters with multiple sideholes, such as the Gensini and Sones, are preferred by others for advancement without guidewire manipulation but are more prone to myocardial staining during ventriculography due to their straight configuration and open end-hole. Severe aortic stenosis may preclude the retrograde catheter approach. Lengthy, unsuccessful attempts to cross the valve increase the risk of complications such as intimal damage or embolism and result in an excess of radiation exposure to patient and personnel. It is therefore prudent to set a time limit for such manipulations. One may then resort to the transseptal technique, which uses a long needle within a catheter advanced from the femoral vein. The interatrial septum is punctured with subsequent catheter advancement into the left atrium or ventricle.[51]

Balloon catheters with no end-hole but multiple sideholes proximal to the balloon are used in pediatric cardiac angiography. Angiographic balloon occlusion catheters with an end-hole distal to the balloon (similar to the Swan–Ganz catheter) have been advocated for subselective pulmonary artery injections. Similarly, the Swan–Ganz catheter itself has been used for bedside pulmonary angiography in certain instances such as the detection of a suspected large embolus which does not require a large and rapid contrast injection.

There has been a recent trend toward the use of very thin-walled, small diameter catheters for angiography. These are particularly suitable for use with the digital subtraction technique because of the latter's greater ability to detect small amounts of contrast. Because catheters with outer dimensions corresponding to 4F or 5F may deliver injection rates of up to 28 cc per second, they are often adequate for selective pulmonary angiography, aortography, and ventriculography. Similar small caliber catheters also have been introduced for selective coronary angiography. However, their major disadvantage lies in the low torque control which makes catheter maneuverability more difficult.

INJECTION RATES

The magnitude of blood flow in both the aorta and pulmonary artery is high, being equivalent to total cardiac output. To opacify these large vessels and their branches for anatomic detail, contrast volumes of 60 to 70 cc at injection rates of 30 to 35 cc per second are required. When aortic root injection is performed with the purpose of evaluating valvular incompetence, however, such high flow rates are not advisable as they may cause factitious incompetence. A total volume of 40 cc at a rate of 20 cc per second is sufficient. Similar combinations apply for injections into the main pulmonary artery. However, because most pulmonary arteriograms are performed selectively in either the right or left lung, they accordingly require reduced rates of approximately 40 cc at 20 cc per second. Judgement of fluoroscopically observed contrast runoff following test injection and knowledge of pulmonary arterial pressure and inferred pulmonary resistance may be used for further adjustment of the contrast injection values. Cardiac ventriculography on either side, in the adult patient, usually practiced as selective left ventriculography, requires 30 to 45 cc of contrast volume, but the injection rate is kept as low as 8 to 15 cc per second because faster rates induce increased premature contractions which interfere with wall motion analysis and also may cause artifactual mitral valve incompetence. Pediatric contrast doses are determined in relation to the patient's size according to the general rule of 1 to 1.5 cc per kilogram of body weight for each injection, delivered in 2 seconds or less. The presence of a large shunt such as a ventricular septal defect may require larger volumes. The advised upper limit for total dose per study is 4 to 6 cc per kilogram of body weight.

Digital subtraction technique, because of its image contrast enhancement capabilities, poses fewer demands on contrast agent delivery. When injected in the arterial system, the contrast can be diluted to approximately 25% of its original concentration and still provide adequate opacification. Alternatively, one may choose to reduce the total contrast volume, keeping the usual concentration to make use of smaller, less traumatic catheters.

For intravenous angiography using digital subtraction technique, it is recommended to inject 30 to 50 cc of contrast at rates of 20 to 30 cc per second in a central location such as the superior vena cava or right atrium. The quality of the contrast bolus arriving in the left heart and the systemic arterial circulation is dependent on the patient's hemodynamic status. The more normal the cardiac output, the more compact and dense the bolus will be, and the better the angiogram. In patients with poor cardiac function, the success of intravenous angiography may be disappointing because the bolus is greatly diluted. This appears to be one of the main causative factors for nondiagnostic angiographic results with the intravenous digital subtraction technique.

PHYSIOLOGIC MONITORING

All patients undergoing angiography should be placed on an electrocardiographic monitor. Arterial blood pressure should be recorded at least periodically. Continuous blood pressure readout of an arterial line is frequently incorporated in a complete cardiac catheterization procedure. Arteriography permits pressure recording through the angiographic catheter for which purpose a three-way connector leading to a pressure transducer can be used conveniently. Pulmonary angiography, ventriculography, and coronary angiography require continuous pressure monitoring capability. Depending on the complexity of the simultaneously occurring hemodynamic evaluation, multichannel pressure transducers and equipment for cardiac output determinations and blood samples for oxymetry should be available.

Some specific technical precautions regarding angiography are worth mentioning. Patients with preexisting left bundle branch block should not be subjected to right heart catheterization for pulmonary angiography without the immediate access to a pacing catheter. This is an important precaution against total atrioventricular block, should right bundle branch block develop during the course of passage through the ventricle.[51a] Pressure measurements in the pulmonary artery before pulmonary angiography are indicated, as the contrast injection can be expected to elevate existing pressures by at least 10 mm Hg. If there is evidence of significant pulmonary hypertension, the study should be performed selectively, to limit the contrast volume for each injection and to avoid exposure of the entire pulmonary vasculature at one time.

RADIOGRAPHIC TECHNIQUE

Angiography of the cardiac chambers and great vessels can be performed with two different radiographic recording systems: direct large film radiography in rapid series or image intensifier cinematography. These should not be looked upon as being competing modalities, as preference for one over the other is related to the clinical indication for the study and they may be supplementary in given situations.

Cineangiography is the most versatile modality for cardiac imaging purposes as it is capable not only of recording the anatomic details of the chamber or vessel being studied, but also of capturing the dynamics of blood flow or wall motion, which is often a crucial aspect of the pathologic diagnosis. For example, a supravalvular aortogram for evaluation of aortic valve dysfunction is ideally done using cine technique because of its greater ability to perform dynamic analysis. Similarly, wall motion analysis for diagnosis of regional abnormalities in a selective angiogram of the left ventricle is much more easily accomplished when viewing a motion picture projection than it would be by examining static films, albeit the latter may be superior in detail and contrast. Although for an angiographic study of the thoracic and abdominal aorta, large film size series are preferred because of the significantly greater image resolution and larger field, the use of cine in the study of an aortic dissection may provide insight into the flow patterns existing in the true and false lumen. The same holds for a pulmonary angiogram in which a cine film recording may disclose more convincingly the filling defect representing a small, fragmented embolus. Cine does have some drawbacks, however, the most important being the necessarily smaller field size, determined by the input surface of the image intensifier, which for the most common image intensifiers in use (5 to 9 inches in diameter) is too small to include the entire thoracic aorta or even the total heart shadow and therefore requires panning. As this is not possible in pulmonary angiography, large size rapid film series are clearly the technique of choice for this procedure.

Typical examples of angiographic studies requiring demonstration of anatomic details include thoracic aortography for aortic dissection, traumatic lacerations, and aneurysm, but also include ventriculography for intracardiac lesions such as congenital membranous stenosis, hypertrophic ridges, and small septal defects. The superior resolution and the ability to place the entire area of interest in one field have also been used with great advantage for coronary arteriography, demonstrating anatomy and vascular disease in great detail. Cinematography, however, once obtaining the quality level of modern cesium iodide image intensifiers, became the favored modality for the recording of selective coronary injections as it permits with much greater convenience and safety the performance of multidirectional projections and also shows much better the dynamic events of filling and clearing.

The so-called spot film camera technique represents basically an intermediate imaging method making use of the electronic image intensifier but substituting the cine camera with one that records the images on films sized 100 or 105 mm. Their resolution capability is somewhat superior to that of cine film technique but the exposure rate is limited although exceeding that of larger size film changers.

DIGITAL SUBTRACTION ANGIOGRAPHY

Digital subtraction angiography is based on the well-known concept of radiographic image manipulation, which involves the superimposition of a negative copy on the original, resulting in a complete disappearance of all image information. If one of the subtracted films contains angiographic information not present in the other, this process makes the contrast-filled structures stand out more clearly without interference of the non-angiographic background information. Modern electronic and computer technology has been substituted for this originally photographic film technique and has made it available in practically push-button design for convenient use in any radiographic laboratory. Because this complementary add-on equipment makes use of the images derived from the image intensifier, it suffers from limitations of field size. The image quality is governed by that of the image intensifier itself, the x-ray equipment components, the television system, and finally the digital matrix.

The advantage of digital subtraction technique lies in its ability to enhance contrast at any given level of the image gray scale. This increases its sensitivity for demonstrating marginal contrast filling and offers the option either to decrease the amount of contrast agent, or to perform the injection less selectively, allowing the use of smaller catheters. Examples of clinical studies making use of this technique are intravenous injection for carotid artery demonstration, intravenous pulmonary angiography, and renal arteriography, among others.

Conversely, subtraction technique is subject to serious image degradation in the event of imperfect film mask match. Involuntary partial movement or uncooperative individuals are the major reason for the relatively high rate of suboptimal results. Because of these problems, cardiac angiographic applications of subtraction techniques have been slow in coming. Intravenous injections for cardiac ventriculography have been used and are shown to be in reasonable agreement with the results of selective catheter ventriculograms or radionuclide angiograms, but have not substituted for these clinically well-established techniques to any degree. Similar approaches to coronary angiography and demonstration of coronary bypass grafts are unrewarding, but the technique holds some promise for semiselective or selective injections of low concentration contrast agents using more lenient and smaller catheters, thus opening the possibility of performance of some angiograms in the form of an outpatient procedure.

ANGIOGRAPHY IN CONGENITAL HEART DISEASE

NORMAL AND ABNORMAL ANGIOGRAPHIC ANATOMY

Cardiac angiography is performed to define the normal and abnormal anatomy. Usually, physical examination and clinical presentation, noninvasive procedures such as the chest x-ray, electrocardiography, echocardiography and nuclide scan will have suggested a fairly accurate presumptive diagnosis. Thus, angiography is usually performed to answer a specific question and optimal views may be preselected for each injection.

RADIOGRAPHIC POSITIONING

Because of the position of the heart in the chest, and the oblique orientation of its long axis, traditional anteroposteror and lateral views may not display the septal surfaces, separate the cardiac chambers, or demonstrate the great vessel relations to best advantage. Accordingly, the concept of more appropriate oblique and later on axial cardiac angiographic projections was developed. Combinations of projection angulations in all these dimensions allow optimal demonstration of any conceivable cardiac structure or abnormality (Figure 14.4).

Such an undertaking is easiest when using multidirectional C-arm stands currently available, eliminating the cumbersome special positioning of the patient within the stationary anteroposterior and lateral oriented traditional equipment. For example, to demonstrate the posterior portion of the interventricular septum and the adjacent area of the endocardial cushions, so important for precise differentiation of certain shunt lesions, one might choose a 50- to 60-degree left anterior oblique (LAO) view with cranial angulation, effectively separating the cardiac cavities and descriptively named the four-chamber view. For visualization of the more anterior portion of the membranous or the muscular septum, a somewhat steeper 60- to 70-degree LAO may be required, usually with less cranial angulation. Similar optimal combinations of projection angulations exist for a number of special indications such as the pulmonary artery bifurcation, atrial septum, cardiac valves, or ventricular wall contours.[52–54]

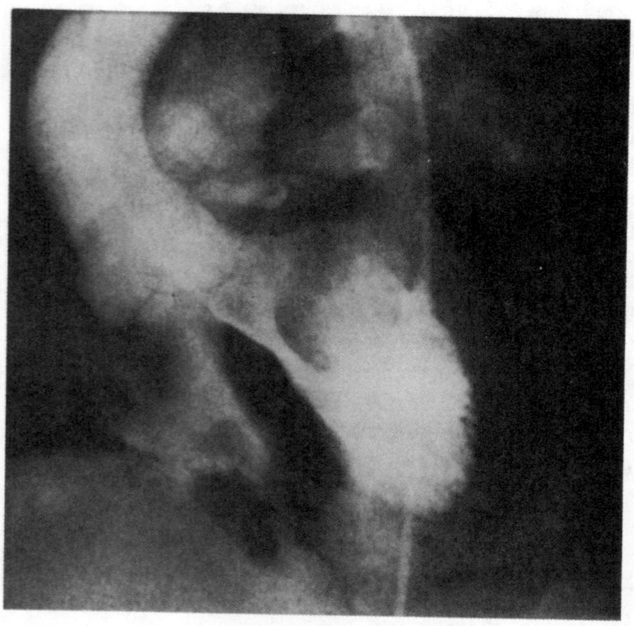

Figure 14.4. Left ventriculogram in a patient with tetralogy of Fallot. Left anterior oblique view with cranial angulation demonstrates the aortic override and left to right ventricular shunting caused by the malalignment ventricular septal defect. The muscular septum is intact.

THE SEGMENTAL APPROACH

The most practical way to analyze the angiographic findings is to use the segmental approach.[55–57] This requires identification of the visceroatrial situs, the atrioventricular relations, and the size and origin of the great vessels as well as their relations to each other. A complete description of angiographic findings in all forms of congenital heart disease would be beyond the scope of this chapter. In the following sections, segmental anatomy and some pathological examples will be included to illustrate the angiographic approach to congenital heart disease.

THE ATRIA

The location of the right atrium is often suggested on the plain film, because it, along with the inferior vena cava, is usually on the same side as the liver. Although its appendage is somewhat distinctive, being broad and triangular, the most reliable identifying feature of the right atrium is its connection to the hepatic portion of the inferior vena cava, which is usually constant even when the infrahepatic inferior vena cava is interrupted as in polysplenia syndrome.[40]

Angiographically the left atrium is a triangular chamber that normally receives two pulmonary veins on either side. This criterion, however, may be invalid in the presence of partial or total anomalous pulmonary venous return. Precise demonstration of the abnormal pulmonary venous anatomy and the status of the atrial septum may require selective injections into the right or left pulmonary arteries.

Although the presence of an uncomplicated atrial septal defect does not mandate angiographic confirmation, such a study may be called for in more complex situations or when involvement of the atrioventricular valves is suspected. In the latter situation, left ventriculography is usually performed.

Direct injection into either atrium may be useful in the evaluation of atresia of either the tricuspid[58] or mitral valve,[59,60] in which case the blind atrium spills immediately to its neighbor and then into the corresponding ventricle, reflecting the existing abnormal blood flow.

THE VENTRICLES

Angiographic identification of a right or left ventricle is better determined by ventricular morphology than by location, orientation or connection, any of which could be misleading, as they would be, for example, in transposition of the great vessels. Good anatomic definition requires direct selective injection into a ventricular chamber, easily performed on the right side with the venous catheter. Morphologic characteristics of a right ventricle include its prominent trabeculations and triangular shape with inlet portion, body, and typical outlet portion also known as the infundibulum or conus. The atrioventricular valve is tricuspid, having a septal leaflet and two mural leaflets. Normally the tricuspid valve and the pulmonary valve are separated from each other by the conus portion of the right ventricle. This differs from the left ventricular anatomy where mitral and aortic valve are in close proximity.

Right ventriculography is frequently performed for evaluation of obstructions to pulmonary flow, which may exist in isolated form or in combination with intracardiac communications (Figure 14.5). When the ventricular septum is intact, pulmonary obstruction can range from mild to critical valvar stenosis to complete pulmonary atresia.[61,62] The right ventricle may be severely hypertrophied, its extremely small chamber generating suprasystemic pressures, at times of a degree to cause reversal of flow through the Thebesian veins into the coronary arterial system with reversed flow direction and runoff into the aorta.[63] If the tricuspid valve is incompetent, the ventricle may assume a more normal size.

When pulmonary obstruction is associated with a ventricular septal defect, it usually represents an abnormality within the tetralogy of Fallot spectrum. A right ventricular contrast injection usually causes direct filling of the aorta, a feature that reflects both the overriding position of the aorta with respect to the ventricular septum, and the increased resistance to runoff in the pulmonary circulation. The ventricular septal defect is caused by a malalignment of the conal septum with the ventricular septum, also being responsible for the luminal compromise of the right ventricular outflow in the form of infundibular stenosis. Varying degrees of abnormality of the pulmonary valve and pulmonary arteries themselves may be associated.[64]

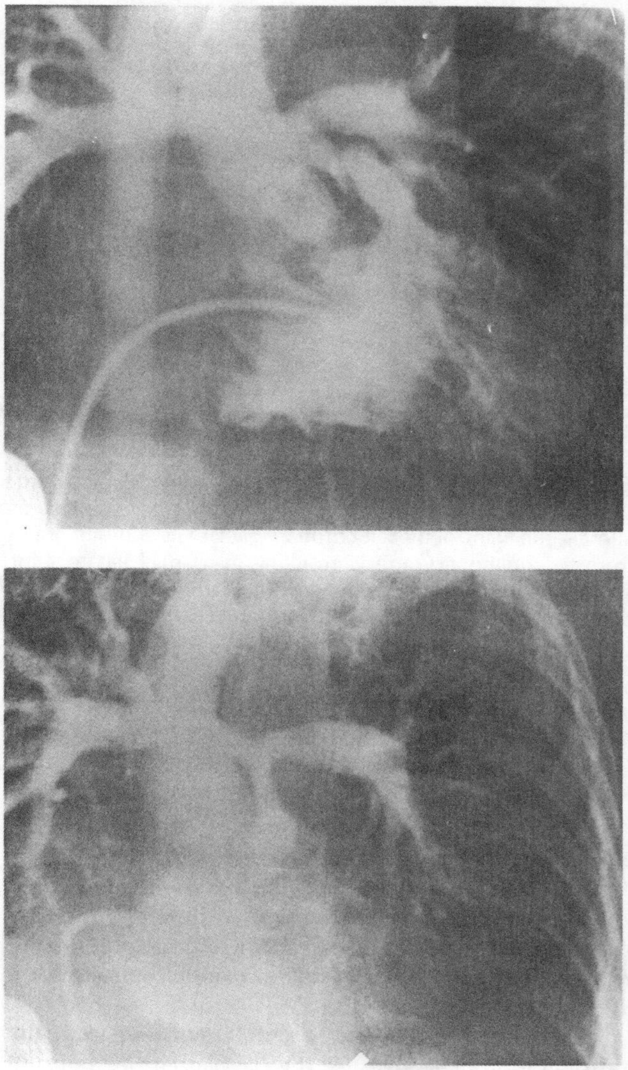

Figure 14.5. *Top,* Tetralogy of Fallot. Right anterior oblique right ventriculogram demonstrates infundibular narrowing caused by conal malalignment, dysplastic pulmonary valve, and pulmonary arterial narrowing. Right-to-left shunting into the overriding right-sided aorta is seen. *Bottom,* Left anterior oblique view with cranial angulation displays to better advantage the narrowed, dysplastic pulmonary artery bifurcation.

Direct left ventricular injection in an infant or child can often be done with a transvenous catheter passed across the atrial septum, through a patent foramen ovale or atrial septal defect. Because the left ventricle has more densely packed trabeculations, its walls appear smoother angiographically than those of the right ventricle. The septal surface of the left ventricle is muscular from the apex to the subaortic area where it becomes the smooth, thin, atrioventricular septum separating the left ventricle from both right atrium and right ventricle. The mitral valve, normally, is in fibrous continuity with the aortic valve in the area of the atrioventricular septum.

Left ventriculography may be indicated to identify and locate septal defects, and to demonstrate the position and function of the mitral valve and the subaortic area. The LAO cranial, so-called four-chamber view is particularly helpful in evaluating defects involving the atrioventricular septum, especially when a common atrioventricular valve is present.[53]

Left ventriculography is also useful when evaluating the subaortic area and the entire thoracic aorta for obstructions potentially occurring at various levels and ranging from subvalvar stenosis to coarctation.[65] When aortic atresia is present, ventriculography is not possible due to severe hypoplasia of the ventricular chamber. In such cases, injection of an umbilical artery catheter advanced into the aorta up to the thoracic level may be done at the bedside and will demonstrate retrograde filling of the hypoplastic arch back to the coronary arteries themselves[66] (Figure 14.6). Mitral atresia is best demonstrated by left atrial injection if possible, which usually shows left-to-right atrial shunting and, through a ventricular septal defect, filling of the small left ventricle and aorta.

GREAT VESSELS

After identification of the ventricular morphology, one must locate and determine the origin of both great vessels and their relation to each other. This includes assessment of the semilunar valves, the ascending aorta, the pulmonary artery and its main branches, and any abnormal communications such as a patent ductus arteriosus.[67] The location of the aortic arch to the right or left side of the trachea and the sequence of origin of the great vessels are important for complete evaluation of complex congenital abnormalities, but in practical terms may also be important to the surgeon planning the operative approach for a Blalock–Taussig shunt for palliation of insufficient pulmonary flow. Likewise, precise delineation of the available pulmonary vasculature, particularly with respect to continuity between right and left sides, as well as the size of the main trunk, is important when planning complete repair.

The principle of selective angiography for optimal result cannot always be maintained. For example, in pulmonary atresia, a selective pulmonary angiogram is im-

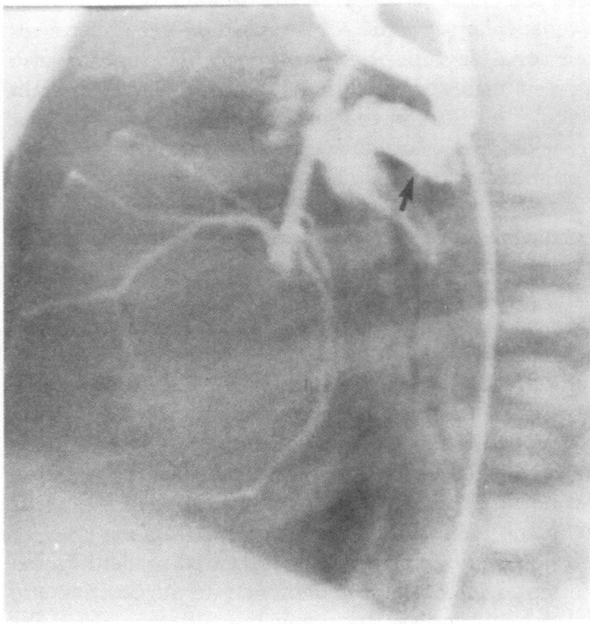

Figure 14.6. Lateral view of umbilical artery catheter injected just proximal to the level of the ductus (*arrow*). The transverse arch and three great vessels are nearly normal in size. The tiny ascending aorta fills retrogradely down to its atretic valve and into the coronary arteries. Diagnosis is aortic atresia.

possible, but a thoracic aortogram will provide for indirect opacification of the pulmonary arterial tree with contrast arriving through a patent ductus arteriosus or segmental collaterals. Retrograde balloon wedge injections into the pulmonary veins may opacify the pulmonary arteries in instances in which systemic collaterals are insufficient to do so. In tetralogy of Fallot, the ascending aorta may be directly entered with the catheter from the right ventricle through the ventricular septal defect because of the aortic override. Should visualization of the aorta be inadequate, retrograde arterial catheterization for selective aortography has to be considered, weighing the known increased risks of arterial intervention in a child against the benefits of the diagnostic study.

CORONARY ARTERIES

Although much less frequently the subject of investigation in children as compared with adult patients, the coronary arteries may sometimes harbor disease that deserves surgical and clinical consideration.[68,69] Rarely, if ever, is a selective injection technique necessary. In most instances a technically well performed contrast injection in the aortic root will result in sufficient contrast delivery to the coronary artery circulation in the presence of arteriovenous fistulas, aberrant coronary artery origin from the pulmonary artery (Figure 14.7), or major coronary artery distribution abnormalities coexisting with congenital cardiac malformations. Among the latter the high incidence of the origin of the left anterior descending artery from the right coronary in tetralogy makes it mandatory that the coronary arteries be visualized preoperatively to prevent unintentional injury during cardiac surgery.[70]

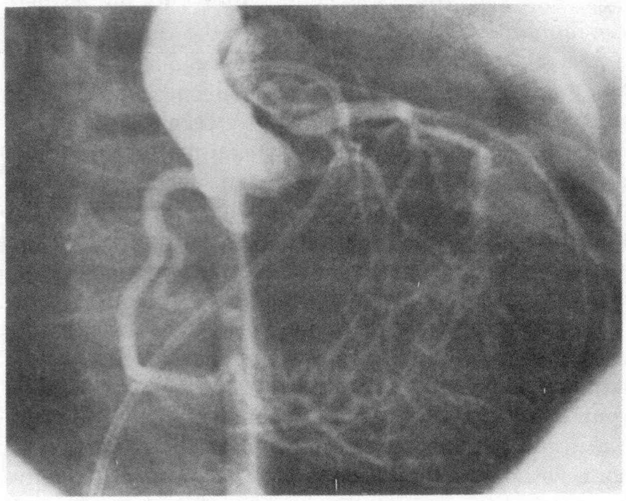

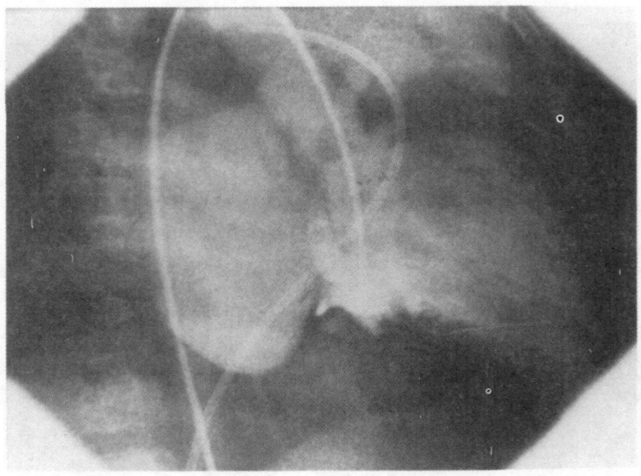

Figure 14.7. *Top*, Retrograde injection in the thoracic aorta shows filling of a large right coronary artery, and via septal collaterals, the filling of the left coronary back to its aberrant origin from the pulmonary artery, resulting in a small left to right shunt. *Bottom,* Retrograde left ventriculogram shows dysfunctional left ventricle secondary to ischemia, with massive mitral regurgitation.

PULMONARY ANGIOGRAPHY

ANGIOGRAPHIC ANATOMY AND POSITIONING

The main pulmonary artery arises anteriorly from the pulmonary infundibulum and courses posteriorly before it bifurcates at a rather acute angle into the right and left main pulmonary arteries. At this point the left pulmonary artery continues posteriorly over the left main bronchus, whereas the right takes a nearly horizontal course toward the right hilum.

In the lung, the pulmonary arterial branches essentially mirror the bronchi. Because the basal branches fan out anteriorly and posteriorly, they are partially superimposed in the anteroposterior projection, and often are better delineated in the respective posterior oblique projection, which also displays the lingular and middle lobe arteries fairly well (Figure 14.8). The superior segmental arteries, projecting due posteriorly, are best demonstrated in the lateral view. A useful approach when searching for

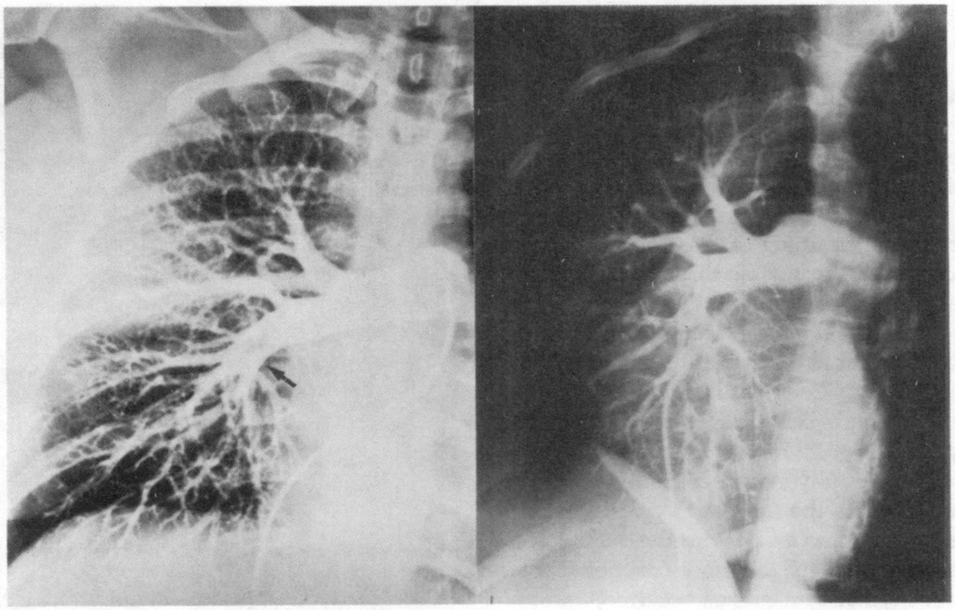

Figure 14.8. *Left,* Selective right pulmonary artery injection in posteroanterior projection shows a suggestion of clot in right lower lobe branches (*arrow*). *Right*, Right posterior oblique projection demonstrates the extent of involvement of the lower lobe branches to better advantage, due to less vessel overlap.

pulmonary emboli is to use the information from a preceding perfusion lung scan as a guide for the optimal projection to be used for the first injection.[71] Such an approach reduces the need for additional injections and allows the immediate choice of a more selective catheter position for injection without preceding angiographic delineation of both pulmonary arteries and their branches.

When pulmonary angiography is being performed for anatomic definition of the main pulmonary artery and branches, for example, to demonstrate bifurcation or branch stenoses, pulmonary artery sling, the anteroposterior projection, often with cranial angulation, is most favorable for clear delineation without superimposition by a large main pulmonary trunk.[53,54,64] The central pulmonary veins are also best demonstrated in the frontal projection, where they are seen entering the left atrium from a lateral direction, two on each side. As the injected contrast agent for a pulmonary angiogram will be followed by its passage through the left heart, the opportunity should not be ignored to depict on the films the left atrium, left ventricle and aorta, the size and appearance of which may provide valuable information.

CLINICAL INDICATIONS FOR PULMONARY ANGIOGRAPHY

The most common indication for pulmonary angiography in the adult patient is suspected pulmonary embolism. Usually, patients are referred for angiography when the findings of the perfusion lung scan are equivocal or if the chest x-ray suggests other abnormalities as the cause of the defects. A technically complete and normal lung scan eliminates the need for pulmonary arteriography. In the event of a high probability finding for pulmonary embolism on the scan, angiographic confirmation may still be considered a necessity in patients who are to be recipients of a vena caval umbrella or thrombolytic therapy. When a serious contraindication to heparin therapy exists in a patient, angiographic confirmation may be necessary to avoid unnecessary or inappropriate therapy with possible deleterious consequences.

The most reliable angiographic sign for embolism is an intraluminal filling defect (Figure 14.9). Complete vessel cutoff is less conclusive; however, careful analysis of the

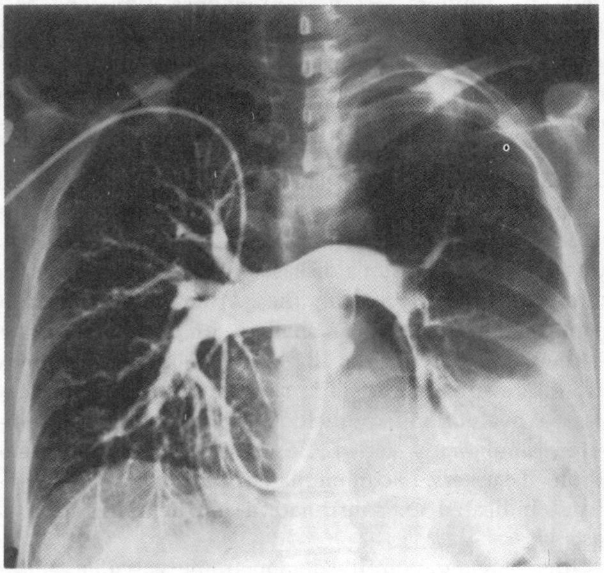

Figure 14.9. Proximal right pulmonary artery injection fills both right and left lungs and demonstrates large clot occluding multiple vessels to the left lung. Note large pleural effusion and parenchymal infiltrate due to pulmonary infarction and hemorrhage.

entire film series will frequently demonstrate the proximal portion of the clot surrounded by some contrast and confirm the diagnosis. Regional crowding of vessels, abnormalities in arterial filling, and defects in peripheral perfusion as well as delayed venous return may be seen in embolic disease, but they can also occur in other conditions with high resistance vessels, for example, in association with atelectasis and pneumonia. Webs, strands, mural irregularities and pruning of distal vessels are angiographic evidence of organizing thrombi adherent to the wall or recanalized vessels and may be seen in chronic embolic disease, not infrequently accompanied by significantly elevated pulmonary arterial pressure.[72]

The evaluation of a patient with chronic obstructive airway disease and emphysema rarely requires angiography. When surgical bullectomy is contemplated, however, pulmonary angiography may be indicated to provide an anatomic road map for the surgeon. Typically, vessels will be displaced around and away from the bullous areas of lung and "redistributed" to the more functional areas. If sufficient parenchymal damage has occurred, and pulmonary hypertension is present, enlargement of the central and main pulmonary arteries may exist as well.[73]

Pulmonary angiography is most suitable for the delineation of pulmonary arteriovenous malformations (AVM). These may be large or small, single or multiple, abnormal connections between the pulmonary artery branches and their corresponding pulmonary veins (Figure 14.10). Blood flow through these lesions is rapid and may result in a significant right to left shunt causing arterial desaturation and posing a high risk for paradoxical embolization. More than half of these patients have hereditary telangiectasia (Osler–Weber–Rendu disease) and may have other arteriovenous malformations in the brain, liver, and mesenteric circulation as well.[74] Other etiologies of pulmonary arteriovenous communication include perforating trauma, schistosomiasis, and vascular metastatic tumors. Accurate demonstration of these malformations is a prerequisite for their treatment, which can be effected by surgical resection or catheter embolotherapy using selective placement of detachable balloons.[75]

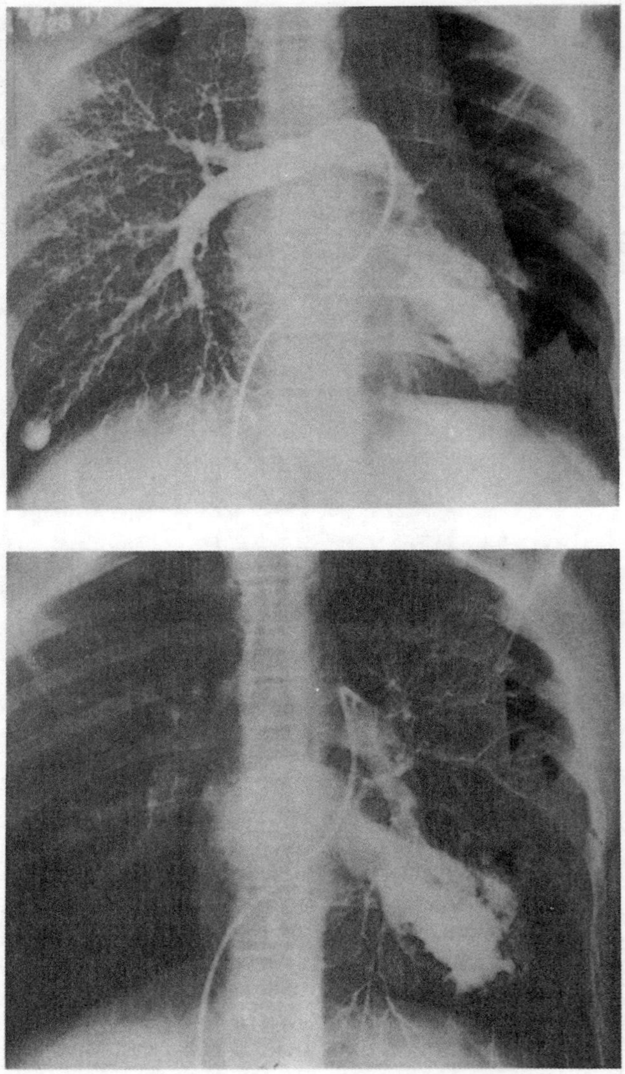

Figure 14.10. *Top,* Right pulmonary artery injection demonstrates small arteriovenous malformation (AVM) in the right lower lobe. *Bottom,* Left pulmonary artery injection demonstrates massive, complex AVM in the left lower lobe, with rapid shunting to the left atrium. This cyanotic patient had Osler-Weber-Rendu disease.

PULMONARY ARTERY ANEURYSMS

Pulmonary arterial aneurysms are relatively rare and may be secondary to septic embolization, tuberculosis, fungal disease, Marfan's disease, Takayasu's arteritis, or trauma.[76,77] When present, they often become initially manifest as abnormal mass shadows on plain chest x-ray. As they may present clinically with hemoptysis, they may lead to the erroneous diagnosis of tumor or inflammatory disease. Evaluation may include contrast-enhanced computed tomography and disclose the local vascular dilatation. If surgery is contemplated, pulmonary angiography is indicated for confirmation and demonstration of vascular detail.

Other angiographically demonstrable vascular abnormalities in the pulmonary circulation may be due to extrinsic compression caused by primary pulmonary and mediastinal tumors or inflammatory processes, although the latter are rare. Pulmonary angiography, however, is rarely practiced in these conditons, unless they raise problems in differential diagnosis in that they clinically simulate pulmonary embolism.

Multiple peripheral pulmonary stenoses of different length and degree are probably manifestations of pulmonary arteritis, including Takayasu's arteritis[78] as well as infectious agents such as maternal rubella. Similar findings have been noted in areas of the lung exposed to radiation therapy. The clinical history in such cases should be decisive for proper interpretation.

THORACIC AORTOGRAPHY

ANGIOGRAPHIC ANATOMY AND POSITIONING

Because of the orientation of the aorta in the chest, it is customary to film the thoracic aorta in the oblique position, as if viewed from the front with the left shoulder elevated. This projection corresponds to the left anterior oblique view for cardiac projections.* This position fully displays the opened aortic arch and demonstrates to best advantage the origins of the great vessels, which are subject to many anatomic variations or pathologic processes. This view is useful for displaying, for example, the site of coarctation of the isthmus of the aorta just distal to the subclavian artery takeoff. It also has the highest yield for demonstrating a traumatic rupture of the aorta following a rapid deceleration injury and the points of intimal damage in aortic dissection. Abnormalities involving the aortic ostium and adjacent supra- and subvalvular regions are also well demonstrated in the projection especially if a cranial angulation is added.

CLINICAL USES FOR THORACIC AORTOGRAPHY

Thoracic aortography is practiced in two settings: the supravalvular injection as an integral part of cardiac catheterization for aortic valve disease and the thoracic aortogram, mainly addressing disease processes involving the central aorta and the arterial branches arising from it. Whereas in the former setting, 35-mm cine equipment is most suited to answer the most commonly occurring questions regarding aortic valve motion or valve incompetence, other clinical situations that require a thoracic aortogram are more appropriately delineated with large format film series. In the following examples, the most common indications for performance of thoracic aortography using either modality will be commented upon.

AORTIC ANEURYSMS

Atherosclerotic aneurysms may involve any portion of the thoracic aorta as well as the abdominal aorta,[79] whereas syphilitic aneurysms are more common in the ascending aorta, involving the coronary ostia as a late manifestation. Mycotic aneurysms, due to either hematogenous spread of bacteria or direct extension from adjacent pulmonary or mediastinal infections, may involve the aorta itself or its great vessel branches and usually present in a saccular fashion (Figure 14.11). Likewise, this septicemia in the form of bacterial endocarditis may involve the aortic valve or cause abscess formation with fistulization into any of the four cardiac chambers.[80]

Angiographic contrast injection opacifies only the blood-filled lumen of the aneurysm, which, if lined with thrombus, may be significantly larger than the contrast-filled portion. In the chest, a thickened or clot-lined aortic wall is visible beyond the contrast shadow because it is adjacent to air-containing lung. Wall thickening greater than 8 to 10 mm measured as the distance between the angiographic border and the outer wall is usually due to more than simple atherosclerotic change and is likely to represent a mural hematoma or chronic dissection.[81,82]

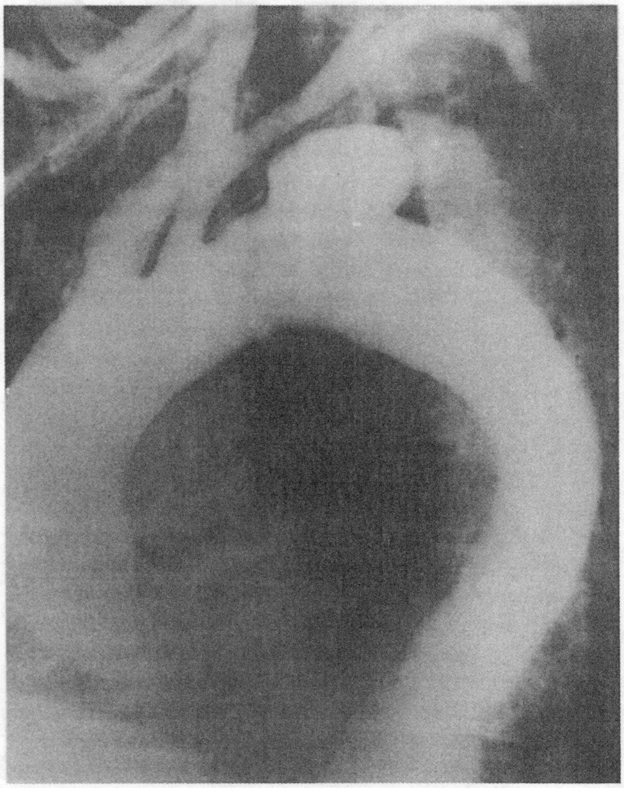

Figure 14.11. Right posterior oblique thoracic aortogram demonstrates saccular, mycotic aneurysm.

Abnormalities of the aortic media include degeneration in the form of cystic medial necrosis, dissecting aneurysm, or hematoma (Figure 14.12). Angiography plays an important role in determining the exact location of the intimal and medial defects, as the choice of medical versus surgical treatment depends on this determination. When the false lumen is clot filled or only partly patent, angiography may define a dissection less well than may computed tomography.

A characteristic traumatic injury to the aortic arch is caused by rapid deceleration, usually in conjunction with motor vehicle accidents. The typical injury is located just distal to the ligamentum arteriosum, as a result of the inertia forces generated by the sizable blood column in the descending aorta. Often this injury results in complete transection, the aorta being held together only with adventitia, which angiographically gives the appearance of a false aneurysm or occasionally resembles a local dissection (Figure 14.13). The topographic relation of such lesions to the great vessels is important for planning the appropriate surgical approach and is an important indication for angiography.[83,84]

AORTIC STENOSIS

When a patient with aortic stenosis is to be examined angiographically, either by a left ventricular or aortic injection, pressure measurements will have been obtained for documentation of a gradient between the left ventricle and the aorta. Angiography then serves to define the anatomy of the aortic valve and the adjacent areas.

If the stenosis is valvular, ie, if it involves the valve

---

*Radiographic terminology depends on the direction of the x-ray through the patient and refers to the position of the body with respect to the recording device. Thus, using large size film changer located in an under table position, LAO becomes an RPO (right posterior oblique) projection.

The posteroanterior and right anterior oblique positions (anteroposterior and left posterior oblique for large film technique) both cause degrees of foreshortening of the arch; nevertheless, they may be useful if a second view is required to clarify a suspected abnormality. The lateral view "unfolds" the arch, similar to the LAO projection, but is limited in its usefulness because it is difficult to penetrate adequately the dense shoulder regions. In infants and children, however, this view is useful for evaluation of coarctation and patent ductus arteriosus.

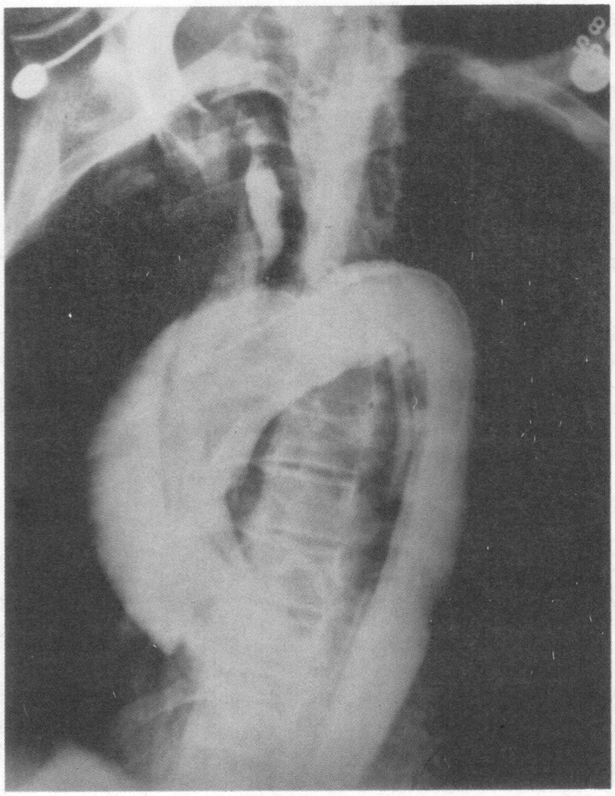

Figure 14.12. Right posterior oblique thoracic aortogram demonstrates thoracic aortic dissection beginning just above the aortic valve and extending into the descending thoracic aorta. Multiple intimal lines are seen and involve the origins of the great vessels.

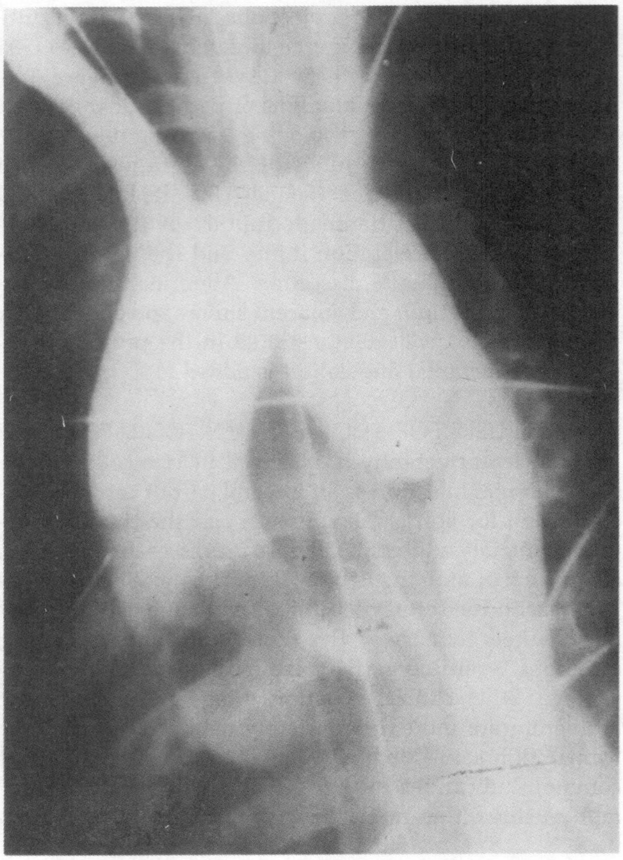

Figure 14.13. Right posterior oblique thoracic aortogram demonstrates complete transection (caused by motor vehicle accident) in the typical location just distal to the left subclavian. The two ends of the aorta are distracted by several centimeters, being held only by adventitia, this area being seen angiographically as a false aneurysm.

leaflets directly, the aortogram delineates the number and morphologic aspects of the aortic sinuses, the movement of the leaflets, as well as the degree of associated regurgitation. For example, a bicuspid valve, a congenital developmental abnormality, typically has a large noncoronary cusp with some degree of fusion between the right and left cusps.[85] Filmed in two different projections, the jet through the bicuspid valve appears spear-like in one and fan-like in the other, although the motion of the free cusps may be relatively preserved (Figure 14.14). In acquired stenosis, the leaflets are thickened, poorly mobile, and usually calcified. In severe cases, identification of three discrete cusps becomes difficult or impossible. Poststenotic dilatation of the ascending aorta may be present in either of these lesions, but is most marked in association with bicuspid valve, because of its longstanding presence.[86,87]

In patients in whom the primary lesion involves the subvalvular area, there is a high incidence of aortic valve abnormality as well, often with thickening of the leaflets due to turbulence, which not infrequently causes valve incompetence to a degree that a supravalvular contrast injection may outline the subaortic chamber lesion as well. Poststenotic dilatation in the ascending aorta as a result of a subaortic lesion is unusual.

Supravalvular stenosis, a rare congenital lesion, represents a spectrum of angiographic appearances including a thin membrane, a discrete ridge projecting into the lumen, or a long tubular narrowing in the ascending aorta beginning immediately above the aortic sinuses.[87] The aortogram demonstrates a variable waist just above the origin of the coronary arteries, which are characteristically large. The valve itself may be normal, but is sometimes biscupid. It is associated with abnormalities of the pulmonic valve, stenoses of the pulmonary branches, great vessels, and visceral vessels, sometimes in association with the syndrome of mental retardation, hypercalcemia, and elfin facies, and is known as the Williams or Beuren syndrome.[88,89]

AORTIC INSUFFICIENCY

The most reliable and clinically practical way to demonstrate and quantify aortic insufficiency is supravalvular injection of contrast. Proper catheter placement a few centimeters above the valve is important to avoid either factitious regurgitation due to interference with valve closure by the catheter or underestimation of regurgitation due to excessive distance from the valve. A specific radiographic projection is of lesser importance, but the field should encompass the entire left ventricular cavity, which is essential for grading purposes. If associated mitral incompetence is suspected, the right anterior oblique projection may be preferred for better assessment of contrast

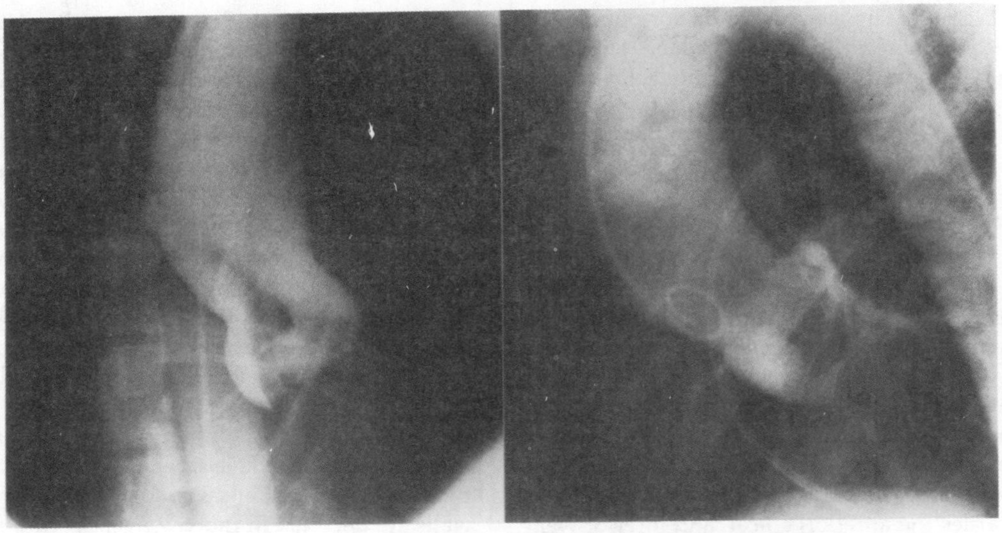

Figure 14.14. *Left*, Bicuspid aortic valve with stenosis. This systolic frame shows the spear-like jet of unopacified blood coming through the stenotic bicuspid valve. *Right,* Viewed laterally, the jet is fan-like in appearance. Note poststenotic dilation.

escape from the ventricle to the atrium. Aortic insufficiency is graded subjectively from the projected cine films. A widely used system denotes a competent aortic valve as zero, whereas massive contrast regurgitation with filling of the entire left ventricle within one heartbeat is represented by the maximal score of 4+, and grades 2+ and 3+ are subjectively judged to be somewhere between these two extremes (Figure 14.15). Although the practical value of such a simple grading scale is apparent, its potential sources of error, eg, differences in exposure and ventricular size, speed, and volume of contrast injection and catheter position, need to be recognized, should the results of other hemodynamic parameters be in conflict.[90]

Evaluation of a prosthetic valve for suspected incompetence may be preceded by fluoroscopy or cinematography of the valve motion without contrast and may demonstrate an abnormal rocking motion suggesting a paravalvular problem.[91,92] Supravalvular aortography in this setting not only discloses malfunction of the prosthesis itself, but also could identify a paravalvular leak or fistulization from the aortic root into any of the cardiac chambers, a situation that occurs in the presence of abscess formation due to bacterial endocarditis.[93]

AORTOGRAPHY AFTER CORONARY ARTERY BYPASS GRAFTING

Usually angiography of aortocoronary bypass grafts is performed selectively along with selective arteriography of the native coronary arteries. On occasion, it may be difficult or impossible to place the catheter in the graft selectively even if the point of proximal anastomosis is marked with a metallic indicator. Before concluding that the inability to visualize a graft indicates occlusion, it is prudent to perform supravalvular aortography that is likely to show some, albeit faint, opacification should patency exist. Identification of a blind nipple at the proximal end of the graft is conclusive for occlusion.

OTHER INDICATIONS FOR THORACIC AORTOGRAPHY

Thoracic aortography is also useful in evaluating complex congenital aortopulmonary connections such as truncus arteriosus, aortopulmonary window, and sequestra-

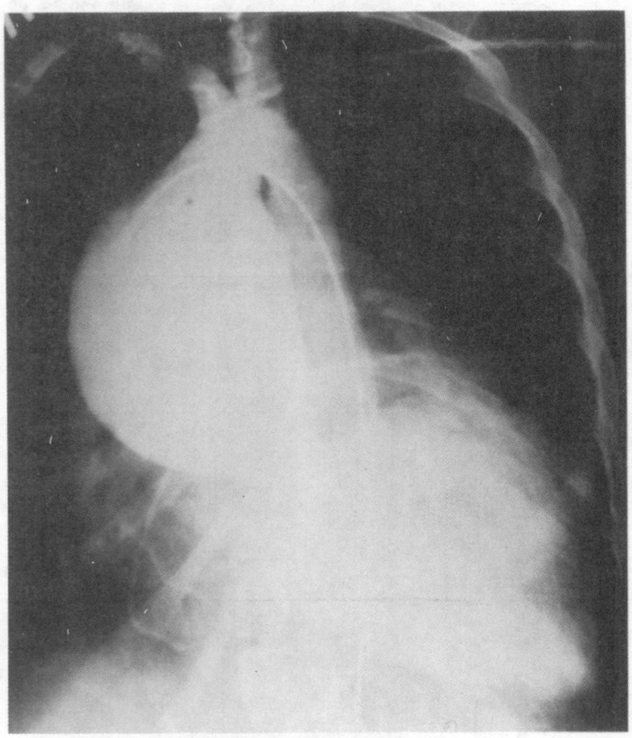

Figure 14.15. Anteroposterior thoracic aortogram in patient with cystic medial necrosis shows massive aortic dilatation confined to the ascending aorta. This was associated with 4+ aortic insufficiency with ventricular dilatation, resulting in secondary mitral regurgitation. The latter resolved after aortic repair.

tion (Figure 14.16).[94] The more common aortopulmonary connection, patent ductus, if not associated with other defects, may be diagnosed clinically without the need for aortography.

VENTRICULOGRAPHY

ANGIOGRAPHIC ANATOMY AND POSITIONING

Ventriculography in the adult is performed most commonly on the left side as an evaluation of the left ventricle's most important pump function on which basically the entire circulation depends. Because of the anatomical position of the heart in the chest, anteroposterior and lateral imaging of the left ventricle does not profile optimally the most important wall structures. If one has to resort to single plane technique, the 30-degree right anterior oblique view appears to render the highest yield as it profiles the anterior, apical, and inferior walls, which are the most common sites of myocardial infarction. This view also demonstrates the mitral valve tangentially, which is optimal for accurate identification of regurgitation or prolapse.

The significant limitations of a single projection ventriculogram and the advantages of biplane technique are indisputable. It is mostly for economic reasons that only single plane equipment is present in most cardiac angiographic laboratories. Should special indications exist, an additional injection may be performed in the left anterior oblique projection for evaluation of previously concealed profiles, for example, the interventricular septum and the lateral walls. Considering the relatively horizontal position of the heart in the chest, the ellipsoid cavity of the left ventricle will project in a significantly foreshortened image. By using an additional cranial angulation of the x-ray equipment, the left ventricle will be displayed perpendicularly to its long axis, so that both septal and lateral walls are depicted in much longer profiles (Figure 14.17). This view is very useful for the diagnosis and precise

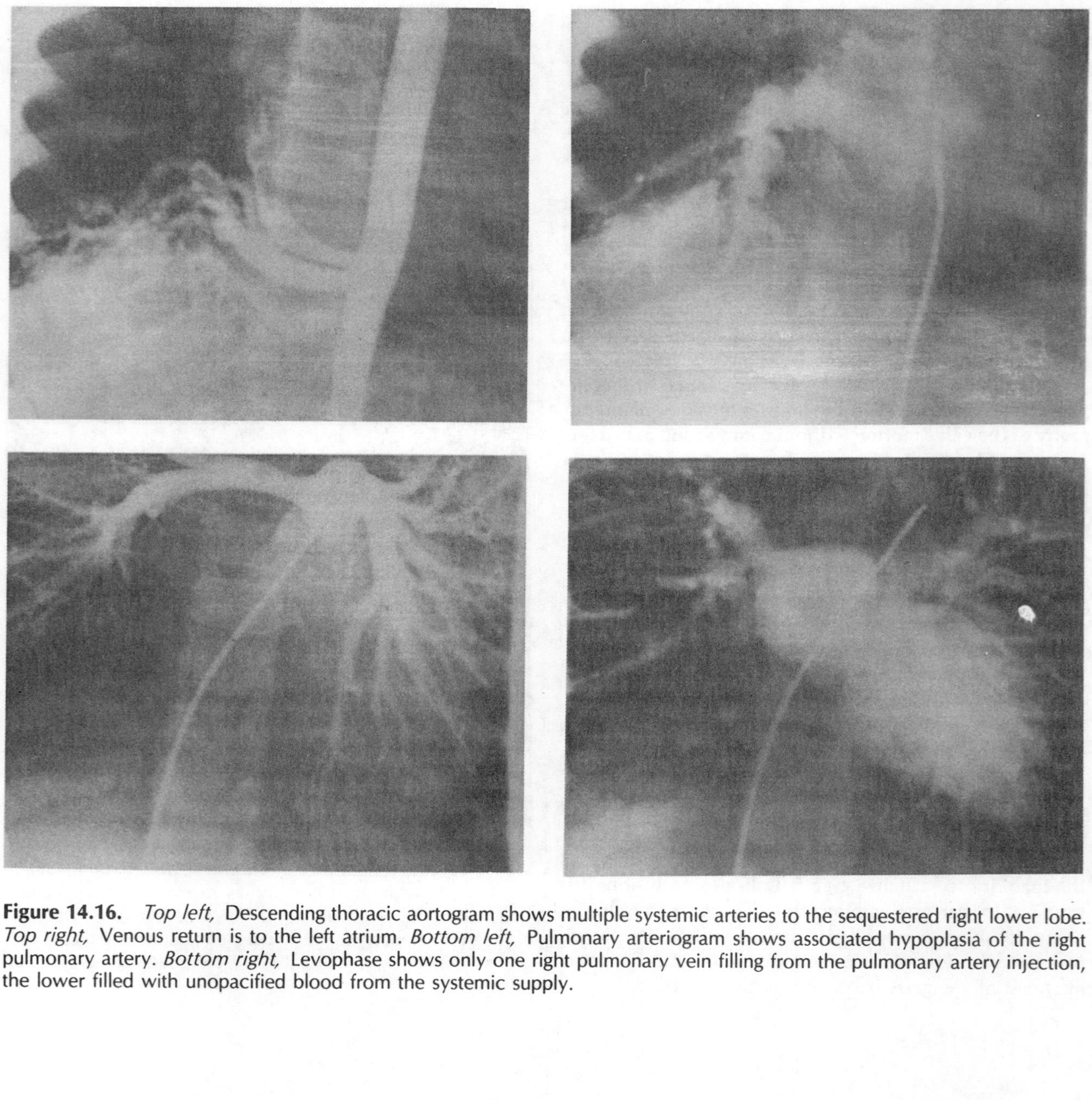

Figure 14.16. *Top left,* Descending thoracic aortogram shows multiple systemic arteries to the sequestered right lower lobe. *Top right,* Venous return is to the left atrium. *Bottom left,* Pulmonary arteriogram shows associated hypoplasia of the right pulmonary artery. *Bottom right,* Levophase shows only one right pulmonary vein filling from the pulmonary artery injection, the lower filled with unopacified blood from the systemic supply.

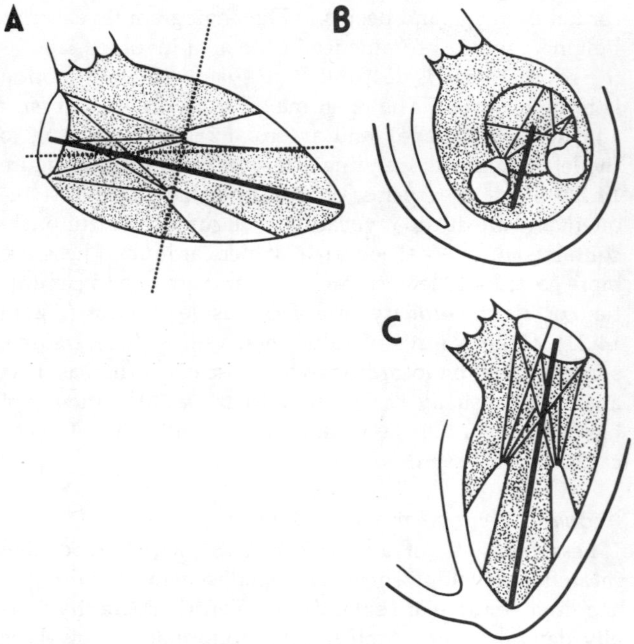

Figure 14.17. *A,* Diagram of a typical right anterior oblique projection, profiling the anterior, apical, and inferior walls, as well as the mitral valve and papillary muscles. *B,* The view at right angles to the right anterior oblique view is the straight left anterior oblique view. Note the foreshortening of the papillary muscles and posterior and septal surfaces as well as the subaortic area. *C,* The left anterior oblique view with cranial angulation places these structures in profile and more clearly delineates the anterior from the posterior leaflets of the mitral valve. (Reproduced with permission from Paulin S: Tilted views in cardiac angiography. *Medicamundi* 1979; 24[1]:2–9.)

localization of defects in the membranous or muscular portion of the septum, local septal hypertrophy and hypertrophic cardiomyopathy, and abnormality of the mitral valve leaflets, particularly prolapse.[95,96]

CLINICAL USES OF VENTRICULOGRAPHY

Wall Motion Analysis

Presently, by far the most common use of left ventriculography in the adult patient is the evaluation of myocardial function in ischemic heart disease. Ideally the ventriculogram should visualize all portions of the myocardial wall in profile. For practical technical reasons, such an ideal situation does not exist and the angiogram is performed in single or biplane projections. The simultaneous right and left anterior oblique axial views are considered optimal for this purpose[97] (Figure 14.18).

The degree and extent of regional myocardial dysfunction are related to the presence of coronary arterial obstruction and both of these factors must be evaluated in order to plan a meaningful approach to therapeutic surgical revascularization. Regional hypokinetic or akinetic wall motion in the cineangiogram is typical for a myocardial infarction and correlates well with the presence of a high grade stenosis or occlusion in the corresponding coronary artery (Figure 14.19). Transient is-

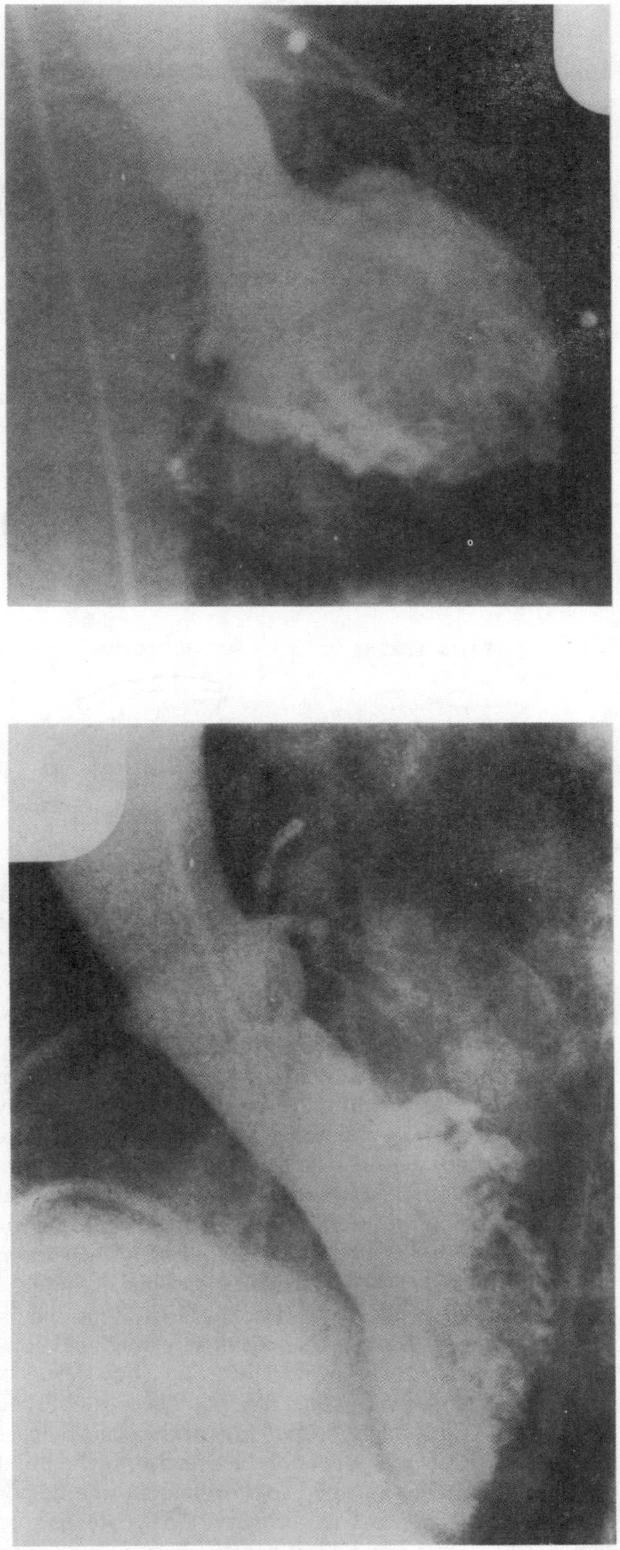

Figure 14.18. *Top*, This right anterior oblique ventriculogram in a patient with mitral stenosis gives the false impression of mild ventricular dilatation. *Bottom*, The left anterior oblique with cranial angulation profiles both the posterior and septal walls, and clearly shows what is really a small left ventricle with leftward deviation of the septum and flattening of the chamber as a result of a large right ventricle.

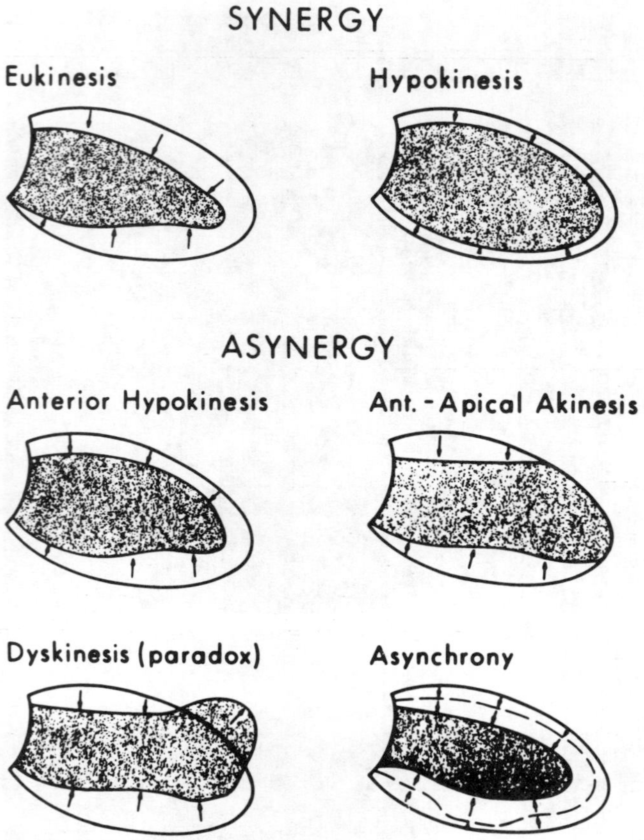

Figure 14.19. This diagram depicts the commonly used terminology for various forms of focal and global ventricular dysfunction. (Modified from Herman MV, Gorlin R: Implications of left ventricular asynergy. *Am J Cardiol* 1969; 23: 538-547. With permission.)

chemia as the cause of angina pectoris will also result in abnormal wall motion, but it is rarely documented in an angiogram as catheterization and angiography are usually performed in the non-challenged patient at rest. Extensive regions of absolute akinesia suggest the presence of a transmural infarction, a finding which would indicate that a surgical revascularization in this territory would be futile. In such situations, repeat angiography with reduced afterload (nitroglycerine effect) or pacemaker-induced augmented post-extrasystolic beat has been advocated by some in order to disclose the existence of regional contractile reserve.[98,99] These procedures are, however, not widely used and their value has not been established conclusively. Conversely, stimulation of the heart by pacing-induced heart rate elevation or exercise to the point of regional ischemia can be used to illustrate the hemodynamic consequences of coronary artery stenosis as demonstrated on a second left ventriculogram. However, such evaluation is performed more safely and more conveniently with radionuclide imaging techniques.

Left Ventricular Aneurysm

A left ventricular aneurysm, analogous to the terms used for vessels, is a regional thinning, stretching, and bulging of the myocardial wall, usually caused by myocardial ischemia and necrosis. The angiogram reveals this bulging contour prominence in the area involved, and as the myocardium is destroyed, no systolic inward motion is to be expected. The great majority are true aneurysms and involve the apex and anterolateral wall, relating to the left anterior descending artery or its branches (Figure 14.20). False aneurysms, on the other hand, are less frequent and are due to myocardial wall rupture, fortuitously contained in a localized area of pericardium. These are more commonly located inferiorly and are due to circumflex or right coronary artery occlusive disease (Figure 14.21). Other causes of false aneurysm include trauma, surgery, and endocarditis with abscess. Whereas true aneurysms usually have a broad base, a false aneurysm has typically a narrow neck reflecting the point of myocardial rupture.[100]

Acquired Ventricular Septal Defects

Less than 1% of all patients with acute myocardial infarction develop ventricular septal ischemia resulting in acquired ventricular septal defect. Ventriculography usually demonstrates a wall motion abnormality as well as the septal perforation. Relatively common locations for the defect are either posterior, near the mitral valve, or anterior, near the apex.[101] Good axial ventriculograms are necessary to demonstrate the location as accurately as possible.

Mitral Valve

The normal function of the mitral valve is dependent on the integrity of the leaflets, the chordae, and the contraction and orientation of the papillary muscles to which they attach. Marked ventricular dilatation alone may change the orientation of the papillary muscles to a degree that coaptation of the leaflets becomes incomplete and mitral insufficiency ensues, although usually of only a mild degree.[102] Angiographically one sees a dilated ventricle without localized wall motion abnormalities. The valve leaflets are neither calcified nor prolapsing. If the underlying cause of ventricular dilatation, for example, aortic insufficiency, is surgically remedied, the mitral regurgitation may become insignificant or disappear.

Ischemia involving the papillary muscles may occur as a complication of acute myocardial infarction. Although complete rupture is rare, rupture of the head of one papillary muscle, which serves chordae to both leaflets, will cause dysfunction to some degree in both anterior and posterior leaflets, resulting in severe mitral regurgitation.[103] The chordae themselves are fairly avascular, but are subject to injury or rupture, usually caused by bacterial endocarditis, rheumatic fever, or other connective tissue weakness.[104] Although one cannot see the chordae angiographically, the resulting flail mitral leaflet and severe mitral regurgitation are obviously strong indirect signs for such chordal rupture.

The spectrum of morphologic changes that are found in mitral valve prolapse includes a dilated anulus, degenerative floppy leaflets, and elongated chordae that are subject to rupture.[105] Although mitral prolapse may occur in an otherwise normal heart, it is frequently associated

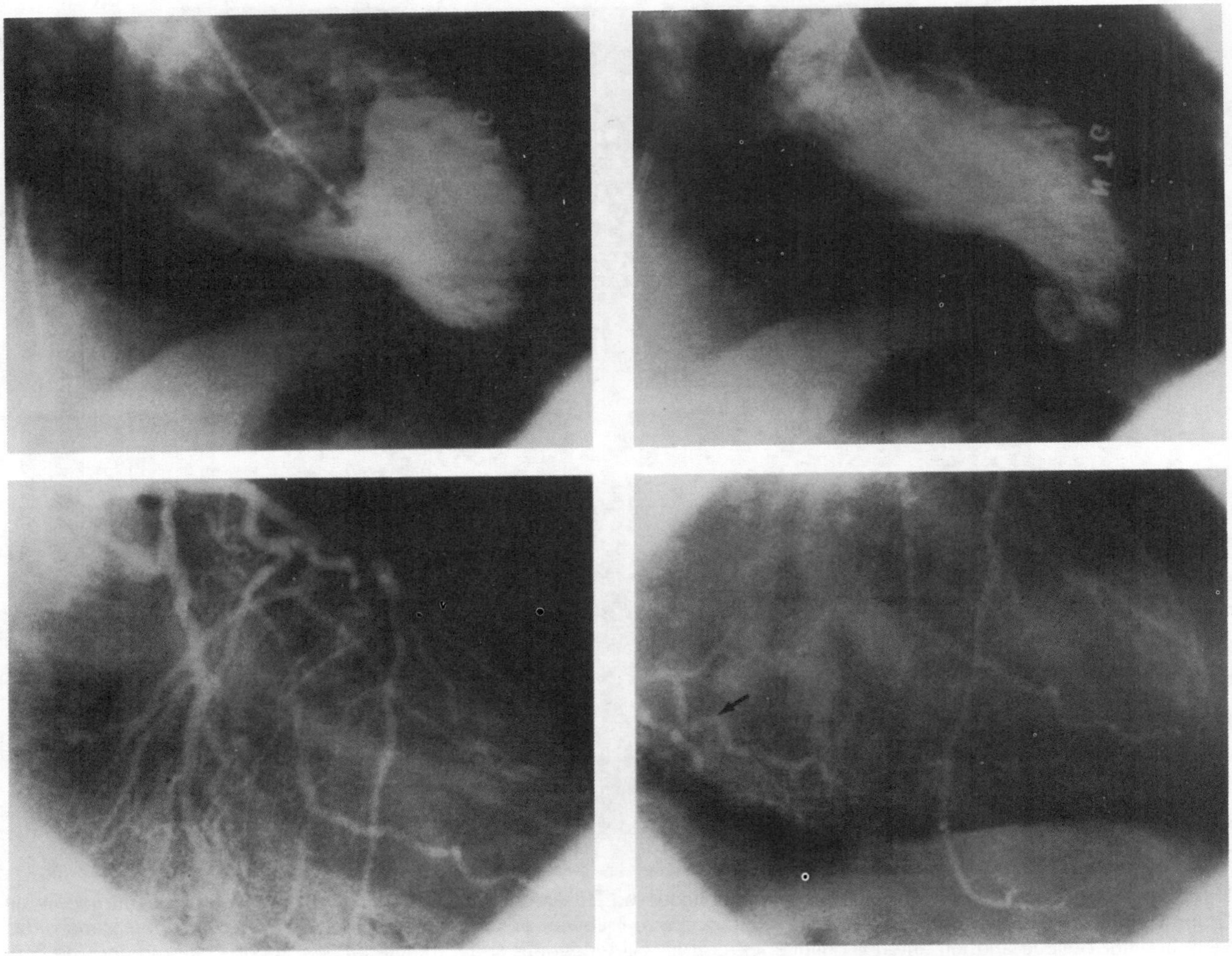

Figure 14.20. *Top left,* This diastolic frame shows an apical bulge, which in systole (*Top right*) is dyskinetic. The anterior wall is akinetic, with some preservation of motion at the base. The inferior wall is severely hypokinetic. *Bottom left,* Shallow right anterior oblique coronary arteriogram shows the expected left anterior descending artery occlusion with local collateralization. *Bottom right,* Visualization of the distal right (*arrow*) implies right coronary artery occlusion, which explains the inferior wall dysfunction.

with Marfan's syndrome[106] and found occasionally together with other congenital abnormalities, particularly atrial septal defect. The clinical diagnosis of mitral valve prolapse is most often made echocardiographically. The reliability of such diagnoses and the criteria on which they are established has been criticized and debated in light of a large echocardiographic survey with an incidence of mitral prolapse to some degree in 20% of a normal and apparently healthy population.[107,108]

Angiographically, mitral prolapse is seen as protrusion of the valve apparatus behind the plane of the mitral anulus into the left atrium. To demonstrate this accurately, one must profile the mitral valve precisely in the right anterior oblique projection. The complementary cranial left anterior oblique view provides additional insight into the pathologic morphology as it allows separation of anterior from posterior leaflet prolapse.[96] It has been reported that 10% to 20% of normal left ventriculograms have 1 to 2 mm posterior motion of the leaflets on the right anterior oblique ventriculogram, a finding that therefore is considered inconsequential, but excursions greater than this are well correlated with clinical signs of abnormal mitral function.[109] Not rarely this coincides with some degree of contrast regurgitation into the left atrium.

Rheumatic mitral valve involvement may result in either valvular insufficiency, stenosis, or both. Pathologically, the chordae shorten, and the free edges of the leaflets scar and contract, precluding adequate tissue for coaptation. The valve leaflets may become markedly immobile, which may be best appreciated in the left anterior oblique ventriculogram. Although a common feature of rheumatic valvular disease is leaflet calcification, it should be recognized that severe hemodynamic obstruction may be present with little calcification and only a subtle angiographic motion abnormality. In such situations, the typical dome shape of the billowing leaflets fused together at the commissures is seen. When the free edges are severely rolled up and the chordae shortened, stenosis may be accompanied by insufficiency.[110]

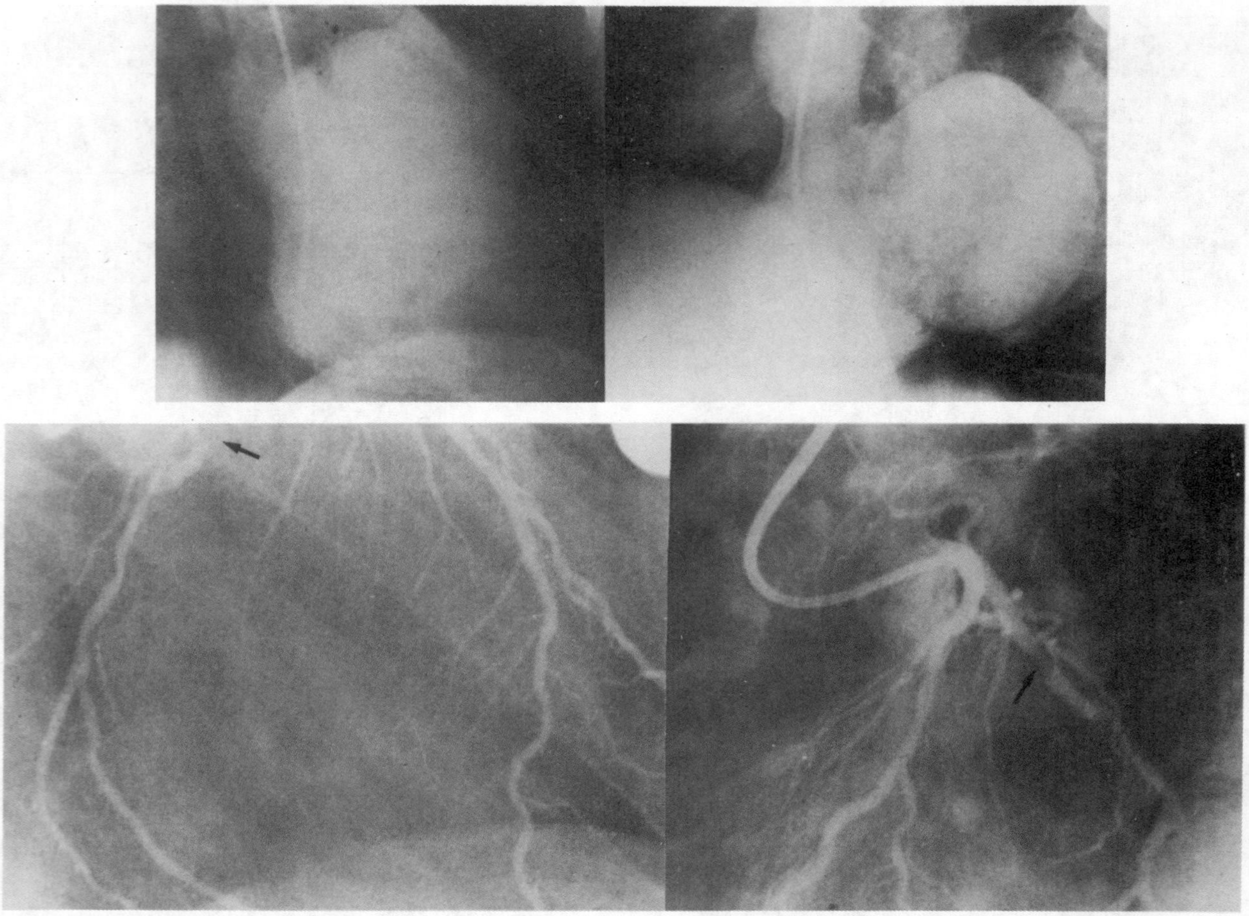

Figure 14.21. *Top left and right,* Right anterior oblique and left anterior oblique views of a left ventriculogram show an enormous posteriorly located false aneurysm, which occurred following an acute myocardial infarction. *Bottom left and right,* Right anterior oblique and left anterior oblique left coronary arteriograms show the circumflex stenosis (*arrow*) and the bare area corresponding to the aneurysm itself and one or more occluded marginal branches.

Left Ventricular Outlet Abnormality

Abnormalities in the subaortic area, such as membranous subaortic stenosis, and idiopathic hypertrophic subaortic stenosis (IHSS) are best visualized on axial left anterior oblique ventriculography, because standard LAO ventriculography may fail to adequately visualize the immediate subaortic area if the ventricle is foreshortened.[96] If aortic regurgitation is present, as it commonly is, an aortic root injection may fill the subaortic chamber outlining the obstruction.

Idiopathic hypertrophic subaortic stenoses may be a subtle angiographic lesion[111] and may also be difficult to document physiologically without provocative testing. For example, isoproterenol administration to elicit maximal contraction and to accentuate the gradient is frequently practiced. Angiographically one sees a thick-walled ventricle with a near obliteration of the ventricular cavity during systole. The proximal septal surface is prominent and obstructive to the ventricular outflow tract, an effect that is compounded by abnormal movement of the anterior leaflet of the mitral valve during systole.[112] Membranous or discrete subaortic stenosis is found more often in the pediatric age group (Figure 14.22). It may be an isolated abnormality or part of a syndrome that includes a parachute mitral valve, subaortic stenosis, and coarctation.[113] Because of the turbulence created, there is often secondary damage and thickening to the aortic valve leaflets themselves, which may result in insufficiency. Although not common, poststenotic dilatation in the ascending aorta can be seen.

DIGITAL TECHNIQUE

With the advent of digital subtraction, intravenous ventriculography has gained a potential role as a noninvasive imaging technique to study cardiac function and anatomy (Figure 14.23). The procedure still requires contrast administration in volumes of 30 to 50 cc, either in a peripheral vein or more centrally in the superior or inferior vena cava via a percutaneously introduced small catheter.

A number of studies have been reported in which digital intravenous left ventriculography has been performed using various contrast enhancement programs, different mask modes, and frame rates, as well as different views. It has been shown, for example, that ventriculograms performed before and after atrial pacing are comparable in their results to exercise radionuclide studies as predictors of significant coronary disease. Left ventricular volume

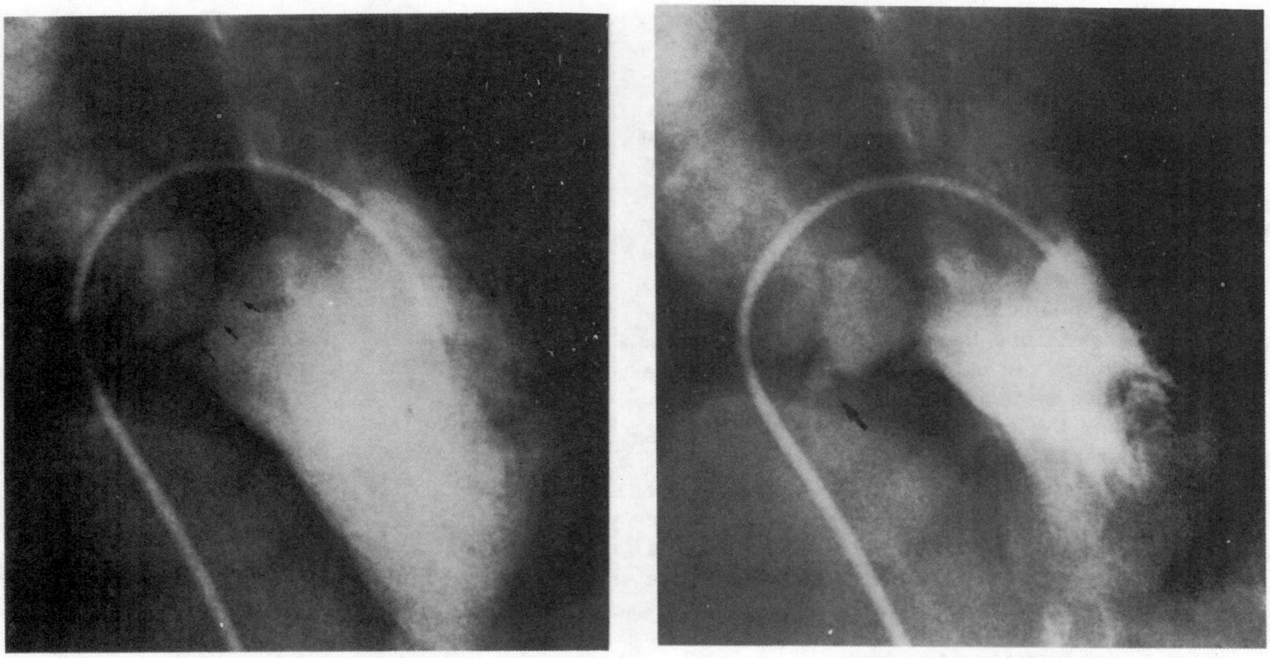

Figure 14.22. *Left,* Left ventriculogram in left anterior oblique projection with cranial angulation demonstrates discrete subaortic membrane (*small arrows*) as seen in diastole. *Right,* In systole the subaortic area is even more obviously narrowed. A small membranous ventricular septal defect is present (*arrow*).

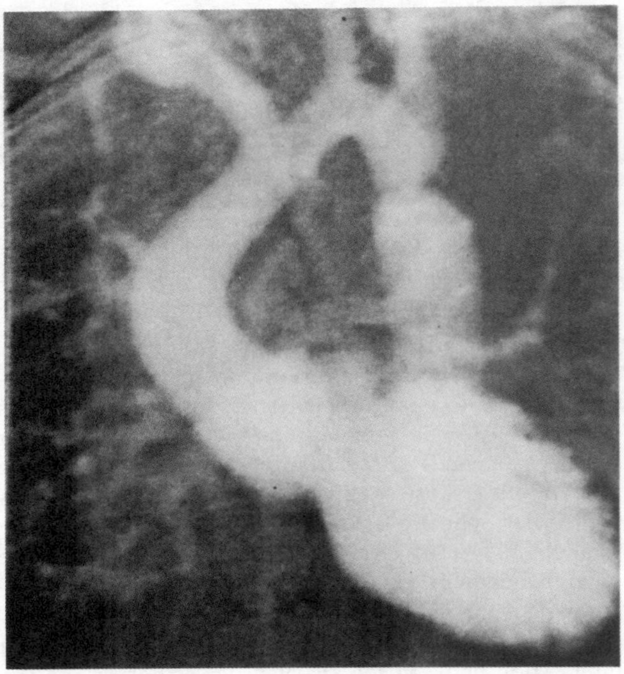

Figure 14.23. This is an intravenous digital study done on an outpatient basis in a child with coarctation of the aorta. Note the dilated ascending aorta, due to coexisting bicuspid valve and the coarctation itself as well as its relation to the great vessels.

and cardiac output determinations by digital ventriculography using computer algorithms compare well with selective cineventriculography and with thermodilution techniques for flow.[10,12,114–116]

An interesting digital method for analysis of ventricular function is the production of an ejection shell image, which is the result of subtracting the end-systolic from the end-diastolic image. The ejection shell normally shows symmetrical displacement of the left ventricular walls during contraction. In some patients with ischemia, for example, the ejection shell will display the area of focal abnormality corresponding to the area of ventricular ischemia.

The availability of digital image recording systems in an angiographic laboratory may become an adjunct to cineangiography, as it reduces the need for the use of large contrast loads in the performance of repeated ventriculograms following pharmacologic intervention, electrical stimulation, or exercise. Also, digital software programs for wall motion analysis and computation of ejection fraction based on densitometry may simplify postcatheterization data calculation. The possibility of using a digital imaging technique for coronary arteriography has been explored but as yet does not compete with the present technique of selective angiography and 35 mm cine film angiography.

CORONARY ARTERIOGRAPHY

ANGIOGRAPHIC ANATOMY AND POSITIONING

Both coronary arteries arise from their corresponding aortic valve sinuses in almost diametrically opposite direction. The right coronary artery runs in the right atrioventricular groove between the free wall of the right ventricle and the right atrium toward the crux of the heart, and in most instances, beyond this point to supply a varying number of branches to the posterior left ventricular wall. The left main coronary artery, initially directed slightly posteriorly, makes a gentle curve in an anterior direction before it bifurcates into its main branches, the left anterior descending artery, which runs anteriorly in the interventricular groove, most frequently reaching and surrounding the cardiac apex, and into the left circumflex artery arising at almost a right angle to continue for a variable distance in the left-sided atrioventricular groove. Thus, the two coronary arteries form an almost complete vascular ring around the base of the heart, from which apically directed branches, the left anterior descending, the posterior descending, and a varying number of right and left marginal branches surround the ellipsoid-shaped free walls of both ventricles. These basics of coronary artery topography, reminiscent of the appearance of a crown, explain the names given by the classical anatomists, the "coronary" arteries (Figure 14.24).

Imaging of all portions of the constantly moving coronary arteries, portions of which will assume any conceivable direction in all three dimensions, has always been an angiographic challenge. From the outset it became apparent that in addition to frontal and lateral views, multiple oblique projections would be necessary to adequately demonstrate the coronary circulation, and hence right anterior and left anterior oblique views (RAO and LAO) became standard projections for the coronary arteriogram (Figure 14.25). As equipment design was limited to obliquities in relation to the patient's long axis, shortcomings were soon encountered in certain important anatomic vascular regions that defied optimal perpendicular depiction. The concept of cranial or caudal x-ray beam angulation to overcome these deficiencies became more imperative in the early 1970s and led to the use of special positioning arrangements achieved by changing the patient's position, for example, the "sitting up" view. This was followed by the development of imaging equipment supports that permit special projections in all three-dimensional directions with great convenience (Figure 14.26). Today, such a multidirectional projection approach for coronary arteriography is considered to be routine and standard.[117–123]

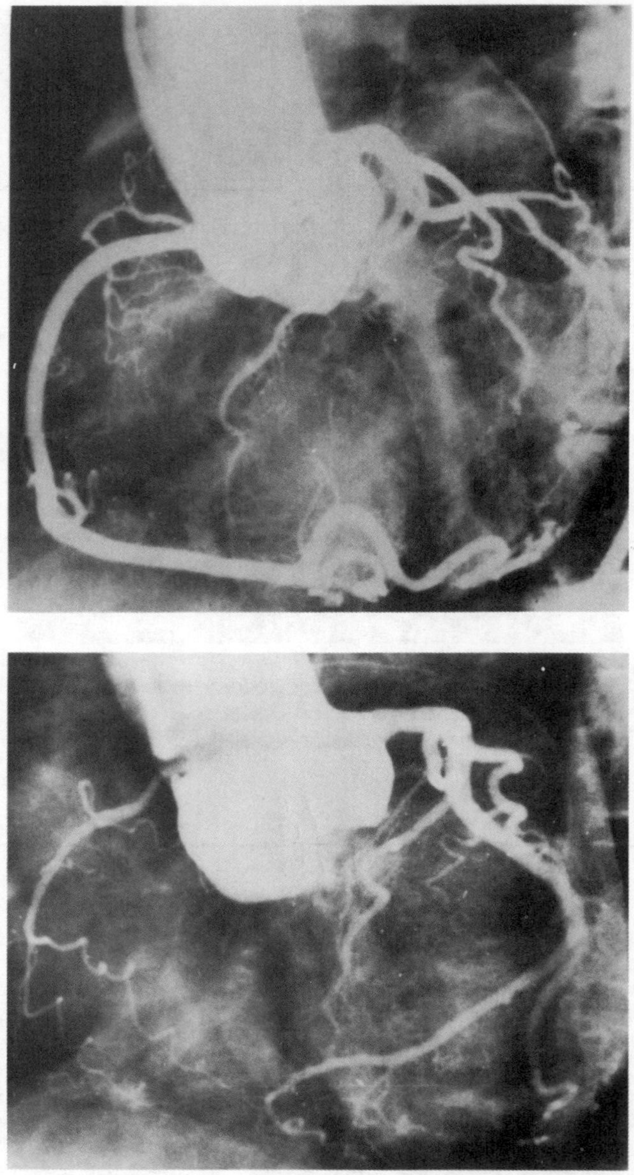

Figure 14.24. Nonselective injections in the aortic root demonstrate normal coronary anatomy. *Top,* Right preponderant system. *Bottom,* Left preponderant system.

VASCULAR TERRITORIES AND CORONARY DISTRIBUTION

Although great individual variations can be expected, the typical territorial relation between right and left coronary artery in the human circulation can be characterized as follows. The right coronary artery surrounds in a semicircle the base of the heart on the right side and accounts for vascular supply to the right ventricular free wall, the posterior interventricular area including the posterior third of the interventricular septum, and a varying region of the posterior left ventricular wall adjacent to it. The left coronary artery and its major division into left circumflex and left anterior descending arteries provide arterial flow to the major portion of the interventricular septum, the anterolateral wall of the left ventricle, including the apex, and the remaining territory of the posterolateral wall. Atrial branches arising from either side are relatively small commensurate with the much lesser nutritive demands of the atrial myocardium. Among the atrial arteries, those supplying the sinus node and atrioventricular node are the largest.

The widely used terms of coronary artery dominance or preponderance are based on the topographic interrelation between right and left coronary artery extension[123] (Figure 14.24). If the right coronary reaches the crux, the intersection between the atrioventricular border and the interventricular groove at the inferior and posterior surface of the heart, it is denoted as dominant. This occurs in about 85% of human hearts. This term should not be misconstrued to denote the magnitude of relative coronary flow, which in spite of this arterial distribution con-

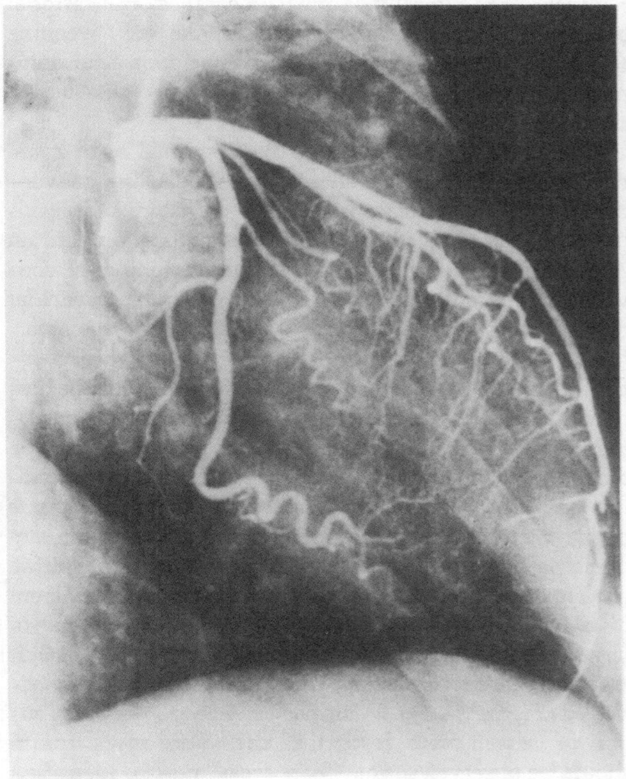

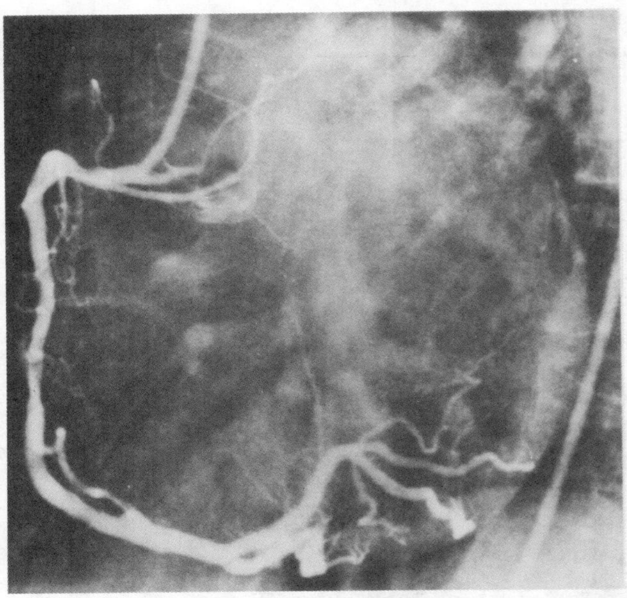

Figure 14.25. *Top,* Selective left coronary injection in right anterior oblique projection. *Bottom,* Selective right coronary injection in left anterior oblique projection.

cept almost always is larger in the left coronary artery. This is easily explained by the fact that the major arterial blood supply of the more metabolically demanding left ventricular myocardium derives from the left coronary artery and its branches.

Whereas extreme cases of right coronary artery preponderance in which the right supplies more than half of the left ventricular wall territory are relatively rare, the presence of a topographic left coronary artery preponderance which implies exclusion of the right coronary

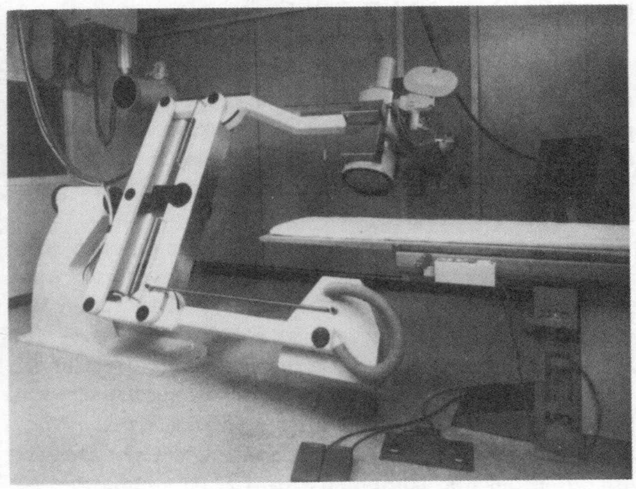

Figure 14.26. Modern C-arm parallelogram system, which can achieve oblique as well as cranial and caudal views without moving the patient.

artery from the supply of the left ventricular myocardium occurs in approximately 7% to 10% of human hearts. In such situations, the presence of a critical obliteration of the left main stem is obviously more ominous, in particular because the availability of intercoronary anastomoses and collaterals is more limited.

Not incorporated in the concept of coronary dominance, but by no means less important, are variations between the left anterior descending and the posterior descending artery in the supply of the cardiac apex and adjacent areas. A very long left anterior descending artery surrounding the apex and extending significantly onto the posterior inferior wall may be accountable for ischemic wall damage in the inferior diaphragmatic area, and correspondingly, lesions in an extremely long posterior descending artery may account for an infarction in the apicolateral region of the left ventricular wall.

By convention, left-sided branches to the left anterior descending artery extending over the entire wall are denoted as diagonal branches, whereas branches of the left circumflex artery are identified as marginal branches. They may vary significantly in number and size but accomplish an even distribution of secondary and tertiary vessels in subepicardial location over the entire wall surface. Relatively commonly (a third of the cases), a major branch may arise directly from the bifurcation, resulting in a left main artery trifurcation, this vessel occupying an intermediate territory between the anterior and posterior free wall of the left ventricle. The term *intermediate artery* or *ramus medianus* is used in such situations. Additional relatively common variations are bifurcations of the left anterior descending artery into almost equal sized branches, the so-called *twin trunk*, early bifurcations of the left main trunk giving the impression of almost two orifices, unusually large first septal perforator branches, the existence of a separately arising right-sided pulmonary conus branch (50%), and mild degrees of ectopic position of both coronary arteries, the latter sometimes posing difficulties when attempting selective injections.

RADIOGRAPHIC PROJECTIONS

Optimal projections for proper identification of particular lesions require great flexibility of the radiographic equipment to compensate for these numerous arterial topographic variations as well as those occurring in relation to cardiac position within the chest. In the following, some of the more frequently encountered challenging situations are exemplified.

Demonstrations of lesions in the left main stem may require special projections, as this vessel curves from posterior to anterior before it bifurcates. Whereas tangential demonstration of the orifice may require a moderate left anterior oblique projection with some cranial angulation, the artery's midportion is most favorably seen in straight frontal projection. Stenoses close to or directly involving the bifurcation are optimally delineated in right anterior oblique projection combined with caudal angulation. As the latter is most frequently encountered in coronary arteriosclerosis, this projection is preferred for the initial run in patients suspected to have a left main lesion. This projection also demonstrates most favorably the proximal portions of the left circumflex artery which in conventional right anterior oblique view would be significantly foreshortened.

Lesions in the proximal portion of the left anterior descending artery are frequently identified in the conventional right anterior oblique projection; however, they are sometimes superimposed by diagonal branches. The latter dilemma can be avoided in the left anterior oblique projection particularly when an additional cranial angulation of 30 degrees more compensates for the extremely anterior direction of the left anterior descending artery in its first third (Figure 14.27). Similarly, a cranial angulation in shallow right anterior oblique projection may separate most favorably the large first septal branches from the left anterior descending and diagonal branches.

An additional favorable projection of the left main bifurcation and the proximal circumflex artery consists of the left anterior oblique view with caudal angulation. Because of the typically draping appearance of the arterial branches, it is also known as the "spider" or "weeping willow" view (Figure 14.28). This projection also demonstrates well the most distal left anterior descending artery as it surrounds the apex.

Angiographic delineation of the proximal right coronary artery is usually well accomplished using conventional right and left anterior oblique projections. To evaluate the origin of the posterior descending branch, an AP-cranial view overcomes the foreshortening in conventional left anterior oblique projection and in particular demonstrates properly arterial bifurcations in this area.

The common practice of performing a selective left ventriculogram just before the angiographic study of the coronary arteries helps to direct attention to areas of suspected ischemia. The presence of abnormal wall motion should intensify the search for a lesion in the corresponding territorial vessel, and make one reluctant to accept a negative finding in the suspect artery lest a significant operable lesion be missed. One important potential pitfall is a flush occlusion of a vessel with poor or nonexistent distal collateralization. For example, a sizable septal or large diagonal may be mistakenly identified as the left anterior descending artery when the latter is flush occluded (Figure 14.29). With each injection, the distribution of vessels with respect to the entire myocardium should be observed so that "bare areas" may be identified appropriately.

CORONARY VARIATIONS AND ANOMALIES

For practical considerations, it might be advisable to distinguish between common anatomic variations present in more than 1% of the population and of a type already discussed, and more striking anomalies occurring less frequently. The overall incidence of such anomalies in the coronary artery circulation was recorded as 1.2% in a large angiographic series.[124]

The most common is the origin of the left circumflex coronary artery from either the right sinus of Valsalva or

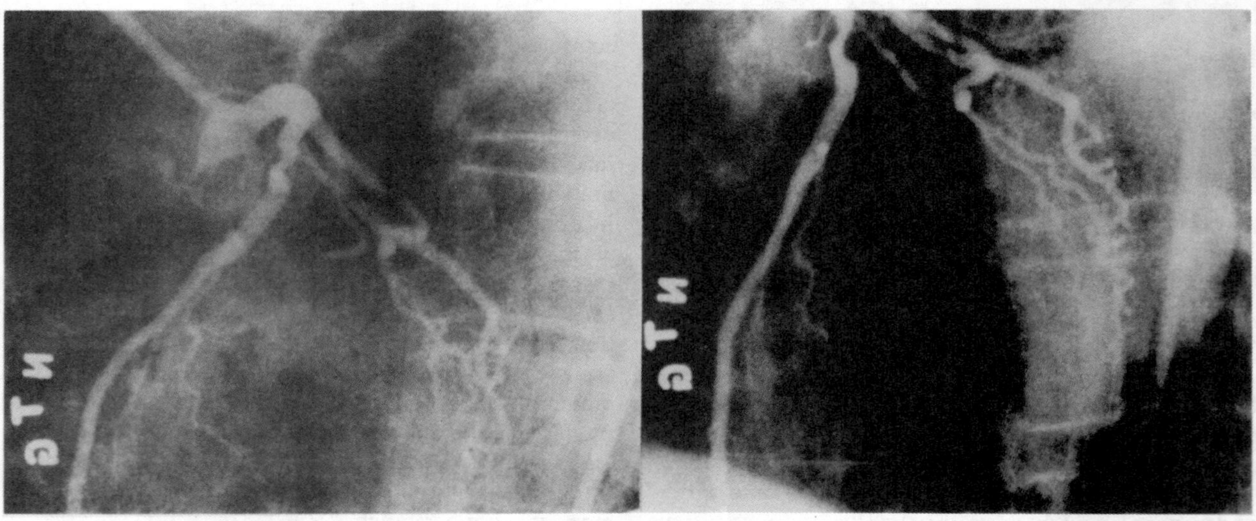

Figure 14.27. *Left,* Standard left anterior oblique view of the left coronary causes foreshortening of the left anterior descending artery (LAD). *Right,* Left anterior oblique with cranial angulation allows the proximal LAD and diagonals to be seen more clearly. In this case, the LAD lesion and a severe stenosis of the first diagonal are much better shown.

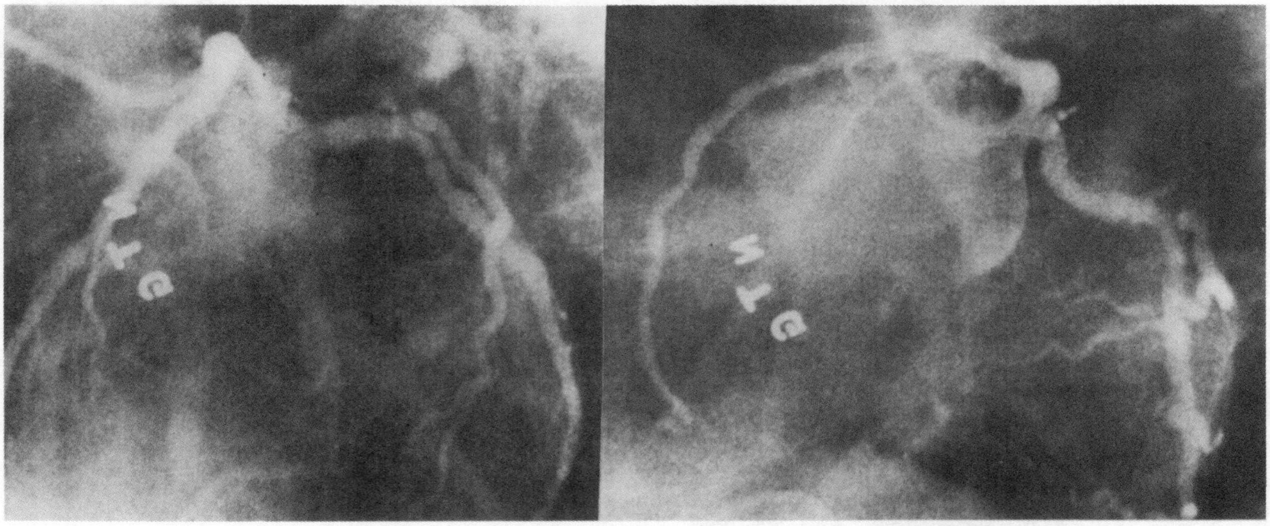

Figure 14.28. *Left,* This standard left anterior oblique view causes overlap and foreshortening in the region of the left main bifurcation and proximal circumflex. *Right,* This caudally angulated left anterior oblique "spider" or "weeping willow" view shows these areas much more clearly.

the proximal right coronary artery itself[125] (Figure 14.30). Its course posterior to the aorta is considered to be of no pathophysiologic significance and the distribution of the circumflex artery branches is practically identical with the normal. Translocation of coronary artery orifices, the right coronary artery arising from the left or the left coronary artery from the right sinus, are relatively rare. These anomalies are also believed to be of little, if any, clinical significance unless the artery passes between the aorta and main pulmonary artery, where its potential compression by these two large vessels may cause regional ischemia. This mechanism has been proposed as the cause of sudden cardiac death, particularly when found in young individuals performing athletic stress.[126] The existence of a double coronary orifice in the left sinus with a clearly separate origin of the left circumflex and left anterior descending artery occurs in slightly less than 1% of human hearts and poses problems for selective catheterization similar to those encountered with an extremely short left coronary main stem.

Other rare abnormalities include single right or left coronary artery, origin of a branch from a noncoronary cusp, and origin of the left anterior descending artery from the right coronary artery. Although compatible with normal arterial supply of the myocardium, these conditions have a tendency to coexist with other congenital cardiac abnormalities.[127]

CLINICAL INDICATIONS

Selective coronary arteriography is most frequently performed in adult patients with suspected or manifested symptoms of ischemic heart disease. It identifies and char-

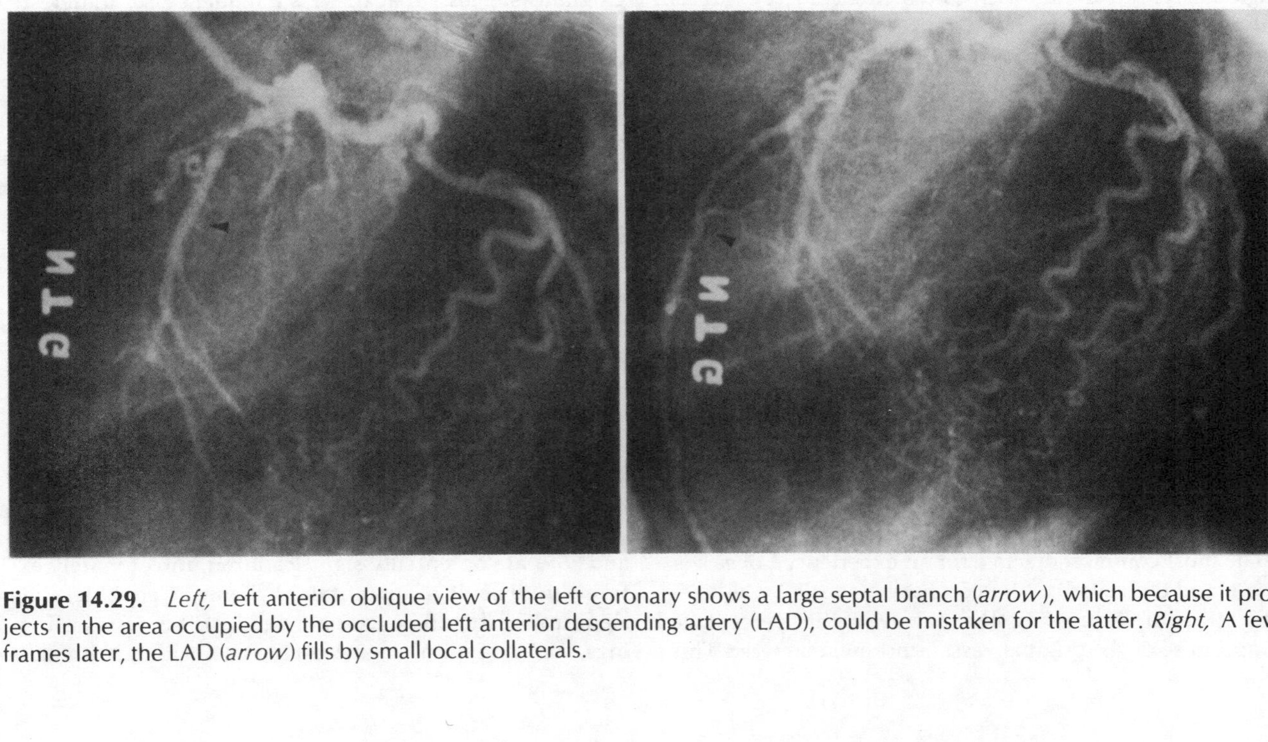

Figure 14.29. *Left,* Left anterior oblique view of the left coronary shows a large septal branch (*arrow*), which because it projects in the area occupied by the occluded left anterior descending artery (LAD), could be mistaken for the latter. *Right,* A few frames later, the LAD (*arrow*) fills by small local collaterals.

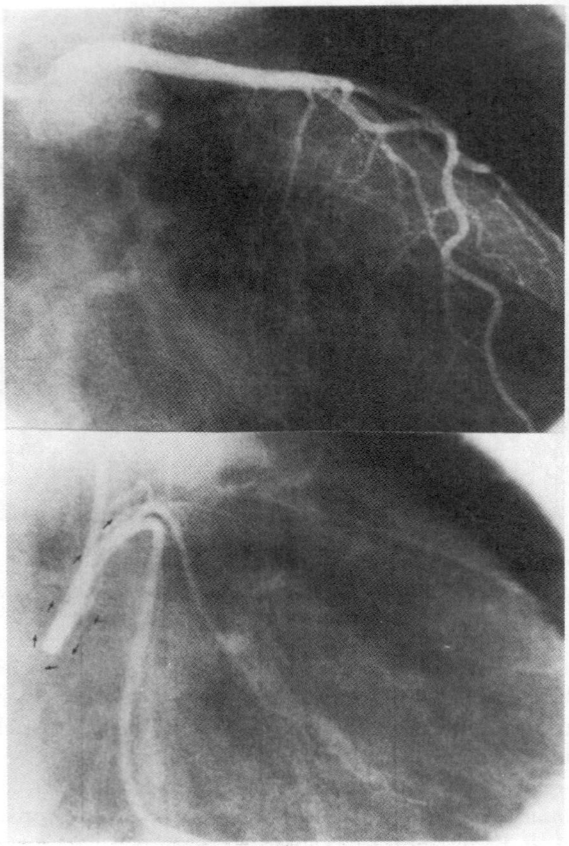

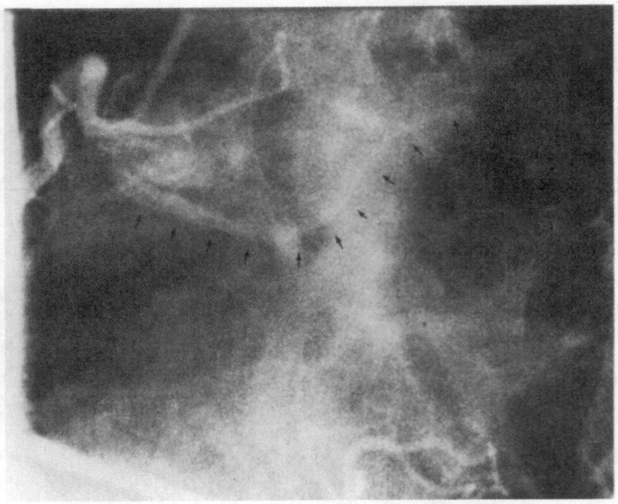

Figure 14.30. *Top left,* Right anterior oblique view of a left coronary injection shows the left anterior descending artery and branches, but no circumflex artery. A search in the left cusp was unrewarding. *Top right,* Left anterior oblique view of the right coronary injection flash fills the circumflex (*arrows*). *Bottom left,* Right anterior oblique view of the injection of the circumflex, which shared a common orifice with the right coronary. Note its posterior course (*arrows*).

acterizes obstructive lesions, whether arteriosclerotic stenoses, thrombosis, embolic occlusions, or spasm. In addition to identifying the presence and extent of coronary artery disease, the angiogram is evaluated in an effort to assess the functional impairment of the circulation. For this purpose, the angiogram serves to grade the severity of luminal compromise, evaluate contrast filling and runoff distal to a stenosis, determine the adequacy of collateral supply, and identify the suitability for bypass or angioplasty. In patients with convincing clinical evidence for myocardial ischemia and no fixed anatomic arterial lesions, additional coronary angiograms under ergonovine challenge may be able to bring out coronary spasm.[128]

Coronary arteriography is increasingly used in acute myocardial infarction to identify a thrombotic occlusion and to monitor the efficacy of selective or intravenous administration of thrombolytic agents. It also identifies underlying stenotic lesions that may require subsequent interventions in the form of angioplasty or bypass surgery.

Selective coronary arteriography may also be performed when ischemic heart disease is not suspected, to document the status of the coronary arteries preoperatively in patients undergoing valve replacement or repair of congenital defects.

DETERMINATION OF THE SIGNIFICANCE OF STENOSIS

The most common practice for an experienced observer is to grade the severity of a coronary stenosis by subjective estimate, expressing the narrowing in percentage compromise of the original vessel's normal diameter. This method suffers from inaccuracies and known inter- and intraobserver variations.[129] One cause for error is the frequently eccentric nature of these lesions, which might be underestimated if not viewed in profile and in several projections. Other important causes are the presence of multiple lesions, varying length of the stenosis, involvement of side branch takeoffs, and last but not least, technical factors related to exposure and intensity of contrast filling. Postmortem correlation with in vivo coronary angiograms suggests that there is a tendency for underestimation of lesions in the clinically performed examination.[130,131]

Assuming a perfectly concentric lesion, a 50% diameter reduction reduces the cross-sectional area of a vessel by 75%, and a 75% diameter reduction correspondingly by 90%. Although it has been shown experimentally that an 85% diameter reduction is required to reduce regional flow in the resting state,[132,133] it can be confidently assumed that lesser degrees of stenosis may cause transient ischemia during situations of increased flow, for example, physical exercise. Based on results of numerous experimental studies as well as correlations of clinical symptoms with angiographic findings, lesions of 75% or greater diameter reduction are considered significant. If they are associated with visibly delayed or decreased contrast flow in the distal vessel, they should be considered to impair arterial flow at rest as well.[134,135]

Lesions of lesser degree and judged to be between 50% and 75% are potentially significant but unfortunately extremely difficult to quantitate. Whenever possible, their significance should be corroborated by other tests or findings, such as typical angina pectoris coinciding with electrocardiographic changes or myocardial scanning with thallium 201 during exercise and rest. Lesions interpreted as less than 50% are considered to be not significant for clinical manifestations of regional myocardial ischemia, unless their diameter reduction has been underestimated due to generalized narrowing of the entire vessel.[136,137]

Clearly, a more precise method to identify the hemodynamic significance of coronary arterial stenosis would be desirable. Efforts in this direction have been made for more precise measurement of arterial calibers and luminal dimensions using computerized densitometry.[138–140]

REFERENCES

1. Christensen EE, Curry TS, Dowdy JE: *An Introduction to the Physics of Diagnostic Radiology*, ed 3. Philadelphia, Lea & Febiger, 1984.
2. Friesinger GC, Adams DF, Bourassa MG, Carlsson E, Elliott LP, Gessner IH, Greenspan RH, Grossman W, Judkins MP, Kennedy JW, Sheldon WC: Report of the Inter-Society Commission for Heart Disease Resources. Optimal resources for examination of the heart and lungs: cardiac catheterization and radiographic facilities. *Circulation* 1983; 68: 893A-930A.
3. Levin D, Dunham L: Angiography: principles underlying proper utilization of radiologic and cineangiographic equipment, in Grossman W (ed): *Cardiac Catheterization and Angiography,* ed 2. Philadelphia, Lea & Febiger, 1980, pp 11–24.
4. Marco R, Paulin S: Angiography: principles underlying utilization of radiologic and cineangiographic equipment, in Grossman W (ed): *Cardiac Catheterization and Angiography,* ed 3. Philadelphia, Lea & Febiger, 1986, pp 14–29.
5. Levin DC, Schapiro RM, Boxt LM, Dunham L, Harrington DP, Ergun DL: Digital subtraction angiography: principles and pitfalls of image improvement techniques. *Am J Roentgenol* 1984; 143:447–454.
6. Harrington DP, Boxt LM, Murray PD: Digital subtraction angiography: overview of technical principles. *Am J Roentgenol* 1982; 139:781–786.
7. Moore RJ: *The Physics of Cardiac Angiography.* Riverside, California, Myrle Co Enterprises Inc, 1985, pp 1–12.
8. Bogren HG, Bursch JH: Digital angiography in the diagnosis of congenital heart disease. *Cardiovasc Intervent Radiol* 1984; 7:180–188.
9. Buonocore E, Pavlicek W, Modic MT, Meaney TF, O'Donovan PB, Grossman LB, Moodie DS, Yiannikas J: Anatomic and functional imaging of congenital heart disease with digital subtraction angiography. *Radiology* 1983; 147:647–654.
10. Carey PH, Slutsky RA, Ashburn WL, Higgins CB: Validation of cardiac output estimates by digital video subtraction angiography in dogs. *Radiology* 1984; 143:623–626.
11. Higgins CB, Norris BL, Gerber KH: Quantitation of left ventricular dimensions and function by digital video subtraction angiography. *Radiology* 1982; 144:461–469.
12. Wasserman AG, Johnson RA, Katz RJ, Leiboff RH, Bren GB, Varghese J, Ross AM: Detection of left ventricular wall motion abnormalities for the diagnosis of coronary artery disease: a comparison of exercise radionuclide and pacing intravenous digital ventriculography. *Am J Cardiol* 1984; 54:497–501.
13. Engels PHC, Ludwig JW, Verhoeven LAJ: Left ventricle evaluation by digital video subtraction angiocardiography. *Radiology* 1982; 144:471–474.
14. Kruger RA: A method for time domain filtering using computerized fluoroscopy. *Med Phys* 1981; 8:466–470.
15. Brody W, Macovski A: Dual-complete energy digital radiography. *Diagn Imaging* 1981: 3:18–25.
16. Riederer SJ, Enzmann DR, Brody WR, Hall AL: The application of matched filtering to contrast material dose reduction in digital subtraction angiography. *Radiology* 1983; 147:853–858.
17. Riederer SJ, Brody WR, Enzmann DR, Hall AL, Maier JK: Work in progress: the application of temporal filtering techniques to hybrid subtraction in digital subtraction angiography. *Radiology* 1983: 147:859–862.
18. Kruger RA, Nelson JA, Ghosh-Roy D, Miller FJ, Anderson RE, Liu P: Dynamic tomographic digital subtraction angiography using temporal filtration. *Radiology* 1983; 147:863–867.
19. Moore RJ: *The Physics of Cardiac Angiography*. Riverside, California, Myrle Co Enterprises, Inc, 1985, pp 7, 8.
20. Balter S, Sones FM, Brancato R: Radiation exposure to the operator performing cardiac angiography with U-arm systems. *Circulation* 1978; 58:925–932.
21. Reuter FG: Physician and patient exposure during cardiac catheterization. *Circulation* 1978; 58:134–139.
22. Freeman LM, Blaufox MD (eds): *Physicians' Desk Reference for Radiology and Nuclear Medicine 1979/1980.* Oradell, NJ, Medical Economics Co, 1979.
23. Malsky SJ, Roswit B, Reid CB, Haft J: Radiation exposure to personnel during cardiac catheterization. *Radiology* 1971; 100:671–674.
24. Wholey MH: Clinical dosimety during the angiographic examination. Comments on coronary arteriography. *Circulation* 50:627–631.
25. Iseri LT, Kaplan MA, Evans MJ: Effect of concentrated contrast media during angiography on plasma volume and plasma osmolality. *Am Heart J* 1965; 69:154–158.
26. Hammermeister KE, Warbasse JR: Immediate hemodyanmic effects of cardiac angiography in man. *Am J Cardiol* 1973; 31:307–314.
27. Cohn PF, Horn HR, Teichholz LE: Effects of angiographic contrast medium on left ventricular function in coronary artery disease. Comparison with static and dynamic exercise. *Am J Cardiol* 1973; 32:21–26.
28. Fischer HW: Hemodynamic reactions to angiographic media: a survey and commentary. *Radiology* 1968; 91:66–73.
29. Wolf GL, Draft L, Kilzer K: Contrast agents lower ventricular fibrillation threshold. *Radiology* 1978; 29:215–217.
30. Adams DF, Paulin S: Effect of radiographic contrast media in selective injections into the sinus node artery. An experimental study in dogs. *Radiology* 1968; 91:719–724.
31. Gensini GG, Di Giorgi S: Myocardial toxicity of contrast agents used in angiography. *Radiology* 1964; 82:24-33.
32. Paulin S, Adams DF: Increased ventricular fibrillation during coronary arteriography with a new contrast preparation. *Radiology* 1971; 101:45–50.
33. Swartz RD, Rubin JE, Leeming BW, Silva P: Renal failure following major angiography. *Am J Med* 1978; 65:31–37.

33a. Taliercio CP, Vliestra RE, Fisher LD, Burnett JC: Risks for renal dysfunction with cardiac angiography. *Ann Intern Med* 1986; 104:501–504.

34. Ansell G: Adverse reactions to contrast agents. Scope of problem. *Invest Radiol* 1970; 5:374–385.
35. Rappaport S, Bookstein JJ, Higgins CB, Carey PH, Sovak T, Lasser EC: Experience with metrizamide in patients with previous severe anaphylactoid reactions to ionic contrast agents. *Radiology* 1982; 143:321–325.
36. Almen T: Development of nonionic contrast media. *Invest Radiol* 1985; 20(suppl):1–9.
37. Bjork L, Eldh P, Paulin S: Non-ionic and dimeric contrast media in coronary angiography. *Acta Radiol (Diagn) (Stock)* 1977; 18:235–240.
38. Serur JR, Als AV, Miner-Green J, Paulin S: Comparative effects of three radiographic contrast agents in isolated normal and ischemic canine hearts. *Invest Radiol* 1980; 15(6 suppl):s196–202.
39. Serur JR, Als AV, Paulin S: Experimental myocardial ischemia. II. Radiographic contrast media toxicity. *Cardiovasc Intervent Radiol* 1982; 5:211–218.
40. Putman CE, (ed): A worldwide clinical assessment of a new nonionic contrast medium: Iohexol. *Invest Radiol* 1985: 20:s1–s121.
41. Adams DF, Fraser DB, Abrams HL: The complications of coronary arteriography. *Circulation* 1973; 48:609–617.
42. Kennedy JW, Baxley WA, Bunnel IL, Gensini GG, Messer JV, Mudd JG, Noto TJ, Paulin S, Pichard AD, Sheldon WC, Cohen M: Complications associated with cardiac catheterization and angiography. *Cathet Cardiovasc Diagn* 1982; 8:5–11.
43. Judkins MP, Gander MP: Prevention of complications of coronary arteriography. *Circulation* 1974; 49:599–602.
44. Bourassa MG, Noble J: Complication rate of coronary arteriography. A review of 5250 cases studied by a percutaneous femoral technique. *Circulation* 1976; 53:106–114.
45. Adams DF, Abrams HL: Complications of coronary arteriography: a follow-up report. *Cardiovasc Radiol* 1979; 2:83–96.
46. Gupta PK, Haft JI: Complete heart block complicating cardiac catheterization. *Chest* 1972: 61:185–187.
47. Eyer KM: Complications of transfemoral coronary arteriography and their prevention using heparin. *Am Heart J* 1973; 86:428.
48. Davis K, Kennedy JR, Kemp HG: Complications of coronary arteriography from the collaborative study of coronary artery surgery (CASS). *Circulation* 1979; 59:1105–1112.
49. Grossman W, Cardiac catheterization by direct exposure of artery and vein, in Grossman W (ed): *Cardiac Catheterization and Angiography*, ed 3. Philadelphia, Lea & Febiger, 1986, pp 45–59.
50. Seldinger SI: Catheter replacement of the needle in percutaneous arteriography. *Acta Radiol* 1953; 39:368–376.
51. Brockenbrough EC, Braunwald E: A new technic for left ventricular angiocardiography and transseptal left heart catheterization. *Am J Cardiol* 1960; 6:1062–1064.

51a. Cheng TO, Bashour T, Kelser GA: Complete heart block occurring during right heart catheterization in a patient with left bundle branch block and a prolonged PR interval studied by bundle of His recording and atrial pacing. *Med Annals of Dist Columbia* 1972; 41:742–743.

52. Bargeron LM, Elliott LP, Soto B, Bream PR, Curry GC: Axial cinean-

giography in congenital heart disease. Sect I. Concept, technical and anatomic considerations. *Circulation* 1977; 56:1075–1083.

53. Elliot LP, Bargeron LM, Bream PR, Soto B, Curry GC: Axial cineangiography in congenital heart diease. Sect II. Specific lesions. *Circulation* 1977; 56:1084–1093.
54. Fellows KE, Keane JR, Freed MD: Angled view in cineangiography of congenital heart disease. *Circulation* 1977; 56:485–490.
55. Van Praagh R, Weinberg PM, Van Praagh S: Malposition of the heart, in AJ Moss, Adams FH, Emmanoulides GC (eds): *Heart Disease in Infants, Children and Adolescents,* ed 3. Baltimore, Williams & Wilkins, 1983, pp 422–458.
56. Van Praagh R: The segmental approach to diagnosis in congenital heart disease. *Birth Defects* 1972; 8:4.
57. Shinebourne EA, Macartney FJ, Anderson RH: Sequential chamber localization: logical approach to diagnosis in congenital heart disease. *Br Heart J* 1976; 38:327–340.
58. Campbell M, Hillis TH: Angiocardiography in cyanotic congenital heart disease. *Br Heart J* 1950; 12:65–72.
59. Noonan JA, Nada AS: The hypoplastic left heart syndrome. *Pediat Clin North Am* 1958; 5:1029.
60. Noonan JA: Hypoplastic left ventricle, in, Moss AJ, Adams FH, Emmanoulides GC (eds): *Heart Disease in Infants, Children and Adolescents,* ed 2. Baltimore, Williams & Wilkins, 1977, pp 430–436.
61. Elliot LP, Adams P Jr, Edwards JE: Pulmonary atresia with intact ventricular septum. *Br Heart J* 1963; 25:489–501.
62. Ellis K, Casarella WJ, Hayes CJ, Gersong WM, Bowman FO, Malm JR: Pulmonary atresia with intact ventricular septum. *Am J Roentgenol* 1972; 116:501–513.
63. Lauer RM, Fink HP, Petry EL, Dunn MI, Diehl AM: Angiographic demonstration of intramyocardial sinusoids in pulmonary valve atresia with intact ventricular septum and hypoplastic right ventricle. *N Engl J Med* 1964; 271:68–72.
64. Fellows KE, Smith J, Keane JF: Preoperative angiocardiography in infants with tetrad of Fallot. Review of 36 cases. *Am J Cardiol* 1981; 47:1279–1285.
65. Freedom RM, Culham JAG, Rowe RD: Angiocardiography of subaortic obstruction in infancy. *Am J Roentgenol* 1977; 29:813–824.
66. Rosengart R, Jarmakani JM, Emmanoulides GC: Single film retrograde umbilical aortography in the diagnosis of hypoplastic left heart syndrome with aortic atresia. *Circulation* 1976; 54:345-357.
67. Jönsson G, Brodén B, Karnell J: Thoracic aortography, with special reference to its value in patent ductus arteriosus and coarctation of the aorta. *Acta Radiol* 1951; suppl 89:1–17.
68. Neufeld HN, Lester RG, Adams P Jr, Anderson RC, Lillehei CW, Edwards JE: Congenital communications of a coronary artery with a cardiac chamber or the pulmonary trunk. *Circulation* 1961; 24:171–179.
69. Edwards JE: The direction of blood flow in coronary arteries arising from the pulmonary trunk. *Circulation* 1964; 29:163–166.
70. White RJ: The nature and significance of anomalous coronary arteries in tetrology of Fallot. *Am J Roentgenol* 1972; 114:350–354.
71. Moses D, Silver T, Bookstein J: The complementary roles of chest radiography, lung scanning and selective pulmonary angiography in the diagnosis of pulmonary embolism. *Circulation* 1974; 49:179–188.
72. Bookstein JJ, Silver TM: The angiographic differential diagnosis of acute pulmonary embolism. *Radiology* 1974; 110:25–33.
73. Miscall L, Duffy RW: Surgical treatment of bullous emphysema: contributions of angiocardiography. *Dis Chest* 1953; 24:489.
74. Dines D, Arms R, Bernetz P, Gomes M: Pulmonary arteriovenous fistulas. *Mayo Clin Proc* 1974; 49:460–465.
75. White RI, Kaufman SL, Barth KH, DeCaprioV, Strandbert JD: Embolotherapy with detachable silicone balloons. *Radiology* 1979; 131:619–627.
76. Jaffe R, Condon V: Mycotic aneurysms of the pulmonary artery and aorta. *Radiology* 1975; 116:291–298.
77. Monchik R, Wilkins E Jr: Solitary aneurysm of the middle lobe artery. A case report and review of solitary peripheral pulmonary artery aneurysms. *Ann Thorac Surg* 1974; 17:496–504.
78. Lupi HE, Sanchez TH, Horowitz S, Gutierrez E: Pulmonary artery involvement in Takayasu's arteritis. *Chest* 1975; 67:69–74.
79. Sprayregen S: Radiologic spectrum of arteriosclerotic aneurysms of the aortic arch. *NY State J Med* 1978; 78:2198–2204.
80. Conde CA, Meller J, Donoso E, Dack S: Bacterial endocarditis with ruptured sinus of valsalva and aortocardiac fistula. *Am J Cardiol* 1975; 35:912–917.
81. Elsen S, Elliott LP: The roentgenology of cystic medial necrosis of the ascending aorta. *Radiol Clin North Am* 1968: 6:437–450.
82. Itzchak Y, Rosenthal T, Adar R, Zallman JR, Lieberman Y, Deutsch V: Dissecting aneurysm of thoracic aorta: reappraisal of radiologic diagnosis. *Am J Roentgenol* 1975: 125:559–570.
83. Gazzaniga AB, Khuri El, Mir-Sepasi HM, Bartlett RH: Rupture of the thoracic aorta following blunt trauma. *Arch Surg* 1975; 110:1119–1123.
84. Sanborn J, Heitzman E, Markarian B: Traumatic rupture of the thoracic aorta: roentgenographic-pathologic correlations. *Radiology* 1970; 95:293–298.
85. Baron MG: The angiocardiographic diagnosis of valvular stenosis. *Circulation* 1971; 44:143–154.
86. Roberts WC, Elliott LP: Lesions complicating the congenitally bicuspid aortic valve. Anatomic and radiographic features. *Radio Clin North Am* 1968; 6:409–421.
87. Roberts WC: Valvular, subvalvular and supravalvular aortic stenosis. Morphologic features. *Cardiovasc Clin* 1973; 5(1):97–126.
88. Beuren AJ, Schulze C, Eberle P, Harmjanz D, Apitz J: The syndrome of supravalvular aortic stenosis, peripheral pulmonary stenosis, mental retardation and similar facial appearance. *Am J Cardiol* 1964; 13:471–483.
89. Kurlander GJ, Petry EL, Taybi H, Lurie Pr, Campbell JA: Supravalvar aortic stenosis. Roentgen analysis of twenty-seven cases. *Am J Roentgenol* 1966; 98:782–799.
90. Lehman JS, Boyle JJ, Debbas JN: Quantitation of aortic valvular insufficiency by catheter thoracic aortography. *Radiology* 1962; 79:361–370.
91. Wilson WJ, Amplatz K, Everhart F: Cinefluorographic study of prosthetic cardiac valves. *Radiology* 1967; 88:779–783.
92. Cihak RJ, Dinsmore RE: A simple method of recording and measuring prosthetic cardiac valve motion. *Radiology* 1971; 98:187–189.
93. Hipona RA, Lerona PT, Paredes S: Radiologic diagnosis of late complications associated with cardiac valve surgery in acquired heart disease. *Radiol Clin North Am* 1971; 9:265–283.
94. Ferris EJ, Smith PL, Mirza FH, Fungar WT, Seiber JJ, Kalderon A, Jeminez JF: Intralobar pulmonary sequestration: Value of aortography and pulmonary angiography. *Cardiovasc Intervent Radiol* 1981; 4:17–23.
95. Als AV, Paulin S, Aroesty JM: Biplane angiographic volumetry using the right anterior oblique and half-axial left anterior oblique technique. *Radiology* 1978; 126:511–514.
96. Elliott LP, Green SE, Rogers MJ, Hood WP, Mantle JA, Papapietro SE: Advantages of the caudocranial left anterior oblique left ventriculogram in adult heart disease. *Am J Cardiol* 1982; 49:369–380.
97. Sandor T, Paulin S, Hanlon WB: Left ventricular wall motion analysis using operator-independent contour positioning. *Comput Biomed Res* 1984; 17:129–142.
98. Dyke SH, Cohn PF, Gorlin R, Sonnenblick EH: Detection of residual myocardial function in coronary artery disease using post-extrasystolic potentiation. *Circulation* 1974; 50:694–699.
99. Pasternac A, Gorlin R, Sonnenblick EH, Kemp HG: Abnormalities of ventricular motion induced by atrial pacing in coronary artery disease. *Circulation* 1972; 45:1195–1205.
100. Vlodaver Z, Coe JI, Edwards JE: True and false ventricular aneurysms. Propensity for the latter to rupture. *Circulation* 1975; 51:567–572.
101. Miller SW, Dinsmore RE, Greene RE, Daggett WM: Coronary, ventricular and pulmonary abnormalities associated with rupture of the interventricular septum complicating myocardial infarction. *Am J Roentgenol* 1978; 131:571–577.
102. Burch GE DePasquale NP, Phillips JH: The syndrome of papillary muscle dysfunction. *Am Heart J* 1968; 75:399–415.
103. Morrow AG, Cohen LS, Roberts WC, Braunwald NS, Braunwald E: Severe mitral regurgitation following acute myocardial infarction and ruptured papillary muscle. Hemodyamic findings and results of operative treatment in four patients. *Circulation* 1968; 37(suppl 2): II-124–II-132.
104. Buonocore E, Acker JJ, Blake HA: Non-rheumatic acute mitral insufficiency caused by ruptured chordae tendineae. *Am J Roentgenol* 1976; 12:336–343.
105. Davies MJ, Moore BP, Braimbridge MV: The floppy mitral valve. Study of incidence, pathology and complications in surgical, necropsy and forensic material. *Br Heart J* 1978; 40:468–481.
106. Anderson RE, Grondin C, Amplatz K: The mitral valve in Marfan's syndrome. *Radiology* 1968; 91:910–914.
107. Jeresaty RM: Ballooning of the mitral valve leaflets. *Radiology* 1971; 100:45–52.
108. Markiewicz W, Stoner J, London E, Hunt SA, Popp RL: Mitral valve prolapse in one hundred presumably healthy young females. *Circulation* 1976; 53:464–473.
109. Ranganathen RN, Silver MD, Robinson TI, Wilson JK: Idiopathic prolapsed mitral leaflet syndrome. Angiographic clinical correlations. *Circulation* 1976; 54:707–716.
110. Demany MA, Kay EB, Zimmerman HA: An angiocardiographic sign for the evaluation of the stenotic mitral valve. *Am J Cardiol* 1966; 18:843–846.
111. Adelman AG, McLoughlin MJ, Marquis Y, Auger P, Wigle ED: Left ventricular cineangiographic observations in muscular subaortic stenosis. *Am J Cardiol* 1969; 24:689–697.
112. Braunwald E, Morrow AG, Cornell WP, Aygen MM, Hilbish TF: Idiopathic hypertrophic subaortic stenosis. Clinical, hemodynamic and angiographic manifestations. *Am J Med* 1960; 29:924–945.
113. Shone JD, Sellers RD, Anderson RC, Adam P, Lillehei CW, Edwards JE: The developmental complex of "parachute mitral valve" supravalvular ring of left atrium, subaortic stenosis, and coarctation of aorta. *Am J Cardiol* 1963; 11:715–725.

114. Nonogi HM, Sasayama S, Sakurai T, Kawai C, Fujita M, Eiho S, Kuwahara M: Intravenous left ventriculography utilizing digital subtraction technique. *Jpn Circ J* 1984; 48:559–566.
115. Goldberg HL, Moses JW, Borer JS, Fisher J, Tamari I, Skelly NT, Cohen B: Exercise left ventriculography utilizing intravenous digital angiography. *Am J Coll Cardiol* 1983: 2:1092–1098.
116. Johnson RA, Wasserman AG, Leiboff RH, Katz RJ, Bren GB, Varghese J, Ross AM: Intravenous digital left ventriculography at rest and with atrial pacing as a screening procedure for coronary artery disease. *Am Coll Cardiol* 1983: 2:905–910.
117. Levin DC, Baltaxe HA: Angiographic demonstration of important anatomic variations of the posterior descending coronary artery. *Am J Roentgenol* 1972; 116:41–49.
118. Bunnell IL, Greene DG, Tandon RN, Arana DT: The half-axial projection. A new look at the proximal left coronary artery. *Circulation* 1973; 48:1151–1156.
119. Lesperance J, Saltiel J, Petitclerc R, Bourassa MG: Angulated views in the sagittal plane for improved accuracy of cinecoronary angiograph. *Am J Roentgenol* 1974; 121:565–574.
120. Sos T, Lee JG, Levin DC, Baltaxe HA: New lordotic projection for improved visualization of the left coronary artery and its branches. *Am J Roentgenol* 1974; 121:575–582.
121. Elliott LP, Bream PR, Soto B, Russell RO, Rogers WJ, Mantle RJ, Hood WP Jr: Significance of the caudal left-anterior-oblique view in analyzing the left main coronary artery and its major branches. *Radiology* 1981; 139:39–43.
122. Elliott LP, Green CE, Rogers WJ, Mantle JA, Papapietro SE, Hood WP, Russel RO: Advantage of the cranial-right anterior oblique view in diagnosing mid left anterior descending and distal right coronary artery disease. *Am J Cardiol* 1981; 48:754–764.
123. Banchi A: Mortfologia della arteriae coronarial cordis. *Arch Ital Anat Embriol* 1904; 3:87.
124. Engel HJ, Toerres C, and Page HLR: Major variations in anatomical origin of the coronary arteries: angiographic observations in 4250 patients without associated congenital heart disease. *Cathet Cardiovasc Diagn* 1975; 1:157–169.
125. Page HL, Engle HJ, Campbell WB, Thomas CS: Anomalous origin of the left circumflex coronary artery. Recognition, angiographic demonstration and clinical significance. *Circulation* 1974; 50:768–773.
126. Benson PA: Anomalous aortic origin of coronary artery with sudden death: case report and review. *Am Heart J* 1970; 79:254–257.
127. Kelley MJ, Wolfson S, and Marshall R: Single coronary artery from the right sinus of Valsalva: angiography, anatomy, and clinical significance. *Am J Roentgenol* 1977; 128:257–262.
128. Rich S, Ford LE, Al-Sadir J: The angiographic effect of ergonovine and nifedipine in coronary artery spasm. *Circulation* 1980; 62:1127–1130.
129. Zir LM, Miller SW, Dinsmore RE, Gilbert JP, Harthorne JW: Interobserver variability in coronary angiography. *Circulation* 1976; 53:627–632.
130. Staiger J, Dieckmann H, Adler CP, Adler CP, Barmeyer J: Postmortem angiographic and pathologic–anatomic findings in coronary heart disease: a comparative study using planimetry. *Cardiovasc Interven Radiol* 1980; 3:1–143.
131. Vlodaver Z, Frech R, Van Tassel RA, Edwards JE: Correlation of the antemortem coronary arteriogram and the postmortem specimen. *Circulation* 1973; 47:162–169.
132. Gould KL, Lipscomb K: Effects of coronary stenoses on coronary flow reserve and resistance. *Am J Cardiol* 1974; 34:48–55.
133. Gould KL, Lipscomb K, Hamilton GW: Physiologic basis for assessing critical coronary stenosis. *Am J Cardiol* 1974; 33:87–94.
134. Robbins SL, Bentor J: The kinetics of viscous flow in a model. Effect of stenoses of varying size, shape and length. *Lab Invest* 1967; 16:864–874.
135. Feldman RL, Nichols WW, Penpine CJ, Conti CR: Hemodynamic significance of the length of a coronary arterial narrowing. *Am J Cardiol* 1978; 41:865–871.
136. Paulin S: Functional alterations in the coronary circulation as mirrored in the angiogram. *Cardiovasc Intervent Radiol* 1982; 5:177–185.
137. Paulin S: Grading and measuring coronary artery stenoses. *Cath Cardiovasc Diagn* 1979; 5:213–218.
138. Sandor T, Sridhar B, Paulin S: Remote densitometric analysis of stenotic lesions. *Int J Biomed Comput* 1979; 10(1):15–22.
139. Nichols AB, Gabrieli CFO, Fenoglio JJ Jr, Esser PD: Quantification of relative coronary arterial stenosis by cinevideodensitometric analysis of coronary arteriograms. *Circulation* 1984; 69:512–522.
140. Spears JR, Sandor T, Als AV, Malagold M, Markis JE, Grossman W, Serur JR, Paulin S: Computerized image analysis for quantitative measurement of vessel diameter from cineangiograms. *Circulation* 1983; 68:453–461.

15 Cardiovascular Applied Physiology and Pathophysiology

Richard J. Bing, MD

Advances in cardiac pathophysiology over the last 30 years have been made primarily in two directions: cardiac metabolism and cardiac contractility. These terms are used here in a general sense. For example, cardiac metabolism covers such divergent fields as myocardial utilization of foodstuffs, intracellular pathways of proteins, and carbohydrate and lipid utilization in relation to cellular structure; it also includes biochemistry and the function of cellular membrane structures that are closely connected to calcium movements.[1-4] These play an important role in the process of excitation-contraction coupling and hence in cardiac contractility and myocardial failure. Functions of membrane structures as related to calcium transport have become a most rewarding and rapidly expanding field in the study of the physiologic and pathophysiologic aspects of heart muscle. Beginning with Ringer's discovery of the role of calcium in cardiac excitation, the study of cellular membrane systems of the cardiac muscle cell has finally begun to yield some clues as to the mechanisms of myocardial failure.[5] As in any coherent organic structure, all metabolic functions are interdependent. Intermediary metabolism and the functions of membranes and contractile proteins represent an organic unit. Any functional disturbance in these structures leads to malfunction of the whole organ and the family of organs, the organism.

This chapter is mainly concerned with mechanisms that form the basis of myocardial failure and myocardial ischemia. These topics were selected because they affect all phases of cardiac metabolism, including membrane function and myocardial contractility. They also involve various facets of the pathophysiologic aspects of the heart. Therefore, no attempt was made to separate physiologic from pathologic processes. The keys to their understanding are identical.

MYOCARDIAL FAILURE

HISTORICAL CONSIDERATIONS

Failure of the circulation has been described for more than 200 years, and only recently has a beginning been made in the understanding of its underlying cellular mechanisms. In contrast, the fundamental cellular aspects of myocardial ischemia and myocardial infarction could be accurately defined during the last 20 years because myocardial ischemia has a specific and well-defined cause. In addition, animal models for the study of regional myocardial ischemia are easily available, but myocardial failure is difficult to reproduce in animals, and no models exist that resemble the picture of congestive heart failure as seen under clinical conditions. Knowledge of myocardial failure (clinically expressed as congestive heart failure) has passed through three stages. The first is represented by the work of the great clinicians of the last century and the beginning of this one, among them Lancisi, Hope Lewis, Harrison, White, and McMichael.[6-11a] The second phase was ushered in by the cardiac catheter, which has made possible the exploration of pressure and flow relations.[12] The third phase, which is still under way, began with studies in cardiac metabolism, first using intubation of the coronary sinus and later biochemical and biophysical studies including the role of Ca^{++} and cellular membrane systems.[13] Knowledge of myocardial failure derived in the precatheterization era is well represented in a chapter on congestive heart failure by White[10] in 1937, where he summarizes the clinical impression that "heart failure is shown by congestion behind the weakened chamber."

The advent of the cardiac catheter in the 1940s placed emphasis on hemodynamic measurements, specifically cardiac output, venous pressure, and peripheral vasoconstriction.[11a,12] This was also the period in which salt and water retention by the kidney was first emphasized.[14] Recordings of right ventricular and pulmonary artery pressure led Cournand and Richards[12] to state that incomplete emptying during systole is a characteristic feature of congestive heart failure in man, a finding that was later extended to direct measurements of the residual volume in the right ventricle.[15] Determination of ejection fraction has currently become an important noninvasive procedure.

Coronary sinus intubation revealed that extraction of foodstuffs by the heart of patients in congestive heart failure is not different from that by the nonfailing heart; this suggested the absence of major disturbances in cardiac energy production, a finding that was later confirmed.[16]

The third period is concerned with the role of Ca^{++} transport in heart muscle cells and with the regulatory role of cellular membrane systems, primarily sarcolemma and sarcoplasmic reticulum.[17,18] Movement of Ca^{++} across the sarcolemma of myocardial cells is an essential event in excitation-contraction coupling.[1] Ca^{++} enters the myocardial cell mainly by a slow influx of Ca^{++} during the plateau phase of the action potential.[19] Ca^{++} antagonists reduce the transmembrane Ca^{++} influx through the slow channel selectively. Myocardial beta-receptor stimulation results in promotion of slow inward Ca^{++} current. Usually beta$_1$-agonists bind with a protein receptor in the sarcolemmal membrane. This stimulates a cascade of events, leading to activation of adenylate cyclase and an increase in cyclic AMP (c-AMP); protein kinases are activated, and phosphorylation of sarcolemmal proteins results, with a subsequent increase in the number of functionally operating Ca^{++} channels, a rise in the slow inward Ca^{++} current, and a release of Ca^{++} from intracellular stores, resulting in the activation of myofilaments and contraction.[20] The central role of c-AMP controlled by the activation of adenylate cyclase or of phosphodiesterase is crucial in this scheme.[21,22] Interrelated events, from beta$_1$-agonist receptors to adenylate cyclase, c-AMP to phosphorylation of sarcolemmal proteins and opening of Ca^{++} channels, are important in understanding the action of beta$_1$-agonists and other cardiotonic agents. Caffeine and theophylline, like amrinone, increase c-AMP by inhibiting phosphodiesterase.[23–25,25a] Ca^{++} must be leaving the cell to prevent overloading. Heart sarcolemma possesses systems responsible for pumping Ca^{++} out of the cell: an Na^{+}/Ca^{++} exchange and a Ca^{++} pumping ATPase (Ca^{++}/Mg^{++} ATPase).[26,27] This subject will be discussed in the paragraphs dealing with the effect of cardiac glycosides and catecholamines.

MEMBRANE PROPERTIES AND CA++ TRANSPORT

Cell membranes possess definite enzyme patterns that make it possible to check the purity of a specific membrane preparation.[26–29] Some of these enzymes are active in sarcolemmal membranes only, such as (Na^{+}/K^{+}) ATPase, adenylate cyclase, and K^{+}-stimulated p-nitrophenylphosphate (K^{+}-pNPPase).[30] Mitochondria membranes are distinguished by the presence of succinate cytochrome c reductase.[30] A model is available to investigate Ca^{++} transfer across sarcolemmal or sarcoplasmic reticulum membranes in vitro.[31,32] Sarcolemmal vesicles are prepared from heart muscle and are formed and sealed in one of two orientations: either right-side out or inside out. This difference in orientation is important because enzymes may be located only on the inner side of the prepared sarcolemmal vesicle. To determine the sidedness of vesicle preparations, adenylate cyclase activity is usually measured using both untreated and alamethicin-preincubated sarcolemmal preparations.[33] Because adenylate cyclase is an inner-membrane enzyme, its activity can only be measured in inside-out or leaky vesicles. Preincubation with alamethicin, a channel-forming ionophore, disrupts normal membrane barriers, permitting free passage of chemicals and unmasking the activity of enzymes located at the inner membrane of right-side out vesicles. By comparing the levels of adenylate cyclase activity obtained with and without alamethicin, the sidedness of vesicles can be estimated.[33]

Membranes of the sarcoplasmic reticulum possess certain similarities to those of sarcolemma, but they differ in many important respects, particularly in the proteins that are phosphorylated to regulate Ca^{++} translocation.[20,34] This difference is indicated, as already described, by the enzyme system contained in sarcolemmal membranes. Because (Na^{+}/K^{+}) ATPase is absent, slow Ca^{++} channels for movement of Ca^{++} across the sarcolemmal membranes do not exist. Sarcoplasmic reticulum is devoid of ATP-dependent Ca^{++} uptake, which is responsible for the fine tuning of intracellular Ca^{++} concentrations by maintaining low diastolic Ca^{++} concentrations. Most important, sarcoplasmic reticulum has no mechanism for Na^{+}/K^{+} exchange, which in sarcolemma allows the sodium pump to participate in the regulation of myocardial contractility. These differences are the result of the specific role of sarcoplasmic reticulum in Ca^{++} accumulation and release, initiating contraction and relaxation of cardiac muscle.[35] ATP-dependent Ca^{++} accumulation in the absence and presence of permanent ions, such as oxalate, is termed Ca^{++} binding and Ca^{++} uptake, respectively.[35] As in sarcolemma, vesicles of sarcoplasmic reticulum can be prepared in pure form in vitro. These vesicles can serve as useful models.[29,30]

As compared with different Ca^{++} transport mechanisms through the sarcolemmal membrane that regulate Ca^{++} balance between extracellular fluid and the cytosol of the whole cell, sarcoplasmic reticulum membranes serve primarily the purpose of quick storage and release of Ca^{++} during the cardiac cycle. Ca^{++} transport mechanisms across the sarcoplasmic reticulum membranes and are therefore less diverse.[20,36] Sarcoplasmic reticulum has a Ca^{++} pumping ATPase that serves as an energy transducer that translocates Ca^{++} across the sarcoplasmic reticulum membrane.[26,37] Regulation of this ATPase and of the transport of Ca^{++} by parallel c-AMP and calmodulin-dependent protein kinases has received much attention.[37a] Calmodulin binds to Ca^{++}, activating a protein kinase, thus phosphorylating another enzyme or protein. Also involved in the Ca^{++} translocation is a protein discovered by Tada and Katz,[20] phospholamban, which is phosphorylated and catalyzed by an endogenous protein kinase. This protein is a major phosphorylation site at which c-AMP-PK acts in cardiac sarcoplasmic reticulum. The chain of events in Ca^{++} transport in sarcoplasmic reticulum, therefore, involves c-AMP, protein kinase, phospholamban, and Ca^{++} pumping ATPase.[20]

Mitochondria also appear to participate in Ca^{++} regulation of the intracellular concentration of Ca^{++}, but at a slower rate than either sarcolemma or sarcoplasmic reticulum. Mitochondria accumulate Ca^{++}.[34] An abnormally high uptake of Ca^{++} after ischemia and reperfusion ("reperfusion syndrome") depresses mitochondrial respiration.[38] Mitochondrial uptake of Ca^{++} occurs apparently in a manner different from that of sarcolemma and sarcoplasmic reticulum.

CONTRACTILITY IN MYOCARDIAL FAILURE

The essential feature of myocardial failure is depression of contractility.[39-41] Several means have been employed to measure cardiac dynamics, such as force-velocity relation, maximal developed tension (P_0), maximal rate of tension development (dp/dt_{max}), and time to peak tension (t_o).[42,43] Following the example of Szent-Gyorgyi, investigators used the glycerinated heart muscle fibers from normal and failing hearts.[44] In this technique, thin muscle strips are immersed into a glycerin-containing solution and stored for several weeks at −20°C. Fiber bundles are then dissected and suspended in a trough containing relaxing solution. Determination of force-velocity relation and of P_0, dp/dt_{max}, and t_o, and resting (passive) and active length-tension relation is then carried out using quick release and a servo system.[42] The force-velocity relation originally described the relative stable tetanic contraction of frog sartorius muscle; it characterizes the dynamic situation during contraction of cardiac muscle. Katz[22] summarized the controversies focused on the force-velocity relation that led to abandonment of V_{max} for quantifying the state of the myocardium in patients with heart disease. However, these controversies do not apply to the determination of V_{max} in isolated muscle fibers obtained from normal and failing heart muscle.

Cardiac contractions are triggered by Ca^{++}. Tropomyosin, a contractile protein, is able to regulate the interaction between actin and myosin.[22] Troponin, another muscle protein, together with tropomyosin sensitizes actomyosin to changes in micromolar concentration of Ca^{++}. Of importance is the close correlation between the rate of ATP hydrolysis by myosin, which possesses ATPase activity. As Katz[22] has stated, the direct relation between myosin ATPase activity and the maximal shortening velocity of conduction (V_{max}) represents a firm basis for the understanding of myocardial contractility.

MOLECULAR BASIS OF MYOCARDIAL FAILURE

Where then does the break in the chain of events leading to myocardial failure occur? It must be stressed again that the solution to this problem is handicapped by a lack of suitable animal models. In a particular strain of golden hamsters, a congenital cardiomyopathy exists that has been used for the study of myocardial failure.[45] Yet this model is not easily available and may differ in important aspects from myocardial failure in human subjects. Furthermore, congestive heart failure is not a uniform clinical entity; it is a term that is based on a clinical picture. The causes may vary, but the final cause is probably the disturbance in excitation-contraction coupling or of protein synthesis. It has been suggested that redirection of protein synthesis may lead to the appearance of a myosin isoenzyme with low ATPase activity and subtle alterations in amino acid sequence,[46-48] but this attractive theory awaits further proof. As first stated by Meerson[49] in 1962 and later confirmed by Zühlke et al,[50] however, a heart subjected to functional strain passes through a series of metabolic alterations, characterized by changes in myocardial protein synthesis. During the final stages of failure, protein synthesis is inhibited, interfering with the renewal of the energy-producing and contractile structures of the myocardium. Zühlke et al[50] were able to show that substances interfering with protein synthesis induce cardiac failure when administered during experimentally produced cardiac hypertrophy. In all likelihood, doxorubicin produces myocardial failure in a similar fashion.

In a minority of patients, prolonged alcohol ingestion results in severe cardiomyopathy with myocardial failure.[40,51] There is damage to cellular myocardial membrane systems, indicated by inhibition of (N^+/K^+)-activated ATPase. There is loss of contractility as shown in depression of V_{max}, P_0, and dp/dt of glycerinated heart muscle fibers from animals exposed to chronic ethanol.[42] In addition, however, discrete biochemical lesions are discernible such as diminished mitochondrial respiratory function and reduced mitochondrial Ca^{++} uptake and binding.[51] Disturbances in Ca^{++} uptake and binding are also noticeable in sarcoplasmic reticulum. There is diminished fatty acid oxidation with increased esterification.[51] These alterations are reversible following cessation of alcohol administration.[52] Despite these experimentally produced biochemical disturbances, cardiac failure due to chronic alcohol administration has not been produced in animals.

CALCIUM AND MYOCARDIAL FAILURE

What changes in Ca^{++} transfer are present in myocardial failure? In the cardiomyopathic hamster, disturbances in the ATP hydrolyzing ability of sarcolemma are found.[53] Ca^{++}/Mg^{++} ATPase as well as Na^+/K^+ ATPase activity may be affected,[35] but again the lack of a suitable model makes projections to clinical heart failure difficult. Another defect that relates to a disturbance in membrane function is adenylate cyclase activity.[35] This enzyme may be inhibited in experimental left heart failure due to aortic constriction.[35]

Changes in sarcoplasmic reticulum have also been noted in myocardial failure. These changes were detected in spontaneously failing hearts in the heart-lung preparation,[54] but this type of failure is atypical, probably the result of depletion of catecholamines.[55] Relevant are the findings of Harigaya and Schwartz[56] and Lindenmayer et al[57] on heart muscle of patients with congestive heart failure due to ischemic or valvular heart disease. In these conditions either the rate of Ca^{++} uptake or the Ca^{++} uptake capacity by sarcoplasmic reticulum was diminished. A similar situation was encountered by Lee et al[58] in dogs with myocardial ischemia. In cardiomyopathic hamsters, reduction in Ca^{++} uptake by sarcoplasmic reticulum was also noted.

A variety of changes in Ca^{++} uptake by mitochondria of failing hearts have been described. For instance, mitochondria from failing human hearts showed diminished Ca^{++} uptake.[57,59] Dhalla et al[35] concluded that "cardiac contractile failure is associated with dysfunction of one or more membrane systems." It is possible, however, that disturbances in Ca^{++} movement are not the primary cause, but they occur secondary to deficient intracellular protein synthesis.[48] In any case, myocardial failure on the molecular level is a protean condition, with many underlying causes, just as the clinical history of "congestive heart failure" varies. The end result of these events is failure of contractility with deficient emptying of the cardiac chamber and venous engorgement.

MECHANISM OF CARDIOTONIC DRUGS

The mechanism of cardiotonic drugs is intimately concerned with Ca^{++} transport. Digitalis glycosides have remained important in the treatment of myocardial failure. The positive inotropic action of cardiac glycosides is based on its effect on Ca^{++} movement across the sarcolemmal membranes, with a resulting increase in intracellular Ca^{++}. Fozzard and Sheets[60] and Katz[61] recently summarized these effects. As already mentioned, several processes are involved in Ca^{++} transport across the sarcolemmal membranes: the Na^+/Ca^{++} exchange and the Na^+/K^+ ATPase. Another mechanism in the outward transport of Ca^{++} is the Ca^{++} pumping ATPase. This enzyme is partially involved in Ca^{++} ejection during diastole.[37] In the intact cell, this enzyme is responsible for the maintenance of low diastolic Ca^{++} concentrations.[62] The enzyme has a higher Ca^{++} affinity and lower maximal Ca^{++} transport capacity than do Na^+/Ca^{++} exchange mechanisms.[27] Little is known about the effect of glycosides on the activity of Ca^{++}-dependent ATPase.

The Na^+/Ca^{++} exchange is fundamental, because it allows the sodium pump to participate in the regulation of myocardial contractility. It is a countertransport, utilizing the energy available from the movement of Na^+ into the cell to power the transport of Ca^{++} out of the cell against a large electrochemical gradient. The Na^+/Ca^{++} exchange mechanism is characteristic of sarcolemmal membranes; it is not present in membranes prepared from sarcoplasmic reticulum. The velocity of the Na^+/Ca^{++} exchange of sarcolemmal membranes is very high, about 30-fold higher than that of sarcolemmal Ca^{++}/Mg^{++} ATPase.[27]

The Na^+/Ca^{++} exchange mechanism represents the most important means by which Ca^{++} is expelled from the heart muscle cell.[27] Katz[61] has stated that a reduction in the Na^+ gradient can inhibit Ca^{++} influx and lead to a net gain in Ca^{++} in the myocardial cell.

Cardiac glycosides inhibit specifically the activity of Na^+/K^+ adenosine triphosphatase. This enzyme hydrolyzes ATP and transfers the energy derived from ATP hydrolysis to *active* Na^+ and K^+ transport across the sarcolemma.[61] It is now well established that cardiac glycosides, through inhibition of Na^+/K^+ ATPase, increase intracellular Na^+, resulting in a net gain in intracellular Ca^{++}. This increase in intracellular Na^+ interferes with Na^+/Ca^{++} exchange, specifically with the transport of Na^+ out of the cell. Therefore, intracellular Ca^{++} is increased, resulting in positive inotropic action of cardiac glycosides.[61] K^+ decreases the binding of cardiac glycosides to the sodium pump through inhibition of Na^+/K^+ ATPase. These inhibitory effects of cardiac glycosides are partially reversed when extracellular K^+ concentration is increased. Therefore, increasing serum K^+ diminishes intracellular Ca^{++} and relieves the toxic effects of digitalis overdose.[61]

Other positive inotropic agents, such as amrinone and milrinone, or inhibitors of angiotensin converting enzyme, such as captopril or beta-adrenergic drugs, have come to the fore. Of potential but not yet proven value are other beta-adrenergic drugs such as TA-064 and prenalterol.[30,63] Apparently c-AMP is involved in the direct inotropic action of amrinone, increasing c-AMP-activated protein kinases and phosphorylation of membrane proteins, opening Ca^{++} channels, and increasing Ca^{++} flux.[64] Honerjager[64] showed that amrinone produced a three- to four-fold increase in c-AMP content of guinea pig papillary muscle, accomplished by inhibition of phosphodiesterase.

Clinically, $beta_1$-agonists are useful when a rapid increase in myocardial contractility is needed, but there is some question as to their chronic use in myocardial failure. It is doubtful whether the chronically failing heart should be stimulated by beta-adrenergic compounds. LeJemtel and Sonnenblick[65] maintain that short-term administration of a positive inotropic agent can increase ventricular irritation.[65] Continuous positive inotropic therapy may exhaust the limited energy supply of the depressed myocardium.[66] Conversely, partial beta-agonists such as TA-064 have been successfully used in the treatment of chronic heart failure.[67]

CYCLIC AMP AND THE POSITIVE INOTROPIC EFFECT

Partial beta-agonists may have a place in the treatment of chronic myocardial failure. A distinction must be made between partial and full $beta_1$-agonists.[63,68] Isoproterenol belongs to the latter group, TA-064 and prenalterol to the former.[63,68,69] Partial agonists possess only part of the inotropic effect of full agonists. The full agonists generate 90% of the maximal response, with only 57% of the receptors remaining unoccupied (spare receptors).[69a] Relevant is the fact that full agonists generate a more pronounced c-AMP stimulus than partial agonists.[70] For a partial $beta_1$-agonist, such as prenalterol, the efficacy of receptor-effector coupling is about 200-fold lower than that for isoproterenol.[69] This may be related to the fact that TA-064, a new $beta_1$-agonist, has cardiac inotropic effect but induces only limited activity of myocardial adenylate cyclase.[63] Reference has already been made to the cascade of events, occurring after administration of a beta-agonist in the sarcolemma: the beta-agonist combines with a beta$_1$-receptor, leading to activation of adenylate cyclase and an increase in c-AMP. Secondary biochemical responses include activation of c-AMP–dependent protein kinase, phosphorylation of protein molecules with the opening of Ca^{++} channels, and activation of Ca^{++}/Mg^{++}-dependent ATPase. The latter is responsible for the finely tuned release of Ca^{++} from the sarcolemma. Nayler[71] demonstrated that the positive inotropic effect exerted by some beta-adrenoceptor *antagonists* can be used to establish dose-response curves for their partial beta-agonistic properties.[71]

Why are some cardiotonic agents powerful inotropic agents, without comparable activation of adenylate cyclase? Chemnitius and Bing[68] summarized these possible mechanisms: (1) For partial beta-agonists, c-AMP may not be the second messenger, but only an indicator for beta-adrenergic stimulation. (2) The concentration of c-AMP in subcellular compartments may differ. (3) Myocardial beta-receptors may be desensitized through beta-agonist–induced protein kinases. This could protect the myocardium from overstimulation. (4) Even small quantities of c-AMP are sufficient to initiate an increase in phosphorylation of target proteins. (5) There may be downgrading of receptors. These questions remain as yet unsolved.

The fact that partial beta-agonists produce little activation of adenylate cyclase may have important clinical consequences. Opie et al[72,73] have examined the relation between c-AMP and irritability of the heart. They consider it possible that c-AMP may play a role in provoking arrhythmias by decreasing the fibrillation threshold.[72,73] Cyclic AMP may alter potassium permeability, changing the threshold of cardiac conductive tissue. It may produce lipolysis or produce afterpotentials, causing automaticity. The probability exists that partial beta-agonists may have as yet unrecognized advantages over full beta-agonists, which could make them useful in the treatment of myocardial failure.

MYOCARDIAL ISCHEMIA

METABOLIC PATHWAYS IN ISCHEMIA

In contrast to myocardial failure, both cause and effect of myocardial ischemia are well defined. Much has been written on the metabolic difference between the effect of global versus regional ischemia or global hypoxia. (In global hypoxia the oxygen tension of the perfusate is reduced, but coronary flow remains constant; global anoxia is the total absence of oxygen in the perfusate; in regional ischemia blood flow through specific areas of the heart is reduced by varying degrees).[74] Although the differences are of interest for the general field of cardiac metabolism, global anoxia and hypoxia do not occur in clinical settings or in the intact animal because of the compensatory increase in coronary flow. Only in perfused heart preparations, when flow can be maintained and controlled in the presence of a reduced oxygen load, can these conditions be reproduced. The present discussion deals primarily with regional ischemia occurring in the experimental animal after ligation of the coronary arteries or in patients who have had a myocardial infarct.

Inhibition of rate-limiting enzymes within the glycolytic pathway represents an important biochemical manifestation of myocardial ischemia. Among rate-limiting enzymes are phosphofructokinase and glyceraldehyde-3-phosphate-dehydrogenase.[75] Phosphofructokinase catalyzes the formation of fructose-1,6-diphosphate from fructose-6-phosphate. Glyceraldehyde-3-phosphate-dehydrogenase catalyzes the oxidation of glyceraldehyde-3-phosphate to 1,3-diphosphoglycerate. The inhibition of these glycolytic enzymes restricts total glycolytic flux and reduces the rate of glycolysis.[1,75] Phosphofructokinase activity is increased by high levels of adenosine diphosphate (ADP), adenosine monophosphate (AMP), and inorganic phosphate (P_i), all of which increase when energy demands are not met.[1] In addition, phosphofructokinase is activated by fructose-1,6-diphosphate and cyclic AMP. The latter is of importance in mediating the ability of catecholamines to stimulate anaerobic glycolysis.[1]

As blood flow and myocardial oxidation are impaired, the ratio reduced nicotinamide adenine dinucleotide/NAD increases. These changes can be monitored by comparing the ratios of lactate to pyruvate of α-glycerophosphate to dihydroxyacetone phosphate, and of β-hydroxybutyrate to acetoacetate. Regional myocardial ischemia produces an increase in both lactate/pyruvate and α-glycerophosphate to dihydroxyacetone phosphate ratios. It affects other biochemical patterns as well. In mitochondria, the ability to provide sufficient adenosine triphosphate is compromised.[1] This is the result of deficiencies in the electron transport chain with subsequent defective phosphorylation.[76–78] The integrity of oxidative phosphorylation mechanisms is ascertained by examining the ADP:O ratio, which represents the number of nanomoles of ATP produced per number of nano-atoms of oxygen consumed.[79,80] Oxygen consumption of mitochondria declines after one hour of ischemia. Other indicators of mitochondrial respiration also diminish. Mitochondrial membrane function is also affected. As a result, the shuttle system whereby reducing equivalents are transferred across the membrane by way of carrier molecules is malfunctioning.[1] This applies particularly to the malate-aspartate shuttle, which is the predominant pathway for disposing of cytoplasmic NADH.[1]

FATTY ACID METABOLISM IN ISCHEMIA

Because of the defect in mitochondrial membrane, fatty acid metabolism in ischemia is deficient. Increased norepinephrine levels in the blood of patients with myocardial infarction result in an increase in total free fatty acids. Fatty acids must be activated before entry into mitochondria. This is accomplished through activation of membrane acyl-CoA synthetase. Carnitine replaces CoA in the fatty acid structure and permits the fatty acid to penetrate the inner mitochondrial membrane. This process is catalyzed by a transferase mechanism.[81,82] These changes in fatty acid metabolism are of considerable importance in myocardial ischemia. They cause changes in ion permeability and (Na^{+}/K^{+}) ATPase activity in sarcolemma interfering with Ca^{++} transport and resulting in changes in cardiac cell function. Lipid abnormalities may lead to further myocardial damage. Several possible reasons for the extension of ischemic damage by membrane-derived lipids have been proposed.[17] For instance, palmitoyl carnitine might have a detergent effect on cell membranes; lysophosphatides, which in the ischemic heart are almost entirely derived from phospholipid hydrolysis, may further damage membrane structure in the ischemic heart.[17] Increased levels of acyl-CoA affect adenosine nucleotide and carnitine palmitoyl-CoA transferase.[83,84] The former is responsible for the exchange of extramitochondrial ADP for intramitochondrial adenosine triphosphate. The decrease in pH of the heart muscle is the result of increased lactate levels. This, together with the elevation of free fatty acids, contributes to the inhibition of phosphofructokinase just described. Such an inhibition is demonstrated by increasing levels of hexose monophosphate and a corresponding decrease in fructose-1,6-diphosphate. As acidosis progresses and ATP levels decline, contractility diminishes. Reddy et al[85] have also demonstrated a marked deficiency in regulatory proteins (troponine and tropomyosin) in the ischemic regions of the dog heart. Weishaar et al[86] demonstrated that in vitro contractility of glycerinated fibers from ischemic heart muscle diminished after one to three hours.

As the myocardium heals, leukocytes, fibroblasts, and monocytes migrate into the necrotic tissue. These cells are active in protein synthesis and in the formation of collagen and mucopolysaccharides. The activity of the hexose monophosphate shunt increases.[87] Therefore, a multiplicity of factors are responsible for a diminution of contractility in ischemic heart muscle. To reiterate, disturbances in the glycolytic pathway with acidosis, changes in mitochondrial function with diminished ATP production, defective fatty acid metabolism with increased free fatty acids in plasma, and changes in membrane function of sarcolemma, sarcoplasmic reticulum, and mitochondria take place. These changes depend on the severity and duration of ischemia.

NUCLEAR MAGNETIC RESONANCE AND MYOCARDIAL ISCHEMIA

The preceding discussion stressed the importance of high energy phosphates in myocardial ischemia. To determine these levels, analysis of quick frozen heart muscle specimens obtained by freeze clamp techniques is necessary because these compounds exchange or are unstable. This precludes consecutive analysis of these compounds in heart muscle biopsy. Nuclear magnetic resonance (NMR) has made noninvasive continuous observations possible. The discovery by Bloch[88] and Purcell et al[89] in the 1940s has laid the cornerstone. Nuclear magnetic resonance has now been applied to biochemistry and medicine in two forms: three-dimensional imaging with high-resolution tomography, and a noninvasive spectroscopic technique to allow separation and identification of chemical forms that contain a sensitive nucleus, such as ^{31}P or ^{13}C. Only the results of NMR spectroscopy will be discussed here, because it carries considerable promise for metabolic studies on normal and ischemic heart muscle. The physical basis for NMR will not be discussed in detail. Suffice it to state that each nucleus has a unique resonant frequency in any given magnetic field, so that when radio waves are transmitted to nuclei within a sample at their resonant frequency, they will absorb the radio frequency energy and will be tipped away from their initial aligned position.[90] When radio frequency energy ceases, the displaced nuclei release the absorbed radio frequency energy and return (by "relaxation") to their initial aligned state. This relaxation can occur by longitudinal (spin lattice) relaxation, referred to as T_1, and by transverse relaxation (T_2, spin-spin relaxation).[90] Both can be assessed by NMR spectroscopy or by imaging. In NMR spectroscopy, the resonant frequency is affected by the chemical environment. This makes possible spectroscopic separation of chemical structures containing the sensitive nucleus, such as that of the naturally occurring nucleus of ^{31}P. The phosphate compounds occurring in myocardium such as ATP, ADP, phosphocreatine, and P_i resonate at different frequencies. The concentration of the individual phosphorus compounds in the spectrum is related to the area under each peak. Intracellular pH can be monitored by the relative position of the P_i peak to the phosphocreatine (PCr) peak.[91]

Up to the present, NMR spectroscopy has been primarily used in isolated perfused heart, kidney, and liver preparations using ^{31}P spectrum, although ^{13}C has considerable potential. For in vivo use, topical magnetic resonance or surface coils have been developed.[92,93] With these and other focusing techniques, it will soon be possible to obtain spectra from specific regions of the heart muscle by placing the surface coil on the chest surface without thoracotomy.

Peaks in NMR spectrum of heart muscle can be assigned to the resonances of ATP, PCr, P_i and sugar phosphates (mainly glucose-6-phosphate). There are three signals corresponding to the phosphates of ATP: β:α:γ. They are in the ratio of 0.5:1.5:0.9. This implies contribution to peak intensities from other phosphorus compounds. In fact, the γ phosphate peak of ATP contains resonances from other pyrophosphates as well as NAD/NADH.

Figure 15.1 shows two spectra from a normal and ischemic heart. The first is from a rabbit heart perfused with Krebs-Henseleit solution. It presents the characteristic findings of ischemia (large P_i, small PCr peaks, Figure 15.1A). In contrast, in a rabbit heart perfused with a perfluorochemical (FC-43, Green Cross, Osaka, Japan), these signs of ischemia are not present (Figure 15.1B).

Several papers on the effect of myocardial ischemia on magnetic resonance spectroscopy have been published.[94–97] To understand the effect of ischemia on resonances of APT, PCr, and P_i, it is necessary to recollect the equilibrium existing between PCr, ADP, and ATP, as catalyzed by creatine kinase: creatine–P^{2-} + $MgADP^-$ + H^+ $\rightleftarrows$ creatine + $MgATP^{2-}$.

Consequently, PCr acts as a rapid accessible reservoir for the conversion of ADP to ATP. It is therefore not surprising that in ischemia, as PCr levels drop rapidly to maintain the ATP level, the P_i level increases in direct proportion.[98,99] Sugar phosphate levels are raised because of activation of glycogenolysis during the ischemic period. Only P_i, sugar phosphate, and nucleotide monophosphate signals are detectable. The chemical shift of the

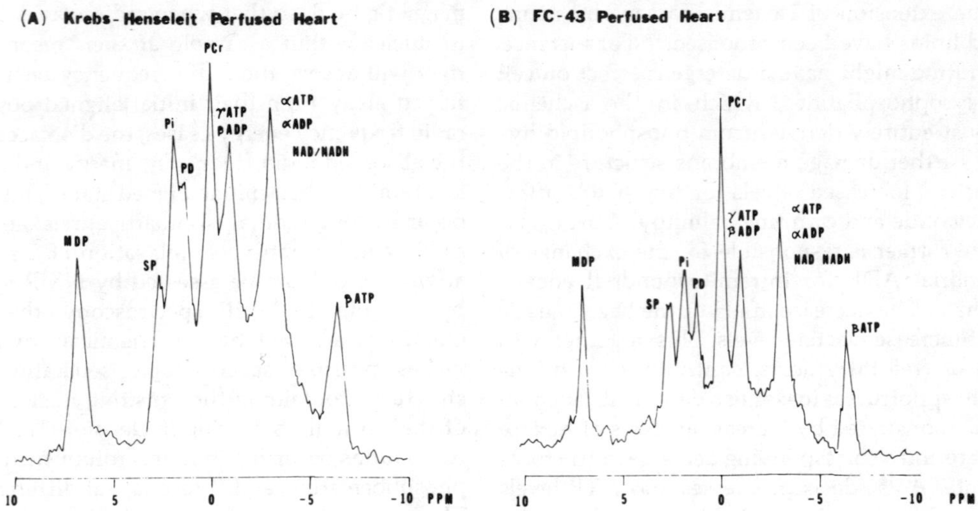

Figure 15.1. [31]P nuclear magnetic resonance spectroscopic findings[102] in an ischemic (A) and a non-ischemic (B) heart. See text for explanation.

latter changes as the pH in the cell decreases due to the production of lactate.

By carrying out repetitive interruptions in perfusion of the guinea pig heart and overlaying the data, Brooks and Willis[100] have been able to improve the time resolution for the acquisition of ^{31}P spectra to 12 seconds in ischemic hearts. As expected, PCr levels decrease, P_i increases, and the chemical shift of the inorganic phosphate peak measuring pH moves upfield. ATP shows no decrease during the 12-second ischemic period, being maintained by the activity of creatine kinase. No ADP can be detected either before or during the period of ischemia. During the recovery period, PCr and P_i return quickly to normal.

Reference was made to the increased rate of healing of the infarcted tissue by insulin.[87] Seymour et al,[101] using ^{31}P-NMR, also discovered that insulin-treated hearts may be protected from transient ischemia by decreasing the rate of depletion of their intracellular ATP content during ischemia. This work represents an example of the potential use of NMR spectroscopy in assessing the efficiency of certain substances in protecting the ischemic myocardium. This subject is of considerable clinical interest, but it has been hindered by a lack of suitable quantitative techniques. With NMR spectroscopy, it will finally be possible to evaluate procedures reported to influence and promote healing of myocardial infarction.

Acknowledgment: This work was supported by grants from the Council for Tobacco Research, USA, Inc; The Margaret W. and Herbert Hoover, Jr. Foundation; and The Charles A. Lindbergh Fund, Inc. The excellent secretarial help of Cheryl Dix and the assistance of Drs. Maythem Saeed and Dominique Freeman in the preparation of this manuscript are greatly appreciated.

REFERENCES

1. Bing RJ: Cardiac metabolism, in Fowler NO (ed): *Cardiac Diagnosis and Treatment.* Philadelphia, Harper & Row, 1980, pp 281–296.
2. Opie LH: *The Heart — Physiology, Metabolism, Pharmacology and Therapy.* London and New York, Grune & Stratton, 1984.
3. Katz AM: *Physiology of the Heart.* New York, Raven Press, 1977.
4. Sperelakis N (ed): *Physiology and Pathophysiology of the Heart.* Boston, Martinus Nijhoff, 1984.
5. Ringer S: A further contribution regarding the influence of different constituents of the blood on the contraction of the heart. *J Physiol* 1882; 4:29–42.
6. Lancisi GM: *De motu cordis et aneurysmatibus, opus post humum in duas partes divisum.* Romae, JM Salvioni, 1728.
7. Hope J: *A Treatise on the Diseases of the Heart and Great Vessels, Comprising a New View of the Physiology of the Heart's Action, According to Which the Physical Signs are Explained.* London, W Kidd, 1832.
8. Lewis T: *Diseases of the Heart.* London, Macmillan, 1933.
9. Harrison TR: *Failure of the Circulation.* Baltimore, Williams & Wilkins, 1935.
10. White PD: *Heart Disease.* New York, Macmillan, 1937.
11. McMichael J, Sharpey-Schafer EP: Cardiac output in man by direct Fick method. Effects of posture, venous pressure change, atropine and adrenaline. *Br Heart J* 1944; 6:33–40.
11a. McMichael J, Sharpey-Schafer EP: Action of intravenous digoxin in man. *Quart J Med* 1944; 13:123–135.
12. Cournand AF, Riley RL, Breed ES, Baldwin EF, Richards DW: Measurement of cardiac output in man using the technique of catheterization of the right auricle or ventricle. *J Clin Invest* 1945; 24:106–116.
13. Bing RJ, Hammond M, Handelsmann JC, Powers RC, Spencer FC, Eckenhoff J, Goodale WT, Hafkenschiel JH, Kety SS: The measurement of coronary blood flow, oxygen consumption and efficiency of the left ventricle in man. *Am Heart J* 1949; 38:1–24.
14. Warren JV, Stead EA: Fluid dynamics in chronic congestive heart failure; interpretation of the mechanism producing the edema, increased plasma volume and elevated venous pressure in certain patients with prolonged congestive failure. *Arch Intern Med* 1944; 73:138–147.
15. Bing RJ, Heimbecker RO, Falholt W, Friedlich A, Carroll D: Method for approximation of residual volume of blood in right ventricle. *Am J Physiol* 1950; 163:698.
16. Bing RJ: *Metabolism of the Heart.* Harvey Lecture Series I. New York, Academic Press, 1954–1955, p 27.
17. Katz AM: Membrane derived lipids and the pathogenesis of ischemic myocardial damage. *J Mol Cell Cardiol* 1982; 14:627–632.
18. Katz AM, Repke DI, Upshaw JE, Polascik MA: Characterization of dog cardiac microsomes. Use of zonal centrifugation to fractionate fragmented sarcoplasmic reticulum ($Na^+ + K^+$). *Biochim Biophys Acta* 1970; 205:473–490.
19. Fleckenstein A: Calcium antagonist in heart and smooth muscle. *Experimental Facts and Therapeutic Prospects.* New York, John Wiley & Sons, 1983.
20. Tada M, Katz AM: Phosphorylation of the sarcoplasmic reticulum and sarcolemma. *Ann Rev Physiol* 1982; 24:401–423.
21. Murad F, Chi Y-M, Sutherland EW: Adenyl cyclase III. The effect of catecholamines and choline esters on the formation of adenosine 3',5' phosphate by preparations from cardiac muscle and liver. *J Biol Chem* 1962; 237:1233–1238.
22. Katz AM: Regulation of myocardial contractility 1958-1983: an odyssey. *J Am Coll Cardiol* 1983; 1:42–51.
23. Scholz M: Effects of beta- and alpha-adrenoceptor activators and adrenergic transmitter releasing agents on the mechanical activity of the heart, in Szekeres L (ed): *Handbook of Experimental Pharmacology.* I. Adrenergic activators and inhibitors, Part I. New York, Springer-Verlag, 1980, vol 54, pp 651–733.

24. Honerjager P, Schafer-Korting M, Reiter M: Involvement of cyclic AMP in the direct inotropic action of amrinone. *Naunyn Schmiedebergs Arch Pharmacol* 1981; 318:112–120.
25. Leier CV, Dalpiaz K, Huss P, Hermiller JB, Magorien RD, Bashore TM, Unverterth DV: Amrinone therapy for congestive heart failure in outpatients with idiopathic dilated cardiomyopathy. *Am J Cardiol* 1983; 52:304–308.
25a. Endo M, Yamashita S, Taira N: Positive inotropic effect of amrinone in relation to cyclic nucleotide metabolism in the canine ventricular muscle. *J Pharmacol Exp Ther* 1982; 221:775–783.
26. Caroni P, Carafoli E: The Ca^{++}-pumping ATPase of heart sarcolemma. Characterization, Calmodulin dependence, and partial purification. *J Biol Chem* 1981; 256:3263–3270.
27. Chemnitius JM, Sasaki Y, Burger W, Bing RJ: The effect of ischemia and reperfusion on sarcolemmal function in perfused canine hearts. *J Mol Cell Cardiol* 1985; 17:1139–1150.
28. Church JG, Sen AK: Regulation of canine heart sarcolemmal Ca^{++}-pumping ATPase by cyclic GMP. *Biochim Biophys Acta* 1983; 728:191–200.
29. Bers DM, Philipson KD, Nishimoto AY: Sodium-calcium exchange and sidedness of isolated sarcolemmal vesicles. *Biochim Biophys Acta* 1980; 601:358–371.
30. Bing RJ, Sasaki Y, Burger W, Chemnitius JM: Cardiac inotropic response of a new β-1-agonist (TA-064) with low sarcolemmal adenylate cyclase activation. *Curr Ther Res* 1984; 36:1127–1144.
31. Jones LR, Besch HR Jr, Fleming JW, McConnanghey MM, Watanabe AM: Separation of vesicles of cardiac sarcolemma from vesicles of cardiac sarcoplasmic reticulum. Comparative biochemical analysis of component activities. *J Biol Chem* 1979; 254:530–539.
32. Reinlib L, Caroni P, Carafoli E: Studies on heart sarcolemma: vesicles of opposite orientation and the effect of ATP on the Na^{+}/Ca^{++} exchange. *FEBS Lett* 1981; 126:74–76.
33. Besch HR Jr, Jones LR, Fleming JW, Watanabe AM: Parallel unmasking of latent adenylate cyclase and (Na^{+}/K^{+}) ATPase activities in cardiac sarcolemmal vesicles. A new use of the channel-forming ionophore alamethicin. *J Biol Chem* 1977; 252:7905–7908.
34. Dhalla NS, Ziegelhoffer A, Harrow JAC: Regulatory role of membrane systems in heart function. *Can J Physiol Pharmacol* 1977; 55:1211–1234.
35. Dhalla NS, Das RK, Sharma GP: Subcellular basis of cardiac contractile failure. *J Mol Cell Cardiol* 1978; 10:363–384.
36. Katz AM: Cyclic adenosine monophosphate effects on the myocardium: a man who blows hot and cold with one breath. *J Am Coll Cardiol* 1983; 2:143–149.
37. Caroni P, Carafoli E: An ATP-dependent Ca^{++}-pumping system in dog heart sarcolemma. *Nature* 1980; 283:765–767.
37a. Le Peuch AM, Le Peuch CJ, DeMaille JG: Concerted regulations of cardiac sarcoplasmic reticulum. Calcium transport by cyclic adenosine monophosphate-dependent and calcium-calmodulin-dependent phosphorylations. *Biochemistry* 1979; 18:5150–5157.
38. Chance B: The energy-linked reaction of calcium with mitochondria. *J Biol Chem* 1965; 240:2729–2748.
39. Bing RJ: The biochemical basis of myocardial failure. *Hosp Pract* 1983; 18:93–112.
40. Bing RJ: Cardiac metabolism: its contributions to alcoholic heart disease and myocardial failure. *Circulation* 1978; 58:965–970.
41. Danforth WH, Ballard FB, Kako K, Choudhury JD, Bing RJ: Metabolism of heart in failure. *Circulation* 1960; 21:112–123.
42. Sarma JSM, Ikeda S, Fisher R, Maruyama Y, Weishaar R, Bing RJ: Biochemical and contractile properties of heart muscle after prolonged alcohol administration. *J Mol Cell Cardiol* 1976; 8:951–972.
43. Julian FJ: The effect of calcium on the force-velocity relation of briefly glycerinated frog muscle fibers. *J Physiol* 1971; 218:117–145.
44. Szent-Gyorgyi A: Free energy relations and contraction of actomyosin. *Biol Bull* 1949; 96:140–161.
45. Bajusz E, Baker JR, Nixon CW, Homburger F: Spontaneous hereditary myocardial degeneration and congestive heart failure in a strain of syrian hamsters. *Ann NY Acad Sci* 1969; 156:105–129.
46. Alpert NR, Mulieri LA: Heat, mechanics and myosin ATPase in normal and hypertrophied heart muscle. *Fed Proc* 1982; 41:192–198.
47. Lompre AM, Schwartz K, Albis AD, Lacombe G, Van Thiem N, Swynghedauw B: Myosin isozyme redistribution in chronic heart overload. *Nature* 1979; 282:105–107.
48. Malhotra A, Karell M, Scheuer J: Multiple cardiac contractile protein abnormalities in myopathic syrian hamsters (Bio 53:58). *J Mol Cell Cardiol* 1985; 17:95–107.
49. Meerson FZ: Compensatory hyperfunction of the heart and cardiac insufficiency. *Circ Res* 1962; 10:250–258.
50. Zühlke V, du Mesnil de Rochemont W, Gudbjarnason S, Bing RJ: Inhibition of protein synthesis in cardiac hypertrophy and its relation to myocardial failure. *Circ Res* 1966; 18:558–572.
51. Bing RJ: Effect of alcohol on the heart and cardiac metabolism. *Fed Proc* 1982; 41:2443–2446.
52. Weishaar R, Sarma JSM, Maruyama Y, Fisher R, Bertuglia S, Bing RJ: Reversibility of mitochondrial contractile changes in the myocardium after cessation of prolonged ethanol intake. *Am J Cardiol* 1977; 40:556–562.
53. Dhalla NS, Singh JN, Bajusz E, Jasmin G: Comparison of heart sarcolemmal enzyme activities in normal and cardiomyopathic (UM-X7.1) hamsters. *Clin Sci Mol Med* 1976; 51:233–242.
54. Gertz EW, Hess ML, Lain RF, Briggs FN: Activity of ventricular calcium pump in the spontaneously failing heart-lung preparation. *Circ Res* 1967; 20:477–484.
55. Kako K, Choudhury JD, Bing RJ: Possible mechanism of the decline in mechanical efficiency of the isolated heart. *J Pharmacol Exp Ther* 1960; 130:46–52.
56. Harigaya SC, Schwartz A: Rate of calcium binding and uptake in normal and failing human cardiac muscle. Membrane vesicles (relaxing system and mitochondria). *Circ Res* 1969; 35:781–794.
57. Lindenmayer GE, Sorbahl LA, Harigaya S, Allen JC, Besch HR, Schwarz A: Some biochemical studies on subcellular systems isolated from fresh recipient human cardiac tissue obtained during transplantation. *Am J Cardiol* 1971; 27:277–283.
58. Lee KS, Ladinsky H, Stuckey JH: Decreased Ca^{++} uptake by sarcoplasmic reticulum after coronary artery occlusion for 60 and 90 minutes. *Circ Res* 1967; 21:439–444.
59. Dhalla NS, Sulake PV, Khandelwal RL, Olson RE: Adenyl cyclase activity in the perfused rat heart made to fail by substrate-lack. *Cardiovasc Res* 1972; 6:344–352.
60. Fozard HA, Sheets MF: Cellular mechanism of action of cardiac glycosides. *J Am Coll Cardiol* 1985; 5:10A–15A.
61. Katz AM: Effects of digitalis on cell biochemistry: sodium pump inhibition. *J Am Coll Cardiol* 1985; 5:16A–21A.
62. Caroni P, Reinlib L, Carafoli E: Charge movements during the $Na^{+}-Ca^{++}$ exchange in heart sarcolemmal vesicles. *Proc Natl Acad Sci USA* 1980; 77:6354–6358.
63. Bing RJ, Burger W, Chemnitius JM, Sugihara J, Sasaki Y: The effects of a new cardiotonic drug (TA-064) on normal and failing heart preparations. *Curr Ther Res* 1984; 36:133–147.
64. Honerjager P, Schafer-Korting M, Reiter M: Involvement of cyclic AMP in the direct inotropic action of amrinone. *Naunyn Schmiedebergs Arch Pharmacol* 1981; 318:112–120.
65. LeJemtel TH, Sonnenblick EH: Should the failing heart be stimulated? *N Engl J Med* 1984; 310:1384–1385.
66. Katz AM: A new inotropic drug: its promise and a caution. *N Engl J Med* 1978; 299:1409–1410.
67. Kino M, Hirota Y, Yamamoto S, Sawada K, Moriguchi M, Kotaka M, Kubo S, Kawamura K: Cardiovascular effects of a newly synthesized cardiotonic agent (TA-064) on normal and diseased hearts. *Am J Cardiol* 1983; 51:802–810.
68. Chemnitius JM, Bing RJ: Beta-1-adrenoceptor agonists with low adenylate cyclase activation: theoretical and clinical implication. *Can J Cardiol* 1985; 1(3):186–188.
69. Hedberg A, Carlsson E, Fellenius E, Lundgren B: Cardiostimulatory effects of Prenalterol, a beta-1-adrenoceptor partial agonist, in vivo and in vitro. Correlation between physiological effects and adenylate cyclase activity. *Nauyn Schmiedebergs Arch Pharmacol* 1982; 318:185–191.
69a. Venter JC: High efficiency coupling between beta-adrenergic receptors and cardiac contractility: direct evidence for "spare" beta-adrenergic receptors. *Mol Pharmacol* 1979; 16:429–440.
70. Levitzki A: *Receptors - A Quantitative Approach.* Menlo Park, Benjamin/Cummings, 1984.
71. Nayler W: Comparative partial agonist activity of beta-adrenoceptor antagonists. *Br J Pharmacol* 1972; 45:382–384.
72. Opie LH: Role of cyclic nucleotides in heart metabolism. *Cardiovasc Res* 1982; 16:483–507.
73. Podzuweit T, Dalby AJ, Cherry GW, Opie LH. Cyclic AMP levels in ischaemic and non-ischaemic myocardium following coronary artery ligation: relation to ventricular fibrillation. *J Mol Cell Cardiol* 1978; 10:81–94.
74. Neely JR, Whitmer JT, Rovetto MJ: Effect of coronary blood flow on glycolytic flux and intracellular pH in isolated rat heart. *Circ Res* 1975; 37:733–741.
75. Kubler W, Spieckermann PG: Regulation of glycolysis in the schemic and the anoxic myocardium. *J Mol Cell Cardiol* 1970; 1:351–377.
76. Estabrook RW: Mitochondrial respiratory control and the polarographic measurement of ADP:0 ratios, in Estabrook RW, Pullman MM (eds): *Methods in Enzymology*, vol 10. New York, Academic Press, 1967, pp 41–47.
77. Chance B, Williams GR: The respiratory chain and oxidative phosphorylation. *Adv Enzymol* 1956; 17:65–134.
78. Lehninger AL: Oxidative phosphorylation. Harvey Lecture Series XIL. New York, Academic Press, 1955.
79. Wilson DF, Dutton PL, Wagner M: Energy-transducing components in mitochondrial respiration, in Sanadi DR, Packer L (eds): *Current Topics in Bio-energetics* Vol 5. New York, Academic Press, 1973 pp 234–265.

80. Lehninger AL: *The Mitochondrion: Molecular Basis of Structure and Function.* Menlo Park, WA Benjamin, 1964.
81. Fritz IB, Yue KTN: Long-chain carnitine acyltransferase and the role of acylcarnitine derivatives in the catalytic increase of fatty acid induced by carnitine. *J Lipid Res* 1963; 4:279–288.
82. Hoppel CL, Tomec RJ: Carnitine palmityltransferase. Location of two enzymatic activities in rat liver mitochondria. *J Biol Chem* 1972; 247:832–841.
83. Bremer J, Norum KR: Mechanism of substrate inhibition of palmityl coenzyme A: carnitine palmityltransferase by palmityl coenzyme A. *J Biol Chem* 1967; 242:1744–1748.
84. Lerner E, Shug AL, Elson C, Shrago E: Reversible inhibition of adenine nucleotide translocation by long chain fatty acyl coenzyme A esters in liver mitochondria of diabetic and hibernating animals. *J Biol Chem* 1972; 247:1513–1519.
85. Reddy YS, Wyborny L, Lewis RM, Schwartz A: Biochemical and morphological correlates of cardiac ischemia: contractile proteins. *Cardiovasc Res* 1976; 10:129–135.
86. Weishaar R, Sarma JSM, Maruyama Y, Fischer R, Bing RJ: Regional blood flow, contractility and metabolism in early myocardial infarction. *Cardiology* 1977; 62:2–20.
87. Gudbjarnason S, De Schryver C, Chiba C, Yamanaka J, Bing RJ: Protein and nucleic acid synthesis during the reparative processes following myocardial infarction. *Circ Res* 1964; 15:320–326.
88. Bloch F: Nuclear induction. *Phys Rev* 1946; 70:460–474.
89. Purcell EM, Torrey HC, Pound RV: Resonance absorption by nuclear magnetic moments in a solid. *Phys Rev* 1946; 69:37–38.
90. Pohost GM, Ratner AV: Nuclear magnetic resonance: potential applications in clinical cardiology. *JAMA* 1984; 1304–1309.
91. Moon RB, Richards JH: Determination of intracellular pH by ^{31}P NMR. *J Biol Chem* 1973; 248:7276–7278.
92. Ackerman JJH, Grove TH, Wong GG, Gadian DG, Radda GK: Mapping of metabolites in whole animals by ^{31}P NMR surface coils. *Nature* 1980; 283:167–170.
93. Balaban RS, Gadian DG, Radda GK: Phosphorus nuclear magnetic resonance study of the rat kidney in vivo. *Kidney Int* 1981; 20:575–579.
94. Gadian DG, Hoult DI, Radda GK, Seeley PJ, Chance B, Barlow C: Phosphorus nuclear magnetic resonance studies on normoxic and ischemic cardiac tissue. *Proc Natl Acad Sci USA* 1976; 73:4446–4448.
95. Nunally RL, Bottomley PA: Assessment of pharmacological treatment of myocardial infarction by phosphorus-31 NMR with surface coils. *Science* 1981; 211:177–180.
96. Williams ES, Kaplan JI, Thatcher F, Zimmerman G, Knoebel SB: Prolongation of proton spin lattice relaxation times in regionally ischemic tissue from dog hearts. *J Nucl Med* 1980; 21:449–453.
97. Flaherty JT, Weisfeldt ML, Bulkley BH, Gardner TJ, Gott VL, Jacobus WE: Mechanisms of ischemic myocardial cell damage assessed by phosphorus-31 nuclear magnetic resonance. *Circulation* 1982; 65(3):561–571.
98. Radda GK, Bore PJ, Gadian DG, Ross BD, Styles P, Taylor DJ, Morgan-Hughes J: ^{31}P-NMR examination of 2 patients with NADH-COQ reductase deficiency. *Nature* 1982; 295:608–609.
99. Gadian D, Radda A, Ross B, Hockaday J, Bore P, Taylor D, Styles P: Examination of a myopathy by ^{31}P NMR. *Lancet* 1981; 2:774–775.
100. Brooks WM, Willis RJ: ^{31}P nuclear magnetic resonance study of the recovery characteristics of high energy phosphate compounds and intracellular pH after global ischaemia in the perfused guinea-pig heart. *J Mol Cell Cardiol* 1983; 15:495–502.
101. Seymour A-ML, Bailey IA, Radda GK: A protective effect of insulin on reperfusing the ischaemic rat heart shown using ^{31}P NMR. *Biochim Biophys Acta* 1983; 762:525–530.
102. Mayr H, Freeman D, Bing RJ, Roberts J: Advantages of perfluorochemical perfusion in the working rabbit heart preparation using ^{31}P NMR spectroscopy (abstr). Society of Magnetic Resonance in Medicine, 4th Annual Meeting, London, August 1985.

16 Congestive Heart Failure: Mechanisms, Evaluation, and Management

Dean T. Mason, MD, Ming C. Chan, MD, and Garrett Lee, MD

Heart failure is the abnormal condition in which disturbed cardiac performance is primarily responsible for the inability of the heart to pump blood at a rate commensurate with systemic metabolic requirements. Heart failure is considered to be compensated when cardiac output is maintained at a normal level by reserve systems principally inherent in the ventricle, often with congestive features and other signs and symptoms attending the operation of these adaptive processes. Decompensated congestive heart failure evolves with chronic low cardiac output despite maximal activity of cardiocirculatory protective mechanisms.

PATHOPHYSIOLOGIC MECHANISMS

The function of the intact heart is governed by intimate integration of four principal determinants[1] that regulate stroke volume and cardiac output: (1) preload (ventricular end-diastolic volume), (2) afterload (intraventricular systolic tension during ejection), (3) contractility (variable force of ventricular contraction independent of loading), and (4) heart rate (frequency of contraction). Preload and contractility are fundamental intrinsic mechanisms inherent in the contractile machinery of the myocardium, whereas afterload and heart rate are largely under extrinsic autonomic modulation. The term *cardiac function* is used in the general sense to refer to the combined action of these determinants of cardiac output and not necessarily to the single determinant, contractility itself.

The disturbed mechanisms operative in all types of clinical heart disease can be evaluated and accurately characterized within the framework of isolated or composite disorders of these four major determinants of cardiac performance. The development of improved techniques[2] and concepts[3] for the assessment of cardiac function in patients by both hemodynamic methods and myocardial mechanics has provided the means for differential analyses of the nature and degree of the roles of each of these fundamental determinants and their interrelations with cardiac compensatory mechanisms governing stroke output in heart failure.

FUNDAMENTAL CAUSES OF HEART FAILURE

Clinical heart disease can be broadly classified on a pathophysiologic basis[3] according to three general forms of cardiac functional abnormalities: (1) primary contractility disturbance, as in idiopathic or ischemic myocardial disease; (2) diastolic mechanical inhibition of cardiac performance (ventricular underloading) in which ventricular hypertrophy does not develop, as in restricted ventricular filling in mitral stenosis or pericardial tamponade; and (3) systolic mechanical overloading of the ventricle characterized by excessive pressure loading, as in aortic stenosis or essential hypertension, or increased volume loading, as in mitral or aortic regurgitation. In systolic ventricular overloading and in primary inotropic disorders, congestive heart failure occurs when there is substantial depression of contractility; decompensation ensues when impairment of the contractile state becomes particularly severe.

PRECIPITATING CAUSES OF HEART FAILURE

In congestive heart failure that is unresponsive to standard medical therapy, in addition to the systematic evaluation of the nature and degree of heart disease, careful consideration of the possibility of noncardiac conditions simulating or perpetuating cardiac dysfunction is essential.[4] The abnormalities that mimic heart disease include pulmonary embolism, other bronchopulmonary disorders, thyrotoxicosis, pheochromocytoma, adrenal tumors and insufficiency, metastatic carcinoma, various forms of anemia, and hepatic and renal disease.

Several conditions may contribute to the persistence of the congestive heart failure state in any type of heart disease: hyperthyroidism, hypothyroidism, anemia, atrial fibrillation and other tachyarrhythmias, heart block, pulmonary embolism, bacterial endocarditis, pulmonary and urinary tract infections, hepatic and renal diseases, hypertension, ingestion of large quantities of alcohol, obesity, excessive physical activity, increased salt and water intake, electrolyte disturbances, abnormalities of acid–base balance, and excessive use of opiates. Finally, complications of cardiovascular drug therapy may perpetuate or worsen pump function, such as cardiac depression due to large doses of antiarrhythmic agents, relatively low blood volume because of too vigorous diuretic therapy, and rhythm and conduction disturbances induced by digitalis toxicity.

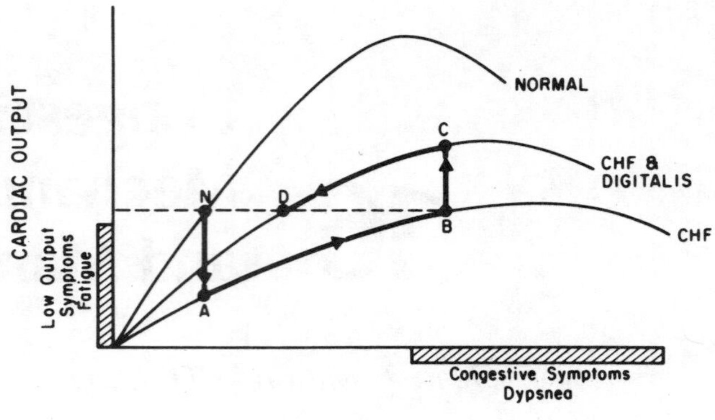

Figure 16.1. Operation of the Frank-Starling mechanism in the preload compensation for heart failure. The three curves represent ventricular function curves in normal, congestive heart failure (CHF), and heart failure after treatment with digitalis. Points N through D indicate in sequence: depression of contractility with decompensated heart failure (A), Frank-Starling compensation (B), increase in contractility with digitalis (C), and reduction in the use of Frank-Starling preload compensation which digitalis allows (D). Points N, D, and B indicate the same cardiac output on the vertical axis, but each point is at a different end-diastolic pressure on the horizontal axis. The excessive end-diastolic pressures causing congestive symptoms and the decreased levels of cardiac performance resulting in low output symptoms are shown by the hatched areas. (From Mason,[3] with permission.)

CARDIAC COMPENSATORY MECHANISMS

When systolic hemodynamic overloading or a primary defect in contractility is imposed on the heart, there are three principal compensatory mechanisms[3] available to it that provide a limited amount of ventricular reserve for the direct support of cardiac function and its fundamental goal of maintaining a normal level of cardiac output: (1) the Frank-Starling principle, (2) ventricular hypertrophy, and (3) the sympathetic nervous system. Deleterious symptoms necessarily accompany the operation of these compensatory mechanisms in their primary role of sustaining stroke volume, and these symptoms restrict the extent to which the adaptive systems can be used.

Ventricular Dilation

The Frank-Starling preload mechanism of ventricular dilation is immediately used to aid the ventricle in maintenance of cardiac output in the presence of an excessive systolic hemodynamic (particularly volume) overload or primary inotropic disturbance (Figure 16.1). The increased end-diastolic volume permits more forceful contraction, and the greater ventricular size allows ejection of a larger stroke volume with less shortening of the circumferential fibers. Conversely, the effectiveness and reserve capacity of the Frank-Starling system are encroached on when the contractile state is diminished, because its ascending limb becomes less steep and flattened with its apex decreased in amplitude so that the reduced maximal stroke volume possible must be delivered at an abnormally high level of end-diastolic pressure. Therefore, the failing ventricle has a lowered and depressed function curve and exhibits decreased systolic response to preload increments. Furthermore, operation of the Frank-Starling preload mechanism by the ventricles for maintaining cardiac output is obligatorily associated with pulmonary and systemic congestion and increased myocardial systolic tension; thereby, the price for use of this reserve system is dyspnea and peripheral edema, along with increased cardiac oxygen needs.

Ventricular Hypertrophy

An increase in the number of contractile units by development of ventricular hypertrophy provides a relatively quickly responsive second compensatory system in support of cardiac output in systolic mechanical (particularly pressure) overloading and in contractile state impairment. Thus, protein synthesis is stimulated by excessive intramyocardial tension, which appears to serve as the mechanical–biochemical transducer or coupling mechanism responsible for accelerated production of ventricular mass. Because extensive ventricular hypertrophy results in relative myocardial ischemia due to cardiac oxygen demands in excess of delivery capacity of even the normal coronary circulation, angina pectoris may attend marked use of the reserve mechanism of hypertrophy.

In addition to the increase in oxygen requirements because of greater muscle mass, myocardial oxygen utilization is also enhanced by the Frank-Starling and adrenergic adaptive mechanisms. Thus, at a given ventricular mass, myocardial oxygen consumption[5] is principally determined directly by three hemodynamic-related variables (Figure 16.2): (1) intramyocardial systolic tension (governed by systolic pressure and cardiac size), (2) heart rate, and (3) contractile state. Ventricular dilation and increased sympathetic activity raise the first two of these factors above normal levels in congestive heart failure.

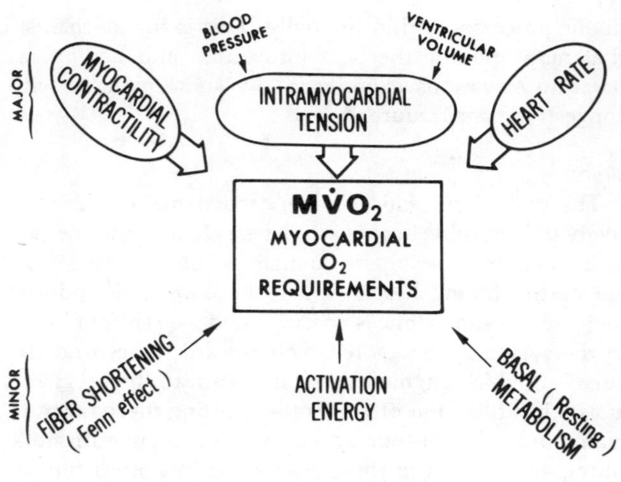

Figure 16.2. Major and minor determinants of myocardial oxygen consumption (MVO_2). In addition to the three major determinants described in the text, external work or ventricular shortening (Fenn effect), energy of activation-relaxation, and basal diastolic energy requirements contribute to a relatively minor degree to overall myocardial oxygen requirements. (From Mason et al,[20] with permission.)

Adrenergic Activity

Besides ventricular dilation and hypertrophy reserves, the dysfunctioning heart has immediately available some inotropic support provided by adrenergic activity. Thus, the ventricles are richly innervated by sympathetic fibers in which increased impulse traffic, through release of its endogenous neurotransmitter, norepinephrine, and consequent myocardial beta-receptor stimulation, is capable of improving contractility and increasing frequency of contraction. There is abundant evidence that sympathetic activity is augmented in congestive heart failure.[6] Paradoxically, however, norepinephrine is reduced in the hypertrophied myocardium (Figure 16.3) because of its defective synthesis, and the dysfunctioning ventricle is largely deprived of this rapidly responsive compensatory mechanism.[7] Conversely, adrenergic support is partially

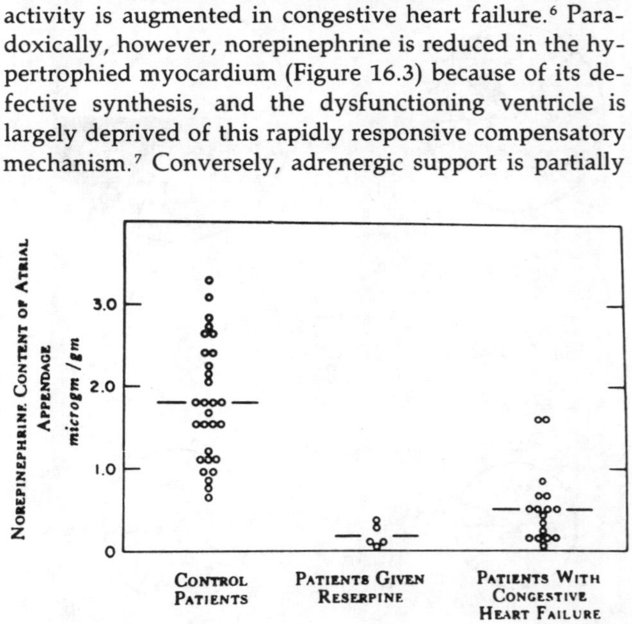

Figure 16.3. Concentration of norepinephrine in the atrial appendages excised at operation in 29 control patients who had not been in congestive heart failure, in five patients who had been treated with reserpine, and in 17 patients who had been in congestive heart failure. (From Chidsey et al,[7] with permission of the *New England Journal of Medicine*.)

restored to the failing heart as the result of increased circulating norepinephrine because of its increased synthesis in the peripheral vasculature (Figure 16.4) and adrenal medulla.[8] The symptoms accompanying utilization of sympathetic assistance include tachycardia, tachyarrhythmias, and those due to redistribution of peripheral blood flow such as excessive sweating, cool skin, and oliguria.

EXTRACARDIAC COMPENSATORY MECHANISMS

It is clear that a state of systemic arteriolar and venous constriction is characteristic of human congestive heart failure.[9] This vasoconstriction compensates for the reduced performance of the heart in support of central and peripheral circulatory function.

Arteries

The increase in total systemic vascular resistance provides a peripheral circulatory mechanism by which arterial pressure is maintained in the presence of low cardiac output. This arteriolar constriction in congestive heart failure is produced mainly by increased sympathetic nervous activity and by a stiffness component in the arteriolar wall (Figure 16.5). In contrast to the failing myocardium, there are increased labile stores of norepinephrine in the arteriolar beds of skeletal muscle in patients with congestive heart failure. The altered mechanical properties of the arterioles in congestive heart failure result from in-

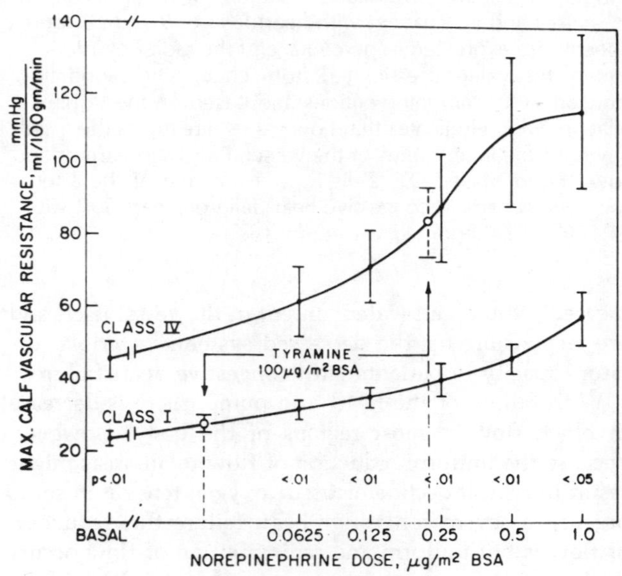

Figure 16.4. Norepinephrine dose-response curves in patients without heart failure (class I) and in those with heart failure (class IV). The average peak values of vascular resistance ($\pm$ standard error of the mean) elicited by intraarterial injections of graded doses of norepinephrine are shown. The probability values indicate the significance of the difference of the responses between the two groups. The mean maximal resistance in response to tyramine (*open circles and vertical broken lines*) is positioned on the appropriate curve, providing an expression of the tyramine response in terms of norepinephrine-equivalent dose. BSA = body surface area. (From Kramer et al,[8] by permission of the American Heart Association, Inc.)

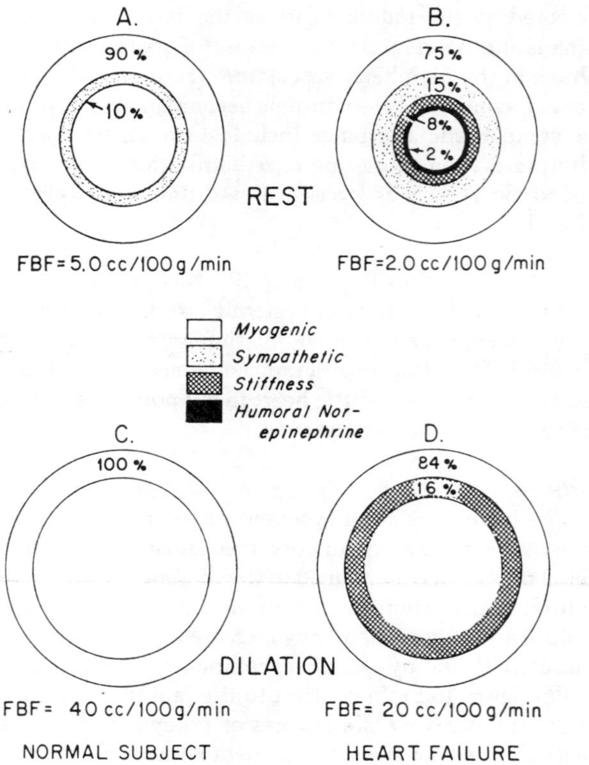

Figure 16.5. Diagram represents the components of vascular resistance in the arterioles of the forearm at rest (*A* and *B*) and during maximal vasodilation (*C* and *D*) in a normal patient (*A* and *C*) and in a patient with heart failure (*B* and *D*). Components are expressed as percentage of the radius of arteriolar lumen; the value is estimated from changes in blood flow induced by certain interventions and based on the Poiseuille relation, which indicates that flow varies directly as the fourth power of the inner radius of the vessel. FBF = forearm blood flow. (From Mason DT, Zelis R: The function of the arterial and venous beds in congestive heart failure. *Heart Bull* 1968; 17:109–112. Reprinted with permission.)

creased sodium and water content in the vessel itself and are responsible for the decreased systemic arteriolar dilator capacity in patients with congestive heart failure.[10]

With failure of the heart as a pump, there is decrease in blood flow to most regions of the body. However, because the uniform reduction of flow to all areas might result in critical decline of tissue oxygen tension in some organs, in severe congestive heart failure this reduction of flow is not uniform and redistribution of flow occurs (Figure 16.6). In advanced congestive heart failure, blood flow to the renal and cutaneous circulations is reduced disproportionately more than that to other areas.[11] At the same time, coronary blood flow remains normal at all stages of congestive heart failure in the absence of coronary arterial disease, and blood flow to skeletal muscle and brain tends to be preserved except with marked congestive heart failure. Thus, adrenergic-mediated vasoconstriction occurs in the kidneys and skin and thereby blood is diverted to the heart, brain, and skeletal muscle, which have high metabolic requirements relative to flow. As a consequence of these regional adjustments in heart failure, there is deterioration of renal function and impairment of the dissipation of heat generated by the metabolic processes within the body. This is the mechanism that may underlie the heat intolerance and body temperature elevations experienced by some patients with congestive heart failure.

Veins

The overall systemic venous capacitance bed is relatively indistensible in congestive heart failure and thereby affords another peripheral circulatory mechanism for the aid of the failing heart.[9] Thus, the adrenergic-induced increase of venous tone is accompanied by a shift of blood in the systemic venous reservoir toward the central circulation, which augments venous return to the heart and assists in utilization of the Frank-Starling mechanism to maintain cardiac output by elevating ventricular diastolic filling. In addition to these alterations in venous tone at rest in congestive heart failure, during exercise there is an excessive increase in venous tone and central venous pressure mediated by increased sympathetic nervous activity and thereby enhanced return of blood to the impaired ventricle.

Kidneys

By their influence on total blood volume through action on salt and water balance, renal mechanisms contribute actively to the altered hemodynamics comprising the heart failure state. Thus, with reduced renal blood flow, which may occur before reduction of cardiac output due to increased adrenergic activity and redistribution of total blood flow, the kidneys retain sodium and water (Figure 16.7), which increases the intravascular volume, thereby

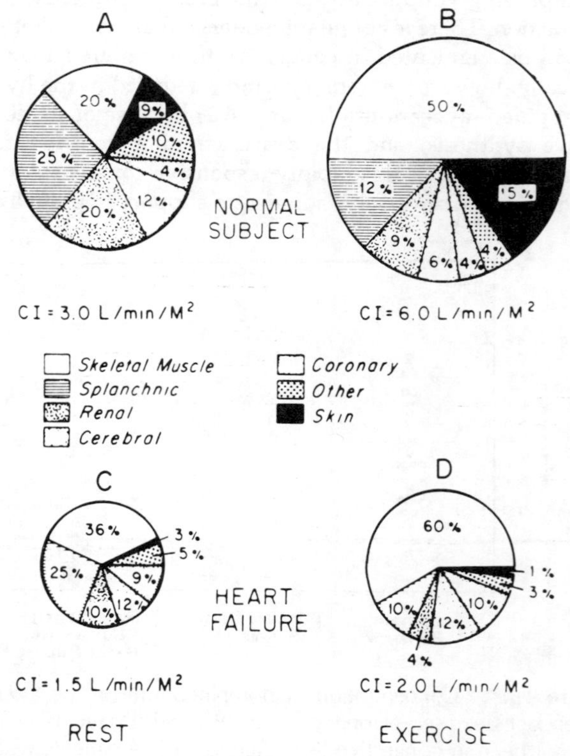

Figure 16.6. Regional distribution of blood flow at rest and during exercise in normal subjects and in patients with heart failure. CI = cardiac index. (From Mason,[9] by permission of the American Heart Association, Inc.)

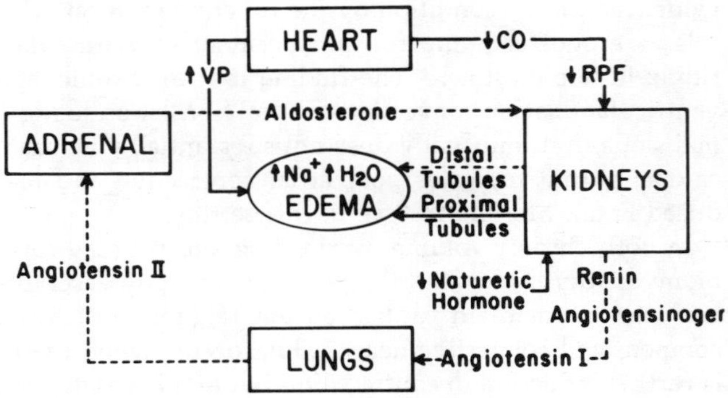

Figure 16.7. Schematic representation of factors producing sodium and water retention in congestive heart failure. Cardiac dysfunction leads to decreased cardiac output (CO) with concomitant reduction in renal plasma flow (RPF), thereby causing increased reabsorption of sodium (Na^+) and water (H_2O) from the proximal renal tubules. These events focused on ↓RPF (factor I) are shown by the solid clockwise arrows. Reduced RPF and related influences activate the renal secretion of renin, which ultimately results in increased adrenal secretion of aldosterone, thus producing increased Na^+ and H_2O reabsorption from the distal renal tubules. These events centered on the elaboration of aldosterone (factor II) are demonstrated by the broken clockwise arrows. In addition, deficiency of a humoral natriuretic substance (factor III) is shown influencing the kidneys to allow greater Na^+ and H_2O reabsorption from the proximal tubules. Finally, the hemodynamic effect of elevated venous pressure (VP) on edema formation is depicted by the solid counterclockwise arrow. (From Tonkon et al,[12] with permission.)

enhancing ventricular filling and the use of the Frank-Starling mechanism for control of cardiac output.[12]

The detection and quantification of occult impairment of sodium excretion in patients with heart disease constitute the basis of the oral sodium tolerance test.[13] Early in congestive heart failure, blood flow to the kidney is reduced to a greater extent than is the glomerular filtration rate; thereby, the filtration fraction is increased and the reabsorption of sodium rises in the proximal convoluted tubules. It is speculated that this increased reabsorption of sodium in congestive heart failure is the result, in part, of insufficiency of an undefined hormonal substance that normally causes proximal renal tubular sodium rejection. In addition, with more advanced congestive heart failure, the renin-angiotensin-aldosterone system is activated, and inappropriate increased secretion of antidiuretic hormone occurs as well, thus leading to enhanced sodium and water reabsorption in the distal tubules. Unlike normal subjects who exhibit diuresis with adrenergic blockade,[14] in persons with congestive heart failure any tendency for an antiadrenergic effect to enhance sodium excretion is overcome by worsening of the depressed cardiocirculatory status, which produces further retention of sodium and water.

FUNCTIONAL CLASSIFICATION

The primary objective of the compensatory mechanisms in clinical heart failure is to maintain basal cardiac output at a normal level. Therefore, initial heart failure symptoms are related to unfavorable side effects necessarily resulting from the action of these mechanisms in performance of their role. Late congestive heart failure symptoms are due to low cardiac output, which is the last hemodynamic variable to become abnormal when cardiac function is reduced.[3]

From these observations, the clinical manifestations of advancing heart failure develop initially (class II functional classification of the New York Heart Association) with dyspnea on exertion (early use of the Frank-Starling mechanism), fatigue with more than ordinary activity (reduced response of cardiac output with exercise due to diminished cardiac contractility), exertional angina pectoris (ventricular hypertrophy with consequent increased myocardial oxygen demands), and excessive tachycardia and sweating with exercise (augmented sympathetic discharge). In the next phase, as the condition worsens (class III), dyspnea, fatigue, angina, tachycardia, and sweating occur with ordinary activity (further depression of contractility with increased use of compensatory mechanisms). These result finally in deterioration (class IV) with weakness, cachexia, mental confusion, oliguria, and hypotension in addition to the other symptoms at rest (caused by reduced basal cardiac output and poor organ perfusion despite maximal use of compensatory mechanisms).

There may be considerable overlap between the relations of altered hemodynamics and clinical features. Thus, when diuretic treatment reduces congestive symptoms and concurrently reduces availability of the Frank-Starling mechanism, class III symptoms may be converted to class II with reduced cardiac output at rest. Furthermore, these functional classes comprise a continuum rather than discrete categories. In class II (congestion with moderate activity) and class III (congestion with mild activity), heart failure is compensated (normal basal cardiac output), and in class IV (congestion at rest) decompensation (low basal cardiac output) occurs. It is evident from this consideration of the correlation of clinical signs and symptoms with pathophysiologic mechanisms that the traditional clinical classification of congestive heart failure is principally based on deleterious expressions of the activity of compensatory mechanisms[3] and not directly on the evaluation of this condition's fundamental hemodynamic variable (cardiac output), the maintenance of which is responsible for congestive heart failure symptoms.

PRIMARY VERSUS SECONDARY HYPERTROPHY

The inotropic state and compensatory mechanisms in primary cardiomyopathy have been compared with those in ventricular hypertrophy secondary to chronic pressure overloading in aortic stenosis.[15] It was considered that quantitative differences in contractility and utilization of reserve mechanisms exist between the primarily and secondarily hypertrophied ventricles. Thus, the contractile state and compensatory systems for cardiac output maintenance are compared in patients with these two lesions (Figure 16.8). In response to pressure overload in compensated aortic stenosis, the ventricle principally employs the hypertrophy mechanism for supporting cardiac output. Although the inotropic state of this secondarily hypertrophied muscle is somewhat diminished, cardiac output is sustained in chronic excessive pressure loading by

	V_{max}	LVEDV	LVH
CARDIOMYOPATHY (primary LV inotropic defect)	↓↓↓	↑	↑
MITRAL REGURGITATION (primary LV volume overload)	↓↓	↑↑	↑
AORTIC STENOSIS (primary LV pressure overload)	↓	0	↑↑↑

Figure 16.8. Compensatory mechanisms for maintaining normal cardiac output in chronic primary and secondary left ventricular hypertrophy (LVH). LV = left ventricle; LVEDV = left ventricular end-diastolic volume. (From Mason,[3] with permission.)

development of more contractile units without increasing end-diastolic volume.

In contrast, in patients with compensated cardiomyopathy who have depressed inotropism as the basic derangement, cardiac output is maintained by operation of both the Frank-Starling and hypertrophy compensatory mechanisms (Figure 16.8). In these patients, normal cardiac output and thereby compensation are accomplished, although the contractile state is more greatly depressed than that in aortic stenosis, because in cardiomyopathy the ventricle does not eject against a severe mechanical abnormality opposing the velocity and extent of fiber shortening.[15] In decompensated congestive heart failure due to primary myocardial disease, cardiac output is reduced when the contractile state becomes further depressed to a low level despite additional maximal utilization of dilation and hypertrophy compensation. In aortic stenosis there is decompensation with decline of cardiac output when the adverse effects of chronic left ventricular outflow obstruction on the myocardium reduce contractility more than in the compensated state, despite further marked hypertrophy and, with the onset of decompensated failure, the development of ventricular dilation. Thus, compensation is maintained in cardiomyopathy and aortic stenosis by relatively dissimilar degrees of the use of preload and hypertrophy reserve mechanisms.[3] Decompensation occurs when normal basal cardiac output cannot be delivered because the contractile state has fallen below a certain critical level in both primary hypertrophy and hypertrophy secondary to chronic pressure overloading; this critical level is lower in primary cardiomyopathy.

Pressure Versus Volume Overload

In further clinical studies, contractility and compensatory mechanisms have been compared in adult patients with chronic ventricular pressure and volume overloading.[3] In compensated volume overload due to long-standing mitral regurgitation, contractility is more depressed than in chronic aortic stenosis (Figure 16.8). In addition, in long-term volume overload, cardiac output is maintained by the mechanisms of both dilation and hypertrophy, whereas compensation is obtained by marked use of hypertrophy reserve alone in aortic stenosis. However, preload remains highly important for maintenance of cardiac output in the hypertrophied nondilated ventricle, as evidenced in this condition by the function of atrial systole as a booster pump for enhancement of ventricular filling in late diastole.[16] The finding that in chronic left ventricular dilation conversion of atrial fibrillation to normal sinus rhythm usually does not substantially increase cardiac output indicates poor atrial contraction and reduced Frank-Starling reserve in this setting.

In both chronic volume overloading and primary cardiomyopathy, Frank-Starling and hypertrophy reserves are used to maintain cardiac output (Figure 16.8). Decompensated congestive heart failure occurs when there is further reduction in contractility, but to a lesser degree in volume overloading than in cardiomyopathy. Therefore, resting cardiac output cannot be maintained at a normal level when contractile state declines to a precarious value. This crucial inotropic level is lowest in primary cardiomyopathy, intermediate in chronic volume overloading, and least reduced compared to normal in chronic excessive ventricular pressure overloading.

Comparison of Volume Overloads

The recognition that alterations in instantaneous impedance to ejection and ventricular fiber tension during ejection (afterload) are important determinants of the dynamics of cardiac contraction has provided appreciation of differences in cardiac performance in conditions of systolic mechanical volume overloading. Therefore, in mitral compared to aortic regurgitation with equivalent total and effective stroke volumes, left ventricular function is more disturbed with greater end-diastolic pressure and volume in aortic regurgitation.[17] In the latter entity, the entire total stroke volume must be delivered into the physiologically high-pressure ascending aorta, whereas the regurgitant volume in mitral insufficiency is immediately ejected into the low-pressure left atrium. These findings concerning the greater afterload burden operative on the left ventricle in aortic incompetence emphasize the clinical observation of poorer cardiac tolerance chronically present in this condition with marked extent of utilization of preload and hypertrophy reserves, in contrast to chronic mitral insufficiency, in which similar systolic volume overload is accompanied by considerably less ventricular mass and systolic tension.

In additional studies on differences in cardiac performance in systolic volume overloading, it was shown that left ventricular function is substantially less compromised in ventricular septal defect than in patent ductus arteriosus at the same level of abnormally increased pulmonary blood flow.[18] Therefore, in ventricular septal defect, the shunted flow is ejected directly into the low-pressure right ventricle, whereas in patent ductus arteriosus the entire left ventricular stroke output must be ejected into the high-pressure aorta before shunting. Therefore, at identically elevated pulmonary-to-systemic flow ratios, in patent ductus arteriosus the left ventricular end-diastolic pressure and volume are greater, duration of ejection is more prolonged and ventricular ejection rate and fraction are less increased, and there is greater ventricular midwall systolic tension, contractile element work, and power than in ventricular septal defect (Figure 16.9). In ventricular septal defect, the lesser increase in

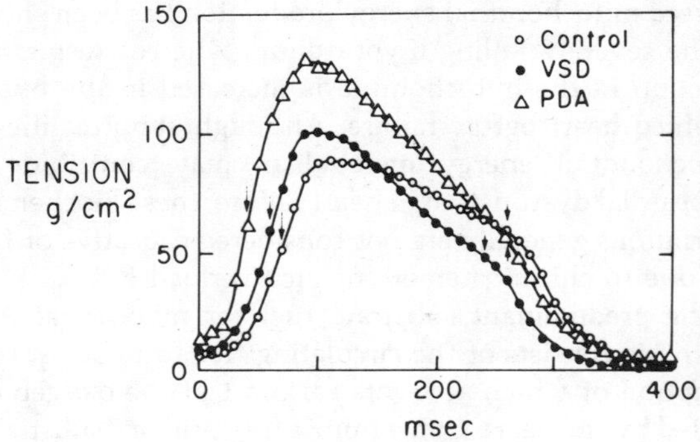

Figure 16.9. Comparison of instantaneous left ventricular wall tension at 5-ms intervals in a normal heart, ventricular septal defect (VSD), and patent ductus arteriosus (PDA) in an open chest canine preparation using external left-to-right shunts. The VSD and patent ductus arteriosus were separately, acutely induced and compared at equal 2 to 1 pulmonary-to-systemic flow ratios. Aortic valve opening is indicated by the solid arrows (*left*) and aortic closure by the broken arrows (*right*). (From Mason,[3] with permission.)

end-diastolic pressure and volume, greater increase in ejection rate and fraction, lesser increase in tension early in systole and in contractile element work and power throughout systole, in contrast to patent ductus arteriosus, and the shorter ejection period with more rapid decrease in tension than normal in ventricular septal defect, are all the result of greater reduction in instantaneous impedance to left ventricular emptying in ventricular septal defect than in patent ductus arteriosus.

From these observations concerning the dynamics of ventricular contraction, ventricular septal defect is similar to mitral regurgitation and patent ductus arteriosus is similar to aortic regurgitation. Therefore, although each of these four conditions of systolic volume overload encroaches on ventricular performance, cardiac function is more disturbed in aortic insufficiency and patent ductus arteriosus. Furthermore, because resistance to ejection is more reduced in mitral regurgitation and ventricular septal defect, their integrated ventricular systolic tension is similar to normal, whereas left ventricular afterload is substantially increased above normal in aortic regurgitation and patent ductus arteriosus. In regard to myocardial oxygen consumption, cardiac energy costs are considerably greater in pressure overloading in which ventricular systolic tension and afterload are markedly more increased than in volume overloading.[19] Furthermore, comparing different types of systolic volume overloads, in those conditions in which impedance offered to ejection is considerably reduced, such as mitral regurgitation and ventricular septal defect, there is a smaller increase in cardiac oxygen requirements than in those conditions in which resistance to ejection is decreased to a smaller degree, as in patent ductus arteriosus and aortic regurgitation.

BIOCHEMICAL–BIOPHYSICAL MECHANISMS

The hemodynamic function of the heart is dependent on the mechanical properties of its myocardium[20] in which the sarcomere is the basic subcellular contractile unit (Figure 16.10). The contractile apparatus of the sarcomere consists of four protein molecular aggregates: the primary interacting (1) actin thin filaments and (2) myosin thick filaments; and the modulator proteins (3) troponin and (4) tropomyosin, which inhibit actomyosin reaction. Resting sarcomere length controls the extent of myofilament overlap, which determines the number of actin–myosin binding sites, the subcellular basis for the active length-tension curve (Figure 16.11) which is the isolated heart muscle equivalent of the Frank-Starling ventricular function curve.[20] The intensity of interaction between thick and thin filaments regulates contractility.

The principal biochemical processes that relate to the ultimate contractile function of the ventricle include those involved in regulation of energy metabolism, contractile machinery of the sarcomere, the muscle relaxing system, electrical and transport activity of the membranes, and protein synthesis within the fiber.[20] It is emphasized that these chemical mechanisms are interrelated, and alterations in any one of them may influence activity in the

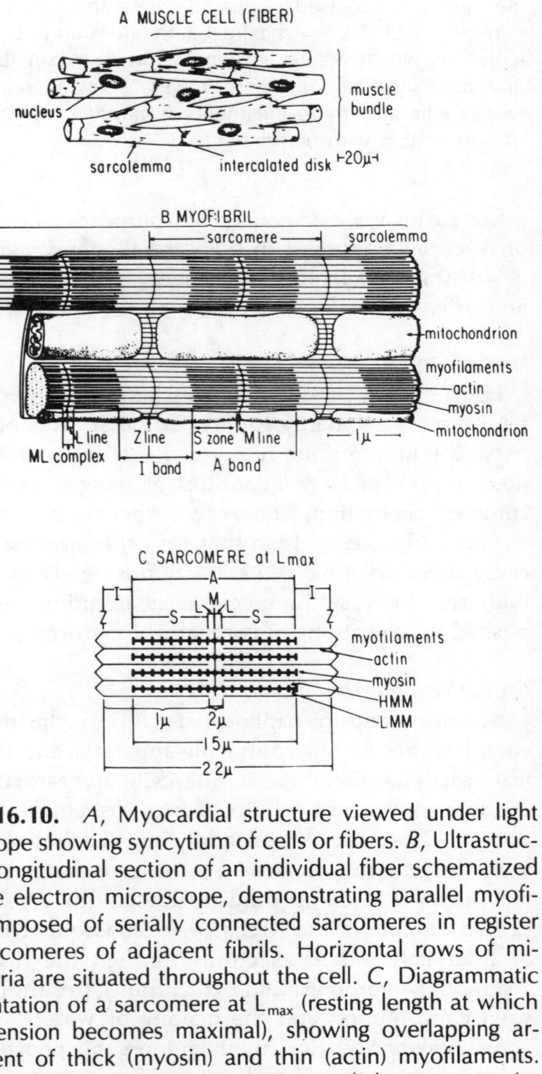

Figure 16.10. *A*, Myocardial structure viewed under light microscope showing syncytium of cells or fibers. *B*, Ultrastructure of longitudinal section of an individual fiber schematized from the electron microscope, demonstrating parallel myofibrils composed of serially connected sarcomeres in register with sarcomeres of adjacent fibrils. Horizontal rows of mitochondria are situated throughout the cell. *C*, Diagrammatic representation of a sarcomere at L_{max} (resting length at which active tension becomes maximal), showing overlapping arrangement of thick (myosin) and thin (actin) myofilaments. HMM = heavy meromyosin; LMM = light meromyosin; S = S zone (area of actin-myosin overlap). (From Mason et al,[20] with permission.)

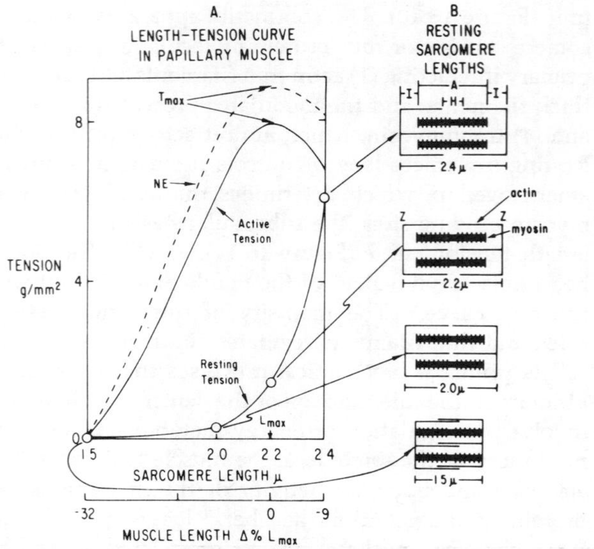

Figure 16.11. *A*, Relations between active and resting (passive) tension development and sarcomere and papillary muscle length of the feline right ventricle. The active tension curve is elevated by increased contractile state induced by norepinephrine (NE). T_{max} = maximal active tension at L_{max} (resting length at which active tension becomes maximal). *B*, Diagrammatic resting sarcomere lengths showing relations between actin and myosin filaments at different preloads. (From Mason et al,[20] with permission.)

other pathways. For conceptual purposes, the sequence of reactions important in myocardial energy metabolism is substrate availability and energy production, storage, and utilization.

MYOCARDIAL ENERGETICS

Heart muscle is uniquely dependent on aerobic metabolism for its energy supply. To satisfy this obligatory need, the myocardium requires the delivery of a continuous supply of large quantities of oxygen through the coronary circulation. The oxygen demand of the heart is considerably greater than that for other organs, and because myocardial oxygen extraction is nearly maximal at body rest, increases in oxygen need are primarily accomplished by elevations in coronary blood flow.

Oxidative Phosphorylation

Because adenosine triphosphate (ATP) is the immediate energy source for the contractile apparatus and biochemical reactions elsewhere in the cell, myocardial energy metabolism normally is directed toward aerobic production of ATP in the mitochondria[20] by substrate oxidation (dehydrogenation of citric acid intermediates requiring nicotinamide adenine dinucleotide), with discharge of carbon dioxide in the Krebs cycle, consequent transport of hydrogen and its electrons through the respiratory chain of flavoproteins and cytochromes (resulting in oxygen consumption and the making of water), and oxidative phosphorylation in which inorganic phosphate acquires a high-energy bond and combines with adenosine diphosphate (ADP) to form ATP (Figure 16.12). Depressed mitochondrial energy production has been shown in the severely failing myocardium, whereas respiratory function in the mitochondria is increased in the hypertrophied heart before failure. Although abnormalities in mitochondrial energy metabolism may contribute to myocardial dysfunction in heart failure, these biochemical aberrations generally are not considered causative of failure due to chronic hemodynamic overload.[20]

The predominant substrate fuel for myocardial ATP synthesis consists of the circulating free fatty acids, consumption of which accounts for most of the oxygen extracted by the heart. Concerning other primary substrates, normally blood glucose is used preferentially in the postprandial state. Circulating lactate also is an important fuel, particularly when its blood concentration is elevated by prolonged skeletal muscle exercise. Blood pyruvate, like glucose, lactate, and free fatty acids, is readily taken up by the myocardium in proportion to its arterial blood concentration. Conversion of the substrate fuels into acetyl-coenzyme A is necessary for their entry into the citric acid cycle for aerobic ATP production (Figure 16.12). Concerning blood glucose as substrate in myocardial energy systems, after the substance is transported across the sarcolemma-transtubular membranes and metabolized to glucose-6-phosphate under the influence of insulin, it may be stored as glycogen or undergo anaerobic glycolysis to pyruvate in the sarcoplasm. In normal conditions, pyruvate is oxidized to acetyl-coenzyme A and undergoes aerobic metabolism in the citric acid cycle within the mitochondria. In the absence of hypoxia, the heart does not produce lactate.

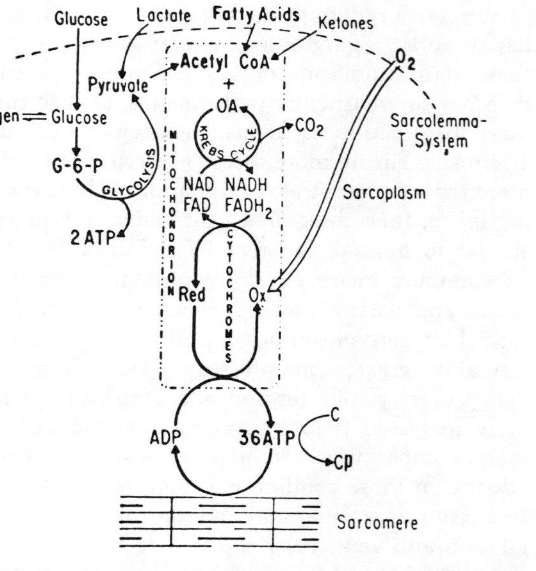

Figure 16.12. Metabolic pathways for energy (ATP) production shown diagrammatically within the cardiac cell. C = creatine; CP = creatine phosphate; FAD = flavin adenine dinucleotide; $FADH_2$ = reduced FAD; G-6-P = glucose-6-phosphate; NAD = nicotinamide adenine dinucleotide; NADH = reduced NAD; Ox = oxidation; Red = reduction. See text for further explanation. (From Mason et al,[20] with permission.)

Anaerobic Glycolysis

The importance of anaerobic glycolysis as a source of energy varies with the state of oxygenation of the myocardium.[20] Normally, glycolysis is of considerably less significance, because this entire process results in only two ATP molecules for each molecule of glucose, whereas each glucose molecule provides 36 molecules of ATP in the aerobic pathways (Figure 16.12). When myocardial oxygen delivery falls, there is increased glycolysis, although this is an ineffective process alone for maintaining energy supply, and ATP levels decline. Also, less pyruvate enters the citric acid cycle during enhanced glycolytic metabolism in myocardial hypoxia. Consequently, in the heart relatively deprived of oxygen, pyruvate is reduced to lactate, and lactate is not extracted; thereby, the hypoxic myocardium may produce more lactate than it consumes, with the result that coronary sinus blood will contain more lactate than systemic arterial blood. In contrast, lactate concentration is greater in arterial blood than in the coronary venous effluent in the normally metabolizing heart owing to myocardial lactate extraction for aerobic synthesis of ATP. By selective catheterization of the coronary sinus, detection of abnormal myocardial lactate metabolism or balance provides a useful biochemical means for the objective identification of myocardial ischemia in patients with coronary artery disease. Furthermore, when the abnormality is not present at rest in patients with angina pectoris, it often can be revealed by increasing the mechanical and metabolic activity of the heart by the performance of exercise, by increasing heart rate with a pacemaker catheter, or by administering isoproterenol.

Creatine Phosphate

In myocardial energy storage, creatine phosphate functions as a limited reservoir of high-energy phosphate to maintain ATP.[20] Therefore, following the cleavage of ATP by myofibrillar ATPase to ADP and inorganic phosphate in the contraction reaction and by the additional myocardial ATPases in other biochemical processes requiring energy utilization, ADP is replenished with a high-energy phosphate from creatine phosphate or by oxidative phosphorylation to reform ATP. Creatine phosphate is resynthesized by oxidative phosphorylation. Although creatine phosphate serves as a ready source of auxiliary chemical energy for ADP, its quantity is relatively small, even in the normal heart. In chronic heart failure, ATP levels are not depleted, although creatine phosphate often is diminished, but this reduction follows rather than precedes abnormal contractile performance.[20]

EXCITATION–CONTRACTION COUPLING

When the stimulating impulse from the cardiac pacemaker arrives at the surface of the myocardial cell, an orderly sequence of events is initiated in which calcium movement is the chief component linking electrical excitation of the fiber with mechanical activation of the contractile machinery in the sarcomere.[20] Excitation of the individual cell proceeds as the depolarization wave spreads throughout the entire fiber along the external sarcolemma and its interior-projecting transtubular (T) membrane system (Figure 16.13). When the depolarizing current in the transtubular system reaches the intimately apposed calcium depots of the intracellular sarcoplasmic reticulum, ionic calcium release is triggered from the sarcoplasmic reticulum into the sarcoplasm. Together with a smaller but crucial quantity of ionic calcium influx across the sarcolemma-transtubular membrane occurring during phase 2 of the transmembrane action potential, this discharged calcium immediately diffuses to the sarcomeres, where it binds to the specific troponin calcium-receptor protein on the thin myofilaments in the overlap region between the thick and thin filaments. Mechanical activation is achieved by the binding of activator-calcium to troponin, which overcomes the troponin–tropomyosin complex inhibition of actin and myosin interaction, with the result that actin–myosin electrostatic cross bridges are formed.[20]

CONTRACTILE PROCESS

The onset of contraction takes place with the development of force and shortening of the contractile elements by the cyclic interaction of actin–myosin linkages pulling the thin filaments along the immobile thick fil-

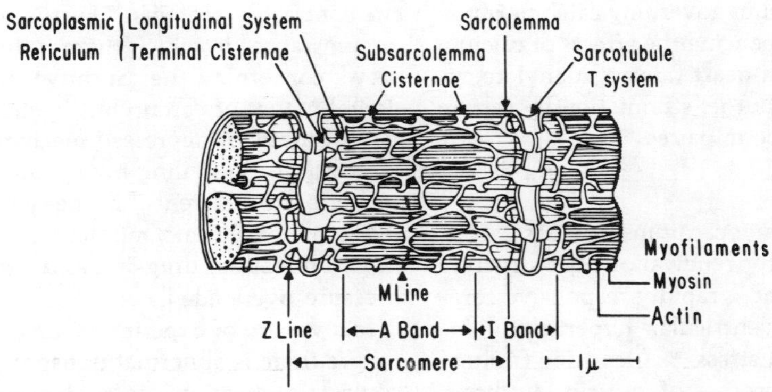

Figure 16.13. Longitudinal diagram of myocardial ultrastructure reconstructed from electron micrographs showing relations between the superficial (sarcolemma and wide T system) and intracellular (sarcoplasmic reticulum) membranes of the cardiac fiber. (From Mason et al,[20] with permission.)

aments.[20] The electrostatic links are broken as myosin ATPase in the myosin heads hydrolyzes ATP, which is diffused to the sarcomeres from closely neighboring mitochondria, to ADP and inorganic phosphate. Thus, a repetitive sequence of making and breaking cross-linkages is established as the actin filament slides past the myosin filament during the entire course of ventricular contraction.

The excitation–contraction coupling process in which calcium is delivered to the contractile apparatus does not require ATP energy. The contractile reaction involving myosin ATPase utilizes the great majority of total myocardial energy, which varies according to the muscle loading conditions and contractile state.[20] Following completion of the active contractile state, the active process of relaxation ensues, with calcium departing from the sarcomere and rapidly binding to the sarcoplasmic reticulum. The cation then is pumped back into the calcium depots of the sarcoplasmic reticulum by sarcotubular calcium pump ATPase (relaxing factor), the total energy needed for relaxation being relatively small.

CYCLIC ADENOSINE MONOPHOSPHATE

Another important biochemical system in heart muscle is that involved with the intracellular regulatory substance cyclic adenosine monophosphate (AMP).[20] Cyclic AMP is synthesized in the sarcoplasm from ATP by stimulation of the enzyme adenylate cyclase of the surface sarcolemma and transtubular membranes. The activity of adenylate cyclase is enhanced by beta-adrenergic receptor stimulation located also in these superficial membranes. The positive inotropic action of certain cardiovascular agents is mediated by activation of this process, leading to increased cyclic AMP formation: catecholamines by stimulation of the beta receptor, and glucagon and thyroid hormone by direct action on adenylate cyclase. Furthermore, the increased contractility produced by aminophylline and amrinone has been attributed to the action of these drugs of inhibiting phosphodiesterase, an intracellular enzyme that inactivates cyclic AMP. Concerning the biochemical mechanisms through which cyclic AMP increases cardiac contraction, myocardial cyclic AMP-dependent protein kinase phosphorylates protein components in sarcoplasmic reticulum governing calcium transport to troponin, thereby enhancing the effects of calcium in the contractile reaction. In heart failure, adenylate cyclase activity is not altered, but its stimulation by certain cardiovascular agents may be impaired.[20]

PROTEIN SYNTHESIS

Protein synthesis in the myocardium provides a continuously operative system for renewal of fiber structure and enzymatic machinery and a rapidly responsive compensatory mechanism for ventricular hypertrophy induced by cardiac mechanical stress.[20] Adenosine triphosphate is consumed in the process of protein synthesis. Excessive intramyocardial tension appears to be the transducer coupling mechanical systolic overload with increased activity of protein synthesis pathways. Increased muscle mass resulting from elevated hemodynamic burden is principally due to hypertrophy rather than hyperplasia of myocardial fibers, although there is some proliferation of connective tissue cells. Activation of all stages of protein synthesis occurs rapidly following acute stress, with increased incorporation of amino acids into proteins in myocardial cells. With chronic severe hemodynamic overload, however, there is some diminution of these processes.[20]

Although the induction of ventricular hypertrophy may result from different factors, including pressure overload, volume overload, hormonal influences, exercise, hypoxia, and primary disturbances of contractility, the development of hypertrophy caused by all these conditions is characterized by the initial mechanism of protein synthesis. Because an increase in muscle mass accompanies hypertrophy, ventricular systolic stress is lessened. In this manner the hypertrophy process compensates for an excessive hemodynamic load by producing more sarcomeres and, in some types of hypertrophy, improves cardiac function to normal. An important concept is that of physiologic versus pathologic ventricular hypertrophy in response to disparate settings. Physiologic hypertrophy is signified by a normal or augmented contractile state with concomitant levels of myosin ATPase activity, in contrast to pathologic hypertrophy characterized by depressed contraccility and diminished myosin ATPase function.[21]

IMPAIRED CONTRACTILITY

It is apparent that a number of highly important biochemical processes are operative in the intact ventricle. Their complete integrity of function and proper integration are essential for normal mechanical and hemodynamic performance of the heart. Although aberrations have been identified in certain of these systems in the failing myocardium, the current view is that abnormalities in myocardial energy production, cyclic AMP reactions, and norepinephrine synthesis may contribute by encroaching on compensatory mechanisms but do not play the primary causative role in the onset of congestive heart failure induced by chronic hemodynamic overload.[20] A more promising possibility is that the biochemical defect or constellation of abnormalities resides in the mechanism of excitation–contraction coupling and the function of the contractile proteins.[20] Furthermore, it is likely that in circumstances in which there is divergence of results and views concerning the causative, contributory, or coincidental nature of certain biochemical abnormalities in the pathogenesis of depressed mechanical function and contractility in the failing myocardium, these dissimilarities reflect basic differences in the types of heart failure studied: acute or chronic, mild or severe, experimental or human, idiopathic, drug-induced, ischemic, or volume- or pressure-overloaded.

In a variety of experimental models of congestive heart failure there is abnormal transport of calcium by the sarcoplasmic reticulum, as evidenced by its impairment of calcium uptake, binding, release, and pump ATPase activity.[22] It has been suggested that the early decline of contractility in myocardial ischemia, with attendant intracellular acidosis due to lactate production, results directly from hydrogen ion inhibition of calcium binding to troponin.[23] In the final phase of ischemic heart disease, exhaustion of ATP supply leads to the development of irreversible ventricular contracture, whereas decreased contractility in the earlier stage of ischemia caused by disturbed excitation–contraction coupling may be reversible with reperfusion of the myocardium with oxygenated blood.

Concerning experimental examples of chronic hemodynamic overload in dogs, mild right[24] or left[25] ventricular outflow obstruction causes sustained increases in myosin ATPase and inotropic function for several weeks in the stress-hypertrophied ventricle before eventual depression of such activity (Figure 16.14). In contrast, severe canine pulmonary or aortic stenosis results in immediate progressive declines in myosin ATPase activity and contractility in the stressed hypertrophied ventricle. Thus, differential responses of physiologic versus pathologic hypertrophy in the stressed ventricle are produced by chronic right or left ventricular pressure overloading,[21] the type of hypertrophy being dependent on the severity and duration of the hemodynamic burden.

In further regard to dysfunction of the contractile proteins in heart failure, attention has been focused on the mechanisms of abnormal energy utilization by myosin ATPase. The enzymatic function of myosin in the contractile process is thought to be governed by the subunit composition of whole myosin (Figure 16.15). Thus, myosin light chains within the heads of myosin appear to suppress the ATPase activity contained in the portion of the heavy chains comprising the myosin heads.[20] The normal left ventricle possesses higher levels of myosin ATPase associated with lesser proportions of myosin light to heavy chains, compared with the normal right ventricle. In mild hemodynamic overload, increased myosin enzymatic function has been observed in the early hypertrophied stressed ventricle consequent to the production of relatively more heavy to light myosin subunits.[24] Therefore, in the early period following mild experimental pulmonic stenosis, the myosin of the hypertrophied right ventricle develops the properties of normal left ventricular myosin. Consistent with the concept that myosin light chains modulate the enzymatic performance of myosin are the findings in chronic severe canine aortic stenosis; myosin ATPase is depressed, whereas the proportion of light to heavy chains of myosin increases in the markedly stressed left ventricle.[25] Thus, in severe hemodynamic overload, the myosin in the heavily stressed left ventricle develops the characteristics of right ventricular myosin in the normal heart.

Finally, concerning the myosin molecular alterations causing the kinetic disorders of diminished myosin ATP hydrolysis, thereby less intense actin–myosin interaction responsible for reduced contractility of pathologic hypertrophy resulting in the decreased contractile force of abnormal cardiac function, reduced myosin ATPase activity appears to be due to structural alterations either in the myosin light chains governing myosin ATPase function or in the active site of the myosin head heavy chains containing myosin ATPase.[20] These molecular alterations in heavy and light chain myosins may be due to pathologic hypertrophy-induced changes in specific isoenzymes regulating the synthesis of the different myosin subunit proteins during the course of cardiac hypertrophy. Therefore, the decrease in contractility related to depressed myosin ATPase function with pathologic hypertrophy appears to be due to either the synthesis of modified isoenzymes leading to myosin molecular abnormalities or charge aberrations of myosin, or both.[26]

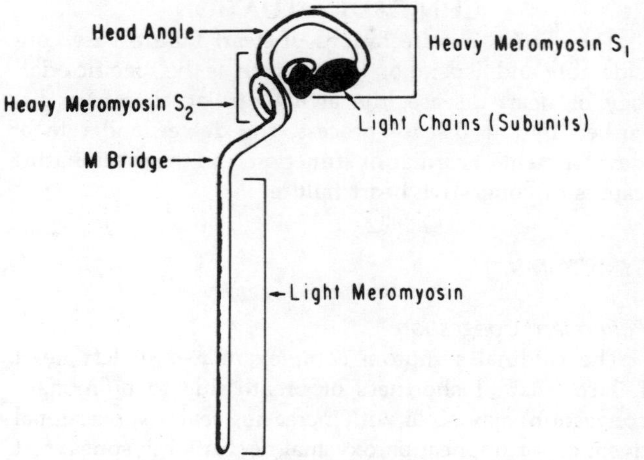

Figure 16.15. Representation of the configuration of one of the two heavy chains of whole myosin. The myosin heavy chain is composed of light meromyosin and heavy meromyosin. The M bridge is between light and heavy meromyosin and the head angle between heavy meromyosin S_1 and heavy meromyosin S_2. In addition, two light chains are bound within the heavy chain myosin head. (From Mason et al,[20] with permission.)

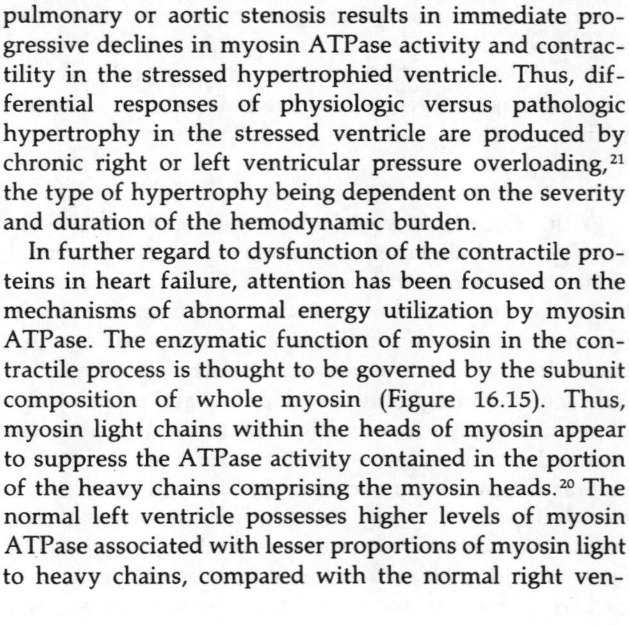

Figure 16.14. Comparison of disparate canine myosin ATPase function from hemodynamically stressed ventricles under different degrees and durations of right and left ventricular outflow obstruction. (From Mason et al,[20] with permission.)

CLINICAL EVALUATION

The clinical manifestations of heart failure vary considerably and depend on factors such as the specific etiology of heart disease, the actual cardiac chambers disturbed by the disease process, the degree and rate of development of cardiac dysfunction, and the precipitating causes of congestive heart failure.

SYMPTOMS

Pulmonary Congestion

The cardinal symptom complex related to left heart failure (that of shortness of breath due to pulmonary congestion) may occur with increasing severity: exertional dyspnea, orthopnea, paroxysmal nocturnal dyspnea, rest dyspnea, and acute pulmonary edema.[27] Progressive degrees of pulmonary capillary and venous distention produce exertional dyspnea, orthopnea (supine dyspnea), and rest dyspnea as engorged vessels encroach upon small airspaces and cause lung stiffness, restricted ventilation, decreased vital capacity and tidal volume, peripheral airway trapping with increased dead space, and ventilation-perfusion alterations with consequent widened alveolar-arterial oxygen difference and hypoxemia. Further, bronchial congestion leads to the dyspnea equivalent of cough, which may become productive when mucus secretion is stimulated. The presence of pulmonary interstitial edema induces attacks of paroxysmal nocturnal dyspnea, and bronchospasm resulting from extravascular swelling of bronchial mucosa causes episodes of cardiac asthma. Alveolar edema with transudation and expectoration of blood-tinged sputum underlies acute pulmonary edema, whereas rupture of distended bronchial capillaries can result in hemoptysis.

Lowered Cardiac Output

Impaired cardiac output response to physical activity brings about easy fatigability, and diminished resting stroke output results in cerebral symptoms and even syncope. Sympathetic-induced redistribution of regional blood flow[28] away from the kidneys during physical activity subsequently leads to the diurnal pattern of nocturia with resting recumbency relatively early in congestive heart failure, whereas oliguria occurs with renal failure and is a late finding in congestive heart failure when basal cardiac output is significantly depressed.

Systemic Congestion

The principal symptoms of right heart failure relate to congestion of the liver and gastrointestinal tract. These include right upper quadrant discomfort, anorexia, nausea, and constipation.

PHYSICAL SIGNS

Depressed Cardiac Contractility

Early impairment of ventricular contractility is usually accompanied by a low-frequency early diastolic gallop (S_3) audible with the stethoscope bell placed lightly over the apex of the appropriate ventricle.[27] Presystolic atrial gallop (S_4) may also be heard with ventricular dysfunction; this finding does not necessarily denote ventricular decompensation but rather represents decreased diastolic compliance of the corresponding ventricle. In sinus tachycardia, third and fourth heart sounds usually merge during diastole to produce a summation gallop. Third heart sounds may be heard in normal adolescents and young adults, and fourth heart sounds are often heard in apparently normal older individuals. Because the rate of left ventricular pressure increase is diminished during isovolumic systole with depressed contractility, there is decreased intensity of the first heart sound in left ventricular failure. Left ventricular ejection may also be delayed with myocardial failure; thus, paradoxical splitting of the second heart sound may occur (pulmonic component of the second sound precedes aortic component) in which second heart sound splitting widens during expiration, in contrast to normal second heart sound splitting increasing with inspiration.

Pulsus Alternans

With severe left ventricular dysfunction, relatively evenly spaced alterations of strong and weak peripheral pulses may occur with each beat. This phenomenon, known as pulsus alternans, is observed most commonly in aortic stenosis, systemic hypertension, cardiomyopathies, and coronary artery disease.[29] Although the precise mechanism leading to the development and perpetuation of pulsus alternans is not firmly established, it is generally regarded that there is alteration of force of ventricular contraction caused by variations in contractility, preload, electrical excitability, and refractoriness. In some patients, pulsus alternans may persist for several days, whereas in other individuals it may be initiated by a premature ventricular contraction and last only a few beats. In general, discrepancy between amplitude of strong and weak beats and duration of the phenomenon are directly related to depression of the left ventricular contractile state.

Dicrotic Pulse

Palpable dicrotic carotid pulsation may occur in left ventricular pump failure.[29] Normally, carotid pulse rises rapidly to its peak or anacrotic shoulder coincident with peak carotid blood flow (percussion wave). The subsequent tidal wave descending limb is interrupted by a dicrotic notch (coincident with aortic valve closure). The dicrotic notch is followed by a small upward diastolic wave (normally not palpable). In left ventricular failure with reduced stroke volume and cardiac output, however, the characteristic decrease in amplitude and rate of increase of the percussion wave result in increased amplitude of dicrotic pulse, which often becomes palpable. Also in left ventricular failure, the carotid pulse ejection period may become shortened because of diminished stroke volume and elevated peripheral vascular resistance.

Elevated Sympathetic Tone

Other abnormalities in the systemic arterial tree are caused by increased sympathetic activity of congestive heart failure. The resting heart rate is increased with excessive rise in pulse rate after minimal exertion, as well as mild diastolic hypertension with narrow pulse pressure. Increased sympathetic tone also produces venoconstriction,[9] which contributes to increased jugular venous pressure. Increased sympathetic activity with low cardiac output in congestive heart failure results in redistribution of peripheral blood flow among the body's organs. Thus, relatively less blood flow is delivered to the cutaneous and renal circulations, causing decreased skin temperature, heat intolerance, and often prerenal azotemia.[28] Distal extremities become cool, increased sweating occurs, and peripheral cyanosis results from increased oxygen extraction with oxygen desaturation in cutaneous veins.

Peripheral Cyanosis

The bluish cutaneous color of cyanosis is best visualized in the oral mucous membranes, tongue and lips, around the mouth, conjunctiva, digital nail beds, fingers, and hands. This abnormal coloration is usually not seen until systemic arterial oxygen saturation becomes less than 85%. Cyanosis is either central or peripheral in origin. Central cyanosis, seen principally in the facial and digital areas, results from intrapulmonary admixture or generalized hypoventilation with diminished ventilation-perfusion and from right-to-left intracardiac shunting in congenital heart disease. Peripheral cyanosis, limited to the extremities, occurs with marked stasis of blood in congestive heart failure with low basal cardiac output, shock states, peripheral arterial or venous obstructive disease, and intense limb vasoconstriction such as cold environment or Raynaud's phenomenon.

Ventricular Hypertrophy

Chronic left ventricular failure ultimately results in progressive left ventricular hypertrophy, which can easily be perceived by precordial palpation. In concentric hypertrophy without dilation, left ventricular hypertrophy produces increased amplitude and duration of the apical pulse with the patient in the left lateral position, often without modification of its location. In hypertrophy with reduced left ventricular compliance, palpation reveals prominent presystolic pulsation caused by left atrial contraction in the presence of diminished ventricular distensibility. With right ventricular hypertrophy, abnormal outward motion along the left sternal border occurs during systole.

Ventricular Dilation

Left ventricular dilation, occurring as a compensatory mechanism to maintain normal resting cardiac output, is appreciated by precordial palpation. With the patient supine, the normal left ventricular impulse occurs during isovolumic systole in the fourth or fifth intercostal space medial to the midclavicular line. An apical impulse lateral to the midclavicular line is indicative of left ventricular dilation. Segmental dyssynergy of the left ventricular anterior wall and apex in coronary heart disease also causes cardiac enlargement with lateral apical pulse sustained in its outward motion during systole. Left ventricular dilation also causes widening of the mitral valve ring and disturbance of papillary muscle function with consequent incompetence of the mitral valve leaflets. Thus, left ventricular dilation itself may lead to some degree of mitral regurgitation which is characterized by an accompanying murmur, commonly pansystolic at the cardiac apex, best heard with the patient in the left lateral decubitus position. Similarly, right ventricular dilation can lead to tricuspid regurgitation with a systolic murmur, often increased in intensity during inspiration, heard best at the left lower sternal border.

Excessive Left Ventricular End-Diastolic Pressure

Left ventricular failure produces an increase in left ventricular end-diastolic pressure and in left atrial pressure, which is transmitted to the pulmonary capillaries through an increase in pulmonary venous pressure. When pulmonary capillary hydrostatic pressure exceeds colloid osmotic pressure, there is fluid transudation into interstitial spaces leading to increased lung extravascular fluid and pulmonary edema. Interstitial edema leads to alveolar edema, with pulmonary rales detectable by chest wall auscultation.

Pleural Effusion

Pleural effusion is also common in chronic congestive heart failure. It is not well recognized that hydrothorax most often occurs with right heart failure or biventricular failure; increased systemic venous pressure is more important than elevated pulmonary capillary pressure in pleural effusion formation.

Valsalva Maneuver

The engorged pulmonary vasculature in left heart failure produces a characteristically abnormal Valsalva response (forceful expiration against closed glottis).[29] Normally a brief initial increase in systemic arterial pressure (representing sudden blood flow from the pulmonary bed into the left heart) occurs, and arterial pressure then decreases (reflecting decreased cardiac output resulting from diminished venous return); this in turn stimulates reflex carotid baroreceptor sympathetic-induced vasoconstriction. With discontinuation of expiration, sudden release of thoracic cavity positive pressure causes a brief additional decrease in arterial pressure. Then, arterial pressure normally rises immediately above pre-Valsalva control arterial pressure accompanied by reflex bradycardia. The striking post-Valsalva arterial pressure overshoot is due principally to continued reflex sympathetic vasoconstriction. In contrast, with left ventricular failure the pulmonary reservoir maintains left ventricular filling throughout the maneuver. Consequently, stroke volume ejected from the impaired left ventricle is maintained and systemic blood pressure remains elevated. Because systemic blood pressure does not decrease, and thus increased baroreceptor stimulation is absent, release of forced expiration results in neither post-Valsalva systemic blood pressure overshoot nor reflex bradycardia.

Excessive Right Ventricular End-Diastolic Pressure

Visual inspection of the jugular veins permits a remarkably accurate estimation of central venous pressure and, in turn, right heart failure, because with elevation of right ventricular end-diastolic pressure right atrial pressure increases. Elevated venous pressure is best observed in the right external and internal jugular veins, with the patient's head elevated so that the top of the blood-oscillating column can easily be noted.[29] With the patient supine, the head of the bed is tilted upward until the jugular veins begin to empty in a pulsating meniscus representing the blood column summit. Central venous pressure is equal in centimeters of water to this meniscus height measured relative to the right atrium, which serves as the column's lowest point or zero level. At the bedside, column height is estimated using the superior sternal angle as reference point, because the right atrium is approximately 5 cm below the sternal angle. With the patient's head elevated approximately 30°, the vertical distance between the sternal angle level to oscillating blood column top is normally less than 3 cm. Thus, this 3 cm plus the 5 cm from the sternal angle to right atrium equals 8 cm of blood, or approximately 5 to 6 mm Hg. The central systemic venous pressure is elevated when the vertical distance between the highest point of the visible pulsation of the jugular vein is greater than 3 cm above the sternal angle.

Peripheral Edema

Peripheral edema is generally found in chronic right heart failure as a result of elevated systemic venous pressure and salt and water retention from diminished renal perfusion. Edema formation occurs in the dependent body portions, usually in the pretibial areas, and can be differentiated from lymphedema by characteristic pitting with mild finger pressure. Noncardiac edema, usually more diffuse in location, is caused by chronic renal disease, profound hypoalbuminemia, Cushing's disease, and premenstrual period. In primary hepatic cirrhosis, ascites is proportionally greater than ankle edema. Facial edema rarely occurs in congestive heart failure and is most commonly the result of superior vena caval obstruction or strenuous respiratory efforts due to chronic obstructive lung disease.

Abdominal Examination

In right heart failure, elevation of right atrial pressure increases venous pressure throughout the entire systemic venous bed. This leads to engorgement of abdominal organs with hepatomegaly and occasionally splenomegaly. These organs are tender with acute congestion. Severe tricuspid regurgitation causes the liver to pulsate during systole. In addition, peripheral edema and ascites occur in severe chronic right heart failure. A useful maneuver to elucidate borderline right ventricular failure is the hepatojugular reflux, in which pressure applied by the open hand to the right upper quadrant increases venous return to the right heart. Because the failing right ventricle is unable to accept this increased venous return, the maneuver elicits an abnormal increase in jugular venous pulse in addition to accentuating the prominent V wave of tricuspid regurgitation.

LABORATORY FINDINGS

Chest Roentgenogram

The frontal chest film serves as a useful screening test for the presence of congestive heart failure by virtue of changes in cardiac size and configuration combined with abnormalities of the lung fields.[27] Normally, in the erect position, there is better perfusion of the lung bases than the apices. When left atrial, pulmonary venous, and capillary pressure becomes elevated, interstitial and perivascular edema develops, particularly in the lung bases where hydrostatic pressure is greatest. The consequent pulmonary vessel compression in the lower lobes causes equalization of vascular size throughout the lung fields with a modest increase in pulmonary capillary pressure. Pulmonary vascular redistribution, manifested by greater prominence of upper lobe vascularity, takes place with moderate elevation of pulmonary capillary pressure. Marked increase in pulmonary capillary pressure leads to interstitial edema characterized by septal Kerley's lines of interlobar interstitial edema, perivascular blunting of peripheral vessels, and subpleural fluid accumulation between the lung and adjacent pleural surface. Severely excessive pulmonary capillary pressure results in alveolar edema and large pleural effusions.

Hemodynamic Performance

In evaluation of the principal determinants of cardiac performance in heart disease, it is possible to measure precisely ventricular preload (end-diastolic pressure, volume, and tension) and afterload (Laplace's relation in which systolic tension is directly equated with the product of ventricular systolic pressure and radius).[30] However, it is considerably more difficult to assess accurately the contractility of the intact human heart. By utilization of cardiac catheterization and noninvasive techniques, there are two general approaches[20] to evaluation of contractility and function of the heart: (1) its pump (hemodynamics) performance characteristics, and (2) its muscle (mechanics) performance characteristics.

In the traditional approach of pump analysis, the contractile state can be estimated qualitatively by standard hemodynamic variables of ventricular function[30] of cardiac output (normal greater than 2.50 L/min/m^2), stroke volume, systolic ejection rate, and left ventricular end-diastolic pressure (normal, less than 13 mm Hg); and the more complex measurements of left ventricular end-diastolic volume, ejection fraction (normal greater than 0.60), stroke work, stroke power, and ventricular mass. Although these hemodynamic variables provide considerable useful information about cardiac function and directional inotropic differences, they are indirect and qualitative indicators of cardiac contractility.[20] The sensitivity of cardiac pump measurements in the evaluation of contractility is increased by determining the hemodynamic response to certain interventions such as exercise and alterations in ventricular loading.[30] Further, inotropic estimation is improved by evaluating hemodynamic responses within the concept of the Frank-Starling principle (ventricular function curve), which relates pump performance characteristics such as cardiac output to left ventricular end-diastolic pressure.[30]

Mechanical Performance

It has become possible to clinically examine contractility in terms of muscle mechanics which describe the force, velocity, and length properties of the ventricular myocardium.[20] In the numerical assessment of the contractile state, the mechanical events occurring during both the isovolumic[31–33] and the ejection[34] phases of systole have been characterized. Thus, mechanical measures of inotropic state have been developed along two general lines: (1) isovolumic indexes using dp/dt (rate of ventricular pressure increase) (Figure 16.16), and (2) ejection indexes employing V_{CF} (circumferential fiber shortening rate). It has been difficult to evaluate the validity and accuracy of these indexes of contractility in the intact heart, because there is no standard measure of this property of the myocardium with which they can be compared. Nevertheless, the mechanical indexes provide qualitative and quantitative estimation of contractility alterations in single patients in response to interventions (Figure 16.17) and of basal contractile state between different patients (Figure 16.18).

MANAGEMENT

It is important to emphasize that cardiac dysfunction should not be allowed to reach refractoriness to medical therapy in congenital heart disease or acquired valvular disorders. Indeed, definitive evaluation by cardiac catheterization and surgery, if appropriate, generally are carried out electively before symptoms in congenital heart disease and when cardiac symptoms occur with ordinary activity (greater than stable class II symptoms by New York Heart Association criteria) in chronic rheumatic valvular heart disease. In severe valvular malfunction, valve replacement should not be delayed to the stage of refractory congestive heart failure, as the secondary abnormalities in ventricular contractility remain after operation corrects the mechanical burden on the ventricle in patients with chronic cardiac symptoms occurring with mild activity (class III) or at rest (class IV) before heart surgery.

GENERAL APPROACH

In patients with chronic congestive heart failure, even if idiopathic cardiomyopathy is the suspected diagnosis, it is our policy to carry out detailed right and left heart catheterization to establish positively the type of heart disease involved and to quantify the extent of cardiac and myocardial dysfunction. In patients with unsuspected congenital or acquired heart disease, corrective or palliative surgery may be possible. In some patients with cardiomyopathies and marked secondary mitral regurgitation, mitral replacement has been helpful despite increased operative risk, prolonged convalescence, and incomplete benefit. In chronic coronary artery disease, elective saphenous vein bypass by itself has not consistently produced improvement in chronic ventricular dysfunction, except in occasional patients with frequent angina in whom satisfactory anastomosis substantially improves blood flow to the ischemic regions of the ventricle. Patients with congestive heart failure caused by chronic coronary artery disease, however, usually do not have prominent anginal symptoms, as they often do not have substantial ischemic potentially normal functioning myo-

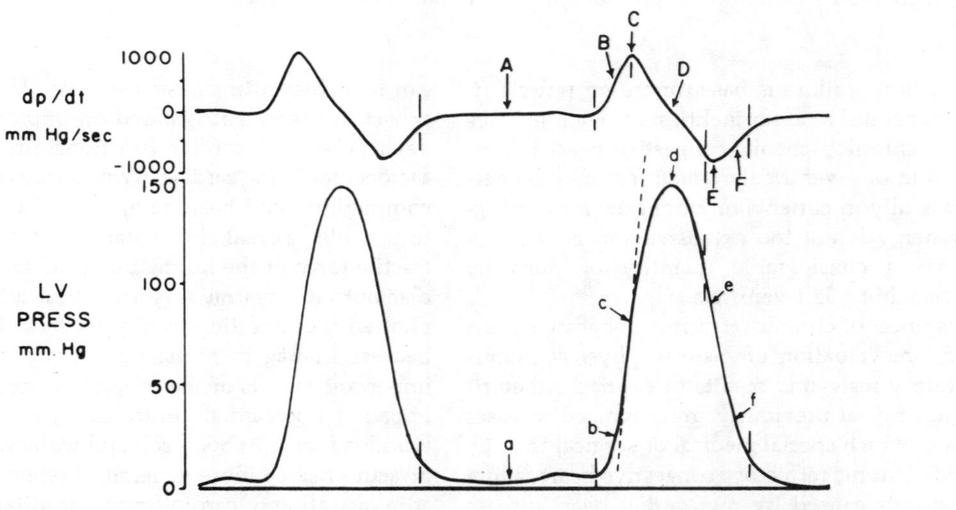

Figure 16.16. Simultaneous recordings of high-fidelity left ventricular pressure (LV) and its first derivative (dp/dt) in a patient with an aortic valve prosthesis. The various portions of the first derivative and corresponding segments of the pressure recording from which they were continuously computed are labeled. During ventricular filling when rate of change of ventricular pressure is minimal, dp/dt is flat at a level near zero (segment A). With the onset of isovolumic contraction, dp/dt rises slowly and then rapidly (segment B) to reach the peak dp/dt (point C), the maximal rate of pressure rise, indicated by slope of the diagonal broken line. Peak dp/dt usually occurs at the instant of opening of the semilunar valves, thus at peak isovolumic ventricular pressure. During early and middle phases of ventricular ejection, dp/dt descends to the baseline, and during late ejection, as intraventricular pressure decreases, dp/dt becomes negative (segment D). The rate of decrease of ventricular pressure is maximal at point E during isovolumic relaxation (segment F). Left ventricular pressure was recorded by direct needle puncture. (From Mason,[31] with permission.)

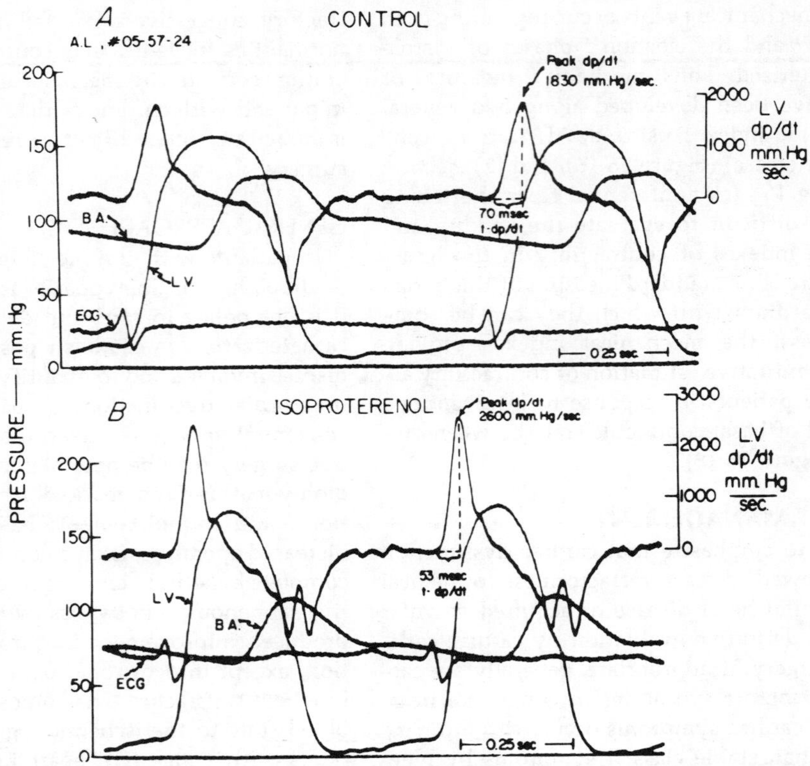

Figure 16.17. Simultaneous recordings of the high-fidelity left ventricular (LV) pressure, its first derivative, and brachial arterial pressure (BA) during the control period (*A*) and after increasing contractility with isoproterenol (*B*) in a patient with an aortic valve prosthesis. The interval from the onset to peak d*p*/d*t* (t-d*p*/d*t*) is indicated. Left ventricular pressure was recorded by direct needle puncture. (From Mason,[31] with permission.)

cardium; their heart failure is based more on muscle fibrosis with generalized abnormalities of wall motion. Conversely, in chronic ischemic congestive heart failure, surgical resection of a ventricular aneurysm may be performed successfully in patients in whom the area of segmental dyssynergy is not too extensive and is well demarcated from a considerable quantity of normally functioning remaining left ventricle.

In many instances of chronic refractory congestive heart failure, careful reevaluation of history, physical examination, laboratory tests, and results of cardiac catheterization does not reveal previously unrecognized diseases or conditions to which special medical or surgical therapy can be applied. Chronic refractory congestive heart failure in such patients is caused by myocardial heart disease (the specific, idiopathic, and ischemic cardiomyopathies) with severe reduction in contractility without primary chronic hemodynamic overload. Ventricular dysfunction may largely be irreversible in these situations. The remainder of this chapter on management of refractory heart failure deals especially with the difficult and relatively incomplete therapeutic modalities that can be used in chronic pump dysfunction resulting mainly from a significantly depressed inotropic state.

Medical therapy is somewhat limited and nonspecific in chronic congestive heart failure caused by primary ventricular muscle dysfunction. Nevertheless, salutary effects can be achieved in most instances. The physiologic approach to treatment is based on improving the principal determinants of cardiac function. Thus, the four major factors regulating cardiac performance (preload, afterload, contractility, and heart rate) are therapeutically adjusted to provide optimal circumstances for the depressed contractile force of the failing pump to deliver a normal cardiac output. Treatment is often best initiated in the hospital with diminution of physical activity and the use of bedrest. Management usually centers on improving three important aspects of the congestive heart failure state: (1) impaired myocardial contractility, (2) excessive cardiac workload, and (3) body salt and water retention. Therapy of acute heart failure generally involves the intravenous administration of cardiotonics, vasodilators, and diuretics guided by central hemodynamic monitoring, whereas treatment of chronic congestive heart failure is focused on the oral preparation of these agents, which can be employed on an ambulatory basis.

DIGITALIS GLYCOSIDES

Because the basic abnormality of the failing myocardium leading to refractory circulatory congestion is marked disturbance of contractile state, the first principle of management is to consider positive inotropic agents for enhancing cardiac performance. Improvement of depressed contractility elevates the entire ventricular func-

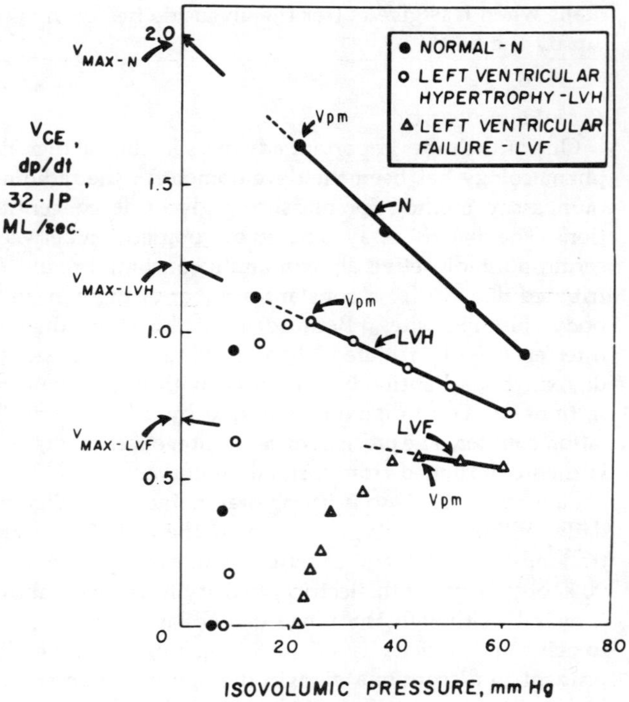

Figure 16.18. Representative comparison of the pressure-velocity relation during isovolumic systole of the left ventricle in a normal individual, in a patient with aortic stenosis with left ventricular hypertrophy in the absence of failure, and in a patient with aortic stenosis with left ventricular hypertrophy and failure. The diagonal broken lines indicate extrapolation of the isovolumic segments to V_{max} at zero load. Vpm = peak measured V_{CE}. IP in the V_{CE} equation and pressure on the horizontal axis are total isovolumic pressure. (From Mason et al,[30] with permission.)

tion curve toward normal, thereby increasing the lowered cardiac output and reducing the excessive left ventricular end-diastolic pressure (Figure 16.1). Rational treatment generally begins with the digitalis glycosides.

Because the beneficial effects of the glycosides stem from their direct stimulatory action on the force of contraction of the myocardium (by increased intracellular calcium influx through sarcolemma membrane reduced sodium-potassium ATPase activity), using these drugs produces some improvement in the depressed contractile state and an increase in low cardiac output. Furthermore, the glycosides exert an overall indirect effect of vasodilation in congestive heart failure[35]; elevated peripheral vascular resistance is reduced by elevation of the diminished cardiac output, thereby allowing withdrawal of sympathetically mediated vasoconstriction which overrides the mild direct vasoconstrictor action of digitalis (Figure 16.19). In regard to myocardial oxygen requirements of the failing heart and digitalis, it is important to point out that, despite the increased oxygen cost of increasing the contractile state per se, the overall glycoside effect is to improve cardiac efficiency and reduce myocardial oxygen consumption, because the predominant indirect action of the agent is to diminish heart size, thereby decreasing intramyocardial systolic tension.[36]

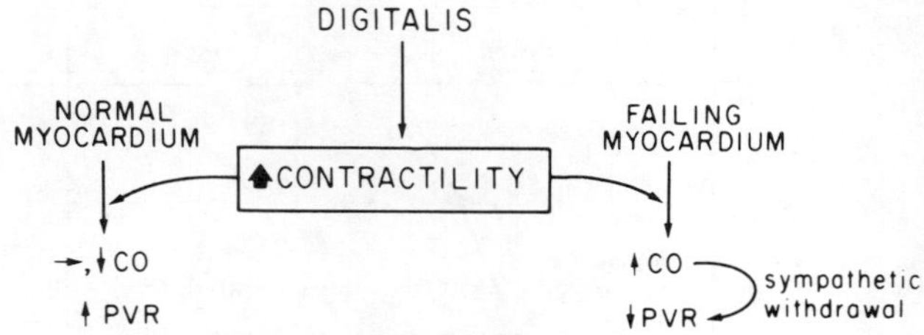

Figure 16.19. Diagrammatic representation of the different hemodynamic translation of the positive cardiac inotropic action of digitalis in the normal heart (*left*) compared with that in the failing heart (*right*). CO = cardiac output; PVR = peripheral vascular resistance. (From Mason et al,[44] with permission.)

Pharmacodynamics

Pharmacodynamic studies of tritiated digoxin have shown that oral digoxin is absorbed considerably better than had previously been appreciated. Eighty percent of an oral dose is absorbed, and therefore the total oral digitalizing dose should now be only 2 mg.[37] In contrast to digitoxin, digoxin is little bound to serum proteins and, therefore, after absorption digoxin is rapidly bound to the myocardium and other tissues, resulting in a myocardial-to-serum ratio of approximately 30 to 1. Digitalis slowly accumulates within the body after institution of a daily maintenance regimen without an initial loading dose. The body retains daily a certain constant percentage of the quantity of systemic glycoside: 30% in the case of digoxin. In normal persons taking 0.5 mg oral tritiated digoxin daily, the plateau concentration of radioactive digoxin in the blood is the same after six days, whether or not an initial loading dose is given.[38] Consequently, only maintenance doses of digoxin (average 0.25 mg) are required to achieve therapeutic concentrations in a few days in nonurgent conditions of heart failure. In situations when rapid digitalization is required, the agent may be given intravenously or intramuscularly. Because parenteral digoxin is completely absorbed, the full digitalizing dose is only 1.50 mg. In such instances, parenteral digoxin is usually given as an initial 0.50-mg dose with subsequent 0.25-mg doses every six hours as necessary.

The traditional concept of the relation between the dose and the positive contractile action of digitalis has been that little contractile benefit is achieved until a certain digitalizing dose is reached, and that the positive contractile action of the glycoside then diminishes as larger doses are administered and toxicity is approached. However, present evidence indicates that there is a linear therapeutic dose-to-contractile response relation.[39] This linear dose-response relation has been shown in isolated cat ventricular papillary muscles for digitoxin, digoxin, ouabain, and acetyl strophanthidin (Figure 16.20). Thus, small or large quantities of the glycosides have the same qualitative contractile action, the extent of which is proportional to the dose employed, and a patient need not receive a maximally tolerated dose of digitalis to achieve some salutary effect. Even small amounts of the glycoside provide some therapeutic action, a point to be kept in

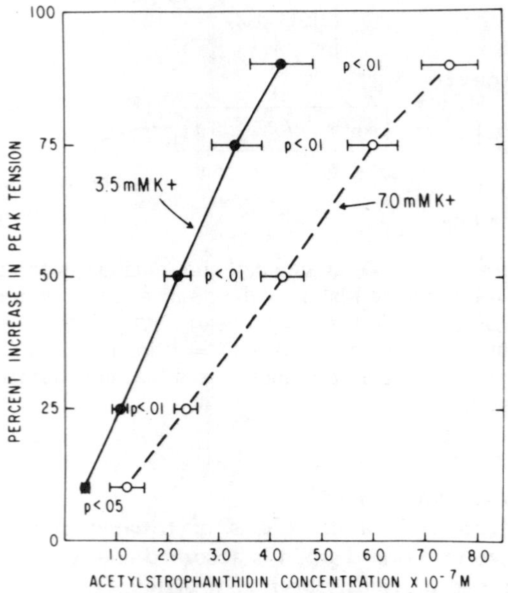

Figure 16.20. Effects of cumulative doses of acetylstrophanthidin on percent increases of peak tension above control peak tension in a 3.5 mM K^+ (*closed circles and continuous lines*) compared with a 7.0 mM K^+ (*open circles and broken lines*) medium. (From Lee et al,[39] with permission.)

mind if the agent is used in patients who may be prone to digitalis toxicity.

Potassium

The serum potassium concentration importantly influences the actions of digitalis. Both the toxic and contractile actions of digitalis are increased when the glycoside is given in the presence of hypokalemia, and these actions are reduced when the glycoside is administered during hyperkalemia. The relation between potassium and the digitalis contractile action has been examined in isolated supported cat papillary muscles.[39] The linear dose-to-contractile response curve for actyl strophanthidin added to the muscle bath with an extracellular potassium concentration of 3.5 mM was significantly depressed when the drug was added to an extracellular bath of 7.0 mM of potassium concentration, showing that digitalis inotropic stimulation is attenuated by pretreatment with potassium (Figure 16.20). In contrast, increasing the extracellular potassium concentration in the muscle bath, from 3.5 to 7.0 mM after pretreatment with digitalis, did not alter the force of cardiac muscle contraction.[39]

From these and related observations, potassium and digitalis seem to compete for myocardial binding sites. However, potassium is bound to the myocardium relatively loosely and it delays subsequent digitalis binding. In contrast, digitalis is firmly bound to myocardial receptors, and thus potassium has little effect on glycoside already attached to the heart before potassium is administered. Translated into the clinical setting, alterations in serum potassium effected before treatment with digitalis have marked influences on the toxic and contractile actions of the glycoside. However, potassium has relatively little influence on the toxic and contractile effects of digitalis when it is given after the glycoside has been taken up by the heart.

Radioimmunoassay

One of the most important advances in clinical digitalis phamacology has been the development of the radioimmunoassay method for measuring glycoside concentrations. The digoxin assay is based on competition between serum nonradioactive digoxin and a constant amount of tritiated digoxin for a constant number of digoxin-antibody binding sites. Because nonradioactive digoxin interferes with tritiated digoxin binding, radioactive digoxin-bound antibody is reduced with higher concentrations of serum digoxin, measured by a liquid scintillation counter. The precise concentration of serum digoxin is then determined from a standard curve.

Patients on 0.25- to 0.50-mg oral maintenance digoxin daily, without toxicity, usually have therapeutic concentrations of 1 to 2 ng/ml of serum, whereas approximately 90% of patients with electrical toxicity have levels above 2 ng/ml. Although the range of overlap between nontoxicity and toxicity is 1.5 to 3.0 ng/ml, it is generally prudent to discontinue digoxin therapy in patients with levels above 2 ng/ml until the serum level falls below this concentration. However, patients with atrial fibrillation, who require more than 0.50 mg of digoxin daily for heart rate control, seem to be relatively insensitive to the development of toxicity, and they may have levels of more than 2 ng/ml. Other conditions in which digitalis dosage may be increased include hyperthyroidism, impaired intestinal absorption in malabsorption syndromes, infancy, altered digitoxin metabolism, and rare instances of digitalis antibodies.

Conversely, there is increased sensitivity to toxicity in ischemic and primary myocardial disease, hypothyroidism, hypoxia, hypokalemia, hypomagnesemia, hypercalcemia, and alkalosis. There is considerable variation in the biologic availability of oral digoxin tablets produced by different manufacturers. Digoxin serum concentrations may vary widely after ingestion of different brands containing the same digoxin content, indicating nonequivalent absorption because of differing product formulation, leading to unequal disintegration and dissolution rates. Lanoxin® is now recognized to be the digoxin brand providing uniform and optimal potency.

Electrophysiologic Effects

The influences of digitalis on the electrophysiologic properties of heart muscle are complex. These effects vary considerably with dose, type of cardiac tissue involved, and autonomic activity.[40] In diastole during intracellular negativity, excitability is raised by the reduced resting potential. Also in diastole, digitalis stimulates automaticity, thereby enhancing subsidiary ectopic pacemakers. In the process of depolarization, the rate of rise of the action potential determining conduction velocity is diminished by digitalis, particularly in the atrioventricular node, thereby leading to various degrees of heart block. Because the speed of depolarization is directly related to the level of resting membrane potential, digitalis depresses membrane responsiveness. The reduction of conduction velocity in the atrioventricular node by digitalis is of major therapeutic significance in slowing the rapid ventricular rate in atrial fibrillation and, thereby, furthering decremental conduction and increasing the functional refractory period of the atrioventricular node. The repolarization process is altered by digitalis, and thus the duration of the action potential in cardiac tissues is shortened, leading to a decrease in refractoriness in myocardial conductive fibers which, in the ventricles, is seen in the narrowing of the QT interval on the surface electrocardiogram. The effects of digitalis on conduction velocity and the refractory period underlie the drug's provocation of reentrant tachyarrhythmias.

Digitalis Toxicity

Although glycoside toxicity can be reversed with digitalis antibodies clinically,[41] this therapeutic modality is not widely available, and a more practical specific antidote is not currently available for the relatively common problem of digitalis intoxication in patients. However, special advantages pertain to the use of potassium, phenytoin, lidocaine, propranolol, bretylium, and cardiac pacing.[40] Although, in experimental animals, the administration of potassium or antiarrhythmic drugs after the onset of electrical toxicity can suppress digitalis-induced tachyarrhythmias, the accumulated dose of digitalis at which these arrhythmias become refractory and fatal is not increased by this treatment.[42] Similarly, in dogs, ventricular overdrive pacing, begun at the onset of ouabain-provoked tachyarrhythmias, can transiently overcome these rhythm disorders, but the maximum tolerated dose of ouabain before death is not altered in comparison with that in control animals receiving digitalis in the same manner.[42] In clinical practice, however, digitalis is discontinued at the onset of toxicity, and antiarrhythmic measures are employed to suppress ectopic activity until the glycoside is excreted or metabolized.

A clinical problem in the use of countershock to electively convert supraventricular arrhythmias has been that life-threatening ventricular arrhythmias attributable to digitalis may be provoked by electrical discharge, even without prior digitalis toxicity.[36] In this case, the amount of discharge energy required to produce ventricular tachycardia is reduced in the digitalized heart. Thus, some clinicians have reduced or withdrawn maintenance digitalis before the use of electroconversion. In contrast, our approach is to continue drug therapy because of the risk of exacerbating heart failure and developing a rapid ventricular rate before cardioversion, and to use small amounts of electrical energy at the time of electroshock.[36] The frequency of ventricular tachyarrhythmias after electroconversion of supraventricular arrhythmias in the presence of digitalis can be reduced, if the shock energy is at the lowest level necessary to achieve conversion. This is done by using initially small, incrementally increasing energy levels of countershock for restoring sinus rhythm and using lidocaine to suppress any premature ventricular contractions occurring with direct current shock.

SYMPATHOMIMETIC AMINES

Isoproterenol

The powerful sympathomimetic, isoproterenol, sometimes is useful in refractory heart failure. Stimulation of contractility and heart rate by the agent is produced by its direct action on beta-adrenergic receptors in the heart. The maximal inotropic effect of isoproterenol usually exceeds that of digitalis before the onset of toxicity.[43] Furthermore, elevation of cardiac output at comparable levels of enhanced contractility is greater with isoproterenol than with digitalis, as the catecholamine produces direct vasodilation by its stimulation of beta receptors in the peripheral arteriolar beds. The influence of isoproterenol on blood pressures varies. When the diseased ventricle is relatively unable to improve its depressed contractile state, the drug produces only a small increase in cardiac output relative to a greater decline in peripheral vascular resistance; therefore, there may be a tendency for blood pressure to decrease.

Because isoproterenol reduces systemic resistance to left ventricular ejection, it may be of special benefit when mitral regurgitation complicates severe cardiomyopathies. Isoproterenol has been more useful in chronic refractory heart failure from causes other than coronary artery disease. The agent is given by slow intravenous drip for several hours at an initial rate of 1 to 3 μg/min.[44] Isoproterenol must be administered cautiously because of the rapid heart rate, ventricular tachyarrhythmias, and hypotension that the agent may provoke. In our experience, it has been a valuable agent in the recovery of patients with the low cardiac output syndrome after cardiac surgery. In addition, for patients with aortic stenosis who have delayed corrective surgery too long, isoproterenol has been useful in causing sufficient reduction of considerably elevated blood urea nitrogen resulting from significantly decreased cardiac output, to allow for safer performance of cardiac catheterization and valve replacement. Isoproterenol may also provide temporary improvement of impaired organ perfusion in chronic cardiomyopathies.

Dopamine

The biologic precursor of norepinephrine, dopamine, possesses certain advantages compared with isoproterenol; therefore, our current choice is dopamine or dobutamine over isoproterenol. The beta receptor–stimulating property of dopamine exerts a positive inotropic effect, and there is mild reduction in total peripheral vascular resistance. Dopamine acts somewhat similarly to epinephrine, with elevation of cardiac output and a directional change of arteriolar resistance intermediate between that of the vasodilation of isoproterenol and the vasoconstriction induced by norepinephrine.[44] In addition, dopamine possesses the beneficial effect of direct non-beta receptor–mediated renal vasodilation. Dopamine is administered slowly by intravenous drip at an initial rate of 2 to 5 μg/kg/min. Epinephrine can be given in the same manner at an initial rate of 1 to 2 μg/min. To obtain the desired effects on cardiac output and blood pressure, the simultaneous use of phentolamine with dopamine or norepinephrine may be more effective than that of the single agent.

Dobutamine

The synthetic sympathomimetic amine, dobutamine, predominantly stimulates $beta_1$-adrenergic cardiac receptors.[45] At equivalent cardiotonic responses, dobutamine effects a weaker $beta_2$-adrenergic action than isoproterenol and less alpha-adrenergic activity than norepinephrine or dopamine. Dobutamine is capable of producing salutary hemodynamic effects sustained for weeks in chronic congestive cardiomyopathy treated for just a few days with the intravenous agent.[46] In addition, the catecholamine may improve cardiac function in chronic ischemic heart failure with infrequent precipitation of tachyarrhythmias. In comparison to dopamine at similar increments of cardiac output, the more cardioselective action of dobutamine appears to effect greater reduction in excessive ventricular preload and less augmentation of heart rate and blood pressure.[47]

Oral Beta-Adrenergic Agonists

A number of orally active sympathomimetics have been shown to possess favorable hemodynamic properties in patients with chronic refractory congestive heart failure. Thus, relative $beta_2$ receptor stimulating agents such as terbutaline, salbutamol, and pirbuterol[48] increase low cardiac output and lower excessive ventricular end-diastolic pressure by virtue of their vasodilator and positive inotropic effects (Figure 16.21). In addition, the relatively cardioselective $beta_1$-adrenergic agonist, prenalterol, improves cardiac function with little increase in heart rate.[49] However, ventricular ectopy and reduced beta-adrenergic responsiveness may occur with long-term use of the oral sympathomimetic agents.

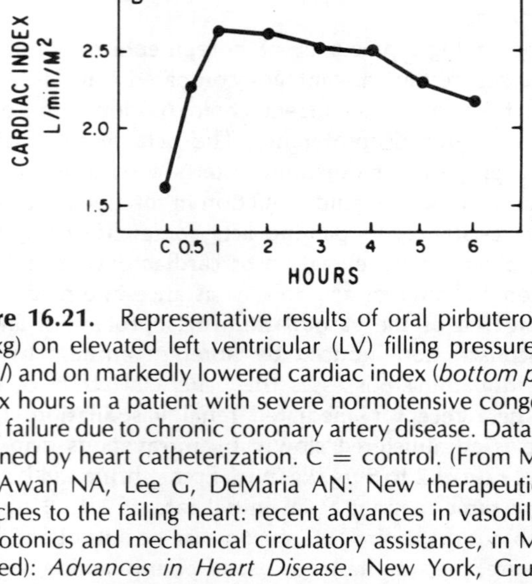

Figure 16.21. Representative results of oral pirbuterol (0.4 mg/kg) on elevated left ventricular (LV) filling pressure (*top panel*) and on markedly lowered cardiac index (*bottom panel*) for six hours in a patient with severe normotensive congestive heart failure due to chronic coronary artery disease. Data were obtained by heart catheterization. C = control. (From Mason DT, Awan NA, Lee G, DeMaria AN: New therapeutic approaches to the failing heart: recent advances in vasodilators, cardiotonics and mechanical circulatory assistance, in Mason DT (ed): *Advances in Heart Disease*. New York, Grune & Stratton, Inc, 1980, vol 3, 403–446. With permission.)

AMRINONE, MILRINONE, AND OTHERS

The recently introduced nonadrenergic compounds, amrinone,[50] milrinone (WIN 47203), MDL-17043 (fenoximone), and related drugs,[51,51a] provide combined cardiotonic and vasodilator properties for the oral and intravenous treatment of severe ventricular dysfunction. By a subcellular mechanism different from digitalis and sympathomimetics, these agents appear to exert their direct positive inotropic action in a manner similar to that of aminophylline. Thus, these agents reduce the activity of the enzyme, phosphodiesterase, that deactivates cyclic AMP, thereby intensifying the action of cyclic AMP on the contractile proteins within the myocardial cell.[51a] Because there is dose-related thrombocytopenia with prolonged use of amrinone, this drug is not recommended for chronic ambulatory therapy. An analog of amrinone, milrinone, appears to be less toxic and therefore may prove suitable for long-term oral use.[52]

DIURETICS

Although it may be difficult to correct the fundamental defect in refractory congestive heart failure by improving a depressed contractile state and relieving an elevated hemodynamic burden, usually it is possible to mobilize excessive body salt and fluid accumulation by rational selection of diuretic agents.[4] Salt restriction is usually not required in early or mild heart failure, as diuretic agents with digitalis suffice. More advanced congestive heart failure, however, does require sodium restriction in the range of 2 g of sodium (5 g of salt) per day. In severe congestive heart failure, it is necessary to restrict sodium to 1 g/day, often limiting daily water intake to below 1 L, with the use of maximum diuretic therapy.

Thiazides

Modern diuretic therapy begins with oral thiazides. These agents interfere with dilution of urine (inhibiting free water formation) in the ascending loop of Henle and distal tubule by preventing reabsorption of sodium, chloride, and potassium with resultant excretion of these ions with water. Hydrochlorothiazide (50 mg) or chlorothiazide (500 mg) is administered once or twice daily.

Aldosterone Antagonists

If the thiazides prove inadequate, an oral aldosterone antagonist should be added. Either spironolactone (25 mg four times daily) or triamterene (100 mg daily) is the agent used. The aldosterone antagonists inhibit the exchange of potassium for sodium in the distal tubules that is produced by aldosterone, excreting sodium while potassium is retained. The aldosterone inhibitors are less powerful than the thiazides, ethacrynic acid, and furosemide, but they promote considerable natriuresis when administered daily for several weeks. An aldosterone antagonist combined with a thiazide makes potassium supplementation hazardous.

Loop Diuretics

If the combination of chlorothiazide with spironolactone or triamterene is unsuccessful, one of the most potent oral diuretics, ethacrynic acid (50 to 100 mg once or twice daily) or furosemide (20 to 80 mg once or twice daily) is substituted for the thiazide. Ethacrynic acid and furosemide block sodium transport from the ascending loop of Henle, thereby interfering with urinary concentrating ability by rendering the renal medullary interstitium less hypertonic for water reabsorption in the collecting ducts. These loop diuretics also possess the thiazide action of inhibiting the dilution of urine in the ascending loop of Henle and the distal tubules. In some refractory conditions, initiation of diuresis appears to be aided by beginning ethacrynic acid (50 mg) or furosemide (40 mg) therapy by the intravenous route.

VASODILATORS

The two significant factors[53] regulating the afterload (ejection tension) of the left ventricle are its radius and systolic pressure, respectively related to chamber volume (preload) and aortic impedance (controlled by arterial compliance and by total peripheral vascular resistance of the systemic arterioles) (Figure 16.22). Because both preload and impedance are increased in heart failure, intramyocardial wall tension (afterload), a principal determinant of myocardial energetics, is also elevated in the failing heart, thereby increasing cardiac oxygen requirements. The cardiac output of the normal heart is mainly governed by systemic venous return (directly related to venous tone), with the left ventricle operating on the steep ascending limb of its function curve (Figure 16.23), aortic impedance being of little importance.[54] In contrast, in the presence of left ventricular dysfunction, arterial resistance is elevated and cardiac output becomes dependent on outflow impedance (Figure 16.23), venous return having minimal influence with the ventricle operating at the apex of its depressed function curve.[54]

The profoundly heightened sympathetic activity in response to decreased cardiac output is excessively operative as an inherent reflex compensatory mechanism attempting to maintain cardiocirculatory integrity in the heart failure state.[55] Because of this, systemic vascular resistance is greater than necessary to sustain arterial pressure with the result that cardiac output is further decreased, thus evoking a deleterious cycle in which pump function is progressively depressed. In addition, systemic venoconstriction is above that required to enhance venous return to the failing ventricle on its flattened function curve characteristic of decreased contractility, thus exacerbating pulmonary edema and excessively increasing myocardial oxygen demand.[55] Importantly, systemic vasodilator therapeutic reduction of both impedance and preload (Figure 16.24) interrupts this harmful sequence by partially counteracting adrenergic overstimulation, thereby augmenting cardiac output, diminishing pulmonary congestion, and improving myocardial energetics.

Vasodilator Spectrum

The vasodilators produce disparate modifications of cardiac function, depending on their differing alterations of preload versus impedance.[56] Nitrates principally cause venodilation (decrease left ventricular filling pressure).[57] In contrast, nitroprusside, phentolamine, and prazosin produce relatively balanced venous and arterial dilation (decrease left ventricular filling pressure and increase cardiac output), provided left ventricular end-diastolic pressure is maintained at its upper limit of normal.[58] The vasodilator spectrum of hemodynamic profiles is completed by hydralazine which predominantly effects arteriolar dilation (increases cardiac output).

Prazosin

Concerning the long-term management of advanced congestive heart failure, orally administered prazosin affords chronic efficacy for several months with addition of this vasodilator to the standard regimen of digitalis and diuretics.[59] Thus, balanced peripheral arterial and venous relaxation (nitroprusside-like effect) of a single dose of prazosin[60] enhances decreased cardiac output (improves fatigue) by decreasing total systemic vascular resistance (impedance), to a similar extent and duration (six to eight hours) as the agent reduces excessive left ventricular filling pressure (preload) (relieves pulmonary congestion and dyspnea) by decreasing venous tone (Figure 16.25); concordantly, myocardial energetics are improved by decline of elevated left ventricular afterload (a preload-impedance product). Prolonged administration of

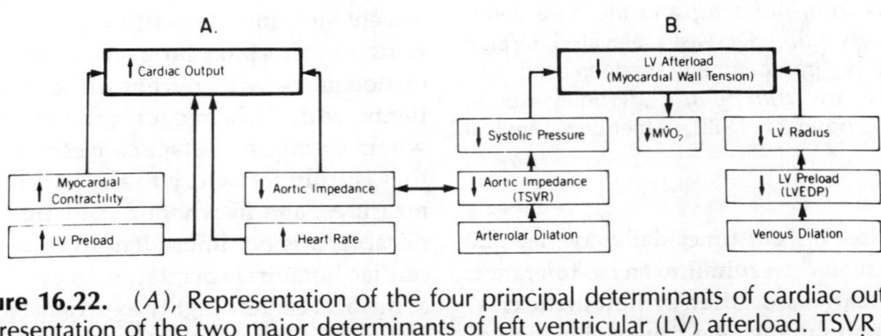

Figure 16.22. (*A*), Representation of the four principal determinants of cardiac output. (*B*), Representation of the two major determinants of left ventricular (LV) afterload. TSVR indicates total systemic vascular resistance; LVEDP, left ventricular end-diastolic pressure; $M\dot{V}O_2$, myocardial oxygen requirements. Arteriolar dilation raises cardiac output (reduces fatigue), decreases LV afterload, and diminishes $M\dot{V}O_2$ (antianginal effect). Venous dilation decreases LVEDP (reduces dyspnea), decreases LV afterload, and diminishes $M\dot{V}O_2$ (antiischemic effect). Combined arteriolar and venous dilation raises cardiac output, decreases LVEDP, diminishes LV afterload, and reduces $M\dot{V}O_2$. (From Mason et al,[55] with permission. Copyright 1980, American Medical Association.)

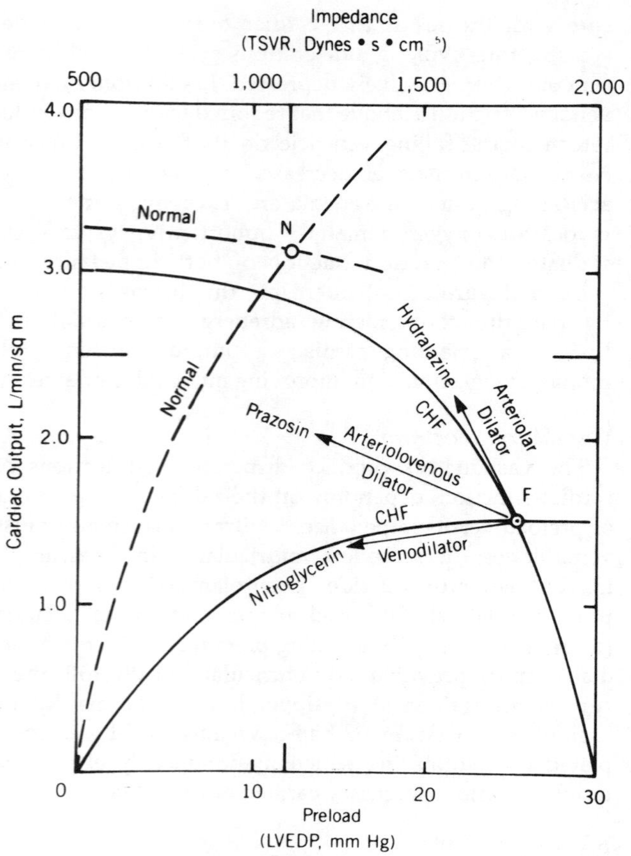

Figure 16.23. Relation of left ventricular preload (LVEDP) and aortic impedance (TSVR) to cardiac output in a normal and a failing left ventricle. In the normal heart (point N), cardiac output is principally regulated by changes in preload (left-to-right ascending broken line relating LVEDP to cardiac output); alterations in impedance are of minor importance (left-to-right horizontal broken line relating TSVR to cardiac output). In contrast, in the failing heart (point F) with congestive heart failure (CHF), cardiac output is principally regulated by changes in impedance (right-to-left ascending unbroken line relating TSVR to cardiac output); alterations in preload are of minor importance (depressed left-to-right horizontal line relating LVEDP to cardiac output). In the failing heart, the pure arteriolodilator, hydralazine, raises decreased cardiac output markedly with a mild decline in elevated LVEDP (*vertical arrow from point F*); the balanced arteriolovenous dilator, prazosin, raises decreased cardiac output and decreases elevated LVEDP (*diagonal arrow from point F*); and the pure venodilator, sublingual nitroglycerin, decreases elevated LVEDP markedly with little or no improvement of decreased cardiac output (*horizontal arrow from point F*). (From Mason et al,[55] with permission. Copyright 1980, American Medical Association.)

prazosin (2 to 7 mg three or four times daily; average, 20 mg/day) provides increased treadmill exercise tolerance, improves New York Heart Association symptomatic classification of dyspnea and fatigue, and causes elevation of reduced scintigraphic and echocardiographic left ventricular ejection fraction.[59] These prolonged salutary effects have been demonstrated by serial testing to be sustained for more than 12 months of continued ambulatory prazosin therapy in patients with chronic coronary heart disease.[61]

With prazosin treatment of congestive heart failure for more than 3 months, late tolerance of the drug may occur in up to one third of patients.[62] This phenomenon may take place with long-term use of any of the vasodilator agents, and appears to be related to accompanying salt and water retention including the vascular wall itself,[10] necessitating increased diuretic requirements of furosemide and especially the aldosterone antagonist spironolactone. Prazosin late tolerance can be circumvented, with full responsiveness of the drug reestablished, by discontinuation of the therapy for a few weeks or by temporary substitution of an alternate vasodilator, such as high-dose hydralazine (75 to 100 mg three or four times daily) plus oral nitrates (isosorbide dinitrate 20 to 40 mg four times daily).[62]

Captopril

Because the renin-angiotensin-aldosterone system is activated in chronic congestive heart failure[12] and the decrease of angiotensin II generation by converting enzyme blockade with intravenous teprotide improves ventricular performance by peripheral vasodilation,[63] the therapeutic efficacy of the oral angiotensin-converting enzyme inhibitor, captopril, has been evaluated in patients with normotensive cardiac dysfunction. Captopril causes nearly balanced systemic venous and arterial relaxation, resulting in marked decline in elevated left ventricular preload and moderate elevation of depressed cardiac output (Figure 16.26).[64] Furthermore, the beneficial cardiocirculatory actions of chronically administered oral captopril (12.5 to 25 mg three times daily) provide prolonged improvement of ventricular function and clinical status in refractory congestive heart failure (Figure 16.27).[65] In addition, long-term therapy with the agent tends to decrease rather than increase diuretic requirements due to prevention of secondary hyperaldosteronism.

CONCLUSIONS

In the ambulatory management of chronic refractory congestive heart failure, it is now our policy to initially augment the therapeutic regimen with captopril when digitalis and diuretics alone are insufficient, and then add conventional vasodilators (prazosin, hydralazine, and nitrates) and finally the new oral cardiotonics. In chronic heart failure intractable to these outpatient measures, relatively sustained benefit may be provided by short periods of inhospital intravenous therapy by dobutamine or dopamine with nitroprusside or by amrinone. In patients with ischemic or primary cardiomyopathies in whom chronic end-stage congestive heart failure develops that is truly refractory to the judicious use of all medical measures, and in whom a palliative operation is not applicable, it is not imprudent to consider the possibility of cardiac homotransplantation in carefully selected patients at medical centers highly experienced with this procedure. However, cardiac homotransplantation is quite restricted in availability and also limited in success. Mechanical cardiac assist devices have not been useful in the management of chronic heart failure, although such devices have provided at least temporary benefit in the treatment of severe cardiac dysfunction caused by acute myocardial infarction. The major inroads in the management of ab-

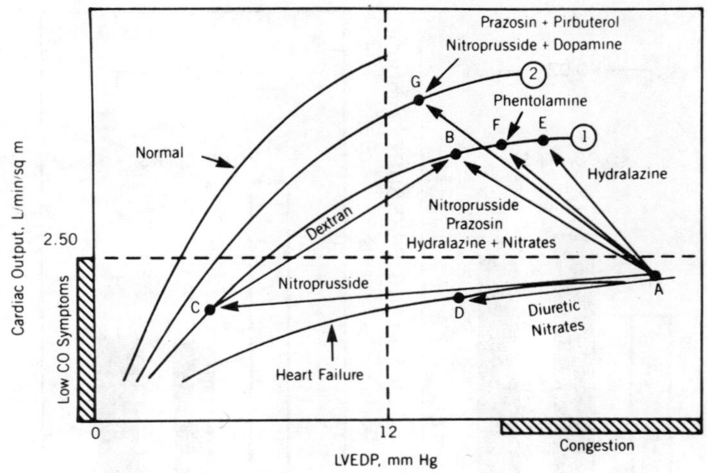

Figure 16.24. Relation between cardiac output (CO) and left ventricular end-diastolic pressure (LVEDP) in a normal subject (*left curve*) and a patient with congestive heart failure (*right curve*). Point A indicates operation of the dysfunctioning left ventricle in CHF. Intermediate curve (1) shows improved relations between CO and LVEDP after administration of hydralazine (point E); nitroprusside, prazosin, or combined hydralazine and nitrates to above LVEDP of 12 mm Hg (point B); and nitroprusside to below LVEDP of 12 mm Hg (point C) with addition of dextran (point B). Enhanced CO and reduced LVEDP following administration of phentolamine are shown by point F. Note that improvements from point A on lowest ventricular function curve to point B on intermediate function curve (1) after administration of nitroprusside, prazosin, or hydralazine and nitrates and to point F after phentolamine are not the result of increased contractility; rather, they are due to an enhanced relation between CO and LVEDP as the result of reduction of impedance to left ventricular ejection produced by these vasodilators. Point D on congestive heart failure curve is LVEDP after diuretic or nitrate therapy. Intermediate curve (2) demonstrates improvement in CO and decrease in LVEDP achieved with combined intravenous nitroprusside and dopamine or dobutamine therapy, or with combined oral prazosin and pirbuterol administration (point G). Horizontal broken line indicates lower limit of normal for CO and vertical broken line indicates upper limit of normal for LVEDP. Congestion indicates pulmonary congestion. (From Mason et al,[55] with permission. Copyright 1980, American Medical Association.)

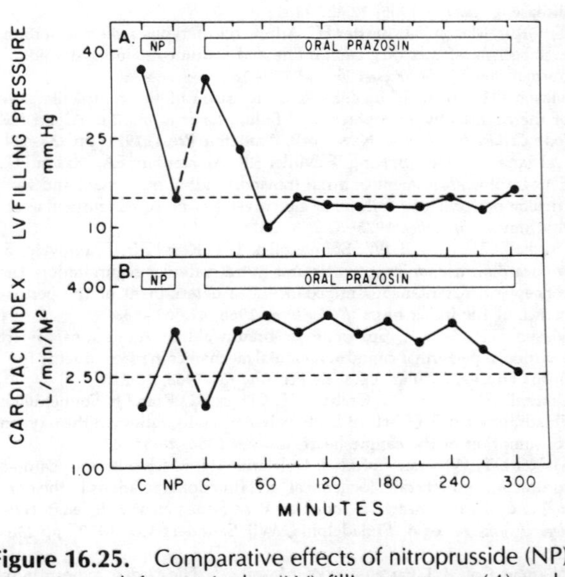

Figure 16.25. Comparative effects of nitroprusside (NP) and prazosin on left ventricular (LV) filling pressure (*A*) and concomitantly on cardiac index (*B*) in a single patient serving as his own control, with severe congestive heart failure due to chronic coronary heart disease. The actions of NP were initially observed, then the infusion discontinued (*diagonal broken lines*), and a 4-mg oral dose of prazosin next given. (From Mason DT, Awan NA, Lee G, DeMaria AN: New therapeutic approaches to the failing heart: recent advances in vasodilators, cardiotonics and mechanical circulatory assistance, in Mason DT (ed): *Advances in Heart Disease*. New York, Grune & Stratton, Inc, 1980, vol 3, pp 403–446. With permission.)

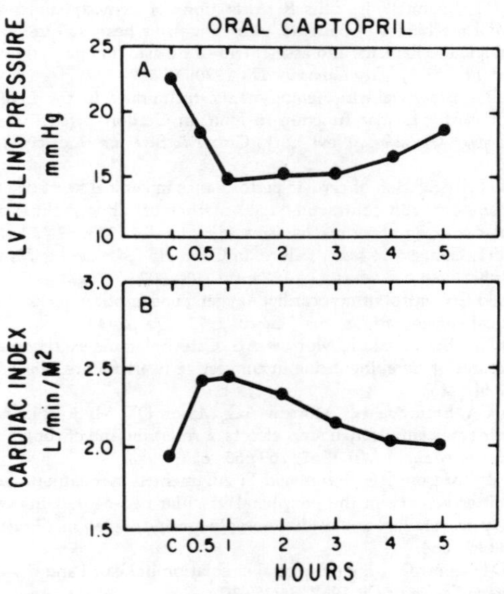

Figure 16.26. Representative results of oral captopril (100 mg) on elevated left ventricular (LV) filling pressure (*top panel*) and on lowered cardiac index (*bottom panel*) for five hours in a patient with severe normotensive congestive heart failure due to chronic coronary artery disease. Data were obtained by heart catheterization. C = control. (From Mason DT, Awan NA, Lee G, De Maria AN: New therapeutic approaches to the failing heart: recent advances in vasodilators, cardiotonics and mechanical circulatory assistance, in Mason DT (ed): *Advances in Heart Disease*. New York, Grune & Stratton, Inc, 1980, vol 3, pp 403–446. With permission.)

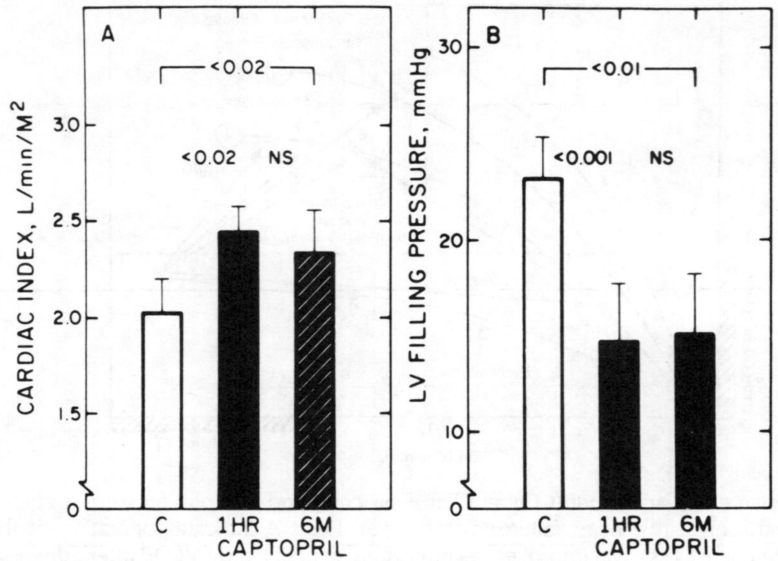

Figure 16.27. Hemodynamic effects of oral captopril in nine patients with severe chronic congestive heart failure on cardiac index (*panel A*) and left ventricular (LV) filling pressure (*panel B*) one hour (1 HR) after initial drug ingestion and after 6 months (6 M) of continuous three-times daily oral therapy. C = control (From Awan et al,[65] with permission.)

solutely intractable myocardial failure incompatible with life in chronic coronary heart disease and the cardiomyopathies must await the development of a successful permanently implantable artificial heart.

Acknowledgment: We gratefully acknowledge the assistance of Leslie J. Silvernail in the preparation of this manuscript.

REFERENCES

1. Mason DT, Spann JF Jr, Zelis R: Alterations of hemodynamics and myocardial mechanics in patients with congestive heart failure: pathophysiologic mechanisms and assessment of cardiac function and ventricular contractility. *Prog Cardiovasc Dis* 1970; 12:507–557.
2. Mason DT, Braunwald E: Hemodynamic techniques in the investigation of cardiovascular function in man, in Gordon B (ed): *Clinical Cardiopulmonary Physiology*. New York, Grune & Stratton, Inc, 1969, pp 153–170.
3. Mason DT: Regulation of cardiac performance in clinical heart disease: interactions between contractile state, mechanical abnormalities and ventricular compensatory mechanisms. *Am J Cardiol* 1973; 32:437–448.
4. Mason DT: Congestive heart failure, in Conn HF (ed): *Current Therapy*. Philadelphia, WB Saunders Co, 1978, pp 195–202.
5. Braunwald E: Control of myocardial oxygen consumption: physiologic and clinical considerations. *Am J Cardiol* 1971; 27:416–432.
6. Chidsey CA, Braunwald E, Morrow AG: Catecholamine excretion and cardiac stores of norepinephrine in congestive heart failure. *Am J Med* 1965; 39:442–451.
7. Chidsey CA, Braunwald E, Morrow AG, Mason DT: Myocardial norepinephrine concentration in man: effects of reserpine and of congestive heart failure. *N Engl J Med* 1963; 269:653–658.
8. Kramer RS, Mason DT, Braunwald E: Augmented sympathetic neurotransmitter activity in the peripheral vascular bed of patients with congestive heart failure and cardiac norepinephrine depletion. *Circulation* 1968; 38:629–634.
9. Mason DT: Control of the peripheral circulation in health and disease. *Mod Concepts Cardiovasc Dis* 1967; 36:25–30.
10. Zelis R, Mason DT, Braunwald E: A comparison of the effects of vasodilator stimuli on peripheral resistance vessels in normal subjects and in patients with congestive heart failure. *J Clin Invest* 1968; 47:960–970.
11. Zelis R, Mason DT, Braunwald E: Partition of blood flow to the cutaneous and muscular beds of the forearm at rest and during leg exercise in normal subjects and in patients with heart failure. *Circ Res* 1969; 24:799–806.
12. Tonkon MJ, Rosen SM, Mason DT: Renal function and edema formation in congestive heart failure, in Mason DT (ed): *Congestive Heart Failure*. New York, Yorke Medical Books, 1976, pp 169-182.
13. Braunwald E, Plauth WH Jr, Morrow AG: A method for the detection and quantification of impaired sodium excretion: results of an oral sodium tolerance test in normal subjects and in patients with heart disease. *Circulation* 1965; 32:223–231.
14. Gill JR Jr, Mason DT, Bartter FC: Adrenergic nervous system in sodium metabolism: effects of guanethidine and sodium-retaining steroids in normal man. *J Clin Invest* 1964; 43:177–184.
15. Mason DT, Spann JF Jr, Zelis R: Comparison of the contractile state of the normal, hypertrophied, and failing heart in man, in Alpert NR (ed): *Cardiac Hypertrophy*. New York, Academic Press, 1971, pp 433-444.
16. DeMaria AN, Lies JE, King JF, Miller RR, Amsterdam EA, Mason DT: Echographic assessment of atrial transport, mitral movement and ventricular performance following electroversion of supraventricular arrhythmias. *Circulation* 1975; 51:273–282.
17. Urschel CW, Covell JW, Sonnenblick EH, Ross J Jr, Braunwald E: Myocardial mechanics in aortic and mitral valvular regurgitation: the concept of instantaneous impedance as a determinant of the performance of the intact heart. *J Clin Invest* 1968; 47:867–883.
18. Mason DT, Zelis R, Spann JF Jr, Braunwald E: Alterations of left ventricular performance and myocardial mechanics in patent ductus arteriosus and ventricular septal defect. *Clin Res* 1968; 16:240.
19. Urschel CW, Covell JW, Graham TP, Clancy RL, Ross J Jr, Sonnenblick EH, Braunwald E: Effects of acute valvular regurgitation on the oxygen consumption of the canine heart. *Circ Res* 1968; 23:33–43.
20. Mason DT, Wikman-Coffelt J, DeMaria AN: Mechanisms of cardiac contraction: structural, biochemical, and functional relations in the normal and diseased heart, in Sodeman WA, Sodeman WA Jr (eds): *Pathologic Physiology*, ed 6. Philadelphia, WB Saunders Co, 1979, pp 230-270.
21. Wikman-Coffelt J, Parmley WW, Mason DT: The cardiac hypertrophy process. Analyses of factors determining pathological vs physiological development. *Circ Res* 1979; 45:697–707.
22. Schwartz A, Sordahl LA, Entman ML, Allen JC, Reddy YS, Goldstein MA, Luchi RJ, Wyborny LE: Abnormal biochemistry in myocardial failure. *Am J Cardio* 1973; 32:407–422.
23. Katz AM: Effects of ischemia on the contractile processes of heart muscle. *Am J Cardiol* 1973; 32:456–460.
24. Wikman-Coffelt J, Fenner C, McPherson J, Zelis R, Mason DT: Alterations of subunit composition and ATPase activity of myosin in early hypertrophied right ventricle of dogs with mild experimental pulmonic stenosis. *J Mol Cell Cardiol* 1975; 7:513–522.
25. Wikman-Coffelt J, Walsh R, Fenner C, Kamiyama T, Salel A, Mason

DT: Effects of severe hemodynamic pressure overload on the properties of canine left ventricular myosin: mechanism by which myosin ATPase activity is lowered during chronic increased hemodynamic stress. *J Mol Cell Biol* 1976; 8:263–270.

26. Wikman-Coffelt J, Parmley WW, Mason DT: Relation of myosin isozymes to the heart as a pump. *Am Heart J* 1982; 103:934-940.
27. Mason DT, Lee G: Congestive heart failure, in Conn RB (ed): *Current Diagnosis*, ed 7. Philadelphia, WB Saunders Co, 1985, pp 397-405.
28. Zelis R, Nelis SH, Longhurst J, Lee G, Mason DT: Abnormalities in the regional circulations accompanying congestive heart failure. *Prog Cardiovasc Dis* 1975; 18:181-199.
29. O'Rourke RA, Crawford MH: Physical findings in heart failure and their physiologic basis, in Mason DT (ed): *Congestive Heart Failure*. New York, Yorke Medical Books, 1976, pp 183-190.
30. Mason DT, Miller RR, Berman DS, Williams DO, DeMaria AN: Cardiac catheterization in the clinical assessment of heart disease and ventricular performance, in Mason DT (ed): *Congestive Heart Failure*. New York, Yorke Medical Books, 1976, pp 225-271.
31. Mason DT: Usefulness and limitations of the rate of rise of intraventricular pressure (dp/dt) in the evaluation of myocardial contractility in man. *Am J Cardiol* 1969; 23:516–527.
32. Mason DT, Spann JF Jr, Zelis R: Quantification of the contractile state of the intact human heart: maximum velocity of contractile element shortening determined by the instantaneous relation between the rate of pressure rise and pressure in the ventricle during isovolumic systole. *Am J Cardiol* 1970; 26:248–257.
33. Mason DT, Braunwald E, Covell JW, Sonnenblick EH, Ross J Jr: Assessment of cardiac contractility: the relation between the rate of pressure rise and ventricular pressure during isovolumic systole. *Circulation* 1971; 44:47–58.
34. Cooper RH, O'Rourke RA, Karliner JS, Peterson KL, Leopold GR: Comparison of ultrasound and cineangiographic measurements of the mean rate of circumferential fiber shortening in man. *Circulation* 1972; 46:914–923.
35. Mason DT, Braunwald E: Studies on digitalis. X. Effects of ouabain on forearm vascular resistance and venous tone in normal subjects and in patients in heart failure. *J Clin Invest* 1964; 43:532–543.
36. Mason DT: Digitalis pharmacology and therapeutics: recent advances. *Ann Intern Med* 1974; 80:520-530.
37. Doherty JE: Digitalis glycosides; pharmacokinetics and their clinical implications. *Ann Intern Med* 1973; 79:229–238.
38. Marcus FI, Burkhalter L, Cuccia C, Pavlovich J, Kapadia GG: Administration of tritiated digoxin with and without a loading dose: a metabolic study. *Circulation* 1966; 34:865–874.
39. Lee G, Zelis R, Mason DT: Linear dose-response and quantitative attenuation by potassium of the inotropic action of acetylstrophanthidin. *Clin Pharmacol Ther* 1977; 22:34-41.
40. Mason DT, Zelis R, Lee G, Hughes JL, Spann JF JR: Current concepts and treatment of digitalis toxicity. *Am J Cardiol* 1971; 27:546-559.
41. Smith TW, Butler VP Jr, Haber E, Fozzard H, Marcus FI, Bremner WF, Schulman IC, Phillips A: Treatment of life-threatening digitalis intoxication with digoxin-specific Fab antibody fragments. Experiences in 26 cases. *N Engl J Med* 1982; 307:1357–1362.
42. Zelis R, Mason DT, Spann JF Jr, Braunwald E: Effects of ventricular stimulation and potassium administration on digitalis-induced arrhythmias. *Am J Cardiol* 1970; 25:428-433.
43. Beiser GD, Epstein SE, Goldstein RE, Stampfer M, Braunwald E: Comparison of the peak inotropic effects of a catecholamine and a digitalis glycoside in the intact canine heart. *Circulation* 1970; 42:805–813.
44. Mason DT, Miller RR, Williams DO, DeMaria AN: Management of chronic refractory congestive heart failure, in Mason DT (ed): *Congestive Heart Failure*. New York, Yorke Medical Books, 1976, pp 293-312.
45. Sonnenblick EH, Frishman WH, LeJemtal TH: Dobutamine: a new synthetic cardioactive sympathetic amine. *N Engl J Med* 1979; 300:17–22.
46. Applefeld MM, Newman KA, Grove WR, Sutton FJ, Roffman DS, Reed WP, Linberg SE: Intermittent continuous outpatient dobutamine infusion in the management of congestive heart failure. *Am J Cardiol* 1983; 51:455–458.
47. Loeb HS, Bredakis J, Gunnar RM: Superiority of dobutamine over dopamine for augmentation of cardiac output in patients with chronic low output cardiac failure. *Circulation* 1977; 55:375–381.
48. Awan NA, Evenson MK, Needham KE, Hermanovich J, Taylor CR, Mason DT: Hemodynamic effects of oral pirbuterol in chronic severe congestive heart failure. *Circulation* 1981; 63:96-101.
49. Awan NA, Needham KE, Evenson MK, Wyn A, Mason DT: Hemodynamic actions of prenalterol in severe congestive heart failure due to chronic coronary disease. *Am Heart J* 1981; 101:158-161.
50. Wynne J, Malacoff RF, Benotti JR, Curfman GC, Grossman W, Holman BL, Smith TW, Braunwald E: Oral amrinone in refractory congestive heart failure. *Am J Cardiol* 1980; 45:1245-1249.
51. Colucci WS, Wright RF, Braunwald E: New positive inotropic agents in the treatment of congestive heart failure. Mechanisms of action and recent clinical developments. *N Engl J Med* 1986; 314:290–299, 349–358.

51a. Braunwald E: Newer positive inotropic agents. *Circulation* 1986; 73(suppl III): III-1–III-239.

52. McDowell A, Baim D, Cherniles J, Bekele T, Braunwald E, Grossman W: Hemodynamic effects of a new inotropic agent (WIN 47203) in patients with refractory heart failure. *J Am Coll Cardiol* 1983; 1:675.
53. Miller RR, Williams DO, DeMaria AN, Mason DT: Ventricular afterload reducing agents in congestive heart failure, in Mason DT (ed): *Congestive Heart Failure*. New York, Yorke Medical Books, 1976, pp 343-364.
54. Mason DT: Afterload reduction and cardiac performance. *Am J Med* 1978; 65:106-125.
55. Mason DT, Awan NA, Joye JA, Lee G, DeMaria AN: Treatment of acute and chronic congestive heart failure by vasodilator-afterload reduction. *Arch Intern Med* 1980; 140:1577-1581.
56. Miller RR, Vismara LA, Williams DO, Amsterdam EA, Mason DT: Pharmacological mechanisms for left ventricular unloading in clinical congestive heart failure: differential effects of nitroprusside, phentolamine, and nitroglycerin on cardiac function and peripheral circulation. *Circ Res* 1976; 39:127–133.
57. Williams DO, Bommer WJ, Miller RR, Mason DT: Hemodynamic assessment of oral peripheral vasodilator therapy in chronic congestive heart failure: prolonged effectiveness of isosorbide dinitrate. *Am J Cardiol* 1977; 39:84-90.
58. Miller RR, Vismara LA, Zelis R, Amsterdam EA, Mason DT: Clinical use of sodium nitroprusside in chronic ischemic heart disease: effects on peripheral vascular resistance and venous tone and on ventricular volume, pump and mechanical performance. *Circulation* 1975; 51:328–336.
59. Awan NA, Miller RR, DeMaria AN, Maxwell KS, Neumann AN, Mason DT: Efficacy of ambulatory systemic vasodilator therapy with oral prazosin in chronic refractory heart failure: concomitant relief of pulmonary congestion and elevation of pump output demonstrated by improvements in symptomatology, exercise tolerance, hemodynamics and echocardiography. *Circulation* 1977; 56:346-354.
60. Awan NA, Miller RR, Mason DT: Comparison of effects of nitroprusside and prazosin on left ventricular function and peripheral circulation in chronic congestive heart failure. *Circulation* 1978; 57:152-159.
61. Awan NA, Mason DT: Oral vasodilator therapy with prazosin in severe congestive heart failure. *Am Heart J* 1981; 101:695-700.
62. Awan NA, DeMaria AN, Mason DT: Ambulatory prazosin treatment of chronic congestive heart failure: development of late tolerance reversible by higher dosage and interrupted substitution therapy. *Am Heart J* 1981; 101:541-547.
63. Gavras H, Faxon DP, Berkoben J, Brunner HR, Ryan TJ: Angiotensin converting enzyme inhibition in patients with congestive heart failure. *Circulation* 1978; 58:770–776.
64. Awan NA, Evenson MK, Needham KE, Wyn A, Mason DT: Efficacy of oral angiotensin-converting enzyme inhibition with captopril therapy in severe chronic normotensive congestive heart failure. *Am Heart J* 1981; 101:22-31.
65. Awan NA, Hermanovich J, Bommer WJ, Needham KE, Mason DT: Long-term hemodynamic and clinical efficacy of captopril therapy in ambulatory management of severe chronic congestive heart failure. *Am Heart J* 1982; 103:474-479.

17 Syncope and Orthostatic Hypotension

Dwight I. Peretz, MD, MSc, FRCP (C), FACP, FACC

Syncope is a sudden and temporary loss of consciousness resulting from an impairment in cerebral function due to a brief deprivation in essential energy substrates, usually the result of decreased cerebral perfusion. The syndrome is short-lived, may be repetitive, and has a multiplicity of causes. It is a symptom complex whose etiology and therapy tax the ingenuity of the diagnostician. Presyncope, near syncope, and "grey-outs" are less well defined, but represent lesser degrees of the same pathophysiologic phenomena.

In this chapter the cardiovascular causes of syncope including orthostatic hypotension will be discussed. No attention will be paid to epilepsy, post-traumatic loss of consciousness, or other forms of loss of consciousness.

INCIDENCE

There is a tendency, both in the population at large and in the medical profession, to treat most cases of syncope somewhat lightly unless serious consequences ensue. The probable reason for this is that syncope is not an uncommon syndrome, arising once or twice in the lifetime of 50% of the population,[1,2] usually in younger persons as a result of some vasovagal reaction to distasteful stimuli, particularly accidents, the sight of blood, or a hospital environment.[3] It accounts for 1% of emergency room admissions.[2] In 3,000 air force personnel whose average age was 29 years, 7% reported at least one episode of nontraumatic, transient loss of consciousness.[1] In a 26-year prospective study of 5,209 men and women between 30 and 65 years of age in the Framingham study, 3% of men and 3.5% of women had had at least one syncopal episode.[3] This phenomenon seems to have two peaks: one in the teens to the early 20s, the vast majority of these persons having vasovagal syncopal attacks,[4] and the next peak after 50 years of age due generally to a cardiovascular cause, not uncommonly sick sinus syndrome or hypersensitive carotid sinus syndrome.[5]

It cannot be emphasized too strongly that the first attack of syncope can lead to disastrous consequences as a result of serious injury to the patient or others around him, particularly in this ever increasingly active world with automobiles, airplanes, and other controlled devices that if mismanaged as a result of loss of consciousness can affect a large number of people. The first attack of syncope, unless it has some obvious explanation, requires careful evaluation to arrive at a diagnosis, so that the precipitating factor or factors can be avoided or adequate preventive therapy instituted.

ETIOLOGY

Syncope is one of the most vexing problems in diagnosis because in most cases there is no single test or battery of tests or maneuvers that will reliably and consistently reproduce the syncope or hint at its cause. It is easy to make the correct diagnosis in a patient with high grade aortic stenosis who becomes syncopal on running to catch a bus. Unfortunately, most patients with syncope have no such dramatic underlying cause that can be found even with extensive testing.[6,7] Recently, Silverstein et al[8] investigated 108 patients admitted to an intensive care unit with syncope and they found that almost half were undiagnosed at discharge.

Syncope seldom results from cerebrovascular disease unless the pathophysiologic changes are singularly extensive.[9,10] Less severe degrees of vascular obstruction in the cerebrovasculature, however, can result in syncope when decreased perfusion is superimposed.

Upon reviewing the charts of 100 patients admitted to the hospital for evaluation of syncope, Eagle and Black[11] examined the charts for the frequency and benefit of diagnostic tests and their relative cost. In 39% no origin for syncope was found and another 18% were believed to have vasovagal episodes. Twelve patients had dysrhythmia as the cause for syncope. The important point, however, is that most patients underwent a variety of diagnostic tests including cardiac enzyme determinations, brain scans, electroencephalograms, and head CAT scan. In most instances these tests added little useful information to the initial history and physical examination and were performed at great expense to the patient. Their data show, and this is certainly the general experience, that extensive neurologic testing in patients with "routine" syncope is not warranted and the focus of hospitalization should be to rule out potentially life-threatening dysrhythmias.[11] It cannot be emphasized too strongly that a neurologic cause for syncope due to intrinsic disease of the cerebral vessels is a rare phenomenon.

A ball valve obstruction of the aqueduct of Sylvius is thought to cause sudden transient syncope, and serious ischemia or infarction of the brain stem can cause syncope, but this would usually not be short-lived or fall into the usual context of a syncopal attack. For all practical purposes, central nervous system vascular phenomena present themselves as paresis or dysesthesia, or paresthesia or dysphasia. Syncope alone is unusual. There are, however, two vascular problems that can certainly present as syncope: the subclavian steal syndrome[12] and Takayasu's syndrome. In the subclavian steal syndrome blood is shunted past the brain through the circle of Willis to the vertebral and subclavian arteries to supply the active muscles in the involved limb. This shunting can cause a global decrease in substrate to the brain. Again, it usually presents with paresis before unconsciousness. Another cause of syncope due to a global decrease in perfusion is classically portrayed in tussive syncope in which intracranial pressures of 300 mm Hg have been identified with rapid repetitive and violent coughing. When intracranial pressure exceeds systemic perfusing pressure for a few seconds, syncope may result. The Valsalva maneuver may also be operative, as in micturition syncope, causing a decrease in venous return, cardiac output, and hence perfusing pressure.[13]

The patient's history is by far the most important single aspect in arriving at a diagnosis. This is probably more so in the syncopal syndrome than in most other areas of medicine. The exact sequence of events and actions of the patient are of the utmost importance in coming to a correct diagnosis. This requires effort on the physician's part, because oftentimes witnesses will have to be tracked down and questioned personally; secondhand information is certainly not acceptable in most cases.

The position of the patient at the time of the attack must be explored. Syncope occurring with long periods of standing in the same position or suddenly arising from bed or a chair is likely to be due to orthostatic hypotension, whereas that occurring when the patient is sitting or lying down is much more likely due to cardiac dysrhythmia. Careful history must be taken to determine seizure-like activity that would suggest epilepsy rather than syncope. It must be understood, however, that hypoxia as a result of bradydysrhythmia, asystole, or serious tachydysrhythmia, such as ventricular tachycardia and ventricular fibrillation, can cause seizure activity in certain predisposed individuals as a result of cerebral hypoxia, particularly if the dysrhythmia is prolonged.

A history of syncopal attacks and the circumstances in which they occurred is important. Questioning regarding distasteful stimuli such as witnessing an accident or having blood sampled would strongly suggest vasovagal causes. Exercise as a precipitating factor would virtually eliminate vasovagal causes and strongly suggest a cardiac cause, either dysrhythmic or obstructive. Medications that the patient is taking are of major significance and should be determined as completely as possible.

Sudden, unannounced, extremely short-lived syncope with no postictal phase is usually the result of an asystolic episode, occasionally the result of short-lived self-aborting ventricular fibrillation or ventricular tachycardia, and rarely caused by type II or vasodepressor hypersensitive carotid sinus syndrome.[5]

Syncope due to orthostatic hypotension, however, is usually preceded by symptoms of cerebral hypoperfusion such as lightheadedness, visual disturbances, or head and neck aches. There may also be accompanying dyspnea and a feeling of intense fatigue.

CARDIOVASCULAR CAUSES OF SYNCOPE

Cardiac causes account for approximately 25% of syncopal episodes (Table 17.1). Classification is based on the four possible mechanisms that allow an inadequate supply of essential metabolic substrates needed for metab-

Table 17.1. Cardiovascular Causes of Syncope

1. Decreased cardiac output
   - A. *Outflow obstruction*
     - Aortic valve disease*
     - Left ventricular outflow obstruction*
       - Hypertrophic obstructive cardiomyopathy
       - Tumor, thrombus
     - Mitral stenosis
     - Prosthetic valve obstruction*
     - Left atrial myxoma or thrombus*
     - Cor triatriatum
   - B. *Inflow obstruction*
     - Superior and inferior vena caval syndrome
     - Right atrial or ventricular myxoma
     - Tension pneumothorax
     - Pulmonary arterial or venous obstruction
     - Constrictive and restrictive cardiomyopathies
       - Constrictive pericarditis
       - Cardiac tamponade
   - C. *Inadequate inotropism*
     - Cardiomyopathy
       - Hypertrophic
       - Ischemic
       - Restrictive
       - Congestive
       - Infiltrative
     - Myocardial damage
   - D. *Electrical impulse formation and conduction problems*
     - Bradycardia and asystole
       - Ischemia/infarct*†
       - Sick sinus syndrome*†
       - Hypersensitive carotid sinus syndrome*†
       - Sinus bradycardia
       - Atrioventricular nodal block—second and third degree*†
       - Intraventricular conduction block
       - Drugs—beta blockers, verapamil
     - Tachycardia
       - Sinus
       - Supraventricular
         - Atrial fibrillation
         - Atrial flutter
         - Paroxysmal atrial tachycardia

Table 17.1. Cardiovascular Causes of Syncope (*Continued*)

Ventricular
- Tachycardia*†
- Fibrillation*†
- Drugs—atropine, catecholamines, tricyclics

Prolonged QT interval syndrome
- Associated with deafness
- Unassociated with deafness
- Acquired (class 1A antidysrhythmic agents)

2. Decreased cerebral perfusing pressure (orthostatic hypotension)

A. *Volume depletion*†
- True loss—dehydration, hemorrhage, gastrointestinal loss
- Pooled—redistribution
  - Drugs
  - Vasovagal†

B. *Drugs*
- Antihypertensives
- Antidepressants (tricyclics)
- Diuretics
- Alcohol
- Nitrates
- L-dopa
- Tranquilizers
- Afterload reduction agents
- Marijuana

C. *Hypoadrenalism*
- Addison's
- Pituitary
- Hypoaldosteronism

D. *Pregnancy*

E. *Allergic diathesis (histamine, bradykinin)*

F. *Deconditioning (prolonged bedrest)*†

G. *Varicose veins*

H. *Mitral valve prolapse*
- Dysrhythmia
- Autonomic nervous system dysfunction

I. *Autonomic nervous system failure*
- Primary
  - Shy–Drager (multiple system atrophy)
  - Bradbury–Eggleston (idiopathic orthostatic hypotension)
  - Riley–Day (familial dysautonomia)
- Secondary
  - Diabetes mellitus
  - Guillain–Barré
  - Amyloidosis
  - Spinal cord lesion
  - Acute intermittent porphyria
  - Heavy metal poisoning

3. Decreased central nervous system flow due to intrinsic cerebrovascular blood deprivation
- Atherosclerosis
- Takayasu's arteritis
- Subclavian steal syndrome
- Tussive
- ? Micturition
- Hyperventilation

4. Transient inadequate energy substrate
- Glucose
- Oxygen
- Ambient
- Hypoxia
- Right-to-left shunts

* Sudden, unannounced syncope of very short duration.

† Common cause of syncope.

olism in cerebral cells. Syncope is generally not the result of inadequate concentrations of the substrates oxygen and glucose in the perfusing blood, but rather the result of decreased cerebral flow as a result of hypotension, inadequate cardiac output, or both, due to a host of factors including (1) decreased cardiac output, (2) decreased perfusing pressure, (3) intrinsic cerebrovascular blood deprivation, and (4) transient inadequate energy substrate.

DECREASED CARDIAC OUTPUT

Decreased cardiac output can be due to obstruction to forward blood flow through the heart, inadequate venous return, or cardiac dysfunction due to dysrhythmia. Aortic and mitral valve disease and dynamic left ventricular outflow tract obstruction, such as that with hypertrophic obstructive cardiomyopathy, are well-established causes of syncope.[14] Whether the syncope is due to an actual decrease in flow across the obstructed valve or, particularly in the case of left ventricular outflow tract obstruction, to transient dysrhythmia is debatable.[15] A ball valve obstruction due to myxoma or thrombus, on a pedicle, is a well-described cause of syncope in this rare clinical situation.[16] Loss of consciousness is uncommon in myxomas, but when present it is commonly associated with certain body positions and resolves with a change of position such as falling to the ground. An unusual cause of forward flow syncope is obstruction of a mechanical prosthetic valve with holdup of the ball or disk due to thrombus, ball-valve variance, or other problems. These causes are usually discernible on physical examination, eliciting the typical cardiac murmurs of aortic valve disease, left ventricular outflow tract obstruction, or mitral valve disease.

The usual diagnostic criteria for evaluation of the severity of aortic and mitral valve disease should be taken into account. In aortic stenosis the loss of the aortic component of the second heart sound, the late-peaking ejection systolic murmur radiating up into the carotid vessels, and evidence of left ventricular hypertrophy clinically, electrocardiographically, or echocardiographically, and in significant mitral stenosis the long mid-diastolic murmur combined with a short A_2-opening snap interval are important factors to consider, because mild obstructions of these valves do not cause syncope. Clinical, echocardiographic, and echocardiographic Doppler evaluation of left ventricular dynamic outflow tract obstruction and valvular obstruction is reliable.

Myxoma and thrombus formation in the left or right atrium are rarely detectable on physical examination but are easily picked up on echocardiography. Diagnosis is more difficult in the case of prosthetic valve obstruction, because the valve may work well when the patient is conscious, and echocardiographic techniques, even in the best hands, are difficult to use in accurately visualizing the details of disk or ball movement. With the new radiodense markers in most plastic prosthetic valves, fluoroscopy is of value.

Inflow obstruction to returning blood is an important cause of decreased cardiac output. The patient is usually quite ill, except in the case of a right atrial myxoma, which can obstruct the tricuspid valve or even advance and obstruct the pulmonary outflow tract, with no sign of disease between attacks. The superior and inferior vena caval syndromes are identified with venous distention, without cardiac pulsation in the jugular veins, and usually with the other signs of serious infiltrating disease causing the obstruction.

Tension pneumothorax again is diagnosed clinically and radiographically and usually leaves little doubt after examination. Pulmonary hypertension as a result of acute pulmonary embolization or chronic obstructive lung disease is an uncommon cause of syncope but can usually be diagnosed clinically as can the "primary" pulmonary hypertension usually seen in young women.[17,18]

Similarly, constrictive and restrictive cardiomyopathies, constrictive pericarditis, and cardiac tamponade have classic findings with a paradoxic jugular pulse and pulsus paradoxus, low voltage QRS complexes on the electrocardiogram, and soft heart sounds. Echocardiography is a great help in the diagnosis.

Inadequate cardiac output due to decreased inotropism of the myocardium secondary to severe ischemia, restrictive or congestive cardiomyopathies, or some infiltrative process in the myocardium may cause near syncope and syncope when increased metabolic demands are made that cannot be met with increased cardiac output.

In the context of acute myocardial damage, loss of consciousness in any position is usually the result of some serious dysrhythmia. Bradycardia is extremely common in the first few hours following myocardial damage, particularly inferior myocardial infarction. There may be associated episodes of asystole. Serious forms of tachyarrhythmias such as ventricular tachycardia and ventricular fibrillation are also common in the first few hours following myocardial damage. Both of these tachydysrhythmias may be self-terminating, with the patient regaining consciousness, but often the dysrhythmia must be aborted with direct current countershock across the precordium. Provided the patient has not been unconscious for more than 60 to 90 seconds, there is usually prompt return of consciousness, with no postictal phase.

If asystolic episodes are identified or if the sinus bradycardia is symptomatic, atropine should be used immediately, 0.6 mg intravenously, and depending on the response, this dose might be increased. The pharmacologic action of atropine on the cardiac conducting system is rather short-lived, often less than one hour, and may require repeated administration at that interval. Mydriasis and dry mouth may well last for many hours longer. It is important to determine if the symptomatic sinus bradycardia is responsive to atropine, because the bradydysrhythmic aspect of acute myocardial infarction resulting from a sinus mechanism is usually over within the first four or five hours, and then a normal sinus response will ensue. However, if there is a poor response of the sinoatrial node to atropine or if a high degree of atrioventricular block is observed, then temporary transvenous pacing is essential.[19,20]

Sinus bradycardia and asystolic episodes are commonly associated with the sick sinus syndrome, sometimes intermixed with episodes of tachydysrhythmia, usually atrial fibrillation, atrial flutter, or paroxysmal atrial tachycardia. The tachydysrhythmia is usually tolerated by the patient, but the bradydysrhythmia may well cause near syncope or frank syncope,[20a] and this requires treatment with permanent transvenous pacing.[21,22]

A syndrome that is considerably more common than the literature would lead one to believe is the hypersensitive carotid sinus syndrome. Although data from the 1981 world pacing survey show that hypersensitive carotid sinus syndrome accounts for only 0.6% of pacemakers implanted in the United Kingdom and 2.4% of those used in the United States, the implantation rate is considerably higher in countries with a greater awareness of this condition, eg, Austria and West Germany, at 6.1% and 12%, respectively.[22a] In centers in which carotid sinus massage is performed routinely during evaluation of patients with bradycardiac problems, the incidence of hypersensitive carotid sinus syndrome has been reported to be 8 to 28 per million population per year.[22a]

The normal carotid sinus reflex has a significant physiologic role to play by decreasing heart rate and systemic pressure as a result of stimulation of the baroreceptors by increased internal pressure (Figure 17.1). A "hypersensitive" response is elicited when external compression of the carotid sinus produces greater than three seconds of asystole or, without the asystole, a greater than 50-mm Hg decrease in blood pressure.[23,24] There is controversy over whether there is in fact increased vagal traffic as a result of stimulation of the carotid baroreceptors or whether there is increased sensitivity of the sinoatrial and atrioventricular nodal tissue to a normal amount of vagal traffic causing these changes. Some of the cases diagnosed as hypersensitive carotid sinus syndrome may in fact be a sick sinus syndrome variant, but most cases of greater than three seconds of asystole with pressure on the carotid sinus are due to increased vagal traffic to the sinoatrial or atrioventricular nodes causing asystole or third degree atrioventricular block, or both.[5] Recent evidence by Gang,[25] who has made direct recordings of sinus node potentials using a transvenous electrode catheter, showed that sinus node function was normal in these patients before carotid sinus massage.[25]

Hypersensitive carotid sinus syncope is not uncommon. In a 550-bed acute care teaching hospital, an average of seven new cases per year were reported by Peretz and Abdulla.[5] The reason that this syndrome is not diagnosed considerably more frequently is that testing of the carotid sinus mechanism has been poorly and infrequently carried out in patients with syncope. The carotid sinus is high up on the carotid artery at the bifurcation, just under the angle of the jaw. When testing for the carotid sinus response, the head must be turned to the contralateral side 45° to adequately expose the carotid sinus and allow pressure 45° inward to compress the carotid sinus between the massaging finger and the underlining cervical spine. Up-and-down pressure over a 2-cm distance with ever-increasing pressure with the patient under electrocardiographic control will often unmask prolonged periods of asystole (Figure 17.2). The patient must be forewarned that he may be asked to cough (if prolonged asystole ensues) and that this command should be followed immediately. Both carotid arteries should be palpable and free of bruits before testing is carried out. Although a

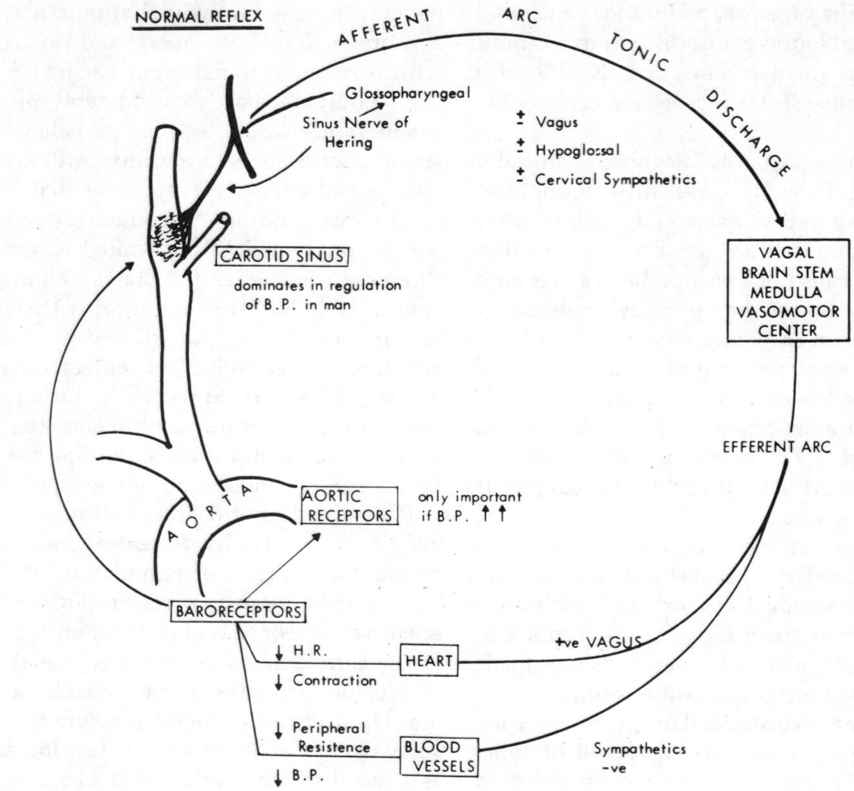

Figure 17.1. Schema of afferent and efferent neurogenic traffic resulting from stimulation of the carotid sinus baroreceptors. (From Peretz and Abdulla,[5] with permission.)

hypersensitive response may be elicited in about 10% of persons over 65 years of age without any history of syncope, unconsciousness need not be produced with the testing maneuver in order to treat those with indications absolutely consistent with asystole: unannounced, sudden, short-lived syncope with complete return of cerebral function instantly on gaining consciousness. This sequence of events is essentially only compatible with asystole or ventricular fibrillation. These patients should have 24-hour ambulatory electrocardiographic monitoring carried out to try to eliminate the possibility of tachycardia as well. Experience has shown that most patients fulfilling these criteria respond well to permanent pacing with a demand rate considerably below their usual intrinsic cardiac rate, but sufficiently high to prevent syncope with severe bradycardia or asystole.[5] Setting the demand rate considerably below the patient's usual intrinsic rate, the demand rate usually being 50 per minute, prevents the so-called "pacemaker syndrome" in which cardiac output decreases if the atrial kick is eliminated as a result of ventricular depolarization being out of synchrony with atrial depolarization. Carotid sinus massage is a safe diagnostic maneuver if performed correctly and with adequate controls. It should always be done with electrocardiographic monitoring.

While electrocardiography is being used to monitor patients suspected of having the hypersensitive carotid syndrome, the blood pressure should also be taken. The type 2, or vasodepressor hypersensitive carotid sinus syndrome, manifests itself as profound hypotension without a significant decrease in cardiac rate.[5] (Table 17.2.) This decrease is due to inhibition of sympathetic traffic to the peripheral vessels mediated through the medullary vasomotor center. It is a rare syndrome, but nonetheless it requires addressing because cardiac pacing will have no effect.[25a] There are a few described cases of combined type 1 (cardioinhibitory) and type 2 (vasodepressor) hypersensitive carotid sinus syndrome. The type 1 case can

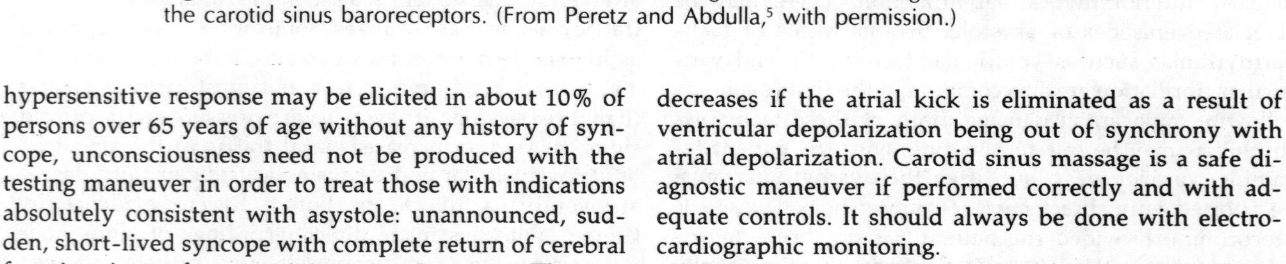

Figure 17.2. Type 1A cardio-inhibitory response to carotid sinus stimulation. (From Peretz and Abdulla,[5] with permission.)

Table 17.2. Classification of Cardioinhibitory and Vasodepressor Response to Carotid Sinus Massage

Type 1 Cardioinhibitory (asystole)
Type 1A Sinoatrial node suppression
Type 1B Atrioventricular node suppression
Type 2 Vasodepressor (peripheral vasodilation without significant bradycardia)
Type 3 Combined

almost always be blocked with atropine, so that if there is a profound decrease in blood pressure, with marked bradycardia, then 1 mg of atropine intravenously should be given and carotid sinus massage attempted again. Hypotension, if due to peripheral vasodilation, will not be prevented by atropine and hence that problem will have to be addressed. The best method currently available for treatment of type 2 (vasodepressor) hypersensitive carotid sinus syncope is surgical denervation of the carotid sinus or section of the glossopharyngeal nerve or nerve of Hering. Radiation to the carotid sinus is also reported to have some therapeutic effect in dampening the response.

The right carotid sinus is usually more sensitive than the left. Men significantly outnumber women in this syndrome and this becomes a much more prominent feature of syncope in older persons. The average age is past the sixth decade.

Atrioventricular and bundle branch block, which may be intermittently bilateral, may cause serious bradydysrhythmia.[26,27] In the subset of chronic bundle branch block, 3% to 5% per year will have syncope.[28] Drugs including beta blockers, certain calcium channel blockers, digitalis, and quinidine overdose may all cause bradycardia or asystole, resulting in loss of consciousness.

With ventricular tachycardia, there is often a forewarning of syncope in that cardiac output and hence blood pressure are maintained for moments, minutes, or even hours depending on the state of the myocardium and the rapidity of the dysrhythmia. With ventricular fibrillation, there also may be sustained near syncope for several moments, particularly if the patient is lying down. This is seen in the cardiac catheterization laboratory where patients will announce that they are going to lose consciousness. Under those circumstances, there is usually about a ten-second delay, the length of time that experimental evidence shows is necessary to cause sufficient hypoxia to bring on total loss of consciousness. The Chinese, with acupuncture anesthesia and hence an awake patient, particularly with open heart procedures, have demonstrated consistently that as the mean arterial pressure decreases below about 50 mm Hg, the patient will lose consciousness in the supine position. This is the first reliable information we have regarding the mean perfusing pressure necessary for cerebral function.

Supraventricular tachydysrhythmias are less likely to cause cerebral symptoms. However, with valvular disease, intrinsic myocardial disease, or coronary artery disease the cardiac output may be sufficiently compromised by any significant tachycardia to cause cerebral symptoms. Atrial fibrillation, atrial flutter, and atrial tachycardia, particularly if an accelerated atrioventricular conduction pathway is available, may have a rapid ventricular response, with a marked decrease in cardiac output.

An electrocardiogram should be taken in all patients with syncope. This may show a prolonged QT interval, a harbinger of torsades des pointes ventricular tachycardia,[29,30] heart block, left ventricular hypertrophy as a result of outflow tract obstruction, sinus arrest, and varying degrees of conduction block. Recent studies showed that the signal-averaged electrocardiography could identify low-amplitude signals in the terminal portion of the QRS complex and ST segment (late potentials) recorded from the body surface, which represent areas of delayed conduction in small areas of diseased myocardium in 11 of 13 patients with ventricular tachycardia and syncope.[30a] The technique is new but does show promise.[30b]

Investigation of both tachydysrhythmias and bradydysrhythmias usually requires ambulatory electrocardiographic monitoring, sometimes repeated on several days.[31–33] If there is a forewarning of the near syncope or syncope, recording devices are available that the patient can apply to the chest wall, press a button, and get a tracing of the dysrhythmia for future evaluation. Ambulatory monitoring of the electrocardiogram is essential and relatively inexpensive if the history and physical examination do not reveal the cause of the syncope. In these patients a surprisingly large number, 10% to 40%, will have transient neurologic symptoms (not always syncope), but in only slightly over half of these can the symptoms noted in the patient's diary be correlated with dysrhythmia. This is important information to have available for correct therapy to be initiated.[31] In addition to having irrefutable evidence of temporally related symptoms and dysrhythmias, episodic nonsymptomatic dysrhythmias may suggest some underlying serious potential dysrhythmias. Couplets or triplets of ventricular ectopy or an R-on-T ventricular premature contraction may forewarn of runs of ventricular tachycardia or ventricular fibrillation.[34–36] Atrial extrasystoles are often the forerunner of atrial fibrillation. Episodes of sinus arrest or varying degrees of heart block may forewarn of asystolic episodes or heart block. Ambulatory electrocardiographic monitoring will provide a diagnosis for the etiology of the syncope in approximately 15% of patients following their first attack.[2]

Electrophysiologic testing requires a sophisticated cardiac catheterization laboratory and trained personnel, is considerably expensive, and is certainly not a routine procedure in a patient with syncope. However, if there is suspicion or confirmation that a serious tachydysrhythmia is causing the syncope, complete electrophysiologic studies should be carried out to demonstrate reproducibility of the dysrhythmia and with reproduction of the dysrhythmia to determine the appropriate medication to combat the problem.[37–40]

DECREASED PERFUSING PRESSURE (ORTHOSTATIC HYPOTENSION)

Orthostatic hypotension is a serious problem that accounts for a significant number of patients who lose consciousness when assuming the upright position. It virtually never occurs on lying down and almost never while sitting. There are a number of conditions that present with orthostatic or postural hypotension. These may be due to nonautonomic nervous system problems or primary or secondary autonomic nervous system failure.

Systemic arterial pressure in the upright posture is maintained by reflex adjustments to the peripheral venous and arterial vascular resistance, cardiac rate, and force of cardiac contraction. Assuming the upright posture, without appropriate neurologic and endocrinologic controls coming into place, would result in pooling of venous and arterial blood due to gravity. A decrease in venous return would therefore decrease the ventricular filling pressure and decrease cardiac output and hence systemic pressure. Upon assuming the upright position, cardiopulmonary volume receptors and arterial baroreceptors, mainly in the aortic arch and carotid sinus area, but also throughout the arterial tree, are stimulated (Figure 17.1). The afferent impulses are carried via the nerve of Hering and glossopharyngeal nerve to the central blood pressure control center in the medulla. The traffic is integrated and an appropriate increase in sympathetic traffic and a decrease in parasympathetic traffic occur, which allow peripheral venoconstriction to increase venous return and cardiac output and arteriolar constriction to increase peripheral resistance. There is also an increase in heart rate and contractility as a result of the sympathetic outflow. At the same time the increase in pressure or volume initiates the renin–angiotensin–aldosterone axis to retain sodium and water, hence increasing blood volume.

Under normal circumstances, therefore, when a person stands up, the blood pressure will decrease by less than 10–15 mm Hg, the diastolic pressure remains the same or tends to rise, and the heart rate will increase by 10 to 12 beats per minute, but if any step of this mechanism is faulty, there may be a severe decrease in blood pressure culminating in inadequate cerebral perfusion and possibly syncope.

The diagnosis of orthostatic (postural) hypotension rests on obtaining an exaggerated decrease in blood pressure from the supine to the upright positions associated with symptoms. As with testing of carotid sinus with massage for a pathologic response, the maneuver of testing the patient's blood pressure standing as well as lying is too often omitted. This is the crucial test for the diagnosis of orthostatic hypotension and very important in the initial examination of a patient with syncope. The pulse rate should be recorded as well as the supine and standing blood pressure, since an increase of less than 10 to 12 beats per minute is the simplest evidence of hypoadrenergic orthostatic hypotension.[40a]

Orthostatic hypotension may be due to true volume depletion from hemorrhage, gastrointestinal loss from diarrhea or vomiting, dehydration, or excessive diuresis. It may also be due to pooled (redistributed) blood which may be due to a host of medications including antihypertensives, tricyclic antidepressants, diuretics, alcohol, and nitrates. Afterload reducing agents are in general use today for intractable congestive cardiac failure and for reduction of blood pressure in hypertensive patients. These agents, captopril, hydralazine, and prazosin, commonly produce postural hypotension due to dampening of the peripheral venous and arterial constricting mechanisms, the goal of the therapy. However, the result may culminate in the patient losing consciousness upon rising. Careful history as to the use of these agents is important. This is probably the most common cause of recurrent, reproducible syncope upon assuming the upright position. It is corrected by withdrawal of the offending agent.

Vasovagal syncope (the common faint) is due to a redistribution of blood and is the most common cause of fainting in teenagers and young adults. Fifteen percent to 25% of young people experience one or more episodes before the age of 30 years.[3] This cause of fainting is unusual to initially occur after that age. A thorough knowledge of the clinical picture of the common faint is critical to the evaluation of patients complaining of syncope. This type of syncope may occur as a response to sudden emotional stress or in a setting of real, threatened, or fancied injury. This is not infrequently brought on by blood letting, the sight of blood, or an accident, or even hearing of surgical manipulation. It has been seen in people just entering a hospital environment. Certain other environmental situations are important, namely, a hot and crowded room, especially if the individual is ill, tired, or intensely hungry. The common faint will take place in the upright posture when systolic blood pressure decreases below about 70 mm Hg. There will be loss of consciousness in the supine position generally when the blood pressure decreases to below 50 mm Hg systolic. The pulse becomes weak or virtually imperceptible, which makes cardiac rate very unreliable from an observer point of view. The cardiac rate may be either slowed or slightly increased. The initial autonomic response is sympathetic with pallor, possible tachycardia, diaphoresis, and sweating as a fight, fright, and flight reaction. When this is not reacted upon, a parasympathetic response is initiated with peripheral vasodilation, bradycardia, and hypotension culminating in loss of consciousness. These attacks are usually aborted by lying down, removal of the offending stimulus, or engaging the patient in conversation.

Hypoadrenalism is a rare cause of postural hypotension, but it should certainly be borne in mind in the hypotensive, thin, "tanned" patient who has a further decrease in blood pressure when assuming the upright position. This may be due to primary adrenal disease or to a decrease in the trophic hormone from the pituitary.

Pregnancy is the other cause, as with atrial myxoma, that can have the patient manifest near syncope or syncope while lying down only to regain consciousness upon assuming another, particularly upright, posture. In pregnancy this is due to obstruction of the inferior vena cava, reducing venous return and thereby decreasing cardiac output with the patient lying down. The obstruction to the inferior vena cava is relieved upon assuming the left decubitus or upright posture, the uterus falling forward and relieving the obstructed inferior vena cava. Lying on the side will be equally effective.

Intense hypotension as a result of an allergic diathesis, with release of histamine, bradykinin, and other vasodilatory and bronchoactive peptides is often accompanied by intense bronchospasm and may result in syncope. This is usually the result of an acute allergic reaction, such as that caused by an insect bite, or the introduction of a parenteral agent such as penicillin or an iodine-containing radiographic contrast material to which the patient is sensitive.

The patient who has been lying in bed for long periods of time and now, more and more, people subjected to prolonged weightlessness may experience syncope upon assuming the upright posture. Certainly lightheaded episodes and near syncope are common under those conditions. Varicose veins may also cause intense pooling peripherally, particularly if the patient has been supine for some time and the blood volume has contracted.

Mitral valve prolapse is a peculiar syndrome which may present with orthostatic hypotension. Echocardiographically, prolapse of the mitral valve cusp is common, particularly in otherwise healthy young females. However, dysrhythmias, chest pain, and chronic fatigue have been attributed to this phenomenon in some individuals.[41,42] Patients with symptomatic mitral valve prolapse often have signs and symptoms of autonomic nervous system dysfunction, and syncope is an occasional symptom. It may be the result of a dysrhythmia or hypotension. Most of these nonautonomic causes of orthostatic hypotension are correctable.

Autonomic nervous system failure may be a primary problem due to a group of rare syndromes or secondary to a number of other disorders. Except for diabetes mellitus, these are all rare.

Patients with autonomic nervous system failure may have scattered complaints depending on the receptor sites and pathways involved in the individual patient. All of those body functions associated with autonomic activity may suffer, including the gastrointestinal tract with constipation or diarrhea, the urinary tract with retention or incontinence, decreased sweating, impaired erections and ejaculation in men, constricted pupils, and nocturia. Many of these patients will have systemic hypertension lying down with hypotension standing up. There is usually an inappropriately small heart rate response to the blood pressure decrease and exercise. If these aspects are brought out in the history and physical findings, then a number of tests are available (Table 17.3) to support the clinical impression.[43] These maneuvers will test the alpha and beta sympathetic system as well as the parasympathetic and baroreceptor moieties. The appropriate tests should be selected for the clinical situation and will quite reliably delineate whether the autonomic nervous system is intact.

Every effort should be made to correct the causes of secondary autonomic nervous system failure. Some of these may be correctable or brought under better control. The primary autonomic nervous system failures are those modalities left after secondary causes have been eliminated. The primary causes are not definitively treatable.

Once the diagnosis is established and all correctable disease processes treated, the orthostatic hypotension often remains and requires symptomatic management with increasing fluid volume by increasing salt intake. Fludrocortisone (nine-alpha-flurohydrocortisone) is remarkably effective in some patients.[43a] They must be instructed to assume the upright position slowly. Patients should get out of bed only after sitting on the side of the bed for a few moments with leg muscle contraction and deep breathing. Elevation of the head of the bed with 3-inch blocks appears to decrease the nocturnal diuresis that patients with autonomic failure may have. Diuretics should be discontinued if at all possible. Mild edema is well tolerated and indicates optimal circulating blood volume. Tension stockings that come right up to the waist can be of value to some patients.

INTRINSIC CEREBROVASCULAR BLOOD DEPRIVATION

Atherosclerosis, Takayasu's arteritis, and subclavian steal may all cause syncope through intrinsic cerebrovascular blood deprivation. Conversely, tussive syncope has been demonstrated to cause a significant increase in intracerebral pressure so that the intracerebral pressure exceeds the perfusing pressure of the blood. Also with coughing there are short-lived repetitive Valsalva maneuvers carried out which limit venous return. With prolonged constant coughing these factors will diminish perfusion of the brain, culminating in syncope. In micturition syncope a decrease in venous return is the major factor.

Table 17.3. Clinical Maneuvers Available to Test Sympathetic and Parasympathetic Autonomic Nervous System Integrity*

Tests	Sympathetic		Parasympathetic	Baroreceptor
	α	β		
Orthostasis test	*		*	*
Phenylephrine test	*		*	*
Cold pressor test	*			
Handgrip test	*			
Forearm vasoconstriction test	*			
Pupillary epinephrine test	*			
Skin wrinkling test	*			
Saliva test	*		*	
Valsalva maneuver	*		*	
Sinus arrhythmia			*	
Atropine test			*	
Isoproterenol test		*		

* Modified from Robertson.[43] Copyright 1981, Williams & Wilkins Co, Baltimore.

This syndrome is generally seen in two different groups. The first of these is seen in otherwise healthy young men who have been out drinking alcohol, gone to bed, and then awakened with a full bladder, groggy, and stand up to urinate. Abdominal pressure is increased to initiate urination and at the same time venous return is decreased due to the Valsalva maneuver. Additionally, there is alcohol-induced peripheral vasodilatation, hypotension, decreased venous return, and hence decreased cardiac output further accentuating the hypotension culminating in syncope. A second group consists of older persons (mean age 60 years) with a preponderance of females with orthostatic hypotension who are taking several medications. Treatment in this latter group must be directed to the orthostasis, often drug-related.[13]

FUNCTIONAL CAUSES

Hysteria and other functional problems can always manifest themselves as unconsciousness, but this syndrome is usually easily detected. The patient rarely hurts himself, is usually under obvious emotional stress, and has other inappropriate psychological behavior.

EVALUATION OF THE PATIENT WITH SYNCOPE

The history is the most important part of the evaluation and will provide the diagnosis in about 25% of the patients with syncope. The events preceding, during, and in the recovery phase of the fainting episode are most important and it is the lucky patient who has an observer who can accurately relay information about these events. It is important to interview the observer at the earliest possible moment. It is impressive how the story changes toward a more dramatic rendition as time goes by. In the vasovagal syncopal episode (simple faint) the patient himself can usually give a good outline of seeing an accident or blood, entering a hospital, or being subjected to laboratory testing. Exertion preceding the syncopal episode speaks strongly for cardiac obstructive disease or dysrhythmia as a cause. The history of drugs taken by the patient can be very important.

In at least 10% of the patients the physical examination will give a clue to the etiology. If patients are included with an unannounced very short-lived syncopal episode, with total recovery instantly on regaining consciousness in a middle-aged or older individual, then physical examination involving testing of the carotid sinus response will account for the clue to the diagnosis in 30% of patients. If a murmur can be heard, suggesting valvular or subvalvular muscular obstruction, echocardiography will be most helpful, and if in the history or on physical examination there is any suggestion of dysrhythmia, then 24-hour ambulatory electrocardiographic monitoring will yield results in another 10% to 15% of patients.[2,31] Examination for the postural effect on blood pressure and cardiac rate is clearly important in determining whether orthostatic hypotension is playing a role.

Unless the cause for the syncope is obvious, with the history and physical examination, ambulatory electrocardiographic monitoring should be carried out in all of these patients as, even if it does not delineate a dysrhythmia compatible with syncope, it may give clues as to the dysrhythmia involved: sinus arrests, atrial extrasystoles occurring frequently as a forerunner to atrial fibrillation, ventricular extra systoles in couplets or triplets or of a multifocal or R-on-T nature suggesting that ventricular tachycardia may be the initiating mechanism for the syncope.[34-36] In the initial workup ambulatory electrocardiographic monitoring will be as effective as physical examination in delineating the cause of the syncope. It should be pointed out that interpretation of ambulatory electrocardiographic monitoring must have correlation of the observed dysrhythmia with symptoms. In at least three studies of patients with syncope, 15% to 46% of patients had additional syncopal episodes during monitoring, but 70% to 80% of these patients had dysrhythmias during the monitoring period, and in only 3% to 14% of the cases was there a significant correlation between the dysrhythmia and the syncopal episode. They must be correlatable to assume that the dysrhythmia has anything to do with the syncope.[32,35,36] It is important that every effort be made to establish that a pacemaker will help the patient. The risk, small as it is, nonetheless exists in the implantation and subsequent years with a pacemaker. The cost is substantial, estimated, including hospital and professional fees, at between $7,700 and $9,000 per implantation.[44]

In the initial workup of the patient echocardiography, in the absence of suspicion of cardiac obstruction abnormalities on the physical examination, is of little value unless myxoma or thrombus (positional syncope or positional loss of syncope) is suspected when the echocardiogram may be diagnostic. One should never resort to echocardiography to detect "silent" mitral valve prolapse.[44a]

Cardiac catheterization is rarely required unless significant valvular lesions can be found with echocardiography and Doppler echocardiography.

An electrocardiogram with a long rhythm strip is indicated in all patients with syncope. It too may reveal sinus arrest, left ventricular hypertrophy, atrial and ventricular ectopy and dysrhythmias, intraventricular conduction block and sinoatrial nodal and atrioventricular nodal block. The short PR interval with delta wave of the Wolff–Parkinson–White syndrome as an initiator of serious tachydysrhythmias may be found. Particular attention must be paid to the QT interval, particularly in children who are deaf and in adults who are on a host of medications particularly class I drugs including quinidine, procainamide, and disopyramide. Low serum potassium, calcium, and magnesium as well as ischemia and phenothiazine derivatives may prolong the QT interval. Bundle branch block and atrioventricular conduction abnormalities have an increased chance of transient complete heart block resulting in syncope.[2] The electrocardiogram also may reveal an acute injury pattern and a small number of acute myocardial infarcts will present with syncope usually due to a tachydysrhythmia or bradydysrhythmia.

The history and physical examination and laboratory tests already outlined, including ambulatory electrocardiographic monitoring for at least two days, will provide the probable diagnosis in approximately 50% of patients.

The remaining 50% of patients will, at this stage, have syncope of unknown etiology and if this workup succeeded their first syncopal episode, further testing will add a small diagnostic yield with vastly added expense. That, combined with the fact that up to 70% of patients will not have a second syncopal attack and consequently the prognosis is excellent,[2,9] suggests further evaluation should be avoided unless there is a recurrence. If the patient is being seen after more than one syncopal attack over a reasonable period of time, neurologic consultation should be sought because even in those patients who do not manifest frank seizure activity the distinct possibility of petit mal and petit absence type of epilepsy has to be considered. Electroencephalography with provocative maneuvers may be necessary.

The majority of the patients remaining after a neurologic cause has been eliminated will have syncope on the basis of a tachydysrhythmia or bradydysrhythmia including asystole. If a distinct hypersensitive reaction can be elicited with carotid sinus massage and the history is compatible with asystole as a cause for the syncope and no other potential cause can be found, then a permanent transvenous pacemaker should be implanted generally at a demand rate below the patient's intrinsic cardiac rate so that it will be essentially in the stand-by mode.[5,45] If hypersensitivity to the carotid sinus testing on several occasions, each several hours apart, does not reveal a hypersensitive reaction, then the distinct possibility of a tachydysrhythmia would also have to be considered. Electrophysiologic studies (EPS) should, if at all possible, be carried out.[37–40,46]

If electrophysiologic studies are not feasible or practical, then using the Lown technique[47,48] of successive Holter monitoring off and on medication, and demanding an 80% reduction in the dysrhythmias with at least two different antidysrhythmic medications, is a reliable method of determining the agents that will correct the dysrhythmia. The problem with this method is that the dysrhythmia causing the problem must be present off and on most days to be able to visualize it on the 24-hour ambulatory monitor. Invasive electrophysiologic studies ultimately are certainly the best method to detect the presence of potential dysrhythmia by inducing it and to detect the correct antidysrhythmic agent to prevent the dysrhythmia. It must be noted, however, that again there has to be reproducibility of the dysrhythmia even with the repeated electrical impulses that are used to generate ventricular tachycardia or ventricular fibrillation. Electrophysiologic studies should be reserved for those patients who have gone through the methods already described, because in the overall pattern of syncope these studies are singularly ineffective in revealing the cause of syncope. In patients with an undiagnosed cause of syncope after history taking, physical examination, electrocardiography, and ambulatory electrocardiographic monitoring, electrophysiologic studies proved to be diagnostic in only a small number of patients. However, this usually led to appropriate therapy that completely relieved symptoms. Kwok et al[45] have analyzed through the literature that of 100,000 people with syncope, 6,100 will undergo EPS to establish the cause of syncope after nondiagnostic electrocardiography and ambulatory electrocardiographic monitoring. In only 1,100 of these patients will EPS be conclusive. Approximately 500 of them will have a tachydysrhythmia and 600 a bradydysrhythmia. In the remaining 5,000 EPS will be unrevealing.[45] Electrophysiologic procedures are most likely to be of benefit in patients who have structural heart disease; overall yield is about 64% in such patients compared with 10% to 15% in those with no structural heart disease.[49]

In slightly less than 50% of patients the cause of syncope will not be determined, and in the remaining diagnosed group the cardiovascular cause will be found in about 50% and a noncardiovascular cause in the other 50%. This is an important distinction to make because, although the overall mortality in the first year of patients diagnosed with syncope is 14%, the mortality in the cardiovascular group is 30% and in the noncardiovascular group 12%, a statistically significant difference. Even more important, in the 50% of patients in whom the syncope is of unknown cause there is a 6% mortality.[6] This was a single study carried out in a hospital setting with a considerable number of acute cardiac problems, which in themselves may have accounted for their high mortality rate.

The epidemiology of syncope in the elderly differs from that in the young. Although a specific cause of syncope is often not able to be established in either the elderly or the young, elderly patients more often have a cardiovascular cause of syncope than the young (33.8% versus 16.8%).[50] Consequently, prolonged electrocardiographic monitoring is more useful in the elderly than in the young in establishing the diagnosis (17% versus 8%). The overall mortality in the elderly with syncope is three times that in the young ($26.9 \pm 3.4\%$ versus $8.3 \pm 2.1\%$) over a two-year period.[50] The evaluation of syncope in the elderly is also more complicated because the elderly often have multiple coexisting medical problems or diseases, are taking multiple medications, and have age-related physiologic changes that can predispose to decreased cerebral perfusion. Therefore, it is important to recognize these differences between the old and the young when making diagnostic and therapeutic plans for patients with syncope.

In summary, every patient presenting with syncope must have thorough history taking. Is the patient old or young? Are there coexisting diseases? Is the patient taking any medicines? Did he or she really faint and lose consciousness? What were the surrounding factors? Was there an aura or any seizure activity? Was a change in position the cause of syncope and is there a reproducible cause that would speak strongly for postural hypotension? Was this a sudden unannounced syncopal attack suggesting asystole, marked bradycardia, or ventricular fibrillation?

On physical examination have all the correctable causes been examined for?

On the laboratory examination far too much attention has been paid to sophisticated and expensive neurologic workups while these rarely will offer a diagnosis to the etiology of syncope and cause great expense to the patient. Every middle-aged or older patient should have carotid sinus massage carried out in a correct fashion to detect if a hypersensitive response may be the clue to asystole as an etiologic factor. Upright blood pressure measurement should always be performed to search for orthostatic hypotension.

We are finally left with the patient who has repeated syncopal attacks of unknown etiology that fulfill the criteria of asystole or ventricular fibrillation: sudden and unannounced syncope of very short-lived duration, measured in seconds, with complete regaining of consciousness immediately with no postictal phase. Should these patients be paced or not? Evidence has been presented that these patients should be offered a permanent transvenous pacemaker set at a demand rate below their usual intrinsic cardiac rate as a stand-by situation to avoid the pacemaker syndrome.

REFERENCES

1. Dermksian G, Lamb LE: Syncope in a population of healthy young adults: incidence, mechanisms and significance. *JAMA* 1958; 168:1200–1207.
2. Kudenchuk PJ, McAnulty JH: Syncope: evaluation and treatment. *Mod Concepts Cardiovasc Dis* 1985; 54:25–29.
3. Boudoulas H, Weissler AM, Lewis RP, Warren JV: The clinical diagnosis of syncope. *Current Prob Cardiol* 1982; 7:7–40.
4. Day SC, Cook EF, Funkenstein H, Goldman L: Evaluation and outcome of emergency room patients with transient loss of consciousness. *Am J Med* 1982; 73:15–23.
5. Peretz DI, Abdulla A: Management of cardioinhibitory hypersensitive carotid sinus syncope with permanent cardiac pacing — a seventeen year prospective study. *Can J Cardiol* 1985; 1:86–91.
6. Kapoor WN, Karpf M, Wieand S, Peterson JR, Levey GS: A prospective evaluation and follow-up of patients with syncope. *N Engl J Med* 1983; 309:197–204.
7. Kapoor WN, Karpf M, Maher Y, Miller RA, Levey GS: Syncope of unknown origin: the need for a more cost-effective approach to its diagnostic evaluation. *JAMA* 1982; 247:2687–2691.
8. Silverstein MD, Singer DE, Mulley AG, Thibault GE, Barnett GO: Patients with syncope admitted to medical intensive care units. *JAMA* 1982; 248:1185–1189.
9. Savage DD, Corwin L, McGee DL, Kannel WB, Wolf PA: Epidemiologic features of isolated syncope: the Framingham study. *Stroke* 1985; 16:626–629.
10. Medina RP, Dreifus LS: Syncope. *Current Prob Cardiol* 1983; 8:1–50.
11. Eagle KA, Black HR: The impact of diagnostic tests in evaluating patients with syncope. *Yale J Biol Med* 1983; 56:1–8.
12. Mannick JA, Suter CG, Hume DM: The "subclavian steal" syndrome: a further documentation. *JAMA* 1962; 182:254–258.
13. Kapoor WN, Peterson JR, Karpf M: Micturition syncope: a reappraisal. *JAMA* 1985; 253:796–798.
14. Schwartz LS, Goldfischer J, Sprague GJ, Schwartz SP: Syncope and sudden death in aortic stenosis. *Am J Cardiol* 1969; 23:647–658.
15. Canedo MI, Frank MJ, Abdulla AM: Rhythm disturbances in hypertrophic cardiomyopathy: prevalence, relation to symptoms and management. *Am J Cardiol* 1980; 45:848–855.
16. Bernstein M, Gerein A, Peretz DI: A case of left ventricular outflow tract tumor obstruction. In association with a bicuspid aortic valve. *J Thorac Cardiovasc Surg* 1969; 60:166–173.
17. Grossman W, Alpert JS, Braunwald E: Pulmonary hypertension, in Braunwald E (ed): *Heart Disease: A Textbook of Cardiovascular Medicine.* Philadelphia, WB Saunders, 1984, pp 823–848.
18. Thames MD, Alpert JS, Dalen JE: Syncope in patients with pulmonary embolism. *JAMA* 1977; 238:2509–2511.
19. Peretz DI: Advanced heart block during acute myocardial infarction treated with an electrode pacing catheter. *Can Med Assoc J* 1967; 96:451–456.
20. Haft JI: Clinical implications of atrioventricular and intraventricular conduction abnormalities. II. Acute myocardial infarction. *Cardiovasc Clinics* 1977; 8(3):65–77.

20a. Barnett HJM, Mohr JP, Stein BM, Yatsu FM: *Stroke: Pathophysiology, Diagnosis, and Management.* New York, Churchill Livingstone, 1986, p 1088.

21. Ferrer MI: The sick sinus syndrome. *Circulation* 1973; 47:635–641.
22. Scarpa WJ: The sick sinus syndrome. *Am Heart J* 1976; 92:648–660.

22a. Morley CA, Perrins EJ, Sutton R: Clinical assessment of the carotid sinus syndrome. *Practical Cardiol* 1986; 12:126–152.

23. Weiss S, Baker JP: The carotid sinus reflex in health and disease—its role in the causation of fainting and convulsions. *Medicine* 1933; 12:297–354.
24. Franke H: *Uber das Karotissinus—Syndrome und der sonenamten hyperaktiven Karotissinusreflex.* Stuttgart, Friedrich-Karl, Schattauer-Verlag, 1966, p 149.
25. Gang ES: Sinus node electrogram in patients with a hypersensitive carotid sinus syndrome. *J Am Coll Cardiol* 1985; 6:1484–1490.

25a. Sugrue DD, Gersh BJ, Holmes DR, Wood DL, Osborn MJ, Hammill SC: Symptomatic "isolated" carotid sinus hypersensitivity: natural history and results of treatment with anticholinergic drugs or pacemaker. *J Am Coll Cardiol* 1986; 7:158-162.

26. Dhingra RC, Denes P, Wu D, Chuquimia R, Amat-y-Leon F, Wyndham C, Rosen KM: Syncope in patients with chronic bifascicular block. Significance, causative mechanisms, and clinical implications. *Ann Intern Med* 1974; 81:302–306.
27. McAnulty JH, Rahimtoola SH, Murphy E, DeMots H, Ritzmann L, Kanarek PE, Kauffman S: Natural history of "high risk" bundle branch block: final report of a prospective study. *N Engl J Med* 1982; 307:137–143.
28. Murphy E, McAnulty JH, Rahimtoola SH: Intraventricular conduction abnormalities associated with coronary artery disease. *Med N Am* 1980; 4:476–490.
29. Steinbrecher UP, Fitchett DH: Torsades de pointes. A cause of syncope with atrioventricular block. *Arch Intern Med* 1980; 140:1223–1226.
30. Soffer J, Dreifus LS, Michelson EL: Polymorphous ventricular tachycardia associated with normal and long Q–T intervals. *Am J Cardiol* 1982; 49:2021–2029.

30a. Kuchar DL, Thorburn CW, Sammel NL: The role of signal averaged electrocardiography in the investigation of unselected patients with syncope. *Aust NZ J Med* 1985; 15:697–703.

30b. Walter PF, Pollak SJ: Technique of QRS signal averaging, in Hurst JW (ed): *The Heart,* ed 6. New York, McGraw-Hill, 1986, pp 1716–1719.

31. Gibson TC, Heltzman MR: Diagnostic efficacy of 24-hour electrocardiographic monitoring for syncope. *Am J Cardiol* 1984; 53:1013–1017.
32. Clarke PI, Glasser SP, Spoto E: Arrhythmias detected by ambulatory monitoring: lack of correlation with symptoms of dizziness and syncope. *Chest* 1980; 77:722–725.
33. Boudoulas H, Schaal SF, Lewis RP, Robinson JL: Superiority of 24-hour outpatient monitoring over multi-stage exercise testing for the evaluation of syncope. *J Electrocardiol* 1979; 12:103–108.
34. Gutiertez MR, Changfoot GH, Peretz DI: Significance of T- wave interruption by premature beats as a cause of sudden death. *Can Med Assoc J* 1968; 98:144–149.
35. Kala R, Viitasalo MT, Toivonen L, Eisalo A: Ambulatory ECG recording in patients referred because of syncope or dizziness. *Acta Med Scand* (Suppl)1982; 668:13–19.
36. Zeldis SM, Levine BJ, Michelson EL, Morganroth J: Cardiovascular complaints— correlation with cardiac arrhythmia on 24-hour electrocardiographic monitoring. *Chest* 1980; 78:456–462.
37. DiMarco JP, Garan H, Harthorne JW, Ruskin JN: Intracardiac electrophysiologic techniques in recurrent syncope of unknown cause. *Ann Intern Med* 1981; 95:542–548.
38. Fisher JD: Role of electrophysiologic testing in the diagnosis and treatment of patients with known and suspected bradycardias and tachycardias. *Prog Cardiovasc Dis* 1981; 24:25–90.
39. Gulamhusein S, Naccarelli GV, Ko PT, Prystowsky EN, Zipes DP, Barnett HJM, Heger JJ, Klein GJ: Value and limitations of clinical electrophysiologic study in assessment of patients with unexplained syncope *Am J Med* 1982; 73:700–705.
40. Hess DS, Morady F, Scheinman MM: Electrophysiologic testing in the evaluation of patients with syncope of undetermined origin. *Am J Cardiol* 1982; 50:1309–1315.

40a. Kuchel O: Orthostatic hypotension: a guide to treatment. *Perspectives in Cardiology* 1986; 2:20–32.

41. Winkle RA, Lopes MG, Fitzgerald JW, Goodman DJ, Schroeder JS, Harrison DC: Arrhythmias in patients with mitral valve prolapse. *Circulation* 1975; 52:73–81.
42. DeMaria AN, Amsterdam EA, Vismara LA, Markson W, Brocchini R, Mason DT: The variable spectrum of rhythm disturbances in the mitral valve prolapse syndrome. *Circulation* 1974; 49–50 (suppl III): III–222.
43. Robertson D: Clinical pharmacology: assessment of autonomic function, in Baughman KL, Greene BM (eds): *Clinical Diagnosis Manual for the Houseofficer.* Baltimore, MD, Williams & Wilkins, 1981, 86–101.

43a. Onrot J, Goldberg MR, Hollister AS, Biaggioni I, Robertson RM, Robertson D: Management of chronic orthostatic hypotension. *Am J Med* 1986; 80:454–464.

44. Case Records of the Massachusettes General Hospital (Case 1— 1982). *N Eng J Med* 1982; 306:32–39.

44a. Prakash R: Mitral valve prolapse diagnosed by echocardiography? *Chest* 1986; 84:474–476.

45. Kwok CK, Beck JR, Pauker SG: Repeated syncope with negative diagnostic evaluation. *Med Decis Making* 1984; 4:351–377.
46. Olshansky B, Mazuz M, Martins JB: Significance of inducible tachycardia in patients with syncope of unknown origin: a long-term follow-up. *J Am Coll Cardiol* 1985; 5:216–223.
47. Lown B: Clinical management of ventricular arrhythmias. *Hosp Practice* 1982; 17:73–86.
48. Lown B, Podrid PJ, DeSilva RA, Graboys TB: Sudden cardiac death — management of the patient at risk. *Current Prob Cardiol* March, 1980; 4(12):1–36.
49. Haddad RM, Sellers TD: Syncope as a symptom. A practical approach to etiologic diagnosis. *Postgrad Med* 1986; 79(2):48–62.
50. Kapoor W, Snustad D, Peterson J, Wieand HS, Cha R, Karpf M: Syncope in the elderly. *Am J Med* 1986; 80:419–428.

18 Clinical and Electrocardiographic Diagnosis of Cardiac Arrhythmias

Leonard S. Dreifus, MD

SINOATRIAL BLOCK

CLINICAL FEATURES

Several disorders of sinoatrial nodal function may result in periods of sinus arrest and, in the absence of a subsidiary or rescuing pacemaker, may produce dizziness or frank syncope. The first demonstration of the Wenckebach structure was due to second degree sinoatrial block, which produced quickening of the pulse (progressively shorter A waves) before the dropped beat (carotid pulse) and failure of atrioventricular (AV) conduction.[1] The sick sinus syndrome, which has come into popular use over the past decade, may represent abnormalities of both impulse formation and conduction in the sinus and perinodal regions.[2] The term *sick sinus syndrome* has been used to encompass a wide variety of abnormalities of impulse formation and conduction involving the sinus node, as well as other specialized cardiac conduction tissue and potential subsidiary pacemakers. Manifestations of the sick sinus syndrome may include: (1) persistent, severe, and inappropriate sinus bradycardia; (2) cessation of sinus rhythm, sinus pauses, or sinus arrest for intervals during which there is also failure of subsidiary escape pacemakers; (3) replacement of the sinus rhythm by an ectopic atrial or junctional pacemaker; (4) paroxysmal or chronic atrial fibrillation, or atrial standstill with total absence of sinus node activity; (5) susceptibility to paroxysmal supraventricular arrhythmia, including atrial fibrillation and junctional tachycardias; (6) prolonged suppression of sinus rhythm after spontaneous or electrical conversion from atrial fibrillation or other supraventricular tachycardias; (7) episodes of sinoatrial exit block following drug (for example, digoxin) therapy; and (8) carotid sinus hypersensitivity resulting in prolonged asystole, high grade AV nodal block, or both.

The sick sinus syndrome has protean presentations and variable degrees of severity. It occurs idiopathically, is a result of various cardiomyopathic, degenerative, or ischemic processes, and often requires escalating therapeutic regimens. Typically, paroxysmal atrial flutter or fibrillation is first treated with drugs (such as digoxin, beta-receptor blocking agents, and more recently verapamil) to slow AV nodal conduction. As episodes increase in frequency, these same drugs may be prescribed prophylactically. After subsequent recurrences of arrhythmia, quinidine or other class I antiarrhythmic drugs may be added. However, at some point in this pharmacologic hierarchy, either primary or posttachycardia symptomatic bradyarrhythmias often become more incapacitating than the tachyarrhythmias, and permanent pacemaker implantation follows. This full-blown constellation of complex tachyarrhythmias and bradyarrhythmias is often referred to as the bradycardia–tachycardia syndrome (Figure 18.1). Actual failure of sinus node automaticity is rather rare, and loss of atrial depolarization may be secondary to exit block of the impulse from the sinus node to the surrounding atrial tissue or repetitive concealed reentries within the perinodal tissues of the sinus node region, preventing subsequent exit of the impulse from the sinoatrial nodal fibers.[3] The bradycardia–tachycardia syndrome represents a subset of the sick sinus syndrome and is characterized by recurrent supraventricular tachyarrhythmias along with periods of bradycardia or actual sinus arrest.[4] Concealed and then manifest sinus node reentry may be one cause of this syndrome, producing periods of both tachyarrhythmia and bradyarrhythmia.[3]

Sinus node automaticity and conduction through the perinodal tissues are analogous to AV disorders. Carotid sinus pressure and drugs such as digitalis and beta- and calcium blocking agents may produce profound effects on sinus node automaticity and conduction. More recently, the introduction of beta-blocking agents for intraocular management of glaucoma has now been recognized as a cause of sinoatrial as well as AV conduction disorders. Sinoatrial disease frequently is associated with both AV nodal as well as His-Purkinje system disease.

ELECTROCARDIOGRAPHIC FEATURES

In patients with sinus node dysfunction, rarely does the sinus rate exceed 90 beats per minute with exercise. Electrophysiologic studies to measure sinus node function include corrected sinus node recovery time, sinoatrial conduction time, as well as direct measurements of sinus node activation using special electrode catheters placed in the region of the sinus node.[5-17] However, electrophysiologic studies are rarely required for clinical diagnosis of sinoatrial rhythm abnormalities, because the studies are frequently associated with inconclusive results for a variety of reasons. Ambulatory Holter monitoring correlating symptoms with electrocardiographic changes is usually diagnostic.[18]

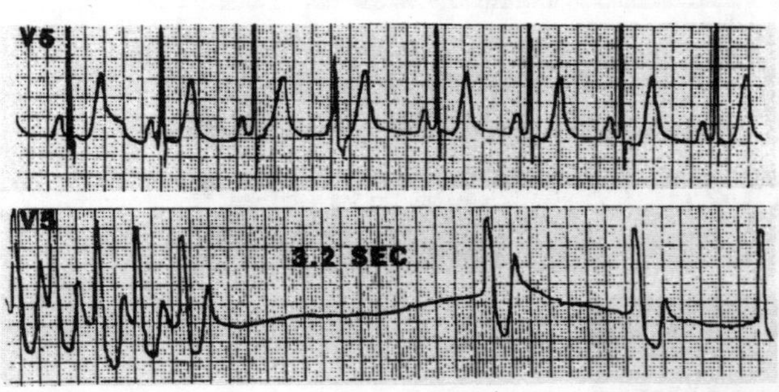

Figure 18.1. Bradycardia-tachycardia, lead V_5. Following a period of tachycardia at a rate of 440 beats per minute, there is a 3-second period of asystole followed by a junctional escape rhythm.

Sinoatrial block may be recognized by characteristic grouped beats (Figure 18.2). Although first degree sinoatrial block cannot be recognized on the surface electrocardiogram, second degree block may have the characteristics of dropped beats appearing in multiples of the sinus rate (Figure 18.3). Furthermore, characteristic Wenckebach periods may be associated with conduction delay from the sinus node to the atrial tissues (Figure 18.2). Third degree sinoatrial block may be manifest only as failure of any P wave to appear and is frequently associated with failure of subsidiary pacemakers to rescue the heart from asystole.

SUPRAVENTRICULAR ARRHYTHMIAS

CLINICAL FEATURES

Supraventricular tachycardias can be classified as in Tables 18.1 and 18.2. Principally, supraventricular tachycardias must first be differentiated from sinus tachycardia. During sinus rhythm, impulses arise in the sinus node and are propagated successfully to the atria and consequently through the AV node to the ventricles via the His-Purkinje system. Rates of 130 beats per minute and greater create the most difficult diagnostic features between sinus tachycardia and supraventricular tachycardias. Rapid sinus rates are usually caused by increased activity of the cardiac sympathetic nerves and withdrawal of vagal inhibitory influences. The maximum heart rate that can be achieved during strenuous exercise varies with age. In healthy young persons the maximum heart rate may reach more than 200 beats per minute, whereas in elderly individuals the maximum rate rarely exceeds 150 to 160 beats per minute. The sinus etiology of the tachycardia is usually recognized by a normal P-wave inscription. P waves are usually upright in leads II, III, and aVF and usually have a uniform, smooth contour without phasic variations such as the dart and dome configuration seen with ectopic mechanisms. Furthermore, even in extreme sinus tachycardia the rate may vary over a considerable range, whereas in paroxysmal supraventricular tachycardia the rate may be rapid but is usually precisely regular.

ATRIAL PREMATURE SYSTOLES

ELECTROCARDIOGRAPHIC FEATURES

Identification of ectopic atrial depolarizations is based on their premature occurrence as well as a P-wave morphology that differs from that of the normal sinus P wave. Usually, the PR interval may increase following an atrial premature systole. A shortened PR interval and inverted P waves in the inferior leads suggest a junctional origin. Frequently, atrial premature systoles occur during inscription of a T wave, and unless the clinician carefully analyzes multiple leads on the electrocardiogram, an early atrial depolarization can be missed (Figure 18.4, *arrow*). Occasionally, premature atrial systoles occur so early in the atrial cycle that conduction to the ventricle fails to occur and only a pause in the ventricular cycle is noted

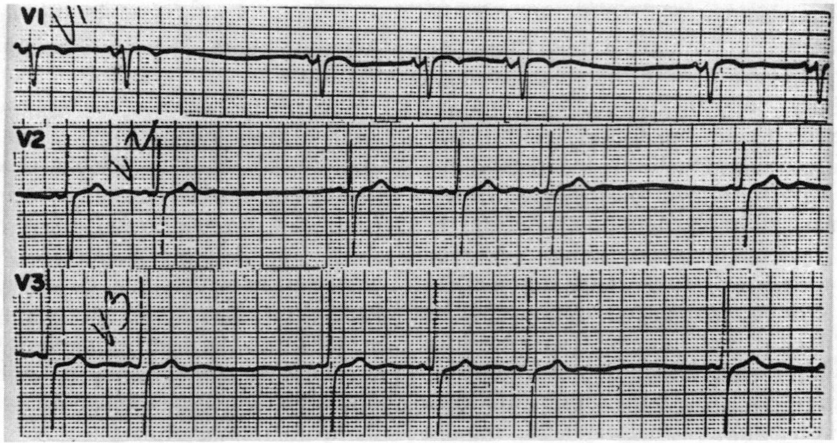

Figure 18.2. Grouped beating showing periods of bigeminy and trigeminy. The PP interval and consequently the RR interval shortened before the pause; this represents 3:2 and 4:3 sinoatrial block.

on the surface electrocardiogram. Furthermore, early atrial premature systoles may not be associated with adequate stroke volume and the stroke rate may be slow and produce neurologic symptoms (Figure 18.4). However, the rhythmicity of the sinus node is offset by the atrial premature systole and suspicion of its presence can then be inferred. Resetting of the sinus node by the premature atrial systole may cause an increase in the interval to the next sinus P wave. In the presence of sinus node dysfunction, the return cycle can be abnormally prolonged (beyond 1.6 seconds). Junctional escape beats occasionally may be seen, which rescue the ventricles from asystole in the presence of sinus node dysfunction. Occasionally, premature atrial systoles will propagate to the His-Purkinje system during the relative refractory period of the right or left bundle branch systems. This is particularly true in the right bundle branch, because this is a longer and thinner group of fibers that demonstrate conduction abnormalities (aberrancy) caused by stress of the premature systole and produce phase 3 conduction block of the right bundle branch variety. Furthermore, the refractory period in the right bundle branch is considerably longer than that in the left. Consequently, aberration of the premature atrial systole showing the right bundle branch block configuration is seen fairly frequently, and these beats must be distinguished from ventricular ectopic complexes and ventricular tachycardia (Figure 18.5). Careful search for a premature atrial systole preceding the wide QRS complex is mandatory to differentiate these ectopic beats from ventricular premature systoles.

PAROXYSMAL SUPRAVENTRICULAR TACHYCARDIA

Paroxysmal supraventricular tachycardias (SVTs) constitute a common group of clinical arrhythmias that may or may not be associated with intrinsic cardiac disease. The attacks are usually sudden in onset and termination. Most have a reentrant mechanism initiated by a fortui-

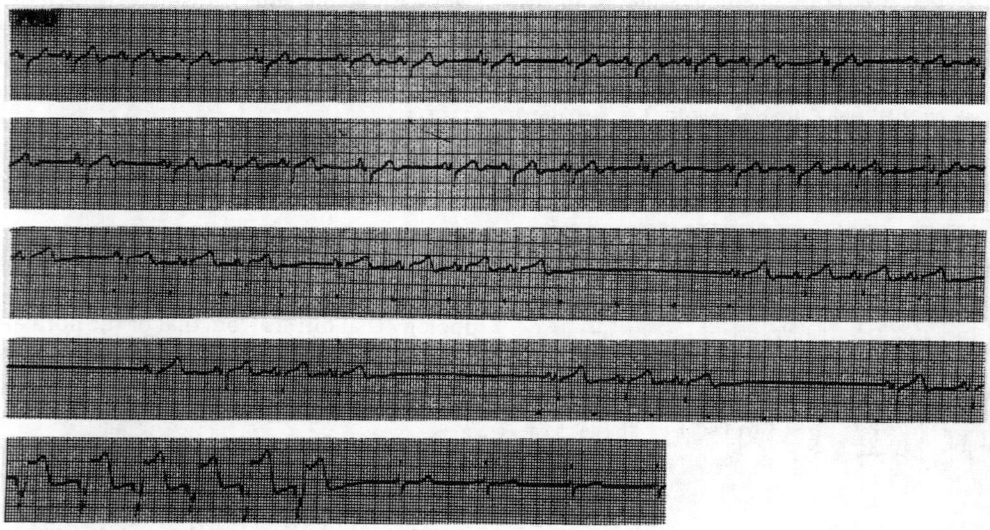

Figure 18.3. Periods of sinus arrest due to sinoatrial block. Sinus cycle length discharges at 760 ms. Dots represent sinus activity and lack of emergence of the sinus node to the atria, causing asystole.

Table 18.1. Supraventricular Tachycardias

Sinoatrial (SA) reentrant tachycardia
Intraatrial reentrant tachycardia
Automatic atrial tachycardia (a) Atrial tachycardia with or without block (PAT) (b) Chaotic atrial tachycardia
Atrioventricular nodal reentrant tachycardia (a) Slow–fast form (b) Fast–slow form
Atrioventricular reentrant tachycardia (a) Wolff–Parkinson–White reentrant tachycardia (b) Concealed bypass type

tously timed premature beat (Figure 18.6, *arrow*). In comparison, the less common types of ectopic or automatic supraventricular tachycardias occur with an initial period of gradual acceleration of the rate and attrition of the rate at the termination of the tachycardia. The rate of paroxysmal, reentrant SVT is usually rapid and regular at 140 to 220 beats per minute. The QRS complexes are typically narrow and are usually less than 100 ms in duration, unless aberrancy develops at the rapid rate or a bundle branch block pattern was also present during sinus rhythm. P waves, if visible on the electrocardiogram, usually remain in a fixed relation to each QRS complex. However, the P waves may vary in their linkage to the QRS complex depending on several important electrophysiologic mechanisms, which will be described briefly. The morphologic characteristics of the P waves are usually clearly different from those of sinus rhythm and they may occur before, simultaneously with, or after the QRS complex. Vagal maneuvers can terminate the tachycardia, but they may not always be successful.

ATRIOVENTRICULAR NODAL REENTRANT TACHYCARDIA: ELECTROCARDIOGRAPHIC FEATURES

SLOW–FAST FORM

Most AV nodal reentrant tachycardias are characterized as the "slow–fast" variety, as will be described below (Figure 18.7). Typically, P waves occur simultaneously with or shortly after the QRS complexes. At times it is difficult to distinguish this variety of SVT from those incorporating a concealed bypass tract. However, electrophysiologic studies can identify antegrade conduction using the normal AV pathway in both instances, but retrograde AV nodal conduction in the former and an AV bypass tract that is extra AV nodal as the retrograde limb of the tachycardia in the latter. It is now generally agreed that functional "longitudinal dissociation" of the AV node or so-called "dual AV nodal pathways" associated

Table 18.2. Differential Diagnosis of Supraventricular Tachycardia

Sinoatrial Nodal Reentrant Supraventricular Tachycardia Initiation and termination by APCs or VPCs independent of interatrial conduction delay or AV conduction delay P waves identical to sinus in morphology and activation sequence PR related to supraventricular tachycardia rate Atrioventricular (AV) nodal block may exist without affecting supraventricular tachycardia Vagal maneuvers slow and then abruptly terminate supraventricular tachycardia
Intraatrial Reentrant Supraventricular Tachycardia Initiation by APCs Atrial activation sequence differs from sinus PR related to supraventricular tachycardia rate Atrioventricular nodal block may exist without affecting supraventricular tachycardia Reentry within Bachmann's bundle can be demonstrated in some instances Vagal maneuvers may not terminate supraventricular tachycardia but may produce AV nodal block
Automatic Atrial Tachycardia **Cannot** initiate or terminate with APCs and is independent of interatrial conduction delay or AV delay Supraventricular tachycardia "warms up": subtle P wave and rate alterations P wave differs from sinus PR varies with supraventricular rate Atrioventricular nodal block may exist without affecting supraventricular rate P-wave morphology may vary with chaotic types Vagal maneuvers do not terminate but produce AV nodal block
Atrioventricular Nodal Reentrant Supraventricular Tachycardia Initiation and termination by APCs or VPCs, or pacing during AV Wenckebach cycles: slow–fast type Initiation dependent on critical increase of AH with shift from fast to slow pathway conduction Retrograde P wave usually buried in QRS or following QRS with long RP Vagal maneuvers slow or abruptly terminate supraventricular tachycardia
Atrioventricular Reentrant Supraventricular Tachycardia (Concealed Bypass) Initiation and termination by APCs or VPCs dependent on critical AV delay but independent of AV nodal delay Retrograde P wave with short RP: atria and ventricles required to initiate and sustain supraventricular tachycardia Ability to preexcite atrium with VPC during supraventricular tachycardia Vagal maneuvers may slow or abruptly terminate supraventricular tachycardia

APCs = atrial premature contractions; VPCs = ventricular premature contractions.

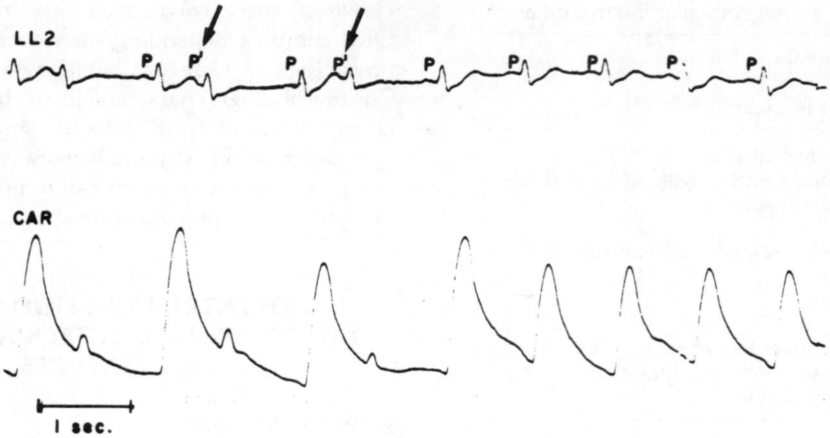

Figure 18.4. Premature atrial systoles P′ occurring early in the diastolic period with a part of ventricular contraction failing to open the atrioventricular valves, producing syncope. LL2 = limb lead 2; CAR = carotid pulse.

with discontinuous AV nodal conduction curves could form the basis for the reentrant circuit in reciprocal tachycardia.[18–24] Under these circumstances the AV node behaves as if there are two pathways with different functional properties. The fast pathway has a longer refractory period, making it more likely to block or fail to conduct if early atrial premature systole occurs. The common form of AV nodal reentry uses the slow pathway (which has a shorter refractory period) for antegrade and the fast pathway for the retrograde conduction. The mechanism of this arrhythmia includes sufficient delay of antegrade conduction in the slow pathway, whereas unidirectional antegrade block occurs in the fast pathway. Critical delay in the slow pathway allows recovery of the previously blocked fast pathway, resulting in a reentry mechanism through retrograde engagement of the fast pathway (Figure 18.7). Initiation of the reentry mechanism can be accomplished either with rapid atrial pacing or by the extrastimulus method in the catheterization laboratory. With either method, SVT is initiated in susceptible patients by producing unidirectional block in the fast pathway and setting up a reentrant mechanism (Figure 18.7). In this form of AV nodal reentry tachycardia, the P waves are usually not visible in the presence of the tachycardia. Most often, the P waves are inscribed simultaneously with the QRS complex (Figure 18.7). Occasionally, the P waves may occur after the QRS complex and are usually inverted in leads II, III, and aVF. Obviously, the relation of the P wave and QRS complex is determined by the conduction time of the retrograde fast pathway.[23] Retrograde dual AV nodal pathways have also been demonstrated. Moe et al[18] and Wu[24] demonstrated discontinuous curves with ventricular extrastimulus testing.

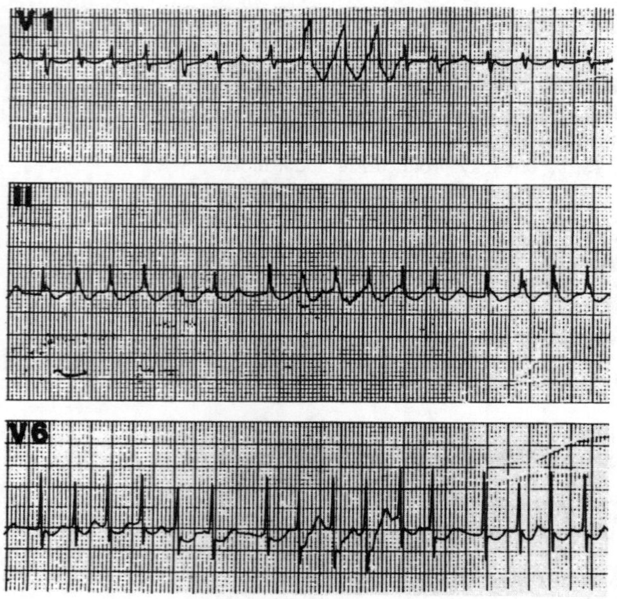

Figure 18.5. Complex atrial tachycardia QRS complexes 8_1 to 10_1 show right bundle branch block in lead V_1, but this conduction delay is not apparent in leads II and V_6. Aberrant beats terminate a short cycle which followed on a longer cycle.

Typically, in the presence of dual pathways, the effective refractory period of the slow pathway is the effective refractory period of the AV node. Furthermore, the functional refractory period of the fast pathway, that is, the shortest H1 to H2 (His to His) interval of the fast pathway curve, is also the AV nodal functional refractory period. The functional refractory period of the slow pathway is not discernible from the slow pathway curve, because by definition, AV nodal conduction is more rapid over the fast pathway. Finally, a relatively prolonged atrial functional refractory period may preclude recognition of dual AV nodal pathways when the atrial extrastimulus method is used.

Anatomic confirmation of dual AV nodal pathways is notably lacking. In experimental preparations, however, Mazgalev et al[25] clearly demonstrated the consequences of the normally occurring, anatomically distinguishable dual inputs to the AV node from the crista terminalis and the interatrial septum. In these studies, mapping of activation patterns suggested that delayed conduction or block within the AV node could allow an impulse to enter

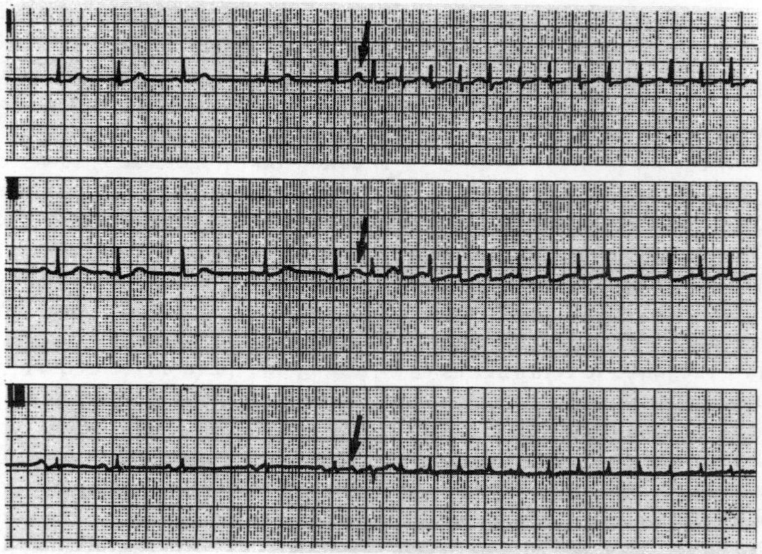

Figure 18.6. Premature atrial systoles (*arrow*) initiating runs of supraventricular tachycardia.

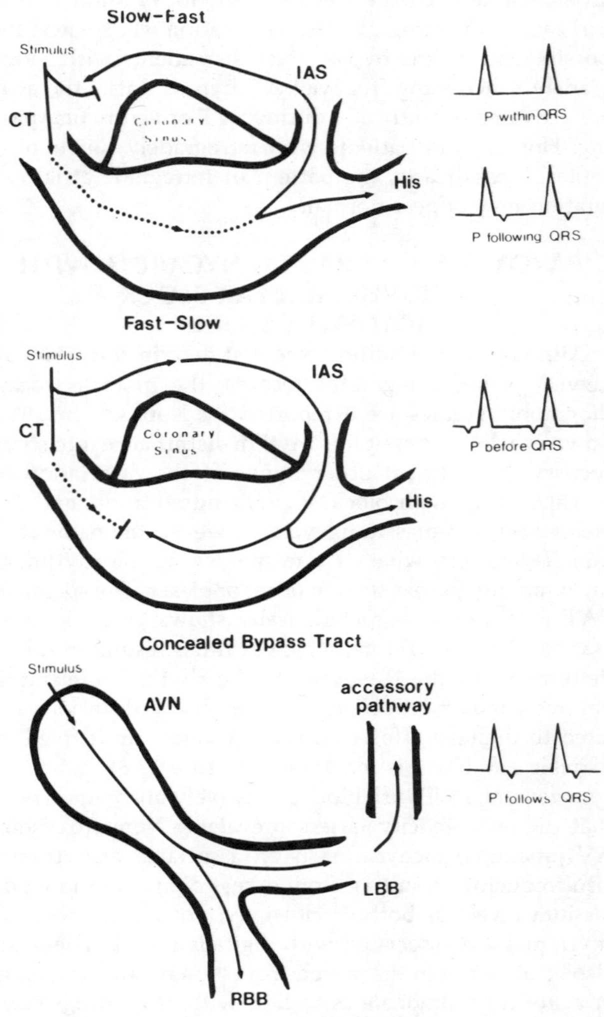

Figure 18.7. Types of supraventricular tachycardia: slow–fast, fast–slow, and concealed retrograde bypass. AVN = atrioventricular node; CT = concealed tract; IAS = interatrial septum; LBB = left bundle branch; RBB = right bundle branch.

one atrionodal input region, emerge from the other atrionodal input region, and conduct through the perinodal fibers to reenter the AV node from the initial input area, thereby completing the reentry circuit[26] (Figure 18.7). Consequently, for the first time an anatomic as well as an electrophysiologic basis for dual pathways could be identified, that is, slow conduction usually within the AV node itself, particularly in the AN and N regions of this structure with fast retrograde conduction through the atrial or perinodal fibers. It is quite clear now that two different structures within the AV nodal area, namely, the AV node itself and the perinodal tissues, could form the basis for dual AV nodal pathways (Figure 18.7). Subsequent studies by Iinuma et al[26] further indicated that the impulse could block in either the slow or fast pathway continuing through the other AV nodal input region to complete the reentry circuit or both types could exist alternatively.

In the basal resting state, normal AV conduction time will increase progressively as the rate of atrial pacing is increased and also when the coupling interval of the extrastimulus (A1–A2) is shortened. Normally, when the plot of the A1–A2 versus A2–H2 or the A1–A2 versus H1–H2 (ie, input versus output) is generated, a smooth AV conduction curve results. In comparison, as suggested by Rosen and his group[21–23] and Wu,[24] a discontinuous A1–A2 versus A2–H2 or A1–A2 versus H1–H2 curve indicates the presence of dual AV nodal pathways. Hence, block in the fast pathway with conduction then occurring solely over the slow pathway, which possesses a shorter refractory period, will produce the phenomenon of a sudden increment in conduction delay. The portion of the curve before this sudden increase in conduction time defines the fast pathway conduction properties. Several variations of this behavior have subsequently been recognized. There may be overlap of the fast and slow conduction pathway curve. Moreover, AV nodal echo beats have been observed in the presence of both continuous as well as discontinuous conduction curves.[26]

Consequently, discontinuous AV nodal refractory curves are not specific for either dual intranodal or extranodal AV pathways.

FAST–SLOW ATRIOVENTRICULAR NODAL REENTRANT TACHYCARDIA

In a minority of instances, the reentrant circuit may be reversed. Under these circumstances, antegrade conduction during paroxysmal SVT occurs through the fast pathway and retrograde conduction through the slow pathway. The P waves (negative in inferior leads) usually precede the QRS complex (Figure 18.7, middle). Electrophysiologic studies are often required to confirm this variety of SVT, although management is usually similar to that of the more common slow–fast variety. In this atypical form of paroxysmal SVT, the slow pathway usually has a relatively long antegrade refractory period and the fast pathway a relatively short refractory period. This form of SVT may occur incessantly and recur with any long-short interval, such as that following most atrial premature complexes or even marked sinus arrhythmia.

SUPRAVENTRICULAR TACHYCARDIA DUE TO SINUS NODE REENTRY

Patterns of conduction and reentry in the sinus node area have been extensively studied by many investigators, as this mechanism can account for some SVTs observed in man. The P waves are usually upright in the limb leads and show no difference in contour from that of sinus-initiated atrial complexes. Clinically, the paroxysms usually show evidence of both sudden offset and onset. Experimental studies by Allessie and Bonke[27] have convincingly demonstrated a point-to-point course of activation during the whole interval between successive atrial responses, indicating a reentrant mechanism. Furthermore, several studies suggest that conduction velocity in the anterior and posterior internodal pathways is faster than that in the middle internodal pathway.[3] It had previously been demonstrated by Hahn et al[28] that a reciprocal rhythm between the atria and sinus node should be possible if the internodal conduction time between successive atrial discharges was greater than the duration of the refractoriness of any element in the circuit. As noted, both the sinus and AV nodes have an important electrophysiologic property of slow conduction that is conducive to the genesis of reentrant arrhythmias.

INTERATRIAL REENTRY

Longitudinal dissociation of Bachmann's bundle has been identified as a mechanism of SVT.[29,30] This phenomenon is characterized by fragmentation of Bachmann's bundle electrograms and is associated with a concomitant reentry within this region. Bachmann's bundle reentry may mimic sinus or AV nodal reentry if the P-wave configuration and the right atrial activation sequence of "high-to-low" or "low-to-high" are the only criteria considered.[30] Therefore, the exact mechanism of this arrhythmia would not be identified unless electrograms were obtained from the region of Bachmann's bundle.

SUPRAVENTRICULAR TACHYCARDIA ASSOCIATED WITH CONCEALED BYPASS TRACTS

A variation of the Wolff–Parkinson–White reentry tachycardia is noted in instances of concealed retrograde conduction (Figure 18.7, lower diagram). Typically, the rate is 140 to 240 beats per minute, and the rhythm is regular, starts abruptly after a premature beat, and terminates suddenly. Tachycardias associated with a concealed retrogradely conducting bypass tract represent the second most commonly seen form of SVT. In these individuals, the accessory pathway will conduct only in a retrograde fashion; consequently, evidence of a delta wave (indicating preexcitation), usually associated with the Wolff–Parkinson–White syndrome, is not observed. Premature ventricular systole may be conducted retrogradely through the accessory pathway but block retrogradely in the AV node. The impulse then returns to the ventricle through the normal AV conduction pathway (orthodromically) and demonstrates a narrow QRS complex. Because retrograde atrial activation proceeds from atrial insertion of the bypass tract, localization of the earliest site of retrograde atrial activation will suggest the possible site of the bypass tract. In patients with retrogradely functioning free wall AV bypass tracts, the atria are activated eccentrically during SVT or ventricular pacing. However, in patients with retrogradely functioning septal bypass tracts, the pattern of retrograde atrial excitation may appear normal.

PAROXYSMAL ATRIAL TACHYCARDIA WITH ATRIOVENTRICULAR BLOCK (PAT WITH BLOCK)

Although this condition was first described in 1909 by Lewis[31] using polygraphic records, the first electrocardiographic studies were reported by Koplik[32] in 1917. Lown et al[33,34] brought this rhythm disturbance into sharp focus with pertinent observations of the association of so-called PAT with block, digitalis intoxication, and decreased serum potassium levels. However, the name *PAT with block* is somewhat of a misnomer, as the rhythm is uncommonly paroxysmal in onset or offset. The so-called PAT with block characteristically shows gradual acceleration of the atrial rate, which at times results in subtle deformities of the P waves. As the rhythm accelerates, various conduction delays may be observed, in part related to digitalis effects on the AV node, until fixed or variable AV block is maintained (Figure 18.8).

In general, PAT with block is relatively uncommon now that digitalis toxicity is less prevalent. Nonparoxysmal AV junctional tachycardia is an associated arrhythmia, also frequently resulting from excess digitalis or low potassium levels or both.[35] However, not all of these arrhythmias are associated with digitalis excess. They can also be observed in the presence of coronary artery disease or acute cor pulmonale as well as with other drugs such as quinidine. PAT with block has occasionally been associated with advanced rheumatic heart disease and may even be a more serious manifestation of atrial disease than atrial fibrillation itself. Obviously, prompt diagnosis of this arrhythmia is mandatory with respect to therapeutic

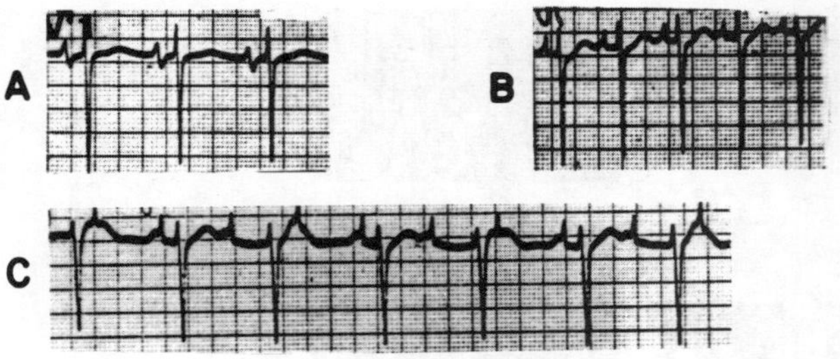

Figure 18.8. Lead V_1. *A*, Sinus rhythm with evidence of biatrial hypertrophy. *B*, Shift of the pacemaker with acceleration of the atrial rate to 120 beats per minute. *C*, Atrial tachycardia with block showing periods of Wenckebach atrioventricular conduction.

implications, particularly in the presence of digitalis excess and lower serum potassium levels. Caution must be exercised in repleting potassium, because AV nodal block may become more acute. A high mortality associated with digitalis arrhythmias has been clearly identified.[35]

Because digitalis and low potassium levels are the most frequently cited causes of this tachycardia, it has been assumed that it is an automatic atrial mechanism. The onset and offset of PAT with block are usually more gradual than sudden, suggesting a gradual shift of the pacemaker focus, although a circus or reentry mechanism cannot be ruled out. Experimental studies have clearly shown that digitalis, especially in the presence of low potassium levels, causes enhanced phase 4 depolarization, which could lead to abnormally enhanced automaticity within certain groups of the atrial fibers. Alternatively, digitalis excess also facilitates so-called oscillatory afterdepolarizations reaching threshold, leading to "triggered" automatic tachyarrhythmias. Diseased tissue may be most susceptible to these arrhythmias.

MULTIFOCAL ATRIAL TACHYCARDIA (CHAOTIC ATRIAL TACHYCARDIA)

Multifocal atrial tachycardia is often associated with various degrees of AV conduction ratios (Figure 18.9). However, these rhythms are closely associated with advanced pulmonary disease, hypoxemia, respiratory acidosis, cardiac decompensation, metabolic derangements, hypokalemia, old age, and general debilitation. Multifocal atrial tachycardia can be diagnosed when there are frequent atrial premature systoles of different contour often occurring in runs and showing marked variations in the PP interval. The P waves differ markedly in character and frequency of discharge (Figure 18.9). Varying degrees of AV conduction block are invariably present. Notably, this form of atrial tachycardia is extremely resistant to conventional doses of digitalis and conversely appears to be aggravated by excessive digitalis or lowered serum potassium levels.

Management of this arrhythmia primarily resides with improvement in pulmonary hygiene. Correction of acid-base balance and pulmonary gas exchange is mandatory. The effects of verapamil either to suppress atrial arrhythmias or to decrease AV nodal conduction are relatively unknown in this situation, and propranolol is usually contraindicated because of the underlying pulmonary disease. However, quinidine or procainamide has occasionally controlled this variety of atrial tachycardia, and intravenous procainamide occasionally results in dramatic improvement.

WOLFF–PARKINSON–WHITE PREEXCITATION SYNDROMES

The Wolff–Parkinson–White (WPW) syndrome was first described as a symptom complex in 1930 by Wolff, Parkinson, and White[36] as abnormally short PR intervals in the presence of a sinus rhythm and a wide QRS complex showing a characteristic delta wave that is usually present.[36–38] These individuals have a tendency to develop paroxysmal SVTs or what is known as WPW tachycardias, which can occur in both healthy as well as diseased hearts. Recently the mechanism of sudden death has been associated with this syndrome in the presence of a short refractory period within the bypass fibers between the atria and ventricles if atrial fibrillation should ensue[39,40] (Figure 18.10). Drugs such as digitalis and verapamil may enhance conduction through the bypass tract, because

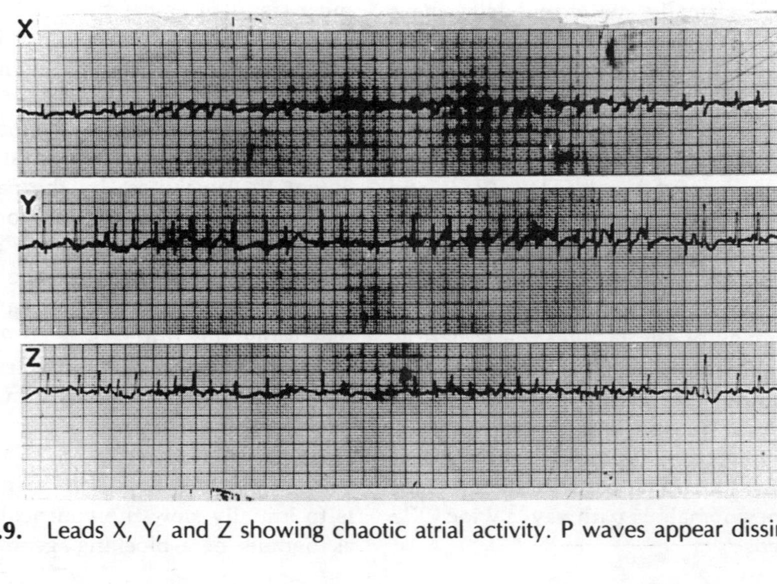

Figure 18.9. Leads X, Y, and Z showing chaotic atrial activity. P waves appear dissimilar in contour.

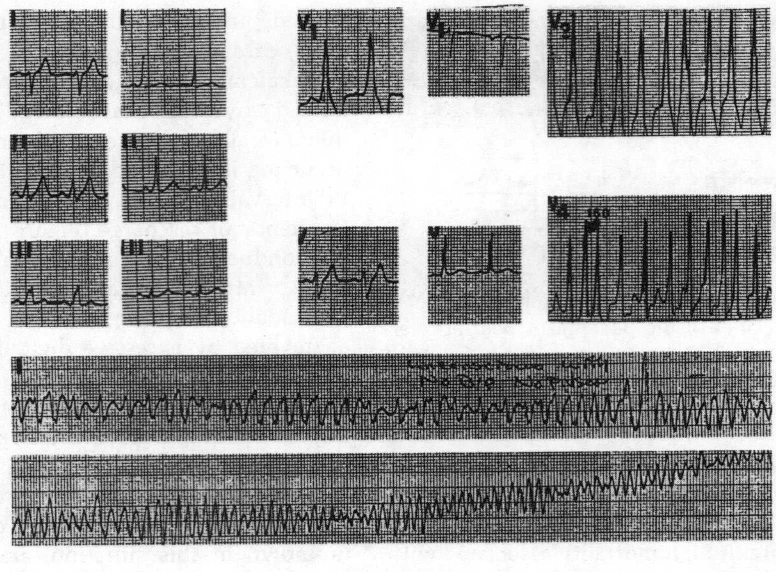

Figure 18.10. Wolff–Parkinson–White configuration. Leads I, II, III, and V_1 demonstrate right axis deviation in the left column, with a normal axis in the right column. Delta waves are seen with both configurations representing at least two bypass tracts. Leads V_2 and V_4 show atrial fibrillation with wide QRS tachycardia with the shortest RR interval representing the refractory period of the bypass tract at 160 ms. Lead II, *lower strip,* shows onset of ventricular fibrillation.

concealed retrograde conduction is limited by these agents.

A typical WPW pattern is produced when an accessory pathway is located usually apart from the normal AV conduction system such as the bundle of Kent. If an atrial impulse is transmitted through the bundle of Kent, early activation of the localized area of the ventricle will produce a delta wave. The remaining ventricle muscle, however, will be depolarized by excitation waves spreading through the normal intraventricular His-Purkinje conduction system after sustaining the usual physiologic delay within the AV junctional tissues. Hence, the characteristic ventricular WPW complex represents a fusion beat and the PJ interval: the interval from the beginning of the P wave to the end of the QRS complex is said to be within 0.2 second in most instances except in certain cases of Mahaim fibers. Ventricular excitation is initiated earlier but terminated normally, with the delta wave solely responsible for the QRS widening. The characteristics of WPW include (1) a PR interval less than 0.12 second, during sinus rhythm; (2) delta wave inscribed at the initial portion of the QRS complex (However, in the presence of posterior septal fibers and Q waves, a delta wave equivalent can be observed in leads II, III, F, and Y.); (3) secondary ST-T–wave changes.

The WPW syndrome is suggested when SVT is associated with the WPW type of QRS configuration. The AV node will serve as one link of the AV reentrant tachycardia; the QRS complex of the tachycardia is narrow if retrograde conduction from the ventricles to the atria occurs through the anomalous pathway (Kent bundle) and antegrade conduction through the AV junction and His bundle. Conversely, if retrograde conduction proceeds through the His and AV junctional tissues and antegrade conduction through the anomalous pathway, a wide QRS tachycardia is observed.

ATRIAL FLUTTER

CLINICAL FEATURES

Atrial flutter is a relatively infrequent atrial arrhythmia that may be observed as either an established or a paroxysmal or transient condition. Rarely is the mechanism chronic in nature and either sinus rhythm is reestablished or atrial fibrillation ensues. Children have been observed to maintain atrial flutter for relatively long periods and reestablishment of sinus arrhythmia usually occurs irrespective of therapy.

Atrial flutter is usually observed with moderately advanced or severe grades of myocardial involvement in patients in the middle and older age groups. Rarely is it observed in normal hearts. Almost any type of trauma, surgical procedure, or active pericardial–myocardial process may be associated with atrial flutter. However, the most frequent association is that with acute myocardial infarction, possibly because of involvement of the atria as well as the ventricles. Rarely is digitalis a cause of atrial flutter.

The symptoms and signs depend mainly on the degree of heart damage, ventricular rate, duration, and to some extent the awareness by the patient of the irregular or rapid rhythm. The most common ventricular rate in atrial flutter is 140 to 150 beats per minute due to a 2:1 AV conduction ratio. However, the use of certain type I antiarrhythmic agents such as quinidine or procainamide may slow the flutter rate to 200 to 230, and 1:1 AV conduction may ensue with acceleration of the ventricular rate. This is especially true in patients who have not previously had digitalis before the initiation of type I antiarrhythmic therapy.

The objective or goal in management of atrial flutter is to initially slow the ventricular rate using drugs such as digitalis, beta-blocking agents, or verapamil. Reversion

:o sinus rhythm can then be achieved with type I antiarrhythmic agents such as quinidine, procainamide, or disopyramide. Rarely is amiodarone necessary to maintain ventricular rates or convert atrial flutter to sinus rhythm. Precordial shock may be necessary in patients demonstrating marked deterioration in cardiac hemodynamics. The etiology of flutter should be immediately reversed, such as electrolyte and metabolic derangements, congestive heart failure, and hemodynamic improvement in the presence of acute myocardial infarction or postoperative open heart surgery.

ELECTROCARDIOGRAPHIC FEATURES

Atrial flutter is usually characterized by sawtooth undulations in the baseline with a rapid atrial rate usually of 300 cycles per minute, a narrow QRS complex, and a ventricular rate of 150 beats per minute due to 2:1 AV conduction ratios (Figure 18.11). Varying conduction ratios such as 3:1, 4:1, or 2:1 alternating with 4:1 give grouped beating and pseudobigeminy (Figure 18.11). Typical sawtooth undulations in the baseline may not be evident particularly in 2:1 conduction ratios, and a wide QRS tachycardia can be confused with ventricular tachycardia (Figure 18.12). However, slight variation in cycle length caused by various degrees of penetration into the AV junction affecting the subsequent FR interval will reveal the true nature of the supraventricular arrhythmia (Figure 18.12).

Following the use of drugs such as digitalis, verapamil, or beta-blocking agents, higher degrees of AV conduction delay are seen. Carotid sinus pressure or other vagal maneuvers frequently will reveal the presence of flutter waves and increase the AV conduction ratio. Occasionally, atrial flutter has been terminated by entrainment of the atrial rate with atrial pacing, or burst pacing may convert flutter to atrial fibrillation with subsequent reversion to sinus rhythm.

ATRIAL FIBRILLATION

CLINICAL FEATURES

Because atrial fibrillation is an extremely common cardiac arrhythmia and is attended with varying ventricular rates, symptoms closely parallel the resulting ventricular rate. The presence of atrial fibrillation usually implies the presence of myocardial or pericardial disease that is most frequently associated with enlargement of the left atrium as seen on echocardiographic studies. Although atrial fibrillation may be paroxysmal, it is usually a chronic stable rhythm and may be the final solution to the so-called sick sinus syndrome when sinus node function becomes extremely slow or nonexistent. Patients usually complain of severe palpitations and weakness in the presence of intermittent atrial fibrillation and may become extremely symptomatic by the constant shifting of cardiac rhythms from sinus to atrial fibrillation. Occasionally intrinsic AV conduction delay may be present and ventricular rates may be in the physiologic range in the absence of drugs that will slow AV conduction such as digitalis, beta blockers, or verapamil. Atrial fibrillation is associated with many forms of heart disease, the most frequent being arteriosclerotic, hypertensive, or rheumatic. Paroxysmal atrial fibrillation may occur because of extreme vagal stimulation such as severe diarrhea or vomiting or in the presence of the so-called "holiday heart" caused by excessive alcohol ingestion. In the presence of untreated atrial fibrillation, the ventricular rates may be quite rapid (160 to 180 per minute) with the sudden onset of hypotension or pulmonary edema. Patients with a large left atrium may be subject to pulmonary or systemic embolization and therefore may require long-term anticoagulant therapy. However, precordial shock is rarely required to terminate atrial fibrillation. Attempts to convert atrial fibrillation to sinus rhythm in the presence of either longstanding atrial fibrillation or a large left atrium are usually unsuccessful.

ELECTROCARDIOGRAPHIC FEATURES

Course undulations are usually seen replacing the baseline and distinct P waves are absent. Rapid irregular atrial activity with cycle lengths of 400 to 800 cycles per minute with a normal QRS duration are usually observed. The ventricular rate in the presence of untreated atrial fibrillation is usually between 150 and 220 beats per minute. The ventricular response is usually grossly irregular unless AV dissociation is present caused by AV conduction block with the ventricles being controlled by an accelerated junctional pacemaker that in itself may show varying

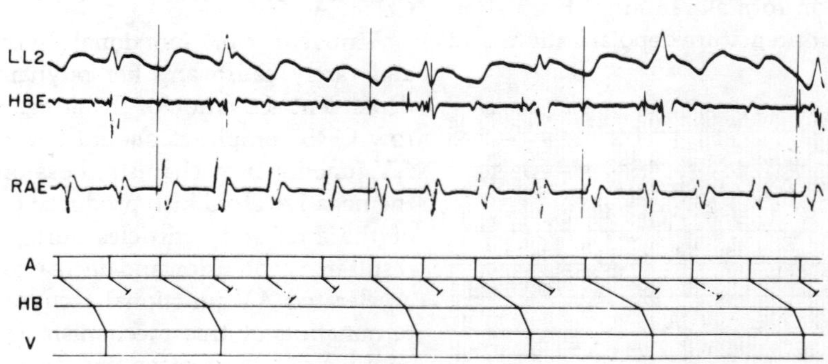

Figure 18.11. Atrial flutter with 2:1 conduction alternating with 4:1 conduction and one period of 3:1 conduction. Note that conduction block occurs above the His bundle, as His bundle complexes are not seen except before each conducted beat. A = atrial activation; HB = His bundle activation; HBE = His bundle electrogram; RAE = right atrial electrogram; V = ventricular activation.

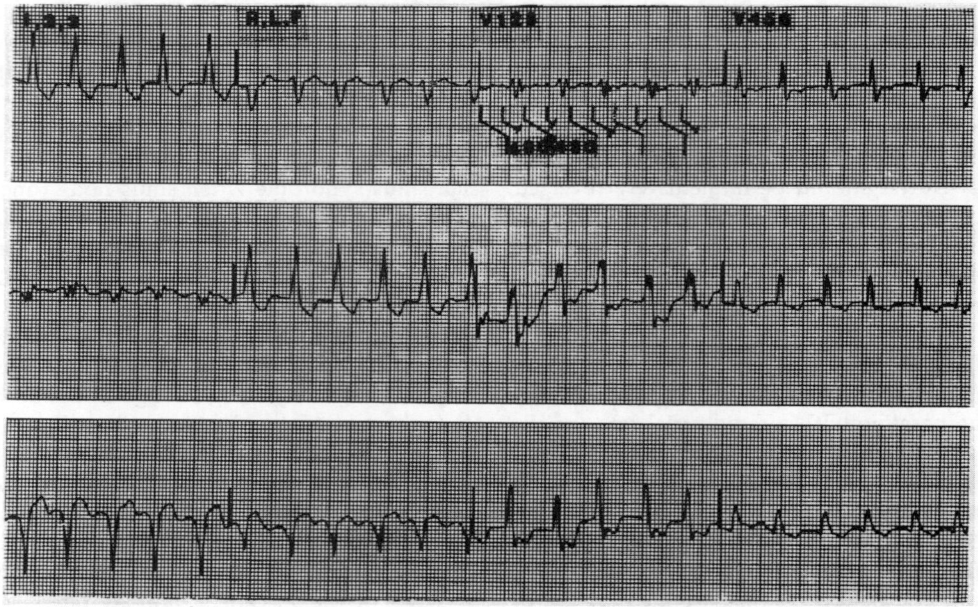

Figure 18.12. Atrial flutter with wide QRS tachycardia present with left axis deviation and inferior infarction. Note there is alternation of RR cycle lengths, 480 versus 430 ms. Deeper penetration of the nonconducted F wave into the atrioventricular (AV) junction produces a prolonged AV conduction time which increases the RR interval to 480 ms. Lack of concealed conduction into the AV junction allows the next conducted F wave to occur without delay and gives a shorter RR interval of 430 ms. Alternation in cycle lengths suggests concealed conduction of supraventricular beats.

conduction ratios to the ventricles and produce grouped beating and an irregular ventricular response.[41,42] It is now known that asynchronous activation of the two principal inputs to the AV node (crista terminalis and interatrial septum) may result in fragmented asynchronous conduction, producing various degrees of concealment of the impulses within the AV node that produces the irregularity of the ventricular rate.[43] Coexisting AV junctional rhythms should be suspected when the RR intervals become regular in a major number of cycle lengths. Digitalis excess is usually responsible for regularization of cycle lengths or the appearance of escape junctional beats due to high-grade AV conduction block. Following the use of digitalis, verapamil, or a beta-blocking agent alone or in combination, the ventricular rate usually slows.

An important distinction to make in atrial fibrillation is that between ventricular premature depolarizations and aberrant ventricular conduction of the supraventricular impulses (Figure 18.13).[44] The wide QRS beats usually follow a short cycle length which was preceded by a longer cycle length. Compensatory pauses are usually not seen because there is no possibility for concealed retrograde conduction from the ventricles into the AV junction to inhibit subsequent atrial impulses in an antegrade direction. These complexes usually have a configuration of right bundle branch block with RSR′ or multiphasic R′ configurations.

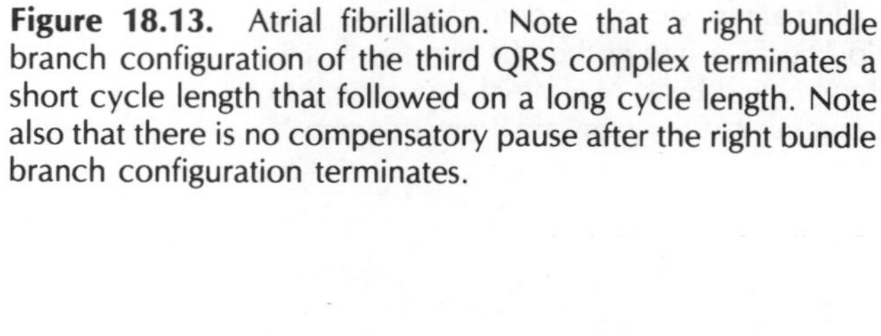

Figure 18.13. Atrial fibrillation. Note that a right bundle branch configuration of the third QRS complex terminates a short cycle length that followed on a long cycle length. Note also that there is no compensatory pause after the right bundle branch configuration terminates.

ATRIOVENTRICULAR JUNCTIONAL ARRHYTHMIAS

CLINICAL FEATURES

Atrioventricular junctional rhythms are usually benign and rarely cause any hemodynamic derangements. Independent activation of the atria and ventricles with narrow QRS complexes should suggest the presence of an AV junctional mechanism. Loss of atrial contribution or the negative atrial kick produced by retrograde activation of the atria and ventricles during the ST segment may result in hypotension and decreased cardiac output. When accelerated AV junctional tachycardia is diagnosed, the termination of this mechanism is necessary, as further administration of offending agents such as digitalis or continuation of hypokalemia may result in more serious cardiac arrhythmias and death. Because the subsidiary rate of the AV junctional pacemaker is usually between 40 and 60 beats per minute, junctional rhythms demonstrating more rapid rates or accelerated junctional mechanisms may result from electrolyte imbalance, ischemia, or excessive drugs such as digitalis.

ELECTROCARDIOGRAPHIC FEATURES

Except for the previously described AV junctional reentrant tachycardias, which have been more recently classified under the supraventricular arrhythmias because the AV node as well as the perinodal fibers are involved in the reentry mechanism, enhanced impulse formation within the AV junctional tissues is rather uncommon.[45] The AV junction is usually defined as part of the specialized conducting system from the so-called approaches to the AV node or the junction between the lower right atrium and the AV node to the bifurcation of the His bundle. Despite its small anatomic dimensions, the AV junction is composed of several different fiber types with dissimilar action potential configurations and conductivity.[45–49] The conduction velocity within the N region of the AV node is extremely slow and is composed of specialized fibers with slow channel properties. The proximal portion above the N region or AN region behaves similarly to the atrial specialized myocardium and the distal or NH region closely resembles that of His bundle activity. Experimental studies showed that enhanced impulse formation can occur within the NH region, particularly in the region of the tricuspid valve.[49] Impulse formation within the AN region has also been observed, whereas enhanced impulse formation within the N region itself is still somewhat undecided, although diastolic depolarization of these fibers has been observed in small experimental preparations of AV nodal tissue. The electrocardiographic characteristics of AV junctional impulses most often represent a QRS configuration of the dominant supraventricular beats. Occasionally, aberrant conduction from impulse formation within the AV node will result in wide QRS complexes as well. Premature narrow QRS complexes can be associated with retrograde P waves either with a short PR interval before the QRS complex, within the QRS complex, or following the QRS complex depending on the relative timing of retrograde conduction to the atrium versus forward conduction to the ventricles. The most common type of junctional beat occurs as an AV junctional escape mechanism (Figure 18.14). These subsidiary pacemakers are frequently seen in patients with normal hearts and may result when automaticity in the sinus node is depressed by excessive vagal stimulation or other mechanisms that will slow the sinus impulse formation. Rescuing AV junctional pacemakers are usually seen in the presence of AV block (Figure 18.15A). Classification of AV junctional impulse formation is shown in Table 18.3. Rarely, concealed AV junctional or His bundle depolarizations may be concealed within the AV junctional tissues but are manifest by failure to conduct subsequent sinus beats to the ventricle, giving the appearance of a type II second degree AV block (pseudo type II AV block). Atrioventricular junctional rhythms may or may not result in AV dissociation (Figure 18.15A and B). Careful analysis of the electrocardiogram to assure linkage between the QRS and P wave is necessary for diagnosis. Exit block, either retrograde or antegrade, can cause irregular atrial or ventricular rates. Rarely AV junctional parasystole can be observed.

ATRIOVENTRICULAR BLOCK

CLINICAL FEATURES

Type I AV block may either be congenital or result from drugs such as digitalis, beta blockers, some calcium blockers, or particularly in the presence of acute inferior wall myocardial infarction. The subsidiary or escape rhythms are usually physiologic in the range of 40 to 60 per minute, and in the presence of an acute process, such as inferior infarction or excessive drugs, pacemakers may not be required (Figure 18.15A). In contrast, type II block is a more sinister type of AV conduction disorder and in more than 95% of cases results in severe symptoms and may culminate in death. Immediate insertion of cardiac pacemakers, both temporary and permanent, is mandatory under these circumstances. In the presence of bifascicular block, usually right bundle branch block plus left anterior hemiblock or left posterior hemiblock associated with acute myocardial infarction, temporary pacemakers, and, if second or third degree block has occurred during the course of the infarction, permanent pacemakers may be required. Patients may experience lightheadedness, dizziness, or frank syncope or drop attacks in the presence of either type of AV heart block. Rarely is it necessary to perform electrophysiologic studies, because type I AV block is usually associated with narrow QRS complexes and type II block with wide QRS complexes. Consequently, clinical decisions can usually be made from the surface electrocardiogram. Furthermore, many signs of AV block are demonstrated at the bedside. First degree AV block is usually associated with a rather soft first heart sound, whereas in type I second degree AV block a quickening of the pulse may be associated with a gradually diminishing first heart sound and a decrease in systolic blood pressure as the PR interval increases. Type I block is usually transitory after acute inferior wall myocardial infarction and rarely requires a temporary or permanent cardiac pacemaker. However, severe hemodynamic consequences can follow long periods of gradual prolongation of the PR interval with the P wave falling within the ST segment of the previous QRS complex.

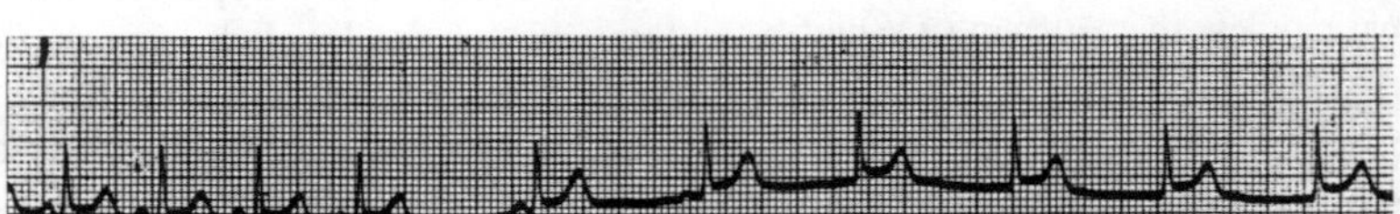

Figure 18.14. A sinus rhythm is present with sinus arrhythmia, and atrioventricular junctional escape beats are seen to the right of the strip, which is a common physiologic phenomenon.

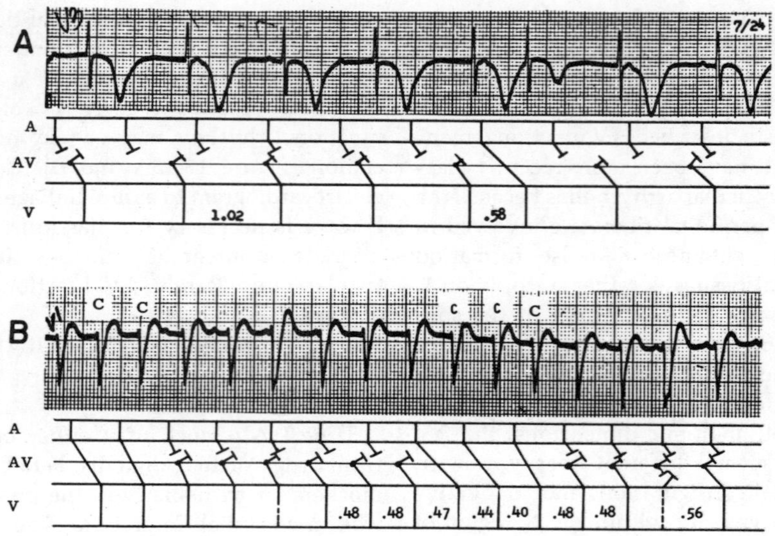

Figure 18.15. Atrioventricular (AV) junctional rhythm. *A,* Atrioventricular junctional escape rhythm with one ventricular capture beat terminating a 0.58 second RR interval. Failure of conduction is mainly due to block. *B,* An accelerated AV junctional rhythm with a cycle length of 470 to 480 ms. Note shorter RR intervals 440 and 400 ms representing ventricular capture.

Invariably these patients require both temporary and occasionally AV sequential pacing. In contrast, type II AV block with wide QRS complexes is invariably associated with syncope, lightheadedness, or congestive failure and almost always requires permanent cardiac pacing. In the presence of acute myocardial infarction with right bundle branch block alone or with left anterior hemiblock, a temporary pacemaker is mandatory. If second degree or higher degrees of block persist, a permanent pacemaker is required.

ELECTROCARDIOGRAPHIC FEATURES

It is customary to divide AV block into first, second, and third degree according to the severity of the conduction disturbance. First degree AV block represents prolongation of AV conduction time (PR interval and the electrocardiogram) beyond the normal range of 0.22 second. However, prolongation of AV conduction may result from a conduction delay within the atria, the AV node,

Table 18.3. Classification of Atrioventricular Junctional Impulse Formation

Intermittent manifestation of atrioventricular (AV) junctional impulse formation
1. Atrioventricular junctional escape beats
2. Atrioventricular junctional premature systoles
   a. Coupled extrasystoles
   b. Parasystole
3. Paroxysmal AV junctional tachycardia

Persistent manifestation of AV junctional impulse formation
1. Atrioventricular junctional rate less than 70/min (AV junctional rhythm)
   a. With dependent activation of atria and ventricles
   b. With independent activation of atria and ventricles
2. Atrioventricular junctional rate greater than 70/min (nonparoxysmal AV junctional tachycardia)
   a. With dependent activation of atria and ventricles
   b. With independent activation of atria and ventricles

or the His-Purkinje system or any combination of the sinus AV transmission system.[50–54] Second degree AV block is diagnosed when some of the impulses originating in either the sinus node or atria die out in certain portions of the AV conduction system and fail to reach the ventricles, whereas third degree AV block represents a condition in which impulse transmission from the atria to the ventricles is almost or entirely blocked and the ventricles are controlled by a subsidiary pacemaker or cardiac arrest occurs. In addition to this classification, second degree block has been further subdivided into two types by the sequence PR intervals in conducted supraventricular beats. This classification is based on the original observations of Wenckebach[1] and Mobitz[55,56] and can simply be stated as follows: When AV conduction times in several successive beats are progressively prolonged, culminating in the dropping out of one ventricular depolarization, type I is diagnosed (Figure 18.16), whereas sudden failure of AV conduction after maintenance of a consistent or constant PR interval is designated as type II (Figure 18.17). It is then understood that this classification can be applied only when more than two sinus or supraventricular impulses are consecutively conducted to the ventricles in the presence of second degree AV block and is not applicable in the presence of third degree block. Recent studies suggest that the clinical course and prognosis as well as the therapy for AV block may depend predominantly on localization of the conduction disturbance within the AV conduction system. Hence, it has become increasingly apparent that AV block should be classified by the level of propagation failure rather than by the consistency or fluctuations of the PR interval.

Unless there is additional subjunctional conduction delay in one or more of the fascicles of the Purkinje system, type I AV block usually occurs within the AV node itself. The QRS complexes are usually narrow and do not exceed 0.11 second in duration (Figure 18.16). In contrast, type

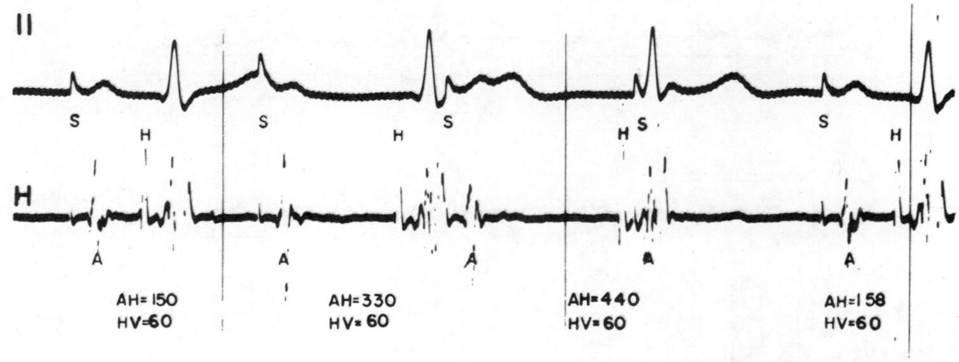

Figure 18.16. Type I atrioventricular block. Increasing AH intervals from 150 to 440 ms before the fourth atrial electrogram and the fourth P wave is not conducted to the ventricles. The HV interval remains constant at 60 ms.

II AV block is invariably associated with wide QRS complexes (0.12 second or greater) and sudden dropping out of the QRS complex without warning or a progressive increase in the PR interval (less than 80 ms) suggests a subjunctional conduction abnormality (Figure 18.17). Several levels of block may coexist and differential diagnoses may be impossible without intracardiac electrode recordings (Figure 18.18). Occasionally, sudden dropping out of the QRS complex without an increase in the PR interval can be associated with narrow QRS complexes. Invariably, the level of block is within His (intra-Hisian block). This type of block is extremely rare and can be diagnosed only with intracardiac recordings, but it has a rather similar significance to type II AV block.

In complete or third degree AV heart block, the level of block may be found either within the AV node or in the subjunctional portion of the His-Purkinje system. When the QRS complexes of the escape rhythm are narrow, block occurs usually in the more proximal portions of the AV node; when the QRS complexes are wide, subjunctional block with escape rhythms within the Purkinje system are usually present.

VENTRICULAR ARRHYTHMIAS

CLINICAL FEATURES

In recent years the detection and management of ventricular arrhythmias have been paramount to preventing cardiovascular catastrophies and sudden death. Ventricular premature systoles are extremely common and are found in almost all segments of the population.[57,58] Consequently, early descriptions of ventricular ectopic beats were given both a benign as well as a malignant prognosis.[59] Patients frequently complain of palpitations, thumping in the chest, or merely pauses. Patients frequently will become terrorized by the presence of an irregular heartbeat when ventricular premature beats are persistent in the bigeminal fashion, and when associated with an inadequate stroke volume, dizziness or syncope. However, most patients with ventricular premature systoles are totally unaware of their presence and emphasis by the physician in the absence of heart disease is discouraged. Most often, however, they are benign and may accompany a variety of cardiovascular problems such as mitral valve prolapse, subaortic stenosis, valvular heart disease, and ischemic cardiomyopathy. Trigger mechanisms may include tobacco, caffeine, alcohol, and especially fatigue.[60]

In the absence of underlying cardiovascular disease the presence of ventricular premature systole usually has no significance and antiarrhythmic drugs clearly are not indicated for cosmetic reasons. Furthermore, it has not been shown that antiarrhythmic therapy given to suppress premature systoles has any clinical merit.[61] In general, the frequency of ventricular premature systole increases with age, and sporadic ventricular premature beats in persons with a normal heart do not seem to be associated with an increased risk or unfavorable prognosis. Conversely,

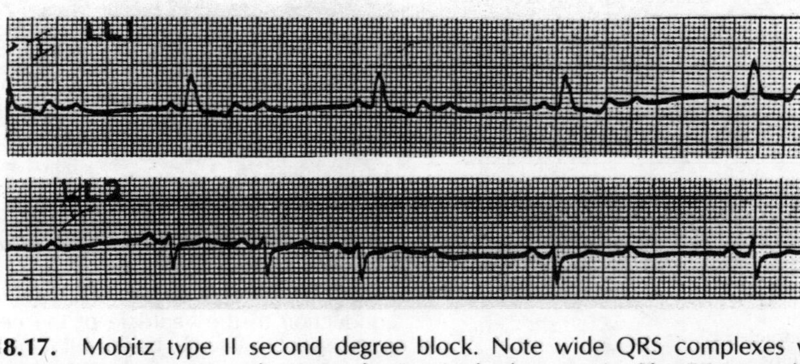

Figure 18.17. Mobitz type II second degree block. Note wide QRS complexes with 2:1 conduction in the upper strip and 4:3 conduction in the lower strip. The PR interval remains constant throughout.

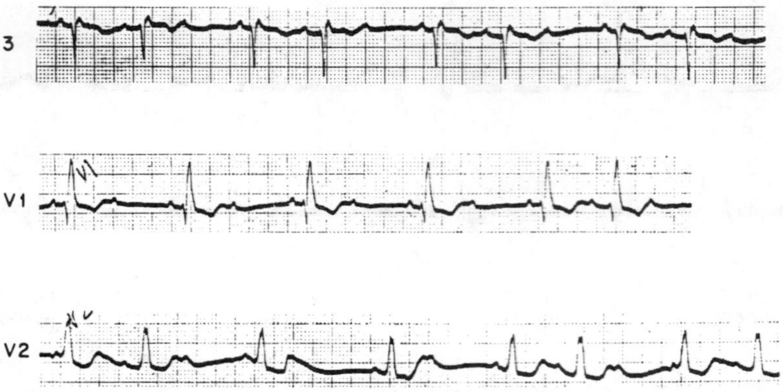

Figure 18.18. Wide QRS complex showing right bundle branch block and right axis deviation, suggesting block in the right bundle branch and left anterior fascicle. In addition, the PR interval gradually increases, suggesting a Wenckebach or type I conduction block in the atrioventricular (AV) node. This represents two levels of AV conduction block.

patients with ischemic heart disease or dilated cardiomyopathies may represent subsets of individuals who are at high risk of sudden death. It has now been recognized that an ejection fraction less than 40% represents an individual risk factor of subsequent cardiac death.[62] In some patients with valvular heart disease and idiopathic subaortic stenosis the incidence of sudden death associated with ventricular arrhythmias is significant.[63] It is now recognized that patients with complex ventricular premature systoles greater than 5 to 10 per minute and multiform or those with sustained or nonsustained ventricular tachycardia as well as the R on T phenomenon associated with cardiac disease are at an exceptionally high risk for cardiac death.[64] Classification of ventricular arrhythmias is usually made according to Lown and Graboys[64] (Table 18.4).

ELECTROCARDIOGRAPHIC FEATURES

Ventricular premature beats are characterized by QRS complexes that are premature, wide, and often bizarre in appearance. Usually the ST segment and T waves are opposite in direction to the main QRS vector forces. P waves, unless coincident, do not precede the QRS complex, although they may be seen to be inscribed retrogradely after the appearance of the ventricular premature systole. The ventricular premature systole may appear anywhere from the end of the refractory period, which is usually coincident with the midportion of the T wave, to the next dominant beat. Ventricular premature systole is usually followed by a pause, especially with retrograde conduction to the atria, which causes the sinus node to be reset and permits time for development of rhythm. Attempted retrograde conduction of the ventricular premature systole may cause the next sinus impulse to be blocked within the AV junction and may also produce a pause (Figure 18.19). Various periods of return of the sinus cycle may be produced by either sinus node reset or collision of the retrograde impulse within the atria or AV junction. Parasystolic ventricular arrhythmia can be detected when the premature ventricular systole is not fixed or related to the dominant rhythm, and it appears that the site of impulse formation within the ventricles or Purkinje system is protected by the dominant rhythm of the heart, so that depolarization of the pacemaker site remains undisturbed (Figure 18.20). Fusion beats are invariably a sign of ventricular ectopic beating. When ventricular premature systole appears at the time of the sinus or dominant QRS complex, various degrees of depolarization of the ventricles by the ectopic ventricular impulse

Table 18.4. Characteristics of Ventricular Premature Beats (VPBs) (Lown Classification)

Grade	Description
0	No ventricular beats
1A	Occasional, isolated VPBs (<30/hour, <1/minute)
1B	Occasional, isolated VPBs (<30/hour, periods of 2 or more per minute)
2	Frequent VPBs (>30/hour)
3	Multiform VPBs
4A	Repetitive VPBs couplets
4B	Repetitive VPBs salvos
5	Early VPBs (ie, abutting or interrupting the T wave)

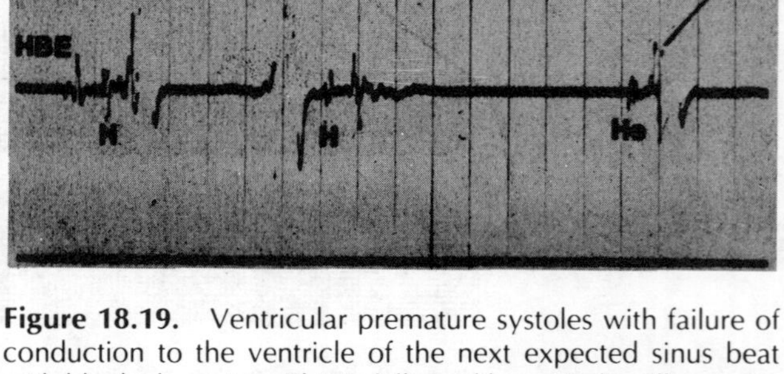

Figure 18.19. Ventricular premature systoles with failure of conduction to the ventricle of the next expected sinus beat with block above His. This is followed by a His bundle escape beat. HRA = high right atrium; HBE = His bundle electrogram; H = His bundle activity.

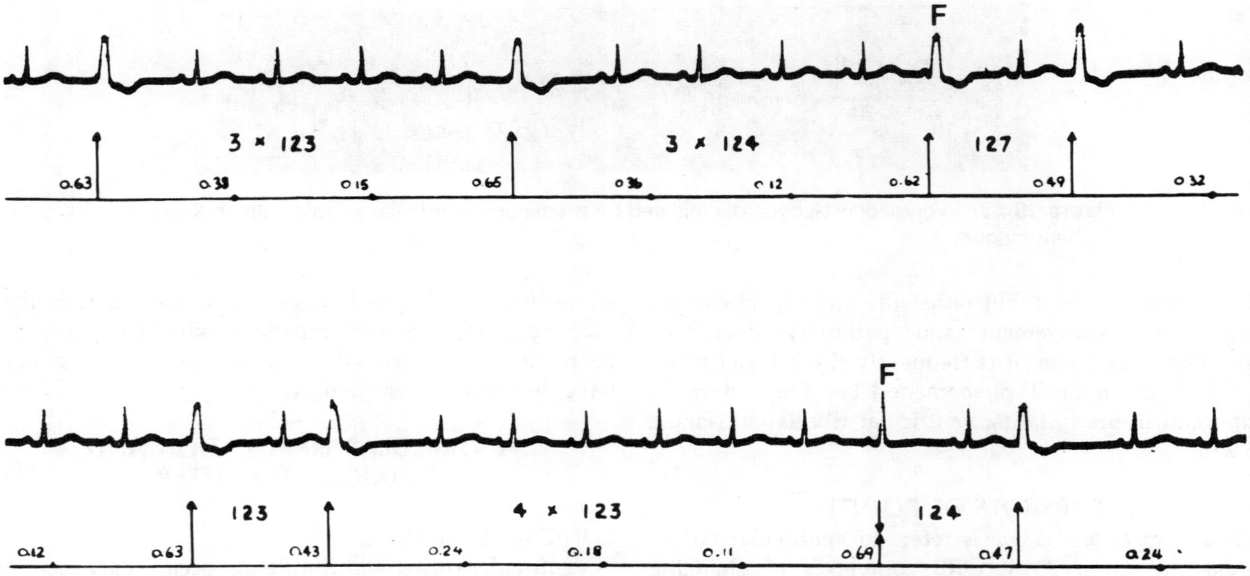

Figure 18.20. Ventricular parasystole and fusion beats (F). Coupling intervals are shown in the line below the electrocardiogram. Appearance of a ventricular ectopic beat occurs only after the refractory period of the ventricle which in this instance measures approximately 430 ms.

and that of the dominant rhythm may occur (Figure 18.20F). Because premature ventricular systoles usually occur earlier in the sinus cycle, fusion complexes are quite uncommon.

VENTRICULAR TACHYCARDIA

Although the normal rate of automatic impulse formation in the Purkinje or ventricular fibers has generally been accepted to be less than 40 beats per minute, the rates of ventricular tachycardia frequently exceed 150 beats per minute. Cycle lengths as short as 180 to 200 ms can frequently be seen. Ventricular tachycardia may be sustained or nonsustained depending on the duration of the tachycardia. Tachycardia lasting more than 15 to 30 seconds is termed *sustained ventricular tachycardia*. Ventricular tachycardia complexes usually show a discordant configuration with a similar contour of QRS in leads V_1 to V_6. More "ugly" tachycardias, which are pleomorphic or multiform, frequently degenerate into ventricular fibrillation. Ventricular tachycardia occasionally may show alternation of QRS complexes, suggesting bidirectional ventricular tachycardia. The electrocardiographic distinction between supraventricular tachycardia with aberration and ventricular tachycardia may at times be impossible without intracardiac leads. However, the presence of fusion beats or capture beats or both may provide evidence for the ventricular origin of the tachycardia. Independent activation of atria and ventricles or retrograde conduction of P waves does not always clearly differentiate ventricular tachycardia from junctional tachycardia. However, AV dissociation during a wide QRS tachycardia is presumptive evidence of the ventricular origin of the mechanism. Left axis deviation is frequently observed in the frontal plane. The QRS complex suggesting a right bundle branch block configuration is usually monophasic or biphasic as opposed to R′ or R′R″ waves in lead V_1 or triphasic configuration. Ventricular tachycardia must be distinguished from supraventricular tachycardia with a wide QRS duration such as can occur with aberrantly conducted supraventricular tachycardia and WPW tachycardia where the impulse travels retrogradely through the AV node and enters the ventricle through an extranodal bypass tract.

Electrophysiologic studies may be necessary to precisely diagnose wide QRS tachycardia (Figure 18.21). Short or negative HV intervals, when present, have been termed bundle branch reentry mechanisms. His bundle deflections are usually not apparent because they are obscured by simultaneous ventricular depolarization. Initiation of ventricular tachycardia by programmed stimulation showing the same contour as the spontaneous beats usually confirms the diagnosis. In acute myocardial ischemia, it is not the coupling interval of ventricular extra-

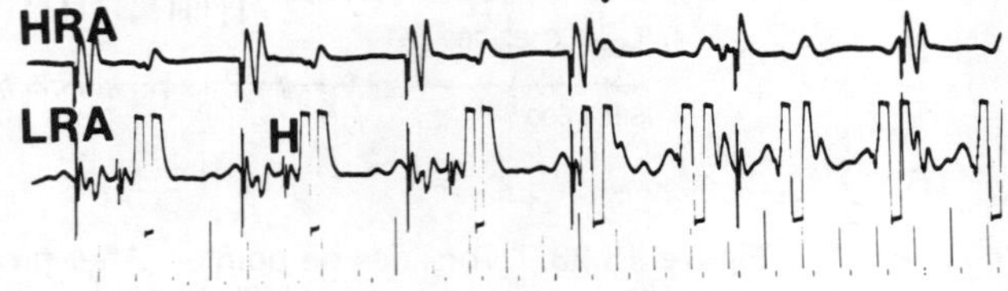

Figure 18.21. Electrophysiologic study. Onset of ventricular tachycardia following atrial pacing (S1S1 = 430 ms). H = His bundle electrogram; HRA = high right atrium; LRA = low right atrium.

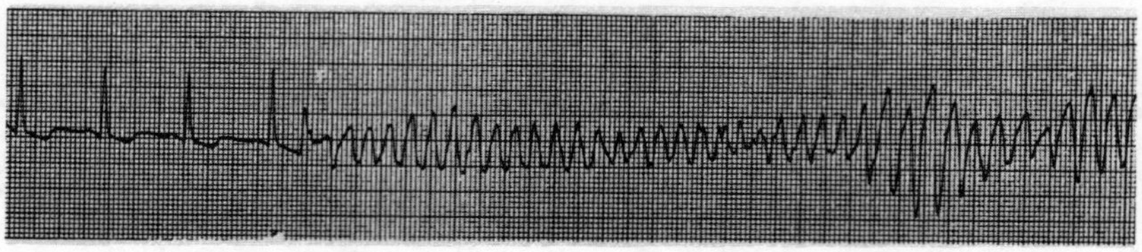

Figure 18.22. Ventricular tachycardia initiated by premature ventricular systole with an R on T phenomenon.

systole that is critical, but rather the underlying electrophysiologic derangement and pathophysiologic arrhythmia mechanism. It is frequently the delayed phase in which the R on T phenomenon becomes extremely important in precipitating ventricular fibrillation (Figure 18.22).

TORSADES DE POINTES

The term *torsades de pointes* refers to ventricular tachycardia characterized by QRS complexes of changing amplitude that appear to twist around the isoelectric line.[65–73] The rates are rather rapid and the QRS complexes quite pleomorphic in character (Figure 18.23). Torsades de pointes frequently occurs in the setting of the long QT interval and may be precipitated by factors that prolong the QT interval such as hypokalemia, type I antiarrhythmic drugs, and bradycardia. This dysrhythmia is frequently initiated by a premature ventricular depolarization occurring late in diastole and associated with a prolonged TU wave. Commonly, spontaneous termination occurs. This rhythm occasionally may degenerate into ventricular fibrillation.[74] The most significant pathophysiologic features of various forms of ventricular tachycardia are not their morphologic features as such but rather their primary association with delayed repolarization, because the initiation of ventricular tachycardia in the setting of a prolonged QT interval has critical implications for therapy. Conversely, polymorphous ventricular tachycardia may be associated with a long QT interval as well. However, the QT interval may be within normal limits and these arrhythmias may respond favorably to type I antiarrhythmic drugs. However, the administration of type I drugs or any agent that further prolongs the QT interval in patients with classic torsades de pointes associated with delayed repolarization may have disastrous consequences.[74,75]

VENTRICULAR FIBRILLATION AND VENTRICULAR FLUTTER

CLINICAL FEATURES

Ventricular flutter and fibrillation occur in a variety of cardiovascular diseases most often associated with acute coronary insufficiency and ischemia. They may result from electrolyte imbalance, hypoxia, or type I antiarrhythmic drugs. Patients who have been resuscitated from sudden death may not show evidence of coronary artery disease.[75–78] Furthermore, individuals who do not show myocardial necrosis even in the presence of coronary artery disease remain at high risk for subsequent ventricular fibrillation. These patients require electrophysiologic studies with the administration of appropriate antiarrhythmic drugs.[77]

ELECTROCARDIOGRAPHIC FEATURES

Except for artifact, no electrocardiographic arrhythmia mimics that of ventricular flutter or fibrillation. These rhythms usually terminate fatally within two to seven minutes unless precordial shock is promptly delivered (Figure 18.22). Ventricular flutter resembles a sine wave, although it can be pleomorphic as well. Frequencies of 152 to 350 per minute are usually observed. Both immediate and delayed onset of ventricular fibrillation has been observed in the animal model. On occlusion of the

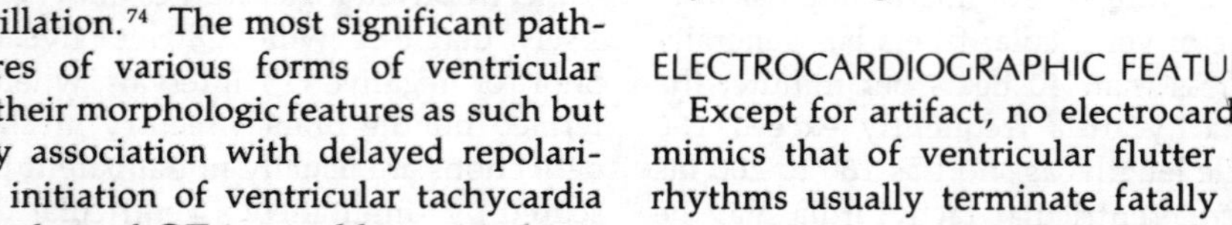

Figure 18.23. Torsades de pointes. After programmed stimulation with an S1S2 of 600 ms, a premature ventricular systole S1S2 is placed at 260 ms. Note the pleomorphic configuration of the ventricular tachycardia which in lead I initially shows inverted complexes followed by upright complexes and then again inverted complexes. In lead V_1, initially upright complexes are followed by inverted complexes and then by upright complexes. This occurred after procainamide 700 mg intravenously, which appeared to aggravate the ventricular tachycardia.

main coronary artery the flurry of ectopic ventricular activity may last between 3 and 12 minutes.[79-82] This is followed by a quiescent period of ten minutes, and a late or delayed flurry of ventricular arrhythmias may culminate in ventricular fibrillation. If reperfusion occurs within 20 to 30 minutes of occlusion, the sudden onset of ventricular fibrillation may follow without any warning arrhythmias. Ventricular fibrillation begins in the border zone between the ischemic and normal myocardium, spreading through the Purkinje system from epicardium to endocardium and finally disorganizing the entire electrical structure of the heart.[79-82]

REFERENCES

1. Wenckebach KF: Beitrage zur Kenntnis der menschlichen Herztatig-keit. *Arch Anat Physiol* 1906; 297:297–354.
2. Ferrer MI: The sick sinus syndrome. *Circulation* 1973; 47:635–641.
3. Satake S, Bianchi J, Dreifus LS, Watanabe Y, Michelson EL: Tachycardia and apparent sinoatrial block due to concealed sinus node reentry. *PACE* 1983; 6:229–237.
4. Dreifus LS, Michelson EL, Kaplinsky E: Bradyarrhythmias: clinical significance and management. *J Am Coll Cardiol* 1983; 1:327–338.
5. Breithardt G, Seipel L: Comparative study of two methods of estimating sinoatrial conduction time in man. *Am J Cardiol* 1978; 42:965–972.
6. Mandel W, Hayakawa H, Danzig R, Marcus HS: Evaluation of sinoatrial node function in man by overdrive suppression. *Circulation* 1971; 44:59–66.
7. Mandel WJ, Hayakawa H, Allen HN, Danzig R, Kermaier AI: Assessment of sinus node function in patients with the sick sinus syndrome. *Circulation* 1972; 46:761–769.
8. Mandel WJ, Laks MM, Obayashi K: Sinus node function; evaluation in patients with and without sinus node disease. *Arch Intern Med* 1975; 135:388–394.
9. Rosen KM, Loeb HS, Sinno MZ, Rahimtoola SH, Gunnar R: Cardiac conduction in patients with symptomatic sinus node disease. *Circulation* 1971; 43:836–844.
10. Strauss HC, Bigger JT Jr, Saroff AL, Giardina EGV: Electrophysiologic evaluation of sinus node function in patients with sinus node dysfunction. *Circulation* 1976; 53:763–776.
11. Dhingra RC, Amat-y-Leon F, Wyndham C, Denes P, Wu D, Miller RH, Rosen KM: Electrophysiologic effects of atropine on sinus node and atrium in patients with sinus nodal dysfunction. *Am J Cardiol* 1976; 38:429–434.
12. Holden W, McAnulty JH, Rahimtoola SH: Characterization of heart rate response to exercise in the sick sinus syndrome. *Br Heart J* 1978; 40:923–930.
13. Jordan J, Yamaguchi I, Mandel WJ: Studies on the mechanism of sinus node dysfunction in the sick sinus syndrome. *Circulation* 1978; 57:217–223.
14. Narula OS, Samet P, Javier RP: Significance of the sinus-node recovery time. *Circulation* 1972; 45:140–158.
15. Kulbertus HE, Leval-Rutten F, Mary L, Casters P: Sinus node recovery time in the elderly. *Br Heart J* 1975; 37:420–425.
16. Breithardt G, Seipel L, Loogen F: Sinus node recovery time and calculated sinoatrial conduction time in normal subjects and patients with sinus node dysfunction. *Circulation* 1977; 56:43–50.
17. Narula OS, Shantha N, Vasquez M, Towne WD, Linhart JW: A new method for measurement of sinoatrial conduction time. *Circulation* 1978; 58:706–714.
18. Moe GK, Preston JB, Burlington H: Physiologic evidence for a dual A-V transmission system. *Circ Res* 1956; 4:357–375.
19. Mendez C, Moe GK: Demonstration of dual A-V nodal conduction system in the isolated rabbit heart. *Circ Res* 1956; 19:378–387.
20. Rosen KM, Metha A, Miller RA: Demonstration of dual atrioventricular nodal pathways in man. *Am J Cardiol* 1974; 33:291–294.
21. Denes P, Wu D, Dhingra RC, Chuquimia R, Rosen KM: Demonstration of dual A-V nodal pathway in patients with paroxysmal supraventricular tachycardia. *Circulation* 1973; 48:549–555.
22. Wu D, Denes P, Dhingra RC, Khan A, Rosen KM: Effect of propranolol on induction of A-V nodal reentrant tachycardia. *Circulation* 1974; 50:665–677.
23. Denes P, Wu D, Dhingra R, Amat-y-Leon F, Wyndham C, Rosen KM: Dual A-V nodal pathways. A common electrophysiologic response. *Br Heart J* 1975; 37:1069–1076.
24. Wu D: Dual atrioventricular nodal pathways: a reappraisal. *PACE* 1982; 5:72–89.
25. Mazgalev T, Dreifus LS, Bianchi J, Michelson EL: The mechanism of AV junctional reentry: role of the atrioventricular junction. *Anat Rec* 1981; 201:179–188.
26. Iinuma H, Dreifus LS, Mazgalev T, Price R, Michelson EL: Role of the perinodal region in atrioventricular reentry: evidence in an isolated rabbit heart preparation. *J Am Coll Cardiol* 1983; 2:465–473.
27. Allessie MA, Bonke FIM: Direct demonstration of sinus node reentry in the rabbit heart. *Circ Res* 1979; 44:557–568.
28. Hahn J, Malozzi AM, Moe GK: Sinoatrial reciprocation in the isolated rabbit heart. *Circ Res* 1968; 22:355–365.
29. Ogawa S, Dreifus LS, Osmick MJ: Longitudinal dissociation of Bachmann's bundle as a mechanism of paroxysmal supraventricular tachycardia. *Am J Cardiol* 1977; 40:915–922.
30. Ogawa S, Dreifus LS, Kitchen JG, Shenoy PN, Osmick MJ: Catheter recording of Bachmann's bundle activation from the right pulmonary artery: a new technique for atrial mapping and the study of supraventricular tachycardia. *Am J Cardiol* 1978; 41:1089–1096.
31. Lewis T: Paroxysmal tachycardia. *Heart* 1909; 1:42–45.
32. Koplik H: Paroxysmal tachycardia in children. *Am J Med Sci* 1917; 154:834–851.
33. Lown B, Marcus JF, Levine H: Digitalis and atrial tachycardias with block; a year's experience. *N Engl J Med* 1959; 260:301–309.
34. Lown B, Wyatt NF, Levine H: Paroxysmal atrial tachycardia with block. *Circulation* 1960; 21:129–143.
35. Dreifus LS, Katz M, Watanabe Y, Likoff W: Clinical significance of disorders of impulse formation and conduction in the atrioventricular junction. *Am J Cardiol* 1963; 11:384–391.
36. Wolff L, Parkinson J, White P: Bundle branch block with short PR interval in healthy young people prone to paroxysmal tachycardia. *Am Heart J* 1930; 5:685–704.
37. Katz LN, Pick A: *Clinical Electrocardiography. Part I. The Arrhythmias.* Philadelphia, Lea & Febiger, 1956, p 679.
38. Ferrer MI: New concepts relating to the preexcitation syndrome. *JAMA* 1967; 201:1038–1039.
39. Dreifus LS, Haiat R, Watanabe Y, Arriaga J, Reitman N: Ventricular fibrillation: a possible mechanism of sudden death in patients with Wolff–Parkinson–White syndrome. *Circulation* 1971; 43:520–527.
40. Dreifus LS, Wellens HJJ, Watanabe Y, Kimbiris D, Truex R: Sinus bradycardia and atrial fibrillation associated with the Wolff–Parkinson–White syndrome. *Am J Cardiol* 1976; 38:149–156.
41. Bellet S: *Clinical Disorders of the Heart Beat.* Philadelphia, Lea & Febiger, 1963, p 133.
42. Friedberg CK: *Diseases of the Heart.* Philadelphia, WB Saunders, 1966, p 526.
43. Mazgalev T, Dreifus LS, Bianchi J, Michelson EL: Atrioventricular nodal conduction during atrial fibrillation in rabbit heart. *Am J Physiol* 1982; 243:H754–760.
44. Gouaux JL, Ashman R: Auricular fibrillation with aberration simulating ventricular paroxysmal tachycardia. *Am Heart J* 1947; 34:366–373.
45. Watanabe Y, Dreifus LS (eds): *Cardiac Arrhythmias. Electrophysiological Basis for Clinical Interpretation.* New York, Grune & Stratton, 1977, p 78.
46. Paes de Carvalho A, de Mello WC, Hoffman BF (eds): *The Specialized Tissues of the Heart.* Amsterdam, Elsevier, 1961, p 115.
47. Truex RC: Anatomical considerations of the human atrioventricular junction, in Dreifus LS, Likoff W (eds): *Mechanisms and Therapy of Cardiac Arrhythmias.* New York, Grune & Stratton, 1966, p 333.
48. Watanabe Y, Dreifus LS: Factors controlling impulse transmission with special reference to A-V conduction. *Am Heart J* 1975; 89:790–803.
49. Watanabe Y, Dreifus LS: Sites of impulse formation within the atrioventricular junction of the rabbit. *Circ Res* 1968; 22:717–727.
50. Watanabe Y, Dreifus LS: Electrophysiologic effects of digitalis on A-V transmission. *Am J Physiol* 1966; 211:1461–1466.
51. Watanabe Y, Dreifus LS: Interactions of quinidine and potassium on atrioventricular transmission. *Circ Res* 1967; 20:434–436.
52. Watanabe Y, Dreifus LS: Interactions of lanatoside C and potassium on atrioventricular conduction in rabbits. *Circ Res* 1970; 27:931–940.
53. Watanabe Y, Dreifus LS: Levels of concealment in second degree and advanced second degree AV block. *Am Heart J* 1972; 84:330–347.
54. Mazgalev T, Dreifus LS, Iinuma H, Michelson EL: Effects of the site and timing of atrioventricular conduction in the isolated perfused heart. *Circulation* 1984; 70:748–759.
55. Mobitz W: Uber die unvollstandige Storung der Erregungsuberleitung zwischen Vorhof und Kammer des menschlichen Herzens. *Z Ges Exp Med* 1924; 41:180–237.
56. Mobitz W: Uber den partiellen Herzblock. *Z Klin Med* 1928; 107:449–462.
57. Hinkle LE, Carver ST, Argyros DC: The prognostic significance of premature contractions in healthy people with coronary heart disease. *Acta Cardiol* 1974; 43:5–32.
58. Brodsky M, Wu D, Denes P, Kanakis C, Rosen KM: Arrhythmias documented by 24 hour continuous electrocardiographic monitoring in 50 male medical students, without apparent heart disease. *Am J Cardiol* 1977; 39:390–395.
59. Kostis JB, McCrone K, Moryea AE, Gotzoyannis S, Aglitz NM, Natarajan

N, Kuo PT: Premature ventricular complexes in the absence of identifiable heart disease. *Circulation* 1981; 63:1351–1356.

60. Dreifus LS, Watanabe Y: Tension drugs and premature systoles. *Am Heart J* 1965; 70:292–294.
61. Dreifus LS, Morganroth J: Antiarrhythmic agents, in Dreifus LS, Brest AN (eds): *Clinical Applications of Cardiovascular Drugs.* The Hague, Martinus Nijhoff, 1980, pp 1–45.
62. Bigger JT Jr, Fleiss JL, Kleiger R, Miller P, Rolnitzky LM, and the Multicenter Post-Infarction Research Group: The relationships among ventricular arrhythmias, left ventricular dysfunction and mortality in the 2 years after myocardial infarction. *Circulation* 1984; 69:250–258.
63. Kowey PR, Eisenberg R, Engel TR: Sustained arrhythmias in hypertrophic obstructive cardiomyopathy. *N Engl J Med* 1984; 310:1566–1569.
64. Lown B, Graboys TB: Ventricular premature beats and sudden cardiac death. *Baylor College of Medicine Cardiology Series* 1980; 3(1):6–24.
65. Dessertenne F: La tachycardie ventriculaire à deux foyers opposés variables. *Arch Mal Coeur* 1966; 59:263–272.
66. Krikler DM, Curry PVL: Torsade de pointes, an atypical ventricular tachycardia. *Br Heart J* 1976; 38:117–120.
67. Kossmann CE: Torsade de pointes: an addition to the nosography of ventricular tachycardia. *Am J Cardiol* 1978; 42:1054–1056.
68. Smith WM, Gallagher JJ: "Les torsades de pointes": an unusual ventricular arrhythmia. *Ann Intern Med* 1980; 93:578–584.
69. Cokkinos DV, Mallios C, Phillias N, Vorides EM: "Torsades de pointe": a distinct entity of ventricular arrhythmia? *Acta Cardiologica* 1978; 33:167–184.
70. Sclarovsky S, Strasberg B, Lewin RF, Agmun J: Polymorphous ventricular tachycardia: clinical features and treatment. *Am J Cardiol* 1979; 44:339–344.
71. Horowitz LN, Greenspan AM, Spielman SR, Josephson ME: Torsades de pointes: electrophysiologic studies in patients without transient pharmacologic or metabolic abnormalities. *Circulation* 1981; 63:1120–1128.
72. Zilcher H, Glogar D, Kaindl F: Torsade de pointes: occurrence in myocardial ischemia as a separate entity. Multiform ventricular tachycardia or not? *Eur Heart J* 1980; 1:63–69.
73. Fontaine G, Frank R, Grosgogeat Y: Torsades de pointes: definition and management. *Mod Concepts Cardiovasc Dis* 1982; 51:103–108.
74. Soffer J, Dreifus LS, Michelson EL: Polymorphous ventricular tachycardia associated with normal and long Q-T intervals. *Am J Cardiol* 1982; 49:2021–2029.
75. Ruskin JN, McGovern B, Garan H, DiMarco JP, Kelly E: Antiarrhythmic drugs: a possible cause of out-of-hospital cardiac arrest. *N Engl J Med* 1983; 309:1302–1306.
76. Eisenberg MS, Hallstrom AP, Copass MK, Bergner L, Short F, Pierce J: Treatment of ventricular fibrillation. *JAMA* 1984; 251:1723–1726.
77. Swerdlow CD, Winkle RA, Mason JW: Determinants of survival in patients with ventricular tachyarrhythmias. *N Engl J Med* 1983; 308:1436–1442.
78. Lesch M, Kehoe RF: Predictability of sudden cardiac death. *N Engl J Med* 1984; 310:255–257.
79. Kaplinsky E, Ogawa S, Balke W, Dreifus LS: Role of endocardial activation in malignant ventricular arrhythmias associated with acute ischemia. *J Electrocardiol* 1979; 12:299–306.
80. Naito M, Michelson EL, Kaplinsky E, Dreifus LS, David D, Blenko TM: Role of early cycle ventricular extrasystoles in initiation of ventricular tachycardia and fibrillation: evaluation of the R on T phenomenon during acute ischemia in a canine model. *Am J Cardiol* 1982; 49:317–322.
81. Kaplinsky E, Ogawa S, Michelson EL, Dreifus LS: Instantaneous and delayed ventricular arrhythmias after reperfusion of acutely ischemic myocardium: evidence for multiple mechanisms. *Circulation* 1981; 63:333–340.
82. Kaplinsky E, Ogawa S, Balke WC, Dreifus LS: Two periods of early ventricular arrhythmia in the canine acute myocardial infarction model. *Circulation* 1979; 60:397–403.

19 Electrophysiologic Diagnosis of Cardiac Arrhythmias

Delon Wu, MD, FACC

The atrioventricular (AV) conducting system consists of several heterogeneous tissues with different functional properties. These involve the sinus node, atria, AV node, His-Purkinje system, and ventricles. Normal cardiac impulse is generated in the sinus node and spreads from the atria to the ventricles in an orderly fashion. The functional integrity of the whole conducting system is essential for normal cardiac rhythm. Generation and transmission of impulse are not directly visualized from the surface electrocardiogram, which depicts the P wave, the PR interval, and the QRS complex. The P wave reflects the activation of the atria; the PR interval, the conduction time from the atria to the ventricles; and the QRS complex, the activation of the ventricles. Abnormalities in impulse formation and transmission are usually implied from the surface electrocardiogram. However, the surface electrocardiogram alone is usually not sufficient to reveal the site or mechanism of abnormalities, or both. Using the recordings of intracardiac electrograms, as well as incremental and premature atrial and ventricular stimulating techniques, a great deal of information can be obtained. This chapter discusses the value and limitation of invasive electrophysiologic testing in the diagnosis of cardiac arrhythmias.

RECORDING AND STIMULATING TECHNIQUES

Recordings of intracardiac electrograms usually require two or more multipolar electrocatheters, depending on the study purpose. A tripolar or quadripolar catheter is percutaneously introduced into the femoral vein, advanced to the right atrium, and placed across the tricuspid valve for recording of the His bundle electrogram.[1–3] A second multipolar catheter is introduced either into an antecubital vein or a femoral vein and advanced to the high right atrium at the junction of the superior vena cava and the right atrium. This catheter is used for right atrial pacing as well as recording of the high right atrial electrogram. When necessary, a third catheter may be placed in the coronary sinus for recording of the left atrial electrogram, and a fourth or even a fifth catheter may be placed in various sites of the right or left ventricle for recordings of local ventricular electrogram or pacing. Multiple surface and intracardiac electrograms are simultaneously displayed and recorded on an oscilloscopic photographic recorder at paper speed of faster than 100 mm per second and with a filter setting between 30 and 500 Hz. The stimulus impulses are usually 2 ms in duration and twice the diastolic threshold. A resting His bundle electrogram is recorded, which depicts an atrial response (A), a His bundle response (H), and a ventricular response (V). In conjunction with the surface electrocardiogram, the PR interval can be subdivided into three subintervals: PA, reflecting conduction time from high to low right atrium; AH, reflecting AV nodal conduction time; and HV, reflecting conduction time in the His bundle and bundle branches (Figure 19.1). These intervals are invisible on the surface electrocardiogram. The normal values of basic intervals are given in Table 19.1.[4–7]

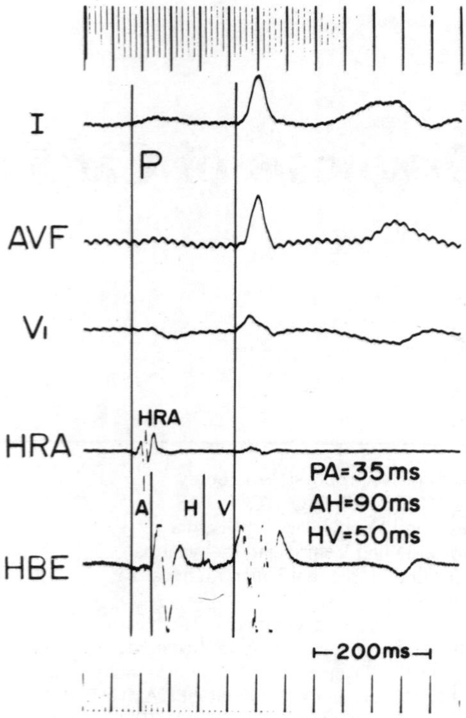

Figure 19.1. Intracardiac recordings. Shown are electrocardiographic leads I, aVF, V_1, bipolar high right atrial electrogram (HRA), and His bundle electrogram (HBE). P = P wave; HRA = high right atrial depolarization; A = low septal right atrial depolarization; H = His bundle depolarization; V = ventricular depolarization. The PA interval is measured from the onset of the P wave to the first rapid deflection of A; the AH interval is measured from the first rapid deflection of A to the first high-frequency component of H; HV is measured from the first high-frequency component of H to the earliest initial deflection of the QRS complex on the surface electrocardiogram.

The antegrade and retrograde properties of the AV conducting system are then evaluated with incremental and extrastimulus pacing techniques.[8-13] The atrium or the ventricle is paced initially at a rate slightly faster than the sinus rate. The pacing rate is then increased progressively to a rate that induced second degree AV or ventriculoatrial (VA) block or higher rates. The extrastimulus testing is performed with an atrial or a ventricular extrastimulus (S_2) coupled to a sinus, an atrial, or a ventricular paced beat (S_1). The coupling interval (S_1–S_2) is progressively shortened until S_2 fails to capture the atrium or the ventricle. A second (S_3) or a third (S_4) extrastimulus may be delivered when necessary. With this technique, both the functional and the effective refractory periods of the AV conducting system can be measured.[8-10] The functional refractory period (FRP) of a tissue is the shortest attainable interval between two impulses, the basic and the premature, traversing that tissue and is measured at a point distal to the tissue. The effective refractory period (ERP) of a tissue is the longest interval between two impulses, the basic and the premature, where the premature impulse fails to traverse the tissue and is measured proximal to the tissue. The normal values of the functional and effective refractory periods among various AV conducting tissues are given in Table 19.2. The functional and effective refractory periods of the atrium, the His bundle, the bundle branches, and the ventricle shorten with decreasing driven cycle length, whereas the effective refractory period of the AV node lengthens with decreasing driven cycle length. The effects of cycle length on AV nodal functional refractory period are variable.[10,14]

Table 19.1. Normal Conduction Intervals in Adults (ms)

	Intervals			
Authors	**PA**	**AH**	**HV**	**H**
Dhingra et al[5]	9–45	54–130	31–55	...
Narula et al[6]	25–60	50–120	35–45	25
Castellanos et al[7]	20–50	50–120	25–55	...

SINUS NODE DISORDERS

Sinus node dysfunction with a prolonged period of ventricular asystole is not an infrequent cause of syncope or severe dizziness. Abnormalities in sinus automaticity or sinoatrial conduction, or both, have been implied as the mechanisms responsible for prolonged asystole.[15-18] Clinically, a sinus node disorder is suggested by electrocardiographic manifestation of persistent sinus bradycardia, sinus arrest, sinoatrial exit block, and inappropriate response to carotid massage, exercise, atropine, propranolol, or isoproterenol. Supraventricular tachyarrhythmias are frequently associated with sinus node dysfunction. Under such circumstances, symptoms of syncope or severe dizziness may relate to the episode of tachyarrhythmias or the time when tachyarrhythmia converts to sinus rhythm. Because the sinus node is repetitively suppressed by the impulses of tachyarrhythmia, a prolonged period of asystole may occur at the moment of conversion.

Serial ambulatory electrocardiographic monitorings are useful in documenting severe sinus node dysfunction and relating the symptoms to the episode of bradycardia. Electrophysiologic testing is usually unnecessary; analysis of clinical data is frequently sufficient in making prognostic and therapeutic decisions in symptomatic patients with sinus node dysfunction. Implantation of a permanent pacemaker is indicated when syncope or severe dizziness is related to the episode of prolonged pauses. However, electrophysiologic testing facilitates the diagnosis of sinus node dysfunction. It can unmask latent sinus node dysfunction in patients with sinus bradycardia in whom the symptoms of syncope or severe dizziness are not clearly related to bradycardia and a decision to implant a permanent pacemaker is equivocal.

The electrophysiologic evaluation of sinus node function includes (1) measurement of sinus node recovery time,[19,20] (2) measurement of sinoatrial conduction time indirectly using extrastimulus or pacing techniques,[21,22] and (3) recording of sinus electrogram with direct analysis of sinoatrial conduction.[23,24] Sinus node recovery time is measured by applying rapid atrial pacing.[19,20,25] With this technique the atria are stimulated at a rate slightly faster than the sinus rate for 30 to 60 seconds. When atrial pacing is suddenly terminated, the sinus node recovery time is measured from the last paced atrial depolarization

Table 19.2. Normal Refractory Periods in Adults (ms)

Authors	ERP Atrium	FRP Atrium	ERP AVN	FRP AVN	ERP HPS	ERP V
Denes et al[10]	150–360	190–390	250–365	350–495	...	...
Schuilenburg[11]	...	...	230–390	330–500	...	...
Akhtar et al[12]	230–330	...	280–430	320–680	340–430	190–290

AVN = atrioventricular node; ERP = effective refractory period; FRP = functional refractory period; HPS = His-Purkinje system; V = ventricular.

to the first sinus recovery cycle. The atrial paced rate is then increased progressively to a rate of 150 beats per minute. The maximum pause from the last atrial paced beat to the first sinus returning beat during atrial pacing at increasing rates is taken as the maximum sinus node recovery time. Normally this interval is less than 1,600 ms. Because sinus node recovery time is directly related to the intrinsic sinus cycle length, many investigators corrected the sinus node recovery time by subtracting the resting sinus cycle length. The normal corrected sinus node recovery time is less than 680 ms. In subjects with normal sinus node function, the corrected sinus node recovery time increases progressively with increasing paced rate and reaches a peak at a paced rate of 130 beats per minute. In patients with sinus node dysfunction, the responses are unpredictable. The first sinus returning cycle may not be prolonged, especially at faster paced rates; unexpected pauses of subsequent sinus cycles are frequently seen.[26] These later pauses are called secondary sinus pauses and are attributed to the conduction abnormalities between the sinus node and the atrium. Although corrected sinus node recovery time corrects the individual variability of intrinsic sinus cycle length, the absolute value of the maximum pause that occurs during sudden termination of atrial pacing or the absolute value of the secondary pauses that occur thereafter may be directly related to the symptoms. Therefore, measurement of all three variables is clinically useful.

Sinoatrial conduction time can be estimated by the responses of sinus returning cycle to an atrial premature depolarization.[21,27] This technique is performed by delivering an atrial premature beat during sinus rhythm. When the premature beat is delivered at coupling intervals close to the sinus cycle length, it collides with the oncoming sinus impulse and fails to reset the sinus impulse. When the premature beat is delivered at a shorter coupling interval, it enters the sinus node and resets the sinus impulse. Therefore, the interval between the premature atrial beat and the returning sinus beat includes the entrance conduction time, the exit conduction time, and the sinus cycle length. By subtracting the sinus cycle length from the interval between the premature atrial beat and the returning sinus beat, a total sinoatrial conduction time is obtained. Assuming that entrance and exit time are equal, the sinoatrial conduction time is equal to half of the total sinoatrial conduction time. In subjects with normal sinus node function, the sinoatrial conduction time estimated indirectly by this technique is usually less than 130 ms, although some investigators have reported a value up to 156 ms. It has also been reported that an inverse relation of sinoatrial conduction time to sinus cycle length exists.[28] However, marked sinus arrhythmia usually invalidates measurement of sinoatrial conduction time, because it cannot be ascertained that the returning sinus cycle is not affected by the premature atrial beat.[29] To avoid the problems of marked sinus arrhythmia, sinoatrial conduction can also be estimated by brief periods (eight beats) of atrial pacing at a rate just above the sinus rate.[22] By subtracting the sinus cycle length from the interval between the last atrial paced beat and the first sinus returning beat, a total sinoatrial conduction time is obtained and the sinoatrial conduction time is equal to half of the total sinoatrial conduction time. The sinoatrial conduction times estimated by these two methods are quite close; however, they are not equivalent. Sinoatrial conduction time is prolonged in patients with sinus node dysfunction. Measurement of sinoatrial conduction time is very sensitive in identifying patients with sinus node dysfunction, but it is not specific in identifying patients for pacemaker implantation.[30–32]

Recordings of sinus node electrogram are frequently successful by placing a multipolar electrocatheter at the junction between the superior vena cava and the right atrium using a filter setting between 0.1 to 50 Hz.[23,24] Careful positioning of the catheter is essential; moving the catheter only a few millimeters away from the critical area usually results in disappearance of the sinus electrogram. Recordings of sinus node electrogram allow direct analysis of sinoatrial conduction as well as direct measurement of sinoatrial conduction time.

Sinoatrial conduction time directly measured from sinus electrogram correlates well with the indirectly measured sinoatrial conduction time, although the latter tends to overestimate the actual sinoatrial conduction time.[24] More importantly, recordings of sinus node electrograms allow accurate measurement of sinoatrial conduction time in patients with marked sinus arrhythmia and allow direct analysis of sinoatrial conduction.[24,33] Several recent studies have shown that sinoatrial exit block rather than suppression of sinus automaticity is responsible for the prolonged episodes of sinus pauses that occur spontaneously or on termination of rapid atrial pacing[24,34,35] (Figure 19.2). In two patients with hypersensitive carotid sinus syndrome, recordings of sinus node electrogram with application of carotid massage reveal prolongation of sinoatrial conduction, as well as slowing in the sinus rate of depolarization at the onset.[36] This is followed by the appearance of sinoatrial exit block and sinus arrest. After termination of carotid massage, sinus node potential does not precede the first atrial impulse and marked prolongation of sinoatrial conduction time with gradual recovery is noted in subsequent beats. Thus, recordings

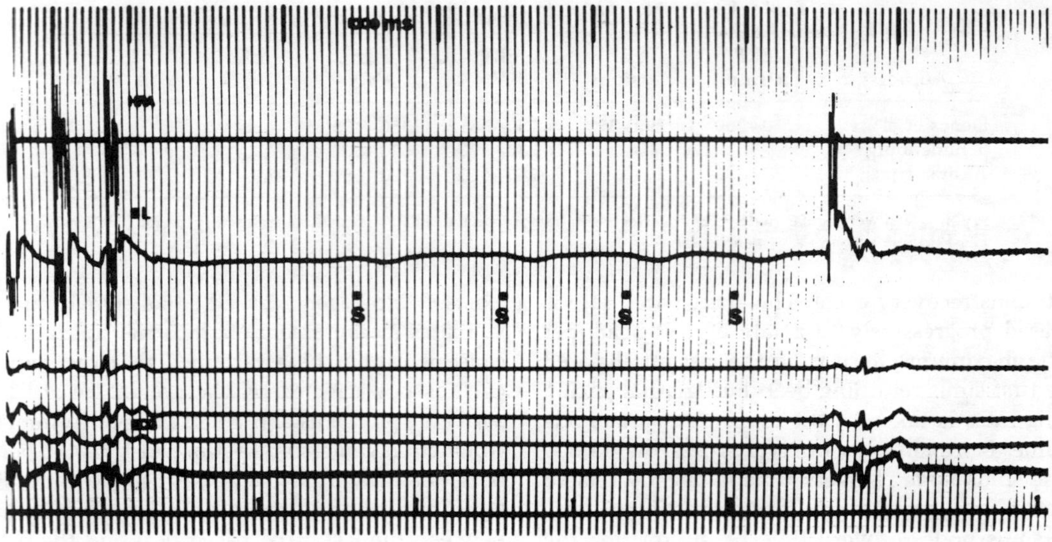

Figure 19.2. Recording of sinus electrogram showing repetitive sinoatrial exit block that occurs after sudden termination of rapid atrial pacing in a patient. From top to bottom: HRA (30 to 250 Hz), SL (sinus lead 0.5 to 30 Hz), and surface electrocardiographic leads I, II, III, and V_1. Four isolated sinus electrograms (S) are clearly seen in SL; a fifth one may be present after the end of the repolarization of the last paced beat. Time mark = 1,000 ms. (From Asseman et al,[35] by permission of the American Heart Association, Inc.)

of sinus node electrograms have contributed significantly to the electrophysiologic mechanisms of sinus node disorders.

The sinus node is under the influence of sympathetic and parasympathetic tone. Neurologic disorder may therefore cause sinus nodal dysfunction. Electrophysiologic evaluation of the sinus node after combined intravenous administration of atropine (0.04 mg/kg) and propranolol (0.2 mg/kg) may allow differentiation of sinus node dysfunction resulting from neurologic dysfunction and those due to intrinsic sinus node disease.[37-39] Evaluation of sinus node function following drug administration may also facilitate the diagnosis of latent sinus node dysfunction. It can also assess the safety of an antiarrhythmic agent when this is indicated in patients with asymptomatic sinus node dysfunction.

ATRIAL DYSRHYTHMIAS

Diagnosis of atrial dysrhythmias such as atrial fibrillation, atrial flutter, atrial tachycardia, or atrial standstill is usually made by analysis of surface electrocardiographic P waves. However, in some patients the surface electrocardiogram may not accurately reflect the underlying arrhythmias, and intracardiac recordings are required for accurate and complete diagnosis. Dissimilar atrial rhythm with fibrillation in one atrium and flutter in the other atrium or standstill in one atrium and fibrillation in the other has been described.[40] Multiple dissimilar atrial rhythm with atrial tachycardia on the surface electrocardiogram, and right atrial standstill with a rapid irregular left atrial rhythm of varying cycle lengths different from the atrial tachycardia on surface electrocardiogram have also been reported[41] (Figure 19.3). In these patients, accurate diagnosis cannot be made without electrophysiologic studies.

Overdrive atrial pacing frequently terminates atrial flutter.[42] However, at paced rates slightly faster than the flutter rate, the flutter rate can be entrained to the paced rate without changes in the morphologic characteristics of the fluttering P waves.[43] Resumption of atrial flutter occurs immediately on termination of atrial pacing. As the pacing rate approaches a critical rate, the morphologic aspects of the fluttering P wave become intermediate between the fluttering P wave and the characteristic P wave

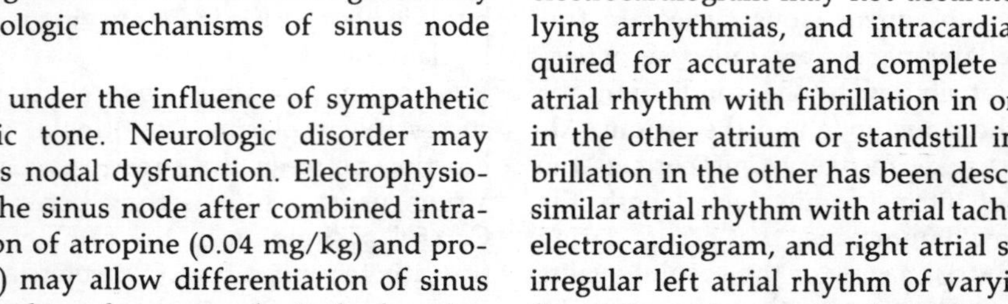

Figure 19.3. Multiple dissimilar atrial rhythm in a patient. Simultaneous recording of lead V_1, high right atrial, and coronary sinus electrograms (HRA and CSA) showing atrial tachycardia (V_1), atrial standstill (HRA), and a rapid irregular left atrial rhythm of varying cycle length (220 ± 380 ms) (CSA). (From Wu et al,[41] with permission.)

from the atrial pacing site. As the pacing rate increases further, complete atrial capture with a total change in P wave morphologic characteristics occurs; atrial flutter may be terminated on termination of pacing. Demonstration of entrainment in some patients with atrial flutter strongly suggests that reentry is the mechanism of atrial flutter in these patients.

ATRIOVENTRICULAR BLOCK

The site of block in patients with AV block is a major prognostic determinant and therapeutic indicator. In most patients, the site of block can be predicted from analysis of the surface electrocardiogram as well as the response to exercise, carotid massage, or administration of atropine. Precise localization, nevertheless, depends on His bundle recording.[6,44] In patients with first degree AV block (PR interval 0.21 second or greater), the AV node is the most common site of conduction delay; however, the delay can also occur in His bundle, bundle branches, atrium, or their combinations. In addition, the upper limit of normal conduction times in the atrium, AV node, His bundle, and bundle branches can produce PR interval prolongation. Atrioventricular nodal delay is manifested by a prolongation of the AH interval; intra-His bundle delay is manifested by split His bundle potentials; delay in the bundle branches is manifested by a prolongation of the HV interval; and intraatrial delay is manifested by a prolongation of the PA interval.[45] First degree AV block alone requires no special therapy.

Second degree AV block can be divided into three types: type I AV block, type II AV block, and high-grade AV block. Type I AV block (Wenckebach block) is characterized by a progressive prolongation of the PR interval until a P wave is blocked. Type I AV block usually reflects AV nodal block and is frequently related to an acute problem such as digitalis intoxication or acute inferior wall myocardial infarction.[46] The block is usually transient, with resumption of conduction within a few days. His bundle recording in patients with type I AV nodal block reveals a progressive lengthening of the AH interval until an atrial electrogram is not followed by a His bundle response. Type I AV block can also occur in the His bundle and bundle branch system. With block in the His bundle, the QRS complex is of normal duration or of bundle branch block pattern. His bundle recording in patients with type I His bundle block reveals split His bundle potentials into an initial H spike and a delayed H' spike with a progressive lengthening of the HH' interval until an H spike is not followed by an H' spike.[47–50] When type I block occurs in the bundle branch system, the QRS complex is of bundle branch block pattern. His bundle recording reveals a progressive lengthening of the HV interval until an H spike is not followed by a QRS complex. Type II AV block is characterized by sudden unexpected block of a P wave without prior lengthening of the PR interval. It often reflects block in the His-Purkinje system; His bundle recording reveals a sudden block distal to the His bundle recording site. High-grade AV block refers to those with 2:1, 3:1, or a higher degree of AV block. It may reflect a block in the AV node, within the His bundle, or in the bundle branch system (Figure 19.4). When the block occurs in the AV node or His bundle, the QRS complex can be of normal duration or of bundle branch block pattern. When the block occurs in the bundle branch system, the QRS complex is of bundle branch block pattern. Precise localization of the site of block requires His bundle recording. Pacemaker implantation is indicated in symptomatic patients with second degree AV block when symptoms of syncope or severe dizziness are related to the bradyarrhythmias. His bundle recording in these patients, although useful, is not crucial in decision making. In asymptomatic patients with second degree AV block, His bundle recording is essential in deciding whether or not permanent pacemaker implantation is necessary. The available data suggest that second degree AV block in the bundle branch system and possibly within the His bundle is associated with a high risk of syncope and sudden death.[47,51] Permanent pacing is justified in this group of patients.

Complete AV block may result from lesions in the AV node, His bundle, or bundle branches.[6,44,51] Complete AV block in the AV node is frequently associated with an effective escape rhythm arising from the distal AV node or His bundle and with a QRS complex of normal duration. His bundle recording reveals that none of the atrial electrograms is followed by a His bundle spike. A His bundle spike with a normal HV interval preceding each escape beat is noted when the escape rhythm arises from the junctional area. Complete His bundle block may be associated with a normal duration or wide QRS complex escape rhythm, depending on whether the subsidiary pacemaker arises from the distal His bundle or ventricles. His bundle recording reveals that each atrial electrogram is followed by a His bundle response. A His bundle spike is also preceding each escape beat when the subsidiary pacemaker arises from the distal His bundle. Complete AV block in the bundle branches is associated with a ventricular escape rhythm showing wide QRS complexes on the surface electrogram. His bundle recording reveals that each atrial electrogram is followed by a His bundle response, whereas a His bundle spike is not preceding the escape ventricular beats. Permanent pacing is unnecessary in asymptomatic patients with complete AV nodal block, although it is indicated in patients with complete His bundle block or complete block in the bundle branches. Complete AV block in both the His bundle and bundle branches is associated with a high incidence of syncope and sudden death.[49–51] His bundle recording in symptomatic patients with complete AV block is not crucial, because these patients need permanent pacing. His bundle recording is essential in a therapeutic decision in patients with asymptomatic complete AV block with either a narrow or wide QRS complex escape rhythm. A site of block in the His bundle or bundle branches suggests the need for permanent pacing.

BUNDLE BRANCH BLOCK

Electrophysiologic studies have contributed significantly to the understanding of bundle branch block. The HV interval reflects the conduction time from the His bundle recording site to the earliest ventricular activation site; prolongation of the HV interval in patients with complete right bundle branch block accompanied by either left anterior or left posterior fascicular block reflects

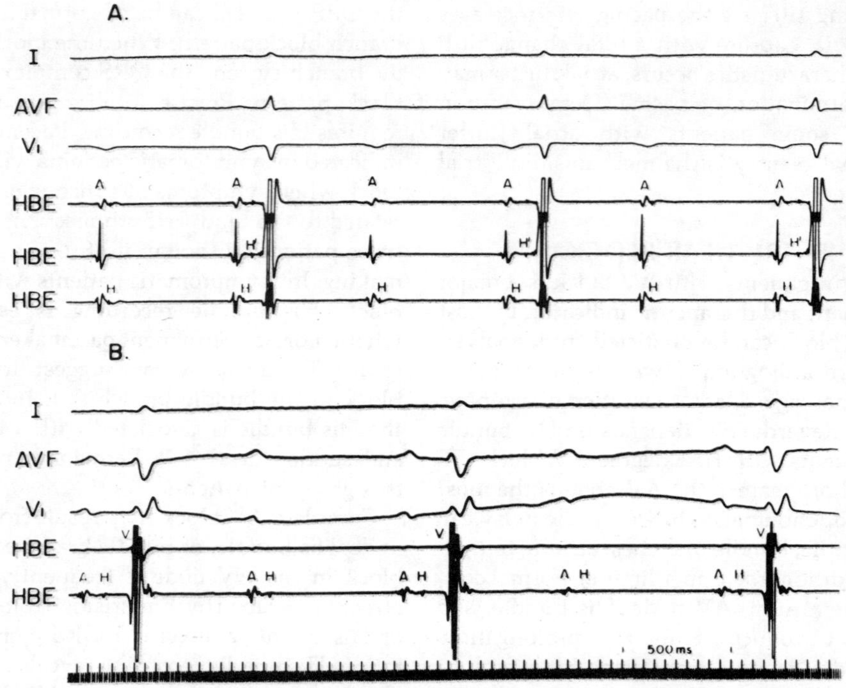

Figure 19.4. His bundle recordings in two patients. *A*, Second degree 2:1 AV block occurring within the His bundle. Three simultaneous His bundle recordings with minor difference in position are shown. Each atrial depolarization is responded with an initial His bundle deflection (H), whereas split His bundle potential with a delay deflection (H′) is seen on each conducted beat. The block occurs between H and H′, that is, within the His bundle. *B*, Second degree 2:1 block occurring distal to the His bundle recording site. The surface electrocardiogram shows complete right bundle branch block. Each atrial depolarization is followed by a His bundle response, whereas a 2:1 block distal to the His bundle recording site is seen. As complete right bundle branch block is present on the surface electrocardiogram, the site of 2:1 block is located in the left bundle branch.

a conduction delay in the remaining fascicle.[52–54] When bundle branch block is accompanied by first degree AV block, prolongation of the AH interval reflecting AV nodal delay is usually present, and additional prolongation of the HV interval is seen in some patients.[45] In patients with alternating bundle branch block, electrophysiologic studies frequently demonstrate incomplete block with a conduction delay in one bundle and a rate-dependent block in the other bundle.[55]

Previous retrospective studies in patients with complete AV block have shown that complete AV block is frequently preceded by bundle branch block. Therefore, patients with bifascicular block, bundle branch block accompanied by first degree AV block, and alternating bundle branch block may be at increased risk of developing complete AV block. Recordings of the HV interval could identify a subgroup of patients in whom progression to high grade or complete AV block is likely to occur. However, the available data from large prospective studies reveal a surprisingly benign course in these patients, especially in young, asymptomatic patients without organic heart disease.[56–58] Despite the fact that an abnormal HV interval (55 ms or longer) in patients with bundle branch block is associated with a higher risk of progression to high-grade AV block, the overall incidence of progression is too low to warrant prophylactic pacemaker implantation in asymptomatic patients.[56]

Even in patients with an HV interval greater than 70 ms, the risk is still small. However, when the HV interval is 100 ms or greater, the risk of progression is 24% over 22 months.[58] In addition, the occurrence of block distal to the His bundle recording site during atrial pacing is associated with a high risk of progression.[59] Therefore, patients with bundle branch block and symptoms of syncope or severe dizziness in whom symptoms are not explained by bradycardia using noninvasive studies, including prolonged ambulatory electrocardiographic monitoring, deserve electrophysiologic testing. Implantation of a permanent pacemaker is indicated when marked prolongation of the HV interval or block distal to the His bundle recording site during atrial pacing, or both, are observed. Awareness of the possibility that in these patients causes other than conduction abnormalities (such as ventricular tachyarrhythmias) could also be responsible for the symptoms is important; therefore, a complete electrophysiologic evaluation with appropriate stimulating protocol should be performed.

CONCEALED CONDUCTION AND PSEUDOATRIOVENTRICULAR BLOCK

Concealed conduction is defined as the effects of a partially penetrating impulse on subsequent impulse conduction and generation. The most common form of concealed conduction is the effects of an interpolated premature atrial or ventricular beat on the conduction of subsequent sinus beat. Under such circumstances, the blocked atrial or ventricular impulse usually penetrates the AV node, causing AH interval prolongation of the subsequent sinus beat. On occasion, the impulse may penetrates the His bundle, causing intra-Hisian delay with split His bundle potentials of the subsequent sinus beat. Concealed conduction can occur at any level in the AV conducting system.

Concealed conduction to the AV node of a nonpropagated junctional extrasystole can produce an electrocardiographic pattern mimicking AV block with (1) a sudden unexpected prolongation of the PR interval, (2) the presence of both type I and type II AV block, (3) the occurrence of type II block with normal QRS complex, and (4) the presence of premature inverted P waves or junctional premature QRS complexes, or both. Although a diagnosis of pseudo-AV block can be obtained by analysis of the surface electrocardiogram, recordings of the His bundle electrogram with demonstration of nonpropagated junctional extrasystole are essential for confirmation of the diagnosis[60] (Figure 19.5). Pseudoatrioventricular block is not an indication for pacemaker insertion.

SUPRAVENTRICULAR TACHYCARDIAS

Supraventricular tachycardia is a common clinical arrhythmia, occurring in patients with or without organic heart disease. The attacks are characterized by sudden onset and sudden termination and are usually initiated by a premature atrial or ventricular beat. The rate of tachycardia ranges between 150 and 220 beats per minute, but it can be as fast as 300 beats per minute in infants and as slow as 100 beats per minute in some patients. The duration of attacks may last from a few seconds to several hours. During attacks of tachycardia, the PR intervals are usually regular and the QRS duration is normal; wide QRS complexes may be seen when functional or preexisting bundle branch block is present. The P waves are usually not visible, but they may be seen behind or in front of the QRS complexes. Vagal maneuvers frequently terminate the tachycardia. Reentry is the mechanism of tachycardia in most patients; enhanced automaticity may be the mechanism of tachycardia in a minority of patients. Electrophysiologic study is useful not only in defining the mechanism of tachycardia, but also in defining an effective therapeutic regimen. The classification of supraventricular tachycardias is given in Table 19.3.

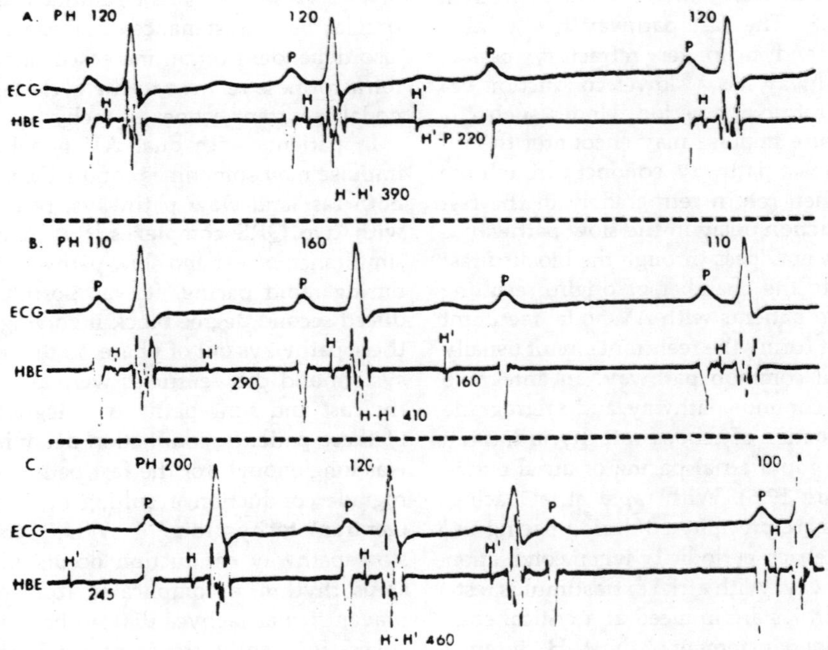

Figure 19.5. Simultaneous recordings of lead II electrocardiogram and His bundle electrogram (HBE) showing the effects of premature His bundle depolarization (H′) on the subsequent sinus beat and also demonstrating the propagation of an H′ to the ventricles. PH intervals are listed at the top of each strip over the cycle it was measured. H′P intervals are listed just under HBE. HH′ intervals are listed on the bottom of each strip. *A*, H′P is 220 ms and the subsequent P wave is blocked. There are both retrograde and antegrade blocks of H′ potentials with no related atrial or ventricular activity. The electrocardiogram resembles Mobitz type II AV block. *B*, The first H′P interval is 290 ms; and the subsequent PH is prolonged to 160 ms. The second H′P is 160 ms with block of the P wave. The electrocardiogram resembles a Wenckebach period, with PR and PH prolongations before the blocked P wave. *C*, The first H′P of 245 ms produced PH prolongation to 200 ms. The second H′ propagates to the ventricle because of a long HH′ interval (460 ms). In tracing *A* and *B*, H′ does not propagate because of a shorter HH′ interval. The P wave following the propagated H′ is blocked because of the short H′P interval. (From Rosen et al,[60] by permission of the American Heart Association, Inc.)

Table 19.3. Supraventricular Tachycardias

Reentrant
AV nodal reentrant tachycardia
Slow–fast form
Fast–slow form
AV reentrant tachycardia
Orthodromic form
Antidromic form
Permanent form with a slowly conducting retrograde paraseptal accessory pathway
Reentry using one accessory pathway for antegrade and another for retrograde conduction
Reentry incorporating Mahaim fibers
Sinus or atrial reentrant tachycardia
Automatic
Atrial tachycardia

AV = atrioventricular.

ATRIOVENTRICULAR NODAL REENTRANT TACHYCARDIA AND DUAL ATRIOVENTRICULAR NODAL PATHWAYS PHENOMENA

At the beginning of this century, reentry was proposed as the mechanism of tachyarrhythmia.[61] In the 1920s, some early investigators[62] implied that it could be a mechanism of supraventricular tachycardia. Subsequently, it was postulated that the AV node could undergo longitudinal dissociation into two pathways with different functional properties.[63] The fast pathway has a faster conduction velocity and a longer refractory period, whereas the slow pathway has a slower conduction velocity and a shorter refractory period. Under such circumstances, a premature impulse may encounter the refractory period of the fast pathway, conduct through the slow pathway, and then return retrogradely in the fast pathway. If the conduction delay in the slow pathway is sufficient, the impulse may pass through the blocked fast pathway and return to the chamber of origin, resulting in an echo response. In patients with AV nodal reentrant tachycardia (slow–fast form), the reentrant circuit usually consists of a proximal common pathway, an antegrade slow pathway, a distal common pathway, and a retrograde fast pathway.[64–68] Induction of echoes or tachycardias can be accomplished with rapid atrial pacing or atrial extrastimulus testing (Figure 19.6). With rapid atrial pacing, echoes or tachycardias are precipitated during pacing-induced atypical Wenckebach periodicity when conduction shifts to the slow pathway. With atrial extrastimulus testing, echoes or tachycardias are induced at a critical coupling interval with sudden increment of the A_2H_2 interval when conduction shifts to the slow pathway. An echo zone can be defined and usually coincides with the coupling intervals at which A_2 is conducted through slow pathway conduction. Nevertheless, achievement of slow pathway conduction may not be sufficient for the initiation of echoes or tachycardia. The conduction delay must be long enough to allow the blocked fast pathway to recover for reexcitation. This critical delay of the slow pathway is called the critical AH interval.[69] The tachycardia can also be initiated by ventricular beats. Retrograde induction of echoes or tachycardias depends on a block in the slow pathway with conduction to the atria through the fast pathway; a critical VA delay is usually not demonstrated.[70]

When AV conduction curves are constructed by plotting the conduction time (AH or A_2H_2) against the pacing cycle length or the coupling intervals of atrial premature beats (AA or A_1A_2), discontinuous AA, AH curves, or A_1A_2, A_2H_2 curves can be demonstrated (Figure 19.7).[66,68,71,72] Demonstration of discontinuous AA, AH, or A_1A_2, A_2H_2 curves suggests a diagnosis of dual AV nodal pathways. Occasionally, the patients may manifest two ranges of nonoverlapping PR or AH intervals during sinus rhythm or at an identical atrial paced cycle length due to fast or slow pathway conduction.[72–74] The occurrence of fast and slow pathway conduction at the same sinus or atrial paced cycle length depends on a long effective refractory period of the fast pathway relative to the sinus or atrial paced cycle length. Shift of conduction from the fast to the slow pathway may be initiated by a premature atrial beat that falls within the effective refractory period of the fast pathway. Repetitive retrograde concealed conduction to the fast pathway keeps the fast pathway refractory and maintains slow pathway conduction. Resumption of fast pathway conduction can be initiated by a premature atrial beat that falls within the effective refractory period of the slow pathway, allowing recovery of the fast pathway for subsequent conduction. Shift of conduction from the fast to the slow pathway or vice versa may also be initiated by a premature ventricular beat. Sustenance of slow pathway conduction is also dependent on an increased retrograde fast pathway refractoriness relative to the cycle length; otherwise, AV nodal reentrant echoes or tachycardias will occur.

In patients with dual AV nodal pathways, an atrial impulse may sometimes conduct simultaneously through both fast and slow pathways, resulting in one P wave with two QRS complexes.[75–78] In most reported cases, simultaneous fast and slow pathway conduction occurred during rapid pacing. It was postulated that pacing-induced second degree block involving both pathways put these pathways out of phase, so that the distal conducting system and the ventricles were able to respond to both the fast and slow pathway antegrade impulse. In some of these patients, conduction delay in the slow pathway was long enough for the fast pathway to recover for retrograde conduction, resulting in initiation of AV nodal reentrant tachycardia.[75,76] When simultaneous fast and slow pathway conduction occurs intermittently during sinus rhythm, a complicated form of nonreentrant supraventricular tachycardia can be seen.[77,78]

Less frequently, the reentrant circuit may be reversed, using the fast pathway for antegrade and the slow pathway for retrograde conduction.[79,80] Electrophysiologic studies in these patients usually demonstrate retrograde discontinuous V_1V_2, V_2A_2 curves (Figure 19.7). The tachycardia is initiated during pacing-induced retrograde atypical Wenckebach periodicity or during ventricular extrastimulus testing when conduction shifts to the slow pathway. A critical VA interval can be demonstrated. The tachycardia can sometimes be initiated with rapid atrial pacing or with atrial extrastimulus testing. Antegrade induction of tachycardia depends on block of the antegrade impulse in the slow pathway and is not related to a critical AH interval. This form of tachycardia is called the fast–slow form AV nodal reentrant tachycardia. Differing

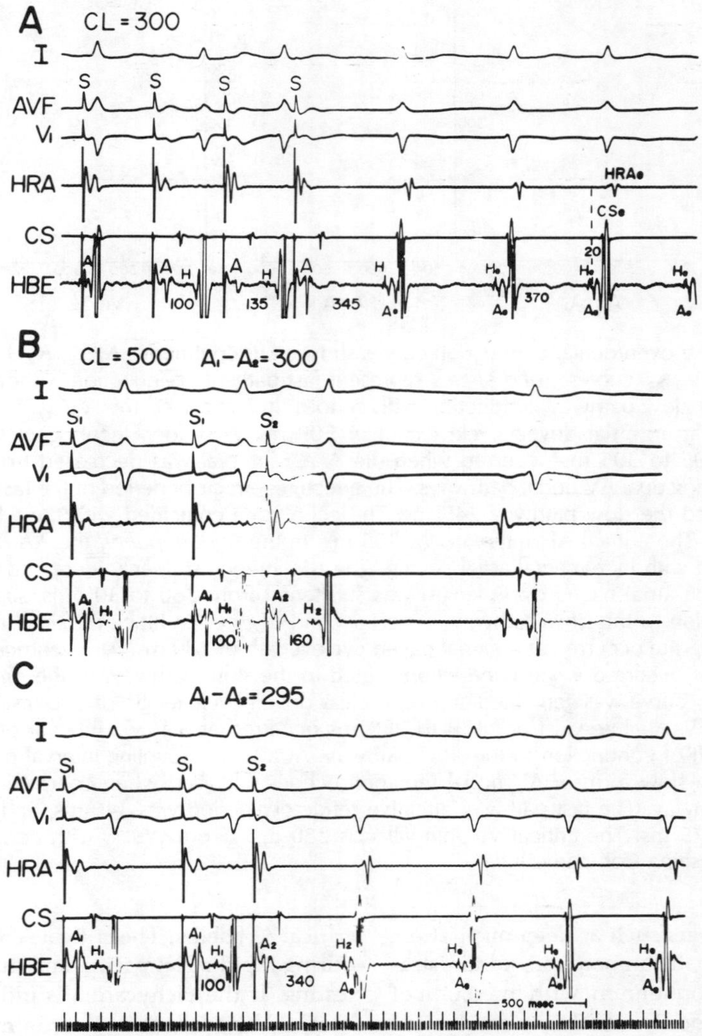

Figure 19.6. Recording showing atypical Wenckebach periodicity, sudden increase of AH interval, and induction of slow-fast form AV nodal reentrant tachycardia. S, A, and H are, respectively, stimulus artifact, low septal right atrial, and His bundle response to atrial pacing. HRAe, CSe, Ae, and He are, respectively, high right atrial, left atrial, low septal right atrial, and His bundle responses of the AV nodal reentrant beats. A_1 and H_1 are, respectively, low septal right atrial and His bundle responses to the basic driven beat (S_1); A_2 and H_2 are, respectively, low septal right atrial and His bundle responses to the extrastimulus (S_2). CS = left atrial electrogram recorded from coronary sinus; paper speed = 100 mm/s. *A*, Atypical Wenckebach periodicity occurred at an atrial paced cycle length of 300 ms. The AH interval suddenly increased from 135 (third paced beat) to 345 ms (fourth paced beat) during the Wenckebach period, suggesting a shift of conduction from the fast to the slow pathway. Atrioventricular nodal reentrant tachycardia was induced following the shift. The cycle length of tachycardia was 390 ms, and the AeHe/HeAe ratio was greater than one (370/20); Ae was earlier than CSe and HRAe. *B & C*, Atrial extrastimulus testing was performed at an atrial driven cycle length of 500 ms. A_1H_1 was 100 ms. In *B*, the A_1A_2 coupling interval and 300 ms; A_2 was conducted through the fast pathway with an A_2H_2 of 160 ms. In *C*, the A_1A_2 coupling interval was 295 ms; A_2 was blocked in the fast pathway and conducted through the slow pathway with a sudden increase of the A_2H_2 interval to 340 ms. Atrioventricular nodal reentrant tachycardia was induced. (From Wu,[68] with permission of the Futura Publishing Company, Inc.)

from the common slow–fast form of AV nodal reentrant tachycardia, the P wave occurs in front of the QRS complex during tachycardia and the ratio of AH and HA is less than one. In the common slow–fast form of AV nodal reentrant tachycardia, the P wave occurs either simultaneously with the QRS complex or immediately after the QRS complex, and the ratio of AH and HA is greater than one.

The sustenance of AV nodal reentrant tachycardia depends on the ability of all components of the reentrant circuit to respond to the circulating impulse repetitively, and therefore, the cycle length of the tachycardia must be longer than the refractory periods of all components of the circuit.[81] The cycle length of the tachycardia is the sum of the conduction times of all components of the circuit. Physiologic or pharmacologic interventions that modify the antegrade or retrograde properties of the fast and slow pathways can depress or enhance AV nodal

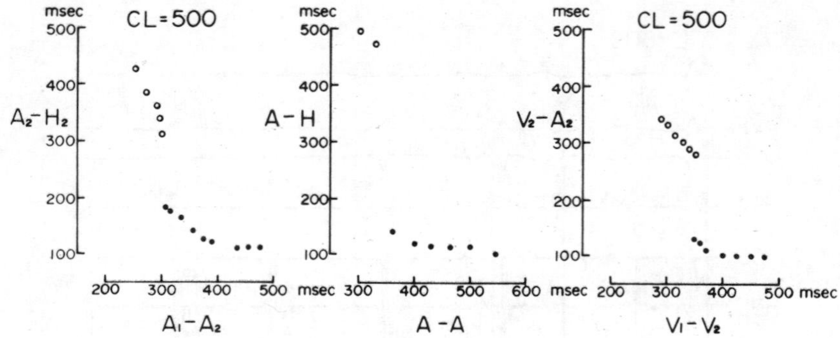

Figure 19.7. Atrioventricular conduction curves showing discontinuous A_1A_2, A_2H_2 and AA, AH and V_1V_2, V_2A_2 curves. *Solid circles* represent fast pathway conduction without echoes, and *open circle* slow pathway conduction with echoes. In *left panel,* the A_1A_2, A_2H_2 curve was generated at an atrial driven cycle length of 500 ms. A sudden increase of the A_2H_2 interval from 195 to 305 ms occurred when the A_1A_2 interval was decreased from 305 to 300 ms, suggesting dual AV nodal pathways. The effective refractory period of the fast pathway was 300 ms, and the slow pathway 245 ms. The echo zone coincided with the whole slow pathway curve. The critical AH interval was 305 ms. In the *middle panel*, the AA, AH curve was constructed with incremental atrial pacing. The AH interval suddenly increased from 145 to 470 ms as the atrial paced cycle length was shortened from 360 to 300 ms, suggesting a shift of conduction to the slow pathway. Type I second degree AV block proximal to the His bundle recording site occurred at an atrial paced cycle length of 280 ms. Atrioventricular nodal reentrant echoes occurred when conduction shifted to the slow pathway. In the *right panel,* the V_1V_2, V_2A_2 curve was generated at a ventricular driven cycle length of 500 ms. A sudden increase of the V_2A_2 interval from 130 to 280 ms occurred at a V_1V_2 interval of 345 ms, suggesting a shift of conduction to the slow pathway. At a V_1V_2 coupling interval of 345 and 280 ms, the fast-slow form of AV nodal reentrant echoes occurred when conduction shifted to the slow pathway. The fast pathway effective refractory period was 340 ms, and the slow pathway was 275 ms. The critical VA interval was 280 ms. (From Wu,[68] with permission of the Futura Publishing Company, Inc.)

reentry. Physiologic maneuvers such as deep inspiration, tilting, carotid massage, eyeball compression, administration of phenylephrine or edrophonium, with induction of vagal reflex, depress antegrade slow pathway conduction and slow the tachycardia.[82,83] Termination of the tachycardia usually results from block in the antegrade slow pathway but may occasionally result from block in the retrograde fast pathway. Atropine shortens the refractory periods, enhances the conduction of the antegrade fast and slow pathways as well as the retrograde fast pathway, and may potentiate the induction of sustained tachycardia.[84] Isoproterenol enhances retrograde fast pathway conduction and facilitates the induction of tachycardia.[85] Digitalis, propranolol, verapamil, diltiazem, and adenosine lengthen the conduction time and refractory periods of both pathways antegradely and may also depress retrograde fast pathway conduction.[86–93] These agents inhibit induction and sustenance of tachycardia. Procainamide, quinidine, disopyramide, and ajmaline selectively increase the refractoriness of the retrograde fast pathway and inhibit the ability to induce or sustain tachycardia.[93–96]

Diagnosis of AV nodal reentrant tachycardia depends on exclusion of atrial reentrant tachycardia or AV reentrant tachycardia incorporating a retrogradely conducting accessory pathway (see subsequent discussion).[67] Induction of atrial reentrant tachycardia is not dependent on achieving a critical AH interval, whereas induction of AV nodal reentrant tachycardia is dependent on achieving a critical AH delay. The critical AH interval is demonstrated during rapid atrial pacing and during atrial extrastimulus testing. If the tachycardia is induced by a blocked atrial beat, AV nodal reentry can almost be excluded. When the tachycardia is induced retrogradely, the activation sequence in atrial reentrant tachycardia is characterized by V→A→A→H sequence, whereas that of the AV nodal reentrant tachycardia is characterized by a V→A→H sequence. Demonstration of a discontinuous AV conduction curve alone does not exclude the possibility of an AV reentrant tachycardia incorporating a retrogradely conducting accessory pathway, as dual AV nodal pathways may be present in these patients. Under such circumstances, demonstration of atrial activation occurring either before or simultaneously with the onset of ventricular activation during tachycardia, or demonstration of His bundle capture (H_2) preceding the atrial capture (A_2) with ventricular extrastimulus (V_2) delivered during the tachycardia suggesting that the change in VA interval (V_2A_2) is dependent on His bundle activation, also supports the diagnosis of AV nodal reentry.

As discontinuity of the AV conduction curve depends on a difference in conduction time of the two pathways, continuous A_1A_2, A_2H_2 curve can possibly occur in patients with AV nodal reentrant tachycardia when the difference in conduction time of the two pathways is minimal.[68] In some patients, the refractory period of the fast pathway may be so prolonged that the fast pathway is available only for retrograde conduction, and a discontinuous curve is not demonstrated. The manifestations of dual AV nodal pathways are summarized in Table 19.4.

PREEXCITATION SYNDROMES

Normally, there is only one conduction pathway between the atria and the ventricles: the AV node and His-Purkinje pathway. In patients with a preexcitation syndrome, there are anomalous connections in addition to the normal pathway.[97,98] These connections consist of an accessory AV muscle connection (Kent bundle), atriofascicular bypass tract (atrio-Hisian fiber), intranodal bypass tract (James fiber), nodoventricular connection (Mahaim fiber), and fasciculoventricular connection (Mahaim fiber). The presence of accessory connections provides anatomic substrates for electrocardiographic manifestation of a short PR interval, delta wave, wide QRS complex, as well as a variety of tachyarrhythmias.

The Wolff–Parkinson–White syndrome is the most common variety of the preexcitation syndrome. Both anatomic and electrophysiologic data indicate that this syndrome is due to an accessory muscle connection between the atrium and the ventricle.[97–99] Impulse transmission in the accessory pathway is much faster than that in the normal pathway. As a consequence, a portion of the ventricle is preexcited, causing a short PR interval and delta wave. The later portion of the QRS complex results from fusion of impulses coming from both the accessory pathway and the normal pathway. Despite a faster conduction velocity, the accessory pathway frequently has a longer refractory period than that of the normal pathway. Therefore, a premature atrial impulse may be blocked in the accessory pathway and conducts to the ventricles solely from the normal pathway. On reaching the ventricle, the impulse returns retrogradely from the accessory pathway to the atria and starts a circus-movement tachycardia. The circus-movement tachycardia may also be initiated by a ventricular premature beat that is blocked in the normal pathway, conducts to the atria through the accessory pathway, and enters the normal pathway antegradely. This type of AV reentrant tachycardia using the normal pathway for antegrade and the accessory pathway for retrograde conduction is called the "orthodromic" form of AV reentrant tachycardia.[67,99–102]

Table 19.4. Manifestations of Dual Atrioventricular (AV) Nodal Pathways

Slow–fast form of AV nodal reentrant tachycardia
Atypical antegrade Wenckebach periodicity
Demonstration of discontinuous AA, AH, or A_1A_2, A_2H_2 curves
Two ranges of nonoverlapping PR intervals during sinus rhythm or AH intervals during atrial pacing at an identical paced rate
One P wave with 2 QRS responses due to simultaneous fast and slow pathway conduction
Fast–slow form of AV nodal reentrant tachycardia
Atypical retrograde Wenckebach periodicity
Demonstration of discontinuous V_1V_2, V_2A_2 curves

Frequently, the accessory pathway may conduct only retrogradely and not antegradely. Under such circumstances, a short PR interval and a delta wave are not seen. However, AV reentrant tachycardia can be initiated by a premature atrial beat that achieves a critical AV delay to allow recovery of the accessory pathway and the atria for reexcitation. This type of accessory pathway is called a concealed accessory pathway.[67,99,103–106]

The accessory pathway can be present in the free wall or the septum, around the tricuspid ring or mitral valve ring. The site of the accessory pathway insertion can be localized by electrophysiologic studies in the catheterization laboratory. The techniques include (1) pacing the atria from different sites,[107,108] and (2) mapping of the atrial activation sequence during an induced episode of AV reentrant tachycardia or during rapid ventricular pacing.[99,109–111] Assuming that the stimulus-delta interval is the shortest and the degree of preexcitation the greatest when pacing is performed at the site of accessory pathway insertion, the right atrium is paced from different sites around the tricuspid ring, whereas the left atrium is paced from different sites in the coronary sinus. However, mapping of the atrial activation sequence during an induced episode of AV reentrant tachycardia or during ventricular pacing provides most accurate information concerning the site of the accessory pathway insertion. This latter technique requires positioning of the catheter at different sites in the coronary sinus and at different sites around the tricuspid valve ring. The earliest site of atrial activation during AV reentrant tachycardia reflects the site of atrial insertion of the accessory pathway, because the accessory pathway is used for retrograde conduction during tachycardia (Figure 19.8).

The presence of an accessory pathway does not imply that the accessory pathway always participates in reentrant tachycardia; the accessory pathway can be a "bystander."[105] The AV reentrant tachycardia is characterized by an eccentric atrial activation sequence and atrial activation that is always occurring after ventricular activation.[67,99,112] When a critically timed ventricular extrastimulus (V_2) is delivered during tachycardia, the atria may be preexcited without activation of the His bundle.[67,99,105,112–114] When ipsilateral bundle branch block develops during tachycardia, the HA interval and the cycle length of tachycardia are lengthened.

The responses of AV reentrant tachycardia to physiologic and pharmacologic maneuvers are analogous to those of AV nodal reentrant tachycardia. Vagal maneuvers and drugs such as verapamil, diltiazem, adenosine, digitalis, and propranolol increase the AV nodal refractory period and are effective in terminating or preventing recurrence of tachycardia.[115–120] Procainamide, quinidine, disopyramide, ajmaline, and amiodarone increase the retrograde accessory pathway refractory period and are effective in preventing recurrence of tachycardia.[121–126]

Rarely, the AV reentrant circuit may be reversed using the accessory pathway for antegrade and the normal pathway for retrograde conduction. As a consequence, the ventricles are activated by the impulse from the accessory

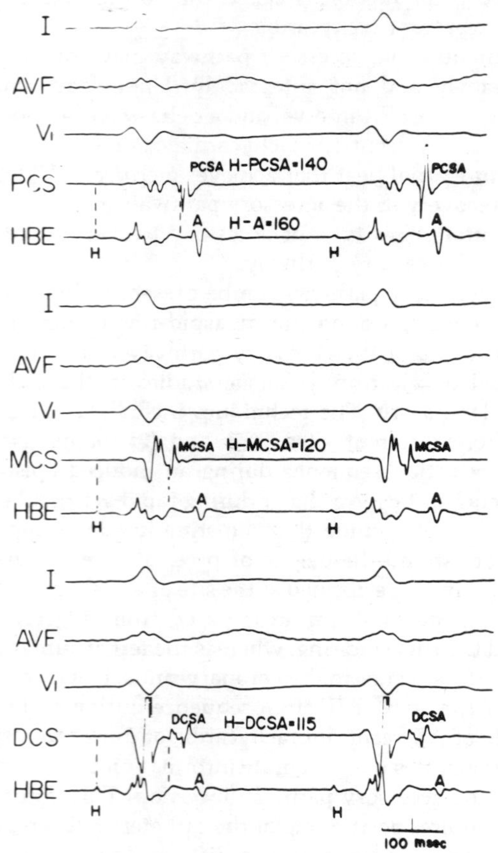

Figure 19.8. Recordings showing AV reentrant tachycardia using the normal pathway for antegrade conduction and a left lateral accessory pathway for retrograde conduction. PCS, MCS, and DCS = proximal, middle, and distal coronary sinus. H-PCSA, H-MCSA, and H-DCSA = interval between the His bundle deflection and the left atrial depolarization recorded from the proximal, middle, and distal coronary sinus. Note that during tachycardia the atrial electrogram recorded from the coronary sinus was activated earlier than that recorded from the His bundle electrogram, and that the earliest atrial activation site was located at the distal coronary sinus.

pathway and the QRS complex is wide and bizarre. This type of tachycardia is called an "antidromic" form of AV reentrant tachycardia.[102,127]

A special type of accessory pathway usually capable of only retrograde conduction and with a slow conduction velocity has been demonstrated in the less common form of supraventricular tachycardia characterized by a long RP and a short PR interval.[102,128–131] This special type of accessory pathway has been shown to be located in the left paraseptal area. Electrophysiologic studies in these patients demonstrated an earliest atrial activation during tachycardia being located in the orifice of the coronary sinus. This type of tachycardia is frequently incessant and drug-resistant and has been called a "permanent" form of AV reentrant tachycardia.

Dual AV nodal pathways can occur in patients with the Wolff–Parkinson–White syndrome.[132] Both the fast and the slow AV nodal pathways may be used as the antegrade limb of the AV reentrant circuit, resulting in changing cycle length of tachycardia or alternation of cycle length during tachycardia. The accessory pathway can be a "bystander" pathway during an episode of AV nodal reentrant tachycardia. In addition, multiple accessory pathways may be present in a patient.[133–136] The presence of multiple accessory pathways may result in multiple reentrant circuits, including using one accessory pathway for antegrade and the other for retrograde conduction (Figure 19.9). Identification of the presence of multiple accessory pathways is extremely important when surgical abolition of the accessory pathway is considered.

There appears to be a higher incidence of atrial fibrillation in patients with the Wolff–Parkinson–White syndrome.[137–139] In these patients, the ventricular rate during atrial fibrillation is usually faster than the rate of AV reentrant tachycardia. Occasionally a rapid ventricular rate with conduction exclusively through the accessory pathway can happen. As a consequence, syncope and ventricular fibrillation can occur. Patients with previously documented ventricular fibrillation have the shortest RR interval during atrial fibrillation of less than 205 ms as well as a short antegrade effective refractory period of the accessory pathway.[138] Electrophysiologic studies with induction of atrial fibrillation and administration of pharmacologic agents are helpful in the management of these patients. Surgical abolition of the accessory pathway is frequently indicated when antiarrhythmic agents fail to modify the property of the accessory pathway.

The combination of a short PR interval, normal QRS complexes, and the presence of paroxysmal tachycardia has been called the Lown–Ganong–Levine syndrome. Although the presence of an atrio-Hisian bypass tract (atriofascicular bypass tract) or an intranodal bypass tract of the James type may be implicated in some patients with this syndrome, previous electrophysiologic studies have shown that the reentrant circuit in these patients is identical to that of dual AV nodal pathways in most patients. Enhanced AV nodal conduction with a short AH interval, subnormal prolongation of the AH interval in response to rapid atrial pacing, and the ability to maintain one-to-one AV conduction at an atrial rate higher than 200 beats per minute are usually found in these patients.[140–143]

The roles of Mahaim fibers in the genesis of cardiac arrhythmias are less well defined.[144,145] Patients with Mahaim fibers may show a short PR interval with an initial slurring of the QRS complex. Only nodoventricular connections have been shown to participate in the reentrant tachycardia that uses the nodoventricular connection for anterograde and the His-Purkinje system for retrograde conduction. The resting electrocardiogram in these patients shows a left bundle branch block QRS morphology, and the electrocardiogram during sustained tachycardia shows the same morphologic characteristics. During tachycardia, there is no His bundle deflection preceding the QRS complex, and a ventriculoatrial dissociation may occur. Patients with fasciculoventricular connections have varying QRS morphologies with either an incomplete left or right bundle branch block pattern. Fasciculoventricular connections have not been shown to participate in reentrant tachycardia, although they can be a

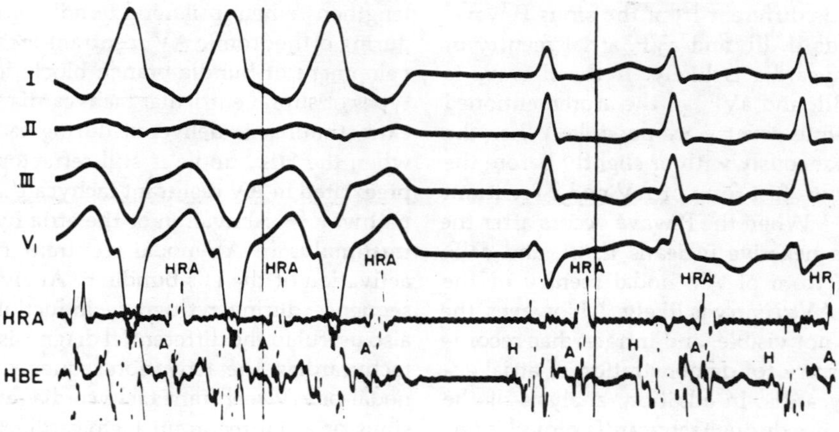

Figure 19.9. Recording showing multiple reentries with spontaneous conversion of wide QRS to narrow QRS tachycardia. The wide QRS tachycardia had a reentrant circuit using a right accessory pathway for antegrade conduction and a left concealed accessory pathway for retrograde conduction and had a rate of 200 beats per minute. The last atrial echo of the wide QRS tachycardia was blocked in the accessory pathway and was conducted antegradely through the AV node His axis with induction of a narrow QRS tachycardia that had a rate of 170 beats per minute. The second beat of the narrow QRS tachycardia showed a functional right bundle branch block aberration. Note that HA conduction time of this beat was identical to the retrograde conduction times of beats 1 and 3 (without right bundle branch block) of the narrow QRS tachycardia. This observation indicates that the reentrant pathway was not located on the right side. Atrioventricular nodal reentry is unlikely, because the change of wide to narrow QRS tachycardia was accompanied by a significant change in rate. This suggests that during both wide and narrow QRS tachycardia, a left-sided accessory pathway was used for retrograde conduction. (From Denes et al,[133] with permission.)

"bystander" during atrial fibrillation or AV nodal reentrant tachycardia.

SINUS AND ATRIAL REENTRANT TACHYCARDIA

The sinus node and the atria may serve as the site of reentry.[67,146,147] Sinus and atrial reentrant tachycardias are initiated by atrial premature beats. The morphology of the P wave is similar to that of the sinus P wave in sinus reentry and different from that of the sinus P wave in atrial reentry. Differing from the AV nodal reentrant tachycardia or AV reentrant tachycardia, a critical AH or AV delay is not required for initiation of sinus or atrial reentrant tachycardia. A premature atrial beat that is blocked proximal to the His bundle recording site can initiate the tachycardia, and AV nodal block can occur during tachycardia. When VA conduction is intact, the tachycardia can also be induced by ventricular pacing. Retrograde induction of sinus or atrial reentrant tachycardia is characterized by an activation sequence of V→A→A→H.[67,147] Similar to other types of supraventricular tachycardias, both sinus and atrial reentrant tachycardias are responsive to carotid massage. Nevertheless, little information is available regarding drug responses. Although these tachycardias appear to be reentrant, the exact mechanism of sinus and atrial reentrant tachycardias is unclear. The possibility of triggered automaticity as the mechanism of tachycardia cannot be excluded.

AUTOMATIC ATRIAL TACHYCARDIA

Repetitive discharge of impulses from an atrial focus because of enhanced automaticity is a mechanism of atrial tachycardia.[67] This type of tachycardia is called "automatic" or "ectopic" atrial tachycardia. The onset of the tachycardia is neither initiated by a premature atrial beat nor terminated by carotid massage. The P wave of the first beat is different from the sinus beat but is identical to the subsequent beat. A period of acceleration in rate may be seen after the onset of tachycardia. Atrioventricular block may be present, particularly with carotid massage. Digitalis overdose is frequently the cause of tachycardia, but it can be seen in patients with chronic obstructive lung disease or cardiomyopathy, and even in patients without organic heart disease.

DIFFERENTIAL DIAGNOSIS

Differentiation among various types of supraventricular tachycardias can be made by analysis of P-wave morphology, the atrial activation sequence, the relation of P wave to QRS complex, the occurrence of AV block during tachycardia, the mode of induction, the demonstration of a critical AH or AV delay, the effect of bundle branch block on the cycle length of tachycardia, and the effect of a ventricular extrastimulus delivered during tachycardia. When the P wave occurs before the QRS complex, the differential diagnosis should include sinus or atrial reentrant tachycardia, fast–slow form of AV nodal reentrant tachycardia, AV reentrant tachycardia using the normal pathway for antegrade and a paraseptal slowly conducting accessory pathway for retrograde conduction, antidromic form of AV reentrant tachycardia, AV reentrant tachycardia using an accessory pathway for antegrade and another accessory pathway for retrograde conduction, and automatic atrial tachycardia.[67,80,99,147] If the P wave is similar to the sinus P wave, sinus reentry is likely. If the P wave is different from the sinus P wave, but is upright in leads II, III, and aVF, atrial reentry or automatic atrial tachycardia is likely. If the P wave is negative in leads II, III, and aVF, all the aforementioned tachycardias except sinus reentry are possible. When the P wave occurs simultaneously with or slightly before the QRS complex, the slow–fast form of AV nodal reentrant tachycardia is likely.[67] When the P wave occurs after the QRS complex and is negative in leads II, III, and aVF, either the slow–fast form of AV nodal reentry or the orthodromic form of AV reentry is likely.[67] However, the P wave is frequently not visible, and intracardiac recordings are usually necessary for demonstration of atrial activation during tachycardia. In addition, analysis of the atrial activation sequence during tachycardia provides important clues regarding the mechanism of tachycardia.[67,99] If the low septal right atrial electrogram recorded from the His bundle catheter precedes all other atrial electrograms, AV nodal reentrant tachycardia (both slow–fast and fast–slow forms) or antidromic AV reentrant tachycardia is likely. If an eccentric retrograde atrial activation sequence is demonstrated, the orthodromic form of AV reentry or AV reentry using an accessory pathway for antegrade and another accessory pathway for retrograde conduction is likely. As the earliest atrial activation site is the site of accessory pathway insertion, the left atrial electrogram recorded from the coronary sinus occurs earlier than other atrial electrograms in patients with a reentrant circuit using a left-sided accessory pathway for retrograde conduction, whereas the atrial electrogram recorded around the tricuspid ring occurs earlier than other atrial electrograms in patients with a reentrant circuit using a right-sided accessory pathway for retrograde conduction. The atrial activation sequence in patients with sinus reentry is from high to low, similar to that of sinus rhythm, whereas the sequence in patients with atrial reentry or automatic atrial tachycardia is variable and depends on the site of the focus.

The occurrence of AV block proximal to or distal to the His bundle recording site can be seen in sinus reentry, atrial reentry, or automatic atrial tachycardia.[67,147] An AV block distal to the His bundle recording site can be seen in AV nodal reentry. However, an AV block proximal to the His bundle recording site should exclude the diagnosis of AV nodal reentry, although block at a site distal to the AV nodal reentrant circuit is theoretically possible.[68] As the normal pathway is part of the reentrant circuit, AV block cannot occur in AV reentry. Carotid massage can also provide clues concerning the mechanism of tachycardia; it may terminate reentrant supraventricular tachycardia, but not automatic atrial tachycardia; it may provoke an AV block in sinus reentry, atrial reentry, and automatic atrial tachycardia, but not in AV nodal reentry and AV reentry.

Although a critical AH delay is required in the induction of AV nodal reentry and a critical AV delay is required in the induction of orthodromic AV reentry, a critical AH or AV delay is not demonstrated in the induction of other forms of supraventricular tachycardia. Because a bundle branch is part of an AV reentrant circuit, the HA interval, as well as the cycle length of tachycardia, lengthens when ipsilateral bundle branch block develops during orthodromic AV reentrant tachycardia.[114] The development of bundle branch block does not affect other types of supraventricular tachycardia. When a ventricular extrastimulus is delivered during tachycardia at a time when the His bundle is still refractory, the atria may be preexcited in AV reentrant tachycardia using an accessory pathway.[105] Activation of the atria by the ventricular extrastimulus in AV nodal reentrant tachycardia requires activation of the His bundle.[67] Analysis of the activation sequence during retrograde induction of tachycardia is also useful in the differential diagnosis of supraventricular tachycardias; the activation sequence is V→A→V in AV nodal or AV reentrant tachycardia, and V→A→A→V in sinus or atrial reentrant tachycardia.[67]

ROLES OF ELECTROPHYSIOLOGIC STUDY

The purposes of electrophysiologic study in patients with supraventricular tachycardia are multiple. First, such study can determine the presence and type of supraventricular tachycardia. For example, in a patient with paroxysms of palpitation without electrocardiographic documentation of arrhythmia, the study can determine whether or not supraventricular tachycardia is the cause of palpitation. In a patient with documented supraventricular tachycardia, the study can determine the type of tachycardia. Second, it can determine the nature and site of reentrant circuit. For example, in a patient with the Wolff–Parkinson–White syndrome, the study not only confirms the presence of an accessory pathway but also determines the location of the accessory pathway and its role in the genesis of tachycardia. Likewise, the site of atrial reentrant or automatic tachycardia can be determined. This information is mandatory when surgical therapy is considered. Third, it can define an effective antiarrhythmic regimen. This is usually achieved by leaving a multipolar electrode catheter in the heart after the initial electrophysiologic study. Subsequent serial drug testings with an intravenous or oral antiarrhythmic agent are performed daily. The patient is then placed on an effective drug regimen based on data gathered during serial drug testings. When the tachycardia is resistant to the antiarrhythmic agent, invasive therapeutic modalities such as surgical intervention or implantation of antitachycardia pacemaker may be considered. Fourth, it can detect the presence of multiple accessory pathways or multiple reentries. The presence of multiple accessory pathways or multiple reentrant circuits has important therapeutic implications and cannot be detected without electrophysiologic studies.

VENTRICULAR TACHYCARDIAS

Automaticity and reentry are the two basic mechanisms of tachycardia.[148–152] Ventricular tachyarrhythmias can result from enhanced normal pacemaker automaticity, from abnormal automaticity in diseased Purkinje or ventricular muscle fibers that have a reduced level of transmembrane potential, or from triggered afterdepolarizations in diseased Purkinje or ventricular fibers that have a reduced level of transmembrane potential. Ventricular tachyarrhythmias can also result from reentry using bundle branches or fascicles as the circuit or from reentry using diseased peripheral Purkinje fibers or ventricular muscle fibers as the circuit. Reentry may occur in tissues with or without a central obstacle; the former is called macroreentry and the latter microreentry. Reflection due to electrotonic interaction in a tissue with delay conduction or conduction block can also be a potential mechanism of ventricular tachyarrhythmia.

Still, there has been no generally accepted classification of ventricular tachycardias. However, there appear to be several different types (Table 19.5): (1) sustained ventricular tachycardia, (2) nonsustained ventricular tachycardia, (3) accelerated idioventricular tachycardia, (4) torsades de pointes, (5) exercise-triggered ventricular tachycardia, and (6) miscellaneous, such as parasystolic or bidirectional ventricular tachycardia. Each type of ventricular tachycardia has a different clinical behavior, although there may be different mechanisms in each tachycardia.

SUSTAINED VENTRICULAR TACHYCARDIA

Sustained ventricular tachycardia refers to tachycardias lasting from minutes to days. Previous myocardial infarction is the most common underlying heart disease in this group of tachycardias. However, sustained ventricular tachycardia can occur in any type of organic heart disease, even without apparent heart disease. Most ventricular tachycardias can be induced by appropriate electrical stimulation by applying single, double, or triple ventricular extrastimuli that are coupled to multiple ventricular-driven cycle lengths.[153-160] Ventricular tachycardias can also be induced by a short burst of rapid ventricular pacing; occasionally, atrial extrastimulus or rapid atrial pacing can also initiate the tachycardia. The right ventricular apex is the usual site of initial stimulation. If ventricular tachycardia is not induced, the right ventricular outflow tract is then stimulated. Induction of ventricular tachycardia sometimes may require left ventricular stimulation.

When studies are appropriately performed, 80% to 90% of clinical ventricular tachycardias can be replicated in the cardiac catheterization laboratory.[153-160] Patients with previous myocardial infarction or without organic heart disease have a higher incidence of reproducibility, whereas those with other forms of heart disease have a lower incidence of reproducibility.[161] More than one QRS morphologic characteristic of ventricular tachycardia may occur in a patient, particularly in those with previous infarction. In some of these patients, tachycardia may arise from a single or close focus with a different exit, whereas in others, tachycardia arises from different foci.[162-167] Endocardial mapping studies are useful in localizing the origin of ventricular tachycardia (Figure 19.10). The techniques include positioning of the electrocatheter at different left and right ventricular sites.[164-167] The ventricular site with an electrogram occurring simultaneously with or slightly earlier than the onset of the QRS complex is taken as the site of origin. This assumption may be erroneous if macroreentry is the mechanism of tachycardia. Under such condition, the site of origin actually involves the whole area of the reentrant circuit.[168] The ventricular site with an electrogram that occurs simultaneously with or slightly earlier than the onset of the QRS complex reflects only the site where the impulse breaks through. Fragmented ventricular electrograms may be recorded at the presumed site of origin.[169] Endocardial mapping is important when surgical intervention with endocardial resection is considered.[170-172] However, hemodynamic deterioration may occur rapidly once a fast ventricular tachycardia is induced, making complete mapping impossible. Technical difficulty in positioning the catheter at different ventricular sites is another problem in performing endocardial mapping. These factors prevent appropriate endocardial mapping studies in the catheterization laboratory in a substantial number of patients.

The ability to replicate clinical ventricular tachycardia in the cardiac catheterization laboratory has allowed serial drug testings for establishing an effective drug regimen in the long-term treatment of patients with recurrent ventricular tachycardia.[173-176] Clinical ventricular tachycardia can be replicated with electrical stimulation in approximately 90% of patients with spontaneous monomorphic and relatively stable tachycardia;[155,157-160] monomorphic sustained ventricular tachycardia is rarely induced in patients without clinical ventricular tachycardia.[157-160] A drug regimen that suppresses the induction of tachycardia will usually suppress spontaneous ventricular tachycardia, whereas a drug regimen that fails to suppress induction of ventricular tachycardia will usually not suppress spontaneous ventricular tachycardia.[175,176] In the case of amiodarone or propafenone, the results of electropharmacologic studies may not predict the clinical responses.[177-180] With these two drugs, suppression of tachycardia induction accurately predicts suppression of spontaneous ventricular tachycardia, whereas failure to suppress tachycardia induction does not necessarily predict ineffectiveness in suppressing spontaneous ventricular tachycardia.

Induction of ventricular tachycardia with programmed stimulation, along with the data obtained from endocardial mapping studies, suggest that reentry is the mechanism responsible for tachycardia. However, definitive evidence has been lacking. Several anecdotal observations have shown that transient entrainment of ventricular tachycardia can be demonstrated with rapid atrial or ventricular pacing at rates faster than the intrinsic rate of ventricular tachycardia but less than the rate that ter-

Table 19.5. Ventricular Tachycardias

Sustained ventricular tachycardia
Nonsustained ventricular tachycardia
Accelerated idioventricular tachycardia
Torsades de pointes associated with a long QT interval
Exercise-triggered ventricular tachycardia
Miscellaneous
Parasystolic ventricular tachycardia
Bidirectional ventricular tachycardia

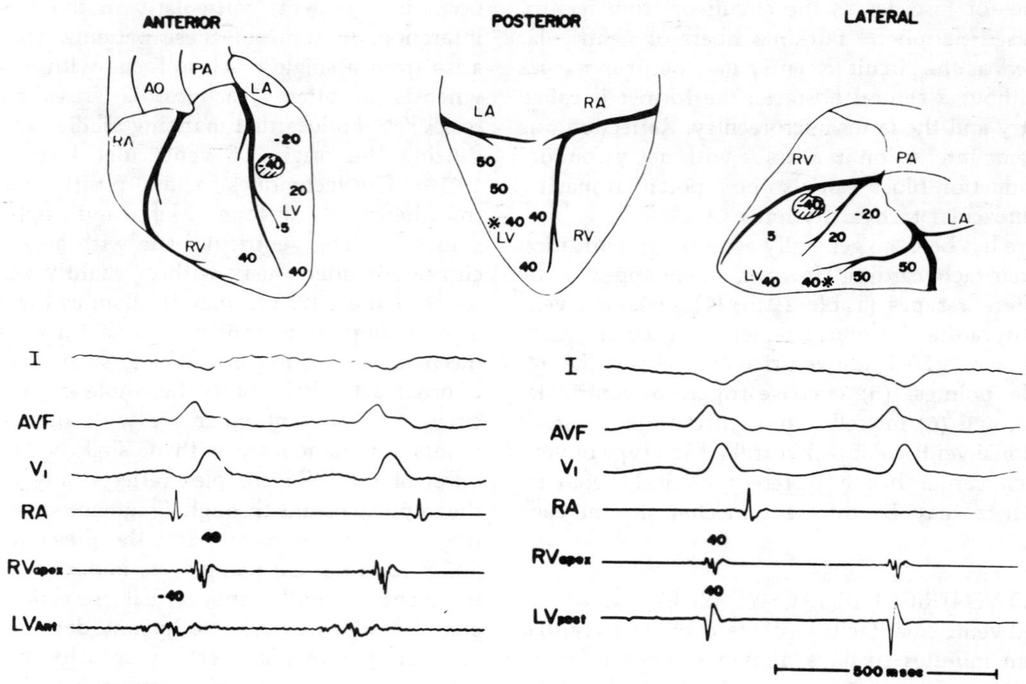

Figure 19.10. Recordings showing endocardial mapping in a patient with sustained ventricular tachycardia of right bundle branch block pattern. RA = right atrial electrogram; RVapex = right apical ventricular electrogram; LVant = left anterior ventricular electrogram; LVpost = left posterior ventricular electrogram. Note the earliest ventricular activation site was recorded at the middle portion of the anterior left ventricle close to the ventricular septum and occurred 40 ms before the onset of the QRS complex. The endocardial activation sequence of the left ventricle is diagrammatically presented in the drawings on top of the tracings. The asterisk indicates the same recording site over the posterior and lateral view.

minates the tachycardia.[181–183] During each episode of entrainment, the focus of ventricular tachycardia is penetrated by the paced impulse and the tachycardia is entrained to the paced rate; the degree of fusion between the paced and the intrinsic ventricular tachycardia complexes increases with increasing paced rate. The last entrained paced beat is always unfused and identical in configuration to the intrinsic ventricular tachycardia complexes; the RR interval between this beat and the preceding beat is identical to the paced cycle length. Termination of ventricular tachycardia occurs only at paced rates at which there is loss of fusion. Demonstration of entrainment provides strong evidence favoring a mechanism of reentry.

A unique type of ventricular tachycardia occurring in young patients without obvious organic heart disease deserves mentioning.[184–186] The electrocardiogram during sinus rhythm in these patients frequently shows a repolarization abnormality over the inferior and lateral precordial leads. The QRS complex during the episode of ventricular tachycardia shows a pattern of right bundle branch block and left axis deviation, whereas the QRS duration during the episode of ventricular tachycardia is relatively narrow and ranges from 0.10 to 0.12 second. The tachycardia can be induced by ventricular as well as atrial stimulation. Exercise can also provoke the tachycardia when a critical sinus rate is achieved. Alternation of cycle length is occasionally seen during tachycardia. Different from the sustained ventricular tachycardias due to other etiologies, this type of ventricular tachycardia is sensitive to verapamil, suggesting that calcium-dependent slow-channel tissue may be involved in the genesis of arrhythmias.[184,186,187]

Sustained ventricular tachycardia can also occur in patients with right ventricular dysplasia, in which the right ventricular musculature is partially or totally replaced by fatty and fibrous tissue.[188–190] Ventricular tachycardia of a left bundle branch configuration frequently occurs in these patients. A 12-lead electrocardiogram during sinus rhythm usually shows T-wave inversion over the right precordial leads; a postexcitation wave may be seen over the right precordial leads when high-amplification and signal-averaging techniques are performed. Induction of tachycardia is similar to that of sustained ventricular tachycardia. Fragmented electrogram with continuous electrical activity may be recorded during tachycardia.[191] This disease is called arrhythmogenic right ventricular dysplasia.

Bundle branch reentry is a rare mechanism of sustained ventricular tachycardia.[192–194] Under such a condition, the QRS complex during tachycardia is identical to that during supraventricular beats with either a left or a right bundle branch block pattern.[194] A His bundle deflection is noted before the QRS complex, with an HV interval equal to or longer than that of sinus beats. The tachycardia may be initiated by atrial stimulation; the atrial induction of tachycardia is dependent on the development of bundle branch block with an HV interval delay. When the tachycardia is induced by ventricular stimulation, it is dependent on a critical VH interval delay. During tachycardia, AV dissociation may occur; the His bundle deflection and the QRS complex may be advanced with a ventricular premature stimulation that either does not affect or may slightly lengthen the HV interval. The tachycardia can be terminated by a ventricular premature beat that is blocked within the bundle branch system.

NONSUSTAINED VENTRICULAR TACHYCARDIA

Nonsustained ventricular tachycardia refers to tachycardia with three or more ventricular complexes; it encompasses different varieties of ventricular tachyarrhythmia. When this occurs in young patients without apparent organic heart disease, it usually presents as a repetitive monomorphic ventricular tachycardia with a QRS morphology of left bundle branch block and inferior axis. Exercise may provoke ventricular tachycardia in some of these patients.[195-198] The electrophysiologic features are consistent with a mechanism of automaticity, and the electrophysiologic study is generally not useful in this group of patients. This arrhythmia is rather benign.

Nonsustained ventricular tachycardia may occur in patients with organic heart disease. It may present with monomorphic or polymorphic ventricular tachycardia. The electrophysiologic mechanisms of these ventricular tachycardias are probably multiple, including reentry, automaticity, and even reflection. The role of electrophysiologic studies in this group of patients is unclear.[157,198,199] Because nonsustained ventricular tachycardia, especially of the polymorphic type, is frequently a nonspecific response to programmed ventricular stimulation, invasive electropharmacologic studies in patients with nonsustained ventricular tachycardia may not be helpful in predicting subsequent clinical responses.

ACCELERATED IDIOVENTRICULAR TACHYCARDIA

Accelerated idioventricular tachycardia frequently complicates acute myocardial infarction or digitalis intoxication. Only rarely does this rhythm occur in other cardiac conditions. Animal studies suggest that the mechanism of accelerated idioventricular tachycardia does not result from enhancement of normal pacemaker activity; rather it results from triggered automaticity due to oscillatory afterdepolarizations.[200,201] Electrophysiologic studies are unnecessary and may not be useful in this arrhythmia.

TORSADES DE POINTES

Torsades de pointes refers to a unique type of repetitive episodes of nonsustained ventricular tachycardia associated with congenital or acquired QT interval prolongation.[202-206] It is characterized by a phasic variation in the electrical polarity of the QRS complex in which the QRS axis undulates and twists around the isoelectric line over runs of usually 5 to 20 beats. The initiating ventricular beat frequently occurs as a characteristic long–short ventricular sequence consisting of a postextrasystolic pause and a premature ventricular beat with a long coupling interval that occurs on top of a prolonged TU wave. Premature ventricular beats as couplets or triplets are frequently seen between the episodes. The tachycardia occasionally may degenerate into ventricular fibrillation. Different from other ventricular arrhythmias, torsades de pointes is usually controlled by overdrive pacing, isoproterenol infusion, or the administration of magnesium sulfate. Type I antiarrhythmic agents not only are ineffective but also frequently aggravate this arrhythmia. The mechanism of this arrhythmia remains unclear. It was initially postulated to result from reentry; however, recent data suggest that this arrhythmia may be related to early afterdepolarization.[202-208] Recording of intraventricular electrograms in a single case with a long QT and multiform ventricular tachycardia has demonstrated a distinct diastolic slow wave of 1.1 mV following the T wave, suggesting that the long QT syndrome is associated with abnormally large afterdepolarizations responsible for tachyarrhythmias.[209]

The presence of QT interval prolongation is essential for the diagnosis of torsades de pointes. Some investigators have labeled polymorphic ventricular tachycardia in patients with a normal QT interval as torsades de pointes.[210] Although some electrocardiographic similarities exist between these two arrhythmias, the electrophysiologic feature of torsades de pointes is completely different from that of polymorphic ventricular tachycardia. Polymorphic ventricular tachycardia is a common nonspecific response to programmed ventricular stimulation,[157] but torsades de pointes is not induced by electrical stimulation. Although type I antiarrhythmic agents aggravate torsades de pointes, these agents are usually effective in polymorphic ventricular tachycardia with a normal QT interval.[199,206] Thus, the distinction has important therapeutic implications.

EXERCISE-TRIGGERED VENTRICULAR TACHYCARDIA

Exercise can provoke ventricular tachycardia through several different mechanisms. For example, in patients with coronary artery disease, exercise may provoke ventricular tachycardia because of increased sympathetic tone, an increase in heart rate, hypoxia, or local acidosis. In patients with ventricular tachycardia induced by atrial pacing at a critical rate, exercise may provoke the tachycardia when the critical rate is achieved during exercise.[185,211]

In patients without organic heart disease in whom paroxysmal ventricular tachycardia developed with a QRS pattern of left bundle branch block and right axis deviation during exercise, the tachycardia can be reproduced with isoproterenol infusion, but not by electrical stimulation.[212,213,213a] In these patients, propranolol effectively terminates and prevents recurrence of the tachycardia. Verapamil effectively terminates the tachycardia but is less effective in preventing exercise-provoked ventricular tachycardia.[212-215] It is postulated that a catecholamine-sensitive calcium-dependent automatic focus is responsible for the tachycardia. Enhanced normal pacemaker automaticity seems unlikely to be the mechanism of tachycardia, because the normal pacemaker automaticity of the Purkinje fibers is independent of the slow inward current and is not likely to respond to verapamil. Whether the tachycardia results from an abnormal automatic focus or a triggered automatic focus cannot be ascertained. The fact that the tachycardia is not inducible with incremental and premature stimulation favors the possibility of an abnormal automaticity. However, repetitive subthreshold oscillatory afterdepolarizations that are triggered by the sinus impulses are equally possible. The subthreshold oscillatory afterdepolarizations may become manifest only when the amplitude is enhanced by the catecholamine of exercise or during isoproterenol infusion.

MISCELLANEOUS VENTRICULAR TACHYCARDIAS

There are other types of ventricular tachycardias such as parasystolic and bidirectional ventricular tachycardias. The focus of a parasystolic ventricular tachycardia is protected with entrance block and may present with a variable degree of exit block. Electrophysiologic mechanisms in this group of patients have not been defined. However, reflection with electrotonic interaction in tissue with a conduction abnormality may be involved in some patients.[144,150,216–218]

Ventricular tachycardia may present rarely with alternating QRS morphology and polarity, resulting in bidirectional ventricular tachycardia. This arrhythmia usually appears in patients with terminal heart failure and digitalis intoxication. Both a supraventricular and a ventricular origin of the arrhythmias has been proposed. However, His bundle recordings in anecdotal patients have demonstrated an origin from the ventricle as well as the junctional area and fascicle.[219–221] The mechanism of this arrhythmia is unclear.

DIFFERENTIAL DIAGNOSIS OF WIDE QRS TACHYCARDIAS

Wide QRS tachycardias embrace several possibilities (Table 19.6), including (1) ventricular tachycardia, (2) atrial fibrillation or atrial flutter with bundle branch block, (3) supraventricular tachycardia (atrial, AV nodal, or AV reentry) with bundle branch block, (4) atrial fibrillation or flutter with conduction over the accessory pathway, (5) atrial tachycardia with conduction over the accessory pathway, (6) antidromic AV reentrant tachycardia, (7) multiple accessory pathways with reentrant tachycardia using antegrade conduction over one and retrograde conduction over the other, (8) reentry associated with Mahaim fibers, (9) AV nodal reentry with conduction of atrial echoes over a "bystander" accessory pathway, (10) AV nodal reentry with AV conduction over "bystander" Mahaim fibers, and (11) atrial fibrillation or flutter over the "bystander" Mahaim fibers. Differentiation among these arrhythmias is frequently possible with careful analysis of the surface electrocardiogram. However, it may require intracardiac recordings with extensive electrophysiologic studies. Atrial fibrillation with bundle branch block or conduction over the accessory pathway usually demonstrates an irregular RR interval, whereas atrial flutter with 2:1 AV conduction or slow atrial flutter with 1:1 AV conduction is accompanied by a regular RR interval. Carotid massage may increase AV block and unmask the fibrillation or flutter when the normal pathway is used for AV conduction; it does not affect conduction when the accessory pathway is used for AV conduction. Likewise, carotid massage may provoke AV block in sinus or atrial reentry with normal pathway conduction and bundle branch block, but not with accessory pathway conduction. Carotid massage also increases the RR interval in atrial fibrillation, atrial flutter, and sinus or atrial tachycardia with "bystander" Mahaim fibers. Carotid massage may terminate supraventricular tachycardia, but usually does not affect ventricular tachycardia, AV reentrant tachycardia using one accessory pathway for antegrade and another accessory pathway for retrograde conduction, or reentrant tachycardia incorporating Mahaim fibers. When AV dissociation or second degree VA block is noted, a diagnosis of ventricular tachycardia or reentry incorporating Mahaim fibers should be considered. The former may be accompanied by capture and fusion beats, whereas the latter is not.

Table 19.6. Differential Diagnosis of Wide QRS Tachycardias

Ventricular tachycardia
Atrial fibrillation or flutter with BBB
Supraventricular tachycardia (atrial, AV nodal, or AV) with BBB
Atrial fibrillation or flutter with conduction over AP
Atrial tachycardia with conduction over AP
Antidromic AV reentrant tachycardia
Reentry using one AP for antegrade and another AP for retrograde conduction
Reentry incorporating Mahaim fibers
AV nodal reentrant tachycardia with conduction of atrial echoes over a "bystander" AP
AV nodal reentrant tachycardia with antegrade conduction over a "bystander" Mahaim fiber
Atrial fibrillation or flutter over a "bystander" Mahaim fiber

AP = Accessory pathway; AV = Atrioventricular; BBB = Bundle branch block.

When the RR interval is regular, the P wave is not visible, or responses to carotid massage are not apparent, electrophysiologic studies are necessary in the differential diagnosis. Recordings of the atrial electrogram will unravel the relation of P wave and QRS complex and facilitate the differentiation among various tachycardias. If a 1:1 relation of P to QRS interval is present, His bundle recording is extremely useful. A His bundle deflection with an HV interval comparable to the supraventricular beat before each QRS complex is seen in patients with supraventricular tachycardias with antegrade normal pathway conduction. A His bundle deflection is not recorded before the QRS complex in ventricular tachycardia; it is usually hidden in the ventricular electrogram when 1:1 retrograde conduction is present. In patients with antidromic AV reentrant tachycardia, the His bundle deflection does not occur before the QRS complex, whereas in patients with reentrant tachycardia using one accessory pathway for antegrade conduction and another accessory pathway for retrograde conduction, or in patients with antegrade conduction over a "bystander" accessory pathway (such as atrial tachycardia or AV nodal reentrant tachycardia), the His bundle deflection either is absent or has a variable HV interval. In these patients, the QRS morphology is identical to that during rapid atrial pacing, the ventricle is activated immediately following the atrial impulse with a short AV interval, and an atrial extrastimulus delivered during tachycardia can advance the QRS complex with similar morphologic characteristics; analysis in the mode of tachycardia induction allows differentiation of tachycardias in these patients. When a "bystander" Mahaim fiber is involved in antegrade conduction, the HV interval is shorter than the normal HV interval and may be variable in the case of a nodoventricular connection; however, the QRS morphology is identical to that during atrial pacing and the ventricles are activated after an AV delay. As stated earlier, reentry incorporating a nodoventricular connection is characterized by no His bundle deflection before the QRS complex that has a left bundle branch block morphology. Atrioventricular dissociation is occasionally seen. The QRS morphology is identical to that during atrial pacing. In patients with ventricular tachycardia using the bundle branch system as the reentrant circuit, the QRS complex is identical to that during atrial pacing and is preceded by a His bundle deflection with an HV interval equal to or longer than that of the sinus beats. Atrioventricular dissociation can occur. Ventricular extrastimulus delivered during tachycardia can advance the His bundle deflection and the QRS complex with no change or a mild prolongation of the HV interval. Careful analysis in the mode of tachycardia induction is mandatory in accurate diagnosis.

SURVIVORS OF OUT-OF-HOSPITAL CARDIAC ARREST

Patients who survive an episode of out-of-hospital cardiac arrest are at high risk of sudden death. Continuous electrocardiographic monitoring in a limited number of patients in whom the event was recorded has demonstrated that ventricular tachycardia preceded ventricular fibrillation in most patients.[222] Electrophysiologic studies in these patients have demonstrated induction of ventricular tachycardia or ventricular fibrillation in 29% to 76%, depending on the aggressiveness of the stimulation protocol.[223-227] A drug regimen that prevents induction of ventricular tachycardia or ventricular fibrillation in patients who have induction of sustained ventricular tachycardia or fibrillation during a control state may prevent subsequent cardiac arrest. Some investigators have also demonstrated that patients surviving an episode of cardiac arrest but having no induction of ventricular tachycardia or fibrillation have a better prognosis than do those having induction of ventricular tachycardia or fibrillation.[226] The pathophysiologic aspects of the latter group of patients is unclear. It has been speculated that some reversible factors such as coronary artery spasm or ischemia may play a role in the genesis of cardiac arrest in these patients.

As mentioned earlier in the discussion of ventricular tachycardia, only a small number of patients with inducible ventricular tachycardia or ventricular fibrillation have responded to a conventional antiarrhythmic agent[175,176]; therefore, alternative therapeutic modalities such as endocardial resection of the focus, implantation of an automatic defibrillator, or electrocoagulation of the focus are required in most of these patients. In addition, failure to respond to amiodarone or propafenone in the catheterization laboratory does not necessarily predict subsequent failure when these agents are administered clinically.[177-180] Nevertheless, electrophysiologic studies with serial drug testings are useful in identifying a subset of patients who respond to less toxic conventional antiarrhythmic drugs with a well-defined pharmacology. Treatment with amiodarone or other experimental agents, implantation of an automatic defibrillator, or cardiac electrosurgery are reserved for those patients who fail to respond to conventional antiarrhythmic agents during electrophysiologic studies. Implantation of an automatic defibrillator or cardiac electrosurgery requires a comprehensive electrophysiologic study.[170,228,229]

PATIENTS WITH ACUTE MYOCARDIAL INFARCTION

Patients with acute myocardial infarction and bundle branch block are at increased risk for developing complete AV block, especially those with newly developed bundle branch block, those with bifascicular block, those with alternating bundle branch block, and those associated with first degree AV block.[230-232] Electrophysiologic studies are helpful in identifying a subgroup of patients at higher risk. The finding of a prolonged HV interval is associated with higher mortality and a higher incidence of progression to advanced AV block.[232] Prophylactic pacing is indicated in these patients. The presence of a normal HV interval is associated with a lower mortality and a minimal risk of developing advanced AV block, and such patients may be observed closely without pacemaker insertion. The roles of electrophysiologic study and implantation of a permanent pacemaker in patients who survive acute myocardial infarction and bundle branch block with progression to advanced AV block have remained unclear at the present time and require further studies.

Several indexes have been identified that are associated with a higher risk of sudden death in patients surviving acute myocardial infarction, but none has been shown to be sufficiently specific to warrant a specific therapy. Demonstration of electrical instability with induction of ventricular tachycardia or fibrillation with programmed ventricular stimulation before the patient is discharged from the hospital has been highly sensitive in identifying a subgroup of patients with subsequent sudden death or the development of spontaneous ventricular tachycardia.[233-235a] However, the technique is too nonspecific to warrant a specific therapy at the present time. Therefore, the role of electrophysiologic study in patients with acute myocardial infarction remains unsettled.

SYNCOPE OF UNEXPLAINED ETIOLOGY

Electrophysiologic studies may identify sinus node dysfunction, AV conduction abnormalities, and tachyarrhythmias in some patients with syncope of unexplained etiology. Some investigators have reported abnormal electrophysiologic findings in up to 56% to 68% of these patients, and that patients responded well to therapy based on electrophysiologic findings during follow-up.[236–239] However, these favorable results may be due in part to bias in patient selection and may not be representative of general patients with syncope of unexplained etiology.[240] Patients without organic heart disease are less likely to have a demonstrable electrophysiologic abnormality during electrophysiologic study. In addition, unexpected sustained monomorphic ventricular tachycardia may be induced in patients with an electrocardiographic abnormality, such as bundle branch block or ventricular preexcitation.[241,242]

INDICATIONS FOR ELECTROPHYSIOLOGIC STUDIES

Although analysis of the surface electrocardiogram along with other noninvasive diagnostic modalities, such as prolonged ambulatory electrocardiographic monitoring, treadmill exercise testing, application of carotid massage, or administration of atropine or isoproterenol are usually sufficient in the diagnosis and management of patients with cardiac arrhythmias, electrophysiologic studies can improve diagnostic, therapeutic, and prognostic decisions. Indications for electrophysiologic studies appear to include the following: (1) asymptomatic patients with chronic second degree AV block, both type I and type II, with or without bundle branch block; (2) asymptomatic patients with complete AV block, with a narrow or wide QRS escape rhythm; (3) patients with chronic bundle branch block and 1:1 AV conduction in whom symptoms of syncope or severe dizziness are unexplained; (4) patients with sinus node dysfunction in whom symptoms of syncope or severe dizziness cannot be related to the bradycardia episode; (5) patients with frequent troublesome paroxysmal supraventricular tachycardia; (6) patients with the Wolff–Parkinson–White syndrome and frequent troublesome paroxysmal supraventricular tachycardia or atrial fibrillation; (7) patients with recurrent ventricular tachycardia; (8) patients with recurrent wide QRS complex tachycardia of undetermined mechanism; (9) patients with tachyarrhythmias in whom invasive therapeutic modalities, such as surgical incision, electrocoagulation, or cryoablation of the focus, or implantation of antitachycardia pacemaker or automatic defibrillator are considered; (10) patients surviving out-of-hospital cardiac arrest; and (11) patients with syncope or severe dizziness in whom the causal mechanism is not defined.

REFERENCES

1. Scherlag BJ, Lau SH, Helfant RH, Berkowitz WD, Stein E, Damato AN: Catheter technique for recording His bundle activity in man. *Circulation* 1969; 39:13–18.
2. Damato AN, Lau SH, Helfant RH, Stein E, Berkowitz WD, Cohen SI: Study of atrioventricular conduction in man using electrode catheter recordings of His bundle activity. *Circulation* 1969; 39:287–296.
3. Narula OS, Scherlag BJ, Samet P: Pervenous pacing of the specialized conducting system in man: His bundle and A-V nodal stimulation. *Circulation* 1970; 41:71–87.
4. Rosen KM: Evaluation of cardiac conduction in the cardiac catheterization laboratory. *Am J Cardiol* 1972; 30:701–703.
5. Dhingra RC, Rosen KM, Rahimtoola SH: Normal conduction intervals and responses in 61 patients using His bundle recording and atrial pacing. *Chest* 1973; 64:55–59.
6. Narula OS, Scherlag BJ, Samet P, Javier RP: Atrioventricular block: localization and classification by His bundle recordings. *Am J Med* 1971; 50:146–165.
7. Castellanos A Jr, Castillo C, Agha A: Contribution of His bundle recording to the understanding of clinical arrhythmias. *Am J Cardiol* 1971; 28:499–509.
8. Wit AL, Weiss MB, Berkowitz WD, Rosen KM, Stein C, Damato AN: Patterns of atrioventricular conduction in the human heart. *Circ Res* 1970; 27:345–359.
9. Wit AL, Damato AN, Weiss MB, Steiner C: Phenomenon of the gap in atrioventricular conduction in the human heart. *Circ Res* 1970; 27:679–689.
10. Denes P, Wu D, Dhingra R, Pietras RJ, Rosen KM: The effects of cycle length on cardiac refractory periods in man. *Circulation* 1974; 49:32–41.
11. Schuilenburg RM: Patterns of V-A conduction in the human heart in the presence of normal and abnormal A-V conduction, in Wellens HJJ, Lie KI, Janse MJ, (eds): *The Conduction System of the Heart.* Philadelphia, Lea & Febiger, 1976, pp 485–503.
12. Akhtar M, Damato AN, Batsford WP, Ruskin JN, Ogunkelu JB: A comparative analysis of antegrade and retrograde conduction patterns in man. *Circulation* 1975; 52:766–778.
13. Narula OS: Retrograde pre-excitation. Comparison of antegrade and retrograde conduction intervals in man. *Circulation* 1974; 50:1129–1143.
14. Schuilenburg RM, Durrer D: Rate-dependency of functional block in the human His bundle and bundle branch-Purkinje system. *Circulation* 1973; 48:526–540.
15. Ferrer MI: The sick sinus syndrome. Its status after ten years (editorial). *Chest* 1977; 72:554–555.
16. Kaplan BM: Sick sinus syndrome (editorial). *Arch Intern Med* 1978; 138:28.
17. Bower PJ: Sick sinus syndrome. *Arch Intern Med* 1978; 138:133–137.
18. Kaplan BM: The tachycardia-bradycardia syndrome. *Med Clin North Am* 1976; 60:81–89.
19. Mandel WJ, Hayakawa H, Danzig R, Marcus HS: Evaluation of sinoatrial node function in man by overdrive pacing. *Circulation* 1971; 44:59–65.
20. Narula OS, Samet P, Javier RP: Significance of the sinus-node recovery time. *Circulation* 1972; 45:140–156.
21. Strauss HC, Saroff AL, Bigger JT Jr, Giardina EGV: Premature atrial stimulation as a key to the understanding of sinoatrial conduction in man. *Circulation* 1973; 47:86–93.
22. Narula OS, Shantha N, Vasquez M, Towne WD, Linhart JW: A new method for measurement of sinoatrial conduction time. *Circulation* 1978; 58:706–714.
23. Hariman RJ, Krongrad E, Boxer RA, Weiss MB, Steeg CN, Hoffman BF: Method for recording electrical activity of the sinoatrial node and automatic atrial foci during cardiac catheterization in human subjects. *Am J Cardiol* 1980; 45:775–781.
24. Reiffel JA, Gang E, Gliklich J, Weiss MB, Davis JC, Patton JN, Bigger JT Jr: The human sinus node electrogram: a transvenous catheter technique and a comparison of directly measured and indirectly estimated sinoatrial conduction time in adults. *Circulation* 1980; 62:1324–1335.
25. Mandel WJ, Hayakawa H, Allen HN, Danzig R, Kermair AI: Assessment of sinus node function in patients with the sick sinus syndrome. *Circulation* 1972; 46:761–769.
26. Benditt DG, Strauss HC, Scheinman MM, Behar VS, Wallace AG: Analysis of secondary pauses following termination of rapid atrial pacing in man. *Circulation* 1976; 54:436–441.
27. Dhingra RC, Wyndham C, Amat-y-Leon F, Denes P, Wu D, Rosen KM: Sinus nodal responses to atrial extrastimuli in patients without apparent sinus node disease. *Am J Cardiol* 1975; 36:445–452.
28. Reiffel JA, Bigger JT Jr, Kontam MA: The relationship between sinoatrial conduction time and sinus cycle length during spontaneous sinus arrhythmias in adults. *Circulation* 1974; 50:924–934.
29. Breithardt G, Seipel L: The effect of premature atrial depolarization on sinus node automaticity in man. *Circulation* 1976; 53:920–925.
30. Strauss HC, Bigger JT Jr, Saroff AL, Giardina EGV: Electrophysiologic evaluation of sinus node function in patients with sinus node dysfunction. *Circulation* 1976; 53:763–776.
31. Dhingra RC, Amat-y-Leon F, Wyndham C, Deedwania PC, Wu D, Denes P, Rosen KM: Clinical significance of prolonged sinoatrial conduction time. *Circulation* 1977; 55:8–15.
32. Gann D, Tolentino A, Samet P: Electrophysiologic evaluation of elderly patients with sinus bradycardia. *Ann Intern Med* 1979; 90:24–29.

33. Gomes JAC, Hariman RI, Chowdry IA: New application of direct sinus node recordings in man: assessment of sinus node recovery time. *Circulation* 1984; 70:663–671.
34. Castillo-Fenoy A, Achard TF, Langenhagen B: Etude du mécanisme de la pause auriculaire par l'enregistrement endocavitaire du potential sinusal chez l'homme. *Arch Mal Coeur* 1980; 73:805–814.
35. Asseman P, Berzin B, Desry D, Vilarem D, Durand P, Delmotte C, Sarkis EH, Lekieffre J, Thery C: Persistent sinus nodal electrograms during abnormally prolonged postpacing atrial pauses in sick sinus syndrome in humans: sinoatrial block vs overdrive suppression. *Circulation* 1983; 68:33–41.
36. Gang ES, Oseran DS, Mandel WJ, Peter T: Sinus node electrogram in patients with the hypersensitive carotid sinus syndrome. *J Am Coll Cardiol* 1985; 5:1484–1490.
37. Jordan JL, Yamaguchi I, Mandel WJ: Studies on the mechanism of sinus node dysfunction in the sick sinus syndrome. *Circulation* 1977; 57:217–222.
38. Kang PS, Gomes JAC, Kelen G, El-Sherif N: Role of autonomic regulatory mechanisms in sinoatrial conduction and sinus node automaticity in sick sinus syndrome. *Circulation* 1981; 64:832–838.
39. Desai JM, Scheinman MM, Strauss HC, Massie B, O'Young J: Electrophysiologic effects of combined autonomic blockade in patients with sinus node disease. *Circulation* 1981; 63:953–960.
40. Zipes DP, Dejoseph RL: Dissimilar atrial rhythms in man and dog. *Am J Cardiol* 1973; 32:618–628.
41. Wu D, Denes P, Amat-y-Leon F, Wyndham C, Chablani RC, Rosen KM: Limitations of the surface electrocardiogram in diagnosis of atrial arrhythmias: further observations on dissimilar atrial rhythm. *Am J Cardiol* 1975; 36:91–97.
42. Vergara GS, Hildner FJ, Schoenfeld CB, Javier RP, Cohen LS, Samet P: Conversion of supraventricular tachycardia with rapid atrial stimulation. *Circulation* 1972; 46:788–793.
43. Waldo AL, Maclean WAH, Karp RB, Kouchoukos NT, James TN: Entrainment and interruption of atrial flutter with atrial pacing: studies in man following open heart surgery. *Circulation* 1977; 56:737–745.
44. Damato AN, Lau SH, Helfant R, Stein E, Patton RD, Scherlag BJ, Berkowitz WD: A study of heart block in man using His bundle recordings. *Circulation* 1969; 39:297–305.
45. Rosen KM, Rahimtoola SH, Chuquimia R, Loeb HS, Gunnar RM: Electrophysiological significance of first degree atrioventricular block with intraventricular conduction. *Circulation* 1971; 43:491–502.
46. Rosen KM, Loeb HS, Chuquimia R, Sinno MZ, Rahimtoola SH, Gunnar RM: Site of heart block in acute myocardial infarction. *Circulation* 1970; 42:925–933.
47. Dhingra RC, Denes P, Wu D, Chuquimia R, Rosen KM: The natural history of second degree A-V block and bundle branch block: observations regarding site and type of block. *Circulation* 1974; 49:638–646.
48. Schuilenburg RM, Durrer D: Conduction disturbances located within His bundle. *Circulation* 1972; 45:612–628.
49. Amat-y-Leon F, Dhingra RC, Denes P, Wu D, Wyndham C, Chuquimia R, Rosen KM: The clinical spectrum of chronic His bundle block. *Chest* 1976; 70:747–754.
50. Guimond C, Puech P: Intra-His bundle blocks (102 cases). *Eur J Cardiol* 1976; 4:481–493.
51. Rosen KM, Dhingra RC, Loeb HS, Rahimtoola SH: Chronic heart block in adults: clinical and electrophysiological observations. *Arch Intern Med* 1973; 131:663–672.
52. Schuilenburg RM, Durrer D: Observation on atrioventricular conduction in patients with bilateral bundle branch block. *Circulation* 1970; 41:967–979.
53. Narula OS, Samet P: Right bundle branch block with normal, left or right axis deviation. *Am J Med* 1971; 51:432–455.
54. Rosen KM, Ehsani A, Rahimtoola SH: H-V intervals in left bundle-branch block: clinical and electrocardiographic correlations. *Circulation* 1972; 46:717–723.
55. Wu D, Denes P, Dhingra R, Amat-y-Leon F, Wyndham D, Chuquimia R, Rosen KM: Electrophysiological and clinical observations in patients with alternating bundle branch block. *Circulation* 1976; 53:456–464.
56. Dhingra RC, Palileo E, Strasberg B, Swiryn S, Bauernfeind RA, Wyndham CRC, Rosen KM: Significance of HV interval in 517 patients with chronic bifascicular block. *Circulation* 1981; 64:1265–1271.
57. McAnulty JH, Rahimtoola SH, Murphy E, DeMots H, Ritzmann L, Kanarek PE, Kaufman S: Natural history of "high risk" bundle branch block. Final report of a prospective study. *N Engl J Med* 1982; 307:137–143.
58. Scheinman MM, Peters RW, Sauve MJ, Desai J, Abott JA, Cogan J, Wohl B, Williams K: Value of the H-Q interval in patients with bundle branch block and the role of prophylactic permanent pacing. *Am J Cardiol* 1982; 50:1316–1322.
59. Dhingra RC, Wyndham C, Bauernfeind R, Swiryn S, Deedwania PC, Smith T, Denes P, Rosen KM: Significance of block distal to the His bundle induced by atrial pacing in patients with chronic bifascicular block. *Circulation* 1979; 60:1455–1464.
60. Rosen KM, Rahimtoola SH, Gunnar RM: Pseudo A-V block secondary to premature nonpropagated His bundle depolarizations: documentation by His bundle electrocardiography. *Circulation* 1970; 42:367–373.
61. Mines GR: On dynamic equilibrium in the heart. *J Physiol* 1913; 46:349–383.
62. Iliescu CC, Sebastiani A: Notes on the effects of quinidine upon paroxysms of tachycardia. *Heart* 1923; 10:223–231.
63. Moe GK, Preston JB, Burlington H: Physiologic evidence for a dual AV transmission system. *Circ Res* 1956; 4:357–375.
64. Schuilenburg RM, Durrer D: Atrial echo beats in the human heart elicited by induced atrial premature beats. *Circulation* 1968; 37:680–692.
65. Schuilenburg RM, Durrer D: Ventricular echo beats in the human heart elicited by induced ventricular premature beats. *Circulation* 1969; 40:337–347.
66. Denes P, Wu D, Dhingra RC, Chuquimia R, Rosen KM: Demonstration of dual AV pathways in patients with paroxysmal supraventricular tachycardia. *Circulation* 1973; 48:549–555.
67. Wu D, Denes P, Amat-y-Leon F, Dhingra R, Wyndham CRC, Bauernfeind R, Latif P, Rosen KM: Clinical, electrocardiographic, and electrophysiologic observations in patients with paroxysmal supraventricular tachycardia. *Am J Cardiol* 1978; 41:1045–1051.
68. Wu D: Dual atrioventricular nodal pathways: a reappraisal. *PACE* 1982; 5:72–89.
69. Goldreyer BN, Damato AN: Essential role of atrioventricular conduction delay in the initiation of paroxysmal supraventricular tachycardia. *Circulation* 1971; 43:679–687.
70. Wu D, Kou HC, Yeh SJ, Lin FC, Hung JS: Determinants of tachycardia induction using ventricular stimulation in dual pathway atrioventricular nodal reentrant tachycardia. *Am Heart J* 1984; 108:44–55.
71. Wu D, Denes P, Wyndham C, Amat-y-Leon F, Dhingra RC, Rosen KM: Demonstration of dual A-V nodal pathways utilizing a ventricular extra-stimulus in patients with A-V nodal reentrant paroxysmal supraventricular tachycardia. *Circulation* 1975; 52:789–798.
72. Wu D, Hung JS, Kou CT: Determinants of sustained slow pathway conduction and relation to reentrant tachycardia in patients with dual atrioventricular nodal transmission. *Am Heart J* 1981; 101:521–528.
73. Rosen KM, Metha A, Miller RA: Demonstration of dual atrioventricular nodal pathways in man. *Am J Cardiol* 1975; 33:291–294.
74. Wu D, Denes P, Dhingra RC, Wyndham C, Rosen KM: Determinants of fast and slow pathway conduction in patients with dual A-V nodal pathways. *Circ Res* 1975; 36:782–790.
75. Lin FC, Yeh SJ, Wu D: Determinants of simultaneous fast and slow pathway conduction in patients with dual atrioventricular nodal pathways. *Am Heart J* 1985; 109:963–970.
76. Gomes JAC, Kang PS, Kelen G, Khan R, El-Sherif N: Simultaneous anterograde fast-slow atrioventricular nodal pathway conduction after procainamide. *Am J Cardiol* 1980; 46:677–684.
77. Csapo G: Paroxysmal non-reentrant tachycardias due to simultaneous conduction in dual atrioventricular nodal pathways. *Am J Cardiol* 1979; 43:1033–1045.
78. Sutton FJ, Lee YC: Supraventricular non-reentrant tachycardia due to simultaneous conduction through dual atrioventricular nodal pathways. *Am J Cardiol* 1983; 51:897–900.
79. Coumel P: Junctional reciprocating tachycardia. The permanent and paroxysmal forms of AV nodal reciprocating tachycardias. *J Electrocardiol* 1975; 8:79–90.
80. Wu D, Denes P, Amat-y-Leon F, Wyndham CRC, Dhingra RC, Rosen KM: An unusual variety of A-V nodal reentry due to retrograde dual A-V nodal pathway. *Circulation* 1977; 56:50–59.
81. Denes P, Wu D, Amat-y-Leon F, Dhingra RC, Wyndham CR, Rosen KM: The determinants of reentrance in patients with dual A-V nodal pathways. *Circulation* 1977; 56:253–259.
82. Josephson ME, Seides SE, Batsford WB, Caracta AR, Damato AN, Kastor JA: The effects of carotid sinus pressure in re-entrant paroxysmal supraventricular tachycardia. *Am Heart J* 1974; 88:694–697.
83. Waxman MB, Bonet JF, Finley JP, Wald RW: Effects of respiration and posture on paroxysmal supraventricular tachycardia. *Circulation* 1980; 62:1011–1020.
84. Wu D, Denes P, Bauernfeind R, Dhingra RC, Wyndham C, Rosen KM: Effects of atropine on induction and maintenance of A-V nodal reentrant tachycardia. *Circulation* 1979; 59:779–788.
85. Hariman RJ, Gomes JAC, El-Sherif N: Catecholamine-dependent atrioventricular nodal reentrant tachycardia. *Circulation* 1983; 67:681–686.
86. Wu D, Wyndham C, Amat-y-Leon F, Denes P, Dhingra RC, Rosen KM: The effects of ouabain on induction of atrioventricular nodal reentrant paroxysmal supraventricular tachycardia. *Circulation* 1975; 52:201–207.
87. Wu D, Denes P, Dhingra R, Kahn A, Rosen KM: The effects of propranolol on induction of A-V nodal reentrant paroxysmal tachycardia. *Circulation* 1974; 50:665–677.
88. Wellens HJJ, Düren DR, Liem KL, Lie KI: Effects of digitalis in patients with paroxysmal atrioventricular nodal tachycardia. *Circulation* 1975; 52:779–788.

89. Rinkenberger RL, Prystowsky EN, Heger JJ, Troup PJ, Jackman WM, Zipes DP: Effects of intravenous and chronic oral verapamil administration in patients with supraventricular tachyarrhythmias. *Circulation* 1980; 62:996–1010.

90. Sung RJ, Elser B, McAllister RG Jr: Intravenous verapamil for termination of re-entrant supraventricular tachycardias. Intracardiac studies correlated with plasma verapamil concentrations. *Ann Intern Med* 1980; 93:682–689.

91. Yeh SJ, Kou HC, Lin FC, Hung JS, Wu D: Effects of oral diltiazem in paroxysmal supraventricular tachycardia. *Am J Cardiol* 1983; 52:271–278.

92. DiMarco JP, Sellers TD, Berne RM, West GA, Belardinelli L: Adenosine: electrophysiologic effects and therapeutic use for terminating paroxysmal supraventricular tachycardia. *Circulation* 1983; 68:1254–1263.

93. Bauernfeind RA, Wyndham CR, Dhingra R, Swiryn SP, Palileo E, Strasberg B, Rosen KM: Serial electrophysiologic testing of multiple drugs in patients with atrioventricular nodal reentrant paroxysmal tachycardia. *Circulation* 1980; 62:1341–1349.

94. Wu D, Denes P, Bauernfeind R, Kehoe R, Amat-y-Leon F, Rosen KM: Effects of procainamide on A-V nodal reentrant paroxysmal tachycardia. *Circulation* 1983; 57:1171–1179.

95. Wu D, Hung JS, Kuo CT, Hsu KS, Shieh WB: Effects of quinidine on atrioventricular nodal reentrant paroxysmal tachycardia. *Circulation* 1981; 64:823–831.

96. Sethi KK, Jaishankar S, Gupta MP: Salutary effects of intravenous ajmaline in patients with paroxysmal supraventricular tachycardia mediated by dual atrioventricular nodal pathways: blockade of the retrograde fast pathway. *Circulation* 1984; 70:876–883.

97. Anderson RH, Becker AE, Brechenmacher C, Davies MJ, Rossi L: Ventricular pre-excitation. A proposed nomenclature for its substrates. *Eur J Cardiol* 1975; 3:27–36.

98. Becker AE, Anderson RH, Durrer D, Wellens HJJ: The anatomical substrates of Wolff–Parkinson–White syndrome. A clinicopathologic correlation in seven patients. *Circulation* 1978; 57:870–879.

99. Gallagher JJ, Pritchett ELC, Sealy WC, Kasell J, Wallace AG: The preexcitation syndromes. *Prog Cardiovasc Dis* 1978; 20:285–327.

100. Durrer D, Schoo L, Schuilenburg RM, Wellens HJJ: The role of premature beats in the initiation and the termination of supraventricular tachycardia in the Wolff-Parkinson-White syndrome. *Circulation* 1967; 36:644–662.

101. Wellens HJJ, Durrer D: The role of an accessory atrioventricular pathway in reciprocal tachycardia: observations in patients with and without the Wolff-Parkinson-White syndrome. *Circulation* 1975; 52:58–72.

102. Coumel P, Attuel P, Flammang D: The role of the conduction system in supraventricular tachycardia, in Wellens HJJ, Lie H, Janse MJ (eds): *The Conduction System of the Heart*. Leiden, HE Stenfert Kroese BV, 1976, pp 424–452.

103. Barold SS, Coumel P: Mechanisms of atrioventricular junctional tachycardia: role of reentry and concealed accessory bypass tracts. *Am J Cardiol* 1977; 39:97–106.

104. Coumel P, Attuel P: Reciprocating tachycardia in overt and latent preexcitation. Influence of bundle branch block on the rate of the tachycardia. *Eur J Cardiol* 1974; 1:423–436.

105. Zipes DP, DeJoseph RL, Rothbaum DA: Unusual properties of accessory pathways. *Circulation* 1974; 49:1200–1211.

106. Neuss H, Schlepper M, Thormann J: Analysis of reentry mechanisms in three patients with concealed Wolff-Parkinson-White syndrome. *Circulation* 1975; 51:75–81.

107. Wellens HJJ, Schuilenberg RM, Durrer D: Electrical stimulation of the heart in patients with Wolff–Parkinson–White syndrome Type A. *Circulation* 1971; 43:99–114.

108. Denes P, Wyndham CR, Amat-y-Leon F, Wu D, Dhingra RC, Miller RH, Rosen KM: Atrial pacing at multiple sites in the Wolff–Parkinson–White syndrome. *Br Heart J* 1977; 39:506–514.

109. Svenson RH, Miller HC, Gallagher JJ, Wallace AG: Electrophysiological evaluation of the Wolff–Parkinson–White syndrome: problems in assessing antegrade and retrograde conduction over the accessory pathway. *Circulation* 1975; 52:552–562.

110. Gallagher JJ, Sealy WC, Wallace AG, Kassel J: Correlation between catheter electrophysiologic studies and findings on mapping of ventricular exitation in the Wolff–Parkinson–White syndrome, in Wellen HJJ, Lie KI, Janse MJ (eds): *The Conduction System of the Heart.* Leiden, HE Stenfert Kroese BV, 1976, pp 588–630.

111. Amat-y-Leon F, Dhingra RC, Wu D, Denes P, Wyndham C, Rosen KM: Catheter mapping of retrograde atrial activation: observations during ventricular pacing and A-V nodal reentrant paroxysmal tachycardia. *Br Heart J* 1976; 38:355–362.

112. Sung RJ, Gelband H, Castellanos A, Aranda JM, Myerburg RJ: Clinical and electrophysiological observations in patients with concealed accessory atrioventricular bypass tracts. *Am J Cardiol* 1977; 40:839–847.

113. Spurrel RAJ, Krikler DM, Sowton E: Retrograde invasion of the bundle branches producing aberration of the QRS complex during supraventricular tachycardia studied by programmed electrical stimulation. *Circulation* 1974; 50:487–495.

114. Kerr CR, Gallagher JJ, German LD: Changes in ventriculoatrial intervals with bundle branch block aberration during reciprocating tachycardia in patients with accessory atrioventricular pathways. *Circulation* 1982; 66:196–201.

115. Wu D, Kou HC, Yeh SJ, Lin FC, Hung JS: Effects of oral verapamil in patients with atrioventricular reentrant tachycardia incorporating an accessory pathway. *Circulation* 1983; 67:425–433.

116. Betriu A, Chaitman BR, Bourassa MG, Brévers G, Scholl JM, Bruneau P, Gagné P, Chabot M: Beneficial effect of intravenous diltiazem in the acute management of supraventricular tachyarrhythmias. *Circulation* 1983; 67:88–94.

117. Wellens HJJ, Durrer D: Effect of digitalis on atrioventricular conduction and circus-movement tachycardias in patients with Wolff–Parkinson–White syndrome. *Circulation* 1973; 47:1229–1233.

118. Wu D, Amat-y-Leon F, Simson RJ, Latif P, Wyndham CR, Denes P, Rosen KM: Electrophysiological studies with multiple drugs in patients with atrioventricular reentrant tachycardias utilizing an extranodal pathway. *Circulation* 1977; 56:727–736.

119. Dhingra RC, Palileo EV, Strasberg B, Swiryn S, Bauernfeind R, Wyndham C, Rosen KM: Electrophysiologic effects of ouabain in patients with preexcitation and circus movement tachycardia. *Am J Cardiol* 1981; 47:139–144.

120. Denes P, Cummings JM, Simpson R, Wu D, Amat-y-Leon F, Dhingra R, Rosen KM: Effects of propranolol on anomalous pathway refractoriness and circus movement tachycardias in patients with preexcitation. *Am J Cardiol* 1978; 41:1061–1067.

121. Wellens HJJ, Durrer D: Effect of procainamide, quinidine, and ajmaline in the Wolff–Parkinson–White syndrome. *Circulation* 1974; 50:114–120.

122. Sellers TD, Campbell RWF, Bashore TM, Gallagher JJ: Effects of procainamide and quinidine sulfate in the Wolff–Parkinson–White syndrome. *Circulation* 1977; 55:15–22.

123. Kou HC, Hung JS, Lee YS, Wu D: Effects of oral disopyramide phosphate on induction and sustenance of atrioventricular reentrant tachycardia incorporating retrograde accessory pathway conduction. *Circulation* 1982; 66:454–462.

124. Kerr CR, Prystowsky EN, Smith WM, Cook L, Gallagher JJ: Electrophysiologic effects of disopyramide phosphate in patients with Wolff–Parkinson–White syndrome. *Circulation* 1982; 65:869–878.

125. Wellens HJJ, Lie KI, Bär FW, Wesdorp JC, Dohmen HJ, Düren DR, Durrer D: Effect of amiodarone in the Wolff–Parkinson–White syndrome. *Am J Cardiol* 1978; 38:189–194.

126. Alboni P, Shantha N, Pirani R, Baggioni F, Scarfo S, Tomasi AM, Masoni A: Effects of amiodarone on supraventricular tachycardia involving bypass tracts. *Am J Cardiol* 1984; 53:93–98.

127. Brady GH, Packer DL, German LD, Gallagher JJ: Preexcited reciprocating tachycardia in patients with Wolff–Parkinson–White syndrome: incidence and mechanisms. *Circulation* 1984; 70:377–391.

128. Brugada P, Bar FWHM, Vanagt EJ, Friedman PL, Wellens HJJ: Observations in patients showing A-V junctional echoes with a shorter P-R than R-P interval: distinction between intranodal reentry or reentry using an accessory pathway with a long conduction time. *Am J Cardiol* 1981; 48:611–622.

129. Gallagher JJ, Sealy WC: The permanent form of junctional reciprocating tachycardia: further elucidation of the underlying mechanism. *Eur J Cardiol* 1978; 8/4–5:413–430.

130. Farre J, Ross D, Wiener I, Bar FW, Vanagt EJ, Wellens HJJ: Reciprocal tachycardias using accessory pathways with long conduction times. *Am J Cardiol* 1979; 44:1099–1109.

131. Guarnieri T, Sealy WC, Kasell JH, German LD, Gallagher JJ: The nonpharmacologic management of the permanent form of junctional reciprocating tachycardia. *Circulation* 1984; 69:269–277.

132. Sung RJ, Styperek J: Electrophysiologic identification of dual atrioventricular nodal pathway conduction in patients with reciprocating tachycardia using anomalous bypass tracts. *Circulation* 1979; 60:1464–1476.

133. Denes P, Amat-y-Leon F, Wyndham C, Wu D, Levitsky S, Rosen KM: Electrophysiologic demonstration of bilateral anomalous pathways in a patient with Wolff–Parkinson–White syndrome (type B preexcitation). *Am J Cardiol* 1976; 37:93–101.

134. Kou HC, Lin FC, Hung JS, Wu D: Demonstration of bilateral anomalous pathways in a patient with the Wolff–Parkinson–White syndrome. *J Form Med Assoc* 1981; 80:457–464.

135. Gallagher JJ, Sealy WC, Kasell J, Wallace AG: Multiple accessory pathways in patients with the pre-excitation syndrome. *Circulation* 1976; 54:571–591.

136. Cinca J, Valle V, Gutierrez L, Figueras J, Rius J: Reciprocating tachycardia using bilateral anomalous pathways: electrophysiologic and clinical implications. *Circulation* 1980; 62:657–661.

137. Campbell RWF, Smith RA, Gallagher JJ, Pritchett El, Wallace AG: Atrial

fibrillation in the preexcitation syndrome. *Am J Cardiol* 1977; 40:514–520.

138. Sellers TD, Bashore TM, Gallagher JJ: Digitalis in the preexcitation syndrome: analysis during atrial fibrillation. *Circulation* 1977; 56:260–267.
139. Sung RJ, Castellanos A, Mallon SM, Bloom MG, Gelband H, Myerburg RJ: Mechanisms of spontaneous alternation between reciprocating tachycardia and atrial flutter-fibrillation in the Wolff–Parkinson–White syndrome. *Circulation* 1977; 56:409–416.
140. Caracta AR, Damato AN, Gallagher JJ, Josephson ME, Varghese PJ, Lau SH, Westura EE: Electrophysiologic studies in the syndrome of short P-R interval, normal QRS complex. *Am J Cardiol* 1973; 31:245–253.
141. Bissett JK, DeSoyza N, Kane JJ, Murphy ML: Altered refractory periods in patients with short P-R intervals and normal QRS complex. *Am J Cardiol* 1975; 35:487–491.
142. Jackman WM, Prystowsky EN, Nacarrelli GV, Fineberg NS, Rahilly GT, Heger JJ, Zipes DP: Reevaluation of enhanced atrioventricular nodal conduction: evidence to suggest a continuum of normal atrioventricular nodal physiology. *Circulation* 1983; 67:441–448.
143. Benditt DG, Pritchett ELC, Smith WM, Wallace AG, Gallagher JJ: Characteristics of atrioventricular conduction and the spectrum of arrhythmias in Lown-Ganong-Levine syndrome. *Circulation* 1978; 57:454–465.
144. Gallagher JJ, Smith WM, Kasell JH, Benson DW, Sterba R, Grant AO: Role of Mahaim fibers in cardiac arrhythmias in man. *Circulation* 1981; 64:176–189.
145. Morady F, Scheinman MM, Gonzalez R, Hess D: His-ventricular dissociation in a patient with reciprocating tachycardia and a nodoventricular bypass tract. *Circulation* 1981; 64:839–844.
146. Narula OS: Sinus node re-entry: a mechanism for supraventricular tachycardia. *Circulation* 1974; 50:1114–1128.
147. Wu D, Amat-y-Leon F, Denes P, Dhingra RC, Pietras RJ, Rosen KM: Demonstration of sustained sinus and atrial reentry as a mechanism of paroxysmal supraventricular tachycardia. *Circulation* 1975; 51:234–243.
148. Hoffman BF, Rosen MR: Cellular mechanisms of cardiac arrhythmias. *Circ Res* 1981; 49:1–14.
149. Antzelevitch C, Jalife J, Moe GK: Characteristics of reflection as a mechanism of reentrant arrhythmias and its relationship to parasystole. *Circulation* 1980; 61:182–191.
150. Antzelevitch C, Moe GK: Electrotonically mediated delayed conduction and reentry in relation to "slow responses" in mammalian ventricular conducting tissue. *Circ Res* 1981; 49:1129–1139.
151. Allessie MA, Bonke FIM, Schopman FJG: Circus movement in rabbit atrial muscle as a mechanism of tachycardia. *Circ Res* 1977; 41:9–18.
152. Wu D: What is the value of calcium antagonist for ventricular tachycardia? *International J Cardiol* 1984; 5:543–547.
153. Wellens HJ, Schiulenburg RM, Durrer D: Electrical stimulation of the heart in patients with ventricular tachycardia. *Circulation* 1972; 46:216–226.
154. Wellens HJJ, Lie KI, Durrer D: Further observations on ventricular tachycardia as studies by electrical stimulation of the heart: chronic recurrent ventricular tachycardia and ventricular tachycardia during acute myocardial infarction. *Circulation* 1974; 49:647–653.
155. Denes P, Wu D, Dhingra RC, Amat-y-Leon F, Wyndham C, Mautner R, Rosen KM: Electrophysiological studies in patients with chronic recurrent ventricular tachycardia. *Circulation* 1976; 54:229–236.
156. Wellens HJJ, Duren DR, Lie KI: Observations on mechanisms of ventricular tachycardia in man. *Circulation* 1976; 54:237–244.
157. Brugada P, Green M, Abdollah H, Wellens HJJ: Significance of ventricular arrhythmias initiated by programmed ventricular stimulation: the importance of the type of ventricular arrhythmia induced and the number of premature stimuli required. *Circulation* 1984; 69:87–92.
158. Mann DE, Luck JC, Griffin JC, Herre JM, Limacher MC, Margo SA, Robertson NW, Wyndham CRC: Induction of clinical ventricular tachycardia using programmed stimulation: value of third and fouth extrastimuli. *Am J Cardiol* 1983; 52:501–506.
159. Buxton AE, Waxman HL, Marchlinski FE, Untereker WJ, Waspe LE, Josephson ME: Role of triple extrastimuli during electrophysiologic study of patients with documented sustained ventricular tachyarrhythmias. *Circulation* 1984; 69:532–540.
160. Morady F, DiCarlo L, Winston S, Davis JC, Scheinman MM: A prospective comparison of triple extrastimuli and left ventricular stimulation in studies of ventricular tachycardia induction. *Circulation* 1984; 70:52–57.
161. Naccarelli GV, Prystowsky EN, Jackman WM, Heger JJ, Rahilly GT, Zipes DP: Role of electrophysiologic testing in managing patients who have ventricular tachycardia unrelated to coronary artery disease. *Am J Cardiol* 1982; 50:165–171.
162. Josephson ME, Horowitz LN, Farshidi A, Spielman SR, Michelson EL, Greenspan AM: Recurrent sustained ventricular tachycardia. 4. Pleomorphism. *Circulation* 1979; 59:459–468.
163. Josephson ME, Horowitz LN, Waxman HL, Cain ME, Spielman SR, Greenspan AM, Marchlinski FE, Ezri MD: Sustained ventricular tachycardia: role of the 12-lead electrocardiogram in localizing site of origin. *Circulation* 1981; 64:257–272.
164. Josephson ME, Horowitz LN, Farshidi A, Spear JF, Kastor JA, Moore EN: Recurrent sustained ventricular tachycardia. 2. Endocardial mapping. *Circulation* 1978; 57:440–447.
165. Horowitz LN, Josephson ME, Harken AH: Endocardial and epicardial activation during sustained ventricular tachycardia in man. *Circulation* 1980; 61:1227–1238.
166. Josephson ME, Horowitz LN, Spielman SR, Greenspan AM, VandePol C, Harken AH: Comparison of endocardial catheter mapping with intraoperative mapping of ventricular tachycardia. *Circulation* 1980; 61:395–404.
167. Waspe LE, Brodman R, Kim SG, Matos JA, Johnston DR, Scavin GM, Fisher JD: Activation mapping in patients with coronary artery disease with multiple ventricular tachycardia configurations: occurrence and therapeutic implications of widely separate apparent sites of origin. *J Am Coll Cardiol* 1985; 5:1075–1086.
168. Gallagher JD, Rossi AJD, Fernandez J, Maranhao V, Strong MD, White M, Gessman LJ: Cryothermal mapping of recurrent ventricular tachycardia in man. *Circulation* 1985; 71:733–739.
169. Josephson ME, Horowitz LN, Farshidi A: Continuous local electrical activity: a mechanism of recurrent ventricular tachycardia. *Circulation* 1978; 57:659–665.
170. Josephson ME, Harken AH, Horowitz LN: Endocardial excision: a new surgical technique for the treatment of recurrent ventricular tachycardia. *Circulation* 1979; 60:1430–1439.
171. Josephson ME, Horowitz LN, Spielman SR, Waxman HL, Greenspan AM: Role of catheter mapping in the preoperative evaluation of ventricular tachycardia. *Am J Cardiol* 1982; 49:207–220.
172. Mason JW, Stinson EB, Winkle RA, Griffin JC, Oyer PE, Ross DL, Derby G: Surgery for ventricular tachycardia: efficacy of left ventricular aneurysm resection compared with operation guided by electrical activation mapping. *Circulation* 1982; 65:1148–1155.
173. Wu D, Wyndham RC, Amat-y-Leon F, Miller R, Dhingra RC, Rosen KM: Chronic electrophysiological study in patients with recurrent paroxysmal tachycardia: a new method for developing successful oral antiarrhythmic therapy, in Kulbertus H (ed): *Reentrant Arrhythmias—Mechanisms and Therapy.* Lancaster, England, MTP Press, 1977, pp 294–311.
174. Fisher JD, Cohen HL, Mehra R, Altschuler H, Escher DJW, Furman S: Cardiac pacing and pacemakers. II. Serial electrophysiologic–pharmacologic testing for control of recurrent tachyarrhthmias. *Am Heart J* 1977; 93:658–668.
175. Horowitz LN, Josephson ME, Kastor JA: Intracardiac electrophysiologic studies as a method for the optimization of drug therapy in chronic ventricular arrhythmia. *Prog Cardiovas Dis* 1980; 23:81–98.
176. Swerdlow CD, Blum J, Winkle RA, Griffin JC, Ross DL, Mason JW: Decreased incidence of antiarrhythmic drug efficacy at electrophysiologic study associated with the use of a third extrastimulus. *Am Heart J* 1982; 104:1004–1011.
177. Heger JJ, Prystowsky EN, Jackman WM, Naccarelli, GV, Warfel KA, Rinkenberger RL, Zipes DP: Amiodarone. Clinical efficacy and electrophysiology during long-term therapy for recurrent ventricular tachycardia or ventricular fibrillation. *N Engl J Med* 1981; 305:539–545.
178. Hamer AW, Finerman WB Jr, Peter T, Mandel WJ: Disparity between the clinical and electrophysiologic effects of amiodarone in the treatment of recurrent ventricular tachyarrhythmias. *Am Heart J* 1981; 102:992–1000.
179. Waxman HL, Groh WC, Marchlinski FE, Buxton AE, Sadowski LM, Horowitz LN, Josephson ME, Kastor JA; Amiodarone for control of sustained ventricular tachyarrhythmias: clinical and electrophysiologic effects in 51 patients *Am J Cardiol* 1982; 50:1066–1074.
180. Chilson DA, Heger JJ, Zipes DP, Browne KF, Prystowsky EN: Electrophysiologic effects and clinical efficacy of oral propafenone therapy in patients with ventricular tachycardia. *J Am Coll Cardiol* 1985; 5:1407–1413.
181. Waldo AL, Henthorn RW, Plumb VJ, MacLean WAH: Demonstration of the mechanism of transient entrainment and interruption of ventricular tachycardia with rapid atrial pacing. *J Am Coll Cardiol* 1984; 3:422–430.
182. Anderson KP, Swerdlow CD, Mason JW: Entrainment of ventricular tachycardia. *Am J Cardiol* 1984; 53:335–340.
183. Mann DE, Lawrie GM, Luck JC, Griffin JC, Margo SA, Wyndham CRC: Importance of pacing site in entrainment of ventricular tachycardia. *J Am Coll Cardiol* 1985; 5:781–787.
184. Lin FC, Finley D, Rahimtoola SH, Wu D: Idiopathic paroxysmal ventricular tachycardia with a QRS pattern of right bundle branch block and left axis deviation: a unique clinical entity with specific properties. *Am J Cardiol* 1983; 52:95–100.

185. Zipes DP, Foster PR, Troup PJ, Pedersen DH: Atrial induction of ventricular tachycardia: reentry versus triggered automaticity. *Am J Cardiol* 1979; 44:1–8.
186. German LD, Packer DL, Bardy GH, Gallagher JJ: Ventricular tachycardia induced by atrial stimulation in patients without symptomatic cardiac disease. *Am J Cardiol* 1983; 52:1202–1207.
187. Mason JW, Swerdlow CD, Mitchell LB: Efficacy of verapamil in chronic, recurrent ventricular tachycardia. *Am J Cardiol* 1983; 51:1614–1617.
188. Marcus FI, Fontaine GH, Guiraudon G, Frank R, Laurenceau JL, Malergue C, Grosgogeat Y: Right ventricular dysplasia: a report of 24 adult cases. *Circulation* 1982; 65:384–398.
189. Cherrier F, Floquet J, Cuillière M, Niemann JL: Right ventricular dysplasia. A report of 7 cases. *Arch Mal Coeur* 1979; 71:963–972.
190. Rossi P, Massumi A, Gillette P, Hall RJ: Arrhythmogenic right ventricular dysplasia: clinical features, diagnostic techniques, and current management. *Am Heart J* 1982; 103:415–420.
191. Rosenfeld LE, Batsford WP: Intraventricular Wenckebach conduction and localized reentry in a case of right ventricular dysplasia with recurrent ventricular tachycardia. *J Am Coll Cardiol* 1983; 2:585–591.
192. Akhtar M, Damato AN, Batsford WP, Ruskin JN, Ogonkelu JB, Vargas G: Demonstration of reentry within the His-Purkinje system in man. *Circulation* 1974; 50:1150–1162.
193. Akhtar M, Gilbert C, Wolf FG, Schmidt DH: Reentry within the His-Purkinje system. Elucidation of reentrant circuit using right bundle branch and His bundle recordings. *Circulation* 1978; 58:295–304.
194. Touboul P, Kirkorian G, Atallah G, Moleur P: Bundle branch reentry: a possible mechanism of ventricular tachycardia. *Circulation* 1983; 67:674–680.
195. Gallavardin L: Extra-systolic ventricular a paroxysmes tachycardiques prolongés. *Arch Mal Coeur* 1922; 15:295–306.
196. Parkinson J, Papp C: Repetitive paroxysmal tachycardia. *Br Heart J* 1947; 9:241–262.
197. Rahilly GT, Prystowsky EN, Zipes DP, Naccarelli GV, Jackman WM, Hegger JJ: Clinical and electrophysiologic findings in patients with repetitive monomorphic ventricular tachycardia and otherwise normal electrocardiogram. *Am J Cardiol* 1982; 50:459–468.
198. Buxton AE, Marchlinski FE, Doherty JU, Cassidy DM, Vassallo JA, Flores BT, Josephson ME: Repetitive, monomorphic ventricular tachycardia: clinical and electrophysiologic characteristics in patients with and patients without organic heart disease. *Am J Cardiol* 1984; 54:997–1002.
199. Buxton AE, Waxman HL, Marchlinski FE, Josephson ME: Electropharmacology of nonsustained ventricular tachycardia: effects of class I antiarrhythmic agents, verapamil and propranolol. *Am J Cardiol* 1984; 53:738–744.
200. Foster PR, Elharrar V, Zipes DP: Accelerated ventricular escapes induced in the intact dog by barium, strontium and calcium. *J Pharm & Exp Ther* 1977; 200:373–383.
201. Vassalle M, Knob RE, Cummings M, Lara GA, Castro C, Stuckey JH: An analysis of fast idioventricular rhythm in the dog. *Circ Res* 1977; 41:218–226.
202. Dessertenne F: La tachycardie ventriculaire à deux foyers opposés variable. *Arch Mal Coeur* 1966; 59:263–272.
203. Krikler DM, Curry PVL: Torsade de pointes, an atypical ventricular tachycardia. *Br Heart J* 1976; 38:117–120.
204. Keren A, Tzivoni D, Gavish D, Levi J, Gottlieb S, Benhorin J, Stern S: Etiology, warning signs and therapy of torsade de pointes: a study of 10 patients. *Circulation* 1981; 64:1167–1174.
205. Kay GN, Plumb VJ, Arciniegas JG, Henthorn RW, Waldo AL: Torsade de pointes: the long-short initiating sequence and other clinical features: observations in 32 patients. *J Am Coll Cardiol* 1983; 2:806–817.
206. Tzivoni D, Keren A, Stern S: Torsade de pointes versus polymorphous ventricular tachycardia. *Am J Cardiol* 1983; 52:639–640.
207. Bardy GH, Ungerleider RM, Smith WM, Ideker RE: A mechanism of torsade de pointes in a canine model. *Circulation* 1983; 67:52–59.
208. Brachmann J, Scherlag BJ, Rosenshtraukh LV, Lazzara R: Bradycardia-dependent triggered activity: relevance to drug-induced multiform ventricular tachycardia. *Circulation* 1983; 68:846–856.
209. Schechter E, Freeman CC, Lazzara R: Afterdepolarizations as a mechanism for the long QT syndrome: electrophysiologic studies of a case. *J Am Coll Cardiol* 1984; 3:1556–1561.
210. Horowitz LN, Greenspan AM, Spielman SR, Josephson ME: Torsade de pointes: electrophysiologic studies in patients without transient pharmacologic or metabolic abnormalities. *Circulation* 1981; 63:1120–1128.
211. Sung RJ, Shen EN, Morady F, Scheinman MM, Hess D, Botvinik EH: Electrophysiologic mechanism of exercise-induced sustained ventricular tachycardia. *Am J Cardiol* 1983; 51:525–530.
212. Wu D, Kou HC, Hung JS: Exercise-triggered paroxysmal ventricular tachycardia. A repetitive rhythmic activity possibly related to afterdepolarization. *Ann Intern Med* 1981; 95:410–414.
213. Palileo EV, Ashley WW, Swiryn S, Bauernfeind RA, Strasberg B, Petropoulos T, Rosen KM: Exercise provocable right ventricular outflow tract tachycardia. *Am Heart J* 1982; 104:185–193.
213a. Higgins JR: Exercise induced sustained ventricular tachycardia in young healthy adults: clinical, electrophysiologic findings and treatment. *J Am Coll Cardiol* 1986; 7(suppl A):223A.
214. Sung RJ, Shapiro WA, Shen EN, Morady F, Davis J: Effects of verapamil on ventricular tachycardias possibly caused by reentry, automaticity, and triggered activity. *J Clin Invest* 1983; 72:350–360.
215. Woelfel A, Foster JR, Simpson RJ Jr, Gettes LS: Reproducibility and treatment of exercise-induced ventricular tachycardia. *Am J Cardiol* 1984; 53:751–756.
216. Moe GK, Jalife J, Mueller WJ, Moe B: A mathematical model of parasystole and its application to clinical arrhythmias. *Circulation* 1977; 56:968–979.
217. Kinoshita S: Mechanisms of ventricular arrhythmias: a theoretical model derived from the concepts of "electrotonic interaction" and "longitudinal dissociation." *Am J Cardiol* 1983; 52:1350–1354.
218. Castellanos A, Luceri RM, Moleiro F, Kayden DS, Trohman RG, Zaman L, Myerburg RJ: Annihilation, entrainment and modulation of ventricular parasystolic rhythms. *Am J Cardiol* 1984; 54:317–322.
219. Kastor JA, Goldreyer BN: Ventricular origin of bidirectional tachycardia. Case report of a patient not toxic from digitalis. *Circulation* 1973; 48:897–903.
220. Cohen SI, Deisseroth A, Hecht HS: Infra-His bundle origin of bidirectional tachycardia. *Circulation* 1973; 47:1260–1266.
221. Schaffer WA, Cobb LA: Recurrent ventricular fibrillation and modes of death in survivors of out-of-hospital ventricular fibrillation. *N Engl J Med* 1975; 293:259–262.
222. Pratt CM, Francis MJ, Luck JC, Wyndham CR, Miller RR, Quinones MA: Analysis of ambulatory electrocardiograms in 15 patients during spontaneous ventricular fibrillation with special reference to preceding arrhythmic events. *J Am Coll Cardiol* 1983; 2:789–797.
223. Myerburg RJ, Conde CA, Sung RJ, Mayorga-Cortes A, Mallon SM, Sheps DS, Appel RA, Castellanos A: Clinical, electrophysiologic and hemodynamic profile of patients resuscitated from prehospital cardiac arrest. *Am J Med* 1980; 68:568–576.
224. Ruskin JN, DiMarco JP, Garan H: Out-of-hospital cardiac arrest. Electrophysiologic observations and selection of long-term antiarrhythmic therapy. *N Engl J Med* 1980; 303:607–613.
225. Josephson ME, Horowitz LN, Spielman SR, Greenspan AM: Electrophysiologic and hemodynamic studies in patients resuscitated from cardiac arrest. *Am J Cardiol* 1980; 46:948–955.
226. Morady F, Scheinman MM, Hess DS, Sung RJ, Shen E, Shapiro W: Electrophysiologic testing in the management of survivors of out-of-hospital cardiac arrest. *Am J Cardiol* 1983; 51:85–89.
227. Benditt DG, Benson DW Jr, Klein GJ, Pritzker MR, Kriett JM, Anderson RW: Prevention of recurrent cardiac arrest: role of provocative electrophysiologic testing. *J Am Coll Cardiol* 1983; 2:418–425.
228. Mirowski M, Reid PR, Winkle RA, Mower MM, Watkins L Jr, Stinson EB, Griffith LSC, Kallman CH, Weisfeldt ML: Mortality in patients with implanted automatic defibrillators. *Ann Intern Med* 1983; 98:585–588.
229. Hartzler GO: Electrode catheter ablation of refractory focal ventricular tachycardia. *J Am Coll Cardiol* 1983; 2:1107–1113.
230. Hindman MC, Wagner GS, JaRo M, Atkins JM, Scheinman MM, DeSanctis RW, Hutter AH Jr, Yeatman L, Ruberfire M, Pujura C, Rubin M, Morris JJ: The clinical significance of bundle branch block complicating acute myocardial infarction. 1. Clinical characteristics, hospital mortality and one-year follow-up. *Circulation* 1978; 58:679–688.
231. Hindman MC, Wagner GS, JaRo M, Atkins JM, Scheinman MM, De Sanctis RW, Hutter AH Jr, Yeatman L, Rubenfire M, Pujura C, Rubin M, Morris JJ: The clinical significance of bundle branch block complicating acute myocardial infarction. 2. Indication for temporary and permanent pacemaker insertion. *Circulation* 1978; 58:689–699.
232. Lie KI, Wellens HJ, Schuilenburg RM: Bundle branch block and acute myocardial infarction, in Wellens HJJ, Lie KI, Janse MJ (eds): *The Conduction System of the Heart.* Leiden, HE Stenfert Kroese BV, 1976, pp 662–672.
233. Hamer A, Vohra J, Hunt D, Sloman G: Prediction of sudden death by electrophysiologic studies in high risk patients surviving acute myocardial infarction. *Am J Cardiol* 1982; 50:223–229.
234. Richards DA, Cody DV, Denniss AR, Russell PA, Young AA, Uther JB: Ventricular electrical instability: a predictor of death after myocardial infarction. *Am J Cardiol* 1983; 51:75–80.
235. Waspe LE, Seinfeld D, Ferrick A, Kim SG, Matos JA, Fisher JD: Prediction of sudden death and spontaneous ventricular tachycardia in survivors of complicated myocardial infarction: value of the response to programmed stimulation using a maximum of three ventricular extrastimuli. *J Am Col Cardiol* 1985; 5:1292–1301.
235a. Kiat H, Richards D, Ross D, Uther J: Prediction of late sustained ventricular tachyarrhythmias after myocardial infarction. *J Am Coll Cardiol* 1986; 7(suppl A):67A.
236. DiMarco JP, Garan H, Harthorne JW, Ruskin JN: Intracardiac electro-

physiologic techniques in recurrent syncope of unknown cause. *Ann Intern Med* 1981; 95:542–548.

237. Hess DS, Morady F, Scheinman MM: Electrophysiologic testing in the evaluation of patients with syncope of undetermined origin. *Am J Cardiol* 1982; 50:1309–1315.
238. Akhtar M, Shenasa M, Denker S, Gilbert CJ, Rizwi N: Role of cardiac electrophysiologic studies in patients with unexplained recurrent syncope. *PACE* 1983; 6:192–201.
239. Morady F, Shen E, Schwartz A, Hess D, Bhandari A, Sung RJ, Scheinman MM: Long-term follow-up of patients with recurrent unexplained syncope evaluated by electrophysiologic testing. *J Am Coll Cardiol* 1983; 2:1053–1059.
240. Dhingra RC, Denes P, Wu D, Chuquimia R, Amat-y-Leon F, Wyndham C, Rosen KM: Syncope in patients with chronic bifascicular block. Significance, causative mechanisms, and clinical implications. *Ann Intern Med* 1974; 81:302–306.
241. Lloyd EA, Hauer RN, Zipes DP, Heger JJ, Prystowsky EN: Syncope and ventricular tachycardia in patients with ventricular preexcitation. *Am J Cardiol* 1983; 52:79–82.
242. Morady F, Higgins J, Peters RW, Schwartz AB, Shen EN, Bhandari A, Scheinman MM, Sauvé J: Electrophysiologic testing in bundle branch block and unexplained syncope. *Am J Cardiol* 1984; 54:587–591.

20 Electrophysiologic Basis for the Treatment of Cardiac Arrhythmias

Yoshio Watanabe, MD

PECULIARITIES OF CARDIAC ARRHYTHMIAS

Cardiac arrhythmias have several peculiarities that must be given due consideration when their treatment is discussed. First, cardiac rhythm disturbances frequently occur in the presence of various organic lesions including ischemic heart disease, cardiomyopathy, myocarditis, valvular heart diseases, and so forth.[1,2] In these cases, treatment of underlying diseases or conditions is of prime importance, as attempts to abolish these arrhythmias may often fail unless overall pathophysiologic abnormalities caused by such diseases can be adequately controlled at the same time. However, almost any kind of arrhythmia can be observed also in the absence of demonstrable cardiac lesions, perhaps as a result of purely functional derangements. Direct antiarrhythmic therapy should naturally be the mainstay in those cases, although a search for factors facilitating arrhythmogenesis with subsequent correction of such factors often leads to more successful management. In this chapter, discussion will be focused on the management of arrhythmias per se, as the treatment of underlying heart disease will be covered in other chapters.

Second, cardiac arrhythmias are classified into more than 30 diagnostic entities,[1-3] and their clinical significance varies widely. For instance, most supraventricular tachyarrhythmias do not carry an immediate risk to the patient's life, whereas ventricular tachyarrhythmias could cause sudden cardiac death, and yet differential diagnosis of these two entities is sometimes difficult on an electrocardiographic record. Hence, precise diagnosis is a prerequisite in the treatment of any rhythm disturbance. Furthermore, even the same type of arrhythmia such as a ventricular premature systole can be associated with diverse prognostic significance, depending on their origin, frequency, accompanying symptoms, underlying cardiac lesions, and the like. Antiarrhythmic therapy, therefore, should ideally be tailored to the individual patient's need, taking all the foregoing factors into consideration.

Third, most rhythm disturbances are transient, being present one moment and gone the next, whereas several varieties such as chronic atrial fibrillation and high grades of atrioventricular (AV) block can be permanent. Intermediate forms are also present, with rather prolonged episodes of either bradycardia or tachycardia. Hence, antiarrhythmic therapy may be directed at either prevention of transient arrhythmia, termination of a long-lasting episode, or improvement of the hemodynamic state and amelioration of symptoms in the presence of chronic arrhythmia, each condition requiring a different approach. Furthermore, certain patients have several varieties of arrhythmia concomitantly, and a given drug may correct one variety but may aggravate another. This is especially true in cases of the so-called bradycardia–tachycardia syndrome, in which most antiarrhythmic agents effective against the tachycardia phase tend to worsen the bradycardia phase.

Lastly, it has become increasingly apparent in recent years that similar arrhythmias can be generated by two or more entirely different electrophysiologic mechanisms. Thus, depending on the causative mechanism, a given arrhythmia in one patient may be abolished by a particular group of antiarrhythmic agents, whereas the same rhythm disturbance in another patient may require different drugs for its suppression. Similar considerations apply to the electrical treatment of arrhythmias as well. For instance, rapid pacing may either readily terminate a tachyarrhythmia, only temporarily slow its rate, or even cause an acceleration in different patients.

COMPLEXITIES OF ANTIARRHYTHMIC THERAPY

In addition to those peculiarities of cardiac arrhythmias, the mechanisms of action of antiarrhythmic therapy are also not straightforward. First, a given drug at one concentration level may produce electrophysiologic changes that are just sufficient in suppressing an arrhythmia, whereas the same drug at higher concentrations may cause much greater electrophysiologic alterations and facilitate arrhythmogenesis.

Second, various pathophysiologic conditions such as ischemia and electrolyte imbalance modify the effects of antiarrhythmic agents at least quantitatively and sometimes even qualitatively. Thus, a drug concentration considered to be therapeutic in one patient or for a group of myocardial cells could be either insufficient or excessive in another patient or for a different cell group, and the presence of any inhomogeneity in the myocardium would be associated with local differences in the cellular response.

Third, it is quite common that an antiarrhythmic agent possesses multiple electrophysiologic actions, concomitantly affecting automaticity, conduction, and refractoriness. Although two or more of these actions may work against the same electrophysiologic mechanism and their combination could sometimes enhance the overall antiarrhythmic efficacy, they may cancel the effects of one another at other times. Furthermore, such diverse responses could result simply from quantitative differences between individual actions, thus rendering the prediction of their net results difficult.

THEORETIC APPROACH TO THE MANAGEMENT OF ARRHYTHMIAS

To logically treat various rhythm disturbances, the following several steps must be followed. The first step obviously is a precise diagnosis of the arrhythmia. In most cases, a good electrocardiographic record would suffice,[3] whereas in certain selected patients, clinical electrophysiologic studies are required.[4] The presence or absence and the type and severity of underlying cardiovascular abnormalities must be fully evaluated in addition.

The second step is the identification of the electrophysiologic mechanism or mechanisms of the arrhythmia. Although this is often difficult in the clinical setting, every effort should be made to use current knowledge of basic electrophysiology in speculating the genesis of individual rhythm disorders. Then, as the third step, the mechanisms of action of pharmacologic and electrical treatment must always be kept in mind, so that selection could be made of a drug or an intervention considered to have the most specific action against those electrophysiologic derangements underlying a given arrhythmia.

Of these three steps, the first step has been covered in detail in chapters 18 and 19. Hence, in this chapter, discussion will focus on the second and third steps. More specifically, several basic electrophysiologic mechanisms causing various cardiac arrhythmias will be reviewed. This will be followed by discussions of the mechanisms of action of antiarrhythmic drugs as well as certain electrical interventions. However, because pharmacologic and electrical treatment of individual arrhythmias will be discussed in detail in subsequent chapters, discussion here will be presented in more basic and theoretic terms so as to lay the groundwork for an in-depth understanding of currently practiced antiarrhythmic therapy.

ELECTROPHYSIOLOGIC MECHANISMS OF CARDIAC ARRHYTHMIAS

In discussing the genesis of cardiac arrhythmias, it is customary to classify the electrophysiologic mechanisms into two major categories, namely, (1) abnormalities of impulse formation and (2) disturbances of conduction of excitation.[5-8] In addition, fibrillation may be discussed as a separate entity.[5]

ABNORMALITIES OF IMPULSE FORMATION

Altered Physiologic Automaticity

Under physiologic conditions, automaticity, or the ability to generate action potentials without extraneous stimuli, is a function of the fibers of the specialized conducting system[3,5-9] including the sinoatrial (SA) node, intraatrial specialized fibers,[10] AV node, His bundle, bundle branches, and peripheral Purkinje network. Therefore, spontaneous impulse formation in these fibers normally results from "physiologic automaticity." The rate of automatic firing in various portions of the AV conducting system, however, is not uniform. The SA node usually shows the most rapid rate of impulse formation, and propagation of sinus impulses discharges all the myocardial fibers. Thus, the SA node assumes the role of pacemaker of the heart. The next highest automaticity is seen in the AV junctional region, followed by the intraventricular conducting system (or Purkinje fibers). Teleologic significance of such a hierarchy of physiologic automaticity is summarized in Table 20.1.

Physiologic automaticity in the fibers of the specialized conducting system is characterized by slow diastolic (phase 4) depolarization.[5-9] More specifically, the transmembrane potential in these fibers attains the highest (most negative) value, called the maximal diastolic potential, immediately after the end of an action potential, and then is gradually decreased (becomes less negative). When reduction of the membrane potential reaches a critical level, called the threshold (or take-off) potential, a smooth transition to a more rapid upstroke of the action potential (phase 0 depolarization) takes place. Subsequent periods of repolarization, often subdivided into phases 1, 2, and 3, bring the membrane potential back to the maximal diastolic potential, and the action potential is completed. In contrast to the fibers of the specialized conducting system, normal working myocardial fibers of the atria and ventricles show no phase 4 depolarization, with their membrane potential remaining constant during electrical diastole.[5-9]

In those automatic fibers, the cycle length of spontaneous impulse formation is determined by (1) the slope of diastolic (phase 4) depolarization, (2) the difference between the maximal diastolic potential and the threshold

Table 20.1. Teleologic Significance of the Normal Hierarchy of Automaticity

Pacemaker Site	Intrinsic Rate	Atrioventricular Delay	Intraventricular Conduction
SA node	Usually adequately rapid (60–100/min)	Usually adequate for ventricular filling	Normal, allowing synchronous depolarization
AV junction	May or may not be adequate (35–70/min)	May or may not be adequate for ventricular filling	Normal, allowing synchronous depolarization
Ventricular conducting system	Often inadequately slow (20–60/min)	Usually inadequate with AV dissociation	Abnormal, causing asynchronous depolarization

potential, and (3) the action potential duration. However, the most important determinant of the rate of impulse formation is probably the slope of diastolic depolarization. Generally, increased sympathetic tone or catecholamines would increase this slope, whereas vagal stimulation or acetylcholine would slow the rate of diastolic depolarization. The SA nodal fibers usually show the steepest slope of phase 4 depolarization; hence, their membrane potential will attain the threshold potential before all other fibers of the specialized conducting system do. This is the reason the SA node acts as the primary pacemaker of the heart. Acceleration of automatic impulse formation in the SA node will cause sinus tachycardia, whereas depression of sinus nodal automaticity will result in sinus bradycardia or even sinus arrest.[3,5–9]

Recently, it has been suggested that the hierarchy of physiologic automaticity, as shown in Table 20.1, is maintained not only by the intrinsically higher rate of impulse formation in the SA node, but also by the phenomenon of overdrive suppression.[11–13] This phenomenon can be described as follows. When an automatic fiber is electrically stimulated at a rate higher than that of its intrinsic impulse formation, a sudden termination of stimulation is often followed by a prolonged pause. This suggests a depression of automaticity by the driving stimuli. In the case of the SA node, demonstration of such a pause by electrical stimulation of the right atrium has been used clinically in the diagnosis of sick sinus syndrome.[14] Nevertheless, in the presence of a sinus rhythm, other fibers of the AV conducting system are continuously discharged (or overdriven) by the sinus impulses, and hence, their automaticity may remain suppressed to levels lower than their intrinsic rhythmicity. In this way, competition between two or more pacemakers with resultant arrhythmias can be prevented, and yet other automatic fibers can generate their own impulses and act as an escape pacemaker if the SA nodal automaticity is markedly depressed or propagation of the SA nodal impulses fails.[3,5]

Under certain pathophysiologic conditions, however, automaticity in certain other areas of the specialized conducting system may be abnormally enhanced, resulting in a higher rate of impulse formation as compared with that of the SA node (Figure 20.1A, *top*). Then, depending on the site of such an increased automaticity, an ectopic pacemaker may control the rhythmicity of either the entire heart or only the ventricles. Varieties of nonparoxysmal ectopic tachycardia are considered to result from this mechanism, including so-called automatic atrial tachycardia, nonparoxysmal AV junctional tachycardia, and nonparoxysmal ventricular tachycardia (idioventricular tachycardia or accelerated idioventricular rhythm). In contrast to the paroxysmal varieties of tachycardia, as will be discussed, nonparoxysmal tachycardias usually have less rapid rates of impulse formation and tend to develop and subside gradually.[3,5]

Occasionally, a group of automatic fibers in an ectopic focus may maintain their rhythmicity without being interrupted by SA nodal or other impulses, presumably because of the presence of an area of protection block surrounding the focus. This is the mechanism of parasystole and produces premature systoles with variable coupling intervals.[1–3,5,15–17]

When automaticity in all portions of the specialized conducting system is depressed (Figure 20.1A, *bottom*), the pacemaker may progressively move downward from the SA node to the AV junction and to a ventricular focus, culminating in ventricular standstill. This is called the downward displacement of pacemaker,[18] and, when combined with a significant AV conduction disturbance in particular, it constitutes one of the most serious bradyarrhythmias. Therefore, both an enhancement and a depression of physiologic automaticity will cause various arrhythmias.

Development of Abnormal Automaticity

In contrast to physiologic automaticity, as just described, the term abnormal automaticity may include several varieties such as (1) depolarization-induced automaticity and (2) afterdepolarizations and triggered activity.

Depolarization-induced Automaticity.[8,19–22] Depolarization-induced automaticity can be subdivided into two types. First, the working myocardial fibers of the atria and the ventricles may develop automaticity under abnormal conditions. Those conditions include perfusion with $K^+ \cdot Ca^{++}$-free solution[23] and the application of a depolarizing current across the cell membrane.[24] Under these conditions, the atrial or ventricular muscle fibers develop diastolic depolarization and show spontaneous firing. Although the first of the foregoing two conditions cannot be expected in the human heart, a condition similar to the second intervention may well occur clinically. For instance, in the presence of acute myocardial infarc-

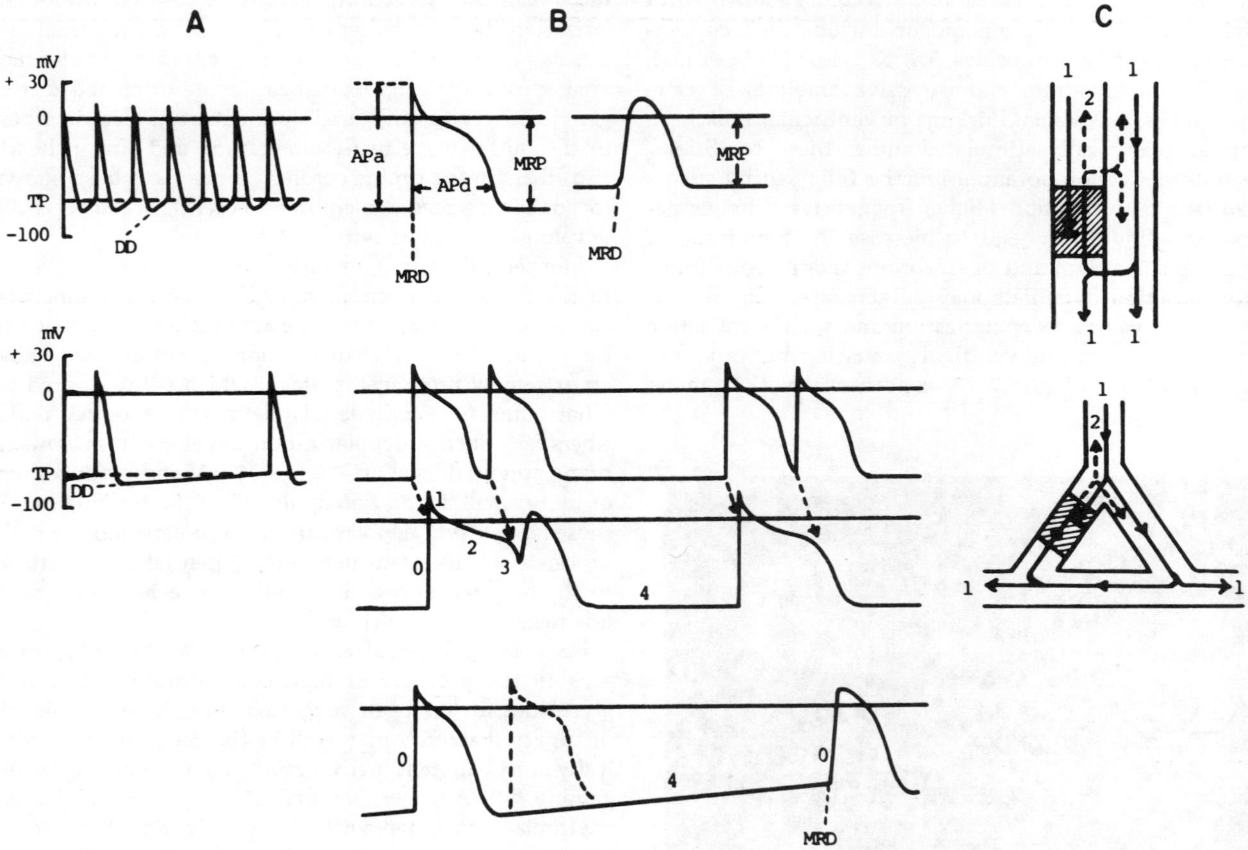

Figure 20.1. Electrophysiologic mechanisms of cardiac arrhythmias are diagrammatically shown. In *A,* enhanced physiologic automaticity with an increased slope of diastolic depolarization (DD) is shown at the top, and depressed automaticity with a much slower rate of diastolic depolarization is shown at the bottom. TP: threshold potential. In *B,* the *top left panel* illustrates a fast response action potential of the Purkinje fiber with a deep membrane resting potential (MRP), a large action potential amplitude (APa), and a rapid maximal rate of depolarization (MRD). APd denotes action potential duration. The *top right panel* shows a slow response action potential as seen in partially depolarized fast response fibers or SA and AV nodal fibers. In the *second panel,* premature responses in the upstream fiber show almost normal action potential characteristics as the action potential duration and the refractory period are relatively short and the fiber has recovered from the preceding depolarization by the time of premature stimulation. The downstream fiber having a much longer action potential duration, however, either responds with reduced amplitude and rate of rise (*left*) or does not respond at all (*right*), causing a conduction block of the phase 3 variety. The *bottom panel* in *B* shows that a propagated action potential in late diastole (*far right*) is accompanied by a markedly reduced rate of phase 0 depolarization because of the loss of membrane potential due to phase 4 depolarization (phase 4 block), whereas a premature response produced immediately after the end of an action potential (*broken line*) arises from the most negative membrane potential and shows a normal phase 0 upstroke. In *C,* either functional, longitudinal dissociation of the conducting pathway (*top*) or two anatomically separate pathways (*bottom*) and the presence of an area of depressed conduction with the property of unidirectional block (*shaded area*) produce a reentry movement, resulting in reexcitation of the initially depolarized tissue (*broken lines*).

tion, K^+ efflux from the injured cardiac cells would cause an elevation of extracellular K^+ concentration in the ischemic area. Combined with hypoxia and acidosis known to supervene in the infarcted zone, high K^+-induced partial depolarization of the cell membrane may well induce diastolic depolarization and impulse formation in the working myocardium.[20–22,25] Prevalence of fibers with reduced membrane potentials and automatic firing in diseased human atrial tissue has also been reported.[8,26,27]

The second type of depolarization-induced automaticity can be seen in partially depolarized Purkinje fibers.[19] Under physiologic conditions, phase 4 depolarization in the Purkinje fiber starts from the maximal diastolic potential of −85 to −90 mV. When their membrane potential is decreased to −50 mV or less negative levels, Purkinje fibers often show higher rates of spontaneous firing with an apparent diastolic depolarization. Hence, it is possible that this mechanism plays some role in ectopic impulse formation occurring in the peripheral Purkinje network located within the ischemic zone.

Afterdepolarizations and Triggered Activity.[19,28–33] There are two different varieties of afterdepolarizations, delayed afterdepolarization and early afterdepolarization. The former refers to a transient reduction in the transmembrane potential after the completion of repolarization when the membrane potential either has returned to the original diastolic level or has become even more negative (called an early afterhyperpolarization).[19] Factors known to be associated with this phenomenon include high concentrations of cardiac glycosides, low K^+, low Na^+, or high Ca^{++} concentration, and excessive amounts of catecholamines.[28-33] When Purkinje or ventricular muscle fibers are electrically stimulated under these conditions, each driven action potential may be followed by such a transient depolarization. Higher frequencies or longer periods of stimulation tend to increase the amplitude of afterdepolarization, and one or more spontaneous (nondriven) action potentials may be generated. Figure 20.2 shows delayed afterdepolarization and such extra action potentials in a canine ventricular muscle fiber produced by low K^+ plus high Ca^{++} concentrations (Watanabe, unpublished observation). Because a delayed afterdepolarization always requires a preceding action potential that acts as a trigger, those spontaneous, extra action potentials arising from the afterdepolarization are often called triggered activity (or triggered automaticity). Certain fibers in the mitral valve leaflets of canine and simian hearts and fibers in the canine coronary sinus have been shown to possess decreased membrane potentials and to easily develop triggered activities.[19,33,34]

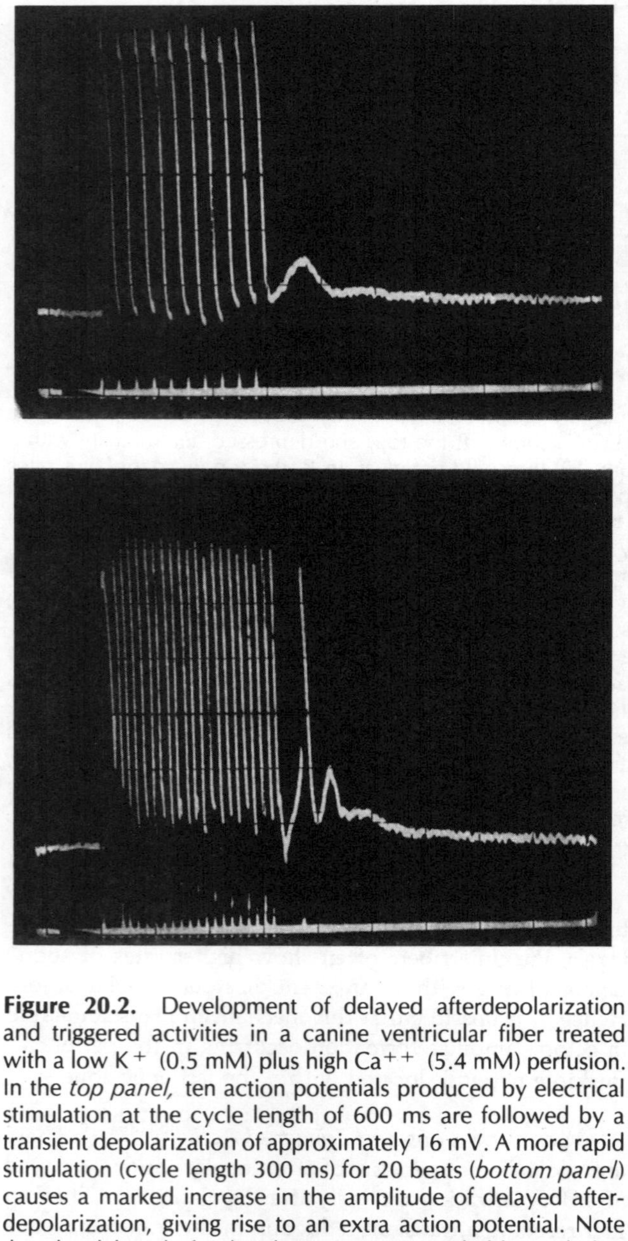

Figure 20.2. Development of delayed afterdepolarization and triggered activities in a canine ventricular fiber treated with a low K^+ (0.5 mM) plus high Ca^{++} (5.4 mM) perfusion. In the *top panel,* ten action potentials produced by electrical stimulation at the cycle length of 600 ms are followed by a transient depolarization of approximately 16 mV. A more rapid stimulation (cycle length 300 ms) for 20 beats (*bottom panel*) causes a marked increase in the amplitude of delayed afterdepolarization, giving rise to an extra action potential. Note that the delayed afterdepolarization is preceded by early hyperpolarization and followed by another, smaller transient depolarization (Watanabe, unpublished observation).

The second variety, or early afterdepolarization, refers to the following phenomenon. Under certain abnormal conditions, especially after the application of aconitine or Ba^{++}, atrial or ventricular action potentials may show an extremely prolonged plateau, which is interrupted by what mimics diastolic depolarization in SA or AV nodal fibers.[19,35] Such a depolarization develops from a membrane potential level of −20 to −30 mV and produces one or more small action potentials. After the termination of those repetitive depolarizations, repolarization finally proceeds and the transmembrane potential either returns to the original level or is stabilized at a new and much less negative level such as −50 mV.

Because a delayed afterdepolarization is most typically seen in the presence of high concentrations of cardiac glycosides, it has been suggested that the phenomenon of triggered activity may well be the cause of those clinically seen "digitalis arrhythmias" such as ventricular bigeminy.[31,32] Another possibility is that ventricular arrhythmias associated with increased sympathetic tones result from this mechanism. Delayed afterdepolarizations appear to depend on increased intracellular Ca^{++} concentration.[32] Contrariwise, whether early afterdepolarizations could also play a role in generating clinical arrhythmias is still uncertain, as those conditions producing this phenomenon are grossly unphysiologic.

DISTURBANCES OF CONDUCTION OF EXCITATION

Delay and Failure of Conduction (Conduction Block)

When an action potential is generated in a myocardial fiber, an inward current flows across the cell membrane. At the same time, a current flows through the nexus to the adjoining cell and depolarizes the latter. In this manner, cell to cell conduction proceeds. The most important determinants of conduction velocity are the maximal rate of phase 0 depolarization (or the upstroke velocity of the action potential) and the action potential amplitude; the greater these values, the faster is the conduction (Figure 20.1B, *top*).[9] Because the maximal rate of depolarization is greater when the action potential arises from deeper membrane potentials, working myocardial fibers of the atria and ventricles as well as Purkinje fibers having physiologically deep membrane potentials show rapid upstroke velocity of the action potential.[9] Their phase 0 depolarization is dependent on a rapid transmembrane influx of Na^+ ions (the fast Na^+ current), and conduction in these fibers is rapid. These action potentials are thus called the fast response.

Contrariwise, in the SA and AV nodal fibers, the membrane potential is much less negative, and the upstroke phase of their action potential is significantly slower.[9,11]

Hence, their action potentials are termed the slow response. Phase 0 depolarization of these fibers is predominantly dependent on the slow inward current[36,37] carried mainly by Ca^{++} and partially by Na^{+}, although the fast Na^{+} current also plays a minor role.[38–41] Consequently, conduction is extremely slow and its margin of safety lower in these two nodal tissues. Catecholamines increase the slow inward current; hence, an increased sympathetic tone tends to improve AV nodal conduction, whereas vagal stimulation has the opposite effect.[42,43]

When the cell membrane in Purkinje, atrial, or ventricular fibers is partially depolarized by various factors such as ischemia and high extracellular K^{+} concentration, their fast Na^{+} channel is inactivated and the action potential upstroke becomes increasingly dependent on the slow inward current. Resultant slow responses in these fast response fibers (Figure 20.1B, *top*) are considered to play a major role in the development of delay and failure of conduction and also reentry movements.[8,19]

One other factor affecting conduction of excitation is the interval at which a second stimulus is applied to a myocardial fiber.[5–9,44] For instance, if a sudden shortening of the stimulus cycle length occurs for some reason, an impulse may arrive at the downstream fibers before the end of their action potential. Then, because of the refractory period, these fibers either show no response, resulting in failure of conduction, or respond with a slowly rising, small action potential, causing a conduction delay (Figure 20.1B, *middle*). Rosenbaum et al[45] termed this mechanism phase 3 block on the premise that the stimulus encroached on phase 3 repolarization of the preceding action potential. In this case, the fast Na^{+} channel is partially inactivated because of the decreased membrane potential (voltage-dependent inactivation), and hence the fibers are refractory. However, in the presence of excessive class 1A antiarrhythmic drugs or certain other conditions, the refractory period sometimes outlasts the action potential, extending into phase 4 or electrical diastole (so-called postrepolarization refractoriness). The reason is that recovery of the fast Na^{+} channel is dependent also on the time after its activation during phase 0, and it may remain partially inactivated even after the end of phase 3 repolarization (time-dependent inactivation). Phase 3 block is therefore not a precise term, but it is often used in clinical arrhythmology because of its compactness as compared with the term *conduction block due to refractory periods.*

Rosenbaum et al[45] also introduced the term phase 4 block. This term refers to the delay or failure of conduction of a stimulus applied in late diastole to fibers showing phase 4 depolarization.[46] Because the membrane potential has become much less negative toward the end of diastole, the fast Na^{+} channel has sustained voltage-dependent inactivation, contributing to the occurrence of a conduction disturbance (Figure 20.1B, *bottom*). The role of phase 3 and phase 4 blocks in the genesis of various bradyarrhythmias and tachyarrhythmias is summarized in Table 20.2.[47,48] Regardless of the mechanisms of conduction block, failure of propagation of sinus impulses in the specialized conducting system could cause bradyarrhythmias such as SA block and AV block.

Table 20.2. Possible Role of Phase 3 and Phase 4 Block in Cardiac Arrhythmias

Phase 3 Block

1. Aberrant intraventricular conduction of supraventricular premature systoles (especially those showing the Ashman phenomenon)
2. Nonconducted supraventricular premature systoles
3. Tachycardia-dependent bundle branch block
4. Gap phenomena in AV conduction
5. So-called dual AV nodal pathways causing paroxysmal AV junctional tachycardia
6. Vulnerability causing repetitive responses and fibrillation

Phase 4 Block

1. Aberrant intraventricular conduction of supraventricular escape beats
2. Bradycardia-dependent bundle branch block
3. Exit block from ectopic pacemakers
4. Protection of parasystolic pacemakers
5. Reentrant premature systoles, especially those showing the rule of bigeminy
6. Certain instances of supernormal AV conduction
7. So-called paroxysmal AV block

Reentry and Reflection

One mechanism by which conduction disturbances could produce tachyarrhythmias is reentry.[49] The occurrence of a reentry movement is predicated on the following three conditions: (1) There are two anatomically or functionally separate pathways capable of forming a circuit. (2) In one of these pathways, an area of depressed conduction exists, which has the property of unidirectional block permitting conduction of excitation only in one direction and not in the other. (3) The time required for the excitation front to make a complete circuit is longer than the refractory period of any portion of the reentrant loop (Figure 20.1C).[5–8]

When the three conditions are satisfied and reexcitation of the initially discharged myocardial tissue occurs once, a coupled premature systole (or a premature systole having a fixed time relation with the preceding beat) will be generated, whereas repetitive reentry along such a circuit (called a circus movement) will cause paroxysmal tachycardia.

The best example of paroxysmal tachycardia using two anatomically separate pathways is Wolff–Parkinson–White (WPW) tachycardia.[50,51] In this case, the reentrant movement most commonly proceeds from the atrial tissue through the AV node, His-Purkinje system, ventricular muscle, bundle of Kent, and back to the atria, thus forming a macroreentry. In paroxysmal AV junctional tachycardia, on the other hand, either functional longitudinal dissociation of the AV nodal tissue[52] or the existence of so-called dual AV nodal pathways has been postulated as the mechanism of reentry.[53–56] However, more recent studies indicate that there are two atrial inputs into the AV node (one through the crista terminalis and the other through the interatrial septum), and a reciprocating tachycardia could develop when antegrade conduction in one of these inputs is blocked.[57,58]

These reentrant tachycardias are commonly initiated by either a spontaneously occurring premature systole or an extrastimulus applied during clinical electrophysiologic studies. Such an observation is explained as follows. If those two pathways have grossly different refractory periods, an appropriately timed premature stimulus may find one pathway still refractory while the other pathway has already recovered from the preceding discharge and is responsive. When the excitation front depolarizing the peripheral tissue through the latter pathway invades the former from the distal end, this pathway is now out of its refractory period and permits retrograde conduction. It is currently believed that most paroxysmal atrial and ventricular tachycardias are also caused by reentrant movements.[3,4,50]

If an abnormal potential difference exists in localized myocardial tissue, a current flow between two fiber groups may reexcite one of them.[7,8,59] For instance, in the presence of marked inhomogeneity of repolarization, fibers having a shorter action potential duration may be depolarized again at the end of phase 3 by a current flow from the adjacent fibers still undergoing repolarization. It has also been shown that reexcitation can occur in a small strand of fibers. In our experiment using canine Purkinje fibers, conduction in the middle portion of the false tendon was depressed by high K^+ concentration. When a stimulus given at the proximal end of this preparation was able to traverse the depressed area, perhaps by an electrotonic spread, and produce an action potential at the distal end, the excitation front apparently returned to the proximal portion, causing a second depolarization. In these instances, no distinct reentry "circuit" could be identified and the excitation wave appeared to move back and forth along the same pathway. Hence, such a phenomenon has been termed *reflection*[19,60] rather than *reentry*. Although the role played by this mechanism in generating clinical arrhythmias cannot be readily demonstrated, ischemia or other organic lesions may well produce localized potential differences facilitating reflection.[59,60]

FIBRILLATION

The atria and ventricles normally are depolarized by a smooth wavefront of excitation and undergo a well-organized excitation. In fibrillation, however, myocardial fibers of the atria or ventricles show entirely disorganized, asynchronous electrical activities.[61,62] Classically, two theories, ectopic impulse formation and reentry, were used in an attempt to explain the genesis of fibrillation.[5] However, it must be pointed out that mechanisms initiating fibrillation and those sustaining this arrhythmia may not be identical.[61] For each of these electrophysiologic mechanisms, various experimental observations have been reported, and controversies still exist between different theories. If a simplified view is to be presented, it is this author's opinion that irregular, disorganized spread of excitation associated with numerous microreentries plays a major role in the maintenance of fibrillation.[5,63] The term random reentry movements has been suggested in describing such microreentries as contrasted to an organized reentry typically seen in Wolff–Parkinson–White tachycardia. It is possible that the aforementioned phenomenon of reflection contributes to such random reentries. Regardng the mechanisms of initiation of fibrillation, reports are available for both rapid ectopic impulse formation and reentry, and clarification of this issue still awaits further studies. Perhaps it will suffice to point out here that the distinction between ectopic impulse formation and stable microreentry movement will be difficult, if not impossible, especially in the clinical setting.

IDENTIFICATION OF ELECTROPHYSIOLOGIC MECHANISMS

Based on the foregoing considerations, the electrophysiologic mechanisms of various arrhythmias may be summarized as in Table 20.3, although limitations in identifying some of these mechanisms have previously been stressed. In this regard, an additional comment is in order on the coexistence of several mechanisms in certain cases. An electrocardiogram from a patient with mitral stenosis is shown in Figure 20.3 to illustrate this point.

In this tracing, no P waves are visible, and the presence of chronic atrial fibrillation has been verified by serial records. However, the RR intervals show some regularity, which can best be explained by assuming the combination of a high grade AV nodal block and AV junctional impulse formation with exit block as diagrammed below lead V_4. The cycle length of this AV junctional rhythm ranges between 0.44 and 0.46 second, corresponding to

Table 20.3. Electrophysiologic Mechanisms of Cardiac Arrhythmias

Arrhythmia	Mechanism
Bradyarrhythmias	
1. Sinus bradycardia	Depressed physiologic automaticity in the SA node
2. Sinus arrest	Depressed physiologic automaticity in the SA node (some associated with conduction block?)
3. SA block	Conduction block
4. AV block	Conduction block
5. Escape rhythm	Physiologic automaticity in a subsidiary focus (sometimes associated with exit block)
6. Downward displacement of the pacemaker	Depressed physiologic automaticity throughout the specialized conducting system
Tachyarrhythmias	
1. Sinus tachycardia	Enhanced physiologic automaticity in the SA node
2. Nonparoxysmal tachycardias	Enhanced physiologic automaticity in an ectopic focus (some due to abnormal automaticity?)
3. Paroxysmal tachycardias	Macro- or microreentry; some due to triggered activity
4. Coupled premature systoles	Microreentry or reflection; some due to triggered activity
5. Parasystole	Physiologic automaticity in an ectopic focus with conduction (protection) block
6. Flutter	Mostly macroreentry; some due to ectopic impulse formation (either due to abnormal automaticity or microreentry?)
7. Fibrillation	Microreentries (plus ectopic impulse formation?)

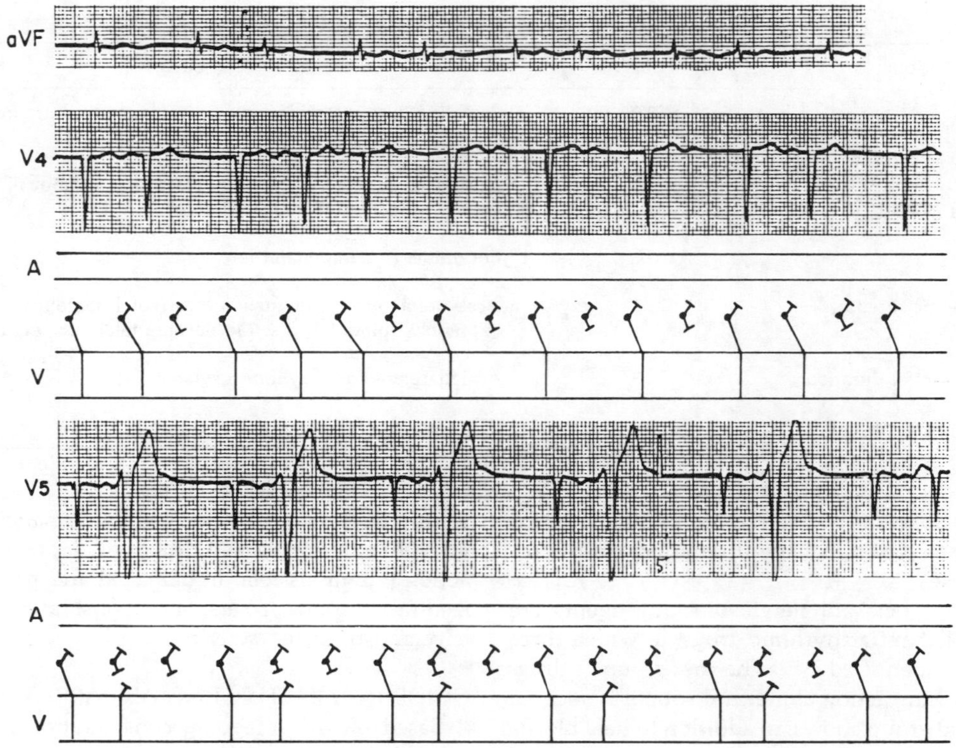

Figure 20.3. Electrocardiographic record showing a complex arrhythmia in which several different electrophysiologic mechanisms must be invoked. In the ladder diagram, A and V denote atrial and ventricular activations, respectively. Detailed discussion in text.

the rate of 130 to 135 per minute; hence, nonparoxysmal AV junctional tachycardia[3,64] is diagnosed. In addition, ventricular premature systoles in the form of bigeminy are seen in lead V_5. Thus, in this case, the following five electrophysiologic mechanisms can be identified: (1) atrial fibrillation probably involving numerous microreentries in the atria, (2) depression and failure of conduction in the AV node, (3) enhanced physiologic automaticity in the AV junction (the NH region of the AV node or the His bundle), (4) exit block from this junctional pacemaker probably due to phase 4 block,[5,48] and (5) ventricular premature systoles caused either by reentry or by delayed afterdepolarization and triggered activity. Mitral stenosis with its hemodynamic consequences and digitalis excess[65] should further be identified as underlying pathophysiologic derangements.

BASIC CONSIDERATIONS IN ANTIARRHYTHMIC DRUG THERAPY

CLASSIFICATION OF ANTIARRHYTHMIC DRUGS

The list of antiarrhythmic drugs has been greatly expanded in the last three decades through the development of newer drugs. Several classifications of these agents have so far been proposed by different investigators, each one having certain advantages as well as shortcomings. Of these, the classification published by Vaughan Williams[66] in 1970, with subsequent additions and modifications, is perhaps most widely accepted today. Hence, in this chapter, the effects of various antiarrhythmic drugs and their indications will be discussed according to this classification (Table 20.4).

Although individual antiarrhythmic agents often have multiple electrophysiologic actions as described previously, the classification is based on their major actions. Hence, those major actions shared by the drugs belonging to the same class will be briefly reviewed first. There are numerous agents in class 1 of Vaughan Williams' classification, including the most classical antiarrhythmic drug, quinidine. All these drugs are considered to block the fast Na^+ current and decrease the maximal rate of phase 0 depolarization and conduction velocity in those fast response fibers. These class 1 agents are thus termed Na^+ channel blockers. However, the potency of this action varies widely between different drugs, and this class has been subdivided into groups A, B, and C. Class 1A drugs such as quinidine, procainamide, and disopyramide moderately depress phase 0 depolarization, whereas this action in class 1B drugs, including lidocaine, diphenylhydantoin, and mexiletine, is much less prominent.[67,68] Agents belonging to class 1C, the most recently added subdivision, are most potent in blocking the fast Na^+ channel and markedly depress conduction in atrial, ventricular, and Purkinje fibers.[69–71]

Aside from their action on phase 0, class 1A drugs depress automaticity in Purkinje fibers and prolong the action potential duration and refractory period in all fast response fibers. In contrast, class 1B drugs shorten the

Table 20.4. Classification of Antiarrhythmic Drugs

Major Actions	Class	Drugs
Blocks the fast Na^+ current (myocardial depressant, membrane stabilizing action)	1A	Ajmaline, disopyramide, procainamide, and quinidine
	1B	Aprindine, diphenylhydantoin, etafenone, ethmozin, lidocaine, mexiletine, propafenone, and tocainide
	1C	Encainide, flecainide, and lorcainide
Blocks beta-adrenergic receptors	2	Acebutolol, alprenolol, atenolol, carteolol, metoprolol, nadolol, oxprenolol, pindolol, practolol, propranolol, sotalol, and timolol
Prolongs action potential duration	3	Amiodarone and bretylium tosylate
Blocks the slow inward current	4	Diltiazem, prenylamine, and verapamil

action potential duration and refractory period, whereas class 1C drugs are stated to have little effect on the repolarization phase.

Next, numerous beta-adrenergic blocking agents are classified as class 2 antiarrhythmic drugs, in which three subgroups can be identified.[72–75] The first group of drugs possess beta blocking action alone, and sotalol is such an agent. The second group shows, in addition to beta blocking action, a direct membrane action similar to that of class 1 drugs. Most typical of these drugs is propranolol, and bupranolol, adobiol, and the like belong to this group. The third group, including pindolol, carteolol, and practolol, exhibits intrinsic beta-adrenergic stimulating action when the sympathetic tone is low or the role of catecholamines has been reduced by reserpine. Drugs such as alprenolol and oxprenolol possess all three actions.

Because of beta-adrenergic blockade, all these class 2 agents tend to depress automaticity in the SA node and Purkinje fibers and depress AV nodal conduction,[76–78] although shortening of the AV nodal conduction time has been occasionally observed.[79,80] Drugs that have a direct membrane action such as propranolol would block the fast Na^+ current and depress conduction in atrial, ventricular, and Purkinje fibers. On the action potential duration and refractory period, these drugs either have no significant effect or tend to shorten them. Whether the intrinsic beta stimulating action of some of the class 2 agents contributes to their antiarrhythmic effects is not known.

Class 3 antiarrhythmic drugs include amiodarone and bretylium tosylate. Both these drugs significantly prolong the action potential duration and refractory period of Purkinje fibers as well as atrial and ventricular muscle, but they appear to have little effect on conduction in these fast response fibers.[81–85] Atrioventricular nodal conduction tends to be depressed by these agents. However, as will be discussed, bretylium tosylate may improve conduction in fibers whose membrane has been partially depolarized by factors such as hypoxia.[86,87] Whether amiodarone has a similar effect is yet to be clarified.

The last group of antiarrhythmic drugs, belonging to class 4, are so-called Ca^{++} antagonists.[88–91] Because these agents block the slow inward current, they significantly depress conduction (and automaticity) in the AV node. In addition, class 4 drugs will depress slow response action potentials seen in damaged and partially depolarized fast response fibers, and abolish abnormal automaticity and triggered activity.

GUIDELINES IN SELECTING ANTIARRHYTHMIC DRUGS

Based on the foregoing considerations, the following general guidelines in the selection of various antiarrhythmic drugs may be derived.[92] First, in the treatment of nonparoxysmal ectopic tachycardias caused by enhanced physiologic automaticity, class 1 and class 2 antiarrhythmic drugs would be effective by depressing diastolic depolarization of AV junctional and Purkinje fibers. Sinus tachycardia usually does not have to be treated, but in a few cases requiring therapy, class 2 (beta blocking) drugs are the most effective.

Second, reentry is considered to play a major role in many tachyarrhythmias including so-called coupled premature systoles, paroxysmal tachycardias, flutter, and fibrillation. The following several mechanisms may successfully interrupt such reentry movements: (1) If a drug depresses conduction, the area of conduction disturbance having the property of unidirectional block may be converted to one of bidirectional block. Reentrant movement will then be abolished. (2) When a drug significantly prolongs the refractory period, the reentrant impulse may find the initially depolarized fibers still refractory, and reexcitation will be prevented. Drugs belonging to class 1A have both these effects on Purkinje, atrial, and ventricular fibers and are therefore indicated against reentrant arrhythmias. Class 1B and 1C agents possess only the first action, whereas class 3 agents would work mainly through the second action. Class 1A and class 3 antiarrhythmic drugs exert these actions also on the bundle of Kent and are effective against WPW tachycardia and the WPW syndrome with atrial fibrillation.[3,82,92] Theoretically, drugs capable of improving conduction may also prevent reentry by eradicating the area of unidirectional block. The possibility of bretylium tosylate exhibiting this action will be discussed.[86,87]

Because paroxysmal AV junctional tachycardia is dependent on a reentry movement in the AV nodal tissue, drugs that depress AV nodal conduction should be used against this arrhythmia. Class 2 and class 4 agents are therefore the drugs of choice (in addition to the classic medication of cardiac glycosides).[93,94] These drugs are also frequently used to control the ventricular rate in the presence of atrial flutter or fibrillation.

If certain cases of nonparoxysmal ectopic tachycardia result from depolarization-induced automaticity in the working myocardium or Purkinje fibers, Ca^{++} antagonists (class 4 agents) should be effective. Likewise, premature systoles and paroxysmal tachycardias caused by delayed afterdepolarization and triggered activity can best be treated with class 4 drugs.[19,90,95] However, it must be reemphasized here that in the clinical setting, distinction between those several mechanisms of tachyarrhythmia is difficult. Hence, it has often been suggested that tachyarrhythmias responding to class 1 agents are probably dependent on reentry movements, whereas those successfully treated with class 4 agents are due to abnormal automaticity or triggered activity. Pitfalls in this kind of statement must be kept in mind and, as will be shown herein, some class 1A drugs may well suppress triggered activities.[96]

Bradyarrhythmias caused by either depressed automaticity or delay and failure of conduction should theoretically be treated with drugs enhancing automaticity and improving conduction. Atropine and isoproterenol are the two currently available drugs with such actions, but frequent side effects limit their clinical use. Therefore, electrical pacing is currently considered the treatment of choice against those bradyarrhythmias.

ELECTROPHARMACOLOGIC ASPECTS OF INDIVIDUAL ANTIARRHYTHMIC DRUGS

As was pointed out earlier, most antiarrhythmic drugs exert multiple actions on cellular electrophysiology, and their classification is based only on one or two major actions shared by several drugs. Those drugs belonging to the same class may therefore possess other actions slightly different from one another. Furthermore, the same single drug may exert dissimilar effects depending on the fiber types and on various pathophysiologic conditions. Because these considerations may well affect the clinical use of individual agents, various electropharmacologic aspects of several representative drugs will be discussed mainly on the basis of our own experimental studies.

Class 1 Antiarrhythmic Drugs

Class 1A Agents. Class 1A agents include quinidine and procainamide, the two classic antiarrhythmic drugs in use since the pre-war days. Reports on their electrophysiologic effects consequently are numerous. However, in this section, disopyramide will be discussed as an example of this class.

In canine Purkinje fibers perfused in a tissue bath, disopyramide (5 μg/ml) significantly decreased the action potential amplitude, overshoot, and maximal rate of phase 0 depolarization.[97] When the false tendon preparation was impaled by two microelectrodes and the conduction time between these two points was determined, it was prolonged by 30% after 30 minutes of drug perfusion. Thus, depression of conduction by disopyramide was evident. Washout of the drug returned all these measurements toward control levels. The action potential duration at 50% of repolarization was significantly shortened by disopyramide, whereas that at 80% repolarization was essentially unchanged during drug perfusion and significantly prolonged after washout of the drug. An interesting finding on the drug effect on the Purkinje repolarization process is presented in Figure 20.4. When drug-induced changes in the action potential duration at 80% repolarization in 40 Purkinje fibers were plotted, this duration was shortened in fibers initially having durations of 280 ms or longer and prolonged in fibers with initial values of 240 ms or shorter (Figure 20.4, *bottom*). Therefore, inhomogeneity of repolarization was greatly reduced by the addition of disopyramide.[97] The ratio between the effective refractory period and action potential duration at 80% repolarization was increased by this drug, indicating relative prolongation of the refractory period.

Interactions of hypoxia and disopyramide were then studied, again using canine Purkinje fibers, and the following observations were made. Perfusion of the false tendon preparation with a hypoxic solution caused significant reduction in the action potential amplitude, the maximal rate of depolarization, and the action potential duration at 50% repolarization. Subsequent addition of disopyramide exaggerated these changes. On the other hand, the action potential duration at 100% repolarization was shortened by hypoxia alone, and the addition of this drug significantly prolonged it despite the maintenance of hypoxic perfusion.

Thus, by assuming the prevalence of similar effects in ventricular muscle fibers, the mechanisms of action of disopyramide against various ventricular tachyarrhythmias can be suggested as follows. First, this drug definitely depressed conduction under both normoxic and hypoxic conditions. This action will convert unidirectional block to bidirectional block and interrupt reentry movements. Second, the drug appeared to decrease the inhomogeneity of Purkinje repolarizations (Figure 20.4), and similar findings were also reported by another group of investigators.[98] If a similar phenomenon should occur in ventricular muscle fibers, it will decrease ventricular vulnerability and help prevent the development of paroxysmal ventricular tachycardia and fibrillation, but this has not been demonstrated to date. However, the increased uniformity of action potential duration caused by disopyramide would allow a more organized propagation of a premature impulse throughout the Purkinje network and reduce the likelihood of setting up reentry circuits. Third, this drug caused a slight prolongation of the effective refractory period relative to the action potential duration. As a result, the membrane potential at the end of the effective refractory period became more negative. Propagation of the earliest premature response will then be improved, and repetitive reentry movements can be prevented. This action is shared by many antiarrhythmic

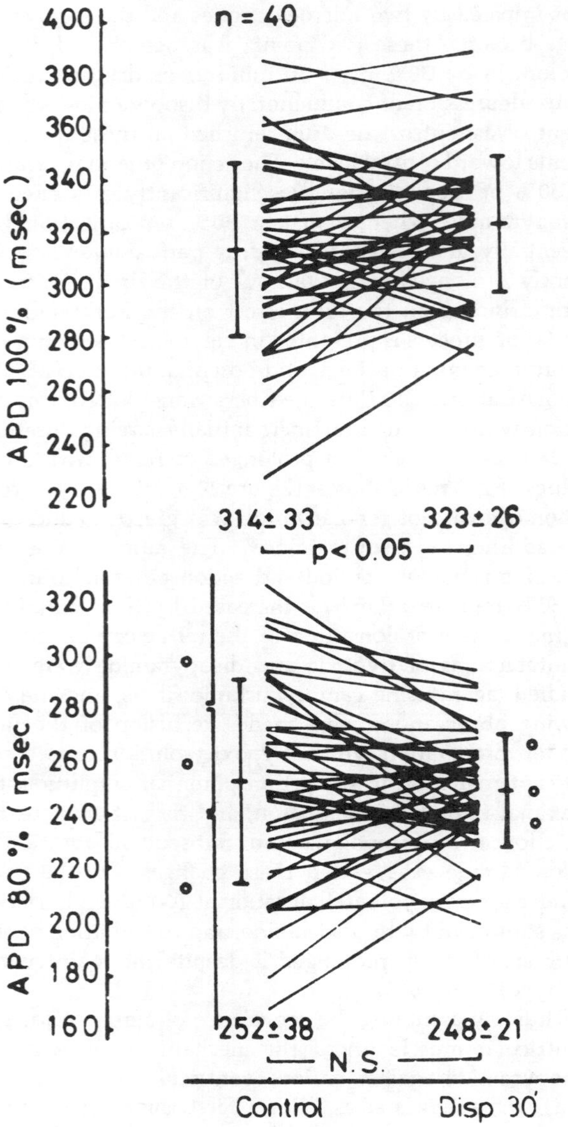

Figure 20.4. Effects of disopyramide on the action potential duration (APD) at 100% (*top*) and 80% repolarization (*bottom*) of canine Purkinje fibers. Note a marked reduction in the variation of action potential duration after a 30-minute perfusion with disopyramide (Disp) at a concentration of 5 μg/ml. *Vertical bars* indicate mean values with 1 standard deviation. *Small open circles* in the *bottom panel* indicate mean values for fibers having initial action potential duration longer than 280 ms, shorter than 240 ms, and between these two values. See discussion in text. (From Yamada et al,[97] p 34, with permission.)

drugs and may be regarded as an important property in the treatment of reentrant tachyarrhythmias.[79,99] Indeed, we have shown that disopyramide can often convert sustained ventricular fibrillation in isolated, perfused rabbit hearts to normal sinus rhythm, perhaps by interrupting microreentry movements.[100]

In one experiment (Figure 20.5A), the canine Purkinje fiber preparation was perfused with 1.75 mg/L of desacetyl-lanatoside C and was electrically driven at the cycle length of 250 ms 20 times. Sudden termination of stimulation was followed by delayed afterdepolarization, producing two slowly rising action potentials. After a longer period of lanatoside C perfusion (Figure 20.5B), ten driven action potentials were followed by five triggered action potentials. After the addition of disopyramide (5 mg/L) to the perfusate, termination of stimulation caused only a small afterdepolarization and no triggered action potentials were produced (Figure 20.5C).[96] Hence, class 1A antiarrhythmic drugs may well be effective against tachyarrhythmias caused by this mechanism. This action may be explained as follows. Bcause class 1 antiarrhythmic drugs block the fast Na^{++} current and decrease the Na^{+} influx during phase 0 depolarization, intracellular Na^{+} concentration can be decreased. Through the operation of the Na^{+}–Ca^{++} exchange mechanism, intracellular Ca^{++} concentration would then be reduced. This reduction will depress delayed afterdepolarization, which is facilitated by increased intracellular Ca^{++} concentration.

The effects of disopyramide on the AV node were studied in small AV nodal preparations (0.2 by 0.2 by

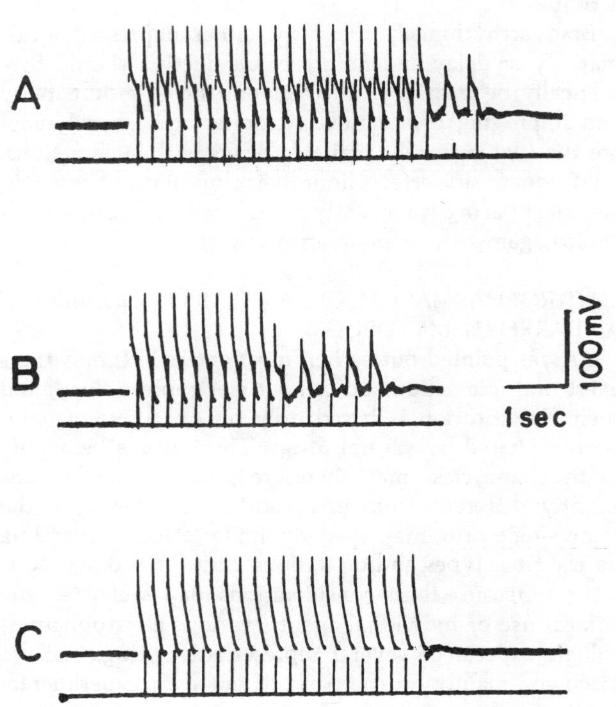

Figure 20.5. Suppression of delayed afterdepolarization and triggered activities by disopyramide. In *A,* the canine Purkinje fiber treated with 1.75 mg/L of desacetyl lanatoside C was electrically driven at the cycle length of 250 ms 20 times. Termination of stimulation was followed by delayed afterdepolarization, producing two slowly rising, spontaneous action potentials. Note markedly decreased maximal rate of depolarization in these two action potentials as shown in the differentiated signal (*bottom record*). In *B,* after a longer period of lanatoside C perfusion, ten driven action potentials were followed by five triggered action potentials. In *C,* after the addition of disopyramide to the perfusate at a concentration of 5 mg/L, termination of rapid stimulation caused only a small afterdepolarization and no triggered action potentials were produced. (Watanabe, unpublished observation.)

0.1 mm) of the rabbit by recording the action potential and studying the membrane currents with voltage clamp techniques.[101] These small preparations exhibit spontaneous firing, with a prominent diastolic depolarization.[102] When disopyramide was added to the perfusate at a concentration of 2.5 μg/ml, the cycle length of firing was prolonged, the maximal rate of depolarization was decreased, and the action potential duration at 100% repolarization was prolonged. Progressive increase of the drug concentration to 5.0 and 10.0 μg/ml exaggerated all these changes. Because these effects were observed in preparations pretreated with tetrodotoxin or atropine, they were considered to represent the direct membrane action of this drug depressing the slow inward current. However, it must be reemphasized that disopyramide and other class 1A drugs depress conduction predominantly in those fast response fibers rather than in the slow response fibers of the AV node.

Perfusion of such a preparation with physostigmine (0.65 μg/ml) markedly depressed its automaticity, and the spontaneous activity almost ceased (Figure 20.6). Subsequent addition of disopyramide at 0.05 μg/ml caused occasional firing of action potentials, and higher concentrations of the drug (0.5 and 2.5 μg/ml) further enhanced the automaticity.[101] This indicates that inhibition of AV nodal automaticity by increased vagal tone can be reversed by the anticholinergic action of disopyramide. Of particular importance in this observation is that such an anticholinergic action appears at a much lower concentration than that producing the direct membrane action. It then follows that administration of a small amount of disopyramide to a patient with increased vagal tone may enhance AV nodal automaticity through the anticholinergic action, whereas a larger dose of this drug in a patient with a relatively low vagal tone may depress automaticity by its direct membrane action. This is probably the reason for the rather inconsistent reports on the effects of this drug on AV junctional arrhythmias. Nevertheless, disopyramide in many respects resembles quinidine, the most classic antiarrhythmic drug in class 1A. Procainamide appears to have much weaker anticholinergic action.

Regarding factors modifying the electrophysiologic effects of class 1A agents, only two of them will be briefly discussed here. First, these drugs appear to decrease the rate of phase 0 depolarization and depress conduction more markedly in ischemic or hypoxic fibers than in normal fibers. This implies that slow conduction in partially depolarized fast response fibers, which is dependent on the "residual" (or depressed) fast Na^+ channel, may readily be blocked by these drugs, thereby interrupting reentry movements in the ischemic myocardium. Second, the depressing action of class 1 antiarrhythmic drugs on the maximal rate of depolarization and conduction in fast response fibers is antagonized by low extracellular K^+ concentrations and is enhanced by high K^+.[103,104] Hence, the clinical efficacy of these drugs can be significantly reduced in the presence of hypokalemia, whereas hyperkalemia may facilitate the development of toxicity. The importance of maintaining normal serum electrolyte levels in antiarrhythmic drug therapy is thus emphasized.

Class 1B Agents. Most typical of class 1B antiarrhythmic drugs is probably lidocaine, although its orally active analogs such as mexiletine[105–107] and several other agents such as diphenylhydantoin[99,108] are also frequently used

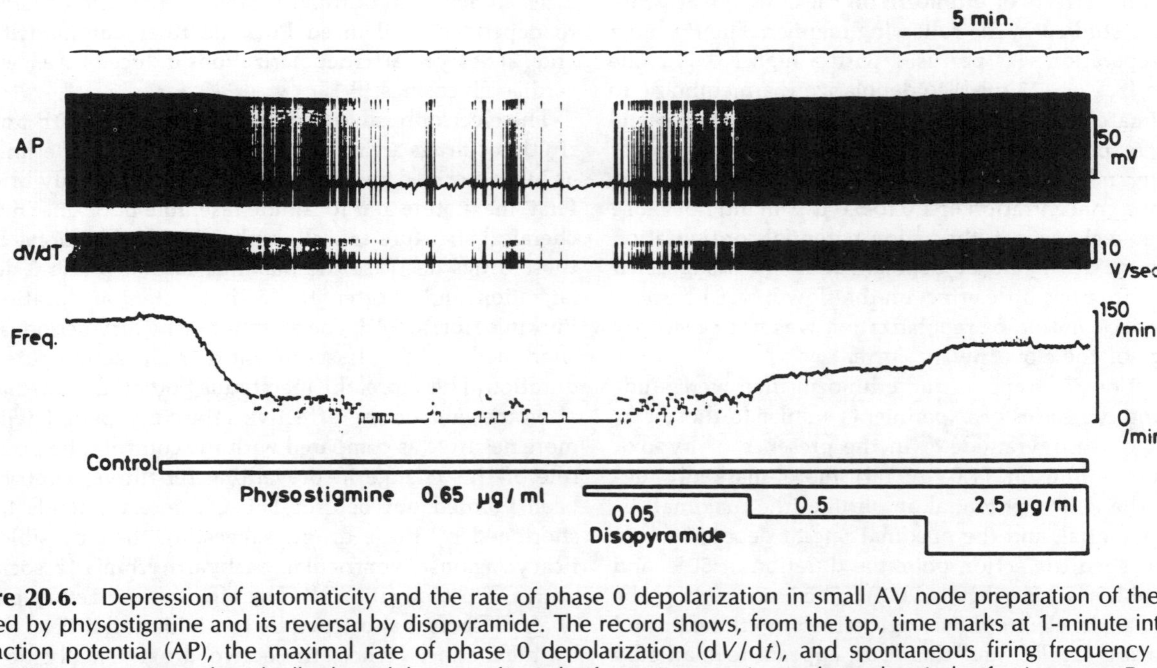

Figure 20.6. Depression of automaticity and the rate of phase 0 depolarization in small AV node preparation of the rabbit caused by physostigmine and its reversal by disopyramide. The record shows, from the top, time marks at 1-minute intervals, the action potential (AP), the maximal rate of phase 0 depolarization (dV/dt), and spontaneous firing frequency (Freq). Physostigmine 0.65 μg/ml markedly slowed the rate of impulse formation, causing prolonged periods of quiescence. Reduction in the action potential amplitude as well as the rate of phase 0 depolarization was also noted. Subsequent addition of disopyramide at progressively higher concentrations partially restored the spontaneous firing frequency toward the control level, associated with some increase in the action potential amplitude. Therefore, anticholinergic action of disopyramide appears to enhance AV nodal automaticity and conduction (Nishimura and Watanabe, unpublished observation).

in clinical practice. In this section, however, our studies on the electrophysiologic effects of ethmozin will be presented to illustrate some class 1B actions.[109] The experiment was carried out on canine Purkinje fibers superfused in a tissue bath, with a protocol similar to that used in studying the disopyramide effects. When ethmozin was added to the perfusate at increasing concentrations of 0.05, 0.2, and 1.0 μg/ml, the maximal rate of phase 0 depolarization was decreased at the lowest concentration (0.05 μg/ml). A higher concentration of 0.2 μg/ml produced significant reductions in the action potential amplitude and overshoot, and shortened the action potential duration at both 50% and 90% repolarization. Conversely, the maximal diastolic potential remained essentially unaffected. Thus, the reduction in the rate of phase 0 depolarization was considered to result from blockage of the fast Na^+ channel and not from membrane depolarization. The shortening of action potential duration was accompanied by a shortening of the effective refractory period. However, the latter was less marked than the former, and the ratio between the effective refractory period and the action potential duration at 90% repolarization was slightly increased after ethmozin perfusion. This action appears to be shared by most class 1B agents.[79,99]

When the membrane responsiveness curve was obtained by correlating the level of membrane potential and the maximal rate of depolarization before and after the addition of ethmozin in the perfusate, the curve was shifted by ethmozin toward higher membrane potentials by several millivolts. Hence, the ethmozin-induced reduction in the rate of phase 0 depolarization was considered to result from an increased inactivation of the fast Na^+ current at all potential levels. On the other hand, the possible effects of ethmozin on the slow inward current were studied in the following manner. The Purkinje fiber preparation was perfused with a high K^+ Tyrode solution (K^+ = 22 mM) to depolarize the membrane to approximately −40 mV, and slow response action potentials were produced by the addition of *l*-isoproterenol (0.025 μg/ml). Because the subsequent addition of ethmozin at a concentration of 1.0 to 5.0 μg/ml did not cause appreciable changes in the action potential configuration and the maximal rate of depolarization, it is suggested that this drug has little effect on the slow inward current, and the acceleration of repolarization was not caused by blockage of the slow inward current.

Interactions of hypoxia and ethmozin then were studied in another series of experiments similar to those carried out on disopyramide.[97] In the presence of hypoxic perfusion, ethmozin (1.0 μg/ml) more markedly decreased the action potential amplitude, the maximal diastolic potential, and the maximal rate of depolarization, and shortened the action potential duration at 50% and 90% repolarization (Figure 20.7). This can perhaps be expected as the electrophysiologic effects of ethmozin and hypoxia are similar, and this drug appears to markedly depress conduction and accelerate repolarization in the ischemic myocardium.[109]

On the basis of these observations and available literature,[110] the mechanisms of action of ethmozin against

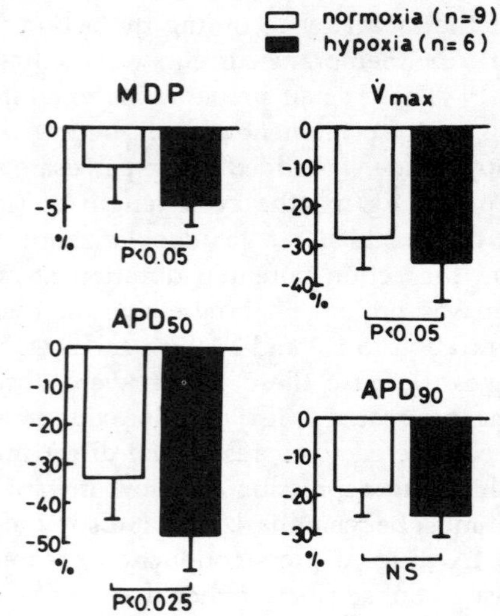

Figure 20.7. Comparison of ethmozin-induced changes in various parameters of canine Purkinje fiber action potential in the presence of normoxic versus hypoxic perfusion. Ethmozin concentration was 1.0 μg/ml. APD_{50} and APD_{90}=action potential duration at 50% and 90% repolarization, respectively; MDP=maximal diastolic potential; NS=not significant; $\dot{V}max$=maximal rate of phase 0 depolarization (From Tsuji et al,[109] with permission).

ventricular tachyarrhythmia are probably ascribed to (1) depression of conduction with conversion of unidirectional block to bidirectional block in the reentry circuit, and (2) relative prolongation of the effective refractory period with reference to the action potential duration. Available literature indicates that this drug can also suppress (1) those ventricular tachyarrhythmias occurring after an acute myocardial infarction that are considered to depend on enhanced Purkinje fiber automaticity,[110] and (2) delayed afterdepolarizations induced by excessive cardiac glycosides.[111]

The electrophysiologic effects of other class 1B antiarrhythmic drugs are naturally similar to those of ethmozin as just described and hence will be reviewed only briefly. First, mexiletine and tocainide resemble lidocaine in their chemical structure as well as pharmacologic actions. Both these drugs decrease the maximal rate of phase 0 depolarization and shorten the action potential duration in Purkinje fibers.[106,112] The effective refractory period is also shortened, but to a lesser extent than the action potential duration. Therefore, the membrane potential immediately after the end of the effective refractory period will be more negative as compared with the control. The possible role of this change in preventing repetitive reentry has been pointed out before. The QT interval tends to be shortened by these drugs, suggesting their possible efficacy against ventricular tachyarrhythmia associated with QT prolongation.[113] The effective refractory period of atrial fibers is shortened by tocainide and little affected by mexiletine. Hence, these two drugs usually do not exhibit significant antiarrhythmic effects against atrial tachyarrhythmias such as atrial fibrillation.

Aprindine has also been classified as a class 1B agent, depressing the rate of phase 0 depolarization and shortening the action potential as well as the effective refractory period of Purkinje fibers.[114] This drug, however, is said to prolong the effective refractory period of atrial fibers, in sharp contrast to mexiletine, and to be effective against certain supraventricular tachyarrhythmias and WPW tachycardia.[106]

Use-dependent Block of the Fast Na^+ Channel. With reference to the major difference between the effects of class 1A and class 1B drugs, or their effects on the refractory period, the concept of use-dependent block of the fast Na^+ channel must be discussed. According to Hondeghem and Katzung and others,[115–117] all class 1 antiarrhythmic drugs are bound to the membrane Na^+ channel and thereby block the fast Na^+ current. This mechanism has often been referred to as a local anesthetic action. More specifically, in the presence of these drugs, the amount of fast Na^+ current flowing at a given membrane potential is reduced, and a higher (more negative) membrane potential is required to obtain the original amount of current. When the drugs are dissociated from the membrane, the Na^+ channel is unblocked and the inflow of the fast Na^+ current is once again restored to the normal level. The speed of such binding as well as dissociation is modulated by (and differs among) the three states of the channel, ie, resting state, activated state, and inactivated state, with the transition from one state to another being governed by the Hodgkin–Huxley equation.[115–117] Generally, drugs are rapidly bound to the channel in the activated state (simplistically, during phase 0 of an action potential), and are much more slowly dissociated in the resting state (roughly during the electrical diastole or phase 4).

By postulating different rate constants of binding and dissociation for individual drugs, the aforementioned investigators were able to simulate the observed effects of quinidine (a prototype class 1A drug) and lidocaine (a prototype class 1B drug) on phase 0 depolarization, thereby substantiating the validity of their hypothesis.[115] As a result, it can be stated that as lidocaine has a rapid rate of dissociation, the Na^+ channel is almost completely unblocked after each action potential, and hence, with repetitive stimulation, the maximal rate of phase 0 depolarization is well maintained. Contrariwise, the rate of dissociation of quinidine is 20 times slower than that of lidocaine. Hence, even after a fairly long electrical diastole, the fast Na^+ channel is still partially blocked by the drug, and repetitive stimulation causes a progressive reduction in the rate of depolarization.[115–117] This is called a use-dependent block and is considered to play some role in the phenomenon of post-repolarization refractoriness mentioned with reference to the term *phase 3 block*. It will then be readily anticipated that the higher the frequency of stimulation, the greater the slowing of the action potential upstroke. (Actual records showing this phenomenon will be presented later with reference to propranolol.) This implies that, during tachycardia, class 1A drugs will cause a greater depression of conduction than class 1B drugs.

It also follows that in atrial fibers having a much shorter action potential duration than Purkinje or ventricular muscle fibers, the duration of electrical diastole (phase 4) is longer, and a sufficient time will be available for unblocking of the Na^+ channel, especially for lidocaine and other class 1B agents. Conversely, quinidine and other class 1A drugs will keep the Na^+ channel still partially blocked during phase 4 of even the atrial action potential. This is probably the reason class 1B drugs are usually less effective in suppressing atrial tachyarrhythmias as compared with class 1A drugs. It is interesting to note that aprindine, unlike lidocaine, appears to show a use-dependent block and, in this regard, acts more like a class 1A agent.[16,118]

Class 1C Agents. This subdivision of class 1 antiarrhythmic drugs has most recently been added to the classification. Because we have not carried out experimental studies on these drugs, the available literature will be briefly reviewed. Generally, drugs belonging to this group are characterized by a potent depressing effect on phase 0 depolarization of fast response fibers.[69–71] Especially in the ventricles, a marked reduction in the conduction velocity by these class 1C drugs often prolongs the QRS duration even when the ventricular rate is reasonably slow as in normal sinus rhythm, whereas such a widening of the QRS interval is seen only during tachycardia when class 1A drugs are administered. Encainide, for instance, has been shown to decrease the maximal rate of depolarization of the ventricular muscle and Purkinje fibers. The action potential duration was slightly shortened in Purkinje fibers but not in ventricular muscle. At higher concentrations, encainide depressed phase 4 depolarization in Purkinje fibers and slowed their impulse formation. Flecainide similarly decreases the maximal rate of phase 0 depolarization in Purkinje fibers and tends to shorten the action potential duration. However, the refractory period appears to be prolonged in ventricular muscle fibers and the bundle of Kent and, to a lesser extent, in the atria and AV node as well.[119]

These observations suggest that the antiarrhythmic mechanism of class 1C agents is mainly through their Na^+ channel blocking action and depression of conduction, leading to the abolition of reentry movement in those fast response fibers. Indeed, class 1C agents are effective in eliminating premature systoles.[120] However, because of such a potent depressing action, these drugs may well facilitate the production of arrhythmias in certain instances.

Class 2 Antiarrhythmic Drugs

A prototype of beta-adrenergic blocking drugs is perhaps propranolol. In this section, however, the result of our experimental studies on carteolol (OPC-1085), another beta blocker with an intrinsic beta stimulating action, will be presented to illustrate the electropharmacologic aspects of class 2 drugs, supplemented by some comparison with propranolol.[80] First, the effects of this drug on SA nodal automaticity were studied using an overdrive suppression test in isolated, perfused rabbit hearts, and a representative example is shown in Figure 20.8. In this experiment, the right atrium was electrically stimulated for 20 seconds at a cycle length of 320 ms

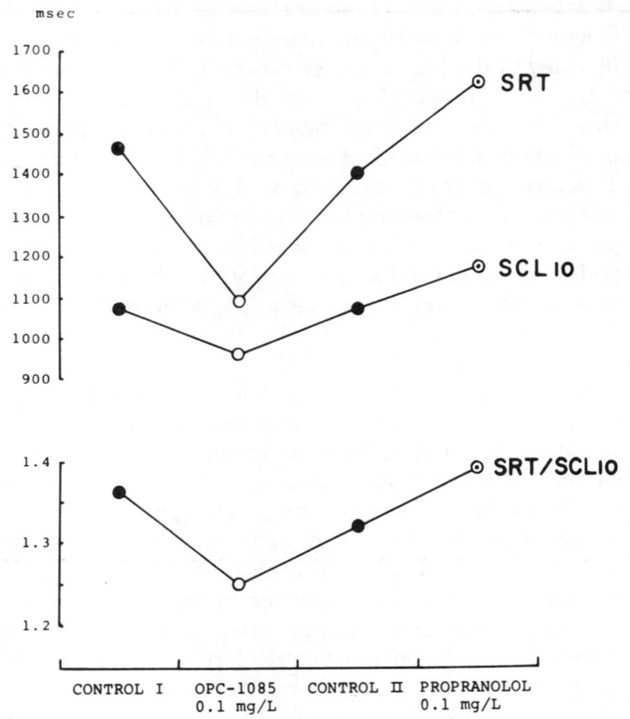

Figure 20.8. Comparison of the effects of carteolol (OPC-1085) and propranolol on overdrive suppression of the rabbit SA node. SCL10=average sinus cycle length in ten spontaneous sinus beats immediately before the overdrive pacing; SRT=sinus node recovery time.

through a close bipolar electrode positioned near the SA node, and the sinus node recovery time (SRT, or the interval from the termination of electrical drive to the appearance of the first postpacing sinus beat) was determined. In the absence of this drug (control I), the sinus node recovery time measured 1,460 ms, whereas the sinus cycle length before the overdrive was 1,070 ms (an average of ten cycles). The difference between these two values (1,460 − 1,070 = 390 ms) represents the so-called corrected sinus node recovery time (CSRT). After the addition of 0.1 mg/L of carteolol, both the sinus cycle length and the sinus node recovery time were shortened, to 950 and 1,090 ms, with a marked shortening of the CSRT to 140 ms. When a similar test was repeated with propranolol (0.1 mg/L) after a washout of carteolol (control II), the CSRT was prolonged to 450 ms. Thus, carteolol appeared to enhance, whereas propranolol depressed SA nodal automaticity.

Conversely, isoproterenol-induced automaticity in the canine Purkinje fiber preparation was clearly depressed by carteolol (0.2 mg/L), apparently to a greater extent than that by the same concentration of propranolol. Such contradictory findings may be explained as follows. In overdrive suppression tests carried out in the presence of a normal sinus rhythm, the sympathetic activity was initially low; hence, the intrinsic beta stimulating action of carteolol may have predominated and directly enhanced SA nodal automaticity, as a reflex sympathetic discharge caused by blood pressure changes cannot be invoked in isolated, perfused rabbit hearts. Against catecholamine-enhanced Purkinje automaticity, only the beta blocking action will be operative, and hence, carteolol, which is considered to have a stronger beta blocking action than propranolol, may have caused a greater depression.

In canine Purkinje fibers, carteolol (5 to 20 mg/L) slightly shortened the action potential duration at 80% repolarization, but tended to prolong the effective refractory period. The action potential amplitude, the maximal diastolic potential, and the maximal rate of depolarization were essentially unchanged at a drug concentration of 5 mg/L, but they were decreased at 20 mg/L. At the latter concentration, conduction at the Purkinje–ventricular muscle junction was clearly depressed, and a reduction in the maximal following frequency was noted. These findings are probably in agreement with the general trend that the concentration of various beta blocking drugs directly affecting the action potential characteristics is usually much higher than the concentration at which the beta blocking action manifests itself.[75,121]

As pointed out earlier, propranolol and some other beta blockers have a direct membrane action similar to that of class 1 drugs. This is illustrated in Figure 20.9, with experimental records obtained from a Purkinje fiber preparation perfused in the tissue bath (Watanabe, unpublished observation). The left panels show the action potential and the maximal rate of depolarization during control perfusion (top) and after the addition of 1 mg/L of propranolol (bottom), while the preparation was being stimulated at 1 Hz. It is clearly seen that propranolol decreased the action potential amplitude without affecting the maximal diastolic potential, and it reduced the maximal rate of phase 0 depolarization. The rightward shift of the record of the maximal rate of depolarization indicates a later arrival of the excitation front at this recording site, and hence, depression of conduction after propranolol. The action potential duration was shortened at both 50% and 90% repolarization, with a lowering of the plateau. In the right panels, the effects of a sudden shortening of the driving cycle length on the maximal rate of depolarization are shown. During control perfusion, the rate of depolarization was only minimally decreased by the rapid drive. Contrariwise, the rapid pacing caused a progressive reduction in the rate of depolarization after propranolol perfusion, a good example of use-dependent block of the fast Na^+ channel. Therefore, slow dissociation of propranolol from the channel may be speculated. This may also explain a relative prolongation of the effective refractory period even though the action potential duration tends to be shortened.

Needless to say, beta blockade will reduce the slow inward current and depress AV nodal conduction. Therefore, class 2 drugs are frequently used to terminate paroxysmal AV junctional tachycardia and to control the ventricular response to atrial flutter or fibrillation.[122–124]

From these observations, it may well be expected that different beta-adrenergic blocking agents may show qualitatively different antiarrhythmic effects depending on the presence or absence of direct membrane action and beta stimulating action. However, in clinical practice, all the beta blockers appear to be effective against similar types of arrhythmia regardless of their actions other than

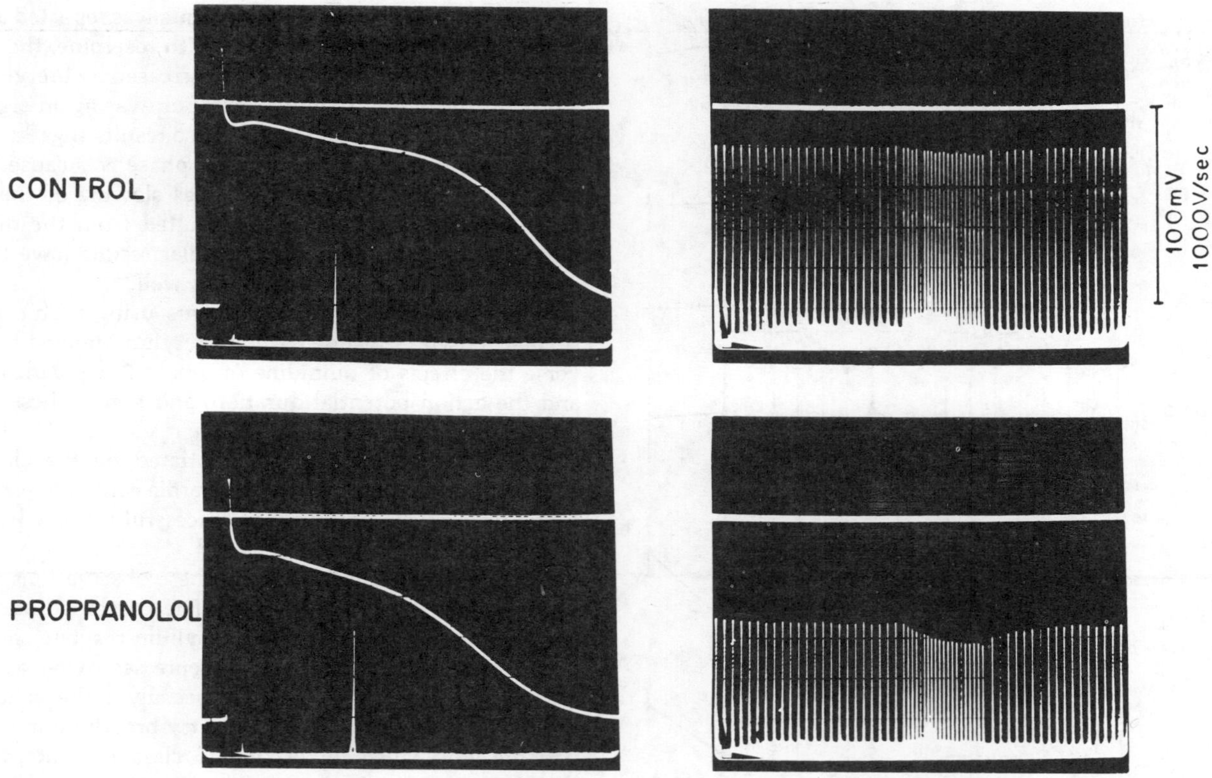

Figure 20.9. Effects of propranolol on the action potential characteristics of the canine Purkinje fiber and on the use-dependent block of the fast Na^+ channel. In the *left panels,* the records show, from the top, zero reference potential, action potential, and dV/dt of phase 0 representing the maximal rate of depolarization. In the *right panels,* sequential changes in the dV/dt record during a sudden shortening of the driving cycle length from 1,000 to 500 ms are shown. Note that there was little change in dV/dt during the control (*top*), whereas in the presence of propranolol the rapid stimulation caused a progressive reduction in the rate of depolarization (*bottom*) (Watanabe, unpublished observation).

beta blockade. For this reason, certain investigators appear to believe that the antiarrhythmic mechanism of class 2 agents is almost solely dependent on their beta blocking action. Class 2 drugs may also be effective against delayed afterdepolarization and triggered activity enhanced by catecholamines or an increased sympathetic tone.

Class 3 Antiarrhythmic Drugs

Class 3 antiarrhythmic drugs include amiodarone and bretylium tosylate.[81–87] Of these, amiodarone is much more extensively used than bretylium tosylate in the treatment of various supraventricular and ventricular tachyarrhythmias. In this section, however, our experimental results on bretylium tosylate will be presented first, followed by a review of the literature on amiodarone.

The electrophysiologic effects of bretylium were studied using canine Purkinje fibers under both normoxic and hypoxic conditions.[87] When bretylium was added to the perfusate at a concentration of 20 mg/L, the action potential duration at 50% and 90% repolarization was significantly prolonged and so was the effective refractory period. The action potential amplitude, the maximal diastolic potential, and the maximal rate of depolarization were unaffected. Washout of the drug with a new control perfusate did not shorten the action potential duration and the refractory period. Bretylium did not affect the membrane responsiveness curve, substantiating the lack of significant changes in the maximal rate of phase 0 depolarization as just described.

Figure 20.10 summarizes the results of our experiment on the interactions between hypoxia and bretylium tosylate using canine Purkinje fibers. When we first tested the effects of hypoxia alone for 60 minutes, the action potential amplitude, the maximal diastolic potential, and the maximal rate of depolarization were all decreased significantly in the first 20 minutes, with subsequent partial recovery. The action potential duration was shortened. After restoration of all parameters to the control level with a return to the normal oxygenation, a second 60-minute hypoxic perfusion was carried out, during the last half of which bretylium was added to the perfusate. The drug significantly increased the action potential amplitude and the maximal diastolic potential. The maximal rate of phase 0 depolarization was also increased 10 to 30 minutes after the addition of bretylium, although the changes were statistically insignificant due to a dissimilar time course of such an increase in different fibers. The maximal rate of depolarization, however, was further reduced in additional control experiments in which bretylium was not added during the last 30 minutes of the hypoxic period. This indicates that the bretylium-induced increase in the maximal rate of depolarization tends to antagonize the development of conduction disturbance

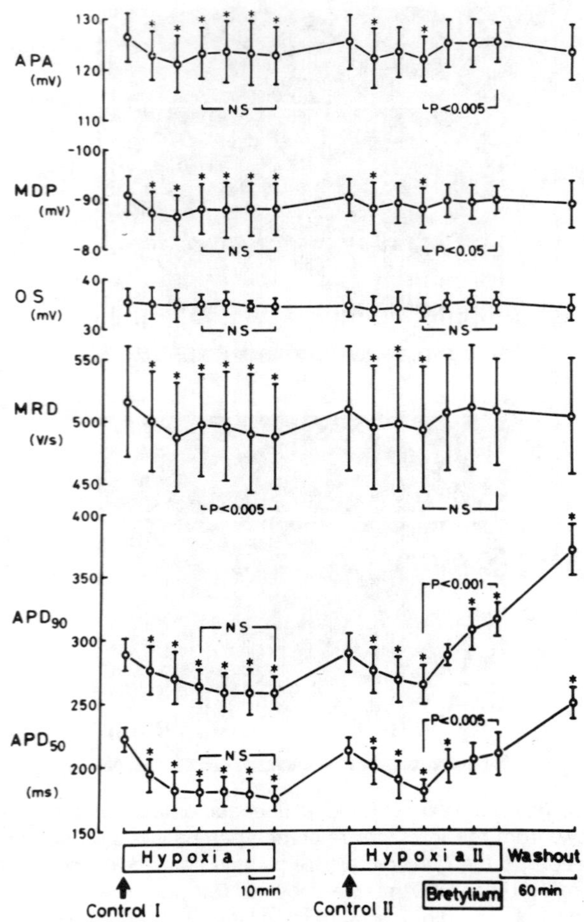

Figure 20.10. Effects of hypoxia alone and of hypoxia plus bretylium tosylate on various action potential measurements in the canine Purkinje fiber. Statistical analyses were made on six experiments using nonreserpinized preparations. APA= action potential amplitude; APD_{90} and APD_{50}=action potential duration at 90% and 50% repolarization, respectively; MDP=maximal diastolic potential; MRD=maximal rate of phase 0 depolarization; OS=overshoot. *Open circles* with vertical bars represent mean values ± standard deviation. Asterisks indicate that the values are significantly different (at 5% level) from either Control I or Control II measurements. Probability values with brackets denote statistical significance on comparing individual measurements after 30 minutes of hypoxia with those after 60 minutes of hypoxia. NS=not significant (From Nishimura et al.[87] Reprinted with permission from the American College of Cardiology).

due to hypoxia. The action potential duration also was increased by bretylium in the presence of hypoxic perfusion (Figure 20.10, *bottom*). Hence, bretylium appeared to reverse all the deleterious effects of hypoxia on both depolarization and repolarization.

Such a combination of improved phase 0 parameters (improved conduction) and prolonged action potential duration (or the refractory period) would be beneficial in interrupting reentry movements in the ischemic ventricles, and this may well be the reason for the reported clinical efficacy of bretylium in the treatment of intractable ventricular fibrillation in acute myocardial infarction.[125-127]

When a similar series of experiments was repeated after pretreatment of the preparations with reserpine, the rate of phase 0 depolarization was not increased by bretylium, although the action potential duration was again significantly prolonged (not shown). These results suggest that improvement in the depolarization phase was caused by a release of catecholamines, whereas slowing of the repolarization phase most likely resulted from the direct membrane action of the drug. Similar results have been published by other investigators as well.[86]

In an earlier series of experiments using rabbit ventricular muscle, we showed that bretylium tended to reverse the effects of quinidine on phase 0 depolarization and the action potential duration, and hence, these two drugs appear antagonistic in their electrophysiologic effects.[128] This was later substantiated by the clinical observation that ventricular tachycardia caused by excessive quinidine medication was successfully treated with bretylium.[129]

Finally, clinical implications of these observations may be summarized as follows.[87] (1) The combined administration of class 1 agents and bretylium tosylate should be avoided because the former depresses, whereas the latter may improve conduction, especially in the ischemic heart. (2) It may be worthwhile to try bretylium in those patients who failed to respond to class 1 agents, after withdrawal of the latter. (3) Bretylium may be used to treat toxic manifestations of quinidine (and possibly other class 1 drugs) as already suggested.

Amiodarone, on the other hand, has a unique property. When administered orally, its effective blood level will not be reached for two to four weeks, and its antiarrhythmic efficacy often lasts more than six weeks after discontinuation of therapy.[130,131] Electrophysiologically, amiodarone markedly prolonged the action potential duration of ventricular muscle fibers without reducing the membrane resting potential and the maximal rate of depolarization.[81,130] Regarding the ionic mechanisms for prolongation of the action potential duration, it is still not clear whether the drug (1) selectively decreases the membrane K^+ conductance, (2) increases the time constant of inactivation of the slow inward current, or (3) causes both these changes.[132] Nevertheless, such a marked prolongation of the action potential duration is accompanied by a significant prolongation of the refractory period, and hence, reexcitation of fibers at a rapid rate will be prevented. Amiodarone appears to depress conduction through the AV node, although the ionic mechanism for this action has not been elucidated.

These observations probably account for the reported clinical efficacy of amiodarone against most varieties of reentrant tachyarrhythmia, including supraventricular and ventricular premature systoles, paroxysmal supraventricular tachycardia, and WPW tachycardia.[82,130,133,134] In the presence of atrial flutter or atrial fibrillation, this drug can be used either to terminate these arrhythmias or to control the ventricular response. This drug appears to be effective in preventing ventricular tachycardia with oral administration, perhaps abolishing premature systoles,[135,136] whereas intravenous amiodarone appears less effective in interrupting episodes of ventricular tachycardia. Clinical reports on this latter mode of administration, however, are certainly available.[137,138]

Class 4 Antiarrhythmic Drugs

Class 4 antiarrhythmic drugs block the slow inward current that plays a major role in the generation of so-called slow response action potentials. Because the slow inward current is carried mainly by Ca^{++} ions, these drugs are usually called Ca^{++} antagonists.[90,91,139] It has earlier been pointed out that those slow responses occur in myocardial fibers partially depolarized by factors such as injury or high K^+ concentrations, and also in the SA and AV nodes under physiologic conditions. In AV nodal fibers, part of the slow inward current appears to be carried by Na^+ ions,[39-41] and hence, it might be more appropriate to call these drugs slow channel blockers. Of various Ca^{++} antagonists, verapamil and diltiazem are the two drugs effectively used in the treatment of arrhythmias, and we have studied the electrophysiologic effects of verapamil on the AV node of rabbits.

When small preparations of the rabbit AV node (in the size of 0.2 × 0.2 × 0.1 mm) were perfused in a tissue chamber as in those experiments on disopyramide (Figure 20.6), and verapamil was added to the perfusate at a concentration of 0.05 μg/ml (5×10^{-8} g/ml), the spontaneous firing frequency did not show consistent changes, with some specimens showing slowing and others showing acceleration. Here, prolongation of the cycle length (depression of automaticity) was caused by a reduction in the slope of diastolic depolarization, which probably resulted from a decreased slow inward current. Contrariwise, shortening of the cycle length (enhancement of automaticity) was explained by a decrease in the outward K^+ current and outward background current.[41] Regardless of these variations in its effects on automaticity, verapamil always caused a reduction in the maximal rate of phase 0 depolarization. This latter action was concentration dependent (Figure 20.11). A slight but statistically significant decrease in the rate of depolarization was observed even at a low concentration of 2×10^{-9} g/ml, and spontaneous firing ceased at a verapamil concentration of 10^{-6} g/ml. These observations suggest that verapamil would definitely depress conduction in the AV node.

Figure 20.12 more directly illustrates the AV conduction disorder caused by verapamil.[39] In this experiment using an isolated, perfused rabbit heart, a His bundle electrogram was recorded from the His bundle region simultaneously with a bipolar electrocardiogram. After a control record (top) was obtained, verapamil (0.5 mg/L) was added to the perfusate. This caused the development of 2° AV block of the Wenckebach variety with a 3:2 conduction ratio (second panel). Failure of propagation within the AV node is indicated by the absence of the His deflection in the third beat. When the Na^+ concentration in the perfusate was elevated from 145 to 172 mM in the presence of verapamil, 1:1 AV conduction was restored with a marked shortening of the AH interval (bottom panel). The possible mechanisms for such an interaction may be explained as follows. Verapamil de-

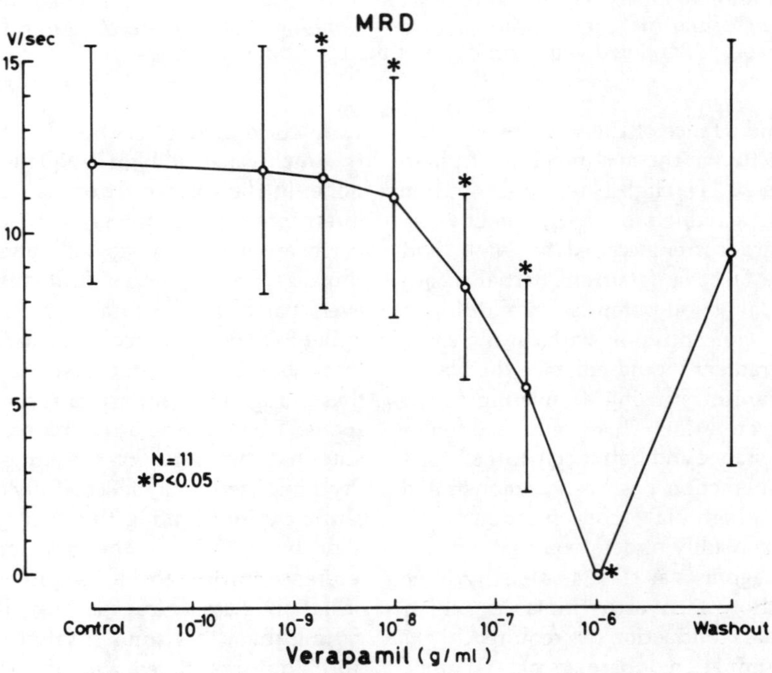

Figure 20.11. Concentration-response curve showing changes in the maximal rate of depolarization (MRD) of spontaneously beating rabbit AV nodal cells produced by progressively higher concentrations of verapamil in the perfusate. At a concentration of 10^{-6} g/ml, spontaneous firing ceased. *Open circles* with vertical bars represent mean values ± standard deviation. Asterisks denote statistical significance compared with the control values (Nishimura and Watanabe, unpublished observation).

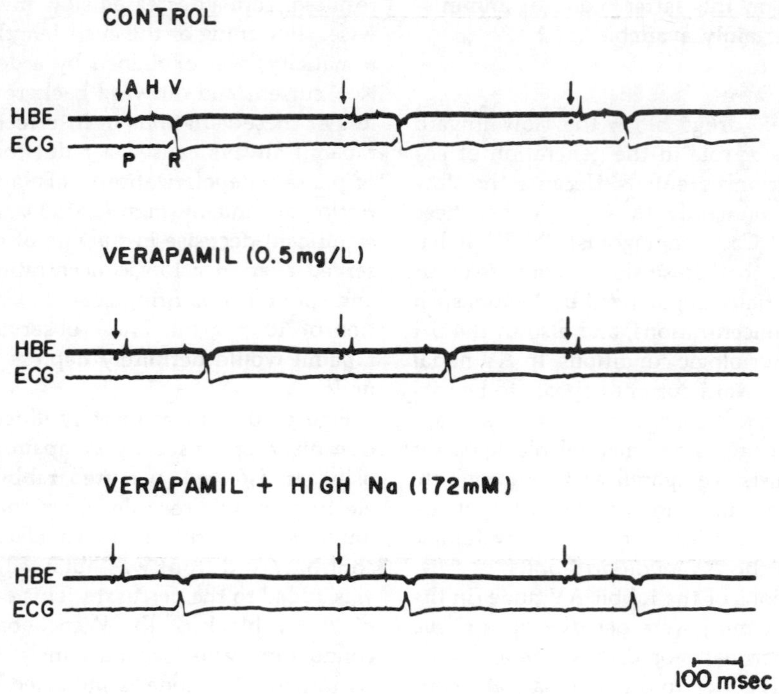

Figure 20.12. Interactions of verapamil and high Na^+ concentration on AV conduction in an isolated, perfused rabbit heart. ECG=bipolar electrocardiogram; HBE=His bundle electrogram. *Arrows* indicate the time of stimulation near the SA node. A, H, and V in the His bundle records represent excitation of the lower right atrium, the His bundle, and interventricular septum, respectively. P and R in the electrocardiogram correspond to atrial and ventricular activation, respectively. Note a second degree AV nodal block with a 3:2 conduction ratio after verapamil perfusion (*middle record*) and restoration of 1:1 conduction and a marked shortening of the AH interval with high Na^+ perfusion (*bottom record*). (From Watanabe.[39] Reprinted with permission of the C. V. Mosby Company).

creases the maximal conductance of the slow inward current ($\bar{g}_s$) causing a reduction in the maximal rate of phase 0 depolarization (Figure 20.11). High Na^+ concentration would antagonize such a reduction of $\bar{g}_s$, thereby increasing the slow inward current carried by Na^+, and also would increase the fast Na^+ current partially contributing to the AV nodal action potential. In addition, a high extracellular Na^+ concentration with an increased transmembrane Na^+ gradient would enhance the Na^+–Ca^{++} exchange mechanism, causing a lowering of the intracellular Ca^{++} concentration. This would lead to decreased intercellular resistance and better cell-to-cell conduction.[140] A similar interaction has been demonstrated between diltiazem and a high Na^+ concentration.[39]

Nevertheless, it can be readily understood that a major indication of Ca^{++} antagonists as class 4 antiarrhythmic drugs will be against those tachyarrhythmias in which depression of AV nodal conduction is required.[141–143] More specifically, (1) termination of paroxysmal AV junctional tachycardia caused by reentry movements in the AV nodal region, and (2) reduction of the ventricular rate in the presence of atrial flutter or fibrillation are the two most common indications of these agents, being associated with a high rate of success. Verapamil has also been shown to exhibit a use-dependent block of the slow inward current, an effect beneficial for these two modes of treatment against high frequency discharge of the AV node. In the former action, AV nodal reentry is usually interrupted in the antegrade limb of the dual AV nodal pathway having a slower conduction velocity and a shorter refractory period (called the α pathway).[143] However, paroxysmal supraventricular tachycardias due to either SA nodal reentry or intraatrial reentry often do not respond to Ca^{++} antagonist drugs,[68,142] probably because these drugs have little depressing action on the fast response fibers in the atria and tend to shorten the action potential duration. For the same reason, class 4 antiarrhythmic agents may successfully terminate a WPW tachycardia by interrupting the reentry movement in the AV node but seldom in the accessory pathway.[144,145] With reference to the second indication for atrial flutter or fibrillation, class 4 drugs are usually unsuccessful in converting them to a sinus rhythm.[146,147] Especially in atrial fibrillation associated with the WPW syndrome, Ca^{++} antagonists do not depress conduction in the bundle of Kent and even tend to shorten its refractory period, often leading to a faster ventricular response and an increased risk of ventricular fibrillation.[148] Hence, class 4 drugs should not be used in such cases.

Because Ca^{++} antagonists block the slow inward current and tend to decrease intracellular Ca^{++} concentration, they will be theoretically effective against ventricular arrhythmias as well, if those arrhythmias are dependent on either (1) slow conduction and reentry occurring in partially depolarized myocardial fibers, or (2) delayed afterdepolarization and triggered activity.[19,90,91] However, as pointed out earlier, it is difficult to identify these mechanisms in the clinical setting, and hence, class 4 antiarrhythmic drugs have been used against ventricular tachyarrhythmias mostly in a trial and error fashion and without much success. In certain selected cases including so-called idiopathic ventricular tachycardia with a QRS pattern of right bundle branch block and left axis deviation,[149,150] Ca^{++} antagonists were shown to be effective. Whether the ventricular tachycardia in those cases was indeed caused by the aforementioned mechanisms can not be determined at this moment. It has further been shown that verapamil often increased the frequency of cellular discharge during sustained ventricular fibrillation in isolated, perfused rabbit hearts produced by rapid electrical stimulation.[100] Hence, class 4 antiarrhythmic agents must be used with caution against ventricular tachyarrhythmias.

MECHANISMS OF ACTION OF PACING AGAINST CARDIAC ARRHYTHMIAS

CARDIAC PACING AGAINST BRADYARRHYTHMIAS

The technology of cardiac pacing has made truly remarkable progress in recent years, expanding its indications to the control of tachyarrhythmias. Yet, even today, various bradyarrhythmias account for a majority of pacemaker implantations in the world. According to statistics compiled in Europe in 1980, for instance, the electrocardiographic findings before pacemaker implantation were AV conduction disturbances in 50% of cases and sick sinus syndrome in 24%.[151] Patients with bundle branch blocks for whom prophylactic pacemaker implantation was indicated against the possible development of serious AV block accounted for most of the remaining population, whereas implantation of various antitachycardia devices occupied only about 1%. Hence, the mechanisms of action of pacing against bradyarrhythmias will be discussed first, although pacing in the treatment of tachyarrhythmias is gaining widespread attention.

Genesis of Bradyarrhythmias and Their Hemodynamic Consequences

As summarized earlier in Table 20.3, the genesis of bradyarrhythmias includes the following: (1) Depression of automaticity in the SA node, or the primary, physiologic pacemaker, would cause sinus bradycardia or sinus arrest. (2) Failure of conduction of sinus impulses along the specialized conducting system would take the form of either SA block or AV block. In the presence of any of the foregoing conditions, certain fibers of the conducting system (most often in the AV junction, followed by the Purkinje system) usually develop diastolic depolarization and generate their own impulses at a rate slower than that of the normal sinus rhythm. This will produce an escape beat or escape rhythm and prevent prolonged ventricular asystole.[3,5] (3) However, depression of SA nodal automaticity or failure of conduction of sinus impulses may sometimes be accompanied by an inefficient escape mechanism. Reduction of the ventricular rate will then be more marked, and serious bradyarrhythmias may ensue. There are several varieties belonging to this category. For instance, the reason certain cases of so-called sick sinus syndrome develop prolonged ventricular asystole and syncope is that a subsidiary pacemaker fails to immediately take over the control of the ventricles, and a more widespread distribution of degenerative changes involving both the SA node and the AV junctional tissue has been suggested in those cases.[152,153] Another example is the occurrence of exit block from a subsidiary pacemaker. Because the rate of impulse formation in those subsidiary foci is intrinsically slower than the sinus rate, such an exit block can cause marked prolongation of the RR interval. An entity termed *downward displacement of the pacemaker* mentioned earlier[18] constitutes another example, where physiologic automaticity is depressed not only in the SA node but also throughout the specialized conducting system, so that the pacemaking site is gradually shifted downward from the SA node to the AV junction and to the Purkinje system. This condition often occurs as a terminal event and causes progressive slowing of the rhythm with increasingly widened QRS complexes, culminating in ventricular standstill.

Nevertheless, these bradyarrhythmias could adversely affect cardiac hemodynamics in two ways: (1) In the presence of supraventricular bradyarrhythmia with an appropriate PR interval, the stroke output could be increased because of a longer diastole. However, if the rhythm is too slow, this increase in the stroke output can be offset, resulting in decreased cardiac output. (2) If, on the other hand, the activity of the subsidiary pacemaker produces asynchrony between atrial and ventricular excitation, or there is AV synchrony with a fixed but inappropriate PR interval, the loss of atrial contribution to ventricular filling and mitral as well as pulmonary venous regurgitation would markedly decrease the stroke volume, further aggravating the reduction of cardiac output.[154]

Mechanisms of Action of Pacing Against Bradyarrhythmias

To correct these hemodynamic problems, the first possibility is ventricular pacing, such as the VVI (noncompetitive demand ventricular) mode, which simulates an idioventricular escape rhythm and increases the ventricular rate so that cardiac output will be increased. However, this mode of pacing produces AV asynchrony and decreased stroke volume. Contrariwise, atrial pacing such as the AAI (noncompetitive, atrial demand) mode would prevent the appearance of atrial asystole, acting as a supraventricular escape rhythm. This mode is therefore more physiologic, but maintenance of an adequate AV sequence must rely on the presence of a normal AV conducting system.

In this regard, AV sequential pacing, such as the DDD (fully automatic, atrioventricular universal dual chamber) mode, takes over the physiologic functions of the specialized conducting system in both impulse formation and AV conduction, restoring normal rhythmicity and an adequate AV sequence. This is the reason the latter mode is called physiologic pacing and has been used more widely in recent years.

CARDIAC PACING AGAINST TACHYARRHYTHMIAS

Genesis of Tachyarrhythmias and Their Hemodynamic Consequences

The genesis of tachyarrhythmias can again be summarized here briefly. (1) Enhanced physiologic automaticity in the SA node or a group of fibers in the specialized conducting system will cause sinus tachycardia or a nonparoxysmal ectopic tachycardia. (2) Development of abnormal automaticity such as triggered activities and depolarization-induced automaticity may account for some instances of premature systoles, paroxysmal tachycardias, and possibly also nonparoxysmal tachycardias. (3) Reentry with either a relatively large circuit (macroreentry) or a smaller circuit (microreentry) is considered to play a major role in generating various premature systoles, paroxysmal tachycardias, flutter, and fibrillation (Table 20.3).

Hemodynamic consequences of these tachyarrhythmias also should be discussed separately for supraventricular and ventricular varieties. In cases of supraventricular tachyarrhythmias producing rapid ventricular responses, reduction of stroke volume due to markedly shortened mechanical diastole may overshadow the increased heart rate and decrease cardiac output.[155] Ventricular tachyarrhythmias tend to produce greater hemodynamic derangements than supraventricular varieties even at a similar ventricular rate,[155] because in most instances the loss of atrial contribution due to AV asynchrony further compromises ventricular filling.[154] Abnormal spread of ventricular excitation may also reduce the efficacy of ventricular contraction. Therefore, even in those simple cases of fully compensated ventricular premature systoles in which ventricular rate equals the sinus rate, most premature systoles are associated with hardly any ejection of blood, thus causing a decrease in blood pressure and cardiac output.

Mechanisms of Action of Pacing Against Tachyarrhythmias

Whereas in the pacemaker treatment of bradyarrhythmias, discussed in the previous section, pacing simply provides a substitute for the physiologic escape pacemaker without directly correcting the cause of the arrhythmia per se, pacing against tachyarrhythmias attempts to correct the electrophysiologic mechanisms underlying the arrhythmia in most instances. Hence, the mechanisms of action of pacing should be discussed for individual electrophysiologic derangements, irrespective of their supraventricular versus ventricular origin.

Pacing Against Enhanced Physiologic Automaticity. As pointed out earlier, electrical stimulation at rates faster than the rate of automatic impulse formation can produce the phenomenon of overdrive suppression when the stimulation is abruptly terminated. However, sinus tachycardia or nonparoxysmal ectopic tachycardia caused by enhanced physiologic automaticity is usually not associated with significant hemodynamic derangements because of its relatively slow rate, and hence, does not require immediate correction, except perhaps in the presence of acute myocardial infarction. Furthermore, the suppressing effects of rapid overdrive pacing are usually transient, and the rate of impulse formation of the ectopic automatic focus will soon return to the original level. For these reasons, this mode of pacing is seldom used as a therapeutic measure.

A unique approach to this problem is the use of paired atrial pacing in which the second stimulus of the pair is blocked in the AV node because of its physiologic refractoriness. In this way, the ventricular rate can be effectively reduced to an adequate level, thus improving cardiac hemodynamics.[156]

Pacing Against Abnormal Automaticity. It has been demonstrated experimentally that repetitive firing of the myocardium resulting from a triggered activity can be abruptly terminated by the application of a single extrastimulus.[19] In this regard, triggered activity resembles reentry movements. Hence, if a paroxysmal tachycardia has been produced by this mechanism, it could theoretically be treated with extrastimuli (or possibly by a burst pacing). However, it seems that, unlike reentry movements, the response of triggered activity to extrastimuli is inconsistent and unpredictable, with a critically timed premature stimulus being able to successfully terminate the repetitive responses at one moment but not at the next. Both an extrastimulus and rapid pacing are also known to increase the amplitude of delayed afterdepolarizations and facilitate the production of triggered activities.[19,28,29] Furthermore, tachyarrhythmias caused by excessive cardiac glycosides or divalent cations (Ca^{++}, Ba^{++}, and the like) tend to show the phenomenon of overdrive acceleration.[157–159] More specifically, termination of rapid stimulation is followed by a shorter escape interval than that before the pacing, and hence, the rhythm can be worsened by such a pacing technique. On the other hand, the effects of extrastimuli and rapid pacing on depolarization-induced automaticity are still not well delineated. For these reasons, application of various pacing techniques to those tachyarrhythmias possibly caused by an abnormal automaticity is not readily envisioned.

Pacing Against Reentry or Circus Movement. If one subscribes to the classic concept of reentry, an "excitable gap" must necessarily be present in the circuit between the advancing wavefront of excitation and the refractory tissue left in the wake of a preceding depolarization in order for the circus movement to be sustained. Premature discharge of such an excitable gap by an extrastimulus or burst pacing will render the entire reentry circuit refractory and interrupt the circus movement. Indeed, a majority of clinically observed paroxysmal atrial as well as AV junctional tachycardias and atrial flutter can successfully be terminated by atrial pacing.[160–162] For this purpose, techniques such as (1) electrical stimulation at a rate slower than the tachycardia rate with the expectation of a fortuitous occurrence of one of the stimuli during the excitable gap (so-called underdrive pacing), (2) a short period of burst pacing, often activated by the patient with a radiofrequency unit, or (3) a more sophisticated, automatic scanning device that senses the occurrence of paroxysmal tachycardia and applies a series of extrastimuli at progressively shorter coupling intervals, and others are available.[163–166]

In certain cases of AV reciprocating tachycardia, AV sequential pacing has been more efficacious than atrial pacing.[167,168] Such an observation can be explained by (1) a greater chance for the engagement of the excitable gap by either antegrade or retrograde impulses, and (2) prevention of the development of reciprocal movement by maintaining an adequately short PR interval. In the latter case, even when two pathways potentially forming a reentry circuit (such as dual AV nodal pathways or an accessory pathway) are available, reciprocating tachycardia cannot occur because either (1) one of the pathways blocked for antegrade conduction has insufficient time to be out of its longer refractory period and does not allow retrograde conduction, or (2) a retrogradely conducted impulse may find the atrial tissue still in its refractory period. Nevertheless, interruption of reentry movements is the major indication of pacemaker treatment currently practiced against tachyarrhythmias.

It must be pointed out, however, that the foregoing discussion applies mainly to those tachyarrhythmias dependent on a macroreentry movement such as WPW tachycardia,[169,170] paroxysmal AV junctional tachycardia, and some cases of atrial flutter, as the excitable gap in their reentry circuit may more easily be engaged by the electrical stimuli. Generally speaking, pacing stimuli applied closer to the localization of reentry circuit are more effective with a greater chance to invade the circuit. Conversely, microreentry movements are probably more difficult to be interrupted by pacing techniques. Hence, failure of an extrastimulus to terminate an episode of tachycardia may not necessarily rule out reentry and suggest abnormal automaticity or triggered activity. An extreme case is perhaps fibrillation, in which numerous random reentry movements are considered to be present. Pacing cannot successfully terminate this arrhythmia.

Occasionally, atrial flutter or atrial tachycardia has been converted to atrial fibrillation by burst pacing,[171,172] because (1) the latter is often transient and spontaneously reverts to a sinus rhythm, and (2) it is easier to control the ventricular response by antiarrhythmic drugs in the presence of atrial fibrillation. In this case, the high frequency stimulation is used to cause an irregular spread of excitation from the pacing site and set up numerous microreentry movements rather than to interrupt reentry.

Several investigators have applied the pacing technique in the treatment of paroxysmal ventricular tachycardia as well, again attempting to interrupt the reentry circuit.[173] However, extreme caution must be exercised in this mode of treatment, as the risk of producing ventricular fibrillation is always present.

CARDIAC PACING AGAINST BRADYCARDIA–TACHYCARDIA SYNDROME

Genesis of Bradycardia–Tachycardia Syndrome

The term bradycardia-tachycardia syndrome was introduced to describe certain cases of so-called sick sinus syndrome in which periods of sinus bradycardia, sinus arrest, or SA block often alternate with various atrial tachyarrhythmias.[174–176] In those instances, the genesis of both bradycardia and tachycardia may very well be explained by histopathologic changes, as postmortem examination often revealed the presence of extensive fibrosis or fatty infiltration involving the SA node as well as the atrial tissue. A marked reduction in the number of SA nodal fibers, with those few surviving cells capable of spontaneous impulse formation being surrounded by massive connective tissue, could lead to bradycardia due to both slower automatic impulse formation and SA block. Degenerative changes in the atrial tissue, on the other hand, would cause inhomogeneous conduction and refractoriness, thus setting the stage for reentry movements and tachyarrhythmias.[26,27]

However, in addition to these anatomic factors, certain purely electrophysiologic mechanisms may facilitate the alternation of bradycardia and tachycardia, as will be discussed herein. First, supraventricular tachyarrhythmias such as paroxysmal atrial tachycardia, atrial flutter, and fibrillation exert overdrive suppression on the SA node and subsidiary pacemakers.[11–14] Hence, sudden termination of these arrhythmias can be followed by a prolonged period of bradycardia. Second, it has been known that in certain cases bradycardia tends to be associated with an increased incidence of premature systoles, and this observation was termed *the rule of bigeminy.*[177] Such a facilitation of premature systoles by longer cycle lengths can be ascribed to (1) loss of membrane potential in some fibers of the specialized conducting system due to diastolic depolarization, which produces phase 4 block[45,46] and a localized conduction disorder, and (2) an increased disparity of the action potential duration and the refractory period,[178] which causes abnormal local potential differences and possible reexcitation. Premature systoles thus produced may well initiate episodes of tachyarrhythmias.

Similar electrophysiologic changes could occur within the ventricles, and indeed, some cases of ventricular arrhythmias may show alternation of bradycardia and tachycardia. For instance, runs of ventricular premature systoles and nonsustained ventricular tachycardia are occasionally observed in cases of high grade AV block with a slow escape rhythm, apparently producing a ventricular variety of the bradycardia–tachycardia syndrome.[179]

Mechanisms of Action of Pacing Against Bradycardia–Tachycardia Syndrome

The major mechanisms of action of cardiac pacing against bradycardia–tachycardia syndrome are basically similar to those already discussed for bradyarrhythmias or tachyarrhythmias alone. However, to successfully control both the bradycardia phase and the tachycardia phase

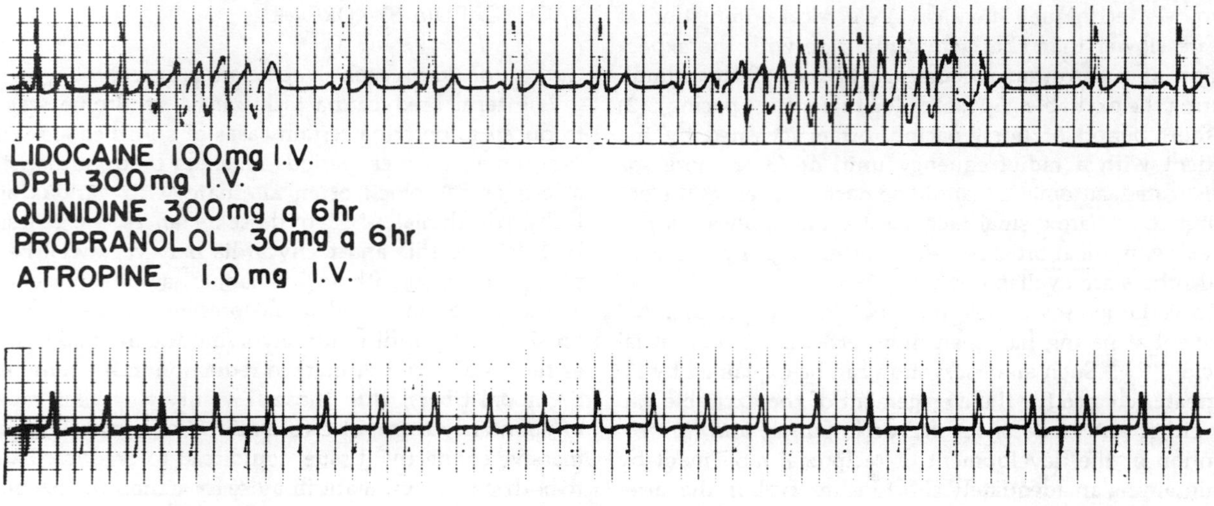

Figure 20.13. A case of recurrent, nonsustained ventricular tachycardia refractory to pharmacologic treatment, which responded to atrial pacing at a rate of approximately 97 beats per minute. Drugs used against this arrhythmia are listed below the top electrocardiogram.

with a pacemaker, it must have those newer and more sophisticated functions of various antitachycardia devices. However, it must be pointed out here that the use of a simpler, less sophisticated model such as the AAI[180] or VVI[181] pacing may still have a place in the treatment of bradycardia–tachycardia syndrome in the following two manners.

First, in view of the rule of bigeminy, prevention of marked bradycardia with pacing immediately after the end of tachyarrhythmias, or a moderate acceleration of the basic ventricular rate, could secondarily reduce the likelihood of another episode of tachyarrhythmia. One such clinical example is shown in Figure 20.13, in which a drug-resistant, recurrent nonsustained ventricular tachycardia was successfully controlled by atrial pacing. Second, drugs such as atropine and isoproterenol used to increase the basic heart rate may often aggravate the tachycardia phase.[175,181] Conversely, because many antiarrhythmic drugs tend to depress physiologic automaticity and also conduction, their use in the control of the tachycardia phase often exaggerates the bradycardia phase and may cause a serious problem. The use of a simple demand pacemaker to prevent the development of marked bradycardia allows the administration of potent antiarrhythmic drugs without these risks. Therefore, a combination of cardiac pacing and pharmacologic therapy constitutes an important approach in the management of the bradycardia–tachycardia syndrome.[181–183]

Acknowledgment: This work was supported in part by grants-in-aid from the Ministry of Education, Science and Culture, and research grants from Fujita Gakuen University, Toyoake, Aichi, Japan.

REFERENCES

1. Bellet S: *Clinical Disorders of the Heart Beat,* ed 3. Philadelphia, Lea & Febiger, 1971.
2. Katz LN, Pick A: *Clinical Electrocardiography. Part I. The Arrhythmias.* Philadelphia, Lea & Febiger, 1956.
3. Watanabe Y, Dreifus LS: *Cardiac Arrhythmias. Electrophysiologic Basis for Clinical Interpretation.* New York, Grune & Stratton, 1977.
4. Josephson ME, Seides SF: *Clinical Cardiac Electrophysiology. Techniques and Interpretation.* Philadelphia, Lea & Febiger, 1979.
5. Watanabe Y, Dreifus LS: Newer concepts in the genesis of cardiac arrhythmias. *Am Heart J* 1968; 76:114–135.
6. Bigger JT Jr: Electrical properties of cardiac muscle and possible causes of cardiac arrhythmias, in Dreifus LS, Likoff W (eds): *Cardiac Arrhythmias.* New York, Grune & Stratton, 1973, pp 97–111.
7. Hoffman BF, Rosen MR: Cellular mechanisms for cardiac arrhythmias. *Circ Res* 1981; 49:1–15.
8. Singer DH, Baumgarten CM, Ten Eick RE: Cellular electrophysiology of ventricular and other dysrhythmias: studies on diseased and ischemic heart. *Prog Cardiovasc Dis* 1981; 24:97–156.
9. Hoffman BF, Cranefield PF: *Electrophysiology of the Heart.* New York, McGraw-Hill Book Co, 1960.
10. Hogan PM, Davis LD: Evidence for specialized fibers in the canine right atrium. *Circ Res* 1968; 23:387–396.
11. Brooks CMc, Lu HH: *Sinoatrial Pacemaker of the Heart.* Springfield, Ill, Charles C Thomas, 1972.
12. Vassalle M: The relationship among cardiac pacemakers. Overdrive suppression. *Circ Res* 1977; 41:269–277.
13. Kodama I, Goto J, Ando S, Toyama J, Yamada K: Effects of rapid stimulation on the transmembrane action potentials of rabbit sinus node pacemaker cells. *Circ Res* 1980; 46:90–99.
14. Mandel W, Hayakawa H, Danzig R, Marcus HS: Evaluation of sinoatrial node function in man by overdrive suppression. *Circulation* 1971; 44:59–66.
15. Watanabe Y: Reassessment of parasystole. *Am Heart J* 1971; 81:451–466.
16. Watanabe Y: Extrasystoles and parasystole. Mechanisms involved. *Triangle* 1973; 12:69–74.
17. Singer DH, Parameswaran R, Drake FT, Meyers SN, DeBoer AA: Ventricular parasystole and re-entry: clinical–electrophysiological correlations. *Am Heart J* 1974; 88:79–87.
18. Hellerstein HK, Turell DJ: The mode of death in coronary artery disease. An electrocardiographic and clinicopathological correlation, in Surawicz B, Pellegrino ED (eds): *Sudden Cardiac Death.* New York, Grune & Stratton, 1964, pp 17–36.
19. Cranefield PF: *The Conduction of the Cardiac Impulse.* Mount Kisco, NY, Futura Publishing Co, 1975.
20. Imanishi S, Surawicz B: Automatic activity in depolarized guinea pig ventricular myocardium. Characteristics and mechanisms. *Circ Res* 1976; 39:751–759.

21. Katzung BG, Morgenstern JA: Effects of extracellular potassium on ventricular automaticity and evidence for a pacemaker current in mammalian ventricular myocardium. *Circ Res* 1977; 40:105–111.
22. Surawicz B: Depolarization-induced automaticity in atrial and ventricular myocardial fibers, in Zipes DP, Bailey JC, Elharrar V (eds): *The Slow Inward Current and Cardiac Arrhythmias.* The Hague, Martinus Nijhoff, 1980, pp 375–396.
23. Müller P: Ca- and K-free solution and pacemaker activity in mammalian myocardium. *Helv Physiol Acta* 1965; 23:C38–40.
24. Arita M, Nagamoto Y, Saikawa T: Automaticity and time-dependent conduction disturbance produced in canine ventricular myocardium. New aspects for initiation of ventricular arrhythmias. *Jpn Circ J* 1976; 40:1409–1418.
25. Katzung BG, Hondeghem IM, Grant AO: Cardiac ventricular automaticity induced by current of injury. *Pfluegers Arch* 1975; 360:193–197.
26. Singer DH, Ten Eick RE, DeBoer AA: Electrophysiologic correlates of human atrial tachyarrhythmias, in Dreifus LS, Likoff W (eds): *Cardiac Arrhythmias.* New York, Grune & Stratton, 1973, pp 97–111.
27. Ten Eick RE, Singer DH: Electrophysiologic properties of diseased human atrium. I. Low diastolic potential and altered cellular response to potassium. *Circ Res* 1979; 44:545–557.
28. Hashimoto K, Moe GK: Transient depolarizations induced by acetylstrophanthidin in specialized tissue of dog atrium and ventricle. *Circ Res* 1973; 32:618–624.
29. Cranefield PF, Aronson RS: Initiation of sustained rhythmic activity by single propagated action potentials in canine cardiac Purkinje fibers exposed to sodium-free solution or to ouabain. *Circ Res* 1974; 34:477–481.
30. Cranefield PF: Action potentials, afterpotentials and arrhythmias. *Circ Res* 1977; 41:415–423.
31. Ferrier GR: Digitalis arrhythmias. Role of oscillatory afterpotentials. *Prog Cardiovasc Dis* 1977; 19:459–474.
32. Ferrier GR, Moe GK: Effect of calcium on acetylstrophanthidin-induced transient depolarizations in canine Purkinje tissue. *Circ Res* 1973; 33:508–515.
33. Wit AL, Fenoglio JJ Jr, Wagner BM, Bassett AL: Electrophysiologic properties of cardiac muscle in the anterior mitral valve leaflet and the adjacent atrium in the dog. Possible implications for the genesis of atrial dysrhythmias. *Circ Res* 1973; 32:731–745.
34. Wit AL, Cranefield PF: Triggered and automatic activity in the canine coronary sinus. *Circ Res* 1977; 41:435–445.
35. Matsuda K, Hoshi T, Kameyama S: Effects of aconitine on the cardiac membrane potential of the dog. *Jpn J Physiol* 1959; 9:419–429.
36. Rougier O, Vassort D, Gargouil YM, Coraboeuf E: Existence and role of a slow inward current during the frog atrial action potential. *Pfluegers Arch* 1964; 308:91–110.
37. Kohlhardt M, Bauer B, Krause H, Fleckenstein A: Differentiation of the transmembrane Na and Ca channels in mammalian cardiac fibers by the use of specific inhibitors. *Pfluegers Arch* 1972; 335:309–322.
38. Noma A, Irisawa H, Kokubun S, Kotake H, Nishimura M, Watanabe Y: Slow inward current systems in the A-V node of the rabbit heart. *Nature* 1980; 285:228–229.
39. Watanabe Y: Effects of calcium and sodium concentrations on atrioventricular conduction: experimental study in rabbit hearts with clinical implications on heart block and slow calcium channel blocking agent usage. *Am Heart J* 1981; 102:883–891.
40. Kokubun S, Nishimura M, Noma A, Irisawa H: Membrane currents in the rabbit atrioventricular node cell. *Pfluegers Arch* 1982; 393:15–22.
41. Nishimura M, Watanabe Y: Effects of slow channel and fast channel blockers on automaticity and action potential characteristics of the rabbit atrioventricular node (abstr). *Am J Cardiol* 1982; 49:921.
42. Nishimura M, Tsuji Y, Hiromasa S, Sugiura M, Katoh T, Watanabe Y: Electrophysiologic effects of adrenaline on the spontaneous action potential of the rabbit atrioventricular node. *J Fujita Gakuen Med Soc* 1983; 7:101–104.
43. Hiromasa S, Nishimura M, Tsuji Y, Watanabe Y: Electrophysiologic demonstration of acetylcholine receptors and acetylcholine effects in the rabbit atrioventricular node (abstr). *J Am Coll Cardiol* 1983; 1:730.
44. Watanabe Y, Dreifus LS: Factors controlling impulse transmission with special reference to A-V conduction. *Am Heart J* 1975; 89:790–803.
45. Rosenbaum MB, Lazzari JO, Eilzari MV: The role of phase 3 and phase 4 block in clinical electrocardiography, in Wellens HJJ, Lie KI, Janse MJ (eds): *The Conduction System of the Heart.* Leiden, HE Stenfert Kroese BV, 1976, pp 126–142.
46. Singer DH, Lazzara R, Hoffman BF: Interrelationships between automaticity and conduction in Purkinje fibers. *Circ Res* 1967; 21:537–558.
47. Watanabe Y, Nishimura M: Terminology and electrophysiologic concepts in cardiac arrhythmias. V. Phase 3 block and phase 4 block. Part 1. *PACE* 1979; 2:335–344.
48. Watanabe Y, Nishimura M: Terminology and electrophysiologic concepts in cardiac arrhythmias. VI. Phase 3 block and phase 4 block. Part 2. *PACE* 2:624–633.
49. Schmitt FO, Erlanger J: Directional difference in the conduction of the impulse through heart muscle and their possible relation to extrasystolic and fibrillary contractions. *Am J Physiol* 1928–1929; 87:326–347.
50. Kulbertus HE (ed): *Re-entrant Arrhythmias.* Baltimore, University Park Press, 1977.
51. Sherf L, Neufeld HN: *The Pre-excitation Syndrome: Facts and Theories.* New York, Yorke Medical Books, 1978.
52. Watanabe Y, Dreifus LS: Inhomogeneous conduction in the A-V node. A model for re-entry. *Am Heart J* 1965; 70:505–514.
53. Moe GK, Preston JB, Burlington H: Physiologic evidence for a dual A-V transmission system. *Circ Res* 1956; 4:357–375.
54. Mendez C, Moe GK: Demonstration of a dual A-V nodal conduction in the isolated rabbit heart. *Circ Res* 1966; 19:378–393.
55. Rosen KM, Mehta A, Miller RA: Demonstration of dual atrioventricular nodal pathways in man. *Am J Cardiol* 1974; 33:291–294.
56. Wu D, Denes P, Wyndham C, Amat-y-Leon F, Dhingra RC, Rosen KM: Demonstration of dual atrioventricular nodal pathways utilizing a ventricular extrastimulus in patients with atrioventricular nodal re-entrant paroxysmal supraventricular tachycardia. *Circulation* 1975; 52:789–798.
57. Mazgalev T, Dreifus LS, Bianchi J, Michelson EL: The mechanism of AV junctional reentry: role of the atrionodal junction. *Anat Rec* 1981; 201:179–188.
58. Iinuma H, Dreifus LS, Mazgalev T, Price R, Michelson EL: Role of the perinodal region in atrioventricular nodal reentry. Evidence in an isolated rabbit heart preparation. *J Am Coll Cardiol* 1983; 2:465–473.
59. Janse MJ, Van Capelle FJL, Morsink H, Kléber AG, Wilms-Schopman F, Cardinal R, D'Alnoncourt CN, Durrer D: Flow of "injury" current and patterns of excitation during early ventricular arrhythmias in acute regional myocardial ischemia in isolated porcine and canine hearts. Evidence for two different arrhythmogenic mechanisms. *Circ Res* 1980; 47:151–165.
60. Antzelevitch C, Jalife J, Moe GK: Characteristics of reflection as a mechanism of reentrant arrhythmias and its relationship to parasystole. *Circulation* 1980; 61:182–191.
61. Moe GK, Abildskov JA: Atrial fibrillation as a self-sustaining arrhythmia independent of focal discharge. *Am Heart J* 1959; 58:59–70.
62. Watanabe Y, Dreifus LS: Mechanisms of ventricular fibrillation. *Jpn Heart J* 1966; 7:110–120.
63. Watanabe Y: Antifibrillatory action of several antiarrhythmic agents, in Hayase S, Murao S (eds): *Cardiology. Proceedings of the VIII World Congress of Cardiology.* Amsterdam, Excerpta Medica, 1979, pp 924–928.
64. de Azevedo IM, Watanabe Y, Dreifus LS: Reassessment of AV junctional rhythms. *Heart & Lung* 1972; 1:626–638.
65. Dreifus LS, Katz M, Watanabe Y, Likoff W: Clinical significance of disorders of impulse formation and conduction in the atrioventricular junction. *Am J Cardiol* 1963; 11:384–391.
66. Vaughan Williams EM: Classification of antiarrhythmic drugs, in Sandøe E, Flensted Jensen E, Olesen KH (eds): *Symposium on Cardiac Arrhythmias.* Södertälje, Sweden, AB Astra, 1970, pp 449–472.
67. Singh BN, Hauswirth O: Comparative mechanisms of action of antiarrhythmic drugs. *Am Heart J* 1974; 87:367–382.
68. Singh BN, Collett JJ, Chew CYC: New perspectives in the pharmacologic therapy of cardiac arrhythmias. *Prog Cardiovasc Dis* 1980; 22:243–301.
69. Elharrar V, Zipes DP: Effects of encainide and metabolites (MJ 14030 and MJ 9444) on canine Purkinje and ventricular fibers. *J Pharmacol Exp Ther* 1982; 220:440–447.
70. Cowen JC, Vaughan Williams EM: Characterization of a new oral antiarrhythmic drug, flecainide (R 818). *Eur J Pharmacol* 1981; 73:333–342.
71. Borchard U, Boisten N: Effect of flecainide on action potentials and alternating current-induced arrhythmias in mammalian myocardium. *J Cardiovasc Pharmacol* 1982; 4:205–212.
72. Lucchesi BR, Whitsitt LS, Stickney JL: Antiarrhythmic effects of beta adrenergic blocking agents. *Ann NY Acad Sci* 1967; 139:940–951.
73. Lucchesi BR, Whitsitt LS: The pharmacology of beta-adrenergic blocking agents. *Prog Cardiovasc Dis* 1969; 11:410–430.
74. Abrams WB, Davies RO: The antiarrhythmic mechanisms of beta-adrenergic blocking agents, in Dreifus LS, Likoff W (eds); *Cardiac Arrhythmias.* New York, Grune & Stratton, 1973, pp 517–530.
75. Wit AL, Hoffman BF, Rosen MR: Electrophysiology and pharmacology of cardiac arrhythmias. IX. Cardiac electrophysiologic effects of beta-adrenergic receptor stimulation and blockade. Part C. *Am Heart J* 1975; 90:795–803.
76. Whitsitt LS, Lucchesi BR: Effects of beta-receptor blockade and glucagon on the atrioventricular transmission system in the dog. *Circ Res* 1968; 23:585–595.
77. Berkowitz WD, Wit AL, Lau SH, Steiner C, Damato AN: The effects of propranolol on cardiac conduction. *Circulation* 1969; 40:855–862.
78. Smithen CS, Balcon R, Sowton E: Use of bundle of His potentials to

assess changes in atrioventricular conduction produced by a series of beta-adrenergic blocking agents. *Br Heart J* 1970; 33:955–961.

79. Pamintuan JC, Dreifus LS, Watanabe Y: Comparative mechanisms of antiarrhythmic agents. *Am J Cardiol* 1970; 26:512–519.
80. Watanabe Y, Toda H, Ozawa M: Cardiac electrophysiologic action of carteolol hydrochloride (OPC-1085), a new beta-adrenergic blocking agent. *PACE* 1978; 1:292–305.
81. Singh BN, Vaughan Williams EM: The effect of amiodarone, a new antianginal drug, on intracellular potentials and other properties of isolated cardiac muscle. *Br J Pharmacol* 1970; 39:657–667.
82. Rosenbaum MB, Chiale PA, Ryba D, Elizari MV: Control of tachyarrhythmias associated with Wolff–Parkinson–White syndrome by amiodarone hydrochloride. *Am J Cardiol* 1974; 34:215–223.
83. Papp JGY, Vaughan Williams EM: The effect of bretylium tosylate on intracellular cardiac action potentials in relation to its antiarrhythmic and local anesthetic activity. *Br J Pharmacol* 1969; 37:380–390.
84. Wit AL, Steiner C, Damato AN: Electrophysiologic effects of bretylium tosylate on single fibers of the canine specialized conducting system and ventricle. *J Pharmacol Exp Ther* 1970; 173:344–356.
85. Bigger JT Jr, Jaffe CC: The effect of bretylium tosylate on the electrophysiologic properties of ventricular muscle and Purkinje fibers. *Am J Cardiol* 1971; 27:82–92.
86. Cardinal R, Sasyniuk BI: Electrophysiological effect of bretylium tosylate on subendocardial Purkinje fibers from infarcted canine hearts. *J Pharmacol Exp Ther* 1978; 204:159–174.
87. Nishimura M, Watanabe Y: Membrane action and catecholamine release action of bretylium tosylate in normoxic and hypoxic canine Purkinje fibers. *J Am Coll Cardiol* 1983; 2:287–295.
88. Zipes DP, Fischer JC: Effects of agents which inhibit the slow channel on sinus node automaticity and atrioventricular conduction in the dog. *Circ Res* 1974; 34:184–192.
89. Wit AL, Cranefield PF: Effect of verapamil on the sinoatrial and atrioventricular nodes of the rabbit and the mechanisms by which it arrests reentrant atrioventricular nodal tachycardia. *Circ Res* 1974; 35:413–425.
90. Fleckenstein A, Roskamm H: *Calcium-Antagonismus.* Berlin, Springer-Verlag, 1980.
91. Watanabe Y, Hayakawa H (eds): *Ca^{++} Antagonists and Cardiac Arrhythmias.* Tokyo, Ishiyaku Publishing Co, 1985.
92. Watanabe Y, Nishimura M, Yamada S, Tsuji Y: Genesis of cardiac arrhythmias and antiarrhythmic drugs, in Hashiba K, Mori H (eds): *Mechanisms and Clinical Aspects of Arrhythmias.* Tokyo, Maruzen Co, 1985, pp 239–267.
93. Watanabe Y, Dreifus LS: Electrophysiologic effects of digitalis on A-V transmission. *Am J Physiol* 1967; 211:1461–1466.
94. Watanabe Y, Dreifus LS: Interactions of lanatoside C and potassium on atrioventricular conduction in rabbits. *Circ Res* 1970; 27:931–940.
95. Gough WB, Zeiler RH, El-Sherif N: Effects of nifedipine on triggered activity in 1-day-old myocardial infarction in dogs. *Am J Cardiol* 1984; 53:303–306.
96. Watanabe Y: Significance of the use of multiple experimental approaches. *Heart* 1984; 16:513–523.
97. Yamada S, Nishimura M, Watanabe Y: Electrophysiologic effects of disopyramide studied in a hypoxic canine Purkinje fiber model. *J Electrocardiol* 1982; 15:31–40.
98. Kus T, Sasyniuk BI: Electrophysiological actions of disopyramide phosphate on canine ventricular muscle and Purkinje fibers. *Circ Res* 1975; 37:844–854.
99. Bigger JT Jr, Basset AL, Hoffman BF: Electrophysiological effects of diphenylhydantoin on canine Purkinje fibers. *Circ Res* 1968; 22:221–236.
100. Watanabe Y: Contrasting effects of disopyramide and verapamil in chemical defibrillation of perfused rabbit hearts (abstr). *J Am Coll Cardiol* 1983; 1:647.
101. Nishimura M, Watanabe Y: Direct membrane action and anticholinergic action of disopyramide phosphate on the spontaneous action potential of the rabbit atrioventricular node. (In preparation.)
102. Kokubun S, Nishimura M, Noma A, Irisawa H: The spontaneous action potential of rabbit atrioventricular node. *Jpn J Physiol* 1980; 30:529–540.
103. Watanabe Y, Dreifus LS, Likoff W: Electrophysiologic antagonism and synergism of potassium and antiarrhythmic agents. *Am J Cardiol* 1963; 12:702–710.
104. Watanabe Y, Dreifus LS: Interactions of quinidine and potassium on atrioventricular transmission. *Circ Res* 1967; 20:434–446.
105. Talbot RG, Julian DG, Prescott LF: Long-term treatment of ventricular arrhythmias with oral mexiletine. *Am Heart J* 1976; 91:58–65.
106. Zipes DP, Troup PJ: New antiarrhythmic agents. Amiodarone, aprindine, disopyramide, ethmozin, mexiletine, tocainide, verapamil. *Am J Cardiol* 1978; 41:1005–1024.
107. Horowitz JD, Anavekar SN, Morris PM, Goble AJ, Doyle AE, Louis WJ: Comparative trial of mexiletine and lidocaine in the treatment of early ventricular tachyarrhythmias after acute myocardial infarction. *J Cardiovasc Pharmacol* 1981; 3:409–419.
108. Dreifus LS, Watanabe Y: Current status of diphenylhydantoin. *Am Heart J* 1970; 80:709–713.
109. Tsuji Y, Nishimura M, Osada M, Watanabe Y: Membrane action of ethmozin on normoxic and hypoxic canine Purkinje fibers. *J Cardiovasc Pharmacol* 1983; 5:961–967.
110. Danilo P, Langan WB, Rosen MR, Hoffman BF: Effects of phenothiazine analog, EN-313, on ventricular arrhythmias in the dog. *Eur J Pharmacol* 1977; 45:127–139.
111. Hewett K, Rosen MR: Effects of ethmozin and procainamide on ouabain-induced afterdepolarizations (abstr). *Fed Proc* 1980; 46:814.
112. Yamaguchi I, Singh B, Mandel WJ: Electrophysiological actions of mexiletine on isolated rabbit atria and canine ventricular muscle and Purkinje fibers. *Cardiovasc Res* 1979; 13:288–296.
113. Maloney JD, Nissen RG, McColgan JM: Open clinical studies at a referral center: Chronic maintenance tocainide therapy in patients with recurrent sustained ventricular tachycardia refractory to conventional antiarrhythmic agents. *Am Heart J* 1980; 100:1023–1030.
114. Verdonck F, Vereecke J, Vleugels A: Electrophysiologic effects of aprindine on isolated heart preparations. *Eur J Pharmacol* 1974; 26:338–347.
115. Hondeghem L, Katzung BG: Test of a model of antiarrhythmic drug action. Effects of quinidine and lidocaine on myocardial conduction. *Circulation* 1980; 61:1217–1224.
116. Courtney KR: Interval-dependent effects of small antiarrhythmic drugs on excitability of guinea-pig myocardium. *J Moll Cell Cardiol* 1980; 12:1273–1286.
117. Campbell TJ: Resting and rate-dependent depression of maximum rate of depolarization (Vmax) in guinea pig ventricular action potentials by mexiletine, disopyramide, and encainide. *J Cardiovasc Pharmacol* 1983; 5:291–296.
118. Kodama I, Anno T: Effects of antiarrhythmic drugs on the conducting system. *Jpn J Clin Med* 1985; 43:2397–2403.
119. Hellestrand KJ, Bexton RS, Nathan AW, Spurrell RAJ, Camm AJ: Acute electrophysiological effects of flecainide acetate on cardiac conduction and refractoriness in man. *Br Heart J* 1982; 48:140–148.
120. Salerno DM, Hodges M, Granrud G, Sharkey P: Comparison of flecainide with quinidine for suppression of chronic stable ventricular ectopic depolarizations: a double-blind, randomized study in ambulatory out-patients. *Ann Intern Med* 1983; 98:455–460.
121. Vaughan Williams EM: Mode of action of beta receptor antagonists on cardiac muscle. *Am J Cardiol* 1966; 18:399–405.
122. Gibson D, Sowton E: The use of beta-adrenergic receptor blocking drugs in dysrhythmias. *Prog Cardiovasc Dis* 1969; 12:16–39.
123. Stook JPP: Beta adrenergic blocking drugs in the clinical management of cardiac arrhythmias. *Am J Cardiol* 1966; 18:444–449.
124. Gettes LS, Yoshonıs KF: Rapidly recurring supraventricular tachycardia. A manifestation of reciprocating tachycardia and an indication for propranolol therapy. *Circulation* 1970; 41:689–700.
125. Bacaner MB: Treatment of ventricular fibrillation and other acute arrhythmias with bretylium tosylate. *Am J Cardiol* 1968; 21:530–543.
126. Bacaner M: Experimental and clinical effects of bretylium tosylate on ventricular fibrillation, arrhythmias and heart block. *Geriatrics* 1971; 26:132–148.
127. Bernstein JG, Koch-Weser J: Effectiveness of bretylium tosylate against refractory ventricular arrhythmias. *Circulation* 1972; 45:1024–1034.
128. de Azevedo IM, Watanabe Y, Dreifus LS: Electrophysiologic antagonism of quinidine and bretylium tosylate. *Am J Cardiol* 1974; 33:633–638.
129. Vander Ark CR, Raynolds EW, Khan DR, Tullet G: Quinidine syncope. A report of successful treatment with bretylium tosylate. *J Thorac Cardiovasc Surg* 1976; 72:464–467.
130. Rosenbaum MB, Chiale PA, Halpern MS, Nau GJ, Przybylski J, Levi RJ, Lazzari JO, Elizari MV: Clinical efficacy of amiodarone as an antiarrhythmic agent. *Am J Cardiol* 1976; 38:934–944.
131. Broekhuysen J, Laurel R, Sion R: Etude comparee du transit et du metabolisme de l'amiodarone chez diverses especes animales et chez l'homme. *Arch Int Pharmacodyn Ther* 1969; 177:340–359.
132. Goupil N, Lenfant J: The effects of amiodarone on the sinus node activity of the rabbit heart. *Eur J Pharmacol* 1976; 39:23–31.
133. Wellens HJJ, Lie KI, Bär FW, Wesdorp JC, Dohmen HJ, Düren DR, Durrer D: Effect of amiodarone in the Wolff-Parkinson-White syndrome. *Am J Cardiol* 1976; 38:189–194.
134. Swan JH, Chisholm AW: Control of recurrent supraventricular tachycardia with amiodarone hydrochloride. *Can Med Assoc J* 1976; 144:43–44.
135. Hegger JJ, Prystowsky EN, Jackman WM, Nacarelli GW, Warfel KA, Rinkenberger RI, Zipes DP: Amiodarone, clinical efficacy and electrophysiology during long-term therapy for recurrent ventricular tachycardia or ventricular fibrillation. *N Engl J Med* 1981; 305:539–544.
136. Saksena S, Rothbart ST, Cappello G: Chronic effects of amiodarone in patients with refractory ventricular tachycardia. *Int J Cardiol* 1983; 3:339–352.
137. Morady F, Scheinman MM, Shen E, Shapiro W, Sung RJ, DiCarlo L:

Intravenous amiodarone in the acute treatment of recurrent symptomatic ventricular tachycardia. *Am J Cardiol* 1983; 51:156–159.

138. Watanabe Y, Katoh T: Amiodarone. *Jpn J Clin Med* 1983; 41:2766–2770.
139. Fleckenstein A: *Calcium Antagonism in Heart and Smooth Muscle. Experimental Facts and Therapeutic Prospects.* New York, John Wiley & Sons, 1983.
140. Loewenstein WR: Junctional intercellular communication: the cell-to-cell membrane channel. *Physiol Rev* 1981; 61:829–913.
141. Schamroth L: The clinical use of intravenous verapamil. *Am Heart J* 1980; 100:1070–1075.
142. Rinkenberger RL, Prystowsky EN, Heger JJ, Troup PJ, Jackman WM, Zipes DP: Effects of intravenous and chronic oral verapamil administration in patients with supraventricular tachyarrhythmias. *Circulation* 1980; 62:996–1010.
143. Hamer A, Peter T, Mandel W: Atrioventricular node reentry: intravenous verapamil as a method of defining multiple electrophysiologic types. *Am Heart J* 1983; 105:629–642.
144. Spurrell RAJ, Krikler DM, Sowton E: Effects of verapamil on electrophysiological properties of anomalous atrioventricular connexion in Wolff–Parkinson–White syndrome. *Br Heart J* 1974; 36:256–264.
145. Tai DY, Chang MS, Svinarich JT, Chiang BN, Sung RJ: Mechanisms of verapamil-induced conduction block in anomalous atrioventricular bypass tracts. *J Am Coll Cardiol* 1985; 5:311–317.
146. Schamroth L: Immediate effects of intravenous verapamil on atrial fibrillation. *Cardiovasc Res* 1971; 5:419–424.
147. Krikler DM, Spurrel RAJ: Verapamil in the treatment of paroxysmal supraventricular tachycardia. *Postgrad Med J* 1974; 50:447–453.
148. Gulamhusein S, Ko P, Carruthers SG, Klein GJ: Acceleration of the ventricular response during atrial fibrillation in the Wolff–Parkinson–White syndrome after verapamil. *Circulation* 1982; 65:348–354.
149. Belhassen B, Rotmensch HH, Laniado S: Response of recurrent sustained ventricular tachycardia to verapamil. *Br Heart J* 1981; 46:679–682.
150. Lin F-C, Finley CD, Rahimtoola SH, Wu D: Idiopathic paroxysmal ventricular tachycardia with a QRS pattern of right bundle branch block and left axis deviation: a unique clinical entity with specific properties. *Am J Cardiol* 1983; 52:95–100.
151. Feruglio GA, Steinbach K: Cardiac pacing in Europe after two decades: a comprehensive survey, in Feruglio GA (ed): *Cardiac Pacing, Electrophysiology and Pacemaker Technology.* Padova, Italy, Piccin Medical Books, 1982, pp 1-13.
152. Rosen KM, Loeb HS, Sinno MZ, Rahimtoola SH, Gunnar RM: Cardiac conduction in patients with symptomatic sinus node disease. *Circulation* 1971; 43:836–844.
153. Narula OS: Atrioventricular conduction defects in patients with sinus bradycardia. Analysis by His bundle recordings. *Circulation* 1971; 44: 1096–1110.
154. Naito M, Miyairi M, Asato T, Nagoshi H, Honda M, Michelson EL, Dreifus LS: Relative contributions of mitral and pulmonary venous regurgitation to the adverse hemodynamic consequences of various cardiac arrhythmias, in Steinbach K (ed): *Cardiac Pacing. Proceedings of the VIIth World Symposium on Cardiac Pacing.* Darmstadt, Steinkopf Verlag, 1983, pp 697–702.
155. Nakano J: Effects of atrial and ventricular tachycardias on the cardiovascular dynamics. *Am J Physiol* 1964; 206:547–552.
156. Cheng TO: Atrial pacing: its diagnostic and therapeutic applications. *Prog Cardiovasc Dis* 1971; 14:230–247.
157. Wittenberg SM, Streuli F, Klocke FJ: Acceleration of ventricular pacemakers by transient increases in heart rate in dogs during ouabain administration. *Circ Res* 1970; 26:705–716.
158. Zipes DP, Arbel E, Knope RF, Moe GK: Accelerated cardiac escape rhythms caused by ouabain intoxication. *Am J Cardiol* 1974; 33:248–253.
159. Foster PR, Elharrar V, Zipes DP: Accelerated ventricular escapes induced in the intact dog by barium, strontium and calcium. *J Pharmacol Exp Ther* 1977; 200:373–383.
160. Gulotta SJ, Aronson AL: Cardioversion of atrial tachycardia and flutter by atrial stimulation. *Am J Cardiol* 1970; 26:262–269.
161. Vergara GS, Hildner FJ, Schoenfeld CB, Javier RP, Cohen LS, Samet P: Conversion of supraventricular tachycardias with rapid atrial stimulation. *Circulation* 1972; 46:788–793.
162. Haft JI, Kosowsky BD, Lau SH, Stein E, Damato AN: Termination of atrial flutter by rapid electrical pacing of the atrium. *Am J Cardiol* 1967; 20:239–244.
163. Dreifus LS, Arriaga J, Watanabe Y, Downing D, Haiat R, Morse D: Recurrent Wolff–Parkinson–White tachycardia in an infant. Successful treatment by a radio-frequency pacemaker. *Am J Cardiol* 1971; 28:586–591.
164. Kahn A, Morris JJ, Citron P: Patient-initiated rapid atrial pacing to manage supraventricular tachycardia. *Am J Cardiol* 1976; 38:200–204.
165. Mandel WJ, Laks MM, Yamaguchi I, Fields J, Berkovits B: Recurrent reciprocating tachycardias in the Wolff–Parkinson–White syndrome. Control by the use of a scanning pacemaker. *Chest* 1976; 69:769–774.
166. Spurrell RAJ, Sowton E: Management of paroxysmal supraventricular tachycardia using a scanning pacing system (abstr). *Br Heart J* 1976; 38:536.
167. Dreifus LS, Berkovits B, Kimbiris D, Moghadam K: Use of atrial and bifocal cardiac pacemakers for treating resistant dysrhythmias. *Eur J Cardiol* 1975; 3:257–266.
168. Krikler D, Curry P, Buffet J: Dual-demand pacing for reciprocating atrioventricular tachycardia. *Br Med J* 1976; 1:1114–1116.
169. Massumi RA, Kistin AD, Tawakkol AA: Termination of reciprocating tachycardia by atrial stimulation. *Circulation* 1967; 36:637–643.
170. Preston TA, Kirsh MM: Permanent pacing of the left atrium for treatment of Wolff–Parkinson–White tachycardia. *Circulation* 1970; 42:1073–1077.
171. Weiner L, Dwyer EM Jr: Electrical induction of atrial fibrillation. An approach to intractable atrial tachycardia. *Am J Cardiol* 1968; 21:731–734.
172. Cohen HE, Meltzer LE, Lattimer G, Linares H, Agrin R: Treatment of refractory supraventricular arrhythmias with induced permanent atrial fibrillation. *Am J Cardiol* 1971; 28:472–474.
173. Fisher JD, Furman S, Mehra M: Termination of ventricular tachycardia by bursts of rapid ventricular pacing, in Watanabe Y (ed): *Cardiac Pacing.* Amsterdam, Excerpta Medica, 1977, pp 194–199.
174. Short DS: The syndrome of alternating bradycardia and tachycardia. *Br Heart J* 1954; 16:208–214.
175. Rubenstein JJ, Schulman CL, Yurchak PM, DeSanctis RW: Clinical spectrum of the sick sinus syndrome. *Circulation* 1972; 46:5–13
176. Bouman LN, Jongsma HJ: Structure and function of the sino-atrial node. A review. *Euro Heart J* 1986; 7:94–104.
177. Langendorf R, Pick A, Winternitz M: Mechanisms of intermittent ventricular bigeminy. I. Appearance of ectopic beats dependent upon length of the ventricular cycle, the "rule of bigeminy." *Circulation* 1955; 11:422–430.
178. Han J, Millet D, Chizzonitti B, Moe GK: Temporal dispersion of recovery of excitability in atrium and ventricle as a function of heart rate. *Am Heart J* 1966; 71:481–487.
179. Linenthal AJ, Zoll PM: Prevention of ventricular tachycardia and fibrillation by intravenous isoproterenol and epinephrine. *Circulation* 1963; 27:5–11.
180. Bellinder G, Nordlander R, Pehrsson SK, Aström H: Atrial pacing in the management of sick sinus syndrome. Long-term observation for conduction disturbances and supraventricular tachyarrhythmias. *Euro Heart J* 1986; 7:105–109.
181. Cheng TO: Transvenous ventricular pacing in the treatment of paroxysmal atrial tachyarrhythmias alternating with sinus bradycardia and standstill. *Am J Cardiol* 1968; 22:874–879.
182. Cohen HE, Kahn M, Donoso E: Treatment of supraventricular tachycardias with catheter and permanent pacemakers. *Am J Cardiol* 1967; 20:735–738.
183. Adelman AG, Wigle ED: The bradycardia, tachycardia, asystole syndrome: treatment by a pacemaker. *Can Med Assoc J* 1969; 100:75–77.

21 Management of Cardiac Arrhythmias

Bramah N. Singh, MD, D Phil (Oxon), FRCP (London) and Koonlawee Nademanee, MD

The rational approach to the control of cardiac arrhythmias presupposes a reasonably precise knowledge of the origin of cardiac dysrhythmias and an understanding of the fundamental mechanisms of antiarrhythmic intervention.[1-8] The increasing application in man of electrophysiologic investigations, especially programmed electrical stimulation, has permitted the elucidation of the nature of many clinical cardiac arrhythmias[9]; it has also allowed the actions of antiarrhythmic compounds to be interpreted from their effects on various electrophysiologic parameters.[10] There have also been major developments in the area of new antiarrhythmic compounds.[5,7,11]

New developments in antiarrhythmic therapy have also occurred in the area of nonpharmacologic therapy. For example, in arrhythmias that are resistant to antiarrhythmic drugs, automatic or patient-activated implantable pacemakers or defibrillators currently under development are becoming realistic therapeutic modalities in selected patients.[12] Another encouraging advance is the development of various surgical techniques in the treatment of drug-resistant tachyarrhythmias.[13,14] This is particularly so in life-threatening ventricular tachyarrhythmias, although greater successes have been achieved in patients with the Wolff–Parkinson–White syndrome.[15,16] In patients being submitted to surgery, preoperative and intraoperative mapping of the activation sequence has permitted accurate localization and interruption of the reentrant pathways involved in such arrhythmias.[14]

Newer developments suggest that it may be possible to establish more objective and clinically meaningful end points of antiarrhythmic therapy than previously possible. For example, the availability of techniques for continuous electrocardiographic monitoring and semiautomated analysis of arrhythmias allows the response of individual dysrhythmias to a particular intervention to be evaluated quantitatively, especially in relation to dose and plasma levels of drugs if pharmacologic therapy is used. Long-term prognostic indexes then can be developed relative to suppression of the spontaneously occurring arrhythmias. It is now known that such indexes may also be developed on the basis of the suppressibility of electrically induced arrhythmias.[17]

This chapter reviews the basis on which a rational approach might be developed for the management of cardiac arrhythmias with particular reference to the newer developments.

ELECTROPHYSIOLOGIC CONSIDERATIONS

A knowledge of the sequence of ionic changes mediating rapid depolarization, repolarization, and spontaneous diastolic depolarization during inscription of the action potential (AP) in pacemaking and nonpacemaking tissues is essential to an understanding of the origin of arrhythmias and how antiarrhythmic drugs exert their salutary effects.

The cardiac AP is a phasic electrical phenomenon that may be separated into five phases. Phase 0, representing sudden depolarization when the membrane potential (MP) is brought to threshold, is mediated by a kinetically fast current (fast response) and a kinetically slow current (slow response). The fast response, mediated by sodium ions, is sudden and brief, lasting only a few milliseconds; its intensity is a function of the MP from which the AP is generated. The study of this relation, commonly known as membrane responsiveness, has shown that until the membrane is repolarized to −55 mV or so, it cannot be reactivated irrespective of the stimulus strength. This level of repolarization thus defines the end of the absolute refractory period (ARP), a parameter that is voltage dependent and varies in length with the action potential duration (APD). Thus, any intervention that lengthens the APD (eg, bradycardia, hypocalcemia, and hypothyroidism) prolongs the ARP; conversely, those that shorten the APD (eg, halothane, anoxia, and tachycardia) tend to abbreviate the ARP. The ARP of cardiac muscle needs to be distinguished from the effective refractory period (ERP), which is the main determinant of the number of propagated impulses that the heart is able to generate per unit of time. It is therefore longer in duration than the ARP, and because generation of a propagated impulse is critically dependent on the recovery of excitability, the ERP, under certain circumstances, may outlast the entire duration of cardiac repolarization. The recovery of excitability in this context is related to the recovery of the sodium-carrier mechanism to a finite degree; inhibition of the fast response as might be produced by local anesthetic drugs may markedly lengthen the ERP with a trivial or no change in the overall APD (and hence the ARP).

In contrast, the second (slow) inward current is carried essentially by calcium ions; the threshold for the activation of this channel is about −35 mV. Therefore, normally it is activated as the fast channel depolarizes the cell. The slow channel in ventricular muscle begins to inactivate at about 500 ms from the onset of depolarization, so that the slow current only starts to attenuate near the end of the plateau phase of the action potential.

Slow response action potentials are normally found in the normal sinus and atrioventricular (AV) nodes and in pathologic situations in which the fast response has been inactivated and the presence of a slow response is associated with depressed conduction velocity.

In contrast to the depolarization phase of the cardiac AP, the repolarization phases are less well understood in terms of the ionic conductances[2] involved. Phase 1, or rapid repolarization, is believed to result in part from the inactivation of sodium conductance occurring at the voltage near 0 mV and is partially related to a chloride current activated at about −10 mV. Phase 2 in Purkinje fibers represents the plateau of the action potential, during which there is little net current flow, being mostly the slow current carried essentially by calcium. The final repolarization (phase 3) of the cardiac action potential is primarily the function of an outward current carried largely by potassium ($^{i}X_1$) and having important time- as well as voltage-dependent properties. It is activated very slowly, in the plateau range of potentials, but its magnitude increases as inactivation of the slow calcium current commences to repolarize the membrane. As the membrane potential becomes more and more negative, the outward potassium current tends to increase and repolarization is accelerated. The second potassium current ($^{i}K_1$), which is voltage dependent only, also appears to contribute to repolarization.

The pacemaker current in Purkinje fibers in the past has been designated as $^{i}K_2$. Unlike the fast response, $^{i}K_2$ is controlled only by a single process, which is activated during depolarization and inactivated when repolarization takes place. It is to be emphasized that, as suggested by recent data, the ionic basis of the pacemaker current is exceedingly complex and may not all be due to a potassium current. There is increasing evidence that at least in part the slow inward calcium current may mediate pacemaker activity in the mammalian heart. As far as pacemaker phenomena in cardiac tissues in general are concerned, it should be emphasized that although the pacemaker potential of Purkinje fiber has been the best studied,[2] increasing evidence points to the possibility that pacemaker activity in the sinoatrial node or pacemaker phenomena in ectopic cardiac arrhythmias may have distinctly different ionic mechanisms. Pacemaker activity in the normal sinus node may be mediated, at least in part, by the slow response. This is suggested by the fact that manganese can block pacemaker activity and depolarize frog atrial fibers; therefore, the second inward current may play a significant role in the generation of pacemaker potentials.[2] Such a mechanism may also mediate the genesis of certain types of abnormal automatic rhythms under pathologic conditions, an understanding of which is clearly of much importance in the control by such pharmacologic interventions as specific calcium antagonists.

MECHANISMS OF CARDIAC ARRHYTHMIAS

Most arrhythmias appear to result from disturbances in impulse generation (ectopic tachyarrhythmias) and impulse conduction (reentrant arrhythmias) or from a combination of both processes.[3,4] A third possibility has recently been considered in the form of "triggered automaticity."[18] In Table 21.1 the mechanisms underlying different experimentally induced arrhythmias are listed in relation to the potential clinical counterparts of the various automatic, reentrant, and triggered tachyarrhythmias.

It is known that latent pacemakers may accelerate in frequency and potential pacemaking cells may develop phase 4 depolarization as a result of stimuli from anoxia, stretch, and edema or excessive sympathetic stimulation. It is possible that certain regenerative pacemaker potentials may be mediated entirely by abnormalities of calcium currents, an inference that is drawn from the effects of selective inhibitors.

The fundamental requirements for reentry are appro-

Table 21.1. Potential Mechanisms of Clinically Occurring Cardiac Arrhythmias

Disorders of impulse formation
Enhanced automaticity
Ectopic supraventricular tachycardia
Idioventricular rhythm
Parasystolic rhythm
Certain types of ventricular ectopic beats and tachycardia
Triggered automaticity
Due to early afterdepolarization: exercised-induced tachycardia; torsades de pointes
Due to late afterdepolarization: digitalis-induced tachyarrhythmias
Disorders of impulse conduction
Reentry
Paroxysmal supraventricular tachycardia (ordered)
Circus movement tachycardia (ordered)
Ventricular ectopics and tachycardia (? ordered)
Ventricular and atrial fibrillation (random)

priate anatomic pathways and slow conduction velocity with unidirectional block in the transmission of cardiac impulse. This permits longitudinal dissociation of the excitation wavefront with return of impulse retrogradely through the region of depressed conduction, further and continuing excitation occurring in a repetitive manner on the basis of a reentrant circuit. For example, in the human AV conduction system, there are fibers capable of conducting impulses at varying frequencies in relation to their refractoriness, a situation that satisfies the requirements for reentry.[4] Most supraventricular tachycardias are due to AV nodal reentry; this appears to result from longitudinal dissociation of the sinus impulse at a time when the dual pathways have significantly different refractory periods. Similarly, in the various preexcitation syndromes, accessory pathways and the AV node may constitute a reentry circuit, with antegrade conduction occurring in the AV node with return of the impulse to the atria retrogradely through the anomalous tract during reciprocating supraventricular tachycardias complicating the syndrome of accelerated conduction.[10] The reciprocation may occur in the reverse direction, although less frequently. Reentry may also occur in the sinus node and in the atria in rarer cases of supraventricular tachycardias.[10] The most common forms of paroxysmal supraventricular tachycardia are indicated in Table 21.2. Programmed stimulation of the heart[9,10] has suggested that reentry is probably the underlying mechanism of most life-threatening ventricular tachycardias found in clinical practice.

Alterations in the repolarization phase of the cardiac AP independently of changes in depolarization may, under certain conditions, be arrhythmogenic. For example, oscillation of the MP during repolarization in damaged myocardium may be brought to threshold by endogenously liberated catecholamines resulting in sustained tachyarrhythmias.[18] This may be one of the mechanisms for the origin of arrhythmias in acute myocardial ischemia. Disparity in the rates of repolarization in adjacent myocardial fibers may also be a source of focal reexcitation and reentry, a function of temporal dispersion in the recovery of excitability as a consequence of differing APDs in subjacent myocardial fibers. Because the ARP is a function of the APD, marked acceleration of repolarization would increase excitability and produce arrhythmias. This is clearly in line with the observation that acetylcholine, anoxia, or halothane shortens the APD and may all produce cardiac arrhythmias.[19] The converse also appears to hold. Homogeneous prolongation of the APD is accompanied by a corresponding lengthening of the ARP with a consequent reduction in the excitability

Table 21.2. Mechanisms Responsible for Paroxysmal Supraventricular Tachycardia

1. Ectopic tachycardia
2. Reentrant tachycardia
    - Without bypass tracts
        - AV nodal reentry (slow–fast; fast–slow)
        - Sinus node reentry
    - With bypass tracts
        - Orthodromic tachycardia
        - Antidromic tachycardia

of the myocardial cell, an antiarrhythmic mechanism. However, it should be mentioned that a number of disease states and syndromes associated with prolongation of repolarization (QT_c interval) lead to life-threatening arrhythmias.[20] From this it is to be inferred that in these conditions, an overall delayed repolarization is not a uniform process, and inhomogeneities of recovery of excitability must be a significant feature in those clinical entities exhibiting arrhythmias in association with an abnormally long QT_c interval on the electrocardiogram.

The role of triggered automaticity in the genesis of clinical arrhythmias is still unclear.[18] A nondriven action potential that arises from an afterdepolarization following an antecedent action potential has been referred to as triggered[4,18]; it can also be triggered in a quiescent fiber by a single excitatory stimulus but, unlike reentrant rhythms, triggered activity may demonstrate the phenomenon of overdrive acceleration rather than suppression or termination following electrical pacing. It is possible that many digitalis-induced arrhythmias and some late ischemic ventricular tachyarrhythmias may arise on the basis of triggered automaticity.[18]

CONTROL OF CARDIAC ARRHYTHMIAS

In the management of cardiac arrhythmias, it is clearly of importance to establish the nature of the arrhythmia and to define its prognostic significance. It is also of significance to examine whether treatment is being embarked on solely to alleviate symptoms (eg, palpitations and syncope) or to prolong survival, or both. For example, the treatment of most supraventricular arrhythmias is usually undertaken for the relief of symptoms. However, it is known that atrial flutter and fibrillation complicating the Wolff–Parkinson–White syndrome, if untreated, may produce not only syncope but also sudden death from ventricular fibrillation.[15,16] Similarly, even asymptomatic episodes of atrial fibrillation in a patient with heart disease and cardiomegaly may be a predisposition to the development of potentially serious embolic phenomena, thus requiring either permanent anticoagulation or adequate suppression of atrial fibrillation. Whether arrhythmias are treated essentially for the relief symptoms or to avert the development of sudden arrhythmic death becomes of paramount importance in the approach to the control of ventricular tachyarrhythmias. It is becoming increasingly clear, for example, that although premature ventricular contractions occur commonly in otherwise healthy individuals[21] as well as those with a varying spectrum of severity of cardiac disease especially of ischemic origin,[22] only in the latter may they be of prognostic import. Finally, it is of obvious importance to identify the cost–benefit ratio of any antiarrhythmic regimen, because not all arrhythmias need aggressive therapy and many regimens, especially pharmacologic, may be associated with a significant potentially life-threatening arrhythmogenic potential.[23]

Approaches to the control of cardiac arrhythmias may be considered under the following categories: *general measures*: (1) exclusion of precipitating causes (including drugs); (2) treatment of underlying cardiac disease (eg, coronary artery spasm); and (3) correction of electrolyte derangements; *specific measures*: (1) pharmacologic therapy;

(2) pacemakers, cardioverters, and defibrillators; and (3) surgery.

PHARMACOLOGIC APPROACHES

Although the ideal antiarrhythmic drug remains to be developed, recent advances in the synthesis of new compounds warrant optimism. The pharmacology of the conventional and newer antiarrhythmic agents will be discussed in chapter 63. It is likely that in the control of cardiac arrhythmias, pharmacologic suppression, especially prophylactic, will remain the mainstay of antiarrhythmic therapy; the use of implantable devices and surgery is likely to be reserved for recalcitrant tachyarrhythmias.

PACEMAKING AND IMPLANTABLE DEVICES

In certain patients, cardiac pacing in a variety of modes may be employed for both acute termination as well as long-term prevention of many types of arrhythmias.[24-27] For the acute interruption of an arrhythmia, a temporary pacing electrode can readily be placed in the patient, and a number of pacing techniques have been used[25] since the initial report of Haft et al[24] on the termination of atrial flutter by pacing. Those techniques included single random extrastimuli, simultaneous AV sequential pacing, dual demand pacing, orthorhythmic pacing, and programmed scanning. Fisher et al[25] recently demonstrated the more frequent effectiveness of bursts of rapid atrial or ventricular stimulation at a rate higher than that of the tachyarrhythmia. Recent developments have taken the form of transvenous intraventricular cardioverters.

Of particular interest is the role of cardiac pacing in the prophylactic management of recurrent arrhythmias. Selected patients can now be offered the use of patient-activated implantable units capable of delivering bursts of rapid atrial stimuli that can terminate recurrences of supraventricular as well as ventricular tachyarrhythmias.[25] Custom-built automatically activated burst pacemakers, although superior to patient-activated devices, have not achieved popularity, probably because such units do not allow flexibility in subsequent pacemaker performance because they are not programmable. Two recent developments are especially encouraging, however. The first is the use of an automatic multiprogrammable tachycardia-terminating pacemaker in patients with reentrant supraventricular tachyarrhythmias.[27] The other is the development of an implantable defibrillator capable of sensing and defibrillating ventricular tachycardia or fibrillation or both. Preliminary reports by Mirowski et al[28] suggest a role for such a device in patients with recurrent cardiac arrests. Although such techniques for sensing and terminating tachyarrhythmias by the use of implantable devices are in the early stages of development, they appear to hold much promise for patients in whom drug therapy is unsatisfactory. Major developments are likely to occur in this modality of antiarrhythmic therapy in the future.[12]

ANTIARRHYTHMIC SURGERY

The main surgical approaches and their indications in the control of refractory arrhythmias are listed in Table 21.3. The subject will be dealt with at length in chapter 22. A variety of surgical approaches are available in selected arrhythmias. It has long been known that sympathetic hyperexcitability may play a dominant role in the genesis of ventricular tachyarrhythmias in some patients. For this reason, from time to time, cardiac sympathectomy has been undertaken in patients with truly refractory ventricular tachyarrhythmias.[29] With the advent of beta blockers and other antiarrhythmic agents, sympathetic ablation is now rarely, if ever, performed. However, it is known that in some patients with the long QT_c interval syndrome, recurrent ventricular tachycardia and even ventricular fibrillation may occur. In this syndrome there appears to be an asymmetry between left and right sympathetic nerve activity; left-sided cervicothoracic sympathectomy, including stellate ganglionectomy, has been reported to normalize the QT interval and prevent potentially fatal recurrent ventricular arrhythmias.[30]

Table 21.3. Surgical Approaches to the Control of Recalcitrant Cardiac Arrhythmias

1. Local ablation, eg, surgical or cryosurgical interruption of AV node or bypass tracts, for reciprocating or AV nodal reentrant tachycardia; local excision of tissue in right ventricular dysplasia
2. Ablation of sources of sympathetic transmitters to the heart
   a. Regional cardiac sympathectomy for intractable ventricular tachycardia
   b. Left stellate ganglionectomy (for recurrent ventricular tachycardia/fibrillation in the context of long QT_c interval syndromes)
3. Myocardial revascularization (occasionally successful in ventricular tachycardia)
4. Aneurysmectomy (for ventricular tachycardia)
5. Encircling endocardial ventriculotomy (for ventricular tachycardia)
6. Endocardial excision (for ventricular tachycardia/fibrillation)
7. Electrode catheter ablation of arrhythmia focus or circuit

Coronary artery bypass grafting has also been suggested as a method of treatment of ventricular tachycardia in patients with ischemic heart disease. However, numerous reports have suggested that myocardial revascularization, alone or in combination with ventricular resection, is usually not effective in the control of recurrent ventricular tachyarrhythmias.[13] In contrast, recurrent tachycardia that invariably occurs in association with acute ischemic episodes may be eliminated by revascularization. However, myocardial revascularization generally plays a minor role in the control of recurrent tachycardia.

In the past, AV nodal transmission was interrupted by either direct surgery or cryosurgical techniques in patients with resistant atrial flutter or paroxysmal supraventricular tachycardias, ventricular rhythm being governed thereafter by artificial pacemaking. Again, the advent of potent antiarrhythmic agents such as amiodarone has made ablation of the AV node a rare therapeutic modality.

Two major syndromes currently account for the largest number of indications for surgery designed to prevent recurrent tachyarrhythmias. These are the Wolff–Parkinson–White syndrome complicated by atrial flutter or fibrillation and paroxysmal ventricular tachycardia.[13-16] In both instances, the approach is based on the application of electrophysiologic study techniques for the preoperative documentation of the sites of origin of the arrhythmias or anomalous conduction pathways, for intraoperative delineation of the same target abnormalities, and for postoperative evaluation of the effectiveness of the surgical procedure. In the Wolff–Parkinson–White syndrome, the surgical approach is keyed to division of the anomalous pathways by endocardial dissection of the AV grooves in the appropriate location.[15,16] Cure rates in experienced centers now exceed 95%, with an overall operative risk of 1% to 2%, which is often related to the associated cardiac disease.

Surgery for ventricular tachycardia is also dependent on the preoperative demonstration of sustained ventricular tachycardia by programmed electrical stimulation.[13,14] The basic goal of the surgical procedure is to identify by direct mapping the site of origin of arrhythmias during induced tachycardia, as indicated by the earliest site of electrical activity. The subendocardial region containing this focus of earliest electrical activity is then resected. The effectiveness of the surgical procedure is reassessed by further attempts to induce the ventricular arrhythmia. The success rate with this technique has been variable, but most centers that employ the method consider it superior to aneurysmectomy without endocardial mapping.[13,14,31] The alternative technique for ventricular tachycardia is encircling endocardial ventriculotomy introduced in France by Guiraudon et al.[32] The method involves visual identification of the border of the postinfarction scar and an incision encircling the entire border, passing from the endocardium to just below the epicardial surface. It is believed that ventriculotomy of this magnitude obliterates potential arrhythmogenic focus or reentry circuits around the scar border.

GENERAL PRINCIPLES IN ANTIARRHYTHMIC THERAPY

In the ensuing chapters, the main resources—antiarrhythmic drugs, pacemakers and defibrillators, and surgery—available to the clinician for the control of cardiac arrhythmias will be outlined in greater detail. In this section the general principles that govern antiarrhythmic therapy are discussed.

The principles that govern acute termination of an arrhythmia may differ from those deemed appropriate for the chronic prophylaxis of recurrent tachyarrhythmias. For example, it is clearly necessary to promptly terminate a tachyarrhythmia irrespective of its origin (whether ventricular or supraventricular) if it is associated with significant and advancing hemodynamic or clinical deterioration. The most appropriate method under these circumstances is usually electrical conversion (defibrillation or cardioversion), rather than trial and error in the use of multiple antiarrhythmic drugs, either empirically or after a lengthy procedure undertaken to elucidate the nature of the arrhythmia. In contrast, for chronic prophylaxis of the same arrhythmia it is clearly important to determine precisely the nature of the arrhythmia before rational therapy aimed at preventing the dysrhythmia can be instituted. It is known, for instance, that paroxysmal supraventricular tachycardia with aberrant ventricular conduction can closely mimic (at least electrocardiographically) ventricular tachycardia; both tachyarrhythmias can be terminated predictably by electrical conversion. For prophylactic control, however, drug therapy for the two types of arrhythmias may be markedly different, emphasizing the need to elucidate the nature of the arrhythmia before prophylactic therapy is initiated. This information, which can now be obtained by intracavitary recordings and by arrhythmia induction techniques,[9,10] is clearly less crucial if termination is all that is required as an urgent clinical indication. Adherence to well-defined principles of antiarrhythmic therapy is particularly rewarding in the management of recurrent cardiac arrhythmias; here, a carefully designed and executed approach may ensure a high degree of success in the treatment of apparently refractory arrhythmias. We generally adopt the following steps in the development of a therapeutic regimen for the treatment of arrhythmia.

1. *Identification of the nature and the severity of the arrhythmia*: Although historical features may sometimes indicate the nature of an arrhythmia, electrocardiographic documentation of the abnormality is nearly always imperative. A 12-lead electrocardiogram during the rhythm disorder is helpful, as is the mode of onset and termination of the spontaneous arrhythmia. This may sometimes be obtained during 24-hour Holter recordings. The 24-hour Holter recordings are particularly valuable in the evaluation of ventricular arrhythmias, and such recordings are generally superior to exercise testing in detecting ventricular ectopy or ventricular tachycardia. It should also be emphasized that whenever possible, Holter recordings are best obtained before treatment is initiated; in "resistant" tachyarrhythmias, all antiarrhythmic agents should be discontinued during monitoring so that the nature and severity of the arrhythmias can be evaluated under as controlled a condition as possible. In arrhythmias that cannot be documented electrocardiographically, on either Holter recording or exercise testing, electrode catheter induction may be undertaken if, on other grounds, the suspected arrhythmia is deemed clinically significant and requiring therapy.

2. *Determination of the nature and severity of the underlying heart disease (if any)*: This is particularly relevant to the issue of whether an arrhythmia (especially an asymptomatic one) merits treatment; the underlying cardiac disease is usually the crucial determinant of the prognostic significance of the arrhythmia itself. The prognosis of most arrhythmias in patients with normal hearts is rarely influenced by the arrhythmia itself.[33] The level of ventricular function may also dictate the type of antiarrhythmic therapy that might be appropriate. For example, a potentially negative inotropic agent such as disopyramide is contraindicated in patients with previous cardiac failure.

3. *Exclusion of precipitating and reversible causes of the arrhythmia*: There are instances in which a patient normally not prone to cardiac arrhythmia may develop one after a potentially arrhythmogenic intervention. Disturbances of electrolyte balance (eg, severe hypokalemia, digitalis, and liquid protein diets), certain drugs (thioridazine, tricyclic antidepressant agents, and lithium carbonate) and episodic myocardial ischemia (eg, Prinzmetal angina) may all precipitate potentially serious cardiac arrhythmias in certain patients. Attempts to control such arrhythmias without correcting the underlying abnormalities are unlikely

to be readily successful and may aggravate the rhythm disorder.

4. *Establishment of the rationale and goal of antiarrhythmic therapy*: In many patients, a clear rationale for the long-term treatment of certain arrhythmias may be difficult to establish. For example, aggressive protracted ventricular ectopy in patients without manifest heart disease is difficult to justify. Similarly, patients with recurrent paroxysmal supraventricular tachycardia occurring once or twice a year and terminating readily with vagal maneuvers undoubtedly do not require continuous drug prophylaxis. However, once the decision for prophylactic treatment has been made, it is mandatory to establish reasonably clear goals of therapy. For an individual patient, it is helpful to define whether antiarrhythmic therapy is being undertaken solely for the relief of symptoms associated with the arrhythmia (an easily measurable index), or whether it is being executed in the expectation of prolonging survival. The parameters for judging the efficacy of therapy in this regard are less well established.

5. *Choice of antiarrhythmic regimen and documentation that the goal of therapy is attained*: Once the reversible and precipitating causes of an arrhythmia have been dealt with, drug therapy is usually the first line of treatment that is considered. Whenever possible, antiarrhythmic agents are selected on the basis of the known mechanisms of the origin of the dysrhythmia relative to the fundamental mode of action of the drug to be used. For example, beta-adrenergic blocking drugs (class II agents) are likely to be most effective in controlling arrhythmias that depend on sympathetic activation (eg, exercise-induced ventricular tachycardia) or those that are due to myocardial ischemia precipitated by increases in myocardial oxygen demand.[34] Similarly, ventricular tachyarrhythmias that result as a direct consequence of coronary vasospasm are likely to, and indeed do, respond most effectively to coronary vasodilators, particularly slow channel blocking drugs (class IV agents).[35,36]

In the overall use of antiarrhythmic drugs, we have found little advantage in combining agents from the same antiarrhythmic class; often such a practice (eg, combining disopyramide and quinidine) is associated with a greater incidence of side effects than that when single agents are used. However, the possibility that small doses of two drugs from the same electrophysiologic class may be combined with advantage has not been excluded and such combination regimens are being used widely even though rigorous studies have not been performed to establish their efficacy and safety. Our own practice is to use a single agent in appropriate doses to "therapeutically acceptable" plasma levels before abandoning it in favor of an alternative agent. If a partial response toward a predefined therapeutic goal is obtained, combination therapy may be considered, but the agent must be from a different antiarrhythmic class if the interaction between the two antiarrhythmic compounds does not preclude the use of the combination. Moreover, in the use of antiarrhythmic compounds, appropriate consideration must be given to the design of the regimen in relation to the pharmacokinetic properties of the drug being used and the clinical status of the patient with the arrhythmia. Failure of pharmacologic therapy is accepted when a single or appropriate combination regimen of antiarrhythmic drug is ineffective in meeting the predetermined goals of therapy or when side effects preclude the continued use of drugs. Other modes of therapy, such as pacemakers, defibrillators, and surgery, are then considered, although on rare occasions such approaches are employed before an exhaustive trial with pharmacologic therapy.

CONTROL OF COMMON CARDIAC ARRHYTHMIAS

What follows is not meant to be used as the only approach to control cardiac arrhythmias. An attempt is made to provide general guidelines in the knowledge that departures from them are likely and indeed are common in individual cases. The two categories of arrhythmias to be discussed are those of supraventricular origin and those arising from the ventricles. Specific dosages and regimens are mentioned in passing and should be obtained from other reference sources or elsewhere in this volume. Details of the conventional and newer drugs are found in recent reports.[1,5,7,8,11,37–44]

SUPRAVENTRICULAR ARRHYTHMIAS

Supraventricular arrhythmias include premature atrial or junctional contractions, atrial flutter and fibrillation, ectopic or reentrant supraventricular tachycardias, multifocal atrial tachycardia, atrial tachycardia with varying AV block, and the arrhythmias complicating the Wolff–Parkinson–White syndrome. These include orthodromic and antidromic paroxysmal supraventricular tachycardias and atrial flutter and fibrillation with varying input of the atrial impulses into the bypass tracts.

Premature Atrial or Junctional Contractions

These are common in healthy subjects and rarely need aggressive medical therapy; if symptomatically troublesome, they may need suppression if not responsive to general measures. Similarly, if they are harbingers of atrial fibrillation in the setting of mitral valve disease or thyrotoxicosis, their suppression by agents such as quinidine and beta blockers may prevent the development of paroxysmal sustained atrial arrhythmias. Therefore, if the underlying disease cannot be corrected, prophylactic drug therapy may be advisable.

Atrial Flutter and Fibrillation

The treatment of these arrhythmias will depend on the clinical setting in which they occur, symptoms and hemodynamic perturbations that they may create, and the chronicity of their occurrence. In each individual case, the decision is made whether the object of therapy is merely to slow the ventricular response or effect conversion to sinus rhythm. The latter approach is adopted if, on clinical grounds, there appears to be a reasonable prospect that the arrhythmia relapse will be prevented by continuous antiarrhythmic therapy or by the elimination of the underlying condition (eg, thyrotoxicosis).

The acute conversion of atrial flutter to sinus rhythm as might be necessary for hemodynamic reasons is best effected by electrical cardioversion. In atrial flutters, if an indwelling pacing electrode is available, sinus rhythm may be restored in most cases by rapid atrial pacing. In atrial fibrillation as well as atrial flutter, intravenous procainamide (up to 1,000 mg) given slowly may produce conversion to sinus rhythm in a significant number of cases. Although data are limited, intravenous administration of class III antiarrhythmic agents such as sotalol and N-acetylprocainamide may also be effective in producing chemical cardioversion. However, the most reliable and consistent method of producing elective cardioversion in atrial flutter and fibrillation is direct current electroversion, although multiple oral doses of quinidine, procainamide, or disopyramide can be used when electroversion is not available. These agents, either alone or in combination with beta blockers, are often effective in maintaining stability of sinus rhythm after cardioversion; preliminary data suggest that class III antiarrhythmic agents (amiodarone, sotalol, and N-acetylprocainamide) may be of greater prophylactic value in this regard.

When the decision is made to merely maintain a controlled ventricular response, prophylactic digoxin therapy continues to be the mainstay of treatment. However, digoxin is relatively ineffective in attenuating exercise-induced increases in rate, and beta blockers or calcium antagonists such as verapamil or diltiazem may be added or used alone to provide smoother control of the resting as well as the exercise-induced heart rate.[44a]

Atrial Flutter and Fibrillation Complicating the Wolff–Parkinson–White Syndrome

Atrial fibrillation complicating the preexcitation syndrome is shown in Figure 21.1. In atrial flutter the response is usually 1:1 and the ventricular response over 300 per minute. The rapid ventricular response in either of these arrhythmias is the usual cause of sudden death in patients with the Wolff–Parkinson–White syndrome, because such rapid rates predispose to the development of ventricular fibrillation. It is clear that any intervention that impedes AV conduction across the AV node in this situation is unlikely to slow the ventricular response. Furthermore, if the fibrillatory impulses are being transmitted over the bypass tract as well as over the AV node, increased AV nodal block may enhance the ventricular response and prove lethal. This may occur with vagal maneuvers, after the administration of calcium antagonists, beta blockers, and especially cardiac glycosides (which also shorten the refractory period of the bypass tracts). Therefore, both acutely as well as prophylactically, the most rational therapy in atrial fibrillation or flutter complicating preexcitation is one that blocks bypass tract conduction and enhances refractoriness. Intravenous class 1 agents (procainamide, profanenone, disopyramide, and rarely lidocaine) may be effective for the conversion of acute episodes, but we prefer cardioversion at the earliest opportunity because of the inherently dan-

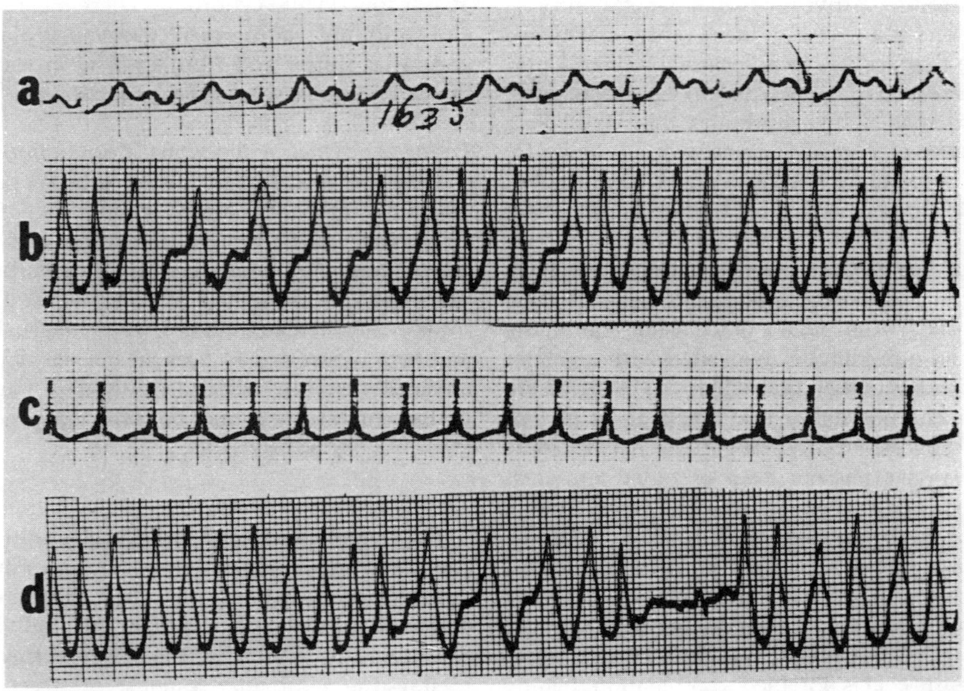

Figure 21.1. An example of arrhythmias that may occur in a patient with the Wolff–Parkinson–White (WPW) syndrome. *A,* Sinus rhythm with normal PR interval but with a small delta (preexcitation) wave indicating minimal "input" of the depolarization wave through the bypass tract. *B,* Atrial fibrillation with all fibrillatory impulses being transmitted to the ventricles through the bypass tract. *C,* Paroxysmal supraventricular tachycardia (with retrograde P wave) with narrow QRS complexes consistent with reentrant loop using the AV node for antegrade conduction. *D,* Further episode of atrial fibrillation using bypass tract; note one sinus complex preceding the sixth complex from the end of the strip. The tracings illustrate the variable RR intervals during atrial fibrillation complicating the WPW syndrome.

gerous nature of the arrhythmia. Numerous agents are now available for prophylaxis after agents such as quinidine, procainamide, or disopyramide fail or are not tolerated. Of particular value are amiodarone, sotalol, encainide, and propafenone. Surgical treatment aimed at identification (by electrophysiologic evaluation) and division of the bypass tract may also be considered in selected cases, especially if drugs prove ineffective and not tolerated.[15,16]

Paroxysmal Supraventricular Tachycardia

The presumed mechanisms of the various types of paroxysmal supraventricular tachycardias are shown in Table 21.2. Examples of the commonly occurring ones are illustrated in Figure 21.2. It will be apparent that in the first four types (A through D) of arrhythmia shown, the QRS complexes are narrow, consistent with ventricular activation occurring through a normal AV nodal activation sequence; in circus movement tachycardias, both concealed (C) as well as overt (D), the QRS complexes are followed immediately by a retrograde P wave in contrast to the "fast-slow" AV nodal reentrant tachycardia in which the RP interval is longer than the PR interval during sinus rhythm. It should be emphasized that in both AV nodal reentrant tachycardia and circus movement (orthodromic) tachycardia, the rational treatment for converting the arrhythmia to sinus rhythm is to block antegrade (vagal maneuvers, beta blockers, digoxin, and par excellence intravenous verapamil or adenosine) or retrograde (intravenous procainamide and other class I agents) AV conduction; prophylaxis is aimed at either eliminating atrial or ventricular ectopy, which initiates the tachycardia, or increasing AV nodal refractoriness, which may preclude both the initiation as well as the perpetuation of the arrhythmia. In our experience, increasing AV nodal refractoriness (by beta blockers, digoxin, sotalol, verapamil, and amiodarone) is more effective prophylaxis for paroxysmal supraventricular tachycardia than is attempting to eliminate ventricular or supraventricular ectopy (eg, the use of quinidine, procainamide, or disopyramide). Narrow QRS reentrant paroxysmal supraventricular tachycardias must be distinguished from the wide QRS paroxysmal supraventricular tachycardia (not due simply to ventricular aberration) due

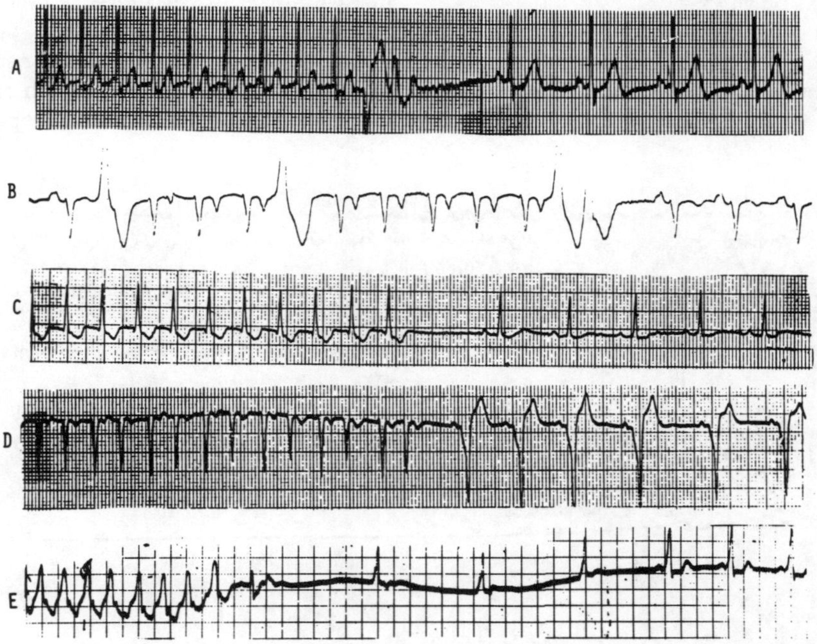

Figure 21.2. Different forms of reentrant paroxysmal supraventricular tachycardia (PSVT). *A,* "Slow-fast" intranodal PSVT. Atria and ventricles are activated almost simultaneously and the slow intranodal pathway constituting the antegrade limb and the fast pathway the retrograde limb of the tachycardia. *B,* "Fast-slow" intranodal PSVT, the converse of that shown in *A*. The tachycardia is initiated by one PVC, is not terminated by a subsequent PVC, but is terminated by PVCs occurring in a pair. Note the delayed retrograde activation of the atria (over slow pathway). *C,* Reentrant PSVT with retrograde atrial activation through a concealed bypass tract. The antegrade limb of the tachycardia is constituted by the AV node. Note the retrograde P wave immediately following the QRS complexes during the tachycardia. Termination of the tachycardia reveals no evidence of preexcitation because conduction over the bypass tract occurs solely in a retrograde direction. *D,* Circus movement tachycardia with the Wolff–Parkinson–White syndrome. During tachycardia, ventricular activation occurs through the AV node, with the retrograde P wave succeeding each QRS complex. Termination of the tachycardia is preceded by cycle length alternation. *E,* Antidromic tachycardia. The reentrant loop is formed by antegrade conduction over bypass tract and retrograde through the AV node.

to circus movement involving antegrade conduction over the bypass tract and retrograde conduction over the AV node (Figure 21.2). Such an arrhythmia (antidromic tachycardia) is unlikely to respond to maneuvers that depress antegrade AV nodal conduction; it is a rare form of paroxysmal supraventricular tachycardia that is best treated acutely by either cardioversion or intravenously administered class I drugs, which depress bypass tract conduction (procainamide, disopyramide, propafenone, and possibly lidocaine). Prophylactically, oral quinidine, disopyramide, propafenone, procainamide, and especially amiodarone and sotalol are variably effective.

Other Forms of Supraventricular Tachyarrhythmias

Treatment of ectopic supraventricular tachycardia is less clearly defined. Agents that depress phase 4 depolarization, particularly class I and II agents and amiodarone, are variably effective in the prophylaxis of recurrent ectopic supraventricular tachycardia. The role of calcium antagonists is uncertain. Multifocal atrial tachycardia is generally nonresponsive to pharmacologic therapy.

VENTRICULAR ARRHYTHMIAS

In treatment of no other tachyarrhythmia is it as important to identify the objectives and the end points of treatment as it is in ventricular arrhythmias. The spectrum of significance of these tachyarrhythmias may be considered as: (1) premature ventricular contractions; (2) nonsustained ventricular tachycardia; (3) sustained ventricular tachycardia; (4) polymorphic ventricular tachycardia or torsades de pointes; and (5) ventricular flutter/fibrillation. In patients with serious cardiac disease, these arrhythmias may constitute a continuum.

Premature Ventricular Contractions

There is little evidence to suggest that in patients who do not have clinical heart disease, the mere presence of premature ventricular contractions (PVCs), even nonsymptomatic runs of ventricular tachycardia, increases the incidence of sudden arrhythmic death.[33] Therefore, if the goal of therapy is designed to reduce the probability of sudden death, therapy in this regard is unlikely to benefit the patient if the PVCs are nonsymptomatic. However, if such patients have troublesome symptoms that do not respond to simple measures (eg, reduction in coffee, tea, and alcohol intake), antiarrhythmic therapy may be contemplated, especially if it can be achieved without producing significant side effects. We generally do not treat asymptomatic PVCs in patients without manifest heart disease. In these, the presence of PVCs does not appear to constitute a significant risk factor for sudden arrhythmic death.[33] In contrast, in patients with significant cardiac disease (eg, patients with myocardial infarction, dilated or hypertrophic cardiomyopathy, and mitral valve

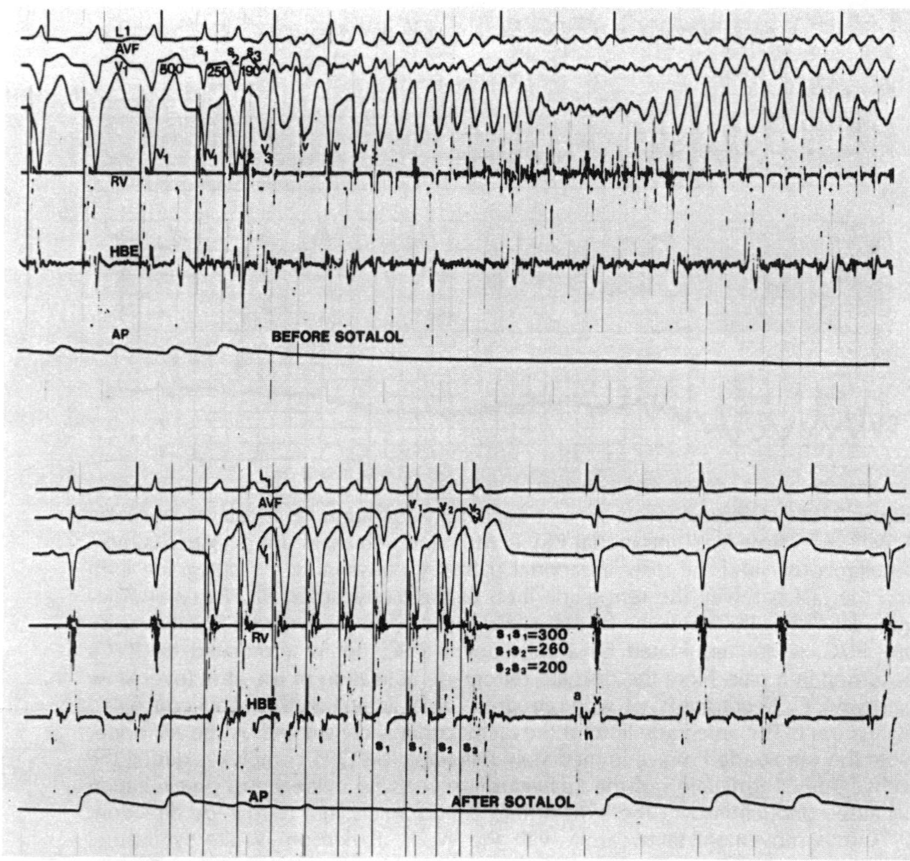

Figure 21.3. Example of the prevention of ventricular tachycardia/fibrillation inducible by programmed electrical stimulation of the heart by the administration of intravenous sotalol (1.5 mg/kg). Double stimuli were used to produce the arrhythmia that was no longer inducible (based on data reported by Nademanee et al[43]).

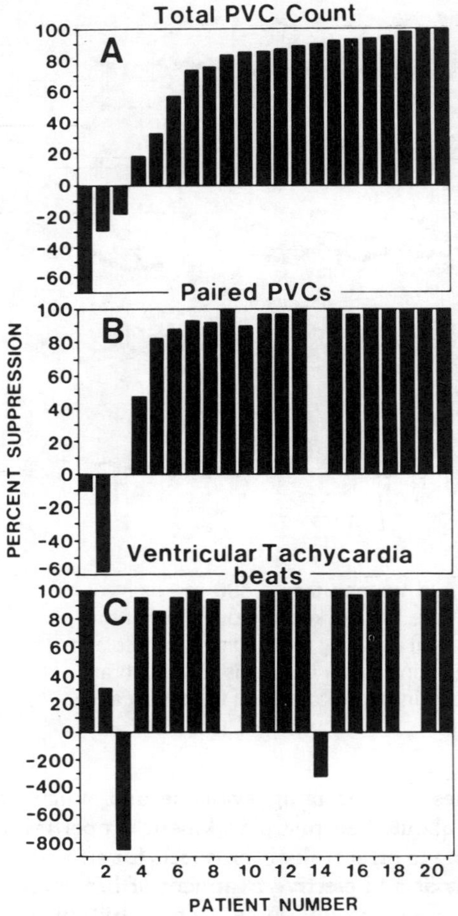

Figure 21.4. Effects of orally administered sotalol on total, paired, and repetitive ventricular ectopic beats in 21 patients with life-threatening ventricular tachyarrhythmias. Note that sotalol is more effective in suppressing complex premature ventricular contractions, a phenomenon that appears to correlate with prognosis and one that is a common feature of many antiarrhythmic agents (based on data from Nademanee et al[43]).

prolapse) the presence of PVCs is associated with a significant increase in the risk for sudden death. It is particularly striking in patients with a history of myocardial infarction.[22] However, data are still lacking to show that suppression of PVCs in these patients may enhance survival, although extrapolation from the experience of Graboys et al[45] in patients with life-threatening ventricular arrhythmias suggests that complex PVCs and nonsustained ventricular tachycardia should be suppressed pharmacologically. Furthermore, data suggest that the end point should be elimination of complex PVCs, rather than an arbitrarily chosen percentage reduction in the total PVC counts, which so far has not been shown to be related to a change in mortality.

Life-Threatening Ventricular Arrhythmias

Under this category, two major groups of ventricular tachyarrhythmias have been identified: (1) symptomatic sustained ventricular tachycardia and (2) ventricular tachycardia and fibrillation occurring in survivors of sudden arrhythmic death. In both groups, patients almost invariably have significant cardiac disease (over two thirds have coronary artery disease) with depressed ventricular ejection fraction. In both groups, over 80% have complex PVCs and runs of ventricular tachycardia on prolonged ambulatory monitoring and about 90% exhibit ventricular tachycardia or fibrillation on programmed electrical stimulation of the heart.[46,47] In a small subset both methods fail to reveal evidence of electrical instability.

Three approaches have been developed as potential therapeutic modalities. First, it has been suggested that for certain antiarrhythmic drugs such as quinidine and procainamide, the attainment of "therapeutic" serum levels may "protect" the patient from recurrent cardiac arrest while exerting little or no influence on ventricular ectopy.[47] Second, there is evidence also that antiarrhythmic agents that abolish the tendency for ventricular tachycardia/fibrillation (VT/VF) to be induced by programmed stimulation of the heart, when given acutely (Figure 21.3), may reliably confer protection against the recurrence of spontaneous VT/VF long-term.[17,43,46] However, most recent data indicate that the converse may not be true. For example, with compounds such as amiodarone[37] and propafenone,[44] failure of suppression of ventricular tachycardia inducible by programmed electrical stimulation does not preclude the possibility of a favorable long-term clinical outcome. Finally, as initially suggested by Graboys et al[45] in the case of conventional agents and further supported by experience with amiodarone,[37] the elimination of complex ventricular ectopy (Figure 21.4) and runs of ventricular tachycardia on Holter recordings during the early phases of therapy appears to accurately predict long-term antiarrhythmic therapy in the case of life-threatening ventricular tachyarrhythmias. Our own recent experience with the drug suggests that with certain antiarrhythmic agents, the effects on spontaneously occurring arrhythmias and those induced by programmed electrical stimulation may be concordant.[43] Although controlled studies remain to be done, the effects of the newer agents indicate that a well-executed medical regimen in patients with life-threatening ventricular arrhythmias may make an inroad into the figures of arrhythmic deaths.

Control of Torsades de Pointes

Torsades de pointes (Figure 21.5) occurs almost invariably in the context of abnormal but heterogeneously lengthened repolarization (QT_c or QU_c interval of the ECG) as might be produced by certain drugs in toxic doses (quinidine, procainamide, Norpace®, and Mellaril®),[48,49] extreme hypokalemia or hypomagnesemia,[48,49] liquid protein diets,[50] and certain hereditary long QT interval syndromes.[20] Thus, torsades is likely to be aggravated by interventions that further lengthen myocardial repolarization. It is therefore of interest that in the present case procainamide converted self-limiting episodes of torsades to sustained tachycardia, and Dilantin®, which shortens repolarization time, was effective in preventing recurrences. The importance of correctly identifying torsades lies in the fact that certain conventional antiarrhythmic drugs such as quinidine, procainamide, and disopyramide are ineffective in this situation and may even aggravate

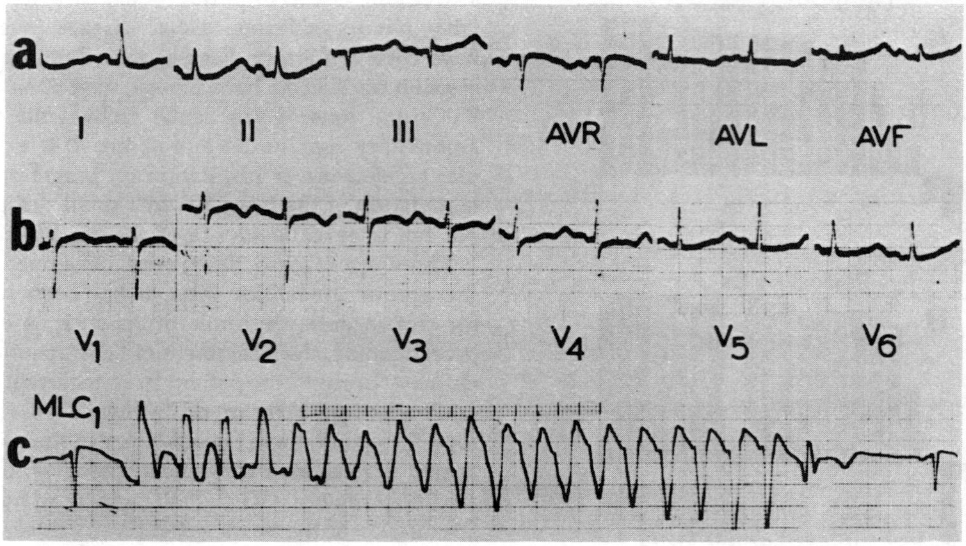

Figure 21.5. Electrocardiographic changes in a 62-year-old woman taking 800 mg daily of thioridazine (Mellaril) presenting with recurrent syncope. Note the marked prolongation of the QU interval (*A* and *B*) and the late cycle ventricular ectopic beat initiating the atypical ventricular tachycardia (torsades de pointes) with an unstable and changing mean QRS axis (*C*). Such an arrhythmia, thought to be due to reentry, characteristically occurs in the context of pathologically and heterogeneously lengthened myocardial repolarization.

it; interventions that shorten repolarization (Dilantin) or produce more synchronous ventricular activation by enhancing rate (pacemaking or isoproterenol) are likely to be more effective[48,49] either alone or in combination with drugs that shorten repolarization. However, these interventions are only used while the "offending" reversible abnormality is being corrected. In the hereditary long QT_c interval syndrome, phenytoin sodium, beta blockers, or left stellate ganglionectomy may all be effective in different patients.[51]

CONCLUSIONS

Major advances in antiarrhythmic therapy have occurred particularly in recent years, and further advances are expected in the future. New developments have followed closely in the wake of advances in clinical and experimental cardiac electrophysiology. The opportunity now exists to test the relevance of experimental data in the clinical laboratory regarding the nature of clinical arrhythmias and the mechanism of action of antiarrhythmic interventions. Drugs with diverse electrophysiologic properties are becoming available and much has been learned about their pharmacokinetic properties; they are beginning to offer realistic prospects for effective and safe prophylaxis and elective treatment of life-threatening as well as other troublesome tachyarrhythmias. Clinical electrophysiologic studies not only have provided a better understanding of arrhythmia mechanisms in man, but also have been valuable in the development of optimal drug regimens and in planning surgical and electrical techniques for controlling dysrhythmias and for placing implantable defibrillators and antitachycardia devices. It appears that therapy based on the precise identity of the arrhythmia, the context in which it occurs, and an understanding of the mechanism of the salutary effects of the proposed intervention can be attended by a high degree of success, even in the so-called refractory and troublesome disorders of cardiac rhythm.

Acknowledgment: This work was supported in part by grants from the Medical Research Service of the Veterans Administration and the American Heart Association, the Greater Los Angeles Affiliate.

REFERENCES

1. Singh BN: Rational basis of antiarrhythmic therapy: clinical pharmacology of commonly used antiarrhythmic drugs. *Angiology* 1978; 29:206–242.
2. Hauswirth O, Singh BN: Ionic mechanisms in heart muscle in relation to the genesis and the pharmacological control of cardiac arrhythmias. *Pharmacol Rev* 1978; 30:5–63.
3. Arnsdorf MF: Membrane factors in arrhythmogenesis: concepts and definitions. *Prog Cardiovasc Dis* 1977; 19:413–429.
4. Hoffman BF, Rosen MR: Cellular mechanisms for cardiac arrhythmias. *Circ Res* 1981; 49:1–15.
5. Singh BN, Collett JT, Chew CYC: New perspectives in the pharmacologic therapy of cardiac arrhythmias. *Prog Cardiovasc Dis* 1980; 22:243–301.
6. Vaughan Williams EM: *Antiarrhythmic Action and the Puzzle of Perhexiline.* London, Academic Press, 1980, pp 1–135.
7. Zipes DP, Troup PJ: New antiarrhythmic agents. Amiodarone, aprindine, disopyramide, ethmozin, mexiletine, tocainide, verapamil. *Am J Cardiol* 1978; 41:1005–1024.
8. Singh BN, Cho YW, Kuemmerle HP: Clinical pharmacology of antiarrhythmic drugs: a review and overview. Part I. *Int J Clin Pharmacol Ther Toxicol* 1981; 19:139–151.
9. Wellens HJJ: Value and limitations of programmed electrical stimulation of the heart in the study and treatment of tachycardias. *Circulation* 1978; 57:845–853.
10. Josephson ME, Seides SF: *Clinical Electrophysiology: Techniques and Interpretations.* Philadelphia, Lea & Febiger, 1979, pp 1–318.
11. Harrison DC, Meffin PJ, Winkle RA: Clinical pharmacokinetics of antiarrhythmic drugs. *Prog Cardiovasc Dis* 1977; 20:217–242.
12. Zipes DP: New approaches to antiarrhythmic therapy. *N Engl J Med* 1981; 304:475–476.

13. Waldo AL, Arciniegas JG, Klein H: Surgical treatment of life-threatening ventricular arrhythmias: the role of intraoperative mapping and consideration of the presently available surgical techniques. *Prog Cardiovasc Dis* 1981; 23:247–264.
14. Horowitz LN, Harken AH, Kastor JA, Josephson ME: Ventricular resection guided by epicardial and endocardial mapping for treatment of recurrent ventricular tachycardia. *N Engl J Med* 1980; 302:589–593.
15. Sealy WC, Gallagher JJ, Pritchett ELC: The surgical anatomy of Kent bundles based on electrophysiological mapping and surgical exploration. *J Thorac Cardiovasc Surg* 1978; 76:804–815.
16. Gallagher JJ, Pritchett ELC, Sealy WC, Kasell J, Wallace AG: The preexcitation syndromes. *Prog Cardiovasc Dis* 1978; 20:285–327.
17. Mason JW, Winkle RA: Accuracy of the ventricular tachycardia-induction study for predicting long-term efficacy and inefficacy of antiarrhythmic drugs. *N Engl J Med* 1980; 303:1073–1077.
18. Rosen MR, Reder RF: Does triggered activity have a role in the genesis of cardiac arrhythmias? *Ann Intern Med* 1981; 94:794–801.
19. Singh BN, Hauswirth O: Comparative mechanisms of action of antiarrhythmic drugs. *Am Heart J* 1974; 87:367–382.
20. Moss AJ, Schwartz PJ: Sudden death and the idiopathic long QT syndrome. *Am J Med* 1979; 66:6–7.
21. Kennedy HL, Underhill SJ: Frequent or complex ventricular ectopy in apparently healthy subjects. A clinical study of 25 cases. *Am J Cardiol* 1976; 38:141–148.
22. Bigger JT Jr: Antiarrhythmic treatment: an overview. *Am J Cardiol* 1984; 53:8B–16B.
23. Velebit V, Podrid P, Lown B, Cohen BH, Graboys TB: Aggravation and provocation of ventricular arrhythmias by antiarrhythmic drugs. *Circulation* 1982; 65:886–894.
24. Haft JI, Kosowsky BD, Lau SH, Stein E, Damato AN: Termination of atrial flutter by rapid atrial pacing of the atrium. *Am J Cardiol* 1967; 20:239–244.
25. Fisher JD, Mehra R, Furman S: Termination of ventricular tachycardia with bursts of rapid ventricular pacing. *Am J Cardiol* 1978; 41:94–102.
26. Cooper TB, MacLean WA, Waldo AL: Overdrive pacing for supraventricular tachycardia: a review of theoretical implications and therapeutic techniques. *PACE* 1978; 1:196–221.
27. Griffin JC, Mason JW, Calfee RV: Clinical use of an implantable automatic tachycardia-terminating pacemaker. *Am Heart J* 1980; 100:1093–1096.
28. Mirowski M, Reid PR, Mower MM, Watkins L, Gott VL, Schauble JF, Langer A, Heilman MS, Kolenik SA, Fischell RE, Weisfeldt ML: Termination of malignant ventricular arrhythmias with an implanted automatic defibrillator in human beings. *N Engl J Med* 1980; 303:322–324.
29. Estes EH, Izlar HL Jr: Recurrent ventricular tachycardia. A case successfully treated by bilateral cardiac sympathectomy. *Am J Med* 1961; 31:491–497.
30. Schwartz PJ, Periti M, Malliani A: The long QT syndrome. *Am Heart J* 1975; 89:378–390.
31. Wittig JH, Boineau JP: Surgical treatment of ventricular arrhythmias using epicardial, transmural, and endocardial mapping. *Ann Thorac Surg* 1975; 20:117–126.
32. Guiraudon G, Fontaine G, Frank R, Escande G, Etievent P, Cabrol C: Encircling endocardial ventriculotomy: a new surgical treatment for life-threatening ventricular tachycardias resistant to medical treatment following myocardial infarction. *Ann Thorac Surg* 1978; 26:438–444.
33. Barrett PA, Peter CT, Swan HJC, Singh BN, Mandel WJ: The frequency and prognostic significance of electrocardiographic abnormalities in clinically normal individuals. *Prog Cardiovasc Dis* 1981; 23:299–319.
34. Singh BN, Jewitt DE: Beta-adrenergic receptor blocking drugs in cardiac arrhythmias. *Drugs* 1974; 7:426–461.
35. Singh BN, Vaughan Williams EM: A fourth class of antidysrhythmic action? Effect of verapamil on ouabain toxicity, on atrial and ventricular intracellular potentials, and on other features of cardiac function. *Cardiovasc Res* 1972; 6:109–119.
36. Singh BN, Ellrodt G, Peter CT: Verapamil: a review of its pharmacological properties and therapeutic use. *Drugs* 1978; 15:169–197.
37. Nademanee K, Singh BN, Hendrickson J, Intarachot V, Lopez B, Feld G, Cannom DS, Weiss JL: Amiodarone in refractory life-threatening ventricular arrhythmias. *Ann Intern Med* 1983; 98:577–584.
38. Singh BN, Vaughan Williams EM: The effect of amiodarone, a new antianginal drug, on cardiac muscle. *Br J Pharmacol* 1970; 39:657–667.
39. Nademanee K, Hendrickson JA, Cannom DS, Goldreyer BN, Singh BN: Control of refractory life-threatening ventricular arrhythmias by amiodarone. *Am Heart J* 1981; 101:759–768.
40. Heger JJ, Prystowsky EN, Jackman WM, Naccarelli GV, Warfel KA, Rinkenberger RL, Zipes DP: Amiodarone. Clinical efficacy and electrophysiology during long-term therapy for recurrent ventricular tachycardia or ventricular fibrillation. *N Engl J Med* 1981; 305:539–545.
41. Bigger JT: Symposium on flecainide acetate. *Am J Cardiol* 1984; 53:1B–122B.
42. Harrison DC, Winkle R, Sami M, Mason J: Encainide: a new and potent antiarrhythmic agent. *Am Heart J* 1980; 100:1046–1054.
43. Nademanee K, Feld G, Hendrickson JA, Singh PN, Singh BN: Electrophysiologic and antiarrhythmic effects of sotalol in patients with life-threatening ventricular tachyarrhythmias. *Circulation* 1985; 72:555–564.
44. Zipes DP: Recent advances in antiarrhythmic therapy: symposium on propafenone. *Am J Cardiol* 1984; 54:1D–73D.
44a. Roth A, Harrison E, Mitani G, Freidenberger L, Rahimtoola SH, Elkayam U: Diltiazem vs digoxin for heart rate control in patients with chronic atrial fibrillation. *J Am Coll Cardiol* 1986; 7:69A.
45. Graboys TB, Lown B, Podrid PJ, DeSilva R: Long-term survival of patients with malignant ventricular arrhythmia treated with antiarrhythmic drugs. *Am J Cardiol* 1982; 50:437–443.
46. Ruskin JN, DiMarco JP, Garan H: Out-of-hospital cardiac arrest: electrophysiologic observations and selection of long-term antiarrhythmic therapy. *N Engl J Med* 1980; 303:607–613.
47. Myerburg RJ, Conde C, Sheps DS, Appel RA, Kiem I, Sung RJ, Castellanos A: Antiarrhythmic drug therapy in survivors of prehospital cardiac arrest: comparison of effects on chronic ventricular arrhythmias and recurrent cardiac arrest. *Circulation* 1979; 59:855–863.
48. Krikler DM, Curry PVL: Torsade de pointes, an atypical ventricular tachycardia. *Br Heart J* 1976; 38:117–120.
49. Smith WM, Gallagher JJ: "Les torsades de pointes": an unusual ventricular arrhythmia. *Ann Intern Med* 1980; 93:578–584.
50. Singh BN, Gaarder TD, Kanegee T, Goldstein M, Montgomerie JZ, Mills H: Liquid protein diets and torsades de pointes. *JAMA* 1978; 240:115–119.
51. Schwartz PJ: Idiopathic long QT syndrome: progress and questions. *Am Heart J* 1985; 109:399–415.

22 Surgical Treatment of Cardiac Arrhythmias

W. Clark Hargrove III, MD and Alden H. Harken, MD

Although most tachyarrhythmias are successfully controlled by drugs, there are a number of patients in whom all conventional and experimental medications fail. Advances in electrophysiology and surgery have led to the development of a specialized area of cardiac surgery which is applicable for arrhythmia control in an increasing number of patients.

Mines[1] in 1913 unwittingly predicted that one day arrhythmias might be induced and treated surgically. In describing his reciprocating rhythm in the ring preparations from auricles of large rays, he noted that "but by the application of several stimuli in succession, it is sometimes possible to start a wave in one direction while the tissue on the other side of the point stimulated is still refractory.... The wave circulates and may continue to do so for 50 revolutions or more." In the same paper he also stated that "the best test for circulating excitation is to cut through the ring at one point. The vigorous circulating wave and its instantaneous arrest by the section of the ring is a sight not easily forgotten." In 1930 Wolff, Parkinson, and White[2] described a syndrome in young persons manifested by bundle branch block, short PR intervals, and paroxysmal tachycardia. In 1933 Wolferth and Wood[3] postulated reentry as the mechanism for the tachycardia. The circuit used an accessory bundle of atrioventricular (AV) conduction (bundle of Kent) as the retrograde pathway and the AV node–His bundle as the antegrade pathway (Figure 22.1). They also postulated the reason for the short PR interval and delta wave (preexcitation) (Figure 22.1). Electrophysiologic studies later confirmed this, and in 1968 Sealy[4] divided an accessory bundle in a patient with the Wolff-Parkinson-White syndrome and incessant circus movement tachycardia, resulting in cure of the tachycardia. Thus, the field of electrophysiologic surgery began. Advances in His bundle recording and later programmed stimulation brought us into the current age of electrophysiologic surgery.

It is, therefore, inducibility and sustaining of arrhythmias by the reentrant mechanism that allows a diagnostic map and surgical correction of certain tachycardias. Although automatic arrhythmias occasionally may be treated surgically, the chances of success are much smaller because of the inconsistent inducibility in the electrophysiologic laboratory and the operating room. In this chapter, we will deal only with those reentrant arrhythmias that can be induced by programmed stimulation.

SURGERY FOR SUPRAVENTRICULAR ARRHYTHMIAS

The most common indication for the surgical management of supraventricular tachyarrhythmias is the treatment of the Wolff–Parkinson–White (WPW) syndrome. There is now a standard approach to the management of these arrhythmias which involves division of the accessory bundle of Kent. Symptomatic paroxysmal supraventricular tachycardia is what brings most patients with this syndrome to medical attention. In 95% of cases this supraventricular tachycardia uses the normal atrioventricular conduction system as the antegrade pathway and the bypass tract as the retrograde pathway, so-called orthodromic tachycardia. In 5% of cases the bypass tract is the antegrade pathway (antidromic tachycardia). About 20% of patients will present with atrial fibrillation and rapid ventricular response. These patients are subject to ventricular fibrillation. The operative indication in most cases is failure to control the supraventricular tachycardia with medication. Patients with atrial fibrillation and rapid ventricular response are more urgent operative candidates because of the possibility of sudden death. Preoperative electrophysiologic testing is necessary to (1) localize and characterize the accessory pathway, (2) demonstrate other accessory pathways, (3) rule out some other mechanism for supraventricular tachycardia and symptoms (eg, AV nodal reentry).[5] Preoperative mapping can localize the bypass tract in 90% to 95% of cases. Never-

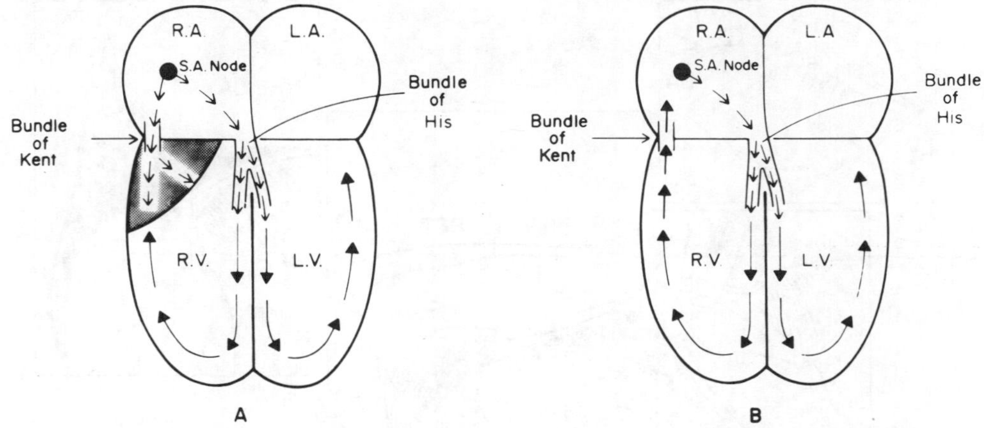

Figure 22.1. *A,* Wolferth and Wood's now proven hypothesis for preexcitation. The atrial impulse traveling over the bundle of Kent results in depolarization of an area of ventricular myocardium earlier than would occur through the His-Purkinje system. This results in a short PR interval and delta wave. The majority of the ventricle is depolarized normally. *B,* Wolferth and Wood's hypothesis (also now proven) for the mechanism of reentrant supraventricular tachycardia using the His-Purkinje system as the antegrade pathway and the bypass tract as the retrograde pathway (orthodromic supraventricular tachycardia). (From Wolferth and Wood,[2] with permission of CV Mosby Co.)

theless, we consider intraoperative mapping essential to define the exact anatomic location of the bundle of Kent and additionally to determine whether more than one bypass tract is present. Multiple bypass tracts occur in about 15% to 20% of patients. To the surgeon, the classic division of the Wolff-Parkinson-White syndrome into two types, A and B, is useless. From an operative standpoint they can be divided into left free wall, right free wall, and septal tracts. The left free wall tracts are approached through the left atrium. Division of the tract is accomplished by dissecting the epicardial space from the left fibrous trigone to the posterior superior process of the left ventricle. The epicardial attachment is left intact (Figure 22.2).[6] The septal and right free wall tracts are approached through the right atrium. The bundle of His should be identified in all cases to avoid damaging the normal conduction system. Injury to the normal conduction system is most likely to occur in the posterior septal dissection. The posterior septal space is anatomically complex. However, the anatomy has been well defined by Sealy and Gallagher.[7] Again the dissection is carried to the epicardial reflection to divide the ventricular attachment of the bypass tract. In a recent personal series reported by Cox et al[8] of 149 bypass tracts in 118 patients there was 100% division of bypass tracts. In this series of bypass tracts there were 86 left free wall (58%), 36 posterior septal (24%), 19 right free wall (13%), and 8 anterior septal (5%). The incidence of heart block was 2.5% and mortality rate was 5%. All deaths were in patients with other heart disease present. Technical points emphasized by Cox are (1) exclusive use of the endocardial approach, (2) optical magnification, (3) wider margin of the surgical dissection with identification of spatial boundaries, (4) sharp dissection with division of only the ventricular insertion of the accessory pathway, and (5) internal identification of the epicardial reflection. Recently Guiraudon et al[9] described a method whereby left free wall tracts are dissected epicardially and endocardial resection is unnecessary. This method is attractive because cardioplegic arrest is not necessary and AV conduction is continuously monitored. This method has also been applied in the division of posterior septal pathways (G. M. Guiraudon, personal communication, 1985). Recently a cryosurgical technique was used by Russian surgeons for ablation of both the left and right parietal and septal accessory atrioventricular connections without the use of extracorporeal circulation and cardiotomy.[10,11] Long-term follow-up is needed before either of these techniques can be confirmed. The endocardial-to-epicardial resection as defined by Sealy and Cox would have to be called the gold standard to which all other operations must be matched.

The surgical treatment of other types of supraventricular tachycardia has also evolved in recent years. A number of these patients have so-called "concealed" accessory pathways. They have a variant of the WPW syndrome with no preexcitation because conduction occurs only in a retrograde fashion over the bypass tract. The substrate for reentry is present, but the bypass tract is "concealed" because there is no preexcitation. Medical refractoriness is the indication for operation in this group, because with no antegrade conduction there is no risk of rapid ventricular response even if atrial fibrillation occurs. Electrophysiologic study and preoperative mapping confirm the presence of the bypass tract.

Intraoperative localization of the concealed pathway is achieved by ventricular pacing and induction of supraventricular tachycardia. The surgical approach is the same as that in all patients with the WPW syndrome.

Ablation of the His bundle is an alternative in all patients with the WPW syndrome. Originally this was accomplished by surgery and more recently by catheter techniques.[12,13] The reentry substrate is eliminated and therefore supraventricular tachycardia is no longer a prob-

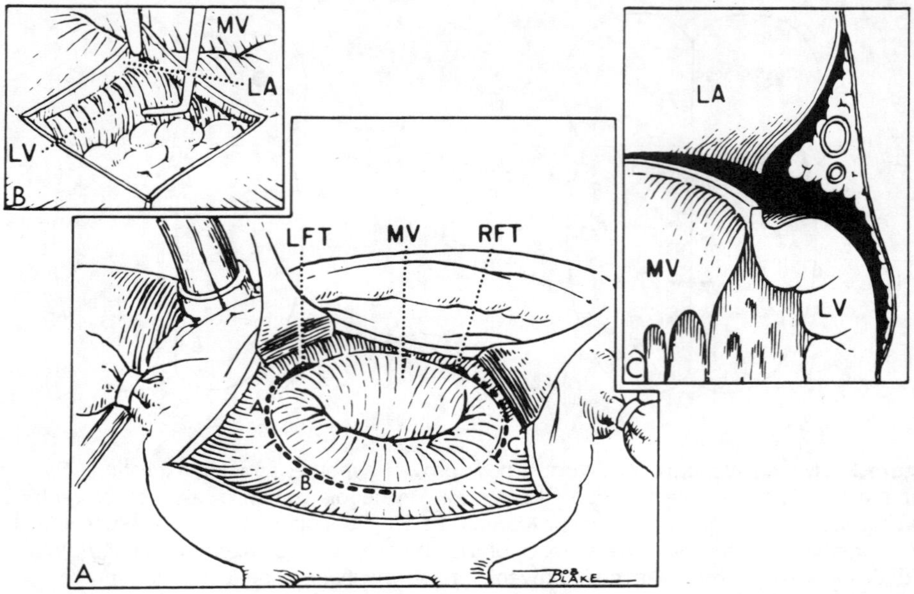

Figure 22.2. Transatrial approach for surgical division of left free wall bypass tracts. In *A*, the left atrium is opened and the mitral valve (MV) and other anatomic landmarks are identified. The incision required for a pathway next to the left fibrous trigone (LFT) is shown by dashed line A. Dashed line B would be used for the usual free wall pathway, whereas dashed line C would be for a second stage in a posterior septal pathway beginning at the right fibrous trigone (RFT). In *B*, dissection is carried out by cleaning the epicardial fat off the left ventricular (LV) and left atrial (LA) myocardium, thus interrupting any bypass tracts. The epicardial reflection is left intact, as illustrated in *C*. (From Sealy WC, Gallagher JJ, Pritchett ELC: The surgical anatomy of Kent bundles based on electrophysiological mapping and surgical exploration. *J Thorac Cardiovasc Surg* 1978; 76:804–815 by permission of the CV Mosby Co.)

lem, but a permanent pacemaker is then necessary. If, however, the patient has a short effective refractory period of the bypass tract, then the risk of rapid ventricular response to atrial fibrillation is still present. Therefore, only in surgical failures would we recommend His bundle division as an alternative method of treatment of the WPW syndrome.

A few patients with AV nodal reentry tachycardia have been treated surgically when uncontrolled by medical management. The substrate for reentry is dual AV nodal pathways. Application of the cryoprobe in the area of the AV node alters the node in some way and the reentry substrate is upset.[14] This procedure currently is experimental. Catheter His bundle ablation and insertion of a backup pacemaker is an alternative.

Left atrial isolation in the management of atrial flutter and fibrillation has been reported.[15] The flutter or fibrillation must be demonstrated to arise from the left atrium. Left atrial isolation might also be applicable in patients with atrial fibrillation or flutter arising from a hypertrophied left atrium in mitral stenosis. Further work is necessary to determine the long-term benefit of this procedure versus His bundle ablation and pacemaker insertion when rapid ventricular response to atrial fibrillation is the primary problem.

Ectopic (automatic) atrial tachycardias can occasionally be treated by excision of the automatic focus when it is possible to initiate the tachycardia and map in the operating room.[16] Because this frequently is not possible, left atrial disarticulation is also a therapeutic option in this difficult-to-manage group of patients.

In summary, when reentrant mechanisms can be demonstrated to initiate supraventricular tachycardias, particularly in the WPW syndrome, well-defined surgical options are present. Rather than subjecting a young person to a lifetime of medication, we consider surgery to be a conservative alternative.

SURGERY FOR VENTRICULAR ARRHYTHMIAS

Malignant ventricular arrhythmias from ischemic heart disease take two basic forms. A group of patients with ventricular tachycardia and ventricular fibrillation in the presence of acute ischemia or exercise represents the minority of patients. They can be treated by coronary bypass grafting alone with acceptable results.[17] Much more commonly malignant arrhythmias arise in patients after infarction. This may occur in the setting of acute infarct but more commonly some time later. Most of these patients have had a large myocardial infarction with aneurysm formation and have a depressed ejection fraction. Indirect operations such as coronary bypass or coronary bypass plus aneurysmectomy resulted in a relatively high operative mortality rate and low overall cure rates (Table 22.1). The definition of operable patients has evolved with the development of programmed electrical stimulation.

Current criteria for operability in patients with is-

Table 22.1. Results of Indirect Surgical Procedures in the Treatment of Refractory Ischemic Ventricular Tachycardia*

Procedure	Patients (*n*)	Operative Mortality (%)	Intractable Arrhythmia Recurrence (%)	Overall Success (%)
Sympathectomy	12	25	17	58
Coronary arterial bypass	45	22	22	56
Aneurysmectomy or infarct-ectomy	95	24	17	59
Aortocoronary bypass plus aneurysmectomy	27	41	4	55
Total	179	26	16	58

* From Boineau and Cox,[18] with permission.

chemia-related malignant ventricular arrhythmias include the presence of an inducible, sustained (greater than 30 seconds) tachycardia of uniform morphology which is refractory to medical therapy. Most patients have had failure of all conventional antiarrhythmic agents and several experimental drugs. Although the exact reentry substrate is difficult to define, it is probably based on microreentry at the borders of the old infarction at the aneurysm site.[18] This led Guiraudon et al[19] in 1978 to develop an arrhythmia isolation operation called encircling endocardial ventriculotomy. In this operation the arrhythmogenic area is isolated from the rest of the ventricle by a nontransmural endocardial-to-epicardial incision, sparing only the epicardium. Although this results in control of the arrhythmia, ventriculotomy depressed left ventricular function in a group of patients who already had severely compromised hemodynamics.[20] Therefore, the procedure as originally described has largely been abandoned. More recently, Guiraudon (personal communication, 1985) has performed a similar procedure using cryoablation, but results are preliminary. In 1980 Harken et al[21] described map-guided subendocardial resection in this group of patients with remarkable success. Preoperative and intraoperative electrophysiologic studies led to the definition of the site of origin of a tachycardia (the area having the earliest presystolic electrogram in the latter half of diastole). Alteration of this area has resulted in obliteration of the tachycardia. They were able to achieve an operative mortality of approximately 10% and cure rates from the arrhythmia of about 85%. Moran et al[22] then performed what they called extended endocardial resection whereby little mapping was done, but all scar within the left ventricle was removed. This included papillary muscles when necessary, and therefore mitral valve replacement was sometimes part of the procedure. Moran's operative mortality rate was 10% and cure rates from tachycardia 85% to 90%. Currently, 160 patients (148 with ischemic heart disease) have undergone operative management of ventricular tachycardia at the Hospital of the University of Pennsylvania, using map-guided subendocardial resection with occasional adjunctive cryoablation. The overall mortality was 10%. All operative survivors undergo postoperative programmed stimulation, 66% of whom have had no inducible ventricular tachycardia. An additional 26% have no ventricular tachycardia on previously ineffective antiarrhythmic drugs, yielding a 92% overall success rate in operative survivors. Results have been similar in patients both early and late after myocardial infarction.[23] Debate currently centers around proper management of patients with inferior wall infarctions and ventricular tachycardia. This subgroup has a lower surgical cure rate. Moran et al[24] continue to advocate papillary muscle excision and mitral valve replacement in this group. We and others[25] believe that endocardial resection and the use of the cryoprobe around the papillary muscles is the proper choice. Further studies will be necessary before the proper method of management is known.

Surgery for malignant ventricular arrhythmia continues to be an investigative process. Aneurysmectomy with some type of wide subendocardial resection would probably provide adequate surgical results in most cases. However, we believe that continued mapping and intraoperative investigation are the best setting for studying the mechanisms of sudden death. Although worldwide over 1,000 patients have benefited from these procedures, continued definition of the reentry substrate in mapping studies might have an impact on the larger public health problem of sudden death from which 200,000 to 300,000 Americans die every year.

Another group of patients without ischemic heart disease but with malignant ventricular arrhythmias arising from the right ventricle has been successfully managed with surgical intervention. These patients have so-called arrhythmogenic right ventricular dysplasia. Excision of the arrhythmogenic focus or right ventricular disarticulation, or both, has resulted in control of the arrhythmia.[26] In patients with tetralogy of Fallot and right ventricular outflow patches, ventricular arrhythmias arising from this area have also been treated by excision or cryoablation.[27]

Other ventricular arrhythmias such as polymorphic ventricular tachycardia and ventricular fibrillation cannot be treated by surgery alone. Implantation of the automatic internal defibrillator has application in some of these patients, either alone[28] or as a supplement to endocardial resection.[29] In addition, other forms of pacing and pacing cardioversion may be applicable in the future.

In summary, a number of surgical options are available in patients with ischemic ventricular arrhythmia and inducible uniform ventricular tachycardia. These operations can control these arrhythmias with acceptable operative mortality and morbidity rates.

REFERENCES

1. Mines GR: On dynamic equilibrium in the heart. *Proc Physiol Soc London* 1913; 46:349–383.
2. Wolff L, Parkinson J, White PD: Bundle-branch block with short P-R interval in healthy young people prone to paroxysmal tachycardia. *Am Heart J* 1930; 5:685–704.
3. Wolferth CC, Wood FC: The mechanism of production of short P-R intervals and prolonged QRS complexes in patients with presumably undamaged hearts: hypothesis of an accessory pathway of auriculo-ventricular conduction (bundle of Kent). *Am Heart J* 1933; 8:297–311.
4. Sealy WC, Hattler BG, Blumenschein SD, Cobb FR: Surgical treatment of Wolff–Parkinson–White syndrome. *Ann Thorac Surg* 1969; 8:1–11.
5. Gallagher JJ, Pritchett ELC, Sealy WC, Kasell J, Wallace AG: The preexcitation syndromes. *Prog Cardiovasc Dis* 1978; 20:285–327.
6. Sealy WC, Gallagher JJ: Surgical treatment of left free wall accessory pathways of atrioventricular conduction of the Kent type. *J Thorac Cardiovasc Surg* 1981; 81:698–706.
7. Sealy WC, Gallagher JJ: The surgical approach to the septal area of the heart based on experiences with 45 patients with Kent bundles. *J Thorac Cardiovasc Surg* 1980; 79:542–551.
8. Cox JL, Gallagher JJ, Cain ME: Experience with 118 consecutive patients undergoing operation for the Wolff–Parkinson–White syndrome. *J Thorac Cardiovasc Surg* 1985; 90:490–501.
9. Guiraudon GM, Klein GT, Gulamhusein S, Jones DL, Yee R, Perkins DG, Jarvis E: Surgical repair of Wolff–Parkinson–White syndrome: a new closed heart technique. *Ann Thorac Surg* 1984; 37:67–71.
10. Bredikis J, Bredikis A: Cryosurgical ablation of left parietal wall accessory atrioventricular connections through the coronary sinus without the use of extracorporeal circulation. *J Thorac Cardiovasc Surg* 1985; 90:199–205.
11. Bredikis J, Bukauskas F, Zebrauskas R, Sakalauskas J, Loschilov V, Nevsky V, Bredikis A, Liakas R: Cryosurgical ablation of right parietal and septal accessory atrioventricular connections without the use of extracorporeal circulation. A new surgical technique. *J Thorac Cardiovasc Surg* 1985; 90:206–211.
12. Sealy WC, Gallagher JJ, Kasell J: His bundle interruption for control of inappropriate ventricular responses to atrial arrhythmias. *Ann Thorac Surg* 1981; 32:429–438.
13. Gallagher JJ, Svenson RH, Kasell JH, German LD, Bardy GH, Broughton A, Critelli G: Catheter technique for closed chest ablation of the atrioventricular conduction system. *N Engl J Med* 1982; 306:194–200.
14. Holman WL, Ikeshita M, Lease JG, Smith PK, Ferguson TB, Cox JL: Elective prolongation of atrioventricular conduction by multiple discrete cryolesions: a new technique for the treatment of paroxysmal supraventricular tachycardia. *J Thorac Cardiovasc Surg* 1982; 84:554–559.
15. Williams JM, Ungerleider RM, Lofland GK, Cox JL: Left atrial isolation. New technique for the treatment of supraventricular arrhythmias. *J Thorac Cardiovasc Surg* 1980; 80:373–380.
16. Gillette PC, Garson A, Hesslein PS, Karpawich PP, Tierney RC, Cooley DA, McNamara DG: Successful surgical treatment of atrial, junctional and ventricular tachycardia unassociated with accessory connections in infants and children. *Am Heart J* 1981; 102:984–991.
17. Bryson AL, Parisi AF, Schechter E, Wolfson S: Life-threatening ventricular arrhythmias induced by exercise: cessation after coronary bypass surgery. *Am J Cardiol* 1973; 32:995–999.
18. Boineau JP, Cox JL: Rationale for a direct surgical approach to control ventricular arrhythmias. Relation of specific intraoperative techniques to mechanism and location of arrhythmic circuit. *Am J Cardiol* 1982; 49:381–396.
19. Guiraudon G, Fontaine G, Frank R, Eschande G, Etievent P, Cabrol C: Encircling endocardial ventriculotomy: a new surgical treatment for life-threatening ventricular tachycardias resistant to medical treatment following myocardial infarction. *Ann Thorac Surg* 1978; 26:438–444.
20. Ungerleider RM, Holman WL, Calcagno D, Williams JM, Lofland GK, Smith PK, Stanley TE III, Quick G, Cox JL: Encircling endocardial ventriculotomy for ischemic ventricular tachycardia. III. Effects on regional left ventricular function. *J Thorac Cardiovasc Surg* 1982; 83:857–864.
21. Harken AH, Horowitz LN, Josephson ME: Comparison of standard aneurysmectomy and aneurysmectomy with directed endocardial resection for the treatment of recurrent sustained ventricular tachycardia. *J Thorac Cardiovasc Surg* 1980; 80:527–534.
22. Moran JM, Kehoe RF, Loeb JM, Lichtenthal PR, Sanders JH, Michaelis LL: Extended endocardial resection for the treatment of ventricular tachycardia and ventricular fibrillation. *Ann Thorac Surg* 1982; 34:538–552.
23. Miller JM, Marchlinski FE, Harken AH, Hargrove WC, Josephson ME: Subendocardial resection for sustained ventricular tachycardia in the early period after acute myocardial infarction. *Am J Cardiol* 1985; 55:980–984.
24. Moran JM, Kehoe RF, Loeb JM, Frederickson JW, Zheutlin TA, Sanders JH, Michaelis LL: The role of papillary muscle resection and mitral valve replacement in the control of refractory ventricular arrhythmia. *Circulation* 1983; 68 (suppl II):II-154–II-160.
25. Ivey TD, Brady GH, Misbach GA, Greene HL: Surgical management of refractory ventricular arrhythmias in patients with prior inferior myocardial infarction. *J Thorac Cardiovasc Surg* 1985; 89:369–377.
26. Fontaine G, Guiraudon G, Frank R, Fillette F, Cabrol C, Grosgogeat Y: Surgical management of ventricular tachycardia unrelated to myocardial ischemia or infarction. *Am J Cardiol* 1982; 49:397–410.
27. Horowitz LN, Vetter VL, Harken AH, Josephson ME: Electrophysiologic characteristics of sustained ventricular tachycardia occurring after repair of tetralogy of Fallot. *Am J Cardiol* 1980; 46:446–452.
28. Mirowski M, Reid PR, Winkle RA, Mower, MM, Watkins L Jr, Stinson EB, Griffith LSC, Kallman CH, Weisfeldt ML: Mortality in patients with implanted automatic defibrillators. *Ann Intern Med* 1983; 98:585–588.
29. Platia EV, Griffith LSC, Watkins L Jr, Mower MM, Guarnieri T, Mirowski M, Reid PR: Treatment of malignant ventricular arrhythmias with endocardial resection and implantation of the automatic cardioverter-defibrillator. *N Engl J Med* 1986; 314:213–216.

23 Cardiac Pacing

J. Warren Harthorne, MD

HISTORICAL BACKGROUND

Man's awareness of the primacy of the heart in the maintenance of life no doubt dates back to the prehistoric times of the early cavemen. An early depiction of an animal heart, which dates from 50,000 years before Christ, can be found in a cave dweller's drawing in Altamira, Spain (Figure 23.1). Although such anatomic wisdom likely arose from trial and error methods of bringing down an edible member of the animal kingdom with bow and arrow, it focused attention on the role of the heart in sustaining life. Our medical counterparts in earlier days observed the variation of the peripheral pulse that attended altered states of health. Wang Chu Ho devoted ten volumes to the study of the pulse in the year 280 BC.[1] Early medieval woodcuts depict methods of pulse palpation. Nonetheless, it was not until Harvey[2] in 1628 published his elaborate anatomic studies (De Motu Cordis) that the interrelation between the central and peripheral circulatory system was fully understood. Interest in reanimation of the dead became a subject of intense study during the 17th and 18th centuries. The writings of Aldini,[3] Bichat,[4] and Schechter[5] depict the intense interest in the origins of life itself and the extreme studies conducted in an effort to restore it among decapitated victims of the French revolution. Concurrent dissection of the heart and its conduction system led to a clearer understanding of the contractile process. Although numerous investigators contributed to this study of cardiac anatomy, the names of Tawara,[6] His,[7] Wenckebach,[8] Keith and Flack,[9] Purkinje,[10] Kent,[11] and Aschoff[12] are those that remain familiar to most physicians today.

Investigations into electricity and magnetism and their origins in all likelihood also date back to prerecorded time. One can imagine the wonderment caused by lightning bolts from the heavens causing fires. Reference to the use of various electric fishes in the treatment of a host of physical and mental disorders predates the Christian era.[13] The development of the compound electric cell by Allessandro Volta in 1799 offered portability to experiments in electrotherapy. Early proponents and practitioners of electrical treatment of multiple disorders included the American statesman, Benjamin Franklin, the French physician, Charcot, and the founder of the Methodist religion, John Wesley.[14] Although amusing and often dangerous misuses of these treatment modalities were practiced, intriguing reports became available in the latter part of the 19th century in the work of Von Ziemssen[15] regarding the direct stimulation of the heart of Catherine Serafin.

Recognition of the relation between a slow pulse and attacks of loss of consciousness dates from the early to mid-part of the 18th century in the Western literature. The clear accounts of Stokes[16] and Adams[17] in the 1800s led to the designation of these attacks as Stokes-Adams attacks, although it must be noted that the reports of Spens, Holberton, Morgagni, and others preceded them. Purposeful stimulation of the heart in such circumstances was not clinically practiced until 1929[18] when an Australian physician and engineer developed and used a stimulator in a young child. The subsequent experience of Hyman[19] and the designation of his device as an "artificial cardiac pacemaker" have gained wider recognition. However, public opinion was as yet not ready to accept such techniques, and even when Zoll[20] reported on the use of transthoracic pacing in 1952, there were those who deemed this as being "against God's will." The ease and

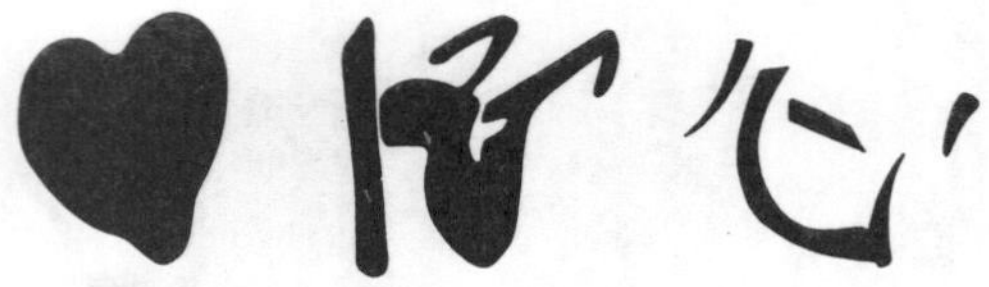

Figure 23.1. Early representations of the heart. Upper Paleolithic painting circa 50,000 BC from the Cave of Pindal, Altamira, Spain (*left*). Egyptian hieroglyph circa 1750 BC (*middle*). Ancient Chinese ideogram (*right*). (From Schechter et al,[1] with permission.)

simplicity of implanting the pacemaker device of today obscure the somewhat long and torturous path that preceded their widespread availability.

MODES OF CARDIAC STIMULATION

In the era before cardiac pacing, most patients with symptomatic heart block died of the repetitive epileptiform seizures that accompanied their erratic rhythms. Approximately 40% of such patients died during the first year and 80% within 4 years of the onset of symptoms despite medical treatment. The earliest cardiac pacemakers were designed to stimulate the ventricles only and provided effective seizure relief. The relative bulk of these early systems and unsophisticated electronic circuitry did not encourage enthusiasm for dual chamber devices. Nonetheless, an atrial triggered ventricular pacing device was described as early as 1958 by Folkman and Watkins[21] and the Cordis Corporation introduced an implantable version in 1963.[22] As newer options of programmability, telemetry, dual chamber pacing and sensing, and tachyarrhythmia functions came along, it became apparent that a code that designates individual pacemaker performance was needed. Such a code has evolved over the past 10 years, and although imperfect, it is in widespread use throughout the world. The reader is encouraged to become familiar with this code as it will be used throughout this chapter. The code, which originally consisted of three positions, was extended in 1982 to five positions to accommodate the designation of programmability, telemetry, and tachycardia functions.[23]

Five position code:

1	2	3	4	5

Position 1 designates the chamber of the heart that is paced: A = atrium, V = ventricle, and D = dual (atrium and ventricle). *Position 2* designates the chamber of the heart that is electronically sensed by the sensing amplifier of the pacemaker circuit: A = atrium, V = ventricle, D = dual (atrium and ventricle), and O = no chamber is sensed as in a fixed rate or asynchronous device. *Position 3* designates the type of pacing function that a sensed event initiates: I = inhibition of output, T = triggering of output as when a sensed atrial event triggers a pacemaker output to the ventricle, D = dual types of sensing function with inhibition or triggering, or both, as the clinical circumstances warrant, O = no sensing function as in an asynchronous pacemaker, and R = reverse pacing as in some antitachycardia devices that inhibit during physiologic rates but stimulate asynchronously during tachycardia. *Position 4* designates the extent of programmability or telemetry options, or both, available in the pacemaker: O = nonprogrammable, P = simple programmable (two options of rate and output), M = multiprogrammable, and C = communicating as in a device that has telemetry to transmit certain stored information. All such systems are multiprogrammable. *Position 5* designates certain antitachycardia functions. Although not yet widely available, a number of such systems are entering clinical practice. The code, at present, is incomplete for all possible options: B = burst pacing, S = scanning pacing, and E = externally activated (by the patient or physician).

Most publications do not include the fourth and fifth positions, as the major functions of most pacemaker devices can be described by the first three positions of the code. When the fourth and fifth positions are used, it is customary to separate them from the first three positions by a comma.

Examples: VOO,OO: This would describe a pacemaker that stimulates the ventricle (V in position 1), does not sense any chamber (O in position 2), has no sensing function (O in position 3), is nonprogrammable (O in position 4), and has no antitachycardia function (O in position 5).

VVI,MO: This describes a pacemaker that stimulates the ventricle (V in position 1), senses the ventricle (V in position 2), inhibits in response to a sensed ventricular event (I in position 3), is multiprogrammable (M in position 4), but has no antitachycardia function (O in position 5).

DDD,CB: This describes a dual chamber pacemaker that is capable of stimulating both chambers of the heart (D in position 1), senses both chambers of the heart (D in position 2), has two types of sensing function (D in position 3), offers telemetry (ie, communication) and multiprogrammability (C in position 4), and provides burst antitachycardia function (B in position 5).

For reasons of brevity, only the first three positions of the pacemaker code are commonly used. A list of representative types of pacing systems follows.

Pacer Code	Conventional Name
Single chamber devices:	
VOO	Fixed rate, asynchronous, ventricular pacemaker
VVI	Noncompetitive, demand ventricular pacemaker
VVT	Noncompetitive, ventricular triggered or ventricular synchronous pacemaker (seldom used except for antitachycardia purposes)
AOO	Fixed rate, asynchronous atrial pacemaker
AAI	Noncompetitive, atrial demand pacemaker
AAT	Noncompetitive, atrial synchronous or atrial triggered pacemaker (seldom used except for antitachycardia purposes)

(List continues next page)

Dual chamber devices:

VAT	Atrial triggered or P-wave triggered ventricular pacemaker
VDD	Atrial triggered, ventricular inhibited pacemaker (Detection of a P wave through the atrial lead triggers a ventricular paced event, whereas detection of a spontaneous ventricular event inhibits the output of the ventricular channel. This device differs from the DDD system in that it does not offer stimulation of the atrium in the presence of slow rates.)
DVI	Atrioventricular sequential pacemaker (This device offers stimulation of both chambers of the heart but only senses in the ventricle. In the presence of a sensed ventricular event, it will inhibit either the atrial or the ventricular output depending upon timing.)
DDD	Fully automatic, atrioventricular universal dual chamber pacemaker (This device offers pacing in both chambers of the heart, provides electronic sensing of both chambers of the heart, and has two types of sensing function. A sensed atrial event will inhibit the output of the atrial circuit and trigger the output of the ventricular circuit. The latter circuit inhibits its output in response to sensing of a ventricular event.)

PROGRAMMABILITY

A further feature of most of today's pacemaker devices is the concept of programmability. This feature allows the user to select those electronic features that the manufacturer has designed into the pacemaker device which best suit the need of the individual patient and to "program" them through a radio frequency or an electromagnetic signal transfer through the intact skin to the implanted pacemaker device. The simple programmable pacemaker (P in position 4) has relatively few options available in contrast to the multiprogrammable pacemaker (M in position 4) wherein the selection may run into quintillions of possibilities. The use of multiprogrammable devices reduces the need for the hospital to store multiple devices that have limited options and offers the opportunity to correct deficiencies in implanted units without requiring further surgery. It is appropriate to emphasize that a device that is manufactured with a specific designation often has several or many other possible modes of function that are obtainable through the simple intervention of programmability (Figure 23.2). Although a single chamber VVI pacemaker can never be programmed to be a DDD device because of the lack of a second circuit and lead to the atrium, a DDD device can be programmed to any number of alternate modes of function by selectively programming on or off its various available parameters. This offers the physician the flexibility of selective alteration of mode whenever a change in the patient's cardiac condition warrants such a change. Although more costly at implant, the multiprogrammable device averts the need for further surgery when limited performance characteristics of nonprogrammable devices

ORIGINAL FACTORY SETTING

PACER TYPE →	VVI	VDD	DVI	DDD	
AVAILABLE PROGRAMMABLE OPTIONS	VVT	VVI	VVI	AAI	VDD
	VOO	VVT	VVT	AAT	VAT
		VOO	VOO	AOO	DVI
			DOO	VVI	DAD*
				VVT	DDI*
				VOO	DDX*
					DOO

Figure 23.2. Available modes of cardiac stimulation in current day programmable pacemakers. Note the limited options in the "simple" programmable single chamber devices. Those modes indicated by an asterisk are specific to certain manufacturers for specialized functions and are not universally available.

prove inadequate for patient needs and require generator replacement.

The programming intervention is accomplished by the use of a device that may be handheld or in the form of a table console. The physician identifies the type of pacemaker that the patient has and the desired option of programming to be utilized. The programming device or devices offer some type of keyboard or pressure-sensitive switches which, when activated, set up the desired programming change. Programming is accomplished by positioning some type of "wand" or handheld device over the implanted generator and activating the programming switch. If an undesirable change has been initiated or if pacemaker capture is momentarily lost, a "panic" button allows immediate adjustment of the device to a safe setting while a more suitable program is established. In some manufacturers' systems, the implanted device must be interrogated through telemetry before programming can be accomplished. This reduces the possibility of misprogramming through transmission of a programming signal designed for another model device. The signal transfer to the implanted pacemaker is accomplished through a radiotelemetric or electromagnetic train of signals that are coded for each available programming intervention.[24] With most current programming devices, the external unit must receive recognition from the pacemaker first to minimize the possibility of "false programming" from environmental signals. A programming intervention may be carried out electively as when one programs down the stimulus output after the initial threshold has stabilized in order to preserve battery life and thereby extend system longevity. An alternative reason for programming arises when some type of device malfunction is identified such as abnormal sensing or capture. By selective modification of the output or sensitivity of the appropriate channel of the pacemaker, the malfunction can often be repaired and the need for further surgery averted. A list of typical programmable options in a representative modern-day dual chamber (DDD) device is found in Table 23.1.

Table 23.1. Representative Programmable Options in a Modern Day DDD Pacemaker

Channel	Rate	Output (pulse width/MA)	Sensitivity (mv)	Refractory (ms)	Atrioventricular Delay (ms)	Pacing Mode	
One	Off	0.2/2.0	0.5	200	0	AOO	VDD
	↓	0.3/3.0	...	250	...		
	30	0.4/4.0	1.3	300	75	AAT	VAT
	↓	0.5/5.0	...	350	...		
	35	0.6/6.0	2.5	400	100	AAI	DVI
	↓	0.8/8.0	...	500	...		
	40	1.0/10.0	Off	...	125	VOO	DDD
	↓	2.0/12.0	...	...	...		
	45	...	...	...	150	VVT	DOO
Two	↓	0.2/3.0	0.5	200	...		
	50	0.3/3.0	...	250	175	VVI	DAD
	↓	0.4/4.0	1.3	300	...		
	55	0.5/5.0	...	350	200	DDT/I	DDT
	↓	0.6/6.0	2.5	400	...		
	Etc	0.8/8.0	...	500	250	DAT	Off
	↓	1.0/10.0	Off	...	...		
	150	2.0/12.0	...	...	...	...	...

PATHOLOGIC BASIS OF CARDIAC CONDUCTION SYSTEM DISEASE

Most recipients of cardiac pacing systems in North America and western Europe have degenerative diseases of the conduction system. However, there are large segments of the world population that are afflicted with inflammatory or toxic and metabolic disorders that warrant consideration. For purposes of organization, this brief review of the pathologic conditions of the conduction system will be discussed under the familiar headings of congenital, traumatic, inflammatory, toxic/metabolic, neoplastic, and degenerative.

CONGENITAL ANOMALIES

The incidence of congenital heart block no doubt varies according to the population under study, the intensity of observation, and whether those with accompanying structural heart disease are included. Approximately 50% of these children will have associated congenital cardiac anomalies in addition to the conduction system disturbance, whereas the remainder present with isolated heart block of variable degree. It has been noted that half the children with congenital heart block are born of mothers with disseminated lupus erythematosus, suggesting a possible transplacental autoimmune impact on the developing conduction system.[25] The infant mortality among those with congenital heart block is high, and those children who survive the newborn era and come to attention for pacemaker implantation probably represent a "survival of the fittest" phenomenon. The difficulties encountered in adapting the relatively large pacing equipment designed for adults to such diminutive infants contributes to their morbidity. Nonetheless, successes in stabilizing the heart rate through pacing in such tiny infants do occur. The indications for pacing in this group of patients are not well defined and are often based more on the physician's perception of stability and the physiologic adequacy of the child's escape rhythm.

The occurrence of familial conduction system disease, although not congenital in the strict sense, has been widely reported[26,27] and is familiar to most physicians who handle sizable populations of patients with pacemakers. This often presents as the history of several members of a family requiring pacemakers or as the documented occurrence of variable fascicular blocks or sinus node disease, or both, occurring among related family members, some of whom eventually develop complete heart block. The inheritance pathway has been the subject of several studies and doctoral theses.[28]

TRAUMATIC INJURY

The predominant traumatic cause of conduction system damage in the western world is damage incurred at the time of cardiac surgery. The sinoatrial node is often traumatized at the time of cannulation for cardiopulmonary bypass or following the Mustard operation for transposition of the great arteries,[28a] which probably contributes to the frequency of postoperative atrial arrhythmias. The atrioventricular (AV) node and bundle of His receive their arterial blood supply from the AV nodal artery which arises from the right coronary artery at the crux of the heart in 90% of the population. Right coronary artery endarterectomy may shear off the origin of this vessel with resultant ischemia and infarction and Mobitz type I AV block. The AV node and the His bundle lie within the intersections of the cardiac skeleton between the mitral and tricuspid valve anuli and beneath the noncoronary cusp of the aortic valve. Surgical trauma of these structures or sutures placed for valve replacement may create temporary or permanent damage to antegrade conduction. In some instances, this may resolve as postoperative edema subsides around the conduction system, but, more commonly, permanent heart block or serious sinus node dysfunction results and cardiac pacing is required[28a] (Figure 23.3).

Isolated case reports of heart block due to stab or bullet wounds of the chest or deceleration chest impact injuries have been reported. Similarly, in patients who have acquired left bundle branch block, passage of an intracardiac pressure monitoring catheter or pacing lead may cause

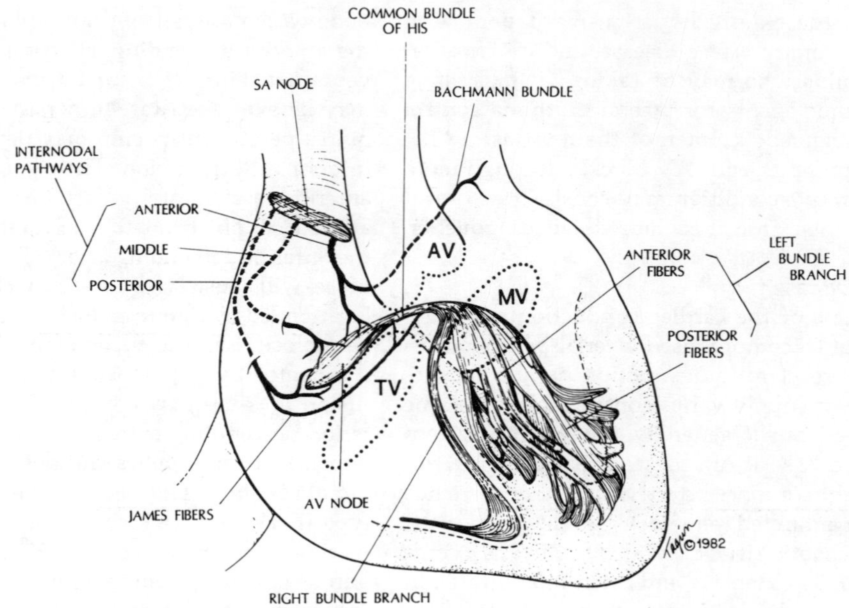

Figure 23.3. Surgical anatomy of the cardiac conduction system. Note that the sinus node may be traumatized during cannulation for cardiopulmonary bypass or during closure of a sinus venosus atrial septal defect. The atrioventricular (AV) node and bundle of His are vulnerable to repair of an ostium primum atrial septal defect or to cardiac valve replacement. AV = aortic valve; MV = mitral valve; TV = tricuspid valve. (From *Intelligence Reports in Cardiac Pacing and Electrophysiology*, vol 1, September 1982, with permission of Dr David Steinhaus and Health Scan Inc)

traumatic block of the right bundle branch with consequent complete heart block. Catheterization of such patients should always be preceded by the insertion of a temporary pacing electrode to avert sudden asystolic arrest.

INFLAMMATORY DISEASE

Perhaps the most common cause of inflammatory heart block today is infestation with trypanasoma Cruzi.[29] This disease is associated with diffuse myocardial fibrosis with concurrent involvement of the conduction system. Because congestive heart failure due to myocardial fibrosis may be an accompanying feature, such patients afflicted with heart block may best be treated by dual chamber pacing systems for restoration of properly timed atrial transport. Earlier causes of inflammatory myocarditis included diphtheria and rheumatic fever, but these conditions have become rare in North America and Europe. Viral myocarditis primarily due to Coxsackie virus[30] is probably more common than appreciated but requires endomyocardial biopsy for confirmation. Syphilitic gummas and tuberculomas were more common in the past but are now rarely seen.

TOXIC AND METABOLIC DISTURBANCES

Although difficult to prove, physicians likely create more heart block through pharmacologic means than they cure through pacing. The greatest offender has been the use of digitalis, particularly in patients in whom the gap between the therapeutic and toxic dose is narrow. The effect on AV node conduction may be manifest as simple first degree heart block without symptoms or life-threatening bradycardia accompanied by extreme ventricular irritability. Treatment often requires the intervention of temporary pacing until offending drug levels subside and normal conduction is restored. Similarly, with quinidine excess, atrial activation is depressed, and QRS complexes widen, often accompanied by bradycardia and "torsades de pointes" for which temporary pacing may be required. The more recent use of beta-adrenergic or calcium blocking agents and other type one antiarrhythmic drugs may be attended by varying degrees of impaired AV conduction such that temporary or permanent pacing, or both, may be required. Similarly, certain antimalarial agents such as chloroquine and antiparasitic antimony compounds are known to cause damage to the cardiac conduction system.

NEOPLASTIC DISEASE

Neoplasms do involve the myocardium but usually as a preterminal phase of metastatic extension of remote or adjoining tumors. A "benign" tumor, which may cause fatal heart block because of its location, is a mesothelioma of the AV node.[31]

DEGENERATIVE PROCESSES

In the western world, the most common cause of conduction system dysfunction by far that requires pacing is associated with degenerative disorders of the heart. Because of the concurrence of several possible causes of disturbed conduction in an elderly patient, it is often impossible to ascribe with certainty a specific etiologic basis. Therefore, the elderly hypertensive patient with aortic stenosis, coronary artery disease, and calcification of the mitral anulus who may be taking digitalis along with antiarrhythmic agents for tachyarrhythmia control challenges the diagnostic acumen of the most astute clinician when he presents with AV block. Although more than one degenerative condition may coexist, it is useful to subcategorize them into their individual components.

Ischemic Heart Disease

Ischemic necrosis of the cardiac conduction system is almost solely due to compromised arterial perfusion resulting from atherosclerotic obstruction of nutrient arteries. The vascular supply varies considerably from one patient to another, but it generally follows the pattern depicted in Figure 23.4. It can be seen that proximal occlusion of the right coronary artery may render the sinus node ischemic or infarcted, and such patients may manifest a variety of chaotic atrial tachyarrhythmias as a complication of a usually extensive and often fatal infarct. In the early days of cardiac surgery, when proximal right coronary endarterectomy was practiced, the origin of the sinus node artery was often damaged with consequent postoperative disorders of sinus node function. The artery to the AV node and proximal bundle of His derives from the distal right coronary artery in 90% of patients. Atheromatous obstruction of the right coronary artery, which is proximal to the origin of this branch and which becomes occluded, may result in inferior wall infarction complicated by Mobitz type I or Wenckebach AV block. The presence of a collateral arterial supply to the AV node which arises from the septal perforating branch of the anterior descending left coronary artery usually prevents actual infarction, and eventual return of conduction may be expected. Rarely, persistent heart block that requires permanent pacing may develop in a patient with inferior wall infarction. The right bundle branch and the anterior fascicle of the left bundle branch derive their arterial supply from the perforating septal branches of the anterior descending artery. Proximal occlusion of this vessel will cause large anterior wall infarction which may be attended by right bundle branch block and left anterior hemiblock. Because such extensive infarcts are often accompanied by hypotension, the resultant decline in perfusion pressure may compromise flow through the posterior descending branch of the right coronary artery which in turn supplies the posterior fascicle of the left bundle branch. This sets up the mechanism for Mobitz type II AV block which carries with it a high mortality (variously estimated at up to 85%). When damage to the bundle branch system becomes evident, temporary pacing in such patients is mandatory, and most observers believe that such patients should receive permanent pacemakers before hospital discharge. Because the infarct damage is extensive, with associated compromise of ventricular function, AV dual-chamber devices are usually recommended.

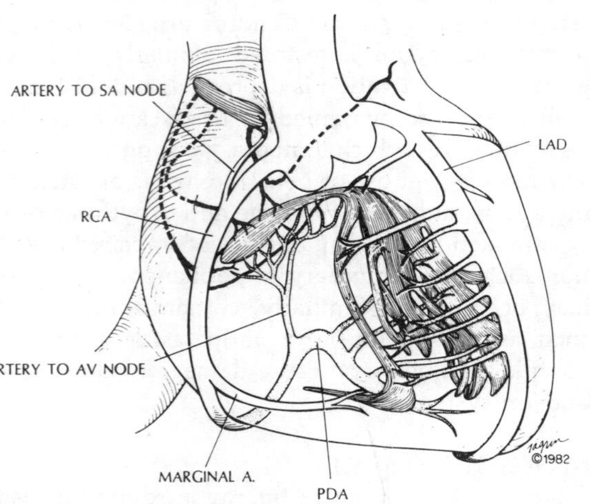

Figure 23.4. Vascular supply of the cardiac conduction system. The artery to the sinoatrial (SA) node arises from the proximal right coronary artery (RCA) in 60% of patients. The artery to the atrioventricular (AV) node arises from the distal RCA in 90% of patients. The right bundle branch and the anterior division of the left bundle are supplied by the septal perforating branches of the anterior descending (LAD) branch of the left coronary artery. The posterior division of the left bundle receives its blood supply from the posterior septal perforating branches of the posterior descending artery (PDA). (From *Intelligence Reports in Cardiac Pacing and Electrophysiology*, vol 1, with permission of Dr David Steinhaus and Health Scan Inc.)

Anular Calcification

As seen from Figure 23.3, the AV node and proximal bundle of His lie within the area circumscribed by the anuli of the semilunar and AV valves. Calcification of these structures as a consequence of chronic rheumatic valvulitis may have impact on and interrupt the continuity of the conduction system. Similarly, isolated calcification of the mitral anulus, which occurs more commonly in elderly women, may have a similar effect.[32]

Bundle Branch Fibrosis

Bundle branch fibrosis is the predominant cause of conduction system disorders in an elderly population. These patients often have preceding hypertension. Although coronary artery disease may coexist, it is not generally thought to be causative. In some instances a familial basis may be identified. The disorders known as Lev's syndrome[33] and Lenegre's disease,[34] although pathologically distinct, are often indistinguishable clinically.

Infiltrative Disorders

Systemic amyloidosis[35] is perhaps the best known infiltrative disorder in which disturbances in AV conduction may arise that eventually require pacing. Similarly, patients with sarcoid heart disease[36] occasionally require permanent pacing for restoration of stable cardiac rhythm.

INDICATIONS FOR CARDIAC PACEMAKER IMPLANTATION

TEMPORARY PACING

The indications for temporary pacing depend primarily on the urgency of the clinical condition of the patient and the perceived likelihood that a demonstrated or threatened bradyarrhythmia may cause cardiovascular instability. In most instances, temporary pacing is employed to avert bradycardia, although occasionally resting hemodynamics improve through dual chamber pacing. In specific instances, pacing may also be used for tachyarrhythmia control. Although considerable overlap exists, temporary pacing is generally considered in the following clinical circumstances.

Acute Myocardial Infarction

As noted in Figure 23.4, the AV node may be rendered ischemic when an atherosclerotic lesion proximal to the origin of the AV nodal artery becomes obstructed, resulting in inferior wall infarction. The resultant effect is the appearance of a Mobitz I or Wenckebach type AV block. This phenomenon is usually transitory with a stable nodal escape rhythm. Temporary pacing is seldom required unless the escape rhythm is consistently below 45 beats per minute or hemodynamic function is compromised. The situation with anterior wall infarction tends to be considerably less stable. Occlusion of the proximal anterior descending branch of the left coronary artery may render the right bundle branch and anterior division of the left bundle branch ischemic, with right bundle branch block and left anterior hemiblock. These infarcts usually involve an extensive area of myocardium, and hypotension and congestive heart failure often coexist. Transient impairment of circulation to the posterior fascicle of the left bundle branch sets up the mechanism for Mobitz type II heart block, which is attended by a high mortality. In most institutions, it is advised that patients with anterior wall infarction accompanied by new fascicular block receive a temporary pacemaker. The indications for temporary pacing are less established in a patient with chronic left bundle branch block who is hospitalized with clinical signs of acute infarction. The timing of pacemaker insertion depends on several factors such as the availability of personnel skilled in performing the procedure and the stability of the patient.

Chronic Bradycardia

Again, the urgency of the patient's clinical situation determines the need for insertion of a temporary pacemaker. For the patient who presents with Stokes-Adams attacks, stabilization with a temporary pacemaker may be appropriate. For others in whom long-standing bradycardia is a chronic problem, it may be reasonable to proceed directly with permanent pacing. When bradycardia is a consequence of drug overdose or occurs in advance of major general surgery, a short period of temporary pacing is often advisable. Several studies, however, have disproved the need for temporary perioperative pacing in patients with chronic unifascicular or bifascicular block.[37]

PERMANENT PACING

Few subjects have generated more interest and controversy in recent years. When these devices were first introduced into clinical practice 25 years ago, the only indication for their use was the Stokes-Adams syndrome caused by complete cardiac standstill. With time, clinical indications were expanded to include less obvious disorders in which bradycardia is episodic or of unclear relation to symptoms. To clarify the general indications for pacing, the Joint Task Force of the American Heart Association and American College of Cardiology published the guidelines[38] itemized in Table 23.2. These guidelines are broken into the following categories: Class I includes conditions generally agreed to warrant permanent pacing; Class II includes conditions for which permanent pacemakers are frequently used, but divergence of opinion exists; Class III includes conditions generally agreed not to warrant permanent pacing.

It is further emphasized that certain clinical descriptors may influence the eventual clinical decision, including (1) the overall clinical condition of the patient including the absence of immediate life-threatening disease; (2) the presence of concomitant cardiac or neurologic disease which may be aggravated by bradycardia; (3) the patient's desire to operate a motor vehicle; (4) remoteness of medical care, extensive travel, and living alone; (5) the need for concomitant medication which impairs conduction or induces slowing of the basic escape rate; and (6) the desires of the patient and family.

As is obvious to the experienced clinician, no "formula" can substitute for careful clinical judgment. However, it must be emphasized that adequate documentation of the offending arrhythmia should be entered into the patient's record whenever possible. Once the decision to proceed with pacemaker insertion has been rendered, the advantages and disadvantages of the various pacing modalities (ie, single versus dual chamber) must be considered. Although many social, economic, and technical factors contribute to the eventual choice of pacing device, the basic difference relates to the physiology of cardiac pacing.

HEMODYNAMICS OF CARDIAC PACING

One of the earliest lessons of cardiac physiology taught in medical school is that cardiac output is determined by the product of heart rate and stroke volume. Figure 23.5 illustrates this principle and emphasizes the interplay of associated factors such as peripheral resistance and neuroendocrine hormonal influence. There is no pacemaker device, either temporary or permanent, that exactly simulates the normal cardiovascular system in all of its remarkable complexity and autoregulation. The conventional, single chamber devices that have served well during the past 20 years offered rate control and avoidance of bradycardia-induced symptoms. In most instances, this was accomplished by a more-or-less arbitrary adjustment of the base pacing rate. Those patients who retained the ability to elevate their heart rates in response to stress above the basic pacing rate could be expected to preserve "normal" exercise physiology in comparison with age- and disease-matched patients. Those whose heart rates remained at all times under the control of the pacing device could respond to stress only through the Frank-Starling mechanism of improved myocardial contractility and improvements in stroke volume. Early physiologic studies of patients with ventricular pacemakers for control of complete heart block showed maximal improvement in cardiac output when the pre-pacing idio-

Table 23.2. Indications for Pacing*

Class I: Pacer Indicated	Class II: Pacer May Be Indicated	Class III: Pacer Not Indicated
Acquired symptomatic AV block	Acquired asymptomatic complete heart block	Syncope of undetermined cause
Congenital symptomatic AV block	Congenital heart block with uncertain symptoms	Asymptomatic sinus bradycardia
Mobitz II 2° block (symptomatic)	Bifascicular or trifascicular block when all other causes of syncope are excluded	Asymptomatic SA block or sinus arrest
Mobitz I 2° block if severely symptomatic	Following myocardial infarction accompanied by transient Mobitz II or complete heart block	Isolated prolonged pauses in atrial fibrillation
Sinus bradycardia with *documented* associated severe symptoms; HR below 50	Asymptomatic 2° Mobitz II AV block	Bradycardia during sleep
Sinus bradycardia of lesser severity if clearly symptomatic; HR above 50	Substantial sinus bradycardia (<40) due to necessary concurrent drugs	Bifascicular block without syncope or signs of AV block
Symptomatic sinus bradycardia due to necessary drugs	"Overdrive" pacing for control of ventricular tachycardia	Asymptomatic Mobitz type I block
Symptomatic sinus bradycardia as a component of brady/tachy syndrome		
Sinus bradycardia accompanied by serious ventricular arrhythmias		
Carotid sinus sensitivity when accompanied by significant bradycardia		

* The reader is strongly advised not to use this abbreviated table of indications but to consult the original publication for details.

AV = atrioventricular; HR = heart rate; SA = sinoatrial.

ventricular rate was raised to a paced rate of 60.[39] Further increases in paced ventricular rate up to 110 achieved only a 12% improvement in cardiac output, demonstrating that as the rate was increased, the stroke volume decreased with minimal change in resting cardiac output. The same study confirmed variable improvements in cardiac output in response to exercise when the ventricular rate was fixed through pacing, again demonstrating dependence on the integrity of myocardial contractility for improvements in stroke volume (Figure 23.6). Restoration of a properly timed atrial contractile mechanism has been of interest for many years before the advent of cardiac pacing. Early studies of temporary AV pacing[40,41] confirmed an improvement in cardiac dynamics, and these techniques came into use in the management of the critically ill patient following myocardial infarction or cardiac surgery before suitable systems were available for implantation. The era of microelectronics offered a significant reduction in circuit size with a simultaneous increase in complexity. Coincident with these developments came the recognition that certain patients with ventricular pacemakers demonstrated altered cardiovascular hemodynamics ranging

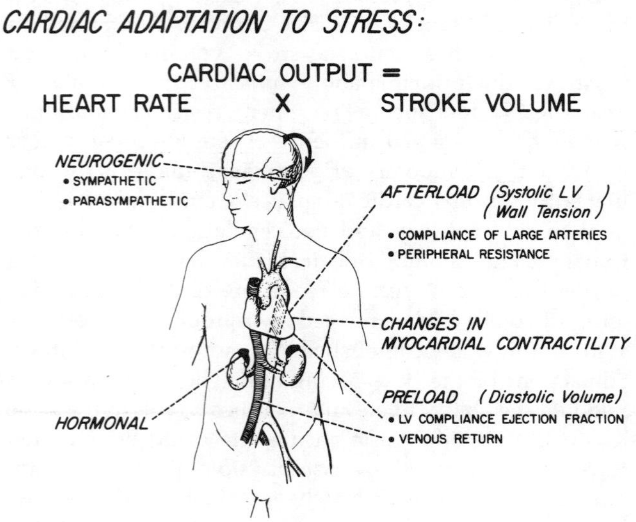

Figure 23.5. Hemodynamic determinants of cardiac output. A conventional, single chamber pacemaker affects only the heart rate, whereas a dual chamber device modifies the rate and the stroke volume through restoration of properly timed atrial transport.

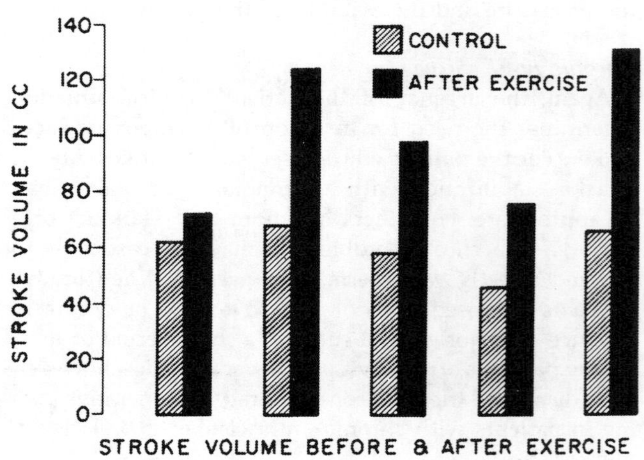

Figure 23.6. Hemodynamic response of five patients to exercise when the heart rate was maintained constant through ventricular pacing. Note the variation from one patient to another which reflects differences in the integrity of myocardial contraction. (From Judge et al,[39] with permission of the *New England Journal of Medicine.*)

from subtle fatigue to cardiovascular collapse induced by pacing.[42,43] Ventriculoatrial conduction had been recognized many years earlier[44] and remained familiar to those involved in arrhythmia management. Its occurrence after a paced ventricular beat (Figure 23.7) was somewhat of a surprise, and it is now recognized as an important marker of altered hemodynamic response to ventricular pacing. Recent studies[45] emphasize that approximately 50% of all patients who receive ventricular pacemakers will demonstrate this phenomenon. Among those patients with predominant sinus node disease, the incidence increases to 85%. Even patients with complete antegrade heart block can be expected to demonstrate this phenomenon in 15% of cases. An important Doppler study by Stewart et al[46] demonstrated that cardiac output increased an average of 19% when patients with dual chamber pacemakers were programmed from the single chamber to the dual chamber mode. For those who demonstrated ventriculoatrial conduction during ventricular pacing, the improvement was 30% (Figure 23.8). Similar findings have been reported by others in the literature. Therefore, it can be said that dual chamber pacing increases cardiac output in patients with preserved sinus rhythm and heart block and that the maximum improvement occurs in those with demonstrable ventriculoatrial conduction during ventricular pacing.

Studies of exercise capacity[47,48] in patients programmed back and forth between the single chamber and dual chamber mode of pacing confirm improvements in circulation time, exercise duration, work capacity, and cardiac output accompanied by a decrease in cardiothoracic ratio and exercise atrial rate. Quality of life questionnaires, although subject to many variables, tended to favor the dual chamber mode of pacing.

In chronic atrial fibrillation or an unstable atrial contractile mechanism accompanied by intermittent or sustained bradycardia, a single chamber ventricular pacemaker is appropriate. For those whose atria retain normal contractile function, the choice of dual chamber versus single chamber pacing becomes a socioeconomic as well as medical issue. For patients who are physically active or who have demonstrated an intolerance to ventricular pacing, the dual chamber devices offer improved hemodynamics.

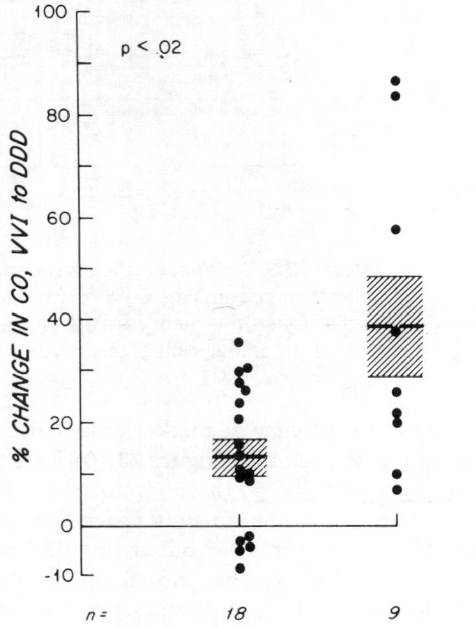

Figure 23.8. In this study, 29 patients with DDD pacemaker devices were randomly programmed from the single chamber ventricular mode to the dual chamber DDD mode. Cardiac output (CO) was recorded by the Doppler technique and the results were plotted according to the presence or absence of ventriculoatrial conduction. Note that the percentage improvement in cardiac output in programming from the VVI to DDD mode of pacing among patients without VA conduction was 17% whereas among patients with VA conduction, it measured 33%. (From Stewart et al,[46] with permission.)

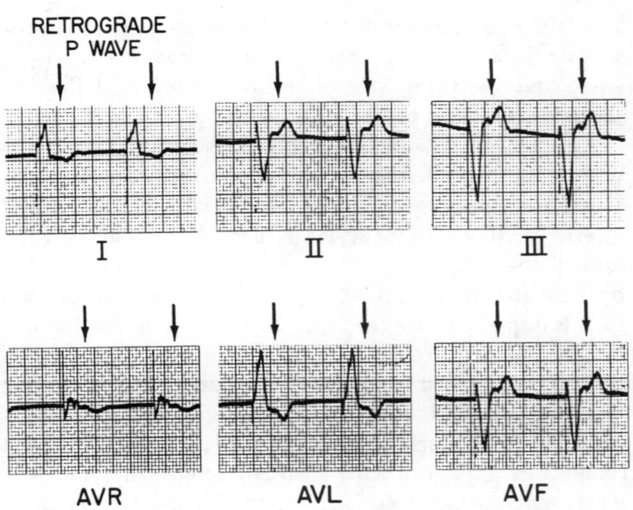

Figure 23.7. Ventriculoatrial conduction during ventricular pacing. Note the retrogradely conducted P waves following each paced ventricular complex. The resultant atrial contraction against a closed atrioventricular valve may be associated with a symptom complex of reduced cardiac output known as "the pacemaker syndrome."

TACHYARRHYTHMIA PACING

Most pacemaker procedures are performed because of bradycardia. The ability to interrupt a reentrant form of tachycardia by an ectopic stimulus has been known for many years and is widely practiced in electrophysiology laboratories. Devices that are manually operated by the patient for this purpose have been employed occasionally for many years. Automatic systems avert the need for patient interaction (Figure 23.9). The availability of microprocessor-based circuitry has enhanced the options for automated tachyarrhythmia devices. Such systems are designed to identify a tachycardia by specific criteria of rate, or suddenness of onset, or both. The pacemaker device may be programmed to emit a series of stimuli in a predetermined pattern which may fire in a single chamber burst or scanning modality or dual chamber underdrive.

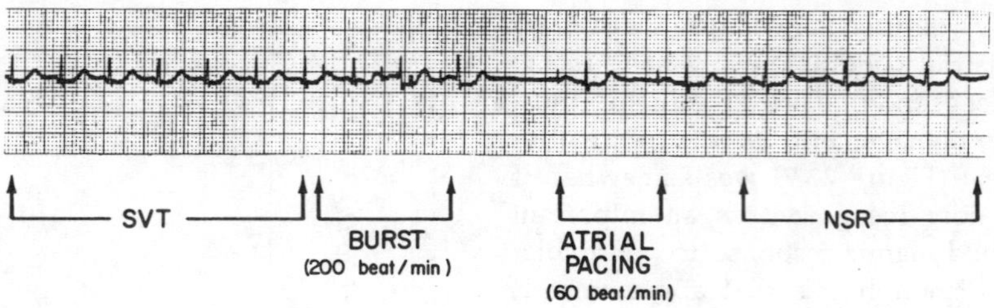

Figure 23.9. Electrocardiogram demonstrating the antitachycardia function of an Intermedics Cybertach pacemaker used for the automatic conversion of recurrent supraventricular tachycardia. Once the tachycardia has been converted, the device functions in a backup demand AAI mode until spontaneous rhythm is restored.

The addition of telemetry of marker pulses aids electrocardiographic interpretation (Figure 23.10). This technology is changing rapidly, so that it is not yet clear which mode of stimulation will ultimately prove most effective. For patients with prior episodes of out-of-hospital sudden death syndromes, interest has grown in the use of the implantable defibrillator and cardioverter (Figure 23.11). It is likely that future units will offer an array of automated tachyarrhythmia interruption algorithms with the backup option of defibrillation if hemodynamic collapse should occur.

TECHNIQUE OF PACEMAKER INSERTION

The pacemaker implantation physician must have basic familiarity with the cardiac anatomy and preferably some ability in cardiac catheterization. In temporary pacing, the procedures may be conducted during emergency cardiac arrest at the bedside or in the more relaxed environment of a fluoroscopic suite. Venous access may be gained either by direct cutdown on a suitable vein or more usually by percutaneous puncture of the subclavian or internal jugular vein. If fluoroscopy is available, right heart catheterization is employed to gain access to the right ventricle. When "blind" insertion is required, guidance as to electrode position may be obtained by recording of the intracardiac electrogram (Figure 23.12). Permanent procedures may be conducted in a catheterization laboratory, radiology suite, or operating room with available fluoroscopic equipment. Customary operating room sterility precautions are mandatory and all personnel should be properly gowned and masked. Fluoroscopy must be available. All procedures are performed using local anesthesia. Venous access is obtained through the right or left chest with the choice dependent on individual preference, patient hobbies, or local chest wall considerations (ie, mastectomy). Meticulous skin preparation of the surgical field is performed using surgical soap, povidone-iodine (Pharmadine, Sherwood Pharmaceuticals, Mahwah, NJ), a degreasing agent, followed by application of sterile drapes and an adhesive skin drape (Steridrape, 3M, Minneapolis, MN). The pacing lead or leads are inserted by direct cutdown on the cephalic vein, if available, or by subclavian vein puncture. It is our practice to position the ventricular lead first by prolapsing it across the tricuspid valve and "working" the flanged or tined lead tip into the trabeculations of the right ventricle.

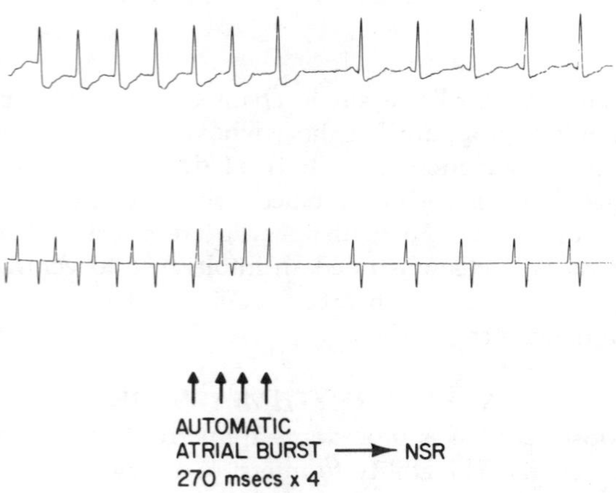

Figure 23.10. This recording demonstrates the simultaneous use of telemetry of a marker signal (*lower tracing*) which indicates pacemaker function during conversion of spontaneous supraventricular tachycardia (*upper tracing*). The marker channel depicts atrial events as positive deflections and ventricular events as negative deflections. Sensed events are recorded as smaller amplitude deflections, whereas pacing is indicated by the taller deflections. In this bipolar Medtronic Symbios (model 7008) DDD pacemaker, the pacing stimuli are not visible on the surface electrocardiogram. The fact that this is a reentrant arrhythmia can readily be perceived by the relation of the atrial to the ventricular marker signals. With return of sinus rhythm, this relation returns to normal.

An active fixation type lead may be selected for patients with smooth-walled right ventricles or those with associated tricuspid regurgitation. The atrial J lead is usually inserted with a straight stylet in place. When this is withdrawn, the lead assumes its preformed J shape and the tip will usually snag in the appendage when withdrawn to the upper part of the right atrium. Considerable experience is required to ascertain correct positioning. An active fixation lead is preferable for patients in whom the atrial appendage is missing because of prior cardiac surgery. When properly positioned, the lead or leads should retain a gentle curve with adequate length to avoid displacement during deep inspiration (Figure 23.13). Once suitable stimulation thresholds and intracavitary signal strengths have been achieved, the leads are carefully anchored at their point of venous entry using the anchoring sleeves provided. A "pocket" is created deep to the subcutaneous fat and superficial to the pectoralis fascia, into which the pulse generator with its attached lead or leads

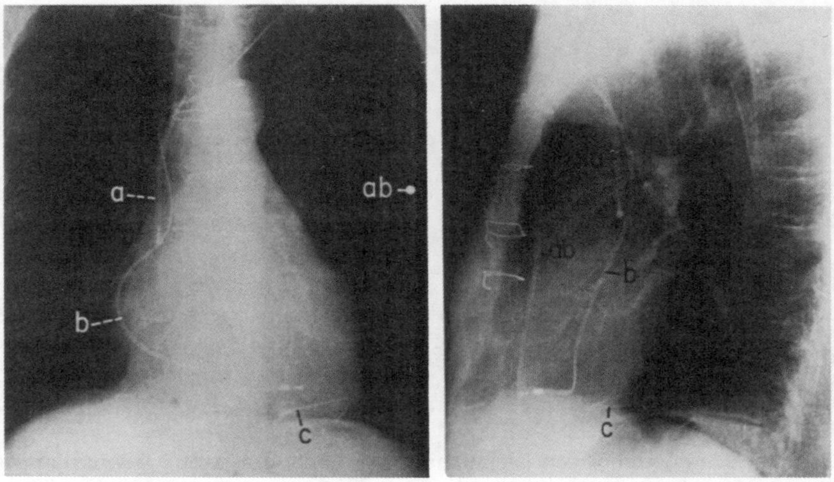

Figure 23.11. Anteroposterior and lateral x-ray films of a patient with an implantable defibrillator. a = transvenous anode positioned in the superior cava/right atrium; b = transvenous ventricular sensing lead; c = epicardial patch cathode; ab = subcutaneous portion of transvenous leads tunneled to abdominal power pack and defibrillator (not shown). The defibrillation shock occurs between the transvenous anode (a) and the epicardial cathode (c).

is inserted. Wound closure is accomplished in several layers using interrupted catgut or synthetic suture material, and a dry sterile dressing with local antibiotic ointment is applied. Prophylactic antibiotics are administered the day before, the day of, and three days after the procedure.

The foregoing description of operative technique is offered only as a guide and it should be emphasized that there is no substitute for a period of apprentice training with one who is already experienced in the technique.

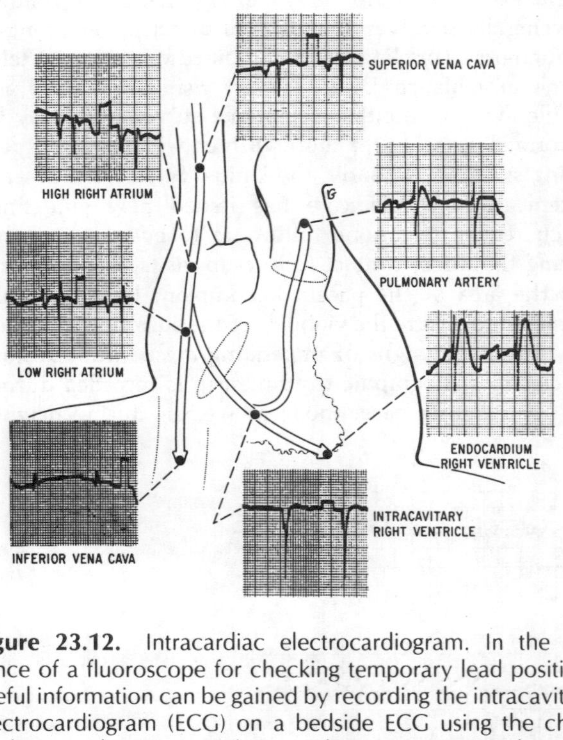

Figure 23.12. Intracardiac electrocardiogram. In the absence of a fluoroscope for checking temporary lead position, useful information can be gained by recording the intracavitary electrocardiogram (ECG) on a bedside ECG using the chest lead. Note the current of injury that accompanies the ventricular electrocardiogram. (From Harthorne JW, McDermott J, Poulin FK: Cardiac pacing, in Johnson RA, Haber E, Austen G (eds): *The Practice of Cardiology*. Boston, Little, Brown & Co, 1980, with permission.)

COMPLICATIONS OF CARDIAC PACING

The patients who undergo temporary or permanent pacemaker insertion are prone to cardiac instability by the nature of their disease. The pacemaker laboratory team must be ever cognizant of the potential for unexpected asystole or ventricular tachyarrhythmias for which cardioversion may be necessary. With proper precautions, perioperative death rate should be below 1%. The consequences of subclavian vein puncture may include venous air embolism, pneumothorax, or arterial puncture which may cause hemothorax or hemopneumothorax. During manipulation of the leads within the heart, various arrhythmias are to be expected. These include cath-

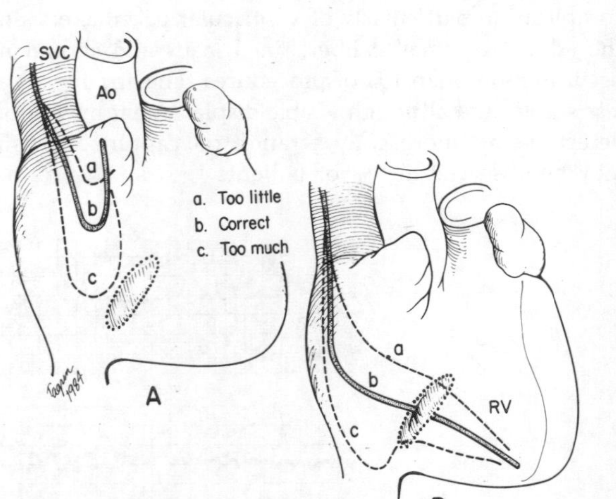

Figure 23.13. The proper position of atrial or ventricular leads, or both, as seen on the fluoroscope. (From *Intelligence Reports in Cardiac Pacing and Electrophysiology*, vol 2. With permission of Dr Andrew Eisenhauer and Health Scan Inc.)

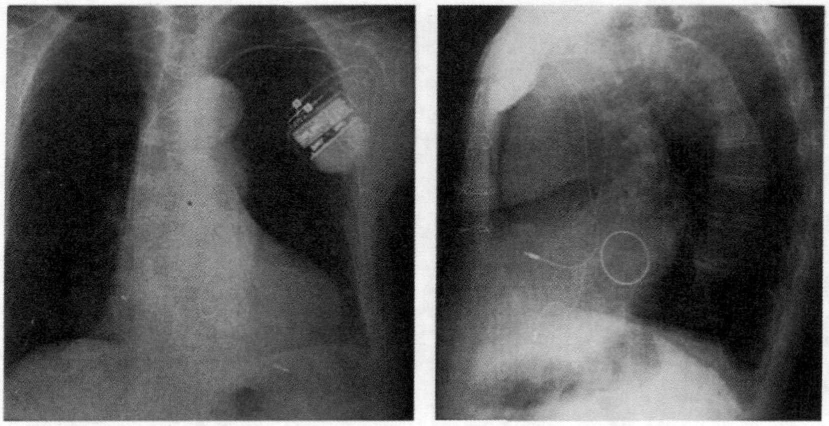

Figure 23.14. Anteroposterior and lateral chest x-ray films of a patient with a transvenous dual chamber pacemaker implanted during the postoperative convalescence from mitral valve replacement because of persistent complete heart block. Note that the atrial lead is an active fixation screw-tipped lead. The ring-shaped stent of the mitral prosthesis is apparent.

eter-induced atrial premature beats, atrial fibrillation, ventricular premature beats, ventricular tachycardia, and ventricular fibrillation. The operating team must anticipate the need for cardiac resuscitation, while maintaining sterility of the operative field.

In patients who are undergoing permanent pacemaker insertion, meticulous attention to hemostasis before pocket closure and careful assessment of clotting function before the procedure will reduce the incidence of pocket hematoma formation. Nonetheless, impaired capillary fragility in an elderly population or the recent use of platelet-inhibiting agents may still result in local accumulation of blood. Unless accompanied by severe pain or the threat of wound dehiscence, this is usually best left alone and will often dissipate into the surrounding tissues within a matter of days. Sepsis of the pacemaker pocket is the consequence of poor surgical technique or secondary intervention, occurs rarely, and requires removal of the entire pacing system including the leads.

Displacement of pacing leads has become an infrequent complication particularly of ventricular pacemakers since the advent of small caliber, tined leads and should not occur in more than 1% of procedures. The atrial leads are less stable, and although visible displacement may not be detectable by fluoroscopy, erratic atrial capture or sensing may be observed in 5% of patients.

FOLLOW-UP OF THE PACEMAKER PATIENT

Follow-up begins when the final suture is placed after initial pacemaker insertion. Beyond detection of the obvious perioperative complications already noted, the monitoring physician must be competent in electrocardiographic analysis and have a confident understanding of how the pacemaker system is intended to function. The frequency and method of follow-up depend on multiple factors beyond the pacemaker device itself. The patient with concurrent unstable medical problems may require closer surveillance than those with isolated conduction system disease alone. The method of follow-up generally involves a mixture of direct patient contact through office or clinic visits combined with interim telephone surveillance. Direct contact visits are usually advisable every 6 months. Telephone surveillance may be performed monthly for those with end-of-life or suspect pacing systems. Recently, the United States Health Care system through Medicare has issued new guidelines which reduce telephone follow-up to every 2 months. During the direct contact follow-up visits, it is essential that the area of the pacemaker implant be thoroughly examined to ensure the viability of the surrounding tissue and to look for signs of impending mechanical erosion. An electrocardiographic rhythm strip is recorded during the free running pacer mode as well as during magnet

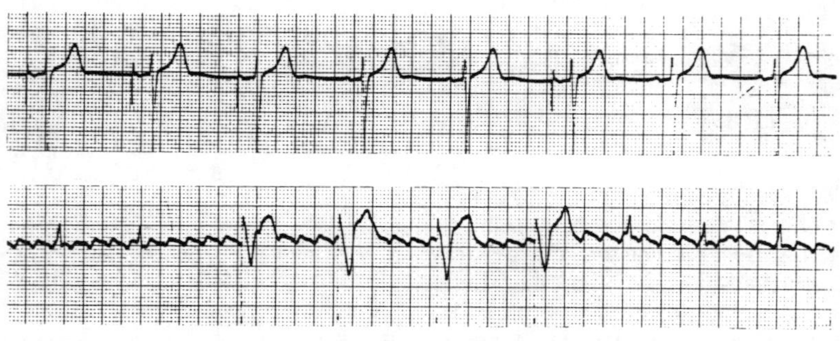

Figure 23.15. Single chamber "demand" pacing of the atrium (AAI above) and ventricle (VVI below). The timing and sensing circuits function continuously. The detection of spontaneous P or R waves through the pacing lead causes inhibition of the output circuit and avoids competition.

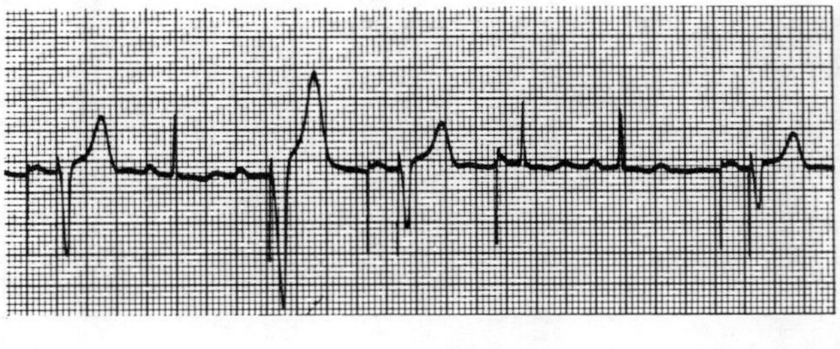

Figure 23.16. Dual chamber, fully automatic DDD pacemaker electrocardiogram. Note that each cardiac cycle presents a new sequence of sensing, timing, and pacing when appropriate. All events are timed from the preceding R wave. Spontaneous P waves initiate an AV counter and pacing at the programmed AV delay will follow if normal conduction does not interrupt it. If spontaneous P waves do not appear, the atrial output circuit will discharge and initiate the AV delay counter.

application. In many pacing systems, it is the magnet rate that reflects residual battery output voltage. This rate should be recorded using an electronic interval counter. All patients should have baseline chest x-ray films to confirm proper lead position (Figure 23.14).

The pulse generator consists of a power source (the batteries), the electronic circuit, and the surrounding housing which protects the inner compartment from the corrosive effects of body fluids. The pacemaker lead connects the heart with the pulse generator. Interruption of proper pacemaker function may result from erratic performance of any of these subcomponents of the pacemaker system.

In its simplest form, a pacemaker circuit consists of an output circuit which modifies the energy emanating from the power supply into an impulse that has identifiable characteristics of duration, amplitude, and rate. The rate of pacing is determined by a timing circuit. In a fixed rate or asynchronous device, the stimulus is emitted in a repetitive fashion regardless of the intrinsic rhythm. The noncompetitive "demand" pacemaker offers a sensing circuit (sensing amplifier) which serves to detect endogenous depolarizations by way of the pacing lead. Therefore, the pacing lead may be thought of as resembling the afferent and efferent fibers of a spinal reflex arc. Spontaneous QRS- or P-wave complexes that are detected in the sensing circuit by way of the lead will inhibit the output circuit (Figure 23.15). A DDD pacemaker may be thought of as two demand pacemakers that are responsible for sustaining atrial and ventricular rhythm, respectively. The two circuits are joined by a logic circuit, so that the events in one electronic channel may be related to those of the other. In the absence of spontaneous P waves, the output circuit of channel one will elicit a paced atrial contraction. This event starts the timing of the AV delay. If after the programmed AV delay "times out" a conducted QRS has not occurred, the output circuit of channel two discharges and creates a paced ventricular complex. Similarly, a spontaneous P wave will cause inhibition of the stimulus from channel one, but the sensed P wave initiates the AV delay timer and ventricular stimulation will be initiated or inhibited depending on events occurring in the ventricle (Figure 23.16).

The predominant abnormalities of pacemaker function to be looked for during follow-up consist of varying degrees of erratic capture or sensing. Failure to detect an intracavitary signal due to an amplitude that is below the sensitivity setting of the pacemaker will result in competitive pacing (Figure 23.17). This may result from perforation of the right ventricular wall by the lead tip or chronic perielectrode fibrosis. Programming to a higher sensitivity may correct the problem. Competitive pacing seldom causes clinical problems in the setting of chronic heart block, but it may induce lethal arrhythmias in patients with recent myocardial infarction or recent cardiac surgery (Figure 23.18).

Loss of capture by the atrial or ventricular output circuit occurs most frequently during the early period after surgery when the implantation threshold rises acutely (Figure 23.19). This acute increase in threshold usually resolves within the first ten days and normal pacemaker function may be restored without surgical intervention. Programming to a higher output setting during the interim is often effective.

Follow-up of patients with dual chamber pacemakers entails the same principles of assessing effectiveness of capture or sensing, or both. Faulty sensing of spontaneous P waves by the atrial channel of dual chamber DDD devices due to subthreshold P waves may be found in approximately 5% of patients. This is usually episodic with random P waves that are "missed" (Figure 23.20). Oversensing of myopectoral contractions in the vicinity of unipolar generators is an occasional cause of recurrent syncope in pacemaker patients (Figure 23.21). With dual chamber devices programmed to the DDD mode, the onset of an atrial tachyarrhythmia may trigger the unit to stimulate the ventricles at the programmed upper tracking rate (Figure 23.22). Judicious choice of programmable pa-

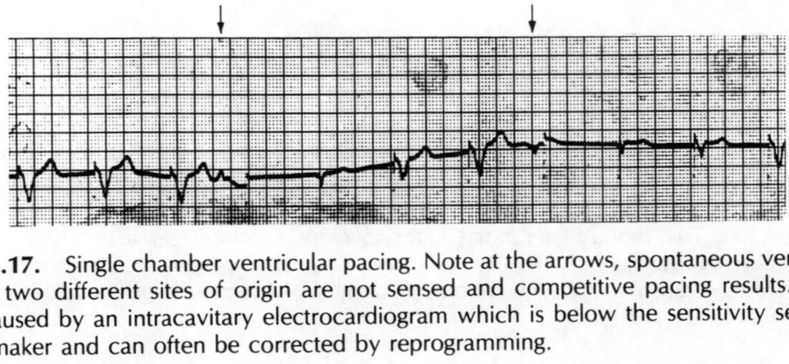

Figure 23.17. Single chamber ventricular pacing. Note at the arrows, spontaneous ventricular events of two different sites of origin are not sensed and competitive pacing results. This is usually caused by an intracavitary electrocardiogram which is below the sensitivity setting of the pacemaker and can often be corrected by reprogramming.

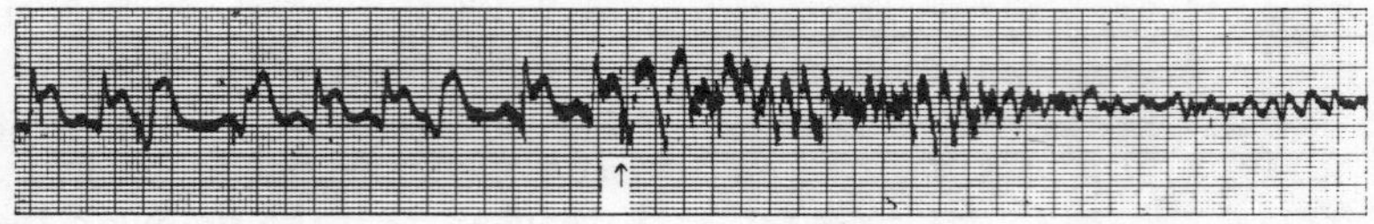

Figure 23.18. Competitive pacing in the setting of acute myocardial infarction may cause ventricular tachycardia or, as in this case, ventricular fibrillation.

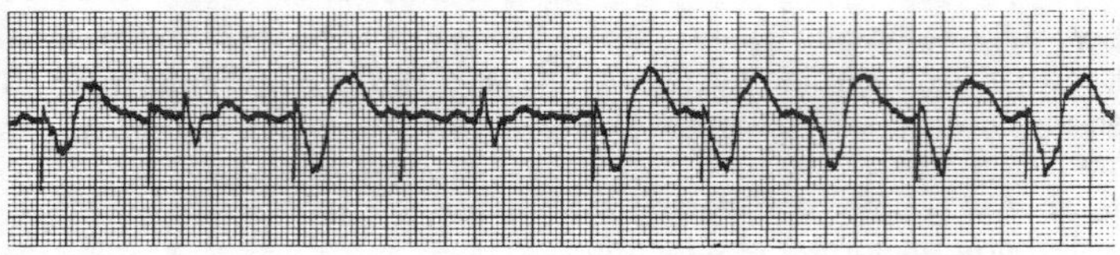

Figure 23.19. Erratic capture is most common during the immediate postimplantation convalescence when the initial threshold rises acutely. Note that the second and fourth stimuli fail to depolarize the myocardium. The difference in pacing interval between the second and third stimuli is caused by sensing of the intervening QRS complex. Reprogramming the output temporarily to a higher setting often corrects this problem.

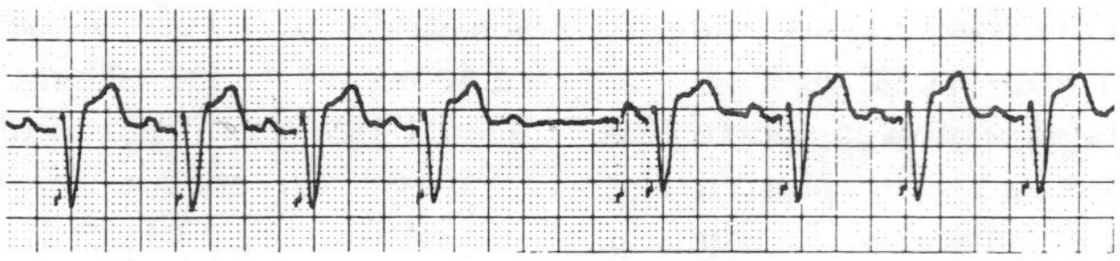

Figure 23.20. Erratic sensing of the P wave is not uncommon with DDD pacemakers because of the narrow gap between the endocardial P-wave amplitude and the available sensitivity setting of the pacemaker device. The first four complexes show proper P-triggered ventricular pacing. The fifth P wave is not sensed by the atrial sense amplifier. When the programmed base rate (50 beats per minute) "times out," AV pacing occurs. The final three complexes show a return of normal P-wave sensing.

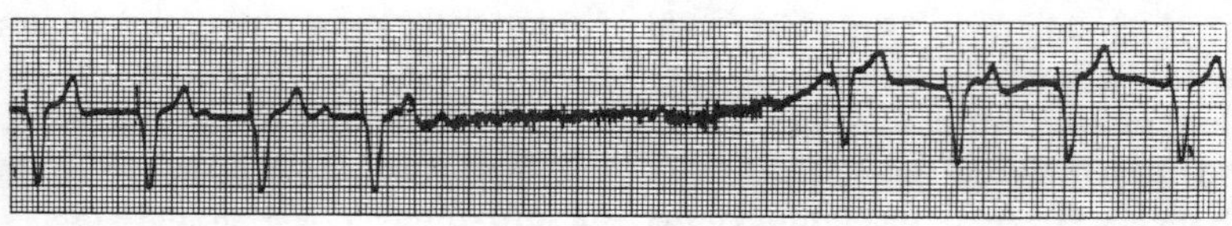

Figure 23.21. Myopectoral inhibition. Note the baseline artifact in the center of the tracing and the absence of pacing caused by detection of skeletal muscle potentials in the vicinity of the pulse generator. This only affects unipolar pacing devices and can often be corrected by reprogramming the sensitivity or choosing a different mode.

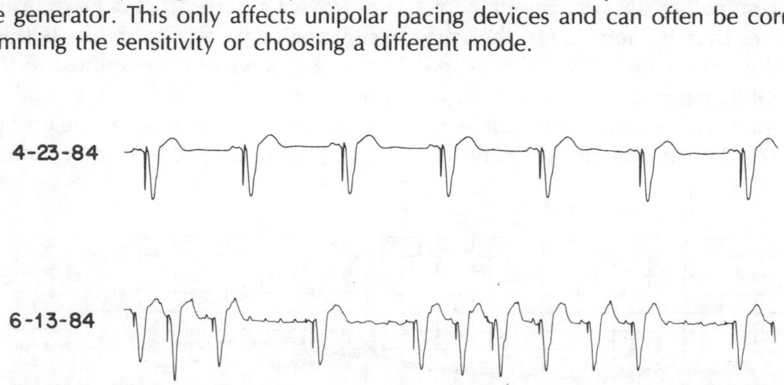

Figure 23.22. A form of pacemaker-mediated tachycardia. In the upper panel, normal DDD pacing is present. Two months later, atrial flutter develops and the pacemaker follows the flutter waves variably due to slight changes in intracavitary signal amplitude. The device paces at its programmed base rate in the absence of sensing or at its programmed upper tracking rate when the flutter waves are detected.

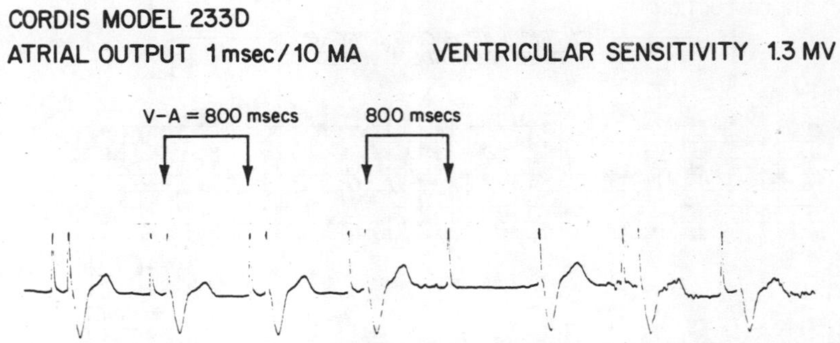

Figure 23.23. Electrocardiographic rhythm strip which demonstrates "cross talk." Note that the identity of the atrial stimulus can be determined by measuring the ventriculoatrial time-out from the preceding R wave. A ventricular stimulus fails to appear in complex 5 because of inhibition of ventricular output consequent to sensing of the atrial stimulus.

rameters combined with careful follow-up avoids most of these occurrences.

The problems of fractured pacing leads, which were not uncommon in the past, have diminished significantly with the newer multistrand leads. Degradation of one recent polyurethane-coated lead created concerns over the biocompatibility of this material. This was related to a specific manufacturing process and has not been observed with leads from other manufacturers. Although random component failure is an occasional cause of erratic circuit function, electronic "runaway" which was seen in the past is almost never observed.

Thrombosis of the ipsilateral vein through which lead insertion is accomplished is a common occurrence[49] that may infrequently cause swelling of the arm. Pulmonary thromboembolism related to transvenous pacing systems is a rare event that has produced an occasional case report.[50,51] Two subtle abnormalities of dual chamber pacing that have been recognized include the phenomena of cross talk and pacemaker-mediated tachycardia. The expression "cross talk" is an engineering term coined to refer to the detection by the sensing circuit of one channel of a dual chamber pacemaker of the output stimulus of the other channel. Therefore, if the amplitude of the atrial output circuit is programmed to a relatively high level and the sensitivity of the ventricular channel set to a high level, detection of the atrial output stimulus may result in inhibition of ventricular stimulation (Figure 23.23). This phenomenon is seldom seen clinically because of an electronic technique of "blanking" the ventricular sensing circuit for a brief instant when the atrial output circuit discharges.

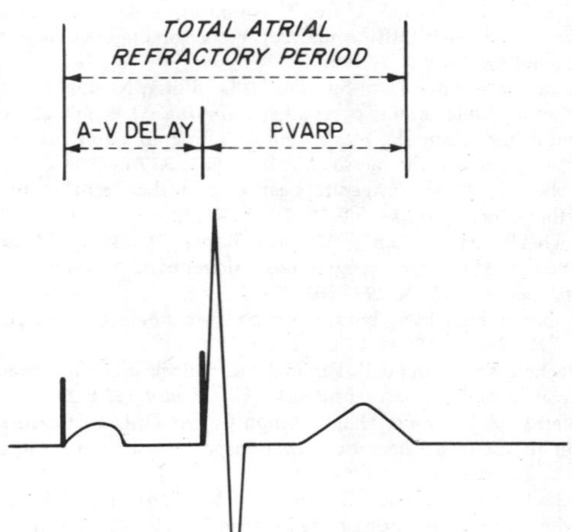

Figure 23.24. Diagrammatic representation of the components of the atrial refractory period of a typical dual chamber pacemaker device. The total atrial refractory period is the sum of the atrioventricular (AV) delay and the postventricular atrial refractory period (PVARP). It is this total interval that determines the upper tracking rate of the pacemaker device in the DDD mode.

The other peculiarity of dual chamber devices that are programmed to the fully automatic DDD mode is the possible detection by the atrial channel of signals other than spontaneous, antegrade P waves. The atrial sensing circuit is refractory for a certain portion of the timing cycle after initiation of a paced P wave or sensing of a spontaneous P wave. This refractory period extends through the AV delay and for a programmable interval beyond the QRS complex (Figure 23.24). Any signals detected by the atrial sensing circuit outside this atrial refractory period will initiate a new paced ventricular event after the programmed AV delay. This may include retrograde P waves, myopectoral contraction signals, or various atrial tachyarrhythmias. The rate of the resultant "pacemaker-mediated tachycardia" will be determined by the rate of the detected signal and by the programmed upper tracking rate of the pacemaker device (Figure 23.25). A variety of innovations are coming along to minimize the occurrence and clinical significance of this phenomenon.

CONCLUSIONS

The current pacemaker device is vastly superior to that of former years. The innovation of microchip technology in which each circuit is an identical "clone" of a master electronic breadboard has markedly reduced the incidence

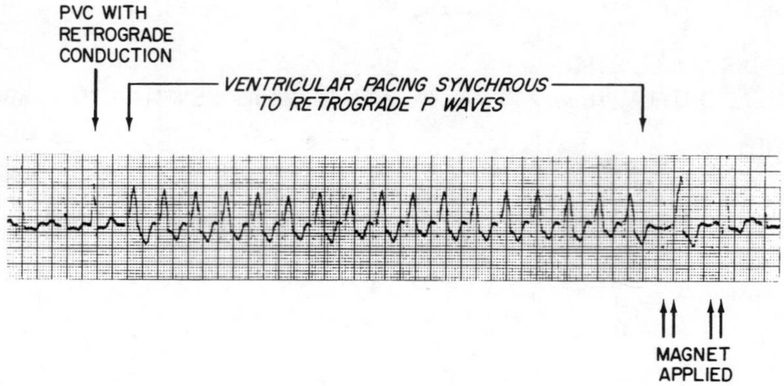

Figure 23.25. An example of a pacemaker-mediated tachycardia caused by a retrograde P wave which is then sensed by the atrial sensing channel. This cycle will continue until retrograde block occurs, or the pacemaker is deactivated by application of a magnet or reprogramming.

of circuit failure which plagued early solid-state devices in which individual components were hand soldered. Such circuits are far more efficient in energy conservation, which contributes to the ultimate longevity of the system. When combined with a lithium power source, stable pacing function for many years can be anticipated. Variations in individual pacing threshold, percentage of time pacing, and differences in programmed setting make it difficult to project "average" longevity for any pacing device. Most modern single chamber systems will provide 7 to 9 years of dependable performance. Dual chamber devices consume more energy because of twin circuits, but they are expected to offer 6 to 8 years of effective battery life. The longevity of systems that offer antitachyarrhythmia functions remains unknown. Rising concerns over cost containment in medical care have focused increasing attention on the indications for use of the more expensive high technology devices and have rejuvenated interest in the reuse of normally functioning units that have been explanted from previous recipients.

REFERENCES

1. Schechter DC, Lillehei CW, Soffer A: History of sphygmology and of heart block. *Dis Chest* 1969; 55(suppl 1):534–579.
2. Harvey W: *The Circulation of the Blood and Other Writings*. London, JM Dent & Sons, Ltd, 1953.
3. Aldini J: *General Views on the Application of Galvanism to Medical Purposes: Principally in Cases of Suspended Animation*. London, J Callow, 1819.
4. Bichat X: *Recherches Physiologiques sur la Vie et la Mort*. Paris, Brosson, Gabon, & Cie, 1800.
5. Schechter DC: Background of clinical cardiac electrostimulation. I. Responsiveness of quiescent bare heart to electricity. *NY State J Med* 1971; 71:2575–2581.
6. Tawara S: *Das Reizleitungsystem des Saugetierherzens*. Jena, Fischer, 1906.
7. His W Jr: Die Thatigheit des embryonalen Herzens und deren Bedeutung für die Lehre von der Herzbewegung bein Erwachsenen. *Arb Med Klin* (Leipzig) 1893; 14–49.
8. Wenckebach KF: Zur Analyse des unregelmassigen Pulses. *Z Klin Med* 1899; 36:181–199.
9. Keith A, Flack MW: The form and nature of the muscular connections between the primary divisions of the vertebrate heart. *J Anat and Physiol* 1906-1907; 41:172–189.
10. Policki B: De Musculari Cordis Structura. Breslau, Inaugural Dissertation, 1839.
11. Kent AFS: Researches on the structure and function of the mammalian heart. *J Physiol* 1893; 15:233–254.
12. Aschoff L, Tawara S: *Die heutige Lehre vonden pathologisch-anatomischen Grundlagen der Herzschache*. Jena, Fischer, 1906.
13. Kellaway P: The part played by electric fish in early history of bioelectricity and electrotherapy. *Bull Hist Med* 1946; 20:112–137.
14. Schechter DC: Origins of electrotherapy. Part I. *NY State J Med* 1971; 71:997–1008.
15. Von Ziemssen H: Studien ueber die bewegungsvorgaenge am menschlichen herzen sowie ueber die mechanische und elektrische erregbarkeit des herzens und des nervus phrenicus, angestellt an dem freiliegenden herzen der Catherina Serafin. *Arch Klin Med* 1882; 30:270–285.
16. Stokes W: Observations on some cases of permanently slow pulse. *Dublin Q J Med Sci* 1846; 2:73–83.
17. Adams R: Cases of diseases of the heart accompanied with pathological observations. *Dublin Hosp Rep* 1827; 4:353–453.
18. Mond HG, Sloman JG, Edwards RH: The first pacemaker. *PACE* 1982; 5:278–282.
19. Hyman AS: Resuscitation of stopped heart by intracardial therapy: further use of the artificial pacemaker. *US Naval Med Bull* 1935; 33:205–214.
20. Zoll PM: Resuscitation of the heart in ventricular standstill by electric stimulation. *N Engl J Med* 1952; 247:768–771.
21. Folkman MJ, Watkins E: An artificial conduction system for the management of experimental complete heart block. *S Forum* 1958; 8:331–334.
22. Keller JW, Nathan DA, Center S: An implantable synchronous cardiac pacer. *Digest* 1962; 15th Annual Conference on Engineering in Medicine and Biology, Nov 5–7, 1962.
23. Parsonnet V, Furman S, Smythe NPD, Bilitch M: Optimal resources for implantable cardiac pacemakers. *Circulation* 1983; 68:227A–244A.
24. Gold RD, Saulson SH, MacGregor DC: Programmable pacing systems: the medium and the message. *PACE* 1982; 5:776–780.
25. Esscher E, Scott JS: Congenital heart block and maternal systemic lupus erythematosus. *Br Med J* 1979; 1:1235–1238.
26. Lynch HT, Mohiuddin S, Moran J, Kaplan A, Sketch M, Zencka A, Runco V: Hereditary progressive atrioventricular conduction defect. *Am J Cardiol* 1975; 36:297–301.
27. Stephan E: Hereditary bundle branch system defect: a new genetic entity? *Am Heart J* 1979; 97:708–718.
28. Sarachek NS, Leonard JJ: Familial heart block and sinus bradycardia. Classification and natural history. *Am J Cardiol* 1972; 29:451–458.

28a. Gillette PC, Wampler DG, Shannon C, Ott D: Use of cardiac pacing after the Mustard operation for transposition of the great arteries. *J Am Coll Cardiol* 1986; 7:138–141.

29. Andrade ZA, Andrade SG, Oliviera GB, Alonzo DR: Histopathology of the conducting tissue of the heart in Chagas' myocarditis. *Am Heart J* 1978; 95:316–324.
30. Davies MJ, Anderson RH, Becker AE: Conduction tissues in systemic disease, in *The Conduction System of the Heart*. London, England, Butterworths, 1983, chap 11.
31. Bharati S, Bicoff JP, Fridman JL, Lev M, Rosen KM: Sudden death caused by benign tumor of the atrioventricular node. *Arch Intern Med* 1976; 136:224–228.
32. Korn D, DeSanctis RW, Sell S: Massive calcification of the mitral annulus: a clinicopathological study of 14 cases. *N Engl J Med* 1962; 267:900–909.
33. Lev M: The pathology of complete atrioventricular block. *Prog Cardiovasc Dis* 1964; 6:317–326.
34. Lenegre J: Etiology and pathology of bilateral bundle branch block in relation to complete heart block. *Prog Cardiovasc Dis* 1964; 6:409–444.

35. Brownstein MH: Cardiac amyloidosis and complete heart block. *NY State J Med* 1966; 66:397–399.
36. Morales AR, Levy S, Davis J, Fine G: Sarcoidosis and the heart, in Sommers SC (ed): *Pathology Annual.* New York, Appleton-Century-Crofts, 1974, p 139.
37. Pastore JO, Yurchak PM, Janis KM, Murphy JD, Zir LM: The risk of advanced heart block in surgical patients with right bundle branch block and left axis deviation. *Circulation* 1974; 49–50(suppl III): III–57.
38. Joint American College of Cardiology/American Heart Association Task Force on Assessment of Cardiovascular Procedures: Guidelines for Permanent Pacemaker Implantation, May 1984. *J Am Coll Cardiol* 1984; 4:434–442.
39. Judge RD, Wilson WS, Siegel JH: Hemodynamic studies in patients with implanted cardiac pacemakers. *N Engl J Med* 1964; 270:1391–1395.
40. Chamberlain DA, Leinbach RC, Vassaux CE, Kastor JA, DeSanctis RW, Sanders CA: Sequential atrioventricular pacing in heart block complicating acute myocardial infarction. *N Engl J Med* 1970; 282:577–582.
41. Leinbach RC, Chamberlain DA, Kastor JA, Harthorne JW, Sanders CA: A comparison of the hemodynamic effects of ventricular and sequential A-V pacing in patients with heart block. *Am Heart J* 1969; 78:502–508.
42. Alicandri C, Fouad FM, Tarazi RC, Castle L, Morant L: Three cases of hypotension and syncope with ventricular pacing. Possible role of atrial reflexes. *Am J Cardiol* 1978; 42:137–142.
43. Haas JM, Strait GB: Pacemaker induced cardiovascular failure: Hemodynamic and angiographic observations. *Am J Cardiol* 1974; 33:295–299.
44. Mines GR: On dynamic equilibrium in cardiac muscle. *Arch J Physiol* 1913; 46:349–383.
45. Hayes DL, Furman S: Atrioventricular and ventriculoatrial conduction times in patients undergoing pacemaker implant. *PACE* 1983; 6:38–46.
46. Stewart WJ, DiCola VC, Harthorne JW, Gillam LD, Weyman AE: Doppler ultrasound measurement of cardiac output in patients with physiologic pacemakers: effects of left ventricular function and retrograde ventriculoatrial conduction. *Am J Cardiol* 1984; 54:308–312.
47. Kruse I, Arnman K, Conradson TB, Ryden L: A comparison of the acute and long-term hemodynamics of ventricular inhibited and atrial synchronous ventricular inhibited pacing. *Circulation* 1982; 65:846–855.
48. DiCola VC, Hand R, Boucher CA, Kanarek DJ, Okada R, Pohost GM, Harthorne JW: Exercise cardiopulmonary assessment with dual chamber versus ventricular pacing. 7th World Congress of Cardiac Pacing, Vienna, Austria, May 1983. *PACE* 1983; 6:300.
49. Stoney W, Addlestone R, Alford W, Burrus G, Frist R, Thomas C: The incidence of venous thrombosis following long term transvenous pacing. *Ann Thorac Surg* 1976; 22:166–170.
50. Kinney E, Allen R, Weidner W, Peirce W, Leaman D, Zelis R: Recurrent pulmonary emboli secondary to right atrium thrombus around a permanent pacing catheter: a case report and review of the literature. *PACE* 1979; 2:196–202.
51. Pasquariello JL, Hariman RJ, Yudelman IM, Feit A, Gomes JAC, El-Sherif N: Recurrent pulmonary embolization following implantation of transvenous pacemaker. *PACE* 1984; 7:790–793.

24 Sudden Cardiac Death

Thomas N. James, MD, MACP

Sudden cardiac death knows no geographic or political boundaries, it affects both sexes at any and every age, and it spares no ethnic or cultural group anywhere. The exact etiology of sudden death may differ and its statistical rank among all medical problems varies from one place to another, but every citizen of the world is vulnerable to some degree.

In the United States about 400,000 sudden cardiac deaths occur annually. Even by the most optimistic estimates fewer than 1% of these may be prevented by the active application of every presently known means available for the purpose. Any hope of reducing this awesome toll will require the urgent acquisition of much more knowledge about the pathogenesis of sudden cardiac death. At both of two recent international meetings dedicated to an examination of the question of sudden cardiac death (the Fifteenth Bethesda Conference of the American College of Cardiology[1] and a Working Group on Sudden Cardiac Death convened by the World Health Organization[2]) it was concluded that the paramount present need is more knowledge about the basic underlying mechanisms leading to lethal instability of the electrical activity of the heart, which is thought by all to be the most prevalent terminal event.

One important principle for understanding sudden cardiac death is to place the matter of coronary disease in an appropriate conceptual context. Contrary to popular assertion, these two subjects are not synonymous; that mistaken belief serves as a regrettable distraction and leads to some erroneous deductions. Most patients with coronary disease do not die suddenly. Indeed, most of them live long and useful lives with a large number dying eventually of something other than coronary disease. Coronary disease is only very slowly progressive, often over a period of decades. What happened at one given moment in a decades-long progression to cause sudden death? What is different about the equally severe coronary disease in two patients, one of whom died suddenly and the other did not? Suggested answers have included changes in coronary tone (spasm), transient or more prolonged thromboses or platelet aggregations, and changes in autonomic neural control of the heart. Undoubtedly these events may contribute to an explanation, but in a given case they are often difficult to assess. By focusing too much attention upon coronary atherosclerosis we neglect what may be much more treatable problems, and ones that may have at least as devastating immediate effects.

Although it cannot be denied that the presence of coronary disease contributes to an unstable milieu in the heart, it is not alone in this effect. Yet, postmortem studies of the heart from victims of sudden cardiac death are too often limited to a search for obstruction in one or more of the major coronary arteries. It is unusual for similar attention to be directed to the *small coronary arteries*, even though these include the specific blood supply to the conduction system. Careful examination of the *conduction system* itself is so rarely performed that the number of laboratories in the world that are seriously dedicated to this purpose can probably be counted on the fingers of two hands. For moment-to-moment influence upon cardiac performance (including its electrical activity) the *nerves and ganglia* of the heart are even more dominant than the coronary arteries, yet it is rare to hear or read of any description of them. *Left ventricular hypertrophy* may be noted by the prosector in passing, but in sudden cardiac death it is one of the most frequent anatomic abnormalities. It is well established that greater myocardial mass increases the hazard of electrical instability.

For heuristic purposes as well as for scientific honesty we should ask whether severe coronary disease, even when present, is or is not the major contributing abnormality to sudden cardiac death. At least equal consideration must be awarded to the presence or absence of appropriate abnormalities in small coronary arteries,[3] to the presence or absence of ventricular hypertrophy with focal fibrosis, to abnormalities of cardiac nerves and ganglia collectively termed cardioneuropathies,[4] to normal and abnormal structural variations in the cardiac conduction system,[5] and to the interplay of all of these with each other and with diseases of the large coronary arteries.

If the broad question of sudden cardiac death is studied, an inescapable lesson is that it occurs in a surprisingly large variety of diseases that have little or no relation to coronary atherosclerosis. These include scleroderma,[6] amyloidosis,[7] sarcoidosis,[8] and many other systemic diseases. For such studies of the pathogenesis of sudden death one attractive advantage is the distinctive histologic characteristics that permit accurate determination of whether the underlying disease involved the heart, particularly the sinus node or atrioventricular (AV) node or His bundle, including their vascular and neural elements. From such information one can retrospectively construct reasonable hypotheses as to what the terminal electrical events may have been. One excellent example is the benign congenital polycystic tumor of the AV node (so-called mesothelioma) which causes heart block and eventually sudden death, but even there it is a puzzle why death occurs when it does, sometimes as late as the seventh or eighth decade of life.[9] Whether the underlying abnormality in any of these systemic diseases proves to be some focal destruction of a component of the cardiac conduction system or its blood supply or innervation, or whether it is the increased ventricular myocardial mass intermingled with focal fibrosis, we must ask how often are any or all of these same types of abnormalities present in the patient who dies with extensive coronary disease? It is just the kind of systematic and comprehensive study that badly needs to be done, but to my best knowledge it has never been attempted. To illustrate these generally neglected but fundamentally important subjects, the following sections will review each of them separately.

THE CONDUCTION SYSTEM OF THE HEART

The growth of knowledge about normal sinus impulse formation and its propagation within the heart comprises a fascinating chapter in the history of our ideas in medicine and cardiology.[10] Many elements of the heart participate in electrical conduction, which ultimately reaches virtually every myocyte. As a corollary, it is generally thought that many different places in the heart may serve as its source of cardiac rhythm given appropriate circumstances. However, this discussion will be limited to the sinus node and to the AV node plus His bundle for the following reasons. All normal rhythm originates within the sinus node, and all normal conduction traverses the AV node and His bundle. Furthermore, the most effective stable escape rhythm in man probably originates near the junction of the AV node and His bundle just as it does experimentally in the dog.[11] This is not to say that other subsidiary ectopic rhythms do not occur, nor that aberrant conduction is never a problem, but only that for the usual or most frequently encountered circumstances it is the sinus node and the AV junctional structures that are the most important.

In man the sinus node contains two special kinds of myocytes[12] which are organized into an interweaving lattice of distinctive cell clusters (P cells) connected by slender fibers (transitional cells). The entire sinus node contains a normally dense collagenous framework surrounding a conspicuously large central artery (Figure 24.1). There are abundant nerves within the sinus node but rarely any ganglia. However, ganglia are numerous at the margins of the sinus node, particularly near its posterior margin. Either normally variant structural changes or influences of disease can affect any of these components of the sinus node, or the sinus node as a whole. For example, advanced amyloidosis virtually destroys the entire sinus node and leaves only sparse collections of recognizable myoctyes (Figure 24.2). A similar process is characteristic of scleroderma heart disease wherein dense scirrhous fibrosis may entirely replace the sinus node (Figure 24.1). In lupus erythematosus the periarterial inflammation may serve as a centrifugally sweeping wave of tissue necrosis that destroys the sinus node (Figure 24.3).

Because of its anatomic proximity to the epicardium (less than 1 mm), the sinus node is anatomically involved in most cases of pericarditis.[13] This involvement includes not only portions of the myocytes of the node but also neighboring neural elements, whereby it may contribute to the pathogenesis of atrial arrhythmias. Either as part of other abnormalities in the sinus node or as separate

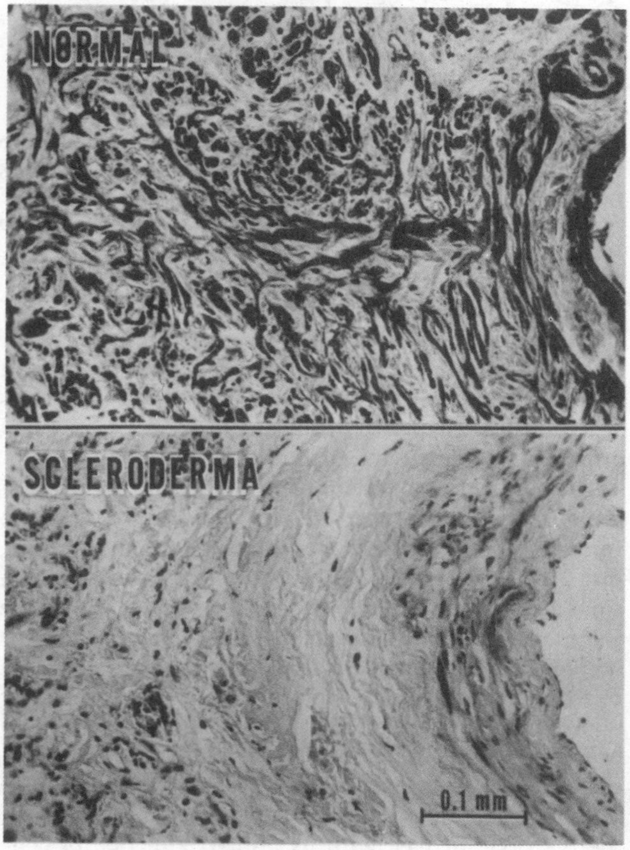

Figure 24.1. These two photomicrographs of human sinus node illustrate its usual architecture as normally seen (*top*) to contrast with the obliterative fibrosis characteristic of the sinus node in scleroderma heart disease (*bottom*) (Goldner trichrome stain; magnifications shown with reference bar; both are the same magnification).

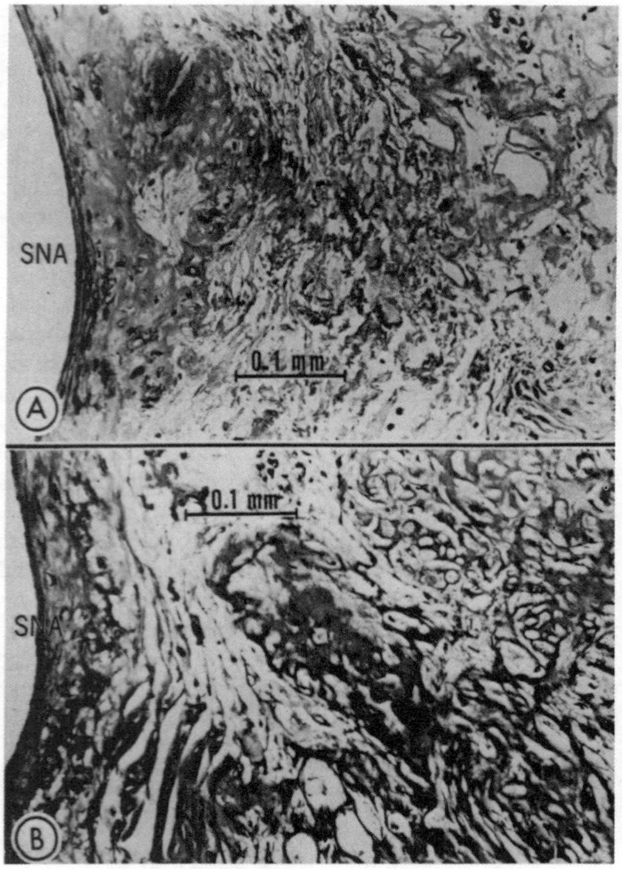

Figure 24.2. In cardiac amyloidosis the sinus node is often completely replaced. These two sections are from the sinus node of a man dying of atrial arrhythmias and amyloidosis. SNA is sinus node artery and all remaining area is the replaced sinus node. *A,* Goldner trichrome stain; *B*, congo red; magnifications are shown with a reference bar.

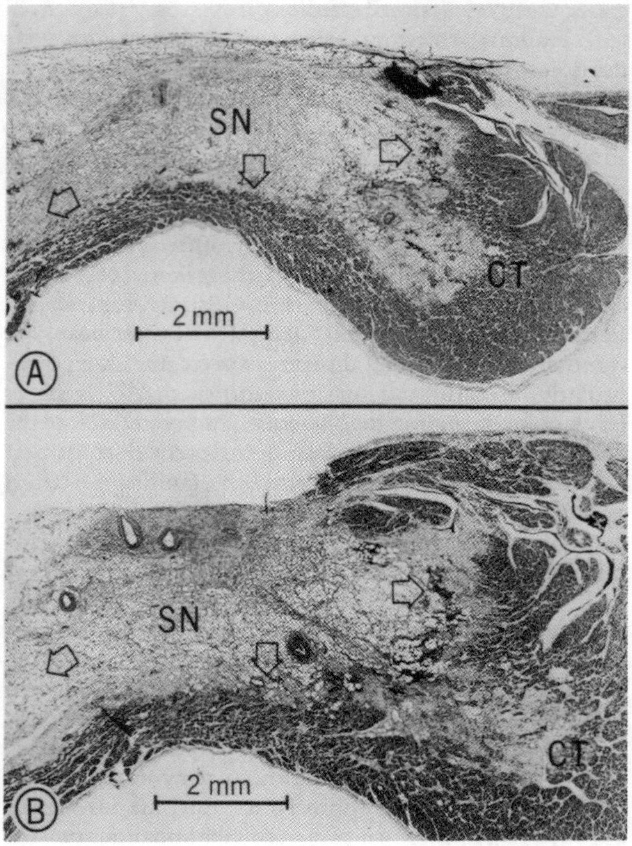

Figure 24.3. Two sections of sinus node (SN) from the heart of a patient with lupus erythematosus who died with atrial arrhythmias. Margins of a centrifugal inflammatory destructive process (*open arrows*) extend away from the sinus node artery into the adjacent crista terminalis (CT) of the right atrium (Goldner trichrome stain; magnifications shown with reference bar).

important components of some systemic disease, both the sinus node artery and the node's neural elements may be damaged or destroyed, but these will be dealt with elsewhere in this chapter by dedicated discussions of small arteries of the heart and of cardioneuropathies.

At the junction of the interatrial and interventricular septa of the human heart the AV node and His bundle form contiguous structures, with the former funneling into the latter (Figure 24.4). In the AV node as in the sinus node, there are two types of myocytes, but there is a much less dense collagenous framework and there is no regularly placed central artery. Furthermore, there are fewer P cells than in the sinus node and proportionately more transitional cells.[14] Because P cells are thought to be the normal site of impulse formation[15] and transitional cells probably serve mainly as electrical distributors of this impulse,[16] the different cytologic characteristics of the AV node fit well with its primary function of conduction. The His bundle is composed principally of longitudinally arrayed strands of Purkinje-type cells with the strands divided from each other by thin collagen sheaths.[17]

It is possible for normal AV conduction to be interrupted by congenital discontinuities of the AV node and His bundle, and some of these anomalous situations may be heritable.[18] Various acquired diseases may produce similar disruption of anatomic continuity and of AV conduction and sometimes they are associated with sudden cardiac death. Examples include tumors such as fibromas[19] or "mesotheliomas."[9] Focal inflammation or necrosis or fibrosis within the conduction system may be the consequence of any of the arteritic diseases[20,21] or scleroderma[6] or focal ischemic degeneration as is observed in congenital homocystinuria.[22] A special affinity for the AV node and His bundle may exist in hemachromatosis when it involves the heart, which may explain the increased incidence of heart block in such patients.[23] As with the sinus node, the local nutrient arteries and neural elements are often the site of important disease, but these will be included in the separate discussion of those topics.

Finally, there is an assortment of normal variations in the morphologic aspects of the AV node and His bundle which cannot be considered pathologic but which may nevertheless be functionally significant relative to the electrical activity of the heart.[24] The widely dispersed and fragmented AV node and His bundle, which are completely normal in the heart of the human fetus, are pro-

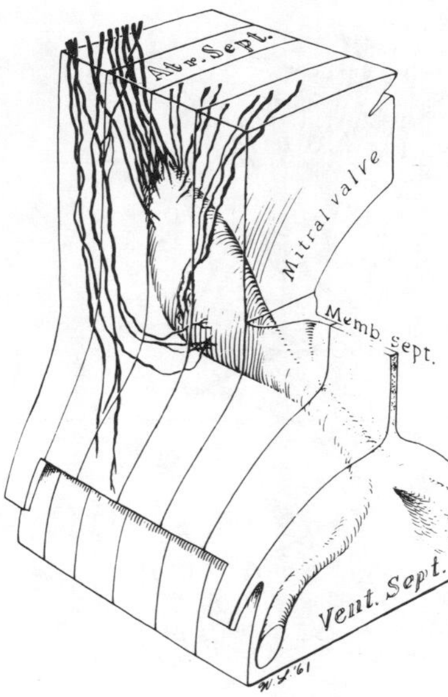

Figure 24.4. Schematic drawing of the atrioventricular (AV) node and His bundle of the human heart. Dark wavy lines represent normal input to the AV node from the internodal pathways. See Figures 6 to 8 for description of functionally important normal variations in this regional anatomy, as discussed in the text. Atr sept=atrial septum; memb sept=membranous septum; vent sept=ventricular septum.

gressively transformed during an important postnatal molding and shaping process which may take several years but is usually completed in early childhood. Although these are normal and ubiquitous events which result in the more smoothly outlined adult AV nodes and His bundles, they may nevertheless be associated with episodes of electrical instability and thereby contribute to the pathogenesis of sudden death in infants (so-called crib death).[25] In some persons this postnatal morphogenesis is never completed, leaving the AV node and His bundle with persistent fetal dispersion of their fibers (Figure 24.5) which may in turn contribute to fractionation of conduction, or pre-excitation, or the development of parasystole or re-entrant tachycardia (Figures 24.6 to 24.8).[26] An opposite form of derangement in postnatal morphogenetic abnormality is the excessive (rather than deficient) events that end in fibrotic destruction of the AV node or His bundle with anatomic discontinuity ending in complete heart block.[27]

CARDIONEUROPATHIES

In every postmortem examination of the heart the major coronary arteries are inspected with care, particularly in cases of sudden death. Such examination is of obvious importance, given that narrowing or occlusion of the major coronary arteries can produce both mechanical and electrical instability of the heart. However, for moment-to-moment control of the factors governing cardiac rhythm, conduction, and repolarization there is at least as powerful an influence exerted by its nerves. Neural

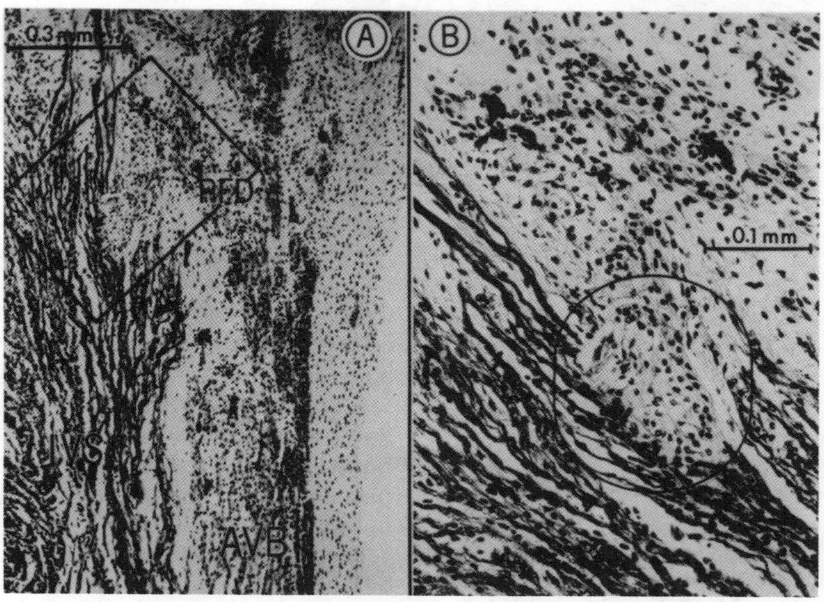

Figure 24.5. Persistent fetal dispersion (PFD) of the atrioventricular node or His bundle (AVB) is a normal variation of postnatal morphogenesis of these structures, shown here from the heart of a child who died suddenly. Area boxed in *A* is presented at a higher magnification in *B* where the cells encircled are seen attached to the crest of the interventricular septum (IVS) but are separated from other conduction tissue. Such cells forming a protected nest of specialized tissue are in an ideal location to function as sources of parasystolic rhythm (Goldner trichrome stain; magnifications shown with reference bar).

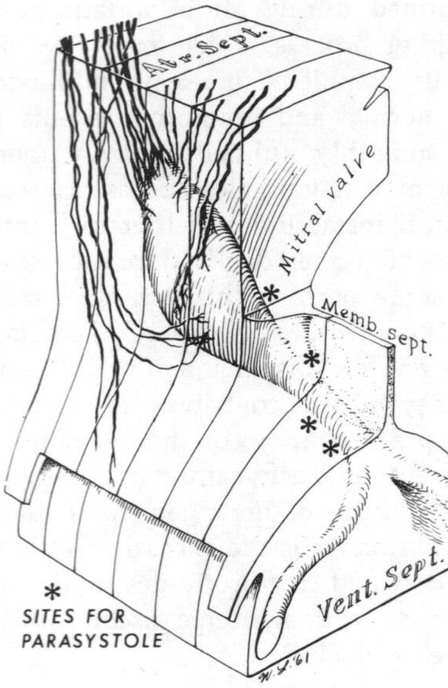

Figure 24.6. Fragments of conduction tissue from the atrioventricular node and His bundle can be found sequestered at any of the sites marked with asterisks, and can serve as the foci from which parasystolic rhythms may originate. Atr sept=atrial septum; memb sept=membranous septum; vent sept=ventricular septum.

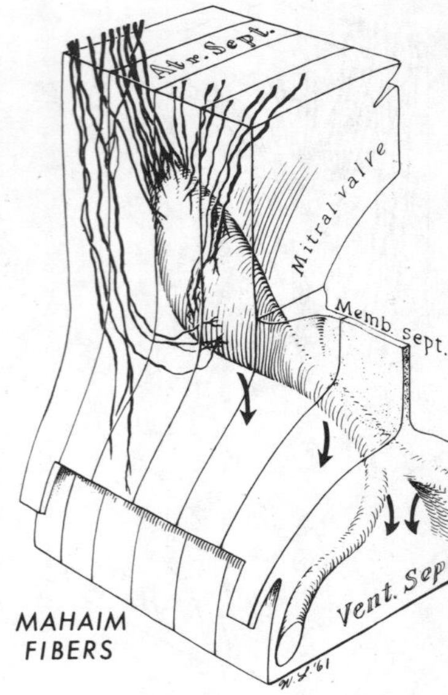

Figure 24.8. Mahaim fibers may course from either the atrioventricular (AV) node or His bundle or proximal segments of a bundle branch directly to the crest of the interventricular septum. Although they may serve to excite ventricular myocardium in an abnormal sequence, they cannot alone cause preexcitation because they originate distal to the probable point of normal AV nodal delay. Atr sept=atrial septum; memb sept=membranous septum; vent septum=ventricular septum.

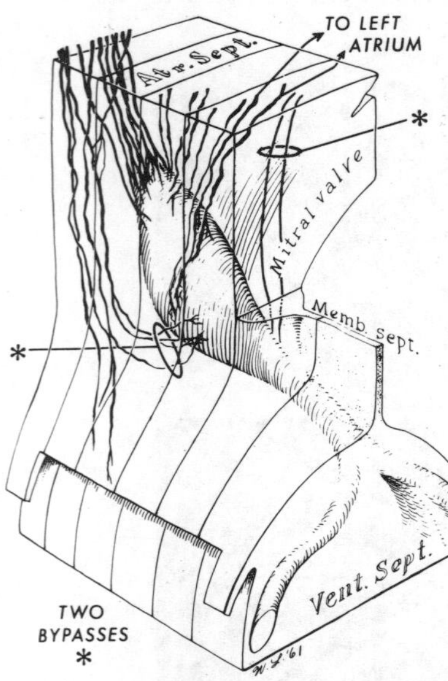

Figure 24.7. Two routes by which normal conduction through the atrioventricular (AV) node may be bypassed are indicated. Fibers from the posterior internodal pathway normally lie beneath the right atrial endocardium (*left asterisk*) overlying the AV node in all human hearts. In rare hearts some fibers (*right asterisk*) penetrate from the interatrial septum directly through the mitral annulus and central fibrous body to join the His bundle. Conduction by either route may contribute to the pathogenesis of preexcitation and reentrant tachycardias. Atr sept=atrial septum; memb sept=membranous septum; vent sept=ventricular septum.

control of the heart occurs not only through the intracardiac nerves and ganglia but also by way of those neural pathways responsible for all afferent and efferent traffic to and from the heart. Any of these neural elements may be the site of morphologic abnormalities with profound functional significance and each of them merits some consideration in evaluating any case of sudden unexpected death not otherwise explained. However, to assess for the heart the exact functional significance of a lesion in the brain or spinal cord would be difficult even for an experienced neuropathologist and may not presently be a practical routine. However, inspection of the major intrathoracic neural pathways such as the vagus or sympathetic trunks is feasible and some investigators have already begun such studies in association with their investigation of sudden death.[28] Even with our present knowledge of cardiac neurophysiology and anatomy, however, it should be expected that the intracardiac neural elements be examined in every case of sudden unexpected death.

Within the normal heart there is an enormous number of myelinated and unmyelinated nerves as well as many ganglia. These are particularly abundant in the vicinity of the cardiac conduction system,[29] but they are also present near the origin of the aorta and main pulmonary artery where there are additionally special neuroreceptors. A neuroreceptor, which may be particularly important relative to the stability of cardiac performance, is composed of one or more small clusters of specialized cells, all of which receive their blood supply from the proximal left coronary circulation, usually the main left coronary artery.[30] In both man and the dog the gross anatomy, histology, and ultrastructure of this tissue are remarkably similar.[31] Because experimental studies in the dog have established that the coronary chemoreceptor is the source of a powerful cardiogenic hypertensive chemoreflex which includes major effects upon cardiac electrical stability, any structural abnormalities of the coronary chemoreceptor in the human heart merit concern for their possible influence in the pathogenesis of sudden cardiac death. In a preliminary study[32] I found just such lesions in ten of eleven human hearts examined from cases of sudden death (Figures 24.9 and 24.10). Of course, each of these same hearts also exhibited an assortment of inflammatory and degenerative lesions in local nerves and ganglia within the region and elsewhere in the myocardium, as would be expected for most possible causes of cardioneuropathy.[4]

Abnormalities of intracardiac nerves, ganglia, or neuroreceptors may be the source of many different distortions within the neural control of the heart, particularly including its electrical activity. Early in the course of any cardioneuropathy the local influence may be excitatory or stimulative, leading to the generation of afferent neural signals. Then or subsequently there may also be some

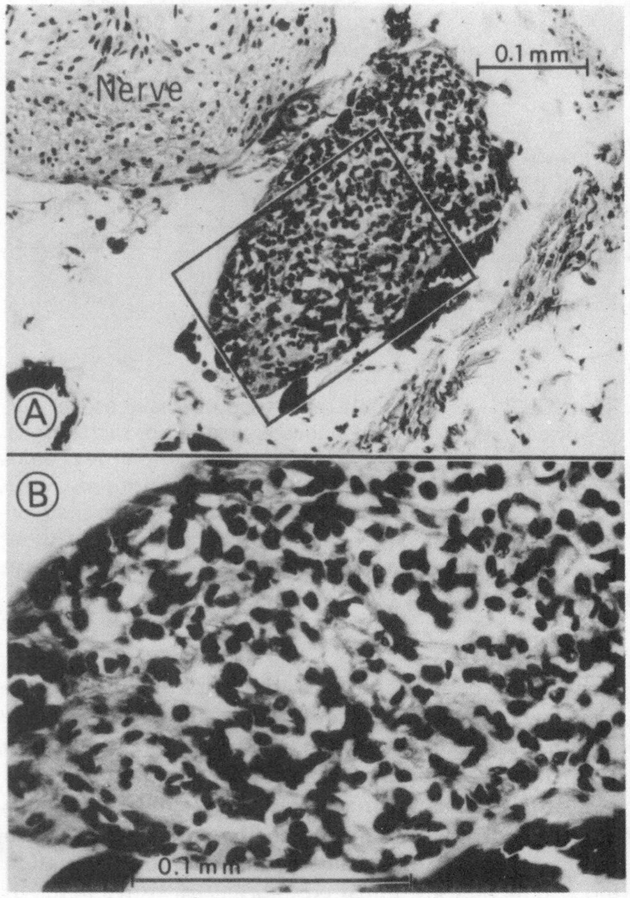

Figure 24.10. A different example of inflammatory destruction of the coronary chemoreceptor from another heart. Note extensive round cell infiltration throughout the chemoreceptor tissue. Area boxed in *A* is seen at a higher magnification in *B* (Goldner trichrome stain; magnifications shown with reference bar).

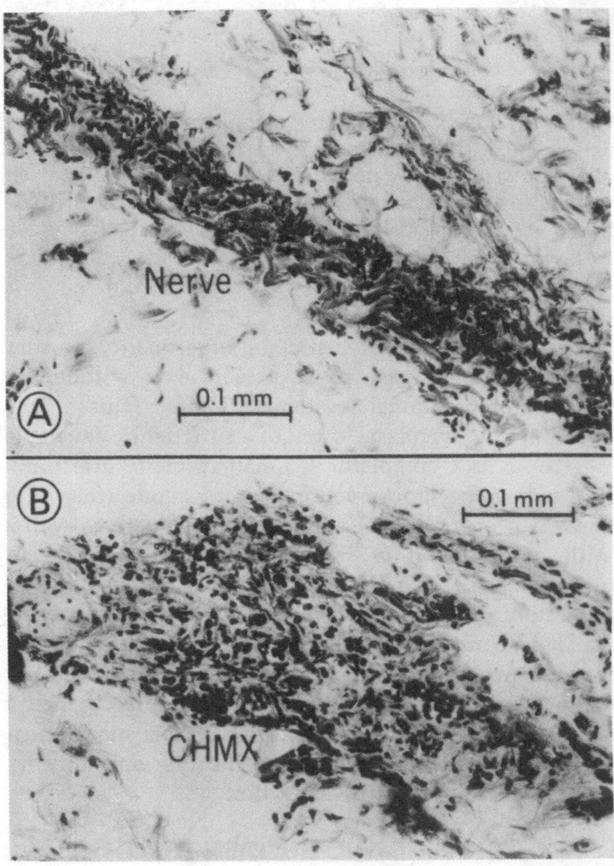

Figure 24.9. Inflammatory degeneration involving a cardiac nerve (*A*) and the coronary chemoreceptor "CHMX" (*B*) in a case of sudden death (Goldner trichrome stain; magnifications shown with reference bar).

distortion of efferent neural activity which could have originated either within the heart or elsewhere, including the brain. When neural traffic to the heart is interrupted, cardiac responses to cognitive processes and emotions become distorted. As a consequence there may be serious or even fatal changes in cardiac rhythm or conduction. Much more needs to be learned about this special subject.

SMALL ARTERIES OF THE HEART

There are at least three reasons why the careful examination of small coronary arteries is necessary in any postmortem attempt to assess the cause of sudden death (Figure 24.11). First, all the blood flow through major coronary arteries normally continues through its smaller branches (defined, for the purpose of discussion, as those 0.1 to 1.0 mm in diameter). Second, vessels of this size comprise most of the potentially effective coronary anastomoses. Third, both the sinus node artery and AV node artery belong in this category. Therefore, even if a large coronary artery is fully patent but its terminating branches are narrowed or occluded, the end result is focal ischemia, degeneration, and eventual fibrosis. If enough

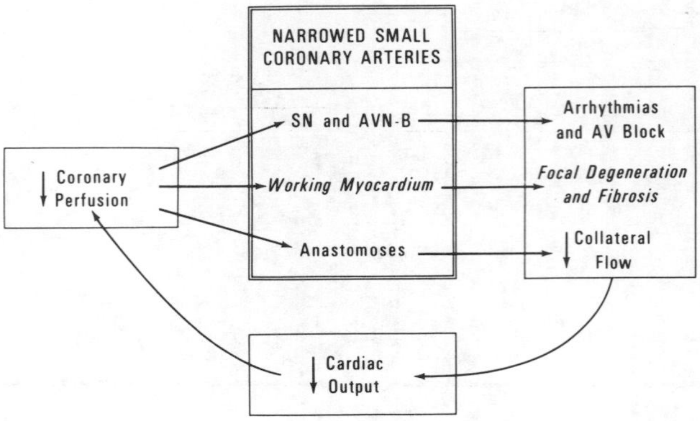

Figure 24.11. Functional significance of small coronary artery disease is depicted using three categories of such vessels: those of the conduction system (sinus node [SN] and atrioventricular node–His bundle [AVN-B]), those perfusing working myocardium of atria and ventricles, and all the intercoronary anastomoses. Progressive narrowing of any of these groups has a cascading effect, compounding the significance in all categories.

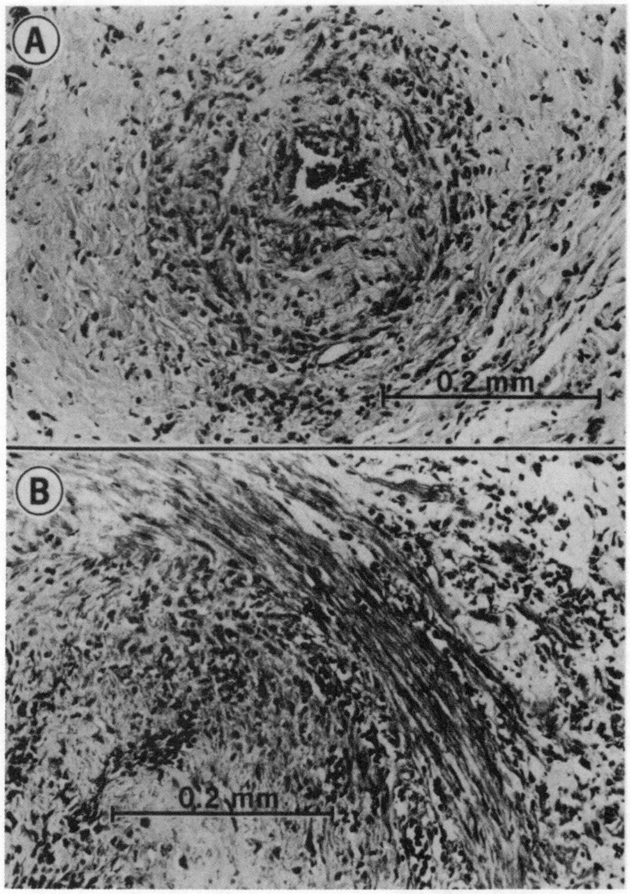

Figure 24.12. Two photomicrographs illustrating marked narrowing of the sinus node artery (*A*) and atrioventricular node artery (*B*) in a fatal case of polyarteritis nodosa with terminal events including atrial arrhythmias and heart block (Goldner trichrome stain; magnifications shown with reference bar).

such vessels become involved, the extent of fibrosis becomes widespread and confluent scars appear. If the anastomoses become narrowed, then collateral circulation is impaired and any additional cause of focal or general myocardial ischemia produces a compounded effect. If either or both of the arteries to the conduction system become narrowed or occluded, then impulse formation and conduction are impaired and electrical instability is often the result.

Assessment of the significance of disease of the small coronary arteries is made difficult in part by their large number, particularly in the ventricular myocardium, but it is nevertheless feasible.[3] For studies of sudden cardiac death it should be mandatory that at least those small arteries supplying the sinus node, AV node, and His bundle be carefully examined. As a corollary, the presence and exact location of any obstructive lesions within the large epicardial coronary branches should take into consideration whether these are proximal or distal to the origin of the small nutrient vessels of the conduction system.[33]

A wide variety of pathologic processes may be responsible for obstruction of small coronary arteries, including those diseases that may cause abnormalities in coagulation such as disseminated intravascular coagulation,[34] thrombotic thrombocytopenic purpura,[35] and congenital homocystinuria.[22] Every collagen disease in some persons afflicted will have an effect upon the small coronary arteries (Figure 24.12), examples including disseminated lupus erythematosus,[36] polyarteritis nodosa,[20] and rheumatoid arthritis.[21] Each of these diseases may also involve large coronary artery branches as well as the pericardium and in many cases the cardiac valves or nerves and ganglia. Certain infiltrative diseases such as amyloidosis[7] or granulomatoses such as sarcoidosis[8] may also cause the small coronary arteries to become narrowed. It need hardly be added that for each of these diseases sudden cardiac death is not a rare terminal event.

There is one special histologic abnormality of small coronary arteries that may be present even without any of the aforementioned systemic diseases. This is focal fibromuscular dysplasia, often of a sufficiently severe degree to occlude completely a small coronary artery. Examples have been observed in the sinus node artery (Figure 24.13) of victims of sudden cardiac death as well as in the AV node artery (Figure 24.14). A remarkable feature of these lesions is the absence of conspicuous degeneration or a local inflammatory response, suggesting that it is a primary proliferative dysplasia rather than a consequence of other local disease. An attractive alternative explanation may be some local disturbance in neural control with or without detectable morphologic abnormalities of the responsible nerves, and this hypothesis merits future investigation.

CHANCE AND SUDDEN DEATH

One frequently encountered source of confusion in discussions or reviews of the subject of sudden death is the tendency (perhaps more honestly a wish) to define a single or only a few responsible factors. For example, the

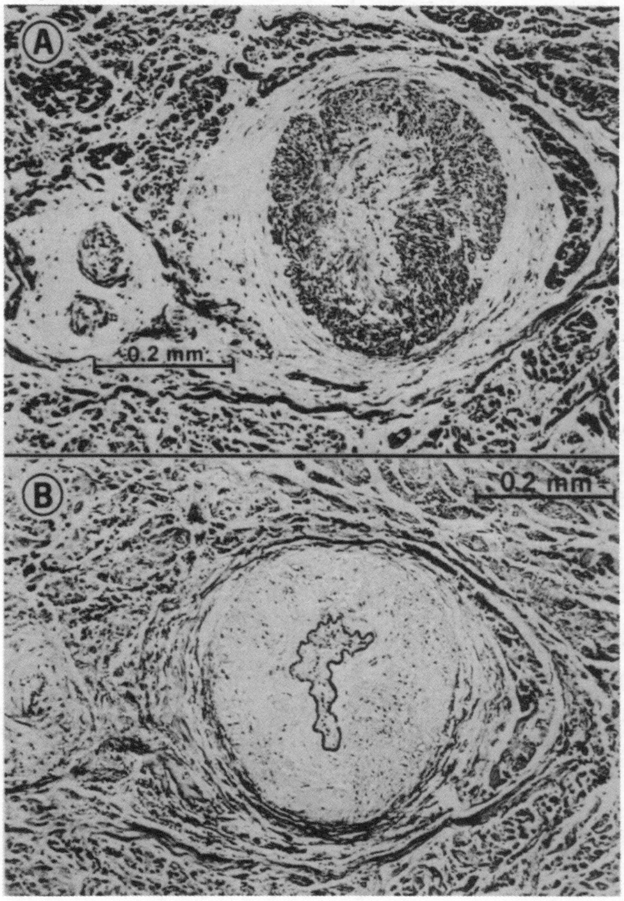

Figure 24.13. Focal fibromuscular dysplasia of the sinus node artery depicted with two adjacent histologic sections in a case of sudden death in a young athlete. The entire lumen of the vessel is obliterated. *A,* Goldner trichrome stain; *B,* Verhoeff-Van Gieson elastic stain; magnifications shown with reference bar.

distracting tendency to make sudden death and coronary artery disease synonymous subjects for discussion does a disservice to both questions. Although it is true that they often coexist, and equally true that coronary artery disease has many ways in which it may predispose to sudden death, what remains unknown and rarely sought is the great number of other contributing factors that coexist in the hearts of victims of sudden death. Such factors, which often also coexist with coronary artery disease, include left ventricular hypertrophy, small coronary artery disease (not itself a form of atherosclerosis, at least as conventionally defined), and cardioneuropathies, as well as a broad array of additional factors (Table 24.1). The surest lesson from careful thought about this multiplicity of factors is that the etiology of sudden cardiac death is more often than not a very complex matter. Rather than one or a few, the usual situation is a mosaic pattern of factors, many of which come and go or change unpredictably.

As I previously admonished in considering sudden death,[37] the scientific mind abhors uncertainty of this nature and will in every way possible reject complicating circumstances in favor of simpler ones, so long as that can honestly be done. Unfortunately, the weight of evidence indicates that the subject is inescapably complex, particularly as to etiology, so that it behooves us to work with that situation as best we can. In every case of sudden cardiac death multiple contributing factors most likely led to the end result. Some of these factors may still have been operative at the time of death, whereas others had come and gone but were nevertheless materially important. Some of the factors may currently be recognizable by anatomic, biochemical, or other currently available methods, but others will require new methods. From each case of sudden cardiac death suitably investigated there is much to learn, regardless of whether the death was

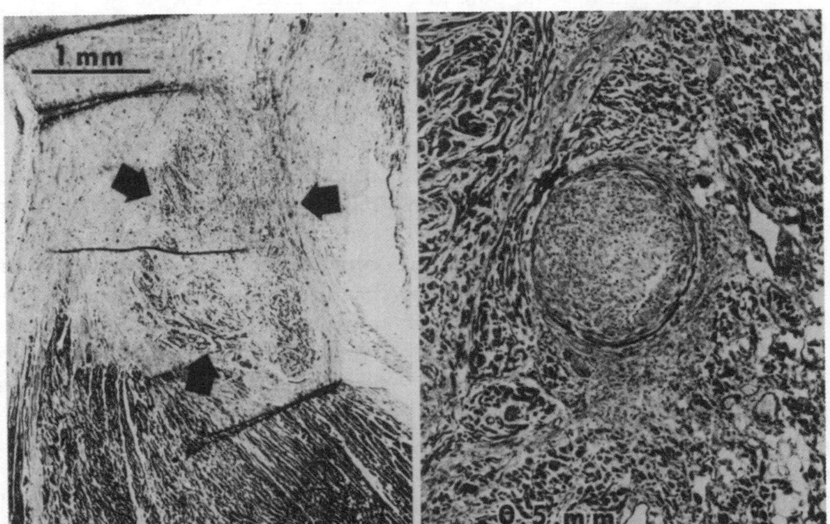

Figure 24.14. Focal fibromuscular dysplasia may also involve the atrioventricular (AV) node artery and lead to destructive fibrosis of the proximal portion of the His bundle (*black arrows on left*) which it normally supplies. The responsible artery is shown within the same patient's AV node on the *right*. Complete heart block was present (Goldner trichrome stain; magnifications shown with reference bar).

Table 24.1. Partial Listing of Acute and Chronic Factors Known or Suspected to Participate in the Pathogenesis of Sudden Cardiac Death*

Acute Factors	Chronic Factors
Platelet aggregations	Left ventricular hypertrophy
Excitatory or inhibitory reflexes	Coronary atherosclerosis
Coronary spasm	Persistent fetal dispersion of AV node, His bundle or both
Cardioneuropathy	Cardioneuropathy
Myocarditis	Myocarditis
Fright	Grief
Arteritis	Sustained hypertension
Sepsis	Infiltrative diseases (amyloidosis, hemachromatosis, sarcoidosis, etc)
Coronary thrombosis	Focal fibrosis (scleroderma, chronic ischemia)
Acute myocardial infarction	Medications (by physician or other)
Acute focal ischemia	Endocrinopathies (thyroid, adrenal)
Acute hypertension	Long QT interval
Sudden hypotension	Malnutrition
Arrhythmias or heart block	Ethanol
Long QT interval	Tobacco smoking
Hypoxia	Small coronary artery disease
Acidosis or alkalosis	Diurnal rhythms
Ion imbalance (especially K+, Ca++)	Climatic changes
Fever	Obesity
Dehydration	Valvular heart disease
Medications (by physician or other)	Cardiomyopathy
Ethanol	
Dysautonomia	
Physical stress	

* Not presented in any order of priority or known relative importance. Two or more of these factors are likely to coexist or to follow sequentially. Some factors exist as both acute and chronic influences.

witnessed or not, whether it occurred within seconds, minutes, or hours, and whether any associated known cardiac or noncardiac disease was present. To restrict or limit the definition of sudden death for research purposes may suit some needs, eg, large epidemiologic programs, but such restriction inevitably diminishes the potential value of postmortem anatomic investigations and may exclude the discovery of findings potentially valuable for all forms of nonepidemiologic research.

It is not nihilistic to admit that chance plays a large role in the pathogenesis of sudden cardiac death. On the contrary, if that is the truth, as the weight of present evidence suggests, then it is only by investigating the determinants of each factor contributing to the final fatal aggregation of circumstances that we can ever hope to mount optimally successful programs aimed at better diagnosis and prevention of as many such factors as possible.

FUTURE STUDIES

When estimating that less than 1% of all sudden cardiac deaths can possibly be prevented or reversed by all currently available methods for the purpose, it is not my intent to suggest that those methods should be ignored. On the contrary, one type of future effort should be the better application of known methods and the improvement of ones now available. However, if we are to recruit new methods and more effective approaches, the larger need is for more research into the panorama of etiologic factors involved. The lengthy list that may currently be tabulated (Table 24.1) gives some idea of the enormity of the work to be done, but even that list is almost certainly incomplete.

From the vantage point of personal work and experience, I suggest that one of the more promising areas for better study is the autopsy. Every serious investigation of the hearts of victims of sudden cardiac death should require careful examination of the cardiac conduction system, of small coronary arteries including those nutrient to the sinus node and AV node, and of nerves and ganglia with particular attention to those in the vicinity of the conduction system, and of the coronary chemoreceptor (Figures 24.9, 24.10). Although special immunofluorescent or other histochemical approaches, electron microscopy, and biochemical measurements all indisputably have their role in such studies, the sad truth is that for most of the proposed examinations even simple light microscopic histologic investigation has been neglected and ignored. From better performance of these simple histologic investigations we can hope to derive more accurately designed and more effective forms of sophisticated (and more expensive) research.

Sudden unexpected death is not limited to the affliction of man but may occur in a wide variety of other animals. It is probably ubiquitous in the fauna of nature. Several instructive examples have been recognized in the dog,[38-40] and more attention should be directed to the investigation of such examples from this readily available species. The accumulation of knowledge about sudden death in dogs will not only enlarge our understanding of the human problem but also contribute to the improvement of breeding methods and health care of the dogs. Some dogs and horses are incredibly valuable financial investments and the preservation of them has large monetary dimensions. When one of them dies suddenly, the event is always newsworthy but regrettably too rarely taken as a special opportunity for research. On an even broader scale, livestock and other domestic animals constitute an enormous economic resource in both highly developed and less developed countries, and the prevention of their sudden death can offer both financial and other rewards, such as better human nutrition and the facilitation of agricultural methods.

Finally, there are special forms of sudden death that appear limited to special geographic regions of the world or perhaps are only best recognized there. A better understanding of these regional examples may provide unexpected enlightenment concerning sudden death in far regions. Just as it has been emphasized that the factors leading to sudden death are usually multiple and often unpredictable, there are some factors that may be present in previously unsuspected frequency and in many different places or countries throughout the world. A systematic method for sharing such work and the knowledge obtained from such collaborative studies could provide rich dividends for all involved. Not the least of these would be a worldwide effort with a humanitarian purpose and leading to international benefits as well as good will.

SUMMARY

Sudden cardiac death is a worldwide problem. Its study can be approached from several directions, but one of the most useful is careful postmortem examination of the heart, the findings from which can lead to many precise additional avenues of investigation. Although coronary artery disease is often associated with sudden cardiac death, the proof of its causative role remains vague and in many cases unsatisfactory. On the basis of a large personal experience with clinicopathologic correlative studies in cases of sudden cardiac death, other elements of the postmortem examination of the heart are discussed and their more frequent use encouraged. These include the cardiac conduction system, small arteries of the heart, and the neural elements within the heart such as nerves, ganglia, and special neuroreceptors. In most cases of sudden cardiac death more than one important cause contributes to its pathogenesis, and the concurrence of these factors is most often by chance. This element of chance and its role in sudden death must be recognized and duly considered in the planning of future research directed at the discovery of means to prevent as many components of the pathogenesis as possible.

Acknowledgment: This work was supported by grants from the National Heart, Lung, and Blood Institute (HL 11,310 and HL 17,667), National Institutes of Health, Bethesda, Maryland, and by the Daniel Webster Cline Memorial Fund for Cardiovascular Research, Birmingham, Alabama.

REFERENCES

1. Fifteenth Bethesda Conference: Sudden Cardiac Death. *J Am Coll Cardiol*(suppl), 1985; 5:1B–198B.
2. Report of a WHO Scientific Group on Sudden Cardiac Death. WHO Technical Report Series, 1985 (in press).
3. James TN: Small arteries of the heart. The 36th George E. Brown Memorial Lecture. *Circulation* 1977; 56:2–14.
4. James TN: Primary and secondary cardioneuropathies and their functional significance. *J Am Coll Cardiol* 1983; 2:983–1002.
5. James TN: Normal and abnormal variations in morphology of the atrioventricular node and His bundle: Functional significance relative to sudden death, NIH Publication No. 84. Third USA-USSR Joint Symposium on Sudden Cardiac Death, 1984, vol 1604, pp 1–23.
6. James TN: De Subitaneis Mortibus. VIII. Coronary arteries and conduction system in scleroderma heart disease. *Circulation* 1974; 50:844–856.
7. James TN: Pathology of the cardiac conduction system in amyloidosis. *Ann Intern Med* 1966; 65:28–36.
8. James TN: De Subitaneis Mortibus. XXV. Sarcoid heart disease. *Circulation* 1977; 56:320–326.
9. James TN, Galakhov I: De Subitaneis Mortibus. XXVI. Fatal electrical instability of the heart associated with benign congenital polycystic tumor of the atrioventricular node. *Circulation* 1977; 56:667–678.
10. James TN: The development of ideas concerning the conduction system of the heart. The Campbell Oration, 1982. *Ulster Med J* 1982; 51:81–97.
11. James TN, Isobe JH, Urthaler F: Correlative electrophysiological and anatomical studies concerning the site of origin of escape rhythm during complete atrioventricular block in the dog. *Circ Res* 1979; 45: 108–119.
12. James TN: The sinus node. *Am J Cardiol* 1977; 40:965–986.
13. James TN: Pericarditis and the sinus node. *Arch Intern Med* 1962; 110:301–311.
14. James TN: Structure and function of the AV junction. The Mikamo Lecture for 1982. *Jpn Circ J* 1983; 47:1–47.
15. Woods WT, Urthaler F, James TN: Spontaneous action potentials of cells in the canine sinus node. *Circ Res* 1976; 39:76–82.
16. Sherf L, James TN, Woods WT: Function of the atrioventricular node considered on the basis of observed histology and fine structure. *J Am Coll Cardiol* 1985; 5:770–780.
17. James TN, Sherf L: Fine structure of the His bundle. *Circulation* 1971; 44:9–28.
18. James TN, McKone RC, Hudspeth AS: De Subitaneis Mortibus. X. Familial congenital heart block. *Circulation* 1975; 51:379–388.
19. James TN, Carson DJL, Marshall TK: De Subitaneis Mortibus. I. Fibroma compressing His bundle. *Circulation* 1973; 48:428–433.
20. James TN, Birk RE: Pathology of the cardiac conduction system in polyarteritis nodosa and its variants. *Arch Intern Med* 1966; 177:561–567.
21. James TN: De Subitaneis Mortibus. XXIII. Rheumatoid arthritis and ankylosing spondylitis. *Circulation* 1977; 55:669–677.
22. James TN, Carson NAJ, Froggatt P: De Subitaneis Mortibus. IV. Coronary vessels and conduction system in homocystinuria. *Circulation* 1974; 49:367–374.
23. James TN: Pathology of the cardiac conduction system in hemachromatosis. *N Engl J Med* 1964; 271:92–94.
24. James TN, Marshall TK: De Subitaneis Mortibus. XVIII. Persistent fetal dispersion of AV node and His bundle within central fibrous body. *Circulation* 1976; 53:1026–1034.
25. James TN: Sudden death in babies: new observations in the heart. *Am J Cardiol* 1968; 22:479–506.
26. James TN: Normal and abnormal variations in anatomy of the atrioventricular node and His bundle and their relevance to the pathogenesis of re-entrant tachycardias and parasystolic rhythms, in Zipes DP, Jalife J(eds): *Cardiac Electrophysiology and Arrhythmias.* New York, Grune & Stratton, 1985, chap 33.
27. James TN, Spencer MS, Kloepfer JC: De Subitaneis Mortibus. XXI. Adult onset syncope, with comments on the nature of congenital heart block and the morphogenesis of the human atrioventricular septal junction. *Circulation* 1976; 54:1001–1009.
28. Rossi L: Cardioneuropathies and extracardiac neural disease. *J Am Coll Cardiol (suppl)* 1985; 5:66B–70B.
29. James TN: Cardiac innervation: anatomic and pharmacologic relations. *Bull NY Acad Med* 1967; 43:1041–1086.
30. James TN, Isobe JH, Urthaler F: Analysis of components in a hypertensive cardiogenic chemoreflex. *Circulation* 1975; 52:179–192.
31. Imamura K, James TN, Scully KT, Hageman GR, Urthaler F: Ultrastructure of a coronary chemoreceptor of dogs and cats. *J Mol Cell Cardiol* 1982; 14:711–724.
32. James TN: Degenerative lesions of a coronary chemoreceptor and nearby neural elements in the hearts of victims of sudden death. Proceedings of the Fourth USA-USSR Symposium on Sudden Death (in press).
33. James TN: *Anatomy of the Coronary Arteries.* Hagerstown, Md, Harper & Row Publishers Inc, 1961.
34. James TN, Marshall ML, Craig MW: De Subitaneis Mortibus. VII. Disseminated intravascular coagulation and paroxysmal atrial tachycardia. *Circulation* 1974; 50:395–401.

35. James TN, Monto RW: Pathology of the cardiac conduction system in thrombotic thrombocytopenic purpura. *Ann Intern Med* 1966; 65:37–43.
36. James TN, Rupe CE, Monto RW: Pathology of the cardiac conduction system in systemic lupus erythematosus. *Ann Intern Med* 1965; 63:402–410.
37. James TN: Chance and sudden death. *J Am Coll Cardiol* 1983; 1:164–183.
38. James TN, Drake EH: Sudden death in Doberman Pinschers. *Ann Intern Med* 1968; 68:821–829.
39. James TN: Congenital deafness and cardiac arrhythmias. *Am J Cardiol* 1967; 19:627–643.
40. James TN, Robertson BT, Waldo AL, Branch CE: De Subitaneis Mortibus. XV. Hereditary stenosis of the His bundle in Pug dogs. *Circulation* 1975; 52:1152–1160.

25 Cardiopulmonary Resuscitation: Recent Advances

James T. Niemann, MD and J. Michael Criley, MD

In the United States, nearly half a million people fall victim to sudden cardiac death each year.[1] The overwhelming majority of victims (90%) have significant underlying coronary artery disease[2] and sudden cardiac death, like atherosclerotic coronary artery disease, is largely encountered in industrialized nations. The prevalence of this "disease" in such nations has had a substantial financial impact, not only in terms of the sophistication of medical care (coronary care units and prehospital cardiac life support) and research directions, but also in terms of life expectancy and productivity of the populations at risk.

Sudden cardiac death is associated with acute coronary occlusion or fresh myocardial infarction, or both, in only 20% to 30% of victims (survivors and nonsurvivors).[3] In most instances, sudden death is the result of a malignant rhythm disturbance facilitated by chronic ischemic heart disease. Early and effective treatment of such rhythm disturbances could reduce the mortality from this manifestation of atherosclerotic coronary artery disease. Cardiopulmonary resuscitation (CPR), which provides artificial circulatory and ventilatory support during cardiopulmonary arrest, combined with pharmacologic and electrical treatment of rhythm disturbances, is an effective means of treating sudden death due to arrhythmias if used early.[4]

In this chapter, we will review recent advances and knowledge of systemic perfusion during closed-chest CPR, recently described closed-chest artificial circulatory support techniques that could improve outcome from cardiac arrest, and contemporary observations of drug effects during cardiac arrest and CPR.

MECHANISM OF BLOOD FLOW DURING CLOSED-CHEST CARDIOPULMONARY RESUSCITATION

The currently practiced technique of closed-chest artificial circulatory support used worldwide is largely the byproduct of feasibility studies of closed-chest defibrillation undertaken by Kouwenhoven et al.[5] These investigators noted that closed-chest or transthoracic countershock of ventricular fibrillation was unlikely to result in a spontaneous perfusing rhythm if defibrillation was not attempted within three minutes of the onset of fibrillation. However, if the thorax of experimental animals was rhythmically compressed during circulatory arrest, transthoracic countershock after up to 30 minutes of ventricular fibrillation could result in a spontaneous perfusing cardiac rhythm.

Thoracic compression during arrest produced arterial pressure fluctuations and flow and were presumed to result from "cardiac massage." It was postulated that the cardiac ventricles were selectively massaged or compressed between the boney structures of the thorax. Ventricular compression would result in predictable hemodynamic effects, leading to ventricular outflow, and pulmonary and systemic perfusion (Figure 25.1). In many respects, ventricular massage during cardiac arrest and thoracic compression were envisioned to produce hemodynamic changes and cardiac anatomic effects that approximated or duplicated those of spontaneous cardiac systoles. Although postulated, such a mechanism was never proven; nonetheless, the effects were impressive and did not require thoracotomy to maintain circulation and restore cardiac function. These noninvasive tech-

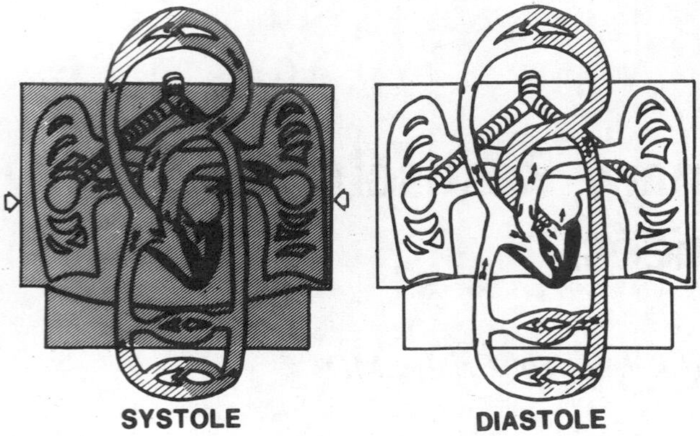

Figure 25.1. Closed-chest CPR hemodynamics: an alternative mechanism for systemic perfusion. During chest compression (CPR systole), there is an abrupt increase in intrathoracic pressure which is directly transmitted to all intrathoracic vascular compartments, the peripheral arterial bed, and the vascular compartments of the abdomen (shaded cross-hatched areas). Comparable increases in intraabdominal arterial and venous pressures are due to right heart reflex and diaphragmatic descent due to pressurization of the thorax. Lower venous pressures are maintained in the brachiocephalic and subdiaphragmatic extraabdominal venous beds due to venous valve closure. During CPR systole, the pulmonic valve closes, but the tricuspid valve is incompetent, resulting in right heart to inferior vena caval reflux (*arrows*). During chest compression, the mitral and aortic valves are open and blood flows (*arrows*) from the pulmonary venous reservoir to peripheral capillary beds protected by venous valves (unshaded cross-hatched areas), ie, brain and lower extremities. During the relaxation phase (CPR diastole), intrathoracic pressure decreases abruptly, the diaphragm ascends, and peripheral venous to right heart return occurs (*arrows*). The pulmonic valve opens and the pulmonary vascular reservoir refills (*arrows*). The aortic valve closes and during diastole an aortic-right atrial pressure difference exists to perfuse the myocardium (*large open arrow*).

niques for cardiac resuscitation, ie, closed-chest cardiac massage and countershock, were quickly embraced by clinicians in the United States and abroad.

Soon after its introduction into clinical practice, the purported mechanism of blood flow during "external cardiac massage" was questioned by the international medical community. Weale and Rothwell-Jackson[6] and MacKenzie et al[7] in the United Kingdom reported nearly identical arterial and venous pressures during cardiac arrest and closed-chest cardiac massage in experimental animals and patients. The absence of a substantial arteriovenous pressure gradient during closed-chest CPR would limit systemic perfusion and it suggested that the ventricles were not selectively compressed or massaged. In investigations in Nuremberg, Gall[8] demonstrated that competence of the atrioventricular valve during arrest and cardiac massage was critically dependent upon selective ventricular compression. Atrial compression produced venous pressures similar to those noted by Weale and MacKenzie. Thus, within five years of its introduction and widespread clinical use, the proposed mechanism of blood flow during closed-chest CPR was seriously questioned, but the issue was not addressed again for two decades.

In 1976, Criley et al[9] demonstrated that vigorous coughing during ventricular fibrillation resulted in arterial pressure fluctuations. This observation was made in patients in whom nonperfusing rhythm disturbances developed following the intracoronary injection of contrast medium. In the monitored setting, vigorous coughing prior to loss of consciousness resulted in peak aortic pressures comparable to those measured during closed-chest CPR when the latter technique had to be employed. Subsequent investigations demonstrated that cough-induced pressure fluctuations were associated with left heart outflow and arterial blood flow.[10] Hemodynamic findings during coughing supported an earlier hypothesis suggested by Weale and Rothwell-Jackson,[6] namely, that blood flow during closed-chest CPR might be the result of intrathoracic pressure changes rather than direct heart massage.

This alternative hypothesis for the mechanism of blood flow during closed-chest CPR has been supported by recent studies. Rudikoff et al[11] demonstrated that pressures recorded in intrathoracic vascular compartments (cardiac chambers and great vessels) were nearly equal during closed-chest CPR systole (thoracic compression) and that these pressures closely approximated intrapleural pressure fluctuations. Higher or more positive peak intrathoracic pressures during CPR systole were accompanied by greater arterial pressures and carotid arterial flows. Although chest compression did not produce an intrathoracic arteriovenous pressure gradient, an extrathoracic gradient was demonstrated between the great arteries and the jugular vein. Such a gradient would facilitate cerebral perfusion during cardiac arrest and closed-chest CPR. The lower pressure in the jugular venous bed was initially ascribed to collapse of the thin-walled veins at the superior thoracic inlet.

In our laboratory, a pressure-synchronized cineangiographic technique was used to study both the hemodynamic and the anatomic effects of closed-chest CPR.[12] A close correlation between arterial and intrathoracic pressure fluctuations and the absence of an intrathoracic arteriovenous pressure gradient area were again demonstrated. In addition, sternal depression (CPR systole) did not produce left heart compression, and closure of the atrioventricular valves did not occur during sternal depression. Pressures recorded in the intrathoracic great vessels and cardiac chambers were consistently greater than those measured in the brachiocephalic venous circulation. During chest compression and pressure-synchronized contrast studies, the abrupt increase in right atrial and central venous pressure resulted in closure of competent venous valves in the extrathoracic brachiocephalic venous bed. The cerebral perfusion gradient (arterial pressure minus jugular venous pressure) and left heart outflow during CPR systole were shown to be directly related to intrathoracic pressure changes, ie, the intrathoracic pressure generated during CPR systole was directly transmitted to the peripheral arterial bed, but the increase in right atrial pressure resulted in closure of venous valves in those venous beds in close proximity to the right heart. Some of these hemodynamic findings have been documented in the clinical population.[11,12] The cardiac anatomic changes that accompany sternal depression in patients have been described by Werner et al[13] using two-dimensional echocardiography and confirm experimental observations. In patients, the atrioventricular valves are open during chest compression and selective compression of the cardiac ventricles is minimal.

If selective ventricular compression occurred during cardiac arrest and closed-chest CPR, certain hemodynamic and anatomic events could be expected or predicted (Table 25.1). Actual observations in the experimental laboratory and in a limited clinical population are also summarized in Table 25.1. The disparity between the expected and the observed is obvious. This disparity supports an alternative mechanism for blood flow during CPR chest compression, namely, that blood flow is the result of phasic alterations in intrathoracic pressure.

REGIONAL BLOOD FLOW DURING CARDIOPULMONARY RESUSCITATION

Kouwenhoven et al[5] remarked that during closed-chest CPR, "adequate circulation for periods as long as 30 minutes was easily maintained with the dog in ventricular fibrillation. A closed-chest defibrillating shock would result in the immediate return of normal sinus rhythm in such animals." Adequacy of circulation was defined only in terms of response to countershock.

Contemporary investigations using state of the art techniques to measure regional blood flow (radiolabeled microspheres) indicate that vital organ perfusion during conventional closed-chest CPR is low, especially when CPR regional flow is compared to pre-arrest or control values.

Available data obtained in different experimental models, using nonstandardized conventional closed-chest CPR techniques during arrest and CPR periods of various durations, indicate that myocardial blood flow during ventricular fibrillation and CPR averages 1% to 40% of control values and cerebral blood flow 3% to 90% of control.[14-20] This wide variation in observed values may be explained by wide variations in control or "normal" values, differences in chest compression techniques (especially force and duration), and the timing of regional flow measurements.[21] Subdiaphragmatic visceral perfusion has consistently been reported to be less than 5% of control. The microsphere technique itself has been well validated in the setting of circulatory arrest and closed-chest CPR.[16] When expressed as a percentage of "normal" or control, or when presented as absolute numbers, CPR flow values appear "inadequate." However, the adequacy of CPR perfusion is only now being addressed from a clinically relevant viewpoint, ie, response to countershock or drug management of arrest rhythm disturbances, or both, and long-term survival.

Ralston et al[18] and Michael et al[20] recently demonstrated that myocardial blood flow of only about 20 ml/min per 100 g of tissue during CPR is enough to facilitate successful defibrillation and to restore spontaneous circulation after prolonged ventricular fibrillation. Such values can be attained with closed-chest CPR alone or combined with alpha-adrenergic agonist support. In our laboratory, myocardial flows of only 15 to 18 ml/min per 100 g of tissue during conventional closed-chest CPR are capable of restoring circulation after postcountershock asystole or pulseless bradycardia.[22] Although these values are low when compared with control values, they indeed appear to be adequate in restoring circulation after circulatory arrest and CPR. Minimal or adequate flow to assure neuronal viability during arrest and CPR has not been determined in appropriately designed studies assessing long-term neurologic outcome. Such information is needed to fully assess the efficacy of CPR as it is currently practiced.

Observations in experimental animals indicate that marked differences in cerebral and myocardial perfusion exist during closed-chest CPR.[23] This difference in regional flow can largely be explained by differences in the perfusion gradients across the resistance vessels of the brain and heart (Figure 25.2). During chest compression or CPR systole, aortic and right atrial pressures are nearly identical and the coronary perfusion gradient (aortic pressure minus right atrial pressure) is nearly zero. Peak aortic and right atrial pressure approximates peak intrathoracic pressure. During the relaxation phase or CPR diastole, a small pressure difference between the aorta and right atrium serves as the driving force for coronary arterial flow and myocardial perfusion.

In contrast, during CPR systole, a substantial pressure difference between the arterial system (aorta and carotid artery) and the jugular vein is usually seen. This cerebral perfusion gradient results from closure of competent venous valves in the jugular veins and direct transmission of developed intrathoracic pressure to the peripheral arterial system. The cerebral perfusion gradient can be increased by mechanical manipulations that increase intrathoracic pressure (see subsequently). Myocardial flow during arrest and CPR is largely a diastolic event and "passive." To effectively increase coronary flow during

Table 25.1. Expected Versus Observed Hemodynamic and Anatomic Findings During Closed-Chest "Cardiac Massage"

Expected	Observed
1. Ventricular pressures > atrial pressures during CPR systole	1. Ventricular pressures = atrial pressures during CPR systole
2. Atrioventricular valves closed during CPR systole	2. Atrioventricular valves open during CPR systole
3. Semilunar valves open during CPR systole	3. Ao valve open and pulmonic valve closed during CPR systole
4. Ao pressure > RA pressure during CPR systole	4. Ao pressure = RA pressure during CPR systole
5. Venae caval pressures < RA pressure during CPR systole	5. Venae caval pressures = RA pressure during CPR systole
6. Jugular venous and intracranial pressure < RA pressure during CPR systole	6. Jugular venous and intracranial pressure < RA pressure during CPR systole
7. Peripheral venous to right heart inflow during CPR systole and diastole	7. Peripheral venous to right heart inflow only during CPR diastole

Ao = aortic; RA= right atrial; CPR systole = closed chest compression; CPR diastole = relaxation phase.

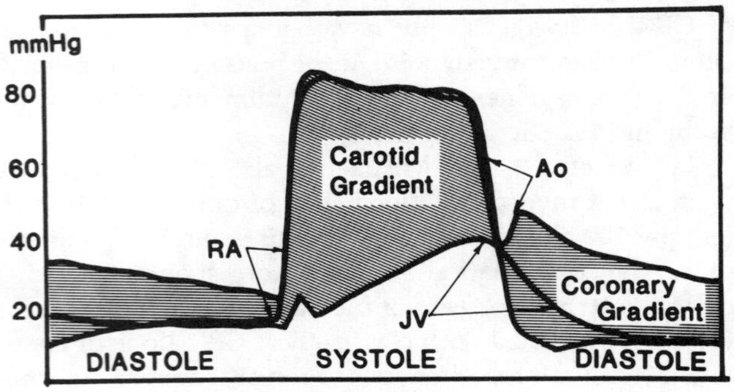

Figure 25.2. CPR pressure and gradients. Typical simultaneous pressures measured in the ascending aorta (Ao), jugular vein (JV), and right atrium (RA) during CPR systole (closed-chest thoracic compression) and diastole (the relaxation phase) during cardiac arrest and conventional CPR are shown. During systole, Ao and RA pressures are nearly identical and the absence of a demonstrable Ao-RA pressure difference precludes coronary flow during compression. However, there is a substantial pressure difference between the aorta and jugular vein (carotid perfusion gradient) to facilitate cerebral flow. In general, there is a closer correlation between the Ao-JV pressure difference and cerebral flow. During CPR diastole, intravascular pressures decrease abruptly. The JV-RA pressure difference is associated with right heart inflow. During relaxation, a small pressure difference between the Ao and RA serves as the driving force for coronary flow and myocardial perfusion (coronary gradient). The largest Ao-RA pressure difference is seen during early diastole and is associated with the majority of CPR myocardial flow.

CPR, diastolic aortic pressure would have to be increased selectively, as vascular resistance should be minimal and right atrial pressure is usually less than 10 mm Hg. Interventions that prolong CPR systole would favor increased cerebral perfusion but would decrease coronary flow. These perfusion gradient differences have received renewed attention in research studies, as they may be "competitive" and limit the overall effectiveness of "new CPR" techniques.

NEW CLOSED-CHEST CARDIOPULMONARY RESUSCITATION TECHNIQUES

New closed-chest CPR techniques have recently been described and investigated in the experimental laboratory (Table 25.2). Most exploit the physiologic principles of the thoracic pump mechanism for blood flow during rhythmic thoracic compression and relaxation. Implicit in this mechanism are the observations that the thoracic and abdominal compartments, separated only by the mobile diaphragm, function as a single unit and are subjected to similar pressure changes during thoracic compression, and that intrathoracic pressure fluctuations are a major determinant of arterial pressure (Figure 25.1).

Simultaneous chest compression and positive-pressure lung inflation (simultaneous compression-ventilation CPR or SCV-CPR) has been well studied in several laboratories with similar results.[11,12,15,16,20] During SCV-CPR, the thorax is usually compressed at a rate of 40 compression/relaxation cycles per minute. Chest compression is usually maintained for 0.9 second (60% of the cycle) and is followed by a relaxation phase of 0.6 second in duration (40% of the cycle). At the onset of chest compression, the airway is simultaneously inflated to pressures of 40 to 110 mm Hg. At the onset of the relaxation phase, the airway is abruptly opened to the atmosphere. Thus, 40 chest compressions and positive-pressure lung inflations are administered each minute. This technique produces dramatic increases in cerebral perfusion during cardiac arrest when compared with chest compression with asynchronous ventilation. However, its effects on myocardial flow are insignificant.[15,16] Improved cerebral flow is largely the result of an improved cerebral perfusion gradient. The myocardial perfusion gradient is not significantly improved. Reported complications have been limited to induced respiratory alkalemia. Barotrauma due to high airway pressure has not been reported by most investigators. Although this method may improve cerebral flow, it has not facilitated restoration of spontaneous circulation after prolonged ventricular fibrillation and CPR. More rapid compression rates and shorter compression durations have not been well studied. The chosen rate and duration for study would tend to favor cerebral flow at the expense of myocardial perfusion. This CPR method, when combined with abdominal binding, did not improve outcome from prehospital cardiac arrest in a recently concluded clinical study (M. Weisfeldt, personal communication).

Abdominal binding during conventional CPR increases intraabdominal pressure and limits the extent of diaphragmatic descent during chest compression.[24] Dia-

Table 25.2. Effects of Modified Cardiopulmonary Resuscitation Techniques in Animal Models

	Arterial Pressure	Cardiac Output	Cerebral Perfusion	Myocardial Perfusion	Survival* (Lab/Clinical)
Simultaneous compression-ventilation CPR (SCV-CPR)	↑	↑	↑	NC	NS/NC
Abdominal binding during conventional CPR	↑	↑ or NC	↑	NS	NS/NS
Abdominal counterpulsation during conventional CPR (IAC-CPR)	↑	↑	↑	NC	NS/NC
Military antishock trousers during CPR (MAST-CPR)	↑	NS	NS	NS	NS/NC
Volume loading during conventional CPR	↑	↑	↓	↓	NS/NS
High Impulse CPR	↑	↑	↑	↑	NC/NS
Pneumatic CPR (vest and binder CPR)	↑	↑	↑	NC	↑/NS

↑ = increased; ↓ = decreased; NC = no change; NS = not studied; * = survival in experimental laboratory or clinical study.

phragmatic excursions during CPR are due to fluctuations in intrathoracic pressure, and movement of the diaphragm is a passive event. Limiting diaphragmatic descent during chest compression would prevent or limit dissipation of developed intrathoracic pressure during chest compression (CPR systole). A given chest compression force should result in more greatly developed intrathoracic pressure and arterial pressures. The cerebral perfusion gradient improves, but the myocardial perfusion gradient is unaffected or decreased because of a greater increase in right atrial CPR diastolic pressure than in aortic diastolic pressure. Abdominal binding during conventional CPR or during SCV-CPR improves cerebral flow, but it has not been demonstrated to improve resuscitation outcome. Binding does not decrease right heart reflux during chest compression nor does it improve subdiaphragmatic venous return.[24]

Abdominal "counterpulsation" during conventional CPR exploits the thoracoabdominal unit and may also produce aortic compression. This method has come to be called interposed abdominal compression CPR or IAC-CPR.[19] The chest is compressed at a rate of 60 compression/relaxation cycles per minute. Artificial ventilation is administered after every fifth chest compression. During the brief period of chest relaxation, the abdomen is compressed with a force of about 80 mm Hg. Because IAC-CPR is a manual CPR technique that does not require specialized equipment, it might be of value in the prehospital arrest setting. This technique produces an increase in cardiac output and cerebral perfusion during ventricular fibrillation and CPR, but it does not improve myocardial blood flow. In experimental animals, it does not improve resuscitation outcome. In a clinical study of prehospital cardiac arrest, IAC-CPR offered no advantage over conventional CPR with respect to resuscitation outcome.[25]

Use of military antishock trousers during conventional CPR (MAST CPR) has been advocated as a means of improving systemic arterial pressure and, by inference, vital organ perfusion during cardiac arrest and artificial circulatory support. Past and contemporary experimental laboratory animal studies (see below) have demonstrated the importance of peripheral arterial tone, with or without alpha-agonist drug support, in the maintenance of vital organ flow and "survival" both during brady/asystolic cardiac arrest produced by asphyxia and during ventricular fibrillation and prolonged artificial circulatory support. Other studies indicate that contrary to initial conjecture, the use of pneumatic external counterpressure (MAST) produces minimal, if any, autotransfusion and that MAST inflation largely increases arterial pressure through an increase in peripheral vascular resistance.[26] In many respects, MAST use during CPR may have physiologic effects similar to those of infusions of alpha-agonist drugs in current use. Use of MAST CPR would appear to be logically supported as a nonpharmacologic means of increasing peripheral vascular tone and, presumably, vital organ perfusion during cardiac arrest. However, MAST CPR has never been shown to improve cerebral or myocardial perfusion in experimental animal models of cardiac arrest and resuscitation. Although MAST use during conventional CPR increases intravascular pressure and common carotid blood flow during cardiac arrest in animals,[27] regional blood flow has never been assessed using the technique nor has resuscitability or survival. In the only large clinical study available for analysis, MAST use during CPR in the prehospital setting had no effect on long-term outcome when compared with CPR without MAST use, regardless of the initially encountered rhythm.[28] Although application of the MAST apparatus may improve arterial pressure during CPR, this effect is probably the sole result of abdominal binding afforded by inflation of the abdominal compartment of the presently used multicompartment garment.

The value of volume loading during CPR was originally thought to be due to an increase in intravascular pressure and an expected increase in left heart outflow. This theoretic benefit could easily be accomplished by crystalloid infusion. However, recent data indicate that volume infusions during CPR increase arterial pressure but decrease vital organ perfusion during CPR.[17] Decreased perfusion is largely the result of an increase in venous pressure and decreases in vital organ arteriovenous pressure gradients that occur after volume infusion. An increase in venous pressure which exceeds that produced in the arterial tree will decrease both the cerebral and the myocardial perfusion gradients (Figure 25.2).

Increasing the depth or force of sternal compression, or both, during CPR or the rate of sternal depressions (high impulse CPR) may increase cardiac output and cerebral and myocardial flow.[29] The salutory effects of increased force can be ascribed to greater developed intrathoracic pressure. The benefit of increased compression rate has not been well delineated physiologically. In the experimental laboratory, increased compression rate does not improve survival after prolonged ventricular fibrillation and artificial circulatory support.[30]

In our laboratory we have studied the hemodynamic and cardiac anatomic effects of circulatory support using a pneumatic vest and abdominal binder with simultaneous high-pressure airway inflation during cardiac arrest (vest and binder CPR).[31] This apparatus most closely mimics the physiologic and hemodynamic events that occur during spontaneous coughing (high intrathoracic and intraabdominal pressures during systole, low intrathoracic and intraabdominal pressures during diastole). In our experience this artificial perfusion and ventilation technique is not associated with significant complications, and it favors improved long-term outcome when compared with conventional CPR. This CPR technique improves not only hemodynamic variables, but also the long-term outcome of prolonged ventricular fibrillation. This technique and device have not been studied in the clinical population but they offer some advantages.

CLINICAL APPLICATION AND USE OF NEW CARDIOPULMONARY RESUSCITATION TECHNIQUES

Renewed interest in the physiology of blood flow during CPR has resulted in the description and study of modified closed-chest artificial perfusion techniques that may improve regional perfusion but that have not been demonstrated to improve outcome from prehospital sudden cardiac death. These modified or new CPR techniques improve cerebral flow but do not improve myocardial perfusion and the likelihood of successful cardiac resuscitation. Currently, no recently described modified closed-chest CPR technique offers any advantage over conventional CPR as practiced world wide.

THE PHARMACOLOGY OF RESUSCITATION

ADRENERGIC AGONISTS

Recent investigations in the experimental laboratory confirm that peripheral arterial tone, reflected by resting or CPR diastolic pressure, is an important determinant of resuscitation outcome.[18,20,32] In general, the higher the aortic pressure during the chest relaxation phase of CPR, the greater the coronary perfusion pressure and myocardial perfusion. Countershock outcome and restoration of spontaneous circulation have been correlated with the magnitude of the coronary perfusion gradient and myocardial perfusion during prolonged cardiac arrest and CPR.

During cardiac arrest and CPR, the beneficial effects of adrenergic drugs with predominant peripheral alpha-agonist actions are largely explained by effects on peripheral vascular resistance. The early work of Redding and Pearson[33] indicates that any drug with alpha-agonist properties is capable of improving the resuscitation outcome.

Epinephrine hydrochloride is the alpha agent most commonly used in clinical practice. It is recommended in the treatment of "refractory" ventricular fibrillation, asystole, and pulseless bradyarrhythmias. It also can be used as a vasopressor agent, if needed, after the return of spontaneous rhythm. During cardiac arrest, the beta-agonist effects of the drug have not been shown to be essential in the restoration of circulation.[34] Recent studies indicate that epinephrine improves not only myocardial blood flow but also cerebral blood flow during cardiac arrest and CPR.[18,20] The effect on cerebral perfusion is due to a redistribution of extracranial arterial flow. Currently, no other alpha agonist offers a real and substantial advantage over epinephrine.

Isoproterenol hydrochloride is a pure beta-agonist with direct myocardial and peripheral vascular effects. The known beta-1 effects of this agent have led to its recommended but unproven benefit in asystole and pulseless bradyarrhythmias. Unfortunately, potent beta-2 effects produce peripheral vasodilatation and may decrease myocardial flow when such an effect is least desired. In the early work of Redding and Pearson,[33] no experimental animal in cardiac arrest survived after receiving isoproterenol. Contemporary investigations suggest that isoproterenol is of limited value in the setting of cardiac arrest because of effects on regional blood flow.[22,34,35] This agent offers no advantage over epinephrine, which also has beta-1 agonist properties. Selective beta-1 agonists (eg, dobutamine) are likewise of limited value in experimental brady-asystolic arrest.[36]

CALCIUM CHLORIDE

The inotropic properties of calcium ions have long been recognized, particularly when calcium is administered in the clinical or experimental setting of hypocalcemia, ie, decreased ionized calcium concentration.[37] The known inotropic properties of this ion led to its early recommendation and current use as an agent to be used in cardiac arrest, particularly when it is due to asystole or pulseless rhythms. However, recognition of the role intracellular calcium accumulation plays in irreversible cellular injury and death during and following ischemia[38,39] has resulted in a reevaluation of the use of calcium chloride in cardiac arrest.

Several retrospective and prospective clinical studies of prehospital cardiac arrest suggest that calcium administration is of limited value in asystole and pulseless bradyarrhythmias and does not improve long-term resuscitation outcome.[40,41] Whether calcium use is actually detrimental has not been established, but it is more than of theoretic concern. Contributions from the international resuscitation research community indicate that the use of calcium blocking agents immediately after restoration of spontaneous circulation improves neuronal viability and neurologic recovery following arrest.[39] Although untested, calcium administration during CPR may attenuate this favorable response to a new class of resuscitation drugs of considerable promise in preventing the short- and long-term effects of brief cerebral anoxia/ischemia. The continued use of calcium in resuscitation pharmacology is an active area of investigation. There are currently no data to support its continued use in the setting of cardiac arrest, except in known or suspected hypocalcemia or hyperkalemia

CALCIUM BLOCKING AGENTS AND ION CHELATORS

The pathobiologic aspects of neuronal injury and death due to anoxia/ischemia are evolving and being defined and redefined.[39] At present, considerable evidence exists to suggest that neuronal injury and death may continue or occur after reperfusion, ie, restoration of circulation after cardiac arrest. Following restoration of cerebral flow, there is a gradual increase in cerebrovascular resistance and a decline in regional cerebral perfusion. This cerebral "no reflow" phenomenon has most recently been ascribed to cerebral vasospasm and was shown to be attenuated or alleviated by postreperfusion treatment with calcium blocking agents (lidoflazine, flunarizine, and nimodepine). The cerebral no-reflow phenomenon appears unrelated to changes in intracranial pressure and to small vessel intravascular coagulation (thrombosis). Limited and uncontrolled studies in the clinical population suggest that calcium blocking agents may improve neurologic recovery after circulatory arrest.[42] A multinational clinical trial is currently in progress to assess the use of such agents in a well-controlled fashion.[43]

Recent experimental data suggest that decompartmentalization of cellular iron stores may also play a role in cell membrane peroxidation after ischemia.[44] Preliminary observations suggest that desferoxamine may be of value in improving the long-term neurologic outcome after arrest and successful resuscitation. Further studies seem warranted and are in progress.

CONCLUSIONS

The science of resuscitation is one of international concern. During the last decade, the mechanism of blood flow during closed-chest CPR was redefined and modifications of current CPR techniques were studied in an attempt to improve vital organ perfusion. In addition, it was recently recognized that cellular injury and death may continue after restoration of spontaneous circulation and that this continued insult substantially limits long-term survival. Preliminary data suggest that such postreperfusion injury can be attenuated pharmacologically. In the future, post-resuscitation care will be as important as the CPR technique used during arrest and the enlightened use of a limited armamentarium of drugs used to treat encountered rhythm disturbances. Early CPR and definitive treatment of ventricular fibrillation (electrical countershock) currently are recognized life-saving interventions that should be supported and encouraged by the medical community.

REFERENCES

1. Lown B: Sudden cardiac death: the major challenge confronting contemporary cardiology. *Am J Cardiol* 1979; 43:313–328.
2. Perper JA, Kuller LH, Cooper M: Arteriosclerosis of coronary arteries in sudden, unexpected deaths. *Circulation* 1975; 52 (suppl 3):27–33.
3. Guerci A: Sudden death. *West J Med* 1980; 133:313–320.
4. Cummins RO, Eisenberg MS: Prehospital cardiopulmonary resuscitation: Is it effective? *JAMA* 1985; 253:2408–2412.
5. Kouwenhoven WB, Jude JR, Knickerbocker GG: Closed-chest cardiac massage. *JAMA* 1960; 173:1064–1067.
6. Weale FE, Rothwell-Jackson RL: The efficiency of cardiac massage. *Lancet* 1962; 1:990–992.
7. MacKenzie GJ, Taylor SH, McDonald AH, Donald KW: Haemodynamic effects of external cardiac compression. *Lancet* 1964; 1:1342–1345.
8. Gall F: Incompetence of the atrioventricular valves during cardiac massage. *J Cardiovasc Surg* 1965; 16:356–360.
9. Criley JM, Blaufuss AH, Kissel GL: Cough-induced cardiac compression. Self-administered form of cardiopulmonary resuscitation. *JAMA* 1976; 236:1246–1250.
10. Niemann JT, Rosborough JP, Hausknecht M, Brown D, Criley JM: Cough CPR: documentation of systemic perfusion in man and in an experimental model; a "window" to the mechanism of blood flow in external CPR. *Crit Care Med* 1980; 8:141–146.
11. Rudikoff MT, Maughan WL, Effron M, Freund P, Weisfeldt ML: Mechanisms of blood flow during cardiopulmonary resuscitation. *Circulation* 1980; 61:345–352.
12. Niemann JT, Rosborough JP, Hausknecht M, Garner D, Criley JM: Pressure-synchronized cineangiography during experimental cardiopulmonary resuscitation. *Circulation* 1981; 64:985–991.
13. Werner JA, Greene HL, Janko CL, Cobb LA: Visualization of cardiac valve motion in man during external chest compression using two-dimensional echocardiography. Implications regarding the mechanism of blood flow. *Circulation* 1981; 63:1417–1421.
14. Voorhees WD, Babbs CF, Tacker WA: Regional blood flow during cardiopulmonary resuscitation in dogs. *Crit Care Med* 1980; 8:134–136.
15. Luce JM, Ross BK, O'Quin RJ, Culver BH, Sivarajan M, Amory DW, Niskanen RA, Alferness CA, Kirk WL, Pierson LB, Butler J: Regional blood flow during cardiopulmonary resuscitation in dogs using simultaneous and nonsimultaneous compression and ventilation. *Circulation* 1983; 67:258–265.
16. Koehler RC, Chandra N, Guerci AD, Tsitlik J, Traystman RJ, Rodgers MC, Weisfeldt ML: Augmentation of cerebral perfusion by simultaneous chest compression and lung inflation with abdominal binding after cardiac arrest in dogs. *Circulation* 1983; 67:266–275.
17. Ditchey RV, Lindenfeld J: Potential adverse effects of volume loading on perfusion of vital organs during closed-chest resuscitation. *Circulation* 1984; 69:181–189.
18. Ralston SH, Voorhees WD, Babbs CF: Intrapulmonary epinephrine during prolonged cardiopulmonary resuscitation: improved regional flow and resuscitation in dogs. *Ann Emerg Med* 1984; 13:79–86.
19. Voorhees WD, Ralston SH, Babbs CF: Regional blood flow during cardiopulmonary resuscitation with abdominal counterpulsation in dogs. *Am J Emerg Med* 1984; 2:128–135.
20. Michael JR, Guerci AD, Koehler RC, Shi AY, Tsitlik J, Chandra N, Niedermeyer E, Rogers MC, Traystman RJ, Weisfeldt ML: Mechanisms by which epinephrine augments cerebral and myocardial perfusion during cardiopulmonary resuscitation in dogs. *Circulation* 1984; 69:822–835.
21. Niemann JT: Artificial perfusion techniques during cardiac arrest: questions of experimental focus vs. clinical need. *Ann Emerg Med* 1985; 14:761–768.
22. Haynes K, Niemann JT, Garner D, Rennie C, Jagles G: Post-countershock asystole/pulseless bradycardias: response to CPR, adrenergic agonists, and glucagon, a non-adrenergic stimulator of adenyl cyclase. *Ann Emerg Med* 1985; 14:496.
23. Niemann JT: Differences in cerebral and myocardial perfusion during closed-chest resuscitation. *Ann Emerg Med* 1984; 13:849–853.
24. Niemann JT, Rosborough JP, Ung S, Criley JM: Hemodynamic effects of continuous abdominal binding during cardiac arrest and resuscitation. *Am J Cardiol* 1984; 53:269–274.
25. Mateer JR, Stueven HA, Thompson BM, Aprahamian C, Darin JC: Interposed abdominal compression CPR versus standard CPR in prehospital cardiopulmonary arrest: preliminary results. *Ann Emerg Med* 1984; 13:764–766.
26. Niemann JT, Stapczynski JS, Rosborough JP, Rothstein RJ: Hemodynamic effects of pneumatic external counterpressure in canine hemorrhagic shock. *Ann Emerg Med* 1983; 12:661–667.
27. Bircher N, Safar P, Stewart R: A comparison of standard, "MAST"-augmented, and open-chest CPR in dogs, *Crit Care Med* 1980; 8:147–152.
28. Mahoney BD, Mirick MJ: Efficacy of pneumatic trousers in refractory prehospital cardiopulmonary arrest. *Ann Emerg Med* 1983; 12:27–31.
29. Maier GW, Tyson GS, Olsen CO, Kernstein KH, Davis JW, Conn EH, Sabiston DC Jr, Rankin JS: The physiology of external cardiac massage: high-impulse cardiopulmonary resuscitation. *Circulation* 1984; 70:86–101.
30. Kern KB, Carter AB, Showen L, Tacker WA, Ewy GA: Resuscitation and twenty-four hour survival among three different modes of manual cardiopulmonary resuscitation (abstr): *Clin Res* 1985; 33:10A.
31. Niemann JT, Rosborough JP, Niskanen RA, Alferness CA, Criley JM: Mechanical "cough" cardiopulmonary resuscitation during cardiac arrest in dogs. *Am J Cardiol* 1985; 55:199–205.
32. Niemann JT, Rosborough JP, Criley JM, Niskanen RA, Alferness CA: Predictive indices of successful cardiac resuscitation during cardiac arrest and experimental cardiopulmonary resuscitation. *Ann Emerg Med* 1985; 14:521–528.
33. Redding JS, Pearson JW: Evaluation of drugs for cardiac resuscitation. *Anesthesiology* 1963; 24:203–207.
34. Otto CW, Yakaitas RW, Blitt CD: Mechanism of action of epinephrine in resuscitation from asphyxial arrest. *Crit Care Med* 1981; 9:321–324.
35. Holmes HR, Babbs CF, Vorhees WD, Tacker WA, DeCaravilla B: Influence of adrenergic drugs upon vital organ perfusion during CPR. *Crit Care Med* 1980; 8:137–140.
36. Yakaitas RW, Otto CW, Blitt CD: Relative importance of alpha and beta adrenergic receptors during resuscitation. *Crit Care Med* 1979; 7:293–296.
37. Drop LJ, Geffin GA, O'Keefe DD, Newell JB, Jacobs ML, Fowler BN, Daggett WM: Relation between ionized calcium concentration and ventricular pump performance in the dog under hemodynamically controlled conditions. *Am J Cardiol* 1981; 47:1041–1051.
38. Katz AM, Reuter H: Cellular calcium and cardiac cell death. *Am J Cardiol* 1979; 44:188–190.
39. White BC, Wiegenstein JG, Winegar CD: Brain ischemia anoxia. Mechanisms of injury. *JAMA* 1984; 251:1586–1590.
40. Stueven HA, Thompson BM, Aprahamian C, Tonsfeldt DJ: Calcium chloride: reassessment of use in asystole. *Ann Emerg Med* 1984; 13:820–822.
41. Harrison EE, Amey BD: Use of calcium in electromechanical dissociation. *Ann Emerg Med* 1984; 13:844–845.
42. Schwartz AC: Neurological recovery after cardiac arrest: clinical feasibility trial of calcium blockers. *Am J Emerg Med* 1985; 3:1–10.
43. Safar P: Recent advances in cardiopulmonary-cerebral resuscitation: a review. *Ann Emerg Med* 1984; 13:856–862.
44. White BC, Aust SD, Arfors KE, Aronson LD: Brain injury by ischemic anoxia hypothesis extension: a tale of two ions? *Ann Emerg Med* 1984; 13:862–867.

26 Congenital Heart Disease in Infants and Children

Mary Allen Engle, MD

Congenital heart disease is present at birth although it may not be recognized until later in childhood or even in adult life. Conversely, some malformations are so severe as to be incompatible even with fetal life and are responsible for some miscarriages. The period of greatest risk of symptoms and death from the anomaly is the first few months of life.

Throughout the world, the incidence of congenital heart disease reported in most studies ranges from 8 to 10 per 1,000 live births. If patients with conditions such as a bicuspid aortic valve, which may become thickened and calcified with age so that stenosis or regurgitation occurs, and the apical systolic click–murmur syndrome due to mitral valve prolapse are included in the statistics, the incidence of congenital heart disease probably exceeds 1 per 100 live births. Although the overall incidence is similar, the frequency of some anomalies differs. In the Oriental population, subpulmonary ventricular septal defect is more common and coarctation of the aorta less common than in other peoples. Because of the care tendered by pediatric cardiologists and cardiac surgeons in the past 30 to 40 years, the prevalence of congenital heart disease in adults is steadily rising. (See also chapter 27, Congenital Heart Disease in the Adult.)

ETIOLOGY

Embryologic studies of the heart indicate that the defect or anomaly develops in the first 6 to 8 weeks of fetal life, when the cardiovascular structures are forming. A possible exception is patent ductus arteriosus, a channel that is normal in the fetus. Its failure to close in the first few hours or days after birth is the abnormality.

In about 95% of affected babies, the cause of the anomaly is unknown. Most parents were healthy adults with the mother of the usual childbearing age. Inquiries about past events, such as exposure to radiation or living at high altitudes, have usually been answered negatively. Although many women had taken various medications, not always on a physician's advice, it was rarely possible to relate the occurrence of congenital heart disease to a specific medication. Some women on long-term anticonvulsant medication, such as trimethadione and paramethadione, and some receiving progesterone early in pregnancy for threatened miscarriage have had a higher-than-average percentage of babies with heart disease, and a few of the infants with malformed limbs caused by thalidomide ingestion by their mothers in pregnancy also had congenital heart disease. Chronically excessive maternal alcoholic intake can result in infants with the fetal alcoholism syndrome, which can include congenital heart disease.

Among the 5% of cases with an identifiable cause of congenital heart disease, a few are due to maternal infection with rubella in the first trimester of pregnancy (now a preventable situation) and a portion are due to genetic factors or chromosomal abnormalities. Certain families exhibit clustering of a particular malformation in sibships or members of more than one generation. Examples include hypertrophic cardiomyopathy as well as atrial septal defect. Some heritable forms of cardiovascular disease occur in syndromes such as the Holt–Oram, Marfan, Ellis–van Creveld, and Noonan syndromes. (See also chapter 28, Genetics and the Cardiovascular System.)

Atrial septal defect (ASD) is the major cardiovascular manifestation associated with skeletal upper limb defects in the Holt–Oram syndrome. A common atrium is common with the chondrodystrophic dwarfism, nail dysplasia, and polydactyly of the Ellis–van Creveld syndrome. Pulmonary valve stenosis and dysplasia accompany webbed neck, pectus excavatum, and cryptorchism in the Noonan syndrome. Chromosomal abnormalities with cardiovascular involvement include the trisomies, such as Down's syndrome (trisomy 21), and other far less common ones, such as trisomy 18; and monosomy, namely, the Turner syndrome (45 XO). Because the key to prevention is understanding the causation, it is clear that we are unable to prevent most forms of congenital heart disease. Therefore, we must be alert to recognize the condition, assess its mild nature or severity, and offer the best in medical or surgical management at the right time.

PATHOPHYSIOLOGY

Congenital cardiovascular anomalies of the heart and major blood vessels produce their effects by rerouting or impairing blood flow. Minor lesions produce no symptoms and are well tolerated, whereas severe anomalies produce major derangements that result in symptoms and signs that are usually recognizable and often treatable soon after birth. Moderately severe anomalies tend to produce few symptoms in childhood, but the gradual effects of their continuing presence may cause problems in later life.

Conditions that impair the normal course of blood flow most often obstruct ventricular outflow: pulmonary or aortic stenosis (at, above, or below the valve) or coarctation of the aorta. The severity of obstruction and the precise location determine the signs and symptoms. The pressure load on the ventricle leads to concentric hypertrophy of the wall of that chamber, but the hypertrophied ventricle is able to maintain an adequate output at rest and on exercise unless the obstruction is severe. At that time, the coronary arterial blood supply to the hypertrophied muscle may be inadequate.

Whereas cardiac chamber enlargement is noted on physical examination and by cardiac series of chest roentgenograms, hypertrophy of the wall is indicated better by the electrocardiogram. With increasingly severe obstruction to pulmonary or aortic flow, the electrocardiogram changes from mild to moderate ventricular hypertrophy by voltage criteria. It progresses to hypertrophy with strain (depression of ST segments and flattening or inversion of T waves) when a coronary arterial imbalance of supply and demand occurs. Dilatation of the hypertrophied chamber and failure of the ventricle are next in the progression of severity. When such dilatation of the chamber occurs, the workload on the ventricle is evident not only by electrocardiographic evidence of hypertrophy, but also by radiologic signs of enlargement.

Malformations that reroute the flow of blood, such as those that produce a left-to-right shunt, result in a volume load on the atria or ventricles and pulmonary vessels. These anomalies cause a murmur characteristic of the leak and cardiac chamber enlargement that are detectable on physical examination, roentgenogram, electrocardiogram, and echocardiogram. Left-to-right shunts increase pulmonary blood flow and thus the size of the main pulmonary artery and its branches. This is evident on roentgenogram unless the shunt is small.

Cardiac failure from large or chronic volume overload may occur at any age, but characteristically a large ventricular septal defect or patent ductus arteriosus causes the heart to fail in the first 2 or 3 months of life, whereas an atrial septal defect causes the heart to fail in later adulthood. Longstanding left-to-right shunts at the atrial level can lead to pulmonary hypertension through pulmonary arterial obstructive disease. With an atrial septal defect, this usually occurs in early adulthood, whereas large shunts at the ventricular or aorticopulmonary level produce adverse effects in early childhood, even by the second or third year.

The anomalies that reroute blood flow often combine features of abnormal mixing because of defective septa plus impairment of blood flow. They cause a right-to-left shunt, resulting in cyanosis with attendant problems of fatigue and breathlessness on exertion. Cyanosis and clubbing of fingers and toes are cosmetic handicaps, as is scoliosis which, by adolescence, is common and sometimes rapidly progressive. There is a special hazard of cerebral complication in the form of a brain abscess or cerebrovascular thrombosis or embolism. It is thought that poor dental structure with defective enamel and dental caries contributes to the risk of brain abscess. Polycythemia, a sequel to hypoxia of the right-to-left shunt, is associated with headache and problems of bleeding or clotting. Some patients with red cell breakdown and hyperuricemia have gout. If the hypoxic, polycythemic woman is able to become pregnant, there is a greater-than-normal risk that the pregnancy will result in abortion or in a baby who has intrauterine growth retardation and is at risk of dying. Cardiac failure or renal impairment are late consequences of the unrelieved cardiac burden and hypoxia. Sudden death is not an uncommon event in some cyanotic patients, such as those with Ebstein's anomaly or pulmonary vascular obstructive disease.

The pathophysiologic aspects of specific anomalies in the three major categories of congenital heart disease with no shunt, left-to-right shunt, or right-to-left shunt will be discussed under Specific Malformations.

CLINICAL MANIFESTATIONS

When interpreting the history and symptoms of a patient with suspected congenital heart disease, it is important to remember that someone born with a malformation has never known what it is like to feel "normal" and so may minimize or fail to recognize symptoms that often are appreciated only in retrospect, after successful surgery. Furthermore, adolescents and adults cannot remember events in the first 3 years of life, often the most difficult period for a patient with congenital heart disease, and they may recall inaccurately events that may provide the cardiologist with important information. In addition, in young infants, symptoms due to cardiac difficulties may simulate other illnesses, such as attacks of "pneumonia," feeding problems, and failure to thrive. Growth lag in weight and height is often a significant symptom of heart disease in a patient with a left-to-right shunt as well as the cyanotic patient. Fatigability, breathlessness on exertion, susceptibility to upper respiratory tract infections, dizziness, syncope, headache, and leg pains are symptoms that often indicate cardiac disability. The history should include questions about a familial history of congenital heart disease as well as the possibility of ingestion of drugs or exposure to possible teratogens before or early in pregnancy. Most growing children, unless they are cyanotic or have a severe malformation, have no symptoms.

PHYSICAL EXAMINATION

Much can be learned from inspection of the patient, noting body build and comparing height and weight with growth chart standards for the age. Respiratory effort; position of comfort; fullness and pulsations of neck veins; exaggerated arterial pulsations in the suprasternal notch, carotids, or pulmonary area; as well as overactivity or bulging of the precordium signify abnormality. The observation of marked arterial pulsations in the suprasternal notch may suggest aortic runoff from a large patent ductus with wide pulse pressure or may be due to a dilated ascending aorta proximal to coarctation of the aorta. The nodding head of a patient with aortic regurgitation may point to that diagnosis. Visible pulsations of intercostal arteries over the posterior chest wall may be important evidence of coarctation of the aorta.

Especially in children, the configuration of the chest wall denotes enlargement of individual cardiac chambers: right ventricular enlargement indicated by a bulge of the lower left sternal border, left ventricular enlargement by a bulge in the lateral chest wall overlying the apex. Retraction of the suprasternal notch and grooving of the lower rib cage due to vigorous excursion of the diaphragm are common in infants and young children with pulmonary vascular engorgement.

Cyanosis of the lips and nailbeds due to arterial oxygen desaturation is accompanied by clubbing of the fingers and toes. Upper and lower extremities should be compared for cyanosis of unequal distribution. The diagnosis of shunt reversal through a patent ductus arteriosus can be made in the patient with cyanosis and clubbing of the toes but with pink lips and fingers of the right hand. The diagnosis of tetralogy of Fallot is strongly suggested if a cyanotic child assumes the squatting position for relief of exertional dyspnea and fatigue. Chronic venous stasis, such as may occur in a patient with severe pulmonic stenosis and intact septa, causes peripheral cyanosis because arterialized blood in the capillary bed resembles venous blood when oxygen is maximally extracted by the tissues.

Edema in an ambulatory subject is dependent and is evident as pedal, pretibial, or sacral edema, but in a young infant who cannot yet sit alone, it is generalized. Its presence may then first be detected as puffiness of the eyelids or by a sudden, "too-good" weight gain. Petechiae, nodules, rash, the skeletal deformities of Marfan's syndrome, and the stigmas of Down's or other syndromes with cardiovascular involvement are among the many significant observations from inspection alone.

Palpation adds to the information being accumulated. A thrill may be felt over the heart or arteries of the neck or over vessels of collateral circulation in the posterior chest. A cardiac thrust of a heaving quality suggests volume overload, whereas a tap along the lower sternal border implies right ventricular enlargement. An impulse may be felt in the pulmonic area that coincides with the exaggerated second sound of pulmonary hypertension. All peripheral pulses should be palpated. It is important to palpate simultaneously the peripheral pulses in the two arms and in the arm and leg and to note the quality and pulse pressure as well as the relation of the arm to the leg pulsations. The detection of strong radial pulses and feeble or impalpable pulsations in the femoral, dorsalis pedis, and posterior tibial arteries strongly suggests the diagnosis of coarctation of the aorta. A water-hammer pulse may be the clue to aortic regurgitation or another lesion associated with a wide pulse pressure, such as a large patent ductus or an arteriovenous fistula. The plateau type pulse of aortic stenosis can easily be recognized. Palpation of the abdomen for enlargement of the liver or spleen adds to the information about the patient's heart. An enlarged and pulsatile liver suggests tricuspid insufficiency.

Correlation of auscultation with phonocardiograms and physiologic measurements has added increased precision and meaningfulness to the sounds the physician hears. The timing, location, radiation, and postural variation of heart murmurs have especial significance in diagnosis of congenital heart disease. A holosystolic murmur at the lower left sternal border is the hallmark of a ventricular septal defect, whereas such a murmur at the apex means mitral regurgitation. Ejection type systolic murmurs of pulmonic origin are loudest in the second left interspace (the pulmonic area), and they radiate to the lung fields posteriorly, whereas those of aortic origin are heard best in the aortic area (the second right interspace) and suprasternal notch, and they radiate to the arteries of the neck. A mid-diastolic to late-diastolic murmur along the lower left sternal border is due to tricuspid overflow or stenosis, and one at the apex is due to excessive flow of blood across the mitral valve or to real stenosis of that atrioventricular valve. An early decrescendo diastolic murmur at the second left interspace, with radiation down the left sternal border, is due to semilunar valve regurgitation. With pulmonic regurgitation and normal pulmonary pressure, the murmur is low-pitched and heard better with the patient supine than erect. The murmur of aortic regurgitation is higher in pitch and is heard better in the upright position. A continuous systolic and diastolic murmur is due to an arteriovenous communication. Localized to the second left interspace, this signifies a patent ductus. A thrill is palpable when the murmur is grade four or more (out of six) in intensity.

The heart sounds also are important signs in diagnosis, especially the second sound in the second left interspace. Normally, this sound is split, and the aortic component precedes the pulmonic. These two sounds separate in inspiration and come closer together on expiration. Changes in splitting and in intensity correlate with pulmonary flow and pressure. In general, the louder the pulmonic component and the narrower the splitting, the greater the pulmonary artery pressure. Conversely, delay and diminution of the pulmonic component, even to the point of inaudibility, signify increasingly severe pulmonic stenosis. Wide and fixed splitting of the second heart sound is heard when there is pulmonic valve stenosis and also when there is greatly increased pulmonary blood flow with normal pulmonary artery pressure, as in atrial septal defect.

When an ejection type systolic murmur from aortic or pulmonic stenosis is heard at the base of the heart, an early systolic ejection sound indicates that the stenosis is valvular rather than subvalvular or supravalvular. Such sounds can also be heard when the aorta or pulmonary artery is dilated. Midsystolic click in association with a late systolic murmur at the apex characterizes the mitral click syndrome with prolapsing valve. (See also chapter 31, Mitral Valve Billowing and Prolapse.) A third heart sound at the apex is heard in many normal children. It is often present with mitral insufficiency. A fourth heart sound is pathologic. In the failing heart, these become the third heart sound, fourth heart sound, or summation gallops.

When measuring blood pressure, especially in infants, children, and obese patients, it is important to choose a cuff of appropriate size for the patient, one that covers at least one half and preferably two thirds of the surface of the upper arm or leg. Blood pressure should be measured in both arms and in the leg in patients suspected of having congenital heart disease and in those with hypertension. Blood pressure higher in the arms than in the legs is an important sign of coarctation. Arterial pulse pressure is narrow in children with severe aortic stenosis and in cyanotic, polycythemic persons.

LABORATORY STUDIES

CARDIAC SERIES OF CHEST ROENTGENOGRAMS

Cardiac series of chest roentgenograms consist of 6-foot films in frontal, right anterior oblique, left anterior oblique, and lateral views with barium swallow in all four views. The four views help to evaluate not only the overall heart size and position but also the size of each cardiac chamber, the ascending and descending aorta, the possibility of retroesophageal vessels, the main pulmonary artery, and the extent of pulmonary vascular markings. Barium in the esophagus delineates the course of the aortic arch and descending aorta, which deviates around retroesophageal vessels and curves posteriorly and laterally if the left atrium is enlarged. The cardiothoracic ratio does not normally exceed 50% except in the first few days of neonatal life. Unusual convexity of the main pulmonary artery indicates enlargement from poststenotic dilatation, high flow, or high pressure, whereas concavity indicates that the pulmonary artery is hypoplastic, absent, or misplaced. The pulmonary arterial tree appears engorged if pulmonary blood flow is increased by a large left-to-right shunt. Excessively clear lung fields and hypoplastic pulmonary arterial branches indicate severe pulmonary stenosis. A disturbance in the distribution of pulmonary arterial flow occurs in obstructive pulmonary hypertension; the main pulmonary artery and the right and left branches are enlarged in the hilar regions but are "cut off" there, so that the periphery is abnormally translucent. Evidence of pulmonary venous congestion or edema can also be detected as a haziness or a perihilar vascular stippling.

ELECTROCARDIOGRAPHY

The electrocardiogram provides information concerning rhythm, rate, conduction, electrical axis, cardiac chamber dilatation or hypertrophy, and strain. The findings must be interpreted in comparison with the normal standards for infants, children, and adults.

The electrocardiogram of the newborn in the first week of life shows right axis deviation with a QRS frontal axis of around 120°, right ventricular dominance (prominent R wave in leads aVR and V_3R, V_1, and often a prominent S wave in leads V_5 to V_6), and frequently left ventricular strain (inverted T wave in leads V_5 to V_6 and lead I and often an upright T wave in lead V_1). After 1 week of age, T waves are positive in leads V_5 to V_6 and leads I and II. By 1 month of age, the decrease in right ventricular wall thickness, in response to lowering of pulmonary vascular resistance, is manifested by a decreasing R wave in lead V_1 and by the appearance of a right ventricular conduction delay (rsR' or rsr') in lead V_1. When this conduction delay is confined to lead V_1 or V_3R, or both, it is normal throughout the childhood years. The electrical QRS axis changes from around 120° to about 90° and then 60°. By 1 month, the left ventricular muscle fibers have enlarged in response to pumping blood at a systemic pressure, so from this time on, left ventricular forces are greater than right ventricular forces (R in lead V_5 taller than R in lead V_1).

Right ventricular hypertrophy is evidenced by persistence of the R and S relations normal for a newborn or by an abnormally large voltage of the R wave in right precordial leads and in lead aVR. The additional finding of deep inversion of T waves and depression of ST segments in right precordial leads and leads aVF, II, and III indicates right ventricular strain and a suprasystemic pressure in the right ventricle.

Right ventricular conduction delay is abnormal when an rsr' or rsR' in the right precordial leads is associated with a slurring of R and S waves in all limb and precordial leads. This usually signifies right ventricular dilatation, such as occurs with atrial septal defect. Complete right bundle branch block with prolonged QRS duration is always abnormal.

Left ventricular hypertrophy in the electrocardiogram of pediatric subjects is interpreted on the basis of voltage criteria. If the algebraic sum of the negative deflection in lead V_1 and positive deflection in lead V_5 exceeds 40 mm in children, left ventricular hypertrophy usually is present. Furthermore, unusually tall R waves, greater than 35 mm in lead V_5 or 20 mm in lead aVF, suggest left ventricular hypertrophy.

If left ventricular strain accompanies left ventricular hypertrophy, T waves in leads V_5 to V_6, aVF, II, and III are inverted or flattened. This represents a severe stage of left ventricular hypertrophy (Figure 26.1). Such a tracing may be found with severe aortic stenosis or endocardial fibroelastosis.

An atrial abnormality is indicated by the form of the P waves. An abnormally high, peaked P wave (greater than 2.5 mm in amplitude in lead II, or a large, initially positive P wave in lead V_1) indicates right atrial enlargement, whereas wide, low, notched P waves in lead II or marked terminal negativity of the biphasic P wave in lead V_1 is evidence of left atrial enlargement. Inversion of P waves in lead I suggests atrial inversion, as in mirror image dextrocardia, or else, an ectopic atrial pacemaker.

CONTINUOUS AMBULATORY ELECTROCARDIOGRAPHY

Continuous ambulatory electrocardiographic recordings are used when an arrhythmia is suspected or proved and to observe the effects of antiarrhythmic medication.

ECHOCARDIOGRAPHY

The echocardiogram is an informative, noninvasive technique that is valuable in initial diagnosis and follow-up. The M-mode and two-dimensional echocardiogram translates intracardiac anatomy and function into a display of "slices" of the beating heart. The many pieces of information that can thereby be analyzed are the presence or absence of septa; abnormalities of position and size of the great arteries; overriding aorta; aortic-mitral continuity; straddling, stenotic, or absent atrioventricular valves; enlargement of either ventricle or atrium; and the presence of pericardial fluid.

Systolic time intervals often are measured together with the M-mode echocardiogram to provide information about preejection and ejection periods of the heart and especially to evaluate pulmonary hypertension.

Two-dimensional echocardiography is uniquely applicable to the analysis of problems posed by patients with congenital heart disease. Addition of Doppler methodology gives an assessment of gradients across a stenosis or of flow through a defect or an incompetent valve.

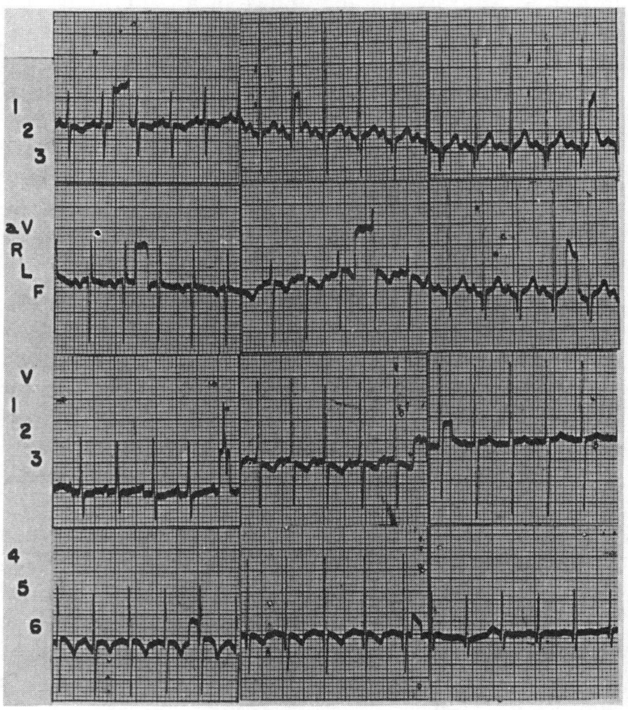

Figure 26.1. Electrocardiogram of a 2-month-old infant in cardiac failure from a large patent ductus arteriosus. Leads V_2 to V_6 are taken at half standardization because of unusually large voltage. Abnormalities are the electrical axis of 90°, persistence of right ventricular hypertrophy (tall R wave in lead V_1), and the presence of left ventricular hypertrophy and strain.

EXERCISE STRESS TEST

An exercise stress test is useful when it is important to evaluate the response to standardized exercise of graded degree in the unoperated or postoperative subject. Isotonic exercise on a treadmill or using a bicycle ergometer simulates a volume load on the heart and is the form of exercise testing we employ. Isometric exercise by sustained handgrip simulates a pressure load on the heart. Arrhythmias can be evaluated before, during, or on recovery from an exercise stress test. Information concerning exercise performance and arrhythmias is important in preoperative evaluation and postoperative follow-up as well as in the assessment of the nonoperative patient with congenital heart disease.

BLOOD TESTS

Blood tests include hemoglobin, hematocrit, and red blood cell count. These are often higher in the cyanotic patient. Before cardiac surgery, screening for bleeding–clotting abnormalities is performed by careful history and by prothrombin time and plasma thromboplastin time. A comprehensive coagulation survey is carried out if an abnormality is suspected.

CARDIAC CATHETERIZATION AND ANGIOGRAPHY

Cardiac catheterization with selective contrast visualization using angled views affords dynamic analysis of cardiovascular structures and function. Not only can pressures, flows, and resistances be measured, but also ventricular volume and function can be assessed. In the well-equipped and well-staffed laboratory, with personnel experienced in design and interpretation of the study, this investigation affords precise information to confirm or to clarify a diagnosis and to evaluate a patient before and after cardiac surgery. A His bundle electrocardiogram can be obtained for delineation of complex arrhythmias and disorders of conduction.

RADIONUCLIDE CINEANGIOGRAPHY

Radionuclide cineangiography at rest and with exercise offers a new modality to evaluate structure and myocardial performance.

DIGITAL SUBTRACTION ANGIOGRAPHY

Digital subtraction angiography with injection in or near the point of interest provides an image with less radiation and with a smaller dose of contrast medium.

NUCLEAR MAGNETIC RESONANCE IMAGING

Nuclear magnetic resonance imaging offers a new method of providing an image of the cardiovascular structures. It employs no ionizing radiation or radiopaque contrast medium, yet offers a great degree of tissue contrast in two or three dimensions. The principle applies the fact that certain atomic nuclei, when placed in a magnetic field and stimulated by radio waves of a particular frequency, will reemit some of the absorbed energy in the form of radio signals. The phenomenon is known as nuclear magnetic resonance (NMR). The images produced permit visualization of cardiac defects, ventricular hypoplasia, valvular thickening, abnormal great vessels, and surgical shunts. The full potential of this new and still expensive methodology has not yet been realized.

SPECIFIC MALFORMATIONS

When congenital malformation is suspected, precise diagnosis of the particular lesion and assessment of its severity need to be made. Preliminary diagnosis and differential diagnosis are based on the presence or absence of cyanosis, the amount of pulmonary blood flow, and the evidence of chamber enlargement or hypertrophy from electrocardiogram and cardiac series of chest roentgenograms. Table 26.1 shows these data for some common anomalies. Then, additional informative studies are selected.

NO SHUNT

Obstruction to Ventricular Outflow

Coarctation of the aorta is recognized at the bedside by palpating stronger pulses proximal to the obstruction than distal. In the usual situation, the coarctation is just beyond the origin of the left subclavian artery (Figure 26.2), so

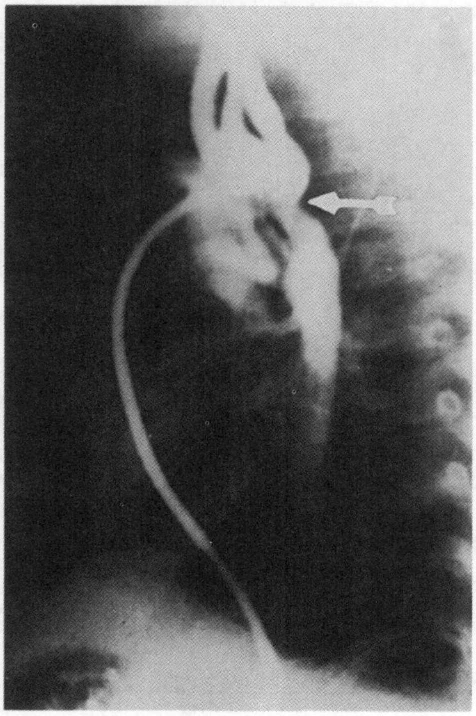

Figure 26.2. Aortogram of baby with coarctation of the aorta (*arrow*). Persistent patent ductus arteriosus adjacent to coarctation permits simultaneous opacification of the pulmonary artery. On chest roentgenogram this lateral margin of aorta above, at, and just below the coarctation produces the "3" sign.

the pulses and blood pressure in the arms exceed those in the legs. The arm pressure may not be much elevated if the coarctation is mild or if collateral circulation is rich (Figure 26.3). It is those vessels that account for a characteristic sign of coarctation: notching of the undersurfaces of the ribs by tortuous intercostal arteries. Often, a systolic murmur is heard posteriorly over the descending aorta at the site of the coarctation. In its usual location

Table 26.1. Differential Diagnosis of Common Congenital Cardiac Anomalies

Category	No Shunt	Left-to-Right Shunt	Right-to-Left Shunt With Pulmonic Stenosis	Right-to-Left Shunt Without Pulmonic Stenosis
Cyanosis	0	0	+	+
Pulmonary blood flow	Average	Increased	Decreased	Increased
Left ventricle, enlarged	Coarctation Aortic Stenosis	Patent ductus arteriosus Ventricular septal defect	Tricuspid atresia	
Right ventricle, enlarged	Pulmonic stenosis	Atrial septal defect	Tetralogy of Fallot Pulmonic stenosis with right-to-left atrial shunt	Complete transposition of great arteries Eisenmenger's syndrome
Both ventricles, enlarged		Atrioventricular septal defect Ventricular septal defect	Truncus arteriosus	

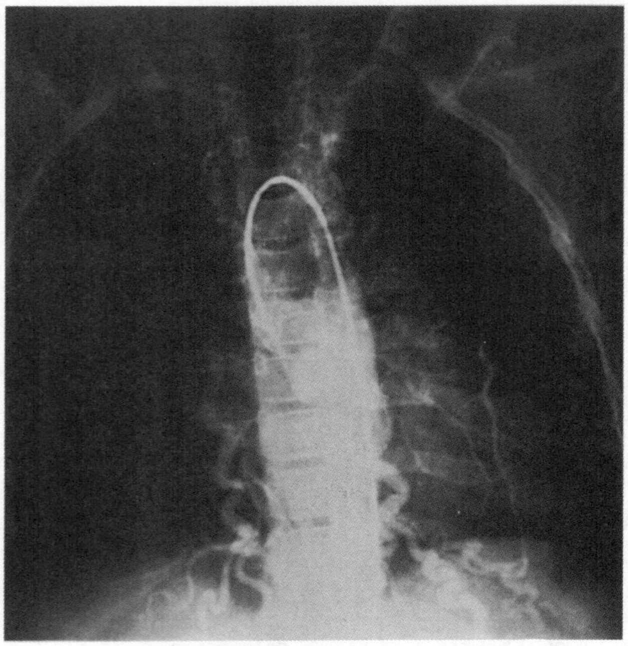

Figure 26.3. Aortic injection in a child opacifies the coarctation of the aorta with the reasons for the "E" and "3" radiologic signs of coarctation evident from the contour of the medial and lateral aspects of the descending aorta. Abundant vessels of collateral circulation are seen.

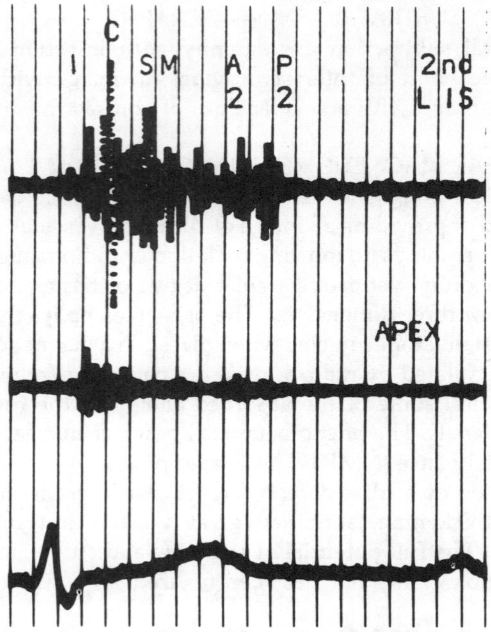

Figure 26.4. Phonocardiogram of a child with severe valvular pulmonic stenosis shows a diamond-shaped systolic murmur with early systolic ejection click (c) in second left interspace (pulmonary area). Second component of second heart sound (P2) is delayed.

the coarctation produces radiologic signs: the "3" sign of the aorta with a proximal segment, constriction, then poststenotic dilatation, and the "E" sign on barium swallow, when the esophagus curves about the prestenotic and poststenotic segments.

Aortic stenosis is usually valvular, with two leaflets of unequal size, fused at one or both commissures. Poststenotic dilatation of the ascending aorta and an early systolic ejection sound are common in valvular stenosis. When stenosis is supravalvular, it is often associated with other features that constitute a syndrome: the supravalvular syndrome of elfin facies, mental retardation, friendly personality, and sometimes in infancy, hypercalcemia. Subaortic stenosis may be due to a discrete fibromuscular membrane just beneath the aortic valve, or it may be muscular, as in hypertrophic cardiomyopathy or a tunnel type of obstruction. Aortic regurgitation often follows discrete subvalvular or supravalvular stenosis.

Pulmonic stenosis is frequently valvular, with an early systolic ejection sound (Figure 26.4) and poststenotic dilatation of the main pulmonary artery (Figure 26.5). Increasing severity of pulmonic stenosis is usually reflected in the electrocardiogram by increasing degrees of right ventricular hypertrophy and strain (Figure 26.6). Dyspnea and fatigue on exertion are symptoms of severe obstruction. When stenosis is severe, hypertrophied muscles of the crista supraventricularis impart a secondary hypertrophic infundibular, subpulmonic stenosis. A discrete band or anomalous muscle bundle may also cause subpulmonic stenosis. Constriction of the main pulmonary artery or branches causes supravalvular or branch pul-

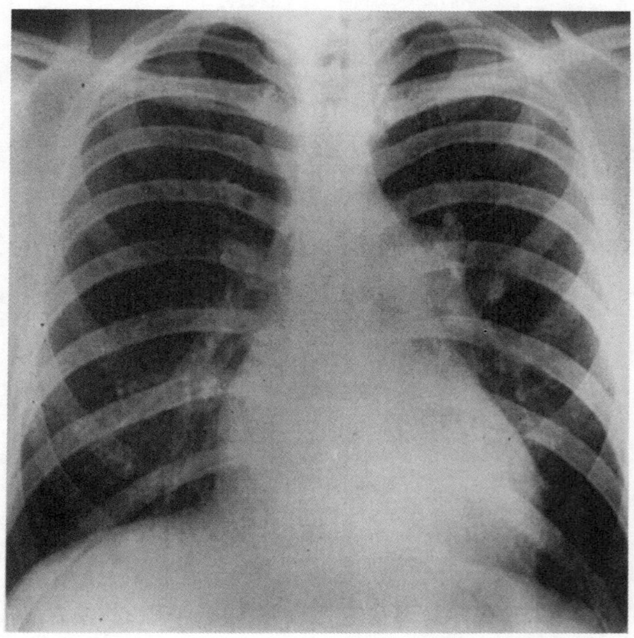

Figure 26.5. Roentgenogram of adolescent boy with severe valvular pulmonic stenosis shows poststenotic dilatation of the main pulmonary artery. The right atrium and ventricle are enlarged, causing the cardiothoracic ratio to be greater than 50%. Hilar pulmonary arteries are well seen, but markings are diminished in the periphery of lung fields.

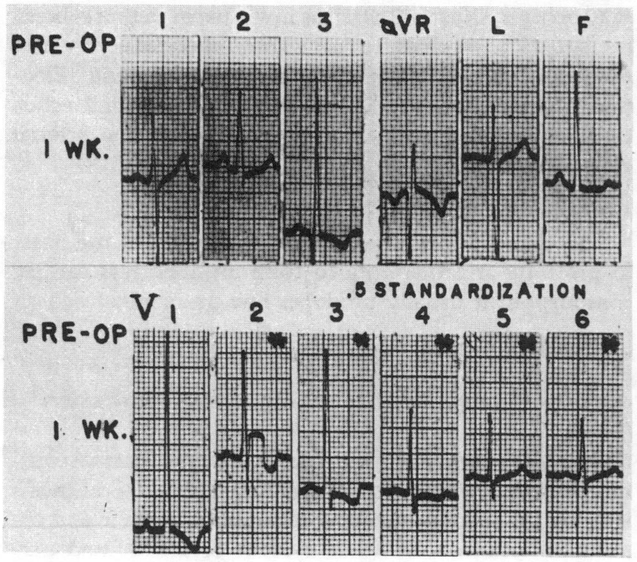

Figure 26.6. Electrocardiogram of a child with extreme pulmonic stenosis and suprasystemic pressure in right ventricle shows right ventricular hypertrophy and strain. Note tall R wave of 37 mm in lead V_1 and deeply inverted T waves in leads V_1 through V_4. *half standardization

monary stenosis. This can be part of the supravalvular syndrome mentioned in the discussion of aortic stenosis.

Primary pulmonary hypertension is a rare congenital cardiac condition. It is due to obstruction to pulmonary blood flow with pulmonary arterial obstructive changes. The echocardiogram gives indirect evidence of pulmonary hypertension in the abnormal values for systolic time intervals.

The indication for additional studies, such as cardiac catheterization, in patients with obstruction to ventricular outflow is the judgment that the obstruction is moderate or severe. Surgery is considered under those circumstances, and to measure pressures and visualize the anatomy become important in the patient's management.

Obstruction to Ventricular Inflow

Obstruction to ventricular inflow is rare. Causes of such obstruction include congenital tricuspid stenosis on the right side and mitral stenosis, cor triatriatum, or supravalvular ring on the left side. When severe, elevated pressure in the atrium proximal to the stenosis is followed by venous distension and edema.

Congenital mitral stenosis causes a late diastolic (presystolic) murmur at the apex of the heart. Sometimes an opening snap is audible there. The pulmonic component of the second heart sound is accentuated. The heart is usually not enlarged until the right ventricle fails. First, it hypertrophies in response to the pulmonary venous, capillary, and arterial hypertension that occurs when obstruction to left atrial outlet is compromised by the stenosis. The left atrium is enlarged, and both the electrocardiogram and the esophagram with barium indicate this, as does the echocardiogram. M-mode echocardiography displays the abnormal slope of mitral valve opening, and two-dimensional echocardiography may further define the nature of the stenosis, such as a parachute mitral valve with a single papillary muscle or a double orifice mitral valve.

Cor triatriatum is a rare malformation that can produce obstruction to ventricular inflow through obstruction to pulmonary venous return. The anomaly is due to failure of resorption of the common pulmonary vein. This results in a partitioning of the left atrium into a proximal chamber that receives pulmonary venous return and a distal chamber in continuity with the mitral valve. Severity of stenosis depends on the size of the orifice in the membrane dividing the left atrium. This membrane can usually be imaged on echocardiography and can be demonstrated on angiocardiography.

Congenital tricuspid stenosis is a great rarity as an isolated anomaly with no cyanosis. More often it occurs with an atrial septal defect and underdeveloped right ventricle as a cyanotic condition.

Ebstein's anomaly of the tricuspid valve is another uncommon anomaly that interferes with normal forward flow of blood. There is downward displacement of the leaflets and thinning of the atrialized right ventricle, which can become markedly dilated. The precordium is quiet. Often, right-sided third and fourth heart sounds are audible, along with a systolic and sometimes a mid- or late diastolic murmur with a scratchy sound. The electrocardiogram shows low voltage in leads V_1 and V_3R with a right ventricular conduction delay or right bundle branch block. The degree of downward displacement determines the size of the right heart; marked displacement causes great enlargement. Echocardiography, especially two-dimensional, shows the abnormal position of the tricuspid valve and the dilatation of the right atrium and atrialized right ventricle. Patency of the foramen ovale is common, and the patient is then cyanotic.

Valvular Regurgitation

Even less common are congenital pulmonic, mitral, or aortic regurgitation. The rare aortico–left ventricular tunnel or channel from right coronary through the upper ventricular septum into the left ventricle functionally resembles aortic insufficiency. The regurgitant murmurs and volume load on the respective ventricle are characteristic for each valve area. It may be that prolapsing mitral valve is a congenital anomaly.

Endomyocardial Abnormality

In unusual instances the mural and sometimes the valvular endocardium is thickened because of endocardial fibroelastosis which affects chiefly the left side of the heart. The electrocardiogram shows left ventricular hypertrophy and strain. The chamber wall is hypertrophied, and the chamber itself may be either restricted and small or, more often, dilated. This condition presents and performs as a cardiomyopathy, usually resulting in death in infancy. Some children survive early heart failure and even lose the cardiomegaly. However, we have followed a few who around the age of 10 years again developed heart failure and died.

"Corrected" Transposition of the Great Arteries

"Corrected" transposition of the great arteries is that position of the arteries in which the aorta is anterolateral and the pulmonary artery posteromedial, the reverse of normal. Because the aorta is to the left of the pulmonary artery, this is also called L-transposition. The aortic and pulmonic valves are appropriate for the great artery. Although venous inflow to the heart is normal at the atrial level, the atrioventricular valves and ventricles are inverted. The right atrium sends blood across a mitral valve to an inverted anatomic left ventricle on the right side, and this physiologically "right" ventricle ejects into the posteromedial great artery, which is the pulmonary artery. Similarly, arterial blood flows in the physiologic direction across the left-sided tricuspid valve and inverted, anatomic right ventricle into the anterolateral aorta.

If no other malformation exists, this individual functions normally. The diagnosis can be suspected from the accentuated second heart sound in the "pulmonic" area (actually the aortic valvular area) in the second left interspace. Additional diagnostic studies, such as echocardiography and digital subtraction angiocardiography, can establish the diagnosis.

Often, however, there are other frequently associated anomalies that affect function. Common among these are ventricular septal defect and pulmonic stenosis. It is not unusual for the patient to be born with, or to acquire, high-grade and even complete heart block.

Congenital Complete Heart Block

Congenital complete heart block is another type of congenital cardiac anomaly that delays the passage of blood through the slow rate of ventricular emptying. The slow ventricular rate is associated with a large diastolic volume and, thus often, with slight to moderate cardiomegaly. On the electrocardiogram, the QRS is usually narrow, indicating block within or proximal to the His bundle, and P waves are often high and peaked, consistent with right atrial hypertrophy. This is probably due to the effort of the atria as they attempt to pump blood through incompletely opened atrioventricular valves. Usually, there is no other cardiac anomaly. If there is, the prognosis is less favorable. Corrected or L-transposition of the great arteries is the anomaly most often associated with congenital heart block. The period of greatest risk of death from the anomaly is the first week of life.

Pacemakers are usually not needed in infants unless they are in heart failure and are usually not needed in children. The first syncopal episode is an indication for a pacemaker. Patients are restricted from unusually strenuous, competitive sports.

Abnormalities of Cardiac Position

These have no pathophysiologic consequence but often are associated with other cardiac anomalies. The heart and viscera normally are in situs solitus, but there may be abnormalities of position of one or both. For instance, there may be dextrocardia due to inversion (mirror image-dextrocardia) or to rotation of the heart (dextroversion or mesoversion), and these abnormal positions of the heart may occur in situs solitus, situs inversus, or in that mixed-up situation referred to as visceral heterotaxy. Chest roentgenogram confirms the abnormal position. Electrocardiogram helps to define atrial position, and echocardiogram helps analyze atrial, ventricular, and arterial connections.

Pericardial Defect

This defect allows the underlying portion of the heart to protrude and therefore to form an abnormal cardiac contour, but it usually produces few problems.

LEFT-TO-RIGHT SHUNT

Abnormal Communications at the Aortico–Pulmonary Level

Patent ductus arteriosus is the most common abnormal communication at the aortico–pulmonary area. The diagnosis is made on auscultation of a continuous systolic and diastolic murmur, with a late systolic crescendo and diastolic decrescendo, localized to the second and third left parasternal spaces (Figure 26.7).

Ductal blood flow is determined by systemic and pulmonary artery pressure and resistance relations and by the size of the ductus itself. With large shunts, the systemic pulse pressure widens, a diastolic mitral valve flow murmur may be heard, and left ventricular and left atrial enlargement is usually present on roentgenogram along with a prominent ascending aorta and main pulmonary artery and with pulmonary vascular engorgement. Electrocardiogram then shows left ventricular hypertrophy. Echocardiographic determination of left ventricular and left atrial size provides important information concerning the approximate magnitude of left-to-right shunting.

Other abnormal communications at the aortico–pulmonary level that produce a continuous murmur include an aortico–pulmonary window (sometimes called an aortic septal defect) between the ascending aorta and pulmonary artery and a coronary arteriovenous fistula into the pulmonary artery or right heart chamber. Anomalous origin of the left coronary artery from the pulmonary artery often behaves more as a cardiomyopathy than as a left-to-right shunt. In patients with anomalous origin of the left coronary artery, blood flows from the aorta to the right coronary artery, then through collateral vessels to the left coronary artery, and back into the pulmonary artery. The diagnosis may be suspected in the baby with cardiomegaly and cardiac failure, by electrocardiographic evidence of an anterolateral myocardial infarction, or by the presence of an apical systolic murmur at the apex. This mitral regurgitation is due to ischemia or infarction of the papillary muscle. Echocardiography supports the diagnosis. Selective injection of contrast medium at cardiac catheterization identifies these abnormal connections between the aorta and pulmonary bed. Approximately 30% of patients survive the first year of life.

Abnormal Communications at the Ventricular Level

Ventricular septal defect: At the ventricular level, the left-to-right shunt is due to a ventricular septal defect or absent ventricular septum. The ventricular septal defect

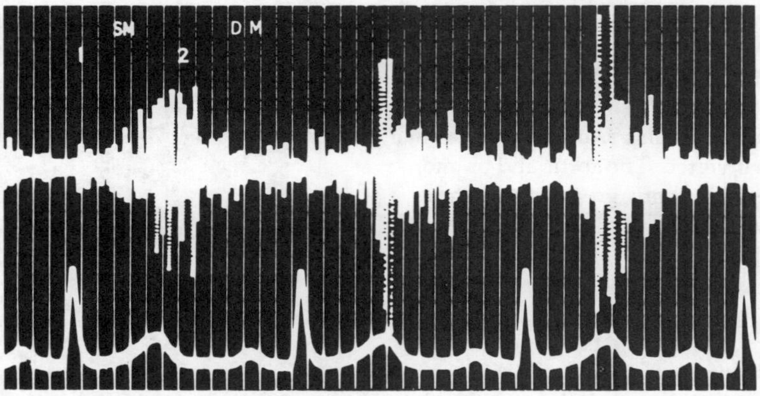

Figure 26.7. Phonocardiogram of a child with patent ductus arteriosus records the characteristic continuous murmur in the pulmonary area: late systolic crescendo and diastolic decrescendo with second heart sound covered by murmur.

is the most common congenital cardiac defect at birth. Most often, the defect is single and high in the membranous septum (infracristal defect, perimembranous defect); sometimes, the opening is subpulmonic (supracristal or subpulmonic ventricular septal defect); or there may be a defect in the muscular septum. Rarely, there is a left ventricular–right atrial shunt. Defects may be multiple. It is the size of the defect more than the location or number that determines the pathophysiologic aspects. A small, restrictive ventricular septal defect causes no cardiac or pulmonary burden. A large, nonrestrictive defect permits equalization of systolic pressure in the two ventricles; the effect is tantamount to a single ventricle. Then, if pulmonary resistance to flow is normally low, torrential pulmonary flow, hyperkinetic pulmonary hypertension, and cardiac failure result. This usually happens by 6 to 8 weeks of age. Increase in obstruction to pulmonary flow, either within the right ventricle or in the pulmonary arterial tree, restricts this left-to-right shunt somewhat. Marked pulmonary vascular obstruction converts the flow through the defect to minimal shunting or to a right-to-left shunt (Eisenmenger's syndrome). Development of marked infundibular pulmonic stenosis converts the condition into acyanotic and then cyanotic congenital heart disease in the form of tetralogy of Fallot.

The hallmark of a ventricular septal defect is the holosystolic murmur at the lower left sternal border. If the defect permits a large shunt, an apical mid-diastolic murmur of the excessive flow across the mitral valve is heard. The pulmonic component of the second heart sound becomes louder and splitting of the second heart sound becomes narrower as the pulmonary pressure becomes higher.

Radiologic signs of a large shunt include enlargement not only of the main pulmonary artery and branches but also of the left atrium and ventricle and right ventricle (Figure 26.8). The electrocardiogram then shows left ventricular hypertrophy and may also show a right ventricular conduction delay or hypertrophy as well as P-wave abnormalities of left or right atrial enlargement, or both. If the shunt is small and pressures are normal, both the electrocardiogram and roentgenogram are normal. If the defect is small, two-dimensional echocardiography is likely not to identify it except by Doppler studies. However, medium or large defects cause dropout of echoes, thus permitting sizing and localization of the defect.

Cardiac catheterization is indicated chiefly as a preliminary to surgery when the defect has produced a cardiopulmonary burden. Measurement of flows and determinations of pulmonary and systemic vascular resistance contribute to the selection of patients for surgery.

Ventricular septal defect with origin of both great arteries from the right ventricle (double outlet right ventricle) is an unusual variety of ventricular septal defect that may be associated with only a left-to-right shunt if the defect is subaortic or if a large, uncommitted ventricular septal defect permits preferential left ventricular-aortic flow. If the ventricular septal defect is subpulmonic or if pulmonic stenosis or pulmonary vascular obstruction coexists and is marked, the complex falls into the cyanotic category.

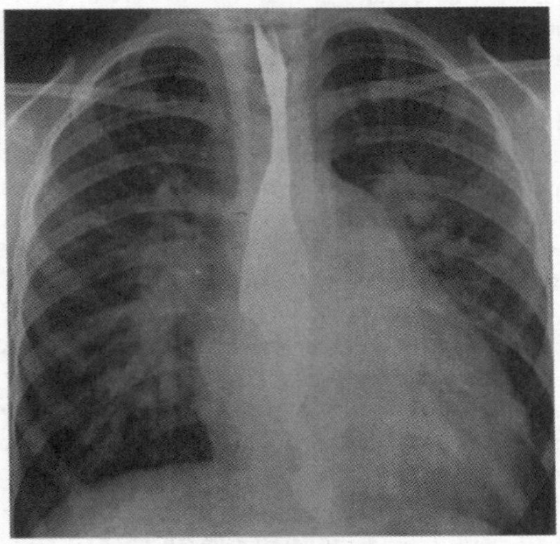

Figure 26.8. Roentgenogram of 3-month-old infant in cardiac failure from large ventricular septal defect. Note cardiomegaly, abnormally convex main pulmonary artery, and engorged pulmonary arterial markings that extend out to the periphery of lung fields.

In double outlet right ventricle, the aorta and pulmonary artery may be in the normal anteroposterior and side-to-side relation, but they may also rotate to side-by-side or transposed (aorta to the right or aorta to the left) relation. Similarly, ventricular situs may be normal or the ventricles may be inverted. The aortic and pulmonic valves are at the same level; both great arteries have a conus beneath the valve.

To analyze this complex anomaly, which can mimic a simple, large ventricular septal defect, requires ingenuity and skill. Echocardiography, especially two-dimensional, contributes greatly. At cardiac catheterization, measurement of systemic systolic pressure in the systemic venous ventricle is a clue to diagnosis. Angled views with selective injection of contrast medium define the relations.

Atrioventricular septal defect, often called *atrioventricular canal*, combines features of both atrial septal defect and ventricular septal defect, but in addition, mitral and tricuspid valvular abnormality and mitral or tricuspid regurgitation may be present. Functionally, the shunt at either level or valvular regurgitation may predominate. A left ventricular-to-right atrial shunt may occur. The electrocardiogram is characteristic of this anomaly. There is a superior QRS axis (marked left axis deviation) with a right ventricular conduction delay, and prolonged atrioventricular conduction (long PR) also is often present. Ventricular hypertrophy depends on the amount of volume or pressure load. The angiocardiographic diagnostic feature is a "gooseneck" deformity of the outflow tract of the left ventricle in the frontal view. Two-dimensional echocardiography can also detect this abnormality as well as the defective septa and atrioventricular valves. In the complete form, an atrioventricular septal defect causes cardiac failure early in infancy and may lead to early pulmonary vascular obstruction in those who survive. This is the most common anomaly in Down's syndrome.

Univentricular heart, common ventricle, and single ventricle are variously used to describe a condition in which there is no demonstrable anatomic partition of venous and arterial blood at the ventricular level. When pulmonary flow is excessive, the patient may appear acyanotic and function as though he has a large ventricular septal defect. In differential diagnosis, the electrocardiogram tends to be unusual for a simple ventricular septal defect. Echocardiography differentiates the two, although sometimes it is difficult to distinguish between a muscle bundle and a remnant of septum. On echocardiography as well as angiocardiography, it is important to map out atrial situs and the number and character of atrioventricular valves and their attachments as well as arterial outlet. When pulmonic stenosis or high resistance to pulmonary flow occurs, then cyanosis is present. This condition will be discussed in more detail in the section on right-to-left shunts.

Abnormal Communications at the Atrial Level

Atrial septal defect: Shunts at the atrial level are most often through a secundum type of atrial septal defect in the fossa ovalis region (Figure 26.9), but they may occur through an ostium primum defect, just above the atrioventricular valves, or a sinus venosus defect, high in the atrium near the orifice of the superior vena cava. In the last situation, partial anomalous pulmonary venous return from the right lung is usually present.

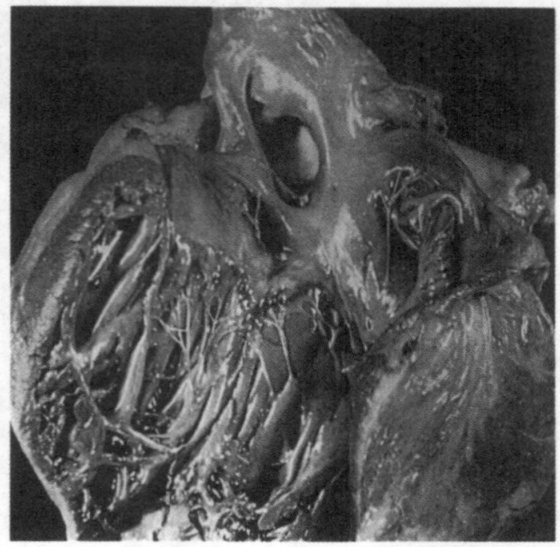

Figure 26.9. Postmortem specimen of adult who died in cardiac failure from a large, secundum-type atrial septal defect, without benefit of surgical closure during childhood.

Total anomalous pulmonary venous return may occur above or below the diaphragm. Supradiaphragmatic drainage occurs into a left vertical vein, superior vena cava, coronary sinus, or right atrium. Infradiaphragmatic drainage involves a long route for the common pulmonary vein to traverse before piercing the diaphragm to drain into a remnant of sinus venosus. Such drainage is regularly obstructed when infradiaphragmatic and is occasionally so when supradiaphragmatic. Obstructed return causes pulmonary hypertension, right ventricular hypertrophy, and predominant right-to-left shunt.

In these shunts at the atrial level, the right atrium and right ventricle and the pulmonary markings are enlarged, but not the left heart chambers or aorta. The electrocardiogram shows an abnormal amount of right ventricular conduction delay and sometimes a long PR interval. There is a systolic murmur, without a thrill, in the pulmonic area and wide, often fixed splitting of the second heart sound. A mid-diastolic murmur at the lower left sternal border is heard when the volume of shunted blood that crosses the tricuspid valve is large. A superior QRS axis on the electrocardiogram is characteristic of ostium primum defects. M-mode echocardiography shows volume load of the right ventricle and flattened or reversed ventricular septal motion. In young children, the two-dimensional echocardiogram in the subxiphoid view distinguishes the low-lying ostium primum defect from secundum and sinus venosus defects. Visualization of the pulmonary veins entering the left atrium helps to rule out anomalous pulmonary venous return.

The roentgenogram often gives information about the site of anomalous pulmonary venous drainage. If it occurs into a left vertical vein, that vessel is prominent, as is the superior vena cava, creating a snowman appearance (Figures 26.10 and 26.11). If drainage occurs into the superior vena cava, that structure is enlarged. Obstructed return appears as stippling throughout the lung fields.

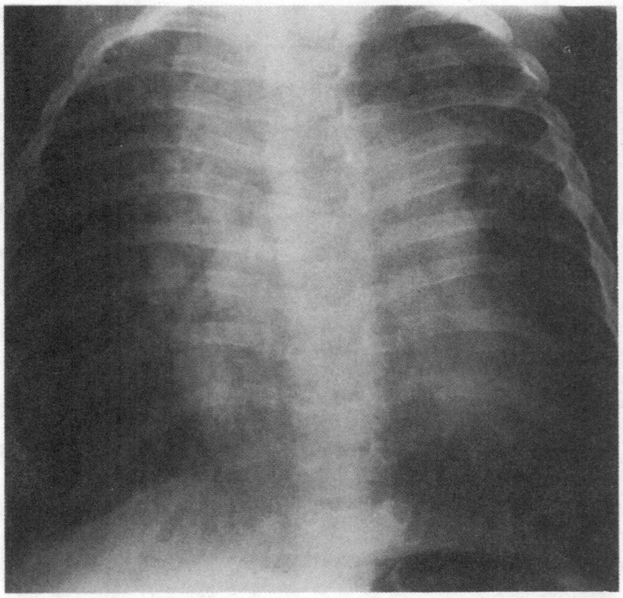

Figure 26.10. Roentgenogram of baby in cardiac failure from total anomalous pulmonary venous return to a left vertical vein, the dilated structure visible laterally and superiorly to the shadow of the prominently convex main pulmonary artery. The superior vena cava on the right base of the heart is also dilated. This vascular collar about the base of the heart, together with the enlarged right atrium and ventricle, gives the impression of a snowman. See Figure 26.11 for angiocardiogram of this patient.

Common atrium is a rare malformation. However, it is the expected anomaly in the Ellis–van Creveld syndrome. When there is common mixing of systemic and pulmonary venous returns, the predominant shunt is left-to-right unless some condition that provokes right ventricular hypertrophy coexists, in the form of pulmonic stenosis or pulmonary vascular obstruction. Physical findings and roentgenograms are those of atrial septal defect, but often the electrocardiogram has an ectopic atrial pacemaker or a superior axis, or both. The two-dimensional echocardiogram identifies no atrial septum.

RIGHT-TO-LEFT SHUNT

Right-to-left shunts combine an abnormal connection between the two circulations with a severe intracardiac or intrapulmonary obstruction to pulmonary flow, so that venous blood enters the aorta, or with obligatory veno-arterial shunting because of common mixing (common truncus arteriosus, common ventricle, or common atrium) or abnormal connection of vessels, such as complete transposition of the great arteries or total anomalous pulmonary venous return. Additional features depend on whether the anomaly results in diminished or excessive pulmonary blood flow. Pulmonary blood flow may be diminished because of pulmonary stenosis or atresia (as in tetralogy of Fallot or tricuspid stenosis or atresia together with a rudimentary right ventricle) or because of inadequacy of the right heart as a pump, as in Ebstein's anomaly with a defect in the atrial septum. In such anomalies, the shunted portion of blood bypasses the lungs.

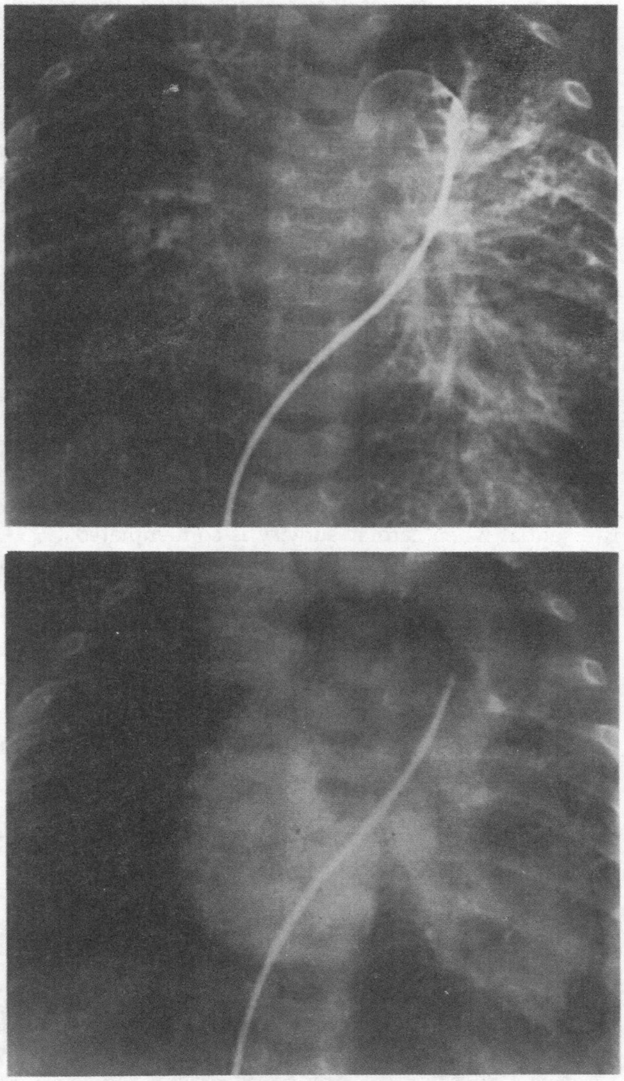

Figure 26.11. Selective injection of contrast medium into main pulmonary artery is followed by opacification of smaller pulmonary arteries and capillaries (*above*) and then by the confluence of opacified pulmonary veins to enter the left vertical vein and continue as the vascular collar about the base of the heart to enter the superior vena cava and right atrium.

The patient may be deeply cyanotic and experience shortness of breath and fatigue on exertion but rarely has cardiac failure. In contrast, when pulmonary flow is excessive and a right-to-left shunt is predominant, the patient may be only minimally cyanotic, yet have considerable cardiac enlargement and, often, cardiac failure early in life until pulmonary vascular obstruction develops and dampens the left-to-right shunt.

With Decreased Pulmonary Blood Flow

Tetralogy of Fallot is the most common of the cyanotic group. Its four features include a ventricular septal defect large enough to equalize systolic pressures in the two ventricles, pulmonic stenosis of such severity that pulmonary artery pressure is normal or below normal, overriding of the aorta due to the disproportionate size of the two great arteries or to rotation of the aortic origin, and right ventricular hypertrophy (Figures 26.12 to 26.14). Some patients are born with all four features, whereas others acquire the last three as infundibular pulmonic stenosis. The systolic murmur is due to pulmonic stenosis rather than the ventricular septal defect. The second heart sound often is single and represents aortic closure. On chest roentgenogram, the average-sized heart is boot-shaped (coeur en sabot), and pulmonary arterial markings are diminished (Figure 26.15). A right aortic arch is present in about 25%; it is readily identified by barium swallow. The electrocardiogram shows right axis deviation and right ventricular hypertrophy with reversal of R and S relations across the precordium (Figure 26.16). Echocardiography diagnoses the ventricular septal defect and aortic override, and tells the size of the right ventricular outflow tract and pulmonary artery. However, I believe that selective right and left ventricular angiocardiography is essential when cardiac surgery is contemplated.

Pseudotruncus arteriosus is a term for tetralogy of Fallot with pulmonary atresia and collateral circulation from the aorta to pulmonary branches, causing the distinctive clinical feature of this malformation, namely, a continuous, humming murmur over one or both lung fields. Selective injection of contrast medium into each collateral vessel is needed to identify the pulmonary blood supply routes

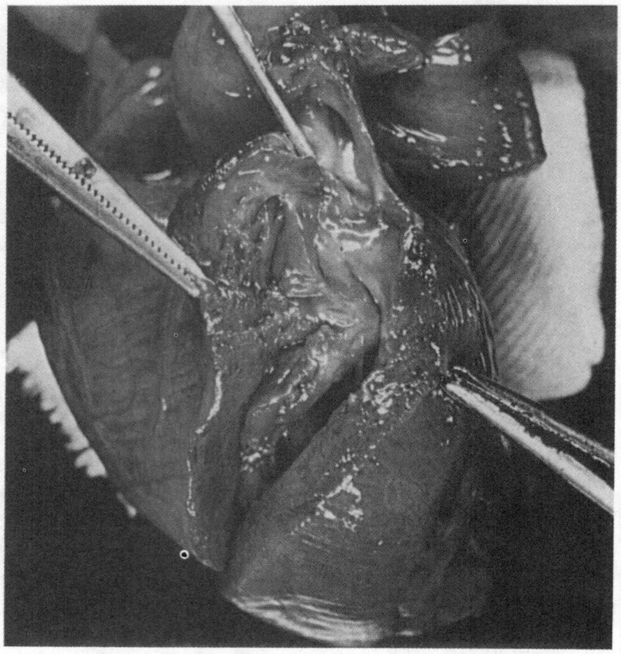

Figure 26.13. Opening the right ventricle in a specimen of tetralogy of Fallot reveals marked infundibular pulmonic stenosis with hypertrophy of the right ventricular wall proximal to the stenosis and thinness of the wall distal in the infundibular chamber. The main pulmonary artery is small.

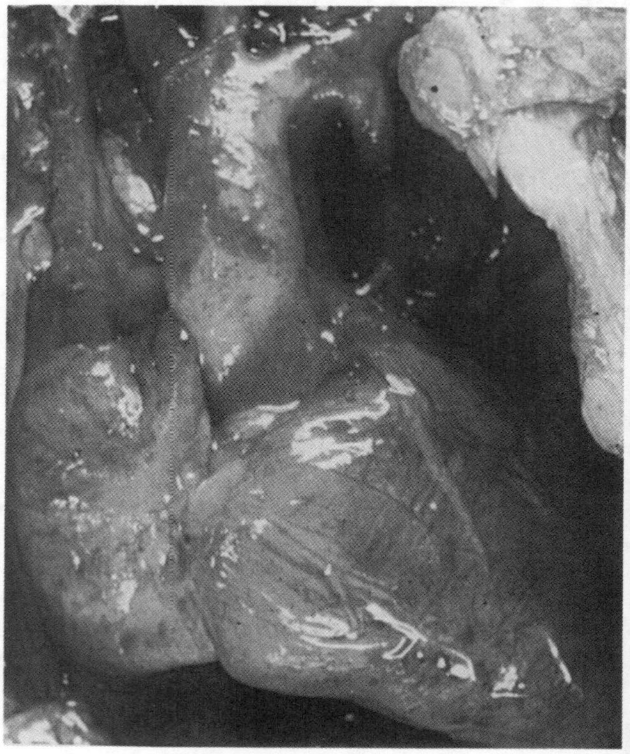

Figure 26.12. Postmortem specimen of newborn infant with tetralogy of Fallot shows the boot-shaped heart so typically seen in chest x-ray films. (See Figure 26.15.) The concavity in the region of the main pulmonary artery that contributes to the boot shape is due to the small size (hypoplasia) of the main pulmonary artery distal to the severe subvalvular pulmonic stenosis. (See Figure 26.13.)

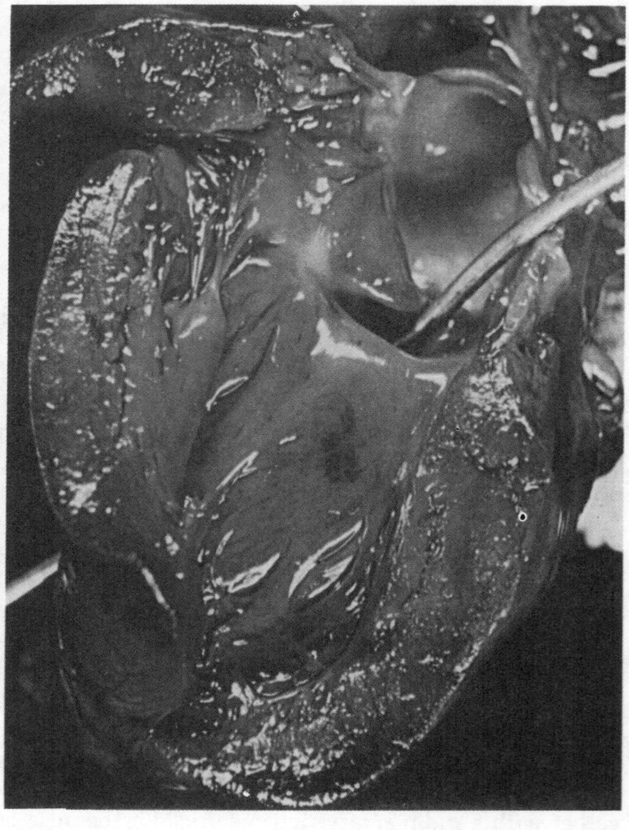

Figure 26.14. Opened left ventricle shows probe through the large, high ventricular septal defect and the overriding aorta.

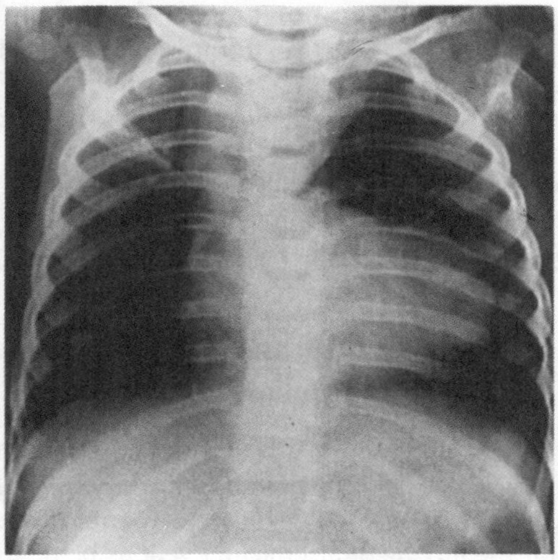

Figure 26.15. Boot-shaped heart with concave main pulmonary artery and tip-tilted apex and exceedingly clear lung fields with practically no visible pulmonary arteries in a baby with severe tetralogy of Fallot.

and to determine if there is continuity between right and left pulmonary arteries and if there is a main pulmonary artery.

Other tetralogy-like conditions that require echocardiography and cardiac catheterization with angiocardiography for differentiation include conditions such as tetralogy with absent pulmonic valve and a grossly dilated main pulmonary artery, tetralogy with an atrial septal defect (pentalogy), and ventricular septal defect with transposition of the great arteries and pulmonary stenosis or atresia, as well as single ventricle with pulmonary stenosis.

Rudimentary right ventricle with tricuspid and pulmonic atresia or stenosis and atrial septal defect or patent foramen ovale are conditions in which the systemic venous return passes through the defect in the atrial septum to mix in the left atrium with the pulmonary venous return, so that the mixed blood enters the left ventricle and aorta. Blood flows to the lungs by one of several routes. If the tricuspid and pulmonic valves are stenotic rather than atretic, venous blood enters the rudimentary right ventricle directly and is pumped to the lungs. If the tricuspid valve is atretic, but a ventricular septal defect is present, mixed blood from the left ventricle goes to the right ventricle and thence to the lungs. If the ventricular septal defect becomes too small, pulmonary flow is decreased. Blood from the aorta may go to the pulmonary circulation through a patent ductus arteriosus or vessels of collateral circulation. All three portions of the right ventricle may be present but hypoplastic: the inflow, mid, and outflow portions. More often, the last two are present. The pulmonic anulus, valve, and main pulmonary artery are often average in size. The effective pulmonic stenosis occurs proximal to the valve, through a restricted atrial septal defect or ventricular septal defect or the rudimentary right ventricle.

The electrocardiogram shows high, peaked P waves of right atrial hypertrophy, left axis deviation, and, in the precordial leads, deep S waves over the right side of the precordium and pure R waves over the left side. Echocardiography and angiocardiography depict the abnormal course of the circulation.

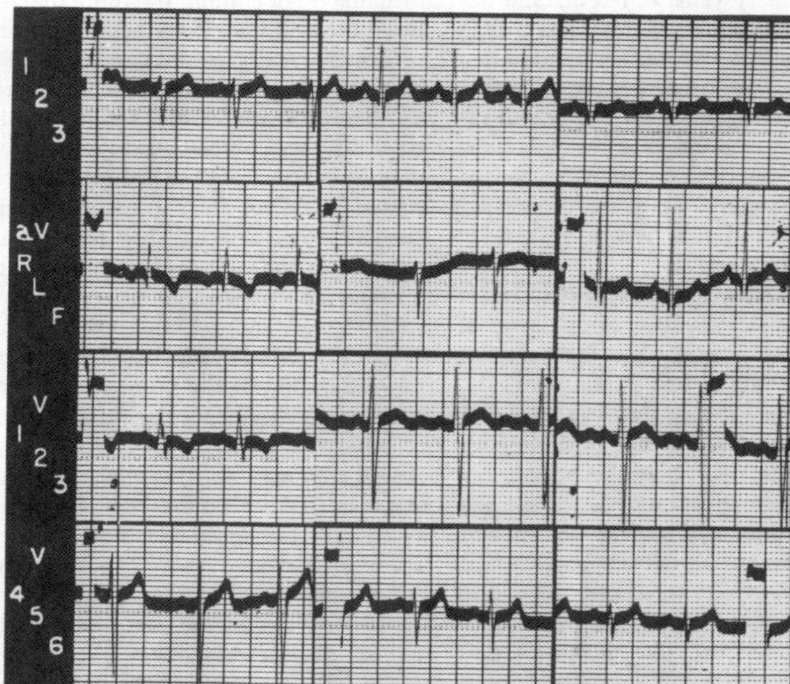

Figure 26.16. Electrocardiogram in tetralogy of Fallot shows right axis deviation and right ventricular hypertrophy with reversal of the usual R and S wave pattern across the precordium.

Pulmonic stenosis with patent foramen ovale or a defect in the atrial septum: The stenosis must be severe to be associated with a right-to-left shunt at the atrial level when the ventricular septum is intact. The systolic pressure in the right ventricle is usually suprasystemic, in excess of aortic pressure. The electrocardiogram shows not only right ventricular hypertrophy but also strain. Remarkably, even with such elevated pressures, the heart may not appear enlarged on the roentgenogram. Except for cyanosis, the clinical features resemble those of pulmonic stenosis with intact septa.

Ebstein's anomaly with patent foramen ovale or atrial septal defect: The deformed leaflets of the tricuspid valve are displaced a variable distance downward into the right ventricle, and the atrialized portion of the ventricle proximal to the free edges of the valve is abnormally thin, whereas the distal wall of the right ventricle is of normal thickness. Heart size and symptoms are related to the degree of downward displacement, which governs the proportions of the functioning right ventricle and atrialized region. Right-sided enlargement may be enormous. Cardiac action is quiet, and scratchy tricuspid systolic and sometimes diastolic murmurs may be heard, with a cadence of heart sounds that includes a third or a fourth heart sound, or both. The electrocardiogram shows right bundle branch block, with low voltage in lead V_1 and high and peaked P waves. Some patients have the Wolff–Parkinson–White syndrome. Supraventricular and ventricular arrhythmias are a problem for a few patients. The chief symptom is fatigability. The echocardiogram is diagnostic. We do not recommend cardiac catheterization.

Anomalous systemic venous return to the left atrium and pulmonary arteriovenous fistula are rare anomalies that decrease pulmonary blood flow by the portion of unoxygenated blood that shunts into the pulmonary veins or left atrium. Because they are so uncommon, diagnosis requires a high index of suspicion when cyanosis is being evaluated in a patient who may not even have a heart murmur. Echocardiography helps by excluding other anomalies, but selective injection of contrast medium into the left antecubital vein or near the left vertical vein may be needed for supradiaphragmatic anomalous systemic venous return, or into the inferior vena cava or hepatic system for infradiaphragmatic anomalous drainage.

Pulmonary arteriovenous fistula is identified at cardiac catheterization by selective injection of a contrast agent into the main pulmonary artery and following its detour into the pulmonary vein or left atrium.

Right-to-left shunt with obstruction to blood flow through the lungs (Eisenmenger's syndrome): The problem is due to pulmonary vascular obstruction with markedly elevated pulmonary vascular resistance plus a communication between the two circulations. The precapillary vascular obstruction may be present from birth but usually is acquired in childhood and manifested symptomatically in young adulthood. Left-to-right shunts reverse, and the stage of Eisenmenger's syndrome is reached. The murmur shortens, and the pulmonic component of the second heart sound becomes loud. It is sometimes followed by an early diastolic murmur of pulmonic regurgitation. Even though the right ventricle is hypertrophied, the overall heart size is average until cardiac output decreases and right-sided heart failure occurs. An electrocardiogram shows right ventricular hypertrophy. Echocardiography with systolic time intervals to estimate pulmonary hypertension and to identify the shunt site is helpful. It is much to be preferred over cardiac catheterization, which may be difficult and dangerous in Eisenmenger's syndrome. Fainting episodes and dyspnea on exertion, as well as sudden death, may occur.

Right-to-left Shunt with Increased Pulmonary Blood Flow

Complete transposition of the great arteries: In simple complete transposition of the great arteries, the aorta arises from the right ventricle and the pulmonary artery from the left ventricle. Survival is possible only when some mechanism exists for the mixing of arterial and venous blood. Infants die of anoxia or in heart failure unless intervention is immediate.

The newborn's findings include cyanosis persisting for a few hours, often with no murmur, with an electrocardiogram that shows the usual right ventricular dominance for a newborn and with a characteristic roentgenogram. When the aorta arises transposed to the right and in front of the pulmonary artery (called dextro- or D-transposition), the vascular pedicle in the frontal view is narrow and it widens in the right anterior oblique projection (Figure 26.17). Echocardiography offers immediate confirmation by showing the anterior aorta and the posterior pulmonary artery, which bifurcates (Figure 26.18). Emergency cardiac catheterization is indicated, so that balloon atrial septostomy may be performed as palliation to permit the mixing of arterial and venous blood at the atrial level. A few months after the balloon septostomy, we recommend operation to reroute the venous return to the heart for physiologic correction of the anomaly.

Complex forms of transposition of the great arteries occur. A coexisting large ventricular septal defect permits survival but leads to early cardiac failure and to pulmonary vascular disease. Complete transposition of the great arteries may also occur with a rudimentary right ventricle, tricuspid atresia or stenosis, atrial septal defect, and ventricular septal defect. When transposed, the aorta originates from the rudimentary right ventricle and is small, whereas the pulmonary artery originates unobstructed from the left ventricle and receives excessive pulmonary blood flow. Mild cyanosis and severe cardiac failure occur early. Banding of the pulmonary artery can palliate the condition by reducing the excess flow.

Taussig-Bing syndrome (double outlet right ventricle with transposition of the aorta and a subpulmonic ventricular septal defect): In this form of double outlet right ventricle, the subpulmonic location of the ventricular septal defect accounts for the cyanosis characteristic of this anomaly. The pulmonary artery receives the highly oxygenated blood from the left ventricle, whereas the aorta receives the mixed venous and shunted arterial blood. When the great arteries are in the usual anatomic position, the ventricular septal defect is anterior and subpulmonic. However, if the great arteries are transposed, the ventricular septal defect is in the posterior position below the pulmonic valve. Iden-

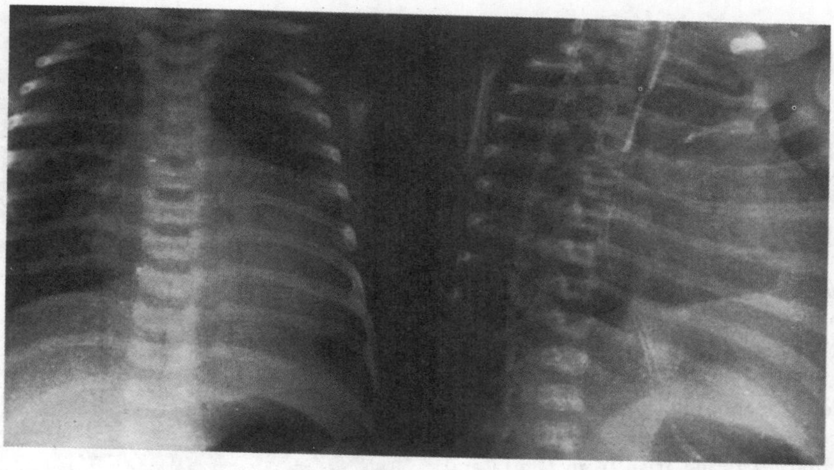

Figure 26.17. Roentgenograms in frontal and right anterior oblique projection of newborn infant with cardiac failure and complete transposition of great arteries. In the frontal view, the heart is enlarged, with a concave main pulmonary artery, but heavy hilar markings, and a narrow base that widens to double that size in the oblique view. This heart shape is referred to as one resembling an egg on its side.

tification of the double conus by echocardiography or by angiocardiography is needed for the diagnosis.

Common mixing with right-to-left shunt with increased pulmonary flow can occur at the atrial, ventricular, or aorticopulmonary level.

(1) *Total anomalous pulmonary venous return* is an uncommon condition that can be amenable to surgery. All pulmonary veins connect to the right atrium or a tributary thereof, and the systemic circulation is supplied by the portion of the mixed arterial and venous blood that shunts from the right to the left atrium through the atrial septal defect. Therefore, there is both a left-to-right and a right-to-left shunt. The patient's degree of cyanosis depends chiefly on the volume of blood reaching the lungs: the greater the pulmonary blood flow and the less obstructed the return, the less cyanosis. The color may even appear normal, as we noted earlier. The anomalous connection is supradiaphragmatic (into a left vertical vein, superior vena cava, coronary sinus, or right atrium) or infradiaphragmatic (into the inferior vena cava, ductus venosus, or hepatic vein). Infradiaphragmatic anomalous drainage is consistently obstructed, and death in infancy is usual. When the veins drain into a distended superior vena cava, they produce a characteristic radiologic appearance, the "snowman heart." When they enter a left vertical vein that continues as a vascular collar around the base of the heart, a "cottage loaf" appearance is seen.

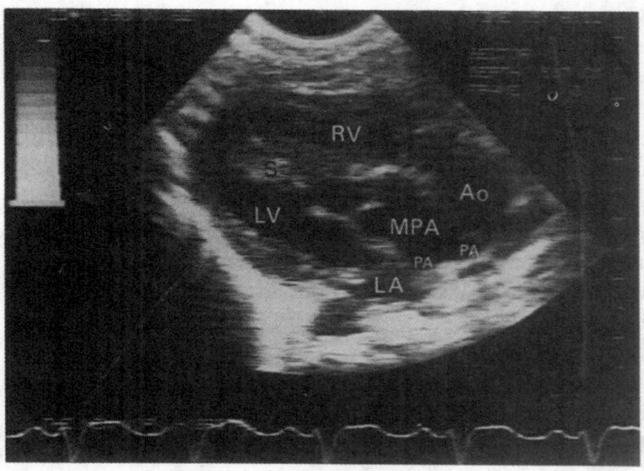

Figure 26.18. Two-dimensional echocardiogram of a newborn with complete transposition of the great arteries in this long-axis view shows simultaneous opacification of two roots, the anterior aorta (Ao) from the right ventricle (RV) and the posterior pulmonary (MPA), which bifurcates (PA) from the left (posterior) ventricle (LV). S indicates ventricular septum.

(2) *Common atrium* is unusual. It is suspected when there is bidirectional shunting at the atrial level and full saturation of the pulmonary veins. It is sometimes found in patients with the Ellis–van Creveld syndrome. This has been described under the section on left-to-right shunts.

(3) *Single or common ventricle* occurs in several versions with different nomenclature. A recent effort to clarify confusion in what to call this condition considers the atrioventricular connections. In the normal heart, two atria connect appropriately to the two ventricles. The term *univentricular atrioventricular connection* was proposed to describe the condition in which the atria connect to only one ventricle. It includes conditions of two atrioventricular valves (double inlet ventricle) or with atresia of one atrioventricular valve.

The most common form is that in which both atrioventricular valves connect with a ventricle that is anatomically a left ventricle. The left ventricle, in turn, connects with a rudimentary right ventricle, a condition often referred to as single ventricle with rudimentary outlet chamber. The semilunar valves and respective great arteries may arise in the usual manner, posteromedial aorta from the left ventricle and anterolateral pulmonary artery from the "right ventricle," or they may be in D- or L-transposition. Both may arise from the main body of the single ventricle or both from the "right ventricular" chamber. There may be a common truncus. Either pulmonic or aortic stenosis may be present.

Function of the patient depends on the balance of pulmonary and systemic blood flows and resistances and on the adequacy of forward flow. Stenosis or insufficiency of the atrioventricular or semilunar valves seriously impairs function with one main ventricular pump. In diagnosis, echocardiography and selective angiography are needed.

(4) *Common truncus arteriosus* is classified into four types, based on the point of origin of the pulmonary arteries. In type I, the common pulmonary trunk exits from the lateral aspect of the truncus near the valve. In type II, there is a separate takeoff of the right and left pulmonary arteries from the posterior aspect of the ascending trunk. In type III, the pulmonary arteries arise from the lateral aspect of the ascending aorta or from brachiocephalic arteries or a ductus-like structure from the transverse arch. In type IV, which resembles the condition of pseudotruncus arteriosus, a variant of tetralogy of Fallot, discussed earlier, the lung vessels derive from systemic arteries leaving the descending aorta. Usually there are two ventricles, although one of them may be underdeveloped, and sometimes there is but one ventricle. The truncus valve may be incompetent or, rarely, stenotic.

When pulmonary flow is unobstructed, the early neonatal decrease in pulmonary vascular resistance leads to excessive pulmonary blood flow and to cardiac failure. Medical management may save a life but at the expense of early development of high pulmonary vascular resistance (Eisenmenger's syndrome).

Diagnosis utilizes the same tools as already described and relies heavily on two-dimensional echocardiography and cardiac catheterization with angiocardiography.

(5) *Hypoplastic left heart syndrome* is usually incompatible with life for more than a few days. The mitral and aortic valves, left ventricle, and ascending aorta are underdeveloped or atretic, and the right ventricle temporarily supplies not only the pulmonary circulation but also, via a patent ductus, the descending aorta and some of the ascending aorta as well (Figure 26.19). Echocardiography (Figures 26.20 and 26.21) has become useful in distinguishing this condition from other more potentially salvageable conditions.

The usual presentation in the newborn period is one of increasing tachypnea and dyspnea with grayish color. The radial and carotid pulses are feeble. If the ductus is patent, femoral pulses may be more easily felt. The precordium is overly active with an enlarged heart and a systolic murmur. Signs of left- and right-sided congestive failure appear early and are followed by shock and death.

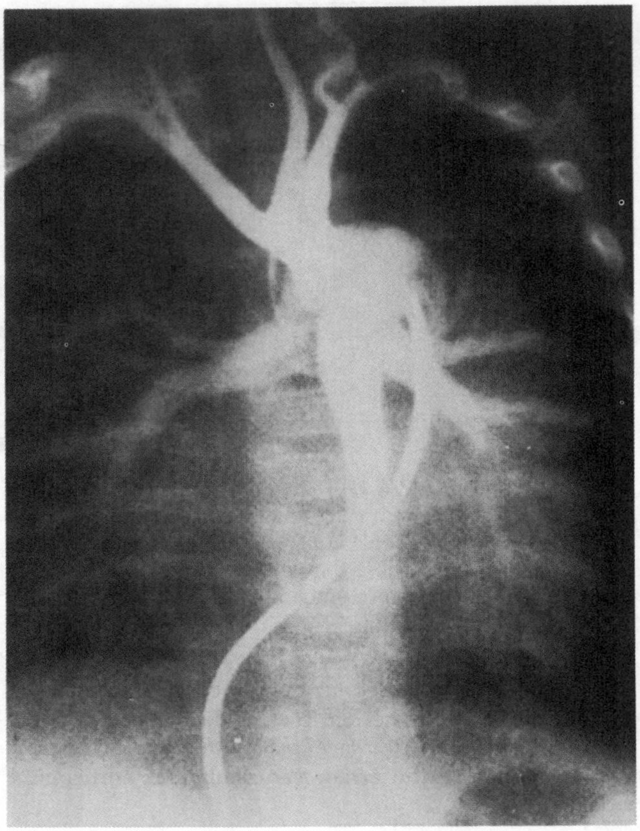

Figure 26.19. Cardiac catheterization of newborn with hypoplastic left heart syndrome shows catheter positioned in large main pulmonary artery. Contrast injection opacifies not only the main pulmonary artery and branches but also, through a patent ductus arteriosus, the descending aorta and, in retrograde fashion, the transverse aortic arch and brachiocephalic arteries and then the slender, thread-like ascending aortic arch.

NATURAL HISTORY AND PROGNOSIS

By the time the natural history of congenital heart disease could be assessed from large numbers of accurately diagnosed cases, it was already being changed by medical and surgical therapy. The greatest risk of morbidity and mortality from congenital heart disease of all kinds was, and still is, the period of early infancy.

Hypoxia and cardiac failure, the two chief causes of death, both respond to treatment, and often their cause can be alleviated or removed. Respiratory tract infections to which patients with excess pulmonary blood flow are susceptible can be combatted with antibiotics. Infective endocarditis can be prevented by antibiotics in therapeutic doses to treat the bacteremia that may occur with dental extractions or genitourinary tract instrumentation. Spontaneously occurring endocarditis can be treated. Brain abscess in the cyanotic child or adult can be accurately diagnosed by brain scan or nuclear magnetic resonance and can be treated with antibiotics and surgical drainage. Cerebrovascular thrombosis or embolism continues to be a threat for cyanotic patients, as is hemoptysis.

Congenital heart disease is not static, and spontaneous changes may modify prognosis. For example, in a patient born with a ventricular septal defect, the hole may remain large and the patient may die in cardiac failure; or the patient's condition may improve because the shunt decreases as infundibular hypertrophy develops or pulmonary arterial obstruction begins, or, conversely, as the ventricular septal defect decreases in size or closes spontaneously. Aneurysm formation of the membranous septum and plastering down of the septal leaflet of the tri-

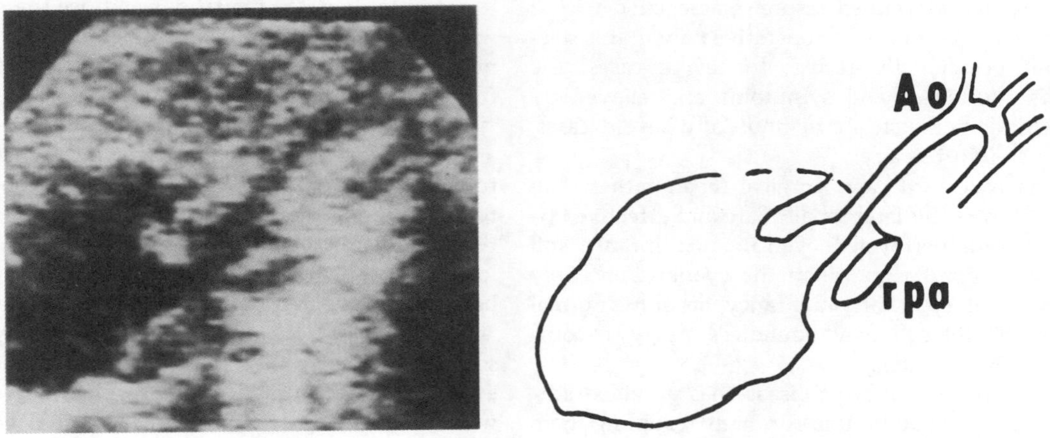

Figure 26.20. Two-dimensional echocardiogram in long-axis view shows the hypoplastic left ventricle with mitral and aortic atresia and small ascending aorta. The large ventricular chamber imaged is the right ventricle. The left ventricle below it is diminutive.

cuspid valve over the defect, as well as fibrous ingrowth, are all mechanisms of spontaneous closure.

In general, the prognosis for good health, normal activity, marriage and children, employment, and insurability is excellent for those with physiologically insignificant lesions, such as a small ventricular septal defect or mild pulmonic stenosis, and for those whose anomalies have been surgically repaired without residua or sequelae.

MANAGEMENT

Optimum management depends on accurate diagnosis and good judgment in choice of medical or surgical treatment, or both. Good judgment is the result of experience and alertness to new developments. Lifelong medical supervision is indicated for those whose anomalies have not been completely corrected surgically (eg, suture ligation of a patent ductus arteriosus) or naturally (spontaneous closure of a ventricular septal defect). Attention to prevention of complications, such as endocarditis, is indicated for all with organic heart disease, even after excellent functional repair. Management of complications such as cardiac failure is standard and should continue unless the cause for the failure has been corrected.

A smooth transition to adulthood is aided by the patient's gaining self-confidence and independence by participating in normal play and school-time activities and attaining some understanding of the nature of the anomaly. Those with surgically remediable lesions are operated on in infancy if the condition is severe and in childhood if it is moderately severe.

Surgical mortality is now low (0% to 5%) for most operable congenital anomalies, and morbidity is at a minimum in children. One common postoperative complication following surgery is the postpericardiotomy syndrome. It occurs as a febrile illness, with a pericardial and often a pleural reaction in about 25% of children but less than 5% of infants under 2 years. It appears to be an

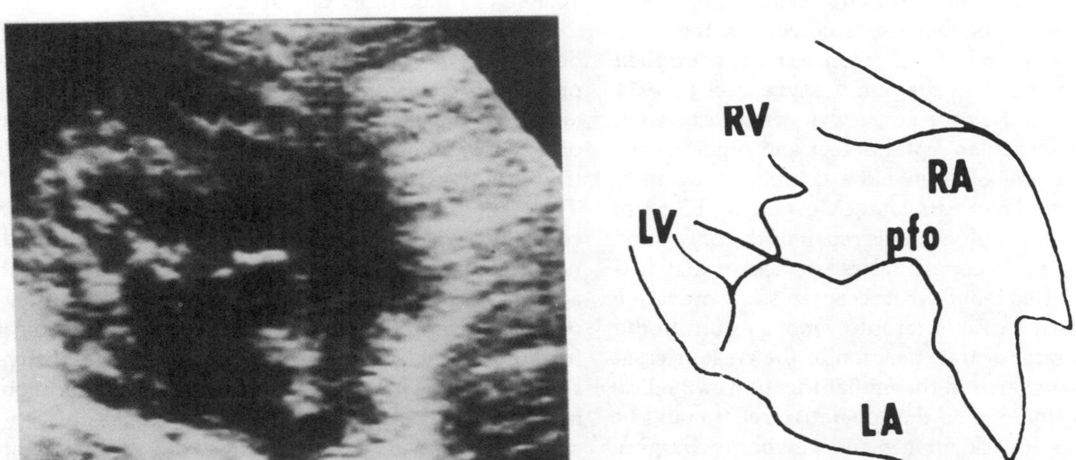

Figure 26.21. Echocardiographic view of left and right atria in same infant as in Figure 26.20 shows enlarged left atrium and bulging of atrial septum and foramen ovale into right atrium.

immunologically determined response associated with a viral illness acquired in the perioperative period. It is self-limited but occasionally recurs. In severe cases, the duration is shortened, and symptoms are relieved by salicylates, indomethacin, or in unusually severe cases, short-term steroid therapy.

The trend is toward early surgical repair rather than palliation followed by later repair. Safe and effective operations are being performed, even in small infants, and the results are gratifying. When the cyanotic or sickly baby has surgical repair early in infancy, his or her normal rate of growth, pink color, and boundless energy are comparable to those of peers.

Surgery for congenital heart disease has provided dramatic and lasting rehabilitation for many, enabling them to live longer and enjoy it more. However, in addition to the benefits they derive, some residua and sequelae deserve attention as well. Most of these people should continue to have lifelong medical surveillance that includes antibiotic prophylaxis at times of possible risk of endocarditis.

What each patient can do postoperatively depends not only on the severity of the anomaly and the age at surgery, but also on the "learning curve" for that particular operation and on what the operation could accomplish in terms of repair. Only two conditions, simple uncomplicated secundum atrial septal defect and patent ductus arteriosus, can be completely corrected.

Let me illustrate the learning curve with a review of the developments in cardiac surgery. It was in 1938 that a patent ductus arteriosus was closed by Dr Robert Gross of Boston, Massachusetts. In November 1944, the first "blue baby" operation, the Blalock–Taussig operation, was carried out in Baltimore, Maryland. The next year, coarctation of the aorta was repaired in the experimental surgical laboratory by Gross and in a patient by Crafoord of Sweden. In 1948, the Blalock–Hanlon operation was introduced for palliation of transposition of the great arteries through creation of an atrial septal defect. That same year, Brock and Sellors independently in England reported on closed pulmonary valvotomy. Open pulmonary valvotomy and closure of atrial septal defect were popularized by Swan of Denver, Colorado, in the early 1950s. It was C. Walton Lillehei's pioneering of controlled cross-circulation and then the pump oxygenator in 1954 that opened up the field of surgery under direct vision for closure of ventricular septal defect and repair of tetralogy of Fallot and of even more complex congenital cardiac anomalies. Ten years later, Mustard of Toronto, Canada, accomplished physiologic repair of the only common kind of cyanotic congenital heart disease that had until that time defied relief, with acceptably low operative risk: the intraatrial baffle to reroute venous return to the atria to compensate for transposition of the great arteries. The early 1970s ushered in the miniaturization of medical and surgical technology so that operative relief could be offered to critically sick infants and newborns. Surgical techniques for increasingly complex anomalies developed, among them the use of external valved conduits to form a channel for blood flow that heretofore did not exist, the Fontan operation for tricuspid atresia-type anomalies to separate the two circulations and use the right atrium with or without the rudimentary right ventricle to achieve pulmonary blood flow, and the arterial switch operation for transposed great arteries.

All of these operations seemed more difficult and had a higher morbidity and mortality rate when first performed by the originator and by the surgeons who soon followed the leader than later in the "learning curve." In time, the cardiologic and surgical analysis of early and long-term results led to improved selection of cases and better operative and perioperative management.

As we follow our patients postoperatively, it is reasonable to expect that those recently operated on will experience fewer complications, residua, and sequelae and will enjoy lasting relief of the congenital heart disease that led to performance of the operation.

LONG-TERM FOLLOW-UP AFTER CARDIAC SURGERY

Among the lessons we have learned during these four and a half decades of the cardiac surgical era is that these patients should continue under long-term, informed follow-up. The results of surgery for the patients, as they see themselves function, and for the cardiologist, who continues to be interested in them, do not always coincide when ratings of excellent, good, fair, or poor are made. Happily, most results are good to excellent. We believe that these patients should be encouraged to be active, to think of themselves as healthy, while the competent cardiologist quietly continues his surveillance, alert to unrelieved conditions and to late occurrence of new murmurs, of arrhythmias, or of the unexpected events we continue to learn about. All the while, he reminds them of the importance of antibiotic prophylaxis for oral surgical procedures or genitourinary instrumentation that might provoke bacteremia and, if the patient is unprotected, infective endocarditis.

To assess the long-term results of cardiac surgery, we need to consider whether the operation was corrective, reparative, or palliative.

TOTAL CORRECTION OF DEFECT

Although the term *total correction* is often applied to the description of an operation or to reports in the literature of a surgical procedure, in truth there is only one operation that is totally corrective. This is surgical obliteration of a simple patent ductus arteriosus. As luck would have it, this is the first operation ever performed successfully. That was in 1938 by Dr Robert Gross after his pediatric colleague, without benefit of any of our modern diagnostic tools except his stethoscope, made the correct diagnosis in a child. By 10 years later, that operation had become so simple, safe, and effective that the indication for surgery became the diagnosis itself, irrespective of symptoms. The most recent development in this anomaly has been the recognition in the last decade of the importance of patent ductus arteriosus in small, immature, premature babies on ventilators. Even though many of these weigh less than 1,000 g, surgery can be carried out safely and effectively to close the ductus.

The early judgment about operation has stood the test

of time. It remains the "gold standard" against which other operations are compared. The correction of this anomaly, usually by suture ligation, restores the heart to normal and the patient is left with normal heart size and heart sounds, no heart murmur, and a normal electrocardiogram and roentgenogram.

REPAIR OF ANOMALY

The next most correctable anomaly is atrial septal defect. This lesion had to await the development of the heart–lung machine in the mid-1950s before the defect in the atrial septum could be visualized and closed directly by sutures or by insertion of a patch. It took about 5 years for problems to be identified and corrected and for this condition to take its place alongside patent ductus arteriosus as one for which surgery is recommended in the asymptomatic child to prevent, if possible, some problems that adults with unoperated atrial septal defect face. The mortality rate for both of these conditions, when uncomplicated, is close to zero, and the benefits are real. Cardiomegaly shrinks to normal size and cardiac murmurs disappear. The second heart sound begins to split physiologically, and the electrocardiogram loses its right ventricular conduction delay.

For many patients, this is the happy ending. They are cured. They and the people with closed patent ductus arteriosus no longer need antibiotic prophylaxis at times of predictable risk of bacteremia, and after a few years of postoperative follow-up to confirm their normalcy, they no longer require long-term follow-up in adulthood.

Some people operated on for atrial septal defect are not quite so fortunate, however. One serious complication occurred early in the "learning curve" and is preventable. This happened when the defect extended to the mouth of the inferior vena cava and the defect was not closed securely in that area. This oversight permitted systemic venous blood to drain into the left atrium, caused cyanosis, and required a second operation.

Another cause for concern in some postoperative atrial septal defect patients has been the early or late occurrence of arrhythmias. Those with the rare sinus venosus type of atrial septal defect, high near the mouth of the superior vena cava and close to the sinoatrial node, are at risk for sinus bradycardia and the sick sinus syndrome. Surgical entry per se into the atrium can be followed by atrial arrhythmias that may not appear till years later.

Finally, those with an ostium primum type of atrial septal defect have an associated lesion: abnormal formation of the mitral valve, sometimes referred to as a cleft. Whether left untouched or, as is more often the case, unfurled with suturing of the edges of the "cleft," these individuals are left with a structural abnormality that may be silent to auscultation and that may function without stenosis, but that can be a site for infective endocarditis. These people deserve antibiotic protection on indication, and they benefit from long-term cardiologic follow-up.

Additionally, the location of their defect in proximity to the atrioventricular node can lead to injury when the patch is placed and thus to early or later appearance of high-grade or complete heart block.

The third best congenital anomaly for repair is valvular pulmonic stenosis, moderate or severe. Although the benefits to the patient are real and sometimes dramatic, and he feels "cured," he still retains a thickened, malformed valve (now able to open), and he continues to have a heart murmur, albeit softer than that before operation. He may even have added the early diastolic murmur of pulmonic insufficiency. This is a small price to pay for having a valve that no longer is stenotic due to commissural fusion. Pulmonic regurgitation in the low-pressure right side of the heart is well tolerated and functionally insignificant. The poststenotic dilatation of the main pulmonary artery usually persists but is unimportant. The electrocardiogram does show regression of hypertrophy, and if the right ventricle were enlarged on x-ray before operation, it usually returns to a normal size when obstruction to right ventricular outflow is relieved. The infundibular pulmonic stenosis due to a hypertrophied musculature almost always spontaneously regresses. In those with severe stenosis and a right-to-left shunt through a patent foramen ovale, cyanosis is relieved when the afterload is removed by open valvotomy under direct vision. For the past 30 years, that has been the treatment of choice in patients with moderate or severe stenosis. The success rate is as high as that for the first two conditions, patent ductus arteriosus and atrial septal defect, and long-term results are excellent. The patients' conditions are not "totally corrected," however, and they benefit from continued surveillance every few years and from antibiotic prophylaxis for oral surgery.

The newly introduced treatment for moderate and severe pulmonic stenosis by balloon dilatation has met with the same early success in carefully selected cases in short-term follow-up as occurred around 1954 when open pulmonic valvotomy under direct vision was first introduced and widely adopted.

Fourth on my list for excellence of repair in long-term follow-up is patch-closure of a large ventricular septal defect. For the first 20 years of this operation, the surgery was carried out in children, most of them over the age of 3 years. The indication for surgery was the presence of a large defect that produced a cardiopulmonary burden with a volume overload on the left and right ventricles and pulmonary circulation. Benefits of abolishing the left-to-right shunt were early apparent: decrease in heart size and pulmonary vascular markings, softening but often not disappearance of the holosystolic murmur, and increase in the child's energy and rate of growth. Highly reparative but not totally corrective, this operation regularly resulted in a pattern of right bundle branch block on the electrocardiogram. Early in the "learning curve," the surgical induction of complete heart block was feared. Without permanent pacemaker therapy, that patient was at high risk of sudden death.

Delay of surgical treatment till around the age of 3 years meant that some patients had already developed pulmonary vascular changes with greater than normal resistance to pulmonary blood flow. We learned that abolition of the shunt could result in a decrease in pulmonary arterial hypertension, but rarely a decrease in pulmonary vascular resistance. In some postoperative children and adolescents, pulmonary pressure began to climb, even though the shunt had been eliminated.

To overcome this problem, earlier surgery was needed. This also would permit successful open repair of the large ventricular septal defect that caused cardiac failure in infancy and sometimes called for a preliminary palliative operation to band the pulmonary artery and cut down the excessive pulmonary blood flow. The cardiac and surgical team collaborated to make early open heart surgery safe enough for babies who needed it. The 1970s saw this accomplished.

The major long-term problem in surgery for ventricular septal defect, aside from that already mentioned of pulmonary hypertension, is the late development of ventricular arrhythmias and the occasional report of sudden death. We hope that during long-term follow-up the patient at risk can be recognized and treated with antiarrhythmic medication. Further, the "learning curve" is a help, because more attention is now paid to meticulous and gentle handling of cardiac tissues and to preservation of ischemic myocardium. We hope that this will prevent such problems.

The remaining conditions stack up slightly less satisfactorily in terms of near completeness of relief. In decreasing order, from fifth down to eighth place, I would rank them as follows: (5) Mustard operation for simple transposition of the great arteries, (6) coarctation operations, (7) repair of tetralogy of Fallot, and (8) aortic valvotomy.

Life for some babies born with transposed great arteries became possible in 1948 when the Blalock–Hanlon operation of atrial septectomy established an opportunity for mixing of venous return and thus palliation. However, Rashkind balloon atrial septostomy, carried out in the first hours of life as soon as this common form of cyanotic congenital heart disease is recognized and before shock, acidosis, and death occur, has afforded consistently successful palliation and benefits can usually be depended on for about 5 or 6 months.

So it is our practice to recommend a venous-switch operation at 3 or 4 months of age, when cyanosis begins to increase and the hemoglobin and hematocrit to rise. Because of the early lessons of the "learning curve" for that operation, our surgeons in 1972 modified the Mustard operation in an attempt to prevent the supraventricular tachyarrhythmias and sick sinus syndrome that were so common. In the long-term follow-up we have been pleased with the excellent results and the low incidence of arrhythmias. The babies begin to gain and to grow and develop like normal children when cyanosis is corrected at such an early age.

The chief problem with the Mustard operation is obstruction to superior vena caval flow, either transiently in the first few days after surgery or later in the next few months. Maintenance of the infant in a head-elevated position as collateral circulation develops through the azygous system has made this only a temporary problem.

We have been so satisfied with the Mustard operation that we have not changed to the other venous switch operation (the Senning operation) or to the arterial switch operation introduced by Jatene in Argentina and used with early success by Yacoub and Stark in England. The advantage of the Senning operation over the Mustard operation is the lesser incidence of caval obstruction. The incidence of atrial arrhythmias has not been reduced. Mortality rates for both are low, about 4% to 5%. The advantage of the arterial-switch operation is that it makes the left ventricle into the systemic ventricle and the right ventricle into the pulmonary pump. Hence, the result is more nearly anatomically correct, and the ability of the right ventricle to serve as a systemic ventricle for many decades need not be a concern. The disadvantages are that the mortality rate is still high. Further, the operation must be carried out when the left ventricle is hypertrophied and able to sustain systemic blood flow in the presence of high vascular resistance. Hence, it must be done in the first days of life or else in the presence of congenital pulmonic stenosis or of a preliminary operation to band the pulmonary artery. Long-term results are not yet available. There is some concern for coronary arterial adequacy with growth and worry about the mismatch of size of the pulmonary arterial root that is often larger than the slender aorta sutured onto it in the switch. Aortic regurgitation has been observed in short-term follow-up.

Repair of coarctation of the aorta followed early upon the success of closure of a ductus as a direct approach to relief of a problem. It offered a "cure" for hypertension and the promise of normalization of the cardiovascular system. Now after 40 years, we still see articles favoring one type of surgical approach over another and questioning the ideal time for surgery. This is because there is not yet the perfect correction for this common condition nor has the ideal time for repair been defined. It is encouraging, however, that clever surgeons still direct their attention to the problem and that cardiologists continue to analyze and to report on the long-term results of the different operations. Our patients are fortunate that the variations in their anatomy can be handled by more than a single surgical technique.

The goals of the operation are to relieve the obstruction to aortic blood flow below the point of maximal narrowing and to do this before degenerative changes have occurred in the aorta itself (about the coarctation or in the ascending aorta), in the systemic arterial bed, or in the aortic valve. At the same time, the aorta should be large enough that the suture line, if it fails to enlarge with growth of the child, does not create a new coarctation.

The ideal candidate is a child aged 5 to 10 or 15 years with a discrete coarctation below the left subclavian artery, with adequate collateral circulation to prevent spinal cord damage when the aorta is cross-clamped, and with a proximal aortic segment of adequate size that the aorta after repair has a reasonable lumen and minimal mismatch that might create turbulence.

These criteria are often met, and the patient does well after resection of the coarctation and end-to-end anastomosis with interrupted sutures on the anterior row. Variations are needed when the coarctation is diffuse and the proximal segment is hypoplastic. Interposition of a tubular graft and turndown of a subclavian artery that has been slit along its length both permit enlargement of such an area of hypoplasia.

Infants in cardiac failure may not be able to wait till the ideal age for their surgery. Carried out early and on this indication, the operation can be lifesaving and one should not be too disappointed if another operation is needed electively around the age of 10 years.

Not every patient comes to medical attention between 5 to 10 years of age. If not, he should not be denied surgery even though the risk of persistent or recurrent and generalized hypertension is greater in the adult than for children.

Part of the problem in long-term follow-up in patients with coarctation is that associated lesions in the ascending aorta, which dilates, and in the aortic valve, which can become stenotic or incompetent, lead to complications as years go by. This group of patients especially needs long-term surveillance and they need antibiotic prophylaxis when surgery or instrumentation is to be carried out in parts of the body that cannot be sterilized.

A truly dramatic breakthrough 30 years ago was the open repair for tetralogy of Fallot introduced by Lillehei. The two important components of tetralogy that need repair are the high ventricular septal defect and the tight infundibular (and sometimes valvular and supravalvular) stenosis. To patch the defect and to remove the obstructing fibromuscular tissue in the infundibulum and enlarge the valvular–supravalvular orifice means that the overriding aorta and right ventricular hypertrophy are also fixed. To see any blue baby become pink because the shunt route has been eliminated is always a thrill. The clubbing goes, growth accelerates, and the ability to exercise without breathlessness appears.

These long-term benefits prevail, but two problems need long-term, continuing surveillance and sometimes medical or surgical treatment. One of these is the fact that surgical relief of pulmonic stenosis is rarely complete and that pulmonic insufficiency often follows an outflow tract patch to enlarge that constricted area. Closure of the ventricular septal defect is not always complete either. The combination of some or all of these residua or sequelae places a volume or pressure load, or both, on the right ventricle. Some patients develop aneurysmal dilatation of the outflow tract of the right ventricle, an additional impairment to right ventricular function.

The second cause for long-term care is that ventricular arrhythmia can develop and be life-threatening. The group at Hammersmith in London reported that older age at operation contributed significantly to the occurrence of these postoperative arrhythmias. It seems prudent to use antiarrhythmic therapy in the group who demonstrate high-grade ventricular ectopy on exercise or at rest.

The last condition we shall discuss is aortic stenosis. Although the operation involves direct repair of the valvular, subvalvular, supravalvular severe stenosis, the anatomy of the malformation itself dictates that no matter how talented the surgeon, the best the patient gets is palliation. Valvular stenosis is the most common form of obstruction to left ventricular outflow. The region of commissural fusion can be opened almost to the anulus, so as to provide some relief of obstruction without causing regurgitation.

Discrete fibromuscular subaortic stenosis can be excised but may recur. In this condition and in supravalvular aortic stenosis, aortic insufficiency may be an accompaniment or a sequel. Nonetheless, albeit imperfect, an operation that lessens critically severe aortic stenosis benefits most patients. Valvotomy is preferable over valve replacement as the first operation for valvular stenosis. Long-term follow-up into adulthood has shown that some require valve replacement later.

REPAIR OR PALLIATION

I shall not rank the Fontan operation in the foregoing grouping of cure or repair, for it has not been in use long enough to permit assessment of its benefits and deficiencies over many years. It is an ingenious method for eliminating cyanosis and establishing pulmonary blood flow in patients who function with a physiologically univentricular heart. It is employed most often in children over the age of 5 or 6 years. It connects the hypertrophied right atrium to the pulmonary artery, sometimes as a direct connection of atrial appendage to main pulmonary artery or sometimes by means of an external-valved or unvalved conduit. In some children with tricuspid atresia who have a functional although small right ventricle, the right atrium is connected to the right ventricle so that flow is more nearly physiologic with atrial and then ventricular systole contributing to pulmonary blood flow. Closure of the atrial septal defect, which had been vital for those with tricuspid atresia up to the moment of the Fontan operation, removes the opportunity for right-to-left shunting and cyanosis. Questions remain concerning the ability of the right atrium, with or without a portion of ventricle in the system, to provide for systemic venous return to reach the pulmonary circulation for many decades. It has already been learned that the development of atrial arrhythmias, although undesirable, can occur without being lethal.

Some cardiologists and surgeons consider this operation as palliation rather than repair, and I have placed it in an intermediate position. Certainly, the removal of the right-to-left shunt is of great benefit, not only cosmetically but also functionally and from the standpoint of removing the hazards of polycythemia and brain abscess.

PALLIATION

To Increase Pulmonary Blood Flow

The first operation to increase pulmonary blood flow in blue babies with severe pulmonic stenosis or atresia is still the most satisfactory in 40 years of use: the Blalock–Taussig operation of subclavian-to-pulmonary artery anastomosis. It is still our first choice if the cyanotic infant's anatomy dictates palliation rather than repair. The Potts anastomosis between the left descending aorta and adjacent pulmonary artery branch has the disadvantage that it enlarges and can produce excessive pulmonary blood flow, cardiac failure, and later pulmonary hypertension due to pulmonary vascular disease. Furthermore, it is difficult to take down if the patient later becomes a candidate for direct repair. The Glenn procedure anastomoses the superior vena cava to the distal end of the divided right pulmonary artery. Over years it tends to shrivel and become less adequate. However, it is still sometimes used in preparation for the Fontan operation. The Waterston shunt, a direct anastomosis between ascending aorta and right pulmonary artery, has the same disadvantages as the Potts anastomosis in that it may be made or may become too large. Its peculiar disadvantage is that it kinks, so that the shunt is directed preferentially into the right lung and less and less into the left.

To Decrease Pulmonary Flow

The other major form of palliation is to decrease excessive pulmonary blood flow by banding the main pulmonary artery. This procedure was developed by Drs Muller and Dammann before the heart–lung machine was perfected and closure of ventricular septal defects became a reality in 1954. Long-term follow-up is rarely more than a few years. Since most bands are placed in early infancy because of intractable cardiac failure, growth into early childhood causes increasingly severe pulmonic stenosis that requires removal of the band. Nevertheless, the operation is still useful as palliation in infants with conditions such as a single ventricle. Selectively, it is used in the preparation of the left ventricle for the arterial-switch operation in transposed great arteries.

To Provide an Accessory Route for Blood Flow

External conduits can be used to connect the right ventricle to the pulmonary arteries or the apex of the left ventricle to the descending aorta to provide a passageway that did not exist for blood flow. The conduit provides adequate outflow for a variable period. It was known in advance that it cannot grow and so could produce stenosis as a child grows. It was unexpected that a peel would develop in some instances that would narrow the lumen or that could come loose and acutely obstruct the flow.

To Provide a Valve to Replace a Stenotic or Regurgitant One

Artificial valves, both mechanical and tissue, provide palliation for the life of that valve. They cause slight stenosis that is tolerated. However, they have a limited life expectancy, which is improving as biomechanical engineers and surgeons collaborate to make valves that work well for many years. Tissue valves, especially in the mitral position, degenerate, sometimes within only a few years. Biomedical engineers are at work on this problem as well.

To Pace the Heart

Surgically induced complete heart block calls for a permanent artificial pacemaker. Some infants born with complete heart block need pacemakers, as do a few who have the sick sinus syndrome. Generations of pacemakers have come into being in the last 30 years, with increasing length of battery life, more miniaturization, and greater sophistication for choice of modes. These pacemakers are models of engineering and electrophysiologic expertise that offer palliation and require long-term attention for the patients who use them.

SUMMARY

In summary, although we cannot prevent congenital heart disease, we can help each baby to be as healthy as possible through precise diagnosis and medical and often surgical management. Long-term surveillance of these infants and children into adulthood is recommended.

BIBLIOGRAPHY

Adams FH, Emmanouilides GC: *Moss' Heart Disease in Infants, Children and Adolescents,* ed 3. Baltimore, Williams & Wilkins, 1983, 795 pp.

Becker AE, Anderson RH: *Cardiac Pathology: An Integrated Text and Colour Atlas.* New York, Raven Press, 1982, 245 pp.

Doyle EF, Engle MA, Gersony W, Rashkind WJ, Talner NS: *Pediatric Cardiology.* New York, Springer-Verlag, 1986, 1,340 pp.

Engle MA: *Pediatric Cardiovascular Disease. Cardiovascular Clinics* 11/2. Philadelphia, FA Davis, 1981, 462 pp.

Engle MA, Perloff JK: *Congenital Heart Disease After Surgery: Benefits, Residua, Sequelae.* New York, Yorke Medical Books, 1983, 419 pp.

Liebman J, Plonsey PE, Gillette PC: *Pediatric Electrocardiography.* Baltimore, Williams & Wilkins, 1982, 354 pp.

Sahn DJ, Anderson F: *An Atlas for Echocardiographers: Two-Dimensional Anatomy of the Heart.* New York, John Wiley & Sons, 1982, 461 pp.

Zuberbuhler JR: *Clinical Diagnosis in Pediatric Cardiology. Modern Pediatric Cardiology.* New York, Churchill Livingstone, 1981, 183 pp.

27 Congenital Heart Disease in the Adult

Dan G. McNamara, MD and Michael R. Nihill, MB, BS, MS, MRCP

In the decade of the 1980s, a new spectrum of congenital heart disease in the adult patient confronts the internist. In prior years, these patients turned up rarely in an adult cardiac clinic. Benign defects were undoubtedly seen in the past by internists but were seldom identified because noninvasive definitive diagnosis using ultrasound technique was not well developed until the past few years, and patients were seldom referred for cardiac catheterization just to confirm a functionally benign cardiac defect.

Patients with the lethal anomalies, transposition of the great arteries, severe tetralogy of Fallot, total anomaly of pulmonary venous return, tricuspid atresia, truncus arteriosus, and severe atrioventricular canal rarely survived infancy, let alone childhood and adolescence. Operations devised from 1938 through 1958 changed the number and type of birth defects that would permit survival after childhood. Definitive closed repair of ductus arteriosus (1938) and of coarctation of the aorta (1944) and pulmonary valve stenosis (1949) assured these individuals a chance at a normal life span.

Palliative procedures, including the Blalock–Taussig anastomosis (1944), the Potts anastomosis (1945), the Blalock–Hanlon creation of an atrial septal defect (1949), and the Muller–Dammann pulmonary artery banding (1952),[1] meant that infants who would have died were now surviving infancy, some long enough to be able to benefit from later definitive surgery. Many others reached adult life still improved from only a palliative procedure.[2]

The development of cardiopulmonary bypass and of profound hypothermia made it possible to repair intracardiac anomalies, such as isolated septal defects and cyanotic lesions including tetralogy of Fallot, transposition of the great arteries, and total anomalous pulmonary venous return. In recent years, with the use of conduits and partitioning procedures, the outlook is good for definitive repair of highly complex anomalies such as truncus arteriosus, complex transposition, tricuspid atresia, and single ventricle, and now operations are being investigated for hypoplastic left heart syndrome.[3]

New drugs for cardiovascular disease, developed since 1950, have improved the chance of recovery in infants both with and without cardiac surgery. These agents include furosemide, digoxin, and dopamine for the treatment of myocardial insufficiency; indomethacin for closure of the ductus in the premature; and prostaglandin for keeping the ductus open (until operation can be performed) in the neonate with a ductus-dependent congenital heart anomaly.

About half the infants born with a cardiac defect have severe critical disease in the first year of life, and without medical or surgical treatment, or both, probably 90% of them die before their first birthday. A conservative estimate based on the current annual U.S. birth rate of 3.2 million indicates that 26,000 infants are born each year with congenital heart disease and 13,000 of them will have a life-threatening defect. In the pretreatment period before 1950, only 10% of the critically ill patients, or about 1,300 patients per year, could have improved spontaneously or with only supportive therapy to be able to reach adult life. Some 90% of the 13,000 patients (or about 11,700) with a less severe defect could undoubtedly reach adult life, so that only half of all individuals born with congenital heart disease, or about 13,000 (90% of the benign ones and 10% of the critical ones), could have survived childhood in the first half of this century.

Since 1960, virtually every infant and child in the United States has had access to one of the cardiac centers because of the Crippled Children's program, the availability of private insurance, and the Medicaid program. A fair estimate is that, beginning in 1980, 90% of the critically ill infants have survived because of modern treatment and are reaching adult life at a rate of 11,000 to 12,000 per year. Now among the adult patients with congenital heart disease, 75% will have postoperative congenital heart disease and only about 25% unoperated anomalies, some of which are minor, some potentially important, and some severe disabling defects.

Internists are seeing more and more patients with surgically repaired (although not always cured) congenital heart disease. Patients with anomalies once known only to the pediatrician, and indeed sometimes only to the neonatologist, are now adults and are beginning to appear at the office of the internist in a postoperative state. Their symptoms, signs, problems, and outlook are quite unlike those of the preoperative patient with the same anomaly.

Historically, there has been only scattered and superficial interest in cardiac anomalies on the part of physicians who treat adult patients with heart disease. This is understandable, considering the preponderance of coronary, hypertensive, and acquired valvular disease in adults requiring the time, attention, and efforts of the internist.

For the past 25 to 40 years, most of the defects that allowed survival to at least early adult life in the untreated state, such as patent ductus arteriosus, atrial septal defect, and coarctation of the aorta, have usually been corrected surgically well before 21 years of age. Many of these patients, presumed to be surgically freed of any existing or potential cardiovascular problem, were dismissed from further follow-up by their pediatric cardiologist and cardiac surgeon. In our experience, early dismissal from further follow-up of the patient with an apparent good surgical result was often recommended to emphasize to the parents and to the child that a normal life could now begin. There is some merit in this approach, but subsequent experience teaches us that late-appearing residual defects, sequelae, and complications must be watched for on a long-term basis.

Patients who still need follow-up despite a corrective operation and those who have uncorrected congenital disease often choose to remain under the care of the physicians (pediatric cardiologist and surgeon) who have been treating them since infancy or childhood.

Training programs in adult cardiovascular disease rarely include experience with the diagnosis and treatment of congenital heart disease in either the child or the adult. Consequently, when the patient reaches the age of 21 years, the choice must be made between changing to the adult cardiologist, who often lacks familiarity with congenital heart defects and has little interest in taking on the responsibility, or continuing to see the pediatric cardiologist, who feels capable of managing the cardiac problems of the adult patient but whose admitting privileges may be limited to a pediatric hospital and whose waiting room, filled with crying infants and active children, is likely to disturb the older patient.

It is the purpose of this chapter to encourage the internist to assume more responsibility for the cardiac care of the adult patient with congenital heart disease and to urge adult cardiology training programs to include "pediatric and congenital heart disease" in their curriculum so that the adult cardiologist of the future will be ready to receive this growing population of patients.

CLASSIFICATION OF ADULTS WITH CONGENITAL HEART DEFECTS

There are too many congenital heart defects (several hundred to date) to cover all of them in any single chapter. In fact, each of the eight well-known common defects (patent ductus arteriosus, atrial septal defect, ventricular septal defect, pulmonary stenosis, aortic stenosis, coarctation, tetralogy of Fallot, and transposition of the great arteries) varies considerably in severity, presentation, outlook, and response to treatment. The "typical" manifestations of some of these anomalies (for example, tetralogy of Fallot) are not always the most common form of the anomaly, but often the best known or most clinically striking.

Furthermore, "new" (that is, previously unrecognized or unreported) defects appear in large clinics for congenital heart disease several times a month. Thus, the physician dealing with congenital heart anomalies must be prepared to identify and manage unique and rare anomalies. There are many patients with rare defects who can be helped and they need the same attention and care that patients with a common defect receive.

Because of the complexity in recognition and treatment of the infinite variety of congenital heart anomalies, we have to first evaluate the patient from a broad functional standpoint. Thus, the types of patient that will be seen in adult life are presented in this chapter from the standpoint of the following categories: (1) benign anomalies, (2) important unoperated anomalies, and (3) postoperative congenital heart disease, both palliative and definitive operations, further subdivided into those with a good result and those with a poor result. Examples are given in each category, but no effort is made to make a complete list of all the possible anomalies that could be seen in a given category. In fact, the reader will find that the same anomaly may appear in more than one functional category, the classification being constructed according to the manner that the adult patient presents to the internist–cardiologist. Also, we review the types of problems that might be encountered in either the benign or the serious defects, whether or not surgical treatment has been performed. Lastly, we propose a plan of follow-up for long-term care of problems that arise as well as a program of preventive cardiology in these patients.

TYPES OF PATIENTS WITH CONGENITAL HEART DISEASE THE INTERNIST MIGHT ENCOUNTER

UNOPERATED CONGENITAL HEART DISEASE

Benign Congenital Heart Anomalies

Benign lesions for the most part have escaped the attention of internists. Perhaps this is beneficial, saving the patients anxiety, time, and money and saving the physicians the frustration of feeling that the search for a minor as well as a rare and obscure defect is required of them. Conversely, most patients usually want to know what abnormality they have, no matter how benign. Furthermore, a few benign lesions become more severe with age and the patient should be checked occasionally to detect early changes. Other defects remain hemodynamically stable for a full lifetime, but the patient may be susceptible to subacute bacterial endocarditis, an additional reason to identify all cardiovascular anomalies, assuming that recognition can be carried out safely and economically and without causing anxiety in the patient.

Hemodynamically benign lesions are often more difficult to suspect or to diagnose than severe lesions. Without symptoms, enlargement of the heart, and other clearly abnormal functional measurements, the hemodynamically unimportant defects are often overlooked in the child and the adult until some complication, perhaps a preventable one, develops. They may be detected primarily by one of the following: (1) auscultation of the heart; (2) the chance detection by x-ray, echocardiogram, or angiogram obtained for some other purpose; (3) the family screen done because a first degree relative proves to have a defect that has a high incidence of familial occurrence (eg, mitral leaflet prolapse); (4) study of the patient with infective endocarditis to search for the etiologic basis of the infection.

The benign lesions of childhood and adult life have the following characteristics.

1. No cardiac chamber (atrial or ventricular) enlargement by physical examination, electrocardiogram (ECG), chest radiograph, or echocardiogram. Dilation of the pulmonary trunk, pulmonary veins, or aorta may occur as an isolated primary, stable, and benign phenomenon.

2. Absence of bona fide subjective cardiac symptoms due to hemodynamic abnormality. Arrhythmias with or without symptoms are not inconsistent with one of the structurally benign congenital anomalies.

3. No large right-to-left shunt as determined by either physical examination, arterial oxygen saturation, dye indicator curve, or contrast echocardiogram.

4. No large left-to-right shunt. Large left-to-right shunts invariably produce cardiac chamber dilatation, hypertrophy, and increased size of pulmonary vessels radiographically, and usually ventricular hypertrophy by ECG, each of which would exclude the patient from the benign category.

5. No elevation of pressure in the pulmonary artery, aorta, or atria and no elevation of ventricular end-diastolic pressure. Some patients with a benign defect may have a slight ventricular resting peak systolic pressure gradient (equal to or less than 20 mm Hg) because of mild semilunar valve obstruction. Intracavitary and intravascular pressure is best assessed by cardiac catheterization, but if a meticulous cardiovascular examination, expertly interpreted ECG, chest radiograph, and echocardiogram reveal no sign of cardiac overwork, then important elevation of pressure is unlikely.

There are several benign defects that might be detected only by murmur or abnormal heart sound or an unusual x-ray shadow. They fall into the following categories:

Small Left-to-Right Shunts. This group of anomalies includes the following.

1. Small atrial septal defects (ASD) including secundum, fenestration of the valve of foramen ovale, sinus venosus ASD, inferior vena cava position of ASD, and ostium primum type of ASD with a minor cleft of the mitral valve. Except for ostium primum defect, which usually has a mitral regurgitant murmur at the apex of the heart, each of the different types of ASD produces a similar soft blowing ejection type of murmur at the left second space and, depending on the volume of the shunt, a widely split S_2. Unless a right ventricular-to-pulmonary artery pressure gradient of 20 mm Hg or more has developed, the murmur of ASD is less impressive than the split S_2; therefore, the defect is easily missed in the asymptomatic young child who normally has prominent S_2 splitting and often a basal innocent murmur. The patient with ASD often reaches adult life without the defect having been spotted on numerous examinations in childhood. The defect is often detected only on chest radiograph obtained for some other purpose.

In a study by Seldon et al[4] in Australia in which mass x-ray screening for lung or heart disease was undertaken in 502,000 people over 14 years of age, 25 cases of ASD previously unknown to the patient were encountered. Subjects whose films were suggestive of heart disease were referred to a cardiologist for examination. A questionnaire was also sent to 67 patients with known ASD and who happened to have been part of the mass x-ray screening. The questionnaire asked if their defect had been reported to them as a result of the screening. In 53 of the 67 patients (79%) the defect had been suspected by mass x-ray screening. In the 21% in whom the anomaly had not been suspected by mass x-ray screening, the left-to-right shunt was known to be small.

The investigators estimated that the incidence of uncorrected ASD between 14 and 60 years of age was about 1 in 5,700 people. Seldon quotes Carlgren, in Sweden, who estimated ASD in the adult population as 1 in 2,500. Furthermore, Seldon et al[4] calculated that 40% of all ASD patients had been undiagnosed during childhood.

2. Partial anomaly of pulmonary venous return, including single anomalous pulmonary vein to right superior vena cava or to left superior vena cava. In this malformation the defect may go undetected for a full lifetime. However, it may be suspected by a faint murmur in the right or left upper mediastinum, and if the shunt is of moderate size, a pulmonary area systolic flow murmur could be heard much like that of ASD. It is unlikely that the shunt would be large enough from a single anomalous pulmonary vein to produce a tricuspid area diastolic flow murmur. The defect may be detected on echocardiography and it could be suspected by an unusual shadow on the chest radiograph.

3. Small ventricular septal defect (VSD). Characteristically the murmur of VSD is loud and plateau in shape, but the very small VSD allows only a small shunt and thus may produce only a low intensity murmur. Unlike the large VSD with increased pulmonary blood flow in which the murmur is plateau, the murmur of the very small VSD is ejection in shape. In the young child with a thin chest wall this murmur is easy to hear, but in the adult with a thick chest wall the very small VSD murmur can be missed entirely. However, it can usually be exaggerated by having the patient exercise.

Because a prominent murmur from early infancy characterizes the small VSD, usually the adult with the small

VSD has known about the defect from childhood and his parents probably knew about it from early infancy. If the patient has been to a pediatric cardiology center, there is a good possibility that the benign nature of the anomaly as well as the need for lifetime prophylaxis against infective endocarditis has been explained to the family. The only life-threatening complication that the patient may encounter as an adult is the small chance of infective endocarditis (see section on Prevention of Infective Endocarditis). The other indirect complication is a psychologic one. The patient may have been made excessively and unnecessarily conscious of his heart defect, to the point that anxiety and fear of a cardiac problem may interfere with a normal adjustment to life. While frequent examinations by the cardiologist imply an unstated concern on the part of the physician and may exaggerate the anxiety, only occasional visits, such as one every 2 to 3 years, may serve to reassure the patient that all is well.

4. Small patent ductus arteriosus (PDA). The large PDA of 5 to 8 mm in diameter is the one that produces the easy-to-hear continuous machinery murmur well known to almost all physicians. However, the very small 1- to 2-mm PDA allows only a small left-to-right, aorta-to-pulmonary artery shunt and thus only a faint murmur. In fact, the murmur may be missed entirely in the child or adult if the patient is examined while sitting or standing. To increase the intensity of a faint ductus murmur, auscultation should be carried out after exercise with the patient supine.

In a long, tortuous PDA the continuous murmur may be quite intermittent, changing with position, and at times not heard at all.[5] This anomaly is easily missed in childhood.

5. Arterial blood supply to a lobe of the lung ("sequestered lobe"). This anomaly produces a faint murmur over the lower part of the chest anteriorly or over the liver, but it usually is associated with other defects and therefore the murmur of the fistula may be obscured by that of another defect. If the abdominal aortic origin of the arterial supply to the lobe is deep within the abdominal cavity, the murmur could be missed entirely. An aortogram is required to identify this anomaly. The shunt may be small, imposing no great strain on the circulation, and therefore treatment—lobectomy—would be worse than the disease.

6. A small peripheral arteriovenous fistula usually produces a continuous murmur and a palpable thrill if the fistula is close enough to the surface to be palpated. If the anomaly produces only a small shunt, no cardiac overload is present and the defect would be recognized only by a continuous thrill or murmur. When the fistula involves the vertebral artery and a tributary of the jugular vein, the thrill and murmur are identified in the neck just below the mastoid process. It requires aortography to demonstrate the anatomic details to decide about the feasibility and necessity for surgical repair.

Asymptomatic Small Right-to-Left Shunt. This group of anomalies, often overlooked throughout a normal and active childhood, may be detected only by unusual heart sounds, ECG, or chest radiograph, because a small right-to-left shunt is defined as one that does not produce visible cyanosis. The right-to-left shunt may be detected only by an indicator dye curve or contrast echocardiogram. The resting arterial oxygen saturation may be in the normal range, but it may decrease with exercise. Because the right-to-left shunt is small, the patient usually mentions no symptoms at rest or with exercise. Even a small shunt, however, is capable of allowing a paradoxic embolus or brain abscess to occur.

Some anomalies that produce an asymptomatic small right-to-left shunt include the following.

1. Persistent eustachian valve with open foramen ovale or small ASD.[6] A small right-to-left shunt may be detectable only during a forced Valsalva maneuver[7] or during exercise using (1) arterial oxygen saturation and (2) contrast echocardiography (the indicator, such as saline, must be injected into the leg rather than the arm vein for eustachian-valve–directed shunt across the patent foramen ovale or small ASD). If cardiac catheterization is performed, then either dye indicator curve or angiocardiogram performed from the inferior vena cava or low right atrium may be necessary to demonstrate the right-to-left shunting.

2. Left superior vena cava to left atrium.[8] This anomaly is often associated with other defects. If the anomalously connected left cava is small and if there is an associated ASD with left-to-right shunt, visible cyanosis would be lacking or slight. It could be identified by an echocardiogram, and right-to-left shunting might be demonstrated by contrast echocardiography providing the indicator is injected into a left arm vein. If there is a left innominate vein carrying jugular and subclavian venous blood to the right heart, the anomalous left vena cava can simply be ligated surgically to cure the patient. Right superior vena cava to left atrium produces a larger right-to-left shunt, but in one adult patient with an active childhood and adolescence,[9] there was no symptom until the appearance of brain abscess prompted etiologic investigation. This anomaly requires injection of indicator substance into the right arm for identification.

3. Small pulmonary arteriovenous (AV) fistula. The small fistula lacks the typical continuous murmur characteristic of large pulmonary AV fistulas. In fact, the anomaly may be suspected only by fortuitous appearance on the chest radiograph as a small area of increased density and confirmed only by pulmonary arteriography. The right-to-left shunt may be too small to produce noticeable arterial oxygen desaturation.

Right-Sided Lesions Without Intracardiac Communication. These lesions include the following.

1. Atrial septal aneurysm.[10] The phenomenon of an atrial septal aneurysm may be congenital or acquired and may be associated with anomalies that have a large left atrial-to-right atrial pressure gradient. One might expect to see bulging of the atrial septum toward the left in anomalies in which the right atrial pressure is high (as in tricuspid atresia). The bulge would be toward the right atrium in anomalies in which left atrial pressure is high (as in mitral stenosis).

Isolated aneurysms of the atrial septum occur, however, in the absence of obvious causes.[11] They often occur as a silent phenomenon and are discovered only by chance at autopsy in the patient whose death was unrelated or in cardiac examination for a murmur that might be innocent or otherwise not connected to the atrial septal aneurysm. Clots have been found attached to either the right or the left side of the atrial septal aneurysm. If the aneurysm is large, it could obstruct the atrioventricular valve. It has been questioned as a cause of arrhythmia. It is not known if the atrial septal aneurysm could be the site of infective endocarditis, but if clots can form on it, undoubtedly it could.

2. Congenital isolated tricuspid regurgitation. This rare anomaly can be suspected by a long plateau systolic murmur, but it may be faint. Identification might be confirmed by Doppler flow analysis sampling in the low right atrium. The anomaly may result from a cleft in the tricuspid valve or tricuspid valve prolapse.

3. The mild form of Ebstein's malformation of the tricuspid valve may produce characteristic quadruple heart sounds that are distant, and often a scratchy type of diastolic murmur is heard that resembles a friction rub. The right bundle branch block on the ECG may be the tip-off, with a small amplitude of the R′ deflection. The diagnosis on echocardiogram is usually quite certain; therefore, heart catheterization can often be avoided. The mild form of Ebstein's malformation without right-to-left shunt requires no treatment, and good heart function can be anticipated indefinitely, except in patients with atrial tachyarrhythmias.

4. Mild pulmonary valve stenosis (defined as right ventricular-to-pulmonary artery peak systolic pressure gradient less than or equal to 20 mm Hg). The low intensity pulmonary stenosis ejection murmur indicates the unimportant degree of obstruction and the ejection click may overshadow the murmur.

The pulmonary area innocent murmur (pulmonary valve "flow" murmur) heard in many healthy children, adolescents, and young adults with thin chest walls resembles that of mild pulmonary stenosis, but the innocent murmur lacks a click and the intensity diminishes or disappears entirely while the patient stands and with slight held inspiration.

5. Mild isolated pulmonary artery branch stenosis (proximal-to-distal pulmonary artery peak systolic pressure gradient less than or equal to 20 mm Hg). The stenosis can occur in the right main or left main branch and the murmur is therefore heard best anteriorly in the infraclavicular area. The stenosis may be located in the right main pulmonary artery and the murmur resembles that of mild aortic stenosis, or in the left main pulmonary artery and the murmur resembles pulmonary valve stenosis. If the stenosis is in the secondary or tertiary branches of the pulmonary arteries, then the ejection systolic murmur is heard best in the axillae and in the posterior aspect of the chest. The location of the murmur has to do with the site of obstruction, but the intensity of the murmur has to do with the severity of obstruction, the cardiac output, and the thickness of the chest wall.

Eldredge et al[12] studied 70 patients with pulmonary artery branch stenosis who had serial cardiac catheterizations ranging in time from 2 to 12 years. In seven patients there was no associated defect, and in two of them there was no change in pressure between the serial catheterizations. In an additional four patients the pressure decreased at the time of the second heart catheterization. As an isolated malformation, pulmonary artery branch stenosis is the most common cardiovascular consequence of maternal rubella syndrome. In most patients with pulmonary branch stenosis due to maternal rubella, the stenosis becomes progressively milder with age. Thus, it is likely that we will see frequent instances of pulmonary branch stenosis in the adult patient.

6. Idiopathic dilatation of the pulmonary artery. The pulmonary artery appears quite dilated, but the right ventricle is not enlarged. The systolic murmur is faint and there may or may not be an associated ejection click. If the right ventricular-to-main pulmonary artery pressure gradient is measured by cardiac catheterization (or estimated by Doppler), the peak systolic gradient usually is 10 mm Hg or less. The radiographic appearance of a dilated main pulmonary artery can be alarming, but the patient should be reassured that a large pulmonary artery is functionally unimportant.

7. Bicuspid pulmonary valve. The bicuspid pulmonary valve usually occurs with other anomalies, but as an isolated defect it is benign. It can cause a faint pulmonary systolic murmur and may infrequently cause a pulmonary insufficiency murmur of no functional importance. Whether isolated bicuspid pulmonary valve is subject to infective endocarditis or not is not known. Vegetations of infective endocarditis can occur in the presumably normal pulmonary valve in the patient with ASD.[13]

8. Quadricuspid pulmonary valve. This valve usually functions normally, but it could be the site of infective endocarditis. The anomaly usually occurs with another cardiac defect.

Benign Left Heart Lesions. Many left heart lesions are benign except for susceptibility to infective endocarditis and may be quiescent in childhood. In the adult, the defect produces either a murmur, a radiographic abnormality, or infective endocarditis, any of which can bring the anomaly to the physician's attention. The late appearance of signs or symptoms often leads to the mistaken impression of acquired heart disease.

1. Aneurysmal dilatation of pulmonary veins. Nelson et al[14] described the findings in four healthy military servicemen whose chest films were suggestive of pulmonary AV fistulas. Angiograms demonstrated idiopathic dilatation of one or more normally draining pulmonary veins (Figure 27.1). There was no disease of the left heart to account for the phenomenon.

Platzker et al[15] reported a similar radiographic appearance of what proved to be a normally draining, although aneurysmally dilated, pulmonary vein.

2. Isolated mitral leaflet prolapse. This anomaly is so common among the general healthy population that in its benign and isolated form (ie, neither secondary to other heart disease or connective tissue disease such as Marfan's syndrome nor associated with mitral regurgitation), it can be considered a variation of normal, largely to be ignored. The patient need not be subjected to limited physical activity, to prophylaxis against infective endocarditis, or to increased premium for life and health insurance. Given these criteria for benign isolated mitral leaflet prolapse,

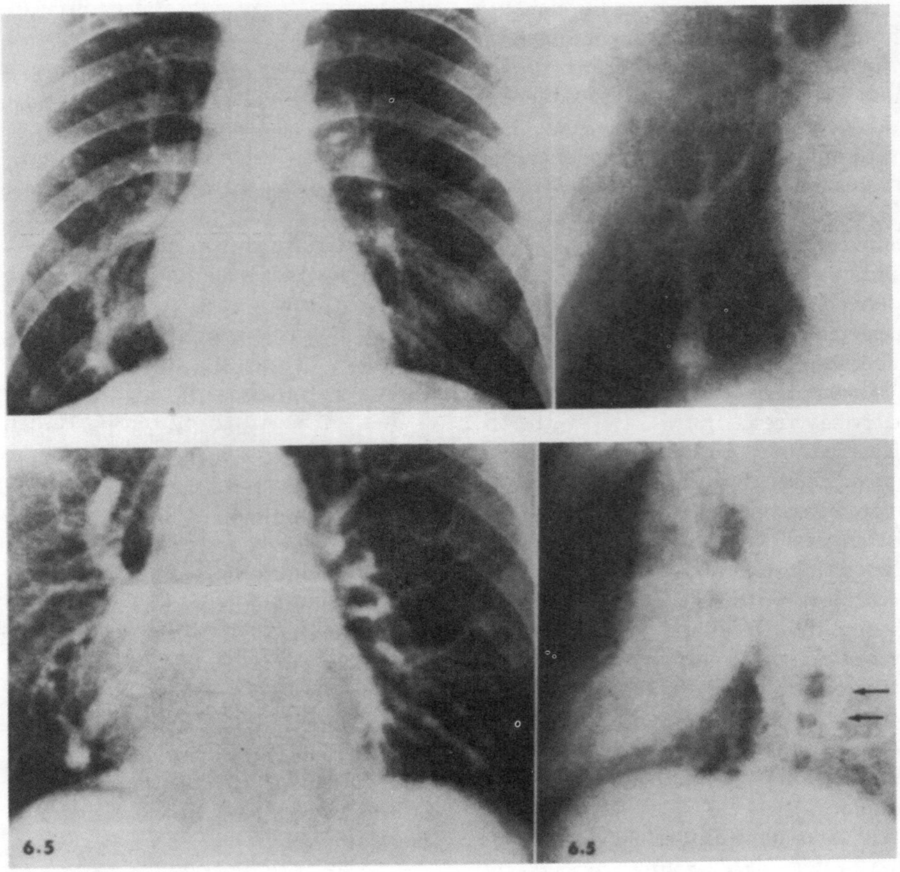

Figure 27.1. *Top,* Chest radiograph in a 19-year-old, asymptomatic military man in whom an abnormal shadow suggesting pulmonary arteriovenous fistula in the right lower lobe was seen on the film. Tomographic view on the right further suggested the fistula. *Bottom,* A pulmonary angiogram in levo-phase shows dilated and normally draining pulmonary veins not associated with heart disease. (From Nelson et al[14] with permission.)

the phenomenon (not a true congenital defect) is an auscultatory event and an echocardiographic variation of normal.

Hickey et al[16] found that among individuals with mitral valve prolapse there is an increased risk of subacute bacterial endocarditis only if there is a mitral regurgitant murmur. They estimate that among 100,000 adults with mitral valve prolapse (and a mitral systolic murmur), infective endocarditis develops in 14 in one year of follow-up and in only 3 patients per 100,000 of the general population.

3. Isolated mitral leaflet cleft. This anomaly is usually associated with ASD of the ostium primum type. It does permit varying degrees of mitral regurgitation depending on the size of the cleft. The benign form creates only a faint murmur of mitral regurgitation, but no enlargement of heart chambers on ECG, chest radiograph, or echocardiogram. The patient is susceptible to infective endocarditis, but otherwise the anomaly causes no functional difficulty. Examination every 1 to 3 years to assure that all is well is probably advisable.

4. Left ventricular false tendon. Perry et al[17] describe false tendons and indicate that they are believed to be a totally benign curiosity capable only of producing a vibratory murmur as well as an unusual and now widely recognized distinctive echocardiographic shadow. Among 3,847 echocardiographic examinations, false tendon was found 31 times (incidence of 0.8%). In 30 cases, the tendon was connected to the papillary muscle on one side and to the ventricular septum on the other. In one case the tendon stretched from one free wall to the other. Half the patients with false tendon had associated heart disease. Of the 16 without heart disease, 15 had a murmur, and in 14 of these 15 patients the murmur was typical of a Still's murmur. Among the 31 patients, 5 had arrhythmia and 3 of the 5 had no heart disease. It is uncertain if the false tendon has any connection with the arrhythmia or any other functional disturbance. The tendon will be noted only on the echocardiogram or as a chance finding at autopsy. Patients who learn that they have a false tendon should be advised that it is a nonsignificant echocardiographic curiosity and need not and should not be followed to watch the natural course.

5. Bicuspid aortic valve. This is the most common malformation of the cardiovascular system, if we exclude the benign isolated type of mitral valve prolapse as an anomaly. Congenital lesions of the aortic valve, of which the bicuspid aortic valve occupies the overwhelming component, occur in 2% of the adult general population[18] (Figure 27.2).

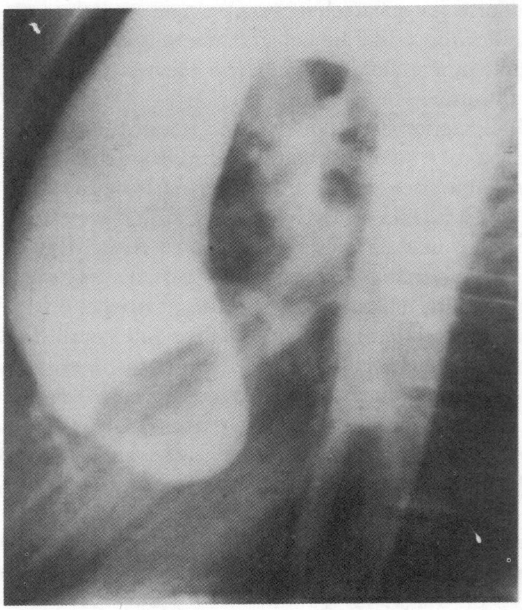

Figure 27.2. Bicuspid aortic valve and nonobstructive "coarctation." Angiogram in aortic root in a 29-year-old physician who was asymptomatic. He was referred for cardiac evaluation because of a faint murmur and a "musical heart sound," which proved to be a systolic ejection click. The leg pressure by auscultation was about 10 mm Hg lower than that in the arm, but the femoral pulse was strong. On angiogram, there was a bicuspid aortic valve, dilated ascending aorta, and a dilated and tortuous aorta just distal to the arch. No pressure gradient could be demonstrated between the left ventricle and the ascending thoracic aorta.

The isolated bicuspid aortic valve is usually not recognized in the child or even the adult until fibrosis or calcification, or both, cause stenosis or insufficiency or the valve serves as a site of infective endocarditis. Another way the bicuspid aortic valve is suspected is by its association with coarctation of the aorta, in which approximately 85% of patients have a bicuspid aortic valve. Curiously enough, although Roberts[18] reported that fully three fourths of specimens with bicuspid aortic valve at autopsy had associated aortic stenosis, aortic stenosis is infrequent (estimated 5%) in the patient with coarctation of the aorta. Folger and Stein[19] explained this by the difference in the structure of the bicuspid aortic valve when it is associated with coarctation and when it is not. Usually, the bicuspid aortic valve has two leaflets of unequal size, but in most patients with coarctation who have a bicuspid aortic valve, the two leaflets are of equal size. It is the inequality in size and shape of the two valve cusps that leads to the turbulence thought to be responsible for valve trauma with deposition of thrombin and platelets leading to valve fibrosis. Ultimately, calcification takes place. Therefore, the valve with little turbulence may remain free of degenerative change.

Bicuspid aortic valve may be suspected in persons in whom calcific aortic stenosis develops at a young age (less than 40 years) or aortic regurgitation develops for no apparent reason. It may be suspected in the patient in whom infective endocarditis develops and who has no clearly obvious intracardiac or valvular congenital heart disease.

Patients with bicuspid aortic valve, whether associated with coarctation of the aorta or not, require regular examinations to insure that infective endocarditis prophylaxis is being followed and that there is no evidence of calcific aortic stenosis or aortic insufficiency. Only about 15% of patients who had bicuspid aortic valve on autopsy examination in Roberts' study[20] had been known to have a normally functioning valve before death.

6. Quadricuspid aortic valve. This is less common than quadricuspid pulmonary valve, but the quadricuspid pulmonary valve usually functions normally, whereas the four-cusp aortic valve causes either stenosis or insufficiency in about half the cases in adults.[21] Only recently the echocardiographic features of quadricuspid aortic valve were described[22] (Figure 27.3), so that perhaps only the functionally significant lesions had been diagnosed

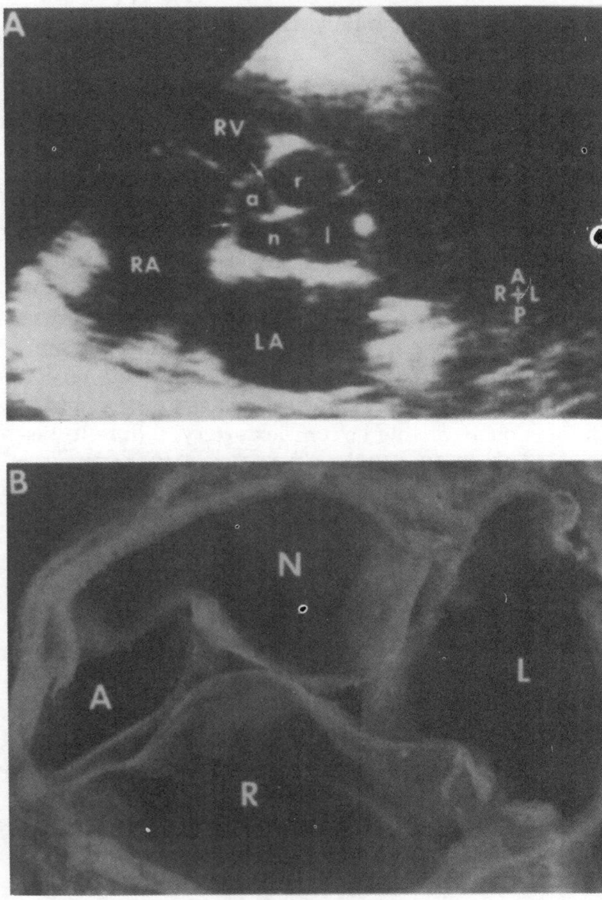

Figure 27.3. *A*, Two-dimensional echocardiogram in parasternal short-axis view. The aortic valve in diastole is seen to have four cusps. An accessory cusp (a) is between the right (r) and the noncoronary (n) cusps. The left coronary cusp is marked (l). The three *arrows* indicate the commissures. In the normal aortic valve the commissural lines make a Y, but in the quadricuspid valve the lines form an X. *B*, Autopsy specimen of quadricuspid valve with similar orientation as depicted in the echocardiographic picture. The accessory cusp (A) is between the noncoronary cusp (N) and the right cusp (R). LA = left atrium; RA = right atrium; RV = right ventricle.

previously, whereas the normally functioning ones had remained undetected.

7. Benign congenital coronary artery anomalies. These anomalies are usually identified fortuitously in the course of angiographic investigation of the patient for either congenital or acquired heart disease.

Because of the frequency of anomalous coronary artery origin and distribution in patients with tetralogy of Fallot, truncus arteriosus, transposition of the great arteries, and ventricular inversion, it is essential to include coronary arteriography in the angiographic study of patients with one of these anomalies who are to undergo surgery. This is especially important if ventriculotomy is going to be necessary to carry out the operation. In about 5% to 10% of patients with tetralogy of Fallot, the left anterior descending coronary artery arises from the right anterior sinus or the right coronary artery and courses along the outflow tract of the right ventricle.[23] This position of the vessel precludes the usual ventriculotomy for repair of the defects associated with tetralogy of Fallot and truncus arteriosus. The anomaly is otherwise functionally unimportant.

The most common variation of coronary artery anatomy in persons with an otherwise normal heart is the origin of the circumflex coronary artery from the right sinus of Valsalva or the right coronary artery itself. The vessel then courses along the posterior aspect of the heart to give off its distribution in the normal manner. This functionally benign anomaly becomes important in performing coronary arteriography for the study of coronary artery disease. Injection into the left main coronary artery would not fill the circumflex branch. Furthermore, in the same case in angiography of the right coronary artery, if the angiographic catheter is placed distal to the origin of the anomalously arising circumflex artery, failure to visualize the circumflex from either the right or the left coronary artery gives the false impression that the circumflex artery is occluded. Also, during cardiopulmonary bypass for open heart surgery, placing a perfusion catheter into the right coronary artery distal to the origin of the circumflex artery could exclude perfusion of the distribution of the anomalously arising circumflex artery.

Other anomalies that may be clinically silent for many years include origin of both coronary arteries from the right aortic sinus of Valsalva, the left coronary artery then passing across the outflow tract of the heart and coursing between the pulmonary artery and the aorta. This anomaly has been associated in a few reported cases of sudden death in athletes.[24] It has been proposed that the coronary artery becomes compressed by dilatation of the aorta and pulmonary artery which occurs physiologically with exercise. It is more likely that the ostium of the coronary artery bends toward a right angle as the aorta becomes dilated with strenuous exercise. Origin of the right coronary artery likewise can take place from the left coronary artery or the left sinus of Valsalva, but its association with ischemia or sudden death is less clear.

Origin of the left coronary artery from the pulmonary artery will be discussed under the anomalies that may be well tolerated in the adult but are functionally important in the infant. A fistula between a coronary artery and any one of the cardiac chambers produces a large left-to-right shunt and will be listed in the section on important anomalies in the child and in the adult with a large left-to-right shunt.

8. Mild "nonobstructive" coarctation of the aorta. This anomaly may remain benign and stable or there may be progression to severe coarctation in late adolescence or early adult life. In a study by Soto et al,[25] nonobstructive coarctation was defined as a lesion in which there is reduction of less than 50% of the lumen diameter compared with the adjacent aorta. Because the obstruction is mild, there are no collateral vessels and the peak systolic blood pressure gradient is equal to 20 mm Hg or less. No rib notching is noted on chest radiograph. These investigators reported seven patients ranging from 44 to 64 years of age. During the period when these seven patients were seen with insignificant coarctation of the aorta, they saw ten adults with true coarctation who ranged from 25 to 33 years of age. In some patients there was no gradient at all and in others the gradient was as high as 19 mm Hg. Five of the seven patients had aortic valve abnormality, either aortic stenosis or aortic insufficiency, and there was a high incidence of dominance of the left coronary artery system, just as there is in severe typical coarctation. Two of the patients had bicuspid aortic valves, and although the aortic valve was tricuspid in four, there was asymmetry of the valve in three of the four.

It is important to recognize that this benign anomaly does not require surgical treatment. Indeed, cross-clamping the aorta long enough to excise the mild stenotic area could prove disastrous, because there are no collateral vessels to supply the spinal cord. Restriction of physical activity is not called for, but the anomaly does theoretically predispose to infective endocarditis and the usual precautions are needed to avoid that complication.

9. Aortic arch anomalies. Nizankowski et al[26] examined the branches of the aortic arch in 453 specimens and found 15 examples of abnormal branching, representing six different types of abnormality. In reviewing publications, they found an additional 19 types of arch vessel anomalies (not including right aortic arch, double aortic arch, isolation from the aorta of arch vessels, or interruption of aortic arch).

The six types that Nizankowski et al[26] found in individuals free of other cardiovascular anomalies, in order of decreasing frequency, were:

(a) Origin of the left vertebral artery directly from the aorta (four branches from the arch).

(b) Origin of the left common carotid, right common carotid, and right subclavian artery from the brachiocephalic trunk; the left subclavian artery arises normally (separately) from the arch (two branches from the arch).

(c) Separate origin of the right common carotid and right subclavian artery in the following order: right subclavian, right common carotid, left common carotid, and left subclavian artery (no brachiocephalic trunk, four vessels from the arch).

(d) Left common carotid artery off the brachiocephalic, left vertebral separate, and left subclavian arteries (three vessels off the arch).

(e) Vessels arising from the arch in this order: right

common carotid, left common carotid, left subclavian, and right subclavian arteries as the final branch passing retroesophageal, crossing the midline to end up at the right arm (no brachiocephalic trunk, four vessels from the arch).

(f) Origin of the brachiocephalic trunk off the descending thoracic aorta with separate origin of the left vertebral artery branching in the following order: left common carotid, left vertebral, left subclavian artery, brachiocephalic trunk passing retroesophageal and branching into the right subclavian and right common carotid artery.

Other possible arch anomalies include the following, but not in order of frequency: a single arterial trunk off the aorta[27]; several types of isolation, including isolation of the left subclavian artery from the aorta, isolation of the right subclavian artery from the aorta, and isolation of the left innominate artery in the right aortic arch.

Any of the isolation anomalies that involve the subclavian artery could lead to subclavian steal symptoms in the adult, although this consequence seems uncommon in the child.

McDowell et al[27] reported on a patient with arterial occlusive disease of the carotid and vertebral arteries who also had a single arterial trunk (common brachiocephalic trunk), which the investigators claim was the "first report" of this anomaly. The anomaly is characteristic of aortic arch in the dog, but is said to be unique in man. The anomaly is functionally benign and presumably was unrelated to the arterial occlusive disease in McDowell's patient.

Another possible arch anomaly is the right aortic arch. According to Barron,[28] there are two types of right aortic arch. Right aortic arch is known to be associated with tetralogy of Fallot in 25% of patients, with truncus arteriosus in 30%, and with isolated VSD in 5%. Right aortic arch associated with congenital heart disease is important mainly to the surgeon who might be performing a Blalock–Taussig anastomosis for tetralogy of Fallot, tricuspid atresia, and other anomalies with pulmonary stenosis. The subclavian artery that arises from the innominate artery is the one that must be used for the anastomosis to achieve an unkinked connection to the pulmonary artery. The right aortic arch is also of importance when retroesophageal subclavian artery occurs and traverses from the descending aorta to the arm; it is the left subclavian artery that is retroesophageal in right aortic arch and the right subclavian artery that is retroesophageal when it occurs with a normal left aortic arch. This vessel creates an unusual indentation in the barium-filled esophagus, but it does not usually cause symptoms. The radial pulse on the side of the right subclavian artery may have slightly smaller pulse pressure than the pulse on the opposite side.

Right aortic arch associated with vascular ring is characterized by a large posterior diverticulum, which displaces the esophagus anteriorly. The retroesophageal subclavian artery arises from this diverticulum and completes the vascular ring. This is one of the aortic arch anomalies that is likely to cause airway obstruction in the infant and esophageal obstruction (dysphagia lusoria) in the adult.

There are several types of cervical aortic arch; some cause tracheal compression with resulting symptoms of airway obstruction or pneumonia, but symptoms may develop late in adult life.[29]

Benign, Quiescent, or Well-tolerated Defects in Adults That Had Been Hemodynamically Severe Defects in Infancy

1. Spontaneous closure or decrease in the size of a large ASD, VSD, or PDA. Any of these three malformations can allow a large left-to-right shunt in early infancy, but reduce in size or spontaneously close in late infancy, childhood, or adolescence. Spontaneous regression in size of complete closure is less common in ASD than in VSD.[30] Spontaneous closure of VSD has been recognized for many years and may occur in as high as 30% of infants seen in the first month of life. Approximately an equal number of patients will show a decrease in size from a large VSD to a small VSD, usually during the first 2 years of life. Spontaneous closure has, however, been observed in childhood and even in early adolescence. The adult patient may present with clinical signs of benign VSD, ie, only a murmur and no cardiac enlargement or other dysfunction, even though the history clearly indicated a severe anomaly in infancy or early childhood.[31]

Spontaneous closure of ductus arteriosus is more likely to occur in the premature infant who recovers from respiratory distress syndrome than in the full-term infant whose patent ductus is an isolated anomaly rather than one simply being held open by the pulmonary hypertension of pulmonary parenchymal disease. Spontaneous closure of a large isolated patent ductus must be exceedingly rare. We have observed large, long, and tortuous ductus arteriosus in which the murmur and the shunt can be demonstrated at one time but not at another and may vary with the patient's position. Disappearance of the murmur could lead to the false impression of spontaneous closure in this type of ductus.[5]

2. Spontaneous decrease in pressure gradient in pulmonary valve stenosis or pulmonary artery branch stenosis. An unexplained decrease in the severity of the pulmonary valve or pulmonary branch stenosis has been observed. Perhaps growth of the valve anulus dilates the stenotic orifice, and likewise pulmonary artery growth increases the lumen diameter of the pulmonary branch obstruction. Spontaneous improvement in pulmonary branch stenosis due to the maternal rubella syndrome has been observed between early infancy and adolescence.

3. The infant with anomalous origin of the left coronary artery from the pulmonary artery is usually in severe failure in the first few months of life and often early death occurs. However, in a few cases, improvement occurs in conjunction with medical treatment and patients may then reach adult life with a relatively normal heart size, with minimal or subtle signs of an old left ventricular myocardial infarction. At least half the survivors of infancy who show remarkable improvement and reach adult life have the murmur of mitral regurgitation because of papillary muscle dysfunction acquired during the stage of left heart failure.

Important Defects in Adulthood That Were Known or Presumed to Have Been Benign in Childhood

1. Asymptomatic nonobstructive bicuspid aortic valve in the child that becomes severe, calcific aortic stenosis in the adult. This apparently occurs in about 75% of patients who have bicuspid aortic valve. It is said to develop less commonly in the bicuspid aortic valve associated with coarctation of the aorta than in the isolated bicuspid aortic valve.

2. Mild to moderate aortic stenosis, either valvular, subvalvular, or supravalvular, in the child can develop a severe pressure gradient unrelated to calcification of the valve cusp in adult life. An increase in body size alone can lead to an increase in the severity of the pressure gradient in the patient moving from childhood to adolescence to adult life. Mild to moderate aortic stenosis in the young patient must be carefully observed in adolescence and adult life as growth increases to watch for the development of a severe pressure gradient before the onset of subjective symptoms.[32,33]

3. Quadricuspid aortic valve is quiescent and benign in the child but usually develops stenosis or insufficiency in the adult.

4. Restrictive VSD with quiescent anomaly of the aortic valve cusp that develops "acquired" aortic regurgitation in late childhood, adolescence, or adult life. Although an anomaly of the aortic cusp is a congenital deformity, the aortic insufficiency that develops in this valve usually occurs late in adult life and may become a progressively severe lesion. In some cases, however, the lesion is stable and no change occurs.[34]

5. Asymptomatic coarctation of the aorta unrecognized, mild, or well tolerated in the child that becomes severe, hypertensive coarctation in the adult (Figure 27.4). When coarctation is diagnosed for the first time in the adult, it is often assumed that the pediatrician failed to recognize it, but there is good evidence that mild coarctation in the child, allowing good femoral pulses, may progress to severe obstruction in the adult with loss of pulses.

6. Asymptomatic ASD in childhood and adolescence in which atrial fibrillation develops followed by congestive heart failure in the adult. In the study by Seldon et al,[4] an estimated 40% of patients with ASD were not recognized in childhood. Atrial septal defect can be extremely difficult to recognize in the child, because the systolic murmur is not loud and the faint diastolic murmur is difficult to learn how to hear. Furthermore, symptoms are subtle or lacking until heart failure brought on by tachydysrhythmia develops in the adult.

Important Defects in Childhood and Adulthood with Unusually Long Survival

1. Cyanotic lesions

a. Pulmonary hypertension, Eisenmenger's reaction, and pulmonary vascular obstructive disease: Irreversible small muscular pulmonary artery obstructive disease includes severe anomalies such as ASD, VSD, PDA, transposition of the great arteries, truncus arteriosus, single ventricle, and atrioventricular canal. The only defect in this group that may be improved by an operation, the palliative Mustard or Senning procedure, is transposition of the great arteries with large VSD and pulmonary vascular obstructive disease.

The basis for the Eisenmenger syndrome is an obstructive lesion in the small- and medium-sized muscular pulmonary arteries. It is believed that these changes occur in response to long-standing high pulmonary artery pressure from early infancy combined initially with a large

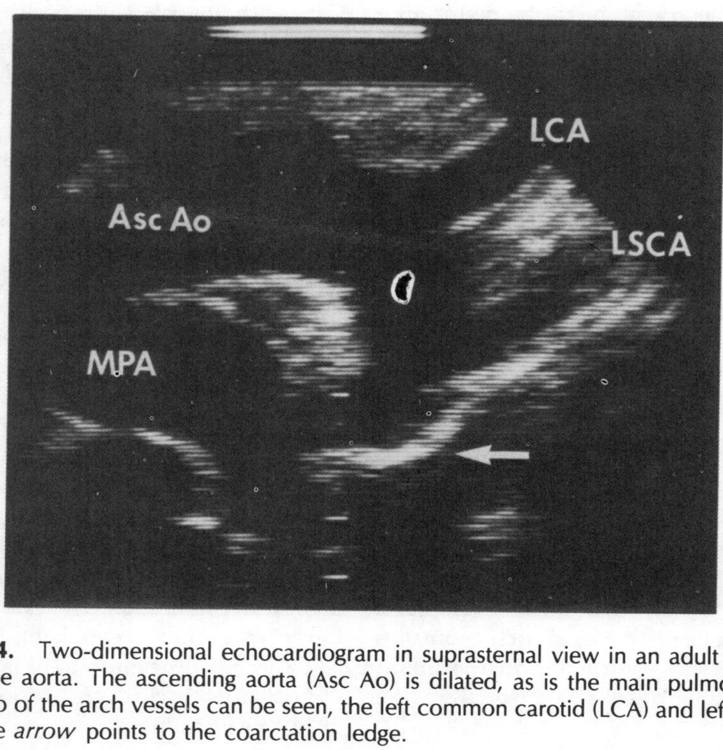

Figure 27.4. Two-dimensional echocardiogram in suprasternal view in an adult with coarctation of the aorta. The ascending aorta (Asc Ao) is dilated, as is the main pulmonary artery (MPA). Two of the arch vessels can be seen, the left common carotid (LCA) and left subclavian (LSCA). The *arrow* points to the coarctation ledge.

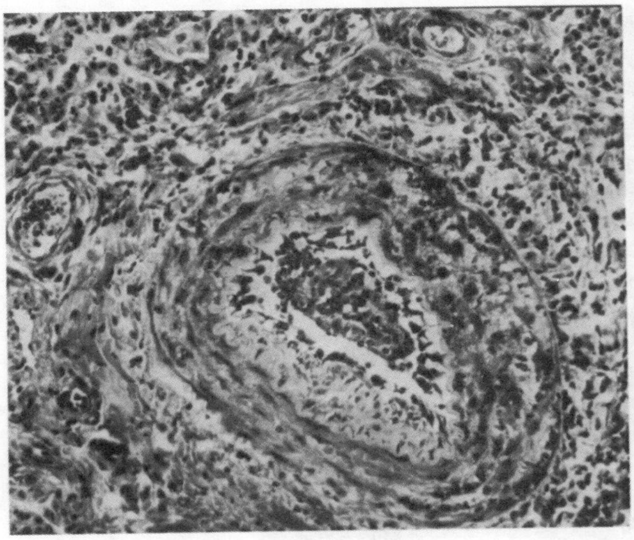

Figure 27.5. Photomicrograph of a muscular pulmonary artery showing advanced pulmonary vascular obstructive disease secondary to large ventricular septal defect. Medial hypertrophy is severe and especially well seen in the somewhat ovoid-shaped vessel between 5 o'clock and 11 o'clock. Internal to the media in the same location, intimal hyperplasia and fibrosis are apparent (grade III changes). Between 10 o'clock and 5 o'clock necrosis and cellular infiltration are evident (grade IV changes).

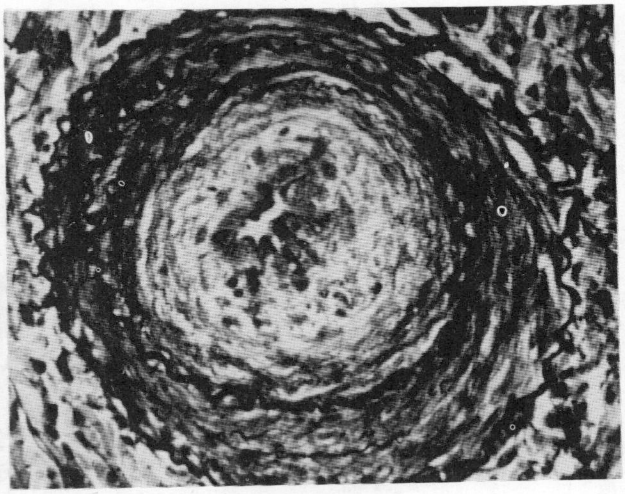

Figure 27.6. The same case as in Figure 27.5. Another muscular pulmonary artery shows almost complete obliteration of the lumen by dense concentric fibrosis and severe medial hypertrophy. The sum of the two radii of the media occupies 70% of the total diameter of the vessel (in the normal, less than 8% of the vessel diameter is made up of the two medial radii).

increase in pulmonary blood flow. Ultimately, pulmonary blood flow decreases as the obstruction becomes more severe.

The histologic features of pulmonary vascular disease have been classified by Heath and Edwards[35] (Figures 27.5 through 27.9). Although the presence of severe vascular disease can usually be suspected on clinical grounds, mild to moderate changes may be difficult to interpret, even with cardiac catheterization and conventional angiography. Although pulmonary biopsy may reveal changes that help to decide about surgical repair, the vessels available for study in the biopsy specimen may be too few to allow conclusions to be drawn. The morbidity associated with lung biopsy must be considered.

One of us (MRN)[36] devised a means of visualizing the caliber of the small muscular pulmonary artery at the time of diagnostic heart catheterization using magnification

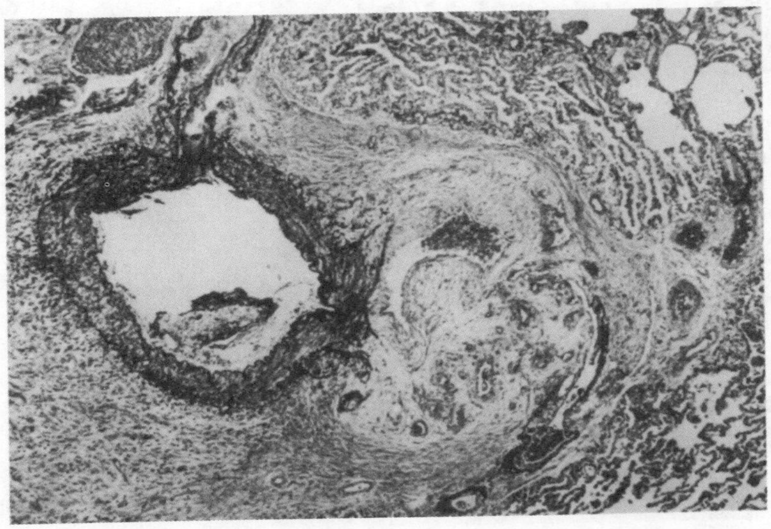

Figure 27.7. In a young adult with primary pulmonary hypertension, another type of severe pulmonary vascular obstructive disease, a plexiform lesion, is seen. Toward the left of the field lies the muscular artery with moderate medial hypertrophy. At 4 o'clock a plexiform lesion arises from the artery. It consists of a tortuous dilated lumen with cellular infiltrate. Identical lesions are seen in congenital malformations in which high pressure and increased pulmonary blood flow coexist from early infancy.

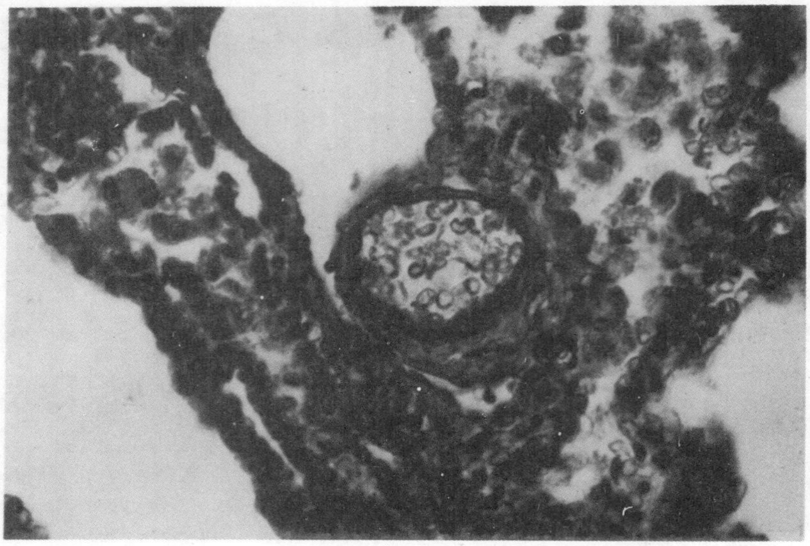

Figure 27.8. Normal small muscular pulmonary artery. The thickness of the muscular layer between the internal and external elastic membranes (two *black lines* seen best at about 11 o'clock to 2 o'clock) measures about 5% of the vessel diameter. The small 100 μ vessel lies adjacent to a bronchiole.

pulmonary artery wedge angiography. The technique can be safely employed in evaluating the patient who might have pulmonary vascular obstructive disease (Figures 27.10 to 27.12). An illustrative case of Eisenmenger's is shown in Figure 27.13.

Pulmonary hypertension secondary to pulmonary venous obstruction, for example due to cor triatriatum or congenital mitral stenosis, is usually correctable by operation, even in the adult (Figure 27.14). It is remarkable how late in life, adolescence or early adult life, the correct diagnosis is made in these patients. This is because there is often no murmur or only a faint one, plus the fact that the symptoms are pulmonary and the physician suspects asthma or other chronic airway obstructive disease. The diagnosis usually can be made by two-dimensional echocardiography.

b. Pulmonary infundibular, valvular, or main trunk stenosis or pulmonary valve or trunk atresia with large, nonrestrictive VSD: This includes tetralogy of Fallot, pseudotruncus (VSD and pulmonary trunk atresia), tri-

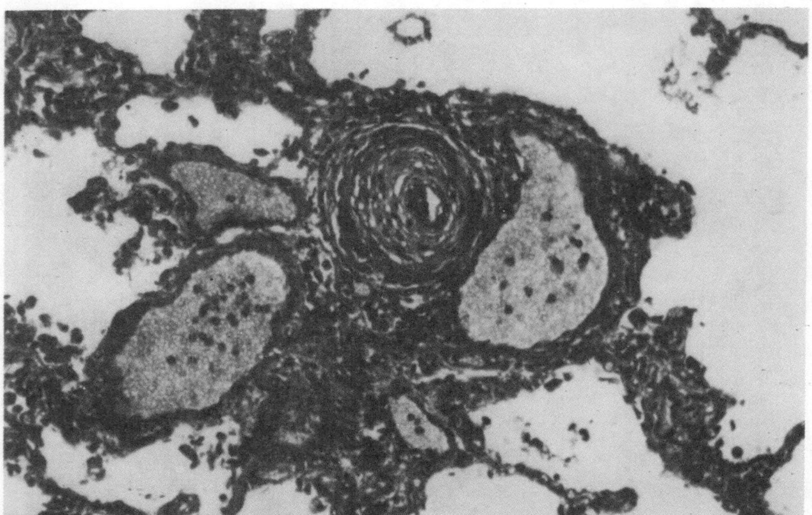

Figure 27.9. Dilatation lesion. Photomicrograph of a small muscular pulmonary artery from a patient with transposition and large ventricular septal defect. There is almost complete occlusion of the lumen due to intimal sclerosis, in addition to the pronounced medial hypertrophy. Three secondary dilatation lesions are seen surrounding the vessel and may serve as bypass arteries.

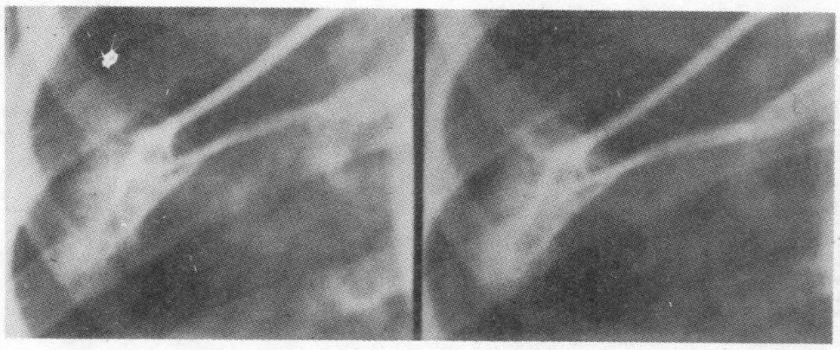

Figure 27.10. Magnification pulmonary artery wedge angiogram. Normal pulmonary vessels in a patient with ventricular septal defect without pulmonary hypertension. On the left, the "early phase" after injection reveals the pulmonary artery above the pulmonary vein below. The artery and vein are of approximately equal caliber. The artery shows gradual tapering and gives off many small vessels (the small muscular pulmonary arteries). On the right, the "mid phase" shows the capillary "blush" with the characteristic ground glass appearance of the normal vascular tree.

cuspid atresia with pulmonary stenosis or pulmonary atresia, single ventricle with pulmonary stenosis or pulmonary atresia (double inlet right or left ventricle), transposition of the great arteries with VSD plus pulmonary stenosis, "corrected" transposition (levotransposition) with VSD, pulmonary stenosis, and diminutive "right ventricle."

c. Right ventricular inflow or outflow stenosis or atresia; pulmonary valve, trunk, or branch stenosis; pulmonary valve atresia with ASD (or patent foramen ovale) but no VSD: This group includes Ebstein's malformation, which is a type of inflow obstruction to pulmonary blood flow. Cyanosis depends on presence of atrial communication (Figure 27.15).

d. Partial anomaly of systemic venous return to the left atrium[9]: This anomaly is also listed under "benign" (silent) defects with small right-to-left shunts, because the severity varies.

2. "Acyanotic" (no visible cyanosis, but some have slight arterial oxygen desaturation).

a. Left-to-right shunt without pulmonary hypertension (that is, no fixed pulmonary vascular obstructive disease), but some have elevated pulmonary artery pressure but low pulmonary vascular resistance.

(1) Large ASD
(2) Total anomalous pulmonary venous return
(3) Fistula from coronary artery to right atrium or right ventricle
(4) Large VSD with only mild to moderate elevation of pulmonary artery pressure
(5) Large PDA with only mild to moderate elevation of pulmonary artery pressure (Figure 27.16)

b. Isolated severe right-sided lesions without VSD, ASD, or patent foramen ovale

(1) Ebstein's malformation with right ventricular outflow obstruction
(2) Pulmonary valve stenosis
(3) Right ventricular infundibular stenosis
(4) Pulmonary artery branch stenosis

c. Severe left-sided obstructive lesion with no right-to-left shunt, but a severe form of left-sided lesion could lead to pulmonary edema with cyanosis or some degree of arterial oxygen desaturation resulting from ventilatory insufficiency.

(1) Individual pulmonary vein stenosis[37]
(2) Stenosis of common pulmonary vein (cor triatriatum)
(3) Congenital mitral stenosis
(4) Congenital mitral valve regurgitation
(5) Hypertrophic-obstructive-nondilated and dilated-congestive cardiomyopathy
(6) Left ventricular outflow obstructive lesion (aortic stenosis: valvular, subvalvular discrete membranous, tunnel stenosis, and supravalvular)
(7) Severe coarctation of aorta in childhood and adulthood

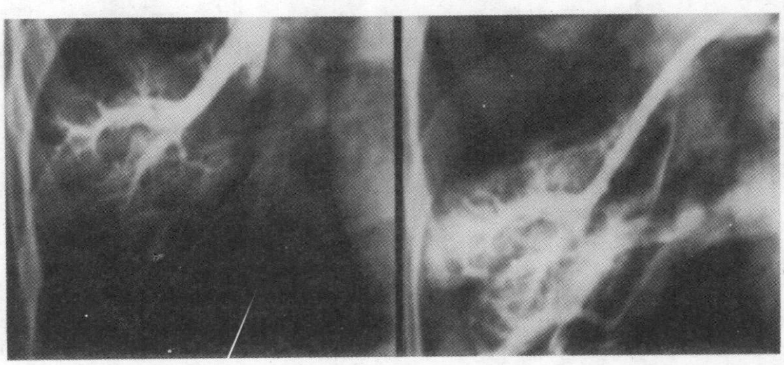

Figure 27.11. Pulmonary artery wedge angiogram in a patient with ventricular septal defect and pulmonary hypertension, but only moderately severe vascular disease and a large left-to-right shunt. Comparing this angiogram with that in Figure 27.10, there is rapid tapering of the dilated artery in the early phase frame on the left. There is a paucity of right angle branches (small muscular arteries). In the "late phase" on the right, the capillary blush is complete. The vascular disease was assumed to be less than a grade III change and proved to be no contraindication to surgical closure of the ventricular septal defect.

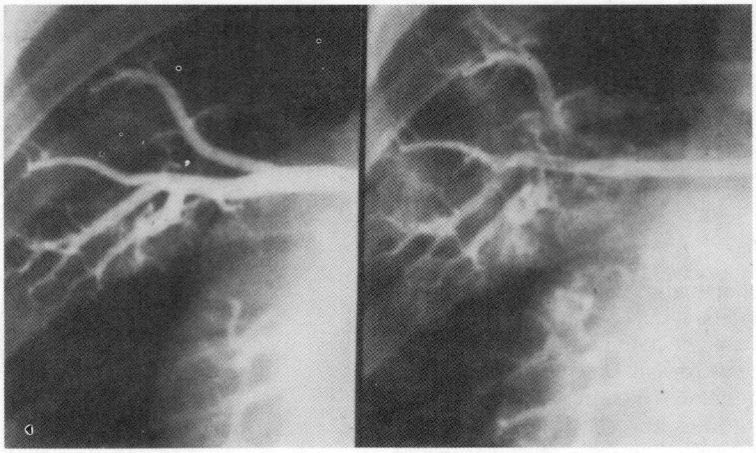

Figure 27.12. Pulmonary artery wedge angiogram in a patient with Eisenmenger's syndrome and severe pulmonary vascular obstructive disease, which renders surgical closure of large ventricular septal defect implausible. The angiographic characteristics of this lesion include an appearance of a bare tree (tree-in-winter), abrupt tapering, few small muscular vessels, and an incompatible blush phase.

POSTOPERATIVE CONGENITAL HEART DISEASE IN THE ADULT

Palliative Operations

1. Shunts for tetralogy of Fallot, tricuspid atresia with pulmonary stenosis, single ventricle with pulmonary stenosis, corrected transposition with VSD, and pulmonary stenosis (Figure 27.17). Currently, the best management for the patient who has had a shunt performed for any of these lesions is to correct the anomaly and close the shunt. However, some adult patients with a functioning shunt will undoubtedly seek the opinion of the cardiologist many years after the palliative procedure. Some are functioning quite well as adults.[38] Unless pulmonary vascular obstructive disease has developed because of a large shunt (such as the Potts), repair can often be carried out in the adult.

The shunts that may be encountered include: (a) Blalock–Taussig anastomosis; (b) Potts anastomosis (Figure 27.18); (c) Waterston extrapericardial anastomosis; and (d) Cooley intrapericardial ascending aorta-to-pulmonary artery anastomosis.

2. Banding of pulmonary artery (Dammann-Muller operation) for VSD, atrioventricular canal, transposition of the great arteries with VSD and pulmonary hypertension, truncus and other anomalies with large VSD, and pulmonary hypertension in infancy (Figure 27.19).

3. Surgical creation of ASD (Blalock-Hanlon operation)

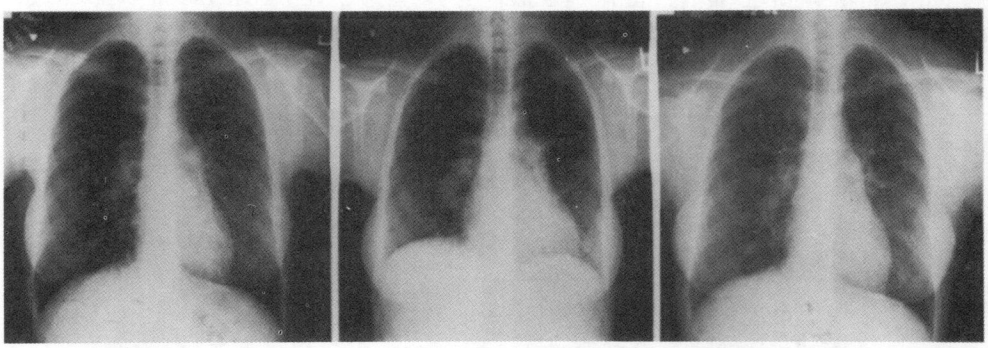

Figure 27.13. Chest radiograph of a 43-year-old woman with ventricular septal defect and Eisenmenger's complex followed by the authors for 30 years. A heart murmur present from birth disappeared at about 12 years of age. Cyanosis appeared at the same time and progressively increased during the next several years, but it has since remained stable. Despite cyanosis and shortness of breath, she maintains a full-time, highly responsible executive position. She is married and lives a normal, although physically limited, life. The patient requests phlebotomy two or three times per year from which she usually obtains symptomatic relief for periods ranging from weeks to months. The chest film reveals large proximal right and left main pulmonary arteries, the contour of right ventricular hypertrophy. In the middle film, at age 38, the heart dilated slightly when excessive phlebotomy produced transient anemia and fluid retention, but in the film at 25 years (on the left) and at 42 years (on the right) the heart is not dilated.

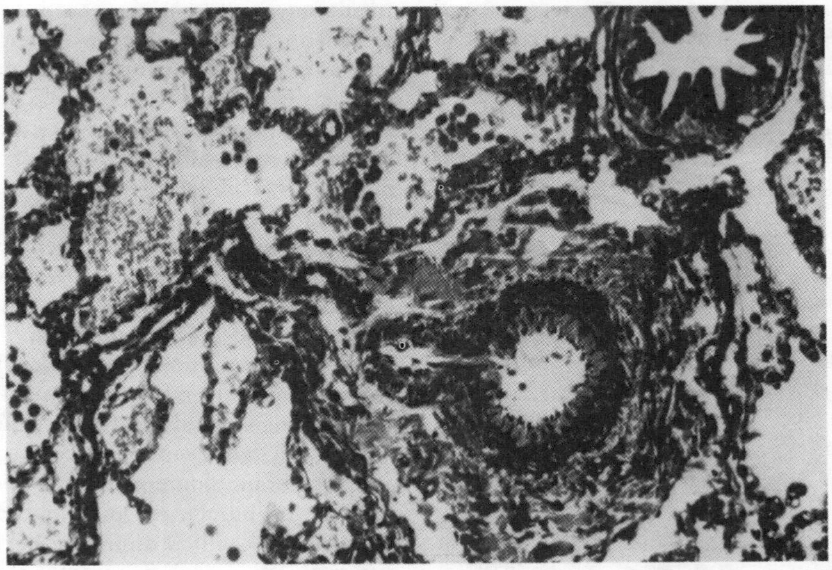

Figure 27.14. Arterial lesion secondary to left heart obstruction. The patient had cor triatriatum with resulting pulmonary hypertension. The hypertrophied media seen in the vessel in the lower portion of the photomicrograph has produced a sphincter-like constriction around the orifice of a dilatation lesion arising at 9 o'clock. This type of pulmonary vascular obstructive disease is reversible once the etiologic lesion is corrected.

for transposition of the great arteries or for inoperable left-sided obstructive lesions to relieve pulmonary venous hypertension.

4. Palliative Mustard atrial baffle repair for improvement of transposition of the great arteries, large VSD with pulmonary vascular obstructive disease (Lindesmith's operation).[39] This is probably the only anomaly with severe cyanosis and pulmonary vascular obstructive disease in which surgical palliation is helpful. The Mustard[40] or Senning[41] atrial baffle procedure is performed leaving the VSD open, which provides symptomatic improvement and increases arterial oxygen saturation.

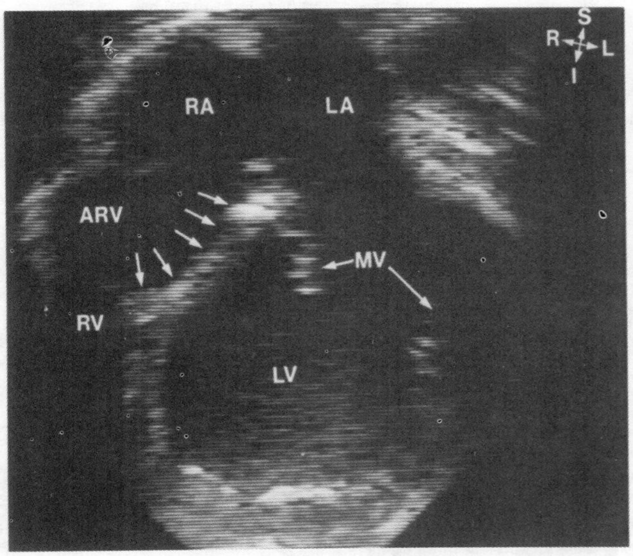

Figure 27.15. Two-dimensional echocardiogram. Apical four-chamber view in a 20-year-old man with Ebstein's malformation of the tricuspid valve. The five *arrows* point to the displaced valve within the atrialized right ventricle (ARV) just inferior to the enlarged right atrium (RA). The left ventricle (LV) is greatly dilated and the patient appears to have also a left ventricular cardiomyopathy. I = inferior; L = left; LA = left atrium; MV = mitral valve; R = right; S = superior.

Palliative Catheterization Intervention for Creation of ASD

1. Creation of larger ASD for inadequate size ASD
   a. Rashkind balloon atrial septostomy[42]
   b. Park blade/balloon atrial septostomy[43]
2. Creation of ASD in a patient with intact atrial septum
   a. Mullins transseptal blade-balloon atrial septostomy[44]

Definitive Operation with Total Correction[45]

1. Secundum ASD
2. Sinus venosus ASD
3. Persistent eustachian valve with ASD
4. Total anomalous pulmonary venous return to left vertical vein
5. Aorticopulmonary window without pulmonary hypertension (rare; this anomaly usually has systemic pressure in pulmonary artery)
6. PDA without pulmonary hypertension
7. Localized pulmonary AV fistula
8. Cor triatriatum
9. Mustard or Senning baffle repair of simple D-transposition (preoperative intact ventricular septum and no pulmonary stenosis or pulmonary hypertension) (Figure 27.20)

Definitive Repair but Residual Defect

1. Ostium primum closure, but persistence of mitral valve cleft or deformity

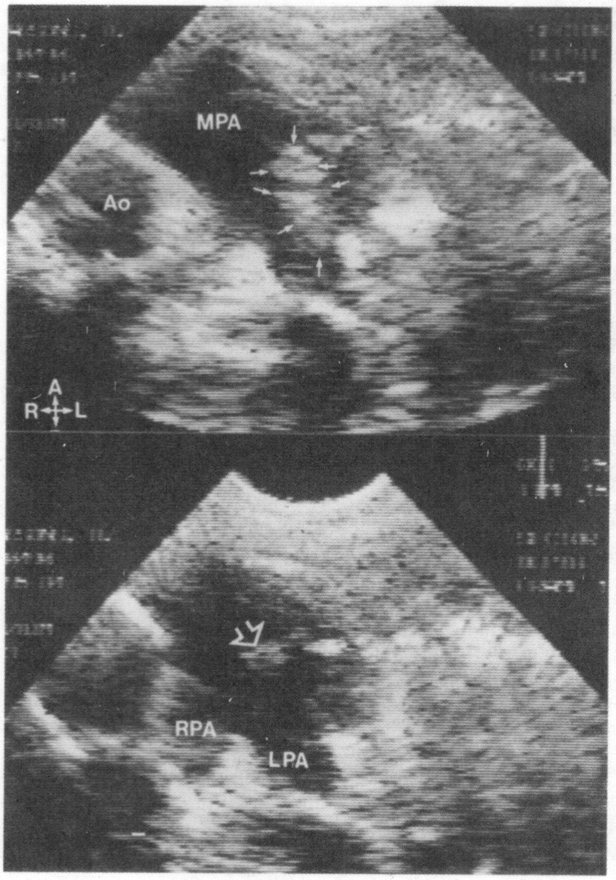

Figure 27.16. Two-dimensional echocardiogram from suprasternal view in adult patient with large patent ductus and infective endocarditis. A prominent vegetation (*upper panel*) is surrounded by small solid *arrows*. The main pulmonary artery (MPA) is dilated. A portion of the root of the aorta (Ao) is seen inferiorly and to the right of the MPA. In the *lower panel* an open *arrow* points to a portion of the vegetation located near the origin of the right (RPA) and left pulmonary artery (LPA). A = anterior; L = left; R = right.

2. Coarctation of aorta is repaired, but bicuspid aortic valve persists in about 85% of patients. Various types of anomaly of the mitral valve are present in a high percentage of patients with coarctation of the aorta. Many of these are minor and require no special treatment.

3. VSD and aortic valve regurgitation. Some deformity of the aortic valve persists whether or not surgical repair is attempted.[34]

4. Other anomalies in which two or more defects typically are associated, and operation repairs only one defect

Definitive Repair but Unavoidable Sequelae

1. Mustard baffle repair of transposition of the great arteries often unavoidably damages sinoatrial node with resulting sinus node dysfunction (sick sinus syndrome, bradytachydysrhythmia syndrome).[46] Occasionally, operation to repair large ostium secundum ASD or sinus venosus ASD may cause sinus node dysfunction.

2. Ventriculotomy performed for repair of VSD and tetralogy of Fallot, to name two anomalies, leaves a ventriculotomy scar that may be the site of arrhythmia or rare aneurysm formation. In some cases the ventriculotomy scar or obscure coronary artery trauma leads to ventricular dysfunction. Right bundle branch block develops as either a proximal (due to ventriculotomy) or a distal (due to dissecting and suturing near or on the right bundle branch) type of intraventricular conduction defect. Although postoperative bundle branch block has no known functional significance, it renders the ECG unreliable in future interpretation of hypertrophy by this modality.

3. Pulmonary valvotomy for pulmonary valve stenosis leaves some degree of pulmonary valve insufficiency. This may lead to no more problem than a postoperative diastolic murmur, but in some patients there is elevated right ventricular end-diastolic pressure and both the right atrium and right ventricle may become slightly dilated after operation. Some patients with a fairly pronounced murmur of pulmonary insufficiency and dilated right ventricle and right atrium are the ones who tire with exercise. Although the treadmill tests are well tolerated in that no important dysrhythmia occurs, the study can help to confirm true exercise-induced fatigue.

4. Aortic valvotomy. Similar to pulmonary insufficiency after pulmonary stenosis surgery, there is usually some degree of aortic insufficiency after aortic valvotomy. Unlike pulmonary insufficiency, aortic insufficiency is potentially a serious problem. When aortic insufficiency is mild, the condition is benign, but annual checkups are advised because it may progress. A mild to moderate degree of aortic insufficiency is preferable to an aortic valve prosthesis. In the adult patient with aortic stenosis who requires surgery, aortic valve replacement rather than valvotomy is virtually always required. Calcific deposits pre-

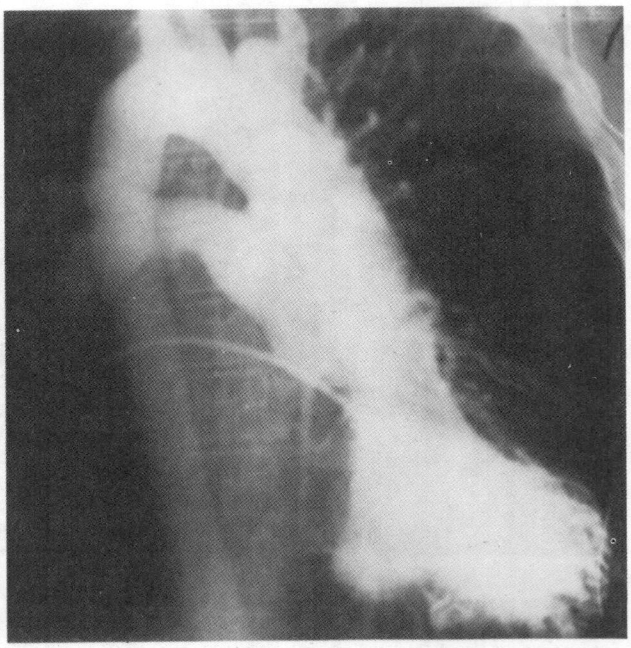

Figure 27.17. Left ventricular angiogram in a 45-year-old intensely cyanotic man, a successful investor, married, and father of two children. Diagnosis: ventricular inversion, double inlet left ventricle, pulmonary stenosis, postoperative Blalock–Taussig anastomosis.

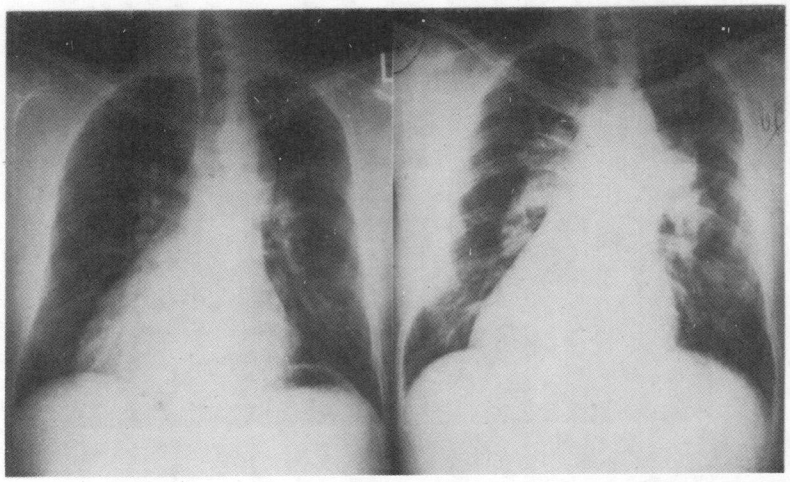

Figure 27.18. Serial chest films in an adult male at 24 years on the left and 26 years on the right. Diagnosis: dextrocardia (isolated; stomach bubble on patient's left), single ventricle, pulmonary stenosis, 20 years postoperative Potts anastomosis (aorta-to-pulmonary artery shunt). Between the two films the patient had developed pulmonary vascular obstructive disease with pulmonary pressure increasing from 20/10 to 90/60 mm Hg. This frequent, although not invariable, complication of the large Potts shunt makes this palliative procedure undesirable.

vent successful valvotomy, but in the adolescent patient 10% or fewer must have valve replacement. Among the adult patients who had aortic valvotomy in infancy and childhood, an estimated 30% will require aortic valve replacement.

Incomplete Repair of Defect but Good Functional Result

Some incompletely repaired anomalies, despite persistent murmur, abnormal radiographic or electrocardiographic features, and bizarre angiographic findings, may nevertheless have functionally adequate if not totally normal resting hemodynamics at postoperative cardiac catheterization. If so, and the exercise test and 24-hour ambulatory electrocardiographic monitor are satisfactory, these patients can be allowed to have a fully normal, active life. The exception is the need for continued follow-up every 1 to 3 years and prophylaxis against infective endocarditis.

1. Ventricular septal defect. In about one third of patients who have repair of VSD, a small interventricular communication persists. This produces a VSD murmur, but if the left-to-right shunt is small, the defect can be left, not requiring additional surgery. The patient should know before operation that a murmur and a small defect may persist. Whether the shunt is small or large postoperatively, infective endocarditis prophylaxis is needed.

2. Aortic or pulmonary valve stenosis. Relief of severe pressure gradient is the goal of the operation. In some instances *no* systolic pressure gradient can be recorded after aortic or pulmonary valvotomy, but in most patients some minor pressure gradient (equal to or less than 20 mm Hg) persists and this produces a murmur, but it may be of no functional significance. It does mean, however, that continued follow-up, including infective endocarditis prophylaxis, is advisable and at more frequent intervals than if there were no gradient at all. Patients should be advised that a murmur will not only persist after operation, but a new murmur, that of valve insufficiency, will be heard.

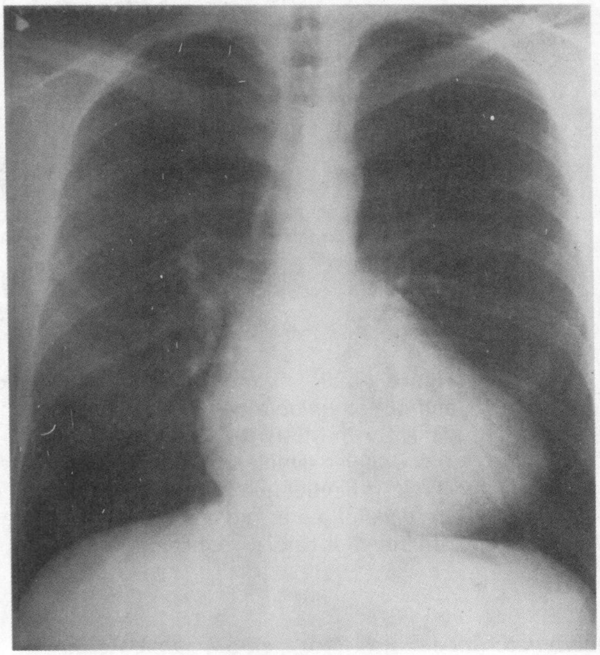

Figure 27.19. Plain chest film in a cyanotic 20-year-old man, height 6 feet 3 inches, weight 195 pounds, with severe limitation of exercise tolerance. Diagnosis: pulmonary hypertension associated with single ventricle (double inlet left ventricle) and ventricular inversion. Pulmonary artery banding at 6 years of age had reduced excessive blood flow to lungs and gave symptomatic improvement until late teens. A systemic-to-pulmonary artery anastomosis at 20 years gave further improvement.

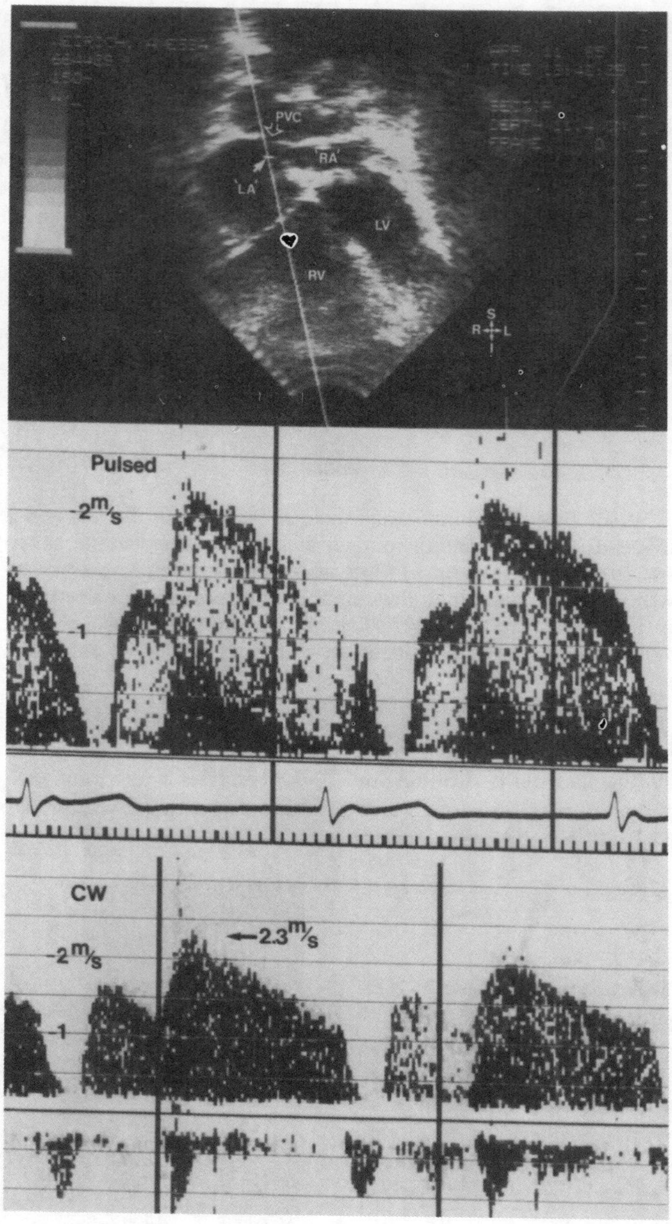

Figure 27.20. Two-dimensional echocardiogram in apical four-chamber view (*upper panel*) and pulsed (*middle panel*) and continuous wave (CW) (*lower panel*) Doppler recording in a patient with Mustard operation (atrial baffle) performed for transposition of the great arteries. The Doppler sample site is at the closed arrow just inferior to pulmonary venous confluence (PVC) within the new left atrium (LA). The pulsed and continuous wave Doppler documented presence of a pressure gradient between the PVC and "LA," estimated to be 21 mm Hg, was confirmed at cardiac catheterization.

Incomplete Repair with Poor Hemodynamic Result

1. Persistent large left-to-right shunt may exist after an attempt to repair one of the complex VSDs such as multiple VSDs or a large VSD in a difficult position to repair (eg, large posterior septal defects). If a large left-to-right shunt persists postoperatively, especially if right ventricular pressure remains elevated because of the shunt, reoperation may have to be performed. In explaining the first operation to the patient, one possible outcome is that the operation may be unsuccessful and must be repeated. Second operations for a repairable defect surprisingly enough have had a high chance of success.

2. Tetralogy of Fallot, unsuccessful repair. Depending on the criteria selected for a poor result from tetralogy of Fallot repair, the chance that such will result ranges from 8% to 34%.[47,48]

In patients examined after tetralogy of Fallot repair at the Texas Children's Hospital, we found that a poor result can be missed from only a clinical and noninvasive evaluation. Therefore, cardiac catheterization should be performed in all patients and we recommend that it be done within a year of operation.[49]

Right ventricular pressure may remain elevated because of persistent large VSD, unrelieved obstruction to right ventricular outflow tract including the pulmonary valve, and unrelieved congenital obstruction in the pulmonary artery branches. Because persistent high right ventricular pressure after repair of tetralogy of Fallot predisposes to arrhythmias and sudden death, reoperation must be performed if the persistent right ventricular hypertension can be surgically relieved.[50]

Complete Repair of Defect with Poor Result Due to Preoperatively Existing Acquired Complications

1. Pulmonary vascular obstructive disease due to arterial thrombi in a polycythemic patient. The obstruction is easily missed in the patient with preoperative tetralogy of Fallot because the right ventricular outflow tract stenosis and low pulmonary blood flow prevent high pressure from being recorded in the pulmonary artery. Postoperatively, however, all the systemic venous return must now pass through the pulmonary arteries. Because the outflow stenosis is removed, the obstructive pulmonary arterial lesion becomes manifest.

Small muscular pulmonary arterial vascular obstructive disease also can result from a long-standing large anastomosis such as the Potts aorta-to-left pulmonary artery shunt.[51] However, pulmonary artery pressure in these patients would have been elevated before intracardiac repair was performed.

Pulmonary vascular obstructive disease develops more commonly before operation in patients with a large congenital left-to-right shunt with systemic pressure in the pulmonary arteries such as may occur with VSD, large ductus, large AV canal, or truncus arteriosus. If the operation is performed in the infant and young child, secondary vascular changes in the small pulmonary arteries usually can be avoided. It may not be known until a year or two after operation that this complication has not been prevented by repair of the defect. In this instance, repairing the defect will create greater problems with the patient, because ultimately right heart failure develops when there is no longer an escape mechanism for the right-sided blood to reach the systemic circulation (Figure 27.21).

2. Preoperatively acquired myocardial damage. Long-standing elevated intraventricular pressure is known to lead to myocardial damage, especially if the ventricle is dilated as well. In left heart anomaly such as critical aortic stenosis or severe coarctation of aorta with severe systemic hypertension, papillary muscle necrosis can develop with subsequent mitral leaflet prolapse and mitral valve regurgitation. In addition, reduced pumping function may result from the combination of pressure overload on left ventricle. High right ventricular pressure from severe valvular pulmonary stenosis may similarly interfere with right ventricular pump function. A long-standing volume overload, however, appears to be well tolerated and usually reversal to normal heart size can be expected after surgical removal of the large volume overload.

Defects Repaired by Catheterization Interventional Procedures

1. Pulmonary valvuloplasty by balloon dilatation for isolated pulmonary valve stenosis.[52] Decrease in right ventricular-to-pulmonary artery pressure gradient has proved successful and safe. Drs Charles Mullins and Michael Nihill have carried out this procedure at Texas Children's Hospital in 39 patients with a right ventricular-to-pulmonary artery peak systolic pressure gradient ranging from 25 to 105 mm Hg (average 53). After balloon valvuloplasty, the average gradient measured 17 mm Hg with a range of 5 to 60 mm Hg. In all but one patient the peak gradient was 25 mm Hg or less and in ten patients it was 10 mm Hg or less. These patients must be followed over a period of several years to know what the final outcome will be, but the early results are as good as those of surgical valvotomy.

2. Balloon angioplasty for coarctation of the aorta.[53] This procedure has been used for restenosis (or persistent stenosis) after operation for coarctation as well as for native coarctation. The early relief of pressure gradient in 40 patients is encouraging (mean 46 mm Hg [range 14 to 88] decreased to a mean of 11 mm Hg [range 0 to 30]) and we must wait for long-term follow-up before recommending this procedure in *all* patients.

3. Ductus occlusion with the umbrella device of Rashkind.[54] Dr Charles Mullins has closed the ductus by venous catheter introduction of Rashkind's device, which is a double umbrella structure with hinged "legs" supporting two polyethylene sponges. Among 62 attempts, the procedure was totally successful in 39 (63%). In some the ductus was too large for the available device. Modifications in design have made the method more successful and in more recent patients there have been 29 successful occlusions in 32 attempts. These patients ranged in age from 4 months to 42 years. One might predict for the future that a large number of patients with patent ductus arteriosus will have obliteration of the ductus by this technique.

LONG-TERM CARE OF THE ADULT PATIENT WITH CONGENITAL HEART DISEASE

ASSESSMENT OF THE POSTOPERATIVE PATIENT

When the patient with postoperative congenital heart disease consults the internist–cardiologist, the question will arise to what extent, if any, is participation in a normal life excluded. The areas of interest to the adult patient may include: (1) Vocational plans: physically or mentally stressful jobs? (2) Sports: competitive or otherwise? (3) Marriage and family: (a) Is pregnancy permissible for the wife? (b) Is the husband or wife solely capable of serving as an effective head of the family? (c) Can the defect be passed on to the offspring? (4) Long-term outlook, including insurability. If the patient does not bring up these questions, the physician should do so,

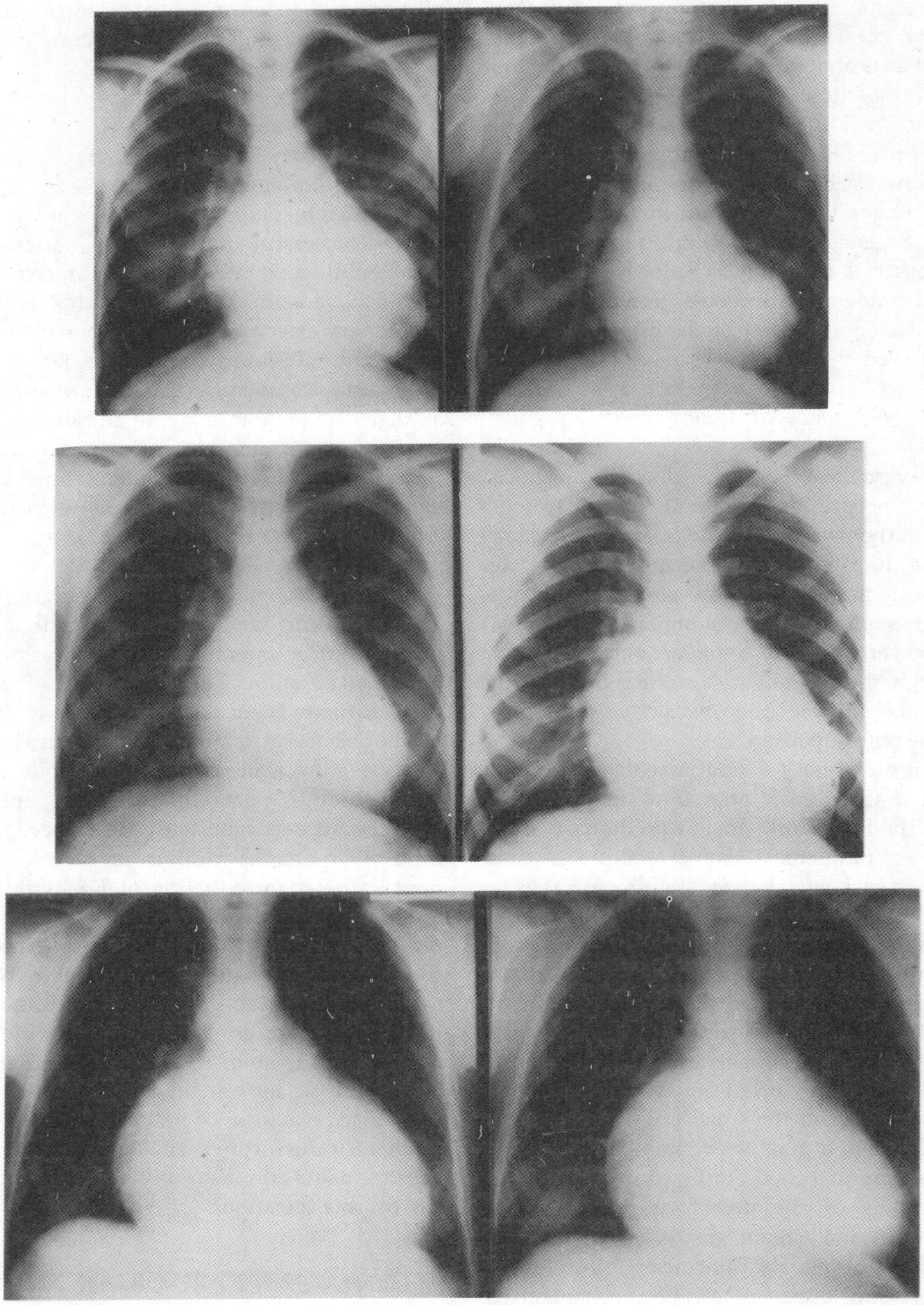

Figure 27.21. Series of chest films in an adult woman whom we had expected to have reversible pulmonary hypertension due to a large ventricular septal defect (VSD) and had surgical closure at age 16. *Top*, Film on left, preoperative repair of large VSD with equal pulmonary artery and aortic pressures and large left-to-right shunt. There is dilation of the left ventricle and right ventricle and increased pulmonary vascular markings. On the right: 6-month postoperative film shows decrease in pulmonary vascular markings and heart size is somewhat smaller. *Middle*, Film on left, 3 years postoperative. Patient has become very short of breath and heart size is slightly larger. Catheterization revealed systemic pressure in the pulmonary artery and elevated right ventricular filling pressure. In the film on the right, $5\frac{1}{2}$ years postoperative, the right ventricle has become dilated and the patient was more symptomatic. *Bottom*, The film on the left was obtained 9 years after operation. The right ventricle and right atrium are greatly dilated. Cardiac catheterization revealed that pulmonary artery pressure exceeds systemic pressure during infusion of isoproterenol. Blade and balloon atrial septostomy resulted in cyanosis, but there was slight symptomatic improvement. Film on the right, 2 months after creation of an atrial septal defect, shows slight decrease in heart size. Since then the patient has had uncomplicated surgery for cholecystectomy and then for tubal ligation for birth control.

because every postoperative patient will want to discuss each point.

The physician needs certain minimal information to be able to discuss these questions, to answer them, or to obtain the answer from the patient's cardiologist:

1. What was (were) the original defect(s) and what was the operation performed?

2. What was the original indication for operation and was the purpose of operation achieved?

3. What is the patient's current exercise tolerance? Is there other important history (for example, syncope)?

4. What is the current medication?

5. What are the findings of a cardiovascular physical examination, including response to exercise?

6. What is the electrocardiographic rate and rhythm? Is there hypertrophy or bundle branch block?

7. What is the finding of the 24-hour ambulatory electrocardiographic monitor?

8. What is the result of the exercise stress test?

9. What are the findings on ultrasonic examination, including two-dimensional and Doppler analysis of pressure gradient and abnormal blood flow?

10. What does the chest radiograph show, including heart size and character of pulmonary vessels?

11. Does the patient require postoperative heart catheterization? Postoperative heart catheterization is usually required for any patient who is not doing well and for those patients who had preoperative pulmonary hypertension. Or, if the results of the previous 10 points are significantly abnormal, heart catheterization should be performed. Catheterization is also indicated in patients with severe preoperative obstructive lesions, especially if a loud murmur persists postoperatively, or if there is an important arrhythmia, cardiac dilatation, or other evidence of inadequate surgical relief of the obstruction.

In assessing the patient for full normal activities, there should be (1) no more than slight enlargement of the ventricles or atria, (2) clinical or echocardiographic signs of normal ventricular filling pressure and mild or no ventricular-to-great vessel pressure gradient, (3) normal exercise test, (4) freedom from significant arrhythmia on 24-hour monitor, (5) normal arterial oxygen saturation, and (6) no large left-to-right shunt. If so, whatever the operation was, the patient can usually be allowed a perfectly normal life, including unlimited educational plans, participation in sports (which must be individualized), and, for women, pregnancy.

According to a study by Whittemore et al,[55] among the offspring of women with congenital heart disease, about 14% had a congenital cardiovascular anomaly and in about half of them the defect was the same as that in the mother. The incidence of congenital anomalies among the offspring of the father who has congenital heart disease was not assessed in this study.

In a review of Nora et al,[56] only about 3% to 5% of the offspring of an affected parent (mother or father) had heart defects. It may be that the study by Whittemore et al[55] turned up a larger number than did that of Nora et al,[56] because Whittemore personally examined every child. Also, her study was prospective and had the benefit of ultrasound for more sensitive and specific detection of heart defects.

PREVENTIVE CARDIOLOGY PROGRAM

General Considerations

The following principles should be adhered to in planning for follow-up of the adult with congenital heart disease:

1. Psychologic encouragement and support on the part of the physician.

2. Assistance in obtaining education, work, and life insurance.

3. Meticulous attention to regular dental hygiene and other measures aimed at prophylaxis against infective endocarditis.

4. Avoid the anxiety and harm of well meant but excessive medical overconcern, overprotection, and oversolicitous follow-up.

5. Provide up-to-date reevaluation for the patient with uncorrected important heart disease who has been denied surgical or medical treatment previously. New developments appear every year in technology, pharmacology, interventional catheterization procedures, and surgical technique. Frequent reevaluation should be made, with the possibility that the new technology might provide a chance for improvement of the patient.

Care of the Cyanotic Patient

Special attention must be given to the cyanotic, polycythemic patient who is currently inoperable. These patients are especially prone to infective endocarditis, brain abscess and pulmonary emboli, hemoptysis, other bleeding diathesis, and thrombotic tendency. Regular, good dental care; prompt eradication of infection, including surgical drainage if needed; and bacteriologically guided specific antibiotic treatment of infections should be carried out.

Compensatory polycythemia is needed to maintain optimal oxygen content in the arterial blood, but hematocrit beyond 65% may accomplish little, because the increased viscosity above this level may decrease vital organ flow. Phlebotomy or erythropheresis may be performed for relief of symptoms of "fullness," fatigue, headache, increasing exertional dyspnea, persistent hemoptysis, and other bleeding tendencies.

We have recommended phlebotomy electively when the centrifuged hematocrit is persistently above 65% or if symptoms occur when the hematocrit is between 61% and 65%. Phlebotomy should always be accompanied by intravenous replacement of an equal amount of isosmolar fluid. A reduction in blood volume alone will result in an increase in the effective blood viscosity for several hours until equilibration can take place by oral fluid intake.

The amount of blood to be withdrawn can be calculated according to the following formula (Patients with secondary polycythemia have an increased blood volume [90 to 100 ml/kg] due to an increase in red blood cell mass, and this must be taken into account when calculating the amount of blood to be withdrawn and replaced):

$$100 \text{ ml} \times \text{weight (kg)} \times \frac{\text{observed hematocrit} - \text{desired hematocrit}}{\text{observed hematocrit}}$$

The desired hematocrit should be 58% to 60% depending on the desired oxygen content and oxygen delivery, which can be determined by the patient's arterial oxygen saturation. The replacement fluid should be isosmolar with plasma. We have used 5% albumin in buffered Ringer's lactate or saline solution.

If the patient weighs 70 kg, the hematocrit is 70%, and the desired hematocrit is 60%, the calculation is as follows:

$$100 \times 70\ (= 7{,}000) \times \frac{70 - 60}{70} = 7{,}000 \times 0.14 = 980.$$

No more than 500 to 700 ml of blood should be removed at one time, so remove 500 ml one day and repeat the following day.

The goal of phlebotomy is to make the patient feel better. The effect normally lasts 2 to 4 months and sometimes longer. The probable benefit, although not proven, is to reduce a bleeding tendency, such as hemoptysis, that may develop. If the patient with severe polycythemia is to have surgery, especially ear, nose, throat, or dental surgery, bleeding tests should be performed. If the platelet count is low, the fibrinogen level is low, and the clot is friable, phlebotomy one to two days before the operation may reduce the bleeding diathesis.

Patients who have had frequent phlebotomies should be checked for signs of iron deficiency, which can be present despite severe polycythemia. A centrifuged hematocrit determination is a better indication of the true hematocrit rather than an automated machine calculation from the measured hemoglobin. The centrifuged hematocrit should be about three times the measured hemoglobin value and any discrepancy might indicate the presence of a microcytic hypochromic anemia. Iron-deficient cyanotic patients often have symptoms of malaise and fatigue out of proportion to the apparent polycythemia. These symptoms are rapidly improved by the administration of oral iron therapy.

Erythropheresis is most often used in patients with pulmonary hypertension due to fixed pulmonary vascular obstructive disease. In patients with severe pulmonary stenosis or atresia, as well as in those with Eisenmenger's syndrome, great care must be taken not to decrease the hematocrit and blood viscosity too much, because systemic resistance will be lowered more than the effective pulmonary resistance and may result in an increase in the amount of right-to-left shunting.

Management of the cyanotic female patient of childbearing age involves special precautions. In general, pregnancy is ill-advised for several reasons. The chance of spontaneous abortion is high, and aside from the psychic trauma of an abortion to both the wife and the husband, there is potential danger to the life of the mother because of the tendency to bleeding, thrombosis, pulmonary and cerebral emboli, as well as septicemia and infective endocarditis.

Despite precautions in the preceding paragraph, if the woman with cyanotic heart disease without congestive failure or pulmonary hypertension wishes to become pregnant, she should be advised of the best available statistics and allowed to make the choice. Whittemore et al[55] studied the outcome of 42 pregnancies in 22 cyanotic women. Only 23 of the 42 (55%) pregnancies resulted in a live birth and only 2% of these 23 infants were full term and of average birth weight. Among the 42 pregnancies in cyanotic mothers, only 6 (14%) had spontaneous abortion, which is not higher than the national average among all women; however, 13 had a therapeutic abortion, so some of those 13 may have had spontaneous abortions if left alone. If such were the case, then the rate would have been 19 of 42, or 45%. Among cyanotic women who had had no operation, only 42% of their pregnancies resulted in a live birth; this figure was 72% for those mothers who had had palliative surgery but remained cyanotic; in the patients whose cyanosis had been relieved by definitive repair, 78% of the pregnancies ended in a live birth and most were normal-sized babies. Despite the theoretic risk to the mother just expressed, none of the mothers had infective endocarditis, brain abscess, or stroke and there was no maternal mortality.

In 6 of the 41 infants born to cyanotic mothers, there was a cardiac defect (14.6%). The incidence of cardiac defects was no higher in the cyanotic than in the acyanotic group and was the same as that in those who had had successful surgery. Among the total of 372 infants born to 233 women with different types of congenital heart defects with and without cardiac surgery, 16% had a congenital defect. Excluding seven mothers who had a syndrome known to be associated with congenital heart disease, the incidence was 14%. The incidence of heart defect in the infants was 25% in mothers who had aortic stenosis. One half the infants with a heart defect had the same anomaly as the mother.

Physicians responsible for the care of the cyanotic patient should encourage the patient to lead a life that is as normal as possible. Although many believe that pregnancy should be discouraged, marriage should be encouraged, providing both partners understand the limitation that heart disease might impose.

Birth control pills are contraindicated in cyanotic, polycythemic patients because they predispose to leg vein thrombosis and to the development of pulmonary emboli. Likewise, birth control pills in any patient with systemic hypertension should be avoided. The intrauterine device for birth control may cause infection, increasing the chance of infective endocarditis. The diaphragm, with spermicidal jelly, is the best accepted device for many couples. Tubal ligation has been used with success. The risk of surgery has been low and it has been performed without general anesthesia.

Insurability

Most of the large, reputable life insurance companies have become sophisticated and up to date in their view of the patient with congenital heart disease, including postoperative congenital heart disease. Patients often are discouraged by their company's insurance representative or by a local insurance agent from applying for life insurance if the individual has had heart surgery. Some insurance companies' medical departments are inadequately informed or misinformed about the outlook for the patient with postoperative or benign unoperated congenital heart disease. It often happens that the patient and family have just been told by the pediatric or adult cardiologist that all is well after surgery, only to then be devastated by a letter from the life insurance company denying the patient's application for coverage.

Today, in well-informed companies, once the patient has fully recovered from definitive (not palliative) surgery and is free of important complications from the operation, life insurance can be obtained with either no or only a slight increase in premium. This includes postoperative patients with defects that can be cured (eg, secundum ASD and PDA without pulmonary hypertension) or virtually cured (eg, VSDs with pulmonary hypertension). In some anomalies in which clinical and noninvasive evaluation may not reveal the current state of the hemodynamic condition, postoperative heart catheterization may help to guide the insurance office. If the heart is enlarged, intracavitary pressures are abnormal, or septal defects persist, even if mild in degree, then the premium may be increased. It is helpful for the physician who knows and understands the patient's hemodynamic condition to write a special letter to the insurance company, adding information about the exercise stress test and other data that would help to define the patient's low risk.

Prevention of Infective Endocarditis

A major preventable complication in patients with congenital heart disease, whether benign or serious, is infective endocarditis. Some defects are said to have a low risk for infective endocarditis, such as ASD and pulmonary valve stenosis. Although the risk is low, infective endocarditis has been reported in both of these anomalies,[57] so many physicians, including the authors, give antibiotic prophylaxis. However, the recent American Heart Association recommendations exclude secundum ASD from the need for prophylaxis against infective endocarditis.[58] On the other hand, other defects, including VSD, PDA, mitral valve regurgitation, and bicuspid aortic valve, have a high risk of infective endocarditis.

In some rare anomalies we have little information about the tendency of the patients to develop infective endocarditis. Likewise, there is uncertainty about the need for prophylaxis against infective endocarditis for lesions such as the benign form of isolated mitral valve prolapse with only a midsystolic click. Patients with the mitral regurgitation murmur associated with mitral leaflet prolapse clearly need protection against infective endocarditis. When in doubt, it is better to use penicillin prophylaxis in all patients with cardiovascular anomalies who undergo a surgical procedure or dental manipulation in which bacteremia is possible.

Now that oral penicillin prophylaxis is of proven value compared with intramuscular route, many objections to the routine use of penicillin have disappeared. Many patients and a few physicians and dentists are a little confused about the development of resistance by individuals to penicillin. To increase patient compliance for antibiotic prophylaxis, physicians should emphasize that only certain organisms (alpha streptococcus, not beta streptococcus) become resistant to penicillin rather than the individual who is receiving the drug. It takes about three days of therapeutic penicillin to develop a resistant strain and another two to three days for the mouth to acquire a new colony of "healthy" (nonpenicillin-resistant) alpha streptococci. Therefore, patients and dentists can use this information to guide therapy if they are unable to locate an American Heart Association schedule that outlines antibiotic prophylaxis for all dental and certain surgical procedures and manipulation.[58]

Because the etiologic factor in a large number of patients with infective endocarditis is asymptomatic gum or root disease, regular twice-yearly meticulous dental examination is highly important in infective endocarditis prevention. Dental check-ups usually include cleaning the teeth; thus, penicillin prophylaxis is needed at that time. For many years physicians have warned the patient to make sure that penicillin prophylaxis is taken before dental procedures, but we have failed to urge the patient to make sure that dental examinations are performed regularly twice a year! Recent information from the American Heart Association[58] indicates that the first dose of penicillin-V should be given only 30 to 60 minutes before the actual procedure commences. The adult patient takes 2 g orally of penicillin-V and subsequently 1 g six hours later. For intramuscular use, give aqueous penicillin-G 2 million units 30 to 60 minutes before and 1 million units six hours later. Allergy to penicillin is not so common as once thought, but, if present, an antibiotic such as erythromycin or cephalosporin should be substituted. Tetracycline is not protective, nor is sulfadiazine. Some physicians like to select their own favorite antibiotic for their allergic patients in place of penicillin, but it is better to adhere to the recommendations of the American Heart Association[58] committee, which has studied this matter in great detail and has obtained the best expert opinions.

The functionally important anomalies that are at high risk for infective endocarditis include postoperative patients with an artificial valve, any conduits, or patches. In addition, the cyanotic lesion with a functioning systemic-to-pulmonary artery anastomosis places the patient at high risk for infective endocarditis. Also, despite successful definitive repair of some defects, prophylaxis is continued for a lifetime. Exceptions may be 6 months or longer after surgically corrected PDA, ASD, and total anomalous pulmonary venous return in which no persistent additional defect can be identified.[59] However, in the first 6 months after any type of heart surgery, prophylaxis is continued if a dental or another type of bacteremia-associated procedure is performed. The American

Heart Association[58] recommends no antibiotic prophylaxis for patients who have had coronary artery bypass surgery.

SUMMARY

Congenital heart defects are just recently beginning to receive the attention from internal medicine diagnostic and treatment centers for cardiovascular disease in the adult patient. Once internists and cardiologists are faced with the increasing numbers of challenging and intellectually stimulating problems brought up by these patients, appropriate attention will surely result. This ideally would include adding pediatric and congenital heart diseases to the adult cardiology training program curriculum. In the meantime, the care of the adult patient with congenital heart disease will likely continue to be the province of the pediatric cardiologist.

The need for overall encouragement and psychic support is especially important in the adult patient who may have been under almost continuous cardiac care since early infancy. The great majority (80% to 90%) of patients with congenital heart disease can now be helped and can be expected to reach adult life as a productive individual with normal intellect and capable of most vocational, social, and recreational activities. These patients can usually plan to marry, have a family, and look forward to an active life. Postoperative congenital heart disease is going to be three times more common than unoperated congenital heart disease. Some persons who have had surgery are virtually cured; others, who have been helped but not cured, still are able to live a relatively normal, if not physically active, life. Some patients who have incomplete repair or a poor result are going to require close cardiac care for their lifetimes.

REFERENCES

1. Muller WH, Dammann JF: The treatment of certain congenital malformations of the heart by the creation of pulmonary stenosis to reduce pulmonary hypertension and excessive blood flow. *Surg Gynecol Obstet* 1952; 95:213–216.
2. White BD, McNamara DG, Bauersfeld SR, Taussig HB: Five year postoperative results of first 500 patients with Blalock–Taussig anastomosis for pulmonary stenosis or pulmonary atresia. *Circulation* 1956; 14:512–520.
3. Norwood WI, Lang P, Castaneda AR, Campbell DN: Experience with operations for hypoplastic left heart syndrome. *J Thorac Cardiovasc Surg* 1981; 82:511–519.
4. Seldon WA, Rubinstein C, Fraser AA: The incidence of atrial septal defect in adults. *Br Heart J* 1962; 24:557–560.
5. Kohler CM, McNamara DG: Elongated patent ductus arteriosus with intermittent shunting. *Pediatrics* 1967; 37:446–448.
6. Bashour T, Kabbani S, Saalouke M, Cheng TO: Persistent Eustachian valve causing severe cyanosis in atrial septal defect with normal right heart pressures. *Angiology* 1983; 34:79–83.
7. Cheng TO: Paradoxical embolism. A diagnostic challenge and its detection during life. *Circulation* 1976; 53:565–568.
8. Raghib G, Ruttenberg HD, Anderson RC, Amplatz K, Adams P, Edwards JE: Termination of left superior vena cava in left atrium, atrial septal defect, and absence of coronary sinus. A developmental complex. *Circulation* 1965; 31:906–918.
9. Park H, Summerer MH, Preuss K, Armstrong WF, Mahomed Y, Hamilton DJ: Anomalous drainage of the right superior vena cava into the left atrium. *J Am Coll Cardiol* 1983; 2:358–362.
10. Hauser AM, Timmis GC, Stewart JR, Ramos RG, Gangadharan V, Westveer DC, Gordon S: Aneurysm of the atrial septum as diagnosed by echocardiography: analysis of 11 patients. *Am J Cardiol* 1984; 53:1401–1402.
11. Wysham DG, McPherson DD, Kerber RE: Asymptomatic aneurysm of the atrial septum. *J Am Coll Cardiol* 1984; 4:1311–1314.
12. Eldredge WJ, Tingelstad JB, Robertson LW, Mauck HP, McCue CM: Observations on the natural history of pulmonary artery coarctation. *Circulation* 1972; 45:404-409.
13. Garcia R, Taber RE: Bacterial endocarditis of the pulmonic valve. *Am J Cardiol* 1966; 18:275–280.
14. Nelson WP, Hall RJ, Garcia E: Varicosities of the pulmonary veins simulating arteriovenous fistulas. *JAMA* 1966; 195:13–17.
15. Platkzer J, Goldhammer E, Simon J, Abinader E: Pulmonary varices, benign congenital anomalies simulating perihilar masses of various etiologies. *Clin Cardiol* 1984; 7:295–298.
16. Hickey AJ, MacMahan SW, Wilcken DEL: Mitral valve prolapse and bacterial endocarditis: When is antibiotic prophylaxis necessary? *Am Heart J* 1985; 109:431–435.
17. Perry LW, Ruckman RN, Shapiro SR, Kuehl KS, Galioto FM, Scott LP: Left ventricular false tendons in children. *Am J Cardiol* 1983; 52:1264–1266.
18. Roberts WC: The structure of the aortic valve in clinically isolated aortic stenosis: an autopsy study of 162 patients over 15 years of age. *Circulation* 1970; 42:91–97.
19. Folger GM, Stein PD: Bicuspid aortic valve morphology when associated with coarctation of the aorta. *Cathet Cardiovasc Diag* 1984; 10:17–25.
20. Roberts WC: The congenitally bicuspid aortic valve: a study of 85 autopsied patients. *Am J Cardiol* 1970; 26:72–79.
21. Hurwitz LE: Quadricuspid semilunar valve. *Am J Cardiol* 1973; 31:623-626.
22. Chandrasekaran K, Tajik AJ, Edwards WD, Seward JB: Two-dimensional echocardiographic diagnosis of quadricuspid aortic valve. *Am J Cardiol* 1984; 53:1732–1733.
23. Hurwitz RA, Smith W, King H, Girod DA, Caldwell RL: Tetralogy of Fallot with abnormal coronary artery: 1967 to 1977. *J Thorac Cardiovasc Surg* 1980; 80:129–134.
24. Moodie DS, Gill C, Loop FD, Sheldon WC: Anomalous left main coronary artery originating from the right sinus of Valsalva. Pathophysiology, angiographic definition, and surgical approaches. *J Thorac Cardiovasc Surg* 1980; 80:198–205.
25. Soto B, Shin MS, Papapietro SE: Nonobstructive coarctation. *Cardiovasc Radiol* 1979; 2:231–237.
26. Nizankowski C, Rajchel Z, Ziolkowski M: Abnormal origin of arteries from the aortic arch in man. *Folia Morphol* 1975; 34:109–116.
27. McDowell DE, Grant MA, Gustafson RA: Single arterial trunk arising from the aortic arch. *Circulation* 1979; 62:181–182.
28. Barron MG: Right aortic arch. *Circulation* 1971; 44:1137–1145.
29. Mullins CE, Gillette PC, McNamara DG: The complex of cervical aortic arch. *Pediatrics* 1973; 51:210–215.
30. El-Said G, Galioto FM Jr, Williams RL, McNamara DG: Spontaneous functional closure of isolated atrial septal defect. *Am J Dis Child* 1971; 122:353–355.
31. Hoffman JIE: Natural history of congenital heart disease. Problems in its assessment with special reference to ventricular septal defects. *Circulation* 1968; 37:97–125.
32. El-Said G, Galioto FM Jr, Mullins CE, McNamara DG: The natural hemodynamic history of congenital aortic stenosis in childhood. *Am J Cardiol* 1972; 30:6–12.
33. Friedman WF, Modlinger J, Morgan JR: Serial hemodynamic observations in asymptomatic children with valvar aortic stenosis. *Circulation* 1971; 43:91–97.
34. Karpawich PP, Duff DF, Mullins CE, Cooley DA, McNamara DG: Ventricular septal defect with associated aortic valve insufficiency. Progression of insufficiency and operative results in young children. *J Thorac Cardiovasc Surg* 1981; 82:182–189.
35. Heath D, Edwards JE: The pathology of hypertensive pulmonary vascular disease. *Circulation* 1958; 10:533–542.
36. Nihill MR, McNamara DG: Magnification pulmonary wedge angiography in the evaluation of congenital heart disease and pulmonary hypertension. *Circulation* 1978; 58:1094–1106.
37. Driscoll DJ, Hesslein PS, Mullins CE: Congenital stenosis of individual pulmonary veins: clinical spectrum and unsuccessful treatment by transvenous balloon dilation. *Am J Cardiol* 1982; 49:1767–1772.
38. Taussig HB, Crocetti A, Eshaghpour E, Keinonen R, Yap KN, Bachman D, Momberger N, Kirk H: Long-time observations on the Blalock–Taussig operation. I. Results of first operation. *Johns Hopkins Med J* 1971; 129:243–259.
39. Lindesmith GG, Stiles QR, Tucker BL, Gallaher ME, Stanton RE, Meyer BW: The Mustard operation as a palliative procedure. *J Thorac Cardiovasc Surg* 1972; 63:75–85.
40. Mustard WT: Successful two-stage correction of transposition of the great vessels. *Surgery* 1964; 55:469–472.
41. Senning A: Surgical correction of transposition of the great vessels. *Surgery* 1959; 45:966–980.

42. Rashkind WJ, Miller WW: Creation of an atrial septal defect without thoracotomy: a palliative approach to complete transposition of the great vessels. *JAMA* 1966; 196:991–992.
43. Park SC, Neches WH, Mullins CE, Girod DA, Olley PM, Falkowski G, Garibjan VA, Matthews RA, Fricker FJ, Beerman LB, Lenox CC, Zuberbuhler JR: Blade atrial septostomy: collaborative study. *Circulation* 1982; 66:258–266.
44. Mullins CE: Transseptal left heart catheterization: Experience with a new technique in 520 pediatric and adult patients. *Pediatr Cardiol* 1983; 4:239–246.
45. Morriss JH, McNamara DG: Residuae, sequelae and complications of surgery for congenital heart disease. *Prog Cardiovasc Dis* 1975; 18:1–25.
46. Gillette PC, El-Said GM, Sivarajan N, Mullins CE, Williams RL, McNamara DG: Electrophysiologic abnormalities after Mustard's operation for transposition of the great arteries. *Br Heart J* 1974; 36:186–191.
47. Ruzyllo W, Nihill MR, Mullins CE, McNamara DG: Hemodynamic evaluation of 221 patients after intracardiac repair of tetralogy of Fallot. *Am J Cardiol* 1974; 34:565–576.
48. Clayman JA, Ankeney JL, Liebman J: Results of complete repair of tetralogy of Fallot in 156 consecutive patients. *Am J Surg* 1975; 130:601–612.
49. Garson A Jr, McNamara DG, Cooley DA: Tetralogy of Fallot in adults, in Roberts WC (ed): *Congenital Heart Disease in Adults, Cardiovascular Clinics.* Philadelphia, FA Davis Co, 1979, pp 341–364.
50. Garson A Jr, McNamara DG: Postoperative tetralogy of Fallot, in Engle MA, Brest AN (eds): *Pediatric Cardiovascular Disease, Cardiovascular Clinics.* Philadelphia, FA Davis Co, 1981, pp 407–429.
51. Von Bermuth G, Ritter DG, Frye RL: Evaluation of patients with tetralogy of Fallot and Potts anastomosis. *Am J Cardiol* 1971; 27:259–264.
52. Kan JS, White RI, Mitchell SE, Garoner TJ: Percutaneous balloon valvuloplasty: a new method for treating congenital pulmonary valve stenosis. *N Engl J Med* 1982; 370:540–543.
53. Lock JE, Niemi T, Burke BA, Einzig S, Castaneda-Zuniga W: Transcutaneous angioplasty of experimental aortic coarctation. *Circulation* 1982; 66:1280–1286.
54. Rashkind WJ, Cuaso CC: Transcatheter closure of patent ductus arteriosus: successful use in a 3.5 kilogram infant. *Pediatric Cardiol* 1979; 1:3–8.
55. Whittemore R, Hobbins JC, Engle MA: Pregnancy and its outcome in women with and without surgical treatment of congenital heart disease. *Am J Cardiol* 1982; 50:641–651.
56. Nora JJ, Dodd PF, McNamara DG, Hattwick MAW, Leachman RD, Cooley DA: Risk to offspring of parents with congenital heart defects. *JAMA* 1969; 209:2052–2054.
57. Casling RS, Rogler WC, McManus R: Isolated pulmonic valve infective endocarditis: a diagnostically elusive entity. *Am Heart J* 1985; 109:558–567.
58. Shulman ST, Amren DP, Bisno AL, Dajani AS, Durack DT, Gerber MA, Kaplan EL, Millard HD, Sanders WE, Schwartz RH, Watanakunakorn C: Prevention of bacterial endocarditis. *Am J Dis Child* 1985; 139:232–235. The identical article by the same authors was also published in *Circulation* 1984; 70:1123A–1127A.
59. Chadwick EG, Shulman ST: Prevention of infective endocarditis. *Mod Concepts Cardiovasc Dis* 1986; 55:11–15.

28 Genetics and the Cardiovascular System

James J. Nora, MD, MPH

Almost all cardiovascular diseases have an important genetic component.[1] Although congenital heart disease (CHD) has been designated as the major topic of this presentation, it is useful first to place CHD within the perspective of the four major categories of cardiovascular disease. Figure 28.1 is a device we have used and frequently modified to provide a current overview of where the various etiologic categories fit in the continuum between the poles of heredity and environment. Visualize the genetic-environmental interaction and consider that in the United States, for example, there have been moderate to significant changes in risk factors during the past decade, hence the need to revise this figure.

For coronary heart disease, the attack on environmental risk factors has been substantial, leaving the genetic contribution in a more prominent position, whereas for congenital heart disease, environmental risk factors are becoming increasingly recognized. Therefore, Figure 28.1 shows congenital heart disease stretching closer to the pole of environment. Essential hypertension appears to have a relatively stronger genetic component in the United States, although the experience in Japan may be different. Finally, rheumatic fever, as important as the genetic contribution is, still requires a group A beta-hemolytic streptococcal infection to become manifest. Thus, rheumatic fever extends all the way to the right to touch the pole of environment.

WHAT SPECIFICALLY CAUSES CONGENITAL HEART DISEASES?

The percentage of cases in our series, best explained by one etiologic mode versus another, has varied slightly over the years. By way of illustration, our congenital heart clinic population of rubella-caused defects was considerably higher in the 1950s and 1960s than it is now. Furthermore, as we learn the specific genetic basis of a disease entity of previously undetermined origin, the etiologic category to which it belongs is increased as a percentage of the whole. For example, demonstrating that Noonan's syndrome (Turner phenotype, Ullrich-Noonan syndrome) conformed to autosomal dominant inheritance almost doubled the number of patients we were seeing in our congenital heart clinic as having a mendelian disorder of any kind. Table 28.1 reveals the etiologic categories encountered in a survey at our congenital heart clinic.[2] This distribution differs from the incidence of CHD in liveborn infants (many with chromosomal anomalies) who do not survive to become part of a clinic population.[3] We will discuss this in more detail when we discuss chromosomal etiology.

MULTIFACTORIAL INHERITANCE AND CONGENITAL HEART DISEASE

As Table 28.1 illustrates, multifactorial inheritance is the most common etiologic category in CHD.[4] Essential components of cardiovascular maldevelopment include: (1) a genetic predisposition to react adversely to one or more environmental triggers; (2) a genetic predisposition to one or more forms of maldevelopment; and (3) exposure to an environmental influence at a vulnerable period of embryogenesis.

Figure 28.2 appears in essentially all of our presentations on the genetics of cardiovascular diseases, and it unavoidably must be discussed here, because it reveals the central concepts of the multifactorial inheritance of congenital heart defects. The curves and thresholds in

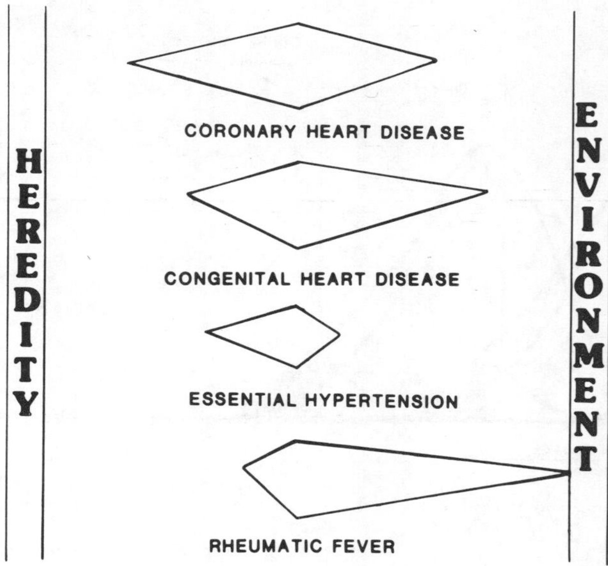

Figure 28.1. The interaction of heredity and environment in the major categories of cardiovascular diseases.

this figure refer to genetic-environmental interactions within families. In the typical low risk (type B) family, the threshold of malformation may be crossed by a symmetrical curve of polygenic predisposition or by a slightly skewed curve (dashed line) in which there are families with mendelian risks (hatched area). In the type C high risk family, the curve of predisposition moves to the right. It is absolutely necessary to recognize that the risks in a given family must be specifically identified as high or low on the basis of the individual pedigree.[5] We cannot simply rely on a general idea of how much increase in risk is to be expected.

At the far left is the curve of the type A family, which suggests the concept that there are families whose curves of genetic predisposition lie so far to the left that it is most unlikely that the thresholds of malformation may be pushed far enough to the left by environmental factors to produce cardiac maldevelopment, even under the influence of the most hazardous teratogens. The curve to the far right (the type C family) suggests that the severe polygenic predisposition (and the rare mutant genes) requires little or no environmental interaction to produce congenital cardiovascular anomalies in a limited number of families. The addition of environmental factors pushes the threshold to the left and greatly increases the risk in type C families with a polygenic predisposition. To repeat, it is critical in counseling to recognize the high risk families.

Table 28.1. Etiologic Categories of Congenital Heart Disease in a Pediatric Cardiology Clinic

Genetic–environmental interaction (multifactorial inheritance)	90%
Primary genetic factors	
Chromosomal	5%
Single mutant gene	3%

However, it is the curve in the middle, the type B family, that represents the great majority of families who have congenital heart disease in a proband and a moderate increase in risk of subsequent congenital heart disease in the family. The specific recurrence risks in relatives of affected probands will be detailed in a subsequent section. What is important in all models of multifactorial inheritance is the relation of the threshold to the curve.

Genetic predisposition to environmental influences is where there is a great deal of activity in our growing knowledge of genetic predisposition to maldevelopment of any kind. It is now becoming possible to move from population level concepts of genetic predisposition to the cellular level and to the biochemical nature of genetic predisposition relating to environmental teratogens (mutagens and carcinogens). One such example that has important implications for congenital heart disease is the work of Nebert and Bigelow.[6] The mechanism for the clearance of many drugs and chemicals involves cytosolic receptors, phase I oxidative enzymes (of which cytochrome P-450 is a prototype), reactive intermediates, and phase II conjugating enzymes. When a chemical enters the body, it has to be eliminated. Take, for example, hydrocarbons, such as benzopyrene or exogenous steroid hormones. These chemicals circulate in the body, enter individual cells, and have the potential of participating in biochemical functions. There is a dynamic body chemistry for chemicals as well as nutrients, in which there is a transformation-utilization-excretion cycle.

If there is a genetic abnormality or breakdown in the cycle and chemicals that should be excreted accumulate, damage results. An aromatic hydrocarbon entering a cell forms a complex with a cytosolic receptor. This complex activates gene loci to induce cytochrome P-450, which metabolizes the chemical to the point at which it becomes a reactive intermediate, such as a toxic epoxide, which can produce cellular damage running the spectrum from carcinogenesis and mutagenesis to teratogenesis. The urgent need of the cell to maintain its integrity is met in most cases by a further step using phase II enzymes to render the chemical product biologically harmless to the host and to lead to its excretion.

Certain strains of mice (and human families) respond vigorously to the message initiated by the hydrocarbon-receptor complex to manufacture phase I enzymes to handle the chemical exposure. The strains of mice that respond vigorously are appropriately called responders. They possess a responsive form of the gene. Other strains do not respond by making large amounts of enzyme to handle the sudden influx of chemical and are therefore termed genetic nonresponders. The ability to respond is transmitted following mendelian laws. Parents may transmit the trait of responsiveness or nonresponsiveness to their offspring. To illustrate, a nonresponsive mother carrying a responsive fetus is exposed to a load of aromatic hydrocarbons. What should be the outcome? Certainly it appears useful for the organism to be able to biotransform in a rapid and efficient manner chemicals in preparation for excretion. Unfortunately, the responsiveness that helps an adult cope with chemicals in the environment may not be useful for a developing fetus that may only

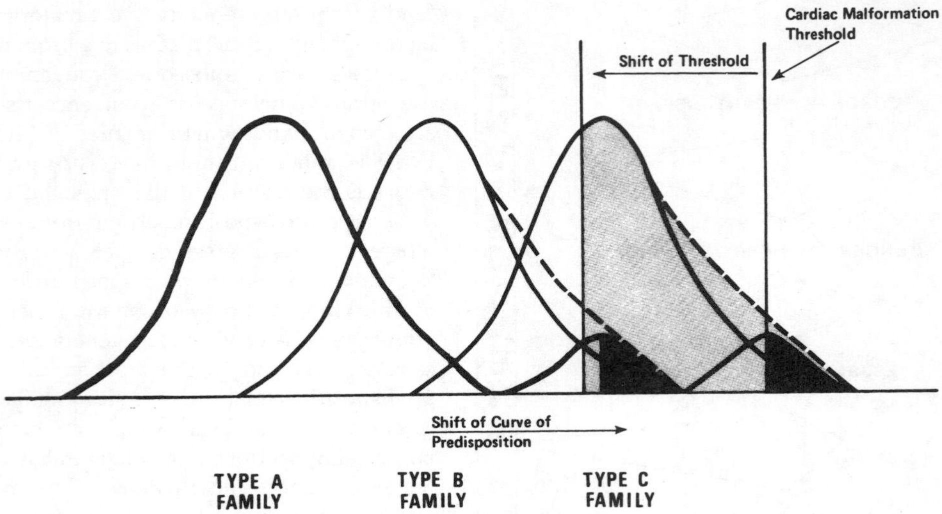

Figure 28.2. The concept of curves of genetic predisposition and environmental influence on the threshold of cardiac malformation. (See text.) (Figures 28.2–28.9 are from Nora JJ, Fraser FC: *Medical Genetics: Principles and Practice,* ed 2. Philadelphia, Lea & Febiger, 1981, and are used with permission.)

be efficient in carrying the biotransformation through phase I, but then may be unable to proceed promptly enough through its immature systems (eg, glutathione limiting) to the second phase of detoxifying the reactive intermediates.

Here in the reactive intermediates lies an important potential for cellular damage. Intuitively, the body is not likely to have the capacity to create an entirely new receptor to handle each new chemical that enters the environment. Pharmaceutical companies may make small changes in a basic chemical structure for various reasons and thus own the new variant. However, the body is not required to develop entirely new biotransformation systems to take care of each new synthetic chemical variant if the cytosolic receptors are multipotential and capable of handling related chemicals as if they were identical. There is an irony in all of this, however: the genetic traits that help an adult escape chemical poisoning may predispose a developing fetus to birth defects, such as cardiovascular malformations.[7]

From the brief exploration of one small portion of genetic predisposition (in this case one involving a major gene and a threshold), it should be clear how essential is the interaction between heredity and environment in maldevelopment. There are, of course, many mechanisms of teratogenesis, which exceed the scope of this presentation. A necessary understanding in the context of what is being presented in this section is that in the early stages of development, morphogenesis is progressing so rapidly that a minor environmental stimulus can produce major maldevelopment.

The second essential component of cardiovascular maldevelopment is that congenital heart diseases as a general category of anomalies run in families and specific heart defects cluster in families. For example, 30% to 60% of affected sibs of patients with ventricular septal defect (VSD) also have VSD.[8] This is similar to what we found in C57BL/6J mice subjected to maternal exposure to dextroamphetamines on day 8 of gestation.[9] In this study, 61% of offspring examined histologically had VSD. Conversely, 39% had other cardiovascular lesions of other types. Fraser[8] in a sizable series reported developmentally related anomalies recurring in families. If 30% to 60% of affected sibs of probands with VSD also have VSD, it means that 40% to 70% have a different heart lesion. Why should this be? We cannot be sure in a single case what the core lesion that is "running in the family" really is. The same teratogenic exposure at day 27 of gestation may be capable of producing tetralogy of Fallot, on day 36 it could cause VSD, and on day 45 produce an atrial septal defect, all on the basis of the same genetic predisposition and environmental interactions. If we encounter a family having tetralogy of Fallot and VSD, we would regard the VSD as a forme fruste of the tetralogy. Our assumption is that heart lesions in first degree relatives are more likely to be related to the same developmental abnormalities rather than to different ones. Clusters of related anomalies in families appear to support this assumption. A familial recurrence of a heart lesion that apparently bears no developmental relation to a previously encountered defect may indeed be unrelated, or it may be a manifestation of a common mechanism of maldevelopment that is obscure to the observer.

Finally, exposure at a vulnerable period of embryogenesis is the third critical component in the process of maldevelopment. This is the area in which we would predict that the earliest significant impact in prevention of congenital heart diseases should take place. Starting with the assumption that a genetic predisposition is acted upon by environmental triggers to produce malformations, a logical strategy would be to identify environmental factors that represent a high risk either to individuals or to the population because of widespread use, even if the individual risk is low.

Examples to illustrate these points are as follows. For rubella[10] and thalidomide,[11] both the individual risks and the population risks were high, because the rate of malformation following exposures at vulnerable periods of embryogenesis was of the order of 50%, and the rate of exposure in many countries was so high as to produce a large number of cases. For a drug such as lithium carbonate,[12] the risk to the individual is high, but the risk to the population is relatively low, because the use of this drug is now generally restricted to patients with manic-depressive psychoses. Conversely, female sex steroids carry with them a small individual risk, but because of the large number of exposures during early pregnancy, the risk to the population may be exceedingly high.[13]

Table 28.2 is derived from several sources including our own studies, but it is particularly indebted to the pioneering work of Lenz.[11] Limits will vary with the teratogenic agent. For example, thalidomide appears to act within a narrower range than does rubella virus. We also know that although the usual time for spontaneous closure of the ventricular septum is 44 days of conceptional age, spontaneous closure is not uncommon in infancy and occasionally occurs later in childhood and even early adult life. Conversely, it is difficult to visualize how truncus arteriosus, transposition of the great arteries, tetralogy of Fallot, double outlet right ventricle, and other truncoconal malformations can occur after truncoconal septation is completed at 34 days of conception. Therefore, the vulnerable period for maldevelopment of these structures should be firm. A corollary of this observation would be that if a patient has a truncoconal anomaly related to a teratogen, we should look for the exposure very early in pregnancy. The treacherous aspect of this problem is that the exposure is likely to occur when the mother is not yet aware that she is pregnant.

Rubella virus has not been implicated in the production of patent ductus arteriosus in exposures later than the second trimester. However, it is theoretically possible for an environmental agent to cause persistent patency with later exposure. In fact, the ministrations (eg, intravenous fluids) that premature infants receive in intensive care nurseries illustrate how the postnatal environment may contribute to patency of the ductus. Peripheral pulmonary artery stenosis (secondary to rubella) and aortic stenosis (secondary to type IIa homozygous hyperlipoproteinemia) are examples of structural lesions that progress after birth. We would infer that certain agents could also act on semilunar or atrioventricular valves and on systemic and pulmonary arteries in later trimesters of intrauterine life. The concept of vulnerable periods is useful when applied to some structures and related to certain teratogens, but it is not inviolable. In fact, in many instances, it may be preferable to think in terms of critical events such as developmental processes that are particularly susceptible to derangement by environmental agents.

What Lenz was able to demonstrate with regard to human heart anomalies was that teratogenic exposures to thalidomide occur from five to 15 days before completion of the embryonic event. We learned that in trying to evaluate the teratogenicity of various agents in the mouse, we have to provide, for example, an exposure to dextroamphetamine three to five days before septal closure to produce VSD.[9] However, for antiheart antibody the teratogen could be given considerably later and still produce a VSD.[14] Both embryologic considerations and epidemiologic evidence support the concept that teratogenic exposure before implantation of the fertilized human ovum does not lead to malformation. If the teratogenic insult is of major proportion, viability is not maintained. Implantation and differentiation must progress to about 14 days conceptional age before maldevelopment may be produced by teratogens. The critical flaw in many studies of teratogen-related cardiac malformations is that the data are irreparably diluted by taking as the vulnerable period of cardiogenesis the entire first trimester rather than the vulnerable period (eg, the third and fourth weeks for transposition of the great arteries).

Critical decisions must be made regarding the use of drugs during pregnancy. The patient must be an informed participant in the decision-making process. Preventive options are available regarding avoidable and unavoidable drug exposures, maternal conditions, and infections. Within the limitations of this presentation, selected important maternal conditions and infections and drug exposures can only be listed (Table 28.3).

It is unlikely that there are any agents currently in our environment capable of the devastating damage of rubella or thalidomide, although the unfortunate possibility exists that another devastating drug like thalidomide could reach the public through inadequate testing procedures.

Table 28.2. Presumed Vulnerable Period for Teratogenic Influence on Cardiovascular Development

Abnormality	Embryonic Event Completed (days)	Limits of Vulnerable Period (days)	Most Sensitive Vulnerable Period (days)
Truncoconal septation	34	14–34	18–29
Endocardial cushions	38	14–38	18–33
Ventricular septum	38–44	14–?	18–39
Atrial septum secundum	55	14–?	18–50
Semilunar valves	55	14–?	18–50
Ductus arteriosus		14–?	18–60
Coarctation of aorta		14–?	18–60

Table 28.3. Selected Potential Cardiovascular (CV) Teratogens

Potential Teratogen	Frequency of CV Disease (excluding frequency of other anomalies) (%)	Most Common CV Lesion Produced by Agent
Drugs		
Alcohol	25–30	Ventricular septal defect (VSD), patent ductus arteriosus (PDA), atrial septal defect (ASD)
Amphetamines	?5–10	VSD, PDA, ASD, transposition of great arteries (TGA)
Anticonvulsants		
Hydantoin	2–3	Pulmonary stenosis (PS), aortic stenosis (AS), coarctation of aorta, PDA
Trimethadione	15–30	TGA, tetralogy, hypoplastic left heart
Lithium	10	Ebstein's anomaly, tricuspid atresia, ASD
Retinoic acid (Accutane)	5–10	VSD
Sex hormones	2–4	VSD, TGA, tetralogy
Thalidomide	5–10	Tetralogy, VSD, ASD, truncus
Infections		
Rubella	35	Peripheral pulmonary artery stenosis, PDA, VSD, ASD
Maternal conditions		
Diabetes	3–5	TGA, VSD, coarctation of aorta
Phenylketonuria	?10–25	Tetralogy, VSD, ASD
Systemic lupus	?40	Complete heart block

However, the area to concentrate on at this time would appear to be low-level teratogens. There may indeed be many agents, such as sex hormones, that may produce malformations in only a small percentage of exposures, but because of the large number of exposures, they may be responsible for more maldevelopment in the general population than a thalidomide. For example, if a cardiovascular teratogen is in such common use that there are exposures during vulnerable periods of 300,000 pregnancies per year, then a risk as small as 1% could produce 3,000 infants with congenital heart disease annually. (These are actual projections we made for hormone production of CHD in the United States in the early 1970s.)

Thalidomide and rubella are probably not truly representative of cardiovascular teratogens in general, in that they may require little genetic predisposition and are capable of causing such a high frequency of maldevelopment (in 50% exposures or more at the vulnerable period of development). There also may be many agents, which are of little consequence to the general population, but may be of grave consequence to individual families or groups with an unusual genetic predisposition. There is considerable precedence for this concept in the discipline of pharmacogenetics. The point here is that in obtaining the genetic and teratogenic history in a family with a patient having a cardiovascular anomaly, the physician should counsel avoidance of nonessential agents to which there has been documented maternal exposure during cardiogenesis in an affected offspring. As a general rule, elimination of exposure to all drugs that can be avoided during pregnancy should be encouraged. A large number of agents have been suspected because they produce malformations in animal models. However, documentation in the human is the definitive criterion that teratogens cause malformation in human subjects. Examples that illustrate the need for precise human studies are: (1) although thalidomide is catastrophic in humans, it fails to produce malformations in commonly used test animals; (2) although cortisone is a good agent to produce cleft palate in the A/J mouse, it does not appear to represent a significant risk for cleft palate in the human.

The possibility of genetic predisposition to one or more malformations should be kept in mind when looking for teratogenic explanations for congenital heart defect. What may be obscured in population studies is the value of unusual patterns or subgroups of anomalies. In the thalidomide syndrome, it was the increase in the frequency of the rare anomaly, phocomelia. A moderate increase in congenital malformations was not the tip-off on the teratogenicity of lithium; it was that the heart was disproportionately attacked and that a relatively rare defect, Ebstein's anomaly, was the lesion most often associated with lithium exposure.[13] Although it is necessary for epidemiologists to debate whether it is anticonvulsants or epilepsy itself that is teratogenic, the clinician is frequently able to distinguish differences in the pattern of anomalies for trimethadione as opposed to hydantoin or phenobarbital or both. The alert practitioner has been and will continue to be the major resource in the recognition of teratogens.

Just as hydantoin or progestogen may produce malformations in more than one simultaneously developing structure and produce a recognizable syndrome, a common teratogenic effect of these agents is seen on a single organ. If the abnormality is rare, such as Ebstein's anomaly, then the chances are greatly increased for implicating a teratogen, such as lithium. If the anomaly is common, such as VSD, the difficulty in identifying a specific environmental cause is greatly increased. Epidemiologists have often despaired that it is impossible to identify a teratogen that is very common in the environment if it produces a common malformation in only a small percentage of exposures. This is no longer a reason for despair; studies can be designed to attack this admittedly difficult problem. A simple way is to eliminate one feature of the problem by identifying rare rather than common defects (eg, Ebstein's anomaly or phocomelia), but that really avoids the issue. Path analysis should be used more widely in studies of congenital heart disease. Moreover, straightforward epidemiologic designs that set out to look for 1% or 2% increases in malformation rates related to specific common potential teratogens are not really difficult to achieve. What slow down the process of epidemiologic advancement are investigations that, because they fail to show a great increase in risk (of the degree found with thalidomide), assume that the agent under investigation is not important. A teratogen may not be "important" in a population sense if the exposure rate is only 1 in 100,000 pregnancies. However, if the rate is one in ten pregnancies, the teratogen may be extremely important, even if it is hard to identify in studies not specifically designed to discover low risk teratogens.

Etiologic considerations for 15 different cardiovascular malformations are summarized in Tables 28.4 and 28.5. Although many more abnormalities exist in anatomic and pathophysiologic classifications, these are the most commonly encountered. From an etiologic point of view there may be considerable overlap. For example, truncus arteriosus, transposition of the great arteries, and tetralogy of Fallot (and other truncoconal anomalies) are probably on a continuum. That one child in a family could have transposition and another tetralogy likely reflects small variations in the genetic-environmental interaction, particularly the time of the environmental insult. What should be stressed is that in only 11 of the 15 lesions is the recurrence risk for a first-degree relative higher than the "sporadic risk" in the general population. From a broad perspective, this statement is correct. From the point of view of specific families this statement must be made with caution. For example, we are aware of families in Mexico with unusually frequent recurrences of Ebstein's anomaly. This is why family-specific counseling must always be emphasized.[5] In these exceptional families we must entertain the possibility of extraordinary genetic or environmental factors.

Table 28.4. Recurrence Risks Given One Sib Who Has a Cardiovascular Anomaly: Personal Series and Suggested Risks Derived From Combined Data*

Anomaly	Probands	No. Affected	Combined Suggested Risk (%)
VSD	306	28/672	3
PDA	220	12/516	3
ASD	172	11/380	2.5
Tetralogy	180	11/366	2.5
PS	166	10/375	2
Coarctation	131	5/281	2
AS	155	8/361	2
Transposition	116	4/229	2
ECD	73	4/151	2
EFE	119	11/286	4
Tricuspid atresia	52	1/98	1
Ebstein's anomaly	47	1/105	1
Truncus	43	1/86	1
Pulmonary atresia	36	1/80	1
Hypoplastic left heart	164	8/370	2

* Adapted from Nora and Nora.[1]

AS = aortic stenosis; ASD = atrial septal defect; ECD = endocardial cushion defect; EFE = endocardial fibroelastosis; PDA = patent ductus arteriosus; PS = pulmonic stenosis; VSD = ventricular septal defect.

Table 28.5. Affected Offspring: Given One Parent with a Congenital Heart Defect*

Anomaly	Personal and Combined Data: Number	Suggested Risk (%)
VSD	7/174	4
PDA	6/139	4
ASD	5/199	2.5
Tetralogy	6/141	4
PS	4/111	3.5
Coarctation	7/253	2
AS	4/103	4

* Adapted from Nora and Nora.[1]

AS = aortic stenosis; ASD = atrial septal defect; PDA = patent ductus arteriosus; PS = pulmonic stenosis, VSD = ventricular septal defect.

At this stage of our knowledge, genetic counseling is one of the more useful methods for preventing congenital heart disease. Four basic concepts for specific levels of risk within the mode of multifactorial inheritance should be kept in mind.

First, the more common the lesion, the more likely it is to recur in first-degree relatives. This is consistent with, and is predicted by, various models of multifactorial inheritance. The risk of ventricular septal defect recurring in a family should be much greater than the risk of tricuspid atresia (Table 28.4).

Second, if two first-degree relatives are affected, the recurrence risk for the next child becomes two to three times as great. If there are three affected first-degree relatives, the recurrence risk is greatly increased. These are the type C families illustrated in Figure 28.2. We counsel that the recurrence risk is likely to be what has already been experienced in the family.

Third, the risk is slightly higher for recurrence if it is a parent who has the defect rather than a sibling (Table 28.5).

Fourth, for lesions such as VSD for which there is evidence that 30% to 75% close spontaneously, it is possible that there has been spontaneous closure in presumably normal parents of affected children. Moreover, we have some historical evidence of "disappearing murmurs" in such parents. To illustrate, in multifactorial inheritance, for a heart defect with 80% heritability and a population frequency of 0.1%, if there are two affected parents, the risk of having an affected child exceeds 60%. These are initially covert type C families.

Putting these observations together, if a family has one child with a heart defect that has an empiric risk of 3%, we would propose 3% as the recurrence risk for the next child. If they have had two children with the same or a related heart defect, we would suggest a recurrence risk of the order of 10%. If they have had three children with apparently related heart defects, we have no way of assuring them that the high risk they have been experiencing will not continue. We would also look carefully for present or historical evidence of congenital heart disease in both parents, stigmas of autosomal dominant syndromes, and unusual environmental factors.

CHROMOSOMAL CAUSES OF CONGENITAL HEART DISEASE

The second most common cause of congenital heart disease after multifactorial inheritance is chromosomal abnormality. Approximately 5% of the patients in our pediatric cardiology clinic have a chromosomal anomaly. In a newborn population, as high as 10% of patients with congenital heart disease have chromosomal problems. The high mortality rates in chromosomal syndromes in the first weeks and months of life account for this difference in prevalence.

Before the chromosomal anomaly was recognized in certain common clinical syndromes, such as Down's syndrome and Turner's syndrome, it was appreciated that an important feature was congenital heart disease. When a discovery as important as the method for clinical study of the human chromosomes became available to investigators, there was a flurry of activity to explore the limits of the new methodology. After some of the common syndromes were defined, it was thought that nonsyndromic, discrete cardiac malformations might also be found in association with gross chromosomal aberrations. This was not to be the case. However, the newer banding techniques have not been fully exploited in this connection. Although it is unlikely that such an association (in the absence of other abnormalities) will be disclosed, the possibility has not been entirely excluded.

Chromosomal syndromes caused by small deletions and partial trisomies have proliferated at a rapid rate during the past decade because of banding techniques, which represent another major advance in karyotyping. The uncommon syndromes are still inadequately described from a cardiovascular point of view, and the cardiovascular problems in the common syndromes are so well known that we must reach a compromise concerning the selection of information to be presented. The first point is that at this stage of our knowledge, when we think of a chromosomal disorder in the origin of a congenital heart lesion, we should think of a syndrome. There should clearly be other manifestations of maldevelopment. If it is a common syndrome, the clinician should recognize it, be able to name it, and be prepared to find the cardiovascular abnormalities most often reported. If it is uncommon, but the pattern of anomalies points to a chromosomal disorder, then a karyotype will be required. For counseling, direct familial transmission of chromosomal anomalies producing congenital heart defects (plus other syndromic features) is relatively rare. However, isochromosomes, translocations, ring chromosomes, and structural abnormalities will be accompanied by variable increases in familial recurrence risk. It is understood that counseling must relate to the karyotype, so we will not repeat for each chromosomal anomaly that there is increased risk in the presence of translocation, etc.

That familial recurrence is uncommon does not negate the value in clinical genetics of diagnosing correctly chromosomal syndromes with associated congenital cardiovascular diseases. The more a physician knows about what his patient has (or is likely to have), the more effective will be his management, including that aspect of the art of medicine that Hippocrates valued the highest: prognosis. It is also imperative to have a sound clinical and laboratory basis for presenting the best approximation of recurrence risk and options for prevention. We have now reached the point at which prenatal diagnosis, including amniocentesis and ultrasound, may be used to reduce the frequency of occurrence of chromosomal syndromes and their associated cardiac anomalies. Table 28.6 summarizes the occurrence of cardiovascular disease in chromosomal disorders responsible for the great majority of causes of such association. The frequency of associated heart disease ranges from as high as 99+% in 18 trisomy to a minimal, if any, increase in Klinefelter's syndrome. The three defects found most often in each syndrome are listed in order, if this is known. It will be appreciated that the cardiovascular abnormalities most frequently found in the general population are usually the most common in the autosomal anomalies as well. Aberrations of the X chromosome, however, are accompanied by a malformation more commonly found in males in a syndrome that has an absent X chromosome (Turner's syndrome), and a malformation more common to females when there is an excess of X chromosomes, as found in the XXXXY syndrome.

Table 28.6. Congenital Heart Diseases in Selected Chromosomal Aberrations

Population Studied	Incidence of CHD (%)	Most Common Lesions 1	2	3
General population	1	VSD	PDA	ASD
21 trisomy	50	ECD	VSD	ASD
18 trisomy	99+	VSD	PDA	PS
13 trisomy	90	VSD	PDA	Dex
22 trisomy	67	ASD	VSD	PDA
22 partial trisomy complex	40	TAPVR	VSD	ASD
4p-	40	ASD	VSD	PDA
5p- (cri-du-chat)	20	VSD	PDA	ASD
8 trisomy (mosaic)	50	VSD	ASD	PDA
9 trisomy (mosaic)	50	VSD	Coarc	DORV
13q-	25	VSD	...	...
+14q-	50	PDA	ASD	Tet
18q-	50	VSD	...	...
XO Turner	35	Coarc	AS	ASD
XXXXY	15	PDA	ASD	ARCA

ARCA = anomalous right coronary artery; ASD = atrial septal defect; Dex = dextroversion; DORV = double outlet right ventricle; ECD = endocardial cushion defect; PDA = patent ductus arteriosus; TAPVR = total anomalous pulmonary venous return; VSD = ventricular septal defect.

A detailed discussion of all of the clinical features of the chromosomal syndromes is not within the purview of this presentation. Rather we will offer only a brief description of general diagnostic features and a review of the cardiovascular aspects. In some instances, our conclusions regarding frequency rates, most common lesions, and other details may conflict slightly with information found in the references we have cited. These discrepancies reflect the addition of some of our experience (which has not previously been published) and the disagreements among various published reports.

AUTOSOMAL ANOMALIES

21 TRISOMY (DOWN'S SYNDROME)

Of all autosomal abnormalities, Down's syndrome is the most common and has a population frequency of about 1:1,000. The general clinical features are summarized in Table 28.7 and are apparent in the photograph in Figure 28.3. About 50% of patients with Down's syndrome have a congenital heart anomaly, which is a major determinant of survival. However, the disagreement is more apparent than real (complete AV canal and VSD are approximately equal in frequency). Most cardiologists believe that the characteristic cardiovascular lesion of Down's syndrome is the complete AV canal. This is certainly the lesion that causes the greatest trouble clinically and is recognized earliest in the critically ill patient with 21 trisomy.

Other common lesions are atrial septal defect (ASD), primum and secundum, patent ductus arteriosus (PDA), isolated or associated with AV canal or VSD, and tetralogy of Fallot. The real discrepancies between the cardiovascular abnormalities in Down's syndrome as opposed to the general population are the great overrepresentation of complete and incomplete endocardial cushion defects and apparent underrepresentation of transposition of the great vessels.

Table 28.7. Clinical Features of Trisomy 21

General	Equal sex distribution; variable lengths of survival
Neurologic	Hypotonic, psychomotor retardation
Head	Characteristic facies: patients look more like other patients with trisomy 21 than like their sibs; flat occiput
Eyes	"Mongoloid slant"; epicanthic folds; Brushfield spots
Ears	Small, frequently low set
Nose	Low nasal bridge
Mouth and chin	Protruding fissured tongue secondary to maxillary hypoplasia and narrow palate
Neck	Broad, frequently webbed
Heart	Congenital heart lesions in 50%, VSD and AV canal most common
Abdomen	Diastasis recti; umbilical hernia; duodenal atresia
Hands	Short hands and fingers; clinodactyly of fifth finger
Feet	Gap between first and second toes with plantar furrow
Urogenital	Occasional cryptorchism
X-ray	Pelvic x-rays iliac index 60°; hypoplasia midphalanx fifth finger
Dermatoglyphics	Simian line; distal axial triradius; ten ulnar loops or radial loops on fourth and fifth fingers
Incidence	1 in 1,000

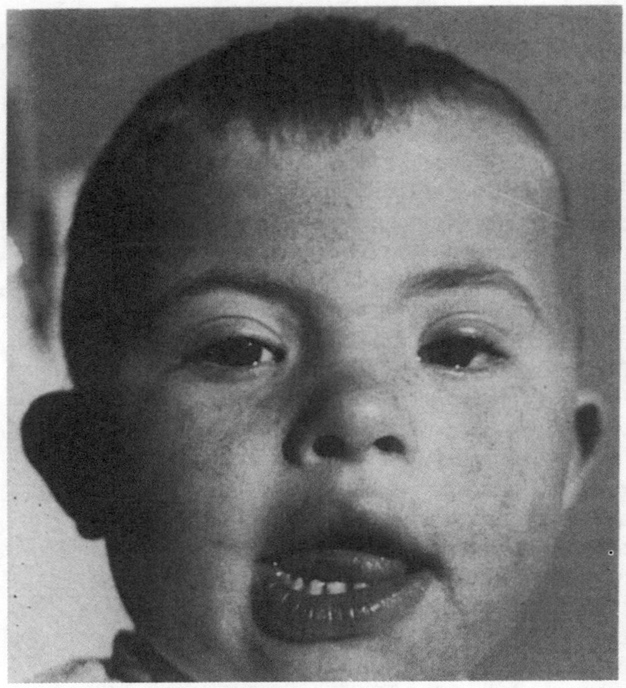

Figure 28.3. Facial features in Down's syndrome. (See text and Table 28.7.)

When following patients with Down's syndrome and congenital heart disease, the physician or counselor should be aware of certain special problems. These children have a tendency to develop pulmonary hypertension more rapidly than do other children with the same apparent anatomic abnormality. One possible explanation is that they do not truly have the same anatomic defect, that an unsuspected PDA contributes high flow under high pressure to the lungs of children who have been followed before heart catheterization as having only VSD or AV canal. However, we have seen enough children with isolated VSD or AV canal in whom pulmonary hypertension rapidly developed without the contribution of patent ductus arteriosus. The point is that if surgery is to be considered, it may require a much earlier and more aggressive approach than that in children without Down's syndrome.

Another precaution is that what appears to be a straightforward diagnosis often is not. Usually left axis deviation on the electrocardiogram will sort out the endocardial cushion defects from other shunting lesions. However, there are many exceptions, which can damage the ego of the diagnostician. We have seen endocardial cushion defects without the sentinel finding of left axis deviation and have found patients with ostium secundum ASD, PDA, and VSD (Becu types 2 and 4 as well as 3) who had left axis deviation.

The first question of the parents, before the questions of etiology and familial recurrence, regards the management of heart disease in their child. This is a very personal and a difficult problem. The parents should be full participants in the decision-making, and trusted family advisors should be welcome. We have seen families literally travel almost halfway around the world with a child having Down's syndrome, severe heart disease, retardation, and the additional handicap of being a deaf mute. The trip was made with no guarantees, but only with the hope that heart surgery would be possible. We have seen other families living within a short distance of the medical center who declined even to have diagnostic cardiac catheterization for their child. In some families the child with Down's syndrome is an integral and beloved family member, and this is the reason given for desiring surgery or wishing to avoid the not inconsiderable risk of surgery. In other situations the abnormal infant or child has become a burden that threatens to destroy the family unit, and surgery is desired or declined in that particular context ("kill him or cure him" or "we can't handle the financial or emotional stress of surgery").

If the heart defect is a simple VSD, ASD, or PDA unaccompanied by severe pulmonary hypertension, the prognosis after surgery can be optimistic for longevity and the opportunity afforded the patient to achieve maximal physical potential. If the anatomic or physiologic derangement of the heart is more complex, the prognosis must be more guarded.

No large series are available to contradict the current impression that the type of heart defect and the natural history of this defect are the same in Down's syndrome produced by complete 21 trisomy, translocation, or mosaicism. The frequency of heart defects may be lower with partial trisomies or mosaics. A distinction must be made in counseling. The recurrence risk of complete 21 trisomy (normal parents) or unbalanced translocation (if the father has balanced translocation) is about 2%. Therefore, the recurrence risk of congenital heart disease in such families is about the same as in the general population (ie, 1%). However, if the mother is the carrier of a balanced translocation, the recurrence risk is about 15% for the syndrome and 7.5% for congenital heart disease (remembering that about 50% of patients with Down's syndrome have CHD). The risk for familial recurrence in offspring of mothers who have mosaicism in which there is a 47,XX,+21 cell line is increased, but there are insufficient data to define the level of increased risk. We are always wary of the young, not-too-bright mother of a patient with Down's syndrome. Even in the absence of any physical stigmas of trisomy 21, a Walker dermal index is a valuable step in assessing possible mosaicism in a parent. Certainly if the Walker index is abnormal, a karyotype is indicated before definitive counseling is given.

18 TRISOMY

This second most common autosomal trisomic syndrome has a population incidence of 1:3,500 to 1:8,000. The clinical features are summarized in Table 28.8 and some are illustrated in Figure 28.4. Congenital heart disease is almost invariably found. (We are aware of only one case in which heart disease was absent.) The most common heart lesions are VSD, PDA, pulmonary stenosis, atrial septal defect (ASD), and coarctation of the aorta. It is the rule rather than the exception for an infant with this syndrome to have more than one heart defect (eg, VSD plus PDA plus ASD). The course of the disease may be more benign in partial trisomies and mosaics and the risk of congenital heart disease appears to be less than that in complete 18 trisomy, but most of these infants also have heart lesions.

Life expectancy in this syndrome is only a few months, which introduces a problem regarding the desirable approach to medical management of the patient and the heart disease. We take the position that cardiac catheterization and aggressive therapy are unjustified. This position must coincide with prevailing laws.

Table 28.8. Clinical Features of Trisomy 18

General	Female sex preponderance (M,1:F,3); low birth weight for gestational age; failure to thrive; early death
Neurologic	Mental and growth retardation; hypertonic
Head	Prominent occiput
Eyes	Epicanthic folds; small palpebral fissures
Ears	Low set; malformed
Mouth and chin	Micrognathia, narrow palatal arch, microstomia; infrequently, cleft lip and/or palate
Thorax	Short sternum; eventration of diaphragm
Heart	Congenital heart anomalies in 99%, most often VSD or PDA
Abdomen	Meckel's diverticulum; inguinal hernia
Hands	Third and fourth fingers clenched against palm with second and fifth fingers overlapping them
Feet	Rocker-bottom shape; great toe dorsiflexed
Pelvis	Small pelvis; limited hip abduction
Urogenital	Renal anomalies; cryptorchism
X-ray	Hypoplastic sternum; thin tapered ribs; hypoplastic mandible; "antimongoloid" pelvis
Dermatoglyphics	Characteristic digital pattern of 6 to 10 low arches; high axial triradius; single flexion crease on digits
Incidence	1 in 3,500 to 1 in 8,000

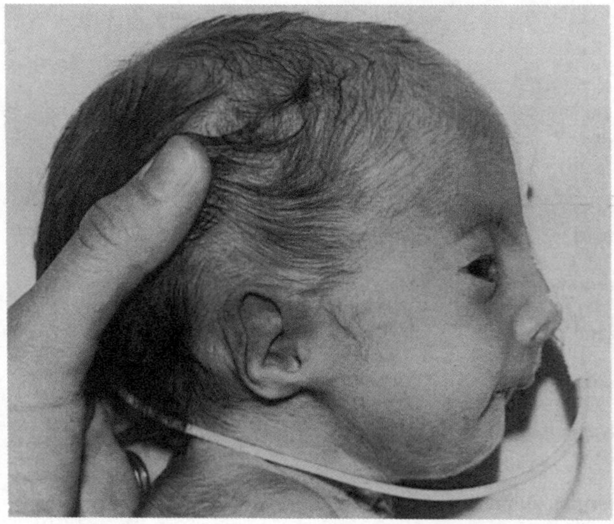

Figure 28.4. Facial features in trisomy 18. (See text and Table 28.8.)

Counseling in this syndrome is that the risk of recurrence of complete 18 trisomy in a given family is negligible. However, familial cases of partial trisomies have been reported. Phenocopies with normal chromosomes, partial trisomies, and mosaics are common enough to require that the physician obtain a karyotype before diagnostic conclusions are reached and before therapeutic and counseling courses are undertaken. It should be noted that the recurrence of phenocopies of 18 trisomy in siblings who have normal chromosomes has raised the question of autosomal recessive inheritance in these patients.

13 TRISOMY

Next most common among the complete trisomies is chromosome 13. The population frequency rate is approximately 1:4,000 to 1:15,000. Table 28.9 presents the clinical features and Figure 28.5 illustrates some of these. Congenital heart disease is found in about 90% of infants with this syndrome. Ventricular septal defect, PDA, complex dextroversion, and ASD are the most common abnormalities of the cardiovascular system. As in 18 trisomy, the coexistence of more than one heart lesion is the rule. Although complex dextroversion is not the most common anomaly, it is sufficiently rare in the general population and so common in this group of patients that it may be looked upon as a characteristic cardiovascular malformation in 13 trisomy. Complex dextroversion, in addition to dextroposition of the heart with normal situs of the abdominal organs, often includes single ventricle, L-transposition of the great arteries, single atrium, total anomalous pulmonary venous return, and pulmonary stenosis (in some combination). The mirror image of the aforementioned conditions may also occur (ie, normal position of the heart with abdominal situs inversus and cardiac anomalies). How well any of the heart lesions are tolerated depends on the hemodynamic state of cardiac output and oxygenation that is ultimately reached. If the shunt is balanced and the output is satisfactory in complex dextroversion, this may be tolerated better than a large left-to-right shunt through a simple PDA.

Table 28.9. Clinical Features of Trisomy 13

General	Equal sex distribution; failure to thrive; apneic spells; early death
Neurologic	Mental and motor retardation; hypertonic or hypotonic; defects of the forebrain (holoprosencephaly, arhinencephaly)
Head	Sloping forehead; scalp defects; microcephaly
Eyes	Colobomata; microphthalmia; anophthalmia
Ears	Low set; malformed
Mouth and chin	Usually cleft lip and/or palate; micrognathia
Heart	Congenital heart lesions in 88%, most often VSD, PDA, and rotational anomalies
Abdomen	Rotational anomalies; hernias, absent spleen; accessory spleens
Hands	Polydactyly; frequently third and fourth fingers clenched against palm with second and fifth fingers overlapping; hyperconvex nails
Feet	Polydactyly; frequently rocker-bottom shape
Urogenital	Polycystic kidneys; hydronephrosis; cryptorchism; bicornuate uterus
Dermatoglyphics	Ridge hypoplasia, radial loops and arches; high triradius, single palmar flexion crease; hallucal arch fibular or fibular-S pattern
Incidence	1 in 4,000 to 1 in 15,000

The most frequent translocation in the general population is t(DqDq). This occurs in about 1:1,000. The great majority of individuals having a D/D translocation are balanced carriers. The risk of an unbalanced translocation occurring among the offspring of a D/D carrier is 1% or slightly higher. In any case, amniocentesis should be recommended in a family in which one parent has a balanced

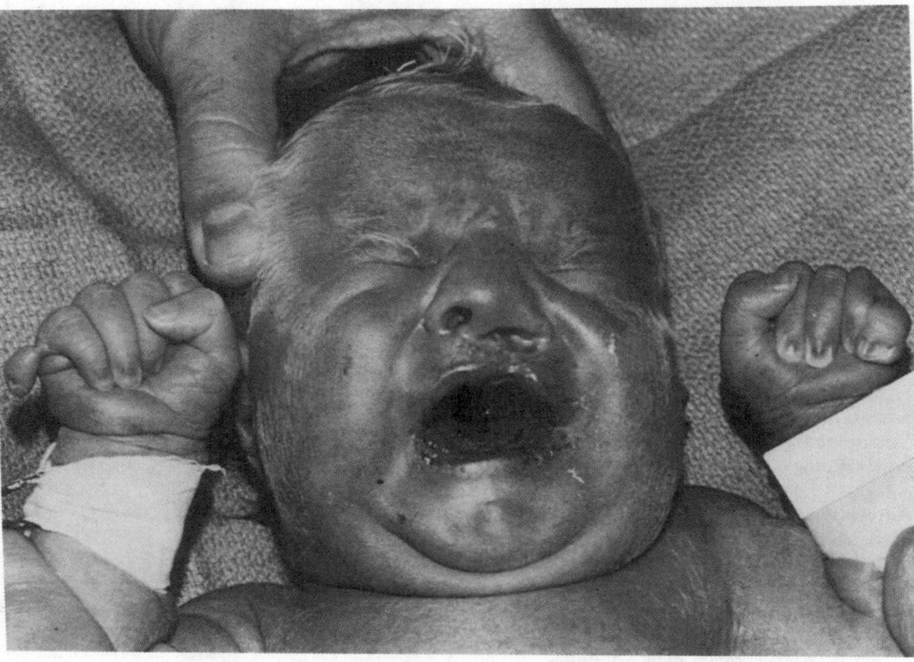

Figure 28.5. Trisomy 13. Note facial and finger anomalies. (See Table 28.9.)

t(DqDq). The heart anomalies and severity of the syndrome appear to be the same whether the karyotype is complete trisomy or translocation. Nonfamilial "phenocopies" with normal chromosomes have also been found and have similar heart lesions.

The risk of recurrence in a family after the birth of a child with a complete 13 trisomy is negligible. We advocate the same nonaggressive diagnostic and therapeutic approach to these patients as to patients with 18 trisomy.

CHROMOSOME 22

Trisomy 22 may actually be ll qter trisomy as suggested by extensive banding studies. The incidence in the population is not known. Clinical features are presented in Table 28.10 and some are illustrated in Figure 28.6. About 67% of patients with this syndrome appear to have congenital heart disease, usually of the less life-threatening variety. Atrial septal defect is most common, followed by VSD and PDA. Familial recurrence of the syndrome has been reported in offspring of a mother who had mosaicism involving a 22 trisomic cell line, but no recurrences have been reported in the presence of normal parental karyotypes. The prognosis for longevity is variable and retardation is usually severe. The decision regarding heart surgery is similar to that in Down's syndrome. The physician may certainly present the possibility of surgery to the parents, if a low risk heart operation could make a child more comfortable and medical management more effective. The very personal decision may be made for or against surgery in the context of fully informed options.

There is also a syndrome produced by the addition to the normal chromosome complement of a small acrocentric chromosome, which has been confirmed by banding techniques as representing partial trisomy 22. A 3:1 preponderance of females is found. The main differences between this partial trisomy and complete "22 trisomy" are the presence in the cat-eye syndrome of coloboma (Figure 28.7) of the iris (hence, the name *cat-eye*) and anal-atresia. Cleft palate and somewhat more severe mental retardation characterize "complete trisomy." From the cardiovascular point of view there is a very important difference: heart disease in cat-eye syndrome is more severe and life-threatening when present. About 40% of patients with partial 22 trisomy have congenital heart disease and in most cases it is accompanied by cyanosis. Complex total anomalous pulmonary venous return associated with other abnormalities such as tricuspid atresia is the most common defect of the cardiovascular system. Ventricular septal defect and ASD are also found as isolated lesions. There are now enough cases to make it seem unlikely that this provocative finding is a sampling error. A similar pattern of anomalies not caused by a chromosomal abnormality has been referred to under the acronym CHARGE (C-coloboma, H-heart disease, A-atresia choanae, R-retarded growth and mental development, G-genital hypoplasia, E-ear anomalies or deafness) association.[15]

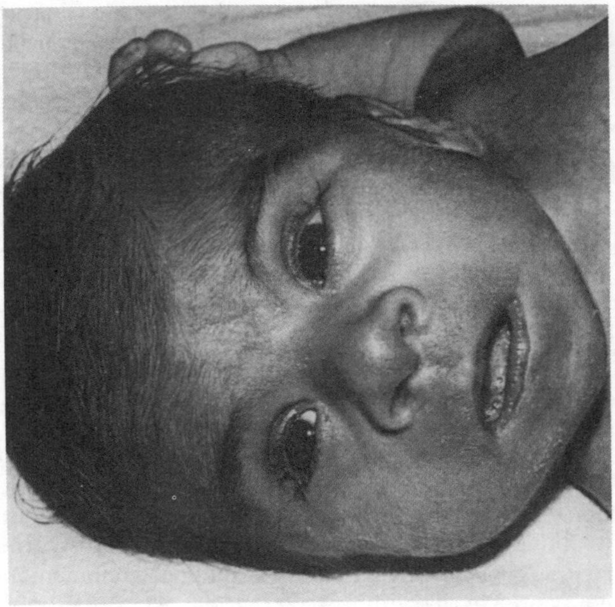

Figure 28.6. Trisomy 22. (See Table 28.10.)

UNCOMMON AUTOSOMAL ANOMALIES

Many more chromosomal aberrations have been described in such small numbers of patients that it is difficult to assign frequency of occurrence of cardiovascular disease. It is probably more realistic to use greater than 50%, approximately 50%, or less than 50% until enough cases are described to justify a closer estimate. Some patients have been less completely studied from a cardiovascular point of view than others, making the exact cardiac diagnosis uncertain. It does not represent a real advance to lump these chromosomal syndromes together,

Table 28.10. Clinical Features of Trisomy 22

General	Equal sex ratio; failure to thrive
Neurologic	Mental and growth retardation
Head	Microcephaly
Ears	Low set, angled, malformed; preauricular tags
Nose	Anteverted nares
Mouth and chin	Cleft palate; micrognathia
Neck	Redundant skin folds
Heart	Anomalies in 67%
Extremities	Abnormal thumbs (digitated or broad); cubitus valgus; dislocation of the hip
Dermatoglyphics	Excess of whorls; distal axial triradius
Incidence	Unknown

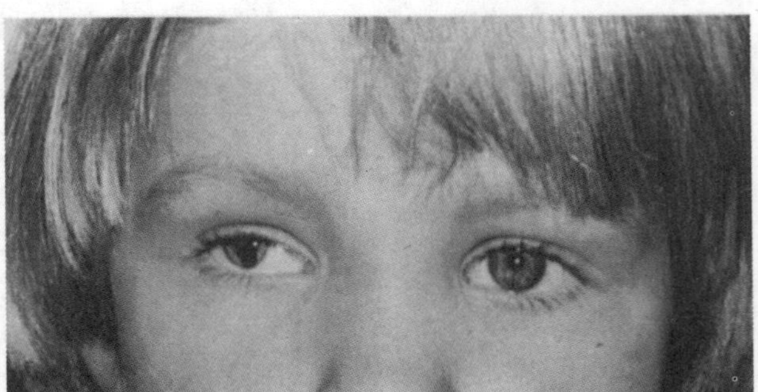

Figure 28.7. Cat-eye syndrome. Note right eye. (See text.)

but if there are no clear differences in the heart problems, then in the interest of economy of space they may be listed as they are in Table 28.6.

As to the clinical diagnosis of these uncommon syndromes, not many physicians feel confident of doing better than proposing a differential, which might include the correct cytogenetic diagnosis. Many clinical features are shared by a large number of syndromes. Further confounding comes from the fact that mosaicism, ring chromosomes, partial trisomies, and partial deletions may yield a different quantity of genetic material in one patient than in another with the same general cytogenetic aberration. A patient with an aneuploid-euploid ratio of 20/80 would predictably have less developmental disruption than would one with a ratio of 80/20.

A few years ago the dictum obtained that if you seek to find a complete trisomy that is viable to term, you should concentrate on the small autosomes. The larger amount of genetic material in a large autosome, if present in triplicate, would be lethal. The dictum is still valid. The new chromosomal syndromes involving large chromosomes are mainly found in patients with mosaic cell lines and partial trisomies and deletions.

SEX CHROMOSOMAL ANOMALIES

45,X TURNER'S SYNDROME

Turner's syndrome, from a cardiovascular point of view, is the most important of the sex chromosomal anomalies. The clinical features of this syndrome are reviewed in Table 28.11 and some features are illustrated in Figure 28.8. Approximately 1 in 2,500 females have a 45,X chromosomal constitution. Of these, about 35% have cardiovascular disease including 5% to 10% who have significant hypertension unrelated to coarctation of the aorta.

There is such an overlap between the phenotypes of XO Turner's syndrome and Noonan's syndrome that they are often indistinguishable in females on the basis of external features. A useful diagnostic dichotomy does exist, however. If the patient has coarctation of the aorta, she almost invariably has Turner's syndrome; if the patient has pulmonary valve stenosis, she has, with almost no exceptions, Noonan's syndrome. Structural anomalies of the X chromosome associated with Turner's syndrome, such as isochromosomes of the long arm, may be accompanied by the same cardiovascular abnormalities as are found in the complete 45,X anomaly. However, XO/XX mosaics may have either pulmonary stenosis or coarctation of the aorta. An explanation for this could be that those with pulmonary stenosis had a 46,XX constitution (and the dominant gene mutation of Noonan's syndrome) up to the point of second cell division, at which time two viable cell lines became established.

Although coarctation of the aorta accounts for two thirds of cardiovascular disease in these patients, other common malformations occur such as VSD, ASD, aortic stenosis, and PDA. Caution must be voiced regarding hypertension in Turner's syndrome. Coarctation of the aorta and renal disease or essential hypertension may coexist, and renal disease or essential hypertension may be present in the absence of coarctation of the aorta. Before scheduling surgical repair of what may appear to be straightforward coarctation of the aorta, it is prudent to have a renal evaluation and to perform cardiac catheterization with angiocardiography. The coarctation is usually juxtaductal and the collateral arteries are also usually satisfactory. Also, if there is a clear discrepancy between the blood pressure and pulse in the upper and lower extremities, there is usually enough anatomic disease to require resection. However, we have all seen patients who, because of systemic hypertension and a clear pressure and pulse differential, were considered to be certain candidates for surgery, but who proved to have minimal anatomic involvement of the aorta. Conversely, we have seen patients with only borderline hypertension and modest pressure and pulse differentials whose severe anatomic restriction was compensated for and obscured by an excellent collateral circulation. We have also seen patients whose elevated systolic blood pressures were unimproved after demonstrable successful coarctectomies, because of the presence of hypertension of other etiology. All of these cases are the exception rather than the rule. However, the best way to avoid problems in these areas is to be certain that the preoperative evaluation is optimal

Table 28.11. Clinical Features of Turner's Syndrome

General	Female. Normal life expectancy may be altered by cardiovascular or renal disease. Invariably small stature for age with eventual height attainment rarely exceeding 60 inches; chromatin-negative
Neurologic	Intellectual development is generally good but is usually below the attainment of siblings; perceptive hearing loss is common
Skin	Frequent pigmented nevi
Head	Characteristic facies; narrow maxilla; small mandible
Eyes	Frequent epicanthic folds; occasional ptosis; infrequent hypertelorism
Ears	Usually normal, sometimes prominent
Mouth	Sharklike-curved upper lip, straight lower lip
Neck	Low posterior hairline; webbed in about 50% of patients
Chest	Shield shaped; widely spaced hypoplastic nipples; underdevelopment of the breasts
Cardiovascular	Anomalies in approximately 35%; coarctation of the aorta is most common; pulmonic stenosis rarely if ever occurs; occasional idiopathic hypertension
Extremities	Cubitus valgus; lymphedema of dorsum of hands and feet in infancy; dystrophic nails; short fourth and fifth metacarpals; short fifth finger with clinodactyly; medial tibial exostosis
Urogenital	Ovarian dysgenesis with infertility (only 6 reported instances of fertility)
Roentgenogram	Hypoplasia of lateral ends of clavicles and sacral wings; platyspondylia; metaphyseal dysplasia of long bones; "positive metacarpal sign" (short fourth and fifth metacarpals)
Dermatoglyphics	Distal axial triradius in 20% to 30%; higher than average ridge count
Incidence	1:5,000 (1:2,500 females)

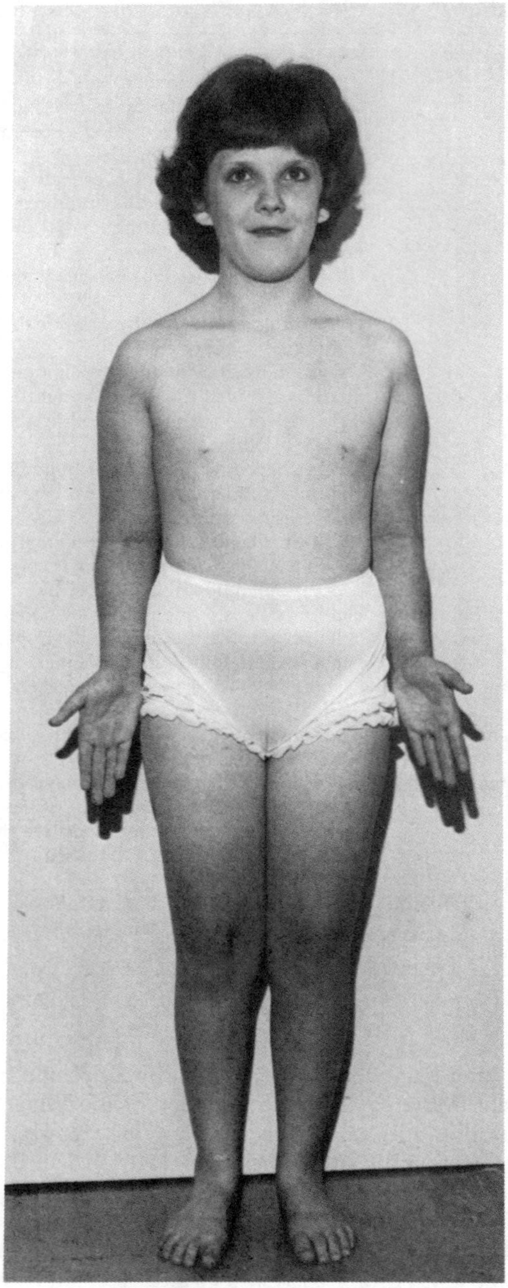

Figure 28.8. 45,X Turner's syndrome. (See text and Table 28.11.)

and that the possibility of confounding variables is shared with the family.

Familial recurrence risk of the 45,X genotype depends on the karyotype. Following a sporadic case, the risk of some form of nondisjunction is probably greater than that in the general population. Finally, how does the number of X chromosomes influence the type of cardiovascular maldevelopment? Coarctation of the aorta is expressed in males twice as often as in females. Patients with the 45,X genotype are phenotypically female, but lack the full female chromosome complement. One can speculate that the so-called inactivated X chromosome in the 46,XX genotype may produce some gene products that have a modest role in cardiovascular development.

XXXXY SYNDROME

The other syndrome of sex chromosomal aberration that has important cardiovascular implications is the XXXXY syndrome (Table 28.12 and Figure 28.9). About 14% have cardiovascular disease and the most common lesion (almost all cases) is PDA. The only other lesions described are ASD and anomalous right coronary artery. The caution here is that just because there is a continuous murmur at the left base does not mean that the patient has a PDA. Fortunately, we catheterized our patient, who turned out to have an anomalous right coronary artery and were prepared to restore a two coronary artery system rather than ligate a PDA.

The interesting etiologic consideration is that these patients with an overabundance of X chromosomes have a malformation (PDA) that is usually expressed twice as commonly in females as in males. As more cases are surveyed, the frequency of PDA decreases, so that at 14%, XXXXY syndrome has a relatively low rate of cardiovascular disease when compared with other chromosomal aberrations. A corollary question could be raised as to why there is no obvious increase in PDA in patients with the XXX and XXXX anomalies. There have been so few cases in the XXXXY syndrome that the frequency of PDA in one of six cases is still difficult to interpret.

OTHER SEX CHROMOSOMAL ANOMALIES

Klinefelter's XXY syndrome has been reported in occasional patients with congenital heart disease. If there is a true increase in risk, it is small. The XXX and XXXX aneuploidies do not appear to have an increased risk and the XXXXY syndrome has been reported to have PDA in one of six cases. A second case had a murmur, diagnosis unspecified. Based on the cases reported so far, the XXXXY, XYY, and XXYY anomalies do not have a significant increase in risk of cardiovascular disease.

Table 28.12. Clinical Features of XXXXY Syndrome

General	Phenotypic males may have some genital ambiguity; small stature
Neurologic	Retarded: IQ between 25 and 50; moderate hypotonia and joint laxity
Head	Characteristic facies (often confused with Down's syndrome); low nasal bridge; protruding mandible; occasional flat occiput
Eyes	Epicanthic folds, slant; occasional Brushfield spots; strabismus
Ears	Malformed; low-set
Neck	Short; occasionally webbed
Cardiovascular	About 15% have congenital heart lesions (eg, PDA)
Extremities	Limited elbow pronation; genu valgum; clinodactyly of fifth finger
Urogenital	Small penis and testes; frequent cryptorchism
Roentgenogram	Radioulnar synostosis
Dermatoglyphics	Average ridge count is low (60%); frequent low arches; occasional simian line
Incidence	Undetermined; relatively uncommon

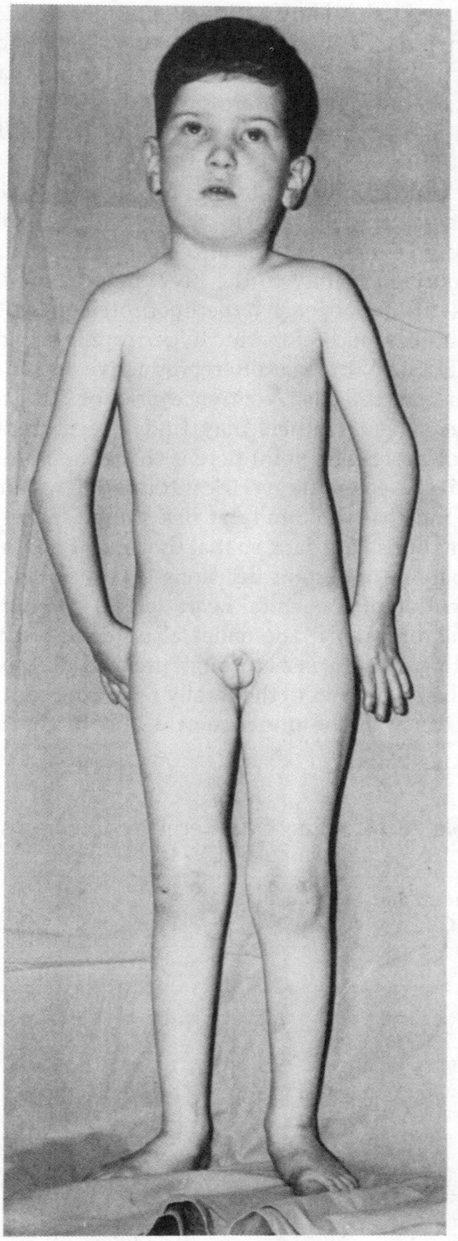

Figure 28.9. 49,XXXXY syndrome. Note facies, arms, and genitalia. (See text and Table 28.12.)

SINGLE MUTANT GENE DISORDERS

It is not possible in a presentation of this size to do more than tabulate a few single gene mutations that produce cardiovascular disease as a feature of a syndrome or as a discrete abnormality. The genetics of many other syndromes (plus a few discrete lesions) have not been clearly established. These will also be briefly tabulated. Some cardiovascular problems are categorized in the literature as mendelian on the basis of only one or two interesting families. Such categorization appears to be valid if there is a rare or unique anomaly or pattern, but it is difficult to defend for common and discrete defects. We will try to reveal areas of disagreement, but ultimately we must assign the etiologic designation that seems to us to best fit the available data.

Counseling for risk of recurrence of the syndrome or discrete lesion is fairly straightforward (eg, 50% autosomal dominant and 25% autosomal recessive) with a few exceptions attributable to penetrance. These exceptions will be noted as they occur. The hardest information to gain from the literature is how frequently cardiovascular diseases are found in many of these syndromes. We have had to draw heavily from our own impressions and experience in many instances. Sometimes the data are firm enough to allow us to offer a percentage risk of cardiovascular disease (or penetrance of the cardiovascular abnormality). Sometimes the data are so imprecise that "low," "moderate," or "high" frequencies are the best approximations we can offer. Obviously we would not include syndromes in which the risk of cardiovascular disease does not appear to exceed the risk in the general population.

As is the case in chromosomal anomalies in the etiology of cardiovascular maldevelopment, when considering single mutant gene causation, it is best (with few exceptions) to look for a syndrome of multiple abnormalities. The format of presentation in this section will be to tabulate selected syndromes or discrete disorders alphabetically under several headings: autosomal dominant, autosomal recessive, and syndromes of undetermined etiology. A problem that plagues clinical geneticists is how much "lumping" and how much "splitting" to accept. For example, our family studies lead us to believe that Aarskog's syndrome is an emphasis on certain features of Noonan's syndrome and that the Lewis syndrome emphasizes merely a feature of Holt-Oram syndrome. Therefore, our tables do not show Aarskog's or Lewis syndrome.

AUTOSOMAL DOMINANT DISORDERS

Autosomal dominant disorders are directly transmitted from a person with the disease to half of their children, on average. There is a high mutation rate in some dominant disorders, so it is common to find a patient whose parents do not have the disease. However, once the mutant gene is in the family, the chance of passing it on becomes 50%. In Table 28.13, the risk of cardiovascular disease as part of the syndrome will be given as 100% if all individuals with the syndrome have cardiovascular involvement. If only half the patients with the syndrome have heart involvement (as in Noonan's syndrome), the cardiovascular risk will be given as 50%. If the question is, what is the chance of recurrence of heart disease in the child of a patient with Noonan's syndrome, the answer is 25%: 50% chance to have the syndrome multiplied by 50% to have heart disease in the presence of the syndrome.

AUTOSOMAL RECESSIVE DISORDERS

In autosomal recessive disease, neither parent has the disease, but both parents are carriers and the recurrence risk for the syndrome occurring in subsequent children is 25%. The frequency of heart disease in patients who have the syndrome is given in Table 28.14, and the risk of heart disease recurring in the family is the risk of

Table 28.13. Autosomal Dominant Conditions with Cardiovascular (CV) Involvement

Condition and Frequency of CV Involvement	Types of CV Involvement
Apert (≈10%)	Ventricular septal defect (VSD), tetralogy of Fallot (TOF), coarctation of aorta (CA)
Ehlers–Danlos, several types (5% to 50%)	AV valve regurgitation, rupture of large blood vessels, eg, carotids, dissecting aneurysms of aorta
Holt–Oram (≈50%)	Atrial septal defect (ASD), VSD
Idiopathic hypertrophic subaortic stenosis (100% by definition)	Myocardial disease
Marfan (60% to 80%)	Mitral and aortic disease
Mitral click murmur (100%)	Mitral insufficiency, dysrhythmias (some families with dominant inheritance)
Myotonic dystrophy, Steinert (65%)	Conduction defects, myocardial disease
Neurofibromatosis (5% to 10%)	Pulmonic stenosis (PS), pheochromocytomia with hypertension, CA
Noonan (50%)	PS, ASD, left ventricular disease
Osteogenesis imperfecta (5% to 10%)	Aortic incompetence
Romano–Ward (100%)	Prolonged QT, syncope, sudden death
Supravalvular aortic stenosis (with or without elfin facies) (100%)	Supravalvular aortic and pulmonic stenosis, peripheral pulmonary artery stenosis
Treacher Collins (≈10%)	VSD, PDA, ASD

having the syndrome (25%) multiplied by the frequency of heart disease associated with the syndrome.

X-LINKED DISORDERS

These diseases are commonly transmitted from an unaffected carrier female to half of her male offspring, on average. There are also X-linked dominant diseases that are lethal in the male. Only a small number of X-linked disorders have cardiovascular involvement and these are of sufficient rarity and complexity as to prohibit simple tabulation.

SYNDROMES AND DISORDERS OF UNDETERMINED ETIOLOGY

Table 28.15 presents a number of conditions in which there is cardiovascular disease, most often as part of a syndrome. Most of these conditions have been observed in families and, to some observers, the formal genetics may be clear. Placing the disorders in this section expresses some continued uncertainty about the etiology.

PREVENTION

Although there is intrinsic value in understanding the genetic and environmental contributions to the production of congenital heart disease, the ultimate goal of our studies is prevention. The clearest strategy for prevention at this time is identification of the individual and family at increased risk, identification of environmental triggers, and prophylactic intervention based on this knowledge. Genetic risk identification and preventive approaches for individuals and families are presently pursued through current practice in clinical genetics, including diagnosis and counseling. Single mutant gene disorders and the usually concomitant syndromes consequent to the effect of a major gene are recognized by clinical examination and pedigree analysis. It is also clear that certain conditions confined mainly to the heart may be mendelizing, such as the monogenic hyperlipoproteinemias, ASD in some families, and idiopathic hypertrophic subaortic stenosis (IHSS). With regard to reproductive decisions, some families may consider recurrence risks of 50% to be acceptable, whereas others may find a recurrence risk of 3% intolerable. The point here is that genetic counseling should be based on the specific information within a given family and that the family at risk should have access to accurate counseling data, so that they may knowledgeably participate in important decisions regarding risks.

Prevention of congenital heart defects that are secondary to chromosomal anomalies also begins with genetic counseling and proceeds through prenatal diagnosis to an option being offered to the family regarding continuation of pregnancy in the presence of a known chromosomal

Table 28.14. Autosomal Recessive Conditions with Cardiovascular (CV) Involvement

Condition and Frequency of CV Involvement	Types of CV Involvement
Carpenter (≈20%)	Patent ductus arteriosus (PDA), ventricular septal defect (VSD), pulmonic stenosis (PS), transposition of great arteries (TGA)
Ellis–van Creveld (50%)	Atrial septal defect (ASD), most commonly single atrium, other congenital heart lesions
Friedreich ataxia (75% to 90%)	Myocardiopathy and conduction defects
Glycogenosis IIa, Pompe, (≈100%)	Myocardiopathy
Glycogenosis III (Cori) and IV (Anderson)	Myocardiopathy (moderate)
Ivemark (100% by definition)	Asplenia with cardiovascular anomalies (some families are recessive)
Jervell and Lange–Nielsen (≈100%)	Prolonged QT, sudden death
Meckel-Gruber (> 25%)	Both complex and simple structural defects
Pseudoxanthoma elasticum (≈100%)	Generalized vascular disease, coronary insufficiency, mitral insufficiency, hypertension
Refsum (> 50%)	Atrioventricular conduction defects
Smith–Lemli–Opitz (≈15%)	VSD, PDA, and other congenital heart diseases
Thrombocytopenia absent radius, TAR (30%)	ASD, tetralogy, dextrocardia
Weill–Marchesani (≈15%)	PS, VSD
Zellweger (low)	PDA, VSD, ASD

Table 28.15. Disorders of Undetermined Etiology That Have Associated Cardiovascular (CV) Disease

Abnormality and Frequency of Associated CV Disease	Types of Associated CV Disease
Arthrogryposis multiplex congenita (10% to 25%)	Patent ductus arteriosus (PDA), ventricular septal defect (VSD), coarctation of the aorta (CA), aortic stenosis (AS)
Asymmetric crying face (3%)	Tetralogy of Fallot (TOF), VSD
Atrial myxoma, familial (highly variable)	Myxoma, rheumatic fever
Biliary-hepatic and cardiovascular disease (≈50%)	Peripheral pulmonary artery stenosis (PPAS), PDA, VSD
Cardioauditory syndrome of Sanchez–Cascos (100% by definition)	? myocardial disease
DeLange syndrome (20%)	VSD, TOF, PDA, double outlet right ventricle
DiGeorge syndrome (85% to 95%)	VSD, interrupted aortic arch, truncus
Goldenhar syndrome (≈50%)	TOF, VSD, atrial septal defect (ASD)
Kartegener syndrome (100% in full syndrome)	Dextrocardia
Klippel–Feil syndrome (25% to 40%)	VSD with pulmonary hypertension, total anomalous pulmonary venous return (TAPVR), transposition of great arteries (TGA), TOF, ASD, PDA
Mitral click murmur (100%)	Mitral prolapse or redundancy
Ophthalmoplegia with AV block (100% by definition)	First, second, or third degree AV block, fascicular blocks
Poland syndrome (10%)	CA, VSD
Rubenstein–Taybi (25%)	PDA, ASD, VSD
Silver syndrome (10% to 20%)	TOF, VSD
Williams syndrome (>90%)	Supravalvar aortic and pulmonic stenosis, PPAS

abnormality. As many as 10% of liveborn infants with CHD have their cardiac maldevelopments as a consequence of a chromosomal disorder. Through amniocentesis this component of risk is already being reduced in many developed countries. Although there are eventual logistic limitations, prenatal diagnosis is still generally underutilized. Ultrasound diagnosis of congenital heart disease in the fetus is progressing to the point that clinical decisions are becoming possible as technology advances.

Reduction of congenital cardiac defects by identifying and eliminating human teratogens has, in some instances, been highly rewarding, as in the experience with rubella and thalidomide. For the most part, however, this approach has been disappointing. Problems with traditional epidemiologic studies have been reviewed, and although it must be acknowledged that it is not easy to discover teratogens that cause only a small increase in cardiac defects (particularly common malformations), it also must be pointed out that there have been serious and unnecessary flaws in clinical teratogenic studies that invalidate much of the data in the literature. What has made these flaws unnecessary is that the guidelines for reasonably accurate teratogen-risk evaluation were determined in the thalidomide investigations two decades ago. They simply have not been strictly applied. By using the tools we have at the moment, much more can be learned about environmental triggers and how they act on genetically predisposed embryos. Major genes that participate in how the body responds to chemicals should become an even broader investigative area than it is today. It should be technically possible to screen individuals and families for genetic susceptibility to chemical teratogens.

In the near future, we should see clinical applications of the techniques of cell biology based on the knowledge of what is going on at the molecular level. The clinical parameters of recombinant DNA technology have yet to be explored in more than a preliminary fashion. For now, it is appropriate not only to look to future developments, but also to insist on rigorous applications of knowledge and techniques that are already available. We must improve our abilities to identify individuals and families at high genetic and environmental risk to devise sound biologic approaches to the elimination of these risks. Heart disease will not disappear from human populations, but the prospect for significant reduction in both the near and long term is entirely feasible. The goal of prevention should be vigorously pursued.

REFERENCES

1. Nora JJ, Nora AH: *Genetics and Counseling in Cardiovascular Diseases.* Springfield, Ill, Charles C Thomas, 1978, pp 1–227.
2. Nora JJ, Nora AH: Genetic epidemiology of congenital heart diseases, in Steinberg AG, Bearn AG, Motulsky AG, Childs B (eds): *Progress in Medical Genetics.* Philadelphia, WB Saunders, 1983, Vol 5, pp 91–138.
3. Hoffman JIE, Christianson R: Congenital heart disease in a cohort of 19,502 births with long-term follow-up. *Am J Cardiol* 1978; 42:641–647.
4. Nora JJ: Multifactorial inheritance hypothesis for the etiology of congenital heart diseases: the genetic-environmental interaction. *Circulation* 1968; 38:604–617.
5. Nora JJ, Nora AH: The evolution of specific genetic and environmental counseling in congenital heart diseases. *Circulation* 1978; 57:205–213.
6. Nebert DW, Bigelow SW: Genetic control of drug metabolism: relationship to birth defects. *Semin Perinatol* 1982; 6:105–115.
7. Kretchmer N: Perspectives in teratologic research. *Teratology* 1978; 17:203–211.
8. Fraser FC, Hunter ADW: Etiologic relations among categories of congenital heart malformations. *Am J Cardiol* 1975; 36:793–796.
9. Nora JJ, Sommerville RJ, Fraser FC: Homologies for congenital heart diseases. *Teratology* 1968; 1:413–416.
10. Cooper LZ, Krugman S: Diagnosis and management of the congenital rubella syndrome. *Pediatrics* 1966; 37:335–442.
11. Lenz W: Chemicals and malformations in man, in *Proceedings of the Second International Conference on Congenital Malformations.* New York, The International Medical Congress Ltd, 1964, pp 263–276.
12. Nora JJ, Nora AH, Toews WH: Lithium, Ebstein's anomaly and other congenital heart defects. *Lancet* 1974; 2:594–595.
13. Nora JJ, Nora AH, Blu J, Ingram EJ, Fountain A, Peterson MJ, Lortscher RH, Kimberling WJ: Exogenous progestogen and estrogen implicated in birth defects. *JAMA* 1978; 240:837–843.
14. Nora JJ, Nihill MR, Miles VN, Morriss JH, Weishuhn EJ: Antiheart antibody production of cardiovascular malformations in the mouse. *Teratology* 1974; 9:143–150.
15. Clark EB: Cardiac embryology. Its relevance to congenital heart disease. *Am J Dis Children* 1986; 140:41–44.

29 Rheumatic Fever: A Model for the Pathologic Consequences of Microbial-Host Mimicry

John B. Zabriskie, MD, Allan Gibofsky, MD, Ashwani Khanna, PhD, and Eva Kemeny, MD

Although the incidence of rheumatic fever has markedly decreased in this country as in most of the industrialized world, one need only visit any of the "developing" or Third World countries to realize that this disease is still one of the major public health problems in the world. It is estimated that 15 to 20 million *new* cases will appear each year in these countries. Perhaps most important from a public health point of view is that most patients survive the acute carditis and then go on to chronic rheumatic valvular disease with all of its severe cardiologic manifestations and complications.

Despite intensive investigation over the years, we still do not have a clear picture of the pathogenic mechanisms involved in this disease process. There are several reasons for this dilemma. First, there is a long latent period from the streptococcal infection to the onset of disease, making prospective studies difficult. In addition, the number of cellular and extracellular structures and toxins associated with the streptococcal organism makes it difficult to decipher which structure or toxin is important in the disease process. Finally, the lack of a suitable experimental model for studying the disease process severely limits the number of studies that can be performed.

To better understand the disease process itself, some of the salient features of the morphology and structure of the streptococcus will first be reviewed. The host's immune response to these structures must also be considered, and finally we must examine in detail those streptococcal antigens that share antigenic determinants with mammalian tissue antigens. Knowledge concerning these areas of microbial–host interactions will hopefully lead to a greater understanding of the clinical and laboratory findings of the disease itself.

STREPTOCOCCAL STRUCTURES

Each streptococcal cell is surrounded by several layers (Figure 29.1). The M protein, seen on the outer surface as fimbria, is the most extensively studied protein antigen and will be discussed in some detail. This antigen serves as a marker for the immunologic subclassification of group A streptococci into specific types. The next layer consists of carbohydrate and contains the specific moiety responsible for the grouping of streptococci, and for group A organisms this is N-acetylglucosamine. Beneath this is a mucopeptide layer, and these three layers make up the cell wall of the streptococcus. Finally, there is the innermost layer, called the protoplast membrane, a lipoprotein structure that will be discussed in further detail. Although chemically these layers appear as discrete separate structures, a truer representation is that cell wall structures in some manner anchor to or are intertwined with membrane structures.

The M proteins are among the most important surface antigens. There are over 80 serologic types of M protein, each of which is capable of stimulating specific protective antibodies as well as sharing a common property, that of being able to avoid phagocytosis by the host's immune system. An important consideration concerning streptococcal vaccines is that a large number of group A streptococcal types can cause rheumatic fever. In contrast, strains associated with poststreptococcal glomerulonephritis appear to be limited to a few types.

Perhaps the most interesting new development in our knowledge of the M-protein moiety has been the work of Manjula and Fischetti.[1] They noted marked structural homology between the M-protein molecule and the muscle protein tropomyosin. More recently, Dale and Beachey[2] showed that antibodies raised against the pepsin fragment of the type 5 M-protein moiety not only were protective in the opsonic assay but also cross-reacted with sarcolemmal tissue. Extending these findings, they noted that there may be as many as three M-protein epitopes cross-reactive with heart tissue, some of which are shared by other M-protein moieties. It also should be noted that there are M-protein moieties (pep 24) that do not appear to have any cross-reactive epitopes.[3]

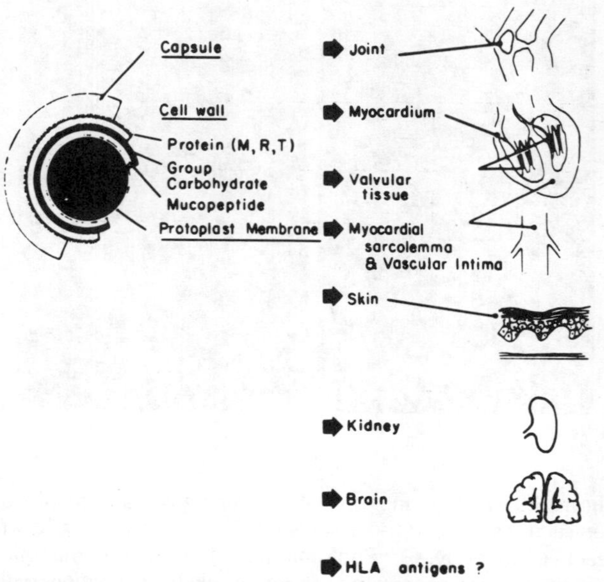

Figure 29.1. Schematic illustration of the components of the streptococcal cell and its cross-reactions with various mammalian tissue components.

Another important cross-reaction involves the group A carbohydrate moiety N-acetylglucosamine and mammalian valvular glycoproteins.[4] In a series of reports Goldstein et al[4] showed that rabbit serum samples raised against the group A carbohydrate cross-react with these valvular glycoproteins and that the shared antigenic determinant is the N-acetylglucosamine of the group A streptococcus and a similar antigen in the valvular glycoprotein material. As will be pointed out herein, this cross-reaction may be important in the pathogenesis of valvular disease in the patient with rheumatic fever.

Current work suggests that cell wall mucopeptide complex may be partly responsible for the chronic, remitting, nodular lesions in connective tissue following a single injection of disrupted group A streptococci.[5] Injection of this material in rats causes chronic relapsing arthritis and synovitis reminiscent of human rheumatoid arthritis,[6] but there is little evidence to suggest that it plays a major role in rheumatic fever.

The final inner layer of the streptococcal cell is a complex lipoprotein containing approximately 72% protein, 25% lipid, and 2% carbohydrate by weight. This structure does not contain cell wall carbohydrates and its antigens are different from those in the streptococcal cell wall. Group A streptococcal membrane structures and mammalian tissues share common antigenic determinants. These findings may be summarized as follows: (1) Cell membranes and extracts from group A streptococci cross-react with human glomerular basement membrane antigens.[7] (2) Rabbit antisera to these streptococcal membrane structures will bind to rabbit and human muscle sarcolemmal membrane antigens (including cardiac muscle).[8,9] They also bind to the smooth muscle of blood vessel walls but not to uterine muscle. (3) Guinea pigs immunized with different types of group A streptococci developed a sensitivity indistinguishable from that produced by sensitization with allogeneic tissues,[10] and there is a close biochemical similarity between mammalian histocompatibility antigens, certain structural glycoproteins, and streptococcal membrane antigens.[11]

Although we have dealt primarily with cross-reactive antigens related to heart or valves, two other streptococcal mammalian tissue reactions are worthy of discussion. Patients with rheumatic chorea possess an antibody that stains caudate nuclei and can be absorbed by streptococcal membrane antigens,[12] indicating that streptococcal antigens share antigenic determinants with brain antigens.[13] Antisera bind to skin fibroblasts as well as to thymocytes.[14] The latter cross-reactivity could be important in the host's immunoregulation to streptococcal antigens.

Concerning these cross-reactions, a word of caution should be introduced. Group A streptococci have immunoglobulin molecule Fc (crystallizable) receptors on their surface, as do tissue antigens.[15] Although many of these cross-reactions just cited are real and have included the appropriate controls, each report of streptococcal cross-reactivity should be carefullly studied for the possibility that the presumed antigen–antibody reaction is *not* due to nonspecific Fc receptor binding.

PATHOGENETIC CONCEPTS OF RHEUMATIC FEVER

Given these myriad microbial–host cross-reactions, what are the pathogenic mechanisms involved in these cross-reactions that might lead to the disease state? There are three main theories concerning the pathogenesis of rheumatic fever and they are listed in Table 29.1. Concerning the first theory, there is really no evidence to support the hypothesis that streptococci persist in the tissues of individuals with rheumatic fever. Repeated attempts to culture organisms from diseased valves have been unsuccessful[16] and a variety of techniques designed to localize bacteria in tissues have also been unsuccessful. The concept that toxins may play a role in disease pathogenesis has been considered by many investigators.[17] However, in general, animal studies showing the various effects of different streptococcal toxins have not been convincing. Yet, the possibility that one or more toxins may produce effects on target organs or vessels, thereby permitting an immunologic insult to the target organ, is certainly feasible but difficult to prove.

Most investigators concerned with the pathogenesis of rheumatic fever therefore now favor the third concept, namely, that the disease is a result of an abnormal immune response (humoral or cellular or both) on the part of the host to a given streptococcal infection. For instance, patients with rheumatic fever have higher antibody titers to streptococcal antigens such as streptolysin O (ASO) than do patients without rheumatic fever.[18] In addition, serum samples of patients with acute rheumatic fever

Table 29.1. Theories of Pathogenesis of Rheumatic Fever

I. Persistence of streptococci or antigens thereof in target tissues
II. Direct cardiac damage by toxin or toxins
III. Abnormal immune response to streptococcal antigens

contain antibodies that react with constituents of human heart tissue.[19,20] Antibodies are present in low titers or absent in uncomplicated streptococcal infections. Elevated antibody titers of antibodies to streptococcal antigens may reflect a greater antigenic challenge, although it should be emphasized that an asymptomatic streptococcal infection, so mild that the patient cannot recall symptoms of pharyngitis, will precipitate an attack of rheumatic fever.

Several observations support the idea that cell-mediated immunity is also important in the rheumatic process. (1) The rare occurrence of the disease before the age of 4 years suggests that several infections with the streptococcus are needed to sensitize the susceptible individual.[21] (2) Streptococcal antigens can be shown to induce delayed hypersensitivity in both animals and man.[22] (3) Examination of the human heart from persons with acute rheumatic fever reveals numerous lymphocytic infiltrates, both perivascular and between muscle bundles (GE Murphy, personal communication, 1985).

Bearing these background remarks in mind, let us now turn to the clinical manifestations of rheumatic fever and examine whether or not humoral and cellular immunity to streptococcal antigens cross-reactive with mammalian antigens play a role in the disease process.

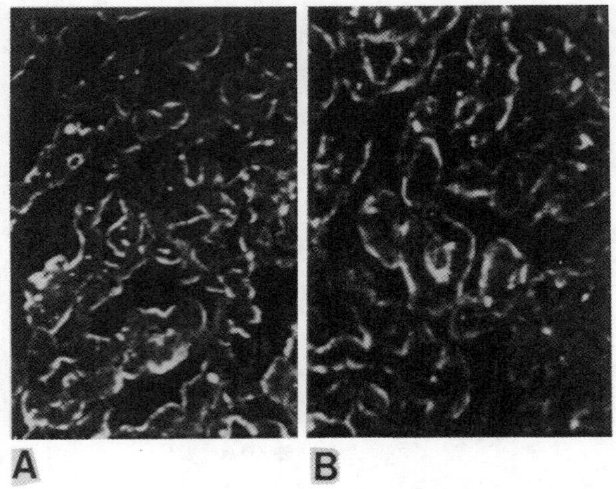

Figure 29.2. Immunofluorescent staining of patterns of frozen sections of heart tissue stained with sera containing heart-reactive antibody. *A*, Photomicrograph of the immunofluorescent pattern seen with a serum sample from a patient with acute rheumatic fever. *B*, Similar pattern obtained with a serum sample from a rabbit immunized with group A streptococcal membranes.

HUMORAL IMMUNITY

The finding that components of the group A streptococcus, when used as immunizing antigens, had the capacity to elicit an antibody that bound to cardiac tissue led to a search for similar antibodies in the serum samples of patients with recent streptococcal infections and their sequelae. When the serum from a patient with acute rheumatic fever is layered over a cardiac section and stained with a fluorescent conjugated anti-IgG antiserum, the staining pattern bears a striking resemblance to the pattern observed with antiserum samples of rabbits immunized with group A streptococci (Figure 29.2).

Examination of serum samples (Table 29.2) from patients with recent streptococcal infections and their sequelae revealed heart-staining antibody in most of them. As can be seen, three to four weeks after the onset of an uncomplicated streptococcal infection, serum samples from these patients had little or no heart-reactive antibody, whereas serum samples from patients with acute rheumatic fever had antibodies detectable at a tenfold dilution. The presence of these high titers of heart-reactive antibodies in the serum samples of patients with acute rheumatic fever has been an important additional diagnostic tool in cases of suspected rheumatic fever. Bright fluorescent staining of cardiac tissue at dilutions of serum greater than 1:10 is considered indicative of acute rheumatic fever. Furthermore, the absence of any significant levels of heart-reactive antibody in patients with other arthritic diseases coupled with the characteristic nuclear staining of serum samples from patients with lupus erythematosus has been helpful in the differential diagnosis of other rheumatic disorders.[19] Serial studies of serum samples obtained from patients with acute rheumatic fever reveal that the antibody declines rapidly during the first three to six months after the initial attack, then more gradually over the next two to three years. At the end of five years the vast majority of patients have little or no detectable antibody present in their serum unless there is intercurrent streptococcal infection or a recurrence of rheumatic fever. When viewed in light of the clinical observation that most rheumatic recurrences occur within the first two years after the initial attack and are rare after five years,[23] the presence of a heart-reactive antibody appears to have more than a casual relation to the disease process.

Table 29.2. Presence of Heart-Staining Antibody in Serum Samples of Patients with Streptococcal Infections

Diagnosis	No. of Patients	Dilutions of Sera Obtained in First 1-2 Weeks			Dilutions of Sera Obtained at Onset of Rheumatic Fever		
		1:5	1:10	1:20	1:5	1:10	1:20
Scarlet fever	25	++*	+	0	+	0	0
Scarlet fever with rheumatic fever	25	+++	++	0	++++	++	+
Other diseases†	28				0	0	0

* Refers to the intensity of immunofluorescent staining of heart tissue.

† Includes patients with rheumatoid arthritis and lupus erythematosus. These serum samples were obtained during active disease.

Our observations of long intervals between attacks and the appearance of heart-reactive antibody in the serum before a recurrence make it tempting to speculate that repeated streptococcal infections (perhaps with subclinical symptoms of disease) may be necessary to stimulate the production of heart-reactive antibodies. Only when the titers are sufficiently elevated does the full-blown disease complex appear. Examination of a small number of rheumatic fever recurrences has indicated that in each case elevated heart-reactive antibody titers were present at the time or just before the second attack.

If this increase in heart-reactive antibody in the serum is related to rheumatic heart disease, then one should be able to demonstrate gamma globulin in the rheumatic heart. Gamma globulin has been demonstrated to be bound to the sarcolemma of the heart of patients with rheumatic fever at the site of histologic damage. Knowledge concerning the nature and specificity of this immunoglobulin will be crucial to our further understanding of the role these antibodies play in the pathologic process.

With respect to valvulitis, serum samples of patients with rheumatic fever and rheumatic heart disease have been shown to contain antibodies that bind to N-acetylglucosamine, the carbohydrate specific to the group A streptococcus. Patients with valvular disease have higher titers of this antibody than do patients without valvular disease, and these antibodies persist for years after the initial attack.[24] In contrast, the titers of patients without valvular disease decline rapidly after the initial rheumatic insult. Persistence of high titers in patients with rheumatic valvular disease may be related to the slow and sustained release of valvular cross-reactive glycoproteins, thus perpetrating the valvular damage. It remains to be seen whether the presence of these antibodies is specific to patients with rheumatic fever or whether they also occur in patients with advancing arteriosclerotic heart disease and other forms of nonrheumatic heart disease.

Swelling of the major joints has always been one of the major features of rheumatic fever. Yet even this manifestation appears to vary from area to area. It has been our own experience, as well as that of other investigators, that incipient carditis without arthritis is often the major clinical manifestation of the disease in tropical areas of the world. Analysis of the synovial fluid in patients with well-documented rheumatic fever with arthritis[25] generally reveals a decrease in the complement components C1q, C3, and C4, indicating their consumption of immune complexes in the joint fluid.

More recently, we have noted the presence of high levels of circulating immune complexes in serum samples of patients with well-documented acute rheumatic fever,[26] which persists for several months after the acute attack. Friedman et al[27] in our laboratory have isolated these complexes and raised antibodies to them in the rabbit. The anti-complex antibody gives a reaction against extracellular products of a rheumatogenic strain, which is distinctly different from that seen with rabbit serum samples raised against complexes obtained from patients with poststreptococcal nephritis. These results also demonstrate that circulating complexes in patients with acute rheumatic fever do indeed contain streptococcal antigens within the complex. However, the nature of the antigens and their relation to the disease complex remain unknown.

Another mechanism for the observed synovitis in rheumatic fever could be antibodies to streptococcal antigens that bind to the smooth muscle of blood vessel walls.[9] Thus, one might envision vasculitis of the vessels secondary to streptococcal antibodies cross-reactive with smooth muscle cells of vessel walls, perhaps augmented by the circulating immune complexes in the serum samples of these patients. The fact that host immunoglobulins have been noted in the blood vessel wall in these patients makes this concept attractive, but still unproven.

The clinical syndrome of rheumatic chorea has always been an enigma to investigators studying the disease, because its major presenting signs are neurologic, not cardiologic in nature. However, recent data have demonstrated that serum samples of patients with Sydenham's chorea contain an antibody that binds to the cytoplasm of caudate nuclei in the thalamic and subthalamic area of the brain.[12] The appearance of this antibody also correlates well with the clinical course of the disease. The relation of this antibody to certain streptococcal cross-reactive antigens has been firmly established by the observation that streptococcal group A membranes completely abolished the immunofluorescent staining, whereas other streptococcal antigens did not. Unpublished data by our group also reveal that this antibody was present in spinal fluid in five well-documented cases of *acute* rheumatic chorea.

CELLULAR IMMUNITY

The question of whether cellular hypersensitivity to streptococci and their products plays a role in the pathogenesis of the nonsuppurative sequelae has been the subject of investigation for many years. Using skin tests as an index of delayed sensitivity to streptococcal products, several investigators have agreed that hypersensitivity to streptococci and their products is a common occurrence in man and increases in intensity with the age of the individual tested.[28] These reactions were also more intense in subjects with rheumatic disease than in nonrheumatic control subjects; the greatest number of positive reactions were obtained with autogenous streptococci, suggesting type specificity to the reaction.[29] Repeated streptococcal infections and exposure to their products may be vital to the disease process in view of the rarity of rheumatic fever before age 3 to 4 years.

During the past five years,[30] our laboratory has been reexploring this question of cellular reactivity to streptococcal antigens in patients with known sequelae of streptococcal infections, namely, rheumatic fever and poststreptococcal glomerulonephritis. Using two in vitro techniques of cellular reactivity to streptococcal antigens, our results to date indicate that patients with acute rheumatic fever have an increased cellular response compared with that of the controls, and this reactivity was primarily to membranes of those streptococcal strains commonly associated with rheumatic fever in Trinidad (Figure 29.3). This reaction persists for at least two years after the initial attack. Because this reactivity was not seen in patients with acute poststreptococcal glomerulonephritis (data not shown), a specific reactivity to these antigens in patients

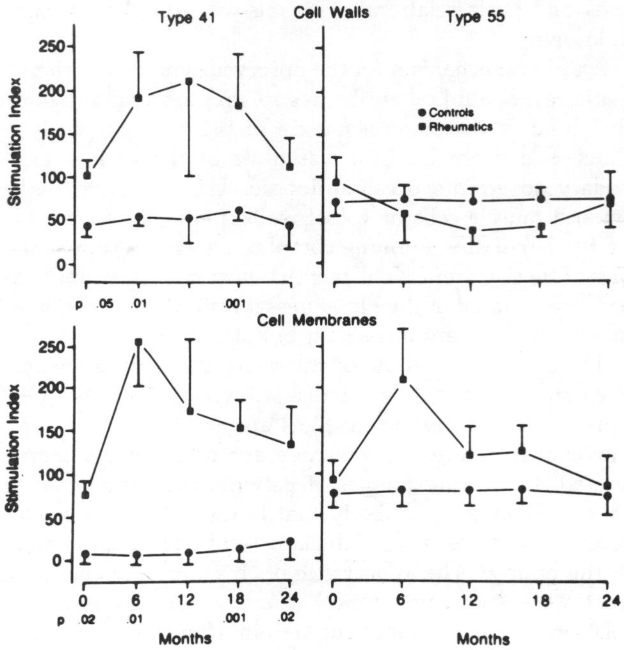

Figure 29.3. Stimulation indexes of mononuclear cell populations obtained from patients with rheumatic fever and control subjects to type 41 and type 55 streptococcal cell wall and membrane antigens. Note the prolonged heightened reactivity to type 41 antigens (*left side*) when compared with the lack of reactivity to type 55 antigens (*right side*).

with rheumatic fever is suggested. The exact nature of the antigen or antigens responsible for the observed reactivity is currently unknown.

Although these results strongly suggest a heightened response to streptococcal antigens in rheumatic individuals, the exact role these sensitized cells play in this disease process remains unknown. The present finding that there is abnormal *cellular* response to membrane antigens coupled with previous reports of an abnormal *humoral* response to the streptococcal membrane could argue strongly for a crucial role of this cell structure in the pathogenesis of rheumatic fever. The cross-reactive properties of these antigens might result in autosensitization to tissue antigens with cytotoxic effects in the host tissues. This concept agrees with the histologic findings in a large number of lymphocytic cells in and near the pathologic heart lesions of rheumatic fever. More recently, Raizada et al[31] also showed that most of the lymphocytes present in these pathologic lesions are of the T_4 helper subset of lymphocytes.

Concerning the cytotoxic activity of these sensitized cells, there are actually few reports that demonstrate target specific killing of these sensitized cells. Experimentally, Yang et al[32] showed that lymphocytes obtained from guinea pigs sensitized to group A streptococcal membrane streptococcus (and not to group A cell walls or group C membranes) were cytotoxic for guinea pig embryonic heart cell monolayers. A crucial and important point in these studies was their observation that guinea pig serum samples containing heart reactive antibody did *not* enhance the cytotoxicity, indicating that the observed cytotoxicity was an antibody independent cell-mediated reaction.

In terms of acute rheumatic fever, only the work of Hutto and Ayoub[33] in a small number of patients has demonstrated that mononuclear cell populations obtained from these patients were indeed cytotoxic for human heart cell monolayers. However, Gowrishankar and Agarwal[34] noted that lymphocytes obtained from patients with acute rheumatic fever exhibited heightened reactions to both streptococcal antigens and heart tissue, indicating that cells sensitized to both streptococcal and tissue antigens are present in these patients.

GENETICS

No discussion of rheumatic fever would be complete without reference to the possibility that individuals with rheumatic fever are perhaps genetically programmed to respond abnormally to a streptococcal infection. A little more than 80 years ago, it was pointed out that rheumatic fever frequently occurred in more than one member of an affected family.[35] Since that time, numerous investigators have postulated that there is an inherited susceptibility to rheumatic fever, but neither the mode of inheritance nor the methods of its expression have been satisfactorily delineated.

Although our efforts to find an association with gene products of either the HLA A or B locus were unsuccessful,[36] recent work in conjunction with that of Patarroyo et al[37] lends strong support to the existence of a genetic marker in patients with rheumatic fever. Using a serum containing a B-cell alloantibody called 883+, a positive reaction was found with the B cells of approximately 72% of all patients with rheumatic fever studied in either New York or Bogota, Colombia, suggesting that this genetic marker was worldwide in its distribution. Screening against a panel of known HLA A, B, C, and DR (D-related) specificities also indicated that this marker was not associated with any of the known HLA phenotypes.

Unfortunately, just when important questions concerning the nature and role of this antigenic marker in the disease process were being asked, the supply of this particular alloantiserum became exhausted, and attempts to find another multiparous serum with similar characteristics were unsuccessful. In an effort to remedy this situation, we have spent the past few years making hybridoma antibodies to the B-cell alloantigen isolated from patients who were originally designated 883+ by the 883+ serum. Our results to date have been successful (Table 29.3). Clone 83S19.23 identifies (with one exception) all patients originally described as 883+ by the multiparous alloantiserum. In addition, clone 256S10 identified five of the seven patients with rheumatic fever originally defined as 883− by the human alloantiserum. Therefore, the use of the two monoclonal antibodies has permitted us to correctly identify approximately 92% of all patients with rheumatic fever. In a preliminary survey of the frequency of the marker 83S19.23 in patients with rheumatic fever from different geographic areas, we noted that the frequency of this B-cell alloantigen is remarkably constant in patients with rheumatic fever for these areas (60% in New Delhi, 72% in New York, and 77% in New

Table 29.3. Comparison of the Original 883+ Rheumatic Fever Patients With Hybridoma Clones 83S19.23 and 256S10

Monoclonal Antibody	Patients with Rheumatic Fever (24)	Normal Subjects (24)
83S19.23*	17/24	5/24
256S10†	5/7	5/24

* Hybridoma clone isolated from animals immunized with B cells from 883+ rheumatic fever patients.

† Hybridoma clone isolated from animals immunized with B cells from 883− rheumatic fever patients.

Note: Assays were carried out by both immunofluorescence and cytotoxicity techniques.

Mexico) and suggests a worldwide distribution of the antigen. This marker is present in approximately 10% to 15% of the normal population, making this group of individuals at high risk of contracting the disease. Because studies of attack rates of rheumatic fever rarely exceed 5% in a given population, factors such as the virulence of the infection, the sensitivity state of the susceptible individual, and the host's response to the infection at the time must also contribute to the actual development of the disease in the susceptible individual.

To further refine our monoclonal genetic markers, a third clone called D8/17 has now been produced whose properties are somewhat different from those characterized by clones 83S19.23 and 256S10. In these experiments, we screened for an antibody that would identify a B-cell alloantigen present in *all* patients with rheumatic fever. Our data are quite promising, and Table 29.4 shows that all patients with rheumatic fever tested to date exhibit a marker present on their B cells. Once again this antigen does not appear to be a product of the HLA A, B, C, or DR loci. The presence of this marker is approximately 10% in the normal population.

Whether or not this antigen is present in other cells or acts as a streptococcal antigen receptor is currently unknown. Neither are we sure of the exact role of the B-cell marker in the production of the pathologic damage seen in rheumatic fever. However, the presence of a genetic marker, which indicates a high risk factor of contracting the disease, has broad public health implications.

AVENUES FOR FUTURE RESEARCH

Although current evidence strongly implicates an abnormal humoral and cellular response on the part of the host to the streptococcal antigens cross-reactive with host tissue, complete details leading to the final pathologic damage are still not completely resolved. However, a

Table 29.4. Frequency of the D8/17 Antigen in Patients With Rheumatic Fever, Normal Subjects, and Those With Other Diseases

Patients with rheumatic fever	69	69	100%
Normal subjects	40	4	10%
Patients with other diseases*	18	1	6%

* Including neurologic disease, poststreptococcal nephritis, and rheumatoid arthritis.

working hypothesis of the pathogenetic mechanisms involved in rheumatic fever is beginning to evolve and may be summarized briefly in the following manner. Exposure in a genetically susceptible individual to infection with the group A streptococcus gives rise to an exaggerated humoral and cellular response to those streptococcal antigens cross-reactive with human cardiac and muscle tissue. This reaction could be augmented or abetted by the uncovering of "buried" cross-reactive determinants in the host, perhaps as a result of a direct toxic effect on the tissues during the early stages of the infection (ie, the latent period). At a critical level of the exaggerated response, tolerance to the host's "self" antigens is broken. There is a direct attack on the host's tissues by cells sensitized to streptococcal antigens that are cross-reactive with heart, brain, or smooth muscle tissues. Experimental data suggest that circulating heart reactive antibody does not play a role in the cytotoxic effects of this cross-reaction. Data confirming these findings in human patients are still unproven.

What is now needed is a more thorough understanding at a molecular level of the exact nature of these cross-reactions. Work now in progress is aimed at isolating in pure form the streptococcal and sarcolemmal antigens responsible for the cross-reaction. Hopefully, sequence data of these proteins will more clearly define the homology between the two antigens and their relation to the M-protein cross-reactive antigens. In addition, knowledge concerning the nature of cardiac antigens responsible for binding of the patient's heart reactive antibody may provide answers as to whether the heart reactive antibody is in reality directed against membrane receptors such as the beta-adrenergic receptors. In the context of any contemplated vaccines, knowledge concerning these cross-reactions will be crucial to avoid sensitizing the individual with rheumatic fever to those tissue components that may actually lead to the disease process.

Turning to the question of the arthritic manifestations of the disease, circulating complexes containing streptococcal antigen and antibodies with perhaps a particular affinity for synovial receptors could account for this clinical manifestation of the disease. However, it cannot be forgotten that antibodies that bind to smooth muscle cells of blood vessel walls are also potentially capable of causing a generalized vasculitis with subsequent effects on joints, myocarditis, skin, and even mesenteric structures. More precise knowledge concerning the nature of the streptococcal antigens within the circulating complexes is needed to determine whether a specific antigen–antibody complex has an affinity for synovial cells or endothelial cells of blood vessel walls or both.

The question of the role of the 883+ marker in the disease process is still a moot point. Among the hypotheses to be considered are the following: (1) The antigen may be a receptor for streptococcal antigens and the immune response thereto. Preliminary work by Williams et al[38] has indicated that the receptors for streptococcal *membrane* antigens and the B-cell alloantigen (883+) are not the same. However, cell wall antigens and extracellular products were not tested in these studies, and the D8/17 antigen may be a specific receptor for these antigens. (2) The D8/17 antigen may be expressed on the heart and other tissues (tonsillar cells) that may be involved in the pathologic process. Persistence of these antigens in the individual susceptible to rheumatic fever (embryonic, minor histocompatibility antigens) might be more closely related to the streptococcal cross-reactive antigen and thus elicit a more vigorous immune response to the host's antigens. Experiments in progress will attempt to determine whether the D8/17 antigen exists on tissues other than lymphocytes such as the heart and smooth muscle.

As noted, although we still do not know the exact role of this genetic marker in the disease process, the ability to identify a group of individuals at risk has broad public health implications. For example, in Third World countries where budgets for health programs are limited, treatment of high risk individuals would be a priority in terms of both prevention of rheumatic fever and candidacy for any contemplated vaccine. In addition, if evidence accrues that only high risk individuals actually get rheumatic fever, the length of penicillin treatment for streptococcal infections in those individuals not bearing the B-cell alloantigens might be changed. It should be emphasized that these studies have not been carried out yet, so that the present regimen of treatment of all streptococcal infections is still advised.

In conclusion, the disease still presents a challenge that will require the continuing best efforts and thoughts of clinicians, epidemiologists, and basic researchers if we are eventually to completely understand this fascinating and as yet unsolved microbial–host interaction.

REFERENCES

1. Manjula BN, Fischetti VA: Tropomyosin-like seven residue periodicity in three immunologically distinct streptococcal M proteins and its implications for the antiphagocytic property of the molecule. *J Exp Med* 1980; 151:695–708.
2. Dale JB, Beachey EH: Protective antigenic determinant of streptococcal M protein shared with sarcolemmal membrane protein of human heart. *J Exp Med* 1982; 156:1165–1176.
3. Dale JB, Beachey EH: Epitopes of streptococcal M proteins shared with cardiac myosin. *J Exp Med* 1985; 162:583–591.
4. Goldstein I, Rebeyrotte P, Parlebas J, Halpern B: Isolation from heart valves of glycopeptides which share immunological properties with streptococcus haemolyticus group A polysaccharides. *Nature* 1968; 219:866–868.
5. Cromartie WH, Schwab JH, Craddock JG: The effect of a toxic cellular component of Group A streptococci on connective tissue. *Am J Pathol* 1960; 37:79–99.
6. Cromartie WJ, Craddock JG, Schwab JH, Anderle SK, Yang CH: Arthritis in rats after systemic injection of streptococcal cells or cell walls. *J Exp Med* 1977; 146:1585–1602.
7. Rapaport FT, Markowitz AS, McCluskey RT, Hanaoka T, Shimada T: Induction of renal disease with antisera to group A streptococcal membranes. *Transplant Proc* 1969; 1:981–984.
8. Kaplan MH, Frengley JD: Autoimmunity to the heart in cardiac disease. Current concepts of the relation of autoimmunity to rheumatic fever, postcardiotomy and postinfarction syndromes and cardiomyopathies. *Am J Cardiol* 1969; 24:459–473.
9. Zabriskie JB, Freimer EH: An immunological relationship between the group A streptococcus and mammalian muscle. *J Exp Med* 1966; 124:661–678.
10. Rapaport FT, Chase RM Jr: Homograft sensitivity induction by group A streptococci. *Science* 1964; 145:407–408.
11. Robert L, Fayolle J, Derouette S, Zabriskie J: Homology of aminoacid composition of structural glycoproteins, transplantation antigens, cell wall glycoproteins, and streptococcus A cell membrane. *Transplant Proc* 1972; 4:415–418.
12. Husby G, van de Rijn I, Zabriskie JB, Abdin ZH, Williams RC Jr: Antibodies reacting with cytoplasm of subthalamic and caudate nuclei neurons in chorea and acute rheumatic fever. *J Exp Med* 1976; 144:1094–1110.
13. Kingston D, Glynn LE: Anti-streptococcal antibodies reacting with brain tissue. I. Immunofluorescent studies. *Br J Exp Pathol* 1976; 57:114–128.
14. Lyampert IM, Kolesnikova VJ, Gnezditskaya EV, Danilova TA, Beletskaya LV, Borodiyuk NA: Cross-reactive antigens of group-A streptococci: their role in the autoimmune process, in Parker TM (ed): *Pathogenic Streptococci.* Chertsey, Surrey, England, Reedbooks, Ltd, 1979, pp 105–106.
15. Holm SE, Christensen P, Schalen C: Alternative interpretations of cross-reactions between streptococci and human tissues, in Parker TM (ed): *Pathogenic Streptococci.* Chertsey, Surrey, England, Reedbooks, Ltd, 1979, pp 72–74.
16. Watson RF, Hirsch GK, Lancefield RC: Bacteriological studies of cardiac tissues obtained at autopsy from eleven patients dying of rheumatic fever. *Arthritis Rheumat* 1961; 4:74–85.
17. Ginsberg I: Mechanisms of cell and tissue injury induced by group A streptococci: relation to post streptococcal sequelae. *J Infect Dis* 1972; 126:294–340.
18. Stollerman GH: *Rheumatic Fever and Streptococcal Infection.* New York, Grune & Stratton, 1975, pp 181–208.
19. Zabriskie JB, Hsu KC, Seegal BC: Heart-reactive antibody associated with rheumatic fever: characterization and diagnostic significance. *Clin Exp Immunol* 1970; 7:147–159.
20. Kaplan MH, Meyerserian M, Kushner I: Immunologic studies of heart tissue. IV. Serologic reactions with human heart tissue as revealed by immunofluorescent methods: isoimmune, Wassermann, and autoimmune reactions. *J Exp Med* 1961; 113:17–36.
21. Rantz LA, Maroney M, DiCaprio JM: Hemolytic streptococcal infection in childhood. *Pediatrics* 1953; 12:498–515.
22. Francis TC, Oppenheim JJ, Barile MF: Lymphocyte transformation by streptococcal antigens in guinea pigs and man, in Rieke WO (ed): *Proceedings of Third Annual Leucocyte Culture Conference.* New York, Appleton-Century-Crofts, 1969, pp 501–518.
23. Stollerman GH: *Rheumatic Fever and Streptococcal Infection.* New York, Grune & Stratton, 1975, pp 218–219.
24. Dudding BA, Ayoub EM: Persistence of streptococcal group A antibody in patients with rheumatic valvular disease. *J Exp Med* 1968; 128:1081–1098.
25. Svartman M, Potter EV, Poon-King T, Earle D: Immunoglobins and complement components in synovial fluid of patients with acute rheumatic fever. *J Clin Invest* 1975; 56:111–117.
26. Van de Rijn I, Fillit H, Brandeis WE, Reid H, Poon-King T, McCarty M, Day NK, Zabriskie JB: Serial studies on circulating immune complexes in post-streptococcal sequelae. *Clin Exp Immunol* 1978; 34:318–325.
27. Friedman J, van de Rijn I, Ohkuni H, Fischetti VA, Zabriskie JB: Immunological studies of post-streptococcal sequelae. Evidence for presence of streptococcal antigens in circulating immune complexes. *J Clin Invest* 1984; 74:1027–1034.
28. Read SE, Zabriskie JB: Immunological concepts in rheumatic fever pathogenesis, in Miescher PA, Müller-Eberhard HJ (eds): *Textbook of Immunopathology.* New York, Grune & Stratton, 1976, pp 471–487.
29. Plate JM, Amos DB: Studies on a lymphocyte activating factor from group A streptococci, in Rieke WO (ed): *Proceedings of Third Annual Leucocyte Culture Conference.* New York, Appleton-Century-Crofts, 1969, pp 485–499.
30. Read SE, Fischetti VA, Utermohlen V, Falk RE, Zabriskie JB: Cellular reactivity studies to streptococcal antigens. Migration inhibition studies in patients with streptococcal infections and rheumatic fever. *J Clin Invest* 1974; 54:439–450.
31. Raizada V, Williams RC Jr, Chopra P, Gopinath N, Prakash K, Sharma KB, Cherian KM, Panday S, Aurora R, Nigam M, Zabriskie JB, Husby G: Tissue distribution of lymphocytes in rheumatic heart valves as defined by monoclonal anti-T cell antibodies. *Am J Med* 1983; 74:90–96.
32. Yang LC, Soprey PR, Whittner MK, Fox EN: Streptococcal-induced cell-mediated-immune destruction of cardiac fibers in vitro. *J Exp Med* 1977; 146:344–360.
33. Hutto JH, Ayoub EM: Cytotoxicity of lymphocytes from patients with rheumatic carditis to cardiac cells in vitro, in Read SE, Zabriskie JB (eds): *Streptococcal Diseases and the Immune Response.* New York, Academic Press, 1980, pp 733–738.
34. Gowrishankar R, Agarwal SC: Leucocyte migration inhibition with human heart valve glycoproteins and group A streptococcal ribonucleic acid proteins in rheumatic heart disese and post-streptococcal glomerulonephritis. *Clin Exp Immunol* 1980; 39:519–525.
35. Cheadle WB: Harveian lectures on the various manifestations of the rheumatic state as exemplified in childhood and early life. *Lancet* 1889; 1:821–827, 871–877, 921–927.
36. Falk JA, Fleischman JL, Zabriskie JB, Falk RE: A study of HLA antigen phenotype in rheumatic fever and rheumatic heart disease patients. *Tissue Antigens* 1973; 3:173–178.
37. Patarroyo ME, Winchester RJ, Vejerano A, Gibofsky A, Chalem F, Zabriskie JB, Kunkel HG: Association of a B-cell alloantigen with susceptibility to rheumatic fever. *Nature* 1979; 278:173–174.
38. Williams RC Jr, Raizada V, Prakash K, Sharma KB, Anand I, Ganguly NK, Zabriskie JB: Studies of streptococcal membrane antigen-binding cells in acute rheumatic fever. *J Lab Clin Med* 1985; 105:531–536.

30 Rheumatic Heart Disease

K.G. Nair, MD, PhD and S. Sharma, MD

Rheumatic heart disease (RHD) is one of the most common cardiovascular conditions in hospitalized patients in the tropics. This is in contrast to the United States, Europe, and Australia where better living conditions and medical care have drastically reduced its incidence.[1] In the subcontinent of India with 700 million persons, about six children per 1,000 are stricken with rheumatic fever. Similar figures are found in the Middle East (Egypt, Sudan, Israel, and Iran); Far East (Burma, Indonesia, Thailand, Polynesia, and the Philippines); Latin America (Mexico, Peru, and Colombia); and in Mongolia and some parts of China. As four fifths of the world's children live in these areas, the magnitude of the problem may well be imagined. Prophylactic measures against RHD, therefore, will need the highest priority in any health program in these countries.[1a]

RHEUMATIC FEVER

Rheumatic fever is the sequel to a *Streptococcus pyogenes* infection. A preceding streptococcal sore throat infection is often found in about 50% to 60% of the patients. The prevalent view is that rheumatic fever is due to a hyperimmune response to a bacterial antigen that affects the connective tissues. The joints and heart are particularly affected. There is no doubt about a relation between infection with hemolytic streptococci of Lancefield's group A and rheumatic fever. It is possible that valvular heart disease may be further aggravated by cardiotropic viruses of the coxsackie B and echo group.

Two or three weeks following a streptococcal sore throat, serologic evidence of infection becomes manifest. Antistreptolysin-O (ASO) titers of 250 Todd units or more are considered indicative of the infection. Other specific antibody tests include antihyaluronidase, antistreptokinase, antinicotinamide-adenine dinucleotidase, and antideoxyribonuclease B.[1b] An antistreptozyme test (ASTZ) is available as a slide agglutination test.[1b] Several commercially available kits have now been developed for the rapid detection of group A streptococci from throat swabs.[1c]

Acute rheumatic fever is usually diagnosed by the modified Jones criteria.[2] These are as follows: *major criteria:* (1) carditis, (2) polyarthritis, (3) chorea, (4) subcutaneous nodules (Figure 30.1), and (5) erythema marginatum; *minor criteria:* (1) fever, (2) arthralgia, (3) prolonged PR interval, (4) elevated erythrocyte sedimentation rate, C-reactive protein, or leukocytosis, (5) evidence of preceding beta-hemolytic streptococcal sore throat infection, and (6) previous history of rheumatic fever or the presence of inactive RHD. Two major criteria or one major plus two minor criteria suggest a high probability of rheumatic fever. Currently, there is a strong trend to include arthralgia in the list of major criteria.[3]

ACUTE RHEUMATIC CARDITIS

DIAGNOSIS

Rheumatic carditis is the most serious manifestation of acute rheumatic fever; when severe, death may result from acute heart failure. More commonly, rheumatic carditis has no symptoms and it is diagnosed during examination of a patient who seeks medical attention because of arthritis or chorea. Patients whose rheumatic illness consists of asymptomatic carditis may develop RHD despite the absence of a medical history of recognized rheumatic fever.[4]

Clinically, patients with acute rheumatic carditis may have endocarditis, myocarditis, pericarditis, or any combination of them. Endocardial involvement is suggested by one or more of the following three murmurs:

1. A significant apical systolic murmur (mitral regurgitation) that is long, high-pitched, blowing, and at least grade II/VI in intensity.[2] It must be distinguished from the click-murmur syndrome associated with mitral valve prolapse and functional (innocent) murmurs.
2. An apical mid-diastolic murmur (Carey-Coombs murmur). It must be differentiated from the apical crescendo, presystolic rumble followed by an accentuated mitral first heart sound, which is indicative of established mitral stenosis rather than acute carditis.
3. A basal diastolic murmur (aortic insufficiency), especially in someone with no history of rheumatic fever. Care must also be taken to exclude a congenital bicuspid aortic valve.

Myocardial involvement is suggested by unequivocal cardiomegaly in a patient with no history of rheumatic fever, by an obvious increase in cardiac size in a patient with a history of RHD, or by congestive heart failure. Pericarditis is manifested by a friction rub, pericardial effusion (clinical, electrocardiographic, or echocardiographic), and rarely cardiac tamponade.[5]

TREATMENT

During the attack, benzathine penicillin G 1.2 million units intramuscularly or penicillin G 200,000 to 300,000 units every six hours for ten days should be given. Salicylates (100 to 150 mg/kg in children or 75 to 100 mg/kg in adults) or ibuprofen (400 to 800 mg, three times a day) are good antiinflammatory agents. Although most authorities endorse the use of steroids in patients with moderate to severe carditis, it is unclear whether they should be given to patients with milder forms of the disease, nor is it settled whether continuous steroid treatment for three weeks[6] or alternate day treatment for six weeks[7] is equally effective.

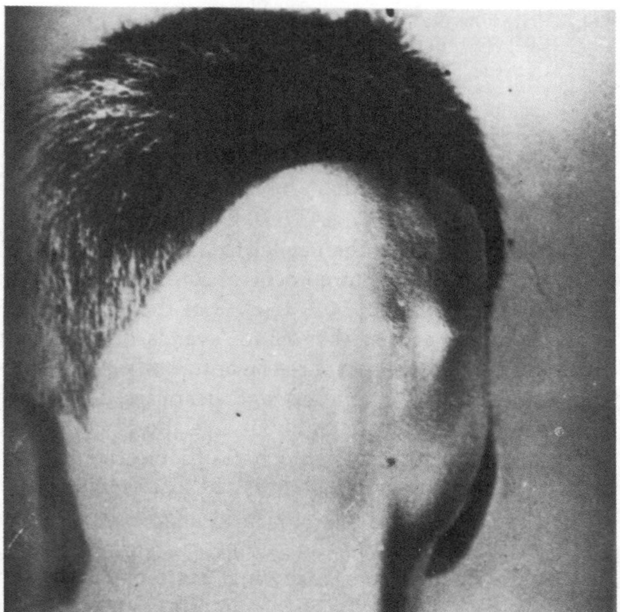

Figure 30.1. Rheumatic subcutaneous nodule on the scalp.

RHEUMATIC HEART DISEASE

Rheumatic heart disease involves principally the mitral and aortic valves. Tricuspid valve lesions are seen in about 10% of cases. The pulmonary valve is rarely involved.[8]

Varying degrees of myocardial damage and pericardial inflammation occur in all cases. About 10% of cases of rheumatic fever become manifest as acute pericarditis, always with underlying valvular involvement. Table 30.1 shows the frequency of valvular involvement in an autopsy study of 500 cases at King Edward VII Memorial Hospital in Bombay, by Kinare.[8]

MITRAL STENOSIS

PATHOLOGY

Rheumatic mitral stenosis is due to fusion of the valve commissures, thickening of the cusps, and pathologic distortion of the subvalvar apparatus. Fusion and contraction of the chordae tendineae, fibrosis, and calcification of the valve cusps occur in severe cases. The effective valve area may be reduced to 0.5 to 1.0 cm^2, leading to enlargement of the left atrium by pressure overload with varying degrees of compliance failure. A mural thrombus may be

Table 30.1. Frequency of Valvular Involvement in Rheumatic Fever

Valve	Percentage of Involvement
Mitral	99.6
Aortic	57.0
Tricuspid	42.7
Pulmonary	7.7
Isolated mitral	45.1
Isolated aortic	0.4
Mitral + aortic + tricuspid	19.6
Mitral + aortic	20.5
Mitral + tricuspid	6.6
Mitral + pulmonary	0.6
Mitral + aortic + pulmonary	0.6
Mitral + tricuspid + pulmonary	0.8
All four valves	5.7

present, usually above the fibrosed posterior cusp and involving the free wall of the left atrium (MacCallum's patch[9]). Narrowing of the mitral valve causes back-up pressure with pulmonary venous congestion, secondary pulmonary hypertension, and right ventricular pressure overload. Tricuspid and pulmonary valve incompetence is secondary to severe pressure overload on the right side of the heart. Lymphatic stasis and hemosiderosis of the lung accompany pulmonary venous congestion. Depending on the severity of the lesion, varying degrees of intimal thickening, medial hyperplasia, and even fibrinoid necrosis are seen in the pulmonary arteriolar bed. In very advanced cases, pulmonary thrombosis and calcification may be seen.

HEMODYNAMIC FEATURES

There are two disturbances in mitral stenosis: the primary problem is that of impaired left ventricular filling and the secondary problem is that of left atrial compliance failure. Impaired left ventricular filling results not only from narrowing of the mitral valvar orifice but also from restricted left ventricular cavity size due to thickening and distortion of the whole mitral subvalvar apparatus. Furthermore, the septum may be distorted and abut the left ventricular cavity when there is gross right ventricular hypertrophy. Both systolic and diastolic properties of the left ventricle are thus affected as judged by the decrease in stroke output, lower peak dp/dt, and prolonged isovolumic relaxation time with reduced peak filling rate. Dyskinesia of the posterior wall of the left ventricle is not infrequent.

Chronic left atrial pressure overload with compliance failure results in elevation of pulmonary capillary pressure. This elevation causes increased transudation of fluid as plasma oncotic pressure is exceeded in the capillaries. Lymphatic stasis, chronic venous congestion, and secondary pulmonary hypertension are the consequences. Multiple, small intrapulmonary hemorrhages cause hemosiderosis. The pulmonary arteriolar resistance rises as pathologic changes of pulmonary hypertension occur in the arteriolar bed. In addition, there is an element of vasoconstriction which further increases pulmonary vascular impedance. The right ventricular pressure must increase to provide the necessary forward flow. As pulmonary artery and right ventricular pressures rise, pulmonic and tricuspid valve regurgitation set in. Reflux into the right atrium causes right atrial volume overload with back-up pressure in the superior and inferior vena cava. Thus, there is systemic venous congestion.

If left ventricular size is above normal in a patient with mitral stenosis, the following associated conditions in descending order of frequency must be suspected: (1) mitral regurgitation, (2) aortic regurgitation, (3) ischemic heart disease, (4) hypertension, and (5) cardiomyopathy (eg, endomyocardial fibrosis). Systemic hypertension may result from embolization of renal vessels, and ischemic heart disease can also result from coronary artery embolization.[10] The source of the embolus is the left atrium.[10]

Severe, late-stage mitral stenosis may be mistaken for cardiomyopathy when the transmitral flow is markedly reduced and causes a faint diastolic murmur.

CLINICAL FEATURES

Symptoms

The symptoms of mitral stenosis may appear insidiously in the adult. However, in young children, the entire disease process may assume a malignant form with accelerated clinical signs and symptoms.

Dyspnea on effort is the first symptom. Fatigability is present, especially in those with atrial fibrillation, because of an inappropriate ventricular response to exercise. In the course of the disease, paroxysmal nocturnal dyspnea, cough with recurrent chest infection, and winter bronchitis will occur. Florid pulmonary edema may appear suddenly. Hemoptysis may be due to a variety of causes: chest infection, pulmonary infarction, pulmonary edema, or rupture of small lung vessels. Systemic emboli from the left atrium to the cerebral, renal, splenic, mesenteric, or limb vessels can occur. Pulmonary embolization may also occur from clots in the right atrium or venous plexus in the pelvis or legs.

Systemic venous congestion results in salt and water retention, oliguria, peripheral edema, pleural effusion, and ascites. Nocturia may be the first sign of reversal of the diurnal rhythm of sodium excretion.

Physical Examination

The patient is usually emaciated because of low cardiac output. A malar flush may be seen in light-skinned subjects. The pulse is of low amplitude and the rhythm may be irregular because of atrial fibrillation. A good volume pulse in the presence of mitral stenosis suggests coexisting aortic insufficiency. Previous embolization may cause an absence of pulse in one of the limbs. The jugular venous pulse should be examined for evidence of coexisting tricuspid valvular disease. A prominent a wave with a v wave showing a slow y descent indicates tricuspid stenosis. A large v wave with a rapid decrease suggests tricuspid insufficiency.

The precordial apical impulse is "tapping" because of a palpable first sound. Occasionally an opening snap may also be palpable. Pulmonary valve closure in severe cases may present as a diastolic shock. A left parasternal heave is usually due to an enlarged right ventricle with tricuspid regurgitation. Sometimes, an enlarged left atrium may push the right ventricle anteriorly and cause parasternal heaving. A sustained apical pulsation suggests coexisting left-sided disease or a large hypertrophied right ventricle. With the latter situation, the murmur of tricuspid regurgitation is usually present. Furthermore, an enlarged right ventricle will cause the lower half of the sternum to be dull on percussion.

Auscultatory findings are generally classic, and recognized, as Sir Thomas Lewis said, "like the bark of one's pet dog." The first sound is loud except in advanced cases in which the valve is unable to move rapidly because of severe fibrosis and calcification. It varies in intensity when there is atrial fibrillation. In sinus rhythm, a harsh presystolic murmur heralds the loud first sound. A loud second sound (pulmonary component) is followed by a sharp opening snap. The intensity of the opening snap depends on the pliancy of the anterior mitral cusp. The distance between the aortic closure sound (A_2) and the opening snap depends on the height of the left atrial pressure and the heart rate. The higher the left atrial pressure, the shorter the A_2-opening snap interval. The longer the prior diastolic cycle length, the wider the A_2-opening snap interval. However, when the latter becomes fixed irrespective of the preceding cycle length, a nonpliable stenotic mitral valve is usually present.[11] The opening snap is followed by a diastolic rumble. The presystolic murmur can easily be accentuated by exercise. Auscultation in the left lateral position is recommended.

A musical systolic murmur that increases on inspiration suggests tricuspid insufficiency. This murmur may be confused with that of mitral insufficiency, but its character, relation to the respiratory phase, and lack of radiation to the axilla will deny it. Liver pulsations will support the diagnosis of tricuspid insufficiency.

The presence of coexisting pulmonary insufficiency may be picked up by auscultating the upper left parasternal area, with the patient sitting up and in quiet expiration. The early diastolic murmur of Graham Steell is localized to the left sternal border. Before committing oneself to this diagnosis, all signs of aortic insufficiency, which may mimic the picture, must be carefully ruled out. Peripheral signs may be helpful in differentiating an aortic from a pulmonic origin.[12,13]

JUVENILE MITRAL STENOSIS

It is common to see young children with severe mitral stenosis in the hospitals of the Indian subcontinent. The appearance is typical (Figure 30.2). Their emaciated looks, retarded growth, and history of frequent sore throats cannot be missed.[14] The precordium bulges because of the enlarged heart. The loud S_1 and S_2 may even be evident on palpation. Acute or subacute rheumatic carditis is not infrequent. Severe pulmonary hypertension is a common feature. The disease may indeed take on a "malignant" form, requiring valvotomy during the teenage years.[15] Nearly 32% of patients die before the age of 20 years. Indeed, as much as 10% of mitral valve surgery is performed in patients under 20 years of age in the Indian subcontinent.[8,16]

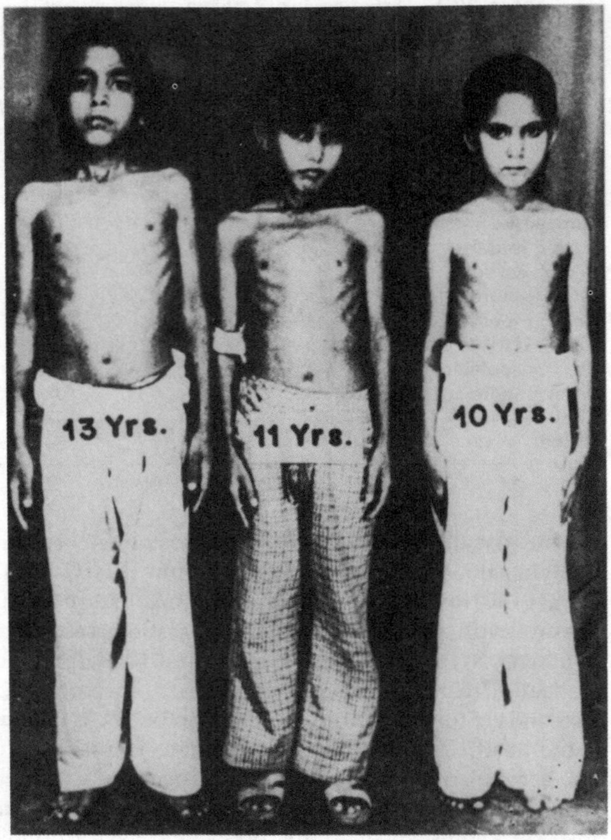

Figure 30.2. Typical growth retardation with emaciation in juvenile rheumatic heart disease.

ELECTROCARDIOGRAPHY

In mild cases the electrocardiogram may be normal. Early signs include a bifid P wave (P mitrale) most prominent in lead II, with a conspicuous negative deflection in lead V_1.[17] The P wave tends to be broad and occupies more than half the PR interval. It becomes peaked in the presence of tricuspid stenosis. When atrial fibrillation supervenes, the P wave is replaced by coarse fibrillary waves.

The QRS axis is generally vertical and points to the right with increasing pulmonary hypertension. A dominant R wave may be present in lead V_1. However, these electrocardiographic changes may not be clear even if there is underlying right ventricular hypertrophy. Palpation of the precordium may be a more reliable index of right ventricular hypertrophy.

In juvenile mitral stenosis with "malignant" progress, the right ventricular hypertrophy is usually severe with tall R waves in leads V_1 to V_4 and deep T-wave inversion due to right ventricular "strain" (Figure 30.3).

CHEST X-RAY

The x-ray appearance, like the auscultatory findings, is typical (Figure 30.4). The ventricular size may be normal or increased. Selective enlargement of the left atrium with straightening of the left heart border is the first sign. A penetrated posteroanterior film will reveal a double outline on the right side, the shadow within being that of

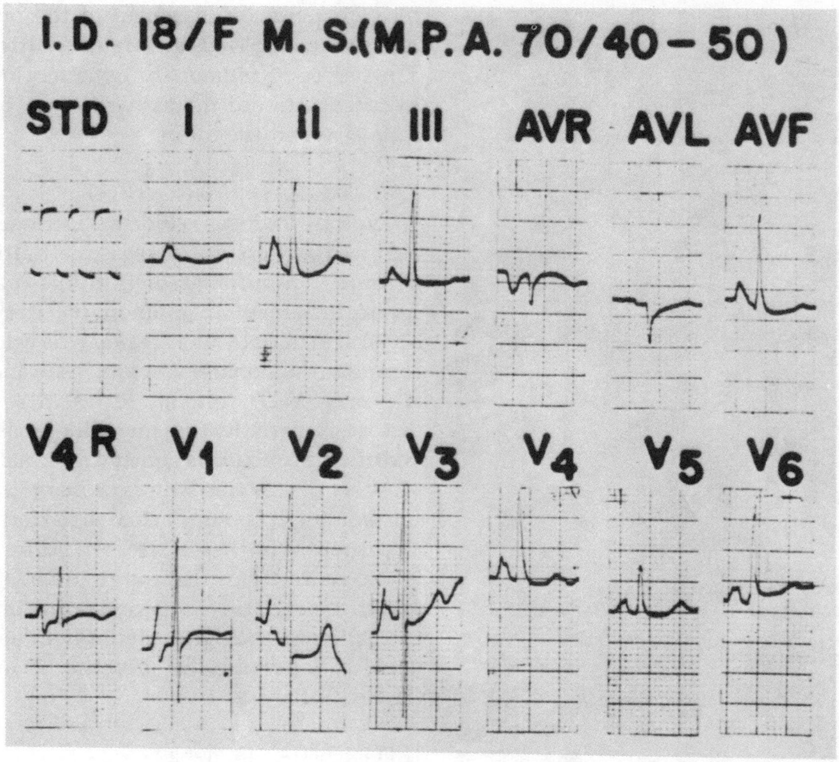

Figure 30.3. Typical electrocardiogram in juvenile mitral stenosis. Note severe right ventricular hypertrophy and biatrial enlargement.

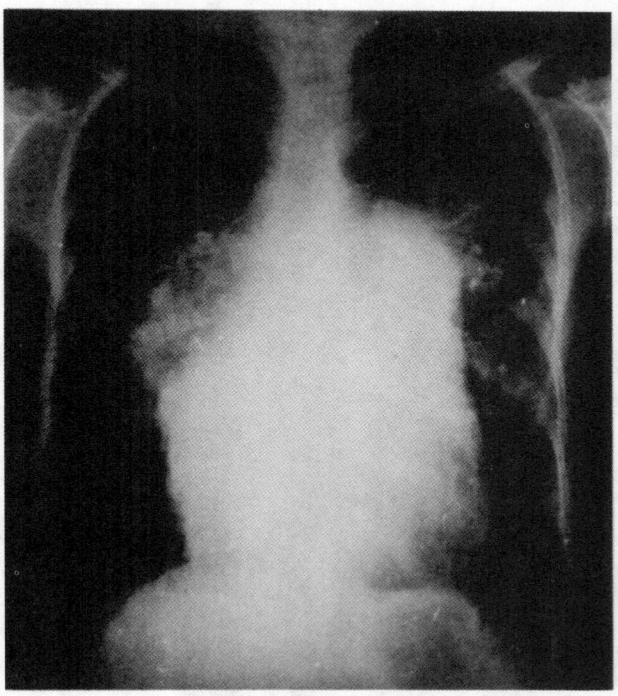

Figure 30.4. Typical x-ray silhouette of the heart and lungs in a young subject with severe mitral stenosis and pulmonary hypertension.

the enlarged left atrium. The left bronchus is raised, giving a wide carinal angle, and barium swallow will reveal indentation of the esophagus by the left atrium. Screening under image intensification may show mitral valve calcification. In the lungs, the upper lobe pulmonary veins are prominent. An increase in the width of the pulmonary artery indicates pulmonary hypertension. With left atrial pressures reaching 25 mm Hg or above, lymphatic lines (Kerley's B lines) show up at the bases. Also, basal pleural effusion, hazy shadowing, and pulmonary edema may be present. In severe cases hemosiderosis and even bone formation may be seen.

ECHOCARDIOGRAPHY

M-mode echocardiography will immediately reveal a reduction in the EF slope which represents the mid-diastolic closure rate (Figure 30.5). A slope of 35 mm per second or less represents moderate mitral stenosis, whereas 0 to 20 mm per second indicates a severe form.[18] The posterior cusp movement is forward in diastole, because of fusion. Thus, the two cusps move in the same direction. Thick echoes with poor amplitude of valve excursion indicate fibrosis and calcification of the valve (Figure 30.6). Two-dimensional echocardiography, in the short-axis view, gives a direct estimate of the valve area. In the long-axis parasternal view the anterior cusp usually has a "hockey-stick" deformity and its restricted motion can be appreciated. Atrial thrombi may be noted in about 60% of cases. Left ventricular wall motion analysis will reveal abnormalities in filling. Obstruction to diastolic filling can also be picked up on Doppler echocardiogra-

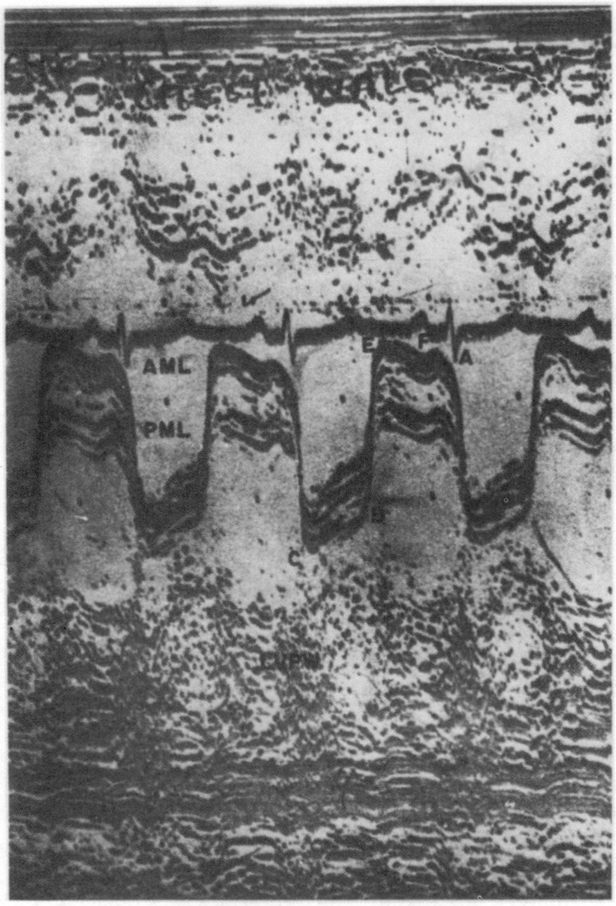

Figure 30.5. M-mode echocardiogram demonstrating a flat EF slope with paradoxic movement of the posterior mitral cusp.

phy. Posterior displacement of the interventricular septum indirectly suggests right ventricular hypertrophy. The degree of pulmonary hypertension may be assessed by attenuation of the early diastolic posterior motion of the valve and the a dip.

CARDIAC CATHETERIZATION

Typical findings include an increase in pulmonary artery wedge pressure, increased left atrial pressure with a definite transmitral gradient in diastole, and a commensurate increment in pulmonary artery pressure (Figure 30.7). The mitral valve area may be calculated by Gorlin's formula. Pulmonary vascular resistance is usually high and may reach systemic levels in severe forms of the disease, especially the juvenile "malignant" type. Left ventricular function is generally normal, but in adults over 40 years of age coexisting coronary artery disease is not uncommon. It is our practice to perform routine coronary angiography in these cases. An aortic root dye injection is also routinely carried out to define the degree of aortic insufficiency, if any. Left ventricular injection of dye with the patient in the right anterior oblique position is always used to determine the presence of mitral insufficiency (Figure 30.8).

DIFFERENTIAL DIAGNOSIS

Diagnosis includes left atrial myxoma, cor triatriatum, and, rarely, pulmonary venoocclusive disease. Also, an Austin-Flint murmur can sometimes be misleading.

Left atrial myxoma produces a variable diastolic murmur dependent on body position, raised erythrocyte sedimentation rate, fever, altered plasma proteins, and systemic embolization. The two-dimensional echocardiographic picture will instantly reveal the mass, and the

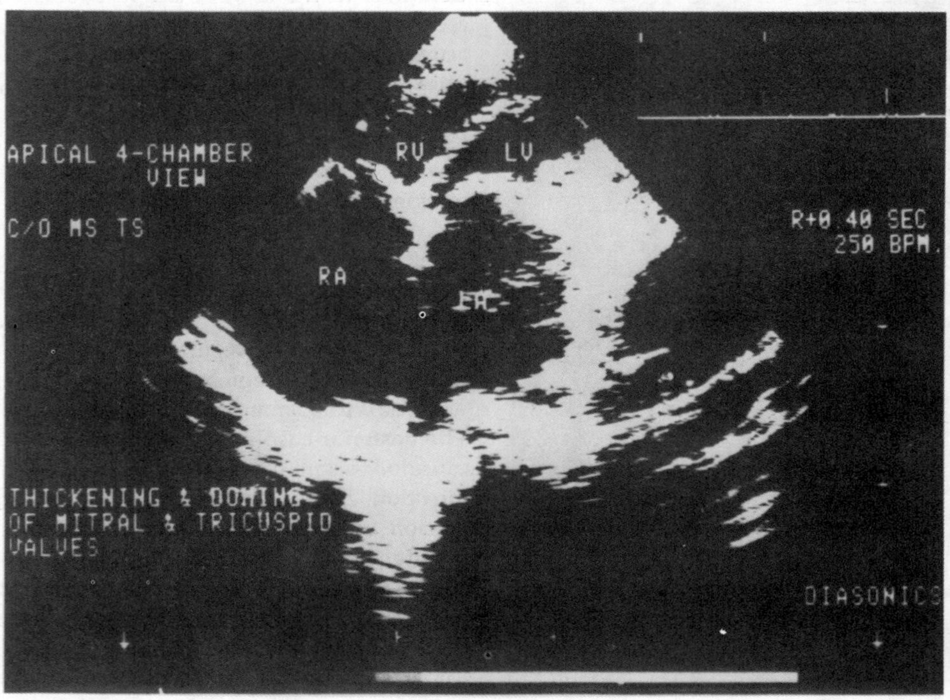

Figure 30.6. Apical four-chamber view in mitral stenosis with tricuspid stenosis. Note thickening and doming of both atrioventricular valves.

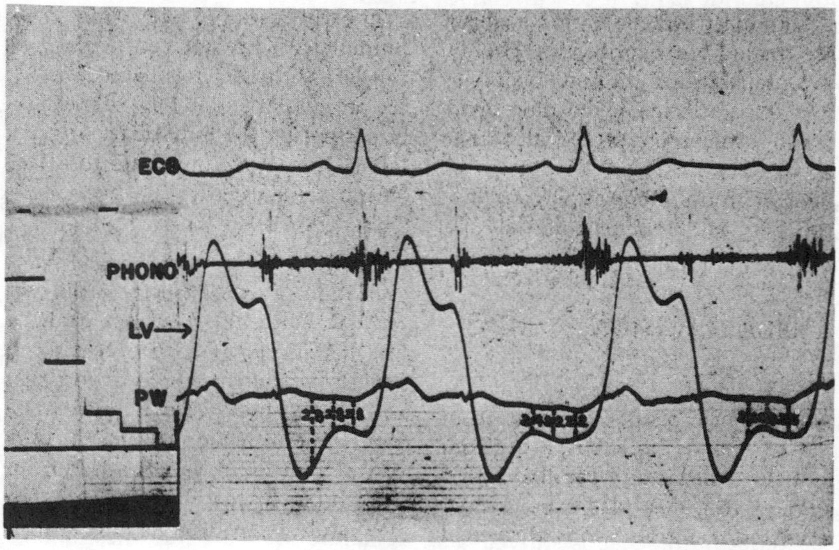

Figure 30.7. Diastolic transmitral gradient in mitral stenosis. LV = left ventricular pressure; PW = pulmonary artery wedge pressure.

M-mode echocardiographic study shows the dense bands of echoes behind the mitral valve in diastole.

An Austin-Flint murmur is usually heard in severe aortic insufficiency. S_1 may be loud and the murmur in diastole may have a presystolic accentuation. However, an opening snap is never present and an echocardiographic study will reveal the flutter of the anterior mitral cusp with a normal EF slope of the valve.

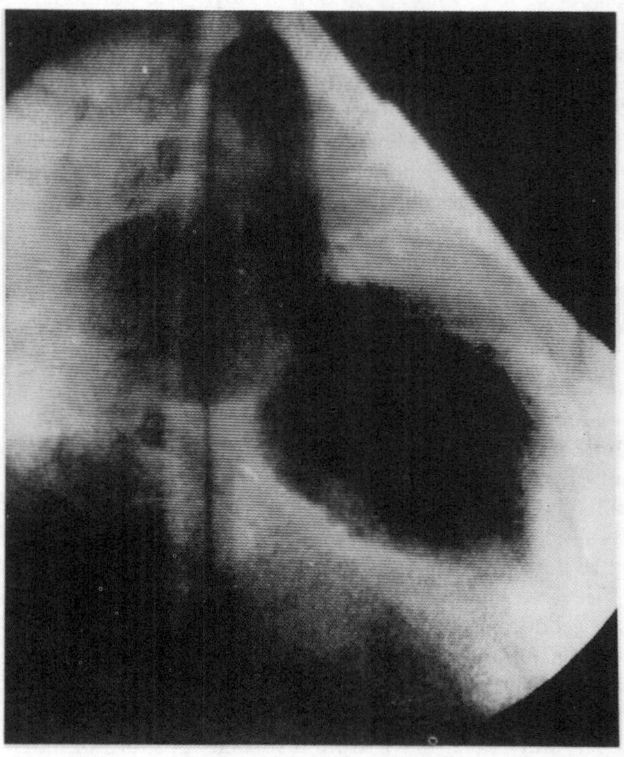

Figure 30.8. Cineangiocardiogram in mitral regurgitation. Note massive systolic reflux of contrast material into left atrium.

When mitral stenosis coexists with an atrial septal defect (Lutembacher's complex), the heart size is usually large with pulmonary plethora, and atrial fibrillation is not uncommon.

TREATMENT

Medical management cannot relieve the obstruction in mitral stenosis. Therefore, efforts should be directed at prevention of rheumatic fever and infective endocarditis. Penicillin is the drug of choice for prophylaxis. Benzathine penicillin, 0.6 million units for children and 1.2 million units for adults, is to be given every three weeks by deep intramuscular injection. Prophylaxis is desirable up to late adult life. It should be noted that, for rheumatic fever chemoprophylaxis in developing countries, administration of benzathine penicillin injections should be once every 3 rather than 4 weeks as recommended by World Health Organization,[1a] regardless of patient age and weight. Prophylaxis is also necessary after cardiac surgery to prevent relapses. Oral phenoxymethyl penicillin (penicillin V), 125 to 250 mg four times a day, is an alternative to injection therapy, but somewhat unreliable because of missed doses.

Penicillin allergy is a known phenomenon and needs to be watched for. Injection adrenaline should be available at the time of injection. Allergic subjects may be given 1 g of sulfadimidine or sulfadiazine orally. Erythromycin, 250 mg twice a day, is also an alternative choice. None of these methods is as satisfactory as intramuscular benzathine penicillin. Prophylaxis of infective endocarditis for dental procedures and other situations associated with transient bacteremia should be followed (see chapter 46 on Infective Endocarditis).

Digitalis preparation is the drug of choice to control the ventricular rate in atrial fibrillation. Verapamil is useful in controlling the irregular response. Prenylamine lactate also slows the ventricular response and improves ventricular filling. Diuretic therapy is essential to prevent fluid retention; potassium chloride is given concurrently to avoid hypokalemia. Pulmonary infection and tonsillitis should be appropriately treated with antibiotics. Highly immunogenic M protein preparations are now available. It may be soon possible for a vaccine to be developed that is specifically useful against streptococcal throat infections.

The surgical treatment of mitral stenosis will be discussed in chapter 32 on Surgical Treatment of Valvular Heart Disease.

MITRAL REGURGITATION

PATHOLOGY

Mitral valvular incompetence results directly from shortening and fibrosis of one or both cusps or from shortening and fusion of the chordae and papillary muscles. Dilatation of the valve ring may also cause regurgitation. Typically the posterior mitral cusp is shrivelled up and the valve ring is dilated. In late cases calcification may occur. Varying degrees of mitral stenosis may coexist with mitral incompetence.

HEMODYNAMIC FEATURES

The left ventricle has an opportunity to regurgitate blood through a low resistance orifice into the left atrium (Figure 30.8). The relative amount that flows backward into the left atrium (regurgitant volume) depends on the relative resistance to forward flow. The pressure buildup in the left atrium depends on its compliance: in a large or giant left atrium secondary to longstanding mitral regurgitation, the pressure will be normal or low,[19] whereas in acute severe mitral regurgitation into a normal or small tight left atrium, high venous pressures may build up.[20] High left atrial pressures lead to pulmonary hypertension. Left ventricular volume overload results in dilatation and hypertrophy of the chamber. In pure mitral regurgitation the stroke output is increased, and if the systemic resistance is decreased, the pulse may acquire a "small water-hammer" character.

CLINICAL FEATURES

In early cases the patients are in sinus rhythm. Later, and especially in patients with a large left atrium, atrial fibrillation supervenes. A history of palpitations is not uncommon. The pulse has a rapid upstroke and is usually rapid. The apex impulse is prominent because of volume overload. It is dynamic but not sustained; S_3 may be palpable. There may also be a left parasternal heave caused by an enlarged left atrium pushing the right ventricle forward. S_1 is either normal or reduced in intensity. A pansystolic murmur of varying intensity is present, radiating to the left axilla and terminating at the origin of the S_2. This is followed by an S_3 which may be high pitched in a nondilated active left ventricle or low pitched in a large, failing left ventricle.

Because of the "shortchanging" of the forward output and reflux into the left atrium, aortic closure may appear earlier than normal. Splitting of the S_2 is therefore easily appreciable. Increased left atrial pressure results in pulmonary hypertension; thus, P_2 is accentuated.

CHEST X-RAY

In early cases the left atrium is enlarged, filling up the pulmonary bay. Left ventricular volume overload causes the left ventricle to enlarge also. The pulmonary veins are prominent and in long-standing cases with pulmonary hypertension the pulmonary artery is prominent. A giant left atrium may contribute to a large cardiac silhouette. Mitral valve calcification may be present.

ELECTROCARDIOGRAM

In mild cases the electrocardiogram shows nothing abnormal. With increased left ventricular volume overload and left atrial pressure overload, changes reflecting left atrial enlargement and left ventricular hypertrophy begin to appear. The P wave is bifid in standard leads and has a negative deflection in lead V_1. In late stages conduction disturbances such as left anterior hemiblock, left bundle branch block, and 1° heart block may appear. Ventricular premature beats are not uncommon.

ECHOCARDIOGRAM

In an M-mode study the valve excursion will be higher than normal. The early diastolic opening slope is more rapid. The two-dimensional echocardiographic study will show poor leaflet coaptation and a volume overloaded enlarged left ventricle. Occasionally, clots in the left atrium may be detected. However, regurgitant flow is best judged by the Doppler technique.[20a,20b]

CARDIAC CATHETERIZATION AND ANGIOGRAPHY

The left atrial pressure tracing will reveal tall V waves because of the systolic regurgitant flow. The pulmonary capillary wedge pressure is usually elevated, and correspondingly there is pulmonary arterial hypertension. In some cases the pulmonary artery pressure may even reach systemic levels. Left ventricular angiography demonstrates reflux of dye into the left atrium. Mitral valve prolapse and calcification may be noted. Depending on the degree of valvular insufficiency, the size of the left ventricle may be normal or grossly enlarged.

A giant left atrium may be seen in advanced cases. Intramural clots are better detected by angiography than by two-dimensional echocardiography.

DIFFERENTIAL DIAGNOSIS

A congenital ventricular septal defect may superficially mimic the physical signs of mitral insufficiency. The murmur of a ventricular septal defect does not radiate to the axilla. Furthermore, an x-ray film of the chest would reveal active pulmonary plethora in cases of ventricular septal defects.

Tricuspid insufficiency with an enlarged right ventricle may produce an apical systolic murmur. However, the murmur increases on inspiration and generally has a musical quality. In endomyocardial fibrosis, the large right atrium may push the right ventricle downwards and to the left and a musical tricuspid insufficiency murmur may be heard only at the apex. Here, a two-dimensional echocardiographic study will immediately clarify the picture. Obliteration of the outflow tract of the right ventricle, the apical clot, and the Doppler study of flow across the mitral and tricuspid valves are all very characteristic of endomyocardial fibrosis.

Nonrheumatic mitral regurgitation due to mitral valve prolapse, myoxmatous degeneration of the valve, ruptured papillary muscle, and papillary muscle dysfunction due to coronary diseases can also present a problem in differential diagnosis. With mitral valve prolapse the heart sounds are usually clear and loud and a typical nonejection midsystolic click may be heard. Furthermore, the apical murmur is late systolic, not pansystolic, unless the prolapse is severe. With papillary muscle rupture the clinical progress is acute and downhill. Pulmonary edema followed by cardiogenic shock is the end result.

Heavy calcification of the mitral valve anulus is generally seen in elderly women and is a known cause of mitral regurgitation. Conduction abnormalities such as atrioventricular block or bundle branch block may be present. Two-dimensional echocardiographic study will demonstrate intense band-like echoes just behind the posterior mitral cusp.

TREATMENT

Apart from penicillin prophylaxis, mild mitral regurgitation does not need any special treatment. As the disease progresses, digitalis and diuretics will be needed. Vasodilator therapy is also useful in promoting forward flow and improving cardiac performance. Several drugs including nitroprusside,[21] hydralazine,[22] and verapamil[23] have been tried with various degrees of success and also some adverse side effects. In severe cases mitral valve repair[24,25] or replacement is the only answer. In patients who are unable to follow anticoagulant therapy after surgery, a bioprosthetic valve is the valve of choice. For further discussion, please refer to chapter 32 on Surgical Treatment of Valvular Heart Disease.

AORTIC INCOMPETENCE

Rheumatic aortic incompetence occurs in about 30% of patients with RHD admitted to the hospital. It is frequently associated with mitral or aortic stenosis. In some cases of mitral stenosis, the associated aortic insufficiency may be mild and it may be detected only by angiocardiography or Doppler echocardiographic studies.

PATHOPHYSIOLOGY

With regurgitant flow the stroke volume increases proportionately and it may be accompanied by vasodilatation, which helps forward flow. The powerful percussion wave in the aorta followed by the rapid upstroke of the radial pulse is most characteristic of the condition. The pulse is of large volume and collapses quickly, giving a "water hammer" effect. Standing waves in the large blood vessels may generate a "pistol shot" sound. Additional aortic stenosis confers a bisferious quality to the brachial pulse. Left ventricular hypertrophy with cavity dilatation occurs because of the volume overload. Finally, left ventricular failure supervenes.

CLINICAL FEATURES

Most patients tolerate aortic regurgitation well and remain asymptomatic for many years. Early symptoms include palpitation and breathlessness. Exertional or paroxysmal nocturnal dyspnea signifies elevated left ventricular end-diastolic pressure. Chest pain is usually due to reduced coronary perfusion in diastole or coexisting coronary artery disease.

The physical findings of aortic regurgitation are typical. The pulse is collapsing in nature (Corrigan's sign) and is best appreciated in the carotid artery. Capillary pulsation in the nail beds (Quincke's sign), nodding of the head with the heartbeat (de Musset's sign), and Duroziez's murmur are all characteristic of aortic insufficiency. Duroziez's murmur is elicited by compressing the femoral artery with the chest-piece of the stethoscope and listening for the retrograde flow murmur in diastole.

The left ventricular impulse is hyperactive because of volume overload, but it is never sustained unless there is coexisting aortic stenosis. On auscultation, the S_1 is normal or soft, S_2 is split, and an early or immediate diastolic murmur is heard along the left sternal edge. It is best heard with the patient sitting up and in quiet expiration. P_2 is loud only if there is pulmonary hypertension caused by elevated left ventricular end-diastolic pressure.

Regurgitant flow causes the anterior mitral cusp to go into a flutter, producing the Austin-Flint murmur, a murmur in mid-diastole that mimics mitral stenosis but there is no associated opening snap.

CHEST X-RAY

The left ventricle is generally enlarged because of volume overload. The aortic root is dilated. The aortic valve may be calcified, especially with associated aortic stenosis. The pulmonary vasculature is normal until the late stage, when because of elevated left ventricular end-diastolic pressure, pulmonary venous congestion develops.

ELECTROCARDIOGRAM

The electrocardiogram reveals left ventricular hypertrophy. Tall R waves with peaked T waves in left precordial leads indicate left ventricular diastolic overload. In severe cases there is left ventricular "strain" and the T waves are inverted in the left-sided precordial leads. Left bundle branch block and 1° atrioventricular block may develop. Left anterior hemiblock is also not uncommon.

ECHOCARDIOGRAM

Left ventricular cavity size is enlarged. The diastolic fluttering of the anterior cusp of the mitral valve is the echocardiographic counterpart of the Austin Flint murmur on auscultation. Elevated left ventricular end-diastolic pressure may cause mitral valve pre-closure. Premature opening of the aortic valve cusps, before the onset of ejection, may be noted. Two-dimensional echocardiography gives a measure of aortic root size, a value often required by the surgeon. Doppler echocardiography is ideal for quantification of the regurgitant flow and for detecting early aortic insufficiency sometimes not detected by auscultation.[25a,25b]

CARDIAC CATHETERIZATION AND ANGIOGRAPHY

Regurgitant flow is best demonstrated by cineangiocardiography, with dye injection in the aortic root, or by digital subtraction angiography. Although digital subtraction angiography generally yielded results comparable to those of conventional cineangiography in the quantitation of mitral regurgitation, it tended to overestimate the severity of aortic regurgitation.[26] Left ventricular end-diastolic pressure is usually normal until the late stage of the disease. A coexisting transmitral diastolic gradient may be detected in the presence of mitral stenosis. Varying degrees of aortic stenosis may produce a transaortic systolic gradient, although a small early systolic gradient in the presence of marked aortic regurgitation could be "functional" in nature.

DIFFERENTIAL DIAGNOSIS

Other causes of a rapid aortic run-off include patent ductus arteriosus, ruptured aneurysm of the sinus of Valsalva, and ventricular septal defect with aortic incompetence. Rarely, a coronary arteriovenous fistula or coronary-cameral fistula may mimic the picture. Cineangiography will almost always provide the answer.

TREATMENT

Mild to moderate aortic insufficiency is so well tolerated that surgical intervention is usually not warranted. Only penicillin prophylaxis is recommended. Vasodilator agents, including nitroprusside,[27] hydralazine,[28] prazosin,[29] nifedipine,[30] and verapamil,[23] have been used with various degrees of success. Their usefulness on a long-term basis, however, requires further study.[31]

Increasing left ventricular size with the presence of symptoms indicates the need for valve replacement. Unfortunately in a subset of such patients irreversible changes in left ventricular function have already occurred, so that even after successful surgical correction of aortic regurgitation congestive heart failure or persistent cardiomegaly as well as depressed left ventricular function may develop.[32] Preoperative evaluation of ejection fraction and left ventricular pressure/volume relation at rest and following exercise by radionuclide ventriculography[32–36] and of end-systolic dimension, left ventricular fractional shortening, and end-systolic stress-percent fractional shortening relation by M-mode echocardiography[32,36,37] may help to identify patients who, while still asymptomatic or minimally symptomatic, require surgical intervention. A recent report[37a] showed that aortic valve replacement is superior to medical therapy, with or without long-term hydralazine, in patients with symptomatic chronic aortic regurgitation. For surgical treatment please see chapter 32 on Surgical Treatment of Valvular Heart Disease.

AORTIC STENOSIS

PATHOLOGY

Pure rheumatic aortic stenosis occurs in 0.4% of all cases of RHD. However, it seldom exists as an isolated lesion. Indeed, a case of pure aortic stenosis is more likely to be one of congenital bicuspid aortic valve.[37b] In cases of rheumatic origin it is frequently associated with aortic insufficiency and a mitral valvular lesion.

PATHOPHYSIOLOGY

The presence of fixed outflow tract obstruction like aortic stenosis leads to a systolic pressure gradient between the left ventricle and the aorta. The gradient may rise steeply on exertion. Due to pressure overload the left ventricle develops concentric hypertrophy. Increased diastolic stiffness of the ventricle causes the left atrial filling pressure to increase, resulting in pulmonary hypertension. In late cases the ventricular chamber dilates and there is pulmonary congestion. The aortic valve may undergo calcification which, due to mitral aortic continuity, may spread to the mitral valve. The PR interval may become prolonged when the adjacent atrioventricular node is involved in the calcific process.

Coexisting coronary artery disease may further affect left ventricular function adversely.

CLINICAL FEATURES

Dyspnea on exertion, chest pain, and a history of syncope are common in hemodynamically significant cases. As left ventricular end-diastolic pressure becomes elevated in the late stages of the disease, the patient develops paroxysmal nocturnal dyspnea. Anginal chest pain may be due to inappropriate coronary flow in a hypertrophied ventricle or to coexisting coronary artery disease. Although there is a 50:50 chance of significant coronary artery disease in patients with aortic stenosis who have angina, the absence of angina in these patients practically excludes the possibility of coronary artery disease.[38] The cause of syncope in aortic stenosis remains uncertain. Suggested mechanisms include carotid sinus reflex hypersensitivity,[39] arrhythmias,[40] acute left ventricular failure,[41] and left ventricular baroreceptor activation.[42,43] In severe cases, sudden death may occur, usually caused by a short burst of ventricular tachycardia or fibrillation.

PHYSICAL EXAMINATION

The brachial pulse is of a slow rising character. With associated aortic incompetence it may assume a bisferious quality. In the carotid artery, a systolic thrill may be felt. The jugular pulse is usually normal, but in severe cases with pulmonary hypertension a small a wave is noted, probably due to altered compliance of the right ventricle because of a bulging interventricular septum.

The apex beat is forceful and well sustained. An additional thrust caused by a palpable left-sided atrial gallop may be felt. On auscultation S_1 is normal or reduced in intensity and is preceded by a loud S_4. The S_2 is single or paradoxically split. When pulmonary hypertension due to elevated left ventricular end-diastolic pressure is present, P_2 is loud.

A typical midsystolic ejection murmur is heard over the aortic area radiating along the left sternal edge to the apex and also to the carotid artery. In severe cases the murmur may be heard even in the elbow, over the olecranon process, because of bone conduction. In advanced cases the murmur may not be loud because of a low cardiac output. In such "burnt-out" cases, aortic stenosis may be missed and the case may be wrongly diagnosed as one of cardiomyopathy. In most cases an early or immediate diastolic murmur may be heard because of associated aortic regurgitation.

CHEST X-RAY

With concentric hypertrophy, the heart size is increased. When left ventricular end-diastolic pressure is elevated, the pulmonary veins will be engorged. The aortic root is usually dilated (poststenotic dilatation). Aortic valve calcification may be present and is best seen by image intensification fluoroscopy.

ECHOCARDIOGRAM

In early cases echocardiographic study may show nothing abnormal. With advancing years, the mobility of the valve becomes reduced. The M-mode study reveals a characteristic box-like contour of the aortic cusps. Dense reflections due to calcium may appear. Two-dimensional echocardiographic study will clearly show immobility of the valve and the reduced orifice size. Left ventricular and septal hypertrophy with scattered areas of fibrosis can be detected. In severe cases there may be apical cavity obliteration. Because of a noncompliant myocardium, the diastolic properties of the left ventricle are altered. This, in itself, would affect the mitral valve diastolic closure rate, but the posterior cusp will move in the opposite direction to the anterior cusp, unlike the case in mitral stenosis where both cusps move in the same direction in diastole. By using certain assumptions it is possible to assess the aortic valve area using Doppler echocardiography.[43a,43b,43c,43d,43e]

CARDIAC CATHETERIZATION AND ANGIOCARDIOGRAPHY

The transaortic pressure gradient and left ventricular end-diastolic pressure can be accurately measured by cardiac catheterization. Left atrial pressure is also elevated and correspondingly an increase in pulmonary artery pressure may be noted. Angiocardiography will reveal the extent of concentric hypertrophy and coexisting cavity dilatation, if any. Frequently, additional aortic regurgitation is present and is best detected by an aortic root injection of contrast substance. In subjects over the age of 40 years it is customary to perform coronary angiography to exclude the possibility of coexisting coronary heart disease.

DIFFERENTIAL DIAGNOSIS

This includes hypertrophic cardiomyopathy, supravalvular aortic stenosis and papillary muscle dysfunction. With hypertrophic cardiomyopathy the arterial pulse is jerky and not slow rising. The systolic murmur is generally present in the fourth and fifth intercostal space. The echocardiographic features of massive and asymmetric septal hypertrophy and systolic anterior motion of the anterior mitral cusp are fairly pathognomonic.

Supravalvular aortic stenosis is a rare condition, generally seen in mentally deficient children. Inequality of the two carotid pulses due to the tendency of a jet stream to adhere to a boundary wall (Coanda effect)[44] may be felt.

The murmur of posterior papillary muscle dysfunction, being nonholosystolic and conducted to the left sternal edge, may occasionally mimic aortic stenosis. However, the left ventricular impulse is never dynamic and sustained in the latter condition.

TREATMENT

Penicillin prophylaxis, as in all other forms of RHD, is recommended. With advanced cases digitalis and diuretics are needed. In symptomatic patients the disease is advanced enough to warrant surgery. Valve replacement with a prosthetic valve is recommended. The valve should have a low profile so as not to interfere with the ejection characteristics of the concentrically hypertrophied myocardium. Recently percutaneous balloon aortic valvuloplasty has been proposed as a possible alternative to aortic valve replacement in elderly and/or high risk patients. However, its long term results need to be determined before it can be applied on a large scale.

TRICUSPID VALVE DISEASE

Rheumatic tricuspid valve disease, which occurs far more frequently in Indians than in Westerners,[45] does not occur in isolated form; it usually exists with mitral stenosis. Roughly 5% to 8% of cases of mitral stenosis have associated tricuspid stenosis. Whereas tricuspid stenosis is always organic in nature, tricuspid regurgitation is usually functional due to right ventricular dilatation.

TRICUSPID STENOSIS

CLINICAL FEATURES

Signs of coexisting tricuspid stenosis must be specifically looked for in every case of mitral stenosis. Due to low cardiac output there may be peripheral cyanosis. A prominent a wave in the neck, with a slow y descent of the v wave, should suggest the diagnosis. The a wave may also be noted in the liver pulsation. On auscultation a separate mid-diastolic rumble, increasing with inspiration, may be audible in the xiphisternal region. A tricuspid opening snap occurring after the mitral opening snap may sometimes be audible; it is better documented phonocardiographically.

CHEST X-RAY

Right atrial enlargement is clearly seen. It may be seen to the right of the left atrial shadow. In late cases with ascites, the domes of the diaphragm are elevated.

ELECTROCARDIOGRAM

The electrocardiogram reveals pointed P waves in leads II, III, and aVF. In lead V_1, there may be a qR complex due to picking up of septal forces through an enlarged right atrial cavity. Indeed, a peaked P wave with a "small" qR complex in lead V_1 strongly points to the coexistence of tricuspid stenosis.

ECHOCARDIOGRAM

The diastolic opening slope of the tricuspid valve is reduced. Two-dimensional studies will reveal doming of the valve into the right ventricle during diastole. An echocardiographic study is recommended in every case of mitral stenosis so as not to miss mild to moderate degrees of coexisting tricuspid stenosis.

CARDIAC CATHETERIZATION AND ANGIOGRAPHY

Transtricuspid valve diastolic gradients in the range of 3 to 10 mm Hg are usually present. The cardiac output is low. Prominent a waves are seen in the right atrium and the v waves have a slow y descent due to the "braking" effect of the narrow orifice. The use of right atrial angiography in demonstrating the thickened tricuspid valve with a narrow jet across the stenotic orifice has been reported from India[46] and Kuwait.[47] Tricuspid stenosis is often combined with tricuspid regurgitation[47] which may be confirmed by right ventriculography. Coexisting mitral stenosis is almost invariably present. Rarely, aortic stenosis may also be present.

DIFFERENTIAL DIAGNOSIS

Right ventricular endomyocardial fibrosis and Ebstein's disease may closely mimic tricuspid stenosis. In endomyocardial fibrosis, right ventricular cavity obliteration and clot formation in the apex are characteristic. Also, there will not be an associated mitral valvular lesion. In Ebstein's disease, multiple heart sounds due to S_3 and S_4 gallop, scratchy systolic murmur along the left sternal edge, electrocardiographic evidence of right bundle branch block or intraventricular conduction defect, type B Wolff-Parkinson-White syndrome, and typical hemodynamic and electrophysiologic studies of the atrialized right ventricle at the low level of the tricuspid valve are indeed pathognomonic.

Rarely, carcinoid heart disease may mimic the picture of rheumatic tricuspid stenosis, but the syndrome of telangiectasia, flushing, bronchospasm, and diarrhea points to the diagnosis. Furthermore, carcinoid involvement of the tricuspid valve results in tricuspid regurgitation, seldom stenosis.[48]

TREATMENT

Tricuspid valvotomy and tricuspid valve replacement in severe cases are the recommended treatments.

TRICUSPID REGURGITATION

Tricuspid incompetence is generally functional and secondary to elevated right ventricular pressure. It is seen in about 40% of all cases; however, only 10% to 12% of cases are severe enough to warrant anuloplasty. Definite cuspal involvement due to rheumatic vegetations and leading to tricuspid incompetence severe enough for valve replacement is rare.

CLINICAL FEATURES

Chronic elevation of systemic venous pressure leads to edema, pleural effusion, and ascites. Cardiac output is usually low and the patient generally complains of fatigue. Hepatic enlargement is obvious with systolic pulsations due to the regurgitant wave. Upper abdominal pain due to distention of the liver capsule, poor appetite, and abdominal bloating are usually present. Chronically elevated venous pressure may also cause protein-losing enteropathy.[49] Mild jaundice associated with a greyish pigmentation gives the patient a characteristic appearance.

On auscultation, the main feature is a musical pansystolic murmur along the left sternal edge. With marked right ventricular hypertrophy and consequent displacement of the tricuspid valve, the murmur may be heard at the apex. However, its musical nature and its increase on inspiration (Rivero-Carvallo's sign)[50] are typical. Furthermore, this murmur does not radiate into the axilla.

CHEST X-RAY

The cardiac silhouette is enlarged. The right atrium may be giant-sized in some cases. Associated signs of mitral or aortic valve disease, or both, are almost always present.

ELECTROCARDIOGRAM

There is right ventricular hypertrophy with enlargement of the right atrium. Atrial fibrillation is a common event.

ECHOCARDIOGRAM

The right ventricular cavity size is large. Tricuspid valve motion is rapid. Right ventricular volume overload also causes reversal of septal wall motion. Injection of small air bubbles by using standard contrast echocardiography techniques shows the appearance of contrast material in the inferior vena cava after an injection in the peripheral vein. Doppler techniques are even superior in detecting reversed flow across the tricuspid valve.[51]

CARDIAC CATHETERIZATION

Right atrial tracings reveal an exaggerated v wave. The y descent is sharp. It may be difficult to enter the right ventricle with a Goodale-Lubin or Cournand catheter; the regurgitant thrust is powerful. A stiffer catheter such as the National Institutes of Health type is used to negotiate the tricuspid valve. Right ventricular pressures are high as is the pulmonary artery pressure. Pulmonary valvular regurgitation may also be present. Transvalvular diastolic gradients of over 3 mm Hg suggest coexisting tricuspid stenosis.

DIFFERENTIAL DIAGNOSIS

These include dilated cardiomyopathy, endomyocardial fibrosis, and Ebstein's disease. The characteristic features of these diseases have already been discussed.

TREATMENT

Medical therapy includes bedrest, low sodium diet, digitalis, and diuretics. Vasodilator therapy with prazosin and the judicious use of captopril are frequently lifesaving. Ascitic and pleural tapping is beneficial. Nifedipine may also be used to reduce pulmonary artery pressure and to provide suitable afterload reduction.

In severe cases, tricuspid anuloplasty or valve replacement is the only treatment. In selected cases tricuspid valve repair, as advocated by Carpentier,[24] has been helpful.

PULMONARY VALVE DISEASE

Although the pulmonary valve was involved in 12.5% of cases in an autopsy study, clinical manifestations of valvular involvement are seldom, if ever, present.

MULTIVALVULAR DISEASE

Multiple valvular involvement is common in RHD. It is vital to recognize multivalvular involvement if surgical treatment is contemplated, because failure to correct all significant valvular defects at operation results in increased mortality. In general, clinical manifestations produced by the more proximal of two valvular lesions, such as the mitral valve in combined mitral and aortic stenosis and the tricuspid valve in combined tricuspid and mitral stenosis, are more prominent than, and tend to mask, those produced by the distal lesion. For this reason all patients suspected of multivalvular disease should undergo complete preoperative evaluation including not only thorough noninvasive studies, especially two-dimensional echocardiography, but also both right and left heart catheterization combined with angiocardiography.

CONCLUSIONS

It cannot be overemphasized that rheumatic heart disease (RHD) continues to be a serious problem in the tropics. About one third of the patients in whom chronic RHD develops die before the age of 20 years. In over 90% of cases the mitral valve is involved and in many of them subvalvular disease is severe enough to warrant early surgery. Redo operations for the second or even the third time are not uncommon. A third of the cases of mitral stenosis have associated aortic insufficiency. Aortic valve replacement may be necessary in 20% of these cases. Rheumatic activity is seen in 35% of all cases. It is sometimes of a simmering nature and may be missed during clinical examination. All attempts must be made to identify and control rheumatic carditis before submitting the patient to surgery.

Severe pulmonary hypertension is common and presents some risk, especially in multivalvular disease. The postoperative course may indeed be stormy.

REFERENCES

1. Gillum RF: Trends in acute rheumatic fever and chronic rheumatic heart disease: a national perspective. *Am Heart J* 1986; 111:430–432.
1a. Padmavati S: Rheumatic fever and rheumatic heart disease in developing countries. *Bul WHO* 1978; 56:543–550.
1b. Stollerman GH: Acute rheumatic fever and its management, in Hurst JW (ed): *The Heart,* ed 6. New York, McGraw-Hill, 1986, pp 1306–1313.
1c. Editorial: Rapid detection of beta hemolytic streptococci. *Lancet* 1986; 1:247–248.
2. Ad Hoc Committee to revise the Jones Criteria (modified) of the Council on Rheumatic Fever and Congenital Heart Disease of the American Heart Association (1965) and the Committee on Rheumatic Fever and Bacterial Endocarditis (1982): Jones criteria (revised) for guidance in the diagnosis of rheumatic fever. *Circulation* 1984; 69:203A–208A.
3. Cherian J: Acute rheumatic fever—the Jones criteria: a review and a case for polyarthralgia. *J Assoc Phys India* 1979; 27:453–457.
4. Taranta A: Rheumatic fever, in McCarty DJ (ed): *Arthritis and Allied Conditions.* Philadelphia, Lea & Febiger, 1985, pp 1052–1072.
5. Tan ATH, Mah PK, Chia BL: Cardiac tamponade in acute rheumatic carditis. *Ann Rheum Dis* 1983; 42:699–701.
6. Human DG, Hill ID, Fraser CB: Treatment choice in acute rheumatic carditis. *Arch Dis Child* 1984; 59:410–413.
7. Etzioni A, Vardi P, Levy J, Benderly A: Treatment choice in acute rheumatic carditis. *Arch Dis Child* 1984; 59:1198–1199.
8. Kinare SG: Rheumatic heart disease in young: pathological aspects. *Indian Heart J* 1983; 35:135–138.
9. MacCallum WG: Rheumatic lesions of the left auricle of the heart. *Bull Johns Hopkins Hosp* 1924; 35:329.
10. Cheng JTO, Cahill WJ, Foley EF: Coronary embolism. *JAMA* 1953; 153:211–213.
11. Cheng TO: Phonocardiographic sign for pliability of a stenotic mitral valve. *Circulation* 1966; 34:III–72.
12. Rackley CE, Edwards JE, Karp RB: Mitral valve disease, in Hurst JW (ed): *The Heart,* ed 6. New York, McGraw-Hill, 1986, pp 754–784.
13. McArthur JD, Sukumar IP, Munsi SC, Krishnaswami S, Cherian G: Reassessment of Graham Steell murmur using platinum electrode technique. *Br Heart J* 1974; 36:1023–1027.
14. Nair KG: Rheumatic fever, in Weatherall DJ, Ledingham JGG, Warrell DA (eds): *Oxford Textbook of Medicine.* Oxford, Oxford University Press, 1983, pp 13.148–13.151.
15. Cherian G, Vytilingam KI, Sukumar IP, Gopinath N: Mitral valvotomy in young patients. *Br Heart J* 1964; 26:157–166.
16. Roy SB, Bhatia ML, Lazaro EJ, Ramalingaswami V: Juvenile mitral stenosis in India. *Lancet* 1963; ii:1193–1196.
17. Saunders JL, Calatayud JB, Schulz KJ, Maranhao V, Gooch AS, Goldberg H: Evaluation of ECG criteria for P-wave abnormalities. *Am Heart J* 1967; 74:757–765.
18. Cope GD, Kisslo JA, Johnson ML, Behar VS: A reassessment of the echocardiogram in mitral stenosis. *Circulation* 1975; 52:664–670.
19. Braunwald E, Awe WC: The syndrome of severe mitral regurgitation with normal left atrial pressure. *Circulation* 1963; 27:29–35.
20. Roberts WC, Braunwald E, Morrow AG: Acute severe mitral regurgitation secondary to ruptured chordae tendineae. Clinical, hemodynamic, and pathologic considerations. *Circulation* 1966; 33:58–70.
20a. Miyatake K, Izumi S, Okamoto M, Kinoshita N, Asonuma H, Nakagawa H, Yamamoto K, Takamiya M, Sakakibara H, Nimura Y: Semiquantitative grading of mitral regurgitation by real-time two-dimensional Doppler flow imaging technique. *J Am Coll Cardiol* 1986; 7:82–88.
20b. Meyers DG, McCall D, Sears TD, Olson TS, Felix GL: Duplex pulsed Doppler echocardiography in mitral regurgitation. *J Clin Ultrasound* 1986; 14:117–121.
21. Goodman DJ, Rossen RM, Holloway EL, Alderman EL, Harrison DC: Effect of nitroprusside on left ventricular dynamics in mitral regurgitation. *Circulation* 1974; 50:1025–1032.
22. Greenberg BH, DeMots H, Murphy E, Rahimtoola SH: Arterial dilators in mitral regurgitation: effects on rest and exercise hemodynamics and longterm clinical followup. *Circulation* 1982; 65:181–187.
23. Butman SM, Eagan J, Olson HG: Hemodynamic effects of verapamil in left ventricular valvular volume overload. *Am Heart J* 1985; 110:416–426.
24. Carpentier A: Cardiac valve surgery — the "French correction." *J Thorac Cardiovasc Surg* 1983; 86:323–337.
25. Spencer FC, Colvin SB, Culliford AT, Isom OW: Experiences with the Carpentier techniques of mitral valve reconstruction in 103 patients (1980–1985). *J Thorac Cardiovasc Surg* 1985; 90:341–350.
25a. Zhang Y, Nitter-Hauge S, Ihlen H, Rootwelt K, Myhre E: Measurement of aortic regurgitation by Doppler echocardiography. *Br Heart J* 1986; 55:32–38.
25b. Masuyama T, Kodama K, Kitabatake A, Nanto S, Sato H, Uematsu M, Inoue M, Kamada T: Noninvasive evaluation of aortic regurgitation by continuous-wave Doppler echocardiography. *Circulation* 1986; 73:460–466.
26. Booth DC, Nissen S, DeMaria AN: Assessment of the severity of valvular regurgitation by digital subtraction angiography compared to cineangiography. *Am Heart J* 1985; 110:409–416.
27. Miller RR, Vismara LA, DeMaria AN, Salel AF, Mason DT: Afterload reduction therapy with nitroprusside in severe aortic regurgitation: improved cardiac performance and reduced regurgitant volume. *Am J Cardiol* 1976; 38:564–567.
28. Elkayam U, McKay CR, Weber L, Eisenberg D, Rahimtoola SH: Favorable effects of hydralazine on the hemodynamic response to isometric exercise in chronic severe aortic regurgitation. *Am J Cardiol* 1984; 53:1603–1607.
29. Strauss MH, Chan YK, Burns R, Leenen FH: Long term prazosin in asymptomatic aortic insufficiency. *Circulation* 1985; 72:III–152.
30. Shen WF, Roubin GS, Hirasawa K, Uren RF, Hutton BF, Harris PJ, Fletcher PJ, Kelly DT: Abnormal left ventricular response to isometric exercise in pure, isolated aortic regurgitation: beneficial effects of nifedipine. *Am J Cardiol* 1984; 54:605–609.
31. Greenberg BH, Rahimtoola SH: Usefulness of vasodilator therapy in acute and chronic valvular regurgitation. *Curr Probl Cardiol* 1984; 9:1–46.
32. Bonow RO, Picone AL, McIntosh CL, Jones M, Rosing DR, Maron BJ, Lakatos E, Clark RE, Epstein SE: Survival and functional results after valve replacement for aortic regurgitation from 1976 to 1983: impact of preoperative left ventricular function. *Circulation* 1985; 72:1244–1256.
33. Gee DS, Juni JE, Santinga JT, Buda AJ: Prognostic significance of exercise-induced left ventricular dysfunction in chronic aortic regurgitation. *Am J Cardiol* 1985; 56:605–609.
34. Wilson RA, Greenberg B, Siemienzuk D, Bristow D, Cheitlin M, Broudy D, Krishnamurthy G, Thomas D: Relationship between ejection fraction and the end-systolic pressure-volume ratio in chronic aortic regurgitation (abstr). *Circulation* 1985; 72:III–152.
35. Iskandrian AS, Hakki A-H, Kane-Marsch S: Left ventricular pressure/volume relationship in aortic regurgitation. *Am Heart J* 1985; 110:1026–1032.

36. Huxley RL, Gaffney FA, Corbett JR, Firth BG, Peshock R, Nicod P, Rellas JS, Curry G, Lewis SE, Willerson JT: Early detection of left ventricular dysfunction in chronic aortic regurgitation as assessed by contrast angiography, echocardiography, and rest and exercise scintigraphy. *Am J Cardiol* 1983; 51:1542–1550.
37. Weiss RJ, Buda AJ, LeMire MS, Pitt B: Assessment of dysfunction in aortic regurgitation by stress-shortening relationship. *Inter J Cardiol* 1985; 8:475–486.
37a. McKay CR, Nanna M, Reid CL, Kawanishi DT, Stiles Q, Elkayam U, Rahimtoola SH: Superiority of aortic valve replacement over arteriolar dilator therapy for symptomatic chronic severe aortic regurgitation. *Clin Research* 1986; 34:12A.
37b. Subramanian R, Olson LJ, Edwards WD: Surgical pathology of combined aortic stenosis and insufficiency: a study of 213 cases. *Mayo Clin Proc* 1985; 60:247–254.
38. Exadactylos N, Sugrue DD, Oakley CM: Prevalence of coronary artery disease in patients with isolated aortic valve stenosis. *Br Heart J* 1984; 51:121–124.
39. Marvin HM, Sullivan AG: Clinical observations upon syncope and sudden death in relation to aortic stenosis. *Am Heart J* 1935; 10:705–735.
40. Schwartz LS, Goldfischer J, Sprague GJ, Schwartz SP: Syncope and sudden death in aortic stenosis. *Am J Cardiol* 1969; 23:647–658.
41. Flamm MD, Braniff BA, Kimball R, Hancock EW: Mechanism of effort syncope in aortic stenosis (abstr). *Circulation* 1967; 36:II–109.
42. Johnson AM: Aortic stenosis, sudden death, and the left ventricular baroreceptors. *Br Heart J* 1971; 33:1–5.
43. Richards AM, Nicholls MG, Ikram H, Hamilton EJ, Richards RD: Syncope in aortic valvular stenosis. *Lancet* 1984; 2:1113–1116.
43a. Smith MD, Dawson PL, Elion JL, Wisenbaugh T, Kwan OL, Handshee S, DeMaria AN: Systematic correlation of continuous-wave Doppler and hemodynamic measurements in patients with aortic stenosis. *Am Heart J* 1986; 111:245–252.
43b. Zhang Y, Ihlen H, Nitter-Hauge S: Estimation of the peak-to-peak pressure gradient in aortic stenosis by Doppler echocardiography. *Internat J Cardiol* 1986; 10:197–212.
43c. Ohlsson J, Wranne B: Noninvasive assessment of valve area in patients with aortic stenosis. *J Am Coll Cardiol* 1986; 7:501–508.
43d. Otto CM, Pearlman AS, Comess KA, Reamer RP, Janko CL, Huntsman LL: Determination of the stenotic aortic valve area in adults using Doppler echocardiography. *J Am Coll Cardiol* 1986; 7:509–517.
43e. Zoghbi WA, Farmer KL, Soto JG, Nelson JG, Quinones MA: Accurate noninvasive quantification of stenotic aortic valve area by Doppler echocardiography. *Circulation* 1986; 73:452–459.
44. French JW, Guntheroth WG: An explanation of asymmetric upper extremity blood pressures in supravalvular aortic stenosis: the Coanda effect. *Circulation* 1970; 42:31–36.
45. Datta BN, Nagrani B, Khattri HN, Sapru RP, Bidwai PS, Suri PK, Gujral JS, Wahi PL: Rheumatic heart disease at autopsy: an analysis of 260 cases in Chandigarh. *Indian Heart J* 1978; 30:39–46.
46. Abraham KA, Cherian G, Durairaj M, Balaji NK, Sukumar IP, John S: Clinical and hemodynamic appraisal of rheumatic tricuspid stenosis. *Indian Heart J* 1977; 25:341–346.
47. Yousof AM, Shafei MZ, Endrys G, Khan N, Simo M, Cherian G: Tricuspid stenosis and regurgitation in rheumatic heart disease: a prospective cardiac catheterization study in 525 patients. *Am Heart J* 1985; 110:60–64.
48. Ross EM, Roberts WC: The carcinoid syndrome: comparison of 21 necropsy subjects with carcinoid heart disease to 15 necropsy subjects without carcinoid heart disease. *Am J Med* 1985; 79:339–354.
49. Waldmann TA: Protein-losing gastroenteropathies, in Berk JE (ed): *Bockus Gastroenterology*, ed 4. Philadelphia, WB Saunders, 1985, pp 1814–1837.
50. Rivero Carvallo JM: Signo para el diagnostico de las insuficiencias tricuspideas. *Arch Inst Cardiol Mexico* 1946; 16:531–539.
51. Curtius JM, Thyssen M, Breuer HM, Loogen F: Doppler versus contrast echocardiography for diagnosis of tricuspid regurgitation. *Am J Cardiol* 1985; 56:333–336.

31 Mitral Valve Billowing and Prolapse

John B. Barlow, MD and Tsung O. Cheng, MD

So-called mitral valve prolapse has aroused much interest for more than two decades, and there is a vast amount of literature pertaining to all aspects. In this chapter, some of this literature will be reviewed. We have both had a long-standing interest in the subject and have independently made a number of observations based on personal clinical experience. We shall discuss in more detail features with which one or both of us have had meaningful experience. Some important problems, albeit partially unresolved, will be emphasized.

Mitral valve prolapse (MVP) has become a widely accepted term for this common cardiac condition. We shall give reasons for our reservations regarding the overall use of MVP to describe a spectrum of a mitral valve anomaly that ranges from extremely mild to very severe. The term *billowing mitral leaflet* (BML) is more appropriate to describe the milder forms of this anomaly when mitral regurgitation is not associated. Nonetheless, to reduce confusion and to improve simplification, we shall use the abbreviation MVP alone when we intend MVP or BML, or both. The abbreviation BML alone will be used only when a comment refers specifically to an aspect of the mitral valve anomaly in which associated mitral regurgitation is absent. The terms *floppy* and *flail* will also be clarified.

HISTORICAL BACKGROUND

There are not many "new diseases."[1] In most instances, the individual physician has not read or heard about the condition which he has not previously encountered and which he may favor has hitherto not been reported. Alternatively the previous recognition and description may have related to different aspects. Both Wooley[2,2a] and Bartecchi[3] recently suggested that some symptomatic patients with MVP were almost certainly encountered by physicians in the 19th and early 20th centuries, but their condition was termed neurocirculatory asthenia, soldier's heart, irritable heart, effort syndrome, or DaCosta's syndrome. During the last two or three decades a "publication explosion"[4] relating to MVP has resulted essentially from two principal observations. The first pertained to confirmation of a mitral valve origin[5] of an apical late systolic murmur and midsystolic click. The second, and probably the one of wider interest, was the recognition of symptoms, clinical signs, and other features associated with the mitral valve anomaly which justified the recognition of a specific syndrome.[6]

At the end of the last century Griffith[7] and later Hall[8] in 1903 suggested that an apical late systolic murmur denoted mitral regurgitation. However, following the teachings of Lewis[9] and MacKenzie,[10] systolic murmurs unaccompanied by other evidence of heart disease were regarded as of little consequence. The British cardiologist, William Evans,[11] both during and after World War II, emphasized that late systolic murmurs were innocent and this view was widely accepted. The common association of a mid-late systolic click with a late systolic murmur had also been recognized. In 1913, Gallavardin[12] attributed such clicks to pleuropericardial adhesions, and the theory of an extracardiac origin became so firmly established[12–15] that McKusick[16] regarded clicks as evidence of a similar origin of late systolic murmurs. An exception to the general trend of opinion was pronounced by the renowned American cardiologist, Paul White,[17] who suggested in 1937 that midsystolic sounds might sometimes arise from abnormal chordae tendineae.

In 1961, the South African, John Reid,[18] revived the hypothesis that these clicks and late systolic murmurs were of mitral valve origin. Reid suggested that the clicks arose from the chordae and he used the term *chordal snap.* Shortly thereafter, Barlow et al[5] demonstrated mitral regurgitation on left ventricular cineangiocardiography in four patients who had murmurs confined to late systole on phonocardiography. A much larger number of Barlow's patients with late systolic murmurs and clicks were not subjected to cardiac catheterization but were studied by means of vasoactive maneuvers; the effects of amyl nitrite, the Valsalva maneuver, and other hemodynamic alterations were compatible with the behavior of a regurgitant systolic murmur of mitral incompetence. The behavior of systolic clicks was also compatible with an intracardiac origin. Because these clicks were shown to move to early systole, or sometimes to be confined to early systole (Figure 31.1), the term *nonejection* systolic click was introduced[6] to differentiate them from aortic and pulmonary ejection clicks or sounds.

Although it was important to demonstrate that nonejection clicks and apical late systolic murmurs have a mitral valve origin, it has been the symptoms and other physical features occurring with the mitral valve anomaly that have caused widespread interest. In 1962, Humphries and McKusick[19] observed an association between a late systolic murmur or systolic click on auscultation with T-wave changes on the electrocardiogram. Some of their patients had a history of anterior chest pain. Humphries and McKusick therefore recognized a "characteristic electrocardiographic-auscultatory syndrome" that "mimics the syndrome of angina pectoris due to coronary insufficiency," but they postulated that previous pericarditis was the explanation. After the mitral valve anomaly was recognized as an integral part of the "syndrome,"[20–22] a plethora of observations and studies of different aspects ensued and widespread interest continues.

Although early publications[20,23] recognized that numerous pathologic conditions could affect the mitral valve mechanism and result in the auscultatory features of a late systolic murmur and nonejection systolic click, some confusion resulted from failure to emphasize the necessity of differentiating primary from secondary MVP.[24,25] The importance of distinguishing secondary from primary MVP will be discussed subsequently in this chapter.

DEFINITION AND NOMENCLATURE

Primary MVP is a degenerative condition of leaflets and chordae. Wooley's group in Ohio[26] recently described the essential histologic features as collagen dissolution with myxomatous degeneration in the principal supporting structures of the valve, so-called discollagenosis. As emphasized by Roberts,[27] this results in redundant leaflet tissue, sometimes associated with excessive length of chordae tendineae. The process may be focal, involving only one scallop, or it may be diffuse, involving both leaflets (Figures 31.2, 31.3, and 31.4). The increase in transverse dimension results in the circumference of the leaflets being larger than the circumference of the mitral valve anulus. Roberts[27] draws an analogy between the normal mitral valve which, when opened, is flat and smooth with appearances similar to that of the mucosa of the ileum, whereas leaflets of MVP have an undulating surface and simulate the mucosa of the jejunum.

The reason for the onset of this degenerative condition is poorly understood. It may commence in childhood, but most pathologists have limited experience with the condition in children and young adults. However, according to Pomerance,[28] myxomatous degeneration is common in the elderly. The condition may be familial, and associated pectus excavatum or other abnormalities of the bony thorax sometimes suggest a generalized disorder of connective tissue. Primary MVP should be regarded as a common forme fruste of the "floppy valve syndrome"[29] with or without skeletal manifestations of Marfan's syndrome.

The term *prolapse* was introduced in 1966 by Criley et

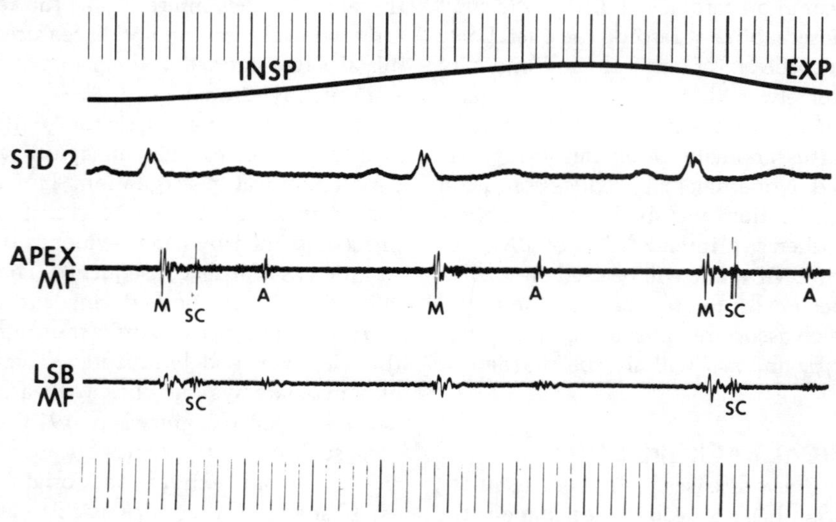

Figure 31.1. Phonocardiogram during respiration demonstrating a nonejection systolic click (SC) occurring early in systole. The systolic click is absent in the second complex. EXP = expiration; INSP = inspiration; LSB = left sternal border; MF = medium frequency; M = mitral closure sound; A = aortic closure sound.

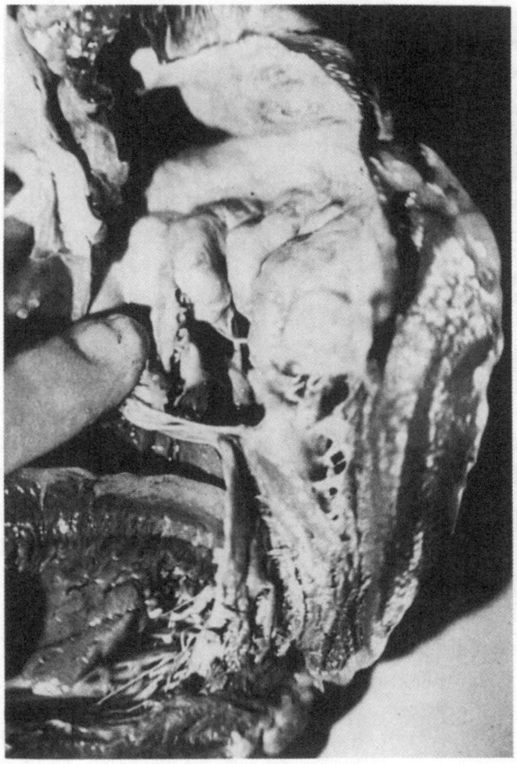

Figure 31.2. Mitral valve of a 24-year-old woman with marked mitral valve prolapse who died suddenly. Redundant leaflets with interchordal hooding are demonstrated.

al[30] when they clarified the cineangiocardiographic appearances of this entity. Drawing an analogy with prolapse of the rectum or uterus, prolapse is regarded by many patients as "abnormal" and sometimes, in both English and Chinese (Tuo Chui, 脱垂), to have an ominous meaning.[31] Nonetheless, prolapse is now widely used irrespective of whether or not the valve anomaly is anatomically mild, echocardiographically demonstrable, or functionally normal. This has contributed to the general confusion, and it seems to us that it is more than a matter of semantics for the terms *billowing, prolapse, floppy,* and *flail* to be defined. Such definitions should be based essentially on the functional anatomy, or pathology, of the mitral valve mechanism. Auscultatory, echocardiographic, cineangiocardiographic, and other clinical features should then be correlated with the probable functional anatomy. It is, after all, the functional anatomy of the mitral valve mechanism that we attempt to assess by all invasive or noninvasive investigations.

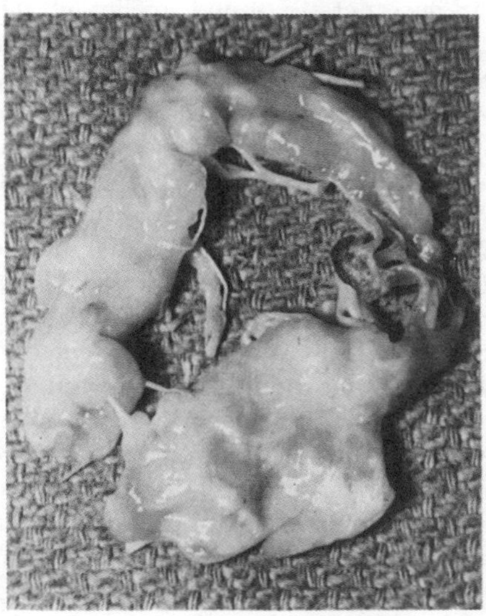

Figure 31.3. Floppy mitral valve excised from a 51-year-old woman who underwent mitral valve replacement for prolapsing mitral valve with progressive mitral regurgitation.

The concept propounded originally by the French cardiac surgeon, Alain Carpentier, defines the essential and important differences between prolapse and billowing.[32] Carpentier restricts the use of the term *prolapse* to failure of the leaflet edges to appose normally. Such partial loss of apposition may occur with or without abnormal billowing of the bellies of the leaflets and some, albeit mild or even minimal, mitral regurgitation will inevitably result. This concept of prolapse implies that the valve function is abnormal, which is, in fact, both appropriate and correct. Any cardiac valve, provided there is no hole in the leaflet, remains competent while there is sustained coaptation of the leaflets. Prevention of apposition may occur if one or more leaflets are fibrosed or retracted. When leaflets are normal in size, or larger, failure of sustained apposition will result in prolapse. On the basis of Carpentier's understanding of mitral valve prolapse, Barlow and Pocock[33] expanded the concept and suggested that the following terminology, which reflects normal and abnormal mitral valve functional anatomy, should alleviate the current confusion.

The normal mitral leaflets billow slightly, after closure, into the left atrial cavity (Figure 31.5A). Exaggeration of this billowing (Figure 31.5B), which may range from marked and diffuse to mild and involving only one scallop or even part of a scallop, should be termed a *billowing mitral leaflet* (BML). This BML may produce a nonejection click, but conclusive evidence of mild BML will not necessarily be detected on echocardiography or cineangiocardiography. If BML progresses, failure of leaflet edge apposition may supervene and then there is prolapse (Figure 31.5C). With prolapse, there has to be some mitral regurgitation which is reflected clinically by a mitral systolic murmur. Because the BML is more marked, it may be confirmed on echocardiography, but that technique, whether M-mode or two-dimensional, detects systolic displacement of the body of a leaflet. If the BML is extreme with voluminous leaflets and elongated chordae, the term *floppy* is appropriate. Some prolapse is almost always present with a floppy valve (Figure 31.5D), and the mitral regurgitation is often holosystolic. The floppy leaflets are readily detected on echocardiography. Echocardiography alone, however, seldom demonstrates the prolapse nor therefore the mitral regurgitation, irrespective of whether the valve has a BML or is floppy. Echocardiographic confirmation of prolapse would entail the demonstration that the leaflet edges are disengaged, but this is not apparent until the prolapse is severe. Progression of severe prolapse, whether with a BML or a floppy

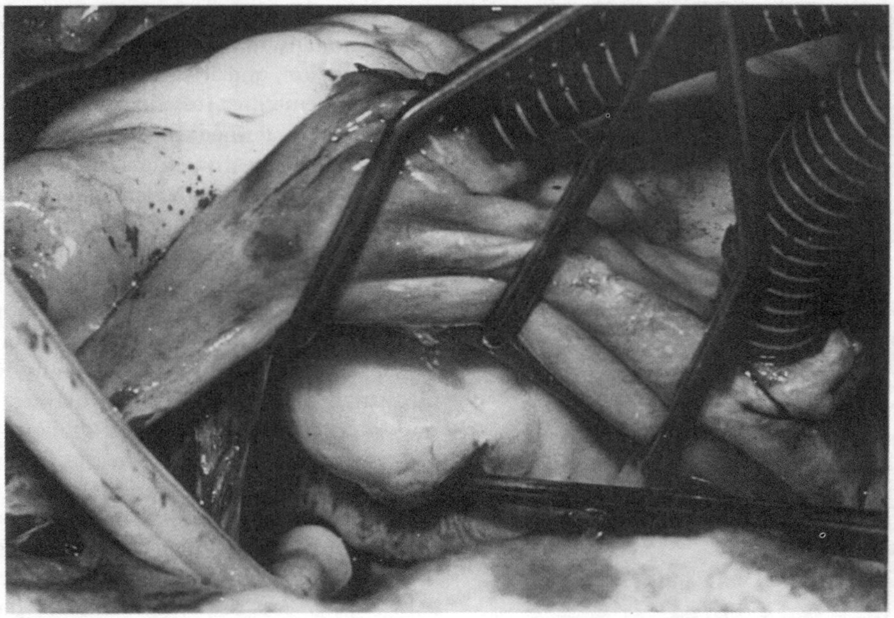

Figure 31.4. Prolapsing mitral valve viewed from left atrium during open heart operation. (From Cheng,[36] with permission of the American College of Chest Physicians.)

valve, will result in ruptured, or at least grossly elongated, chordae and part of the leaflet will then be *flail* (Figure 31.5E). Mitral regurgitation is now hemodynamically significant and displacement of the leaflet edge is readily apparent on echocardiography. Thus, although there is overlap and the dividing margins somewhat ill-defined, floppy is the extreme of a marked BML and flail that of severe prolapse.

SECONDARY MITRAL VALVE BILLOWING OR PROLAPSE AND ASSOCIATED CONDITIONS

The mitral valve mechanism is complex and any condition affecting the papillary muscles, chordae tendineae, anulus, leaflets, or the size of the left ventricular cavity could result in MVP. Many conditions[24,32,34–80c] have been associated with or causative of MVP (Table 31.1). When MVP is a secondary or an associated entity, clinical and other features as well as the prognosis are determined as much or more by the underlying or coexistent condition as by the valve anomaly itself. This will readily be apparent, for example, if MVP is secondary to hypertrophic cardiomyopathy or occlusive coronary artery disease.[20,25,38–43,81–84] Auscultatory features of MVP are common, and it is often uncertain in patients with ischemic heart disease, cardiomyopathy, systemic hypertension, or congenital heart disease whether they reflect MVP secondary to the principal pathologic condition or are an unrelated feature.[32]

Although this chapter is concerned mainly with primary MVP, which should be regarded as a highly prevalent forme fruste of floppy valve syndrome, with or without the skeletal manifestations of Marfan's syndrome, it is relevant to mention briefly a unifying concept concerning the pathophysiologic aspects of MVP.[43] In MVP the underlying mechanism has one common denominator, namely, the suspension apparatus of the mitral valve is too big, either absolutely or relatively, for the left ventricular cavity to contain (Figure 31.6). There is "too much" valve apparatus in primary MVP, floppy valve syndrome, Marfan's syndrome, rheumatic endocarditis,[85] and coronary artery disease with papillary muscle dysfunction or following trauma. "Too little" cavity size, as in idiopathic hypertrophic cardiomyopathy, atrial septal defect, straight back syndrome, pectus excavatum, chronic right ventricular overload,[86] and possibly some normal females and highly trained athletes, may allow systolic billowing of anatomically normal mitral leaflets. Indeed, Markiewicz et al[87] found smaller left ventricular end-diastolic dimensions and volumes on echocardiograms among healthy females with MVP than in those without MVP. The apparent decrease in frequency of MVP among older persons may be due to a gradual increase in left ventricular dimension which "corrects" the ventricular-valvular disproportion and thus minimizes or even eliminates MVP.[80] Similarly, the diminution of MVP during pregnancy could be explained by hypervolemia increasing left ventricular dimensions.[88]

As indicated in Table 31.1, MVP has been associated with many extracardiac conditions. Although in some the relation is probably coincidental, in many they are causally related. Embryologically the mitral valve differentiates into its final form during the sixth week of fetal life, which is the time when the vertebral column and thoracic cage are beginning their chondrification and ossification.[89,90] Therefore, any interference with growth at this stage of development may affect both the mitral valve and the bony skeleton, thus explaining the high incidence of skeletal abnormalities[44–46] in patients with MVP. An-

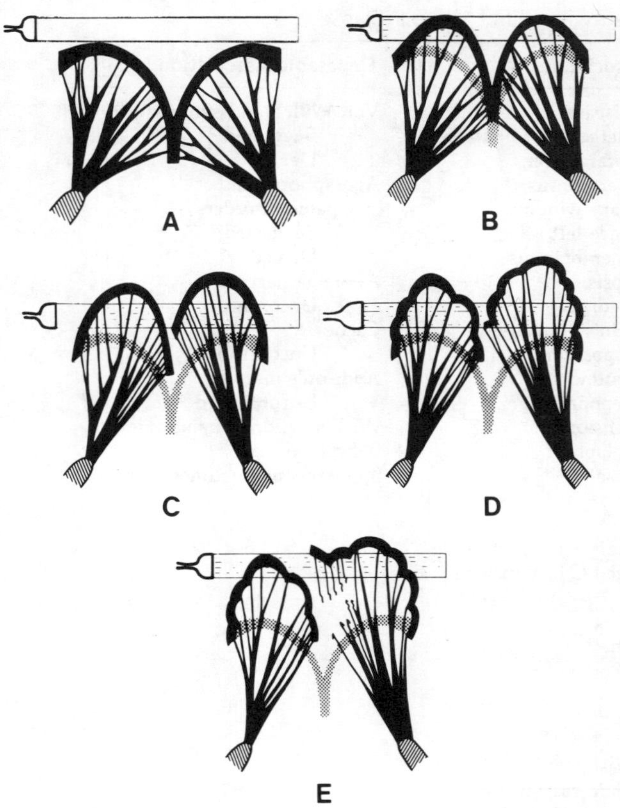

Figure 31.5. Billowing (BML), floppy, prolapsed, and flail mitral valves with schematic representation of an echocardiographic beam. *A*, Normal mitral valve showing papillary muscles, chordae tendineae, and apposed leaflet edges. *B*, BML; the chordae are lengthened, and the voluminous leaflets "billow" into the left atrium and may be detected echocardiographically. In this and subsequent drawings, the positions of normal leaflets are superimposed with a stippled pattern. *C*, BML with prolapse; the valve is incompetent, but failure of leaflet edge apposition is not detected echocardiographically. *D*, Floppy valve with prolapse; the voluminous floppy leaflets are readily demonstrated on echocardiography. *E*, Floppy valve and flail leaflet; marked regurgitation is present and the flail leaflet edge should be demonstrated echocardiographically.

other explanation for the association is that MVP is a manifestation of a forme fruste of Marfan's syndrome with a basic connective tissue disorder affecting the skeleton, the connective tissue, and the mitral valve. Supporting the contention that there is a widespread connective tissue and collagen abnormality are the findings of a frequent association between primary MVP and various connective tissue and collagen diseases (Table 31.1), an increased incidence of herniorrhaphy in men with MVP reported from Manchester, England,[37] and a prevalence of concomitant prolapse of the tricuspid[51–55] and aortic valves.[52–54,91] Development of the mitral and tricuspid leaflets, chordae, anulus, and the septum secundum as well as the thoracic vertebrae, ribs, and sternum all proceeds simultaneously between days 42 and 49 of embryonic life.[89,90] This might contribute to the association of MVP with a secundum atrial septal defect,[43,92–98] in addition to the hemodynamic effects of chronic underloading of the left ventricle[43] and chronic overloading of the right ventricle, both of which decrease left ventricular cavity size and cause the coaptation zone of the mitral leaflets to become distorted.[43,94,99]

AUSCULTATORY FEATURES OF MITRAL VALVE PROLAPSE AND BILLOWING

Auscultation remains the most sensitive method of detecting MVP. An isolated nonejection systolic click (NESC) reflects BML, which may be extremely mild or localized to part of a scallop. The NESC is usually mid- or late systolic and may be single or multiple (Figure 31.7). When a late NESC is loud, it may be mistaken for a second sound and an associated late systolic murmur may incorrectly be assessed as an early diastolic murmur (Figure 31.8). More rarely, the NESC may occur in early systole.[6,100,101] Nonejection systolic clicks vary in intensity and timing either spontaneously (Figure 31.1) or with hemodynamic alterations (Figures 31.9, 31.10, and 31.11). It is of clinical importance that an NESC may be audible only after a postural change. Repeated auscultation in the supine, left lateral, sitting, standing, and squatting positions may be necessary to detect an NESC. The clinical significance of an inconstant NESC will be considered later. Criley et al[30] demonstrated from cineangiocardiographic studies that a billowing posterior mitral leaflet reached its peak at the time of the NESC. It is therefore possible that the NESC results from elongated, and functionally unequal, chordae being stretched at the time of such maximal billow. Dock[102] postulated that an NESC arises in the leaflets themselves at the time of maximal billow.

The presence of a diastolic click has been reported with MVP[22,36,103–106] (Figure 31.12), but a reported incidence varying between 8%[105] and 15%[22] seems unduly high and has not been in accord with our clinical experience. The diastolic click in MVP may represent continued reverse ballooning of the prolapsed mitral leaflet, which returns during early left ventricular relaxation.[36,105,106] Far more commonly will be a physiologic third heart sound, especially in young persons. When significant mitral regurgitation supervenes, a third heart sound is one of the characteristic auscultatory features.

When mitral regurgitation occurs with a BML, then leaflet edges have failed to appose and true prolapse is present.[33] The classical and generally accepted systolic murmur occurs in late systole. There may also be a holosystolic murmur, and this reflects more severe prolapse and mitral regurgitation. The late systolic murmur of MVP is usually loudest at the apex and best heard in the left lateral position. The murmur is seldom louder than grade III/VI and the effect of respiration may be variable. The intensity is sometimes increased during inspiration, which suggests a functional anatomic alteration[6] rather than a hemodynamic explanation. Phonocardiography confirms that the murmur is crescendo-decrescendo in shape with maximal accentuation in the middle or latter part of the murmur.[20] The murmur extends to the aortic component of the second heart sound, and vibrations may pass through that sound.[20,106] It is possible that the early

Table 31.1. Conditions Associated with Mitral Valve Prolapse

Definite Association	Probable Association	Debatable Association
Primary MVP[24]	Congenital heart disease	Von Willebrand syndrome
Floppy valve syndrome[24,35a]	(atrial septal defect,	Suggested[73]
Connective tissue disorders	ventricular septal defect,	Denied[74]
Marfan's syndrome[24]	patent ductus arteriosus,	Agoraphobia and
Ehlers-Danlos syndrome[34]	aortic-pulmonary window,	panic disorders
Pseudoxanthoma elasticum[24]	complete absence left	Suggested[75–77]
Turner syndrome[24]	pericardium, membranous	Denied[78,79]
Relapsing polychondritis[24]	subaortic stenosis,	Anorexia nervosa
Joint hypermobility syndrome[35]	supravalvular aortic	Unconfirmed[80]
Collagen diseases	stenosis, Ebstein's anomaly,	Cachexia
Rheumatic endocarditis[24,35a]	corrected transposition,	Unconfirmed[80]
Mitral stenosis[36]	infundibular pulmonary	Addison's disease
Lupus erythematosus[24]	stenosis, Uhl's anomaly)[32]	Unconfirmed[80]
Hernia[37]	Pulmonary hypertension[49,50]	Wiskott-Aldrich syndrome[80a]
Coronary artery disease[38–42]	Tricuspid valve prolapse[51–56]	Behcet's disease[80b]
Cardiomyopathy	Aortic valve prolapse[52–54,56]	Spontaneous pneumothorax[80c]
Hypertrophic[24,43]	Bicuspid aortic valve[57]	
Congestive[24]	Athletes[24,32,43]	
Myocarditis[24]	Noonan's syndrome[32]	
Mitral commissurotomy[41]	Congenital prolonged QT syndrome[32]	
Trauma[43]	Keratoconus[58]	
Left atrial myxoma[24]	Hyperthyroidism[32]	
Left ventricular aneurysm[24]	Rheumatoid arthritis[59]	
Muscular dystrophy[24]	Sickle cell disease[60]	
Wolff-Parkinson-White syndrome[24]	Hypomastia[61]	
Skeletal abnormalities	Stickler's syndrome[62]	
Straight back syndrome[44]	Migraine[63]	
Pectus excavatum[44]	Coronary artery spasm[64,65]	
Scoliosis[45]	Absent or hypoplastic circumflex[43,66]	
Other anomalies[46]	Variations in coronary origins[67]	
Pulmonary emphysema[32]	Fragile X-syndrome[68]	
Osteogenesis imperfecta[32,46a]	Klinefelter's syndrome[69]	
Inherited disorders of metabolism	Hypomagnesemia[32]	
(Hunter's and Hurler's syndrome,	Dysautonomia[70,71]	
San Fillipo syndrome, Fabry's	Intracranial aneurysm[72]	
disease, Sandhoff's disease)[32]	Neuroectomesodermal histodysplasia[32]	
Orthostatic hypotension[47,48]	Irritable bowel syndrome[72a]	
	Down's syndrome[72b]	

Note: Direct references are given only for conditions that were not mentioned in Barlow and Pocock.[24,32]

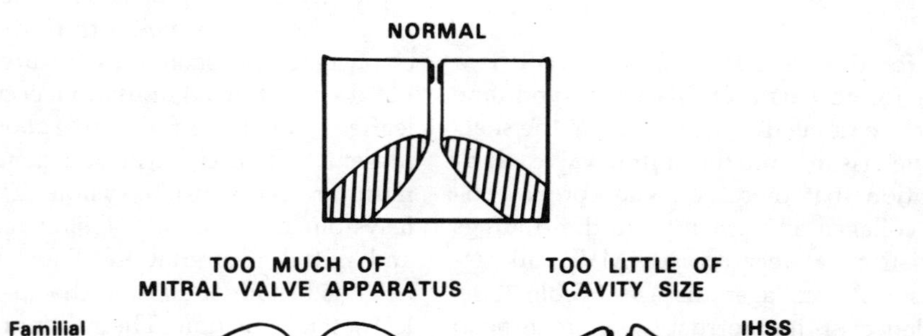

Figure 31.6. Pathophysiology of mitral valve prolapse. IHSS = idiopathic hypertrophic subaortic stenosis. (From Cheng,[43] with permission of the American College of Chest Physicians.)

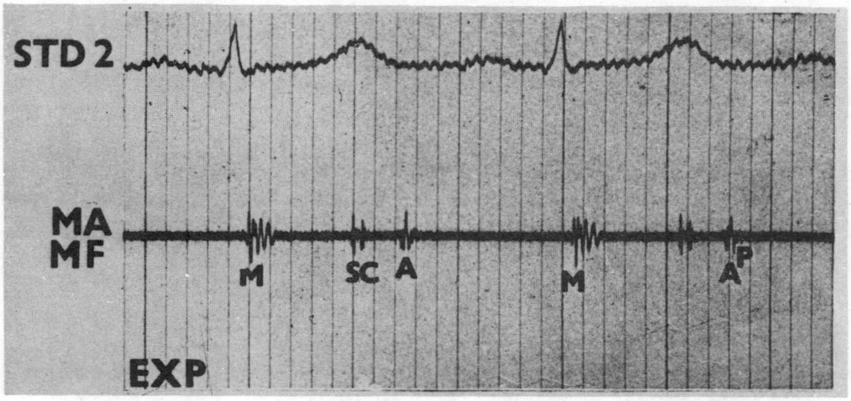

Figure 31.7. Medium frequency (MF) phonocardiogram recorded at the mitral area (MA), demonstrating two nonejection systolic clicks of constant timing. EXP = expiration; M = mitral closure sound; A = aortic closure sound; P = pulmonic closure sound.

diastolic decrescendo murmur described by Wei and Fortuin[105] is sometimes a reflection of this mechanism.

Vasoactive maneuvers or other alterations affecting the functional anatomy of the mitral valve mechanism will affect the timing and intensity of late systolic murmurs.[5,6,20] The murmur may become pansystolic with a ventricular extrasystole (Figure 31.13), louder but remain in late systole after phenylephrine injection (Figure 31.13), but it has a variable change in timing and intensity when alterations in blood pressure as well as end-diastolic left ventricular volume occur. Amyl nitrite inhalation (Figure 31.14), the straining phase of the Valsalva maneuver and the adoption of the erect posture, all of which result in a decreased left ventricular end-diastolic volume, cause late systolic murmurs to move earlier in systole. In the former two instances, the murmur becomes softer, presumably because of the accompanying hypotension. With the adoption of the erect posture, however, the murmur may become both louder and longer. This change may depend on the augmented force of ventricular contraction produced by increased sympathetic activity in that position as well as, in some instances, increased MVP as a result of the decrease in left ventricular end-diastolic volume.[20] A late systolic murmur of MVP may also become earlier, longer, and louder during acute anxiety or after intravenous infusion of the sympathomimetic drug isoproterenol.[107] It is noteworthy that phenylephrine, which produces systemic hypertension but has little inotropic action or effect on left ventricular end-diastolic volume, causes the late systolic murmur to become louder without significantly changing its configuration or timing (Figure 31.13). Dynamic auscultation should be employed not only to bring about the midsystolic click or late systolic murmur, or both, but also to differentiate MVP from other causes of late systolic murmur such as rheumatic mitral regurgitation, idiopathic hypertrophic subaortic stenosis, aortic valvular stenosis, and papillary muscle dysfunction (Table 31.2).

An apical early nonpansystolic murmur, which is decrescendo on a phonocardiogram (Figure 31.9), has been emphasized by Barlow and Pocock[107] as also denoting mitral regurgitation. These early systolic murmurs are oc-

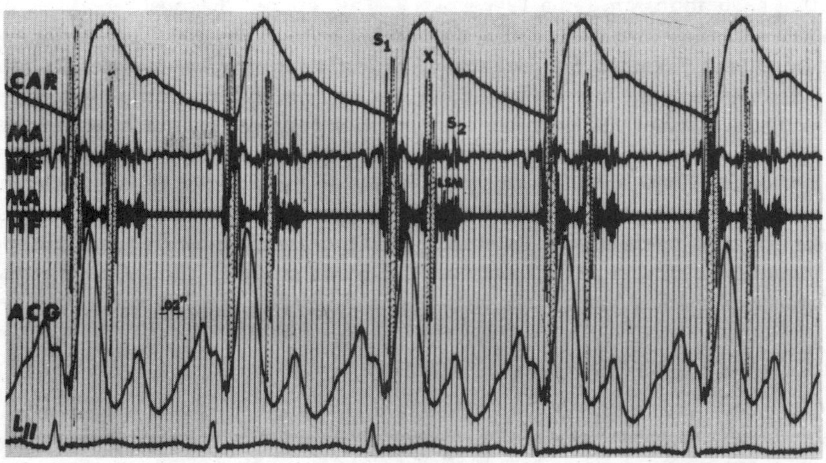

Figure 31.8. A loud late systolic click (X) being possibly mistaken for the second heart sound (S_2) and consequently the late systolic murmur (LSM) mistaken as an early diastolic murmur. The click coincides with the midsystolic dip or retraction in the apexcardiogram (ACG). CAR = carotid pulse; HF = high frequency; MA = mitral area; MF = medium frequency; S_1 = first heart sound. (Modified from Cheng.[39])

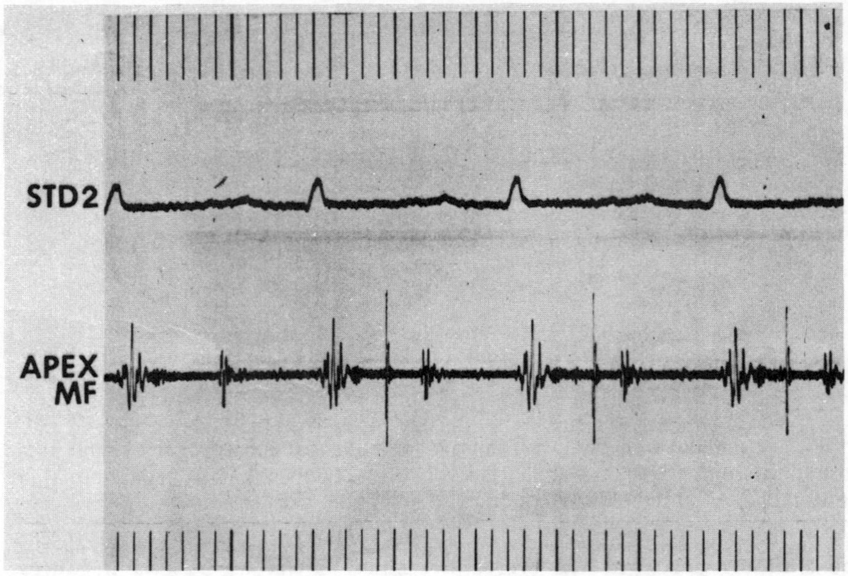

Figure 31.9. Phonocardiogram of a teenaged girl showing a nonejection click varying in position and absent in the first complex. In addition, a soft early nonpansystolic murmur of mitral regurgitation can be seen. MF = medium frequency.

casionally observed to become late on standing or to move spontaneously to late systole during examination. Barlow and Pocock[24] consider that this apical early systolic murmur should be regarded as having similar significance to that of the more easily detected and assessed late systolic murmur.

Like murmurs arising at other sites in the heart, mitral systolic murmurs may develop a musical intonation. The musical vibrations may occur throughout systole or may be confined to early or late systole (Figure 31.15). They frequently vary markedly in intensity and may be loudest during inspiration.[6] At times, the murmur may assume a quality simulating the honk of a goose[108,109] or the whoop in pertussis.[109] Musical murmurs may be extremely loud and audible to the patient[110,111] or to persons in close proximity.[111,112] Of historical interest was the report by Osler in 1880 of such an instance in a 12-year-old girl whose "remarkable whistling sound was distinctly audible at a distance of 3 feet 2 inches by measurement."[112] Osler stated that there were times when the murmur completely disappeared. It has also been our experience that the musical intonation of a murmur often disappears after days or weeks. These mitral "whoops" do not appear to have an ominous significance, and we have not observed them either to precede valve rupture or to develop more commonly during or after infective endocarditis.[107] The response of musical late systolic murmurs to amyl nitrite and phenylephrine is similar to that of other late systolic murmurs.

ECHOCARDIOGRAPHIC FEATURES OF BILLOWING AND PROLAPSED MITRAL VALVES

The development of echocardiography has constituted one of the milestones in the clinical detection of MVP. Regrettably, much of the literature has created confusion because it is seldom clear whether patients with only a BML as opposed to true prolapse are being studied. At the present time, numerous patients are referred for echocardiographic examination to confirm or exclude the presence of MVP.[113] Such examinations will remain misleading unless, or until, the limitations of echocardiography in relation to billowing, prolapse, floppy, or flail leaflets are understood.[33]

The reputed diagnostic features of MVP on M-mode echocardiography are: (1) posterior excursion of the leaflet or leaflets during late systole, (2) holosystolic hammocking of one or both mitral leaflets, (3) systolic anterior motion followed by notching in midsystole and late systolic posterior motion,[114,115] and (4) sudden posterior collapse of the anterior mitral leaflet in early systole as it attempts to contact the prolapsing posterior leaflet.[116] The first two are the most frequent and specific signs. A recent M-mode study[117] concluded that these two major echocardiographic signs, namely, late systolic posterior mo-

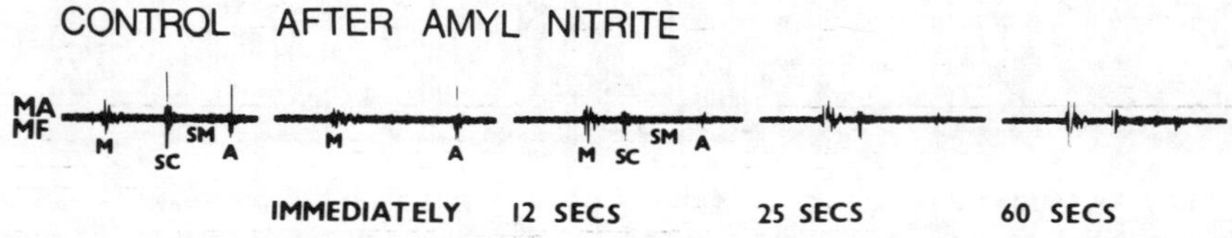

Figure 31.10. Phonocardiogram showing the earlier movement and decreased intensity of a nonejection systolic click (SC) after inhalation of amyl nitrite. Immediately after inhalation the click has disappeared. MA = mitral area; MF = medium frequency; SM = systolic murmur.

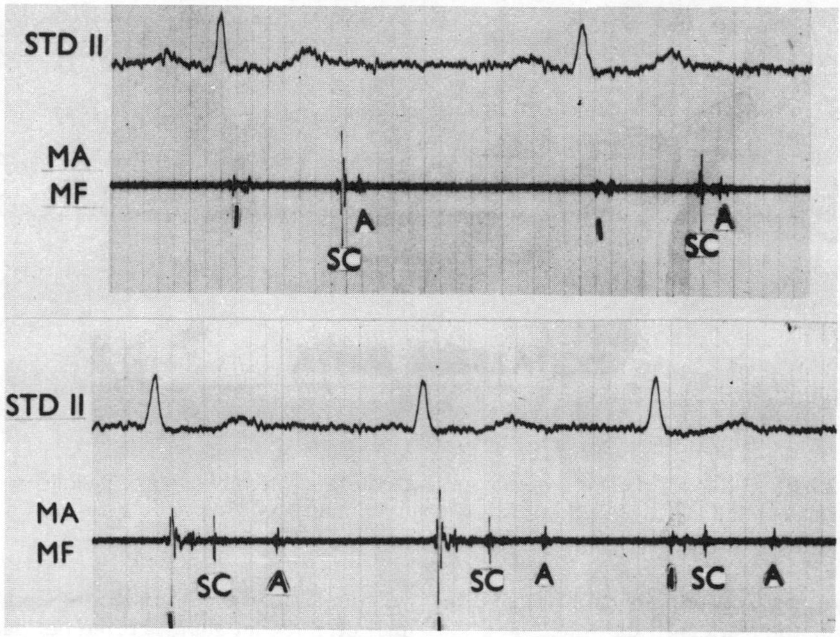

Figure 31.11. Phonocardiograms of a middle-aged woman recorded during sinus rhythm (*top*) and later during atrial fibrillation (*bottom*). The systolic click (SC) occurs earlier in systole during atrial fibrillation. MA = mitral area; MF = medium frequency.

tion and holosystolic hammocking of the mitral leaflets, when combined as a single criterion, had a sensitivity of 85% and a specificity of 99%. Other signs, including systolic echoes in the mid left atrium, systolic anterior motion, early diastolic anterior motion of the posterior mitral leaflet, and shaggy or heavy cascading linear diastolic echoes posterior to the mitral valve, although highly specific, are less common and occur always in combination with late systolic posterior motion or holosystolic hammocking.[117]

The finding of late systolic billowing or midsystolic buckling of the mitral valve has withstood the test of time and has proved quite specific with rare exception.[117a] Occasionally apparent posterior displacement of the mitral valve in patients with pericardial effusion due to systolic posterior swinging of the heart[118] or in patients with dilated congestive cardiomyopathy[119,120] may superficially resemble, but should not be confused with, MVP. Echocardiographic MVP has also been reported during premature ventricular contractions in apparently normal subjects but not with sinus beats.[121]

Although M-mode echocardiography has been a boon in the diagnosis of MPV, especially in its worldwide application in epidemiologic surveys, it has also created some confusion and controversies. The confusion arises from the observation that it is possible to produce "echocardiographic MVP" by an abnormal inferiorly directed orientation of the transducer[122] and that minor degrees of late systolic posterior motion of the body of the leaflet are common in normal subjects.[123] Controversies also resulted from arbitrarily proposed criteria of using 2-, 3-, or 5-mm systolic posterior motion of the mitral valve

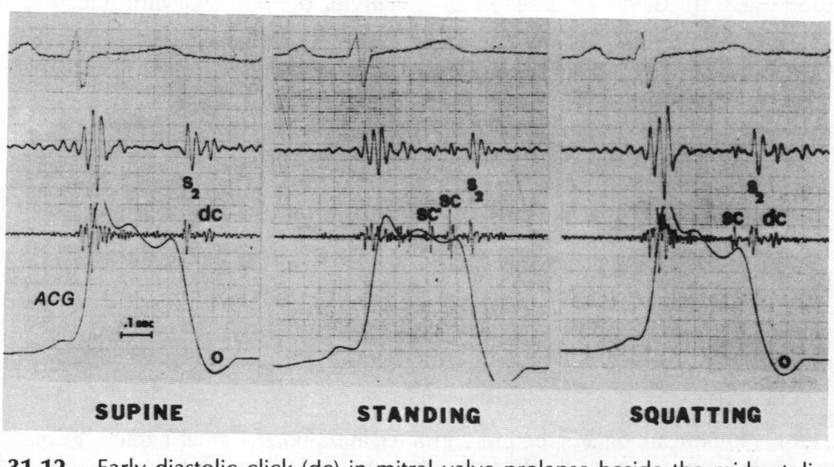

Figure 31.12. Early diastolic click (dc) in mitral valve prolapse beside the midsystolic clicks (SC′, SC). Phonocardiograms recorded in both low (*upper channel*) and medium (*lower channel*) frequencies. ACG = apexcardiogram; S_2 = second heart sound.

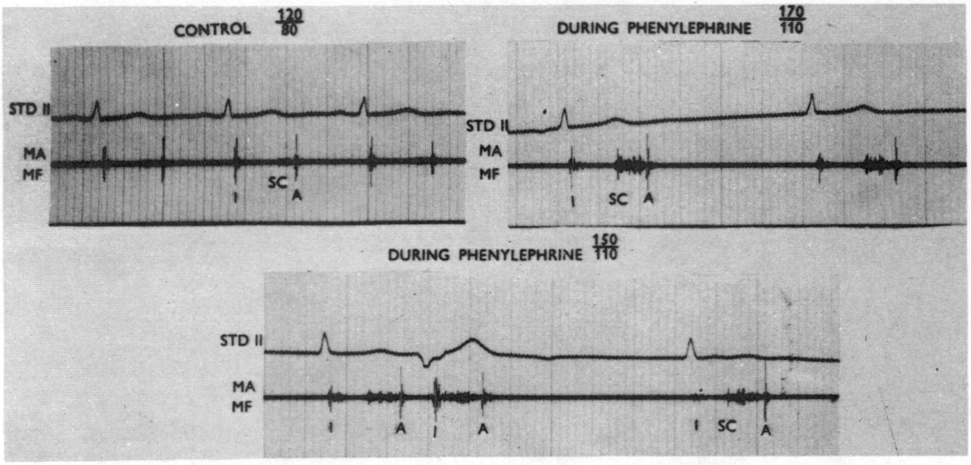

Figure 31.13. Phonocardiograms demonstrating increased intensity of a late systolic murmur after phenylephrine injection and the late systolic murmur becoming pansystolic with a ventricular extrasystole. (From Barlow,[6] with permission.)

below a line connecting the closure point of leaflets with the point of opening of the leaflets in diastole.[100,120,124]

Because of the confusion and controversies introduced by the M-mode echocardiogram which visualizes only part, an "icepick" view, of the mitral valve, it is not surprising that the advent of two-dimensional (2-D) echocardiography with its spatial orientation was hailed with great enthusiasm in the diagnosis of MVP where it has been considered by some[125–127] to be superior to M-mode echocardiography. Superior arching of the mitral leaflets above the plane of the atrioventricular ring, as represented by a line extending from the base of the aortic valve to the atrioventricular junction, is an accepted 2-D echocardiographic indication of an abnormal BML, except perhaps in children.[128] When both the long axis and four-chamber views are used (Figure 31.16), diagnostic accuracy is increased.[129,129a]

We repeat that although echocardiography has provided objective evidence of the mitral valve anomaly, criteria and conclusions have been confused by the lack of clarity concerning terminology. Echocardiography, either M-mode or 2-D, demonstrates a BML or a floppy leaflet. It will not demonstrate failure of leaflet edge coaptation, which is true prolapse, until the MVP is severe or a leaflet is flail.[33] Both types of echocardiography should therefore be reassessed in accord with the concept of the functional anatomy of billowing and prolapse.[33] Billowing mitral leaflet alone is often not demonstrable on echocardiography in patients with an isolated NESC. When an associated systolic murmur is present, echocardiography will usually confirm the "billowing bodies of the leaflets," that is BML, because the valve anomaly is more severe. It does not show, however, whether or not mitral regurgitation is present unless the prolapse has become severe and a leaflet is partly flail. Patients with a holosystolic murmur have marked BML or even a floppy valve, and these will be readily demonstrated on either M-mode or 2-D echocardiography.[32] The role of Doppler in the diagnosis of MVP awaits further study.[127]

ANGIOCARDIOGRAPHIC FEATURES OF BILLOWING AND PROLAPSED MITRAL VALVES

Left ventricular cineangiography has been a yardstick for the diagnosis of MVP. Typically there is end-systolic billowing of one or both mitral leaflets with or without varying degrees of mitral regurgitation (Figure 31.17). However, more recent studies[130,131] noted an inordinately high incidence of angiographic evidence of BML, especially of the posterior mitral leaflet, in a variety of cardiac disorders, yielding a large discrepancy between clinical, echocardiographic, and angiographic findings. Particular

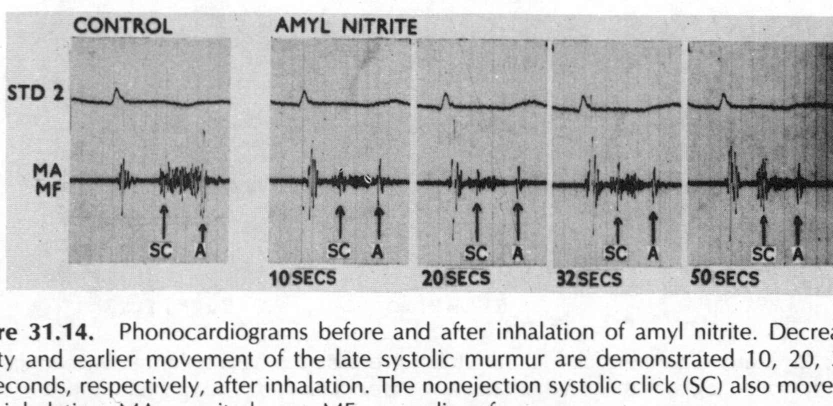

Figure 31.14. Phonocardiograms before and after inhalation of amyl nitrite. Decreased intensity and earlier movement of the late systolic murmur are demonstrated 10, 20, 32, and 50 seconds, respectively, after inhalation. The nonejection systolic click (SC) also moves earlier after inhalation. MA = mitral area; MF = medium frequency.

Table 31.2. Differential Diagnosis of Late Systolic Murmurs

	MVP	RMR	IHSS	AS	PMD
Systolic click	Mid-late	0	Rare	Early	Transient
First sound	↔*	↓	↔	↔	↑
Diastolic sound	Early click	S_3	S_4	S_4	$S_3 + S_4$
Post PVC	↓	↔	↑	↑	↓
Inspiration	↑↓	↓	↓	↓	↑
Valsalva maneuver	↓	↓	↑	↓	↓
Handgrip	↓	↑	↓	↓	↑
Squatting	↓	↑	↓	↑	↑
Standing	↑	↓	↑	↓	↓
Amyl nitrite	↓	↓	↑	↑	↑

*Except in early-onset MVP where first sound may be accentuated. From Tei C, Shah PM, Cherian G, Wong M, Ormiston JA: The correlates of an abnormal first heart sound in mitral-valve-prolapse syndromes. *N Engl J Med* 1982; 307:334–339.

AS = aortic-valvular stenosis; IHSS = idiopathic hypertrophic subaortic stenosis; MVP = mitral valve prolapse; 0 = absent; Post PVC = beat after premature ventricular contraction; PMD = papillary muscle dysfunction; RMR = rheumatic mitral regurgitation; S_3 = diastolic gallop; S_4 = presystolic gallop; $S_3 + S_4$ = both diastolic and presystolic gallops; ↓ = decrease; ↑ = increase; ↑↓ = variable; ↔ = no change.

attention to the mitral fulcrum and fornix is important. The mitral fulcrum is the point of attachment of the mitral leaflets to the anulus, and the fornix is that part of the left ventricle between the fulcrum and papillary muscles. The mitral fulcrum is identifiable angiographically in the right anterior oblique projection by contrast substance trapped in the recess between the leaflet and the adjacent endocardium[132] (Figure 31.18). The diagnosis of BML is made when there is posterior and inferior paraanular displacement of the mitral leaflet beyond the level of the mitral fulcrum during systole. More recent reports[132–134] further underscored the importance, which was emphasized in 1966 by Barlow and Bosman,[21] of the disappearance in diastole of these protrusions in true MVP, whereas the contrast-filled contour remains unchanged in this normal fulcrum during the following diastole in pseudoprolapse (Figure 31.18). A useful technique to demonstrate a BML is negative contrast left atriography which circumvents altogether the issue of the left ventricular fulcrum (Figure 31.19).

The posterior leaflet, which is a triscalloped structure (Figure 31.17), is the more commonly involved in MVP on both anatomic and angiographic studies.[135,136] Pathologic studies indicated that combined leaflet prolapse is frequently present, whereas isolated anterior leaflet prolapse is unusual.[137] Although the optimal angiographic projection for visualization of posterior leaflet billowing is the conventional 30° right anterior oblique view, billowing of the anterior leaflet is more difficult to see in this view because of overlapping and superposition by the opacified aortic valve. The left anterior oblique projection is more useful for identification of billowing of the anterior leaflet. In this view, the two mitral leaflets do not overlap; thus, the billowing anterior leaflet may be seen as a convexity lying in close proximity to the aortic root, protruding into the left atrium, and occupying the anterosuperior segment of the mitral anulus (Figure 31.20).

Other abnormalities noted on left ventricular cineangiography include segmental contractile abnormalities located predominantly in the basal, mid, and anterolateral segments,[92,138,139] an increased mean rate of left ventricular circumferential fiber shortening,[138] a dilated mitral anulus,[140] and mitral regurgitation of various degrees. These contraction abnormalities have been proposed as evidence of a primary cardiomyopathy causing or associated with MVP. We believe that they are secondary to MVP, as evidenced by their normalization following surgical replacement of the prolapsed mitral valve.[106]

In view of the high prevalence and frequent association of both coronary artery disease and MVP in many populations, because patients with primary MVP often present with chest pain that sometimes is indistinguishable from angina due to coronary artery disease, and because coronary artery disease and MVP have divergent prognostic implications, selective coronary arteriography may be indicated in some cases. In patients with primary MVP, coronary arteriograms have invariably been normal unless coexistent occlusive coronary artery disease was coincidentally present.[25] It was shown by Cheng[141] that primary MVP can often be differentiated from MVP secondary to coronary artery disease by the ventriculographic appearance of the MVP. In his experience, the mitral valve in primary MVP simulates a "beak" of a bird, whereas in coronary artery disease it is like a

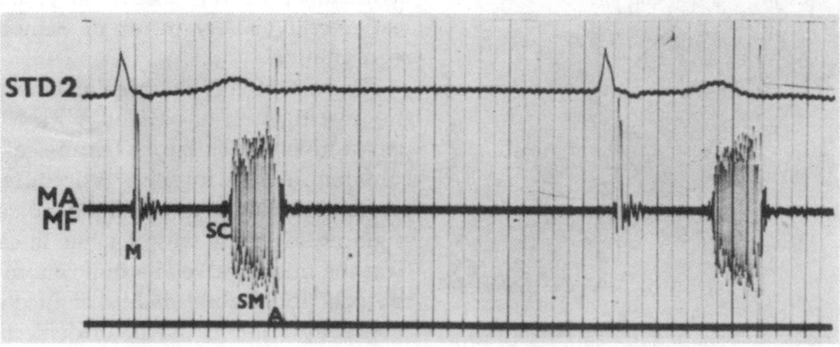

Figure 31.15. Phonocardiogram demonstrating a loud musical late systolic murmur (SM). A = aortic closure; M = mitral closure; MA = mitral area; MF = medium frequency; SC = systolic click.

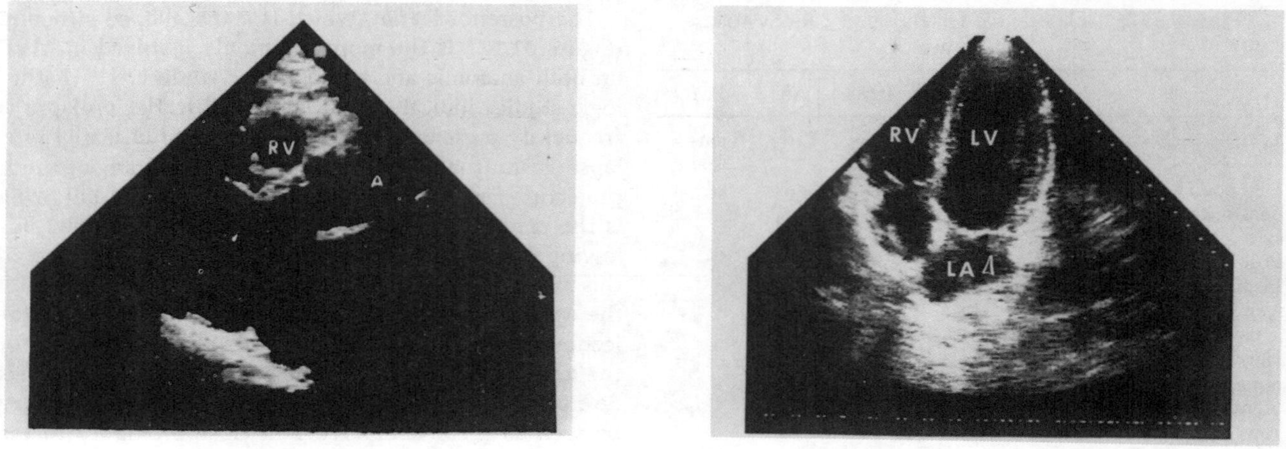

Figure 31.16. Long axis (*left*) and four-chamber (*right*) two-dimensional echocardiograms showing prolapse of both mitral leaflets, especially the posterior one (*arrowhead*). Ao = aorta; LA = left atrium; LV = left ventricle; RV = right ventricle.

"nipple."[141] Cheng considers that this difference in angiographic appearance of the MVP, which has subsequently been observed by others,[142,143] is explained by the fact that chordae tendineae are uniformly elongated in primary MVP, whereas they are more unevenly tethered in papillary muscle dysfunction secondary to coronary artery disease.

Additional observations during angiography in the diagnostic evaluation of patients with MVP have related to the detection of associated prolapse of other cardiac valves. Tricuspid valve prolapse was detected by right ventriculography in approximately 50% of patients with MVP studied by Gooch et al.[144] Although angiographic diagnosis of tricuspid valve prolapse is fraught with considerable difficulty because of possible distortion of the tricuspid valve by the transvalvular placement of the angiographic catheter and the known variability of the angiographic appearance of the normal tricuspid valve and anulus, such a high association is supported by both echocardiographic[51–53,55,145,146] and pathologic[37,137] studies. The clinical relevance of these cineangiocardiographic observations of a high prevalence of associated tricuspid valve prolapse remains uncertain. Isolated significant organic tricuspid regurgitation presumably does not develop because of low pressures on the right side of the heart. It remains possible that infective endocarditis affecting the tricuspid valve, which certainly does result in severe regurgitation, may in some instances have occurred on a prolapsed tricuspid valve. Associated aortic valve prolapse has seldom been observed in studies relating to the mitral valve,[29,147] but this may relate to the nature of the population investigated. Triple valve prolapse has been reported in Marfan's syndrome.[147a] The clinical syndrome of aortic regurgitation due to aortic leaflet prolapse recently described by Lakier et al,[148] Allen et al,[149] and Bellitt et al[149a] is probably a similar pathologic entity to primary MVP. However, because of the different functional anatomy of the aortic valve, prolapse of an aortic leaflet will usually result in hemodynamically marked regurgitation.

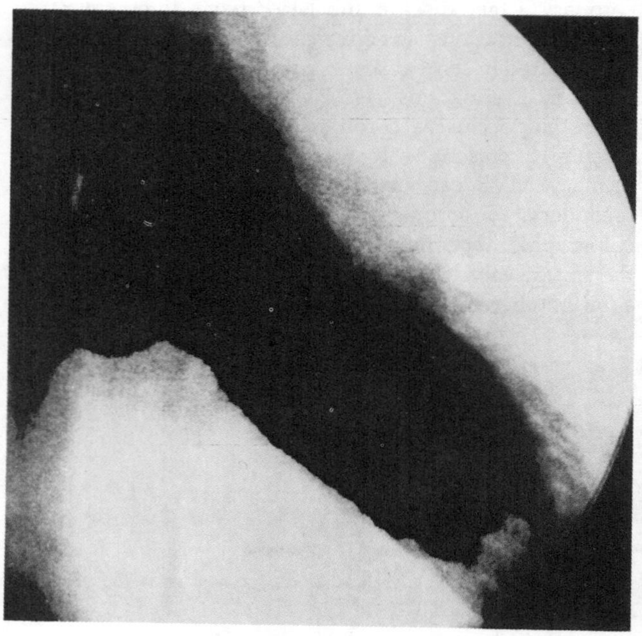

Figure 31.17. Typical doughnut-shaped appearance of prolapsing triscalloped posterior leaflet and anterior leaflet of the mitral valve demonstrated on left ventriculography in right anterior oblique projection.

The role of left ventricular cineangiocardiography in the investigation of patients with MVP must be seen in perspective. Auscultatory features of MVP are extremely common and an invasive procedure such as cineangiocardiography should seldom be indicated. Left ventricular angiocardiography was of value in earlier studies to confirm the mitral valve anatomic anomaly of billowing and the functional abnormality of incompetence. Angiocardiography remains useful in demonstrating a BML that may be marked, moderate, or confined to one scallop. It will also confirm mitral regurgitation, if that is deemed necessary, in patients with mitral systolic murmurs, but

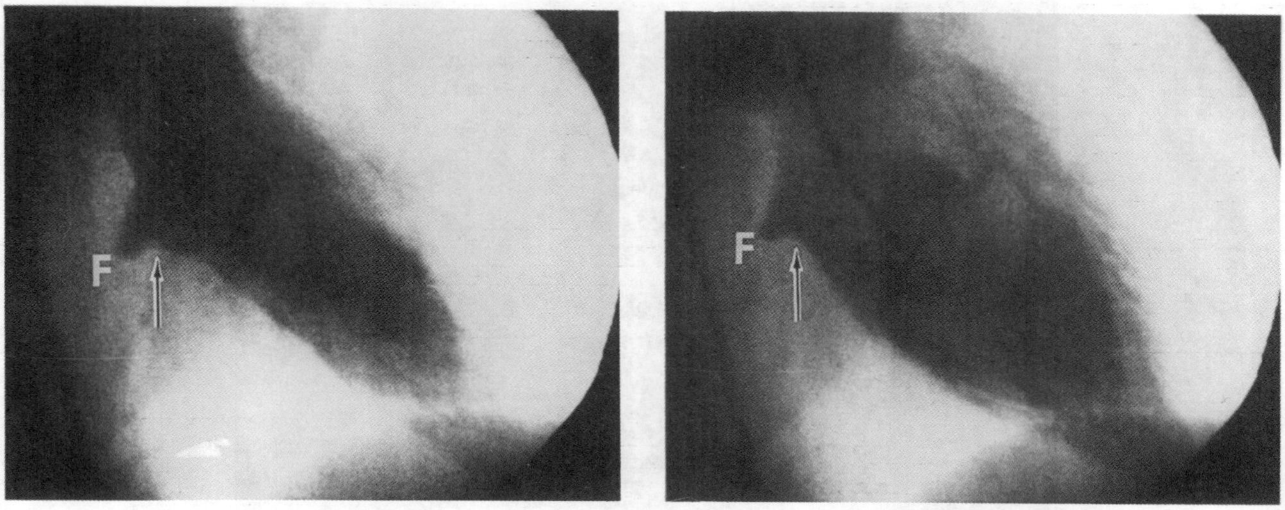

Figure 31.18. Pseudoprolapse simulated by the posterior mitral fulcrum (F), which is present during both systole (*left*) and diastole (*right*), adjacent to a concave fornix (*arrow*).

it will not demonstrate lack of leaflet edge apposition until the prolapse becomes extremely severe or a leaflet is flail.

PRIMARY MITRAL VALVE PROLAPSE (BARLOW'S) SYNDROME

Despite the large number of subjects, asymptomatic and otherwise completely normal, with auscultatory, echocardiographic, and angiocardiographic evidence of primary MVP, the experience of cardiologists with numerous similar patients who complain of chest pain, palpitations, dizziness, or syncope has been convincing and has resulted in the recognition of a specific syndrome. The term *syndrome* is justified because there may be many associated features including symptoms, electrocardiographic changes, arrhythmias, conduction defects, systemic emboli, autonomic disorders, and possibly myocardial dysfunction. The importance of making the diagnosis of primary MVP syndrome relates in most cases to the contribution of reassurance that serious heart disease is not present, that symptoms are of nuisance value only, and that the prognosis for life is excellent.[24,32,107]

PREVALENCE OF PRIMARY MITRAL VALVE PROLAPSE

Motulsky's comments made in 1978[150] that, "for every patient with symptomatic mitral valve prolapse . . ., there are hundreds of asymptomatic persons," remain pertinent. The prevalence of MVP in population surveys has depended on the nature of the population studied[128,151–153] as well as the relative significance attached to ausculta-

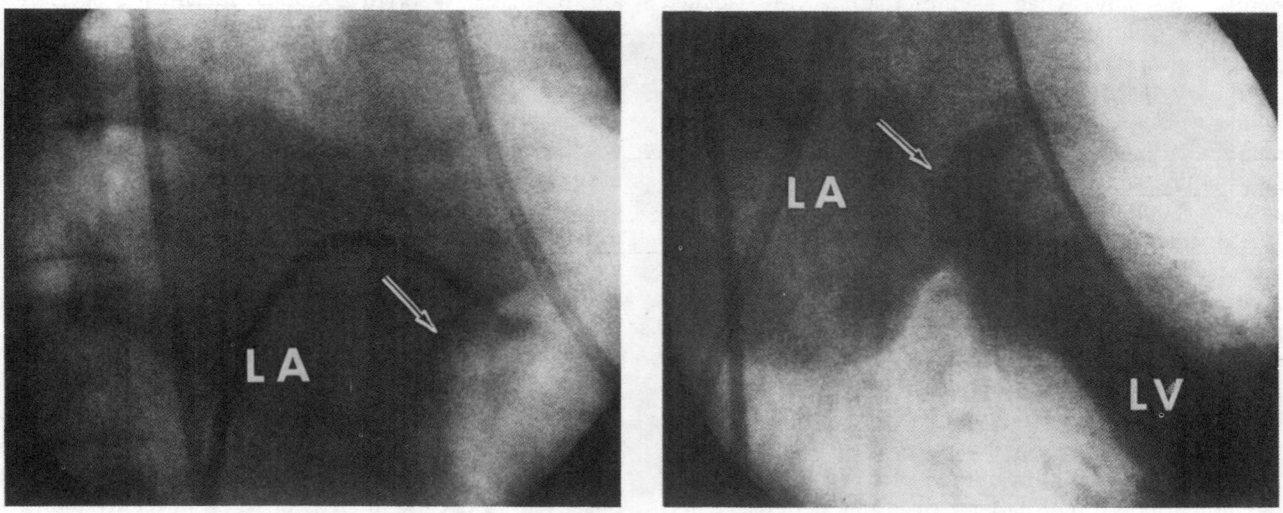

Figure 31.19. Left atrial (LA) injection through a transseptal catheter in the right anterior oblique projection (*left*), showing a prolapsed mitral valve (*arrow*) as a negative contrast. Subsequent left ventricular (LV) injection in the same projection (*right*), showing the same prolapsed mitral valve (*arrow*) as a positive contrast accompanied by marked mitral regurgitation outlining the entire left atrium (LA).

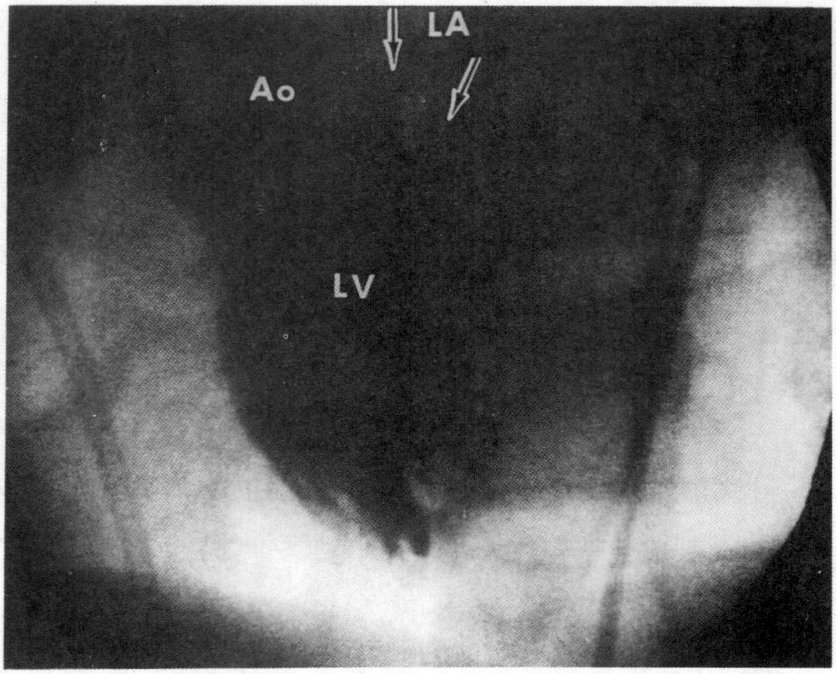

Figure 31.20. Left ventriculogram (LV) in left anterior oblique projection of the same patient in Figure 31.19, showing anterior mitral valve prolapse as a convexity (*vertical arrow*) protruding into the left atrium (LA) in close proximity to the root of the aorta (Ao), and also prolapse of the posterior mitral leaflet (*oblique arrow*). Significant mitral regurgitation was present.

tion, echocardiography,[125,154,155] angiography,[81,130] or necropsy.[154,155a,156] Mitral valve prolapse is the most frequently diagnosed valve disorder in the United States, but it is also a universal disease and has been described in nearly every country in the world. Survey of the literature relating to prevalence shows a range from 1% to 24%[32,37,87,125,151–174b] (Table 31.3). It is important to judge these high numbers in perspective and it is unlikely that significant "pathology" is present in most instances. Patients, especially when asymptomatic, with isolated NESCs or "echo only" MVP can possibly be regarded as subjects at one end of a normal distribution curve.[32]

Primary MVP is as prevalent in blacks as in whites,[152,153,170a] more common in women than men,[128,151–153,156,159,166,170] and the Framingham epidemiologic study suggested a diminished occurrence in the aged.[174] Young women in the Framingham study had a 17% incidence of MVP, whereas the anomaly was detected in only 1% of women aged 80 years or over.[174] Men had a prevalence of about 3% at all ages.[174] Why MVP is more common in females than in males is not entirely clear. Smaller left ventricular size[43,173] and lower body weight[175] in women may play a role. The secondary fibrosis of the mitral leaflets and chordae tendineae, which was observed in some pathologic series[156] and also suggested by decreasing magnitude of MVP on echocardiographic follow-up of patients over long periods,[176] may explain the reduced frequency of MVP diagnosed in older patients.

Mitral valve prolapse was detected echocardiographically in 7% of stable newborn girls[177] and in 5% of a pediatric population.[178] It is also very prevalent on echocardiographic examination in athletes.[158a,165] Mitral valve prolapse has been reported as the main cause of sport-associated cardiologic morbidity, especially syncope,[179] in the British Army.[180]

INHERITANCE AND GENETICS OF PRIMARY MITRAL VALVE PROLAPSE

Since its first recognition in the early 1960s, the familial occurrence of MVP gained ready acceptance. After Barlow and Bosman[21] reported a kindred in which 6 of 17 relatives studied were affected, several families of affected kindreds in two or three generations have been documented,[181–183] including the "all in the family" phenomenon.[107,184] An autosomal dominant mode of inheritance was first suggested in 1969 by Hunt and Sloman[185] who used mainly auscultation for detection of MVP. Subsequently, 40% to 50% of first degree relatives were found to be affected in several echocardiographic studies.[186–189] Evidence for autosomal dominant inheritance was provided by three further studies.[186,188,190]

Expression of the MVP gene appears to be affected by both sex and age. Females have a higher incidence of MVP in the cumulative findings of available population surveys.[87,157,173,174,191] Similarly, more first degree female relatives, 56%[192] to 60%,[186] than male relatives, 23%[192] to 27%,[186] were affected. There is also an age-dependent onset with a decline in signs of MVP in relatives of increasing age.[187,189,192]

An increased frequency of HLA antigens in patients with MVP was found by two groups,[193,194] but not by two others.[195,196] Studies of other genetic markers such as dermal arches[196,197] have been even less conclusive.

Table 31.3. Prevalence of Mitral Valve Prolapse Around the World

Country	Male	Female	Overall
Australia[157]	4%	4%	4%
Brazil[158]	...	...	4%
Britain[125]*	...	2%	...
Britain[37]	...	...	5%
Britain[156†]	3.9%	5.2%	4.5%
Canada[158a]	...	...	22%
China (Hans in Sichuan)[159]*	2.2%	6.3%	4.3%
China (Kazaks in Xinjiang)[151]	2.8%	7.7%	5.3%
China (schoolchildren in Guangdong)[160]	...	...	1.9%
Denmark[161]*	...	...	7%
Germany[162]*	6.89%	13.84%	9.8%
Hong Kong (Chinese)[154]	7.2%*; 5.4%†	8%*; 6.4%†	7.7%*; 5.8%†
India (outpatient)[162a]	...	2.7%	...
India[163]	...	16%*	...
Israel[164]	...	...	5%
Italy[152]	0.7%	3.3%	1.8%
Italy (blacks)[152]	...	...	1.4%
Italy (athletes)[165]	...	...	10%
Japan (schoolchildren)[166]	0.78%	1.26%	1%
Japan[155a†]	1 x‡	4 x‡	7.5%
Japan[155*]	11%	8%	11%
Korea[167]	3.3%	10%	6.7%
Poland[168]	...	...	4%
Russia[169]	...	...	2.64± 0.36%
Spain[170]	1 x‡	2 x‡	4.3%
South Africa[32]	...	...	14.3%
South Africa (blacks)[170a]	...	...	17.9%
Sweden[171]	7%	8%	7.4%
Turkey[172]	...	...	7.6%
USA[87,173,174]	3%	6.2%–17%	...
USA (blacks)[153]	9%	24%	17%
USA (health survey)[174a]	...	15.4%	...
USA (non-care-seeking adolescents)[174b]	2.25%	6.16%	4.18%

* Echocardiographic studies.

† Autopsy studies.

‡ Expressed as a ratio.

MYOCARDIAL DYSFUNCTION IN PRIMARY MITRAL VALVE PROLAPSE

Controversy continues as to whether there is a generalized myocardial disorder in some patients with the primary MVP syndrome, especially those complaining of chest pain and those with an abnormal electrocardiogram. Evidence of a diffuse myocardial abnormality has been supported by biopsy studies and histochemical analysis.[198,199] Malcolm[200] reviewed the data in 1980 and judged that a metabolic or biochemical mechanism was a likely explanation for some symptoms, especially the chest pain. Conclusions drawn from radionuclide studies of left ventricular function in the primary MVP syndrome have also been contradictory.[201–210] To our knowledge, no necropsy evidence supporting "a myocardial factor" has been produced. We do not understand why myocardial function should be significantly affected in the primary MVP syndrome, but this possibility requires clarification. The regional abnormalities of left ventricular wall motion that have been detected[211,211a] cineangiocardiographically in both systole and diastole can probably be attributed to abnormal tension, in both systole and diastole, on chordae and papillary muscles from the billowing mitral leaflets.

MANIFESTATIONS AND MANAGEMENT OF PRIMARY MITRAL VALVE PROLAPSE SYNDROME

ASYMPTOMATIC PRIMARY MITRAL VALVE PROLAPSE

Primary MVP in asymptomatic persons may be recognized during routine examination, including that for employment or life insurance, or in surveys of schools and other institutions. The condition is sometimes detected because of an abnormal electrocardiogram, which may have been performed under similar circumstances. The asymptomatic subject may have been informed of the abnormality and must then be regarded as a "patient." Irrespective of whether the MVP is in a subject or a patient, the following practical approach to management is suggested:

An isolated nonejection systolic click on auscultation or echocardiographic evidence only of "mitral valve prolapse": Irrespective of whether the electrocardiogram shows T-wave changes, a large number of asymptomatic subjects are detected during routine examinations as having auscultatory or echocardiographic evidence of a BML. The auscultatory evidence will be an isolated, albeit sometimes intermittent, nonejection click. In the absence of a systolic murmur, echocardiographic evidence of billowing is rare in our experience, but the entity of "echo only" MVP is nonetheless reputedly common.[212] In many such instances, either auscultation has presumably been hurried and inadequate or else the echocardiographic findings are open to criticism and due to faulty transducer angulation. The asymptomatic subject or patient should either not be informed about the "valve anomaly" or, if he knows it already, should be strongly reassured that it is virtually a normal variant that occurs in a large number of healthy people. There should be valid reasons before a stress electrocardiogram or Holter monitoring is performed in such subjects. An effort electrocardiogram is indicated if the individual is employed in an important public service capacity, such as an airline pilot. A stress electrocardiogram is also indicated if the BML is detected during examination for a life insurance policy. Adults undergoing a routine check-up are often subjected to an effort test, irrespective of the presence of BML, to exclude occlusive coronary artery disease. Although asymptomatic subjects with a BML may occasionally develop arrhythmias after effort, the prognostic significance of this observation remains uncertain. It is rare to encounter an important arrhythmia such as supraventricular tachycardia or multifocal ventricular extrasystoles in such subjects.[213] Even if multifocal extrasystoles are detected in an asymptomatic subject and there is no other evidence, including electrocardiographic, of occlusive coronary artery disease, there is little evidence to suggest that antiarrhythmic therapy is indicated.[214] It is seldom warranted, and often not practicable, for most other asymptomatic subjects with auscultatory or echocardiographic evidence of a BML detected during routine surveys to be subjected to a stress electrocardiogram. This pertains, for example, to school children, students, or employees in a factory.

The management of patients with MVP with regard to prophylaxis against infective endocarditis remains controversial.[215–219] The confusion has been compounded because investigators have not always clarified whether mitral regurgitation was associated. Although occasional cases of infective endocarditis in patients with an isolated nonejection systolic click have been documented,[220,221] not only is prophylaxis against infective endocarditis in the large number of subjects involved impracticable, but also the overall benefit derived from it is questionable. Antibiotic prophylaxis against infective endocarditis in patients with an isolated NESC or with "echo only" evidence of MVP is not recommended.

Systolic murmur of mitral regurgitation: If a late systolic murmur, albeit intermittent, is detected, this denotes mitral regurgitation and the risk of infective endocarditis is almost certainly greater. The subject should be informed of the MVP and advised to take prophylactic antibiotics before dental treatment or other procedure of "risk." Policy regarding the detection and management of arrhythmias should be the same as that already described for asymptomatic subjects with an isolated NESC or "echo only" MVP.

Most subjects with a constant late systolic murmur on auscultation can be shown to have BML on echocardiography. The BML is confined to late systole on M-mode echocardiography, and this timing can be confirmed on 2-D echocardiography. An asymptomatic subject with a late systolic murmur should be assessed annually for evidence of progression of the MVP on auscultation and of increase of the extent of the BML on echocardiography. In our experience, most late systolic murmurs do not change over many years.

It is more difficult to define a definite policy in subjects who have an early nonpansystolic apical murmur. These murmurs have received little attention in the literature, but it is probable, particularly when they are confined to the apex and associated with an NESC, that they denote mild mitral regurgitation and therefore some prolapse.[24,107] Subjects with a mitral early systolic murmur should thus be managed on the same lines as those with a late systolic murmur.

Asymptomatic subjects with a holosystolic murmur of mitral regurgitation are easily recognized on auscultation, and echocardiography will invariably confirm the billowing of the bodies of the leaflets. The extent of the mitral regurgitation is still assessed as mild provided there is no clinical, electrocardiographic, or radiologic evidence of left ventricular or left atrial enlargement, splitting of the second sound is normal, and an associated third heart sound is judged "physiologic." Physiologic third heart sounds are extremely common in children, young adults, and physically fit older subjects. Prophylaxis against infective endocarditis is indicated and regular clinical and echocardiographic examination should be undertaken to assess the increase in the severity of mitral regurgitation. Maximal, or submaximal, stress testing is also advisable, but if the patient is truly asymptomatic, the development of ventricular ectopy, provided it is not present in triplets or showing the R on T phenomenon, can probably be managed in a similar manner to that of asymptomatic patients with isolated NESCs or nonpansystolic murmurs.

It is difficult to generalize in patients with mild mitral regurgitation who have pansystolic murmurs as far as a policy toward strenuous physical exercise is concerned. Some cardiologists would advise against very strenuous sport because the exercise may cause deterioration in the valve lesion or worsening of complex ventricular arrhythmias.[221a]

SYMPTOMATIC PRIMARY MITRAL VALVE PROLAPSE SYNDROME

Most patients with primary MVP encountered in clinical cardiac departments are symptomatic. Whether or not the clinician believes that some or none of the symptoms can be attributed to the primary MVP, the symptoms are of concern to the patient who is seeking assistance. Many of these symptomatic patients are anxious and the anxiety may be responsible for, or certainly aggravate, some symptoms. For example, breathlessness is a common symptom, yet this cannot be explained on an organic basis. Although the chest pain, which is often sharp, severe, localized, and fleeting, often probably does have a causal relation to the mitral valve anomaly, some physicians do not agree with that sentiment. Similar chest pain occurs in other patients, particularly anxious patients, without definite evidence of MVP. Irrespective of whether the physician considers that symptoms or other manifestations of the primary MVP syndrome can be attributed to the mitral valve anomaly, an approach to the management of these features is necessary.

Anxiety

The large number of patients with primary MVP who suffer from anxiety is noteworthy and is not always understood. So-called "panic attacks," which may be associated with chest pain, have also been described.[75–77] In some patients with MVP, anxiety supervenes after an incorrect diagnosis of occlusive coronary artery disease has been made.[107] In others, anxiety in a genuinely symptomatic patient may be caused or aggravated by the insistence of medical attendants that no organic disease is present. It is not "reassuring" to patients with disturbing symptoms, such as chest pain, dizziness, or palpitations, to be told that they are "neurotic." The anxiety associated with the primary MVP syndrome invariably has a cardiac connotation in that there is fear of serious heart disease or sudden death. The symptomatic presentation is therefore similar to, if not identical with, so-called irritable heart, neurocirculatory asthenia, soldier's heart, DaCosta's syndrome, the atypical chest pain syndrome, and similar disorders.[222] Some studies[78,79] have not confirmed a definite association of MVP with anxiety or panic disorder.

These patients require much reassurance. We have found it consoling to most patients to be informed that they have "a very common but mild valve anomaly, that valve function is normal or very mildly abnormal, and that other associated symptoms are genuine, although not completely understood, and are of nuisance value only." Administration of a beta-receptor blocking agent alleviates the systemic effects of anxiety whether or not it also directly affects the underlying causes, such as arrhythmia or myocardial contractility, of other symptoms.

Several studies have provided evidence of abnormal autonomic function in some symptomatic patients with the MVP syndrome, and a hyperadrenergic state or catecholamine sensitivity has been postulated.[223,223a] The observation of symptomatic orthostatic hypotension[47] and of ischemic-appearing ST segments in response to forced hyperventilation also suggests autonomic dysfunction. However, the exact relation of these findings to anxiety remains uncertain. It is difficult to understand why an anomaly of a cardiac valve should correlate with autonomic dysfunction. We believe that the various autonomic disturbances reflect manifestations of anxiety rather than a direct correlation with the valve anomaly. The anxiety, in turn, is often a reaction to the disabling symptoms of chest pain, palpitations, presyncope, or even syncope and is worsened by unsympathetic medical advisors.

Chest Pain

Despite the large number of anxious patients with the primary MVP syndrome and chest pain, a presentation of chest pain, sometimes severe and disabling, in somewhat stoical subjects who were previously unaware of having MVP or any other cardiac abnormality has impressed many clinicians. Although so-called "atypical" chest pain is a symptom that may have many causes, we believe that MVP is one of them. The chest pain may be more frequent in patients with MVP who have an abnormal electrocardiogram,[211] but the electrocardiogram, both at rest and after effort, may be normal.[107] The mechanism of production of the pain is poorly understood. Cobbs and King,[106] Cobbs,[224] Jeresaty[225] as well as Pocock and Barlow[226] independently suggested that increased traction from chordae tendineae may tug on a papillary muscle and produce pain. Following their angiocardiographic observations of regional left ventricular wall movement abnormalities in patients with MVP, Gibson and Brown[211] also considered the possibility that regional subendocardial ischemia may be a factor in causing both pain and arrhythmias.

The pain is usually sharp, fleeting, left-sided, and localized to the apical region. There is seldom a relation to exercise or emotion. Some patients insist that they have to sit or even lie down. The pain may be sufficiently severe to cause considerable anxiety or a feeling of "impending doom." It may occur in bed at night but seldom wakes the patient. Holter monitoring has not demonstrated a correlation between transient T-wave changes and chest pain. These characteristics have left some clinicians unconvinced that the chest pain is cardiac, or indeed organic, in origin. Other patients, invariably with associated anxiety, complain of a constant localized chest pain lasting for hours or even days. We do not dispute that anxiety is an aggravating factor, and in some instances probably the principal factor, which contributes to chest pain in symptomatic patients with the primary MVP syndrome.

A few patients complain of chest pain indistinguishable from angina. It is possible that some have learned of the nature of true angina pectoris from other patients or medical attendants. In our experience, a stress electrocardiogram is highly contributory in excluding occlusive coronary artery disease but, depending on the context of the situation, selective coronary arteriography or radionuclide studies may be necessary for confirmation. The problem is obviously easier to resolve in, for example, a 20-year-old woman as opposed to a middle-aged man. It is among this group of patients with "typical angina" that a possible causal relation between primary MVP and myocardial ischemia or infarction in the presence of anatomically normal or near-normal coronary arteries arises. In 1976, Chesler et al[227] reported on four patients with primary MVP, myocardial infarction, and anatomically normal coronary arteries and postulated that coronary artery spasm or coronary artery emboli may be causally related to MVP. One of those four patients, a 23-year-old man, had a small parietal lobe infarct, presumably embolic, about 22 months after a myocardial infarction. Although a few observers[64,65,142,228–233] have confirmed an association between coronary artery spasm and MVP, the possibility of a causal relation between primary MVP and myocardial ischemia or infarction has not to date aroused much interest.

We continue to favor a causal relation between primary MVP and myocardial ischemia or infarction, possibly induced by coronary artery spasm which in turn may be provoked by coronary emboli. The chest pain of MVP can be differentiated in most instances from angina due to coronary artery disease. However, true angina may be atypical and have "widely variable expression," whereas the chest pain of some patients with MVP may closely simulate angina. We have encountered a relatively small group of patients in whom stress electrocardiography, selective coronary arteriography, and, most importantly, the recording of an electrocardiogram during the pain have singly or in combination been essential to clarify the assessment.

It needs to be emphasized that a possibility of coronary artery spasm arises in only a small minority of patients with the primary MVP syndrome who complain of chest pain. Although ergonovine injection may have a role in provoking coronary artery spasm in such patients, we consider that the most valuable method of excluding the possibility of coronary artery spasm is to record an electrocardiogram during an attack of the "typical angina pectoris."

Reassurance is again important in the management of patients with primary MVP syndrome who complain of chest pain. Beta-receptor blocking agents are often also contributory, irrespective of their effect on anxiety. In the small number of patients in whom coronary artery spasm may be a factor, calcium channel blockers such as nifedipine should be effective. As will be discussed later, small emboli from the voluminous prolapsing mitral valve are a feature of MVP, although cerebral emboli have received most attention. When coronary emboli are suspected, antithrombotic therapy with aspirin and dipyridamole is indicated.[32]

Systemic Emboli

Cerebral emboli, usually small, are a rare but generally recognized complication of the primary MVP syndrome. We are well aware of the high prevalence of MVP in both asymptomatic and symptomatic subjects and therefore of the possible fallacy in attributing systemic emboli to a relatively minor valve abnormality, which is so common. Nevertheless, Pomerance[28] observed thrombus formation on ballooning mitral valves and Chesler et al[234] described aggregates of platelets and fibrin in the angle between the posterior mitral leaflet and the left atrial wall. A potential source of bland emboli is therefore apparent. Barnett et al[235] detected a significantly high incidence of MVP in patients under 45 years of age with transient ischemic attacks, and similar evidence was provided in the European literature.[236–238] An association between MVP and migraine[239] has been reported, and increased platelet aggregability[240–242a] or a hypercoagulable state[242b] may be the pathophysiologic mechanism. The occurrence of systemic emboli in patients with MVP has also been described in the South African literature.[143,243]

Our own ongoing clinical observations strongly favor an association between bland cerebral emboli and MVP. The vast majority of these patients had previously been asymptomatic, and it does not seem practicable to prescribe antithrombotic therapy routinely to patients with MVP. Patients who have had embolic events, however, have invariably responded well to antithrombotic (usually aspirin and dipyridamole) therapy.

The possible role of coronary emboli in primary MVP syndrome has already been discussed in this chapter under the section on chest pain.

Progressive Mitral Regurgitation

It remains unknown how to predict with certainty the future course of an individual patient with the primary MVP syndrome as regards progression to significant mitral regurgitation in the absence of infective endocarditis. Part of the problem has related to confusion from terminology. The term "mitral valve prolapse" has been used to describe the functionally normal valves of asymptomatic subjects,[87] on the one hand, and the severely incompetent valves of patients requiring mitral valve replacement,[244] on the other. Some follow-up studies over 10 to 40 years[245–250] have suggested progression to significant mitral regurgitation in 3% to 9% of patients. However, such progression sometimes related to onset of infective endocarditis or included patients with Marfan's syndrome. Recent literature[251–253] emphasizes the role of MVP as a cause of severe mitral regurgitation, but the prevalence of this complication is not clarified. Similarly, Tresch et al,[254] in their description of 30 patients with "mitral valve prolapse requiring surgery," emphasized that many of their patients had had a long history of a systolic murmur, but the incidence in which such patients rupture chordae and develop severe mitral regurgitation remains unclear. The 4-year follow-up of 139 South African black schoolchildren by Cohen et al[170a] revealed the development of significant mitral regurgitation in only one subject.

We have observed patients with MVP and a late systolic murmur advance to a pansystolic murmur during a 10- to 20-year period, but rapid progression is very unusual in the absence of infective endocarditis or Marfan's syndrome. A few patients with a late systolic murmur are presumably suffering from "the floppy valve syndrome" without skeletal manifestations of Marfan's syndrome, but we find it difficult, or impossible, to identify these with certainty. Obvious BML on echocardiography does not mean that marked MVP with severe regurgitation will inevitably ensue. It is clear that some, especially middle-aged or elderly men, will develop severe mitral regurgitation associated with rupture of chordae to the posterior leaflet. We have observed this progression, but infrequently. Middle-aged or elderly Caucasian patients with floppy valves or the syndrome of "idiopathic rupture of chordae"[255] requiring mitral valve surgery are not uncommon. As a matter of fact, MVP is probably the most common cause of spontaneous chordal rupture.[256–258] However, although 11% of patients with MVP have echocardiographic evidence of ruptured chordae, most of them (71%) do not have symptomatic deterioration.[259]

We conclude that most patients, irrespective of age or sex, who have a late or early nonpansystolic murmur of MVP associated with BML on echocardiography will have a favorable course and will not progress to severe mitral regurgitation. The prognosis in a patient with a pansystolic murmur and pansystolic billowing on echocardiography is less favorable, but progression to severe mitral regurgitation in the absence of Marfan's syndrome or infective endocarditis also has seldom been observed.

Infective Endocarditis

The risk of infective endocarditis for any valvular or other cardiac lesion must relate significantly to social customs, particularly dental hygiene, in the relevant population. As far as the primary MVP syndrome is concerned, risk has surely to depend on whether or not mitral regurgitation is associated. This aspect has not always been readily apparent from previous literature. Clemens and Stanton[260] estimated that the risk for patients with MVP is eight times that for patients without underlying heart disease. Indications for prophylaxis against infective endocarditis in MVP remain somewhat controversial[215–218,260a] and have already been discussed. We repeat that there would be less confusion if patients with mitral regurgitation on auscultation were evaluated separately from those who have an isolated NESC or "echo only" MVP. It is neither practicable nor desirable to recommend prophylaxis in every patient who has auscultatory or echocardiographic evidence of a BML in the absence of mitral regurgitation. Although the efficacy of antibiotic prophylaxis against infective endocarditis is not entirely proven,[261–264,264a] it remains generally accepted that patients with mitral regurgitation should receive such prophylaxis.

The microbial agents causing infective endocarditis on prolapsing mitral valve are similar to those that infect valves deformed by congenital or rheumatic processes.

Although viridans streptococci are the most common organisms, coagulase-negative staphylococcal endocarditis is not an infrequent occurrence in patients with MVP.[220,264b] Recognition of the occurrence of endocarditis due to coagulase-negative staphylococci in patients with MVP is important for several reasons. First, blood cultures positive for these organisms are frequently disregarded in patients without prosthetic heart valves or intravascular catheters. Second, the indolent course of some coagulase-negative staphylococcal endocarditis may delay consideration of the correct diagnosis, particularly in patients without congenital or rheumatic heart disease. Finally, even with effective antimicrobial therapy on the basis of in vitro studies, the clinical course may be prolonged and characterized by multiple responses to and relapses following drug withdrawal.[264b]

Electrocardiographic ST-segment and T-wave Changes

The prevalence of electrocardiographic abnormalities in the primary MVP syndrome varies in different series, depending on the selection of patients, but they may range from about 30%[265] to 40%.[266] Fifty-three (37%) of 144 patients, most of whom were symptomatic, reported by Barlow and Pocock[107] in 1975 had an abnormal electrocardiogram. The most widely recognized pattern is an inverted or partially inverted T wave in leads II, III, and AVF with resultant abnormally wide mean frontal plane QRS-T angle. Similar T-wave abnormalities occur in the anterior leads (Figure 31.21) which may or may not be associated with changes in the inferior leads. T-wave inversion may be complete or partial, involving either the initial or terminal portion. Deepening of the notch, until the T wave is completely inverted, may develop in the absence of obvious cause or after effort. The ECG may alter spontaneously (Figure 31.22) and this change may take place within minutes. Adoption of the erect position may also invert T waves. Prominent upright U waves are quite common, especially in the right precordial leads. Prolongation of the QT interval has also been observed in MVP and may be important because of a reputed association with ventricular arrhythmias.[267]

The shape and behavior of the ST-segment and T-wave changes of the primary MVP syndrome show no essential differences from ST-segment and T-wave changes regarded as "nonspecific"[32] which have been associated with or attributed to atypical chest pain syndrome, autonomic disturbances, athletes heart, DaCosta's syndrome, hyperventilation, anxiety, and other causes. Q waves simulating myocardial infarction have also been observed.[21,268,269] A narrow posteroanterior chest diameter may have been responsible for some cases in which electrocardiographic patterns simulated anterior infarction. In other cases, however, true infarction (Figure 31.23), albeit with normal coronary arteries, may be associated with MVP.[227]

The mechanism of these ST-segment and T-wave changes has not been fully clarified. The possibility of increased traction by chordae tendineae on the papillary muscles and underlying myocardium has previously been mentioned.[224–226] For similar reasons, Gibson and Brown[211] discussed the possibility of regional subendocardial ischemia following their angiocardiographic observations of regional left ventricular wall movement abnormalities in patients with MVP. Because of normalization of the ST-segment and T-wave changes following propranolol administration, an autonomic imbalance has been suggested.[270] The possibility remains that the abnormal electrocardiographic patterns reflect a cardiomyopathy in some patients with MVP.[200,271]

Because chest pain and an abnormal electrocardiogram are prominent features of both the primary MVP syndrome and occlusive coronary artery disease, the differentiation of these two conditions is an extremely common problem in clinical practice. As previously stated, this differentiation is clearly more difficult in a middle-aged man than in a young woman. Although both conditions may occur in the same patient, in most cases a careful history and stress electrocardiogram will usually serve to resolve the problem with confidence. Radionuclide studies or selective coronary arteriography combined with left ventriculography should be indicated in a minority of patients.

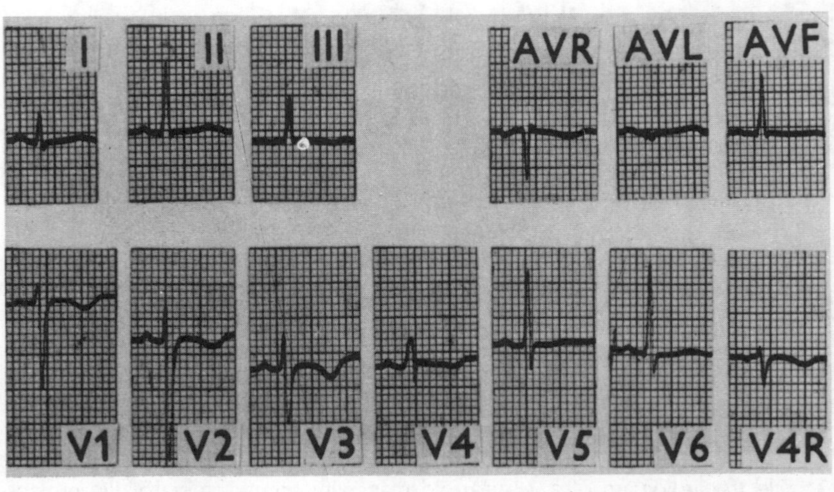

Figure 31.21. Electrocardiogram of an asymptomatic 20-year-old woman with a nonejection systolic click. Abnormal T-wave inversion is demonstrated in the anterior chest leads.

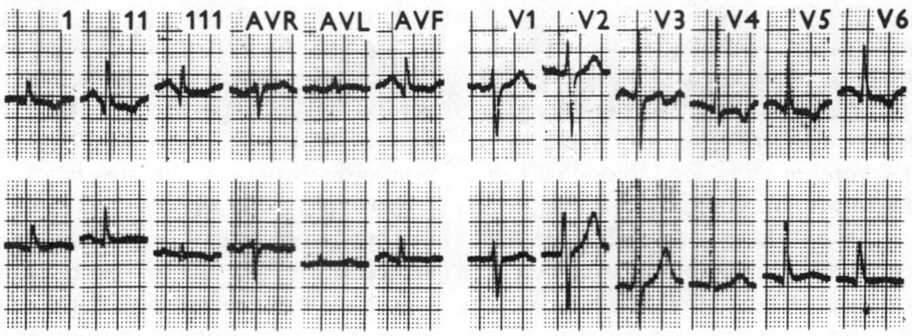

Figure 31.22. Electrocardiograms of a 22-year-old woman with mitral valve prolapse. The lower tracing is recorded 24 hours after the upper tracing and shows spontaneous "normalization" of the inverted T waves in leads V_3 through V_6.

Arrhythmias and Conduction Defects

Symptoms such as palpitations, lightheadedness, dizziness, or syncope suggest the presence of arrhythmias or conduction defects, but exercise electrocardiography or ambulatory monitoring may be necessary for confirmation. Arrhythmias may occasionally occur without symptoms and, conversely, dizziness and palpitations have been prominent complaints at times when electrocardiographic monitoring or clinical examination provided no objective explanation.[107,267] Orthostatic hypotension should be excluded in all patients with these symptoms,[47] particularly if 24-hour ambulatory monitoring is negative.

A wide variety of arrhythmias[107,267,271a] has been encountered in association with the primary MVP syndrome and includes supraventricular tachycardia, atrial fibrillation, atrial flutter, atrial ectopic beats, ventricular tachycardia, and ventricular fibrillation. Ventricular extrasystoles are the most common rhythm disturbance, may be unifocal or multifocal, and may display the R on T phenomenon. They are often precipitated or aggravated by emotion and exercise. Ventricular extrasystoles may occur with an otherwise normal electrocardiogram, irrespective of whether they are uni- or multifocal or whether they are present at rest or only after exercise (Figure 31.24).[24] The cause of the arrhythmias is speculative. Ventricular arrhythmias may result from abnormal tension on papillary muscles, with secondary papillary muscle and adjacent myocardial ischemia.[211] Endocardial friction lesions, produced by contact between the chordae and left ventricular endocardium, have been emphasized by Chesler et al[234] to be associated with myxomatous mitral valves, and the friction responsible for the lesions may be a cause of the ventricular dysrhythmias. Furthermore, traction on the papillary muscles[106] or "diastolic dumping" of the voluminous leaflets[272] may also produce endocardial irritability and dysrhythmias. Deposits of fibrin and platelets found in the angle between the posterior mitral leaflet and the left atrial wall could be a cause of coronary embolism,[234] again possibly leading to ventricular arrhythmias. Associated coronary artery spasm may be a possible cause of ventricular tachyarrhythmia.[65]

Atrial arrhythmias could not be explained by these mechanisms, but an abnormal stretch of the BML may still be pertinent.[273,274] The latter theory is particularly attractive because mitral leaflets have been demonstrated to contain muscle fibers in direct continuity with left atrial

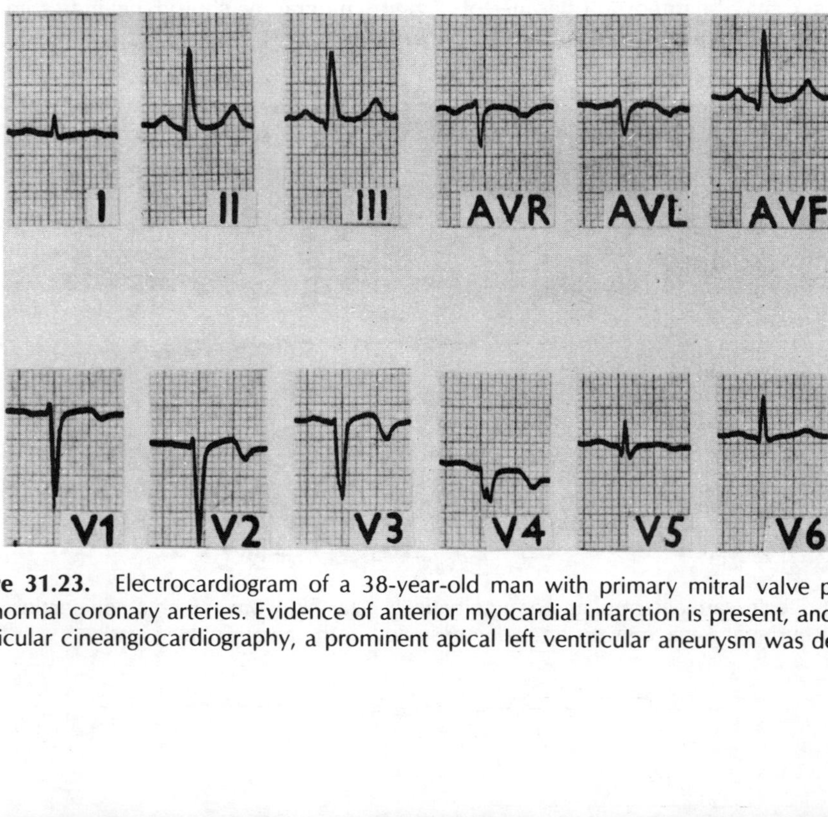

Figure 31.23. Electrocardiogram of a 38-year-old man with primary mitral valve prolapse and normal coronary arteries. Evidence of anterior myocardial infarction is present, and on left ventricular cineangiocardiography, a prominent apical left ventricular aneurysm was detected.

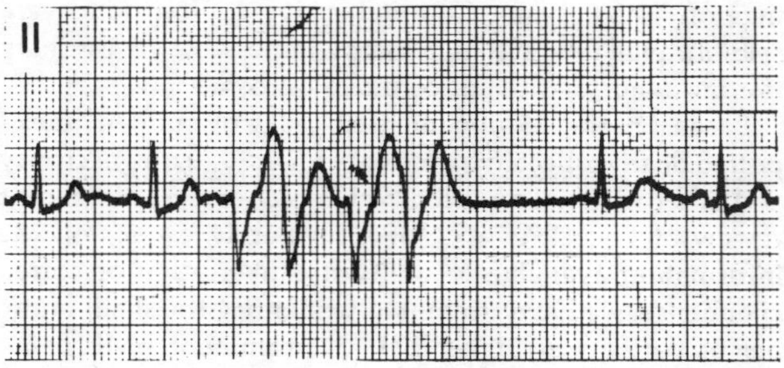

Figure 31.24. Standard lead II recorded three minutes after exercise in a 28-year-old woman with primary mitral valve prolapse who complained of palpitations. Multiple ventricular extrasystoles are demonstrated comprising a short run of ventricular tachycardia.

myocardium. Spontaneous phase 4 depolarization of these muscle fibers in response to stretch may generate action potentials that propagate to the left atrial wall.[275,276] These properties may set the stage for left-sided bypass tracts and for reentrant supraventricular tachyarrhythmia which is a common sustained tachyarrhythmia in MVP.[277] Finally, progressive left atrial and left ventricular dilatation from hemodynamically significant mitral regurgitation secondary to more advanced MVP further enhances the incidence of atrial and ventricular arrhythmias.[278–280] The Framingham study[281] indicated a high prevalence of complex or frequent ventricular dysrhythmias during 24-hour ambulatory electrocardiographic monitoring in subjects with MVP: more than 50% of the subjects with echocardiographically detected MVP had complex or frequent ventricular premature beats (Lown grade 2 or higher[282]), and 28% of such subjects had supraventricular tachycardias during such monitoring. However, these dysrhythmias were also prevalent in subjects without MVP in the Framingham study, and this excess of dysrhythmias in those with MVP did not reach statistical significance.[281]

Conduction disturbances include sinoatrial block, left and right bundle branch block, left anterior hemiblock, and atrioventricular block of varying degrees.[107,267,283] Conduction system abnormalities in MVP have also been investigated by electrophysiologic studies.[284] The mechanism of the conduction disturbances has not been clarified. Trent et al[285] described interruption of the conduction system as a result of fibrosis in the myocardium in one patient. Bharati et al[286] in 1981 made a detailed study of the conduction system in three cases of BML and observed premature aging and sclerosis of the atrioventricular node and trifascicular conduction system, thrombosis of the sinoatrial nodal artery, and fatty infiltration in the approach to the sinoatrial and atrioventricular nodes. In 1967 James[287] had described in Marfan's syndrome a degenerative process of small coronary vessels supplying the sinus and atrioventricular nodes, the His bundle, and its branches. The relevance of these histologic findings in the pathogenesis of conduction defects needs elucidation. Whatever the mechanism of conduction disturbances in MVP, a conduction disturbance as the possible cause of palpitations or syncope should be excluded before starting treatment with antiarrhythmic drugs, especially beta-receptor blocking agents.

The management of conduction defects or supraventricular arrhythmias in patients with the primary MVP syndrome does not differ from that of patients without MVP and will not be further discussed. The detection and management of ventricular arrhythmias are probably the most important challenge for the clinician who is confronted with symptomatic patients with the primary MVP syndrome. The symptoms suggestive of episodes of arrhythmia are palpitations, lightheadedness or dizziness, and syncope. All patients with such symptoms should be subjected to 24-hour Holter monitoring or to a stress electrocardiogram. If the rhythm remains normal or unifocal ventricular ectopic beats develop, our policy is to treat symptoms with firm reassurance and sometimes a beta-receptor blocking agent. A good response can be anticipated. If Lown[282] grade 3, 4A, 4B, or 5 ventricular ectopy is detected, then the arrhythmia should be treated until control is achieved or symptoms considerably improve. Beta-receptor blocking agents are again the standby of drug therapy and the addition of diphenylhydantoin is sometimes effective.[106,226] The beta-receptor blocking agent, sotalol, is unique in that it also has class III antiarrhythmic activity.[288] One of us (JBB) has had favorable results over several years using this beta-receptor blocking agent in the treatment of supraventricular and ventricular arrhythmias due to any underlying pathologic condition. Aprindine may be considered in patients who do not respond to other antiarrhythmic drugs.[289,290] Overdrive coronary sinus pacing has been used in refractory ventricular tachycardia and fibrillation.[291] Overdrive atrioventricular sequential pacing would now probably be preferred.

The surprising recent observation of Saltissi et al[292] from St. Thomas' Hospital in London of the beneficial effects of digoxin on chest pain and arrhythmias in MVP deserves further investigation.

All effective antidysrhythmic drugs may have serious or dangerous side effects. Side effects of disopyramide and quinidine have led us almost to abandon their use. Amiodarone is the most effective antiarrhythmic agent that we have used to date in the treatment of refractory ventricular tachyarrhythmias. The potentially serious side effects of that drug mitigate against its use, except in severe cases intractable to other therapy.

SUDDEN DEATH IN PRIMARY MITRAL VALVE PROLAPSE SYNDROME

In 1970 Pocock and Barlow[226] subjected 12 patients with the primary MVP syndrome to a submaximal effort test and detected multifocal ventricular extrasystoles in three. They therefore emphasized the importance of exercise in precipitating premature ventricular contractions and warned of a potential risk of sudden death should multifocal ventricular ectopy develop. At that time, sudden death was not a recognized complication of the MVP syndrome, although one such patient had been reported by Hancock and Cohn[22] in 1966 and another by Barlow et al[20] in 1968. Following that original warning, however, numerous studies throughout the world revealed that the MVP syndrome was highly prevalent. Furthermore, despite detection of potentially lethal ventricular ectopy after exercise or on 24-hour Holter monitoring, reports of sudden death were scanty and clinical details or necropsy findings were usually absent or incomplete. It therefore became widely accepted that primary MVP is a benign condition with a generally excellent prognosis. The problem of sudden death has been compounded by the probability in some instances that the MVP was a secondary or associated feature. The arrhythmogenic effect of drugs, notably quinidine, may well have been responsible for sudden death in other cases. In addition, sudden unexpected death, with or without preceding observation of potentially fatal ventricular arrhythmias, has occasionally been encountered in young adults in whom necropsy neither showed evidence of an MVP nor provided a satisfactory explanation for the cause of death.

It regrettably should now be generally accepted and recognized that sudden death may indeed occur in patients with primary MVP, but that data currently available indicate that the incidence is extremely rare. Although it is highly probable that an arrhythmia, presumably ventricular fibrillation,[292a] is usually responsible, bradycardia and asystole have been observed in patients with MVP.[293] In addition, because of the association between myocardial ischemia or infarction with anatomically normal coronary arteries and primary MVP, this mechanism will also be an occasional cause of sudden death. Coronary artery spasm,[64,65,142,227–233] possibly initiated by coronary emboli, may be the mechanism of production of myocardial infarction in some cases of primary MVP. The finding of accessory atrioventricular pathways by Vesterby et al[294] may be related to an arrhythmic cause of sudden death in MVP.

It should again be emphasized that most symptomatic patients with the primary MVP syndrome have complaints largely attributable to anxiety with no confirmation, including on Holter monitoring and stress electrocardiography, of potentially fatal ventricular ectopy. Nonetheless, the demonstration of multifocal ventricular extrasystoles, especially when showing the R on T phenomenon or causing appropriate symptoms, cannot be ignored irrespective of whether an underlying or associated cardiac condition, including MVP, is present. The nature of the cardiac condition, the presence of relevant symptoms, and the context of the situation in which the ventricular ectopy is detected are crucial factors in assessing an individual patient. It is difficult to generalize. Few cardiologists would dispute that patients with multifocal ventricular extrasystoles and coronary artery disease or hypertrophic cardiomyopathy are at significant risk of sudden death. Conversely, the prognosis of patients with multiform ventricular ectopy occurring with MVP or without detectable underlying cardiac disease is generally good.[214,295] Because of our known interest in the MVP syndrome, we have received information from other centers on unpublished cases of unexpected sudden death in which MVP or floppy leaflets were detected at necropsy. Chesler et al[234] recently reported necropsy findings of similar cases. Comprehensive clinical data were seldom available and it remains impossible to estimate the incidence of this unfortunate outcome.

Based on the 25 documented cases of sudden unexpected death collected by Jeresaty[296] in 1979, the necropsy and other material reported by Chesler et al,[234] the recent review of Pocock et al[297] of a further 17 cases, and the information available to us from conversation or correspondence, we have attempted to identify the small number of patients at higher risk. A prominent BML demonstrated on M-mode or 2-D echocardiography and indisputable mitral prolapse, confirmed clinically by a constant apical late systolic murmur that becomes louder and longer on standing, are pertinent features especially if detected at an early age. Abnormal T waves and ventricular ectopy on the resting electrocardiogram are other probable risk factors. Sudden unexpected death has a preponderance in women, often in their third decade. Regrettably, there are exceptions to all those "higher risk" features. Nonetheless, until more data allow a more accurate profile of the patient at risk to be obtained, a policy has to be formulated that will not create anxiety, even cardiac neurosis, in the large number of asymptomatic subjects or symptomatic patients. On current evidence we suggest that symptomatic patients with ventricular ectopy at rest, especially when there is a convincing history of palpitations, syncope, or even presyncope, be subjected to 24-hour ambulatory monitoring, or if facilities are not readily available, to a strenuous stress test. Those in whom multiform ventricular extrasystoles or other potentially dangerous arrhythmias develop should be maintained on antiarrhythmic drugs with regular monitoring to ensure that control is adequate. Any beta-receptor blocking agent may be contributory, but we have already suggested the advantages of giving sotalol, which has class III antiarrhythmic activity, in some cases. Amiodarone should be used for intractable and serious ventricular arrhythmias. If patients continue to exhibit dangerous arrhythmias despite sotalol, amiodarone, or other antiarrhythmic agents, overdrive atrioventricular sequential pacing is probably indicated.

The role of mitral valve surgery also has to be considered. Cobbs and King[106] subjected a patient with MVP and recurrent ventricular fibrillation to mitral valve replacement in 1973 and observed improvement following surgery. In 1979 Kay et al[298] reported improvement after mitral valve repair in six symptomatic patients with severe billowing but mild mitral regurgitation. Kay emphasized that the indication for mitral valve surgery related to the disabling symptoms and the arrhythmias and not to the hemodynamically mild mitral regurgitation. Kay (personal communication, 1984) has now extended this experience and remains satisfied with the long-term results. A policy of surgical treatment for ventricular arrhythmias or symptoms in patients with the primary MVP syndrome without significant mitral regurgitation may seem unduly aggressive. However, uncontrollable and potentially fatal arrhythmias in an appropriately symptomatic patient cannot be ignored. It seems justifiable to regard the combination of an advanced BML or floppy mitral valve demonstrated echocardiographically and confirmed angiocardiographically, important symptoms such as presyncope or syncope, and documented dangerous ventricular arrhythmias, unresponsive to treatment with antiarrhythmic agents or overdrive pacing, as an indication for mitral valve repair despite the absence of hemodynamically significant mitral regurgitation. Good results have been reported recently.[299]

REFERENCES

1. Hardison JE: Quest for a new disease. *Am J Med* 1984; 76:1.
2. Wooley CF: From irritable heart to mitral valve prolapse: the Osler connection. *Am J Cardiol* 1984; 53:870–874.

2a. Wooley CF: From irritable heart to mitral valve prolapse: British Army medical reports, 1860 to 1870. *Am J Cardiol* 1985; 55:1107–1109.

3. Bartecchi CE: Historical beginnings of the mitral valve prolapse syndrome. *Am J Cardiol* 1984; 54:1165–1166.
4. Devereux RB, Perloff JK, Reichek N, Josephson ME: Mitral valve prolapse. *Circulation* 1976; 54:3–14.
5. Barlow JB, Pocock WA, Marchand P, Denny M: The significance of late systolic murmurs. *Am Heart J* 1963; 66:443–452.
6. Barlow JB: Conjoint clinic on the clinical significance of late systolic murmurs and nonejection systolic clicks. *J Chron Dis* 1965; 18:665–673.
7. Griffith JPC: Midsystolic and late systolic mitral murmurs. *Am J Med Sci* 1892; 104:285–294.
8. Hall JN: Late systolic mitral murmurs. *Am J Med Sci* 1903; 125:663–666.
9. Lewis T: *Diseases of the Heart*, ed 4. London, Macmillan & Co, Ltd, 1949, p 154.
10. MacKenzie J: *Diseases of the Heart*, ed 4. London, Oxford University Press, 1925, p 357.
11. Evans W: Mitral systolic murmurs. *Br Med J* 1943; 1:8–9.
12. Gallavardin L: Pseudo-dedoublement du deuxième bruit du coeur simulant le dedoublement mitral par bruit extracardiaque telesystolique surajoute. *Lyon Med* 1913; 121:409–477.
13. McKusick VA, Kline EW, Webb GN: Spectral phonocardiographic demonstration of selected varieties of cardiovascular sounds. *Am Heart J* 1955; 49:911–933.
14. McKusick VA: *Cardiovascular Sound in Health and Disease*. Baltimore, Williams & Wilkins Co, 1958, pp 190–191, 417–418.
15. Leatham A: Systolic murmur. *Circulation* 1958; 17:601–611.
16. McKusick VA: Symposium on cardiovascular sound. *Circulation* 1957; 16:424–427.
17. White PD: *Heart Disease*, ed 2. New York, Macmillan, 1937, p 211.
18. Reid JV: Mid-systolic clicks. *S Afr Med J* 1961; 35:353–355.
19. Humphries JO, McKusick VA: The differentiation of organic and "innocent" systolic murmurs. *Prog Cardiovasc Dis* 1962; 5:152–171.
20. Barlow JB, Bosman CK, Pocock WA, Marchand P: Late systolic murmurs and nonejection ("mid-late") systolic clicks. An analysis of 90 patients. *Br Heart J* 1968; 30:203–218.
21. Barlow JB, Bosman CK: Aneurysmal protrusion of the posterior leaflet of the mitral valve. An auscultatory-electrocardiographic syndrome. *Am Heart J* 1966; 71:166–178.
22. Hancock EW, Cohn K: The syndrome associated with midsystolic click and late systolic murmur. *Am J Med* 1966; 41:183–196.
23. Pocock WA, Barlow JB: Etiology and electrocardiographic features of the billowing posterior mitral leaflet syndrome. *Am J Med* 1971; 51:731–739.
24. Barlow JB, Pocock WA: Mitral valve prolapse, the specific billowing mitral leaflet syndrome, or an insignificant non-ejection systolic click. *Am Heart J* 1979; 97:277–285.
25. Barlow JB, Pocock WA, Obel IWP: Mitral valve prolapse: primary, secondary, both or neither? *Am Heart J* 1981; 102:140–143.
26. King BD, Clark MA, Baba N, Kilman JW, Wooley CF: "Myxomatous" mitral valves: collagen dissolution as the primary defect. *Circulation* 1982; 66:288–296.
27. Roberts WC: Congenital cardiovascular abnormalities usually "silent" until adulthood: morphologic features of the floppy mitral valve, valvular aortic stenosis, discrete subvalvar aortic stenosis, hypertrophic cardiomyopathy, sinus of Valsalva aneurysm, and the Marfan syndrome, in Roberts WC (ed): *Congenital Heart Disease in Adults*. Philadelphia, FA Davis, 1979, pp 407–453.
28. Pomerance A: Ballooning deformity (mucoid degeneration) of atrioventricular valves. *Br Heart J* 1969; 31:343–351.
29. Read RC, Thal AP, Wendt VE: Symptomatic valvular myxomatous transformation (the floppy valve syndrome). A possible forme fruste of the Marfan syndrome. *Circulation* 1965; 32:897–910.
30. Criley JM, Lewis KB, Humphries JO, Ross RS: Prolapse of the mitral valve: clinical and cine-angiocardiographic findings. *Br Heart J* 1966; 28:488–496.
31. Hurst JW: Words—good and bad. *Am J Cardiol* 1984; 54:444–445.
32. Barlow JB, Pocock WA: The mitral valve prolapse enigma: two decades later. *Mod Concepts Cardiovasc Dis* 1984; 53:13–17.
33. Barlow JB, Pocock WA: Billowing, floppy, prolapsed or flail mitral valves? *Am J Cardiol* 1985; 55:501–502.
34. Brandt KD, Sumner RD, Ryan TJ, Cohen AS: Herniation of mitral leaflets in the Ehlers-Danlos syndrome. *Am J Cardiol* 1975; 36:524–528.
35. Grahame R, Child A: Mitral valve prolapse. *Br Med J* 1984; 289:317.

35a. Marcus R, Sareli P, Antunes M, Magalhaes M, Meyer T, Grieve T, Barlow J: Functional pathology of mitral regurgitation in active rheumatic carditis—surgical and echocardiographic observations. *J Am Coll Cardiol* 1986; 7(suppl A):8A.

36. Cheng TO: Coexistent mitral valve prolapse and mitral stenosis. *Chest* 1982; 81:526–527.
37. Beton DC, Brear SG, Edwards JD, Leonard JC: Mitral valve prolapse: an assessment of clinical features, associated conditions and prognosis. *Quart J Med* 1983; 52:150–164.
38. Cheng TO: Some new observations on the syndrome of papillary muscle dysfunction. *Am J Med* 1969; 47:924–945.
39. Cheng TO: Late systolic murmur in coronary artery disease. *Chest* 1972; 61:346–356.
40. Cheng TO: Midsystolic clicks and coronary heart disease. *Chest* 1973; 63:298.
41. Cheng TO: The systolic click: Is it a syndrome, a diagnostic sign or a benign curiosity? *Mod Med* 1976; 44:58–59.
42. Cheng TO: Mitral valve prolapse. *Chungking Med* 1980; 3:32–38.
43. Cheng TO: The click-murmur syndrome. A medical pendulum and a unifying concept. *Chest* 1976; 70:569–572.
44. Bon Tempo CP, Ronan JA, de Leon AC, Twigg HL: Radiographic appearance of the thorax in systolic click-late systolic murmur syndrome. *Am J Cardiol* 1975; 36:27–31.
45. Russo L, Aloisi B, Ierna A, Centaro A, Negro R, Brancate B: Scoliosis and mitral valve prolapse: an epidemiological and etiopathogenetic screening. *G Ital Cardiol* 1980; 10:1001–1005.
46. Albert J, Ekoe JM, Lemetayer P, Ott H: Prolapse de la valve mitrale. Association a des anomalies squelettiques. *Presse Med* 1984; 13:441–442.

46a. Hortop J, Tsipouras P, Hanley JA, Maron BJ, Shapiro JR: Cardiovascular involvement in osteogenesis imperfecta. *Circulation* 1986; 73:54–61.

47. Santos AD, Mathew PK, Hilal A, Wallace WA: Orthostatic hypotension: a common unrecognized cause of symptoms in mitral valve prolapse. *Am J Med* 1981; 71:746–750.
48. Honkala M, Pirttiaho H, Salmela P, Ikaheimo M, Lilja M: Mitraaliprolapsiin Liittyva vaikea ortostaattinen hypotonia nuorella naisella. *Duodecim* 1984; 100:351–354.
49. Goodman DJ, Harrison DC, Popp RL: Echocardiographic features of primary pulmonary hypertension. *Am J Cardiol* 1974; 33:438–443.
50. Garcia-Dorado AD, Bello L, Edez-Aviles F, Rodriquez JA: Right ventricular enlargement and mitral valve prolapse (abstr). *Eur Heart J* 1984; 5(suppl 1):337.
51. Schlamowitz RA, Gross S, Keating E, Pitt W, Mazur J: Tricuspid valve prolapse: a common occurrence with the click-murmur syndrome. *J Clin Ultrasound* 1982; 10:435–439.
52. Ogawa S, Hayashi J, Sasaki H, Tani M, Akaishi M, Mitamura H, Sano M, Hoshino T, Handa S, Nakamura Y: Evaluation of combined valvular prolapse syndrome by two dimensional echocardiography. *Circulation* 1982; 65:174–180.
53. Morganroth J, Jones RH, Chen CC, Naito M: Two dimensional echocardiography in mitral, aortic and tricuspid valve prolapse. The clinical problem, cardiac nuclear imaging considerations and a proposed standard for diagnosis. *Am J Cardiol* 1980; 46:1164–1177.
54. Wolff JE, Denis B, Machecourt J, Contamin C, Hadjian O, Bourlard P, Page E, Martin-Noel P: Aortic and tricuspid valve involvement associated with mitral valve prolapse. *Arch Mal Coeur* 1983; 76:1362–1367.
55. Brown AK, Anderson V: Two dimensional echocardiography and the tricuspid valve. Leaflet definition and prolapse. *Br Heart J* 1983; 49:495–500.
56. Malcolm AD: Mitral valve prolapse associated with other disorders: casual coincidence, common link, or fundamental genetic disturbance? *Br Heart J* 1985; 53:353–362.
57. Chisholm JC Jr: Mitral valve prolapse syndrome associated with congenital bicuspid aortic valve. *J Natl Med Assoc* 1981; 73:921–923.
58. Braunwald E: *Heart Disease. A Textbook of Cardiovascular Medicine*, ed 2. Philadelphia, WB Saunders, 1984, p 1090.
59. Flores M, Agosti J, Damborenea C, Aguirre C: Rheumatoid arthritis with severe aortic insufficiency and prolapse of the mitral valve. *Scan J Rheumatol* 1984; 13:28–32.

60. Lippman SM, Ginzton LE, Thigpen T, Tanaka KR, Laks MM: Mitral valve prolapse in sickle cell disease. Presumptive evidence for a linked connective tissue disorder. *Arch Intern Med* 1985; 145:435–438.
61. Rosenberg CA, Derman GH, Grabb WC, Buda AJ: Hypomastia and mitral-valve prolapse. Evidence of a linked embryologic and mesenchymal dysplasia. *N Engl J Med* 1983; 309:1230–1232.
62. Liberfarb RM, Altshuler EE, Goldblatt A: Hypomastia and mitral-valve prolapse. *N Engl J Med* 1984; 310:1054.
63. Gamberini G, D'Alessandro R, Labriola E, Poggi V, Manzoni GC, Carpeggiana P, Sacquegna T: Further evidence on the association of mitral valve prolapse and migraine. *Headache* 1984; 24:39–40.
64. Cheng TO: Mitral valve prolapse and coronary artery spasm. *Br Heart J* 1982; 48:301.
65. Sakuma T, Kakihana M, Togo T, Matsuda M, Ogawa T, Sugishita Y, Ito I, Kurusu T: Mitral valve prolapse syndrome with coronary artery spasm: a possible cause of recurrent ventricular tachyarrhythmia. *Clin Cardiol* 1985; 8:306–308.
66. Gentzler RD, Gault JH, Liedtke AJ, McCann WD, Mann RH, Hunter AS: Congenital absence of the left circumflex coronary artery in the systolic click syndrome. *Circulation* 1975; 52:490–496.
67. Hinterauer L, Tartini R: Major variations in origin of coronary arteries and mitral valve prolapse (abstr). *Eur Heart J* 1984; 5:(suppl 1):291.
68. Hagerman RJ, Synhorst DP: Mitral valve prolapse and aortic dilatation in the fragile X syndrome. *Am J Med Genet* 1984; 17:123–131.
69. Fricke GR, Mattern HJ, Schweikert HU, Schwanitz G: Klinefelter's syndrome and mitral valve prolapse. An echocardiographic study in twenty-two patients. *Biomed Pharmacother* 1984; 38:88–97.
70. Coghlan HC, Phares P, Cowley M, Copley D, James TN: Dysautonomia in mitral valve prolapse. *Am J Med* 1979; 67:236–244.
71. Gordon IB, Rassokhin VM, Nikitina TN, Koryakin AM, Gordon AI, Suvorova TY, Gorbatovsky AY, Eremenko SN, Dantsiter OV, Trifonova NF: Constitutional (genetically determined) vegetative dystonia and connective tissue dysplasia in idiopathic mitral valve prolapse. *Klin Med* 1984; 62:63–67.
72. Jackson AC: Association of mitral valve prolapse and intracranial aneurysms. *South Med J* 1983; 76:712–713.
72a. Sataline L: Irritable bowel syndrome and mitral valve prolapse syndrome. *JAMA* 1985; 253:41.
72b. Goldhaber SZ, Rubin IL, Brown W, Robertson N, Stubblefield F, Sloss LJ: Valvular heart disease (aortic regurgitation and mitral valve prolapse) among institutionalized adults with Down's syndrome. *Am J Cardiol* 1986; 57:278–281.
73. Pickering NJ, Brody JI, Barrett MJ: Von Willebrand syndromes and mitral valve prolapse: linked mesenchymal dysplasias. *N Eng J Med* 1981; 305:131–134.
74. Kuhsel LC, Polster J, Rudiger HW: An investigation into the frequency of mitral valve prolapse in von Willebrand disease. *Clin Genet* 1983; 24:128–131.
75. Kantor JS, Zitrin CM, Zeldis SM: Mitral valve prolapse syndrome in agoraphobic patients. *Am J Psychiat* 1980; 137:467–469.
76. Grunhaus L, Gloger S, Rein A: Mitral-valve prolapse and panic disorders. *Isr J Med Sci* 1982; 18:221–223.
76a. Nesse RM, Cameron OG, Buda AJ, McCann DS, Curtis GC, Huber-Smith MJ: Urinary catecholamines and mitral valve prolapse in panic-anxiety patients. *Psychiat Res* 1985; 14:67–74.
77. Zuo CY: Panic attack and mitral valve prolapse. *Chin J Neuropsychiatry* 1983; 16:244–245.
78. Hickey AJ, Andrews G, Wilcken DEL: Independence of mitral valve prolapse and neurosis. *Br Heart J* 1983; 50:333–336.
79. Shear MK, Devereaux RB, Kramer-Fox R, Mann JJ, Frances A: Low prevalence of mitral valve prolapse in patients with panic disorder. *Am J Psychiatry* 1984; 141:302–303.
80. Levine HJ, Isner JM, Salem DN: Primary versus secondary mitral valve prolapse: clinical features and implications. *Clin Cardiol* 1982; 5:371–375.
80a. Johnson CD: Mitral valve prolapse and Wiskott-Aldrich syndrome. *Cardiovasc Rev Rep* 1985; 6:874–879.
80b. Shen LL, Cui GG, Liang RL: Valve prolapse in Behcet's disease. *Br Heart J* 1985; 54:100–101.
80c. Margaliot SZ, Barzilay J, Bar-David M, Lewis BS, Froom P, Forecast D, Gross M: Spontaneous pneumothorax and mitral valve prolapse. *Chest* 1986; 89:93–94.
81. Verani MS, Carroll RJ, Falsetti HL: Mitral valve prolapse in coronary artery disease. *Am J Cardiol* 1976; 37:1–6.
82. Aranda JM, Befeler B, Lazzara R, Embi A, Machado H: Mitral valve prolapse and coronary artery disease. Clinical hemodynamic and angiographic correlation. *Circulation* 1975; 52:245–253.
83. Steelman RB, White RS, Hill JC, Nagle JP, Cheitlin MD: Midsystolic clicks in arteriosclerotic heart disease. A new facet in the clinical syndrome of papillary muscle dysfunction. *Circulation* 1971; 44:503–515.
84. Crawford MH: Mitral valve prolapse due to coronary artery disease. *Am J Med* 1977; 62:447–451.
85. Kinsley RH, Girdwood RW, Milner S: Surgical treatment during acute phase of rheumatic carditis. *Surg Ann* 1981; 13:299–323.
86. Nagata S, Park YD, Nakanishi N, Beppu S, Sakakibara H, Nimura Y: Mitral valve abnormalities in patients with right ventricular pressure overload. Analysis by real time cross sectional echocardiography. *Br Heart J* 1984; 52:186–190.
87. Markiewicz W, Stoner J, London E, Hunt SA, Popp RL: Mitral valve prolapse in one hundred presumably healthy young females. *Circulation* 1976; 53:464–473.
88. Lutas EM, Devereux RB, Kramer-Fox R, Spitzer M: Disappearance of mitral valve prolapse during pregnancy. *J Cardiovasc Ultrason* 1984; 3:183–186.
89. Davies J: *Human Developmental Anatomy*. New York, Ronald Press, 1963, pp 81, 276, 278.
90. Arey LB: *Developmental Anatomy. A Textbook and Laboratory Manual of Embryology*, ed 7. Philadelphia, WB Saunders, 1974, pp 404–410.
91. Mardelli TJ, Morganroth J, Naito M, Chen CC: Cross-sectional echocardiographic detection of aortic valve prolapse. *Am Heart J* 1980; 100:295–301.
92. Pocock WA, Barlow JB: An association between the billowing posterior mitral leaflet syndrome and congenital heart disease, particularly atrial septal defect. *Am Heart J* 1971; 81:720–721.
93. McDonald A, Harris A, Jefferson K, Marshall J, McDonald L: Association of prolapse of posterior cusp of mitral valve and atrial septal defect. *Br Heart J* 1971; 33:383–387.
94. Schreiber TL, Feigenbaum H, Weyman AE: Effect of atrial septal defect repair on left ventricular geometry and degree of mitral valve prolapse. *Circulation* 1980; 61:888–896.
95. Kambe T, Ichimiya S, Toguchi M, Hibi N, Fukui Y, Nishimura K: Cross-sectional echocardiographic study on the mitral valve prolapse associated with secundum atrial septal defect. *Jpn Circ J* 1981; 45:260–267.
96. Nagata S, Nimura Y, Sakakibara H, Beppu S, Park Y-D, Kawazoe K, Fujita T: Mitral valve lesion associated with secundum atrial septal defect. Analysis by real-time two dimensional echocardiography. *Br Heart J* 1983; 49:51–58.
97. Ballester M, Presbitero P, Foale R, Rickards A, McDonald L: Prolapse of the mitral valve in secundum atrial septal defect: a functional mechanism. *Eur Heart J* 1983; 4:472–476.
98. Raju PK, Rajani M, Shrivastava S: Mitral valve prolapse associated with secundum atrial septal defect: clinical, hemodynamic and angiographic correlations. *J Assoc Physicians India* 1983; 31:709–713.
99. Crawford MH, O'Rouske RA: Mitral valve prolapse: a cardiomyopathic state? *Progr Cardiovasc Dis* 1984; 27:133–139.
100. Cheitlin MD, Byrd RC: Prolapsed mitral valve: the commonest valve disease? *Curr Prob Cardiol* 1984; 8:7–54.
101. Hutter AM, Dinsmore RE, Willerson JT, DeSanctis RW: Early systolic clicks due to mitral valve prolapse. *Circulation* 1971; 44:516–522.
102. Dock W: Production mode of systolic clicks due to mitral cusp prolapse. *Arch Intern Med* 1973; 132:118–125.
103. Bonner AJ, Noble RJ, Feigenbaum H: Early diastolic sound associated with mitral valve prolapse. *Arch Intern Med* 1976; 136:347–349.
104. Cheng TO: Diastolic click in mitral valve prolapse. *Arch Intern Med* 1977; 137:696.
105. Wei JY, Fortuin NJ: Diastolic sounds and murmurs associated with mitral valve prolapse. *Circulation* 1981; 63:559–564.
106. Cobbs BW Jr, King SB III: Ventricular buckling: a factor in the abnormal ventriculogram and peculiar hemodynamics associated with mitral valve prolapse. *Am Heart J* 1977; 93:741–758.
107. Barlow JB, Pocock WA: The problem of nonejection systolic clicks and associated mitral systolic murmurs: emphasis on the billowing mitral leaflet syndrome. *Am Heart J* 1975; 90:636–655.
108. Rackley CE, Whalen RE, Floyd WL: The precordial honk. *Am J Cardiol* 1966; 17:509–515.
109. Behar VS, Whalen RE, McIntosh HD: The ballooning mitral valve in patients with the "precordial honk" or "whoop." *Am J Cardiol* 1967; 20:789–795.
110. Lababidi Z: Floppy mitral whistle heard across the room. *Am Heart J* 1976; 91:825.
111. Segall HN: Autoauscultation in a patient with floppy mitral valve syndrome. *Am Heart J* 1976; 91:269–272.
112. Osler W: On a remarkable heart murmur heard at a distance from the chest wall. *Can Med Surg J* 1879–1880; 8:518–519.
113. Shah PM: Update of mitral valve prolapse syndrome: When is echo prolapse a pathological prolapse? *Echocardiography A Review of Cardiovascular Ultrasound* 1984; 1:87–95.
114. DeMaria AN, Neumann A, Lee G, Mason D: Echocardiographic identification of the mitral valve prolapse syndrome. *Am J Med* 1977; 62:819–829.
115. Gardin JM, Talano JV, Stephanides MS, Fizzano BS, Lesch MD: Systolic anterior motion in the absence of asymmetric septal hypertrophy: a buckling phenomenon of the chordae tendineae. *Circulation* 1981; 63:181–187.

116. O'Rourke RA, Crawford MH: The systolic click-murmur syndrome: clinical recognition and management. *Curr Prob Cardiol* 1976; 1:1–60.
117. Haikal M, Alpert MA, Whiting RB, Ahmad M, Kelly D: Sensitivity and specificity of M mode echocardiographic signs of mitral valve prolapse. *Am J Cardiol* 1982; 50:185–190.
117a. Feigenbaum H: *Echocardiography*, ed 4. Philadelphia, Lea & Febiger, 1986, p 269.
118. Levisman JA, Abbasi AA: Abnormal motion of the mitral valve with pericardial effusion: pseudo-prolapse of the mitral valve. *Am Heart J* 1976; 91:18–20.
119. Felner JM, Schlant RC: *Echocardiography: A Teaching Atlas*. New York, Grune & Stratton, 1976, p 364.
120. Sahn DJ, Wood J, Allen HD, Peoples W, Goldberg SJ: Echocardiographic spectrum of mitral valve motion in children with and without mitral valve prolapse: the nature of false positive diagnosis. *Am J Cardiol* 1977; 39:422–431.
121. Chandraratna PAN, Lopes JM, Littman BB, Gupta JD, Samet P: Abnormal mitral valve motion during ventricular extrasystoles. An echocardiographic study. *Am J Cardiol* 1974; 34:783–786.
122. Markiewicz W, London E, Popp RL: Effect of transducer placement on echocardiographic mitral valve motion. *Am Heart J* 1978; 96:555–556.
123. Sahn DJ, Allen HD, Goldberg SJ, Friedman WF: Mitral valve prolapse in children. A problem defined by real-time cross-sectional echocardiography. *Circulation* 1976; 53:651–657.
124. Bloch A, Vignola PA, Walker H, Kaplan AD, Chiotellis PN, Lees RS, Myers GS: Echocardiographic spectrum of posterior systolic motion of the mitral valve in the general population. *JCU* 1977; 5:243–247.
125. Wann LS, Grove JR, Hess TR, Glisch L, Ptacin MJ, Hughes CV, Gross CM: Prevalence of mitral prolapse by two dimensional echocardiography in health young women. *Br Heart J* 1983; 49:334–340.
126. Brown AK, Anderson V: M-mode and cross-sectional (2D) echocardiograms in the diagnosis of mitral valve prolapse. *Eur Heart J* 1981; 2:147–154.
127. Abbasi AS, DeCristofaro D, Anabtawi J, Irwin L: Mitral valve prolapse: comparative value of M-mode, two-dimensional and Doppler echocardiography. *J Am Coll Cardiol* 1983; 2:1219–1223.
128. Warth DC, King ME, Cohen JM, Tesoriero VL, Marcus E, Weyman AE: Prevalence of mitral valve prolapse in normal children. *J Am Coll Cardiol* 1985; 5:1173–1177.
129. Alpert MA, Carney RJ, Flaker GC, Sanfelippo JF, Webel RR, Kelly DL: Sensitivity and specificity of two-dimensional echocardiographic signs of mitral valve prolapse. *Am J Cardiol* 1984; 54:792–796.
129a. Levine RA, Triulzi MO, Harrigan P, Weyman AE: In vivo validation of a nonplanar mitral anular shape: implications for the diagnosis of mitral valve prolapse. *J Am Coll Cardiol* 1986; 7(suppl A):7A.
130. Smith ER, Fraser DB, Purdy JW, Anderson RN: Angiographic diagnosis of mitral valve prolapse: correlation with echocardiography. *Am J Cardiol* 1977; 40:165–170.
131. Somerville J, Kaku S, Saravalli O: Prolapsed mitral cusps in atrial septal defect. An erroneous radiological interpretation. *Br Heart J* 1978; 40:58–63.
132. Spindola-Franco H, Bjork L, Adams DF, Abrams HL: Classification of the radiological morphology of the mitral valve. Differentiation between true and pseudo prolapse. *Br Heart J* 1980; 44:30–36.
133. Chiddo A, Mastrangelo D, Morrone A, Iliceto S, Rizzon P: Diagnosi angiografica di prolasso della mitrale: errorie limiti. *G Ital Cardiol* 1983; 13:283–290.
134. Engle PJ, Hickman JR, Cowley MJ: Angiographic diagnosis of posterior mitral leaflet prolapse. *J Am Coll Cardiol* 1984; 3:1085–1091.
135. Ranganathan N, Silver MD, Robinson TI, Kostuk WJ, Felderhof CH, Patt NL, Wilson JK, Wigle ED: Angiographic-morphologic correlation in patients with severe mitral regurgitation due to prolapse of the posterior mitral valve leaflet. *Circulation* 1973; 48:514–518.
136. Ranganathan N, Silver MD, Robinson TI, Wilson JK: Idiopathic prolapsed mitral leaflet syndrome. Angiographic-clinical correlation. *Circulation* 1976; 54:707–716.
137. Lucas RV Jr, Edwards JE: The floppy mitral valve. *Curr Probl Cardiol* 1982; 7:1–48.
138. Cipriano PR, Kline SA, Baltaxe HA: An angiographic assessment of left ventricular function in isolated mitral valvular prolapse. *Invest Radiol* 1980; 15:293–298.
139. Dubriel JP: Idiopathic mitral valve posterior leaflet prolapse: hemodynamic and angiocardiographic studies. *PrzegL Lek* 1983; 40:423–430.
140. Leachman RD, DeFrancheschi A, Zamalloa O: Late systolic murmurs and clicks associated with abnormal mitral valve ring. *Am J Cardiol* 1969; 23:679–683.
141. Cheng TO: Primary versus secondary mitral valve prolapse. *Am Heart J* 1981; 102:946.
142. Huckell VF: Mitral valve prolapse and coronary artery spasm. *Br Heart J* 1982; 48:301.
143. Przybojewski JZ, Tredoux JG, van der Walt JJ, Tiedt FAC: Mitral valve prolapse complicated by acute cerebral embolism, arrhythmias and painless myocardial infarction. A case presentation and overview. *S Afr Med J* 1984; 65:390–396.
144. Gooch AS, Maranhao V, Scampardonis G, Cha SD, Yang SS: Prolapse of both mitral and tricuspid leaflets in systolic murmur-click syndrome. *N Engl J Med* 1972; 287:1218–1222.
145. Werner JA, Schiller NB, Frasquier R: Occurrence and significance of echocardiographically demonstrated tricuspid valve prolapse. *Am Heart J* 1978; 96:180–186.
146. Mardelli TJ, Morganroth J, Chen CC, Naito M, Vergel J: Tricuspid valve prolapse diagnosed by cross-sectional echocardiography. *Chest* 1981; 79:201–205.
147. McKay R, Yacoub MH: Clinical and pathological findings in patients with "floppy" valves treated surgically. *Circulation* 1973; 48(supp III):III-63–III-73.
147a. Petitalot JP, Chaix AF, Barraine R: Echocardiographic features of triple valve prolapse with incompetent foramen ovale in Marfan's syndrome. *Am Heart J* 1986; 111:187–189.
148. Lakier JB, Copans H, Rosman HS, Lam R, Fine G, Khaja F, Goldstein S: Idiopathic degeneration of the aortic valve. A common cause of isolated aortic regurgitation. *J Am Coll Cardiol* 1985; 5:347–351.
149. Allen WM, Matloff JM, Fishbein MC: Myxoid degeneration of the aortic valve and isolated severe aortic regurgitation. *Am J Cardiol* 1985; 55:439–444.
149a. Bellitti R, Caruso A, Festa M, Mazzei V, Iesu S, Falco A, Cotrufo M, Agozzino L: Prolapse of the "floppy" aortic valve as a cause of aortic regurgitation. A clinico-morphologic study. *Int J Cardiol* 1985: 9:399–410.
150. Motulsky AG: Biased ascertainment and the natural history of diseases. *N Engl J Med* 1978; 298:1196–1197.
151. Zhou Y, Zu Z, Wang J, Jiang L, Wong C: Prevalence of mitral valve prolapse: click murmur syndrome among 2001 Kazaks in Xinjiang. *Chin J Cardiol* 1983; 11:82.
152. Rizzon P, Biasco G, Brindicci G: Epidemiologia e criteri diagnostici del prolasso della mitrale. *G Ital Cardiol* 1979; 9(suppl 1):3.
153. Savage DD, Devereux RB, Donahue R, Joiner G, Anderson SJ, Rosen RA, Wilson P, Kramer R, Brown WT, Garrison R, Castelli WP, Feinleib M: Mitral valve prolapse in blacks. *J Natl Med Assoc* 1982; 74:895–900.
154. Chen WC, Ng WL, Chow SF, Wong HC: Prevalence of mitral valve prolapse in Hong Kong Chinese. A clinical and autopsy study. *Chin Med J* 1984; 97:352–356.
155. Sasaki H, Ogawa S, Handa S, Nakamura Y, Yamada R: Two dimensional echocardiographic diagnosis of mitral valve prolapse syndrome in presumably healthy young students. *J Cardiogr* 1982; 12:23–31.
155a. Sugiura M, Matsushita S, Ueda K: A clinicopathological study on valvular diseases in 3000 consecutive autopsies of the aged. *Jpn Circ J* 1982; 46:337–345.
156. Davies MJ, Moore BP, Braimbridge MV: The floppy mitral valve. Study of incidence, pathology, and complications in surgical, necropsy and forensic material. *Br Heart J* 1978; 40:468–481.
157. Hickey AJ, Wolfers J, Wilcken DL: Mitral-valve prolapse. Prevalence in an Australian population. *Med J Aust* 1981; 1:31–33.
158. Lion MF, Schubsky V, Ortiz J, Sousa JEMR, Batlouni M, Decourt LV: Prolapso valvular mitral—simposio. *Arq Bras Cardiol* 1980; 35:63–79.
158a. Laurenceau JL, Turcot J, Dumesnil JG: Echocardiographic study of Olympic athletes, in Lubich T, Venerando A (eds): *Sports Cardiology International Conference, Rome, April 1978*. Bologna, Aulo Gaggi Publisher, 1980, p 705.
159. Du CL, Liu YD, Wu ZX, Wen RL: Prevalence of mitral valve prolapse syndrome among 1600 healthy youngsters in Chengdu, Sichuan, China. *New Med* 1982; 13:10–11.
160. Prevention and Treatment Region for Cardiovascular Diseases, Fanyu County, Guangdong: Epidemiologic study of heart disease in 7168 school children. *Chin J Cardiol* 1983; 11:33–35.
161. Egeblad H, Sorensen PS: Prevalence of mitral valve prolapse in younger patients with cerebral ischemic attacks. A blinded controlled study. *Acta Med Scand* 1984; 216:385–391.
162. Heni HE, Ibrahim Z: Echokardiographische untersuchung zur haufigkeit des idiopathischen mitralklappenprolaps (click syndrom). *Med Welt* 1980; 31:595–597.
162a. Antani J, Rao MS, Biradar NS, Nanjappa H, Thankur DS: Incidence and clinical profile of click-murmur syndrome in Indian females. *Indian Heart J* 1982; 34:285.
163. Nambiar U, Alurkar VM, Durairaj M, Saini P, Narayanan GR: Mitral valve prolapse in apparently healthy Indian women. *Indian Heart J* 1982; 34:285.
164. Neufeld HN: Personal communication, 1984.
165. Meloni L, Cherchi A, Fonzo R, Bina P, Bonomo P: Prolasso della mitrale in giovani atlete. *G Ital Cardiol* 1979; 9 (suppl 1):85.
166. Sakamoto T, Hada Y, Amano K, Yamaguchi T, Takenaka K: Population study of mitral valve prolapse in the young: eight years' experiences. *Circulation* 1984; 70(suppl II):II-162.
167. Lee WR, Sheikh MU, Lee KJ: Prevalence of mitral valve prolapse in presumably healthy Korean adults. *Clin Cardiol* 1985; 8:356–358.

168. Ostrowska B: Mitral valve prolapse as a cause of pseudoneurotic symptoms in young men. *Kardiol Pol* 1983; 26:559–564.
169. Bochkova DN: Incidence of mitral valve prolapse among the population of Moscow. *Kardiologiia* 1983; 23:40–43.
170. Cortina-Llosa A, Simarro-Garcia C, Simmaro-Martin E, Prieto-Granda J, Gonzalez-Camino F: Mitral valve prolapse: incidence, clinical aspects and diagnostic data. *Rev Esp Cardiol* 1980; 33:317–326.
170a. Cohen M, Pocock WA, Lakier JB, McLaren MJ, Lachman AS, Barlow JB: Four year follow-up of black school children with non-ejection clicks and mitral systolic murmurs. *Am Heart J* 1978; 95:697–701.
171. Bryhn M, Persson S: The prevalence of mitral valve prolapse in healthy men and women in Sweden. *Acta Med Scand* 1984; 215:157–160.
172. Saraclar M, Ozme S, Ozkutlu S, Usanmaz I: The frequency of mitral valve prolapse in electrocardiographic disturbances of unknown origin. *Turk J Pediatr* 1981; 23:23–28.
173. Procacci PM, Savran SV, Schreiter SL, Bryson AL: Prevalence of clinical mitral-valve prolapse in 1169 young women. *N Engl J Med* 1976; 294:1086–1088.
174. Savage DD, Garrison RJ, Devereux RB, Castelli WP, Anderson SJ, Levy D, McNamara PM, Stokes J III, Kannel WB, Feinleib M: Mitral valve prolapse in the general population. I. Epidemiologic features: The Framingham Study. *Am Heart J* 1983; 106:571–576.
174a. Cheng TO: Recent development in cardiology. *Chin Med J* 1983; 96:499–506.
174b. Lachman AS, Schulman P, Arfken CL, Farrish GCM, Slowik DS, McLaren MJ: Prevalence of mitral valve prolapse in non-care-seeking adolescents. *J Am Coll Cardiol* 1986; 7(suppl A):42A.
175. Devereux RB, Brown WT, Lutas EM, Kramer-Fox R, Laragh JH: Association of mitral-valve prolapse with low body-weight and low blood pressure. *Lancet* 1982; 2:792–795.
176. Devereux RB, Sachs I, Kramer-Fox R, Brown WT: Evolution of echocardiographic findings in patients with mitral valve prolapse. *J Cardiovasc Ultrasound* 1983; 2:29–34.
177. Chandraratan PAN, Vlahovich G, Kong Y, Wilson D: Incidence of mitral valve prolapse in one hundred clinically stable newborn baby girls: an echocardiographic study. *Am Heart J* 1979; 98:312–314.
178. Greenwood RD: Mitral valve prolapse. Incidence and clinical course in a pediatric population. *Clin Pediatr* 1984; 23:318–320.
179. Lynch P, Ineson N: Syncope and mitral valve prolapse. *Br Med J* 1984; 288:1538.
180. Lynch P: Cardiological problems in sport. *Br J Hosp Med* 1983; 30:82.
181. Stannard M, Sloman JG, Hare WSC, Goble AJ: Prolapse of the posterior leaflet of the mitral valve. A clinical, familial and cineangiographic study. *Br Med J* 1967; 3:71–74.
182. Shell WE, Walton JA, Clifford ME, Willis PW III: The familial occurrence of the syndrome of mid-late systolic click and late systolic murmur. *Circulation* 1969; 39:327–337.
183. Rizzon P, Biasco G, Brindioci G, Mauro F: Familial syndrome of midsystolic click and late systolic murmur. *Br Heart J* 1973; 35:245–259.
184. Desser KB, Bokhari SI, Benchimol A, Romney D: All in the family: matrimonial mitral valve clicks. *Angiology* 1981; 32:355–360.
185. Hunt D, Sloman G: Prolapse of the posterior leaflet of the mitral valve occurring in eleven members of a family. *Am Heart J* 1969; 78:149–153.
186. Weiss AN, Mimbs JW, Ludbrook PA, Sobel BE: Echocardiographic detection of mitral valve prolapse. Exclusion of false positive diagnosis and determination of inheritance. *Circulation* 1975; 52:1091–1096.
187. Fortuin NJ, Strahan NV, Come PC, Humphries JO, Murphy EA: Inheritance of the mitral valve prolapse syndrome. *Clin Res* 1977; 25:470A.
188. Devereux RB, Brown WT, Kramer R, Sachs I: Inheritance of mitral valve prolapse: autosomal dominant with reduced expression in children and adult males. *Clin Res* 1981; 29:512A.
189. Strahan NV, Murphy EA, Fortuin NJ, Come PC, Humphries JO: Inheritance of the mitral valve prolapse syndrome. Discussion of a three-dimensional penetration model. *Am J Med* 1983; 74:967–972.
190. Scheele W, Allen HN, Krans R, Rubin PJ: Familial prevalence and genetic transmission of mitral valve prolapse. *Circulation* 1976; 54:III-111.
191. Sbarbaro JA, Mehlman DJ, Wu L, Brooks HL: A prospective study of mitral valve prolapse in young men. *Chest* 1979; 75:555–559.
192. Devereux RB, Brown WT, Kramer-Fox R, Sachs I: Inheritance of mitral valve prolapse: effect of age and sex on gene expression. *Ann Intern Med* 1982; 97:826–832.
193. Braun WE, Ronan J, Schacter B, Gardin J, Isner J, Grececk J: HLA antigens in mitral valve prolapse. *Transplant Proc* 1977; 9:1862–1871.
194. Kachru RB, Telischi M, Cruz JB, Patel R, Towne WD: The HLA antigens and ABO blood groups in an American black population with mitral valve prolapse. *Tissue Antigens* 1979; 14:256–260.
195. Jeannet M, Bloch A: HLA types in mitral valve prolapse. *N Engl J Med* 1979; 301:108.
196. Rice GPA, Boughner DR, Stiller C, Ebers GC: Familial stroke syndrome associated with mitral valve prolapse. *Ann Neurol* 1980; 7:130–134.
197. Kramer R, Brown WT, Devereux RB: Mitral valve prolapse: association with anxiety neurosis (panic attacks) and dermal arches. *Am J Hum Genet* 1980; 32:115A.
198. Mason JW, Koch FH, Billingham ME, Winkle RA: Cardiac biopsy evidence for a cardiomyopathy associated with symptomatic mitral valve prolapse. *Am J Cardiol* 1978; 42:557–562.
199. Malcolm AD, Cankovic-Darracott S, Chayen J, Jenkins BS, Webb-Peploe MM: Biopsy evidence of left ventricular myocardial abnormality in patients with mitral leaflet prolapse and chest pain. *Lancet* 1979; I:1052–1055.
200. Malcolm AD: Myocardial mysteries surrounding mitral leaflet prolapse. *Am Heart J* 1980; 100:265–267.
201. Gaffney FA, Wohl AJ, Blomqvist CG, Parkey RW, Willerson JT: Thallium-201 myocardial perfusion studies in patients with the mitral valve prolapse syndrome. *Am J Med* 1978; 64:21–26.
202. Massie B, Botvinick EH, Shames D, Taradash M, Werner J, Schiller N: Myocardial perfusion scintigraphy in patients with mitral valve prolapse. Its advantage over stress electrocardiography in diagnosing associated coronary artery disease and its implication for the etiology of chest pain. *Circulation* 1978; 57:19–26.
203. Klein GJ, Kostuck WJ, Boughner DR, Chamberlain MJ: Stress myocardial imaging in mitral leaflet prolapse syndrome. *Am J Cardiol* 1978; 42: 746–750.
204. Greenspan M, Iskandrian AS, Mintz GS, Croll MN, Segal BL, Kimbiris D, Bemis CE: Exercise myocardial scintigraphy with ^{201}thallium-use in patients with mitral valve prolapse without associated coronary artery disease. *Chest* 1980; 77:47–52.
205. Newman GE, Gibbons RJ, Jones RH: Cardiac function during rest and exercise in patients with mitral valve prolapse. Role of radionuclear angiocardiography. *Am J Cardiol* 1981; 47:14–19.
206. Gottdiener JS, Borer JS, Bacharach SL, Green MV, Epstein SE: Left ventricular function in mitral valve prolapse: assessment with radionuclide cineangiography. *Am J Cardiol* 1981; 47:7–13.
207. de Moraes AG, Sousa JEMR, Thom AF, Martins LRF, Meneghello RS, Pimentel WA, Marioni H, Gimenes VML, Pontes SC Jr: Cintigrafia do miocardio com talio-201 em pacientes com prolapso da valva mitral, com e sem coronariopatia. *Arg Bras Cardiol* 1981; 36:377–386.
208. Tresch DD, Soin JS, Siegel R, Love M, Keelan MH Jr: Mitral valve prolapse: evidence for a myocardial perfusion abnormality. *Am J Cardiol* 1978; 41:441.
209. Butman S, Chandraratna PAN, Milne N: Stress myocardial imaging in patients with mitral valve prolapse: evidence of a perfusion abnormality. *Cathet Cardiovasc Diagn* 1982; 8:243–252.
210. Ahmad M, Haibach H: Left ventricular function in patients with mitral valve prolapse. A radionuclide evaluation. *Clin Nucl Med* 1982; 7:562–567.
211. Gibson DG, Brown DJ: Abnormal left ventricular wall movement in patients with chest pain and normal coronary arteriograms. Relation to inferior T wave changes and mitral prolapse. *Br Heart J* 1979; 41:385–391.
211a. Colle JP, LeGoff G, Ohayon J, Bonnet J, Bricaud H, Basse P: Quantitative frame by frame analysis of regional contraction and lengthening on left ventricular cineangiograms: application to the study of normal left ventricles and left ventricles with mitral valve prolapse. *Clin Cardiol* 1986; 9:43–51.
212. Oakley CM: Mitral valve prolapse: harbinger of death or variant of normal? *Br Med J* 1984; 288:1853–1854.
213. Barlow JB, Pocock WA: Mitral valve prolapse, the athlete's heart, physical activity and sudden death. *Int J Sports Cardiol* 1984; 1:9–24.
214. Montague TJ, McPherson DD, MacKenzie BR, Spencer CA, Nanton MA, Horacek BM: Frequent ventricular ectopic activity without underlying cardiac disease: analysis of 45 subjects. *Am J Cardiol* 1983; 52:980–984.
215. Clemens JD, Ransohoff DF: A quantitative assessment of pre-dental antibiotic prophylaxis for patients with mitral-valve prolapse. *J Chron Dis* 1984; 37:531–544.
216. Bor DH, Himmelstein DU: Endocarditis prophylaxis for patients with mitral valve prolapse. A quantitative analysis. *Am J Med* 1984; 76:711–717.
217. Retchin SM, Fletcher RH, Waugh RA: Endocarditis and mitral valve prolapse: What is the "risk"? *Int J Cardiol* 1984; 5:653–659.
218. Hickey AJ, MacMahon SW, Wilcken DEL: Mitral valve prolapse and bacterial endocarditis: When is antibiotic prophylaxis necessary? *Am Heart J* 1985; 109:431–435.
219. Kowalski SE: Mitral valve prolapse. *Can Anaesth Soc J* 1985; 32:138–141.
220. Lachman AS, Bramwell-Jones DM, Lakier JB, Pocock WA, Barlow JB: Infective endocarditis in the billowing mitral leaflet syndrome. *Br Heart J* 1975; 37:326–330.
221. LeBauer EJ, Perloff JK, Keliher TF: The isolated systolic click with bacterial endocarditis. *Am Heart J* 1967; 73:534–537.
221a. Jeresaty RM: Mitral valve prolapse: definition and implications in athletes. *J Am Coll Cardiol* 1986; 7:231–236.
222. Wooley CF: Where are the diseases of yesteryear? DaCosta's syndrome, soldiers heart, the effort syndrome, neurocirculatory asthenia and the mitral valve prolapse syndrome. *Circulation* 1976; 53:749–751.
223. Boudoulas H, Reynolds JC, Mazzaferri E, Wooley CF: Mitral valve prolapse syndrome: the effect of adrenergic stimulation. *J Am Coll Cardiol* 1983; 2:638–644.

223a. Pasternac A, Kouz S, Gutkowska J, Petitclerc R, Vellas B, de Champlain J, Cantin M, Bourasse MG: Abnormal plasma levels of atrial natriuretic factor (ANF) in patients with symptomatic mitral valve prolapse. *J Am Coll Cardiol* 1986; 7(suppl A):169A.
224. Cobbs BW Jr: Clinical recognition and medical management of rheumatic heart disease and other acquired valvular disease, in Hurst JW, Logue RB (eds): *The Heart*, ed 2. New York, McGraw-Hill Book Company, Inc, 1970, p 813.
225. Jeresaty RM: Mitral valve prolapse-click syndrome. *Progr Cardiovas Dis* 1973; 15:623–652.
226. Pocock WA, Barlow JB: Postexercise arrhythmias in the billowing posterior mitral leaflet syndrome. *Am Heart J* 1970; 80:740–745.
227. Chesler E, Matisonn RE, Lakier JB, Pocock WA, Obel IWP, Barlow JB: Acute myocardial infarction with normal coronary arteries: a possible manifestation of the billowing mitral leaflet syndrome. *Circulation* 1976; 54:203–209.
228. Rippe JM, Singh JB, Jarvais N, Adams E, Erkkilä K: Mitral valve prolapse and spasm of normal coronary arteries: report of four cases and review of the literature. *Angiology* 1984; 35:300–307.
229. Makino H, Al-Sadir J: Myocardial infarction in patients with mitral valve prolapse and normal coronary arteries. *J Am Coll Cardiol* 1983; 1:661.
230. Buda AJ, Levene DL, Myers MG, Chisholm AW, Shane SJ: Coronary artery spasm and mitral valve prolapse. *Am Heart J* 1978; 95:457–462.
231. Mautner RK, Katz GE, Iteld BJ, Phillips JH: Coronary artery spasm: a mechanism for chest pain in selected patients with the mitral valve prolapse syndrome. *Chest* 1981; 79:449–453.
232. Kawasaki K, Hosoda S: Epidemiology of coronary spasm. *Nippon Rinsho* 1984; 41:315—320.
233. Cheng TO: Coronary artery spasm - 1984. *Chest* 1984; 86:918–926.
234. Chesler E, King RA, Edwards JE: The myxomatous mitral valve and sudden death. *Circulation* 1983; 67:632–639.
235. Barnett HJM, Boughner DR, Taylor DW, Cooper PE, Kostuk WJ, Nichol PM: Further evidence relating mitral valve prolapse to cerebral ischemic events. *N Engl J Med* 1980; 302:139–144.
236. Larbi E, Mehlman DJ, Talano JV: Increased neurological events in subtypes of mitral valve prolapse (abstr). *Eur Heart J* 1984; 5(suppl I):225.
237. Fieschi C, Francia A, Allori L, Argentino C, Bernadi S, Bertazzoni G, Carpinteri F, Di Piero V, Ferroluzzi M, Lenzi GL, Prencipe M, Servi M, Zanette E: Mitral valve prolapse as a risk factor for TIA. A study with echocardiography and dynamic ECG. *Eur Neurol* 1983; 22:233–239.
238. Barletta GA, Gagliardi R, Benvenuti L, Fantini F: Cerebral ischemic attacks as a complication of aortic and mitral valve prolapse. *Stroke* 1985; 16:219–223.
239. Litman GI, Friedman HM: Migraine and the mitral valve prolapse syndrome. *Am Heart J* 1978; 96:610–614.
240. Scharf RE, Hennerici M, Bluschke V, Lueck J, Kladetzky RG: Cerebral ischemia in young patients: Is it associated with mitral valve prolapse and abnormal platelet activity in vivo? *Stroke* 1982; 13:454–458.
241. Walsh PN, Kansu TA, Corbett JJ, Savino PJ, Goldburgh WP, Schatz NJ: Platelets, thromboembolism and mitral valve prolapse. *Circulation* 1981; 63:552–559.
242. Steele P, Weily H, Rainwater J, Vogel R: Platelet survival time and thromboembolism in patients with mitral valve prolapse. *Circulation* 1979; 60:43–45.
242a. Pasternac A, Latour J-G, Kouz S, Gauthier C, Petitclerc R, de Champlain J, Vellas B, Goulet C: Increased platelet release products and aggregation in symptomatic mitral valve prolapse (MVP). *J Am Coll Cardiol* 1986; 7(suppl A):28A.
242b. Elam MB, Viar MJ, Ratts TE, Chesney CM: Mitral valve prolapse in women with oral contraceptive-related cerebrovascular insufficiency: associated persistent hypercoagulable state. *Arch Intern Med* 1986; 146:73–77.
243. Hirsowitz GS, Saffer D: Hemiplegia and the billowing mitral leaflet syndrome. *J Neurol Neurosurg Psychiatry* 1978; 41:381–383.
244. Waller BF, Maron BJ, Del Negro AA, Gottdiener JS, Roberts WC: Frequency and significance of M-mode echocardiographic evidence of mitral valve prolapse in clinically isolated pure mitral regurgitation. Analysis of 65 patients having mitral valve replacement. *Am J Cardiol* 1984; 53:139–147.
245. Belardi J, Lardani H, Manubens S, Sheldon WC, Moreyra A: Idiopathic prolapse of the mitral valve: a follow up study in 137 patients studied by angiography. *Am J Cardiol* 1976; 37:120.
246. Hill DG, Davies MJ, Braimbridge MV: The natural history and surgical management of the redundant cusp syndrome (floppy mitral valve). *J Thorac Cardiovasc Surg* 1974; 67:519–525.
247. Koch FH, Hancock EW: Ten year follow-up of forty patients with the midsystolic click/late systolic murmur syndrome. *Am J Cardiol* 1976; 37:149.
248. Allen H, Harris A, Leatham A: Significance and prognosis of an isolated late systolic murmur. A 9- to 22-year follow up. *Br Heart J* 1974; 36:525–532.
249. Appelblatt NH, Willis PW III, Lenhart JA, Shulman JI, Walton JA: Ten to 40 year follow-up of 69 patients with systolic click with or without apical late systolic murmur. *Am J Cardiol* 1975; 35:119.
250. Mills P, Rose J, Hollingsworth J, Amara I, Craige E: Long-term prognosis of mitral-valve prolapse. *N Engl J Med* 1977; 297:13–18.
251. Kolibash AJ, Bush CA, Fontana MB, Ryan JM, Kilman J, Wooley CF: Mitral valve prolapse syndrome: analysis of 62 patients aged 60 years and older. *Am J Cardiol* 1983; 52:534–539.
252. DePace NL, Nestico PF, Morganroth J: Acute severe mitral regurgitation. Pathophysiology, clinical recognition and management. *Am J Med* 1985; 78:293–306.
253. Penkoske PA, Ellis FH Jr, Alexander S, Watkins E Jr: Results of valve reconstruction for mitral regurgitation secondary to mitral valve prolapse. *Am J Cardiol* 1985; 55:735–738.
254. Tresch DD, Doyle TP, Bonchek LI, Siegel R, Keelan MH, Olinger GN, Brooks HL: Mitral valve prolapse requiring surgery. Clinical and pathological study. *Am J Med* 1985; 78:245–250.
255. Marchand P, Barlow JB, du Plessis LA, Webster I: Mitral regurgitation with rupture of normal chordae tendineae. *Br Heart J* 1966; 28:746–758.
256. Jeresaty RM, Edwards JE, Chawla SK: Mitral valve prolapse and ruptured chordae tendineae. *Am J Cardiol* 1985; 55:138–142.
257. Ren JF, Panidis IP, Kotler MN, Mintz GS, Goel I, Ross J: Flail mitral valve syndrome: comparison with chronic mitral regurgitation of other etiologies. *Am Heart J* 1985; 109:435–442.
258. Hickey AJ, Wilcken DEL, Wright JS, Warren BA: Primary (spontaneous) chordal rupture: relation to myxomatous valve disease and mitral valve prolapse. *J Am Coll Cardiol* 1985; 5:1341–1346.
259. Grenadier E, Keidar S, Sahn DJ, Alpan G, Goldberg SJ, Valdez Cruz LM, Lima CO, Barron JV, Allen HD, Palant A: Ruptured mitral chordae tendinae may be a frequent and insignificant complication in the mitral valve prolapse syndrome. *Eur Heart J* 1985; 6:1006–1015.
260. Clemens JD, Stanton BF: What is the risk of infective endocarditis in mitral valve prolapse? *J Cardiovasc Med* 1984; 9:465–469.
260a. Baddour LM, Bisno AL: Infective endocarditis complicating mitral valve prolapse: epidemiologic, clinical, and microbiologic aspects. *Rev Infect Dis* 1986; 8:117–137.
261. Bayliss R, Clarke C, Oakley C, Somerville W, Whitefield AGW: The teeth and infective endocarditis. *Br Heart J* 1983; 50:506–512.
262. Bayliss R, Clark C, Oakley CM, Somerville W, Whitfield AGW, Young SEJ: The bowel, the genitourinary tract, and infective endocarditis. *Br Heart J* 1984; 51:339–345.
263. Guntheroth WG: How important are dental procedures as a cause of infective endocarditis? *Am J Cardiol* 1984; 54:798–801.
264. Baltch AL, Schaffer C, Hammer MC, Sutphen NT, Smith RP, Conroy J, Shayegani M: Bacteremia following dental cleaning in patients with and without penicillin prophylaxis. *Am Heart J* 1982; 104:1335–1339.
264a. Harris P, Tingelstad J, Kavey R-E, Thomas J, Perry J, Chung K, Manning J: Infective endocarditis in pediatric mitral valve prolapse patients: a multicenter review. *Clin Research* 1986; 34:233A.
264b. Baddour LM, Phillips, TN, Bisno AL: Coagulase-negative staphylococcal endocarditis. Occurrence in patients with mitral valve prolapse. *Arch Intern Med* 1986; 146:119–121.
265. Engle PJ, Alpert BL, Hickman JR: The nature and prevalence of the abnormal exercise ECG in mitral valve prolapse. *Am Heart J* 1979; 98:716–724.
266. Abinader EG: The effect of beta blockade on the abnormal exercise test in patients with mitral valve prolapse. *J Cardiac Rehabil* 1984; 4:95–100.
267. Winkle RA, Lopes MG, Fitzgerald JW, Gordman DJ, Schroeder JS, Harrison DC: Arrhythmias in patients with mitral valve prolapse. *Circulation* 1975; 52:73–81.
268. Lobstein HD, Horwitz LD, Curry GC, Mullins CB: Electrocardiographic abnormalities and coronary arteriograms in the mitral click-murmur syndrome. *N Engl J Med* 1973; 289:127–131.
269. Tuqan SK, Mau RD, Schwartz MJ: Anterior myocardial infarction patterns in the mitral valve prolapse-systolic click syndrome. *Am J Med* 1975; 58:719–723.
270. Abinader EG: Adrenergic beta blockade and ECG changes in the systolic click murmur syndrome. *Am Heart J* 1976; 91:297–302.
271. Gulotta SJ, Gulco L, Padmanabhan V, Miller S: The syndrome of systolic click, murmur and mitral valve prolapse—a cardiomyopathy? *Circulation* 1974; 49:717–728.
271a. Kavey REW, Blackman MS, Sondheimer HM, Byrum CJ: Anti-arrhythmic therapy in children with mitral valve prolapse. *J Am Coll Cardiol* 1985; 5:430.
272. Criley JM, Heger J: Prolapsed mitral leaflet syndrome. *Cardiovasc Clin* 1979; 10:213–233.
273. Criley JM, Zeilenga DW, Morgan MT: Mitral dysfunction. A possible cause of arrhythmias in the prolapsing mitral leaflet syndrome. *Trans Am Clin Climatol Assoc* 1973; 85:44–53.
274. Leclercq JF, Malergue MC, Milosevic D, Rosengarten MD, Attuel P, Coumel P: Troubles du rythme ventriculaires et prolapsus mitral. A propos de 35 observations. *Arch Mal Coeur* 1980; 73:276–287.

275. Witt AL, Fenoglio JJ, Wagner BM, Bassett AL: Electrophysiological properties of cardiac muscle in the anterior mitral valve leaflet and the adjacent atrium in the dog. Possible implications for the genesis of atrial dysrhythmias. *Circ Res* 1973; 32:731–745.
276. Witt AL, Fenoglio JJ, Hordof AJ, Reemtsma K: Ultrastructure and transmembrane potentials of cardiac muscle in the human anterior mitral leaflet. *Circulation* 1979; 59:1284–1292.
277. Josephson ME, Horowitz LN, Kastor JA: Paroxysmal supraventricular tachycardia in patients with mitral valve prolapse. *Circulation* 1978; 57:111–115.
278. Shah AA, Quinones MA, Waggoner AD, Barndt R, Miller RR: Pulsed Doppler echocardiographic detection of mitral regurgitation in mitral valve prolapse: correlation with cardiac arrhythmias. *Cathet Cardiovasc Diagn* 1982; 8:437–444.
279. Hochreiter C, Kramer HM, Kligfield P, Kramer-Fox R, Devereux RB, Borer JS: Arrhythmias in mitral valve prolapse: effect of additional mitral regurgitation. *J Am Coll Cardiol* 1983; 1:607.
280. Kligfield P, Hochreiter C, Kramer H, Devereux RB, Niles N, Kramer-Fox R, Borer JS: Complex arrhythmias in mitral regurgitation with and without mitral valve prolapse: contrast to arrhythmias in mitral valve prolapse without mitral regurgitation. *Am J Cardiol* 1985; 55:1545–1549.
281. Savage DD, Levy D, Garrison RJ, Castelli WP, Kligfield P, Devereux RB, Kannel WB, Feinleib M: Mitral valve prolapse in the general population. 3. Dysrhythmias: The Framingham Study. *Am Heart J* 1983; 106:582–586.
282. Lown B, Wolf M: Approaches to sudden death from coronary heart disease. *Circulation* 1971; 44:130–142.
283. Swartz MH, Teichholz LE, Donoso E: Mitral valve prolapse. A review of associated arrhythmias. *Am J Med* 1977; 62:377–389.
284. Ware JA, Magro SA, Luck JC, Mann DE, Nielsen AP, Rosen KM, Wyndham CRC: Conduction system abnormalities in symptomatic mitral valve prolapse: an electrophysiologic analysis of 60 patients. *Am J Cardiol* 1984; 53:1075–1078.
285. Trent JK, Adelman AC, Wigle ED, Silver MD: Morphology of a prolapsed mitral valve leaflet. *Am Heart J* 1970; 79:539–543.
286. Bharati S, Granston AS, Liebson PR, Loeb HS, Rosen KM, Lev M: The conduction system in mitral valve prolapse syndrome with sudden death. *Am Heart J* 1981; 101:667–670.
287. James TN: Pathology of small coronary arteries. *Am J Cardiol* 1967; 20:679–691.
288. McKibbin JK, Pocock WA, Barlow JB, Scott Millar RN, Obel IWP: Sotalol, hypokalaemia, syncope, and torsade de pointes. *Br Heart J* 1984; 51:157–162.
289. Troup PJ, Zipes DP: Aprindine treatment of recurrent ventricular tachycardia in patients with mitral valve prolapse. *Am Heart J* 1979; 97:322–328.
290. Vlay SC, Kallman CH, Reid PR: The utility of aprindine blood levels in the management of ventricular arrhythmias. *J Am Coll Cardiol* 1985; 5:738–743.
291. Ritchie JL, Hammermeister KE, Kennedy JW: Refractory ventricular tachycardia and fibrillation in a patient with the prolapsing mitral leaflet syndrome: successful control with overdrive pacing. *Am J Cardiol* 1976; 37:314–316.
292. Saltissi S, Crowther A, Byrne C, Clarke S, Jenkins BS, Webb-Peploe MM: The effects of oral digoxin therapy in primary mitral leaflet prolapse. *Eur Heart J* 1983; 4:828–837.
292a. Boudoulas H, Schaal SF, Stang JM, Fontana ME, Kolibash AJ, Wooley CF: Mitral valve prolapse—sudden death with long-term survival. *J Am Coll Cardiol* 1986; 7(suppl A):29A.
293. Leichtman D, Nelson R, Gobel FL, Alexander CS, Cohn JN: Bradycardia with mitral valve prolapse. A potential mechanism of sudden death. *Ann Intern Med* 1976; 85:453–457.
294. Vesterby A, Bjerregaard P, Gregersen M, Fode K: Sudden death in mitral valve prolapse: associated accessory atrioventricular pathways. *Forensic Sci Int* 1982; 19:125–133.
295. Fleg JL, Lakatta EG: Prevalence and prognosis of exercise-induced nonsustained ventricular tachycardia in apparently healthy volunteers. *Am J Cardiol* 1984; 54:762–764.
296. Jeresaty RM: *Mitral Valve Prolapse*. New York, Raven Press, 1979, p 142.
297. Pocock WA, Bosman CK, Chesler E, Barlow JB, Edwards JE: Sudden death in primary mitral valve prolapse. *Am Heart J* 1984; 107:378–382.
298. Kay JH, Krohn BG, Zubiate P, Hoffman RL: Surgical correction of severe mitral prolapse without mitral insufficiency but with pronounced cardiac arrhythmias. *J Thorac Cardiovasc Surg* 1979; 78:259–267.
299. Reece IJ, Cooley DA, Painvin A, Okereke OUJ, Powers PL, Pechacek LW, Frazier OH: Surgical treatment of mitral systolic click syndrome: results in 37 patients. *Ann Thorac Surg* 1985; 39:155–158.

32 Surgical Treatment of Valvular Heart Disease

Viking O. Björk, MD

Acquired cardiac disorders, by definition, develop after birth, in contradistinction to congenital malformations of the heart. The dividing line is sometimes blurred, however. For example, aortic valve stenosis in a middle-aged or elderly person may be secondary to calcification of a congenital bicuspid valve.

The principal cause of acquired cardiac disease formerly was rheumatic fever. With the virtual disappearance of rheumatic fever in many countries, however, other causes have come to predominate, including infections, degenerative processes, and various connective-tissue diseases.

MITRAL STENOSIS

ETIOLOGY

Congenital mitral stenosis is uncommon and is mostly seen in combination with mitral incompetence. Often the chordae tendineae arise from a single, fused papillary muscle (parachute type deformity), which prevents full opening of the cusps in diastole.

The most common cause of mitral stenosis is rheumatic fever, although only about half of the patients have a history of this disease. The endocarditis of rheumatic fever deforms the valve, leading to adhesion of the commissures and thickening of the leaflets. Progressive fibrosis and calcification often finally produce a rigid, calcified plate with a central orifice. Because many patients have had pancarditis in the acute stage of the disease, the myocardium may be affected.

PATHOPHYSIOLOGY

The mitral valve orifice normally is 4 to 6 cm^2 when fully opened. Reduction of this area to 2 cm^2 implies a hindrance to cardiac output, and an area of less than 1.5 cm^2 is associated with distinct symptoms in many cases. Three hemodynamic changes occur in severe mitral stenosis: pressure increase in the left atrium and pulmonary veins, increase in pulmonary vascular resistance, and diminution in stroke volume. The pressure in the left atrium does not normally exceed 10 mm Hg. In mitral stenosis it increases to double or more. When the left atrial pressure is higher than the osmotic pressure of plasma, ie, 25 to 30 mm Hg, there is a risk of pulmonary edema.

Hypertension in the pulmonary veins evokes reflex spasm in the fine pulmonary arteries. The resistance in these vessels increases and leads to pulmonary hypertension. If this state persists, the right ventricle will show hypertrophy, insufficiency, and dilation, changes that can lead to secondary tricuspid insufficiency (present in about 20% of cases).

Another characteristic complication of chronic mitral stenosis is thromboembolism. The risk is greatest in patients with left atrial enlargement and fibrillation. The thrombi usually derive from the auricle of the left atrium.

SYMPTOMS

The most common symptom of mitral stenosis is exertional dyspnea. The causal effort initially is extreme, but it gradually diminishes to simple movements such as those involved in dressing. Other common symptoms are cough, palpitation, paroxysmal nocturnal dyspnea, and hemoptysis. Right ventricular failure results in enlargement of the liver and peripheral edema. Arterial emboli give rise to sudden neural deficit such as hemiplegia, restriction of visual fields, or other manifestations of abrupt circulatory disturbance.

DIAGNOSIS

In typical cases a low-pitched diastolic murmur is localized to the apex and heralded by an opening snap, and the first heart sound is accentuated. Auscultation of the lungs often reveals rhonchi and crepitations as signs of pulmonary venous hypertension.

In exceptional cases of mitral stenosis no murmur can be heard. The condition then is grave, with stroke volume inadequate for hemodynamic prerequisites of an audible murmur. The diagnosis in such cases can be suspected from the abnormal heart sounds and the severity of other symptoms.

Chest radiograms characteristically show enlargement of the left atrium, best seen on lateral films in which the atrium bulges backwards and displaces the esophagus. The anteroposterior films show signs of pulmonary venous engorgement, and pulmonary hypertension produces prominence of the pulmonary artery and enlargement of the right atrium and ventricle. In chronic, severe mitral stenosis the relative heart volume sometimes exceeds 1,000 ml/m^2. Evidence of valvular calcification can give guidance in the diagnosis and choice of treatment.

The electrocardiogram demonstrates dilation or hypertrophy of the left atrium with characteristically bifid P waves (P mitrale). Atrial fibrillation is present in at least 50% of cases. Often it is the change from sinus rhythm to atrial fibrillation that causes patients to seek medical advice. At echocardiography the cusps are thickened and rigid, with impaired motility and delayed closure.

Heart catheterization is unnecessary for the diagnosis of typical mitral stenosis. In apparently mild cases, however, or if there are complicating factors, catheterization can be helpful in assessing the degree of stenosis. The pressure gradient across the valve must then be determined simultaneously with the cardiac output. Pulmonary vascular resistance should also be calculated. Angiocardiography provides no additional information in uncomplicated cases.

DIFFERENTIAL DIAGNOSIS

In cases with no history of rheumatic fever and with short duration of symptoms and maintained sinus rhythm, the possibility of left atrial myxoma must be considered in diagnostic differentiation. An echocardiogram will readily resolve the issue.

TREATMENT

Mild stenosis (valve orifice area greater than 2 cm^2) with few symptoms should be conservatively managed. In more severe narrowing (valve orifice area less than 1.5 cm^2), surgery is recommended, particularly if the patient has troublesome dyspnea or if embolism has occurred.

CLOSED METHOD FOR OPERATION OF MITRAL STENOSIS

Several operations can be performed to relieve mitral stenosis. The oldest, transventricular dilation of the valve, is feasible only if the adherent leaflets are pliable and without calcification. With the steeply declining incidence of rheumatic fever, however, such cases have become rare, and this has led to gradual abandonment of closed mitral dilation. An advantage of the operation is that cardiopulmonary bypass is not required; however, the result is relatively unreliable.

The closed method for treatment of mitral stenosis with transventricular dilatation will give good results only in selected cases. The operative mortality is around 2%; the procedure is fast and inexpensive.

With the patient lying on his right side, the left side of the chest is entered subcostally under the fifth rib. The pericardium is opened in front of the phrenic nerve. The Tubbs dilator is introduced through the apex of the left ventricle and under guidance of the index finger in the left atrium through the appendix, advanced to an optimal position, and opened about 4 cm in a man and 3.5 cm in a woman (Figure 32.1). The result achieved is then evaluated with the finger.

In areas where acute rheumatic fever has disappeared,

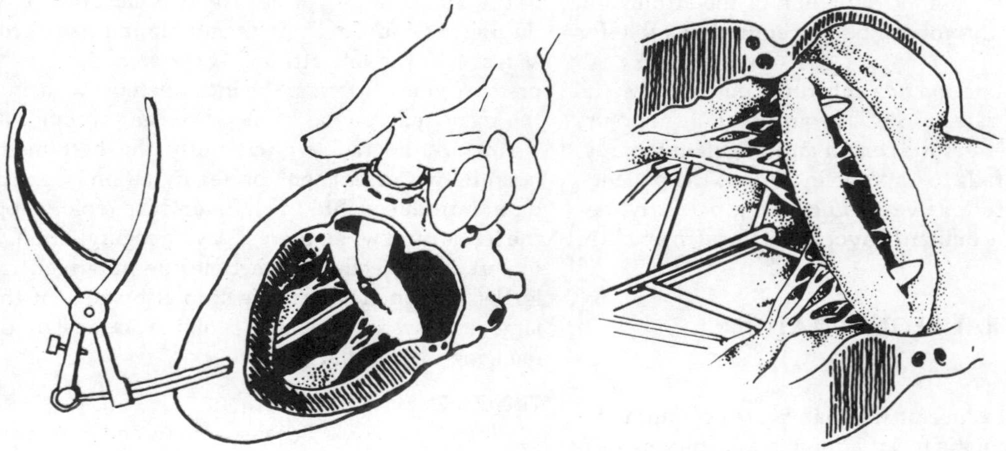

Figure 32.1. Diagram of a dilator introduced through the left ventricle under guidance of the index finger in the left atrium through the appendix to an optimal position (left) and opened (right).

many cases are not suitable. The closed method has been abandoned there in favor of an open procedure, which otherwise had to be performed as an emergency in 5% in connection with dilatation and in 20% during a ten-year follow-up. With a closed procedure, the preoperative selection has to be more careful to obtain these good results, with a left ventricular angiogram to exclude mitral insufficiency in combination with shortened chordae tendineae and fusion of the top of the papillary muscles directly to the mitral leaflets.

OPEN MITRAL COMMISSUROTOMY

For the reasons cited, closed dilation was gradually superseded by open mitral commissurotomy, performed under direct visual control with the use of cardiopulmonary bypass. The fused commissures are divided and any adherent chordae are separated. The functional result is reliable. If commissurotomy proves to be impracticable, a prosthetic valve can be inserted at the same operation.

MITRAL RECONSTRUCTION IN PREDOMINANT MITRAL STENOSIS

In the presence of a stenotic mitral orifice, both a nondistensible left atrium and a giant left atrium are incapable of generating or maintaining an efficient mitral gradient. Under these circumstances, surgery has to avoid a residual gradient; therefore, reconstructive surgery can only be used when a good functioning valve can be achieved. Residual insufficiency will also be poorly tolerated. In the presence of good atrial compliance an imperfect reconstruction can improve the patient's condition, but this same anatomic result in a patient with rigid or giant left atrium may be disastrous.

Intraoperative careful identification of each element of the mitral apparatus is essential and requires good visibility, patience, and judgment. The atriotomy incision is large and carried just behind the interatrial groove; it is prolonged upwards beyond and behind the superior vena cava and curved backwards behind the inferior vena cava so that the valve can be clearly studied. The use of nerve hooks to separate and elevate the leaflets is advantageous. The anulus, leaflets, commissures, chordae, and papillary muscles must be systematically inspected and their pathology identified. Some obvious limitations to reconstruction are apparent immediately, some not so readily. In the presence of a predominant stenotic lesion with retracted leaflets, anuloplasty after commissurotomy will result in a valve that is competent but has a residual gradient. Accepted reconstructive techniques include sectioning of the fused commissures, sectioning of thickened secondary chordae, and longitudinal incision of the papillary muscles which will remarkably increase the mobility of the mitral apparatus. The chordae can be shortened by pulling them downward into a split papillary muscle. Selective reduction of the anulus can be performed with the help of prosthetic flexible rings. Techniques such as cusp extension and chordal replacement currently cannot be recommended.

In conclusion, reconstructive surgery represents a new approach that significantly reduces the number of valve replacements. The difficulty resides, however, in the need for a variety of techniques tailored to the requirements of each valve. The limiting factors must clearly be established, so that too bold an approach resulting in malfunctioning valves may be avoided.

Mitral valve replacement has become the most widely used operation for mitral stenosis largely because the valve in most patients who now come to surgery is so destroyed that conservative valvuloplasty is not feasible. During valve replacement, the auricle of the left atrium is ligated as prophylaxis against thromboembolism. The operation is associated with a 3% to 5% mortality rate. Life-long, well-monitored anticoagulant medication is required postoperatively.

PROGNOSIS

A number of factors determine the outlook in mitral stenosis. Slight to moderate stenosis without thromboembolism is compatible with a good prognosis even if not surgically treated. The patient must adjust to a quiet life-style. Enlargement and fibrillation of the atrium and the occurrence of thromboembolism are unfavorable for the prognosis.

Following implantation of a substitute mitral valve, the five-year survival rate is 75%. Thromboembolism occurs in 5% of these cases despite correct anticoagulant therapy. Physical capacity fails to improve in 20% of the patients, even if the substitute valve is functioning perfectly, because there is concomitant myocardial insufficiency in most cases.

MITRAL REGURGITATION

ETIOLOGY

The commonest cause of the many cases of mitral regurgitation is rheumatic fever, although a history of such disease can be elicited in only a small proportion of cases. Often, the incompetence is combined with stenosis due to scarring and calcification of the valve. Another common form of mitral incompetence is caused by degenerative changes in the valve leaflets and chordae tendineae. These changes produce backward bulging of the whole valve, but especially its anterior leaflet, into the atrium during systole ("ballooning" or "billowing" mitral valve or mitral valve prolapse). The chordae may even rupture; chordal rupture may be spontaneous or frequently happens during exertion. Bacterial endocarditis can cause valvular destruction and severe regurgitation. Other possible causes are papillary muscle dysfunction, when a myocardial infarction has involved the papillary muscles, and left ventricular dilation due to myocardial failure.

PATHOPHYSIOLOGY

Insufficiency of the mitral valve results in regurgitation of blood from the left ventricle to the left atrium in each systole. As a result, there is added volume load on the left ventricle during diastole and increased pressure in the left atrium. The systolic pressure waves can sometimes reach 40 to 70 mm Hg. Pulmonary edema nevertheless is seldom seen in these cases.

SYMPTOMS

Even severe mitral regurgitation with left ventricular enlargement often produces surprisingly few symptoms. Gradually, however, the patient experiences dyspnea on effort and general fatigue. The onset of atrial fibrillation usually is remarked by the patient as palpitation.

DIAGNOSIS

A high-pitched systolic murmur is audible over the apex, and especially in the rheumatic form of mitral regurgitation, it is transmitted to the left axilla. Radiologically there is enlargement of the left cardiac chambers. Calcification of the valve is unusual, as is severe pulmonary congestion.

The electrocardiogram sometimes gives evidence of left ventricular hypertrophy. Atrial fibrillation can be demonstrated in slightly less than half of the patients. Echocardiography reflects dilation of the left atrium and ventricle, but gives no more specific picture.

Heart catheterization is useful for assessing the state of the circulation. Typically, there is elevation of the end-diastolic pressure in the left ventricle and also a prominent V wave in the left atrium. There sometimes is a minor pressure gradient across the incompetent valve, indicating the increased volume of blood passing through it.

Angiocardiography is currently the best method for quantitative assessment of regurgitation. Contrast medium introduced into the left ventricle rapidly appears in the left atrium when there is severe regurgitation. Filming in certain projections sometimes permits registration of leaflet motion. The investigation also shows if there is a large end-systolic residual volume as a sign of commencing myocardial failure.

TREATMENT

When symptoms become severe and cardiac volume shows a tendency to increase, surgical treatment is advisable. In most cases, deformity of the leaflets precludes valvuloplasty. Mitral valve replacement is then necessary. The associated mortality is 3% to 5%.

VALVE RECONSTRUCTION IN PREDOMINANT MITRAL VALVE INCOMPETENCE

The aim of valvular reconstruction is to restore the function rather than the anatomy of the valvular apparatus. It involves either limiting or increasing leaflet motion in addition to remodeling the anulus by prosthetic ring anuloplasty.

Correction of Leaflet Prolapse

A. Posterior leaflet prolapse. Prolapse of the posterior leaflet is usually due to ruptured or elongated chordae. This prolapse will require a quadrangular resection of the leaflet with suture of its edges and a prosthetic ring anuloplasty to reinforce the repair.

B. Anterior leaflet prolapse. Extensive prolapse of the anterior mitral leaflet due to major chordae rupture cannot be repaired. Only limited central prolapse of the middle portion can be treated with a triangular resection and the edges sutured with interrupted 6–0 sutures. Extensive prolapse of the anterior mitral leaflet due to chordal elongation may be treated by chordal shortening. This technique consists of burying the extra length of elongated chordae in a trench created in the tip of the corresponding papillary muscle.

C. Anulus dilatation. Anulus dilatation in combination with mitral valve incompetence in certain cases can be treated with a suitable prosthetic ring, if it will allow restoration of a normal shape and an optimal orifice area, and prevent recurrent dilatation of the anulus. A good and stable result may be achieved if a good surface of coaptation and good pliability of the leaflets have been restored.

MITRAL VALVE REPLACEMENT

See Choice of Substitute Valve.

PROGNOSIS

Slight degrees of mitral regurgitation carry a favorable prognosis. The more severe forms involve gradual and possibly serious deterioration of left ventricular function. In such cases, therefore, it is important to avoid undue delay in surgical treatment.

AORTIC STENOSIS

Not until functioning valvular prostheses became available were acceptable results obtained from surgery of the aortic valve. Early experience with valvotomy and decalcification was discouraging. The first clinically suitable ball valve was introduced by Starr and Edwards in 1961 in the United States.

ETIOLOGY

Aortic stenosis usually is a congenital anomaly with a bicuspid valve. When the valve calcifies and becomes rigid, symptoms arise from the obstruction. A history of rheumatic fever is found in only a few cases. Arteriosclerosis occasionally causes calcification of the valve, with resultant stenosis.

PATHOPHYSIOLOGY

Aortic obstruction increases the demands made on left ventricular work. To begin with, the heart can compensate for the stenosis by hypertrophy of the ventricular muscle. As the hypertrophy increases, however, the coronary blood flow becomes inadequate to sustain the ventricular work, and myocardial ischemia is manifest as angina pectoris or possibly even small infarctions. The filling pressure (the pressure required to distend the ventricle in diastole) increases with an ensuing increase in atrial pressure, particularly during exertion. In a few cases the aortic pressure fails to increase as usual in response to effort, which can lead to serious cardiac arrhythmia and syncope.

SYMPTOMS

Mild aortic stenosis (valve orifice greater than 1 cm^2), as a rule, is asymptomatic. More severe narrowing is associated with anginal pain and dyspnea on exertion. In some elderly patients the presenting picture is one of left ventricular failure and pulmonary congestion. Syncope or dizzy spells are serious symptoms that should prompt immediate investigation.

DIAGNOSIS

The classic sign is a systolic ejection murmur in the second intercostal space to the right of the sternum, transmitted along the carotid arteries but audible also at the apex. A high-pitched, protracted murmur suggests severe stenosis.

At radiologic examination the heart size usually is normal. Prominence of the left ventricle on lateral films can suggest hypertrophy. Poststenotic widening of the ascending aorta is seen in 50% of these patients. Advanced stenosis, particularly in elderly persons, can produce enlargement of the left ventricle and the entire heart, and signs of pulmonary congestion. Calcification of the valve is present in most cases, but often it is not discernible on conventional films. Calcifications are best visualized from filming of heart movements through an image intensifier.

The electrocardiogram in many cases shows left ventricular hypertrophy. Some of these patients also have left bundle branch block. Atrial fibrillation is uncommon. Echocardiography may demonstrate calcification of the aortic valve, hypertrophy of the left ventricle, dilation of the aorta, and the like, but it gives no direct information on the degree of stenosis.

Heart catheterization is not required when physical findings are clear and calcification is radiologically visible. In uncertain cases, however, particularly if the symptoms are uncharacteristic, measurement of the severity of stenosis can be important. This is most easily achieved in connection with angiocardiography, by means of a pull-out pressure curve. When contrast medium has been instilled into the left ventricle, the catheter is retracted to the aorta, while pressure and stroke volume of the heart are recorded. If possible, end-diastolic pressure in the ventricle is determined to assess the state of the myocardium.

Angiocardiography should be performed in doubtful cases and in cases in which anginal pain seems disproportionate to the severity of aortic stenosis. Selective coronary angiography in these cases will indicate any significant coronary stenosis. In other cases, injection of contrast medium into the ascending aorta can suffice. If the catheter can be manipulated into the left ventricle, the contrast will aid in the assessment of myocardial function.

TREATMENT

Surgery in principle is indicated in all patients with symptomatic aortic stenosis. In clinically doubtful cases, guidance is obtained from assessment of stenosis at heart catheterization. Surgery generally is advised when the valve orifice is smaller than 1 cm^2.

Operation is performed with cardiopulmonary bypass through a median sternotomy. Valvular calcifications are always too extensive to permit conservative reconstruction. Extirpation of the valve and implantation of a substitute is the only possible procedure. Careful removal of all calcifications is important to provide reliable tissue attachments for the replacement valve. Postoperative anticoagulant therapy must be given to prevent thromboembolism. Surgical mortality is 3% to 4%.

Advanced age no longer contraindicates aortic valve replacement, which considerably relieves the load on the left ventricle. If the patient's general health is good, the operation can be performed in patients up to the age of 85 years.

PROGNOSIS

Symptomatic aortic stenosis without surgical treatment carries a 50% five-year death rate, including a 20% rate of sudden deaths. Most patients are symptom-free after valve replacement and can lead a normal life. About 90% are still alive 5 years postoperatively, and 60% after 15 years.

AORTIC REGURGITATION

ETIOLOGY

The most common cause of aortic valve incompetence formerly was rheumatic fever, leading to scarring and thickening of the cusps. Most cases now are due to bacterial endocarditis which, in its acute phase, can cause septic perforation of the cusps. Degenerative systemic diseases, some hereditary connective-tissue disorders (eg, Marfan's syndrome), and dissecting aortic aneurysm are among the other causes. In the latter conditions, damage to the cusp attachments causes prolapse.

PATHOPHYSIOLOGY

Because the aortic valve is incompetent, much (sometimes more than 50%) of the blood that is pumped into the aorta leaks back into the left ventricle, which becomes dilated and hypertrophied. The stroke volume increases, producing characteristically bounding pulsations in the aorta and the peripheral arteries. The residual volume of blood in the left ventricle gradually increases while the atrial pressure rises, especially during exertion.

SYMPTOMS

As long as the left ventricle can compensate for the leak, the patient has no obvious symptoms. Dyspnea of effort gradually appears, and sometimes there is anginal chest pain. A few patients experience discomfort from the increased pulsations.

DIAGNOSIS

Aortic regurgitation is readily missed at clinical examination, as the diastolic murmur it produces can be relatively faint. The murmur is of high frequency and best heard in the third left intercostal space when the patient is seated and leaning slightly forward. The large stroke volume often produces a systolic ejection murmur over the aorta. The conspicuous pulsations also give diagnostic guidance. Measurement of the blood pressure shows increased pulse amplitude, with low diastolic pressure (usually about 50 mm Hg).

The electrocardiogram may show left axis deviation and signs of left ventricular hypertrophy. Atrioventricular block of variable degree is sometimes seen. Atrial fibrillation can occur at later stages.

At radiologic examination there is enlargement of the left ventricle with downward-lateral displacement of the apex. Measurement of the cardiac volume is useful for observing the course of aortic incompetence. As the incompetence progresses, the heart volume increases.

Echocardiography shows fluttering motion of the anterior mitral valve leaflet as it encounters the backflow from the aortic valve. The size of the left ventricle is some indication of the degree of aortic insufficiency.

Heart catheterization is sometimes performed to assess the state of the circulation. Pressure should preferably be measured both at rest and during exercise. If an increase in end-diastolic pressure in the left ventricle during exercise is accompanied by an increase in left atrial pressure, this signals the beginning of left ventricular failure.

Angiocardiography is used to study the degree of regurgitation and also to clarify anatomic conditions. In sepsis, for instance, abscess may be demonstrable in the aortic root. When contrast medium is injected into the aorta, a variable amount leaks back into the left ventricle, which in many cases is dilated. Secondary mitral insufficiency is sometimes demonstrable when there is a large amount of aortic leakage with left ventricular dilation.

TREATMENT

Young patients may tolerate considerable aortic regurgitation for as long as 10 to 20 years without appreciable symptoms. Surgery needs to be considered only when symptoms appear and the volume of the left atrium and ventricle shows signs of increase. Once this increase begins, progression may be rapid and require surgical alleviation.

Patients with acute septic endocarditis present special problems. The infection preferably should be eradicated and an interval of 5 to 6 weeks allowed before operation to permit consolidation of the tissues in the aortic root. If the patient's condition does not permit this delay, earlier operation will be necessary, possibly even while the infection is active.

The principle of surgery is the same as that for aortic stenosis. The damaged valve is extirpated and a substitute implanted. Hemodynamic improvement is immediate, with disappearance of pathologic pulsations. Subsequently, there is also regression of the left ventricular dilation.

The mortality associated with elective aortic valve replacement is 3% to 4%. The figure is considerably higher when the indication is more urgent, as in septic insufficiency of the valve.

PROGNOSIS

As mentioned, most patients with slight aortic regurgitation do well without surgery. For most patients with more severe valvular incompetence, operation will sooner or later be necessary, though precise figures are difficult to obtain. When there is massive left ventricular dilation with secondary mitral regurgitation, operation should proceed without delay.

The 5-year postoperative survival rate is around 70% and 50% are living after 15 years. In a few cases (1%–3%), inadequate healing following valve implantation results in paravalvular leakage, necessitating a second operation.

TRICUSPID REGURGITATION AND STENOSIS

ETIOLOGY

Insufficiency of the tricuspid valve most often is caused by secondary dilation of the right ventricle associated with mitral stenosis. Because the valvular ring is widened, the leaflets are not opposed during systole. Congenital cardiac anomalies with right ventricular enlargement can also lead to tricuspid regurgitation. Organic changes in the leaflets as such are seldom the cause of incompetence or stenosis, and are seen most likely after rheumatic fever. Stenosis of the tricuspid valve is extremely rare and is usually seen only after rheumatic fever or with septic vegetations in drug addicts. In the former instance, it usually coexists with mitral stenosis.

PATHOPHYSIOLOGY

Defective closure of the valve permits leakage of blood from ventricle to atrium during systole. Mean atrial pressure increases and a pathologic V wave appears on the pressure curve.

SYMPTOMS

Elevated pressure in the venous system can produce swelling of the liver and peripheral edema. Cirrhosis of the liver and ascites are extreme manifestations.

DIAGNOSIS

A large systolic wave with increased filling of neck veins usually indicates the diagnosis. Examination for venous congestion should be performed with the patient reclining at a 45° angle. The murmur in tricuspid regurgitation is low-pitched and best heard toward the base of the sternum. It tends to be louder during inspiration. The diastolic murmur from tricuspid stenosis is often masked by the concomitant mitral valve stenosis.

Radiograms show right atrial enlargement, and atrial fibrillation usually is demonstrated on the electrocardiogram. Right ventricular dilation is found at echocardiography. Findings at heart catheterization include elevated mean pressure in the right atrium and a pathologic V wave of varying appearance. These findings usually are accentuated by exercise.

At angiocardiography, contrast medium leaks from the right ventricle into the right atrium. In addition, there is often regurgitation to the inferior vena cava, in which the blood flow is reversed during systole.

Tricuspid incompetence can best be assessed by perioperative palpation of the valve simply done by introducing the index finger through a small incision in the auricle of the right atrium. In significant regurgitation, the finger encounters a strong jet of blood during systole.

TREATMENT

A short period of rest and diuretic medication suffices to relieve secondary tricuspid insufficiency in many cases. Equally often, however, it is necessary to control the regurgitation surgically while treating the primary lesion or lesions. The best procedure then is anuloplasty, ie, plication of the valvular ring by strategically placed sutures. The aim then is to bring the two major leaflets, posterior and anterior, into apposition during systole. The result is checked by renewed palpation through the auricle after the heart has resumed its circulatory function.

When there are advanced organic changes of the valve, such as stenosis or scarring of the cusps, that would make anuloplasty ineffective, valve replacement becomes necessary. A tricuspid valve with septic vegetations is resected without primary valve replacement at first. At a later stage, when there is no risk of infection, valve replacement can be performed in patients cured from drug addiction.

PROGNOSIS

The underlying cause of the tricuspid incompetence determines the prognosis in most cases. When a certain stage has been reached, return to competence is not achievable, even if the pressure in the right ventricle has been reduced. In mild cases, however, regression of valvular failure can be anticipated when right ventricular pressure decreases.

COMBINED VALVULAR LESIONS

Rheumatic fever often attacks more than one cardiac valve. Combined aortic-mitral and mitral-tricuspid valve lesions are common. One problem is that the hemodynamic changes produced by one of the lesions readily lead to underestimation of the concomitant pathologic condition. An example is mitral stenosis occurring together with aortic stenosis. Because of diminished stroke volume due to mitral narrowing, the severity of the aortic obstruction may not be apparent. Also difficult to evaluate is the combination of aortic regurgitation and mitral stenosis, because the diastolic murmur produced by the aortic leak may easily mask the murmur caused by the mitral narrowing. Only by careful preoperative investigation under the guidance of an experienced cardiologist can the various components of such complex cardiac disorders be correctly evaluated.

Exceptionally there may be organic changes at all three valve sites, aortic, mitral, and tricuspid. Triple valve replacement may then be necessary to improve the patient's condition. Even after such extensive and apparently drastic operations, however, a good long-term result may be obtained.

CHOICE OF SUBSTITUTE VALVE

Valves used for replacement fall into two main categories: biologic and mechanical. Both have advantages and disadvantages that can make the choice between them difficult. The main disadvantage of mechanical valves is their association with thromboembolism. Deposits of fibrin and platelets, mainly on the metal surfaces, may be flung off as emboli or enlarge to thrombi that can impair the function of the valve. Patients therefore must receive life-long and carefully monitored anticoagulant therapy. Anticoagulation reduces the risk of embolism from 10% to less than 1% when the valve is in the aortic position, and from 25% to between 2% and 5% when the valve is in the mitral position.

BIOLOGIC VALVE SUBSTITUTES

Numerous tissues have been tested for use in valve replacement including homografts, autologous fascia lata, and xenografts of porcine aorta, dura mater, and calf pericardium. Mimicking of normal aortic valves was usually attempted by forming three pocket-shaped cusps on a plastic or steel frame. Outside of the orifice ring is a suture ring resembling that in mechanical prostheses. To denature the protein in the valve substance and to increase its stability, the tissue generally is fixed in glutaraldehyde, which also has some sterilizing effect.

Approximately ten different types of valvular bioprostheses are commercially available. They are all made of xenogenic biologic tissues preserved in buffered glutaraldehyde of which the concentration is almost identical, varying from 0.2% to 0.8%. The additional use of formalin in solution storage is intended to improve the sterility of the biologic tissues. Differences among the various valves include the type of tissues (porcine valve or bovine pericardium), the stent design, and the method of mounting.

Valve bioprosthesis was introduced in clinical practice in 1971 by Alain Carpentier of Paris. The principal disadvantage of biologic valve substitutes is their relatively limited durability. The mechanical stress is excessive in a small proportion of these valves, which then rupture after a short time. Calcification of many valves will necessitate valve replacement after 6 to 8 years. The incidence of infection is somewhat higher with biologic than with mechanical valves. The great advantage of tissue valves is that the patients as a rule do not require maintenance anticoagulation.

Tissue valves are not totally free from thromboembolic complications. During the first 3 months after surgery the risk of thromboembolism is similar to that with mechanical valves because the synthetic material of the valve is exposed to blood before fibrin covering occurs. Therefore, anticoagulants should systematically be given for 3 months to patients with a bioprosthesis. However, many surgeons prefer to continue anticoagulation in patients with poor myocardial function, calcified or thrombosed left atrium, and atrial fibrillation. Neither do tissue valves tend to produce disturbing murmurs.

Because of rapid calcification of the biologic valves in growing children, their use is contraindicated in young people below the age of 20. As biologic valves can be used without anticoagulants, they are preferred in young women planning to have children, in patients in whom for some reason anticoagulation treatment cannot adequately be continued throughout their lifetime, and in some elderly patients.

MECHANICAL HEART VALVES

More than 30 years ago, Hufnagel and Harvey[1] showed that an acrylic caged ball valve prosthesis could be tolerated in the bloodstream and function satisfactorily in the descending aorta in many patients for up to 18 years. About the same time, Robicsek[2] demonstrated the feasibility of allograft replacement of one tricuspid leaflet in a series of 16 surviving dogs.

For more than 20 years, direct replacement of malfunctioning mitral and aortic valves has been accomplished and is now an accepted routine procedure. Many developments in design and manufacture of artificial heart valves have been considered, but few of these designs have survived the 10-year clinical time test. Therefore, only those mechanical valves still most commonly in clinical use, with which I have had personal experience, will be discussed.

PRINCIPAL MECHANICAL VALVE DESIGNS

THREE PLIABLE LEAFLET VALVES

The first artificial heart valve design I used clinically was made of Teflon® and copied the natural aortic valves. The three leaflets were individually sutured in place (Bahnson) or as a prepared unit in a Teflon cage (Muller), replacing the aortic valves. Within 1 to 1½ years, these Teflon leaflets were covered with a fibrin envelope containing a great amount of calcium causing tissue fatigue with rupture, usually at the center of the cusp (Figure 32.2, top). A trial to prevent calcium deposits and tissue ingrowth by covering a Teflon mesh with silicone still resulted in cusp rupture within 1 year (Hufnagel). To use the natural three-leaflet valve design, it is necessary for researchers in the field of polymer science first to develop a genuinely biocompatible man-made flexible membrane of adequate strength to withstand 40 million cycles a year. No three-leaflet artificial valve design is currently in clinical use. Similar complications are found in biologic valves after longer observation (Figure 32.2, bottom).

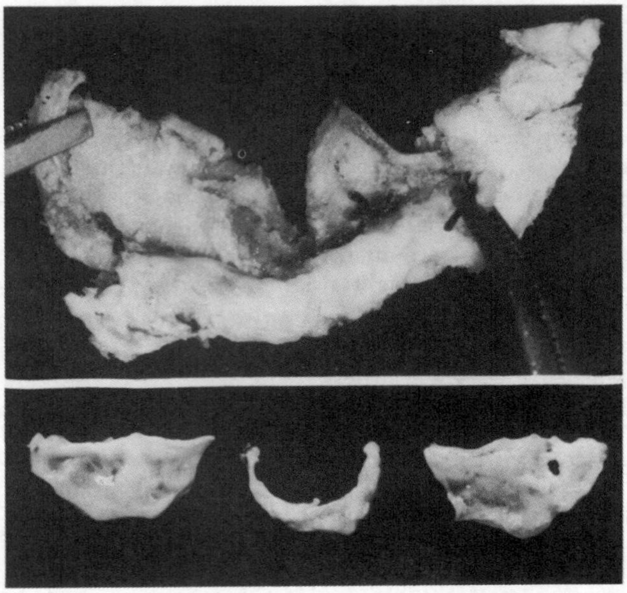

Figure 32.2. *Top*, Explanted Teflon aortic valve leaflet that ruptured after 1 year; it is covered with a fibrin envelope with a calcium deposit. *Bottom*, Isolated aortic leaflet (in the middle) made of the patient's own fascia lata explanted after 4½ years because of shrinkage with insufficiency.

CENTRAL OCCLUDING POPPET VALVES

Ball Valves

Harken et al[3] were the first to insert a caged ball valve into the aortic orifice. Starr et al[4] in 1960 developed the ball valve further, incorporating a sewing ring and simplifying the cage, using this prosthesis first for mitral valve replacement and then for aortic valve replacement (Figure 32.3). The overall design of this valve with a silicone poppet has not been changed over the years and is still in use in some centers. This Starr-Edwards ball valve design uses an overlapping closing mechanism, as the ball occluder hits the valve ring on closure. In contrast to this design, the non-overlapping Smeloff-Cutter valve has a ball slightly smaller than the orifice. A subcage on the proximal side of the valve retains the ball in the closed position with its equator in the plane of the sewing ring. A small clearance around the ball ensures easy passage of the ball into the orifice, giving rise to mild regurgitation which was thought to diminish the risk of thrombus formation. The Smeloff-Cutter valve is still in use. The Magovern valve is a standard ball and cage valve that incorporates two rows of interlocking mechanical teeth around the orifice ring activated by removing a special valve holder once the valve is located correctly during insertion. This valve is no longer in use because of the hazard of dislocation by imperfect placement or calcification. In my series of 120 patients in whom the Starr-Edwards ball valve was used, careful follow-up with repeat transseptal heart catheterization at rest and during exercise was performed in 46 cases.[5] Residual obstruction, with gradients of 50 to 70 mm Hg, was found in patients

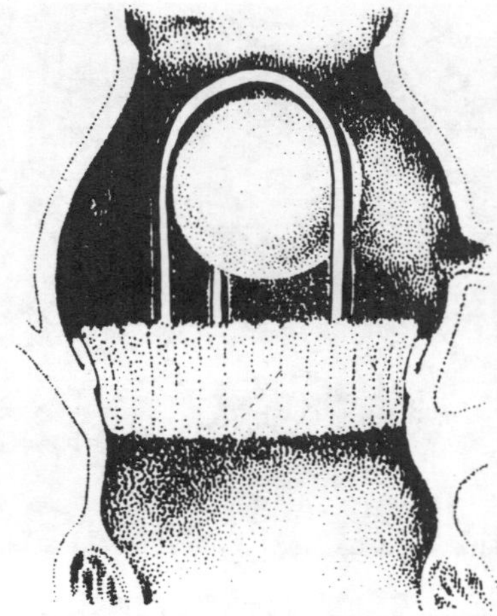

Figure 32.3. The Starr-Edwards ball valve showed too high a residual obstruction at transseptal heart catheterization at rest and during exercise, especially in patients with a narrow aortic root.

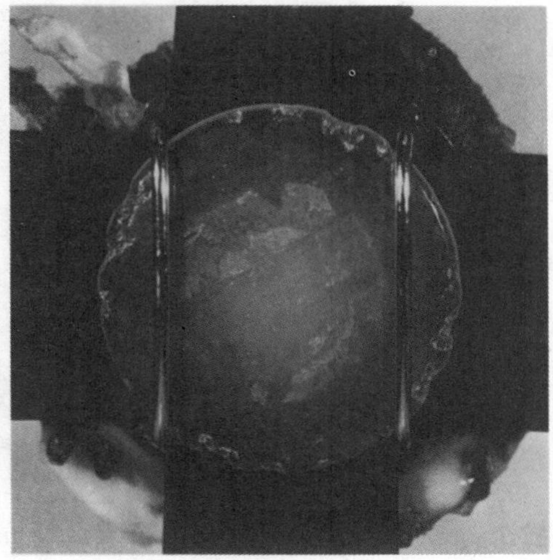

Figure 32.5. Explanted Kay-Shiley disk valve after 12 years demonstrates good function but has grooves in the edges of the disk.

with a narrow aortic root, necessitating a search for an improvement in valve design. After mitral valve replacement for mitral stenosis with a small left ventricle, the ball valve caused outflow obstruction and impinged on the interventricular septum, sometimes giving rise to arrhythmia (Figure 32.4).

Caged Disk Valves

Using a flat disk as occluder permitted considerable height reduction of the cage as in the Beall, Starr-Edwards, and Kay-Shiley valves.[6] This was considered important in mitral valve replacement, especially in patients with a small left ventricle. In a personal series of 88 patients with Kay-Shiley aortic valve replacement, we noted the same high transvalvular pressure gradients as with the ball valves. Subsequently, I do not recommend caged disk valves. The quality of Kay-Shiley disks was very good with only edge notching, but perfect function, when explanted after 12 years (Figure 32.5).

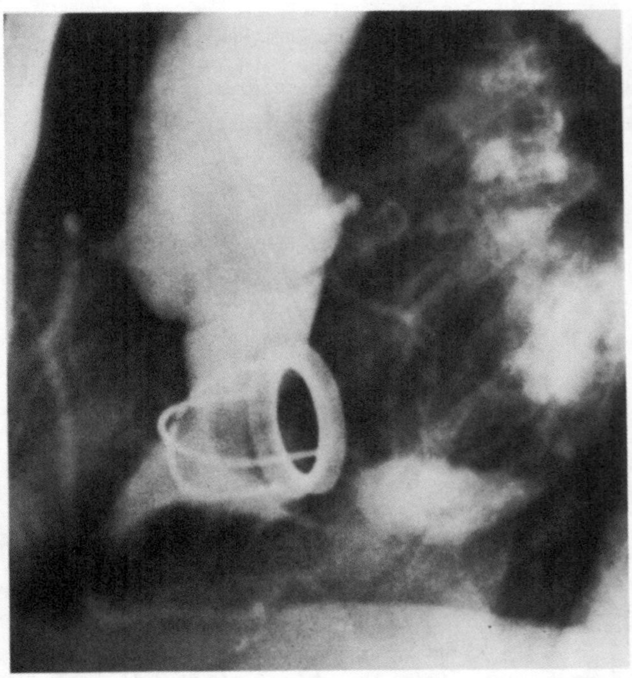

Figure 32.4. In patients with mitral stenosis and a small left ventricle, the Starr-Edwards ball valve caused left ventricular outflow obstruction and arrhythmia as the cage impinged on the interventricular septum.

TILTING DISK VALVES

In vitro tests show that after aortic valve replacement, the high pressure gradient could significantly be diminished by permitting the disk to tilt open. A limited clinical trial with a Wada valve[7] with a hinged Teflon disk confirmed the concept and the gradient diminished nearly 50% in comparison with that of the central occluding valves (Figure 32.6). However, these same clinical trials demonstrated that in principle the hinge itself was the weak area. Subsequent investigations indicated that all wear was concentrated in the hinge area (Figure 32.7); as a result, the disk soon malfunctioned with embolization. This dysfunction occurred in all valves, sooner in the larger valves. Therefore, it became obvious that a hinge design should be avoided, as a low flow area was pro-

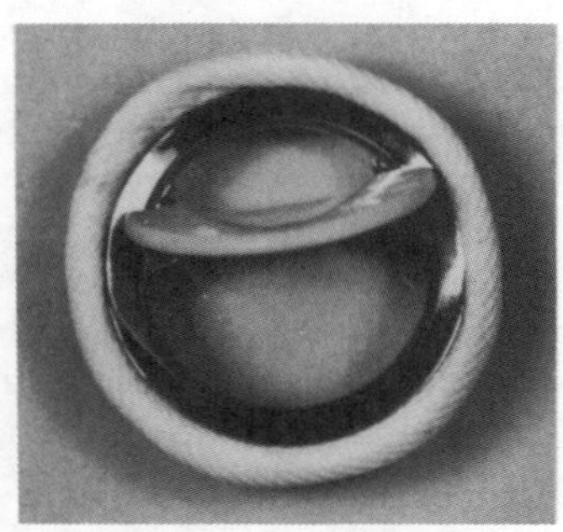

Figure 32.6. The Wada valve with hinged Teflon disk, which tilted open, diminished the gradient nearly 50% in comparison with the central occluding valves.

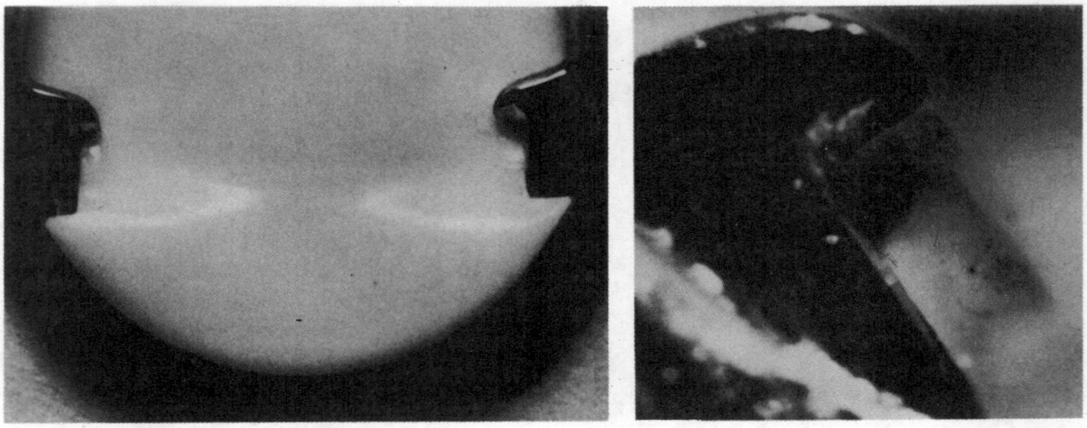

Figure 32.7. *Left*, The wear was concentrated in the hinge area, causing malfunction and disk embolization of the Wada valve. *Right*, Close-up of the hinge area deformation through wear.

duced behind the hinge that was very sensitive to wear and thrombosis. In cooperation with Shiley, a free-floating tilting disk valve was developed in 1968. After comparing the Shiley valve with other valves in pulse duplicator studies, I accepted the valve for clinical use on January 16, 1969.[8] The first disks were made of Delrin® (Dupont), which has a seven times greater resistance to wear than Teflon. As the disk rotated and was free floating, the wear was well distributed, and studies of valves explanted after 12 years suggest a durability of approximately 30 years. The first 140 aortic valve replacements showed a 55% 15-year actual survival, not including a 6.6% operative mortality. Another tilting disk valve, later in clinical use, was the Lillehei-Kaster valve. The disk in this valve overlapped the valve cage, effecting greater hemolysis and a higher gradient; as the internal diameter was 2 mm smaller for the same outer diameter as the Björk-Shiley valve, it therefore is no longer recommended. The Hall-Kaster valve is a relatively new tilting disk valve, whereby the disk is guided by an arm through a central hole in the disk. This valve, currently used under the name Medtronic-Hall, has an acceptable gradient and good durability, and hemolysis is reported to be slight but consistent. Another new valve, the Omniscience tilting disk valve, is not widely accepted because of the reportedly high thromboembolic complication rate.

BILEAFLET VALVES

The St. Jude valve design incorporates two semicircular hinged pyrolytic carbon occluders in a pyrolytic carbon ring.[9] This valve also has a low gradient and is viewed with optimism, but its long-term durability remains to be proven as clinical experience exceeds 5 years in only a minority of patients. The two pairs of hinges make this valve sensitive to trauma and thrombosis, with nonsynchronous leaflet movement or leaflet embolization already reported in five cases.[10] Current studies indicate this valve will need lifetime anticoagulation therapy as do all other mechanical valves.

THE OPTIMUM TILTING DISK VALVE

During 17 years[1] experience with more than 4,000 valve replacements with the Björk-Shiley tilting disk valve, the same principal design has been retained with a stepwise improvement regarding (1) hemodynamics, (2) thromboembolic complications, and (3) durability. These different factors have been optimized and combined into the monostrut valve, which is considered the next generation of the Björk-Shiley valve.

OPTIMAL HEMODYNAMICS

To obtain optimal valve function, the following applies: (1) The disk opening angle at 70° gives so low a gradient that little will be gained by a further increase in the disk opening angle (Figure 32.8). At an angle greater than 70°, the increased pulsatile regurgitation will constitute a greater functional loss than that gained by slightly decreasing the gradient[11] (Figure 32.9).

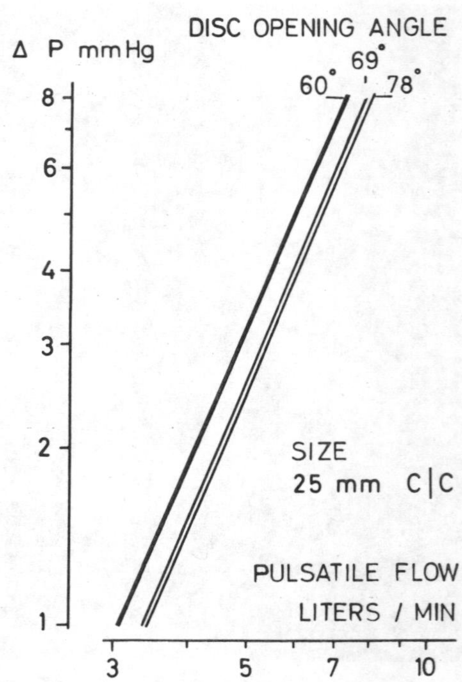

Figure 32.8. The optimal opening angle of the Björk-Shiley (BS) tilting disk valve was 70°, and little was gained by a larger opening angle.

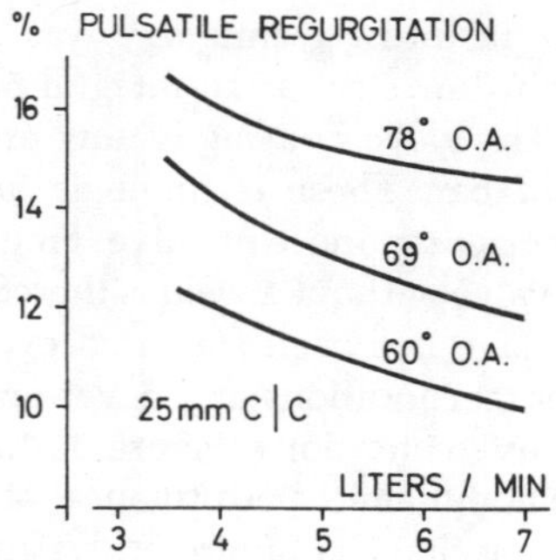

Figure 32.9. Pulsatile regurgitation at a 78° opening angle (OA) increased more than the amount gained by further decreasing the transvalvular gradient.

(2) The convexo-concave shape of the disk and cage design, permitting the disk to come out 2.5 mm from the valve ring in the open position, will in itself diminish the gradient 15% (Figures 32.10 and 32.11).[12] A further 10% decrease in the transvalvular gradient was obtained by employing the Björk-Shiley monostrut valve with a 70° opening angle (Figures 32.8, 32.10, and 32.11), as there is no vortex formation behind the smaller opening.[13]

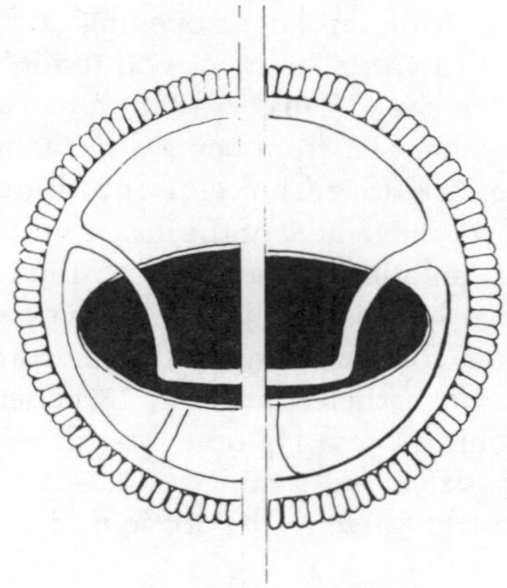

Figure 32.11. Diagram of the 70° Björk-Shiley monostrut (*right*) having one arm of the outflow strut as well as one partition of the opening less than the 60° convexo-concave valve (*left*).

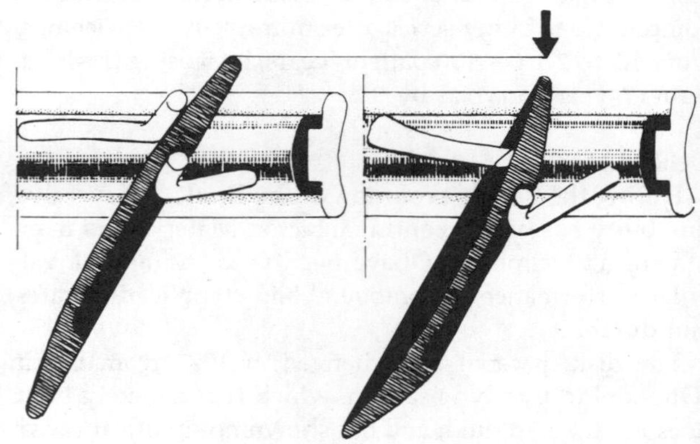

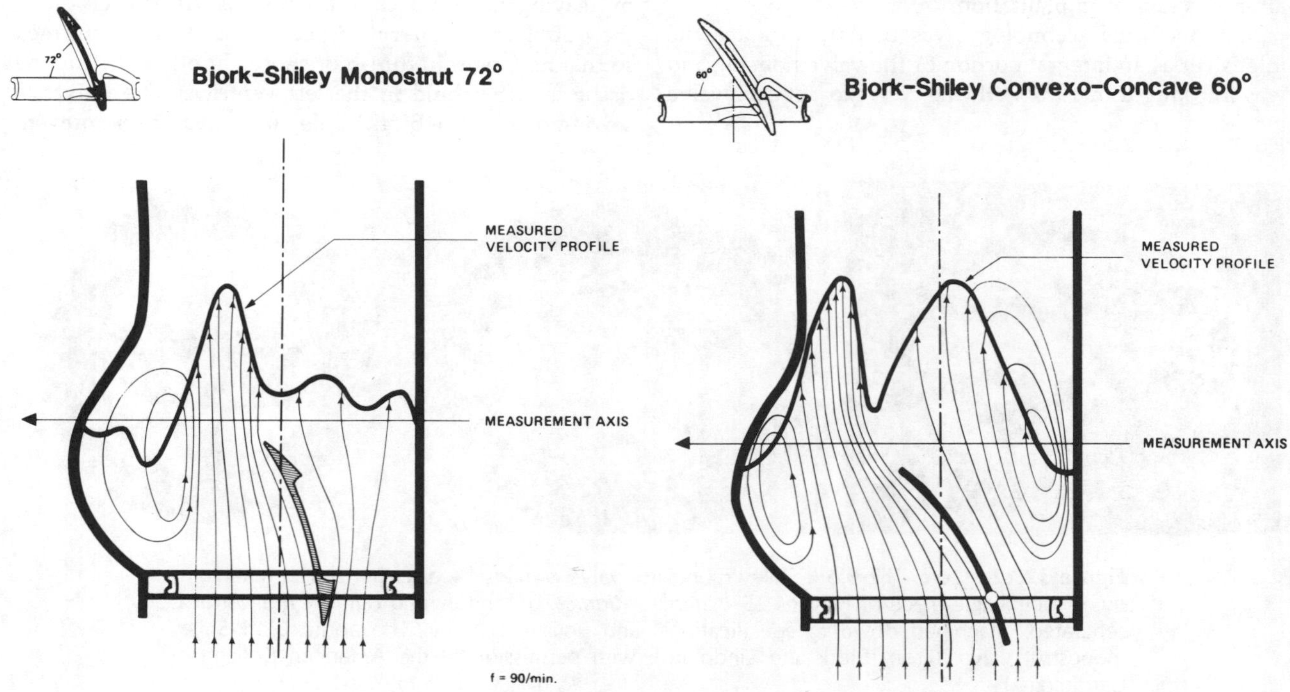

Figure 32.10. *Top*, The convexo-concave (CC) shape of the disk (*arrow*) permitted the disk to slide out 2.5 mm from the valve ring in the open position. To the left is the standard or flat disk. *Bottom*, Diagram of the 70° Björk-Shiley monostrut valve (*left*) giving less vortex formation behind the smaller opening in comparison with the 60° convexo-concave valve (*right*). (From Björk and Lindblom[22] with permission of the American College of Cardiology.)

(3) Orientation of the larger opening away from the aorta in mitral valve replacement will diminish the gradient during exercise.[14] This orientation will also prevent an aortic regurgitant jet from being directed into the left atrium by the disk. (See Choice of Substitute Valve.)

Naturally, free movement of the disk is most important, and optimal orientation in the aortic position is obtained when the large hole is against the convex wall of the ascending aorta, corresponding to the noncoronary cusp. Transseptal heart catheterization in 17 patients showed gradients of only 11 mm Hg or a 1.4-cm^2 effective area in the 21-mm valve and 9 mm in a 2.0-cm^2 area in the 23-mm monostrut valve in the aortic position.[15]

THROMBOEMBOLIC COMPLICATIONS

As the edge of the straight disk in the open position touched the valve ring, a downstream low flow area was created at that point. In this area, thrombosis tended to begin when anticoagulation therapy was not effective. To avoid this problem, the convexo-concave disk was introduced, which in the open position moves out from the valve ring approximately 2.5 mm, creating a space between the disk edge and the valve ring. Thus, the low flow area behind the disk was diminished by 50% corresponding to a simultaneous decrease in thromboembolic complications in my series after mitral valve replacement from 4.1 to 2.1 per 100 patient-years, increasing the long-term (7-year) survival by 9%.[16–18]

DURABILITY

During the design evolution of the Björk-Shiley valve, durability has been a continual factor. Material and manufacturing technologies have been used to improve valvular performance, thromboembolic complication rates, and durability.

The disk material was changed in 1971 from Delrin (Dupont) to pyrolytic carbon, which is completely inert, does not take up fluid, and has shown no significant wear after 13 years of implantation.[19, 20]

Manufacturing technology was used to produce the inlet strut as an integral portion of the valve housing and was introduced in 1977 with the convexo-concave valve model.

In 1982, manufacturing technology was successful in producing the outflow strut as an integral portion of the valve housing. The valve housing is now produced from a single piece of bar. These technologic improvements resulted in the current monostrut valve (Figure 32.12).[21,22] The monostrut valve without a weld is therefore so strong that the struts have not been fractured even under extreme experimental conditions and never under maximal physiologic loading conditions (Figure 32.13).

Excellent hemodynamic performance at recatheterization[22] and no mechanical failure or dysfunction of this Björk-Shiley monostrut valve have been experienced during a 4-year period with more than 900 cases in Stockholm.

COMPLICATIONS OF VALVE REPLACEMENT

MECHANICAL VALVE DYSFUNCTION

Some of the reported dysfunctions of mechanical valves can be avoided by the surgeon with experience; other dysfunctions can only be avoided by further design development.

Obstruction of the Poppet Movement

A few of the ball valves underwent degenerative changes with the passage of time. The so-called "ball variance" could cause grooving or cracking of the ball, which could be obstructed when the crack slipped into an arm of the cage. Subsequently, regurgitation with hemolysis and hemolytic anemia occurred.

All tilting disk valves need a careful implantation technique, because they are sensitive to obstruction of the disk movement. If, in the aortic area, a suture is cut too long and is being caught between the disk and the valve ring, the disk movement is obstructed. Immediate reexploration cutting the suture short is the only way to restore function.

In the mitral area, disk obstruction is usually caused by leaving behind a chorda tendinea. After excision of the mitral valve, careful inspection has to be performed so that no long thin thread or chorda or other obstructing tissue is left behind in the left ventricle. The universal sewing ring on the Björk-Shiley mitral valve will prevent

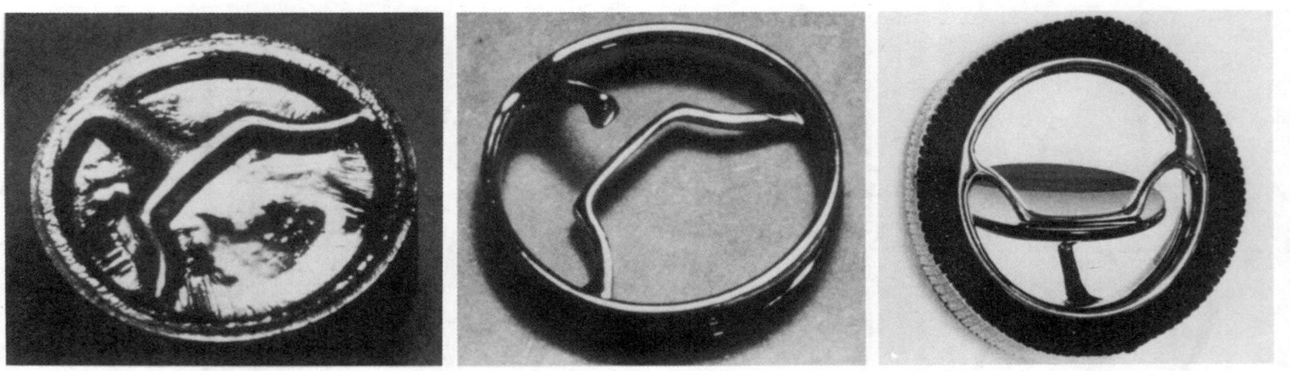

Figure 32.12. *Left*, The Björk-Shiley monostrut valve is made by electrochemical machining out of one single piece of Haynes 25 material. *Middle*, The inflow and outflow monostrut is separated, machined down to specifications, and polished. *Right*, The aortic Björk-Shiley monostrut valve. (From Björk and Lindblom[22] with permission of the American College of Cardiology.)

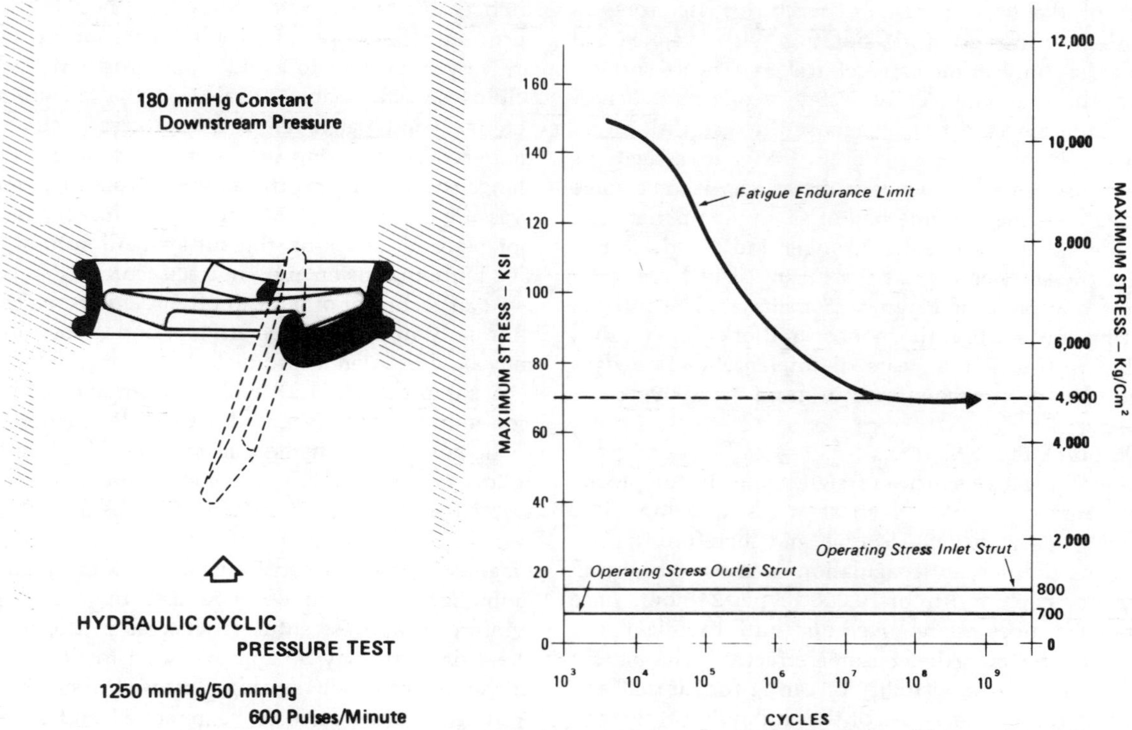

Figure 32.13. *Left*, The Björk-Shiley monostrut hydraulic fatigue test. The monostrut valve operates 1250 mm Hg at 600 pulses per minute without failure. *Right*, The fatigue endurance limit of the Björk-Shiley monostrut valve is ten times higher than the operating stress under normal physiologic conditions. (From Björk and Lindblom[22] with permission of the American College of Cardiology.)

any suture from coming close to the disk. The valvular rim is placed between the two flanges of the sewing ring so that the sutures are completely covered by the atrial flange of the sewing ring. Furthermore, the lower or ventricular sewing ring will act as a muscle guard to prevent tissue ingrowth or to keep ventricular muscle from coming too close to the moving disk, if the left ventricle is diminishing in size over the years (Figure 32.14). A supraanular suture ring is, however, easier to use. Before closing the left atrium the surgeon must convince himself about the free movement of the disk and, if at all possible, rotate the valve with the valve holder so that the large opening of the Björk-Shiley valve is away from the aortic orifice, in a posterior to inferior orientation, wherever the space for the disk seems best. An anterior orientation of the large hole in the mitral position will cause extra regurgitation into the left atrium if there is aortic insufficiency and will increase the transvalvular gradient on exercise because of the inward movement of the upper portion of the interventricular septum during diastole.

Escape of the Poppet

In ball valves, wear of the ball or ball variance has been the cause of escape of the ball in Starr-Edwards and Braunwald-Cutter ball valves. Wear of the cage has been the cause of ball escape in the DeBakey ball valve. Wear of the disk caused escape of the disk in the caged disk valves of Beall and Cross-Jones.

Among the tilting disk valves, wear of the disk caused its escape in the Wada valves, whereas T fracture of the welded outflow strut in earlier Björk-Shiley valves caused the disk to escape. Among the hinged bileaflet St. Jude valves, escape of one of the two leaflets has already been reported in five cases and is probably due to wear of the hinge.[10]

Most valves having mechanical dysfunction have disappeared from the market. However, there is no way to

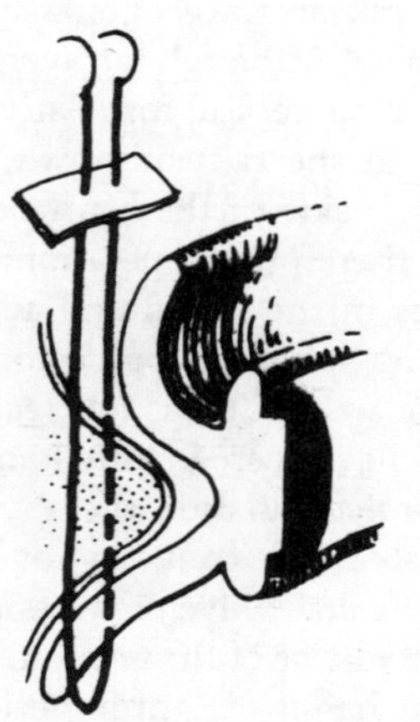

Figure 32.14. Diagram of the universal sewing ring whereby the upper flange will cover the sutures, preventing them from coming too close to the disk. The lower sewing ring on the ventricular side of the valvular rim acts as a muscle guard and prevents tissue ingrowth or sticking to the left ventricular wall as the heart diminishes in size during the years after the operation.

predict or diagnose a pending fracture. Therefore, in the patient with sudden deterioration with dyspnea and tachycardia, only immediate referral to a heart surgical unit can be lifesaving. Only a stethoscope and a chest x-ray film are necessary to diagnose the disk dislocation or outflow strut fracture, or both. Other investigations are a waste of crucial time as reoperation with exchange of the valve is the only method of saving the patient. To make the valve consistently stronger and avoid a weld, the outflow strut as well as the inflow strut have to be made of one piece of Haynes 25 material. The integral valve ring now exists as the monostrut Björk-Shiley valve, and during the first 4 years of implantation, no dysfunction has been encountered in more than 900 cases.

THROMBOEMBOLISM

All mechanical valves are foreign bodies in the bloodstream causing turbulence, shear stress, and low flow areas with a tendency to clotting, and therefore the patient needs lifetime anticoagulation therapy. I begin an intravenous heparin drip of 20,000 IU per 24 hours once the drainage tubes are removed and until the dicumarol or warfarin treatment has become effective. The patient should have the responsibility of caring for himself and learning to follow the values of the thrombotest, thereby helping the physician to carry on a well-conducted anticoagulation program. Thromboembolic complications are usually more frequent: 2.1 per 100 patient-years after mitral valve replacement and 1.1 per 100 patient-years after aortic valve replacement. The common occurrence of chronic atrial fibrillation is another contributing factor to the increased rate of thromboembolic complications after mitral valve replacement.

THE CLOTTED PROSTHESIS

The incorporation of a radioopaque tantalum ring marker in the disk has helped to diagnose restricted disk motion under noninvasive examination such as cineradiography or fluoroscopy. The symptoms are those of a partially obstructed valve orifice, and it is important for the attending physician to recognize and treat this condition without delay. Although intravenous streptokinase treatment has been successful for relatively recent thrombosis of a valve in the tricuspid area, it is not recommended on the left side of the heart because of the risk of embolization; therefore, reoperation is required for all clotted prostheses in the mitral and aortic area with re-replacement of the valve. Thrombectomy may be sufficient in the aortic area, but it is not recommended in the mitral position. I have seen a clotted aortic valve only in cases in which anticoagulation therapy was not used or suddenly terminated. The convexo-concave design of the Björk-Shiley tilting disk valve prosthesis has significantly diminished the incidence of thromboembolic episodes and in my experience has made thrombotic obstruction extremely rare.

PARAPROSTHETIC LEAKAGE

Prosthetic valve fixation takes approximately half a year until tissue ingrowth in the suturing is complete. During this time, the valve is dependent on the suture fixation. Therefore, multiple point fixation of the prosthetic valve by means of interrupted nonabsorbable sutures and the prophylactic administration of antibiotics are very important to avoid a paraprosthetic leak. If the anulus is weak, friable, or calcified, the calcium has to be removed and patch-reinforced sutures used. With the universal sewing ring in the mitral position, the lower flange is placed below the anulus so that high ventricular pressure will press the suture ring against the anulus and not place all stress on the sutures. All sutures must be tied without tension and knotted securely. Paraprosthetic leaks of technical origin can often be detected by a murmur early in the postoperative period. Subsequent leaks may be due to endocarditis.

A paraprosthetic leak will cause an audible regurgitation murmur, and increased red cell destruction will lead to hemolysis and hemolytic anemia. Heart failure will follow if the leak is of hemodynamic significance. Increased serum lactic dehydrogenase, as a sign of hemolysis, is a significant indication for reoperation, but the diagnosis should be confirmed by angiocardiographic examination. Repair can often be made by a series of patch-reinforced mattress sutures, whereas in the mitral area, the atrial wall may be approximated to the atrial flange of the universal sewing ring. Diseased tissue and abscess walls sometimes have to be removed and a new valve inserted. If endocarditis is present, one should be prepared to repeat the operation several times.

ENDOCARDITIS

Postoperative endocarditis is a serious, sometimes fatal complication. The prosthesis is a foreign body in the bloodstream and is therefore sensitive to infection; at most centers, it is reported to be 2% or less, independent of which valve substitute is used. For optimal antibiotic treatment, it is important to identify the infecting organism as soon as possible by blood cultures. If antibiotic treatment in septic doses for 6 weeks is not effective, reoperation may be necessary to excise necrotic tissue and insert a new valve, accepting a high mortality.

HEMOLYSIS

With the nonoverlapping disk in the Björk-Shiley tilting disk valve, the serum lactic dehydrogenase level as the most sensitive sign of hemolysis will usually be within the normal range or slightly above the upper limit after single and double valve replacement. As the disk will close with significant impact 40 million times a year, the design of the disk hitting as small an area as possible is favorable in the long run. Any increased hemolysis will indicate some malfunction such as a paravalvular leak or an obstruction that has to be investigated.

RUPTURE OF THE LEFT VENTRICLE

A rare, but often fatal complication after mitral valve replacement is rupture of the posterior wall of the left ventricle (Figure 32.15). If rupture occurs before the chest is closed, most patients can be saved. Extracorporeal circulation must be instituted as rapidly as possible so that repair can be performed on the relaxed left ventricle (Figure 32.16).

To prevent this most severe complication, the following technical points should be observed:

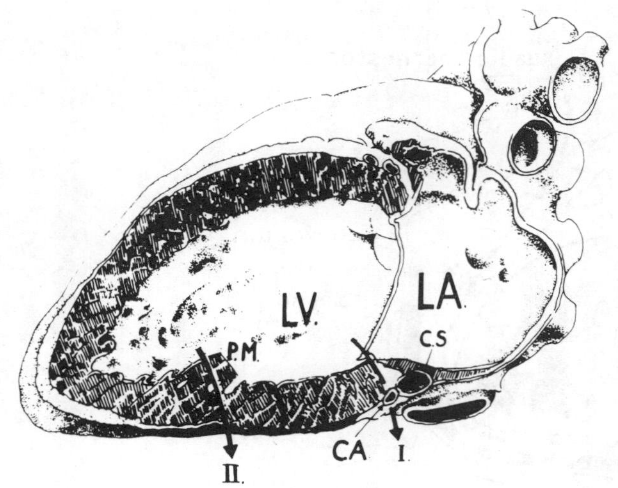

Figure 32.15. Left ventricular (LV) rupture after mitral valve replacement may occur in the atrioventricular plane (I) or half way down the posterior left ventricular wall (II). CA = coronary artery; CS = coronary sinus; LA = left atrium; PM = papillary muscle.

In the relaxed heart during cardioplegia, the papillary muscles should not be tilted up too high when divided, to avoid creating a thin area half way down on the posterior wall which may rupture.

To avoid rupture in the posterior atrioventricular groove, the following are recommended:

- The removal of calcium should not be too radical through the anulus.
- The prosthetic valve should not be too large for the anulus. Measurement of the anulus during cardioplegia may indicate too large a size. When in doubt, use the next smaller valve, because there is no reason from a hemodynamic point of view to use the larger valve in the mitral orifice.

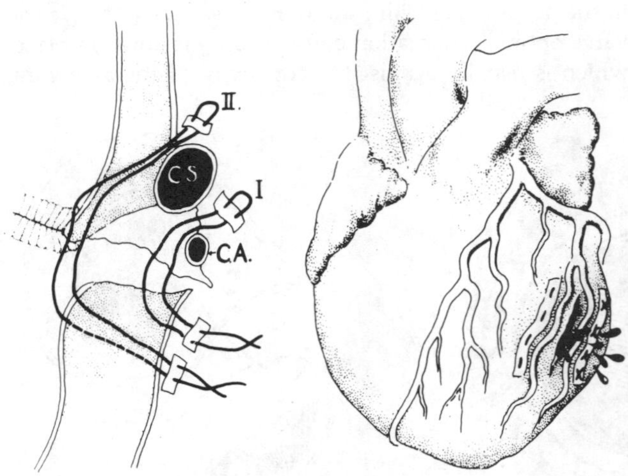

Figure 32.16. *Left*, After immediate institution of extracorporeal circulation, repair can be performed on the flaccid heart with patched sutures, including the sewing ring and avoiding the circumflex coronary artery (CA) and coronary sinus (CS). *Right*, In the posterior left ventricular wall, it may be difficult to avoid inclusion of some circumflex coronary artery branches during repair.

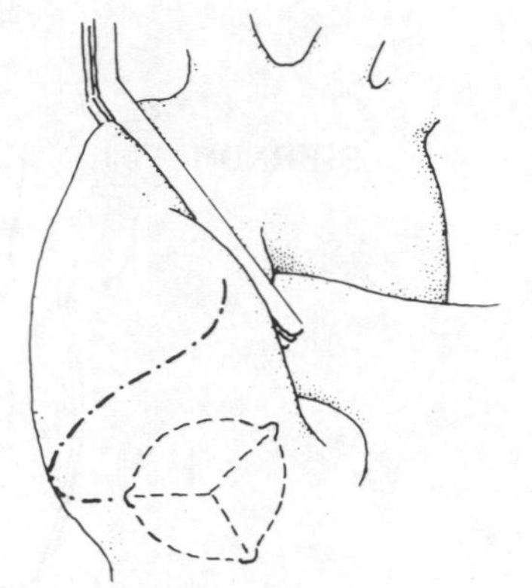

Figure 32.17. The aorta is opened by an oblique incision ending above the commissure between the left and the noncoronary cusp.

- Never drain the apex of the left ventricle.
- Never lift up the left ventricle after the mitral valve is sutured in place; so doing may cause rupture in the atrioventricular groove.

THE OPERATION

Practically all valvular surgery is performed through a median sternotomy incision with extracorporeal circulation using hemodilution and perfusion hypothermia between 25° and 30°C. The ascending aorta and the right atrium are cannulated.

Aortic Valve Replacement

For aortic valve replacement, a single venous cannula draining both the inferior vena cava and the right atrium inserted through the atrial appendix is used. First, a brief period of cooling perfusion is used. If the heart fibrillates and there is pure aortic stenosis, cold potassium cardioplegic solution is given in the aortic root. If there is aortic insufficiency or the heart does not fibrillate, it can be electrically fibrillated; the aorta can be cross-clamped and then opened through an oblique incision, ending above the commissure between the left and the noncoronary cusp (Figure 32.17). Cardioplegia is then achieved by selectively perfusing first the left and then the right coronary artery. In aortic valvular disease it is most important to cool the hypertrophic left ventricle; therefore, most of the solution is given in the left coronary artery. However, cardioplegia must also be achieved in the right coronary artery to diminish postperfusion arrhythmia. The myocardial temperature should be decreased to between 10° and 15°C and kept well below 20°C throughout the procedure. An isolation pad behind the heart and local cooling will help keep the myocardial temperature down (Figure 32.18).

A stenosed aortic valve can be removed in one piece starting in the noncoronary cusp. When the valves are heavily calcified, blunt dissection is used to separate the calcium from the sinus wall and to reach the valvular base, especially in the area of the commissures. Time must be taken to remove all calcium, piece by piece, with blunt neurosurgical dissectors or other suitable instruments to prevent the calcium pieces from falling into the ventricular cavity.

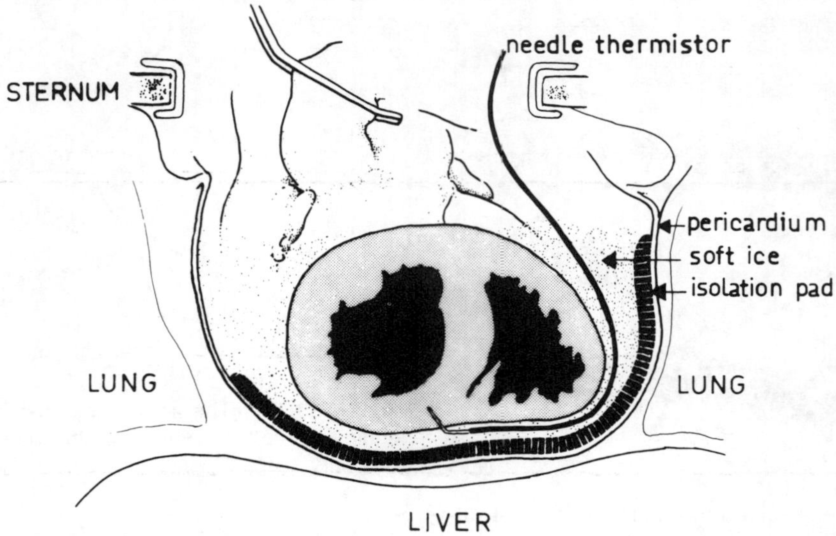

Figure 32.18. An isolation pad behind the heart and local cooling with soft ice will help to keep the myocardial temperature down.

The tissue anulus is then measured with sizers, accepting the valve corresponding to the largest possible sizer that can pass down into the ventricle. I have never used an aortic valve smaller than 21 mm. If the 21-mm valve seems too big in an adult patient, it is easy to enlarge the aortic incision with an outflow patch. In children, much greater enlargement can be achieved with the Konno procedure, so that a 21- or 23-mm valve can be introduced. The 21-mm monostrut valve gives a gradient of only 11 mm Hg and an area of 1.4 cm^2, and the 23-mm valve has a gradient of 9 mm Hg corresponding to an effective area of 2.0 cm^2.

The valve is first dipped into a solution of heparin and penicillin to prevent infection and is then placed on the valve holder and subsequently rotated ten times in each direction so that it rotates easily. This practice will facilitate the exact orientation of the valve, if it becomes necessary to rotate the valve in situ after it has been implanted. If, during rotation, the process still feels difficult, the sewing ring should be kept stationary with a clamp to prevent the sutures from cutting through. Only the valve holder should be used to rotate the valve, as any other instrument may damage the valve and change the disk to strut clearance with the risk of disk embolization.

In patients with narrow aortic roots, I usually use about 30 isolated over-and-over 2–0 Ti-cron sutures to prevent constriction of the anulus and get the largest possible valve in place (Figure 32.19, left and middle). If the orifice is wide and the tissue of the anulus is weak or brittle, patch-reinforced mattress sutures are employed (Figure 32.19, right). The sewing ring sutures should not be placed too deep into the sewing ring to avoid the inner circular cord, which can make rotation of the valve in situ more difficult. Before placing the valve, it is again immersed in the heparin-penicillin solution. I always try to give the valve optimal orientation before sliding it down in place, which is usually against the convexity of the ascending

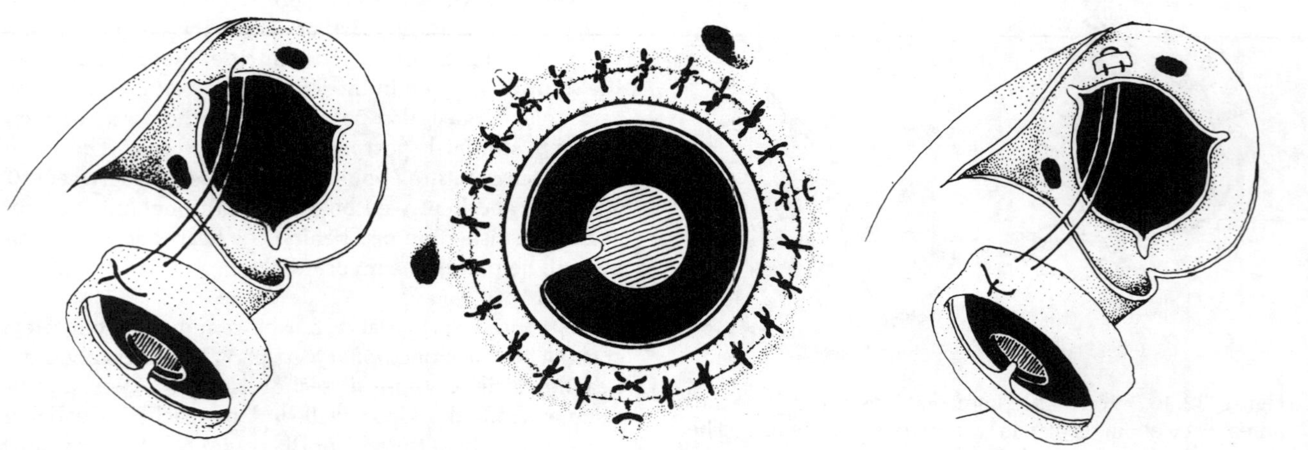

Figure 32.19. *Left*, For fixation of an aortic valve in a narrow anulus, about 30 isolated over-and-over 2-0 Ti-cron sutures are used and placed well away from the disk in the sewing ring. *Middle*, The knot is placed as far as possible from the disk and the sutures are cut short. *Right*, When the anulus tissue is weak or brittle, patch-reinforced mattress sutures are used.

aorta or toward the noncoronary sinus (Figure 32.20). I first tie the sutures corresponding to the left coronary sinus, and then to the right to be sure that the coronary ostia are not obstructed by the sewing ring. If there is difficulty in seating the valve, the suture ring can be placed on top of the noncoronary anulus.

It is important to cut the tied sutures short, to make sure they cannot be caught between the disk and the ring, and to verify that no structure can obstruct the free movement of the disk. The left ventricle can be drained by a catheter through the right superior pulmonary vein or through the aortic valve. Rewarming is started while the sutures are being tied. Air is evacuated from the heart and the ascending aorta as the aortic incision is closed with two layers of 4–0 prolene® sutures and the cross-clamp is removed during temporary reduction of bypass flow with the patient in the head down or Trendelenburg position. After about 15 minutes of reperfusion, the heart is usually ready to take over the circulation.

Mitral Valve Replacement

For mitral valve replacement, both the superior and inferior venae cavae are usually cannulated as the tricuspid valve often requires anuloplasty. I always use the double-flanged or supraanular sewing ring. Twenty isolated mattress sutures are passed, first from the ventricular side of the lower flange of the sewing ring and then through the mitral anulus from the ventricular side (Figure 32.21). If necessary, the sutures can be tied over patches on the atrial side and covered by the atrial flange. The supraanular suture ring is faster and easier to use.

The larger hole of the valve should be oriented against the posterior or inferior part of the left ventricle, away from the aortic orifice to achieve optimal function (Figure 32.22, left). In this posterior orientation, the transvalvular gradient during exercise is smaller than that in an anterior orientation. The reason is that during diastolic filling of the ventricle, the proximal septal portion moves inwards and narrows an anterior inflow but not a posterior inflow

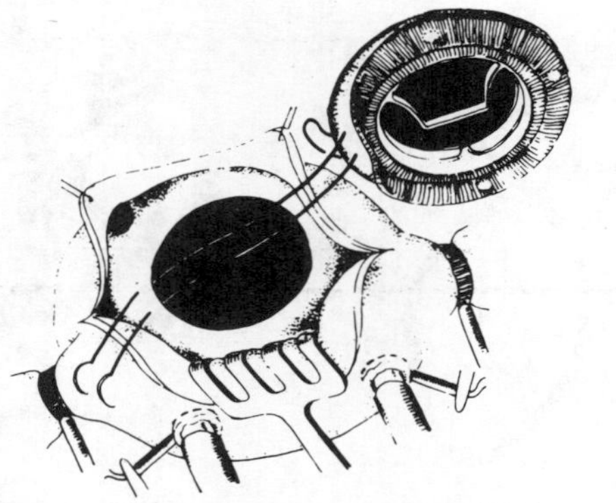

Figure 32.21. About 20 2–0 Ti-cron mattress sutures are passed from the ventricular side of the lower sewing ring and from the ventricular side of the valvular rim.

(Figure 32.22, left and middle). Furthermore, a regurgitant jet from the aortic ostium may hit the anteriorly oriented disk, be directed into the left atrium, and delay disk closure, thereby causing mitral insufficiency (Figure 32.22, right). Even if the ideal orientation is desirable, completely free mobility of the tilting disk has absolute priority.

Tricuspid Valve Replacement

Tricuspid valve replacement is seldom used, as conservative procedures are often possible. If a tilting disk valve has to be used in the tricuspid position, as sometimes in Ebstein's disease, orientation with the large hole toward the diaphragmatic surface of the right ventricle is preferred. The valve is then introduced with the same technique as that in the mitral position.

ANTICOAGULATION

A careful anticoagulation program is of great importance, and sudden interruption is often followed by thromboembolic complications and must be avoided if at all possible. At this time, all patients with mechanical heart valves need lifelong anticoagulation therapy. Serious hemorrhagic complications from this treatment are less than 1.0 per 100 patient-years in our series.

We begin anticoagulation therapy as early as possible after the operation when the chest drainage tubes are removed, usually on the second postoperative day with a continuous intravenous infusion of 20,000 IU of heparin per 24 hours until effective prothrombin depression can be achieved. The patient should wear an identity tag indicating the anticoagulation program. The dosage should be reduced to reach slightly above normal therapeutic levels before elective surgery or dental extraction. In pregnant women approaching 2 weeks before delivery, we switch to heparin, which does not cross the placental barrier to the fetus.

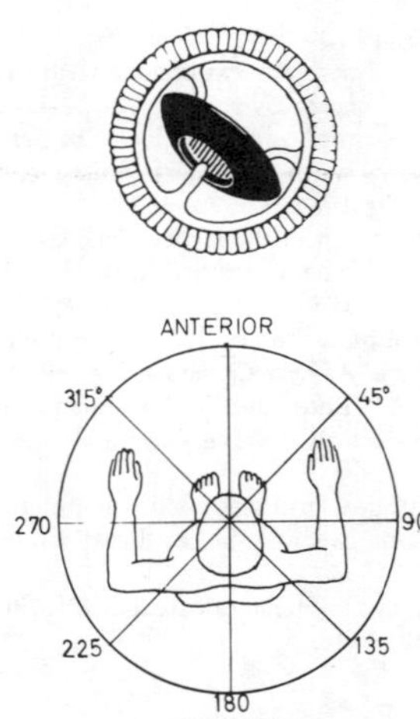

Figure 32.20. If free movement of the disk can be obtained, the large opening of the valve is oriented towards the convexity of the ascending aorta or anterior and slightly to the right. (From Björk and Lindblom[22] with permission of the American College of Cardiology.)

ANTIBIOTIC TREATMENT

We have used intravenous antibiotics in high doses the day before, during, and for three to five days after the operation with a combination of benzylpenicillin and cloxacillin to be followed by oral benzylpenicillin for 3 months. We added the prolonged oral treatment to prevent late endocarditis with paravalvular leakage. For den-

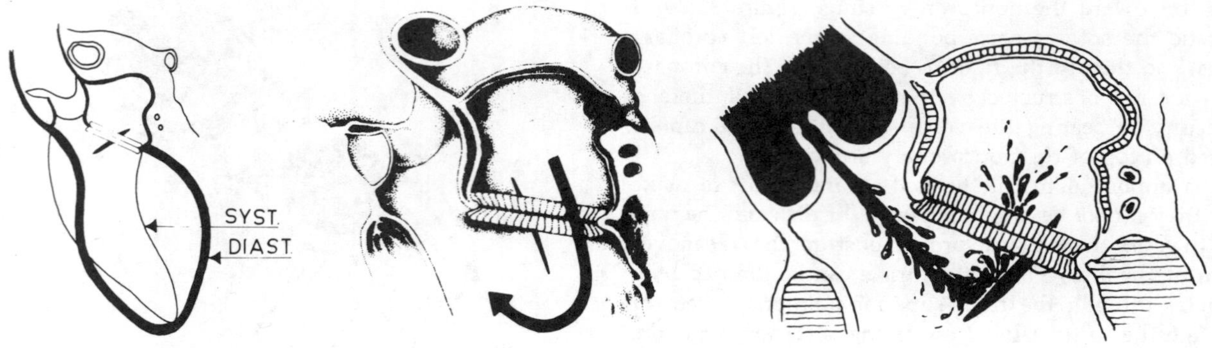

Figure 32.22. *Left*, The inward movement of the upper portion of the interventricular septum during diastole will narrow the anterior inflow from the left atrium. Diast = diastole; syst = systole. *Middle*, If free movement of the disk is to be obtained, the large opening of the valve should be oriented away from the aortic ostium, the disk then having the position of the anterior mitral leaflet. *Right*, A regurgitant jet from the aortic ostium may hit the anteriorly oriented disk and be directed into the left atrium, delaying closure and causing mitral insufficiency. (From Björk and Lindblom[22] with permission of the American College of Cardiology.)

tal treatment or surgery of the urinary tract, all patients with prosthetic valves should be given antibiotic prophylaxis. (See also chapter 46 on Infective Endocarditis.)

CONCLUSIONS

The Björk-Shiley monostrut valve has such strength that it has not been fractured under extreme experimental conditions and never under physiologic conditions in vivo. Therefore, this valve is now used in eight of ten totally artificial hearts, especially in pneumatically driven hearts in which high pressures may be encountered on increasing the heart rate. The goal of having a mechanical heart valve without the need for anticoagulation therapy has currently stimulated a variety of research efforts. With improved technology, further advances may one day be expected. New material and surfaces may permit new designs in artificial heart valves. Because many patients with biologic valves have to be reoperated on between 5 and 10 years, mechanical valves are preferred in areas where the medical profession can handle anticoagulation and the patient will cooperate.

REFERENCES

1. Hufnagel CA, Harvey WP: The surgical correction of aortic regurgitation. *Bull Georgetown Univ Med Cent* 1953; 6:60–61.
2. Robicsek F: Cardiac valve transplantation. *Acta Med Acad Sci Hung* 1954; 5:81–91.
3. Harken DE, Soroff HS, Taylor WJ, Lefemine AA, Gupta SK, Lunzer S: Partial and complete prostheses in aortic insufficiency. *J Thorac Cardiovasc Surg* 1960; 40:744–762.
4. Starr A, Edwards ML, McCord CW, Griswold HE: Aortic replacement. Clinical experience with a semirigid ball valve prosthesis. *Circulation* 1963; 22:779–783.
5. Rodriguez L: Hemodynamic and angiographic findings in patients with isolated aortic valvular disease before and after insertion of a Starr-Edwards aortic ball-valve prosthesis. *Scand J Thorac Cardiovasc Surg* 1970; 5(suppl):5–39.
6. Kay JH, Kawashima Y, Kagawa Y, Tsuji HK, Redington JV: Experimental mitral valve replacement with a new disc valve. *Ann Thorac Surg* 1966; 2:485–498.
7. Wada J, Komatsu S, Ikeda K, Kitaya T, Tanaka N, Yamada H: A new hingeless valve, in Brewer LA III (ed): *Prosthetic Heart Valves*. Springfield, IL, Charles C Thomas, 1969, pp 304–314.
8. Björk VO: A new tilting disc valve prosthesis. *Scand J Thorac Cardiovasc Surg* 1969; 3:1–10.
9. Nicoloff DM, Emery RW, Arom KV, Northrup WF III, Jorgensen CR, Wang Y, Lindsay WG: Clinical and hemodynamic results with the St. Jude medical cardiac valve prosthesis. A three year experience. *J Thorac Cardiovasc Surg* 1981; 82:674–683.
10. Hjelms E: Escape of a leaflet from a St. Jude medical prosthesis in the mitral position. *Thorac Cardiovasc Surg* 1983; 81:310–312.
11. Björk VO: The optimal opening angle of the Björk-Shiley tilting disc valve prosthesis. *Scand J Thorac Cardiovasc Surg* 1981; 15:223–227.
12. Björk VO: The improved Björk-Shiley tilting disc valve prosthesis. *Scand J Thorac Cardiovasc Surg* 1978; 12:81–84.
13. Björk VO: Advantages and long-term results of the Björk-Shiley valve. *Cardiovasc Med* 1982; 1:293–304.
14. Björk VO: Optimal orientation of the 60° and the 70° Björk-Shiley tilting disc valves. *Scand J Thorac Cardiovasc Surg* 1982; 16:113–118.
15. Björk VO, Lindblom D, Henze A: The monostrut strength. *Scand J Thorac Cardiovasc Surg* 1985; 19:13–19.
16. Björk VO, Henze A: Ten years' experience with the Björk-Shiley tilting disc valve. *J Thorac Cardiovasc Surg* 1979; 78:331–342.
17. Marshall WG Jr, Kouchoukos NT, Pollock SB, Bradley EL: Early results of valve replacements with the Björk-Shiley convexo-concave prosthesis. *Ann Thorac Surg* 1984; 37:398–403.
18. Yoganathan AP, Corcoran WH, Harrison EC, Carl JR: The Björk-Shiley aortic prosthesis: flow characteristics, thrombus formation and tissue overgrowth. *Circulation* 1978; 58:70–76.
19. Björk VO: The pyrolitic carbon occluder for the Björk-Shiley tilting disc valve prosthesis. *Scand J Thorac Cardiovasc Surg* 1972; 6:109–113.
20. Björk VO, Henze A, Hindmarsh T: Radiopaque marker in the tilting disc of the Björk-Shiley heart valve. *J Thorac Cardiovasc Surg* 1977; 73:563–569.
21. Björk VO: Metallurgical and design development in response to mechanical dysfunctions in Björk-Shiley heart valves. *Scand J Thorac Cardiovasc Surg* 1985; 19:1–12.
22. Björk VO, Lindblom D: The monostrut Björk-Shiley valve. *J Am Coll Cardiol* 1985; 6:1142–1148.

33 Hypertension and Hypertensive Heart Disease

Jay M. Sullivan, MD

The World Health Organization defines an arterial blood pressure of 160/95 mm Hg or greater as hypertension and blood pressure between 140/90 and 160/95 mm Hg as borderline hypertension.[1] Systolic hypertension indicates a systolic pressure above 160 mm Hg and diastolic pressure of 90 mm Hg or less. Using these criteria, several populations have been studied to determine the prevalence of hypertension in various parts of the world. In the United States, 18% of the population has diastolic hypertension by WHO criteria. However, the prevalence of hypertension varies with age, sex, race, education, socioeconomic class, and geographic region. For example, in the United States, the prevalence of hypertension increases with age, is higher in blacks than in whites, and is more frequently found in males than in females until middle age, at which time the ratio reverses (Figure 33.1). Data collected by the National Health Examination Survey of the Public Health Service on a random sample of the adult US population between the ages of 18 and 79 years showed that 16% of white adults and 30% of black adults had diastolic blood pressures higher than 90 mm Hg.[2] Using a diastolic pressure of 95 mm Hg as a cutoff point showed 9% of white adults and 22% of black adults above this level. This survey revealed that the prevalence of hypertension was roughly two times as high in blacks as in whites. When hypertension was found in blacks, blood pressure levels tended to be higher than those in whites. As a consequence, hypertensive heart disease, defined as the presence of left ventricular hypertrophy or failure,[3] was present from three to nine times more frequently in various subgroups of the black population than in comparable white subgroups.[4] The distribution of blood pressure among western European populations resembles that found in the United States.

Extensive hypertension screening has been carried out in the widely divergent regions and populations of the People's Republic of China. Overall, 4.85% of the population were found to have hypertension and another 2.88% to have borderline hypertension.[5] Considerable variation was found among regions, varying from a high of 17.76% in Lhasa, Tibet, and 9.53% in Beijing, to lows around 2.7% in Guangdong and Guizhou. In general, the prevalence was higher in North and Northeast China than in the southern provinces, and higher among urban than rural populations. When the frequency of hypertension among different population groups living in the same region was compared, those groups that traditionally had a high sodium diet had a higher prevalence of hypertension. For example, in Inner Mongolia, hypertension was found in 9.7% of nomadic Mongols, who make extensive use of salt in preserving and preparing food.[6,7] In contrast, the Hans of Inner Mongolia, who use less salt, have a prevalence of only 6.5%.

Hypertension screening in northern India has shown a prevalence of 4.91% in males and 5.44% in females. The frequency of hypertension was higher in urban populations (6.4%) than in rural populations (3.6%) and was highest in India's most populous cities, around 10%.[8] As in other countries, the prevalence of hypertension in India increases with age. This phenomenon was particularly marked in a Nigerian survey[8a] that found a frequency of hypertension of 5% in women between the ages of 15 and 24 years, which increased to 64% among those between 65 and 74 years.

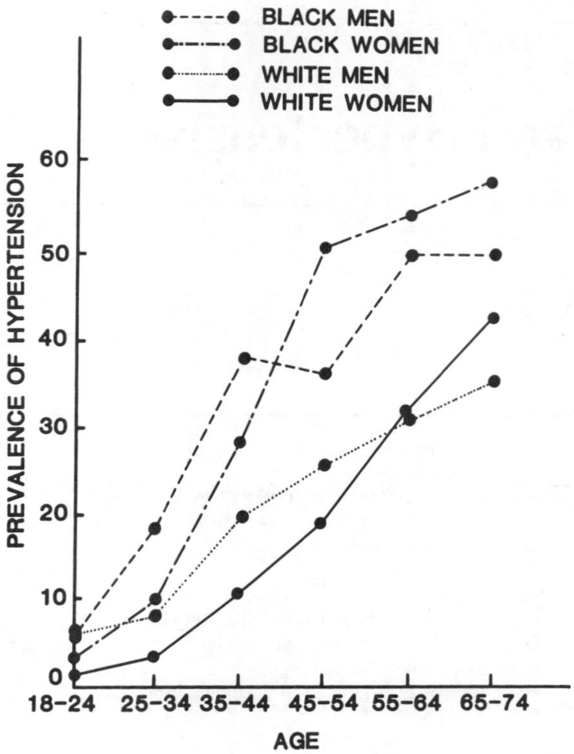

Figure 33.1. Prevalence of hypertension in the United States defined as the percentage of persons with systolic blood pressure of at least 160 mm Hg or diastolic blood pressure of at least 95 mm Hg. (Data from the Health and Nutrition Examination Survey, 1971–1974. Source: Advance Data, Vital and Health Statistics of the National Center for Health Statistics, No. 1, Oct 18, 1976.)

Although the WHO criteria of 160/95 mm Hg are a convenient "cutpoint" for epidemiologic surveys, they leave unsolved two major clinical problems in dealing with individual subjects. First, an individual's blood pressure varies continually throughout the day, increasing with activity, anxiety, discomfort, and even concentration, and decreasing with relaxation or sleep (Figure 33.2). Although the severely hypertensive patient might have a consistent elevation of diastolic blood pressure to levels of 115 mm Hg or above, given his variability, how can we fit an individual into relatively narrow categories of borderline, mild (diastolic pressures between 90 and 104 mm Hg), or moderate (diastolic pressures between 105 and 114 mm Hg) hypertension? To begin, multiple measurements of blood pressure should be made, in triplicate, on at least on three separate days to allow estimation of a patient's representative blood pressure and a decision regarding management. It must be kept in mind that even transient elevation of blood pressure on casual measurements has been found to be associated with subsequent cardiovascular disease.[9,10]

Next, attention must be paid to the technique of blood pressure measurement. The WHO recommends measurement of blood pressure with the patient seated comfortably in a quiet room with the forearm supported and the arm muscles relaxed.[1] The upper arm should be exposed and a cuff of suitable size used, ie, a cuff width of 13 to 15 cm for the adult of average size. The cuff should be inflated while the brachial or radial pulse is palpated until the pulse disappears. A stethoscope is then used to auscultate the Korotkoff sounds over the brachial artery. Phase IV diastolic pressure is measured when the sounds muffle and phase V when sound disappears. Because most studies relating diastolic pressure to risk have used phase V pressures, these should be used to assess the need for

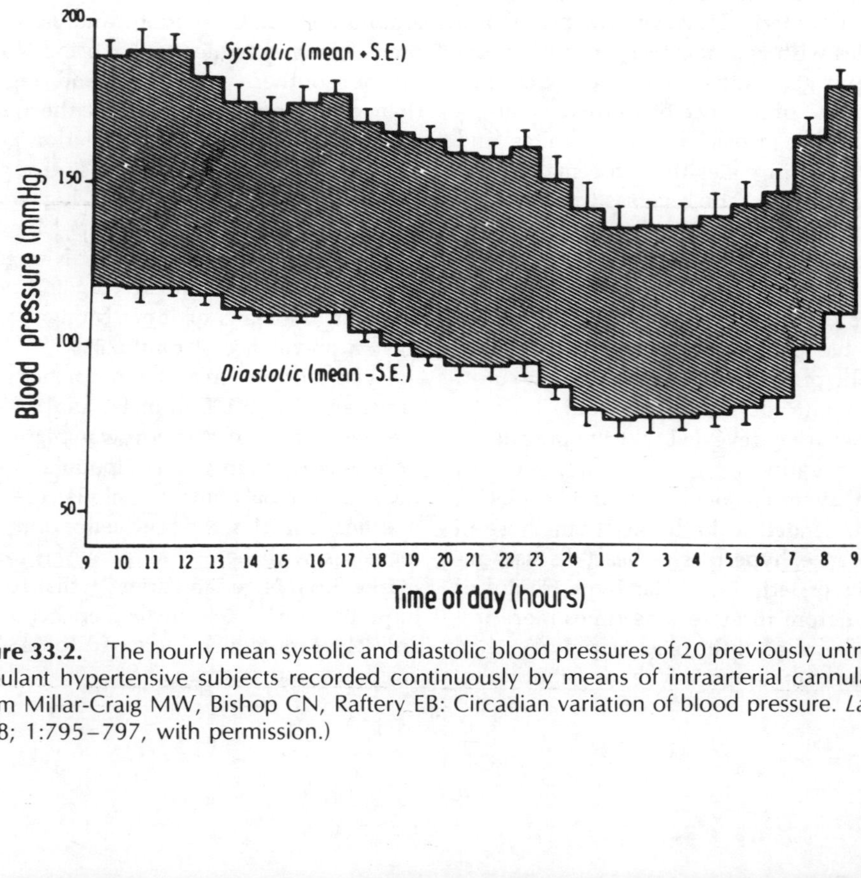

Figure 33.2. The hourly mean systolic and diastolic blood pressures of 20 previously untreated ambulant hypertensive subjects recorded continuously by means of intraarterial cannulation. (From Millar-Craig MW, Bishop CN, Raftery EB: Circadian variation of blood pressure. *Lancet* 1978; 1:795–797, with permission.)

treatment. Pressures should be made in triplicate over a period of at least three minutes and the lowest of the three measurements recorded.

The second problem related to the clinical assessment of individual patients is due to the fact that hypertension is associated with an increased risk of cardiovascular morbidity and mortality, and insurance actuarial data have clearly shown that this increased risk begins at levels of arterial pressure well beneath 160/95 mm Hg.[10] For example, at diastolic pressures between 88 and 92 mm Hg, excess mortality over 20 years of follow-up was increased 36% in men and 32% in women. Similiarly, the Framingham study showed that subjects whose blood pressure was between 140/90 and 160/95 had a twofold greater risk of developing cardiovascular disease over a follow-up period of 18 years.[11] The lower the cutpoint that is used, the higher is the prevalence of hypertension (Figure 33.3) and the greater is the magnitude of the public health problem posed by detecting and treating so many individuals. When hypertension is defined as a blood pressure of 140/90 mm Hg or greater, fully 38% of the population of the United States is hypertensive.[12] Do all of these individuals, as well as those elsewhere in the world, require a lifetime of antihypertensive therapy? Subsequent sections will consider the consequences of untreated hypertension of varying degrees of severity and the evidence that the benefits of antihypertensive therapy outweighs the risks in mild, moderate, and severely hypertensive patients.

ESSENTIAL VERSUS SECONDARY HYPERTENSION

Essential hypertension refers to patients who do not have a detectable cause for their blood pressure elevation. Secondary hypertension includes blood pressure elevation due to the many other disease processes listed in Table 33.1. Discovery of an underlying cause can lead to surgical correction, thus eliminating the need of a lifetime of pharmacologic therapy. The timing of a workup to

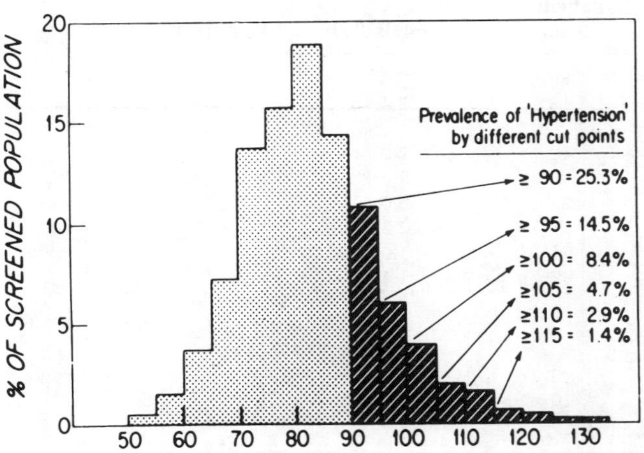

Figure 33.3. Frequency distribution of diastolic blood pressure at home screen of 158,906 persons, 30 to 69 years of age, HDFP, 1974. (From The Hypertension Detection and Follow-up Program: A progress report, Hypertension Detection and Follow-up Program Cooperative Group. *Circ Res* 1977; 40[suppl I]:I-106–I-109, by permission of the American Heart Association, Inc.)

Table 33.1. Types of Hypertension*

I. Systolic and diastolic hypertension
  A. Primary, essential, or idiopathic
  B. Secondary
    1. Renal
      a. Renal parenchymal disease
        (1) Acute glomerulonephritis
        (2) Chronic nephritis
        (3) Polycystic disease
        (4) Connective tissue diseases
        (5) Diabetic nephropathy
        (6) Hydronephrosis
      b. Renovascular
      c. Renin-producing tumors
      d. Renoprival
      e. Primary sodium retention (Liddle's syndrome, Gordon's syndrome)
    2. Endocrine
      a. Acromegaly
      b. Hypothyroidism
      c. Hypercalcemia
      d. Hyperthyroidism
      e. Adrenal
        (1) Cortical
          (a) Cushing's syndrome
          (b) Primary aldosteronism
          (c) Congenital adrenal hyperplasia
        (2) Medullary: pheochromocytoma
      f. Extraadrenal chromaffin tumor
      g. Carcinoid
      h. Exogenous hormones
        (1) Estrogen
        (2) Glucocorticoids
        (3) Mineralocorticoids: licorice, carbenexolone
        (4) Sympathomimetics
        (5) Tyramine-containing foods and MAO inhibitors
    3. Coarctation of the aorta
    4. Pregnancy-induced hypertension
    5. Neurologic disorders
      a. Increased intracranial pressure
        (1) Brain tumor
        (2) Encephalitis
        (3) Respiratory acidosis: lung or central nervous system disease
      b. Quadriplegia
      c. Acute porphyria
      d. Familial dysautonomia
      e. Lead poisoning
      f. Guillain-Barré syndrome
    6. Acute stress, including surgery
      a. Psychogenic hyperventilation
      b. Hypoglycemia
      c. Burns
      d. Pancreatitis
      e. Alcohol withdrawal
      f. Sickle cell crisis
      g. Postresuscitation
      h. Postoperative
    7. Increased intravascular volume
    8. Drugs and other substances
II. Systolic hypertension
  A. Increased cardiac output
    1. Aortic valvular regurgitation
    2. Arteriovenous fistula, patent ductus
    3. Thyrotoxicosis
    4. Paget's disease of bone
    5. Beriberi
    6. Hyperkinetic circulation
  B. Rigidity of aorta

*From Kaplan NM: Systemic hypertension: mechanisms and diagnosis, in Braunwald, E (ed): *Heart Disease, A Textbook of Cardiovascular Medicine,* ed 2. Philadelphia, WB Saunders, 1984, with permission.

detect secondary hypertension must be determined on an individual basis.

It is estimated that 80% of patients referred to a major medical center with hypertension that is severe or resistant to therapy have essential hypertension, whereas in a community practice 90% to 95% of patients with blood pressure elevation usually have essential hypertension. In a group of patients referred to a medical center because of resistant hypertension, underlying renal disease was the cause of blood pressure elevation in approximately 14%. Of the total group, 5% of these patients had renal artery stenosis; 2%, unilateral pyelonephritis; and 1%, a unilateral hypoplastic kidney.[13] Thus, approximately one half of the patients with hypertension due to renal disease were potential candidates for surgical cure of hypertension (Table 33.2).

About 4% of patients with resistant hypertension had adrenal causes of blood pressure elevation and less than 1% of the patients had coarctation of the aorta. Thus, among patients with severe hypertension, the yield of surgically curable forms is relatively high, around 10% of the total. Therefore, patients with diastolic pressures above 115 mm Hg or those who show evidence of target organ damage probably should be evaluated for underlying causes of hypertension when they are first detected.

At present, efforts are being directed toward early detection and treatment of patients with mild blood pressure elevation to prevent cardiovascular morbidity. In these patients, the yield of surgically curable secondary forms of hypertension is much lower (Table 33.3). Thus, it is reasonable to limit the initial evaluation of a patient with mild hypertension to history, physical examination, and a small number of laboratory studies and to pursue a more extensive evaluation of those patients who fail to respond to antihypertensive therapy.

Table 33.3. Causes of Hypertension in Office Practice*

	Canada (%)	Scandinavia (%)
Essential	94	95.3
Chronic renal disease	5	2.4
Renovascular disease	0.2	1.0
Coarctation	0.2	0
Primary aldosteronism	0	0.1
Cushing's syndrome	0.2	0.1
Pheochromocytoma	0	0.2
Oral contraception	0.2	0.8
Total patients (No.)	665	1,000

* Adapted from Rudnick KV, Sackett DL, Hirst S, Holmes C: Hypertension in a family practice. *Can Med Assoc J* 1977; 117:492-497 and Danielson M, Dammström B: The prevalence of secondary and curable hypertension. *Acta Med Scand* 1981; 209:451-455.

CONSEQUENCES OF ELEVATED BLOOD PRESSURE

To evolve a rationale for treating patients with blood pressure elevation, the effects of hypertension on the cardiovascular system that lead to the accelerated development of vascular disease must be examined (Figure 33.4). Since the development in 1898 of methods for indirect measurement of blood pressure, extensive data have been collected.[14] During the next 60 years, of necessity patients were followed without effective antihypertensive therapy. It soon became clear that severely elevated blood pressure was associated with a grave prognosis. Patients with diastolic blood pressure of 130 mm Hg or greater had a short time to survive when the elevated pressure was associated with evidence of significant target organ damage, papilledema, retinal hemorrhages and exudates, congestive heart failure, or diminished renal function. The most frequent symptoms in

Table 33.2. Workup of 500 Hypertensive Patients at Peter Bent Brigham Hospital, Boston, Massachusetts*

Type	Cause	Patients (No.)	Subtotals (%)	Total (%)
Essential	Benign	386	77.2	
	Malignant	12	2.4	79.6
Renal	Unilateral pyelonephritis	10	2.0	
	Bilateral pyelonephritis	8	1.6	
	Renal artery stenosis	25	5.0	
	Chronic glomerulonephritis	11	2.2	
	Hypoplastic kidney	5	1.0	
	Polycystic kidney	7	1.4	
	Kimmelstiel-Wilson disease	2	0.4	
	Juxtaglomerular cell tumor	1	0.2	13.8
Adrenal	Cushing's	5	1.0	
	Primary aldosteronism	10	2.0	
	Pheochromocytoma	5	1.0	4.0
Miscellaneous	Hyperkinetic heart syndrome	4	0.8	
	Coarctation of the aorta	3	0.6	
	Others	1	0.2	
	Unclassified	5	1.0	2.6

* From Sullivan JM: Arterial hypertension, in Blacklow RS (ed): *McBryde's Signs and Symptoms*, ed 6. Philadelphia, JB Lippincott, 1983, with permission.

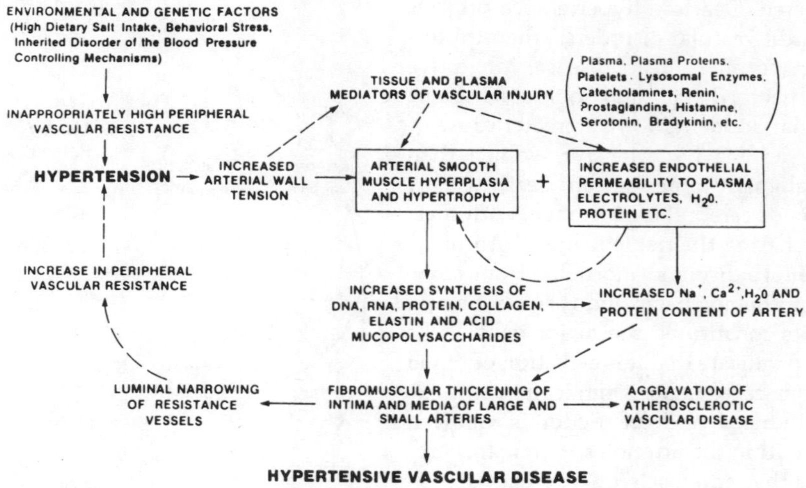

Figure 33.4. A unified concept of the causes and results of hypertensive vascular disease. (From Hollander W: Role of hypertension in atherosclerosis and cardiovascular disease. *Am J Cardiol* 1976; 38:786–800, with permission.)

such patients were visual impairment, headache, gross hematuria, dyspnea, edema, nausea, vomiting, epigastric pain, and malaise.[15] In one series of 105 cases, it was noted that most patients died within 4 months, and that few patients survived longer than 16 months.[16] In these patients, the malignant phase of elevated blood pressure was either essential or associated with diseases of the renal parenchyma. In a postmortem series of 124 cases, chronic pyelonephritis was found in 21% and chronic glomerulonephritis in 15%.[17]

With the development of effective treatment, it became apparent that prognosis was improved by the use of antihypertensive agents. The results of several studies suggested that antihypertensive therapy lengthened the half-time of survival of patients with malignant hypertension from approximately six months to about two and a half years. Patients with prior renal damage did not show as great an improvement in survival with treatment as did patients with well-preserved renal function because of progression of underlying renal disease.[18] Patients with impaired renal function, ie, endogenous creatinine clearance less than 45 ml per minute, did not do as well with treatment. Only four of fifteen patients with reduced clearance were alive one year after the initiation of therapy, whereas eight of 11 patients with better preserved clearance were alive one year after beginning therapy.[19] The prognosis for these patients has been improved by the increasing availability of chronic hemodialysis and renal transplantation, which allow support of renal function.[20]

Hodge and Smirk[21] noted that treated hypertensive patients ultimately died from complications that differed from those responsible for the deaths of untreated patients. Before the era of antihypertensive therapy, 32% of hypertensive patients died with cerebrovascular accidents, 22% from congestive heart failure, 21% from coronary artery disease, 1.4% from uremia, and 24% from other causes. After the development of antihypertensive therapy, 42% of patients died from coronary disease, 23% from cerebrovascular accidents, 9.5% from uremia, 6% from congestive heart failure, and 20% from other causes.

These data suggest that even partial control of severe hypertension improved prognosis, but those patients who had residual blood pressure elevation continued to develop target organ damage. The findings pointed out the need for additional study of the harmful effects of less severe levels of blood pressure elevation. In 1959, the Build and Blood Pressure Study of the United States Society of Actuaries found that blood pressure and longevity were inversely related, starting at levels of around 90/60 mm Hg.[22] These observations were confirmed by the study of 1979.[11]

In 1954, 5,127 residents of Framingham, Massachusetts[23] began to participate in a long-term study of cardiovascular morbidity and mortality. This investigation was observational, and no therapeutic interventions were initiated. The participants underwent physical and laboratory examination followed by reevaluation at two-year intervals. Of the men and women between 30 and 60 years of age who entered the study, 18% of the men and 16% of the women had systolic blood pressures greater than 160 or diastolic pressures greater than 95 mm Hg. Forty-one percent of the men had blood pressure elevations above 140 systolic and 90 mm Hg diastolic, whereas 48% of the women were in this range. For patients with moderate elevation of blood pressure, the risk of developing congestive heart failure was found to be six times greater than that in subjects with a blood pressure less than 140/90 mm Hg. The risk of developing a stroke was three to five times as great and the risk of having a fatal heart attack was two to three times as great. The higher the blood pressure, the shorter was the life expectancy. The risk of developing cardiovascular disease was incremental with the level of blood pressure. These observations applied to women as well as to men, were independent of age at the time of initial examination, and held even when other risk factors, such as abnormal lipid levels, obesity, diabetes, and electrocardiographic abnormalities were considered. Death in hypertensive subjects was due to several cardiovascular disorders: atherothrombotic brain infarction, coronary heart disease, congestive heart failure, and hemorrhagic and nonhemorrhagic stroke. Cerebrovascular accidents were a greater cause of death and disability among hypertensive women than among men.[24] In malignant hypertension, death usually occurred from uremia or cerebral hemorrhage, with male and female patients sharing the risk equally. With moderate hypertension, morbidity and mortality from coronary heart disease and hemorrhagic and thrombotic cerebrovascular accidents constituted the major risks.

There is evidence to indicate that it is elevation of blood pressure itself that causes vascular complications. In experimental animals, induced vasoconstriction is followed by sclerotic changes within the arterioles.[25] In man, three observations indicate that atherosclerotic changes are related to the level of blood pressure. In patients with coarctation of the aorta, atherosclerotic lesions are found in the high pressure areas of the aorta but not in the low pressure area beyond the coarctation.[26] Patients with congenital heart disease and with long-standing pulmonary hypertension develop atherosclerotic lesions in the pulmonary arterial tree.[27] In patients with renal artery stenosis and associated hypertension, nephrosclerotic changes develop in the "healthy kidney," whereas the vascular tree distal to the stenosis in the ischemic kidney is usually protected from the development of nephrosclerosis.[28] The complications of hypertension are directly related to the level of high blood pressure, but the risk imposed by a given level of arterial pressure is increased by the concomitant presence of additional risk factors such as smoking, hypercholesterolemia, diabetes mellitus, and a family history of cardiovascular disease.

PATHOPHYSIOLOGY OF ESSENTIAL HYPERTENSION

CONTROL OF THE CIRCULATION

The circulatory system allows absorption of oxygen from the atmosphere and food products from the gut, distributes these compounds to cells throughout the body, and transports water, carbon dioxide, and other waste products from the cells to lung, kidney, and skin for excretion (Figure 33.5). This function is served by the circulation of blood throughout the body under the driving force of pressure generated by the heart. To fully understand the problems of arterial hypertension, one must be informed about the basic components of the circulatory system: the ventricles, pressure-generating pumps; the aorta and other large elastic and muscular arteries, which serve as conduits; the resistance arterioles, which regulate the flow of blood out of the arterial tree into the capillaries, which allow diffusion of materials into and out of cells. The venules, veins, and atria serve as capacitance vessels, ie, chambers capable of storing a wide range of blood volumes without large changes in pressure.[29] The circulatory system is capable of intrinsic regulation due to the physical properties of its components and autoregulation in each of the tissues it serves and is under the overall integrative control of the autonomic

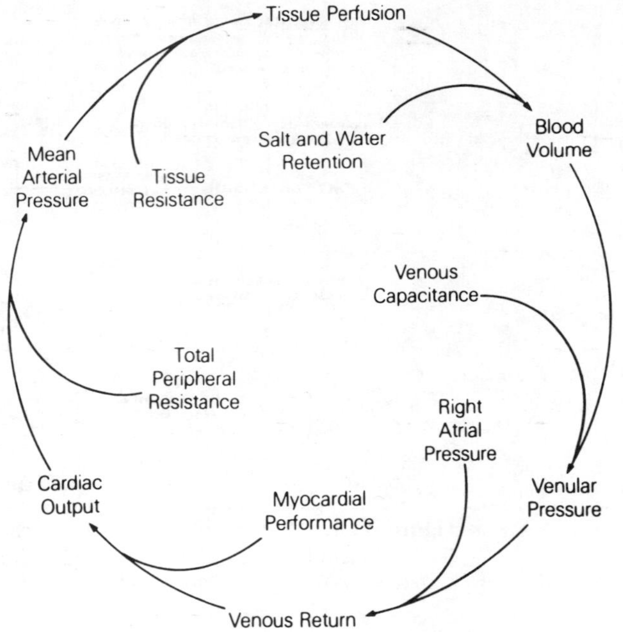

Figure 33.5. Regulation of the circulation: interplay of factors to maintain arterial pressure and tissue perfusion. (From Sullivan JM: Arterial hypertension, in Blacklow RS (ed): *McBryde's Signs and Symptoms,* ed 6. New York, J Lippincott, 1983, with permission.)

nervous system, which regulates function in response to changing physiologic circumstances.

The hemodynamic expression of Ohm's law helps one to understand how the circulation is controlled. Ohm stated that electrical voltage equaled the product of current (amperage) and resistance (ohms). Similarly, the Poiseuille equation for flow of homogeneous fluids states that as vessel length and blood viscosity usually do not vary greatly in a given individual, this equation can be simplified to state: flow = pressure/resistance, or arterial pressure = cardiac output × total peripheral resistance.

Resistance is a ratio, relating pressure and flow, and reflects the vasomotor tone of vascular smooth muscle fibers in resistance arterioles. These arterioles are influenced by both remote and local factors[30] (Figure 33.6).

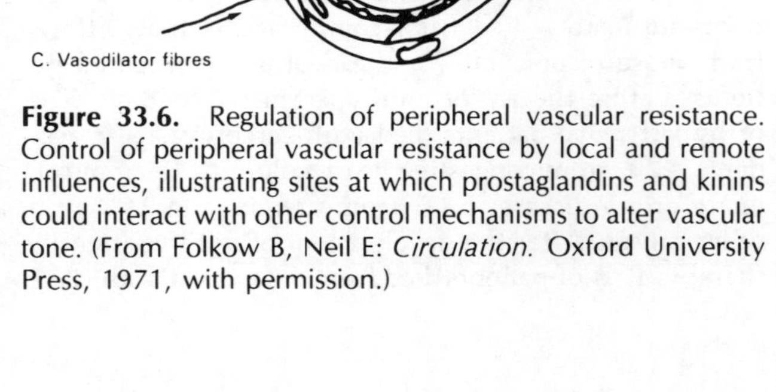

Figure 33.6. Regulation of peripheral vascular resistance. Control of peripheral vascular resistance by local and remote influences, illustrating sites at which prostaglandins and kinins could interact with other control mechanisms to alter vascular tone. (From Folkow B, Neil E: *Circulation.* Oxford University Press, 1971, with permission.)

Impulses traveling through the vasoconstrictor fibers of the sympathetic nervous system increase resistance, whereas fibers in the parasympathetic nervous system have a weak vasodilatory effect. The circulation also carries and delivers to the resistance arterioles vasoactive compounds such as catecholamines, angiotensin II, vasopressin, serotonin, histamine, bradykinin, and certain prostaglandins which act directly to alter vasomotor tone.

Local factors have important effects on vascular smooth muscle. In metabolically active tissues, the release of adenosine, hydrogen, and potassium ion and the consumption of oxygen are associated with vasodilatation as the tissue autoregulates local blood flow. Adenosine is a very powerful vasodilator, which is particularly important in the regulation of coronary blood flow. Vascular smooth muscle cells are myogenically active and display slow, rhythmic contraction due to spontaneous depolarization. The stretching effect of arterial blood pressure also stimulates contraction of vascular smooth muscles, an effect originally described by Bayliss.[31] Finally, accumulation of sodium ion in vascular smooth muscle increases sensitivity to circulating angiotensin II and catecholamines[32] and contributes to an elevated vascular resistance.

The second major component in the regulation of blood pressure is cardiac output, the product of heart rate and stroke volume. Heart rate is determined by the intrinsic rate of spontaneous depolarization and repolarization of the sinoatrial node of the heart and regulated by the counterbalancing influences of the stimulatory sympathetic and inhibitory parasympathetic nervous systems. Blood-borne substances, such as the catecholamines, also influence the heart rate.

The other determinant of cardiac output is stroke volume, which, in turn, is determined by the size of the left ventricle at the end of diastole and the extent of myocardial fiber shortening during systole. Fiber shortening is determined by three factors: preload, afterload, and contractility. Preload can be defined as the degree of stretch of the myocardial fibers at the end of diastole. This results from the compliance characteristics of the ventricle and the filling pressure. The latter reflects both venous tone and intravascular volume. As the ventricle increases in size, the amount of blood ejected increases until a plateau is reached at which point further increases in size fail to increase ventricular performance. Contractility relates ventricular performance to end-diastolic length. When a heart fails, a given fiber length elicits a less than normal contraction, thus contractility is increased when catecholamines stimulate the heart, the same degree of stretch leads to greater contraction, and contractility is said to be increased. In the intact heart, afterload refers to systolic myocardial wall tension, which is determined by intraventricular pressure and ventricular size. When preload and contractility are held constant, decreased afterload increases myocardial fiber shortening. A decrease in venous return reduces preload and left ventricular systolic pressure. Thus, afterload can be altered in either of two ways: (1) decreasing arterial blood pressure, and (2) reducing ventricular size, usually by decreasing intravascular volume or by inducing venous dilatation.

HEMODYNAMICS OF HYPERTENSION AND HYPERTENSIVE HEART DISEASE

Several investigators have observed that patients with mild to moderate essential hypertension usually have a normal cardiac output.[33] Thus, the increase in blood pressure is accompanied by an increase in total peripheral resistance, the hemodynamic characteristic of established human essential hypertension.

Certain hypertensive patients have transient elevation of blood pressure to levels above 140/90 mm Hg but are normal at other times. This has been designated borderline hypertension. Several laboratories have studied the hemodynamic status of this group of hypertensive patients and have found that they differ from those with mild to moderate fixed essential hypertension. The first observations in this area were reported by Widimsky et al,[34] who studied young patients and found that as a group, these individuals had an elevated cardiac output at rest, a calculated total peripheral resistance which fell within the normal range, and an elevated blood pressure which was due to the increase in cardiac output. Eich et al[35] studied an older group of patients with borderline hypertension and also found an elevated cardiac output with vascular resistance within the normal range. Subsequently, several other laboratories have confirmed the finding of an elevated cardiac output in patients of similiar description and have also noted that such individuals tend to have a higher left ventricular systolic ejection rate and a faster heart rate, leading several to propose that a disorder of the autonomic nervous system might be involved in the pathogenesis of borderline hypertension. Julius et al[36] found a spectrum of hemodynamic changes present in individuals with borderline hypertension, ranging from those with high cardiac output to those whose cardiac output was relatively reduced. It has been proposed that borderline hypertension is the initial phase of a disease process that eventually leads to sustained elevation of blood pressure and vascular resistance.

Studies have been carried out attempting to find a reason for the elevation in cardiac output. Ulrych et al[37] found that although such individuals did not have an increase in intravascular volume to explain the increased output, the volume appeared to be redistributed towards the central circulation. Thus, an increased amount of blood was present in the cardiopulmonary circulation, increasing venous return to the heart and stimulating an increase in cardiac output via the Starling mechanism.

Another explanation for the increased cardiac output could be increased activity of the autonomic nervous system. The evidence in favor of this proposal is the fact that such individuals have an increased heart rate and an increased rate of left ventricular ejection. Julius et al[38] studied the effect of beta-adrenergic blockade and parasympathetic inhibition in young patients with hypertension secondary to an elevated cardiac output and found that this dual blockade resulted in a return of cardiac output to normal levels. They also studied the effect of interventions such as sitting, mild exercise, and infusion of dextran on the hemodynamics of individuals with borderline hypertension and found that peripheral vascular resistance during any intervention was higher in the labile hypertensives than in the normotensive individuals. Similarly, Sannerstedt et al[39] studied the degree to which cardiac output and vascular resistance change with exercise in patients with labile hypertension in comparison with normals and found that the slope of the line relating output to resistance was shifted, indicating that peripheral vascular resistance was inappropriately elevated in individuals with mild labile hypertension.

Takeshita and Mark[40] studied the effect of stimuli causing maximum reactive hyperemia on forearm blood flow and resistance in normal subjects and subjects with borderline hypertension and demonstrated that forearm vascular resistance fails to decrease as greatly during maximum reactive hyperemia in labile hypertensives. It has also been observed that such patients have altered diastolic properties of the left ventricle[41] and attenuation of the conjunctival microvasculature.[42]

Thus, patients with borderline hypertension are characterized by an increased cardiac output, a central redistribution of blood volume, and evidence of enhanced activity of the autonomic nervous system leading to an increased heart rate, an increase in left ventricular ejection rate, and an inability to decrease forearm vascular resistance adequately in response to circumstances leading to an increase in blood flow.

Essential hypertension can be further subdivided into categories of mild, moderate, and severe, depending on the degree of elevation of diastolic pressure and the extent of involvement of target organs: the brain, the heart, the kidneys, and the peripheral vasculature. The hemodynamic pattern found in each of these subgroups appears to be determined by the interplay of three factors. The first relates to the degree of increase of peripheral vascular resistance and blood pressure. The second involves the degree of cardiac hypertrophy compensating for the elevated blood pressure and later the degree of impairment of cardiac function. The third factor relates to the extent to which pressure diuresis has taken place, resulting in a gradual contraction of intravascular volume and a redistribution of fluid volumes.

Meerson[43] postulated that ventricular function undergoes three stages of change during the development of hypertension. As afterload increases gradually, a stage of enhanced function of the ventricle occurs due to hypertrophy, during which time the heart can perform increased work. During this phase, the heart has been affected by the increased blood pressure, but it can still function normally. Later, hypertrophy no longer suffices to compensate for the increased afterload and the function of the left ventricle becomes impaired. Initially, this impaired function is subtle and requires sensitive techniques to detect.

Early in the natural history of hypertension no evidence of cardiac involvement is apparent on electrocardiogram or chest x-ray. Hemodynamic studies have shown that cardiac output remains normal. However, because vascular resistance and arterial pressure are higher, the ventricular workload is increased. Heart rate tends to be increased whereas stroke volume and left ventricular ejection rate, a reflection of ventricular contractility, are normal.

If the hypertensive process continues without treatment, the first evidence of cardiac involvement on physical examination emerges, with the appearance of a fourth heart sound. The electrocardiogram may reveal evidence of left atrial enlargement. Systolic time intervals show that the preejection period is prolonged at this stage. Heart rate remains elevated and cardiac output remains normal, although ventricular ejection rate begins to decrease. At this point, even though the chest x-ray might not reveal cardiac enlargement, echocardiographic techniques can demonstrate increased thickness of the left ventricular wall.

The progression of the hypertensive process leads to the development of cardiac enlargement on chest x-ray and the appearance of voltage and other criteria for left ventricular hypertrophy on the electrocardiogram. At this point, hemodynamic studies reveal further increases in total peripheral resistance and arterial pressure, cardiac output is reduced, even at rest, and systolic ejection rate decreases further.

Another factor that has profound influence upon the hemodynamics of severe hypertension is the redistribution of fluid volumes. In human hypertension, studies have not revealed a change in either total body water or in intracellular fluid volume. Thus, attention has focused on the distribution of extracellular fluid.

Over the years, a number of physiologic studies have pointed out that the kidney will increase its output of urine as arterial pressure rises, thus reducing intravascular volume and decreasing arterial pressure to the prior level.[44] Guyton et al[45] proposed that an impairment of the kidney's ability to respond appropriately to pressure is a major factor in the genesis of essential hypertension (Figure 33.7). In the hypertensive patient, it has been postulated that the kidney is set to begin pressure diuresis at a higher level. Thus, an individual with an expanded intravascular volume, eg, secondary to a high sodium diet, would initially increase cardiac output, thus stimulating autoregulation in individual organs throughout the body, leading to an increase in local, then total peripheral resistance, an increase in blood pressure, and an increase in urinary excretion of sodium and water, restoring cardiac output and intravascular volume to normal at the price of a higher vascular resistance and arterial blood pressure.

Changes in pressure within the blood vessels also serve to redistribute intravascular volume. An increase in intravascular pressure tends to increase the transport of water across capillary walls into the interstitial fluid, thus reducing intravascular volume. Similarly, a reduction of pressure is associated with an expansion of intravascular volume as fluid returns from the interstitial spaces. Measurement of interstitial fluid volume in patients with essential hypertension has usually shown that the ratio of plasma volume to interstitial fluid volume is reduced, suggesting transcapillary passage of fluid into the interstitial spaces due to the high intravascular pressure.

Tarazi[46] studied fluid compartments in several forms of clinical hypertension, demonstrating that as blood pressure increases in the presence of normal renal function, intravascular volume decreases on the basis of a

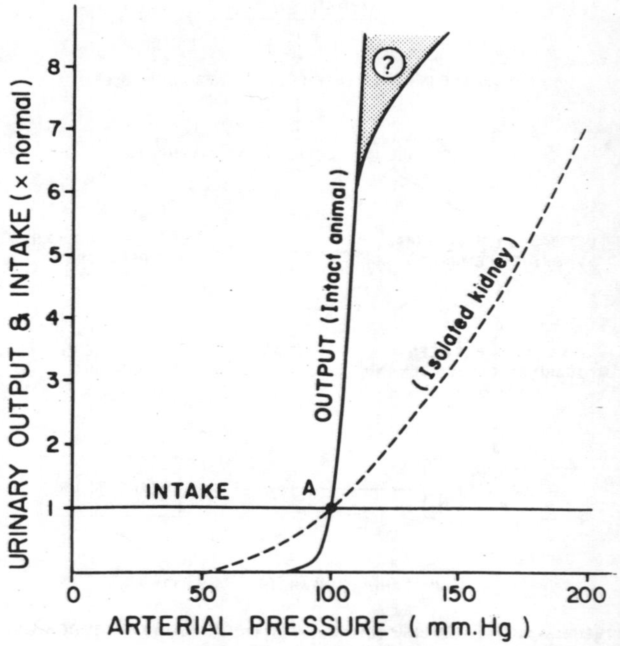

Figure 33.7. Graphic procedure for analyzing the long-term level of arterial pressure, based on the renal-body fluid mechanism for pressure control. The steep solid curve is the normal urinary output curve in an intact animal. (From Guyton AC: Regulation of arterial pressure. II. The renal-body fluid system for long-term pressure control. Mechanisms of hypertension, in *Textbook of Medical Physiology,* ed 5. Philadelphia, WB Saunders, 1976, with permission.)

decrease in plasma volume. The higher the pressure, the lower the intravascular volume, unless significant parenchymal renal disease is present, in which case the level of blood pressure elevation is directly proportional to the plasma volume (Figure 33.8). Thus, individuals with severe hypertension presenting for urgent treatment might be anticipated to have a significantly contracted intravascular volume if they are free of renal failure. Therefore, excessive use of diuretic therapy in such individuals is inappropriate. Similarly, antihypertensive therapy based on the use of vasodilating agents can be anticipated to decrease intravascular pressure, allowing the return of fluid from the interstitium into the vascular tree, leading to a blunting of the antihypertensive effect or pseudotolerance. Thus, careful use of diuretic agents to counter this effect after the initiation of antihypertensive therapy is appropriate.

Increasing degrees of severity of essential hypertension are marked by increases in peripheral vascular resistance. The phase of increased cardiac output, characteristic of young borderline hypertensive patients, may sometimes persist into the phase of mild essential hypertension and, less frequently, is found in the severely hypertensive patient.[47] Alternatively, cardiac output may be normal in the mildly hypertensive patient. Such individuals do not have clinically measurable damage involving the heart, kidneys, or brain. At times, patients in this group are found to have redistribution of blood volume to the cardiopulmonary circulation. Such hypertensive subjects also have an increased heart rate and evidence of increased

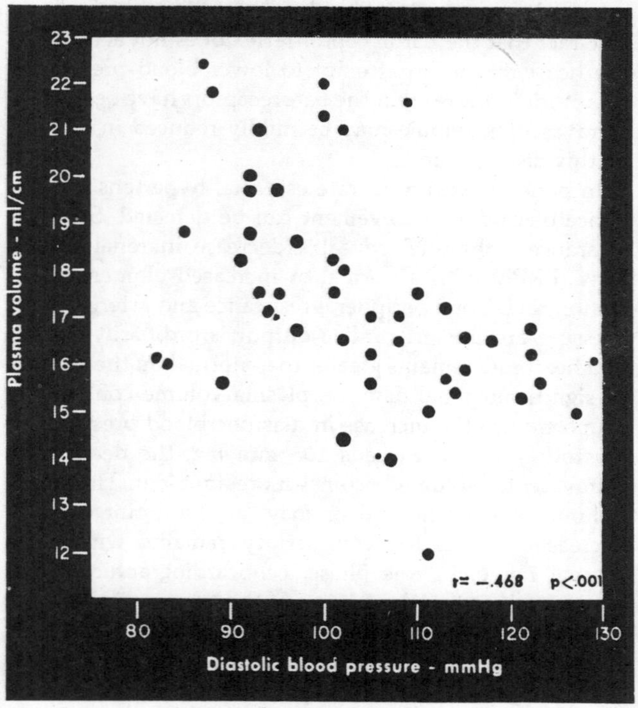

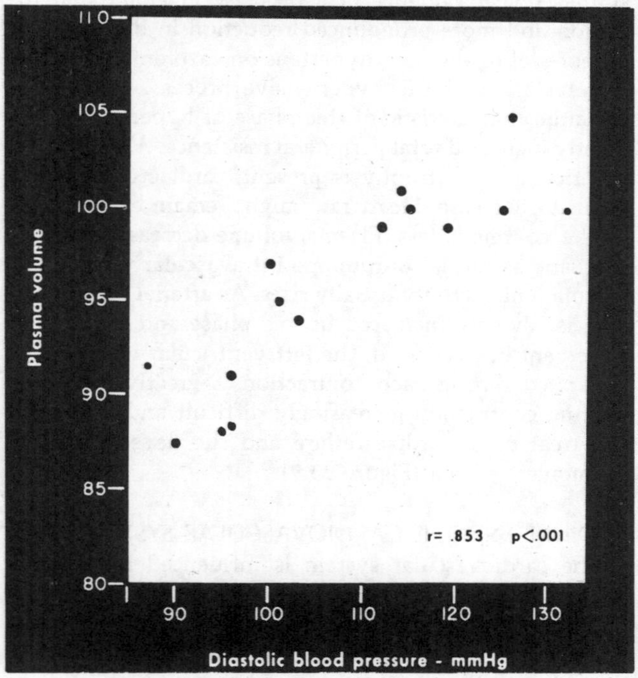

Figure 33.8. *Top*, A highly significant inverse relation between plasma volume and diastolic arterial pressure (average for week) in 47 men with essential hypertension. *Bottom,* A direct relation between plasma volume (expressed in percentage of normal to allow comparison of values for men and women) and diastolic pressure in 16 patients with hypertension accompanying renal parenchymal disease. (From Tarazi RC, Dustan HP, Frohlich ED, Gifford RW Jr, Hoffman GC: Plasma volume and chronic hypertension. Relationship to arterial pressure levels in different hypertensive diseases. *Arch Intern Med* 1970; 125:835–842. Copyright 1970, American Medical Association, with permission.)

myocardial contractility with a normal stroke volume. The fact that the baroreceptor reflex does not act to slow the heart rate in an attempt to lower blood pressure at this point indicates that the baroreceptors have been reset. Intravascular volume may be mildly reduced in patients of this description.

In patients with moderate essential hypertension, evidence of cardiac involvement can be detected. Standard clearance techniques reveal a decrease in renal plasma flow (ERPF) with a normal or increased glomerular filtration rate. Total peripheral resistance and arterial blood pressure are higher, cardiac output is ordinarily normal and heart rate remains greater than normal. In the absence of significant renal damage, plasma volume contracts in proportion to the increase in diastolic blood pressure. As diastolic pressure exceeds 105 mm Hg, the decrease in intravascular volume becomes more apparent. The stroke volume remains normal or may, at this point, start to decrease. Myocardial contractility remains within the normal range. In this phase, echocardiographic studies may reveal increased thickness of the left ventricular wall.

Severe essential hypertension develops as diastolic pressure increases still further and evidence of target organ damage emerges clinically. The chest roentgenogram and electrocardiogram begin to reveal evidence of cardiac enlargement and ventricular hypertrophy. Renal function studies reveal evidence of a decrease in glomerular filtration and more pronounced reduction in ERPF. In the absence of malignant hypertension, azotemia is a late manifestation of the hypertensive process. The hemodynamic characteristic of this phase of hypertension is a greatly increased total peripheral resistance. Although left ventricular hypertrophy is present, cardiac output may begin to decrease. Heart rate might remain elevated but stroke volume is less. Plasma volume decreases still further, and as cardiac output and intravascular volume fall, plasma renin activity usually rises. As arterial blood pressure is severely increased in this phase and cardiac enlargement has occurred, the left ventricular wall tension generated during each contraction is greatly increased, making contraction increasingly difficult and leading, if not treated, to cardiac failure and the development of pulmonary edema (Figure 33.9).

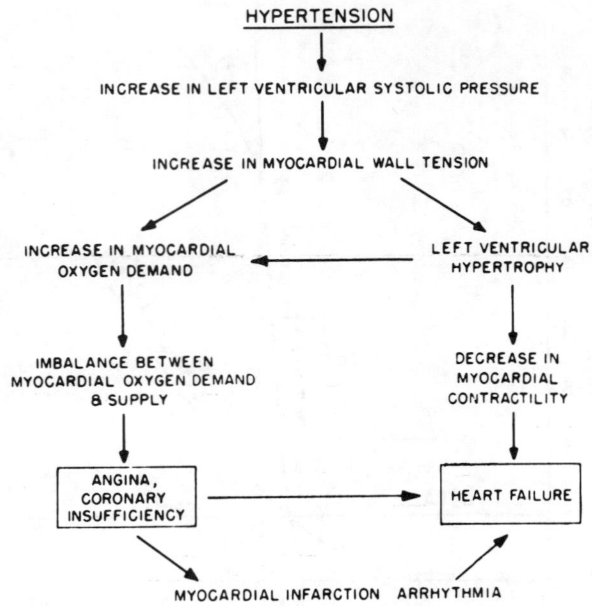

Figure 33.9. Adverse effects of hypertension on myocardial function. (From Hollander W: Role of hypertension in atherosclerosis and cardiovascular disease. *Am J Cardiol* 1976; 38:786–800, with permission.)

SODIUM AND THE CARDIOVASCULAR SYSTEM

The cardiovascular system is influenced by sodium. Dietary intake of this cation has been proposed to be an important influence in the development of high blood pressure[48] which, if untreated, affects the heart by predisposing to the development of left ventricular hypertrophy, congestive heart failure, coronary artery disease, and other cardiovascular disorders. The prevalence of hypertension has been shown to vary directly with sodium intake in a number of populations. However, even in populations consuming relatively large quantities of sodium, eg, in northern Japan where the average daily intake of sodium is 25 g, 60% to 65% of individuals do not become hypertensive.[49] It has been shown that extreme sodium restriction sometimes reduces blood pressure[50] and extracellular fluid.[51] It has also been observed that moderate salt restriction decreases average blood pressure by about 8/4 mm Hg.[52] However, all individuals do not respond to sodium restriction with a decrease in blood pressure.[53] These observations suggest that certain individuals are more sensitive to sodium than others. At present, we lack the clinical means to identify reliably the sodium-sensitive individual.

The mechanism by which sodium chloride ingestion results in blood pressure elevation has not been determined. One proposal, derived from a number of lines of experimental evidence, suggests that excessive intake of sodium chloride leads to sodium and water retention, expansion of extracellular fluid and intravascular volume, increased venous return, and elevated cardiac index. As elevated blood flow to the tissues continues, whole body autoregulation takes place, with subsequent increase in total peripheral resistance and the eventual development of hypertension.[54] The elevated blood pressure leads to increased urine output and restoration of extracellular fluid and cardiac index to normal, whereas hypertension is sustained because of the elevated vascular resistance (Figure 33.10). Guyton et al[45] applied systems analysis to study this problem and have derived data supporting this general outline. In studies of the relative effects of the various feedback loops involved in blood pressure control, they concluded that chronic blood pressure elevation will not occur unless the kidney fails to increase salt and water excretion appropriately and therefore does not reduce extracellular fluid or arterial blood pressure back to normal.

Certain animal experiments have supported this proposal. Coleman and Guyton have shown that sodium and water loading of dogs with reduced renal mass causes a chronic expansion of extracellular fluid, followed by a series of events similar to those observed in rats with renovascular hypertension by Ledingham, with sequential elevation of cardiac index, vascular resistance, and blood

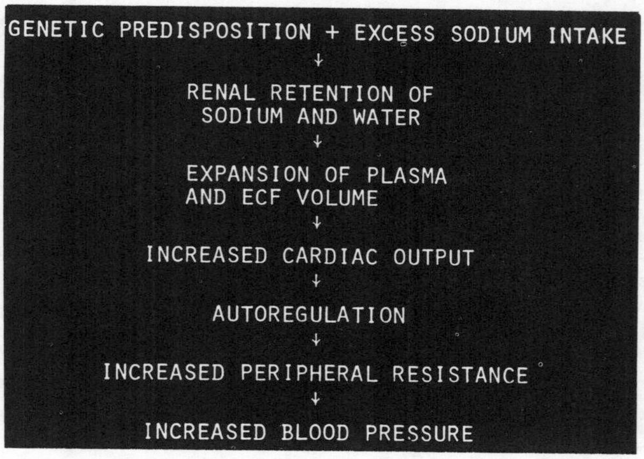

Figure 33.10. Possible sequence of events leading to the development of chronic essential hypertension in sodium-sensitive individuals.

pressure. Increased urine output ultimately lowers extracellular fluid.[54] Dahl[55] has selectively inbred strains of rats to produce groups that invariably develop hypertension when fed salt and others resistant to hypertension despite sodium loading, a circumstance similar to the human experience. Bianchi[56] and Dahl[57] have transplanted the kidneys of sodium-resistant rats into hypertensive sodium-sensitive rats who subsequently became normotensive. Transplantation of kidneys from hypertensive rats has succeeded in making sodium-resistant rats sodium-sensitive, thus suggesting that the genetic predisposition to sodium sensitivity resides in the kidney. However, in parabiotic experiments, Dahl et al[58] demonstrated transmittal of a humoral factor from the plasma of sodium-sensitive animals which raises the blood pressure of sodium-resistant rats. Tobian et al[59] have produced chronic hypertension in rats fed 8% sodium for four months,[59] and have observed that the kidneys of sodium-sensitive rats require a higher level of perfusion pressure for a given amount of sodium excretion. Ganguli et al[60] have studied the hemodynamic effects of sodium loading in Dahl "S" (sensitive) and "R" (resistant) rats, observing that the sodium-resistant rats responded with vasodilation, which allowed blood pressure to remain normal despite an increased cardiac index. In contrast, the sodium-sensitive rats responded with an increase in blood pressure, cardiac index, and vascular resistance, the latter increasing with time as the cardiac index fell to control levels. The elevated blood pressure was maintained by the increased vascular resistance.

Cardiac function and sodium homeostasis are interrelated in a number of ways that might influence the way that an individual responds to sodium. One of the most interesting recent findings in this area has been the discovery of atrial natriuretic factor. Granular structures in the atria, interposed among myocytes, were described by Kisch[61] in 1956. DeBold[62] later observed that these granules were altered by changes in water and electrolyte balance and, with his coworkers, that atrial extracts caused a rapid and potent natriuretic response.[63] Recent studies have shown that the several peptide atrial natriuretic factors isolated to date have molecular weights ranging from 5,000 to 30,000 daltons, relax vascular and intestinal smooth muscle, decrease blood pressure, and do not inhibit Na-K ATPase or change glomerular filtration rate. Natriuresis takes place because atrial natriuretic factor inhibits resorption of Na, K, Cl, and water in the renal tubule, probably distal to the loop of Henle.[64] Atrial natriuretic factor has also been found to have an inhibitory effect on renin and aldosterone secretion[64a] and on vasopressin release.[64b] A deficiency of this factor could underlie sodium sensitivity.

In addition to their hormonal function, the left atrium and posterior left ventricle also contain stretch receptors[65] which respond to sodium-induced changes in blood volume and heart size. As left atrial size increases, the receptors are activated, vagal afferent nerve traffic increases, and heart rate, total peripheral resistance, and blood pressure decrease. Further, the release of antidiuretic hormone is inhibited and water excretion increases, thus reducing heart size. Renal blood flow, glomerular filtration rate, and sodium excretion increase as stimulation of the stretch receptors also results in decreased efferent nerve traffic to the kidney, which in turn reduces renin release, angiotensin II formation, and aldosterone secretion. With chronic increases in heart size, the sensitivity of atrial and ventricular receptors decreases, thereby reducing the capacity to restore fluid components to normal levels. Impaired receptor function could explain why vascular resistance does not decrease appropriately in sodium-sensitive individuals when heart size is increased by a high sodium intake.

Expansion of intravascular volume by sodium-loading in volume-dependent forms of experimental hypertension leads to the appearance of plasma of a digoxin-like substance, endoxin.[66] This nonpeptide compound, of less than 500 dalton molecular weight, inhibits Na-K ATPase, thus preventing resorption of sodium throughout the renal tubule and causing natriuresis. However, by inhibiting Na-K ATPase throughout the body, particularly in vascular smooth muscle, endoxin leads to intracellular accumulation of sodium, then of calcium, thus causing vasoconstriction and elevation of blood pressure.[67] Hamlyn et al[68] have observed that plasma levels of an Na-K ATPase inhibitor are proportional to the level of blood pressure in patients with essential hypertension. Such a substance could have an important influence on the way in which an individual responds to dietary sodium.

In studies of normotensive volunteers, Kirkendall et al[69] found that a 400-mEq sodium diet resulted in increased forearm blood flow without an increase in blood pressure or in right atrial pressure, thus suggesting that local vasodilatation took place. Mark et al[70] found that patients with borderline hypertension decreased forearm blood flow when salt loaded, suggesting that sodium acts to cause vasoconstriction in such patients. Studies of patients with labile[71] or mild essential hypertension[72] have shown normal extracellular fluid or plasma volumes, or both, but have demonstrated elevated cardiac index and normal vascular resistance, suggesting that these patients are in but one phase of hypertension development and will later develop elevated vascular resistance if their tissues undergo autoregulation. Whether sodium intake contributes to this elevation of cardiac index in man is not known.

Sullivan et al,[73] using echocardiographic techniques, have made serial measurements of cardiac index during states of high and low sodium intake. First, they observed that a high sodium diet increased heart size[73] (Figure 33.11). A 200-mEq sodium diet, given after a period of sodium restriction, resulted in a 5% or greater increase in mean blood pressure in about 40% of borderline hypertensive subjects but in only 22% of normal subjects.[74] The normal subjects responded to sodium repletion with an increase in cardiac index and a decrease in total peripheral resistance. The response in the hypertensive subjects was more variable; of those showing an increase in blood pressure, 50% did so because of an increase in cardiac index without an adequate decrease in vascular resistance, and 50% on the basis of an increase in vascular resistance, suggesting that the human population of North America is far less genetically homogeneous than the Dahl sodium-sensitive rat. Whether these changes persist, and which, if any, are associated with the eventual development of hypertension are important unanswered questions. Sullivan and Ratts[75] found that increased cardiac index and decreased vascular resistance persist more than 12 months in sodium-resistant subjects (Figure 33.12) and have found that blood pressure remained elevated at six months in sodium-sensitive subjects because of an inadequate decrease in resistance.

This heterogeneity of response has been found by other investigators under different circumstances. In patients requiring chronic hemodialysis, Onesti et al[76] found that expansion of extracellular fluid did not cause an increase in vascular resistance or blood pressure in previously normotensive subjects, whereas blood pressure rose along with resistance in 60% or with cardiac index in 20% of the hypertensive patients. Similarly, Bravo et al[77] found that mineralocorticoid-induced hypertension in the dog was in some cases associated with an increased resistance and in other cases with an increased cardiac index. Berecek and Bohr[78] made similar observations in the pig. Luft et al[79] studied the hemodynamic and metabolic response of normal subjects to extremes of sodium intake, 10 to 1,500 mEq daily. They found that an intake of 800 mEq or more was associated with a significant increase in average blood pressure and in cardiac index.

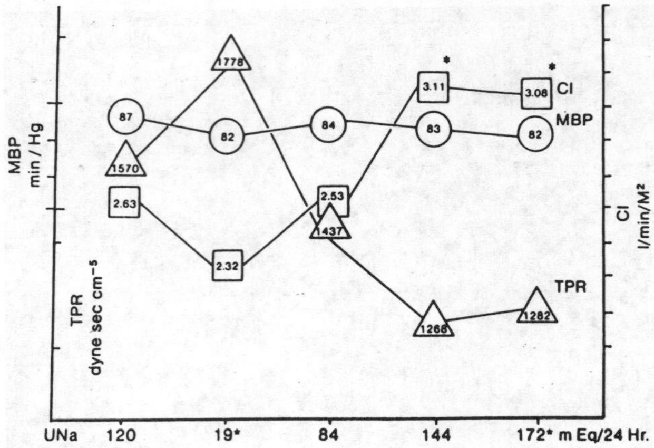

Figure 33.12. Adaptation to daily sodium intake of approximately 200 mEq by ten normotensive sodium-resistant subjects. The first three observations were five days apart, whereas period 4 (144 mEq sodium excretion) was 6 months later and period 5 (172 mEq sodium) was 1 year later. (Adapted from Sullivan JM, Ratts TR: Hemodynamic mechanisms of adaptation to chronic high sodium intake in normal humans. *Hypertension* 1983; 5:814–820, by permission of the American Heart Association, Inc.)

Epidemiologic studies also suggest a link between potassium deficiency sodium intake and hypertension.[80,80a] Direct infusion of potassium chloride or slight increases in serum potassium concentration have been found to have a vasodilatory effect in several vascular beds in man and in experimental animals.[81,82] Evidence has been presented to suggest that this effect is attenuated in hypertensive human subjects.[83] Potassium has natriuretic effects because of decreased tubular absorption of sodium. Luft et al[84] reported that potassium replacement promotes saluresis and reduces the blood pressure elevating effects of sodium in normal subjects, and MacGregor et al[85] found that potassium supplementation decreases blood pressure in hypertensive subjects. Recently, Tobian et al[86] presented evidence that although a high potassium diet did not prevent the development of hypertension in the salt-sensitive rat, the hypertensive rats developed fewer cardiovascular accidents when given potassium supplements. Thus, potassium might be an important modifier of the effects of sodium on the cardiovascular system.

Alterations in intracellular calcium are hypothesized to be involved in the pathogenesis of essential hyperten-

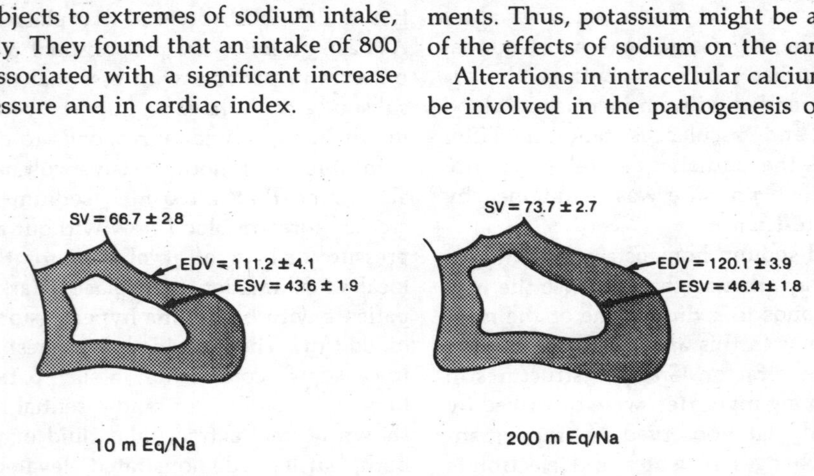

Figure 33.11. Effect of sodium intake on heart size and stroke volume. (From Sullivan JM: Sodium and the heart, in Messerli FH [ed]: *The Heart and Hypertension.* New York, Yorke Medical Group, 1986, with permission.)

sion,[86a] but whether this is a secondary association or a causal relation is unresolved. Studies of dietary calcium intake and blood pressure yielded contradictory results. Pietinen et al[86b] pointed out that both the hypertension rate and calcium intake in Finland are among the highest in the world. Lau et al[86c] offered experimental evidence against the role of calcium deficiency in genetic hypertension in spontaneously hypertensive rats. However, within populations several groups have reported an association between low calcium intake and raised blood pressure.[86d–g] But the correlations are weak in the extreme, and the calcium hypothesis requires careful testing with intervention studies of adequate size and duration before calcium supplementation can be recommended for therapy in hypertensive patients.[86h]

Impaired left ventricular diastolic function has been found in patients with cardiac hypertrophy.[87] The maximum left ventricular filling rates in young, borderline hypertensive patients without left ventricular hypertrophy was not found to vary as heart size was altered by variations in sodium intake in the same way as in normal subjects.[41] Recently, Ratts et al[88] reported that a group of patients presenting with chronic hypertension and heart failure of recent onset contained only 39% who had echocardiographic evidence of impaired left ventricular function, and of these, 91% had a history of alcoholism, previous myocardial infarction, or other illness which could cause abnormal left ventricular function. Fully 61% had normal systolic shortening despite hypertrophied ventricles, suggesting that sodium-induced volume overload, plus a stiff left ventricle with abnormal diastolic relaxation, possibly explained the development of pulmonary congestion.

Thus, in normal, sodium-resistant individuals, a high sodium diet results in an increase in left ventricular end-diastolic and end-systolic size, an increase in stroke volume and in cardiac index, which is accommodated by a decrease in total peripheral resistance, which in turn maintains arterial blood pressure at usual levels. The sodium-sensitive individual usually shows the same cardiac response, but does not have a lower vascular resistance to the same degree or even has vasoconstriction; therefore, blood pressure rises. The reason for this abnormal interplay between flow and resistance remains to be discovered.

These observations suggest that perhaps as many as 40% of patients with chronic essential hypertension are sodium sensitive and the efforts to correct the contraction of plasma volume, which can be anticipated to accompany chronic hypertension, will result in further elevation of blood pressure. In addition, the relatively noncompliant left ventricle with impaired diastolic function that is found in otherwise healthy individuals with chronic hypertension will cause an accentuated rise in left ventricular filling pressure and pulmonary capillary pressure if such individuals receive a sudden saline load, such as an aggressive attempt to correct intravascular volume contraction.

Although aging is associated with increased arterial stiffness and a higher prevalence of hypertension, in unacculturated societies with low dietary sodium intake arterial pressure rises to a lesser degree with increasing age, and prevalence of hypertension is markedly less than in Western societies with regular salt intake.[88a,88b] Recent studies from China[88c,88d] and Australia[88e] have shown that arterial stiffness (measured as aortic pulse wave velocity) is also dependent on dietary sodium intake and that the relation between arterial stiffness and sodium intake is independent of, and additional to, the relation between stiffness and mean arterial pressure. Thus even in normotensive subjects, reduced sodium intake has a beneficial effect in improving arterial distensibility which is independent of its antihypertensive action.

MEMBRANE TRANSPORT AND THE CONTROL OF BLOOD PRESSURE

Considerable evidence has been accumulated in recent years to suggest that the apparent genetic predisposition to hypertension in human beings might be due to abnormalities of electrolyte transport across cell membranes. In 1975, Edmundson[89] reported that the rate of extrusion of sodium from the white blood cells of patients with essential hypertension was impaired, resulting in an increased concentration of sodium within the white blood cell. Since this time, evidence has been uncovered demonstrating that there are at least three systems of sodium transport in the wall of erythrocytes, which have been used widely as an experimental model because of their availability. One is an energy-requiring sodium-potassium pump which requires lysis of adenosine triphosphate for activity, ie, it is energy dependent. This system is inhibited by ouabain and by endoxin, the digoxin-like substance that appears in the circulation of animals and man subjected to volume overload. Sodium-potassium cotransport is a second system which results in a coupled transmembrane efflux and influx of sodium and potassium. This system is inhibited by furosemide. Third, a lithium-sodium exchange or countertransport system exists which results in an exchange of sodium or lithium for sodium across the plasma membrane. The latter two systems are not inhibited by ouabain.

Garay et al[90] have studied sodium-potassium cotransport in normal subjects and subjects with essential hypertension or with secondary hypertension and found that outward transport of both sodium and potassium was reduced in the red cells of most patients with essential hypertension and in the normotensive offspring of hypertensive parents. Patients with secondary forms of hypertension were not found to have the same impairment of cotransport. These observations have stimulated considerable research about possible abnormalities of the sodium-potassium cotransport system in various populations, with conflicting results. Three studies[90–92] have found impaired sodium-potassium cotransport, whereas three others[93–95] have not confirmed the presence of an abnormality. However, considerably different methods were used in the various studies.

Adragna et al[96] demonstrated elevated red blood cell sodium-potassium cotransport in white subjects with essential hypertension, whereas Tuck et al[97] found reduced cotransport in black normotensive subjects.

Ghione et al[91] and Cusi et al[92] demonstrated impaired

sodium-potassium cotransport in the red blood cells of patients with essential hypertension. In contrast, Walter and Distler[94], Swarts et al,[93] and Duhm et al[95] failed to show an abnormality of cotransport in patients with essential hypertension.

Cannasa et al[98] studied sodium-lithium countertransport in red cells of patients with essential hypertension and found that increased activity characterizes this particular sodium transport system in the hypertensive subject. The countertransport system was also found to be abnormal in normotensive first degree relatives of the patients with essential hypertension. Most other studies of sodium-lithium cotransport, by Woods et al,[99] Travisan et al,[100] and Brugnara et al[101] also showed abnormalities in the erythrocytes of subjects with essential hypertension. However, Duhm and Gobel[102] and Isben et al,[103] using modified methods, failed to confirm the presence of abnormal sodium-lithium countertransport in hypertensive patients.

Thus, the weight of evidence points to the existence of abnormalites of sodium transport in the cell membranes of hypertensive subjects, although the exact nature and distribution of this abnormality await additional research and further standardization of techniques. Present data suggest that the most reproducible abnormality is that of sodium-lithium countertransport.

Blaustein[67] has postulated that if an abnormality of sodium transport exists that results in reduced extrusion of sodium from the intracellular space and accumulation of sodium therein, this would in turn result in enhanced sodium calcium exchange across cell membranes, causing a net increase of intracellular calcium concentration. In the case of contractile cells, such as vascular smooth muscle in the resistance arteriole, or cardiac muscle, this sequence of events would result in enhanced contractility. A relatively increased cardiac output against a relatively fixed vascular resistance would in turn result in an elevation of blood pressure.

ACTIVITY OF THE SYMPATHETIC NERVOUS SYSTEM IN HYPERTENSION

Many inconclusive reports, published over several years, continue to prompt a search for evidence linking the sympathetic nervous system to either the initiation or the maintenance of essential hypertension. Several lines of evidence contribute to this continuing interest. The first is that patients with pheochromocytoma and high serum levels of epinephrine/norepinephrine have high blood pressure which usually returns to normal when the tumor is removed and catecholamine levels return to normal. Second, patients with essential hypertension have higher resting pulse rates than patients with normal blood pressure.[71] Third, patients with essential hypertension respond favorably to therapy with agents which interfere with the action of the sympathetic nervous system at several different levels. Fourth, several studies have found elevated levels of norepinephrine in the plasma of certain patients with essential hypertension, but the overlap with normotensive patients was quite extensive.[104–106] Fifth, plasma levels of dopamine-β-hydroxylase, which are believed to reflect the activity of peripheral sympathetic nerve endings, correlate closely with diastolic blood pressure levels in hypertensive subjects.[107,108]

Part of the difficulty in establishing a role for the sympathetic nervous system or eliminating this possibility has been methodologic. Early studies relied on relatively insensitive bioassay or spectrophotofluorometric techniques to measure catecholamines. More recent studies, carried out with more sensitive double isotope techniques, have supported a role for the sympathetic nervous system, although this point has not been established conclusively.[109] Louis et al[108] measured plasma norepinephrine levels in 31 patients with essential hypertension and found a significant individual correlation between plasma norephinephrine concentration and simultaneous arterial pressure. They also found an impressive correlation between plasma norepinephrine levels and the effects of treatment with ganglionic blocking agents on systolic arterial pressure. These are the most convincing correlations available but still do not prove the point that the sympathetic nervous system is overactive in those patients with essential hypertension when compared with normal subjects.

It has been assumed that excretion of the metabolic breakdown products of epinephrine and norepinephrine are reflections of endogenous sympathetic nervous system activity, even though these levels do not allow quantitation of the amount of norepinephrine that undergoes reuptake by the nerve endings after stimulus and release. In support of this postulate is the observation that urinary excretion of metabolites increases with posture or after sympathetic or ganglionic blockade. A review of studies in which these compounds have been measured in patients with essential hypertension shows conflicting results.[110] Vanillylmandelic acid excretion has been found to be elevated in one study, unchanged in two others, and down in a fourth study. Total metanephrine excretion has also been inconsistent, with two studies finding normal levels and two groups observing an elevation. Likewise, norepinephrine excretion has been found to be normal in ten studies, up in two and down in one, whereas dopamine excretion was found to be normal in two studies and decreased in one. Gitlow et al[111] found elevated plasma norepinephrine clearance rates in patients with essential hypertension, but DeQuattro and Sjoerdsma[112] usually found normal rates except in patients who also had elevated urinary norepinephrine levels.

At centers in which accurate measurement of plasma norepinephrine levels can be obtained and the normal range well established, therapy can be planned, when elevated levels are found, to take advantage of the effects of the centrally acting alpha$_2$ receptor agonists or agents that block the sympathetic nervous system peripherally. In theory, beta-adrenergic receptor blockers should not be effective in this group, because the alpha-adrenergic receptors would not be blocked and would respond to elevated norepinephrine levels by increasing peripheral vascular resistance. However, if the elevated blood pressure is due primarily to an elevated cardiac output, blockade of beta$_1$ receptors should decrease pressure.

In clinics that do not have access to plasma norepinephrine determinations, a clue to the presence of elevated activity of the sympathetic nervous system can be provided by a rapid heart rate, a hyperdynamic precordium, or the finding of orthostatic hypertension. When mean arterial blood pressure climbs by 10 mm Hg or more when the patient assumes an upright position, orthostatic hypertension is present and suggests overactivity of the sympathetic nervous system.

THE RENIN-ANGIOTENSIN-ALDOSTERONE SYSTEM

The long-known association between nephritis and hypertension led Tigerstadt and Bergman[113] to search for pressor substances in the kidney. In 1898, they described the hemodynamic effects of crude saline extracts of rabbit kidney, showing that such a preparation caused an increase in blood pressure within 10 seconds, which peaked at two minutes and disappeared by 20 minutes. In 1934, Goldblatt[114] produced hypertension by partial occlusion of the renal artery of the dog. In 1939, Page[115] observed that renin, mixed with saline and injected into an ear vessel, did not cause vasoconstriction, but was a vasoconstrictor when mixed with blood, suggesting that renin must interact with a component of blood before a pressor substance is formed. The same year, Braun-Menendez[116] found a pressor substance in renal vein blood that did not have the physical properties of renin and eventually proved to be angiotensin. In 1953, Simpson et al[117] purified aldosterone. In 1955, as a result of work from a number of laboratories, angiotensins I and II were isolated and angiotensin-converting enzyme described. In 1960, Laragh et al[118] and Genest et al[119] observed elevated aldosterone excretion in patients with malignant hypertension, and Laragh observed that infusion of angiotension II caused increased urinary aldosterone excretion. Thus, the components forming a negative feedback loop were uncovered (Figure 33.13). The liver synthesizes renin substrate, a glycoprotein that is released into the circulation. Renin, a proteolytic enzyme released by the juxtaglomerular cells of the kidney cleaves a decapeptide, angiotensin I, from the substrate molecule. During passage through the pulmonary circulation, angiotensin I is lysed by converting enzyme, leaving the octapeptide angiotensin II, a potent vasopressor, which is eventually destroyed by angiotensinases. Angiotensin II has several effects, among which are vasoconstriction, facilitation of norepinephrine release and aldosterone release, which in turn causes sodium retention in the distal tubules of the kidney. Evidence exists that the aldosterone effect might also be mediated by a heptapeptide, angiotensin III.[120]

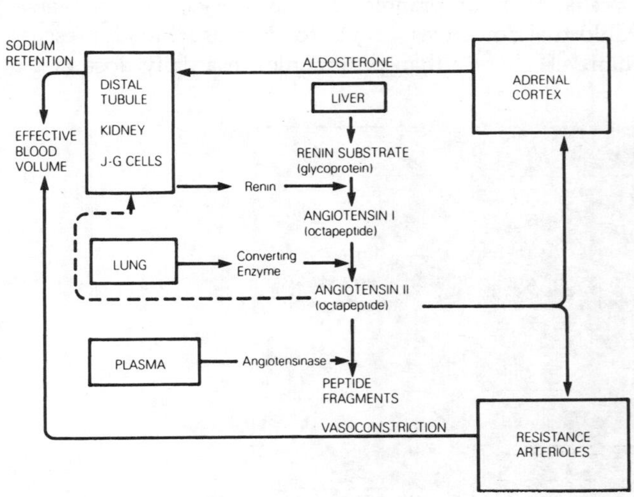

Figure 33.13. The renin-angiotensin-aldosterone negative feedback loop for the regulation of effective blood volume. (Reproduced with permission from Sullivan JM: Arterial hypertension, in Blacklow RS [ed]: *McBryde's Signs and Symptoms,* ed 6. New York, JP Lippincott, 1983, with permission.)

The renin–angiotensin system acts to maintain blood pressure in two major ways: by increasing effective blood volume and by increasing peripheral vascular resistance. In addition, angiotensin II acts directly on the juxtaglomerular cells to inhibit renin release, thus acting as a control on the system. Any manipulation that tends to decrease blood pressure, blood volume, or sodium concentration tends to activate the feedback loop. Hemorrhage, hypotension, sodium depletion, gastrointestinal fluid loss, upright posture, and renal artery stenosis all stimulate renin release.

The control of renin release is complicated and involves the interplay of a number of factors. The major factors involved are: the vascular receptor in the afferent renal arteriole, the macula densa, the sympathetic nervous system, and several blood-borne substances.[121] The vascular receptor is comprised of the juxtaglomerular cells and portions of the afferent glomerular arteriole. This receptor responds to changes in wall tension caused by changes in perfusion pressure,[122] sympathetic nerve activity,[123] and intrinsic changes in vascular smooth muscle during renal autoregulation.[124] The macula densa responds to changes in the rate of sodium delivery,[125] but the relative importance of this mechanism in the control of renin release is not clear. A number of agents are known to effect renin release, including sodium,[126] potassium,[127] angiotensin II,[128] catecholamines,[129] estrogens,[130] adrenal steroids,[131] ADH,[132] and prostaglandins.[133,134]

Although the renal sympathetic nerves are an important modulating factor in the control of renin release, they are not essential. Increased renin secretion in response to sodium depletion has been demonstrated in dogs with bilateral renal denervation.[135] In experimental animals, it has been shown that beta-adrenergic receptor blockade prevents the increase in renin secretion produced by hypoglycemia,[136] brain stem stimulation,[137] infusion of catecholamines,[138] acute hemorrhage, adrenalectomy, chronic salt depletion, and acute renal artery constriction.[139] Although evidence has been presented to show that renin secretion is also prevented by alpha-adrenergic receptor blockade,[138] other laboratories have observed that agents that block alpha-adrenergic receptors actually potentiate stimulated renin release.[140,141] Human studies have shown that small intravenous doses of propranolol promptly suppress renin release,[142] whereas studies of longer duration have yielded variable results. Oral propranolol has been reported to decrease blood pressure and plasma renin activity proportionately,[143] to lower renin activity without affecting blood pressure in patients with renovascular hypertension,[144] to block the rise in plasma renin activity that follows diuretic therapy or upright posture,[145] and to lower blood pressure without affecting renin activity in patients receiving diuretics.[146,147]

Aldosterone and angiotensin II are the two effector compounds in this system that act directly on target tissues. Potassium and ACTH stimulate aldosterone secretion, as does angiotensin II, whereas large increases in plasma sodium concentration inhibit aldosterone release.

The main clinical use for measurement of components of the renin–angiotensin system is for the diagnosis of secondary hypertension. Patients with primary aldosteronism have suppressed plasma renin activity, and measurement of differential renal vein renin activity in patients with renovascular lesions helps to predict the outcome of surgery, although not with complete accuracy.[148]

If plasma renin activity is measured in a group of normal subjects of comparable age, under standard conditions of posture, activity, diet, and time of day, values will fall within a relatively narrow range, especially if the measurements are made in the controlled environment of a metabolic study ward. Outpatient studies offer less precision because it is difficult for an outpatient to adhere to a constant metabolic diet. An attempt has been made to solve this difficulty by taking advantage of the fact that plasma renin activity reflects recent sodium intake. Thus, Brunner et al[149] collected a 24-hour urine sample for measurement of sodium excretion on the day that blood was drawn for measurement of plasma renin activity, after their subjects had been up and about for the morning.[149] Other investigators have subdivided patients on the basis of plasma renin activity after administration of a diuretic.[150] Drayer[151] found that measurement of plasma renin activity after five days of chlorthalidone therapy provides an alternative and inexpensive way to characterize hypertensive patients by renin level (Figure 33.14).

When renin activity is measured in patients with essential hypertension, the values spread over a much wider range than that seen in normal subjects. Roughly 30% of the patients will have renin activity lower than normal, and around 10% to 15% will have activity higher than normal. Thus, patients with essential hypertension can be subdivided on the basis of high, normal, or low plasma renin activity. After several years of intensive research, the cause of low renin hypertension is not clear.[152] The physiologic aspects of renin release suggest that patients with low renin hypertension might be relatively volume overloaded, as are patients with primary aldosteronism, whereas those with high renin activity might be volume depleted and relatively vasoconstricted because of high circulating angiotensin II levels, as found in patients with malignant or renovascular hypertension. Thus, concepts of "volume dependent" or low renin hypertension, and "vasoconstrictor dependent" or high renin hypertension, have evolved.[153] As shown in Table 33.4, most types of hypertension can be classified in this manner.

The effects of various antihypertensive agents have been studied in low renin hypertension to test the hypothesis that blood pressure elevation in such patients is volume dependent. Most workers now agree that these patients respond well to aminoglutethimide which blocks the synthesis of mineralocorticoids,[154] to thiazide diuretics,[153] or to spironolactone, an aldosterone antagonist.[155]

Patients with high renin hypertension have been treated with propranolol, a beta-adrenergic blocking agent that blocks the release of renin. It has been reported that patients with high renin hypertension respond unusually well to this form of therapy, but the observation remains controversial.[143] Woods et al[156] examined this problem with a prospective, double-blind crossover study of 54 patients with low and normal renin essential hypertension. The patients were classified by three methods, ie, upright plasma renin activity versus 24-hour urinary sodium excretion on an ad libitum diet, plasma renin activity after furosemide diuresis and upright posture, and plasma renin activity after seven days on a 65 mEq sodium diet versus 24-hour sodium excretion. Although a good correlation was found among the methods, the three did not exactly identify the same patients with low renin activity. All patients then received chlorthalidone for 18 weeks, then propranolol for 18 weeks, or vice versa. Chlorthalidone was found to decrease blood pressure more effectively than propranolol in a daily dose of 3.5

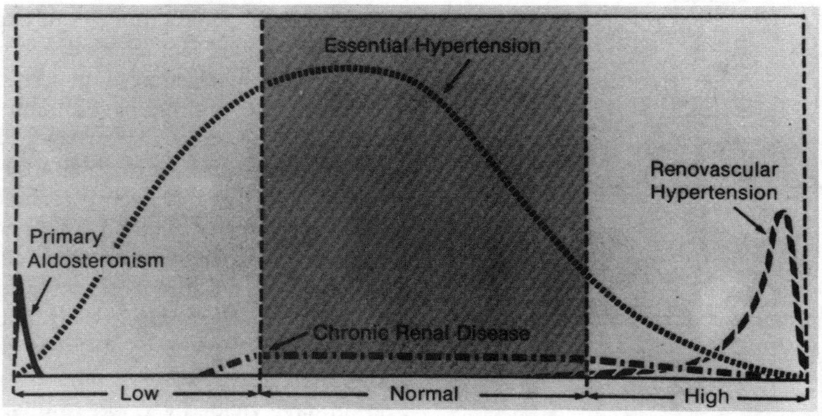

Figure 33.14. Schematic representation of plasma renin activity in various hypertensive diseases. The expected number of patients with each type of hypertension is indicated along with their proportion of low, normal, or high renin levels. (From Kaplan NM: Renin profiles: the unfulfilled promises. *JAMA* 1977; 238:613. Copyright 1977, the American Medical Association, with permission.)

Table 33.4. Angiotensin II Generation in Hypertensive Vascular Disease*

Low Plasma Renin Activity	Normal Plasma Renin Activity	High Plasma Renin Activity
A. Aldosteronism	A. Normal aldosterone secretion	A. Secondary aldosteronism
1. Primary	1. Normal renin essential hypertension	1. Malignant or severe hypertension
2. Pseudoprimary	2. Unilateral renal disease†	2. Unilateral renal disease with severe hypertension
3. Tertiary?	3. Bilateral renal vascular or parenchymal disease†	3. Bilateral renal vascular or parenchymal disease†
4. Glucocorticoid suppressible	4. Cushing's syndrome	4. High renin essential hypertension
B. Mineralocorticoidism	5. Coarctation of the aorta	5. Renin-secreting kidney tumors
1. 11-beta hydroxylase deficiency	6. Pheochromocytoma	6. Iatrogenic: oral contraceptive use
2. 17-alpha hydroxylase deficiency		B. Without secondary aldosteronism
3. Adrenal carcinoma		1. Potassium depleted patients with foregoing disorders
4. Ectopic ACTH-secreting tumors		
5. Excess 18-OH DOC?		
C. No clearly demonstrable adrenal-cortical disease		
1. Low renin essential hypertension		
2. Parenchymal renal disease†		
3. Liddle's syndrome		
4. Gordon's hyperkalemic patient		
5. Iatrogenic: mineralocorticoid or licorice ingestion		

* Laragh JH, Baer L, Brunner HR, Buhler FR, Sealey JE, Vaughan ED Jr: Renin, angiotensin and aldosterone systems in pathogenesis and management of hypertensive vascular disease. *Am J Med* 1972; 52:633–652, with permission of Dun-Donnelley Publishing Corp.

† Note: Patients with parenchymal or renal vascular (unilateral or bilateral) disease may exhibit low, normal, or high circulating plasma renin activity.

mg/kg. As a group, patients with low renin activity had no greater reduction in pressure after chlorthalidone than did patients with normal renin activity. Also, patients with normal renin hypertension did not have a greater reduction in blood pressure in response to propranolol than did patients with low renin hypertension. However, when the distribution of blood pressure responses within the groups was analyzed, it was found that chlorthalidone reduced blood pressure to normal in a larger percentage of patients with either low or normal plasma renin activity than did propranolol and that chlorthalidone was particularly effective in the low renin group. The investigators concluded that renin measurements were of limited benefit in selecting antihypertensive therapy and recommended initiating therapy with diuretics in the usual patient.

Roughly one third of patients with essential hypertension have low renin or volume-dependent hypertension, and another 60% have normal renin activity, which has been interpreted to suggest that they too have a volume component involved in their blood pressure elevation. Thus, 80% to 90% of patients with hypertension might be expected to respond to diuretic therapy. Because those patients who fail to respond to diuretic therapy are ordinarily placed on sympatholytic drugs, which tend to decrease renin release[157] in practice, a conventional stepped-care therapeutic approach will eventually cover the spectrum of high to low renin hypertension.

Compounds have been developed that either block converting enzyme activity, thus preventing the formation of angiotension II, for example, teprotide (a nonapeptide),[158] captopril,[159] enalapril,[160,160a] and lisinopril,[161] or which block angiotensin II receptors (saralasin, a synthetic octapeptide).[162] These agents, used sequentially with diuretics, allow more precise estimation of the relative contribution of the renal pressor system and that of effective blood volume to the production of hypertension in a given patient. For example, intravenous infusion of saralasin or a converting enzyme inhibitor will be followed by a decrease in blood pressure if the patient has a renin-dependent form of hypertension. The administration of a diuretic then reveals the contribution of the volume component in part but is masked by reactive hypereninemia caused by the administration of the diuretic. If the blocking compound is then given a second time, the contribution of effective blood volume can then be assessed.[153] These agents have been useful in identifying patients with renovascular hypertension.[163] Plasma renin activity has also been found to play a role in the antihypertensive effect of calcium channel blockers. Patients with low renin activity show a more pronounced decrease in blood pressure than patients whose renin activity is relatively high.[164]

Certain data have suggested that renin is an additional risk factor in the development of cardiovascular disease.[149] Thus, for a given level of blood pressure elevation, a patient with low renin activity would have less of a tendency to develop the cardiovascular complications of hypertension than does a patient with the same level of blood pressure but normal or high renin activity. This concept has not received confirmation and should not form the basis for a decision exempting patients with low renin hypertension from adequate therapy.

Despite the rational appeal of this renin-profile approach, the results are often disappointing.[156,165] Although pathophysiologic profiling of hypertensive subjects remains an interesting area for research, there is at present no compelling evidence that such a characterization is of significant help in routinely selecting therapy for patients with hypertension.

PROSTAGLANDINS AND HYPERTENSION

Contained within the cardiovascular system are several control points at which disorders of prostaglandin metabolism might contribute to alterations in blood pressure. As mentioned earlier, elevated blood pressure reflects a disturbed relation between cardiac output and peripheral vascular resistance, and patients with uncomplicated essential hypertension usually have a normal cardiac output and an elevated vascular resistance. The interplay of intrinsic and extrinsic factors in the control of resistance offers multiple sites for interactions with prostaglandins, which might result in a disturbance of blood pressure regulation by either an excess of prohypertensive factors or inadequate antihypertensive influences.

Total peripheral resistance is influenced by several blood-borne substances. For example, vasoconstriction can be affected by circulating angiotensin II or catecholamines. As prostaglandins function primarily as local hormones, they oppose the actions of circulating hormones by virtue of their synthesis at the site of action of the circulating hormone in vascular smooth muscle.

Another mechanism that affects vascular resistance is local release of norepinephrine from nerve endings, which results in vasoconstriction and is an important component of the overall integrated function of the central nervous system in circulatory control. Local production of PGE_2 influences vascular tone by interfering with release of norepinephrine from nerve endings.[166] Genetic or environmental influences that might impair local PGE_2 or PGI_2 production or hasten destruction of these compounds might play a role in the enhanced vascular reactivity known to occur in the earliest phases of essential hypertension.

There are three intrinsic mechanisms that are important in the regulation of vascular resistance[30]: basal vascular tone, the Bayliss effect,[31] and, perhaps most important relative to the production of prostaglandins, the influence of local tissue metabolites on vascular resistance. As tissue perfusion falls, oxygen delivery becomes inadequate, local adenosine triphosphate breakdown exceeds synthesis, and vasodilator substances accumulate. Which compound, if any, bears the greatest influence on local autoregulation has not been established. It is at this point that prostaglandins undoubtedly exert an important effect on overall circulatory regulation. Local production of PGI_2 and of PGE_2 would result in vasodilatation, whereas production of thromboxane and $PGF_{2\alpha}$ would contribute to vasoconstriction.

The other major component in the regulation of blood pressure is cardiac output. Young patients with labile hypertension often have a hyperkinetic circulation characterized by a high cardiac output.[34] Although this finding has been attributed to overactivity of the sympathetic nervous system, it is conceivable that deficient prostaglandin synthesis, or increased destruction, would remove their modulating effect on norepinephrine release, thus resulting in a higher heart rate, which could contribute to an increased cardiac output as well as an inadequate decrease in vascular resistance.

The prostaglandins are potentially important in regulating both myocardial preload and afterload. $PGF_{2\alpha}$ is a venoconstrictor,[167] increased production of which would result in increased venous return and a subsequent increase in cardiac output. The vasodilator effects of PGI_2 and PGE_2 would decrease afterload and might contribute to decreased preload by dilating veins. Conversely, the vasoconstrictor effect of $PGF_{2\alpha}$ and of thromboxane A_2 may increase both preload and afterload.

In experimental animals, prostaglandins have variable effects on myocardial contractility, depending on experimental conditions and species. Most studies have shown that prostaglandins of the E and A series increase cardiac output and have a positive inotropic effect.[168] In man, infusions of PGE_1 increase stroke volume and heart rate, thus increasing cardiac output. Conceivably, excess synthesis of prostaglandins of the E series could contribute to a hyperkinetic circulatory state which in turn could initiate a chain of events leading to hypertension.[169] Blood pressure also depends on the volume of blood contained within the vascular tree. A large body of evidence now exists linking renal prostaglandin metabolism to the regulation and distribution of renal blood flow.

Prostaglandins and Blood Vessels

The mechanisms by which prostaglandins influence peripheral vascular resistance fall into three general categories. The first is the direct vasodilating or vasoconstricting effects of locally synthesized prostaglandins,[170] eg, PGE_2, PGI_2, and $PGF_{2\alpha}$. The second mechanism is modulation of the actions of other vasoactive substances by locally synthesized compounds. For example, locally synthesized PGE_2 impairs release of norepinephrine from nerve terminals.[166] Third is by the indirect effects of prostaglandins synthesized elsewhere, eg, synthesis of PGE_2 is important in maintaining renal blood flow, particularly to the inner cortex and medulla.[171] Prostaglandins also play a role in salt and water excretion, in part by interfering with the action of ADH on the collecting tubules.[172] Prostaglandins synthesized in the kidney can influence total body sodium and water, thus influencing plasma and intracellular fluid volume and sodium balance and thereby the reactivity of vascular smooth muscle to pressor agents. Recent studies suggest that PGI_2 is released into the circulation from the pulmonary vascular bed.[173,174] Unlike other prostaglandins, PGI_2 is not destroyed on passage through the lungs[175,176] and could influence peripheral arteriolar tone.

Piper and Vane[177] reported that one or more substances released from guinea pig lung during anaphylaxis contracted the rabbit aorta. Later, it was found that indomethacin blocked the formation of "rabbit aorta contracting material" (RCS), suggesting that RCS might be related to a precursor of prostaglandins. The eventual discovery of the endoperoxides and their isolation in pure form enabled them to be distinguished from RCS by their longer half-life in aqueous solution. In a series of experiments involving the synthesis of prostaglandins in blood platelets, Hamberg and Samuelsson[178] found that endoperoxides within platelets are converted into a hemiacetal derivative with an oxane structure, plus malondialdehyde and a C_{17}-hydroxy acid (Figure 33.15). The first compound, now designated thromboxane B_2, is the breakdown product of A_2, an unstable intermediate. The TxA_2, formed in platelets and in other tissues subjected to injury, contributes to platelet aggregation and produces vasoconstriction.[179]

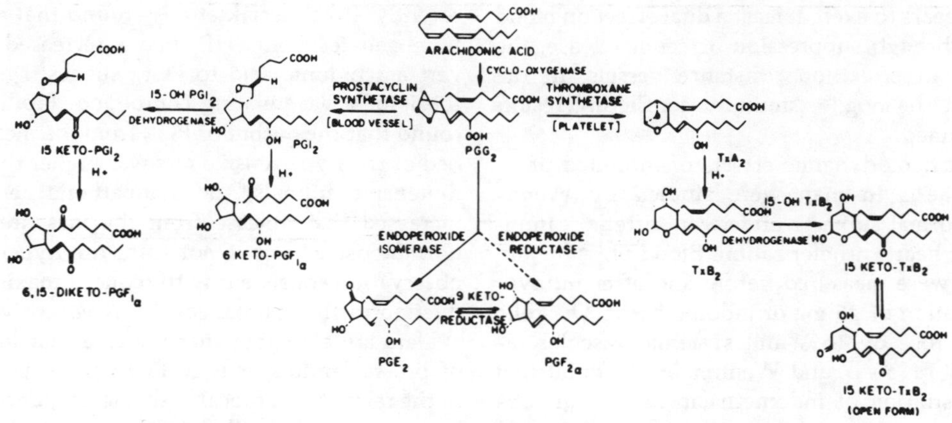

Figure 33.15. Metabolism of arachidonic acid by the prostaglandin synthetase complex. A major product of vascular tissues is prostacyclin (PGI_2) and a major product of blood platelets is thromboxane A_2 (TxA_2). (From Sullivan JM, McGiff JC: Kallikrein-kinin and prostaglandin systems in hypertension, in Rosenthal J [ed]: *Arterial Hypertension, Pathogenesis, Diagnosis and Therapy.* New York, Springer-Verlag, 1982, with permission.)

Bunting et al[180] demonstrated another unstable product of the transformation of the endoperoxides. The structure of this substance has been elucidated and the compound has been designated PGI_2 or prostacyclin (Figure 33.15). This compound, which is produced by blood vessels, has two important biologic effects, vasodilatation and inhibition of platelet aggregation. Moncada et al[181] demonstrated that vascular rings from human colic or gastric blood vessels can synthesize PGI_2, the veins producing more than the arteries. The effect occurs spontaneously but disappears with time or with washing of the specimens. Incubation of washed vascular tissue with arachidonate then restores production of prostacyclin. This production can be blocked in two ways: first, by the addition of indomethacin which, by inhibiting cyclooxygenase, prevents the conversion of arachidonic acid into endoperoxides, and second, by the addition of 15-hydroxy-peroxy-arachidonic acid, which blocks the conversion of endoperoxides to prostacyclin by inhibiting the prostacyclin synthetase step.

The addition of prostacyclin-synthesizing vascular rings to platelet-rich plasma inhibits platelet aggregation. It is possible that endothelial production of prostacyclin is the mechanism by which the body prevents thrombus formation throughout the healthy vascular tree. Vascular tissue, injured either by trauma such as abrupt elevation of blood pressure during a hypertensive crisis or by atherosclerosis, might not be able to synthesize prostacyclin adequately, thus allowing the deposition of platelets, formation of thrombi, and perhaps initiation or acceleration of atherosclerosis. It can also be postulated that failure to synthesize PGI_2 might result in elevated vascular resistance.

As noted previously, local synthesis of PGE_2 in the vessel wall can interfere with adrenergic transmission, primarily by inhibiting the release of norepinephrine from nerve terminals.[166] This would result in vasodilatation or at least diminished vasoconstriction, thus playing a potentially important role in local or systemic regulation of blood flow and pressure. In addition, local synthesis of PGE_2 and PGI_2 in vascular walls antagonizes the effect of both norepinephrine and angiotensin II and may play a role in angiotensin tachyphylaxis. Aiken[182] used femoral and celiac arterial strips to study the effects of angiotensin II. Doses repeated every 30 minutes continued to contract the femoral strips but had progressively less effect on the celiac artery strips. When inhibitors of cyclooxygenase were given, tachyphylaxis did not develop in the celiac strips. The addition of PGE_2 had no effect on the contraction of femoral arterial strips evoked by angiotensin II, but reduced its effect on the celiac arterial strips. The experiments of Aiken[182] suggested that angiotensin II can stimulate and release prostaglandins in the vascular wall, thus blunting its own vasoconstrictor effect, at least in the mesenteric vascular bed. Angiotensin II has been reported to stimulate the release of PGI_2 from the kidney,[183] the lung, blood vessels,[184] and the heart.[185] These observations may explain the loss of sensitivity to angiotensin II which takes place in normal pregnancy. Both PGE_2 and PGI_2 have been shown to attenuate the pressor responses to norepinephrine and to angiotensin II.[186] Thus, failure of an organ to synthesize adequate amounts of PGE_2 or PGI_2 in response to a pressor stimulus is a potential mechanism for the development of elevated vascular resistance and hypertension.[186]

Attempts have been made to produce hypertension by treating experimental animals with inhibitors of cyclooxygenase. These experiments have yielded conflicting results. Beilin and Bhattacharya[187] and Colina-Chourio et al[188] observed an elevation of blood pressure in rabbits treated with indomethacin, whereas Muirhead et al[189] did not. Romero and Strong[190] administered indomethacin to rabbits with one-clip, two-kidney renovascular hypertension and found no effect on blood pressure in rabbits with normal renal blood flow and normal plasma renin activity, whereas hypertension was aggravated in animals with low renal blood flow and elevated plasma renin activity. Although plasma renin activity initially fell in both groups, it did not remain suppressed in those animals whose blood pressure increased. Thus, in the rabbit, indomethacin appears to exert at least a dual effect on blood pressure, one through suppression of renin release, the other through an effect on resistance vessels. In the rat[191,192] and in the dog,[193] similarly conflicting results have been obtained.

The systemic hemodynamic effects of inhibited prostaglandin synthesis in man were studied by Wennmalm.[194] Six normal subjects underwent arterial cannulation and right heart catheterization. Blood pressure and cardiac output were measured before and after intravenous administration of 25 mg of indomethacin. Diastolic blood pressure rose by 16% and systemic vascular resistance by 49%. Nowak and Wennmalm[195] found that chronic administration of indomethacin in normal subjects results in a modest elevation of blood pressure, whereas other investigators have failed to produce such an elevation.[196] Patak et al[197] reported that indomethacin aggravated hypertension in man and antagonized the effects of furosemide. Durão et al[198] observed that indomethacin counteracted the antihypertensive effects of both pindolol and propranolol in seven hypertensive patients whose hypertension had previously been controlled by beta blockade. In view of current knowledge, several explanations are possible. Intravenous indomethacin might have prevented the formation of vascular PGE_2 or PGI_2, thereby allowing vasoconstriction to take place unimpeded by the modulating influence of the prostaglandins, or the inhibiting effects of PGE_2 on norepinephrine release might have been removed, allowing adrenergically induced vasoconstriction to take place. Another mechanism is suggested by the observations of De Jong et al,[199] who noted that indomethacin actually decreased blood pressure in two siblings with renin-dependent hypertension, while also decreasing plasma renin activity and plasma aldosterone concentration. These studies point to the important role of the prostaglandin system in the regulation of blood pressure in man. However, the conflicting reports indicate that the matter requires additional investigation.

With the information that blood vessels have the capacity to synthesize two compounds with potentially important antihypertensive effects, it is a logical step to apply the model of an enzyme deficiency disease and propose that hypertension might follow inadequate synthesis of either PGI_2 or PGE_2. However, when this hypothesis has been examined in spontaneously hypertensive animals or animals made hypertensive by renal artery constriction or DOCA-salt, the opposite was found to be the case, ie, while blood pressure was elevated, increased prostaglandin synthesis was found.

Rioux et al[200] studied the release of prostaglandin-like material from the aortas of normal rats, spontaneously hypertensive rats (SHR), and rats in whom hypertension had been induced by either renal artery constriction or the administration of DOCA and salt. Increased release of prostaglandins was observed in all three forms of hypertension. Furthermore, prostaglandin release returned to normal levels when hypertension was reversed in the latter group. Similarly, Limas and Limas[201] observed increased levels of prostaglandin synthetase activity in the microsomal fraction of the renal medulla of SHRs. More recently, Pace-Asciak et al[202] found that aortic rings and homogenates from SHRs had a decreased ability to convert arachidonic acid to PGI_2, suggesting impaired synthesis of a vasodilating compound. Pipili and Poyser[203] found that the output of PGI_2 from the mesenteric arterial bed of the hypertensive rats was higher than that of normotensive animals, and sympathetic nerve stimulation increased PGI_2 release from the mesenteric bed of the normotensive rat but not from the hypertensive rat, an observation consistent with reduced maximum PGI_2 production in the spontaneously hypertensive rat.

Data are emerging that indicate that local production of prostaglandins, mainly PGI_2, plays an important role in the regulation of local vascular resistance. Several studies have shown that blockade of prostaglandin synthesis in the kidney reduces the concentration of prostaglandin-like material in renal venous blood and decreases total renal blood flow.[204–206] Studies of the effect of blockade of prostaglandin synthesis on blood flow in extremities have yielded conflicting results. Aiken and Vane[205] found no significant increase in hindlimb vascular resistance in the dog hindlimb after treatment with indomethacin. However, Lonigro et al[206] and more recently Beaty and Donald[207] found that treatment with indomethacin or meclofenamate was followed by an increase in resting vascular resistance in the dog hindlimb. Beaty and Donald[207] further noted that blockade of prostaglandin synthesis had no effect on blood flow in the exercising hindlimb but did affect reactive hyperemia which progressively diminished the longer the vascular occlusion was maintained. This suggests that the local accumulation of metabolites during exercise or in tissues distal to a vascular occlusion was capable of overriding the relative vasoconstriction that occurred when prostaglandin synthesis was blocked.

Ishii et al[208] studied plasma levels of PG-6-keto-$F_{1\alpha}$, a breakdown product of PGI_2, in normal subjects and in patients with essential hypertension and compared the effect of intravenous infusions of norepinephrine on hemodynamics and PG-6-keto-$F_{1\alpha}$ levels. They found reduced levels of PG-6-keto-$F_{1\alpha}$ in the plasma of essential hypertensive patients. In response to norepinephrine, the normal subjects had an increase in both cardiac index and total peripheral resistance, whereas in patients with essential hypertension only cardiac output increased. Norepinephrine infusion resulted in an increase in plasma levels of PG-6-keto-$F_{1\alpha}$, which was greater in normal subjects than in patients with hypertension. Ishii et al concluded that prostaglandin metabolism was altered in patients with essential hypertension, resulting in impaired production of a vasodilating prostaglandin.

Chaignon et al[209] studied the effect of intravenous infusions of prostaglandin I_2 in patients with severe hypertension. Treatment with PGI_2 resulted in a decrease in mean blood pressure from 154 to 120 mm Hg and of total peripheral resistance of 45%. Concomitantly, cardiac index rose 40%. Plasma norepinephrine and plasma renin activity also increased during PGI_2 infusions. Measurements of blood volumes during PGI_2 infusions revealed a central translocation of blood. Thus, PGI_2 is an effective vasodilator that lowers blood pressure, but the antihypertensive effect is blunted by the increase in cardiac output.

Lima and Turner[210] studied the effect of prostacyclin on lymphocyte cyclic-AMP production before and after beta blockade with propranolol. They found that prior treatment with a beta-blocking agent significantly increased the amount of prostacyclin-induced cyclic-AMP production and suggested that prostaglandin causes vasodilatation of vascular beds during beta-adrenergic blockade, thus contributing to the antihypertensive effect.

The Blood Platelets and Prostaglandins

As knowledge of the pathways of prostaglandin metabolism has evolved, it has become apparent that compounds having different actions are synthesized from the same precursors in blood vessels and in blood platelets, and these products of the endoperoxides, TxA_2 of platelets and prostacyclin of vascular tissues, play counterbalancing roles (Figure 33.16). In the blood vessel wall, conversion of the cyclic endoperoxides into prostacyclin results in the formation of a product that prevents platelet aggregation and promotes vasodilatation.[181] Conversely, in the aggregating platelet the endoperoxides PGG_2 and PGH_2 are converted largely to TxA_2, a potent vasoconstrictor whose formation is associated with platelet aggregation. This compound, TxA_2, has a half-life in aqueous solution of only 30 seconds and is a vasoconstrictor.[179] Both aspirin and indomethacin inhibit cyclooxygenase activity, thus preventing the conversion of arachidonic acid to endoperoxides, and thereby their breakdown products, TxA_2, PGI_2, and PGE_2.

Despite TxA_2's potency as a vasoconstrictor, there is no evidence to date that this compound is present in circulating plasma or that enhanced release of thromboxane contributes to elevated vascular resistance in any experimental model. As mentioned previously, there is evidence that PGI_2 is released into the circulation after synthesis in the vasculature of the lung. Gryglewski et al[173] and Moncada et al[174] demonstrated that arterial blood contains an unstable disaggregating substance that enhances the effect of exogenous PGI_2 and that is present in greater amounts in arterial than in venous blood. Although this substance may serve to reduce platelet aggregation during turbulent flow in a high pressure system, impaired release might also be associated with increased vascular resistance. This area remains speculative, however, as vascular tissues have been reported to contain sufficient prostaglandin dehydrogenase activity to inactivate PGI_2 within the vessel wall.[211]

Whether or not PGI_2 functions as a circulating hormone remains a matter for additional investigation. Several observations support the conclusion that PGI_2 is released from the pulmonary endothelium into the pulmonary capillary circulation. Hensby et al[212] demonstrated higher concentrations of 6-oxo-$PGF_{1\alpha}$, a breakdown product of PGI_2, in the left ventricle than in the pulmonary arteries of five human subjects. Recent evidence supports the concept that a breakdown product of PGI_2 might mediate some of PGI_2's properties. Szczeklik et al[213] demonstrated that both blood pressure and platelet response to ADP were suppressed for one hour after inhalation of PGI_2,

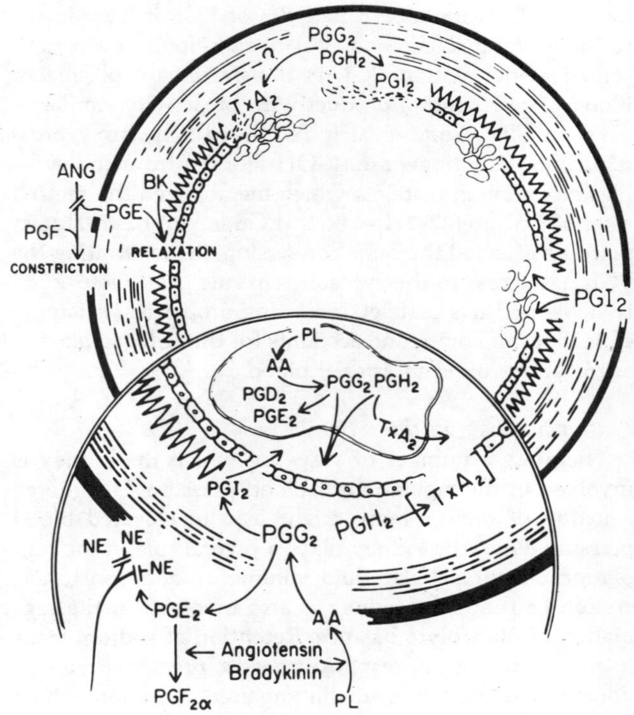

Figure 33.16. Cross-section of the vascular wall showing possible interactions of prostaglandins and vasoactive hormones. Magnification of the vascular wall, interfaced with blood and a circulating platelet, is shown at the lower portion of the figure. At the endothelial surface and the subendothelial zone of vascular tissues, the major product of arachidonic acid (AA) metabolism arising from tissue stores of phospholipids (PL) is prostacyclin (PGI_2). A major product of arachidonic acid metabolism within the aggregating platelet is thromboxane A_2 (TxA_2). Formation of TxA_2 within the vasculature may occur only under pathologic conditions. Angiotensin and bradykinin, which activate acylhydrolases within the vascular wall, promote prostaglandin synthesis. In addition to PGI_2, PGE_2 is a major product of arachidonic acid metabolism in the vascular wall. Its main function may be to modulate release of the adrenergic neurotransmitter, norepinephrine (NE). Further, PGE_2 may be converted to $PGF_{2\alpha}$ on activation of the enzyme PGE-9-ketoreductase by either angiotensin or bradykinin. Outside the area of magnification additional interactions of prostaglandins are shown. *On the right,* the formation of PGI_2 repels aggregating platelets. *At the top,* the failure of formation of PGI_2 in an area of damaged endothelium results in platelet aggregation, which may be related to the evolution of atherosclerosis. On injury of vascular tissues, formation of PGI_2 may be compromised and thromboxane A_2 formation, by both platelets and vascular tissue, may predominate (*top*). *On the left,* possible interactions of angiotensin (ANG) and bradykinin (BK) with prostaglandins are indicated: PGE_2 may contribute to the vasodilator effects of bradykinin (relaxation). In contrast, PGE_2 usually antagonizes the vasoconstrictor effect of angiotensin, whereas $PGF_{2\alpha}$ may facilitate this action of angiotensin. (Reproduced with permission from Sullivan JM, McGiff JC: Kallikrein-kinin and prostaglandin systems in hypertension, in Rosenthal J [ed]: *Arterial Hypertension, Pathogenesis, Diagnosis and Therapy.* New York, Springer-Verlag, 1982, with permission.)

far exceeding the known half-life of PGI_2 in blood, two to three minutes. Gimeno et al[214] and Hoult et al[215] presented evidence that PGI_2 is transferred by plasma or blood platelets into a product with bioactivity similar to 6-keto-PGE_1. Wong et al[216] recovered 9-hydroxy prostaglandin dehydrogenase (9-OH PGDH) from the cytoplasm of human platelets which metabolized the methyl ester of PGI_2 to (22-3H)-6-keto-PGE_1 methyl ester. Intact platelets effected the same conversion, demonstrating the PGI_2 has access to the cytosolic enzyme. As 6-keto-PGF_1 is stable and has platelet-inhibiting properties, it is possible that this compound accounts for the reduced platelet aggregation found in arterial blood.

Prostaglandins and the Kidney

There are a number of ways by which the kidney is involved in the regulation of blood pressure. Disordered function of one or more might lead to elevated blood pressure. First, the kidney plays a pivotal role in the regulation of extracellular fluid volume. In addition to excretion of fluid, the kidney is also involved in the regulation of electrolyte balance. Retention of sodium leads to enhanced vascular responsiveness to pressor stimuli.[217] Potassium depletion results in impaired dilatation, which in turn might lead to hypertension.[218] The kidney releases pressor substances that affect vascular resistance. Angiotensin I may function as a vasoconstricting agent within the kidney[219]; it is converted to the pressor angiotensin II primarily during passage across the lungs.[220] The kidney also produces antihypertensive substances, such as vasodepressor neutral lipids[221] and prostaglandins.[222]

As prostaglandins are involved in the regulation of renal function, evidence linking prostaglandin synthesis and degradation to hypertension has been sought. However, the evidence derived from experiments using surgically or pharmacologically induced hypertension in animals has questionable relevance to human hypertension, and studies of spontaneously hypertensive rats have yielded conflicting results. For example, Dunn[223] and Limas and Limas[201] found increased prostaglandin synthetase activity in the renal medullas of spontaneously hypertensive rats, whereas Pace-Asciak[224] and Limas and Limas[201] found decreased 15-prostaglandin dehydrogenase activity, which degrades prostaglandins, in the renal cortex of SHRs, and Stygles et al[225] found no change in renal PGE_2 production in the renomedullary tissues of SHRs, even after the development of hypertension. Ahnfelt-Ronne and Arrigoni-Martelli[226] found evidence of increased $PGF_{2\alpha}$ synthesis in the renal papillas of Wistar-Kyoto-Okamoto rats, whereas Armstrong et al[227] have not found this to be the case in New Zealand SHRs. In studies of human subjects with essential hypertension, Tan et al[228] found evidence of impaired renal production of prostaglandin E_2 which, through reduction of renal blood flow and retention of sodium and water, could result in elevated blood pressure.

Prostaglandins play a role in the regulation of renal blood flow, particularly when renal function is challenged.[229] McGiff et al[230] showed that antidiuresis and renal vasoconstriction evoked by angiotensin II were diminished by intrarenal release of PGE_2, the principal product of prostaglandin synthesis in the kidney that can attenuate the action of antidiuretic hormone.[172] Later, Aiken and Vane[205] showed that indomethacin administration resulted in enhanced vasoconstrictor effects of angiotensin II in the kidney.

Inhibition of prostaglandin cyclooxygenase results in reduction of all products formed downstream from this step (Figure 33.15). Not only is production of the vasodilator and natriuretic agent, PGE_2, diminished, but also that of the vasoconstrictor, $PGF_{2\alpha}$. Synthesis of PGI_2 and thromboxane A_2 is also inhibited.[180] Experiments using either indomethacin, meclofenamate, aspirin, ibuprofen, or other nonsteroidal antiinflammatory agents result in diminished production of all the products of arachidonic acid metabolism that have markedly different physiologic effects. Therefore, the effects of cyclooxygenase inhibitors on the renal circulation vary widely with experimental conditions. Indomethacin does not affect renal blood flow in either the anesthetized or conscious dog.[171] However, when the anesthetized dog is acutely stressed by laparotomy, a large increase in renal prostaglandin release occurs. Under these conditions, administration of indomethacin results in greatly increased renovascular resistance and a decrease in renal venous prostaglandin levels to those observed in the conscious dog. Any stress will increase prostaglandin release several-fold. This increase is associated with maintenance of renal blood flow at normal levels. When indomethacin is administered under these conditions, a precipitous decrease in renal blood flow results.

A prostaglandin-dependent mechanism is involved not only in the regulation of renal blood flow during stress, but also in the intrarenal distribution of blood flow. In studies using the isolated dog kidney, it has been shown that blood levels of PGE_2 correlated with increased fractional blood flow to the inner cortex, whereas indomethacin caused a disproportionate reduction of blood flow to the inner cortex, which resulted in a redistribution of renal blood flow.[231] A possible clinical correlation of these findings is the nephropathy of analgesic abuse. This condition has been suggested to be due to medullary ischemia secondary to reduced synthesis of one or more vasodilator prostaglandins. However, the capacity to synthesize prostaglandins is shared by a number of structures in all zones of the kidney. Larsson and Anggard[232] demonstrated synthesis of prostaglandins in the renal cortex. Cyclooxygenase is known to be present in three different tissues in the kidney. The interstitial cells of the renal medulla have the ability to synthesize prostaglandins,[221] as do the vascular structures of the kidney[233] and the cells lining the distal nephron and collecting ducts.[234] The latter location accords with the known interrelations between prostaglandins and ADH. ADH causes a greater concentration of urinary solute if given after treatment with indomethacin.[235] Thus, a prostaglandin of the E series blunts the effects of ADH[172] and favors the excretion of free water.[235]

Tobian et al[236] reported reduced levels of PGE_2 in the renal papillas of Dahl salt-sensitive rats and further noted that salt loading resulted in a lesser increase in PGE_2 than was observed in Dahl salt-resistant rats. By feeding Dahl

S rats a diet high in linoleic acid, a precursor of arachidonic acid, it was possible to restore renal PGE_2 levels to normal and prevent the sodium-related increase in blood pressure.

Interrelation of Prostaglandins and the Renin-Angiotensin System

There are complex interrelations of the prostaglandin and the renin-angiotensin-aldosterone systems. Infusion of angiotensin II results in release of renal prostaglandins.[230] Arachidonic acid, the precursor of renal prostaglandins, enhances renin release.[133] Indomethacin decreases plasma renin activity and prevents the effects of arachidonic acid. Indomethacin also prevents prostaglandin release in response to angiotensin. Thus, a prostaglandin mechanism appears to participate in the regulation of renin release, whereas generation of angiotensin after release of renin can in turn stimulate prostaglandin synthesis. Frolich et al[237] studied prostaglandin mechanisms in the regulation of plasma renin activity in man. They found that indomethacin administration is followed by diminished plasma renin activity, plasma aldosterone concentration, and urinary sodium and prostaglandin excretion in both normal and hypertensive subjects. As angiotensin infusion continues to stimulate aldosterone secretion after the administration of indomethacin, the effect of the latter compound on aldosterone secretion is due presumably to diminished generation of angiotensin. They have also noted that indomethacin prevents the immediate increase in plasma renin activity which ordinarily follows administration of furosemide. Indomethacin has two effects, which might explain these observations. First, it interferes with the synthesis of prostaglandins. Secondly, indomethacin causes sodium and fluid retention. Thus, the relative contribution of inhibition of prostaglandin synthesis and of sodium retention to the decrease in plasma renin activity that ordinarily follows indomethacin administration is not clear.

Weber et al[238] demonstrated that PGE_2, the principal product of renal prostaglandin synthesis, did not directly affect renin release from renal slices. However, a metabolic intermediate in the production of PGE_2, the endoperoxide PGG_2, was shown to increase renin release. These data suggest that inhibition of PGE_2 synthesis does not affect renin release directly; rather, suppression of prostaglandin endoperoxide synthesis, or one of its breakdown products, may be the determining factor. Whorton et al[239] demonstrated release of renin from rabbit renal cortical slices incubated with PGI_2. A linear response was observed over 30 minutes of incubation, which suggested that a breakdown product of PGI_2 might be involved, in view of the short half-life of PGI_2, in aqueous solution. However, the hydrolysis product of PGI_2, 6-keto-$PGF_{1\alpha}$, was not active. Hoult and Moore[240] subsequently found 9-hydroxy-prostaglandin dehydrogenase (9-OH PGDH) activity in the kidney, the product of which, 6-keto-PGE_1, is stable and was demonstrated to be a potent stimulator of renin release by Spokas et al.[241] Jackson et al[242] examined renin secretion rates after infusion of either PGI_2 or 6-keto-PGE_1 into the renal artery of the dog and found 6-keto-PGE_1 to be five times more potent than PGI_2.

The multiplicity of effects of indomethacin and other nonsteroidal antiinflammatory agents on arachidonic acid metabolism in the kidney must be recognized. The first step in prostaglandin synthesis is the release of arachidonic acid by the action of several phospholipases. The second is the cyclooxygenase step which leads to production of the cyclic endoperoxides. This step is inhibited by indomethacin and similar compounds. Downstream from generation of endoperoxides is the formation of a number of vasoactive products in different cellular elements within the kidney. Within the vascular wall, stimulation of cyclooxygenase results primarily in the production of PGI_2, a compound that prevents aggregation of platelets and causes vasodilatation.[233] Within the interstitial cells of the renal medulla, stimulation of the cyclooxygenase step results primarily in the production of PGE_2.[243] Within the collecting tubules, prostaglandin synthesis becomes intimately involved with the kallikrein-kinin system and with the antidiuretic hormone. Furthermore, these are products of the prostaglandin endoperoxides which require special conditions for their synthesis. Thus, thromboxane A_2, a potent vasoconstrictor, is synthesized in negligible quantities by the normal kidney. However, renal injury, eg, ureteral ligation, results in the synthesis of large amounts of thromboxane within the kidney.

It has been proposed that a deficiency in renal prostaglandin production is involved in the pathogenesis of essential hypertension. Campbell et al[244] investigated normotensive and hypertensive black and white women and found that sodium depletion resulted in increases in urinary $PGF_{2\alpha}$ and thromboxane B_2 production in normotensive subjects but not in hypertensive patients. Race and renin status also influenced prostaglandin $F_{2\alpha}$ excretion. The increase in urinary prostaglandin $F_{2\alpha}$ excretion was seen only in black and normal renin hypertensive patients and not in white or low renin hypertensive patients. With sodium loading, there were no consistent changes in excretion of any of the three compounds measured; however, urinary kallikrein excretion did rise with sodium intake. Thus, the only difference between hypertensive and normotensive subjects was an attenuation in the increase in excretion of prostaglandins that was ordinarily seen during sodium depletion.

Lebel and Grose[245] examined urinary excretion of prostaglandin E_2 and $F_{2\alpha}$ in normal and hypertensive subjects and found that 12% of hypertensive patients had extremely low levels of urinary prostaglandin E_2, but the average values for the normal and hypertensive patients were not significantly different. There was no relation between urinary prostaglandins and the level of blood pressure, plasma renin activity, or sodium excretion.

Ruilope et al[246] studied urinary prostaglandin E_2 excretion in normal subjects and hypertensive patients and found elevated prostaglandin E_2 excretion in normal renin essential hypertension, whereas patients with low renin essential hypertension excreted values lower than did normal subjects. In this study, plasma renin activity and urinary prostaglandin E_2 excretion were found to be significantly related. Indomethacin reduced excretion of PGE_2 in normal subjects and normal renin hypertensive subjects but not in low renin essential hypertensive subjects. In addition, indomethacin resulted in further increases in blood pressure in normal renin essential hypertensive patients.

Sato et al[247] studied the effect of dietary sodium intake on renal metabolism of prostaglandins and found that a low sodium intake increased urinary excretion of the main metabolites of prostaglandin $F_{2\alpha}$ but not of prostaglandin E or $F_{2\alpha}$ itself. A high sodium intake resulted in increased urinary excretion of prostaglandin E. Increasing dietary intake of potassium did not affect urinary excretion of prostaglandins.

Rathaus and Bernheim[248] studied the effect of propranolol on urinary excretion of prostaglandins E_2 and $F_{2\alpha}$ in normal subjects and patients with essential hypertension. They found that urinary excretion of prostaglandin E_2 increased significantly after propranolol, whereas that of prostaglandin $F_{2\alpha}$ did not change. After intravenous furosemide, treatment with propranolol resulted in an increased prostaglandin E_2 response. Prostaglandin $F_{2\alpha}$ increased in response to furosemide before propranolol treatment, but after beta blockade there was no effect.

THE KALLIKREIN-KININ SYSTEM

Interrelations of Prostaglandins and the Kallikrein-Kinin System

Bradykinin is a potent vasodilator peptide. When infused into the renal artery, it causes natriuresis and diuresis[249,250] which might be secondary to changes in renal blood flow. Two separate systems exist in man for the formation of kinins.[251] In plasma, prekallikrein, synthesized in the liver,[252] is acted on by prekallikrein activators to form active kallikrein. This proteolytic enzyme in turn acts on plasma kininogens to generate bradykinin. The active peptide is lysed by kininases in plasma and tissues.

The cells of the distal renal tubule synthesize urinary kallikrein.[253,254] In the distal segments of the nephron, this enzyme acts on kininogen to generate lysyl-bradykinin[253] which in turn is cleaved to form bradykinin by an aminopeptidase.[251] Although little bradykinin infused into the renal artery or proximal tubules is recovered in the urine,[255,256] bradykinin infused into the distal tubule is almost completely recovered.

Although the physiologic role of the kallikrein-kinin system remains incompletely understood, two facts appear to be well established: (1) Urinary kallikrein excretion is increased by sodium-retaining hormones which can be interpreted as evidence supporting a role of kinins in the regulation of salt and water balance.[257,258] (2) Interventions that alter extracellular fluid volume affect plasma renin activity and plasma bradykinin levels similarly.[258–261] A rise in bradykinin levels, at a time when angiotensin II levels are high, might serve to protect against excessive vasoconstriction during circumstances of salt depletion or volume loss. It can be further proposed that either excess activity of pressor elements in this balance or inadequate activity of vasodepressor elements can result in hypertension. Prostaglandins interact with both elements, reinforcing the activity of the kallikrein-kinin system and blunting the influence of the renin-angiotensin system.[262]

Kinins can be involved in the action of prostaglandins in several ways. Bradykinin activates a phospholipase[263] which releases arachidonic acid and leads to increased synthesis of prostaglandins.[264] Kinins also stimulate PGE-9-ketoreductase[265] which results in the conversion of PGE_2 to $PGF_{2\alpha}$.[170] These two actions may explain the venoconstrictor effect of the kinins.

Prostaglandins and kinins may also interact locally, within the tissue in which they are formed. The vasodilation evoked by bradykinin in vascular tissue is an example of modulation of the action of kinins by prostaglandins,[266] whereas the venoconstrictor effect of the kinins in mesenteric veins[170] and the actions of the kinins on urine concentration[267] are examples of prostaglandin release mediating the effects of kinins. Finally, the level of activity of the kallikrein-kinin system may influence the basal generation of prostaglandins, which contributes to the maintenance of normal blood flow in the kidney.[171,268]

Interrelations of the Renin-Angiotensin and Kallikrein-Kinin Systems

There are many similarities between the two systems (Figure 33.17). Both renin and kallikrein are proteolytic enzymes formed and stored within the kidney, both may be released by the autonomic nervous system, and both act on plasma globulins to release decapeptides, angiotensin I, and lysylbradykinin. Each decapeptide is converted to an octapeptide by angiotensin-converting enzyme or kininase II,[269] which profoundly affects its activity, angiotensin I undergoing conversion to angi-

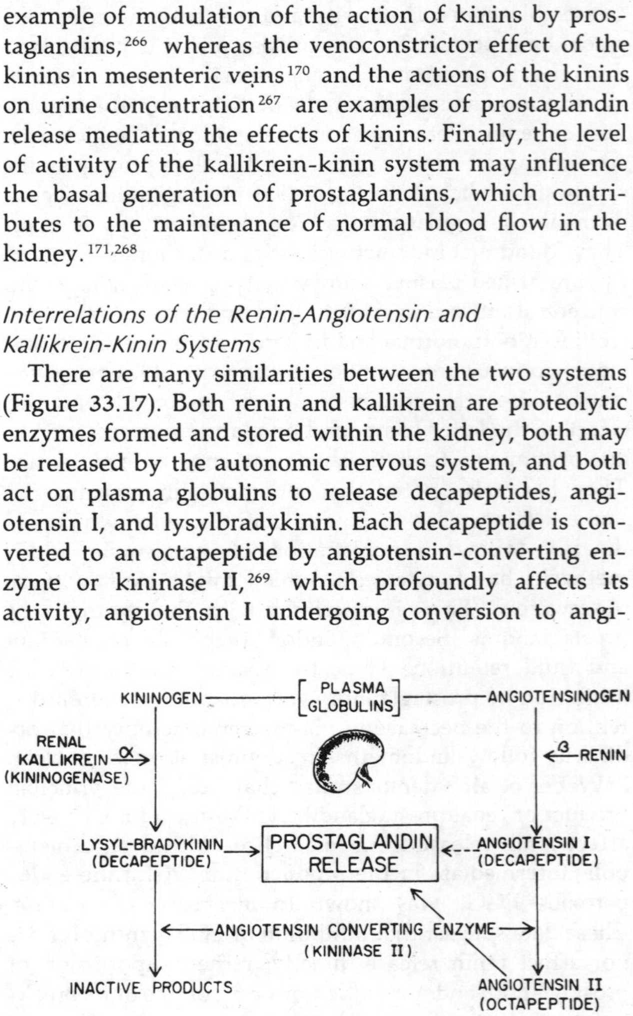

Figure 33.17. Comparison of the renal kallikrein-kinin and renin-angiotensin systems. The symbols α and β above the arrows proceeding from kallikrein and kinin, respectively, refer to adrenergic mechanisms that participate in the regulation of kallikrein (α) and renin (β) release. The major products of each system are capable of releasing prostaglandins. Angiotensin-converting enzyme, which increases the activity of the renin-angiotensin system by conversion of angiotensin I to the more active angiotensin II, correspondingly reduces the activity of the kallikrein-kinin system by degrading lysylbradykinin to inactive products. (Reproduced with permission from Sullivan JM, McGiff JC: Kallikrein-kinin and prostaglandin systems in hypertension. in Rosenthal J [ed]: *Arterial Hypertension, Pathogenesis, Diagnosis and Therapy*. New York, Springer-Verlag, 1982, pp 170–186.)

otensin II whereas bradykinin undergoes degradation.[270] Both bradykinin and angiotensin II release prostaglandins from several tissues, eg, infusion of either elevates renal venous prostaglandin concentrations to 10% to 50% above control levels.[222,271] The effector compounds in the two systems, angiotensin II and bradykinin, have opposite pressor effects, which may serve to balance one another. Several clinical studies have demonstrated parallel increases in the activity of the renin-angiotensin and kallikrein-kinin system[258,259] in response to stimuli that alter effective intravascular volume such as salt depletion and upright posture.

Kallikrein-Kinin System in Human Hypertension

Urinary excretion of kallikrein is decreased in human and experimental forms of hypertension.[272,273] The development of a radiochemical assay for urinary kallikrein[274] has made possible the application of this method to the study of large populations of hypertensive subjects and their families.[275,276] Many subjects with essential hypertension excrete less kallikrein than normotensive subjects and have decreased responsiveness to stimuli, which increases kallikrein excretion.[257] The lower secretory rates are found in hypertensive black subjects, although normotensive black subjects show decreased kallikrein excretion when compared with normal white subjects matched for age and sex.[275] These differences were not related to variations in urinary sodium and potassium excretion or volume.

Examination of the relations among urinary kallikrein, plasma renin activity, and renal blood flow suggests that a vasodilator system, the kallikrein-kinin-prostaglandin, participates in the regulation of vascular resistance in the kidney, together with the renin-angiotensin system. Decreased kallikrein excretion in the dog with renal arterial stenosis correlates with renal blood flow, not with changes in either urinary volume or sodium excretion.[277] Both vasoconstrictor and vasodilator agents can release renal kallikrein. The signal for kallikrein release is probably a change in transmural pressure, as blunting of kallikrein release has been reported after renal compliance was reduced by wrapping the kidney with latex.[278] A study of hypertensive patients with unilateral renal arterial stenosis provides additional evidence for depressed activity of the kallikrein-kinin system in the ischemic kidney, and an inverse relation between the activities of the renin-angiotensin and kallikrein-kinin systems.[279] In this study, plasma renin activity was elevated and kinin levels were depressed in the venous effluent of the diseased kidney, whereas the reverse obtained for the contralateral kidney.

Studies of kallikrein excretion in hypertension have made important contributions to our understanding of the pathogenesis and inheritance of hypertension.[280] Decreased urinary concentration of kallikrein has been shown in both black children and black adults. As these children were not clinically hypertensive, a relation was sought between urinary kallikrein and the level of blood pressure within these families. Both diastolic and systolic blood pressures in the families with the lowest urinary kallikrein concentrations were significantly higher than those in families showing the highest urinary kallikrein concentrations. The measurements were repeated three years later in the same population, confirming the original results.[276] These studies support the hypothesis that a deficiency of the kallikrein-kinin system contributes to the development of high blood pressure in a susceptible population.

O'Connor[281] studied urinary kallikrein activity in patients with essential hypertension treated with propranolol and found that this beta-blocking agent diminished urinary kallikrein excretion at the same time that renal blood flow and blood pressure were reduced. However, the change in renal blood flow did not correlate with the change in kallikrein excretion. O'Connor et al[282] also studied urinary kallikrein excretion after renal transplantation and found that urinary kallikrein appeared to originate in the transplanted kidney. Urinary excretion of kallikrein was lower in hypertensive transplant recipients than in normotensive subjects. Patients in whom acute tubular necrosis or rejection developed also excreted less kallikrein than did those in whom it did not.

Saruta and Kondo[283] studied urinary kallikrein excretion and other endocrine factors in young patients with essential hypertension. Most of these individuals had normal plasma renin activity. However, when subjects were grouped into low, normal, and high renin groups, urinary excretion of kallikrein was increased in the high renin group and reduced in the low renin group.

The major exception to the conclusion that hypertension is usually associated with deficient kallikrein excretion is mineralocorticoid-induced hypertension[284]; aldosteronism is associated with increased excretion of kallikrein. Kallikrein excretion is also elevated in normotensive subjects when mineralocorticoid activity is augmented by administration of sodium-retaining steroids or sodium restriction. The demonstration that elevated kallikrein excretion, induced by a low sodium diet, can be decreased by spironolactone led to the proposal that the concentration of mineralocorticoids determines the rate of kallikrein excretion.[284] An alternative explanation is that a consequence of elevated mineralocorticoid activity, such as increased potassium excretion, may play a role in increasing kallikrein-kinin activity. Urinary kallikrein concentration has been positively correlated with potassium excretion[280] but not with sodium excretion. Decreased extracellular potassium, resulting from increased excretion, may result in enhanced renal prostaglandin synthesis, which may augment the activity of the renal kallikrein-kinin system. Changes in extracellular potassium concentration can affect renal prostaglandin synthesis,[243,285] which in turn affects kallikrein release or kinin generation or both, perhaps by operating through a kallikrein-releasing mechanism similar to the prostaglandin mechanism that regulates renin release.[286]

The relation between sodium excretion and the activity of the renal kallikrein-kinin system is uncertain. The intrarenal kinin levels may be of greater importance than kallikrein excretion. In most of the studies that addressed the effects of altered activity of the renal kallikrein-kinin system on salt and water excretion, changes in kallikrein excretion were measured rather than changes in kinin levels. However, Marin-Grez et al[287] measured changes in urinary kallikrein excretion and kinin levels in caval blood of the dog in response to acute expansion of extracellular fluid volume induced by sodium. They found a positive correlation between changes in blood levels of kinins of renal origin and changes in sodium excretion induced by saline administration. Three studies suggest that the renal kallikrein-kinin system, perhaps in concert with renal prostaglandins, participates in regulating sodium chloride excretion. First, Nasjletti et al[288] demonstrated a relation between the transient decrease in urinary sodium in the conscious rat produced by the kallikrein inhibitor, aprotinin, and the immediate reduction in PGE excretion. Secondly, in the dog, enhancement of the activity of the renal kallikrein-kinin system by inhibition of the degradative enzyme, kininase II, was associated with natriuresis.[255] Thirdly, in the rat, antibodies of bradykinin have been shown to attenuate the enhanced excretion of sodium chloride in response to acute isotonic saline loading.[289]

As changes in kinin generation have profound effects on prostaglandin levels within the kidney,[290] and as prostaglandins may contribute to the effects of kinins on salt and water excretion,[267] prostaglandins should be measured simultaneously with the components of the kallikrein-kinin system to assess the effects of changes in either on salt and water excretion. In view of the wide distribution of prostaglandin-synthesizing enzymes among the cellular elements of the kidney,[234] it is important to recognize that compartmentalization of kinin and prostaglandin metabolism may have important consequences for renal function. The functional result of the interactions of the renal kallikrein-kinin and prostaglandin systems may be restricted to the urinary compartment. Entry of kallikrein into the distal tubules[291] and subsequent formation of kinin then may result in kinin-mediated generation of prostaglandins in the distal nephron and collecting ducts, the latter affecting the excretion of free water.[267] A study by Weber et al[292] indicates that a major prostaglandin-metabolizing enzyme, PGE-9-ketoreductase, which converts PGE_2 to $PGF_{2\alpha}$, is influenced by sodium balance. Thus, retention of a water load and conservation of sodium are facilitated by increased activity of this enzyme, which lowers levels of PGE_2 intrarenally by favoring formation of $PGF_{2\alpha}$. As prostaglandins of the E series inhibit ADH activity,[172] their conversion to PGF facilitates reabsorption of water. Kinins can also influence PGE-9-ketoreductase activity.[265] This interaction may explain the effects of kinins on free water generation. When prostaglandins are released through the actions of kinins, free water is generated if PGE_2 is the principal product, whereas when $PGF_{2\alpha}$ is released in response to kinin, water conservation occurs. The activity of PGE-9-ketoreductase, modified by kinins, may be a function of the state of sodium chloride balance. It is here that a hypertensive mechanism may be operative; deficient intrarenal generation of kinins or prostaglandins in response to salt intake may result in inappropriate expansion of extracellular fluid volume, a recognized factor in the pathogenesis of hypertension.[45]

Although the physiologic role of the kallikrein-kinin system in the kidney has not been proved, it appears to be related to renovascular dilatation and natriuresis. Both kallikrein and kinin are excreted in the urine but not always in relation to each other. The excretion of kallikrein is influenced by changes in activity of the renin-angiotensin-aldosterone system as well as by changes in diet. Hypertension appears to reduce kallikrein excretion, particularly renal parenchymal hypertension. Kallikrein excretion rises when dietary sodium is restricted. Similarly, kallikrein excretion rises when thiazide diuretics are administered.[293] O'Connor[293] found that individuals who respond to thiazides have a greater increase in urinary kallikrein excretion than do those who failed to respond, which suggests that the renal kallikreins may be involved in the antihypertensive effects of thiazide diuretics.

VASODEPRESSOR LIPIDS

Recent research suggests that the kidney influences blood pressure in yet another way, through the release of vasodepressor lipids. Muirhead[294] showed that interstitial cells from the renal medulla grown in tissue culture elaborate lipid compounds that result in a reduction in arterial pressure. It has been shown that transplanted renal medullary tissue from normotensive animals will protect against the development of renoprival, one-kidney, one-clip, sodium-overload hypertension and genetic hypertension.[295] However, transplants of renocortical tissue or other nonrenal tissues do not have the same protective effect. Renal interstitial cells, grown in tissue culture, have been transplanted and also found to protect against the development of hypertension.[296] Tobian et al,[297] Manthorpe,[298] and Susic et al[299] have confirmed this antihypertensive function of the kidney. Gothberg et al[300] published data suggesting that the release of vasodepressor lipids is responsible for a rapid decrease in blood pressure in rats with two-kidney, one-clip hypertension after removal of the clip.

Muirhead et al[301] distinguished two types of antihypertensive medullary lipids which differ in solubility and chromatographic behavior. One is a highly polar glycerophospholipid which has been designated antihypertensive polar renal medullary lipid. The other, antihypertensive neutral medullary lipid, differs from the former in that it does not require chemical reduction to become biologically active. Both compounds, given intravenously, decrease blood pressure. The antihypertensive polar renal medullary lipid, when given intravenously to hypertensive rats, decreased peripheral vascular resistance. The antihypertensive neutral renal medullary lipid lowers blood pressure while reducing heart rate and increasing efferent renal nerve activity, which suggests that a central nervous system action is involved in the antihypertensive effect of this compound. Faber et al[302] recently studied the regional hemodynamic effects of both antihypertensive renal medullary lipids in conscious rats. Both compounds were given both intravenously and into the central nervous system of rats with and without sinoaortic deafferentation. The results suggested that neither lipid had an effect mediated through the central nervous system. Nonetheless, both lipids were again shown to be potent vasodepressor agents. The antihypertensive polar renal medullary lipid was found to have potent peripheral vasodilatory effects and also reduced the response to vasoconstrictor agents.

These observations have led Muirhead[303] to propose that a deficiency in elaboration of antihypertensive radiomedullary lipids plays a role, perhaps permissive, in the development of hypertension.

MANAGEMENT OF THE HYPERTENSIVE PATIENT

RATIONALE FOR TREATMENT

The long-term goal in the treatment of hypertension is to prevent the premature development of cardiovascular disease. The complications of hypertension can be divided into those due solely to elevated blood pressure per se: further progression of hypertension, renal failure, hemorrhagic stroke, congestive heart failure, and dissecting aneurysm. Other complications are related to the accelerated atherosclerosis associated with hypertension: acute myocardial infarction, atherothrombotic cerebral infarction, and intermittent claudication. Even patients with minimal blood pressure elevation are subject to the development of these atheromatous complications.[11]

In the 1950s, it was found that pharmacologic reduction of blood pressure prevented the development of necrotic and sclerotic changes in the arterioles of animals with experimental hypertension.[304] In the clinic, it soon became evident that patients with malignant hypertension benefited from therapy.[305,306] Improved prognosis was limited by the presence of renal damage or underlying renal parenchymal disease. Patients with severely reduced renal function due to advanced nephrosclerosis, that is, endogenous creatinine clearance less than 45 ml per minute and estimated renal plasma flow less than 150 ml per minute, did not do as well even with treatment. Only 4 of 15 patients with lower clearance were alive one year after the initiation of therapy, whereas 8 of 11 patients with clearance higher than 45 ml per minute were alive one year after beginning therapy.[307] Although it soon became apparent that patients with accelerated or malignant hypertension benefited from treatment, it was not known whether patients with diastolic blood pressures between 90 and 129 mm Hg had anything to gain from the expense and inconvenience of chronic antihypertensive therapy or whether risks of therapy outweighed the benefits of lowering blood pressure. In 1964, Hamilton et al[308] reported the results of an eight-year prospective study which found that only 4% of an effectively treated group of hypertensive subjects developed the complications of hypertension. In 1966, Wolff and Lindeman[309] reported a controlled two-year study of 87 patients, which also showed only 33% as many cardiovascular complications in a treated group as in a group receiving placebo.

A landmark investigation of this problem was the Veterans Administration Cooperative Study of Antihypertensive Agents.[310,311] In this project, male veterans were hospitalized for evaluation. Those with diastolic blood pressures above 129 mm Hg, those with secondary hypertension, and those whose blood pressures dropped beneath 90 mm Hg without therapy were excluded from the study. Patients who already had evidence of cardiovascular complications were included in the trial. After a placebo lead-in period, the patients were randomized blindly into two groups. One group received placebo and the other group received hydrochlorothiazide, reserpine, and hydralazine added stepwise as needed to control blood pressure.

It soon became apparent that complications were developing rapidly in the subgroup of patients with the highest blood pressures. As a result, the 143 patients who entered the study with diastolic blood pressures between 115 and 129 mm Hg were analyzed after a period of about 20 months (Table 33.5). Analysis of events in the untreated group showed that several patients had developed advanced grades of retinopathy, accelerated hypertension, renal failure, dissecting aneurysm, retinopathy with congestive heart failure, strokes, sudden death, and myocardial infarction. In contrast, one patient in the treated group developed a drug reaction and one patient had a minor stroke. The difference between the two groups was highly significant, and it was proved that antihypertensive therapy benefited male patients with diastolic blood pressures between 115 and 129 mm Hg.

There remained a subgroup of 380 patients who had entered the study with average, resting diastolic pressures between 90 and 114 mm Hg during the initial hospitalization. These patients were followed for as long as five years, with an average follow-up of 3.3 years. There were 35 terminating morbid events in the control group as opposed to 9 in the treated group; 21 nonterminating cardiovascular events in the control group as opposed to 13 in the treated group; and 20 instances of accelerated hypertension in the control group as opposed to none in the treated group (Table 33.6). The fatalities consisted of seven strokes in the control group and none in the treated group; three myocardial infarctions in the control group and two in the treated group; eight instances of sudden death in the control group as opposed to four in the treated group; and one instance of ruptured arteriosclerotic aneurysm in the treated group. There was a significant reduction of nonfatal strokes and congestive heart failure in the treated group, but the incidence of coronary heart disease did not differ significantly between the two groups.

Table 33.5. Incidence of Mortality and Morbidity*

	Placebo-Treated Patients	Actively Treated Patients
Deaths	4	0
Class A events	10	0
Subtotal	14	0
Other treatment failure	7	1
Total terminating events	21	1
Class B events (nonterminating)	6	1
Total	27	2

* From Veterans Administration Cooperative Study Group on Antihypertensive Agents: Effects of treatment on morbidity pressures in hypertension. Results in patients with diastolic blood pressures averaging 115 through 129 mm Hg. *JAMA* 1967; 202:1028–1034.

Table 33.6. Causes of Death and other Terminating Morbid Events*

Cause	Control Group	Treated Group
Deaths due to class A events†		
Cerebrovascular hemorrhage	3	0
Subarachnoid hemorrhage	1	0
Dissecting aneurysm	1	0
Deaths due to class B events†		
Myocardial infarction	3	2
Sudden death	8	4
Cerebrovascular thrombosis	3	1
Ruptured atherosclerotic aneurysm	0	1
Total related deaths‡	19	8
Terminating morbid events other than death		
Class A events		
Uncontrolled cardiac failure	5	0
Dissecting aortic aneurysm	1	0
Subarachnoid hemorrhage	1	0
Fundi, striate hemorrhages	1	0
Acute hypertensive encephalopathy	1	0
Subtotal	9	0
Treatment failures		
Cerebrovascular thrombosis, severe	4	0
Progressive azotemia	1	0
Fundi, one striate hemorrhage and ? early papilledema	1	0
Fundi, one striate hemorrhage and ? encephalopathy	1	0
Hypotension	0	1
Subtotal	7	1
Total	16	1

* From the Veterans Administration Cooperative Study Group on Antihypertensive Agents: Effects of treatment on morbidity in hypertension. II. Results in patients with diastolic pressure averaging 90 through 114 mm Hg, *JAMA* 1970; 213:1143–1152.

† Class A events refer to hypertensive complications; class B events refer to atherosclerotic complications.

‡ Does not include four unrelated deaths, two in the control group and two in the treated group.

Analyzing the data from the subgroup of patients with diastolic blood pressures between 90 and 114 mm Hg, it was found that the risk of developing a morbid cardiovascular event during a five-year period was reduced from 55% in the group receiving a placebo to only 18% in the group on active treatment.[312] The difference between the treated and untreated group was statistically significant for patients with initial diastolic blood pressures of 105 mm Hg or more. For those patients who entered the trial with lower pressures, the risk of developing a cardiovascular event was not as great and the benefit from antihypertensive therapy was not as marked, although the patients in this subgroup also appeared to benefit from treatment. In no instance did it appear that antihypertensive therapy increased morbidity or mortality and indeed this study suggests that long-term antihypertensive therapy is relatively benign.

The Veterans Administration study established that treatment of male patients with a diastolic blood pressures above 105 mm Hg conveys significant benefit to the patient. Women were not studied. Thus, there was no proof that they would benefit equally from therapy. Physicians remained cautious about applying the results of this trial for several reasons. The starting blood pressures were defined as the average of the resting diastolic pressures from the fourth through the sixth day of hospitalization. Patients with significant levels of diastolic hypertension, when placed in the hospital, often became normotensive or nearly so by the fourth day. Thus, those patients participating in the Veterans Administration study probably had more sustained hypertension. Secondly, although patients with mild blood pressure elevation are at risk of developing cardiovascular damage, they have less risk than patients with higher levels of blood pressure. The Veterans Administration study showed that patients with levels of diastolic blood pressure between 90 and 104 mm Hg benefited less from antihypertensive therapy than their counterparts with higher blood pressures. Thus, when treating patients with mild elevations of blood pressure, it was advisable to weigh the limited benefit of therapy against the greater inconvenience, greater expense, and greater risk of side effects from antihypertensive therapy. The risk–benefit ratio in this group did not appear to be as favorable as it was in those individuals who had persistent diastolic blood pressures above 105 mm Hg.

Considering the data from the Build and Blood Pressure Study of 1959, from Framingham, from the Veterans Administration study, and from other sources, many authorities at the time conservatively recommended that patients with sustained diastolic blood pressures between 90 and 104 mm Hg receive treatment on an individualized basis. A very important factor in reaching a decision to prescribe antihypertensive medications for such patients was the presence or absence of additional cardiovascular risk factors. As these factors appear to be additive, a patient with a slight risk imposed by a minor elevation of blood pressure has a much greater chance of developing cardiovascular disease if he or she also smokes cigarettes or has diabetes mellitus, elevated serum cholesterol, or a family history of premature cardiovascular disease. In such a case, an attempt should be made to reduce as many risk factors as possible including the mildly elevated blood pressure.

The results of the Veterans Administration study have been extended in an important way by the recent findings of the Hypertension Detection and Follow-up Program (HDFP), a five-year, 14-center study involving 10,900 patients, which provided the first convincing evidence that mortality in patients with a diastolic blood pressures of 90 to 104 mm Hg was reduced by effective antihypertensive therapy.[313]

The participants in HDFP ranged in age from 30 to 69 years and included both males and females. Over 70% of the cohort had diastolic blood pressures between 90 and 104 mm Hg. The patients were stratified on the basis of age, sex, race, organ involvement, and prior treatment history and randomized into one of two groups. One group received treatment from their usual source of medical care, the other received intensive antihypertensive therapy at special centers where free medications were given, waiting time was short, extensive patient education measures used, and lost patients retrieved. Stepped-care therapy was used in the centers, consisting of thiazide diuretic, with the addition of reserpine, methyldopa, or, less frequently, propranolol, if needed. Hydralazine and then guanethidine were added in sequence if goal blood pressure had not been reached. The therapeutic goal of the centers was to lower diastolic blood pressure to levels beneath 90 mm Hg or by 10 mm Hg, whichever was lower. By the end of five years, the goal had been achieved in 64.9% of the center care patients and in 43.6% of the referred care group. Thus, both groups received antihypertensive treatment. The difference lay in the degree of effectiveness. Although the average starting diastolic blood pressure was about 101 mm Hg in both groups, after five years blood pressure had fallen to 84.1 mm Hg in the center-care group, while falling to only 89.1 mm Hg in the referred care patients. Mortality from all causes was 17% lower in the center-care group, 20% lower in patients whose pretreatment diastolic pressure was 90 to 104 mm Hg. The difference was highly significant ($P < .01$). Similarly, effective treatment decreased death from cerebrovascular disease by 45% and from acute myocardial infarction by 46%. It should be noted that most other studies have not observed a reduction of myocardial infarction with antihypertensive therapy. Overall, there was a 15% reduction in the death rate from ischemic heart disease in the center-care group.

Similarly, an Australian trial of therapy in 3,427 patients with mild hypertension has demonstrated a beneficial effect of treatment of individuals whose pretreatment diastolic blood pressure ranged between 95 and 109 mm Hg.[314] In this trial, mortality from cardiovascular disease was reduced by two thirds over a four-year period. A somewhat similar result was reported more recently by the European Working Party on High Blood Pressure in the Elderly.[314a] Both of these trials included a blinded control group treated with placebo, which makes their conclusions particularly convincing. The existence of the placebo group made possible the interesting and important observation that fully 45% of placebo-treated Australian patients experienced a decrease in diastolic pressure to levels beneath 95 mm Hg over a three-year period, suggesting that patients with mild hypertension can be followed for a time while intake of sodium and calories is reduced and levels of exercise increased before a decision is reached regarding the use of antihypertensive drugs.

Thus, there is now strong evidence to support decreasing of blood pressure in asymptomatic individuals with diastolic blood pressures between 90 to 95 and 104 mm Hg, even if they are free of end organ damage and even if they are relatively old (some of the participants in HDFP were 74 at its conclusion). For those individuals with deceptively "mild" hypertension, treatment might appropriately begin with weight reduction, salt restriction, and regular exercise with pharmacologic agents added when these measures are unsuccessful.

BORDERLINE HYPERTENSION

The criteria for entry into the Veterans Administration study and the Hypertension Detection and Follow-up Program and the Australian Trial required sustained diastolic hypertension. As a result, we have no firm data to prove that therapy of labile or borderline hypertension ultimately benefits the patient, although we do have information suggesting that borderline hypertension places the patient at risk.

A diagnosis of borderline hypertension creates both diagnostic and therapeutic problems. A patient can have transient elevation of blood pressure to levels above 140/90 mm Hg if in pain or discomfort or if anxious. It is necessary to determine how often elevation of blood pressure occurs. Frequent determinations over a period of three to six months can help resolve the question. Checking the pressure after rest, and having a nonphysician or family member check the pressure at home may give information about whether the patient's pressure has returned to normal or whether it is fluctuating around a mildly elevated average.

Data from the Society of Actuaries suggests that even mildly elevated casual blood pressure is associated with increased risk.[11] The group with mild elevation of blood pressure had shortened longevity and was composed of patients with both fixed and labile hypertension. The findings of the Framingham study were also based on casual blood pressure determinations and did not separate persons with mild fixed hypertension from those with mild labile hypertension. However, when the Framingham data were analyzed to assess the impact of lability, it was found that for any given average pressure, the degree of variability of the pressure did not affect the risk of cardiovascular event.[315] Thus, it is the average pressure around which repeated readings vary that determines risk.

Borderline hypertension can follow several courses: some return to normal blood pressure levels, some continue to have labile blood pressure elevations, and others develop fixed hypertension.[316] The discovery of borderline hypertension demands that the patient continue to be under medical surveillance so that the shortest possible time will elapse between the possible later development of fixed elevation of blood pressure and the initiation of effective antihypertensive therapy. Some authorities advocate the initiation of antihypertensives for most patients with borderline hypertension, since they are likely to develop fixed hypertension and early therapy might avoid years of slowly progressive target organ damage. However, as yet there has not been a controlled study demonstrating that antihypertensive therapy of borderline hypertension has any benefit.

Virtually all available antihypertensive agents serve to decrease pressure in patients with mild, transient elevation. Such patients respond to diuretic therapy. Because hemodynamic studies in some of these patients show a hyperkinetic circulation, they have been treated successfully with beta-adrenergic receptor blocking agents and can often respond to very low doses.[317] However, before deciding to treat, efforts must be made to evaluate the degree of risk faced by a patient with borderline hypertension, that is, the degree, frequency, and duration of pressure elevation. Hypertensive damage is increased by the presence of other risk factors, and attention must be paid to use of cigarettes, family history, blood lipid levels, and glucose intolerance. When several risk factors are present, therapeutic intervention appears to be reasonable.

SYSTOLIC HYPERTENSION

Isolated systolic hypertension (greater than 160 mm Hg) is often seen in older patients. Ejection of blood from the left ventricle into a rigid aorta causes a wide pulse pressure and an elevated systolic pressure. A few patients with elevated systolic pressure have disorders associated with high cardiac output, such as thyrotoxicosis, anemia, or arteriovenous fistulas. Because systolic hypertension is thought to reflect underlying atherosclerosis, it has not been an indication for antihypertensive therapy. However, in the Build and Blood Pressure Study, mortality increased with each increment of systolic pressure at any given level of diastolic pressure for both men and women regardless of age.[10]

Multivariate analysis of the data from Framingham also shows that systolic blood pressure correlates with the risk of coronary heart disease even better than diastolic or mean pressure. This observation applied equally to men and women over 45; however, diastolic pressure seemed to be the strongest determinant of risk in younger men.[318]

In a study of older patients with isolated systolic hypertension, Colandrea et al[319] found an increased incidence of coronary artery disease, strokes, and overall mortality during an eight-month period of observation. However, many patients with systolic pressure elevation also had diabetes mellitus, so the systolic hypertension might have been a reflection of increased susceptibility to vascular damage or of the presence of atherosclerosis in the elderly. The possibility exists that systolic hypertension, even though caused by atherosclerosis, may still act to further accelerate atherosclerosis, precipitate congestive heart failure, and thus contribute to morbidity and mortality. At present, we can conclude that such patients are at risk and reach decisions regarding antihypertensive therapy on an individual basis. However, when elderly patients are treated, antihypertensive agents should be started at a low dose and increased gradually with careful monitoring. A clinical trial is underway to determine the desirability and feasibility of drug therapy for isolated systolic hypertension in the elderly.

THERAPEUTIC GOALS

There is no clear dividing line between normal and elevated blood pressure. The lower the blood pressure, the lower the risk of cardiovascular disease. There is no absolute goal in blood pressure, but rather one that must be individualized for each patient. Based on the results of the Veterans Administration studies,[310,311] the Australian Trial of Mild Hypertension,[312] and the HDFP,[313] the Joint National Committee on Detection, Evaluation and Treatment of High Blood Pressure in its 1984 report (JNC III)[320] has recommended that individuals under 60 with diastolic pressures of 95 mm Hg or more have pharmacologic therapy if necessary, whereas those with diastolic pressures between 90 and 94 mm Hg, if otherwise at low risk, undergo careful follow-up with nonpharmacologic therapy. If pressures remain above 90 mm Hg despite nonpharmacologic measures, and risk factors such as male sex, cigarette smoking, diabetes, or hypercholesterolemia are present, the HDFP data suggest that the benefit of drug therapy outweighs the known risks. The JNC III advises that, "The initial goal of antihypertensive therapy is to achieve and maintain diastolic pressures at lower than 90 mm Hg if feasible. A reasonable further goal is the lowest diastolic pressure consistent with safety and tolerance."

When compared with a group treated until an average diastolic pressure of about 90 mm Hg was obtained, the results of the HDFP suggest that patients have fewer cardiovascular complications when diastolic pressures are lowered to 85 mm Hg or less. Thus, the HDFP has changed not only our indications for administering antihypertensive therapy, but also our therapeutic goals.

Reaching an ideal blood pressure must be weighed against the side effects of the drugs required to reach that goal. Persons can have blood pressure reduced to 140/90 mm Hg on relatively moderate doses of medications and may be entirely free of side effects. Yet, when medications are increased in an attempt to lower the pressure further, the patient may be unacceptably sleepy or fatigued and may find that the medications are interfering with the quality of life. Here, the physician must use skill to match medication to patient, and judgment in measuring other risk factors to assess how much danger the remaining minor elevation of blood pressure poses for the patient. If untoward effects occur that cannot be tolerated or avoided by changing antihypertensive agents, a compromise must be made. Data from the Veterans Administration study suggest that even partial blood pressure control is beneficial.[321]

When arteriosclerosis narrows a blood vessel, flow across the stenosis depends on perfusion pressure. If arterial pressure falls, perfusion of the area distal to the lesion decreases. In the brain, this leads to symptoms of cerebrovascular insufficiency; in the heart, to angina pectoris; in the extremities, to claudication; and in the kidneys, to diminished renal function. In a patient with a history, physical findings, or laboratory tests that suggest the presence of underlying vascular disease, blood pressure must be decreased carefully, while looking for evidence of potentially adverse effects of the reduced pressure. It is somewhat reassuring to note that the hypertensive survivors of strokes, when treated with antihypertensive agents, do not develop an increased rate of recurrence of stroke. In addition, antihypertensive therapy significantly decreases the development of congestive heart failure in such patients.[322]

EVALUATION OF THE PATIENT WITH HYPERTENSION

History and Physical Examination: General Considerations

In the evaluation of patients with elevated blood pressure, the physician has three major goals. The first is to estimate the severity and rate of progression of the hypertensive process, the second is to assess target organ damage, and the third is to find curable forms of hypertension. A complete history and physical examination are essential steps in reaching these goals.

An attempt must be made to date the onset of hypertension. Records should be obtained for confirmation of blood pressure readings. It should be established whether the point of muffling or the point of disappearance of Korotkoff sounds was used to determine the diastolic pressure. The point of muffling tends to overestimate the true diastolic intraarterial pressure, whereas the point of disappearance tends to underestimate the true diastolic pressure and is influenced by arm thickness, length of stethoscope tubing, background noise, and acoustic ability.[323]

It is important to establish whether the patient has had frequent mild labile elevations when under periods of stress that have always returned to normal, or whether evidence suggests a clear and relentless increase in blood pressure, which may not be greatly elevated, but has been climbing steadily for years and has now clearly reached a point requiring treatment.

The history should be evaluated for evidence of target organ damage. Ordinarily, moderate levels of blood pressure elevation are asymptomatic until an event occurs that reflects cardiovascular or renal disease. One study has suggested that symptoms of headache and dizziness most often develop after patients have been informed of their blood pressure elevation and now have reason to be concerned about hypertension. However, patients with diastolic levels above 130 noted headache and those above 110 noted dizziness even before learning of their problem.[324,325]

Symptoms of hypertensive central nervous system damage reflect overlapping pathologic events. One includes the coma, convulsions, and mental obtundation associated with the encephalopathy of severe hypertension. Another reflects destruction of central nervous system tissue either by hemorrhage from a ruptured subarachnoid aneurysm or from a small Charcot–Bouchard aneurysm at the bifurcation of an intracerebral blood vessel. A third includes signs of ischemic damage that follows thrombotic occlusion of atherosclerotic lesions in the cerebral vessels. Finally, widespread atherosclerosis of cerebral vessels, which occurs prematurely in hypertensive patients, is reflected by symptoms such as memory loss and emotional instability.

Aching in the lower extremities while walking, which disappears with rest, suggests intermittent claudication secondary to atherosclerotic involvement of the vascular supply of the lower extremities.

Symptoms of renal impairment include loss of appetite, nausea, polyuria, ankle edema, hematuria, flank pain, and proteinuria. A history of urinary tract infections is suggested by back pain, fever, urinary frequency, urgency, and dysuria.

Inquiry should be made about symptoms suggesting secondary hypertension. Renal parenchymal disease is the most common secondary cause of hypertension; it is suggested by a history of recurrent urinary tract infections and chronic pyelonephritis, or by episodes of edema, hematuria, and proteinuria in childhood, suggesting acute glomerulonephritis. The most common surgically curable form of secondary hypertension is renal vascular disease, which is suspected when the hypertension suddenly appears before the age of 35 or after the age of 55, or if the hypertension begins with flank pain or hematuria. Evidence of a source of emboli that might lodge in the renal artery also suggests a renal cause of hypertension and is suggested by a history of rheumatic fever, heart murmurs (especially the murmur of mitral stenosis), cardiac arrhythmias, or cardiomyopathy.

To investigate adrenal causes of hypertension, one searches for symptoms of pheochromocytoma. These chromaffin cell tumors usually release mixtures of epinephrine and norepinephrine, and the symptoms depend on the relative amount of each catecholamine released. Patients who release norepinephrine show signs of intense alpha-adrenergic stimulation: blanching of the skin, sweating, headache, and reflex slowing of the heart rate. Patients with tumors secreting epinephrine display the signs of beta-adrenergic receptor stimulation: flushing, tachycardia, and, at times, hypotension. Patients with pheochromocytoma frequently have postural hypotension. Because an undetected pheochromocytoma can have a fatal outcome, it is essential to keep this diagnostic possibility in mind.

Primary aldosteronism presents with less specific symptoms. The diagnostic hallmark is hypokalemia, which is frequently asymptomatic. When symptoms are present, they consist of episodic muscle weakness, polyuria, polydipsia, nocturia, paresthesia, and tetany.

Cushing's syndrome is usually suspected from the physical examination. The clinical history includes the development of truncal obesity, bone pain, easy bruising, increasing hair growth, and the development of a round, florid face.

Patients with coarctation of the aorta are frequently asymptomatic. When the coarctation is severe, the patient may complain of intermittent claudication or may have headaches because of the elevated blood pressure in the upper part of the body. This diagnosis should be considered in young patients, usually male, with mild hypertension and a "functional" heart murmur.

Patients with hyperparathyroidism may also develop hypertension.[326] Points in the history that suggest this diagnosis are depression, constipation, peptic ulcer, and renal calculi.

Space-occupying intracerebral lesions can also present with blood pressure elevation. Most often this consists of systolic hypertension with a wide pulse pressure and a slow pulse rate. The examiner should direct appropriate questions about localizing neurologic symptoms to evaluate this possibility.

Patients with acute intermittent porphyria may display hypertension during an acute attack. Positive historical features include episodic hypertension, abdominal cramps, and precipitation by drugs such as the barbiturates.

It is now well established that the use of oral contraceptive agents can cause hypertension and that blood pressure elevation may take as long as six months to resolve.[327] Other pharmacologic agents that can elevate blood pressure are: sympathomimetics in asthma, hay fever, and cold preparations; steroids; and nonsteroidal antiinflammatory agents.[328]

Knowledge of the patient's family history is important. Although a strict genetic mode of inheritance of hypertension has not been found, blood pressure elevation tends to run in families. The children of two hypertensive parents are especially prone to develop hypertension. Patients often do not know whether their relatives have hypertension and should be questioned for evidence of premature death or vascular disease.

Examination of the Cardiovascular System

It is essential to measure blood pressure in both arms because atherosclerotic lesions or preductal coarctation of the aorta can result in asymmetric pressures. This might cause the physician to make a falsely low estimate of the central arterial pressure or miss the fact that atherosclerotic lesions are present. A difference in arm readings of 20 mm Hg strongly suggests obstruction. The next step is examination of the neck. The jugular venous pulse is inspected to determine whether it is distended, reflecting an elevated pressure, or whether the contour is abnormal. The carotid arteries must be examined. First, the neck is inspected visually for abnormal pulsations. Next, the arteries are palpated and their relative contour assessed. In the hyperkinetic circulation of young patients with labile hypertension, the upstroke is brisk. Older patients who might have atherosclerotic lesions somewhere between the aortic valve and the jaw may have a slow upstroke. The presence of carotid or subclavian bruits should be noted. On auscultation of the thorax and lungs, the examiner listens for basilar rales, indicative of congestive heart failure, and for extracardiac bruits, which might point to underlying coarctation of the aorta. In young hypertensive patients, cardiac examination can reveal vigorous precordial pulsations and a systolic ejection murmur, which together suggest a hyperkinetic circulation.

The examiner also looks for evidence of hypertensive heart disease. Inspection of the chest wall and palpation of the cardiac apex can disclose a palpable atrial gallop or S_4, a sign that the ventricle has begun to hypertrophy and that its compliance characteristics have changed; this results in the development of an audible sound as the left atrium forcefully ejects blood into the left ventricle.

Cardiac auscultation can reveal an S_3 gallop which usually indicates cardiac dilatation and failure. However, an S_3 can be a physiologic finding in the young, athletic subject with a slow heart rate and a large stroke volume. Systolic ejection murmurs in the older hypertensive suggest calcification of the aortic valve, an apical holosystolic regurgitant murmur suggests dilatation of the left ventricle with valvular insufficiency, and in severe hypertension the decrescendo diastolic murmur of aortic insufficiency suggests dilatation of the aorta and aortic valve ring.

Examination of the cardiovascular system extends to the abdomen, where the presence of systolic bruits indicates underlying atherosclerosis of the aorta and bruits occupying both systole and diastole suggest renal artery stenosis. Physical examination should include palpation and auscultation of the femoral pulses for evidence of atherosclerosis or coarctation of the aorta. When significant coarctation of the aorta exists, the femoral pulse is diminished, the peak of the pulse is delayed relative to the pulse at the radial artery, and arterial pressure is lower in the legs than in the arms. The popliteal, posterial tibial, and dorsalis pedis pulses should be examined for evidence of peripheral atherosclerosis.

Neurologic examination should search for focal lesions, either as a cause of the hypertension or as manifestation of previous intracerebral hemorrhage or infarction.

Retinal Examination

The changes that take place in the optic fundus can be divided into those due to arteriolosclerosis and those due to elevated blood pressure. Retinal exudates can result from other disorders, such as diabetes mellitus, emboli, malignancy, arteritis, hematologic malignancies, and primary renal disease.

The central artery of the retina is a muscular artery. After passing through the lamina cribosa of the sclera, the internal elastic lamina of the artery thins and usually disappears by the first bifurcation. The muscularis decreases in thickness as the vessels course away from the optic disk.[329] Thus, most of the vessels visualized are true arterioles, at least those beyond one or two disk diameters from the optic disk. The most characteristic change is vasoconstriction, but structural changes also take place in the intimal and muscular layers.

Keith et al[330] described four groups of arteriolar and retinal changes in patients with hypertension, each associated with decreased survival. Patients with group 1 changes, focal or segmental arteriolar narrowing, survived reasonably well. Prognosis was worse in groups 2, 3 and 4. Group 2 changes refer to narrowing at the point at which the retinal vein crosses behind a thickened arterioles. Group 3 changes also include retinal hemorrhages and exudates, and group 4 changes include papilledema.

Scheie[331] has proposed a new classification that takes into account the fact that certain retinal changes are arteriolosclerotic and that some are specifically due to hypertension. The major difference between this classification and that of Keith et al is the designation of arteriovenous nicking as a nonhypertensive change.

Because hypertension is the most common predisposing factor for the development of arteriolosclerosis, the hypertensive patient might be expected to show the changes of both processes. Arteriolosclerosis can also develop in the absence of hypertension but in the presence of diabetes mellitus, old age, or hyperlipidema. In general, arteriolosclerotic changes correlate roughly with the duration of the blood pressure elevation, and the degree of the hypertensive changes corresponds with the severity of hypertension.[332]

Arteriolosclerosis is a diffuse process that involves thickening of the vessel walls.[333] This process begins with the deposition of hyaline material and lipid beneath the endothelium. The muscular layer is involved, and the adventitial layers are eventually involved. These changes are reflected by a wide arteriolar light reflex, a silver or copper-wire appearance, arteriovenous crossing changes, and increased arteriolar tortuosity. Healthy young persons can also show tortuous arterioles in the absence of underlying arteriolosclerotic disease. Arteriolovenous nicking begins with mild depression of the vein, followed by obliteration for short distances on either side of the arteriole, and later by thickening of the vessel distal to the crossing.

The most striking hypertensive change is retinal hemorrhage, which is associated with severe hypertension and characteristically occurs near the optic disk. The lesions are usually flame-shaped because they occur in the nerve fiber layer and extend between the fibers.

Other forms of hemorrhage can occur in hypertension, but can be associated with other disease entities. When the hemorrhage is located in the periphery and is solitary and round in shape, it may be a sign of advanced arteriolosclerosis or of arteriolar or venous occlusion. Patients with diabetes mellitus develop capillary aneurysms and may occlude small vessels leading to ischemic areas of hemorrhage. Patients with diabetes, stroke, trauma, leukemia, and normal subjects can develop hemorrhages in the deep layer of the retina. These hemorrhages are usually raised, bright red, and large with sharp borders.

Two types of retinal exudates can be seen on ophthalmoscopic examination. "Hard" exudates have a sharp margin and are thought to represent the residua of hemorrhages in layers deep to the retinal vessels. These exudates often appear after the initiation of antihypertensive therapy and can take as long as a year to resolve.[333]

The other common type of retinal exudate is the "cotton wool" or "soft" exudate, which appears suddenly and rapidly increases in size. With the initiation of antihypertensive treatment, the exudates become coarsely granular, develop small red microaneurysms, and gradually disappear. Such exudates are usually located near the optic disk and are believed by some to represent ischemic infarcts.

The appearance of soft exudates with flame hemorrhages suggests that the hypertensive process is accelerating. These retinal changes can heal completely when the blood pressure is lowered and the exudates often disappear in several days. Although soft exudates are ordinarily associated with severe hypertension, they can also be seen in lupus erythematosus and dermatomyositis and after occlusion of the central retinal vein. The appearance of soft exudates and striate hemorrhages can also be associated with the development of retinal edema. One manifestation of retinal edema is the star figure that forms around the macula of hypertensive patients and resolves slowly with antihypertensive therapy.

When soft exudates and striate hemorrhages are accompanied by papilledema, malignant hypertension is present and the patient's prognosis is grave because of impending renal failure. The development of papilledema can be gradual. The patient may develop, in sequence, loss of physiologic cupping of the optic disk, blurring of the nasal margins of the disk, distention of the retinal veins, blurring of the temporal margins, and finally elevation of the optic disk. With successful antihypertensive therapy, papilledema usually disappears in two to three months, although some irregularity around the edges of the optic disk may persist for a year. When papilledema appears, other causes such as brain tumors, cerebral swelling secondary to trauma, intracerebral hemorrhage, pseudotumor cerebri, and lead poisoning should be considered.

Controversy continues to exist over the role of vasospasm in producing the retinal changes of hypertension. There is agreement that acute forms of hypertension, such as eclampsia or acute glomerulonephritis, are accompanied by severe retinal arteriolar vasoconstriction. With chronic hypertension, it is difficult to distinguish sclerotic changes from acute vasoconstrictive changes if the vessels do not dilate and constrict during the examination or change acutely in response to therapy. Irregularity of the vessel outline suggests chronic, sclerotic changes.

The development of hemorrhages or exudates signals a serious progression of hypertension. This progression from grade 2 to grade 3 retinal changes demands more aggressive management of the elevated blood pressure, often requiring prompt hospitalization.

Laboratory Evaluation

The findings of the HDFP suggest that persons with diastolic blood pressure higher than 90 mm Hg should be detected and treated.[313] Approximately 37 million Americans fit this description. Should they all have a costly work-up before being treated? In the 10,900 participants of the HDFP, the incidence of secondary hypertension was found to be less than 1%. Thus, an extensive laboratory evaluation to detect secondary causes of hypertension would not be cost effective. Procedures such as the intravenous urogram or digital subtraction renal angiograms, measurement of plasma or urinary catecholamines or their metabolites, and assay of the renin-angiotensin-aldosterone system should be ordered only when specific indications are uncovered by history or physical examination.

However, before the institution of antihypertensive therapy, every patient should undergo a limited number of baseline laboratory studies. The studies recommended by the Joint National Committee on Detection, Evaluation and Treatment of Hypertension[320] are listed in Table 33.7. If the clinical history is suggestive, additional studies should be performed to rule out curable forms of hypertension. Suggested screening and definitive studies for

Table 33.7. Initial Evaluation of the Hypertensive Patient*

Medical History
Physical Examination
Laboratory Studies

1. To determine severity of vascular disease and possible causes of hypertension:
   - A. Hemoglobin
   - B. Hematocrit
   - C. Complete urinalysis
   - D. Serum potassium
   - E. Serum creatinine
   - F. Electrocardiogram
2. To assess cardiovascular risk factors and provide baseline for following possible adverse effect of antihypertensive medications:
   - A. Total cholesterol
   - B. High density lipoprotein cholesterol
   - C. Fasting plasma glucose
   - D. Serum uric acid

*Modified from the 1984 Report of the Joint National Committee on Detection, Evaluation, and Treatment of High Blood Pressure.

the most common forms of secondary hypertension are given in Table 33.8.

Cardiovascular Evaluation

Electrocardiogram: The electrocardiogram can suggest the presence and the severity of left ventricular hypertrophy in the following ways[334]: (1) increased voltage, duration, and direction of the main QRS vector; (2) prolonged onset of intrinsicoid deflection in the left precordial leads; (3) leftward and posterior change in direction of the initial (0.02 second) QRS vector; (4) altered repolarization with more anterior and rightward direction of ST segment and T-wave vector; (5) left atrial abnormality or altered terminal P-wave vector. It is postulated that some of these abnormalities are directly related to increased left ventricular muscle mass.

Increased left ventricular surface area and closer proximity of the enlarged heart to the chest wall account for increased voltage. As the left ventricle enlarges, a greater proportion of the total QRS voltage is composed of left ventricular potentials. Because the left ventricle occupies a posterior position, the mean QRS becomes more posteriorly directed. A greater period of time is required to depolarize the increased mass of left ventricular wall, resulting in increased duration of the QRS, increased duration of endocardial to epicardial activation, and prolongation of the onset of intrinsicoid deflection in the left precordial leads. Other electrocardiographic changes do not appear to be related to the increase in left ventricular mass.

The initial 0.02 second of the QRS reflects septal depolarization. Alteration of these forces can be caused by septal fibrosis and subsequent block in the branches or fascicles of the left bundle. Such a block can also cause superior displacement of the mean QRS vector. Increasing amounts of septal fibrosis can manifest as altered initial forces, superior and leftward displacement of the mean QRS vector, marked left axis deviation, widening of the QRS, or even complete left bundle branch block. The initial QRS vector can be displaced so far posteriorly that the initial R wave is lost in the right precordial leads, mimicking anterior myocardial infarction.

Left atrial abnormality may be present in any disorder of the left ventricle. This finding may be transient, due to altered conduction caused by elevated left atrial pressure, or permanent, as a result of left atrial dilatation and fibrosis.

The altered time course of repolarization in left ventricular hypertrophy causes nondiagnostic ST- and T-wave abnormalities. Similar changes are caused by other factors, such as digitalis, electrolyte disturbance, and myocardial ischemia. ST-segment elevation and upright T waves in leads V_1 and V_2, and ST depression with inverted T waves in leads V_5 to V_6, I, and aVL is referred to as a left ventricular "strain" pattern. The combination of altered depolarization and repolarization results in a wide QRS-T angle, normally less than 90 degrees in any one plane. A QRS-T angle greater than 120 degrees can be seen in left ventricular hypertrophy.

Despite characteristic electrocardiographic features, the electrocardiogram is a relatively insensitive means for detecting left ventricular hypertrophy. Romhilt et al[335] examined 33 electrocardiographic criteria in 360 prospective autopsy specimens. Each criterion was compared for sensitivity in detecting left ventricular hypertrophy in 160 specimens and for presence in the absence of left ventricular hypertrophy in 200 (Table 33.9). It should be noted that the point-score system, which will be discussed more fully, is as sensitive and is more specific than any individual measure.

Combinations of increased precordial voltage were the most sensitive abnormality, but they were present in less than 60% of patients with left ventricular hypertrophy and in about 10% of specimens without hypertrophy. Delayed onset of intrinsicoid deflection in leads V_5 to V_6 greater than 0.05 and increased voltage in the limb leads are more specific but are present less frequently.

Left axis deviation was present in 24% of specimens with left ventricular hypertrophy, but is frequently seen in the absence of hypertrophy.

Combining voltage, QRS duration, delayed intrinsicoid deflection, left axis deviation, ST-T wave abnormalities, and left atrial involvement, Romhilt and Estes[336] devised a weighted system for the detection of left ventricular hypertrophy with high sensitivity but without the high incidence of false-positive results seen when voltage criteria were used alone (Table 33.10). The vectorcardiogram has shown only slightly higher correlative values than the scalar electrocardiogram.

In a study by Dern et al,[337] 43 to 44 patients showed

Table 33.8. Screening Tests for Most Common Forms of Secondary Hypertension

Disorder	Primary Screen	Definitive Screen
1. Renal artery stenosis	Transvenous digital subtraction renal angiogram or rapid sequence intravenous pyelogram	Renal arteriogram and renal vein renins
2. Renal parenchymal disease	Dipstick urinalysis, creatinine	Creatinine clearance, ultrasound, renal biopsy when indicated
3. Pheochromocytoma	Urine vanillylmandelic acid, metanephrines, or catecholamines	Adrenal CAT scan or arteriograms
4. Primary aldosteronism	Serum potassium	Plasma renin activity and aldosterone after Na^+ restriction, adrenal vein sampling
5. Cushing's syndrome	Rapid, overnight dexamethasone suppression	Longer dexamethasone suppression test, adrenal arteriograms
6. Coarctation of aorta	Cuff blood pressure in legs	Aortogram

Table 33.9. Sensitivity and Specificity of Electrocardiographic Criteria for Left Ventricular Hypertrophy (LVH)*

Electrocardiographic Criterion	LVH Detected (%)	Present in Absence of LVH(%)
$S_{V1-2} + R_{V5} \geqq 35$ mm	56.3	12.5
$S_{V1} + R_{V5-6} > 30$ mm	55.6	10.5
$S_{V1-2} + R_{V5-6} > 35$ mm	55.6	11.5
$S_{V2} + R_{V4-5} > 35$ mm	55.6	14.5
R + S > 40 mm†	55	13.5
Point-score system	54	3
Delayed onset intrinsicoid V_5 or $V_6 \geqq$ 0.05 s	29	0.5
R_{V_5} or $R_{V_6} > 26$ mm	25	1.5
Left axis - 30° or greater	24.4	13
$R_{aVL} \geqq 10$ mm	13.1	0.5
$R_I > 13$ mm	10.6	0
$R_I + S_{III} > 25$ mm	10.6	0

* From Romhilt DW, Bove KE, Norris RJ, Conyers E, Conradi S, Rowlands DT, Scott RC: A critical appraisal of the electrocardiographic criteria for the diagnosis of left ventricular hypertrophy. *Circulation* 1969; 40:185–195, by permission of the American Heart Association, Inc.

†The greatest R in any precordial lead plus the greatest S in any precordial lead.

a reduction in precordial voltage during antihypertensive therapy. The mean QRS vector in the frontal plane did not change significantly, suggesting that QRS alterations in this plane are permanent and probably related to septal fibrosis. Leftward and superior mean QRS orientation was noted in patients with the highest systolic pressures, whereas more posterior QRS orientation was seen in patients with higher diastolic pressures. Repolarization changes showed early reversibility with therapy. Because of the nonspecific nature of these changes, the significance of their reversal is not clear.

Table 33.10. Point-Score System*

Electrocardiographic Criteria	Score
Amplitude	3 points
Any of the following:	
Largest R or S wave in the limb leads ≧20 mm	
S wave in lead V_1 or $V_2 \geqq 30$ mm	
R wave in lead V_5 or $V_6 \geqq 30$ mm	
ST-T segment changes (pattern of left ventricular strain)	
Without digitalis	3 points
With digitalis	(1) point
Left atrial abnormality	3 points
Terminal negativity of the P wave in lead V_1 1 mm or more in depth and duration 0.04 s or more	
Left axis deviation −30° or more	2 points
QRS duration 0.09 s or more	1 point
Intrinsicoid deflection in lead V_5, $V_6 \geqq 0.05$ s	1 point
Left ventricular hypertrophy	5 points
Probable left ventricular hypertrophy	4 points

* From Romhilt DW, Estes EH: A point-score system for the ECG diagnosis of left ventricular hypertrophy. *Am Heart J* 1968; 75:752–758, with permission of CV Mosby.

Chest radiograph: The routine posteroanterior and lateral chest radiographs are important in evaluating cardiac size, left ventricular and left atrial enlargement, pulmonary venous congestion, enlargement of the aortic root, tortuosity and calcification of the thoracic aorta, and signs of coarctation of the aorta.

Early left ventricular enlargement does not produce significant change in the cardiac silhouette or cardiothoracic ratio. With developing hypertrophy, there is increasing convexity to the left heart border due to enlargement of the left ventricular outflow tract. The lower left heart border enlarges leftward, and the apex points downward.

Dilatation, tortuosity, or elongation of the aortic root can result in a widened mediastinal shadow. Uncoiling or tortuosity of the aorta is present in fewer than 3% of persons under 40 years of age; therefore, its presence suggests target organ involvement. In older patients, tortuosity is usually due to atherosclerosis.

In the lateral projection, significant left ventricular enlargement is suggested if its posterior border extends more than 2 cm beyond the shadow of the inferior vena cava. Slight left atrial enlargement is commonly seen in patients with hypertension and is apparent when the posterior left atrial wall indents the barium-filled esophagus.

The left anterior oblique view suggests left ventricular enlargement when posterior displacement of the cardiac border causes the spine to be overlapped.

The chest radiograph suggests coarctation of the aorta when the shadow of the dilated left subclavian artery on the upper mediastinal border, or rib notching due to dilated intercostal arteries, is seen. Lateral views with barium swallow can demonstrate aortic dilatation proximal to the coarctation. The "reversed-three sign" or "E-sign" due to the aortic dilatation proximal to and distal to the coarctation is another characteristic radiographic finding.

Echocardiography: Although the presence of electrocardiographic evidence of left ventricular hypertrophy (LVH) carries a considerable increase in cardiovascular morbidity and mortality, especially if repolarization abnormalities are present, it is clear that relatively few patients with hypertension meet electrocardiographic criteria for LVH. In the HDFP, only 5% of the mild to moderately hypertensive participants had LVH on electrocardiogram.[313] In the Framingham study, LVH on electrocardiogram was present in 50% of patients whose systolic blood pressure was 180 mm Hg or more.[338] However, the introduction of echocardiography to the study of hypertensive patients has revealed a much higher frequency of left ventricular involvement. The echocardiograph allows measurement not only of wall thickness but also of chamber dimensions, thickness to radius ratios, left ventricular mass, and left ventricular wall stress. Devereaux and Reichek[339] compared echocardiographic measurements of left venticular mass with postmortem measurements in 34 patients, found a correlation coefficient of 0.96 ($P < .001$), a sensitivity of 93%, and a specificity of 95%. These observations have subsequently been confirmed in a larger group of 86 patients[340] and by other investigators.[341,342] Applying echocardiography studies to hypertensive subjects, it was found that of a group of hypertensive subjects, only 3% of whom had electrocardiographic evidence of LVH, fully 48%

had increased left ventricular mass or wall thickness on echocardiogram.[343]

Although it is clear that electrocardiographic evidence of LVH is associated with shortened longevity, it has not yet been established that evidence of increased left ventricular mass by echocardiography is associated with increased cardiovascular morbidity or mortality. When a muscle is presented with an increased workload, it first undergoes adaptive hypertrophy. If the increased workload is continued and is beyond the capacity of the muscle to adapt, muscle failure results. When blood pressure first rises, the thickness and mass of the left ventricle increase so that the stress per unit of mass is normalized. As mentioned earlier, to contract the left ventricle must develop sufficient tension to overcome the afterload that it faces during shortening. Myocardial wall tension, according to the law of LaPlace, is a direct function of intracavity pressure and ventricular radius, and inversely related to wall thickness. Thus, tension $= P \times R/2h$, where P equals pressure, R equals left ventricular radius, and h equals left ventricular wall thickness. Indeed, it has been shown that left ventricular mass does not correlate with arterial blood pressure as well as with left ventricular stress.[344]

An important area of contemporary investigation has been the problem of separating physiologic, adaptive hypertrophy from pathologic hypertrophy. Data derived from experimental and clinical studies suggest that the increased left ventricular mass of early adaptive hypertrophy is accompanied by hypercontractility.[345] This is followed by a period of sustained adaptive hyperfunction. Later, contractility becomes reduced, even before ventricular function is impaired. Subsequently, left ventricular failure ensues.

Abi-Samra et al[346] examined patterns of left ventricular hypertrophy in 43 hypertensive patients with left ventricular hypertrophy and demonstrated several patterns of hypertrophy. Concentric hypertrophy was observed in 20.3%, asymmetric septal hypertrophy in 21.6%, and combined hypertrophy and dilatation in 16.2%. Cardiac performance was inversely related to end-systolic stress and directly related to the ratio of end-systolic pressure to end-systolic volume.

In recent years, attention has been turned to the effect of antihypertensive therapy on left ventricular hypertrophy and function in addition to the effect of pharmacologic agents on blood pressure. In the spontaneously hypertensive rat, it was found that reversal of hypertrophy could be obtained by treatment with methyldopa, captopril, or a combination of reserpine, hydralazine, and hydrochlorothiazide, whereas treatment with hydralazine alone did not reverse hypertrophy despite control of blood pressure, and treatment with minoxidil alone actually increased hypertrophy.[347] In contrast, it has been observed that ventricular hypertrophy in the renovascular hypertensive rat could be reversed by either unilateral nephrectomy, converting enzyme inhibition, or calcium blockers.[348] These observations suggest that the factors producing hypertrophy, other than increased afterload, differ in different forms of hypertension and that the activity of the adrenergic nervous system may play an important role in the production and reversal of ventricular hypertrophy.[348a]

Radionuclide studies: Borer et al[349] used intravenous technetium-99m equilibrium radionuclide cineangiography to study left ventricular function at rest and during exercise in 60 patients with essential hypertension and 26 with aortic stenosis. The object of their investigation was to determine if left ventricular performance was independent of loading stresses in such patients and how removal of the loading stress affected ventricular behavior. In the patients with hypertension, a significant but weak direct relation was found between systolic arterial pressure and ejection fraction and an inverse relation between systolic pressure and the degree of change in ejection fraction with exercise. A strong correlation was found between systolic fractional shortening on echocardiogram and resting end-systolic wall stress. However, neither this relation nor arterial pressure predicted the result of exercise, suggesting that some patients with hypertension have changes in left ventricular function that are independent of systolic pressure.

The 26 patients with aortic stenosis were studied before and after valve replacement. It was found that ejection fraction could increase with exercise to a much greater extent after surgery, showing that functional improvement of a hypertrophied myocardium can take place when abnormally elevated afterload is corrected.

The abnormal ventricular responses to exercise noted by Borer et al[349] in certain of their hypertensive patients may be explained by the observation of Francis et al[350] who subdivided their hypertensive patients into groups with and without electrocardiographic evidence of coronary artery disease. Each patient underwent measurement of ventricular function at rest and during upright bicycle exercise with first-pass radionuclide angiocardiograms. No abnormalities of resting or exercise ejection fraction, nor regional wall motion, were found in the patients without electrocardiographic abnormalities, suggesting coronary artery disease. Even those patients with LVH on electrocardiogram had a normal response to exercise. In contrast, 19 of 23 of those patients whose electrocardiograms indicated the presence of coronary artery disease had an abnormally blunted increase or even a decrease in ejection fraction with exercise. These observations suggest that left ventricular systolic functional reserve is maintained in most patients with essential hypertension as long as they remain free from significant coronary artery disease.

Echocardiographic studies of ventricular function during different phases of the cardiac cycle have given new insights into the pathophysiologic aspects of hypertensive heart disease. For decades, it has been believed that unrelieved systemic arterial hypertension results in ventricular hypertrophy, eventually leading to dilation and failure. Accelerated coronary atherosclerosis with myocardial ischemia has also been thought to play an important role in the genesis of congestive heart failure in the hypertensive patient. However, in 1984, Ratts et al[88] reported that hypertensive patients presenting with pulmonary edema could be separated into two distinct groups by echocardiography: those with dilated ventricles and poor systolic function, who usually also had either a history of prior myocardial infarction or chronic alcoholism, and those with hypertrophied ventricles with small or normally sized ventricular cavities and well-preserved systolic function, who were postulated to have impaired diastolic compliance, resulting in high ventricular filling pressures. In 1985, Topol et al[351] demonstrated that patients in the latter group had abnormal diastolic function with a prolonged early diastolic filling period and reduced peak diastolic dimension increase. Such patients were usually elderly black women who sometimes responded to vasodilator therapy with severe hypotensive reactions.

The studies of Ratts et al[88] and Topol et al[351] point out the need for distinguishing between the two groups of patients, as those with dilated ventricles and impaired systolic function should benefit from careful afterload reduction whereas those whose systolic function is well preserved but whose pulmonary capillary wedge pressures are high because of impaired diastolic function should benefit most from cautious reduction of venous return or even from the use of negative inotropic agents.

Renal Evaluation

Routine urinalysis: In the initial evaluation of a patient with newly discovered hypertension, one of the earliest considerations should be the possible presence of undetected renal disease, because chronic parenchymal renal disease is the most common cause of secondary hypertension. Additionally, the intrarenal vasculature and glomerular capillaries are susceptible to hypertensive damage, resulting in a loss of function.

Routine urinalysis is useful in assessing these possibilities. A clean-catch midstream specimen is less likely to contain contaminants causing misleading results. The osmolality or specific gravity screens for loss of concentrating ability. Urine should be collected when the patient is relatively dehydrated, eg, the second voiding after rising. Severe proteinuria and glycosuria can cause elevated specific gravity. The finding of proteinuria should lead to further evaluation. With the semiquantitative methods used in screening examinations, trace amounts may reflect no more than a normal amount of protein. A 1+ designation is abnormal in properly collected specimens and indicates protein concentrations of 10 to 30 mg/100 ml. Such patients should have quantitative protein excretion measured.

Patients with glycosuria should be evaluated for diabetes mellitus, because glomerulosclerosis is associated with renal insufficiency and hypertension.

Microscopic examination of the urine sediment is an important part of the evaluation. A normal urine sediment contains few formed elements, for example, one or two red blood cells, one to two white blood cells, occasional hyaline casts, and a few epithelial cells. Casts indicate parenchymal renal damage if present in an abnormal amount or type. Red blood cell or hemoglobin casts indicate active glomerular injury. Large amounts of white blood cells and bacteria indicate an infection in the urinary tract.

Renal function tests: Costly laboratory tests are not required in the evaluation of patients with hypertension. The serum creatinine is an excellent qualitative measure of glomerular filtration (GFR). When the serum creatinine reaches a value twice that of the mean control level, the GFR is approximately 50%. The endogenous creatinine clearance may be obtained to semiquantitate the degree of impairment of glomerular filtration rate but adds little to practical value in patient management when the serum value is normal.

Quantitative measurement of glomerular filtration and renal plasma flow are possible through measurement of inulin and paraaminohippuric acid (PHA) clearances; however, these are seldom accomplished in the evaluation of most hypertensive patients.

DIAGNOSTIC STUDIES FOR SECONDARY HYPERTENSION

Renal Parenchymal Disease

Although renal parenchymal disease is the most common cause of secondary hypertension, the way in which this disorder results in hypertension is not clear.[352] The possibilities include abnormal stimulation of the renin-angiotensin system with inadequate response to the negative feedback signals due to renal damage, inadequate control of sodium homeostasis, and impaired production of renal vasodepressor substances.[294]

Although the pathogenesis may differ, the approach to treatment of patients with renal parenchymal disease is much the same as that of patients with essential hypertension, except for a few considerations.[353] Drugs that affect renal function adversely should be used with caution in patients with more than mild to moderate reduction of glomerular filtration, that is, those with a serum creatinine above 2.0 mg %. Thiazide diuretics, chlorthalidone, spironolactone, triamterene, metolazone, and guanethidine all increase nitrogen retention.

The second consideration regards adjustment of dosage. Furosemide and ethacrynic acid are useful in treating patients with severe renal insufficiency, but a larger dose is required as function decreases. Failure to respond to antihypertensive therapy is often due to an inadequate dose of diuretic or to excessive sodium intake. The gastrointestinal side effects seen with large doses of ethacrynic acid limits its usefulness in renal failure. Drugs that depend on renal excretion, such as methyldopa, must be given in smaller doses as renal function deteriorates.

Renovascular Hypertension

In 1914, Volhard[354] postulated that hypertension was caused by stenotic small arteries throughout the renal parenchyma with systemic arterial hypertension developing as the circulation attempted to drive blood through the kidneys' purification system. In 1934, Goldblatt[355] demonstrated that stenosis of the canine renal artery resulted in systemic arterial hypertension and that removal of the stenosis returned blood pressure to control levels. Since this time, a number of studies have demonstrated that renal artery stenosis is a cause of hypertension in man and that correction of the stenosis frequently cures the hypertension. Renal artery stenosis is probably the most common surgically correctable cause of hypertension in man.

There are two major forms of renal artery stenosis. The first is fibromuscular dysplasia, a disorder with destruction of vascular smooth muscle and fibrous proliferation within the wall of the artery.[356] This condition affects females more often than males by a ratio of about 3 to 1 and often appears in younger patients. The lesions are usually present in the distal two thirds of the renal artery, although they may also involve other sections. On microscopic grounds, these lesions can be subdivided into four subgroups, based on which layer of the arterial wall has the greatest involvement (Table 33.11).

The second major type of renal artery stenosis is caused by atherosclerosis. This lesion occurs more often in males by a 2 to 1 ratio, characteristically occurs in older age groups, and usually involves the proximal third of the renal artery.

The clinical history is rarely of great help in diagnosing renovascular hypertension. However, items that are consistent with a renovascular origin are: hypertension with a diastolic pressure above 130 mm Hg; sudden onset of hypertension with a diastolic pressure above 110 mm Hg in patients less than 30 years old; accelerated hypertension with hemorrhages, exudates, or papilledema; prior history of flank pain, hematuria, or renal trauma; hypertension remaining resistant to pharmacologic therapy; and the presence of epigastric or flank bruits throughout systole and diastole. Diastolic bruits are more specific than systolic.

Rapid-sequence intravenous urograms are probably the best way to screen patients for renal artery stenosis.[357] However, transvenous digital subtraction renal angiography may eventually prove to be superior. The best indicator of unilateral stenosis is the late appearance of contrast material on the ischemic side. Another indication is a difference in renal size. As the left kidney is normally 0.5 cm longer than the right, a difference of 1.5 cm or greater when the left kidney is larger, or 0.5 cm or more when the right kidney is larger, is significant. Because the ischemic kidney reabsorbs filtered water in excess of contrast material, delayed hyperconcentration is another sign of unilateral stenosis, as is scalloping along the course of the ureter, secondary to enlargement of collateral ureteric blood vessels.

The radioactive renogram and renal scan provide an alternative means of screening. The renogram has a higher incidence of false-positive results and does not reveal the anatomic details yielded by intravenous urography, such as hydronephrosis, pyelonephrotic scarring, and reduction in size secondary to glomerulonephritis. A multicenter cooperative study of renovascular hypertension found that about 10% of patients with essential hypertension have abnormal intravenous urograms, whereas 22% of patients with surgically correctable renovascular hypertension have normal urograms.[358] Patients with hypertension and abnormal urograms have about a 50% chance of the presence of surgically correctable renovascular hypertension. Digital subtraction intravenous angiography, a newly developed but not yet widely available technique, offers the potential to improve detection of significant lesions without the risk of more invasive angiographic procedures.

Although average peripheral vein renin activity is higher in patients with renovascular hypertension than in patients with essential hypertension, there is so much overlap of individual values within the two groups that peripheral renin activity is not very useful in screening patients for renovascular hypertension.[359]

However, the blood pressure elevation in patients with renal artery stenosis is related to increased activity of the renin-angiotensin system, and it has been shown that intravenous infusion of the angiotensin II receptor blocking agent saralasin lowers pressure to normal in patients with true renovascular hypertension, thus providing an additional way to screen for or assess the clinical significance of renal artery stenosis.[360,361]

When an abnormal intravenous urogram or radioactive renogram has been obtained, the next diagnostic step is usually renal arteriography. This shows the anatomy of the lesion, if present. In postmortem studies, however, it has been found that about 40% of patients with renal artery stenosis were normotensive. Thus, functional assessment of a stenotic lesion is important. The most widely used method is measurement of renal vein renin activity in both renal veins. Elevated activity on the is-

Table 33.11. Classification of Idiopathic Fibromuscular Stenosis of Renal Artery*

Cleveland Clinic (1958–1969)	Mayo Clinic (1962–1969)	Combined: Cleveland Clinic and Mayo Clinic (1970)
	Intima	
(Idiopathic stenosis) Intimal fibroplasia	Intimal fibrous stenosis	Intimal fibroplasia
	Media	
Fibromuscular hyperplasia	(Fibromuscular stenosis) Fibromuscular dysplasia (focal, multifocal, or tubular stenosis with or without aneurysm)	Fibromuscular dysplasia (focal, multifocal, or tubular stenosis with or without aneursym)
	Fibromuscular dysplasia with medial thickening	Medial fibroplasia Medial hyperplasia
Medial fibrolasia with aneurysm (mural fibrosis) Subadventitial fibroplasia Dissecting aneurysm	Fibromuscular dysplasia with dissecting aneurysm	Perimedial fibroplasia Medial dissection
	Adventitia	
	Periarterial fibrous stenosis	Periarterial fibroplasia

* From Harrison EG Jr, McCormack LJ: Pathologic classification of renal arterial disease in renovascular hypertension. *Mayo Clin Proc* 1971; 46:161–167, with permission.

chemic side and a renal vein renin ratio of ischemic to uninvolved side of 1.5 or greater allows correct prediction of the results of surgery in about 80% of cases.[362] When bilateral renal artery stenosis is present, this procedure is less valuable, although it may provide an estimate of which kidney is contributing most importantly to the elevation in blood pressure.

Studies by Strong et al[363] demonstrated that the sensitivity of renal vein renin measurement can be enhanced by sodium depletion. Low sodium diet plus full doses of oral diuretics for three days before measurement of renal vein renin activity improved the predictive value of the test from 35% to 90%. It is the impression of many that agents that act to reduce renin release tend to decrease the sensitivity of the test.

In experienced hands, bilateral ureteral catheterization and split renal function tests were once of limited value in predicting the results of surgery, but the predictive value is not as great as that of renal vein renin ratios and there is rarely an indication at present to proceed with such a study.

An abnormal intravenous urogram, arterial stenosis on arteriography, and a renal vein renin ratio of greater than 1.5 do not automatically indicate surgical correction. Many patients respond to pharmacologic therapy and many are high-risk surgical candidates.

In a retrospective study of 24 patients who responded favorably to therapy, it was found that 7 patients with fibromuscular dysplasia taking diuretics plus reserpine or methyldopa had an average decrease in diastolic blood pressure of 20 mm Hg, whereas 17 of the other patients with arteriosclerotic lesions had a similar decrease in blood pressure, but required additional vasodilator therapy.[364] Presently, many such patients can be controlled with angiotensin-converting enzyme inhibitors.

Corrective renovascular surgery in patients with significant extrarenal arteriosclerosis may improve blood pressure, but may not prolong life.[365] Thus, individual judgment must be applied to each case. It is reasonable to limit renal artery surgery to these patients who fail to respond to pharmacologic therapy. The recently developed technique, percutaneous transluminal angioplasty, offers a less invasive way to relieve renal ischemia.[366] Unfortunately, not all stenotic lesions can be dilated successfully with a balloon-tipped catheter and many become restenosed after an initially successful intervention. However, in some patients, periodic redilatation may offer a lower risk of complications and mortality than surgical bypass.[366a]

Pheochromocytoma

Pheochromocytomas are usually nonmalignant tumors of chromaffin cells of adrenal medulla or sympathetic ganglia. Neuroblastomas and ganglioneuromas arising from ganglion cells and chemodectomas arising from chemoreceptor cells are related tumors. Pheochromocytomas also occur in association with familial neurocutaneous disorders, thyroid medullary carcinoma, and hyperparathyroidism.

Pheochromocytomas contain the enzymes needed to metabolize tyrosine to catecholamine. After uptake, tyrosine is hydroxylated to dihydroxphenylalanine (dopa) by the rate-limiting tyrosine hydroxylase step. Dopa is decarboxylated to dihydroxphenethylamine (dopamine), which in turn is oxidized to norepinephrine in storage granules. In tissues containing phenethanolamine-N-methyl-transferase, norepinephrine is methylated to form epinephrine. This enzymatic step is usually confined to the adrenal medulla.[367]

Symptoms of pheochromocytoma occur as catecholamine mixtures are released into the circulation. The Valsalva maneuver, exercise, pregnancy, overeating, urination, and ingestion of tyramine-containing foods have all precipitated attacks. The most common symptoms are headache, sweating, palpitation, pallor, and nausea.[368] More than half the patients with pheochromocytoma have persistent hypertension with spikes; the remainder have intermittent hypertension. It is not unusual for such patients to be followed for several years before a diagnosis is reached. Postural hypotension is found in approximately two thirds of patients. The cardiovascular effects of catecholamines result in most of the symptoms. Norepinephrine stimulates alpha-adrenergic receptors, causing systolic and diastolic hypertension, bradycardia, and cardiac arrhythmias. Epinephrine stimulates both alpha- and beta-receptors, causing tachycardia, elevated cardiac output, arrhythmias, and either hypotension or systolic hypertension. Both compounds decrease gastrointestinal motility, inhibit insulin release, and elevate blood sugar, free fatty acids, lactic acid, and basal metabolic rate. Norepinephrine is the major compound produced by most tumors, although predominant production of epinephrine has been reported.[369] Although the two types of tumors usually cannot be separated clinically, it is a reasonable assumption that attacks associated with bradycardia are norepinephrine mediated, whereas attacks associated with hypotension are epinephrine mediated.

The main problems in the management of patients with pheochromocytoma are to confirm the diagnosis by biochemical tests, to locate the tumor, and to remove it with adequate monitoring after appropriate preparation of the patient.

Biochemical tests for urinary catecholamines or their metabolites form the mainstay of diagnosis.[370] Values twice normal or higher are usually found in the urine of affected patients. After release of catecholamines, relatively small amounts are excreted unchanged in the urine. Circulating catecholamines are converted to metanephrine and normetanephrine by hepatic catechol-o-methyl transferase (COMT). These products are excreted in the urine or metabolized throughout the body by monoamine oxidase to vanillylmandelic acid. Small amounts of norepinephrine are metabolized to dihydroxymandelic acid within the neuron and converted to vanillylmandelic acid by COMT.

Urinary (and plasma) catecholamines are present in small amounts and are difficult to measure. Elevated values are found in patients receiving methyldopa, levodopa, or any catecholamine-containing medication. Measurement of urinary total metanephrine is a more reliable technique in many laboratories. Elevated values are found in patients receiving monoamine oxidase inhibitors. Vanillylmandelic acid can be measured by a colorimetric phenolic acid reaction, but results are elevated by ingestion of phenol-containing foods. A more specific spectrophotometric method is not influenced by diet, but it is lowered by monoamine oxidase inhibitors or clofibrate, and falsely elevated by nalidixic acid.[371] If urinary levels of one product are elevated, a separate collection should be made and a different product found to be elevated before the patient is subjected to surgery. All urine collections should be made in an acid-containing bottle to prevent breakdown of catecholamine metabolites.

Bravo et al[372] compared the newer radioenzymatic assays of plasma catecholamines with 24-hour urinary vanillylmandelic acid and metanephrine in 24 patients with pheochromocytoma and 40 without pheochromocytoma. They found false-negative results in one patient using the radioimmunoassay, in 11 using vanillylmandelic acid, and in five using metanephrine excretion. However, meticulous attention to patient preparation and specimen handling appeared to be essential.

The diagnosis of pheochromocytoma should never be made solely on the basis of pharmacologic testing. Provocative tests, that is, those causing an elevation in blood pressure after the administration of histamine, tyramine, or glucagon, or blocking tests, inducing a decrease in pressure after administration of phentolamine, have a significant number of false-positive and false-negative results and also have an associated risk. However, pharmacologic testing is sometimes useful in clarifying equivocal biochemical results.

When the diagnosis of pheochromocytoma has been confirmed, the surgeon is faced with the problem of locating the tumor. Approximately 80% of these tumors arise in the adrenals, most on the right. Another 10% to 15% arise from intraabdominal sympathetic ganglia or from the organs of Zuckerkandl. Most extraabdominal tumors arise from the thoracic sympathetic chain and can be seen on oblique chest films. Cervical tumors are usually palpable or cause local symptoms. Intravenous urograms or adrenal tomograms show displacement of the kidney by a suprarenal mass in 50% of cases.

Arteriography can localize tumors but can also precipitate acute attacks.[373] Patients should be prepared for study with alpha-adrenergic blocking agents for one week before arteriography. Finding one tumor on arteriography does not rule out the presence of others, which are found in 15% to 20% of patients. Vena caval catheterization with catecholamine measurement at several sites is at times useful in localizing tumors. More recently, computerized axial tomography, echograms, and scintigraphy by ^{131}I-meta-iodobenzylguanidine have been used successfully to locate pheochromocytomas.[374,375]

Because N-methyl transferase is usually limited to the adrenal medulla, it was hoped that the presence of significant amounts of epinephrine in the blood or urine placed the tumor in the adrenal glands.[376] Several case reports have now shown that epinephrine can be formed by extraadrenal tumors.

Preoperative management of the patient with pheochromocytoma is based on pharmacologic stabilization for one or two weeks with alpha-adrenergic blockade.[377] Additional beta-adrenergic blockade is indicated when cardiac arrhythmia or serious tachycardia develops, but it should not be used routinely because of the risk of inducing heart failure in patients who might have catecholamine cardiomyopathy. Alpha-methylparatyrosine, an inhibitor of tyrosine hydroxylase, can eliminate symptoms by interfering with catecholamine synthesis and has proved to be useful in the preoperative treatment of patients with pheochromocytoma or in controlling the symptoms of those with inoperable or metastatic tumors.[377a]

Primary Aldosteronism

In 1953, Simpson et al[378] described the isolation of a potent adrenal mineralocorticoid. In 1955, Conn[379] studied a patient with signs of mineralocorticoid excess, and reported the first case of an adrenal adenoma producing the syndrome of primary aldosteronism.

Aldosterone causes resorption of sodium and secretion of potassium and hydrogen in the distal renal tubule. This leads to the characteristics of primary aldosteronism: hypertension and depletion of body potassium stores. Potassium depletion causes symptoms of muscle weakness and fatigue, and leads to the development of nephropathy with symptoms of polyuria and nocturia. The hypertension associated with primary hyperaldosteronism is ordinarily mild and well tolerated, although cases of more severe hypertension have been reported. Malignant hypertension secondary to primary aldosteronism is believed to be very rare.

At present, the most useful screening test for primary aldosteronism is measurement of serum potassium, which is usually less than 3.5 mEq per liter in such patients. Because some patients with hyperaldosteronism have mild or borderline hypokalemia, it is advisable to repeat measurement of serum potassium in patients with borderline values. To rely on serum potassium for screening, it is necessary to be certain that the patient has not been taking potassium supplement nor restricting dietary sodium. When less sodium is presented to the distal renal tubules, less is exchanged for potassium, and thus serum potassium levels remain relatively normal.

Many circumstances other than primary aldosteronism result in hypokalemia. The most common is prior use of diuretic agents. Other causes are potassium-wasting renal disease, Cushing's syndrome, and aldosteronism secondary to renovascular or renal parenchymal disease. The last category includes a syndrome of hypertension associated with hyponatremia, hypokalemia, thirst, polyuria, polydipsia, and weight loss, called the hyponatremic hypertensive syndrome.[379a,379b] Although the most common cause is renal artery disease, it may also develop after diuretic treatment, in malignant hypertension, or during hemodialysis.[379b] Smoking may be a predisposing factor.[379a] Clinicians should be alert to the possible existence of the hyponatremic hypertensive syndrome; hyponatremia in a hypertensive patient suggests secondary rather than primary hyperaldosteronism. The features of this syndrome can be controlled either by use of converting enzyme inhibitors or by surgical intervention.[379a,379b]

Plasma renin activity should be measured under well-defined conditions in patients with unexplained hypokalemia.[380] Patients with primary aldosteronism have retained sodium and water but "escape" before developing edema. Because of volume overexpansion, plasma renin levels are usually suppressed. Our practice has been to place patients on a low sodium diet (10 mEq Na, 100 mEq K) for four days and to obtain a blood sample for measurement of renin at around noon on the morning of the fourth day, after the patient has been up and about all morning. The combination of upright posture and sodium depletion acts to stimulate renin release; however, in patients with primary aldosteronism, because of volume overexpansion, plasma renin activity remains suppressed.

A patient with suppressed renin activity has either aldosteronism or "low renin" hypertension. (See section on the renin-angiotensin system for a discussion of "low-renin" hypertension.) Definitive diagnosis of primary aldosteronism requires hospitalization for precise metabolic studies. The presence of a low plasma renin activity despite volume depletion must be confirmed, and elevated plasma or urinary aldosterone, which is not suppressed physiologically when the patient receives a salt load, must be demonstrated. Once the biochemical diagnosis of primary aldosteronism has been made, an attempt is made to locate the tumor by computed tomography, which can detect bilateral enlargement or adenomas as small as 1 cm,[381] by bilateral adrenal venography and sampling of adrenal venous blood for assay of plasma aldosterone levels, or by surgical exploration of both adrenal glands.

Primary aldosteronism, although frequently caused by a single adenoma, can also result from three other causes: idiopathic hyperaldosteronism, indeterminate hyperaldosteronism, and glucocorticoid-remediable hyperaldosteronism.[382] Surgical excision of an adrenal adenoma producing aldosterone ordinarily leads to correction of both hypertension and electrolyte abnormality. Some patients with biochemical evidence of aldosteronism have been found to have bilateral nodular hyperplasia of the adrenal cortex. Bilateral adrenalectomy results in correction of electrolyte abnormalities, but hypertension persists.[383] Although these two groups of patients show some differences in the way in which they respond to manipulations of salt and fluid balance, until recently there has been no certain way to separate the two groups before surgery, other than demonstration of a single adenoma by adrenal venography or demonstration of elevated levels of aldosterone in both adrenal veins. It now appears that patients with bilateral nodular hyperplasia excrete abnormally high levels of an adrenal glomerulosa cell stimulating factor in the urine.[384]

A third group of patients has been described in whom signs and biochemical evidence of aldosteronism are present but who respond to the administration of deoxycorticosterone (DOCA) by suppressing urinary aldosterone secretion to normal levels.[385]

A fourth group of patients has glucocorticoid-remediable hyperaldosteronism. This rare disorder is found in children more often than in adults. The patients present signs, symptoms, and biochemical evidence of aldosteronism, but the administration of replacement doses of glucocorticoid results in correction of the blood pressure, suppression of urinary aldosterone secretion, and correction of electrolyte levels.[386]

Cushing's Syndrome

In patients with syndromes of excessive cortisol secretion, either from adrenocortical hyperplasia or adrenocortical tumor, hypertension frequently develops. Ordinarily, Cushing's syndrome is apparent on physical examination, with the patient displaying truncal obesity, round face, buffalo hump, purple striae, multiple bruises over thin skin, and bone pain. To pursue the diagnosis, the next step should be a rapid dexamethasone suppression test.[387] The patient receives 1 mg of dexamethasone at midnight. This is perceived by the hypothalamus as an elevation of plasma corticosteroids, which leads to diminished pituitary ACTH release and diminished adrenal secretion of corticosteroids. In normal subjects, measurement of plasma cortisol at 8:00 AM the next morning should reveal marked suppression of less than 5 g/100 ml. Patients with various forms of Cushing's syndrome fail to sustain cortisol suppression and require hospitalization for further evaluation.[388]

Treatment of Cushing's syndrome depends on the nature of the tumors. Benign or surgically approachable tumors are treated by resection, which results in improvement or cure of the hypertension. Unfortunately, many tumors causing Cushing's syndrome are not resectable. For medical (palliative) therapy, several drugs have been used to decrease adrenal production of steroids including mitotane, aminoglutethimide, metyrapone, trilostane, and ketoconazole.[388a]

Adrenocortical Enzyme Deficiencies

Congenital disorders exist in which one of the hydroxylase enzymes necessary for the production of corticosteroids is absent, resulting in diminished serum levels of corticosteroids and elevated pituitary secretion of ACTH.[389] Because steroid synthesis cannot proceed through the normal pathways, the compensatory drive results in production of excess amounts of other steroid compounds, including some with salt-retaining properties. The syndrome more frequently seen in adults involves deficiency of 17-hydroxylase, which catalyzes conversion of progesterone to 17-hydroxyprogesterone.[390] When this enzyme is missing, glucocorticoid, estrogen, and androgen production are impaired. The clinical syndrome consists of primary amenorrhea, hypertension, and defeminization. The diagnosis is suspected when urinary excretion of 17-ketosteroids and 17-hydroxysteroids is low or absent, despite hypertension. Dexamethasone, 1 mg daily for 7 to 14 days, should result in correction of the hypertension.

Oral Contraceptive Hypertension

In the late 1960s, investigators noted a decrease in blood pressure when certain hypertensive women discontinued oral contraceptive agents, and that reinstitution of oral contraceptive therapy was followed by a reappearance of hypertension.[391,392] Later, prospective studies demonstrated that the administration of oral contraceptives causes a statistically significant rise in systolic blood pressure, which increased 7 mm Hg, whereas diastolic pressure tended to rise about 2 mm Hg.[393] The incidence of hypertension in users of oral contraceptive agents varies from 1% to 18% in various series.[394] An association has not been found between duration of treatment and incidence of hypertension. Blood pressure usually returns to pretreatment levels when contraceptives are discontinued, but the process may take as long as six months.

The pathophysiologic aspects of oral contraceptive hypertension are not yet fully understood. The estrogenic component stimulates increased hepatic synthesis of several proteins, including renin substrate. As substrate levels rise, plasma renin activity remains constant, and plasma renin concentration should fall as enzyme release is inhibited. These events occur in both normotensive and hypertensive women and therefore have not been firmly implicated as the cause of hypertension; other studies have implicated the progestogens.

Patients in whom hypertension is found to develop must use other means of contraception. If blood pressure is significantly elevated, the patient should be treated with antihypertensive agents for about six months. The dosage should then be reduced or the drug discontinued to determine if it is still necessary. If blood pressure elevation is mild, the patient can be observed for a six-month period before deciding to institute antihypertensive therapy or workup for other secondary causes of hypertension.

Certain patients are at greater risk of developing hypertension while receiving oral contraceptive agents: the elderly, the obese, those with a history of hypertensive pregnancies, and those with a family history of hypertension. Although these patients may cautiously start oral contraceptives, they must remain under careful medical observation, with blood pressure measured at least every two months for the first year, then two or three times a year. Malignant hypertension with irreversible renal failure has been reported due to oral contraceptive agents.[395]

Licorice Ingestion

Licorice contains a salt-retaining compound, glycyrrhizic acid. Ingestion of large amounts of licorice on a daily basis results in sodium retention, potassium excretion, hypertension, and hypokalemia.[396] Because intravascular volume is expanded, plasma renin activity and plasma urinary levels of aldosterone are low.

Hyperparathyroidism

In a series of 40 patients with primary hyperthyroidism studied by Rosenthal and Roy,[397] 13 were found to be hypertensive. Nine patients initially presented with hypertension, of whom seven were discovered to have hyperparathyroidism through serum calcium determinations. In this series, the prevalence of primary hyperparathyroidism in hypertensive patients was 7.6%, whereas the frequency ranges between 0.1% and 0.2% in the general population. In a series of 80 patients reported on by Madhavan et al,[398] 17.5% were hypertensive, and one half of these experienced significant improvement in their hypertension after parathyroidectomy. This possibility should be considered in patients presenting with a history of depression, recurrent peptic ulcer, bone pain, renal calculus formation, and constipation.

Coarctation of the Aorta

Coarctation of the aorta causes hypertension in the upper extremities either by mechanical means or through an effect on renal blood flow. Although patients with coarctation of the aorta are ordinarily asymptomatic, certain symptoms, such as pain and coldness of the extremities on exercise, epistaxis, and headache, should suggest this diagnosis. On physical examination, there is a decrease, absence, or delayed peak of pulsation in the femoral arteries in comparison with the radial pulse. Measurement of blood pressure with a large cuff in the legs reveals a gradient. Radiographic examination of the chest may show the findings discussed earlier. Physical examination may reveal pulsations in the intercostal spaces, in the axilla, and in the interscapular space. A midsystolic murmur is frequently audible on the anterior chest, which radiates to the back. Murmurs may also be heard along the lateral chest wall over dilated collateral vessels.[399]

Coarctation of the aorta is often associated with other congenital cardiac abnormalities, most often bicuspid aortic valve, patent ductus arteriosus, ventricular septal defect, or valvular aortic stenosis.

Unless contraindications exist, surgical correction is recommended to prevent complications of severe hypertension, rupture of cerebral aneurysms or of the aorta, left ventricular failure, and bacterial endocarditis.[400]

ANTIHYPERTENSIVE THERAPY

Nonpharmacologic Measures

Mild blood pressure elevation gradually causes vascular damage with time. Successful long-term therapy demands that the patient fully understand the risk imposed by untreated hypertension and the need for lifelong therapy.

Changes in life-style: Contemporary therapy emphasizes early detection and treatment of mild hypertension. This approach gives rise to concern about the effects of antihypertensive agents when given for a lifetime. Because the risk-benefit ratio cannot be calculated precisely, consideration should be given to nonpharmacologic therapy of mild hypertension before hypotensive drugs are prescribed.

Stress: Hypertension can be provoked by subjecting experimental animals to recurrent stress. Emotional stress elevates blood pressure, even in persons whose blood pressure is ordinarily within normal limits. Constant monitoring of blood pressure shows elevation during periods of activity.

Unfortunately, it is difficult to do anything about stress. Major life changes, such as retirement from active professional life, can be followed by improved blood pressure, but most often this is not a practical approach. Regular periods of rest during the day have not proved to be very effective in controlling blood pressure, nor has sedation or tranquilizers.

It has been found that regular elicitation of the relaxation response for periods of 20 minutes, twice a day, results in lower blood pressure in some persons.[401] However, the therapeutic value of this approach appears to be limited.

Exercise: Strenuous activity and isometric exercise tend to elevate blood pressure. It is unwise for hypertensive patients or patients in the coronary age group to attempt strenuous exercise without prior conditioning, and isometric exercises, such as weight-lifting, should be avoided. Regular, moderate isotonic exercise is beneficial. Hypertensive patients on standard antihypertensive agents have been found to have better blood pressure control when following a program of regular exercise.[402] Boyer and Kasch[403] observed an average decrease in diastolic pressure of 11.8 mm Hg in a group of 24 hypertensive men participating in a walk-jog program.

Obesity: Weight is positively correlated with blood pressure.[404] Although weight loss is not invariably followed by a great reduction in blood pressure, elimination of obesity is advisable for general medical reasons, such as control of hyperlipidemias.[404a] Furthermore, control of obesity is important not only for the treatment of hypertension, but also for the prevention of left ventricular hypertrophy.[404b] Even in normal-weight subjects with hypertension, weight loss can induce a fall in blood pressure that leads to a reduction in antihypertensive medication; a 4-kg weight loss has been shown to be equivalent to the amount of antihypertensive medication required for effective control of mild hypertension.[404c]

Tobacco: Cigarette smoking increases blood pressure transiently. On the average, smokers tend to have lower blood pressure than nonsmokers. However, cigarette smoking is definitely a risk factor in the development of cardiovascular disease, which, when combined with hypertension, represents a potent combination. Moderate pipe or cigar smoking does not appear to have an adverse effect on cardiovascular mortality.

Alcohol: Moderate use of alcohol does not increase blood pressure. However, blood pressure rises as alcohol use increases.[405,405a,405b,405c] Patients should also be aware of the caloric implications of alcohol, the adverse effect on the control of type 4 hyperlipidemia, and the dangers of adding the sedative effects of alcohol to those of antihypertensive sympatholytic agents. Therefore, moderation in alcohol consumption to less than 2 ounces of ethanol daily for patients with hypertension is recommended.[405d]

Salt: Populations with high average daily sodium intake contain a large number of hypertensive persons.[406] Kempner[407] showed that improvement of severe hypertension required extreme salt restriction, less than 8 mEq of sodium daily. This is a difficult diet to follow and requires special salt-free foods. More recent studies have shown that mild to moderate hypertension improves when sodium intake is lowered from 150 to 200 mEq to 50 to 90 mEq per day.[52,408,409] Although recent studies indicate that people vary considerably in their response to sodium,[74] until convenient and reliable methods are developed for the detection of salt-sensitive patients, it is prudent to advise the hypertensive patient to follow a no-added-salt diet. Although recent research has uncovered suggestions that blood pressure may be influenced by dietary intake of potassium,[80a] calcium,[409a] or magnesium,[409b] or a combination of these, further evidence is needed to clarify these relations. At present, it would be premature to recommend changes in dietary consumption of these cations.

Pharmacologic Agents

A wide variety of antihypertensive agents and combinations of agents have been placed on the market over the past two and a half decades. As physicians have gained familiarity with these compounds and their side effects, the number in general use has come to be reduced to a relatively small group: thiazide diuretics, agents that block the sympathetic nervous system, vasodilators, and the newly introduced agents that block the renin-angiotensin system. Interest is also growing in the use of calcium channel blocking agents. It has become generally understood that the use of a large dose of a single antihypertensive agent tends to produce more side effects for a given hypotensive effect than does the combined use of smaller doses of two or three antihypertensive agents with different mechanisms of action: As a result, the concept of "stepped-care" has emerged, which has been recommended by the Joint National Committee on Detection, Evaluation and Treatment of Hypertension[320] (Table 33.12).

Unless contraindications exist, therapy is usually initiated with a thiazide diuretic or a beta-blocking compound dependent on the patient's age and race. Loop diuretics should be reserved for selected patients, such as those with renal failure. If the goal blood pressure has not been reached by two to four weeks of full-dose therapy, a sympatholytic agent, such as one listed here, is

Table 33.12. Stepped-Care Approach to Drug Therapy*

Step	Drug Regimens
1	Begin with less than a full dose of either a thiazide-type diuretic or a beta blocker†; proceed to full dose if necessary and desirable
2	If blood pressure control is not achieved, either add a small dose of an adrenergic-inhibiting agent‡ or a small dose of thiazide-type diuretic; proceed to full dose if necessary and desirable§; additional substitutions may be made at this point
3	If blood pressure control is not achieved, add a vasodilator, hydralazine hydrochloride, or minoxidil for resistant cases.
4	If blood pressure control is not achieved, add guanethidine monosulfate

* From The Joint National Committee on Detection, Evaluation, and Treatment of High Blood Pressure, The 1984 Report of the Joint National Committee on Detection, Evaluation, and Treatment of High Blood Pressure, *Arch Intern Med* 1984; 44:1045–57.

† Beta blockers include atenolol, metoprolol tartrate, nadolol, oxprenolol hydrochloride, pindolol, propranolol hydrochloride, and timolol maleate.

‡ These include centrally acting adrenergic inhibitors (clonidine hydrochloride, guanabenz acetate, and methyldopa), peripherally acting adrenergic inhibitors (guanadrel sulfate and reserpine), and an $alpha_1$-adrenergic blocker (prazosin hydrochloride).

§ A high percentage (70% to 80%) of patients with mild hypertension will respond to the foregoing regimen using steps 1 and 2.

An angiotensin-converting enzyme inhibitor may be substituted at steps 2 through 4 if side effects limit use of other agents or if other agents are ineffective. Slow channel calcium-entry blockers (diltiazem hydrochloride, nifedipine, and verapamil hydrochloride) have not been approved for therapy in hypertension but may be acceptable as steps 2 or 3 drug.

added and gradually increased to a maximum tolerated dose or a diuretic is added if initial therapy consisted of a beta blocker. It is important to bear in mind that the step 2 agents are approximately the same in potency when given in the maximum recommended dose. However, all have side effects and potentially adverse effects (Table 33.13).

The art of successful antihypertensive therapy involves the careful matching of medication to patient, for example, selecting beta-blocking agents for patients with angina pectoris or with a history of recent acute myocardial infarction while avoiding them in the treatment of hypertensive patients with asthma, heart failure, or advanced degrees of heart block.[410] Similarly, methyldopa should be avoided in treating patients with liver diseases; reserpine, in depressed patients; clonidine and methyldopa in patients with chronic fatigue, and so on.

If a patient cannot tolerate the first step 2 agent selected, others should be tried before proceeding to step 3. If the combination of sympatholytic and diuretic therapy is not completely effective, hydralazine or minoxidil, direct-acting vasodilators, are added to the antihypertensive program and gradually increased to a full dose. Prazosin hydrochloride may be used instead of hydralazine hydrochloride if it was not selected as the step 2 agent. Minoxidil is a potent vasodilator, which carries side effects of fluid retention, pericardial effusion, hirsutism, and headache.[411]

For some time, the potent adrenergic blocking agent guanethidine has been the mainstay of step 4 treatment of resistant hypertension. The introduction of angiotensin-converting enzyme inhibitors offers an additional option for steps 1 through 4. Captopril, one of these agents, has possible side effects of skin rash, proteinuria, granulocytopenia, and loss of taste.[412,413] Calcium channel blockers also lower blood pressure, but the various compounds in this group have side effects such as tachycardia, fluid retention, impaired atrioventricular conduction, and reduced myocardial contractility.[413a] Thus, none of the antihypertensive agents is ideal, and a choice must be made based on individual considerations.

In most patients, control of blood pressure can be obtained with a simple program of antihypertensive agents

Table 33.13. Adverse Drug Effects*

Drugs	Side Effects	Precautions and Special Considerations
Diuretics		
Thiazides and related sulfonamides	Hypokalemia, hyperuricemia, glucose intolerance, hypercholesterolemia, hypertriglyceridemia, and sexual dysfunction	May be ineffective in renal failure; hypokalemia increases digitalis toxicity; and hyperuricemia may precipitate acute gout
Loop diuretics	Same as for thiazides	Effective in chronic renal failure; cautions regarding hypokalemia and hyperuricemia same as above; and hyponatremia may be found, especially in the elderly
Potassium-sparing agents	Hyperkalemia	Danger of hyperkalemia in patients with renal failure
Amiloride hydrochloride	Sexual dysfunction	...
Spironolactone	Gynecomastia, mastodynia, and sexual dysfunction	...
Triamterene	...	...
Adrenergic Antagonists		
β-Adrenergic blockers†	Bradycardia, fatigue, insomnia, bizarre dreams, sexual dysfunction, hypertriglyceridemia, decreased high-density lipoprotein cholesterol	Should not be used in patients with asthma, chronic obstructive pulmonary disease, congestive failure, heart block (greater than first degree), and sick sinus syndrome; use with caution in patients with diabetes and peripheral vascular disease
Central-acting adrenergic inhibitors	Drowsiness, dry mouth, fatigue, and sexual dysfunction	...
Clonidine hydrochloride	...	Rebound hypertension may occur following abrupt discontinuance
Guanabenz acetate	...	Same as for clonidine
Methyldopa	...	May cause liver damage and positive direct Coombs' test result
Peripheral-acting adrenergic inhibitors	Sexual dysfunction and nasal congestion	...
Guanadrel sulfate	Orthostatic hypotension and diarrhea	Use cautiously in elderly patients because of orthostatic hypotension
Guanethidine monosulfate	Same as for guanadrel	Same as for guanadrel
Rauwolfia alkaloids	Lethargy	Contraindicated in patients with a history of mental depression; use with caution in patients with a history of peptic ulcer

Table 33.13. Adverse Drug Effects* (*Continued*)

Drugs	Side Effects	Precautions and Special Considerations
Reserpine		
α_1-Adrenergic blocker	Same as for *Rauwolfia* alkaloids	Same as for *Rauwolfia* alkaloids
Prazosin hydrochloride	"First dose" syncope, orthostatic hypotension, weakness, and palpitations	Use cautiously in elderly patients because of orthostatic hypotension
Combined α- and β-adrenergic blockers		
Labetalol hydrochloride‡	Asthma, nausea, fatigue, dizziness, and headache	Contraindicated in cardiac failure, chronic obstructive pulmonary disease, sick sinus syndrome, and heart block (greater than first degree); use with caution in patients with diabetes
Vasodilators	Headache, tachycardia, and fluid retention	May precipitate angina in patients with coronary heart disease
Hydralazine hydrochloride	Positive antinuclear antibody (without other changes)	Lupus syndrome may occur (rare at recommended doses)
Minoxidil	Hypertrichosis, ascites (rare)	May cause or aggravate pleural and pericardial effusions
Angiotensin-Converting Enzyme Inhibitors	Rash and dysgeusia (rare at recommended doses)	Can cause reversible, acute renal failure in patients with bilateral renal arterial stenosis; neutropenia may occur in patients with autoimmune-collagen disorders; and proteinuria (rare at recommended doses)
Slow Channel Calcium-Entry Blocking Agents §	Headache, hypotension, and dizziness	...
Diltiazem hydrochloride	Nausea	Use with caution in patients with congestive failure or heart block
Nifedipine	...	...
Verapamil hydrochloride	Flushing, edema, and constipation	Same as for diltiazem

* From The 1984 Report of the Joint National Committee on Detection, Evaluation, and Treatment of High Blood Pressure. *Arch Intern Med* 1984; 144:1045–1057.

† Sudden withdrawal of these drugs may be hazardous in patients with heart disease.

‡ This drug has not yet been approved by the Food and Drug Administration.

§ These drugs have not yet been approved by the FDA for the treatment of hypertension.

with few side effects. Unless selected on demographic grounds, around 50% of patients respond to diuretic or beta blocker therapy alone. Therefore, unless the hypertension is severe, therapy should be started with diuretics or beta blockers and additions made as needed. When diastolic pressure is greater than 115 mm Hg, a diuretic and a step 2 agent should be started simultaneously.

The pharmacologic properties of most antihypertensive agents are summarized in Table 33.14.

HYPERTENSIVE EMERGENCIES AND URGENCIES

In about 10% of patients, an accelerated or malignant phase occurs as a complication of almost all types of primary and secondary hypertension. Severe diastolic hypertension, group 3 or group 4 retinopathy, and progressive renal failure are the features characterizing this phase. Hypertensive encephalopathy, cerebral hemorrhage, left ventricular failure, and fluid retention are other common findings. Malignant hypertension is associated with a poor prognosis unless successfully treated before the vascular damage has taken place.[18]

Pathophysiology

The control system for maintaining normal blood pressure involves several negative feedback loops. Normally, as blood pressure rises, a stimulus is created that decreases the output of one or more of the forces maintaining the pressure. Negative feedback loops are known to exist, which involve the renin-angiotensin-aldosterone system and the sympathetic nervous system among others.

Although the pathogenesis of the malignant phase is not completely understood, it has been proposed that conversion to a malignant phase occurs when increasing levels of blood pressure and an accelerating rate of vascular damage cause a normal negative feedback loop to become a positive loop. For example, plasma renin activity is usually elevated in patients with malignant hypertension, which is inappropriate because a rising pressure should be associated with a falling renin level as the body attempts to maintain pressure homeostasis. Because renin levels are high, angiotensin II and aldosterone levels rise and, as a result, sodium and water are retained, effective blood volume increases, and plasma renin levels should fall. However, high pressure injures the kidney, renin continues to be released despite the increased effective blood volume and blood pressure, and thus a negative feedback loop becomes a positive factor in further elevating arterial pressure.

The malignant phase of hypertension can be reversed by aggressive antihypertensive therapy, which arrests progressive vascular damage. Therefore, during the malignant phase of hypertension, there is an urgent

Table 33.14. Antihypertensive Agents*

Type of Drug	Dosage Range (mg/day) Initial	Dosage Range (mg/day) Maximum	Plasma Half-Life (h)	Onset of Action (h)	Peak Action (h)	Duration of Action (h)	Frequency of Dosage (per day)
Diuretics							
Thiazides and related sulfonamide diuretics							
Bendroflumethiazide	2.5	5	3–4	2	4	6–12	1
Benzthiazide	25.0	50	1-2	2	4	12–18	2–4
Chlorothiazide sodium	250.0	500	1.5+.2	2	4	6–12	1–2
Chlorthalidone	25.0	50	44+10	2	4	6–12	1
Cyclothiazide	1.0	2	1–2	<6	7–12	18–24	1–3
Hydrochlorothiazide	25.0	50	2.5+.2	2	6	12	1–3
Hydroflumethiazide	25.0	50	17	2	4	6–12	2
Indapamide	2.5	5	14	1–2	2	8–12	1
Methyclothiazide	2.5	5	1–2	2	6	24	1
Metolazone	2.5	5	8	1	2	12–24	1
Polythiazide	2.0	4	25.7	2	4	36	1
Quinethazone	50.0	100		2	6	18–24	1
Trichlormethiazide	2.0	4	1–2	2	4	24	1
Loop diuretics							
Bumetanide	0.5	10	1–1.5	1	1–2	4–6	1
Ethacrynic acid	50.0	200	1	.5	2	6–8	1–2
Furosemide	80.0	480	.85+.17	1	1–2	6–8	2
Potassium-sparing agents							
Amiloride hydrochloride	5.0	10	6–9	2	6–10	24	1
Spironolactone	50.0	100	13–24	24–48	2–4	48–72	1–4
Triamterene	50.0	100	2.8+.9	2–4		7–9	2
Adrenergic inhibitors							
Beta-adrenergic blockers							
Atenolol	25.0	100	6–9	1	2–4	24	1
Metoprolol tartrate	50.0	300	3–4	1	1.5	3–4	1
Nadolol	20.0	120	20–24		3–4	20–24	1
Oxprenolol hydrochloride	160.0	480	2		1–2		2
Pindolol	20.0	60	3–4		1	3–4	2
Propranolol hydrochloride	40.0	480	3.9 ± .4		2	2–3	2
Propranolol, long-acting (LA)	80.0	480	10		6		1
Timolol maleate	20.0	60	4	.5	1–2	4–5	2
Central-acting adrenergic inhibitors							
Clonidine hydrochloride	0.2	1.2	8.5 ± 2	.5–1	.33	8–24	2
Guanabenz acetate	8.0	32	6	1	2–4	<12	2
Methyldopa	500.0	2,000	1.8 ± .2		4–6	8–24	2
Peripheral-acting adrenergic antagonists							
Guanadrel sulfate	10.0	150	10	2	4–6	4–14	2–4
Guanethidine monosulfate	10.0	300	98–185		6–8	240–336	1
Rauwolfia alkaloids							
Rauwolfia (whole root)	50.0	100					
Reserpine	0.05	0.25		1	24	2–3 wks	1
Alpha$_1$-adrenergic blocker							
Prazosin hydrochloride	1.0	20	2.9 ± .8	1.5	3	8–12	2
Combined alpha- and beta-adrenergic blockers							
Labetalol	200.0	1,200	6–8	1–2	2–4	8–12	2
Vasodilators							
Hydralazine hydrochloride	50.00	300	2.5		.25–.33	6	2–4
Minoxidil	5.0	100	4	.5	2–3	75	1
Angiotensin-converting enzyme inhibitors							
Captopril	37.5	150	4.5	15–30	1–1.5		3
Enalapril maleate	10.0	40	<2	1–2	4–6	12–16	1–2
Slow channel calcium-entry blocking agents							
Diltiazem hydrochloride	120.0	240	3.5	.5–1	2–3	2–6	3–4
Nifedipine	30.0	180	2	.15	.5	3–5	3
Verapamil hydrochloride	240.0	480	2.8–12		1–2	8–10	3–4

*Modified from The Joint National Committee on Detection, Evaluation, and Treatment of High Blood Pressure, The 1984 Report of the Joint National Committee on Detection, Evaluation, and Treatment of High Blood Pressure. *Arch Intern Med* 1984; 144:1045–1057.

need for the reduction of blood pressure to normotensive levels.[414]

Differential Diagnosis

There are several hypertensive emergencies that require early, expert, and intensive treatment (Table 33.15). These include subarachnoid hemorrhage, intracerebral hemorrhage, hypertensive encephalopathy, acute left ventricular failure due to hypertension, dissecting aneurysm, and acute and advancing renal insufficiency due to hypertension, eclampsia, and pheochromocytoma.

In addition to these hypertensive emergencies, there are less obvious situations that also require urgent therapy. Patients often experience a period of acceleration of hypertension in which the manifestations of vascular damage are not proportionate in all target organs. For example, patients may present with hypertensive encephalopathy in the absence of papilledema, hemorrhages, or exudates. Other patients may present with blurred vision, retinal hemorrhages, and exudates, yet may have neither impairment of consciousness nor renal function. It is important to realize that the urgency of blood pressure reduction varies with the hypertensive emergency and that the approach to treatment and the agent used vary.[415] Severely hypertensive patients with subarachnoid hemorrhage or patients with acute left venticular failure and pulmonary edema secondary to hypertension require more immediate blood pressure reduction than does an otherwise asymptomatic hypertensive patient with group 3 hypertensive retinopathy and severely elevated diastolic pressure. The clinical signs and symptoms associated with a hypertensive crisis are listed in Table 33.16.

Principles of Therapy

The primary aim in the management of hypertensive emergencies is the reduction of diastolic blood pressure to a normal range. This should be attempted with constant attention to maintaining perfusion of vital organs. Patients without preexisting symptoms of vascular insufficiency rarely develop such complications when blood pressure is reduced, although a transient decrease in urine output with a slight rise in serum creatinine or blood urea nitrogen is often noted. In the presence of significant coronary or cerebrovascular insufficiency, angina, electrocardiographic signs of ischemia, frank myocardial infarction, transient cerebral ischemia, convulsions, and cerebral infarction can occur, primarily as a result of precipitous decrease in arterial pressure. This can usually be avoided if a more controlled reduction of pressure is achieved with close monitoring of vital organ functions. Persistence is often more important than speed of reduction.

Table 33.15. Hypertensive Emergencies*

1. Malignant hypertension
2. Hypertensive retinopathy with fundal hemorrhages and symptomatic reduction in visual acuity
3. Hypertensive encephalopathy
4. Acute left heart failure due to hypertension
5. Dissecting aneurysm with hypertension
6. Subarachnoid hemorrhage with hypertension
7. Intracerebral hemorrhage with severe hypertension
8. Acute or advancing renal insufficiency with severe hypertension
9. Hypertensive crisis in pheochromocytoma
10. Eclampsia

* From Sullivan JM: Arterial hypertension, in Blacklow RS (ed): *McBryde's Signs and Symptoms,* ed 6. Philadelphia, JB Lippincott, 1983, with permission.

Table 33.16. Clinical Characteristics of Hypertensive Crisis*

Blood pressure: Usually >140 mm Hg diastolic
Funduscopic findings: Hemorrhages, exudates, papilledema
Neurologic status: Headache, confusion, somnolence, stupor, visual loss, focal deficits, seizures, coma
Cardiac findings: Prominent apical impulse, cardiac enlargement, congestive failure
Renal: Oliguria, azotemia
Gastrointestinal: Nausea, vomiting

* From Kaplan NM: *Clinical Hypertension,* ed 3. Baltimore, Williams & Wilkins, 1982, with permission.

Parenteral therapy falls into two categories. The first includes agents with a relatively long duration of action, which are given as a bolus followed by a blood pressure response of considerable variation in degree and duration. The second category comprises drugs with a short duration of action that require constant intravenous infusion and close supervision to effect a controlled and smooth decrease in blood pressure.[416] Gentle diuretic therapy should be employed in most cases to potentiate the effect of other agents and to prevent secondary retention of salt and water, but should not be given to the point of inducing intravascular volume depletion, reflex vasoconstriction, and additional renin release and angiotensin II generation.[417] Oral antihypertensive therapy should be started as soon as possible, because it will be required eventually and the onset of action is relatively slow.

Nine antihypertensive agents are available in the United States for parenteral use in the treatment of hypertensive emergencies and urgencies. Their dosages, onsets of action, and potential adverse effects are summarized in Table 33.17. It is our opinion that vasodilator drugs are the agents of choice in the treatment of hypertensive emergencies other than those associated with pheochromocytoma, where alpha-adrenergic receptor blockers are indicated; dissecting aneurysm, where beta-adrenergic receptor blockers are necessary; and perhaps subarachnoid or intracerebral hemorrhage, where vasodilatation might aggravate bleeding. The reason for this recommendation is the observation that most hypertensive emergencies are associated with marked elevation of total peripheral resistance, which falls, allowing cardiac output and organ perfusion to rise when vasodilators are administered (Figure 33.18). In contrast, agents other than peripheral alpha receptor blockers, which interfere with the activity of the sympathetic nervous system, result in a reduction in cardiac output which, in the presence of diuretic-induced volume depletion or intravascular volume depletion due to pressure diuresis, can lead to compensatory vasoconstriction and potentially to further impairment of organ perfusion (Figure 33.19).

Table 33.17. Drugs for Managing Hypertensive Emergencies and Urgencies[*]

Drugs	Intramuscular Dose (mg)[†]	Intravenous: Single Dose (mg)	Intravenous: Continuous Infusion[‡]	Onset of Action	Adverse Drug Effects
Direct vasodilators					
Diazoxide		50–100 bolus[§]	15–30 mg/min over 20–30 min	3–5 min	Nausea, vomiting, hyperglycemia, hyperuricemia, hypotension, flushing, tachycardia, and chest pain
Sodium nitroprusside			50–100 mg/L	Instantaneous	Nausea, vomiting, muscle twitching, sweating, thiocyanate intoxication, and apprehension
Hydralazine hydrochloride	10–50	10–20[‖]	200 mg/L	Intramuscularly 20–30 min; intravenously 10–12 min	Tachycardia, palpitations, flushing, headache, vomiting, and aggravation of angina
Nitroglycerine			0.5–10 μg/kg/min	2–5 min	Bradycardia, tachycardia, flushing, headache, vomiting, and methemoglobinemia
Sympathetic blocking agents					
Reserpine	1–5			2–3 h	Drowsiness, stupor, bradycardia, hypotension, and activation of peptic ulcer
Labetalol hydrochloride		20–80 IV bolus	2 mg/min	5–10 min	Vomiting, nausea, scalp tingling, burning in throat and groin, pain at injection site, postural hypotension, and dizziness
Methyldopate hydrochloride		250–500[¶]		2–3 h	Drowsiness
Trimethaphan camsylate			1,000 mg/L	5–10 min	Paresis of bowel and bladder, orthostatic hypotension, blurred vision, and dry mouth
Alpha-receptor blocking agents	5–15	5–15 (rapid injection essential)	200–400 mg/L	Instantaneous	Tachycardia and flushing

[*] From The 1984 Report of the Joint National Committee on Detection, Evaluation, and Treatment of High Blood Pressure.[320]

[†] Start with the smallest dose shown. Subsequent doses and intervals of administration should be adjusted according to the response of blood pressure (BP).

[‡] Start infusion slowly and adjust rate according to response of BP. Constant surveillance is mandatory. Concentration of solution can be adjusted according to patient's fluid requirements.

[§] To be given at intervals of five to ten minutes.

[‖] The total dosage should be contained in a volume of at least 20 ml and the solution should be administered from a 20- or 50-ml syringe. Blood pressure should be monitored continuously while the injection is being made. Rate of injection should not exceed 0.5 ml/min. To avoid hypotension, the injection should be stopped frequently when the BP is falling.

[¶] Diluted up to 100 ml and injected during a 30- to 60-minute period.

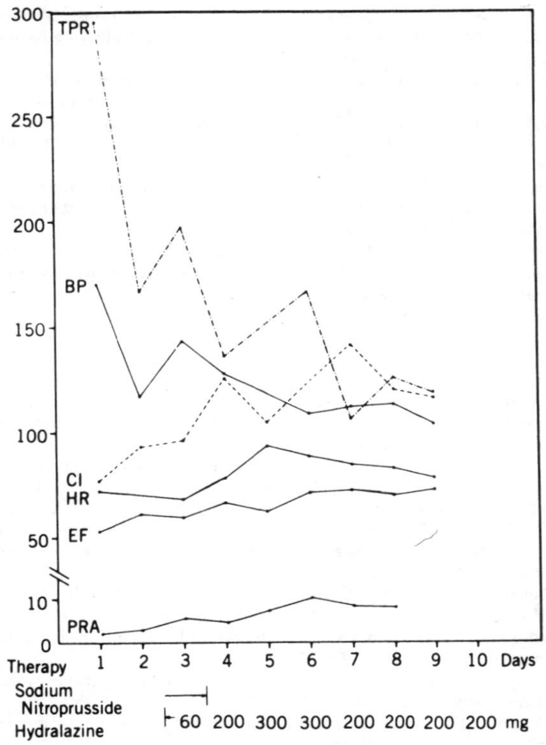

Figure 33.18. Effect of vasodilator agents on hemodynamic variables and plasma renin activity (PRA, ng/mL/h) in patient 1 with severe hypertension. BP = mean arterial blood pressure (mm Hg); CI = cardiac index (mL/s); EF, ejection fraction (%); HR = heart rate (beats/min); TPR indicates total peripheral resistance (dyne-s-cm^{-5} $\times$ 10^{-1}). Note rise in PRA, CI, HR, and EF as TPR and BP fall. (From Sullivan JM, Schoeneberger AA, Ratts TE, Palmer ET, Samaha JK, Mance CJ, Muirhead EE: Short-term therapy of severe hypertension. Hemodynamic correlates of the antihypertensive response in man. *Arch Intern Med* 1979; 139:1233–1239. Copyright 1979, American Medical Association, with permission.)

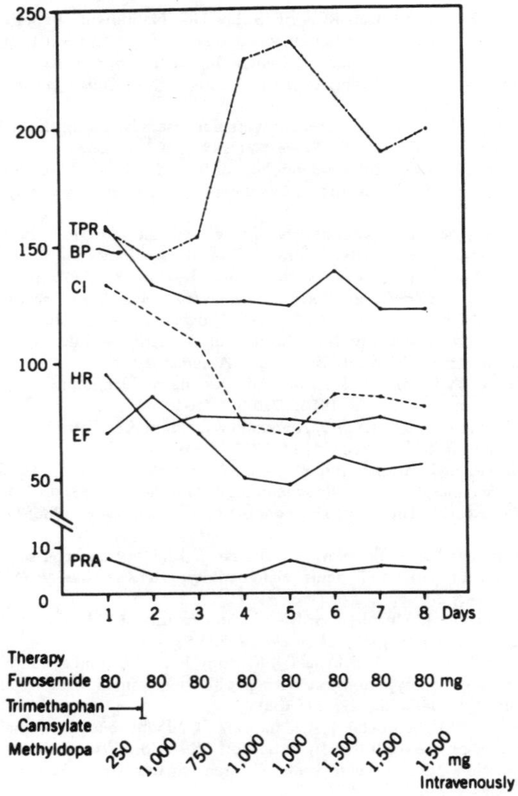

Figure 33.19. Combined sympatholytic-diuretic therapy of patient 8 with severe hypertension. Reductions in blood pressure (BP) are accompanied by a decrease in cardiac index (CI), which was elevated initially, whereas total peripheral resistance (TPR) actually rises. Pretreatment CI was normal in this group, but also fell after initiation of therapy. EF = ejection fraction (%); HR = heart rate (beats/min); PRA = plasma renin activity (ng/mL/h). (From Sullivan JM, Schoeneberger AA, Ratts TE, Palmer ET, Samaha JK, Mance CJ, Muirhead EE: Short-term therapy of severe hypertension. Hemodynamic correlates of the antihypertensive response in man. *Arch Intern Med* 1979; 139:1233–1239. Copyright 1979, American Medical Association, with permission.)

Hypertensive crises with concomitant renal failure present special management problems.[20] Not only do patients with malignant hypertension present with oliguria and renal failure, but also patients with dissecting aneurysms can develop oliguria due to obstruction of the renal arteries and patients with acute glomerulonephritis can develop acute renal failure. These patients retain salt and water, which makes them less sensitive to antihypertensive agents and can lead to problems with congestive heart failure. Effective hemodialysis can correct these problems and can sustain life while fibrinoid necrosis of renal arterioles resolves.[418] Some patients recover enough renal function to be able to live without chronic dialysis.

A few patients with end-stage renal failure become resistant to antihypertensive agents despite removal of salt and water by dialysis. Such patients have extremely high levels of plasma renin activity and become normotensive when the kidneys are removed. It has become apparent that malignant hypertension does not contraindicate successful long-term dialysis and transplantation. The results obtained in such patients are comparable to those obtained in patients with renal failure secondary to glomerulonephritis.

Acknowledgment: I am indebted to Dr James C. Hunt for his thoughtful review and helpful suggestions and to Mrs Patricia Hopkins for her expert assistance in the preparation of this manuscript. This work was supported in part by Grants HL-21523, National Heart, Lung, and Blood Institute and RR-0211, General Clinical Research Center, US Public Health Service.

I am grateful for permission from the Year Book Medical Publishers to quote freely from background material concerning the pathogenesis of hypertension gathered in preparation of the book *Hypertension and Pregnancy* by Jay M. Sullivan, MD (Copyright 1986 by Year Book Medical Publishers).

REFERENCES

1. Guidelines for the treatment of mild hypertension: Memorandum from a WHO/ISH meeting. *Hypertension* 1983; 5:394–397.
2. Rowland M, Roberts J: Blood pressure levels in persons 6–74 years. United States, 1976–80. Advance Data. National Center for Health Statistics #84. US Department of Health & Human Services, PHS Oct 8, 1982.
3. The Criteria Committee of the New York Heart Association: *Nomenclature and Criteria for Diagnosis of Diseases of the Heart and Great Vessels,* ed 7. Boston, Little, Brown & Co, 1973, p 15.
4. Stamler J, Kjelsberg M, Hall Y: Epidemiologic studies on cardiovascular-renal disease. I. Analysis of mortality by age-race-sex-occupation. *J Chron Dis* 1960; 12:440–455.

5. Wu YK, Lu CQ, Gao RC, Yu JS, Liu GC: Nationwide hypertension screening in China during 1979–80. *Chin Med J* 1982; 95:101–108.
6. Zhou JC, Chen YJ, Ma YD: Geographic distribution of hypertensive subjects in Inner Mongolia autonomous region. *Chin J Cardiol* 1983; 11:35.
7. Cheng TO: Prevalence of cardiovascular diseases among the national minorities of China. *Ann Intern Med* 1984; 101:562–563.
8. Gupta SP, Siwach SB: Epidemiology of hypertension in a North Indian population. Based on rural-urban community surveys. *Jpn Heart J* 1984; 25:65–73.
8a. Akinkugbe OO: Epidemiology of hypertension and stroke in Africa, in Hatano S, Shigematsu I, Strasser T (eds): *Hypertension and Stroke Control in the Community.* Geneva, World Health Organization, 1976, pp 28–42.
9. Dawber TR: *The Framingham Study: The Epidemiology of Atherosclerotic Disease.* Cambridge, Massachusetts, Harvard University Press, 1980.
10. Blood Pressure Study 1979. Society of Actuaries and Association of Life Insurance Medical Directors of America, 1979.
11. Kannel WB: Some lessons in cardiovascular epidemiology from Framingham. *Am J Cardiol* 1976; 37:269–82.
12. Itskovitz HD, Kochar MS, Anderson AJ, Rimm AA: Patterns of blood pressure in Milwaukee. *JAMA* 1977; 238:864–868.
13. Sullivan JM: Arterial hypertension, in Blacklow RS (ed): *MacBryde's Signs and Symptoms,* ed 6. Philadelphia, JB Lippincott, 1983, pp 261–294.
14. Riva-Rocci S: Un nuovo sfigmonometro. *Gazz med Torino* 1986; 47:981–1001.
15. Schottstaedt MF, Sokolow M: The natural history and course of hypertension with papilledema (malignant hypertension). *Am Heart J* 1953; 45:331–362.
16. McMichael J, Murphy EA: Methonium treatment of severe and malignant hypertension. *J Chron Dis* 1955; 1:527–535.
17. Kincaid-Smith P, McMichael J, Murphy EA: The clinical course and pathology of hypertension with papilloedema (malignant hypertension). *Q J Med* 1958; 27:117–153.
18. Perry HM Jr, Schroeder HA, Catanzara FJ, Moore-Jones D, Camel GH: Studies on the control of hypertension. VIII. Mortality, morbidity, and remission during twelve years of intensive therapy. *Circulation* 1966; 33:958–972.
19. Sokolow M, Perloff D: Five year survival of consecutive patients with malignant hypertension treated with antihypertensive agents. *Am J Cardiol* 1960; 6:858–863.
20. Woods JW, Blythe WB: Management of malignant hypertension complicated by renal insufficiency. *N Engl J Med* 1967; 277:57–61.
21. Hodge JV, Smirk FH: The effect of drug treatment of hypertension on the distribution of deaths from various causes. A study of 173 deaths among hypertensive patients in the years 1959 to 1964 inclusive. *Am Heart J* 1967; 73:441–452.
22. Build and Blood Pressure Study, Chicago Society of Actuaries, vol 2, 1959.
23. Kannel WB, Castelli WP, McNamara PM, Sorlie D: The Framingham study: Some factors affecting morbidity and mortality in hypertension. *Milbank Mem Fund Q* 1969; 47:116–142.
24. Kannel WB, Schwartz MJ, McNamara PM: Blood pressure and risk of coronary heart disease. The Framingham study. *Dis Chest* 1969; 56:43–52.
25. Byrom FB: Pathogenesis of hypertensive encephalopathy and relation to malignant phase of hypertension: experimental evidence from hypertensive rat. *Lancet* 1954; 2:201–211.
26. Sako Y: Effect of turbulent blood flow and hypertension on experimental atherosclerosis. *JAMA* 1962; 179:36–40.
27. Heath D, Wood EH, Dushane JW, Edwards JE: The relation of age and blood pressure to atheroma in the pulmonary arteries and thoracic aorta in congenital heart disease. *Lab Invest* 1960; 9:259–272.
28. Brust AA, Ferris EB: Diagnostic approach to hypertension due to unilateral kidney disease. *Ann Intern Med* 1957; 47:1049–1066.
29. Rushmer RF: *Structure and Function of the Cardiovascular System.* Philadelphia, WB Saunders, 1972.
30. Mellander S, Johannsson B: Control of resistance, exchange and capacitance function of the peripheral circulation. *Pharmacol Res* 1968; 20:117–196.
31. Bayliss WM: On the local reaction of the arterial wall to changes of internal pressure. *J Physiol* 1902; 28:220–231.
32. Folkow B, Neil E: *Circulation,* New York, Oxford University Press, 1971.
33. Frohlich ED: Hemodynamics of hypertension, in Genest J, Koiw E, Kuchel O (eds): *Hypertension.* New York, McGraw-Hill, 1977, pp 15–49.
34. Widimsky J, Fejfarova MD, Fejfar A: Changes of cardiac output in hypertensive disease. *Cardiologia* 1957; 31:381–389.
35. Eich RJ, Peters RJ, Cuddy RP, Smulyan H, Lyons RH: Hemodynamics in labile hypertension. *Am Heart J* 1962; 63:188–195.
36. Julius S, Randall OS, Esler MD, Kashima T, Ellis C, Bennett J: Altered cardiac responsiveness and regulation in the normal cardiac output type of borderline hypertension. *Circ Res* 1975; 36(suppl 1):I-199–I-207.
37. Ulrych M, Frohlich ED, Dustan HP, Page IH: Cardiac output and distribution of blood volume in central and peripheral circulations in hypertensive and normotensive man. *Br Heart J* 1969; 31:570–574.
38. Julius S, Pascual AV, Sannerstedt R, Mitchell C: Relationship between cardiac output and peripheral resistance in borderline hypertension. *Circulation* 1971; 43:382–390.
39. Sannerstedt R: Hemodynamic response to exercise in patients with arterial hypertension. *Acta Med Scand* 1966; 180(suppl 458):1–13.
40. Takeshita A, Mark AL: Decreased vasodilator capacity of forearm resistance vessels in borderline hypertension. *Hypertension* 1980; 2:610–616.
41. Al-Aouar ZR, Ratts TE, Cunningham BR, Sullivan JM: Altered ventricular diastolic properties in borderline hypertension: effect of sodium intake. *Circulation* 1981; 64(IV):IV-322.
42. Sullivan JM, Prewitt RL, Josephs JA: Attenuation of the microcirculation in young patients with high output labile hypertension. *Hypertension* 1983; 5:844–851.
43. Meerson F: The myocardium in hyperfunction, hypertrophy, and failure. *Circ Res* 1969; 25(suppl 2):1–54.
44. Ledingham JM, Cohen RD: The role of the heart in the pathogenesis of renal hypertension. *Lancet* 1963; 2:979–981.
45. Guyton AC, Granger HJ, Coleman TG: Autoregulation of the total systemic circulation and its relation to control of cardiac output and arterial pressure. *Circ Res* 1971; 28(suppl 1):93–97.
46. Tarazi RC: Hemodynamic role of extracellular fluid in hypertension. *Circ Res* 1976; 38(suppl II):II-73–II-83.
47. Sullivan JM, Schoeneberger AA, Ratts E, Palmer ET, Samaha JK, Mance CH, Muirhead EE: Short-term therapy of severe hypertension. Hemodynamic correlates of the antihypertensive response in man. *Arch Intern Med* 1979; 139:1233–1239.
48. Ambard L, Beaujard E: Causes de l'hypertension arterielle. *Arch Gen Med* 1904; 1:520–533.
49. Sasaki N: The relationship of salt intake to hypertension in the Japanese. *Geriatrics* 1964; 19:735–744.
50. Kempner W: Treatment of kidney disease and hypertensive vascular disease with rice diet. *N Carolina Med J* 1944; 5:125–133.
51. Murphy RJF: The effect of "rice diet" on plasma volume and extracellular fluid space in hypertensive subjects. *J Clin Invest* 1950; 29:912–917.
52. Parijs J, Joosens JV, Vander Linden L, Verstreken G, Amery AKPC: Moderate sodium restriction and diuretics in the treatment of hypertension. *Am Heart J* 1973; 85:22–34.
53. Luft FC, Weinberger MH, Grim CE, Fineberg NS, Miller JZ: Sodium sensitivity in normotensive human subjects. *Ann Intern Med* 1983; 98:758–762.
54. Coleman TG, Guyton AC: Hypertension caused by salt loading in the dog. III. Onset transients of cardiac output and other variables. *Circ Res* 1969; 25:153–160.
55. Dahl LK: Salt and hypertension. *Am J Clin Nutr* 1972; 25:231–244.
56. Bianchi G, Fox U, DiFrancesco GF, Giovanetti AM, Patetti D: Blood pressure changes produced by kidney cross-transplantation between spontaneously hypertensive rats (SHR) and normotensive rats (NR). *Clin Sci Mol Med* 1974; 47:435–448.
57. Dahl LK, Heine M, Thompson K: Genetic influence of the kidneys on blood pressure. Evidence from chronic renal homografts in rats with opposite predispositions to hypertension. *Circ Res* 1974; 34:94–101.
58. Dahl LK, Knudsen KD, Iwai J: Humoral transmission of hypertension: evidence from parabiosis. *Circ Res* 1969; 24(suppl):I21–I33.
59. Tobian L, Ishii M, Duke M: Relationship of cytoplasmic granules in renal papillary interstitial cells to "post-salt" hypertension. *J Lab Clin Med* 1969; 73:309–319.
60. Ganguli M, Tobian L, Iwai J: Cardiac output and peripheral resistance in strains of rats sensitive and resistant to NaCl hypertension. *Hypertension* 1979; 1:3–7.
61. Kisch B: Electron microscopy of the atrium of the heart. *Exp Med Surg* 1956; 14:99–112.
62. deBold AJ: Heart atria granularity effects changes in water-electrolyte balance. *Proc Soc Exp Biol Med* 1979; 161:508–511.
63. deBold AJ, Borenstein HB, Veress AT, Sonnenberg H: A rapid and potent natriuretic response to intravenous injection of atrial myocardial extract in rats. *Life Sci* 1981; 28:89–94.
64. Sonnenberg H, Cupples WA, deBold AJ, Veress AT: Intrarenal localization of the natriuretic effect of cardiac atrial extract. *Can J Physiol Pharmacol* 1982; 60:1149–1152.
64a. deBold AJ: Atrial natriuretic factor: a hormone produced by the heart. *Science* 1985; 230:767–770.
64b. Samson WK: Atrial natriuretic factor inhibits dehydration and hemorrhage-induced vasopressin release. *Neuroendocrinology* 1985; 40:277–279.
65. Mark AL: The Bezold-Jarisch reflex revisited: clinical implications of inhibitory reflexes originating in the heart. *J Am Coll Cardiol* 1983; 1:90–102.
66. De Wardener HE, Clarkson EM: The natriuretic hormone: recent developments. *Clin Sci* 1982; 63:415–420.
67. Blaustein MP: Sodium ions, calcium ions, blood pressure regulation, and hypertension: a reassessment and a hypothesis. *Am J Physiol* 1977; 232:C165–C173.
68. Hamlyn JM, Ringel R, Schaeffer J, Levinson PD, Hamilton BP, Ko-

warski AA, Blaustein MP: A circulating inhibitor of (Na + K) ATPase associated with essential hypertension. *Nature* 1982; 300:650–652.
69. Kirkendall WM, Connor WE, Abboud F, Rastogi SP, Anderson TA, Fry M: The effect of dietary sodium on the blood pressure of normal man, in Genest J, Koiw E (eds): *Hypertension '72.* Berlin, Springer-Verlag, 1972, pp 360–374.
70. Mark AL, Lawton WJ, Abboud FM, Fitz AE, Connor WE, Heistad DD: Effects of high and low sodium intake on arterial pressure and forearm vascular resistance in borderline hypertension. *Circ Res* 1975; 36(suppl 1):I-194–I-198.
71. Frohlich ED, Tarazi RC, Dustan HP: Re-examination of the hemodynamics of hypertension. *Am J Med Sci* 1969; 257:9–23.
72. Julius S, Pascual AV, Reilly K, London R: Abnormalities of plasma volume in borderline hypertension. *Arch Intern Med* 1971; 127:116–119.
73. Sullivan JM, Ratts TE, Schoeneberger AA, Samaha JK, Palmer ET: The effect of diet on echocardiographic left ventricular dimensions in normal man. *Am J Clin Nutr* 1979; 32:2410–2415.
74. Sullivan JM, Ratts TE, Taylor JC, Kraus DH, Barton BR, Patrick DR, Reed SW: Hemodynamic effects of dietary sodium in man. A preliminary report. *Hypertension* 1980; 2:506–514.
75. Sullivan JM, Ratts TE: Hemodynamic mechanisms of adaptation to chronic high sodium intake in normal humans. *Hypertension* 1983; 5:814–820.
76. Onesti G, Kim KE, Greco JA, del Guercioz ET, Fernandes M, Swartz C: Blood pressure regulation in end-stage renal disease and anephric man. *Circ Res* 1975; 36(suppl 1):I-145–I-152.
77. Bravo E, Tarazi R, Dustan H: Multifactorial analysis of chronic hypertension induced by electrolyte-active steroids in trained unanesthetized dogs. *Circ Res* 1977; 40(suppl 1):I-140–I-145.
78. Berecek K, Bohr D: Whole body vascular reactivity during the development of deoxycorticosterone acetate hypertension in the pig. *Circ Res* 1978; 42:764–771.
79. Luft FC, Weinberger MH, Grim CE: Sodium sensitivity and resistance in normotensive humans. *Am J Med* 1982; 72:726–736.
80. Langford HG: Dietary potassium and epidemiologic data. *Ann Intern Med* 1983; 98:770–772.
80a. Bulpitt CJ, Broughton PMG, Markowe HLJ, Marmot MG, Rosc G, Semmence A, Shipley MJ: The relationship between both sodium and potassium intake and blood pressure in London civil servants. A report from the Whitehall Department of Environmental Study. *J Chronic Dis* 1986; 39:211–219.
81. Emanuel DA, Scott JB, Haddy FJ: Effect of potassium on small and large blood vessels of the dog forelimb. *Am J Physiol* 1959; 197:637–642.
82. Lowe RD, Thompson JW: The effect of intra-arterial potassium chloride infusion upon forearm blood flow in man. *J Physiol (Lond)* 1962; 162:69P–70P.
83. Overbeck HW, Derifield RS, Pamnani MB: Attenuated vasodilator responses to K in essential hypertensive men. *J Clin Invest* 1974; 53:678–686.
84. Luft FC, Rankin LI, Bloch R, Weyman AE, Willis LR, Murray RH, Grim CE, Weinberger MH: Cardiovascular and humoral responses to extremes of sodium intake in normal black and white men. *Circulation* 1979; 60:697–706.
85. MacGregor GA, Smith SJ, Marhandu ND, Banks RA, Sagnella GA: Moderate potassium supplementation in essential hypertension. *Lancet* 1982; 2:567–570.
86. Tobian L, Lance J, Ulm K, Iwai J: Dietary K supplements prevent strokes in stroke-prone SHR. *Clin Res* 1984; 32:555A.
86a. Folsom AR, Smith CL, Prineas RJ, Grimm RH Jr: Serum calcium fractions in essential hypertension and matched normotensive subjects. *Hypertension* 1986; 8:11–15.
86b. Pietinen P, Dougherty R, Mutanen M, Leino U, Moisio S, Iacono J, Ruska P: Dietary intervention study among 30 free-living families in Finland. *J Am Diet Assoc* 1984; 84:313–318.
86c. Lau K, Gafter U, Rydell D, Eby B, Pesigan M, Tropp I, Garno J, Zikas D: Evidence against the role of calcium deficiency in genetic hypertension. *Hypertension* 1986; 8:45–49.
86d. McCarron DA, Morris CD, Henry HJ, Stanton JL: Blood pressure and nutrient intake in the United States. *Science* 1984; 224:1392–1398.
86e. Harlan WR, Hull AL, Schmouder RL, Landis JR, Thompson FE, Larkin FA: Blood pressure and nutrition in adults. The National Health and Nutrition Examination Survey. *Am J Epidemiol* 1984; 120:17–27.
86f. Garcia-Palmieri MR, Costas R, Cruz-Vidal M, Sorlie PD, Tillotson J, Havlik RJ: Milk consumption, calcium intake, and decreased hypertension in Puerto Rico. Puerto Rico Heart Health Program study. *Hypertension* 1984; 6:322–328.
86g. Gruchow HW, Sobocinski KA, Barboriak JJ: Alcohol nutrient intake and hypertension in US adults. *JAMA* 1985; 253:1567–1570.
86h. Hypertension: is there a place for calcium? *Lancet* 1986; 1:359–361.
87. Gibson DG, Trail TA, Hall RJC, Brown DJ: Echocardiographic features of secondary left ventricular hypertrophy. *Br Heart J* 1979; 41:54–59.
88. Ratts TE, Addington B, Gerlach P, Conway L, Sullivan JM: Echocardiographic-clinical correlation of heart failure in hypertension. *J Am Coll Cardiol* 1984; 3:592.
88a. Oliver WJ: Sodium homeostasis and low blood pressure populations, in Kesteloot H, Jossens JV (eds): *Epidemiology of Arterial Pressure.* The Hague, Martinus Nijhoff, 1980, pp 229–241.
88b. Taylor R, Zimmer P, Levy S, Collins V: Group comparisons of blood pressure and indices of obesity and salt intake in Pacific populations. *Med J Aust* 1985; 142:499–501.
88c. Avolio AP, Chen SG, Wang RP, Zhang CL, Li MF, O'Rourke MF: Effects of aging on changing arterial compliance and left ventricular load in a northern Chinese urban community. *Circulation* 1983; 68:50–58.
88d. Avolio AP, Deng FQ, Li WQ, Luo YF, Huang ZD, Xing LF, O'Rourke MF: Effects of aging on arterial distensibility in populations with high and low prevalence of hypertension: comparisons between urban and rural communities in China. *Circulation* 1985; 71:202–210.
88e. Avolio AP, Clyde KM, Beard TC, Cooke HM, Ho KKL, O'Rourke MF: Improved arterial distensibility in normotensive subjects on a low salt diet. *Arteriosclerosis* 1986; 6:166–169.
89. Edmondson R, Hilton P, Jones W: Abnormal leucocyte composition and sodium transport in essential hypertension. *Lancet* 1975; 1:1003–1005.
90. Garay RP, Elghozi JL, Dagher G, Meyer P: Laboratory distinction between essential and secondary hypertension by measurement of erythrocyte cation fluxes. *N Engl J Med* 1980; 302:769–771.
91. Ghione S, Buzzxigoli G, Bartolini V, Balzan S, Donato L: Comparison of outward and inward Na+/K+ cotransport-mediated fluexes in erythrocytes of essential hypertensive patients. Preliminary results. *Clin Exp Hypertension* 1981; 3:809–814.
92. Cusi D, Barlassina C, Ferrandi M, Lupi P, Ferrari P, Bianchi G: Familial aggregation of cation transport abnormalities and essential hypertension. *Clin Exp Hypertension* 1981; 3:871–884.
93. Swarts HG, Bonting SL, de Pont JJ, Schuurmans-Stekhoven FMAH, Thien TA, Van T, Laar A: Cation fluexes in Na+-K+-activated ATPase activity in erythrocytes of patients with essential hypertension. *Hypertension* 1981; 3:641–649.
94. Walter U, Distler A: Abnormal sodium efflux in erythrocytes of patients with essential hypertension. *Hypertension* 1982; 4:205–210.
95. Duhm J, Gobel BO, Lorenz R, Weber PG: Sodium-lithium exchange and sodium-potassium cotransport in human erythrocytes. Part 2. A simple uptake test applied to normotensive and essential hypertensive individuals. *Hypertension* 1982; 4:477–482.
96. Adragna NC, Canessa ML, Solomon H, Slater E, Tostenson DC: Red cell lithium-sodium countertransport and sodium-potassium cotransport in patients with essential hypertension. *Hypertension* 1982; 4:795–804.
97. Tuck ML, Gross C, Maxwell MH, Brickman AS, Krasnoshtein G, Mayes D: Erythrocyte Na+, K+ cotransport and Na+, K+ pump in black and Caucasian hypertensive patients. *Hypertension,* 1984; 6:536–544.
98. Cannasa MN, Adragna N, Soloman HS, Connolly TM, Tosteson DC: Increased sodium-lithium counter-transport in red cells of patients with essential hypertension. *N Engl J Med* 1980; 302:772–776.
99. Woods JW, Falk RJ, Pittman AW, Klemmer PJ, Watson BS, Nambookiri K: Increased red-cell sodium-lithium countertransport in normotensive sons of hypertensive parents. *N Engl J Med* 1982; 306:593–595.
100. Trevisan M, Ostrow D, Cooper R, Liu K, Sparks S, Okonek A, Stevens E, Marquardt J, Stamler J: Abnormal red cell ion transport and hypertension. The People's Gas Study. *Hypertension* 1983; 5:363–367.
101. Brugnara C, Corrocher R, Foroni L, Steinmayr M, Bonfanti F, DeSandre G: Lithium-sodium countertransport in erythrocytes of normal and hypertensive subjects. *Hypertension* 1983; 5:529–534.
102. Duhm J, Gobel OB: Sodium-lithium exchange and sodium-potassium cotransport in human erythrocytes. Part 1. Evaluation of a simple uptake test to assess the activity of the two transport systems. *Hypertension* 1982; 4:468–476.
103. Isben KK, Jensen HE, Wieth JO, Funder J: Sodium-lithium countertransport in erythrocytes from patients and from children having one hypertensive parent. *Hypertension* 1982; 4:703–709.
104. Engelman K, Portnoy B, Sjoerdsma A: Plasma catecholamine concentration in patients with hypertension. *Circ Res* 1970; 27:I-141–I-146.
105. DeQuatro V, Chan S: Raised plasma-catecholamines in some patients with primary hypertension. *Lancet* 1972; 1:806–809.
106. Louis WJ, Doyle AE, Anavekar S: Plasma norepinephrine levels in essential hypertension. *N Engl J Med* 1973; 288:599–601.
107. Stone RA, Gunnells JC, Robinson RR, Schanberg SM, Kirshner N: Dopamine-beta-hydroxylase in primary and secondary hypertension. *Circ Res* 1974; 34:I-47–I-56.
108. Louis WJ, Doyle AE, Anavekar SN, Johnston CI, Geffen LB, Rush R: Plasma catecholamine, dopamine-beta-hydroxylase and renin levels in essential hypertension. *Circ Res* 1974; 34:1–57.
109. Engelman K, Portnoy B, Lovenberg W: A sensitive and specific double isotope derivative method for the determination of catecholamine in biological specimens. *Am J Med Sci* 1968; 255:259–268.
110. DeQuattro V, Miura J: Neurogenic factors in human hypertension. Mechanism or myth? in Laragh JH (ed): *Hypertension Manual.* New York, Yorke Medical Books, 1972, pp 277–312.

111. Gitlow SE, Mendlowitz M, Wilk EK, Wilk S, Wolf RL, Naftchi NE: Plasma clearance of dl-beta-H3-norepinephrine in normal human subjects and patients with essential hypertension. *J Clin Invest* 1964; 43:2009–2015.
112. DeQuattro V, Sjoerdsma A: Catecholamine turnovers in normotensive and hypertensive man: effects of antiadrenergic drug. *J Clin Invest* 1968; 47:2359–2373.
113. Tigerstadt R, Bergman PG: Niere and Dreishauf. *Skand Arch Physiol* 1898; 8:223–271.
114. Goldblatt H, Lynch J, Hanzal RF, Summerville WW: Studies on experimental hypertension. I. The production of persistent elevation of systolic blood pressure by means of renal ischemia. *J Exp Med* 1934; 59:347–379.
115. Page, IH: On the nature of the pressor action of renin. *J Exp Med* 1939; 70:521–542.
116. Braun-Menendez E, Fasciolo JC, Leloir LF, Munoz JM: La substancia hipertensora de la sangre del rinon isquemiado. *Rev Soc Argent Biol* 1939; 15:420–425.
117. Simpson SA, Tait JF, Wettstein A, Neher R, von Euw J, Reichstein T: Isolierung eines neuen kristallisierten Hormons aus Nebennieren mit besonders hoher Wieksamkeit aus den Meneral-Stofswechsel. *Experientia* (Basel) 1953; 9:333–335.
118. Laragh JH, Angers M, Kelly WG, Lieberman S: Hypotensive agents and pressor substances. The effect of epinephrine, norepinephrine, angiotensin II and others on the secretory rate of aldosterone in man. *JAMA* 1960; 174:234–240.
119. Genest J, Nowaczynski W, Koiw E, Sandor T, Biron P: Adrenocorticoid function in essential hypertension, in Boch KD, Cottier PT (eds): *Essential Hypertension.* Berlin, Springer-Verlag, 1960, pp 126–146.
120. Blair-West JR, Coghlan JP, Denton DA, Funder JW, Scoggins BA, Wright RD: The effect of heptapeptide (2-8) and hexapeptide (3-8) fragments of angiotensin II on aldosterone secretion. *J Clin Endocrinol Metab* 1971; 32:575–578.
121. Davis JO: What signals the kidney to release renin? *Circ Res* 1971; 28:301–306.
122. Tobian L, Tomboulian A, Janecek J: Effect of high perfusion pressures on the granulation of juxtaglomerular cells in an isolated kidney. *J Clin Invest* 1959; 38:605–610.
123. Vander AJ: Effect of catecholamines and the renal nerves on renin secretion in anesthetized dogs. *Am J Physiol* 1965; 209:659–662.
124. Skinner SL, McCubbin JW, Page IH: Control of renin secretion. *Circ Res* 1964; 15:64–76.
125. Vander AJ, Miller R: Control of renin secretion in the anesthetized dog. *Am J Physiol* 1964; 207:537–546.
126. Brown JJ, Davies DL, Lever AR, Robertson JIS: Plasma renin concentration in human hypertension. I. Relationship between renin, sodium, and potassium. *Br Med J* 1965; 3:144–148.
127. Veyrat R, Brunner HR, Manning EL, Muller AF: Inhibition de l'activité de la rénine plasmatique par le potassium. *J Urol Nephrol (Paris)* 1967; 73:271–275.
128. Vander AJ, Geelhoed GW: Inhibition of renin secretion by angiotensin II. *Proc Soc Exp Biol Med* 1965; 120:399–403.
129. Wathen RL, Kingsbury WS, Stouder DA, Schneider EG, Rostorfer HH: Effects of infusion of catecholamines and angiotensin II on renin release in anesthetized dogs. *Am J Physiol* 1965; 209:1012–1024.
130. Helmer OM, Griffith RS: The effect of the administration of estrogens on the renin-substrate (hypertensinogen) content of rat plasma. *Endocrinology* 1952; 51:421–426.
131. Robb CA, Davis JO, Johnson CI, Hartreoft PM: Effect of deoxycorticosterone on plasma renin activity in conscious dogs. *Am J Physiol* 1969; 216:884–889.
132. Vander AJ: Inhibition of renin release in the dog by vasopressin and vasotocin. *Circ Res* 1968; 23:605–609.
133. Larsson C, Weber P, Anggard E: Arachidonic acid increases and indomethacine decreases plasma renin activity in the rabbit. *Eur J Pharmacol* 1974; 28:391–394.
134. Henrich WL: Role of the prostaglandins in renin secretion. *Kidney Int* 1981; 19:822–830.
135. Gotshall RW, Davis JO, Shade RE, Spielman W, Johnson JA, Beaverman B: Effects of renal denervation on renin release in sodium depleted dogs. *Am J Physiol* 1973; 225:344–349.
136. Assaykeen TA, Clayton PL, Goldfien A, Ganong WF: Effect of alpha- and beta-adrenergic blocking agents on the renin response to hypoglycemia and epinephrine in dogs. *Endocrinology* 1970; 87:1318–1322.
137. Passo SS, Assaykeen TA, Goldfien A, Ganong WF: Effect of alpha and beta adrenergic blocking agents on the increase in renin secretion production by stimulation of the medulla oblongata. *Neuroendocrinology* 1971; 7:97–104.
138. Winer N, Walkerkorst WG: Effect of cyclic AMP, sympathomimetic amines and adrenergic antagonists on renin secretion. *Circ Res* 1971; 29:239–248.
139. Winer N: Mechanism of increased renin secretion associated with adrenalectomy, hemorrhage, renal artery constriction and sodium depletion, in Genest J, Koiw E (eds): *Hypertension '72.* Berlin, Heidelberg, New York, Springer-Verlag, 1972, pp 25–36.
140. Tanigawa H, Allison DJ, Assaykeen TA: A comparison of the effects of various catecholamines on plasma renina activity alone and in the presence of adrenergic blocking agents, in Genest J, Koiw E (eds): *Hypertension '72*. Berlin, Heidelberg, New York, Springer-Verlag, 1972, pp 37–44.
141. Ganong WF: Effect of sympathetic activity and ACTH on renin and aldosterone secretion, in Genest J, Koiw E (eds): *Hypertension '72.* Berlin, Heidelberg, New York, Springer-Verlag, 1972, pp 4–13.
142. Sullivan JM, Adams DF, Hollenberg NK: Beta-adrenergic blockade in essential hypertension. Reduced renin release despite renal vasoconstriction. *Circ Res* 1976; 39:532–536.
143. Buhler FR, Laragh JH, Baer L, Vaughan ED Jr, Brunner HR: Propranolol inhibition of renin secretion. *N Engl J Med* 1972; 287:1209–1214.
144. Michelakis AM, McAllister RG: The effect of chronic adrenergic receptor blockade on plasma renin activity in man. *J Clin Endocrinol* 1972; 34:386–394.
145. Winer N, Chokski DS, Yoon MS, Freedman AD: Adrenergic receptor mediation of renin secretion. *J Clin Endocrinol* 1969; 29:1168–1175.
146. Bravo EL, Tarazi RC, Dustan HP: Beta-adrenergic blockade in diuretic-treated patients with essential hypertension. *N Engl J Med* 1975; 292:66–70.
147. Bravo EL, Tarazi RC, Dustan HP: On the mechanism of suppressed plasma renin activity during beta-adrenergic blockade with propranolol. *J Lab Clin Med* 1974; 83:119–128.
148. Couch NP, Sullivan JM, Crane C: The predictive accuracy of renal vein renin activity in the surgery of renovascular hypertension. *Surgery* 1976; 79:70–76.
149. Brunner HR, Laragh JH, Baer L, Newton MA, Goodwin FT, Krakoff LR, Bard RH, Buhler FR: Essential hypertension: renin and aldosterone, heart attack and stroke. *N Engl J Med* 1972; 286:441–449.
150. Channick BJ, Adlin EV, Marks AD: Suppressed plasma renin activity in hypertension. *Arch Intern Med* 1969; 123:131–140.
151. Drayer JIM, Kloppenborg PWC, Benraad TJ: Detection of low-renin hypertension: evaluation of out-patient renin-stimulating methods. *Clin Sci Mol Med* 1975; 48:91–96.
152. Dunn MJ, Tanner RL: Low-renin hypertension. *Kidney Int* 1974; 5:317–325.
153. Laragh JH: Vasoconstriction-volume analysis for understanding and treating hypertension: the use of renin and aldosterone profiles. *Am J Med* 1973; 55:261–274.
154. Woods JW, Liddle GW, Stant EG Jr, Michelakis AM, Brill AB: Effect of an adrenal inhibitor in hypertensive patients with suppressed renin. *Arch Intern Med* 1969; 123:366–370.
155. Carey RM, Douglas JG, Schjweikert JR, Liddle GW: The syndrome of essential hypertension and suppressed plasma renin activity: normalization of blood pressure with spironolactone. *Arch Intern Med* 1972; 130:849–854.
156. Woods JW, Pittman AW, Pulliam CC, Werk EE, Waider W, Allen CA: Renin profiling in hypertension and its use in treatment with propranolol and chlorthalidone. *N Engl J Med* 1976; 294:1137–1143.
157. Weidman P, Hirsch D, Maxwell MH, Okun R: Plasma renin and blood pressure during treatment with methyldopa. *Am J Cardiol* 1974; 34:671–676.
158. Green LJ, Camargo ACM, Krieger EM, Stewart JM, Ferreira SH: Inhibition of the conversion of angiotensin I to II and potentiation of bradykinin by small peptides present in Bothrops jararaca venom. *Circ Res* 1972; 31(suppl 2):62–71.
159. Ondetti MA, Rubin R, Cushman DW: Design of specific inhibitors or angiotensin-converting enzyme: new class of orally active antihypertensive agents. *Science* 1977; 196:441–444.
160. Sweet CS, Gross DM, Arbegast PT, Gaul JL, Britt PM, Ludden CT, Weitz D, Stone CA: Antihypertensive activity of N-{(S)-1-(Ethoxycarbonyl)-3-phenylporopyl}-L-ala-L-pro (MK-42), an orally active converting enzyme inhibitor. *J Pharmacol Exp Ther* 1981; 216:63–69.
160a. Todd PT, Heel RC: Enalapril. A review of its pharmacodynamic and pharmacokinetic properties, and therapeutic use in hypertension and congested heart failure. *Drugs* 1986; 31:198–248.
161. Ulm EH, Hichens M, Gomez HJ, Till AE, Hand E, Vassil TC, Biollaz J, Brunner HR, Schelling JL: Enalapril maleate and a lysine analogue (MK-521) disposition in man. *Br J Clin Pharmacol* 1982; 14:357–362.
162. Pals DT, Mascucci FD, Sipos F, Denning GS Jr: A specific competitive antagonist of the vascular action of angiotensin II. *Circ Res* 1971; 29:664–672.
163. Streeten DHP, Anderson GH, Dalakos TG: Angiotensin blockade: its clinical significance. *Am J Med* 1976; 60:817–824.
164. Resnick LM, Sealey JE, Laragh JH: Calcium metabolism and the renin-aldosterone system determine the acute blood pressure response to calcium channel blockade. *Circulation* 1982; 66:II-107.
165. Kaplan NM: Renin profiles: The unfulfilled promises. *JAMA* 1977; 238:611–613.
166. Hedqvist P: Studies on the effect of prostaglandins E1 and E2 on the sympathetic neuromuscular transmission in some animal tissues. *Acta Physiol Scand (Suppl)* 1970; 345:1–40.
167. DuCharme DW, Weeks JR, Montgomery RG: Studies on the mech-

anism of the hypertensive effect of prostaglandin $F_{2\alpha}$. *J Pharmacol Exp Ther* 1968; 160:1–10.
168. Malik KU, McGiff JC: Cardiovascular actions of prostaglandins, in Varim SMM (ed): *Prostaglandins: Physiological, Pharmacological and Pathological Aspects.* England, MTP Press Ltd, 1976, pp 103–200.
169. Nakano JM, McCurdy JR: Cardiovascular effects of prostaglandin El. *J Pharmacol Exp Ther* 1967; 156:538–586.
170. Terragno DA, Crowshaw K, Terragno NA, McGiff JC: Prostaglandin synthesis by bovine mesenteric arteries and veins. *Circ Res* 1975; 36–37(suppl I):I-76–I-80.
171. Terragno NA, Terragno DA, McGiff JC: Contribution of prostaglandins to the renal circulation in conscious, anesthetized and laparotomized dogs. *Circ Res* 1977; 40:590–595.
172. Grantham JJ, Orloff J: Effect of prostaglandin E1 on the permeability response of the isolated collecting tubule to vasopressin, adenosine 3′, 5′-monophosphate, and theophylline. *J Clin Invest* 1968; 47:1154–1161.
173. Gryglewski RJ, Korbut R, Ocetkiewicz A: Generation of prostacyclin by lungs in vivo and its release into the arterial circulation. *Nature* 1978;273:765–767.
174. Moncada S, Korbut R, Bunting S, Vane JR: Prostacyclin is a circulating hormone. *Nature* 1978; 273:767–768.
175. Armstrong JM, Lattimer N, Moncada S, Vane JR: Comparison of the vasodepressor effects of prostacyclin and 6-oxo-prostaglandin F_1-alpha with those of prostaglandin E_2 in rats and rabbits. *Br J Pharmacol* 1978; 62:125–130.
176. Dusting GJ, Moncada S, Vane JR: Recirculation of prostacyclin (PGI_2) in the dog. *Br J Pharmacol* 1978; 64:315–320.
177. Piper PJ, Vane JR: Release of additional factors in anaphylaxis and its antagonism by anti-inflammatory drugs. *Nature* 1969; 223:29–35.
178. Hamberg M, Samuelsson B: Prostaglandin endoperoxides. Novel transformations of arachidonic acid in human platelets. *Proc Natl Acad Sci USA* 1974; 71:3400–3404.
179. Hamberg M, Svensson J, Samuelsson B: Thromboxanes: a new group of biologically active compounds derived from prostaglandin endoperoxides. *Proc Natl Acad Sci USA* 1975; 72:2994–2998.
180. Bunting S, Gryglewski R, Moncada S, Vane JR: Arterial walls generate from prostaglandin endoperoxides, a substance (prostaglandin X) which relaxes strips of mesenteric and coeliac arteries and inhibits platelet aggregation. *Prostaglandins* 1976; 12:897–913.
181. Moncada S, Higgs EA, Vane JR: Human arterial and venous tissues generate prostacyclin (prostaglandin X), a potent inhibitor of platelet aggregation. *Lancet* 1977; 1:18–20.
182. Aiken JW: Effects of prostaglandin synthesis inhibitors on angiotensin tachyphylaxis in the isolated coeliac and mesenteric arteries of the rabbit. *Pol J Pharmacol Pharm* 1974; 26:217–227.
183. Mullane KM, Moncada S: Prostacyclin release and the modulation of some vasoactive hormones. *Prostaglandins* 1980; 20:25–49.
184. Grodzinska L, Gruglewski RJ: Angiotensin-induced release of prostacyclin from perfused organs. *Pharmac Res Commun* 1980; 12:339–347.
185. Needleman P, Bronson SD, Wyche A, Sivakoff M, Nicolaou KC: Cardiac and renal prostaglandin I_2. Biosynthesis and biological effects in isolated perfused rabbit tissue. *J Clin Invest* 1978; 61:839–849.
186. Nasjletti A, Malik KU: Interrelations between prostaglandins and vasoconstrictor hormones: contribution to blood pressure regulation. *Med Clin North Am* 1981; 65:881–889.
187. Beilin LJ, Bhattacharya J: The effect of prostaglandin synthesis inhibitors on renal blood flow distribution in conscious rabbits. *J Physiol* 1977; 269:395–405.
188. Colina-Chourio J, McGiff JC, Nasjletti A: Effect of indomethacin on blood pressure in the normotensive unanesthetized rabbit: possible relation to prostaglandin synthesis inhibition. *Clin Sci* 1979; 57:359–365.
189. Muirhead EE, Brooks B, Brosius WL: Indomethacin and blood pressure control. *J Lab Clin Med* 1976; 88:578–583.
190. Romero JC, Strong JC: The effect of indomethacin blockade of prostaglandin synthesis on blood pressure of normal rabbits and rabbits with renovascular hypertension. *Circ Res* 1977; 40:35–41.
191. Chrysant SG, Townsend SM, Morgan PR: The effects of salt and meclofenamate administration on the hypertension of spontaneously hypertensive rats. *Clin Exp Hypertension* 1978; 1:381–391.
192. McQueen D, Bell K: The effects of prostaglandin E_1 and sodium meclofenamate on blood pressure in renal hypertensive rats. *Eur J Pharmacol* 1976; 37:223–235.
193. Yun J, Kelly G, Bartter FC: Effect of indomethacin on renal function and plasma renin activity in dogs with chronic renovascular hypertension. *Nephron* 1979; 24:278–282.
194. Wennmalm A: Hypertensive effect of the prostaglandin synthesis inhibitor indomethacin. *IRCS* (Research on: Endocrine System) 1974; 2:1099.
195. Nowak J, Wennmalm A: Influence of indomethacin and prostaglandin E1 on total and regional blood flow in man. *Acta Physiol Scand* 1978; 102:484–491.
196. Negus P, Tannen RL, Dunn MJ: Indomethacin potentiates the vasoconstrictor actions of angiotensin II in normal man. *Prostaglandins* 1976; 12:175–180.
197. Patak RB, Mookerjee C, Bentzel P, Hysert P, Babe M, Lee J: Antagonism of the effects of furosemide by indomethacin in normal and hypertensive man. *Prostaglandins* 1975; 10:649–659.
198. Durão V, Prata MM, Goncalves LMP: Modification of antihypertensive effect of beta-adrenoceptor-blocking agents by inhibition of endogenous prostaglandin synthesis. *Lancet* 1977; 2:1005–1007.
199. De Jong PE, Donker AJM, Vand der Wall E, Erkelens DW, Van Derhem GK, Doorenbos H: Effect of indomethacin in two siblings with a renin-dependent hypertension, hyperaldosteronism and hypokalemia. *Nephron* 1980; 25:47–52.
200. Rioux F, Quirion R, Regoli D: The role of prostaglandins in hypertension. I. The release of prostaglandins by aortic strips of renal, DOCA-salt, and spontaneously hypertensive rats. *Can J Physiol Pharmacol* 1977; 55:1330–1338.
201. Limas CJ, Limas C: Prostaglandin metabolism in the kidneys of spontaneously hypertensive rats. *Am J Physiol* 1977; 233:H87–H92.
202. Pace-Asciak CR, Carrara MC, Rangaraj G, Nicolaou KC: Enhanced formation of PGI2, a potent hypotensive substance, by aortic rings and homogenates of the spontaneously hypertensive rat. *Prostaglandins* 1978; 15:1005–1012.
203. Pipili E, Poyser NL: Release of prostaglandins I_2 and E_2 from the perfused mesenteric arterial bed of normotensive and hypertensive rats. Effects of sympathetic nerve stimulation and norepinephrine administration. *Prostaglandins* 1982; 23:543–549.
204. McGiff JC, Crowshaw K, Terragno NA: Renal prostaglandins: possible regulators of the renal actions of pressor hormones. *Nature* 1970; 227:1255–1257.
205. Aiken JW, Vane JR: Intrarenal prostaglandin release attenuates the renal vasoconstrictor activity of angiotensin. *J Pharmacol Exp Ther* 1973; 183:678–687.
206. Lonigro AJ, Itskovitz HD, Crowshaw K, McGiff JC: Dependency of renal blood flow on prostaglandin synthesis in the dog. *Circ Res* 1973; 32:712–717.
207. Beaty O III, Donald DE: Contribution of prostaglandins to muscle blood flow in anesthetized dogs at rest, during exercise, and following inflow occlusion. *Circ Res* 1979; 44:67–75.
208. Ishii M, Uehara Y, Hirata Y, Atarashi K, Ikeda T, Sugimoto T, Takeda T, Murao S: Effects of norepinephrine infusion on systemic hemodynamics and plasma 6-keto-prostaglandin $F_{1\alpha}$ in normotensive subjects and patients with essential hypertension. *Jpn Circ J* 1982; 46:494–502.
209. Chaignon M, Ruffie ML, Lucsko M, Cuche JL, Guedon J: Prostacyclin infusion in hypertension: acute hemodynamic and hormonal effects. *N Engl J Med* 1982; 307:559.
210. Lima DR, Turner P: Beta-blocking drugs increase responsiveness to prostacyclin in hypertensive patients. *Lancet* 1982; 2:444.
211. Wong PY-K, Sun FF, McGiff JC: Metabolism of prostacyclin in blood vessels. *J Biol Chem* 1978; 253:5555–5557.
212. Hensby CN, Barnes PJ, Dollery CT, Dargie H: Production of 6-oxo-$PGF_{1\alpha}$ by human lung in vivo. *Lancet* 1979; 2:1162–1163.
213. Szczeklik A, Gryglewski RJ, Nizankowska E, Nizankowski R: Pulmonary and anti-platelet effects of intravenous and inhaled prostacyclin in man. *Prostaglandins* 1978; 16:651–659.
214. Gimeno MF, Sterin-Borda L, Borda ES, Lazzari MA, Gimeno AL: Human plasma transforms prostacyclin (PGI_2) into a platelet antiaggregatory substance which contracts isolated bovine coronary arteries. *Prostaglandins* 1980; 19:907–916.
215. Hoult JRS, Lofts FJ, Moore PK: Stability of prostacyclin in plasma and its transformation by platelets to a stable spasmogenic product. *Br J Pharmacol* 1981; 73:218P.
216. Wong PY-K, Lee WH, Chao PH-W, Reiss RF, McGiff JC: Metabolism of prostacyclin by 9-hydroxyprostaglandin dehydrogenase in human platelets. Formation of a potent inhibitor of platelet aggregation and enzyme purification. *J Biol Chem* 1980; 255:9021–9024.
217. Hollenberg NK, Solomon HS, Adams DF, Abrams HL, Merrill JP: Renal vascular responses to angiotensin and norepinephrine in normal man. *Circ Res* 1972; 31:750–757.
218. Meneely GR, Ball COT, Youmans JB: Chronic sodium chloride toxicity: the protective effect of added potassium chloride. *Ann Intern Med* 1957; 47:263–273.
219. Itskovitz HD, McGiff JC: Hormonal regulation of the renal circulation. *Circ Res* 1974; 34(suppl I):I-65–73.
220. Vane JR: The release and fate of vasoactive hormones in the circulation. *Br J Pharmacol* 1969; 35:209–242.
221. Muirhead EE, Leach BC, Byers LW, Brooks B, Daniels EG, Hinman JW: Antihypertensive neutral renomedullary lipids (ANRL), in Fisher JW (ed): *Kidney Hormones.* New York, Academic Press, 1971, pp 485–506.
222. McGiff JC, Crowshaw K, Terragno NA, Lonigro AJ: Renal prostaglandins: possible regulators of the renal actions of pressor hormones. *Nature* 1970; 227:1255–1257.
223. Dunn MJ: Renal prostaglandin synthesis in the spontaneously hypertensive rat. *J Clin Invest* 1976; 58:862–870.

224. Pace-Asciak CP: Decreased renal prostaglandin catabolism precedes onset of hypertension in the developing spontaneously hypertensive rat. *Nature* 1976; 263:510–512.
225. Stygles VG, Reinke DA, Rickert DE, Hook JB: Increased blood pressure in the SHR is not related to a deficit in renomedullary PGE_2. *Experientia* 1978; 34:1025–1026.
226. Ahnfelt-Ronne I, Arrigoni-Martelli E: Increase $PGF_{2\alpha}$ synthesis in renal papilla of spontaneously hypertensive rats. *Biochem Pharmacol* 1978; 27:2363–2367.
227. Armstrong JM, Blackwell GJ, Flower RJ, McGiff JC, Mullane KM, Vane JR: Genetic hypertension in rats is accompanied by a defect in renal prostaglandin catabolism. *Nature* (London) 1976; 260:582–586.
228. Tan SY, Sweet P, Mulrow PJ: Impaired renal production of prostaglandin E_2: a newly identified lesion in human essential hypertension. *Prostaglandins* 1978; 15:139–150.
229. Clive DM, Stoff JS: Renal syndromes associated with nonsteroidal antiinflammatory drugs. *N Engl J Med* 1984; 310:563–572.
230. McGiff JC, Crowshaw K, Terragno NA, Lonigro AJ: Release of a prostaglandin-like substance into renal venous blood in response to angiotensin II. *Circ Res* 1970; 26,27(suppl I):I-121–I-130.
231. Itskovitz HD, Terragno NA, McGiff JC: Effect of a renal prostaglandin on distribution of blood flow in the isolated canine kidney. *Circ Res* 1974; 3:770–776.
232. Larsson C, Anggard E: Regional differences in the formation and metabolism of prostaglandins in the rabbit kidney. *Eur J Pharmacol* 1973; 21:30–36.
233. Terragno NA, McGiff JC, Terragno A: Synthesis of prostaglandin by vascular and nonvascular renal tissues and the presence of an endogenous prostaglandin synthesis inhibitor in the cortex, in Vargastig BB (ed): *Advances in Pharmacology and Therapeutics* (vol 4). *Prostaglandins and Immunopharmacology*. Oxford, Pergamon Press, 1978, pp 39–46.
234. Janszen FHA, Nugteren DH: Histochemical localisation of prostaglandin synthetase. *Histochemie* 1971; 27:159–164.
235. Berl T, Raz A, Wald H, Horowitz J, Czacakes W: Prostaglandin synthesis inhibition and the action of vasopressin: studies in man and rat. *Am J Physiol* 1977; 232:F529–F537.
236. Tobian L, Ganguli M, Johnson MA, Iwai J: Influence of renal prostaglandins and dietary lineoleate on hypertension in Dahl S rats. *Hypertension* 1982; 4:325–328.
237. Frolich JC, Hollifield JW, Dormois JC, Frolich BL, Seyberth H, Michaelakis AM, Oates JA: Suppression of plasma renin activity by indomethacin in man. *Clin Res* 1976; 39:447–452.
238. Weber PC, Larsson C, Anggard E, Hamberg M, Corey EJ, Nicolaow KC, Sameulsson B: Stimulation of renin release from rabbit renal cortex by arachidonic acid and prostaglandin endoperoxides. *Circ Res* 1976; 39:868–874.
239. Whorton AR, Misono K, Hollifield J, Frolich JC, Inagami T, Oates JA: Prostaglandins and renin release: stimulation of renin release from rabbit renal cortical slices by PGI2. *Prostaglandins* 1977; 14:1095–1104.
240. Hoult JR, Moore PK: Pathways of prostaglandin $F_{2\alpha}$ metabolism in mammalian kidneys. *Br J Pharmacol* 1977; 61:615–616.
241. Spokas EG, Ferreri NR, Wong PY-K, McGiff JC: Effect of 6-keto prostaglandin E_1 (6-keto-PGE_1) on renin release from rabbit renal cortical slices. *Circulation* 1980; 62:III-287.
242. Jackson EK, Herzer WA, Zimmerman JB, Branch RA, Oates JA, Gerkens JF: 6-keto prostaglandin E_1 is more potent than prostaglandin I_2 as a renal vasodilator and renin secretagogue. *J Pharmacol Exper Ther* 1981; 216:24–27.
243. Zusman RM, Keiser HR: Prostaglandin biosynthesis by rabbit renomedullary interstitial cells in tissue culture. *J Clin Invest* 1977; 60:215–223.
244. Campbell WB, Holland OB, Adams BV, Gomez-Sanchez CE: Urinary excretion of prostaglandin E_2, prostaglandin $F_{2\alpha}$, and thromboxane B_2 in normotensive and hypertensive subjects on varying sodium intakes. *Hypertension* 1982; 4:735–741.
245. Lebel M, Grose JH: Renal prostaglandins in borderline and sustained essential hypertension. *Prostaglandins-Leukotrienes-Med* 1982; 8:409–418.
246. Ruilope L, Garcia-Robles R, Barrietos A, Bernis C, Alcazar J, Tresguerres JA, Rodicio J: The role of urinary PGE_2 and renin-angiotensin-aldosterone system in the pathogenesis of essential hypertension. *Clin Exp Hypertension* 1982; 4:989–1000.
247. Sato M, Abe K, Haruyama T, Yasujima M, Sato K, Chiba S, Imai Y, Hiwatari M, Kasai Y, Tajima J, Itoh S, Seino M, Goto T, Yoshinaga K: Effect of dietary sodium intake on the metabolism of prostaglandins in the kidney in hypertensive patients. *Prostaglandins-Leukotrienes-Med* 1982; 8:199–219.
248. Rathaus M, Bernheim J: Effect of propranolol treatment on the urinary excretion of prostaglandins E_2 and $F_{2\alpha}$ in patients with essential hypertension. *Isr J Med Sci* 1982; 18:231–234.
249. Willis LR, Ludens JH, Hook JB, Williamson HE: Mechanism of natriuretic action of bradykinin. *Am J Physiol* 1969; 217:1–5.
250. Stein JH, Congbalay RC, Karsh DL, Osgood RW, Ferris TF: The effect of bradykinin on proximal tubular sodium reabsorption in the dog: evidence for functional nephron heterogeneity. *J Clin Invest* 1972; 51:1709–1721.
251. Pierce JV, Webster ME: Human plasma kallidins: isolation and chemical studies. *Biochem Biophys Res Commun* 1961; 5:353–357.
252. Coleman RW: Formation of human plasma kinin. *N Engl J Med* 1974; 291:509–515.
253. Ward PE, Gedney CD, Dowben RM, Erdos EG: Isolation of membrane bound renal kallikrein and kininase. *Biochem J* 1975; 151:755–758.
254. Orstavik TB, Nustad K, Brandtzaeg P, Pierce JV: Cellular origin of urinary kallikreins. *J Histochem Cytochem* 1976; 24:1037–1039.
255. Nasjletti A, Colina-Chourio J, McGiff JC: Disappearance of bradykinin in the renal circulation of dogs. Effect of kininase inhibition. *Circ Res* 1975; 37:59–65.
256. Carone FA, Pullman TN, Oparil S, Nakamura S: Micropuncture evidence of rapid hydrolysis of bradykinin by rat proximal tubule. *Am J Physiol* 1976; 230:1420–1424.
257. Margolius HS, Horwitz D, Pisano JJ, Keiser HR: Urinary kallikrein excretion in hypertensive man. Relationships to sodium intake and sodium-retaining steroids. *Circ Res* 1974; 35:820–825.
258. Streeten DHP, Kerr LP, Kerr CB, Prior JC, Dalakos TG: Hyperbradykininism: a new orthostatic syndrome. *Lancet* 1972; 2:1048–1053.
259. Wong PY, Talamo RC, Williams GH, Coleman RW: Response of the kallikrein-kinin and renin-angiotensin systems to saline infusion and upright posture. *J Clin Invest* 1975; 55:691–698.
260. Mersey JH, Williams GH, Hollenberg NK, Dluhy RG: Relationship between aldosterone and bradykinin. *Circ Res* 1977; 40(suppl I):84–88.
261. Vinci JM, Zusman RM, Izzo JL, Bowden RE, Horwitz D, Pisano JJ, Keiser HR: Human urinary and plasma kinins. Relationship to sodium-retaining steroids and plasma renin activity. *Circ Res* 1979; 44:228–237.
262. Vane JR, McGiff JC: Possible contributions of endogenous prostaglandins to the control of blood pressure. *Circ Res* 1975; 36-37(suppl I):I-68–I-75.
263. Hong SL, Levine L: Stimulation of prostaglandin synthesis by bradykinin and thrombin and their mechanism of action on MC5-5 fibroblasts. *J Biol Chem* 1976; 251:5814–5816.
264. Damas J, Bourdon V: Liberation dacide arachidonique par la bradykinine. *Comptes Rend Seances Société Biol Filiales* 1974; 168:1445–1448.
265. Wong PY-K, Terragno DA, Terragno NA, McGiff JC: Dual effects of bradykinin on prostaglandin metabolism: relationship to the dissimilar vascular actions of kinins. *Prostaglandins* 1977; 13:1113–1125.
266. Messina EJ, Weiner R, Kaley G: Inhibition of bradykinin vasodilation and potentiation of norepinephrine and angiotensin vasoconstriction by inhibitors of prostaglandin synthesis in rat skeletal muscle. *Circ Res* 1975; 37:430–437.
267. McGiff JC, Itskovitz HD, Terragno NA: The action of bradykinin and eledoisin in the canine isolated kidney; relationships to prostaglandin. *Clin Sci Mol Med* 1975; 49:125–131.
268. Beilin LJ, Bhattacharya J: The effects of prostaglandin synthesis inhibitors on renal blood flow distribution in conscious rabbits. *J Physiol* 1977; 269:395–405.
269. Erdos EG: The kinins. A status report. *Biochem Pharmacol* 1976; 25:1563–1569.
270. Erdos EG: Angiotensin I converting enzyme. *Circ Res* 1975; 36:247–255.
271. McGiff JC, Terragno NA, Malik KU, Lonigro AJ: Release of a prostaglandin E-like substance from canine kidney by bradykinin. *Circ Res* 1972; 31:36–43.
272. Margolius HS, Geller R, de Jong W, Pisano JJ, Sjoerdsma A: Altered urinary kallikrein excretion in rats with hypertension. *Circ Res* 1972; 30:358–362.
273. Elliot AH, Nuzum FR: Urinary excretion of a depressor substance (kallikrein of Frey and Kraut) in arterial hypertension. *Endocrinology* 1934; 18:462–474.
274. Bevan VH, Pierce JV, Pisano JJ: A sensitive isotopic procedure for the assay of esterase activity: measurement of human urinary kallikrein. *Clin Chem Acta* 1971; 32:67–73.
275. Levy SB, Lilley JJ, Frigon RP, Stone RA: Urinary kallikrein and plasma renin activity as determinants of renal blood flow; the influence of race and dietary sodium intake. *J Clin Invest* 1977; 60:129–138.
276. Zinner SH, Margolius HS, Rosner B, Kass EH: Eight year longitudinal study of blood pressure and urinary kallikrein in childhood. *Clin Res* 1977; 25:266A.
277. Keiser HR, Andrews MJ Jr, Guyton RA, Margolius HS, Pisano JJ: Urinary kallikrein in dogs with constriction of one renal artery. *Proc Soc Exp Biol Med* 1976; 151:53–56.
278. Mills IH, MacFarlane NAA, Ward PE: The renal kallikrein-kinin system and the regulation of salt and water excretion. *Fed Proc* 1976; 35:181–188.
279. Hulthen UL, Lecerof H, Hokfelt B: Renal venous output of kinins in patients with hypertension and unilateral renal artery stenosis. *Acta Med Scand* 1977; 202:189–191.
280. Zinner SH, Margolius HS, Rosner B, Keiser HR, Kass EG: Familial

aggregation of urinary kallikrein concentration in childhood: relation to blood pressure, race and urinary electrolytes. *Am J Epidemiol* 1976; 104:124–132.

281. O'Connor DT: Response of the renal kallikrein-kinin system, intravascular volume, and renal hemodynamics to sodium restriction and diuretic treatment in essential hypertension. *Hypertension* 1982; 4(suppl III):III-72–III-78.
282. O'Connor DT, Bars AP, Amend W, Vincenti F: Urinary kallikrein excretion after renal transplantation: relationship to hypertension, graft source, and renal function. *Am J Med* 1982; 73:475–481.
283. Saruta T, Kondo K: Endocrine factors in juvenile essential hypertension. *Jpn J Med* 1982; 21:152–154.
284. Margolius HS, Horwitz D, Pisano JJ, Kaiser HR: Relationships among urinary kallikrein, mineralocorticoids and human hypertensive disease. *Fed Proc* 1976; 35:203–206.
285. Galvez OG, Bay WH, Roberts BW, Ferris TF: The hemodynamic effects of potassium deficiency in the dog. *Circ Res* 1977; 40:I-11–I-16.
286. McGiff JC: Bartter's syndrome results from an imbalance of vasoactive hormones. *Ann Intern Med* 1977; 87:369–372.
287. Marin-Grez M, Cottone P, Carretero A: Evidence for an involvement of kinins in regulation of sodium excretion. *Am J Physiol* 1972; 223:794–796.
288. Nasjletti A, McGiff JC, Colina-Chourio J: Interrelationships of the renal kallikrein-kinin and prostaglandin systems in the conscious rat: influence of mineralocorticoids. *Circ Res* 1978; 43:799–807.
289. Marin-Grez M: The influence of antibodies against bradykinin on isotonic saline diuresis in the rat. *Pflugers Arch* 1974; 350:231–239.
290. Colina-Chourio J, McGiff JC, Miller MP, Nasjletti A: Possible influence of intrarenal generation of kinins on prostaglandin release from the rabbit perfused kidney. *Br J Pharmacol* 1976; 58:165–172.
291. Carretero OA, Scicli AG: Renal kallikrein: its localization and possible role in renal function. *Fed Proc* 1976; 35:194–198.
292. Weber PC, Larsson C, Scherer B: Prostaglandin E_2-9-ketoreductase as a mediator of salt intake-related prostaglandin-renin interaction. *Nature* 1977; 266:65–66.
293. O'Connor DT: Response of the renal kallikrein-kinin system, intravascular volume, and renal hemodynamics to sodium restriction and diuretic treatment in essential hypertension. *Hypertension* 1982; 4:II-172–II-177.
294. Muirhead EE: Antihypertensive functions of the kidney. *Hypertension* 1980; 2:444–464.
295. Muirhead EE, Stirman JA, Jones F: Renal autotransplantation and protection against renoprival hypertensive cardiovascular disease and hemolysis. *J Clin Invest* 1960; 39:266–281.
296. Muirhead EE, Rightsel WA, Leach BE, Byers LW, Pitcock JA, Brooks B: Reversal of hypertension by transplants and lipid extracts of cultured renomedullary interstitial cells. *Lab Invest* 1977; 36:162–172.
297. Tobian L, Azasr S: Antihypertensive and other functions of the renal papilla. *Trans Assoc Am Physicians* 1971; 84:281–288.
298. Manthorpe T: Antihypertensive and hypertensive effects of the kidney. *Acta Path Microbiol Scand* 1975; 83A:395–405.
299. Susic D, Sparks JC, Machado EA, Kentera D: The mechanisms of renomedullary antihypertensive action: haemodynamic studies in hydronephrotic rats with one-clip hypertension. *Clin Sci Mol Med* 1978; 54:361–367.
300. Gothberg G, Lundin S, Folkow B: Acute vasodepressor effect in normotensive rats following extracorporeal perfusion of the declipped kidney of two-kidney, one clip hypertensive rats. *Hypertension* 1982; 4(suppl II):II-101–II-105.
301. Muirhead EE, Folkow B, Byers LW, Desiderio DM, Thoren P, Gothberg G, Daw AW, Brooks B: Cardiovascular effects of antihypertensive polar and neutral renomedullary lipids. *Hypertension* 1983; 5(suppl I):I-112–I-118.
302. Faber JE, Barron KW, Bonham AC, Lappe R, Muirhead EE, Brody MI: Regional hemodynamic effects of antihypertensive renomedullary lipids in conscious rats. *Hypertension* 1984; 6:494–502.
303. Muirhead EE: Case for a renomedullary blood pressure lowering hormone. *Contrib Nephrol* 1978; 12:69–81.
304. Gaunt R, Antonchak N, Miller GJ, Renzi AA: Effect of reserpine (Serpasil) and hydralazine (Apresoline) on experimental steroid hypertension. *Am J Physiol* 1955; 182:63–68.
305. Perry HM Jr, Schroeder HA: The effect of treatment on mortality rates in severe hypertension. A comparison of medical and surgical regimens. *Arch Intern Med* 1958; 102:418–428.
306. Dustan HP, Schneckloth RE, Corcoran AC, Page IH: The effectiveness of long-term treatment of malignant hypertension. *Circulation* 1958; 18:644–651.
307. Sokolow M, Perloff D: Five year survival of consecutive patients with malignant hypertension treated with antihypertensive agents. *Am J Cardiol* 1960; 6:858–863.
308. Hamilton M, Thompson EN, Wisniewski TKM: The role of blood pressure control in preventing complications of hypertension. *Lancet* 1964; 1:235–238.
309. Wolff FW, Lindeman RD: Effects of treatment on hypertension: results of a controlled study. *J Chron Dis* 1966; 19:227–240.
310. Veterans Administration Cooperative Study Group on Antihypertensive Agents: Effect of treatment on morbidity: results in patients with diastolic blood pressures averaging 115 through 129 mm Hg. *JAMA* 1970; 213:1143–1152.
311. Veterans Administration Cooperative Study Group on Antihypertensive Agents: Effect of treatment on morbidity: results in patients with diastolic blood pressure averaging 90 through 114 mm Hg. *JAMA* 1970; 213:1143–1152.
312. Veterans Administration Cooperative Study Group on Antihypertensive Agents: Effects of treatment on morbidity in hypertension. III. Influence of age, diastolic pressure, and prior cardiovascular disease, further analysis of side effects. *Circulation* 1972; 45:991–1004.
313. Hypertension Detection and Follow-Up Program Cooperative Group: Four Year Findings of the Hypertension Detection and Follow-up Program. 1. Reduction in mortality of persons with high blood pressure, including mild hypertension. *JAMA* 1979; 242:2562–2571.
314. The Australian Therapeutic Trial in Mild Hypertension. Report by the Management Committee. *Lancet* 1980; 1:1261–1267.
314a. Amery A, Birkenhager W, Brixko P, Bulpitt C, Clement D, Deruyttere M, DeSchaepdryver A, Dollery C, Fagard R, Forette F, Forte J, Hamdy R, Henry JF, Joossens, Leonetti G, Lund-Johansen P, O'Malley K, Petrie J, Strasser T, Tuomilehto J, Williams B: Mortality and morbidity results from European Working Party on High Blood Pressure in the Elderly Trial. *Lancet* 1985; 1:1349–1354.
315. Kannell WB, Sorlie P, Gordon T: Labile hypertension: a faulty concept. The Framingham Study. *Circulation* 1980; 61:1183–1187.
316. Harlan WR, Oberman A, Mitchell RE, Graybiel A: A 30 year study of blood pressure in a white male cohort, in Onesti G (ed): *Hypertension Mechanism and Management*. New York, Grune & Stratton, 1973, pp 85–91.
317. Frohlich ED, Kozul VJ, Tarazi RC, Dustan HP: Physiological comparison of labile and essential hypertension. *Circ Res* 1970; 27(suppl I):55–69.
318. Kannel WB, Gorden T, Schwartz MJ: Systolic versus diastolic blood pressure and risk of coronary heart disease: The Framingham study. *Am J Cardiol* 1971; 27:335–346.
319. Colandrea MA, Friedman GD, Nichaman MZ, Lynd CN: Systolic hypertension in the elderly: an epidemiologic assessment. *Circulation* 1970; 41:239–245.
320. The Joint National Committee on Detection, Evaluation and Treatment of High Blood Pressure: The 1984 Report of the Joint National Committee on Detection, Evaluation and Treatment of High Blood Pressure. *Arch Intern Med* 1984; 144:1045–1057.
321. Freis ED: How far should blood pressure be lowered in treating hypertension? *JAMA* 1975; 232:1017–1018.
322. Hypertension-Stroke Cooperative Study Group: Effect of antihypertensive treatment on stroke recurrence. *JAMA* 1974; 229:409–418.
323. Kirkendall WM, Burton AC, Epstein FH, Freis ED: Recommendations for human blood pressure determination by sphygmomanometers. *Circulation* 1967; 36:980–988.
324. Bandran RHA, Weir RJ, McGuiness JB: Hypertension and headache. *Scott Med J* 1970; 15:48–51.
325. Weiss NS: Relation of high blood pressure to headache, epistaxis and selected other symptoms: The United States health examination survey of adults. *N Engl J Med* 1972; 287:631–633.
326. Rosenthal FD, Roy S: Hypertension and hyperparathyroidism. *Br Med J* 1972; 4:396–397.
327. Romney B: Oral contraceptive hypertension. *Cardiovasc Rev Rep* 1981; 2:75–79.
328. Messerli FH, Frohlich ED: High blood pressure. A side effect of drugs, poisons and foods. *Arch Intern Med* 1979; 139:682–687.
329. Friedenwald JS: Retinal and choroidal arteriosclerosis, in Ridley F, Sorsby A (eds): *Modern Trends in Ophthalmology*. New York, Paul B Hoeber, 1940, p 77.
330. Keith NM, Wagener HP, Barker NW: Some different types of essential hypertension: their courses and prognosis. *Am J Med Sci* 1939; 197:332–343.
331. Scheie HG: Evaluation of ophthalmoscopic changes of hypertension and arteriolar sclerosis. *Arch Ophthalmol* 1953; 49:117–138.
332. Kirkendall WM, Armstrong ML: Vascular changes in the eye of the treated and untreated patient with essential hypertension. *Am J Cardiol* 1962; 9:663–668.
333. Diseases of the ocular blood vessels, in Friedenwald JS, Wilder HC, Maumenee AE, Sanders TE, Keyes JEL, Hogan MJ, Owens WC, Owens EU (eds): *Ophthalmic Pathology—An Atlas and Textbook*. Philadelphia, WB Saunders, 1952, p 310.
334. Kossmann CE, Burchell HB, Pruitt RD, Scott RC: The electrocardiogram in ventricular hypertrophy and bundle-branch block. *Circulation* 1962; 26:1336–1351.
335. Romhilt DW, Bove KE, Norris RJ, Conyers E, Conradi S, Rowlands DT, Scott RC: A critical appraisal of the electrocardiogram criteria for

the diagnosis of left ventricular hypertrophy. *Circulation* 1969; 40:185–195.

336. Romhilt DW, Estes EH: A point-score system for the ECG diagnosis of left ventricular hypertrophy. *Am Heart J* 1968; 75:752–758.
337. Dern PL, Pryor R, Walker SH, Searls DT: Serial electrocardiographic changes in treated hypertensive patients with reference to voltage criteria, mean QRS vectors, and the QRS-T angle. *Circulation* 1967; 36:823–829.
338. Kannel WB: Prevalence and natural history of electrocardiographic left ventricular hypertrophy. *Am J Med* 1983; 75(suppl 3A):4–11.
339. Devereux RB, Reichek N: Echocardiographic determination of left ventricular mass in man. Anatomic validation of the method. *Circulation* 1977; 55:613–618.
340. Devereux RB, Alsonso DR, Lutas EM: Sensitivity of echocardiography for detection of left ventricular hypertrophy, in Keurs HEDJ, Schipperheyn JJ (eds): *Cardiac Left Ventricular Hypertrophy.* Martinus Nijhoff, The Hague, 1983, pp 16–37.
341. McFarland TM, Alam M, Goldstein S, Pickard SD, Stein PD: Echocardiographic diagnosis of left ventricular hypertrophy. *Circulation* 1978; 57:1140–1144.
342. Ditchey RB, Schuler G, Peterson KL: Reliability of echocardiographic and electrocardiographic parameters in assessing serial changes in left ventricular mass. *Am J Med* 1981; 70:1042–1050.
343. Savage DD, Garrison RJ, Kannel WB, Castelli WP, Anderson SJ, Stokes J III, Padget S, Feinleib M: Prevalence, characteristics and correlates of echocardiographic left ventricular hypertrophy in a population-based sample—preliminary findings: the Framingham study. *Circulation* 1982; 66(suppl II):11–63.
344. Reichek N: Echocardiographic assessment of left ventricular structure and function in hypertension: methodology. *Am J Med* 1983; 75(suppl 3A):19–25.
345. Frohlich ED: Physiologic considerations in left ventricular hypertrophy. *Am J Med* 1983; 75(suppl 3A):12–18.
346. Abi-Samra F, Fouad FM, Tarazi RC: Determinants of left ventricular hypertrophy and function in hypertensive patients. An echocardiographic study. *Am J Med* 1983; 75(suppl 3A):26–33.
347. Sen S, Tarazi RC, Bumpus FM: Cardiac hypertrophy and antihypertensive therapies. *Cardiovasc Res* 1977; 11:427–433.
348. Sen S, Tarazi RC, Bumpus FM: Reversal of cardiac hypertrophy in renal hypertensive rats: medicine vs surgical therapy. *Am J Physiol* 1981; 240:H408–H412.

348a. Fouad FM, Tarazi RC: Restoration of cardiac function and structure by converting inhibition possibilities and limitations of long-term treatment in hypertension and heart failure. *J Cardiovasc Pharmacol* 1986; 8(suppl 1):S53–S57.

349. Borer JS, Jason M, Devereux RB, Fisher J, Green MV, Bacharach SL, Pickering T, Laragh JH: Function of the hypertrophied left ventricle at rest and during exercise. Hypertension and aortic stenosis. *Am J Med* 1983; 75(suppl 3A):34–39.
350. Francis CK, Cleman M, Berger HJ, Davies RA, Giles RW, Black HR, Vita N, Zito RA, Zaret BL: Left ventricular systolic performance during upright bicycle exercise in patients with essential hypertension. *Am J Med* 1983; 75(suppl 3A):40–46.
351. Topol EJ, Traill TA, Fortuin NJ: Hypertensive hypertrophic cardiomyopathy of the elderly. *N Engl J Med* 1985; 312:277–282.
352. Tobian L: A viewpoint concerning the enigma of hypertension. *Am J Med* 1972; 52:595–609.
353. Hunt JC, Strong CG, Harrison EG Jr, Furlow WL, Leary FJ: Management of hypertension of renal origin. *Am J Cardiol* 1970; 26:280–288.
354. Volhard F, Fahr T: *Die Brightsche Nierenkrankheit, Klinik, Pathologie und Attas.* Berlin, Springer-Verlag, 1914.
355. Goldblatt H, Lynch J, Hanzal RF, Summerville WW: Studies on experimental hypertension. I. The production of persistent elevation of systolic blood pressure by means of renal ischemia. *J Exp Med* 1934; 59:347–379.
356. Kincaid OW, David GD, Hallerman RJ, Hunt JC: Fibromuscular dysplagia of the renal arteries: arteriographic features, classification and observations on the natural history of the disease. *Am J Roentgenol* 1968; 104:271–282.
357. Hunt JC, Strong CG, Sheps SG, Bernatz PE: Diagnosis and management of renovascular hypertension. *Am J Cardiol* 1969; 23:434–445.
358. Bookstein JJ, Abrams HL, Buenger RE, Reiss MD, Lecky JW, Franklin SS, Bleifer KH, Varady PD, Maxwell MH: Radiologic aspects of renovascular hypertension. 3. Appraisal of arteriography. *JAMA* 1972; 221:368–374.
359. Amsterdam EA, Couch NP, Christlieb AR, Harrison JH, Crane C, Dobrzinsky SS, Hickler RB: Renal vein renin activity in the prognosis of surgery of renovascular hypertension. *Am J Med* 1969; 47:860–868.
360. Brunner HR, Gavras H, Laragh JH, Keenan R: Hypertension in man: exposure of the renin and sodium components using angiotensin II blockade. *Circ Res* 1974; 34(suppl I):I-35–I-43.
361. Streeten DHP, Anderson GH, Freiberg JM, Dalakos TG: Use of an angiotensin II antagonist (Saralasin) in the recognition of "angiotensinogenic" hypertension. *N Engl J Med* 1975; 292:657–662.
362. Couch NP, Sullivan JM, Crane C: The predictive accuracy of renal vein renin activity in the surgery of renovascular hypertension. *Surgery* 1976; 79:70–76.
363. Strong CG, Hunt JC, Sheps SG, Tucker RM, Bernatz PE: Renal venous renin activity: enhancement of sensitivity of lateralization by sodium depletion. *Am J Cardiol* 1971; 27:602–611.
364. Chassin MRG, Sullivan JR: Pharmacologic management of renovascular hypertension. *JAMA* 1974; 227:421–423.
365. Kjellbo H, Lund N, Bergentz SE, Hood B: Renal artery stenosis. III. Follow-up observations in operated and nonoperated patients. *Scand J Urol Nephrol* 1970; 4:49–57.
366. Gruntzig A, Vetter W, Meier B, Kuhlmann LL, Lutolf U, Siegenthaler W: Treatment of renovascular hypertension with percutaneous transluminal dilatation of a renal artery stenosis. *Lancet* 1978; 1:801–802.

366a. Brenner BM, Rector FC: *The Kidney,* ed 3. Philadelphia, W B Saunders, 1986, p 1232.

367. Wurtman RJ: Catecholamines. *N Engl J Med* 1965; 273:637–646, 693–700, 746–753.
368. Thomas JE, Rooke ED, Krale WF: The neurologists' experience with pheochromocytoma. *JAMA* 1966; 197:754–758.
369. Page LB, Raker JW, Berberich FR: Pheochromocytoma with predominant epinephrine secretion. *Am J Med* 1969; 47:648–652.
370. Sjoerdsma A, Engleman K, Waldmann TA, Cooperman LH, Hammond WG: Pheochromocytoma: current concepts of diagnosis and treatment. *Ann Intern Med* 1966; 65:1302–1326.
371. Rayfield EJ, Cain JP, Casey MP, Williams GH, Sullivan JM: Influence of diet on urinary VMA excretion. *JAMA* 1972; 221:704–705.
372. Bravo EL, Tarazi RC, Gifford RW, Stewart BH: Circulating and urinary catecholamines in pheochromocytoma: diagnostic and pathophysiologic implications. *N Engl J Med* 1979; 301:682–686.
373. Rossi P, Young IS, Panke WF: Techniques, usefulness, and hazards of arteriography of pheochromocytoma. *JAMA* 1968; 205:547–553.
374. Epstein AJ, Patel SK, Petasnick JP: Computerized tomography of the adrenal gland. *JAMA* 1979; 242:2791–2794.
375. Sisson JC, Frager MS, Valk TW, Gross MD, Swanson DP, Wieland DM, Tobes MC, Beierwaltes WH, Thompson NW: Scintigraphic localization of pheochromocytoma. *N Engl J Med* 1981; 305:12–17.
376. Sullivan JM: Pheochromocytoma. *Arch Surg* 1972; 104:130–131.
377. Pertsemlidis D, Gitlow SE, Siegel WC, Kark AE: Pheochromocytoma. 1. Specificity of laboratory, diagnostic tests. 2. Safeguards during operative removal. *Ann Surg* 1969; 169:376–385.

377a. Hurst JW: *The Heart,* ed 6. New York, McGraw-Hill, 1986, pp 1083–1084.

378. Simpson SA, Tait JF, Wettstein A, Neher R, von Euw J, Reichstein T: Isolierung eines neuen kristallisierten Hormons aus Nebennieren mit besonders hoher Wieksamkeit aus den Mineralstoffweschel. *Experientia* (Basel) 1953; 9:333–335.
379. Conn JW: Presidential address. II. Primary aldosteronism, a new clinical syndrome. *J Lab Clin Med* 1955; 45:6–17.

379a. Heslop H, Richards AM, Nicholls MG, Espiner EA, Ikram H, Maslowski AH: Hyponatraemic-hypertensive syndrome due to unilateral renal ischemia in women who smoke heavily. *NZ Med J* 1985; 98:739–742.

379b. Hyponatraemic hypertensive syndrome, editorial. *Lancet* 1986; 1:718–719.

380. Conn JW, Cohen EL, Rovner DR: Suppression of plasma renin activity in primary aldosteronism. *JAMA* 1964; 190:213–221.
381. Dunnick NR, Schaner EG, Doppman JF, Strott CA, Gill JR, Javadpour N: Computed tomography in adrenal tumors. *Am J Roentgenol* 1979; 132:43–46.
382. Biglieri EG, Stockigt JR, Schambelan M: Adrenal mineralocorticoids causing hypertension. *Am J Med* 1972; 52:623–632.
383. Laragh JH, Ledingham JGG, Sommers SC: Secondary aldosteronism and reduced plasma renin in hypertensive disease. *Trans Assoc Am Physicians* 1967; 80:168–182.
384. Bravo EL, Sen S, Bumpus FM, Fouad FM, Tarazi RC, Gill J: Regulation of a new aldosterone-stimulating factor in primary aldosteronism. *Hypertension* 1984; 6:780.
385. Biglieri EG, Slaton PE, Kronfield SF, Schambelan M: Diagnosis of an aldosterone-producing adenoma in primary aldosteronism: an evaluative maneuver. *JAMA* 1967; 201:510–514.
386. Sutherland DJA, Ruse JL, Laidlaw JC: Hypertension, increased aldosterone secretion, and low plasma renin activity relieved by dexamethasone. *Can Med Assoc J* 1966; 95:1109–1119.
387. Tucci JR, Jagger PI, Lauler DP, Thorn GW: Rapid dexamethasone suppression test for Cushing's syndrome. *JAMA* 1967; 199:374–382.
388. Herrera MG, Cahill GF, Thorn GW: Cushing's syndrome: diagnosis and treatment. *Am J Surg* 1964; 107:144–152.

388a. Gomez-Sanchez CE: Cushing's syndrome and hypertension. *Hypertension* 1986; 8:258–264.

389. Bongiovznni AM, Root AW: The adrenogenital syndrome. *N Engl J Med* 1963; 268:1283–1289, 1342–1351, 1391–1399.
390. Biglieri EG, Herron MA, Brust N: 17-hydroxylation deficiency in man. *J Clin Invest* 1966; 45:1946–1954.

391. Laragh JH, Sealey JE, Ledingham JGC, Newton MA: Oral contraceptives: renin, aldosterone, and high blood pressure. *JAMA* 1967; 201:918–922.
392. Woods JW: Oral contraceptives and hypertension. *Lancet* 1967; 2:653.
393. Fisch IR, Freedman SH, Myatt AV: Oral contraceptives, pregnancy and blood pressure. *JAMA* 1972; 222:1507–1510.
394. Editorial: Blood pressure and the pill. *Br Med J* 1973; 1:693.
395. Zacherle BJ, Richardson JA: Irreversible renal failure secondary to hypertension induced by oral contraceptives. *Ann Intern Med* 1972; 77:83–85.
396. Koster M, David EK: Reversible severe hypertension due to licorice. *N Engl J Med* 1968; 278:1381–1383.
397. Rosenthal FD, Roy S: Hypertension and hyperparathyroidism. *Br Med J* 1972; 4:396–397.
398. Madhavan T, Frame B, Block MA: Influence of surgical correction of primary hyperparathyroidism on associated hypertension. *Arch Surg* 1970; 100:212–214.
399. Campbell M: Natural history of coarctation of the aorta. *Br Heart J* 1970; 32:633–640.
400. March HW, Hultgren HN, Gerbode F: Immediate and remote effects of resection on the hypertension in coarctation of the aorta. *Br Heart J* 1960; 22:361–373.
401. Benson H, Marzetta BR, Rosner BA: Decreased blood pressure associated with the regular elicitation of the relaxation response: a study of hypertensive subjects, in Eliot RS (ed): *Contemporary Problems in Cardiology. Stress and the Heart.* New York, Futura, 1974, vol 1, p 293.
402. Hanson JS, Nedde WH: Preliminary observations on physical training for hypertensive males. *Circ Res* 1970; 27:149–53.
403. Boyer JL, Kasch FW: Exercise therapy in hypertensive men. *JAMA* 1970; 211:1668–1671.
404. Tyroler HA, Heyden S, Hames CG: Weight and hypertension: Evans County studies of blacks and whites, in Paul O (ed): *Epidemiology and Control of Hypertension.* New York, Stratton International Medical Book Conference, 1975, pp 177–201.
404a. Jackson R, Beaglehole R, Stewart A, Stokes Y: Serum lipids, body mass, and exercise levels in Auckland, 1982. *NZ Med J* 1986; 99:97–100.
404b. MacMahon SW, Wilcken DEL, Macdonald GJ: The effect of weight reduction on left ventricular mass. A randomized controlled trial in young overweight hypertensive patients. *N Engl J Med* 1986; 314:334–339.
404c. Imai Y, Sato K, Abe K, Sasaki S, Nihei M, Yoshinaga K, Sekino H: Effect of weight loss on blood pressure and drug consumption in normal weight patients. *Hypertension* 1986; 8:223–228.
405. Arkwright PD, Beilin LJ, Rouse I, Armstrong BK, Phil D, Vandongen R: Effects of alcohol use and other aspects of lifestyle on blood pressure levels and prevalence of hypertension in a working population. *Circulation* 1982; 66:60–66.
405a. Gruchow HW, Sobocinski KA, Barboriak JJ: Alcohol, nutrient intake, and hypertension in US adults. *JAMA* 1985; 253:1567–1570.
405b. Paulin JM, Simpson FO, Waal-Manning HJ: Alcohol consumption and blood pressure in a New Zealand community study. *NZ Med J* 1985; 98:425–428.
405c. Klatsky AL, Friedman GD, Armstrong MA: The relationships between alcoholic beverage use and other traits to blood pressure: a new Kaiser Permanente study. *Circulation* 1986; 73:628–636.
405d. Final Report of the Subcommittee on Nonpharmacological Therapy of the 1984 Joint National Committee on Detection, Evaluation, and Treatment of High Blood Pressure: Nonpharmacological approaches to the control of high blood pressure. *Hypertension* 1986; 8:444–467.
406. Dahl LK: Salt intake and salt need. *N Engl J Med* 1958; 258:1152–1157, 1205–1208.
407. Kempner W: Treatment of hypertensive vascular disease with rice diet. *Am J Med* 1948; 4:545–577.
408. Carney S, Morgan T, Wilson M, Matthews G, Roberts R: Sodium restriction and thiazide diuretics in the treatment of hypertension. *Med J Aust* 1975; I:803–807.
409. Magnani B, Ambrosioni E, Agosta R, Racco F: Comparison of the effects of pharmacological therapy and a low-sodium diet on mild hypertension. *Clin Sci Mol Med* 1976; 51(suppl III):625s–626s.
409a. McCarron DA, Morris CD: Blood pressure response to oral calcium in persons with mild to moderate hypertension: a randomized double-blind placebo-controlled crossover trial. *Ann Intern Med* 1985; 103:825–831.
409b. Altura BM, Altura BT: Interactions of Mg and K on blood vessels—aspects in view of hypertension. Review of present status and new findings. *Magnesium* 1984; 3:175–194.
410. Beta-blocker Heart Attack Study Group: The beta-blocker heart attack trial. *JAMA* 1981; 246:2073–2074.
411. Dormois JC, Young JL, Nies AS: Minoxidil in severe hypertension: value when conventional drugs have failed. *Am Heart J* 1975; 90:360–368.
412. Gavras H, Brunner HR, Turini GA, Kershaw GR, Tifft CP, Cuttelod S, Gavras I, Vukovich RA, McKinstry DN: Antihypertensive effect of the oral angiotensin converting-enzyme inhibitor SQ 14,225 in man. *N Engl J Med* 1978; 298:991–995.
413. Sullivan JM, Ginsburg BA, Ratts TE, Johnson JG, Barton BR, Kraus DH, McKinstry DN, Muirhead EE: Hemodynamic and antihypertensive effects of captopril, an orally active angiotensin converting enzyme inhibitor. *Hypertension* 1979; 1:397–401.
413a. Halperin AK, Cubeddu LX: The role of calcium channel blockers in the treatment of hypertension. *Am Heart J* 1986; 11:363–381.
414. Report of Inter-society Commission for Heart Disease Resources Hypertension Study Group, J. Edwin Wood, MD, Chairman: Resources for the Management of Emergencies in Hypertension. *Circulation* 1971; 43A:157–160.
415. Finnerty FA: Hypertensive encephalopathy. *Am J Med* 1972; 521:672–678.
416. Bhatia SK, Frohlich ED: Hemodynamic comparison of agents useful in hypertensive emergencies. *Am Heart J* 1973; 85:367–373.
417. Sullivan JM, Schoeneberger AA, Ratts TE, Palmer ET, Samaha JK, Mance CJ, Muirhead EE: Short-term therapy of severe hypertension: hemodynamic correlates of the antihypertensive response in man. *Arch Intern Med* 1979; 139:1233–1239.
418. Woods JW, Blythe WB, Huffines WD: Management of malignant hypertension complicated by renal insufficiency. A follow-up study. *N Engl J Med* 1974; 291:10–14.

34 Hyperlipidemia and Atherosclerosis

Peter T. Kuo, MD

Atherosclerotic cardiovascular disease constitutes a major public health problem in many parts of the world. In the past 30 years, investigators have used a wide range of disciplines to obtain information on the causative or associated factors of atherosclerosis in general and coronary artery disease (CAD) in particular. Early experimental production of hypercholesterolemia and atherosclerotic arterial lesions by cholesterol-oil feeding in rabbits[1] and in higher animal models[2] suggested a possible association between high cholesterol-high fat diet and hypercholesterolemia in human atherosclerosis. However, there is reason to cast doubt on the transfer of information obtained in animals to human subjects. The logical approach to the problem is to test the diet–hyperlipidemia–heart-disease hypothesis in human subjects by: (1) epidemiologic identification of CAD risk factors,[3,4] (2) dietary modification of institutionalized and free-living populations,[5-8] and (3) evaluation of the effect of hypocholesterolemic diet-drug therapy on the progression of CAD by serial coronary arteriography.[9-13] A definitive answer to the hyperlipidemic and atherosclerosis connection finally came in 1984 with the publication of the results of The Lipid Research Clinics Coronary Primary Prevention Trial.[14] The trial is a multicenter, double-blind, randomized, and placebo control study. This study of 3,806 men lasting over seven years was designed to evaluate the combined use of low-cholesterol-fat diet and bile acid sequestrant treatment of hypercholesterolemia. The treated group maintained an average 8% reduction in serum cholesterol as compared with the placebo group, and a 19% reduction in the incidence of myocardial infarction and sudden death. These reductions in the incidence of CAD were closely correlated with a reduction in serum cholesterol and especially in low density lipoproteins (LDL). The relationship between elevated LDL cholesterol and CAD in a free-living asymptomatic population of older men was further confirmed by the recently published results of the Lipid Research Clinics Program Prevalence Study.[14a]

On the basis of the aggregate information obtained from various investigations, clinicians, cardiologists, and health professionals will assuredly begin to pay attention to early detection, referral, and treatment of atherosclerogenic-prone hyperlipidemia to prevent and reduce the morbidity and mortality of CAD.

TYPES OF HYPERLIPIDEMIA

Different types of hyperlipidemia in various degrees of severity are frequently encountered in the practice of internal medicine and cardiology. The practical step is to define them as either primary or secondary types of hyperlipidemia.

PRIMARY HYPERLIPIDEMIA

Years of investigation have delineated several primary hyperlipidemias, ie, those that do not constitute one manifestion of a known metabolic or systemic disease by: (1) genetic analysis of plasma lipoprotein–lipids in family members of hyperlipidemic patients with CHD,[8] (2) a history of premature CHD in first degree family members, (3) the demonstration of cutaneous and tendinous xanthomas and premature corneal arcus, and (4) general resistance to nonpharmacologic therapy.

Fredrickson et al[15] classified their hyperlipidemic patients according to increases in one or the other four classes of plasma lipoproteins into types I to V hyperlipoproteinemia. This classification was later modified by the World Health Organization by subdividing type II into IIa and IIb.[16] The phenotype type IIa lipoprotein abnormality, for example, corresponds well to a well-defined genetic entity of familial hypercholesterolemia, but this and all the other lipoprotein phenotypes are not genetically specific. Accordingly, Goldstein et al[17] and

Goldstein and Brown[17a] initiated familial studies to identify a specific genetic basis of primary hyperlipidemia in an attempt to obtain a better understanding of the underlying metabolic defect or defects that would provide useful information on prognosis and treatment. Since then, several fairly well but still imperfectly defined primary types of hyperlipidemia have been identified.[18,19] A simplified correlation between the phenotypic and genetic typing systems based on either plasma lipoproteins or plasma lipid elevations is presented in Table 34.1.

SECONDARY HYPERLIPIDEMIA

When elevated plasma lipid levels are produced as one manifestation of a systemic and metabolic disease, they are considered as secondary hyperlipidemias. Physicians should make every effort to diagnose and treat the basic disease of these patients. It is worthwhile to emphasize that in most instances the secondary forms of hyperlipidemia are indistinguishable from the primary (genetic) types solely by plasma lipid–lipoprotein analyses. Examples of the more common causes of secondary hyperlipidemia are faulty dietary habits, unhealthy life-style, excessive alcohol consumption, and the use of contraceptives, steroids, and hormones. A list of better known causes of secondary hyperlipidemia is presented in Table 34.2.

The obvious first step in treatment should be directed towards the basic disease problem or problems. If there is a coexisting primary disturbance in lipid metabolism, it can then be properly diagnosed to provide information for prescribing a specifically efficacious hypolipemic treatment.

DIAGNOSIS OF HYPERLIPIDEMIA (HYPERLIPOPROTEINEMIA); APOLIPOPROTEIN ABNORMALITIES

Hyperlipidemia is diagnosed by measuring the two major lipid components of plasma lipoproteins, namely, cholesterol and triglycerides, after a 12- to 14-hour fast. Epidemiologic study indicates that the relation between the plasma cholesterol level and the risk of CAD is a continuum with no clearcut point of distinction between healthy and CAD-prone populations.[4] Furthermore, plasma lipid levels are known to exhibit a wide range of variabilities between different populations because of complex interactions of genetic, cultural, and economic factors. Despite the lack of "healthy" baseline values, epidemiologic survey and consensus experience suggest that the threshold point of serum cholesterol level for raising the risk of CAD is in the range of 200 to 220 mg/dl, and that a triglyceride concentration no higher than 250 mg/dl[20] should be considered an acceptable range for Americans between 40 and 60 years of age. Average serum cholesterol for oriental populations with a low incidence of CAD is in the 150 to 170 mg/dl range.

Table 34.1. Correlation of Hyperlipidemias with Hyperlipoproteinemias

Hyperlipoproteinemias (Genetic or Sporadic)	Phenotypes	Elevated Lipoprotein Class
Familial hyperlipemia (lipoprotein lipase deficiency); apoprotein CII deficiency	Type I	Chylomicron
Familial hypercholesterolemia	Type IIa	LDL
Combined hyperlipidemia	Type IIb	LDL and VLDL
Remnant hyperlipidemia (dysbetalipoproteinemia)	Type III	IDL
Familial hypertriglyceridemia	Type IV	VLDL
Mixed hyperlipemia	Type V	VLDL and chylomicron

IDL = intermediate density lipoprotein; LDL = low density lipoprotein; VLDL = very low density lipoprotein.

Table 34.2. Hyperlipidemia Secondary to Altered Metabolism and Disease States

1. Metabolic and Physiologic
   (a) Weight gain after middle age
   (b) Pregnancy, after second trimester
   (c) Sedentary life-style
2. Dietary Habits
   (a) High saturated fat intake
   (b) High simple carbohydrate intake
   (c) High alcohol consumption
3. Drug-Induced
   (a) Steroids and hormones; estrogens; contraceptives
   (b) Thiazide diuretics
   (c) Beta adrenergic blocking agents
4. Disease States
   (a) Hypothyroidism
   (b) Diabetes mellitus
   (c) Renal diseases (nephrosis)
   (d) Hepatic disease (obstructive jaundice)
   (e) Porphyria
   (f) Dysgammaglobulinemia

Earlier studies in "apparently" healthy subjects suggest that plasma lipid levels rise with advancing age. By application of more stringent methods for diagnosis of CAD, a high percentage of latent atherosclerosis has been uncovered in the older age population. Therefore, upward adjustment of plasma lipid levels with increasing age to delineate a CAD-free population may not be desirable.

The association between hypertriglyceridemia and atherosclerosis[7,21–23] may, at least in part, be operative through the high density lipoprotein effect. An inverse relation between high density lipoprotein cholesterol (HDL-C) and very low density lipoprotein triglyceride (VLDL-TG) as well as an association of a high VLDL-TG/HDL-C ratio with CAD has been demonstrated.[24] Thus, depressed HDL-C may be reflected in defective triglyceride transport and utilization to account for elevated VLDL or triglyceride levels.[25] Furthermore, epidemiologic and clinical studies suggest that HDL may facilitate the removal of cholesterol from peripheral tissue cells, presumably from lipid-laden cells in the arterial wall, to reduce the incidence of CAD.[26–28] In view of these observations, study of hyperlipidemia and atherosclerosis should include HDL-C determination. A suggested "apparently normal" plasma lipid profile is presented in Table 34.3.

The discussions presented in the previous section indicate that measuring the two major lipid components of plasma lipoproteins, cholesterol and triglycerides, would

Table 34.3. Suggested "Normal" Plasma Lipid Profile

Lipid	Concentration (mg/dL)
Total cholesterol	Equal to or less than 200
Triglyceride	Equal to or less than 250
Low density lipoprotein-cholesterol	Equal to or less than 120
High density lipoprotein-cholesterol	Equal to or greater than 50

usually provide adequate information on most hyperlipidemic patients seen in clinical practice. However, to distinguish the lipoprotein fractions from which the two major plasma lipids fractions are derived can help to reveal the basic genetic-metabolic abnormalities of hyperlipidemia in certain cases.[15] For example, moderately high plasma cholesterol levels may be due to elevated HDL-C, a desirable antiatherosclerosis metabolic state. High density lipoprotein cholesterol is usually measured by precipitating VLDL and LDL with heparin and manganese.[29] Low density lipoprotein cholesterol is calculated by the difference between total cholesterol and HDL-C plus VLDL-triglyceride/5.[30] Serum lipoprotein pattern analysis is also helpful in the diagnosis of chylomicronemia, although hyperchylomicronemia can also be diagnosed by grossly turbid (milky) fasting plasma and separation of a creamy top layer after refrigeration.

Recently, interest has been growing in the diagnostic potential of the apoprotein component of plasma lipoproteins. Apolipoproteins A-I and A-II are the major protein constituents of HDL, and Apo B is the principal protein moiety of LDL. Early investigations have shown that apoprotein estimations may broaden the scope in the assessment of risk for CAD beyond the capability of lipid and lipoprotein determinations.[30a] They may help to identify an increased susceptibility to premature atherosclerosis in the absence of either hyperlipidemia or hyperlipoproteinemia.[30b]

CONTROL OF HYPERLIPIDEMIA

The primary objective in treating hyperlipidemia is either to prevent its development or to retard–stabilize the progression of atherosclerotic vascular disease. Secondary objectives are to control (1) arthritis-like symptoms due to tendinous xanthomas, (2) eruptive and palmar xanthomas that may cause localized mucocutaneous symptoms and cosmetic disturbance, and (3) attacks of acute abdominal pain and pancreatitis induced by chylomicronemia.

Glueck et al[31] and Kwiterovich[32] have emphasized the importance of early diagnosis and treatment of childhood hyperlipidemia to prevent premature development of atherosclerosis. They suggest screening children between ages one and 19 for hyperlipidemia, if their parents are known to have: (1) high cholesterol or triglycerides levels or both, (2) myocardial infarction or a stroke before 50, and (3) a history of diabetes, hypertension, and gout. In a given child with a positive family history, the diagnosis of an inherited disturbance is established by the demonstration of either persistent hypercholesterolemia (greater than 200 mg/dl), and high LDL-C (greater than 120 mg/dl) and/or hypertriglyceridemia (greater than 250 mg/dl).

Those hyperlipidemic states that are secondary to various metabolic abnormalities, organ dysfunction, and ulty living habits can be successfully controlled by appropriate management of the basic disorders. The recommendation for diet-drug therapy in patients with primary disturbances in lipid metabolism is outlined next.

TREATMENT OF PRIMARY HYPERLIPIDEMIA

DIET TREATMENT

Appropriate dietary modification constitutes the important first step and should be continued indefinitely to complement drug treatment in all types of hyperlipidemia. The diet is designed to increase the polyunsaturated:saturated fat ratio and to reduce daily dietary cholesterol content to less than 300 mg. Table 34.4 provides basic suggestions on the use of fats, proteins, and carbohydrates in the "therapeutic" diet as modified from the recommendations made by the American Heart Association.

For patients with CAD who are motivated to follow more stringent restrictions, an "alternative diet" as devised by Connor and Connor[33] which lowers the total fat content to 20% and saturated fat to 5% of the total daily caloric intake, respectively, while reducing the dietary cholesterol to 100 mg per day, can be used to maximize plasma lipid lowering effects by diet.

DRUG TREATMENT

The use of hypolipemic drugs should be considered in atherosclerosis-prone individuals and in patients whose hyperlipidemia is resistant to dietary treatment. A sizable list of drugs has been developed and used for control of various types of hyperlipidemia. This discussion will be limited to preparations that are known to have a high plasma lipid-lowering effect but low undesirable reactions. Hypolipemic drugs can be loosely divided into two major groups based on their principal action: (1) to lower triglycerides[34] (nicotinic acid, clofibrate, and gemfibrozil) or (2) to lower cholesterol (cholestyramine, colestipol, and probucol). This arbitrary differentiation is made to provide a rationale for the choice of drugs with the under-

Table 34.4. A Modified American Heart Association Recommended Diet for Hyperlipidemia Control (in % Total Daily Caloric Intake)

Fats:
1. Reduce saturated fats to 5% to 10%
2. Poly- and monounsaturates of 20% to 25%

Carbohydrates
1. Increase to about 55%
2. Increase complex carbohydrates–starches
   Decrease simple carbohydrates–sugars

Proteins
1. About 20%, with high biologic value
   (mainly fish, fowl, and shellfish with low cholesterol content)

Cholesterol
1. Less than 300 mg/day

standing that these drugs have multiple and overlapping pharmacologic activities.

Clofibrate (Atromid-S®)

This is a branched-chain fatty acid ester believed to act primarily to reduce triglyceride-rich VLDL production and to facilitate VLDL catabolism. The effect of Atromid-S on LDL may vary from one patient to another.[35,36] Therefore, in most cases, the drug would lower serum triglycerides, but it would exert a variable effect on the plasma cholesterol level. Additionally, it is moderately effective in raising the plasma HDL level.

Side effects: Clofibrate is generally well tolerated. However, on prolonged administration, the Coronary Drug Project reported about a twofold increase in gallstone incidence and significant increases in cardiovascular symptoms and signs in CAD patients receiving clofibrate treatment.[37] The European Collaborative Study[38] reported a small incidence of hepatic and intestinal disease in patients taking Atromid on a long-term basis.

Dosage and use: Clofibrate is the drug of choice in treating patients with type III hyperlipoproteinemia (dyslipoproteinemia) characterized by an IDL increase. It is generally prescribed in a dosage of 1.5 to 2.0 g per day in two to three divided doses.

Gemfibrozil (Lopid®)

This is a substituted aliphatic acid preparation similar to clofibrate. Preliminary information obtained from a study of human subjects with types IIa, IIb, and IV hyperlipoproteinemia shows the drug to be most effective in reducing serum triglycerides and only mildly effective in lowering serum cholesterol.[39] As VLDL is being suppressed, there is a concomitant increase in HDL-C.[40,40a]

Side effects: So far no serious adverse effects from drug use have been encountered. Some patients complain of abdominal pain and distension when taking the drug in a fasting state. A minimal change in glucose tolerance has been reported.[39–41]

Dosage and use: Gemfibrozil is usually given in dosages of 1.2 g per day in two divided doses. In clinical trials, it has been given to patients with phenotypes IIa, IIb, and IV hyperlipoproteinemia. To date the drug is prescribed for most clinical types of hyperlipidemia, but its effect is mainly on triglycerides. The Helsinki Heart Study is designed to evaluate its value in prevention and management of CAD.[41] The results of this clinical trial will be forthcoming in the near future.

Nicotinic Acid (Niacin)

This is a member of B vitamins with an antipellagra effect. In large doses it inhibits lipolysis from adipose tissue and suppresses free fatty acid flux to the liver for VLDL synthesis.[35] This action results in reduction of plasma triglyceride-rich VLDL and its availability for conversion to LDL.

Side effects: The most disturbing effect of niacin is the initial flushing and pruritis (prostaglandin release, which can be partially suppressed by aspirin). In most cases this reaction would subside after one to two weeks. Niacin can also cause gastrointestinal symptoms if it is taken in the fasting state. Its other undesirable serious side effects are hepatic dysfunction, cholestatic jaundice, hyperglycemia, hyperuricemia, and gouty arthritis.[42]

Dosage and use: Niacin is a potent lipid-lowering agent. In 3 to 7 g per day in divided dosages to be taken with meals, it is prescribed for the control of hypertriglyceridemia (VLDL elevation) as well as hypercholesterolemia (LDL elevation).[34,35] In the Coronary Drug Project[42] it accomplished a borderline reduction in the five-year incidence of CHD death and reinfarction.

Cholestyramine (Questran®) and Colestipol (Colestid®)

Both are anion exchange resins. They are insoluble in water and act to bind bile acids (the degradation products of cholesterol) to increase fecal bile acid excretion. This series of biologic events stimulates increased cholesterol and LDL catabolism as well as increased cholesterol biosynthesis. In human subjects, the increased LDL-cholesterol catabolic rate is higher than the compensatory biosynthetic rate.[43] The net result is a lowering of plasma LDL-cholesterol. As the demand for cholesterol is increased, resulting from the drug-mediated cholesterol loss, hepatic cells are stimulated to produce increased numbers of LDL receptors. Thus the resins treatment provides partial correction of the cellular LDL receptor defect as demonstrated by Brown and Goldstein[44] in familial hypercholesterolemia.

Side effects: Constipation is the most common side effect, but it is readily controllable by stool softeners. Other minor gastrointestinal symptoms of nausea, distension and cramps would improve after a period of adjustment. Their long-term administration is well tolerated with no significant impairment in the absorption of fat or fat soluble vitamins.

Dosage and use: Levy et al[45] reported a 20% reduction in plasma cholesterol and a 27% reduction in LDL in patients with heterozygous familial hypercholesterolemia on 16 g of cholestyramine per day. We have reported a little more pronounced plasma cholesterol reduction in familial hypercholesterolemic patients on a combined diet–30 g colestipol per day regimen.[9] Cholestyramine was used to reduce the incidence of CAD in the Lipid Research Clinics Coronary Primary Prevention Trial.[14]

Probucol (Lorelco®)

Probucol is a sulfur-containing butylphenol compound. Unlike bile acid sequestrants, it is absorbed through the portal circulation and appears to exert its primary action by inhibiting cholesterol biosynthesis.[46] At the same time the drug acts to enhance the synthesis and excretion of bile acids. The drug decreases not only plasma cholesterol (LDL) but also HDL-cholesterol.[47]

Side effects: The main side effect of probucol is loose stools with occasional episodes of disturbing diarrhea. The drug tends to cause lengthening of the QT interval on the electrocardiogram without increasing susceptibility to cardiac arrhythmia. So far, no serious adverse effect of the drug has been reported.

Dosage and use: Probucol 1.0 g per day is usually administered in two divided doses to lower the serum cholesterol level of patients with heterozygous familial hypercholesterolemia by about 20% from the average baseline values.[48] High density lipoprotein cholesterol is decreased almost by a similar degree. This latter effect has caused some concern, because HDL is believed to have an antiatherogenic effect. However, long-term administration of probucol has resulted in regression of cutaneous and tendinous xanthomas[48] and in a suggestive reduction of clinical cardiovascular events.[49,50]

Combined Hypolipemic Therapy

Decreasing abnormally elevated serum lipid levels (triglycerides and cholesterol) to suggested "normal" levels in most patients with primary hyperlipidemia may not be easy to accomplish with mono-drug therapy. A number of investigators have employed combinations of drugs with complementary serum lipid-lowering mechanisms in an attempt to obtain control of resistant primary hyperlipidemias. The therapeutic design is to prescribe a drug that would facilitate degradation–excretion of cholesterol, coupling it with another preparation to block the heightened lipid biosynthesis. Examples of fairly well-studied combination therapies are the use of colestipol or cholestyramine in combination with either niacin or probucol. The dosage of one or the other drug in a given combination therapy may be adjusted according to the long-term response pattern of the patient.[51–53] Several investigators have presented angiographic evidence indicating the feasibility to arrest the progression of atherosclerotic lesion through optimal control of hyperlipidemia with combined drug regimen.[9–12,54] Two examples of stabilizing CAD progression for five to six years with hypolipemic therapy are shown in Figures 34.1 and 34.2.

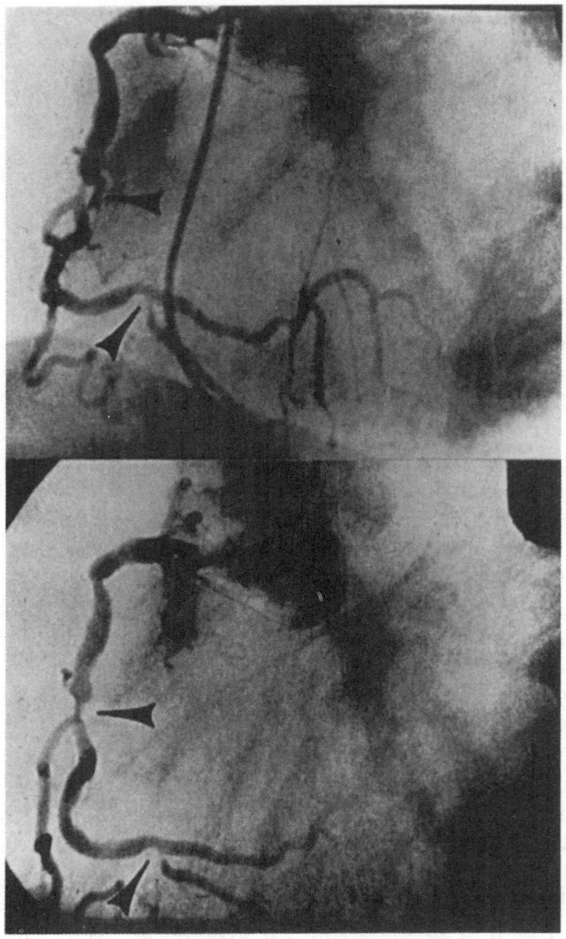

Figure 34.1. Right coronary arteriograms in patient AS performed five and a half years apart. *Top*, Before hypolipemic therapy. *Bottom*, Five and a half years after hypolipemic therapy.

Inhibitors of 3-hydroxy-3-methylglutaryl-CoA (HMG-CoA) reductase such as compactin and mevinolin are still in the investigational stage. Either of them can be used in combination with a bile acid sequestrant to reduce LDL-C in patients with familial hypercholesterolemia.[55,56]

Measures Helpful in Increasing High Density Lipoprotein

Most hygienic measures including weight reduction, stop smoking, regular aerobic exercise,[57,58] and alcohol[59,60] in moderation (about 60 ml per day) are helpful in increasing the HDL level. Hypolipemic drugs known to exert a salutary effect on HDL concentration when administered in adequate dosages are listed in the order of their HDL enhancement potential as follows: nicotinic acid, gemfibrozil, and clofibrate.

COMMENTS

Hyperlipidemia has long been recognized as a major CAD risk factor based on the observation made in a number of experimental, epidemiologic, population, and clinical studies. However, many medical professionals and most of the lay public have remained unconvinced before conclusive scientific proof was available. This long-awaited "proof" has recently been announced to the public by the publication of the Lipid Research Clinics Coronary Primary Prevention Trial data.[14] Results obtained from this nationwide well-controlled study provide strong support for the use of diet-drug treatment of hypercholesterolemia (LDL elevation) to prevent early development of CAD and its complications.

In clinical practice, the initial step in dealing with hyperlipidemic patients is to differentiate the condition into primary and secondary types. In patients in the latter category, attention is directed to the management of the basic disease and not to the hyperlipidemia per se. Although five of six types of primary hyperlipoproteinemias have been associated with atherosclerosis, experiences indicate that in most instances the demonstration of elevation in either plasma cholesterol or triglyceride or both (lipid components of lipoproteins) would suffice in prescribing treatment and in assessing prognosis. Nevertheless, some knowledge of the atherosclerotic low density lipoproteins (VDL, IDL, and LDL) and the suggested salutary effect of atherosclerosis-protective HDL is useful in the management of certain special groups of hyperlipidemic patients. For example, moderate elevations in serum total cholesterol must be interpreted with caution, because a contribution from HDL-C must be taken into consideration, especially in young female patients.

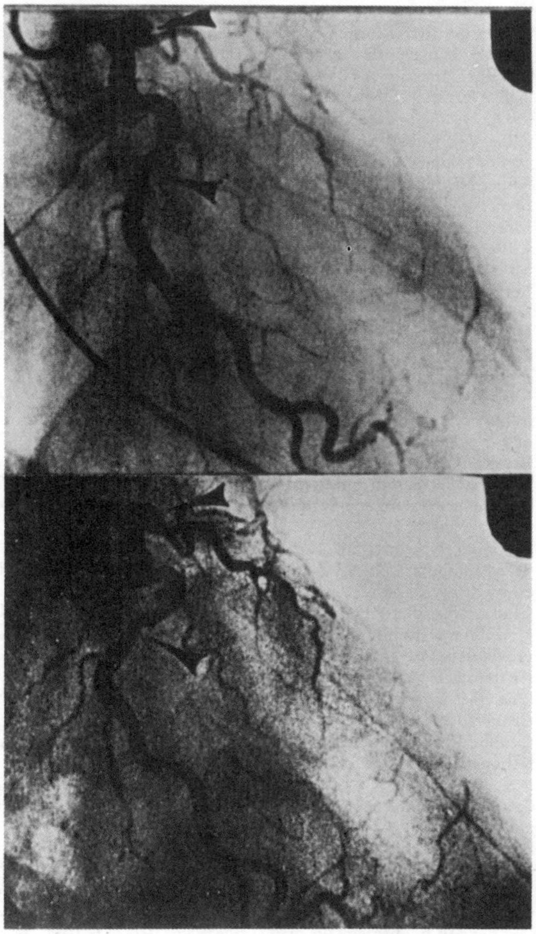

Figure 34.2. Left coronary arteriograms in patient LA performed six years apart. *Top*, Before hypolipemic therapy. *Bottom*, Six years after hypolipemic therapy.

Clinically, hyperlipidemia in a major portion of the patient population is attributable to faulty dietary habit and unhealthy life-style. Even when a genetic abnormality is partly or predominantly responsible for the hyperlipidemia, treatment should still begin with dietary intervention. The patient and the family members should be educated on the principles of "therapeutic" diet for life-long modification of the family's eating habit. Habitual adherence to the "therapeutic" diet will result in variable degrees of improvement in lipid metabolism and will act to complement the hypolipemic effect of drug therapy when indicated.

Drug treatment is invariably required in patients with primary hyperlipidemia (hyperlipoproteinemia). Although the ease of administration and relative freedom from unpleasant side effects are important factors, drug selection should be made primarily on: (1) its mode of action, which is specific for the hyperlipidemia in a given patient; (2) the knowledge that it is nontoxic or relatively free from undesirable side effects on long-term administration.

Results of the National Heart, Lung, and Blood Institute-sponsored Coronary Prevention Trial[14] combined with data obtained by a number of investigators,[9-13] have provided a consensus for a reduction in elevated plasma cholesterol or triglycerides or both (LDL, VLDL, LDL and VLDL) to reduce the incidence of mortality and morbidity from CAD.[61] In addition, several investigators have performed serial coronary and peripheral arteriograms to demonstrate that well-controlled hypolipemic therapy can help to stabilize or retard the progression and even promote regression of atherosclerotic arterial lesions in human subjects.[9-12] There is reason to believe that if identification and modification of this major CAD risk factor were made in the incipient stages of atherogenesis, a substantial reduction in CAD could be accomplished.

SUMMARY

1. The recently completed National Heart, Lung, and Blood Institute-sponsored multicenter double-blind Coronary Heart Disease Prevention Trial has provided the long sought-after proof that hyperlipidemia is a major CAD risk factor and that the incidence of CAD and its complications can be modified favorably by control of hyperlipidemia with appropriate diet-drug therapy. This nationwide study confirms and validates the earlier reports on the feasibility of stabilizing or promoting regression of atherosclerotic arterial lesions through hyperlipidemia control.

2. Current investigations suggest that in most instances, simple differentiation of hyperlipidemia into hypercholesterolemia and hypertriglyceridemia (major components of LDL and VLDL) can supply adequate information for use in clinical practice. In a few special conditions the application of lipoprotein analysis may provide insight into the underlying genetic/metabolic abnormality in the selection of a specific therapeutic modality.

3. Before considering hypolipemic therapy, attempts should be made to exclude secondary hyperlipidemia. In those cases, treatment should be directed at the primary disease or diseases for control of hyperlipidemia.

4. Life-long dietary modification is the key to treatment of all types of hyperlipidemia including primary hyperlipidemia. Both the patients and their family members should be educated in the principles and importance of dietary modification to boost compliance.

5. In a given familial hyperlipidemia, a specifically effective hypolipemic drug or a combination of drugs with minimal or no long-term toxic side effects should be prescribed to augment the therapeutic diet for decreasing elevated plasma lipid levels, and maintaining them in the "normal" range in a given population.

6. Early detection and control of atherosclerosis-prone hyperlipidemia in children and young adults should be vigorously promoted to reduce the high incidence of atherosclerotic cardiovascular disease.

Acknowledgment: This work was supported in part by research grants from the Leola Detwiler Research Foundation and the American Heart Association, Somerset–Hunterdon Chapter and New Jersey Affiliate. Alan C. Wilson, MD, and Randee Goldstein were responsible for accurate lipid–lipoprotein analyses. We wish to thank Merrell Dow Pharmaceutical Inc, Cincinnati, Ohio, for their support and the supply of probucol, the Upjohn Company, Kalamazoo, Michigan, for a long-term supply of colestipol, and The Best Food Company, Union, New Jersey, for the corn oil and peanut butter used in our research studies.

REFERENCES

1. Anitschkow N, Chalatow S: Ueber experimentelle Cholesterinsteatose und ihre Bedeutung für die Entstehung einiger pathologischer Prozesse. *Centralbl Path path Anat Jena* 1913; 24:1–9.
2. Armstrong ML, Connor WE, Warner ED: Tissue cholesterol concentration in the hypercholesterolemic rhesus monkey. *Arch Path* 1969; 87:87–92.
3. Key A: Coronary heart disease: the global picture. *Atherosclerosis* 1975; 22:149–192.
4. Kannel WB, Castelli WP, Gordon T, McNamara PM: Serum cholesterol, lipoproteins and risk of coronary artery disease. The Framingham Study. *Ann Intern Med* 1971; 74:1–12.
5. Dayton S, Pearch ML, Hashimoto S, Dixon WJ, Tomiyasu U: A clinical trial of a diet high in unsaturated fat in preventing complication of atherosclerosis. *Circulation* 1969; 40(suppl II): 1–63.
6. Turpeinen O, Miettenen M, Karvonen MJ, Roine P, Pekkarinen M, Lehtosuo EJ, Alivirta P: Dietary prevention of coronary heart disease: long-term experiment. *Am J Clin Nutr* 1968; 21:255–276.
7. Hjermann I, Velve Byre K, Holme I, Leren P: Effect of diet and smoking intervention on the incidence of coronary heart disease. *Lancet* 1981; 2:1303–1310.
8. Hazzard WR, Goldstein JL, Schrott HG, Motulsky AG, Bierman EL: Hyperlipidemia in coronary heart disease. III. Evaluation of lipoprotein phenotypes of 156 genetically defined survivors of myocardial infarction. *J Clin Invest* 1973; 52:1569–1577.
9. Kuo PT, Hayase K, Kostis JB, Moreyra AE: Use of combined diet and colestipol in long-term (7–7½years) treatment of patients with type II hyperlipoproteinemia. *Circulation* 1979; 59:199–211.
10. Kuo PT, Kostis JB, Moreyra AE, Hayes JA: Familial type II hyperlipoproteinemia with coronary heart disease. Effect of diet-colestipol-nicotinic acid treatment. *Chest* 1981; 79:286–291.
11. Blankenhorn DH, Brooks SH, Selzer RH, Barndt R Jr: The rate of atherosclerosis change during treatment of hyperlipoproteinemia. *Circulation* 1977; 57:355–361.
12. Nikkila EA, Viikinkoski P, Valle M, Frick MH: Prevention of progression of coronary atherosclerosis by treatment of hyperlipidemia: a seven year prospective angiographic study. *Br Med J* 1984; 289:220–223.

12a. Kanamori K, Nishijima H, Kojima S, Matsumura N, Sato I, Murakami R, Minami M, Yasuda H: Relationship between lipids and angiographically defined coronary artery disease in Japanese patients. *Am Heart J* 1984; 108:1207–1211.

12b. Arntzenius AC, Kromhout D, Barth JD, Reiber JHC, Bruschke AVG, Buis B, Van Gent CM, Kempen-Voogd N, Strikwerda S, Van Der Velde EA: Diet, lipoproteins, and the progression of coronary atherosclerosis. The Leiden intervention trial. *N Engl J Med* 1985; 312:805–811.

13. Gotto AM, Gorry GA, Thompson JR, Cole JS, Trost R, Yeshurun D, DeBakey ME: Relationship between plasma lipid concentrations and coronary artery disease in 496 patients. *Circulation* 1977; 56:875–883.
14. Lipid Research Clinics Program: The lipid research clinics coronary primary prevention trial results. I. Reduction in incidence of coronary heart disease. II. The relationship of reduction in incidence of coronary disease in cholesterol lowering. *JAMA* 1984; 251:351–364, 365–374.

14a. Rubenstein C, Romhilt D, Segal P, Heiss G, Chambless LE, Boyle KE, Ekelund L-G, Adolph R, Sheffield LT: Dyslipoproteinemias and manifestations of coronary heart disease. The Lipid Research Clinics Program Prevalance Study. *Circulation* 1986; 73 (suppl I):I-91–I-99.

15. Fredrickson DS, Goldstein JL, Brown MS: Familial hyperlipoproteinemias, in Stanbury JB, Wyngaarden JB, Fredrickson DS, (eds): *The Metabolic Basis of Inherited Disease.* New York, McGraw-Hill, 1978, pp 604–655.
16. Beaumont JL, Carlson LA, Cooper GR, Feijfar Z, Fredrickson DS, Strasser T: Classifications of hyperlipidemias and hyperlipoproteinemias. *Bull WHO* 1970; 43:891–908.
17. Goldstein JL, Schrott HG, Hazzard WR, Bierman EL, Motulsky AG: Hyperlipidemia in coronary heart disease. II. Genetic analysis of lipid levels in 176 families and delineation of a new inherited disorder combined hyperlipidemia. *J Clin Invest* 1973; 52:1544–1568.

17a. Goldstein JL, Brown MS: Familial hypercholesterolemia: a genetic receptor disease. *Hospital Practice* 1985; 20(11):35–46.

18. Havel RJ: Classification of the hyperlipidemias. *Ann Rev Med* 1977; 28:195–209.
19. Havel RJ: Approach to the patient with hyperlipidemia. *Med Clin North Am* 1982; 66:319–333.
20. Consensus Conference, NHLBI: Treatment of hypertriglyceridemia. *JAMA* 1984; 251:1196–1200.
21. Albrink MJ, Man EB: Serum triglycerides in coronary artery disease. *Arch Intern Med* 1959; 103:4–8.
22. Kuo PT: Hypertriglyceridemia in coronary artery disease and its management. *JAMA* 1967; 201:87–94.
23. Lippel K, Tyroler H, Eder H, Gotto A Jr, Vahouny G: Relationship of hypertriglyceridemia to atherosclerosis. *Arteriosclerosis* 1981; 1:406–417.
24. Phillips NR, Havel RJ, Kane JP: Levels and interrelationships of serum and lipoprotein cholesterol and triglycerides. Association with adiposity and the consumption of ethanol, tobacco and beverages containing caffeine. *Arteriosclerosis* 1981; 1:13–24.
25. Tall AR, Small DM: Plasma high-density lipoproteins. *N Engl J Med* 1978; 299:1232–1236.
26. Miller GJ, Miller NE: Plasma high density lipoprotein concentration and development of ischemic heart disease. *Lancet* 1975; 1:16–19.
27. Miller NE, Thelle DS, Forde OH, Mjos OD: The Tromso heart study, high-density lipoprotein and coronary heart disease: a prospective case-control study. *Lancet* 1977; 1:965–967.
28. Castelli W, Doyle JT, Gordon T, Hames CG, Hjortland MC, Hulley SB, Kagan A, Zukel WJ: HDL cholesterol and other lipids in coronary heart disease. The cooperative lipoprotein phenotyping study. *Circulation* 1977; 55:767–772.
29. Warnick GR, Albers JJ: A comprehensive evaluation of the heparin-manganese precipitation procedure for estimating high density lipoprotein cholesterol. *J Lipid Res* 1978; 19:65–76.
30. Friedewald WT, Levy RI, Fredrickson DS: Estimation of the concentration of low-density lipoprotein cholesterol in plasma without use of the preparative ultracentrifuge. *Clin Chem* 1972; 18:499–502.

30a. Kesteloot H. Huang DX, Yang XS, Claes J, Rosseneu M, Geboers J, Joossens JV: Serum lipids in the People's Republic of China. Comparison of Western and Eastern populations. *Arteriosclerosis* 1985; 5:427–433.

30b. Maciejko JJ, Holmes DR, Kottke BA, Zinsmeister AR, Dinh DM, Mao SJT: Apolipoprotein A-I as a marker of angiographically assessed coronary artery disease. *N Engl J Med* 1983; 309:385–389.

31. Glueck CJ, Fallat RW, Tsang R: Hypercholesterolemia and hypertriglyceridemia in children: a pediatric approach to primary atherosclerosis prevention. *Am J Dis Child* 1974; 128:569–577.
32. Kwiterovich PO Jr: Pediatric aspects of hyperlipoproteinemia, in Rifkind BM, Levy RI (eds): *Hyperlipidemia, Diagnosis and Therapy.* New York, Grune & Stratton, 1977.
33. Connor WE, Connor SL: The dietary treatment of hyperlipidemia. Rationale, technique, and efficacy. *Med Clin North Am* 1982; 66:485–518.
34. Grundy SM: Hypertriglyceridemia: mechanisms, clinical significance, and treatment. *Med Clin North Am* 1982; 66:519–535.
35. Levy RI, Morganroth J, Rifkin BM: Treatment of hyperlipidemia. *N Engl J Med* 1974; 290:1295–1301.
36. Wilson DE, Lees RS: Metabolic relationships among the plasma lipoproteins. Reciprocal changes in the concentrations of very low and low density lipoproteins in man. *J Clin Invest* 1972; 51: 1051–1057.
37. Coronary Drug Project Research Group: Gallbladder disease as a side effect of drugs influencing lipid metabolism *N Engl J Med* 1977; 296: 1185–1190.
38. Committee of Principal Investigators: A cooperative trial in the primary prevention of ischemic heart disease using clofibrate. *Br Heart J* 1978; 40:1069–1118.
39. Samuel P: Effects of gemfibrozil on serum lipids. *Am J Med* 1983; 74(5A):23–27.
40. Glueck CJ: Influence of gemfibrozil on high-density lipoproteins. *Am J Cardiol* 1983; 52:31B–34B).

40a. Vega GL, Grundy SM: Gemfibrozil therapy in primary hypertriglyceridemia associated with coronary heart disease. Effects on metabolism of low-density lipoproteins. *JAMA* 1985; 253:2398–2403.

41. Manninen V: Clinical results with gemfibrozil and background to the Helsinki heart study. *Am J Cardiol* 1983; 52:35B–38B.
42. The Coronary Drug Project Research Group: Clofibrate and niacin in coronary heart disease. *JAMA* 1975; 231:360–381.
43. Levy RI, Langer T: Hypolipidemic drugs and lipoprotein metabolism. *Adv Exp Med Biol* 1972; 26:155–163.
44. Brown MS, Goldstein JL: Receptor-mediated control of cholesterol metabolism. Study of human mutants has disclosed how cells regulate a substance that is both vital and lethal. *Science* 1976; 191:150–154.
45. Levy RI, Fredrickson DS, Stone NJ, Bilheimer DW, Brown WV, Glueck CJ, Gotto AM, Herbert PN, Kwiterovich PO, Langer T, LaRosa J, Lux SE, Rider AK, Shulman RS, Sloan HR: Cholestyramine in type II hyperlipoproteinemia. *Ann Intern Med* 1973; 79:51–58.
46. Barnhart JW, Sefranka JA, McIntosh DD: Hypocholesterolemic effect of 4,4-(iso-propylidenedithio)-bis (2,6-di-t-butylphenol) (Probucol) *Am J Clin Nutr* 1970; 23:1229–1233.
47. Gagne C, Lupien PJ, Brun D, Moorjani S, Toussaint M: Probucol and high-density-lipoprotein cholesterol. *Can Med Assoc J* 1980; 123:356.
48. Yamamoto A, Matsuzawa Y, Kishino B, Hayashi R, Hirobe K, Kikkawa T: Effects of probucol on homozygous cases of familial hypercholesterolemia. *Atherosclerosis* 1983; 48:157–166.
49. Miettinen TA, Huttunen JK, Strandberg T, Naukkarinen V, Mattila S, Kumlin T: Lowered HDL cholesterol and incidence of ischemic heart disease. *Lancet* 1981; 2:478.
50. Tedeschi RE, Taylor HL, Martz BL: Clinical experience of the safety and cholesterol-lowering action of probucol, in Noseda G, Lewis B,

Paoletti R (eds.): *Diet and Drugs in Atherosclerosis.* New York, Raven Press, 1980, p 199.

51. Kane JP, Malloy MJ, Tun P, Phillips NR, Freedman DD, Williams ML, Rowe JS, Havel RJ: Normalization of low-density-lipoprotein levels in heterozygous familial hypercholesterolemia with a combined drug regimen. *N Engl J Med* 1981; 304:251–258.
52. Nestel PJ: Cholestyramine and probucol synergism. *Ann Intern Med* 1982; 97:622.
53. Dujovne CA, Krehbiel P, Decoursey S, Jackson B, Chernoff SB, Pitterman A, Garty M: Probucol with colestipol in the treatment of hypercholesterolemia. *Am Intern Med* 1984; 100:477–482.
54. Kuo PT, Wilson AC, Kostis JB, Moreyra AE, Goldstein R: Effect of combined probucol and colestipol treatment in patients with familial hypercholesterolemia and coronary artery disease. *Chest* 1984; 86:284.
55. Mabuchi H, Sakai T, Sakai Y, Yoshimura A, Watenabe A, Wakasugi T, Koizumi J, Takeda R: Reduction of serum cholesterol in heterozygous patients with familial hypercholesterolemia. Additive effects of compactin and cholestyramine. *N Engl J Med* 1983; 308:609–613.
56. Bilheimer DW, Grundy SM, Brown MS, Goldstein JL: Mevinolin and colestipol stimulate receptor-mediated clearance of low density lipoprotein from plasma in familial hypercholesterolemia heterozygotes. *Proc Natl Acad Sci USA* 1983; 80:4124–4128.
57. Wood PH, Haskell W, Klein H, Lewis S, Stern MP, Farquhar JW: The distribution of plasma lipoproteins in middle-aged male runners. *Metabolism* 1976; 25:1249–1257.
58. Huttunen JK, Lansimies E, Voutilainen E, Ehnholm C, Hietanen E, Penttila I, Siitonen O, Rauramaa R: Effect of moderate exercise on serum lipoproteins. A controlled clinical trial with special reference to serum high-density lipoproteins. *Circulation* 1980; 60:1220–1229.
59. Castelli WP, Doyle JT, Gordon T, Hames CG, Hjortland MC, Hulley SB, Kagan A, Zukel WJ: Alcohol and blood lipids. *Lancet* 1977; 2:153–155.
60. Hartung GH, Foreyt JP, Mitchell RE, Mitchell JG, Reeves RS, Gotto AM: Effect of alcohol intake on high-density lipoprotein cholesterol levels in runners and inactive men. *JAMA* 1983; 249:747–750.
61. Consensus Conference: Lowering blood cholesterol to prevent heart disease. *JAMA* 1985; 253:2080–2086.

35 Medical Aspects of Coronary Artery Disease

William C. Sheldon, MD

Coronary artery disease remains the leading cause of death in industrialized nations and is of growing concern in developing countries. The medical aspects of coronary artery disease will be discussed in this chapter. Myocardial infarction, coronary artery spasm, surgical and other interventional aspects of coronary artery disease are discussed elsewhere.

Although William Heberden in 1768 is credited with the first description of angina pectoris, its association with coronary atherosclerosis was suspected by Edward Jenner in 1786. Jenner recognized the symptoms of angina pectoris in his friend John Hunter and predicted that he had coronary artery disease. This was proved correct by postmortem study when Hunter died in 1793. In the meanwhile Caleb Parry noted severe coronary artery disease at autopsy in a man with angina pectoris, and quite independently in 1793 Samuel Black also noted severe coronary artery disease at autopsy in a patient who had angina pectoris and died with symptoms suggesting myocardial infarction.[1-3] Although this formulation of angina pectoris and its relation to coronary atherosclerosis evolved between 1768 and 1793, more than 100 years elapsed before the syndrome of acute myocardial infarction was linked with coronary artery occlusion by James Herrick in 1912.[4] Herrick described a case of acute myocardial infarction in a 55-year-old man who died 52 hours after the onset of pain. He also recognized that death may be "sudden, seemingly instantaneous and perhaps painless," or that it may occur within minutes from shock associated with severe anginal pain. He also recognized, as Heberden had suggested, nonfatal cases with mild angina resulting in patchy fibrosis due to coronary atherosclerosis, particularly involving small vessels.

In 1940 Blumgart, Schlesinger, and Davis[5] described the relation between angina pectoris, coronary thrombosis, and myocardial infarction and the importance of the intercoronary collateral circulation. In 1958 Sones and Shirey[6] extended the principles of left heart catheterization and cineangiography to visualize the coronary arteries, first by aortic root injections and subsequently by selective injection of contrast media directly into the right or left coronary artery. This paved the way for the definitive diagnosis of coronary artery disease in living patients, the correlation of symptoms with anatomy,[7-9] the delineation of prognostic parameters as assessed by the clinical course of patients with angiographically proven coronary artery disease,[10-13] and the development of specific surgical and nonsurgical interventional procedures to correct specific coronary artery obstructions.[14-16]

ETIOLOGY OF CORONARY ATHEROSCLEROSIS

Despite our understanding of the anatomy, pathophysiology, clinical manifestations, and therapeutic concepts as they have evolved over the past 200 years, the etiology of coronary atherosclerosis remains obscure. Atherosclerosis and abnormalities of lipid metabolism are discussed in another chapter. The importance of lipid deposition in the arterial wall was recognized by Virchow[17] in 1856. Anitschkow and Chalatow[18] described an experimental model in which an atherosclerotic-like lesion was induced in rabbits with a cholesterol-rich diet, and the lesion regressed after termination of the experimental diet. Studies of the relation between blood lipids and coronary atherosclerosis have yielded contradictory results because of the observations that many patients with coronary artery disease had seemingly normal levels of blood cholesterol, and that in autopsy series cholesterol levels were similar in patients who died of coronary heart disease compared with those who died accidentally. Other studies showed a tendency for increased levels of cholesterol in patients with clinical coronary disease, and cholesterol has gradually emerged as a definite associated factor in coronary atherosclerosis. In the 1950s several epidemiologic studies in the United States underscored the importance of cholesterol as a risk factor, and studies of the relation between cholesterol consumption and coronary heart disease in other countries seemed to support the concept of cholesterol as an important risk factor.[19,20] Other factors associated with coronary atherosclerosis have also emerged: family history, hypertension, and cigarette smoking.

Current thinking integrates all these factors into a mosaic theory encompassing host-related factors (age, sex, heredity, endocrine abnormalities, and disorders of lipid metabolism), vascular factors (vascular injury due to hypertension, smoking, etc), and environmental factors (diet, stress, and exercise) (Figure 35.1).

CLINICAL MANIFESTATIONS AND PATHOPHYSIOLOGY OF CORONARY ARTERY DISEASE

Although the hallmark symptoms of coronary artery disease are angina pectoris and acute myocardial infarction, it is important to recognize that many patients do not recognize prodromal symptoms, and nearly half of the initial presenting events are catastrophic, ie, acute myocardial infarction or sudden death. In the Framingham study,[21] only 38% of men and 61% of women had angina pectoris as the presenting symptom. If the angina is typical, over 94% of patients have significant (50%) narrowing of at least one coronary artery, and half have total occlusion of one or more vessels. At least 50% have involvement of two or more arteries. If the presenting symptom is myocardial infarction, 98% of patients have significant coronary arterial narrowing, two thirds of patients have multivessel disease, and at least 60% have at least one totally occluded vessel.[7]

Angina pectoris and myocardial infarction are late manifestations of a pathologic process that has evolved gradually over many years before reaching a critical threshold of myocardial ischemia sufficient to produce symptoms or trigger cardiac arrhythmia and sudden death (Figure 35.2). After a long period of latency, clinical awareness frequently results from a sudden and unpredictable mechanical event, ie, the development of severe stenosis or total occlusion from (1) thrombus formation at the site of an intimal plaque; (2) superficial injury, disruption, or dissection of an arteriosclerotic plaque with subintimal hemorrhage; (3) coronary spasm related to mechanical or possibly neurohumoral events or both; or (4) combinations of these events (Table 35.1). The secondary myocardial sequelae of this process depend on the location of the coronary lesion and the size of the area of myocardium perfused by the involved artery, the anatomic distribution of coronary arteries and the propensity for adjacent branches to perfuse branches distal to the obstruction through intercoronary collateral communications, and the extent of arteriosclerotic involvement of neighboring arteries that may compromise blood flow through collateral channels (Table 35.2). If the arteriosclerotic process develops gradually without major intercurrent mechanical events such as those just described, it is possible for advanced and diffuse arteriosclerotic narrowing to occur diffusely with little or no myocardial scarring. However, the effect of this arterial process on the myocardium also depends on factors related to myocardial work and its metabolic requirements. Increased myocardial metabolic demand from physical activity, other forms of stress that influence arterial pressure and pulse rate (hypertension or hyperthyroidism), and associated valvular or other cardiac disease including myocardial hypertrophy may tax the blood supply or coronary flow reserve. This may result in the appearance of symptoms relatively early in the natural course of the arteriosclerotic process. In some patients myocardial responses other than acute myocardial infarction may develop, such as hypertrophy, depression

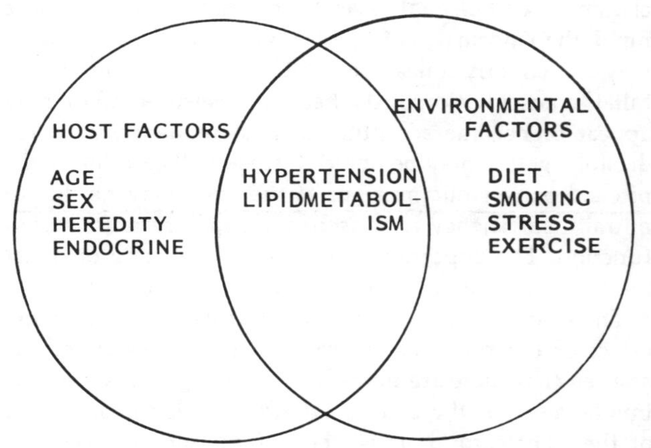

Figure 35.1. Interrelation of host and environmental factors in the etiology of coronary atherosclerosis. (See text.)

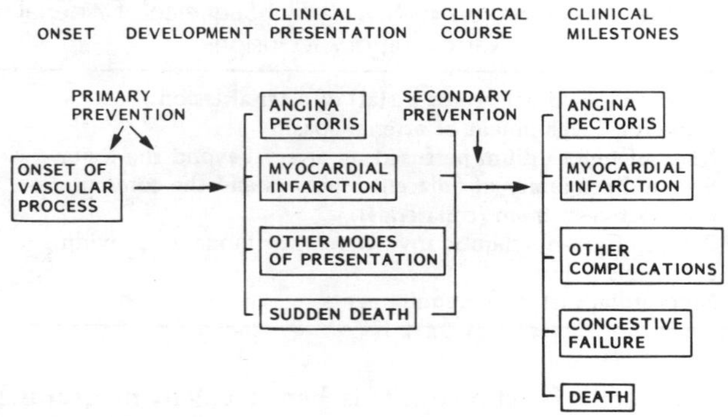

Figure 35.2. Time course of coronary atherosclerosis before and after clinical appearance. (See text for discussion.)

Table 35.1. Factors in the Development of Arterial Narrowing or Occlusion

- Gradual build-up of arteriosclerotic plaque
- Thrombus formation
- Disruption of plaque with subintimal hemorrhage
- Spasm of artery at site of plaque

Table 35.2. Factors in Myocardial Sequelae of Arterial Narrowing or Occlusion

- Location (proximal versus distal) of arterial lesion
- Time for development of arterial spasm
- Mass of myocardium perfused by artery beyond the lesion
- Size and proximity of adjacent branches and the communications between them (collaterals)
- Extent of arteriosclerotic involvement of branches providing collaterals
- Myocardial metabolic requirements

of contractile function due to ischemia, patchy myocardial fibrosis, cardiac arrhythmias, or combinations of these effects.

CLINICAL FEATURES OF ANGINA PECTORIS

When Heberden[2] in 1768 described the syndrome of angina pectoris, he was unaware of its cause and referred to a sense of strangling and anxiety with a fear of impending death. He noted that the pain was paroxysmal in nature and that those afflicted sometimes died suddenly. Angina pectoris is not an entity in itself, but rather it is a term applied to a symptom complex (Table 35.3). It occurs intermittently and is usually brief in duration. Typically, it is produced by a physical activity that the patient may have previously been able to perform without difficulty. The discomfort begins mildly, so as to be scarcely perceptible and gradually increases in intensity. Although it may be mild, after a few recurrences it cannot usually be ignored. It is not well localized and may be felt anywhere between the upper abdomen and the jaw. Occasionally it may be felt most clearly in either or both elbows, wrists, mandible, or teeth. If there has been a previous injury to an arm or shoulder, this may become the focus of the discomfort. As the discomfort builds in intensity, the zone of sensation may expand. Hence, discomfort that may have begun in the upper portion of the chest may encompass a larger area or extend to the neck, shoulders, or arms and sometimes the interscapular area. Pain that began in the arms may spread across the chest. There is usually a sense of uneasiness in the chest and this is accompanied by fear or apprehension. There may be associated weakness, heaviness of the arms, slight air hunger, nausea, or clamminess.

The discomfort is usually not described as painful. More commonly it is described in terms of pressure, tightness, heaviness, burning, or indigestion. As it builds in intensity, the patient either consciously or subconsciously reduces or ceases activity and he soon learns how to pace his activity to avoid the discomfort or to rest or cease activity to control it. Occasionally he will find it necessary to stand quietly or lean against a tree to bring relief. The upright position is preferred to recumbency. He will recognize that it is more likely to occur when he is active following meals or in cold weather. He will also note its occurrence when there is physical activity associated with emotion, ie, sexual intercourse, or when hurrying, as to catch an airplane or meet a deadline, or during an argument. Sometimes, as the condition progresses, the symptom will also occur at rest, but even this may be associated with circulatory changes mimicking those that occur during exercise: first reclining after the activity of preparing for bed, during sleep (in relation to dreams or nightmares), or with the first activity after arising from sleep. Occasionally the discomfort will occur at rest, totally unrelated to any evident generalized circulatory changes or mental or physical activity. It is thought that such episodes may be the result of spontaneous changes in coronary artery vascular tone or coronary artery spasm.

Table 35.3. Ten Important Characteristics in the Evaluation of Chest Pain (Discomfort)

1. Character (sharp, dull, tight, aching, pressure, burning, etc)
2. Location/distribution
3. Severity
4. Frequency
5. Duration
6. Radiation
7. Associated symptoms
8. Precipitating factors
9. Relieving factors
10. Preventative factors

Sometimes the patient will discover that performing the Valsalva maneuver will bring relief. He may have used sublingual nitroglycerin, which usually results in abatement of the attack within two to three minutes. In the later stages of the disease, larger and more frequent doses of nitroglycerin may be required. Early in the course of the disease, patients are likely to avoid the use of nitroglycerin because of the headache it sometimes produces. After the attack has subsided completely, the patient feels quite well and without residual effects. He may be able to continue activities quite normally, and indeed he may be able to achieve a higher level of physical activity than that which provoked the attack, the so-called "second-wind" phenomenon.

PHYSICAL SIGNS ACCOMPANYING ANGINA PECTORIS

If one has the opportunity to examine a patient during an anginal attack, the first sign is often a subtle but definite change in the patient's demeanor. As the discomfort begins, he may appear preoccupied or distracted from conversation and appear somewhat anxious. He may exhibit slight pallor and the skin may become cool and clammy. The pulse rate even at rest may be slightly more rapid than normal or irregular, and the blood pressure may rise slightly unless the attack is severe, when it may fall. On auscultation of the heart a presystolic gallop may appear or become accentuated; less frequently a protodiastolic gallop may be noted. Occasionally a faint, high-pitched pansystolic murmur at the apex may be due to mitral insufficiency from ischemic papillary muscle dysfunction. The appearance of ventricular ectopy or moist rales in the lung base are particularly ominous signs.

The examiner may have an opportunity to observe the effect of carotid sinus massage on the attack. If one is assured that there are no bruits indicating arteriosclerotic involvement of the carotid arteries, gentle massage first of the right carotid sinus, then of the left if necessary, will often produce reflex bradycardia and sometimes dramatic resolution of the anginal attack. In examining the patient other findings that are associated with coronary artery disease may also be noted such as obesity, hypertension, xanthelasma, tendon or tuberous xanthomas, or ear lobe creases.

It is sometimes desirable to obtain an electrocardiogram as early in the attack as possible. Apart from any baseline abnormalities, the ST segments are usually depressed by at least 1 mm and are flat or downsloping. Elevation of the ST segment would suggest the injury current of early infarction or the phenomenon of coronary artery spasm producing severe regional ischemia. If the electrocardiogram can be observed at the beginning of the attack, ST-segment alterations may be observed one to three minutes before the patient recognizes the earliest symptom, and as the ST segments gradually return to the baseline, the attack subsides. Rarely is cardiac fluoroscopy performed or chest x-rays obtained during the course of an anginal attack, and subtle changes in heart size could not be identified without preanginal films for comparison. However, when angina has been provoked by exercise, a slight increase in heart size occurs.

CLINICAL COURSE: ANGINA PECTORIS AND RELATED CLINICAL SYNDROMES

Anginal episodes may occur infrequently or at a rather predictable level of activity without increasing in frequency or severity. However, when the angina is of recent onset, its future course is highly uncertain. Its sudden appearance is suggestive of a recent mechanical event involving one of the coronary arteries, ie, disruption of an arteriosclerotic plaque, mural thrombus formation, spasm or occlusion of a smaller branch, or possibly even occlusion of a major branch with collateral perfusion of distal branches. The same mechanical event in another patient may result in acute myocardial infarction, depending on the relation between the metabolic requirements of the myocardium and its perfusion. Angina pectoris of recent onset should never be considered stable, chronic, or benign. Frequently it is progressive in both frequency and intensity, leading to infarction within weeks if not hours, or it may crescendo and then decrescendo in the course of a few days or weeks, suggesting possible coronary occlusion without infarction. The patient with recent onset angina should be treated as if he were in a preinfarctional state, and he should be examined frequently until his symptoms begin to subside. In one study[22] one third of patients with angina of recent onset (three months) had acute myocardial infarction within four months and 9% died. Half remained symptomatic and one third were free of symptoms after a two-year follow-up. When studied angiographically, half had multiple vessel involvement.

Approximately half the patients with new onset angina continue to experience angina pectoris of a more or less stable variety. Many will modify their life-styles and successfully adapt to their symptoms. Others will require more radical changes in their daily life, or more aggressive drug treatment to control their symptoms. The likelihood of an abrupt worsening of symptoms diminishes during the months after recent onset angina, and the patient may remain stable for many years. However, after two to five years there is an increasing likelihood of exacerbation of symptoms or complications.

The time course of coronary artery disease is punctuated by milestones that relate symptoms to pathophysiologic events (Figure 35.2). As noted previously, myocardial infarction or sudden death is the initial manifestation in more than half the men.[21] Angina, when present, may not always conform to the pattern just described. The initial episode may be sudden, severe, and prolonged, unrelated to physical activities, and without clinical evidence of myocardial infarction (coronary failure, coronary insufficiency, or the intermediate syndrome). Less frequently, angina appears abruptly but recurs frequently, without apparent provocation, often at rest. A variant of angina pectoris was described by Prinzmetal, in which episodes of rest pain occurred in clusters, accompanied by ST-segment elevation and disturbances of heart rhythm with ventricular ectopy or ventricular tachycardia. This syndrome has been associated with coronary spasm. Although it usually occurs in the setting of severe fixed coronary obstructions, it may occur with only mild atherosclerotic involvement.[23,24]

After initial presentation with angina, coronary failure, or myocardial infarction heralding the existence of coronary disease, the patient may experience a period of time during which he is free of symptoms, or with relatively mild, controllable symptoms (chronic stable angina). This may last for several years before he experiences an exacerbation of symptoms or other complications of the disease.

The term *unstable angina pectoris* includes not only recent onset angina but also crescendo angina or prolonged severe pain (coronary failure), whether this is a presenting manifestation or occurs late in the setting of chronic previously stable angina (Table 35.4). Unstable angina pectoris implies an anatomic change in the coronary circulation disrupting any homeostatic mechanisms that may have been achieved. This may represent a completed event, ie, coronary occlusion without infarction, or an incomplete event, ie, sudden severe narrowing from a partially ruptured plaque, subintimal hemorrhage, or nonocclusive thrombus. The patient with unstable angina, as with recent onset angina, requires close observation and thoughtful evaluation for therapeutic alternatives.

Another clinical category is represented by the patient who has recently sustained a myocardial infarction. Prodromal anginal symptoms are not always recognized before infarction. Acute myocardial infarction is the first indication of coronary artery disease in 20% to 40% of patients. Patients who have had angina before their infarction may or may not experience these symptoms following infarction, depending on the level of their activ-

Table 35.4. Types of Unstable Angina

- Angina of recent onset
- Increasing frequency or severity of angina
- New onset of rest angina or prolonged angina unresponsive to usual measures
- Recurrent angina at rest
- Recurrent angina early after myocardial infarction

ities and the presence of regions of residual myocardial ischemia. With or without postinfarction angina, it is unwise to assume that the infarction was a completed event and that further complications will not occur. As for patients with recent onset angina and coronary failure, the likelihood of complications diminishes after the first few months following infarction, but the incidence of recurrent myocardial infarction and sudden death is the highest during the early postinfarction months. This group of patients also requires prudent evaluation and follow-up.

Two small but important groups of patients in whom coronary artery disease may ultimately be detected include survivors of sudden cardiac death or cardiac arrest, and individuals with an abnormal stress test during routine testing. The former group, although quite small, has a high incidence of advanced coronary artery disease when studied arteriographically. The latter group, unique to those environments where electrocardiographic stress testing is performed routinely, has a somewhat lower but rather variable incidence of coronary artery disease when studied arteriographically, depending on the population being tested.

The clinical diagnosis of coronary artery disease depends fundamentally on the recognition of angina pectoris or acute myocardial infarction. The presence of other risk factors may help the physician in estimating the probability of coronary atherosclerosis, but they are of little value in deciding if or how to treat the condition. When the diagnosis is uncertain, a period of observation is sometimes useful. Symptoms may sometimes become more typical or subside. The suspicion of coronary artery disease should not be permitted to continue without confirmation for more than a few days or weeks, however, for a delay in diagnosis may be hazardous and may delay important treatment or lead to inappropriate treatment. Whether confronted by a patient with an initial manifestation of coronary artery disease or with a new milestone in a patient with previously recognized disease, the physician should determine whether the recent event is complete (ie, arterial occlusion) or incomplete. Usually the diagnosis can be clarified with the help of ancillary yet simple diagnostic tests.

DIAGNOSTIC AIDS

The diagnosis of coronary artery disease can be facilitated through a variety of methods.

ELECTROCARDIOGRAM

The electrocardiogram is most useful (and is over 98% reliable), particularly if it shows evidence of previous myocardial infarction. Other abnormalities in the resting electrocardiogram are less helpful, including atrial arrhythmias, ventricular ectopy, conduction abnormalities, left ventricular hypertrophy, and resting nonspecific ST-T–wave abnormalities.

ELECTROCARDIOGRAPHIC STRESS TESTING

Despite the development of standardized protocols for electrocardiographic stress testing, the diagnostic accuracy has not been sufficiently high to justify its use as a routine screening procedure. Asymptomatic population groups that are not dependent on physician referral for screening lead to only moderately high sensitivity and specificity in results of electrocardiographic stress testing, compared with populations consisting of those referred for cardiac diagnostic evaluation in whom electrocardiographic stress testing is associated with high sensitivity and only moderate specificity.[25] The diagnostic accuracy of electrocardiographic stress testing is enhanced by using all the information that can be obtained in these studies.[26] Most valuable is the precipitation of angina during exercise or the observation of flat or downsloping ST-segment depression of 2 mm or more. An increase of R-wave voltage, instead of the mild decrease that usually occurs in response to exercise, is suggestive of myocardial ischemia, as is exercise-induced reduction of blood pressure. The occurrence of these abnormalities at a low level of exercise lends weight to the diagnostic accuracy of the study. Baseline electrocardiographic abnormalities confound the interpretation and diminish the value of this diagnostic modality.

RADIONUCLIDE EXAMINATION OF THE HEART

A number of radioisotopes have been used to help assess cardiac anatomy and function. These may be grouped according to their individual characteristics and the manner in which they are used. In the first-pass technique the heart is imaged as an isotope is injected as a bolus, and a series of scans are obtained as the isotope passes through the heart and lungs. In the multiple gated acquisition technique (MUGA scan)[27] a series of images of the heart are built up as scans are obtained, respectively, at specific times (gates) in the heart cycle, the recording device being controlled by the electrocardiogram. When displayed in sequence, these scans show cardiac motion and reflect changes in the intracardiac blood pool that occur during the heart cycle. Both global and regional analyses of wall motion can be carried out.

Several isotopes are metabolically active and, when taken up by myocardial tissue, can be used to obtain a scintigraphic image of the heart by the scanning camera. Cesium-131 and thallium-201 are taken up by normal myocardium, whereas technetium-99 is absorbed only when there is myocardial injury. Thallium-201 has been used more frequently, particularly in conjunction with exercise testing.[28] During the high metabolic turnover of stress, thallium-201 is rapidly taken up by normal nonischemic myocardium, whereas its uptake is delayed in areas that are ischemic. This differential can be observed by comparing scans obtained immediately after the intravenous injection of thallium-201 at peak exercise with those obtained three to four hours later after equilibration has been achieved between myocardial and blood pool thallium. Fibrotic areas will fail to take up the isotope at all and appear as a "cold spot." One of the more important applications of thallium perfusion scanning in conjunction with electrocardiographic stress testing is to assess the significance of questionable or borderline lesions detected by coronary arteriography in the patient with atypical symptoms. Technetium pyrophosphate is absorbed by inflamed or injured myocardium and appears as a "hot spot."

Certain radioisotopes produce positrons,[29] and after injection and equilibration with nonradioactive elements of the body, they can produce a chemical map of the distribution of specific elements within the body. Positron emission tomograms provide information regarding biochemical activity as well as distribution of these elements. Magnetic resonance imaging offers another promising approach to the study of myocardial metabolism. None of these radionuclear methods provides direct information regarding coronary artery anatomy, but rather they provide indirect information with regard to myocardial perfusion and wall motion.

CORONARY ARTERIOGRAPHY

Coronary arteriography[2,30] is the definitive method for determining the presence or absence of coronary artery disease and assessing the adequacy of myocardial perfusion as well as prognostic implications.

In most cases the diagnosis of coronary artery disease can be obtained by clinical evaluation, aided perhaps by simple clinical tests. Coronary arteriography is employed not only to establish or rule out the diagnosis when this cannot be accomplished confidently by other means, but also to provide guidance with regard to treatment. With the availability of medical, surgical, and nonsurgical interventional alternatives in the management of coronary artery disease, coronary arteriography plays an increasingly important role. In this chapter we will not attempt to discuss the role of bypass graft surgery, balloon coronary angioplasty, or thrombolytic therapy in the management of the patient with coronary artery disease, except to state that these measures have proven safe and feasible in selected patients. Both balloon coronary angioplasty[16,31] and bypass graft surgery have been proven effective in relieving angina pectoris, and bypass graft surgery is of proven value in prolonging life in certain high risk subsets of patients.[32-37] Coronary arteriography then is indicated when there is a need to know with certainty whether or not significant coronary disease exists and when there is a need to exercise choices among the growing number of medical and surgical therapeutic alternatives.

Coronary arteriography is accomplished through catheterization of the brachial artery (Sones technique) or the femoral artery (Judkins technique). Under fluoroscopic control, the specially designed catheter is placed in the orifice of the right or left coronary artery. During continuous electrocardiographic monitoring, contrast material is injected into the artery and the process is photographed on motion picture film. The right and left coronary arteries are visualized in several projections and usually before and after the administration of sublingual nitroglycerin. Occasionally, other pharmacologic agents are employed to test for provocative coronary artery spasm. A left ventriculogram is an essential component of a coronary arteriographic study.

The coronary arteriographic examination can be accomplished in 20 to 30 minutes in most centers and is frequently employed as an outpatient procedure. Although complications relate to the age and clinical status of the patient, in most centers coronary arteriography can be accomplished with a mortality rate of less than 0.01%.

MEDICAL MANAGEMENT OF CORONARY ARTERY DISEASE

The treatment of coronary artery disease requires consideration of three important principles: (1) assurance of adequate myocardial perfusion, (2) achieving a reasonable balance between (a) reducing myocardial energy requirements and (b) maintaining a normal life-style through judicious control of host and environmental factors (diet, activities, blood pressure, and smoking) as well as drug therapy, and (3) reasonable attempts to control the atherosclerotic process by retarding if not preventing its progression. The goal of treatment is to preserve normal activities, control symptoms, and optimize longevity. There is no single treatment or combinations thereof that guarantee that these goals can be accomplished (Table 35.5).

Unless incapacitated from left ventricular myocardial insufficiency from previous infarction, the patient should be encouraged to maintain normal activities insofar as possible without precipitating anginal symptoms. After recognizing anginal symptoms he will usually learn how to control them. The only absolute restriction is to avoid those activities and circumstances that are likely to produce symptoms. There are many *relative* restrictions including (1) avoidance of sudden bursts of strenuous exertion, (2) avoidance of exercise without a warm-up, (3) avoidance of physical exertion after meals or in cold weather, and (4) avoidance of combinations of physical and emotional stress.

Control of other environmental and host factors should be undertaken, including weight reduction, if appropriate, to achieve normal body weight, control of hypertension if present, control of diabetes, and discontinuance of smoking.

It is desirable to obtain daily physical exercise provided this is not inconsistent with the individual's tolerance for physical activities. Although there is no consistent evidence that this alters prognosis or prevents complications in patients with manifest coronary heart disease, the sense

Table 35.5. Fundamentals of Medical Management

1. Understanding of the disease process
2. Control of risk-factor variables
    - Hypertension
    - Smoking
    - Diabetes mellitus
    - Obesity
    - Hyperlipidemia
3. Daily exercise
4. Coronary artery dilators
    - Nitrates
    - Calcium channel blockers
5. Control of myocardial metabolic requirements
    - Control of activity
    - Beta-adrenergic blockers
6. Modification of clotting mechanisms
    - Thromboxane A_2 inhibitors
    - Antithrombin agents

of well-being is improved through exercise. Moreover, it may help to control body weight and hyperlipidemia.

The patient with coronary artery disease should abstain from smoking cigarettes and probably from the use of nicotine in any form. In addition to being a vasoconstrictor, nicotine decreases the level of high density lipoproteins. Smoking also promotes platelet aggregation and reduces platelet survival. It is clearly associated with an increased risk for the development of coronary artery disease, myocardial infarction, and sudden death. Stopping smoking lessens these risks.[38–40]

Although there is a wealth of information linking abnormal lipid metabolism to the risk of developing coronary artery disease,[19,20,41] there is only scant information that modification of lipid levels will prevent the development of critical coronary artery disease,[42,43] or that this is of benefit in the presence of manifest coronary atherosclerosis, ie, secondary prevention.[44–46] Nevertheless, as a general principle, it seems prudent to attempt to control plasma lipids, particularly in younger individuals with abnormally high lipid levels.[47]

The consumption of saturated fatty acids should be reduced. This is best accomplished by reducing the proportion of animal fats, including dairy products, in the diet and substituting polyunsaturated fats or vegetable oil. There is evidence that weight control, abstinence from smoking, and exercise may help to increase the proportion of plasma high density lipoproteins, whereas reduction in animal fats in the diet and substitution with polyunsaturated fatty acids will help to lower total cholesterol and low density lipoproteins. If hyperlipidemia persists despite these measures, pharmacologic intervention may be considered.

The selection of drugs or combinations thereof in the treatment of diet-refractory hyperlipidemia depends on the specific type of lipid abnormality that is present. Fredrickson et al[48,49] have classified the disorders of lipid metabolism according to the lipoprotein electrophoretic characteristics (Table 35.6):

1. Type I hyperlipidemia is characterized by increased levels of chylomicra in the plasma and is not considered to be an important factor in the development of atherosclerosis.

2. Type II hyperlipidemia is associated with increased levels of beta lipoproteins, and because cholesterol is carried prominently in the beta lipoprotein fraction, there are high cholesterol levels. This is frequently familial and is associated with a high risk of coronary artery disease. In type IIa hyperlipidemia only the cholesterol is elevated. In type IIb the triglyceride concentration is also increased. Both are more likely to respond to resins that bind bile acids in the intestine, inhibit the absorption, and promote the breakdown of cholesterol. Such bile acids include cholestyramine and cholestipol. These may be used alone or in combination with nicotinic acid (Table 35.7). Probucol may be helpful in lowering cholesterol levels in type IIa.

3. Type III hyperlipidemia is infrequent and is associated with elevations of both cholesterol and triglycerides. It is distinguished from type IIb by cloudiness of the fasting plasma and a broad beta band on lipoprotein electrophoresis and is associated with a high risk for coronary artery disease. It is best treated with clofibrate.

Table 35.6. Classification of Hyperlipoproteinemias

		Types				
	Normal	I	II	III	IV	V
Lipoprotein characteristics		Increased chylomicra	Increased beta	Broad beta band	Increased pre-beta	Increased chylomicra and pre-beta
Appearance of fasting plasma	Clear	Creamy layer	Clear	Cloudy	Cloudy	Creamy layer and cloudy
Cholesterol	2+	2+	4+	4+	3+	3+
Triglyceride	1+	4+	(a) 2+ (b) 4+	4+	4+	4+
Abnormal glucose tolerance	—	—	—	±	+	+
Prevalence	—	Rare	Common	Infrequent	Very common	Rare
Risk of coronary artery disease	—	Low	Very high	Very high	High	Low
Symptoms and signs	—					
Obesity		...	...	...	+	+
Abdominal pain		+	...	...	±	...
Accelerated atherosclerosis		...	+	...	...	...
Xanthelasma		...	+	...	...	...
Eruptive xanthomas		+	...	...	...	...
Palmar and tuberoeruptive xanthomas		...	...	+	...	...
Tendon and tuberous xanthomas		...	+	...	...	...
Lipemia retinalis		+	...	...	...	+
Hepatosplenomegaly		+	...	...	...	+
Corneal arcus		...	+	...	...	...

Table 35.7. Drug Therapy of the Hyperlipidemias*

Type	Resin (Cholestyramine or Cholestipol)	Clofibrate or Gemfibrozil	Probucol	Nicotinic Acid
1	. . .	. . .	. . .	. . .
2a	1	. . .	2	2
2b	1	2	. . .	2
3	. . .	1	. . .	2
4	. . .	1	2	2
5	. . .	. . .	. . .	1

* Author's choice.

4. Type IV hyperlipidemia is probably the most common in the United States and is associated with a band of pre-beta lipoproteins containing very low density lipoproteins. It is typical of patients with diabetes mellitus and abnormal carbohydrate tolerance but is seen in others as well. If not controlled with weight reduction and restriction of animal fats and free sugar in the diet as well as alcohol, it may be treated with drugs like clofibrate, gemfibrozil, or probucol, either alone or in conjunction with cholestyramine.[50]

5. Type V hyperlipidemia is rare and is associated with increased chylomicra as well as the pre-beta band including triglycerides. The incidence of coronary disease is low in such patients, but when present type V hyperlipidemia is best treated with clofibrate or nicotinic acid.

Not mentioned in the list of agents useful in treating hyperlipidemias is dextrothyroxine. This may be useful in patients with type II and III hyperlipidemia, although it is probably contraindicated in patients with coronary artery disease because of its potential for aggravating angina or cardiac arrhythmia. Probably the most important factor in the management of these hyperlipidemias is the quality and frequency of medical followup. Nonadherence to diet or drug treatment, or both, is high and the patient may become quite dependent on the physician for reassurance and motivational reinforcement.

MANAGEMENT OF ANGINA PECTORIS

The single most useful agent in angina pectoris is nitroglycerin. Administered sublingually in doses of 0.16 to 0.4 mg (1/400 to 1/150 gr) the anginal attack usually begins to subside within one to two minutes and is completely relieved within two to five minutes. Occasionally a second or third nitroglycerin tablet may be necessary. There is no longer doubt that nitroglycerin works by its combined effects on producing coronary vasodilatation and reducing myocardial requirement. The latter is accomplished by reducing afterload by decreasing systemic arterial pressure and reducing preload through peripheral venous pooling. When he recognizes the anginal discomfort, the patient should be instructed to use nitroglycerin promptly if rest with cessation of activity in the upright position does not produce an immediate diminution in its intensity. Nitroglycerin tablets have a tendency to lose potency over time, particularly when stored in light at room temperature. When fresh, nitroglycerin often causes a slight stinging sensation or "bite" when placed under the tongue. It is best stored in a cool environment or refrigerator in a glass bottle. The supply should be replenished every six months. Tablets that the patient may keep with him, stored at room temperature, should be replenished more frequently. Vascular headache is a common side effect with nitroglycerin and is frequently severe enough to discourage patients from using this medication. Often it is necessary to titrate the dose, finding the lowest effective dose that will relieve angina without producing headache. The patient may be instructed to use it preventatively, if he anticipates an activity that is likely to produce symptoms. He should be cautioned against using nitroglycerin prophylactically to permit exertion that is unwise or otherwise avoidable.

A number of long-acting nitrates are available that may be helpful and used prophylactically in patients who are experiencing frequent symptoms as well as patients with known severe coronary atherosclerosis who may not be capable of recognizing anginal symptoms. Isosorbide dinitrate, dipyridamole, and nitroglycerin ointment or nitroglycerin patches have been shown to elevate the anginal threshold in stress testing for periods in excess of one hour, but there is considerable individual variability in the duration of this effect. Oral nitrate-containing medications are usually prescribed at intervals of 6 to 12 hours and the cutaneous forms at intervals of 12 to 24 hours. Treatment should be tailored to meet individual patient requirements. Side effects are similar to those with nitroglycerin.

The metabolic requirements of the myocardium may be reduced with the use of a class of drugs known as beta-adrenergic blocking agents. The beta-adrenergic responses increase the heart rate and velocity of myocardial shortening, increasing the energy requirements of the myocardium. Alpha-adrenergic responses increase peripheral arterial tone and systemic arterial resistance. Beta-adrenergic blocking agents reduce the force and velocity of myocardial contraction, as well as heart rate, and attenuate these responses to the stimulus of fright or exercise. They have proved very useful, therefore, in the management of patients with angina pectoris, particularly in conjunction with nitrates. Propranolol was the first of these agents to be used, and the prototype of beta-blocking agents. In doses of 10 to 40 mg four times daily propranolol has been helpful in reducing the frequency of anginal attacks, particularly when used in conjunction with a vasodilator (nitrate). The negative chronotropic and inotropic effects of propranolol are the result of its ability to block the $beta_1$-adrenergic receptors that are located chiefly in the heart. It also has a blocking effect on $beta_2$-adrenergic receptors that are located in bronchial and vascular musculature. Propranolol is therefore referred to as "nonselective" in its beta-blocking effects. The $beta_2$-blocking effect may produce bronchial constriction and trigger bronchial asthma in susceptible patients, and beta-adrenergic blocking agents are generally contraindicated in such patients. Other examples of nonselective beta blockers include nadolol, pindolol, and timolol. Examples of cardioselective (primarily $beta_1$) adrenergic blocking agents include metoprolol and atenolol. Beta-blocking agents also may have varying degrees of sympathomimetic activity, and also a membrane-stabilizing effect. The latter may be useful for some cardiac arrhythmias (Table 35.8).

Although the efficacy of beta-adrenergic blockers in reducing the frequency of anginal episodes is well established, the benefit of these drugs in preventing myocardial infarction and in long-term survival is less clear, except in the postinfarction patient. Several clinical trials suggested a short-term reduction in mortality, primarily sudden death, when beta-adrenergic blockers were initiated early in the course of acute myocardial infarction.[51–53] In the beta blocker heart attack trial (BHAT) sponsored by the National Heart, Lung, and Blood Institute in the United States,[52] mortality from coronary heart disease was 6.2% among patients in whom propranolol was initiated five to 21 days after acute myocardial infarction, compared with 8.5% in a placebo group, after an average follow-up period of 25 months. Nonfatal reinfarction occurred in 4.4% of patients in the propranolol group, compared with 5.3% in the placebo group. In a randomized trial from Sweden using metoprolol, initiated as soon as possible after hospitalization for suspected acute myocardial infarction, total mortality at 90 days was 5.7% in the metoprolol group and 8.9% in the placebo group.[53] In a Norwegian multicenter study using timolol initiated seven to 28 days after infarction, the cumulative mortality at 33 months was 13.3% in the treatment group, compared with 21.9% in the placebo group.[51] The sudden death rate was 7.7% in the treatment group, compared with 13.9% in the placebo group. The reinfarction rate was 14.4% in the treatment group and 20.1% in the placebo group. It is not clear how long the protective effects of beta blockers may persist in postinfarction patients, but the BHAT and Norwegian studies suggested a benefit for up to three years.

Another class of therapeutic agents useful in the management of coronary artery disease, based on their ability to block the flux of calcium across the cell membrane of the vascular musculature, is the calcium channel blocking agents. These agents reduce the force and velocity of smooth muscle contraction and produce vasodilatation. They may also reduce blood pressure, reduce cardiac contractility, and retard atrioventricular (AV) conduction (Table 35.9). The first of this class to be studied was nifedipine, which proved to be effective in the treatment of variant angina pectoris due to coronary artery spasm. In addition to being potent vasodilators, these agents tend to have a negative inotropic effect and a somewhat variable depressant effect on AV conduction. Studied initially in patients with the syndrome of coronary artery spasm, nifedipine[54] was associated with a striking reduction in the frequency of spontaneous anginal episodes. A benefit was observed when nifedipine was administered also to patients with exercise-induced angina. The frequency of exercise-induced episodes was diminished, and studies using stress testing and pacing-induced angina have demonstrated an elevated angina threshold in association with calcium channel blockade.[55–57] These agents may be used independently or in conjunction with nitrates or beta-adrenergic blockers, or both, but when combination treatment is used, careful follow-up is necessary because of the potential for drug interactions, particularly sinus node depression and AV conduction abnormalities. Edema of the lower extremities is a common side effect with nifedipine because of its vasodilatory effect and venous pooling. This can usually be controlled by titrating the dose or adding a diuretic.

Recent interest in thrombolytic therapy for acute myocardial infarction has confirmed the high incidence of total occlusion of the infarct-related artery by fresh thrombus.[58–60] When these studies were extended to patients with unstable angina, a similar high incidence of apparent intracoronary thrombus formation was observed.[61–63] Localized intimal injury may initiate platelet aggregation. The aggregated platelets in turn release thromboxane A_2, which stimulates further platelet aggregation unless this is inhibited by prostacyclin. The latter may be deficient at these sites because of intimal thickening. It has been suggested that this may initiate the syndrome of unstable angina pectoris and its sequelae.[64,65] This lends impetus to the study not only of thrombolytic agents in acute coronary syndromes, but also to pharmacologic prophylaxis in patients with other manifestations of coronary artery disease, including those of angina pectoris. Drugs that inhibit platelet cyclooxygenase may be beneficial in preventing these episodes. Aspirin and sulfinpyrazone have been studied in postinfarction patients as well as in those with unstable angina.[66–68] Results have been mixed in postinfarction patients. A recent study of unstable angina pectoris suggested that the incidence of nonfatal acute myocardial infarction was lower in patients treated with aspirin, and the combined incidence of death or nonfatal acute infarction was lower in the treatment group. The reduction in mortality alone in the aspirin group did not achieve

Table 35.8. Variable Effects of Beta Blockers

Agent	Cardioselective (Primary $Beta_1$ Blocking)	Noncardioselective ($Beta_1$ and $Beta_2$ Blocking)	Intrinsic Sympathomimetic Activity	Membrane-Stabilizing Activity
Propranolol	–	+	–	+
Nadolol	–	+	–	–
Timolol	–	+	–	–
Pindolol	–	+	+	+
Metoprolol	+	–	–	+
Atenolol	+	–	–	–

Table 35.9. Calcium Channel Blocking Agents

Agent	Effects				
	Blood Pressure	Heart Rate	AV Conduction	Contractility	Coronary Dilatation
Nifedipine	↓↓↓	↑	0	0	↑↑
Verapamil	↓↓	↓↑	↓↓↓	↓↓	↑↑
Diltiazem	↓	0-↓	↓↓	0-↓	↑↑↑

statistical significance.[66] Of interest is that some beta-adrenergic blockers also appear to have a mild inhibitory effect on thromboxane synthesis and platelet aggregation.[69]

Various other medications have been employed in the treatment of coronary artery disease. Clinical trials employing anticoagulant prophylaxis following acute myocardial infarction with coumarin-like agents have produced conflicting results. It is possible that short-term benefit might be derived in high risk patients, ie, those in whom early ambulation cannot be achieved, those with prolonged hypotension or shock, and those with atrial arrhythmia or suspected ventricular aneurysm. Aminophylline as an adjunct to nitrates is sometimes helpful in patients with angina decubitus. Poorly absorbed from the upper gastrointestinal tract, an 0.5-g rectal suppository taken at bedtime, along with elevation of the head of the bed approximately 6 inches to reduce venous return and preload, may help to prevent nocturnal episodes. A diuretic may have the same effect for patients with angina decubitus by attenuating the increase in circulating plasma volume and preload that occurs during recumbency. Digitalis is not ordinarily helpful unless there is evidence of diminished myocardial reserve. Digitalization may benefit nocturnal episodes in such patients. The judicious use of sedatives and tranquilizers may be helpful. In severe angina that is refractory to treatment, thyroid suppression with the thyroid suppressant propylthiouracil may be considered.

The management of the patient with coronary artery disease may test the skill, ingenuity, and patience of the physician. At best, coronary artery disease is a chronic, gradually progressive disorder. At worst, it is punctuated by one or more crises, ranging from recurrent episodes of coronary insufficiency or waxing or waning of the anginal syndrome to acute myocardial infarction or sudden death. Therapy must be continually monitored and periodically adjusted. As stated previously, the goal of treatment is to allow the patient to lead as nearly normal a life as possible, with a minimum of restrictions and medications. In the natural course of the disease there is an inevitable tendency to restrict activities progressively and add medication upon medication. This practice is rarely necessary and is to be discouraged. Regular reassessment of treatment requires consideration of all the therapeutic alternatives that may be available, both medical and surgical.

CLINICAL COURSE OF MEDICALLY MANAGED CORONARY ARTERY DISEASE

During the past 25 years, with the availability of coronary arteriography and growing interest in coronary artery bypass graft surgery, great interest has emerged in the so-called natural history or clinical course of patients with coronary artery disease. Several studies were initiated before the availability of coronary artery bypass graft surgery and several have been undertaken as part of randomized trials of bypass surgery. None is a natural history study in the strict sense, in that these nonsurgical patients were treated by general medical principles, without uniformity or control. Herein lies an implicit acceptance that these general medical measures have little if any impact on long-term survival. Nevertheless, these studies do reflect, in a general sense, the outcome that could be anticipated with medical measures by which patients were generally treated in the 1960s and 1970s. However, these observations are confounded by the declining mortality from coronary heart disease that began to occur in the United States in the mid-1960s.[70] The reasons for this declining mortality are both multiple and poorly understood. A population that is more alert to good health habits, more effective control of blood pressure in patients with hypertension, and subtle changes in diet and the smoking habits of the American population have undoubtedly contributed.[71] Proudfit et al[8,9,13,72] followed a group of patients with angiographically defined coronary atherosclerosis for more than 15 years. These studies have underscored the importance of two major anatomic descriptors of disease on prognosis: the extent of disease or the number of vessels involved, and the status of the left ventricle at the time of baseline angiography. The duration of symptoms, which is related to the extent of disease, is a factor in long-term survival, but not in severity of symptoms. Certain clinical descriptors of left ventricular function, such as cardiac enlargement or electrocardiographic evidence of left ventricular hypertrophy, myocardial infarction, and ST- or T-wave changes were also linked to survival. Two clinical parameters not directly related to coronary anatomy or left ventricular status that influenced survival were hypertension and arteriosclerosis obliterans.

The 15-year survival rates for patients with single-, double-, triple-, and left main coronary artery disease were 48%, 28%, 18%, and 9%, respectively (Figure 35.3). The 15-year survival rate according to the angiographic status of the left ventricle ranged from about 42%, when the baseline left ventriculogram was normal, to 15% in the presence of a ventricular aneurysm or diffuse contractile impairment (Figure 35.4).

Randomized coronary artery surgical trials provide another view of the clinical course of candidates for surgical treatment that are randomized to medical management. Although medically treated patients from these trials are not comparable because of baseline differences, they do

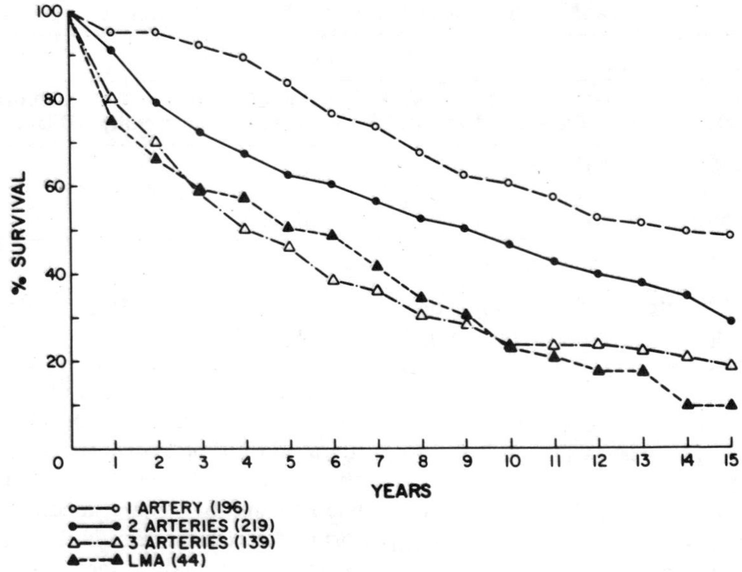

Figure 35.3. Actuarial survival of patients with coronary artery disease according to extent of disease; medical treatment, surgical, and nonsurgical candidates. (From Proudfit,[72] by permission of the American Heart Association.)

reflect the range of survival that could be anticipated with such patients in the 1970s. Among these patients, five-year survival with single-vessel disease ranged from 88% to 93%, double-vessel disease, 85% to 94%, and triple-vessel disease, 75% to 89%. When Proudfit in his 1963–1965 series analyzed survival of patients who qualified for surgical candidacy, he found five-year survival rates of 83% for single-vessel disease, 68% for double-vessel disease, and 54% for triple-vessel disease. It is not clear whether the lower five-year survival rates for patients in the early 1960s are due to baseline differences in populations selected for study or to other factors contributing to the generally declining mortality from coronary artery disease during these years. Nevertheless, these figures portray the evolving prognosis for patients with medically managed coronary artery disease in the 1960s and 1970s.

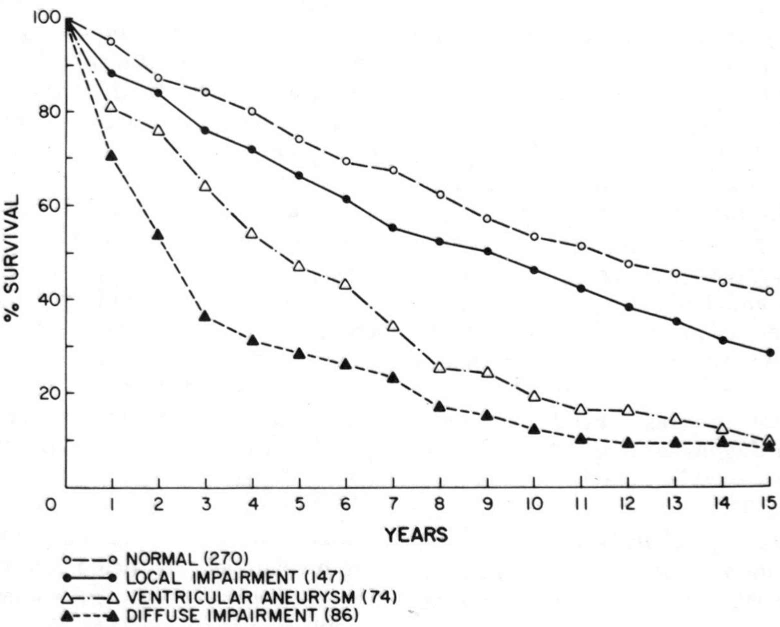

Figure 35.4. Actuarial survival of patients with coronary artery disease according to status of left ventricle by ventriculography: medical treatment, surgical, and nonsurgical candidates. (From Proudfit,[72] by permission of the American Heart Association.)

PROGRESSION OF CORONARY ATHEROSCLEROSIS

Fundamental to the understanding of the clinical course of coronary atherosclerosis is the recognition that mortality is rarely the result of the clinical or anatomic status of the patient at the time of the baseline study. Patients die invariably as a consequence of the future course of the disease, ie, progression of the atherosclerotic process. In analyzing the relation between the risk factors at the time of baseline study and evidence of progression in subsequent angiographic studies, Kramer et al[73] found that baseline risk factors were not helpful in predicting progression. The same applies to risk factors at the time of a second arteriographic study. Although progression occurs at all ages, progression occurred significantly more frequently than nonprogression in the younger patients (aged 30 to 39). Time is a powerful predictor of progression, 42% of patients demonstrating progression within five years of the baseline time, compared with 77% in studies performed after five years. Other risk factors, including family history, weight, smoking, diabetes, cholesterol, and triglyceride levels, were not helpful in predicting progression.[73,74] Other recent studies have suggested a relation between lipid-lowering therapy and progression of disease.[45,46] In analyzing specific coronary arterial segments for progression of disease, Kramer et al[73] found that the likelihood of finding a new arterial occlusion during follow-up study was related to the severity of the lesion at the initial study and was not related to the time interval. If segments that became occluded are excluded, progression of the lesion to more severe degrees of obstruction was related not only to the severity of the lesion at the initial study, but also to time. In interpreting these studies on progression, however, it must be emphasized that only patients who survived to have a follow-up coronary arteriogram could be included, and estimates of progression in survivors may be underestimated, having excluded patients who died as a consequence of progression. However, among survivors, symptomatic patients are more likely to undergo follow-up arteriography, leading to an overestimate of the rate of progression.

It has been 200 years since coronary atherosclerosis was identified as the cause of angina pectoris. The past 25 years have witnessed an explosion of new knowledge regarding the pathophysiology, clinical course, and treatment of coronary artery disease. Although the recent decline in mortality that has occurred in the United States is encouraging, coronary heart disease remains the leading cause of death. Coincident with the urbanization and industrialization of Third World countries, coronary heart disease is emerging as an important public health issue. It is hoped that the knowledge gained in the United States during the past 25 years may be useful to developing nations in controlling the impact of coronary heart disease on their populations.

REFERENCES

1. Proudfit WL: Origin of concept of ischaemic heart disease. *Br Heart J* 1983; 50:209–212.
2. Heberden W: Some account of a disorder of the breast. *Medical Transactions*. London, Royal College of Physicians, 1772; pp 59–67.
3. Parry CH: *An Inquiry into the Symptoms and Causes of the Syncope Anginosa, Commonly Called Angina Pectoris*. Bath, England, R Crutwell, 1799.
4. Herrick JB: Clinical features of sudden obstruction of the coronary arteries. *JAMA* 1912; 59:2015–2020.
5. Blumgart HL, Schlesinger MJ, Davis D: Studies on the relation of the clinical manifestations of angina pectoris, coronary thrombosis and myocardial infarction to the pathologic findings. *Am Heart J* 1940; 19:1–19.
6. Sones FM Jr, Shirey EK: Cine coronary arteriography. *Mod Concepts Cardiovasc Dis* 1962; 31:737–738.
7. Proudfit WL, Shirey EK, Sones FM Jr: Selective cine coronary arteriographic: correlation with clinical findings in 1000 patients. *Circulation* 1966; 33:901–910.
8. Bruschke AVG, Proudfit WL, Sones FM: Progress study of 590 consecutive nonsurgical cases of coronary disease followed 5 to 9 years. I. Arteriographic correlations. *Circulation* 1973; 47:1147–1153.
9. Bruschke AVG, Proudfit WL, Sones FM: Progress study of 590 consecutive nonsurgical cases of coronary disease followed 5 to 9 years. II. Ventriculographic and other correlations. *Circulation* 1973; 47:1154–1163.
10. Humphries JO, Kuller L, Ross RS, Friesinger CG, Page EE: Natural history of ischemic heart disease in relation to arteriographic findings. A twelve-year study of 224 patients. *Circulation* 1974; 49:489–497.
11. Webster JS, Moberg C, Rincon G: Natural history of severe proximal coronary disease as documented by coronary cine angiography. *Am J Cardiol* 1974; 33:195–200.
12. Reeves TJ, Oberman A, Jones WB, Sheffield LT: Natural history of angina pectoris. *Am J Cardiol* 1984; 33:423–430.
13. Proudfit WL, Bruschke AVG, Sones FM Jr: Natural history of obstructive coronary artery disease: ten-year study of 601 nonsurgical cases. *Prog Cardiovasc Dis* 1978; 21:53–78.
14. Favaloro RG: Saphenous vein autograft replacement of severe segmental coronary artery occlusion. *Ann Thorac Surg* 1968; 5:334–339.
15. Johnson WD, Flemma RJ, Lepley D Jr, Ellison EH: Extended treatment of severe coronary artery disease: a total surgical approach. *Ann Surg* 1969; 170:460–470.
16. Gruentzig AR, Senning A, Siegenthaler WE: Nonoperative dilatation of coronary-artery stenosis. Percutaneous transluminal coronary angioplasty. *N Engl J Med* 1979; 301:61–68.
17. Virchow R: Endarteriitis deformans und einfache fettmetamorphose der gefasswand. *Gesammelte Abhandlungen zur Wissenschaftlichen Medizin*. Frankfurt-Main, Federal Republic of Germany, Verlag von Meidinger, Sohn und Comp, 1856, pp. 499–513.
18. Anitschkow N, Chalatow S: Ueber experimentelle Cholesterinsteatose und ihre Bedeutung für die Entstehung einiger pathologischer Prozesse. *Zentralbl Allg Pathol* 1913; 24:1–9.
19. Keys A: Atherosclerosis: a problem in newer public health. *J Mt Sinai Hosp* 1953; 20:118–139.
20. Keys A: Epidemiologic aspects of coronary artery disease. *J Chronic Dis* 1957; 6:552–559.
21. Kannel WB, Feinleib M: Natural history of angina pectoris in the Framingham study. *Am J Cardiol* 1972; 29:154–163.
22. Bertolasi CA, Tronge JE, Mon GA, Turri D, Lugones MI: Clinical spectrum of "unstable angina." *Clin Cardiol* 1979; 2:113–120.
23. Prinzmetal M, Kennamer R, Merliss R, Wada T, Bor N: Angina pectoris. I. A variant form of angina pectoris. Preliminary report. *Am J Med* 1959; 27:375–388.
24. Bott-Silverman C, Heupler FA Jr, Yiannikas J: Variant angina—comparison of patients with and without fixed severe obstruction coronary artery disease. *Am J Cardiol* 1984; 54:1173–1175.
25. McNeer JF, Margolis JR, Lee XL, Kisslo JA, Peter RH, Kong Y, Behar VS, Wallace AG, McCants CB, Rosati R: The role of the exercise test in the evaluation of patients for ischemic heart disease. *Circulation* 1978; 57:64–70.
26. Ellestad MH: *Stress Testing, Principles and Practice*, ed 3. Philadelphia, FA Davis, 1986.
27. Borer JS, Bacharach SL, Green MV, Kent KM, Epstein SE, Johnston GS: Real-time radionuclide cineangiography in the noninvasive evaluation of global and regional left ventricular function at rest and during exercise in patients with coronary-artery disease. *N Engl J Med* 1977; 296:839–844.
28. Massie BM, Botvinick EH, Bristow JD: Myocardial perfusion scintigraphy with thallium-201: current status and future prospects, in Yu PN, Goodwin JF (eds): *Progress in Cardiology*, vol 11. Philadelphia, Lea & Febiger, 1982, pp 19–55.
29. Goldstein RA, Mullani NA, Gould KL: Quantitative myocardial imaging with positron emitters, in: Yu PN, Goodwin JF (eds): *Progress in Cardiology*, vol 12. Philadelphia, Lea & Febiger, 1983, pp 147–191.
30. Judkins MP: Selective coronary arteriography. I. Percutaneous transfemoral technique. *Radiology* 1967; 89:815–824.

31. Kent NM, Bentivoglio LG, Block PC, Cowley MJ, Dorros G, Gosselin AJ, Gruentzig A, Myler RK, Simpson J, Stertzer SH, Williams DO, Fisher L, Gillespie MJ, Kelsey S, Mullin SM, Mock MB: Percutaneous transluminal coronary angioplasty: report from the Registry of the National Heart, Lung, and Blood Institute. *Am J Cardiol* 1982; 49:2011–2020.
32. Sheldon WC: Coronary artery bypass graft surgery. The Cleveland Clinic experience, 1967–1983. *Postgrad Med* 1984; 75(6): 108–121.
33. Takaro T, Hultgren HN, Lipton MJ, Detre KM, Participants in the Study Group: The VA cooperative randomized study of surgery for coronary arterial occlusive disease. II. Subgroup with significant left main lesions. *Circulation* 1976; 54(suppl 3):107–117.
34. European Coronary Surgery Study Group: Long-term results of prospective randomized study of coronary artery bypass surgery in stable angina. *Lancet* 1982; 2:1173–1180.
35. Veterans Administration Coronary Artery Bypass Surgery Cooperative Study Group: Eleven-year survival in the Veterans Administration randomized trial of coronary bypass surgery for stable angina. *N Engl J Med* 1984; 311:1333–1339.
36. CASS Principal Investigators and Their Associates: Coronary artery surgery study (CASS): a randomized trial of coronary artery bypass surgery. Survival data. *Circulation* 1983; 68:939–950.
37. Passamani E, Davis KB, Gillespie MS, Killip T, the CASS Principal Investigators and Their Associates: A randomized trial of coronary bypass surgery. Survival of patients with a low ejection fraction. *N Eng J Med* 1985; 312:1665–1671.
38. Wilhelmsson C, Vedin JA, Elmfeldt D, Tibblin G, Wilhelmsen L: Smoking and myocardial infarction. *Lancet* 1975; 1:415–419.
39. Garrison RJ, Feinleib M, Castelli WP, McNamara PM: Cigarette smoking as a confounder of the relationship between relative weight and long-term mortality. The Framingham Heart Study. *JAMA* 1983; 249:2199–2203.
40. Libow M, Schlant RC: Smoking and heart disease, in Yu PN, Goodwin JF (eds): *Progress in Cardiology*, vol 11. Philadelphia, Lea & Febiger, 1982, pp 131–161.
41. Kannel WB, Castelli WP, Gordon T, McNamara PM: Serum cholesterol, lipoproteins, and the risk of coronary heart disease: the Framingham Study. *Ann Intern Med* 1971; 74:1–12.
42. Turpeinen O, Karvonen MJ, Pekkarinen M, Miettinen M, Elosuo R, Paavilainen E: Dietary prevention of coronary heart disease: the Finnish Mental Hospital Study. *Int J Epidemiol* 1979; 8:99–118.
43. Lipid Research Clinics Program: The Lipid Research Clinics Coronary Primary Prevention Trial results. I. Reduction in incidence of coronary heart disease. *JAMA* 1984; 251:351–364; and II. The relationship of reduction in incidence of coronary heart disease to cholesterol lowering. *JAMA* 1984; 251:365–374.
44. Coronary Drug Project Research Group: The Coronary Drug Project: clofibrate and niacin in coronary heart disease. *JAMA* 1975; 231:360–381.
45. Brensike JF, Levy RI, Kelsey SF, Passaimani ER, Richardson JM, Loh IK, Stone NJ, Aldrich RF, Battaglini JW, Moriarty DJ, Fisher MR, Friedman L, Friedewald W, Detre KM, Epstein SE: Effects of therapy with cholestyramine in progression of coronary atherosclerosis: results of the NHLBI Type II Coronary Intervention Study. *Circulation* 1984; 69:313–324.
46. Arntzenius AC, Knomhout D, Barth JD, Reiber JHC, Bruschke AVG, Buis B, Van Gent CM, Kempen-Voogd N, Strikwerda S, Van der Velde EA: Diet, lipoproteins and the progression of coronary atherosclerosis. The Leiden Interventional Trial. *N Engl J Med* 1985; 312:806–810.
47. National Institutes of Health Consensus Development Conference Statement: Lowering blood cholesterol to prevent heart disease. *JAMA* 1985; 253:2080–2086.
48. Fredrickson DS, Levy RI, Lees RS: Fat transport and lipoproteins—an integrated approach to mechanisms and disorders. *N Engl J Med* 1967; 276:34–44, 94–103, 148–156, 215–225, 273–281.
49. Fredrickson DS: A physician's guide to hyperlipidemia. *Mod Concepts Cardiovasc Dis* 1972; 41:31–36.
50. NHLBI Consensus Development Panel: Treatment of hypertriglyceridemia. *JAMA* 1984; 251:1196–1200.
51. The Norwegian Multicenter Study Group. Timolol-induced reduction in mortality and reinfarction in patients surviving acute myocardial infarction. *N Engl J Med* 1981; 304:801–807.
52. Beta-blocker Heart Attack Trial Research Group. A randomized trial of propranolol in patients with acute myocardial infarction. I. Mortality results. *JAMA* 1982; 247:1707–1714.
53. Hjalmarson A, Elmfeldt D, Herlitz J, Holmberg S, Malek I, Nyberg G, Ryden I, Swedberg K, Vedin A, Waagstein F, Waldenstrom A, Waldenstrom J, Wedel H, Wilhelmsen I, Wilhelmsen C: Effect on mortality of metoprolol in acute myocardial infarction. *Lancet* 1981; 2:823–827.
54. Antman E, Muller J, Goldberg S, MacAlpin R, Rubenfine M, Tabatznik B, Liang C, Heupler F, Achuff S, Reichek N, Geltman E, Zerin NZ, Neff RK, Braunwald E: Nifidepine therapy for coronary artery spasm. Experience in 127 patients. *N Engl J Med* 1980; 302:1269–1273.
55. Emanuelsson H, Holmberg S: Mechanism of angina relief after nifedipine: hemodynamic and myocardial metabolic study. *Circulation* 1983; 68:124–130.
56. Subramanian VB, Bowles MJ, Khurmi NS, Davies AB, Raftery EB: Rationale for the choice of calcium antagonists in chronic stable angina: objective double-blind placebo-controlled comparison of nifedipine and verapamil. *Am J Cardiol* 1982; 50:1173–1179.
57. Hung J, Lamb IH, Connolly SJ, Jutzy KR, Goris ML, Schroeder JS: Effect of diltiazem and propranolol alone on exercise performance and left ventricular function in patients with stable effort angina: double-blind, randomized, and placebo-controlled study. *Circulation* 1983; 68:560–567.
58. DeWood M, Spores J, Hensley GR, Simpson CS, Engster GS, Sutherland KI, Grunnewald RP, Shields JP: Coronary arteriographic findings in acute transmural myocardial infarction. *Circulation* 1983; 68(suppl I):39–49.
59. Ganz W, Buchbinder N, Marcus H, Mondkar A, Maddahi J, Charuzi Y, O'Connor L, Shell W, Fishbein MC, Kass R, Miyamoto A, Swan HJC: Intracoronary thrombolysis in evolving myocardial infarction. *Am Heart J* 1981; 101:4–13.
60. Kennedy JW, Ritchie JL, Davis KB, Fritz JK: Western Washington randomized trial of intracoronary streptokinase in acute myocardial infarction. *N Engl J Med* 1983; 309:1477–1482.
61. Vetrovec CW, Leinbach RL, Gold HK, Cowley MJ: Intracoronary thrombolysis in syndromes of unstable ischemia: angiographic and clinical results. *Am Heart J* 1982; 104:946–952.
62. Mandelkorn JB, Wolf NM, Singh S, Schechter JA, Kersh RI, Rodgers DM, Workman MB, Bentivoglio LG, LaPorte SM, Meister SG: Intracoronary thrombus in nontransmural myocardial infarction and in unstable angina pectoris. *Am J Cardiol* 1983; 52:1–6.
63. Epstein SE, Palmeri ST: Mechanisms contributing to precipitation of unstable angina and acute myocardial infarction: implications regarding therapy. *Am J Cardiol* 1984; 54:1245–1252.
64. Willerson JT, Campbell WB, Winniford MD, Schmitz J, Apprill P, Firth BG, Ashton J, Smitherman T, Bush L, Buja LM: Conversion from chronic to acute coronary artery disease: Speculation regarding mechanisms. *Am J Cardiol* 1984; 54:1349–1354.
65. Hinch PD, Hillis LD, Campbell WB, Firth BG, Willerson JT: Release of prostaglandins and thromboxane into the coronary circulation in patients with ischemic heart disease. *N Engl J Med* 1981; 304:685–691.
66. Lewis HD, Davis JW, Archibald DG, Steinke W, Smitherman TC, Doherty JE III, Schnaper HW, LeWinter MM, Linares E, Pouget JM, Sabhabwal SC, Chesler E, Demots H: Protective effects of aspirin against acute myocardial infarction and death in men with unstable angina. *N Engl J Med* 1983; 309:396–403.
67. Elwood PC, Cochrane AL, Burr ML, Sweetnam PM, Williams G, Welsby E, Hughes SJ, Renton R: A randomized controlled trial of acetyl salicylic acid in the secondary prevention of mortality from myocardial infarction. *Br Med J* 1974; 1:436–440.
68. The Anturane Reinfarction Trial Research Group: Sulfinpyrazone in the prevention of cardiac death after myocardial infarction. *N Engl J Med* 1978; 298:289–295.
69. Campbell WB, Johnson AR, Callahan KS, Graham RM: Antiplatelet activity of β-adrenergic antagonists: inhibition of thromboxane synthesis and platelet aggregation in patients receiving long-term propranolol treatment. *Lancet* 1981; 2:1382–1384.
70. Cooper R, Stamler J, Dyer A, Garside D: The decline in mortality from coronary heart disease, U.S.A., 1968–1975. *J Chronic Dis* 1978; 31:709–720.
71. Goldman L, Cook EF: The decline in ischemic heart disease mortality rates. An analysis of the comparative effects of medical interventions and changes in lifestyle. *Ann Intern Med* 1984; 101:825–836.
72. Proudfit WL, Bruschke AVG, MacMillan JP, Williams GW, Sones FM Jr: Fifteen-year survival study of patients with obstructive coronary artery disease. *Circulation* 1983; 68:986–997.
73. Kramer JR, Kitazume H, Proudfit WL, Matsuda Y, Williams GW, Sones FM Jr: Progression and regression of coronary atherosclerosis: relation to risk factors. *Am Heart J* 1983; 105:134–144.
74. Kramer JR, Kitazume H, Proudfit WL, Matsuda Y, Goormastic M, Williams GW, Sones FM Jr: Segmental analysis of the rate of progression in patients with progressive coronary atherosclerosis. *Am Heart J* 1983; 106:1427–1431.

36 Coronary Artery Spasm

Tsung O. Cheng, MD and Hirofumi Yasue, MD

Coronary artery spasm (CAS), like the click-murmur syndrome of mitral valve prolapse,[1] is another problem on the medical pendulum that has made several opposite swings in past decades. Although Osler[2] in 1910 first suggested that spasm of a coronary artery was responsible for an acute attack of angina pectoris, his hypothesis was soon discarded after Blumgart et al[3] and French and Dock[4] in the early 1940s showed that coronary insufficiency arose chiefly from mechanical obstruction of the coronary artery due to atherosclerosis. In 1959 Prinzmetal et al[5] then described an entity called variant angina in patients who developed ST-segment elevation on the electrocardiagram (ECG) during nonexertional angina; because the angina occurred spontaneously without an increased myocardial oxygen demand, the theory of coronary spasm causing a decreased supply was invoked. However, their theory did not receive much attention, because such spasm had never actually been observed or documented and because many of their patients had significant atherosclerosis at autopsy. In the early 1970s Cheng et al[6] demonstrated by selective coronary arteriography the existence of reversible coronary vasospasm even in the absence of atherosclerosis. It was not until the work of Maseri et al[7] that the impact of CAS was really appreciated. With the introduction of calcium slow-channel blockers as a new, definitive, and effective class of therapeutic agents against CAS, the approach to the management of patients with coronary artery disease entered a new era in the 1980s.

ARTERIOGRAPHIC FINDINGS OF CORONARY ARTERY SPASM

Coronary arteries are able to dilate and constrict as a means to regulate coronary blood flow. Changes in the diameter of coronary arteries can readily be demonstrated by sublingual administration of nitroglycerin in the cardiac catheterization laboratory. These are normal physiologic changes of the vasomotor tone of the large coronary arteries. Coronary artery spasm, however, is a transient constriction of a large coronary artery, which results in myocardial ischemia.

Yasue[8] and Yasue et al[9] performed coronary arteriography in 85 patients during 96 attacks of CAS, 69 associated with ST-segment elevation and 27 with ST-segment depression in the ECG. The locations[10] and degrees of spasm are shown diagrammatically in Figure 36.1. Of the 69 attacks of spasm with ST-segment elevation, 42 caused total occlusion, 25 subtotal occlusion (99% of luminal diameter), and 2 diffuse narrowing (60% to 90% of luminal diameter) of a large coronary artery. Total occlusion was generally associated with more severe ST-segment elevation than was subtotal occlusion or diffuse narrowing. Therefore, most attacks (60.9%) of spasm with ST-segment elevation were associated with total occlusion of a large coronary artery.

Of the 27 attacks of spasm with ST-segment depression, 9 caused subtotal occlusion and 12 caused diffuse narrowing of a large coronary artery. In three patients with attacks associated with ST-segment depression, cor-

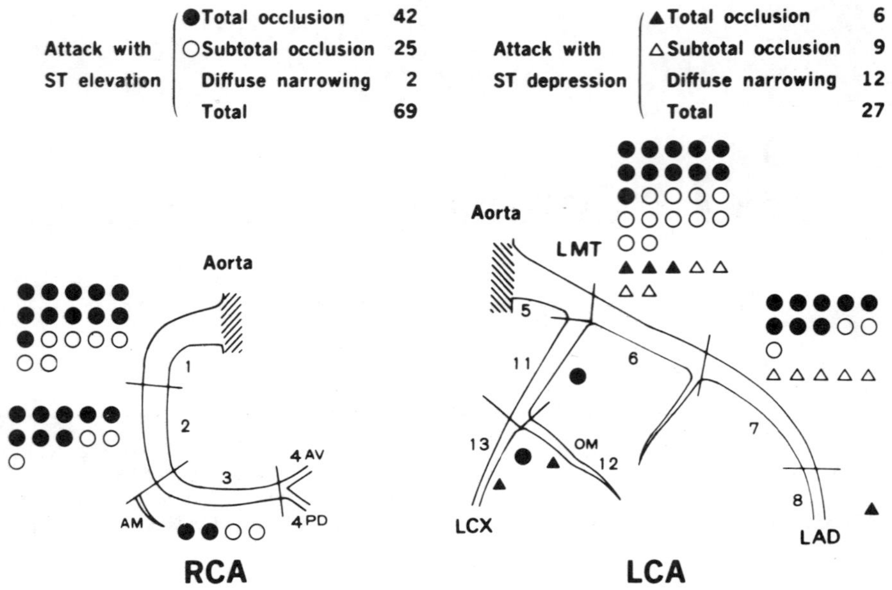

Figure 36.1. Coronary arteriographic findings during an attack of coronary artery spasm with ST-segment elevation and an attack with ST-segment depression. Coronary arteries were divided into 15 segments according to the American Heart Association Committee Report,[10] as shown by the numbers on the diagram of coronary arteries. AM = acute marginal branch; AV = atrioventricular nodal branch; LAD = left anterior descending artery; LCA = left coronary artery; LCX = left circumflex artery; LMT = left main trunk; OM = obtuse marginal branch; PD = posterior descending branch; RCA = right coronary artery. (From Yasue,[8] with permission.)

onary spasm caused total occlusion of the left anterior descending artery at the proximal segment during the attack, but there was a rich supply of collateral vessels to the distal segment. In two patients whose attacks were associated with either ST-segment elevation or ST-segment depression in the same leads, coronary arteriograms were obtained during both types of attack. In both patients, angina with ST-segment elevation was associated with total occlusion of a large coronary artery, whereas angina with ST-segment depression was associated with either subtotal occlusion (Figure 36.2) or diffuse narrowing of the same artery.

Most attacks (77.8%) of coronary spasm with ST-segment depression were therefore associated with either subtotal occlusion or diffuse narrowing of a large coronary artery. When the attack with ST-segment depression was associated with total occlusion, the occlusion by spasm occurred either at a proximal segment of a large coronary artery that received a rich supply of collateral vessels to its periphery or at a distal segment of a large coronary artery.[8,9]

The results of this study in humans are in agreement with the data from animal experiments,[11] indicating that angina pectoris with ST-segment elevation is associated with more severe myocardial ischemia than is angina pectoris with ST-segment depression, the former representing transmural ischemia and the latter subendocardial ischemia. Occasionally, ST-segment depression and ST-segment elevation may occur simultaneously in the same patient (Figure 36.3), because of combined subendocardial and transmural ischemia following vasospastic narrowing of different severity in various branches.

Coronary spasm can occur either alone or superimposed on atherosclerosis. The frequency with which spasm occurs in an angiographically normal coronary artery varies among different reported series[6,12–17] (Table 36.1). Four of the five patients reported on in Cheng's initial series[6] in 1973 had normal coronary arteriograms; one of them at autopsy had normal coronary arteries. In the latest series reported by Cheng,[17] 60 of 80 patients (75%) referred for study because of a diagnosis of variant angina had angiographically normal coronary arteries. In the series reported by Endo et al,[14] 19 of their 35 patients (54%) had coronary artery disease. In all 22 patients reported on by Heupler,[16] none had coronary atherosclerosis. In the series reported by Shubrooks et al[13] from the Coronary Care Unit of the Massachusetts General Hospital, most of their patients had unstable angina or preinfarction angina and it was therefore a mixed group containing many patients with atherosclerotic coronary obstructive disease. Of the 126 patients reported on by Yasue et al,[8] 37 (29.3%) had normal coronary arteries, 66 (52.4%) had one-vessel disease, 16 (12.7%) had two-vessel disease, and 7 (5.6%) had three-vessel disease. The degree of fixed narrowing of arteries involved or presumed to have been involved in spasm were examined. Two patients had spasm of both the right coronary artery and the left anterior descending artery. Of the 128 coronary arteries involved or presumed to have been involved in spasm, 33 (25.8%) were normal, 15 (11.7%) had 25% narrowing, 21 (16.4%) had 50% narrowing, 19 (14.8%) had 75% narrowing, 29 (22.7%) had 90% narrowing, and 11 (8.6%) had 99% fixed stenosis of the luminal diameter. Spasm usually appeared at the site of atherosclerotic stenosis,

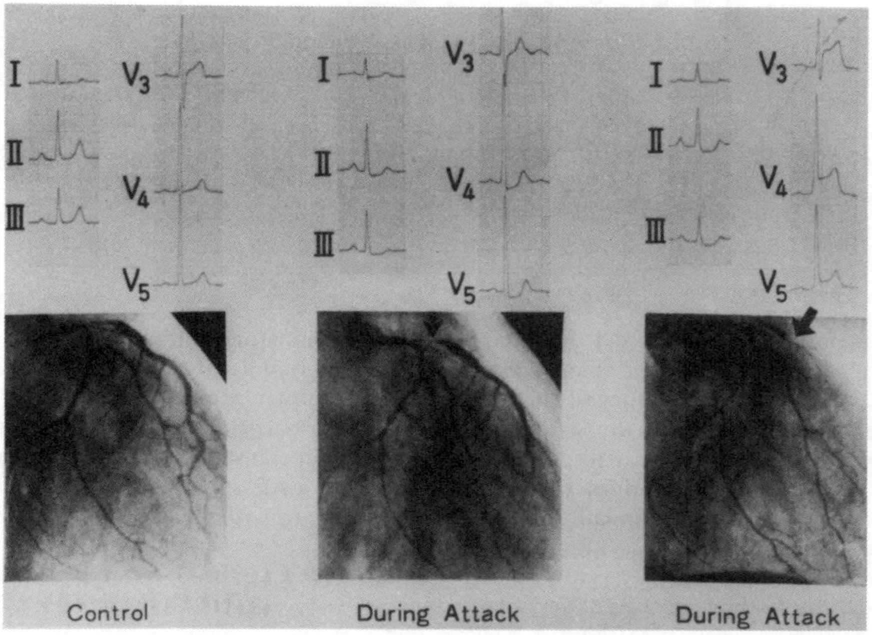

Figure 36.2. Coronary arteriograms and corresponding electrocardiograms during attacks of coronary artery spasm with either ST-segment elevation or depression in the precordial leads. During an attack with ST-segment elevation, spasm totally occluded the left anterior descending artery (*right*). During an attack with ST-segment depression, spasm subtotally occluded the same artery at the same site (*center*). The *left panel* shows the control. (From Yasue et al,[9] with permission.)

but there were some exceptions, as were also reported by MacAlpin.[18]

When the coronary artery involved or presumed to have been involved in spasm was normal or almost normal (less than 50% stenosis of the luminal diameter), spasm occurred more often at the right than at the left coronary artery. Of the 48 normal or almost normal coronary arteries involved or presumed to have been involved in spasm, 33 (68.7%) were the right coronary artery, 12 (25.0%) the left anterior descending artery, and 3 (6.3%) the left circumflex artery.[8]

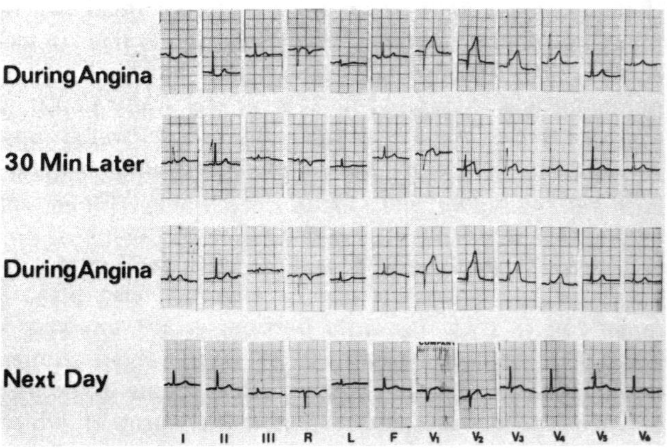

Figure 36.3. Simultaneous ST-segment depression and ST-segment elevation in variant angina. During the initial attack of angina (*top panel*), ST-segment elevation occurred in precordial leads V_1 to V_4 and ST-segment depression occurred in limb leads I, II, and L; coronary arteriograms showed total spastic occlusion of the proximal left anterior descending artery involving the origin of its first diagonal branch. During the next episode of angina (*third panel*), ST-segment elevation occurred in precordial leads V_1 to V_3 without ST-segment depression in limb leads; coronary arteriography at this time showed a shorter segment of total spastic occlusion of the proximal left anterior descending artery distal to the origin of its first diagonal branch, which was not involved.

These results indicate that CAS can occur in normal coronary arteries as well as in atherosclerotic vessels and that the main cause of variant angina is not atherosclerotic obstruction.

INCIDENCE AND PREVALENCE

Although the incidence of coronary artery spasm and the prevalence of variant angina seem to be much higher in the Japanese than in Occidentals[19] (in Japan variant angina is present in 23% of all patients with angina[20]), the large number of papers on the subject published in recent years in the United States,[21] Canada,[22] France,[23]

Table 36.1. Incidence of Coronary Artery Disease in Patients with Variant Angina

Authors	Patients	Yes	No: No.	No: %
Cheng et al[6] (1973)	5	1	4	80
MacAlpin et al[12] (1973)	19	17	2	10
Shubrooks et al[13] (1975)	20	17	3	15
Endo et al[14] (1975)	35	16	19	54
Selzer et al[15] (1976)	29	20	9	31
Heupler[16] (1980)	22	0	22	100
Yasue[8] (1983)	126	89	37	29
Cheng[17] (1984)	80	20	60	75

Table 36.2. Comparison of Severity of Coronary Artery Lesion in Cases of Variant Angina in Japan and Western Countries

Country	No. of Cases	Coronary Stenosis 50% or Less	Coronary Stenosis More Than 50%
Japan	162	70 (43.2%)	92 (56.8%)
USA, France, and Italy	174	41 (23.6%)	133 (76.4%) (X^2 test, $p <$ 0.001)

Adapted from Kimura,[20] with permission.

Germany,[24] Switzerland,[25] Italy,[7] United Kingdom,[26] Denmark,[27] Russia,[28] Israel,[29] Poland,[30] Spain,[31] South Africa,[32] Austrialia,[33] and Argentina[34] suggest that there is, in fact, no geographic difference of any significance. Even in China where the entity was virtually unknown until 1973 when, following Sino-American rapprochement mutual exchange of medical information was resumed and coronary arteriography was introduced in China[35], case reports began to appear in recent years.[36,37]

Coronary arteriographic findings in cases of variant angina in Japan and in Western countries show that differences exist in the prevalence of variant angina without organic stenosis; there is a higher incidence in Japan than in the Western countries.[19] As a matter of fact, Kimura,[20] who himself had this disorder, noted a statistically significant difference between the incidence of variant angina accompanied by a coronary lesion in Western countries and that in Japan (Table 36.2). The reason for this difference may be explained, in part, by the greater prevalence of coronary atherosclerosis in the United States than in Japan[38,39] and the higher incidence in Japanese who had migrated to the United States than in those living in Japan.[19] However, it is extremely difficult to explain why spasm in patients without significant coronary atherosclerosis is more frequently observed in Japanese than in Western people and, for that matter, in people in China, a close neighbor of Japan. One reason may be that the concept of variant angina is more popularized, and provocative tests for coronary spasm such as ergonovine or hyperventilation test are more frequently performed in Japan than in other countries. Further investigation is necessary to answer this question, especially because coronary arteriography is now being more frequently employed in China.[40]

ROLE OF SPASM IN ISCHEMIC CORONARY SYNDROMES

Although CAS is now clearly established as the cause of Prinzmetal's variant angina, "variant of the variant,"[6] and angina at rest, there is increasing recognition that CAS may be a significant factor in a broad spectrum of other ischemic coronary artery syndromes, including classic effort angina, unstable angina, acute myocardial infarction, and sudden death (Table 36.3). The first instance of acute inferior wall myocardial infarction due to severe spasm of the left circumflex artery was reported in 1972.[41] Further support for the role of CAS in angina and acute myocardial infarction is provided by the observations of Lange et al[42] that some munition workers experienced Monday morning angina following withdrawal from chronic industrial nitroglycerin exposure, acute myocardial infarction developed in a few, and all had normal or nearly normal coronary arteries on coronary arteriography. Of particular importance is the interesting observation that transient Q waves may appear and then disappear in CAS, supporting the concept of the "stunned" myocardium without permanent necrosis.[43]

OTHER CLINICAL SYNDROMES ASSOCIATED WITH CORONARY SPASM

Of interest is the recently reported connection between mitral valve prolapse and CAS.[44,45] One of the most perplexing problems in current cardiologic practice is the management, both diagnostic and therapeutic, of patients who have chest pain associated with mitral valve prolapse.[46] Mitral valve prolapse, which may result from coronary artery disease,[46,47] may also itself be responsible for CAS.[44] Increased alpha-adrenergic tone appears to play an important role in both patients with mitral valve prolapse and those with CAS.[48] Therefore, it is not difficult to see the connection between the two.

Recent study also links variant angina, migraine headache, and Raynaud's phenomenon. Miller et al[22] found that patients with variant angina had an incidence of migraine of 26% compared with 6% in cardiac control subjects and 10% in normal subjects. Raynaud's phenomenon was diagnosed in 24% of the study group as opposed to 5% and 3% in the respective control groups. At least one of the disorders was present in 24 patients with variant angina, and 11% of the patients with variant angina had both migraine and Raynaud's phenomenon.

Emotional stress, which is known to be a factor in Raynaud's phenomenon and in migraine, also plays a major role in CAS. Recently Bashour et al[49] analyzed a detailed psychologic profile in 27 middle-aged women with angina and normal coronary arteriograms, and found 9 with typical vasospastic angina, the onset of which

Table 36.3. Syndromes Associated with Coronary Artery Spasm

1. Prinzmetal's variant angina
2. Variant of the variant
3. Angina at rest
4. Unstable angina
5. Effort angina
6. Acute myocardial infarction
7. Sudden death
8. Monday morning angina in nitroglycerin workers
9. Mitral valve prolapse

Adapted from Cheng,[17] with permission.

coincided with sudden worsening of a tense but contained emotional imbalance due to an erupting traumatic experience commonly centered around sexuality. Three of the nine patients had Raynaud's phenomenon and four had migraine. Their study, therefore, strongly supports a causal relation between emotional distress and attacks of CAS and the earlier findings of an increased association between CAS, migraine, and Raynaud's phenomenon.

CORONARY SPASM, CARDIAC ARRHYTHMIAS, AND SUDDEN DEATH

Various forms of arrhythmia often appear during attacks of coronary spasm. Yasue[8] reported the incidence and types of arrhythmias during attacks in 88 patients with variant angina (Table 36.4). Ventricular arrhythmias such as ventricular premature contractions or ventricular tachycardia were the most frequent: ventricular premature contractions were found in 31 (35.2%), ventricular tachycardia in 15 (17.1%), and ventricular fibrillation in 5 (5.7%) of the 88 patients. Sinus bradycardia (heart rate less than 50 beats per minute) was found in 15 (17.1%), supraventricular premature contractions in 13 (14.8%), and atrioventricular block of high degree (second or third degree) in 9 (10.2%). Ventricular premature contractions, ventricular tachycardia, and supraventricular premature contractions appeared more often when ST-segment elevation occurred in the anterior leads than when ST-segment elevation occurred in the inferior leads (Table 36.4). However, sinus bradycardia, sinoatrial block and/or sinus arrest, and atrioventricular block appeared more frequently when ST-segment elevation occurred in the inferior leads (Table 36.4). Figure 36.4 shows an example.

Arrhythmias during attacks of variant angina are more likely to occur at the peak of an attack or when the attack is severe or prolonged. Therefore, the incidence of arrhythmia depends largely on the severity of the attack, the time of recording of the ECG (whether taken at the beginning, at the peak, or near the end of the attack), and the duration of the ECG recording (whether continuous monitoring was made). The incidence of arrhythmia in Yasue's series was calculated from the ECG taken during the most severe attack in each patient. The severity of the attack of acute myocardial ischemia can be gauged by the magnitude of ST-segment elevation and the incidence of arrhythmia is higher in patients with greater ST-segment elevation than in patients with lesser degrees of ST-segment elevation, irrespective of the location of myocardial ischemia represented by ST-segment elevation.[8]

Coronary artery spasm is also given prominent consideration in the causation of sudden death.[50] Serious, and often fatal, cardiac arrhythmias may occur during an attack of variant angina. The association of an advanced degree of heart block with ventricular tachycardia and ventricular fibrillation has been well documented in patients with variant angina[6] (Figure 36.5). Other reports noted an incidence of ventricular fibrillation of 10%[51] and of cardiac arrest of 22%[52] among patients with variant angina. Although ventricular dysrhythmias have generally been considered as the mechanism of sudden death in patients with CAS, recent work found another hitherto unrecognized mechanism, namely, sinus node dysfunction[53,54] (Figure 36.6). That three patients were encountered over a relatively short time suggests that it is not an isolated, rare event but one that may occur more frequently than commonly recognized. The observation that CAS was the mechanism of sinus node dysfunction in patients with variant angina has direct clinical rele-

Table 36.4. Incidence and Types of Arrhythmia During Attacks in 88 Patients with Variant Angina.*

	Electrocardiographic Leads with ST-Segment Elevation							
	Anterior		Inferior		Anterior and Inferior		Total	
	No.	%	No.	%	No.	%	No.	%
VPC	24	51.1	5	13.5	2	50.0	31	35.2
VT	11	23.4	3	8.1	1	25.0	15	17.1
VF	2	4.3	2	5.4	1	25.0	5	5.7
AV block (first degree)	1	2.1	3	8.1	1	25.0	5	5.7
AV block (second & third degree)	1	2.1	7	18.9	1	25.0	9	10.2
SA block and sinus arrest	1	2.1	5	13.5	0	0.0	6	6.8
Sinus bradycardia	0	0.0	15	40.5	0	0.0	15	17.1
Sinus tachycardia	3	6.4	0	0.0	0	0.0	3	3.4
SVPC	11	23.4	2	5.4	0	0.0	13	14.8
AF and MFAT	3	6.4	1	2.7	0	0.0	4	4.6
No arrhythmia	18	38.3	12	32.4	1	25.0	31	35.2
Total no. of patients	47		37		4		88	

* From Yasue,[8] with permission.

AF = atrial fibrillation; AV = atrioventricular; MFAT = multifocal atrial tachycardia; SA = sinoatrial; SVPC = supraventricular premature contraction; VPC = ventricular premature contraction; VF = ventricular fibrillation; VT = ventricular tachycardia.

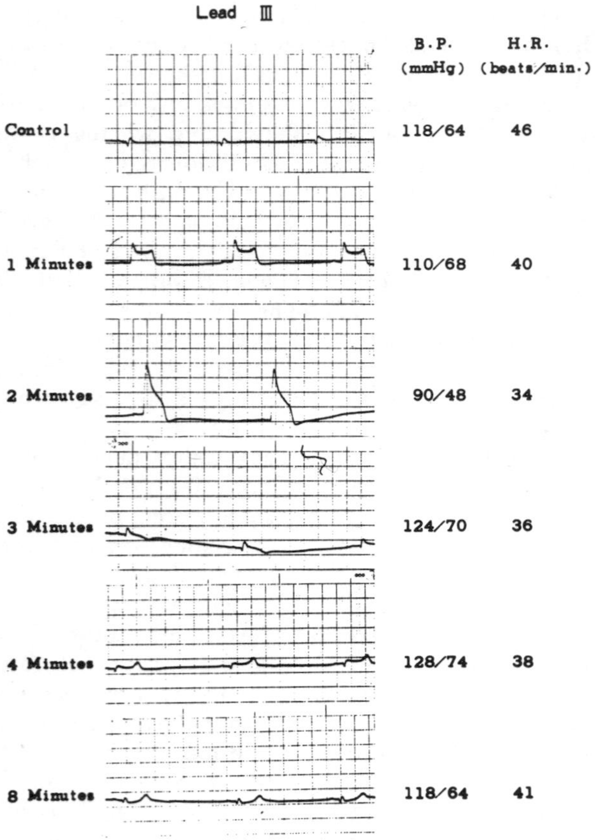

Figure 36.4. Heart rate and blood pressure during an attack of coronary artery spasm with ST-segment elevation in the inferior leads. Marked sinus bradycardia (34 beats per minute) and hypotension (90/48 mm Hg) appeared at the peak of the attack. BP = blood pressure; HR = heart rate. (From Yasue,[8] with permission.)

vance in two respects. First, just as in other patients with sinus node dysfunction, pacemaker therapy[55] may be an important consideration in the therapeutic armamentarium for a subset of patients with CAS. Second, some drugs used to treat CAS, such as verapamil (vide infra), should be avoided in the presence of proven or suspected sinus node dysfunction.[54]

PATHOGENESIS OF CORONARY ARTERY SPASM

The exact pathogenetic mechanism for and the etiology of CAS are not known. However, several factors or agents that precipitate CAS have been identified. These include cold,[56,57] hyperventilation,[58,59] alkalosis,[60] exercise,[6,61,62] methacholine,[63,64] epinephrine,[63,65] ergot alkaloids,[66,67] cocaine,[68,69] oral contraceptives,[70] cigarettes,[70,71] alcohol,[72–74] and thromboxane A_2.[75]

The relation between CAS and the autonomic nervous system has been not only recognized for some time, but also extensively investigated more recently. Stimulation of alpha-adrenergic receptors results in coronary vasoconstriction, and large coronary arteries are richly supplied with alpha-receptors.[76,77] Indeed, stimulation of alpha-receptors by injection of epinephrine after beta-blockade with propranolol causes coronary spasm,[65] and phentolamine, an alpha-blocking agent, suppresses coronary spasm in some patients.[78] Coronary artery spasm can also be induced by injection of methacholine,[63,64] a parasympathomimetic agent; and atropine, which blocks the parasympathetic nerve activity, suppresses the attack of variant angina in some patients.[63,79] The activity of parasympathetic nerve is increased at rest and is decreased during activity. Coronary artery spasm most often occurs at rest and is not usually induced by exercise in the daytime.[80] Thus, parasympathetic as well as sympathetic nerve activity seems to play a role in the pathogenesis of CAS.[50]

However, alpha-adrenergic activity or parasympathetic nerve activity, or both, may not be the sole factor responsible for CAS because whether CAS can be induced by alpha-stimulation or by injection of methacholine, or both, depends largely on the time of day or night. The nearer the time of alpha-stimulation or of injection of methacholine to the time zone of spontaneous attacks of CAS, which is usually from midnight to early morning, the easier it is for these stimuli to induce CAS. Therefore, even a slight degree of sympathetic discharge caused by such activities as walking, straining at stool or urination, cleaning teeth or shaving, exposure to cold, or smoking may induce CAS in the early morning. However, in the afternoon even a higher degree of sympathetic discharge such as strenuous exercise may not induce CAS.[80] Pharmacologic agents such as epinephrine, methacholine, or ergonovine in small doses can easily induce CAS in the early morning, but they may not induce spasm even in large doses in the afternoon.

There is therefore a circadian variation in the reactivity of the large coronary artery to adrenergic and muscarinic stimulation, which is probably related to circadian variation in tone of the large coronary artery in most patients with CAS. There are also daily, weekly, monthly, and yearly variations in the reactivity of the large coronary artery in most patients with CAS.[78]

The relation between attacks of variant angina and alcohol ingestion is interesting and one that has recently been examined by Takizawa et al.[74] Because alcohol is commonly taken in daily life around the world, the demonstration that alcohol may induce coronary vasospastic angina in a significant number of patients with variant angina has very important clinical implications. As a matter of fact, the third patient in the original series of variant angina with normal coronary arteriograms reported by Cheng et al[6] has relapses of variant angina only when he indulges in excessive alcohol consumption, whether or not he becomes inebriated (unpublished observation by TOC). Although the precise mechanism of alcohol-induced CAS remains to be elucidated, it is possible that alcohol is metabolized in the liver to acetaldehyde, which releases catecholamines that in turn induce coronary vasospasm through alpha-adrenergic receptors present in large coronary arteries.[76,77]

The possible role of serotonin in the genesis of coronary vasospasm had also been considered, because serotonin (5-hydroxytryptamine) is known to contract isolated cor-

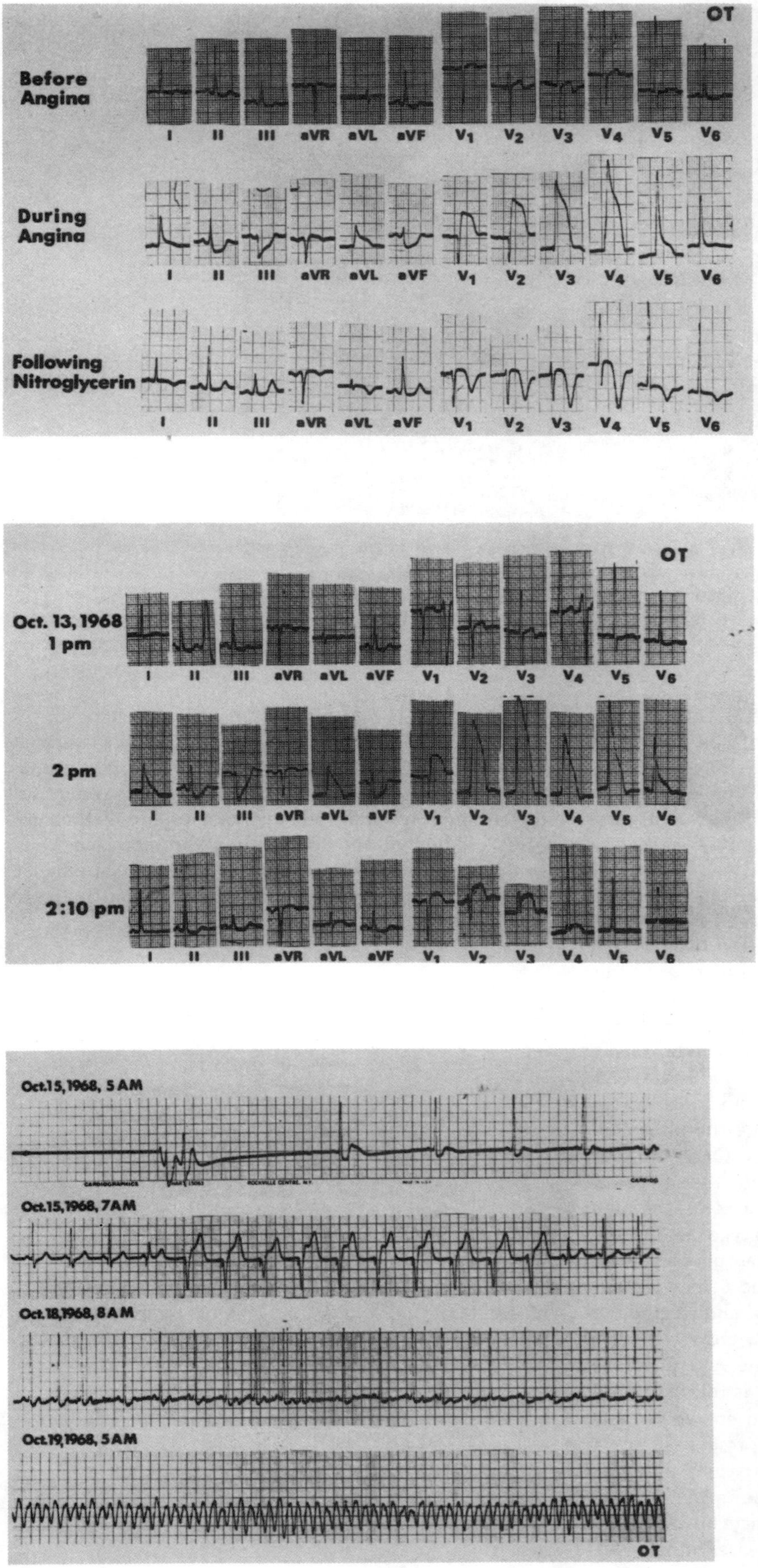

Figure 36.5. Typical electrocardiographic changes during variant angina (*top*) and without angina (*middle*). In the same patient an advanced degree of heart block later developed (*bottom, upper panel*); a temporary transvenous right ventricular endocardial electrode-pacemaker (*bottom, second panel*) was inserted and then removed 3 days later (*bottom, third panel*); the patient subsequently died of ventricular tachycardia and fibrillation (*bottom, fourth panel*). (From Cheng,[17] with permission.)

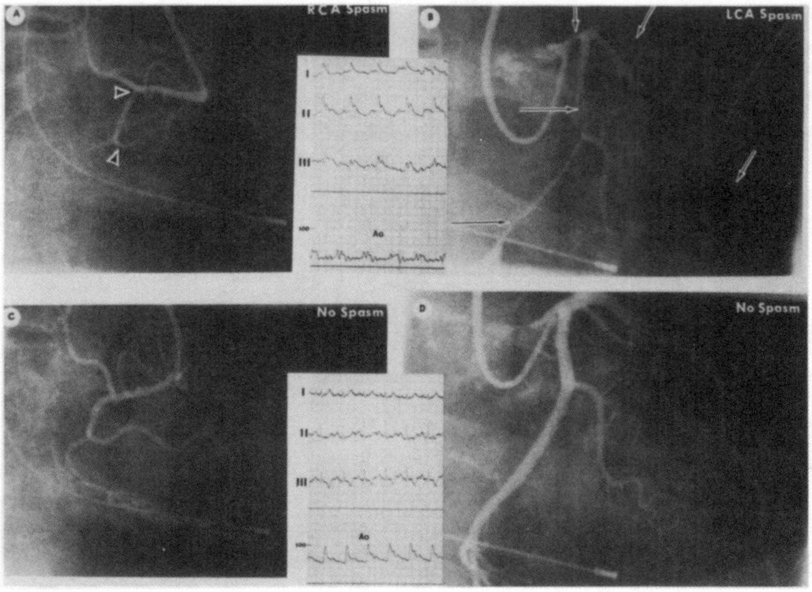

Figure 36.6. In a patient with coronary vasospastic angina complicated by recurrent syncope, sinus node dysfunction was demonstrated during coronary artery spasm (CAS) when demand pacing ensued (*top*), and normal sinus mechanism was present when there was no CAS (*bottom*). (From Cheng,[17] with permission.)

onary arteries in vitro.[81–83] However, it was refuted in recent studies of ketanserin, a specific serotonin(HT_2)-receptor blocker, which revealed no consistent differences in the number of ischemic episodes and nitroglycerin consumption between ketanserin- and placebo-treated patients with Prinzmetal's angina.[84]

The recent discovery of thromboxane A_2, a potent vasoconstrictor released by the aggregating platelets, and prostacyclin, a potent vasodilator produced by the vascular endothelial cells, opens a new field of research on the mechanisms that control local vascular tone. Work on the interrelation of prostaglandins and platelet function has further helped in understanding the involvement of platelets in thrombosis, coronary artery disease, and CAS.[84a] The most abundant prostaglandin precursor is arachidonic acid, which is present among the phospholipids of all mammalian cell membranes. Once released from the cell membrane by the action of the activated enzyme phospholipase A_2, arachidonic acid can be metabolized in one of two pathways into oxygenated products by cyclo-oxygenase (also known as prostaglandin synthetase) and thus converted into the stable prostaglandins with two double bonds of the E and F series, as well as into two unstable products with great and contradictory biologic activity: thromboxane A_2 and prostacyclin (Figure 36.7). Thromboxane A_2 is formed in the presence of thromboxane synthetase, an enzyme found in platelets. Prostacyclin is formed in the presence of prostacyclin synthetase, an enzyme abundantly present in the vascular endothelium. A relative increase in the level of thromboxane A_2 or a decrease in prostacyclin may play an etiologic role in CAS. Indeed, increases in platelet aggregation[85] and in thromboxane A_2 [75] and beta-thromboglobulin[85a] in coronary sinus blood have both recently been demonstrated during attacks of CAS in variant angina, although there is some question as to whether increased production of coronary sinus thromboxane A_2 is a cause or a result of vasospastic angina.[86] Antiplatelet agents like aspirin, dipyridamole, indomethacin, and sul-

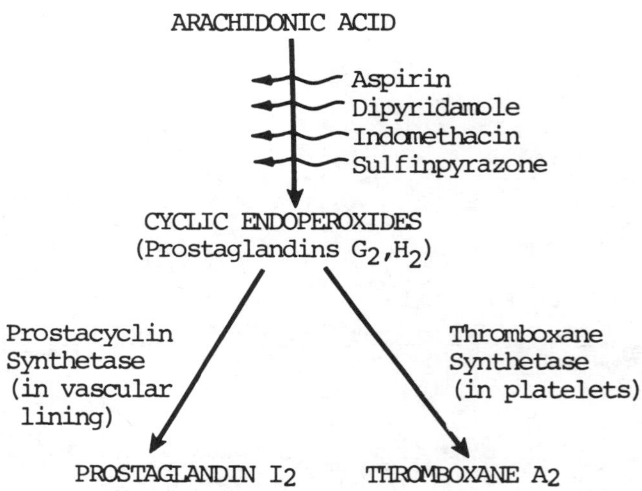

Figure 36.7. Metabolic pathway of arachidonic acid, synthesis of prostacyclin and thromboxane A_2, and sites of inhibition by certain antiplatelet drugs. (From Cheng[17] with permission.)

finpyrazone have inhibitory effects on prostaglandin metabolism and formation of thromboxane A_2. However, their role in the management of CAS is unclear and controversial. Some investigators have suggested that because aspirin, dipyridamole, indomethacin, and sulfinpyrazone block the conversion of arachidonic acid to cyclic endoperoxides, generation of thromboxane A_2 as well as prostacyclin may be inhibited. That these drugs block prostacyclin synthesis may account for the absence of dramatic improvement. As a matter of fact, aspirin[87] and indomethacin[88] may sometimes aggravate CAS in variant angina. However, other investigators have proposed that because prostacyclin is formed in the vascular lining, coronary arteries with significant atherosclerosis may be incapable of prostacyclin synthesis.[50,89] Therefore, these agents may block only thromboxane A_2 generation with consequent beneficial effect. Nevertheless, at this time, therapy of CAS with antiplatelet agents has not been shown conclusively to be of benefit.

DIAGNOSIS OF CORONARY ARTERY SPASM

The diagnosis of CAS is clinically important not only because it may play a role in the pathogenesis of several well-known coronary syndromes, but also because specific treatment with various drugs including the recently introduced calcium slow-channel blockers (vide infra) is now available. The diagnosis is usually obvious if typical electrocardiographic changes in the form of ST-segment elevation over the site corresponding to the coronary artery in spasm are observed during an attack (Figure 36.5, *top*.) Unfortunately some of these patients may have no angina during the period of ST-segment elevation (Figure 36.5, *middle*, "variant angina without angina"[6]); therefore, unless continuous 12-lead ECGs are obtained, the diagnosis may often be missed. Many patients with variant angina have infrequent attacks and consequently ambulatory Holter monitoring is a low-yield procedure. Similarly, radionuclide studies are often not helpful because of the transient and unpredictable nature of the attacks; thallium scan may reveal either perfusion defects or excess uptake.[90]

The only certain method of diagnosing CAS is, of course, coronary arteriography. However, angiographic observations of CAS during routine studies in the cardiac catheterization laboratory are rare, and they are usually made by chance except when contrast injections are performed during an episode of variant angina. The incidence of CAS observed during routine angiographic studies is low, because of (1) frequent occurrence of "benign" catheter-induced spasm, especially of the right coronary artery; (2) the common practice of premedicating patients with atropine, which tends to mask coronary spasm[79]; (3) the routine use of nitroglycerin for repeat left ventriculography preceding coronary arteriography; (4) delay in exchanging a preformed coronary catheter when the coronary artery in spasm is not the one for which the catheter is designed; (5) concern over repeat injections of the spastic coronary arteries during angina with alarming electrocardiographic changes and reflex reaction of prompt nitroglycerin administration; (6) the relatively small statistical chance of occurrence at angiography of transient CAS in a sedated patient, unless one is patient enough to wait for its spontaneous occurrence or it is induced; (7) lower coronary artery tone in the afternoon than in the morning due to the circadian variation in variant angina.[80,91,92]

Provocative testing is therefore usually indicated to establish a diagnosis. In the United States the most commonly used agent is ergonovine maleate (Ergotrate®),[66] an ergot alkaloid and smooth muscle constrictor. Ergonovine maleate, which is a lysergic acid and amine alkaloid, rather than ergotamine tartrate (Gynergen®), which is an amino acid alkaloid, is to be used in provocative testing, because of less tendency for endothelial damage or excessive uterine contraction[93] and also less risk of inducing acute myocardial infarction.[67] Several protocols of ergonovine testing have been proposed; common to all reported protocols is coronary arteriography and evaluation of baseline left ventricular hemodynamic function prior to ergonovine administration, intravenous administration of ergonovine in incremental doses (0.05, 0.10, 0.20, 0.30, and in some cases 0.40 mg) with continuous hemodynamic and electrocardiographic monitoring, and standby freshly prepared nitroglycerin solution for intravenous or intracoronary administration for prompt reversal of induced CAS. For the results of an ergonovine test to be positive, all of the following three criteria—typical angina, a focal CAS of greater than 40%, and ST-segment elevations (Figure 36.8)—must be met, as esophageal spasm may result from ergonovine stimulation and may produce pain indistinguishable from angina.[93] Transient U-wave inversion with or without ST-segment elevation has also been reported in attacks of variant angina induced by ergonovine maleate, especially in spasm of the left anterior descending coronary artery.[94,95] The U wave may either remain inverted in some cases in the recovery phase when the ST-segment elevation has already subsided[94,95] or precede ST-segment elevation in other cases.[94] Even transient T-wave abnormalities (peaking, flattening, or a diphasic T wave) can represent an "abortive attack" of variant angina caused by incomplete or transient CAS, or both.[96] These two observations have an important clinical implication, particularly with regard to provocative tests performed with electrocardiographic monitoring only. Their appearance without, or before, the emergence of ST-segment elevation may forestall the additional administration of ergonovine maleate and thus avoid possible complications usually associated with larger doses of the drug.

It is therefore obvious that ergonovine testing should only be performed in a coronary arteriographic laboratory, although in some centers ergonovine testing has been performed in a coronary care unit in patients whose coronary anatomy is known from a recently performed coronary arteriogram. Contraindications are the same whether or not coronary arteriography is performed and they include multiple critical organic stenoses, severe left ventricular dysfunction or heart failure, recent myocardial infarction, recent prolonged myocardial ischemic pain, significant hypertension, uncontrolled ventricular arrhythmias, cerebrovascular disease, and pregnancy. Although other provocative tests have been proposed such

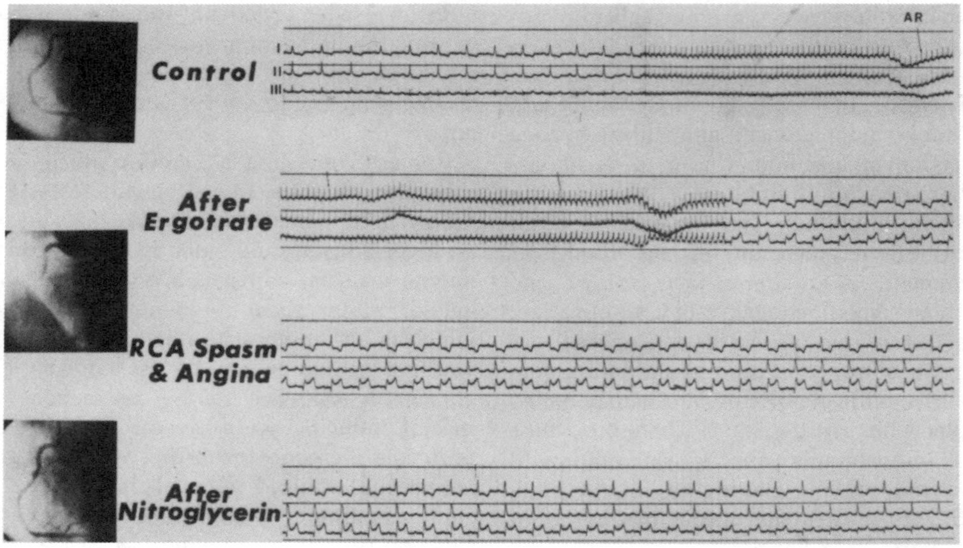

Figure 36.8. Induction of right coronary artery (RCA) spasm, angina, and ST-segment elevation by ergonovine maleate and subsequent resolution after sublingual nitroglycerin administration in a patient with variant angina. (From Cheng,[17] with permission.)

as methacholine injection,[63,64] the cold pressor test,[57] atrial pacing[6] (Figure 36.9), and exercise[6,61,62,97] (Figure 36.10), ergonovine testing remains the most sensitive and specific method for diagnosis of CAS[98] and is safe provided there is strict adherence to the protocol just outlined.[99]

HEMODYNAMIC CONSEQUENCES OF CORONARY ARTERY SPASM

Continuous monitoring of patients with variant angina revealed no consistent increase in heart rate, blood pressure, or dP/dt in any patient before the onset of ST-segment elevation.[7] Immediately after ST-segment elevation and chest pain, there was an increase in left ventricular end-diastolic pressure[6] (Figure 36.11).

Reports concerning the effect of coronary spasm on the left ventriculogram have been few. Endo et al[64] observed on left ventriculography that asynergy of the left ventricle appeared during an attack in one patient with variant angina. Yasue et al[8] performed left ventriculography before and during attacks of CAS in four patients. In two patients CAS involved the left anterior descending artery; in the other two patients, it involved the right coronary artery. Left ventriculograms during the attack of CAS revealed marked wall motion abnormalities that involved primarily the anterolateral and apical segments in the two patients who had spasm of the left anterior descending artery and the diaphragmatic and posterobasal segments in the two patients who had spasm of the right coronary artery. An example is shown in Figure 36.12. Spasm appeared at the proximal segment of the left anterior descending artery and occluded it completely. Left ventriculograms at the time of CAS revealed marked wall motion abnormalities involving predominantly the anterolateral and apical segments. In the two patients with spasm of the left anterior descending artery, left ventricular ejection fraction decreased from 82% and 78% before spasm to 56% and 50% during spasm, respectively. In the two patients with spasm of the right coronary artery, ejection fractions were 68% and 64% before spasm and 52% and 59% during spasm, respectively. Therefore, spasm of a large coronary artery resulted in abnormalities

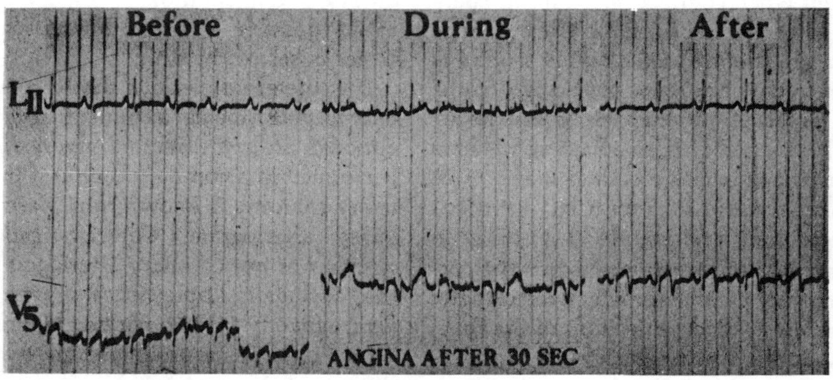

Figure 36.9. Atrial-pacing-induced ST-segment elevation and angina in a patient with variant angina. (From Cheng,[17] with permission.)

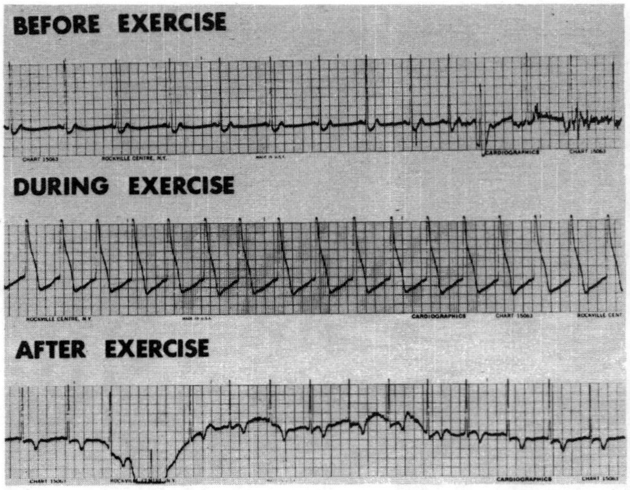

Figure 36.10. Exercise-induced ST-segment elevation in a patient with variant angina whose other electrocardiograms are illustrated in Figure 36.5. Note the inappropriately slow increase in heart rate with exercise. (From Cheng,[17] with permission.)

of segmental wall contraction corresponding to the blood supply distribution of the artery. Spasm of the left anterior descending artery produced a more profound effect on global left ventricular function as reflected by a greater decrease in ejection fraction during spasm than did that of the right coronary artery. Spasm also produces variable degrees of mitral regurgitation[64] due to papillary muscle dysfunction.[6,44,47,100,101] Myocardial ischemia not only alters the contractile properties of the heart but also impairs ventricular relaxation as evidenced by a decreased peak diastolic left ventricular dP/dt.[8]

ROLE OF CALCIUM IN CORONARY ARTERY SPASM

The human epicardial coronary artery is not just a passive conduit through which blood flows, but it is a highly reactive vessel in constant motion with cyclical periods of contraction and relaxation. This phenomenon of vasomotion is most probably a part of the normal process of autoregulation and is a calcium-mediated event.[102] Coronary artery spasm can be regarded as strong contraction of smooth muscle induced by an increase in intracellular calcium ions. Such increases in intracellular calcium ions occur in response to stimulation of the artery with an agonist, such as alpha-adrenergic stimulation with norepinephrine. The calcium ion acts as the excitation signal for the muscle cells of the artery to couple and contract. When the cells are stimulated to contract by any of the neurohormonal substances that have this ability, an influx of calcium takes place. Calcium, on entering the cell through voltage-dependent channels, first binds to calmodulin, a calcium-binding protein in smooth muscle, and the calcium-calmodulin complex activates the enzyme myosin-kinase that catalyzes the transfer of phosphate to myosin. In this form, myosin can interact with actin to produce muscle contraction and arteriolar constriction. Additional receptor-operated Ca^{++} channels can be recruited as a consequence of activation of alpha-adrenergic receptors in the sarcolemma.

CALCIUM CHANNEL BLOCKER THERAPY

From the foregoing description, greatly simplified, it seems obvious that there are several points at which the excitation-contraction coupling by calcium can be interrupted or inhibited. Calcium fluxes can be cut off at the surface of the cell membrane, or within the calcium "slow" channel or channels in this membrane, or between the membrane and the sarcoplasmic reticulum, or in such a way as to prevent release or uptake of calcium by the sarcoplasmic reticulum, or, finally, by preventing the binding of calcium to the regulatory proteins. This basically is what the various calcium channel blockers do. Calcium channel blockers offer a whole new approach to

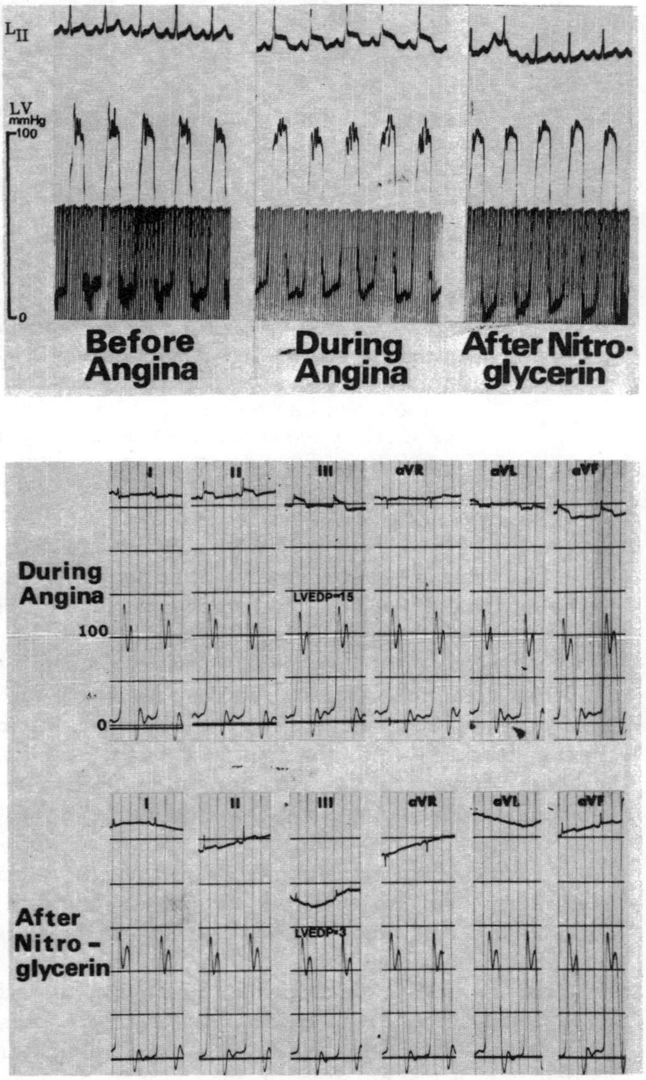

Figure 36.11. Left ventricular (LV) hemodynamic responses before, during, and after an attack of variant angina in two patients. During angina with ST-segment elevation the left ventricular end-diastolic pressure (LVEDP) increased with a concomitant decrease in systolic pressure. (From Cheng et al,[6] by permission of the American Heart Association, Inc.)

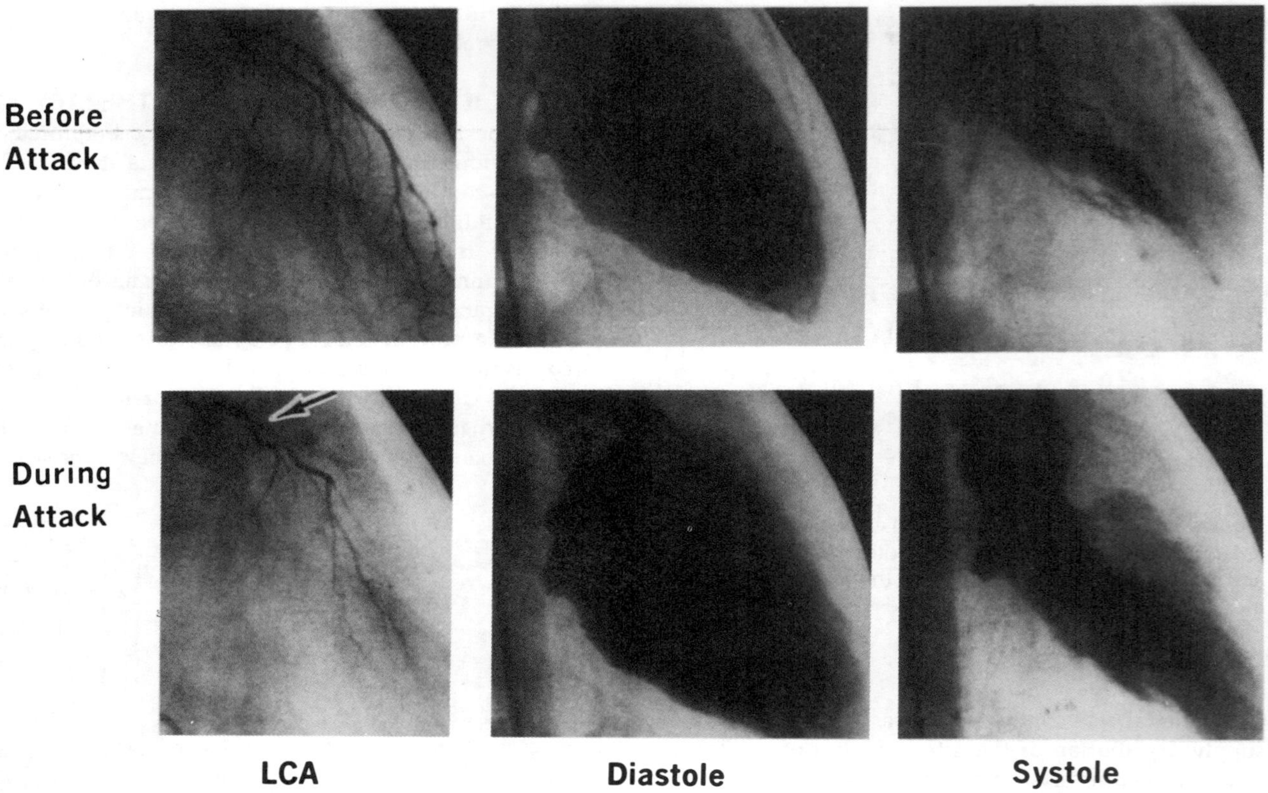

Figure 36.12. Coronary arteriograms and left ventriculograms during coronary artery spasm. Spasm completely occluded the left anterior descending artery at the proximal site (*arrow, lower left panel*). Left ventriculograms revealed marked wall motion abnormalities involving predominantly the anterolateral and apical segments during spasm (*lower middle and right*). The ejection fraction decreased from 82% before spasm to 56% during spasm. The upper panels show the control coronary arteriogram and left ventriculograms. LCA = left coronary arteriogram. (From Yasue,[8] with permission.)

the therapy of CAS. They are a giant step forward in the 1980s in the management of vasospastic angina analogous to the introduction of beta-blockers in the treatment of classical exertional angina in the 1960s.

In the United States three calcium channel blockers are available: nifedipine, verapamil, and diltiazem. Although they are grouped under the general heading of calcium channel blockers, each drug has a different chemical structure—nifedipine, a dihydropyridine derivative; verapamil, a papaverine derivative; diltiazem, a benzothiazepine derivative—and its own specific pharmacologic and pharmacokinetic mechanisms of action and adverse reactions and, therefore, its specific clinical indications and contraindications. However, all three are very effective against CAS.

Nifedipine is effective against CAS in a usual dosage of 30 to 120 mg per day in divided doses every six hours. Its principal side effect is pedal edema due to peripheral vasodilation. It has no effect on the conduction system and can be given safely with beta-blockers and nitrates.

Verapamil is very effective in CAS, especially if there are coexistent supraventricular tachyarrhythmias. The standard dosage is 80 to 480 mg/day in divided doses every six to eight hours. Side effects include constipation, muscle cramps, rash, nausea, and vomiting. It can be given along with nitrates or cautiously with beta-blockers, but it should not be given to patients with conduction disturbances, sinus node dysfunction (vide supra), or congestive heart failure.

Diltiazem is also effective against CAS, and at its usual dosage of 240 to 360 mg/day in divided doses every six hours, it is practically devoid of any adverse reactions. It can be given safely with beta-blockers or nitrates, but it is contraindicated in atrioventricular conduction disease and severe left ventricular failure.

There are other calcium channel blockers, eg, lidoflazine, mioflazine, bepridil, dilazep, nicardipine, nitrendipine, nisoldipine, and tiapamil, that are either being tested in the United States or being used in other countries. However, there is no convincing evidence thus far that would make them competitive with nifedipine, verapamil, and diltiazem.

The effectiveness of calcium channel blockers in treating CAS has now changed the diagnostic approach to patients with Prinzmetal's variant angina. In some centers, the therapeutic response to a calcium channel blocker is frequently used as an alternative to establishing a diagnosis by ergonovine testing. With effective calcium channel blocker therapy, the ergonovine test often gives negative results (Figure 36.13).

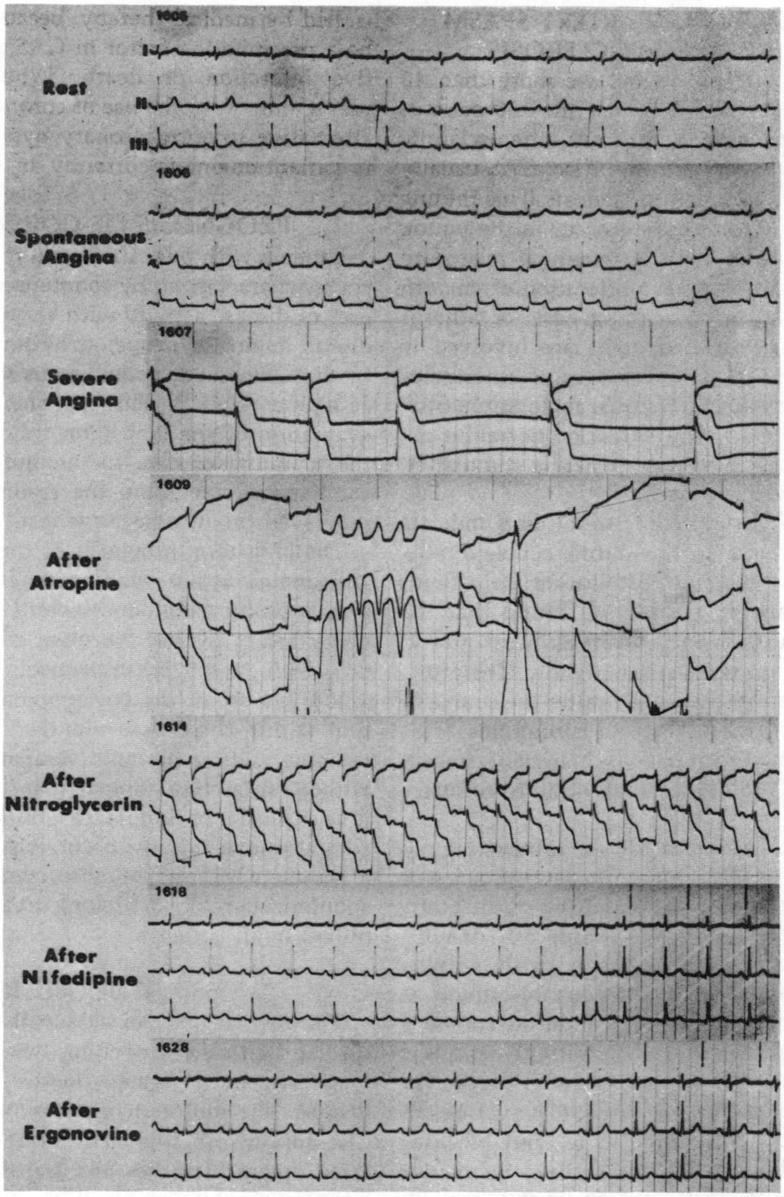

Figure 36.13. During cardiac catheterization (*first panel*) angina and ST-segment elevation spontaneously developed in leads II and III with reciprocal ST-segment depression in lead I due to right coronary artery spasm (*second panel*), accompanied by sinus bradycardia (*third panel*) and ventricular tachycardia (*fourth panel*), unrelieved by two sublingual 0.4-mg nitroglycerin tablets (*fifth panel*), but promptly relieved by chewing 10 mg of nifedipine (*sixth panel*). Thereafter, intravenous ergonovine maleate in incremental doses up to 0.6 mg failed to provoke coronary artery spasm, angina, or electrocardiographic changes (*seventh panel*). The time of each event is indicated in left upper corner of each panel. (From Cheng,[17] with permission.)

USE OF BETA-BLOCKERS IN CORONARY ARTERY SPASM

Patients who have CAS without significant coronary atherosclerosis generally respond exceedingly well to calcium channel blocker therapy. Those who have CAS superimposed on fixed atherosclerotic coronary artery disease may occasionally require the addition of beta-blockers to reduce myocardial oxygen demand. Beta-blockers alone are not effective in the treatment of CAS, and they in fact may exacerbate clinical symptoms by increasing alpha-adrenergic activity. However, if nitrates or calcium channel blockers, or both, are used simultaneously, beta-blockers, especially propranolol because of its antiplatelet effects, may be administered with impunity.

RELATION OF CORONARY ARTERY SPASM TO CORONARY ATHEROSCLEROSIS

Most patients with variant angina are more than 40 years of age (in Yasue's series,[8] 127 of the 130 patients were more than 40) and have significant atherosclerotic stenosis of the large coronary arteries. Also, CAS usually appears at the site of atherosclerotic stenosis. This finding seems to indicate that CAS does not occur in the young and normal coronary artery and is somehow related to atherosclerosis. It is known that proliferation of smooth muscle cells is essential in the pathogenesis of atherosclerosis.[103] All coronary arteries that are involved in spasm may probably be in various stages of atherosclerosis, although some may appear normal angiographically. A recent report indicates that atherosclerotic rabbit arteries are more sensitive to alpha-adrenergic stimulation and ergonovine than normal arteries.[104]

Reports of animals fed high-cholesterol diets indicate that calcium blockers can alter the natural course of atherosclerotic disease.[102] Ginsburg[102] followed up patients on diltiazem more than two years and found that the number of cardiovascular events, such as heart attack, sudden death, and angina, decreased markedly. Therefore, calcium channel blockers may actually alter the course of the disease process as well as relieve symptoms. This observation assumes a new significance in light of a recent report that prolonged CAS may actually lead to coronary atherosclerosis.[105]

Marzilli et al[105] recently reported on an interesting patient whose spontaneous CAS 8 months later progressed to fixed arteriosclerotic narrowing, requiring coronary artery bypass surgery. However, angiographically demonstrable CAS could be provoked repeatedly by the administration of intracoronary or intravenous histamine to miniature swine with experimentally induced coronary atherosclerosis and would subside after nitroglycerin was given or be prevented by a calcium channel blocker or an agent that blocks histamine H_1 receptors such as diphenhydramine, but not a histamine H_2 receptor blocking agent such as cimetidine.[106] Therefore, two distinctive mechanisms are currently postulated to be involved in the pathogenesis of ischemic coronary heart disease: (1) fixed organic obstruction by progressive atherosclerosis of the coronary arteries, and (2) dynamic functional obstruction by transient coronary vasospasm. Heretofore, these two mechanisms have been thought to be unrelated. Now it has been well shown not only that fixed atherosclerotic narrowing can often be a nidus for superimposed coronary vasospasm, but also that coronary spasm itself can lead to subsequent development of fixed atherosclerotic coronary obstructions.

SURGICAL THERAPY OF CORONARY ARTERY SPASM

Medical therapy is the treatment of choice in patients with documented or presumed CAS irrespective of the presence or absence of significant atherosclerotic stenosis. Coronary artery bypass grafting may be indicated in those patients with significant atherosclerotic lesions and resultant organic stenoses.[107] However, the operation should be deferred until spasm has been completely controlled by medical therapy, because operation itself may be a precipitating factor in CAS, resulting in perioperative infarction or death. Whether the addition of plexectomy[108] or the use of coronary angioplasty[109] as an alternative to aortocoronary bypass surgery is effective in variant angina is currently an unsettled issue.

PROGNOSIS OF CORONARY SPASM

Patients with pure CAS tend to have a chronic clinical course characterized by spontaneous variations in the degree of disease activity with varying degrees of disability due to angina, syncope, arrhythmia, and myocardial infarction. However, spontaneous remission is frequent, in as high as 45%.[110] This fact should be considered in an evaluation of the long-term results of treatment and in the planning of care for an individual patient; during spontaneous remission the ergonovine provocative test may even produce negative results.[111,112]

The long-term prognosis of treated patients with variant angina is not yet known, but it seems to depend greatly on the extent and severity of existing organic coronary artery disease. Survival at 1, 2, and 3 years was 95%, 90%, and 87%, respectively.[113] These patients have a 20% chance of the development of myocardial infarction within the first 3 months.[7,113] Treatment with nifedipine, diltiazem, and verapamil improved survival without infarction compared to treatment with perhexiline maleate or long-acting nitrates alone.[113] Because complications usually occur within the first 3 months after diagnosis and because symptoms often disappear spontaneously,[111,113] lifelong treatment may not be required in all patients.

CONCLUSION

The revival of CAS as a pathogenetic mechanism in cardiac ischemia is opening new horizons for research, diagnosis, and treatment in the field of ischemic heart disease. The clinical manifestations of ischemic heart disease appear to be the result of a variable combination of fixed organic stenoses and transient functional changes in the coronary lumen resulting from vasoconstriction and intravascular obstruction by blood elements. Variant angina represents only one aspect of a continuous spectrum of vasospastic myocardial ischemia. At one end of the spectrum is a normal coronary artery that is so susceptible to vasoconstrictive stimuli that spasm can be elicited by a host of stimuli, even of relatively low intensity; this hypersensitivity is efficiently reduced by nitrates and calcium channel blockers. At the other end of the spectrum is advanced coronary atherosclerosis that may be so severe as to require coronary bypass surgery for effective myocardial revascularization. In between these two extremes exist various combinations of the two. The triggering stimuli responsible for local vascular hypersensitivity remain to be elucidated, although recent studies which eliminated potential suspects such as alpha-adrenergic stimuli,[114] thromboxane,[115] prostacyclin deficiency,[116] and serotonin[117] seem to narrow the field in the search for the elusive underlying mechanism. The recent finding that coronary tissue from cardiac patients contains stores of histamine that are substantially increased above values in noncardiac patients suggests that a sudden release of vasoactive material due to injury, platelet aggregation,[118,119] or an "allergic" response as occurs in an antigen-antibody type reaction, could be responsible for CAS.[120] The recent report from Japan on selective thromboxane A_2 synthetase inhibition in vasospastic angina may also have important clinical implications.[121]

REFERENCES

1. Cheng TO: The click-murmur syndrome. A medical pendulum and a unifying concept. *Chest* 1976; 70:569–572.
2. Osler W: Lumleian lectures on angina pectoris. *Lancet* 1910; 1:697–702.
3. Blumgart HL, Schlesinger MJ, Davis D: Studies on the relation of the clinical manifestations of angina pectoris, coronary thrombosis, and myocardial infarction to the pathologic findings with particular reference to the significance of the collateral circulation. *Am Heart J* 1940; 19:1–91.
4. French AJ, Dock W: Fatal coronary arteriosclerosis in young soldiers. *JAMA* 1944; 124:1233–1237.
5. Prinzmetal M, Kennamer R, Merliss R, Wada T, Bor N: Angina pectoris. I. A variant form of angina pectoris. Preliminary report. *Am J Med* 1959; 27:375–388.
6. Cheng TO, Bashour T, Kelser GA, Weiss L, Bacos J: Variant angina of Prinzmetal with normal coronary arteriograms. A variant of the variant. *Circulation* 1973; 47:476–485.
7. Maseri A, Severi S, Nes MD, L'Abbate A, Chierchia S, Marzilli M, Ballestra AM, Parodi O, Biasini A, Distante A: Variant angina, one aspect of a continuous spectrum of vasospastic myocardial ischemia. Pathogenetic mechanisms, estimated incidence and clinical and coronary arteriographic findings in 139 patients. *Am J Cardiol* 1978; 42:1019–1035.
8. Yasue H: Electrocardiographic, hemodynamic and angiographic consequences, in Chahine RA (ed): *Coronary Artery Spasm*. Mt Kisco, NY, Futura Publishing Co, 1983, pp 85–118.
9. Yasue H, Omote S, Takizawa A, Masao N, Hyon H, Nishida S, Horie M: Comparison of coronary arteriographic findings during angina pectoris associated with ST elevation or depression. *Am J Cardiol* 1981; 47:539–546.
10. AHA Committee Report: A reporting system on patients evaluated for coronary artery disease. *Circulation* 1975; 51(April):5.
11. Ekmekci A, Toyoshima H, Kwoczynski JK, Nagaya T, Prinzmetal M: Angina pectoris. IV. Clinical and experimental difference between ischemia with ST elevation and ischemia with ST depression. *Am J Cardiol* 1961; 7:412–426.
12. MacAlpin RN, Kattus A, Alvaro AB: Angina pectoris at rest with preservation of exercise capacity. Prinzmetal's variant angina. *Circulation* 1973; 47:946–958.
13. Shubrooks SJ, Bete JM, Hutter AM, Block PC, Buckley MJ, Dagget WM, Mundth ED: Variant angina pectoris: Clinical and anatomic spectrum and results of coronary bypass surgery. *Am J Cardiol* 1975; 36:142–147.
14. Endo M, Kanda I, Hosoda S, Hayashi H, Hirosawa K, Konno S: Prinzmetal's variant form of angina pectoris. Re-evaluation of mechanisms. *Circulation* 1975; 52:33–37.
15. Selzer A, Langston M, Ruggeroli C, Cohn K: Clinical syndrome of variant angina with normal coronary arteriogram. *N Engl J Med* 1976; 295:1343–1347.
16. Heupler F: Syndrome of symptomatic coronary arterial spasm with nearly normal coronary arteriograms. *Am J Cardiol* 1980; 45:873–881.
17. Cheng TO: Coronary artery spasm — 1984. *Chest* 1984; 86:918–926.
18. MacAlpin RN: Relation of coronary arterial spasm to sites of organic stenosis. *Am J Cardiol* 1980; 46:143–153.
19. Kimura E, Kishida H: Treatment of variant angina with drugs: A survey of 11 cardiology institutes in Japan. *Circulation* 1981; 63:844–848.
20. Kimura E: Variant form of angina pectoris. Its clinical features and treatment. *Jpn Heart J* 1980; 21:131–139.
21. Schroeder JS, Feldman RL, Giles TD, Friedman MJ, DeMaria AN, Kinney EL, Mallon SM, Pitt B, Meyer R, Basta LL, Curry RC, Groves BM, MacAlpin RN: Multiclinic controlled trial of diltiazem for Prinzmetal's angina. *Am J Med* 1982; 72:227–232.
22. Miller D, Waters DD, Warnica W, Szlachcic J, Kreeft J, Theroux P: Is variant angina the coronary manifestation of a generalized vasospastic disorder? *N Engl J Med* 1981; 304:763–766.
23. Bertrand ME, Lablanche JM, Tilmant PY, Thieuleux FA: Le spasme arteriel coronaire. A propos de 165 observations. *Arch Mal Coeur* 1983; 76:713–721.
24. Kaltenbach M, Krehan L, Kober G, Becker H-J: Coronarographic findings in patients with ST elevation in exercise ECG and Prinzmetal angina, in Lichtlen PR (ed): *Coronary Angiography and Angina Pectoris*. Stuttgart, Germany, Georg Thieme, 1976, pp 76–83.
25. Burkart F: Die medikamentose Therapie der Angina Pectoris. *Schweiz Med Wachenschr* 1983; 113:1898–1903.
26. Dart AM, Alban-Davis H, Lowndes RH, Dalal JJ, Ruttley MR, Henderson AH: Ergometrine induced 'angina'—a diagnostic pitfall. *Br Heart J* 1980; 43:104.
27. Sandoe E, Vilhelmsen R, Efsen F: Prinzmetal's variant angina. *Acta Med Scand [Suppl]* 1981; 644:34–41.
28. Khomaziuk AI: Spazm koronarnykh sosudov (obzor literatury). *Vrach Delo* 1983; 12(December):10–18.
29. Drory Y, Kariv I: Variant (Prinzmetal) angian pectoris. *Harefuah* 1982; 103:163–168.
30. Opolski G, Korewicki J, Ostrzycki A, Stanislawska J, Zielenski T: Wykorzystanie proby z ergonowina do diagnostyki i oceny terapii anginy Prinzmetala. *Kardiol Pol* 1982; 25:485–489.
31. Delcan Dominguez JL, Abeytua Jimenez M: Diagnostico y tratamiento de la angina vasoespastica. *Rev Esp Cardiol* 1982; 35:(pt II) 43–51.
32. Maze SS, Opie LH, Lloyd EA: The role of coronary artery spasm in anginal syndromes. *S Afr Med J* 1982; 61:161–164.
33. Brown JM, Radford DJ: Coronary artery spasm causing myocardial infarction and ventricular fibrillation. *Med J Aust* 1981; 2:34–36.
34. Girotti AL, Rutitzky B, Schmidberg J, Crosatto J, Rosenbaum MB: Spontaneous remission in variant angina. *Br Heart J* 1981; 45:517–521.
35. Cheng TO: Cardiology in People's Republic of China — Paul D. White Lecture, in Russek HI (ed): *New Horizons in Cardiovascular Practice*. Baltimore, University Park Press, 1975, pp 1–27.
36. Gong LS, Qian JA, Wang GY: Variant angina complicated by third-degree A-V block and Adams-Stokes syndrome. *Shanghai Med J* 1980; 3:119.
37. Chen Z, Bai M, Xu Y, Yao K, Chen K, Tao S: The role of coronary arterial spasm in the progress of coronary heart disease. *Chin J Intern Med* 1981; 20:412–414.
38. Keys A (ed): Coronary heart disease in seven countries. *Circulation* 1970; 41(suppl I): I-1–I-211.
39. Kimura N, Nakayama Y: Natural history of heart disease from epidemiological investigation. *Jpn Circ J* 1972; 36:11–14.
40. Cheng TO: Cardiology in China revisited. *Am J Cardiol* 1978; 42:700–702.
41. Cheng TO, Bashour T, Singh BK, Kelser GA: Myocardial infarction in the absence of coronary arteriosclerosis: result of coronary spasm(?). *Am J Cardiol* 1972; 30:680–682.
42. Lange RL, Reid MS, Tresch DD, Keelan MH, Bernhard VM, Coolidge G: Nonatheromatous ischemic heart disease following withdrawal from chronic industrial nitroglycerin exposure. *Circulation* 1972; 46:666–678.
43. Bashour TT, Kabbani SS, Brewster HP, Wald SH, Hanna ES, Cheng TO: Transient Q waves and reversible cardiac failure during myocardial ischemia: electrical and mechanical stunning of the heart. *Am Heart J* 1983; 106:780–783.
44. Cheng TO: Mitral valve prolapse and coronary artery spasm. *Br Heart J* 1982; 48:301.
45. Rippe JM, Singh JB, Jarvais N, Adams E, Erkkila K: Mitral valve prolapse and spasm of normal coronary arteries: report of four cases and review of the literature. *Angiology* 1984; 35:300–307.
46. Cheng TO: Primary versus secondary mitral valve prolapse. *Am Heart J* 1981; 102:946.
47. Cheng TO: Late systolic murmur in coronary artery disease. *Chest* 1972; 61:346–356.
48. Chierchia S: The role of alpha-adrenergic receptors in the pathogenesis of coronary spasm. *Clin Cardiol* 1983; 6:496–500.
49. Bashour TT, Hakim O, Cheng TO: Coronary spastic angina in middle-aged women: a psychosomatic disorder? *Am Heart J* 1983; 106:609–613.
50. Shepherd JT, Vanhoutte PM: Spasm of the coronary arteries: causes and consequences (the scientist's viewpoint). *Mayo Clin Proc* 1985; 60:33–46.
51. MacAlpin RN: Is coronary artery spasm causing your patient's angina? *Mod Med* 1979; 47:32–46.
52. Conti CR: Coronary artery spasm. *Cardiovasc Rev Rep* 1980; 1:17–26.
53. Bashour TT, Hakim O, Ennis AL, Cheng TO: Coronary artery spasm with sinus node dysfunction and syncope. *Arch Intern Med* 1982; 142:1719–1721.
54. Bashour TT, Kabbani SS, Brewster HP, Wald SH, Hanna ES, Cheng TO: Sinus node dysfunction during coronary vasospastic angina. *Am Heart J* 1984; 108:1056–1059.
55. Cheng TO: Transvenous ventricular pacing in the treatment of paroxysmal atrial tachyarrhythmias alternating with sinus bradycardia and standstill. *Am J Cardiol* 1968; 22:875–879.
56. Hilal H, Massumi R: Variant angina pectoris. *Am J Cardiol* 1967; 19:607–608.

57. Raizner AE, Chahine RA, Ishimori T, Verani MS, Zacca N, Jamal N, Miller RR, Luchi RJ: Provocation of coronary artery spasm by the cold pressor test. Hemodynamic, arteriographic and quantitative angiographic observation. *Circulation* 1980; 62:925–932.
58. Yasue H, Nagao M, Omote S, Takizawa A, Miwa K, Tanaka S: Coronary arterial spasm and Prinzmetal's variant form of angina induced by hyperventilation and Tris-buffer infusion. *Circulation* 1978; 58:56–62.
59. Hisano K, Matsuguchi T, Ootsubo H, Nakagaki O, Tomoike H, Takeshita A, Nakamura M: Hyperventilation-induced variant angina with ventricular tachycardia. *Am Heart J* 1984; 108:423–425.
60. Yasue H, Omote S, Takizawa A, Nagao M, Nosaka K, Nakajima H: Alkalosis-induced coronary vasoconstriction: effects of calcium, diltiazem, nitroglycerin and propranolol. *Am Heart J* 1981; 102:206–210.
61. Yasue H, Omote S, Takizawa N, Nago M, Miwa K, Tanaka S: Exertional angina pectoris caused by coronary arterial spasm: effects of various drugs. *Am J Cardiol* 1979; 43:647–652.
62. Specchia G, De Servi S, Falcone C, Bramucci E, Angoli L, Mussini A, Marinoni GP, Montemartini C, Bobba P: Coronary arterial spasm as a cause of exercise-induced ST-segment elevation in patients with variant angina. *Circulation* 1979; 59:948–954.
63. Yasue H, Touyama M, Shimamoto M, Kato H, Tanaka S, Akiyama F: Role of autonomic nervous system in the pathogenesis of Prinzmetal's variant form of angina. *Circulation* 1974; 50:534–539.
64. Endo M, Hirosawa K, Kaneko N, Hase K, Inoue Y, Konno S: Prinzmetal's variant angina. Coronary arteriogram and left ventriculogram during attack induced by methacholine. *N Engl J Med* 1976; 294:252–255.
65. Yasue H, Touyama M, Kato H, Tanaka S, Akiyama F: Prinzmetal's variant form of angina as a manifestation of alpha-adrenergic receptor-mediated coronary arterial spasm: documentation by coronary arteriography. *Am Heart J* 1976; 91:148–155.
66. Cheng TO: Ergotrate in coronary artery spasm. *Circulation* 1976; 53:585–586.
67. Yasue H, Omote S, Takizawa A, Nagao M: Acute myocardial infarction induced by ergotamine tartrate: possible role of coronary arterial spasm. *Angiology* 1981; 32:414–418.
68. Schachne JS, Roberts BH, Thompson PD: Coronary artery spasm and myocardial infarction associated with cocaine use. *N Engl J Med* 1984; 310:1665–1666.
69. Kossowsky WA, Lyon AF: Cocaine and acute myocardial infarction. A probable connection. *Chest* 1984; 86:729–731.
70. Jugdutt BI, Stevens GF, Zacks DJ, Lee SJK, Taylor RF: Myocardial infarction, oral contraception, cigarette smoking and coronary artery spasm in young women. *Am Heart J* 1983; 106:757–761.
71. Maouad J, Fernandez F, Barrillon A, Gerbaux A, Gay J: Diffuse or segmental narrowing (spasm) of the coronary arteries during smoking demonstrated on angiography. *Am J Cardiol* 1984; 53:354–355.
72. Fernandez D, Rosenthal JE, Cohen LS, Hammond G, Wolfson S: Alcohol-induced Prinzmetal variant angina. *Am J Cardiol* 1973; 32:238–239.
73. Arikawa K, Kashima T, Imamura M, Ariyama T, Tanaka H: Alcohol-induced Prinzmetal's variant angina. *J Jpn Coll Angiol* 1980; 20:265–267.
74. Takizawa A, Yasue H, Omote S, Nagao M, Hyon H, Nashida S, Horie M: Variant angina induced by alcohol ingestion. *Am Heart J* 1984; 107:25–27.
75. Ohmori M, Tada M, Kuzuya T, Yamagishi M, Matsuda H, Inoue M, Abe H, Kodama K: Thromboxane A_2 as a precipitating factor in coronary arterial spasm of variant angina. *Circulation* 1983; 68:III–22.
76. Zuberbuhler RC, Bohr DF: Response of coronary smooth muscle to catecholamines. *Circ Res* 1965; 16:431–440.
77. Bohr DF: Adrenergic receptors in coronary arteries. *Ann NY Acad Sci* 1967; 39:799–807.
78. Yasue H: Pathophysiology and treatment of coronary arterial spasm. *Chest* 1980; 78:216–223.
79. Cheng TO: Against routine use of atropine during coronary arteriography. *Cathet Cardiovasc Diagn* 1981; 7:459.
80. Yasue H, Omote S, Takizawa A, Nagao M, Miwa K, Tanaka S: Circadian variation of exercise capacity in patients with Prinzmetal's variant angina: role of exercise-induced coronary arterial spasm. *Circulation* 1979; 59:938–948.
81. Brazenor RM, Angus JA: Ergometrine contracts isolated canine coronary arteries by a serotonergic mechanism: no role for alpha adrenoceptors. *J Pharmacol Exp Ther* 1981; 218:530–536.
82. Bentley KI, Henry PD: Serotonin, a potent constrictor of human coronary artery. *Circulation* 1981; 64:446A.
83. Yokoyama M, Henry PD: Supersensitivity of atherosclerotic arteries to ergonovine partially mediated by a serotonergic mechanism. *Circulation* 1979; 59-60 (suppl II): II–387.
84. De Caterina R, Carpeggiani C, L'Abbate A: A double-blind, placebo-controlled study of ketanserin in patients with Prinzmetal's angina. Evidence against a role for serotonin in the genesis of coronary vasospasm. *Circulation* 1984; 69:889–894.
84a. Vane J: Prostacyclin—From discovery to clinic. *Circulation* 1985; 72 (suppl. III):IIIB–IIIC.
85. Robertson RM, Robertson D, Friesinger GC, Timmons S, Hawiger J: Platelet aggregates in peripheral and coronary sinus blood in patients with spontaneous coronary artery spasm. *Lancet* 1980; 2:829–831.
85a. Ogasawara K, Aizawa T, Nishimura K, Satoh H, Fujii J, Katoh K: Beta-thromboglobulin release within coronary circulation—a potential role of platelets in ergonovine-induced coronary vasospasm. *Intern J Cardiol* 1986; 10:15–22.
86. Yui Y, Hattori R, Takatsu Y, Kadota K, Kambara H, Nakajima H, Murakami T, Kawai C: Is increased coronary sinus thromboxane A_2 production a cause or a result of vasospastic angina? *Circulation* 1983; 68:III–397.
87. Miwa K, Kambara H, Kawai C: Effect of aspirin in large doses on attacks of variant angina. *Am Heart J* 1983; 105:351–355.
88. Cheng TO: Angina aggravator. *Mod Med* 1983; 51:234.
89. Vane JR: Prostaglandins and the cardiovascular system. *Br Heart J* 1983; 49:405–409.
90. Kronenberg MW, Robertson RM, Born ML, Steckley RA, Robertson D, Friesinger GC: Thallium-201 uptake in variant angina. Probable demonstration of myocardial reactive hyperemia in man. *Circulation* 1982; 66:1332–1338.
91. Araki H, Koiwaya Y, Nakagaki O, Nakamura M: Diurnal distribution of ST-segment elevation and related arrhythmias in patients with variant angina: a study by ambulatory ECG monitoring. *Circulation* 1983; 67:995–1000.
92. Waters DD, Miller DD, Bouchard A, Bosch X, Theroux P: Circadian variation in variant angina. *Am J Cardiol* 1984; 54:61–64.
93. Cheng TO: Esophageal function in patients with angina and normal coronary arteriograms. *Ann Surg* 1984; 119:123.
94. Miwa K, Murakami T, Kambara H, Kawai C: U wave inversion during attacks of variant angina. *Br Heart J* 1983; 50:378–382.
95. Matsuguchi T, Koiwaya Y, Nakagaki O, Takeshita A, Nakamura M: Transient U wave inversion during variant angina. *Am Heart J* 1984; 108:899–904.
96. Rovai D, Distante A, Moscarelli E, Morales MA, Picano E, Palombo C, L'Abbate A: Transient myocardial ischemia with minimal electrocardiographic changes: an echocardiographic study in patients with Prinzmetal's angina. *Am Heart J* 1985; 109:78–83.
97. Sato I, Tomobuchi Y, Funahashi T, Ohe T, Kamakura S, Matsuhisa M, Haze K, Shimomura K: Poor responsiveness of heart rate to treadmill exercise in vasospastic angina. *Clin Cardiol* 1985; 8:206–212.
98. Waters DD, Szlachcic J, Bonan R, Miller DD, Dauwe F, Theroux P: Comparative sensitivity of exercise, cold pressor and ergonovine testing in provoking attacks of variant angina in patients with active disease. *Circulation* 1983; 67:310–315.
99. Cheng TO: Irreversible coronary occlusion and ergonovine. *Circulation* 1982; 65:640.
100. Cheng TO: Some new observations on the syndrome of papillary muscle dysfunction. *Am J Med* 1969; 47:924–945.
101. Cheng TO: Coronary artery spasm. *Chin J Intern Med* 1984; 23:179–184.
102. Ginsburg R: Coronary artery spasm: clinical experience and implications. *Hosp Pract* 1983; 18:165–176.
103. Ross R, Glomset JA: The pathogenesis of atherosclerosis. *N Engl J Med* 1976; 295:369–377.
104. Yokoyama M, Goldman M, Henry PD: Supersensitivity of atherosclerotic rabbit arteries to α-adrenergic stimulation and ergonovine. *Circulation* 1978; 58(suppl II): II-57.
105. Marzilli M, Goldstein S, Trivella MG, Palumbo C, Maseri A: Some clinical considerations regarding the relation of coronary vasospasm to coronary atherosclerosis: a hypothetical pathogenesis. *Am J Cardiol* 1980; 45:882–886.
106. Shimokawa H, Tomoike H, Nabeyama S, Yamamoto H, Araki H, Nakamura M, Ishii Y, Tanaka K: Coronary artery spasm induced in atherosclerotic miniature swine. *Science* 1983; 221:560–562.
107. Johnson AD, Stroud HA, Vieweg WVR, Ross J: Coronary angiographic patterns and results of medical and surgical therapy in 42 consecutive patients with variant angina pectoris, in Kaltenbach M, Lichtlen P, Balcon R, Bussman W (eds): *Coronary Heart Disease*, 3rd International Symposium, Frankfurt. Stuttgart, Germany, Georg Thieme, 1978, pp 181–190.
108. Bertrand ME, Lablanche JM, Rousseau MF, Warembourg HH, Stankowtak C, Soots G: Surgical treatment of variant angina: Use of plexectomy with aortocoronary bypass. *Circulation* 1980; 61:877–882.
109. Corcos T, David PR, Bourassa MG, Val PG, Robert J, Mata LA, Waters DD: Percutaneous transluminal coronary angioplasty for the treatment of variant angina. *J Am Coll Cardiol* 1985; 5:1046–1054.
110. Waters DD, Bouchard A, Theroux P: Spontaneous remission is a frequent outcome of variant angina. *J Am Coll Cardiol* 1983; 2:195–199.
111. Waters DD, Szlachcic J, Theroux P, Dauwe F, Mizgala HF: Ergonovine testing to detect spontaneous remissions of variant angina during long-term treatment with calcium antagonist drugs. *Am J Cardiol* 1981; 47:179–184.

112. Dalal JJ, Griffiths BE, Ruttley MST, Henderson AH: Remission of coronary spasm confirmed by angiography and ergometrine provocation: two case reports. *Eur Heart J* 1981; 2:475–478.
113. Waters DD, Miller DD, Szlachcic J, Bouchard A, Methe M, Kreeft J, Theroux P: Factors influencing the long-term prognosis of treated patients with variant angina. *Circulation* 1983; 68:258–265.
114. Chierchia S, Davies G, Berkenboom G, Crea F, Crean P, Maseri A: α-Adrenergic receptors and coronary spasm: an elusive link. *Circulation* 1984; 69:8–14.
115. Chierchia S, de Caterina R, Crea F, Patrono C, Maseri A: Failure of thromboxane A_2 blockade to prevent attacks of vasospastic angina. *Circulation* 1982; 66:702–705.
116. Chierchia S, Patrono C, Crea F, Ciabattoni G, De Caterina R, Cinotti GA, Distante A, Maseri A: Effects of intravenous prostacyclin in variant angina. *Circulation* 1982; 65:470–477.
117. Freedman SB, Chierchia S, Rodriguez-Plaza L, Bugiardini R, Smith G, Maseri A: Ergonovine-induced myocardial ischemia: no role for serotonergic receptors? *Circulation* 1984; 70:178–183.
118. Mullane KM, Bradley G, Moncada S: The interactions of platelet-derived mediators on isolated canine coronary arteries. *Eur J Pharmacol* 1982; 84:115–118.
119. Moulds RFW, Iwanov V, Young MJ: Vasoactive effects of platelet aggregates. *N Engl J Med* 1984; 311:198–199.
120. Kalsner S, Richards R: Coronary arteries of cardiac patients are hyperreactive and contain stores of amines: a mechanism for coronary spasm. *Science* 1984; 223:1435–1437.
121. Yui Y, Hattori R, Takatsu Y, Kawai C: Selective thromboxane A_2 synthetase inhibition in vasospastic angina pectoris. *J Am Coll Cardiol* 1986; 7:25–29.

37 Percutaneous Transluminal Coronary Angioplasty

Peter C. Block, MD

HISTORY OF ANGIOPLASTY

Angioplasty was the term used by Dotter and Judkins[1] in 1964 to describe the use of a coaxial catheter system for dilation of atherosclerotic peripheral arteries. With this technique, a wire guide is advanced through the atherosclerotic stenosis. An 8F catheter is then followed over the wire guide and finally a 12F catheter is introduced over the 8F catheter, gradually dilating the atherosclerotic stenosis. Staple[2] later developed a single 8F or 10F catheter with a gradually tapering tip, which produced the same result. However, high complication rates, such as intimal damage to arteries at the site of stenosis and local complications at the insertion site of large catheters, were common and therefore the technique never gained wide acceptance.

Zeitler et al[3] used the procedure extensively in Germany. The technique was modified by Gruentzig and Hopff[4] who developed a balloon dilation catheter; a noncompliant balloon attached near the tip allowed a small catheter to be introduced percutaneously. This development diminished the rate of complications at the insertion site and still allowed wide dilation of any atherosclerotic stenosis. The balloon could be inflated to a predetermined outer diameter at a pressure of 4 to 5 atm, but the balloon did not expand beyond that. This catheter could traverse more stenotic segments of peripheral vessels, and it produced a lateral force against the atherosclerotic plaque as balloon inflation occurred, rather than the combination longitudinal/lateral force that was produced by earlier coaxial catheter systems (Figure 37.1). Initial and follow-up studies in 1977 in patients who had undergone angioplasty of peripheral atherosclerotic lesions[5] established this therapeutic technique as effective treatment for atherosclerotic stenoses in the iliofemoral vasculature.

Miniaturization of catheters to sizes that allow passage through stenotic coronary arteries was a prerequisite for transluminal coronary angioplasty. Because the normal size of most proximal coronary arteries is between 3 and 4 mm, most stenoses that are hemodynamically significant are less than 1.5 mm in diameter. Guiding catheters are needed so that the small dilating balloon catheters can be introduced into the appropriate coronary artery (Figure 37.1). Animal experiments[6] showed that transluminal coronary angioplasty could be performed with safety and demonstrated its feasibility for use in human subjects.

Coronary angioplasty was performed first in vivo at distal coronary artery stenoses at the time of coronary artery bypass graft surgery. A short dilating catheter was introduced into the open coronary artery during bypass surgery and was passed through distal coronary stenoses. Dilations were successful, without the development of myocardial infarction or peripheral embolization. Embolization of atherosclerotic material occurs in about 3%

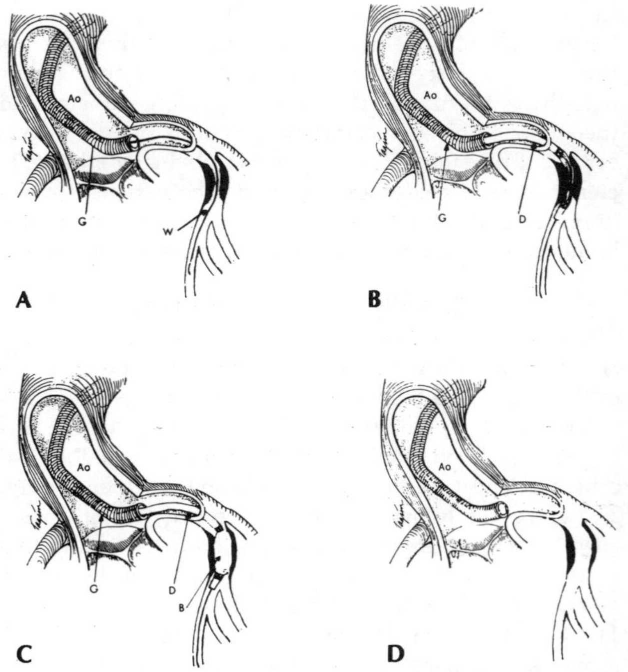

Figure 37.1. Schematic drawing of percutaneous transluminal coronary angioplasty. *A*, The guiding catheter (G) is positioned at the coronary ostium and the steerable wire guide (W) is passed through the stenosis and into the distal coronary artery. *B*, The dilating catheter (D) is then passed over the wire guide and through the stenotic segment so that the dilating balloon lies within the area of stenosis. *C*, The balloon (B) is inflated. *D*, The balloon is deflated and the dilating catheter is removed. Repeat angiography is then performed to evaluate the size of the improved lumen. Ao = aorta. Compare with Figure 37.2.

of angioplasties performed in peripheral arteries,[5] but this is not a clinical problem for coronary angioplasty. Gruentzig performed the first percutaneous transluminal coronary angioplasty (PTCA) in 1977 in Switzerland. His preliminary communication[7] initiated widespread clinical investigation and further development of the technique into an effective treatment for coronary atherosclerotic stenoses in certain patients with angina pectoris.

TECHNIQUE

Careful evaluation of a coronary stenosis to determine if it is treatable by angioplasty is important. During cineangiographic evaluation, intravenous nitroglycerin should be given to evaluate the stenotic area more completely and to exclude the possibility that coronary spasm is responsible for the patient's symptoms.

Following coronary angiography, a guiding catheter is introduced percutaneously in place of the angiographic catheter. This can be done at the puncture site of the femoral artery (or brachial artery using a cutdown procedure). The guiding catheter is advanced under fluoroscopic control to the appropriate coronary ostium. Pressure monitoring from the tip of the guiding catheter allows the operator to avoid occluding the coronary orifice with the catheter tip, assuring adequate coronary flow as the dilating catheter is introduced subselectively through the guiding catheter and into the coronary circulation.

The dilating catheter, within which is a movable, steerable wire guide, is advanced through the guiding catheter. The wire guide is then carefully advanced under fluoroscopic control down the appropriate coronary artery and through the coronary stenosis. It is passed distally into the coronary circulation, avoiding entrance into side branches. The dilating balloon catheter is then advanced over the wire guide. This technique minimizes the risk of plaque dissection or perforation (Figure 37.1). If a balloon catheter must be exchanged after the coronary stenosis is traversed, the use of a long exchange wire to accomplish this minimizes the risk of plaque dissection. Contrast medium can be injected intermittently through the dilating catheter or the guiding catheter at the coronary orifice as the wire guide is advanced to and through the coronary stenosis to assure its proper position. This allows precise positioning of the balloon within the coronary stenosis before the balloon is inflated (Figure 37.1). Balloon diameters used in the coronary circulation vary between 2 and 3.7 mm. Selection of balloon size is important so that the diameter of the undiseased portion of the coronary artery adjacent to the stenosis is not exceeded by the diameter of the inflated dilating balloon, thereby minimizing overstretching of the vessel and the risk of vessel rupture.[8] The maximum outer diameter of most PTCA balloons is reached when the pressure within the balloon is approximately 5 atm. Higher inflation pressures may slightly deform some balloons and expand them further, although the change is small.

The dilating balloon is inflated with a mixture of contrast material and 5% dextrose in water, allowing fluoroscopic visualization and cineangiographic recording of balloon inflation and deflation (Figure 37.2). If intracoronary pressure is measured from the tip of the dilating catheter, the pressure decreases as the tip of the catheter crosses the coronary stenosis and enters the artery distal to the stenosis (Figure 37.3). Once the balloon is positioned at the coronary stenosis, a small amount of contrast material can be injected into the distal coronary artery through the dilating catheter or through the guiding catheter to document both the intraluminal position of the dilating catheter tip and its precise position within the coronary stenosis. Inflation of the balloon to 4 to 6 atm usually allows full balloon expansion. The balloon should be kept inflated for at least 15 seconds and preferably 30 to 60 seconds. Longer inflation times may diminish the elastic recoil of the outer layers of the coronary artery and improve the initial as well as the long-term results. If the plaque is resistant and the balloon does not expand fully at 4 to 6 atm, a second inflation with higher pressures to 10 to 12 atm almost always succeeds in inflating the balloon fully even when calcium is present in the arterial wall.

After deflation of the dilating balloon, pressure in the distal coronary artery increases as blood flow is restored (Figure 37.3). One measure of the success of the PTCA procedure is an increase in distal coronary perfusion pressure compared with the pre-PTCA pressure (a loss of the

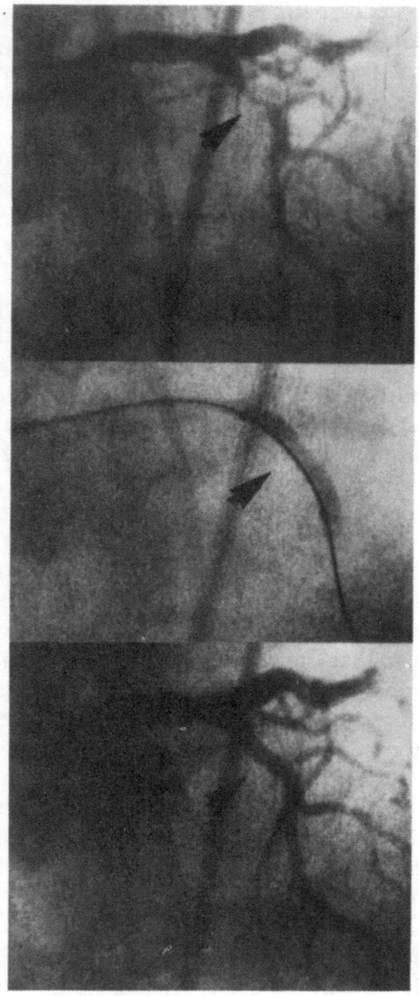

Figure 37.2. Frames from a left anterior oblique coronary cineangiogram taken before, during balloon inflation, and after percutaneous transluminal coronary angioplasty (PTCA). *A*, The coronary stenosis (*arrow*) is in the midportion of the left anterior descending coronary artery. *B*, The dilating balloon is inflated within the coronary stenosis. *C*, Angiogram taken at the completion of PTCA. The previously stenotic segment (*arrow*) is now widely patent.

pressure gradient across the stenosis). Even if the first dilation abolishes the pressure gradient across the coronary stenosis, two or three inflations are usually performed. If the gradient is not initially abolished, the second and third inflations may frequently diminish the pressure gradient further and produce a better PTCA result (Figure 37.3).

The dilating catheter is across the residual stenosis when the final pressure gradient is measured. Therefore, some contribution of its size to the pressure gradient is expected. It is unusual for successful PTCA to completely obliterate the pressure gradient. A final pressure gradient of 10 to 20 mm Hg across the coronary stenosis is common.

After PTCA, the dilating catheter is withdrawn into the guiding catheter. The wire guide can be left across the stenosis if the result of the PTCA is uncertain, allowing safe advancement of the balloon catheter across the stenosis a second time if necessary. Repeat angiography is performed through the guiding catheter and the angiographic appearance of the coronary artery is recorded. If the site of PTCA appears well dilated, the catheters and wire guides are removed. The patient is monitored carefully for 6 to 12 hours. Most patients return home to normal activity 24 hours after the procedure.

MECHANISM OF ANGIOPLASTY

Successful angioplasty is accompanied by disruption and splitting of the atheromatous plaque. When the size of the inflated balloon and the vessel is similar, as occurs in only mild to moderate stenosis, inflation of the angioplasty balloon results in desquamation of endothelial cells and shearing of superficial plaque elements only. Therefore, the lumen of the artery is only slightly widened. However, exposure of subendothelial connective tissue elements to the bloodstream results in deposition of platelets where the dilating balloon was inflated.[9–11] The local injury to the area of mild stenosis produces a restenosis rate after PTCA that is identical to that of more severe stenoses.[12] If the angioplasty balloon is inflated in an area of more severe stenosis, full inflation of the dilating balloon produces splitting of the atheromatous plaque.[13,14] As the expansile force of the inflating balloon exceeds the strength of the nonelastic plaque, the plaque splits at its weakest, thinnest portion (Figure 37.4). Sections of the coronary arteries of autopsied human hearts in which angioplasty was performed postmortem,[15] experimental studies of transluminal angioplasty in the coronary arteries of normal dogs,[10] experimental studies in an atherosclerotic model in rabbits,[9,15] and pathologic specimens studied after successful angioplasty of femoral and coronary arteries in human subjects[16–18] (Figure 37.5) all support this concept.

The split in the plaque usually extends to the external elastic membrane.[9,13,15,16] After the intima and inner media of the atheromatous plaque are split, the outer layers of the artery are stretched over the expanding circumference of the dilating balloon. The outer media and adventitia are elastic and are easily stretched circumferentially. As the media and adventitia stretch, the split in the atherosclerotic plaque widens. Maintenance of inflation of the dilating balloon longer than 30 seconds may diminish elastic recoil of the outer layers of the artery and also injure the muscle cells of the outer media, which produces a more permanent, effective angioplasty.

Despite the controlled injury to the atheromatous plaque and artery that is produced by PTCA, embolization of atheromatous material, except for rare endothelial cells, has not been demonstrated experimentally and has not been a problem clinically.[19,20]

Angiography of the coronary artery immediately after successful PTCA shows enlargement in luminal diameter. Almost always one or the other view will demonstrate an irregular outline of contrast material in the area of the PTCA (Figures 37.6 and 37.7) caused by contrast medium flowing within the split in the atheromatous plaque.[13,21]

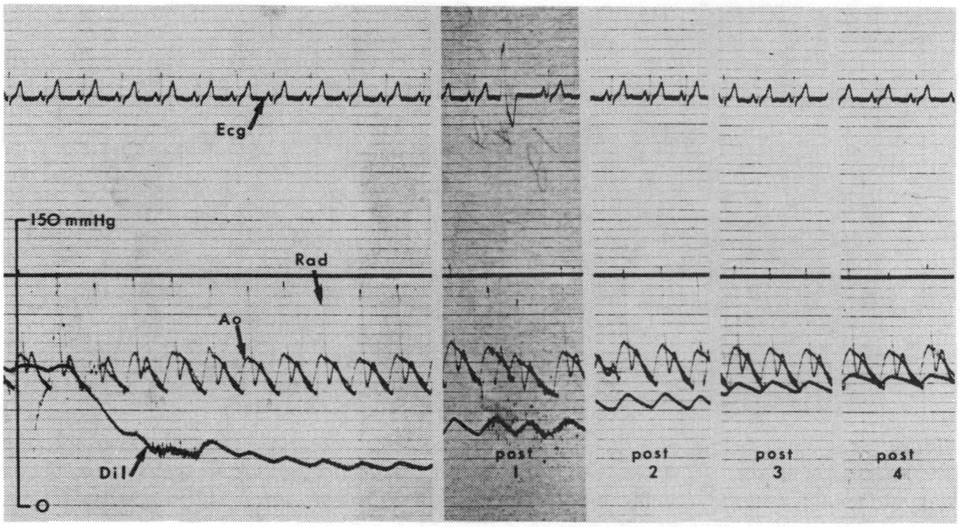

Figure 37.3. Pressure recordings from the radial artery (Rad), the central aorta (Ao), and the tip of the dilating catheter (Dil) during percutaneous transluminal coronary angioplasty. As the tip of the dilating catheter is advanced through the coronary stenosis, pressure recorded from the tip of the dilating catheter decreases. After the first balloon deflation (post 1), the gradient across the stenosis is diminished. Three more inflations (post 2, post 3, and post 4) almost abolish the gradient completely.

It may appear as a localized area of coronary dissection. Contrast density at the site of PTCA may be less than that in the normal coronary artery because there is always residual irregularity of the lumen due to the split plaque. This may produce a "ground glass" appearance during angiography at the PTCA site.[22]

The repair mechanism after PTCA is complex. A normal appearance and smooth lining of the vessel are frequently seen on angiograms taken 6 weeks or longer after the procedure. Pathologic studies show multiple ways in which the split plaque heals. Endothelialization of the split plaque, remodeling of the plaque material, and fibrous retraction of the split plaque may all contribute to improvement in luminal size after PTCA. Focal injury in some instances may accelerate the atheromatous process.[23] Platelet deposition within the split plaque and thrombus formation with organization may contribute to recurrent stenoses in some patients early after PTCA. Such restenosis occurs in 20% to 30% of patients after successful PTCA.[24]

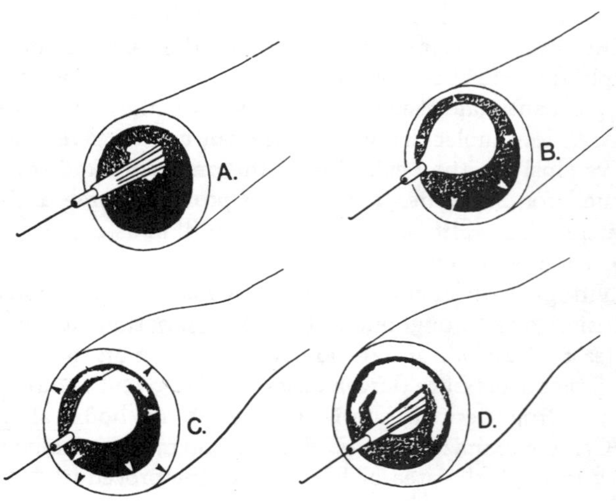

Figure 37.4. Schematic diagram of the mechanism of transluminal angioplasty. The deflated dilating catheter lies within the coronary stenosis (*A*). As the balloon is inflated, the atheromatous plaque resists stretching (*B*). With higher inflation pressures, the atherosclerotic plaque splits at its weakest point and the elastic outer media and adventitia are stretched, enlarging the lumen (*C*). The balloon is deflated and withdrawn, leaving a stretched, dilated vessel with an enlarged lumen (*D*).

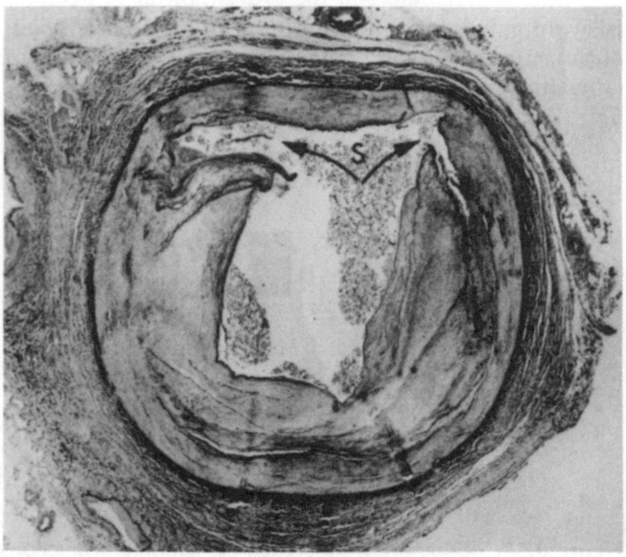

Figure 37.5. Section of femoral artery at the site of angioplasty, revealing splits (S) of the fibrous intimal plaque extending to the internal elastic lamina and circumferentially following it (*arrows*). The original lumen has been enlarged by the splits in the plaque. (From Block et al,[16] reprinted by permission of the *New England Journal of Medicine*.)

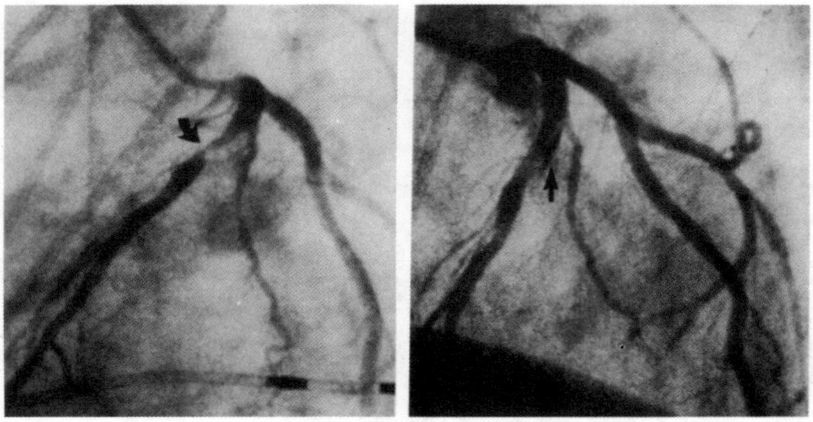

Figure 37.6. Angiogram of a stenosis of a left anterior descending coronary artery before (*left*) and after (*right*) PTCA. Note the split in the atheromatous plaque which is seen as a separate area of opacification by angiographic dye (*right, straight arrow*). Compare with Figure 37.7. (From Block,[21] reprinted by permission of Lea & Febiger.)

PHARMACOLOGIC AGENTS USED IN PATIENTS UNDERGOING PERCUTANEOUS TRANSLUMINAL CORONARY ANGIOPLASTY

DRUGS USED BEFORE PERCUTANEOUS TRANSLUMINAL CORONARY ANGIOPLASTY

Because of the platelet deposition that occurs at the time of PTCA due to exposure of subendothelial vessel wall components to blood elements, "antiplatelet" agents should be given the day before PTCA and continued afterwards (Figure 37.8). Aspirin ideally should be given the day before the procedure. A dose of 300 mg once or twice a day is probably adequate. Dipyridamole may add to aspirin's effect of reducing platelet adhesiveness and should also be given in dosages of at least 50 to 75 mg three times a day. The efficacy of pretreatment with aspirin and dipyridamole in the prevention of acute coronary thrombus formation during PTCA has been well-documented.[24a] Giving antiplatelet therapy before PTCA raises the potential problem of a bleeding diathesis if the patient requires emergency coronary artery bypass graft surgery because of a complication of PTCA. However, the incidence of emergency surgery is low enough and the bleeding diathesis is usually controllable, so that these are not major practical problems.

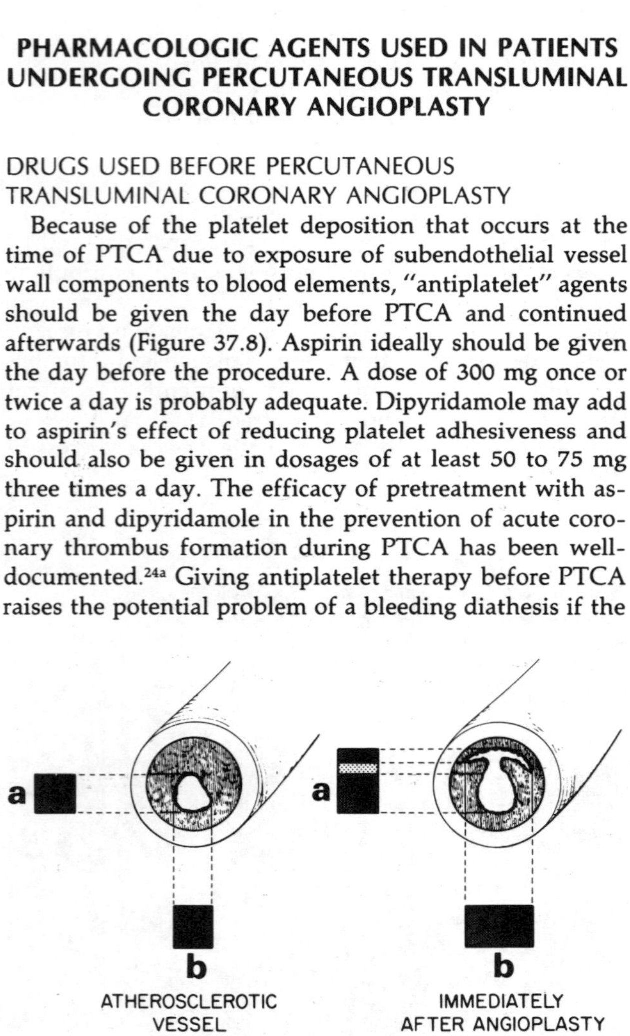

Figure 37.7. Diagram of theoretic angiographic projections of an atherosclerotic artery before (*left*) and after (*right*) PTCA. Intimal splitting produced by successful PTCA enlarges the lumen. Angiographically the lumen appears enlarged in both projections (a and b) but only in projection "a" can the split be seen. Compare with Figure 37.6. (From Block,[21] reprinted by permission of Lea & Febiger.)

DRUGS USED DURING PERCUTANEOUS TRANSLUMINAL CORONARY ANGIOPLASTY

The most important medication given to patients during PTCA is heparin. Heparin should be given at the beginning of the procedure in relatively large doses, approximately 100 U/kg intravenously. If heparin is discontinued at the end of PTCA, it is rarely necessary to reverse its effect with protamine before removing the arterial catheter. If PTCA produces a long "split" in the artery that can be seen angiographically, or if the area that was dilated is a particularly long segment of the coronary artery, heparin should be continued in a constant intravenous infusion to maintain the partial thromboplastin time at one and a half to two times the normal range. If antiplatelet agents cannot be given the day before PTCA, low molecular weight dextran can be given intravenously at the beginning of the procedure and continued for 24 hours. The dextran provides some antiplatelet effect, although its efficacy in diminishing acute occlusion or restenosis is unknown.[11,24]

Nitroglycerin should be given at a constant intravenous infusion rate throughout PTCA. It is important to give at least 25 μg/min intravenously; depending on the systolic blood pressure, larger doses can be given. Intravenous nitroglycerin is continued four to six hours after PTCA to maximize coronary dilation and maximize blood flow through the area of PTCA after the procedure.

DRUGS GIVEN AFTER PERCUTANEOUS TRANSLUMINAL CORONARY ANGIOPLASTY

Intravenous nitrates and low molecular weight dextran (if given) are continued approximately 6 and 24 hours after PTCA, respectively. Dipyridamole is also continued. After all arterial catheters are removed, aspirin therapy is reinstituted. Calcium channel blockers are begun im-

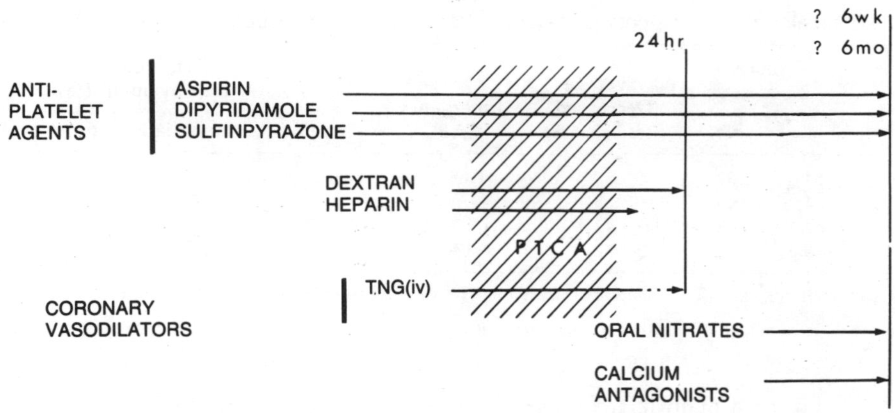

Figure 37.8. Schematic diagram of drugs given before, during, and after PTCA. The shaded area represents the time of PTCA. (From Block,[21] reprinted by permission of Lea & Febiger.)

mediately after successful PTCA to maximize coronary flow. Long-acting nitrates are given for the same reason. Whether these medications are effective in promoting the effect of angioplasty and minimizing the rate of restenosis is unclear.

The length of time that calcium channel blockers, nitrates, and dipyridamole should be given is not established. Most centers continue these medications 1 to 3 months. If at that time the patient remains asymptomatic, medications are discontinued. The patient is maintained on aspirin therapy at least 1 year.

INDICATIONS FOR PERCUTANEOUS TRANSLUMINAL CORONARY ANGIOPLASTY

Although some patients with coronary stenosis can be treated solely with PTCA, PTCA should be considered only one part of the treatment of coronary disease. Patients considered for PTCA should have angina pectoris due to coronary stenosis that cannot easily be controlled with medical therapy, be intolerant of medical therapy, or be in severe jeopardy from the coronary stenosis. Noninvasive evaluation of patients before and after PTCA using exercise testing, thallium scintigraphy with exercise, or gated cardiac blood pool scintigraphy with exercise all are useful to evaluate the patient before PTCA and for comparison after PTCA.

The patients best suited for PTCA have proximal coronary artery stenoses that are discrete, concentric, and greater than 50% of the vessel's transverse diameter.[25–28] The coronary stenosis should not be longer than 10 mm and preferably shorter than 5 mm. Because most dilating catheters have balloon segments only 20 to 25 mm in length, longer lesions are more difficult to dilate successfully. It may be difficult to advance the dilating catheter smoothly through an eccentric lesion. Dilating an eccentric lesion may affect the relatively normal side of the artery and leave the atherosclerotic plaque relatively unchanged.[29] Calcification of a coronary stenosis is not a contraindication to PTCA. Balloon material tolerates pressure high enough to dilate even calcified lesions successfully. It is rare that a balloon inflated to more than 8 or 9 atm of pressure will continue to have a "dog bone" appearance, with the ends of the balloon inflated on either side of a stenosis, whereas the midportion remains compressed by an unyielding atherosclerotic plaque. It is rarely necessary to increase inflation pressure to 12 or 13 atm to fully inflate the balloon.

The appearance of stenosis on angiography does not predict the ease of successful PTCA. Stenoses that appear too narrow to allow passage of the dilating catheter may be easily traversed and successfully dilated. Luminal irregularities within a stenosis may make it difficult to pass the wire guide and the dilating catheter through the stenosis. If standard dilating catheters cannot traverse the stenosis, small, low-profile catheters can be used and will successfully traverse an extremely tight stenosis. Initial dilation with a catheter of small diameter is then followed by a second dilation with a larger catheter placed over an exchange wire.

REPRESENTATIVE CLINICAL SERIES

Percutaneous transluminal coronary angioplasty is useful therapy in selected patients with refractory angina.[30,31] Data from representative clinical series are summarized in Table 37.1. Most early studies reported a primary success rate between 60% and 80% and a restenosis rate of 20% to 33% at 1 year of follow-up. In most series approximately 90% of patients whose PTCA appeared successful on angiography had improvement in symptoms and in functional status of at least one New York Heart Association (NYHA) class. Exercise testing documented an improvement in mean working capacity for 53% to 80% of the predicted working capacity following successful PTCA.[30,31]

NATIONAL HEART, LUNG, AND BLOOD INSTITUTE PTCA REGISTRY

From 1979 to 1982, 3079 patients undergoing PTCA were enrolled in a voluntary National Heart, Lung, and Blood Institute (NHLBI) Registry.[31a] Most patients (72.5%) had single-vessel coronary disease, 25% had multivessel disease, and 2.5% had main left coronary stenosis. Almost all patients (92%) had normal left ventricular function. There were 3,441 dilations attempted; 62% were dilations of the left anterior descending coronary artery, 26% of the right coronary, 7% of the circumflex,

Table 37.1. Clinical Series of Patients Undergoing Percutaneous Transluminal Coronary Angioplasty

Study	No.	Primary Success %	Primary Success No.	Average Decreased Stenosis (%)	Emergency CABGS	MI (%)	Symptomatic Improvement (%) Immediate	Symptomatic Improvement (%) 6 mo	Restenosis (%)
Gruentzig, 1979[30]	50	64	32	50	10% (5)	12	90	78	11 (9 mo)
Scholl, 1982[27]	70	64	45	55	NA	6	91	55	30 (6 mo)
Kent, 1982[44]	59	64	38	43	5% (3)	2	79	50	29 (6 mo)
NHLBI, 1984[31a]	3,079	66.6		52	3%	5.5	92	54	33 (1 yr)

CABGS = coronary artery bypass graft surgery; MI = myocardial infarction; NA = not available; NHLBI = National Heart, Lung, and Blood Institute; No. = number of patients.

4% of a bypass graft, and 1% of a main left coronary artery.

Results and Predictors of Success

Primary angiographic success with PTCA (defined as greater than 20% improvement in luminal diameter angiographically) was achieved in 67% of the attempts. There was a mean reduction in stenosis after PTCA of 52% following successful dilation. The most important reason for failure of PTCA was an inability to traverse the stenosis with a dilating catheter. This accounted for 63% of failures and was related to an inability either to cross a stenosis or to reach a lesion distal to a sharp curve in the coronary artery. Inability to dilate the lesion once it had been traversed by the dilating catheter was another reason for failure.[27,32]

These data represent an average of the many clinical centers that contributed data to the NHLBI Registry. The centers had varying levels of experience, and all centers underwent a learning curve.[32] The fact that there is a marked learning curve associated with PTCA is supported by an increase in the primary success rate from 60% in the first year of the Registry to more than 80% in the last year of the Registry.[33] In addition, new guiding catheter technology, smaller dilating catheters, the introduction of steerable floppy-tipped wire guides, and improved balloon material have improved success rates. At present the primary success rate in experienced hands should reach 90% or more[34] (Table 37.2).

Complications

Table 37.3 summarizes the most common complications in patients entered in the NHLBI Registry.[35] Major complications (death, nonfatal myocardial infarction, or the need for emergency coronary artery bypass graft surgery) occurred in 9.4% of all attempts. The overall mortality rate directly attributable to PTCA was 0.6%. Mortality was increased in patients with main left coronary artery disease (3.8%), prior coronary artery bypass graft surgery (2.9%), female gender (1.8%), and age greater than 60 years (1.7%).

Emergency coronary artery surgery was needed in 6.6% of patients. The major indications for coronary artery bypass surgery were coronary dissection (46%), coronary occlusion (20%), and prolonged angina pectoris (14%). Of patients who had urgent coronary artery bypass graft surgery, nonfatal myocardial infarction occurred in 41%.[36,37] The incidence of nonfatal myocardial infarction during emergency coronary artery surgery after failed PTCA is significantly reduced by early use of the intraaortic balloon pump placed in the catheterization laboratory at the time of failed PTCA.[38,39,39a] The intraaortic balloon pump frequently stabilizes the condition of patients with ongoing myocardial ischemia after blood vessel closure and allows surgery at a lower risk. The frequency of all coronary events, prolonged angina, myocardial infarction, and coronary spasm diminishes as investigator experience with angioplasty increases. Of note is that coronary occlusion or coronary dissection does not decrease significantly with increasing operator experience. This is explained by the fact that PTCA causes splitting of the atheromatous plaque. Immediate thrombotic occlusion or focal dissection or both occur in a small number of patients regardless of investigator experience.

Factors associated with a higher incidence of complications include (1) female gender, (2) lesion severity of greater than 90%, (3) PTCA attempt of the right coronary

Table 37.2. Outcome of Initial Percutaneous Transluminal Coronary Angioplasty

	NHLBI Registry 1980	NHLBI Registry 1981	Present
Primary Success	59%	63%	85–90%
MI	4%	5%	2–5%
Emergency CABG	6%	7%	2–5%
In-hospital Death	1%	1%	<1%

For abbreviations, see Table 37.1.

Table 37.3. Summary of Complications of Percutaneous Transluminal Coronary Angioplasty: National Heart, Lung, and Blood Institute Registry Data

Complication	Percent*
Prolonged angina	6.8
Myocardial infarction	5.5
Coronary occlusion	4.9
Coronary dissection	4.4
Coronary spasm	4.2
Ventricular fibrillation	1.8
Hypotension	1.5
Bradycardia	1.4
Peripheral arterial	0.7
PTCA-related deaths	0.6

*Overall frequency of complications = 21.2%.

artery, (4) unstable angina pectoris, and (5) age greater than 60 years.

Intimal disruptions or splits were initially classified as coronary dissection in the NHLBI Registry and considered a complication. Investigation of the mechanism of successful PTCA reveals that splitting of the atheromatous plaque accompanies a successful result.[9] Consequently, coronary dissection should be defined as a complication only in patients in whom it is associated with major luminal obstruction, coronary occlusion, myocardial infarction, or deterioration of flow requiring emergency coronary artery surgery. Intimal tearing or dissection was reported in 13% of patients in the NHLBI Registry, but true coronary dissection only occurred in one third of these patients. Intimal coronary dissection occurs more often in women and in patients with PTCA of the right coronary artery, multivessel disease, eccentric lesions, and nondiscrete lesions.[40]

EVALUATION OF SUCCESSFUL PERCUTANEOUS TRANSLUMINAL CORONARY ANGIOPLASTY

Improved angiographic appearance of the coronary artery and an increase in functional classification of the patient are the most desirable end points after successful PTCA. Other methods should be used to objectively document the efficacy of PTCA in improving coronary flow. The exercise electrocardiogram, thallium scintigraphy after exercise testing, and blood pool scintigraphy after exercise all improve after successful PTCA.[27,28,30,41–45] Thallium exercise scintigraphy after PTCA is most often used to follow patients. The presence of a thallium defect after exercise, even in asymptomatic patients, is highly predictive of restenosis following successful PTCA.[46,46a] About half the patients (52%) still have an abnormal radionuclide cineangiographic study after successful PTCA. Because PTCA does not obliterate the stenosis but only improves flow, sensitive tests such as blood pool radionuclide scintigraphy after exercise may continue to show abnormalities of left ventricular function with stress.

Of patients with successful PTCA, 84% return to work following the procedure. Although this figure is not significantly different from that of patients who have undergone coronary bypass graft surgery, the length of time until return to work is shorter (7 days versus 73 days).[47]

Objective measurements of coronary sinus blood flow[48] show increases in coronary blood flow after successful PTCA. These data substantiate that improved working capacity, improved functional class, disappearance of thallium reperfusion defects after exercise, and improved left ventricular contractility with exercise are all due to increases in coronary blood flow after successful PTCA.

LONG-TERM FOLLOW-UP

A subset of 1,397 patients from the NHLBI Registry from 65 centers has been followed for at least one year after successful PTCA.[31] The duration of follow-up was one year in 906 patients, two years in 349, three years in 108, and four years in 34.

Seventy-four percent of the patients did not require another procedure, and 62% were symptom free. A second PTCA was necessary in 11.4% of patients; 65% of these patients were symptom-free at follow-up. Overall, therefore, 85% of patients did not require coronary artery bypass graft surgery. Of patients in whom restenosis developed, 12.9% chose coronary artery bypass surgery rather than repeat PTCA. The annual mortality rate after PTCA in patients with single-vessel disease was less than 1% per year and with multivessel disease 3% per year. Important predictors of late cardiac death were multivessel and left main coronary artery disease. Both predict a relatively high risk group in the years after PTCA. Late cardiac deaths occurred at the same rate whether patients underwent subsequent coronary artery bypass graft after unsuccessful PTCA during either the same or a subsequent hospitalization. However, mortality was greater when PTCA was unsuccessful and no subsequent coronary artery bypass graft was performed (Table 37.4).

A second PTCA can be performed with a high degree of success (85%) and a low complication rate. Major complications occur in only 3% and emergency bypass surgery is needed in 2%. Of the patients in the NHLBI Registry who had repeat PTCA, none died during the repeat procedure.

If PTCA alleviates symptoms for 1 year, the prognosis for continued asymptomatic status is excellent. At 2, 3, and 4 years after successful PTCA, patients from the NHLBI Registry had no increase in the incidence of recurrent symptoms. This indicates that the dilated vessel remains open. This long-lasting beneficial effect was further confirmed in a 5-year follow-up report from Switzerland.[48a] Recurrence of symptoms 1 year or more after PTCA is more likely due to progression of disease in other locations in the coronary arteries than at the site of the previous PTCA.[48b]

SPECIAL APPLICATIONS OF PTCA

Although the best patients for PTCA are patients with isolated single-vessel coronary stenoses, evaluation by many investigators of other groups of patients that

Table 37.4. Follow-Up Data After Initial Percutaneous Transluminal Coronary Angioplasty Success: National Heart, Lung, and Blood Institute Registry Data*

Data	Percent
No additional revascularization (neither repeat PTCA nor CABGS)	74
Repeat PTCA	11.4
CABGS required	12.9
MI	3.6 (2%/yr)
Death	1.8 (1%/yr)
MI or death	5.4 (3%/yr)
Anginal status at last follow-up:	
No angina	71
Improved	20
Unchanged	6
Worse	3

* Mean follow-up time = 18 months; 906 were followed up for 1 year, 349 for 2 years, 108 for 3 years, and 34 for 4 years.

For abbreviations, see Table 37.1.

can be helped by PTCA has expanded its use (Table 37.5).[48,49–61]

UNSTABLE ANGINA PECTORIS

Percutaneous transluminal coronary angioplasty is useful in selected patients with unstable angina pectoris.[49,50] Comparison of patients with unstable angina pectoris treated by PTCA with similar patients with stable angina showed that the combined 18-month mortality and myocardial infarction rate was low in both groups (10.8% and 9.5%, respectively). No differences were observed in mortality and myocardial infarction rates between patients with unstable angina treated surgically or with PTCA. Primary angiographic and clinical success is the same as that in patients undergoing PTCA for stable angina.[50] Recurrent angina may be less in patients treated with PTCA than in those treated with coronary artery bypass graft.[51] Successful PTCA in patients with unstable angina produces normalization of hemodynamic and myocardial response to stress. Therefore, PTCA can be performed as safely and successfully in patients with unstable angina as in those with stable angina. The procedure is associated with low mortality and morbidity. Marked improvement in symptoms and myocardial response to stress can be demonstrated. Appropriate anatomic criteria for PTCA must be met before patients with unstable angina are considered candidates for the procedure.

MULTIVESSEL DISEASE

Although patients with multivessel disease are potential candidates for PTCA,[52–54] many are not good candidates. Percutaneous transluminal coronary angioplasty cannot reestablish blood flow through long segments of coronary occlusion and it may have a higher risk in complex atherosclerotic disease where there are multiple occlusions in the coronary vasculature or segments of severe atherosclerotic narrowing that are longer than 2 cm. Multiple PTCAs in the same patient in one setting must have a progressively higher risk of emergency coronary artery bypass graft.[55] This may not be as high as anticipated if complication rates requiring surgery are patient related rather than lesion related. The restenosis rates of multivessel PTCA must also be partially cumulative. However, the appeal of PTCA in selected patients with multivessel disease makes some patients with multiple coronary stenoses attractive candidates for the procedure. In considering patients with multivessel disease candidates for PTCA, it is important to consider whether it is better to attempt PTCA of only the most stenotic lesion or to attempt PTCA of all stenotic coronary arteries. Given the well-proved efficacy of coronary artery bypass graft surgery in patients with multivessel coronary disease, it would be premature to consider the use of PTCA as the primary mode of therapy in these patients. Whether the increased complication rates of PTCA in patients with multivessel disease are acceptable and whether long-term follow-up studies show results comparable to those achieved with coronary artery bypass graft surgery are awaited with interest.

STENOSES IN CORONARY ARTERY BYPASS GRAFTS

Autogenous saphenous vein bypass grafts are frequently narrowed by scarred venous valves or by atherosclerosis. These are the predominant causes of late graft closure after coronary artery bypass graft.[56] Approximately 60% of bypass grafts remain patent between 10 and 12 years after surgery. Because bypass graft narrowing is due primarily to intimal proliferative or atherosclerotic occlusive changes, PTCA can be used as an alternative to repeat coronary artery bypass graft surgery. Angiographic improvement was achieved in 60% of patients in the PTCA Registry and in 78% and 84% of the most recent series of graft-PTCA reported.[57,57a] The success rate is high because there are no side branches into which the tip of the dilating catheter can be advanced and because the stenoses can usually be easily traversed by the dilating catheter. The complication rate is low (2.5% for emergency coronary artery bypass graft). Successful angioplasty of proximal aortic-bypass graft anastomotic sites and stenoses of the proximal portion of bypass grafts is associated with a restenosis rate of 50% or more. Percutaneous transluminal coronary angioplasty of stenoses in the distal portion of the bypass grafts and at the bypass graft–coronary artery anastomotic site has a restenosis rate similar to that in native coronary PTCA.[57a]

Coronary bypass grafts that have been in place more than 5 years may develop degenerative atherosclerotic plaques. These plaques are composed of friable atherosclerotic material. Passage of a dilating catheter and

Table 37.5. Special Applications of Percutaneous Transluminal Coronary Angioplasty

Study	No.	Primary Success %	Primary Success No.	Average Decreased Stenosis (%)	Emergency CABGS (%)	MI (%)	Symptomatic Improvement (%) Immediate	Symptomatic Improvement (%) 6 mo	Restenosis (%)
Williams, 1981[48] (unstable angina)	17	76	13	46	6 (1)	0	100	92	8 (3 mo)
Stertzer, 1981[51a] (left main)	8	100	8	43	0	0	100	62	25 (1 yr)
David, 1982[60] (variant angina)	5	80	4	45	0	0	25	50	50 (4 mo)
Block, 1984[57] (bypass grafts)	40	78	31	52	2.5	0	NA	58	38 (8 mo)
Dervan, 1983[61] (total occlusion)	13	54	7	59	0	0	NA	NA	43

CABGS = coronary artery bypass graft surgery; MI = myocardial infarction; NA = not available; No. = number of patients.

angioplasty of such stenoses may cause peripheral embolization of atherosclerotic material dislodged by the expanding angioplasty balloon. Recognition of such degenerative lesions can be made angiographically. Degenerative plaques are usually long, have an irregular contour, and may have superimposed thrombus. In contrast, fibrous plaques, which are smooth and relatively discrete, do not contain degenerative atherosclerotic material and can be treated with angioplasty.

VARIANT ANGINA

Variant angina due to coronary artery spasm without underlying obstructive coronary artery disease should not be treated with PTCA.[57b] However, most patients with variant angina have associated underlying obstructive coronary artery disease.[58,59] It is assumed that an increase in coronary vasomotor tone in a coronary artery partially obstructed by atherosclerotic plaque may cause reversible obstruction at the site of the organic stenosis. For this reason, PTCA can be used to treat this kind of variant angina. In a small series of patients, an 80% primary angiographic success was achieved.[60] However, despite angiographic success, symptomatic improvement occurred in only 25% of patients and there was a high incidence of restenosis. Therefore, it appears that the efficacy of PTCA in variant angina is limited. Unless the underlying obstructive atherosclerotic lesion is at least 50%, PTCA should not be considered.

TOTALLY OCCLUDED CORONARY ARTERIES

Low profile catheters and steerable, floppy-tipped guide wire systems allow PTCA in some patients in whom total coronary occlusion is present.[61,62] Angina pectoris associated with total coronary artery occlusion is usually due to inadequate collateral circulation to viable myocardium originally served by the occluded vessel. This may occur without previous myocardial infarction. Because the involved vessel is already occluded and collateral flow is present, PTCA can be performed with little risk of precipitating ischemia or necessitating emergency coronary bypass graft surgery. To minimize the risk of vessel perforation, a floppy-tipped guide wire is first advanced through the occluded coronary artery into the distal vessel. The guide wire seems to follow the occluded true lumen rather than tunnel through the atheroma. The incidence of intimal dissection and immediate reclosure is not greater in patients with total occlusion than in those with subtotal occlusion. Distal embolization, coronary perforation, or myocardial infarction have not been clinically apparent.[61] The restenosis rate, however, is higher than that observed after conventional PTCA, and the success rate is lower.[63,63a] Patients in whom occlusion has developed within 6 months of angioplasty are more likely to have an initially successful primary result.

PERCUTANEOUS TRANSLUMINAL CORONARY ANGIOPLASTY IN ACUTE MYOCARDIAL INFARCTION IN COMBINATION WITH THROMBOLYTIC THERAPY

Although thrombolytic therapy with streptokinase or other thrombolytic agents may restore coronary patency rapidly enough to interrupt myocardial infarction, up to one third of patients do not show reflow and in approximately one third in whom reflow occurs reocclusion develops.[64] Percutaneous transluminal coronary angioplasty is successful in opening total occlusion in almost 70% of cases of thrombolytic failure and increases the overall reflow rate from 66% to 77%. Similar experiences have recently been reported from the Mayo Clinic.[64a]

The frequency of recurrent ischemic events in patients who have had successful thrombolytic therapy but residual stenosis of 90% or greater is high (76%). In contrast, if the residual stenosis after successful thrombolysis is less than 90%, only 14% of patients have recurrent ischemic events. Only 6% of patients had recurrent ischemic events after PTCA performed for severe residual stenosis. Late restenosis or reocclusion, however, occurs frequently (45% of successful PTCA cases). Although immediate PTCA after thrombolytic therapy produces increased clinical stability in the hospital, late restenosis is common and repeat PTCA may be necessary.

PERCUTANEOUS TRANSLUMINAL CORONARY ANGIOPLASTY USED ALONE IN ACUTE MYOCARDIAL INFARCTION

Percutaneous transluminal coronary angioplasty can be used to reestablish blood flow to an area of acute myocardial infarction.[65] Both subtotal and total occlusion can be successfully opened. Distal embolization is rarely observed. Cardiac catheterization performed ten days later in 123 patients[65] showed improved left ventricular function in 100 patients (81%). There was an 81% mean increase in ejection fraction from 41% prior to PTCA to 59% after PTCA. Ten percent of the entire group of 222 patients reoccluded the infarct artery in the post-PTCA period. Eighty-two percent of the patients were in stable condition at the time of discharge. If an occluded vessel in the setting of acute myocardial infarction does not appear to contain extensive thrombus, PTCA may be the preferred initial approach to the occluded artery because it can be performed quickly. Early restoration of blood flow most likely maximizes myocardial viability in the infarct zone.

RESTENOSIS AFTER SUCCESSFUL PERCUTANEOUS TRANSLUMINAL CORONARY ANGIOPLASTY

The major problem after successful PTCA is restenosis of the dilated segment. Using the criterion of recurrence of angina pectoris for which additional revascularization procedures (either repeat PTCA or coronary bypass surgery) were performed, restenosis occurred in 24% of patients in the NHLBI Registry who had an initially successful PTCA.[46] Recurrence appears most often within the first 6 months after successful PTCA.

In patients who have follow-up angiography, restenosis is defined in two ways: (1) a greater than 30% worsening of the luminal diameter from the immediate post–PTCA lumen size; (2) a loss of more than 50% of the angiographic improvement produced by the PTCA found in angiograms taken immediately after PTCA.

Restenosis occurred in 30% of patients using the first definition and in 33% of patients using the second. Angiographic restenosis occurs more frequently than clinical restenosis, and is not always associated with recurrence of symptoms. Restenosis occurs more commonly in men, in patients who had bypass graft stenoses dilated, in patients who initially are NYHA class III or IV, and in patients without previous myocardial infarction.[65a] It also occurs more commonly if the pressure gradient measured across the coronary stenosis before PTCA is more than 40 mm Hg, and if the final pressure gradient measured immediately after PTCA is greater than 20 mm Hg. So far, there has been little effect of post–PTCA treatment regimens (antiplatelet therapy, calcium antagonists, and the like). Aspirin used after PTCA, however, seems to be more useful than warfarin in preventing restenosis.[66]

Restenosis rates vary.[27,30,45] Currently, a restenosis rate of 25% to 35% can be expected 1 year after successful PTCA. The recurrence of symptoms after successful PTCA correlates highly with the presence of restenosis. If patients develop recurrent angina, restenosis is present in 56%. In patients without chest pain after successful PTCA, restenosis is found angiographically in only 14%.[45]

Although the incidence of restenosis after successful PTCA is high, repeat PTCA can be used to treat restenosis with a high degree of success. The success rate in the NHLBI Registry among patients undergoing a second PTCA is 85% versus 63% in patients undergoing an initial PTCA.[67,68] The complication rate of a second PTCA is low. The myocardial infarction rate is 1.5% and emergency coronary artery bypass graft rate is only 2%. None of the patients in the NHLBI Registry who underwent a second PTCA for restenosis died as a consequence of the procedure.[46]

Table 37.6. Percutaneous Transluminal Coronary Angioplasty (PTCA): Indications and Contraindications

Indications/Eligibility

1. Disabling angina, refractory to medical treatment, with objective evidence of ischemia, CABG candidate, with appropriate angiographic findings:
   A. One-vessel CAD, relatively discrete, subtotal noncalcified stenosis, not at branch point.
   B. Two-vessel CAD, amenable lesion (as above) in both.
   C. Three-vessel CAD, focal lesions.
   D. S/P CABG with subtotal stenosis of graft (preferably not proximal), accessible by PTCA.
2. Following successful thrombolysis in acute MI with residual high-grade stenosis amenable to PTCA.
3. Recently occluded vessel, without other significant CAD, with disabling angina and objective evidence of ischemia in the collateralized zone.
4. Left main stenosis with life-threatening ischemia, not eligible for CABG.
5. Multivessel disease or suboptimal anatomy with disabling angina, not eligible for CABG.

Relative Contraindications

1. Left main coronary artery stenosis.
2. Multivessel CAD with disabling angina, diffuse disease.
3. Variant angina (Prinzmetal's).
4. Poor LV function.

CABG = coronary artery bypass graft surgery; CAD = coronary artery disease; LV = left ventricular; S/P = status post.

SUMMARY

Percutaneous transluminal coronary angioplasty is established as one way of treating patients with coronary artery atherosclerosis. Its use has been greatly expanded by major technical improvements and operator experience. However, PTCA must be offered in the perspective of alternative medical and surgical therapy. If a patient has little myocardial ischemia or jeopardy from a coronary stenosis and can tolerate angina pectoris with medical therapy, PTCA is unnecessary. For patients in whom medical therapy is inadequate to control symptoms or if objectively documented ischemia is present despite the absence of symptoms, PTCA may be an option. The possibility of emergency coronary artery bypass surgery due to a complication of PTCA may influence a recommendation of this mode of therapy in specific patients. The choice for PTCA in each patient should be made after careful assessment of the risk/benefit ratio of PTCA versus medical therapy versus coronary artery bypass surgery. Because it improves symptoms, has the unique advantage of a short hospital stay, is associated with minimal discomfort and rapid convalescence, and has a relatively low cost[69,70] as well as low risk, PTCA should be recommended if interventional therapy is indicated and if the coronary anatomy is suitable (Table 37.6). "PTCA is here to stay"[71] and will constitute an increasingly important part of the workload for all active cardiac catheterization laboratories and cardiac surgical units throughout the world.

REFERENCES

1. Dotter CT, Judkins MP: Transluminal treatment of arteriosclerotic obstruction. Description of a new technique and a preliminary report of its application. *Circulation* 1964; 30:654–662.
2. Staple TW: Modified catheter for percutaneous transluminal treatment of atherosclerotic obstructions. *Radiology* 1968; 91:1041–1043.
3. Zeitler E, Gruentzig AR, Schoop W (eds): *Percutaneous Vascular Recanalization.* Heidelberg, Springer, 1978.
4. Gruentzig AR, Hopff H: Perkutane Rekanalisation chronischer arterieller Verschlusse mit einer neuen Dilatations-Katheter. *Deutsch Med Wochenschr* 1974; 99:2502–2510.
5. Gruentzig AR: *Die perkutane transluminale Rekanalisation chronischer Arterienverschlusse mit einer neuen Dilatationstechnik.* Baden-Baden, G Witzstrock Verlag, 1977.
6. Gruentzig AR, Turina MI, Schneider JA: Experimental percutaneous dilatation of coronary artery stenosis. *Circulation* 1976; 54:II–81.
7. Gruentzig AR: Transluminal dilatation of coronary artery stenosis. *Lancet* 1978; 1:263.
8. Saffitz JE, Rose TE, Oaks JB, Roberts WC: Coronary arterial rupture during coronary angioplasty. *Am J Cardiol* 1983; 51:902–904.
9. Block PB, Fallon JT, Elmer D: Experimental angioplasty: lessons from the laboratory. *Am J Roentgenol* 1980; 135:907–912.
10. Pasternak RC, Baughman KL, Fallon JT, Block PC: Scanning electron microscopy after transluminal angioplasty of normal canine coronary arteries. *Am J Cardiol* 1980; 45:591–598.
11. O'Gara PT, Guerrero JL, Feldman B, Fallon JT, Block PC: Effect of dextran and aspirin on platelet adherence following transluminal angioplasty of normal canine coronary arteries. *Am J Cardiol* 1984; 53:1695–1698.
12. Ischinger T, Gruentzig AR, Hollman J, King S III, Douglas J, Meier B, Bradford J, Tankersley R: Should coronary arteries with less than 60% diameter stenosis be treated by angioplasty? *Circulation* 1983; 68:148–154.
13. Block PC, Baughman KL, Pasternak RC, Fallon JT: Transluminal angioplasty: correlation of morphological and angiographic findings in an experimental model. *Circulation* 1980; 61:785–788.
14. Castaneda-Zuniga R, Formanek A, Tadavarthy M, Vlodaver Z, Edwards JE, Zollikofer C, Amplatz K: The mechanism of balloon angioplasty. *Radiology* 1980; 135:565–571.

15. Baughman KL, Pasternak RC, Fallon JT, Block PC: Transluminal coronary angioplasty of postmortem human hearts. *Am J Cardiol* 1981; 48:1044–1047.
16. Block PC, Myler RK, Stertzer S, Fallon JT: Morphology after transluminal angioplasty in human beings. *N Eng J Med* 1981; 305:382–400.
17. Block PC: Mechanism of transluminal angioplasty. *Am J Cardiol* 1984; 53:69C–71C.
18. Waller BF: Early and late morphologic changes in human coronary arteries after percutaneous transluminal coronary angioplasty. *Clin Cardiol* 1983; 6:363–372.
19. Block PC, Elmer D, Fallon JT: Release of atherosclerotic debris after transluminal angioplasty. *Circulation* 1982; 65:950–952.
20. Sanborn TA, Faxon DP, Waugh D, Small DM, Haudenschild C, Gottsman SB, Ryan TJ: Transluminal angioplasty in experimental atherosclerosis. *Circulation* 1982; 66:917–922.
21. Block PC: Percutaneous transluminal coronary angioplasty, in Yu PN, Goodwin JF (eds): *Progress in Cardiology,* vol 11. Philadelphia, Lea & Febiger, 1982, pp 1–15.
22. Holmes DR Jr, Vlietstra RE, Mock MB, Reeder GS, Smith HC, Bove AA, Bresnahan JF, Piehler JM, Schaff HV, Orszulak TA: Angiographic changes produced by percutaneous transluminal coronary angioplasty. *Am J Cardiol* 1983; 51:676–683.
23. Ross R, Glomset JA: The pathogenesis of atherosclerosis. *N Engl J Med* 1976; 285:369–377, 420–425.
24. Faxon DP, Sanborn TA, Haudenschild CC, Ryan TJ: Effect of antiplatelet therapy on restenosis after experimental angioplasty. *Am J Cardiol* 1984; 53:72C–76C.
24a. Barnathan E, Laskey WK, Kleaveland JP, Kussmaul WG, Hirshfeld JW Jr: Aspirin and dipyridamole pretreatment in the prevention of acute thrombus formation during coronary angioplasty. *J Am Coll Cardiol* 1986; 7:64A.
25. Cowley MJ, Block PC: Percutaneous transluminal coronary angioplasty. *Mod Concepts Cardiovasc Dis* 1981; 50:25–29.
26. Kent KM, Banka V, Bentivoglio LG, Block PC, Cowley M, Diamond G, Dorros G, Ellestad M, Faxon D, Fiedotin A, Goldberg S, Gruentzig A, Hamby R, Hirshfeld J, Kaltenbach M, Kober G, Lach R, Leatherman L, Lee G, Meyer J, Myler R, Ockene I, Robert E, Rosing D, Simpson J, Sosa J, Spring D, Stertzer S, Vlietstra R, Walton J, Williams D, Fisher L, Gillespie M, Mullin S, Mock M: Percutaneous transluminal coronary angioplasty (PTCA): update from the NHLBI Registry. *Circulation* 1980; 62(Suppl III):III–160.
27. Scholl JM, Chaitman BR, David PR, Dupras G, Brevers G, Val PG, Crepeau J, Lesperance J, Bourassa MG: Exercise electrocardiography and myocardial scintigraphy in the serial evaluation of the results of PTCA. *Circulation* 1982; 66:380–390.
28. Block PC: Percutaneous coronary angioplasty. *Am J Roetgenol* 1980; 135:955–957.
29. Meier B, Gruentzig AR, Hollman J, Ischinger T, Bradford JM: Does length or eccentricity of coronary stenoses influence the outcome of transluminal dilatation? *Circulation* 1983; 67:497–499.
30. Gruentzig AR, Senning A, Siegenthaler WE: Non-operative dilatation of coronary artery stenosis. Percutaneous transluminal coronary angioplasty. *N Engl J Med* 1979; 301:61–68.
31. Kent KM, Bentivoglio LG, Block PC, Cowley MJ, Dorros G, Gosselin AJ, Gruentzig A, Myler RK, Simpson J, Stertzer SH, Williams DO, Fisher L, Gillespie MJ, Detre K, Kelsey S, Mullin SM, Mock M: Percutaneous transluminal coronary angioplasty. Report from the NHLBI Registry. *Am J Cardiol* 1982; 49:2011–2020.
31a. Cowley MJ, Block PC: A review of the NHLBI PTCA Registry data, in Jang GD (ed): *Angioplasty*. New York, McGraw-Hill, 1986, pp 368–378.
32. Meier B, Gruentzig AR: Learning curve for PTCA: skill, technology or patient selection. *Am J Cardiol* 1984; 53:65C–66C.
33. Kelsey SF, Mullin SM, Detre KM, Mitchell H, Cowley MJ, Gruentzig AR, Dent KM: Effect of investigator experience on percutaneous transluminal coronary angioplasty. *Am J Cardiol* 1984; 53:56C–64C.
34. Block PC: Percutaneous transluminal coronary angioplasty: role in the treatment of coronary artery disease. *Circulation* 1985; 72(suppl V):V-161–V-165.
35. Dorros G, Cowley M, Simpson J, Bentivoglio L, Block P, Bourasa M, Detre K, Gosselin A, Gruentzig A, Kelsey S, Kent K, Mock M, Mullin S, Myler R, Passamani E, Stertzer S, Williams D: Percutaneous transluminal coronary angioplasty: report of complications from the National Heart, Lung, and Blood Institute PTCA registry. *Circulation* 1983; 67:723–730.
36. Dorros G, Cowley MJ, Janke L, Kelsey SF, Mullin SM, Van Raden M: In-hospital mortality rate in the National Heart, Lung, and Blood Institute PTCA Registry. *Am J Cardiol* 1984; 53:17C–21C.
37. Cowley MJ, Dorros G, Kelsey SF, Van Raden M, Detre KM: Emergency CABG after coronary angioplasty: the National Heart, Lung, and Blood Institute's PTCA Registry experience. *Am J Cardiol* 1984; 53:22C–26C.
38. Akins CW, Block PC: Surgical intervention for failed percutaneous transluminal coronary angioplasty. *Am J Cardiol* 1984; 53:108C–112C.
39. Murphy DA, Craver JM, Jones EL, Gruentzig AR, King SB III, Hatcher CR Jr: Surgical revascularization following unsuccessful percutaneous transluminal coronary angioplasty. *J Thorac Cardiovasc Surg* 1982; 84:342–348.
39a. Block PC: Emergency surgery after percutaneous transluminal coronary angioplasty: he who calls the tune may have to pay the piper. *Ann Thorac Surg* 1985; 40:1–3.
40. Cowley MJ, Dorros G, Kelsey SF, Van Raden M, Detre KM: Acute coronary events associated with percutaneous transluminal coronary angioplasty. *Am J Cardiol* 1984; 53:12C–16C.
41. Hirzel HO, Nuesch K, Gruentzig AR, Luetolf UM: Short and long term changes in myocardial perfusion after PTCA assessed by thallium-201 exercise scintigraphy. *Circulation* 1981; 63:1001–1006.
42. Meier B, Gruentzig AR, Siegenthaler WE, Schlumpf M: Long term exercise performance after PTCA and CABG. *Circulation* 1983; 68:796–802.
43. Okada RD, Boucher CA, Strauss HW, Pohost GM: Exercise radionuclide imaging approaches to coronary artery disease. *Am J Cardiol* 1980; 46:1188–1204.
44. Kent KM, Bonow RO, Rosing DR, Ewels CJ, Lipson LC, McIntosh CL, Bacharach S, Green M, Epstein SE: Improved myocardial function during exercise after successful PTCA. *N Engl J Med* 1982; 306:441–446.
45. Rosing DR, Van Raden MJ, Mincemoyer RM, Bonow RO, Bourassa MG, David PR, Ewels CJ, Detre KM, Kent KM: Exercise, electrocardiographic and functional responses after percutaneous transluminal coronary angioplasty. *Am J Cardiol* 1984; 53:36C–41C.
46. Holmes DR, Vlietstra RE, Smith HC, Vetrovec GW, Kent KM, Cowley MJ, Faxon DP, Gruentzig AR, Kelsey SF, Detre KM, Van Raden MJ, Mock MB: Restenosis after PTCA: a report from the National Registry of the National Heart, Lung, and Blood Institute. *Am J Cardiol* 1984; 53:77C–81C.
46a. Stuckey TD, Beller GA, Gibson RS, Watson DD, Tedesco CL, Nygaard TW, Burwell LR: Multivariate analysis of clinical, angiographic and exercise TL-201 variables for the prediction of recurrent angina after percutaneous transluminal coronary angioplasty. *J Am Coll Cardiol* 1986; 7:106A.
47. Holmes DR, Van Raden MJ, Reeder GS, Vlietstra RE, Jang GC, Kent KM, Vetrovec GW, Cowley MJ, Dorros G, Kelsey SF, Detre KM, Mock MB: Return to work after coronary angioplasty: a report from the National Heart, Lung, and Blood Institute Percutaneous Transluminal Coronary Angioplasty Registry. *Am J Cardiol* 1984; 53:48C–51C.
48. Williams DO, Riley RS, Singh AK, Gewirtz H, Most AS: Evaluation of the role of coronary angioplasty in patients with unstable angina pectoris. *Am Heart J* 1981; 102:1–9.
48a. Hirzel HO, Eichhorn P, Kappenberger L, Gander MP, Schlumpf M, Gruentzig AR: Percutaneous transluminal coronary angioplasty: late results at 5 years following intervention. *Am Heart J* 1985; 109:575–581.
48b. Robert EW, Ricks WB, Rossen RM, Nagel MR, Green SE, Koransky A, Thomas T: Late recurrence of angina following coronary angioplasty: the role of new atherosclerotic disease. *J Am Coll Cardiol* 1986; 7:21A.
49. Meyer J, Schmitz HJ, Kiesslich T, Erbel R, Krebs W, Schulz W, Bardos P, Minale C, Messmer BJ, Effert S: Percutaneous transluminal coronary angioplasty in patients with stable and unstable angina pectoris: analysis of early and late results. *Am Heart J* 1983; 106:973–980.
50. Plotnick CD: Aproach to the management of unstable angina. *Am Heart J* 1979; 98:243–248.
51. Faxon DP, Detre KM, McCabe CH, Fisher L, Holmes DR, Cowley MJ, Bourassa MG, Van Raden M, Ryan TJ: Role of percutaneous transluminal coronary angioplasty in the treatment of unstable angina: report from the National Heart, Lung, and Blood Institute PTCA and Coronary Artery Surgery Study Registries. *Am J Cardiol* 1984; 53:131C–135C.
51a. Stertzer SH, Wallsh E, Bruno MS: Evaluation of transluminal coronary angioplasty in left main coronary artery stenosis (abstr.) *Am J Cardiol* 1981; 47:396.
52. Vlietstra RE, Holmes DR Jr, Reeder GS, Mock MB, Smith HC, Bove AA, Bresnahan JF, Piehler JM: Balloon angioplasty in multivessel coronary artery disease. *Mayo Clin Proc* 1983; 58:563–567.
53. Mock MB, Holmes DR, Vlietstra RE, Gersh BJ, Detre KM, Kelsey SF, Orszulak TA, Schaff HV, Piehler JM, Van Raden MJ, Passamani ER, Kent KM, Gruentzig AR: PTCA in the elderly patient: experience in the National Heart, Lung, and Blood Institute PTCA Registry. *Am J Cardiol* 1984; 53:89C–91C.
54. McNamara JJ, Norenburg RG, Goebert HW, Soeter JR: Distribution and severity of atherosclerosis in the coronary arteries. *J Thorac Cardiovasc Surg* 1976; 71:637–640.
55. Dorros G, Stertzer SH, Cowley MJ, Myler RK: Complex coronary artery angioplasty: multiple coronary dilatations. *Am J Cardiol* 1984; 53:126C–130C.
56. Bourassa MG, Enjalbert M, Campeau L, Lesperance J: Progression of atherosclerosis in coronary arteries and bypass grafts: 10 years later. *Am J Cardiol* 1984; 53:102C–107C.
57. Block PC, Cowley MJ, Kaltenbach M, Kent KM, Simpson J: Treatment

of coronary bypass graft stenoses with percutaneous angioplasty: an alternative to repeat surgery. *Am J Cardiol* 1984; 53:666–668.

57a. Reeder GS, Bresnahan JF, Holmes DR, Mock MB, Orszulak TA, Smith HC, Vlietstra RE: Angioplasty for aortocoronary bypass graft stenosis. *Mayo Clin Proc* 1986; 61:14–19.

57b. Abi-Mansour P, Roubin G, Gruentzig AR: Coronary angioplasty: which patients will now benefit? *J Crit Illness* 1986; 1(2):52–60.

58. Macalain AN: Relation of coronary arterial spasm to site of organic stenosis. *Am J Cardiol* 1980; 46:143–146.

59. Shubrooks SJ Jr, Bete JM, Hutter AM Jr, Block PC, Buckley MJ, Daggett NM, Mundth ED: Variant angina pectoris: clinical and anatomic spectrum and results of coronary bypass graft surgery. *Circulation* 1975; 36:142–147.

60. David PR, Walters DD, Scholl JM, Crepeau J, Szlachcic J, Lesperance J, Hudon G, Bourassa MG: Percutaneous transluminal coronary angioplasty in patients with variant angina. *Circulation* 1982; 66:695–702.

61. Dervan JP, Baim DS, Cherniles J, Grossman W: Transluminal angioplasty of occluded coronary arteries: use of a moveable guide wire system. *Circulation* 1983; 68:776–784.

62. Holmes DR Jr, Vlietstra RE, Reeder GS, Bresnahan JF, Smith HC, Bove AA, Schaff HV: Angioplasty in total coronary artery occlusion. *J Am Coll Cardiol* 1984; 3:845–849.

63. Holmes DR Jr, Vlietstra RE, Reeder GS: Elective PTCA of total coronary arterial occlusions not associated with acute infarction. *J Am Coll Cardiol* 1983; 1:656–661.

63a. Bonan R, Kouz S, Crepeau J, Lesperance J, Theroux P: Coronary angioplasty (PTCA) for total coronary occlusion: success rate and follow-up. *J Am Coll Cardiol* 1986; 7:238A.

64. Gold KH, Cowley MJ, Palacios IP, Vetrovec GW, Akins CW, Block PC, Leinbach RC: Combined intracoronary Streptokinase infusion and coronary angioplasty during acute myocardial infarction. *Am J Cardiol* 1984; 53:122C–125C.

64a. Holmes DR Jr, Smith HC, Vlietstra RE, Nishimura RA, Reeder GS, Bove AA, Bresnahan JF, Chesebro JH, Piehler JM: Percutaneous transluminal coronary angioplasty, alone or in combination with streptokinase therapy, during acute myocardial infarction. *Mayo Clin Proc* 1985; 60:449–456.

65. Rutherford BD, Hartzler GO, McConahay DR, Johnson WL Jr: Direct balloon angioplasty in acute myocardial infarction without prior use of streptokinase. *J Am Coll Cardiol* 1986; 7:149A.

65a. Block PC: Setting parameters for percutaneous transluminal coronary angioplasty. *Cardiovasc Med* 1985; 10(3):4–6.

66. Thornton MA, Gruentzig AR, Hollman J, King SB, Douglas JS: Coumadin and aspirin in prevention of recurrence after transluminal coronary angioplasty: a randomized study. *Circulation* 1984; 69:721–727.

67. Williams DO, Gruentzig AR, Kent KM, Detre KM, Kelsey SF, To T: Efficacy of repeat percutaneous transluminal coronary angioplasty for coronary restenosis. *Am J Cardiol* 1984; 53:32C–35C.

68. Kent KM, Bentivoglio LG, Block PC, Bourassa MG, Cowley MJ, Dorros G, Detre KM, Gosselin AJ, Gruentzig AR, Kelsey SF, Mock MB, Mullin SM, Passamani ER, Myler RK, Simpson J, Stertzer SH, Van Raden MJ, Williams DO: Long-term efficacy of percutaneous transluminal coronary angioplasty (PTCA): Report from the National Heart, Lung, and Blood Institute PTCA Registry. *Am J Cardiol* 1984; 53:27C–31C.

69. Jang GC, Block PC, Cowley MJ, Gruentzig AR, Dorros G, Holmes DR, Kent KM, Leatherman LL, Myler RK, Sjolander SME, Stertzer SH, Vetrovec GW, Willis WH, Williams DO: Relative cost of coronary angioplasty and bypass surgery in a one vessel disease model. *Am J Cardiol* 1984; 53:52C–55C.

70. Wilson JM, Dunn EJ, Wright CB, Bailey WW, Callard GM, Melvin DB, Mitts DL, Will RJ, Flege JB Jr: The cost of simultaneous surgical standby for percutaneous transluminal coronary angioplasty. *J Thorac Cardiovasc Surg* 1986; 91:362–370.

71. The expanding scope of coronary angioplasty, editorial. *Lancet* 1985; 1:1307–1308.

38 Surgical Treatment of Coronary Artery Disease

Altagracia M. Chavez, MD and Floyd D. Loop, MD

The death rate from cardiovascular disease has shown a continued and progressive decline since 1970.[1] Among industrialized nations, the United States ranks seventh in the mortality rate for coronary artery disease. Death rates for all major categories of cardiovascular disease have declined, and downward trends have been recorded for all four major sex-color groups. A parallel decrease in mortality from all causes has been noted. Although these findings are intriguing, they are unexplained. The effect of changes in the life-style of the population, such as better control of hypertension, reduced consumption of saturated fats, a decline in cigarette smoking, and an increase in exercise, is considered responsible for these trends in mortality.[2,3] Certainly medical and surgical therapeutic innovations cannot account for these results, because the deceleration began before modern methods of treatment became available.

Nonetheless, cardiovascular disease is the most common cause of death in the United States. An estimated 5 to 6 million persons in this country have symptomatic coronary atherosclerosis and an undetermined number have silent disease. Coronary artery disease accounts for one third of all deaths in persons between the ages of 35 and 64 years and remains the single most important reason for full disability allowances before age 65. It also is the single most important cause of hospitalization.[4]

The introduction of coronary arteriography 25 years ago[5] heralded a new era in the treatment of ischemic heart disease. Direct coronary artery surgery soon became a therapeutic reality, and innovations in this field over the intervening years have made bypass grafting an acceptable option in the treatment of patients with coronary artery disease. Progress is anticipated in the medical management of coronary atherosclerosis through improved drug therapy, greater recognition of high-risk patients, emphasis on risk factor intervention, and the advent of balloon angioplasty.

DIAGNOSIS

Coronary arteriography is the best means of defining the pathologic anatomy of patients with coronary artery disease. The extent of coronary atherosclerosis and left ventricular function are important and independent prognostic indicators which permit stratification into subsets of varying risk. For patients with coronary artery disease, findings at catheterization correlate better with survival than do symptoms, electrocardiographic findings, results of stress testing, or clinical risk factors.

This does not imply that all patients with chest pain should be subjected to coronary angiography as the initial diagnostic procedure. In the CASS registry, 28% of the patients evaluated for suspected coronary atherosclerosis had normal results or minimal disease.[6] Forty percent of women catheterized had normal coronary arteries and another 10% had only mild narrowing. Among the men in the group, 12% had normal arteries and 5% had minimal disease.[7] Noninvasive techniques, including exercise tolerance tests and radionuclide studies, have some usefulness in selecting appropriate patients for coronary angiography, but improved methods of screening are needed to reduce the number of normal arteriograms obtained.

Coronary arteriography has significant limitations. The hydraulic characteristics of coronary arterial stenoses are grossly oversimplified by the angiographic interpretation of the percentage of stenosis.[8] Epicardial Doppler flow transducers used intraoperatively have documented discrepancies between angiographic estimation of the percentage of obstruction and the functional significance of coronary arterial narrowing during reactive hyperemia.[9] In addition, one postmortem study found that 97% of vessels reported angiographically to have less than 50% narrowing had at least a 75% reduction in luminal cross-sectional diameter.[10] Evaluation of vessel size distal to coronary artery obstruction and the functional evaluation of intercoronary collaterals are often poorly defined by coronary arteriography.[11]

Despite these limitations, coronary arteriography currently remains the best means of defining coronary anatomy and is a necessary procedure in patients who may be referred for coronary bypass grafting. Included in this group might be survivors of acute myocardial infarction who have residual severe left ventricular impairment (ejection fraction less than 30%)[12]; patients whose post-infarction course is complicated by angina, congestive heart failure, or intractable arrhythmias[13]; patients with unstable angina[14]; patients with unacceptable symptoms on maximal medical therapy; and patients with classic angina who demonstrate marked ischemia or worsening ejection fraction during stress exercise testing.

Survivors of sudden cardiovascular collapse constitute a special group of patients in whom coronary arteriography should be considered. In the Seattle Heart Watch experience, the percentage of successful initial resuscitations of such patients has doubled over the past decade.[15] Although most of these patients have not had acute infarction,[16] about 75% of such arrests are due to coronary heart disease and the recurrence rate in survivors approaches 30% within the first year.[17] Aggressive evaluation and therapy in these patients seem warranted.

SURVIVAL AFTER MEDICAL THERAPY

As noted previously, findings at cardiac catheterization are the best predictors of survival in patients with coronary artery disease. Patients grouped according to the number of diseased vessels, impairment of left ventricular function, and presence or absence of left main coronary artery obstruction show wide variations in five-year survival. This factor may complicate direct comparison of survival rates between medical and surgical therapy.

Differences in studies attempting to estimate the natural history of coronary artery disease may be affected by selection criteria, changing medical therapy, completeness of follow-up, and duration of symptoms. Simply reporting average annual mortality is inaccurate, because mortality from coronary disease is not linear. Inconsistent relations between baseline symptoms, extent of disease, and prognosis have been described. In addition, the poorer survival of medically treated patients with left main coronary artery obstruction is well recognized[18]; hence, these patients are generally excluded from such studies.

Patients with no or mild (30% or less narrowing) coronary atherosclerosis have five-year survival rates of 95% and 98%, respectively.[19,20] This excellent survival is not surprising in view of experimental data showing that occlusions of 30% are required to reduce maximal coronary flow but that resting flow is not affected until 85% obstruction is reached.[21]

Table 38.1 summarizes five-year survival data from large studies of patients treated medically (nonoperatively). These include the prospective Veterans Administration[22] and European Cooperative Study,[23] the group-matched Seattle Heart Watch experience,[24] and data from Johns Hopkins University,[25] Duke University,[26] the Coronary Artery Surgery Study,[20,27] Ontario,[28] and the Cleveland Clinic.[29] The patients included in these studies had severe atherosclerosis (defined as greater than 50% to greater than 70% narrowing) and represent groups compiled in the 1960s and 1970s. The largest series comes from the CASS registry of nearly 13,000 medically treated patients.[20]

Table 38.1. Five-Year Survival of Nonoperative (Medical) Treatment†

Study Group	Extent of Disease		
	One-Vessel	**Two-Vessel**	**Three-Vessel**
VA Cooperative[22]	88	87	76
European Cooperative[23]	...	88	82
Seattle Heart Watch[24]	92	78	58
Johns Hopkins[25]	100	88	60
Duke University[26]	90	82	65
CASS[20]	89	82	62
CASS[27*]	68	57	46
Ontario[28]	92	65	55
Cleveland Clinic[29]	88	68	57

*CASS[27] reported these results from a subgroup of patients who had an estimated 70% or greater proximal narrowing in one or more major coronary arteries.

†Tables 38.1 and 38.2 are from Loop FD: Progress in surgical treatment of coronary atherosclerosis. Part 1. *Chest* 1983; 84:611–624. Used with permission.

These studies show improved five-year survival in patients followed up in the 1970s[22,23,26] compared with those followed up in the 1960s.[28,29] The exception was the CASS subgroup with an estimated proximal arterial narrowing of 70% or greater[27] in whom survival appeared to be lower than that reported in the older studies.[28,29] The investigators concluded that proximal obstruction carried a worse prognosis than did obstruction at other sites, excluding left main coronary artery disease. Severity of left ventricular impairment had an adverse effect on survival in all subgroups in each of these studies. Left ventricular performance is recognized as the most important isolated predictor of survival.[26]

Five-year survival of medically treated patients with one-vessel disease reported on more recently ranged from 92% to 96%.[30] Overall, patients with right coronary artery disease had the best prognosis. Patients with lesions of the anterior descending coronary artery before the first septal perforator had a 90% five-year survival compared with 98% in the group with more distal lesions; this probably reflects the greater amount of jeopardized myocardium in the former. These investigators also found that nearly 20% of the medically treated patients had had either nonfatal myocardial infarction or cardiac death at five years. This rate was not significantly affected by which of the three major coronary arteries was involved.

A report from Duke[31] on 1,214 medically treated patients with symptomatic coronary artery disease studied between 1969 and 1978 indicated that nonfatal infarction accounted for about one third of the initial cardiac events. In patients with one- or two-vessel disease and normal left ventricular function, nonfatal infarcts were responsible for as much as two thirds of the initial events. Ventricular function was an important predictor of survival, but the number of diseased vessels was an important predictor of ischemic events. The probability of surviving an ischemic event is strongly influenced by the quality of left ventricular function and the presence of left main coronary artery disease.

Proudfit et al[32] reported on a group of 598 patients in whom coronary arteriography was performed between 1963 and 1965. These patients all had greater than 50% obstruction of one or more major coronary arteries, all were initially treated medically, and all were followed up a minimum of 15 years. None had surgery for coronary artery disease within five years of catheterization, but 60 patients eventually did undergo bypass grafting. Total survival at 15 years was 48% for one-vessel disease, 28% for two-vessel disease, 18% for three-vessel disease, and 9% for left main coronary artery disease. Ninety-five percent of all deaths during the first five years were due to coronary artery disease; the percentage decreased to 84% and 64% for the second and third five-year periods. At 15 years, cardiac survival in the group with one-vessel disease was 66% for the right coronary artery, 64% for the circumflex, and 46% for the anterior descending artery. Poor left ventricular function, duration of symptoms of 60 months or more, multivessel disease, and peripheral atherosclerosis all correlated with poor survival when patients with left main coronary artery disease were excluded.

CURRENT MYOCARDIAL REVASCULARIZATION

INDICATIONS

The indications for coronary artery bypass surgery have been a subject of considerable study and debate. Most bypass operations currently are performed for relief of anginal symptoms or to prolong life, or both, especially in higher risk patients such as those with left main, three-vessel, or two-vessel disease. Currently recognized indications include[33] (1) stable disabling angina that interferes with life-style despite therapy; (2) angina with left main, three-vessel, or two-vessel disease; (3) severe narrowing of a proximal anterior descending artery supplying a large area of myocardium; (4) postinfarction angina; (5) variant angina associated with persistent anatomic obstruction; (6) evidence of severe ischemia at low work loads on exercise testing in asymptomatic patients; and (7) obstructive coronary anatomy in patients having valve surgery.

The foregoing indications are not universally agreed upon nor are they the only reasons patients might be referred for bypass surgery. In 15 CASS participating centers, myocardial jeopardy (a composite score of the relation of proximal lesions to retained wall motion in anterior and inferior left ventricular segments) was the most important determinant of referral for coronary surgery.[34] Anterior wall jeopardy (ie, the left anterior descending arterial distribution) was a substantially more important reason for referral than was inferior wall risk. Clinical factors that also were found to influence referral included severity of angina, number of operable vessels, change in activity, unstable angina, and left main coronary artery disease. Although heterogeneity of therapy was noted among the participating centers, certain trends emerged. Between 1974 and 1979, the number of patients operated on for mild angina with single-vessel disease decreased, whereas the number of patients operated on for left main coronary artery disease increased. These trends find support in the literature which indicates that symptoms and longevity were improved by surgical therapy in patients with left main and three-vessel disease.[18,23]

Patients with single-vessel coronary artery disease are not a homogeneous group. As noted before, proximal stenosis of the left anterior descending coronary artery carries a worse prognosis than does either isolated stenosis of the right or circumflex coronary artery or more distal anterior descending coronary artery stenosis.[35,36] Therefore, the site and severity of stenosis and the amount of myocardium at risk[37] need to be considered in evaluating these patients. It must be remembered that 20% of sudden death victims and 15% to 20% of patients with left ventricular aneurysms have one-vessel disease.

Asymptomatic or mildly symptomatic patients with one- or two-vessel disease are generally not referred for coronary artery bypass. Investigators at the National Heart, Lung, and Blood Institute[38,39] found that such patients have low rates of sudden death or acute myocardial infarction, and they recommended withholding operation until symptoms worsen. Patients with no or mild symptoms and three-vessel disease had a different prognosis: those with good exercise capacity had a 4% annual mortality rate, whereas those with poor exercise capacity had a rate of 9%. Follow-up of these patients was only 26 months. The CASS randomized trial[6] found no survival advantage at five years for medical or surgical treatment in patients with either mild or no symptoms after acute infarction. The investigators concluded that for such patients operative intervention could be delayed until symptoms worsened.

Coronary surgery for patients who survive acute myocardial infarction has been recommended for the subgroup that is at high risk of death. This group includes patients with recurrent or persistent angina, patients who have sustained large infarcts (especially those with complex ventricular dysrhythmias), patients with ischemia at low work loads on stress testing, and those with nontransmural infarction. Epstein et al[12] found that 20% of survivors of acute infarction have an ejection fraction of less than 30%. The first-year mortality rate among this group with severe left ventricular impairment ranged from 25% to 45% and these constituted the majority of deaths in the first year. Exercise stress testing in the remaining 80% of patients identified a high-risk ischemic group which had a first-year mortality of 15% to 20%. These patients should undergo arteriography to determine if they are candidates for bypass grafting or angioplasty.

OPERATIVE RISK

Since 1967, when direct myocardial revascularization by coronary artery bypass grafting was introduced, morbidity and mortality have declined markedly and patterns of patient-related risk factors have changed. Technologic achievements that have increased the safety of operation include (1) better preoperative hemodynamic management; (2) greater operative experience; (3) improvements in cardiac anesthetic management; (4) myocardial protection afforded by cold chemical cardioplegia; (5) more complete revascularization; (6) blood conservation; and (7) improved postoperative monitoring and management.

Experience from various centers reporting on large numbers of patients documents the improved survival.[40–42] The mortality rate for coronary artery bypass grafting is currently about 2% despite the findings that patients referred for coronary artery surgery in the 1980s are generally older, have more extensive coronary atherosclerosis, have worse preoperative left ventricular function, and have more associated medical problems. Therefore, the better results are not due to selection of lower risk patients.[43]

Several studies have analyzed the changing risk factors for coronary artery surgery. Miller et al[44] divided the Stanford experience into two groups: those operated on between 1971 and 1975 and those who underwent operation between 1977 and 1979. The later group was older, contained more women, and the patients had more extensive atherosclerosis, more severe angina, and more left ventricular impairment. Using multivariate analysis, the investigators found that in the early group the priority of operation, presence of left main coronary artery disease, severity of congestive heart failure, hypertension, and mitral regurgitation were all independent predictors of operative mortality. Similar analysis for the group operated on between 1977 and 1979 showed that only emergency operation and congestive heart failure remained independent determinants of operative mortality.

A CASS review of 6,176 cases from 1975 to 1978[45] pooling operative results from 15 participating centers found that overall operative mortality was 2.3% but ranged from 0.3% to 6.6%. Therefore, the experience of the surgeon or surgical team emerged as the principal risk factor. Other predictors of operative risk included advanced age, female gender, heart failure, left main coronary artery disease, impaired left ventricular function, and emergency operation. Another CASS review[46] found that in the subset of patients with left main coronary artery disease, operative risk was increased by advanced age, female gender, duration and severity of angina, emergency operation, left coronary dominance, severity of left main coronary artery stenosis, and left ventricular impairment.

The Cleveland Clinic experience with patients undergoing primary myocardial revascularization from 1970 through 1982 was recently reviewed.[47] The patients were divided into four groups based on date of operation. Analysis revealed that the more recent groups had older patients, a higher proportion of women, more diabetic patients, more extensive coronary atherosclerosis, and more frequent left ventricular impairment. Operative mortality was 0.8% for the group operated on in the 1980s. Each group was independently analyzed for variables that increased operative mortality, and some interesting trends emerged: (1) left main coronary artery disease, the number of grafts placed, and poor left ventricular function were no longer significant risk factors in the cohort operated on from 1980 to 1982; (2) emergency operation, female gender, congestive heart failure, and increased age persisted as risk factors; (3) incomplete revascularization and an abnormal electrocardiogram emerged as new independent risk factors in the recent group.

The influence of gender on operative mortality has been analyzed separately.[48,49] Increased operative risk in women is accounted for by smaller size, which is probably associated with coronary arteries of smaller diameter. Men and women of the same size (defined by body surface area) having the same clinical and angiographic risk variables do not have a significantly different risk of operative death.

Morbidity from coronary artery surgery has also decreased in incidence during the past ten years. Although the risk of stroke has remained about the same (1% to 2%),[47] the incidence of myocardial infarction has shown a significant downward trend.[44,49] This improvement is due to better intraoperative hemodynamic and anesthetic management and to the widespread use of cold chemical cardioplegia for myocardial protection. Cold solutions containing potassium (20 to 30 mEq/L) produce diastolic arrest and decrease the metabolic demands of the myocardium,[50] thereby sparing stores of energy-rich phosphate compounds during the period of aortic cross-clamping.[51] Delivery of the cardioplegia solution may be suboptimal distal to atherosclerotic obstruction, leaving certain areas poorly protected and subject to ischemic injury. Temperature mapping confirms differences in hypothermia after injection of cardioplegia solution. Maneuvers to provide more uniform cooling and protection include injecting cardioplegia solution through the grafts (after distal anastomoses are constructed) and into the aorta at a controlled pressure and volume.[52] Blood cardioplegia may be advantageous in patients who require long periods of cross-clamping.[53–55] The enhanced myocardial protection afforded by chemical cardioplegia has been documented in numerous clinical and experimental studies.[56,57] Inadequate myocardial protection rather than graft closure is responsible for most perioperative myocardial infarctions.[58]

Other causes of morbidity after coronary artery surgery include supraventricular arrhythmias (reported in 10% to 30% of patients), reoperation for bleeding, respiratory insufficiency, and wound disruption or infection. The incidence of most of these has decreased significantly in recent years.[43,47] New ventricular dysrhythmias in the postoperative period are almost always associated with underlying myocardial injury.

LONG-TERM RESULTS AFTER OPERATION

GRAFT PATENCY AND LEFT VENTRICULAR FUNCTION

Improvement in myocardial function in areas in which perfusion was increased by saphenous vein grafts was demonstrated by Chatterjee et al.[59] The same investigators found that improvement in left ventricular ejection fraction and indexes of myocardial contractility did not correlate with increased coronary blood flow, oxygen delivery, or oxygen consumption despite a higher heart rate and rate-pressure product achieved during postoperative pacing stress.[60] Therefore, improved regional and global function and metabolism may be due to redistribution of blood flow to ischemic and nonischemic myocardium.

Other studies have shown that left ventricular function is frequently improved by patent grafts, whereas occluded grafts may depress left ventricular function.[61] One study found that asynergic left ventricular segments were improved in 25%, unchanged in 72%, and worsened in 3%.[62] Ejection fraction during exercise and exercise-induced wall motion abnormalities also were improved in most postoperative patients who benefited clinically.[63]

Factors that affect early patency of saphenous vein grafts include (1) preservation of vein endothelium during procurement, preparation, and storage; (2) operative technique; (3) relation of vein to coronary artery diameter; (4) recipient arterial runoff; (5) antiplatelet therapy; and (6) the coronary artery grafted, ie, anterior descending grafts consistently show higher patency compared with circumflex or right coronary artery grafts. Clinical reports document improved graft patency with greater operative experience.[43,64-67] Patency at one year is 80% to 90% in most series.[68] Grafts to moderately obstructed (40% to 50%) vessels have the same patency as do those to more severely obstructed vessels.[69] Women have lower vein graft patency rates than do men.[49] Cephalic vein[70] and cryo-preserved vein allografts[71] have inferior patency rates when compared with those of saphenous vein autografts.

Sequential grafts have the theoretic advantage of increasing distal runoff, thereby perhaps improving patency. Other advantages are that vein graft length is conserved and there are fewer proximal anastomoses. The disadvantages of sequential grafts are that they are more demanding to construct[72] and that occlusion of the conduit may endanger a large myocardial mass. Early patency rates for sequential grafts appear to be the same or higher than those for grafts with single distal anastomoses.[73-75]

Coronary endarterectomy with saphenous vein graft placement may be a useful adjunct to revascularization of diffusely diseased coronary arteries. A higher incidence of perioperative myocardial infarction (4.5% versus 2.4%)[44,76] and a slightly lower patency rate (85% at one year and 77% at 3.5 years)[77] are seen when endarterectomy is combined with saphenous vein grafting. Operative mortality, survival, and clinical results are not different with or without endarterectomy.

The use of anticoagulants or antiplatelet drugs to improve graft patency has been studied with contradictory results.[78-83] In a recent Mayo Clinic experience,[84] the administration of antiplatelet drugs was begun preoperatively and early results showed a 3% graft closure rate in the treatment group versus 10% in the placebo group. Cardiac catheterization after one year confirmed the favorable result with 8% of the vein grafts in the treatment group occluded versus 28% in the placebo group.[85]

Several groups have studied the progression of coronary atherosclerosis after bypass grafting.[86-88] Although such progression has occurred in most bypassed arteries with severe occlusion, the progression is found predominantly in the coronary segment proximal to the graft. Progression in the distal segment is relatively infrequent and proceeds at a rate similar to that in ungrafted vessels. No recognized risk factors have been found to correlate with the progression of disease.[89] It is of interest that proximal arterial closure is less frequent when an internal mammary artery is used to bypass a greater than 50% obstruction than when a saphenous vein conduit is used (37% versus 55%).[69,90]

Later on, especially after the fifth to seventh postoperative year, graft atherosclerosis is the most important cause of late graft occlusion. A report from the Montreal group[91] reviewed serial catheterizations in 82 patients over 10 to 12 years. They showed changes suggestive of vein graft atherosclerosis in 17% of the grafts at five to seven years and in 49% at 10 to 12 years. Because only angiographically visible grafts were evaluated, these findings would tend to underestimate the true incidence of vein graft atherosclerosis. Development of atherosclerotic lesions in the grafts was not related to age, clinical risk factors, extent of preoperative coronary disease, or progression of disease in ungrafted arteries. The Montreal group has found that levels of high-density lipoproteins were lower and triglyceride levels higher in patients in whom new lesions developed during follow-up,[92] although other observers have reported no correlation between lipid levels and the development of graft occlusion.

The internal mammary artery graft is emerging as the conduit of choice for coronary artery bypass grafting. Exercise testing[93,94] and clinical improvement[75,95] have documented the efficacy of this conduit. The mammary artery in necropsy studies has been spared from the progressive intimal thickening noted in coronary arteries with increasing age.[96] The one-year patency rate of 92% to 97%[97,98] and the 90% late patency rate[99] are consistently superior to reported rates for saphenous vein grafts. Lytle et al[100] recently reviewed graft patency in patients who underwent arteriography within five years (mean 15 months) and again more than five years (mean 88 months) after operation. Ninety-seven percent of the internal mammary grafts showed no stenosis at early study, and 96% of these were unchanged at late study. The corresponding figures for vein grafts in this series were 82% and 55%, respectively.

ANGINA RELIEF

Bypass grafting has been shown to be superior to medical therapy in alleviating or improving angina.[101] Table 38.2, summarizing data from four prospective randomized studies of chronic angina, shows significantly more improvement in functional class, fewer symptoms during sexual activity, less use of antianginal medication, and a higher rate of uneventful course in the surgical patients.

Postoperative relief of angina correlates with revascularization completeness, graft patency, and progressive atherosclerosis. Factors that influence graft patency have been discussed. Studies of patients in whom angina recurs postoperatively have found the recurrence rate after the first year to be 3% to 4% per year.[102-104] In one study,[103] changes in a graft or coronary artery were noted in 64% of patients with clinical deterioration but in only 18%

Table 38.2. Incidence of Various Clinical Features in Patients Treated Medically and Surgically*

Clinical Feature	Medical Therapy (%)	Surgical Therapy† (%)
Functional class		
Improved:		
Asymptomatic	0–9‡	33–55
Better	48–52	76–90
Worse	3–21	5–6
Angina at rest	45–55	18–20
Uneventful course up to 7 yr	12	50
Symptoms during sexual activity		
None	30	50
Angina	45	16
Therapy		
Nitroglycerin	59–67	21–27
Propranolol	60–75	7–20

* Data from four prospective randomized studies of chronic angina from Rahimtoola,[101] used with permission.

† All differences between medical and surgical patients were statistically significant.

‡ In the European Coronary Surgery Study, 14% of medical patients became asymptomatic. However, many of the asymptomatic patients in the medically treated group received surgery.

without it. Another study reported graft closure in 22% of patients with recurring symptoms but in only 4% of those who remained angina-free.[105]

Completeness of revascularization is defined as grafts performed to all major coronary arteries greater than 1 mm in diameter that demonstrate an estimated 50% to 70% or greater narrowing on preoperative angiography. There is a significant difference in angina relief in patients with complete versus incomplete revascularization even when all grafts remain patent: 87% for complete compared with 42% for incomplete revascularization.[106] Jones et al[107] in a review of patients with three-vessel disease found that the completely revascularized group had an 88.5% five-year survival compared with 83.5% in the incompletely revascularized group. The former also had a higher rate of employment, and 70% were angina-free compared with 58% in the latter group. Improved long-term survival has been found in completely revascularized patients in virtually all five- and ten-year analyses.

SURVIVAL

The major issue is whether or not bypass grafting prolongs life. Tables 38.3 and 38.4 summarize the results of various series reporting ten- and five-year survival after coronary artery surgery. In comparing survival in medically and surgically treated cohorts, it is necessary to refer to specific subsets of patients with coronary artery disease.

Patients with significant left main coronary artery obstruction have improved survival after surgical therapy. One early series cited five- and ten-year survival rates of 88% and 68%, respectively, in these patients.[121] An early randomized study reported 30-month survival of 88% after surgical therapy and 65% with medical management.[22] The CASS report of patients with left main coronary artery disease noted four-year survival rates of 88% in the surgical group and 63% in the medical group.[122] Older age, left ventricular dysfunction, congestive heart failure, severity of left main coronary artery stenosis, and the pattern of coronary dominance affected the survival rates, but the trend toward longer survival with operative intervention was seen in all of these groups.

The European Coronary Surgery Study Group[23] randomly placed 768 men with mild to moderate angina and good left ventricular function into medical or surgical therapy groups. Randomized patients with three-vessel disease showed a 94% five-year survival after surgery compared with 82% in the medically treated group. Left ventricular dysfunction had an adverse effect on survival in both groups. Left main and proximal left anterior descending arterial obstruction in patients with two- or three-vessel disease was indicative of high risk. Other independent risk factors identified in this study were peripheral arterial disease, ST-segment depression on exercise testing, ischemic changes on the resting electrocardiogram, and increasing age. The investigators concluded that survival in the high-risk groups was better with surgical than with medical treatment.

The CASS randomized trial of patients with mild or no angina after myocardial infarction found no significant difference in five-year survival between the groups assigned to medical or surgical treatment.[6] Overall survival was 92% in the medical group and 95% in the surgical group. Survival for subgroups with one-, two-, or three-vessel disease was not significantly different regardless of therapeutic assignment. Patients with ejection fractions greater than 50% had a 95% five-year survival with either medical or surgical therapy. For patients with an ejection fraction less than 50%, survival was 84% in the medical group and 92% in the surgical group, not a statistically significant difference. Despite the small numbers, further analysis showed that for patients with impaired ventricular function and three-vessel disease, bypass grafting offers a significant survival advantage compared with medical therapy.[123]

The investigators in the CASS trial concluded that for patients similar to those in the study (ie, those with mild or no symptoms after infarction), surgery may be deferred until symptoms worsen without increasing mortality. Important caveats in extrapolating from these data include: (1) the study group was strictly defined in terms of clinical status; (2) almost 75% of the patients had a normal ejection fraction; (3) patients with left main coronary artery disease were excluded; (4) crossover from medical to surgical therapy during the five years of observation ranged from 10% among patients with one-vessel disease to 38% among patients with three-vessel disease; and (5) for survival calculation, patients remained in their originally assigned groups, eg, a medical patient who later had surgery was analyzed in the medical group.

Proudfit et al[124] retrospectively analyzed survival in a group of 408 medically treated patients chosen to closely match the CASS randomization criteria. Overall five-year survival was 88.5%, but when subgroups defined by ejection fraction, anginal status, and number of diseased vessels were compared with the CASS data, these investigators found lower survival in multivessel disease cohorts (Table 38.5). Their five-year survival was similar to that

Table 38.3. Ten-Year Survival After Coronary Artery Surgery

Study Group	Patients (No.)	Series Year	Ten-Year Survival (%)
Baylor College of Medicine[108]	500	1968–1971	65*
The Cleveland Clinic[49]	2,000	1971–1972	78.6
St. Luke's (NYC)[102]	748	1970–1973	79
Texas Heart Institute[109]	22,284	1970–1981	70.2
Salt Lake City[110]	761	1969–1980	81.4†
Houston Veterans Administration[111]	56	1972–1974	66

* Estimated from one-, two-, and three-vessel subsets.

† Cardiac deaths only.

From Loop FD: Progress in surgical treatment of coronary atherosclerosis. Part 2. *Chest* 1983; 84:740–755. Used with permission.

of the medical patients with two- and three-vessel disease in the European Cooperative Study. These differences, despite the clinical comparability of the two study groups, are surprising and raise questions about the applicability of the results from the CASS trial. Results in the community may be different from those obtained by the CASS investigators.

Patients with one- and two-vessel disease have good reported long-term survival. Randomized studies of such patients with only mild angina and normal left ventricular function fail to show an advantage of either medical or surgical therapy.[23] Five-year survival of 96% and ten-year survival of 82% have been reported in surgical patients with one-vessel disease.[49] The higher risk for patients with proximal obstruction of the anterior descending coronary system has already been discussed.

Preoperative left ventricular function has an important influence on long-term survival. Poor left ventricular performance is generally defined as an ejection fraction of 30% to 35% or less. In the Stanford experience, the five-year survival of comparable medically and surgically treated patients with poor left ventricular function was 18% and 66%, respectively.[125] Operative mortality in this group of patients treated between 1972 and 1978 was 9% and the strongest determinant of survival was the presence or absence of preoperative congestive heart failure. Another study of patients with impaired left ventricular function[126] reported a 2.1% operative mortality, a two-year survival of approximately 90%, and angina relief in 77%. An intraaortic balloon pump was used in 9% of these patients and the low operative mortality was attributed to better myocardial protection and other technical factors.

A recent review from the Cleveland Clinic addressed the question of whether the type of conduit used influences long-term survival after bypass grafting.[127] Two groups of patients were studied: (1) patients who received an internal mammary artery graft alone or combined with saphenous vein grafts; (2) patients who received saphenous vein bypass grafts only. Multivariate analysis showed that the internal mammary artery graft was second only to ventricular function as a predictor of survival. Survival at ten years in the group with internal mammary artery grafts was 86.6% compared with 75.9% in the group with vein grafts. In the group with internal mammary artery grafts, the ten-year survival was 93.4% for one-vessel disease, 90.0% for two-vessel disease, and 82.6% for three-vessel disease. Rates for the saphenous vein graft

Table 38.4. Five-Year Survival After Coronary Artery Surgery

Study Group	Patients (No.)	Series Year	Five-Year Survival (%)
The Cleveland Clinic Foundation[112]	741	1967–1970	89.0
Baylor College of Medicine[113]	1,144	1969–1971	88.6
Hospital of the Good Samaritan (LA)[114]	1,532	1969–1974	83.6
Salt Lake City[110]	761	1969–1980	91.6
St. Louis University[115]	1,733	1970–1977	88.1
Texas Heart Institute[109]	22,284	1970–1981	89.6
St. Louis Park and Hennepin County Medical Centers, Minneapolis[116]	304	1971–1978	88.0
Veterans Administration Cooperative[117]	332	1972–1974	83.0
Hines Veterans Administration, Loyola University[118]	71	1968–1974	87.4
Seattle Heart Watch[119]	1,880	1968–1974	86.3
The Cleveland Clinic Foundation[†49]	5,000	1973–1977	94.2
Buffalo General Hospital[120]	1,051	1973–1977	94.0
Emory University[42]	3,433	1973–1979	89.0
European Coronary Surgery Study Group[23]	368	1973–1976	92.4‡

* Cardiac deaths only.

† From 1973–1977, the first 1,000 patients operated on each year.

‡ Men with mild-moderate angina and good left ventricular function.

From Loop FD: Progress in surgical treatment of coronary atherosclerosis. Part 2. *Chest* 1983; 84:740–755. Used with permission.

Table 38.5. Comparison of Five-Year Survival in Medically Treated Patients

Indications	CASS[6] (%)	Proudfit[124] (%)
Mild angina, EF ≥ 0.5	95	91.3
One-vessel	95	94.5
Two-vessel	97	89.0
Three-vessel	94	82.7
Mild angina, EF <0.5	85	71.9
Postinfarction, no angina	89	85.4
One-vessel disease	93	94.5
Two-vessel disease	94	88.0
Three-vessel disease	89	80.3

EF = ejection fraction.

cohort were 88.0%, 79.5%, and 71.0%, respectively (Figure 38.1). In addition, patients receiving internal mammary artery grafts had overall significantly fewer cardiac events and rehospitalizations than did the group with vein grafts only.

Older age has an adverse effect on survival after bypass surgery. A CASS report on patients aged 65 or older who underwent coronary artery surgery[128] found an operative mortality of 5% and a five-year cumulative survival of 83%. Survival at five years was 84% in patients aged 65 to 69 years, 80% for those aged 70 to 74, and 70% for those aged 75 or older. Left ventricular dysfunction and associated medical disease had further adverse effects on survival.

The influence of perioperative myocardial infarction on survival formed the basis of another CASS report.[129] These investigators found a 5.7% incidence of perioperative infarction in the pooled series. Complicated perioperative infarcts were defined by congestive heart failure, shock, dysrhythmia, or arrest. Five-year survival was not significantly different in patients without perioperative infarcts than in patients with uncomplicated perioperative infarcts (92% versus 89% for those discharged from the hospital). Patients with complicated perioperative infarcts had a hospital mortality of 45.2% and, of the hospital survivors, only 73% were alive at five years, a significant difference. In another report of patients with perioperative infarction, 76% survived five years compared with 90% of those without such infarcts.[130] A third study found no difference between patients with and those without perioperative infarction in either clinical status or survival.[131]

Cardiac events are reduced in frequency after bypass surgery. The Seattle Heart Watch found a 26% reduction in cardiovascular hospitalizations for their surgically treated cohort compared with the medical group. The rate of hospitalization for myocardial infarction was 1.1% per year in the surgical group versus 2.6% per year in the medical group after a mean follow-up of six years.[132] When perioperative infarction was considered, the overall infarction rate was not significantly different between the two groups. Mason et al[133] found that both the incidence and fatal outcome of acute myocardial infarction were lower in surgical patients.

The favorable influence of bypass surgery on the incidence of sudden death has been documented.[134,135] In one study of patients with two- and three-vessel disease,

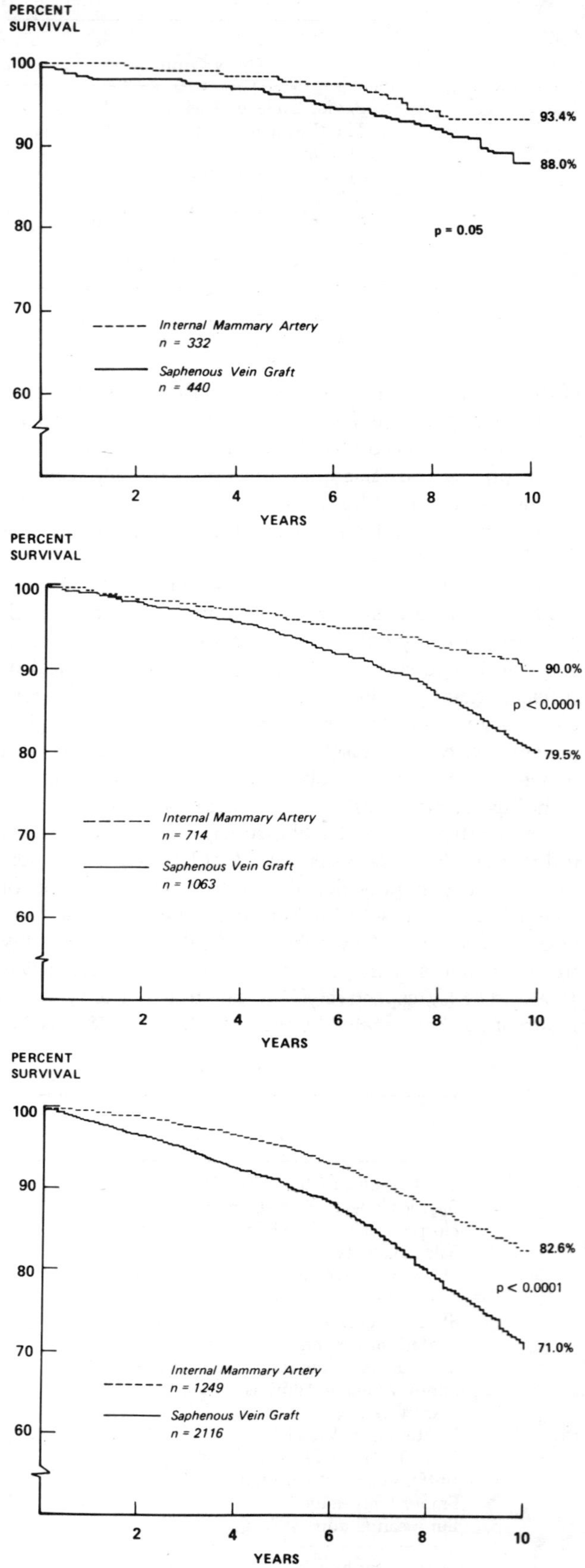

Figure 38.1. Survival curves for internal mammary artery versus saphenous vein graft groups: *top*, one-vessel disease; *middle*, two-vessel disease; *bottom*, three-vessel disease. (From Loop et al[127] with permission.)

6% of the surgical patients and 24% of the medical patients died suddenly (mean 39 months).

The effect of coronary grafting on malignant ventricular dysrhythmias has been more difficult to define. Most investigators have found no consistent improvement in the frequency or severity of ventricular dysrhythmias that occur at rest or with exercise.[136,137]

RETURN TO WORK

There are many factors that influence whether or not a patient will return to work after coronary artery surgery. Although most patients are symptomatically improved, reports have identified other factors that influence postoperative employment (Table 38.6). Preoperative employment, postoperative clinical status, and age are the strongest predictors of return to work. A report from Montreal noted that an increasing percentage of patients are returning to work after coronary artery surgery. In patients operated on between 1969 and 1972, the rate was 69%; between 1973 and 1978, 76%; and in 1979 and 1980, 89%.[141] Clearly, this issue has important economic ramifications.

UNSTABLE ANGINA

The term "unstable angina" is imprecise but includes patients with recent onset of angina, recent progressive angina, and a changing pattern of angina either at rest or with effort. Coronary arteriography has been recommended in all patients with unstable angina[14] to identify those with high risk pathoanatomy (left main and three-vessel disease) and to evaluate patients for coronary bypass grafting or angioplasty in the event that symptoms continue or recur despite maximal medical therapy.

The initial therapy of patients with unstable angina should include intensive medical management to achieve hemodynamic stability. The finding of a 4% operative mortality and an 18% perioperative infarction rate in patients without an organized preoperative stabilization period emphasizes this recommendation.[142] Early management may include the use of nitrates, beta blockers, calcium antagonists, hemodynamic monitoring with adjustment of preload and afterload, and, if needed, intraaortic balloon pumping. Such therapy will stabilize the majority of patients and reduce the risk in those for whom surgical intervention is indicated. More recent reports[143–146] cite operative mortality of 1.2% to 3%, perioperative infarct rates of 2% to 13%, and good long-term survival with reduced symptoms in selected patients with unstable angina.

Table 38.6. Factors Affecting Return to Work Cited in Two or More Studies*

Positive Factors	Negative Factors
Employed preoperatively	Unemployed preoperatively
Age <55 yr	Age >55 yr
High income	Low income
Male	Female
Self-employed worker	Blue-collar worker
White-collar worker	Presence of cardiac symptoms
College education	Number of chronic medical problems
Relief of symptoms	Physician advice
Good LV performance	Receipt of disability compensation
College education	

* This information was abstracted largely from references 138 to 140.
LV = left ventricular.
From Loop FD: Progress in surgical treatment of coronary atherosclerosis. Part 2. *Chest* 1983; 84:740–755. Used with permission.

About 36% of patients with unstable angina for whom early medical management is successful will undergo operation in the first 30 months.[147] Discriminant analysis has found that multiple vessel involvement, frequent angina, prolonged pain, heart failure, and hypertension are clinical markers for the crossover group.[148]

ACUTE INFARCTION

Patients with acute myocardial infarction face a risk of in-hospital death of between 30% and 40%.[149] Although early mortality is higher in patients with transmural infarction, about 43% of patients with nontransmural infarction will have extension of their infarcts within two weeks.[150] Because approximately 60% of patients in the nontransmural infarction group have two- or three-vessel disease, they are considered by some to be candidates for coronary arteriography.[151] Patients in whom postinfarction angina develops face mortality rates that may be 50% or higher.[152,153] Subsets of patients who survive transmural infarction face high first-year mortality rates if they have either severe left ventricular impairment or they demonstrate ischemia during exercise stress testing.[12] Extent of disease and degree of left ventricular impairment have been correlated with prognosis in the first three years after infarction.[154]

Nevertheless, myocardial infarction per se is not generally accepted as an indication for either coronary arteriography or emergency revascularization. This is probably because reports from groups that perform such emergency operations make it clear that timing is critical for a successful outcome.[155,156] The Spokane group,[157] reviewed earlier, has the most extensive experience in this area. Operative mortality for patients with nontransmural infarcts was 3.1%. The rate in patients with transmural infarcts operated on within six hours of the onset of symptoms was 3.8%, whereas the rate in the subset of patients undergoing subsequent revascularization was 8%. At ten-year follow-up, the survival rate was 92% for the early revascularization group and 79% for those who underwent subsequent revascularization. Although impressive, these data do not support the concept that early revascularization is beneficial in all patients with acute infarction, because such benefit could only be demonstrated in a randomized trial.

REOPERATION

Reoperations for coronary artery disease are increasing in frequency. In the early years of coronary artery surgery, reoperation was performed most often for early graft closure or incomplete revascularization. Today, late graft closure, often secondary to vein graft atherosclerosis, and progressive coronary atherosclerosis account for most reoperations. Greater operative experience, better myocardial protection, and better blood conservation measures have improved the results of reoperation for coronary disease.[158] The experience with coronary reoperations from the Cleveland Clinic has been reviewed.[159] Patient-related risk factors for reoperation were little different from those in patients undergoing first-time coronary operation with the exception that insulin-dependent diabetic patients were more numerous in the reoperation group (19% versus 9%). Coronary atherosclerosis before reoperation was more extensive than before the primary operation. Three-vessel disease was seen in 79% and left main coronary artery disease in 22%. Similarly, left ventricular dysfunction was worse in that 60% of patients had left ventricular impairment and one third lost previously normal left ventricular function in the interval between operations. The rate of reoperation for graft failure increased from 26% during 1969 to 1976 to 40% during 1981 to 1982. In contrast, reoperation for progressive atherosclerosis in the native circulation declined from 62% in 1969 to 1976 to 23% in 1981 to 1982, presumably because of more complete revascularization at the initial procedure in the later group and greater use of the internal mammary artery graft.

Mortality for reoperation was 2% in the more recent group, and major perioperative morbidity also decreased significantly in the later years. The number of grafts per patient increased from 1.4 to 2.3 and complete revascularization increased from 65% to 76%.

Vein graft patency rates were essentially the same as those for primary operations and the superior patency of internal mammary artery conduits was also seen in the reoperation group. Complete relief of symptoms occurred five years postoperatively in 50% of patients undergoing reoperation compared with 60% to 70% of those undergoing primary operation, a finding attributed to more diffuse disease and left ventricular dysfunction in the patients undergoing a second coronary procedure. Survival in the reoperation group was 89% at five years and was influenced by the extent of disease and left ventricular function. Survival was not significantly different among the groups with angiographic indications, ie, those operated on for graft closure, progressive disease, or both, fared equally well.

REFERENCES

1. McGinnis JM: Recent health gains for adults. *N Engl J Med* 1982; 306:671–673.
2. Kannel WB: Meaning of the downward trend in cardiovascular mortality. *JAMA* 1982; 247:877–880.
3. Stamler J: The marked decline in coronary heart disease mortality rates in the United States, 1968-1981; summary of findings and possible explanations. *Cardiology* 1985; 72:11–22.
4. Working Group on Heart Disease Epidemiology: The National Heart, Lung and Blood Institute. NIH Publication No. (NIH) 79-1667, National Heart, Lung and Blood Institute, Bethesda, MD, June 1979
5. Sones FM Jr, Shirey EK: Cine coronary arteriography. *Mod Concepts Cardiovasc Dis* 1962; 31:735–738.
6. CASS Principal Investigators and Their Associates: Coronary Artery Surgery Study (CASS): A randomized trial of coronary artery bypass surgery: survival data. *Circulation* 1983; 68:939–950.
7. Killip T, and the Principal Investigators of CASS and Their Associates: The National Heart, Lung, and Blood Institute Coronary Artery Surgery Study (CASS). *Circulation* 1981; 63(suppl I):1–39.
8. Gould KL: Dynamic coronary stenosis. *Am J Cardiol* 1980; 45:286–292.
9. Wright C, Doty D, Eastham C, Laughlin D, Krumm P, Marcus M: A method for assessing the physiologic significance of coronary obstructions in man at cardiac surgery. *Circulation* 1980; 62(suppl I)I-111–I-115.
10. Waller BF, Roberts WC: Amount of narrowing by atherosclerotic plaque in 44 nonbypassed and 52 bypassed major epicardial coronary arteries in 32 necropsy patients who died within 1 month of aortocoronary bypass grafting. *Am J Cardiol* 1980; 46:956–962.
11. Levin DC, Cohn LH, Koster JK Jr, Collins JJ Jr: The reliability of angiography in predicting quality and caliber of the distal coronary artery lumen in preparation for bypass surgery. *Circulation* 1983; 68(suppl II)II-185–II-189.
12. Epstein SE, Palmeri ST, Patterson RE: Evaluation of patients after acute myocardial infarction: indications for cardiac catheterization and surgical intervention. *N Engl J Med* 1982; 307:1487–1492.
13. Rogers WJ, Mantle JA, Rackley CE: Is coronary bypass surgery feasible in evolving MI? *J Cardiovasc Med* 1982; 7:835–850.
14. Russell RO, Rackley CE, Kouchoukos NT: Unstable angina pectoris: management based on available information. *Circulation* 1982; 65(suppl II):II-72–II-77.
15. Eisenberg MS, Hallstrom A, Bergner L: Long-term survival after out-of-hospital cardiac arrest. *N Engl J Med* 1982; 306:1340–1343.
16. Baum RS, Alvarez H, Cobb LA: Survival after resuscitation from out of hospital ventricular fibrillation. *Circulation* 1974; 50:1231–1235.
17. Ruskin JN, DiMarco JP, Garan H: Out-of-hospital cardiac arrest: electrophysiologic observation and selection of long term anti-arrhythmic therapy. *N Engl J Med* 1980; 303:607–613.
18. Takaro T, Hultgren HN, Lipton MJ, Detre KM, and Participants in the Study Group: The VA cooperative randomized study of surgery for coronary arterial occlusive disease. II. Subgroup with significant left main lesions. *Circulation* 1976; 54(suppl III):III-107–III-117.
19. Proudfit WL, Bruschke AVG, Sones FM Jr: Clinical course of patients with normal or slightly or moderately abnormal coronary arteriograms: 10-year follow-up of 521 patients. *Circulation* 1980; 62:712–717.
20. Mock MB, Ringqvist I, Fisher LD, Davis KB, Chaitman BR, Kouchoukos NT, Kaiser GC, Alderman E, Ryan TJ, Russell RO Jr, Mullin S, Fray D, Killip T III, and Participants in the Coronary Artery Surgery Study: Survival of medically treated patients in the Coronary Artery Surgery Study (CASS) Registry. *Circulation* 1982; 66:562–568.
21. Gould KL, Lipscomb K, Hamilton GW: Physiologic basis for assessing critical coronary stenosis: instantaneous flow response and regional distribution during coronary hyperemia as measures of coronary flow reserve. *Am J Cardiol* 1974; 33:87-94.
22. Takaro T, Hultgren HN, Detre KM, Peduzzi P: The Veterans Administration Cooperative Study of stable angina: current status. *Circulation* 1982; 65(suppl II):II-60–II-67.
23. European Coronary Surgery Study Group: Long-term results of prospective randomised study of coronary artery bypass surgery in stable angina pectoris. *Lancet* 1982; 2:1173–1180.
24. Hammermeister KE: Survival analyses: summation and clinical implications, in Hammermeister KE (ed): *Coronary Bypass Surgery. The Late Results*. New York; Praeger Publishers, 1983, pp 251–261.
25. Platia EV, Grunwald L, Mellits ED, Humphries JO, Griffith LSC: Clinical and arteriographic variables predictive of survival in coronary artery disease. *Am J Cardiol* 1980; 46:543–552.
26. Harris PJ, Harrell FE Jr, Lee KL, Behar VS, Rosati RA: Survival in medically treated coronary artery disease. *Circulation* 1979; 60:1259–1269.
27. Mock MB, Fisher L, Killip T, Alderman EL, Austen WG, Bourassa MA, Brooks H, Cohen LS, Frommer PL, Frye RL, Glassman E, Gosselin AJ, Harthorne JW, Judkins MP, Kaiser GC, Kemp HG Jr, McKneally MF, Mudd JF, Myers W, Passamani E, Ringqvist I, Rogers WJ, Russel RO Jr, Ryan TJ, Sautter RD, Sheffield T, Sosa JA, Tristani F, Fray D: The natural history of nonoperated patients with ischemic heart disease: The CASS experience, in Hammermeister KE (ed): *Coronary Bypass Surgery. The Late Results.* New York, Praeger Publishers, 1983, pp 83–98.
28. Burggraf GW, Parker JO: Prognosis in coronary artery disease: angiographic, hemodynamic, and clinical factors. *Circulation* 1975; 51:146–156.
29. Proudfit WL, Bruschke AVG, Sones FM Jr: Natural history of obstructive coronary artery disease: ten-year study of 601 nonsurgical cases. *Prog Cardiovasc Dis* 1978; 21:53–78.
30. Califf RM, Tomabechi Y, Lee KL, Phillips H, Pryor DB, Harrell FE Jr, Harris PJ, Peter RH, Behar VS, Kong Y, Rosati RA: Outcome in one-vessel coronary artery disease. *Circulation* 1983; 67:283–290.
31. Harris PJ, Lee KL, Harrell FE, Behar VS, Rosati RA: Outcome in medically treated coronary artery disease. Ischemic events: nonfatal infarction and death. *Circulation* 1980; 62:718–726.
32. Proudfit WL, Bruschke AVG, MacMillan JP, Williams GW, Sones FM Jr: Fifteen-year survival study of patients with obstructive coronary artery disease. *Circulation* 1983; 68:986–997.
33. Corday E, Swan HJC, Corday SR: Medical versus surgical treatment of coronary artery disease - 1981. *Cardiovasc Rev Rep* 1981; 2:281–288.
34. Alderman EL, Fisher L, Maynard C, Mock MB, Ringqvist I, Bourassa MG, Kaiser GC, Gillespie MJ: Determinants of coronary surgery in a consecutive patient series from geographically dispersed medical cen-

ters: The Coronary Artery Surgery Study. *Circulation* 1982; 66(suppl I):I-6–I-15.

35. Leong K, Jones RH: Influence of the location of left anterior descending coronary artery stenosis on left ventricular function during exercise. *Circulation* 1982; 65:109–114.
36. Brooks N, Cattell M, Jennings K, Balcon R, Honey M, Layton C: Isolated disease of left anterior descending coronary artery. *Br Heart J* 1982; 47:71–77.
37. Abedin Z, Dack S: Isolated left anterior descending coronary artery disease: choice of therapy. *Am J Cardiol* 1977; 40:654–657.
38. Epstein SE, Kent KM, Goldstein RE, Borer JS, Rosing DR: Strategy for evaluation and surgical treatment of the asymptomatic or mildly symptomatic patient with coronary artery disease. *Am J Cardiol* 1979; 43:1015–1025.
39. Kent KM, Rosing DR, Ewels CJ, Lipson L, Bonow R, Epstein SE: Prognosis of asymptomatic or mildly symptomatic patients with coronary artery disease. *Am J Cardiol* 1982; 49:1823–1831.
40. Kouchoukos NT, Oberman A, Kirklin JW, Russell RO Jr, Karp RB, Pacifico AD, Zorn GL: Coronary bypass surgery: analysis of factors affecting hospital mortality. *Circulation* 1980; 62(suppl I): I-84–I-89.
41. Rahimtoola SH, Grunkemeier GL, Teply JF, Lambert LE, Thomas DR, Suen YF, Starr A: Changes in coronary bypass surgery leading to improved survival. *JAMA* 1981; 246:1912–1916.
42. Jones EL, Craver JM, King SB III, Douglas JS, Bradford JM, Brown CM, Bone DK, Hatcher CR Jr: Clinical, anatomic and functional descriptors influencing morbidity, survival and adequacy of revascularization following coronary bypass. *Ann Surg* 1980; 192:390–402.
43. Loop FD, Cosgrove DM, Lytle BW, Thurer RL, Simpfendorfer C, Taylor PC, Proudfit WL: An 11 year evolution of coronary arterial surgery (1967-1978). *Ann Surg* 1979; 190:444–455.
44. Miller DC, Stinson EB, Oyer PE, Jamieson SW, Mitchell RS, Reitz BA, Baumgartner WA, Shumway NE: Discriminant analysis of the changing risks of coronary artery operations: 1971-1979. *J Thorac Cardiovasc Surg* 1983; 85:197–213.
45. Kennedy JW, Kaiser GC, Fisher LD, Maynard C, Fritz JK, Myers W, Mudd JG, Ryan TJ, Coggin J: Multivariate discriminant analysis of the clinical and angiographic predictors of operative mortality from the Collaborative Study in Coronary Artery Surgery (CASS). *J Thorac Cardiovasc Surg* 1980; 80:876–887.
46. Chaitman BR, Rogers WJ, Davis K, Tyras DH, Berger R, Bourassa MG, Fisher L, StoverHertzberg V, Judkins MP, Mock MB, Killip T: Operative risk factors in patients with left main coronary-artery disease. *N Engl J Med* 1980; 303:953–957.
47. Cosgrove DM, Loop FD, Lytle BW, Baillot R, Gill CC, Golding LAR, Taylor PC, Goormastic M: Primary myocardial revascularization: trends in surgical mortality. *J Thorac Cardiovasc Surg* 1984; 88:673–684.
48. Fisher LD, Kennedy JW, Davis KB, Maynard C, Fritz JK, Kaiser G, Myers WO, and the Participating CASS Clinics: Association of sex, physical size, and operative mortality after coronary artery bypass in the Coronary Artery Surgery Study (CASS). *J Thorac Cardiovasc Surg* 1982; 84:334–341.
49. Loop FD, Golding LR, MacMillan JP, Cosgrove DM, Lytle BW, Sheldon WC: Coronary artery surgery in women compared with men: analyses of risks and long-term results. *J Am Coll Cardiol* 1983; 1:383–390.
50. Engelman RM, Rousou JH, Lemeshow S, Dobbs WA: The metabolic consequences of blood and crystalloid cardioplegia. *Circulation* 1981; 64(suppl II):II-67–II-74.
51. Levitsky S, Feinberg H: Techniques for administering clinical cardioplegia-crystalloid cardioplegia, in Engelman RE, Levitsky S (eds): *A Textbook of Clinical Cardioplegia.* Mount Kisco, NY, Futura Publishers, 1982, pp 297–304.
52. Daggett WM, Jacocks MA, Coleman WS, Johnson RG, Lowenstein E, Vander Salm TJ: Myocardial temperature mapping: improved intraoperative myocardial preservation. *J Thorac Cardiovasc Surg* 1981. 82:883–888.
53. Roberts AJ, Moran JM, Sanders JH, Spies SM, Lichtenthal PR, Kaplan KJ, Michaelis LL: Clinical evaluation of the relative effectiveness of multidose crystalloid and cold blood potassium cardioplegia in coronary artery bypass graft surgery: a nonrandomized matched-pair analysis. *Ann Thorac Surg* 1982; 33:421–433.
54. Cunningham JN Jr, Adams PX, Knopp EA, Baumann FG, Snively SL, Gross RI, Nathan IM, Spencer FC: Preservation of ATP, ultrastructure, and ventricular function after aortic cross-clamping and reperfusion: clinical use of blood potassium cardioplegia. *J Thorac Cardiovasc Surg* 1979; 78:708–720.
55. Buckberg GD: Progress in myocardial protection during cardiac operations. *Cardiovasc Clin* 1982; 12:9–30.
56. Berger RL, Davis KB, Kaiser GC, Foster ED, Hammond GL, Tong TGL, Kennedy JW, Sheffield T, Ringqvist I, Wiens RD, Chaitman BR, Mock M: Preservation of the myocardium during coronary artery bypass grafting. *Circulation* 1981; 64(suppl II):II-61–II-66.
57. Moore GW, Hutchins GM: Coronary artery bypass grafts in 109 autopsied patients: statistical analysis of graft and anastomosis patency and regional myocardial injury. *JAMA* 1981: 246:1785–1789.
58. Bulkley BH, Hutchins GM: Myocardial consequences of coronary artery bypass graft surgery: the paradox of necrosis in areas of revascularization. *Circulation* 1977; 56:906–913.
59. Chatterjee K, Swan HJC, Parmley WW, Sustaita H, Marcus H, Matloff J: Depression of left ventricular function due to acute myocardial ischemia and its reversal after aortocoronary saphenous-vein bypass. *N Engl J Med* 1972; 286:1117–1122.
60. Chatterjee K, Matloff JM, Swan HJC, Ganz W, Kaushik VS, Magnusson P, Henis MM, Forrester JS: Abnormal regional metabolism and mechanical function in patients with ischemic heart disease: improvement after successful regional revascularization by aortocoronary bypass. *Circulation* 1975; 52:390–399.
61. Wolf NM, Kreulen TH, Bove AA, McDonough MT, Kessler KM, Strong M, LeMole G, Spann JF: Left ventricular function following coronary bypass surgery. *Circulation* 1978: 58:63–70.
62. Zir LM, Dinsmore R, Vexeridis M, Singh JB, Harthorne JW, Daggett WM: Effects of coronary bypass grafting on resting left ventricular contraction in patients studied 1 to 2 years after operation. *Am J Cardiol* 1979; 44:601–606.
63. Kent KM, Borer JS, Green MV, Bacharach SL, McIntosh CL, Conkle DM, Epstein SE: Effects of coronary-artery bypass on global and regional left ventricular function during exercise. *N Engl J Med* 1978; 298:1434–1439.
64. Campeau L, Lespérance J, Corbara F, Hermann J, Grondin CM, Bourassa MG: Aortocoronary saphenous vein bypass graft changes 5 to 7 years after surgery. *Circulation* 1978; 58(suppl I):I-170–I-175.
65. Kouchoukos NT, Karp RB, Oberman A, Russell RO Jr, Alison HW, Holt JH Jr: Long-term patency of saphenous veins for coronary bypass grafting. *Circulation* 1978; 58(suppl I):I-96–I-99.
66. Campeau L, Crochet D, Lespérance J, Bourassa MG, Grondin CM: Postoperative changes in aortocoronary saphenous vein grafts revisited: angiographic studies at two weeks and at one year in two series of consecutive patients. *Circulation* 1975; 52:369–377.
67. Bourassa MG, Campeau L, Lespérance J, Grondin CM: Changes in grafts and in coronary arteries after saphenous vein aortocoronary bypass surgery, in Hammermeister KE (ed): *Coronary Bypass Surgery. The Late Results.* New York, Praeger Publishers, 1983, pp 293–310.
68. Lawrie GM, Morris GC Jr, Chapman DW, Winters WL, Lie JT: Patterns of patency of 596 vein grafts up to seven years after aorta-coronary bypass. *J Thorac Cardiovasc Surg* 1977; 73:443–448.
69. Cosgrove DM, Loop FD, Saunders CR, Lytle BW, Kramer JR: Should coronary arteries with less than fifty percent stenosis be bypassed? *J Thorac Cardiovasc Surg* 1981; 82:520–530.
70. Siefert D, Bircks W, Jehle J, Schulte HD: Aorto-coronary bypass grafts using cephalic veins. *Thorac Cardiovasc Surg* 1982; 30:15(A).
71. Bical O, Bachet J, Laurian C, Camilleri JP, Goudot B, Menu P, Guilmet D: Aortocoronary bypass with homologous saphenous vein: long-term results. *Ann Thorac Surg* 1980; 30:550–557.
72. Grondin CM, Limet R: Sequential anastomoses in coronary artery grafting: technical aspects and early and late angiographic results. *Ann Thorac Surg* 1977; 23:1–8.
73. Grondin CM, Vouhé P, Bourassa MG, Lespérance J, Bouvier M, Campeau L: Optimal patency rates obtained in coronary artery grafting with circular vein grafts. *J Thorac Cardiovasc Surg* 1978; 75:161–167.
74. Sewell WH: Should we do Y- and sequential grafts for coronary bypass? *Ann Thorac Surg* 1979; 27:397–398.
75. Yeh TJ, Heidary D, Shelton L: Y-grafts and sequential grafts in coronary bypass surgery: a critical evaluation of patency rates. *Ann Thorac Surg* 1979; 27:409–412.
76. Halim MA, Qureshi SA, Towers MK, Yacoub MH: Early and late results of combined endarterectomy and coronary bypass grafting for diffuse coronary disease. *Am J Cardiol* 1982; 49:1623–1626.
77. Miller DC, Stinson EB, Oyer PE, Reitz BA, Jamieson SW, Moreno-Cabral RJ: Long-term clinical assessment of the efficacy of adjunctive coronary endarterectomy. *J Thorac Cardiovasc Surg* 1981; 81:21–29.
78. Pantely GA, Goodnight SH Jr, Rahimtoola SH, Harlan BJ, DeMots H, Calvin L, Rosch J: Failure of antiplatelet and anticoagulant therapy to improve patency of grafts after coronary-artery bypass: a controlled, randomized study. *N Engl J Med* 1979; 301:962–966.
79. Mayer JE, Lindsay WG, Castaneda W, Nicoloff DM: Influence of aspirin and dipyridamole on patency of coronary artery bypass grafts. *Ann Thorac Surg* 1981; 31:204–210.
80. Baur HR, VanTassel RA, Pierach CA, Gobel FL: Effects of sulfinpyrazone on early graft closure after myocardial revascularization. *Am J Cardiol* 1982; 49:420–424.
81. Metke MP, Lie JT, Fuster V, Josa M, Kaye MP: Reduction of intimal thickening in canine coronary bypass vein grafts with dipyridamole and aspirin. *Am J Cardiol* 1979; 43:1144–1148.
82. Steele PP, Rainwater JO, Vogel RA: Sulfinpyrazone decreases vein graft occlusion in patients following coronary artery bypass surgery. *Am J Cardiol* 1980; 45:425(A).
83. McEnany MT, Salzman EW, Mundth ED, DeSanctis RW, Harthorne JW, Weintraub RM, Gates S, Austen WG: The effect of antithrombotic

therapy on patency rates of saphenous vein coronary artery bypass grafts. *J Thorac Cardiovasc Surg* 1982; 83:81–89.

84. Chesebro JH, Clements IP, Fuster V, Elveback LR, Smith HC, Bardsley WT, Frye RL, Holmes DR Jr, Vlietstra RE, Pluth JR, Wallace RB, Puga FJ, Orszulak TA, Piehler JM, Schaff HV, Danielson GK: A platelet-inhibitor-drug trial in coronary-artery bypass operations: benefit of perioperative dipyridamole and aspirin therapy on early postoperative vein-graft patency. *N Engl J Med* 1982; 307:73–78.
85. Chesebro JH, Fuster V, Clements IP, Elveback LR, Smith HC, Frye RL, Pluth JR, Schaff HV: Perioperative dipyridamole plus aspirin therapy improves early aortocoronary vein graft patency with a continued late effect on individual grafts. *J Am Coll Cardiol* 1983; 1:618(A).
86. Bourassa MG, Lespérance J, Corbara F, Saltiel J, Campeau L: Progression of obstructive coronary artery disease 5 to 7 years after aortocoronary bypass surgery. *Circulation* 1978; 58(suppl I):I-100–I-106.
87. Frick MH, Valle M, Harjola PT, Korhola O: Changes in native coronary arteries after coronary bypass surgery: role of graft patency, serum lipids and hypertension. *Am J Cardiol* 1975; 36:744–750.
88. Palac RT, Hwang MH, Meadows WR, Croke RP, Pifarre R, Loeb HS, Gunnar RM: Progression of coronary artery disease in medically and surgically treated patients 5 years after randomization. *Circulation* 1981; 64(suppl II):II-17–II-21.
89. Kramer JR, Matsuda Y, Mulligan JC, Aronow M, Proudfit WL: Progression of coronary atherosclerosis. *Circulation* 1981; 63:519–526.
90. Loop FD, Irarrazaval MJ, Bredee JJ, Siegel W, Taylor PC, Sheldon WC: Internal mammary artery graft for ischemic heart disease: effect of revascularization on clinical status and survival. *Am J Cardiol* 1977; 39:516–522.
91. Campeau L, Enjalbert M, Lespérance J, Vaislic C, Grondin CM, Bourassa MG: Atherosclerosis and late closure of aortocoronary saphenous vein grafts: sequential angiographic studies at 2 weeks, 1 year, 5-7 years, and at 10-12 years after surgery. *Circulation* 1983; 68(suppl II):II-1–II-7.
92. Campeau L, Enjalbert M, Lespérance J, Bourassa MG, Kwiterovich P, Wacholder S, Sniderman A: The relation of risk factors to the development of atherosclerosis in saphenous vein bypass grafts and the progression of disease in the native circulation. *N Engl J Med* 1984; 311:1329–1332.
93. Siegel W, Loop FD: Comparison of internal mammary artery and saphenous vein bypass grafts for myocardial revascularization: exercise test and angiographic correlations. *Circulation* 1976; 54(suppl III):III-1–III-3.
94. Vogel JHK, McFadden RB, Spence R, Jahnke EJ Jr, Love JW: Quantitative assessment of myocardial performance and graft patency following coronary bypass with the internal mammary artery. *J Thorac Cardiovasc Surg* 1978; 75:487–498.
95. Tector AJ, Schmahl TM, Janson B, Kallies JR, Johnson G: The internal mammary artery graft: its longevity after coronary bypass. *JAMA* 1981; 246:2181–2183.
96. Sims FH: A comparison of coronary and internal mammary arteries and implications of the results in the etiology of arteriosclerosis. *Am Heart J* 1983; 106:560–566.
97. Loop FD, Sheldon WC, Lytle BW, Cosgrove DM, Proudfit WL: The efficacy of coronary artery surgery. *Am Heart J* 1981; 101:86–96.
98. Barner HB, Swartz MT, Mudd JG, Tyras DH: Late patency of the internal mammary artery as a coronary bypass conduit. *Ann Thorac Surg* 1982; 34:408–412.
99. Lytle BW, Cosgrove DM, Saltus GL, Taylor PC, Loop FD: Multivessel coronary revascularization without saphenous vein: long-term results of bilateral internal mammary artery grafting. *Ann Thorac Surg* 1983; 36:540–547.
100. Lytle BW, Loop FD, Cosgrove DM, Ratliff NB, Easley K, Taylor PC: Long-term (5 to 12 years) serial studies of internal mammary artery and saphenous vein coronary bypass grafts. *J Thorac Cardiovasc Surg* 1985; 89:248–258.
101. Rahimtoola SH: Coronary bypass surgery for chronic angina — 1981: a perspective. *Circulation* 1982; 65:225–241.
102. Cameron A, Kemp HG, Shimomura S, Santilli E, Green GE, Hutchinson JE, Mekhjian H: Coronary bypass surgery, a ten year follow-up. *Circulation* 1982; 66(suppl II):II-245(A).
103. Campeau L, Lespérance J, Hermann J, Corbara F, Grondin CM, Bourassa MG: Loss of the improvement of angina between 1 and 7 years after aortocoronary bypass surgery: correlations with changes in vein grafts and in coronary arteries. *Circulation* 1979; 60(suppl I):I-1–I-5.
104. Frick MH, Harjola PT, Valle M: Persistent improvement after coronary bypass surgery: ergometric and angiographic correlations at five years. *Circulation* 1983; 67:491–496.
105. Palac RT, Meadows WR, Hwang MH, Loeb HS, Pifarre R, Gunnar RM: Risk factors related to progressive narrowing in aortocoronary vein grafts studied 1 and 5 years after surgery. *Circulation* 1982; 66(suppl I):I-40–I-44.
106. Cukingnan RA, Carey JS, Wittig JH, Brown BG: Influence of complete coronary revascularization on relief of angina. *J Thorac Cardiovasc Surg* 1980; 79:188–193.
107. Jones EL, Craver JM, Guyton RA, Bone DK, Hatcher CR Jr, Riechwald N: Importance of complete revascularization in performance of the coronary bypass operation. *Am J Cardiol* 1983; 51:7–12.
108. Lawrie GM, Morris GC Jr, Calhoon JH, Safi H, Zamora JL, Beltengady M, Baron A, Silvers A, Chapman DW: Clinical results of coronary bypass in 500 patients at least 10 years after operation. *Circulation* 1982; 66(suppl I):I-1–I-5.
109. Hall RJ, Elayda MA, Gray A, Mathur VS, Garcia E, DeCastro CM, Massumi A, Cooley DA: Coronary artery bypass: long-term follow-up of 22,284 consecutive patients. *Circulation* 1983; 68(suppl II):II-20–II-26.
110. Liddle HV: Perspectives in coronary artery surgery. *J Thorac Cardiovasc Surg* 1981; 81:1–10.
111. Mathur VS, Guinn GA: Prospective randomized study to evaluate coronary bypass surgery: 10 year follow-up. *Circulation* 1982; 66(suppl II):II-219(A).
112. Sheldon WC, Rincon G, Pichard AD, Razavi M, Cheanvechai C, Loop FD: Surgical treatment of coronary artery disease: pure graft operations, with a study of 741 patients followed 3–7 yr. *Prog Cardiovasc Dis* 1975; 18:237–253.
113. Lawrie GM, Morris GC Jr, Howell JF, Ogura JW, Spencer WH III, Cashion WR, Winters WL, Beazley HL, Chapman DW, Peterson PK, Lie JT: Results of coronary bypass more than 5 years after operation in 434 patients. *Am J Cardiol* 1977; 40:665–672.
114. Stiles QR, Lindesmith GG, Tucker BL, Hughes RK, Meyer BW: Long-term follow-up of patients with coronary artery bypass grafts. *Circulation* 1976; 54(suppl III):III-32–III-34.
115. Tyras DH, Barner HB, Kaiser GC, Codd JE, Laks H, Pennington DG, Willman VL: Long-term results of myocardial revascularization. *Am J Cardiol* 1979; 44:1290–1296.
116. Peterson CR, Helseth HK: Survival after coronary artery bypass surgery: significance of preoperative left-ventricular function. *Minn Med* 1979; 62:813–821.
117. Takaro T, and the Participants in the VA Cooperative Study of Surgery for Coronary Arterial Occlusive Disease: Results of a randomized study of medical and surgical management of angina pectoris. *World J Surg* 1978; 2:797–807.
118. Gunnar RM, Loeb HS, Palac R, Pifarre R: Improved survival in patients with chronic angina pectoris treated surgically: report of a randomized prospective study of aortocoronary bypass from Hines, Illinois, in Hurst JW (ed): *The Heart. Update II.* New York, McGraw-Hill Book Co, 1980, pp 205–220.
119. Hammermeister KE, DeRouen TA, Zia M, Dodge HT: Survival of surgically treated coronary artery disease patients in the Seattle Heart Watch angiography registry, in Hammermeister KE (ed): *Coronary Bypass Surgery. The Late Results.* New York, Praeger Publishers, 1983, pp 195–218.
120. Greene DG, Bunnell IL, Arani DT, Schimert G, Lajos TZ, Lee AB, Tandon RN, Zimdahl WT, Bozer JM, Kohn RM, Visco JP, Dean DC, Smith GL: Long-term survival after coronary bypass surgery: comparison of various subsets of patients with general population. *Br Heart J* 1981; 45:417–426.
121. Loop FD, Lytle BW, Cosgrove DM, Sheldon WC, Irarrazaval M, Taylor PC, Groves LK, Pichard AD: Atherosclerosis of the left main coronary artery: 5 year results of surgical treatment. *Am J Cardiol* 1979; 44:195–201.
122. Chaitman BR, Fisher LD, Bourassa MG, Davis K, Rogers WJ, Maynard C, Tyras DH, Berger RL, Judkins MP, Ringqvist I, Mock MB, Killip T, and participating CASS medical centers: Effect of coronary bypass surgery on survival patterns in subsets of patients with left main coronary artery disease: report of the Collaborative Study in Coronary Artery Surgery (CASS). *Am J Cardiol* 1981; 48:765–777.
123. Passamani E, Davis KB, Gillespie MJ, Killip T, and CASS Principal Investigators and Their Associates: A randomized trial of coronary artery bypass surgery: survival of patients with a low ejection fraction. *N Engl J Med* 1985; 312:1665–1671.
124. Proudfit WL, Kramer JR, Bott-Silverman C, Goormastic M: Survival of nonsurgical patients with mild angina or myocardial infarction without angina (in press).
125. Miller DC, Stinson EB, Alderman EL: Surgical treatment of ischemic cardiomyopathy: is it ever too late? *Am J Surg* 1981; 141:688–693.
126. Jones EL, Craver JM, Kaplan JA, King SB III, Douglas JS, Morgan EA, Hatcher CR Jr: Criteria for operability and reduction of surgical mortality in patients with severe left ventricular ischemia and dysfunction. *Ann Thorac Surg* 1978; 25:413–424.
127. Loop FD, Lytle BW, Cosgrove DM, Stewart RW, Goormastic M, Williams GW, Golding LAR, Gill CC, Taylor PC, Sheldon WC, Proudfit WL: Influence of the internal-mammary-artery-graft on 10-year survival and other cardiac events. *N Engl J Med* 1986; 314:1–6.
128. Gersh BJ, Kronmal RA, Schaff HV, Frye RL, Ryan TJ, Myers WO, Athearn MW, Gosselin AJ, Kaiser GC, Killip T III: Long-term (5-year) results of coronary bypass surgery in patients aged 65 years old or older: a report from the Coronary Artery Surgery Study. *Circulation* 1983; 68(suppl II):II-190–II-199.

129. Schaff HV, Gersh BJ, Fisher LD, Frye RL, Mock MB, Ryan TJ, Ells RB, Chaitman BR, Alderman EL, Kaiser GC, Faxon DP, Bourassa MG, and Participants in the Coronary Artery Surgery Study: Detrimental effect of perioperative myocardial infarction on late survival after coronary artery bypass: report from the Coronary Artery Surgery Study - CASS. *J Thorac Cardiovasc Surg* 1984; 88:972–981.
130. Namay DL, Hammermeister KE, Zia MS, DeRouen TA, Dodge HT, Namay K: Effect of perioperative myocardial infarction on late survival in patients undergoing coronary artery bypass surgery. *Circulation* 1982; 65:1066–1071.
131. Gray RJ, Matloff JM, Conklin CM, Ganz W, Charuzi Y, Wolfstein R, Swan HJC: Perioperative myocardial infarction: late clinical course after coronary artery bypass surgery. *Circulation* 1982, 66:1185–1189.
132. Hamilton WM, Hammermeister KE, DeRouen TA, Zia MS, Dodge HT: Effect of coronary artery bypass grafting on subsequent hospitalization. *Am J Cardiol* 1983; 51:353–360.
133. Mason DT, Amsterdam EA, DeMaria AN, Smith JL, Lee G, Joye JA, Vera Z, Awan NA: The prevention of myocardial infarction by coronary bypass surgery, in Hurst JW (ed): *The Heart. Update II*. New York, McGraw-Hill Book Co, 1980, pp 103–114.
134. Hammermeister KE, DeRouen TA, Murray JA, Dodge HT: Effect of aortocoronary saphenous vein bypass grafting on death and sudden death: comparison of nonrandomized medically and surgically treated cohorts with comparable coronary disease and left ventricular function. *Am J Cardiol* 1977; 39:925–934.
135. Vismara LA, Miller RR, Price JE, Karem R, DeMaria AN, Mason DT: Improved longevity due to reduction of sudden death by aortocoronary bypass in coronary atherosclerosis: prospective evaluation of medical versus surgical therapy in matched patients with multivessel disease. *Am J Cardiol* 1977; 39:919–924.
136. Garan H, Ruskin JN, DiMarco JP, Derkac WM, Akins CW, Daggett WM, Austen WG, Buckley MJ: Electrophysiologic studies before and after myocardial revascularization in patients with life-threatening ventricular arrhythmias. *Am J Cardiol* 1983; 51:519–524.
137. Lehrman KL, Tilkian AG, Hultgren HN, Fowles RE: Effect of coronary arterial bypass surgery on exercise-induced ventricular arrhythmias: long-term follow-up of a prospective randomized study. *Am J Cardiol* 1979; 44:1056–1061.
138. Stanton BA, Jenkins CD, Denlinger P, Savageau JA, Weintraub RM, Goldstein RL: Predictors of employment status after cardiac surgery. *JAMA* 1983; 249:907–911.
139. Barnes GK, Ray MJ, Oberman A, Kouchoukos NT: Changes in working status of patients following coronary bypass surgery. *JAMA* 1977; 238:1259–1262.
140. Oberman A, Wayne JB, Kouchoukos NT, Charles ED, Russell RO, Rogers WJ: Employment status after coronary artery bypass surgery. *Circulation* 1982; 65(suppl II):II-115–II-119.
141. Boulay FM, David PP, Bourassa MG: Strategies for improving the work status of patients after coronary artery bypass surgery. *Circulation* 1982; 66(suppl III):III-43–III-49.
142. Golding LAR, Loop FD, Sheldon WC, Taylor PC, Groves LK, Cosgrove DM: Emergency revascularization for unstable angina. *Circulation* 1978; 58:1163–1166.
143. Levine FH, Gold HK, Leinbach RC, Daggett WM, Austen WG, Buckley MJ: Management of acute myocardial ischemia with intraaortic balloon pumping and coronary bypass surgery. *Circulation* 1978; 58(suppl I):I-69–I-72.
144. Jones EL, Waites TF, Craver JM, Bone DK, Hatcher CR Jr, Thompkins T: Unstable angina pectoris: comparison with the National Cooperative Study. *Ann Thorac Surg* 1982; 34:427–434.
145. Hultgren HN, Shettigar UR, Miller DC: Medical versus surgical treatment of unstable angina. *Am J Cardiol* 1982; 50:663–670.
146. Rahimtoola SH, Nunley D, Grunkemeier G, Tepley J, Lambert L, Starr A: Ten-year survival after coronary bypass surgery for unstable angina. *N Engl J Med* 1983; 308:676–681.
147. National Cooperative Study Group: Unstable angina pectoris: National Cooperative Study Group to compare medical and surgical therapy. I. Report of protocol and patient population. *Am J Cardiol* 1976; 37:896–902.
148. Kronenfeld JJ, Charles ED Jr, Wayne JB, Oberman A, Kouchoukos NT, Rogers WJ, Mantle JA, Rackley CE, Russell RO Jr: Unstable angina pectoris: an examination of modes and costs of therapy. *Circulation* 1979; 60(suppl I):I-16–I-22.
149. Goldman L, Cook F, Hashimoto B, Stone P, Muller J, Loscalzo A: Evidence that hospital care for acute myocardial infarction has not contributed to the decline in coronary mortality between 1973–1974 and 1978–1979. *Circulation* 1982; 65:936–942.
150. Marmor A, Sobel BE, Roberts R: Factors presaging early recurrent myocardial infarction ("extension"). *Am J Cardiol* 1981; 48:603–610.
151. Madigan NP, Rutherford BD, Frye RL: The clinical course, early prognosis and coronary anatomy of subendocardial infarction. *Am J Med* 1976; 60:634–641.
152. Schuster EH, Bulkley BH: Early post-infarction angina: ischemia at a distance and ischemia in the infarct zone. *N Engl J Med* 1981; 305:1101–1105.
153. Chaturvedi NC, Walsh MJ, Evans A, Munro P, Boyle DM, Barber JM: Selection of patients for early discharge after acute myocardial infarction. *Br Heart J* 1974; 36:533–535.
154. Sanz G, Castaner A, Betriu A, Magrina J, Roig E, Coll S, Paré JC, Navarro-López F: Determinants of prognosis in survivors of myocardial infarction: a prospective clinical angiographic study. *N Engl J Med* 1982; 306:1065–1070.
155. Berg R, Kendall RW, Duvoisin GE, Ganji JH, Rudy LW, Everhart FJ: Acute myocardial infarction: a surgical emergency. *J Thorac Cardiovasc Surg* 1975; 70:432–439.
156. Phillips SJ, Kongtahworn C, Zeff RH, Benson M, Iannone L, Brown T, Gordon DF: Emergency coronary artery revascularization: a possible therapy for acute myocardial infarction. *Circulation* 1979; 60:241–246.
157. DeWood MA, Spores J, Berg R Jr, Kendall RW, Grunwald RP, Selinger SL, Hensley GR, Sutherland KI, Shields JP: Acute myocardial infarction: a decade of experience with surgical reperfusion in 701 patients. *Circulation* 1983; 68(suppl II):II-8–II-16.
158. Loop FD, Cosgrove DM, Kramer JR, Lytle BW, Taylor PC, Golding LAR, Groves LK: Late clinical and arteriographic results in 500 coronary artery reoperations. *J Thorac Cardiovasc Surg* 1981; 81:675–685.
159. Loop FD, Lytle BW, Gill CC, Golding LAR, Cosgrove DM, Taylor PC: Trends in selection and results of coronary artery reoperations. *Ann Thorac Surg* 1983; 36:380–388.

39 Lasers in Cardiovascular Disease

Daniel S. J. Choy, MD, FACP

In 1958, C.H. Townes of Columbia University invented the MASER (acronym for Microwave Amplification by Stimulated Emission of Radiation). In 1959, in collaboration with A. Schawlow of Bell Telephone Laboratories, Townes proposed the LASER, for Light Amplification by Stimulated Emission of Radiation. In 1960, the first working laser, based on a ruby crystal, was devised by T.H. Maiman of Hughes Aircraft. Since then, numerous types of lasers, based on liquid, gas, and crystal gain media, with wavelengths from x-ray to infrared, have been demonstrated. Of these, only the lasers relevant to medicine will be discussed.

PHYSICS

LASERS

A typical laser is represented in Figure 39.1. The resonator chamber containing the gas, liquid, or crystal medium is terminated at one end by a mirror and at the other with a semitransparent mirror. In gas lasers, an electric discharge generated by the electrodes at the sides of the chamber "pumps" or raises the atoms of the medium to an excited quantum level. When each atom falls back to its ground level, a photon is emitted. In steady-state operation, photons are reflected back and forth between the end mirrors and stimulate the emission of just enough additional photons to provide the optical output power from the semitransparent mirror. The photon wavelength is determined by the energy difference between the ground and the excited quantum levels. The laser thus converts electrical power into highly monochromatic optical power. The laser output takes the form of a well-collimated pencil beam (Figure 39.2). The laser energy may be emitted as single pulses, with a duration expressed in nano- (10^{-9}) or microseconds (10^{-6}), or as a continuous wave (cw). The power of a laser beam is expressed in watts; the total energy, or watts $\times$ time (seconds) as joules. Power density is expressed as watts per square centimeter and incident energy density as joules per square centimeter. "Q" switching is a method of generating short energetic pulses by means of an optical switch inside the resonator that holds off laser action until a large number of excited atoms are stored. Opening the switch then produces a sudden burst of stimulated emission. The term "Q" derives from standard radio and microwave terminology and refers to the quality factor of a resonating system. Peak laser power ranges from miliwatts to megawatts over pulse lengths in the microsecond range.

The lasers with relevance to medicine are listed with their wavelengths (1 nm = 10^{-9} m = 10 angstroms):

Helium–neon	632.3 nm
Ruby	694.3 nm
Argon	488 nm and 514.5 nm
Neodymium: YAG	1060 and 1318 (Yttrium aluminum garnet)
Carbon dioxide	10,600 nm
Dye	various, 630 nm
Excimer (UV)	193, 248, 308, 330 nm

WAVE GUIDES

The laser has been adapted to endoscopic use in the body only because of the existence of the optical fiber. An optical fiber (Figure 39.3) consists of a silica glass core with a glass cladding of slightly lower refractive index surrounding it. A light beam entering one end of an optical fiber is internally reflected within the core until it emerges from the distal end. When a fiber is bent beyond a critical radius ($\pm$1.0 cm), the incident angle of a light beam at the curve exceeds a critical angle beyond which internal reflection cannot occur, and light will be refracted through the cladding. Optical fibers used in medical lasers typically have core diameters ranging from 80 to 600 μm

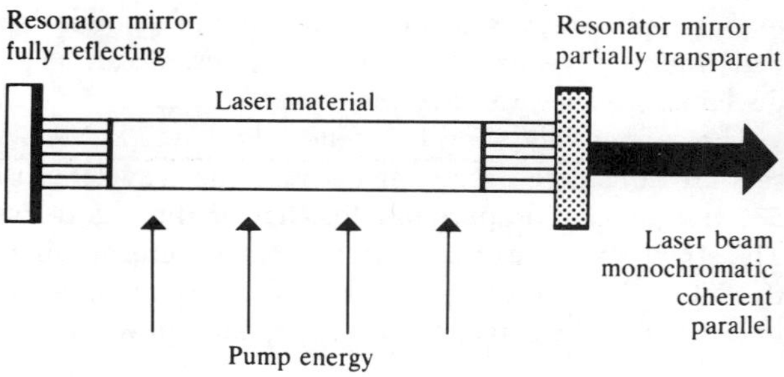

Figure 39.1. Basic elements of a laser. (Figures 39.1, 39.2 and 39.4 are reproduced from Hofstetter A, Frank F: *The Neodymium-YAG Laser in Urology.* Basle, Switzerland, Editiones "Roche," 1980. Copyright 1980 by F Hoffmann-La Roche and Co. Reprinted with permission.)

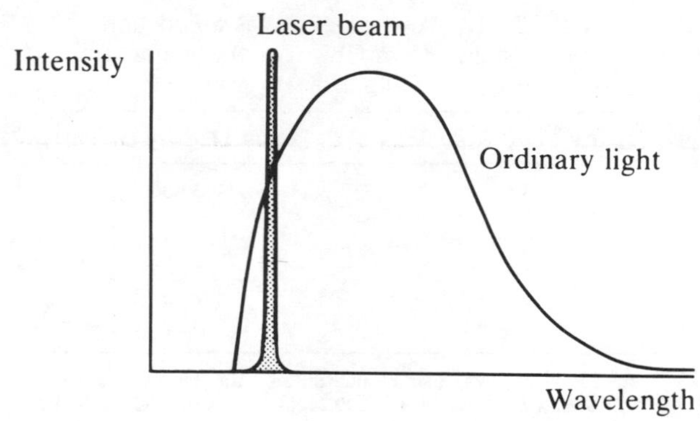

Figure 39.2. Ordinary light is noncoherent. A laser beam consists of light waves that are coherent.

(10^{-6}m). With increasing core diameter, power density and fiber flexibility decrease. Power density outside the fiber is also affected by beam divergence and distance from the fiber tip (Table 39.1).

Certain laser wavelengths, such as CO_2, are difficult to transmit through optical fibers and must be delivered along line-of-sight optical paths with articulating mirrors. Each mirror interface absorbs some energy, resulting in energy loss. Delivery systems for the CO_2 laser are therefore designed with the minimum number of mirrors that will still allow sufficient maneuverability of the handheld applicator. Despite recent reports,[1,2] there is as yet no practical optical fiber for the CO_2 laser. The excimer (from excited dimer) laser resembles the CO_2 laser in this respect. The 193-nm wavelength cannot be transmitted through a silica fiber, although fibers are transparent to somewhat longer wavelengths.[3]

INTERACTION OF DIFFERENT LASERS WITH TISSUE

In general, lasers produce a thermal and a nonthermal effect on tissues. The nonthermal effects[4] associated with pulsed laser systems, such as Raman scattering and shock waves, with the exception of photo dissociation (to be further discussed), are chiefly of interest to physicists.

Thermal effects vary according to (1) wavelength of the laser, (2) color of and color-related energy absorption by the target tissue, (3) power delivered, (4) local cooling factors, such as capillary blood flow and infused saline, and (5) thermal relaxation time, in the case of pulsed laser energy delivery. Laser destruction of tissue, with the exception of the excimer laser, is achieved by almost instantaneous heating of the target tissue to a temperature in excess of 100°C, with vaporization of all tissue components.

The tissue interaction effects of the specific lasers of importance in clinical medicine are listed as follows:

The CO_2 laser emits at the infrared end of the spectrum and acts by vaporizing water. Cellular water is boiled off and the tissue evaporates. The color of the tissue is unrelated to energy absorption at this wavelength. Because CO_2 laser energy is strongly absorbed by water, tissue penetration is low. The cutting effect is pronounced.

The Nd:YAG laser at 1,060 nm has greater tissue penetration and forward scatter than the CO_2 and argon

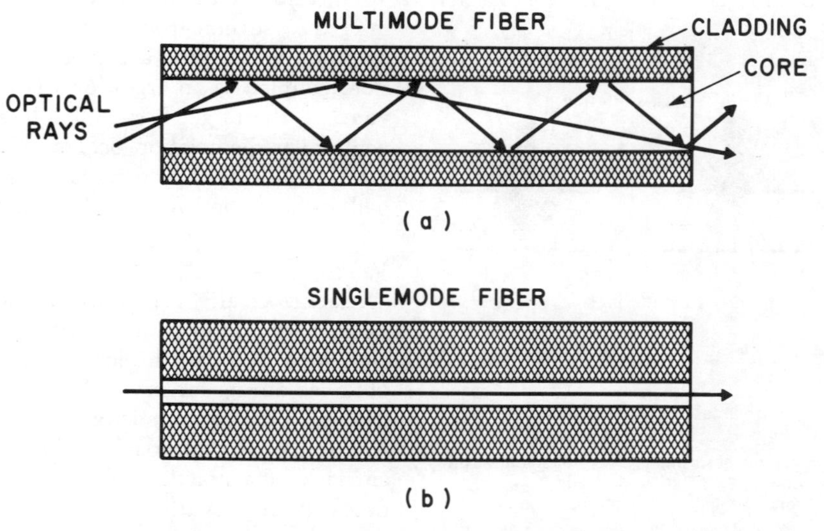

Figure 39.3. Typical optical fiber. High refractive index glass core is surrounded by lower refractive index cladding. (From Henry PS: Introduction to light wave transmission. *IEEE Communications Magazine* 1985; 23(5):12–16. Copyright 1985 IEEE. Used with permission.)

Table 39.1. Power Density as a Function of Distance from Fiber Tip, Assuming a Power Output of 10 Watts*

Distance (mm) from Tip	Power Density (w/cm^2)
0	3,536
1	372
2	132
3	67
4	41
5	27

*From Choy DSJ: Vascular recanalization with the laser catheter. *IEEE J Quantum Electronics* 1984; QE20:1420–1426. Copyright 1984 by IEEE. Reproduced with permission.

lasers (Figure 39.4). There is more protein coagulation than seen with the argon laser. There is greater absorption of Nd:YAG laser energy by darker colored tissues.

The Nd:YAG line at 1,318 nm as compared with the line at 1,060 nm is associated with lower coagulative effects and both higher cutting and evaporative tissue effects.[4]

The Q switched form of the Nd:YAG laser produces extremely short pulses with high peak power that causes vaporization of thin cell layers. This effect is exploited in posterior capsulotomy.

The argon laser emits a blue-green light that is transmitted through water and preferentially absorbed by tissues of complementary colors, ie, red. It is completely absorbed even by dilute blood.[5] It produces greater evaporative effects and less forward scatter than the Nd:YAG. For equal power it results in a zone of coagulation narrower than that associated with the Nd:YAG.

The excimer laser at shorter wavelengths (193 nm) produces photo dissociation or disruption of molecular bonds with exquisite precision (Figure 39.5). There is increasing thermal effect with longer wavelengths. The excimer laser is absorbed by water and has not as yet been used in vivo. Its potential in medicine lies in its nonthermal effect and great precision.

The dye laser, at 630 nm, is a red light. This laser is

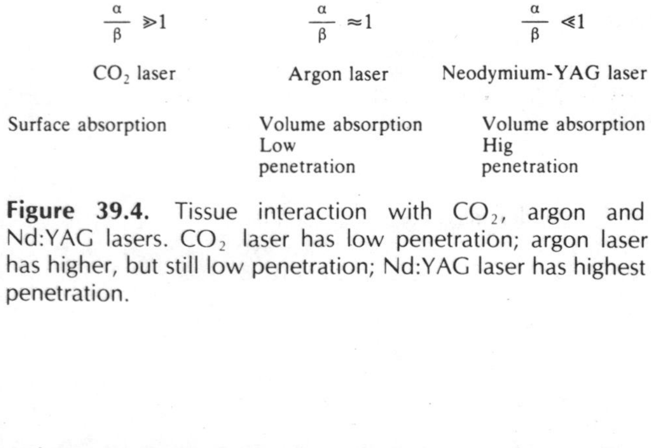

Figure 39.4. Tissue interaction with CO_2, argon and Nd:YAG lasers. CO_2 laser has low penetration; argon laser has higher, but still low penetration; Nd:YAG laser has highest penetration.

useful in photodynamic therapy because of its high tissue penetration. Dye lasers of other wavelengths can be produced by varying the dye medium.

The copper vapor and frequency-doubled Nd:YAG lasers are considered together because the wavelength of 530 nm generated approximates that of the argon laser. The effect on tissue of these two lasers is therefore similar to that of the argon laser. These lasers may become more important in the future because of greater power output.

LASERS IN MEDICINE

Lasers found their first medical application in ophthalmology, because the lens is a natural window for the transmission of laser light into the body. For over a decade, argon laser photocoagulation for diabetic retinopathy has been standard therapy. Posterior capsulotomy has already been mentioned. Newer therapeutic applications include vocal cord polypectomy in otolaryngology; upper gastrointestinal bleeding,[6] esophageal tumors,[7] and condyloma acuminata[8] in gastroenterology; meningiomas[9] and arteriovenous malformations[10] in neurosurgery; endometriosis,[11] Fallopian tube reconstruction,[12] and cervical dysplasia[13] in gynecology; hemangiomas,[14] tattoo removal,[15] and malignant tumors[16] in dermatology; bladder tumors[17] and urethral tumors[18] in urology; photodynamic therapy of tumors sensitized by hematoporphyrin and accessible to light,[19] and ablation of obstructive tumors in the bronchial tree in oncology. With increasing understanding of tissue interaction with laser light, the list of applications continues to expand.

LASERS IN CARDIOVASCULAR DISEASE

The existence of the low transmission loss, flexible optical fiber made possible the application of laser energy to the cardiovascular area.

ABLATION OF PATHOLOGIC TISSUES

Conductive Tissues

The canine bundle of His has been successfully ablated in vivo by several groups.[20,21] Using standard endocardial mapping techniques, a catheter incorporating an optical fiber coupled to an argon or a Nd:YAG laser is maneuvered to the target tissue. The laser is fired until atrioventricular dissociation occurs. A clinical application of great value would be percutaneous ablation of accessory pathways in the Wolff-Parkinson-White syndrome.

Valves

Macruz et al[22] perforated artificially created stenotic pulmonary valves in dogs with an argon laser. Isner et al[23] vaporized calcific deposits on human aortic valves obtained during surgery and at necropsy with a CO_2 laser through a dissecting microscope. Technical difficulties in transferring this approach to clinical use include the present lack of a practical fiber for the CO_2 laser and the necessity of providing a dry field.

Myocardium

The difficulty of visualizing the myocardium deep in the ventricle complicates myotomy for hypertrophic car-

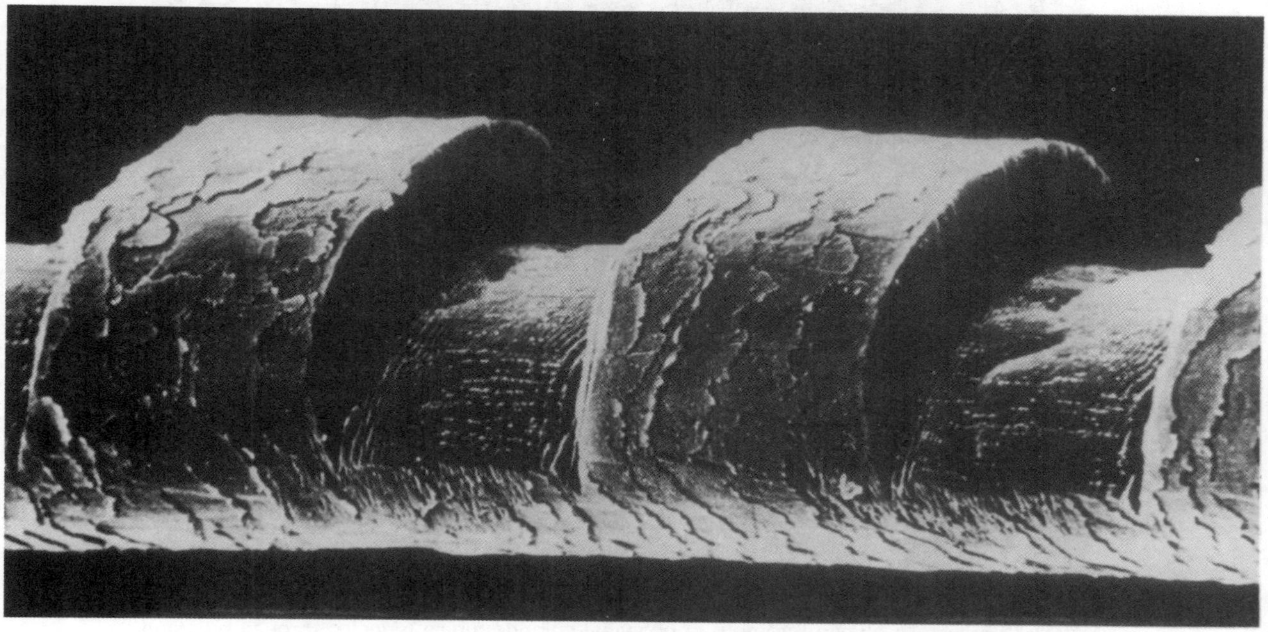

Figure 39.5. Human hair (125 μm) etched by excimer laser. (Work by R. Srinivasan, IBM T. J. Watson Research Center, and Professor W. M. Hess, Brigham Young University. Reproduced with permission.)

diomyopathy. Morrow[24] states that myotomy incisions "must extend to the apical termination of the muscular ridge," and "for this to be accomplished, the knife must be plunged into the septum until it is out of sight, completely." Taking advantage of the laser light illumination of the ventricular wall, and the mating of the argon laser wavelengths of 488 and 514 nm to the absorption spectra of myoglobin of 400 to 650 nm, Isner's group[25] performed argon laser myotomy in a patient with hypertrophic cardiomyopathy in 1984.

Septum

In 1964, Case et al[26-29] demonstrated relief of ischemic left ventricular failure in dogs by creating interatrial septal defects. Our group has proposed the use of the Nd:YAG laser catheter for percutaneous production of interatrial septal defect for treating intractable left ventricular failure in man. Experiments are being planned in this area. The choice of the Nd:YAG laser is based on its great tissue penetration and its partial transmission in blood.

VESSEL ANASTOMOSIS

The pioneering efforts of Neblett,[30] Gomes et al,[31] Jain,[32] and Dew[33] made use of the CO_2, argon, and Nd:YAG lasers at low power outputs. Arteries as small as 0.5 mm in diameter can be "welded" in laser anastomosis. In comparison with suture anastomosis, the laser technique provides applicability to vessels deep in the operative field, relative lack of foreign body reaction, rare reocclusions by thrombi, and a time saving up to fivefold.

ARTERIAL RECANALIZATION

History

In 1980, two groups[34,35] independently proposed the use of laser energy to ablate atherosclerotic plaque obstructions in vivo. Our group had tunneled through a fresh human thrombus (Figure 39.6) with a laser beam from a Coherent Model 900 argon laser in 1978. Subsequently, we performed in vivo recanalization of an artificially thrombosed rabbit aorta and a canine femoral artery with a Coherent Model 1000 argon laser in 1981.[36] Abela et al[37] compared the effects of the CO_2, argon, and Nd:YAG lasers on atherosclerotic plaque. Complete endothelial repair in laser-irradiated swine arteries was reported by Gerrity et al.[38] Lee et al[39] confirmed the efficacy of the argon and Nd:YAG lasers in vaporizing atherosclerotic plaque. A patient faced with amputation for ischemic peripheral vascular disease had the femoral artery recanalized by Ginsburg's group[40] at Stanford University with an argon laser system under fluoroscopic guidance in 1983. Geschwind et al[41] recanalized three femoral arteries with a Nd:YAG laser in 1984. Choy et al[42] performed argon laser recanalization of the coronary artery in five patients during coronary artery bypass surgery at the University of Toulouse in September 1983.

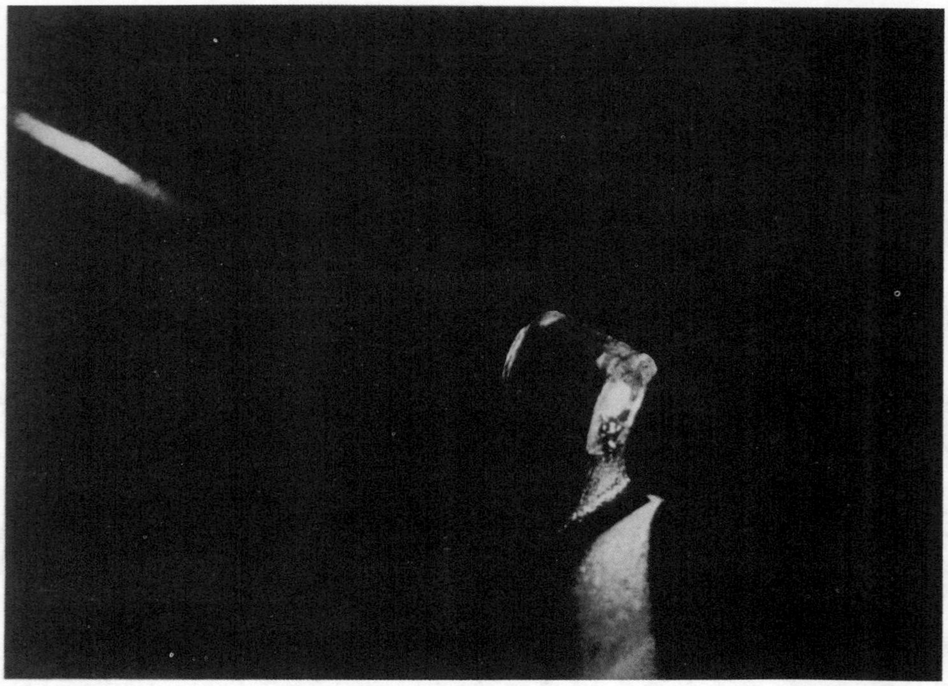

Figure 39.6. Fresh human thrombus in polyvinyl chloride tubing tunneled through by argon laser. Note beam distal to thrombus.

Subsequent human clinical trials by Ginsburg, Geschwind, and Choy will be described subsequently.

In Vitro Data

Analysis of gases generated by vaporization of plaque and thrombi by gas chromatography and absorbance spectroscopy[43] and mass spectroscopy[44] indicates the major constituents to be water vapor, nitrogen, carbon dioxide, hydrogen, and trace amounts of short chain carbon molecules (Table 39.2). No particulate matter was found by Case et al[45] in the effluent of arterial thrombi and plaque vaporized by argon laser. Other investigators[46–48] have confirmed the absence of particulate matter and distal embolization following laser irradiation of plaque and thrombus obstructive lesions. Early inexperience, lack of a coaxial relation between catheter and vessel, and direct mechanical trauma caused by the unprotected fiber contributed to vessel perforations reported by several groups.[49–51] Typical histologic changes caused by laser impact on tissue consist of a superficial zone of carbonization, then a zone of lacunae which may represent pockets of water vapor, followed by a deeper zone of thermally induced protein coagulation (Figure 39.7). These changes are seen with the CO_2, argon, and Nd:YAG lasers used in the cw (continuous wave) mode. Recent work[52] suggests that these lasers, used with extremely short pulses that allow a long thermal relaxation time, may produce the smooth surfaces characteristically seen with the excimer laser.[52a,52b,52c]

Table 39.2. Composition of Vapor Generated by Lasing of Thrombus and Plaque Concentration (Percent by Volume)*

	Thrombus	Plaque
Nitrogen	17.3	24.0
Oxygen	1.16	3.6
Argon	0	0.1
Carbon dioxide	50.0+	29.6
Hydrogen	14.9	15.3
Methane	2.9	13.5
Ethane	1.54	2.3
Ethylene	5.7	4.8
Propane	1.35	1.81
Propylene	3.5	3.9
C4+ hydrocarbons	0.67	1.21
Aromatic hydrocarbons	0.10	0

*From Kaminow et al, with permission of the Optical Society of America.[44]

The excimer laser has received wide publicity, but it has yet to be used in vivo. The current problems are (1) low power per pulse, (2) difficulty of coupling the beam to a fiber, (3) lack of suitable fibers for transmission of ultraviolet at shorter wavelengths (193 nm), and (4) concerns about possible carcinogenicity. The excimer laser could prove to be the laser of choice if these problems can be solved.

Photodynamic therapy of tumors was adapted by Spears et al[53] to the treatment of atherosclerotic plaque on the theory that the smooth muscle cells of plaque will selectively absorb hematoporphyrin derivative (HPD). Exposure of the photosensitized plaque to laser light at 630 nm from a rhodamine dye laser creates singlet oxygen which leads to cell necrosis. The choice of the 630 nm wavelength is based on the high penetration through blood of light at this frequency. Suggestive but not entirely convincing results have been reported using HPD

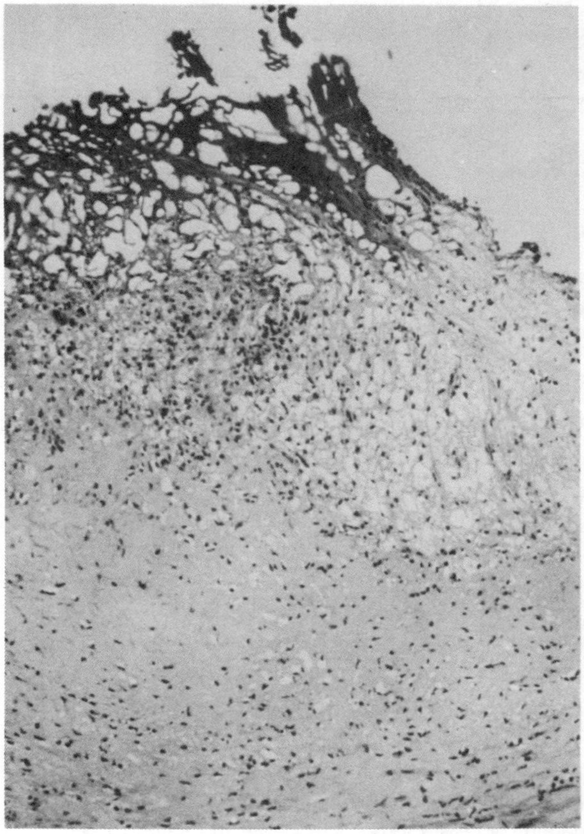

Figure 39.7. Histologic appearance of a lasered surface. Note thin carbonized layer and underlying zones of protein coagulation and multiple lacunae. These last may represent pockets of water vapor.

therapy in high lipid diet-induced atherosclerotic plaque in the rabbit aorta.

Angiograms of a human cadaver coronary artery and a femoral artery from an amputated specimen recanalized with an argon laser catheter are shown in Figures 39.8 and 39.9, respectively. The wall of the laser-treated femoral artery is smooth, whereas the untreated distal artery has a beaded, irregular surface characteristic of diffuse atherosclerotic involvement.

In Vivo Animal Data

Successful in vivo laser recanalizations in both the rabbit and canine models have been reported by Sanborn et al,[50] Lee et al,[54] Abela et al,[49] and our group.[37,55] The Nd:YAG laser, because of its high tissue penetration, produced the largest number of perforations, and the argon laser the least. The atherosclerotic plaques induced in rabbits by a high lipid diet are softer, contain less collagen, are noncalcified, and are therefore not comparable to native human atherosclerotic plaques. Macruz proposed engrafting atherosclerotic human arteries to canine femoral arteries. At least one group in the United States has attempted this procedure.[56]

In Vivo Human Data

Peripheral Arteries. Ginsburg's group[57] at Stanford treated 20 patients with stenotic lesions of the femoral artery with severe symptoms, recommended amputation, and medical contraindications to surgery. The laser source was an argon laser with maximum resonator power of 16 watts. There were two perforations and ten successful procedures. In most cases only a small lumen was achieved (1 mm in 6-mm vessels), and the operations were supplemented by balloon dilatation. The catheter was introduced with the Seldinger technique and guided to the stenotic lesion under fluoroscopy. Whenever possible, the fiber was first passed beyond the lesion and the laser was activated as the fiber was pulled back in a retrograde direction. This "pullback" technique minimizes the chances of perforation by keeping the fiber coaxial to the vessel. Long-term followup data are unavailable.

Geschwind et al[58] performed recanalization in 14 human femoral arteries with a Nd:YAG laser. Supplementary balloon dilatation was necessary in the last ten procedures. Four late reocclusions occurred.

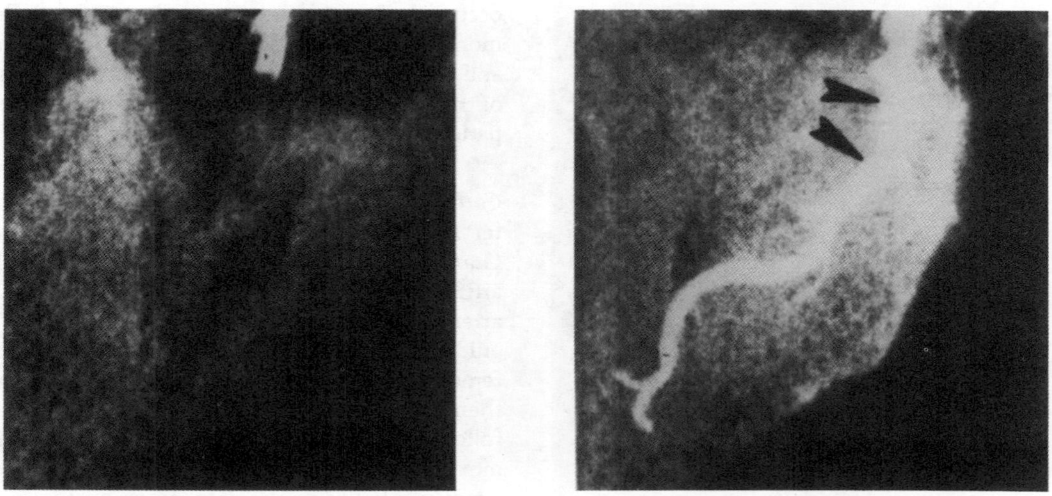

Figure 39.8. Angiograms of cadaver left anterior descending coronary artery showing total occlusion by thrombus, and patency after laser recanalization. *Arrows* indicate site of thrombus.

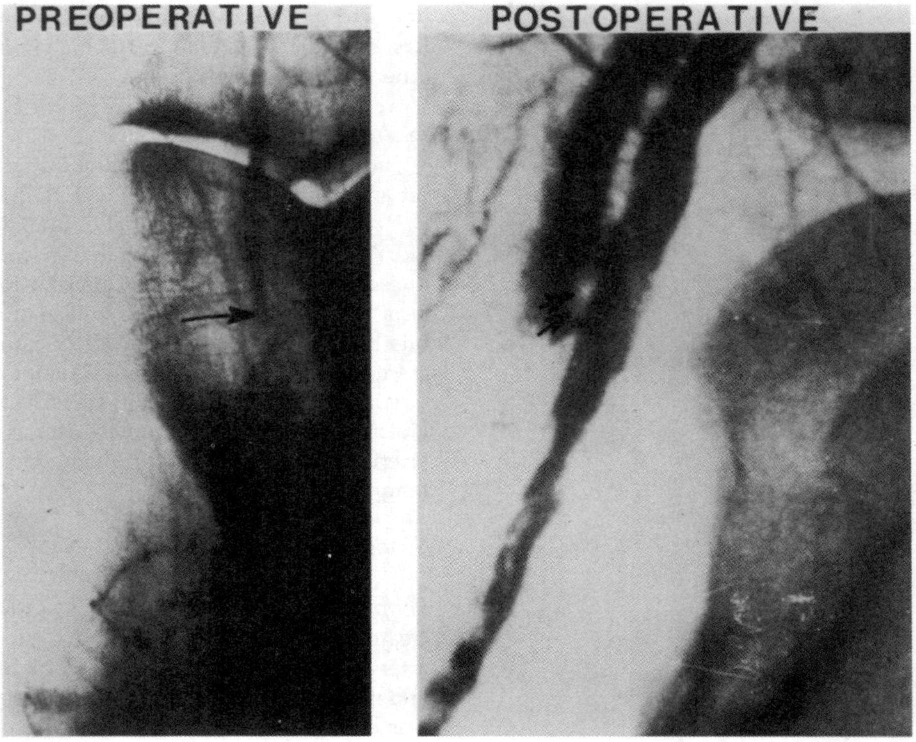

Figure 39.9. Angiograms of femoral and popliteal artery showing total occlusion (*arrow*) preoperatively and patency after laser recanalization. Anastomotic site between popliteal artery and Gortex graft (*double arrow*) has also been opened. Note smooth wall of laser-irradiated artery compared with plaque beaded wall of untreated distal artery.

Coronary Arteries. In September 1983, our group[42] recanalized high grade stenotic coronary arteries (three left anterior descending and two right coronary arteries) in five patients undergoing coronary artery bypass surgery. There was one mechanical perforation, which was immediately repaired. Four arteries were successfully reopened. All five arteries were bypassed with saphenous vein grafts for ethical reasons. One laser-treated artery was immediately excised for histologic study. A new lumen, approximately 70%, was created (Figure 39.10). The pretreatment lumen was estimated to be 5% to 10%. All laser-treated arteries were reoccluded at three months. However, one laser-treated artery was still patent at 25 days (Figure 39.11).

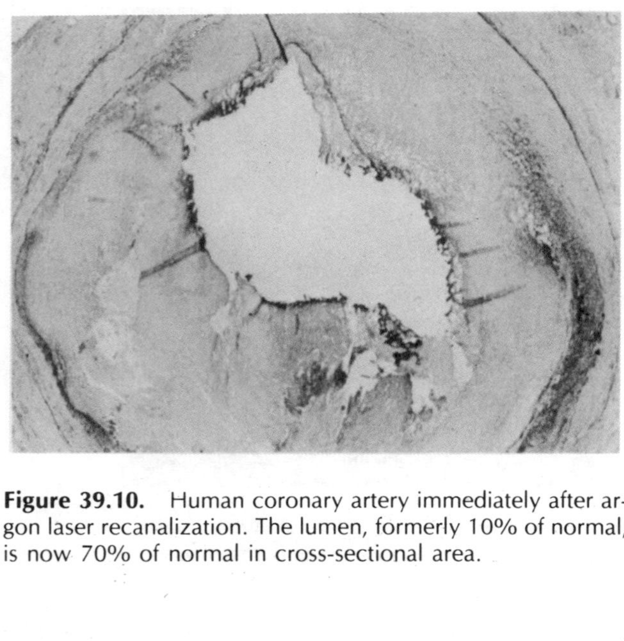

Figure 39.10. Human coronary artery immediately after argon laser recanalization. The lumen, formerly 10% of normal, is now 70% of normal in cross-sectional area.

In January 1984, we recanalized three totally occluded right coronary arteries during coronary bypass surgery for other stenotic arteries.[59] All three patients had sustained transmural infarcts distal to the right coronary artery lesions. These arteries were not bypassed. Although one of the three was heavily calcified, no perforations occurred. Two of the arteries were reoccluded at three months. The third patient refused repeat angiography, and the fate of his right coronary artery is unknown. As of this writing, 31 and 27 months postoperatively, all eight patients are alive and well.

Carotid Arteries. In June 1985, in collaboration with Peter Ascher and Johannes Lammer of the University of Graz, Austria, our group successfully recanalized seven artificially thrombosed and atherosclerotic cadaver carotid arteries, with one perforation, using a fluoroscopically guided laser catheter inserted percutaneously through the femoral artery (Figure 39.12). One human patient was then so treated with an 8 second exposure of argon laser, followed by surgical endarterectomy. An estimated 100 mm^3 of plaque was ablated. The significance of these experiments lies in the demonstration that vital stenotic arteries can be recanalized through a percutaneous approach, guided by fluoroscopy.

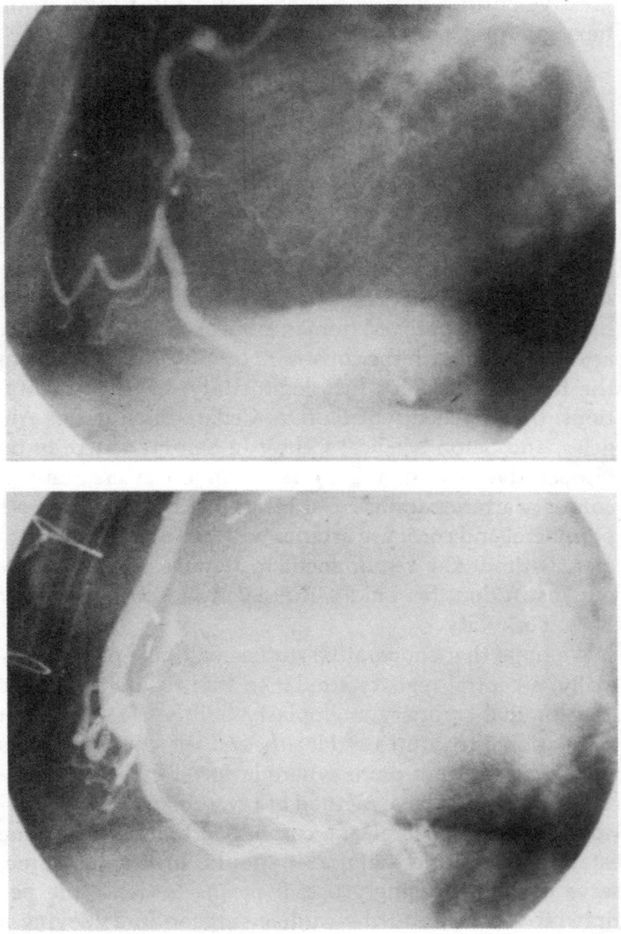

Figure 39.11. Angiograms of human right coronary artery preoperatively showing 95% stenosis, and 25 days after laser recanalization and bypass grafting showing continued patency of the lasered segment. (From Choy et al[42] with permission of Clinical Cardiology Publishing Co, Inc, and the Foundation for Advances in Clinical Medicine.)

CURRENT PROBLEMS

Extensive work by several groups has convincingly demonstrated that distal embolization is not a problem. Of major concern to all investigators is the possibility of vessel perforation. With care in maintaining a coaxial relation between the laser catheter and the vessel, use of the pullback technique, and use of the argon laser, it is possible to minimize the danger of perforation. With intraoperative use, when visual guidance is employed, the vessel should be dissected free so that the entire circumference can be seen. Wall thickness is increased by the presence of plaque; this segment therefore appears darker than normal vessel wall, because there is less light transmission. Laser recanalization is then accomplished by progressively "sculpting" the luminal surface until light transmission is uniform throughout. Protective amber goggles, 50% of the optical density of the standard goggles, should be used. The standard goggles do not permit accurate visual monitoring of the recanalization procedure. In the final analysis, successful laser recanalization depends on operator experience.

Fluoroscopically guided laser recanalization is more difficult because the visual cues of determining wall thickness are absent. An estimate of wall thickness must be made indirectly by relating the diameter of the new lumen to that of the normal vessel proximal to the lesion. The angioscope, in our opinion, is of little value because (1) it provides a distorted two-dimensional image of a three-dimensional situation, (2) it adds to the diameter of the catheter, (3) it decreases the flexibility of the catheter, and (4) it is expensive. We rely on a combination of the pullback technique when dealing with stenotic lesions, and a short exposure, short advance technique in totally occlusive lesions. This consists of three steps performed repetitively: (1) angiography, (2) saline flush, and (3) a 1- to 2-second exposure of the argon laser. The saline flush prevents interaction between the laser and the ra-

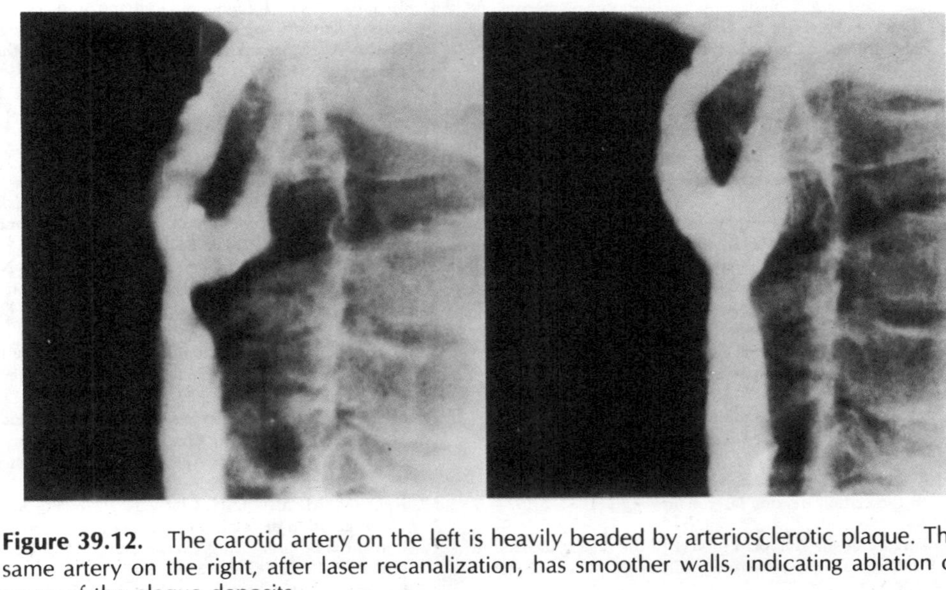

Figure 39.12. The carotid artery on the left is heavily beaded by arteriosclerotic plaque. The same artery on the right, after laser recanalization, has smoother walls, indicating ablation of some of the plaque deposits.

diocontrast material, which produces a precipitate of unknown chemical composition.

Several institutions are investigating the use of nontoxic dyes that selectively adsorb to atherosclerotic plaque and not to intima. These dyes, of color complementary to the laser wavelength, increase the energy absorption by the plaque, in effect differentiating between plaque and normal intima.

If the fiber tip is in contact with the target tissue, and heat dissipation is insufficient, the fiber tip temperature can rise above the ignition point and a phenomenon we call "burnback" occurs. In this situation, the fiber is burned back in a retrograde direction. Various protective shields, a tip with a high flash point and the like, are being studied.

The ability to steer or guide a catheter is important to the laser angiographer. Until a practical system is developed, one must rely on the present technology of preformed tips with memory, guide wires, and guiding catheters. The ideal laser catheter should have a highly flexible tip for ease of following complex curves of the arterial tree, and a built-in method of tip steering that does not add unduly to the catheter diameter.

Reocclusions occurred in 40% of Ginsburg's, four of Geschwind's 14, and all of our cases after laser recanalization. We believe this to be the most serious problem of all. Possible causes are endothelial disruption and attendant increase of thrombogenicity, and reduced blood flow either from inadequate lumen size after recanalization or competition from bypass grafts. Blood flow to infarcted myocardium is known to be markedly decreased.[60] This was the case in our three patients with the totally occluded right coronary arteries. A more aggressive antithrombotic regimen will be instituted in the next group of patients treated.

THE FUTURE

The general enthusiasm with which the new field of laser recanalization has been received by the cardiology community augurs well for the future.[61,62] Since its inception in the late 1970s, laser recanalization has attracted increasing numbers of highly competent investigators. Regulatory agencies have not been far behind in recognizing its potential. The Food and Drug Administration has currently approved human clinical trials in peripheral arteries, albeit with the constraint of immediately excising the treated vessel for histologic study, in three institutions: the University of Florida, Cedars-Sinai in Los Angeles, and Seton Medical Center in San Francisco; in intraoperative use of a CO_2 laser for endarterectomy in coronary arteries at the Texas Heart Institute, and for both peripheral and coronary arteries with the argon laser catheter, without the requirement to remove the vessels, at our institution, St. Luke's-Roosevelt Hospital Center in New York City.

We hope that cooperative studies will take place eventually, a central registry similar to that for percutaneous transluminal coronary angioplasty will be established at the National Institutes of Health, and the chief problems will be solved to a point where laser recanalization as a relatively noninvasive method of revascularization for peripheral, renal, cerebral, and coronary arteries will become established routine therapy. It should, in the meantime, serve as an increasingly useful means to assist the peripheral vascular and the cardiac surgeon in achieving a more complete revascularization of ischemic tissues.

REFERENCES

1. Eldar M, Battler A, Neufeld H, Gaton E, Arieli R, Akselrod S, Levite A, Katzir A: Transluminal carbon dioxide laser catheter angioplasty for dissolution of atherosclerotic plaques. *J Am Coll Cardiol* 1984; 3:135–137.
2. Takahishi K, Yoshida N, Yakota M: Optical fibers for transmitting high powered carbon dioxide laser beam. *Sumitomo Elect Tech Rev* 1984; 23:203–210.
3. Grundfest WS, Litvack F, Forrester JS, Goldenberg TSVI, Swan HJC, Morgenstern L, Fishbein M, McDermid IS, Rider DM, Pacala TJ, Laudenslager JB: Laser ablation of human atherosclerotic plaque without adjacent tissue injury. *J Am Coll Cardiol* 1985; 5:929–933.
4. Goldman L: *The Biomedical Laser: Technology and Clinical Applications.* New York, Springer-Verlag, 1981.
5. Kaplan MD, Case RB, Choy DSJ: Vascular recanalization with the Argon laser: the role of blood in the transmission of laser energy. *Lasers Surg & Med* 1985; 5:275–279.
6. Dwyer RM, Bass M: Laser phototherapy in man using Argon and Nd:YAG lasers. *Gastrointest Endosc* 1978; 24:195–196.
7. Mellow MH, Pinkas H: Endoscopic therapy for esophageal carcinoma with Nd:YAG laser: prospective evaluation of efficacy, complications and survival. *Gastrointest Endosc* 1984; 6:334–339.
8. Scott RS, Castro DJ: Treatment of condyloma acuminata with carbon dioxide laser: a prospective study. *Lasers Surg & Med* 1984; 4:157–162.
9. Cerullo LJ: Laser neurosurgery: past, present, and future. *IEEE J Quant Elect* 1984; 12:1397–1400.
10. Fasano VA: The treatment of vascular malformation of the brain with laser surgery. Presented at Congress of Laser Neurosurgery II, Chicago, Ill, Sept 1982.
11. Bellina JH, Voros JI, Fick AC, Jackson JD: Surgical management of endometriosis with the carbon dioxide laser. *Microsurgery* 1984; 5:197–201.
12. Bellina JH: Microsurgery of the Fallopian tube with the carbon dioxide laser: analysis of 230 cases with a two-year follow-up. *Lasers Surg & Med* 1983; 3:255–260.
13. Anderson MC: Treatment of cervical intraepithelial neoplasia with the carbon dioxide laser: report of 543 patients. *Obstet Gynecol* 1982; 59:720–725.
14. Apfelberg DB, Moser MR, Lasl H: Progress report on extended clinical use of the Argon laser for cutaneous lesions. *Lasers Surg & Med* 1980; 1:71–83.
15. Bailin DS, Katz JL, Levine AL: Removal of tattoos by carbon dioxide laser. *J Dermatol Surg Oncol* 1980; 6:997–1001.
16. Koslov AP, Moskalik KG: Pulsed laser radiation therapy of skin tumors. *Cancer* 1980; 46:2172–2178.
17. Hofstetter A, Frank F, Keiditsch E, Bowering R: Endoscopic Nd:YAG laser application for destroying bladder tumors, clinical papers. *Eur Urol* 1981; 7:278–282.
18. Hofstetter A: Laser application for destroying ureter tumors (abstr). *Lasers Surg & Med* 1983; 3:152.
19. Dougherty TJ, Kaufman JE, Goldfarb A, Weiskaupt KR, Boyle D, Mittleman A: Photoradiation therapy for treatment of malignant tumors. *Cancer Res* 1978; 38:2628–2635.
20. Lee BI, Fletcher RD, Cohen AI, Cutler DJ, Del Negro AA, Singh SN: Transcatheter endocardial ablation—comparison of laser photo ablation and electrode shock ablation (abstr). *J Am Coll Cardiol* 1984; 3(2): 536.
21. Narula OS, Bharati S, Chan MC, Embi AA, Lev M: Laser micro transection of the HIS bundle: a pervenous catheter technique (abstr). *J Am Coll Cardiol* 1984; 3(2):537.
22. Macruz R, Armelin E, Gomes OM, Brum JMG, Fiorelli AI, Ribeiro MP, Mittentag J, Lopes EA, Camargo PR, Madrigano MGC, Pillegi JCF, Decourt LV, Zerbini EJ: Aplicacao do laser no sistema cardiovascular. *Arq Bras Cardiol* 1982; 39:5–10.
23. Isner JM, Michlewitz H, Clarke RH, Donaldson RF, Salem DN: Laser photo ablation of aortic valve calcium: evaluation of argon versus carbon dioxide laser using excised surgical and postmortem specimens (abstr). *J Am Coll Cardiol* 1984; 3:558.
24. Morrow AG: Hypertrophic subaortic stensosis. Operative methods uti-

lized to relieve left ventricular outflow obstruction. *J Thorac Cardiovasc Surg* 1978; 76:423–430.
25. Isner JM, Clarke RH, Pardian NG, Donaldson RF, Salem DN, Konstam MA, Payne DD, Cleveland RJ: Laser myoplasty for hypertrophic cardiomyopathy. In vitro experience in human postmortem hearts and in vivo experience in a canine model (transarterial) and human patient (intraoperative). *Am J Cardiol* 1984; 53:1620–1626.
26. Case RB, Roven RB, Crampton RS: Relief of high left atrial pressure in left ventricular failure. *Lancet* 1964; 2:841–842.
27. Roven RB, Crampton RS, Case RB: Influence of venous shunts on left atrial pressure in left ventricular failure. *Clin Res* 1964; 12:56.
28. Roven RB, Crampton RS, Case RB: Surgical approach to the relief of left ventricular failure. *Circulation* (suppl III) 1964; 29 & 30:III–149.
29. Roven RB, Crampton RS, Case RB: Effect of compromising right ventricular function in left ventricular failure by means of interatrial and other shunts. *Am J Cardiol* 1969; 24:209–219.
30. Neblett CR: Reconstructive vascular surgery with use of the carbon dioxide laser. Presented at the Congress of Laser Neurosurgery II. Chicago, Ill, 1982.
31. Gomes OM, Macruz R, Armelin E, Ribeiro MP, Brum JMG, Bittencourt D, Verginelli G, Zerbini EJ: Vascular anastomosis by Argon laser beam. *Texas Heart Inst J* 1983; 10:145–150.
32. Jain KK: Sutureless microvascular extracranial anastomosis with Nd:YAG laser (abstr). *Lasers Surg & Med* 1984; 3:311–312.
33. Dew DK: Laser microsurgical repair of soft tissue: a demonstration of surgical techniques (abstr). *Lasers Surg & Med* 1984; 3:351.
34. Choy DSJ: Fiberoptic laser tunneling device: the laser catheter. *Beijing/Shanghai Proceedings of an International Conference on Lasers.* New York, Wiley-Interscience, 1980, pp 685–690.
35. Macruz R, Martins JRM, Tupinamba AS, Lopes EA, Vargas H, Pena AM, Carvalho VB, Armelin E, Decourt LV: Possibilidades terapeuticas do raio laser em ateromas. *Arq Bras Cardiol* 1980; 34:9–12.
36. Choy DSJ, Stertzer SH, Rotterdam HZ, Sharrock N, Kaminow IP: Transluminal laser catheter angioplasty. *Am J Cardiol* 1982; 50:1206–1208.
37. Abela GS, Normann S, Cohen D, Feldman RL, Geiser EA, Conti CR: Effects of carbon dioxide, Nd:YAG, and Argon laser radiation on coronary atheromatous plaques. *Am J Cardiol* 1982; 50:1199–1205.
38. Gerrity RG, Loop FD, Golding LAR, Ehrhart LA, Argenyi ZB: Arterial response to laser operation for removal of atherosclerotic plaques. *J Thorac Cardiovasc Surg* 1983; 85:409–421.
39. Lee G, Ikeda RM, Kozina J, Mason DT: Laser dissolution of coronary atherosclerotic obstruction. *Am Heart J* 1981; 102:1074–1075.
40. Ginsburg R, Kim DS, Cuthener D, Toth J, Mitchell RS: Salvage of an ischemic limb by laser angioplasty: description of a new technique. *Clin Cardiol* 1984; 7:54–58.
41. Geschwind H, Boussignac G, Teisseire B, Vielledent C, Gaston A, Becquemin JP, Maviolini P: Percutaneous transluminal laser angioplasty in man. *Lancet* 1984; 1:844.
42. Choy DSJ, Stertzer SH, Myler RK, Marco J, Fournial G: Human coronary laser recanalization. *Clin Cardiol* 1984; 7:377–381.
43. Clarke RH, Donaldson RF, Isner JM: Identification of photoproducts liberated by in vitro laser irradiation of atherosclerotic plaque, calcified valves and myocardium (abstr). *Lasers Surg & Med* 1984; 3:358.
44. Kaminow IP, Wiesenfeld JM, Choy DSJ: Argon laser disintegration of thrombus and atherosclerotic plaque. *Appl Optics* 1984; 23:1301–1302.
45. Case RB, Choy DSJ, Dwyer EM Jr, Silvernail PJ: Absence of distal emboli during in vivo laser recanalization. *Lasers Surg & Med* 1985; 5:281–290.
46. Choy DSJ, Stertzer SH, Myler RK, Marco J, Kaminow IP, Fournial G: Argon laser coronary angioplasty: mass spectrometer evaluation, technetium 99 scintigraphy, human intraoperative evaluation (abstr). *J Am Coll Cardiol* 1984; 3(2):489.
47. Abela GS, Pepine CJ, Conti RC: Effects of laser irradiation on human blood: relation between exposure and debris formation (abstr). *J Am Coll Cardiol* 1984; 3:489.
48. Isner JM, Clarke RH: The current status of lasers in the treatment of cardiovascular disease. *IEEE J Quant Elect* 1984; 12:1406–1419.
49. Abela G, Cohen D, Feldman RL, Geiser EA, Normann S, Conti CR: Use of laser radiation to recanalize stenosed arteries in a live animal model. *Circulation* 1982; 66(suppl. II):II–366.
50. Sanborn TA, Faxon DP, Haudenschild CC, Gottsman SB, Ryan TJ: Angiographic and histopathologic consequences of in vivo laser radiation of atherosclerotic lesions. *Circulation* 1983; 68:III–145.
51. Jain A, Dedhia H, Savrin R, Withers A: Laser angioplasty in chronic occlusion of canine arteries (abstr). *Eur Heart J* 1984; 5:64.
52. Deckelbaum L, Donaldson RF, Isner JM, Bernstein J, Clarke RH: Elimination of pathologic injury associated with laser induced tissue ablation using pulsed energy delivery at low repetition rates. *J Am Coll Cardiol* 1985; 5:408.
52a. Downar E, Butany J, Jares A, Stoicheff BP: Endocardial photo-ablation by excimer laser. *J Am Coll Cardiol* 1986; 7:546–550.
52b. Eldar M, Battler A, Gal D, Rath S, Rotstein Z, Neufeld HN, Akselrod S, Katzir A, Gaton E, Wolman M: The effects of varying lengths and powers of CO_2 laser pulses transmitted through an optical fiber on atherosclerotic plaques. *Clin Cardiol* 1986; 9:89–91.
52c. Deckelbaum LI, Isner JM, Donaldson RF, Laliberte SM, Clarke RH, Salem DN: Use of pulsed energy delivery to minimize tissue injury resulting from carbon dioxide laser irradiation of cardiovascular tissues. *J Am Coll Cardiol* 1986; 7:898–908.
53. Spears JR, Serur J, Shropshire D, Paulin S: Fluorescence of experimental atheromatous plaques with hematoporphyrin derivative. *J Clin Invest* 1983; 71:395–399.
54. Lee G, Ikeda RM, Stobbe D, Ogata C, Embi A, Chan MC, Reis RL, Mason DT: Intraoperative use of dual fiberoptic catheter for simultaneous in vivo visualization and laser vaporization of peripheral atherosclerotic obstructive disease. *Cathet Cardiovasc Diagn* 1984; 10:11–16.
55. Marco J, Silvernail PJ, Fournial G, Choy DSJ, Fajadet J, Case RB: Complete patency in thrombus-occluded arteries two weeks after laser recanalization. *Lasers Surg & Med* 1985; 5:291–296.
56. Abela GS, Normann S, Feldman RL, Conti CR, Pepiñe CJ: A new model for evaluation of transluminal recanalization: human atherosclerotic coronary artery heterografts. *Circulation* 1983; 68 (Suppl III):III–5.
57. Ginsburg R: Personal communication, 1985.
58. Geschwind H, Boussignac G, Teisseire B: Transluminal laser angioplasty in man. *Circulation* 1984; 70(Supp II):II–298.
59. Choy DSJ, Marco J, Fournial G, Stertzer SH: Argon laser recanalization of three totally occluded human right coronary arteries. *Clin Cardiol* 1986; 9:296–298.
60. Prioleau WH, Clark S, Gross A, Voegele LD, Hairston O: Flow in coronary artery bypass grafts to totally and partially occluded left anterior descending coronary arteries. *Ann Thorac Surg* 1982; 34:490–492.
61. Isner JM, Clarke RH: Laser angioplasty: unraveling the Gordian Knot. *J Am Coll Cardiol* 1986; 7:705–708.
62. Forrester JS, Litvack F, Grundfest WS: Laser angioplasty and cardiovascular disease. *Am J Cardiol* 1986; 57:990–992.

40 Acute Myocardial Infarction

H. J. C. Swan, MD, PhD, MACP and Prediman K. Shah, MD, FACC

The past two decades have been characterized by major advances in our knowledge of myocardial ischemia and infarction. This not only has allowed for more effective diagnostic and therapeutic interventions, but also forms a general framework for a broader understanding of the effects of atherosclerosis and thrombosis in the coronary vessels.

The purpose of this chapter is to present facts concerning acute myocardial infarction that are substantively understood and to indicate those areas in which new knowledge is still required. It is also intended to provide a general basis for the treatment of acute myocardial infarction, recognizing that more sophisticated approaches and newer pharmacologic agents will be developed in the future that will have a more specific and a presumably beneficial effect on the disorder.

ETIOLOGY AND PATHOGENESIS OF ACUTE MYOCARDIAL INFARCTION

More than 90% of myocardial infarctions result from complications of atherosclerotic coronary vascular disease. In a small proportion of cases, myocardial infarction may result from nonatherosclerotic causes (Table 40.1).

Coronary vascular disease is a manifestation of atherosclerosis localized to the coronary arteries. It can and not uncommonly does exist concurrently in other portions of the vascular tree. This relation underscores the clinical correlations between such varied conditions as diabetes, hyperlipidemia, hypercholesterolemia, and other states that predispose to the generalized atherosclerotic process, as well as clinical manifestations of vascular disease in other organs, including the peripheral circulation and the carotid arteries. A clear relation between diseases of these organ systems with coronary occlusion and myocardial infarction has been demonstrated.[1]

Atherosclerosis is a general term for one or several different forms of arteriopathy. The actual pathologic lesions vary not only with the pathologic processes, affecting specific individuals, but also with the degree of maturation of the atherosclerotic lesion itself.

In recent years, it has been demonstrated that total or near total occlusion by thrombus formation on preexisting coronary atheroma is the proximate cause of acute myocardial infarction in the overwhelming preponderance of cases.[2] The mechanisms resulting in transition of an atherosclerotic plaque with resultant chronic coronary stenosis into coronary thrombosis with total or near total occlusion of the coronary lumen are not completely known. However, pathologic evidence supports the concept of ulceration of the plaque with exposure of the

Table 40.1. Nonatherosclerotic Factors and Acute Myocardial Infarction

1. Congenital anomalies of the coronary arteries
   - Anomalous origin of left coronary artery
   - Coronary arteriovenous fistula
   - Congenital aneurysm of the coronary arteries
   - Pulmonary hypertension from other congenital causes
2. Coronary embolism
   - Prosthetic valve embolus
   - Atrial fibrillation and left atrial thrombus
   - Paradoxical embolus (pulmonary hypertension interatrial communication)
   - Cardiac myxoma
3. Nonatherosclerotic coronary artery disease
   - Polyarteritis nodosa, rheumatoid arthritis
   - Syphilis
   - Takayasu's disease
   - Mucopolysaccharidosis (Hurler's syndrome)
   - Amyloid arteriopathy
   - Pseudoxanthoma elasticum
   - Homocystinuria
   - Mucocutaneous lymph node disease (Kawasaki's syndrome)
4. Coronary arterial and myocardial trauma
   - Catheter-induced dissection
   - Catheter-induced embolus
   - Coronary-arterial laceration
   - Coronary-arterial or myocardial contusion
5. Diseases of the aorta or aortic valve
   - Acute dissection
   - Marfan's syndrome
   - Aortic stenosis
6. Myocardial infarction with angiographically normal vessels*

* Associated factors in certain of these etiologies appear to be related to sensitivity of coronary arteries, including cigarette smoking, hypercoagulability, contraceptive steroids, polycythemia vera, and effects of pharmacologic agents.

vessel wall to circulating blood elements, mostly platelets, leading to platelet aggregation and subsequent fibrin deposition and thrombus formation. Chemical mediators released by platelets, ie, thromboxane, may perpetuate the process by enhancing platelet aggregation and slow-flow secondary to vasospasm. Whether coronary spasm initiates ulceration of plaque or occurs secondarily after platelet aggregation is not known. Recognition of the relation of an occluding whole blood thrombus allows for a broader understanding of the clinical presentation of the disease, and offers the potential of significant therapeutic intervention. In patients studied by coronary angiography within six hours of the onset of symptoms, 87% had complete (thrombotic) occlusion. In patients studied 12 to 24 hours after the onset of symptoms, complete occlusion occurred in only 65%.[3] Spontaneous lysis of an occluding clot occurs in some patients; up to 25% of late angiograms in patients with myocardial infarction show patent arteries of infarction. Whether the thrombus is composed of platelets only, or of platelet and fibrin, in all instances is not yet clear. When a vessel becomes completely occluded, a pressure differential builds; this may force the occluding "plug" distally, thus relieving the obstruction and symptoms and allowing for spontaneous dispersion of the adherent blood components downstream.[4] If the obstruction remains intact and if the vessel so obstructed is major, then transmural myocardial infarction will result in the area at risk. If early spontaneous thrombolysis or downstream displacement of a localized thrombus occurs within the phase of ischemia, then acute coronary insufficiency without infarct may result. It seems likely that both platelet and whole blood thrombi are soft and may be readily dispersed. If the occluding thrombus is not displaced or spontaneous lysis is delayed beyond three hours, and the area at risk is large, necrosis will commence in 20 to 40 minutes and will proceed from endocardium to epicardium until a high proportion of the area subtending the obstructed vessel has become infarcted. A second atherosclerotic mechanism postulates fixed, unrelenting near maximal (greater than 95%) nonocclusive stenosis with an epicardial steal due to a multitude of metabolic, autonomic, endocrine, and other factors rendering subendocardial blood flow close to zero. Nontransmural infarction is more frequent; electrocardiographic criteria for subendocardial infarction may be present.

EFFECT OF BLOOD FLOW REDUCTION

Progressive reduction in epicardial contraction occurs as flow is caused to decrease from 70% to 30% of control, at which point contraction ceases (Figure 40.1). Concomitantly with this flow reduction, lactate (usually used by contracting myocardium) is produced in excess by contracting ischemic myocardium, and at 20% of resting blood flow, large quantities of lactate are found in the appropriate coronary vein.[5] It can be concluded that maintenance of contraction depends on levels of blood flow that relate closely to that found under normal resting

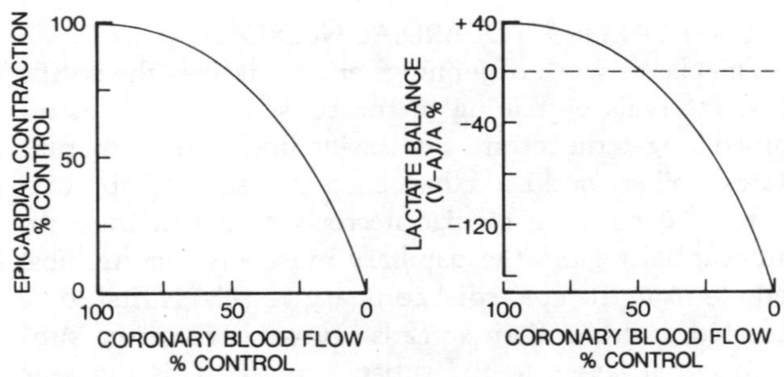

Figure 40.1. Relation of reduction in coronary blood flow to reduction in epicardial contraction (*left panel*) and metabolic state of the myocardium as judged by lactate balance (*right panel*). Epicardial contractility is probably preserved to a greater extent than endocardial contractility for reasons described in the text. Note that at a reduction of blood flow to approximately 50% of control, there is a significant alteration in contractile state and in at least one marker of local substrate utilization. As blood flow approaches 10% to 20%, profound alterations in metabolism and a near absence of contractility pertains. (Figures 40.1, 40.3, 40.4, 40.5, 40.6, and 40.9 reproduced with permission from Swan HJC: Ventricular function in ischemia and infarction and following reperfusion, in Levine HJ, Gaasch WH (eds): *The Ventricle: Basic and Clinical Aspects,* Boston, Martinus Nijhoff Publishing, 1985, pp 271–288.)

conditions (greater than 70%), consistent with the high extraction of oxygen from coronary capillary blood. The contractile activity of the subendocardial or the intermediate layers of myocardium is depressed to an even greater degree for equivalent reductions of flow. In the presence of severely limited coronary flow, there is a significant "steal" of blood from the subendocardial to the subepicardial layers of the myocardium. Therefore, when total coronary blood flow is reduced to 30% of control, epicardial flow is 50%, whereas subendocardial flow may be already less than 10% or approaching zero.

When such experiments are repeated with immediate complete occlusion of the coronary artery, myocardial contraction ceases within 2 to 4 beats. If the duration of complete occlusion is limited to two minutes, rapid normalization of contractile function, intracardiac pressures, and flow can be achieved. At five minutes, regional contraction recovers more slowly, peak ventricular pressure remains slightly depressed, and end-diastolic pressure remains elevated for several minutes. For 20-minute occlusion there is prolonged depression of contractile function, but evidence of necrosis is not seen. For occlusions of 30 to 60 minutes and longer, anatomic and enzymatic evidence of necrosis can be demonstrated. If the coronary circulation is occluded for brief (one to two minutes) intervals but at a high degree of frequency (15 times per hour), function is not restored and abnormal levels of MB-CK are suggestive of focal myocardial necrosis.

In summary, therefore, brief transient occlusions of the coronary arteries 20 minutes or less in duration cause complete cessation of myocardial contractile function with progressive passive stretch of the myocardium involved. Longer occlusions have incomplete recovery, which processes on a time scale inversely proportional to the duration of occlusion (Figure 40.2).

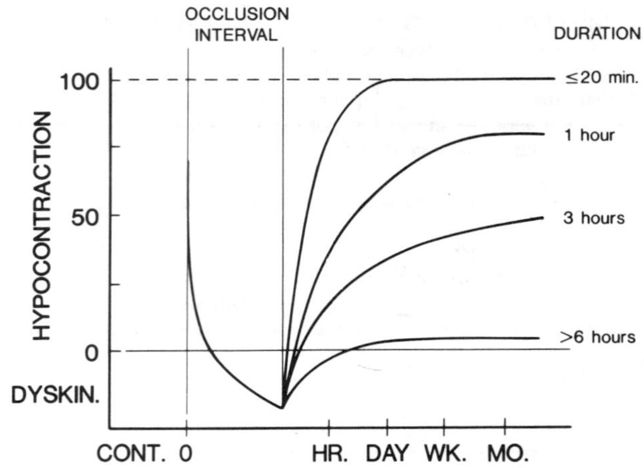

Figure 40.2. Relation of duration of complete coronary occlusion to return of contractile function. Scale on the left represents reduction in contraction measured by magnitude and velocity of wall motion from control (100%). Dyskinesia, or an outward movement of the area of regional ischemia, is the zone below the zero line. The occlusion interval is variable, the individual duration being indicated to the immediate right of the panel. The time scale after the occlusion intervals is indicated as hours, days, weeks, and months. For occlusions of two to five minutes (not shown), there is a prompt restoration of contractile function when blood flow is reestablished. In the case of 1- to 3-hour duration of complete cessation of blood flow, the magnitude of restoration may be significantly affected by relative small contributions from collateral flow. It is possible that function may apparently recover in 3-hour occlusions, principally due to absorption of necrotic tissue and, perhaps, its replacement by compensatory hypertrophy of the remaining myocardial cells.

EVOLUTION OF MYOCARDIAL NECROSIS

The classic work of Jennings et al[6,7] defines the critical time intervals pertaining to the consequences of maintained long-term coronary occlusion under normothermic states. When occlusion has been present for approximately 20 minutes, cardiac necrosis occurs in the subendocardial region: the papillary muscle (structure most remote from the epicardial coronary vessels) is first to be affected; necrosis then spreads outwards from the subendocardial layers to the subepicardium. This dynamic border or "rate of recruitment" possibly reflects the preferential flow of blood to the subepicardial as opposed to the endocardial layers, when total flow available to the epicardial coronary artery is severely reduced to only that entering through collateral channels, as in thrombotic complete coronary occlusion. Nevertheless, patchy areas of myocytes survive within the area of necrosis, even in extensive transmural infarction.

Necrosis is completed in a variable interval (up to four hours or even more) after the onset of total coronary occlusion. In the interval of approximately 20 minutes to three to four hours, an increasing proportion of the area at risk passes from the ischemic state (reversible) to the infarcted myocardium (nonreversible). This proportionality reflects the wavefront of completed necrosis moving from endocardial to epicardial surface (Figure 40.3). Carefully completed experimental studies in the dog suggest that the lateral "border zone," if one truly exists, is small and does not offer significant potential for myocardial salvage per se.[8] Durations of occlusion longer than four to six hours will not increase the magnitude of tissue that becomes necrotic. Infarcted myocardium is clearly incapable of generating cardiac contraction.

Acute myocardial infarction is said to be present when significant necrosis of myocardium dominates the underlying pathologic condition. Initially, at least, extensive ischemia is present in the area at risk, but areas remote from the primary infarct may be perfused by significantly narrow coronary arteries and may become relatively ischemic because of hyperkinesis occasioned by the infarct proper. Myocardial infarction progresses through a series of phases, each of which is associated with significantly abnormal ventricular function. Myocardial infarction occurs in different regions of the heart depending on the actual artery of infarction and the area it perfuses. Complete coronary occlusion due to thrombus formation is the primary precipitating cause of acute myocardial infarction; subcritical (90+%) narrowing with some subsequent infarction is less common. The course may be modified by the presence of preexisting collateral vessels and by the blood pressure response in the individual patient at the onset of acute coronary occlusion. Therefore,

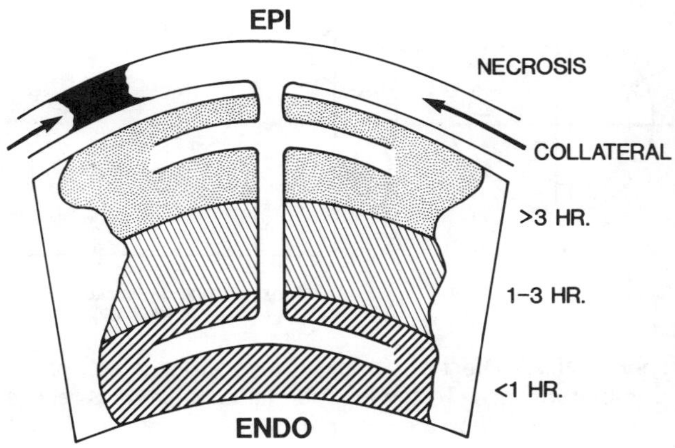

Figure 40.3. Complete occlusion of a coronary artery supplying an area of significant magnitude results in effects on the territory supplied by completely occluded coronary artery. The diagram represents a completely occluded artery (*top left*, coronary flow from left to right). Collateral flow of small magnitude is possible through the remaining coronary bed. There is maximal vasodilatation in both the subendocardial and subepicardial intramyocardial vessels. Any residual blood flow through collaterals will be preferentially directed to the subepicardial layers of the myocardium. Thus, subendocardial flow approaches 0 and subepicardial flow may be 5% to 15% of normal. As a consequence, there is a progressive increase in the proportion of the area at risk, which passes from the ischemic state. An approximate time scale is placed to the right of the figure with maximal myocardial destruction between one and three hours in the example given. The significance of collateral flow will be presented later in Figure 40.9 and in the section on thrombolytic therapy.

hypotension will accelerate the progress from the phase of ischemia and mixed pathology and that of necrosis, whereas hypertension may serve to preserve some degree of collateral flow and thus the subepicardial myocardium. However, if the vessel occluded is small or the collateral circulation generous, the magnitude of infarction will be less than the area originally at risk, or rarely, completely absent.

TECHNIQUES IN THE STUDY OF CARDIAC MECHANICS

Cardiac ischemic injury is essentially regional in nature, excluding the unusual situation of global hypoperfusion or hypoxia, which will not be considered herein. A myriad of techniques have been used in the experimental animal and in man, and will be presented briefly as a further introduction to the clinical consequences of infarction. Each technique has its own particular attributes and disadvantages, and no single technique alone allows for a comprehensive understanding of the mechanics of myocardial ischemia and infarction. However, evaluating the results of a multitude of different approaches allows for a reasonably comprehensive understanding of the whole.

In the animal preparation, length, force, and thickness strain gauges, and implanted markers or ultrasonic crystals are accurate measures of differing dimensions of regional performance. Epicardial length gauges probably reflect only the behavior of a few millimeters of epicardial wall thickness and do not give further information. Implanted crystals can be placed to define motion and velocity in a two-dimensional setting. Similar considerations pertain to measurements of wall thickness. Measurement of mechanics or geometry involves a summary of the behavior of a complex heterogeneous three-dimensional structure of continuously changing shape that thus far allows for only an approximation of the physiologic truth, but sufficient for practical evaluation of the clinical events.

Geometric measurements are the principal bases for the study of cardiac ischemia in man. These methods include left ventriculography of radiographic contrast; scintigraphic technetium-99m ventriculography through either a first pass or equilibrium technique; and M-mode or two-dimensional echocardiographic visualization or secondary derivations of geometry, which are currently incompletely assessed. The latter include measurements of wall thickening, including complex computer modification of the available images. Scintigraphic and echographic techniques are useful because they can be employed without invasive entry to the body and therefore are of particular applicability in man.[9,10] The development of image subtraction technologies, using low-dose radiographic contrast, may allow for wider application of angiography in the diagnostic evaluation of patients with myocardial ischemia and infarction. Virtually all imaging techniques have as their objectives the analysis and reconstruction of geometry and definition of areas of normal or abnormal wall motion. A number of schemes have been derived to numerically quantify these analyses; no uniformity currently exists within or between techniques. Of particular importance is the assessment of the centroid from which measurements are made and conclusions as to whether or not the centroid should be a moving or fixed reference point. However, all such studies are noncontinuous and expensive, require considerable cooperation for a relatively long period by critically ill patients, and require highly skilled technology. Reproducibility and accuracy in the critical care environment still require validation.

Hence, application of radiologic methods in the acute phase of myocardial infarction is limited. Whereas contrast ventriculography in specialized laboratories has been of great value in the development of our knowledge in this field, its invasive nature, as well as its inherent logistic difficulties, and competing noninvasive techniques have caused contrast radiography to fall from favor as a routine method in the evaluation of induced changes in ventricular function in man. However, radionuclide scintigraphy has practical and logistical applicability in the intensive care or coronary care unit; multiple studies of ejection fraction, regional wall motion, and right ventricular function have been published.[11]

Measurements of pressure and flow reflect consequences of changes in regional mechanics and geometry, although the relation is not highly precise. They have the advantage that they may be converted into near continuous or continuous observation and may be rapidly responsive to significant acute changes in regional mechanics. For example, acute cardiac ischemia is promptly reflected by an increase in the pulmonary capillary wedge pressure, a reflection of change in the left ventricular diastolic pressure—itself a manifestation of altered left ventricular volume, contractility, or compliance.[12] Data conventionally obtained by hemodynamic monitoring include stroke volume, systemic and pulmonary vascular resistance, and the filling pressures of each ventricle.[13] They have the further advantage of widespread utilization, application by trained critical care personnel, and relevance to interventions potentially useful in a clinical situation. The practical use of balloon flotation catheters in the management of acute myocardial infarction will be detailed herein.

CONCEPTUAL MECHANICAL MODEL OF THE ISCHEMIC OR INFARCTED HEART

With the recognition in the early 1970s that cardiogenic shock was not accompanied by uniform depression in cardiac wall motion, a model of the heart in acute ischemia or infarction was proposed, consisting of a nondilated nonhypertrophied left ventricle without prior injury.[14] The spherical two-component model included a totally noncontractile ischemic or infarcted noncompliant segment operating in series with a normally perfused area with normal contractility and compliance. This model has been validated in an experimental preparation. The effects of changes in compliance and hypercontraction in the noninjured area will be considered further.

The immediate mechanical alterations are illustrated schematically in Figure 40.4. Assuming a prior normal contractility and an ejection fraction of 0.67 for the normal noninfarcted ventricle, normal volumes and pressures would pertain. A near linear relation exists between ejection fraction and the percentage of myocardial wall involved, although this is not a rigorously proven statement. From this relation (see legend for Figure 40.4) a small area of myocardial involvement (for example, 10%, point a in Figure 40.4) results in a near negligible reduction in ejection fraction, whereas a larger degree of involvement (40%, point b in Figure 40.4) results in an important, and indeed serious, reduction in ejection fraction to approximately 0.40. Examining only the larger area of dysfunction, it is evident that at constant contractility for the remaining myocardium and at a constant end-diastolic volume, stroke volume declines substantively to approximately 40 ml/m². If ejection fraction remains constant, end-diastolic volume must increase to restore stroke volume. Assuming no change in diastolic ventricular volumes or in the compliance of the normal myocardium, the presence of infarct mandates increases in diastolic filling pressure. It can be concluded that as a result of acute severe ischemia in which contraction ceases but diastolic compliance is unchanged in both the injured and uninjured region, the physiologic consequences are a reduction in ejection fraction proportional to the relative perimeter involved by injury, an increase in diastolic pressures, and a decrease in stroke volume and cardiac output of a magnitude related to the area of injury.

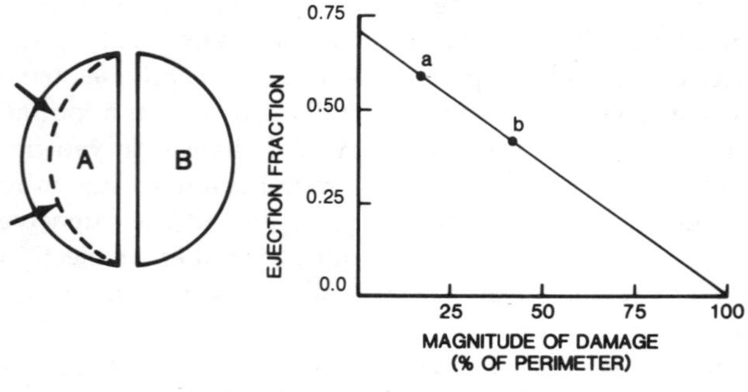

Figure 40.4. Reduction in ejection fraction as a function of magnitude of wall involved. To the left the heart is represented as a sphere, of which portion A has retained normal contraction, and portion B has suffered myocardial ischemia and is rigid and noncontractile. On the right the progressive reduction in ejection fraction (proportion of end-diastolic content ejected during systole) is progressively decreased. See text for details.

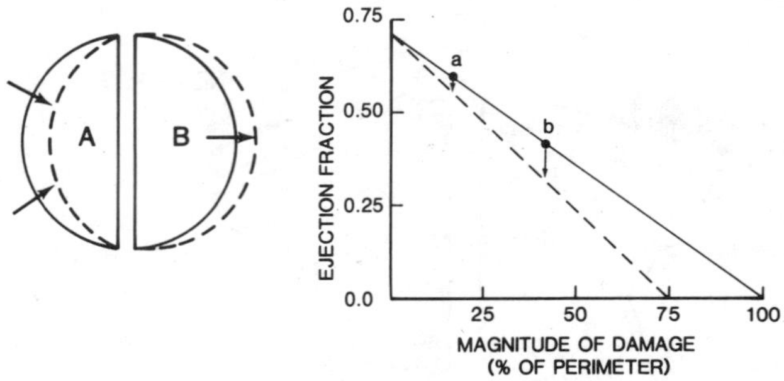

Figure 40.5. Effect of compliant myocardial infarct on cardiac performance. To the left, normal contraction is retained by segment A, but there is paradoxic expansion (outward movement) in the compliant infarcted component indicated by B. In contrast to the prior (Figure 40.4) situation (*right panel*), the resulting ejection fraction (– –) is reduced at all levels. Although this is of no great significance if the infarct is determined by the proportion of perimeter involved, this has a major effect in larger infarcts. See text for details.

However, if the process proceeds to infarction, changes in compliance of the area of injury are likely. Experimental evidence (discussed later) suggests that in the presence of ischemia, there is, at least initially, an increase in diastolic stiffness of the affected area; in the presence of infarction, altered elastic compliance, creep, and stretch affect the physical properties of the infarcted myocardium[15,16] (Figure 40.5). Systolic distention of the compliant myocardium will materially worsen global ventricular function. Thus, for infarcts of similar magnitude, a large compliant infarction will result in further reduction in ejection fraction from 0.40 to 0.27. Stroke volume will be reduced to less than 25 ml/m². The energetics of the normally functioning, or even hyperfunctioning, residual myocardium will be absorbed in the useless distention of the infarcted myocardium. Even with significant increases in end-diastolic volume, ejection fraction values of 0.20 or less are incompatible with maintenance of an adequate stroke volume.

Stroke volume and the magnitude of systolic expansion are highly dependent on ventricular afterload. If afterload is low and diastolic filling pressure is high, then the "wasted" contractile effort is reduced. However, afterload is usually increased by peripheral vasoconstriction due to baroreceptor and chemoreceptor activity, resulting in a further reduction in cardiac output and elevation in end-diastolic ventricular pressure, this despite increases in heart rate and hypercontractility in the adequately perfused residual myocardium.

Alteration in the contractile state of the ventricle, whether spontaneous or caused by exogenous stimuli such as vasoactive drugs, can result in only a minor apparent improvement in overall hemodynamics; added mechanical burdens may cause drastic adverse changes (Figure 40.6). Even if one assumes a 20% enhancement in stroke volume as a result of changes in contractility, this will be effected only in the healthy residual myocardium. The injured territory is incapable of responding and in the case of a compliant or "stretch capable" infarct, the actual effects of increased contractility may be deleterious. This conclusion is well sustained by the essentially negligible improvement in global performance to inotropic interventions in severe heart failure associated with myocardial infarction. On the contrary, increased mechanical burdens such as mitral regurgitation or ventricular septal perforation have a disastrous effect on overall cardiac function in myocardial infarction. Expected symptoms of acute heart failure will result. Even in the presence of a small infarction, forward stroke volume at 10 mm Hg left ventricular filling pressure declines from 55 to 60 ml/m^2 to 30 ml/m^2 with a 50% regurgitant fraction. The validity of this model is supported by the observation that cardiogenic shock can occur in patients with relatively small primary infarcts, but with secondary added mechanical lesions. Recognition of the dire consequences of additional mechanical burdens in such patients has now prompted the concept of emergent surgical intervention.

Thus, infarct size, contractility, compliance, mechanical load, heart size, and other factors are prime determinants in the outcome of patients with myocardial infarction, and similar, although not identical, concepts applied to patients with myocardial ischemia who, incidentally, also may have transient mitral regurgitation due to papillary muscle ischemia. Each of the factors has a temporal course during injury, and each may alter to variable degrees. The specifics will be considered later in other sections of this chapter.

During the early phase of evolving myocardial infarction, the general hemodynamic responses will depend on the magnitude of area involved; in clinical practice, a great variability between patients exists. This has required the development of magnitude concepts: hemodynamic subsets. If the infarct is small (10% of ventricular perimeter), slight increases in heart rate and blood pressure occur. A large infarct (30% to 40% perimeter) results in systolic bulging of the affected area, the myocardium in the injured area fails to thicken during systole, and with continued systolic stress and the failure of cellular integrity and contractile reinforcement during systole, tissue "creep" occurs and thinning of the affected myocardium in both systole and diastole develops. Residual myocardium supplied by nonrestricted coronary vessels demonstrates hyperkinesis, and the magnitude and velocity of systolic wall thickening in these areas appear enhanced.[17] Cardiac chamber volume increases and ejection fraction falls. Heart rate increases and after an initial decrease the blood pressure is restored at a slightly reduced level. In small infarcts blood pressure and cardiac output are preserved. Occasionally they are increased due to catecholamine hyperproduction. In larger infarcts the cardiac output is severely reduced (cardiac index less than 2.2 L/min/m^2), and systemic vascular resistance increases. Although infarcts equivalent to 20% to 30% of perimeter are associated with evidence of heart failure—increased diastolic ventricular pressures, reduced cardiac output, and elevated systemic vascular resistance—recovery is the rule and the signs of severe heart failure do not always

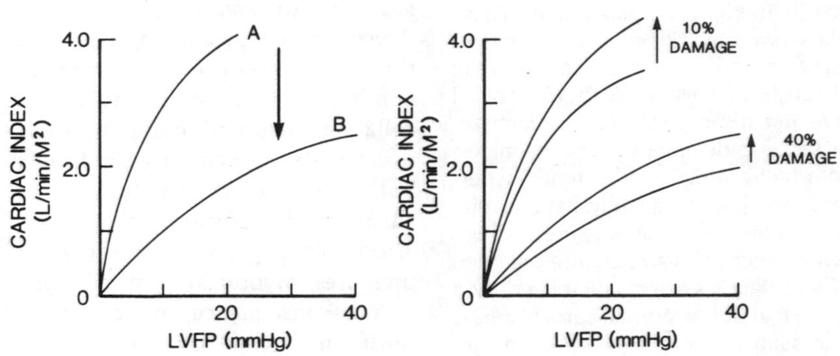

Figure 40.6. Relation of cardiac index to left ventricular filling pressure and its modification in myocardial infarction. *Left panel* indicates the effect of a mechanical lesion, such as acute mitral insufficiency or ventricular septal perforation in a heart, with a previously small infarct and a function curve identified by *A*. Assuming no change in other controlling parameters, the development of 50% regurgitation or shunt results in a "systemic" cardiac performance characterized by curve *B*, with an obligatory increase in left ventricular filling pressure, and a marked reduction in systemic blood flow. The *right panel* shows the effect of maximal inotropic stimulation in a small (10%) damaged and a large (40%) damaged myocardial infarct. Because there is less available healthy perfused contractile myocardium in the larger infarct, the absolute magnitude of change in cardiac index (improvement) is smaller than that when the damage is the less.

persist. Larger infarcts (perimeter involvement greater than 30%) are frequently associated with pulmonary congestion and edema. Profound reduction in cardiac output (cardiac index less than 1.7 L/min/m²) and the clinical syndrome of cardiogenic shock—profound tissue hypoperfusion—develops. Prior myocardial scar or an additional new mechanical lesion adds to the circulatory burden, and short- and long-term prognosis as to survival is generally poor (Figure 40.7).

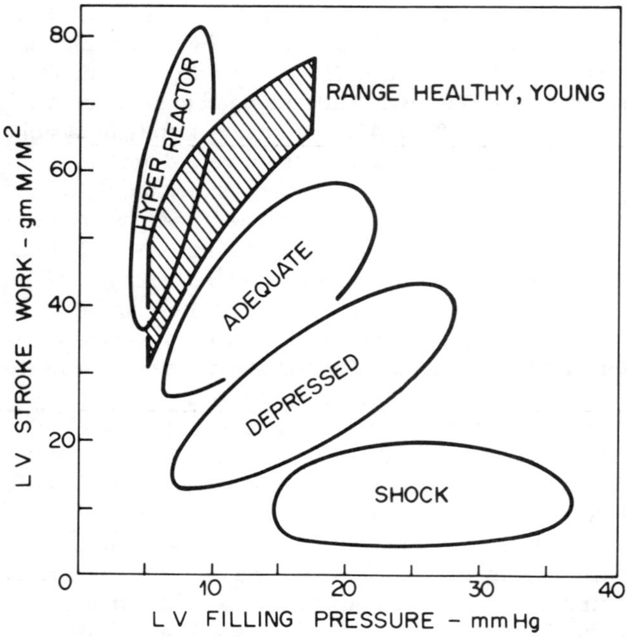

Figure 40.7. Relation of clinical to hemodynamic presentation in patients with acute myocardial infarction. This hypothetical diagram presupposes first infarction of increasing magnitudes (from top to bottom). The parameters of cardiac index and left ventricular filling pressure are presented as indicators of change in hemodynamic state. Certain patients with small infarcts have normal hemodynamic parameters. These patients are frequently those with inferior myocardial infarction, enjoy a good prognosis and have essentially normal hemodynamics. A small subset of these (5% to 10% of all infarcts) exhibit a hyperdynamic response to a small infarction, presumably due to release of endogenous catecholamines. Such patients present with tachycardia, and at times hypertension, agitation, and anxiety. They frequently have a relatively high cardiac output and normal filling pressures. A high proportion of patients with anterior infarction present with pulmonary congestion. These patients are characterized by a high filling pressure and a normal or low normal cardiac index. The principal treatment in such patients is the relief of pulmonary congestion by lowering filling pressures, which may be achieved utilizing diuretics and/or venodilators. Patients with profound depression of cardiac index and a seriously elevated filling pressure have the poorest prognosis and many of these will progress into cardiogenic shock. Not specifically identified in this figure is the relatively small proportion of patients who currently present with hypovolemia. Such patients have low cardiac output, but this is secondary to an extremely low left ventricular filling pressure. At times, the use of powerful diuretics is associated with nausea and vomiting. Such patients may require fluid volume replacement for restoration of cardiac performance.

Parenthetically, human patients with overt ventricular aneurysm may demonstrate apparent involvement of 50% or more of the perimeter; however, as an index of myocardial destruction this may be misleading, because extensive thinning and myocardial creep mask the existence of a considerable quantity (as much as 70% of normal) of contracting myocardium. As convalescence progresses and the tissue of such a functional aneurysm scars and becomes nondistensible, adequate function frequently returns.

In summary, a general deterioration in ventricular systolic and diastolic function occurs in evolving myocardial infarction in man. Wide variations exist in the magnitude of area at risk, the presence of collateral circulation, the initial circulatory, metabolic, and hormonal response to the acute insult, the continued stresses on injured and healing myocardium, and other factors concerned with the healing process.

CLINICAL SIGNIFICANCE OF PATHOPHYSIOLOGY

The term acute myocardial infarction is synonymous with the occurrence of myocardial necrosis of a magnitude sufficient to cause recognizable symptoms, alterations in the electrical activity of the heart, liberation of enzymes from myocardial tissue, and depression of mechanical function. Lesser degrees of myocardial necrosis may occur in other conditions, including unstable angina, prolonged myocardial ischemia, infection, microemboli, and the like. However, under these circumstances, the patient does not manifest the clinical syndrome of important regional myocardial necrosis. As stated, the time course of necrosis is complex and related to absolute levels of residual blood flow, regional regulation of distribution of the limited available blood supply, and cell membrane stability, commencing within 30 minutes in some cases. Longer myocardial survival depends on a number of factors, among which the most important is residual inflow from an incompletely occluded but severely (90+%) stenosed artery supplying the area at risk or from collateral connections—dependent on preexisting developed channels and adequate perfusion pressure. Under the least favorable circumstances, such as sudden acute occlusion, no preformed collateral channels, and arterial hypotension, transmural necrosis will be completed in three hours or less, whereas in the most favorable circumstances, such as subtotal occlusion with preformed collaterals, maintained arterial diastolic blood pressure, and low left ventricular diastolic pressures, myocardium may be preserved completely.

As a consequence, the temporal phases of acute myocardial infarction have been defined (Table 40.2) to include the phase of ischemia, the phase of necrosis, the phase of compensation, and the phase of healing.[18] These temporal phases allow the clinician to relate his diagnostic and therapeutic evaluations and interventions in accord with the underlying pathology and pathophysiology. Severely ischemic myocardium is incapable of mechanical contraction. In addition, necrotic myocardium is deprived of the viable mechanical elements to prevent passive stretch during systole and, hence, is vulnerable to "materials creep," described as the thinning and stretching phase of necrosis. The phase of compensation is associ-

Table 40.2. Temporal Phases in the Genesis of Acute Myocardial Infarction

Phase	Pathology	Duration*
1. Ischemia	Reversible normal	20–60 min
(a) Mixed		
2. Necrosis	Completed infarct	1–5 h
3. Compensation	Absorption-thinning-fibrosis	12 h–2 w
4. Healing	Scar formation and contraction	1–6 mo

* The ranges vary widely.

ated with adjustments in cardiopulmonary, metabolic, and endocrine functions. The phase of healing is characterized by cellular infiltration and reabsorption, the laying down of primitive collagen, and scar formation and maturation. For complete maturation, four to six months or more are required if the scar is large.

CLINICAL SYNDROMES OF ISCHEMIA WITHOUT INFARCTION

The clinical manifestations of myocardial ischemia without infarction may be usefully considered in the classification in Table 40.3 and in detail elsewhere. These clinical syndromes derive from the development of a critical or subcritical level of obstruction of an important branch of a coronary artery. Their consequences are related to the extent of the territory involved in the ischemic process and the severity and duration of the ischemia. Certain of these ischemic syndromes actually may be accompanied by evidence of myocardial necrosis of small magnitude, but insufficient to justify the clinical syndrome to be labeled "myocardial infarction." Valvular dysfunction secondary to ischemia or infarction may cause transient mitral regurgitation and pulmonary congestion. Myocardial ischemia may also be present in the absence of pain, which is implied in the use of the term *angina*. Both electrocardiographic and mechanical alterations in cardiac function occur at a level of reduction of coronary blood flow insufficient to cause the pain syndrome and recur repeatedly during ordinary daily activity in patients with chronic stable angina.

Disorders of ventricular function in the presence of coronary artery disease are regional in nature. Patients with chronic stable angina pectoris without prior infarction will usually demonstrate normality of systolic performance with normal resting left ventricular stroke volume, ejection fraction, and normal regional wall motion.

Table 40.3. Classification of Angina Pectoris

Mechanism	Clinical Title
1. Fixed atherosclerosis (severe)	Chronic stable angina (Heberden's)
2. Fixed atherosclerosis (moderate) with normal vasomotion	Mixed (common) angina
3. Atherosclerosis with plaque instability (endothelial disruption)	Unstable angina
4. Atherosclerosis; severe, moderate with abnormal vasomotion (spasm)	Variant angina (Prinzmetal's)

Minor abnormalities of diastolic function may be present, including a modest elevation in end-diastolic ventricular pressure, and alteration in the filling pattern of the left ventricle consistent with increased stiffness (reduced compliance).[19] The presence of a resting abnormality of regional function is suggestive of preexisting scar due to prior myocardial infarction.

Abnormalities of systolic function can be demonstrated in patients with the ischemic clinical syndromes during angina by exercise or by pacing, or other interventions such as elevation of ventricular afterload. Under stress there is a reduction in ejection fraction during exercise and the development of hypokinesis, akinesis, or even dyskinesis in the territory supplied by the restricted coronary artery.[20] Systolic function is progressively reduced with increasing degrees of abnormality of contraction throughout the territory of ischemia. A decrease in overall ventricular function occurs by progressive recruitment of the areas of lesser dysfunction as exercise progresses. Immediately following exercise, restoration of function in the abnormal tissue occurs, particularly under circumstances in which afterload and preload are promptly reduced.[21] Enhancement of systolic function is usually present in the remote, adequately perfused myocardium.

Diastolic function shows further progressive deterioration during stress. End-diastolic pressure rises, at times to levels consistent with the development of pulmonary congestion and edema. End-systolic and end-diastolic volumes show a marked increase. Mitral regurgitation may substantively enhance the abnormality of pump function, and ultimately cardiac output decreases. Restoration of diastolic function after cessation of stress is likewise prompt. Under conditions of rapid cardiac pacing, elevated diastolic pressure may decrease within a beat of cessation of pacing and achieve normality in 30 to 60 seconds.

In general, the adverse consequences of stress on ventricular function in patients with the more classic Heberden's angina pectoris are transient and reversible. In like manner, dysfunction associated with Prinzmetal's variant angina appears to be short-lived. However, in patients with prolonged coronary insufficiency, a severe manifestation of the anginal syndrome and intermingling with clinical infarction, recovery of myocardial function may be slow. Whether this is due to subclinical myocardial necrosis or to alterations of function associated with a more prolonged ischemic event, such as platelet occlusion with spontaneous reperfusion, is currently unknown. Unstable angina as a prodrome of acute infarction will be discussed later. The prognosis of prolonged coronary insufficiency does not differ greatly from that of infarction per se.[22]

Chronic heart failure is a frequent accompaniment of ischemic heart disease and is usually due to extensive scarring consequent to prior myocardial infarction with or without associated valvular dysfunction. Severe cardiac enlargement, with ejection fraction values varying between 10% to 20%, elevated left ventricular end-diastolic pressures, and the clinical manifestations of heart failure, including pulmonary congestion, shortness of breath, and fatigue are present; the prognosis is very poor. Occasionally this phenomenon may be due largely to extensive myocardial ischemia and surgical restoration of blood flow can result in near miraculous restoration of ventricular function in such individuals.

CLINICAL PRESENTATION OF ACUTE MYOCARDIAL INFARCTION

The clinical manifestations of acute myocardial infarction are variable, although chest pain or pressure is the classic presenting feature. Prior strenuous activity is noted in 5% to 15% of subjects; a far greater proportion have the initiation of symptoms at rest or on awakening from sleep. The most important single issue in regard to the symptom of chest pain is its presence and severity, its nonrelief by cessation of activity or by nitroglycerin, and its associated symptoms of diaphoresis, nausea, weakness, apprehension (fear of impending death), and shortness of breath.[23] Approximately 60% of patients with acute infarction have prior evidence of atherosclerotic vascular disease, angina pectoris, abnormal electrocardiogram, or previous myocardial infarction. A 40% to 60% prevalence of prodromal symptoms of unstable angina, dyspnea, or unusual fatigue has been described one to four weeks preceding acute myocardial infarction by several investigators.[24] In a substantial proportion, the duration of cardiac symptoms is relatively brief. Males are affected more frequently and at an earlier age than females, and risk factors for coronary atherosclerosis may (or may not) be present. The pain pattern itself is varied. It may be acute, sudden, and intense in onset or smoldering for several hours before becoming fixed and continuous. It may wax and wane and then increase acutely in intensity. The classic pain syndrome may be diagnostic of acute myocardial infarction; however, the absence of several of the commonly described features does not exclude this diagnosis.[25] Classically the pain is sudden, intense, and localized to the retrosternal area with a band-like and excruciating character. Nevertheless, there may be lesser degrees of discomfort, including oppression, a sense of heaviness retrosternally, with or without radiation to the classical locations in the left shoulder, left arm, both arms, jaw, neck, back, or epigastrium. The pain may spontaneously devolve over several hours or may require powerful narcotics for its relief. Waxing and waning of a less intense level of discomfort are common. Important associated symptoms include nausea, belching, bloating, or "heartburn" with or without vomiting, a sense of cold in the periphery with extreme weakness, and relatively severe "soaking" sweats with the need to sit or lie down so as to prevent a fainting spell. Palpitations, transient or continuous, a sense of faintness, and at times a sense of impending death also characterize the more classic presentations. Of prime importance is the recognition that none of these manifestations may be sufficiently clear to allow for the diagnosis. This is particularly true of patients admitted to an emergency room for an unexplained episode of weakness or acute sweating without characteristic chest discomfort. Acute shortness of breath may be an early manifestation of myocardial infarction. In about 5% to 10% of cases, the infarction is totally devoid of any symptoms and recognized during an incidental evaluation (silent infarction).[26] In another 5% to 10% of cases in which it is thought to be silent some questioning reveals evidence of atypical symptoms ignored or misinterpreted by the patient.[25] Acute myocardial infarction is the first presenting indication of 20% to 40% of cases of coronary artery disease. Sudden death, most frequently related to ventricular fibrillation, may occur in the prehospital phase within the first couple of hours of onset of coronary occlusion.

Because prompt recognition of acute myocardial infarction today allows for many options as to management, including acute revascularization, a prompt diagnosis is essential. The most important prerequisite is suspicion of the possibility of this diagnosis. This is particularly true in the emergency room setting when patients, particularly males over the age of 50 years with adverse risk factors including prior acute myocardial infarction, presenting with unclear but suggestive complaints must be considered as having possible myocardial infarction until proven otherwise. Causes of confounding chest pain that may be confused with acute myocardial infarction are listed in Table 40.4.

PHYSICAL EXAMINATION

Physical examination may or may not be particularly revealing and abnormalities often relate to the complications associated with myocardial infarction, the coexistence of disease affecting other organs, and alterations in autonomic nervous system caused by infarction or pain and the anxiety and fear associated with it. The specific physical findings associated with complications of acute myocardial infarction will be dealt with under specific sections dealing with complications. When significant heart failure is present, the patient may also be tachypneic. The peripheral pulse may be normal, rapid or slow, and regular or irregular, depending on the status of autonomic tone, arterial pressure, conduction, or rhythm disturbances. Sinus tachycardia is common, particularly accompanying anterior infarctions, whereas in others it may reflect a response to hypotension or heart failure, pain, and anxiety. Sinus or junctional bradycardia tends to be more common in inferior infarction, most likely a manifestation of enhanced parasympathetic activity.

Table 40.4. Common Causes of Chest Pain in Suspect Acute Myocardial Infarction

1. Cardiac ischemia
    - Unstable angina. Prinzmetal's angina
    - Accelerated angina. . . Rest, postprandial angina
    - Prolonged myocardial ischemia
2. Other cardiac and vascular
    - Acute pericarditis
    - Pneumonia
    - Pleurisy
    - Pulmonary embolus
    - Aortic dissection, aortic aneurysm
3. Noncardiac causes
    - Anxiety state
    - Chest wall pain
    - Esophagus, stomach, duodenum, gallbladder disease
    - Renal, biliary colic
    - Herpes zoster

Cold, clammy skin is indicative of vasoconstriction and stimulation of the sweating mechanisms by increased sympathoadrenal activity. The patient may also demonstrate peripheral cyanosis caused by a reduction in skin blood flow with extraction of oxygen to a level so as to produce cyanosis in the capillary blood. The temperature may be normal, or after 18 to 24 hours rise by 1° to 1.5°C, presumably caused by failure of heat loss due to systemic vasoconstriction. The patient is usually alert and mentation is normal in the presenting phases of acute myocardial infarction. Later confusion and coma are manifestations of a profound reduction in cardiac output and severe hypotension. Examination of the vascular system may reveal evidence of additional vascular disease in the retinal arteries, peripheral circulation, and carotid system. In the presenting phase of acute myocardial infarction, the neck veins are usually flat, unless the patient has had prior infarcts and heart failure or has sustained right ventricular infarction. Pulmonary examination may reveal rales depending on the presence of left ventricular dysfunction and its severity.

Precordial examination may be unremarkable or may demonstrate a diffuse apical impulse or a paradoxic apical or juxtapical impulse corresponding to outward systolic bulging of the left ventricular infarcted segment. A palpable thrill is rare on presentation, but it may be felt if ventricular septal rupture occurs. Heart sounds may be normal or diminished in intensity. Paradoxic splitting of S_2 may be heard with or without complications of left bundle branch block, whereas wide splitting of S_2 may occur if right bundle branch block or severe mitral regurgitation is present. Systolic apical murmurs are common after acute myocardial infarction, most often due to papillary muscle dysfunction, but they could also result from rupture of papillary muscle or ventricular septum. Palpable and audible S_4 and S_3 may be evident, especially in the presence of left ventricular dilation or left ventricular failure.

A pericardial friction rub is unusual in the early presentation of acute myocardial infarction, but it may occur later in 10% to 20% of patients. Detection early in the apparent course of the illness is suggestive of the differential diagnosis of primary pericarditis. A persistent rub suggests that the infarct (if confirmed) is of relatively large magnitude. Late in the course of the illness (14 or more days) a new pericardial rub is suggestive of a postmyocardial infarction syndrome.

The blood pressure response is nonspecific. Patients previously normotensive may remain unchanged or become hypertensive or hypotensive. Previously hypertensive patients may become normotensive or hypotensive. Large infarction may normalize blood pressure in a previously hypertensive patient.

Physical examination of other body systems is important when findings are positive. Evidence of peripheral vascular disease strengthens the diagnosis of atherosclerosis; acute embolism is a rare manifestation in the early phase of myocardial infarction; upper quadrant and subxiphoid tenderness may suggest the presence of subdiaphragmatic disease. Acute mesenteric vascular insufficiency with abdominal tenderness and rigidity and absent bowel sounds is a rare initial manifestation of acute myocardial infarction. The association of cerebrovascular and coronary disease allows for the association of stroke with acute evolving myocardial infarction; hypoperfusion associated with hypotension secondary to new myocardial infarction may result in confusion, overt psychosis, or at times coma.

ELECTROCARDIOGRAPHIC FINDINGS

The 12-lead electrocardiogram remains the primary diagnostic tool in the diagnosis of acute myocardial infarction.[27] However, no single electrocardiographic pattern is pathognomonic of the condition; rather the electrocardiogram undergoes evolution in a manner not unlike that described for the differing pathophysiologic phases of evolving myocardial infarction. During the phase of necrosis, transmural myocardial infarction is usually associated with the development of new Q waves or the disappearance or reduction in magnitude of R waves. However, the significance of specific waveforms requires reevaluation because Q waves can be observed in patients with nontransmural infarcts. Classically, nontransmural (subendocardial) myocardial infarction is defined by the presence of persistent ST-segment depression or T-wave inversion without Q waves or both; however, the correctness of this interpretation has been questioned. The anatomic location of the infarct will determine in which leads diagnostic alterations are identified.

It is not within the scope of this chapter to describe the multitude of electrocardiographic manifestations of acute myocardial infarction. For this the reader is referred to chapter 5 on Electrocardiography and Vectorcardiography. Importantly, however, the presence of a Q morphology in appropriate locations may be suggestive of, but not highly specific for, new acute myocardial infarctions; in like manner, the absence of Q morphology does not exclude the possibility of this diagnosis. The sensitivity and specificity of a single electrocardiographic tracing are greatly enhanced by the availability of prior tracings for comparison. Evidence of new Q waves in the inferior (leads II, III, and aVF), anteroseptal and/or anterolateral leads (V_1–V_3, V_3–V_6) is strong evidence that the clinical event is a transmural infarct. Q waves may be associated with other forms of myocardial injury, cardiomyopathies, systemic or pulmonary hypertension, cardiac tumors, amyloidosis, the Wolff–Parkinson–White syndrome, left bundle branch block, ventricular paced rhythm, and the like. Also, ST-T–wave changes are nonspecific and may be associated with pericardial disease, myocarditis, drugs, electrolyte imbalance, hyperventilation, and posture. Acute pulmonary embolism and acute pericarditis may be associated with alteration of R-wave magnitude and ST-T–wave alterations; symptoms may be similar to those of a patient presenting with acute infarction.

SERUM ENZYME ABNORMALITIES

In addition to the electrocardiogram, the presence of abnormal levels of certain "cardiac" enzymes in the blood stream represents important (and at times essential) confirmatory criteria for the diagnosis[28] (Figure 40.8). Myo-

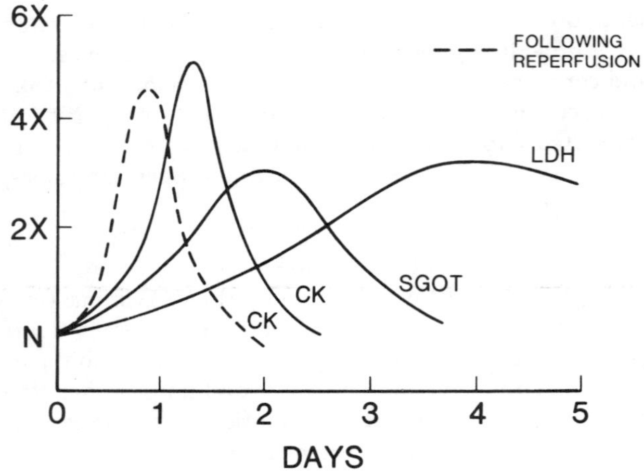

Figure 40.8. Time course of plasma enzyme levels following acute myocardial infarction. *Solid lines* indicate the appearance, magnitude, and clearance of creatine kinase (CK), serum glutamic oxaloacetic transferase (SGOT), and lactic dehydrogenase (LDH). *Note*: CK peaks at approximately 30 hours and ordinarily declines over the next 36 to 72 hours. The rise in LDH is gradual, peaking between 3 and 4 days and slowly returning to baseline. *Broken line* indicates the change in CK associated with reperfusion by thrombolysis or very early cardiac surgery. There is a prompt and rapid release of CK at the time of reperfusion, with peak values occurring at approximately 16 hours with a more rapid washout of CK from the plasma.

cardial necrosis is associated with failure of integrity of the myocardial cell membrane that allows escape of intracellular enzymes. Of these, by far the most important today are the creatine kinases (CK), in particular, the myocardial specific MB fraction.[29] Conventionally, in nonreperfused infarction, serum creatine kinase (CK) levels start to rise in six to ten hours, reach a maximum in 16 to 30 hours, and then decline. Although the exact source and kinetics of elevated levels of serum glutamic oxaloacetic transferase (SGOT) and lactic dehydrogenase (LDH) is unclear, it appears that CK-MB is derived from the necrotic myocardial cells. It is believed that free release of CK indicates cell death; if a cell is dead, it must release its contained CK to the local extracellular space. Total CK and CK-MB levels in the systemic circulation must also reflect "washout" of the "free" enzyme from the extracellular space through myocardial lymphatic drainage or by residual blood flow from collateral or reperfused vessels. If blood flow is restored, then the extracellular myocardial CK is rapidly discharged into the systemic circulation; between 60% and 80% is recovered. If blood flow is not restored, then only approximately 15% of the released enzyme can be recovered in the system circulation. Creatine kinase (MM and BB) is also found in skeletal muscle and brain tissue and may be elevated in primary muscle disease and following intramuscular injections. Serum glutamic oxaloacetic transferase levels are usually increased 12 to 20 hours after the onset of symptoms and peak at 36 to 48 hours. These values return to normal in approximately four days. Lactic dehydrogenase is elevated between 12 and 24 hours after the onset of symptoms, peaks at approximately 72 to 84 hours, and returns to normal on the tenth day. The "battery" estimate of all of these enzymes, common in the past, has now been substantively replaced by measurements of CK only, and, when facilities are available, of the MB fraction. Additional useful information relative to the diagnosis of acute myocardial infarction does not appear to be derived from the measurement of other enzymes.

Estimates of cardiac enzymes are important from two standpoints. First, a rise in CK-MB isoenzyme is a highly specific diagnostic tool in acute myocardial infarction.[30] However, its immediate (within 12 hours) sensitivity is restricted because the rise in enzyme levels fundamentally follows necrosis by a variable time interval and thus fails to provide a prognostic index of use in the initial treatment of the patient. Second, total CK and CK-MB estimations have been used as a "post-facto" quantification of the magnitude of myocardial destruction.[31,32] This concept depends on an estimation of the total amount of enzyme released from the necrotic myocardium, which is then related empirically to the number of grams of tissue that would produce the measured quantity of CK in plasma. The approach depends on a number of assumptions in relation to CK kinetics and the acceptance of a low recovery rate in the serum for tissue loss. Despite the reliance placed by many on enzymatically based infarct size, experimental evidence suggests that the recovery ratio varies considerably.[33] Such estimates should be regarded as approximate at best. Nevertheless, patients who have substantively greater levels of CK or CK-MB identified in serum tend to have larger territories of necrosis and a poorer prognosis. It should be remembered that recanalization of an infarct-related artery can "wash out" CK and give earlier and high peak levels in the blood in comparison with a nonreperfused infarction of identical magnitude (Figure 40.8).

DIAGNOSIS OF ACUTE MYOCARDIAL INFARCTION

It is convenient to regard diagnostic criteria in terms of sensitivity and specificity. The "sensitivity" of a test is the proportion of patients with the disease or condition in whom the diagnostic criteria are positive for the disease. The "specificity" is the proportion of patients without disease in whom the diagnostic criteria are negative. The prior history in regard to risk factors and the presenting symptoms exhibit low sensitivity and specificity in that patients in whom myocardial infarction is evolving may have no prior history and relatively minimal symptoms, whereas patients in whom myocardial infarction is not evolving may present with similar symptoms. The astute physician will effectively relate the totality of presentation to a correct diagnosis. However, because the consequences of failure to diagnose may be serious, it is recommended that patients with suggestive histories be admitted to surveillance for at least 24 hours, even in the presence of an electrocardiogram within normal limits or characterized by "nonspecific" findings, together with serum CK-MB levels that have not yet risen. Diagnosis of myocardial infarction is generally made when there is a characteristic rise and fall in serum levels of CK-MB in association with appropriate electrocardiographic evolution, with or without associated symptoms. In some patients in whom electrocardiographic changes are inconclusive or uninterpretable or enzyme values are ambiguous, technetium pyrophosphate scintigraphy performed two to five days after presumed infarction may reveal the presence and location of myocardial necrosis.

CLINICAL COURSE OF PATIENTS WITH ACUTE MYOCARDIAL INFARCTION

The clinical course of the patient may be relatively uncomplicated[34] or modified by the occurrence of several minor and major complications. The important complications are listed in Table 40.5. Approximately 50% to 75% of patients have a relatively uncomplicated course, whereas in the remainder one or more fatal or nonfatal complications develop.

MANAGEMENT OF ACUTE MYOCARDIAL INFARCTION

The objectives of treatment to assure immediate survival of the patient are to maintain the general comfort and well-being of the patient, to limit necrosis in critically ischemic myocardium (the territory at risk), to optimally manage associated complications, and to assess the risk of postdischarge adverse events to help prevent such events in high-risk patients.

Table 40.5. Complications of Acute Myocardial Infarction

A. *Disturbances of rate or rhythm*
- Bradycardia: sinus, AV nodal, idioventricular
- Ectopic beats: atrial, ventricular
- Tachyarrhythmias: supraventricular (atrial fibrillation, flutter, tachycardia), ventricular (ventricular tachycardia, fibrillation)

B. *Disturbances of conduction*
- AV nodal: 1°, 2°, 3° AV block
- Intraventricular: hemiblocks, bundle branch block, Mobitz II block, 3° AV block

C. *Pump dysfunction*
- Left and/or right ventricular failure
- Pulmonary edema
- Shock

D. *Mechanical*
- Rupture: septal, papillary muscle, free wall
- Aneurysm: true, pseudoaneurysm

E. *Ischemic*
- Postinfarction angina
- Infarct extension

F. *Pericardial*
- Early pericarditis
- Late pericarditis (Dressler's syndrome)

G. *Thromboembolic*
- Mural and systemic
- Venous and pulmonary

H. *Miscellaneous*
- Psychosexual dysfunction
- Deconditioning
- Frozen shoulder

GENERAL PRINCIPLES

Patients with proven acute myocardial infarction should be admitted to the hospital. Although home care has been advocated by some, a minimal period of observation of at least 48 hours in a monitored environment would be prudent, even in uncomplicated myocardial infarction. Clinical evaluation alone may fail to identify patients with a relatively high risk of arrhythmia or hemodynamic complications on initial presentation. Cardiac arrhythmias can be extremely difficult to predict and their consequences can be disastrous.

The patient should be made comfortable, the pain controlled, and reassurance given. The patient should be attached to an electrocardiographic monitor. A 12-lead electrocardiogram should be obtained on admission and 24 hours later, as well as an x-ray of the chest and other investigations as defined by individual patient needs. On the assumption that the patient is not considered appropriate for reperfusion therapy (discussed later), specific pharmacologic treatment should be confined to the relief of pain and anxiety unless other symptom complications become manifest. The patient should have complete bedrest for 24 to 48 hours, but he or she then can be mobilized as his or her condition allows. If the patient has truly uncomplicated myocardial infarction, plans for discharge from the hospital may be made on or about the seventh day following the acute event, and in circumstances of great need for facilities, possibly sooner.

SPECIFIC THERAPY

Specific therapy of acute myocardial infarction revolves around preservation of ischemic myocardium and limitation of infarct size as well as treatment of complications.

Limitation of Infarct Size

Intensive investigation has been directed at the development of pharmacologic measures that would limit or "reduce" infarct size (Table 40.6). Because necrosis is by definition a nonreversible state, a more precise statement as to the objective would be to achieve a reduction in the proportion of myocardium in the territory at risk that passes from the ischemic to the necrotic state. Thus, as just stated herein, limitation of infarct size is only possible during the phase of ischemia or mixed pathology during

Table 40.6. Interventions Designed to Limit Infarct Size

1. Reduce cardiac work
   - Beta-adrenergic blocking agents
   - Nitroglycerin and other nitrates
   - Other vasodilators—sodium nitroprusside
   - Calcium channel blocking agents

2. Improve myocardial perfusion
   - Thrombolysis—intracoronary, intravenous
   - Transluminal coronary angioplasty
   - Coronary artery bypass grafting

3. Improve substrate delivery
   - Hyaluronidase
   - Glucose insulin potassium solutions
   - Antiinflammatory agents—steroids, nonsteroidal agents
   - High oxygen mixtures

which ischemic myocardium is progressively recruited to the necrotic pool. However, additional benefits of the proposed pharmacologic interventions include relief of ischemia at a distance, and the effects on contractility, myocardial irritability, and thrombus formation. Such interventions have been directed most frequently toward the objectives of reducing demand by myocardium for metabolic substrate. Two fundamental problems concerning modification (reduction) of tissue oxygen requirements require consideration. The first of these relates to distribution of available blood flow within the myocardium. In severe coronary disease the subendocardial vessels are in a state of maximal metabolically induced vasodilation, whereas subepicardial vessels may still retain vasomotor tone. Ischemic myocardial cells will use available substrate to preferentially maintain membrane integrity and vital mitochondrial and cytosolic reactions at the absolute expense of contraction. Thus, myocardial cells may survive in the ischemic state, receiving as little as perhaps 10% of their ordinary oxygen supply, provided energy is not diverted to the purposes of contraction.

Limitation of infarct size is not possible in the phases of acute myocardial infarction beyond approximately four to eight hours, depending on the availability of collateral blood flow and the completeness or near completeness of the primary occlusive process (Figure 40.9). Although many interventions in the laboratory were believed to have had significant benefit, variability in the temporal relation of treatment to the onset of ischemia (before, at initiation, and 3 to 24 hours later) does not allow for solid conclusions to be reached. Therefore, despite substantive experience in multiple animal models, and the demonstration of infarct limitation by direct tissue studies, clearly favorable responses in clinical situations have been lacking.[35,36] The effects of many such interventions may only be to delay the process by which ischemic tissue proceeds to necrosis rather than reduce its absolute magnitude.

Discrepancies between the findings in experimental studies and clinical experiences are probably related to variables in the clinical situation that are not amenable to precise control. Clinical end points have been difficult to define with precision and to obtain with exactness. It is not possible to relate immediate and late mortality solely and only to the efficacy of a proposed intervention to limit infarct size. Although careful anatomic studies on the magnitude of "territory at risk" and the resulting area of necrosis at differing times following coronary occlusion have been possible in animal models, only secondary (soft) end points have been applicable in man, including the serum levels of CK or its myocardial specific isoenzyme (CK-MB), derived infarct size indexes,[30–32] and the magnitude and alteration of certain elements of the electrocardiogram. Therefore, absolute values of CK-derived infarct size and magnitudes of change in the degree of elevation of the ST segment or T-wave direction and morphology have been used as indicators of relative changes in infarct size. Precise studies on the kinetics of CK in infarction cast doubt on the validity of such conclusions.[33] Although normalization of the ST segment of the electrocardiogram probably indicates a lessening in

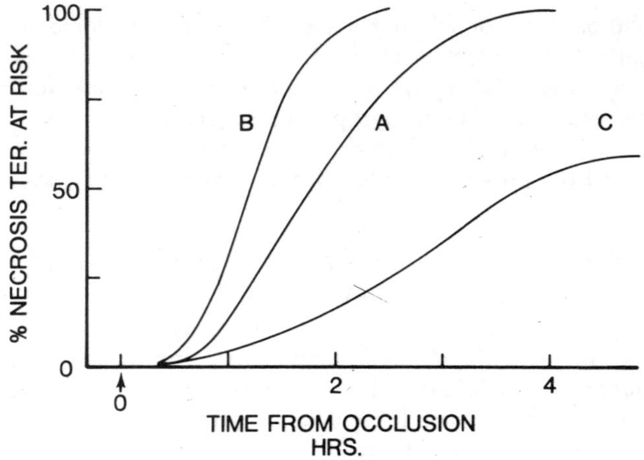

Figure 40.9. Increase in the proportion of myocardium in the area at risk passing to the necrotic state is a function of time. From the onset of complete coronary occlusion and in the absence of substantive collateral flow, necrosis commences at 20 to 30 minutes and progresses to completion in 3 to 5 hours (A). The steepest part of the slope (defining the time of maximal loss of ischemic but still viable tissue) probably lies at approximately 2 hours. The curve to the left (B) indicates a "worse case" situation. This postulates an individual with relatively mild (50 ± % stenosis) coronary artery disease. If such an individual develops an acute thrombus and the area at risk is large, such an individual might be expected to suffer acute cardiac collapse and potentially fatal arrhythmias, and in the absence of preformed collaterals and an adequate perfusion pressure, completed transmural necrosis could potentially develop in 1 to 2 hours. The more favorable case illustrated by the curve to the right (C) defines an individual with preexisting significant coronary disease, continued myocardial ischemia, predeveloped collateral vessels, and a hypertensive response to the acute event. In this situation, preservation of the middle and subepicardial layers of myocardium may be quite prolonged. Occasionally a substantive proportion of myocardium remains viable, and indeed, functional, perfused by collateral vessels alone.

the severity of ischemic damage, it appears imprudent to extrapolate such variables to conclusions regarding limitation of the final extent of necrosis. In man, myocardial perfusion imaging (including technetium uptake) and radionuclide ventriculography have been used in the definition of alterations in perfusion and function in the course of clinical ischemic syndromes and may yet prove useful.

Specific interventions. Several agents have been used in clinical practice to limit infarct size (Table 40.6). Nitrate preparations, particularly nitroglycerin, have been proposed to reduce the role of spasm in the artery of infarction, to increase collateral flow, to increase venous pooling (and thus reduce ventricular volumes and preload), and to achieve a further reduction in arterial blood pressure and in left ventricular wall tension, thereby favorably restoring the apparent transmural imbalance between endocardial and epicardial blood flow so as to provide minimal flow required for myocardial survival. Although several clinical studies have suggested favorable effects, including a reduction in the (sum of) precordial ST-segment elevation, a decrease in left ventricular filling pressures, and a reduction in mortality, the conclusion that such favorable results are related specifically to infarct size limitation cannot be substantiated.

Additional agents for limitation of infarct size include beta-adrenergic blocking agents that may have beneficial effects by their negative inotropic action, reducing myocardial oxygen utilization. Also, heart rate is reduced, diastolic time is increased, and favorable effects on the ST segment and CK release have been reported.

Glucose–insulin–potassium solutions have been used because of their ability to counter the elevation of free fatty acid release during the acute infarction and to provide substrate for anaerobic glycolysis. Corticosteroids and nonsteroidal antiinflammatory agents have been shown to reduce infarct size in the experimental preparation. However, delayed healing associated with many antiinflammatory agents may increase the incidence of myocardial rupture and slow healing of a completed infarct and possibly increase the risk of infarct expansion or rupture.

In summary, concerning infarct size limitation by drugs acting on the cardiovascular system, the conclusion of Rude et al,[35] that "No intervention has yet proved sufficiently efficacious to warrant its routine clinical use" still stands. To limit infarct size, intervention must be applied during the phase of ischemia and mixed pathology. Once necrosis is complete (between three and six hours in most patients, and possibly up to eight hours in a small proportion of cases with preformed collateral vessels or incomplete primary occlusion), it is illogical to anticipate primary salvage of myocardium in the territory at risk. More favorable outcomes may result in some patients from early restoration of coronary blood flow by thrombolysis, angioplasty, or coronary bypass surgery.

Thrombolytic Therapy

As outlined early in this chapter, acute myocardial infarction cannot be regarded as a single pathophysiologic entity.[18] The phase of ischemia is that period during which myocardial salvage may occur as a result of the initiation of reperfusion. The duration of this time window (the interval in which a significant portion of myocardium in the territory at risk remains viable) varies between patients (Figure 40.9). A reasonable ground rule is that in the average patient, perhaps as much as 50% of jeopardized myocardium, particularly in the subepicardial zones of the myocardium, remains viable up to three hours after the onset of continued unrelenting chest pain. However, the proportion of ischemic myocardium at three hours may be smaller or larger and progression to complete necrosis in the territory at risk may be complete in as short a period of two hours or as long as four to six hours. Nevertheless, for revascularization therapies to be intelligently applied, a short time window must be assumed in all cases and therapy initiated as soon as possible after the onset of symptoms. Although many forms of revascularization are available to the physician, including intracoronary thrombolytic therapy,[37] acute angioplasty,[38] and acute myocardial revascularization by direct bypass surgery,[39] the therapy currently available that appears to offer the option of earliest intervention is intravenous streptokinase[40,40a] or urokinase,[40b] and very likely in the future, of tissue plasminogen activator (tPA)[41,41a] or other suitable thrombolytic agents such as prourokinase[41b] and acylated plasminogen streptokinase complex.[41c] The principles of application of this therapy are outlined in chapter 41. Although, in the opinion of the authors, to be broadly effective, thrombolytic agents must be administered intravenously and at the earliest point in time following the onset of symptoms, much has been learned concerning thrombolytic therapy from the published experiences associated with intracoronary administration of either streptokinase or urokinase. Two such examples of this application are shown in Figures 40.10 and 40.11.

Practical Application. It is our current practice[40] to recommend the administration of thrombolytic therapy in patients who present to our hospital within three hours of the onset of the symptom of continued chest pain and in whom diagnostic electrocardiographic changes are found and no contraindications to thrombolytic anticoagulant therapy exist. It is hoped that therapy in the future may possibly be started at an earlier time in the illness (ie, in the home or ambulance) in many patients. We currently do not favor late application of intravenous thrombolytic therapy, because adverse complications may significantly exceed any potential benefit. A history is sought of prior severe hypertension, stroke, bleeding, recent trauma or surgery, bleeding diathesis, or other known contraindications to thrombolytic therapy. Ongoing randomized trials, which include large numbers of patients treated substantively later than this important time window, will probably add more confusion than clarity to this already complex issue.

At the time of diagnosis, 750,000 to 1.5 million units of streptokinase is infused intravenously over an interval of 15 to 30 minutes. Careful observation with electrocardiographic monitoring for the occurrence of reperfusion arrhythmias, frequent measurement of the arterial blood pressure (by indirect means), and the continuous presence of an experienced physician or specifically trained health aide is essential. Infusion is conducted through a vein in the antecubital fossa or one of the extremities. Central catheterization or vascular puncture is avoided. Attainment of reperfusion is judged by indirect clinical criteria, relief of pain, normalization of the ST segment of the electrocardiogram, and relief of symptoms of dyspnea, as well as by the presence of reperfusion arrhythmias, correction of intraventricular or atrioventricular conduction delays if present, and the prompt (15 to 60 minutes) liberation of relatively large quantities of CK-MB enzyme into the systemic blood stream (on retrospective analysis). We generally confirm the patency of infarct-related artery on coronary angiography performed three to five days later.

Reports[42,43] now indicate that early intravenous therapy can result in a high frequency of primary opening of apparently occluded coronary vessels (greater than 80%). Reperfusion arrhythmias are usually self-terminating and

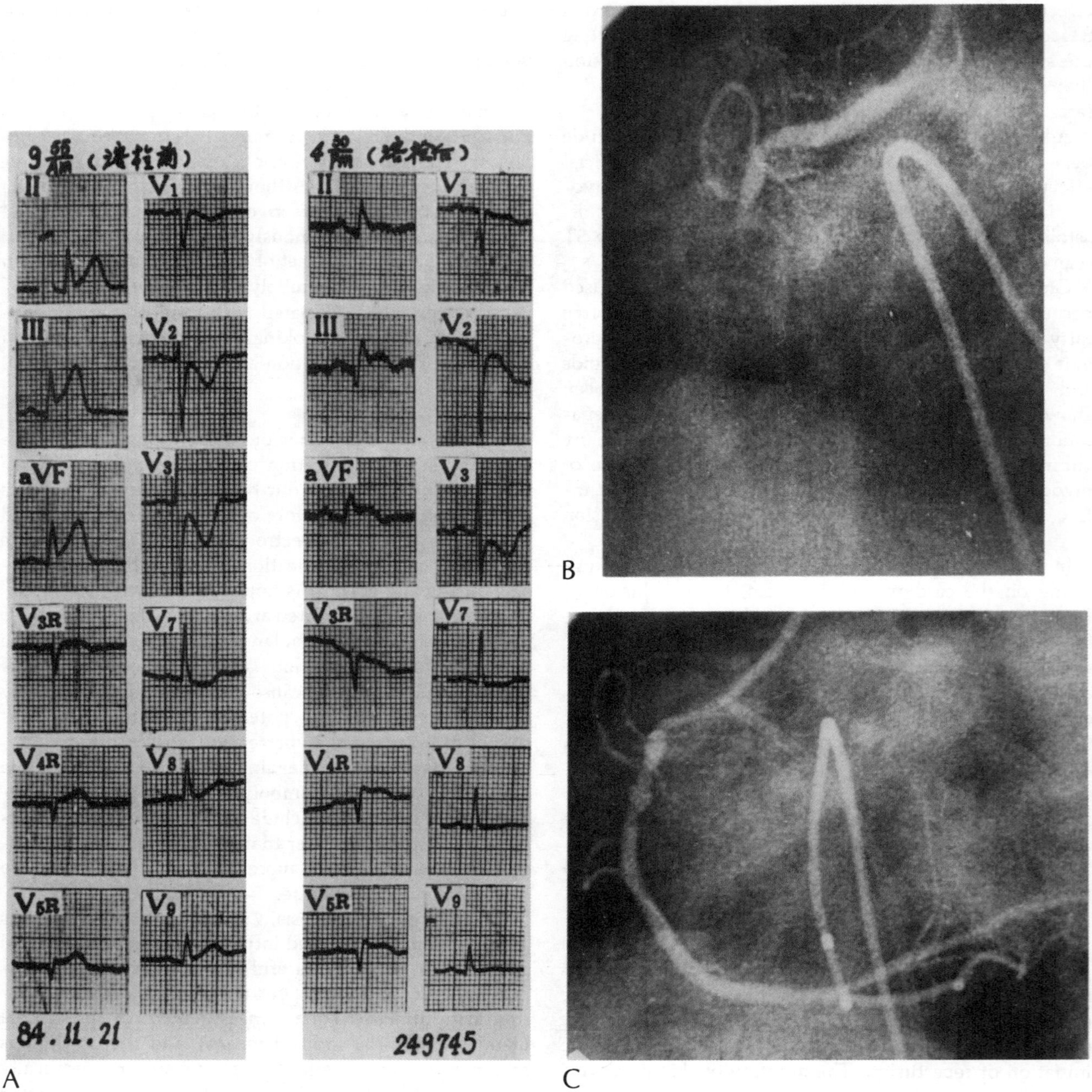

Figure 40.10. The first patient in China treated with intracoronary streptokinase for acute inferior myocardial infarction on November 21, 1984. The patient, a 55-year-old woman, received intracoronary streptokinase 4 hours and 40 minutes after the onset of chest pain. The electrocardiograms before and after streptokinase treatment were shown in *A*. Right coronary arteriogram before thrombolysis (*B*) showed complete proximal obstruction. After streptokinase (*C*) a residual 30% narrowing remained in the middle third of the right coronary artery. The post-streptokinase ECG (right panel in *A*) showed resolution of the marked ST segment elevations in II, III and aVF (left panel in *A*) and no development of pathological Q waves. Elevation of the ST segments in V_{3R} and V_{4R} suggested probable right ventricular involvement. Reperfusion ventricular fibrillation which was successfully treated with defibrillation was the only complication. (Figures 40.10 and 40.11 are courtesy of Dr. S. Q. Tao and Z. J. Chen, Cardiovascular Institute and Fu Wai Hospital, Chinese Academy of Medical Sciences, Peking, China.)

uncommonly require electrocardioversion or antiarrhythmic therapy. Apparent benefits of thrombolytic therapy include early relief of symptoms and a reduction in symptoms with a reduction in the need for narcotics and pain-relieving treatment, preservation of R-wave amplitude on the electrocardiogram and, in some cases, improvement in ventricular function and the size of the perfusion defect on a thallium-201 scintigram, and improvement in perfusion and metabolism on positron emission tomography. Recovery of contractile function of salvaged and virtually nonfunctioning or poorly functioning myocardium may sometimes be delayed by days to weeks despite restoration of coronary patency. We believe that thrombolytic reperfusion, if performed in time, can pre-

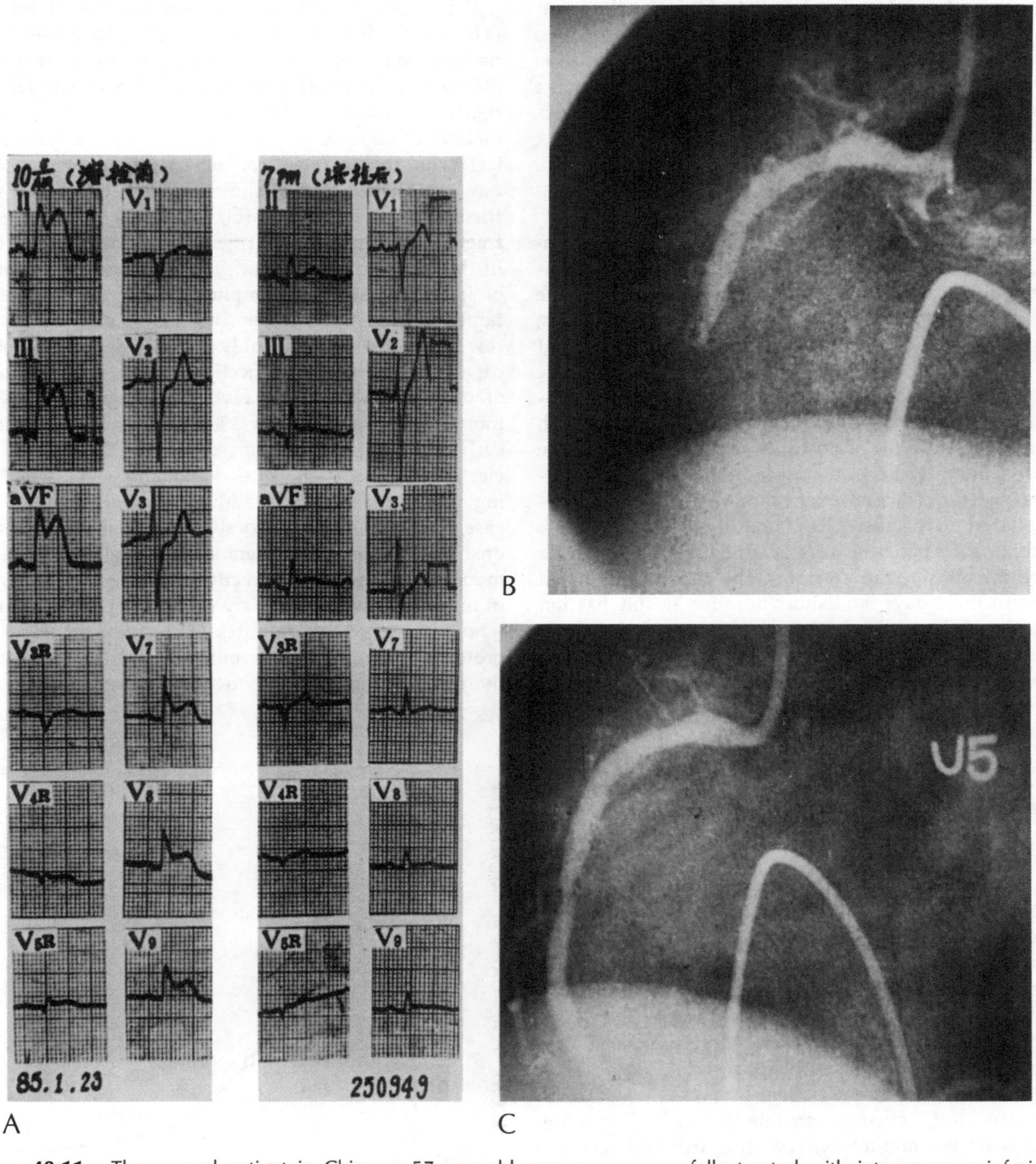

Figure 40.11. The second patient in China, a 57-year-old man, was successfully treated with intracoronary infusion of urokinase for acute inferior myocardial infarction on January 23, 1985. Treatment was started 4 hours and 40 minutes after the onset of chest pain. The electrocardiograms before and after the treatment are shown in *A*. Right coronary arteriogram before treatment (*B*) showed complete obstruction of the mid-portion of the right coronary artery. After urokinase infusion a less than 50% residual stenosis remained (*C*). Limitation of the size of the inferior myocardial infarction was probably achieved as judged from the resolution of the marked ST segment elevations in II, III and aVF with no development of pathological Q waves and normalization of ST segments also in V_{3R}, V_{4R}, V_{5R}, V_7, V_8 and V_9 (*A*). It should be noted that in China the route of administration of thrombolytic agents has also been switched from intracoronary to intravenous with equally impressive results.

vent transmural spread of necrosis, preserving the subepicardial portion of myocardium at risk. Compensatory hypertrophy over the ensuing weeks and months may then occur in some patients, resulting in further restoration of ventricular function.

An important consideration relative to thrombolytic therapy is the state of the residual coronary vessels.[44] Rethrombosis is more common in patients with initially high-grade coronary stenosis.[44a] Restoration of ventricular function appears to be more complete in patients with lesser degrees of residual narrowing or incomplete occlusions. In our experience a significant proportion of patients (up to 35%) require surgical revascularization during the initial hospitalization. In recent months angioplasty, either after or before intracoronary thrombolytic therapy, has been advocated. Whatever the method of therapy, severe obstructive coronary artery disease in patients presenting within the ischemic phase of acute myocardial infarction and treated by thrombolytic therapy cannot be ignored.

MANAGEMENT OF THE CLINICALLY UNCOMPLICATED PATIENT

Uncomplicated myocardial infarction[34] refers to a patient with initially positive diagnostic features for infarction when evaluated 36 to 48 hours following the onset of symptoms, is then pain free without narcotics, has normal vital signs, and has absent S_3 or S_4, absent rales at the lung bases, no radiologic evidence of cardiac enlargement or pulmonary congestion, and no cardiac arrhythmias and conduction abnormalities. Most of such patients have inferior or posterior myocardial infarction; a relative minority have anterior infarctions. The left ventricular ejection fraction may be normal or variably depressed even in the absence of clinically identifiable heart failure. In such patients, electrocardiographic monitoring can be discontinued in 48 hours, the patient ambulated in two to three days, and short-duration hospitalization and early discharge accomplished. However, it is important to recognize that the diagnosis of "completed uncomplicated" myocardial infarction cannot be made before 48 to 72 hours, because many patients require such a time interval "to declare" the relative severity of their illness. Few such patients manifest the late development of heart failure and/or serious cardiac arrhythmias, embolization, or cardiac rupture. A small proportion (5% to 10%) require later reclassification to a "complicated" category because of new ischemia, extension of necrosis, rupture, embolism, or arrhythmias.

If the patient clinically has no complications, ambulation should commence by 48 to 72 hours with walking and preparation for discharge within five to seven days of the acute onset of the illness. This program is suitable only for those with the most favorable short- and intermediate-term prognosis. Therefore, we recommend careful observation of cardiac rhythm to ascertain the absence of arrhythmias during the patient's hospital stay, and a "mini-stress test," raising heart rate by treadmill exercise to 120 beats per minute between the fifth and seventh day following the acute event. If a patient has a normal blood pressure response and is without symptoms and without changes on the electrocardiogram to indicate ischemia, arrhythmias, or conduction abnormalities, his short- and intermediate-term prognosis is generally excellent.[45,46] He should be discharged on the sixth to eighth day, a convalescence at home of approximately one to two weeks is recommended, and early return to work encouraged. Such patients should initially be employed in a manner so as to minimize physical stress levels; in patients in whom this is not possible, return to full-time work should be delayed.

Comprehensive programs of management for patients with uncomplicated acute myocardial infarction require the present establishment of an accurate prognosis by identification of the few patients within this classification who are at higher risk.

We recommend the use of radionuclide scintigraphy (Th-201) to identify abnormalities of perfusion and technetium-99m equilibrium-angiography to determine in quantitative terms the ejection fraction of the left and right ventricles and the location and extent of abnormalities of regional wall motion.[11] Several factors of critical value in the establishment of prognosis have been now established; one of the most important is left ventricular ejection fraction (Figure 40.12).[47] The ejection fraction in a given patient generally is determined early in the course of the illness, in the absence of extension of infarction or other complications. Thus, a value obtained at any time during hospitalization or in the ensuing few weeks gives a reasonably accurate description of the capacity of the ventricle. Ejection fraction values in excess of 0.40 generally have a favorable prognosis: one-year mortality is approximately 3% to 5%. In the presence of early ventricular aneurysm formation[48] with reduced ejection fraction, such values do not apply; yet, after healing and in the absence of additional coronary artery disease, prognosis may be favorable. Additional studies demonstrate that exercise tolerance, a correlate of residual myocardium, correlates directly with long-term prognosis in regard to adverse coronary events. Therefore, patients who can exceed ten minutes of exercise on the Bruce protocol enjoy a favorable outcome. Hence, to establish the prognosis in patients who have apparent uncompli-

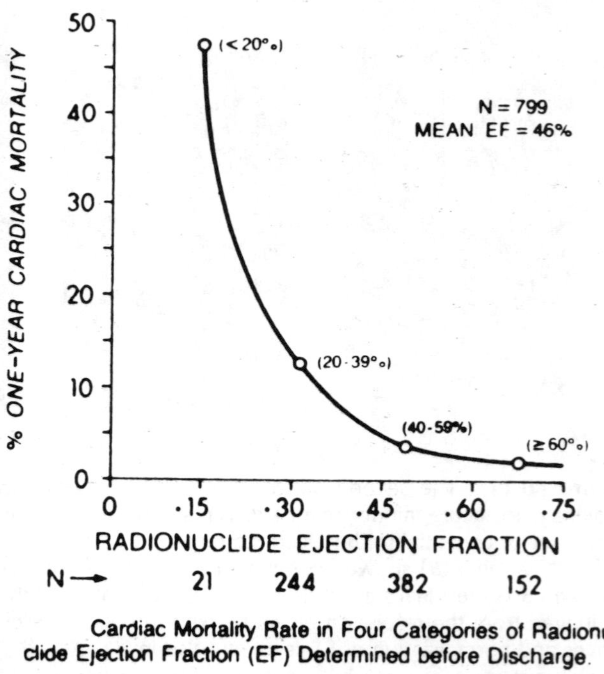

Figure 40.12. Data of the Northeastern Infarct Research Group. Relation of left ventricular ejection value to survival at 20 months. Of a total of 410, 92 patients had myocardial infarction of moderate magnitude. Of patients whose ejection fraction at rest exceeded 0.5, the 20-month survival rate exceeded 96%. Of those patients who had an ejection fraction of less than 0.30, the 20-month survival rate was approximately 70%, and for those with ejection fractions of 0.20 or less, it was 40% to 50%. This demonstrates the significance of myocardial destruction in both short- and long-term outcomes of this clinical syndrome.

cated myocardial infarction, late submaximal exercise testing (four to six weeks), using a formal protocol including at least duration of exercise, heart rate, blood pressure, and electrocardiographic responses, and if possible determination of left ventricular ejection fraction at rest and exercise, should identify those patients with an extremely good prognosis. Such factors would include a duration of exercise of ten minutes or more, a normal blood pressure and heart rate response as related to age, and an ejection fraction at rest in excess of 0.40, increasing by at least 0.05 at peak exercise, without postexercise hypotension or arrhythmias. For such patients, in addition, a prudent life-style with regular physical activity to encourage the concept of "wellness," a return to full-time work, modification in diet so as to maintain adequate weight, abolition of smoking, and control of any tendency to high blood pressure is strongly recommended. In this favorable prognostic group, we do not recommend the routine use of beta blocker drugs other than in the management of hypertension.

MANAGEMENT OF THE COMPLICATED PATIENT

Arrhythmias

This topic is considered in greater detail elsewhere. The common arrhythmias consequent to acute myocardial infarction include supraventricular arrhythmias (premature atrial beats, supraventricular tachycardia, atrial fibrillation, and flutter) and ventricular arrhythmias (ventricular ectopic beats, ventricular tachycardia, and ventricular fibrillation). The specifics of treatment of these arrhythmias are summarized in Table 40.7.

Conduction Abnormalities

Conduction abnormalities due to dysfunction of the AV node occur frequently (15% to 20% cases) in inferior myocardial infarction, ranging from 1° to 2° and 3° AV block. When AV conduction abnormalities occur within the first six to eight hours of acute inferior infarction, they tend to be related to increased vagal tone and hence may respond well to intravenous atropine (1.0 to 2.0 mg). However, AV conduction abnormalities may appear later in the course of inferior infarction, within 24 to 72 hours, tend to progress from 1° to 2° to 3° AV block, rarely respond to atropine, and often require temporary pacing.[49] This delayed AV conduction abnormality may be related to ischemic damage to the AV node rather than to enhanced vagal tone. Temporary pacing is recommended when a persistent slow heart rate due to a high grade AV block is associated with hypotension, heart failure, or escape ventricular arrhythmias. Because AV conduction returns to normal in over 95% of such cases, most often within three to seven days but occasionally as late as two and a half weeks, placement of a permanent pacemaker is seldom necessary.

Intraventricular conduction abnormalities (hemiblock, bundle branch block, Mobitz II block, and complete AV block) tend to occur more often in anterior infarction, are

Table 40.7. Some Drugs Useful in the Management of Arrhythmias

State	Drug	Dose	Adverse Effects	Note
Bradycardia	Atropine	0.5 mg slow IV repeated up to 2 mg	Anticholinergic, tachycardia, paradoxic bradycardia, or AV block	Give if associated with hypotension or use pacing if refractory to drugs
Sinus tachycardia	Propranolol (if no heart failure)	IV 0.5 mg/min up to 0.1 mg/kg	Bradycardia, heart failure, conduction disturbances, bronchospasm	Treat underlying cause, eg, hypovolemia, pain, anxiety, fever, heart failure
Bradycardia, asystolic arrest	Atropine and epinephrine	Epinephrine 0.5 mg slow IV; atropine as above	Tachycardia	Emergency; give at 10-min intervals; infuse isoproterenol; temporary pacemaker insertion
	Isoproterenol	10–60 mg slow IV	Ventricular fibrillation, hypotension	
Ventricular arrhythmias	Lidocaine	IV 50 mg slowly every 5 min to total of 200–300 mg, then infusion of 1–3 mg/min	Few unless heart failure, hepatic failure, > 70 yr	High first-pass metabolism; treat associated causes, eg, electrolyte imbalance, heart failure
Supraventricular arrhythmias	Verapamil	5–10 mg IV	Hypotension, AV block, heart failure	Interactions with digoxin, beta blockers; C^2 may result in hypotension
	Propranolol	IV 0.5–0.75 mg, then orally	As above	
	Digoxin	IV or oral 0.75–1.0 mg; in 24 h; 0.25–0.5 mg/day maintenance	GI symptoms, AV block, ectopy	Best for atrial fibrillation and frank heart failure, elderly, renal function CHF

AV = atrioventricular; CHF = Congestive heart failure; GI = gastrointestinal; IV = intravenous.

often associated with relatively large infarctions with depressed ventricular function, a higher incidence of severe pump failure, and an increased mortality from pump failure or late ventricular fibrillation, especially if conduction abnormalities include bundle branch block or Mobitz II or complete AV block. Temporary pacing is considered for complete AV block, Mobitz II block, and prophylactically in patients with bundle branch block with or without additional fascicular block. Patients with new onset bundle branch block, particularly those with additional hemiblock, have a 20% to 40% risk of development of sudden complete AV block. Some studies have suggested a similar risk for preexisting bundle branch block with supervening acute myocardial infarction as well. The role of permanent pacing in patients who have survived a new transient or persistent bundle branch block or transient high grade AV block, following anterior infarction, is controversial; however, permanent pacing is recommended if high grade AV block persists.

PUMP FAILURE IN ACUTE MYOCARDIAL INFARCTION

Disturbances of contractile function, systolic and diastolic ventricular function, vascular reactivity, and mechanical overload (mitral regurgitation, septal rupture, and cardiac rupture with tamponade) result in changes in ejection fraction, volumes, intracardiac filling pressures, systemic and pulmonary arterial pressures, stroke volume, and cardiac output. Compensatory adjustments may mask the magnitude of dysfunction or they may become clinically manifest. From a pragmatic clinical standpoint it is useful to categorize these patients with pump dysfunction into subsets, which are conceptually useful in understanding the pathophysiology and prognosis and in providing guidelines for therapeutic interventions.

Clinical Subsets

Two commonly used methods of clinical categorization are the Killip[24] and Cedars-Sinai[50] subsets. Although conceptually useful, these classifications require expansion to incorporate pathophysiologic mechanisms. Clinical categorization, although generally consistent with hemodynamic categorization, may show significant discrepancies in 20% to 30% of cases because of "phase lags" between alterations in hemodynamics and the related physical findings, coexistent confounding diseases, and intrinsic physiologic variations due to compensatory adjustments in systolic and diastolic ventricular function.

Hemodynamic Subsets

A frequently used hemodynamic classification is that reported by Forrester et al (Table 40.8, Figure 40.13).[50] Although conceptually useful, providing therapeutic guidelines and strong outcome predictions, it does not incorporate volumetric data relative to either ventricle,[51] function of the right ventricle, or arrhythmias.

A combined clinical and hemodynamic assessment, coupled in selected cases with noninvasive measurement of function, including two-dimensional echocardiography, Doppler flow studies, and radionuclide scintigraphy, can best provide an assessment of presence, severity, and pathophysiologic mechanism of pump dysfunction in acute myocardial infarction.

Hemodynamic Monitoring In Acute Myocardial Infarction. The development in 1970 of the flow-directed, balloon-tipped flotation catheter[52] provided the ability to obtain critical hemodynamic information at the bedside at a sufficiently low risk level to allow for its practical implementation in clinical management of patients with critical illnesses. Balloon flotation catheters are much less stiff than conventional instruments. A balloon, located so as to disperse the forces concentrated on a small tip to a much larger balloon surface, protects the endocardium of the right atrium and right ventricle from stimulation associated with the passage of an unprotected catheter tip across its surface. Such catheters can be inserted at the bedside, in the anesthesia suite, or in the critical care unit with relative ease. The procedures have

Table 40.8. Clinical and Hemodynamic Subsets of Acute Myocardial Infarction

Clinical Subsets

Subset	Pulmonary Congestion	Peripheral Hypoperfusion	Mortality %	Mortality No.	CI	PCP
I	No	No	1	1/75	2.7 ± 0.5	12 ± 7
II	Yes	No	11	4/36	2.3 ± 0.4	23 ± 5
III	No	Yes	18	4/22	1.9 ± 0.4	12 ± 5
IV	Yes	Yes	60	40/67	1.6 ± 0.6	27 ± 8

Hemodynamic Subsets

Subset	PCP > 18 mm Hg	CI <2.2 L/min/m²	Mortality %	Mortality No.
I	No	No	3	2 / 62
II	Yes	No	9	3 / 62
III	No	Yes	23	8 / 35
IV	Yes	Yes	51	36 / 70

CI = cardiac index (L/min/m²); PCP = pulmonary capillary pressure (mm Hg).

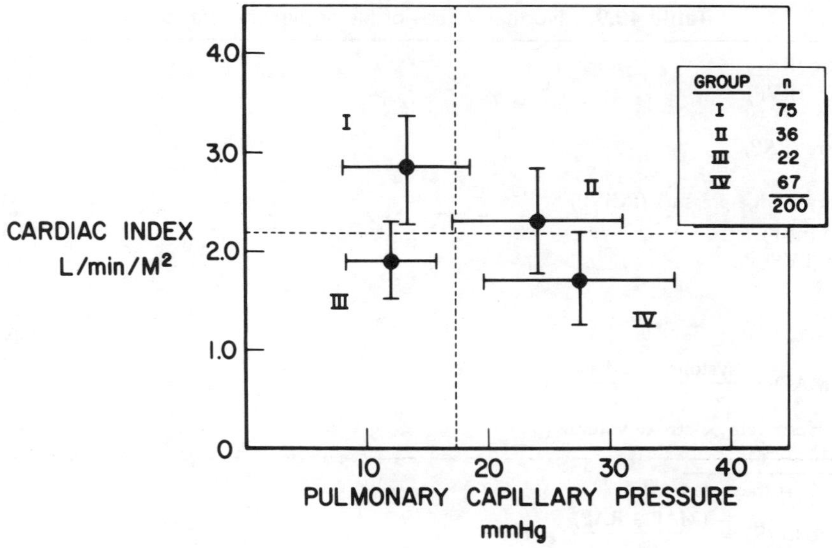

Figure 40.13. Hemodynamic subsets—prognosis and frequency. These data are derived from 200 patients with hemodynamic evaluation in the relatively early course of acute myocardial infarction. Patients were evaluated at an average time of 30 hours after the onset of symptoms. At that time a satisfactory correlation between clinical and hemodynamic evaluation was achieved. In that, 70% of the patients were correctly identified. However, clinical evaluation frequently failed to identify patients with relatively severe elevation in left ventricular filling pressure; on the contrary, patients who had had diuresis and were hemodynamically approaching normal were frequently identified as having severe pulmonary congestion. This is due to the time lag of entry and clearance of fluid into the extravascular pulmonary space. (See text.)

necessary qualities of simplicity and practicality and do not require unusual or specialized levels of skill on the part of participants.

Catheters may be introduced into the vascular system by venous cutdown or percutaneously. The latter is the method of choice. Once the intravenous location of the introduction sheath is confirmed, the flotation catheter is inserted under electrocardiographic and pressure monitoring with fluoroscopic guidance if available. The catheter is advanced into the right atrium, the location of which is denoted by pressure fluctuations coincident with the respiratory cycle. The balloon is then inflated with 1.0 to 1.5 ml of air, and the catheter successively advanced through the right atrium and right ventricle and into the pulmonary artery. Steady advancement allows the recording of the pulmonary artery wedge tracing. Deflation of the balloon requires the catheter to recoil back into a more proximal position in the right, left, or main pulmonary artery. If a further measurement of wedge pressure is required, the balloon is reinflated and allowed to float into the wedge position. In all patients the electrocardiogram and the pressure at the catheter tip are recorded continuously during advancement. It is necessary to obtain a permanent record of pressures within the right-sided intracardiac chambers, and to define the presence and significance of disturbances of cardiac rhythm. Diastolic pulmonary artery pressure may be used to designate wedge pressure if, on initial comparison, these two values approximate closely. In patients with intrinsic pulmonary disease and elevated pulmonary arteriolar resistance, this precludes the use of pulmonary arterial diastolic pressure as a suitable measure of pulmonary wedge pressure, and therefore requires repeated direct measurements of pulmonary wedge pressure by reinflation of the catheter balloon.

Normal values obtained with the balloon flotation catheter are listed in Table 40.9. Thermodilution is the most frequently used technique of cardiac output. When applied with due attention to the specific details of its implementation, the technique is highly reproducible. It is an application of Fick's principle, and a number of small, dedicated, and relatively inexpensive computer devices are available for the incorporation of the transient changes in blood temperature associated with a precisely known quantity of "heat," to allow for calculation of cardiac output. The thermodilution technique is apparently both precise and accurate. In patients who are in a steady state, when the methodology is carefully applied, the total variance appears to be approximately 4%. Directional changes of approximately ± 10% can be estimated accurately with this technique. The measurement of pressures within the right side of the heart are usually good to ± 2 to 3 mm Hg.

Although hemodynamic monitoring can be regarded as a major advance in our ability to assess and care for the critically ill patient, the technique is invasive; therefore, there is a definite, although low, incidence of complications, even in skilled hands.[53] Strict attention to the guidelines presented in Table 40.10 will minimize problems related to inaccurate measurement of data and phys-

Table 40.9. Normal Values of Hemodynamic Variables

Variable	Normal value
Mean right atrial pressure (RAP)	0 to 8 mm Hg
Right ventricular pressure (RVP)	Systolic 20–25 mm Hg Diastolic 4–8 mm Hg
Pulmonary artery pressure (PAP)	Systolic 20–25 mm Hg Diastolic 6–12 mm Hg
Mean pulmonary capillary wedge pressure (PCWP)	6–12 mm Hg
Mean left atrial pressure (LAP)	6–12 mm Hg
Left ventricular pressure (LVP)	Systolic 110–120 mm Hg Diastolic 8–12 mm Hg
Systemic arterial pressure	Systolic 110–120 mm Hg Diastolic 70–80 mm Hg
Mean arterial pressure (MAP) $= \frac{\text{systolic} + 2\ \text{diastolic}}{3}$	
Cardiac output (CO) = Heart rate $\times$ stroke volume (SV)	4–5 L/min
Cardiac index (CI) $= \frac{\text{CO}}{\text{body surface area}}$	2.5–3.5 L/min/m^2
System vascular resistance (SVR) $= \frac{(\text{MAP} - \text{RAP})}{\text{CO}} \times 80$	800–1,200 dynes-s-cm^{-5}
Pulmonary vascular resistance (PVR) $= \frac{\text{mean PAP} - \text{mean PCW}}{\text{CO}} \times 80$	60–100 dynes-s-cm^{-5}
Total pulmonary resistance (TPR) $= \frac{\text{mean PA}}{\text{CO}} \times 80$	200–300 dynes-s-cm^{-5}
Stroke volume (SV) $= \frac{\text{CO}}{\text{HR}}$	55–100 ml/beat
Stroke volume index (SVI) $= \frac{\text{stroke volume}}{\text{BSA}}$	35–45 ml/M^2/beat
Left ventricular stroke work index SWI = (MAP–PCW) $\times$ SVI $\times$ 0.0136	45–75 gm m/M^2/beat

ical complications, which are usually associated with inexperience or failure on the part of the physician or supporting personnel to be aware of the potential for complications. Complications of hemodynamic monitoring are listed in Table 40.11.

Syndrome of Pulmonary Congestion Alone (Forrester II). This syndrome occurs in about 15% to 25% of cases of acute myocardial infarction and is a direct consequence of elevated pulmonary capillary wedge pressure (usually 10 to 25 mm Hg), which in turn is due to an elevated left ventricular end-diastolic pressure. Elevation of left ventricular filling pressure may result predominantly from increased diastolic stiffness in which systolic function (ejection fraction and cardiac output) may be preserved or from systolic dysfunction with left ventricular dilation or both. Mitral regurgitation may also directly contribute to pulmonary capillary hypertension.

These patients have clinical features of pulmonary congestion, ie, basilar pulmonary rales, S_3 gallop, abnormal chest x-ray with pulmonary venous engorgement, and mild hypoxemia. Therapy consists of decreasing pulmonary capillary wedge pressure by slow diuresis using 20 to 40 mg of intravenous furosemide or alternatively afterload and preload reduction with sublingual nitrates (isosorbide dinitrate 2.5 to 10 mg every three to four hours) or nitroglycerin ointment (1 to 2 inches every four to six hours) or in severe cases by using intravenous nitroglycerin or nitroprusside infusion, particularly when mitral regurgitation or hypertension coexist. Hemodynamic monitoring is generally not necessary in most such patients and careful clinical assessment often suffices.

Syndrome of Acute Pulmonary Edema Without Shock. This presentation in 5 to 10% of cases of acute myocardial infarction differs from the syndrome of pulmonary congestion only in the acuteness and severity of clinical manifestations, the degree of pulmonary congestion, and/or transient or persistent mitral regurgitation. There is rapid and marked elevation of pulmonary capillary wedge pressure, resulting in transudation of fluid at rates overwhelming the ability of lymphatic clearance. The pulmonary capillary wedge pressure generally exceeds 25 mm Hg.

This acute syndrome requires intensive therapy with immediate attention to: (1) maintenance of adequate gas exchange by providing supplemental oxygen through a face mask and, if necessary, endotracheal intubation; mechanical ventilation (positive pressure) should be considered if the patient is moribund or has refractory hypoxemia or progressive hypercarbia with a falling pH; (2) immediate restoration of sinus rhythm if persistent supraventricular or ventricular tachyarrhythmias are present; electrocardioversion is indicated; (3) rapid reduction of pulmonary capillary wedge pressure by administration of sublingual nitroglycerin or buccal application of 0.25 to 0.5 inch of 2% nitroglycerin ointment. In resistant cases, intravenous nitroglycerin or nitroprusside may be necessary. Morphine sulfate, 2 to 4 mg, given intravenously is generally used to calm the patient and possibly

Table 40.10. Practical Guidelines for Optimal Data Acquisition

1. Measurement of pressures
   a. Transducer dome, pressure tubing, manifolds, stopcocks, and catheter lumen free of air bubbles or blood clot; no kinks in the catheter or pressure tubing
   b. Transducer, the oscilloscope, and paper recorder calibrated against a mercury manometer. Calibrations repeated 3 to 4 times in a 24-hour period.
   c. Pressure transducer must be placed at the predefined "0" level* and calibration signal should be checked
   d. Immediately before measuring a pressure, "0" level and calibration rechecked
   e. Pressures measured at end-expiration regardless of spontaneous or artificial ventilation
   f. When catheter-whip and ringing artifact are superimposed, pressure waveforms should be recorded on paper and measurements made, eliminating artifactual components

2. Cardiac output determination
   a. Catheter tip should be in a proximal pulmonary artery; right atrial lumen must be in the right atrium before injectate is rejected
   b. Injectate and body temperature should be accurately determined (current models of catheter and computers automatically obtain their values from thermisters)
   c. A constant and accurate volume of injectate (5 to 10 ml)
   d. For good reproducibility, iced injectate (3°C to 5°C) volumes of 5 or 10 ml; room temperature injectate (21°C to 23°C) volumes should be 10 ml
   e. No more than 3 to 4 seconds should be allowed to elapse between the time the syringe bearing the injectate is taken out of a sterile bath, connected to the right atrial post of the Swan–Ganz catheter, and injection made with a smooth, firm, and rapid unhesitating stroke.
   f. Consecutive injections should be made in the same phase of spontaneous or artificial respiration
   g. In general, three consecutive cardiac output values differing by less than 10% are recorded and averaged
   h. The calibration constant on the computer must be adjusted according to the type, temperature, and volume of injectate
   i. Whenever unexpected or widely variable values are obtained, check catheter tip location, right atrial port location, cable and computer system, and the quality of thermodilution curve for inaccuracies.

* Usually one half the distance of anterior sternum to posterior spinal process at the approximate level of the orifice of the tricuspid valve.

produce mild vasodilation. Intravenous diuretics, while effective, may take up to 20 to 30 minutes to act and should be used to supplement the beneficial effects of nitrates. Routine digitalization, aminophylline, or intermittent positive pressure breathing is rarely helpful and best avoided. Nitrates and other vasodilators have rendered tourniquets and phlebotomy generally unnecessary.

After the patient's condition is stabilized, complete assessment of the causative factors is required. If severe mitral regurgitation (intermittent or persistent), septal perforation, or recurrent ischemia is discovered, early cardiac catheterization followed by appropriate surgery is the only effective therapy. Stabilization may be improved by intraaortic balloon counterpulsation.

Syndrome of Low Output State or Shock with Pulmonary Congestion or Edema (Forrester IV). This syndrome reflects a further and most severe stage in the spectrum of pump dysfunction; in addition to pulmonary congestion and edema, the patient exhibits evidence of a persistent low cardiac output state. Clinically there is hypotension (systolic pressure less than 90 mm Hg), mental obtundation, cool clammy skin, thready rapid pulse, hypoxemia, and, in severe cases, metabolic (lactic) acidosis and hypothermia. Hemodynamic monitoring and correction of gas exchange abnormalities, associated arrhythmias or bradycardias, and electrolyte and acid-base abnormalities are essential. Specific measures include raising tissue perfusion by improving cardiac output. A minimal arterial pressure of 90 to 100 mm Hg, while relieving pulmonary congestion by reducing left ventricular filling pressure, is necessary.[54]

Hemodynamic evaluation shows a severely depressed cardiac index (1.8 L/min/m^2 or less), elevated systemic vascular resistance (greater than 2,000 dynes-s-cm^{-5}), a widened arteriovenous oxygen difference, a severely depressed stroke work index (less than 20 gm m/m^2), and elevated pulmonary arterial and wedge pressure. Heart rate is increased (greater than 100 beats per minute) whereas systolic blood pressure is generally 90 mm Hg or less. These are the clinical features of "cardiogenic shock." In the absence of severe mitral regurgitation or ventricular septal rupture, left ventricular function is severely depressed, with 35% or more of the myocardium nonfunctional due to recent infarction or a combination of recent and old infarction. The outlook for survival is poor (80% to 100% mortality) regardless of therapy with three possible exceptions, ie, cases in which this syndrome

Table 40.11. Complications Associated With Invasive Hemodynamic Monitoring

I. Pulmonary artery catheterization
   A. Associated with vein cannulation
      1. Bleeding and hematoma
      2. Local infection and systemic sepsis
      3. Inadvertent arterial puncture
      4. Pneumothorax (subclavian and jugular routes)
      5. Injury to thoracic duct (left internal jugular and subclavian routes)
      6. Transient hoarseness of voice
      7. Air or clot embolism
   B. Associated with catheter passage and placement
      1. Extravascular placement of catheter (intrapleural space, mediastinum)
      2. Thrombosis or phlebitis of vein
      3. Atrial and ventricular arrhythmias
      4. Transient right bundle branch block or complete heart block in patients with preexisting left bundle branch block
      5. Pulmonary embolism and infarction
      6. Pulmonary arterial rupture, bronchopulmonary fistula
      7. Tricuspid and pulmonary valve damage with sterile or infective endocarditis
      8. Coiling and knot formation
      9. Rupture of balloon
   C. Misinterpretation or inaccurate measurement of data
      1. Missed diagnosis or inappropriate diagnosis
      2. Inappropriate therapy
II. Arterial cannulation
   1. Local bleeding, hematoma, false aneurysm
   2. Arterial dissection, spasm, thrombosis, and vascular insufficiency
   3. Local and systemic sepsis
   4. Retrograde cerebral embolization from vigorous flushing

results from severe mitral regurgitation or ventricular septal rupture, or early in the phase of "mixed pathology," in which a considerable proportion of nonfunctioning myocardium is ischemic but still viable. In the latter case, normal function may be restored by early revascularization using nonsurgical (thrombolysis or percutaneous transluminal coronary angioplasty) or surgical techniques. This last group of patients can be identified if shock occurs immediately or soon after the onset of infarction (within one to two hours), and is accompanied by evidence of recurrent or persistent extensive ischemia.

In the first two categories, early cardiac catheterization and surgery can permit a 60% to 70% salvage rate.[55] Intraaortic balloon pumping can be used for stabilization in these patients in preparation for invasive diagnostic testing and throughout surgery to follow.[56]

PHARMACOLOGIC AGENTS USEFUL IN IMPROVING PUMP FUNCTION

Three classes of drugs of value are inotropic agents, peripheral vasodilators, and diuretics.

Inotropic Drugs

The immediate objective of management in cardiogenic shock is to improve cardiac output and to maintain systemic arterial pressure between 90 and 100 mm Hg.

Although the beneficial effects of digitalis, on ventricular performance are well known, acute digitalization is ineffective or only marginally effective in severe pump failure following acute myocardial infarction.[57] Furthermore, acutely ischemic myocardium may be more sensitive to the arrhythmogenic effects of digitalis, and the peripheral vasoconstrictor effects of rapid intravenous administration of digitalis could have deleterious consequences. Therefore, digitalis is of limited use in cardiogenic shock. However, it is of unquestioned value in the management of atrial arrhythmias, such as atrial fibrillation and flutter, complicating myocardial infarction, which should be its main indication in this setting. Whether digoxin therapy in general after myocardial infarction increases mortality remains a controversy. Although reports from three large observational studies of patients after myocardial infarction[57a,57b,57c] seemed to indicate that the mortality rate in digoxin-treated patients was higher than those who did not receive digoxin, the recent findings in the Multicenter Investigation of Limitation of Infarct Size (MILIS) population[57d] failed to support this assertion.

Sympathomimetic inotropic vasoactive agents, most frequently dopamine and dobutamine and occasionally norepinephrine, are used in cardiogenic shock.[54] Isoproterenol is practically never used in this setting.

Dopamine stimulates beta and dopaminergic receptors and also causes release of endogenous norepinephrine from sympathetic nerve endings.[58] At relatively small doses of 2 to 5 μg/kg per minute, $beta_1$-adrenergic–stimulant effects on myocardial contractility are observed to result in improved cardiac output. In addition, increases occur in renal blood flow with redistribution towards the inner third of the cortex, an effect mediated by interaction with dopaminergic-specific receptors. At this dosage, chronotropic and peripheral vasoconstrictor effects are minimal and worsening of myocardial ischemia generally does not occur. With progressively larger doses, there is a greater chronotropic–arrhythmogenic effect, alpha-adrenergically mediated vasoconstrictor and vasopressor actions that may decrease tissue-perfusion and increase pulmonary arterial and left ventricular filling pressures secondary to elevated afterload. At large doses (greater than 15 to 20 μg/kg per minute) myocardial ischemia may actually be provoked when increments in myocardial oxygen consumption due to inotropic, chronotropic, and vasopressor effects exceed any beneficial effects of increased coronary blood flow secondary to direct coronary dilator or arterial pressor effects.

The use of intravenous dopamine infusion in "cardiogenic shock" requires extremely careful titration of dosage, which must be individualized beginning from a small dose (2 to 5 μg/kg per minute), to improve cardiac output and renal and other organ perfusion, while maintaining a systolic blood pressure of 90 to 100 mm Hg. Excessive increases in heart rate (greater than 110 to 115 beats per minute), supraventricular or ventricular arrhythmias, or excessive peripheral vasoconstriction can result and should be avoided. Because of marked individual variations in dose response, it is crucial to use the smallest dose that produces optimal hemodynamic and clinical improvement with the least side effects. Other adverse effects include precipitation or worsening of myocardial ischemia, local gangrene especially when extravascular extravasation occurs, nausea and vomiting, and facilitation of AV conduction in the presence of supraventricular arrhythmias.

Dobutamine is a synthetic sympathomimetic amine that has predominantly beta-adrenergic agonist actions, accounting for its positive inotropic and chronotropic effects, with only minimal alpha-adrenergic agonist effects, accounting for its lack of vasoconstrictor effects even at large doses.[59] Dobutamine does not release endogenous norepinephrine and has no direct renal vasodilator effects. Dose-related increases in stroke volume and cardiac output and reduction in left ventricular filling pressures are notable in acute as well as chronic heart failure with important increases in heart rate being uncommonly observed at infusion rates under 15 to 20 μg/kg per minute.

Dobutamine is preferred over dopamine because it produces equivalent increases in cardiac output but a greater reduction in left ventricular filling pressure and no vasoconstrictor effects. In general, it tends to produce lesser increases in heart rate and arrhythmias compared with dopamine. Also compared with dopamine, dobutamine has weaker pressor effects, making it less useful when systemic blood pressure is very low, ie, less than 70 mm Hg. The dobutamine infusion should begin with a small dose (2 to 5 μg/kg per minute) with rapid titration under careful clinical, electrocardiographic, and hemodynamic monitoring until the cardiac output and clinical status of the patient improve without excessive increases in heart rate, emergence of serious or frequent arrhythmias, or myocardial ischemia. Other adverse effects include nausea, headache, and acceleration of AV conduction in the presence of supraventricular arrhythmias.

Norepinephrine is a naturally occurring catecholamine with potent peripheral vasoconstrictor effects mediated through alpha-adrenergic receptor stimulation.[60] Norepinephrine has weaker $beta_1$-adrenergically mediated myocardial inotropic and chronotropic effects. The profound peripheral vasoconstrictor effects of norepinephrine make it an effective pressor agent with much less overall positive chronotropic or arrhythmogenic effects.[61] Although such effects may be a distinct advantage in terms of maintenance of adequate arterial pressure in severely hypotensive patients, increases in arterial pressure are achieved at the expense of intense peripheral vasoconstriction, with little increase in cardiac output and further compromise of peripheral organ blood flow. However, in a few patients with cardiogenic shock in whom systemic arterial pressure is low (70 mm Hg or less) and pressor doses of dopamine produce tachyarrhythmias, small doses of norepinephrine may be used to maintain systemic arterial pressure at around 90 mm Hg systolic. At small doses, mild inotropic effects of norepinephrine may produce a modest improvement in cardiac output in some patients. The combined use of norepinephrine with an alpha-adrenergic blocking drug, such as phentolamine, or a direct vasodilator, such as nitroglycerin or sodium nitroprusside, may minimize peripheral vasoconstrictor effects and help unmask positive inotropic effects. Norepinephrine infusion should begin with a small dose (1 to 4 μg/min) with titration to optimal clinical and hemodynamic effects. Adverse effects include excessive peripheral vasoconstriction and compromise of organ blood flow, worsening of ventricular function caused by increased afterload, and tissue necrosis and sloughing if extravascular extravasation occurs. In some patients, an excessive increase in blood pressure may produce a slowing of heart rate through baroreceptor-mediated reflex increase in vagal tone.

Vasodilators

The rationale for the use of vasodilators in cardiogenic shock and heart failure rests on their ability to reduce ventricular afterload by dilating the systemic arteriolar bed and to reduce ventricular preload by dilating the peripheral venous bed.[62] Reduction in ventricular afterload decreases impedance to left ventricular ejection, which enhances forward ejection, thereby increasing cardiac output (Figure 40.14). Decreased impedance to ejection into the aorta is particularly helpful in reducing the degree of regurgitation and left–to–right shunt in the presence of mitral regurgitation and ventricular septal rupture, respectively. Preload reduction contributes to the reduction in ventricular filling pressures. Reduced afterload and preload also tend to decrease myocardial oxygen demand and may favor redistribution of perfusion to the subendocardium during diastole, thereby producing a favorable oxygen demand and supply relation in ischemic myocardium. Vasodilators may also shift the left ven-

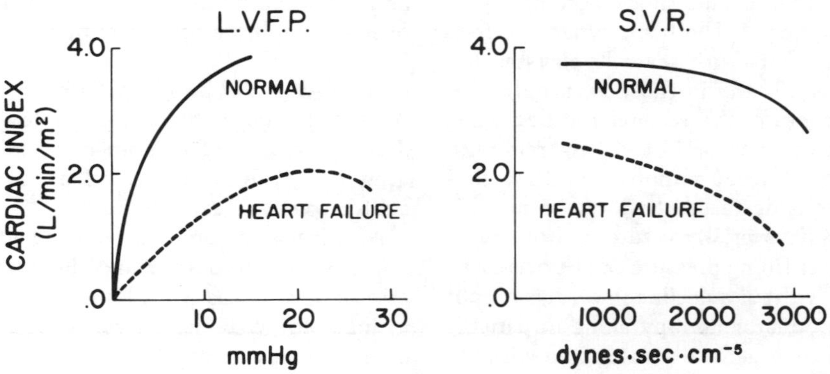

Figure 40.14. Relation of cardiac index to preload and afterload. Cardiac index (L/min/m^2) is defined on the vertical axis. In the *left panel* is shown the relation to left ventricular filling pressure (in mm Hg) and in the *right panel*, to systemic vascular resistance (in dynes-s-cm^{-5}). *Solid lines* indicate the relation of heart with normal contractile capabilities. *Broken line* indicates patients with heart failure from virtually any cause. It is critical to maintain cardiac index as close to 2 L/min/m^2 as possible. Inadequacy of tissue perfusion and the development of cardiogenic shock occurs if cardiac index is maintained below 1.7 L/min/m^2 for any significant period of time. *Left panel* indicates that it is necessary in the patient with heart failure to maintain a left ventricular filling pressure between 15 and 20 mm Hg. Although the normal heart is relatively sensitive to filling pressure changes, adequate cardiac index is maintained at virtually all left ventricular filling pressures down to approximately 4 mm Hg. In the *right panel*, and for a left ventricular filling pressure of between 5 and 10 mm Hg, cardiac index is maintained normally until systemic vascular resistance is greatly increased. Compensatory mechanisms include increase in left ventricular filling pressure. In the heart failure patient, however, an important reduction of cardiac index is seen in the presence of elevated (> 2,000) systemic vascular resistance. Drugs may be used to manipulate systemic vascular resistance to values in the range of 1,000 with a left ventricular filling pressure maintained at approximately 15 to 20 mm Hg. This will then result in a cardiac index that may be optimal for the contractile state of the given heart.

tricular diastolic pressure–volume relation to the right and decrease the filling pressures at a given end-diastolic volume.[63] Excessive hypotension that may compromise myocardial blood flow, particularly through coronary arteries with severe flow-limiting stenosis, remains a complication of vasodilator use. Therefore, decreases in coronary blood flow coupled with reflex tachycardia provoked by hypotension could be deleterious on the oxygen supply–demand relation in ischemic myocardium. Hypotension may also compromise perfusion to other organs such as the brain and kidney. Excessive reduction in left ventricular filling pressures or the use of vasodilators in patients with low or normal filling pressures predispose to hypotension and tachycardia because of a reduced cardiac output. These considerations demand caution and care in the use of vasodilators in critically ill patients and make frequent clinical and hemodynamic evaluation essential. The effects of vasodilator therapy on the outcome in patients with established cardiogenic shock have never been examined in properly controlled studies, although Chatterjee et al[64] reported favorable short-term survival of about 44% in a small number of patients with severe pump failure; however, long-term survival was poor and most survivors continued to have severe heart failure, even in the short term.

Intravenous Vasodilators. *Sodium nitroprusside* infusion produces prompt arteriolar and venular dilation that results in hemodynamic and short-term clinical improvement in severe heart failure and shock accompanying acute myocardial infarction.[65] The hemodynamic effects are more marked in patients with severely elevated left ventricular filling pressures and in those with mitral regurgitation or septal rupture. We recommend beginning therapy at a low-dose infusion of 10 to 20 μg/min with upward titration every 10 to 20 minutes until left ventricular filling pressure is decreased to 15 to 18 mm Hg without allowing systolic arterial pressure to drop below 90 mm Hg. In some cases filling pressure can be decreased to more normal levels without a decline in cardiac output or blood pressure. Vasodilator therapy alone in patients with severe power failure is generally associated with the possible risk of unacceptable arterial hypotension unless combined with an inotropic drug (dopamine or dobutamine) or mechanical circulatory assist with intraaortic balloon counterpulsation.

The adverse effects of nitroprusside therapy include excessive hypotension, reflex tachycardia, possible worsening of myocardial ischemia, accumulation of cyanide, thiocyanate, and toxicity (particularly in renal insufficiency and with prolonged infusions), and worsening of arterial hypoxemia due to increased intrapulmonary ventilation/perfusion mismatch. Limiting the dose and duration of therapy, frequent monitoring of serum thiocyanate levels to avoid exceeding levels of 6 mg%, and the prophylactic use of the cyanide-chelating agent hydroxycobalamin to avoid cyanide toxicity have been recommended.

Intravenous nitroglycerin is a rapidly acting agent that causes a greater reduction in ventricular filling pressures with only modest increases in stroke volume and cardiac output in patients with severe left ventricular failure.[66] These differential effects have been attributed to relatively greater venodilation compared with arteriolar dilation, but significant arteriolar dilation may be observed with increasing doses. Nitroglycerin has been suggested as having more favorable effects on the intramyocardial distribution of coronary blood flow to ischemic myocardium than nitroprusside, but comparative studies in cardiogenic shock have not been performed. Nitroglycerin can produce adverse effects such as hypotension with reflex tachycardia, headaches from cerebral vasodilation and possibly increased intracranial tension, increased intraocular pressure in patients with glaucoma, methemoglobinemia, Wernicke's encephalopathy, and ethanol intoxication (ethanol is the vehicle for many intravenous preparations). Rarely, hypotension and paradoxic profound bradycardia may occur, which generally respond to atropine administration and cessation of nitroglycerin therapy. The safe use of intravenous nitroglycerin in cardiogenic shock may require concomitant use of an inotropic drug (dopamine or dobutamine) or intraaortic balloon counterpulsation to sustain or elevate a low systemic arterial pressure.

Phentolamine not only is a nonselective alpha-adrenergic blocking agent but also has direct smooth muscle relaxant and mild direct inotropic and chronotropic effects as well. In comparison with nitroprusside and nitroglycerin, it produces a relatively greater increase in heart rate and a lesser decrease in filling pressures.[67] It is generally not used except in combination with norepinephrine infusion and to minimize the effects of extravascular extravasation of norepinephrine or dopamine.

Combined Vasodilator and Catecholamine Therapy

Several studies have demonstrated the superior hemodynamic effects of combined vasodilator and inotropic drug therapy in chronic as well as acute low-output states and congestive heart failure.[68]

Afterload- and preload-reducing effects of vasodilators improve cardiac output and decrease ventricular filling pressures, whereas the addition of inotropic drugs helps to maintain systemic arterial pressure. Therefore, combined therapy may offset each drug's adverse effects while augmenting overall ventricular function. The vasodilators frequently used for this purpose are alpha-adrenergic blocking drugs, including phentolamine, and direct vasodilators, including nitroglycerin and sodium nitroprusside. The principal advantage of combining vasodilators and dopamine or dobutamine is that increments in cardiac output are achieved at a lower left ventricular filling pressure and systemic vascular resistance than is possible with inotropic drugs alone. The combined use of dopamine and dobutamine has also been suggested in the treatment of cardiogenic shock as a means of achieving a more favorable acute hemodynamic response at smaller doses.

INTRAAORTIC BALLOON COUNTERPULSATION

Intraaortic balloon pumping is the most commonly used mechanical circulatory assist device in the management of cardiogenic shock.[69] The recent development of a percutaneous insertion technique has made it easier to initiate balloon counterpulsation in a relatively short time.

Balloon counterpulsation decreases left ventricular work and oxygen demand because of its systolic afterload-reducing effect, while the increased diastolic aortic pressure helps to maintain or improve coronary perfusion pressure and subendocardial blood flow. Combined systolic unloading and diastolic augmentation tend to reduce myocardial ischemia, left ventricular filling pressures, mitral regurgitation, and left-to-right shunt across a ventricular septal rupture, while the forward stroke volume and cardiac output may show a modest improvement.

Although patients in cardiogenic shock frequently demonstrate temporary clinical and hemodynamic improvement during intraaortic balloon counterpulsation, short- and long-term mortality remains unchanged[69] unless intraaortic balloon pumping is used for short-term stabilization of the patient in preparation for salvage of still viable ischemic myocardium by coronary revascularization or correction of severe mechanical complications, ie, mitral regurgitation and ventricular septal rupture (to be discussed in more detail in the chapter). Therefore, every attempt should be made to determine the presence of surgically remediable lesions as described earlier, using noninvasive and invasive techniques. We recommend diagnostic cardiac catheterization, usually within 12 to 36 hours of the onset of balloon counterpulsation with surgical intervention for suitable patients. Those patients who are unsuitable for surgery or in whom surgery must be delayed because of intercurrent complications should be weaned if possible from balloon counterpulsation after a period of stabilization of two to four days.

Intraaortic balloon counterpulsation should not be considered a benign procedure, because complications may occur in up to 30% of patients. These complications are mostly vascular, ie, compromise of extremities and abdominal viscera, damage to the femoral artery, and aortic dissection, but also include infection, hemolysis, thrombocytopenia, gas leak, and embolism. Complications are particularly likely in older individuals, particularly older women and those with aortoiliac vascular disease.

EARLY REPERFUSION

Because ventriculopenic shock results from large areas of nonfunctioning left ventricular myocardium, early reperfusion during the "mixed pathology" phase of myocardial infarction, when substantial amounts of nonfunctioning myocardium is still viable, may be the most rational and effective therapy in preventing the otherwise hopeless outcome of cardiogenic shock.[70] Such early reperfusion can restore contractile function of a portion of the myocardium in the area at risk immediately or in a more delayed fashion, render reperfused myocardium more responsive to inotropic agents, and preserve ventricular function. Preliminary reports of thrombolytic therapy, percutaneous transluminal coronary angioplasty, or both in selected patients with cardiogenic shock are encouraging in this regard.

CARDIAC SURGERY

Cardiac surgery may improve the long-term survival of selected patients with shock following acute myocardial infarction.[71] These patients may benefit from coronary revascularization and/or corrective repair of a potentially lethal mechanical complication, ie, severe mitral regurgitation, ventricular septal perforation, or subacute free-wall rupture. Survival rates of 50% to 75% may be achieved with this approach in properly selected cases.

MECHANICAL COMPLICATIONS OF ACUTE MYOCARDIAL INFARCTION

Acute Mitral Regurgitation

Acute mitral regurgitation in acute myocardial infarction may result from papillary muscle ischemia and dysfunction or rupture.

Papillary Muscle Dysfunction

Ischemia, infarction, or rupture of the posteromedial papillary muscle is five to ten times more common than that of anterolateral papillary muscle, possibly because of a more inconsistent and tenuous blood supply coming predominantly from a single artery.

Papillary muscle ischemia or infarction is rarely sufficient to result in mitral regurgitation, unless there is deranged contractile function of the left ventricular myocardium contiguous to the base of the papillary muscle. Mitral regurgitation resulting from papillary muscle dysfunction occurs when papillary muscle contraction fails or occurs along an abnormal axis, shifted inappropriately by coexistent ventricular dilatation and dyssenergy, resulting in failure of the mitral leaflets to coapt appropriately in systole.[72,72a]

Papillary muscle dysfunction complicating acute myocardial infarction causes intermittent or persistent mitral regurgitation demonstrated either by auscultation of a systolic apical murmur of variable intensity, duration, pitch, and radiation, by hemodynamic signs of disproportionately large V waves on pulmonary capillary wedge pressure, or by left ventricular angiography.[72a] However, the murmur may be nondescript, soft or loud; high- or low-pitched; holosystolic or midsystolic; or even completely absent (silent)[73] despite severe mitral regurgitation. Depending on the severity of left ventricular dysfunction and the degree of acute mitral regurgitation, clinical evidence of persistent or intermittent pulmonary congestion, pulmonary edema, hypotension, or a shock state may develop. Recognition of severe mitral regurgitation, persistent or intermittent, requires a high index of clinical suspicion and is aided by bedside Swan–Ganz right heart catheterization. Echocardiography coupled with Doppler flow study may be extremely valuable in making the correct diagnosis.[74] Such patients should be subjected to prompt cardiac catheterization followed by cardiac surgery. In preparation for cardiac catheterization and surgery, the condition of a severely symptomatic patient requires stabilization with pharmacologic unloading with intravenous vasodilators or with mechanical circulatory assist using intraaortic balloon pumping.

Papillary Muscle Rupture

Rupture of the left ventricular papillary muscle (commonly the tip of the posterior papillary muscle) occurs in less than 1% of all infarcts but accounts for 5% of infarcts resulting in death.[75] Papillary muscle rupture tends to occur between two and seven days after infarction, but as many as 20% of cases may occur within 24 hours of the onset of infarction. Most ruptures occur as a complication of inferior or posterior infarction resulting from occlusive disease of the right or circumflex coronary artery. Nearly 50% of patients demonstrate relatively small or subendocardial infarction. Similarly, the extent of coronary artery disease may be mild, with up to 50% of patients having single-vessel disease.

The clinical presentation is dominated by the sudden appearance of a systolic murmur not previously recognized, severe pulmonary congestion, and pulmonary edema; hypotension is frequent, and many patients rapidly progress to shock. The systolic murmur may be early and short in duration (due to rapid equilibration of left atrial and left ventricular pressures in late systole), nondescript, and even completely absent (silent mitral regurgitation) in some patients. The severe respiratory distress and adventitious pulmonary sounds caused by pulmonary edema may make a murmur difficult to hear, even when present. A palpable thrill is rare in papillary muscle rupture. The chest x-ray shows pulmonary congestion or edema, which may be preferentially distributed to the upper lobes of the lungs simulating pulmonary infiltrates. This preferential location may be consequent to the mitral regurgitant jet being directed toward the orifice of the upper lobe pulmonary veins. The left ventricular ejection fraction is often normal or increased because of the limited extent of myocardial necrosis and ventricular unloading in severe mitral regurgitation. The right ventricular ejection fraction may be depressed because of associated acute pulmonary arterial hypertension or coexistent right ventricular ischemic damage.

The diagnosis can be made noninvasively with two-dimensional echocardiography, in the appropriate clinical context. A flail mitral leaflet and hyperdynamic left ventricular wall motion can be demonstrated.[74] When Doppler measurements are employed, the presence and severity of mitral regurgitation can be estimated at the bedside. Hemodynamic evaluation shows elevated pulmonary capillary wedge pressure with tall "V" waves, which may be reflected in the pulmonary arterial pressure. Papillary muscle rupture can be differentiated from ventricular septal rupture by two-dimensional echocardiography, the presence of a palpable thrill (present in 50% of cases of septal rupture but seldom, if ever, in papillary muscle rupture) and right heart catheterization data.

The prognosis is uniformly poor, with a 50% mortality within 24 hours and 94% mortality within eight weeks. Early surgical correction of the mitral leak by valve replacement or repair can salvage 60% to 70% of patients. The catastrophic course, the frequent presence of limited myocardial necrosis and obstructive coronary artery disease, and the favorable results of surgical therapy require early recognition and early surgery in cases of papillary muscle rupture. In preparation for urgent cardiac catheterization and subsequent surgery, patients frequently require intraaortic balloon pumping and additional diuretic, vasodilator, or inotropic therapy, or a combination thereof, for temporary stabilization.

Ventricular Septal Rupture

Interventricular septal rupture is a serious complication of acute myocardial infarction occurring in 0.5% to 2% cases of infarction and responsible for up to 5% of all infarct-related deaths.[76] Although multivessel obstructive coronary artery disease is common, septal rupture may complicate single-vessel disease. Rupture of the septum occurs equally frequently in anterior and in inferior or posterior infarction. Rupture of the septum may occur within the first 24 hours (30%); however, most occur between three and seven days following infarction. Septal rupture produces a left-to-right shunt, causing right ventricular volume overload, increased pulmonary blood flow, and reduced systemic blood flow. Reduction in systemic blood flow results in a low-output hypotensive syndrome that frequently progresses to shock. The left ventricular ejection fraction is usually normal or supernormal, but it may be depressed when the primary infarct is large. The right ventricular ejection fraction may be depressed secondary to right ventricular volume overload, particularly in those patients with inferior infarction who have concomitant ischemic damage of the right ventricle.

Septal rupture produces a new, loud, and harsh holosystolic precordial murmur with widespread radiation associated with a palpable thrill in about 50% of cases. Clinically, the patient often develops chest pain followed by signs and symptoms of a low-output state, hypotension, or shock. Right ventricular volume overload secondary to the shunt, concomitant right ventricular ischemic damage, and tricuspid regurgitation may produce systemic venous congestion out of proportion to pulmonary venous congestion. The diagnosis can be made at the bedside using two-dimensional echocardiography with or without Doppler flow studies. Right heart catheterization using the Swan–Ganz catheter is useful in confirming the diagnosis when a significant step-up of oxygen saturation (10% or more) from the right atrium to right ventricle or proximal pulmonary artery can be demonstrated. The left-to-right shunt usually exceeds 50%. Without surgical therapy, there is a 25% mortality within 24 hours, 50% mortality at one week, 80% mortality at two months, and only 5% to 7% survival at one year. Vasodilators and intraaortic balloon pumping may reduce the degree of left-to-right shunt and produce temporary stabilization. The effective therapy remains early cardiac surgery preceded by cardiac catheterization.[77] During cardiac catheterization the use of a catheter with a tip balloon, which when inflated in the main pulmonary artery effectively bands the pulmonary artery and thereby reduces the shunt across the ventricular septal defect, may be a life-saving measure before immediate corrective surgery can be carried out.[77a] Such an aggressive approach generally results in a 50% to 70% survival rate. Surgical results appear to be more favorable for anteriorly located septal ruptures (complicating anterior infarction) compared with posteriorly located defects (complicating inferior or posterior infarction). Delay in a decision to proceed with surgery simply selects out the low-risk group, whereas the sickest patients have already died in the interim. Early aggressive surgical intervention is strongly recommended.

Free Wall Rupture

Free wall rupture may account for 8% to 24% of infarct-related deaths,[78] occurring in 1.5% to 8% of all transmural myocardial infarcts. Although about 30% of ruptures may occur within 24 hours of the onset of infarction, the peak incidence appears between the second and eighth days after infarction. Rupture occurs mainly in the left ventricle, complicating anterior and inferior infarcts equally frequently, but only rarely in the right ventricle. First infarction, age over 70 years, female sex, and hypertension appear to be risk factors for rupture. The role of early ambulation and the short-term use of antiinflammatory drugs (steroids and indomethacin) and anticoagulants in precipitating cardiac rupture has been suggested but remains unproven.

Most frequently, cardiac rupture presents as a catastrophic syndrome characterized by sudden chest pain, agitation followed by bradycardia, hypotension, distention of neck veins, and electromechanical dissociation. Death often ensues rapidly because of hemopericardium and tamponade. Few patients with this mode of presentation can be salvaged, even with immediate pericardiocentesis, emergency thoracotomy, and surgical repair.

An occasional patient has a subacute course with progressively increasing signs of cardiac tamponade over hours or days; a high index of suspicion can lead to proper investigation, diagnosis, and appropriate surgery. Because the extent of myocardial necrosis can vary from small to large, it is particularly important to recognize this entity, in that surgery can lead to gratifying long-term results. Recently a two-dimensional echocardiographic triad—regional dilatation of the left ventricle, decreased wall thickness in this area throughout the cardiac cycle, and pericardial effusion—was described and said to be diagnostic of impending cardiac rupture.[78a] Therefore, serial two-dimensional echocardiographic studies in patients with acute myocardial infarction might provide evidence of imminent cardiac rupture early enough to allow definitive surgical treatment and thus prevent its usual catastrophic outcome.

Pseudoaneurysm

This rare complication of transmural myocardial infarction results from partial rupture of the infarcted area, most often in the left ventricle, followed by containment of the resulting hemopericardium by adhesions between the pericardium and epicardium.[79] The precise incidence is not known (approximately 0.5%). The pseudoaneurysm tends to communicate with the body of the left ventricle through a narrow neck and may remain small or enlarge progressively and be laminated by a thrombus. Unlike in a true aneurysm, the wall of the pseudoaneurysm is composed of pericardium and adhesions and is devoid of myocardial tissue and coronary arteries. Pseudoaneurysm may be clinically silent and only discovered during routine investigation (echocardiography, radionuclide ventriculography, or angiography) or it may present with clinical manifestations similar to those of a true aneurysm, ie, progressively worsening congestive heart failure, recurrent ventricular arrhythmias, radiographic evidence of cardiomegaly with an abnormal bulge on the cardiac border, and persistent elevation of the ST segment overlying an area of infarction on the electrocardiogram. Systolic and diastolic murmurs may be present, presumably related to to-and-fro movement of blood across the narrow neck of the aneurysm, thus simulating valvular heart disease. Unlike a true aneurysm, the pseudoaneurysm is prone to free rupture with an invariably fatal outcome. Surgical resection is strongly recommended in asymptomatic as well as symptomatic patients because of this risk.

True Ventricular Aneurysm

A true ventricular aneurysm occurs in about 10% of patients surviving acute transmural myocardial infarction and is most frequently observed with anterior infarction involving the left ventricle, the apex, and rarely the posterobasal wall. The aneurysm is a noncontractile outpouching of the left ventricle that forms when the infarcted segment stretches and thins.[80] The aneurysm initially contains necrotic tissue, but with time its walls become more densely fibrotic and may even calcify. Aneurysms vary in size, have a wide base, and are frequently lined with thrombus.

A ventricular aneurysm produces congestive heart failure by a splinting effect on adjacent normal myocardium and by a mechanical disadvantage to normal contracting myocardium. In addition, the high frequency of associated mural thrombosis favors systemic emboli, which are found in nearly 50% of patients with mural thrombi at autopsy, although a much lower incidence (2% to 5%) is recognized clinically. Ventricular aneurysm also predisposes to recurrent ventricular arrhythmias, which are thought to originate from reentry circuits within or around the aneurysm. Rupture of a true aneurysm is extremely rare.

The diagnosis of ventricular aneurysm can be suspected when a patient develops severe heart failure, embolic events, or recurrent ventricular arrhythmias after myocardial infarction and has a diffuse or dyskinetic left ventricular apical impulse, a bulge on the left heart border on chest x-ray, and ST-segment elevation persisting beyond two weeks following acute infarction. A two-dimensional echocardiogram and a radionuclide ventriculogram can confirm the diagnosis and differentiate it from a pseudoaneurysm.

Surgical resection of the aneurysm is indicated in the presence of refractory heart failure, and refractory and recurrent life-threatening arrhythmias, although aneurysm resection does not always eliminate the latter. Anticoagulant therapy or surgical removal is advised for systemic emboli of clinical significance, although controlled studies are lacking. Early intravenous streptokinase and heparin therapy in evolving myocardial infarction may reduce the incidence of mural thrombus formation in anterior transmural infarction.

Shock Syndrome Without Pulmonary Congestion or Pulmonary Edema Resulting From Hypovolemia

The hypovolemic state should be diagnosed when left ventricular filling pressures are low or normal in association with low cardiac output and low systemic blood pressure with clinical evidence of organ hypoperfusion.[81] The causes of hypovolemia in acute infarction include overdiuresis, excessive use of vasodilators, inappropriate peripheral vascular pooling, diaphoresis and vomiting, and mesenteric vascular insufficiency. Many of these patients can be recognized when shock is associated with collapsed neck veins, clear lung fields, and absence of S_3 gallop; however, hemodynamic monitoring is necessary to document low or normal left ventricular filling pressures in some patients. A cardiac index of 2.2 L/min/m^2 or less with a pulmonary capillary wedge pressure 18 mm Hg or lower (Forrester, III[50]) is the typical profile. Many patients with predominant right ventricular dysfunction complicating an acute inferior infarction may exhibit a similar hemodynamic profile (*vide infra*).

Hypovolemic shock responds to rapid volume infusion using aliquots of 50 to 100 ml of fluid (colloid or crystalloid) given under close clinical and hemodynamic control until the pulmonary capillary wedge pressure is elevated to a maximum range of 15 to 18 mm Hg. Further volume infusion may precipitate pulmonary congestion or edema and must be avoided. In some patients, particularly those receiving crystalloid infusions, pulmonary congestion and edema may be precipitated by volume infusion even at lower pressures because of dilutional hypoalbuminemia. For these reasons, careful clinical assessment must be made in addition to hemodynamic monitoring. Some patients fail to have improved pump function despite restoration of pulmonary capillary wedge pressure to seemingly adequate levels. These patients may either have a severe reduction in left ventricular systolic function or alterations in left ventricular compliance.

Predominant Right Ventricular Dysfunction from Ischemia or Infarction

Ischemia or infarction of the right ventricle may occur in 30% to 40% of patients with acute inferior myocardial infarction.[51,82] It is generally associated with posterior septal infarction and variable degrees of inferoposterior left ventricular infarction, because these areas all share a common blood supply from the right coronary artery. In 40% to 50% of cases it is associated with a low-output hypotensive or shock state. The diagnosis of dominant right ventricular infarction should be considered when the patient demonstrates elevated jugular venous pressure during normal respiration or during inspiration (Kussmaul's sign) or during abdominal compression (abdominojugular reflux) with little evidence of pulmonary congestion. A murmur of tricuspid regurgitation occurs in 15% to 25% of cases. In about two thirds of the patients, however, jugular venous pressure may be normal on initial presentation. Some patients also demonstrate pulsus paradoxus, thereby simulating cardiac tamponade. In addition to the changes of acute inferior infarction, the electrocardiogram frequently shows ST-segment elevation in right-sided precordial leads (V_1, V_{3R}, or V_{4R}) or less commonly over leads V_1 to V_5. Such precordial ST-segment elevations may create confusing electrocardiographic patterns simulating concomitant left anterior descending coronary occlusion. Hemodynamic findings include elevation of right atrial and right ven-pressure equal to or above the pulmonary capillary wedge pressure, which may be low, normal, or only modestly tricular end-diastolic pressure equal to or above the pulmonary capillary wedge pressure, which may be low, normal, or only modestly elevated. Other hemodynamic findings may include: a steep Y wave, with a paradoxic increase during inspiration; dip and plateau during diastole in the right ventricular pressure tracing; pulmonary arterial and right ventricular pulsus alternans; and diminished pulse pressure in the right ventricle and pulmonary artery. Many of these hemodynamic changes are found in patients with pulmonary embolism, cardiac tamponade, constrictive pericarditis, or restrictive myocardial disease. In nearly 30% of patients, abnormalities of right atrial pressure may not be detected and may appear later in the course of illness or they may be unmasked during volume infusion. A right-to-left shunt through a stretched patent foramen ovale resulting in severe arterial desaturation may occur on rare occasions. Echocardiography and radionuclide ventriculography demonstrate disproportionate right ventricular dilation,[51] dyssynergy, and a depressed ejection fraction compared with that of the left ventricle, which demonstrates a well-preserved global ejection fraction of 0.45 or greater (Figure 40.15). However, severe left ventricular global and regional dysfunction may coexist in some cases of right ventricular infarction, and such patients should be considered to have severe biventricular dysfunction and categorized separately.

The low-output hypotensive syndrome complicating predominant right ventricular dysfunction results from reduced left ventricular filling caused by depressed right ventricular systolic ejection as well as an increased intrapericardial pressures because of right ventricular dilation.

Volume infusion alone is rarely successful in improving the hemodynamic or clinical state; concomitant use of inotropic or vasoactive drug therapy is generally required. Maintenance of an AV sequence is essential if the patient has bradyarrhythmia, and temporary dual chamber pacing is useful because restoration of atrial contribution results in marked hemodynamic improvement. The overall hospital outcome is favorable in this subset of patients and is partly related to spontaneous improvement in right ventricular function. However, when severe left ventricular dysfunction (hemodynamic evidence of which may remain masked) coexists or papillary muscle or ventricular septal rupture occurs, the outlook becomes grave.

Early Postinfarction Pericarditis

This complication has been reported in about 10% of cases of acute myocardial infarction, the majority developing clinical evidence between 24 and 72 hours thereafter.[83] Pericarditis tends to occur more frequently with larger infarctions; thus, congestive heart failure and atrial and ventricular arrhythmias frequently coexist. Early pericarditis may be asymptomatic and recognized only when the characteristic pericardial friction rub is heard; however, in many patients, recurrent chest pain following acute infarction raises an initial suspicion of pericarditis. The pain of pericarditis is often reported to be different from the pain of infarction, being duller in nature and generally accentuated by breathing, coughing, sneezing, deglutition, truncal movement, and supine posture. The pain may also radiate to the shoulder and the trapezius muscle ridge (trapezius ridge sign). The patient may have

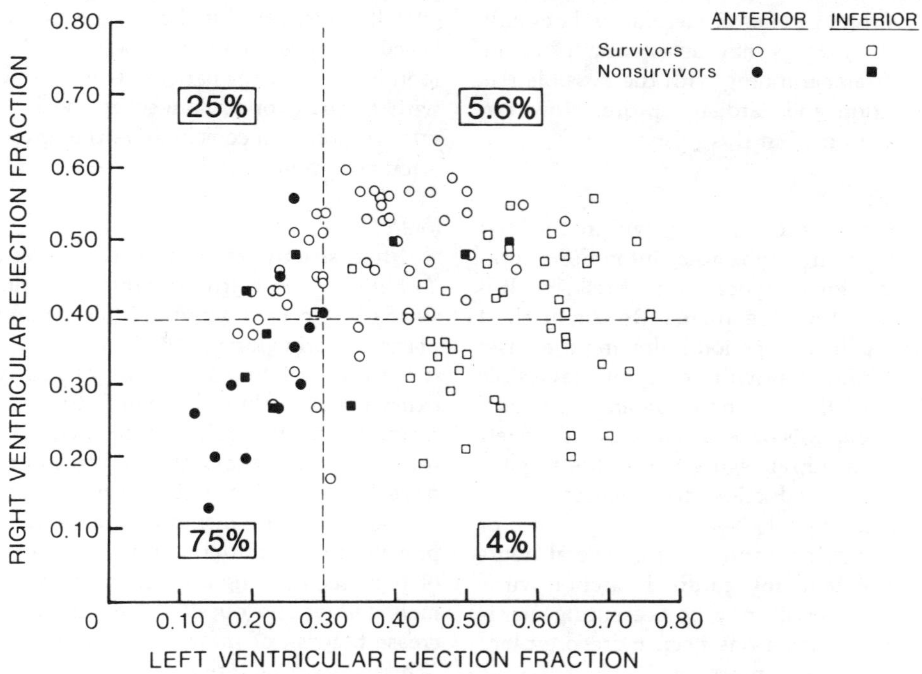

Figure 40.15. The relationship of left and right ventricular ejection fraction to one year mortality in 114 patients with acute myocardial infarction admitted in Killip class I and II is illustrated. The ejection fractions were determined within 24 hours of onset of symptoms. A severely reduced left ventricular ejection fraction (≤ 0.30) was associated with a 25% mortality when the right ventricular ejection fraction was normal and 75% mortality when the right ventricular ejection fraction was depressed. Patients with a left ventricular ejection fraction > 0.30 had a low mortality whether or not right ventricular ejection fraction was depressed. (From Shah et al: Variable spectrum and prognostic implications of left and right ventricular ejection fractions in patients with and without clinical heart failure after acute myocardial infarction. *Am J Cardiol* in press, used with permission.)

a low-grade temperature, but the diagnostic hallmark is the scratchy three-component pericardial friction rub heard along the left sternal border. The friction rub is notoriously evanescent and may easily be missed unless the patient is examined several times a day. It could be confused with a murmur if fewer than three components are present. The echocardiogram may not necessarily be helpful because effusion is uncommon. The electrocardiogram is also generally not useful, because ST-T segments have already been distorted by the process of infarction, making it difficult to detect additional ST-T wave changes.[84]

The symptoms often show a prompt response to analgesic antiinflammatory medications, ie, acetylsalicylic acid (aspirin), indomethacin (Indocin®) or ibuprofen (Motrin®).[85] These drugs may be used three or four times a day, are usually effective in severely symptomatic patients, and can generally be stopped within three to five days. In rare cases in which severe symptoms persist, a single large intravenous dose of steroids may be helpful. Anticoagulants in acute myocardial infarction complicated by early pericarditis are suggested to increase the risk of intrapericardial bleeding. However, personal experience as well as the available literature is not clear on this issue. It is prudent to maintain such a patient under close clinical surveillance for evidence of increasing pericardial effusion. Serial echocardiograms may be valuable in this regard.

Postmyocardial Infarction Syndrome

In 1955, Dressler[85a] described a syndrome characterized by constitutional disturbances including fever, malaise, anorexia, and manifestations of pleurisy, pericarditis, pleuropericardial effusions, pulmonary infiltrates, dyspnea, arthralgia or arthritis, and an elevated sedimentation rate and leukocyte count occurring one to four weeks after infarction in 1% to 3% of cases. Unlike early postinfarction pericarditis, this syndrome tends to have a more prolonged course of weeks to months with remissions and recurrences. Dressler's syndrome has been attributed to immunologic or autoimmune mechanisms. Acute heart antibodies may be observed in the blood in 60% to 80% of cases.

The treatment of Dressler's syndrome follows similar lines as those of early postinfarction pericarditis, ie, the use of nonsteroidal antiinflammatory analgesic agents such as indomethacin and aspirin. In severely symptomatic cases, however, a prolonged course of oral steroid therapy (with subsequent tapering) often produces dramatic resolution. Cardiac tamponade is rare but may be precipitated by anticoagulant therapy, thereby requiring pericardiocentesis. Prolonged use of steroids and possibly other antiinflammatory drugs may delay infarct healing and may result in infarct thinning with the possible risk of aneurysm formation and cardiac rupture. However, there is no conclusive proof in this regard.

Postinfarction Angina

Recurrent ischemia at rest occurring within the first two weeks following acute myocardial infarction represents evidence of additional myocardium at risk.[86,87] It is therefore equivalent to unstable angina. Recurrent chest pain after a variable pain-free period following the onset of acute myocardial infarction with or without reversible ST-T–wave changes on the electrocardiogram or episodic painless ST-T–wave changes or recurrent episodes of left ventricular failure, and mitral regurgitation due to papillary muscle ischemia, conduction disturbances, or arrhythmias accompanied by ST-T–wave changes with or without chest pain or pain continuing for several hours following the onset of acute myocardial infarction without a truly pain-free interval may be presenting manifestations. Recurrent ischemia has been more prevalent in nontransmural myocardial infarction.

Postinfarction ischemia could occur either as a nontransmural infarction threatening to extend transmurally (ischemia in infarct) or due to ischemia in remote myocardial segments (ischemia at a distance). Ischemia in the infarct zone could result when there is preservation of some residual flow to the infarct zone because of subtotal thrombotic occlusion of infarct-related artery or from neighboring collaterals, and this residual flow is intermittently jeopardized. Ischemia at a distance may occur when remote myocardial segments are perfused by coronary arteries with flow-limiting stenoses, when systemic hypotension occurs, when myocardial oxygen demand is increased secondary to ventricular dilation and increased sympathoadrenal activity, or when collateral inflow from an infarct-related artery is jeopardized by the primary coronary occlusion. The long-term prognosis of patients with postinfarction angina due to "ischemia at a distance" is more unfavorable in comparison with that of patients with "ischemia in the infarct."

Differentiation of postinfarction recurrent chest pain from that of pericarditis or impending cardiac rupture is crucial in order to institute appropriate therapy (see sections on "Pericarditis" and "Cardiac Rupture"). A 12-lead electrocardiogram, careful history taking, and physical examination must be carried out immediately in a patient in whom recurrent ischemia is suspected.

The management of such patients is predicated on the potential mechanisms of recurrent ischemia just outlined herein, of which more than one may affect a given patient. Although nitrates, beta blockers, and Ca^{++} channel blockers are frequently used in a manner analogous to that of the treatment of unstable angina to decrease oxygen requirement and increase supply, more rational therapy is the establishment of reperfusion. We recommend urgent cardiac catheterization in all such patients to delineate coronary anatomy and the need for thrombolysis and anticoagulation or for surgical or nonsurgical (angioplasty) revascularization. No large scale clinical trials specifically address this issue; the recommendations are based on current clinical experience. The intraaortic balloon is reserved for patients whose condition is unstable with frequent or prolonged episodes of ischemia and a poor response to conservative therapy, and then only as a temporary measure.

Infarct Extension

When strict criteria are used, ie, recurrent chest pain 24 hours or more after original infarction with new persistent electrocardiographic changes and reevaluation of plasma creatine kinase, the incidence of infarct extension is between 6% and 17%. The pathophysiologic basis of extension is likely to be similar to the one described for recurrent postinfarction ischemia. Extension may be higher in nontransmural than transmural infarcts; others have failed to find a significant difference. The higher incidence in nontransmural infarction may be due to the prevalence of subtotal coronary occlusion in this subset of patients, creating a potentially unstable situation. Female gender and obesity have also been reported to increase the risk of infarct extension.

Infarct extension results in further left ventricular dysfunction and increases both the inhospital as well as long-term mortality.

INTERMEDIATE AND LATE MANAGEMENT OF THE PATIENT WITH ACUTE MYOCARDIAL INFARCTION

GENERAL PROGNOSIS

The more comprehensive programs of management for patients with acute myocardial infarction should logically relate to the establishment of a prognosis that carries a reasonable degree of certainty as to its validity. Although many prognostic profiles have been defined,[88,89] more recent multivaried analyses indicate that the extent of myocardial damage and the presence of abnormalities of the electrocardiogram (additional to manifestations of the infarct itself)[89] are the two most important single prognostic factors. Prior infarction, age, diabetes, hypertension, obesity, cigarette smoking, and other important adjuncts do not appear to be independent additional prognostic features of major importance. Other primary cardiac factors (Table 40.12) are of great individual importance. Clearly the magnitude of myocardial destruction indicates the quantity of myocardium that remains. In establishing a

Table 40.12. Preexisting Conditions That Influence the Management of Acute Myocardial Infarction

Prior myocardial infarction
Prior bypass surgery
Prior vascular surgery
Valvular heart disease
Aortic stenosis, insufficiency; mitral stenosis, insufficiency
Carotid artery disease
Stroke
Serious arrhythmias
Pulmonary, renal diseases

prognosis, it must be realized that specific prognoses of a high degree of favorability (as just described) or a high degree of risk are relatively easy. It is those in the intermediate levels that offer the greatest challenge. The steps in the intermediate and late management of the patient following acute myocardial infarction are outlined in Table 40.13.

We recommend the use of radionuclide angiography to determine in quantitative terms the ejection fraction of the left and right ventricles and the location and extent of abnormalities of regional wall motion. Several factors of critical value in determining prognosis have been now established, one of the most important being left ventricular ejection fraction (Figure 40.10). The ejection fraction in a given patient generally is determined early in the course of the illness, in the absence of extension of infarction or other complications. Thus, a value obtained at any time during hospitalization or in the ensuing few weeks gives a reasonably accurate description of the capacity of the ventricle.

FAVORABLE OUTCOME

Ejection fraction values in excess of 0.55 (within the normal range) have an extremely favorable prognosis; the one-year mortality is approximately 1%. Additional studies demonstrate that exercise tolerance, a correlate of residual myocardium, correlates directly with long-term prognosis in regard to adverse coronary events. Therefore, patients who can exceed ten minutes of exercise on the Bruce protocol enjoy a favorable outcome. Hence, to establish the prognosis in patients with intermediate or uncertain levels of risk, late submaximal testing (four to six weeks) using a formal protocol including duration of exercise, heart rate, blood pressure, and electrocardiographic responses, and if possible determination of left ventricular ejection fraction at rest and exercise, should identify those patients with a good prognosis.[45] Favorable criteria would include a duration of exercise of ten minutes or more, a normal blood pressure and heart rate response as related to age, and an ejection fraction at rest in excess of 0.40, increasing by at least 0.05 at peak exercise, without post-exercise hypotension or arrhythmia. For such patients, in addition, a prudent life-style with regular physical activity to encourage the concept of "wellness," return to full activity, modification in diet so as to maintain adequate weight, no smoking, and control of any tendency to high blood pressure is strongly recommended. In this prognostic group, the routine use of beta blocking agents, Ca^{++} channel blocking agents, nitrates, nitroglycerin patches, or other expensive drugs whose efficacy in a favorable group has never been demonstrated (and probably never can be) is not recommended. Such patients should have an exercise stress test at six months, one year, two years, and four years following their acute event or when symptoms or other changes occur. Only if they demonstrate significant alteration in testing responses should further interventions be considered. The new availability of angioplasty in uncomplicated patients who already have an extremely favorable prognosis may lead to unnecessary (and potentially dangerous) intervention by the aggressive angiographer.

However, in the "uncomplicated" patient, if a significant and unexpected limitation in exercise duration is discovered, arrhythmias associated with exercise develop, and an unchanged or a reduced left ventricular ejection fraction is noted during exercise, then the possibility of additional clinically significant coronary artery disease should be investigated. In these patients a thallium stress test will define a remote area of ischemia and its extent.[90] If extensive, then angiography and an appropriate intervention to correct significant and threatening vascular disease is indicated. In the interim, the patient should be maintained on appropriate doses of beta blocking agents and Ca^{++} channel blocking agents. Work should be restricted and the patient prepared psychologically for intervention to correct important but occult vascular disease.

Table 40.13. Steps in the Intermediate and Late Management of Myocardial Infarction

A.	Ambulation; discharge; convalescence at home Return to work; work levels
B.	Establishment of prognosis; testing
C.	Medications—beta blockers, Ca^{++} channel blockers Antiarrhythmic agents Nitrates Specific management of diabetes, gout, and hyperlipidemia
D.	Tests for cardiac capacity and limitations, extent (if any) of residual ischemia
E.	Specific activities—"Wellness" Work level, job Diet Home activities Sexual activity Walking, jogging, sports
F.	Procedures directed towards modification of atherosclerotic risk Anticoagulants; antiplatelet agents Angioplasty; coronary artery bypass grafting
G.	Psychologic aspects Anxiety, depression Emotional support within family Role model; self-worth

"COMPLICATED" MYOCARDIAL INFARCTION

This category includes patients with prior infarcts and those with new anteroseptal, anterior, anterolateral, and apical infarction, but it also includes some patients with dominant right ventricular infarction. Ejection fraction is below 0.50; values of less than 0.30 have a poor one-year prognosis.[47] The hospital course is characterized by continued tachycardia, and ventricular and atrial ectopy may be found. Dyspnea, orthopnea, cyanosis, cold extremities, mental obtundation, and confusion confirm the diagnosis of pulmonary congestion and systemic hypoperfusion. Systolic blood pressure is not elevated and may be less than 100 mm Hg. (An exception is the uncommon patient with acute elevation of catecholamines with agitation, tachycardia, and moderate systolic hypertension. This "hyperkinetic" subgroup is effectively treated with low-dose beta blockade.)

The principles of management of patients who have

survived myocardial infarction despite serious cardiac arrhythmias and the presence of clear signs of congestive heart failure and perhaps have had other additional complications, are different from those of the uncomplicated patient. Their greatest risk lies in disorders related to extensive myocardial destruction and the possibility of severe additional coronary vascular disease. Ambulation in these patients should be deferred until the seventh day or later, when signs of pulmonary congestion and the presence of cardiac arrhythmias have disappeared or are minimal. Careful inhospital rehabilitation over the ensuing one or two weeks may be necessary. The most useful single test to establish a prognosis is a scintigraphic study to determine the ejection fraction and wall motion abnormality of the left and right ventricles. If the ejection fraction of the left ventricle is 0.30 or less, then the one-year prognosis is seriously limited and a mortality of 25% or greater may be expected.

INTERMEDIATE PROGNOSIS

Management strategies for those with an intermediate prognosis must take into account that such prognoses are developed in terms of a group. Thus, in the uncomplicated patient group, the great majority will survive without any form of treatment. In the group with a poor prognosis, the great majority of patients will fail to survive in the absence of formal treatment. A reasonably high proportion of patients in the intermediate group may enjoy a favorable life-style and survival. The task is to separate this group into those who are at a particularly high (or low) risk and direct appropriate therapy towards them.

Patients in the intermediate prognostic group are those who have evidence of moderate heart failure during the course of myocardial infarction or in whom important and sustained cardiac arrhythmias develop, including, but not limited to, multiple, multifocal, and persistent ectopy, late signs of moderate congestive heart failure, an ejection fraction between 0.35 and 0.40, and additional complicating factors (such as additional valvular heart disease or old myocardial infarction). This patient population is in need of a precise prognosis early following infarction. They may require six days of complete bedrest and 10 to 12 days of hospitalization. Their convalescence should last at least 3 to 4 weeks, and their return to partial work should be slow. Before discharge, the results of a ministress test should be evaluated. The results of the ministress test should determine whether or not angiography is performed before discharge from the hospital. If the stress test results are favorable, including the absence of symptoms, attainment of target heart rate, normal blood pressure response, and absence of electrocardiographic changes, such patients should be allowed to convalesce for approximately 6 to 8 weeks at which time a formal stress test with thallium scan during exercise and at rest (reperfusion) should be carried out (as described herein). In patients who have an unfavorable response to the limited level stress test in the hospital, angiography at that time is recommended for definition of additional and potentially serious coronary artery disease. If this is found, it should be managed appropriately by surgery or angioplasty.

UNFAVORABLE PROGNOSIS

For patients with extremely low ejection fractions (excluding those with obvious ventricular aneurysm), the prognosis progressively worsens. Our recommendation is to gradually ambulate such patients, and with a hospital stay of 14 to 21 days or more according to their condition, conduct a low-level ministress test immediately before planned discharge. If the patient is unable to attain a target heart rate of 110 to 120 beats per minute, if ST-segment deviations occur in response to the minimal stress, if arterial blood pressure decreases during stress, or if clear-cut angina pectoris develops, the patient is taken directly to cardiac catheterization so as to define coronary anatomy and particularly to identify those patients with hazardous additional coronary vascular disease. Myocardial revascularization may be carried out safely at 3 to 4 weeks after infarction (and earlier if necessary) by either angioplasty or coronary artery bypass grafting. These patients are at particular hazard should the residual and jeopardized myocardium undergo further adverse changes; hence, it is important to identify this subgroup clearly as early as feasible and engage in a revascularization protocol when possible. There is little compelling evidence that the use of nitrates, beta blockers, and other agents in this poor prognostic group materially affects outcome. Postoperatively, however, an appropriate regimen of antiplatelet agents and anticoagulants is defined. Life-style modification including diet, limited physical activity, limited workload, and perhaps an altered role within the family structure may be necessary.

Patients who are not suitable for angioplasty or surgical management should be placed on appropriate beta-blocking drugs. Although the prognosis of a large group of patients following myocardial infarction was favorably influenced by propranolol,[91] some patients develop troublesome side effects to this particular beta-blocking drug, including severe bradycardia. A variety of beta-blocking agents is now available. One that minimizes confusion and depression within a patient should be selected. The patient should remain on beta-blocking drugs for at least one year and some patients (those in whom occasional arrhythmias are demonstrated) indefinitely. Many physicians will also employ Ca^{++} channel blocking agents and nitrates (particularly transdermal currently) in such patients. There is no evidence that the addition of these agents materially alters outcome in the asymptomatic patient who has recovered from a complicated acute event and who has minimal additional coronary artery disease.

CARDIAC REHABILITATION

Particular efforts should be made in the field of cardiac rehabilitation,[92] beginning in the acute phase as the state of the patient permits. Specific activities should be encouraged, including regular walking, strict limitation of salt intake, and a modified diet. In the absence of hyperlipidemia, hypertriglyceridemia, hyperuricemia, or diabetes, modification of diet should be directed fundamentally at calorie content. Maintenance of body weight at or below normal for sex, height, and age should be the goal. Beneficial effects of formal training programs have not been demonstrated. If the formal stress test carried out two to three months after the event demonstrates a "stable" myocardium (defined by the absence of reversible ischemia on thallium testing), a "fixed" ejection fraction (which does not decline by more than 5%), and increasing arterial pressure throughout exercise, then such patients may have angiography deferred. Even if disease is present and is not productive of ischemia, it seems possible that these "medical" and behavioral interventions may significantly delay progression of coronary artery disease, facilitate the development of collateral blood flow, improve the general health of the patient, and allow the patient to enjoy an improved life-style. Many of these patients will demonstrate continued progression of coronary artery disease over the years; when that occurs, more definitive interventions become necessary.

In summary then, the steps in the management of intermediate and late phases of myocardial infarction are fundamentally related to prognosis which itself is determined by the magnitude of myocardial destruction, the presence of cardiac arrhythmias, and the state of the residual coronary vascular bed. Each of these three aspects should clearly be understood in the formation of a medical or surgical management program and appropriate testing and physician investigations. A "special circumstance" exists in the presence of a ventricular aneurysm. Many patients with ventricular aneurysm have normal residual coronary vessels. If an aneurysm is detected, it is recommended that angiography be carried out before the patient leaves the hospital to establish the presence or absence of disease in the residual vessels. In the absence of disease, slow convalescence is recommended. If associated atherosclerosis is not evident, then the patient may be carried at low blood pressure levels to minimize stretch on the healing scar tissue. When this matures and contracts, then a relatively long survival and a quality lifestyle may be predicted with a reasonable degree of confidence. The presence of important additional coronary artery stenosis necessitates carefully planned observation and surgical intervention after some maturation of scar has occurred.

REFERENCES

1. Roberts WC: Coronary arteries in fatal acute myocardial infarction. *Circulation* 1972; 45:215–230.
2. Chandler AB, Chapman I, Erhardt LR, Roberts WC, Schwartz CJ, Sinapius D, Spain DM, Sherry S, Ness PM, Simon TL: Coronary thrombosis in myocardial infarction: report of a workshop on the role of coronary thrombosis in the pathogenesis of acute myocardial infarction. *Am J Cardiol* 1974; 34:823–833.
3. DeWood MA, Spores J, Notski R, Mouser LT, Burroughs R, Golden MS, Lang HT: Prevalence of total coronary occlusion during the early hours of transmural myocardial infarction. *N Engl J Med* 1980; 303:897–902.
4. Folts JD, Crowell EB Jr, Rowe GG: Platelet aggregation in partially obstructed vessels and its elimination with aspirin. *Circulation* 1976; 54:365–370.
5. Waters DD, da Luz P, Wyatt HL, Swan HJC, Forrester JS: Early changes in regional and global left ventricular function induced by graded reductions in regional coronary perfusion. *Am J Cardiol* 1977; 39:537–543.
6. Reimer KA, Lowe JE, Rasmussen MM, Jennings RB: The wavefront phenomenon of ischemic cell death. I. Myocardial infarct size vs. duration of coronary occlusion in dogs. *Circulation* 1977; 56:786–794.
7. Reimer KA, Jennings RB: The "wavefront phenomenon" of myocardial ischemic cell death. II. Transmural progression of necrosis within the framework of ischemic bed size (myocardium at risk) and collateral flow. *Lab Invest* 1979; 40:633–644.
8. Hearse DJ, Opie LH, Katzeff IE, Lubbe IVF, van der Werff TJ, Peisach M, Boulle G: Characterization of the "border zone" in acute regional ischemia in the dog. *Am J Cardiol* 1977; 40:716–726.
9. Maurer G, Nanda NC: Two dimensional echocardiographic evaluation of exercise-induced left and right ventricular asynergy: correlation with thallium scanning. *Am J Cardiol* 1981; 48:720–727.
10. Wackers FJTh, Sokole EB, Samson G, Schoot JB, Lie KI, Liem KL, Wellens HJJ: Value and limitations of thallium-201 scintigraphy in the acute phase of myocardial infarction. *N Engl J Med* 1976; 295:1–5.
11. Shah PK, Pichler M, Berman D, Singh BN, Swan HJC: Left ventricular ejection fraction determined by radionuclide ventriculography in early stages of first transmural myocardial infarction: relation to short-term prognosis. *Am J Cardiol* 1980; 45:542–546.
12. Figueras J, Singh BN, Ganz W, Charuzi Y, Swan HJC: Mechanism of rest and nocturnal angina: observations during continuous hemodynamic and electrocardiographic monitoring. *Circulation* 1979; 59:955–968.
13. Swan HJC, Ganz W: Techniques for the investigation of the cardiovascular system in the critically ill patient, in Tinker J, Rapin M (eds): *Care of the Critically Ill Patient*. Berlin, Heidelberg, New York, Springer-Verlag, 1983, pp 933–944.
14. Swan HJC, Forrester JS, Diamond G, Chatterjee K, Parmley WW: Hemodynamic spectrum of myocardial infarction and cardiogenic shock: a conceptual model. *Circulation* 1972; 45:1097–1110.
15. Eaton LW, Bulkley BH: Expansion of acute myocardial infarction: its relationship to infarct morphology in a canine model. *Circ Res* 1981; 49:80–88.
16. Schuster EH, Bulkley BH: Expansion of transmural myocardial infarction: a pathophysiologic factor in cardiac rupture. *Circulation* 1979; 60:1532–1538.
17. Stack RS, Phillips HR, Grierson DS, Behar VS, Kong Y, Peter RH, Swain JL, Greenfield JC Jr: Functional improvement of jeopardized myocardium following intracoronary streptokinase infusion in acute myocardial infarction. *J Clin Invest* 1983; 72:84–95.
18. Swan HJC, Shah PK, Rubin S: Role of vasodilators in the changing phases of acute myocardial infarction. *Am Heart J* 1982; 103:707–715.
19. Barry WH, Brooker JZ, Alderman EL, Harrison DC: Changes in diastolic stiffness and tone of the left ventricle during angina pectoris. *Circulation* 1974; 49:255–263.
20. Reduto LA, Wickemeyer WJ, Young JB, del Ventura LA, Reid JW, Glaeser DH, Quinones MA, Miller RA: Left ventricular diastolic performance at rest and during exercise in patients with coronary artery disease. Assessment with first-pass radionuclide angiography. *Circulation* 1981; 63:1228–1237.
21. Rozanski A, Berman D, Gray R, Diamond G, Raymond M, Prause JA, Maddahi J, Swan HJC, Matloff J: Preoperative prediction of reversible myocardial asynergy by postexercise radionuclide ventriculography. *N Engl J Med* 1982; 307:212–216.
22. Schroeder JS, Lamb IH, Hu M: Do patients in whom myocardial infarction has been ruled out have a better prognosis after hospitalization than those surviving infarction? *N Engl J Med* 1980; 303:1–5.
23. Alonzo AA, Simon AB, Feinleib M: Prodromata of myocardial infarction and sudden death. *Circulation* 1975; 52:1056–1062.
24. Killip T, Kimble JT: Treatment of myocardial infarction in a coronary care unit. A two year experience with 250 patients. *Am J Cardiol* 1967; 20:457–464.
25. Norris NM: *Myocardial Infarction*. Edinburgh, Churchill Livingstone, 1982.
26. Kannel WB, Abbott RD: Incidence and prognosis of unrecognized myocardial infarction. An update on the Framingham study. *N Engl J Med* 1984; 311:1144–1147.
27. Levine HD, Young E, Williams RA: Electrocardiogram and vectorcardiogram in myocardial infarction. *Circulation* 1972; 45:457–470.
28. Sobel BE, Shell WE: Serum enzyme determinations in the diagnosis and assessment of myocardial infarction. *Circulation* 1972; 45:471–482.
29. Roberts R, Sobel BE: Creatine kinase isoenzymes in the assessment of heart disease. *Am Heart J* 1978; 95:521–528.
30. Roberts R, Gowda KS, Ludbrook PA, Sobel BE: Specificity of elevated serum MB creatine phosphokinase activity in the diagnosis of acute myocardial infarction. *Am J Cardiol* 1975; 36:433–437.
31. Grande P, Hansen BF, Christiansen C, Naestoft J: Estimation of acute myocardial infarct size in man by serum CK-MB measurements. *Circulation* 1982; 65:756–764.
32. Bleifeld W, Mathey D, Hanrath P, Buss H, Effert S: Infarct size estimated from serial serum creatine phosphokinase in relation to left ventricular hemodynamics. *Circulation* 1977; 55:303–311.
33. Vatner SF, Baig H, Manders WT, Maroko PR: Effects of coronary artery reperfusion on myocardial infarct size calculated from creatine kinase. *J Clin Invest* 1978; 61:1048–1056.
34. Swan HJC, Blackburn HW, DeSanctis R, Frommer PL, Hurst JW, Paul O, Rapaport E, Wallace A, Weinberg S: Duration of hospitalization in "uncomplicated completed acute myocardial infarction." *Am J Cardiol* 1976; 37:413–419.
35. Rude RE, Muller JE, Braunwald E: Efforts to limit the size of myocardial infarcts. *Ann Intern Med* 1981; 95:736–761.

36. Lange LG, Sobel BE: Pharmacological salvage of myocardium. *Ann Rev Pharmacol Toxicol* 1982; 22:115–143.
37. Rentrop P, Blanke H, Karsch KR, Kaiser H, Kostering H, Leitz K: Selective intracoronary thrombolysis in acute myocardial infarction and unstable angina pectoris. *Circulation* 1981; 63:307–317.
38. Phillips SJ, Kongtahworn C, Zeff RH, Bensen M, Iannone L, Brown T, Gordon DF: Emergency coronary artery revascularization: a possible therapy for acute myocardial infarction. *Circulation* 1979; 60:241–246.
39. Meyer J, Merx W, Dörr R, Lambertz H, Bethge C, Effert S: Successful treatment of acute myocardial infarction shock by combined percutaneous transluminal coronary recanalization (PTCR) and percutaneous transluminal coronary angioplasty (PTCA). *Am Heart J* 1982; 103:132–134.
40. Ganz W, Geft I, Shah PK, Lew AS, Rodriguez L, Weiss T, Maddahi J, Berman DS, Charuzi Y, Swan HJC: Intravenous streptokinase in evolving myocardial infarction. *Am J Cardiol* 1984; 53:1209–1216.
40a. Gruppo Italiano Per Lo Studio Della Streptochinasi Nell'infarto Miocardico (GISSI): Effectiveness of intravenous thrombolytic treatment in acute myocardial infarction. *Lancet* 1986; 1:397–401.
40b. Tennant SN, Dixon J, Venable TC, Page HL, Jr, Roach A, Kaiser AB, Frederiksen R, Tacogue L, Kaplan P, Babu NS, Anderson EE, Wooten E, Jennings HS III, Breinig J, Campbell WB: Intracoronary thrombolysis in patients with acute myocardial infarction: comparison of the efficacy of urokinase with streptokinase. *Circulation* 1984; 69:756–760.
41. TIMI Study Group: The thrombolysis in myocardial infarction (TIMI) trial; phase I findings. *N Engl J Med* 1985; 312:932–936.
41a. Williams DO, Borer J, Braunwald E, Chesebro JH, Cohen LS, Dalen J, Dodge HT, Francis CK, Knatterud G, Ludbrook P, Markis JE, Mueller H, Desvigne-Nickens P, Passamani ER, Powers ER, Rao AK, Roberts R, Ross A, Ryan TJ, Sobel BE, Winniford M, Zaret B and Co-Investigators: Intravenous recombinant tissue-type plasminogen activator in patients with acute myocardial infarction: a report from the NHLBI thrombolysis in myocardial infarction trial. *Circulation* 1986; 73:338–346.
41b. Van de Werf F, Nobuhara M, Collen D: Coronary thrombolysis with human single-chain, urokinase-type plasminogen activator (pro-urokinase) in patients with acute myocardial infarction. *Ann Intern Med* 1986; 104:345–348.
41c. Marder VJ, Rothbard RL, Fitzpatrick PG, Francis CW: Rapid lysis of coronary artery thrombi with anisoylated plasminogen: streptokinase activator complex. Treatment by bolus intravenous injection. *Ann Intern Med* 1986; 104:304–310.
42. Schröder R, Biamino G, Leitner ER, Linderer T, Bruggemann T, Heitz J, Vohringer HF, Wegscheider K: Intravenous short-term infusion of streptokinase in acute myocardial infarction. *Circulation* 1983; 67:536–548.
43. Taylor GJ, Mikell FL, Dove JT, Bachelder JE, Thull A, Hansen S, Wellons HA, Schneider JA: Intravenous versus intracoronary streptokinase therapy for acute myocardial infarction in community hospitals. *Am J Cardiol* 1984; 54:256–260.
44. Swan HJC: Thrombolysis in acute myocardial infarction: treatment of the underlying coronary artery disease. *Circulation* 1982; 66:914–916.
44a. Schröder R: Intravenous streptokinase in acute MI. *Cardiovasc Med* 1986; 11(1):45–52.
45. Theroux P, Waters DD, Halphen C, Debaisieux J-C, Mizgala HF: Prognostic value of exercise testing soon after myocardial infarction. *N Engl J Med* 1979; 301:341–345.
46. Fuller CM, Raizner AE, Verani M, Nahormek PA, Chahine RA, McEntee CW, Miller RA: Early post-myocardial infarction treadmill stress testing. An accurate prediction of multivessel coronary disease and subsequent cardiac events. *Ann Intern Med* 1981; 94:734–738.
47. The Multicenter Postinfarction Research Group: Risk stratification and survival after myocardial infarction. *N Engl J Med* 1983; 309:331–336.
48. Meizlish JL, Berger HJ, Plankey M, Errico D, Levy W, Zaret BL: Functional left ventricular aneurysm formation after acute anterior transmural myocardial infarction. Incidence, natural history and prognostic implications. *N Engl J Med* 1984; 311:1001–1006.
49. Hindman MC, Wagner GS, JaRo M, Atkins JM, Scheinman MM, DeSanctis RW, Hutter AH, Yeatman L, Rubenfire M, Pujura C, Rubin M, Morris JJ: The clinical significance of bundle branch block complicating acute myocardial infarction. 2. Indications for temporary and permanent pacemaker insertion. *Circulation* 1978; 58:689–699.
50. Forrester JS, Diamond GA, Swan HJC: Correlative classification of clinical and hemodynamic function after myocardial infarction. *Am J Cardiol* 1977; 39:137–145.
51. Shah PK, Maddahi J, Berman DS, Pichler M, Swan HJC: Scintigraphically detected predominant right ventricular dysfunction in acute myocardial infarction: clinical and hemodynamic correlates and implications for therapy and prognosis. *J Am Coll Cardiol* 1985; 6:1264–1272.
52. Swan HJC, Ganz W, Forrester J, Marcus H, Diamond G, Chonette D: Catheterization of the heart in man with the use of a flow-directed balloon-tipped catheter. *N Engl J Med* 1970; 283:447–451.
53. Sprung CL: *The Pulmonary Artery Catheter. Methodology and Clinical Applications.* Baltimore, University Park Press, 1983.
54. Forrester JS, Diamond G, Chatterjee K, Swan HJC: Medical therapy of acute myocardial infarction by application of hemodynamic subsets. Parts I and II. *N Engl J Med* 1976; 295:1356–1362 & 1404–1413.
55. Miller DC, Stinson EB: Surgical management of acute mechanical defects secondary to myocardial infarction. *Am J Surg* 1981; 141:677–683.
56. Bregman D, Nichols AB, Weiss MB, Powers ER, Martin EC, Casarella WJ: Percutaneous intraaortic balloon insertion. *Am J Cardiol* 1980; 46:261–264.
57. Morrison J, Coromilas J, Robbins M, Ong L, Eisenberg S, Stechel R, Zema M, Reiser P, Scherr L: Digitalis and myocardial infarction in man. *Circulation* 1980; 62:8–16.
57a. Moss AJ, Davis HT, Conard DL, DeCamilla JJ, Odoroff CL: Digitalis-associated cardiac mortality after myocardial infarction. *Circulation* 1981; 64:1150–1156.
57b. Moss AJ, Davis HT, Odoroff CL, Bigger JT, Multicenter Postinfarction Research Group: Digitalis-associated mortality in postinfarction patients. *Circulation* 1983; 68(suppl 3)III-368.
57c. Bigger JT, Fleiss JL, Rolnitzky LM, Merab JP, Ferrick KJ: Effect of digitalis treatment on survival after acute myocardial infarction. *Am J Cardiol* 1985; 55:623–630.
57d. Mueller JE, Turi ZG, Stone PH, Rude RE, Raabe DS, Jaffe AS, Gold HK, Gustafson N, Poole WK, Passamani E, Smith TW, Braunwald E, The MILIS Study Group: Digoxin therapy and mortality after myocardial infarction. Experience in the MILIS Study. *N Engl J Med* 1986; 314:265–271.
58. Mueller HS, Evans R, Ayres SM: Effect of dopamine on hemodynamics and myocardial metabolism in shock following acute myocardial infarction in man. *Circulation* 1978; 57:361–365.
59. Sonnenblick EH, Frishman WH, LeJemtel TH: Dobutamine: a new synthetic cardioactive sympathetic amine. *N Engl J Med* 1979; 300:17–22.
60. Abrams E, Forrester JS, Chatterjee K, Danzig R, Swan HJC: Variability in response to norepinephrine in acute myocardial infarction. *Am J Cardiol* 1973; 32:919–923.
61. Swan HJC: Effect of noradrenaline on the human circulation. *Lancet* 1949; 2:508–510.
62. Chatterjee K, Parmley WW, Ganz W, Forrester J, Walinsky P, Crexells C, Swan HJC: Hemodynamic and metabolic responses to vasodilator therapy in acute myocardial infarction. *Circulation* 1973; 48:1183–1193.
63. Cohn JN: Progress in vasodilator therapy for heart failure. *N Engl J Med* 1980; 302:1414–1416.
64. Chatterjee K, Swan HJC, Kaushik VS, Jobin G, Magnusson P, Forrester JS: Effects of vasodilator therapy for severe pump failure in acute myocardial infarction on short-term and late prognosis. *Circulation* 1976; 53:797–802.
65. Cohn JN, Franciosa JA, Francis GS, Archibald D, Tristani F, Fletcher R, Montero A, Cintron G, Clarke J, Hager D, Saunders R, Cobb F, Smith R, Loeb H, Settle H: Effect of short-term infusion of sodium nitroprusside on mortality rate in acute myocardial infarction complicated by left ventricular failure. Results of a Veterans Administration cooperative study. *N Engl J Med* 1982; 306:1129–1135.
66. Jaffe AS, Roberts R: The use of intravenous nitroglycerin in cardiovascular disease. *Pharmacotherapy* 1982; 2:273–280.
67. Walinsky P, Chatterjee K, Forrester JS, Parmley WW, Swan HJC: Enhanced left ventricular performance with phentolamine in acute myocardial infarction. *Am J Cardiol* 1974; 33:37–41.
68. Richard C, Ricome JL, Rimailho A, Bottineau G, Auzepy P: Combined hemodynamic effects of dopamine and dobutamine in cardiogenic shock. *Circulation* 1983; 67:620–626.
69. DeWood MA, Notske RN, Hensley GR, Shields JP, O'Grady WP, Spores J, Goldman M, Ganji JH: Intra-aortic balloon counterpulsation with and without reperfusion for myocardial infarction shock. *Circulation* 1980; 61:1105–1112.
70. Lew AS, Weiss AT, Shah PK, Fishbein MC, Berman DS, Maddahl J: Extensive myocardial salvage and reversal of cardiogenic shock after reperfusion of the left main coronary artery by intravenous streptokinase. *Am J Cardiol* 1984; 54:450–452.
71. Gray RJ, Sethna D, Matloff JM: The role of cardiac surgery in acute myocardial infarction. I. With mechanical complications. *Am Heart J* 1983; 106:723–728.
72. Heikkila J: Mitral incompetence complicating acute myocardial infarction. *Br Heart J* 1967; 29:162–169.
72a. Cheng TO: Some new observations on the syndrome of papillary muscle dysfunction. *Am J Med* 1969; 47:924–945.
73. Forrester JS, Diamond G, Freedman S, Allen HN, Parmley WW, Matloff J, Swan HJC: Silent mitral insufficiency in acute myocardial infarction. *Circulation* 1971; 44:877–883.
74. Mintz GS, Victor MF, Kotler MN, Parry WR, Segal BL: Two-dimensional electrocardiographic identification of surgically correctable complications of acute myocardial infarction. *Circulation* 1981; 64:91–96.
75. Nishimura RA, Schaff HV, Shub C, Gersh BJ, Edwards WD, Tajik AJ: Papillary muscle rupture complicating acute myocardial infarction: analysis of 17 patients. *Am J Cardiol* 1983; 51:373–377.

76. Moore CA, Stuckey TD, Nygaard TW, Gibson RS: Post-infarction ventricular septal rupture: the importance of infarct location and right ventricular function in determining survival (abstr). *J Am Coll Cardiol* 1985; 5:400.
77. Fox AC, Glassman E, Isom OW: Surgically remediable complications of myocardial infarction. *Prog Cardiovasc Dis* 1979; 21:461–484.
77a. Grant P, Patel P, Singh SP: Balloon catheter used in the treatment of a ventricular septal rupture following a myocardial infarction. *N Engl J Med* 1986; 314:60–61.
78. Rasmussen S, Leth A, Kjoller E, Pederson A: Cardiac rupture in acute myocardial infarction: a review of 72 consecutive cases. *Acta Med Scand* 1979; 205:11–16.
78a. Hermoni Y, Engel PJ: Two-dimensional echocardiography in cardiac rupture. *Am J Cardiol* 1986; 57:180–181.
79. Knowlton AA, Grauer J, Plehn JF, Liebson PR: Ventricular pseudoaneurysm: a rare but ominous condition. *Cardiovasc Rev Repor* 1985; 6:508–518.
80. Swan HJC, Magnusson PT, Buchbinder NA, Matloff JM, Gray RJ: Aneurysm of the cardiac ventricle. Its management by medical and surgical intervention. *West J Med* 1978; 129:26–40.
81. Russel RO Jr, Rackley CE, Pambo J, Hunt D, Potanin C, Dodge HT: Effects of increasing left ventricular filling pressure in patients with acute myocardial infarction. *J Clin Invest* 1970; 49:1539–1550.
82. Lloyd EA, Gersh BJ, Kennelly BM: Hemodynamic spectrum of "dominant" right ventricular infarction in 19 patients. *Am J Cardiol* 1981; 48:1016–1022.
83. Lichstein E: Early postmyocardial infarction pericarditis. *Pract Cardiol* 1982; 8(2):60–66.
84. Krainin FM, Flessas AP, Spodick DH: Infarction-associated pericarditis: rarity of diagnostic electrocardiogram. *N Engl J Med* 1984; 311:1211–1214.
85. Berman J, Haffajee CI, Alpert JS: Therapy of symptomatic pericarditis after myocardial infarction: retrospective and prospective studies of aspirin, indomethacin, prednisone and spontaneous resolution. *Am Heart J* 1981; 101:750–753.
85a. Dressler W: A complication of myocardial infarction resembling idiopathic, recurrent benign pericarditis (abstr). *Circulation* 1955; 12:697.
86. Hutchins GM, Bulkley BH: Infarct expansion versus extension: two different complications of acute myocardial infarction. *Am J Cardiol* 1978; 41:1127–1132.
87. Schuster EH, Bulkley BH: Ischemia at a distance after acute myocardial infarction: a cause of early postinfarction angina. *Circulation* 1980; 62:509–515.
88. Madsen EB, Hougaard P, Gilpin E: Dynamic evaluation of prognosis from time-dependent variables in acute myocardial infarction. *Am J Cardiol* 1983; 51:1579–1583.
89. Schlant RC, Forman S, Stamler J, Canner PL: The natural history of coronary heart disease: prognostic factors after recovery from myocardial infarction in 2789 men. The five-year finding of the coronary drug project. *Circulation* 1982; 66:401–414.
90. Silverman KJ, Becker LC, Bulkley BH, Burow RD, Mullits D, Kallman CH, Weisfeldt ML: Value of early thallium-201 scintigraphy for predicting mortality in patients with acute myocardial infarction. *Circulation* 1980; 61:996–1003.
91. Beta-blocker Heart Attack Study Group: The beta-blocker heart attack trial. *JAMA* 1981; 246:2073–2074.
92. Wenger NK, Hellerstein HK: *Rehabilitation of the Coronary Patient.* New York, John Wiley & Sons, 1978.

41 Thrombolytic Therapy in Cardiology: Accomplishments and Prospects

E.I. Chazov, MD, PhD

Effective, simple, and safe thrombolytic therapy is an old dream of the clinician, which unfortunately has not yet come true. Myocardial infarction, stroke, pulmonary thromboembolism, thrombosis of mesenteric and renal arteries, venous thromboses of the lower extremities, postoperative and postlabor thromboembolic complications, and occlusion of vascular grafts are only some of the conditions requiring a concerted and effective therapeutic effort.

For a long time there was no theoretic basis for the development of thrombolytic methods. Until the 1950s the understanding of the mechanisms of thrombi formation was predicated on the classic Virchow's triad described in 1887[1] and the fibrin clot formation theory developed in the late 19th century by Schmidt,[2] Hammarstein,[3] and Morawitz.[4] They gave a general description of the processes leading to thrombus formation and could not show rational ways to increase the efficacy of thrombolytic therapy.

The approach to the prevention and treatment of thromboses was purely empiric. These pursuits were doomed to failure, because attempts at intervention in the complex and multicomponent system regulating the fluid state of blood were rough and inadequate. The drugs suggested for correction of thromboses and thromboembolic conditions had a bitter fate; a meteoric rise and seemingly splendid results were followed by disappointment.

In the late 1960s to early 1970s, valuable insights were gained into the mechanisms of hemostasis and fibrin formation because of the development of a new methodology, which revealed the complexity of these processes. Molecular mechanisms of the interplay among the blood clotting system components were established, the role of platelets and vessel wall constituents in thrombogenesis was specified, and understanding of the fibrinolytic system was considerably increased. Simultaneously, physicians accumulated practical experience in the clinical application of anticoagulants, inhibitors of functional platelet activity and fibrolytic enzymes, analyzed the reasons for their inefficacy, and elucidated the pathogenetic mechanisms underlying the side reactions preventing routine use of these preparations.

Both the theoretic premises[5-8] and the accumulated experience in the clinical application of heparin and platelet inhibitors[9-12] indicated that these agents could be used only to prevent or limit intravascular blood coagulation. The absence of enzyme activity, which can dissolve fibrin threads, makes them unable to affect a developed thrombus.

In search of new methods to combat thrombosis and thromboembolism, cardiologists have turned to the agents inducing the lysis of fibrin.

FIBRINOLYTIC THERAPY: THEORETIC PREMISES AND MAJOR REASONS FOR CLINICAL INEFFICACY

Recent years have seen considerable accomplishments in the research into fibrinolytic system components, mechanisms of their interaction, and molecular mechanisms leading to the degradation of fibrin.[13-17] It is currently well known that, along with the blood clotting system and platelets, an important role in the regulation of hemostasis and thrombus formation is played by the enzyme system controlling the rate of stabilized fibrin lysis.

The fibrinolytic system has three main components: (1) *plasminogen*, a protein precursor capable of conversion under certain conditions into plasmin, an active fibrolytic enzyme; (2) *fibrinolysis activators*, enzymes catalyzing the conversion of plasminogen to plasmin (urokinase, tissue activator of fibrinolysis, and blood plasma proteins); (3) *fibrinolysis inhibitors*, high molecular compounds that can rapidly neutralize the activity of plasmin (alpha-1 antiplasmin and alpha-2 macroglobulin) or sharply reduce the rate of plasminogen conversion into plasmin (C_1-inactivator, antithrombin III, urokinase inhibitor, and inhibitor of the tissue activator of fibrinolysis).

Regulation of the rate of fibrinolysis in the organism is a result of a subtle interaction of plasminogen activators with the components capable of neutralizing plasmin and compounds inhibiting the conversion of plasminogen to plasmin.

In response to a vessel wall injury, substantial amounts of urokinase and tissue activator of fibrinolysis[15-17] are discharged simultaneously with an acceleration of the processes leading to the thrombus formation (adhesion, aggregation and platelet release reaction, and a series of cascade reactions resulting in the formation of fibrin threads). Under the influence of fibrinolysis inhibitors, inactive proenzyme plasminogen is converted to active fibrolytic enzyme plasmin, which can selectively break peptide bonds in the fibrin-polymer molecule and thus bring about lysis of the thrombus. This property of plasmin constitutes the basis for its therapeutic effect. Thrombolytic action of fibrinolysis activators (including those of microbial origin, eg, streptokinase) is explained by their ability to sharply increase the rate of plasmin formation.

Failure of anticoagulant therapy is accounted for by the fact that these preparations can be effective, even in theory, only at one stage in the cascade reaction leading to fibrin formation, but not after the formation of threads made of polymeric fibrin molecules. Because the rate of blood clotting is high, all therapeutic measures that attempt to achieve thrombolysis with the help of anticoagulants would be always "belated."

These data made it possible to conclude that fibrinolysin (plasmin) or fibrinolysis activators, those of microbial origin included, have the best prospects if used as the basis for therapeutic agents with thrombolytic activity.

Much experience has now been acquired in the application of plasmin preparations[18,19] and fibrinolysis activators[20,21] in the therapy of thrombosis in various vascular beds. In our clinic, we have used fibrinolytic agents in the treatment of acute myocardial infarction, pulmonary thromboembolism, and thrombosis of veins of the lower extremities for over 20 years. This long-standing experience allows certain conclusions to be drawn as to the expediency of and indications for the use of these preparations, to choose the most rational treatment plan, and to determine its therapeutic efficacy.

Thrombolytic agents should be administered early after the onset of thrombosis and in sufficiently large doses. However, there is a considerable risk of thrombohemorrhagic complications.[5] Significant progress in thrombolytic therapy was made with the combined application of fibrinolytic agents and heparin. Studies carried out in the USSR Cardiology Research Center showed that the most effective way of treating acute myocardial infarction was to imitate the natural anticlotting reaction by the administration of fibrinolytic drugs (fibrinolysin or streptokinase) in combination with heparin. Various patterns of fibrinolytic drug application, specifically in myocardial infarction, have been suggested, and efficacy depends on many factors. The concentration of the drug and consequently its activity are significantly reduced in the coronary vessels compared to the initial concentration in the vein into which it was injected. This is explained by dilution of the agent with blood during circulation. However, the drug is subjected to the action of powerful inhibitory systems blocking the activity of fibrolytic enzymes. Therefore, maximal doses, verging on those causing hemorrhagic complications, are required to achieve successful treatment. In 1974, in an attempt to avoid these adverse effects, we first used an intracoronary pathway for fibrinolytic enzyme administration in the therapy of myocardial infarction. The results of the first trials were reported in 1976 at the European Cardiology Congress in Amsterdam. However, an intravenous administration is still routinely used in most clinics because of certain difficulties in the intracoronary procedure, namely, the need for special equipment and specially trained personnel. At the same time, the time factor should be taken into account. Fibrinolytic therapy in myocardial infarction, unless begun within five hours after the onset of acute coronary insufficiency, proved to be ineffective.

In treating patients with thromboses, physicians currently use both plasmin (fibrinolysin) and plasminogen activators (streptokinase, urokinase, and tissue activator), inducing the formation of active plasmin in the vascular bed or directly in the thrombus.

Native plasmin (fibrinolysin) is seldom used, because of frequent complications and low efficacy. Most widely used preparations now are plasminogen activators (streptokinase [Streptase®], and urokinase). The use of tissue activator is now being examined in the United States. Complex thrombolytic therapy in acute myocardial infarction, thromboses, and thromboembolism of other vascular beds includes a single intravenous administration of 10,000 U of heparin followed by an intravenous (IV) drip infusion of 80,000 to 90,000 U of fibrinolysin or 750,000 to 1,500,000 U of streptokinase (Streptase) diluted in 250 ml of isotonic sodium chloride solution supplemented with 10,000 U of heparin. This mixture is infused over six to ten hours, the infusion being often repeated after an 8 to 12 hour interval (during the treatment of chronic venous and arterial thromboses, thrombolytic therapy sometimes lasts for four to five days). Some researchers advocate infusion of native thrombolytic enzymes over a shorter time, but these "shock" regimens are associated with side effects (allergy, hemorrhage, and recurrent thrombosis). Subsequently, routine heparin therapy is given for five to seven days, the bleeding time being maintained one and a half to twofold higher than normal.

Because of the significant role of coronary thrombosis in the pathogenesis of myocardial infarction, much attention is given to the assessment of the effects of streptokinase in the acute phase of the disease. Our trials showed that mortality in a group of patients who received this complex therapy was twofold lower than that in the control group. However, streptokinase was effective only if therapy was begun within five hours after the onset of symptoms.[5]

Another natural fibrinolysis activator, urokinase, was

also reported to have beneficial effects in acute myocardial infarction as well as in pulmonary embolism, thromboses of cerebral arteries, acute peripheral arterial thrombosis and embolism,[22] venous thrombosis,[23] and venous and arterial thrombosis of the retina.[24]

Comparing the efficacy and side effects of streptokinase and urokinase, some investigators give preference to the latter. Actually, urokinase does have the important advantage of being a less foreign protein to the patient's organism compared to the microbial enzyme. However, urokinase is much more expensive, which hinders its routine clinical application. Currently, researchers are looking for less costly methods of urokinase production, among which the methods of genetic engineering are considered most hopeful.

The foregoing data indicate that the early 1960s saw the formation of a general strategy in thrombolytic therapy, based on stimulation of the fibrinolytic system through the administration of both the active enzyme plasmin (fibrinolysin) and activators of endogenous fibrinolysis. In other words, enzymatic fibrinolysis using streptokinase, urokinase, and fibrinolysin became the foundation of thrombolytic therapy.

In the beginning, clinicians were enthusiastic about these fibrinolytic agents of enzymatic origin. However, as patient data accumulated, it became apparent that a positive specific effect (lysis of a thrombus) was often accompanied by complications (hemorrhage, in up to 80% of cases; recurrent thrombosis and embolism as a result of thrombus fragmentation, in 30%; allergic reactions, in 30%), causing some specialists to be dissatisfied with this therapy.

The side effects of these fibrinolytic preparations are mainly due to a number of objective reasons. Therefore, all the thrombolytic preparations, which are widely used now, are enzymes, and during parenteral administration the "shortcomings" related to their protein nature become manifest. In the systemic circulation, enzymes are promptly inactivated, which does not allow a buildup of the necessary concentration of the agent at the site of thrombus formation without increasing the intravenous doses. Moreover, all the fibrinolytic compounds, except urokinase, have a marked antigenicity. Finally, overdosage of these drugs leads to serious complications such as hemorrhage or recurrent thrombosis or both. Therefore, a prolonged drip intravenous infusion with strict control of hemostasis is required, but even this type of administration fails to rule out side effects in many patients.[25]

Consequently, the injected doses must be limited, which frequently does not allow for a maximally effective concentration at the site of thrombosis. Thus, the factors decreasing clinical efficacy of the preparations add to the inconveniences of practical use.

It stands to reason, therefore, that thrombolytic methods require further elaboration. Our own experience in this field and a number of theoretic premises indicate that the most promising approaches to increased efficacy of thrombolytic enzymes and fewer side effects are as follows: (1) buildup of a high concentration of a fibrinolytic preparation at the site of a forming thrombus through catheterization of the corresponding artery (endovascular therapy); (2) reduction of the rate of fibrinolytic preparation degradation (immobilized enzymes); (3) retention of a fibrinolytic preparation at the site of thrombosis (deposited enzymes); (4) directed transport of drugs to a zone of thrombus formation (directed drug transport).

ENDOVASCULAR THROMBOLYTIC THERAPY IN ACUTE MYOCARDIAL INFARCTION

The efficacy of fibrinolytic therapy depends on multiple factors. One of the decisive factors is the maximal concentration of a fibrinolytic agent at the site of thrombosis, which can be achieved in two ways. One is the intravenous administration of massive doses of fibrinolytic agents that would sharply increase the fibrinolytic activity of blood in the systemic circulation. These doses theoretically might significantly exceed the routinely used therapeutic ones if it were not for the increased probability of massive hemorrhage and other complications. Another way is to administer fibrinolytic agents right near the thrombus. This procedure makes it possible to create a high local concentration without the adverse effects of massive doses. According to our data,[5,25] the time required for clot lysis in this type of administration is several times shorter than that required in the routine application of fibrinolytic agents, the total dose of the preparations, which is also important, being reduced scores of times. These advantages are sufficient compensation for the difficulties presented by local administration of fibrinolytic agents into the pulmonary artery and other vessels during thromboembolism.

Experimental and patient data prove that a new treatment, which was later termed endovascular (catheter) thrombolytic therapy,[26] is promising and expedient. Evidence obtained while studying the effects of thrombolytic administration into the large vessels, eg, pulmonary artery during thromboembolism, on the whole confirmed our opinion that this approach would also be effective in myocardial infarction. Despite the reliable theoretic premises of endovascular thrombolytic therapy in acute myocardial infarction, however, in the 1960s we failed to implement the catheterization of coronary arteries on a wide scale.

The practical development of this procedure in the early 1960s confronted serious difficulties, namely, (1) the impossibility of sufficiently precise regulation of the dose delivered to the coronary arteries, even in intrabulbar administration of the drug at a certain phase in the cardiac cycle. Inaccuracy could dramatically influence the results; too small a dose would be ineffective, whereas an insignificant overdose would lead to unpleasant consequences mainly resulting from a cardiodepressive action of the fibrinolytic preparations; (2) absence of an adequate method to control the actual effect of treatment on the thrombus. Assessment of results by indirect signs, such as ECG and activity of blood enzymes, was not always convincing enough.

These difficulties were mostly overcome with the help of selective catheterization and angiography of coronary arteries. The thrombolytic effect of intracoronary fibrinolysin administration during myocardial infarction was first documented by my colleagues and myself in 1974.

This method has now been used in about 100 cases of acute myocardial infarction.

On the whole, our own data and the results of other investigators indicate that intracoronary administration of fibrinolysin and streptokinase in patients with acute myocardial infarction resulting from coronary artery thrombosis is a more effective method of revascularization than is infusion of enzymes into the systemic circulation. Intracoronary administration of fibrinolysin was especially effective at early stages of the disease.

In many cases we could not determine whether thrombosis had preceded or developed after the onset of infarction, or whether the deposition of thrombotic masses on a preexisting nonobturating thrombus (eg, a hemostatic plug) led to complete occlusion of the coronary artery and the development of myocardial necrosis. However, within two to five hours after an attack of angina, the patient apparently already had coronary artery thrombosis (Figure 41.1, *left*). Moreover, the thrombus was fresh as indicated directly by complete lysis (coronary angiography data) within 50 to 60 minutes after the beginning of local thrombolytic therapy (Figure 41.1, *right*) and indirectly by restoration of sinus rhythm (reperfusion of the sinoatrial node artery during proximal thrombotic occlusion of the right coronary artery) as early as 30 minutes after infusion was begun. Our early experiments showed that such a high lysis rate in a relatively small vessel is possible if the "age" of the thrombus is two to four hours. It is even more probable, for the lysis occurred in human coronary arteries compromised by atherosclerosis, not in the practically normal vessels of an experimental animal.

Results of our studies have completely corroborated the assumption that local administration of fibrinolysin can bring about rapid degradation of the thrombus and restoration of blood flow in a coronary artery. In less than one hour the blood flow was restored not only in the main artery but also in smaller arteries branching from it. This is confirmed by the following facts: (1) sinus rhythm was already restored in patients within 30 minutes after the start of intracoronary infusion. Restoration of normal rhythm indicates that within this time the thrombus was lysed at least to the SA node level, and thrombosis of the artery itself, if it had actually occurred, was eliminated. (2) In the same group of patients, a distinct reaction to a contrast medium injection appeared in the form of a widened and deformed ventricular complex during control coronary arteriography following the intracoronary fibrinolysin infusion, ie, one hour after the start of treatment. In accordance with our previous observations, such an electrocardiographic reaction to an intracoronary contrast medium injection results from the preparation's effect on the myocardium, and only when the patency of both the major and small vessels is satisfactory. In marked stenosis and especially in coronary occlusion, this reaction is absent, as was the case in our patients before treatment.

The obtained data also indicate that intracoronary administration of thrombolytic agents is satisfactorily tolerated after myocardial infarction, and the cardiodepressant effect of fibrinolysin, at the infusion rate and doses used, is moderate.

Special attention is drawn to a sufficiently stable effect of intracoronary fibrinolysin with heparin, followed by therapy with fibrinolysin and heparin as well as indirect anticoagulants given according to our regimen. Control angiograms obtained 1 month after the onset of the disease (revascularization in 90% of cases) indicate good patency of the previously occluded artery. This fact is significant, for it confirms in principal the possibility of maintaining patency of atherosclerotic coronary arteries after revascularization with the help of anticoagulant therapy. There is no reason to believe

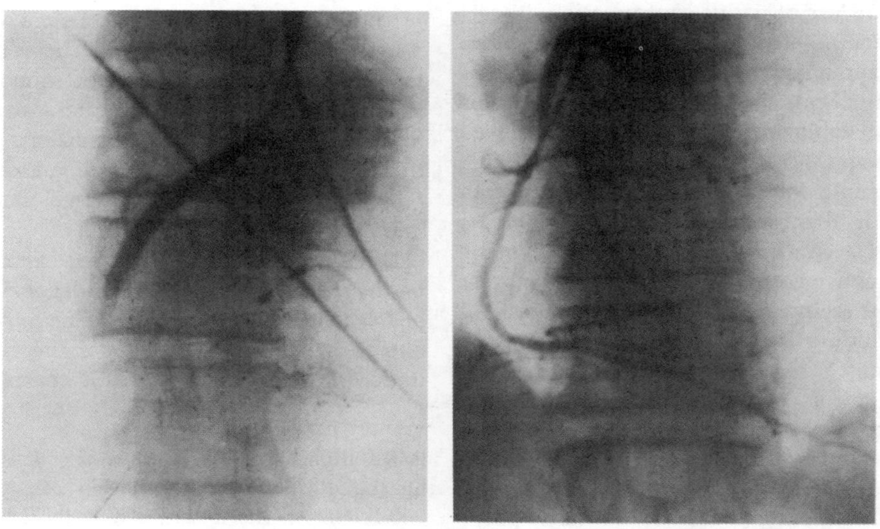

Figure 41.1. Efficacy of intracoronary fibrinolysin administration in acute myocardial infarction. *Left*, Angiogram of the right coronary artery (anterior view) of patient K. Diagnosis: acute myocardial infarction. Occlusion of the proximal part of the artery. *Right*, Angiogram of the right coronary artery (anterior view) of the same patient after intracoronary infusion of fibrinolysin with heparin.

that preventive therapy with anticoagulants would be ineffective if the thrombolytic effect was achieved by routine drug administration.

In our trials with intracoronary fibrinolysin, we did not observe a "usual" side effect of lytic agents such as increased bleeding, which is explained by the use of substantially smaller doses compared to those given in routine intravenous infusion.

Because patient data are scant, we cannot yet arrive at a definite conclusion about the real value of intracoronary administration of fibrinolytic preparations. The dosage and infusion rate chosen empirically should be further analyzed and specified. Future studies will show which of the currently used fibrinolytic agents is preferable, how this treatment affects cardiac function, what can be done to avoid possible complications, and so forth. We believe, however, that even the already available evidence makes it possible to consider this method rather promising.

IMMOBILIZED THROMBOLYTIC ENZYMES: FUNDAMENTALS OF INCREASED EFFICACY OF THROMBOLYTIC THERAPY

Application of the method described in the previous section on intracoronary administration of fibrinolytic agents and endovascular thrombolytic therapy of other vascular beds will not provide a universal solution to the problems of thrombolytic therapy. This method is complicated and requires a network of costly angiographic units and training of highly qualified specialists. Besides, these facilities would be inaccessible to most patients, whereas treatment success, especially in acute thrombosis, largely depends on early intervention. All of that necessitate the search for a simple fibrinolytic therapy accessible even to emergency aid teams.

To eliminate at least some of the shortcomings characteristic of thrombolytic preparations, we have used approaches developed by a relatively new discipline, enzyme engineering. Because inactivation of enzymes is largely related to the loss of native conformation, ie, certain spatial organization, efforts were mainly directed to preservation of enzyme activity. As is known, the conformational stability of proteins can be increased by multipoint binding to a stabilizing carrier. It can be achieved (Figure 41.2) by chemical coupling of an enzyme globule to a soluble or insoluble polymeric carrier, either through copolymerization of the modified protein with some monomer and subsequent incorporation into a polymeric gel matrix or through incorporation into tight polymer gel pores. Each of these methods has its advantages and disadvantages, including those from the viewpoint of medical application.

Because the main goal of our work was to develop immobilized thrombolytic enzymes for administration into the bloodstream, we first had to find a completely biocompatible and biodegradable polymeric carrier. Among many potentially suitable carriers, the native polysaccharide dextran, extensively used in medicine as a plasma substitute, proved to be the most successful option. An inert molecule of dextran can easily be modified, and reactive groups introduced into it can chemically bind protein molecules. Excess reactive groups can easily be

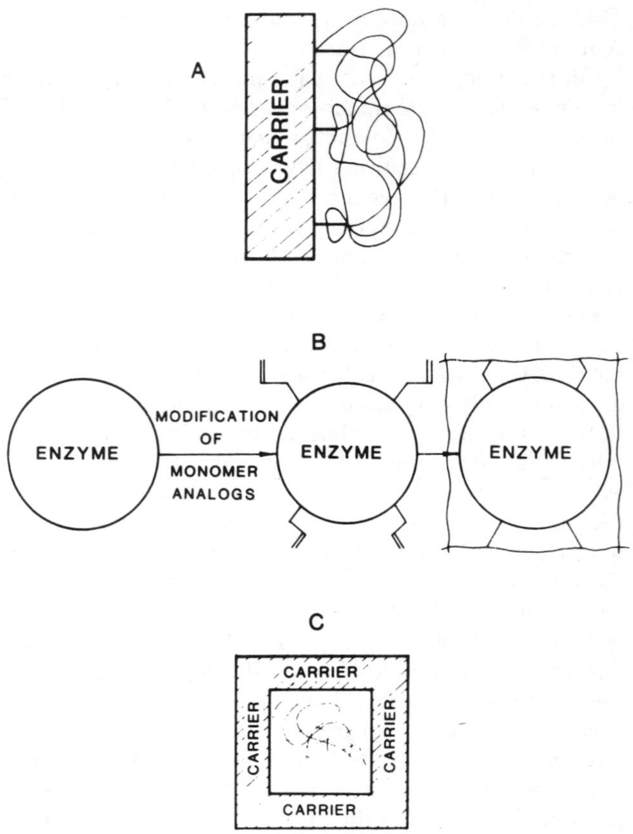

Figure 41.2. Principles of enzyme immobilization (multipoint binding to the carrier). *A*, Coupling of a protein globule with a polymer. *B*, Copolymerization of a modified enzyme with a monomer and its subsequent incorporation into the matrix of a polymer gel. *C*, Incorporation of protein into gel pores.

removed after the protein binding reaction, returning complete inertness and biocompatibility to the carrier molecule.[25,27]

Naturally this and other carriers were preliminarily tested on model enzymes.[28] These tests were neccesary to elucidate the effects of immobilization on biochemical properties of the protein and its stability, and to determine the optimal conditions of immobilization that would guarantee maximal preservation of specific protein properties and increased stability with minimum side reactions.

Under optimal conditions, the carriers had little effect on the specific properties of model enzymes. The catalytic and Michaelis constants describing these properties are altered insignificantly, whereas the stability of proteins under physiologic conditions is sharply increased.[28]

IMMOBILIZED STREPTOKINASE: HISTORY OF DEVELOPMENTAL, EXPERIMENTAL, AND CLINICAL GROUNDS FOR APPLICATION IN CARDIOLOGY

Using the carriers and methods of binding developed in the enzyme engineering laboratory of the USSR Cardiology Research Center, we have obtained a whole set of enzymes, protein inhibitors, hormones, and other compounds immobilized on various carriers which, after appropriate biomedical and pharmacologic trials, may turn into new effective therapeutic agents. However, even now we can state that at least one of the preparations, ie, immobilized streptokinase, had a lucky "fate." The choice of streptokinase can be explained as follows.

First, from the beginning, it was meant as a preparation for application in a cardiology clinic. Second, taking into account the high incidence and danger of diseases caused by or associated with thrombosis, it seemed expedient to develop a thrombolytic preparation. Third, among the thrombolytic enzymes (fibrinolysin, urokinase, and streptokinase), the latter was the most widely used in medical practice because of its relatively low cost. Finally, streptokinase was a good example of the drawbacks of modern enzymatic thrombolytic therapy. Numerous side effects and its complex application limited the possibilities of this treatment. Moreover, streptokinase, being a microbial enzyme, often caused toxic responses in the organism.

The product of covalent binding of a streptokinase molecule to a modified water-soluble matrix of dextran was called streptodecase. The preparation has passed a series of experimental and clinical trials in the USSR Cardiology Research Center. Immobilization of streptokinase on dextran largely eliminates the shortcomings of the native enzyme; as a result of binding to dextran, it became much more stable in the circulation and caused less significant toxic and allergic reactions, its antigenicity being reduced approximately 30-fold.

Despite its sharply increased resistance to endogenous proteases and the loss of antigenic activity, streptokinase binding to dextran does not reduce its fibrinolytic activity.[29,30] Therefore, a study of the effects of streptodecase on the fibrinolytic system of patients with thrombosis of the femoral artery showed that a single intravenous injection of the immobilized enzyme brought about a stable increase in fibrinolytic activity (Figure 41.3). Moreover, streptodecase exerts a "selective" effect on fibrinolysis without inhibiting coagulation, a characteristic of streptokinase.

The results obtained in these trials showed that (1) a single intravenous infusion of 3,000,000 to 6,000,000 FU (fibrinolytic units) of streptodecase causes a prolonged and considerable increase in fibrinolytic activity with a minimal influence on coagulability, ie, a prolonged increase in fibrinolysis (from three to ten days) is not accompanied by "streptase-like" inhibition of coagulation[29]; (2) direct action of the immobilized enzyme on fibrinogen is not manifested, ie, streptodecase does not lyse fibrinogen (typical fibrinogen degradation products are determined in smaller amounts than those found during streptokinase treatment); (3) unlike streptokinase therapy, it does not sharply increase the activity of plasmin inhibitors, the acid-labile inhibitors either disappearing or being converted to activators[30]; (4) during streptodecase treatment, a significant decrease in the platelet count and pathologic alterations in platelet function are absent.[29]

Data obtained in preliminary clinical trials made it possible to assume that streptodecase therapy would eliminate or minimize thrombolytic and hemorrhagic complications. We based this conclusion on extensive clinical evidence, which gave sufficient reasons for wide-scale production of the new thrombolytic preparation.

An industrial technology for production of immobilized streptokinase has been developed in the USSR. It does not require expensive equipment, and the cost of the drug, called streptodecase, is mainly determined by the cost of Streptase. Streptodecase successfully passed clinical trials, and from 1981 its routine use was approved by the Pharmacological Committee of the USSR Ministry of Health.

We currently have at our disposal the data on streptodecase therapy in more than 500 cases (Table 41.1).

The criteria used to assess the preparation included clinical efficacy, convenience of application, tolerability, frequency of complications, and effect on hemostasis. By these criteria, it was compared with the native enzyme preparation, Streptase (Boehring, FRG).

If there were no general contraindications for throm-

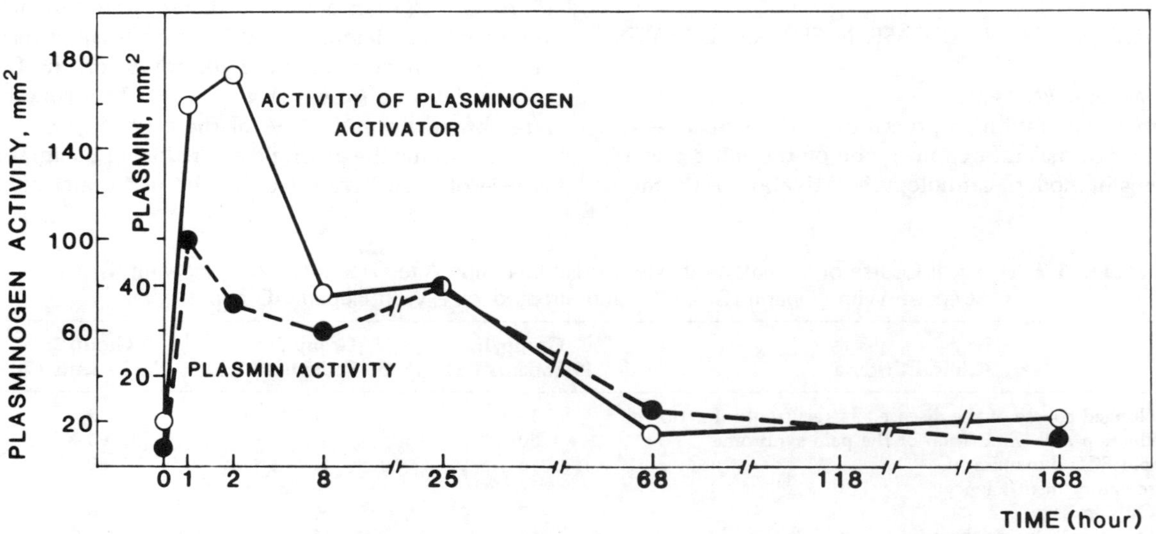

Figure 41.3. Plasminogen activator level (*open circle*) and plasmin activity (*closed circle*) in the blood of patients receiving streptodecase. A single administration of streptodecase brings about a stable increase in fibrinolytic activity.

Table 41.1. Categories of Patients Receiving Streptodecase

Disease	No. of Patients
1. Acute myocardial infarction	200
2. Pulmonary thromboembolism	50
3. Chronic venous thrombosis	25
4. Intraocular hemorrhage	175
5. Retinal vein thrombosis	50

bolytic therapy, patients were given a continuous intravenous infusion of a 2-ml preparation dissolved in physiologic solution containing 300,000 FU necessary for inactivation of possibly existing antibodies. After one hour (the time for testing tolerability), 2,700,000 FU of streptodecase was given in a single intravenous infusion for five minutes, with preliminary dilution of the preparation in 20 ml of saline or reopolyglycine. The total therapeutic dose of the enzyme therefore amounted to 3,000,000 FU, although in some cases 6,000,000 FU was used. During the treatment of systemic thromboses, heparin and antiaggregates were compulsory therapy, starting the first days of treatment.

Naturally, a single intravenous infusion of the entire therapeutic streptodecase dose (3,000,000 FU) has a unique advantage over a drip intravenous infusion of the native enzyme for many hours. It allows therapy to be simplified and to be brought nearer the patient, which is an important requisite of effective treatment of acute thrombosis.

In ophthalmologic practice, a local, ie, subconjunctival, retrobulbar, or, more seldom, intravitreous, administration of streptodecase was used. Usually, 30,000 to 45,000 FU (0.2- to 0.3-ml solution) was used. The number of injections in a therapeutic course varied from one to ten (depending on the efficacy) over a three- to five-day interval.

Clinical trials have confirmed the efficacy of the new thrombolytic agent and revealed certain mechanisms whereby streptodecase exerts effective action on fibrinolysis and blood coagulation.

EFFICACY OF STREPTODECASE IN CERTAIN DISEASES

Acute Myocardial Infarction

Further elaboration of procedures in the treatment of acute myocardial infarction is one of the most pressing problems in modern cardiology.[5] Activation of thrombus formation plays a primary role in the pathogenesis of this disease.[31] Therefore, we thought it worthwhile to analyze the results of streptodecase application with concomitant heparin in 200 patients with acute myocardial infarction. Thirty patients with this disease who received a perfusion of streptokinase and heparin, and 19 patients treated with heparin without a fibrinolytic agent served as the controls in this study.[32]

Table 41.2 reflects the dynamics of alterations of clinical indexes under the effect of this therapy. The obtained data indicate that streptodecase facilitated a more favorable course in acute myocardial infarction: the manifestations of circulatory insufficiency were decreased or completely abolished in nearly all the patients who had them on admission to the hospital; in most cases, chest pain was promptly relieved without recurrence; many patients showed rapid positive electrocardiographic dynamics (return of the R-ST segment to baseline and first inversion of the T wave within one to two days in 64% of patients). Moreover, within the first 24 hours after the onset of infarction, we observed fewer rhythm and conduction disorders. Only in ten patients treated with streptodecase did the disease take an unfavorable course, ending in recurrent myocardial infarction.

Comparison of treatment with streptodecase and that with streptokinase (Table 41.3) with respect to the frequency of side effects showed that streptodecase was well tolerated, especially taking into account that the entire therapeutic dose was given in a single infusion. Table 41.4 demonstrates that the side effects characteristic of native streptokinase (allergic reactions, bleeding, and thromboembolism) were absent. A short-term elevation in temperature was registered in approximately 50% of patients and in most cases did not require special therapy.

Myocardial thallium-201 scanning and radionuclear ventriculography made it possible to assess the effect of streptodecase on the perfusion and contractile function of the left ventricle in patients with acute myocardial infarction. Compared with the results in patients in the control group (no thrombolytic therapy), considerable improvement was demonstrated in myocardial perfusion in the affected regions of the myocardium on the fifth to seventh day in all cases (Figure 41.4). The same results were obtained only in 33% of the control group.

To determine the possibility of reducing the infarct size because of a positive effect on the periinfarct zone, we

Table 41.2. Clinical Course of Patients With Myocardial Infarction After Treatment With Heparin (Group 1), Streptase With Heparin (Group 2), and Streptodecase With Heparin (Group 3)

Clinical Criteria	Group 1: 19 Patients (%)	Group 2: 30 Patients (%)	Group 3: 200 Patients (%)
Prolonged course of the disease and recurrent infarction	15.8	7.7	5
Reduction and elimination of the pain syndrome	50	64	90
Rapid ECG dynamics	16	43	60
Circulatory insufficiency:			
On admission	37	50	56
Developed during therapy	43	13	2.5
By the 14th day of disease			
Disappeared	17	38	82
Decreased	68	42	17

Table 41.3. Specific Complications After Therapy With Streptodecase and Native Streptokinase (Streptase) (%)

Complication	Streptase	Streptodecase
Hemorrhage	50–75	0
Thromboembolism	10–15	0
Allergic reactions	25	15*

*Increased body temperature only.

studied the dynamics of the activity of MB creatine phosphokinase, lactic dehydrogenase, and asparagine and alanine transferases.

Serial determinations of enzyme activity indexes in the blood serum showed that streptodecase-treated patients had more rapid dynamics than did the controls. We also used 35-lead precordial mapping of the myocardium. The data and analysis of both methods suggest that streptodecase has a favorable effect on the periinfarct zone. Such a tendency does not rule out the principal probability of reduction in infarct size under the effect of the immobilized enzyme.

The comparative effects of streptodecase and streptokinase on the clotting and fibrinolytic systems in acute myocardial infarction are also of interest (Figure 41.5). It was established that a continuous intravenous drip infusion of streptokinase in patients with acute myocardial infarction brought about a dramatic inhibition in blood coagulation, simultaneously maintaining high fibrinolytic activity. This apparently was responsible for the development of bleeding in 50% of patients receiving streptokinase (Figure 41.5, *top*).

At the same time, in patients with acute myocardial infarction given a single massive dose of streptodecase, we observed a substantial and prolonged increase (three to ten days) in fibrinolytic activity with a minimal effect on coagulability. The increase in fibrinolytic activity was not accompanied by a "streptase-like" inhibition in coagulation (Figure 41.5, *bottom*) which in theory substantiates the safety of the new thrombolytic therapy.

The data just presented favor the expediency of streptodecase application in acute myocardial infarction. A sharp increase in fibrinolytic activity and the absence of significant alterations in the clotting system apparently facilitate lysis of a thrombus, leading to restoration of blood flow in a clotted coronary artery. Further observations, including those using coronary arteriography, surely are required to confirm this assumption. The results of the trial, however, even now give us reasons to recommend widespread use of streptodecase in acute myocardial infarction.

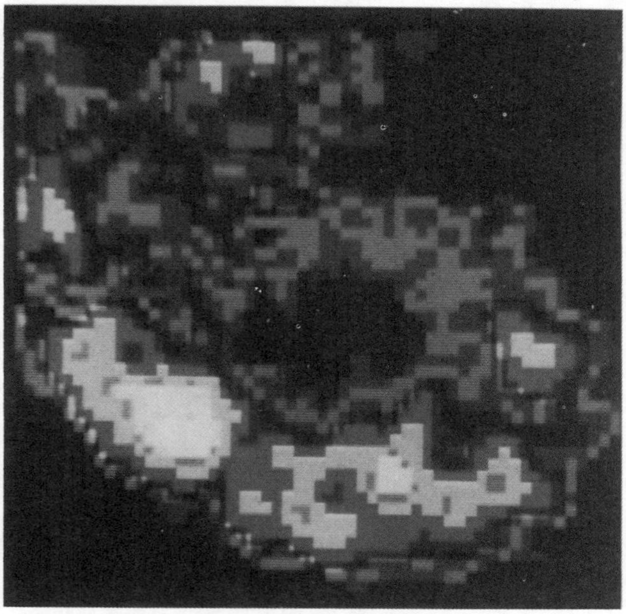

Figure 41.4. Effect of streptodecase on the myocardial perfusion indexes in a 47-year-old patient with a diagnosis of acute myocardial infarction. The myocardial scan taken on the seventh day after streptodecase infusion and the start of combined therapy with heparin. Practically normal radionuclide uptake indicates the restoration of blood supply to the infarct zone.

Pulmonary Thromboembolism

A trial of the clinical efficacy of streptodecase in 50 cases of pulmonary thromboembolism (PTE) showed that 77% of patients had improved clinical symptoms 24 to 48 hours after the administration; dyspnea, tachycardia, cyanosis, and electrocardiographic signs of the right cardiac chamber's overload decreased or disappeared. The improved clinical picture of the disease correlated with the objective dynamics of quantitative thrombosis indexes (Table 41.4). The efficacy of streptodecase in PTE was also confirmed by scanning (Figure 41.6). In most patients, we observed practically complete recovery of pulmonary perfusion.

After streptodecase, partial lysis of the thrombus was observed in all patients and complete revascularization of occluded branches of the pulmonary artery in 33% of

Table 41.4. Dynamics of Quantitative Indexes of Thrombosis in Patients With Massive Thromboembolism of the Pulmonary Artery Receiving Streptodecase

	Time After Start of Therapy					
Index	Before Treatment	1 Wk	2 Wk	1 Mo	3–6 Mo	1 Yr
1. Perfusion deficiency	40.9± 2.2	24.7±3.1	17.5±5.2	16.0±5.3	4.7±3.1	4.2±3.0
2. General Miller index*	23.6± 1.7	—	9.0±2.0	—	—	—
3. Perfusion index	9.8± 0.9	—	3.0±0.8	—	—	—
4. Pulmonary artery systemic pressure	66.0±11.5	35.0±3.5	32.0±6.5	30.0±6.5	—	—

*Quantitative indicator of thrombosis obtained during analysis of lung scans.

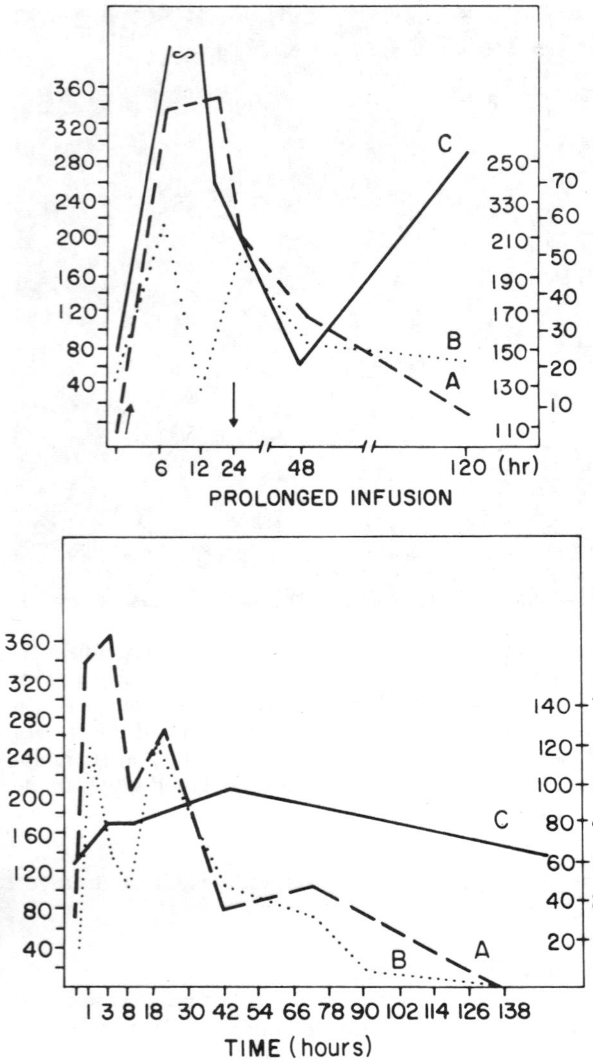

Figure 41.5. Effects of streptokinase (*top*) and streptodecase (*bottom*) on the main clotting and fibrinolytic indexes in patients with acute myocardial infarction. Graph shows the dynamics of activator (A) and plasmin (B) activity, and partial thromboplastin time (C) during streptokinase and streptodecase therapy. *Top,* As seen, to achieve practically the same level of fibrinolysis activation, continuous 24-hour drip IV infusion of streptokinase is required. During this period, coagulation is dramatically inhibited. Partial thromboplastin time increases so that it is practically impossible to measure it. Subsequently, sharp activation of coagulation occurs with decreasing fibrinolysis. *Bottom,* Instant administration of the entire therapeutic dose of streptodecase is accompanied by an equally significant increase in fibrinolysis, but it does not lead to inhibition of coagulation. Curve reflecting partial thromboplastin time practically remains at baseline during the entire period of observation.

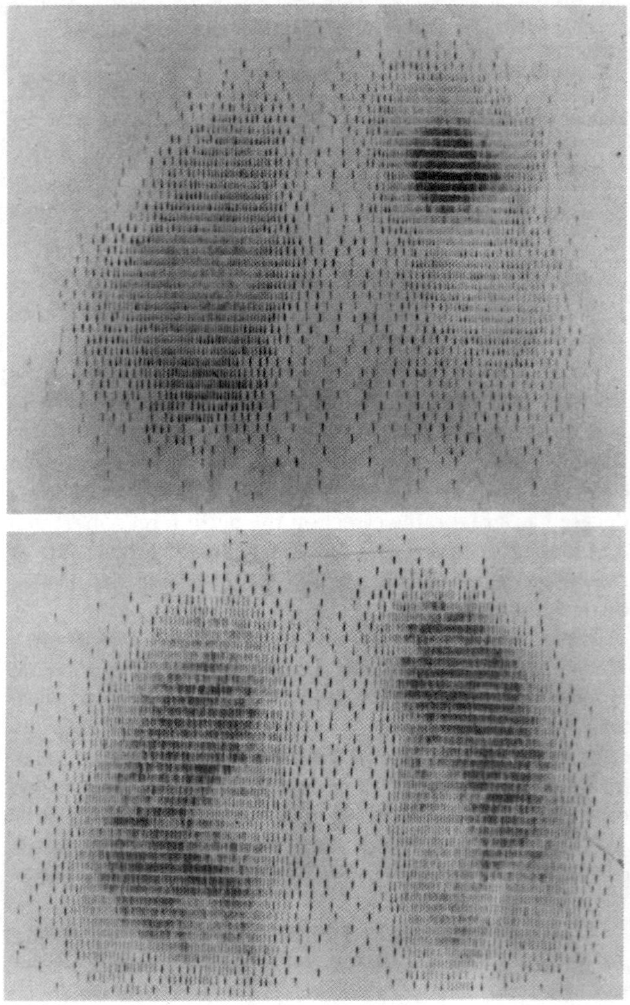

Figure 41.6. Restoration of lung perfusion in a 43-year-old patient with a diagnosis of pulmonary artery thromboembolism. *Top*, Scan taken before treatment (anteroposterior view, perfusion deficiency about 50%). *Bottom*, Lung scan of the same patient taken 6 days after infusion of 6,000,000 fibrinolytic units of streptodecase shows practically complete recovery of pulmonary perfusion.

patients (shown by pulmonary angiography) (Figure 41.7).

The obtained data generally indicate that streptodecase has beneficial effect in PTE, the best results being achieved in nonocclusive obstruction of the pulmonary artery and in the absence of marked hemodynamic disorders.[33]

Vitreous Hemorrhage

Insufficient efficacy of existing thrombolytic preparations makes it difficult to successfully treat patients with intraocular hemorrhage. As it turns out, streptodecase opens up wide avenues for therapy of this disorder. Examination of 175 patients with intraocular hemorrhage showed that treatment is not accompanied by unpleasant sensations; as a rule, no local reaction was observed in the treated eye.[34]

The therapeutic effect was achieved in most cases within two to three days. Maximal lysis of blood was observed within three to eight days of drug administration. In all patients hyphema was completely dissolved in two to three days (Figure 41.8), and the blood in the vitreous body, within seven to eight days (60% of patients). In 30% of patients, blood in the anterior chamber and vitreous body was completely dissolved, as confirmed by ultrasonography (Figure 41.9). The vision remained

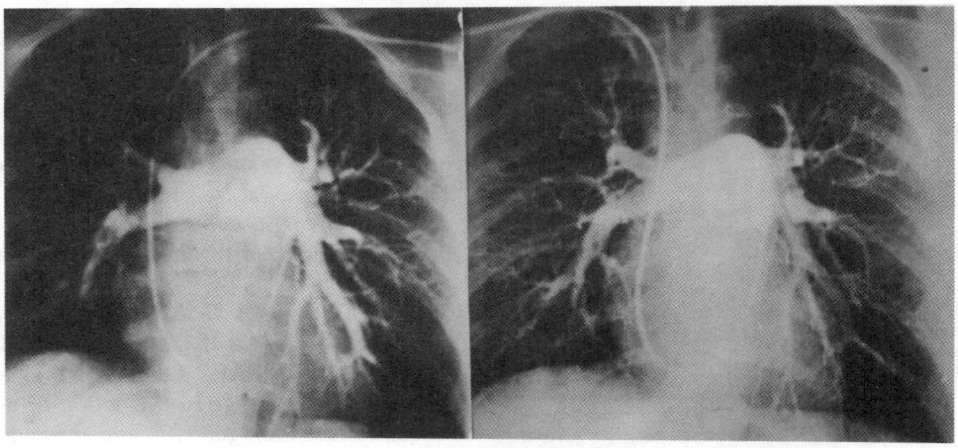

Figure 41.7. Revascularization by streptodecase of the pulmonary artery branches occluded by a thrombus in a 45-year-old patient with a diagnosis of pulmonary thromboembolism. *Left*, Initial angiogram taken before treatment shows thromboembolic occlusion of the right main branch and left upper branch of the pulmonary artery. *Right*, Post-streptodecase angiogram shows complete restoration of patency in the left pulmonary artery branches and in the right pulmonary artery. Only the right medial branch remains occluded.

impaired, however, apparently due to the character of the trauma.

Analysis of patient data shows that streptodecase is more effective in ocular contusion and postoperative bleeding. It was much more effective than any native thrombolytic currently used for therapy of intraocular bleeding. The method is simple, convenient, and does not require additional equipment.

The available evidence makes it possible to conclude that application of streptodecase in intraocular hemorrhage allows maximal increase in the lysis of blood that flows into the vitreous body, avoids specific complications characteristic of native fibrinolytic agents, improves the functional properties of the injured eye, and reduces hospitalization time.

Retinal Vein Thrombosis

Thrombosis of the retinal vein is another widespread ailment that depends on thrombolytic therapy. The native thrombolytic enzymes used up to the present have serious drawbacks, limiting their application in this disease. Multiple infusions are one of them. They are necessary to achieve the maximal thrombolytic effect, but they lead to sensitization and local allergic reaction (hyperemia, edema, and chemosis).

A study of the effects of streptodecase in 50 patients with retinal vein thrombosis showed that treatment resulted in complete or partial lysis of hematoma (depending on the degree of a hemorrhagic component) on the fundus of the eye, a decrease or elimination of edema by activation of the blood flow in the parafoveal vascular network, and restoration of the circulation in previously occluded veins (Figure 41.10). After streptodecase, the acuity of vision in six patients who had only been able to count fingers shown right in front of the face increased to 0.05 to 0.1; in 15 patients, from 0.2 to 0.3 to 0.5 to 0.6; in five patients, from 0.2 to 0.3 to 0.8 to 1.0.

Results in the clinical application of streptodecase for thrombosis of the central retinal vein and its branches are promising, affording recovery even at advanced stages of the pathologic process.

In summary, clinical evidence demonstrated the irre-

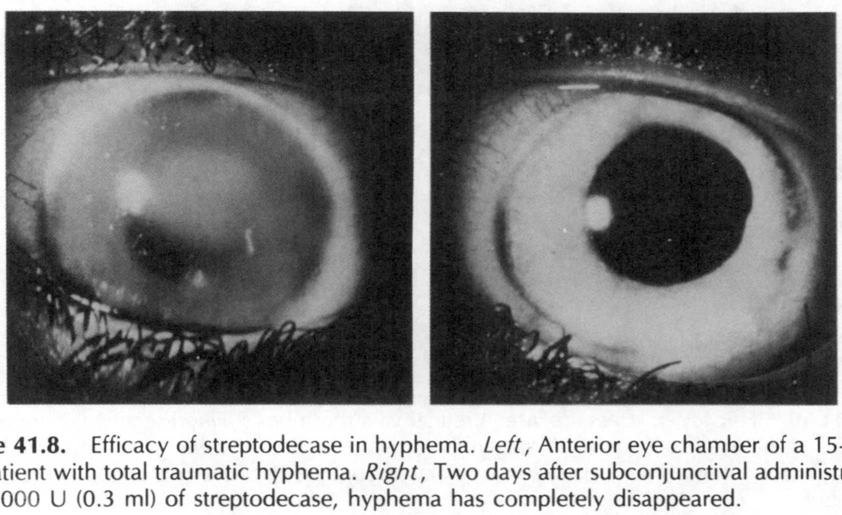

Figure 41.8. Efficacy of streptodecase in hyphema. *Left*, Anterior eye chamber of a 15-year-old patient with total traumatic hyphema. *Right*, Two days after subconjunctival administration of 45,000 U (0.3 ml) of streptodecase, hyphema has completely disappeared.

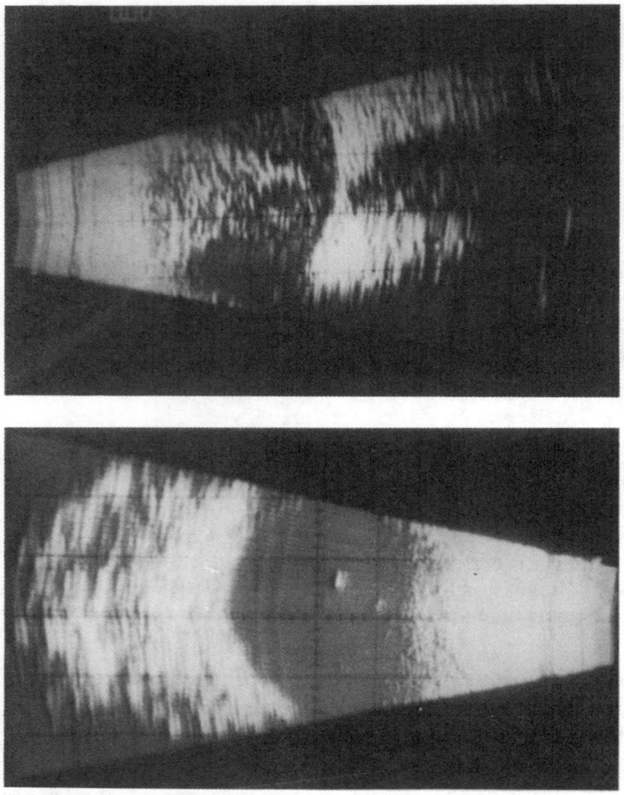

Figure 41.9. Efficacy of streptodecase in vitreous hemorrhage. *Top*, Initial echogram of a patient with traumatic bleeding into the vitreous body after unsuccessful treatment with fibrinolysin, heparin, and corticosteroids (day 15). Vision was only photoperception, ie, blindness, due to the presence of fibrin threads in the vitreous body. *Bottom*, Echogram of the same eye after two injections of 45,000 fibrinolytic units of streptodecase. Only few opacities can be seen, which is fully consistent with recovery of vision to 0.6. The patient resumed work two weeks after the start of treatment.

futable advantages of this preparation over the native enzyme streptase and other thrombolytic agents. Simple and convenient application, a selective effect on fibrinolysis, the absence of a significant influence on the blood clotting system, and, finally a prolonged effect are all properties that make us favor a wide therapeutic application of streptodecase, and we hope that it will pave the way for other representatives of the new family of protein drugs, immobilized thrombolytic enzymes.

DEPOSITION OF IMMOBILIZED ENZYMES FOR LOCAL THROMBOLYSIS: THROMBOLYTIC THERAPY OF THE FUTURE

Increased resistance to the action of endogenous proteases, reduced antigenicity, and few side effects are important factors but not the only conditions that determine the effective application of fibrinolytic enzymes in thrombolytic therapy in cardiology.

The process of thrombus formation is, as a rule, a local event related to alterations in one or, more seldom, several vessels.[31] General predisposition to hemostatic disorders (increased coagulability and reduced fibrinolytic activity) in patients with cardiovascular disease may lead to thrombus formation only if it is accompanied by local disturbances in the vascular structure.[31]

All of these facts gave an impetus to the development of regulated deposition of fibrinolytic preparations at the site of thromboembolic occlusion without increasing their concentration in the systemic circulation.

Endovascular therapy is one way to build up maximal drug concentration at the site of thrombosis (see section on Efficacy of Streptodecase in Certain Diseases). The endovascular therapy, however, does not afford prolonged deposition and optimal therapeutic action, because the existing preparations are water-soluble, cannot be detained in the zone of thrombus, and do not possess a prolonged effect.

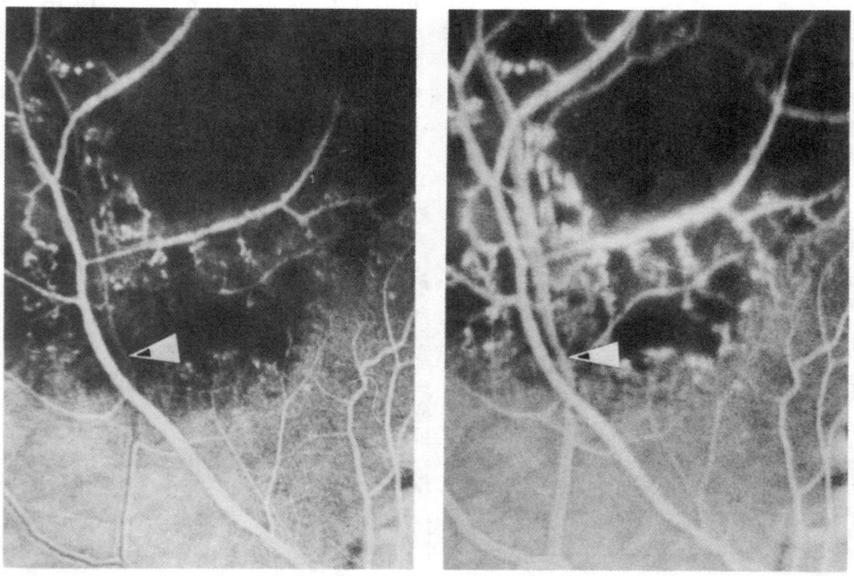

Figure 41.10. Efficacy of streptodecase in retinal vein thrombosis. Fluorescent angiograms of the fundus of the eye in a 68-year-old patient before (*left*) and after (*right*) streptodecase (19th second of examination). After treatment, accelerated contrasting of the occluded vein (*arrow*) was apparent.

We attempted to solve the problem using the method of enzyme engineering, which proved so effective in the development of streptodecase. Instead of the soluble dextran, however, we had to find another carrier which could be localized at a certain part of the vessel bed. Such a carrier had to be biocompatible, biodegradable, and suitable for enzyme immobilization.

The major advantage afforded by local deposition of an immobilized therapeutic agent in the vessel bed is the possibility of achieving a significantly high concentration at the focus of a pathologic process compared to that with administration of a usual soluble preparation into the systemic circulation.

The rate of enzyme release from these biodegradable carriers into the medium will be determined by the rate of carrier breakdown under physiologic conditions and its localization at the site of thrombosis, by mechanical restraint of the carrier in the occluded vessel. It was also assumed that as with dextran in the case of streptodecase, the carrier should stabilize the enzyme molecule and increase its resistance to the action of endogenous proteases and fibrinolytic inhibitors. In addition, the carrier must be able to reduce the adverse effects characteristic of native thrombolytic enzymes.

Bearing all of these requirements in mind, we chose 20 to 40 μm of Sephadex® granules as a carrier. It was established that as a result of periodate oxidation through which protein-reactive carbonyl groups are introduced into the carrier, Sephadex (which consists of coupled dextrans) acquires a capability for slow degradation in aqueous media. The degradation rate depends on the degree of carrier modification and ranges from several hours to several days.[35] Animal experiments showed that it is possible to achieve local deposition of immobilized protein molecules using G-25 Sephadex granules as a carrier (Figure 41.11).

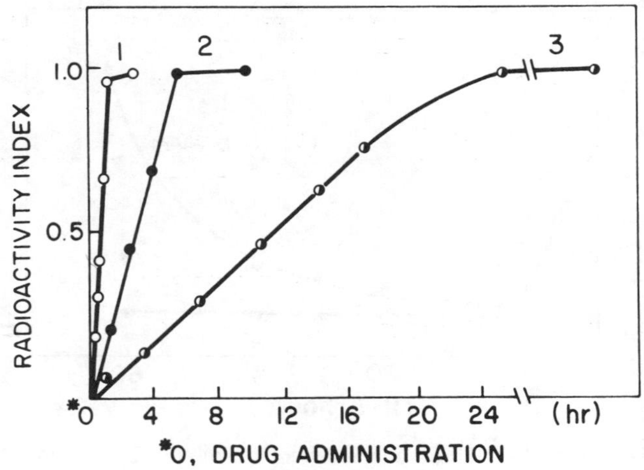

Figure 41.11. Dependence of Sephadex microsphere dissolution rate on the type of preparation. Rate of Sephadex dissolution was measured by ^{131}I-albumin release (radioactivity index) into the bloodstream: (1) native human serum albumin; 2.3, serum albumin covalently bound to aldehyde Sephadex; (2) high degree of oxidation; and (3) low degree of oxidation. Microspheres (2 to 6 mg or 2 to 6 mln microgranules, d = 20 to 40 μm) were administered into the left coronary artery of the dog. Alterations in the labeled Sephadex content were evaluated by the radioactivity index over the abdominal cavity and heart. The obtained ratio levels the error caused by the circulation of the radioactive label in the vascular bed. The period of protein retention at the site of administration is determined by the carrier dissolution rate, ie, less oxidized Sephadex (3) deposited into the myocardium for a considerably longer time compared with a more oxidized and rapidly dissolvable one (2).

Analysis of the dissolution rate of polysaccharide carriers intended to prolong drug action in a long-term experiment showed that the rate of Sephadex microsphere degradation in the organism (Figure 41.11) and under laboratory conditions[35] is similar. Because the rate of carrier breakdown, the amount of carrier-bound preparation, and the dynamics of its release can be regulated, prospects for their clinical application seem rather hopeful.

It was demonstrated on model enzymes that an enzyme does not lose its activity after binding of its protein molecule to Sephadex, but the protein stability increases with respect to autolysis, pH, and temperature. Thus, the coupling of an enzyme molecule to Sephadex does not lead to enzyme inactivation and simultaneously facilitates stabilization of the protein in the bloodstream. Therefore, we chose this approach to develop stabilized thrombolytic preparations.

First, we decided to try fibrinolysin, because its main therapeutic shortcoming was rapid inactivation in the circulation,[5] with the consequent need to administer large doses of the preparation to maintain the therapeutic concentration.

Experiments on dogs showed that the newly developed biodegradable preparations of fibrinolysin (modified G-25 Sephadex microgranules containing 200 mg of enzyme/fibronectin [Koch-Leit, UK]/per 1 g of carrier) exert a marked and prompt thrombolytic effect (dose of 10 mg)[36]: restoration of the blood flow rate (Figure 41.12) and complete normalization of the angiographic picture (Figure 41.13) were observed in animals with experimental thrombosis of the femoral artery.

The results (Figures 41.14 and 41.15) indicate that immobilized fibrinolysin (10 million 40 μm microspheres) possessing prominent fibrinolytic activity cannot bring about a clinically significant blockage of the distal vessel bed. This conclusion was corroborated by the data of another study of perfusion pressure and blood flow in a treated and intact (control) artery.[36]

It was also established that the biodegradable fibrinolysin preparations afford a more significant degree of the required fibrinolytic activity alteration at the site of thrombosis (Figure 41.14). A reciprocal interrelation between plasminogen and plasmin was revealed during low antiplasmin activity (Figure 41.15), which points to an increase in fibrinolytic potential under the effects of immobilized fibrinolysin.

The data generally indicate that practically all the enzyme is concentrated at the site of thrombosis without circulating in the systemic vessel bed; the enzyme "works" directly on the substrate (thrombus), and its inactivation by the natural inhibitors is dramatically decreased. A "therapeutic" dose of the preparation is sig-

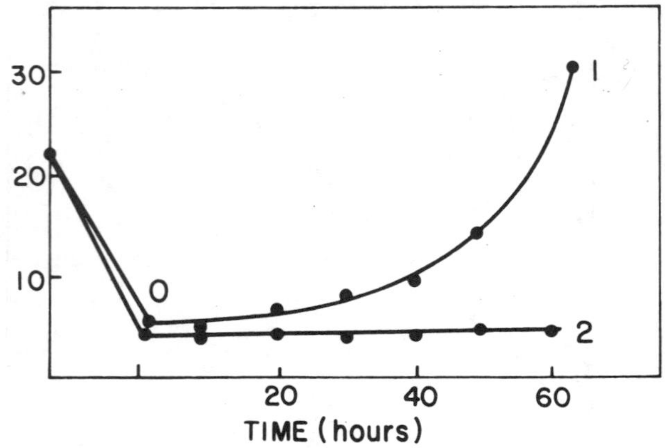

Figure 41.12. Thrombolytic effect of immobilized fibrinolysin (blood flow curve was registered on a Mingograph 34). 0 = time of immobilized fibrinolysin administration; 1 = treated artery (the right one); 2 = untreated artery (the left one). The horizontal axis indicates the time in minutes, and the ordinate indicates the speed of blood flow in milliliters per second.

Under anesthesia, the left and right femoral arteries were isolated and shunted with system with a ball flow meter. Red thrombus was prepared from dog venous blood drawn one hour before the experiment. Both femoral arteries were occluded with equal amounts of thrombotic masses. Thirty minutes after occlusion, 10 mg of fibrinolysin (Koch Leit, UK) covalently coupled to Sephadex G-25 granules was injected into the right femoral artery. Blood flow was completely restored one hour after injection. Control (left femoral) artery remains occluded.

nificantly smaller than the one required for lysis of such a thrombus in the intravenous administration of native fibrinolysin, a single injection being sufficient to achieve lysis of a thrombus.

Coronary artery thrombosis is known to be one of the most frequent direct causes of acute myocardial infarction.[31] Therefore, the final objective of our efforts is to develop thrombolytic preparations effective in coronary artery thrombosis. Arterioles and capillaries in the myocardium and lower extremities have distinctive features.[37] Therefore, the absence of occlusion in the distal parts of the vascular tree does not necessarily mean that injection of 40-μm granules into the coronary artery would not cause ischemia and necrosis of the heart muscle.

To elucidate this question we studied the effect of intracoronary infusion of Sephadex microspheres on microcirculation, electrocardiographic index, and histochemical activity of dog myocardium. We also determined the activity of blood enzymes reflecting early ischemic damage to the myocardium. A scheme of intracoronary perfusion with microspheres is shown in Figure 41.16.

Intracoronary administration of 0.02 g of G-25 Sephadex (20,000 particles per gram of myocardium) apparently causes no damage to intact heart. The morphofunctional peculiarities of the myocardial network afford adequate redistribution of blood flow to compensate for inadequate perfusion of myocardial areas supplied by the arterioles plugged by the carrier granules.

This evidence is far from being conclusive, but in our view it is sufficient to encourage further trials of immobilized fibrinolysin in coronary thrombosis.

On the whole, the results of a series of experiments reported on herein make it possible to state that micro-

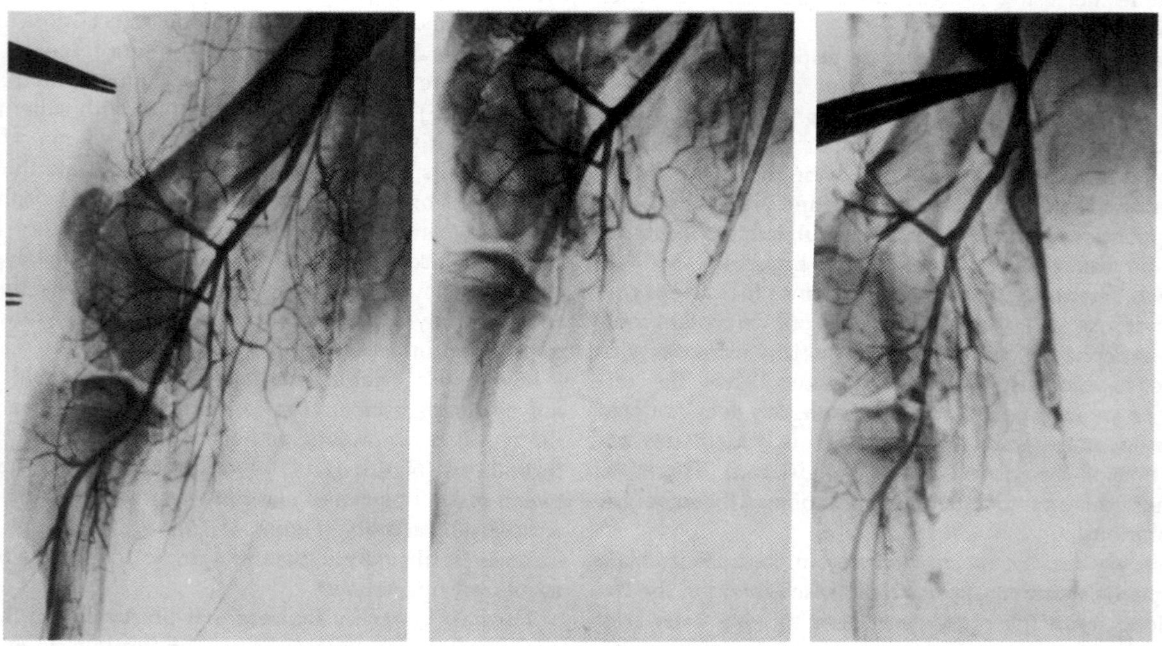

Figure 41.13. Effect of immobilized fibrinolysin on thrombolysis in dogs. Angiograms of dog right femoral artery (*left*) prior to occlusion, (*middle*) experimental thrombotic occlusion of the artery, (*right*) one hour after deposition of immobilized fibrinolysin on the thrombus. There was complete lysis of the thrombus and restored patency.

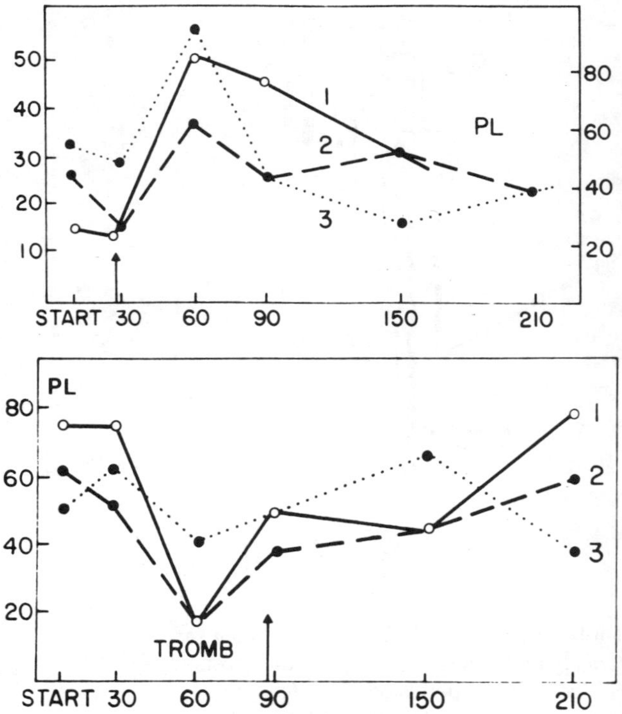

Figure 41.14. Fibrinolytic activity of blood flowing from the site of drug deposition (vein) (1) in the systemic circulation (inferior vena cava) (2), and plasmin activity (PL) in the arterial blood (3) during deposition of fibrinolysin immobilized on microspheres in control dogs (no thrombus) (*top*) and during experimental thrombosis (TROMB) (*bottom*) of the femoral artery (arrow = time of fibrinolysin administration). Data indicate that injection of the preparation (10 mg microspheres, 1,500 fibrinolytic units) into intact canine femoral artery caused a local increase in plasmin activity in the arterial blood, and increased fibrinolytic activity in the blood flowing from the drug deposition site and in the systemic circulation. In experimental thrombosis of the femoral artery, fibrinolytic activity of the whole blood is sharply decreased immediately after occlusion and increases directly after immobilized fibrinolysin infusion.

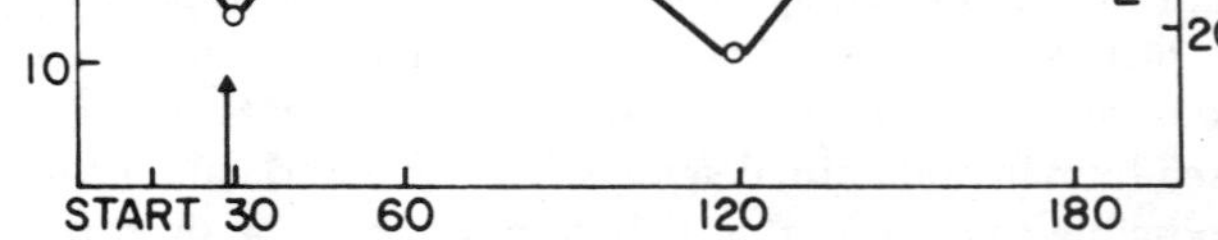

Figure 41.15. Reciprocal relation of plasminogen activator (1) and plasmin (2) activities following deposition of immobilized fibrinolysin. *Right axis*, plasminogen activator activity; *left axis*, plasmin activity (mm^2). *Arrow* = time of immobilized fibrinolysin administration.

spheric carriers (specifically, Sephadex) can successfully be used in the development of immobilized enzymes capable of being deposited in occluded arteries. As was already noted, intravascular administration of fibrinolytic agents has certain drawbacks. In this type of therapy, only an insignificant amount of the enzyme gets into the circulation. It is so small, compared with routine doses, that it may even be disregarded. At the same time, the possibility of enzyme inactivation is dramatically reduced.

Application of thrombolytic enzymes according to the suggested method has considerable advantages. The administration of fibrinolysin immobilized on microspheres of polysaccharide origin substantially increases fibrinolysis at the site of deposition, because of both the enzyme itself and the increased fibrinolytic activity of the blood. There currently are no principal limitations in therapy of peripheral thromboses and thromboembolism, including those of the pulmonary artery, with long-acting fibrinolytic agents.

Data on the diffusive ability of the myocardial capillary bed in ischemia may be regarded as a prerequisite to the application of various therapeutic agents (thrombolytic agents, hyaluronidase, insulin, etc) to therapy of ischemic heart disease via deposition of the agents directly in an ischemic or periinfarct zone.

DIRECTED DRUG TRANSPORT: PROSPECTS FOR APPLICATION IN THE PREVENTION AND TREATMENT OF THROMBOSIS

Thrombolytic therapy is placed in a dilemma. On the one hand, to create a high local concentration of a fibrinolytic agent requires the administration of large doses of the preparation into the systemic circulation. On the other hand, increased dosage is fraught with side effects. We think that a solution to the problem may be afforded by directed drug transport.

The main idea of directed drug transport is to achieve a significant concentration of the preparation in a given place using a vector substance that recognizes a pathologically altered zone due to distinctive features in the chemical structure of the latter.[38,39]

The two systems of directed transport that currently are being developed most intensively are: (1) direct coupling of a therapeutic agent to the vector[40] and (2) conjugation of a drug-bearing "microcontainer" to the vector.[41] Antibodies, certain hormones, lectins, and some other substances are used to specifically recognize lesion zones and deliver drugs or drug-bearing containers there.

Systems of the first type (drug-vector) are mostly intended to increase the efficacy of oncologic therapy. The accent is made on the development of immunotoxins, the complexes containing catalytic units of natural toxins (ricin and diphtheria toxin) bound to the antibodies with a given specificity. The antibodies recognizing the surface of a cancer cell deliver the toxin to the area of malignant growth; the toxins penetrate the cell and affect the ribosomes. Thus, they cause degradation of the tumor and achieve treatment success without affecting uninvolved tissues of the organ.

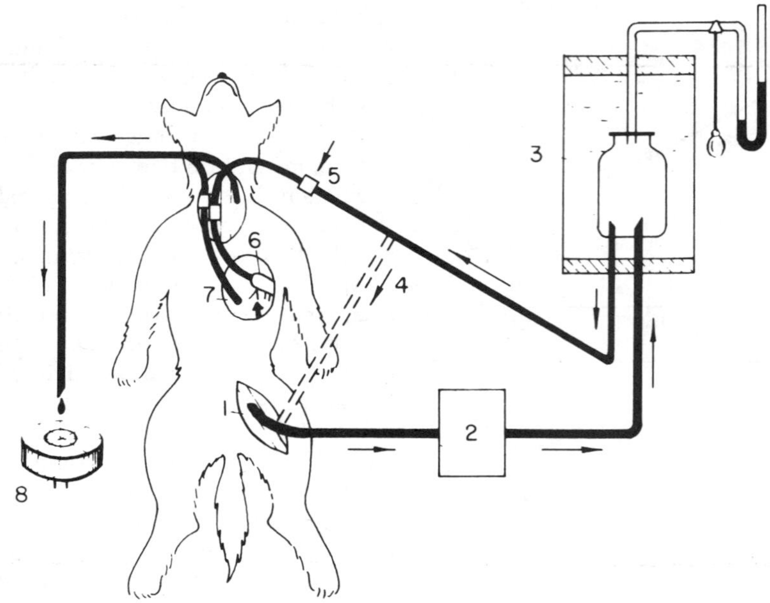

Figure 41.16. Schematic representation of the regulated coronary perfusion experiment (*arrows* show direction of blood flow). (1) femoral artery; (2) perfusion pump; (3) thermostatic vessel with a manometer; (4) shunt for switching the blood flow to perfusion of the left coronary artery; (5) flow meter; (6) left coronary artery; (7) venous coronary sinus; (8) collector for samples of blood flowing from the venous coronary sinus.

Research on the second type of systems has just started, but it is already clear that it has bright prospects in various fields of medicine. In these systems, antibodies to characteristic components of a tissue or organ are used as vectors.[41] The monoclonal antibodies seem to be the most hopeful, because they exhibit the highest degree of specificity in distinguishing the antigenic characteristics of lesion zones from those of healthy tissues.

At present, liposomes[41,42] and red blood cell membranes[43] are considered to be the most suitable containers. The drug encapsulated in a relatively large chamber (compared with the size of a drug molecule) is protected in the circulation from contact with blood by the inert membrane of a red blood cell or liposome. Therefore, the drug does not cause adverse effects. For the same reason, it is not prematurely degraded and exerts its effect only at a designated site.

The development of this new therapeutic approach was facilitated by elaboration of methods for stable fixation of antibody molecules to liposomes[44–47] and erythrocytes.[43] In the USSR Cardiology Research Center, my colleagues have worked out such binding procedures, which are accompanied neither by the loss of antibody properties nor by the destruction of the carrier membrane.

Presently, it is generally accepted that impairment of integrity of the vascular endothelial lining is the initial stage of thrombus formation, leading to denudation of collagen structures[48–50]; restoration of the endothelium does not occur until a thrombus is formed. Therefore, despite adhesion of platelets to this zone and formation of a thrombus head, collagen structures of the intima for a long time remain in contact with the blood.[48,50] Naturally, it is rather tempting to detect such sites of endothelial injury and exert a specific effect on them to prevent platelet adhesion to the denuded collagen (at early stages of thrombus formation) or deliver a fibrinolytic preparation there (at later stages), thus creating its high concentration only in the necessary zones.

To solve this problem we used antibodies to collagen as a vector, and liposomes and red blood cells as containers for directed drug transport to a zone of thrombus formation. We worked out a model of a damaged vessel wall to study its interaction with the systems: (1) liposome antibodies to collagen and (2) red blood cell antibodies to collagen. The model is a culture of endothelial cells derived from human umbilical vein and grown on a fibrillar collagen. By altering the conditions of culture, one can imitate the luminal surface of an unaffected vessel wall, or the one with punctate or vast endothelial damage (Figure 41.17).

To couple the antibodies to the surface of liposomes[41] and red blood cells, we have used the methods developed in the USSR Cardiology Research Center.

It was established in experiments (Table 41.5 and Figure 41.18) and on a model of deendothelialized rabbit aorta[51] that the obtained complexes (antibodies to collagen type I and III: liposomes) specifically recognize those parts of the surface that are not coated with endothelium. Analogous results were obtained in the experiments on perfused human and animal vessels. The obtained data make it possible to assume that this complex may be used for directed drug transport to the zone of a forming thrombus to increase the local concentration of fibrinolytic preparations.

Another system, antibodies to collagen-red blood cell, also seems to have good prospects for prevention and

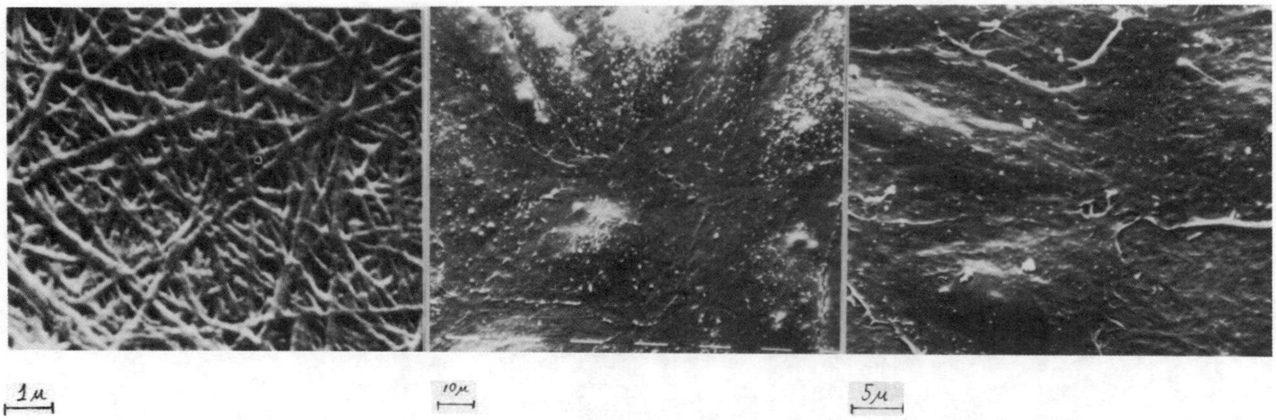

Figure 41.17. Models of the inner surface of a normal and damaged vessel wall. *Left*, Model of vast denudation. The bottom of multiwell wells was coated with fibrillar collagen; original magnification × 9,440. It can be regarded as an imitation of subendothelium in parts of the vessel wall with vast (about 2 cm^2) denuded areas. *Middle*, Model of punctate denudation. Confluent cultures of endothelial cells derived from human umbilical vein were cultured in collagen-coated wells (five days after seeding; original magnification × 1,300). By the third to fifth day in culture, cells covered 40% to 60% of the well bottom; size of intercellular gaps coated with collagen was 1,000 to 15,000 μm^2. The model imitates the structure of the luminal surface after local desquamation of one to ten endothelial cells. *Right*, Model of undamaged endothelium. Confluent cultures of endothelial cells were grown in collagen-coated wells (nine days after seeding; original magnification × 1,180). At confluency, the entire fibrillar collagen was coated with a dense monolayer of endothelial cells. The model imitates the structure of unaffected vascular luminal surface. Unlike animal models in which vast denudation of the subendothelium is performed in vivo using a balloon catheter, this one makes it possible to model different types of damage to the endothelial lining, from a punctate desquamation of one or several cells to vast deendothelialization.

therapy of thromboses. Both under the conditions of culture and in perfused vessel experiments, red blood cells bearing the antibodies to type I collagen effectively bind to deendothelialized vascular zones and uncoated areas in preconfluent endothelial cultures.

On the whole, the obtained evidence indicates that in principle the complexes of liposomes and erythrocytes with antibodies to collagen can be used for directed transport of fibrinolytic enzymes to the site of thrombosis. Surely, extreme caution should be exerted in extrapolating the available data and applying them to real clinical situations. Specifically, the discussed models are only an imitation of the processes occurring during thrombus formation in human arteries in vivo. Thus, for example, it cannot be ruled out that blood proteins may, to a certain extent, "mask" the antigenic collagen determinants. Without experimental verification, we cannot definitely conclude whether or not the in vivo hydrodynamic conditions would affect the "binding" of the complexes to deendothelialized zones. The available data, however, make it possible to assume even now that these effects would hardly be significant.

Specifically, the interaction of "pure" liposomes with collagen practically does not differ from that of the liposome-nonspecific immunoglobulin complexes.[41] At the same time, attachment of the antibodies to liposomes considerably increases the selectivity of their binding to a model deendothelialized vascular surface. Preliminary data also show that the addition of plasma proteins has no effect on the specificity of the liposome-antibody conjugate binding to a collagen substrate.

The experiments on perfused human and animal vessels make it possible to hope that the hydrodynamic factors related to the blood flow rate too would not have much influence on binding. A possibility of the in vivo application of such systems has already been demonstrated in dogs. The antibodies against canine heart muscle myosin covalently bound to liposomes were successfully targeted to a zone of experimental infarction.[52]

There is no doubt that the aforedescribed systems have good prospects, especially in the therapy of thrombosis. Actually, they would be a paragon of thrombolytic therapy affording the maximal concentration of a fibrinolytic agent at the site of thrombosis without side effects on hemostasis in other parts of the vascular tree. Among possible candidates for the application to directed drug transport, I would mention immobilized fibrinolysin,[37] streptodecase,[34] and stabilized urokinase, lately devel-

Table 41.5. Interaction of the Complex (Liposomes-Antibodies to Type I Collagen) with Endothelial Cultures of Different Density and Pure Collagen (Radioactivity Level, Degradation per Minute)

Collagen Type I	Growing Endothelium, Degree of "Coating," 40–50%	Confluent Endothelium, Degree of "Coating," 100%
11,970±616	4,178±320	1,702±74

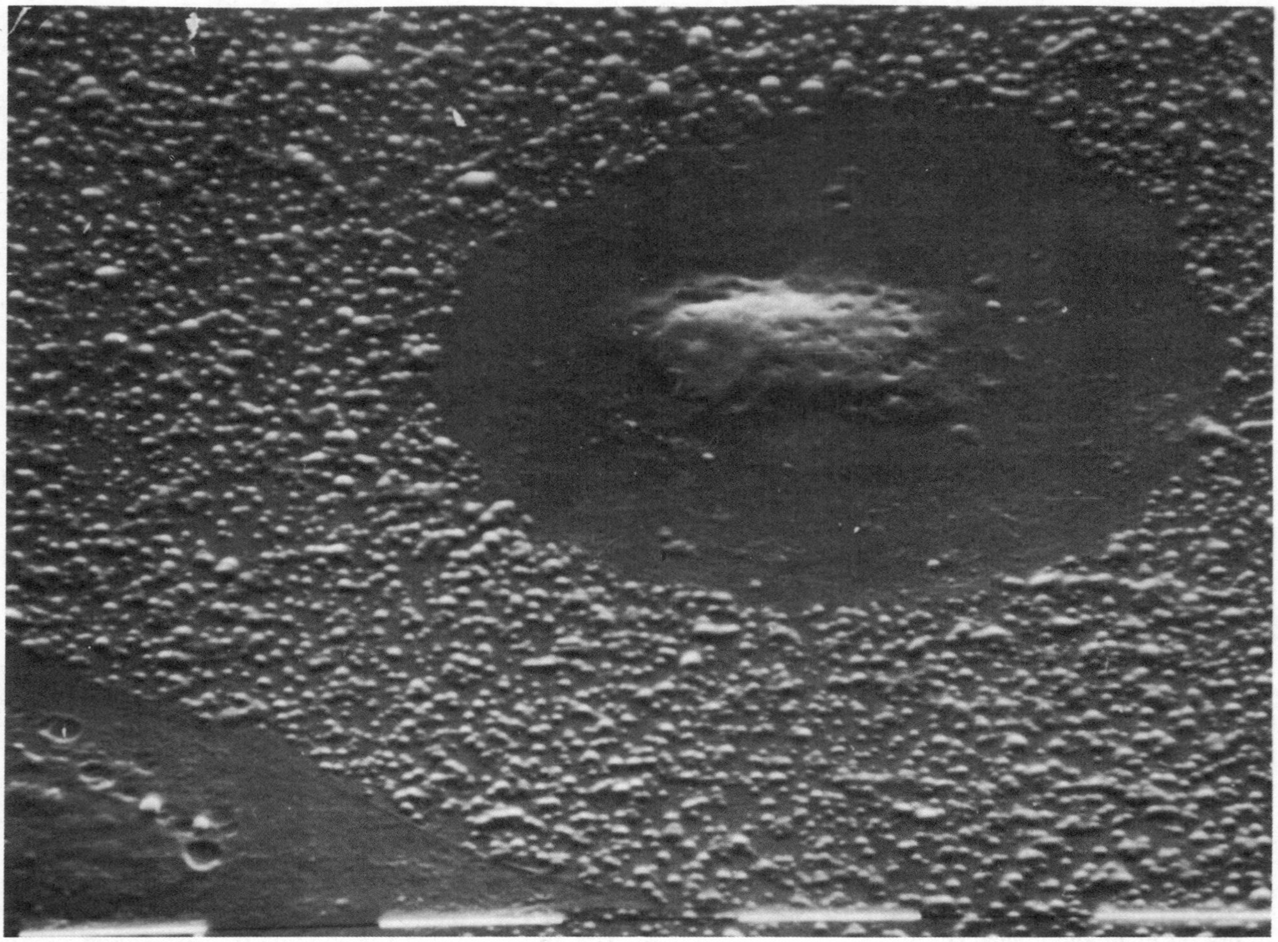

Figure 41.18. Scanning electron micrograph of the liposomes: collagen-specific antibody conjugates. Conjugates are bound to denuded collagen in a preconfluent endothelial culture, but they do not contact the endothelial surface (original magnification × 1,670).

oped in the USSR Cardiology Research Center. To create the most favorable conditions for thrombolysis and arrest the thrombus growth, the containers, in addition to fibrinolytic agents, may be loaded with heparin and the agents inhibiting platelet aggregation. This would considerably increase the efficacy of anticoagulants with direct action and antiaggregates at the site of thrombosis. Simultaneously, their systemic effects on the blood-clotting system and platelets would be abolished or substantially decreased. As is known, the impossibility of meeting these two requirements is mainly responsible for the side reactions caused by anticoagulants and platelet inhibitors, which bars their application to therapy of thrombosis and embolism.

REFERENCES

1. Virchow R: *Gesammelte Abhandlungen zur wissenschaftlichen Medicin*. Frankfurt, Meidinger Sohn u Comp, 1887.
2. Schmidt A: Uber die faserstoff Gerinnung. *Pflugers Arch* 1872; 6:413–428.
3. Hammarstein O: Weitere Beitrage zur Kenntiniss der Fibrinbildung. *Hoppe Seylers Z Physiol Chem* 1849; 28:98–119.
4. Morawitz P: Die Chemie der Blutgerinnung. *Ergeb der Physiol Biol Chem Exp Pharmacol* 1905; 4:307–326.
5. Chazov EI, Lakin KM: *Anticoagulants and Fibrinolytics*. Chicago, London, Year Book Medical Publishers Inc, 1981.
6. Kudryashov BA, Lapina LA: Nonenzymatic fibrinolysis and its role in the organism, in Chazov EI, Smirnov VN (eds): *Thrombosis and Thrombolysis*. New York, Plenum Press, 1984, pp 3–34.
7. Lakin KM, Makarov VA: Platelet aggregation inhibitors, in Chazov EI, Smirnov VN (eds): *Thrombosis and Thrombolysis*. New York, Plenum Press, 1984, pp 82–107.
8. Belitzer VE, Varetskaya TV: Fibrinogen-fibrin transformation, in Chazov EI, Smirnov VN (eds): *Thrombosis and Thrombolysis*. New York, Plenum Press, 1984, pp 1–2.
9. Engelberg H, Brown KD: *Heparin. Metabolism, Physiology and Clinical Application*. Springfield, Ill, Charles C Thomas, 1963.
10. Markwardt F: Gerinnungsphysiologic Analyse der Wirkung synthetischer Trombin inhibitoren. *Thromb Diath Haemorrh*. 1972; 27:99–104.
11. O'Brien JR, Etherington MD, Shuttlarooth RD: Ticlopidine, an antiplatelet drug: effect in human volunteers. *Thromb Res* 1978; 13:245–257.
12. Deutsch E: Vitamin k in medical practice: adults. *Vitam Horm* 1966; 24: 665–679.
13. Castellino FY: Recent advances in the chemistry of the fibrinolytic system. *Chem Rev* 1980; 81:431–446.
14. Collen D, Lijnen NR: The fibrinolytic system in man: an overview, in Verstraete M, Collen D, Lijnen HR (eds). *Thromobolysis: Biological and Therapeutic Properties of New Thrombolytic Agents*. London, Churchill Livingstone, 1985, pp 1–14.
15. Wiman B, Collen D: Molecular mechanisms of physiological fibrinolysis. *Nature* 1979; 272:549–550.
16. Ogston D: Natural activators of plasminogen, in Gaffney PJ, Balkuv-Ulutin S (eds): *Fibrinolysis: Current Fundamental and Clinical Concepts*. London, Academic Press, 1978, pp 1–15.

17. Andreenko IV: *Fibrinolysis (Biochemistry, Physiology, Pathology)*. Moscow, Moscow University Publishers, 1979.
18. Schmutzler R, Koller F: Die Thrombolyse Therapie. *Ergeb Inn Med* 1965; 22:157–162.
19. Jurgens J, Beller FK: *Klinische Methoden der Blutgerinnungsanalyse*. Stuttgart, Thieme, 1959.
20. Binger BR, Reissert J, Beckmann R: Isolation and characterization of a plasminogen activator (PA) from human myocardial tissue. *Thromb Haemost* 1981; 46:414–426.
21. Cole ER, Snopko RM: Physical, chemical and immunological properties of porcine and human plasminogen activator. *Thromb Haemost* 1981; 46:211–232.
22. Fletcher AP, Alkjaersig N, Sherry S, Genton E, Hirch J, Bachmann F: The development of urokinase as thrombolytic agents. *J Lab Clin Med* 1965; 65:713–727.
23. Stetter H: Fibrinolytische Therapie bei Verbrennungen, in Schneider KW (ed): *Fibrinolytische Therapie*. Marburg, Lahn, 1974, pp 105–129.
24. Suyama T, Shibuga Y: Urokinase: Clinico-pharmacological aspects about therapeutic dose in the treatment of thromboembolic disease. *Med Postgrad* 1970; 8:1–8.
25. Torchilin VP, Mazaev AV, Il'ina EV, Goldmacher VS, Smirnov VN, Chazov EI: Chemical aspects of enzyme modification and stabilization for use in therapy, in Wingard LB, Berezin IV, Klyosov AA (eds): *Future Directions for Enzyme Engineering*. New York, Plenum Press, 1979, pp 219–232.
26. Chazov EI, Matweyeva LS, Mazaev AV, Sargin KYe, Sadovskaya GV, Ruda MYa: Intracoronary injection of fibrinolysine during myocardial infarction. *Ter Arkh* 1976; 48:8–19.
27. Chazov EI, Mazaev AV, Torchilin VP, Smirnov VN: Possibilities of use of biocompatible preparations of immobilized enzymes and physiologically active compounds of prolonged action for treatment of thromboses and other diseases of cardiovascular system, in *Urgent Problems of Hemostasiology* (Russian). Moscow, Nauka, 1981, pp 327–336.
28. Torchilin VP, Bobkova AS, Smirnov VN, Chazov EI: Enzyme immobilization on biocompatible carriers. I. Immobilization of alpha-chymotrypsin on modified sephadexes. *Bioorg Chem* 1976; 2:116–124.
29. Chazov EI, Mazaev AV, Suvorova LA, Suvorov AV, Torchilin VP, Smirnov VN: Effect of the new Soviet preparation streptodecase in fibrinolysis system. *Kardiologiia* 1981; 8:18–26.
30. Chazov EI, Mazaev AV, Voronkov YuI, Suvorova LA: Streptodecase, New Soviet thrombolytic preparation of prolonged action. *Ter Arkh* 1981; 9:79–83.
31. Chazov EI: *Thromboses and Embolism in the Clinical Treatment of Internal Disease* (Russian). Moscow, Meditsina, 1967, pp 262–267.
32. Chazov EI, Golikov AP: Use of streptodecase in acute myocardial infarction. *Kardiologiia* 1981; 12:10–18.
33. Ilyin VN, Voronkov YI, Rodionov SV, Savelyev VS, Chazov EI: Successful treatment by streptodecase of massive thromboembolism of pulmonary artery combined with extensive acute myocardial infarction. *Ter Arkh* 1982; 11:140–153.
34. Chazov EI, Gundorova RA, Romashenko AD, Mazaev AV, Torchilin VP: Immobilized streptokinase (streptodecase) in treatment of intraocular hemorrhages. *Vestn Oftalmol* 1982; 4:61–67.
35. Torchilin VP, Rejzer IL, Il'ina EV: Principles of prolongation of enzymatic preparations, in Chazov EI, Morgan H (eds): *Myocardial Metabolism* (Russian). Moscow, Meditsina, 1979, pp 362–367.
36. Bessolitzina LA, Mazaev AV, Suvorov AA, Torchilin VP: Effect of biosoluble microspheres of immobilized fibrinolysin on fibrinolysis system. *Bull Exp Biol Med* 1980; 1:16–19.
37. Mazaev AV, Ginzburg EM, Serebryakova LI, Torchilin VP, Chazov EI: Microcirculation state in myocardial ischemia and its changes after deposition of Sephadex biosoluble microspheres in coronary bed. *Kardiologiia* 1979; 10:45–49.
38. Copley AL: Fibrinogen, platelets, and a new theory of atherosclerosis. *Thromb Res* 1979; 14:249–266.
39. Barnhart MI, Chen S: Vessel wall models for studying interaction capabilities with blood platelets. *Semin Thromb Hemostas* 1978; 5:112–129.
40. Gregoriadis G: Targeting of drugs. *Nature* 1977; 265:407–409.
41. Smirnov VN, Berdichevsky VR, Alexeev AB, Sviridov DD, Torchilin VP: Targeted liposome transport to the reconstituted vessel wall, in Chazov EI, Smirnov VN (eds): *Vessel Wall in Athero- and Thrombogenesis*. Berlin, Heidelberg, New York, Springer-Verlag, 1982, pp 195–206.
42. Sinha D, Karush F: Attachment to membranes of exogenous immunoglobulin conjugated to a hydrophobic anchor. *Biochem Biophys Res Commun* 1980; 90:554–561.
43. Samokhin GP, Smirnov MD, Myzukantov VR, Smirnov VN: Red blood cell targeting to collagen-coated surfaces. *FEBS Lett* 1983; 154:247–253.
44. Torchilin VP, Goldmacher VS, Smirnov VN: Comparative study on covalent and noncovalent immobilization of enzymes on the surface of liposomes. *Biochem Biophys Res Commun* 1978; 85:983–996.
45. Torchilin VP, Klibanov AL: Preliminary hydrophobization of hydrophilic protein improves its binding with liposomes. *Bioorg Khim* 1980; 6:791–803.
46. Heath TD, Robertson D, Birbeck MSC: Covalent attachment of horseradish peroxidase to the outer surface of liposome. *Biochim Biophys Acta* 1980; 599:42–49.
47. Torchilin VP, Khaw BA, Smirnov VN, Haber E: Preservation of antimyosin antibody activity after covalent coupling to liposomes. *Biochem Biophys Res Commun* 1979; 89:114–124.
48. Weiss HJ: Platelet physiology and abnormalities of platelet function. *N Engl J Med* 1975; 293:531–541, 580–588.
49. Gordon JL, Milner AJ: Blood platelets as multifunctional cells, in Gordon JL (ed): *Platelets in Biology and Pathology*. Amsterdam, New York, Oxford, Elsevier/North Holland Biomedical Press, 1976, pp 3–15.
50. Mustard JF, Packham MA: Platelets and thrombosis in the development of atherosclerosis and its complications, in Day HJ, Molony BA, Nishizawa EE (eds): *Thrombosis Animal and Clinical Models*. New York, London, Plenum Press, 1978, pp 7–18.
51. Leytin VL, Sviridov DD: A model for studying platelet interaction with cellular and macromolecular constituents of the vessel wall in vitro, in Chazov EI, Smirnov VN (eds): *Vessel Wall in Athero- and Thrombogenesis*. New York, Springer-Verlag, 1982, pp 173–192.
52. Chazov EI: Advances and perspectives of thrombo- and atherosclerosis. Studies in the USSR, in Chazov EI, Smirnov VN (eds): *Vessel Wall in Athero- and Thrombogenesis*. New York, Springer-Verlag, 1982, pp 216–227.

42 The Randomized Control Trials of Prevention of Myocardial Infarction

Thomas C. Chalmers, MD

The primary prevention of acute myocardial infarction (AMI) is an ideal case study of international cardiologic research because it illustrates so many of the problems and successes of large scale cooperative studies, often carried out across international boundaries. The problem is ideally suited to randomized control trials (RCTs) because the endpoints are few and finite and the treatments are generally based on our current knowledge of the pathophysiologic abnormalities of the disease. Although the reduction in coronary incidence or death rate to be expected from any one therapy is low, the worldwide medical importance of a significant reduction is enormous in terms of total lives saved and money spent for health care. It is therefore most important to document any potential improvements as small as 10% by multiple large scale studies.

Because some RCTs have combined patients who have had a clinically documented infarction with those who have not, and because asymptomatic infarcts are common, this review does not always distinguish between primary and secondary prevention of infarction.

The studies outlined herein illustrate the need for meticulous gathering of data after careful control of blinding in the random assignment of therapies.[1] Another challenging problem is that of using surrogate endpoints that may be more common and therefore determinable by smaller numbers, but it may be less meaningful. Many studies show a reduction in coronary deaths plus nonfatal myocardial infarctions (AMI incidence), but little or no change in the overall death rate.[2–14] The question persists as to whether that is due to the fact that patients were not followed long enough on or off therapy, or if therapy was the cause of death from noncardiovascular causes in some patients while saving others.[4,7] This question often requires the follow-up of patients much longer than they have been up to the present, and the study of many more patients than have been included, even though the numbers are already large.

The existence of multiple studies of the same agent or minor modifications of the same agent in a common disease, and the existence of standardized criteria for diagnosing the disease make this an ideal subject for the new science of meta-analysis.[15,16] By this term is meant the combining of results from multiple research projects so that conclusions can be drawn from all of the studies and their statistical significance determined, when any one individual study is too small or too variant to give a reliable answer. Meta-analysis is useful when the studies show a trend in one direction that only becomes statistically significant when they are combined. It is useful when studies are statistically significantly positive or negative, but there is a need to narrow down the estimate of range of difference between treated and control patients. It is helpful when studies have disparate conclusions, because the discrepancies may be attributable to the differences in quality, for example, efficiency in the control of bias, or to differences in patient material or treatment, all of which can be measured. Finally, meta-analysis in such situations is useful because subgroups of patients (which are almost always too small so conclusions from individual trials are not anticipated) may be combined to suggest meaningful results when all the trials are put together. However, the dangers of drawing conclusions from retrospective analyses must be kept in mind. Meta-analyses of most of the trials to be outlined herein have been carried out.[17–31]

If studies are to be combined, they not only have to be concerned with similar agents in similar patients but also have to be of adequate quality. Methods are now available for assessing the quality of randomized control trials in a quantitative manner, so that those with varying degrees of poor quality can be dropped and a determination made as to whether or not the results are consistent no matter what the quality of the trials.[32] Presumably, bias or other factors may prejudice the outcome sufficiently to distort meta-analysis, and even meta-analyses may suffer from unrecognized biases.[33]

Finally, there is one more technologic point that needs

to be emphasized: the importance of multifactorial trials. It is apparent that different etiologic factors cause AMI and that drugs that attack those factors separately may or may not be cumulatively effective. Studying more than one agent in a factorial study will indicate whether or not there is interaction, and if there is not, the efficacy of each independent therapy can be determined with half the number of patients that would be required to study first one and then the other. However, in secondary prevention, it is now too late to do a factorial designed study of two agents compared with a no-treatment control, because the no-treatment control is no longer justified in most patients. Evidence is strong that at least two different kinds of therapy, antiplatelet drugs and beta blockers, are effective.[14,18,20,23,29,31] However, the less efficient three-arm studies might still be ethically performed

EXAMPLES OF MULTIPLE TYPES OF STUDIES SO FAR PERFORMED

LONG-TERM ANTICOAGULANT THERAPY

Anticoagulants are the oldest drugs used to prevent recurrent AMI. A few studies have shown some effect, but the results have been variable, possibly because of the inadequate quality of the older studies. The summation of effects is barely positive.[26]

THROMBOLYTIC ENZYMES

The administration of thrombolytic enzymes as soon as possible after admission to the hospital for AMI has been the subject of RCTs with long-term follow-up. The situation is complicated by the variable treatment received by patients after the thrombolysis was attempted. Meta-analysis of all the studies, however,[31] shows a highly significant reduction in long-term mortality brought about by early attempts to lyse the thrombus in the coronary arteries. This plus suggestive data on anticoagulant therapy and, as will be shown, the effectiveness of antiplatelet drugs confirms the hypothesis that thrombosis, at least in part, contributes to the myocardial damage that occurs when a coronary artery is plugged.

ANTIPLATELET DRUGS

Aspirin was suggested over 10 years ago as a preventive in this field,[34] but it was not taken seriously until the last 10 years. As reviewed in a meta-analysis by Canner[20] and an unsigned one by Peto,[29] six major studies, although not statistically significantly positive, add up to a real effect by aspirin in prolonging life as well as in reducing the incidence of coronary disease. The difference is small, however, and it has taken a large number of patients to establish.

Other drugs affecting platelets that have been tried in large-scale long-term trials are sulfinpyrazone (Anturane®) and dipyridamole (Persantine®). The latter has been combined with aspirin because the side effects of Persantine in doses large enough to affect platelet function are too great.

The Anturane-Reinfarction Trials[12,13] and the Persantine-Aspirin Reinfarction studies (PARIS)[14,35] are excellent examples of large-scale long-term trials supported by pharmaceutical houses. They can be contrasted because of their method of funding. In the former, the coordinating center and data analysis center were within the pharmaceutical firm that was supporting the study. In the latter, it was an independent operation supported by a grant and supervised by a Policy Advisory Board that made all decisions irrespective of the wishes of the pharmaceutical firm. In the Anturane-Reinfarction Trials, there were many withdrawals after randomization and during analysis for various reasons, and the Food and Drug Administration (FDA) has refused to approve the drug because of the appearance of bias in determining which patients were included and which were removed in the major trial.[36] No such question has arisen in the PARIS trials. The first showed a trend favoring Persantine–aspirin over aspirin and placebo; in the second, when Persantine and aspirin were compared with a placebo in 50% more patients, a statistically significant difference in the incidence of coronary disease was demonstrated, but still there was no difference in overall mortality. None of the side effects in either instance were fatal. Although the largest of the single trials of aspirin, the Aspirin Myocardial Infarction Study (AMIS),[37] was negative, evidence from all studies indicates that patients should be on some antiplatelet drugs after AMI. Whether or not the consistent changes in the incidence of coronary disease will eventually be followed by a reduction in overall mortality remains to be seen. Recent evidence of a long-term effect of nicotinic acid suggests that this effect will occur.[38]

BETA BLOCKERS

Here the evidence is stronger and there are a number of individual studies that are statistically significantly positive. Meta-analysis has confirmed that the drugs were effective in reducing long-term mortality.[17,18,22,25,27,28] However, the contraindications to long-term beta-blocker therapy are serious and fairly well defined, such that about 25% of patients do not qualify according to the present state of our knowledge.

ANTIARRHYTHMIC AGENTS

In contrast to the aforementioned agents, all of whose trials tend to give positive results, in this case the group of drugs tends to have a negative effect on survival.[39] There is no doubt that the drugs diminish the frequency of arrhythmias, but it is most unlikely that they could prolong survival.

CHOLESTEROL-LOWERING THERAPIES

Epidemiologic evidence is overwhelming that AMI is associated with elevated serum cholesterol.[40,41] Whether or not lowering the cholesterol level after an infarction has occurred, by either drugs or diet, will decrease both the incidence of AMI and the overall mortality has been the subject of much debate. The granddaddy of all post-myocardial infarction studies, the Coronary Drug Project, began 20 years ago to investigate the then popular agents, the estrogens, in two doses, clofibrate, T4, and nicotinic acid.[5,6] Only the last had a significant effect on the incidence of AMI, and in the ensuing 10 years, when the patients stopped receiving the drug, the difference in overall mortality had reached statistical significance.[38] This could be a chance event or it could illustrate that if a myocardial infarction is prevented, the patient has a greater likelihood of living longer even though the drug is not continued after that time. More follow-up studies with trends in the incidence of AMI need to be carried out. Clofibrate had essentially no effect and is no longer used because of the long-term primary prevention trial in Europe[7] which showed that although the incidence of AMI was reduced, the rate of cancer and the overall mortality were significantly greater in the patients receiving clofibrate. The effects of diet[2,3,42] or the cholesterol-lowering agent, cholestyramine,[10,11] have been studied with suggestive positive results as primary treatment, but no therapy has shown a reduction in overall mortality among patients who have and have not already had an infarct. In fact, the large Coronary Primary Prevention Trial of the Lipid Research Clinics[10,11] was barely positive even though the patients were in the upper 5% category with regard to cholesterol levels.

The final answer to the question of secondary prevention will be obtainable from the study now going on known as the Program on the Surgical Control of the Hyperlipidemias (POSCH). In this case, half of 800 patients had the serum cholesterol decreased by 30% and the low density lipoprotein cholesterol decreased by 40%[43] as the result of ileal bypass surgery, and they will be followed as long as they or the investigators live to determine whether close to 100% compliance with a procedure that drastically decreases low density lipoprotein cholesterol has any effect on overall mortality.

The final answer to the primary prevention challenge can only be forthcoming if the countries with high rates of coronary disease are willing to support expensive long-term trials of diet and drugs among persons in all risk categories. Most studies so far completed have been undersized.[44]

In summary, drug therapy during and after a first AMI does seem to reduce recurrences. The evidence for primary prevention by diet or effective drugs if any become available is suggestive enough to warrant their use in high risk patients, but there is as yet no proof that changing the diet of all persons in industrialized countries by more than a moderate amount will prolong life. Not enough is known about the long-term side effects of lowering serum cholesterol of those in low risk categories to warrant a drastic change in diet among the young as well as the old. This statement is made in the presence of overwhelming epidemiologic evidence and suggestive trends in controlled trials, because proof ought to be available before all persons are subject to severe changes in lifestyles. The fault lies not in the work of the epidemiologists and those throughout the world who have conducted inconclusive RCTs, but rather with the policymakers and the economists who have been unwilling or unable to recognize that an enormously devastating and expensive epidemic requires for its elimination the bold expenditure of large amounts of money for research, much more than has so far been spent and much less than the disease crying out for prevention costs the public each year.

Acknowledgment: This study was supported in part by Grant No. LM031116 from the National Library of Medicine to Mount Sinai School of Medicine, New York, New York.

REFERENCES

1. Chalmers TC, Celano P, Sacks HS, Smith HS Jr: Bias in treatment assignment in controlled clinical trials. *N Engl J Med* 1983; 309:1358–1361.
2. Leren P: The Oslo diet–heart study. Eleven-year report. *Circulation* 1970; 42:935–942.
3. Dayton S, Pearce ML, Hashimoto S, Dixon WJ, Tomiyasu U: *A controlled clinical trial of a diet high in unsaturated fat in preventing complications of atherosclerosis.* American Heart Association Monograph No. 25:II-1–II-63, 1969.
4. Pearce ML, Dayton S: Incidence of cancer in men on a diet high in polyunsaturated fat. *Lancet* 1971; 1:464–467.
5. Trial of clofibrate in the treatment of ischemic heart disease. Five-year study by a group of physicians of the Newcastle upon Tyne region. *Br Med J* 1971; 4:767–775.
6. Coronary Drug Project Research Group: Clofibrate and niacin in coronary heart disease. *JAMA* 1975; 231:360–381.
7. Oliver MF, Heady JA, Morris JN, Cooper J: WHO cooperative trial on primary prevention of ischemic heart disease using clofibrate to lower serum cholesterol: mortality follow-up. Report of the Committee of Principal Investigators. *Lancet* 1980; 2:379–385.
8. Carlson LA, Danielson M, Ekberg I, Klintemar B, Rosenhamer G: Reduction of myocardial reinfarction by the combined treatment of clofibrate and nicotinic acid. *Atherosclerosis* 1977; 28:81–86.
9. Miettinen M, Turpeinen O, Karvonen MJ, Elosuo R, Paavilainen E: Effect of cholesterol-lowering diet on mortality from coronary heart-disease and other causes. A twelve-year clinical trial in men and women. *Lancet* 1972; 2:835–838.
10. Lipid Research Clinics Program: The Lipid Research Clinics Coronary Primary Prevention Trial results. I. Reduction in incidence of coronary heart disease. *JAMA* 1984; 251:351–364.
11. Lipid Research Clinics Program: The Lipid Research Clinics Primary Prevention Trial Results. II. The relationship of reduction in incidence of coronary heart disease to cholesterol lowering. *JAMA* 1984; 251:365–374.
12. The Anturane Reinfarction Trial Research Group: Sulfinpyrazone in the prevention of sudden death after myocardial infarction. *N Engl J Med* 1980; 302:250–256.
13. Report from the Anturan Reinfarction Italian Study: Sulphinpyrazone in post-myocardial infarction. *Lancet* 1982; 1:237–242.
14. Prepared for the Investigator Group by Klimt CR, Knatterud GL, Stamler J, Meier P: Persantine–Aspirin Reinfarction Study. Part II. Secondary coronary prevention with Persantine and aspirin. *J Am Coll Cardiol* 1986; 7:251–269.
15. Glass GV: Primary, secondary and meta-analysis of research. *Educational Researcher* 1976; 10:3–8.
16. Smith ML, Glass GV: Meta-analysis of psychotherapy overcome studies. *Am Psychol* 1977; 32:752–760.
17. Baber NS, Lewis JA: Confidence in results of beta-blocker postinfarction trials. *Br Med J* 1982; 284:1749–1750.
18. Baber NS, Lewis JA: Beta-adrenoceptor blockade and myocardial infarction: when should treatment start and for how long should it continue? *Circulation* 1983; 67(suppl I):I-71–I-77.
19. Bassan MM, Shalev O, Eliakin A: Improved prognosis during long-term treatment with beta-blockers after myocardial infarction: analysis of randomized trials and pooling of results. *Heart and Lung* 1984; 13(2):164–168.
20. Canner PL: Aspirin in coronary heart disease. Comparison of six clinical trials. *Isr J Med Sci* 1983; 19:413–423.
21. DeSilva RA, Hennekens CH, Lown B, Casscells W: Lignocaine prophylaxis in acute myocardial infarction: an evaluation of randomised trials. *Lancet* 1981; 2:855–858.
22. Furberg CD, Bell R: Effect of beta-blocker therapy on recurrent nonfatal myocardial infarction. *Circulation* 1983; 67 (suppl I):I-83–I-85.
23. Furberg CD, May GS: Effect of long-term prophylactic treatment on survival after myocardial infarction. *Am J Med* 1984; 76:76–83.
24. Goldman L, Batsford WP: Risk–benefit stratification as a guide to lidocaine prophylaxis of primary ventricular fibrillation in acute myocardial infarction: an analytic review. *Yale J Biol Med* 1979; 52:455–466.
25. Frishman WH, Furberg CD, Friedewald WT: Drug therapy: Beta-adrenergic blockade for survivors of acute myocardial infarction. *N Engl J Med* 1984; 310:830–837.
26. Leizorovicz A, Boissel JP: Oral anticoagulant in patients surviving myocardial infarction. A new approach to old data. *Eur J Clin Pharmacol* 1983; 24:333–336.
27. Lewis JA: Beta-blockade after myocardial infarction—A statistical view. *Br J Clin Pharmacol* 1982; 14:15S–21S.
28. Lewis JA, Ellis SH: A statistical appraisal of postinfarction beta-blocker trials. *Prim Cardiol* 1982; (suppl 1):31–37.
29. Peto R: Aspirin after myocardial infarction. *Lancet* 1980; 1:1172–1173.

30. Tran ZV, Weltman A, Glass GV, Mood DP: The effects of exercise on blood lipids and lipoproteins: a meta-analysis of studies. *Med Sci Sports Exerc* 1983; 15:393–402.
31. Stampfer MJ, Goldhaber SZ, Yusuf S, Peto R, Hennekens CH: Effect of intravenous streptokinase on acute myocardial infarction: pooled results from randomized trials. *N Engl J Med* 1982; 307:1180–1182.
32. Chalmers TC, Smith H Jr, Blackburn B, Silverman B, Schroeder B, Reitman D, Ambroz A: A method for assessing the quality of a randomized control trial. *Controlled Clin Trials* 1981; 2:31–49.
33. Kussin PS, Chalmers TC, Reitman D, Messer J, Sacks HS: A saga of meta-analysis. The relationship between steroid therapy and peptic ulcer disease. (Unpublished data, March 1986).
34. Boston Collaborative Drug Surveillance Group: Regular aspirin intake and acute myocardial infarction. *Br Med J* 1974; 1:440–443.
35. The Persantine–Aspirin Reinfarction Study Research Group: Persantine and aspirin in coronary heart disease. *Circulation* 1980; 62:449–461.
36. Temple R, Pledger GW: The FDA's critique of the Anturane Reinfarction Trial. *N Engl J Med* 1980; 303:1488–1492.
37. Aspirin Myocardial Infarction Study Research Group: A randomized, controlled trial of aspirin in persons recovered from myocardial infarction. *JAMA* 1980; 243:661–669.
38. Canner PL for the CDP Research Group: Mortality in Coronary Drug Project patients during a 9-year post-treatment period (abstr). *J Am Coll Cardiol* 1985; 5:442.
39. May GS, Eberlein KA, Furberg CD, Passamani ER, DeMets DL: Secondary prevention after myocardial infarction: a review of long-term trials. *Prog Cardiovasc Dis* 1982; 24:331–352.
40. Keys A (ed): Coronary heart disease in seven countries. *Circulation* 1970; 41(suppl I):1–211.
41. Stamler J, Kaplan NM (eds): *Prevention of Coronary Heart Disease.* Philadelphia, WB Saunders Co, 1983, pp 188–207.
42. Diet–Heart Review Panel of the National Heart Institute. *Mass field trials of the diet–heart question. Their significance, timeliness, feasibility and applicability. An assessment of seven proposed experimental designs.* American Heart Association Monograph 1969; No. 28, pp 1–44.
43. Moore RB, Buchwald H, Varco RL, and Participants on the Surgical Control of the Hyperlipidemias: The effect of partial ileal bypass on plasma liproproteins. *Circulation* 1980; 62:469–476.
44. Freiman JA, Chalmers TC, Smith H Jr, Kuebler RR: The importance of beta, the type II error and sample size in the design and interpretation of the randomized control trial. Survey of 71 "negative" trials. *N Engl J Med* 1978; 299:690–694.

43 Cardiomyopathy and Myocarditis

John F. Goodwin, MD, FRCP, FACP, FACC

DEFINITION OF CARDIOMYOPATHY

Cardiomyopathy is defined as a "disorder of cardiac muscle of unknown cause"[1]; myocardial disorders that are part of a general system disease are defined as specific heart muscle diseases.[2-4] It is important to make this distinction, otherwise true cardiomyopathies become obscured by the large numbers of specific heart muscle diseases. This chapter will concentrate on the cardiomyopathies and on myocarditis and its relation to cardiomyopathy; certain of the rare specific heart muscle diseases will be dealt with briefly to illuminate the contrasts.

CLASSIFICATION OF CARDIOMYOPATHY

The cardiomyopathies are classified into three main groups on the basis of different disorders of structure and function. These include hypertrophic cardiomyopathy, dilated (congestive) cardiomyopathy, and restrictive cardiomyopathy. It should be emphasised that these groups are distinct and do not merge one into the other.

Hypertrophic cardiomyopathy is a genetically determined disorder characterised by massive hypertrophy of the left ventricle (and sometime of the right) with reduced systolic volume, powerful contraction, increased ventricular stiffness, and impaired relaxation. There is commonly asymmetrical hypertrophy of the septum, and systolic pressure gradients are often found within the left ventricle. In some patients, gradients are absent and the hypertrophy is symmetrical. The coronary arteries are large, smooth, and patent.

Dilated (congestive) cardiomyopathy is characterised by severely impaired pump function of both ventricles with dilatation of the ventricular cavities and moderate ventricular hypertrophy. It is a multifactorial syndrome, with congestive heart failure of unknown origin as its principal feature.

Restrictive cardiomyopathy is characterized by restriction of ventricular filling as a result of rigid unyielding endocardial, subendocardial, or myocardial disease that impairs ventricular distention. Initially there is good pump function. The most common cause is endomyocardial fibrosis with or without eosinophilia. Amyloid disease of the heart induces a restrictive syndrome but with marked differences from endomyocardial fibrosis. Apart from these three clearly defined groups, there is a fourth indeterminate group in which lie conditions that cannot with certainty be defined as cardiomyopathies. These include multiple arrhythmias, connective tissue disorders, the long QT syndrome, prolapse of the mitral valve, and angina with "normal" coronary arteries.

Terminology is important. Elimination refers to disappearance of the ventricular cavity by compression and apposition of its walls. Obstruction refers to organic mechanical hindrance to ventricular outflow; resistance to filling refers to hindrance to ventricular filling, caused by a stiff, poorly compliant hypertrophied ventricle that relaxes abnormally. Restriction to filling refers to organic interference resulting from endomyocardial disease of the ventricle with endocardial fibrosis and thrombosis. Obliteration refers to reduction in ventricular cavity size due to organic material within the cavity.

HYPERTROPHIC CARDIOMYOPATHY

PATHOLOGY

Examination of the gross specimen of the heart reveals massive hypertrophy. Often this is asymmetrical, involving the ventricular septum out of proportion to the rest of the ventricular musculature. The bulge of the septum is usually in the proximal part, but it may be diffuse throughout the septum in its midportion or at the apex. The papillary muscles of the mitral valve are large and participate in the hypertrophy. Displacement of the anterior papillary muscle is often prominent. Endocardial thickening beneath the aortic valve is common. Secondary thickening of the valve leaflets may be observed, and, on occasion, calcification has been noted. Patchy fibrosis can be seen throughout the hypertrophied muscle. In severe cases the marked disproportion between massive hypertrophy and the slit-like ventricular cavity is remarkable.

HISTOLOGY

Histological examination shows extreme hypertrophy of the muscle fibers, which are often arranged in short runs with a tendency to form whorls. The nuclei are large, bizarre in shape, and often surrounded by clear, perinuclear haloes. The intramyocardial arterioles usually are normal, although internal thickening may be found in branches in the region of the septum. There may be some thickening of the endocardium. The extramural coronary arteries are normal.

ELECTRON MICROSCOPY

On electron microscopy, myofibrillar disarray is prominent and usually extensive. Histochemical studies show severe accumulation of glycogen. Although myofibrillar disarray occurs in the normal fetal heart at an appropriate stage in its development and has been found in other forms of heart disease, it is much more extensive in hypertrophic cardiomyopathy.[1,3,5] When combined with the changes on light microscopy, the diagnosis can usually be confirmed, but the disease is patchy and biopsy studies may not always sample representative areas.

AETIOLOGY

There is little doubt that hypertrophic cardiomyopathy is a distinct entity and not merely the result of other influences acting on the heart, because it is frequently found in the absence of other heart disease or any cause for myocardial hypertrophy. There may be a link between catecholamines, endocrine disorders, and hypertrophic cardiomyopathy. Administration of nerve growth factor to dogs can cause hypertrophy, pressure gradients, and myocardial fiber disarray. Noradrenalin in subhypertensive doses also causes hypertrophic cardiomyopathy in dogs.[6,7] Clinical investigation reveals that adrenergic stimulation increases pressure gradients and reduces diastolic compliance of the left ventricle, whereas beta-adrenergic blockade reverses these effects. There is an association between disorders of catecholamines and neural crest tissue, on the one hand, and hypertrophic cardiomyopathy, on the other. Systemic hypertension is present in around 10% of patients with hypertrophic cardiomyopathy. Additional evidence of endocrine involvement includes the reversible hypertrophic cardiomyopathy noted in the infants of diabetic mothers and the production of myofibrillar disarray in the hearts of fetuses of pregnant rats given triiodothyroacetic acid (triac).[8] There is an association between hyperthyroidism, hyperinsulinism, and hypertrophic cardiomyopathy. Hypertrophic cardiomyopathy may be a genetically determined disorder of handling of catecholamines by the developing fetal heart.[9,10] It is possible that failure of the normal regression of disproportionate septal thickness and myocardial fibral disarray in foetal life might occur because of faulty interaction between noradrenalin and myocardial receptor sites. The absence or deficiency in amount of some factor necessary for these developmental changes might also be considered.

CLINICAL FEATURES

Hypertrophic cardiomyopathy has a wide spectrum of severity and symptoms. Many patients have no symptoms at all. Symptoms, when they occur, tend to consist of breathlessness on exertion, chest pain of anginal type usually on effort but sometimes at rest, palpitations, dizziness, and syncope. The clinical signs are largely determined by the presence or absence of systolic pressure gradients within the left ventricle and on the presence or absence of significant mitral regurgitation.

When pressure gradients are appreciable and persistent, there are three characteristic physical signs. The first is the character of the arterial pulse which is ill-sustained, jerky, but of normal volume. The second is the characteristic systolic murmur which begins after the first heart sound and is heard maximally at the left sternal edge and the apex[11] (Figure 43.1). It is of the ejection type. The third physical sign is the palpable left atrial beat which can be felt preceding the powerful left ventricular thrust, although it may be necessary to turn the patient onto the

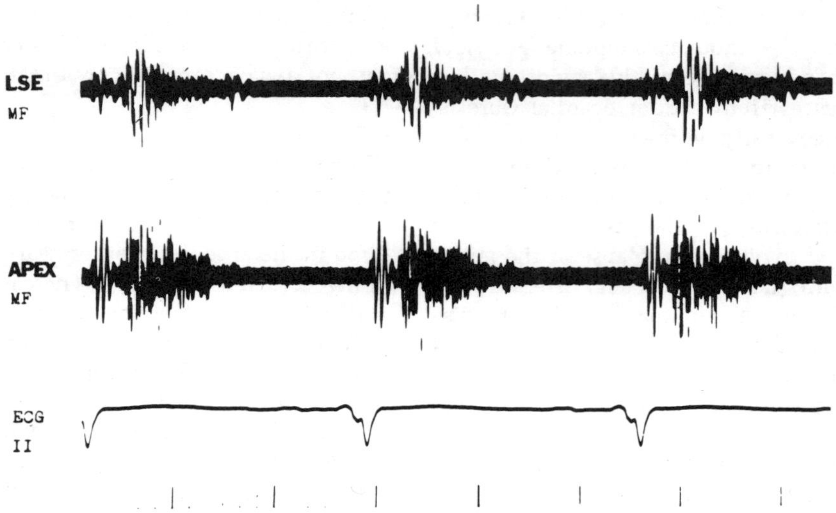

Figure 43.1. Phonocardiograms showing ejection systolic murmur of delayed onset after first heart sound at left sternal edge (LSE) and apex. MF = medium frequency. (From Goodwin,[11] with permission.)

left side to appreciate it. Apart from these physical signs the second heart sound may be single or have a reversed split if aortic valve closure is delayed. There is not infrequently a third sound, but only occasionally a fourth sound; sometimes there may be a soft diastolic rumble at the apex due either to the stiff left ventricle with impaired relaxation or to disproportionate hypertrophy of the septum jutting into the inflow tract of the left ventricle, simulating mitral stenosis. The jugular venous pressure is usually normal, but in patients with right-sided involvement there may be a prominent "a" wave.

In patients with no pressure gradients there may be no abnormal physical signs, but usually the pulse is somewhat ill-sustained and an atrial beat may be felt. Patients are usually remarkable for their excellent physical development. Skeletal abnormalities are unusual and many patients are extremely active despite the disease.

DIFFERENTIAL DIAGNOSIS

The differential diagnosis (Table 43.1) can be very wide indeed. It depends mainly on the clinical features and most importantly, the three clinical signs already mentioned. When there is a systolic murmur of late onset, the main differential diagnosis is of mitral valve prolapse, whereas chordal rupture and papillary muscle failure are also contenders.

When there is a full length systolic murmur, rheumatic mitral regurgitation is to be suspected and is particularly likely to cause confusion if atrial fibrillation and valvular calcification are present. Ventricular septal defects may occasionally cause difficulty, but the murmur is not usually delayed or ejection in type. Both valvular and subvalvular discrete aortic stenosis can cause confusion, particularly because in discrete subvalvular stenosis the arterial pulses may be slightly jerky. However, aortic valve closure is soft and there is usually an early diastolic murmur.

In patients with dominantly right-sided hypertrophic cardiomyopathy, pulmonary stenosis may cause difficulty. With pulmonary valvular stenosis, an early systolic click is heard and pulmonary valve closure is late and soft. Also, there is no evidence of left ventricular involvement.

When the systolic murmur is absent or only trivial, the main problem in differential diagnosis is to distinguish it from coronary artery disease. Some young athletic persons may present with features suggestive of hypertrophic cardiomyopathy including an ejection systolic murmur, a jerky pulse, and evidence suggestive of left ventricular hypertrophy. Full investigation may be needed to make the correct diagnosis.

When in hypertrophic cardiomyopathy there is a mitral diastolic murmur, mitral stenosis is suspected. But the opening snap of mitral stenosis is not present in hypertrophic cardiomyopathy, although a third or fourth heart sound may be. However, the radiologic features can be quite similar. (See section on radiology.)

When there is angina without abnormal physical signs, coronary artery disease is usually suggested. The clue to hypertrophic cardiomyopathy may be found on the electrocardiogram which can show bizarre inverted T waves, left ventricular hypertrophy, left atrial hypertrophy, and Q waves. However, the electrocardiogram may be normal, particularly in young persons. Coronary arteriography is needed to make the differential diagnosis with certainty, although echocardiography is helpful. It is important to remember that hypertrophic cardiomyopathy can mimic many cardiac diseases, and it should be considered when the clinical or electrocardiographic picture suggests severe left ventricular hypertrophy and the signs do not all fit up. Of particular importance is a family history of sudden death. It is also important to remember that hypertrophic cardiomyopathy can occur in association with almost any form of cardiac disease, the most common acquired dis-

Table 43.1. Differential Diagnosis of Hypertrophic Cardiomyopathy (HCM)

Clinical Features	Differential Diagnosis	Notes	Comments
With late onset systolic murmur	Mitral valve prolapse	Murmurs start later in systole; often midsystolic click	
	Chordal rupture	Murmur may be full length	Hypertrophic cardiomyopathy may occur *in association with* any other form of heart disease: *Acquired*: Coronary artery disease Hypertension *Congential*: Aortic stenosis Atrial septal defect
	Papillary muscle failure	Linear calcification in left ventricle on x-ray	
	Ischaemic or other cause		
	Left ventricular endomyocardial disease		
With full length systolic murmur	Rheumatic mitral regurgitation	May require angiogram if atrial fibrillation and valve calcification present	
	Ventricular septal defect	Murmur not ejection type	
	Aortic stenosis		
	Valvular	Systolic click; pulse anacrotic	
	Discrete	A_2 soft	
	subvalvular	Early diastolic murmur common	
	Pulmonic stenosis	Early systolic click; P2 late and soft; no evidence of left heart involvement	
With no or trivial systolic murmur	Coronary artery disease	Coronary arteriography needed	
	Athlete's heart	May have jerky pulse, but left atrial beat not felt; may need angiography	
	Amyloid heart disease	No S_3	
With mitral diastolic murmur	Mitral stenosis	Opening snap not S_3 or S_4 in mitral stenosis	
With angina and normal physical signs	Coronary artery disease	ECG may suggest HCM; bizarre T-wave inversion; LVH, LAH, and Q waves suggest HCM	

ECG = electrocardiogram; LAH = left atrial hypertrophy; LVH = left ventricular hypertrophy.

ease being coronary artery disease and hypertension, and the congenital diseases being aortic stenosis and atrial septal defect (Table 43.1).

HAEMODYNAMIC FINDINGS

There are three major groups of abnormalities: first, the powerful overactive contraction of the left ventricle; second, elimination of the ventricular cavity in systole with apposition of the anterior mitral valve apparatus to the hypertrophied septum; and third, the complex of disorders of diastolic function involving impaired relaxation and abnormal filling. As a background to all these abnormalities there is the striking hypertrophy that may be patchy or generalized and is often associated with variable amounts of fibrosis. The powerful contraction of hypertrophied left ventricle is emphasised by the high ejection fraction, often between 80% and 90%. This powerful contraction is largely responsible (together with the hypertrophy) for the elimination of the left ventricular cavity in later systole. This elimination is associated with systolic pressure gradients in the cavity of the left ventricle, particularly at the site of apposition of the anterior mitral valve apparatus to the hypertrophied septum. These gradients are essentially "flow" gradients and do not indicate true mechanical obstruction. They are largely incidental to the general haemodynamic abnormality and do not necessarily imply that there are two types of hypertrophic cardiomyopathy: those with and those without obstruction.[5,12] The following factors make true obstruction unlikely: (1) the gradients are extremely variable; (2) the contents of the left ventricle are ejected in the first one half to two thirds of systole; (3) the reduced left ventricular end-systolic volume indicates overemptying; (4) the ejection fraction is usually 80% or above; (5) flow continues in the aorta, even when gradients develop; (6) gradients can be produced in any heart by powerful inotropic stimulation or acute ventricular hypovolaemia. However, there is no doubt that in some patients the asymmetric hypertrophy of the septum is sufficiently massive, together with the small left ventricular cavity, as to introduce some anatomic barrier. If the word obstruction is to be used, it is in this type of patient that it is least inappropriate. Such patients may require septal resection.

DIASTOLIC ABNORMALITY

These are by far the most significant aspects of the disease and determine many of its features. There is ample evidence of prolonged and irregular relaxation, together with abnormalities of filling. Left ventricular wall movement is incoordinate, patchy, and not uniform, whereas isovolumic relaxation and the rapid filling phase of diastole are abnormal. Studies of diastolic time intervals with phonocardiography, echocardiography, and M-mode echocardiography have shown that the normal sequence of events in diastole is completely disrupted. Aortic valve closure occurs after the minimum dimension of the left ventricular cavity, and the isovolumic relaxation period (from aortic valve closure to mitral valve opening), although often prolonged, tends to be shortened in patients with gradients. The peak left ventricular filling rate is prolonged as is the time taken to reach the peak ventricular filling rate.

Left ventricular filling tends to be hindered by beta-adrenergic stimulation and improved by beta-adrenergic blockade, as is the case with outflow tract systolic gradients.

SYMPTOMS

The disorders of diastolic function largely explain the symptoms. Dyspnea is due to the high end-diastolic pressure of the left ventricle that causes left atrial and pulmonary venous hypertension. The cause of chest pain is not entirely clear, but it is probably due to impaired coronary artery flow in diastole caused by the poorly relaxing incompliant ventricular muscle. Palpitations are usually due to ectopic rhythms, premature contractions, atrial fibrillation, or ventricular tachycardia.

Syncope is a common symptom in hypertrophic cardiomyopathy and has two main causes, one haemodynamic and the other arrhythmic. The haemodynamic faults are those of difficulty in filling the left ventricle in diastole and elimination of the left ventricular cavity in systole (Figure 43.2). A combination of these events may result in interruption of blood flow through the heart and acute hypotension with loss of consciousness. The problem is likely to be aggravated by tachycardia, which limits the time available for filling of the left ventricle and so potentiates the diastolic fault. Tachycardia also stimulates further the elimination of the left ventricular cavity and tends to increase the magnitude of any intraventricular pressure gradient that is present. The arrhythmic cause of syncope is more common than the haemodynamic cause. It is due to episodes of ventricular arrhythmia, multiform, multiple ventricular ectopic contractions, or runs of ventricular tachycardia. However, both haemodynamic and arrhythmic causes may operate together in the same patient, but the most common cause of sudden death is probably arrhythmia.

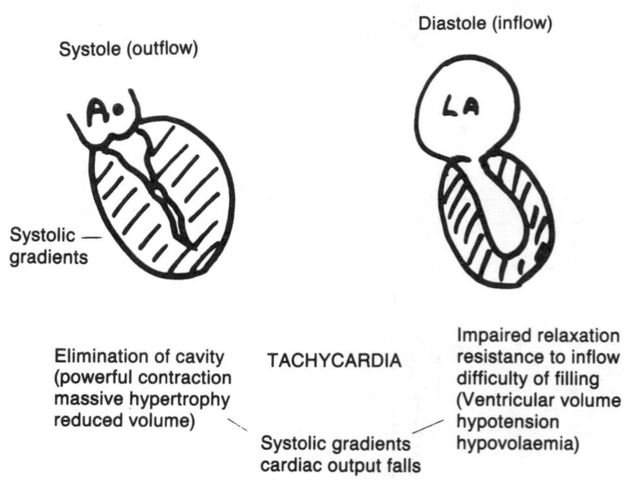

Figure 43.2. Diagram to show interaction between systolic and diastolic functions in hypertrophic cardiomyopathy in relation to syncope and sudden death. (From Goodwin,[11] with permission.)

INVESTIGATIONS

Electrocardiography

Electrocardiography may show virtually a normal appearance, particularly in young persons, but it usually shows definite evidence of left ventricular hypertrophy with increased QRS voltage and T-wave changes. The T waves are often sharply inverted and of increased voltage. There is commonly left axis deviation sufficient to indicate left anterior hemiblock, the PR interval tends to be short, there is left atrial hypertrophy, and frequently Q waves are seen in central and left precordial leads. Occasionally preexcitation is seen and more rarely there may be conduction defects. Biphasic QRS complexes of increased voltage indicating septal and right ventricular hypertrophy are often found in leads V_2, V_3, and V_4. In patients with predominantly right-sided disease the appearances may be those of severe right ventricular hypertrophy.

Radiography of the Chest

The appearances are frequently not striking and the cardiac silhouette may show little, if any, abnormality. However, in a number of cases, there may be a sharply convex left border to the heart, suggesting massive hypertrophy of the left ventricular free wall. Occasionally there may be a bulge of sufficient degree to suggest a cardiac tumour. The most common appearance, however, is that indicating an elevated left atrial pressure with slight left atrial enlargement, distention of vascular markings for the upper lobes with attenuation to the lower lobes, and evidence of interstitial oedema. An unusual but well-recognised complication is calcification of the mitral valve. Thus, the radiologic appearances may, at times, be similar to those of mitral valve disease.

Echocardiography

M-mode echocardiography shows a number of characteristic features in typical patients. These are: reduction in the dimensions of the left ventricular cavity, increased thickness of the ventricular septum in comparison with the posterior wall of the left ventricle in a ratio of 1.5 to 1, reduced rate of closure of the mitral valve, and relative immobility of the ventricle septum with marked contraction of the posterior wall. In patients with systolic pressure gradients there is usually midsystolic closure of the aortic valve and systolic anterior motion of the mitral valve, the anterior valve apparatus touching the septum. Many of these features can be found in other cardiac conditions, particularly those causing left ventricular hypertrophy, and are not, in themselves, specific. However, when all the features are found on the same echocardiogram, the diagnosis becomes extremely likely, but echocardiography should always be interpreted in light of the clinical picture. Two-dimensional echocardiography is valuable in showing the hypertrophied septum eliminating the ventricular cavity in systole and the site and extent of the ventricular hypertrophy. The movement of the ventricular septum may vary from normal to paradoxical. To obtain full value from echocardiography, two-dimensional studies should always be combined with M-mode echocardiography.

Angiocardiography

Angiocardiography reveals a characteristic appearance (Figure 43.3). The shape of the left ventricle is grossly distorted, the massive hypertrophy often encroaching on the cavity, giving it a star-shaped appearance in severe cases. The end-systolic frame shows elimination of the ventricular cavity, leaving only a small triangular portion beneath the aortic valve (Figure 43.3, *left*); in some cases there may be isolation of contrast medium at the apex of the ventricle. The diastolic volume appears normal, but the left ventricle appears angulated mainly because of massive hypertrophy of the papillary muscles (Figure 43.3, *right*). There is usually trivial mitral regurgitation, but occasionally mitral regurgitation may be massive when secondary changes such as calcification or infection have seriously damaged the mitral valve. Aortic valve and aorta usually appear normal. The coronary arteries are smooth bore, widely patent, and large.

Radionuclide Angiography

Gated blood pool scanning reveals the high ejection fraction of 80% to 90% already mentioned.[12] A rather characteristic finding on gated cardiac imaging is the "tear drop sign."[12a] The left ventricle during diastole appears bulbous at the apex and narrowed at the base due to disproportionate septal hypertrophy. Positron emission tomography and nuclear magnetic resonance have still to be evaluated. The latter may be used both to examine the biochemical fluxes within the myocardium and to study systolic and diastolic function.

PROGNOSIS

The prognosis of hypertrophic cardiomyopathy is largely determined by the tendency to sudden death. Half of those who die, die suddenly and usually unexpectedly for the reasons already mentioned in connection with palpitations and syncope. Were it not for the tendency to sudden death, hypertrophic cardiomyopathy would be a relatively benign condition, and indeed many patients with milder forms of the disease do live for many years with few, if any, symptoms. Prognosis is undoubtedly worse in patients in whom the disease is diagnosed in childhood and who have a family history of sudden death and progressive symptoms.

No single haemodynamic or electrocardiographic feature appears to be a particular guide to prognosis. In patients without the adverse features mentioned, the annual death rate is in the region of 2.4%, but in patients who are especially vulnerable, the incidence is more than doubled.

A relation between sudden death and ventricular arrhythmia has now been established.[13] Patients particularly at risk are those who have episodes of ventricular tachycardia or frequent multiform multifocal ventricular ectopic beats detected on ambulatory electrocardiographic monitoring. Usually such arrhythmias are not appreciated by the patient[14] and therefore constitute an occult hazard

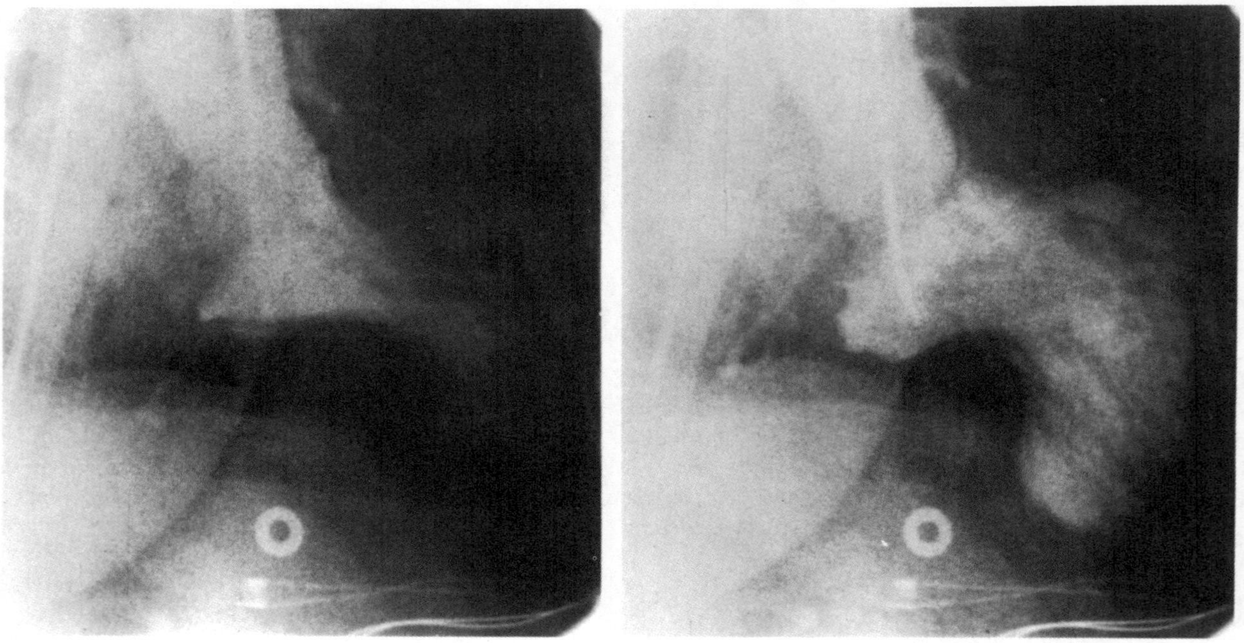

Figure 43.3. Anteroposterior cineangiograms of the left ventricle in hypertrophic cardiomyopathy showing in systolic frame (*left*) elimination of mid- and apical portions of the left ventricle and slight mitral regurgitation, and in diastolic frame (*right*) angulation of the ventricle but normal volume. (From Goodwin,[11] with permission.)

that emphasises the need for regular electrocardiographic monitoring. Supraventricular arrhythmias have not been shown to carry the same risk of sudden death, but atrial fibrillation at a rapid ventricular rate is a serious complication, for it removes the atrial drive necessary to fill the stiff left ventricle and, because of the tachycardia, reduces the time available for filling. Patients in whom atrial fibrillation develops commonly develop a low cardiac output state and may have pulmonary oedema or severe congestive heart failure; occasionally they may die if the arrhythmia is not rapidly controlled. Episodic atrial fibrillation is a prominent cause of deterioration in symptoms, the development of heart failure, and a risk of embolism.

Causes of death other than arrhythmia are congestive heart failure, systemic embolism, infective endocarditis, and massive myocardial infarction. Myocardial infarction has been shown to occur in the absence of disease of the major coronary arteries.[14a]

In contrast to adults, arrhythmias are uncommon in children and adolescents with hypertrophic cardiomyopathy and are not a marker of those at particular risk of sudden death.[14b] This suggests that in children and adolescents with hypertrophic cardiomyopathy the initiating event of sudden death is more likely to be an acute hemodynamic alteration than an arrhythmia.

TREATMENT

Treatment must be directed at improving the major abnormalities of disease, reducing the hazards, limiting symptoms, and preventing progression of the disease. Unfortunately no means of preventing progression is known, but measures can be taken to attack the other problems.

The incidence of sudden death can be reduced by the use of amiodarone to prevent serious ventricular arrhythmias, and this is the single, most important treatment.[15–17] Patients whose ambulatory monitoring studies show episodes of ventricular tachycardia or multiple multiform ventricular ectopic beats should be given amiodarone. The initial dose should be 600 mg daily for five days followed by 400 mg daily five days of the week. The side effects include nausea and dyspepsia during the first few days of treatment and later corneal deposits, pulmonary fibrosis, thyroid function disturbance, photosensitivity, and changes in liver function. Most of the complications are dose related and can be reduced to a minimum by keeping the dose within the limits mentioned. Some patients may break through the accepted maintenance dosage and require more amiodarone, however. In others, regular monitoring may show disappearance of the ventricular arrhythmias and the dose can be safely reduced. No other antiarrhythmic drug has so far been shown to have the same prophylactic effects as amiodarone.[18] The best alternatives are probably quinidine and sotalol, the latter having both a beta-blocking action and an amiodarone-like action. Unfortunately, neither of these drugs is as effective as amiodarone.

The relief of symptoms is best achieved by the use of nonselective beta-adrenergic blockade, propranolol being the drug of choice. It should be started at 10 mg three times a day and increased to 200 to 300 mg a day. Most patients tolerate propranolol well and around 70% will benefit symptomatically. There is no firm evidence that propranolol improves the prognosis. Alternatives to propranolol are oxyprenolol, which may be given in double the dose of propranolol, metoprolol, and atenolol. Metoprolol and atenolol are marginally less effective because they are relatively selective agents, but their advantage is that they can be used in circumstances when nonselective agents are contraindicated, such as peripheral vascular disease, lung disease, or diabetes mellitus.

Much interest has surrounded the use of calcium channel blocking agents. Verapamil has been shown to relieve symptoms and improve exercise tolerance and haemodynamics in some patients[19] but unfortunately in others nonspecific subjective side effects may occur or much more seriously there may be pulmonary oedema or sudden death.[20] Verapamil should not be used as a first-line drug for the relief of symptoms, but it may be tried cautiously in patients who do not have high left atrial pressure or conduction defects.[21] It should be started in the hospital under careful monitoring conditions, using a small dose of 40 mg three times daily initially.

Nifedipine is still under investigation. It has the theoretic disadvantage of producing vasodilatation, which may be disadvantageous because it reduces ventricular volume and increases cavity elimination. However, it has been suggested that its favourable effects on diastolic relaxation of the ventricle outweigh the disadvantageous effects of vasodilatation.[22,23] Nifedipine is still in the experimental stage and should not be used routinely.

Combinations of drugs may be indicated when it is necessary to both prevent arrhythmias and relieve symptoms. In this event, amiodarone and propranolol can be combined, but verapamil should not be given with amiodarone. An alternative to a combination of amiodarone and propranolol is sotalol, but it is much less effective. Disopyramide has been advised both for its negative inotropic effect and for its antiarrhythmic effect. It has not been shown to improve prognosis, but claims have been made that it improves symptoms.

It is important that treatment be adjusted to the individual. Patients at low risk, who have no family history, no symptoms, but signs of only mild disease without arrhythmias on electrocardiographic monitoring probably do not require any treatment at all but merely regular observation which should include electrocardiographic monitoring. Those with both symptoms and ventricular arrhythmias should receive a combination of beta-adrenergic blockade and amiodarone.

Surgically, septal resection is indicated in patients who have severe symptoms that do not respond to medical treatment and who have a gradient of pressure in the left ventricle of at least 50 mm in systole that is persistent and with pronounced asymmetrical hypertrophy of the ventricular septum. There is no evidence that surgical treatment improves prognosis, but it has been shown to reduce gradients, lower left ventricular end-diastolic pressure, and improve symptoms and effort tolerance. The combined early and late mortality in collected series is high, around 16% to 20%, although in some individual series the immediate mortality is much lower. There is a tendency for congestive heart failure to develop late, after the operation, as a result of either surgical treatment or progression of the disease. Mitral valve replacement is indicated only in patients who have extreme mitral regurgitation as a result of secondary damage to the mitral valve. Patients who are extremely breathless and have high left atrial pressure and mitral regurgitation on angiography respond well to mitral valve replacement, which should consist of a low profile mechanical prosthesis or preferably a biologic valve. In patients who have both occlusive coronary artery disease and hypertrophic cardiomyopathy, coronary artery bypass grafting may be indicated in the former,[24] but it is not certain whether septal resection is of value in the latter. The decision as to whether anginal pain originates in hypertrophic cardiomyopathy or in the diseased coronary arteries is extremely difficult without coronary arteriography.[24]

The place of pacemaker treatment has not been fully defined. The pacemaker may be of value in patients in whom extreme bradycardia develops with propranolol, which is otherwise helpful in relieving symptoms. The rare patient who has serious conduction defects needs a pacemaker in his own right, and it is possible that new generation sequential pacemakers may be of value in maintaining atrial contraction to help fill the left ventricle. The main disadvantage of conventional ventricular pacemaking is the loss of effective atrial drive, and this benefit must be set against the possible benefits of the technique. A possible hazard of pacemaking is the induction of arrhythmias.

DILATED (CONGESTIVE) CARDIOMYOPATHY

Dilated cardiomyopathy is characterised by striking dilatation of the ventricles, which have grossly impaired systolic function that leads eventually to progressive intractable congestive heart failure.

PATHOLOGY

The heart is always overweight and may even be double its normal size. The chambers are severely dilated and the heart muscle is pale and flabby. The ventricular walls are usually of normal thickness because, despite hypertrophy, the stretching of the myocardium produced by the dilatation masks the hypertrophy. The endocardium is nonspecifically thickened and thrombus formation is common. Fibrous replacement can be found scattered throughout the myocardium. The coronary arteries are normal. Histologic study shows no specific changes. Myocardial fibres are aligned normally, there are hypertrophic changes in the fibre nuclei, but the diameters of the fibres are normal because of attenuation. The increase in fibrous tissue is due either to an increase in interstitial collagen tissue or to focal replacement of myocardial fibres. The appearances are essentially nonspecific, although occasionally some focal accumulations of inflammatory cells may be found, and in long-standing cases there may be some myocytolysis. Electron microscopy confirms the presence of hypertrophy, showing an increase in the number of mitochondria and degeneration of the cristae of the mitochondria. The pathologic diagnosis is therefore largely one of exclusion.

INCIDENCE

Dilated cardiomyopathy is worldwide in distribution. A study from Malmö, Sweden,[25] suggests that 10 cases per 100,000 of the population per year might be a realistic estimate, although similar studies from other countries have not been made.

CAUSE OF DISEASE

The cause is unknown, but various disorders have been suggested as being "risk" or "conditioning" factors including alcoholism, hypertension, pregnancy and the puerperium, and previous viral infections. Consumption of large amounts of alcohol over long periods of time can result in a syndrome indistinguishable from that of dilated cardiomyopathy. This syndrome, known as alcoholic heart muscle disease, can be reversed if alcohol is discontinued, and alcohol is clearly not the cause of dilated cardiomyopathy because most patients with the disease have not consumed large quantities of alcohol and the disease is common in children. However, alcohol abuse may well aggravate dilated cardiomyopathy. Although hypertension may occasionally be an important factor, most patients with dilated cardiomyopathy do not have any evidence of previous hypertension. A dilated form of heart muscle disease occurs in pregnancy and the puerperium, but no specific factor associated with pregnancy has emerged to account for the cardiomyopathy. The most appealing causation is that of progressive myocardial damage due to disturbance of autoimmunity within the myocardium, set up by a previous viral infection. This will be discussed further in the section under myocarditis.

CLINICAL FEATURES

The symptoms are essentially those of impaired cardiac function. Because the disease is a diffuse one, there may be symptoms suggesting impairment of both right and left ventricular function. Tiredness on effort and undue lassitude, accompanied by dyspnoea on exertion, are usually the initial symptoms. As the disease progresses, paroxysmal nocturnal dyspnoea may occur and symptoms associated with congestive heart failure, such as swelling of the abdomen, pain in the right hypochondrium, and dependent oedema occur.

CLINICAL SIGNS

These are initially those of impaired systolic function with a dilated heart. There is evidence of left ventricular enlargement with dilatation of the left ventricle suggested by a displaced and poor quality thrusting left ventricular apex and a fourth heart sound due to increased left ventricular end-diastolic pressure. Later a filling gallop may be heard and subsequently the jugular venous pressure increases as signs of right heart failure develop. In the early stages, however, the diagnosis may depend on the symptoms and the detection of cardiac enlargement with gallop rhythm. In the late stages of the disease, the clinical picture is one of severe low output cardiac failure with extreme dyspnoea, cold, blue extremities, small volume arterial pulses, elevated jugular venous pressure and evidence of tricuspid regurgitation and extensive oedema of the legs, often accompanied by ascites. There is enlargement of the liver, which frequently pulsates, and examination of the lungs reveals basal rales. There may be sacral oedema.

HAEMODYNAMIC FINDINGS

The haemodynamic findings are essentially those of low output cardiac failure with low cardiac index and ejection fraction, the latter in severe cases varying between 10% and 30%; an increase in left ventricular end-diastolic pressure, which usually results in a modest degree of pulmonary arterial hypertension; and dilatation of the right ventricle and papillary muscles resulting in tricuspid regurgitation, which is frequently severe and demonstrated by a systolic wave in jugular venous pulse. The jugular venous pressure is commonly substantially elevated at least in advanced cases to 20 mm Hg or more above the sternal angle. Blood pressure is normal in the early stages, but in severe cases is usually somewhat low, being between 90 and 110 mm Hg in systole. There is frequently some degree of mitral regurgitation for the same reasons as tricuspid regurgitation. Regurgitation of both atrioventricular valves tends to become less as the condition improves and dilatation of the ventricles diminishes.

INVESTIGATIONS

Electrocardiography

The electrocardiogram is frequently nonspecific, showing repolarisation changes only. In some cases there may be definite evidence of left ventricular hypertrophy. The deep T-wave inversion seen in hypertrophic cardiomyopathy is virtually never found. There may be evidence of left and right atrial hypertrophy and in 10% to 15% of patients there is atrial fibrillation. Left bundle branch block occurs in roughly the same proportion of patients. In a minority of patients there may be Q waves, simulating myocardial infarction and probably due to patchy myocardial cell destruction, which removes the positive vector forces and creates local conduction defects.

Radiography of the Chest

The cardiac silhouette is commonly enlarged. There is usually prominence of the right atrium and evidence of dilatation of the left ventricle. The left atrium may be slightly enlarged and there are commonly signs of elevated left atrial pressure with the usual vascular changes and interstitial oedema. In advanced cases pleural effusions are common, and pericardial effusion may impart a globular shape to the cardiac silhouette. There may be evidence of localised or generalised pulmonary oedema. Valvular calcification is very unusual.

Echocardiography

Echocardiography is essentially a nonspecific demonstration of ventricular dilatation and depressed contractile function. On M-mode studies the dimensions of both ventricles are increased and movement of the posterior wall of the left ventricle is poor. The mitral valve is displaced towards the posterior wall but is otherwise normal. Two-dimensional studies may show thrombus in the ventricles or atria and demonstrate marked ventricular dilatation but modest hypertrophy. Usually there is generalised ventricular hypokinesia, but occasionally areas of global dyskinesia may be found resembling coronary heart disease.

Angiocardiography

Left ventricular angiography shows marked dilatation of the left ventricle with little difference in end-systolic and end-diastolic volumes, both of which are substantially increased. As with echocardiographic viewing, there is usually global hypokinesia, but occasionally regional dyskinesia may be seen. The coronary arteries are normal.

Ambulatory Electrocardiographic Monitoring

As in hypertrophic cardiomyopathy it has become apparent that episodes of ventricular tachycardia and ventricular ectopic beats are common in dilated cardiomyopathy.[26] It is probable that ventricular tachycardia is an important cause of sudden death,[26a] and this matter is being further investigated.

Radioisotope Studies

Gated blood pool scanning confirms low ejection fractions between 10% and 30%.

DIFFERENTIAL DIAGNOSIS

The differential diagnosis depends on exclusion of the usual causes of heart failure, such as hypertension, coronary heart disease, and valvular disease. It is also necessary to exclude specific heart muscle disease and to search diligently for evidence of neurologic disease, collagen vascular disease, and granulomatous disease. Thus, a complete clinical investigation and haematologic and biochemical analyses are necessary. Thyroid function should be estimated in every case. In view of the occasional presentation of pheochromocytoma with heart failure and normotension or hypotension, urinary excretion of vanilmandelic acid should be assayed. If necessary, catecholamine blood levels should be estimated. The most difficult differential diagnosis as a rule is to distinguish it from coronary heart disease without a history of angina or myocardial infarction. Usually the differential diagnosis can be made without coronary arteriography on the basis of the lack of evidence of atherosclerotic disease elsewhere, but occasionally coronary arteriography is essential.

PROGNOSIS

Although it is apparent from retrospective studies that some patients may have the disease for many years, the history is usually a short one; one to two years or a few months of symptoms of heart failure, and once heart failure is established the prognosis is poor. From 30% to 50% of patients have died within five years and 70% at ten years.[27] Some patients, around 20%, may unexpectedly improve and survive much longer.[10] The reason for this improvement is not fully understood. Some patients may die suddenly before the onset of heart failure or after heart failure has become established, the cause of death usually being ventricular arrhythmia. The best indicator of prognosis is haemodynamic, patients with a low cardiac index being among those who do least well.

COMPLICATIONS

The complications are mainly those of severe congestive heart failure. Thrombosis in the dilated poorly contracting left ventricle may give rise to systemic embolism, and if there is atrial fibrillation, thrombus may develop in the left atrium and give rise to the same result. Pulmonary embolism may occur as a result of deep venous or pelvic vein thrombosis consequent to extensive oedema and low cardiac output and immobilisation. Severe mitral regurgitation occurs occasionally but is unusual. Infective endocarditis is exceptional.

TREATMENT

Because the cause of dilated cardiomyopathy is unknown, no specific treatment is available. Treatment should be considered under four headings: (1) treatment of heart failure; (2) prevention and treatment of arrhythmias; (3) prevention and treatment of embolism; and (4) surgical treatment.

Treatment of heart failure differs in no way from that of heart failure from other causes. The introduction of vasodilator therapy has improved the quality of life and diminished symptoms, but it has not prolonged survival.[27a]

In the prevention and treatment of arrhythmia it is essential that regular ambulatory electrocardiographic monitoring be undertaken as for hypertrophic cardiomyopathy. When significant ventricular arrhythmias are revealed, amiodarone is indicated. Amiodarone has the great advantage in dilated cardiomyopathy in that it has no significant negative inotropic effect, giving it a distinct advantage over other antiarrhythmic drugs that do have a negative inotropic effect.[26] Digitalis should be used with care, because especially in the presence of hypokalaemia it may predispose to the very ventricular arrhythmias that treatment is aimed to prevent. Because of doubt as to the long-term effectiveness of digitalis for heart failure with sinus rhythm and the possible unwanted effects, digitalis should not usually be given for more than a few months.

In the prevention and treatment of embolism, anticoagulants are indicated in patients who have paroxysmal or established atrial fibrillation, severe congestive heart failure, or evidence of thrombus in any of the cardiac chambers. Naturally, a history of systemic or pulmonary embolism is also an indication for anticoagulants. Care must be taken with oral anticoagulants because of the impairment of liver function that results from severe heart failure.

As for surgical treatment, although mitral repair or replacement has been attempted in patients who have severe mitral regurgitation, operation is usually unsuccessful because of the severely damaged myocardium. The only consistently effective surgical treatment is cardiac transplantation, which has been shown to significantly improve prognosis in patients with dilated cardiomyopathy.[28] Any patient under the age of 50 years who is extremely symptomatic despite full therapy for severe heart failure should be considered for transplantation.[28a]

Mention must be made of treatment by beta-adrenergic blockade. This has been claimed to improve prognosis significantly, using small incremental doses of metoprolol on an inpatient basis and reducing or discontinuing the treatment at the first sign of deterioration of heart failure. The reasons for improvement are not fully understood, but they may be connected with alteration in the $beta_1$ receptors in the myocardium. However, this treatment must still be regarded as experimental and not to be advised for routine use.

General measures such as rest, prevention of infection, and avoidance of cigarette smoking and alcohol are also important.

RESTRICTIVE CARDIOMYOPATHY

This is the type of cardiomyopathy in which the burden of disease falls upon diastole rather than systole. The haemodynamics are similar to those of constrictive pericarditis with early rapid filling of the ventricles and later slow filling and limitation of filling. The most common cause of restrictive cardiomyopathy is endomyocardial fibrosis, although a similar but not identical picture may be caused by infiltrative conditions that produce a particularly rigid myocardium, such as amyloid disease (to be discussed).

Endomyocardial fibrosis occurs in two forms: the tropical type and the temperate climate variety with eosinophilia originally described by Loeffler. The pathologic findings in the two types are virtually identical, and they have been grouped together under the same general title of eosinophilic endomyocardial disease.[29]

PATHOLOGY

Either ventricle may be involved, usually the right ventricle in 10% to 30% of cases, the left ventricle in 10% to 40%, and both ventricles in 50% to 70%. External examination of the heart shows moderate cardiac enlargement. There is striking endocardial thickening that most frequently involves the inflow tract, apex, and part of the outflow tract of the left ventricle and the inflow tract of the right ventricle. The atrioventricular valves are involved, and in the case of the mitral valve only the anterior apparatus is affected. The atria are seldom involved. As the disease progresses, the degree of endocardial thickening may be such as to obliterate most of the ventricular cavity. The cardiac apex is drawn progressively towards the atrioventricular valves, producing the characteristic external dimple. Thrombi are common overlying the endocardial fibrosis. The coronary arteries are normal. Pericardial thickening may be present and pericardial effusions can occur.

HISTOLOGY

Histologic examination reveals characteristic layering of the thick endocardium. Superficially beneath the thrombus there is collagen tissue often separated into two layers. There is a zone of granulation tissue and a zone of loosely arranged connective tissue in which dilated blood vessels, together with inflammatory cells are plentiful. In the early stages of the disease when the inflammatory process is at its height, the endocardium may be intensely infiltrated with eosinophils. Later the eosinophils may disappear and the cellular infiltration be replaced by granulation and fibrous tissue. Intramyocardial vessels often show severe thickening secondary to the inflammatory changes. The myocardial fibres are normally aligned, but they show some evidence of hypertrophy.

THE EOSINOPHIL

There is evidence that in patients with endomyocardial fibrosis of the temperate climate variety with hypereosinophilia there are clones of immunologically abnormal eosinophils that have vacuolation, and degranulation and extrude cationic protein that damages the myocardium and endocardium. The reasons for the immunologic changes in the eosinophils are unknown, and there may be many different stimuli for the change. Endomyocardial fibrosis is common in the hypereosinophilic syndrome[30] in which eosinophils may also infiltrate other organs. Eosinophilic heart disease may exist in other forms, as in the Churg-Strauss syndrome in which there is eosinophilia, asthma, a dilated form of cardiomyopathy, and commonly pericardial involvement.[30] Endomyocardial fibrosis apparently does not occur. The reasons for these differences are not known.

In the tropical type of endomyocardial fibrosis, eosinophilia is not usually a feature, although studies currently in progress reveal immunologically abnormal eosinophils in some patients. The matter remains open because until recently immunologic studies of eosinophils in tropical patients have not been made. Tropical endomyocardial fibrosis is common in zones around the equatorial belt and therefore it can be found in Central Africa, South America, and India. There are certain differences from the temperate climate variety, such as recurrent episodes of fever (often accompanied by arrhythmia) before the disease becomes established, the higher incidence in the rainy season, and the incidence in humid climates. These differences may merely be those of genetics and environment and do not necessarily suggest two different diseases. Presumably many different stimuli can cause the eosinophil to develop its abnormal characteristics.

CLINICAL FEATURES

The symptoms are essentially those of heart failure. However, it must be realised that the heart failure is of a particular type, that of diastolic impairment, systolic function remaining unimpaired until a late stage, but wherever the fault lies, the effect is to restrict cardiac output and to cause the clinical picture of heart failure. Fatigue on effort and lassitude indicate a low cardiac output, whereas dyspnoea suggests involvement of the left ventricle. When the left ventricle is severely involved, the clinical features are those of left ventricular failure. There are commonly third and fourth heart sounds, and mitral regurgitation is frequent. The systolic murmur tends to die away towards the end of systole and as the valve becomes progressively more competent. When the right ventricle is involved, the appearances suggest constrictive pericarditis. The jugular venous pressure is high and shows an M-shaped pattern with prominent "a" and v waves and sharp x and y descents. The cardiac impulse may be impalpable, and there may be no significant murmurs, although tricuspid regurgitation can occur. Advanced cases demonstrate ascites, hepatic enlargement, and pleural and pericardial effusion. Ascites are often out of proportion to the oedema of the ankles.

HAEMODYNAMIC FINDINGS

The haemodynamic findings are similar to those of constrictive pericarditis. The sudden restriction to filling imposed by the endocardial lesions causes the normal expansion of the ventricles in diastole to cease abruptly. This produces a characteristic dip-and-plateau configuration of the ventricular pressure pulse which shows an early diastolic dip followed by a rapid rise to a plateau well above the zero level. This effect in turn results in the characteristic jugular venous pressure pulse with the dominant "a" wave, the rapid x descent from the v wave, and rapid y descent. The y descent coincides with the early diastolic dip of the ventricular pressure pulse, and it is at this point that the characteristic third heart sound is heard. However, there are certain differences from constrictive pericarditis, notably a tendency for the early diastolic dip not to reach to or below zero and for the pulmonary artery pressure to be elevated, which is unusual in constrictive pericarditis. Pulmonary hypertension in endomyocardial fibrosis is the result of a high left atrial pressure when the left ventricle is also involved.

INVESTIGATIONS

Electrocardiography

The electrocardiogram is essentially nonspecific.

Radiography of the Chest

In right-sided endomyocardial fibrosis there may be massive enlargement of the right atrium, giving the heart an enormous globular silhouette which is accentuated by pericardial effusion in many cases. When the right ventricle is solely or predominantly involved, the lung fields may be unduly clear and the vascular markings attenuated. When the left ventricle is involved, there is not infrequently a linear streak of calcium in the region of the body of the left ventricle because of calcification in overlying thrombus. The left ventricle is enlarged, and when the mitral valve is significantly involved, the left atrium is also. There is frequently the pulmonary vascular pattern of elevated left atrial pressure.

Echocardiography

Two-dimensional echocardiography is of great value, especially the apical four-chamber view that may show obliteration of the apices of one or both ventricles. The left parasternal view tends to show bright echoes in the region of the endocardium and mitral valve. M-mode echocardiography may show impairment of ventricular relaxation in prolongation of the down slope, and the appearance of a plateau in contraction of the posterior wall of the left ventricle.

Angiocardiography

Angiocardiography, when the left ventricle is involved, shows sharp cutoff of the apex of the ventricle, so that the left ventricle may resemble a boxing glove. When the right ventricle is involved, the inflow tract is cut off; in severe cases, there may be complete obliteration of the ventricle except for a small outflow tract sinus. The right atrium tends to be very large, and the left atrium is also enlarged when there is mitral regurgitation.

DIFFERENTIAL DIAGNOSIS

The major differential diagnosis of restrictive cardiomyopathy is constrictive pericarditis, and in the right-sided type of endomyocardial fibrosis the similarity may be close. Differentiation may be extremely difficult. The haemodynamic differences already mentioned are of importance. Calcification in the pericardium points strongly to constrictive pericarditis, but it is often absent in that condition. The presence of an apical systolic murmur suggesting mitral regurgitation strongly favours endomyocardial fibrosis, but it can occasionally be found in constrictive pericarditis for reasons that are uncertain. In difficult cases computed tomographic scanning of the heart may be useful in showing clearly the thickened pericardium in constrictive pericarditis. However, it is not infallible. If doubt still remains, then endomyocardial biopsy or exploratory thoracotomy is fully justified.

DIASTOLIC HEART DISEASE

The term diastolic heart disease has been used to describe conditions in which the main brunt of the disease falls upon diastole. These are hypertrophic cardiomyopathy, endomyocardial fibrosis, amyloid disease of the heart, and constrictive pericarditis. All have some similarities and some differences. As stated, constrictive pericarditis and restrictive cardiomyopathy have considerable similarities. The abnormalities in diastole of hypertrophic cardiomyopathy are very different, reflecting not true restriction to inflow but impaired relaxation, elasticity, and filling of the ventricles. Amyloid disease of the heart has some features similar to those of restrictive cardiomyopathy, but certain marked differences exist. Some form of diastolic heart disease may be suspected clinically when high jugular venous pressure is combined with a small or normal-sized heart and gallop rhythm with or without an apical systolic murmur.

TREATMENT

In the acute inflammatory stage of endomyocardial fibrosis, steroids, hydroxyurea, and vincristine have been helpful. In the later stages, particularly when atrioventricular valve regurgitation is severe, endocardiectomy and valve replacement have shown promise and should certainly be considered.

AMYLOID HEART DISEASE

Amyloid heart disease may exist as an entity within the heart alone or it may involve many other organs. It is not the purpose of this chapter to describe amyloid disease in general, but merely to concentrate on the cardiac manifestations. The amyloid substance surrounds the small blood vessels in the myocardium, producing a degree of ischaemia and also causing the myocardium to become stiff and unyielding, often described as the "stiff heart."[31] The rigidity of the myocardium causes abnormal filling of the ventricles, somewhat resembling constrictive pericarditis and restrictive cardiomyopathy. The main difference, however, is in the pattern of filling. In amyloid disease filling of the ventricles is slow throughout and there is no early rapid filling phase. This prevents the development of a third heart sound, and this is an important point in differentiating it from constrictive pericarditis and restrictive cardiomyopathy.[31] Otherwise the clinical picture may be similar.

Cardiac pain is often a feature of amyloid disease of the heart and tends to cause confusion with coronary heart disease. This confusion is sometimes accentuated by the electrocardiogram which tends to show deep Q waves in precordial leads. Echocardiography shows a "granular sparkling" appearance of the thickened myocardium,[31a] but this is not a specific feature, and similar appearances can show in patients with severe hypertrophy and fibrosis. On occasion amyloid disease of the heart can resemble hypertrophic cardiomyopathy,[31b] and in fact the two conditions have occasionally been found to occur together.

There is virtually no effective treatment for amyloid disease of the heart. When amyloidosis is secondary to long-standing inflammatory or infective disease, every effort should be made to control this disease; however, in this type of secondary amyloidosis the heart is not usually involved. Colchicine may be useful in familial Mediterranean fever and dimethyl sulphoxide has been given by infusion and topical administration to patients with amyloidosis, but the results are uncertain and the drug unpleasant to use.

Confirmation of a clinical diagnosis of amyloidosis is best made by endomyocardial biopsy.

MYOCARDITIS, WITH SPECIAL REFERENCE TO ITS RELATION TO DILATED (CONGESTIVE) CARDIOMYOPATHY

The term myocarditis indicates involvement of heart muscle by a toxic or infective agent and therefore in the widest sense includes damage to the myocardium by drugs and toxins as well as infective agents. However, in the context of this chapter, and in particular in the context of cardiomyopathy, the term myocarditis will refer to an infective process. Viral infections of the heart, which are well recognised, may be due to a number of viruses, particularly coxsackie- and echoviruses. Coxsackieviruses A and B are picornaviruses, having RNA as the nucleic acid core. Echoviruses, however, are enteroviruses, but certain types have been associated with cardiac disease.

In acute viral heart disease in man, the brunt of the attack falls upon the myocardium, although the pericardium is frequently involved also. Endocardial involvement is uncertain and lacks proof.

Confirmation of viral myocarditis in man is difficult, a firm diagnosis often being impossible because of the inability to obtain a tissue diagnosis from the heart and because the virus tends to disappear from heart muscle very rapidly. A high order of probability is present when there is isolation of virus or recovery of labelled virus antibody from the heart. A moderate order of association includes isolation of the virus from the pharynx or faeces and a fourfold rise in type-specific neutralising antibodies or a concomitant titre in the serum of 1/32 or more type-specific IgM. Low order association exists when either virus is isolated from the pharynx or there is a fourfold rise in the type-specific antibodies. Diagnosis, therefore, often depends on the clinical picture, association of symptoms and signs, and probabilities.

CLINICAL MANIFESTATIONS

These include unexplained tiredness, cough, dyspnoea, fainting attacks, and palpitations. If severe, skeletal myalgic pain is also associated with these symptoms, with a febrile illness, the probability of myocarditis becomes greater. The cardiovascular physical signs are those of an inappropriate and persistent tachycardia, gallop rhythm (often summation in type), and evidence of cardiac dilatation. There may be evidence of congestive heart failure in some cases with elevated jugular venous pressure, hepatomegaly, oedema, and rales at the bases of the lungs. Blood pressure is then often low, as is pulse pressure, but there can be considerable difficulty in differentiating between myocarditis and pericarditis, pericarditis often concealing the presence of myocarditis. Chest pain radiating around the scapulae which is worse on breathing, relieved by bending forward, and worse on movement suggests pericarditis. An increase in jugular venous pressure on inspiration and waning of the arterial pulse on inspiration together with pericardial friction indicate pericarditis with effusion. A third heart sound suggests myocardial involvement or progression of acute pericarditis to constrictive pericarditis. A systolic murmur suggests mitral or tricuspid regurgitation due to left or right ventricular dilatation, and it therefore implies involvement of the myocardium.

INVESTIGATIONS

The electrocardiogram may show evidence of pericarditis with widespread ST-segment elevation but otherwise tends to show nonspecific T-wave changes. Arrhythmias may occur, varying from ectopic beats to atrial fibrillation; occasionally heart block is seen.

Echocardiography will reveal pericardial effusion and may show impairment of systolic function of the ventricles, with dilatation.

Radiography of the chest shows cardiomegaly, but this can be due to pericardial effusion rather than cardiac dilatation.

PATHOLOGY

There is focal necrosis of the myocardium and fraying of myofibrils with mononuclear neutrophil cell infiltrates. The replacement fibrosis may be patchy, but it tends to be greater in long-standing cases. In severe cases there is dilatation of the ventricles, but hypertrophy is unusual. The pericardium may show inflammatory changes even with no clinical evidence of pericarditis.

NATURAL HISTORY

The natural history of acute viral myocarditis is not well known, because the diagnosis is often missed and recognition is difficult and uncertain. However, it is probable that the vast majority of patients (over 90%) recover completely. A small percentage of patients, perhaps 1%, develop signs of definite cardiac involvement, and a few may die suddenly of overwhelming infection with or without conduction defects. Some patients may pass into a subacute or chronic phase in which the dominant feature is progressive heart failure of unknown cause following an illness suggesting viral infection. A fourth possible pathway concerns the induction of an autoimmune process in the myocardium by the viral infection that after a latent period leads to progressive myocardial damage and the syndrome of dilated cardiomyopathy. This is the "infectious" immune theory of the causation of dilated cardiomyopathy.

INFECTIOUS IMMUNE THEORY OF DILATED (CONGESTIVE) CARDIOMYOPATHY

The concept of, and evidence for, autoimmune disorders being set up by previous infections and leading to chronic diseases is well known in medicine. Obvious examples in cardiovascular disease are rheumatic heart disease, Chagas' disease, and possibly sarcoidosis.

The experimental induction of virus myocarditis in small animals such as the mouse is relatively easy, especially using the encephalomyocarditis virus. Serial pathologic and histologic studies show the development of cardiac dilatation, heart failure, and progressive fibrosis and myocytolysis in the myocardium. Coxsackie B virus myocarditis in mice has been followed by patchy areas of fibrosis in the myocardium. Viruses are not recoverable from the myocardium after the acute stage, and there are certain differences from the changes seen in chronic myocarditis and dilated cardiomyopathy in man, notably calcification in the myocardium. It is uncertain whether the evidence gained from experiments in mice can be extrapolated to man and it would be wise to be cautious in this regard at the present time. Therefore, in man clinical evidence for the infectious immune theory of dilated cardiomyopathy rests mainly, although not entirely, on the detection of chronic myocardial disease in patients who have had documented acute myocarditis. There are now a number of anecdotal reports of patients developing chronic myocardial disease of the type of dilated cardiomyopathy after a viral infection of the heart. Studies have also shown evidence of very high neutralising antibody titres to coxsackie B1-6 virus in the blood of patients with dilated cardiomyopathy, as compared with controls.[32,33] Therefore, some evidence exists to suggest that patients with dilated cardiomyopathy may have some autoimmune disorder involving the heart. Circulating muscle-specific antimyolemmal antibodies have been found in patients with dilated cardiomyopathy, and in one case endomyocardial biopsy has shown fluorescent virus antibodies in the myocardium in a patient with dilated cardiomyopathy. Also, a patient has been described whose endomyocardial biopsy showed particles resembling herpes virus and whose condition progressed to dilated cardiomyopathy.

In addition to this evidence, there are data from patients with dilated cardiomyopathy who come to cardiac transplantation. The risk of developing lymphoma in these patients is apparently much higher than that in other patients treated by transplantation, whereas a defect in suppressor T-cell function and deficient natural killer cell activity has been shown in patients with dilated cardiomyopathy.[34,35]

Increasing experience of endomyocardial biopsy indicates that 15% to 80% of patients with a clinical diagnosis of dilated cardiomyopathy show cellular infiltration indicative or suggestive of previous myocarditis.[36–38] In the absence of other causes such as drug effects or sensitivity, this is suggestive, although not overwhelming, evidence of previous myocardial infection leading to dilated cardiomyopathy. A further connection between myocarditis and dilated cardiomyopathy is the association in some patients of a short history of congestive heart failure of unknown cause, with evidence of active myocarditis on endomyocardial biopsy. How often this occurs remains to be determined.[38a,38b]

Although it is not suggested that previous myocarditis is the cause of dilated cardiomyopathy in every case, the weight of evidence points to this in at least some patients. Dilated cardiomyopathy may also prove to be the end-result of a variety of other conditioning factors, perhaps in individuals rendered more susceptible by genetic influences. It is well known that dilated cardiomyopathy can occur in families, and the cellular abnormalities could be the result of previous infections, perhaps because a genetic fault predisposes to a virus becoming cardiotropic.

Despite circumstantial evidence linking previous viral infection with dilated cardiomyopathy, the role that primary viral infection might play is uncertain. Selective damage to a subpopulation of suppressor T-cell lymphocytes is possible and might provide a basis for the development of an autoimmune disorder. The trigger mechanism that initiates the cardiomyopathy remains unknown.

SPECIFIC HEART MUSCLE DISEASE

Because these conditions do not come within the definition of cardiomyopathies, they do not strictly come within the scope of this chapter. However, it may be helpful, in order to lend counterpoint to the cardiomyopathies, to describe briefly some of the specific heart muscle diseases. Examples of an infective heart muscle disease (Chagas' disease), a deficiency disease (Keshan disease), a granulomatous disease (sarcoidosis), and a toxic disease (alcohol) will be given. Finally, a short note will be made of a peripartal cardiomyopathy, because its exact place in the classification of cardiomyopathies and specific heart muscle disease is difficult to determine.

The list of rare specific heart muscle diseases is almost inexhaustible. An example, not necessarily complete, is given in Table 43.2.

CHAGAS' DISEASE

Chagas' disease is due to the protozoan *Trypanosoma cruzi*, which causes this most common form of heart disease in some areas of South America, notably Venezuela and Brazil. Nearly 35 million people are exposed to the risk of infection, which is essentially an endemic infection of rural populations. The vector is a triatomid bug that in-

Table 43.2. List of Rare Specific Heart Muscle Diseases

Infective	Endocrine and Metabolic	Infiltrative Diseases	Deficiency and Nutritional Disorders	Connective Tissue Disorders	Granulomas and Neoplasms	Neuromuscular Disorders	Sensitivity and Toxic Reactions
Viral	Thyrotoxicosis	Haemochromatosis	Disturbances of potassium metabolism	Systemic lupus erythematosus	Sarcoidosis	Friedreich's ataxia	Sulphonamides
Rickettsial	Myxoedema	Refsum's disease	Kwashiorkor	Rheumatoid arthritis	Leukaemia	Myotonic dystrophy	Penicillin
Fungal	Phaeochromocytoma	Hurler's syndrome	Magnesium deficiency	Polyarteritis nodosa	Secondary neoplasms	Duchenne's muscular dystrophy	Antimony
Bacterial	Agromegaly	Niemann-Pick disease	Beriberi	Scleroderma	Carcinoid	Facioscapulo-humeral dystrophy	Alcohol
Protozoal	Diabetes	Hand-Schüller-Christian disease		Dermatomyositis			Isoprenalin
		Marquio-Ullrich disease					Adriamycin
							Radiation

habits dwellings, such as poor wooden structures, or may be associated with wild animals. Bugs drop from the ceilings of dwellings, bite the victim, and release the trypanosomes into the blood. Although the lesions affect mainly the heart, they can also involve the gastrointestinal tract, causing megaesophagus and megacolon. Cardiac involvement occurs essentially in three phases: acute, latent, and chronic.

Pathology of the Heart

In the acute phase the heart may be slightly enlarged, overweight, and dilated. Histologic study shows severe myocarditis and many myocardial fibres contain pseudoleishmanial cysts. Degeneration of myocardial fibres and fibrosis is also seen. In the chronic phase the heart is overweight with dilatation of all the cardiac chambers. Lymphatic hyperplasia may be seen following the course of the major coronary vessels. The most characteristic lesion is thinning of the left ventricular wall, usually in the region of the apex, often producing a small aneurysm. Pseudocysts containing the organism can be found even at this late stage. Areas of fibrous replacement and features of healed myocarditis are also evident. Lesions may be found in the autonomic nervous and conducting systems.

Clinical Features

In the acute phase oedema of one or both orbits and skin rashes occur. There is fever, lymphadenopathy, hepatomegaly, splenomegaly, and peripheral oedema. Tachycardia is often a feature. At this stage the electrocardiogram shows prolongation of the PR and QT intervals with nonspecific repolarisation changes. The patient may then pass into the latent phase which may last from 10 to 20 years, and little is known of the changes that occur during this phase. Complement fixation remains positive.

The chronic phase can be divided into three stages. In the first stage there may be no symptoms, but rhythm disturbances producing dizziness and fainting spells can occur. The second stage is noted by the onset of cardiomegaly, and the third stage by congestive heart failure and thromboembolism.

Investigations

Electrocardiography. Changes are not specific in the acute phase, but in the chronic phase multiple multifocal premature ventricular beats, bundle branch block, and heart block may occur. Ambulatory electrocardiographic monitoring is an important investigation for the evaluation of arrhythmias and conduction defects.

Echocardiography. The two-dimensional mode shows segmental dyskinesia and often an apical ventricular aneurysm. Sometimes, in asymptomatic patients, echocardiography may yield the first indication of alteration in contraction of an otherwise apparently normal heart.

Invasive Methods of Investigation. These include haemodynamic studies, angiocardiography, electrophysiologic studies, and endomyocardial biopsy. Haemodynamic studies in the later stages show evidence of poor contractile function. Angiocardiography shows an increase in end-diastolic volume, diminished ejection fraction, and localised asynergy. Intraventricular thrombosis and apical aneurysm may be found in the final stages. Electrophysiologic studies can be used to select patients for special antiarrhythmic treatment or pacemaking. Endomyocardial biopsy is helpful in making an early diagnosis and in following the progress of the disease.[38c]

Prevention

Improvement in housing conditions and socioeconomic situations in general is the major weapon in prevention. Widespread insecticide spraying programmes are also of great value. Early recognition of the disease by sensitive noninvasive techniques of investigation permits early intensive treatment.

Treatment

Treatment consists of two main groups of drugs. The nitrofurane derivatives have largely been superseded by the nitroimidazole derivatives. Treatment is oral, and in acute Chagas' disease it causes rapid remission of fever as well as of the signs and symptoms of the parasitaemia. Antiarrhythmic treatment may also be necessary. Pacemaking is often required and aneurysmectomy may be valuable in treating refractory ventricular tachycardia.

Diagnosis

Diagnosis is aided by a specific complement fixation test (Guerreiro-Machado reaction), but it may be misleading for it can be positive in patients who have been infected but whose hearts are not involved. The test becomes positive in the early phases and remains positive during the later phases of the disease. Recent studies indicate that patients with a positive Guerreiro-Machado reaction show a significantly lower life expectancy than does the control population, but only when clinical and/or electrocardiographic abnormalities coexist.[39]

KESHAN DISEASE

Keshan disease (see chapter 44) is attributed to selenium deficiency and has been described in areas of mainland China since 1950. Selenium intake is markedly reduced in populations from infected areas and the level of selenium in the blood and scalp hair is significantly decreased.

Pathology

The pathologic changes are confined to the heart. Grossly the heart is greatly dilated. Myocardial necrosis and intermingled fibrosis are found. Greyish yellow patches of necrosis and whitish fibrotic areas are seen scattered throughout the myocardium. They are focal but may become confluent. The lesions are particularly prominent in the left ventricular wall, being most severe in the subendocardium. Coagulation necrosis, myocytolysis, and fibrosis are found on histologic study.

Incidence

Keshan disease occurs in 14 provinces of China in a long narrow belt from northeast to southwest. The highest annual incidence is thought to be 33 cases per 100,000 population. Children below the age of 15 years and women of childbearing age are most susceptible.

Clinical Features

Acute Keshan disease commonly has a fulminating onset and a high mortality rate. Cardiogenic shock is frequent with hypotension, dizziness, and restlessness; vomiting is frequent and severe. In patients who survive, the clinical picture is one of dilated cardiomyopathy. Arrhythmias are common; ventricular premature beats, atrial fibrillation, ventricular tachycardia, and conduction defects are frequently seen.

Management

Sodium selenite has been given successfully as a preventive measure and supplementation of the diet on a large scale with oral selenium has resulted in significant reduction in the number of new cases.

SARCOID HEART DISEASE

Sarcoid heart disease has been recognised since 1929. A collection of cases in Great Britain was started by Fleming in 1971. The latest figure is 290 cases, 100 of them with necropsy confirmation.[40]

Pathology

Sarcoid granulomas are found in the heart at necropsy in about 20% of patients. Cardiac deposits mainly involve the distal portion of the ventricular septum, the left ventricular papillary muscles, and adjacent free walls and the right or left ventricular free walls. These sites of involvement are particularly likely to produce conduction disturbances, especially complete heart block with ventricular septal involvement, mitral regurgitation when the left ventricular papillary muscles are involved, and left ventricular aneurysm when the left ventricular free wall is damaged. In addition, ventricular arrhythmias are common and may be intractable. Sudden death is a frequent termination and may be the initial manifestation of sarcoidosis.

Clinical Features

The clinical features depend on the site of the major sarcoid involvement and may be very protean. Several syndromes are recognised; acute severe mitral regurgitation can result from disruption of papillary muscles infiltrated with sarcoid tissue, episodes of cardiac pain and congestive heart failure may suggest coronary heart disease, and the development of left ventricular aneurysm may further compound the difficulty of diagnosis.

The most common presentation is some form of arrhythmia, usually a conduction defect producing Adams-Stokes attacks or episodes of dizziness or palpitations. Repetitive intractable ventricular arrhythmias are also a mode of presentation. The combination of intractable arrhythmias with severe heart failure is well recognised.

Investigations

Electrocardiography. The most common abnormality is some form of tachyarrhythmia followed closely by various forms of heart block. T-wave changes may occur and changes of myocardial infarction have been recorded.

Chest Radiography. This is not usually specific with regard to the heart, although if there is a large cardiac aneurysm, this may be revealed radiologically.

Echocardiography. Echocardiography reveals dilatation of the ventricles and poor contraction, often with asynergy. Intraventricular thrombus may be present. The appearances are not specific for sarcoidosis, however.

Endomyocardial Biopsy. If positive, this is of great value. A negative result should not be regarded as excluding the disease, as sarcoidosis is patchy. Unfortunately the Kviem test is not entirely reliable and examples of severe sarcoid heart disease have been recorded with a persistently negative Kviem test.

Angiocardiography. Angiocardiography does not reveal any specific appearance, but it confirms the findings of echocardiography. The coronary arteries are normal.

Other Organs Usually Involved

The most common organ involved is the lung, but lymph node, skin, eye, spleen, liver, nerves, bone, and parotid have all been described. Occasionally lesions may be found in the uterus, pituitary, meninges, kidney, and thyroid.

Diagnosis

Diagnosis largely depends on keeping the possibility of myocardial sarcoidosis in mind in any patient who has severe repetitive arrhythmias with or without heart block or who has heart failure of unknown cause. Endomyocardial biopsy may give the definitive answer[41] and search should be made for sarcoid involvement in other organs, especially the lungs and liver. Transbronchial pulmonary biopsy may be useful and liver biopsy may be needed. Failure to find evidence of sarcoid disease elsewhere than in the heart does not exclude myocardial sarcoidosis, which is often not part of a florid picture of sarcoidosis. The heart can be massively involved when other organs are only minimally affected.[41]

Treatment

Arrhythmias, heart block, and heart failure must be treated on their own merits. Pacing is required in heart block, but the tachyarrhythmias commonly do not respond to the usual antiarrhythmic drugs. It has been suggested that steroid treatment reduces the incidence of sudden death, but there is no certain evidence of this, although steroids are probably worth trying once the diagnosis has been made. Surgical treatment to ablate arrhythmogenic areas or to resect ventricular aneurysm may have to be considered.

ALCOHOLIC HEART MUSCLE DISEASE

Alcoholic heart muscle disease is diagnosed when low output heart failure with cardiomegaly, dilated ventricles, and poor contractile function occurs in a patient who has taken large quantities of alcohol over a long period and who does not have any reason for heart failure from any other cause. In addition to producing heart failure, alcohol may exert other effects on the heart, notably arrhythmias and possibly hypertension. However, in patients consuming large quantities of alcohol, heart failure may be due not only to the direct effect of alcohol on the myocardium but also to thiamine deficiency. The amount of alcohol necessary to produce heart muscle disease is not exactly known. Probably 40 g of alcohol a day for more than 10 years constitutes a significant risk.

Pathology

The pathology of chronic alcoholic heart muscle disease is not specific and is indistinguishable from that of dilated cardiomyopathy.

Effects of Alcohol on the Heart

Alcohol has a direct effect on the heart, altering the ionic permeability of cardiac cells; potassium, phosphate, and possibly magnesium are lost from the left ventricle. Lipid transport is abnormal, free fatty acid uptake is increased and myofibrillar ATPase activity suggests a direct depressant action on the myocardium. Acetaldehyde may be involved in the process by which alcohol produces myocardial depression. Acute administration of alcohol to normal man produces an increase in cardiac output and heart rate without change in stroke volume. Patients who already have cardiac damage have greater depression of myocardial function on acute alcohol ingestion.

Clinical Features

The earliest stage of alcoholic heart muscle disease may be supraventricular arrhythmia, the most common being paroxysmal atrial flutter or fibrillation. In the early stages also there may be signs suggesting thyroid overaction with tachycardia, sweating, tremor, and mild to moderate hypertension. Later the symptoms are those of biventricular failure with exertional dyspnoea, orthopnoea, palpitations, and fatigue followed by oedema of the extremities and signs of congestive heart failure. Chest pain may occur but is not typical of angina. Although severe alcoholic heart muscle disease causes low output congestive heart failure, in some patients there may be a suggestion of a higher output with dilated veins and warm extremities possibly as a result of coincident alcoholic liver disease.

Laboratory Investigations

An elevated mean corpuscular volume of the erythrocyte together with an elevated gammaglutamyl transpeptidase level are strong pointers to excessive alcohol consumption, although this does not necessarily mean alcoholic heart muscle disease. Further indications are elevated blood uric acid or triglyceride levels. Urinary or blood alcohol estimations may be valuable if long-standing alcohol abuse is suspected.

Electrocardiography. There are no pathognomonic changes in the electrocardiogram. Nonspecific T- and ST-segment changes occur and there may be intraventricular conduction disturbances, bundle branch block, or left ventricular hypertrophy.

Radiography of the Chest. This usually shows cardiomegaly, which tends to regress when the patient stops drinking. This improvement is a valuable pointer to alcohol as the cause of heart muscle disease.

Echocardiography. The echocardiogram may be useful in detecting early disease. A decrease in the velocity of left ventricular fibre shortening with an increase in left ventricular systolic and diastolic dimensions has been reported.

Radioisotope Tests. Gated blood pool scanning can be of value in enabling serial measurements of left ventricular function to be made with and without exercise and before and after cessation of alcohol consumption.

Endomyocardial Biopsy. The findings are similar to those in dilated cardiomyopathy. Myocardial enzyme activities may give some clue to diagnosis. A clear separation has been suggested between dilated cardiomyopathy and alcoholic heart muscle disease in patients who had abstained from alcohol in that creatine phosphokinase and glutamic oxalacetic transaminase were significantly lower in the former.

Diagnosis

The diagnosis often depends on a high index of suspicion in a patient who may have high alcohol consumption and no other reason for heart failure, especially if there is other evidence of alcoholism. A detailed alcohol history clearly is extremely important, but the diagnosis cannot always be sustained unless cessation from alcohol use causes definite regression of heart failure.

Treatment

Treatment essentially consists of complete abstinence from alcohol and it may be very effective. In addition, antiarrhythmic therapy and also therapy for heart failure may be required. Vitamins, especially of the B group, should be given.

PERIPARTAL HEART DISEASE

Peripartal heart disease is defined as unexplained cardiac failure occurring in women during late pregnancy or after childbirth. Peripartal cardiomyopathy has been described from all over the world, but it is common in Africa and in underprivileged Negroes in the United States. The pathology and haemodynamic features are identical to those of dilated cardiomyopathy.

Clinical Features

These are identical to those of dilated cardiomyopathy, but the relation to pregnancy, parturition, and probably lactation is well established. Affected women are usually multiparous and of higher mean age than the general population of pregnant patients. Symptoms and signs of congestive heart failure usually begin after delivery or in the last few weeks of pregnancy. Chest pain may occur and in some cases is attributable to pulmonary embolism. Transient hypertension has been noted on admission to the hospital and subsides following treatment for heart failure. In some patients, however, this hypertension may possibly be the cause of heart failure; therefore, such patients, strictly speaking, are not suffering from peripartal heart disease.

Laboratory Investigations

Electrocardiographic, radiologic, and angiographic features are indistinguishable from those of dilated cardiomyopathy.

Aetiology

The aetiology is unknown, but the following have been suggested: (1) glomerulonephritis, (2) an association with toxaemia in pregnancy, (3) nutrition, and (4) infection. Glomerulonephritis is unlikely as it has rarely been encountered. An association with toxaemia in pregnancy also seems unlikely because massive proteinuria does not occur in peripartal cardiomyopathy. Nutrition may possibly be a factor in patients in Korea in whom thiamine deficiency has been identified. Infection seems possible in that at least some of the patients are suffering from the effects of viral myocarditis, as possibly is the case in dilated cardiomyopathy. Some studies have shown evidence suggesting previous viral myocarditis.

The Special Type of Peripartal Heart Disease in Northern Nigeria

There is a high incidence of severe heart failure in the postpartum period in Hausa women in the northern region of Nigeria.[42] This has been attributed to excessive fluid and salt overload and responds rapidly and usually completely to cessation of overload and diuretic therapy.[43] It is possible that some of these patients have true cardiac failure, but in the majority it seems that the heart failure is simply due to salt and water overload.

Treatment

There is no specific treatment, which should be in general that for heart failure. Important preventive measures are avoidance of further pregnancy if the heart remains enlarged after an episode of peripartal heart failure, maintenance of adequate nutrition, and a public health campaign to eradicate customs that can produce or aggravate heart failure.

REFERENCES

1. Goodwin JF: Congestive and hypertrophic cardiomyopathies: a decade of study. *Lancet* 1970; 1:731–739.
2. Report of the WHO/ISFC Task Force on the definition and classification of cardiomyopathies. *Br Heart J* 1980; 44:672–673.
3. Goodwin JF: The frontiers of cardiomyopathy. *Br Heart J* 1982; 48:1–18.
4. World Health Organization: *Cardiomyopathies: report of a WHO expert committee.* Technical report series 697, WHO, Geneva, 1984.
5. Goodwin JF: Mechanisms in cardiomyopathies. *J Mol Cell Cardiol* 1985; 17(suppl 2): 5–9.
6. Laks MM, Morady F, Swan HJC: Myocardial hypertrophy produced by chronic infusion of subhypertensive doses of norepinephrine in the dog. *Chest* 1973; 64:75–78.
7. Raum WJ, Laks MM, Garner D, Swerdloff RS: β-adrenergic receptor and cyclic AMP alterations in the canine ventricular septum during long-term norepinephrine infusion: implications for hypertrophic cardiomyopathy. *Circulation* 1983; 68:693–699.
8. Olsen EGJ: An endocrine experimental model for myofibrillar disarray as found in hypertrophic cardiomyopathy. *J Mol Cell Cardiol* 1985; 17(suppl 2):35–40.
9. Goodwin JF: An appreciation of hypertrophic cardiomyopathy. *Am J Med* 1980; 68:797–800.
10. Wenger NK, Goodwin JF, Roberts WC: Cardiomyopathy and myocardial involvement in systemic disease, in Hurst JW (ed): *The Heart.* New York, McGraw-Hill, 1986, pp 1181–1248.
11. Goodwin JF: Hypertrophic cardiomyopathy: clinical aspects and investigations, in Goodwin JF (ed): *Heart Muscle Disease.* Lancaster, England, MTP Press, 1985, pp 23–33.
12. Sugrue DD, McKenna WJ, Dickie S, Myers MJ, Lavendar JP, Oakley CM, Goodwin JF: Relation between left ventricular gradient and relative stroke volume ejected in early and late systole in hypertrophic cardiomyopathy. Assessment with radionuclide cineangiography. *Br Heart J* 1984; 52:602–609.

12a. Al-Bahar R, Hayatt N, Mohammed MM, Abdel-Dayem HM: "Tear drop sign" in hypertrophic cardiomyopathy. A finding on gated cardiac imaging. *Clin Nucl Med* 1986; 11:121–122.

13. McKenna WJ, England D, Doi YL, Deanfield JE, Oakley C, Goodwin JF: Arrhythmias in hypertrophic cardiomyopathy. I. Influence on prognosis. *Br Heart J* 1981; 46:168–172.
14. Goodwin JF, Krikler DM: Arrhythmias as a cause of sudden death in hypertrophic cardiomyopathy. *Lancet* 1976; 2:937–940.

14a. O'Gara PT, Bonow RO, Damske BA, Maron BJ, Spirito P, Bacharach SL, Green MB, Larson SM, Epstein SE: Myocardial perfusion abnormalities in patients with hypertrophic cardiomyopathy and normal coronary arteries. *J Am Coll Cardiol* 1986; 7:95A.

14b. McKenna WJ, Deanfield J, Franklin R, Krikler S, Dickie S: Arrhythmia in children and adolescents with hypertrophic cardiomyopathy: incidence and relation to prognosis. *J Am Coll Cardiol* 1986; 7:204A.

15. McKenna WJ, Krikler DM: Clinical evaluation of the efficacy of oral amiodarone. *Br Heart J* 1984; 51:241–242.
16. McKenna WJ, Harris L, Rowland E, Kleinebenne A, Krikler DM, Oakley CM, Goodwin JF: Amiodarone for long-term management of patients with hypertrophic cardiomyopathy. *Am J Cardiol* 1984; 54:802–810.
17. McKenna WJ, Oakley CM, Krikler DM, Goodwin JF: Improved survival with amiodarone in patients with hypertrophic cardiomyopathy and ventricular tachycardia. *Br Heart J* 1985; 53:412–416.
18. McKenna WJ, Harris L, Perez G, Krikler DM, Oakley C, Goodwin JF: Arrhythmias in hypertrophic cardiomyopathy. II. Comparison of amiodarone and verapamil in treatment. *Br Heart J* 1981; 46:173–178.
19. Bonow RO, Dilsizian V, Rosing DR, Maron BJ, Bacharach SL, Green MV: Verapamil-induced improvement in left ventricular diastolic filling and increased exercise tolerance in patients with hypertrophic cardiomyopathy: short- and long-term effects. *Circulation* 1985; 72:853–864.
20. Rosing DR, Condit JR, Maron BJ, Kent KM, Leon MB, Bonow RO, Lipsen LC, Epstein SE: Verapamil therapy: a new approach to the pharmacologic treatment of hypertrophic cardiomyopathy. III. Effects of long-term administration. *Am J Cardiol* 1981; 48:545–553.
21. Rosing DR, Idanpaan-Heikkila U, Maron BJ, Bonow RO, Epstein SE: Use of calcium-channel blocking drugs in hypertrophic cardiomyopathy. *Am J Cardiol* 1985; 55:185B–195B.
22. Lorell BH, Paulus WJ, Grossman W, Wynne J, Cohn PF: Modification of abnormal left ventricular diastolic properties by nifedipine in patients with hypertrophic cardiomyopathy. *Circulation* 1982; 65:499–507.
23. Lorell BH: Use of calcium channel blockers in hypertrophic cardiomyopathy. *Am J Med* 1985; 78(2B):43–54.
24. Cokkinos DV, Krajcer Z, Leachman RD: Coronary artery disease in hypertrophic cardiomyopathy. *Am J Cardiol* 1985; 55:1437–1438.
25. Torp A: Incidence of congestive cardiomyopathy, in Goodwin JF, Hjalmarson A, Olsen EGJ (eds): *Congestive Cardiomyopathy.* Moelndal, Sweden, AB Hassle, 1981, pp 18–22.
26. McKenna WJ, Krikler DM, Goodwin JF: Arrhythmias in dilated and hypertrophic cardiomyopathy. *Med Clin North Am* 1984; 68:983–1000.

26a. Stevenson LW, Fowler MB, Schroeder JS, MacAlpin RN, Dracup KA, Fond V: Unexpected poor survival with dilated cardiomyopathy where transplantation denied due to limited symptoms. *J Am Coll Cardiol* 1986; 7:203A.

27. Fuster V, Gersh BJ, Giuliani ER, Tajik AJ, Brandenburg RO, Frye RL: The natural history of idiopathic dilated cardiomyopathy. *Am J Cardiol* 1981; 47:525–531.

27a. Sheikh MU, Guipta AK, Robinson F, Mills RJ, Dais K, Ali N, Lee WR: Long-term hydralazine therapy in dilated cardiomyopathy: effect on survival. *J Am Coll Cardiol* 1986; 7:94A.

28. Copeland JG, Emery RW, Levinson MM, Copeland J, McAleer MJ, Riley JE: The role of mechanical support and transplantation in treatment of patients with end-stage cardiomyopathy. *Circulation* 1985; 72(suppl II):II-7–II-12.

28a. Editorial: Natural history of dilated cardiomyopathy. *Lancet* 1986; 1:248–249.

29. Olsen EGJ, Spry CJF: The pathogenesis of Löeffler's endomyocardial disease and its relationship to endomyocardial fibrosis, in Yu PN,

Goodwin JF (eds): *Progress in Cardiology*. Philadelphia, Lea & Febiger, 1979, pp 281–303.

30. Spry CJF, Davies J, Tai PC, Olsen EGT, Oakley CM, Goodwin JF: Clinical features of fifteen patients with hypereosinophilic syndrome. *Q J Med* 1983; 52:1–22.
31. Chew CC, Ziady GM, Raphael MJ, Oakley CM: Functional defect in amyloid heart disease. The "stiff heart" syndrome. *Am J Cardiol* 1975; 36:438–444.

31a. Siquiera-Filho AG, Cunha CLP, Tajik AJ, Seward JB, Schattenberg TT, Giuliani ER: M-mode and two-dimensional echocardiographic features in cardiac amyloidosis. *Circulation* 1981; 63:188–196.

31b. Sedlis SP, Saffitz JE, Schwob VS, Jaffe AS: Cardiac amyloidosis simulating hypertrophic cardiomyopathy. *Am J Cardiol* 1984; 53:969–970.

32. Cambridge G, MacArthur CGC, Waterson AP, Goodwin JF, Oakley CM: Antibodies to Coxsackie B viruses in congestive cardiomyopathy. *Br Heart J* 1979; 41:692–696.
33. Yang LD, Chen HZ, Pu SY, Zhu JR, Shi OS, Yang YZ: Possible etiological association of Coxsackie B viruses with idiopathic dilated cardiomyopathy. *Chin J Cardiol* 1984; 12:86–89.
34. Anderson JL, Carlquist JF, Hammond EH: Deficient natural killer cell activity in patients with idiopathic dilated cardiomyopathy. *Lancet* 1982; 2:1124–1127.
35. Anderson JL, Carlquist JF, Higashikubo R: Quantitation of lymphocyte subsets by immunofluorescence flow cytometry in idiopathic dilated cardiomyopathy. *Am J Cardiol* 1985; 55:1550–1554.
36. Mason JW, Billingham ME, Ricci DR: Treatment of acute inflammatory myocarditis assisted by endomyocardial biopsy. *Am J Cardiol* 1980; 45:1037–1044.
37. Zee-Cheng CS, Tsai CC, Palmer DC, Codd JE, Pennington DG, Williams GA: High incidence of myocarditis by endomyocardial biopsy in patients with idiopathic congestive cardiomyopathy. *J Am Coll Cardiol* 1984; 3:63–70.
38. Dec GW Jr, Palacios IF, Fallon JT, Aretz HT, Mills J, Lee DCS, Johnson RA: Active myocarditis in the spectrum of acute dilated cardiomyopathies. Clinical features, histologic correlates, and clinical outcome. *N Engl J Med* 1985; 312:885–890.

38a. Waller BF, Slack JD, Dillon JC, Mirro MJ, Kelly K, Valentine RP, Yum MN, French MLV: Rarity of myocarditis on endomyocardial biopsy in patients with new onset idiopathic congestive heart failure. A histologic and ultrastructural, immunohistochemical and viral serologic analysis of 72 patients. *J Am Coll Cardiol* 1986; 7:120A.

38b. Dec WG, Fallon JT, Schaer JM, Southern J, Palacios IF: Does repeat endomyocardial biopsy aid in the diagnosis of active myocarditis? *J Am Coll Cardiol* 1986; 7:121A.

38c. Pereira Barretto AC, Mady C, Arteaga-Fernandez E, Stolf N, Lopes EA, Higuchi ML, Bellotti G, Pileggi F: Right ventricular endomyocardial biopsy in chronic Chagas' disease. *Am Heart J* 1986; 111:307–312.

39. Espinosa R, Carrasco HA, Belandria F, Fuenmayor AM, Molina C, Gonzalez R, Martinez O: Life expectancy analysis in patients with Chagas' disease: prognosis after one decade (1973–1983). *Intern J Cardiol* 1985; 8:45–56.
40. Fleming HA: Sarcoid heart disease. *Br Med J* 1986; 292:1095–1096.
41. Lemery R, McGoon MD, Edwards WD: Cardiac sarcoidosis: a potentially treatable form of myocarditis. *Mayo Clinc Proc* 1985; 60:549–554.
42. Julian DG, Szekely P: Peripartum cardiomyopathy. *Progr Cardiovasc Dis* 1985; 27:223–240.
43. Homan DC: Peripartum cardiomyopathy. *N Engl J Med* 1985; 312:1432–1437.

44 Keshan Disease

Bo-Qi Gu, MD and Tsung O. Cheng, MD

INCIDENCE AND PREVALENCE

Keshan disease (KSD) (克山病) is an endemic cardiomyopathy of unknown origin. From known data, it was recognized that in the middle of the winter of 1935, many deaths occurred in local inhabitants in Keshan County, Heilongjiang Province, China. As the cause was unknown at that time, the disease was named after the county. Because of the sudden onset, repeated vomiting, and inevitable fatal outcome, local residents called it the "disease of sudden death" or the "disease of emesis of yellow water." According to a local document of Keshan County, this disease had been discovered in the county as far back as 1907. From 1947 to 1952 in northeast China, 4,758 patients died of KSD.[1] In 1938, hundreds of immigrants had this disease in Huanglong District, Shanxi Province. In Chuanxi and Chuxiong, Yunnan, Yi Autonomous State, many pediatric cases of KSD were reported in 1961 and 1966, respectively. In 1975, KSD was identified in Tibet when a number of pediatric cases of subacute KSD were diagnosed in Lhasa Valley. Today it is confirmed that the affected areas of KSD included 14 provinces and autonomous regions in China. Guichou is a highly suspicious endemic area. Except in North Korea (1951) and Japan (Xinzhou myocardial disease), no similar case has been reported elsewhere in the world.[2]

Clinically, based on functional performance of the heart, KSD has been classified into four types: acute, with sudden onset with cardiogenic shock and severe arrhythmia; subacute, with both cardiogenic shock and congestive heart failure; chronic, with marked dilation of the cardiac chambers and congestive heart failure; and latent, with various degrees of cardiomegaly but compensated cardiac function.

Keshan disease is restricted to certain areas in China with strongly leached hill and mountain soils and to some with "black earth" soils, such as the northeast endemic areas, and the endemic areas extend in a broad band across the country, from northeast to southwest (Figure 44.1).

Keshan disease mainly affects the agricultural population, especially those peasants whose staple foods are self-grown. The urban population is always spared.[3,4] The morbidity shows no difference between male and female subjects over 50 years of age; however, weanling and preschool children and women of childbearing age are most susceptible. In southwest districts the disease predominantly affects children. Most acute cases of KSD occur in deep winter from November to February of the next year, whereas chronic and subacute cases are prevalent in early spring and summer (in the southwest districts).

PATHOLOGY

In KSD pathologic changes mainly involve the myocardium. Owing to the spotted distribution of subendomyocardial necrosis, the conduction system is usually affected. Focal necrosis of skeletal muscles, thromboembolic phenomena, and congestion of visceral organs represent the minor pathologic features of KSD.

HEART

Macroscopically, the heart is enlarged and increased in weight. Both ventricles are dilated symmetrically. Because of marked dilatation, cardiac hypertrophy is somewhat overshadowed. The left ventricular wall measured 1.22 $\pm$ 0.27 cm in thickness in adult patients and the right ventricular wall 0.33 $\pm$ 0.11 cm. The dimensions of the

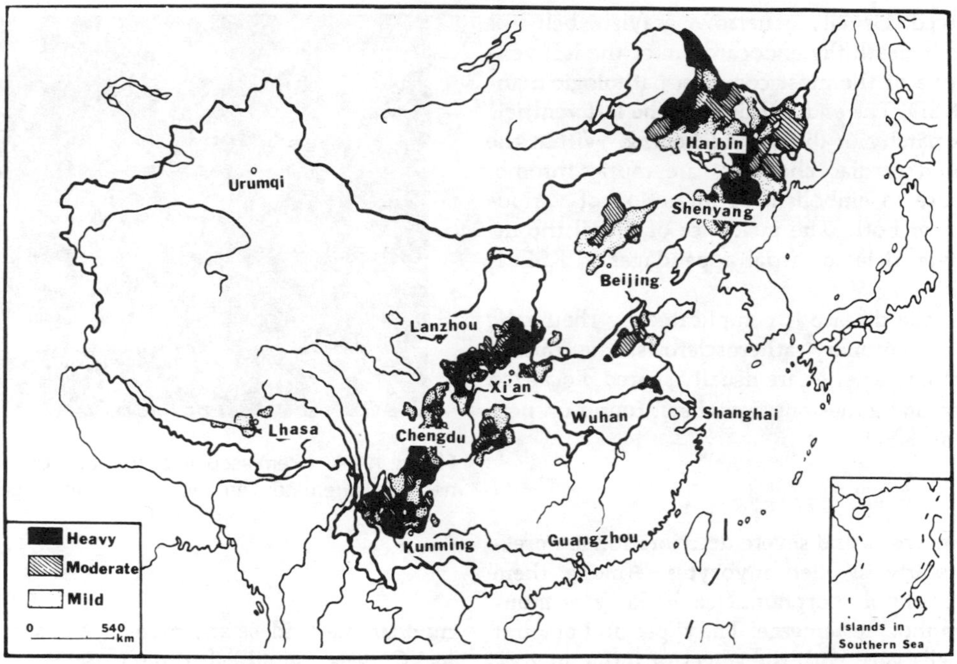

Figure 44.1. The map of distribution of endemic districts of Keshan disease in China. (Modified from *Acta Nutr Sin* 1982; 4:176.)

inflow and outflow tract of both ventricles are higher than those in the control group. Thus, both the longitudinal and transverse diameter of the heart are increased significantly.[5,6] In cases of severe myocardial necrosis the heart weighs from 250 to 350 g. One of the heaviest hearts of long-standing chronic KSD weighed 580 g[7] (Figure 44.2).

In the subendomyocardium, fibrous scar tissue and deteriorated foci of different histologic age intermingle. The myocardium situated nearer to the endocardium is more

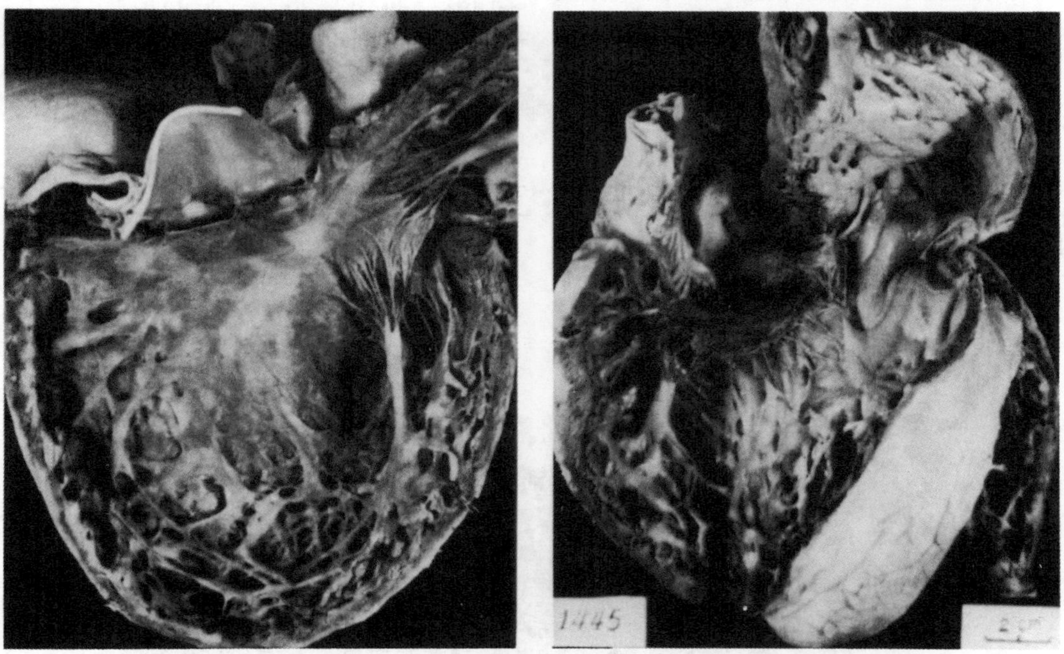

Figure 44.2. Extreme dilatation of the left ventricle and thinning of its wall (*left*); marked dilatation of the right ventricle (*right*) in chronic KSD. This 28-year-old patient had heart palpitations and dyspnea for one year. The electrocardiogram shows right bundle branch block. The patient died of congestive heart failure. At autopsy the heart weighed 510 g.

severely damaged. Usually a narrow, grayish, belt-like lesion is found beneath the endocardium of the left ventricle. This is one of the most common pathologic manifestations of KSD. The endocardium of the left ventricle usually shows patchy or diffuse thickening. Within the markedly dilated cardiac chambers are mural thrombi which predispose to embolism or infarction of various visceral organs, or both. The incidence of mural thrombosis of both ventricles or atrial appendages in KSD is about 13%.[8]

Except when the disease is complicated by rheumatic heart disease or coronary atherosclerosis, the cardiac valves and coronary arteries are usually spared. Localized or diffuse epicardial adhesions have been found on necropsy in Tibetan KSD.

Histopathology

Coagulation necrosis and severe deterioration are present with irregularly swollen myocytes. Among them varying numbers of polymorphonuclear leukocytes, monocytes, and lymphocytes emerge. The types and amount of infiltrating cells vary with the stages of inflammatory processes of the myocardium. Myocytolysis of myocytes results from severe fatty degeneration and hydropic change of myocardial cells, which is another type of myocardial necrosis.

Disseminated miliary multifocal necrosis is the fundamental myocardial lesion of KSD. The myocardial foci usually exhibit a perivascular pattern along the course of mural coronary tributaries. In children these lesions have a much closer relation to small branches of coronary arteries than they do in adults.[9,10] Repair of myocardial lesions mainly depends on condensation of local reticulin fiber of the myocardial interstitial tissue and conversion into scar tissue (noncellular sclerosis) (Figures 44.3 and 44.4).

Histochemical Studies

Acid phosphatase activity was obviously increased in muscle fibers surrounding the necrotic foci probably because of the increased membranous permeability of the myocardial cell organelles, and the succinic dehydrogenase activity was greatly reduced in the damaged myocardial cells. No significant change has been found in monoamine oxidase and myosin ATPase[11] (Harbin Medical College, unpublished data, 1972).

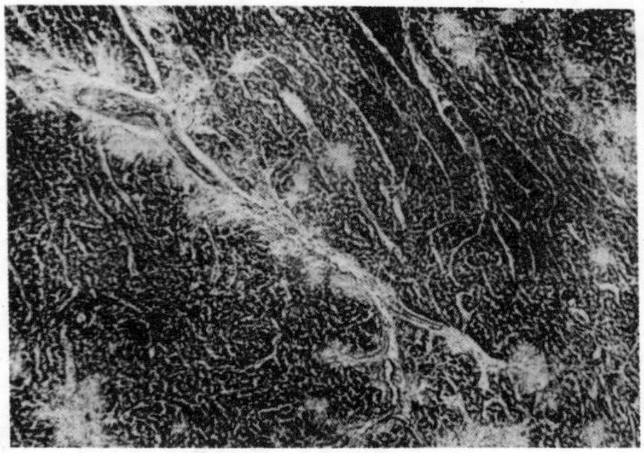

Figure 44.4. Perivascular distribution of foci of myocardial necrosis. (Hematoxylin and eosin stain; original magnification × 44.)

Electronmicroscopic Investigation

In semi-thin sections the cardiac cell hyaline mass is composed of many compacted myofibrils interrupted by numerous minute segments of contraction bands.[12–14] Between two bands are many fat droplets and fine granules with deep blue-tinged groups of cardiac mitochondria. Because of overcontraction and stretching of the myofilaments, the myofibrils disrupt into many hyalinized contraction bands formed by a series of coagulated sarcomeres. Between two bands are noted clumps of dense calcified mitochondia, much dilated sarcoplasmic reticulum, and fatty droplets. The cardiac mitochondria reveal various degrees of swelling, tubular degeneration, and decreased matrix density. Occasionally myelin figures of bizarre shaped giant mitochondria can be seen.

Under light microscope the myocardial cells are juicy and filled with numerous "vesicles." The myofibrils disappear gradually because of the myocytoplasm lytic process. Electronmicroscopically most of the intracytoplasmic vesicles are composed of greatly dilated and degenerated myocardial mitochondria or sarcoplasmic reticulum. In

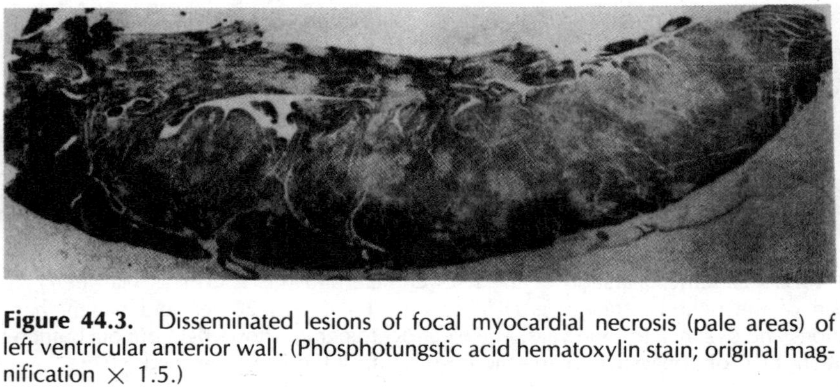

Figure 44.3. Disseminated lesions of focal myocardial necrosis (pale areas) of left ventricular anterior wall. (Phosphotungstic acid hematoxylin stain; original magnification × 1.5.)

the vesicles, debris or segments of mitochondrial cristae can be found. Scattered pieces of myofibril with attenuated, well-preserved myofilaments may be seen in between (Figures 44.5, 44.6, and 44.7).

Pathologic Changes in the Heart Conduction System

Because of the anatomic coincidence of subendocardial localization of the conduction system and myocardial multifocal necrosis in KSD, the conduction system is rarely spared. Arrhythmias are the usual clinical feature in KSD. Histologic examination of the sinoatrial node, atrioventricular node, and His bundle and its branches shows that both bundle branches are severely affected.[15] During penetration into the subendocardium of the right ventricular septum the right bundle branch is usually interrupted by necrosis or fibrosis. The His bundle and atrioventricular node show slight changes. No significant change has been found in the sinoatrial node. However, clinically, in third degree atrioventricular block focal hyaline necrosis, myocytolysis, and inflammatory infiltration of both bundle branches and Purkinje fiber at different levels have been shown pathologically.

OTHER VISCERAL ORGANS

Ascites, pleural effusion, and pericardial effusion are usual in patients with prolonged heart failure. The largest amount of ascitic fluid seen was about 3,000 ml.

Skeletal Muscle

Lesions of the skeletal muscles such as the diaphragm, intercostal and gastrocnemius muscles, and even the tongue have been reported since 1959, with the diaphragm having the most damage. The incidence varies from 16% to 27% in autopsy cases of KSD.[8] The pathologic features of skeletal muscle are hyalinization or waxy degeneration of single myocytes followed by infiltration of polymorphonuclear leukocytes, monocytes, and lymphocytes and active sarcolemmal cell proliferation.

Liver

About 50% of patients with chronic KSD have congestive liver fibrosis. In only 5% does cardiac cirrhosis develop. Persistent cardiogenic shock with prolonged hypotension may lead to centrolobular infarctoid necrosis of the liver.[16]

Respiratory Tract

Acute or chronic pulmonary congestion and pulmonary edema are usual in KSD. At necropsy, pulmonary hemorrhagic infarction was seen in 6% of cases. As many as 70% of the children with KSD in the southern endemic areas have accompanying interstitial pneumonia.[17]

Central Nervous System

Cerebral infarction is not discovered at necropsy, although it is reported by some clinicians as 13%.[18]

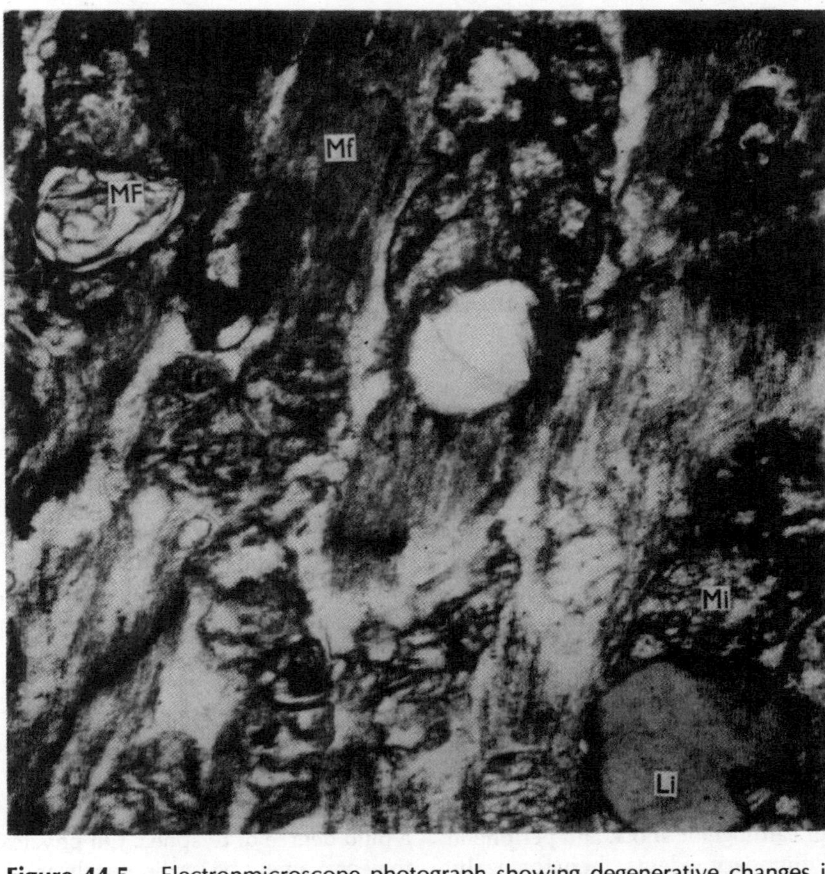

Figure 44.5. Electronmicroscope photograph showing degenerative changes in most of the cardiac mitochondria (Mi) and myelin figure formation (MF) with lipid deposition (Li). Mf = myofibril. (Original magnification × 25,000.)

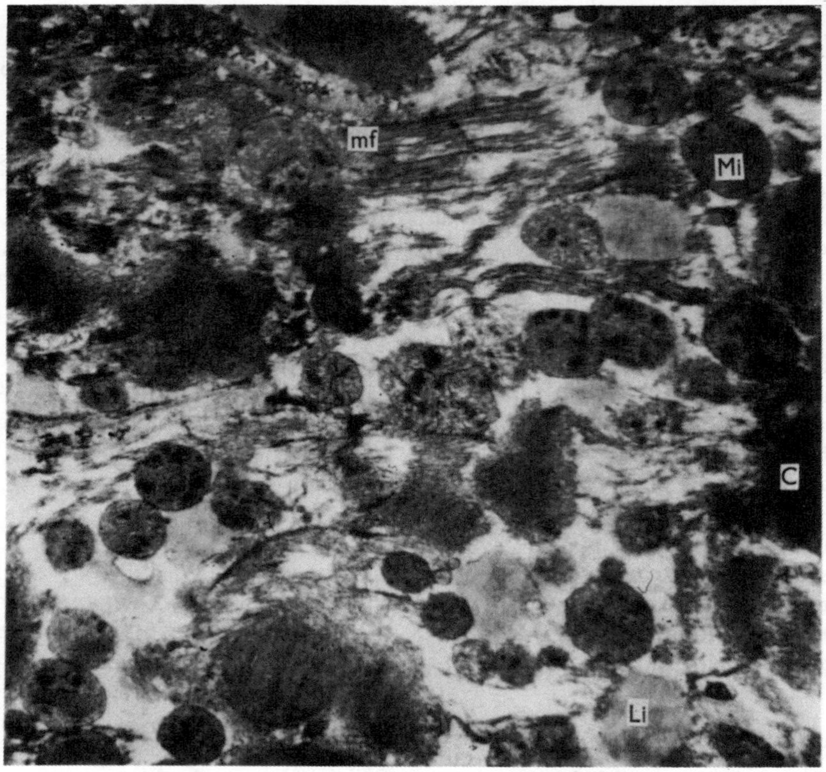

Figure 44.6. Electronmicroscope photograph showing coagulation (C) of myofilaments (mf) and compacted mitochondria (Mi) with dense electron granules. (Original magnification × 9,000.)

FETAL KESHAN DISEASE

Six fetuses with KSD have been reported since 1959. Their mothers had acute or chronic KSD. The morphologic features of fetal KSD are similar to those in adults. The myocardial lesions are situated mostly beneath the endocardium, but contrary to adult KSD, in the fetus the right ventricle is affected more severely than the left. The placenta shows no significant changes. The gestational age of the affected fetus is almost always more than 6 months.[19]

CLINICAL FEATURES

ACUTE KESHAN DISEASE

Acute KSD is characterized by sudden onset, in severe cases, of symptoms due to cardiogenic shock, acute pulmonary edema, and severe arrhythmia. Patients complain of epigastric discomfort, nausea, and intractable repeated vomiting in which even the duodenal contents are evacuated. The mechanism of such vomiting is still not certain (viscerovagal reflex or anoxia). Because of cerebral anoxia, the patients always become restless and finally die of repeated attacks of convulsive seizures. Acute cardiac dilatation may develop gradually within 24 hours. The patients have both signs of cardiogenic shock and peripheral circulatory collapse. Pulmonary edema, hepatomegaly, and edema of the lower extremities appears in the later period. The mortality from acute KSD reached 80% until the use of vitamin C megadose therapy, after which it decreased to below 10% to 20%.

SUBACUTE KESHAN DISEASE

Subacute KSD is characterized by an insidious onset and mainly affects children of 1 to 5 years of age. Patients usually show puffiness of the face and also signs of cardiogenic shock. The degree of shock is somewhat milder than that in acute KSD. They often manifest signs of right-sided or right- and left-sided congestive heart failure. The heart is usually moderately enlarged. Tachycardia and gallop rhythm are the usual findings.

CHRONIC KESHAN DISEASE

Chronic KSD may be derived from acute or subacute KSD. Signs and symptoms of chronic congestive heart failure dominate the clinical picture. Dilatation of both sides of the heart, diminished cardiac sounds, diastolic gallop, and a precordial pansystolic murmur are the usual physical findings.

LATENT KESHAN DISEASE

Latent KSD is usually detected during mass survey for KSD in endemic districts. Most of the patients are asymptomatic. Some patients have palpitations of the heart and a mild degree of dyspnea. On physical examination there may or may not be cardiomegaly and low intensity cardiac sounds. Extrasystolic heart beats and right bundle branch block are the important electrocardiographic findings.

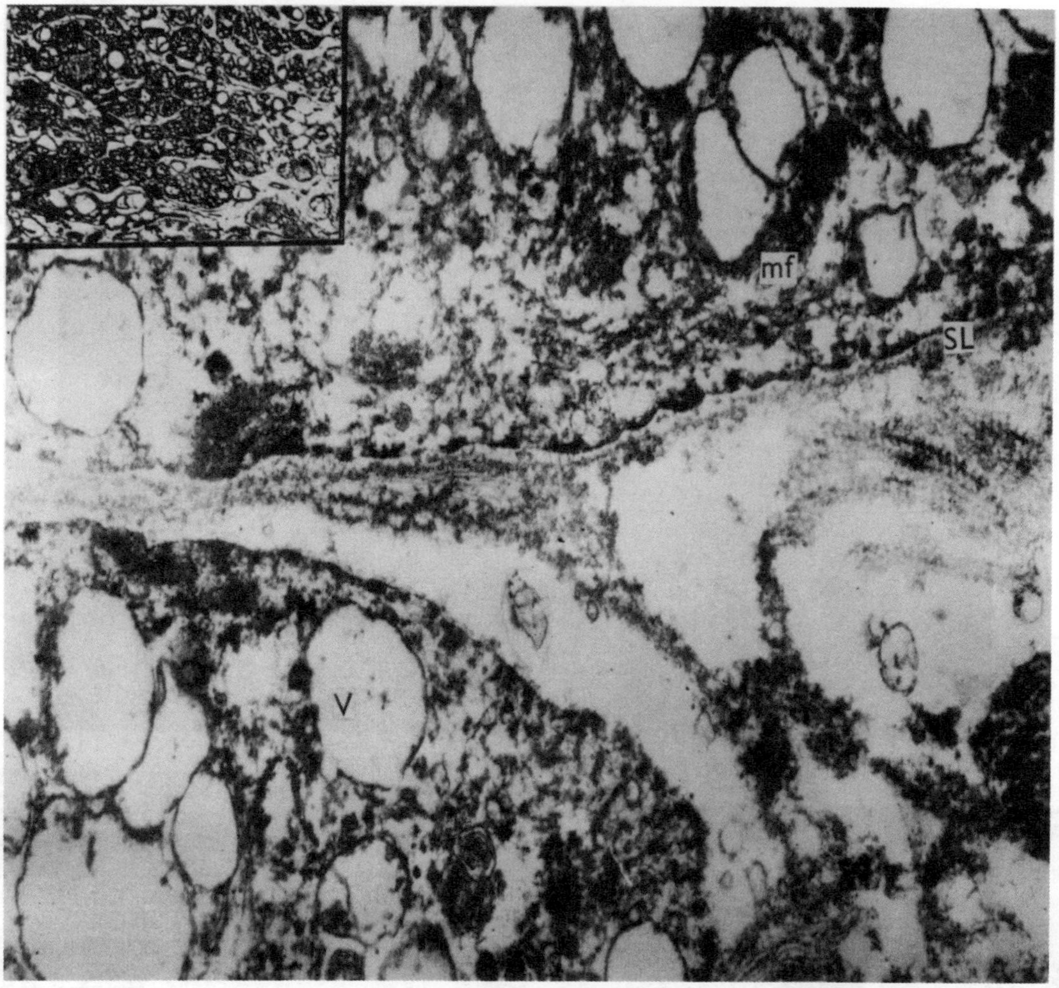

Figure 44.7. Electronmicroscope photograph showing two adjacent myocytes within myocytoplasm and numerous dilated vesicles (V) with myofilament (mf) residue in between. (Original magnification × 35,000.) The inset shows semi-thin section of hydropic change and myocytolysis of myocytes. SL = sarcolemma.

NONINVASIVE DIAGNOSTIC INVESTIGATION

RADIOGRAPHY

Cardiomegaly of various degrees, low tonus of heart contraction, and weakness of cardiac pulsation are the positive findings. The cardiac shadow usually reveals a triangular or bag-like shape with a cardiothoracic ratio of 0.60 to 0.70. Straightening of the lateral border of the left ventricle is sometimes observed (Figures 44.8A, 44.8B). Radiokymographically, the amplitude of the heart contraction waves is greatly reduced or even disappears (Figure 44.8C); abnormal contraction waves are sometimes discovered. To compare the radiographic cardiac features of chronic KSD with those of congestive cardiomyopathy, 40 cases each were studied.[6] In congestive cardiomyopathy the cardiac shadow often showed a ball-like shape on chest film. Its cardiac tonus and compensatory potentiality of the right side seemed to be better than those in KSD. In KSD the pathologic changes usually involve both ventricles. As a result, the redistribution of blood in the upper portion of both lungs occurs more often in congestive cardiomyopathy, whereas diffuse pulmonary interstitial edema is more frequent in KSD.[6]

ELECTROCARDIOGRAPHY

In a ten-year long-term follow-up survey of 659 cases of various types of KSD in Fanrong commune KSD districts, Heilongjiang province, these electrocardiograms were collected and analyzed in detail.[20] The incidence of arrhythmia was 84.4%, bundle branch block 63%, ectopic rhythm 48.1%, sinoatrial node arrhythmia 24.6%, and atrioventricular block 12.6%. Electrocardiographic changes of myocardial injury are particularly common in acute KSD. Once the patient has severe cardiogenic shock, a monophasic current may appear (Figure 44.9). Ectopic rhythm, atrial fibrillation, and bundle branch block are usually found in chronic and latent KSD. Ventricular extrasystolic beats of multifocal origin also indicate that most originate from the left ventricle. The incidence of complete atrioventricular block was 3.3%. An increase of QRS duration greater than 0.12 second also denoted that the idioventricular pacemaker was situated below the bi-

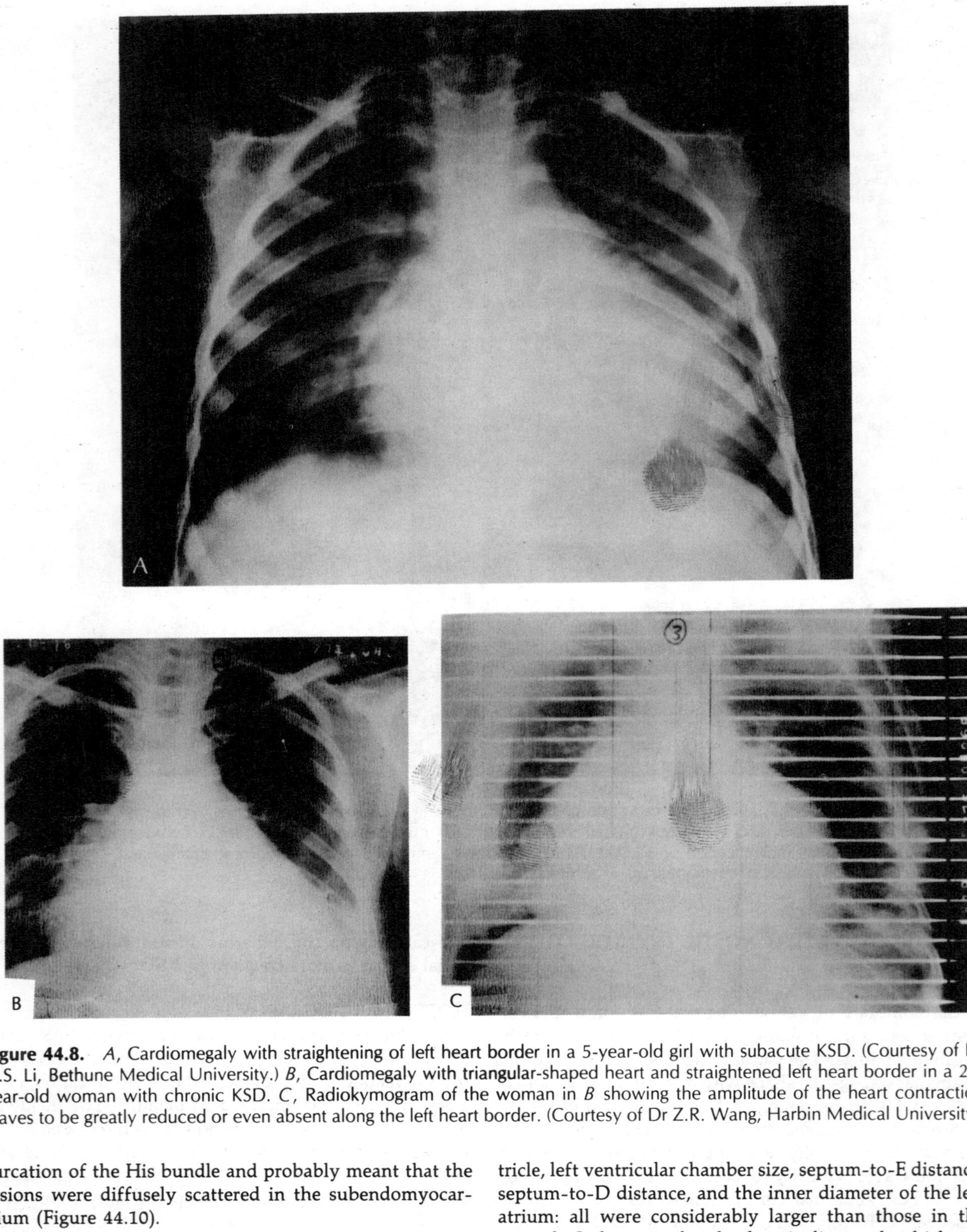

Figure 44.8. *A*, Cardiomegaly with straightening of left heart border in a 5-year-old girl with subacute KSD. (Courtesy of Dr G.S. Li, Bethune Medical University.) *B*, Cardiomegaly with triangular-shaped heart and straightened left heart border in a 29-year-old woman with chronic KSD. *C*, Radiokymogram of the woman in *B* showing the amplitude of the heart contraction waves to be greatly reduced or even absent along the left heart border. (Courtesy of Dr Z.R. Wang, Harbin Medical University.)

furcation of the His bundle and probably meant that the lesions were diffusely scattered in the subendomyocardium (Figure 44.10).

ECHOCARDIOGRAPHY

One hundred twenty-six patients with various types of KSD receiving both M-mode and B-mode echocardiographic examinations were compared with 73 healthy control subjects[21] (Figure 44.11). Differences between the two groups of subjects were very significant statistically ($P < 0.001$) with regard to outflow tract of the left ventricle, left ventricular chamber size, septum-to-E distance, septum-to-D distance, and the inner diameter of the left atrium: all were considerably larger than those in the controls. In latent and early chronic disease the thickness of the ventricular septum was increased (greater than 11 mm), but relative septal thickness, ie, septal-to-posterior wall ratio, was also increased in late chronic disease because of a much dilated left cardiac chamber and greater thinning of the free posterior wall of the left ventricle. Motion of the ventricular septum and posterior wall of the left ventricle was decreased in about 50% of KSD

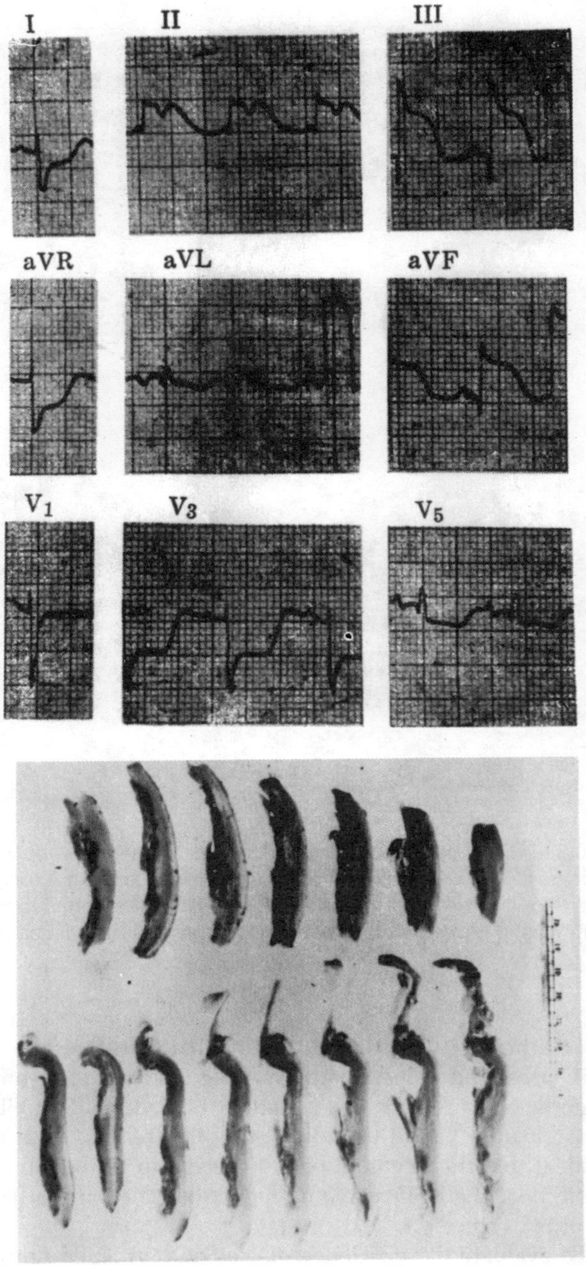

Figure 44.9. Acute KSD in a 4-year-old boy with a history of repeated vomiting accompanied by signs of cardiogenic shock. *Top,* Electrocardiogram shows marked ST segment elevation in leads II, III, and aVF, and ST-segment depression in leads I, aVR, aVL, V_3, and V_5. *Bottom,* At autopsy circumferential subendocardial necrosis and hemorrhage (dark color) are depicted in multiple longitudinal sections of anterior and lateral wall of left ventricle.

patients. Paradoxic motion of the septum was found in 9% of latent and 5% of chronic cases. Systolic thickening of the septum was diminished in 6% of latent and 4% of chronic cases. Kang et al[22] reported similar results on M-mode echocardiographic study in 84 patients with KSD and 57 healthy control subjects (Table 44.1). In a recent report from the Department of Pediatrics, Sichuan Medical College,[23] the marked decrease in contraction of the lower part of the left ventricle and the segmental left ventricular asynergy were found to be characteristic of KSD and helpful in its differentiation from other cardiomyopathies.

INVASIVE DIAGNOSTIC INVESTIGATION

Instead of the conventional endomyocardial bioptome, Sun et al[24] and Chen and Liang[25] used a self-made instrument, a redesigned fibroendoscope bioptome, to perform myocardial biopsy in four patients with chronic and one with latent disease using the right great saphenous vein to get to the right ventricular myocardium. Under the electronmicroscope, the membranous system of myocyte such as an intercalated disk, T tube, and myosarcolemma showed various degrees of dilatation. Proliferation and vesiculation of mitochondria, abnormal bifurcation of myofibrils, and spherical microparticles were observed, but all these electronmicroscopic findings are nonspecific for both KSD and congestive cardiomyopathy.[12,26,27]

ETIOLOGY AND MANAGEMENT

Research work on the origin of KSD has been carried out for about 50 years, and many hypotheses have been suggested. They are mainly biologic (viral infection) and also nonbiologic (selenium deficiency, nutritional imbalance, and intoxication).

VIRAL INFECTION

Over 50 strains of virus have been isolated from the KSD victim's blood and tissues either in southwest or in northeast endemic districts. Most of them were identified to be coxsackie or echo enteroviruses and some were undetermined. However, most specimens were obtained from southwest endemic districts. Because of the divergence in distribution among those virus strains, no significant difference in seroimmunologic test results between residents in endemic and nonendemic districts, and no significant difference in the incidence of detected micro-RNA virus between healthy children in endemic and those in nonendemic districts, the pathogenetic specificities of the isolated virus strain cannot yet be confirmed.[28-30] Owing to the high incidence of enteroviral infection and interstitial viral pneumonia during the summer in southwest endemic districts, many researchers tend to believe that viral infection rather than an etiologic factor may be one of the cofactors in the pathogenesis of KSD. This also serves to explain the seasonal prevalence of KSD in the southwest district.[5,31]

LOW SELENIUM LEVELS AND KESHAN DISEASE

As early as 1964, one of us (BQG) had noted that a coincidence existed between the endemic distribution of KSD and that of the white muscle disease (WMD) of domestic animals and also had found certain similarities in the symptoms, signs, and pathologic changes between them. However, no further investigation was made in this field after therapeutic doses of sodium selenite in a few patients with acute KSD failed to improve the patient's

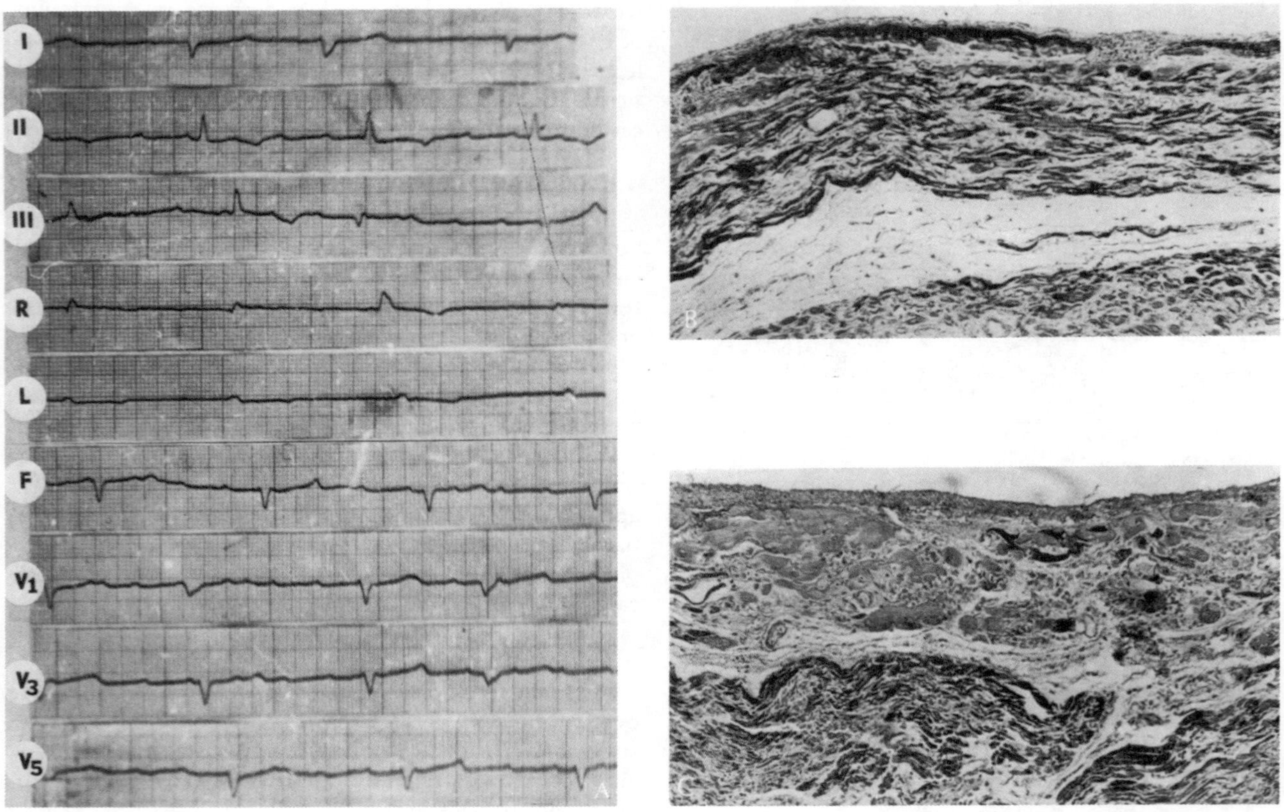

Figure 44.10. Acute KSD in a 39-year-old woman with a history of discomfort in the epigastric region, restlessness for 36 hours, and a blood pressure of 90/70 mm Hg. The electrocardiogram (*left*) showed third degree atrioventricular block. Histologic sections revealed that both anterior (*upper right*) and posterior (*lower right*) fascicles of the left bundle branch and right bundle branch are interrupted by necrotic foci and cellular infiltrations. (Hematoxylin and eosin stain; original magnification × 400.)

condition. In 1965 a farm hospital physician from Shanxi province, who had a similar idea about the etiologic relation between KSD and WMD in animals, administered Na_2SeO_3 to some patients with chronic and latent KSD for either therapeutic or prophylactic purposes. Subsequently, research workers from Xian Medical College, Chinese Academy of Medical Sciences, Institute of Geography of Chinese Academy of Sciences, and many others cooperated to study the etiologic relation between Se and KSD.[32] After many years of investigation of the chemical environment it was found that KSD is mainly distributed in the low selenium content districts (the weighted means of selenium in wheat, rice, and corn is less than 0.025 ppm). These three food grains are the main selenium sources of rural residents in China.[3] The selenium content of scalp hair and staple cereal samples from endemic districts have a much lower selenium level.[33,34] A difference of mean selenium content in scalp hair between endemic districts and nonendemic districts was very significant.[35] The whole blood content of glutathione peroxidase[36] and the amount of 24-hour urinary excretion of selenium[37] between endemic and nonendemic residents were investigated, and statistically significant differences were found between the two groups. However, it was of interest to compare the selenium status of people from other parts of the world with that of subjects in a KSD area, and values were available from at least four regions: New Zealand,[38] Finland,[39] the Federal Republic of Germany,[40] and the United States[41] (Table 44.2). It is evident that the selenium blood levels (5 to 10 ng/ml) in subjects of the KSD area are much lower than any other recorded values.

To evaluate the efficiency of Na_2SeO_3 in KSD a prophylactic study was carried out under strict control among children in Sichuan province endemic districts from 1974 to 1977. The results indicated that Na_2SeO_3 could not only lower the morbidity and mortality of KSD but also alleviate its clinical course[42] (Tables 44.3 and 44.4). Oral selenium supplementation has also been shown to reverse the biochemical evidence of the selenium deficiency state in patients with[43] or without[44] cardiomyopathy in the United States.

Selenium deficiency is a basic but not a unique factor in the pathogenesis of KSD. It cannot explain all the epidemiologic characteristics of this disease: no further decrease in hair selenium content was found during its seasonal prevalence[45]; in affected regions the urban population and families of workers and staff members living in the same rural area are practically secure; in certain low selenium districts no person with KSD has been dis-

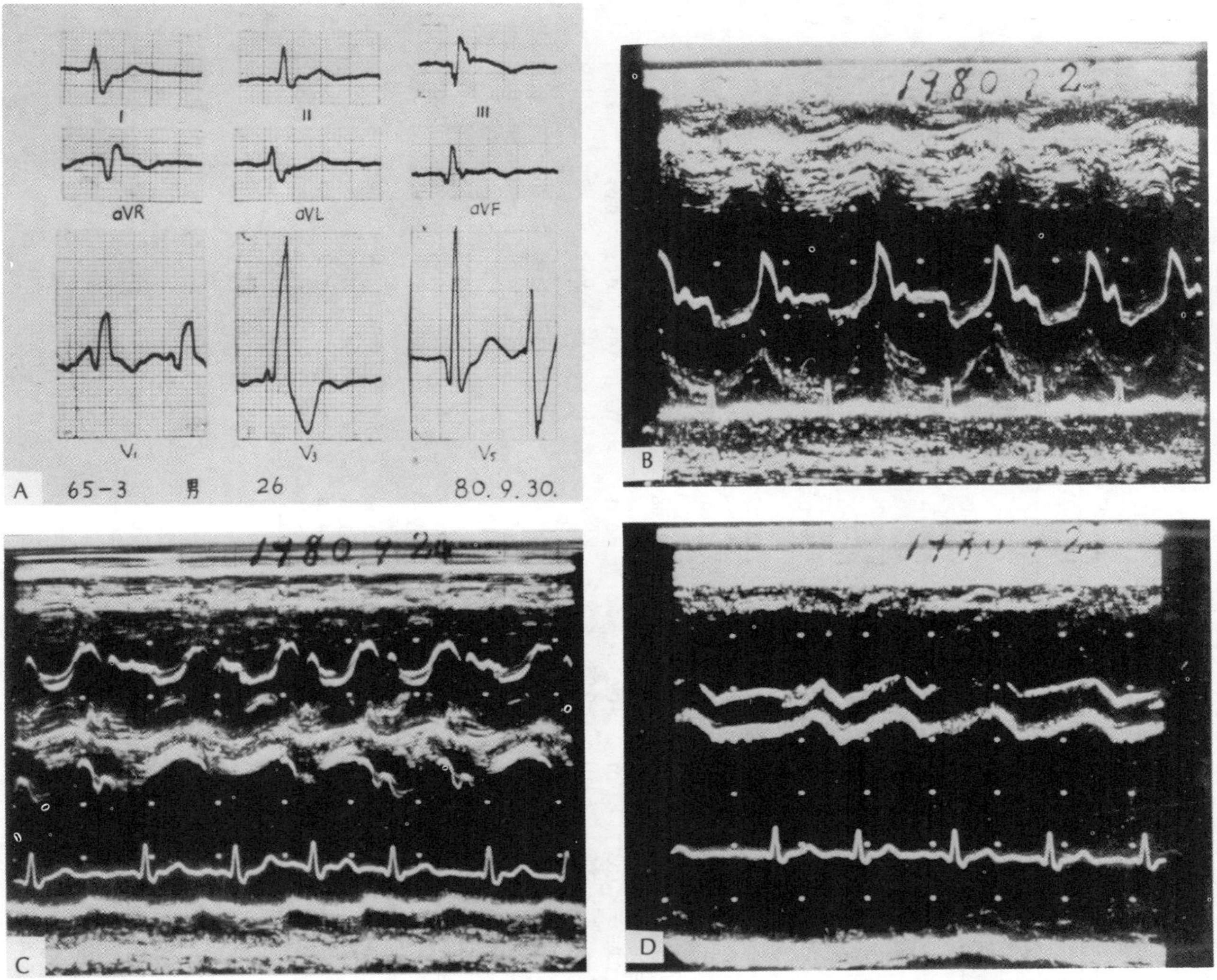

Figure 44.11. Electrocardiogram and echocardiograms of a 26-year-old man with chronic KSD. The electrocardiogram (*A*) shows atrial fibrillation, right bundle branch block, and occasional ventricular premature beats. The echocardiograms show left ventricular dilation with an inlet diameter of 70 mm and paradoxic septal motion (*B*), right ventricular dilation with a right ventricular diameter of 46 mm (*C*), and left atrial dilation with an end-diastolic diameter of 88 mm and subnormal aortic diameter (*D*). (Courtesy of Dr D.Y. Xia, Harbin Medical University.)

covered. Therefore, other influences such as dietary, biologic, and geo-factors other than selenium must not be neglected.[4,31,46,47] Some workers seem to pay much attention to the relation between vitamin E and selenium deficiency in the pathogenesis of KSD, but at the present time there is insufficient evidence to support vitamin E deficiency as one of the KSD pathogenetic cofactors.[46]

OTHER TRACE ELEMENTS

Recently, besides selenium, levels of other trace elements such as Cu, Zn, Mn, Cr, Mo, and Ca were found in scalp hair or blood of KSD patients,[48] and comparative analysis of the contents of 17 amino acids in oats from endemic and nonendemic districts[49,50] was performed. Experiments in animals fed endemic grain to investigate the relation between certain elements and cardiac metabolism were also carried out.[51] Yet further work in these fields is required to explore the actual relation between them.

CONCLUSIONS

Keshan disease, an endemic cardiomyopathy, appears to be a unique myocardial disorder with a history of one century; its mystery is finally being cleared gradually. From epidemiologic, clinical, pathologic, and etiologic points of view, it is quite different from all other types of cardiomyopathy of unknown etiology, such as idiopathic myocarditis, viral myocarditis, cardiac sarcoidosis, various kinds of postinfectious myocarditis, and myocardial disorders due to endocrine disturbances and avitaminosis (eg, vitamin B_1 deficiency).[5,52,53]

We greatly appreciate the decision of the World Health Organization Experts Committee in classifying KSD as a special type of cardiomyopathy distinct from congestive cardiomyopathy.[53] Pathophysiologically, both KSD and congestive cardiomyopathy are characterized clinically by cardiac pump failure. In a broad sense, they both belong to the dilated cardiomyopathy group, but KSD has its

Table 44.1. Echocardiographic Measurements in 84 Cases of Keshan Disease* in mm, mm/s

		Base of the Heart					Mitral Valve							Ventricle				LV Function
		Aorta			LAID		Septum							LVPW		RVD		
							Upper		Lower									
		D_s	A	RVOT	S	D	T	A	T	A	LVOT	RVD	E-F Slope	T	A	S	D	EF (%)
Subacute	#	2	2	2	2	2	2	2	...	...	2	2	2	2	2	2	2	2
	Mean	13.5	6.5	13.0	17.5	14.0	3.5	4.0	...	...	17.5	10.0	60.0	6.5	6.0	40.0	34.0	41.5
Acute (preschool children)	#	21	21	21	21	21	2	1	16	13	20	20	17	19	19	20	20	20
	Mean	15.62	6.57	12.80	17.38	11.76	3.50	7.00	3.19	5.08	19.85	7.50	89.12	6.42	6.84	31.15	29.60	40.91
	Range	14~19	4~9	8~22	11~32	6~22			3~7	2~7	10~34	3~17	48~131	5~9	2~11	24~47	22~41	20.80~65.00
Acute (school children)	#	15	15	15	15	15	...	...	12	10	15	14	15	15	14	15	15	15
	Mean	17.93	7.2	13.67	17.87	11.80	...	...	4.33	4.20	21.40	11.78	81.87	7.33	7.04	40.60	33.67	41.60
	Range	15~21	6~11	10~23	13~25	5~20	...	...	3~7	2~10	16~27	4~21	13~14	5~10	2~11	23~51	23~42	20.80~60.36
	P**	<0.01	<0.01	<0.05	<0.05	<0.01	...	...	<0.05	<0.01	>0.05	>0.05	≤0.01	>0.05	<0.05	>0.05	<0.05	>0.05
Latent (children)	#	18	18	18	18	18	4	4	12	10	17	18	16	17	17	18	18	18
	Mean	17.28	6.56	11.72	17.56	11.94	5.00	5.25	4.25	4.60	23.71	8.44	85.06	7.65	6.53	38.50	32.28	40.67
	Range	12~20	4~8	6~20	12~23	7~16	4~6	5~6	3~6	3~10	13~36	27~50	54~148	4~11	4~9	27~50	23~43	23.40~63.10
	P**	<0.01	<0.01	<0.01	<0.01	<0.01	>0.05	>0.05	<0.05	<0.01	>0.05	<0.01	<0.01	>0.05	>0.05	<0.01	<0.01	>0.05
	P†	>0.05	>0.05	>0.05	>0.05	>0.05	—	—	>0.05	>0.05	>0.05	<0.05	>0.05	>0.05	>0.05	>0.05	>0.05	>0.05
Latent (adult)	#	8	8	8	8	8	1	1	7	6	7	7	7	7	8	8	8	8
	Mean	23.50	8.88	19.25	27.00	16.75	6.00	9.00	4.86	5.17	32.29	15.00	77.00	7.71	7.75	52.00	43.50	44.63
	Range	20~34	6~13	10~30	17~42	11~22	...	...	3~8	3~8	16~25	8~25	43~114	5~10	5~11	38~68	30~61	10.50~73.90
Chronic	#	20	20	19	20	20	6	6	10	7	7	15	19	17	16	16	16	18
	Mean	23.20	7.30	20.74	35.20	28.10	6.33	4.83	5.20	5.14	38.18	11.67	102.84	8.35	7.13	64.81	53.81	27.83
	Range	15~30	3~13	12~30	21~53	14~45	4~10	3~7	2~8	3~10	19~60	4~22	62~175	5~11	2~11	36~82	31~77	10.80~50.10
	P‡	>0.05	>0.05	>0.05	<0.01	<0.01	—	—	>0.05	>0.05	>0.05	>0.05	>0.05	>0.05	>0.05	<0.05	>0.05	<0.05
Normal (school children)	#	57	51	57	57	57	33	23	24	10	56	55	57	55	55	55	55	55
	Mean	19.46	8.82	16.46	20.37	14.58	5.94	6.04	5.71	7.40	23.80	11.29	123.30	7.09	8.35	45.27	38.09	40.18
	SD	1.29	1.84	3.46	3.32	2.98	1.56	1.72	2.19	1.71	4.53	3.95	31.71	1.41	1.59	9.88	5.98	12.88
	SE	0.17	0.26	0.46	0.44	0.39	0.27	0.36	0.45	0.54	0.61	0.53	4.20	0.19	0.21	1.33	0.81	1.74
	Range	16~23	6~16	12~22	12~28	7~20	3~10	2~9	4~10	5~10	14~37	2~18	65~188	5~10	5~13	24~56	18~50	11.80~66.20

* Adapted from Kang et al.[22]

** P value as compared with normal.

† P value as compared with early stage.

‡ P value as compared with late stage.

A = amplitude; D = diastole; D_s = diameter in systole; EF = ejection fraction; LAID = left atrial internal diameter; LVOT = left ventricular outflow tract; LVPW = left ventricular posterior wall; RVD = right ventricular diameter; RVOT = right ventricular outflow tract; S = systole; SD = standard deviation; SE = standard error; T = thickness.

Table 44.2. Dietary Selenium Intake and Blood Selenium Levels Around the World*

Country	Dietary Selenium Intake (μg/day)	Blood Selenium Level (ng/ml)
China (Keshan disease area)	11	8
New Zealand	28	60–83
Finland	30	56–81
Federal Republic of Germany	–	53–130†
United States	62–216	157–265
Venezuela (Caracas)	218	355
China (endemic selenosis area)	4,990	3,180

* Adapted from Levander.[41]

† Calculated from serum selenium levels in Lombeck et al.[40]

specificities in pathologic findings, pathogenesis, and etiology, and a differential diagnosis can still be made in most cases.[5,23,54] From x-ray findings there are also some subtle although definite differences between them.[6] However, on clinical grounds alone, without the epidemiologic history background, it might at times be difficult to make a differential diagnosis between them. Although we have long been acquainted with the pathologic manifestations of various selenium deficiency diseases in animals such as white muscle disease in domestic animals, hemorrhagic diathesis in poultry, and diarrhea in young donkeys, we still were unsure whether the "geo-factor" selenium deficiency—a weak pathogenetic factor—might be the actual cause of cardiac necrosis in human beings. We did not find the answer until two autopsy studies of fatal myocardial necrosis due to prolonged use of parenteral nutrition with gastrointestinal dysfunction were reported recently.[55,56] Histologic study in one case was performed by Dr Ge Keyou, an eminent pathologist in China, who has been engaged in KSD research for many years. From published reports we found that in both cases there were very low selenium levels and also very low glutathione peroxidase activity in both blood and heart muscle. It is interesting that the pathologic characteristics of myocardium closely mimicked those in KSD, so that we know now selenium deficiency may actually cause cardiac necrosis in human beings. These findings led us to consider the similar myocardial changes of patients with fibrocystic disease of the pancreas, which are also similar to those of pediatric KSD, because it is known that in fibrocystic disease due to the lack of pancreatic juice secretion, which results in malignant diarrhea and steatorrhea, all these tend to cause decreased absorption of fat, soluble vitamins, and trace elements.[57] Therefore, selenium and vitamin E deficiency cannot be ruled out as a main cause of cardiac necrosis in this disease.

There are many countries and districts all over the world, such as the United States, Australia, New Zealand, and Egypt, that have the low selenium geologic condition and also the animal selenium deficiency as in China, but KSD has never been reported in these countries. This may be explained by their high percentage of animal protein intake and high population mobility, ie, the actual selenium intake is not low but higher than the so-called minimal requirements of 60 μg/day.[3] This may also serve to explain why KSD is extremely rare in urban residents, officials, nonfarm workers, and businessmen in China.[4] From the early 1970s, the incidence of KSD in China has declined gradually. The reasons may be multiple. No new patients were discovered in many old endemic districts. The incidence of KSD declined continuously in the 1980s. Therefore, it is reasonable to state that rural urbanization has increased the production rate and thus changed the life-style and living standards, especially the dietary components and food supply. Consequently, KSD may disappear forever in China as living conditions further improve.

The Third International Symposium on Selenium in Biology and Medicine was held from May 28 to June 1, 1984 in Beijing. Meanwhile a medal and certificate of Schwartz Prize 1984 were awarded to Chinese scientists from the Chinese Academy of Medical Sciences and Xian Medical College to recognize and encourage their great efforts in KSD research work for many years. Many foreign experts pointed out that it was the Chinese scientific

Table 44.3. Prophylactic Effect of Selenium Supplements Against Keshan Disease*

Year	Total Subjects	No. of Cases	No. Alive	Disease: Latent	Disease: Improved	Disease: Chronic	Deaths
Control Group							
1974	3,985	54	27	16	9	2	27
1975	5,445	52	26	13	10	3	26
1976	212	1	1	0	0	1	0
Treated Group							
1974	4,510	10	10	9	0	1	0
1975	6,767	7	6	6	0	0	1
1976	12,579	4	2	2	0	0	2
1977	12,749	0	0	0	0	0	0

* Adapted from Keshan Disease Research Group.[42]

Table 44.4. Heart X-ray Examination of Patients With and Without Selenium Supplement (1974–1977)*

	Year	No. of Cases	Year of Examination	No. of Cases Examined	Results: Normal	Slight Dilation	Moderate Dilation	Severe Dilation
Untreated Groups								
	1974	54	1974	36	7†	—	29†	—
			1975	29	13	6	4	6
			1976	25	13	5	4	3
			1977	26	14	6	4	2
	1975	52	1975	35	11	4	10	10
			1976	25	12	4	5	4
			1977	25	9	10	5	1
	1976	1	1976	1	0	0	1	0
			1977	1	0	0	0	1
Treated Groups								
	1974	10	1974	8	2†	—	6†	—
			1975	9	7	1	0	1
			1976	9	7	1	0	1
			1977	10	8	1	0	1
	1975	7	1975	6	6	0	0	0
			1976	6	5	1	0	0
			1977	5	4	1	0	0
	1976	4	1976	2	1	1	0	0
			1977	2	2	0	0	0
	1977	0	1977	0	0	0	0	0

* Adapted from Keshan Disease Research Group.[42]

†Examined by fluoroscopy; the results divided into normal and dilated heart.

Note: Cardiothoracic ratio: normal = 0.46 to 0.51, slight dilation = 0.52 to 0.55, moderate dilation = 0.56 to 0.60, and severe dilation over 0.60.

workers who explored the vivid relation between selenium deficiency and the pathogenesis of KSD and Kaschin-Beck disease[58–61] and who really substantiated the interrelations between selenium and health. No doubt it paves a magnificent way of exploring and making advances in the research field of trace elements. Along these lines it may be of particular interest to note the recent report from China's Fourth Military Medical University of a distinct lower selenium level in both blood and hair of patients with non-KSD dilated cardiomyopathy than in normal subjects and other cardiac patients (Table 44.5).[62] Similar findings have been reported from the Federal Republic of Germany.[63,64]

Table 44.5. Blood and Hair Selenium Levels in Patients with Non-KSD Dilated Cardiomyopathy, Normal Subjects, and Patients with Other Cardiac Diseases

Subjects	Blood Selenium (μg/ml)	Hair Selenium (μg/g)
Dilated cardiomyopathy, non-KSD	0.039 ± 0.012	0.280 ± 0.052
Normal	0.086 ± 0.028	0.640 ± 0.160
Other cardiac diseases*	0.089 ± 0.018	0.690 ± 0.210

* Including rheumatic heart disease, coronary heart disease, hypertensive heart disease, etc.

REFERENCES

1. Hong BY: The general conditions of the spreading and endemic districts of Keshan disease, in Hong BY (ed): *Keshan Disease*. Beijing, People's Medical Publishing House, 1957, pp 1–11.
2. Lu YR: Keshan disease, in Wu ZM (ed): *Pathology*. Beijing, People's Medical Publishing House, 1983, pp 163–165.
3. The Study Group of Environmental and Endemic Diseases: The relation of Keshan disease to the natural environment and the background of selenium nutrition. *Acta Nutr Sin* 1982; 4:175–182.
4. Su Y, Yu WH: Nutritional biogeochemical etiology of Keshan disease. *Chin Med J* 1983; 96:594–596.
5. Gu BQ: Pathology of Keshan disease. A comprehensive review. *Chin Med J* 1983; 96:251–261.
6. Wang ZR, Wang Q, Yu SQ, Gu BQ, Zeng XH: A radiographic-pathologic correlative analysis between congestive cardiomyopathy and Keshan disease. *Chin J Roentgenol* 1981; 15:173–177.
7. Lu YR: Pathologic studies of Keshan disease in China in recent 10 years. *Natl Med J Chin* 1959; 45:191–198.
8. Gu BQ, Li CR, Shi DZ, Jia WZ, Guo SS: A study on pathologic changes of heart in Keshan disease. *Chin J Pathol Suppl* 1964; 158–176.
9. Zeng XH, Guo TF, Zhao SX, Zhu XF, Gu BQ: A study of the relationship between distribution of myocardial foci and coronary blood vessels in Keshan disease. I. The pathogenesis of perivascular foci. *Chin J Cardiol* 1982; 10:117–121.
10. Zeng XH, Zhao SX, Zhu XF, Guo TF: A study of the relationship between distribution of myocardial foci and coronary blood vessels in Keshan disease. IV. The vascular supply of the ventricular septum and pathogenesis of myocardial foci. *Chin J Endemiol* 1985; 4:46–48.
11. Ge KY, Chen XS, Xue AN, Bei J, Wang SQ: Morphological and histochemical observation of myocardium of Keshan disease. *Acta Nutr Sin* 1982; 4:91–95.
12. Section of EM, Central Lab, Harbin Medical College: Preliminary observation on the myocardium in Keshan disease. *Scientia Sin* 1974; 17:569–590.
13. Ge KY, Xiu AA, Wang SQ: Ultrastructural changes of myocardial necrosis of Keshan disease. *Natl Med J Chin* 1980; 60:407–409.
14. Gu BQ, Li XZ, Zeng XH, Wu ZD: Comparison of the myocardial changes in Keshan disease under light and electron microscope. *Chin J Endemiol* 1984; 3:153–156.
15. Lu YR, Wang KL: An anatomic–pathological study on conduction system of myocardium in Keshan disease. *Chin J Pathol* 1963; 3:180–187.
16. Gu BQ, Zeng XH: An observation on pathologic changes of liver in Keshan disease. *J Harbin Med Univ* 1975; 1-2:113–117.

17. Wang F, Li GS: A pathological study on Keshan disease among children of northeast and southwest endemic districts. *J Jilin Med Univ* 1976; 3:117–137.
18. Xia DY, Guan ZZ, Ye RX: A clinical analysis on 17 cases of Keshan disease accompanied with cerebral embolism during 15 years in Fangrong Commune, Fu Yu County, Heilongjiang. Symposium on Research on Keshan Disease. *J Harbin Med Univ* 1979; 6:190–192.
19. Li CR: A pathomorphologic study on Keshan disease fetus. *Heilongjiang Yi Kan* 1959; 2:14–19.
20. Department of Research on Keshan Disease, Harbin Medical University: Electrocardiographic characteristics of 659 cases of Keshan disease, Fu Yu County. *J Harbin Med Univ* 1976; 5:30–33.
21. Xia DY, Zhao HX, Guan ZZ, Wang SZ, Wu ZH, Yu WH, Qi ZQ, Yu FQ: A B-mode and M-mode echocardiographic diagnostic study on Keshan disease. *Chin J Cardiol* 1982; 10:133.
22. Kang TJ, Liang JX, Yuan DR, Yong YX: An echocardiographic preliminary observation on 84 cases of Keshan disease. *Chin J Intern Med* 1980; 19:442–445.
23. Tang SC, Liu YX, Jin ZH: Echocardiographic features of Keshan disease in children, in Doyle EF, Engle MA, Gersony WM, Rashkind WJ, Talner NS (eds): *Abstracts of Second World Congress of Pediatric Cardiology*. New York, Springer-Verlag, 1985, p 121.
24. Sun GC, Yang YX, Ye FL, Ding DX, Wang SC: Clinical application of endomyocardial biopsy (report of 36 cases). *Chin J Cardiol* 1984; 12:99–100.
25. Chen JD, Liang LX: A preliminary electron microscopic observation on endomyocardial biopsy specimens of Keshan disease patient. *Nat Med J Chin* 1983; 63:538–540.
26. Knieriem JH: Electron microscopic findings in congestive cardiomyopathy, in Kaltenback M, Loogen F, Olsen EGJ (eds): *Cardiomyopathy and Myocardial Biopsy*. Heidelberg, Springer-Verlag, 1978, pp 71–86.
27. Li XZ, Wang XM, Jin XM, Wang YD, Song YN, Li H, Wang P, Piao ZN, Jin GL: An electron microscopic observation on endomyocardial biopsy specimens of dilated type cardiomyopathy. *Natl Med J Chin* 1984; 64:753–755.
28. Wu ZR, Wang I, Zhou LH, Guan GX, Deng SQ: Preliminary report of viral etiological study of Keshan disease. *Chin J Endemiol* 1984; 3:65–67.
29. Department of Microbiology: A study on viral etiology of Keshan disease. *J Chongging Med Coll* 1978; 2:1–5.
30. Su CQ, Gong QM, Li Q, Chen CZ, Zhou DJ, Jin QX: Preliminary summary of viral etiology of Keshan disease. *Natl Med J Chin* 1979; 59:466–470.
31. Keshan Disease Research Group of Chinese Academy of Medical Sciences: Epidemiologic studies on the etiologic relationship of selenium and Keshan disease. *Chin Med J* 1979; 92:477–482.
32. Yang GQ, Chen JS, Wen ZM, Ge KY, Zhu LZ, Chen XC, Chen XS: The role of selenium in Keshan disease. *Adv Nutr Res* 1984; 6:203–231.
33. Xu KL, Xue ML, Zhang PY, Feng CF, Hong SY, Liang WS: Selenium status and dietary selenium content of populations in the endemic and non-endemic areas of Keshan disease. *Acta Nutr Sin* 1982; 4:183–190.
34. Yang GQ, Wang GY, Yin TA, Sun SZ, Zhou RH, Man RE, Zhai FV, Guo SH, Wang HZ, You DQ: Relationship between the distribution of Keshan disease and selenium status. *Acta Nutr Sin* 1982; 4:191–200.
35. Wang MY: Geographical differentiation of selenium content in hair from children and youngsters in China—a discussion about relationship between selenium deficiency and geographical epidemiology of the Keshan disease. *Act Nutr Sin* 1982; 4:201–207.
36. Zhu LZ, Xia YM, Yang GQ: Blood glutathione peroxidase activities of populations in Keshan disease affected and non-affected areas. *Acta Nutr Sin* 1982; 4:229–233.
37. Yin TA, Sun SZ, Wang HZ, You DQ, Yang GQ: The differences of the content of urinary selenium excretion between the children from endemic and nonendemic areas of Keshan disease. *Chin J Preven Med* 1979; 13:207–210.
38. Thomson CD, Rea HM, Doesburg VM, Robinson MF: Selenium concentrations and glutathione peroxidase activities in whole blood of New Zealand residents. *Br J Nutr* 1977; 37:457–460.
39. Levander OA, Alfthan G, Arvilommi H, Gref CG, Huttunen JK, Kataja M, Koivistoinen P, Pikkarainen J: Bioavailability of selenium to Finnish men as assessed by platelet glutathione peroxidase activity and other blood parameters. *Am J Clin Nutr* 1983; 37:887–897.
40. Lombeck I, Kasperek K, Feinendegen LE, Bremer HJ: The state and supply of selenium in healthy children and dietetically treated patients with inborn errors of metabolism, in Kirchgessner M (ed): *Trace Element Metabolism in Man and Animals—3*. Freising, FRG, Technische Universität München, 1978, pp 312–315.
41. Levander OA: Clinical consequences of low selenium intake and its relationship to vitamin E. *Ann NY Acad Sci* 1982; 393:70–82.
42. Keshan Disease Research Group of Chinese Academy of Medical Sciences: Antiepidemic Station of Sichuan province, Chengdu, Antiepidemic Station of Xichang District, Sichuan, and Antiepidemic Station of Mianning County, Sichuan: Observations on effect of sodium selenite in prevention of Keshan disease. *Chin Med J* 1979; 92:471–476.
43. Collipp PJ, Chen SY: Cardiomyopathy and selenium deficiency in a two-year-old girl. *N Engl J Med* 1981; 304:1304.
44. King WWK, Michel L, Wood WC, Malt RA, Baker SS, Cohen HJ: Reversal of selenium deficiency with oral selenium. *N Engl J Med* 1981; 304:1305.
45. Sun SZ, Yin TA, Wang HZ, You DQ, Yang GQ: The relationship between high prevalence season of Keshan disease and scalp hair selenium level of residents. *Chin J Preven Med* 1980; 14:17–19.
46. Yang GQ: On the etiological relationship between selenium and Keshan disease. *Prog Phys Sci* 1983; 14:313–317.
47. Wang F, Li GS, An RG, Yang TS: A study on the pathogenic factors in the grains from endemic districts of Keshan disease. *Chin J Pathol* 1982; 11:308–312.
48. Zhou BC, Zeng SJ, Che CB, Yu WH: Eight element levels in scalp hair of patients with Keshan disease. *Chin J Endemiol* 1985; 4:41–45.
49. Dong GS, Fu D, Zeng SJ, Feng L: Comparative analysis of the contents of amino acids in oats from endemic and nonendemic areas of Keshan disease. *J Harbin Univ* 1985; 1:12–14.
50. Fu D, Che CB, Zeng SJ, Yu WH: Determination of tryptophan in several grains from endemic and nonendemic areas of Keshan disease. *J Harbin Univ* 1985; 1:15–17.
51. An RG, Li GS, Zhang GT, Zhang LC, Pu FQ: Influence of Keshan disease endemic grains upon certain element metabolism—changes of element contents after injection of isoproterenol. *Chin J Endemiol* 1985; 4:11–15.
52. Wang F, Li GS: From pathomorphologic changes point of view to discuss the etiology of Keshan disease. *Natl Med J Chin* 1962; 48:17–21.
53. Report of a WHO Expert Committee: *Cardiomyopathies*. WHO Technical Report Series 697, Geneva, World Health Organization, 1984, pp 55–58.
54. Zeng XH, Gu BQ: The similarities and dissimilarities between congestive cardiomyopathy and Keshan disease. *Natl Med J Chin* 1981; 61:570.
55. Johnson RA, Bakers SS, Fallon JT, Maynard EP, Ruskin JN, Wen ZM, Ge KY, Cohen HJ: An occidental case of cardiomyopathy and selenium deficiency. *N Engl J Med* 1981; 304:1210–1212.
56. Fleming CR, Lie JT, McCall JT, O'Brien JF, Baillie EE, Thistle JJ: Selenium deficiency and fatal cardiomyopathy in a patient on home parenteral nutrition. *Gastroenterology* 1982; 83:689–693.
57. Nezelof C, Lancret P: Lesions of myocardial fibrosis during fibrocystic disease of pancreas. *Arch Fr Pediatr* 1959; 16:1035–1046.
58. Chu CJ, Tsui TY: Pathologic study of metacarpo–interphalangeal joints in Kaschin-Beck disease. *Chin Med J* 1978; 4:309–318.
59. Yang GQ: Selenium problem concerning human health in China. *Chin J Endemiol* 1984; 1:1–2.
60. Burk RF: Newer understanding of selenium metabolism. *IM-Internal Medicine for the Specialist* 1985; 6:148–153.
61. Yang SY: An endemic cardiomyopathy in China: Keshan disease, in Doyle EF, Engle MA, Gersony WM, Rashkind WJ, Talner NS (eds): *Pediatric Cardiology*. New York, Springer-Verlag, 1986, pp 975–977.
62. Huang YS: Report on selenium and dilated cardiomyopathy. *Chin Med Trib* 1985; 5:37.
63. Oster O, Prellwitz W, Kasper W, Meinertz T: Congestive cardiomyopathy and the selenium content of serum. *Clin Chim Acta* 1983; 128:125–132.
64. Weber MAJ, Hotte C, Zitzmann A, Theisen K, Schrammel D: Selenium deficiency in dilated cardiomyopathy. *Circulation* 1985; 72(Suppl III):III-157.

45 Diseases of the Pericardium

E. William Hancock, MD

Diseases of the pericardium result from a wide range of pathologic processes that cover nearly every area of medicine and surgery.[1-4] In some instances the pericardial disease presents as a specific and primary form of heart disease, but more often it is part of a general systemic disease. Despite the variety of disease processes, pathologic changes in the pericardium can usually be classified into a small number of categories, such as pericardial inflammation (pericarditis), pericardial thickening, pericardial effusion, and adhesion of the pericardium to the heart. These pathologic changes represent the response of the pericardium to injury. The pericardium responds to injury in a relatively small number of ways. Therefore, the term pericarditis is a broad one, indicating that the pericardium has been affected by one of many possible disease processes.

The most important forms of pericarditis the world over are still those caused by infection, particularly viral, bacterial, and tuberculous. In many developed countries, bacterial and tuberculous pericarditis have become rare; the more important forms of pericarditis are now those that represent complications of chronic diseases that are changed in their natural history as a result of advanced forms of medical treatment. For example, neoplastic involvement of the pericardium is no longer a feature only of terminal cancer, but rather it is a complication that can often be treated successfully. Also, uremic pericarditis is no longer a feature only of terminal renal failure, but it represents a problem that frequently arises in patients who live a long time with the aid of dialysis. As a further example, constrictive pericarditis as a late complication of cardiac surgery is now a more common cause of constrictive pericarditis in developed countries than is either tuberculous or bacterial infection. This chapter, in keeping with the emphasis of the volume on the international aspects of cardiology, will emphasize the infective causes of pericarditis around the world, while putting in perspective the problems often seen in developing countries.

ANATOMIC ABNORMALITIES

ANATOMY OF THE PERICARDIUM

The pericardium is a continuous thin layer of tissue that totally surrounds the heart. It is folded upon itself to form parietal and visceral layers. The parietal layer is separated from the heart and is often thought of as being the pericardium proper. The visceral layer, also known as the epicardium, is intimately attached to the heart and represents the surface of the heart. Between the parietal and visceral layers is the pericardial space, normally containing approximately 10 to 20 ml of fluid. The anatomic arrangement is therefore similar to that of the pleural space.

The normal pericardium is only approximately 0.1 mm thick. The thickness of 1 mm that is often stated to be the normal pericardial thickness in clinical imaging studies such as echocardiography or computed tomography (CT) is exaggerated by the limited powers of resolution of these techniques of imaging. The pericardial membrane has only a single layer of mesothelial cells on its surface, with an inner layer of connective tissue. The connective tissue layer is mostly collagen, with a smaller amount of elastic tissue.[5] The predominance of collagen results in a membrane that is tough and inelastic, despite its thinness. The collagen is arranged in wavy bundles that are oriented in differing directions, resulting in a crisscross effect. Straightening of the wavy collagen bundles is probably one mechanism by which the pericardium can stretch when it is distended by an enlarging heart or by pericardial fluid under increased pressure.[6]

The mesothelial cells that form the surface of the pericardium are endowed with a complex arrangement of microvilli, providing them with a surface area that is vastly greater than that expected with a single layer of cells. This promotes rapid and easy exchange of water and small molecules across the pericardium. The mesothelial cells also have a great deal of interdigitation and overlap, so that they are readily able to stretch.

CONGENITAL DEFECTS OF THE PERICARDIUM

Congenital defects of the pericardium are relatively rare, but interesting abnormalities that are clinically significant in some cases. They may be divided into four categories, according to the location of the defect.

The most frequent and important type of defect of the pericardium is that involving the left lateral pericardium, often referred to as pleuropericardial defect.[7] The pleura is also deficient, so that a free opening exists between the pericardial space and the left pleural space. Such defects may be total, or they may be partial of various sizes. Total defects are less important, because they rarely if ever lead to clinical complications. Partial defects create the possibility of herniation of portions of the heart through the defect and hence of strangulation of such herniated portions of the heart.[8] Sudden death may result, possibly caused by compression of a coronary artery involved in the herniation. Nasser[9] described a patient with angina pectoris apparently resulting from chronic compression of the left anterior descending coronary artery by the edge of a partial defect of the left pericardium.

Congenital defect of the left pericardium is usually first detected on plain chest roentgenograms, showing prominence of the shadow of the left atrial appendage in the frontal projection. The left atrial appendage is the portion of the heart that is most likely to prolapse through such a defect. This abnormality can also be detected by echocardiography,[10,11] computed tomographic scanning,[12] and nuclear magnetic resonance imaging.[12a]

Most patients with partial defects of the left pericardium do not develop complications, and surgical treatment is therefore not necessary unless there is evidence of complications. Either closure of the defect, if it is relatively small, or enlargement of the defect so that it becomes equivalent to a total absence of the left pericardium may be carried out. Trauma may cause defects of the left pericardium that are similar to those of congenital origin and that may lead to similar complications.[13–15]

The other types of congenital pericardial defects are those that involve the right pleuropericardium, the diaphragmatic pericardium, or the entire pericardium.[16,17] These are rare, and even more rarely are they a direct cause of clinical complications.

PERICARDIAL CYSTS

Pericardial cysts are probably congenital, although they usually present in adult life as an apparently acquired abnormality. They occur most frequently at the right cardiophrenic angle and are usually first discovered on a roentgenogram of the chest. They are usually asymptomatic and have little or no clinical significance except for the problem of differential diagnosis between solid tumors and other masses that might occur in this region. Echocardiography or computerized tomography is usually sufficient to reveal the cystic nature of the mass and thus to eliminate the need for exploratory surgery.[18,19]

FUNCTION OF THE PERICARDIUM

The pericardium does not have a clearly defined function. Its absence appears to create no obvious defect in the function of the heart.[20] The pericardium, with its small amount of serous fluid in the pericardial space, evidently permits the heart to move with its cycle of filling and emptying with a minimum of friction and a minimum of interaction with the surrounding structures. Such freedom from friction likely reduces the work of the heart; although no such decrease in the work of the heart has been measured, it may simply be that the methods of measuring the work of the heart are not sufficiently accurate to measure relatively small changes.

Resistance to infection that might spread to the heart from the adjacent lung, pleura, and mediastinum has traditionally been suggested as a possible functional role for the pericardium. This remains an unproven thesis.

ROLE IN VENTRICULAR FUNCTION

If the pericardium has an important functional role, it is most likely to be its effect on the filling of the heart and the regulation of the diastolic pressures in the right and left ventricles. Filling of the two ventricles in diastole is influenced by many physiologic variables, one of the most important of which is the intrinsic distensibility, or compliance, of the muscular chambers. Given that a ventricle fills to a certain volume, the diastolic pressure in that ventricle reflects the compliance of the chamber; this is different for the right and left ventricle and also varies widely in various physiologic and pathologic states. Because the pericardium surrounds the two ventricles, it is evident that the compliance of the pericardium can at least potentially influence the effective compliance of the ventricles.

When the heart dilates acutely, particularly in response to a large increase in the circulating blood volume, the pericardium clearly has a restraining action. Its compliance is limited, and the increase in diastolic pressure in the ventricles significantly reflects this limited compliance as well as the limited compliance of the ventricular chambers themselves. This effect is well demonstrated in studies in experimental animals. The effect is more difficult to see in human subjects, but it is probably evident in a few unusual clinical circumstances. Acute severe mitral regurgitation and total correction of tetralogy of Fallot are both circumstances in which there is an acute volume load on the heart and in which elevated filling pressures have occurred that are relieved when a tight pericardium is opened surgically. The common practice in cardiac surgery of leaving the pericardium widely open or only loosely approximated at the conclusion of the operation is based partly on this consideration as well as the more common problem of blood or fluid accumulating in a closed pericardial sac postoperatively.

In addition to its role in the effective diastolic compliance of the ventricular chambers, the pericardium also plays a role in equalizing the volume and diastolic pressure in the right and left ventricles in conditions of acute volume overload.

That the pericardium is an important contributor to compliance of the ventricles in chronic volume overload or in chronic enlargement of the heart due to other causes is doubtful. In chronic conditions the pericardium enlarges as the heart enlarges, and it has been difficult to confirm the possibility that it might play a chronic restraining role. The enlargement of the pericardium that occurs when there is chronic enlargement of the heart appears to occur mainly by hypertrophy of the pericardial tissue; stretching of the existing connective tissue elements appears to play a smaller and short-term role.

ACUTE PERICARDITIS

Acute pericarditis is a clinical syndrome that occurs frequently in pericardial disease of many etiologies.[21,22] The cause may be evident initially, as in patients on chronic renal dialysis or in those with a chronic connective tissue disorder such as systemic lupus erythematosus in which acute pericarditis develops as a complication of a known chronic disease. In other instances, acute pericarditis develops as a new and independent condition; the etiology may or may not be discovered by subsequent studies, the pericarditis remaining as idiopathic acute pericarditis. There are broad similarities in the clinical features of the acute pericarditis syndrome across a wide variety of etiologic circumstances.

SYMPTOMS

The cardinal symptom of acute pericarditis is chest pain. This is a centrally located anterior chest pain that usually develops suddenly and persists many hours or longer. The pain may variously be described as sharp or dull, aching or stabbing, pressure-like or suffocating, and so forth. These characteristics are similar to those of the pain of acute myocardial infarction. The chest pain in acute pericarditis is also usually pleuritic, often strikingly so, and aggravation with inspiration is felt primarily in the substernal area. Most patients with acute pericarditis prefer to sit upright, apparently because the pain is aggravated by the supine position as well as by breathing. The pleuritic and positional features help to differentiate the pain of acute pericarditis from that of acute myocardial infarction in most instances. Also, pleuritic pain due to primary processes in the lung and pleura is usually located primarily on the right or left side of the chest, rather than the midline. Thus, a substernal pleuritic pain of sudden onset is relatively characteristic of acute pericarditis.

PHYSICAL FINDINGS

The cardinal physical finding in acute pericarditis is the pericardial friction rub. The friction rub is like a cardiac murmur in that it is a noise that persists for a perceptible time during a specific phase of the cardiac cycle. Friction rubs are usually of medium frequency, with a variety of frequency components, often giving a "scratchy" impression to the listener. Occasionally, a friction rub has a distinctive "creaky" or "leathery" character, but for the most part the acoustic quality itself does not differentiate a friction rub from a cardiac murmur.

Friction rubs are distinctive in that they typically have three components in time—systolic, early diastolic, and late diastolic—corresponding to the three phases in the cardiac cycle in which the movements of the heart are the most abrupt.[23] The three components may exist all together or in any combination. The most distinctive, and virtually pathognomonic, finding is the triphasic rub, because there is no combination of cardiac murmurs that simulates it. The presystolic component alone is highly characteristic, because it is unlikely that it would be simulated by anything but the murmur of mitral stenosis, and mitral stenosis would almost always have additional auscultatory features. The systolic and early diastolic components of a friction rub produce a to-and-fro effect that could be simulated by to-and-fro aortic murmurs. The systolic component alone is the least distinctive, because many systolic ejection murmurs have a "scratchy" quality. Friction rubs have little correlation with the presence or absence of pericardial fluid or with the amount of fluid that is present.[24]

Pericardial friction rubs are usually heard best at the left sternal border in the third interspace, but they may be heard anywhere over the precordium. They often vary with respiration and position, most frequently being louder in expiration and in the sitting position. However, the respiratory and positional variations are unpredictable, so that a thorough examination for a friction rub should include auscultation in all phases of respiration and in several positions.

ELECTROCARDIOGRAPHIC FINDINGS

The characteristic electrocardiographic finding in acute pericarditis is elevation of the ST segment in all of those leads in which the positive electrode is oriented toward the epicardial surfaces of the right or left ventricle (Figure 45.1). This often includes all of the standard 12 leads except aVR; however, leads V_1, III, and aVL may also be excluded, depending on the QRS axis and the anatomic position of the heart relative to precordial lead placement.

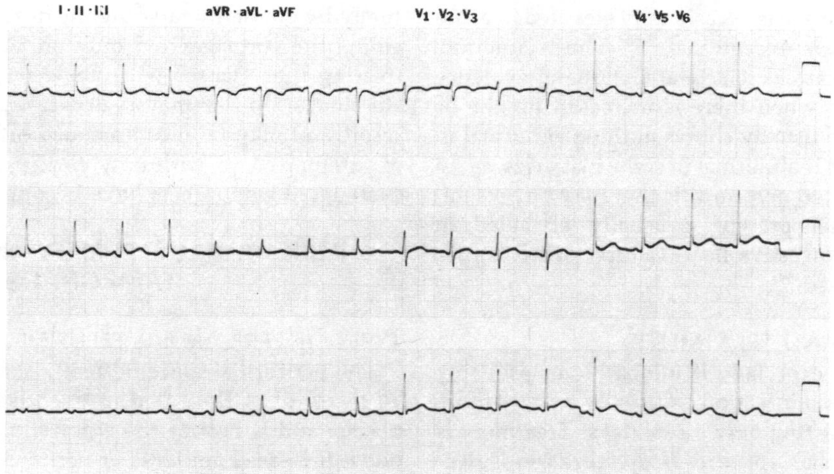

Figure 45.1. Electrocardiogram in acute pericarditis. There is ST-segment elevation in both anterior and inferior leads.

ST-segment elevation in acute pericarditis is usually slight or moderate in degree and has an upward concave form. The foregoing features usually differentiate acute pericarditis from early acute myocardial infarction on the electrocardiogram, because the latter shows ST-segment elevation localized to an anterior, lateral, or inferior group of leads with reciprocal ST-segment depression in the opposite lead groups. Also, the ST-segment elevation of early acute myocardial infarction is often severe and usually shows an upward convex form. The normal variant ST-segment elevation is more difficult to distinguish from that of acute pericarditis, in that it is also present in diffuse leads, with an upward concave form. The normal variant is usually associated with taller T waves in the leads that show prominent ST-segment elevation than is acute pericarditis.[25] In addition, the heart rate is usually normal or slow in the presence of the normal variant ST-segment elevation, which is related to the presence of predominant parasympathetic tone and is normalized by exercise in which a sympathetic neural effect on the heart becomes predominant.

Acute pericarditis is also accompanied frequently by depression of the PR segment (Figure 45.2). This accounts for some or all of the apparent ST-segment elevation in some leads. PR-segment depression is usually seen best in lead II, or any other lead in which there is a prominent upright P wave. It does not occur with the normal variant ST-segment elevation, and therefore it is a helpful point in making this differentiation.

Many cases of acute pericarditis show evolution of electrocardiographic abnormalities, ST-segment elevation being followed by a phase of T-wave inversion before the return to normal. ST-segment elevation generally resolves before the T waves become inverted; therefore, in acute pericarditis there is no stage in which ST-segment elevation and T-wave inversion are both present, whereas in acute myocardial infarction such a stage does typically occur. The normal variant ST-segment elevation is a stable pattern on the resting electrocardiogram.[26]

Cardiac arrhythmias have sometimes been considered to result from pericarditis, especially atrial arrhythmias that have been thought to result from inflammation of the thin-walled atrium. According to Spodick's analysis,[27] however, patients with acute pericarditis who show arrhythmias nearly always have associated organic heart disease, and it is doubtful whether arrhythmias should be ascribed to acute pericarditis alone.

LABORATORY STUDIES

Apart from the laboratory abnormalities that reflect a specific etiology, laboratory studies show only relatively slight and nonspecific findings in acute pericarditis. The erythrocyte sedimentation rate is elevated in a large proportion of cases and the white blood cell count is often mildly increased. Levels of serum enzymes such as creatine kinase and lactic dehydrogenase are typically normal; however, they may be mildly elevated, reflecting some degree of inflammatory myocardial involvement. The MB

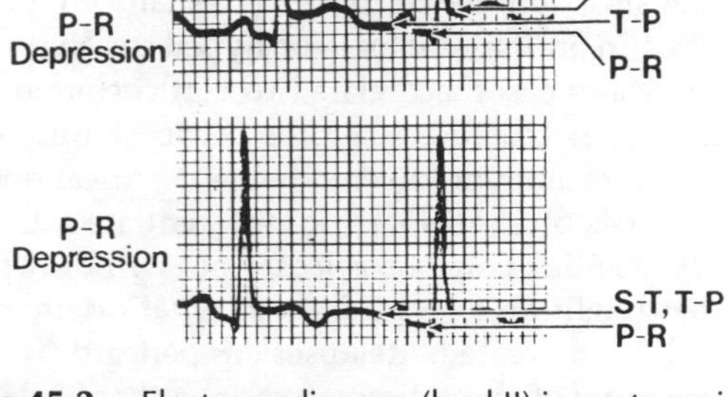

Figure 45.2. Electrocardiogram (lead II) in acute pericarditis. Apparent elevation of the ST segment may be partially (*middle panel*) or almost entirely (*lower panel*) due to depression of the PR segment.

fraction of creatine kinase is occasionally elevated in acute pericarditis, but this is exceptional.[28,29] The technetium pyrophosphate myocardial scintigram, showing evidence of myocardial injury when there is increased uptake of the radionuclide, also usually shows nothing abnormal in acute pericarditis, but is abnormal in some instances, again reflecting the associated myocarditis that may be present. Pleural effusion, when present, is usually left-sided, in contrast to that in congestive heart failure, which is predominantly right-sided.[29a]

CLINICAL COURSE AND TREATMENT

Acute pericarditis, especially if idiopathic or probably the result of acute viral infection, is usually a short-term, self-limited illness, lasting only a few days. Treatment is symptomatic rather than specific. Hospitalization is necessary only when differential diagnosis between acute myocardial infarction and other potentially life-threatening acute conditions is not clear when the patient is examined, or there is evidence of cardiac tamponade from associated pericardial effusion.

The first priority in management, after confirming the diagnosis and ruling out cardiac tamponade, is relief of pain, often achieved with analgesic drugs such as codeine, or morphine if necessary. Aspirin or nonsteroidal antiinflammatory drugs, such as indomethacin and ibuprofen, are also useful.[30] The antiinflammatory drugs are primarily symptomatic, although they are often considered to have a somewhat specific action in suppressing the pericarditis itself. There are insufficient controlled objective clinical trials to assess whether the antiinflammatory drugs are more efficacious than simple analgesic agents.

Therapy with adrenal corticosteroids is often used in patients with acute pericarditis who appear to be severely ill or who do not show a rapid response to simpler therapy. Corticosteroid drugs are probably the most effective antiinflammatory therapy available for acute pericarditis. However, corticosteroids should be used only for strong indications, if at all, because their use may lead to a more difficult problem later if the pericarditis tends to relapse when the corticosteroid is discontinued.[31]

Acute pericarditis follows a persistent course in a few instances. These cases become subacute or chronic, and progress to constrictive pericarditis in some instances. Patients who follow this course can usually be recognized as having unusually severe and persistent pericarditis from the outset.[32]

Chronic recurrent, or relapsing, pericarditis occurs rarely following acute pericarditis of various etiologies. Its mechanism is unknown, but it is usually thought to have a basis in an immunologic or hypersensitivity phenomenon. Many cases are related to corticosteroid therapy, the relapse occurring when the corticosteroid is discontinued or its amount lowered below a critical dose. In these cases it is often difficult to differentiate a true relapse of pericarditis from a corticosteroid withdrawl syndrome that might occur regardless of what original condition had been treated. Relapses of pericarditis often consist primarily of chest discomfort and other ill-defined systemic symptoms, sometimes without any objective signs of active pericarditis.

Relapsing pericarditis can usually be controlled eventually by gradually tapering the dose of corticosteroid, by giving the corticosteroid only on alternate days, and by treating the relapses with analgesics, aspirin, and nonsteroidal antiinflammatory drugs. Pericardiectomy is a last resort and may be recommended after more than a year of attempting to withdraw corticosteroids or when the cushingoid side effects have become excessive.

PERICARDIAL EFFUSION AND CARDIAC TAMPONADE

TYPES OF PERICARDIAL EFFUSION

The pericardial space normally contains approximately 10 to 20 ml of fluid that is essentially an ultrafiltrate of plasma and is part of the extracellular fluid space in the body. Increased amounts of pericardial fluid are likely to develop in any of the great variety of pathologic processes that involve the pericardium.[33] It is useful to categorize the types of pericardial effusion according to the gross appearance of the fluid.

In *serous effusion* the fluid is similar to that which is present normally. This type of effusion occurs frequently in congestive heart failure.[34] It is also frequent in other systemic conditions in which there is retention of sodium and water and expansion of the extracellular fluid space in the body. For example, approximately 40% of women develop pericardial effusion during normal pregnancy.[35]

Serofibrinous effusion is the type most frequently seen when the pericardial effusion is due to the common types of pericarditis, including idiopathic, viral infection, neoplastic, radiation-induced, connective tissue disease, and many others. There is a fibrinous deposit on the pericardial surface in these cases. The fluid is thin and clear, but the protein concentration is higher than that in an ultrafiltrate of plasma, usually in the range of 2.0 to 5.0 g/dl.

Serosanguineous effusion also occurs frequently in many of the same types of pericarditis that usually lead to serofibrinous effusion. Tuberculous and neoplastic pericardial disease have often been considered the usual causes of serosanguineous fluid, but idiopathic pericarditis, radiation-induced, and many others are also likely to cause this type of fluid. The hematocrit ranges up to approximately 10% in fluids that appear grossly serosanguineous.

Bloody pericardial effusion, or hemopericardium, is associated with a hematocrit higher than 10%, often similar to that of the circulating blood. Hemopericardium is essentially due to bleeding into the pericardial space, and the most frequent causes include trauma such as knife or gunshot wounds, perforation of the heart during acute myocardial infarction or as a complication of cardiac catheterization procedures, rupture of aortic dissections into the pericardial space, or defects in coagulation, most frequently those defects secondary to warfarin anticoagulation therapy.

Cholesterol pericardial effusion is a rare condition in which the fluid has a glistening "gold paint" appearance because of a high cholesterol content. It is usually associated with a clinical syndrome of idiopathic chronic pericardial effusion. The high cholesterol concentration may represent the effects of continuing formation and reabsorption of pericardial fluid, with the cholesterol-containing lipoproteins being retained and gradually concentrated because of their large molecular size.[36]

Chylous pericardial effusion is another rare condition that results from a communication between the thoracic duct and the pericardial space. The fluid is milky-white because of a high concentration of chylomicrons laden with triglycerides. Chylous pericardial effusion usually presents as chronic idiopathic pericardial effusion, not associated with chylous fluid in the abdominal or pleural cavities. The reason for the abnormal communication may be unknown, but there is likely to be a background of trauma or of venous or lymphatic obstruction.[37–39]

Iatrogenic pericardial effusion may result from penetration of venous catheters into the pericardial space, with inadvertent infusion of fluids such as saline or mixtures used for partial or total parenteral nutrition.[40,41]

Pneumopericardium, with little or no associated effusion, may also occur and may cause cardiac tamponade.[42] It is usually a complication of closed chest trauma, but it may result from direct extension of pathologic processes in the lung, esophagus, or stomach.

PATHOPHYSIOLOGY OF PERICARDIAL EFFUSION

The principal importance of pericardial effusion is that it may increase the pressure in the pericardial space to such a level that the heart is compressed. Pressure in the pericardial space is normally approximately zero with reference to outside atmospheric pressure and is similar to the pressure in the intrapleural space. As increased amounts of pericardial fluid develop, the pressure in the pericardial space rises, slowly at first and then rapidly as the pericardium reaches its limits of distensibility (Figure 45.3). The pressure-volume relation in the pericardial space is extremely variable, however, and probably depends primarily on how rapidly the fluid develops. When the fluid accumulates over months and years, there may be an immense effusion that is associated with a pericardial pressure within the normal range; this is seen in myxedema, for example, with as much as 2 L of pericardial fluid. Conversely, when the fluid develops over minutes or a few hours, the pericardial pressure may rise steeply when no more than 150 to 200 ml has accumulated; this is seen, for example, in traumatic hemopericardium.

When the pericardial space is free of adhesions and loculations, the pericardial fluid surrounds nearly all of the heart and the same pressure is exerted on all of the cardiac chambers. However, the right-sided chambers, particularly the right atrium, have thinner walls and lower pressures within and are more rapidly compressed than are the left-sided chambers. Thus, pressures in the central veins, right atrium, right ventricle (in diastole), and pericardial space become nearly equilibrated and rise together; when a level of 10 to 12 mm Hg is exceeded, pressures in the pulmonary veins, left atrium, and left ventricle (in diastole) also begin to rise and all of the intracardiac pressures (in diastole) are nearly equilibrated. Compression of the heart reduces its size, limits cardiac output, and necessitates a higher venous pressure to fill the heart. The decrease in arterial pressure is a late secondary effect and represents decompensated tamponade (Figure 45.4).

CLINICAL DETECTION OF PERICARDIAL EFFUSION

History and physical examination offer few or no specific clues to the presence of pericardial effusion. Enlargement of the pericardial sac by fluid does not cause symp-

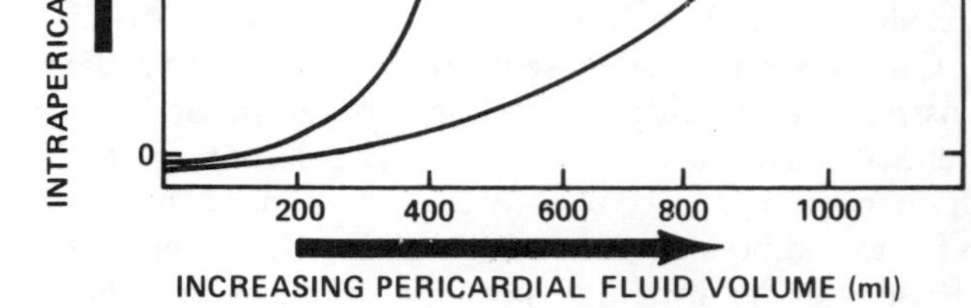

Figure 45.3. Diagrammatic illustration of the relation between pressure and volume in the pericardical space. With a rapidly developing pericardial effusion, the pressure in the pericardial space rises more steeply than it does with a slowly developing effusion. (Figures 45.3, 45.4 and 45.6 are from Hancock EW: Cardiac tamponade. *Med Clin North Am* 1979; 63:223–237, with permission.)

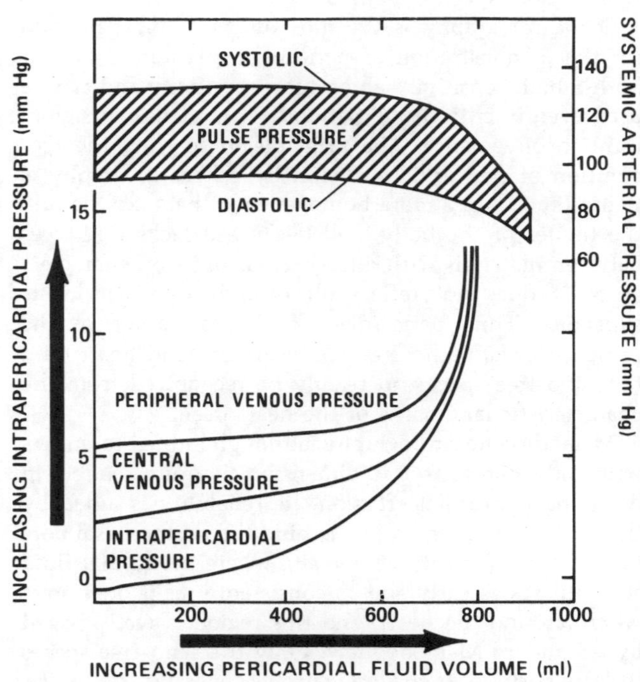

Figure 45.4. Diagrammatic illustration of the response of intravascular pressures to an increasing intrapericardial pressure. Central and peripheral venous pressures become equilibrated. Arterial pressure decreases only after venous pressure has increased significantly.

toms in itself and only rarely would enlargement of the pericardial space be sufficiently great to reduce the volume of the lungs and thereby produce dyspnea. Enlargement of the percussible area of cardiac dullness, without corresponding outward displacement of the cardiac impulse, is characteristic of pericardial effusion, but it is not often sufficiently accurate to be useful.

The electrocardiogram is expected to show reduced QRS voltage in the presence of pericardial effusion. The normal range is large, however, and only approximately 10% of patients with pericardial effusion have abnormally low voltage.[43] Electrical alternans, reflecting a swinging of the heart within a large pericardial effusion with each heartbeat, is a rather specific sign of pericardial effusion, but it is present only in a minority of cases.

The chest roentgenogram is expected to show enlargement of the cardiomediastinal silhouette in the presence of pericardial effusion, and it does indeed show this with effusions of moderate or large size. However, the shape of the cardiomediastinal silhouette is not characteristic and not reliable for diagnosis. One sign in the plain chest roentgenogram that is relatively specific for pericardial effusion is the fat line, usually seen in the lateral projection and based on the principle that a layer of fat on the epicardial surface of the heart has a lower radiodensity than does the myocardium or the pericardial fluid on either side.[44] Fat lines are recognized in only a minority of patients with pericardial effusion. Therefore, although the chest roentgenogram is often the first clue that a patient has pericardial effusion, an enlarged cardiomediastinal silhouette is a nonspecific finding, and the demonstration of pericardial effusion requires further study with a more specific method.

Echocardiography is the most useful clinical method for the demonstration of pericardial effusion[45,46] It has both a high sensitivity and a high specificity and can be used even in critically ill patients without risk or significant inconvenience. The principle underlying the recognition of pericardial effusion by echocardiography is that a liquid has a more homogeneous character than do the tissues of the body, and because it lacks interfaces between materials with differing transmission characteristics, it does not reflect ultrasound from within its substance. Thus, pericardial effusion is marked by the presence of an echo-free space around the heart, and the echo-free space can readily be recognized from the characteristic landmarks of the heart itself.

M-mode echocardiography, although limited to images with only one anatomic dimension, is quite reliable in detecting pericardial effusion. Its reliability is aided by the fact that the region just behind the posterobasal portion of the left ventricle is a site where pericardial fluid accumulates as early and as consistently as it does anywhere around the heart, and this region is well imaged by a standard M-mode view. Only the echo-free spaces that are posterior to the left ventricle generally are specific for pericardial effusion. Echo-free spaces that are anterior to the heart may be due to pericardial effusion, to epicardial fat, or to other mediastinal tissue.[47] The amount of pericardial fluid can be categorized as small, moderate, or large, but more precise quantification is unreliable because of the uneven distribution of the fluid around the heart.

There are several pitfalls in the recognition of pericardial effusion by M-mode echocardiography that must be considered to avoid errors in diagnosis. The echo-free space should be imaged in a view in which the gain setting has temporarily been reduced so as to visualize only the single strongest echo. The single strongest echo should represent the interface of the posterior pericardium and the air-filled lung, and therefore it serves as an important landmark. Pleural effusion on the left side can mimic pericardial effusion closely unless this landmark is correctly located. Pericardial effusion occasionally can also be simulated by conditions such as pericardial thickening, solid masses adjacent to the heart, layers of subepicardial fat, enlarged coronary sinus or descending aorta, or unusually located aneurysms of the left ventricle.[48] Conversely, pericardial effusion can be overlooked on the echocardiogram when the effusion is loculated and present only in a region that is not well visualized. It can also be overlooked when there is a hemopericardium, because blood is less homogeneous and reflects ultrasound from within its substance more than do the usual serofibrinous or serosanguineous fluids.

Two-dimensional echocardiography adds substantially to the echocardiographic assessment of pericardial effusion, because it permits visualization of the presence and the thickness of the layer of fluid all around the circumference of the heart. In some cases the two-dimensional echocardiogram shows pericardial effusion that would be missed in the M-mode study, but the most important addition of the two-dimensional study is the assessment of how much fluid is present in various locations. This information is particularly helpful in planning and carrying out pericardiocentesis.

Computed tomography and nuclear magnetic resonance imaging are also useful in demonstrating pericardial effusion.[49–52] These techniques are more elaborate and more expensive than echocardiography and should be used in difficult cases in which the echocardiogram has been inconclusive. Radionuclide imaging can demonstrate pericardial effusion as well, but the resolution is less than that with either echocardiography, computed tomography, or nuclear magnetic resonance imaging.[53] Ga-67 scintigraphy is more useful in demonstrating myopericarditis rather than pericardial fluid itself.[54]

CLINICAL RECOGNITION OF CARDIAC TAMPONADE

Cardiac tamponade presents in a variety of ways, demonstrating a particular distinction between surgical (often traumatic) and medical cases.[55–58] The definition of cardiac tamponade unfortunately is not a standard one. Some refer to tamponade as a condition in which pericardial effusion under increased pressure produces any measurable hemodynamic abnormality, whereas others use the term tamponade to refer only to situations in which there is "circulatory embarrassment," usually implying a shock-like picture or at least some definite degree of hypotension or reduction in cardiac output, or both. In this chapter, the former definition will be used, and the hypotensive or shock-like picture will be referred to as decompensated cardiac tamponade. The concept of noncritical, or compensated, tamponade is particularly relevant in medical cases in which the tamponade usually develops more gradually and remains compensated for a longer time than is typical in surgical cases.

The essential hemodynamic effect of compression of the heart by fluid under increased pressure is elevation of the central venous pressure, reflecting a similar elevation in right ventricular diastolic pressure and right atrial mean pressure. The level of the central venous pressure is an accurate indicator, within 2 to 4 mm Hg, of the level of intrapericardial pressure in the presence of cardiac tamponade. Unfortunately, central venous pressure is often difficult to estimate on physical examination in patients in whom cardiac tamponade is suspected. Superficial veins such as the external jugular vein are likely to be constricted and hence less visible than usual. If the patient is severely ill, it may be difficult to conduct examination of the neck veins in the several positions that are required for optimal examination. Instrumentation, particularly indwelling jugular venous catheters, may also compromise the examination. Nevertheless, accurate assessment of the central venous pressure is the key to recognizing cardiac tamponade, and if the physical examination is inconclusive on this point, there should be a readiness to measure the central venous pressure directly. The venous pressure waveform shows a prominent systolic (x) descent in cardiac tamponade and is different from that seen in constrictive pericarditis (Figure 45.5).

Cardiac tamponade may exist rarely in the presence of a relatively low or even normal central venous pressure. It may be seen within the first few minutes of tamponade that is produced, for example, by perforation of the heart during cardiac catherization, because systemic venoconstriction and the increase in venous blood volume have not yet had time to develop. Also, patients who have depletion of the circulating blood volume and extracellular fluid volume, because of persistent vomiting, diarrhea, or diminished fluid intake, for example, may have cardiac tamponade with relatively normal central venous pressure.[59] These conditions are rare exceptions to the general rule.

Paradoxical pulse, or an exaggerated decrease in arterial pressure with inspiration, is also expected to be present in nearly all patients with cardiac tamponade. However, it is frequently not detected for several reasons. Paradoxical pulse is usually defined as a decrease of 10 mm Hg or more in the arterial systolic pressure with inspiration, as measured with the conventional sphygmomanometer. However, the value of 10 mm Hg is arbitrary, and it also is probably more applicable to direct arterial recordings than to sphygmomanometric measurements. The pulse pressure decreases as does the systolic pressure (Figure 45.6). Direct arterial recordings usually show substantially greater variation in pressure with respiration than that revealed by the sphygmomanometric reading. Other factors that tend to obscure the presence of the paradoxical pulse include irregular breathing patterns with very brief inspiration, irregular cardiac rhythms, and low arterial pressure with narrow pulse pressure.

The mechanism of paradoxical pulse is still not clearly understood, perhaps because the relative importance of several mechanisms has been difficult to estimate quantitatively. It is known that the decrease in arterial pressure with inspiration reflects a decrease in the stroke volume of the left ventricle. Moreover, the decrease in stroke volume is associated with a decrease in the systolic and diastolic volume of the left ventricle with inspiration, accompanied by a reciprocal increase in the systolic and diastolic volume of the right ventricle. These changes in

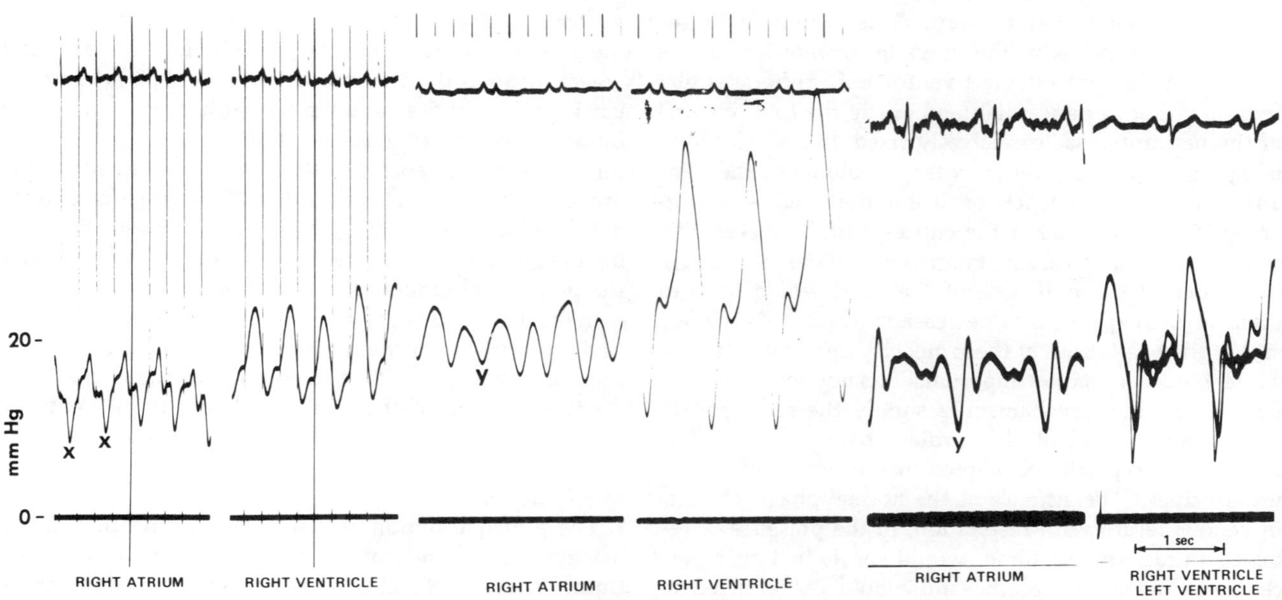

Figure 45.5. Right atrial and right ventricular pressure waveforms in three forms of compressive pericardial disease: *Left*, Cardiac tamponade; *middle*, subacute constrictive pericarditis; *right*, chronic constrictive pericarditis. In cardiac tamponade there is a dominant venous X descent and an elevated beginning diastolic pressure in the right ventricle. In chronic constrictive pericarditis there is a dominant venous Y descent and a prominent dip-plateau diastolic pattern in the right ventricle. The waveforms in subacute constriction are intermediate. (From Hancock EW,[110] with permission.)

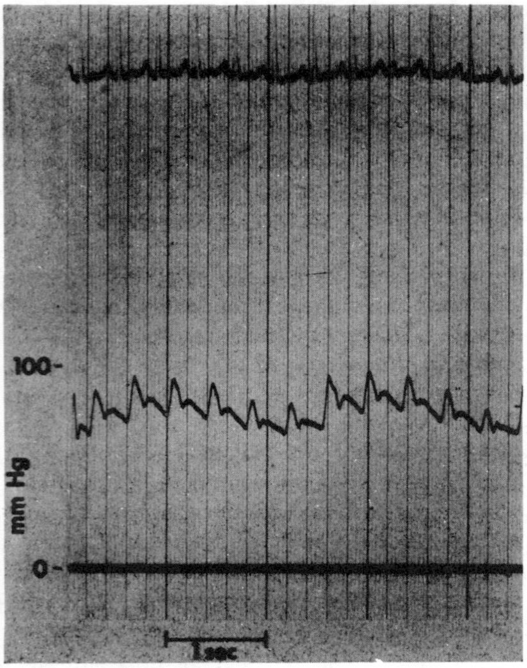

Figure 45.6. Arterial pressure recording in a patient with cardiac tamponade, showing a typical paradoxical pulse.

the volume and output of the ventricles with inspiration reflect phasic changes in the venous return to the heart with respiration and are qualitatively similar in normal physiologic circumstances and in cardiac tamponade. Two mechanisms have traditionally been held to explain the exaggerated variation with respiration in cardiac tamponade. Katz and Gauchat[60] pointed out that the left atrium, but not the pulmonary veins, is compressed by pericardial fluid under pressure and hence that pulmonary venous pressure would decrease with inspiration more than would left atrial pressure. This would favor sequestration of blood in the lungs on inspiration, at the expense of flow into the left ventricle. Dornhorst et al[61] indicated that in pericardial tamponade the total volume of the pericardial sac is relatively fixed. In normal physiologic circumstances the increase in volume of the right atrium and right ventricle on inspiration could result in an increase in volume of the entire heart. However, this could not occur in cardiac tamponade where an increase in volume of the right side of the heart would have to occur at the expense of a decrease in volume of the left side of the heart. Both of these mechanisms probably play a role, but their relative importance has not been assessed. Perhaps another mechanism is simply the reduction in the volumes of all of the cardiac chambers in cardiac tamponade, typically to approximately one half of the usual values.[62] Persistence of the normal phasic changes in venous return with respiration, in the presence of reduced intracardiac volume, would result in larger percentage changes in volume and would be reflected in larger changes in stroke output and arterial pressure.

Because of several factors involved in its genesis, the degree of paradoxical pulse does not correlate well with the severity of cardiac tamponade from one patient to another. Spodick et al[63,64] pointed out that even those cases of pericardial effusion in which the venous pressure is normal may still have subtly increased respiratory variation in the stroke volume of the left ventricle, as inferred from measurements of the systolic time intervals. Finally, paradoxical pulse can also occur in other conditions such as constrictive pericarditis, obstructive airway disease, congestive heart failure, restrictive cardiomyopathy, pulmonary embolism, right ventricular infarction, hypovolemia, shock, intrathoracic tumors, obesity, ascites, and pregnancy.

Kussmaul's sign, or an increase in jugular venous pressure with inspiration, has often been quoted as a sign of cardiac tamponade, but this is an error. Venous pressure either decreases or shows minimal variation with inspiration in cardiac tamponade. Kussmaul's sign does occur in constrictive pericarditis and also in other cardiac disorders in which the venous pressure is markedly elevated.

Although low voltage in the electrocardiogram merely reflects the presence of pericardial effusion, electrical alternans does correlate with the presence of cardiac tamponade in most instances.[65] The reason for this correlation is not clear. The swinging heart is most likely to occur when pericardial effusion is large, when the fluid is of low viscosity, and when there are no adhesions to limit the motion of the heart. These conditions are most often met in cases of neoplastic pericardial invasion, which in fact provide most of the examples of electrical alternans in pericardial effusion. Because neoplastic pericardial disease is usually associated with at least some degree of tamponade, the association of electrical alternans with tamponade may be an indirect one.

Echocardiography may show a variety of signs that tend to indicate that the pericardial effusion is under increased pressure and is producing cardiac tamponade. The most important of these is the inward motion, or "collapse" of the wall of the right atrium and the right ventricle in diastole.[66,67,67a] This sign reflects the fact that the pressure in the pericardial space is elevated to a point where it equals the pressure within the cardiac chambers, particularly at those points in the cardiac cycle where the intracardiac pressure reaches its lowest point (early diastole in the right ventricle, late diastole and early systole in the right atrium). The inward motion sign requires two-dimensional echocardiography for its demonstration, using the apical four-chamber view for the right atrium and the parasternal long-axis view for the right ventricle.

In the more severe cases of cardiac tamponade a reduced cavity dimension of the right ventricle can be seen on the echocardiogram, including standard M-mode studies. The diagnostic value of this is reduced by the difficulty of knowing the normal value for this dimension.

MANAGEMENT

The principal option available to the physician in the management of pericardial effusion is removal of the fluid. Pericardial fluid may be removed by needle pericardiocentesis or by one of several surgical techniques.

The indications for removal of pericardial fluid may be divided into three categories. These are diagnosis with regard to etiology, diagnosis with regard to pathophysiology, and treatment of cardiac tamponade. If the central venous pressure is normal, then diagnosis with regard to etiology is the only indication. If the central venous pressure is elevated, then all three indications are potentially relevant.[68]

The most important etiologic diagnoses that are frequently made from studies of the pericardial fluid are infective (except viral) and neoplastic disease. Hemopericardium is first diagnosed from the pericardial fluid occasionally, and the rare diagnosis of chylopericardium will also be made by obtaining the fluid. Because bacterial and tuberculous infection and neoplastic pericardial invasion usually lead to cardiac tamponade at a relatively early stage, it is unusual to make these diagnoses by a study of pericardial fluid in patients in whom the central venous pressure is normal. Thus, the likelihood of benefit from the purely "diagnostic tap" is relatively low, compared with that of pericardiocentesis in patients who have elevated venous pressure.[69]

The pathophysiologic diagnosis is relevant in many patients with pericardial effusion and elevated venous pressure, because cardiac tamponade is not necessarily present in such patients or it may only be part of the problem. The elevated venous pressure may be due to associated congestive heart failure (especially in patients on chronic renal dialysis), to associated visceral constrictive pericarditis (especially in radiation-induced pericardial disease), or to superior vena caval obstruction (especially in patients with neoplastic disease). When the pericardiocentesis is accompanied by appropriate hemodynamic and angiographic studies, these additional conditions can be evaluated.

The choice between needle pericardiocentesis and one of several surgical methods of removing pericardial fluid is somewhat controversial, with widely differing practices in various medical institutions in the United States as well as around the world. The facilities that are available and the training and experience of the physicians who are involved, as well as the specific medical problem in the patient under consideration, have much to do with the choice of procedure.

Pericardiocentesis has some advantage in simplicity and flexibility with regard to personnel and facilities. Although it should ideally be performed in a cardiac catheterization laboratory, it can be done at the bedside or in other facilities if required by circumstances.[70] Only local anesthesia is needed. The procedure is easily combined with hemodynamic monitoring, which permits assessment of associated congestive heart failure or visceral constrictive pericarditis to be carried out in a critical manner. Pericardiocentesis is more hazardous than most invasive cardiologic procedures; the principal risk is that of hemopericardium from inadvertent puncture of the heart. This complication is guarded against by the use of a monitoring electrocardiogram attached to the needle and also by the use of two-dimensional echocardiography during the procedure to guide the insertion of the needle.[71,72] Echocardiographic contrast injections also aid in determining the position of the needle tip. The determination of the pH of the fluid[73] and the performance of the circulation time[73a] are both quick and simple methods to exclude inadvertent ventricular punctures in bloody pericardiocentesis. A catheter should usually be left indwelling in the pericardial space for several days after the procedure to allow continued drainage if the fluid reforms rapidly.

Surgical drainage of the pericardial fluid is preferred to pericardiocentesis in many institutions for several reasons. The risk of perforating the heart is minimized, and the success of draining the fluid effectively is maximized.[74,75] In addition, a larger drainage tube may be inserted that will be more effective in draining pericardial fluid that is relatively thick. Subxiphoid pericardiostomy can be performed with the patient under local anesthesia and may be as well tolerated as uncomplicated pericardiocentesis. However, subxiphoid pericardiostomy is often performed with general anesthesia, as is the more extensive left lateral thoracotomy with partial pericardiectomy. The term *pericardial window* is often used, but it is not well defined. Surgical procedures for the relief of cardiac tamponade are better defined as subxiphoid pericardiostomy or parietal pericardiectomy of varying extent, performed through a thoracotomy incision.

Acute pulmonary edema or acute dilatation of the heart with congestive heart failure has occurred in rare instances following removal of pericardial fluid.[76,77]

LOCALIZED CARDIAC TAMPONADE

Various types of localized compression of the heart may occur, because of loculated collections of fluid that exert pressure on only a portion of the heart. This compression is seen most frequently in the early recovery period after cardiac surgery, but it may occur as long as 1 year later. It may also occur in the subacute phase of active pericarditis, particularly that due to purulent bacterial infection,[78] and it has also occurred in the pericarditis that complicates acute myocardial infarction.[79] The left atrium or the right atrium and right ventricle are most likely to be compressed. Localized compression of the left atrium is likely to produce a syndrome that is dominated by pulmonary vascular congestion, whereas compression of the right-sided chambers produces a syndrome that is characterized by hypotension and elevation of the venous pressure, without necessarily a prominent paradoxical pulse. Obstruction of the right ventricular outflow tract may also result from a localized pericardial abscess.[80] Echocardiography is less helpful than it is in typical cases of pericardial effusion and tamponade, because the effusion may be difficult to demonstrate (particularly if it is lateral to the right atrium) and also because some pericardial fluid is expected to be present in any case under such clinical circumstances.

The physiologic aspects of compression of individual chambers of the heart are complex. Fowler and Gabel[81] reported experimental studies in which tamponade could be produced only by compression that included the atria, and not by compression solely of the right ventricle or left ventricle; whether their experimental preparation simulated the clinical cases in which localized compression of the right ventricle appeared to cause tamponade is uncertain.

CONSTRICTIVE PERICARDITIS

Constrictive pericarditis is a condition in which the heart is compressed or constrained by a thickened and adherent pericardium. The condition is characterized by elevated pressure during diastole in all of the cardiac chambers, reflecting the increased resistance of the heart to filling because of abnormal restraint by the pericardium. In the classic form, the parietal pericardium is adherent to the visceral pericardium, effectively obliterating the pericardial space. A form of combined pericardial effusion and constriction also occurs in which fluid remains in the pericardial space and the constriction is due solely to the visceral pericardium.

Constrictive pericarditis, like pericardial effusion, can probably result from virtually any of the causes of pericarditis.[82–84] In the past, the most frequent etiology by far was thought to be tuberculous pericarditis. It still is the case in many areas of the world, particularly southern Africa and many tropical areas. In the United States, in many European countries, and in Japan, however, tuberculous pericarditis has become rare as a cause of constrictive pericarditis, and most cases are idiopathic. Most recent cases in China have been idiopathic as well, although tuberculous pericarditis accounts for approximately 40%.[85,86] The prevalence of tuberculous infection as a cause of chronic constrictive pericarditis possibly was exaggerated in the past, because in many cases this etiology was assumed when there was a positive tuberculin skin test or some other evidence of previous tuberculous infection, even though proof of tuberculous involvement of the tissue from the pericardium was lacking. In developed countries in which tuberculous infection is now the exception rather than the rule, most cases of chronic constrictive pericarditis apparently are not tuberculous and must be considered idiopathic.

Several new causes of constrictive pericarditis have appeared in recent years as a result of advances in medical treatment. The most prominent of these is the constrictive pericarditis that follows cardiac surgery, usually coronary artery bypass.[86a] Although these cases involve only a small proportion of patients who undergo coronary artery bypass surgery, the large number of such operations now being performed in many countries have given this cause a prominent place among the known etiologies of constrictive pericarditis.[87–90] The report of a case 20 years after the Beck operation may suggest a continuing late incidence of this complication.[91] Various advances in diagnosis have also revealed other relatively rare causes of constrictive pericarditis.[92–101] (Table 45.1).

Table 45.1. Some Rare Causes of Constrictive Pericarditis, With Representative References

Etiology	Author and Reference
Juvenile rheumatoid arthritis	Pearl[92]
Hypereosinophilic syndrome	Virmani et al[93]
Methysergide	Harbin et al[94]
Idiopathic mediastinal fibrosis	Hanley et al[95]
Procainamide	Browning et al[96]
Mulibrey nanism	Perheentupa et al[97]
Sarcoidosis	Garrett et al[98]
Dialysis	Ptacin[99]
Dressler's syndrome	Haiat[100]
Atrial septal defect	Albers et al[101]

Chronic constrictive pericarditis is notorious for its difficulty of diagnosis. This probably stems from the pathophysiologic characteristics of the condition, which has essentially one prominent feature, the chronic sustained elevation of systemic venous pressure. As compression of the heart gradually develops, the venous pressure increases as a compensatory mechanism and maintains the filling of the heart, the cardiac output, and the arterial pressure within or close to the normal range. Pulmonary venous pressure, being equilibrated with systemic venous pressure, also remains only slightly or moderately elevated in most cases, so that signs and symptoms of pulmonary vascular congestion are minimal.

The predominant effects of the sustained elevation in venous pressure in chronic constrictive pericarditis are hepatomegaly, ascites, and pleural effusion. Edema of the lower extremities occurs as well, but it is surprisingly inconspicuous in many patients with constrictive pericarditis, possibly because they are often younger than most patients with the common forms of congestive heart failure and have normal tissue turgor and more competent venous valves in the lower extremities. Thus, many patients with constrictive pericarditis are suspected for a long time of having chronic liver disease, ascites of various other causes, or pleural effusion of various or unknown causes before the key importance of the elevated jugular venous pressure becomes apparent. The normal appearance of both the heart and the lungs on plain chest roentgenogram and the minimal degree of electrocardiographic abnormality also contribute to the delay in diagnosis that often occurs.

Patients with constrictive pericarditis regularly have several abnormalities on physical examination that usually permit the diagnosis to be suspected. The jugular venous pressure is elevated, and a somewhat characteristic pulsatile waveform is usually present, in which two positive and two negative deflections occur in each cardiac cycle (M or W waveform). In the most classical cases the negative deflection in early diastole (Y descent) is much more prominent than the negative deflection in systole (X descent), a waveform that has been referred to as Freidreich's sign. Kussmaul's sign, or an increase in the jugular venous pressure level with inspiration, may occur as well (Figure 45.7). Conversely, paradoxical pulse is often not prominent in constrictive pericarditis, particularly in classical chronic cases.

The cardiac impulse in constrictive pericarditis is usually visible and palpable (in contrast to that in patients with cardiac tamponade) and often shows a retraction in systole and a prominent outward movement in early diastole (Figure 45.8). The outward movement in early diastole may be so prominent as to merit the term *diastolic heartbeat*.

Another characteristic physical sign in patients with chronic constrictive pericarditis is the abnormal sound in early diastole, often referred to as the "diastolic knock." The early diastolic sound is similar to the S_3 that occurs

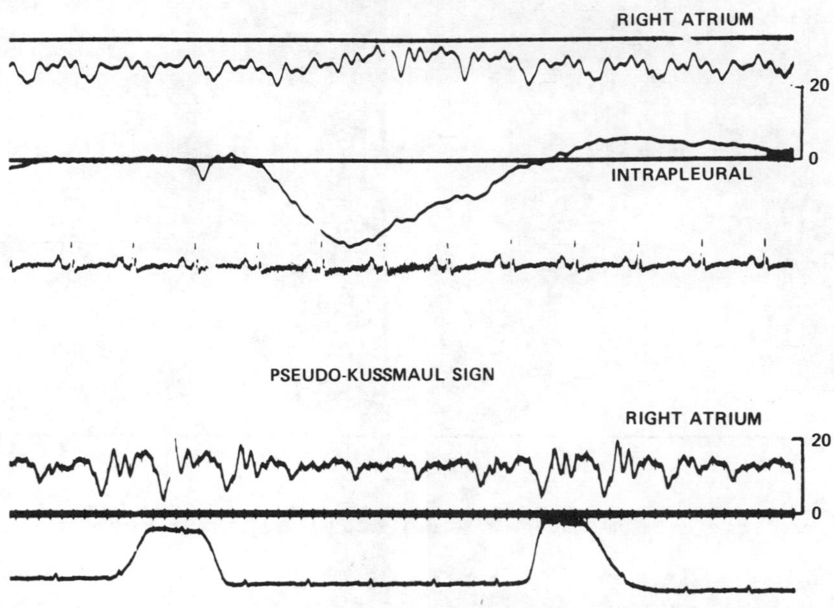

Figure 45.7. The upper panel illustrates Kussmaul's sign, a rise in venous pressure with inspiration. In the lower panel there is an increase in the amplitude of the venous pressure wave forms with inspiration, but not a rise in venous pressure; this may be termed a pseudo-Kussmaul's sign.

in mitral regurgitation and left ventricular failure. The early diastolic sound of constrictive pericarditis is often slightly earlier in timing and higher in pitch than the other varieties of S_3 and may simulate a mitral opening snap or a widely split S_2 (Figure 45.8). However, it frequently simulates S_3 rather closely; the term *knock* has perhaps even been taken to indicate that the sound originates from the calcified pericardium knocking against the chest wall, a doubtful concept. It would be preferable to regard the early diastolic sound as a filling sound, reflecting the termination of a filling phase in which the dimension or pressure within the ventricle, or both, had increased rapidly; this mechanism would be similar to that of both the normal and pathologic S_3.

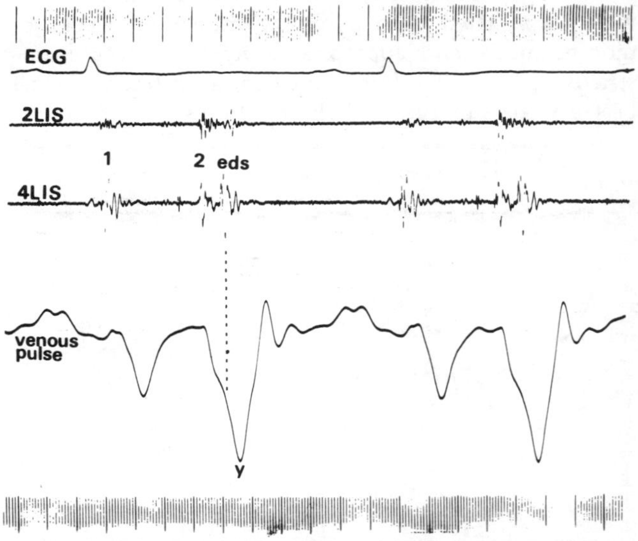

Figure 45.8. Phonocardiograms from the second left interspace (2LIS) and fourth left interspace (4LIS) with indirect jugular venous pressure recording in a patient with chronic constrictive pericarditis. There is a prominent extra sound in early diastole (EDS) that occurs just before the nadir of the deep Y descent in the venous pulse.

The electrocardiogram is usually abnormal in chronic constrictive pericarditis, but the abnormalities are nonspecific. The P waves are often low in amplitude and notched, and 20% to 30% of the patients have chronic atrial fibrillation. QRS voltage is usually average or in the low normal range, rarely abnormally low. There are usually borderline or diffusely abnormal T waves of nonspecific character.

The chest roentgenogram typically shows a normal heart size and is likely to be within normal limits unless pericardial calcification is visible or pleural effusion present (Figure 45.9). Evidence of pulmonary vascular congestion is usually not prominent, even though pulmonary venous pressure is substantially elevated.

Echocardiography is less useful in constrictive pericarditis than in pericardial effusion, but it shows one or more abnormalities in most instances.[102–104] Pericardial thickening usually can be recognized, but this finding does not in itself indicate constriction. Moreover, there is usually some abnormality of the motion of the ventricular septum during the cardiac cycle; the most characteristic abnormality is an increased prominence of the motion of the septum anteriorly in early diastole, followed by an equally prominent movement posteriorly, giving the appearance of a "notch" in the M-mode recording of the motion of the septum. Another feature that may be evident is completion early in diastole of posterior motion of the posterior wall of the left ventricle, with no further motion during the remainder of diastole; this reflects abnormal filling dynamics in which the great predominance of ventricular filling occurs in the initial portion of dias-

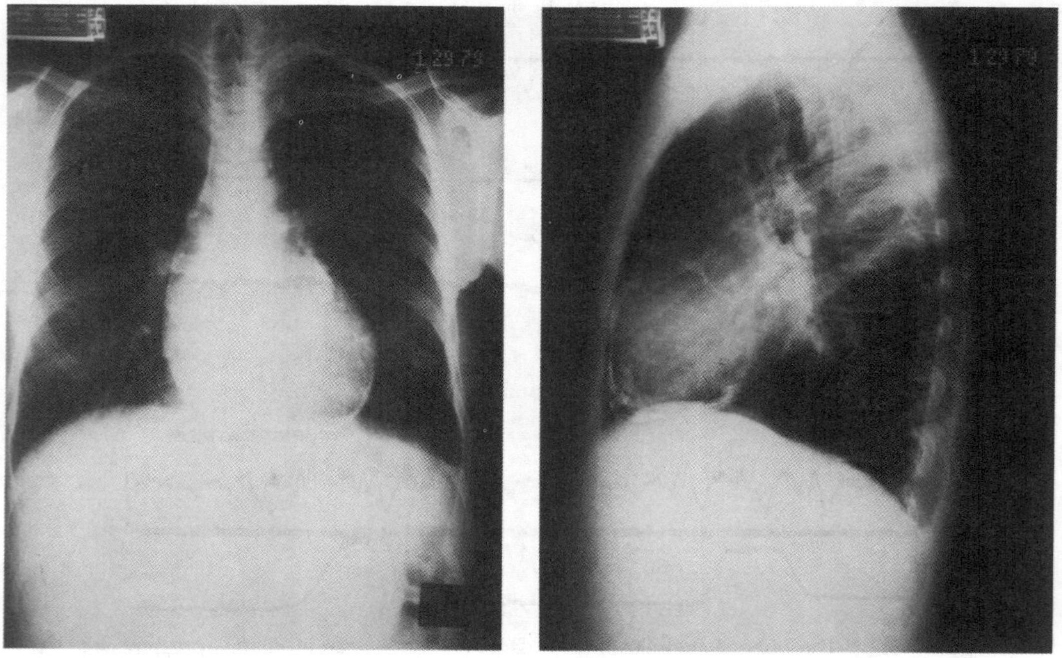

Figure 45.9. Frontal (*left*) and lateral (*right*) chest roentgenograms in a patient with chronic calcific constrictive pericarditis.

tole.[105,106] However, systolic motion is normal, which helps to distinguish constrictive pericarditis from various primary and secondary myocardial diseases.

Doppler ultrasonography has been used to demonstrate the abnormal patterns of blood flow within the heart that are characteristic of chronic constrictive pericarditis.[107] The increased rate of ventricular filling in early diastole, the abrupt cessation of filling, and the short filling period can all be demonstrated by this method.

Computed tomography and nuclear magnetic resonance imaging also demonstrate pericardial thickening and probably have a better resolution for this purpose than echocardiography. However, the pericardium may only be 5 mm thick in a nuclear magnetic resonance study in constrictive pericarditis.[108] Normally sized ventricles, with dilatation of the right atrium, superior and inferior venae cavae, and the hepatic veins, is also a characteristic finding.

Cardiac catheterization to support the diagnosis of constrictive pericarditis is usually advisable. The characteristic findings include elevation of diastolic pressure in all chambers of the heart to a similar level (Figure 45.10). The right ventricular pressure waveform shows a drop to near zero in initial diastole, followed by an abrupt increase to an elevated plateau of pressure during the remainder of diastole; this waveform has often been termed the square root sign. Because right ventricular systolic pressure is not elevated, diastolic pressure is usually equivalent to more than 25% of the systolic pressure; this ratio often serves to differentiate the right ventricular pressure waveform in constrictive pericarditis from that in ordinary congestive heart failure, in which a similar dip-plateau may be seen. In congestive heart failure the systolic pressure usually is elevated as well.

Angiography shows essentially normal chamber volume and contractility in patients with constrictive pericarditis. Therefore, major dilatation or hypocontractility of the left ventricle suggests an additional myocardial abnormality and should question the diagnosis of constrictive pericarditis.

SUBACUTE EFFUSIVE-CONSTRICTIVE PERICARDITIS

The picture of constrictive pericarditis just described is the classical picture of chronic constrictive pericarditis, with an illness that is a year or longer in duration. In modern medical practice, constrictive pericarditis is commonly associated with a history measuring weeks or months and is more appropriately termed subacute constrictive pericarditis. Important clinical differences exist between the subacute and chronic forms.

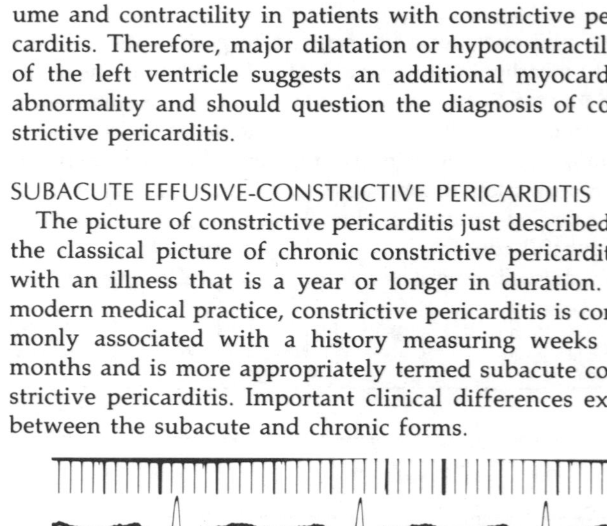

Figure 45.10. Right and left ventricular pressure recorded simultaneously in a patient with constrictive pericarditis. The pressures during diastole in the two ventricles are essentially the same.

Subacute constrictive pericarditis frequently follows a recent episode of active or even acute pericarditis, in which systemic symptoms, fever, and a pericardial friction rub have been present.[109] Pericardial effusion has also been present, and the effusion often persists as the constrictive pericarditis is developing. Thus, the patient is likely to be seen when there is pericardial effusion and simultaneous constriction of the heart by the visceral pericardium (epicardium).

Effusive-constrictive pericarditis has some features more like those of cardiac tamponade than those of chronic constrictive pericarditis. Paradoxical pulse is usually prominent. Pericardial effusion is present, and the cardiomediastinal silhouette is correspondingly enlarged on plain chest roentgenogram. The key to diagnosis of the associated constriction is the information obtained from hemodynamic monitoring during pericardiocentesis. If, by removal of fluid, the intrapericardial pressure is reduced to a normal level, while the central venous pressure decreases no more than 5 mm Hg and remains in excess of 12 mm Hg, associated visceral pericardial constriction is likely to be present. The diagnosis is strengthened if a complete hemodynamic study after fluid removal shows that the diastolic pressure remains essentially equilibrated in all cardiac chambers and that the pressure waveforms are characteristic of constrictive pericarditis.

The natural progression of effusive-constrictive pericarditis is to a more typical noneffusive constriction and ultimately a classical chronic constriction. The effusive-constrictive condition is a phase in the development of classical constriction. However, the constriction is often severe in the effusive-constrictive phase, and a well-developed constriction is not expected to be reversed by anything other than surgical therapy even in this active phase.

Effusive-constrictive pericarditis is most frequently idiopathic or radiation induced in developed countries, whereas infective pericarditis (particularly tuberculous) is most often responsible in less developed and in tropical countries. Rheumatoid arthritis and other connective tissue diseases, neoplasms, chronic renal failure, and other conditions account for a few cases. The natural history is similar for all etiologies except neoplasm, which usually involves advanced encasement of the heart by tumor if the effusive-constrictive syndrome is present.

The resemblance of many features of effusive-constrictive pericarditis to those of cardiac tamponade suggests that this type of constriction is different physiologically from classical chronic constrictive pericarditis.[110] Tamponade could be likened to a continuously acting elastic constriction, whereas classical chronic constriction could be likened to a rigid fixed-volume shell around the heart. The elastic constriction would compress the heart throughout the cardiac cycle, whereas the rigid shell would compress the heart only in mid to late diastole, as the diastolic filling would increase the size of the heart up to that of the rigid shell. Effusive-constrictive pericarditis and also subacute constriction in the absence of effusion act more like the elastic type of constriction. Paradoxical pulse, Kussmaul's sign, and pressure waveforms in the right ventricle and right atrium differ in the two prototypical mechanisms of constriction.

In 1977 Bush et al[110a] described a group of patients with occult constrictive pericardial disease in whom the baseline hemodynamics were normal, but typical pressure pulse morphology of constriction developed following rapid infusion of 1,000 ml of saline over a period of six to eight minutes. All were symptomatic with dramatic improvement after pericardiectomy.

SURGICAL TREATMENT OF CONSTRICTIVE PERICARDITIS

Pericardiectomy generally is the indicated treatment in constrictive pericarditis. Surgery may be unnecessary in some cases of borderline severity, particularly if the patient is elderly or has an illness likely to have a greater impact on the future clinical course than would the constrictive pericarditis.[111] Diuretics may be sufficient to control the symptoms satisfactorily in such mild cases. However, no treatment other than surgery should be expected to reverse the constrictive process itself.

The procedure of pericardiectomy takes several forms, depending on the nature of the pathologic changes. In chronic constrictive pericarditis without effusion, the parietal pericardium is adherent to the visceral pericardium; the two layers may separate along a natural cleavage plane, and "stripping" of the parietal pericardium along such a cleavage plane may adequately relieve the constriction. However, the possible constrictive role of the visceral pericardium must be evaluated, as it too may contribute to constriction and require removal. Stripping of the visceral pericardium is more difficult and requires meticulous sharp dissection. In effusive-constrictive pericarditis, the visceral pericardium clearly is constrictive and sharp dissection is the essence of the operation. Heimbecker et al[112] advocate a "waffling" procedure in which the adherent pericardium is incised into many small sectors without being extensively removed. Whatever the technique, the extent of pericardiectomy determines the success of the operation. Instances in which constrictive pericarditis appeared to recur after pericardiectomy were usually those in which the surgical procedure was not extensive enough, usually because it was limited to parietal pericardiectomy in the presence of a visceral constricting element.[113]

The operative risk in pericardiectomy for constrictive pericarditis is approximately 5%, the most important complications being intraoperative hemorrhage due to laceration of the chambers of the heart. The long-term results are excellent, however. Often, the decrease in central venous pressure does not occur immediately, but it requires several weeks to resolve, the reason for which is unknown.

INFECTIVE PERICARDITIS

VIRAL PERICARDITIS

The prevalence of viral infection as a cause of pericarditis is difficult to assess because of the uncertainty as to whether all or most cases of idiopathic pericarditis are due to viruses. Although viruses are often assumed to be the cause, particularly of idiopathic acute pericarditis, studies of neutralizing antibody titers and attempts to isolate viruses are unrevealing in most instances. It remains for future advances in virology to demonstrate whether viruses are in fact the etiologic agents in most of these cases. Until then, it is preferable to distinguish idiopathic acute pericarditis from definite cases of viral origin.

Documented acute viral infection has often occurred in outbreaks, usually of Coxsackie infection. ECHO viruses are also frequently responsible, and a wide variety of other systemic viral infections may include an element of acute pericarditis. Recently, fibrinous pericarditis with or without effusion has been reported in patients with acquired immune deficiency syndrome (AIDS), a disease caused by a retrovirus.[113a,113b] These cases of documented viral pericarditis have clinical features and a clinical course that are indistinguishable from those of idiopathic acute pericarditis.

TUBERCULOUS PERICARDITIS

Tuberculous pericarditis is still frequent in many areas of the world, although it is much less frequent in many developed countries than it was in the past.[114,115] The pathogenesis of tuberculous pericarditis is somewhat obscure, as it is associated with active pulmonary tuberculosis in a minority of cases. In the United States, it chiefly affects black males or immigrants from less developed countries.

Tuberculous pericarditis usually presents as active pericarditis, although frequently of a more subacute nature than is typical of idiopathic acute pericarditis. Pericardial effusion is usually present, and cardiac tamponade and constrictive pericarditis often develop early in the course. Results of the tuberculin skin test are typically positive, so that negative test results in the absence of a general anergy are usually effective in ruling out a tuberculous etiology in patients with active pericarditis.

The definitive diagnosis depends on demonstration of the tubercle bacillus, usually in cultures of pericardial fluid or pericardial tissue. Demonstration of acid-fast bacilli in smears of pericardial fluid can be done in some instances. Demonstration of caseating granulomas in histologic studies of pericardial tissue is also a useful method of diagnosis. The suspicion of tuberculous pericarditis is one clinical circumstance in which biopsy of the pericardium has a well-defined advantage in diagnosis over studies limited to the pericardial fluid.

Tuberculous pericarditis is effectively treated with antituberculous chemotherapy in most instances. Fowler[4] recommends isoniazide, 300 mg daily, and rifampin, 600 mg daily, with pyridoxine 50 mg daily, for nine months. The addition of corticosteroids has been advocated, but it has not been shown to be clearly beneficial and need not be used routinely. The most difficult decisions in treatment occur in patients in whom cardiac tamponade and constrictive pericarditis develop during the active infective phase. Tamponade may initially be managed with pericardiocentesis, but the likelihood of effusive-constrictive pericarditis is great. If constrictive pericarditis develops, it should be treated surgically for the same indications that would apply to idiopathic subacute constrictive pericarditis, even though the course of antituberculous chemotherapy is still in progress. Deaths in tuberculous pericarditis are most frequently due to the development of constriction during the active phase that was not recognized and operated on soon enough.

BACTERIAL PERICARDITIS

Although still relatively frequent in some tropical and less developed areas of the world, purulent bacterial pericarditis is now relatively rare.[116–118] The entity of pneumococcal pericarditis, developing as a complication of pneumococcal pneumonia, has shown a particularly great decline in incidence since the advent of antibiotics, but it still occurs occasionally.[119,120] Bacterial pericarditis is now seen most often as a complication of systemic infection, often as a complication of thoracic surgery or burns or as a complication of impaired immunity, in patients with neoplasm, chronic renal failure, organ transplants, or corticosteroid therapy.[121]

Any species of bacterium that is infective in man probably can cause bacterial pericarditis. The most frequent organisms in adults include the staphylococcus and various gram-negative strains.[122,123] In children, Hemophilus influenzae is particularly frequent.[124,125] Some of the less frequent infecting strains[126–134a] are listed in Table 45.2.

Bacterial pericarditis usually produces a severe clinical illness in which fever and leukocytosis are prominent. In addition, cardiac tamponade usually develops soon after the onset, and progression to constrictive pericarditis is likely to occur over the next several weeks. Diagnosis

Table 45.2. Some of the Less Common Etiologic Agents in Bacterial Pericarditis, With Representative References

Bacterial Species	Author and Reference
Leptospirosis	Douvier et al[126]
Listeria	Holoshitz et al[127]
Serratia	Khan[128]
Streptococcus anginosus-constellatus	Reder et al[129]
Legionella	Friedland et al[130]
Meningococcus	Rao et al[122]
Salmonella	Theler-Ballmer et al[131]
Tularemia	Meredith[132]
Beta-hemolytic streptococcus	Hanson and Engel[133]
Campylobacter	Lieber et al[134]
Brucella melitensis	Ugartemendia et al[134a]

depends on studies of the pericardial fluid, showing leukocyte counts in excess of 10,000 mm^3 with a predominance of neutrophils and a positive culture for the bacteria. The organisms can also be seen on Gram's stain of the pericardial fluid in most instances.

In addition to appropriate antibiotic therapy, bacterial pericarditis usually requires surgical drainage of the fluid. This procedure may be unnecessary in instances in which the fluid is more serous than purulent, but generally the initial pericardiocentesis that leads to the diagnosis should be followed by surgical pericardiostomy and large tube drainage. Left lateral thoracotomy is preferable to the subxiphoid approach in cases of bacterial infection, because progression to constriction has followed in some cases when only the subxiphoid pericardiostomy was used initially.

FUNGAL PERICARDITIS

Fungal pericarditis is rare and is usually a complication of impaired immunity or contaminated intravenous needles or catheters. Histoplasmosis is an exception, as it may occur as a primary infection in endemic areas.[135,136] Fungal organisms[137–142] that may cause pericarditis are listed in Table 45.3.

PARASITIC INFECTION

Most parasitic infections that are endemic in the tropical areas of the world may cause pericarditis. Those that have been reported[143–148] are listed in Table 45.4.

PERICARDITIS IN INFECTIVE ENDOCARDITIS

Infective endocarditis is associated with a significant incidence of pericardial effusion in both clinical studies using echocardiography and postmortem studies. The pericardial effusion is probably of infective origin, occurring as an extension of the valvular infection; the fluid is not grossly purulent, however, and cardiac tamponade and constriction are the exception rather than the rule. Thus, the clinical picture and course are more like those of idiopathic pericarditis than typical bacterial pericarditis.[149,150]

THE POSTCARDIOTOMY SYNDROME

A syndrome of acute pericarditis that occurs frequently after cardiac surgery has come to be known as the postcardiotomy syndrome.[151,152] It was originally noted in the early days of intracardiac surgery, when most operations were performed for mitral stenosis, and it was thought to represent recurrence of acute rheumatic fever. It subsequently became clear that the syndrome also followed surgery for nonrheumatic heart disease and that the mechanism did not relate to rheumatic fever. Its cause is unknown, but, in common with similar syndromes that may follow myocardial infarction and cardiac trauma with hemopericardium, it probably relates to the presence of blood in the pericardial space.

The postcardiotomy syndrome is characterized chiefly by the presence of pericardial type chest pain. There may also be a pericardial friction rub, pericardial effusion, pleural effusion or pneumonitis, fever, and an elevated erythrocyte sedimentation rate, but these features have a variable incidence. It occurs most frequently within the first few weeks after the operation, but it may occur up to 1 year later. Its natural history usually is similar to that of acute benign pericarditis, but it tends to be more persistent and more likely to return in a recurrent relapsing pattern than is typical acute idiopathic pericarditis. The pericardial effusion is occasionally large enough to lead to cardiac tamponade.[153] Although those patients in whom constrictive pericarditis develops after cardiac surgery have often had a prominent postpericardiotomy reaction, this is not always the case; the relation of the two syndromes is not clear. The mere presence of pericardial effusion does not indicate the presence of the postcardiotomy syndrome, as this is found in most patients in the early postoperative period.[154,155]

Treatment of the postcardiotomy syndrome is similar to that of acute idiopathic pericarditis. Although corticosteroids are often used, it is preferable to use aspirin or nonsteroidal antiinflammatory drugs first. The risk of enhancing the development of the relapsing pericarditis syndrome with corticosteroid dependency is perhaps greater in the postcardiotomy syndrome than in idiopathic acute pericarditis.

Table 45.3. Organisms That May Be Responsible for Fungal Infection of the Pericardium, With Representative References

Fungal Infection	Author and Reference
Actinomycosis	Ramsdale et al[137]
Aspergillosis	Rubin and Moellering[121]
Candidiasis	Eng et al[138]
Coccidioidomycosis	Chapman and Kaplan[139]
Cryptococcosis	Duvall and Carbone[140]
Histoplasmosis	Young et al[141]
Nocardiosis	Susens et al[142]

Table 45.4. Some Parasitic Diseases of the Pericardium, With Representative References

Parasitic Infection	Author and Reference
Amebiasis	Tyagi et al[143]
Dracunculosis	Kinare et al[144]
Filariasis	Charon and Sinha[145]
Hydatid disease	Cheng[146]
Toxoplasmosis	Sagrista-Sanleda et al[147]
Trypanosomiasis	Dupont et al[148]

PERICARDITIS AFTER MYOCARDIAL INFARCTION

Patients with acute myocardial infarction are subject to two types of acute pericarditis during the course of their recovery. The first type occurs within the first seven to ten days after myocardial infarction and represents fibrinous pericarditis in the area overlying the region of acute infarcted myocardium. The second type, also known as Dressler's syndrome, occurs after more than seven to ten days and most probably represents a hypersensitivity reaction, possibly mediated by autoantibodies to substances released from the infarcted myocardium, or possibly a reaction to the presence of blood in the pericardial space.[156] Both types of pericarditis are characterized by acute chest pain, often with a pericardial friction rub, pericardial effusion, and new electrocardiographic abnormalities characteristic of acute pericarditis. Both conditions also create the problem of differential diagnosis between pericarditis, recurrent ischemic cardiac pain or infarction, pulmonary embolism, and pneumonia.

Dressler's syndrome is particularly interesting because of its similarity to the postcardiotomy syndrome and to similar syndromes that occur after trauma to the heart and bleeding into the pericardial space. Bleeding into the pericardial space, with a subsequent hypersensitivity reaction, possibly unites these syndromes with a common mechanism. Dressler's syndrome has become less frequent in the United States in recent years, possibly because of the declining use of anticoagulant therapy in acute myocardial infarction.[157]

As with the postcardiotomy syndrome, the mere demonstration of pericardial effusion by echocardiography after acute myocardial infarction is a nonspecific finding, because it is present in up to one third of patients.[158,159]

Pericarditis after myocardial infarction is probably treated equally effectively with aspirin or nonsteroidal antiinflammatory drugs.[160] As with other forms of pericarditis without a specific cause, corticosteroids are probably more potent, but also more difficult to withdraw later.

A third type of pericarditis after myocardial infarction occurs when there is a secondary bacterial infection of the necrotic region of the myocardium.[161] This is a rare and usually fatal complication.

PERICARDITIS IN PATIENTS WITH NEOPLASMS

SECONDARY NEOPLASTIC PERICARDIAL DISEASE

Involvement of the pericardium by neoplastic disease is frequent and occurs with a great variety of neoplastic disorders.[162] It is more frequently found at autopsy than on clinical examination. The most frequent neoplasms are carcinoma of the lung or the breast. Leukemia and lymphoma are also relatively frequent.[163] The spread to the pericardium may occur by local extension (particularly with lung cancer) or by a lymphatic or hematogenous route (especially with breast cancer).

In most instances the patient in whom neoplastic disease of the pericardium develops has been known to have neoplastic disease. Occasionally, however, the development of pericardial effusion and cardiac tamponade marks the initial presentation of neoplastic disease, most likely lung cancer or other carcinoma such as that of the colon.[164,165]

Neoplastic disease of the pericardium is usually associated with tumor nodules seeded on the pericardial surfaces and leading to pericardial effusion. The effusion is usually relatively thin, even though serosanguineous. Neoplastic pericardial effusion is most likely to give rise to the phenomena of swinging heart and electrical alternans. Occasionally, however, there may be encasement of the heart by solid tumor, with the syndrome of effusive-constrictive pericarditis, or simply noneffusive constriction of the heart by solid tumor.[166]

The diagnosis of neoplastic disease of the pericardium is usually confirmed by cytologic studies of the pericardial fluid, which gives positive results in 80% to 90% of the cases of carcinoma of the lung or breast. Other conditions, particularly lymphoma and leukemia, have a lower percentage of positive cytologic results and are more likely to require histologic study of a pericardial biopsy to confirm the diagnosis. The level of the carcinoembryonic antigen is also elevated in the pericardial fluid in most patients with neoplastic pericardial disease. The percentage of patients with neoplastic pericardial disease who show either positive cytologic results or an elevated level of the carcinoembryonic antigen is probably greater than 90%.[167] Imaging studies of the pericardium, such as echocardiography or computed tomography, may show tumor masses as evidence of the neoplastic basis for pericardial effusion, but this is not often demonstrable.

The choice of treatment for neoplastic pericardial effusion with cardiac tamponade depends on several factors. This condition was once considered to be essentially terminal and unresponsive to treatment, but it is no longer the case. In breast carcinoma, particularly, there may be remissions of many months or longer, even after the neoplasm has spread to the pericardium. Pericardiocentesis is usually indicated as the first procedure, serving to confirm the positive cytologic results and to relieve tamponade initially. When a catheter is left in the pericardial space for drainage over several days after initial pericardiocentesis, there may be no recurrence for many weeks or months, if then. If there is early recurrence, pericardiocentesis may be repeated or surgical pericardiostomy may be resorted to in order to avoid the risk and inconvenience of repeated pericardiocenteses. Chemotherapy and radiation therapy may be helpful.[168]

Instillation of tetracycline into the pericardial space to promote adhesions and minimize recurrence of pericardial effusion is effective in some instances.[169] Instillation of antineoplastic chemotherapeutic agents into the pericardial space is also gaining more use.

PRIMARY NEOPLASM OF THE PERICARDIUM

In contrast with the frequency of secondary neoplastic involvement of the pericardium, primary pericardial neoplasm is rare. The most important primary tumor is mesothelioma of the pericardium.[170,171] It usually presents initially as pericardial effusion and tamponade of unknown origin, with biopsy of the pericardium eventually revealing the true nature of the problem. This tumor is highly malignant.

RADIATION-INDUCED PERICARDITIS

Radiotherapy to the thorax, delivered in doses of approximately 4,000 rads by the techniques commonly used in the 1960s, produced clinically significant pericardial disease in about 5% of patients.[172] Modern techniques, including the use of multiple ports and special shielding of the heart, have reduced this incidence, but the possibility of pericardial disease as a complication of radiotherapy still exists.[173] Because the pericardial disease may first appear years after radiotherapy has been completed, new cases continue to appear, usually in patients with Hodgkin's disease, as this condition is most likely to be associated with prolonged remission after mediastinal radiotherapy.[174]

Radiation-induced pericardial disease may take the

form of acute pericarditis, chronic pericardial effusion with or without tamponade, effusive-constrictive pericarditis, or chronic noneffusive constrictive pericarditis.[172] The disease may progress from one of these forms to another. It most frequently develops during the first year after radiotherapy, but it can occur as long as 25 years later.

The conclusion that pericardial disease is radiation induced is an inference that rests on excluding a neoplastic cause. In general, if the patient does not demonstrate active neoplastic disease anywhere in the body and if cytologic study of the pericardial fluid gives negative results, particularly if the original diagnosis was Hodgkin's disease and no recurrence was noted within the previous 5 years, the pericardial disease is likely to be radiation induced and is not due to recurrent neoplasm.[175]

Patients with radiation-induced pericardial disease can be managed in a manner similar to those with idiopathic pericarditis with the same clinical features. The syndrome of effusive-constrictive pericarditis is particularly frequent in radiation-induced cases; therefore, when a patient with previous radiotherapy presents with pericardial effusion and elevated venous pressure, it is particularly important to perform hemodynamic monitoring in association with pericardiocentesis to detect associated visceral constriction.

Pericardiectomy for radiation-induced constrictive pericarditis gives results that are generally satisfactory and comparable to those in patients with the idiopathic form. However, some patients have associated myocardial fibrosis also secondary to radiation; these patients are likely to have unsatisfactory results of pericardiectomy for this reason. Endomyocardial biopsy may identify such myocardial fibrosis preoperatively; however, if the evidence of constriction is strong, and particularly if the right and left ventricles are not dilated, pericardiectomy is still indicated.

DRUG-INDUCED PERICARDITIS

Pericarditis may be induced by a variety of drugs. These adverse reactions may be grouped into those associated with the systemic lupus erythematosus-like syndrome, the syndromes of myopericarditis associated with antineoplastic chemotherapy, and a miscellaneous group of drugs that appear to cause pericardial effusion.[176,177] Some of the more frequently reported drug-induced forms of pericardial disease[96,178–185] are listed in Table 45.5.

PERICARDITIS IN RHEUMATIC DISEASES

Pericarditis is a relatively frequent feature in all rheumatic diseases, a phenomenon that indicates the importance of the pericardium as an arena for clinically evident hypersensitivity immunologic reactions in the body.[186] Even acute rheumatic fever, although rare in the United States and other developed countries, is still a cause of acute pericarditis and occasionally cardiac tamponade.[187]

Systemic lupus erythematosus is eventually associated with pericarditis in a high percentage of cases, usually in the form of acute pericarditis. This complication usually responds well to corticosteroid therapy. Cardiac tamponade occurs in a few instances and constrictive pericarditis develops rarely. The syndrome of mixed connective tissue disease is similar to classical systemic lupus erythematosus with regard to the complication of pericarditis.[188]

Rheumatoid arthritis has increasingly been recognized as a cause of pericardial disease, particularly chronic pericardial effusion and effusive-constrictive pericarditis. As many as one third of the patients with rheumatoid arthritis have evidence of pericarditis at postmortem examination, usually fibrous adhesive pericarditis.[189,190] Rheumatoid nodules are occasionally present, but the pathologic abnormalities are otherwise nonspecific. Pericardiectomy gives satisfactory results in constrictive pericarditis of rheumatoid origin. Further experience is needed to determine whether the intrapericardial instillation of corticosteroids is useful in these cases.

PERICARDITIS IN UREMIA AND DIALYSIS

True uremic pericarditis, known as a finding associated with the terminal few weeks of renal failure, is now an indication for dialysis. It is seen less often, because patients usually begin dialysis before the onset of this complication. A new form of pericarditis has taken its place, the pericarditis that occurs in patients who are on chronic dialysis.

The pathogenesis of pericarditis in patients on dialysis is unclear, because it occurs even when dialysis is effective. It may represent viral infection in a chronically ill

Table 45.5. Drugs That May Cause Pericarditis and Pericardial Effusion, With Representative References

Drug Actions	Author and Reference
Systemic lupus erythematosus syndrome	
Procainamide	Browning et al[96]
Hydralazine	Carey et al[178]
Isoniazide	Greenberg and Lutcher[179]
Antineoplastic chemotherapy	
Bleomycin	Durkin et al[180]
Cyclophosphamide	Steinherz et al[181]
Cytarabine	Vaickus and Letendre[182]
Anthracyclines	Bristow et al[183]
Miscellaneous	
Captopril	Zatuchni[184]
Methysergide	Harbin et al[94]
Minoxidil	Evans and Tucker[185]

patient with impaired immune mechanism. Because the associated pericardial effusion is usually serosanguineous, another possibility is that the anticoagulation associated with dialysis leads to bleeding into the pericardial space. It has been postulated that certain large molecules normally excreted by the kidney are not effectively dialyzed and are the cause of pericarditis. Whatever the mechanism, it is important to distinguish dialysis pericarditis from the classical uremic pericarditis, because the latter responds readily to dialysis, whereas the former may or may not respond to more intensive dialysis.[191,192]

Dialysis pericarditis, like other forms of acute pericarditis, is clinically characterized chiefly by chest pain, although chest pain is less frequent than in cases of other etiologies. Friction rubs are often present, and there is usually some pericardial effusion. The electrocardiogram is less likely to show typical ST-segment elevation than it is in acute pericarditis of other origins. Paroxysmal atrial tachyarrhythmias are the most frequently encountered arrhythmias.[192a]

The clinical presentation of dialysis pericarditis, if not that of chest pain and pericardial friction rub, is often that of hemodynamic complications such as increasing congestive heart failure or hypotension precipitated by dialysis sessions. Cardiac tamponade presents somewhat differently in these patients, because of their frequent concomitant hypertension, left ventricular hypertrophy, and chronic congestive heart failure. Paradoxical pulse is less frequent, probably because the hypertrophied left ventricle with elevated filling pressures in the left-sided chambers is less easily compressed than is the right ventricle. In the presence of dialysis pericarditis, pericardial effusion, and congestive heart failure with elevated central venous pressure, it is not unusual to find in a hemodynamic study that congestive heart failure with fluid overload is the predominant problem, whereas the pericardial effusion is under only mildly increased pressure, if any. Therefore, a complete hemodynamic study in association with pericardiocentesis is particularly important in dialysis patients.

Aspirin and nonsteroidal antiinflammatory drugs are useful in controlling the symptoms related to active pericarditis. Instillation of triamcinolone, a nonabsorbable corticosteroid, into the pericardial space has been advocated, but it is probably rarely necessary to control the process adequately.[193] The dialysis technique may be switched to peritoneal dialysis rather than hemodialysis, or regional heparinization may be substituted for systemic heparin.

Tamponade due to dialysis pericarditis can usually be controlled by pericardiocentesis, or by subxiphoid pericardiostomy if preferred. Although pericardiectomy is used often in some centers, it can probably be avoided in most instances by the use of the simpler drainage procedures.[194,195] Constrictive pericarditis can occur as a complication of dialysis pericarditis, but it is rare.[99]

REFERENCES

1. Shabetai R: *The Pericardium*. New York, Grune & Stratton, 1981.
2. Reddy PS, Leon DF, Shaver JA (eds): *Pericardial Disease*. New York, Raven Press, 1982.
3. Spodick DH: The normal and diseased pericardium: Current concepts of pericardial physiology, diagnosis and treatment. *J Am Coll Cardiol* 1983; 1:240–251.
4. Fowler NO: *The Pericardium in Health and Disease*. Mount Kisco, New York, Futura Publishing Co, 1985.
5. Ishihara T, Ferrans VJ, Jones M, Boyce SW, Kawanami O, Roberts WC: Histologic and ultrastructural features of normal human parietal pericardium. *Am J Cardiol* 1980; 46:744–753.
6. Wiegner AW, Bing OHL: Mechanical and structural correlates of canine pericardium. With scanning electron microscopy by Borg TK and Caulfield JB. *Circ Res* 1981; 49:807–814.
7. Leguerrier A, Milon J, Marcade E, Rioux C, Logeais Y, Lanchou G: Anatomical basis for the treatment of agenesis of the left pericardium. Three case reports. *Anat Clin* 1982; 3:309–312.
8. Jones JW, McManus BM: Fatal cardiac strangulation by congenital partial pericardial defect. *Am Heart J* 1984; 107:183–185.
9. Nasser WK: Congenital Defects of the Pericardium, in Fowler NO (ed): *The Pericardium in Health and Disease*. Mount Kisco, New York, Futura Publishing Co, 1985, p 51.
10. Nicolosi GL, Borgioni L, Alberti E, Burelli C, Maffesanti M, Marino P, Slavich G, Zanuttini D: M-mode and two-dimensional echocardiography in congenital absence of the pericardium. *Chest* 1982; 81:610–613.
11. Ruys F, Paulus W, Stevens C, Brutsaert D: Expansion of the left atrial appendage is a distinctive cross-sectional echocardiographic feature of congenital defect of the pericardium. *Eur Heart J* 1983; 4:738–741.
12. Hager J, Hammerer I, Egender G: Zur diagnostik angeborener pleuroperikardialer defekte. *ROFO* 1984; 141:172–175.
12a. Schiavone WA, O'Donnell JK: Congenital absence of the left portion of parietal pericardium demonstrated by nuclear magnetic resonance imaging. *Am J Cardiol* 1985; 55:1439–1440.
13. Kron IL, Cox PM Jr: Cardiac injury after chest trauma. *Crit Care Med* 1983; 11:524–526.
14. Roebuck EJ, Minford J: Traumatic rupture of the pericardium with herniation of the heart. *Brit J Radiol* 1983; 56:585–588.
15. Glass JD, McQuillen EN, Hardin NJ: Iatrogenic cardiac herniation: post mortem case. *J Trauma* 1984; 24:632–633.
16. Minocha GK, Falicov RE, Nijensohn E: Partial right-sided congenital pericardial defect with herniation of right atrium and right ventricle. *Chest* 1979; 76:484–486.
17. Casey BM, Nieman H, Gallagher T, DuBois J, Kane L: Syndrome of mesodermal defects involving the abdominal wall, diaphragm, sternum, heart and pericardium. *Br J Radiol* 1975; 48:52–54.
18. Patel BK, Markivee CR, George EA: Pericardial cyst simulating intracardiac mass. *Am J Roentgenol* 1983; 141:292–294.
19. Pezzano A, Belloni A, Faletra F, Binaghi G, Colli A, Rovelli F: Value of two-dimensional echocardiography in the diagnosis of pericardial cysts. *Eur Heart J* 1983; 4:238–246.
20. Shabetai R, Mangiardi L, Bhargava V, Ross J Jr, Higgins CB: The pericardium and cardiac function. *Prog Cardiovasc Dis* 1979; 22:107–134.
21. Dunn M, Rinkberger RL: Clinical aspects of acute pericarditis. *Cardiovasc Clin* 1976; 7(3):131–147.
22. Jin YR, Qian YJ: Etiological analysis of 100 cases of pericarditis. *Chin J Int Med* 1983; 22:131–133.
23. Spodick DH: Pericardial rub. Prospective, multiple observer investigation of pericardial friction in 100 patients. *Am J Cardiol* 1975; 35:357–362.
24. Markiewicz W, Brik A, Brook G, Edoute Y, Monakier I, Markiewicz Y: Pericardial rub in pericardial effusion: lack of correlation with amount of fluid. *Chest* 1980; 77:643–646.
25. Ginzton LE, Laks MM: The differential diagnosis of acute pericarditis from the normal variant: New electrocardiographic criteria. *Circulation* 1982; 65:1004–1009.
26. Wanner WR, Schaal SF, Bashore TM, Norton VJ, Lewis RP, Fulkerson PK: Repolarization variant vs acute pericarditis. A prospective electrocardiographic and echocardiographic evaluation. *Chest* 1983; 83:180–184.
27. Spodick DH: Frequency of arrhythmias in acute pericarditis determined by Holter monitoring. *Am J Card* 1984; 53:842–845.
28. Tiefenbrunn AJ, Roberts R: Elevation of plasma MB creatine kinase and the development of new Q waves in association with pericarditis. *Chest* 1980; 77:438–440.
29. Marmor A, Grenadir E, Keidar A, Edward S, Palant A: The MB fraction of creatine phosphokinase: An indicator of myocardial involvement in acute pericarditis. *Arch Int Med* 1979; 139:819–820.
29a. Cheng TO: Don't overlook pericarditis. *Consultant* 1985; 25:17.
30. Sherry DD, Patterson MWH, Petty RE: The use of indomethacin in the treatment of pericarditis in childhood. *J Pediatr* 1982; 100:995–998.

31. Hancock EW: Management of pericardial disease. *Mod Conc Cardiovasc Dis* 1979; 48:1–6.
32. Horn F, Eichorn P, Wuethrich A, Jenni R, Turina M, Krayenbuhl HP: Diagnosis, etiology and clinical course of acute and chronic pericarditis. *Schweiz Med Wochenshr* 1983; 113:1766–1768.
33. Yang XS, Huang DX: Etiological analysis of 234 autopsied cases with pericardial effusion. *Chin J Int Med* 1983; 22:138–140.
34. Riba AL, Morganroth J: Unsuspected substantial pericardial effusions detected by echocardiography. *JAMA* 1976; 236:2623–2625.
35. Halphen C, Haiat R: Decouverte echocardiographique d'epanchements pericardiques muets au cours de la grossesse normale. *Arch Mal Coeur* 1983; 76:71–76.
36. Brawley RK, Vasko JS, Morrow AG: Cholesterol pericarditis. Considerations of its pathogenesis and treatment. *Am J Med* 1966; 41:235–248.
37. Rose DM, Colvin SB, Danilowicz D, Isom OW: Cardiac tamponade secondary to chylopericardium following cardiac surgery: Case report and review of the literature. *Ann Thor Surg* 1982; 34:333–336.
38. Schwartz C, Lesbre JP, Kalisa A, Jarry G, Fardellone P, Funk F, Simony J: Chylopericardium, chylopneumothorax and cystic lymphangioma. Report on one case and review of the literature. *Poumon-Coeur* 1983; 39:209–213.
39. Chan RMT, Dodek A: Chylopericardium in a drug addict. *Arch Int Med* 1984; 144:1857–1868.
40. Damtew B, Lewandowski B: Hydrothorax, hydromediastinum and pericardial effusion: a complication of intravenous alimentation. *Can Med Assoc J* 1984; 130:1573–1574.
41. Maschke SP, Rogove HJ: Cardiac tamponade associated with a multilumen central venous catheter. *Crit Care Med* 1984; 12:611–613.
42. Cummings RG, Wesly RLR, Adams DH, Lowe JE: Pneumopericardium resulting in cardiac tamponade. *Ann Thor Surg* 1984; 37:511–518.
43. Casale PN, Devereux RB, Kligfield P, Eisenberg RR, Phillips MC: Pericardial effusion: relation of clinical echocardiographic and electrocardiographic findings. *J Electrocardiol* 1984; 17:115–122.
44. Carsky EW, Mauceri RA, Azimi F: The epicardial fat pad sign: Analysis of frontal and lateral chest radiographs in patients with pericardial effusion. *Radiology* 1980; 137:303–308.
45. Chandraratna PA: Echocardiographic evaluation of pericardial disease. *JAMA* 1983; 250:2677–2680.
46. Engel PJ: Echocardiographic findings in pericardial disease, in Fowler NO (ed): *The Pericardium in Health and Disease*, Mt Kisco, New York, Futura Publishing Co, 1985, pp 99–151.
47. Parameswaran R, Goldberg H: Echocardiographic quantitation of pericardial effusion. *Chest* 1983; 83:767–770.
48. Rifkin RD, Isner JM, Carter BL, Bankoff MS: Combined posteroanterior subpericardial fat simulating the echocardiographic diagnosis of pericardial effusion. *J Am Coll Card* 1984; 3:1333–1339.
49. Isner JM, Carter BL, Bankoff MS, Konstam MA, Salem DN: Computed tomography in the diagnosis of pericardial heart disease. *Ann Intern Med* 1982; 97:473–479.
50. Brundage BH, Rich S, Spigos D: Computed tomography of the heart and great vessels: present and future. *Ann Int Med* 1984; 101:801–809.
51. Gouliamis A, Andreou J, Steriotis J, Kalovidouris A, Vlahos L, Papavassiliou C: Detection of pericardial heart disease by computed tomography. *Clin Radiol* 1984; 35:397–400.
52. Stark DD, Higgins CB, Lanzer P, Lipton MJ, Schiller N, Crooks LE, Botvinick EB, Kaufman L: Magnetic resonance imaging of the pericardium: normal and pathologic findings. *Radiology* 1984; 150:469–474.
53. Yeh SH, Liu RS, Liu OK: Pertechnetate (Tc-99m) sequential scintiphotography—Aid in differentiating exudative from transudative pericardial effusions: Concise communication. *J Nucl Med* 1982; 23:386–390.
54. Lin DS, Tipton RE: Ga-67 cardiac uptake. *Clin Nuc Med* 1983; 8:603–604.
55. Robertson JM, Mulder DM: Pericardiectomy: A changing scene. *Am J Surg* 1984; 148:86–92.
56. Guberman BA, Fowler NO, Engel PJ, Gueron M, Allen JM: Cardiac tamponade in medical patients. *Circulation* 1981; 64:633–640.
57. Brodarick S, Paine R, Higa E, Carmichael KA: Pericardial tamponade, a new complication of amyloid heart disease. *Am J Med* 1982; 73:133–135.
58. King TE Jr, Stelzner TJ, Sahn SA: Cardiac tamponade complicating the postpericardiotomy syndrome. *Chest* 1983; 83:500–503.
59. Antman EM, Cargill V, Grossman W: Low-pressure cardiac tamponade. *Ann Int Med* 1979; 91:403–406.
60. Katz LN, Gauchat HW: Observations on pulsus paradoxus (with special reference to pericardial effusions). *Arch Int Med* 1924; 33:371–393.
61. Dornhorst AC, Howard P, Leathart GL: Pulsus paradoxus. *Lancet* 1952; 1:746–748.
62. Manyari DE, Kostuk WJ, Purves P: Effect of pericardiocentesis on right and left ventricular function and volumes in pericardial effusion. *Am J Card* 1983; 52:159–162.
63. Spodick DH, Paladino D, Flessas AP: Respiratory effects on systolic time intervals during pericardial effusion. *Am J Card* 1983; 51:1033–1035.
64. Wayne VS, Bishop RL, Spodick DH: Dynamic effects of pericardial effusion without tamponade. Respiratory responses in the absence of pulsus paradoxus. *Br Heart J* 1984; 51:202–204.
65. Rosoff M, Cohen MV, Grose R, Greenberg MA: Clinical and hemodynamic correlation in patients with pericardial effusion and swinging heart by echocardiography. *J Clin Ultrasound* 1983; 11:477–483.
66. Kronzon I, Cohen ML, Winer HE: Diastolic atrial compression: A sensitive echocardiographic sign of cardiac tamponade. *J Am Coll Card* 1983; 2:770–775.
67. Singh S, Wann LS, Schuchard GH, Klopfenstein HS, Leimgruber PP, Keelan MH Jr, Brooks HL: Right ventricular and right atrial collapse in patients with cardiac tamponade — a combined echocardiographic and hemodynamic study. *Circulation* 1984; 70:966–976.
67a. Klopfenstein HS, Schuchard GH, Wann LS, Palmer TE, Hartz AJ, Gross CM, Singh S, Brooks HL: The relative merits of pulsus paradoxus and right ventricular diastolic collapse in the early detection of cardiac tamponade: an experimental echocardiographic study. *Circulation* 1985; 71:829–833.
68. Krikorian JG, Hancock EW: Pericardiocentesis. *Am J Med* 1978; 65:808–814.
69. Permanyer-Miralda G, Sagrista-Sauleda J, Soler-Soler J: Are "diagnostic" pericardiocentesis and pericardial biopsy warranted in the management of acute pericardial disease? *Circulation* 1984; 70:II-103 (abstract).
70. Callaham M: Pericardiocentesis in traumatic and nontraumatic cardiac tamponade. *Ann Emerg Med* 1984; 13:924–945.
71. Dubourg O, Ferrier A, Gueret P, Farcot JC, Terdjman M, Rocha P, Bourdarias JP: Bidimensional contrast echocardiography in drainage of pericardial blood effusions with tamponade. *Presse Med* 1983; 12:2225–2228.
72. Callahan JA, Seward JB, Nishimura RA, Miller FA Jr, Reeder GS, Shub C, Callahan MJ, Schattenberg TT, Tajik AJ: Two-dimensional echocardiographically guided pericardiocentesis: experience in 117 consecutive patients. *Am J Cardiol* 1985; 55:476–479.
73. Kindig JR, Goodman MR: Clinical utility of pericardial fluid pH determination. *Am J Med* 1983; 75:1077–1079.
73a. Cheng TO: Ventricle or pericardial space. *Ann Intern Med* 1973; 78:461.
74. Alcan KE, Zabetakis PM, Marino ND, Franzone AJ, Michelis MF, Bruno MS: Management of acute cardiac tamponade by subxiphoid pericardiotomy. *JAMA* 1982; 247:1143–1148.
75. Levin BH, Aaron BL: The subxiphoid pericardial window. *Surg Gynecol Obstet* 1982; 155:804–806.
76. Vandyke WH Jr, Cure J, Chakko CS, Gheorghiade M: Pulmonary edema after pericardiocentesis for cardiac tamponade. *New Eng J Med* 1983; 309:595–596.
77. Timmis AD, Daly K, Monaghan M, Jewitt DE: Pericardiocentesis in myocarditis: the protective role of the pericardium in severe heart failure. *Brit Med J* 1983; 287:1348.
78. Laurent JM, Lablanche JM, Prat A, Pladys A, Ducloux G: Diastolic restriction caused by encysted hemopericardium a year after coronary bypass. *Arch Mal Coeur* 1984; 77:343–348.
79. Gore JM, Haffajee CI, Love JC, Dalen JE: Isolated right ventricular tamponade after pericarditis from acute myocardial infarction. *Am J Cardiol* 1984; 53:372–373.
80. Upward JW, Daly K, Jackson G: Pericardial abscess causing right ventricular outflow tract obstruction. Successful surgical correction. *Br Heart J* 1983; 49:507–509.
81. Fowler NO, Gabel M: The hemodynamic efforts of cardiac tamponade: mainly the result of atrial, not ventricular, compression. *Circulation* 1985; 71:154–157.
82. Chen HZ: Pay attention to the pericardial diseases. *Chin J Int Med* 1983; 22:129–130.
83. Blake S, Bonar S, O'Neill H, Hanly P, Drury I, Flanagan M, Garrett J: Aetiology of chronic constrictive pericarditis. *Br Heart J* 1983; 50:273–276.
84. Mizuno A, Asano K: Surgery for chronic pericarditis—thirty years' experience. *Jpn Circ J* 1983; 47:1331–1333.
85. Hu LX, Shi XH, Xu YQ, Ni YF, Zheng GS, Lan ZR: Pericardial constriction. Clinical analysis of 209 cases. *Chin J Int Med* 1983; 22:134–137.
86. Zhou GW, Wang ZS, Lin CX: Constrictive pericarditis: A clinicopathologic analysis of 55 cases. *Chin J Int Med* 1983; 22:144–148.
86a. Kabbani SS, Bashour T, Ellertson DG, Geiger J, Hanna ES, Cheng TO: Constrictive pericarditis following myocardial revascularization: a possible cause of graft occlusion. *Am Heart J* 1985; 110:493–495.
87. Kutcher MA, King SB III, Alimurung BN, Craver JM, Logue RB: Constrictive pericarditis as a complication of cardiac surgery. Recognition of an entity. *Am J Cardiol* 1982; 50:742–748.
88. Boreaux JL, Lemaitre J: Constrictive pericarditis following heart surgery: apropos of 2 cases. *Acta Clin Belg* 1983; 38:236–241.
89. Ribeiro P, Sapsford R, Evans T, Parcharidis G, Oakley C: Constrictive

pericarditis as a complication of coronary artery bypass surgery. *Br Heart J* 1984; 51:205–210.
90. Bensaid J, Delhoume B, Virot P, Doumeix JJ: A new cause of constrictive pericarditis, cardiac surgery (letter). *Press Med* 1984; 13:1748.
91. Fraker TD, Walsh TE, Morgan RJ, Kim K: Constrictive pericarditis late after the Beck operation. *Am J Card* 1984; 54:931.
92. Pearl WR: Constrictive pericarditis in adolescents: a review. *Military Med* 1983; 148:600–602.
93. Virmani R, Chun PKC, Dunn BE, Hartmen D, McAllister HA: Eosinophilic constrictive pericarditis. *Am Heart J* 1984; 107:803–807.
94. Harbin AD, Gerson MC, O'Connell JB: Simulation of acute myopericarditis by constrictive pericardial disease with endomyocardial fibrosis due to methysergide therapy. *J Am Coll Card* 1984; 4:196–199.
95. Hanley PC, Shub C, Lie JT: Constrictive pericarditis associated with combined idiopathic retroperitoneal and mediastinal fibrosis. *Mayo Clin Proc* 1984; 59:300–304.
96. Browning CA, Bishop RL, Heilpern RJ, Singh JB, Spodick DH: Accelerated constrictive pericarditis in procainamide-induced systemic lupus erythematosus. *Am J Cardiol* 1984; 53:376–377.
97. Perheentupa J, Autio S, Leisti S, Raitta C, Tuuteri L: Mulibrey nanism, an autosomal recessive syndrome with pericardial constriction. *Lancet* 1973; 2:351–355.
98. Garrett J, O'Neill H, Blake S: Constrictive pericarditis associated with sarcoidosis. *Am Heart J* 1984; 107:394.
99. Ptacin MJ: Uremic constrictive pericarditis: Case report. *Military Med* 1983; 148:603–605.
100. Haiat R: Post-myocardial infarction constrictive pericarditis (letter). *Am Heart J* 1981; 101:358.
101. Albers WH, Hugenholtz PG, Nadas AS: Constrictive pericarditis and atrial septal defect, secundum type. *Am J Card* 1969; 23:850–857.
102. Chandraratna PAN, Aronow WS, Imaizumi T: Role of echocardiography in detecting the anatomic and physiologic abnormalities of constrictive pericarditis. *Am J Med Sci* 1982; 283:141–146.
103. Tei C, Child JS, Tanaka H, Shah PM: Atrial systolic notch on the interventricular septal echogram: An echocardiographic sign of constrictive pericarditis. *J Am Coll Card* 1983; 1:907–912.
104. Pandian NG, Skorton DJ, Kieso RA, Kerber RE: Diagnosis of constrictive pericarditis by two-dimensional echocardiography: Studies in a new experimental model and in patients. *J Am Coll Card* 1984; 4:1164–1173.
105. M'Zah N, Dobrinski G, Evans JI, Canny M, Chollet D, Bejean-Lebuissan A, Grosgogeat Y: Differential diagnosis between constrictive pericarditis and cardiac amyloidosis by computerized M-mode echocardiography. *Arch Mal Coeur* 1984; 77:625–632.
106. Janos GG, Arjunan K, Meyer RA, Engel P, Kaplan S: Differentiation of constrictive pericarditis and restrictive cardiomyopathy using digitized echocardiography. *J Am Coll Card* 1983; 1:541–549.
107. Agatston AS, Rao A, Price RJ, Kinney EL: Diagnosis of constrictive pericarditis by pulsed Doppler echocardiography. *Am J Card* 1984; 54:929–930.
108. Soulen RL, Stark DD, Higgins CB: Magnetic resonance imaging of constrictive pericardial disease. *Am J Card* 1985; 55:480–484.
109. Hancock EW: Subacute effusive-constrictive pericarditis. *Circulation* 1971; 43:183–192.
110. Hancock EW: On the elastic and rigid forms of constrictive pericarditis. *Am Heart J* 1980; 100:917–923.
110a. Bush CA, Stang JM, Wooley CF, Kilman JW: Occult constrictive pericardial disease. Diagnosis by rapid volume expansion and correction by pericardiectomy. *Circulation* 1977; 56:924–930.
111. Bashour TT, Kabbani SS, Jokhadar M, Hanna ES, Cheng TO: Constrictive pericarditis: Medical versus surgical treatment. *Cardiovasc Rev & Rep* 1983; 4:1337–1340.
112. Heimbecker RO, Smith D, Shimizu S, Kestle J: Surgical technique for the management of constrictive epicarditis complicating constrictive pericarditis (the waffle procedure). *Ann Thor Surg* 1983; 36:605–606.
113. Pick RA, Joswig BC, Bloor CM: Recurrent cardiac constriction after pericardiectomy. *Arch Int Med* 1984; 144:2061–2063.
113a. Cammarosano C, Lewis W: Cardiac lesions in acquired immune deficiency syndrome (AIDS). *J Am Coll Cardiol* 1985; 5:703–706.
113b. Fink L: Cardiac manifestations in the acquired immune deficiency syndrome. *IM* 1985; 6(8):47–59.
114. Strang JIG: Tuberculous pericarditis in Transkei. *Clin Card* 1984; 7:667–670.
115. Faruqui AMA: Heart disease in South Asia: Experience in Pakistan, in Hurst JW (ed): *Clinical Essays on the Heart*, Vol 1. New York, McGraw-Hill, 1983, pp 313–338.
116. Jaiyesimi F, Abioye AA, Antia AU: Infective pericarditis in Nigerian children. *Arch Dis Child* 1979; 54:384–390.
117. Corachan M, Poore P, Hadley GP, Tanner A: Purulent pericarditis in Papua New Guinea: Report on 12 cases and review of the literature in a tropical environment. *Trans R Soc Trop Med Hyg* 1983; 77:341–343.
118. Lawrie J: Tropical Pericarditis (letter). *Trans R Soc Trop Med Hyg* 1983; 77:880–881.
119. Klacsmann PG, Bulkley BH, Hutchins GM: The changed spectrum of purulent pericarditis. An 86 year autopsy experience in 200 patients. *Am J Med* 1977; 63:666–673.
120. Laaban JP, d'Orbcastel OR, Prudent J, de Fenoyl O, Rochemaure J: Primary pneumococcal pericarditis complicated by acute constriction. *Intensive Care Med* 1984; 10:155–156.
121. Rubin RH, Moellering RC Jr: Clinical, microbiologic and therapeutic aspects of purulent pericarditis. *Am J Med* 1975; 59:68–78.
122. Rao VS, Rajashekaraiah KR, Rice T, Riaz M, Towne W, Kallick CA: Primary meningococcal pericarditis. *South Med J* 1980; 73:1276–1278.
123. Graham BS, Reiss TF, Gregory DW: Pericarditis associated with Hemophilus influenzae Type B pneumonia and bacteremia in two adults. *Chest* 1983; 84:48–50.
124. Morgan RJ, Stephenson LW, Woolf PK, Edie RN, Edmunds LH Jr: Surgical treatment of purulent pericarditis in children. *J Thor Cardiovasc Surg* 1983; 85:527–531.
125. Fyfe DA, Hagler DJ, Puga FJ, Driscoll DJ: Clinical and therapeutic aspects of Haemophilus influenzae pericarditis in pediatric patients. *Mayo Clin Proc* 1984; 59:415–422.
126. Douvier JJ, Ledain L, Besse P: Leptospirosis with isolated cardiac manifestations. *Sem Hosp Paris* 1984; 60:701–702.
127. Holoshitz J, Schneider M, Yaretzky A, Bernheim J, Klajman A: Listeria monocytogenes pericarditis in a chronically hemodialyzed patient. *Am J Med Sci* 1984; 288:34–37.
128. Khan MY: Subacute constrictive pericarditis from Seratia marcescens bacteremia. *Hum Pathol* 1983; 14:1089–1091.
129. Reder RF, Raucher H, Cesa M, Mindich BP: Purulent pericarditis caused by Streptococcus anginosus - constellatus. *Mt. Sinai J Med* 1984; 51:295–297.
130. Friedland L, Snydman DR, Weingarden AS, Hedges JR III, Brown R, Busky M: Ocular and pericardial involvement in Legionnaires' disease. *Am J Med* 1984; 77:1105–1107.
131. Theler-Ballmer D, Noseda G, Reiner M, Keller H: Pericarditis and myocarditis in Salmonellosis. *Schweiz Med Wschr* 1980: 110:1394–1401.
132. Meredith HC Jr: Tularemic pericarditis: A report of two cases including one of constrictive pericarditis. *Ann Int Med* 1950; 32:688–699.
133. Hanson G, Engel PJ: Purulent pericarditis caused by beta-hemolytic group C streptococcus. *Arch Int Med* 1981; 141:1351–1353.
134. Lieber IH, Rensimer ER, Ericsson CD: Campylobacter pericarditis in hypothyroidism. *Am Heart J* 1981; 102:462–463.
134a. Ugartemendia MC, Curos-Abadal A, Pujol-Rakosnik M, Pujadas-Capmany R, Escriva-Montserrat E, Jane-Pesquer J: Brucella mellitensis pericarditis. *Am Heart J* 1985; 109:1108.
135. Saslaw S, Norfleet RG, Dapra DJ: Acute histoplasma pericarditis. *Arch Int Med* 1968; 122:162–166.
136. Wheat LJ, Stein L, Corya BC, Wass JL, Norton JA, Grider K, Slama TG, French ML, Kohler RB: Pericarditis as a manifestation of histoplasmosis during two large urban outbreaks. *Medicine* 1983; 62:110–119.
137. Ramsdale DR, Gautam PC, Perera B, Charles RG: Cardiac tamponade due to actinomycosis. *Thorax* 1984; 39:473–474.
138. Eng RJ, Sen P, Browne K, Louria DB: Candida pericarditis. *Am J Med* 1981; 70:867–869.
139. Chapman MG, Kaplan L: Cardiac involvement in coccidioidomycosis. *Am J Med* 1957; 23:87–98.
140. Duvall CP, Carbone PP: Cryptococcus neoformans pericarditis associated with Hodgkin's disease. *Ann Int Med* 1966; 64:850–856.
141. Young EJ, Vainrub B, Musher DM: Pericarditis due to histoplasmosis. *JAMA* 1978; 240:1750–1751.
142. Susens GP, Al-Shamma A, Rowe JC, Herbert CC, Bassis ML, Coggs GC: Purulent constrictive pericarditis caused by Nocardia asteroides. *Ann Int Med* 1967; 67:1021–1032.
143. Tyagi SK, Anand IS, Deodhar SD, Datta DV: A clinical study of amoebic pericarditis. *J Assoc Phys India* 1980; 28:515–519.
144. Kinare SG, Parulkar GB, Sen PK: Constrictive pericarditis resulting from dracunculosis. *Brit Med J* 1962; 1:845.
145. Charan A, Sinha K: Constrictive pericarditis following filarial effusion. *Indian Heart J* 1973; 25:213–215.
146. Cheng W: Hydatid cysts in the pericardium—a new case and review of the literature. *Thorac Cardiovasc Surg* 1982; 30:56–57.
147. Sagrista-Sanleda J, Permanyer-Miralda G, Juste-Sanchez C, De Buen-Sanchez ML, Pujadas-Capmany R, Arcalis-Arce L, Soler-Soler J: Huge chronic pericardial effusion caused by Toxoplasma gondii. *Circulation* 1982; 66:895–897.
148. Dupont B, Charmot G, Lapresle C: Trypanosomiase revelee par des trypanides et compliquee de myopericardite. *Nouv Presse Med* 1979; 8:1579–1581.
149. Ben Ismail M, Hannachi N: Pericardial involvement in infectious endocarditis. Apropos of 11 cases. *Arch Mal Coeur* 1983; 76:893–901.
150. Buchbinder NA, Robers WC: Left-sided valvular infective endocarditis. A study of forty-five necropsy patients. *Am J Med* 1972; 53:20–35.
151. Nishimura RA, Fuster V, Burgert SL, Puga FJ: Clinical features and

long-term natural history of the postpericardiotomy syndrome. *Int J Card* 1983; 4:443–450.

152. Engle MA: Early and late manifestations of the postpericardiotomy syndrome. *Int J Card* 1983; 4:451–454.
153. Ofori-Krakye SK, Tyberg TI, Geha AS, Hammond GL, Cohen LS, Langou RA: Late cardiac tamponade after open heart surgery: Incidence, role of anticoagulants in its pathogenesis and its relationship to the postpericardiotomy syndrome. *Circulation* 1981; 63:1323–1328.
154. Weitzman L, Tinker WP, Kronzon I, Cohen ML, Glassman E, Spencer FC: The incidence and natural history of pericardial effusion after cardiac surgery — an echocardiographic study. *Circulation* 1984; 69:506–511.
155. Stevenson LW, Child JS, Laks H, Kern L: Incidence and significance of early pericardial effusion after cardiac surgery. *Am J Card* 1984; 54:848–851.
156. Dressler W: The post-myocardial-infarction syndrome. *Arch Int Med* 1959; 103:28–42.
157. Lichstein E: The changing spectrum of post-myocardial infarction pericarditis. *Int J Cardiol* 1983; 4:234–237.
158. Wunderink RG: Incidence of pericardial effusions in acute myocardial infarctions. *Chest* 1984; 85:494–496.
159. Kaplan K, Davison R, Parker M, Przybylek J, Light A, Bresnahan D, Ribner H, Talano JV: Frequency of pericardial effusion as determined by M-mode echocardiography in acute myocardial infarction. *Am J Card* 1985; 55:335–337.
160. Berman J, Haffajee CI, Alpert JS: Therapy of symptomatic pericarditis after myocardial infarction: Retrospective and prospective studies of aspirin, indomethacin, prednisone, and spontaneous resolution. *Am Heart J* 1981; 101:750–753.
161. Silliman RA, Peters JD, Ginsberg MB: Infections of the heart complicating acute myocardial infarction. *South Med J* 1984; 77:934–936.
162. Arena FP, Chiaramida A, Cheng G, Jones Z: Neoplastic pericarditis—A retrospective analysis of the Memorial Sloan-Kettering Cancer Center experience 1961–1980. *Proc Am Soc Clin Oncol* 1983; 2:C-7.
163. Acquitella GC, Roura ET, Maury AJ, Stern RO, Acquitella H: High incidence of pericardial effusion in non-Hodgkin's lymphoma: Usefulness of echocardiography. *Eur J Cancer Clin Oncol* 1982; 18:1131–1136.
164. Kacenelenbogen R, Devriendt J, DeReuck M, DePaepe J, Decoodt P, DeRoy G, Schmerber J, Staroukine M: Cardiac tamponade as first manifestation of colonic cancer. *Arch Int Med* 1984; 144:622–623.
165. Chen KTK: Extracardiac malignancy presenting with cardiac tamponade. *J Surg Oncol* 1983; 23:167–168.
166. Kirwan M, Blake S, Neligan M, O'Malley E, Bergin A, Bonar F, Flanagan M, Garrett J, Griffin B, Whelan D: Cardiac constriction due to malignant disease of the pericardium. *Ir J Med Sci* 1983; 152:454–455.
167. Tatsuta M, Yamamura H, Yamamoto R, Ichii M, Iishi H, Noguchi S: Carcinoembryonic antigens in the pericardial fluid of patients with malignant pericarditis. *Oncology* 1984; 41:328–330.
168. Primrose WR, Clee MD, Johnston RN: Malignant pericardial effusion managed with vinblastine. *Clin Oncol* 1983; 9:67–70.
169. Davis S, Rambotti P, Grignani F: Intrapericardial tetracycline sclerosis in the treatment of malignant pericardial effusion: an analysis of thirty three cases. *J Clin Oncol* 1984; 2:631–636.
170. Coplan NL, Kennish AJ, Burgess NL, Deligdish L, Goldman ME: Pericardial mesothelioma masquerading as a benign pericardial effusion. *J Am Coll Cardiol* 1984; 4:1307–1310.
171. Vogelzang NJ, Schultz SM, Iannucci AM, Kennedy BJ: Malignant mesothelioma. The University of Minnesota experience. *Cancer* 1984; 53:377–383.
172. Cohn KE, Stewart JR, Fajardo LF, Hancock EW: Heart disease following radiation. *Medicine* 1967; 46:281–298.
173. Stewart JR, Fajardo LF: Radiation-induced heart disease: An update. *Prog Cardiovasc Dis* 1984; 27:173–194.
174. Applefeld MM, Cole JF, Pollock SH, Sutton FJ, Slawson RG, Singleton RT, Wiernik PH: The late appearance of chronic pericardial disease in patients treated by radiotherapy for Hodgkin's disease. *Ann Int Med* 1981; 94:338–341.
175. Gutierrez CA, Just-Viera JO: Clinical spectrum of radiation induced pericarditis. *Am Surg* 1983; 49:113–115.
176. Kantrowitz NE, Bristow MR: Cardiotoxicity of antitumor agents. *Prog Cardiovasc Dis* 1984; 27:195–200.
177. Ahmed M, Slayton RE: Report on drug-induced pericarditis. *Cancer Treat Rep* 1980; 64:353–355.
178. Carey RM, Coleman M, Feder A: Pericardial tamponade: A major presenting manifestation of hydralazine-induced lupus syndrome. *Am J Med* 1973; 54:84–87.
179. Greenberg JH, Lutcher CL: Drug-induced systemic lupus erythematosus: a case with life-threatening pericardial tamponade. *JAMA* 1972; 222:191–193.
180. Durkin WJ, Pugh RP, Solomon J, Rosen P, Pajek TF, Bateman RJ: Treatment of advanced lymphomas with bleomycin (NSC-125066). *Oncology* 1976; 33:140–145.
181. Steinherz LJ, Steinherz PG, Mangiacasale D, O'Reilly R, Allen J, Sorell M, Miller DR: Cardiac changes with cyclophosphamide. *Med Pediatr Oncol* 1981; 9:417–422.
182. Vaickus L, Letendre L: Pericarditis induced by high-dose cytarabine therapy. *Arch Int Med* 1984; 144:1868–1869.
183. Bristow MR, Thompson PD, Martin RP, Mason JW, Billingham ME, Harrison DC: Early anthracycline cardiotoxity. *Am J Med* 1978; 65:823–832.
184. Zatuchni J: Captopril pericarditis. *JAMA* 1984; 251:343–344.
185. Evans CW, Tucker SC: Pericarditis: A complication of minoxidil therapy. *South Med J* 1983; 76:815–816.
186. Cohen AS, Canoso JJ: Pericarditis in the rheumatologic diseases. *Cardiovasc Clin* 1976; 7(3):237–255.
187. Tan ATH, Mah PK, Chia BL: Cardiac tamponade in acute rheumatic carditis. *Ann Rheum Dis* 1983; 42:699–701.
188. Alpert MA, Goldberg SH, Singsen BH, Durham JB, Sharp GC, Ahmad M, Madigan NP, Hurst DP, Sullivan WD: Cardiovascular manifestations of mixed connective tissue disease in adults. *Circulation* 1983; 68:1182–1193.
189. Kay GN, Bennett JC: The heart in rheumatoid arthritis, in Hurst JW (ed), *Clinical Essays on the Heart*, Vol 3. New York, McGraw-Hill, 1984, pp 83–103.
190. Kahan A, Feldman JL, Menkes CJ, Fontaine JL: Tamponade recidivante au cours d' une polyarthrite juvénile traitée par péricardotomie et corticoïdes. *Nouv Presse Med* 1982; 11(34):2567.
191. Spector D, Alfred H, Siedlecki M, Briefel G: A controlled study of the effect of indomethacin in uremic pericarditis. *Kidney Int* 1983; 24:663–669.
192. DePace NL, Nestico PF, Schwartz AB, Mintz GS, Schwartz JS, Kotler MN, Swartz C: Predicting success of intensive dialysis in the treatment of uremic pericarditis. *Am J Med* 1984; 76:38–46.

192a. Bashour TT, Guha A, Cheng TO, Parrish A, Kramer N: Paroxysmal atrial tachyarrhythmias induced by hemodialysis: an early sign of effusive pericarditis(?). *Clin Research* 1973; 21:403.

193. Peraino RA: Pericardial effusion in patients treated with maintenance dialysis. *Am J Nephrol* 1983; 3:319–322.
194. Frame JR, Lucas SK, Pederson JA, Elkins RC: Surgical treatment of pericarditis in the dialysis patient. *Am J Surg* 1983; 146:800–803.
195. Lazarus JM: Pericardial effusion (letter). *Arch Int Med* 1984; 144:1317.

46 Infective Endocarditis

Harold C. Neu, MD, FACP

In the past decade, infection of heart valves or of other parts of the cardiac system, such as septal defects, mural endocardium, or arterioarterial shunts, has been referred to as infective endocarditis. This term is preferable to the former use of bacterial endocarditis because we now recognize that fungi, Chlamydia, and even Rickettsia can be responsible for valvular abnormalities. Infective endocarditis generally had been classified as acute or subacute based on the progression of untreated disease. The acute form usually followed a fulminant course because it was caused by virulent organisms such as *Staphylococcus aureus, Streptococcus pyogenes, S pneumoniae,* or *Neisseria gonorrhoeae.* The subacute form of the disease in which death did not occur for several weeks or months had a slow, indolent course with fever, weight loss, and a variety of systemic constitutional symptoms. This form of disease was characteristically due to the viridans group of streptococci. As our understanding of the pathophysiologic aspects of endocarditis has progressed, we have come to realize that infective endocarditis should be classified on the basis of the infecting agents because this will have important implications for therapy both with antibacterial agents and in reference to surgery, which has come to play an increasingly important role in the ultimate therapy of this disease.

EPIDEMIOLOGY OF INFECTIVE ENDOCARDITIS

The precise incidence of infective endocarditis is not known because case definitions differ among the many reported series. However, approximately 1 case per 1,000 hospital admissions with a range of 0.1 to 5 cases per 1,000 admissions has been seen in the last two decades in most teaching centers.[1-4] There have been significant changes in the mean age of patients with endocarditis. In the 1920s the median age was less than 30 years.[5] Currently over 50% of the patients are over 50 years of age.[1,2] The disease is uncommon in children at the present time, and with improvements in cardiovascular surgery endocarditis has become even less common in the last several decades.[6,7] Approximately 25% of patients are less than 30 years of age. Most of these younger patients in recent years have been those in whom the disease is secondary to narcotic addiction.[8] The mean age of men generally is six to seven years greater than that of women, and in all series men constitute a larger number of cases in the range of 55% to 70%, so that the mean male–female ratio is approximately 1.7 to 1.[1,2,9] In recent years endocarditis has developed in a significant proportion of patients as a result of nosocomial infections that are secondary to the use of intravenous lines such as intravenous catheters, hyperalimentation lines, pacemakers, or dialysis shunts.[1,2]

The heart valve involved in infective endocarditis depends on the underlying disease (Table 46.1). In patients with natural valve involvement the mitral valve is involved in 25% to 45% of cases, the aortic valve alone in 5% to 35%, and both the aortic and mitral valves in 5% to 35%.[1-3] In normal individuals the tricuspid valve is rarely involved (0 to 5%) and the pulmonary valve rarely, if ever (less than 1%).[10] Both right- and left-sided disease in normal individuals occurs in less than 4% of patients. With an aging population aortic valve involvement is increasing, and most series have noted that the aortic valve is involved in 60% of male patients but in only 30% of female patients.

In narcotic addicts, who in some institutions constitute a significant proportion of patients with endocarditis, the valve involvement is distinctly different from that in normal patients. In narcotic addicts 60% of the patients will have no underlying heart disease, and there is a predilection for involvement of the tricuspid valve.[11-13] The tricuspid valve is involved in approximately 50% of narcotic addicts, the aortic valve in 20%, the mitral valve in 10%, and the aortic and mitral valves in 15%.[11,12]

Virtually any type of structural heart disease may predispose to infective endocarditis if it results in turbulent blood flow. Until the 1960s rheumatic heart disease was the underlying pathologic process in 35% to 75% of the infections with mitral valve involvement and in 85% of the patients with underlying rheumatic heart disease.[13] Congenital heart disease in the past was an important cause of infective endocarditis with patients developing endocarditis on patent ductus arteriosus, ventricular septal defects, coarctation of the aorta, bicuspid aortic valves, and tetralogy of Fallot.[13] Endocarditis characteristically has been uncommon in patients with secundum atrial defects because these lesions result in little turbulence of blood flow.

Degenerative cardiac lesions, such as calcified mitral anulus or calcified valvular defects, have become a more important underlying pathologic predisposing condition in recent years, particularly as a cause of underlying disease in patients who have no demonstrable valvular disease.[14] Idiopathic hypertrophic subaortic stenosis (IHSS) has been recognized in the last few years as a potential underlying lesion that may lead to the development of endocarditis.[15] Infection has occurred in the aortic valve, mitral valve, both valves, and in the subaortic endocardium. In approximately 5% of patients with IHSS, infective endocarditis will develop. Mitral valve prolapse syndrome has been recognized in the last several years to predispose to endocarditis.[16] Endocarditis will develop in approximately 10% of patients with isolated mitral valve prolapse. The patients with this syndrome in whom infective endocarditis develops have had holosystolic murmurs, and none of the patients has had an isolated click without a murmur.[16-18] Interestingly, infective endocarditis in patients with mitral valve prolapse produces symptoms and signs that are more difficult to recognize, and the mortality is lower when compared with that of left-sided endocarditis and other valvular lesions.[17,18]

Table 46.1. Valve Involvement in Endocarditis: Percentage of Infections

Valve	Native Valves	Addicts	Prosthetic Valves
Aortic	35	15–20	60
Mitral	40	15–20	30
Tricuspid	1	50–55	<5
Aortic and mitral	15	5–10	<5
Pulmonary	<1	1	. . .
Congenital defect	5–6	<1	5
Total	100%	100%	100%

Prosthetic valve endocarditis is a relatively recent phenomenon. In the past three decades the incidence of endocarditis after valve replacement has ranged from 1% to 9%.[19-25] Although in the 1960s a higher incidence of endocarditis was noted, in recent years the acute or early onset of endocarditis has markedly decreased.[19-21] The aortic valve appears to be more susceptible to infection than the mitral valve, with 60% of prosthetic valve endocarditis involving an aortic prosthesis versus 30% involving a mitral prosthesis and 10% occurring in patients with multiple prostheses.[22] The incidence of prosthetic valve endocarditis in patients who have porcine heterografts is approximately 2%, and the incidence with mechanical valves 3%.[24,25]

PATHOGENESIS OF INFECTIVE ENDOCARDITIS

PATHOGENESIS OF NATURAL VALVE INFECTIONS

A number of factors are involved in the pathogenesis of infective endocarditis. Basically, these involve a valve or septal lesion which creates turbulent flow from a high to a low pressure area, formation of sterile platelet fibrin thrombi, bacteremia, and affinity of bacteria for valvular tissue and thrombi.[26] Bacteremia by itself is not sufficient to produce endocardial infection.[27] The intravenous injection of large inocula of bacteria into rabbits fails to produce endocarditis, and clinically endocarditis is an extremely rare event in patients who have frequent bacteremia such as the immunocompromised patient. The endocardial surface of the heart valve must be modified to predispose it to colonization by circulating bacteria.[28] Studies of heart valves have shown that there are small platelet–fibrin thrombi along the valvular lines of closure. These develop because of local stresses such as blood turbulence. The formation of microscopic endocardial thrombi, which are referred to as nonbacterial thrombotic endocarditis (NBTE), appears to be a requisite for the development of infective endocarditis. Studies in rabbits have demonstrated that NBTE is useful in the initiation of endocardial infection because infective endocarditis will uniformly develop in animals with nonbacterial thrombi after streptococcal or staphylococcal bacteremia.[29] The formation of thrombi requires alteration of the valvular endothelium so that its ability to trigger the local deposition of platelets or fibrin is increased. In animals it is possible to place a sterile polyethylene catheter across an aortic or tricuspid valve and rapidly induce the formation of platelet thrombi.[27] In patients with rheumatic heart disease, damage to the endothelium occurs either through immune complex deposition or as a result of the hemodynamic abnormalities associated with the valvular deformity. Endocarditis occurs characteristically downstream from where blood flows from a narrow orifice at a high velocity to a low pressure area.[30] For example, infective endocarditis characteristically occurs on the atrial surface of the mitral valve and the ventricular surface of the aortic valve when there is valvular insufficiency. There is a decrease in lateral pressure immediately below the regurgitant flow. Cardiac lesions with a high degree of turbulence, such as small ventricular septal defects, and stenotic valves readily create conditions that lead to bacterial colonization. Cardiac defects in which a large area is involved, such as a large ventricular septal defect, or in low flow lesions, such as an ostium secundum atrial septal defect, or in situations such as atrial fibrillation rarely result in infective endocarditis. Furthermore, the role of hemodynamic factors in both the initiation and maintenance of infective endocarditis is demonstrated by the fact that endocarditis at the site of a patent ductus arteriosus or arteriovenous fistula can be cured by surgical ligation alone.[31]

Once nonbacterial thrombotic lesions have developed on a valve or on the endocardium, transient bacteremia may result in the colonization of these lesions and the development of infective endocarditis. Bacteremia often occurs after trauma to the mucosal surfaces that have large numbers of bacteria. This is true for areas such as the mouth, around the teeth, gastrointestinal, urologic, and gynecologic areas.[32,33] In general, bacteremia is of a low grade nature, less than 10 colony forming units per milliliter, and the blood stream is normally sterile within 30 minutes. Bacteremia is a much more frequent event than most individuals realize. It not only follows dental and medical procedures, such as tooth extraction, tonsillectomy, and sigmoidoscopy, but it is frequent with daily activities such as tooth brushing, chewing hard candy, or the use of oral irrigation devices (Table 46.2).[33] Blood cultures taken during various procedures usually show diphtheroids or *Propionibacterium,* but these organisms rarely cause endocarditis. Indeed, the viridans group of streptococci, a major cause of endocarditis, is isolated only in patients who undergo various surgical procedures. Organisms must have special properties that enable them to colonize valve surfaces. Susceptibility of potential pathogens to complement-mediated bactericidal activity appears to be an important factor in the development of endocarditis. Strains of bacteria resistant to complement's bactericidal properties are more likely to survive during bacteremia and produce infective endocarditis.[34]

It was thought that preformed antibodies facilitated endocardial infection. However, more recent studies have suggested that preformed antibodies can actually reduce the incidence of endocarditis in rabbits infected with the viridans group of streptococci or *S pneumoniae.*[35,36] Immunization results in more rapid clearance of organisms from the blood. A final factor that may be important is the relation of organisms to platelets. Platelets may serve as a barrier to colonization through their role in bacterial clearance. It appears that the ability of certain organisms to adhere to platelet thrombi on valves is a critical step in the development of endocarditis.

Table 46.2. Incidence of Bacteremia After Various Procedures and Bodily Events

Source	Positive Blood Cultures (%)
Dental extraction	15–85
Periodontal surgery	30–85
Chewing hard object	15–50
Tooth brushing	5–25
Water pik	25–40
Respiratory	
Tonsillectomy	25–40
Intubation	15–20
Bronchoscopy	10–15
Gastrointestinal	
Barium enema	0–10
Liver biopsy	5–10
Sigmoidoscopy	0–10
Upper endoscopy	5–15
Urologic	
Cystoscopy	0–15
Prostatic resection, transurethral	15–50
Urethral dilatation	15–30
Obstetric and gynecologic	
Removal of intrauterine device	0–15
Vaginal delivery	0–10

Organisms associated with infective endocarditis, namely, viridans streptococci, enterococci, *S aureus,* and *S epidermidis* adhere more readily to aortic valvular tissue in vitro than do organisms that are uncommon causes of infective endocarditis, such as *Klebsiella pneumoniae* or *Escherichia coli* (Table 46.3).[37,38] Although different factors may be involved in the adherence of bacteria to valves, one clear-cut factor is the bacterial synthesis of extracellular polysaccharides such as dextran. Over 50% of endocarditis-associated strains of streptococci produced dextran whereas most blood isolates of viridans streptococci do not.[39] Streptococcal adherence to platelet-fibrin is proportional to the amount of dextran produced. Furthermore, in vitro streptococci adhere more readily to traumatized canine valves if they produce dextran. Treatment of dextran-producing strains

Table 46.3. Adherence of Bacteria to Valvular Tissue

Organism	Adherence Ratio*
Streptococcus mutans	1,500
Streptococcus bovis	590
Streptococcus miteor	330
Streptococcus sanguis	300
Streptococcus faecalis	180
Streptococcus milleri	140
Staphylococcus aureus	560
Staphylococcus epidermidis	460
Pseudomonas aeruginosa	35
Escherichia coli	2
Klebsiella pneumoniae	4

* Based on lack of adherence of a test organism. If two colonies of *E coli* would adhere to a valve in culture, 1,500 *S mutans* would adhere.

with dextranase markedly reduces their adherence to valves. Other factors that may be important are the presence of fibronectin, a plasma glycoprotein that is a major surface constituent of mammalian cells. Fibronectin may mediate the binding of bacteria to platelet thrombi.[40] *Streptococcus mutans* and *S aureus* bind better to valvular material in the presence of fibronectin.

Following colonization of the valve, the bacteria develop in a vegetation that will enlarge with further deposition of a fibrin platelet material and bacterial proliferation. Bacterial colonies will be found beneath the surface of the vegetation. Hence, they are poorly killed by phagocytic cells because the vegetation provides an environment in which bacterial killing is at a minimum. Very high colony numbers of bacteria, 10^9 to 10^{10} bacteria per gram of valvular tissue, will develop. The bacteria within this fibrin matrix are in a reduced state of metabolic activity.[41] Bacteria adherent to valve surfaces stimulate tissue thromoplastin from the tissue of the valve and activate further coagulation by the extrinsic pathway.[42]

The role of white cells in endocarditis is unclear. It has been suggested that phagocytosis of microorganisms by monocytes at the vegetation will generate tissue thromboplastin formation which acts as a stimulus to further fibrin deposition in the growth of the vegetation.[43] White cells may modulate the course of endocarditis because neutropenic animals tend to have a more aggressive illness with higher levels of bacteremia than do normal animals.[44] Leukocytes may act normally in the vegetation to inhibit bacterial growth provided they reach the vegetations, but further studies are necessary to delineate the true role of the white cells.

PATHOGENESIS OF EARLY PROSTHETIC VALVE ENDOCARDITIS

Prosthetic valve endocarditis has been divided into early and late endocarditis. Early endocarditis refers to endocarditis occurring in the first 60 days after operation. This period of time is a reasonable separation because it requires about 60 days to endothelialize the area at the base of the valve where it has been sewn into the heart.

Staphylococcus epidermidis is the most common cause of early prosthetic valve endocarditis.[19] This probably is a result of valve contamination occurring in the perioperative period as a result of contamination of valvular tissue by microorganisms in the pumped blood during bypass. In the immediate postoperative period, the postoperative valve and the ring site are not endothelialized and are more susceptible to microbial colonization. Patients frequently have many intravascular catheters and pressure monitoring devices going through the skin which may seed microorganisms onto the nonendothelialized area. Furthermore, infection at other extracardiac sites may result in bacteremia producing contamination on the heart valve.

In late prosthetic valve endocarditis, the organisms are the same as those seen in native valve endocarditis, particularly with reference to streptococcal species. Stress and turbulence will produce rough areas either at the site where the artificial valve is sewn into the heart or the porcine valve, allowing microorganisms to aggregate in a manner similar to that which occurs with natural valves.

PATHOLOGY OF INFECTIVE ENDOCARDITIS

Infective endocarditis produces pathologic changes in more organs than just the heart because there may be involvement of the kidney, central nervous system, spleen, lungs, and skin as well. In the heart the vegetations of infective endocarditis are usually located at the line of closure of a valve leaflet at the atrial surface of the atrioventricular valve, and on the ventricular surface of the semilunar valve, such as the aortic valve.[45,46] Vegetations vary in size from a few millimeters to as large as several centimeters with some organisms such as fungi or *Haemophilus parainfluenzae.*

Vegetations may be single or multiple and vary in their consistency and gross appearance. Infective endocarditis vegetation lesions consist of fibrin platelet aggregates and masses of bacteria up to concentrations of 10^9 per gram of tissue. It is rare to see red or white blood cells within the mass of platelets and bacteria. In general, vegetations seen in acute endocarditis tend to be larger, softer, more pliable, and less healed than those in subacute endocarditis. Acute infection may lead to perforation of the valve leaflet, rupture of chordae tendineae, involvement of the interventricular septum by abscess, or involvement in the structure of the papillary muscles. Myocardial infarction may result from fragments of vegetation embolizing to the coronary vessels, or pericarditis may be encountered in endocarditis.[47]

Certain bacteria are more likely to produce abscess formation. For example, staphylococcal endocarditis is more frequently associated with valve ring abscesses and fistula formation into the myocardium. Other lesions such as aneurysms of the valve leaflet or sinus of Valsalva may result from infective endocarditis.[46,47]

In recent years we have become more aware of the involvement of the kidney in infective endocarditis. Several different pathologic processes may be encountered including glomerulonephritis, infarction, or actual abscess formation. Abscesses of the kidney are infrequent and occur primarily with staphylococcal disease. Infarctions have been noted in approximately 50% of autopsy cases. The kidney usually is normal in size but slightly swollen, and multiple petechiae are found in the capsule.

Focal glomerulonephritis is found in 40% to 80% of patients with endocarditis.[48,49] It tends to be a segmental process in which there is mesangial and endothelial proliferation, infiltration of white blood cells, fibrinoid necrosis, and fibrosis. Some patients may have diffuse glomerulonephritis with generalized cellular hyperplasia in most glomerular tufts. Between 10% and 20% of patients with infective endocarditis will develop an immune complex glomerulonephritis that is analogous to that found in collagen vascular disease such as lupus erythematosus.[48,49] Subepithelial deposits, which consist of IgG, IgM, IgA, and complement can be demonstrated by immunofluorescence.

Several different forms of involvement occur in the central nervous system.[50,51] Cerebral emboli have been noted in approximately one third of patients with infective endocarditis. The most commonly affected area is the middle cerebral artery or its branches. In addition to cerebral infarction, abscesses, mycotic aneurysms, intracerebral or subarachnoid hemorrhage, cerebritis, and meningitis all have been noted.[52] Mycotic aneurysms are seen more frequently with viridans group streptococcal endocarditis than with other organisms. The aneurysms occur most frequently at bifurcation points in cerebral vessels but can occur in other vessels of the body.

Another organ that may be involved in infective endocarditis is the spleen in which infarction has been noted in patients at autopsy. Spleen abscess is fairly uncommon but does occur. The patient with right-sided endocarditis may develop pulmonary emboli with or without infarction, lung abscess, pneumonia, pleural effusion, and empyema.

CLINICAL MANIFESTATIONS OF INFECTIVE ENDOCARDITIS

Ironically, although the sources of the infecting bacteria in endocarditis are endogenous seeding from teeth, gums, sinuses, prostate, bladder and the bowel, the precise etiologic factor in many cases of endocarditis is not known. A history of a preceding dental procedure is elicited in 20% of patients with endocarditis caused by streptococci of the viridans type.[1–3] Enterococcal endocarditis may follow urologic or urogenital procedures, but only 50% of patients will have a history of such a preceding procedure.[1–3] Furthermore, patients with staphylococcal endocarditis will produce a history of preceding staphylococcal skin infection in less than 50% of the patients.

The actual interval between the event that produces the bacteremia and the onset of the symptoms of infective endocarditis is usually less than two weeks.[53] What is long, however, is the time from the onset of symptoms to diagnosis, and this in the subacute form of endocarditis may be anywhere from four to eight weeks with a median of five weeks.

The symptoms and signs of infective endocarditis are extremely broad because many organ systems may be involved[54] (Table 46.4). It is important to remember that we are dealing not only with a bacteremic process, but also with a process in which there may be embolization to many organs, and that as a result of the infection an immunologic process is occurring that results in circulating immune complexes that may produce disease in diverse organs.

Table 46.4. Clinical Manifestations of Infective Endocarditis

Symptoms	Percentage	Physical Findings	Percentage
Fever	80–90	Fever	80–90
Weakness	40–50	Heart murmur	85
Chills	20–40	Emboli	50
Dyspnea	20–40	Skin changes	15–50
Night sweats	30–40	Osler's nodes	10–15*
Anorexia	20–25	Petechiae	20–40
Weight loss	20–25	Janeway lesion	5*
Malaise	20–25	Splenomegaly	20–50*
Myalgias	20–25	Clubbing	5*
Skin lesions	20–25	Retinal lesions	5–10
Stroke	15–20		
Headache	10–15		
Confusion	10–15		

*Seen in individuals with symptoms longer than six weeks.

Fever is the most common symptom in patients with infective endocarditis. Nonetheless, in 5% of patients fever may be absent, usually in patients who have renal failure, severe congestive heart failure, markedly advanced age, or general severe debility.[1,4] It is rare for a patient with endocarditis to have a fever greater than 103°F except in acute infective endocarditis, particularly that due to *S aureus.* The fever may be remitting or constant.

There is a variety of generalized, nonspecific symptoms, such as anorexia, weight loss, malaise, chills, emesis, weakness, night sweats, and generalized fatigue. Approximately 40% of patients with infective endocarditis will have musculoskeletal complaints that may occur early in the illness.[55] These may include monoarticular arthralgia, low back pain, diffuse myalgia, and as such may mimic other rheumatic or collagen vascular diseases. Some of the initial symptoms may be related to embolic episodes such as splenic artery emboli, which will result in left upper quadrant pain in the abdomen, or renal infarction, which may be associated with costovertebral angle pain.

Because neurologic manifestations occur in 20% to 40% of patients with endocarditis, these may be much more prominent and focus the attention on the neurologic system rather than on the cardiovascular. Major cerebral emboli producing sensory loss, ataxia, hemiplegia, aphasia, or alteration in mental status may be a presenting event. Some patients with endocarditis actually develop a toxic encephalopathy and personality change. Finally, brain abscess or purulent meningitis can occur with *S aureus* endocarditis and be a presenting symptom.

Cardiac murmurs occur in most patients with endocarditis, although they may be absent in patients with acute endocarditis and particularly in the patient with narcotic-associated endocarditis of the tricuspid valve.[1–4,13] It is distinctly uncommon to encounter changing murmurs or the development of a new murmur such as an aortic insufficiency murmur. Indeed, less than 10% of patients will show either of these particular findings, and when these findings are present, they usually indicate acute staphylococcal endocarditis. The patients may have symptoms and signs of congestive heart failure, particularly if they have what is noted to be a new regurgitant murmur. A pericardial friction rub is a distinctly rare phenomenon.

Other classical manifestations of endocarditis may not be present because their formation is to a certain extent dependent on chronicity of the infection. Indeed, the earlier diagnosis of infective endocarditis in recent years has decreased the incidence of many peripheral manifestations of endocarditis. Clubbing is currently present in at the most 10% to 15% of patients.[1] Hypertrophic osteoarthropathy is exceedingly uncommon today. Splinter hemorrhages are found in the nails of many patients, but it is critical to remember that these are a most nonspecific phenomenon seen in elderly patients and may also be the result of certain work-related trauma. Petechiae are found in 20% to 40% of patients if a long time has elapsed before diagnosis. The petechiae may occur on the extremities, on buccal mucosa, on the palate, and particularly on the conjunctivae. The petechial lesions are initially red, but become brown and barely visible over a two- to three-day period of time.

Osler's nodes are small, nodular lesions found on the pads of the fingers and toes, which are small, painful, and nodular in appearance. They frequently are multiple and may last a few hours or days. Osler's nodes are rare in patients with acute infective endocarditis and occur primarily in patients with long-standing disease, that is, disease for more than six weeks. Even in such patients, only 25% at most will show this interesting phenomenon. Osler's nodes are not a specific indication of infective endocarditis because they can be seen in diseases such as systemic lupus erythematosus, hemolytic anemia, and gonococcal infections. Janeway lesions are larger, nontender, macular, hemorrhagic areas that occur on the palms and soles. These lesions are thought to be embolic in origin and are frequent in acute endocarditis due to staphylococci. Some Osler's nodes appear to be embolic, whereas others are based on local vasculitis due to antigen–antibody complex disease.[56] Roth's spots are small, pale retinal lesions that are surrounded by hemorrhage and located near the optic disk. These lesions are seen in less than 5% of patients with infective endocarditis and are also found in patients with connective tissue disorders, leukemia, and hemolytic anemia.

Splenomegaly is present in 25% to 40% of patients with endocarditis.[1–4] It occurs most commonly when symptoms are prolonged, that is, longer than six weeks, and it is distinctly uncommon in acute endocarditis. Other findings in endocarditis may be the result of embolic phenomena, such as emboli to the spleen, kidneys, or lungs. Major vessel emboli, such as those to the femoral, brachial, popliteal, or radial arteries, are most commonly encountered with fungal endocarditis. Indeed, symptoms of claudication in a young addict should suggest occlusion of the femoral vessels due to *Candida.*

The manifestations of endocarditis in the narcotic addict may be distinctly different from those in patients with natural valve endocarditis.[8,11,12] The tricuspid valve is involved in over 50% of patients with narcotic-associated endocarditis.[8] The signs of tricuspid involvement, however, are present in perhaps only one third of patients. Hence, a systolic regurgitant murmur that is louder with inspiration is usually not heard, nor is there a pulsatile liver or large V waves in the neck. A third of patients with tricuspid valve infection will have symptoms of pleuritic chest pain, and pulmonary complaints and findings will dominate the clinical picture.

Clinical manifestations of prosthetic valve endocarditis also are to some extent different (Table 46.5). Fever is the most common symptom in virtually all patients with prosthetic valve endocarditis.[20,21,57] A change in a heart murmur or development of a new one occurs in approximately 60% of patients, and there is evidence of systemic embolization in approximately 40%. Petechiae are seen in approximately 40% of patients with prosthetic valve endocarditis, but Osler's nodes, Janeway lesions, and Roth's spots are extremely infrequent, occurring in 10% to 15% of patients. On occasion there may be occlusion or malfunction of the prosthetic valve. In either event, a stenosis murmur or marked muffling of the heart sounds may develop.

Table 46.5. Symptoms, Clinical Signs, and Laboratory Findings in Prosthetic Valve Endocarditis

Findings	Percentage
Fever	95
Malaise	60
Anemia	70
Hematuria	55
Leukocytosis	50
New or changed murmur	55
Systemic emboli	40
Petechiae	40
Splenomegaly	30
Cutaneous lesions	10–15

LABORATORY FINDINGS IN INFECTIVE ENDOCARDITIS

Although most patients with infective endocarditis have some abnormality in hematologic parameters, none of these abnormalities can be considered diagnostic because they occur in many other diseases with which endocarditis can be confused. Anemia is present in 70% to 90% of patients with endocarditis.[1–4] The anemia is that seen in chronic diseases, namely, a normochromic, normocytic anemia with a low serum iron and low iron-binding capacity. Anemia tends to be more severe in patients in whom there has been a long period between infection and recognition of the disease. Leukocytosis is present in 20% to 30% of patients with infective endocarditis. Leukocyte counts of 15,000 to 25,000 may be seen in the acute form of endocarditis, particularly in patients with narcotic addiction. The differential count is usually normal, although there may be a predominance of band forms. Although leukopenia may be seen in 10% of patients with endocarditis, it is in no way common and is most frequent in patients with long-term illness associated with splenomegaly. The leukocyte count will be within normal limits in most patients with viridans group streptococcal endocarditis.

It has been stated that mononuclear cells can be detected in the peripheral blood of 25% of patients with endocarditis, particularly if blood is taken from an earlobe puncture. However, such cells are also found in patients with tuberculosis, typhoid fever, typhus, and malaria, which would be chronic illnesses in which unexplained fever, myalgia, and wasting would be noted. The erythrocyte sedimentation rate, which is relatively easy to determine and inexpensive, is elevated in most patients with infective endocarditis. Mean erythrocyte sedimentation rates using the Westgren method have been 50 mm per hour.[2] In acute endocarditis the erythrocyte sedimentation rate may not be elevated. It is usually normal or low in persons with infective endocarditis who have congestive heart failure, disseminated intravascular coagulation, or renal failure. A nonspecific increase in gamma globulin is noted in 20% to 30% of patients with endocarditis. A positive rheumatoid factor latex fixation test is found in 50% of patients whose duration of illness exceeds six weeks.[1-4] Complement levels are elevated in some patients and low in those who have renal involvement. False-positive serologic tests for syphilis are distinctly uncommon in bacterial endocarditis.

Urinalysis frequently gives abnormal results in patients with endocarditis, with fully 50% to 60% of patients having moderate proteinuria. Microscopic hematuria is seen in 30% to 50% of patients. Red cell casts, however, are much less frequent, and hematuria, pyuria, and white blood cell casts are unusual. Urine cultures may be positive in patients with staphylococcal endocarditis, providing a clue to the disease. Urine cultures, however, are negative in patients with viridans streptococcal endocarditis and usually negative as well in patients with enterococcal or endocarditis due to other organisms.

The most important laboratory test in evaluating a patient for infective endocarditis is the blood culture. Bacteremia in endocarditis is a relatively constant phenomenon in which bacteria are discharged at a constant rate from endocardial vegetations.[58] This is not the result of breaking off of infected particles, which is an important fact to consider because it indicates that arterial blood cultures have no demonstrable advantage over venous blood cultures.[59,60] Cultures of blood can be obtained at any time of the day or at any body temperature without particular advantage.[61] If cultures are to be positive, it is likely that all of them will be positive. The successful isolation of bacteria from patients with infective endocarditis depends on the number of blood cultures obtained, the volume of blood cultured, and the techniques used by the laboratory to process the blood cultures.[60] Two to three separate blood samples for culture should be collected within a 24-hour interval from patients who have not received antimicrobial therapy within the preceding two weeks. This number of blood cultures will be sufficient for the isolation of the etiologic agent in at least 96% of previously untreated patients with infective endocarditis. Collection of an additional two or three separate blood samples may be necessary in previously treated patients or in those with endocarditis due to fastidious organisms if the initial blood cultures do not yield growth after 24 to 48 hours of incubation. Indeed, in a study at New York Hospital[58] covering a 15-year period, in streptococcal endocarditis the first blood culture was positive in 96% of cases, and one of the first two cultures was positive in 98%. When antibiotics had been administered in the previous two weeks, the rate of positive cultures declined from 97% to 91%. Other studies have shown that 64% of cultures are positive in patients receiving antibiotics before hospitalization versus 100% in patients without antimicrobial agent exposure.[62]

Most blood cultures contain a few organisms, that is, 1 to 30 bacteria per milliliter. It is recommended that 5 ml of blood be injected into a suitable medium and cultured both aerobically and anaerobically. Some groups, such as the Mayo Clinic, however, recommend a larger volume of blood, insisting that 10 ml of blood should be the minimal essential volume per culture.[60] Supplementation of blood cultures with 15% sucrose or other special techniques have not increased the yield. At least 95% of clinically important bacteria are isolated from blood cultures by the seventh day of incubation. Therefore, a total of seven days of incubation of blood cultures is sufficient. However, some organisms such as *Haemophilus, Cardiobacterium,* or *Actinobacillus* require anywhere from 7 to 21 days for growth.[63] It is critical, therefore, to let the laboratory know that endocarditis is suspected, and if the initial cultures are negative and the clinical situation seems compatible with endocarditis, an arrangement should be made to maintain the cultures a longer time. Some organisms such as vitamin B_6-dependent streptococci, which account for 5% to 6% of episodes of infective endocarditis, may grow on initial blood isolation methods, but will not grow when subcultured.[64] Fungi are particularly difficult to grow, but the use of a biphase medium may increase the yield.[65] If the laboratory is aware of the consideration of endocarditis, attempts will be made to inoculate such organisms onto a proper medium.

Other techniques that may be useful in the diagnosis are antibody associated. Patients with *S aureus* endocarditis may have antibodies against teichoic acid, which is a major constituent of the cell wall of staphylococci. Teichoic acid antibodies have been detected by counterimmunoelectrophoresis in over 95% of patients, but false-positive test results have been found in 10%.[66-69] In general, teichoic acid antibody titers greater than 1:4 are indicative of disseminated staphylococcal disease such as endocarditis or osteomyelitis. Generally, however, the teichoic acid antibody tests should be viewed primarily as confirmatory of other tests. Although circulating immune complexes can be detected in many patients with infective endocarditis, such circulating immune complexes are also found in patients with septicemia and in approximately half of noninfected narcotic addicts.[70,71] Mixed type cryoglobulins are also present in at least 85% of patients with infective endocarditis, but this is also a nonspecific observation. Circulating immune complexes have been found in prosthetic valve endocarditis and are suggested to aid in diagnosis.[72,73]

A variety of other serologic tests have been used in an attempt to more readily make a diagnosis of fungal endocarditis, including the use of anti-*Candida* antibodies. However, the tests for determining antifungal antibodies are poorly standardized and in general have been extremely difficult to interpret. Tests for mannan antigenemia also appear to be unreliable. The same statements may be made for the test for *Aspergillus,* which also may be difficult to diagnose as a cause of endocarditis.

Echocardiography has been used in the diagnosis of infective endocarditis since 1973.[74] It is possible using echocardiograms to identify vegetations on all of the four valves.[74] However, echocardiography has been most successful in left-sided disease. Through the use of two-dimensional cross-sectional real time techniques, it is possible to detect vegetation as small as 2 mm.[75-77] Characteristically there is a shaggy band of irregular echoes in a nonuniform distribution on a leaflet of the valve that has unrestricted motion (see chapter 6 on Echocardiography and Doppler Echocardiography). The technique has been most successful with vegetation on the mitral and aortic valves, although in recent years vegetations on the tricuspid valve have been better visualized.[77a,77b] The echocardiogram may be of particular help in recognizing the large vegetations in fungal endocarditis in which blood cultures may be negative, but it has failed here also.[78] In general, echocardiography has not been as helpful in prosthetic heart valve infection as it has been in natural valve infection.[79] It is important to realize that a negative echocardiogram does not exclude the diagnosis of infective endocarditis.[76] However, false-positive results are rare. What is most helpful, as will be discussed later in this chapter, is the use of echocardiography in evaluating complications of infective endocarditis, particularly those surrounding the aortic valve, and in evaluating the risk for systemic emboli, congestive heart failure, and the need for emergency surgery.[80-83] For example, of 22 patients with vegetations demonstrated by echocardiography, 21 had major complications and 8 died, whereas of 14 patients without vegetations, 8 had complications and only 2 died.[76] Overall, the echocardiogram in the patient with infective endocarditis should be used as added evidence to aid in the management of the patient, rather than be relied on to make a diagnosis.

Although cardiac catheterization with quantitative blood cultures has been used to study the problem of both right-sided and left-sided endocarditis, it is a potentially dangerous technique that may result in a more rapid development of aortic insufficiency. In general, cardiac catheterization should be used not to make a diagnosis, but rather to aid in determining the hemodynamic status of the patient with reference to surgical intervention in the particular situation.

Imaging techniques to detect endocarditis using technetium-99m-labeled antibody have been tried, but the method is not established.[84] There has been little use of computed tomography in bacterial endocarditis, but it has been possible to detect an aortic root abscess.[85]

MICROBIOLOGIC ETIOLOGY OF ENDOCARDITIS

Virtually any species of bacteria is capable of producing infective endocarditis. Nonetheless, streptococci and staphylococci account for 75% to 90% of cases of endocarditis, particularly in community hospitals.[1-3,9,86,87] The infecting organism is, to a major extent, defined by the underlying disease. Thus, organisms in narcotic addicts tend to be different from those in individuals with normal valves and in patients with prosthetic heart valves. The etiology in each situation is given in Table 46.6.

STREPTOCOCCI

Streptococci cause 40% to 80% of cases of endocarditis.[9,86,87] In the past these organisms were referred to as viridans streptococci. Viridans streptococci are a group of organisms and not a true species. These organisms produce alpha hemolysis on blood agar, that is, partial hemolysis of the agar. The most common streptococcal organisms isolated from cases of endocarditis are *S sanguis, S bovis, S mutans,* and *S mitior.*[88] Other streptococcal species such as *S milleri* and *S salivarius* also may be important.

Streptococcus mutans causes 15% of cases of streptococcal endocarditis.[89] This organism is a microaerophilic and somewhat fastidious organism that occasionally will be identified as a group D streptococcal organism and confused with enterococci. This is important because therapy for infection due to this organism need not include two drugs nor be of the duration required for true enterococci. *Streptococcus bovis* occurs in the gastrointestinal tract of human subjects and belongs to Lancefield group D organisms.[90-92] However, it is not a true enterococcus. *Streptococcus bovis* has been associated with carcinoma or polyp lesions of the colon or other parts of the gastrointestinal tract, and any patient with endocarditis due to this organism must have a complete evaluation of the gastrointestinal tract usually requiring colonoscopy and barium enema.[93,94]

Enterococci that belong to the group D family consist primarily of *S faecalis* and *S faecium.* These organisms ac-

Table 46.6. Etiologic Agents of Infective Endocarditis: Percentages

Organisms	Native Valve	Narcotic Addicts	Prosthetic Valves: Early	Prosthetic Valves: Late
Streptococci	60–80	10–20	10	20–45
Viridans streptococci	30–40	10	5	30
Enterococci	10–15	10	5	15
Other*	15–25	<5	<1	5
Staphylococci	20–35	55–60	40–50	30
Staphylococcus aureus	10–25	50–55	20	10
S epidermidis	1–2	5–10	25	20
Fastidious gram-negative bacteria†	1–5	<1	<1	<1
Enterobacteriaceae	1	5	15	<1
Pseudomonas aeruginosa	1	5	10	1–3
Bacillus species	<1	1–2	<1	<1
Diphtheroides	<1	1	10	5
Mixed infections	1–2	5–10	<1	<1
Fungi	<1	3–5	10	1–5
Other organisms	<1	1–5	1–2	1–2
Culture negative	5–20	<1	...	1–5

* Primarily *S bovis*

† *Haemophilus, Actinobacillus, Cardiobacterium.*

count for between 5% and 15% of cases of infective endocarditis and they have become increasingly important in recent years.[91,95] Although disease due to this organism usually is subacute as is that with other streptococcal species, it is important to recognize that the organisms can produce an acute illness. The mean age of patients with enterococcal endocarditis generally is older than that of patients with other streptococcal species. The therapy of infection due to this organism is more complicated and will be discussed subsequently.

Nutritionally deficient streptococci are important organisms because of both the difficulty in growing them and the requirement for combined antimicrobial agents such as a beta-lactam and an aminoglycoside to achieve cure.[64] Other streptococcal species such as the group A streptococcus have been distinctly uncommon in recent years. Group B streptococci may produce a fulminant form of disease, particularly in diabetic patients and, overall, 50% of patients with group B streptococcal disease have had a fatal outcome and major systemic emboli are often encountered.[96] *Streptococcus milleri* accounts for only 5% to 10% of cases of infective endocarditis, but it has a marked predilection for producing subsequent complications involving the liver, brain, lungs, and other areas.[97,98] It also has produced myocardial abscesses and purulent pericarditis.

STAPHYLOCOCCI

Staphylococci account for 20% to 30% of cases of infective endocarditis.[86,87,99–101] Most cases of staphylococcal endocarditis are due to *S aureus,* particularly in normal individuals and in narcotic addicts. *Staphylococcus aureus* can infect valves that have no detectable damage.[99] Indeed, in approximately one third of patients there is no underlying cardiac disease. *Staphylococcus aureus* endocarditis is often a fulminant acute illness, resulting in death in approximately 40% of patients.[102] Interestingly, the infective endocarditis due to *S aureus* seen in narcotic addicts tends to be a less severe disease with mortality rates less than 10% in contrast to the disease seen in patients over the age of 50.[8,102] *Staphylococcus aureus* frequently produces myocardial abscess and valve ring abscess. It also may produce focal abscess within the lung, brain, spleen, kidney, and other organs. Indeed, the extracardiac involvement usually is noted earlier than is the cardiac disease. In the last few years, particularly in narcotic addicts, methicillin-resistant strains of *S aureus* have been encountered in the United States.[103]

Although *S epidermidis* does produce disease in normal individuals, it is fairly infrequent.[104,105] By way of contrast, the most common etiologic microorganism found in prosthetic valve endocarditis is *S epidermidis,* accounting for 25% to 30% of episodes.[106]

FASTIDIOUS GRAM-NEGATIVE BACTERIA

Various *Haemophilus* species have been the cause of infective endocarditis (Table 46.6). However, in contrast to other forms of bacterial disease, the species most frequently involved have been *H parainfluenzae, H paraphrophilus,* and *H aphrophilus.*[107,108] Overall, these organisms account for only 1% to 2% of the cases of endocarditis. However, several important clinical findings are associated with the organisms. *Haemophilus parainfluenzae* in particular has been associated with major central nervous system complications and with emboli to major peripheral arteries.[109,110] *Haemophilus aphrophilus* also may produce central nervous system disease. Other organisms that are related are *Actinobacillus, Actinomycetocomitans,* and *Cardiobacterium hominis.*[63,107,111,112] Overall, these organisms tend to produce subacute infective endocarditis with large friable vegetations, frequent emboli, and the development of congestive heart failure due to extensive valve damage, which requires valve replacement.[112,113] These organisms usually seed previously damaged cardiac valves during bacteremia from a respiratory source. Despite bacteriologic cure, embolization and congestive heart failure are common events. These organisms are particularly important to keep in mind because they may not grow for up to one to three weeks after the initial blood cultures are obtained.

GRAM-NEGATIVE BACILLI

Overall, 1% to 5% of cases of infective endocarditis are due to aerobic gram-negative bacilli.[107,108] These organisms most often produce disease in a select group of patients such as the narcotic addict, patients with prosthetic valves, and patients with cirrhosis. The diagnosis is obviously difficult to make, because gram-negative septicemia is a common event. However, in gram-negative bacillary endocarditis, bacteremia persists despite adequate antimicrobial agents. An etiologic basis for the bacteremia, such as an abscess, must be excluded. The most common gram-negative organisms to cause endocarditis in patients other than narcotic addicts are *Salmonella* species.[107,114,115] Among the *Salmonella, S chloraesuis* and *S typhimurium* account for most cases. However, other species have been involved as well.[115] *Escherichia coli, Citrobacter, Klebsiella, Enterobacter, Serratia, Proteus,* and *Providencia* have all been reported to cause endocarditis. One organism that has been seen in particular in narcotic addicts in the San Francisco area of the United States is *Serratia marcescens.*[116] *Serratia* has also been a cause of endocarditis on prosthetic valves.[107,111,117,118] In most instances, *Serratia* endocarditis is subacute, with the diagnosis made by persistent bacteremia and the use of echocardiography. *Escherichia coli,* although the most common cause of bacteremia, infrequently causes endocarditis.[107,119] Echocardiography should be used when there is persistent bacteremia despite adequate antibiotic therapy. *Proteus* rarely causes endocarditis and *Klebsiella* species have caused endocarditis after cardiac surgery. Other species such as *Providencia, Citrobacter,* and *Enterobacter* rarely cause endocarditis except following cardiac surgery. *Pseudomonas aeruginosa* endocarditis is seen predominantly in men who are intravenous drug abusers.[120,121] *Pseudomonas* may involve normal valves and frequently coexists with gram-positive organisms such as streptococci or staphylococci in the addict.[120] *Pseudomonas* also produces endocarditis in patients with malignancy,[122] in burn patients,[123] and in those who have had cardiac surgery. *Pseudomonas cepacia* is another organism that causes nosocomial endocarditis and endocarditis in narcotic addicts.[124,125]

GRAM-POSITIVE BACILLI

Listeria monocytogenes has caused primarily left-sided endocarditis.[126,127] It has been associated with major emboli and a significant mortality. The average age of patients is 53 years with 71% greater than 50 years. Patients usually have preexisting valvular heart disease. Fever often has been low grade and diagnosis made by multiple blood cultures. Lactobacilli also have caused infective endocarditis, as have bacillus species.[128] *Bacillus* is encountered primarily in narcotic addicts or in patients with underlying malignancy.[129,130] *Corynebacterium* (diphtheroids) are uncommon in normal individuals, but they are an important cause of disease in patients with prosthetic heart valves.[131] *Erysipelothrix rhusiopathiae* is a rare cause of endocarditis.

ANAEROBIC BACTERIA

The most common anaerobic organism involved in endocarditis has been *Bacteroides fragilis.*[132–134] Other species such as *Fusobacterium* and *Clostridium* species have also been reported. The classic picture is one of bacterial endocarditis developing on underlying rheumatic heart disease. In most cases of anaerobic endocarditis, the disease is polymicrobial and one in which microaerophilic or anaerobic streptococci are also involved.[135] The normal portal of entry appears to be the gastrointestinal tract, although both *Fusobacterium* and *Bacteroides oralis* or *B melaninogenicus* can arise from a mouth source. *Eikenella corrodens* has caused late infection of prosthetic valves.[136] Whether anaerobic endocarditis has increased in recent years is unclear, because marked improvements in the isolation techniques for anaerobic organisms have been developed in the past decade.

OTHER BACTERIA

Many other bacteria have been reported as isolated causes of infective endocarditis. These include *Brucella, Vibrio, Acinetobacter, Flavobacterium, Kingella,* and *Bordetella* species, but most are isolated case reports.[137–141]

FUNGI

Fungal endocarditis occurs in several settings. It may follow cardiovascular surgery or prolonged intravenous therapy or it may occur in narcotic addicts.[142–144] Fungal endocarditis that follows cardiac surgery most frequently has been due to *Candida albicans.*[143] This was a significant problem in the 1960s and early 1970s and was in large part related to the extensive use of antimicrobial agents at surgery and to poor attention to the prevention of fungal infection. Endocarditis that follows prolonged intravenous administration or antibiotic use or both usually is due to *C albicans.*

Narcotic-associated fungal endocarditis has been on the decline in recent years. In the late 1960s and 1970s it was a fairly frequent occurrence. In contrast to the other *Candida* forms of endocarditis, the species of *Candida* that cause endocarditis in the narcotic addict are different. *Candida parapsilosis, C gulliermondii,* and *C stellatoidea* are the cause of most cases. The source of these organisms is unknown because they rarely are cultured from drug materials.

Other fungi involved in endocarditis include the *Aspergillus* species, the most common being *Aspergillus fumigatus* followed by *A flavus* and *A niger.*[145,146] Again, *Aspergillus* endocarditis seemed to peak in the late 1960s and early 1970s and was probably related to contamination of air in cardiac surgery operating rooms. *Aspergillus* endocarditis infrequently yields positive blood cultures, and virtually none of the patients with this disease survive.[146] Other organisms of a fungal nature that have caused endocarditis at the time of operation have included *Paecilomyces, Phialophora, Hormodendrum,* and *Penicillium mucor.*[147–149] Other fungi that exist in the environment infrequently will cause infective endocarditis. These include *Histoplasma, Blastomyces, Coccidioides,* and *Cryptococcus.*

OTHER MICROORGANISMS

Coxiella burnetii, Q fever, causes endocarditis in the United Kingdom and Australia and rarely in the United States.[150] Q fever endocarditis occurs most often in males who have a history of preexisting heart disease and in over 80% of cases involves the aortic valve.[151] There frequently is a history of an influenza-like illness in the preceding 6 to 12 months. Most patients have hypergammaglobulinemia and thrombocytopenia, and many will develop immune complex glomerulonephritis. Diagnosis may be made by serologic means and Rickettsia can be demonstrated in valve tissue in 60% to 80% of patients. *Chlamydia psittaci* has been the source of endocarditis in a small number of patients in recent years,[152] and *Legionella pneumophila* has also been reported to cause endocarditis on a prosthetic valve.[153]

CULTURE-NEGATIVE ENDOCARDITIS

Blood cultures have reportedly been sterile in approximately 2% to 30% of cases in most large series of endocarditis.[1–4] Several factors may predispose to this particular phenomenon. If cultures are taken toward the end of a prolonged course, usually longer than three months, if the patient has uremia or right-sided endocarditis, or if fastidious organisms such as the *Haemophilus* species are involved, cultures may prove to be negative.[62,154] Furthermore, as already noted, endocarditis due to fungi, rickettsiae, and chlamydiae characteristically are culture-negative.

MICROORGANISMS IN PROSTHETIC VALVE ENDOCARDITIS

Prosthetic valve endocarditis has characteristically been divided into early infection, less than 60 days, and late infection, greater than 60 days.[19,21,22] The most common etiologic agent in both types of prosthetic valve endocarditis is *S epidermidis,* which accounts for 25% to 30% of cases.[155,156] *Staphylococcus aureus* is more frequent in early prosthetic valve endocarditis, approximately 20% versus 10% in late prosthetic valve endocarditis. In patients in whom endocarditis develops one year or more after implantation of a prosthetic valve, streptococcal species, primarily viridans group streptococci, account for 30% of infections.[156] Diphtheroids are seen most frequently in early prosthetic valve endocarditis, as is *C albicans* and *Aspergillus.*

BACTERIA INVOLVED IN INFECTIVE ENDOCARDITIS IN ADDICTS

Consideration of the organisms involved in infective endocarditis in addicts must take into account the presence or absence of underlying valvular disease or the presence of cardiac disease before the development of endocarditis. In addicts with underlying rheumatic disease or congenital abnormalities of valves, endocarditis will develop on the left side due to organisms found in normal individuals.[157] However, among other patients who use intravenous or subcutaneous injection of narcotics, the most common organism is *S aureus* followed by *P aeruginosa* and then *Candida* species. Narcotic addicts are also a major source of methicillin-resistant *S aureus* endocarditis. The incidence of staphylococcal endocarditis in addicts appears to be related primarily to nasal and oral carriage of *S aureus* and not to contamination of heroin or other narcotic products.[158]

TREATMENT OF ENDOCARDITIS

PRINCIPLES OF THERAPY

To achieve cure of endocarditis, a number of factors must be met. It is necessary to follow a bactericidal drug program that can be continued for a long enough period to achieve sterilization of the vegetations. The drug must be administered in concentrations that can penetrate into vegetations to achieve a cure. Finally, the more rapidly the antibiotics kill bacteria in vitro, the more likely it is that organisms will be eradicated. Animal model experiments have delineated many concepts in the therapy of infection.[159]

Most clinical evidence indicates that peak serum bactericidal concentrations greater than or equal to a 1:8 dilution of the patient's serum correlate with a favorable outcome.[160–162] By bactericidal is meant a reduction in the inoculum or organisms, usually 10^5 per milliliter to less than 10^2 per milliliter in 24 hours of incubation. In general, except for unusual circumstances, which will be indicated, the route of administration of antibiotics to treat endocarditis should be parenteral to achieve adequate absorption of the drug. The susceptibility of microorganisms causing endocarditis should be determined by tube or agar dilution to know the precise minimal inhibitory concentration (MIC) and minimal bactericidal concentration (MBC) so that therapy may be appropriately directed. Furthermore, it is critical that the microbiology laboratory be instructed to save the microorganism to ascertain whether therapy is effective. In general, intravascular catheters should not be used in the treatment of endocarditis because they may cause superinfection with other organisms. Unless there is a major need for their use, anticoagulants are to be avoided in patients with endocarditis because of their association with bleeding complications, in particular subarachnoid hemorrhage.

The initial treatment of infective endocarditis in many cases will be instituted while awaiting the results of cultures. Penicillins, cephalosporins to a lesser degree, and vancomycin are the mainstays of therapy. The program that is selected usually has been directed against the most resistant organism. This in general is enterococci. Hence, programs have combined a penicillin or vancomycin and an aminoglycoside. However, if the course is acute and the patient is a parenteral drug user or has a foreign body in the heart, therapy must be directed against staphylococci. Once the cause is known, therapy should be modified to one of the programs listed for a particular organism.

PENICILLIN-SUSCEPTIBLE STREPTOCOCCAL ENDOCARDITIS

Most strains of the viridans group of streptococci are highly susceptible to penicillin with MICs of less than 0.2 μg/ml. However, 15% to 20% of the viridans group of streptococci are resistant to this concentration of penicillin. In addition, some strains of *S mutans* demonstrate a low MIC to penicillin, but the MBC may be as high as 1 to 32 μg/ml. Hence, these organisms should be considered in the penicillin-resistant category. Three regimens have been widely used and have proved effective for penicillin-susceptible streptococcal endocarditis. The first of these is the administration of aqueous penicillin G intravenously for four weeks at a dosage of 12 to 24 million units daily. A second program is to administer aqueous penicillin G in a dosage of 10 to 20 million units intravenously each day or procaine penicillin G 1.2 million units intramuscularly every six hours for four weeks combined with streptomycin 0.5 g intramuscularly every 12 hours for the first two weeks. A third program used at the Mayo Clinic is a two-week course of procaine penicillin 1.2 million units intramuscularly every six hours or aqueous penicillin G 10 to 20 million units intravenously each day, plus streptomycin 0.5 g intramuscularly every 12 hours. These programs will produce cure rates of at least 98%.[163] A course of penicillin alone at 14 to 16 million units each day for 10 to 14 days yielded cures in 85% with a 15% relapse.[164] Although a four-week course of penicillin has yielded 98% cures.[165,166] The four-week penicillin plus two-week streptomycin therapy has also yielded cures of 98%.[167,168] More recently, Wilson et al[169,170] indicated that two weeks of therapy with penicillin by the intramuscular route and streptomycin also intramuscularly is equally effective with a 2.2% failure rate. Table 46.7 presents a comparison of the different methods.

Most institutions in the past have used the four-week intravenous antimicrobial program. However, a major ad-

Table 46.7. Results of Various Treatment Programs for Penicillin-Susceptible Streptococci*

Program	No. of Patients	Relapse No.	Relapse %
Penicillin, 4 wk IV	107	2	2
Penicillin 4 wk IV and Streptomycin 2 wk IM	185	0	0
Penicillin 2 wk IM or IV and Streptomycin 2 wk IM	224	2	1

* From references 165 to 170.
IM = intramuscularly; IV = intravenously.

vantage of two-week therapy is that it is more cost effective than is four weeks of hospitalization and treatment. The major disadvantage of the two-week program is the risk of streptomycin-associated vestibular toxicity. However, four weeks of intravenous antimicrobial therapy may result in other nosocomial infection because of phlebitis at the intravenous sites. In a patient with a penicillin-susceptible strain of streptococcus in whom the duration of the disease exceeds three months, it is probable that the optimal program is four weeks of penicillin plus an initial two weeks of streptomycin. Such a program probably would also be most satisfactory for *S mutans* endocarditis and for the vitamin B_6-requiring streptococci.[64] In the penicillin-allergic patient, a number of different programs are acceptable. Cephalothin, 2 g intravenously every four hours for four weeks, has been used with success, but cefazolin, 1 to 2 g either intramuscularly or intravenously every six hours for four weeks, would be much more cost effective. It has been suggested that when these programs are used, streptomycin should be administered for the initial two weeks. There is no reason to use a second generation or third generation cephalosporin to treat endocarditis. Conversely, a program of vancomycin, 1 g intravenously every 12 hours administered as a single agent for four weeks, has also proved highly successful. The dosage of vancomycin should be adjusted if the patient has depressed renal function. Table 46.8 lists the various programs.

PENICILLIN-RESISTANT STREPTOCOCCAL ENDOCARDITIS

Endocarditis caused by enterococci has been a particular problem because mortality approximates 20% and relapses occur in 12% to 20% of patients.[171] Enterococci are group D streptococci of which *S faecalis* and *S faecium* are the most common cause of enterococcal endocarditis. Enterococci differ from other streptococci because the concentration of penicillin or ampicillin needed to inhibit them is 0.5 to 2 μg/ml. Furthermore, they are not killed at this concentration, but concentrations of 32 to 64 μg/ml are required for killing. In the past *S faecalis* was susceptible to streptomycin, but this is less likely to be true today.[171] Penicillin or ampicillin alone is inadequate therapy for enterococcal endocarditis and an aminoglycoside must be used as well. In the past, streptomycin was routinely combined with penicillin. However, in the past two decades 40% of enterococci fail to be synergistically inhibited when streptomycin is combined with penicillin, whereas synergy of penicillin or ampicillin is noted when these beta-lactams are combined with gentamicin. Sus-

Table 46.8. Treatment Programs for Streptococcal Endocarditis

Antibiotic	Dosage	Route	Duration (wk)	Comment
Penicillin-susceptible streptococci and S bovis				
Penicillin G	12–24 million units every 4 h divided	IV	4	Preferred if elderly patient, symptoms >6 wk
Penicillin G plus	12–24 million units every 4 h divided	IV	4	Symptoms >6 wk
Streptomycin	500 mg every 12 h	IM	2	
Penicillin G plus	18–24 million units every 4 h divided	IV	2	Use if short period of infection
Streptomycin	500 mg every 12 h	IM	2	
Cefazolin or	1 g every 6 h	IV	4	Use if allergic to penicillin
Vancomycin	1 g every 12 h	IV	4	
Enterococcal Endocarditis or Penicillin-resistant Streptococci				
Penicillin	18–24 million units divided 4 h	IV	4–6*	Follow renal function
or				
Ampicillin plus	12 g divided 4 h	IV	4–6*	
Gentamicin	1 mg/kg every 8 h	IV	4–6*	
Vancomycin ±	500 mg every 6 h	IV	6	If penicillin-allergic, and follow hearing and renal function
Gentamicin	1 mg/kg every 8 h	IV	4	

* Six weeks if long duration of symptoms, if mitral valve involved, or both.

IM = intramuscularly; IV = intravenously.

ceptibility to streptomyin has been arbitrarily defined as an enterococcus, *S faecalis,* which is inhibited by less than 2,000 μg/ml of streptomycin. This simple test will demonstrate which patient should receive penicillin-gentamicin rather than penicillin-streptomycin. In some parts of the world, there are strains of enterococci that are resistant even to gentamicin. Optimal therapy for infective endocarditis due to such strains in unknown.[172,173] Other aminoglycosides such as tobramycin and amikacin should not be used to replace gentamicin because some *S faecalis* and particularly *S faecium* are resistant to these agents.[171]

Enterococcal endocarditis should be treated with a combination of either aqueous penicillin G, 20 million units intravenously a day, combined with streptomycin, 0.5 g intramuscularly every 12 hours for six weeks, or with aqueous penicillin G, 20 million units intravenously per day, combined with gentamicin, 1 mg/kg intramuscularly every eight hours (Table 46.8).[173] Studies from the Mayo Clinic[174] suggest that the major factors in relapse of enterococcal endocarditis are infection that has been present for longer than three months before diagnosis and mitral valve infection, particularly in the patient with a calcific mitral valve.

Some investigators prefer to use ampicillin 2 g intravenously administered every four hours for a total dosage of 12 g per day. Some in vitro studies have shown that mezlocillin combined with gentamicin results in more rapid killing of enterococci than does penicillin G–streptomycin, but there is little clinical experience with this combination.

Patients who do not have a long interval between the onset of symptoms and diagnosis (less than three months) and those without mitral valve involvement can be treated for four weeks.[173,174] Patients with these two risk factors should be treated for six weeks. The dosage of gentamicin should be adjusted on the basis of renal function. If serum aminoglycoside levels exceed 1 μg at a trough period, the dosage may need to be decreased. In a significant number of patients who receive more than 3 mg/kg per day of gentamicin, reversible nephrotoxicity will develop. Irreversible vestibular toxicity will develop in approximately 15% of patients receiving streptomycin for four weeks.

It is critical for the physician to realize that cephalosporins have no role in the treatment of penicillin-resistant streptococcal species, such as enterococci. Enterococci are highly resistant to cephalosporins, and clinical trials have been uniformly unsatisfactory. Vancomycin as a single drug at 0.5 g intravenously every six hours has been used to treat enterococcal endocarditis. Vancomycin has also been combined with gentamicin. Unfortunately, such a combination offers a greater chance of toxicity to the kidney and hearing, and there is no clinical proof of a superiority of the combined program over the use of vancomycin alone. A final alternative program for such patients is penicillin desensitization and subsequent therapy with penicillin and an aminoglycoside.

Endocarditis caused by streptococcal species other than enterococci that are not inhibited by 0.2 μg/ml of penicillin requires therapy with 20 million units of penicillin G intravenously each day plus 0.5 g of streptomycin intramuscularly every 12 hours for two weeks or penicillin G 12 to 24 million units intravenously plus gentamicin at a dose of 3 mg/kg per day administered in three equal doses either intravenously or intramuscularly for two weeks. Streptococci of this type may occur in patients who have been receiving oral penicillins that have selected relatively resistant strains in the oral pharynx. Vancomycin should be used to treat endocarditis in penicillin-allergic patients infected with streptococci with penicillin MICs greater than 0.2 μg/ml.

STAPHYLOCOCCAL ENDOCARDITIS

It frequently is extremely difficult to distinguish staphylococcal bacteremia from true endocarditis. An infection due to *S aureus* can cause persistent bacteremia in 10% to 15% of patients. Bacteremia can produce distant abscesses without being due to endocarditis. However, because *S aureus* can produce endocarditis on normal heart valves, the decision on how long treatment should be continued is a most difficult one. Embolic events in the central nervous system, signs of microembolization, and staphylococcal bacteremia in the presence of narcotic addiction or a prosthetic heart valve should always be assumed to be due to endocarditis even in the absence of a murmur or a new murmur. Staphylococcal bacteremia acquired outside the hospital is more likely to produce endocarditis. Endocarditis will develop in less than 5% of patients with staphylococcal bacteremia if promptly treated. In a patient with no underlying valvular disease in whom staphylococcal bacteremia develops, if a focus of infection is readily identified, brief therapy for the infection is indicated.[175] If bacteremia develops due to an infected intravenous catheter, there is a major risk that endocarditis may develop.[176]

It is unfortunate that there still is a high mortality (approximately 35% to 50%) in acute *S aureus* endocarditis. Mortality is highest in patients over 50 years of age, particularly if they have left-sided heart involvement and have had central nervous system manifestations.[100,177] In general, *S aureus* endocarditis in narcotic addicts has a lower mortality than in nonaddicts.[178] Most *S aureus* is resistant to penicillin G. The current recommendation of therapy (Table 46.9) is a penicillinase-resistant penicillin, such as nafcillin or oxacillin 1.5 to 2 g intravenously every four hours for six weeks, or in penicillin-allergic patients, a cephalosporin, cephalothin, 2 g intravenously every four hours, or cefazolin, 2 g every six hours for six weeks. There is no evidence that one antistaphylococcal penicillin is more effective than another. Therefore, in those countries in which cloxacillin is the agent used intravenously, it has been as effective as oxacillin or nafcillin. Methicillin probably should no longer be considered an appropriate agent because there is an undue incidence of renal toxicity when it is used at large doses for six weeks. Failures have occurred with cefazolin because it is not as effective against staphylococci as is cephalothin. New cephalosporins such as cefamandole, cefuroxime, and cefotaxime should not be used to treat staphylococcal endocarditis. A combination of antistaphylococcal penicillin plus an aminoglycoside, gentamicin, produces a synergistic effect

Table 46.9. Treatment Programs for Staphylococcal Endocarditis

Antibiotic	Dosage	Route	Duration (wk)	Comments
Penicillin-Susceptible Isolates				
Penicillin G	24 million divided 4 hourly	IV	4	Beta-lactamase assay must be performed on isolate
Penicillin-Resistant Isolates				
Nafcillin or Oxacillin	2 g every 4 h	IV	4–6	Addict population can be treated 4 wk
Penicillin-Allergic Patients				
Vancomycin or	500 mg every 6 h	IV	6	...
Cephalothin	2 g every 4 h	IV	6	
Methicillin-Resistant Isolates				
Vancomycin plus	500 mg every 6 h	IV	6	Check serum bactericidal titers
Rifampin	300 mg every 12 h	PO	6	

IM = intramuscularly; IV = intravenously; PO = orally.

against *S aureus* both in vitro and in experimental endocarditis in rabbits. However, clinical studies in man have not demonstrated a benefit of such a program.[102,178] Furthermore, there is a greater incidence of nephrotoxicity without improvement in mortality when an aminoglycoside such as gentamicin is combined with an antistaphylococcal penicillin to treat staphylococcal endocarditis. Oral therapy for staphylococcal endocarditis has been used with success in addicts with right-sided endocarditis,[179] but it is never to be recommended in normal subjects.

It is important to remember that in staphylococcal endocarditis the response to therapy tends to be slower than that with streptococcal disease. Indeed, blood cultures may remain positive for up to a week after initiation of appropriate therapy. Furthermore, the patient may remain febrile for seven to ten days after appropriate therapy has been instituted. In the penicillin-allergic patient, vancomycin 0.5 g every six hours intravenously for six weeks is recommended therapy. Although clindamycin has been used to treat patients with staphylococcal endocarditis, there is a large relapse rate and hence the drug cannot be recommended.

Patients with methicillin-resistant *S aureus* endocarditis should be treated with vancomycin.[180] Some patients with methicillin-resistant endocarditis, particularly narcotic addicts, have been treated with trimethoprim-sulfamethoxazole with success.[181] At the present time, several other agents are under study for treatment of methicillin-resistant endocarditis. One of these is teicoplanin, administered 200 mg daily either intravenously or intramuscularly, and the new quinolone antimicrobial agents such as ciprofloxacin 750 mg administered orally every eight hours. However, it is too early to know whether these latter two agents will be as effective as vancomycin has been.

Some staphylococci are relatively tolerant to the action of beta-lactam antibiotics, that is, the difference between the MIC and the MBC is 32-fold or greater.[182] In such patients, the administration of rifampin, 300 mg orally every 12 hours, may be useful. The addition of rifampin will increase serum bactericidal activity and in most cases in which rifampin has been added to penicillin, cephalosporin, or vancomycin, the clinical response has been superior to that with a single agent.[183] Finally, in some situations the use of three agents, that is, antistaphylococcal penicillin, aminoglycoside, and rifampin, may cure such patients; however, persistence of the organism should prompt a consideration of surgery rather than a continuation of drugs.

Staphylococcus epidermidis endocarditis occurs primarily with prosthetic valves. However, the individual in whom *S epidermidis* endocarditis develops on a natural valve should be treated with oxacillin or nafcillin at a dose of 12 g per day for four to six weeks.[184] If the *S epidermidis* is a methicillin-resistant strain, vancomycin should be used, because such strains will not respond uniformly to cephalosporin therapy.

Although most community-acquired *S epidermidis* is beta-lactam susceptible, patients who acquire *S epidermidis* in the hospital acquire methicillin-resistant strains.[185] Therefore, many cases of *S epidermidis* prosthetic valve endocarditis are due to methicillin-resistant isolates. A retrospective study of 55 patients with prosthetic valve endocarditis caused by methicillin-resistant *S epidermidis* demonstrated that vancomycin was most effective.[106] There was an 81% cure rate among 26 patients receiving vancomycin alone or combined with rifampin compared with a beta-lactam–rifampin cure rate of 50%. The role of surgery must be stressed because it frequently is necessary to remove the valve. The best program would be vancomycin, rifampin, and gentamicin, although this increases the risk of ototoxicity and nephrotoxicity. Because the vancomycin MICs of *S epidermidis* that cause prosthetic valve endocarditis are high, it is necessary to use large doses and to monitor blood levels.

ENDOCARDITIS DUE TO *STREPTOCOCCUS PNEUMONIAE, NEISSERIA GONORRHOEAE,* AND *NEISSERIA MENINGITIDIS*

Endocarditis due to pneumococci, gonococci, or meningococci is uncommon at the present time. Most pneumococcal endocarditis occurs in patients with underlying alcoholism. In such patients pneumococcal pneumonia, pneumococcal arthritis, and endocarditis develop affecting primarily the aortic valve. Therapy of this disease is penicillin, 18 to 24 million units intravenously for four weeks. Gonococcal endocarditis in the penicillin era is a rarity.[186] It usually occurs in patients under 30 years of age who have no history of valvular disease. The aortic valve is most often involved with the development of insufficiency. The proper program for treating gonococcal or meningococcal endocarditis is unknown, but most authorities recommend a program of 18 to 24 million units of penicillin G intravenously for a four-week period.

ENDOCARDITIS DUE TO ENTEROBACTERIACEAE

The therapy of endocarditis due to Enterobacteriaceae organisms depends entirely on the antimicrobial susceptibility of the microorganisms. Infective endocarditis due to *E coli* or *Proteus mirabilis* can be treated with ampicillin 12 g per day intravenously if the organisms are susceptible. New cephalosporin antibiotics, such as cefotaxime, ceftizoxime, or ceftazidime, are preferred because of the markedly lower inhibitory concentrations required to inhibit these organisms, and the small discrepancy between inhibition and killing seen with these new cephalosporin antibiotics.

Serratia marcescens endocarditis occurring on the left side of the heart will not respond to medical therapy, even with third generation cephalosporins or with trimethoprim-sulfamethoxazole. Valve replacement is always required to achieve cure. Right-sided endocarditis due to *S marcescens* will respond to therapy with agents such as cefotaxime or ceftizoxime 2 g intravenously every six hours combined with gentamicin 1 to 1.5 mg/kg every eight hours. Therapy should be given a minimum of four weeks and probably six weeks. Alternatively, trimethoprim-sulfamethoxazole at doses of trimethoprim of 12 to 15 mg/kg per day could be used.

Pseudomonas aeruginosa endocarditis on the tricuspid valve may respond to large doses of azlocillin or piperacillin, 18 to 24 g per day administered in doses of 3 to 4 g every four hours, combined with tobramycin, 1.5 mg/kg administered every eight hours. Both drugs would have to be administered for a six-week period. There is a significant degree of nephrotoxicity associated with this program. It may be necessary to remove the tricuspid valve. New agents that can be used in the penicillin-allergic patient are ceftazidime or aztreonam, 2 g every six hours, combined with an aminoglycoside. Ciprofloxacin 750 mg orally every eight hours has also proved successful.

Medical treatment of *P aeruginosa* infective endocarditis involving the left side of the heart is uniformly unsuccessful. Hence, patients with this disease will require early surgical removal of the valve. Whether the use of new agents such as ciprofloxacin will change this is doubtful.

INFECTIVE ENDOCARDITIS DUE TO *HAEMOPHILUS* AND ASSOCIATED SPECIES

Infective endocarditis due to *Haemophilus* species such as *H parainfluenzae, Cardiobacterium hominis,* or *Actinobacillus* organisms should be treated with ampicillin at a dose of 12 g per day for four weeks. It is recommended that initial therapy be a beta-lactam–aminoglycoside combination using gentamicin as the aminoglycoside at a dose of 1 mg/kg every eight hours. Several of the new third generation cephalosporins such as cefotaxime and ceftizoxime have also proved to be effective therapy for endocarditis due to these species in penicillin-allergic patients or in patients who have failed to respond to the aforementioned therapy. The dosage of cefotaxime should be 2 g every six hours or with ceftriaxone it may be possible to administer 2 g every 12 hours.

ENDOCARDITIS DUE TO ANAEROBIC BACILLI

Although infective endocarditis due to anaerobic bacteria such as *B fragilis* is distinctly uncommon, in the rare patient with this illness the most appropriate therapy would be metronidazole, 500 mg administered every six hours for 30 days. Because of the excellent oral absorption of this drug, it can be administered orally. Other agents that may be effective would be clindamycin, 600 mg intravenously every six hours, or piperacillin or mezlocillin, 4 g intravenously every four hours if the organism is susceptible.

FUNGAL ENDOCARDITIS

The mainstay of therapy for fungal endocarditis is surgery. Although all patients with *Candida* or *Aspergillus* endocarditis should be treated with amphotericin B at a dosage of 0.6 mg/kg per day, none of the patients will be cured by this means. Furthermore, there is no evidence that the combination of amphotericin and 5-fluorocytosine will achieve cure, nor will the combination of amphotericin and rifampin. Once a diagnosis of fungal endocarditis is made, therapy with amphotericin should be instituted. Amphotericin produces numerous side effects. We routinely administer a test dose of 1 mg in 100 ml of 5% dextrose in water. If the patient develops chills and fever, before the next dose we administer an antihistamine 50 mg, meperidine 20 mg, and salicylates 600 mg. Subsequently we administer daily doses of 35 to 50 mg of amphotericin in 200 to 300 ml of fluid over a four-hour period. Although it has been recommended that surgery be delayed for one to two weeks of therapy, we believe this is unwise. The infected valve should be removed as soon as diagnosis is made. Delay in removal of the valve merely results in progression of the illness, making ultimate surgery more difficult. Following removal of the valve, it is necessary to continue amphotericin therapy. Our program has been to give a 2-g total dose of amphotericin over a period of time required to achieve that dosage, administering 0.4 to 0.6 mg/kg per day. With this program we have successfully cured several patients. Other fungi causing endocarditis after surgery must be surgically removed and therapy with amphotericin given after surgery.

Q FEVER ENDOCARDITIS

Because the antibiotics effective against *Coxiella burnetti* are only rickettsiostatic, it is necessary to perform surgery in most cases. Mortality using tetracycline as therapy appears to be at least 70%. Organisms have been found in valve tissue even following lengthy therapy. Currently it is recommended that the valve be replaced and tetracycline be administered for 12 months after removal of the valve.[150]

CULTURE-NEGATIVE ENDOCARDITIS

Optimal therapy for endocarditis, which clinically is highly suggested by physical findings and laboratory tests, but not proven by isolation of a microorganism, should consist of either penicillin, 18 to 24 million units per day administered intravenously, plus gentamicin, 1 mg/kg administered every eight hours, or ampicillin, 12 g per day replacing the penicillin. This program is chosen to provide activity against penicillin-resistant streptococci. It is generally recommended that the aminoglycoside be continued for a minimum of two weeks and that the penicillin or ampicillin be continued for a full six weeks. If staphylococcal disease is suggested, a penicillinase-resistant penicillin such as oxacillin is added to the aforementioned program using three drugs.

PROSTHETIC VALVE ENDOCARDITIS

Antibiotic selection for the treatment of prosthetic valve endocarditis is based on the etiologic microorganism and in vitro susceptibility test results (Table 46.10). As with other forms of endocarditis, bactericidal antibiotics are necessary and combinations of antibiotics frequently are used to achieve a synergistic effect in this difficult-to-treat infection. For penicillin-resistant streptococci it is currently recommended that aqueous penicillin G, 20 million units per day intravenously, plus gentamicin be used for six weeks. A similar program is used for resistant streptococci of the viridans group and for enterococci. In the latter case, in the presence of prosthetic valves, eight weeks of therapy is necessary. Prosthetic valve endocarditis due to *S aureus* should be treated with a beta-lactamase–stable penicillin, such as nafcillin. A combination of nafcillin plus rifampin may have some clinical advantage, although this has not been confirmed by large studies. Because a large number of *S epidermidis* organisms, which cause prosthetic valve endocarditis, are resistant to methicillin and hence to all beta-lactams, the current program recommended is a combination of vancomycin, rifampin, and gentamicin, as already discussed.

The most appropriate therapy for diphtheroid prosthetic valve endocarditis is controversial. Vancomycin in combination with rifampin or gentamicin appears to be the most reasonable program. In patients with prosthetic valve endocarditis, when blood cultures are not positive, the most appropriate therapy is vancomycin plus gentamicin, which will provide activity against streptococcal, staphylococcal, and diphtheroid species. Medical cures of prosthetic valve endocarditis are somewhat disappointing. In many situations, relapse is common and the ultimate therapy is surgical. In our own experience, all patients with gram-negative bacteria, *S epidermidis*, and *S aureus* ultimately have required surgery. We have treated streptococcal endocarditis medically with success when the organisms have been penicillin susceptible.

TEST TO MONITOR ANTIMICROBIAL THERAPY

The preceding comments regarding therapy indicate that it is critical that the MIC and MBC be determined for organisms causing endocarditis. Disk sensitivity testing is not reliable and may be misleading. During therapy, the bactericidal activity of serum against the infecting organism can be monitored by serum bactericidal titers, as originally described by Schlicter and MacLean[187] in 1949. The test has been performed in different ways and, hence, there have been great disagreements regarding the interpretation of results. The optimal time to perform the test is at the peak of antimicrobial activity because it is peak concentrations that correlate best with outcome. In general, a serum bactericidal titer 1:8 or greater correlates with therapeutic success in both patients and rabbit models of endocarditis.[159–161] The serum bactericidal titer should be determined several days into therapy. It is critical to obtain blood cultures during therapy at an antibiotic trough period to be certain that the microorganism has been eradicated. Cultures performed immediately after completing a course of therapy are of little value. Most relapses occur in the first several weeks; therefore, follow-up blood cultures should be performed during this time.

SURGICAL THERAPY OF INFECTIVE ENDOCARDITIS

Surgery currently is performed in 25% to 60% of patients with native valve endocarditis and approximately 75% of patients with prosthetic valve endocarditis.[188–194] The generally accepted indications for surgical removal of the valve during active endocarditis are refractory congestive heart failure, more than one systemic embolic episode, uncontrolled infection, ineffective antimicrobial therapy such as fungal endocarditis, resection of mycotic aneurysms or myocardial abscess, valve dysfunction on fluoroscopy, and most cases of prosthetic valve endocarditis.

The most common causes of death in infective endocarditis currently are congestive heart failure, embolic phenomena and local suppurative complications within the heart, or prosthetic valve endocarditis that has failed to improve with antimicrobial therapy. Patients with aortic valve endocarditis in whom congestive heart failure develops with aortic regurgitation have a significant mortality, and surgery should be performed in such patients. It appears that the hemodynamic state of the patient is critical in deciding whether valve replacement should be performed. Although echocardiography is useful in the evaluation and detection of complications of infective en-

Table 46.10. Treatment of Prosthetic Valve Endocarditis

Organisms	Regimen of Choice*	Alternative Regimen*	Duration (wk)
Streptococci			
Penicillin-susceptible (MIC ≤0.2 μg/ml) including *S bovis*	Penicillin G 20 million units/day IV, in divided doses every 4 h	Vancomycin 30 mg/kg/day IV in divided doses every 6 h, or cephalothin 2 g IV every 4 h	6
	Aqueous penicillin G as above plus streptomycin 500 mg IM every 12 h or gentamicin 1 mg/kg IV every 8 h during first 2 wk	Cephalothin or vancomycin as above plus streptomycin or gentamicin in dosages noted during first 2 wk	6
Enterococci and Penicillin-resistant streptococci (MIC >0.2 μg/ml)	Aqueous penicillin G 20 million units/day IV in divided doses every 4 h plus gentamicin 1 mg/kg IV every 8 h	Vancomycin 30 mg/kg/day IV in divided doses every 6 h plus gentamicin in dosages noted	8
Staphylococci			
S aureus (methicillin-susceptible)	Nafcillin or oxacillin 2.0 g IV every 4 h	Cephalothin 2 g IV every 4 h or vancomycin 30 mg/kg/day IV in divided doses every 6 h	8
S aureus (methicillin-resistant)	Vancomycin 30 mg/kg/day IV in divided doses every 6 h	None	8
S epidermidis (methicillin-susceptible)	Nafcillin 2 g IV every 4 h	Vancomycin 0.5 g IV every 6 h	8
S epidermidis (methicillin-resistant)	Vancomycin 30 mg/kg/day IV in divided doses every 6 h plus rifampin 300 mg orally every 8 h	...	8
	Vancomycin and rifampin in above dosages plus gentamicin 1 mg/kg IV every 8 h for first 2 wk		
Diphtheroids	Vancomycin 30 mg/kg/day in divided doses every 6 h alone or plus gentamicin 1 mg/kg IV every 8 h	Penicillin G 24 million units/day IV in 6 doses if susceptible	8
Fastidious gram-negative†	Ampicillin 12–15 g/day in divided doses every 4 h plus gentamicin 1 mg/kg IV every 8 h	Cefotaxime 2 g IV every 6 h alone	6
Candida	Amphotericin B 0.6 to 1.0 mg/kg/day IV + surgery		...

* Dosages given are for adults with normal renal function; appropriate adjustments must be made for patients with renal insufficiency.
† *Hemophilus* species, *Actinobacillus actinomycetemcomitans*, and *Cardiobacterium hominis*.
In all cases the serum bactericidal titer should be checked.

docarditis,[79,194a] hemodynamic monitoring with a Swan-Ganz balloon-floatation catheter remains the most reliable technique for assessment of ventricular function.[194a] A high left ventricular end-diastolic pressure is an indication for prompt surgery.

The mortality in patients with infective endocarditis who are operated on during active disease is no greater than the mortality in patients who do not undergo surgery.[191] However, operative mortality in infected patients is higher than that in patients with noninfective valvular disease.[191] Overall survival rates of patients undergoing replacement for endocarditis are similar to those of patients who have undergone replacement of heart valves electively. Interestingly, the risk of prosthetic valve endocarditis due to the infecting organism is extremely small after surgical removal of a native valve.[195] There has been increased recognition that little is to be gained from delaying surgery once valve replacement is indicated because of hemodynamic deterioration.[194,195] When congestive heart failure persists despite digoxin, diuretics, and other therapeutic modalities, surgical therapy is indicated. It has been suggested that patients over the age of 50 who have endocarditis of the aortic valve due to *S aureus* should undergo surgery because they have an extremely high likelihood of developing severe congestive heart failure within the next two years and dying of cardiac disease.

This clearly is not true in all cases, but the hemodynamic status of such patients must be watched closely after completing therapy and surgery performed if congestive heart failure develops. In tricuspid endocarditis in drug addicts, tricuspid valvectomy without replacement has been the recommended practice, because not only is there less chance for reinfection following resumption of intravenous drug abuse, but tricuspid valvectomy is also hemodynamically well-tolerated.[195a] However, this approach has recently been challenged.[195b] In the patient with prosthetic valve endocarditis, the risk of recurrence due to the original infecting organism has been a problem in 0 to 15% of patients.[194] Valve replacement is recommended in all patients with prosthetic valve endocarditis in whom moderate to severe heart failure develops. Marked instability of the prosthesis also is an indication for surgery, and patients in whom prosthetic obstruction develops due to large vegetations require emergency surgery.[194,195] The precise length of time a patient should be treated with antibiotics following removal of an infected valve is unknown. Most authorities currently treat for one to three weeks depending on the degree of infection, the operative findings, and the type of organism. In staphylococcal disease or fungal infection, a longer period of therapy is necessary.

It is important to realize that a patient who has class III or IV heart failure and has responded to a course of antimicrobial therapy may still require cardiac valve replacement. Clearly, if the heart failure is unresponsive in 24 to 48 hours, valve replacement should be considered. Those patients who begin the illness with class II heart failure and who deteriorate to class III or IV should undergo cardiac valve replacement.[195] The risk of valve dehiscence and prosthetic valve endocarditis is higher in patients with active endocarditis at the time of operation than in patients who have already had therapy and had the blood stream cleared of microorganisms.[196] If the patient with endocarditis has a relapse following an adequate course of therapy, a second treatment course is acceptable if the microorganism is a nutritional variant streptococcus or an enterococcus. With gram-negative bacteria, however, it is probably necessary to proceed with cardiac valve replacement. Myocardial abscesses at the present time can be followed using two-dimensional echocardiography to guide the decision as to when surgery may be necessary.[197] Some patients with abscesses due to highly susceptible organisms may respond to antimicrobial therapy alone.

MANAGEMENT OF EXTRACARDIAC COMPLICATIONS OF INFECTIVE ENDOCARDITIS

The decisions regarding management of extracardiac complications of endocarditis are complex.[198] Approximately 30% of patients will have clinically apparent emboli. The highest frequency of embolic events occurs with organisms that produce large mobile vegetations such as the *H parainfluenzae,* some other fastidious gram-negative bacilli, and fungi such as *Aspergillus.* If the two-dimensional echocardiography reveals large mobile valve vegetations and the microorganism is one associated with a high risk of embolization, surgical replacement of the valve should be considered.[83] If there are large vegetations caused by microorganisms infrequently associated with embolization, a medical program should be followed. Following an embolism, the presence of a large vegetation should prompt early operation, whereas the absence of vegetations on two-dimensional echocardiography indicates that medical treatment can be continued.[81-83]

Although mycotic aneurysms are an uncommon finding in patients with infective endocarditis, they have been recognized increasingly in recent years and probably constitute between 2% and 6% of intracranial aneurysms.[199] The patient with severe or localized headaches should undergo computed tomographic scanning with contrast material. If this does not delineate the lesion and if there is evidence of a bleeding central nervous system episode, angiography should be performed because it may be possible to remove or wrap an intracerebral mycotic aneurysm.

PROPHYLAXIS OF INFECTIVE ENDOCARDITIS

To develop a practical program for prophylaxis of infective endocarditis, it is necessary to understand the relative risk of bacteremia following various procedures. Table 46.2 indicates the incidence of transient bacteremia after different procedures. Such information can be further evaluated with regard to those procedures that are at significant risk or very low risk. For example, dental procedures likely to cause bleeding, oral surgery involving the teeth or gums, delivery, abortion, or insertion of an intrauterine device, tonsillectomy and adenoidectomy, urinary catheterization or other urinary procedures and drainage of abscesses all are associated with a significant risk of bacteremia. Other procedures such as examination of the teeth or adjustment of orthodontic appliances, cardiac catheterization, endotracheal intubation, or diagnostic procedures such as liver biopsy, bronchoscopy, or barium enema are associated with a very low or negligible risk of bacteremia. It is also necessary to understand those cardiac conditions in which there is a high risk of endocarditis versus those in which the risk is relatively low or negligible (Table 46.11).

Antibiotic prophylaxis should be prescribed for patients who have congenital or valvular heart diseases or a cardiac prosthesis. The procedures that should be covered are those associated with a high risk of bacteremia. In the past, errors have occurred in the administration of antibiotics to prevent endocarditis. These were starting antibiotics too early, which usually resulted in replacement of the normal susceptible oral flora with resistant organisms in the mouth, continuing antimicrobial agents for too long, which also predisposed to resistance, and using small doses of antibiotics that did not significantly reduce the number of microorganisms. The primary goal of prophylaxis is to reduce the number of microorganisms in the circulation and to alter the surface properties of the microorganism by persisting subinhibitory concentrations of the antimicrobial agents, which will decrease the ability of the microorganisms to adhere to valvular tissue.

No controlled trials of prophylaxis have been performed because of the numbers needed to obtain inter-

Table 46.11. Risk for Development of Infective Endocarditis As a Result of Various Cardiac Lesions

Relatively High Risk	Intermediate Risk	Very Low or Negligible Risk
Prosthetic heart valves	Mitral valve prolapse	Atrial septal defect
Aortic valve disease	Isolated mitral stenosis	Arteriosclerotic plaques
Previous infective endocarditis	Calcific aortic sclerosis	Syphilitic aortitis
Mitral insufficiency	Tricuspid valvular disease	Cardiac pacemakers
Patent ductus arteriosus	Pulmonary valvular disease	
Ventricular septal defect	Asymmetric septal hypertrophy	
Coarctation of the aorta	Catheters in right heart	
Marfan's syndrome	Intracardiac prosthetic implants	

pretable results and because of the ethical question of a control group.[200] Endocarditis has developed despite prophylaxis.[201] Most cases (92%) occurred after dental procedures and were primarily due to the viridans group of streptococci. Ironically, in 60% of cases the organism was susceptible to the antibiotic used for prophylaxis. Mitral valve prolapse was found in 33% of cases, congenital lesions in 29%, and rheumatic heart disease in 21%. These data further indicate the importance of mitral valve prolapse as a predisposition to endocarditis.

It is interesting that patients who have had endocarditis are at greater risk of developing endocarditis.[202] Patients with mitral valve prolapse are eight times more likely to develop endocarditis than are normal subjects.[203] However, Clemens and Ransohoff[203] calculated that prophylaxis was not really cost effective.

The rationale for prophylaxis during gastrointestinal procedures is not based on many data because extremely few cases of endocarditis have followed gastrointestinal diagnostic procedures.[204,205]

Current recommendations (Table 46.12)[206] for prophylaxis of endocarditis for dental procedures suggest the use of penicillin, 2 g orally one hour before and 1 g six hours later. For high risk patients undergoing gastrointestinal or genitourinary tract procedures with a high risk of bacteremia, ampicillin, 2 g intramuscularly or intravenously, plus gentamicin 1.5 mg/kg intramuscularly or intravenously one half hour before the procedure. In penicillin-allergic patients, vancomycin at a dose of 1 g administered slowly over one hour before the procedure should prove effective and need not be repeated. If this is not feasible, erythromycin 1 g should be used one hour before the procedure followed by 1 g six hours later.

The recommendations of the British Society of Antimicrobial Chemotherapy are 3 g of oral amoxicillin in a single dose for dental procedures and erythromycin for the penicillin-allergic patient.[207] For genitourinary and gastrointestinal procedures they recommend intramuscular amoxicillin and gentamicin, using vancomycin in the penicillin-allergic patient. The single oral 3-g amox-

Table 46.12. Prophylaxis of Endocarditis*

Standard Regimens	for dental procedures and oral or upper respiratory tract surgery	penicillin V 2.0 g orally 1 h before, then 1.0 g 6 h later†
	oral regimen for penicillin-allergic patients (oral and respiratory tract only)	erythromycin 1.0 g orally 1 h before, then 0.5 g 6 h later†
Special Regimens	parenteral regimen for high risk patients; also for GI or GU tract procedures	ampicillin 2.0 g IM or IV *plus* gentamicin 1.5 mg/kg IM or IV, 0.5 to 1 h before†
	parenteral regimen for penicillin-allergic patients	vancomycin 1.0 g IV slowly over 1 h, starting 1 h before; *add* gentamicin 1.5 mg/kg IM or IV if GI or GU tract involved†
	oral regimen for minor GI or GU tract procedures	amoxicillin 3.0 g orally 1 h before, then 1.5 g 6 h later†
	cardiac surgery, including implantation of prosthetic valves	cefazolin 2.0 g IV at induction of anesthesia, repeated 8 and 16 h later; gentamicin 1.5 mg/kg if gram-negative bacteria a problem in the institution

* (1) These regimens are empiric suggestions; no regimen has been *proven* effective for prevention of endocarditis and prevention failures may occur with any regimen; (2) these regimens are not intended to cover all clinical situations; judgment on safety and cost–benefit issues should be considered in each individual case; (3) one or two additional doses may be given if the period of risk for bacteremia is prolonged.

† *Pediatric dosages*: ampicillin 50 mg/kg; erythromycin 20 mg/kg for first dose, then 10 mg/kg; gentamicin 2.0 mg/kg; penicillin V and amoxicillin, for children who weigh more than 60 pounds, use same as for adults; for children less than 60 pounds, use half the adult dose; vancomycin 20 mg/kg.

icillin regimen would give dentists, who rarely inject antibiotics, one standard simpler method with which they are more prone to comply.[208]

During open heart surgery, an antimicrobial prophylactic program currently is recommended, although good clinical studies have not been performed to establish the value of this prophylaxis.[206] Postcardiotomy endocarditis most frequently would be caused by staphylococci. Hence, prophylaxis should be limited to a short course of an antistaphylococcal agent, such as a cephalosporin, or vancomycin.[209] At the present time the recommended therapy is cefazolin, 2 g intravenously at the induction of anesthesia with repeated doses administered at 8 and 16 hours. For the penicillin-allergic patient, vancomycin 1 g should be administered one hour before induction and then 0.5 g intravenously 8 and 16 hours later. When it is known that there have been gram-negative infections due to *Pseudomonas, Enterobacter,* or *Serratia,* an aminoglycoside such as gentamicin can be administered simultaneously with cefazolin or vancomycin.

REFERENCES

1. Garvey G, Neu HC: Infective endocarditis: an evolving disease. *Medicine* 1978; 57:105–127.
2. Pelletier LL, Petersdorf RG: Infective endocarditis. A review of 125 cases from the University of Washington Hospitals. *Medicine* 1977; 56:287–298.
3. Cherubin CE, Neu HC: Infective endocarditis at The Presbyterian Hospital in New York City from 1938-1967. *Am J Med* 1971; 51:83–96.
4. Von Reym CF, Levy BS, Arbeit RD: Infective endocarditis: an analysis based on strict definitions. *Ann Intern Med* 1982; 94:505–511.
5. Thayer WS: Studies on bacterial (infective) endocarditis. *Johns Hopkins Hosp Rep* 1926; 21:1–7.
6. Johnson CM, Rhodes KH: Pediatric endocarditis. *Mayo Clin Proc* 1982; 57:86–94.
7. Kaplan EL: Infective endocarditis in the pediatric age group: an overview, in Kaplan EL, Taranta AV (eds): *Infective Endocarditis.* Dallas, American Heart Association, 1977, pp 51–54.
8. Chambers HF, Korzeniowski OM, Sande MA, National Collaborative Endocarditis Study Group: *Staphylococcus aureus* endocarditis: clinical manifestations in addicts and non-addicts. *Medicine* 1983; 62:170–177.
9. Venezio FR, Westenfelder GO, Cook FV, Emmerman J, Phair JP: Infective endocarditis in a community hospital. *Arch Intern Med* 1982; 142:789–792.
10. Roberts WC, Buchbinder NA: Right-sided valvular infective endocarditis. A clinicopathological study of 12 necropsy patients. *Am J Med* 1972; 53:7–12.
11. Dreyer NP, Fields BN: Heroin-associated endocarditis. *Ann Intern Med* 1973; 76:699–702.
12. Tuazon CU, Cardella TA, Sheagren JN: Staphylococcal endocarditis in drug users. *Arch Intern Med* 1975; 135:1555–1561.
13. Blumenfeld S, Griffiths SP, Morgan BC: Bacterial endocarditis in children with heart disease: a review based on the literature and experience with 58 cases. *Pediatrics* 1960; 26:993–1017.
14. Moulsdale MT, Eykyn SJ, Phillips I: Infective endocarditis; 1970-1979. A study of culture-positive cases in St. Thomas' Hospital. *Quart J Med* 1980; 49:315–326.
15. Chagnac A, Rudniki C, Loebel H, Zahavi I: Infectious endocarditis in idiopathic hypertrophic subaortic stenosis. Report of three cases and review of the literature. *Chest* 1982; 81:346–349.
16. Corrigan D, Bolen J, Hancock EW, Popp RL: Mitral valve prolapse and infective endocarditis. *Am J Med* 1977; 63:215–222.
17. Clemens JD, Horwitz RI, Jaffe CC: A controlled evaluation of bacterial endocarditis in persons with mitral-valve prolapse. *N Engl J Med* 1982; 307:776–780.
18. Nolan CM, Kane JJ, Grunow WA: Infective endocarditis and mitral valve prolapse: a comparison with other types of endocarditis. *Arch Intern Med* 1982; 14:447–450.
19. Wilson WR, Danielson GK, Guiliani ER, Geraci JE: Prosthetic valve endocarditis. *Mayo Clin Proc* 1982; 57:155–161.
20. Masur H, Johnson WD Jr: Prosthetic valve endocarditis. *J Thorac Cardiovasc Surg* 1980; 80:31–37.
21. Dismukes WE, Karchmer AW, Buckley MJ, Austen WG, Swartz MN: Prosthetic valve endocarditis: analysis of 38 cases. *Circulation* 1973; 48:365–377.
22. Slaughter L, Morris JE, Starr A: Prosthetic valve endocarditis: a 12-year review. *Circulation* 1973; 47:1319–1326.
23. Dismukes WE: Prosthetic valve endocarditis: factors influencing outcome and recommendations for therapy, in Bisno AL (ed): *Treatment of Infective Endocarditis.* New York, Grune & Stratton, 1981, pp 167–181.
24. Wilson WR, Jaumin PM, Danielson GK, Guilliani ER, Washington JA II, Geraci JE: Prosthetic valve endocarditis. *Ann Intern Med* 1975; 82:751–756.
25. Rossiter SJ, Stimson EB, Dyer PE, Miller DC, Schapira JN, Martin RP, Shumway NE: Prosthetic valve endocarditis: comparison of heterograft tissue valves and mechanical valves. *J Thorac Cardiovasc Surg* 1978; 76:795–802.
26. Scheld WM: Pathogenesis and pathophysiology of infective endocarditis, in Sande MA, Kaye D, Root RK (eds): *Endocarditis.* New York, Churchill Livingstone, 1984, pp 1–32.
27. Garrison PK, Freedman LR: Experimental endocarditis. I. Staphylococcal endocarditis in rabbits resulting from placement of a polyethylene catheter in the right side of the heart. *Yale J Biol Med* 1970; 42:399–410.
28. Durack DT, Beeson PB, Petersdorf RG: Experimental bacterial endocarditis. III. Production and progress of the disease in rabbits. *Br J Exp Pathol* 1973; 54:142–151.
29. Freedman LR: The nonbacterial thrombotic vegetation, in *Infective Endocarditis.* New York, Plenum, 1982, pp 9–25.
30. Rodbard S: Blood velocity and endocarditis. *Circulation* 1960; 27:18–28.
31. Angist HA, Oka M: Pathogenesis of bacterial endocarditis. *JAMA* 1983; 183:294–297.
32. Everett ED, Hirschmann JV: Transient bacteremia and endocarditis prophylaxis: a review. *Medicine* 1977; 56:61–72.
33. Rogosa M, Hampp EG, Nevin TA, Wagner HN Jr, Driscoll EJ, Baer PN: Blood sampling and cultural studies in the detection of postoperative bacteremias. *J Am Dent Assoc* 1960; 60:171–180.
34. Durack DT, Beeson PB: Protective role of complement in experimental *Escherichia coli* endocarditis. *Infect Immun* 1977; 16:213–217.
35. Durack DT, Gilliland BC, Petersdorf RG: Effect of immunization on susceptibility to experimental *Streptococcus mutans* and *Streptococcus sanguis* endocarditis. *Infect Immun* 1978; 22:52–56.
36. Adler SW, Selinger DS, Reed WP: Effect of immunization on the genesis of pneumococcal endocarditis in rabbits. *Infect Immun* 1981; 34:55–61.
37. Gould K, Ramirez-Ronda CH, Holmes RK, Sanford JP: Adherence of bacteria to heart valves in vitro. *J Clin Invest* 1975; 56:1364–1370.
38. Scheld WM, Valone JA, Sande MA: Bacterial adherence in the pathogenesis of endocarditis. *J Clin Invest* 1978; 61:1394–1404.
39. Ramirez-Ronda CH: Adherence of glucan-positive and glucan-negative streptococcal strains to normal and damaged heart valves. *J Clin Invest* 1978; 62:805–814.
40. Abraham SN, Beachey EH, Simpson WA: Adherence of *Streptococcus pyogenes, Escherichia coli* and *Pseudomonas aeruginosa* to fibronectin-coated and uncoated epithelial cells. *Infect Immun* 1983; 41:1261–1268.
41. Durack DT, Beeson PB: Experimental bacterial endocarditis. II. Survival of bacteria in endocardial vegetations. *Br J Exp Pathol* 1972; 51:50–62.
42. Drake TA, Rodgers GM, Sande MA: Tissue factor is a major stimulus for vegetation formation in enterococcal endocarditis in rabbits. *J Clin Invest* 1984; 73:1750–1753.
43. VanGirkel CJW, Thorig L, Thompson J, Oh JIH, vanAllen WG: Enhancement of generation of monocyto tissue thromboplastin by bacterial phagocytosis. Possible pathway for fibrin formation on infected vegetations in bacterial endocarditis. *Infect Immun* 1979; 25:388–395.
44. Medders MJM, Thompson J, Bauer WC, VanFurth R: Role of granulocytes and monocytes in experimental *Escherichia coli* endocarditis. *Infect Immun* 1984; 43:491–496.
45. Weinstein L, Schlesinger JJ: Pathoanatomic, pathophysiologic and clinical correlations in endocarditis. *N Engl J Med* 1974; 291:832–837.
46. Krause JR, Levison SP: Pathology of infective endocarditis, in Kaye D (ed): *Infective Endocarditis.* Baltimore, University Park Press, 1976, pp 55–86.
47. Roberts WC: Characteristics and consequences of infective endocarditis (active or healed or both) learned from morphological studies, in Rahimtoola SH (ed): *Infective Endocarditis.* New York, Grune & Stratton, 1978, pp 55–123.
48. Gutman RA, Striker GE, Gilliland BC, Cutler RE: The immune complex glomerulonephritis of bacterial endocarditis. *Medicine* 1972; 51:1–25.
49. Levy RL, Hong R: The immune nature of subacute bacterial endocarditis (SBE) nephritis. *Am J Med* 1973; 54:645–652.
50. Ziment I: Nervous system complications in bacterial endocarditis. *Am J Med* 1969; 47:593–607.
51. Jones HR Jr, Siekert RG, Geraci JE: Neurologic manifestations of bacterial endocarditis. *Ann Intern Med* 1969; 71:21–28.
52. Greenlee JE, Mandell GL: Neurological manifestations of infective endocarditis. A review. *Stroke* 1973; 4:958–969.
53. Starkbaum M, Durack DE, Beeson PB: The "incubation period" of subacute bacterial endocarditis. *Yale J Biol Med* 1977; 50:49–58.

54. Hermans PE: The clinical manifestations of infective endocarditis. *Mayo Clin Proc* 1982; 57:15–21.
55. Churchill MA Jr, Geraci JE, Hunder GG: Musculoskeletal manifestations of bacterial endocarditis. *Ann Intern Med* 1977; 87:754–759.
56. Alpert JS, Krow HF, Dalen JE: Pathogenesis of Osler's nodes. *Ann Intern Med* 1976; 85:471–475.
57. Watanakunakorn C: Prosthetic valve endocarditis. A review. *Prog Cardiovasc Dis* 1979; 22:181–204.
58. Werner AS, Cobbs GE, Kaye D, Hook EW: Studies on the bacteremia of bacterial endocarditis. *JAMA* 1967; 202:199–203.
59. Mallen MS, Hube EL, Brenes M: Comparative study of blood cultures made from artery, vein, and bone marrow in patients with subacute bacterial endocarditis. *Am Heart J* 1947; 33:692–695.
60. Washington JA II: The role of the microbiology laboratory in the diagnosis and antimicrobial treatment of infective endocarditis. *Mayo Clin Proc* 1982; 57:22–32.
61. Weiss H, Ottenberg R: Relation between bacteremia and temperature in subacute bacterial endocarditis. *J Infect Dis* 1932; 50:61–68.
62. Persanti EL, Smith IM: Infective endocarditis with negative blood cultures: an analysis of 52 cases. *Am J Med* 1979; 66:43–50.
63. Geraci JE, Wilson WR, Washington JA II: Infective endocarditis caused by *Actinobacillus actinomycetemcomitans:* report of four cases. *Mayo Clin Proc* 1980; 55:415–419.
64. Roberts RB, Krieger AG, Schiller NL, Gross KC: Viridans streptococcal endocarditis: the role of various species, including pyridoxal-dependent streptococci. *Rev Infect Dis* 1979; 1:955–965.
65. Hall MM, Mueske CA, Istrup DM, Washington JA II: Evaluation of a biphasic medium for blood cultures. *J Clin Microbiol* 1979; 10:673–676.
66. Tuazon CU, Sheagren JN: Teichoic acid antibodies in the diagnosis of serious infections with *Staphylococcus aureus. Ann Intern Med* 1976; 84:543–546.
67. Tenenbaum MJ, Archer GL: Prognostic value of teichoic acid antibodies in *Staphylococcus aureus* bacteremia: a reassessment. *South Med J* 1980; 73:140–143.
68. Wheat LJ, Kohler RB, White A: Teichoic acid antibody determination by agar-gel diffusion: effect of using dilute antigen preparations. *J Clin Microbiol* 1979; 10:138–140.
69. Bayer AS, Tillman DB, Concepcion N, Guze LB: Clinical value of teichoic acid antibody titers in the diagnosis and management of the staphylococcemias. *West J Med* 1980; 132:294–300.
70. Bayer AS, Theofilopoulos AN, Tillman DB, Dixon FJ, Guze LB: Use of circulating immune complex levels in the serodifferentiation of endocarditic and nonendocarditic septicemias. *Am J Med* 1979; 66:58–62.
71. Kauffmann RH, Thompson J, Valentin DM, Daha MR, Van Es LA: The clinical implications and the pathogenetic significance of circulating immune complexes in infective endocarditis. *Am J Med* 1981; 71:17–25.
72. McKenzie PE, Hawke D, Woodroffe AJ, Thompson AJ, Seymour AE, Clarkson AR: Serum and tissue immune complexes in infective endocarditis. *J Clin Lab Immunol* 1980; 4:125–132.
73. Hooper DC, Bayer AC, Karchmer AM, Theofilopoulos AN, Swartz MN: Circulating immune complexes in prosthetic valve endocarditis. *Arch Intern Med* 1983; 143:2081–2084.
74. Dillon JC, Feigenbaum H, Koenecke LL: Echocardiographic manifestations of valvular vegetations. *Am Heart J* 1973; 86:698–706.
75. Ginzton LE, Seigal RJ, Criley JM: Natural history of tricuspid valve endocarditis: a two dimensional echocardiographic study. *Am J Cardiol* 1982; 49:1853–1859.
76. Hickey AJ, Wolfers J, Wilcken DE: Reliability and clinical relevance of detection of vegetations by echocardiography in bacterial endocarditis. *Br Heart J* 1981; 46:624–628.
77. Nagata S, Park YD, Nagae K, Beppu S, Kawazoe K, Fujita T, Sakakibara H, Nimura Y: Echocardiographic features of bioprosthetic valve endocarditis. *Br Heart J* 1984; 51:263–266.
77a. Robbins MJ, Soeiro R, Frishman WH, Strom JA: Right-sided valvular endocarditis: etiology, diagnosis, and an approach to therapy. *Am Heart J* 1986; 111:128–135.
77b. Robbins MJ, Frater RWM, Soeiro R, Frishman WH, Strom JA: Influence of vegetation size on the clinical outcome of right-sided infective endocarditis. *Am J Med* 1986; 80:165–171.
78. Peterson SP, Schiller N, Stricker RB: Failure of two-dimensional echocardiography to detect Aspergillus endocarditis. *Chest* 1984; 85:291–294.
79. Come PC, Isaacs RE, Riley MF: Diagnostic accuracy of M-mode echocardiography in active infective endocarditis and prognostic implications of ultrasound-detectable vegetations. *Am Heart J* 1982; 103:839–847.
80. Scanlan JG, Seward JB, Tajik AJ: Valve ring abscess in infective endocarditis: visualization with wide angle two dimensional echocardiography. *Am J Cardiol* 1982; 149:1794–1800.
81. Davis RS, Strom JA, Frishman W, Becker R, Matsumoto M, Lejentel TH, Sonnenblick EH, Frater RWM: The demonstration of vegetations by echocardiography in bacterial endocarditis: an indication for early surgical intervention. *Am J Med* 1980; 69:57–63.
82. Mintz GS, Kotler MN: Clinical value and limitations of echocardiography. Its use in the study of patients with infectious endocarditis. *Arch Intern Med* 1980; 140:1022–1026.
83. Wong D, Chandraratna HM, Wishnow RM, Dusitnanond V, Nisalasuriya A: Clinical implications of large vegetations in infectious endocarditis. *Arch Intern Med* 1983; 143:1874–1877.
84. Wong DW, Dhawan VK, Tanaka T, Mishkin FS, Reese IC, Thadepalli H: Imaging endocarditis with TC-99m labeled antibody: an experimental study. *J Nucl Med* 1982; 23:229–234.
85. Cowan JC, Patrick D, Reid DS: Aortic root abscess complicating bacterial endocarditis. Demonstration by computed tomography. *Br Heart J* 1984; 52:591–593.
86. Bayliss R, Clarke C, Oakley CM, Somerville W, Whitfield AG, Young SE: The microbiology and pathogenesis of infective endocarditis. *Br Med J* 1983; 50:513–519.
87. Nakamura K, Koyanagi H, Hirosawa K: Spectrum of infective endocarditis in the past five years. *Jpn Circ J* 1982; 46:352–361.
88. Parker MT, Ball LC: Streptococci and aerococci associated with systemic infection in man. *J Med Microbiol* 1976; 9:275–302.
89. Harder EJ, Wilkoswke CJ, Washington JA II: *Streptococcus mutans* endocarditis. *Ann Intern Med* 1974; 80:364–369.
90. Watanakunakorn C: *Streptococcus bovis* endocarditis. *Am J Med* 1974; 56:256–263.
91. Moellering RC, Watson BK, Kunz LJ: Endocarditis due to group D streptococci. Comparison of diseases caused by *Streptococcus bovis* with that produced by enterococci. *Am J Med* 1974; 57:239–250.
92. Hoppes WL, Lerner PI: Nonenterococcal group D streptococcal endocarditis caused by *Streptococcus bovis. Ann Intern Med* 1974; 81:588–592.
93. Steinberg D, Nagger CZ: *Streptococcus bovis* endocarditis with carcinoma of the colon. *N Engl J Med* 1977; 297:115–120.
94. Klein RS, Remco RA, Catalano MT: Association of *Streptococcus bovis* with carcinoma of the colon. *N Engl J Med* 1977; 297:800–803.
95. Mandell GL, Kaye D, Levison ME, Hook EW: Enterococcal endocarditis: an analysis of 38 patients observed at the New York Hospital-Cornell Medical Center. *Arch Intern Med* 1970; 125:238–264.
96. Reid TMS: Group B streptococcal endocarditis. *South Med J* 1977; 22:13–18.
97. Shlaes DM, Lerner PI, Wolinsky E: Infections due to Lancefield group F and related streptococci *(S. milleri, S. angiosus). Medicine* 1981; 60:197–203.
98. Hosea SW: Virulent *Streptococcus viridans* bacterial endocarditis. *Am Heart J* 1981; 101:174–178.
99. Wilson R, Hamburger M: Fifteen years' experience with staphylococcal septicemia in a large city hospital: analysis of fifty-five cases in the Cincinnati General Hospital 1940 to 1954. *Am J Med* 1957; 22:437–457.
100. Watanakunakorn C, Tan JS, Phair JP: Some salient features of *Staphylococcus aureus* endocarditis. *Am J Med* 1973; 54:473–480.
101. Bayer AS: Staphylococcal bacteremia and endocarditis. State of the art. *Arch Intern Med* 1982; 142:1169–1173.
102. Watanakunakorn C, Baird IM: Prognostic factors in *Staphylococcus aureus* endocarditis and results of therapy with a penicillin and gentamicin. *Am J Med Sci* 1977; 273:133–139.
103. Levine DP, Cushing RD, Jui J, Brown WJ: Community acquired methicillin-resistant *Staphylococcus aureus* endocarditis in the Detroit Medical Center. *Ann Intern Med* 1982; 97:330–338.
104. Geraci JE, Hanson KC, Guiliani ER: Endocarditis caused by coagulase negative staphylococci. *Mayo Clin Proc* 1968; 43:420–434.
105. Tuazon CU, Miller H: Clinical and microbiological aspects of serious infections caused by *Staphylococcus epidermidis. Scand J Infect Dis* 1983; 15:347–360.
106. Karchmer AW, Archer GL, Dismukes W: *Staphylococcus epidermidis* causing prosthetic valve endocarditis: microbiological and clinical observations as guides to therapy. *Ann Intern Med* 1983; 98:447–455.
107. Cohen PS, Maguire JH, Weinstein L: Infective endocarditis caused by gram-negative bacteria: a review of the literature 1945-1977. *Prog Cardiovasc Dis* 1980; 22:205–242.
108. Geraci JE, Wilson WR: Endocarditis due to gram-negative bacteria: report of 56 cases. *Mayo Clin Proc* 1982; 57:145–148.
109. Geraci JE, Wilkoswke CJ, Wilson WR, Washington JA II: *Haemophilis* endocarditis: report of 14 patients. *Mayo Clin Proc* 1977; 52:209–215.
110. Lynn DJ, Kane JG, Parker RH: *Haemophilus parainfluenzae* and *influenzae* endocarditis: a review of 40 cases. *Medicine* 1977; 56:115–127.
111. Geraci JE, Greippo PR, Wikoswke CJ, Wilson WR, Washington JA II: *Cardiobacterium hominis* endocarditis: four cases with clinical and laboratory observations. *Mayo Clin Proc* 1978; 53:49–53.
112. Ellner JJ, Rosenthal MS, Lerner PI, McHenry MC: Infective endocarditis caused by slow-growing, fastidious gram-negative bacteria. *Medicine* 1979; 58:145–158.
113. Parker SW, Apicella MA, Fuller CM: *Haemophilus* endocarditis. Two patients with complications. *Arch Intern Med* 1983; 143:48–51.
114. Rich M, St Mary E: Case reports: *Salmonella* subacute endocarditis. *Ann Intern Med* 1956; 44:162–166.
115. Schneider PJ, Nernoff J, Gold JA: Acute *Salmonella* endocarditis: report of a case and review. *Arch Intern Med* 1967; 120:478–482.

116. Mills J, Drew D: *Serratia marcescens* endocarditis. A regional illness associated with intravenous drug abuse. *Ann Intern Med* 1976; 84:29–35.
117. Quintiliani R, Gilford RH: Endocarditis from *Serratia marcescens*. *JAMA* 1969; 208:2055–2059.
118. Williams JC Jr, Johnson JE III: *Serratia marcescens* endocarditis. *Arch Intern Med* 1970; 125:1038–1040.
119. Hansing CE, Allen VD, Cherry JD: *Escherichia coli* endocarditis: a review of the literature and a case study. *Arch Intern Med* 1967; 120:472–477.
120. Reyes MP, Lerner AM: Current problems in the treatment of infective endocarditis due to *Pseudomonas aeruginosa*. *Rev Infect Dis* 1983; 5:114–126.
121. Archer G, Fekety FR, Supena R: *Pseudomonas aeruginosa* endocarditis in drug addicts. *Am Heart J* 1974; 88:570–578.
122. Saroff AL, Armstrong D, Johnson WD: *Pseudomonas* endocarditis. *Am J Cardiol* 1973; 32:234–237.
123. Robinson OG, Hoopes JE, Conn JH: Acute bacterial endocarditis in a burned patient. *Ann Surg* 1964; 30:617–618.
124. Noriega ER, Rubinstein E, Simberkoff MS, Rahal JJ: Subacute and acute endocarditis due to *Pseudomonas cepacia* in heroin addicts. *Am J Med* 1975; 59:29–36.
125. Neu HC, Garvey GJ, Beach MP: Successful treatment of *Pseudomonas cepacia* endocarditis in a heroin addict with trimethoprim-sulfamethoxazole. *J Infect Dis* 1973; 128:S768–770.
126. Bayer AS, Chow AW, Guzel B: *Listeria monocytogenes* endocarditis: report of a case and review of the literature. *Am J Med Sci* 1977; 273:319–326.
127. Nieman RE, Lorber B: Listerosis in adults: a changing pattern. *Rev Infect Dis* 1980; 2:207–227.
128. Tennebaum MJ, Warner JF: *Lactobacillus casei* endocarditis. *Ann Intern Med* 1975; 82:539–541.
129. Ihde DC, Armstrong D: Clinical spectrum of infection due to Bacillus species. *Am J Med* 1973; 55:839–845.
130. Reller B: Endocarditis caused by *Bacillus subtilis*. *Am J Clin Pathol* 1973; 60:714–718.
131. Gerry JL, Greenough WB: Diphtheroid endocarditis: report of nine cases and review of the literature. *Johns Hopkins Med J* 1976; 139:61–68.
132. Nastro LJ, Finegold SM: Endocarditis due to anaerobic gram-negative bacilli. *Am J Med* 1973; 54:482–496.
133. Galgiani JN, Busch DF, Brass C: *Bacteroides fragilis* endocarditis, bacteremia and other infections treated with oral or intravenous metronidazole. *Am J Med* 1978; 65:284–289.
134. Nastro LJ, Sarma RJ: Infective endocarditis due to anaerobic and microaerophilic bacteria. *West Med J* 1982; 137:18–24.
135. Felner JM, Dowell VR Jr: Anaerobic bacterial endocarditis. *N Engl J Med* 1970; 283:1188–1192.
136. Geraci JE, Hermans PE, Washington JA II: *Eikenella corrodens* endocarditis: report of cure in two cases. *Mayo Clin Proc* 1974; 49:950–953.
137. Perry TM, Belter LF: Brucellosis and heart disease. II. Fatal brucellosis. A review of the literature and report of new cases. *J Pathol* 1960; 36:673–693.
138. Pratt DS, Tenny JH, Bjurk CM: Successful treatment of *Brucella mellitensis* endocarditis. *Am J Med* 1978; 64:897–900.
139. Loeb H, Bettag JL, Yung NK: *Vibrio fetus* endocarditis. Report of 2 cases. *Am Heart J* 1966; 71:381–385.
140. Glen RH, Moellering RC, Kunz LJ: Infections with *Acinetobacter calcoaceticus (Herellea vaginocola)*: clinical and laboratory studies. *Medicine* 1977; 56:79–97.
141. Sage MJ, Maslowski AH, MacCulloch D: Bacterial endocarditis due to *Kingella kingae*. *N Zealand Med J* 1983; 96:795–796.
142. Rubenstein E, Noriega ER, Simberkoff MS, Holzman R, Rahal JJ Jr: Fungal endocarditis: analysis of 24 cases and review of the literature. *Medicine* 1975; 54:331–344.
143. Seelig MS, Goldberg P, Kozinn PJ, Berger AR: Fungal endocarditis: patients at risk and their treatment. *Postgrad Med J* 1979; 56:632–641.
144. Levison ME: Therapy of endocarditis due to gram-negative bacteria and fungi, in Sande MA, Kaye D, Root RK (eds): *Endocarditis*. New York, Churchill Livingstone, 1984; pp 151–162.
145. Carrizosa J, Levison ME, Lawrence T, Kaye D: Cure of *Aspergillus ustus* endocarditis on a prosthetic valve. *Arch Intern Med* 1974; 133:486–490.
146. Barst RJ, Prince AS, Neu HC: *Aspergillus* endocarditis in children: a case report and review of the literature. *Pediatrics* 1981; 68:73–81.
147. Silver MD, Tuffnell PG, Bigelow WG: Endocarditis caused by *Paecilomyces varioli* affecting an aortic valve allograft. *J Thorac Cardiovasc Surg* 1971; 61:278–281.
148. Slifkin M, Bowers HM Jr: *Phialophora mutabilis* endocarditis. *Am J Clin Pathol* 1975; 63:120–130.
149. Hall WJ: *Penicillium* endocarditis following open heart surgery and prosthetic valve insertion. *Am Heart J* 1974; 87:501–506.
150. Tobin MJ, Cahill N, Gerty G, Mauer B, Blake S, Daly K, None R: Q fever endocarditis. *Am J Med* 1982; 72:396–400.
151. Haldane EV, Marrie TJ, Faulkner RS, Lee SH, Cooper JH, MacPherson DD, Montague TJ: Endocarditis due to Q fever in Nova Scotia: experience with five patients in 1981-1982. *J Infect Dis* 1983; 148:978–985.
152. Bel-Kahn J, Watanakunakorn C, Menefee MG, Long HD, Dicter R: *Chlamydia trachomatis* endocarditis. *Am Heart J* 1978; 95:627–636.
153. McCabe RE, Baldwin JC, McGregor CA, Miller DC, Vosti KL: Prosthetic valve endocarditis caused by *Legionella pneumophila*. *Ann Intern Med* 1984; 100:525–527.
154. Van Scoy RE: Culture-negative endocarditis. *Mayo Clin Proc* 1982; 57:149–154.
155. Ivert TS, Dismukes WE, Cobbs CG, Blackstone EH, Kiklin JM, Bergdahl LA: Prosthetic valve endocarditis. *Circulation* 1984; 69:223–232.
156. Gnan JW, Dismukes WE: Prosthetic valve endocarditis: an overview. *Herz* 1983; 81:320–331.
157. Neu HC, Srinivasan S: Infective endocarditis increases among narcotic addicts. *J Cardiovasc Med* 1981; 7:675–688.
158. Tuazon CU, Sheagren JN: Increased rate of carriage of *Staphylococcus aureus* among narcotic addicts. *J Infect Dis* 1974; 129:725–727.
159. Drake TA, Sande MA: Antimicrobial treatment: lessons learned from experimental models, in Sande MA, Kaye D, Root RK (eds): *Endocarditis*. New York, Churchill Livingstone, 1984, pp 77–100.
160. Coleman DL, Horwitz RI, Andriole VT: Association between serum inhibitory and bactericidal concentrations and therapeutic outcome in bacterial endocarditis. *Am J Med* 1982; 73:260–267.
161. Jordan GW, Kawachi MM: Analysis of serum bactericidal activity in endocarditis, osteomyelitis and other bacterial infections. *Medicine* 1981; 60:49–61.
162. Stratton CW, Weinstein MP, Reller LB: Correlation of serum bactericidal activity with antimicrobial agent level and minimal bactericidal concentration. *J Infect Dis* 1982; 145:160–168.
163. Wilson WR, Giuliani ER, Geraci JE: Treatment of penicillin-sensitive streptococcal infective endocarditis. *Mayo Clin Proc* 1982; 57:95–100.
164. Hamburger M, Stein L: *Streptococcus viridans* subacute bacterial endocarditis: two week treatment schedule with penicillin. *JAMA* 1952; 149:542–545.
165. Kartchmer AW, Moellering RC Jr, Maki DG, Swartz MN: Single antibiotic therapy for streptococcal endocarditis. *JAMA* 1979; 241:1801–1806.
166. Malacoff RF, Frank E, Andriole VT: Streptococcal endocarditis (nonenterococcal, non-group A): single vs. combination therapy. *JAMA* 1979; 241:1807–1810.
167. Thompsett R, Hurst ML: Bacterial endocarditis: selected aspects of treatment. *Trans Am Clin Climatol Assoc* 1972; 83:95–101.
168. Wolfe JC, Johnson WD Jr: Penicillin-sensitive streptococcal endocarditis: in vitro and clinical observations on penicillin-streptomycin therapy. *Ann Intern Med* 1974; 81:178–181.
169. Wilson WR, Geraci JE, Wilkowske CJ, Washington JA II: Short-term intramuscular therapy with procaine penicillin plus streptomycin for infective endocarditis due to viridans streptococci. *Circulation* 1978; 57:1158–1161.
170. Wilson WR, Thompson RL, Wilkowske CJ, Washington JA II, Giuliani ER, Geraci JE: Short-term therapy for streptococcal infective endocarditis: combined intramuscular administration of penicillin and streptomycin. *JAMA* 1981; 245:360–363.
171. Moellering RC Jr: Treatment of enterococcal endocarditis, in Sande MA, Kaye D, Root RK (eds): *Endocarditis*. New York, Churchill Livingstone, 1984, pp 113–133.
172. Tompsett R, Berman W: Enterococcal endocarditis: duration and mode of treatment. *Trans Am Clin Climatol Assoc* 1977; 89:49–57.
173. Herzstein J, Ryan JL, Mangi RJ, Greco TP, Andriole VT: Optimal therapy for enterococcal endocarditis. *Am J Med* 1984; 76:186–191.
174. Wilson WR, Wilkowske CJ, Wright AJ, Sande MA, Geraci JE: Treatment of streptomycin-susceptible and streptomycin-resistant enterococcal endocarditis. *Ann Intern Med* 1984; 100:816–823.
175. Iannini PB, Crosley K: Therapy of *Staphylococcus aureus* bacteremia associated with a removable focus of infection. *Ann Intern Med* 1976; 84:558–562.
176. Watanakunakorn C, Baird IM: *Staphylococcus aureus* bacteremia and endocarditis associated with a removable infected intravenous device. *Am J Med* 1977; 63:253–258.
177. Thompson RL: Staphylococcal infective endocarditis. *Mayo Clin Proc* 1982; 57:106–114.
178. Korzeniowski O, Sande MA, and the National Collaborative Endocarditis Study Group: Combination antimicrobial therapy for *Staphylococcus aureus* endocarditis in patients addicted to parenteral drugs and in nonaddicts. *Ann Intern Med* 1982; 97:496–503.
179. Parker RH, Fossieck BE: Intravenous followed by oral antimicrobial therapy for staphylococcal endocarditis. *Ann Intern Med* 1980; 93:832–834.
180. Craven DE, Kollisch NR, Hsieh CR, Connolly MG Jr, McCabe WR: Vancomycin treatment of bacteremia caused by oxacillin-resistant *Staphylococcus aureus*: comparison with beta-lactam antibiotic treatment of bacteremia caused by oxacillin-sensitive *Staphylococcus aureus*. *J Infect Dis* 1983; 147:137–143.
181. Markowitz N, Saravolatz L, Pohlod D, Quinn E: Comparative efficacy and toxicity of trimethoprim versus vancomycin in the therapy of serious *S aureus* infection. Abstract 638. 23rd Intersci Conf Antimicrob Agents Chemother, October 1983, Las Vegas, Nevada.

182. Sabath LD, Wheeler N, Laverdiere M, Blazevic D, Wilkinson BJ: A new type of penicillin resistance of *Staphylococcus aureus*. *Lancet* 1977; 1:443–447.
183. Faville RJ, Zaske DE, Kaplan EL, Crossley K, Sabath LD, Quie PG: *Staphylococcus aureus* endocarditis combined therapy with vancomycin and rifampin. *JAMA* 1978; 240:1963–1965.
184. Keys TF, Hewitt WL: Endocarditis due to micrococci and *Staphylococcus epidermidis*. *Arch Intern Med* 1973; 132:216–220.
185. Archer GL, Tenenbaum MJ: Antibiotic-resistant *S. epidermidis* in patients undergoing cardiac surgery. *Antimicrob Agents Chemother* 1980; 17:269–272.
186. Cooke DB, Arensberg D, Felner JM, Rimland D, Lesser LM: Gonococcal endocarditis in the antibiotic era. *Arch Intern Med* 1979; 139:1247–1250.
187. Schlicter JG, MacLean H: A method of determining the effective therapeutic level in the treatment of subacute bacterial endocarditis with penicillin. *Am Heart J* 1947; 34:209–211.
188. Mills SA: Surgical progress: surgical management of infective endocarditis. *Ann Surg* 1982; 195:367–383.
189. Scalia D, Bortolotti U, Milano A, Stritoni P, Panizzon G, Valfria C, Mazzucco G, Gallucci V: Surgical treatment of infectious endocarditis in the active phase. Experience in 40 cases. *G Ital Cardiol* 1981; 11:643–649.
190. Levitsky S, Mammana RB, Silverman NA, Weber F, Hiro S, Wright RN: Acute endocarditis in drug addicts: surgical treatment for gram-negative sepsis. *Circulation* 1982; 66:1135–1138.
191. Lewis BS, Agathangelou NE, Coulsen PR, Antunes M, Kinsley RH: Cardiac operation during active infective endocarditis: results of aortic, mitral and double valve replacement in 94 patients. *J Thorac Cardiovasc Surg* 1982; 84:579–584.
192. Weaver JP, Crawford FA Jr, Kratz JM, Sade MM: Valve replacement for native valve endocarditis. *Ann Surg* 1984; 50:40–42.
193. Haraphongse M, Fraser RS, Callaghan JC, Rossall RE: Infective endocarditis: surgical treatment of 41 patients. *Can J Surg* 1982; 25:138–140.
194. Cobbs CG, Gnann JW Jr: Indications for surgery, in Sande MA, Kaye D, Root RK (eds): *Endocarditis*. New York, Churchill Livingstone, 1984, pp 201–212.
194a. Reid CL, Chandraratna PAN, Rahimtoola SH: Infective endocarditis: improved diagnosis and treatment. *Current Prob Cardiol* 1985; 10(1):6–50.
195. Dinubile MJ: Surgery in active endocarditis. *Ann Intern Med* 1982; 96:650–659.
195a. Arbulu A, Asfaw I: Tricuspid valvulectomy without prosthetic replacement. Ten years of clinical experience. *J Thorac Cardiovasc Surg* 1981; 82:684–691.
195b. Stern HJ, Sisto DA, Strom JA, Soeiro R, Jones SR, Frater RWM: Immediate tricuspid valve replacement for endocarditis: indications and results. *J Thorac Cardiovasc Surg* 1986; 91:163–167.
196. Wilson WR, Danielson GK, Guiliani ER, Washington JA II, Jaumin PM, Geraci JE: Valve replacement in patients with active infective endocarditis. *Circulation* 1978; 58:585–588.
197. Frantz PT, Murray GF, Wilcox BR: Surgical management of left ventricular–aortic discontinuity complicating bacterial endocarditis. *Ann Thorac Surg* 1980; 29:1–7.
198. Wilson WR, Giuliani ER, Danielson GK, Geraci JE: Management of complications of infective endocarditis. *Mayo Clin Proc* 1982; 57:162–170.
199. Wilson WR, Lie JT, Houser OW, Piepgros DG, Geraci JE: The management of patients with mycotic aneurysm. *Curr Clin Top Infect Dis* 1981; 2:151–183.
200. Kaplan EL: Bacterial endocarditis prophylaxis—tradition or necessity? *Am J Cardiol* 1986; 57:478–479.
201. Durack DT, Bisno AL, Kaplan EL: Apparent failures of endocarditis prophylaxis. Analysis of 52 cases submitted to a national registry. *JAMA* 1983; 250:2318–2322.
202. Ivert TSA, Dismukes WE, Cobbs CG, Blackstone EH, Kirklin JW, Bergdahl LA: Prosthetic valve endocarditis. *Circulation* 1984; 69:223–232.
203. Clemens JD, Ransohoff DF: A quantitative assessment of predental antibiotic prophylaxis for patients with mitral valve prolapse. *J Chron Dis* 1984; 37:531–544.
204. Shorvon PJ, Eykn SJ, Cotton PB: Gastrointestinal instrumentation, bacteremia and endocarditis. *Gut* 1983; 24:1078–1093.
205. Bayliss R, Clarke C, Oakley CM, Somerville W, Whitfield AGW, Young SEJ: Incidence, mortality and prevention of infective endocarditis. *J Royal Coll Physicians London* 1986; 20:15–20.
206. Shulman ST, Amren DP, Bisno AL, Dajani AS, Durack DT, Gerber MA, Kaplan EL, Millard HD, Sanders WE, Schwartz RH, Watanakunakorn C: Prevention of bacterial endocarditis. *Circulation* 1984; 70:1123A–1127A.
207. Working party of the British Society for Antimicrobial Chemotherapy: The antibiotic prophylaxis of infective endocarditis. *Lancet* 1982; 2:1323–1326.
208. Kaye D: Prophylaxis for infective endocarditis: an update. *Ann Intern Med* 1986; 104:419–423.
209. Chadwick EG, Shulman ST: Prevention of infective endocarditis. *Mod Concepts Cardiovasc Dis* 1986; 55:11–15.

47 Tumors of the Heart

Zvi Vered, MD and Henry N. Neufeld, MD

Cardiac tumors are the subject of extensive literature and enormous interest, clearly out of all proportion to their prevalence when compared with other much more common heart diseases. The probable reasons for this unusual amount of interest are: (1) clinically, the resemblance of cardiac tumors to other cardiac and often noncardiac diseases; (2) the uncertainty of the nature and pathogenesis of some forms of these tumors; (3) the ability to correctly diagnose and surgically treat and cure many types of cardiac tumors.

CLASSIFICATION

Tumors of the heart may be primary or secondary, benign or malignant. They may arise or involve the pericardium, epicardium, myocardium, or endocardium. The more common forms of cardiac neoplasms are as follows:

A. *Primary Tumors*
  I. *Benign*
    1. Myxoma
    2. Rhabdomyoma
    3. Fibroma
    4. Lipoma
    5. Papilloma
    6. Angioma
    7. Teratoma
    8. Leiomyoma
    9. Xanthoma
    10. Hamartoma
    11. Epithelial inclusion cyst
    12. Neurofibromatosis (involving the heart)
  II. *Malignant*
    1. Sarcomas of all types
    2. Mesothelioma
    3. Rhabdomyosarcoma
    4. Epithelioma

B. *Secondary Tumors*
  I. *Direct invasion from adjacent areas*
    1. Bronchi
    2. Lungs
    3. Pleura
    4. Breast
    5. Thymus
    6. Mediastinum
  II. *Metastatic Spread*
    1. Hematogenous
    2. Lymphatic
  III. *Systemic Neoplasms with Cardiac Involvement*
    1. Leukemia
    2. Hodgkin's disease
    3. Lymphosarcoma
    4. Kaposi's sarcoma
    5. Carcinoid tumor.

INCIDENCE

Based on large pathologic series, the incidence of primary cardiac tumors ranges between 0.0017% and 0.28%.[1-4] Lymburner[5] in a large series found 4 cases in 8,500 autopsies, an incidence of 0.05%. Secondary tumors are more common, being found in 0.25% to 1.0% of autopsies.[6,7] They comprise 5% to 11% of all malignant tumors throughout the body.[8,9]

PATHOLOGY

PRIMARY TUMORS

Three fourths of primary cardiac tumors are benign.[10] Myxoma is by far the most common primary neoplasm, followed by sarcoma and rhabdomyoma. The more common tumors will be described in detail.

Benign Tumors

Myxoma: Myxomas arise in the endocardium. The most common site is the left atrial side of the interatrial septum, close to the mitral valve. However, the tumor may arise from different sites within the left atrium,[11] right atrium, or bilaterally in each atrium,[12,13] in the ventricles, or even simultaneously in the atrium and ventricle.[14] A myxoma of the mitral valve has also been reported.[15]

These tumors are usually pedunculated, polypoid, and friable, although they often may be rounded and have a smooth surface (Figure 47.1). They are usually soft, gelatinous, and mucoid and may have areas of hemorrhage and thrombosis. Myxomas occasionally may be sessile.[16] They are usually 5 to 6 cm in diameter, but may range from 1 to 15 cm.[17]

Microscopic examination reveals a myxoid mucopolysaccharide matrix in which polygonal cells and blood vessels may be observed. Endothelial cells leave the surface and also penetrate the tumor, lining special channels that run from the surface. On the surface, areas of thrombi, hemorrhage, cystic formation, or filium may be found.[17] These pathologic findings may resemble organized thrombus, and indeed one theory suggests that myxomas are not true neoplasms but may represent one form of organized thrombus.[18] The vast majority of investigators, however, consider cardiac myxomas as true neoplastic processes.[3,19–22] Evidence in favor of the neoplastic theory is as follows: (1) ultrastructural studies[23,24] that reveal myxoma cells with intracellular junctions (zonulae adherens), single nuclei, rough endoplasmic reticulum, free ribosome, Golgi apparatus, mitrochondria, and filaments. On scanning electron microscopy, myxomas are covered with endothelium, and endothelium-lined crevices and clefts are often observed, which are not present in atrial thrombi; (2) the production of factor VIII by myxoma cells[25]; (3) on tissue culture, myxoma cells resembling multipotential mesenchymal cells rather than fibroblasts, which characterize thrombi[22]; (4) the possibility of recurrence after surgical removal.

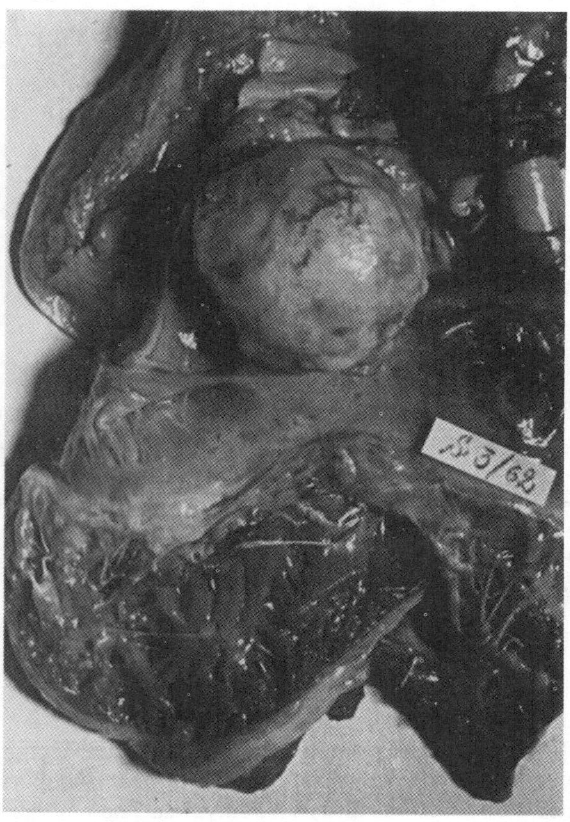

Figure 47.1. Left atrial myxoma. The tumor is rounded, smooth, and firm.

It is generally agreed that myxomas are benign in nature; however, a few reports indicate the possibility of distant implantation as in brain or bone.[14,17–25]

Rhabdomyoma: This is the most common cardiac tumor in infants and children.[26,27] It is probably not a true neoplasm, but rather a hamartoma, without any mitotic activity[27,28] and with a rather typical ultrastructural appearance.[28] It is usually yellow–grey and small in size (1 to 20 mm in diameter). The microscopic features are also typical: the dominant cell contains a central cytoplasmic mass suspended by fine fibrillar processes radiating to the periphery, thus being termed "spider cells."[3] The cytoplasm is rich with glycogen and stains positively with periodic acid-Schiff (PAS) reagent.[17]

The right and left ventricles are the usual sites of these tumors. Most commonly they are multiple. The atria are involved in about 30%. They may obstruct valvular orifices or cause valvular regurgitation on both the left and right side of the heart. Obstruction is often the cause of death.[27] Occasionally diffuse cardiac involvement and enlargement are present without distinctive tumor formation.

A common association of cardiac rhabdomyoma is tuberous sclerosis occurring in up to 50% of these patients. Less commonly associated lesions are adenoma sebaceum and benign tumors of the kidney, most commonly hamartoma and angiomyolipoma.[27]

Fibroma: This tumor also is most common in infants and children, but it may occur at any age.[17,29,30] Males and females are equally affected. It is usually ventricular and intramural in location, and it tends to calcify or even ossify. Up to one third of patients die suddenly from tumor penetration of the conduction system or left ventricular outflow obstruction.[31] Typically, the tumors are grey, not encapsulated, and firm, and measure 3 to 7 cm in diameter.

Microscopic examination reveals elongated fibroblasts admixed with fibrous tissue intermingled with adjacent myocardial fibers at the periphery of the tumor.[32] Fibrous tissue consists of collagen and elastic fibers. These microscopic findings are not typical, and therefore the diagnostic criteria are not uniformly agreed upon and various other terminologies have been employed.[20] As in rhabdomyoma, it is not clear whether fibromas are true neoplasms or rather represent hamartomas.[32]

Papillary tumors of heart valves (fibroelastoma): Papillary tumors are usually located on the cardiac valves or on the endocardium near the valves. Most commonly, they are found coincidentally at surgery or at postmortem examination. However, they may cause valvular insufficiency or coronary and cerebral embolization.[3,17,33,33a] They are usually small, measure up to 3 to 4 cm in diameter, and may be single or multiple. Any valve may be involved, the tricuspid valve being the most frequent location in children as opposed to the aortic valve in adults.[34] Microscopic findings reveal a core of connective tissue consisting of an acid mucopolysaccharide matrix, smooth muscle cells, collagen, and elastic fibers covered by endothelium. These tumors should be distinguished from Lambl's excrescences, which are deposits of cellular matrix covered by a single layer of endothelium. The latter are common findings on heart valves that had had endothelial damage.[35,36]

Lipoma: Lipomas may occur anywhere in the heart and are equally distributed between both sexes. They may vary from 1 cm in size to tumors weighing more than 2 kg.[37] When they are intrapericardial, they may cause pericardial effusion. They may mimic a pericardial cyst or localized effusion or may be discovered on routine chest x-ray films as a silent mediastinal mass.[38,39] Intramyocardial lipomas are usually small and encapsulated.[17] Most tumors are sessile or polypoid. The most common locations are the left ventricle, right atrium, and interatrial septum.[20] On microscopic examination, the tumor is usually encapsulated, the major cell is the typical mature fat cell, and connective tissue, fibrous or muscular tissue, or vacuolated brownish fat, as in the case of hibernoma, may be observed.

Lipomas should be differentiated from lipomatous hypertrophy of the interatrial septum, in which adipose tissue invades the interatrial septum.[17,40,41] These lesions may range from 2 to 8 cm in diameter and may invade and bulge into the atrial cavity. It is more common in elderly, female, and generally obese patients.[41]

Mesothelioma of the atrioventricular node: Mesotheliomas of the atrioventricular node are usually small in size but may measure up to 3 cm in diameter. They are reported to occur at any age[17,42] and are usually cystic or polypoid in appearance. This is the smallest tumor capable of causing complete heart block and sudden death.[42] The exact source of the tumor is not clear, and it is believed to arise as a result of an arrest in development. Other terms have been used to describe them, such as lymphangiepithelioma[42] and congenital polycystic tumor of the atrioventricular node.[43] This tumor always should be sought for in cases of sudden unexpected and unexplained death, especially in the young.

Angiomas: Angiomas are rare cardiac tumors usually discovered at postmortem examination.[44] They may occur all over the heart but are usually intramural and often located in the interventricular septum[10,20]; therefore, they may cause heart block and sudden death[45] and occasionally pericardial effusion and tamponade. They may be found in the right heart chambers. They are usually sessile or polypoid, ranging from 1 to 3 cm in diameter. Microscopic findings include endothelium-lined spaces that may contain blood, lymphatic tissue, or thrombi.

Pericardial cysts: These cysts are the most frequent benign tumors of the pericardium. They are usually discovered on routine chest x-ray films; however, about one third may be symptomatic. They are discovered usually during the second to fourth decade of life and are equally distributed between men and women. They are usually located at the right costophrenic angle[46] but may be found elsewhere. Pericardial cysts develop because of abnormal development of mesenchymal tissue during fetal life. They are usually unilocular and filled with clear liquid.[47] The differential diagnosis of pericardial cysts on chest x-ray films is solid tumors, aneurysms or pseudoaneurysms, or herniation of the omentum or liver through the diaphragm. Two-dimensional echocardiography and computed tomography can help to establish the diagnosis.

Malignant Tumors

These tumors make up about one fourth of primary cardiac neoplasms.[1,3,17] Practically all malignant primary tumors of the heart are sarcomas; therefore, their overall frequency is second only to that of myxomas. They are equally distributed between men and women. They may appear anywhere in the heart, but the right and left atria are the most common sites.[20] Primary sarcomas, especially osteosarcomas[47a] of the heart, may be both intramural and intracavitary. Cardiac sarcomas tend to proliferate and metastasize, early death ensuing within a few weeks to 2 years from the onset of symptoms.[48] The most frequent organs of metastasis are the lungs, thoracic lymph nodes, mediastinum, and vertebral column; however, virtually every organ may be affected. The tumor may invade the pericardial space and cause hemorrhagic pericardial effusion or tamponade. Intracavitary obstruction due to the tumor mass is also common, involving the superior vena cava and thus producing the superior vena caval syndrome.

Angiosarcoma: This is the most frequent cardiac sarcoma and includes a wide variety of pathologic presentations, including Kaposi's sarcoma and angioreticuloendotheliomas, as well as other forms of angiosarcoma. It tends to occur in adults and is more prevalent among men.[49] The right atrium is by far the most common site, often arising from the interatrial septum. They may cause obstruction to right-sided flow or hemorrhagic pericardial effusion.[50,50a] Microscopic examination reveals rather specific anastomotic vascular channels lined with atypical endothelial cells.[51] Electron microscopy reveals immature or primitive endothelial cells, pericysts as well as undifferentiated mesenchymal cells.[52]

Rhabdomyosarcoma: This is the second most common cardiac sarcoma and is more common in males. There is no single chamber predilection and multiple tumors are not infrequent. Significant obstruction of a cardiac valve is present in about 50% of affected patients.[53] This tumor may occasionally be mistaken for myxoma because it may form a polypoid extension into a cardiac chamber. On microscopy, rhabdomyoblasts are the hallmark of this lesion; cross-striations may be observed.[20] Other less characteristic cells are strap cells, tennis racquet cells, and spider cells with periodic acid-Schiff positive cytoplasm.[20]

Fibrosarcoma: Fibrosarcoma is characterized by a soft, whitish, fish flesh appearance (Figure 47.2). Areas of necrosis and hemorrhage may be observed or a thrombus may form and obstruct a cardiac chamber.[3]

Mesothelioma: Mesothelioma is the most frequent malignant tumor of the pericardium.[17] It causes hemorrhagic

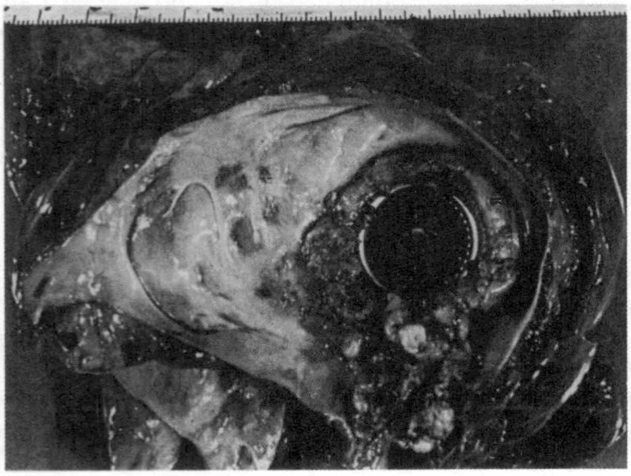

Figure 47.2. An unusual case of a huge fibrosarcoma filling the whole cavity of the left atrium in a patient with a prosthetic mitral valve.

pericardial effusion and less commonly constrictive pericarditis or vena caval obstruction. Males are affected more commonly than females in a ratio of 2:1. The prognosis is poor.

Other malignant tumors: Systemic malignant lymphoma may involve the heart in about one third of the cases; however, primary cardiac lymphoma is rare.[54] Liposarcomas with the characteristic histologic appearance (Figure 47.3) may involve the interatrial septum and obstruct the mitral valve or pulmonary veins or both.[55] A case of malignant fibrous histiocytoma of the left atrium, first mistaken to be a myxoma, has also been described.[56]

SECONDARY TUMORS

Secondary tumors may gain access to the heart through one of four major means: (1) direct penetration from an adjacent structure (Figure 47.4); (2) hematogenous spread (Figure 47.5); (3) lymphatic spread (Figure 47.6); and (4) direct growth along the vena cava (Figure 47.7) or pulmonary veins.[10,57,58]

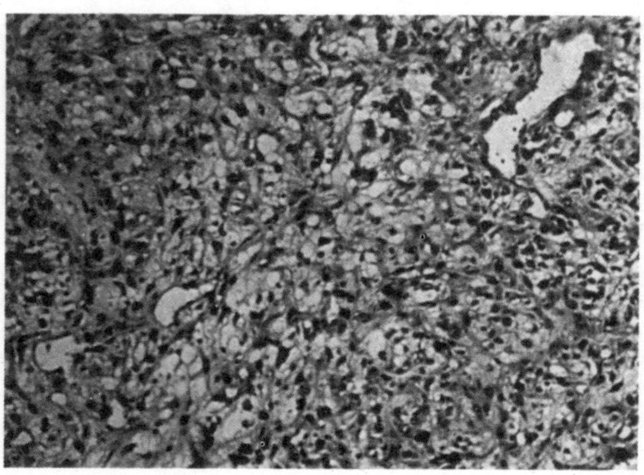

Figure 47.3. Typical histologic appearance of a liposarcoma of the heart.

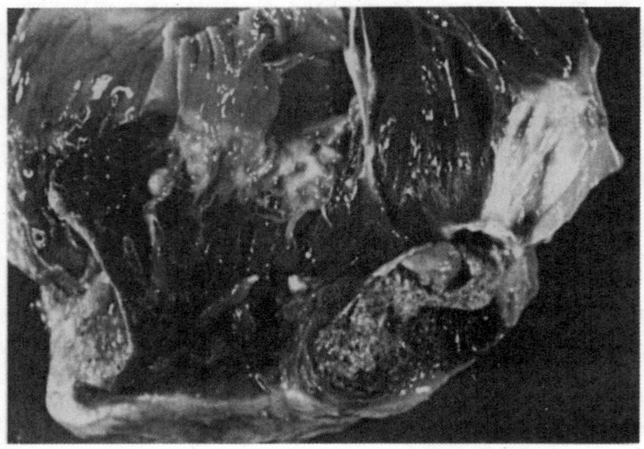

Figure 47.4. Direct penetration of a bronchogenic carcinoma of the heart.

Origin of Secondary Tumors

Metastases to the heart are relatively infrequent, possibly because of the strong active motion of the heart, rapid coronary blood flow, and efficient afferent lymphatic drainage.[10]

All types of primary malignant tumors may metastasize to the heart[59]; however, malignant melanoma seems to have a special tendency, with cardiac involvement in over 50% of the cases.[60] The most frequent cardiac metastases are those from bronchogenic carcinoma and carcinoma of the breast, accounting for approximately 30% of all cardiac metastases. Involvement of the heart occurs in about 50% of cases of leukemia and in about one sixth of cases of lymphoma. Reticulum cell sarcoma shows a somewhat

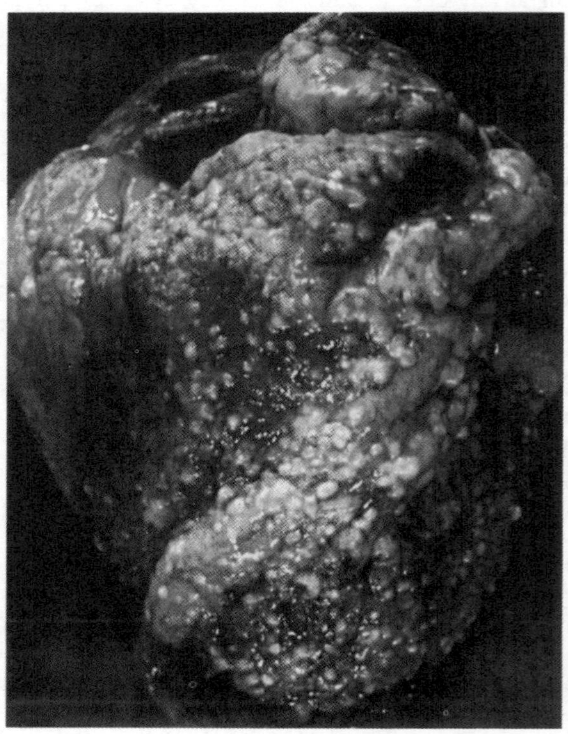

Figure 47.5. Disseminated cardiac metastases.

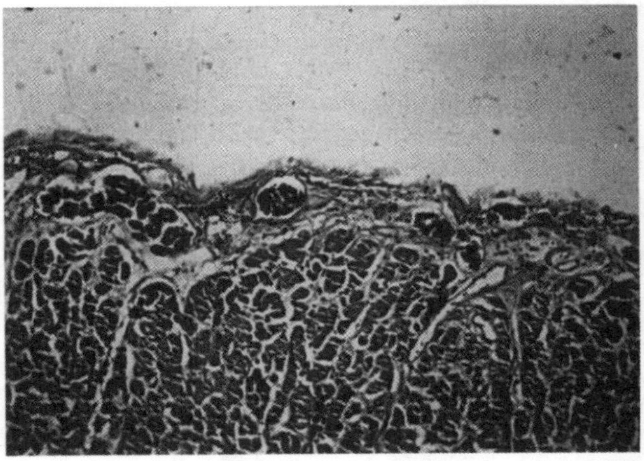

Figure 47.6. Subepicardial lymphatic spread of a bronchogenic carcinoma.

greater tendency to cardiac involvement than the other lymphomas.[54] In these cases there is usually extensive myocardial infiltration and occasionally occlusion of a major coronary vessel.

The presence of cardiac metastases usually indicates widespread metastases. Isolated cardiac metastases are rare.[61] Cardiac metastases are easily observed on macroscopic examination as small firm whitish nodules or masses (Figure 47.5). Microscopic examination usually allows identification of the origin of the metastases.

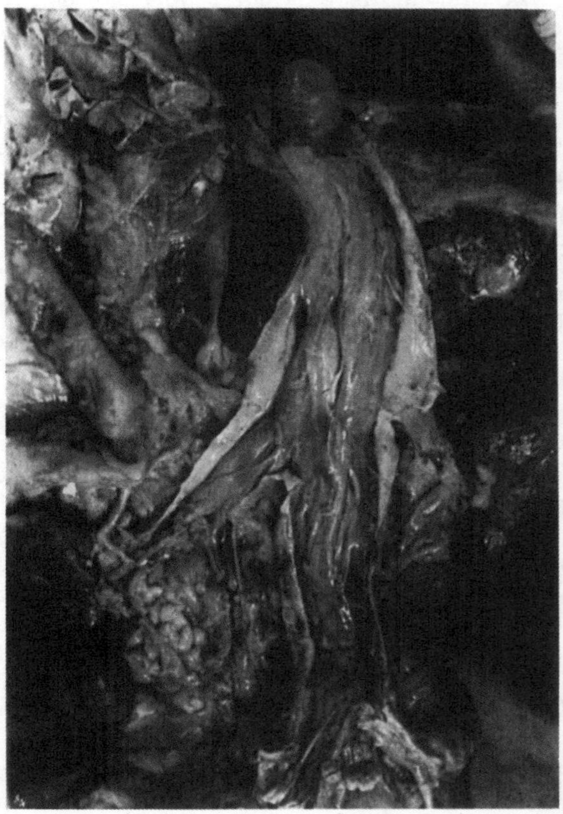

Figure 47.7. Leiomyomatosis of the heart. The tumor is growing along the inferior vena cava.

Sites of Cardiac Metastases

Applefeld et al[62] reported on 2,436 cases of the 12 most common tumors that tend to metastasize to the heart. Of them, 367 (15.1%) had cardiac, 270 (11.1%) pericardial, and 54 (2.2%) cardiac and pericardial metastases.

Pericardial involvement usually causes pericardial effusion, which may be chylous (as in lymphomatous involvement), hemorrhagic, or even normal in appearance. Cardiac tamponade occasionally may occur.[63] Constrictive pericarditis, if present, is more frequent as the result of radiation therapy than the primary tumor.[64]

Obstruction of the superior vena cava may cause the superior vena cava syndrome. The tumors that usually produce this are bronchogenic carcinoma and lymphoma.[65] Obstruction of the inferior vena cava usually results from lymphoma and occasionally from leiomyomatosis (Figure 47.7).

Carcinoid heart disease is a unique phenomenon that will be discussed separately.

CLINICAL MANIFESTATIONS

Both primary and secondary cardiac tumors may have a great variety of clinical presentations. The clinical picture depends on the location of the tumor, its nature, size, and configuration. Generally, cardiac tumors may produce systemic or cardiac signs and symptoms, or both.

SYSTEMIC PRESENTATIONS

A variety of symptoms and signs have been attributed to cardiac tumors. The most important ones include systemic and pulmonary emboli, fever, malaise, cachexia, rash, arthralgia, Raynaud's phenomenon, and unusual behavior.[66–69] Laboratory findings may include an elevated sedimentation rate, anemia, hypergammaglobulinemia, leukocytosis, thrombocytosis, and thrombocytopenia.[66,67,70–72] Several mechanisms have been suggested to explain the systemic manifestations of cardiac tumors. Among them the immunologic basis seems to be the most attractive. Antimyocardial antibodies were found in a patient with myxoma; their level decreased after removal of the tumor.[73] Another patient with myxoma developed multiple myeloma presumably because of continuous immunologic stimulation by the tumor.[74] Despite these facts, the exact mechanism for the variety of systemic presentations of cardiac tumors is yet uncertain. The differential diagnosis includes a systemic infection, malignancy, bacterial endocarditis, and collagen vascular disease.

When recurrent systemic embolization occurs in the absence of mitral valve disease, bacterial endocarditis, or atrial fibrillation, a cardiac tumor should be suspected. Of all cardiac tumors, myxomas most frequently cause embolization; however, other more solid tumors also may occasionally embolize.

The clinical picture of systemic embolization depends on the target organ anywhere in the body, where infarction, hemorrhage, or both occur or occasionally vascular aneurysms may develop.[13,67,75–78] Microscopic examination of the embolus found at operation may lead to a diagnosis of cardiac tumor.[75–78] Similarly, biopsy of the skin or mucous membrane from an area with petechiae may also unmask the diagnosis of a tumor embolus.[67]

Tumors of the right side of the heart (and occasionally the left side when an intracardiac shunt is present) may cause pulmonary embolism.[79–81] This occasionally may lead to pulmonary hypertension and a clinical picture of cor pulmonale.[82] Clinically, pulmonary embolism due to a cardiac tumor cannot be distinguished from general thromboembolism. However, perfusion lung scans may show unusually prolonged discrete perfusion defects, unlike thromboembolism which tends to recanalize and resolve. In addition, scans only occasionally demonstrate total obstruction of blood flow to a lung with normal perfusion to the other one, which is also unusual in cases of thromboembolism.[80]

CARDIAC PRESENTATIONS

The site of the tumor is the most important determinant of its clinical presentation; however, its nature and size are also important.[83]

Left Atrial Tumors

Because myxomas are by far the most common primary cardiac tumor and are usually located in the left atrium, this is the most common intracardiac site of primary cardiac tumors.

The signs and symptoms produced by left atrial tumors are those related to obstruction of the mitral orifice (Figure 47.8) or inadequate closure of the mitral valve resulting in mitral regurgitation. Therefore, the symptoms mimic those of mitral valvular disease[83]: mainly, dyspnea on effort or at rest, orthopnea, paroxysmal nocturnal dyspnea, palpitations, cough, hemoptysis, fatigue, chest pain, or acute pulmonary edema. These may be accompanied by other presentations that are usually not related to mitral valve disease such as sudden death, syncope, pallor, and weight loss.[83] If these symptoms are paroxysmal, sudden in onset, or related to body position, this may serve as a clue to the diagnosis of a tumor rather than mitral valve disease.[83,84] The recent finding of a vasoactive intestinal polypeptide in a patient with left atrial myxoma[84a] suggests a new possible explanation for some of the less well understood systemic manifestations such as hypotension and syncope that are not related to body position.

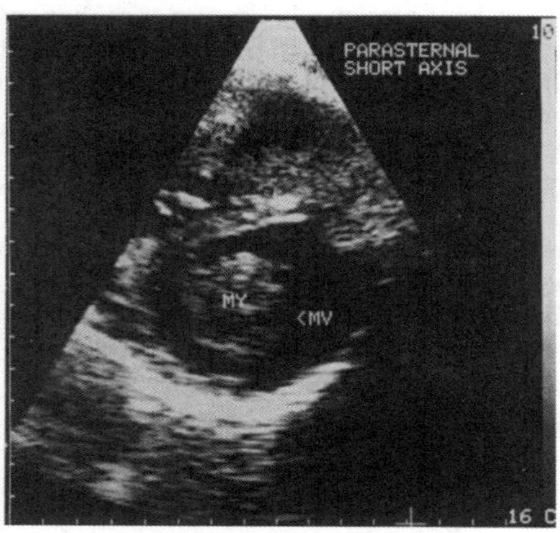

Figure 47.8. Two-dimensional echocardiography viewed from the parasternal short axis, demonstrating complete obstruction of the mitral orifice by a myxoma. MY = myxoma.

Physical examination, however, may resemble mitral valve disease or be nonspecific. Signs of left heart failure, such as pulmonary congestion, are frequent. Cardiac auscultation may reveal a loud and widely split S_1, an S_4, a holosystolic murmur of mitral regurgitation that may change in magnitude or even disappear with a change of body position, and occasionally a diastolic rumbling murmur produced by obstruction to mitral flow. A rather typical finding is an early diastolic tumor "plop" sound that is probably produced by the tumor as it strikes the endocardium.[85] This sound is often mistaken to be an S_3 or an opening snap, although it usually comes earlier and has a distinct rather pathognomonic quality.

Right Atrial Tumors

As in left atrial tumors, most symptoms and signs of right atrial tumors arise from either obstruction of the tricuspid orifice or interference with tricuspid valve closure, resulting in tricuspid regurgitation. Occasionally, traumatic destruction of the tricuspid valve may occur.[86] The most common findings are those of right heart failure: peripheral edema, hepatomegaly, distended neck veins with a prominent "a" wave, ascites, weakness, and fatigue.[80,87] Right heart failure may develop rapidly. Pulmonary embolism and pulmonary hypertension may occur[80,81] and right-to-left shunting through a patent foramen ovale may result in hypoxia, polycythemia, cyanosis, and clubbing.[80,87]

Physical findings may include peripheral edema, hepatomegaly, ascites, distended neck veins, and the superior vena caval syndrome. Cardiac auscultation may reveal a holosystolic murmur of tricuspid regurgitation with or without an early diastolic rumble resembling tricuspid stenosis. These murmurs may change with respiration and may disappear abruptly when the patient's position is changed.[84] A tumor plop as in left atrial tumors has also been described.[88]

The differential diagnosis includes Ebstein's anomaly, tricuspid regurgitation, carcinoid syndrome, constrictive pericarditis, and restrictive cardiomyopathy.[84]

Left Ventricular Tumors

Tumors of the left ventricle may be intramyocardial or intracavitary. When intramyocardial, they are often silent for prolonged periods. Signs and symptoms include left ventricular dysfunction, arrhythmias, and conduction disturbances (including complete heart block). When predominantly intracavitary, these tumors may cause left ventricular outflow tract obstruction resulting in dizziness, chest pain, dyspnea, and syncope. Chest pain may also be caused by coronary obstruction either directly by the tumor or through embolization. Physical findings may include a systolic murmur at the base of the heart that changes with body position. Systolic blood pressure may also vary with body position.[89] The differential diagnosis includes all forms of left ventricular outflow tract obstruction,[90] cardiomyopathy, and coronary artery disease.[91,92]

Right Ventricular Tumors

Right ventricular tumors may protrude into the right ventricular inflow or outflow tracts. The signs and symptoms depend on their location and include right heart failure characterized by elevated venous pressure, peripheral edema, hepatomegaly and ascites (inflow obstruction), or shortness of breath, cyanosis, syncope, and sudden death (outflow obstruction).[93,94] Physical examination may include a systolic ejection murmur at the pulmonary area resembling pulmonary stenosis[95] or a diastolic rumble resembling tricuspid obstruction. Other cardiac findings may include an S_3, delayed P_2, and a low pitched diastolic sound caused by the tumor. Pulmonary hypertension and pulmonary regurgitation may also be present. In the neck veins a prominent "a" wave and Kussmaul's sign may be observed.[96]

The differential diagnosis includes pulmonary stenosis, pulmonary regurgitation, pulmonary thromboembolism, tricuspid regurgitation, and restrictive cardiomyopathy.

Pericardial Tumors

The clinical picture of neoplastic pericarditis may vary from totally asymptomatic cases to severely ill patients or it even may be the cause of death. Although in the past the antemortem diagnosis of pericardial involvement of neoplastic disease was rather infrequent,[97] today with the advent of two-dimensional echocardiography, the diagnosis is usually readily made. The most common symptoms are chest pain, dyspnea, cough, and weakness. Physical findings of pericardial friction rub or distant heart sounds are uncommon. Significant pericardial effusion and even cardiac tamponade requiring pericardiocentesis are more frequent than in acute pericarditis. The prognosis depends primarily on the nature of the tumor.

CARCINOID HEART DISEASE

CARCINOID SYNDROME

The most common site of carcinoid tumors is the gastrointestinal tract. Other less common sites are the bronchus, biliary tract, pancreas, and testes.[98] Occasionally primary ovarian carcinoid tumors have been described.[99] The carcinoid syndrome is usually produced by liver metastasis of ileal carcinoids that contain cytoplasmic granules that in turn take up and reduce silver salts (argentaffinity). The carcinoids contain a high concentration of 5-hydroxytryptamine (5-HT), which produces the well-known urine product of 5-hydroxyindoleacetic acid (5-HIAA), which serves as the diagnostic test for this syndrome. The clinical presentation consists of cutaneous flushing, intestinal hypermobility, bronchial constriction, edema, and cardiac lesions. These result from the vasoactive amines that are released into the systemic circulation. Carcinomas of the bronchus, thyroid, or pancreas occasionally may cause the carcinoid syndrome, although the tumor itself lacks the morphologic and histochemical characteristics of carcinoid tumor.

CARDIAC MANIFESTATION

Primary carcinoid tumors of the heart have not yet been described, and the tumor only rarely metastasizes to the heart.[98] However, the tumor products often cause the distinctive valvular disease. The right side of the heart is the common site of involvement; however, the left side may also be involved, particularly when the tumor is bronchial or an interatrial communication is present. Occasionally when there is extensive right heart involvement, the left heart may also be involved. The macroscopic findings are white–yellow glistening deposits usually over the tricuspid and pulmonic valves, but frequently over the right atrial and right ventricular endocardium as well. When these deposits contract, they may cause tricuspid regurgitation and pulmonary stenosis. They occasionally may cause right-sided restrictive cardiomyopathy.[100] On the left side, mitral stenosis or regurgitation may be present but is usually of no functional significance.[100a] Microscopic examination reveals superficial deposits of fibrous tissue over normal endothelium. Tumor cells are not found. The pathogenesis of cardiac lesions is not clear. Both 5-HT and bradykinins have been implicated.[98]

The clinical findings are related to the valvular lesions. Physical signs may indicate tricuspid regurgitation and right heart failure, especially elevated jugular venous pressure with an accentuated "v" wave, pansystolic lower sternal border murmur accentuated by inspiration, often associated with early diastolic flow murmur, parasternal heave, hepatomegaly with systolic pulsation, ascites, and peripheral edema. These may be associated with findings of pulmonary stenosis presented by an upper sternal systolic murmur with or without a thrill.

The diagnosis depends on a combination of systemic features associated with the characteristic cardiac findings. Although combined lesions of both mitral and aortic valves are fairly common as a consequence of either rheumatic heart disease or infective endocarditis or both, combined lesions of both tricuspid and pulmonic valves are rare, and carcinoid is the only condition in which uniformly both, not just one, right-sided valves are involved together.[100a] Urinary excretion of 5-HIAA is usually markedly elevated. In suspected cases computed axial tomography, ultrasonography, or angiography may help to identify metastases to the liver.[101]

Recent data[100a] refute earlier suggestions that patients with carcinoid heart disease have longer symptomatic illnesses compared with those without carcinoid heart disease: mean survival after the onset of dermal flushing, diarrhea, or wheezing (whichever symptom comes first) was 4.7 years in 21 patients with carcinoid heart disease and 6.3 years in 15 patients without carcinoid heart disease, no difference of statistical significance. Therefore, although carcinoid heart disease frequently is the cause of death in patients with the carcinoid syndrome, the development of carcinoid heart disease is not related to the duration of symptoms of the carcinoid syndrome. Treatment, including valve surgery, is palliative.[101a,101b]

DIAGNOSTIC TECHNIQUES

The noninvasive diagnosis of various forms of heart disease is one of the most rapidly developing areas in cardiology. The feasibility of diagnosing cardiac tumors, a diagnosis that only 20 years ago was rarely made antemortem, serves as a good example of this development.

Although several techniques exist, echocardiography, especially two-dimensional modality, is now recognized as the standard method of providing sensitive and accurate information on intracardiac masses in symptomatic as well as asymptomatic patients.[102,103] In most cardiac centers today, patients with a cardiac tumor are referred for surgery on the basis of two-dimensional echocardiographic diagnosis alone.[104,105]

RADIOLOGIC FINDINGS

The chest roentgenogram may often be normal or nonspecific in patients with cardiac tumors; however, several findings may be observed including cardiac enlargement, enlargement of a specific chamber, alterations in pulmonary vasculature, masses, mediastinal widening, pericardial effusion, and intracardiac calcifications.[106–108] Calcification may occur with many types of cardiac tumor[108,109] and should be differentiated from other structures that may show calcification, such as cardiac valves, anulus, coronary arteries, pericardium, or organized thrombus. Calcification in a child or infant should always raise the question of a cardiac tumor.

When the information obtained from a plain chest roentgenogram is nonspecific, fluoroscopy may offer a better means of localizing and differentiating the roentgenographic findings.

ECHOCARDIOGRAPHY

Left Atrial Tumors

Although more than 15 cases of left atrial tumor have been diagnosed at our Heart Institute in recent years, this diagnosis is always cause for celebration because the vast majority of these tumors were myxomas and the patients were "cured" by operation. Most myxomas are pedunculated, highly mobile, and relatively large; therefore, they are readily detected by both M-mode and two-dimensional modalities.[85,110–115] The classical M-mode characteristics are a reduced EF slope and dense diastolic echoes filling the entire space behind the anterior mitral leaflet. When a continuous scan is obtained from the mitral valve toward the aortic root, the systolic tumor echoes are seen in the left atrial cavity.[110–114] In smaller and less mobile tumors the diagnosis is more difficult. Careful imaging of the left atrium from various angles is required.[116,116a] The differential diagnosis on the M-mode scan includes mitral stenosis, especially in cases of heavy fibrosis and calcification, vegetations, and left atrial thrombi. Patients with mitral valve prolapse or ruptured chordae tendineae occasionally may be misdiagnosed as having a tumor, because the redundant posterior leaflet may appear as a dense mass of echoes on the M-mode tracing.

Most of these problems can be overcome by using two-dimensional modality.[105] This is the preferred technique for the identification, localization, and size estimation of left atrial tumors[104,116a,116b] (Figure 47.9). The differentiation between tumor and thrombus is somewhat more difficult and may at times be impossible.[116c] However, thrombi usually are immobile, may have a layered appearance (which can be more easily detected using a phased-array system), and are localized at the posterior left atrial portion.[117] Areas of hemorrhage have been described in left atrial myxomas, presented as areas of echolucency. This finding may serve as another clue in the differential diagnosis, because it is not observed in cases of thrombi or vegetations.[118] However, that the presence or absence of large sonolucent areas is not always reliable in the distinction of hemorrhages within a myxoma from a thrombus is attested by the recent report of a free-floating left atrial thrombus that contains a sonolucent core[118a] and is confirmed by other workers.[116b]

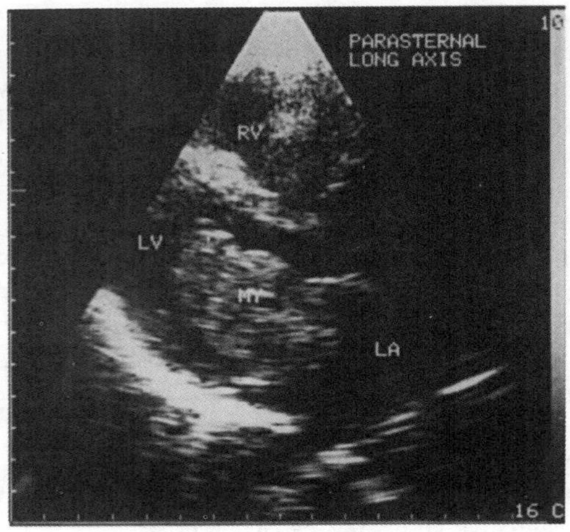

Figure 47.9. Two-dimensional echocardiography viewed from the parasternal long axis, demonstrating a large myxoma penetrating the left ventricle during diastole. LA = left atrium; LV = left ventricle; MY = myxoma; RV = right ventricle.

Right Atrial Tumors

The M-mode characteristics of right atrial tumors resemble those of the left atrium. A mass of echoes is observed behind the tricuspid valve, moving into the right ventricle during diastole.[86] Again, two-dimensional modality enables better visualization of the right atrium and the tricuspid valve from various angles, and therefore it is a more sensitive and accurate technique for diagnosing these lesions.[119] Whenever a left atrial myxoma is diagnosed, careful examination of the right atrium is required, because biatrial lesions are not infrequent.[104,120]

Ventricular Tumors

Tumors of the left or right ventricles may be observed on M-mode echocardiography mainly if they have a prominent intracavitary portion. A mass of echoes is observed in the adjacent ventricle or a paradoxic septal motion can be observed in some of the right ventricular tumors.[96] Two-dimensional echocardiography is the preferred technique for these lesions for all the previously mentioned reasons. In addition, it has the advantage of demonstrating intramural tumors that can only rarely be diagnosed by the single beam M-mode technique. The differential diagnosis between a ventricular tumor and a thrombus may not be easy.[121] Computer assisted tomographic tissue characterization techniques may help to overcome this problem.[122]

Pericardial Tumors

Pericardial tumors can be diagnosed using echocardiography.[123-125] On the M-mode tracing, a thickened pericardium and pericardial effusion are observed.[124] A two-dimensional echocardiogram demonstrates the extent and distribution of the effusion and may demonstrate the intrapericardial tumor mass itself.

This modality has been helpful in diagnosing some of the extracardiac tumors that may compress the pericardium or a cardiac chamber.[126]

OTHER NONINVASIVE METHODS

The older diagnostic techniques, namely phonocardiography, apexcardiography, ballistocardiography, and pressure or carotid pulse analysis are not helpful in the diagnosis of a cardiac tumor. Apart from the rather typical tumor plop that may be detected using phonocardiography,[83] no other sensitive signs exist using these techniques.

The more advanced techniques, however, may provide useful information and may complement or even replace echocardiography, especially when a technically adequate echocardiogram cannot be obtained. Among these, gated blood pool radionuclide imaging[127-129] has been described to be effective. Computed tomography,[130,131,131a] magnetic resonance imaging,[132,132a] and digital subtraction angiography[133] are promising as powerful diagnostic techniques in various aspects of cardiovascular pathology including cardiac tumors. Magnetic resonance imaging is a particularly exciting new modality because it is able to detect metabolic alterations in cardiac tissue[134]; therefore, it may have the potential to differentiate tumor from normal tissue.[134a]

It is beyond the purpose of this chapter to describe each modality in detail, and the reader is referred to more specific literature on this subject.[127-134,134a]

CARDIAC CATHETERIZATION

Cardiac catheterization, as discussed before, is not necessary in many cases of cardiac tumor. Currently, the major indications for the procedure in the case of cardiac tumors are: (1) technically inadequate noninvasive tests: (a) incomplete visualization of the tumor or its attachment and (b) inability to demonstrate other cardiac chambers; (2) the need for additional information, mainly on the presence and extent of coronary heart disease; (3) the need for accurate measurement of pressures, such as pulmonary pressure.

Cardiac catheterization, when performed, should be carried out carefully to avoid the possibility of embolization from a tumor fragment or an associated thrombus.[135] Whenever possible, a thorough noninvasive evaluation of all cardiac chambers is recommended and injections should be made into the chamber proximal to the one where the tumor is located.[107] The transseptal approach should not be used in these cases.[135] Sometimes the diagnosis of atrial myxoma may be suspected by demonstration of tumor vessels at coronary angiography.[136,136a]

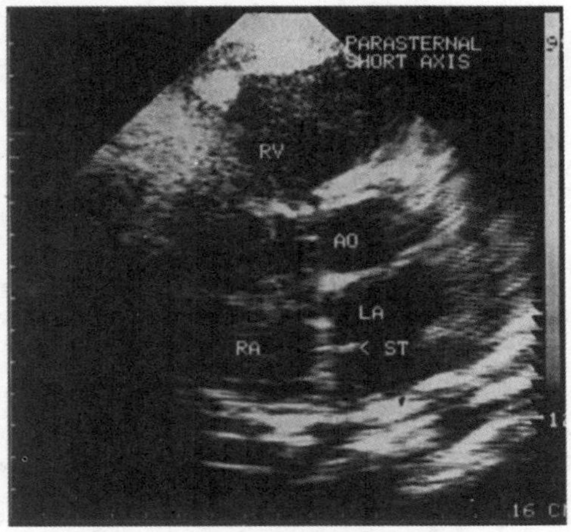

Figure 47.10. Two-dimensional echocardiography from the parasternal short-axis view. The remnant of a stalk (*arrow*) is seen in the left atrium following excision of a myxoma. AO = aorta; ST = stalk. Other abbreviations as in Figure 47.9.

TREATMENT

As a rule, surgical removal of the tumor is indicated whenever possible. In benign tumors, especially cardiac myxoma, a complete cure after resection is expected.[17,137,138,138a] When a cardiac myxoma is diagnosed, the operation should be performed immediately. Although in the past closed operations were performed, today as a rule all cardiac tumors should be removed under direct vision using extracorporeal circulation. Thus, thorough inspection of all four cardiac chambers is possible, and the possibility of tumor fragment embolization is minimized.

In most malignant tumors, either primary or secondary, an operation is not curative. These tumors usually involve a large portion of cardiac tissue and have often already metastasized. Surgery is indicated to exclude the possibility of a benign tumor, or occasionally for palliation, to avoid pressure or obstruction of vital cardiac structures. Additional treatment includes chemotherapy and radiation.[139,140] Although some success has been reported, especially in lymphosarcoma[141] and angiosarcoma,[142] in the vast majority of these tumors therapy does not effect a marked change in the course of the disease.

Periodic clinical and echocardiographic follow-up is indicated in each patient following surgical removal of a tumor, especially myxoma, because recurrences have been reported (Figure 47.10).

REFERENCES

1. Fine G: Neoplasms of the pericardium and heart, in Gould SE (ed): *Pathology of the Heart and Great Vessels*. Springfield, IL, Charles C Thomas, 1968, p 851.
2. Straus R, Merliss R: Primary tumors of the heart. *Arch Pathol* 1945; 39:74–78.
3. Heath D: Pathology of cardiac tumors. *Am J Cardiol* 1968; 21:315–327.
4. McAllister HA Jr: Primary tumors of the heart and pericardium. *Pathol Annu* 1979; 14:325–355.
5. Lymburner RM: Tumors of the heart: histopathological and clinical study. *Can Med Assoc J* 1934; 30:368–373.

6. Scott RW, Garvin CF: Tumors of the heart and pericardium. *Am Heart J* 1939; 17:431–436.
7. Fabian JT, Rose AG: Tumors of the heart. A study of 89 cases. *S Afr Med J* 1982; 61:71–77.
8. Willis RA: *The Spread of Tumors in the Human Body*, ed 2. London, Butterworth & Co, 1952.
9. Gassman HS, Meadows R Jr, Baker LA: Metastatic tumors of the heart. *Am J Med* 1955; 19:357–365.
10. Prichard RW: Tumors of the heart: review of the subject and report of one hundred and fifty cases. *Arch Pathol* 1951; 51:98–128.
11. Jugdutt BI, Rossall RE, Sterns LP: An unusual case of recurrent left atrial myxoma. *Can Med Assoc J* 1975; 112:1099–1100.
12. Dashkoff N, Boersma RB, Nanda NC, Gramiak R, Anderson MN, Subramanian S: Bilateral atrial myxomas: echocardiographic considerations. *Am J Med* 1978; 65:361–366.
13. Leonhardt ETG, Kullenberg KPG: Bilateral atrial myxomas with multiple arterial aneurysms: a syndrome mimicking polyarteritis nodosa. *Am J Med* 1977; 62:792–794.
14. Morgan DL, Palazola J, Reed W, Bell HH, Kindred LH, Beauchamp GD: Left heart myxomas. *Am J Cardiol* 1977; 40:611–614.
15. Sandrasagra FA, Oliver WA, English TAH: Myxoma of the mitral valve. *Br Heart J* 1979; 42:221–223.
16. St. John Sutton MG, Mercier LA, Guiliani ER, Lie JT: Atrial myxomas. A review of clinical experience in 40 patients. *Mayo Clin Proc* 1980; 55:371–376.
17. McAllister HA Jr, Fenoglio JJ Jr: *Tumors of the Cardiovascular Systems*. Washington, DC, Armed Forces Institute of Pathology, 1978.
18. Sayler WR, Page DL, Hutchins GM: The development of cardiac myxomas and papillary endocardial lesions from mural thrombus. *Am Heart J* 1975; 89:4–17.
19. Carney JA: Differences between nonfamilial and familial cardiac myxoma. *Am J Surg Pathol* 1985; 9:53–55.
20. Bloor CM: *Cardiac Pathology*. Philadelphia, JB Lippincott Co, 1978, pp 386–418.
21. Bashey RI, Nochumson S: Cardiac myxoma. Biochemical analysis and evidence for its neoplastic nature. *NY State J Med* 1979; 79:29–32.
22. Glasser SP, Bedynek JL, Hall RJ, Hopeman AR, Treasure RL, McAllister HA Jr, Esterly JA, Manion WC, Sanford HS: Left atrial myxoma. Report of a case including hemodynamic, surgical, histologic and histochemical characteristics. *Am J Med* 1971; 50:113–122.
23. Ferrans VJ, Roberts WC: Structural features of cardiac myxomas. Histology, histochemistry and electron microscopy. *Hum Pathol* 1973; 4:111–146.
24. Wold LE, Lie JT: Scanning electron microscopy of intracardiac myxoma. *Mayo Clin Proc* 1981; 56:198–200.
25. Morales AR, Fine G, Castro A, Nadji M: Cardiac myxoma (endocardioma). An immunocytochemical assessment of histogenesis. *Hum Pathol* 1981; 12:896–899.
26. Gorshevina TI, Nedozorova VK: Rabdomioma serdtsa u 5-mesiachnogo rebenka. *Pediatriia* 1983; 6:72.
27. Fenoglio JJ Jr, McAllister HA Jr, Ferrans VJ: Cardiac rhabdomyoma. A clinicopathologic and electron microscopic study. *Am J Cardiol* 1976; 38:241–251.
28. Bruni C, Prioleau PG, Ivey HH, Nolan SP: New fine structural features of cardiac rhabdomyoma. Report of a case. *Cancer* 1980; 46:2068–2073.
29. Hoen AG, Ellis EJ: Intramural fibroma of the heart. *Am J Cardiol*, 1966; 17:579–584.
30. Reul GJ Jr, Howell JF, Rubio PA, Peterson PK: Successful partial excision of an intramural fibroma of the left ventricle. *Am J Cardiol* 1975; 36:262–265.
31. Oliva PB, Breckinridge JC, Johnson ML, Brantigan CO, O'Meara OP: Left ventricular outflow obstruction produced by a pedunculated fibroma in a newborn. Clinical, angiographic, echocardiographic and surgical observations. *Chest* 1978; 74:590–593.
32. Feldman PS, Meyer MW: Fibroelastic hamartoma (fibroma) of the heart. *Cancer* 1976; 38:314–323.
33. Pomerance A: Papillary "tumours" of the heart valves. *J Pathol Bacteriol* 1961; 81:135–140.
33a. Topol EJ, Biern RO, Reitz BA: Cardiac papillary fibroelastoma and stroke. Echocardiographic diagnosis and guide to excision. *Am J Med* 1986; 80:129–132.
34. Lichtenstein HL, Lee JCK, Stewart S: Papillary tumor of the heart: incidental finding at surgery. *Hum Pathol* 1979; 10:473–475.
35. Lambl VA: Papillare Excrescenzen an der Semilunar-Klappe der Aorta. *Wien Med Wochenschr* 1856; 6:244–247.
36. Cha SD, Incarvito J, Fernandez J, Chang KS, Maranhao V, Gooch AS: Giant Lambl's excrescences of papillary muscle and aortic valve: echocardiographic, angiographic and pathologic findings. *Clin Cardiol* 1981; 4:51–54.
37. Moulton AL, Jaretzki A III, Bowman FO Jr, Silverstein EF, Bregman D: Massive lipoma of heart. *NY State J Med* 1976; 76:1820–1825.
38. Shumacker HB Jr, Leshnower AC: Extracavitary lipoma of the heart. Operative resection. *Ann Thorac Surg* 1974; 18:411–414.
39. Reyes LH, Rubio PA, Korompai FL, Guinn GA: Lipoma of the heart. *Int Surg* 1976; 61:179–180.
40. Reyes CV, Jablokow VR: Lipomatous hypertrophy of the cardiac interatrial septum. A report of 38 cases and review of the literature. *Am J Clin Pathol* 1979; 72:785–788.
41. Prior JT: Lipomatous hypertrophy of cardiac interatrial septum. A lesion resembling hibernoma, lipoblastomatosis and infiltrating lipoma. *Arch Pathol* 1964; 78:11–15.
42. Manion WC, Nelson WP, Hall RJ, Briety RE: Benign tumor of the heart causing complete heart block. *Am Heart J* 1972; 83:535–542.
43. James TN, Galakhow I: De Subitaneis Morbitus. XXVI. Fatal electrical instability of the heart associated with benign congenital polycystic tumor of the atrioventricular node. *Circulation* 1977; 56:667–678.
44. Tabry IF, Nasser VH, Rizk G, Touma A, Dagher IK: Cavernous hemangioma of the heart: case report and review of the literature. *J Thorac Cardiovasc Surg* 1975; 69:415–420.
45. Grant RT, Camp PD: Case of complete heart block due to arterial angioma. *Heart* 1932; 16:137–143.
46. Feigin DS, Fenoglio JJ, McAllister HA, Madewell JE: Pericardial cysts. A radiologic-pathologic correlation and review. *Radiology* 1977; 125:15–20.
47. Maier HC: Diverticulum of the pericardium. With observations on mode of development. *Circulation* 1957; 16:1040–1045.
47a. Reynard JS Jr, Gregoratos G, Gordon MJ, Bloor CM: Primary osteosarcoma of the heart. *Am Heart J* 1985; 109:598–600.
48. Whorton CM: Primary malignant tumors of the heart. Report of a case. *Cancer* 1949; 2:245–260.
49. Glancy DL, Morales JB, Roberts WC: Angiosarcoma of the heart. *Am J Cardiol* 1968; 21:413–419.
50. Strohl KP: Angiosarcoma of the heart: a case study. *Arch Intern Med* 1976; 136:928–929.
50a. Cheng TO, Sutton DC: Primary hemangioendotheliosarcoma of heart, diagnosed by angiocardiography. Review of the literature and report of a case. *Circulation* 1955; 11:456–461.
51. Panella JS, Paige ML, Victor TA, Semerdjian RA, Hueter DC: Angiosarcoma of the heart. Diagnosis by echocardiography. *Chest* 1979; 76:221–223.
52. Yang HY, Wasielewski JF, Lee W, Lee E, Paik YK: Angiosarcoma of the heart: ultrastructural study. *Cancer* 1981; 47:72–80.
53. Van Bruggen HW, de Koning J: Pulmonic stenosis caused by a malignant tumor of the heart. *Am Heart J* 1968; 76:526–533.
54. Roberts WC, Glancy DL, DeVita VT Jr: Heart in malignant lymphoma (Hodgkin's disease, lymphosarcoma, reticulum cell sarcoma and mycosis fungoides). A study of 196 autopsy cases. *Am J Cardiol* 1968; 22:85–107.
55. Case records of the Massachusetts General Hospital weekly clinicopathological exercises. Case 43-1971. *N Engl J Med* 1971; 285:1016–1023.
56. Gabelman C, Al-Sadir J, Lamberti J, Fozzard HA, Laufer E, Replogle RL, Myerowitz PD: Surgical treatment of recurrent primary malignant tumor of the left atrium. *J Thorac Cardiovasc Surg* 1979; 77:914–921.
57. Timmis AD, Smallpeice C, Davies AC, Macarthur AM, Gishen P, Jackson G: Intracardiac spread of intravenous leiomyomatosis with successful surgical excision. *N Engl J Med* 1980; 303:1043–1044.
58. Kadir S, Coulam CM: Intracaval extension of renal cell carcinoma. *Cardiovasc Intervent Radiol* 1980: 3:180–183.
59. Atkinson K, McElwain TJ, Mackay AM: Myeloma of the heart. *Br Heart J* 1974; 36:309–312.
60. Glancy DL, Roberts WC: The heart in malignant melanoma: a study of 70 autopsy cases. *Am J Cardiol* 1968; 21:555–571.
61. Herbut PA, Maisel AL: Secondary tumors of the heart. *Arch Pathol* 1942; 34:358–364.
62. Applefeld MM, Pollock SH: Cardiac disease in patients who have malignancies. *Current Problems in Cardiology*. Chicago, Year Book Medical Publishers, 1980, vol 4, p 5.
63. Simms EB, Katz RJ, DiBianco R, Matthews MJ, Fletcher RD, Minna JD: Conservative management of pericardial tamponade in lung cancer. *Proc Am Assoc Can Res* 1979; 20:410.
64. Applefeld MM, Slawson RG, Spicer KM, Singleton RT, Wesley M, Wiernik PH: Long-term cardiovascular evaluation of patients with Hodgkin's disease treated by thoracic mantle radiation therapy. *Cancer Treat Rep* 1982; 66:1003–1013.
65. Perez CA, Presant CA, Van Amburg AL III: Management of superior vena cava syndrome. *Semin Oncol* 1978; 5:123–134.
66. Goodwin JF: Symposium on Cardiac Tumors. The spectrum of cardiac tumors. *Am J Cardiol* 1968; 21:307–314.
67. Huston KA, Combs JJ Jr, Lie JT, Guiliani ER: Left atrial myxoma stimulating peripheral vasculitis. *Mayo Clin Proc* 1978; 53:752–756.
68. MacGregor GA, Cullen RA: The syndrome of fever, anaemia and high sedimentation rate with an atrial myxoma. *Br Med J* 1959; 2:991–993.
69. Willey RF, Matthews MB, Walbaum PR: An unusual case of large right atrial myxoma. *Br Heart J* 1980; 44:108–110.
70. Levinson JP, Kincaid OW: Myxoma of the right atrium associated with

polycythemia. Report of successful excision. *N Engl J Med* 1961; 264:1187–1192.
71. Vuopio P, Nikkila EA: Hemolytic anemia and thrombocytopenia in a case of left atrial myxoma associated with mitral stenosis. *Am J Cardiol* 1966; 17:585–589.
72. Firor WB, Aldridge HE, Bigelow WG: A follow-up study of three patients after removal of left atrial myxoma five to ten years previously. *J Thorac Cardiovasc Surg* 1966; 51:515–520.
73. Currey HL, Mathews JA, Robinson J: Right atrial myxoma mimicking a rheumatic disorder. *Br Med J* 1967; 1:547–548.
74. Graham SL, Sellers AL: Atrial myxoma with multiple myeloma. *Arch Intern Med* 1979; 139:116–117.
75. Silverman J, Olwin JS, Graettinger JS: Cardiac myxomas with systemic embolization. *Circulation* 1962; 26:99–103.
76. Koikkalainen K, Kostiainen S, Luosto R: Left atrial myxoma revealed by femoral embolectomy. *Scand J Thorac Cardiovasc Surg* 1977; 11:33–35.
77. Schweiger MJ, Hafer JG Jr, Brown R, Gianelly RE: Spontaneous cure of infected left atrial myxoma following embolization. *Am Heart J* 1980; 99:630–634.
78. Cogan DG, Wray SH: Vascular occlusions in the eye from cardiac myxomas. *Am J Ophthalmol* 1975; 80:396–403.
79. Viswanathan B, Luber JM Jr, Bell-Thomson J: Right ventricular myxoma. *Ann Thorac Surg* 1985; 39:280–281.
80. Muroff LR, Johnson PM: Right atrial myxoma presenting as non-resolving pulmonary emboli: case report. *J Nucl Med* 1976; 17:890–892.
81. Gonzales A, Altieri PI, Marquez E, Cox RA, Castillo M: Massive pulmonary embolism associated with a right ventricular myxoma. *Am J Med* 1980; 69:795–798.
82. Heath D, Mackinnon J: Pulmonary hypertension due to myxoma of the right atrium, with special reference to the behavior of emboli of myxoma in the lung. *Am Heart J* 1964; 68:227–235.
83. Harvey WP: Clinical aspects of cardiac tumors. *Am J Cardiol* 1968; 21:328–343.
84. Greenwood WF: Profile of atrial myxoma. *Am J Cardiol* 1968; 21:367–375.
84a. Harrison LH Jr, Said SI, Ezekowitz MD, Krous HF: Vasoactive intestinal polypeptide in cardiac myxoma. *J Thorac Cardiovasc Surg* 1985; 89:800–806.
85. Bass NM, Sharratt GP: Left atrial myxoma diagnosed by echocardiography, with observations on tumor movement. *Br Heart J* 1973; 35:1332–1335.
86. Waxler EB, Kawai N, Kasparian H: Right atrial myxoma: echocardiographic, phonocardiographic, and hemodynamic signs. *Am Heart J* 1972; 83:251–257.
87. Talley RC, Baldwin BJ, Symbas PN, Nutter DO: Right atrial myxoma. Unusual presentation with cyanosis and clubbing. *Am J Med* 1970; 48:256–260.
88. Massumi R: Bedside diagnosis of right heart myxomas through detection of palpable tumor shocks and audible plops. *Am Heart J* 1983; 105:303–310.
89. de Paiva EC, Macieira-Coelho E, Amram SS, Duarte CDS, Coelho E: Intracavity left ventricular myxoma. *Am J Cardiol* 1967; 20:260–262.
90. Vered Z, Schneeweiss A, Meltzer RS, Neufeld HN: Echocardiographic assessment of left ventricular outflow tract obstruction. *Am Heart J* 1983; 106:177–181.
91. Isner JM, Falcone MW, Virmani R, Roberts WC: Cardiac sarcoma causing "ASH" and simulating coronary heart disease. *Am J Med* 1979; 66:1025–1030.
92. Cabin HS, Costello RM, Vasudevan G, Maron BJ, Roberts WC: Cardiac lymphoma mimicking hypertropic cardiomyopathy. *Am Heart J* 1981; 102:466–468.
93. Marin-Garcia J, Fitch CW, Shenefelt RE: Primary right ventricular tumor (fibroma) simulating cyanotic heart disease in a newborn. *J Am Coll Cardiol* 1984; 3:868–871.
94. Hada Y, Wolfe C, Murry GF, Craige E: Right ventricular myxoma. Case report and review of phonocardiographic and auscultatory manifestations. *Am Heart J* 1980; 100:871–877.
95. Goldstein S, Mahoney EB: Right ventricular fibrosarcoma causing pulmonic stenosis. *Am J Cardiol* 1966; 17:570–578.
96. Sasse L, Lorentzen D, Alvarez H: Paradoxical septal motion secondary to right ventricular tumor. *JAMA* 1975; 234:955–956.
97. Thurber DL, Edwards JE, Achor RWP: Secondary malignant tumors of the pericardium. *Circulation* 1962; 26:228–241.
98. Grahame-Smith DG: The carcinoid syndrome. *Am J Cardiol* 1968; 21:376–387.
99. Sworn MJ, Edlin GP, McGill DAF, Mousley JS: Tricuspid valve replacement in carcinoid syndrome due to ovarian primary. *Br Med J* 1980; 280:85–86.
100. McGuire MR, Pugh DM, Dunn MI: Carcinoid heart disease. Restrictive cardiomyopathy as a late complication. *J Kansas Med Soc* 1978; 79:661–665.
100a. Ross EM, Roberts WC: The carcinoid syndrome: comparison of 21 necropsy subjects with carcinoid heart disease to 15 necropsy subjects without carcinoid heart disease. *Am J Med* 1985; 79:339–354.
101. Smevik B, Kolmannskog F, Aakhus T: Computed tomography and angiography in carcinoid liver metastases. *Acta Radiol* 1983; 24:189–193.
101a. Kay JH: Eleven-year follow-up after tricuspid valve replacement and pulmonic valvulotomy in the carcinoid syndrome. *Am J Cardiol* 1984; 53:651.
101b. DiSesa VJ, Mills RM Jr, Collins JJ Jr: Surgical management of carcinoid heart disease. *Chest* 1985; 88:789–791.
102. Galton BB: Left atrial myxoma without significant cardiac manifestations. *J Med Soc NJ* 1979; 76:754–757.
103. Oldershaw PJ, Sutton M St J, Gibson RV: Long asymptomatic period of atrial myxomas. *Thorax* 1980; 35:70–71.
104. Lappe DL, Bulkley BH, Weiss JL: Two-dimensional echocardiographic diagnosis of left atrial myxoma. *Chest* 1978; 74:55–58.
105. Lewis BS, Lewis N, Popp RL, Weiss AT, Borman JB, Gotsman MS: Diagnostic value of cross-sectional echocardiography in left atrial myxoma. *Isr J Med Sci* 1979; 15:426–430.
106. Steiner RE: Radiologic aspects of cardiac tumors. *Am J Cardiol* 1968; 21:344–356.
107. Abrams HL, Adams DF, Grant HA: The radiology of tumors of the heart. *Radiol Clin North Am* 1971; 9:299–326.
108. Sharratt GP, Grover ML, Monro JL: Calcified left atrial myxoma with floppy mitral valve. *Br Heart J* 1979; 42:608–610.
109. Davis GD, Kincaid OW, Hallermann FJ: Roentgen aspects of cardiac tumors. *Semin Roentgenol* 1969; 4:384–394.
110. Liu HY, Cheng KZ, Yang WY, Li ZS, Meng XQ: Diagnosis of intracardiac myxomas by echocardiography. *Chin Med J* 1983; 96:421–428.
111. Finegan RE, Harrison DC: Diagnosis of left atrial myxoma by echocardiography. *N Engl J Med* 1970; 282:1022–1023.
112. Gustafson A, Edler I, Dahlback O, Kaude J, Persson S: Left atrial myxoma diagnosed by ultrasound cardiography. *Angiology* 1973; 24:554–562.
113. Schattenberg TT: Echocardiographic diagnosis of left atrial myxoma. *Mayo Clin Proc* 1968; 43:620–627.
114. Wolfe SB, Popp RL, Feigenbaum H: Diagnosis of atrial tumors by ultrasound. *Circulation* 1969; 39:615–622.
115. Abdulla AM, Stefadouros MA, Mucha E, Moore HV, O'Malley GA: Left atrial myxoma: echocardiographic diagnosis and determination of size. *JAMA* 1977; 238:510–511.
116. Nasser WK, Davis RH, Dillon JC, Tavel ME, Helman CH, Feigenbaum H, Fisch C: Atrial myxoma. I. Clinical and pathologic features in nine cases. II. Phonocardiographic, echocardiographic, hemodynamic and angiographic features in nine cases. *Am Heart J* 1972; 83:694–704, 810–824.
116a. Charuzi Y, Bolger A, Beeder C, Lew AS: A new echocardiographic classification of left atrial myxoma. *Am J Cardiol* 1985; 55:614–615.
116b. Fyke FE III, Seward JB, Edwards WD, Miller FA, Reeder GS, Schattenberg TT, Shub C, Callahan JA, Tajik AJ: Primary cardiac tumors: experience with 30 consecutive patients since the introduction of two-dimensional echocardiography. *J Am Coll Cardiol* 1985; 5:1465–1473.
116c. Kmetzo JJ, Peters RW, Plotnick GD, Carliner NH, Baumgartner WA, Fisher ML: Left atrial mass. Thrombus mimicking myxoma. *Chest* 1985; 88:906–907.
117. Tallury VK, DePasquale NP: Ultrasound cardiography in the diagnosis of left atrial thrombus. *Chest* 1979; 59:501–503.
118. Rahilly GT Jr, Nanda NC: Two-dimensional echographic identification of tumor hemorrhages in atrial myxomas. *Am Heart J* 1981; 101:237–239.
118a. Sherman W, Nozad SE, Stoian A, Madias JE: Free-floating left atrial thrombus and systemic embolization. *Chest* 1985; 87:694–695.
119. Come PC, Kurland GS, Vine HS: Two dimensional echocardiography in differentiating right atrial and tricuspid valve mass lesions. *Am J Cardiol* 1979; 44:1207–1212.
120. Imperio J, Summers D, Krasnow N, Piccone VA Jr: The distribution pattern of biatrial myxomas. *Ann Thorac Surg* 1980; 20:469–473.
121. St John Sutton MG: Echocardiographic features of free floating thrombus mimicking right ventricular myxoma. *Br Heart J* 1983; 50:605.
122. Greenleaf JF, Johnson SA, Lent AH: Measurement of spatial distribution of refractive index in tissues by ultrasonic computer assisted tomography. *Ultrasound Med Biol* 1978; 3:327–339.
123. Farooki ZQ, Hakimi M, Arciniegas E, Green EW: Echocardiographic features in a case of intrapericardial teratoma. *J Clin Ultrasound* 1978; 6:108–110.
124. Lin TK, Steck JM, Eckert WG, Lin JJ, Farha SJ, Hagan CT: Pericardial angiosarcoma simulating pericardial effusion by echocardiography. *Chest* 1978; 73:881–883.
125. Chandraratna PAN, Littman BB, Serafini A, Whayne T, Robinson H: Echocardiographic evaluation of extracardiac masses. *Br Heart J* 1978; 40:741–749.
126. Yoshikawa J, Sabah I, Yanagihara K, Owaki T, Kato H, Tanemoto K: Cross-sectional echocardiographic diagnosis of large left atrial tumor and extracardiac tumor compressing the left atrium. Limitation of M

mode echocardiography in distinguishing the two lesions. *Am J Cardiol* 1978; 42:853–857.
127. Pohost GM, Pastore JO, McKusick KA, Chiotellis PN, Kapeliakis GZ, Myers GS, Dinsmore RE, Block PC: Detection of left atrial myxoma by gated radionuclide cardiac imaging. *Circulation* 1977; 55:88–92.
128. Pitcher D, Wainwright R, Brennand-Roper D, Deverall P, Sowton E, Maisey M: Cardiac tumours: non-invasive detection and assessment by gated blood pool radionuclide imaging. *Br Heart J* 1980; 44:143–149.
129. Winzelberg GG, Rapoport F, Boucher CA, Carey RW, McKusick KA, Strauss HW: Combined gated cardiac blood pool scintigraphy and Ga-citrate scintigraphy for detection of cardiac lymphoproliferative disorders. *Radiology* 1981; 141:191–192.
130. Goodwin JD, Axel L, Adams JR, Schiller NB, Simpson PC Jr, Gertz EW: Computed tomography: a new method for diagnosing tumor of the heart. *Circulation* 1981; 63:448–451.
131. Sutton D, Al-Kutoubi MA, Lipkin DP: Left atrial myxoma diagnosed by computerized tomography. *Br J Radiol* 1982; 55:80–81.
131a. Kawai N, Sotobata I, Iwase M, Shiki K, Yokota M, Tanaka M, Kondo K, Iwamura N, Tsuchida T: Evaluation of left atrial myxoma with transmission computed tomography. *Am Heart J* 1985; 109:1116–1118.
132. Osbakken M, Briggs RW: Nuclear magnetic resonance: theory and review of cardiac applications. *Am Heart J* 1984; 108:574–590.
132a. Pizzarello RA, Goldberg SM, Goldman MA, Gottesman R, Fetten JV, Brown N, Kahn EI, Stein HL: Tumor of the heart diagnosed by magnetic resonance imaging. *J Am Coll Cardiol* 1985; 5:989–991.
133. Crummy AB, Strother CM, Sackett JF, Ergun DL, Shaw CG, Kruger RA, Mistretta CA, Turnipseed WD, Lieberman RP, Myerowitz PD, Ruzicka FF: Computerized fluoroscopy: digital subtraction for intravenous angiocardiography and arteriography. *Am J Roentgenol* 1980; 135:1131–1140.
134. Menasche P, Fauchet M, Fossel ET, Piwnica A: Nuclear magnetic resonance: a new method for noninvasive assessment of cardiac metabolism. *Med Prog Technol* 1982; 8:183–185.
134a. Pflugfelder PW, Wisenberg G, Boughner DR: Detection of atrial myxoma by magnetic resonance imaging. *Am J Cardiol* 1985; 55:242–243.
135. Pindyck F, Pierce EC, Baron MG, Lukban SB: Embolization of left atrial myxoma after transseptal cardiac catheterization. *Am J Cardiol* 1972; 30:569–571.
136. Rasmussen KK, Peeples TC, Nellen JR: Unusual variant in tumor vascularity associated with left atrial myxoma. *Am J Roentgenol* 1983; 141:927–928.
136a. Hinterauer L, Goebel N, Hess O: Demonstration of tumor vessels of a right atrial myxoma by means of coronary angiography. *Fortschr Geb Rontgenstr Nuklearmed* 1985; 142:99–100.
137. Castaneda AR, Varco RL: Tumors of the heart: surgical consideration. *Am J Cardiol* 1968; 21:357–362.
138. Silverman NA: Primary cardiac tumors. *Ann Surg* 1980; 191:127–138.
138a. Hanson EC, Gill CC, Razavi M, Loop FD: The surgical treatment of atrial myxomas. Clinical experience and late results in 33 patients. *J Thorac Cardiovasc Surg* 1985; 89:298–303.
139. Laws JW, Annes GP, Bogren HG: Primary malignant tumors of the heart. *Calif Med* 1973; 118:11–17.
140. Sagerman RH, Hurley E, Bagshaw MA: Successful sterilization of a primary cardiac sarcoma by supervoltage radiation therapy. *Am J Roentgenol* 1964; 92:942–946.
141. Garfein OB: Lymphosarcoma of the right atrium. Angiographic and hemodynamic documentation of response to chemotherapy. *Arch Intern Med* 1975; 135:325–327.
142. Sharma S, Tendolkar A, Parulkar GB: Angiosarcoma of the heart. *Am Heart J* 1985; 109:601–603.

48 Traumatic Heart Disease (Cardiac Injuries)

Richard A. Crass, MD and Donald D. Trunkey, MD

The lethality of cardiac injuries has long been recognized. In the *Iliad* (about 950 BC) it is stated that "Patroklos wounded Sarpedon with a javelin—the insulting victor with disdain bestrode the prostrate prince and on his bosom trod; then drew the weapon from his panting heart, the reeking fibers clinging to the dart. From the wide wound gushed a stream of blood, and the soul issued in the purple flood."[1] In 1642, the concept that cardiac injuries were uniformly fatal was challenged by Tourby who at autopsy found scarring of the heart in a man who had been stabbed in the chest with a sword four years previously.[1] Purple[2] in 1855 summarized the findings in 42 reported cases of cardiac wounds. He found that not all cardiac injuries were immediately fatal, and that the right ventricle was injured most commonly, but patients appeared to survive longer if the left ventricle was the one injured. Fisher in 1868 reported on 452 cardiac injuries, with several patients recovering without incident.[1] The first operation for cardiac injury was performed in 1871 when Collender removed a needle from the heart, and the patient survived.[1] The first attempt at suturing a cardiac wound was made in 1895 by Cappelen.[3] The patient died two days later, but the case attracted attention because of the short-term survival and the fact that the operation was technically successful. Two years later, Rehn[4] reported the first successful suturing of a cardiac injury. Operation on cardiac wounds then became a firmly established practice so that in 1903 Ricketts was able to report success in 20 of 56 repairs of cardiac wounds.[1] The next advance was Beck's description[5] in 1926 of temporary inflow occlusion to achieve a relatively bloodless field. He also detailed the technique of digital occlusion of wounds while sutures were placed. Bigger[6] in 1934 described sternotomy as an approach to cardiac wounds and differentiated for the first time between those patients presenting with tamponade in whom the results were good, and patients with hypovolemic arrests secondary to hemorrhage through the pericardial wound into the chest. Bright and Beck[7] in 1935 presented the first series of cases of blunt cardiac injury in which mortality was almost uniform. The first survival after blunt injury had already been reported in 1895 by Moullin and Mansel, the patient being a football player with traumatic tamponade which was decompressed surgically.[7] Escaude and Bruez[8] in 1917 reported seven operations for intracardiac bullet removal in a series of 14 cases with four survivors. They also reported successful removal of four intracavitary missiles that had migrated to a hypogastric vein. Harken[9] during World War II reported successful removal of 56 foreign bodies from the heart, 13 of which were in the cardiac chamber, with no deaths. He attributed his success to the ready availability of banked blood.

TYPES OF INJURIES

The two broad categories of cardiac injuries include those caused by a penetrating object and blunt cardiac injuries. Penetrating injuries can be due to stabwounds, gunshot wounds, and impalement on objects including one's own fractured ribs. Blunt injuries can be caused by a variety of mechanisms, including direct blows, compression, deceleration, and increased intravascular pressure due to abdominal compression. These mechanisms most characteristically occur in high speed motor vehicle accidents, with the victim being thrown against the steering wheel. There is a definite difference in the incidence of penetrating versus blunt cardiac injuries when comparing urban and rural areas. With the increase in urban crime, the dominant injury in most cities is penetrating cardiac injury, whereas in rural areas, blunt cardiac injury secondary to motor vehicle accidents is more common. It was estimated that in 1973 cardiac trauma occurred in 900,000 of the total of 25 million motor vehicle accidents.[10] Of trauma victims with severe chest wall injuries, including rib and sternal fractures, up to 30% will have associated cardiac trauma.[11,12]

The most common cardiac injury due to penetrating trauma is laceration of the right ventricle, because the right ventricle comprises the largest portion of the anterior exposure of the heart, placing it most at jeopardy in a stabwound of the anterior torso. Less frequently injured, in order of frequency, are the left ventricle, right atrium, and left atrium. Right ventricular injuries have half the mortality of left ventricular injuries, with the overall mortality still ranging from 60% to 80%.[13,14] Stab-wounds generally produce less tissue trauma than do gunshot wounds. The wounding power of a missile in a gunshot wound depends on several factors, one being the amount of energy carried by the missile, as expressed by the formula:

$$KE = 1/2\ MV^2$$

where KE equals kinetic energy, M equals mass, and V equals velocity. Velocity then is the most important determinant of energy of the missile. The other factor is the amount of energy imparted to the wounded tissue. A missile that exits the body without imparting much energy causes much less trauma to tissue than does a deformed, fragmented, or tumbling missile that imparts most of its energy in the tissue. Shotgun wounds are a special case because at close range (less than 3 meters) incredible amounts of energy are imparted to the tissue, whereas at long range (greater than 7 meters) the individual pellets each function as a separate low velocity missile with little wounding power. If the laceration in the ventricle and pericardium is large, rapid exsanguination occurs and survival is rare. Most survivors have a small laceration in both myocardium and pericardium and present with signs and symptoms of pericardial tamponade. A penetrating object can injure anything in its path, so that coronary artery lacerations, septal perforations, valvular lacerations, intracardiac shunts, and lacerations of papillary muscles or chordae tendineae occasionally occur.

The most common blunt cardiac injury is myocardial contusion, occurring in up to 20% of patients with severe chest injury, 16% of autopsied motor vehicle fatalities, and in as high as 76% of selected motor vehicle accident victims with multiple injuries.[10–12] Depending on the extent of the contusion, the pathophysiologic aspects vary from a small contusion with a potential for cardiac dysrhythmia warranting careful monitoring, up to and including a large area of myocardial necrosis with cardiac dysfunction and the potential for delayed rupture of the heart. Other blunt cardiac injuries include myocardial rupture, septal perforation, coronary artery disruption, rupture of valve cusps, papillary muscle, or chordae tendineae, traumatic pericarditis, and pericardial rupture (with potential for cardiac herniation)[15] (Table 48.1).

Table 48.1. Cardiac Injuries

Myocardium
1. Contusion
2. Laceration
3. Infarction
4. Rupture
5. Septal perforation
6. Intracardiac shunts
7. Arrhythmias

Coronary arteries
1. Laceration
2. Intimal disruption
3. Thrombosis
4. Perivascular hematoma

Valves
1. Rupture or laceration of valve cusps
2. Rupture or laceration of papillary muscles or chordae tendineae

Pericardium
1. Hemopericardium, cardiac tamponade
2. Traumatic pericarditis
3. Constrictive pericarditis
4. Pericardial rupture
5. Cardiac herniation

DIAGNOSIS

Penetrating cardiac trauma is easier to diagnose than is blunt cardiac trauma because a precordial wound always suggests to the clinician the possibility of a subjacent cardiac injury. Even penetrating cardiac injuries can be difficult to diagnose depending on whether there is cardiac tamponade, hypovolemia, or, most confusingly, a mixed picture. If there is a large hole in the pericardium with rapid decompression bleeding from the heart, the patient may present in pure hypovolemic shock. If the hole in the pericardium is small, all bleeding will be contained within the pericardium and the patient will present with pure tamponade. Combinations are possible, with a mixed picture presenting first as hypovolemia and tamponade with variable elevation of the central venous pressure after resuscitation. Paradoxical pulse, muffled heart tones, and distended neck veins (Beck's triad) are often absent in patients with acute pericardial tamponade.[16] Because hypovolemia is a much more common cause of shock in the trauma victim, it is easy to overlook the cardiac causes of hypotension, which are seen frequently in trauma. These include tension pneumothorax, cardiac tamponade, and severe myocardial contusion resulting in cardiac dysfunction. A patient with antecedent cardiac dysfunction becomes difficult to assess. Some of these dilemmas can be circumvented by an organized approach to the status of the circulation in the trauma victim. An experienced clinician will always ensure that the airway is adequate or established and that ventilation is occurring. The next priority is to assess the circulation with a few expedient maneuvers. The first maneuver is to feel an extremity to determine if it is warm or cool and clammy. If it is cool and clammy, the patient is assumed to be in shock, and the next maneuver is to rapidly feel a carotid or femoral pulse to ascertain the approximate blood pressure and assess the quality of the pulse. With experience, one can tell whether the pulse is thready (meaning blood pressure approximately 60 mm Hg), normal (meaning a blood pressure of over 100 mm Hg), or somewhere in between. Once shock is established, the next maneuver is to inspect the neck veins (Figure 48.1). In hypovolemic shock, they will be flat, whereas in cardiac causes of shock (in their pure form) the neck veins will be distended. To differentiate between tension pneumothorax and cardiac tamponade, the tracheal position is important. With tension pneumothorax, there will be a deviation of the trachea to the contralateral side, which simplifies the diagnosis. After the presence of pneumothorax with percussion is confirmed, rapid needle evacuation of the appropriate hemithorax is performed. The

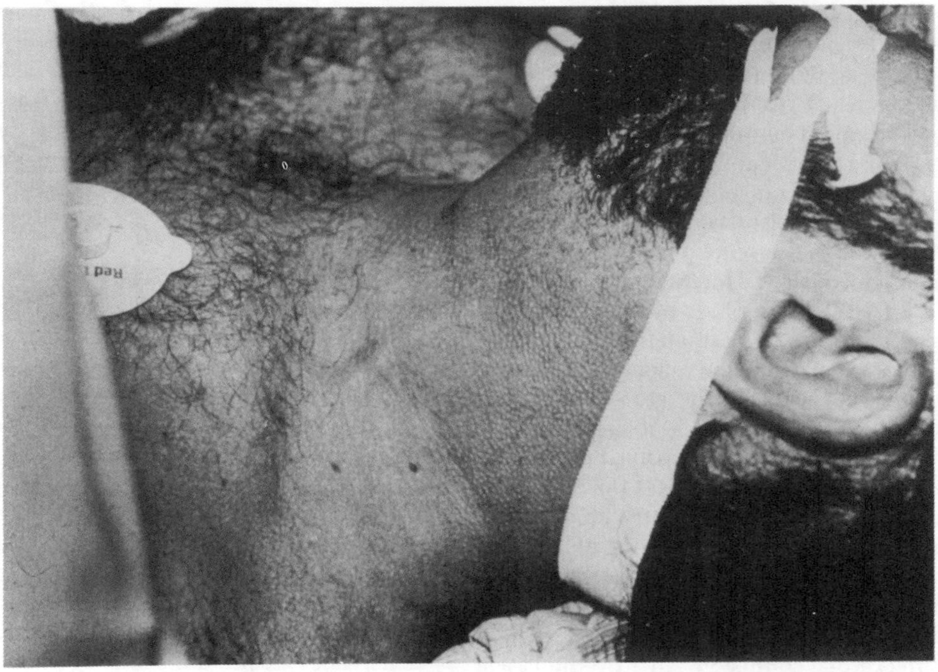

Figure 48.1. This 34-year-old man was stabbed once just to the right of the sternum in the fourth intercostal space. He was in clinical shock and neck veins are obviously distended. Cardiac tamponade was confirmed at thoracotomy and the right ventricular wound was sutured.

neck veins are less useful if the patient presents with a combination of hypovolemia and a cardiac cause of shock, in which case the neck veins may only distend after volume replenishment.

The stability of the patient with suspected cardiac tamponade due to penetrating trauma dictates the nature of the evaluation. Findings on chest radiographs are usually nonspecific (Figure 48.2). If the patient is comatose and in or near cardiac arrest, emergency room thoracotomy is both diagnostic and therapeutic. It should be performed only if immediate surgical consultation is available; otherwise, therapeutic pericardiocentesis should be performed.[17,18] If blood pressure is maintained, evaluation should include insertion of a central venous catheter and consideration of thoracotomy in the operating room if signs of tamponade are present. If available, a two-dimensional echocardiogram is extremely sensitive for detection of free pericardial fluid. In less typical cases, a second choice is diagnostic pericardiocentesis, although there is the potential for myocardial laceration and creation of tamponade where none previously existed. This potential can be minimized by connecting the pericardiocentesis needle to the chest lead of the electrocardiogram and stopping penetration when an injury current appears on the electrocardiogram. However, false-negative and false-positive pericardiocentesis results are obtained in up to one half the cases.[19] Tension pneumothorax can mimic cardiac tamponade, and tracheal position should be checked before any of the aforementioned procedures are contemplated. If pericardial tamponade is diagnosed or temporarily treated by pericardiocentesis, or both, surgical consultation should be obtained, as the consensus currently is that all patients

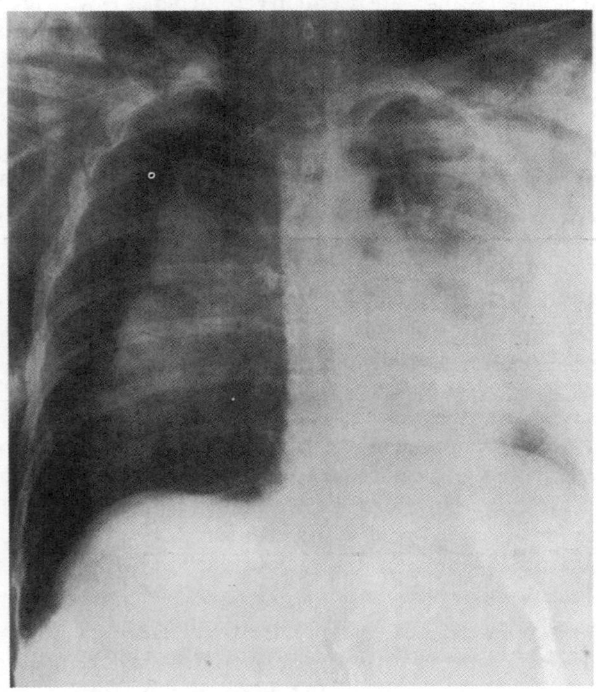

Figure 48.2. This 28-year-old man was involved in a motor vehicle accident. He arrived in the emergency room in profound shock. A single chest film was obtained en route to the operating room. His injuries included lacerations of the right mainstem bronchus and right atrium, and rupture of the spleen. All injuries were repaired.

with traumatic tamponade should have thoracotomy with repair of the cardiac lesion. Tamponade or exsanguination can also be due to laceration of a coronary artery, which can only be distinguished from a cavitary laceration of the heart at thoracotomy. If minimal bleeding occurs from a coronary laceration, the patient may present with myocardial ischemia. Internal derangements of the heart, including septal perforations, fistulas, and valvular injury, are difficult to diagnose in the acute phase. Small fistulas usually seal spontaneously.[20] Internal derangements, when suspected after the acute phase of injury, are generally best diagnosed by cardiac catheterization.

Diagnosis of myocardial contusion following blunt thoracic trauma remains difficult and in less obvious cases is possible only if there is a high index of suspicion. The electrocardiogram may be normal to grossly abnormal depending on the size, location, and nature of the contusion. The ST-T–wave segment may be slightly abnormal in intramyocardial hemorrhage to be indicative of an acute myocardial infarction with full-thickness necrosis in devascularizing injuries. The appearance of any new atrial or ventricular arrhythmia or bundle branch block pattern should suggest myocardial contusion. An arrhythmia will develop in approximately 20% of patients with a myocardial contusion and it may be their only diagnostic clue.[21] The MB isoenzyme fraction has been a disappointing laboratory study in myocardial contusion. It is not as specific for cardiac muscle as previously thought and indeed can be elevated with injury to skeletal muscle and various other tissues that can be injured by blunt trauma. Echocardiography[22] and radionuclide (eg, pyrophosphate) scans[23] are useful in certain patients with areas of myocardial dysfunction, ischemia, or necrosis, but again they may be normal in less severe cardiac contusions. Rarely, right ventricular contusion, like right ventricular infarction, simulates constrictive pericarditis.[24] Although use of the right ventricular Frank-Starling mechanism in patients with traumatic right ventricular contusion generally maintains right ventricular pump function at a level similar to that in traumatized patients without acute myocardial contusion, a concurrent elevation in the pulmonary vascular resistance associated with lung injury or concomitant left ventricular contusion could result in a significant depression of right ventricular pump function at lower levels of right ventricular afterload than otherwise tolerated.[25] If suspicion is high enough, a period of monitoring is appropriate in any patient with significant blunt thoracic trauma and should probably be continued for 72 hours. Hopefully, in the coming years a "gold standard" for early diagnosis of myocardial contusion will be developed to help with this, in many cases, still imprecise diagnosis. Those few patients with cavitary rupture and tamponade or exsanguination who survive to reach the hospital can usually be saved only by emergency room thoracotomy. Some patients with myocardial contusion will develop a more insidious tamponade, and echocardiography or pericardiocentesis may be necessary to diagnose the less obvious cases. Blunt injury to the coronary arteries, such as intimal disruption, is difficult to distinguish from myocardial contusion. Internal blunt derangements of the heart, such as valvular cusp rupture or rupture of papillary muscles or chordae tendineae, as with penetrating internal derangements, are difficult to diagnose acutely and are generally diagnosed by cardiac catheterization following the acute phase when signs suggest their presence. Rupture of the pericardium with cardiac herniation can usually be suggested by the chest radiograph.

TREATMENT

Pericardiocentesis, as well as being diagnostic, can also be therapeutic, at least temporarily. If there is delay before thoracotomy, such as that necessary to assemble the surgical team or to allow transfer to an appropriate facility, a plastic catheter left in the pericardial sac will allow repeated aspirations to be performed. Although approximately 200 cc of fluid in the pericardial sac is necessary to cause hypotension, removal of as little as 10 to 20 cc of fluid may restore normal blood pressure. However, this can give a false sense of security, and complete operative evacuation of clot and definitive repair of the cardiac lesion should be performed.

Emergency room thoracotomy should be performed only if immediate surgical consultation is available and if the patient with suspected cardiac injury is in full arrest or comatose and agonal.[26] Emergency room thoracotomy is best performed through the left fifth intercostal space from the sternal border to the axilla. Division of the sternal cartilaginous attachments of the fourth and fifth ribs allows better exposure. The pericardium should be opened vertically anterior to the phrenic nerve. After clot is evacuated, internal cardiac massage can be performed with digital compression of the aorta, directing cardiac output to the vital coronary and cerebral circulation. Myocardial wounds can be either digitally occluded, with definitive repair performed later in the operating room, or closed with sutures in the emergency room. During placement of such sutures, care should be taken to avoid constricting or occluding coronary arteries. Wounds near coronary arteries are best handled with horizontal mattress sutures passing beneath the coronary artery at risk. Coronary artery lacerations of the distal one third can usually be safely ligated, whereas more proximal injuries should be repaired. In some instances, however, distal lesions may be associated with dysrhythmia when ligated. Coronary artery repair is facilitated by cardiopulmonary bypass with cardiac arrest if available.[27] In anterior cardiac wounds, the posterior surface should be inspected for a through-and-through injury. Defibrillation can be performed with internal paddles set at approximately 40 watt-seconds. If fibrillation recurs, in addition to the usual pharmacologic maneuvers such as correcting acidosis and giving transtracheal or intravenous epinephrine, warm saline solution can be used to bathe the heart, because hypothermia is a common problem in difficult defibrillation in the cardiac trauma victim. If additional exposure is necessary, the sternum can be transected and the incision extended into the right fifth intercostal space.

If the patient's condition is stable, thoracotomy is best performed in the more controlled environment of the operating room. Although left anterolateral thoracotomy is generally the most versatile incision in trauma victims, median sternotomy is advocated in selected patients.[28] If during laparotomy for lower thoracic or multiple stab-wounds, the patient's condition suddenly deteriorates and tamponade is suspected, a pericardial window can rapidly be performed through the central tendon of the diaphragm to rule out tamponade and evacuate any clot. Sternotomy or left thoracotomy can then be performed for definitive repair.

Internal derangements of the heart are generally not addressed during emergency surgery, with repair attempted only of surface injuries of the heart or coronary vessels. During the immediate postoperative period, internal derangements (eg, septal laceration or valvular, papillary muscle, and chordae tendineae injury), if suspected on clinical grounds, can be identified by cardiac catheterization and semielective repair under cardiopulmonary bypass planned. Most intracardiac missiles are also best extracted under cardiopulmonary bypass (Figures 48.3 and 48.4). Intraoperative echocardiography is particularly useful in localizing the missile, thus greatly shortening the pump time on cardiopulmonary bypass.[29]

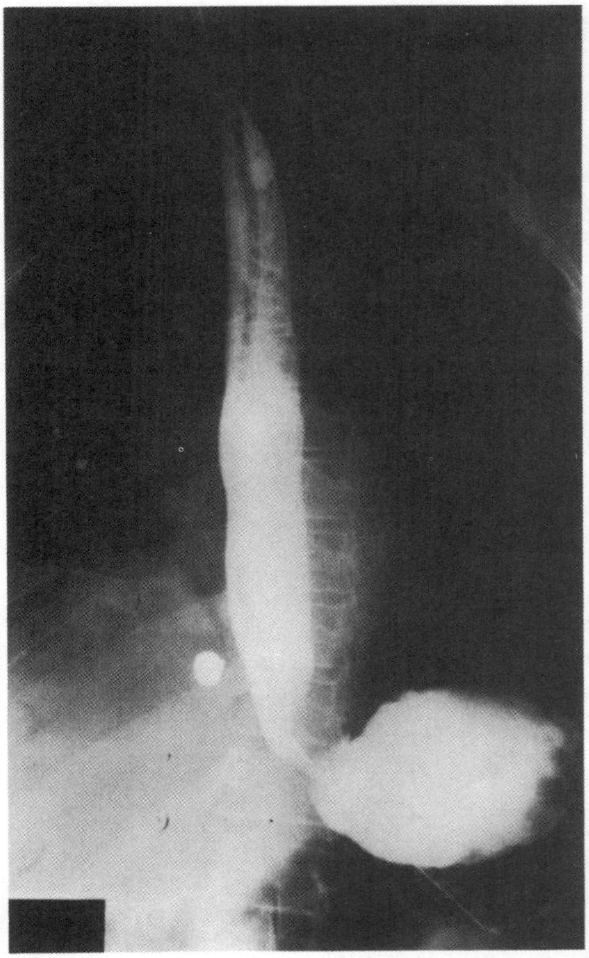

Figure 48.3. This 23-year-old man received a single gunshot wound in the right third intercostal space. His condition was hemodynamically stable. An esophogram was obtained because of the proximity of the missile. During this study it was obvious the missile was "moving," confirming the diagnosis of intracardiac missile. This missile was removed from the right ventricle at thoracotomy and the right atrium repaired.

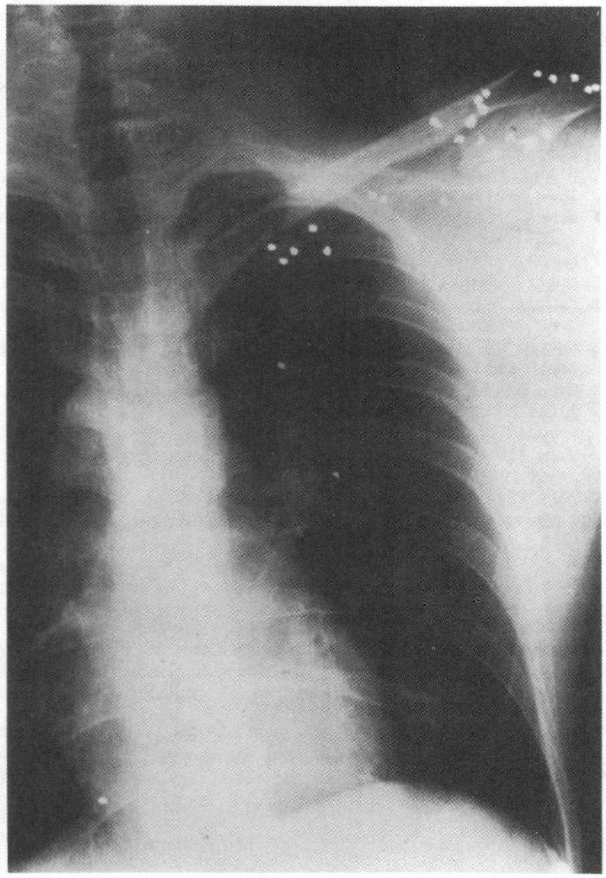

Figure 48.4. This 27-year-old man sustained a single close-range shotgun blast to the left shoulder and face. Chest x-ray shows a single pellet that has embolized to the right ventricle. Surgical removal was not necessary because it was on the right side, and further embolization to the lung is benign. In contrast, small missiles in the left heart can be associated with significant problems when further embolization occurs, such as that to the cerebral circulation, and should be removed.

Treatment of patients with suspected myocardial contusion is identical to that of patients with suspected myocardial infarction. Observation in a monitored environment is the mainstay of therapy, with arrhythmias treated as appropriate.[30] Cardiac dysfunction should be treated with afterload reduction or pressors as dictated by hemodynamics as determined with the aid of an arterial line and a thermodilution cardiac output measurement equipped Swan–Ganz catheter. Echocardiography should be performed early in such unstable patients to search for both free pericardial fluid and areas of dyskinesia. If coronary artery injury is suspected by dyskinesia or electrocardiography, diagnosis is confirmed by coronary angiography. One of the most controversial areas in the management of patients with suspected myocardial contusion is how long monitoring should be performed, but 72 hours is a generally accepted period in patients in whom contusion is "ruled out." We feel that close communication between the trauma surgeon and the cardiologist during this period is important in management.

REFERENCES

1. Meade RH: *A History of Thoracic Surgery*. Springfield, Ill, Charles C Thomas, 1961, pp 413–429.
2. Purple SS: Statistical observations on wounds of the heart and their relation to forensic medicine with a table of forty-two recorded cases. *NY J Med Collat Sci* 1855; 14:411–434.
3. Cappelen A: Vulnus cordis. *Nosrk Mag Laegevidensk* 1895; 6:285.
4. Rehn L: Uebr pentrierende Herz wunden und Herznaht. *Arch Klin Chir* 1897; 55:315–329.
5. Beck CS: Wounds of the heart: the technic of suture. *Arch Surg* 1926; 1:205–207.
6. Bigger IA: Wounds of the heart. *Clin* 1934; 1:133–159.
7. Bright EF, Beck CS: Contusions of the heart. *JAMA* 1935; 104:109–114.
8. Escaude F, Bruez P: Deux cas de projectile inclus dans les parois du coeur et bien tolérés. *Rev Chir* 1917; 53:268–280.
9. Harken DE: Foreign bodies in, and in relation to, the thoracic blood vessels and heart. *Surg Gynec Obstet* 1946; 83:117–125.
10. Jones JW, Hewitt RL, Drapanas T: Cardiac contusion: capricious syndrome. *Ann Surg* 1975; 181:567–574.
11. Kissane RW: Traumatic heart disease. *Circulation* 1952; 6:421–425.
12. Sigler LH: Trauma of the heart due to nonpenetrating chest injuries. *JAMA* 1942; 119:855–861.
13. Beall AC, Patrick TA, Ikies JE, Bricker EL, DeBakey ME: Penetrating wounds of the heart: changing patterns of surgical management. *J Trauma* 1972; 12:468–473.
14. Sugg WL, Rea WJ, Ecker RR, Webb WR, Rose EF, Shaw RR: Penetrating wounds of the heart: an analysis of 459 cases. *J Thorac Cardiovasc Surg* 1968; 56: 531–545.
15. Parmley LF, Manion WC, Mattingly TW: Nonpenetrating traumatic injury to the heart. *Circulation* 1958; 18:371–396.
16. DeGennaro VA, Bonifils-Roberts EA, Ching N, Nealon TF: Aggressive management of potential penetrating cardiac injuries. *J Thorac Cardiovasc Surg* 1980; 79:833–837.
17. Baker CC, Thomas AN, Trunkey DD: The role of emergency room thoracotomy in trauma. *J Trauma* 1980; 20:848–855.
18. Ivatury RR, Shah PM, Ito K, Ramirez-Schon G, Suarez F, Rohman M: Emergency room thoracotomy for the resuscitation of patients with "fatal" penetrating injuries of the heart. *Ann Thorac Surg* 1981; 32:377–385.
19. Symbas PM, Harlattis N, Waldo WJ: Penetrating cardiac wounds: a comparison of different therapeutic methods. *Ann Surg* 1976; 183:377–381.
20. Thandroyen FT, Matisonn RE: Penetrating thoracic trauma producing cardiac shunts. *J Thorac Cardiovasc Surg* 1981; 81:569–573.
21. Doyt DB, Anderson AE, Rose EF: Cardiac trauma: clinical and experimental correlations of myocardial contusion. *Ann Surg* 1974; 180:452–460.
22. Markiewicz W, Best LA, Burstein S, Peleg H: Echocardiographic evaluation after blunt trauma of the chest. *Int J Cardiol* 1985; 8:269–274.
23. Simon TR, Parkey RW, Lewis SE: Role of cardiovascular nuclear medicine in evaluating trauma and the postoperative patient. *Semin Nucl Med* 1983; 13:123–141.
24. Ruder MA, Flaker GC, Alperta MA, Selmon MR: Right ventricular myocardial contusion simulating constrictive pericardial disease. *Am Heart J* 1984; 108:1353–1354.
25. Sutherland GR, Cheung HW, Holliday RL, Driedger AA, Sibbald WJ: Hemodynamic adaptation to acute myocardial contusion complicating blunt chest injury. *Am J Cardiol* 1986; 57:291–297.
26. Schwab CW, Adcock OT, Max MH: Emergency department thoracotomy (EDT). A 26-month experience using an "agonal" protocol. *American Surgeon* 1986; 52:20–29.
27. Espada R, Whisennand HH, Mattox KL, Beall AC: Surgical management of penetrating injuries to the coronary arteries. *Surgery* 1975; 78:755–760.
28. Demetriades D: Cardiac wounds. Experience with 70 patients. *Ann Surg* 1986; 203:315–317.
29. Hasset A, Moran J, Sabiston DC, Kisslo J: Utility of echocardiography in the management of patients with penetrating missile wounds of the heart. *J Am Coll Cardiol* 1986; 7:1151–1156.
30. Schmelzer VM, Wetstein L: Emergency evaluation and therapy of cardiac trauma. *Cardiology Emergency Decisions* 1986; 2:24–28.

49 Diseases of the Aorta and Its Branches

Michael E. DeBakey, MD and Charles H. McCollum, MD

A number of conditions cause aortic disease. These vary according to geographic location of the patients and site of the disease in the aorta. With the control of infections such as syphilis, aortitis has become a much less common cause of aortic disease than formerly. Yet, with the ever-increasing incidence of life expectancy in the western world, atherosclerotic and degenerative diseases of the aorta are the most common causes of aortic disease.

Atherosclerosis is the most frequent form of degenerative disease of the aorta. Lipid depositions or fatty streaks develop as early manifestations of atherosclerosis.[1] Intimal plaques, which contain lipid-rich material, and additional pathologic alterations, consisting in hemorrhage, calcification, ulceration, and thrombosis, eventually develop. The process begins initially in the intima. Progression of the intimal disease or build-up of the thrombus may occlude the lumen of the aorta or the origin of a major branch. Significant pathologic changes eventually develop in the surrounding media, with degeneration of the elastic and smooth muscle fibers. The aorta becomes dilated and elongated as the collagen fibers and mucoid ground substance decrease. Thus, aneurysms may begin to develop. Important risk factors include diabetes, hyperlipidemia, smoking, and hypertension.

Atherosclerotic occlusive disease characteristically affects the terminal abdominal aorta and spares the thoracic aorta. Any of the major branches of the aorta may, however, be affected. Thus, atherosclerosis may develop in the branches of the aortic arch or in the renal and mesenteric arteries of the upper abdominal aorta. Weakness of the aorta, with aneurysmal formation, develops usually in the abdominal aorta, followed in order by the descending thoracic aorta, ascending aorta, aortic arch, and thoracoabdominal aorta. Cystic medial degeneration and myxomatous degeneration are other common forms of degenerative aortic disease. Aortic dissection is caused by cleavage of the aortic media by a dissecting hematoma. The separation of the medial fibers does not usually completely encircle the lumen, but the entire length of the vessel is often involved.

Aortic infection is rarely caused by syphilis. Most aortic infections, secondary to bacterial sepsis, result in mycotic aneurysms or are secondary to infections after surgical procedures or trauma. Several specific inflammatory disorders known as Takayasu's disease or giant-cell aortitis are occasionally encountered.

The most common congenital anomalies of the aorta are coarctation and patent ductus arteriosus. Anomalies of the sinus of Valsalva and aortic arch are less common. Trauma is becoming increasingly important in the pathogenesis of aortic disease. Deceleration injuries and penetrating wounds of the chest may cause aortic disease. Tumors are a rare cause of aortic disease.

CONGENITAL ANOMALIES OF THE AORTA

A brief review of the embryology of the aortic arch system is important for better understanding of congenital anomalies of the aorta. In the early embryo, the six aortic arches connect the ventral aortic sac and the paired dorsal aorta.[2] Normally, the left fourth aortic arch becomes dominant while the caudal segment of the right fourth aortic arch becomes obliterated. The third aortic arch forms the carotid arteries, the sixth aortic arch forms the pulmonary arteries, and the seventh cervical segmental artery supplies the upper limb bud as the subclavian artery. The aorta caudal to the brachial arches becomes fused as the single unpaired dorsal aorta.

If the left aortic arch becomes obliterated and the right aortic arch persists, a mirror image arrangement develops that results in a right aortic arch. A retroesophageal right subclavian artery forms. If the proximal, rather than the distal, right aortic arch becomes obliterated, the right subclavian artery arises from the unpaired aorta. It passes posterior to the esophagus in reaching the right limb bud and forms a retroesophageal right subclavian artery. When both aortic arches persist, a complete aortic ring is formed. The result is a bifid or double aortic arch, which may surround and cause tracheal or esophageal compression. The ductus arteriosus connects the derivative of the sixth aortic arch or pulmonary artery with the left aortic arch. If the left fourth arch becomes obliterated, the ductus arteriosus remains attached to the left dorsal aorta along with the subclavian artery, or the arch may become obliterated distal to the ductus arteriosus.

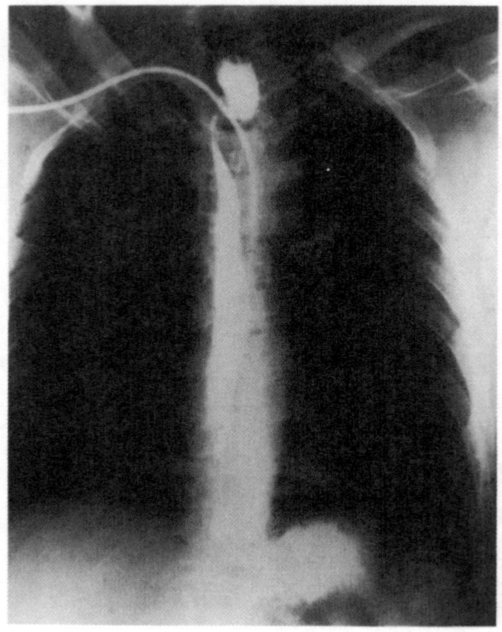

Figure 49.1. Esophagogram of a patient with dysphagia showing esophageal compression by the anomalous right subclavian artery. Catheter introduced through the right brachial artery illustrates the course of the aberrant artery. Division of the right subclavian artery through a right thoracotomy affords relief of symptoms. (From DeBakey and Noon,[5] with permission.)

AORTIC ARCH

Bayford was the first to report a case of a vascular anomaly. In 1794, he described a patient with a retroesophageal right subclavian artery.[3] Gross[4] reported the first successful surgical case in 1945 when he divided a double aortic arch.

Congenital anomalous development of the aortic arch system occurs in various forms and results in displacement or compression of the trachea and esophagus producing "vascular rings."[5] Most common among these maldevelopments are double aortic arch, right aortic arch with ligamentum arteriosum, anomalous innominate artery, anomalous left common carotid artery, and aberrant right subclavian artery. The essential clinical manifestations of these anomalies are produced by tracheal or esophageal obstruction. From anterior compression of the trachea, respiratory distress with stridor and inspiratory retraction of the intercostal and supraclavicular tissue occur. These symptoms tend to appear early in infancy and are often associated with the double or bifid aortic arch. A noisy, "crowing" respiration, which is readily audible, is associated with an increased respiratory rate. Such symptoms are often aggravated by feeding. As a result of aspiration, respiratory infections and bronchial pneumonia may ensue and constitute serious respiratory complications. Vascular rings that produce posterior compression of the esophagus may cause dysphagia lusoria. Some patients may be able to swallow fluids, but not semisolids; in others, the reverse is true. Regurgitation in nursing is common and may be associated with aspiration resulting in frequent respiratory infections.

The diagnosis may be suspected in plain roentgenograms of the chest, which show evidence of pneumonitis. Displacement or constriction of the lower trachea may be seen on bronchography. Roentgenography after ingestion of barium may show posterior indentation or compression of the esophagus (Figure 49.1). When indicated, aortography will confirm the diagnosis.

Symptoms of esophageal or tracheal compression are an indication for surgical treatment. The goal is to relieve the compression without sacrificing a major vital artery. Thus, the carotid circulation should never be permanently interrupted, but an anomalous right subclavian artery producing posterior esophageal compression may be safely divided without restoration of vascular continuity (Figure 49.1). In the presence of a double aortic arch, usually the one on the left anterior side of the trachea is the lesser of the two and may be safely divided between the origins of the left common carotid and the left subclavian artery (Figure 49.2). In other cases, a ligamentum arteriosum plays a role in the formation of the vascular ring and should be divided as part of the reparative procedure (Figure 49.3). Full mobilization of the arch after

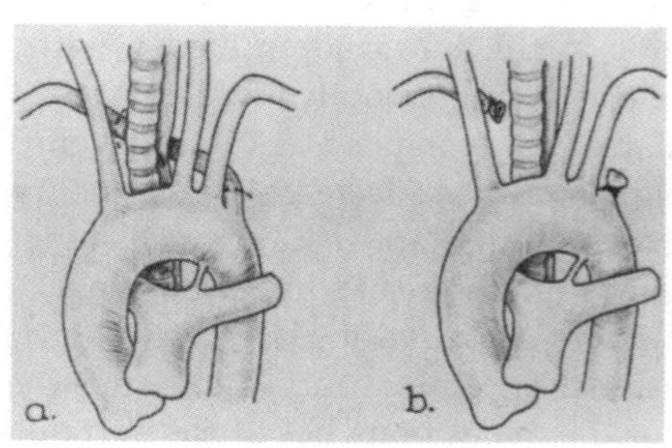

Figure 49.2. *a*, Anomalous retroesophageal right subclavian artery producing incomplete vascular ring. *b*, Division of right subclavian artery relieves esophageal obstruction without causing ischemic symptoms in the arm. (From DeBakey and Noon,[5] with permission.)

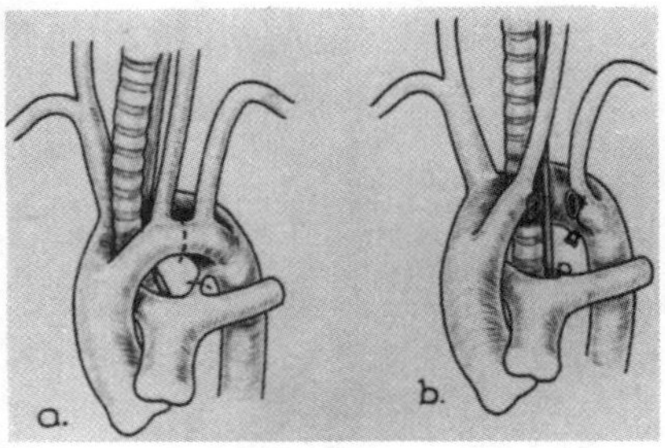

Figure 49.3. Complete vascular ring. *a*, Bifid aortic arch causing tracheal and esophageal compression. *b*, Release of vascular ring by division of left limb between the left common carotid and left subclavian arteries. (From DeBakey and Noon,[5] with permission.)

division of the ligamentum arteriosum is important. Most patients with vascular rings can be treated satisfactorily through left thoracotomy. Usually, relief of the tracheal and esophageal obstruction is associated with dramatic clinical improvement.

PATENT DUCTUS ARTERIOSUS

Gross successfully ligated a patent ductus arteriosus in 1938 and provided a tremendous stimulus to the development of cardiovascular surgery.[6] The ductus connects the left pulmonary artery with the descending thoracic aorta just distal to the left subclavian artery, or to the innominate artery in the case of a right aortic arch. The ductus is almost always on the left side, even when a right aortic arch is present. The left recurrent laryngeal nerve passes under the ductus and aids in its identification.

The ductus arteriosus is important in the fetus to shunt blood from the pulmonary artery to the aorta and systemic circulation. With expansion of the lungs after birth, however, pulmonary vascular resistance decreases. The ductus usually begins to close after birth, except in infants with cyanotic heart disease. If the ductus remains patent, a left-to-right cardiac shunt develops. The severity of the shunt depends on the pulmonary vascular resistance and the size of the shunt. Although the shunt may be well tolerated for many years, eventually pulmonary vascular changes develop leading to pulmonary hypertension. Then, a balanced or a right-to-left shunt results.

These patients may simply show retarded physical growth, or they may have shortness of breath associated with heart failure. If they are not treated, pulmonary hypertension is a late and severe complication. Bacterial endocarditis may develop in a patent ductus arteriosus.

The diagnosis is usually made on the basis of the characteristic continuous murmur in the second left interspace. The heart may appear normal or only slightly enlarged on roentgenography of the chest. If the patient is asymptomatic, results of electrocardiography will be normal. Cardiac catheterization is not necessary for diagnosis but is performed in children with atypical findings or those in whom other cardiac defects are suspected.

Operation is performed through the posterior lateral left fourth intercostal space. The ductus is identified after the mediastinal pleura is opened. Care is taken to avoid injury to the recurrent laryngeal nerve. Simple ligation may be performed. Division and suture are most satisfactory, however, especially if the ductus is large. Surgical correction of a symptomatic patent ductus arteriosus can be safely performed in the neonate. The results of surgical closure of a patent ductus arteriosus are excellent because the work load of the heart is immediately lowered when the shunt is closed.

COARCTATION

Coarctation is a congenital obstruction to the flow of blood through the proximal descending thoracic aorta.[5] It usually occurs in the isthmic region of the aortic arch where it joins the descending thoracic aorta just distal to the origin of the left subclavian artery. The location of the ductus arteriosus or ligamentum provides a useful means of classification. This classification is based on the relation of the coarctation to the ductus arteriosus or ligamentum (Figure 49.4). If the constriction is distal to the level of the ductus, it is a postductile or adult type. Preductal constriction is known as the infantile type. About 10% of patients with coarctation of the aorta have a patent ductus arteriosus, most of whom have preductal or infantile coarctation. This type has a much more unfavorable prognosis, often resulting in early death. These patients also have intracardiac abnormalities that are incompatible with growth and normal development. The most common of these anomalies is ventricular septal defect, but other serious congenital cardiac defects occur, such as mitral valve disease, endocardial fibroelastosis, aortic valvular disease, agenesis of the ascending aorta, or single ventricle with chamber. This type of coarctation tends to be more elongated or diffuse. Because of the striking disturbance of circulation from the coarctation and the associated intracardiac defects, symptoms are usually manifested in infancy.

The more common form of coarctation is the adult or postductal type in which the constriction is distal to the ductus. Because the circulation to the distal segment of the aorta is provided by a rich collateral network of vessels arising from the subclavian branches supplying the shoulder girdle, the ductus is not vital and usually becomes obliterated soon after birth. The intercostal arteries, which receive a major portion of the blood passing through the collateral channels, become dilated and tortuous, pro-

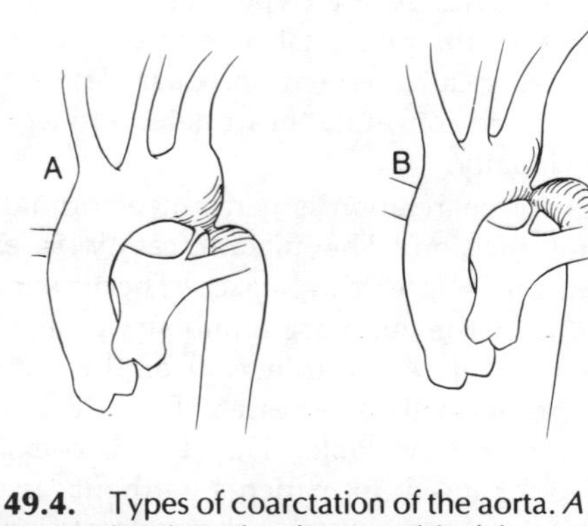

Figure 49.4. Types of coarctation of the aorta. *A*, Postductile (adult); *B*, Preductile (infantile). (Modified from DeBakey and Noon.[5])

ducing secondary manifestations, such as erosion of the undersurface of the ribs. This is a diagnostic feature of this condition in patients five to ten years of age. The postductal type is commonly associated with a bicuspid aortic valve. In the uncomplicated postductal type of coarctation, patients are often asymptomatic, and the diagnosis is made later in life when hypertension or a murmur is detected. Symptoms include headache, shortness of breath, palpitation, or pain in the chest. Weakness or fatigue of the legs may occur, particularly with excessive exercise. Symptoms of congestive failure may develop. A striking physical finding is diminished or absent femoral pulses; there is frequently a delay in the femoral pulse, as compared to the pulses in the arms. Because of brachiocephalic hypertension, prominent pulsations, due to the enlarged collateral circulation, are present over the neck, supraclavicular area, and chest wall. The systolic murmur is heard over the base of the heart or the left hemothorax. The roentgenogram of the chest will usually show cardiomegaly and the characteristic notching of the aorta due to the prominent proximal aorta and the poststenotic dilatation of the aorta distal to the coarctation. One of the most characteristic radiologic signs is notching of the ribs due to dilatation and tortuosity of the intercostal arteries, but it usually is not present until adolescence. The electrocardiogram may show no abnormalities, but significant left ventricular hypertrophy is present after sustained hypertension. Symptoms of preductal or infantile coarctation usually appear early in infancy and are complicated by associated intracardiac abnormalities. Congestive heart failure is the most common presenting symptom. Aortography is seldom necessary for diagnosis but is important in planning the operation if surgical treatment is considered, and in identifying aneurysmal disease associated with the coarctation.

Several factors must be considered in determining the time of operation. The risk of recurrent coarctation is reduced if operation is delayed until late childhood or early adolescence. If the operation is not performed before the end of the second decade of life, however, the risk of serious residual hypertension and its sequela is significantly increased. Our studies indicate that the presence of severe hypertension, as well as the age of the patient, should be considered in selecting the appropriate time for operation.[7] Thus, we would recommend earlier operation in children with severe hypertension and coarctation. Children with severe hypertension or congestive heart failure with the preductal type of coarctation may require early surgical intervention. Coarctation complicated by associated congenital heart defects must be considered individually.

Operation for coarctation is performed through a left posterolateral incision. The pleural cavity is exposed through the fourth intercostal space. The proximal and distal portions of the aorta are immobilized, and care is exercised not to injure the thin wall of the intercostal, bronchial, or other collateral vessels. Four different surgical techniques are available.[5] Direct end-to-end anastomosis may be used in patients without associated aneurysmal disease or local atherosclerotic changes (Figure 49.5). The anastomosis must be done carefully

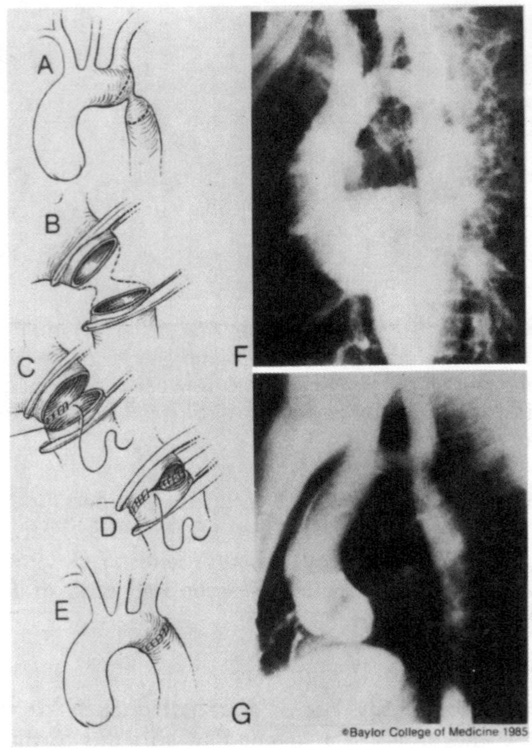

Figure 49.5. Coarctation of the aorta. *A* to *E*, Technique of surgical resection, with end-to-end anastomosis. *F*, Preoperative aortogram showing typical coarctation. *G*, Postoperative aortogram showing patent aortic anastomosis. (From DeBakey and Noon,[5] with permission.)

without undue tension which leads to complications at the site of the anastomosis. The entire aortic constriction should be excised to provide the largest diameter for anastomosis. If end-to-end anastomosis is feasible without excessive tension, it may be done satisfactorily. Although we prefer a continuous over-and-over suture technique, others use interrupted sutures on the anterior surface of the anastomosis.

Patch-graft angioplasty is a simple technique that may be applicable in many patients with coarctation (Figure 49.6). It has the advantage of not requiring resection of the coarctation and thereby of minimizing the operative procedure. The coarctation is isolated, and the proximal and distal occluding clamps are applied. A longitudinal incision is made through the coarctation, extending into normal artery proximally and distally. A patch graft of Dacron® velour is prepared and sewn into place with a continuous Dacron suture. Release of the distal and proximal clamps establishes normal blood flow. A portion of the internal constricting ring of tissue in the coarctation may be resected in some patients in addition to the patch-graft angioplasty.

We perform resection with graft replacement in almost one half of our cases[7] (Figure 49.7). It is indicated in (1) extensive coarctations, as in the preductal or infantile type, (2) coarctations that involve the aortic arch with stenosis extending proximally to the subclavian artery, (3) subisthmic coarctations involving the middle and lower thirds of the thoracic aorta, and (4) any type of

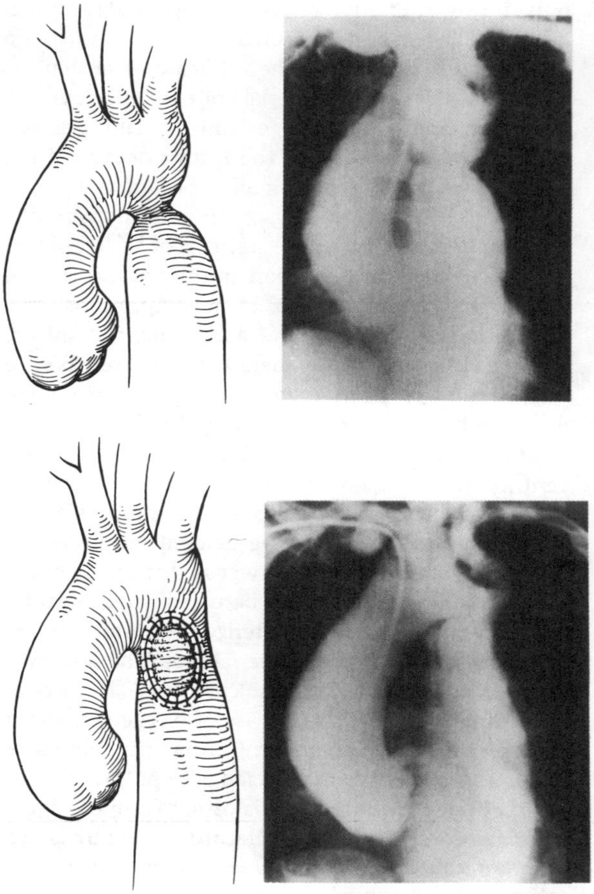

Figure 49.6. *Top*, Preoperative drawing and aortogram of coarctation of aorta. *Bottom*, Postoperative drawing and aortogram demonstrating technique of patch-graft aortoplasty to restore circulation. (From DeBakey and Noon,[5] with permission.)

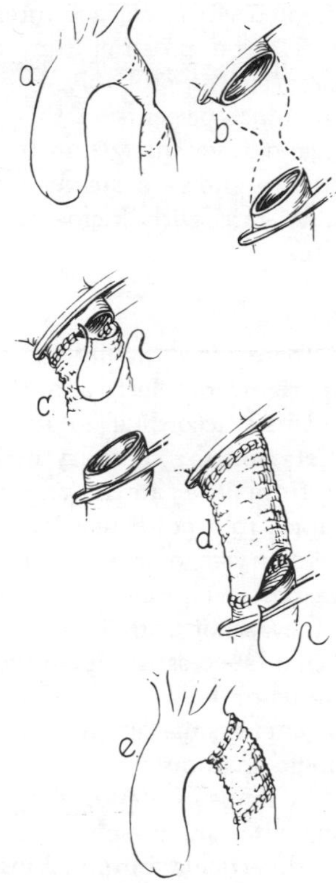

Figure 49.7. Technique of surgical resection and graft replacement of coarctation of aorta. (From DeBakey and Noon,[5] with permission.)

coarctation in which local degenerative changes and aneurysm make anastomosis a hazard. The involved segment of aorta is completely excised, emphasis being placed on removal of the entire constricture with all the associated pathologic conditions. A suitably sized woven Dacron graft is selected, and the proximal end-to-end anastomosis is first performed with a continuous over-and-over suture. The graft is tailored to the appropriate length, and just before completion of the distal end-to-end anastomosis, both proximal and distal occluding clamps should be momentarily released to flush the aorta of possible clots. After completion of the anastomosis, the distal clamp is removed first. This allows inspection of the anastomosis under local arterial pressure and permits air to escape from the graft. The proximal clamp is then gradually released to minimize bleeding through the interstices of the graft and to avoid sudden decrease in blood pressure in the proximal aorta that may lead to disturbances of cardiac or cerebral function. If the coarctation is in the distal aortic arch and involves the origin of the left subclavian artery, graft replacement of the excised segment is necessary for complete repair. Such preductal coarctations are uncommon, but they have been discovered even in young adults and are therefore compatible with survival during infancy. If the coarctation involves the left subclavian artery, the aortic continuity is first reestablished. The circulation in the left subclavian artery is then reestablished by using a smaller graft attached to the larger aortic graft by an end-to-end anastomosis and suturing it end to end to the stump of the subclavian artery.

The fourth technique occasionally used is aortic bypass. It is generally indicated if resection of the coarctation could be hazardous or is undesirable, or if aortic bypass facilitates the expeditious surgical correction in certain poor-risk patients. Appropriate exclusion clamps are applied to a convenient segment of the aortic wall proximally and distally, with aortic blood flow essentially unaltered. A linear incision is then tailored, and the proximal end-to-side anastomosis is completed. A partial occlusion clamp is placed on the distal aortic segment, and another end-to-side anastomosis is performed. As the clamps are slowly released, bleeding from the suture line and from the graft itself soon ceases, and the operative procedure is completed. The bypass operation thus provides the means of obtaining a physiologic cure in the presence of complicating features.

Our surgical experience includes more than 190 cases of coarctation.[7] About half of the patients were in the first two decades of life, with the remainder distributed almost equally among the third, fourth, and fifth decades. The ages ranged from 1 year to 60 years. Two thirds of the patients had severe hypertension. Fifty-eight percent of the patients had radiographic evidence of rib erosion or notching associated with enlarged intercostal arteries.

Some type of Dacron prosthetic graft was used in 65% of our series. This is probably a reflection of the high incidence of older patients in this series with attendant local degenerative changes in the aorta. Analysis of our experience shows a steady reduction in the operative mortality rate with increased application of grafting procedures.

SINUS OF VALSALVA

Anatomically, there are normally three aortic sinuses of Valsalva: the right, the left, and the noncoronary sinus. Each is named according to its relation to the aortic valve leaflets and the coronary ostia. The sinuses extend distally from the aortic annulus as dilated pouches in the aorta to a point usually just beyond the coronary ostia. Aneurysm of a sinus of Valsalva, with rupture into the right ventricle, was first described in 1831 by Hope.[8] It was not until 1957 that Lillehei et al[9] performed the first successful operative repair of an aneurysm of a sinus of Valsalva. We proposed a logical classification of aneurysms of the sinus of Valsalva based on pathologic anatomy.[10]

Anomalies of the sinus of Valsalva may be congenital or acquired. Congenital aneurysms of the sinus of Valsalva are localized diverticular outpouchings of a coronary sinus and are usually confined to one aortic sinus. The pouching eventually protrudes into a cardiac chamber or into the myocardium. Rupture into a cardiac chamber produces an aorto-intracardiac fistula. These aneurysms may be associated with other congenital cardiac defects, the most common being ventricular septal defect. Aortic valvular insufficiency often occurs from distortion or fibrosis of the aortic valve.[11] Sakakibara and Konno[12] proposed a detailed classification of congenital aneurysms of the sinus of Valsalva.

The cause of these congenital aneurysms is not known. Abbott[13] suggested that a weakness at the point of fusion with the aorticopulmonary septum resulted from defective development of the distal bulbar system. Although this explains abnormalities in the right and noncoronary sinus, it does not adequately explain the anomaly in the left coronary sinus. Edwards and Burchell[11] demonstrated separation between the aortic media and the anulus fibrosus of the aortic valve. This resulted in a weakness and subsequent formation of an aneurysm and could account for aneurysms in all three sinuses.

In contrast, acquired aneurysms usually involve more than one sinus of Valsalva, and the ascending aorta as well. These may be due to infection, such as syphilis or endocarditis, as well as disorders of degenerative connective tissue. Rarely, an aneurysm may result from blunt or penetrating trauma. The aortic valvular insufficiency commonly associated with these aneurysms occurs because of valvular or anular distortion. Rupture is usually extracardiac, rather than intracardiac, as in congenital defects.

Aneurysms of the sinus of Valsalva are rare. They represent a small percentage of all congenital cardiovascular disorders that are treated surgically. Typically, these aneurysms are asymptomatic. Early diagnosis is made only during evaluation for other congenital cardiovascular defects. They may be detected earlier if distortion or impairment of function of the intracardiac structures produces symptoms or if bacterial endocarditis develops. The aneurysm gradually enlarges until it ruptures into the ventricle or atrium during the fourth decade of life.

Results of physical examination before rupture are usually normal. After rupture, a continuous murmur develops which is best heard over the sternum or left sternal border. Because of valvular distortion and fibrosis, aortic valvular insufficiency often develops. A new murmur is secondary to the fistula between the aorta and the intracardiac chamber into which the aneurysm ruptures. Before rupture, results of plain roentgenography are nonspecific. After rupture, signs of a left-to-right shunt with cardiac enlargement, increased pulmonary vascularity, and left ventricular enlargement due to aortic valvular insufficiency may be present. Also after rupture, signs of hypertrophy and strain may be evident on electrocardiography. Echocardiography may provide useful noninvasive data, but the diagnosis can be established only by aortography and cardiac catheterization. Aortography will show the jet of contrast material from the aneurysm entering the appropriate cardiac chamber. The left-to-right shunt is produced with increase of oxygen tension in the appropriate cardiac chamber. Cardiac function is normal unless aortic valvular insufficiency or pulmonary outflow obstruction is produced by distortion from the aneurysm. Heart failure secondary to intracardiac rupture is the most common cause of death. The average age at death of patients with congenital aneurysm of the sinus of Valsalva in one report was 33 years, and the mean survival time was only one year.[14]

Only a small portion of patients with aneurysms of the ascending aorta have acquired aneurysms of the sinus of Valsalva. These aneurysms are usually found in men over the age of 30 years. They may be asymptomatic or they may produce a wide variety of symptoms. Cardiac symptoms result primarily from aortic valvular insufficiency due to a deformed aortic valve or anulus. Patients with aneurysms secondary to infection may seek medical advice during the acute or chronic stage. Endocarditis may produce an aneurysm of the sinus of Valsalva by erosion of the sinus and formation of an abscess.

Most of these acquired aneurysms are not detected on physical examination. A murmur is heard on auscultation, which is due to valvular dysfunction from distortion by fibrosis, prolapse from dissection, or distortion or enlargement of the aortic anulus. Fistulas rarely develop in acquired aneurysms of the sinus of Valsalva. The electrocardiogram shows nothing abnormal until the aneurysm ruptures, when evidence of left venticular hypertrophy and strain may be seen. Depending on the size and location of the aneurysm, the results of plain roentgenograms of the chest may vary considerably. In aneurysms due to syphilitic aortitis, calcification in the wall is common as in atherosclerotic aneurysms. Because acquired aneurysms usually involve multiple sinuses and a portion of the ascending aorta, they appear as fusiform or sacciform aneurysms of the ascending aorta. The diagnosis is established by aortography and cardiac catheterization (Figure 49.8). Associated cardiac disease is identified, and the extent of the aneurysm is determined. Coronary cinearteriography should also be performed because most of these patients are in the age group in which coronary artery disease occurs.[15]

Surgical closure of the defect and resection or obliteration of the aneurysm is the primary treatment for congenital aneurysms of the sinus of Valsalva (Figure 49.9). Some authorities believe that sudden death is rare in the natural history of this disease and do not advise operation on patients with asymptomatic congenital aneurysms. Symptoms appear at the time of cardiac rupture, and elective repair can be effective. The defect is repaired by a combined approach through the ascending aorta and the chamber of intracardiac protrusion or rupture. The windsock-like deformity produced by the aneurysm or fistula, or both, is resected and obliterated through the involved cardiac chamber. The defect in the sinus is closed through the aorta to avoid injuring the aortic valve. If required, the aortic valve can be reconstructed or replaced simultaneously.

Since acquired aneurysms rarely involve intracardiac structures except the aortic valve, they can be repaired through the ascending aorta with the use of total cardio-

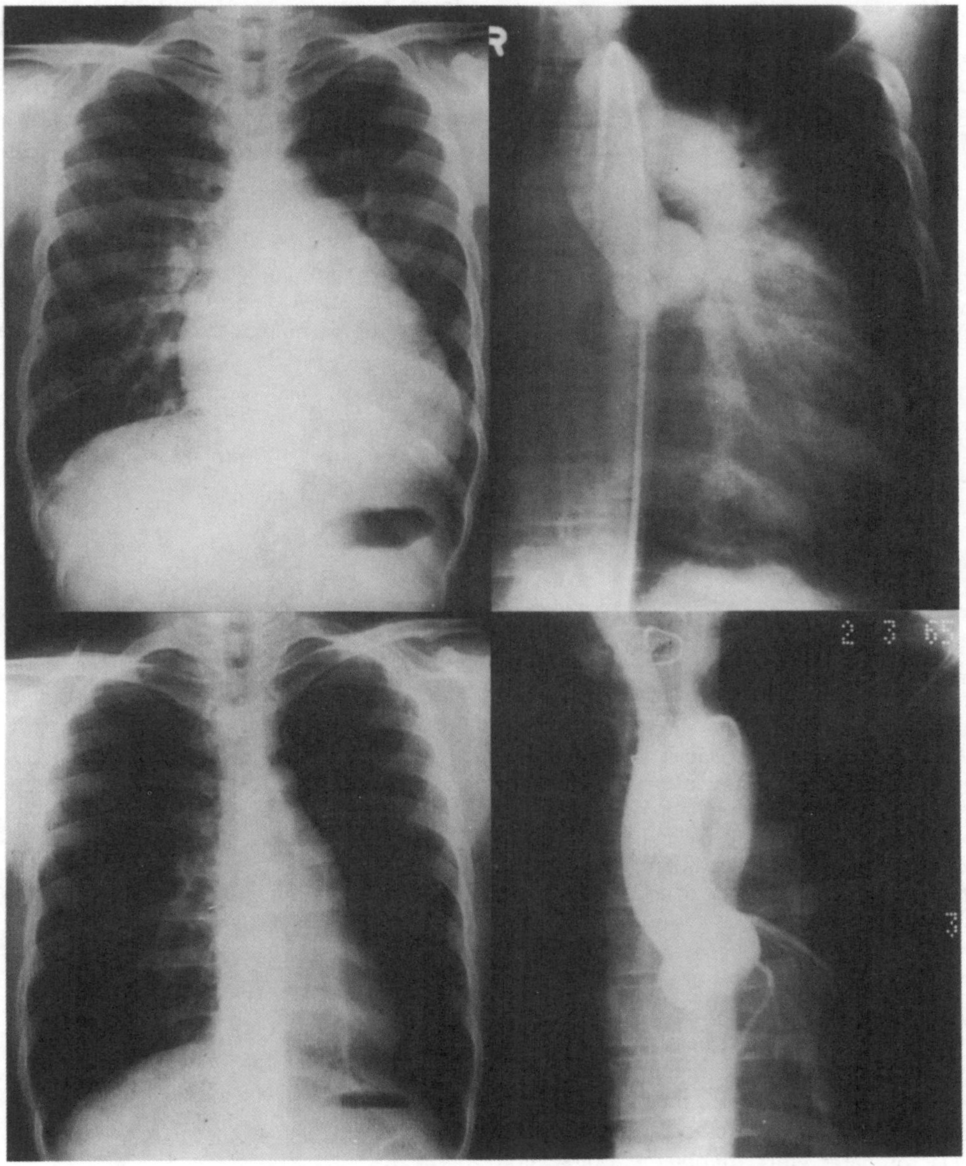

Figure 49.8. *Top left*, Posteroanterior roentgenogram of the chest shows cardiomegaly and increased pulmonary vascularity. *Top right*, Aortic root injection with radiopaque medium shows aneurysm of the right coronary sinus with fistula to the right ventricle immediately below the pulmonary valve. *Bottom left*, After operation, cardiac size and pulmonary vascularity are decreased. *Bottom right*, Aortic root injection with radiopaque medium two years after operation shows absence of the left-to-right shunt. (From DeBakey ME, Noon GP: Aneurysms of the sinuses of Valsalva, in Sabiston DC, Spencer FC (eds): *Gibbon's Surgery of the Chest.* Philadelphia, WB Saunders, 1983, p 948, with permission.)

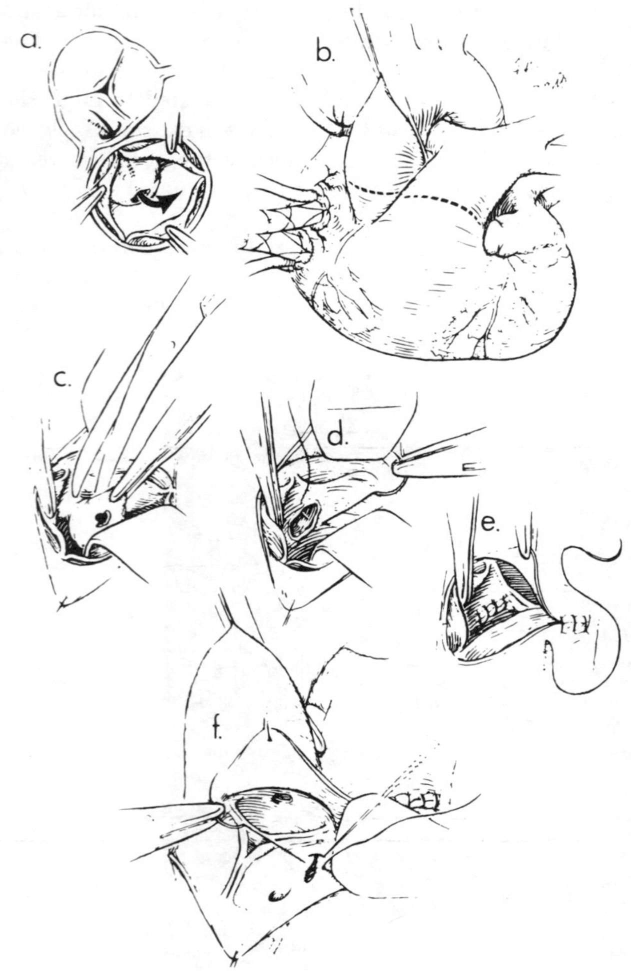

Figure 49.9. Surgical technique for aneurysm of the right coronary sinus with fistula into the right ventricle. *a*, Anatomy of anomaly. *b*, Transverse incision made in pulmonary artery and ascending aorta. *c*, Pulmonary valve retracted and windsock deformity excised. *d*, Fistulous opening into the right ventricle closed with suture. *e*, Suture closure of pulmonary arteriotomy. *f*, Fistula opening in the right coronary sinus closed with suture. (From DeBakey ME, Noon GP: Aneurysms of the sinuses of Valsalva, in Sabiston DC, Spencer FC (eds): *Gibbon's Surgery of the Chest*. Philadelphia, WB Saunders, 1983, p 952, with permission.)

pulmonary bypass and cold cardioplegia solution. The aortic valve often must be replaced because of valvular or anular deformity. The method of repair of the aneurysm depends on its size and location. Small or localized aneurysms may be obliterated or resected and replaced with a woven Dacron patch graft. Involvement of several sinuses in the ascending aorta will require resection of the sinuses and ascending aorta and replacement with a graft (Figure 49.10). This necessitates reimplanting the coronary ostia into the graft and then wrapping the aortic wall around the newly implanted graft by the graft-inclusion technique. If the patient also has atherosclerotic coronary artery disease, concomitant coronary artery bypass grafting can be performed.

The results of surgical correction of aneurysms of the sinus of Valsalva have been gratifying. Mortality and morbidity rates have steadily decreased as experience has been gained. The operative mortality rate for congenital aneurysms has been less than 5%, and for acquired aneurysms, less than 10%.

ANEURYSMS OF THE AORTA

Much has been learned about aneurysms since Dubost[16] performed the first successful surgical resection of an aneurysm more than three decades ago. Certain conceptual developments have evolved that have broadened our understanding of this condition. First, an aneurysm tends to progress and ultimately to produce serious and even lethal complications from rupture or compression of surrounding structures. Rupture is due to weakening or destruction of the media and occurs regardless of the cause of the aneurysm. Thus, the therapeutic objective is complete removal of the aneurysm, but restoration of circulation is desirable and necessary after resection of the aneurysm.

A second concept is that aneurysmal disease has a tendency to assume distinctive patterns with regard to location, extent, and segmental characteristics (Figure 49.11). In most patients, an arterial segment above and below the pathologic process is relatively normal, a char-

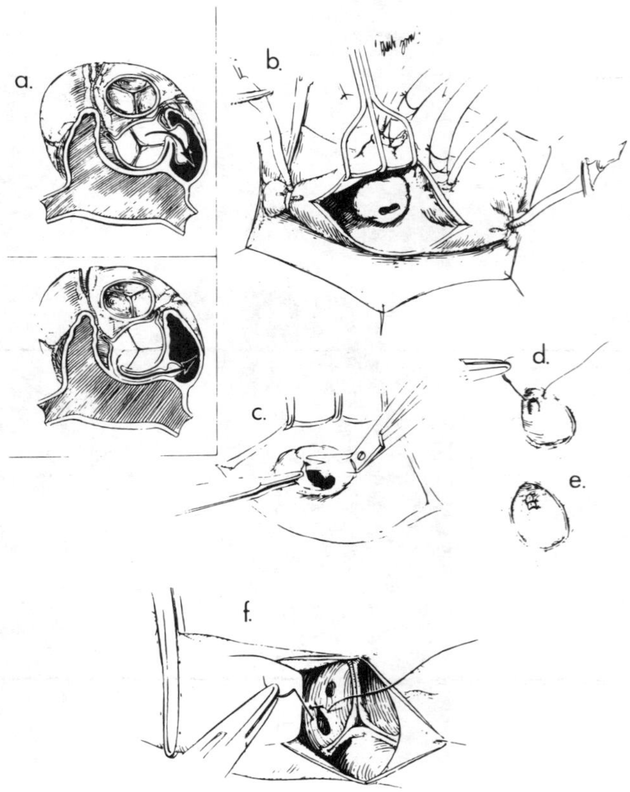

Figure 49.10. *a*, Aneurysm of right or left coronary sinus with fistula into right atrium. *b*,*c*, Aneurysm exposed in right atrium and excised. *d*,*e*, Fistulous opening closed with suture. *f*, Fistula opening in coronary sinus closed through aortotomy. (From DeBakey ME, Noon GP: Aneurysms of the sinuses of Valsalva, in Sabiston DC, Spencer FC (eds): *Gibbon's Surgery of the Chest*, Philadelphia, WB Saunders, 1983, p 952, with permission.)

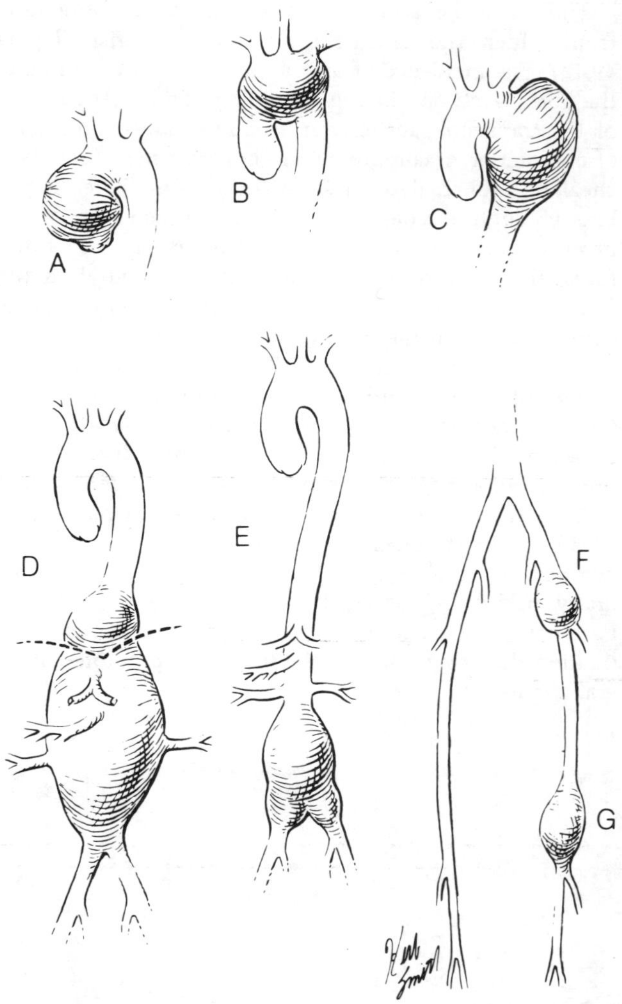

Figure 49.11. Most frequent sites of aneurysms of aorta and major arteries. *A*, Fusiform aneurysm of ascending aorta. *B*, Fusiform aneurysm of the aortic arch involving the brachiocephalic arteries. *C*, Fusiform aneurysm of descending aorta. *D*, Large fusiform thoracoabdominal aneurysm involving the celiac, superior mesenteric, and renal arteries. *E*, Fusiform aneurysm of abdominal aorta and iliac arteries. *F*, Fusiform aneurysm of the femoral artery. *G*, Fusiform aneurysm of the popliteal artery. (From Lindsey et al,[1] with permission.)

acteristic that makes the aneurysm amenable to surgical resection. In general, three surgical methods are used: (1) excision and graft replacement, (2) obliteration by endoaneurysmorrhaphy and restoration of circulation with a bypass, and (3) excision with patch-graft angioplasty for some sacciform aneurysms.[17]

A third concept is the morphologic classification of aneurysms into sacciform, fusiform, or dissecting types. Finally, aneurysms have distinctive patterns with regard to location that provide characteristic features for development of surgical techniques.

ASCENDING AORTA

In most aneurysms of the ascending aorta, the diagnosis is made in an asymptomatic patient by demonstration of an enlarged ascending aorta on routine plain roentgenograms of the chest. The diagnosis may be confirmed by contrast aortography. Some patients have symptoms due to aortic valvular insufficiency and heart failure. They have a murmur of aortic valvular insufficiency. When seen, they may have pain due to expansion of the aneurysm or rupture of the ascending aorta. If the rupture occurs into the pericardium, signs of pericardial tamponade will be present. Pain is commonly associated with a dissecting aneurysm, but it may be due to aortitis or erosion of the sternum or rib from the expanding pulsatile aneurysm. Less frequently, patients have compression or obstruction of adjacent structures. Obstruction of the superior vena cava or innominate vein may produce venous distension over the arms and neck. Patients with aneurysms of the ascending aorta require thorough cardiac evaluation, including cardiac catheterization and cinecoronary arteriograms. Occasionally, a computed tomography scan of the chest is helpful in differentiating a solid mediastinal tumor from an ascending aortic aneurysm.

Morphologically, these ascending aneurysms may be sacciform, fusiform, or dissecting. In the occasional patient with a sacciform aneurysm, tangential excision of the aneurysm with lateral aortorrhaphy or with patch-graft angioplasty may be performed. Segmental resection with graft replacement is necessary in fusiform aneurysms and more extensive sacciform aneurysms. Temporary cardiopulmonary bypass is required. The first successful resection of the entire ascending aorta for an aneurysm was performed in 1956 with use of an aortic homograft and cardiopulmonary bypass.[18] This successful case provided further support to our growing conviction that this method was the most effective for treating these patients and required only the proper application of technical resources.

Improvements in the surgical technique have produced various modifications through the years. The operation is currently performed with the use of cardiopulmonary bypass with arterial cannulation of the common femoral artery or in the aortic arch. Cold potassium cardioplegia and moderate total body hypothermia provide cardiac and cerebral protection. Three separate techniques are available. The aneurysm that is localized to the supracoronary portion of the ascending aorta is simply replaced with a woven Dacron graft by the graft inclusion technique. If the aortic valve is diseased, the valve is resected separately and replaced with a prosthetic valve (Figure 49.12).

Excellent immediate and long-term results have been obtained with overall operative and hospital mortality rates of 4% and 9%.[19] Survival rates by actuarial representation were 69.5% in eight years.

Lastly, an aneurysm of the entire ascending aorta and aortic anulus requires complete resection and replacement with a composite valve graft prosthesis. This necessitates reimplantation of the coronary arteries to the prosthetic graft.

AORTIC ARCH

Aneurysms of the transverse aortic arch presented a strong challenge to the surgeon. The major problem in surgical treatment is concerned with the consequences of arrest of circulation to the brain and heart. In addition, hemorrhagic coagulopathy after operation presented a special group of technical considerations.

The transverse aortic arch is the segment of the aorta from which the brachiocephalic vessels arise (Figure 49.13). The incidence of aneurysms is about the same in the aortic arch and in the ascending aorta.[20] Aneurysms of the transverse aortic arch usually produce symptoms of obstruction or compression of adjacent structures. Tracheal or bronchial obstruction may cause wheezing, a brassy cough, tracheal tug, or pneumonitis secondary to obstruction. Rupture may occur into any of these structures, the pericardium, mediastinum, or pleural cavity. The recurrent laryngeal or phrenic nerves may become compressed from the expanding aneurysm.

Crawford and Crawford[20(p15)] classified these aneurysms into two groups for consideration of treatment. Group I includes aneurysms in the distal arch that can be exposed and isolated between clamps distal to the innominate artery. They can be treated by simple aortic cross-clamping and repair of the aneurysm by patch graft or tubular graft, depending on the amount of aortic circumference involved. Neither cardiac function and coronary perfusion nor cerebral perfusion is interrupted. Peripheral resistance is lowered with intravenous vasodilation therapy to protect the heart and promote collateral circulation.

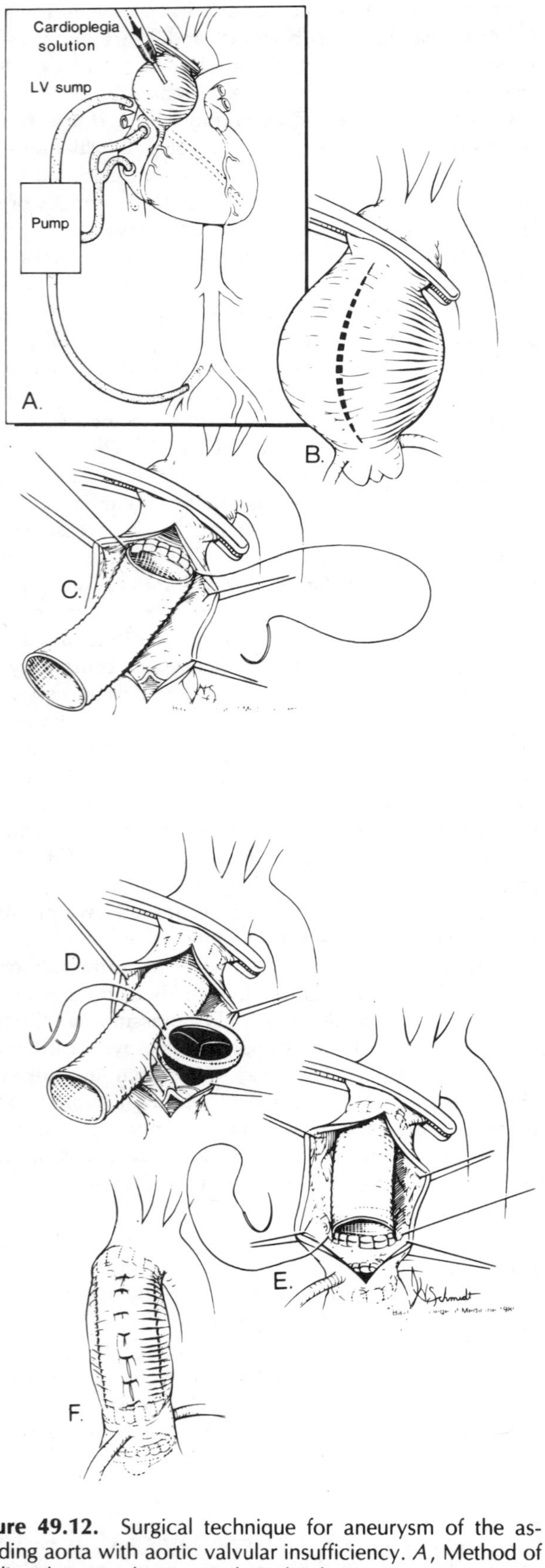

Figure 49.12. Surgical technique for aneurysm of the ascending aorta with aortic valvular insufficiency. *A*, Method of cardiopulmonary bypass and cardioplegia. *B*, Incision in ascending aorta. *C*, Distal aortic suture anastomosis. *D*, Aortic valve replacement. *E*, Proximal aortic anastomosis. *F*, Wrapping of aneurysmal wall about graft.

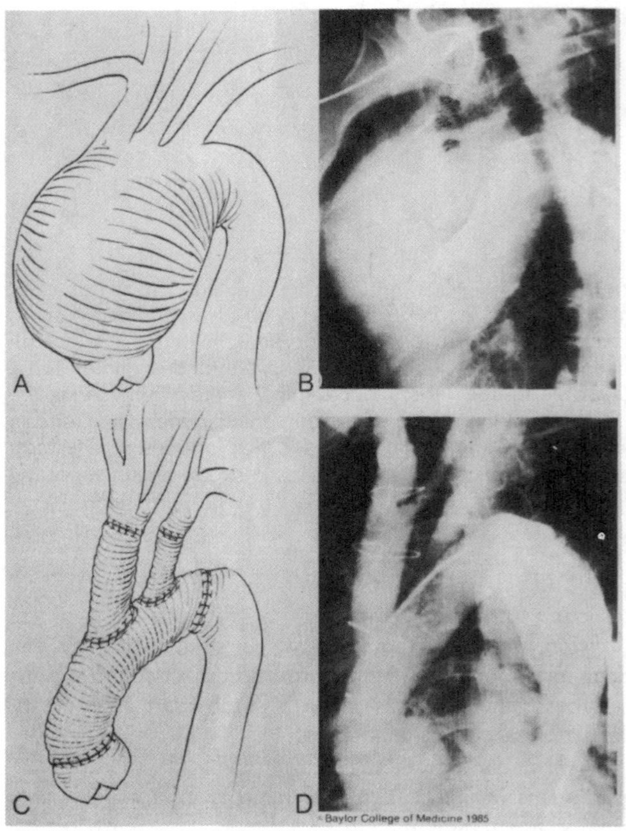

Figure 49.13. *A*, *B*, Preoperative drawing and aortogram in a man with cough and chest pain showing large fusiform aneurysm of ascending aorta and aortic arch. *C*, Technique of resection of aneurysm and Dacron replacement, with use of method of perfusion shown in Figure 49.14. *D*, Aortogram 12 years after surgery illustrating functioning graft. (Modified from DeBakey.[17])

Group II includes those aneurysms requiring clamping of the innominate and left carotid arteries. They are treated by the graft inclusion technique with reattachment of the origin of the brachiocephalic vessel directly into the opening made into the graft. Cardiopulmonary bypass and profound hypothermia (12° to 20°C rectally) are used for cerebral and myocardial protection. Most aneurysms in this group were due to atherosclerosis, were sacciform, were located in the concave side of the distal arch, involved in the entire circumference of the aortic wall, and were secondary to degenerative disease.

Hypothermia and temporary shunts were used in our early efforts to provide circulation during temporary arrest of circulation through the aortic arch. Homografts and later Dacron grafts were used by attaching the temporary grafts to the proximal segment of the ascending aorta to the descending thoracic aorta just distal to the left subclavian artery and to both common carotid arteries. Circulation was arrested in the aortic arch by clamps, and circulation was being maintained to the brain and the rest of the body through the temporary attached grafts. The aortic arch was excised and replaced with a graft, and the temporary bypass grafts were removed. The technical feasibility of this procedure was confirmed by the extremely satisfactory immediate postoperative course in one patient and encouraged us to continue using the procedure.

This technique had certain disadvantages. The necessity of performing and later removing four end-to-side anastomoses of a temporary graft prolonged the operation and increased the surgical risk. Another problem was that in some patients the aneurysm extended proximally to involve the entire ascending aorta, so that it was impossible to attach the proximal end of the shunt. In 1957, one of us (MED) successfully replaced an aneurysm of the ascending aorta and transverse aortic arch with an aortic homograft with use of total cardiopulmonary bypass with separate perfusion of the innominate and left carotid arteries.[21] With subsequent experience, several additional technical modifications were made. Use of coronary artery perfusion reduced cardiac ischemic complications, and insertion of arterial perfusion catheters into both axillary arteries permitted better cerebral perfusion through the right carotid and both vertebral arteries (Figure 49.14). Recent techniques of profound hypothermia and brief periods of circulatory arrest have proved valuable in reducing cerebral complications. They have, however, introduced a problem of excessive bleeding at the anastomosis and through the graft during prolonged warm-up while the patient is heparinized and placed on cardiopulmonary bypass. Graft porosity has been reduced by sterilizing the woven Dacron graft saturated with commercially available human serum albumin or platelet-rich plasma. This procedure produces a more adherent fibrin deposition, which is not easily washed off by exposure to heparinized blood.

Aneurysms of the transverse arch of the aorta involving the innominate and left common carotid artery are exposed through median sternotomy. Venous cannulas are placed in the superior vena cava and the femoral vein.

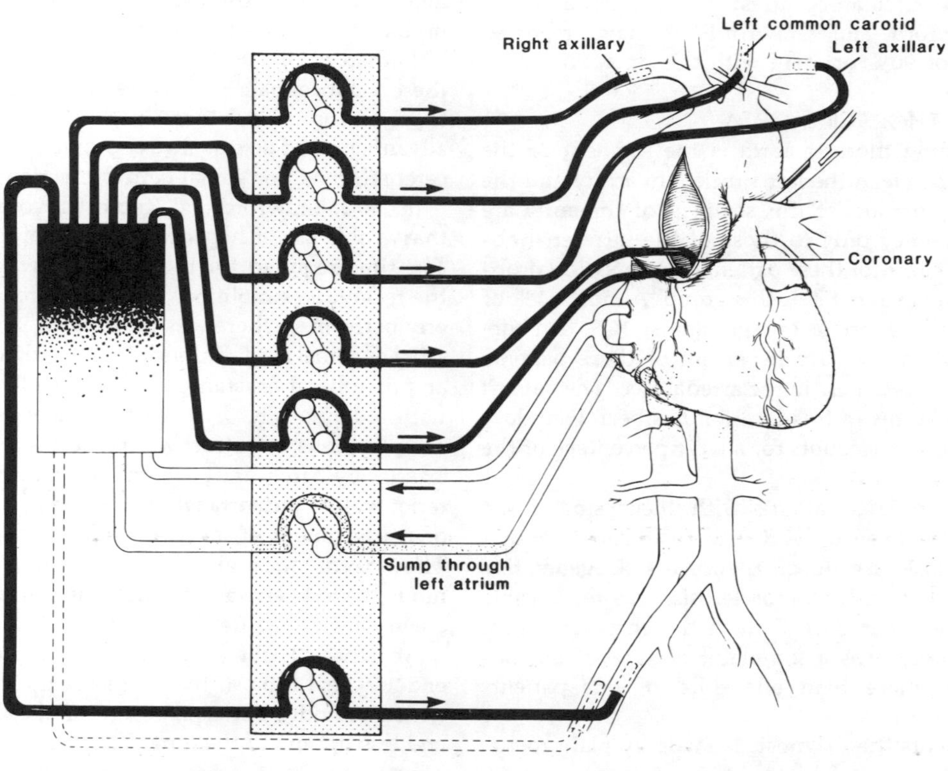

Figure 49.14. Method of perfusion during cardiopulmonary bypass for resection and graft replacement of ascending aorta and aortic arch in patient in Figure 49.13. (From DeBakey,[17] with permission.)

The left ventricle is sumped through the right pulmonary vein. As cardiopulmonary bypass is started, total body cooling is provided by use of a heat exchanger in the cardiopulmonary bypass circuit. Cooling is achieved at a relatively slow rate, depending on the size of the patient, to prevent brain-core gradient. Intravenous administration of nitroprusside enhances perfusion by reducing peripheral resistance. Sludging is avoided by mild hemodilution. Acidosis is prevented by bicarbonate injections.

When profound hypothermia is achieved (12° to 20°C), the distal aortic clamp is applied. The brachiocephalic vessels are clamped to avoid embolism. The aneurysm is excised and a woven Dacron graft, previously soaked in albumin and sterilized, is sutured to the upper descending thoracic aorta by the graft inclusion technique. An oval opening is made along the convex surface of the graft and sutured around the origins of the brachiocephalic vessels. The head is lowered, and the free end of the graft is elevated and filled with blood both from the brachiocephalic vessels and from the distal aorta to expel air. The graft is clamped proximal to the brachiocephalic vessels as the clamps are removed from the distal aorta; in this way, cerebral perfusion is resumed. Rewarming is started at this point. Depending on the proximal extent of the aneurysm, the proximal graft is sutured to the ascending aorta or the aortic root, the composite valve/graft being used if the aortic valve is involved. In this case, coronary reattachment to the graft is necessary. After complete rewarming has occurred, the patient is weaned from cardiopulmonary bypass, and blood component therapy is required to avoid coagulation abnormalities. Using circulatory arrest and profound hypothermia, Crawford and Crawford[20(p15)] have reported survival rates of 90% or more with this operation.

DESCENDING THORACIC AORTA

The descending thoracic aorta is the segment of the thoracic aorta between the left subclavian artery and the diaphragm. Aneurysms of this segment of the aorta are second in frequency only to those of the infrarenal abdominal aorta. Many of these patients have medical problems that are characteristic of this group. Almost 60% of our patients had hypertension and almost 30% had coronary artery disease.[22] Fifteen percent of these patients have aneurysms elsewhere in the arterial tree. The natural history of aneurysms in this location has been well documented.[23] Rupture accounts for a large percentage of the deaths.

In our series of 500 patients with aneurysms of the descending thoracic aorta, 51% had fusiform, 29% dissecting, and 20% sacciform aneurysms. Degenerative disease, associated with atherosclerosis, was responsible for 87% of the aneurysms. Pain in the chest, the most common symptom, was a complaint of 42% of our patients. Slightly more than one third of our patients were asymptomatic.

In most patients the diagnosis is made by plain roentgenograms of the chest. The aneurysm appears as a mass in the posterior mediastinum. Calcification of the aneurysmal wall helps to delineate the aneurysm. Occasionally, computed tomography scanning is helpful in further determining the cause of a posterior mediastinal mass. Compression or displacement of the esophagus or trachea may be identified by contrast studies. Erosion of the spine or ribs may be readily identified on the roentgenogram. Hoarseness may be present with involvement of the left recurrent laryngeal nerve. Compression of the adjacent tracheobronchial tree or esophagus may cause cough, hemoptysis, dysphagia, or hematemesis. Widening of the mediastinum or hemithorax suggests impending rupture of the thoracic aorta. Aortography is essential to confirm the diagnosis and to localize the aneurysm. The appropriate surgical treatment can be planned after the site and extent of the disease in the descending thoracic aorta are determined.

The first successful replacement of an aneurysm of the descending thoracic aorta with an aortic homograft without use of a shunt or bypass was performed in 1953.[24] Since then, the surgical technique has been modified and improved. The problems associated with proximal descending thoracic aortic clamping and surgical resection and replacement of long segments of the descending thoracic aorta have long been identified. Control of afterload of the heart and avoidance of ischemic injuries to the kidneys and spinal cord are major concerns. A number of methods have been used to minimize these problems. Surface hypothermia, left atrial–femoral artery bypass, shunts with use of a pump, left subclavian or axillary artery to distal descending thoracic aorta or common femoral artery shunts with use of a pump, and femoral vein to femoral artery shunts with use of a pump oxygenator have been employed. All these procedures require total heparinization of the patient, which may cause bleeding problems. To avoid total anticoagulation with heparin, Valiathan et al[25] used various direct shunts to alleviate the brachiocephalic hypertension and provide distal arterial perfusion. All these methods, however, have disadvantages and do not always provide the needed cardiac, cerebral, renal, or spinal cord protection.

In 1973, Crawford and Rubio[26] advocated a technique that avoids use of heparin and extracorporeal circulation. The time required for the operation was shortened, and the technique simplified. When the procedure was properly performed, there was no increase in the incidence of renal or spinal cord complications. Cardiac hemodynamics and peripheral resistance are controlled with vasodilators with reduction in, or at least no increase in, spinal cord complications. An effort was made to preserve intercostal arteries by patch-graft aortoplasty, replacement of an anterior wall of the aorta while preserving the posterior wall, or reattachment of large or multiple intercostal arteries. These techniques, along with the graft inclusion technique, have been valuable adjuvants in the treatment of aneurysms of the descending thoracic aorta.

Anesthesia is obtained with a bifurcated, double-lumen endotracheal tube so that the left lung can be collapsed, which provides better exposure of the descending aorta and less trauma to the lung. The chest is opened through a posterolateral thoracotomy, usually through the fifth intercostal space. The uninvolved aorta proximally and distally is dissected free and mobilized. The proximal aortic clamp is applied slowly as pharmacologic manipulation is carried out to decrease peripheral vascular resistance and avoid hypertension in the brachiocephalic vessels and subsequent heart strain (Figure 49.15). The aorta is opened longitudinally. An appropriate-sized woven Dacron graft is selected. Continuous 3–0 Prolene® sutures are used for the proximal anastomosis. Bleeding intercostal vessels are ligated, or intercostal arteries are reattached when appropriate. The distal anastomosis is performed in a manner similar to the proximal anastomosis. Before the distal anastomosis is completed, the patient's head is lowered, and both aortic segments are flushed by temporary release of the clamps. The graft is filled with blood to evacuate air. The aorta is slowly unclamped as the blood volume is replaced with fluids and blood intravenously. The aneurysmal wall of the aorta is tightly sutured around the graft for better hemostasis.

In our personal series, a variety of technical procedures were used before 1970 to avoid brachiocephalic hypertension, heart strain, and ischemia distal to the aortic clamp.[22] Of the 500 patients in the series, 383 (76.6%) had operations with adjuvants to bypass the occluded aortic segment. These techniques included hypothermia (17 patients), femoral vein–femoral artery bypass (two patients), external shunts (13 patients), left atrial-to-femoral artery bypass (349 patients), and right atrial-to-femoral artery bypass (two patients). Adjuvant shunts and bypass procedures were discontinued in 1970. One hundred seventeen patients (23.4%) have had resection without special adjuvants since 1970.

During this period, 470 patients had resection of aneurysms with graft replacement, 20 had resection with patch-graft angioplasty, six had resection with thoracoabdominal bypass, two had resection with primary closure, and two had re-entry procedures. The higher incidence of pulmonary complications, the occasional difficulty with the bypass or shunt procedure, longer operative time, more blood loss, the possibility of air embolism, and occasional femoral artery dissection prompted us to deal with these aneurysms without bypass or shunt procedures. The operative mortality rate dropped impressively from 18.5% when bypass shunts or other adjuvant methods were used before 1970 to 9.4% without bypass techniques since 1970. Moreover, the incidence of the serious postoperative complication of spinal cord ischemia did not significantly change. Paraparesis developed in nine of 383 patients (2.3%) treated before 1970. In only 2.5% (three of 117) of patients treated since 1970 without shunt or bypass techniques did neurologic complications develop.

The overall mortality rates for fusiform, sacciform, and dissecting aneurysms were 17%, 12.1%, and 19.4%, respectively. Almost 42% of the operative deaths were due to myocardial infarction with or without congestive heart failure; 13.5% were due to subsequent dissection with rupture, and another 13.5% were due to pulmonary insufficiency. The leading cause of late deaths was again cardiac, accounting for 29.6% of the late deaths; 22.2% of the late deaths were due to rupture of aneurysms of other parts of the aorta. This emphasizes the need for careful and long-term follow-up of all patients with aneurysms of the aorta. They are definitely prone to development of aneurysms in other areas of the arterial tree or to aneurysmal formation at a later date. The long-term survival rate in our series of 500 patients with aneurysms of the descending thoracic aorta has been gratifying (Figure 49.16).

DISSECTING AORTIC ANEURYSMS

Despite sporadic observations regarding dissecting aortic aneurysms made since the 16th century, confusion existed regarding the pathogenesis of the disease. In his classic treatise in 1934, Shennan[27] did much to clarify the problem. On the basis of extensive investigation, he concluded that medial degeneration was the most significant underlying cause of dissection. On analysis of collected cases, Shennan reported that death occurred within 24 hours in 66% and within one week in another 27% of the patients. This rapidly fatal course of the disease has been confirmed in a number of other published reports on the natural course of the disease. Anagnostopoulos et al[28] in 1972 analyzed a series of 963 patients collected from six different reports. Seventy percent of the patients

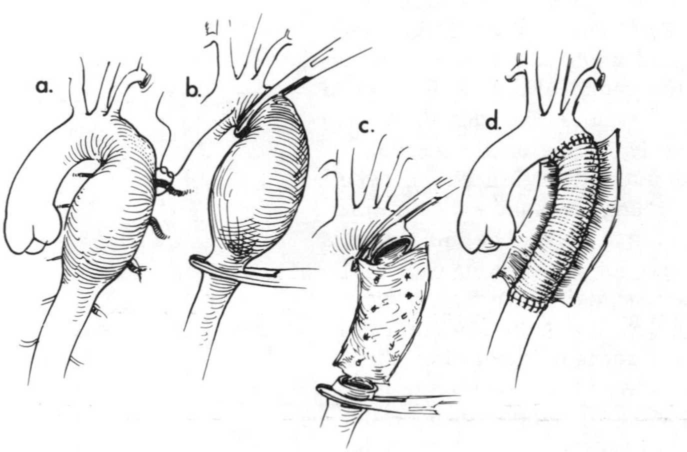

Figure 49.15. Current operative technique for resection of aneurysm of descending thoracic aorta and Dacron graft replacement. (From DeBakey et al,[22] with permission.)

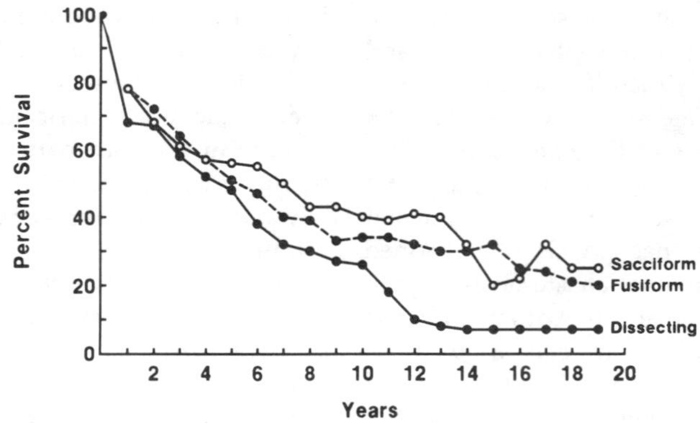

Figure 49.16. Long-term survival rate of 500 patients who had surgical resection of aneurysms of the descending thoracic aorta. (From DeBakey et al,[22] with permission.)

died within one week of onset of dissection and 90% within three months. Only a few patients survived more than one year.

The most common complications of dissecting aortic aneurysm are rupture of the wall of the false aneurysm with fatal hemorrhage; pericardial hemorrhage with progressive tamponade; obstruction of vital branches of the aorta with cerebral, coronary, or visceral ischemia; and severe aortic valvular incompetence with acute heart failure. Medical measures for pain, hypertension, and myocardial contractility may stabilize the acute process but will have little effect on preventing death. Surgical treatment provides a more effective method of controlling the dissection. One of us (MED) performed the first successful repair of a dissecting aneurysm of the descending thoracic aorta in 1955.[29] Since then, a better understanding of anatomic and pathologic patterns of the disease has enabled us to develop certain concepts for more effective surgical treatment. From our experience with patients treated surgically for dissecting aortic aneurysms, we classified the different forms of disease and outlined appropriate surgical treatment for each type.[30]

The classification is based on the anatomic site and extent of the dissecting process. Although the initial intimal tear may occur in any part of the aorta, it usually develops in the ascending or proximal descending aorta. Because of the occurrence of more than one intimal tear, and because retrograde and antegrade dissection occur, the original site of dissection cannot always be determined by clinical or aortographic studies. We identified three types of aortic dissection depending on the segment of aorta involved by the dissection[31] (Figure 49.17). Type I dissections affect the ascending aorta and extend distally into the descending abdominal aorta. The initial tear is usually a transverse opening of the anterior wall of the proximal ascending aorta. The original tear may, however, occur in the aortic arch or descending thoracic aorta, with retrograde dissection to the aortic root and distal dissection throughout the remainder of the aorta (Figure 49.18). Dilatation of the anulus or lack of support of the intimal attachment of the valves resulting from the proximal extension of the dissecting process may produce aortic incompetence.

Type II dissection characteristically originates as an anterior transverse intimal tear just above the aortic valve. The dissection is limited to the ascending aorta and terminates proximal to the origin of the innominate artery. Aortic valvular incompetence is frequently present. The posterior wall of the ascending aorta often remains intact.

Type III dissection develops distal to the origin of the left subclavian artery and may extend distally for a varying distance. In type IIIa, the dissection is limited to the descending thoracic aorta (Figure 49.19). More often, however, the dissection known as type IIIb extends below the diaphragm, affecting the abdominal aorta and the visceral and iliac arteries.

The most common symptom was pain, particularly in types I and III. Hypertension, which was present in about 90% of patients, was the most common physical finding. Other frequent physical signs were congestive heart failure and Marfan's syndrome. Only 10% to 15% of the patients were asymptomatic.

Follow-up studies in patients who survived the acute episode indicated that death occurred in over 29% from rupture of aneurysms that developed after the original treatment.[32] The incidence of subsequent development of aneurysms in the various types of dissection is significantly different (Figure 49.20). Thus, in types I and IIIb, the incidences were 30% and 38%, whereas in type II, it was 14% and in type IIIa, 16%. The importance of control

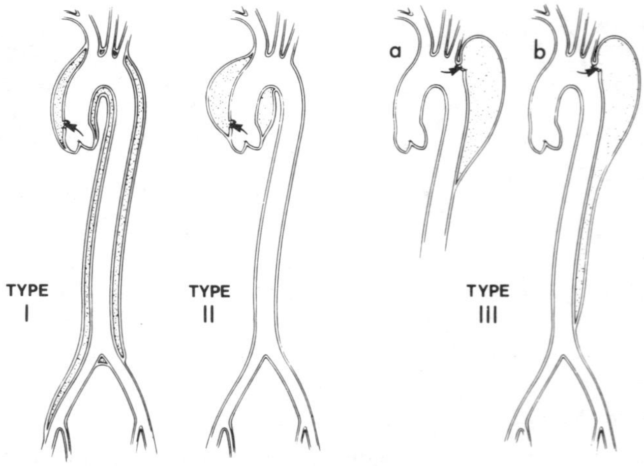

Figure 49.17. Classification of dissecting aneurysms of the aorta into three types. (From DeBakey,[17] with permission.)

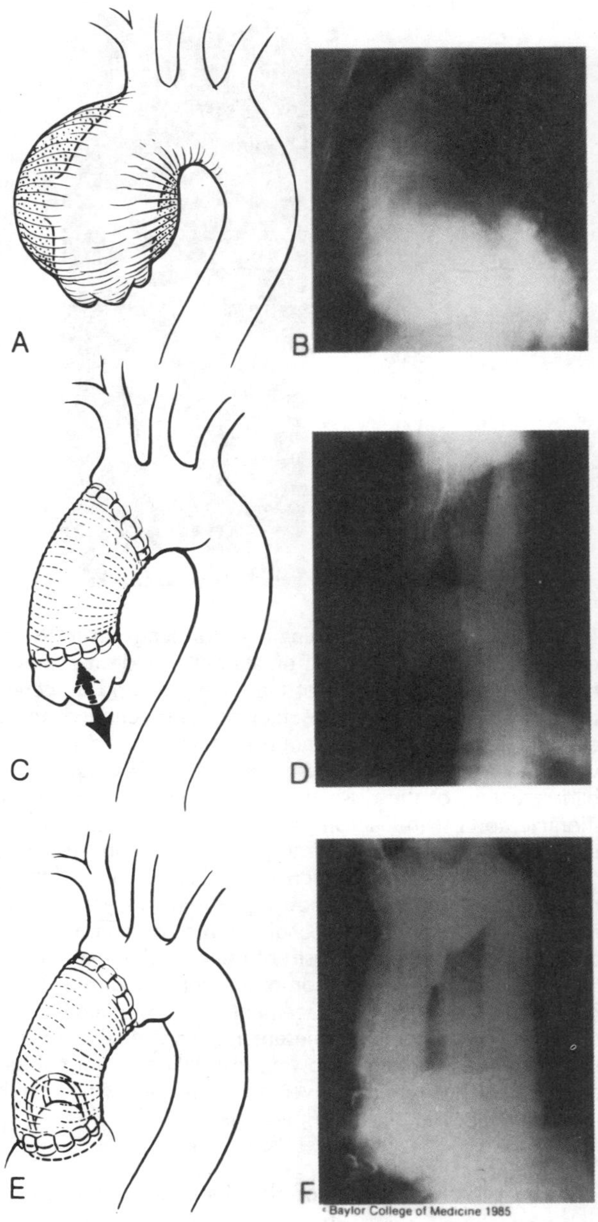

Figure 49.18. *A*, *B*, Preoperative drawing and aortogram in a man with a type II dissecting aortic aneurysm. *C*, *D*, Drawing and aortogram made six years after operation showing functioning graft and severe aortic insufficiency. *E*, Drawing showing subsequent aortic valve replacement. *F*, Aortogram 12 years after aortic valve replacement, and 18 years after resection of aneurysm showing functioning graft. (From DeBakey et al,[32] with permission.)

of hypertension is shown by the fact that subsequent aneurysms developed in 45.5% of patients with uncontrolled hypertension, but in only 17.4% of those with controlled hypertension.

In all types of aortic dissection, the initial treatment consists in medical measures to stabilize the cardiovascular system and in early angiography. The patient's condition is monitored closely with central venous and arterial lines in the intensive care unit. The blood pressure should be reduced to the lowest level compatible with maintenance of cerebral, cardiac, and renal function. The

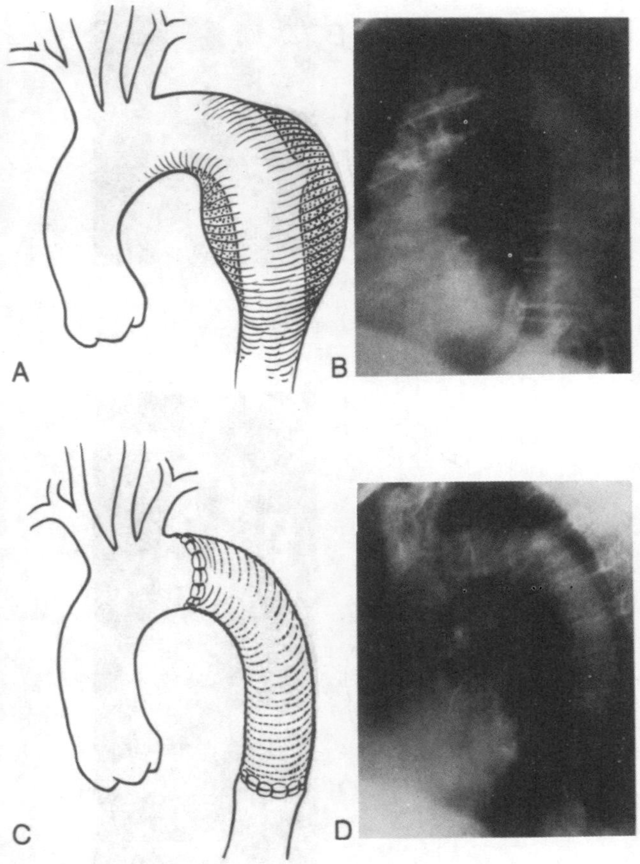

Figure 49.19. *A*, *B*, Preoperative drawing and aortogram of type IIIa dissecting aneurysm of descending thoracic aorta. *C*, Drawing showing method of resection and graft replacement. *D*, Aortogram showing functioning graft 18 years after operation. (Modified from DeBakey et al.[32])

most common agents used are nitroprusside and propranolol. Operation should be performed early because of possible eminent rupture, severe aortic insufficiency, cerebral ischemia, enlarging pericardial effusion, and occlusion of coronary and other vital aortic branches.

The initial tear was in the ascending aorta in 62%, in the transverse arch in 9%, in the isthmus in 16%, in the descending thoracic aorta in 10%, and in the abdominal aorta in 3% of patients.[33] The dissection may spread proximally or distally at varying rates until the entire proximal or descending aorta is involved. Several patterns of dissection are produced. The dissections that begin in the ascending aorta tend to progress distally along the greater curvature of the ascending aorta, transverse arch, and upper descending thoracic aorta. Dissections that begin in the arch or upper descending aorta usually extend distally in the posterolateral aspect of the descending aorta, abdominal aorta, and left iliac artery. Varying degrees of retrograde dissection occur in patients in whom the initial tear is in the transverse arch.

Type I

This type represents a surgical emergency because of the tendency for the development of aortic valvular insufficiency with congestive heart failure, aortic rupture

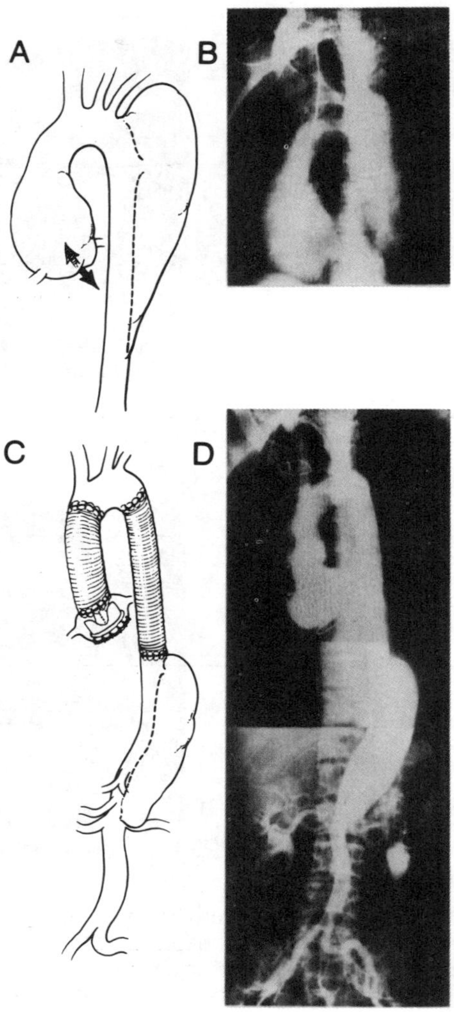

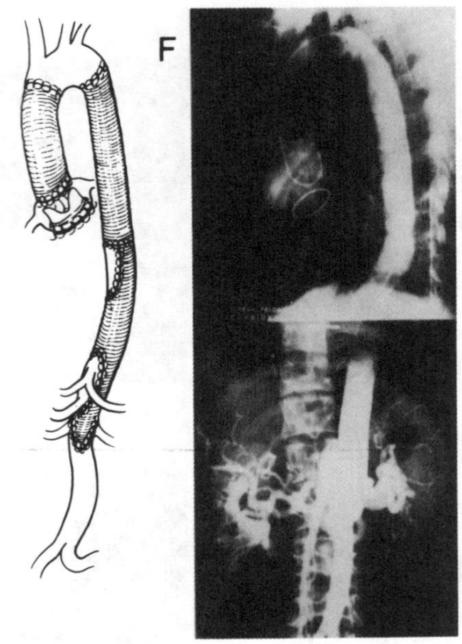

Figure 49.20. *A*, *B*, Drawing and aortogram of a 26-year-old white man with stigmata of Marfan's syndrome showing type I dissecting aneurysm of the ascending and descending thoracic aorta and aortic insufficiency. Resection of the ascending aorta with Dacron graft replacement and aortic valvular replacement was performed. Two weeks later, patient had resection of the dissecting aneurysm of the descending thoracic aorta with Dacron graft replacement after outer and inner layers of false lumen were approximated with attachment of graft distally to normal lumen. *C*, *D*, Drawing and aortogram made eight months later showing satisfactory graft replacement of ascending and descending thoracic aorta, but development of extensive aneurysm of upper abdominal aorta. *E*, Surgical technique of resection of the upper abdominal aneurysm and Dacron graft replacement with restoration of continuity to celiac, superior mesenteric, and renal arteries. *F*, Postoperative aortogram showing restoration of normal function. Patient has remained well and is leading a normal life. (From DeBakey et al,[32] with permission.)

with death, or obstruction to the branches of the aorta with ischemia of the brain, viscera, or limb. After rapid medical stabilization and diagnostic aortography, operation should be performed. Cardiopulmonary bypass may be initiated through the femoral artery and vein, and a median sternotomy is made. Cardiopulmonary bypass, moderate hypothermia, and cold cardioplegia coronary perfusion are instituted. The distal aortic clamp is applied, usually proximal to the innominate artery. A longitudinal incision is made into the aneurysm. The proximal extent of the aneurysm determines the need for concomitant aortic valve replacement or coronary artery reimplantation. The distal anastomosis is performed initially with a woven Dacron graft. Some surgeons impregnate the graft with human serum albumin using a steam autoclave or a platelet-rich solution to reduce porosity. Dacron-felt baffles are used to reinforce the wall of the aorta to improve the strength of the anastomosis. This also obliterates and decompresses the distal false lumen to prevent progression of the dissection and relieve the obstruction to flow of the transverse arch vessels.

If the proximal extent of the dissection does not involve the aortic wall with the coronary arteries or the anulus of the aortic valve, simple supracoronary anastomosis is performed, again with the Dacron-felt baffles. Air and debris are removed before release of the clamps, and coronary flow is restored. As the patient's own heart begins pumping, the patient is weaned off cardiopulmonary bypass.

If the aortic valve is incompetent, it is replaced, usually according to the composite valve/graft technique. The ostia of the coronary artery can be attached separately to the graft. In some patients, the valve apparatus can be suspended so as to maintain the host-valve mechanism.

Type II

This type is corrected by resection of the ascending aorta and replacement with a woven Dacron graft with use of total cardiopulmonary bypass. The aortic valve is usually incompetent, particularly in chronic dissections, so that it usually must be replaced. Therefore, the composite valve/graft is often best. In the acute form, it may be possible to avoid valve replacement by resuspension of the valves.

Type III

In type IIIa dissection, the dissection is limited to the descending thoracic aorta distal to the left subclavian artery and proximal to the diaphragm. Thus, the entire diseased segment can be resected and replaced with a woven Dacron graft through a left thoracotomy. Again, the Dacron baffles are useful in reinforcing the aortic wall at the anastomotic suture line and in using the graft-inclusion technique. The aortic wall can be sutured around the newly inserted graft to provide better hemostasis. Reattachment of the intercostal artery to provide spinal cord flow is generally not successful because of the friability of the undissected aortic wall.

With improvements in preoperative preparation and refinements in surgical techniques, we have noted progressive reduction in the operative mortality rate (Figure 49.21). The mortality rate in the acute stage of the disease is almost twice that of the subacute and chronic stages in all three types. The most common cause of operative death was rupture of the aneurysm (26%).[34] This observation emphasizes the unpredictable and potentially fatal nature of the disease. Twenty-five percent of the deaths were related to myocardial infarction, followed by congestive heart failure (24%) and respiratory failure (10%).

Paraplegia was the most prevalent postoperative complication in type III; this is not surprising since this type has the most extensive aortic dissection. The incidence of spinal cord ischemia in type III has remained about the same since 1970. At that time, we abandoned the various adjuvant shunt and bypass procedures to prevent spinal cord ischemia and concentrated on simplifying and expediting the surgical procedure. The result has been reduction in the mortality rate with essentially the same low incidence of spinal cord ischemia.

In our series, the overall five-year survival rate was 57%, and the ten-year survival rate, 32% (Figure 49.22). These figures are compared with those in a collective series of nonsurgically treated patients in which only 10% survived three months, and none lived longer than three years.

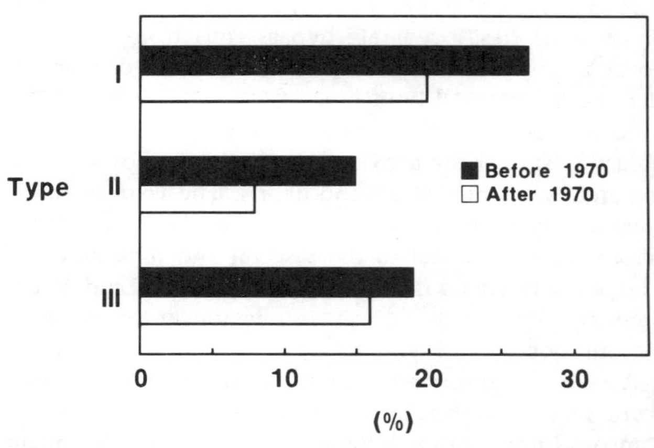

Figure 49.21. Perioperative mortality rate in 527 patients with dissecting aneurysms of the aorta before and after 1970, according to type of dissection. (From DeBakey et al,[34] with permission.)

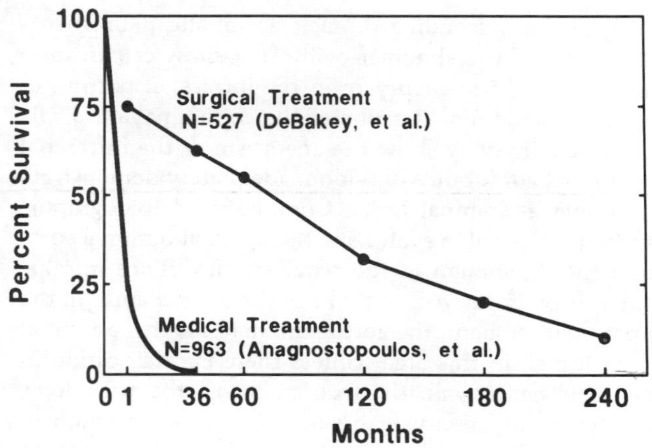

Figure 49.22. Survival curves comparing surgical treatment during a period of 20 years in 527 patients with dissecting aortic aneurysms with a collected series of medically treated patients reported by Anagnostopoulos et al.[28] (From DeBakey et al,[32] with permission.)

THORACOABDOMINAL ANEURYSMS

These aneurysms involve the descending thoracic and abdominal aorta. This segment of the aorta requires special consideration because it includes the upper portion of the abdominal aorta from which arise the mesenteric and renal arteries. These aneurysms are grouped together because of this anatomic characteristic, the thoracoabdominal incision used for exposure, and similar problems of reconstruction. Many serious and challenging problems are encountered including the necessity to manage the cardiac hemodynamics, avoidance of excessive visceral and renal ischemia during operation, the technical difficulties of vascular reconstruction, the danger of spinal cord ischemia and paraplegia, and control of bleeding after operation.

Like aneurysms in any location, rupture and death are a threat. Moreover, compression and erosion into adjacent structures may occur. If the lungs are involved, cough, pulmonary infection, or hemoptysis may develop. If the esophagus, stomach, or duodenum is eroded or compressed, dysphagia or gastrointestinal bleeding may be present. Back pain may develop secondary to erosion of vertebral bodies. Involvement and thrombosis of the spinal arteries may lead to paraplegia. Erosion with rupture into the inferior vena cava or iliac veins can produce an aortovenous fistula and heart failure. Peripheral embolization of the atheromatous debris within the lumen of the aneurysm may cause distal ischemic symptoms. Thoracoabdominal aneurysms may be asymptomatic and may be found on routine roentgenograms of the chest or abdomen.

On physical examination, the diagnosis should be suspected when the proximal portion of a pulsatile abdominal mass extends under the costal margin of the thoracic cage. Plain roentgenograms of the chest may show widening of the descending thoracic aorta, and plain roentgenograms of the abdomen will often show calcification in the wall of the aneurysm in the infrarenal portion or the upper abdominal portion of the abdominal aorta. Ultrasonography may show the aneurysm of the infrarenal abdominal aorta but will seldom adequately demonstrate the upper abdominal aorta. Computerized tomographic scanning is useful in evaluating the upper abdominal aorta from the diaphragm to the renal arteries. Since intraluminal thrombosis frequently lines the dilated aorta in the suprarenal segment, the aortogram may suggest a normal aortic lumen in this area. Unless there is calcification in the aneurysmal wall, the true extent of the pathologic changes in the aneurysmal wall may not be determined. The computerized tomographic scan identifies both the internal and external walls of the aorta and enables precise determination of the size of the aneurysm in the upper abdominal aorta. Contrast aortography is still mandatory in evaluating the extent of the aneurysm and in planning the operation. Associated occlusive disease of the visceral or renal vessels that will require arterial revascularization at operation can also be identified. Twenty percent of patients with thoracoabdominal aneurysms have associated occlusive disease in the visceral or renal arteries.[20(p78)] Patients undergoing extensive aortography should be well hydrated by intravenous administration of fluids before the procedure is performed. A liter of crystalloid therapy and intravenous administration of mannitol before aortography will reduce deterioration secondary to iodinated contrast material.

In the operating room, the patient's condition is monitored carefully with central venous Swan-Ganz catheters to determine pulmonary artery–pulmonary capillary wedge pressure and cardiac output. Additional intravenous cannulization should include central as well as several large-bore peripheral, venous catheters. Rapid volume and blood replacement sometimes becomes necessary. Serial electrolyte and arterial blood gases are determined.

A good anesthesia team is critical in preventing proximal brachiocephalic hypertension and major depression of cardiac function and in maintaining management of peripheral resistance. Since major physiologic changes occur during aortic cross-clamping, proper fluid administration and delivery of sodium nitroprusside are necessary to control these factors. An inhalation anesthetic is administered through a double-lumen endobronchial tube which allows deflation of the left lung and proper ventilation of the right lung. Collapse of the left lung provides better exposure during the thoracotomy and diminishes trauma to the left lung. Excessive cardiac compression is also avoided.

Exposure is achieved through a thoracoabdominal incision. The thoracotomy level depends on the proximal extent of the aneurysm. If the aneurysm affects only the distal thoracic aorta, exposure through the eighth or ninth interspace is adequate. More extensive involvement of the descending thoracic aorta may require incision into the fifth or sixth intercostal space. The incision is extended and directed across the costal margin into the abdomen where it is extended distally in the midline down to the pubis if necessary. The thoracic aorta is easily exposed by medial retraction of the collapsed lung. A radial incision of the diaphragm from the point of division of the costal arch to the aortic hiatus is necessary. The posterior peritoneum is incised with the electrocautery in the relatively avascular plane lateral to the left side of the colon. As the spleen, tail of the pancreas, left kidney, and colon are retracted medially and anteriorly, the entire posterolateral abdominal aorta from the diaphragm to the aortic bifurcation is exposed.

Heparin is administered as the proximal clamp is applied. The anesthesiologist also starts an infusion of nitroprusside to stabilize the proximal blood pressure and cardiac hemodynamics.The aneurysm is opened longitudinally on the posterolateral aspect of the aorta. To help prevent profuse bleeding and minimize the need for excessive blood transfusions, the autotransfusion unit is used to collect blood for subsequent reperfusion. The laminated thrombus and atherosclerotic debris within the aneurysm are removed. Back bleeding from the celiac, superior mesenteric, and renal arteries is controlled by insertion and inflation of a small Fogarty catheter. Whereas small intercostal or lumbar arteries are suture ligated, selected large intercostal or lumbar arteries are preserved for subsequent reattachment to the graft. A woven Dacron tube graft is selected. The proximal aortic anastomosis is performed end to end. The graft is sutured to the inside of the proximal descending thoracic aorta with a continuous suture, according to the graft-inclusion technique. After the anastomosis is completed, hemostasis is checked by temporary release of the aortic clamp. The graft is placed under proper tension, and circular or oval openings are made in the large graft at the appropriate junction of the orifices of the visceral and renal arteries. If the origins of the celiac, superior mesenteric, and both renal arteries are close together, a single anastomosis can be performed between the graft and the aortic wall (Figure 49.23). If the distance separating the origins of these vessels is excessive, up to four openings in the aortic graft are made, and the individual vessels are sutured individually to the aortic graft. If associated occlusive disease affects the origin of these vessels, endarterectomy through the aorta can be performed. Occasionally, because of severe associated distal occlusive disease in the mesenteric or renal arteries, a separate bypass graft from the main aortic graft is necessary for attachment to one or more of the visceral or renal branches.

As the visceral and renal branches are reattached, temporary release of the proximal aortic clamp allows flushing and evacuation of air and debris. The Fogarty catheters are then deflated and removed. A clamp is applied across the graft distal to the visceral and renal vessels. The proximal clamp is slowly released as fluids and blood products are rapidly given intravenously to prevent hypotension.

An opening or openings may also be fashioned in the aortic graft for suture to the posterior aortic wall to encompass intercostal or lumbar arteries to provide spinal cord perfusion. The distal aortic anastomosis is performed end to end to the distal abdominal aorta or with use of a bifurcation graft and attaching the distal limbs to the iliac or femoral arteries. All suture lines are carefully checked for hemostasis. The outer aneurysmal wall,

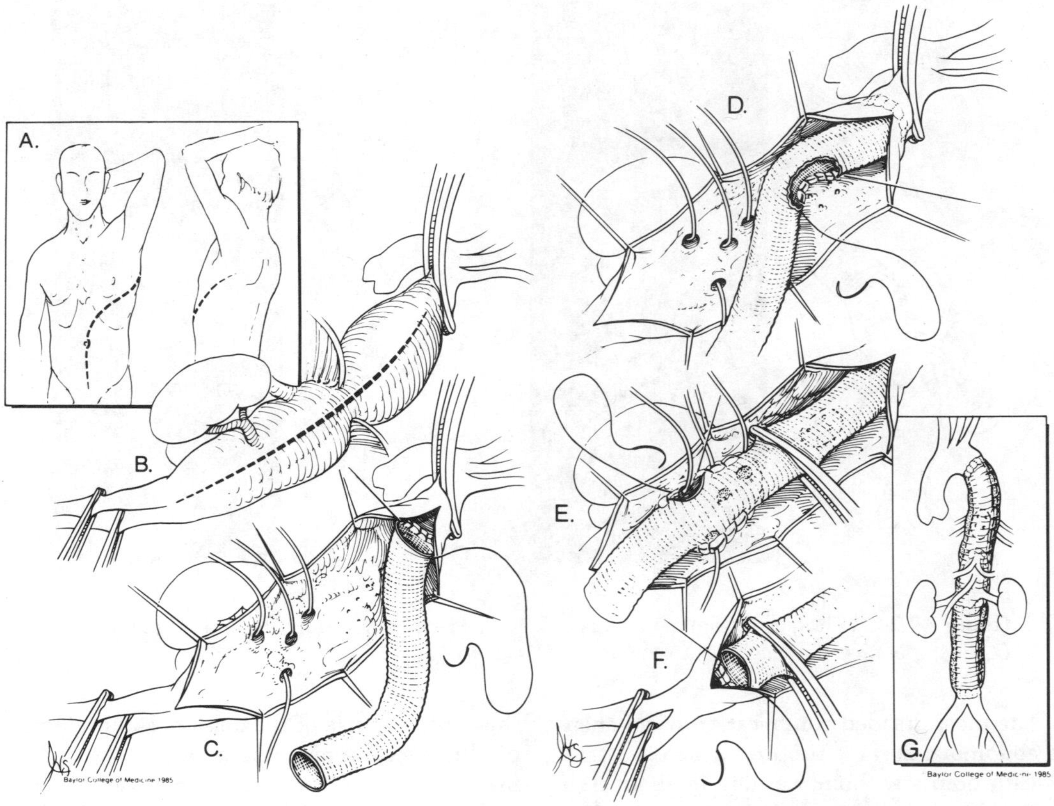

Figure 49.23. Surgical repair of thoracoabdominal aneurysm. *A*, Incision made through lower intercostal space and extended as midline abdominal incision to pubis. *B*, Thoracic and abdominal aorta exposed through a retroperitoneal approach and the diaphragm divided. Vascular clamps were applied and the aneurysm was incised. *C*, Bleeding from renal and visceral arteries controlled with balloon catheters. Proximal anastomosis completed with woven Dacron graft. *D*, Opening made in graft opposite two sets of intercostal arteries and graft sutured over these openings. *E*, Clamp repositioned providing spinal cord circulation. After elliptical opening fashioned in graft, anastomosis performed to island of aorta to provide circulation to celiac, superior mesenteric, and both renal arteries. *F*, Clamp again repositioned to restore visceral and renal circulation. Distal aortic anastomosis completed. *G*, Aortic aneurysmal wall sutured around graft.

which is not excised, is sutured tightly about the aortic graft. This technique minimizes the amount of dissection, provides better hemostasis, and avoids excessive blood loss. The wound is closed in appropriate layers.

Our initial experience with this type of aneurysm was in August 1955, when hypothermia was used in an attempt to prevent the potential ischemic damage to the abdominal viscera. These aneurysms were later managed with use of temporary bypass grafts to provide circulation during aortic cross-clamping. Thus, in the first successful treatment of a patient with a thoracoabdominal aneurysm, these techniques were used to minimize ischemia in the vital organs during resection and graft replacement.[35] After the branches of the graft were anastomosed to the celiac, superior mesenteric, and both renal arteries, the temporary bypass graft was removed. This led to modification of the procedure by combining the bypass principle with a permanent replacement.[36] The Dacron graft was anastomosed proximally to the descending thoracic aorta, end to side, above the aneurysm. The distal abdominal aortic anastomosis was made end to side. Anterograde aortic flow was stopped by the application of an aortic clamp proximal to the descending thoracic aortic aneurysm, mesenteric and renal flow being provided through the aortic graft. Dacron grafts were placed from the main aortic bypass graft to each renal artery and the superior mesenteric and celiac arteries. The aneurysm was then resected, and the ends of the aorta were sutured. This procedure minimizes the ischemic arrest in each of the branch arteries to 10 or 15 minutes, a period that is well tolerated (Figure 49.24).

Among our first 42 patients, 64% have done well up to more than ten years.[37] With newer modifications of the surgical technique, as suggested by Crawford and Crawford,[20(p133)] more than 90% of these patients survived operation. These figures are comparable to results of infrarenal abdominal aortic aneurysmal replacement.

The risk of paraplegia in these patients depends on the extent of the disease. Obviously, when long segments of the descending thoracic aorta are affected, the incidence of neurologic complications is higher. Extensive experience in this area has shown, however, that the incidence of paraplegia should be no more than about 2%.

ABDOMINAL AORTIC ANEURYSMS

The infrarenal abdominal aorta is the most common site for the development of aneurysms. It characteristically arises below the origin of the renal arteries and extends for varying distances to or beyond the aortic

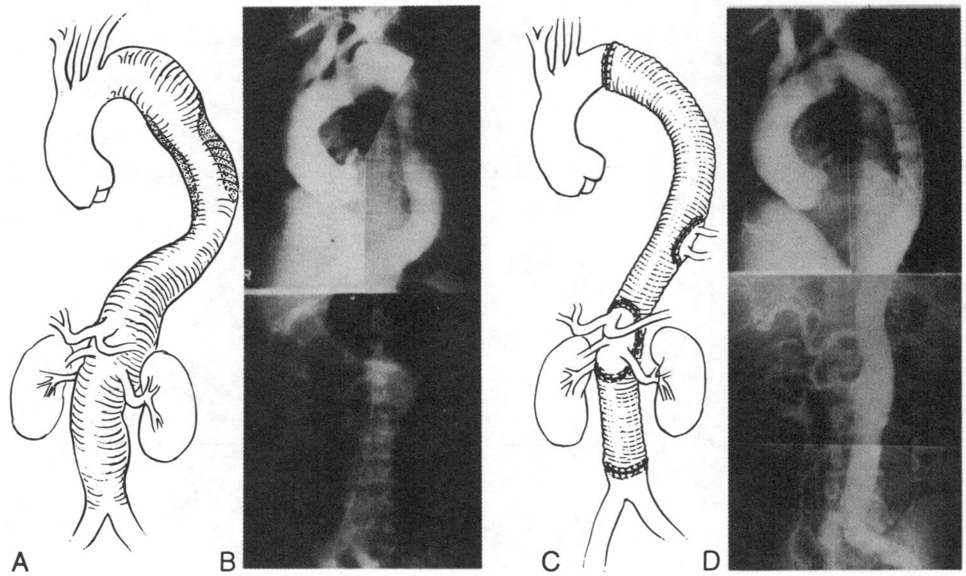

Figure 49.24. Thoracoabdominal aneurysm. *A*, *B*, Preoperative drawing and aortogram. *C*, *D*, Postoperative drawing and aortogram.

bifurcation. The most dreaded complication of an aneurysm of the abdominal aorta is rupture, which is fatal if untreated. Death occurs without warning in about 33% of the patients within one year of diagnosis and in 81% within five years.[38] Since 1952, an effective method of surgical treatment has been available. Dubost[16] was the first to excise an aneurysm of the abdominal aorta successfully and replace it with a homograft. Our first successful excision of an abdominal aortic aneurysm and graft replacement was performed on November 6, 1952.[39] At that time we did not know about Dubost's operation. Since then, we have increased our knowledge of the disease and improved the surgical technique.

Although aneurysms have many causes, most of them are due to atherosclerosis secondary to degenerative changes in the aortic wall. The pathophysiologic aspects of this degenerative process are not well understood, but the effects of hypertension and elastin or collagen deficiency certainly play a role. Other less common causes of abdominal aortic aneurysms are trauma, infection (mycotic), aortitis, dissection, and anastomosis.

It is estimated that abdominal aortic aneurysms may exist in as much as 2% of the elderly in the western world.[40] The incidence of abdominal aortic aneurysms is increasing. One reason for this increase may be that more asymptomatic aneurysms are being diagnosed during routine physical or roentgenographic examinations for other problems. Aneurysms are common in other parts of the arterial tree. Up to 12% of patients with abdominal aortic aneurysms also have aneurysms of the thoracic aorta.[20(p134)]

About 10% to 30% of abdominal aortic aneurysms rupture.[41] Because of the law of Laplace, larger aneurysms are more inclined to rupture than smaller ones. Yet, small abdominal aneurysms may also rupture. At postmortem examination, aneurysms less than 5 cm in diameter ruptured in 18% of the patients.[42] The rate of progression in the natural course of the disease is unpredictable. Results of ultrasonic examination, however, showed that abdominal aortic aneurysms tend to increase by 0.4 cm a year.[43]

The ages of patients with aneurysms of the abdominal aorta range from 30 to over 100 years.[44] The highest incidence is in the seventh decade of life. In our series, over 20% were 70 years or older. The ratio of men to women is 9:1. Twenty-five percent of our patients have associated coronary artery disease, and over 33% of them have hypertension. Segmental occlusive or aneurysmal disease of other parts of the aorta and major arterial trunks occurs not infrequently. Forty percent of patients have aneurysmal or occlusive disease of the aortic bifurcation and iliac arteries.[20(p136)] Significant occlusive disease of the renal artery is present in 19% of patients. Associated visceral mesenteric artery disease is infrequent.

About 75% of abdominal aortic aneurysms are diagnosed by detection of a pulsatile abdominal mass on physical examination during routine roentgenography of body systems or during celiotomy for other reasons. Most patients are asymptomatic. Less than one fourth to one third of the patients seek medical advice because of discomfort in the abdomen or back. Compression or erosion of the vertebral bodies can cause pain in the back. The duodenum may be stretched over an abdominal aortic aneurysm and cause partial intestinal obstruction. If the aneurysm erodes into the gastrointestinal tract, upper gastrointestinal bleeding occurs. Initially, bleeding is intermittent, but catastrophic hemorrhage will ensue if the patient is not treated. An abdominal aortic aneurysm may also erode and rupture into the inferior vena cava and produce dramatic clinical manifestations of congestive heart failure and edema of the legs accompanied by a loud abdominal bruit and widened pulse pressure. Ureteral obstruction may occur and is due to direct pressure from an expanding aneurysm or retroperitoneal fibrosis with "inflammatory" aneurysms.

In patients with large abdominal aortic aneurysms or in small, thin patients, palpation of a pulsatile abdominal mass makes the diagnosis easy. Plain roentgenograms usually show the typically calcified shadow in the wall of the aneurysm. Unsuspected abdominal aortic aneurysms may be discovered during routine urologic or lumbar spine roentgenography. Ultrasonography, a new diagnostic tool, is extremely helpful in evaluating the abdominal aorta. Computerized axial tomography provides accurate diagnostic information, particularly for aneurysms of the upper abdominal aortic segment. Nevertheless, aortography remains the most precise method for diagnosis of aneurysms of the abdominal aorta, including the adjacent thoracic aorta and iliac arteries, as well as for defining occlusive disease in the visceral, renal, or iliac arteries. Retrograde contrast aortography is the most widely used technique. Aortography is especially indicated if one suspects: (1) associated renovascular hypertension, (2) a possible aneurysm of the upper abdominal aorta, (3) intestinal angina, (4) unexplained abdominal bruit, or (5) horseshoe kidney. Digital subtraction arteriography provides more information than digital subtraction venography.

As with any candidate for major abdominal surgery, patients with abdominal aortic aneurysms should have careful preoperative evaluation. Studies include standard electrocardiography, roentgenography of the chest, complete blood count, urinalysis, and determination of blood urea nitrogen, creatinine, and blood sugar levels. Excretory urograms may uncover unsuspected ureteral disease or the rare horseshoe kidney, which would require special surgical techniques.

Because abdominal aortic aneurysm is known to be associated with coronary artery disease, thorough cardiac evaluation, including coronary arteriography when indicated, should be completed. The benefit of previous coronary artery bypass grafting has been well established in patients with significant coronary artery disease.[45] Patients with transient ischemic attacks or stroke should have carotid arteriography. Asymptomatic carotid bruits are evaluated by noninvasive vascular testing. Significant carotid disease should be corrected surgically before an elective abdominal aortic operation is performed. In patients with significant carotid artery disease and a large or tender abdominal aortic aneurysm, the two conditions can be corrected at the same operation.

Current surgical technique is based on more than 30 years' experience with thousands of aneurysms of the abdominal aorta (Figure 49.25). Central venous catheters are inserted, and Swan-Ganz catheters are used in high-risk or known cardiac patients. Arterial pressure is monitored, and arterial blood studies are done frequently. After a general endotracheal anesthetic is administered, exposure is obtained through a xiphoid-to-pubis midline incision. The abdomen is routinely explored. The transverse colon and transverse mesocolon are retracted cephalad. The small intestines are brought out of the abdomen, retracted to the right, and covered with moist towels. Incision is made into the posterior peritoneum to the left of the duodenum. The aneurysm is easily identified. With minimal dissection, the uninvolved aorta above and arterial segments below the aneurysm are exposed. Three to five thousand units of heparin are injected into the lumen of the aneurysm as a proximal aortic clamp is applied above the aneurysm and below the renal arteries. After the distal clamps are applied, the aneurysm is incised longitudinally. The intraluminal clot and intima are removed. Bleeding from the lumbar vessels is controlled with sutures. An appropriate-sized woven Dacron graft is selected. Anastomosis is accomplished end to end into the proximal aorta, according to the graft-inclusion technique. If the aneurysm affects only the abdominal aorta, a tube graft is used, and the distal anastomosis is performed in similar fashion. Before the distal anastomosis is completed, the aortic clamp is temporarily released to flush debris from the proximal aorta and to evacuate the air. Because the interstices of the graft are filled with blood and fibrin, leakage through the graft is avoided. As the clamps are released and blood flow is reestablished, careful monitoring of the blood pressure will prevent the "declamping" shock syndrome. This complication is rare if the aortic clamp is opened slowly and intravenous administration of fluids is accomplished rapidly. The cautious and temporary use of vasopressor agents may be necessary to control excessive hypotension. Intravenous

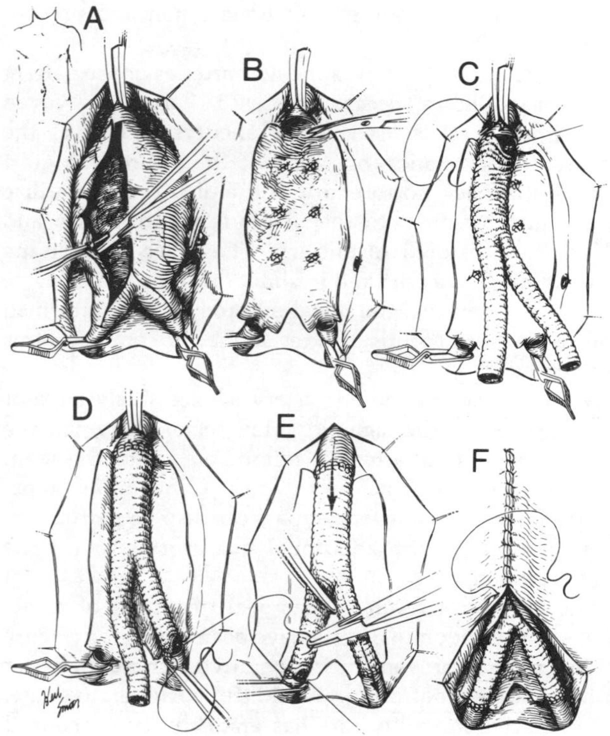

Figure 49.25. Technique of excision and graft replacement of abdominal aortic aneurysm of distal aorta and common iliac arteries. *A*, Midline abdominal incision. Aneurysm opened and thrombus and intima removed. *B*, Lumbar arteries ligated, and proximal aorta trimmed. *C*, Proximal anastomosis performed using Dacron graft. *D*, Left limb of graft anastomosed to left common iliac artery. *E*, Right limb of graft anastomosed to right common iliac artery. *F*, Remaining aneurysmal wall closed over graft and posterior peritoneum closed. (From Garrett et al,[37] with permission.)

administration of sodium bicarbonate helps to prevent acidosis.

If the aneurysm involves the iliac arteries or the patient also has occlusive disease of the iliac artery, a woven bifurcation graft is used. If the aneurysm involves the common iliac arteries, one limb of the bifurcation graft can be attached end to end into the distal common iliac artery just proximal to the iliac artery bifurcation and blood flow restored to one leg. The other limb of the bifurcation graft is sutured in similar fashion. If occlusive disease is extensive, the distal anastomosis is performed end to side into the distal external iliac or common femoral artery.

If the inferior mesenteric artery is excessively large or if circulation to the sigmoid colon seems marginal, the inferior mesenteric artery is reimplanted into the main trunk of the abdominal aortic graft. Concomitant renal artery or mesenteric artery bypass can also be performed, when indicated, with additional side-arm grafts off the main aortic graft.

The long-term results of surgical treatment of aneurysms of the abdominal aorta have been gratifying (Figure 49.26); with improvement in operative technique, better intraoperative monitoring, and skillful postoperative care, the operative mortality rate has gradually been reduced to about 4% or 5% despite an increasing number of older patients and those with significant risk factors. The surgical risk, however, in patients requiring emergency operation for ruptured aneurysm remains high, about 35% in our experience.

A brief comment should be made regarding "inflammatory" aneurysmal disease. Walker et al[46] first described this condition in 1972. Most previous reports had dealt with ureteral obstruction associated with retroperitoneal fibrosis. The reported incidence of this disease has ranged from 5% to 10%.[46,47] Crawford and Crawford[20(p262)] recently called attention to the rarity of this condition with an incidence of only 1.1%. The condition almost always occurs in atherosclerotic infrarenal abdominal aortic aneurysms. Most patients were men with a history of excessive use of tobacco.

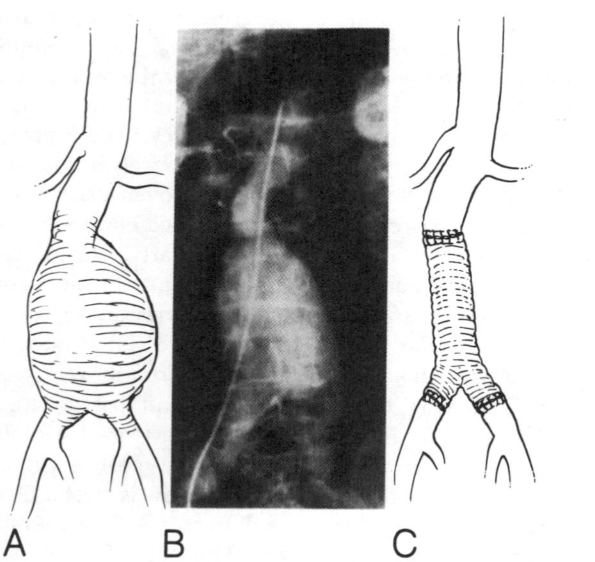

Figure 49.26. *A*, *B*, Preoperative drawing and aortogram showing large fusiform aneurysm of infrarenal aorta. *C*, Postoperative drawing showing resection of aneurysm and Dacron bifurcation graft replacement.

"Inflammatory" aneurysmal disease is characterized by a pulsatile midline inflammatory mass. The overlying adjacent peritoneal surface is inflamed. The inflammatory changes extend laterally, and in most cases the ureter is affected. The aneurysmal wall is greatly thickened from extensive fibrosis and dense inflammatory infiltrate. Most patients, when first seen, have a history of increased pain suggestive of aortic rupture. The computerized axial tomography shows an aneurysm with an excessively thick wall outside the ring of calcification which is usually seen in the outer edge of the aneurysmal wall. Aortography is helpful in the diagnosis, and the excretory urogram may show ureteral involvement with or without hydronephrosis. The sedimentation rate is usually elevated.

Treatment consists in standard excision and graft replacement. Special consideration must be given to proximal control above the level of inflammation and careful avoidance of excessive dissection, which might injure associated structures.

OCCLUSIVE DISEASE OF THE AORTA

Occlusive disease of the aorta may be congenital or acquired. The congenital form consists primarily in coarctation of the aorta and has been discussed in the section on congenital disorders. The acquired form may be caused by a number of pathologic conditions. Thromboobliterative disease, from atherosclerosis, is the most common single significant cause of occlusive disease of the aorta and its branches. Other causes include syphilis, tuberculosis, collagen vascular disease, aortic dissection, and trauma. An important pathologic feature of most occlusive aortic disease is localized and segmental distribution with relatively normal vessels proximal and distal to the occlusive process. This characteristic permits surgical correction of the arterial occlusion.

Acquired arterial occlusive disease is far more important than the congenital form. Characteristic patterns of disease and manifestations of arterial insufficiency can be classified into three subgroups of occlusion: (1) the major branches of the aortic arch, (2) the visceral and renal branches of the abdominal aorta, and (3) the terminal abdominal aorta and iliac arteries.

AORTIC ARCH

Thromboobliterative disease of the major arteries arising from the aortic arch encompasses several clinical entities with various synonyms. These include the aortic arch syndrome, pulseless disease, Takayasu's disease, and Martorell's syndrome. The condition is characterized by partial or complete occlusion in one, two, or three branches of the aortic arch. The disease is segmental and produces manifestations of arterial insufficiency in the arms, face, and cerebrum. It was first described by Broadbent[48] in 1875, and subsequently further described by Takayasu[49] in 1908. It was not until 1951, when Shimizu and Sano[50] described "pulseless disease," however, that attention was focused on the condition. The disease was originally thought to be restricted primarily to oriental countries, but recent reports indicate a more widespread geographic distribution. About 85% of patients with Takayasu's syndrome are female, with onset of the disease between ages 3 and 35 years.[51] The early symptoms in about two thirds of the patients are nonspecific, consisting of fever, myalgia, and anorexia. Clinical manifestations in the chronic phase depend on the extent and location of the disease.

Several types of Takayasu's arteritis are recognized. In one study,[52] type I occurred in about 8% of patients and was limited to the aortic arch and its branches. Type II, which represented 11% of the series, affected the descending thoracic and abdominal aorta. Type III, accounting for about 65% of patients, involved the aortic arch vessels and the abdominal aorta and its branches. Hypertension is common and may be related to aortic coarctation or renal artery stenosis. The neurologic symptoms are most likely associated with hypertension or cerebral ischemia from extracranial occlusive disease.

Our experience suggests that atherosclerosis is the most frequent cause of this condition.[53] The occlusive process develops in the innominate, left carotid, or left subclavian artery and may include all branches or may be limited to only one or two of the branches. The disease is localized and rarely extends beyond the origin of these vessels at the aortic arch. Thus, the distal vessels in the neck are relatively free of disease. The obstruction may be complete or incomplete. Incomplete occlusion is usually segmental and therefore amenable to surgical treatment. The clinical manifestations vary considerably depending on the location and extent of the disease and the development of collateral circulation. Symptoms may be related to ischemia of the brain or arms. Cerebral symptoms may vary from mild headache, vertigo, and syncope to complete paralysis. Ocular symptoms consist in visual disturbances, as diplopia, or amaurosis fugax. In the arm, symptoms are usually mild and consist in weakness, claudication, and easy fatigability.

Analysis of our experience suggests that the disease affects men more often than women and occurs most often in the fourth to seventh decades of life.[54] This age distribution reflects the high incidence of atherosclerosis in our patient population, as opposed to that of others who report a higher incidence of aortitis.

The result of physical examination is striking; the primary finding is absence of peripheral pulses beyond the point of stenosis. Thus, occlusion of the innominate artery is associated with decreased or absent pulses in the right carotid artery and in the right arm, with diminution or absence of blood pressure in the right arm. Occlusion of the left subclavian artery causes decreased or absent pulses in the left arm, with diminution of the blood pressure in this limb. Stenosis of the left common carotid artery reduces left carotid pulse in the neck. Bruits are often heard at the base of the neck and in the supraclavicular region in patients with stenotic disease. Most patients with chronic disease will have a well-developed collateral circulation, so that the distal digits are not impaired. Ischemia, however, including ulceration and gangrene, may develop, particularly in the presence of secondary distal occlusion of the axillary, brachial, radial, or ulnar arteries. Neurologic signs may be present if the patient has actually had a cerebral infarction, secondary to occlusion of the innominate or carotid arteries, from ischemia or thromboembolic disease.

When the diagnosis is suspected, arch aortography provides confirmation and precise information that is essential to proper treatment. This information includes the location of the occlusive disease and its extent, both proximally and distally. The most satisfactory technique is retrograde femoral arch aortography.

The localized or segmental nature of occlusive disease of the origin of the branches of the aortic arch permits application of direct operative techniques designed to restore normal pulsatile flow distal to the occlusion. This results in relief of symptoms and prevents progression of the manifestations of arterial insufficiency in the brain and arm. In general, two surgical techniques are used: endarterectomy and bypass. Endarterectomy has limited application, being used only for disease that is extremely discrete and well-localized to relatively short segments of the artery. In patients with occlusive disease secondary to the acute phase of aortitis, endarterectomy is not indicated because of the high percentage of early failures due to the inflammatory process. In general, conservative measures are in order initially, followed in the chronic phase by an appropriate bypass operation. Localized endarterectomy may be applicable if the patient has only one diseased atherosclerotic vessel.

The bypass technique may be used for patients with more extensive disease and those with multiple arterial occlusive processes (Figure 49.27). Depending on the nature and extent of the occlusion, exposure may be obtained through a limited second intercostal right anterior thoracic incision or a midline sternal splitting incision. Sternotomy is preferable if localized endarterectomy is to be performed, because it provides better distal control of the branches of the aortic arch.

Short, localized occlusive disease of the innominate artery should be approached through a median sternotomy. After vascular clamps are applied, the longitudinal arteriotomy is made, and local endarterectomy is performed. Repair is accomplished by primary arteriorrhaphy or patch-graft angioplasty, and the occlusive clamps are released to restore circulation. An alternative method is segmental resection of the innominate artery and Dacron graft replacement. Right anterior thoracotomy is most applicable in patients in whom bypass is to be used. Application of a specially designed curved lamp to the anterior lateral wall of the ascending aorta permits exclusion of a portion of the aortic wall without interference with aortic circulation. A longitudinal incision is made in the excluded segment of the ascending aorta, and an appropriate-sized knitted Dacron tube graft is anastomosed end to side with a simple, continuous, through-and-through suture. In patients with occlusion of more than one of the major branches of the aortic arch, it is still preferable to use a single tube attached to the ascending aorta in order to avoid several grafts in the thoracic inlet and thus prevent compression or obstruction of the airway

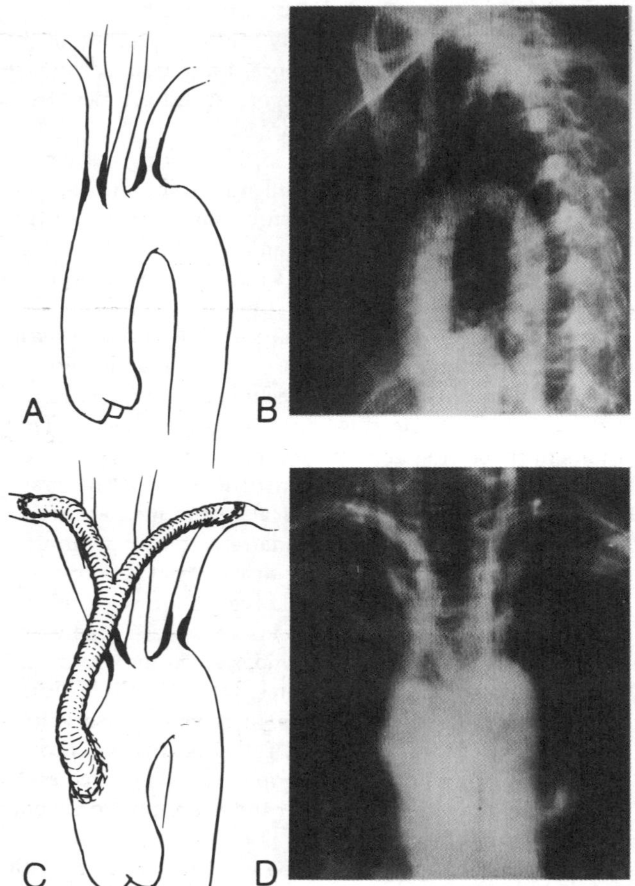

Figure 49.27. *A*, *B*, Drawing and aortogram made before operation showing occlusive disease of innominate and left subclavian arteries manifested by intermittent claudication of both arms and persistent paresis of left arm. *C*, Drawing showing functioning graft. Patient has remained asymptomatic for 15 years after operation. *D*, Aortogram three years after operation illustrating functioning bypass graft.

or venous return. The appropriate distal vessel is exposed through a separate cervical incision. The actual location of the distal anastomosis depends on the extent, location, and number of occluded vessels. Multiple occluded arteries arising from the aortic arch are common, and several bypasses may be required to correct all the obstructions. In such patients, the proximal end of the graft is sutured to the side of the ascending aorta and distally to one of the distal branches. Side limbs are brought off the main graft and sutured to the other appropriate vessels in the neck. The graft passes from the mediastinum through a tunnel made by blunt dissection retrosternally through the thoracic inlet and connecting with the cervical incision.

If the occlusion is limited to the innominate artery and its bifurcation is normal, circulation can be reestablished to both by insertion of a bypass from the ascending aorta to the common carotid or subclavian artery. If the bifurcation of the innominate artery is diseased, distal anastomosis from the ascending aorta to both right common and right subclavian arteries with use of two limbs is necessary. Circulation can be restored to the right common carotid and right subclavian arteries in patients with isolated, single-vessel disease by carotid-subclavian or subclavian-carotid bypass through an extrathoracic approach. The extrathoracic procedure eliminates the risk of thoracotomy, minimizes the operative procedure, and reduces the morbidity and mortality rates.

If the patient has associated disease of the carotid bifurcation, carotid endarterectomy can be performed, and the distal anastomosis from the previously inserted ascending aortic graft can be sutured to the endarterectomized segment at the carotid bifurcation.

A brief comment should be made about the subclavian steal syndrome[55] (Figure 49.28). Patients with segmental occlusion of the proximal left subclavian artery may have claudication of the left arm, or more often, symptoms of vertebrobasilar insufficiency when first seen. They often have reversal of flow in the left vertebral artery. Relief can be obtained by an extrathoracic carotid subclavian bypass graft.

Results of surgical treatment for occlusive disease of branches of the aortic arch have been highly gratifying with restoration of normal pulsatile circulation in the arteries beyond the obstruction, relief of symptoms, and resumption of normal activity.

RENAL ARTERY

Renovascular hypertension from narrowing of the renal arteries, a surgically correctable form of hypertension, is generally thought to represent between 5% and 10% of the hypertensive population. Renovascular hypertension should be considered in all hypertensive patients. Persons particularly prone to this form of hypertension are young people with high blood pressure of recent onset, no family history of high blood pressure, and an abdominal bruit. In our patients, atherosclerosis was the cause of renal artery stenosis in 83%, fibromuscular hyperplasia in 13%, renal aneurysm in 3%, and abdominal coarctation in 1%.[56] Most patients were in the fifth to seventh decades of life, but 23% of our patients were under 40 years of age.[57] Nearly all our patients with fibromuscular hyperplasia were female. In the atherosclerotic group, nearly two thirds were male patients. In a review of a large number of patients with aneurysms, occlusive disease of the distal aorta, iliac and femoral arteries, or both, 44% of the hypertensive patients had occlusive disease of the renal arteries.[57]

Both renal arteries were diseased in 30% of our patients.[56] Atherosclerotic occlusion is usually incomplete and localized to a short segment of the artery at or near the origin of the aorta. In a small number of patients, the occlusive process may be incomplete and involve the major part of the artery up to the primary branches. The atheroma is usually on the left.[58(p434)] In fibromuscular hyperplasia, the middle and distal portions of the artery are usually affected. Localized disease of the renal artery was found in 47% of our patients, and in 53% of the patients, the renal artery lesion was clearly associated with a generalized atherosclerotic process.[59]

In either type, the vessel distal to the occlusive process remained essentially normal and was of sufficient size to

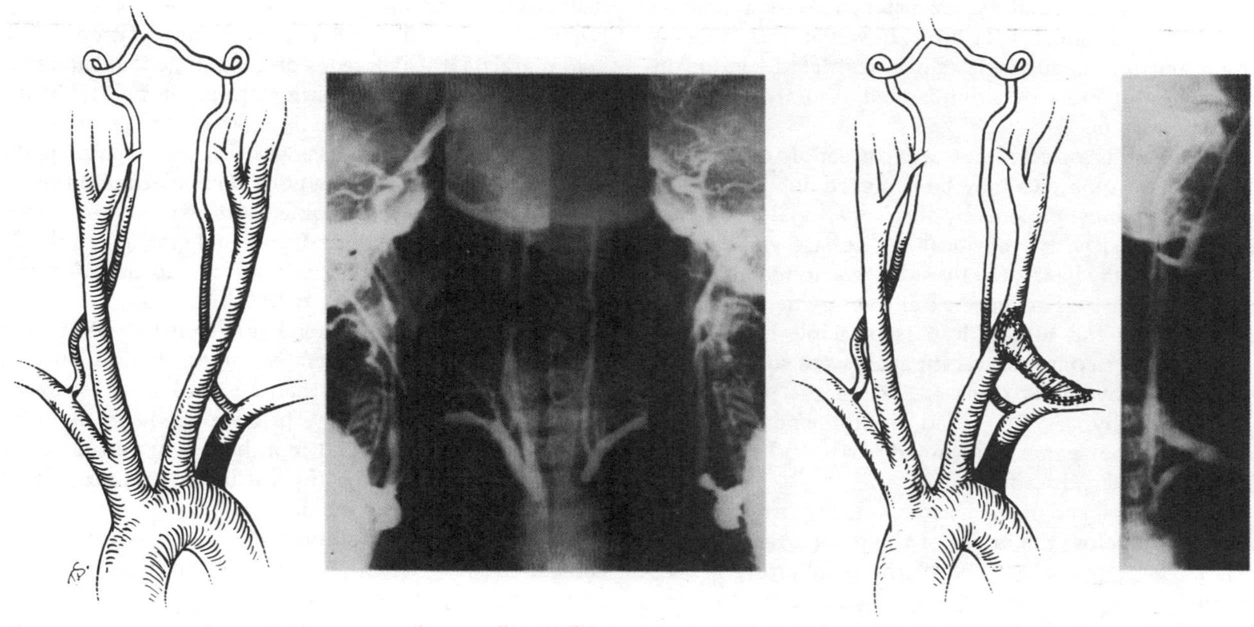

a. b. c. d.

Figure 49.28. *a*, Preoperative drawing in patient with vertebrobasilar insufficiency and left arm claudication. *b*, Arteriogram showing site of occlusion in proximal left subclavian artery (subclavian steal syndrome). *c*, Drawing showing patent, functioning graft. *d*, Arteriogram nine years after operation showing carotid-subclavian artery bypass graft. (From DeBakey and Noon,[57] with permission.)

permit surgical reconstruction. Some patients may have complete obstruction; in most instances, because of the extent of the occlusive process and the atrophied kidney, nephrectomy is required to remove even small remnants of renal tissue that may be responsible for hypertension. If collateral circulation is adequate to maintain patency of the distal arterial segments, the kidney can be saved in some patients.[60] In a few, the occlusive process may involve the branches of the renal artery and may require segmental nephrectomy or the new techniques of ex vivo "bench surgery."

Since about 10% of patients have multiple accessory renal arteries, these accessory vessels become an important consideration. They are small and originate more anteriorly on the aortic circumference. Because of their small size and the extent of the occlusion, surgical reconstruction is often difficult or impossible. Segmental or total nephrectomy is required in these patients.

Hypertension may be identified in patients with a blood pressure of 140 mm Hg systolic and 90 mm Hg diastolic. Renovascular hypertension tends to be a relatively more severe type of high blood pressure. The more severe the hypertension, the higher the probability that it results from a correctable cause, such as renovascular hypertension. Thus, all patients with a diastolic blood pressure higher than 100 mg Hg should be evaluated for renovascular hypertension.

Many patients have no physical signs indicating renal artery stenosis except hypertension. Yet, systolic murmurs can often be heard in the upper part of the abdomen or in the flanks. Many of these patients have evidence of atherosclerosis in other parts of the arterial system. Results of urinalysis are usually normal. Blood urea nitrogen and creatinine levels are normal unless the patient has chronic occlusive renal disease or significant impairment of excretion. The excretory pyelogram may show delay in excretion of contrast material or one smaller kidney, observations suggestive of renal disease. The value of excretory pyelography is somewhat limited as a screening procedure, however, since in about 30% of patients with renal artery stenosis excretory function is normal on pyelography. Rapid sequence excretory pyelography has been suggested to aid in the diagnosis of significant renal artery disease. Difference in renal length of 1.5 cm or more as compared with the contralateral kidney, hyperconcentration of contrast material on late films, and unilateral delay in caliceal appearance time have been considered positive criteria.[58(p440)] Many authors have, however, reported significant false-negative results. Isotope renography has not proved to be a valuable screening tool for identification of renovascular hypertension.

Renal aortography with selective renal arteriography is the best way to identify anatomically significant occlusive disease of the renal artery. The coexistence of renal artery stenosis and hypertension does not, however, establish a causal relation. Functional studies are required to identify functional renal artery stenosis. Split renal function studies have been advocated. A positive result consists of a 40% reduction in urine volume, a 50% increase in creatinine clearance, and a 100% increase in para-aminohippuric acid concentration on the diseased side. Because of technical difficulties, however, most centers have discontinued split renal function studies. Renal vein renin assays have become extremely valuable in identifying functional renovascular hypertension. This technique has many potential sources for error, however, including antihypertensive medications and unrestricted sodium intake. The test must be administered accurately to avoid spurious results.

Treatment is directed toward correction of renal ischemia. This objective may be achieved and renal tissue conserved in most patients by surgical arterial reconstruction.[56] Patients with well-localized disease who are relatively thin may be treated by endarterectomy and patch-graft angioplasty. For more extensive segmental disease, however, the end-to-side bypass principle is more frequently used. In our most recent analysis of surgical treatment for renovascular disease, 75% of the patients had renal artery bypass, 15% had thromboendarterectomy with or without patch-graft angioplasty, and 10% had a variety of other procedures.[59]

The proximal end of the Dacron velour graft is attached to the aorta below the origin of the renal arteries (Figure 49.29). The patent distal end of the renal artery is preferentially exposed by dissection outward from the aorta, although occasionally it may be necessary to reflect the colon medially. The graft is then inserted under direct vision or through a retroperitoneal tunnel made by blunt dissection, and the renal anastomosis is made end to side distal to the occlusive process. In most of our renal artery bypasses, we used the 6 mm or 8 mm knitted Dacron velour graft. Other surgeons prefer autogenous saphenous vein, autologous hypogastric artery, or polytetrafluorethylene grafts. Bifurcation or separate grafts may be used for bilateral disease. Bypass grafting has proved particularly effective in restoring normal circulation to the kidneys. In patients with combined aortoiliac and renal artery disease, the proximal end of the renal graft is attached to the side of the aortic segment of the aortic bifurcation graft.

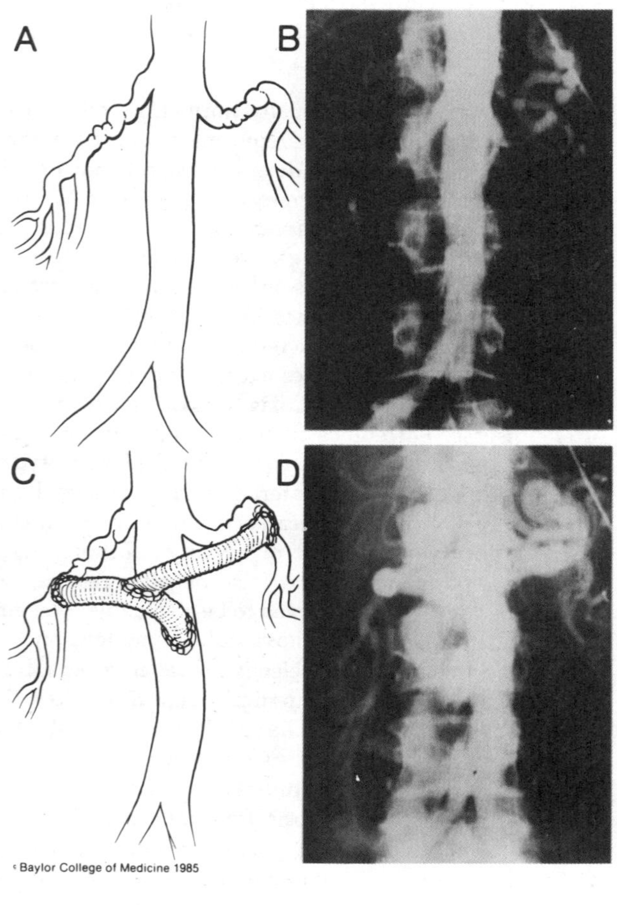

Figure 49.29. *A*, *B*, Preoperative drawing and renal aortogram in young, hypertensive woman showing fibromuscular hyperplasia of both renal arteries. *C*, *D*, Postoperative drawing and aortogram showing functioning bilateral renal artery bypass grafts.

Renal artery reconstruction has been performed in more than 500 patients. The operative mortality rate has gradually been reduced to less than 2%.[59] Blood pressure was normal or improved in 65% of our patients with a mean follow-up interval of 49.3 months. Forty percent of the late deaths were due to myocardial infarction, 19% to stroke, and 9% to carcinoma.

Like others, we have noted that renovascular surgery is most effective when performed in younger patients in whom prolonged, severe hypertension has not yet produced irreversible changes in the vascular bed.[61] An aggressive diagnostic and surgical approach in patients with renovascular hypertension is justified. The low operative mortality rate and the good blood pressure response to surgical treatment make it the procedure of choice in carefully selected patients.

CELIAC/SUPERIOR MESENTERIC ARTERY

Another clinical manifestation of peripheral vascular occlusive disease is mesenteric ischemic syndromes. Much has been done in recent years to delineate these syndromes and to identify the underlying pathophysiologic changes.[62] Unfortunately, the diagnosis of acute mesenteric ischemic syndrome is often delayed until after intestinal gangrene has developed, and the only alternative is resection of the infarcted intestine. Acute mesenteric insufficiency is associated with a high mortality rate. At least 50% of patients in whom acute arterial mesenteric insufficiency develops have preliminary symptoms, but the problem is one of early recognition and diagnosis.[62]

Mesenteric arterial ischemic disease can be classified into acute and chronic syndromes. The most common manifestations of mesenteric ischemia are acute ischemia of the superior mesenteric artery and ischemic disease of the colon. These occur with approximately equal frequency. Most cases of acute occlusion of the mesenteric artery are embolic. Acute mesenteric ischemia often results from low perfusion states such as are associated with myocardial infarction, heart failure, cardiac arrhythmias, or sepsis.

Ischemic disease of the colon represents a wide variety of disorders ranging from ischemia of only the mucosa to gangrene of the entire thickness of the colon. Acute ischemia of the colon may develop after ligation of the inferior mesenteric artery during operation on the abdominal aorta or during resection of the colon. Careful surgical technique to avoid injury to the blood supply of the colon or reanastomosis of the origin of the inferior mesenteric artery during abdominal aortic surgery can prevent this complication. Ischemia of the colon can also occur in low-flow states with similar antecedent conditions of hemodynamic instability as described in the discussion of acute ischemia of the superior mesenteric artery.

The principal problem for the vascular surgeon regarding mesenteric insufficiency is chronic ischemia. According to Goodman,[63] Baccelli first described the term "abdominal angina." In 1958, Shaw and Maynard[64] reported the first successful surgical treatment of chronic mesenteric ischemia. Many patients with acute mesenteric ischemia have had previous symptoms of chronic mesenteric ischemia.

Relatively severe arterial occlusion in several mesenteric arteries is necessary to reduce the blood flow in the gastrointestinal tract and produce symptoms. Sixty-one percent of our patients had occlusion or severe stenosis in at least two of the three arteries.[65] The most frequently occluded was the celiac artery, followed by the superior mesenteric artery. Occlusion may be complete or incomplete, but the disease is limited to the orifice of the occluded vessel or to the first 2 to 3 cm. As in other sites of occlusive arterial disease, the distal arterial segment remains essentially free of disease.

Extensive collateral circulation develops after stenosis or occlusion of the celiac and superior mesenteric arteries. Numerous anastomoses between the celiac and superior mesenteric arteries can develop as can collaterals between the superior mesenteric and the inferior mesenteric arteries. The marginal artery of Drummond is the functional artery in the colon that communicates with branches of the superior and inferior mesenteric artery. One particularly prominent collateral artery, which has been named the meandering artery of Riolan, courses into the root of the mesocolon between the origins of the superior mesenteric and inferior mesenteric arteries. Identification of this artery during aortography should raise the suspicion of possible mesenteric artery ischemia. Damage to the meandering artery of Riolan can produce serious ischemia of the small intestine or colon after aortic or colonic operations.

Atherosclerosis is the basic underlying disease in most patients with chronic mesenteric ischemia. Associated atherosclerotic disease is common. In fact, many of our patients have had associated abdominal aortic aneurysms or occlusive disease of the aortoiliac region or renal arteries.

The clinical manifestations of chronic abdominal angina are typical. Patients complain of crampy, abdominal pain usually immediately after eating. The pain may become so intense in the later stages that the patient severely limits the intake of food. The pain is usually in the epigastrium but may be diffuse or may extend into the back. Anorexia is common. Nearly all patients have moderate to severe loss of weight. Other symptoms include flatulence, bloating, diarrhea, and constipation.

Most of our patients were thin and asthenic, with evidence of loss of weight. A bruit is usually audible over the upper portion of the abdomen. Evidence of atherosclerosis in other areas is common. Steatorrhea may also be present.

The diagnosis initially may be one of exclusion. The major differential diagnosis at first is cancer of the gastrointestinal tract. Symptoms often mimic those of pancreatic cancer. These patients usually have contrast studies of the gastrointestinal tract and even endoscopy. Although results of these studies are usually normal, puddling of the barium may be identified in the intestine. Occult blood is sometimes found in the stool. Results of studies for malabsorption, such as increased fecal fat or decreased excretion D-xylose, are often not helpful.

The diagnosis may be firmly established by aortography. The aortogram must be made with the patient in the lateral position because of the origin of the celiac and superior mesenteric arteries on the anterior aspect of the aorta, which is visualized only in the lateral projection. Additionally, posteroanterior exposure of the aorta is required to identify associated aortoiliac and renal artery occlusive disease. The retrograde catheter technique with use of selective celiac and mesenteric arteries has proved to be extremely valuable in identifying the mesenteric occlusion.

The only effective treatment is an operation designed to restore normal circulation. No other treatment will relieve symptoms and prevent progression of the disease to mesenteric thrombosis and gastrointestinal infarction. Physicians should be alert to the symptoms if the diagnosis is to be made before acute mesenteric insufficiency develops and an elective operation can be performed. Endarterectomy, excision and graft replacement, and bypass graft procedures have all been used. Limitation of the obstruction of the celiac and superior mesenteric arteries usually to the first portion of these vessels makes endarterectomy attractive, but difficulty is encountered in exposure of the upper abdominal aorta which requires a thoracoabdominal incision.

The end-to-side bypass technique has been our preference for many years (Figure 49.30). The operation is performed through a long midline abdominal incision. The infrarenal abdominal aorta is exposed. The proximal end of the graft is attached to the side of the aorta. The graft is passed behind the transverse mesocolon and stomach and is sutured to the side of the enlarged splenic or hepatic artery with celiac artery disease, or directly to the superior mesenteric artery at the base of the mesentery of the small intestine. If two-vessel revascularization is necessary, one end of a second graft is sutured to the side of the initially inserted graft and attached to the second distal vessel. Our preference has been the Dacron velour knitted tube graft, 6 or 8 mm in diameter. Many of these patients will have had previous or concomitant abdominal aortic vascular procedures, and the proximal anastomosis may originate from an abdominal aortic graft.

The results of these procedures have been gratifying.[65] The hospital mortality rate is low (3%). Thirty of our 32 patients (94%) became completely asymptomatic after operation. Most regained their normal weight and had no further postprandial pain.

ABDOMINAL AORTA AND ILIAC ARTERIES

Occlusive disease of the terminal abdominal aorta and proximal common iliac arteries was first reported by Leriche[66] in 1923. Although he did not fully understand the nature of the thrombotic and occlusive process, he did observe that the obliterative disease was localized. He initially recommended lumbar sympathectomy as treat-

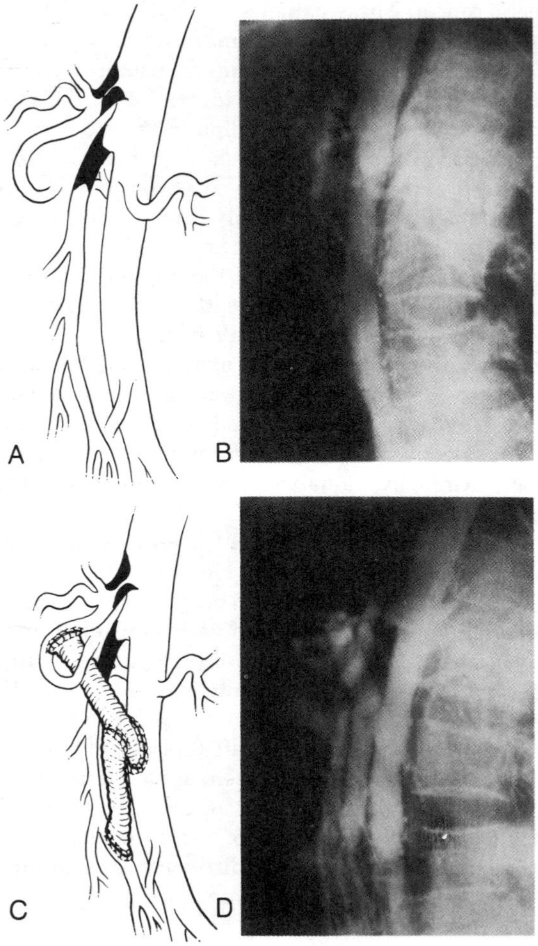

Figure 49.30. *A, B,* Preoperative drawing and lateral aortogram showing occlusive disease in celiac and superior mesenteric arteries in a patient with postprandial abdominal pain, weight loss, and anorexia. *C, D,* Postoperative drawing and aortogram showing splenic and superior mesenteric artery bypass grafts. After operation, the patient became asymptomatic and regained weight.

ment. In 1940[67] and again in 1948,[68] he updated his experience with the syndrome and defined it more precisely. He listed five specific manifestations in the early stages of the disease: (1) sexual impotence, (2) extreme fatigability of the legs on walking, (3) atrophy of the leg muscles, (4) absence of trophic disturbances, and (5) pallor of the legs. He described the absence of femoral and pedal pulses confirmed by oscillometry. In the later stages, cyanosis and ischemic changes of the toes developed.

In 1951, Oudot[69] successfully resected an occluded aortoiliac segment and replaced it with a homograft. Meanwhile, two significant technical developments had occurred in vascular surgery. Thromboendarterectomy was described by dos Santos[70] of Lisbon in 1947, and the bypass principle was developed by Kunlin[71] of France in 1951.

It has been well established pathologically that the occlusive process is caused by atheromatous changes that are usually confined initially to the intimal layer. These changes occur at the origin of the common iliac arteries from the aorta or at the iliac bifurcation. Continued enlargement of the atheromatous process causes increasing constriction of the lumen until the circulation is sufficiently retarded to cause thrombosis and complete obstruction. Depending on the rate and stage of development of these pathologic changes, obstruction of one or both iliac arteries may be incomplete, or occlusion of one may be complete with partial constriction of the other. When both common iliac arteries become completely obstructed, the superimposed thrombus propagates proximally toward the renal arteries and causes complete obstruction of the distal abdominal aorta. In most patients, the thromboobliterative process is well confined to the aortoiliac segment; yet, about 30% of patients have secondary segmental occlusion in the distal arterial tree, usually in the femoral and popliteal arteries. In general, we have observed that patients with distal occlusive disease in the femoropopliteal segment are nearly a decade older than those with aortoiliac occlusive disease. Recognizable patterns of disease occur, depending on the site and extent of the atheromatous occlusive process.

Aortoiliac occlusive disease occurs predominately in men; the ratio of men to women is 10:1.[57] About 90% of patients are in the fifth to seventh decades of life (range, between 23 and 90 years of age). In addition, about one third of the patients operated on for symptomatic aortoiliac occlusive disease have obstruction in the origin of the profunda femoris arteries in the groin. Clinical manifestations vary somewhat with the location, extent, and duration of the occlusive process. In the early stages, the patient may complain of fatigue in the thighs and buttocks. This may progress to intermittent claudication which may be in the lower legs, thighs, and buttocks or a combination of these. Another common complaint is sexual impotence. Isolated aortoiliac occlusive disease is rarely the cause of ischemia at rest or ischemic tissue loss, except by embolization. Yet, as the occlusive process worsens and is associated with more secondary distal occlusive disease, rest pain and trophic changes will eventually occur. Ultimately, these symptoms may be associated with atrophy of muscle and subcutaneous tissue, loss of hair, and hypertrophy of toenails. The most significant physical signs are a systolic bruit over the lower portion of the abdomen extending into the inguinal areas and absence or diminution of pulses in the femoral, popliteal, and pedal regions.

The diagnosis is usually identified on routine physical examination. Noninvasive testing in the vascular laboratory is now available to help confirm these clinical impressions. Ultimately, the diagnosis will need to be confirmed by aortography. With incomplete aortoiliac occlusive disease, retrograde femoral aortography can be performed. Bilateral percutaneous femoral arteriography produces good demonstration of the distal arterial bed and runoff. Translumbar aortography or retrograde transaxillary aortography can be performed in patients with complete aortoiliac occlusive disease. In addition to confirming the diagnosis, arteriography also provides precise information regarding the site and extent of the disease both proximally and distally. This is essential in planning the surgical procedure and in identifying associated occlusive disease and unsuspected aneurysmal disease. Occlusion of the renal or visceral artery may not be anticipated.

The patient's condition should be evaluated preoperatively, with studies for possible concomitant occlusive vascular disease in the extracranial carotid artery or coronary arteries. More than one third of our patients with aortoiliac occlusive disease had significant coronary artery disease. Almost one half had hypertension, and about one tenth had diabetes mellitus. The patient's pulmonary, hepatic, and renal function must also be determined before operation.

Several methods of surgical treatment are now available: bypass surgery, thromboendarterectomy, patch-graft angioplasty, and excision with graft replacement. Selection of the appropriate method or combination of methods depends on the extent and nature of the occlusive process and involvement of the aortic wall. In occasional patients, usually young women in whom the atheroma is extremely well localized to the abdominal aorta, thromboendarterectomy with patch-graft angioplasty may be performed.[72] In still other patients in whom the wall of the abdominal aorta is extensively diseased, as in association with intense inflammatory reaction, periaortic fibrosis, or aneurysmal formation, this segment may require resection. Then, end-to-end anastomosis of the proximal end of the aortic bifurcation graft is performed. The distal anastomosis is performed end to side to the external iliac or common femoral arteries.

Surgical treatment as evolved from our experience has now become reasonably standardized with some variations according to the extent and nature of the disease. The bypass technique, because of its simplicity, avoidance of injury to adjacent structures, and long-term good results, has become our procedure of choice (Figure 49.31). The peritoneal cavity is approached through a midline incision, and the small intestine is retracted to the right. The infrarenal abdominal aorta is exposed through an incision in the overlying peritoneum. If the occlusive process extends up to the renal arteries, these arteries should also be exposed. Heparin is injected into the aorta as a proximal occluding clamp is applied. A 4- to 5-cm vertical incision is made through the anterior aortic wall, several centimeters below the origin of the renal arteries. The thromboatherosclerotic process, which is fairly firm in most patients, is identified. If necessary, localized thromboendarterectomy is performed. If the disease extends proximally to involve the origin of the renal arteries, the abdominal aorta immediately above the level of the renal arteries is temporarily occluded manually after occlusion clamps have been placed on the renal arteries to prevent embolic debris to the renal artery. The thrombotic disease is dissected free. Intermittent release of the pressure on the aorta allows flushing of any retained debris; careful checking is important to be certain that no debris is left in the ostia of the renal arteries. Reapplying the aortic clamp below the renal artery and releasing the renal artery clamps restore renal artery perfusion. Palpation of good pulses in both renal arteries verifies their patency. The proximal end of the thrombotic process is inspected to be sure that there is no possibility of dissection. When satisfied that the occlusive process has been removed completely from the proximal infrarenal abdominal aorta, a suitable-sized DeBakey Dacron knitted bifurcation graft is selected. The aortic end of the graft is attached to the aorta as an end-to-side anastomosis with use of continuous vascular sutures. A clamp is placed across the aortic graft near the anastomosis while the proximal aortic clamp is cautiously released, restoring flow through the native vessel. The anastomosis is inspected for hemostasis.

The site for the distal anastomosis must then be determined. If the preoperative arteriogram and manual palpation suggest that the external iliac artery is suitable for a bypass graft, the anastomosis is done at this level within the abdominal cavity. If, however, significant occlusive disease exists in the external iliac artery, the distal anastomosis must be performed in the common femoral artery in the groin. The external iliac artery is exposed through an opening in the peritoneum overlying this artery in the pelvis. The appropriate limb of the previously inserted bifurcation graft is passed retroperitonealy to the area of the external iliac artery. Clamps are applied proximally and distally on the external iliac artery. A 2- to 3-cm vertical incision is made on the anterior wall of the external iliac artery. The limb of the bifurcation graft is fashioned, and end-to-side anastomosis is performed with the continuous Dacron suture. Before the anastomosis is completed, proximal and distal flushing is performed. The aortic graft is flushed through the nonattached graft. Removal of the clamps restores blood flow through the newly inserted limb of the bifurcation graft. Similar anastomosis is performed on the contralateral side.

If the graft must be attached to the common femoral artery, this artery is exposed through a vertical incision in the groin. The graft is then tunneled posterior to the inguinal ligament into the groin. Anastomosis is accomplished end to side in routine fashion.

Attention must be given to outflow from the common femoral artery. This is particularly true if the superficial femoral artery is occluded. An adequate runoff through the profunda femoris artery is particularly important and may require profundaplasty.[73]

Patients with significant extracranial occlusive disease or coronary artery disease may need carotid endarterectomy or coronary artery bypass grafting before elective aortoiliac reconstruction. Simultaneous procedures are being done with increasing frequency in properly selected patients.[65]

Contraindications to surgical treatment for the Leriche syndrome are related to certain severe or disabling cerebral, cardiac, renal, pulmonary, or malignant diseases that are not amenable to effective treatment and would greatly increase the risk of anesthetization and operation. In such circumstances, moreover, the Leriche syndrome is less important and less life-threatening to the patient, and its treatment is not likely to improve the patient's welfare. In selected patients, however, in whom loss of limb is threatened and associated cardiac or pulmonary disease increases the surgical risk, it may be possible to perform extraanatomic bypass with use of general anesthesia or axillofemoral bypass, or in patients with occlusion of a single iliac artery, femoro-

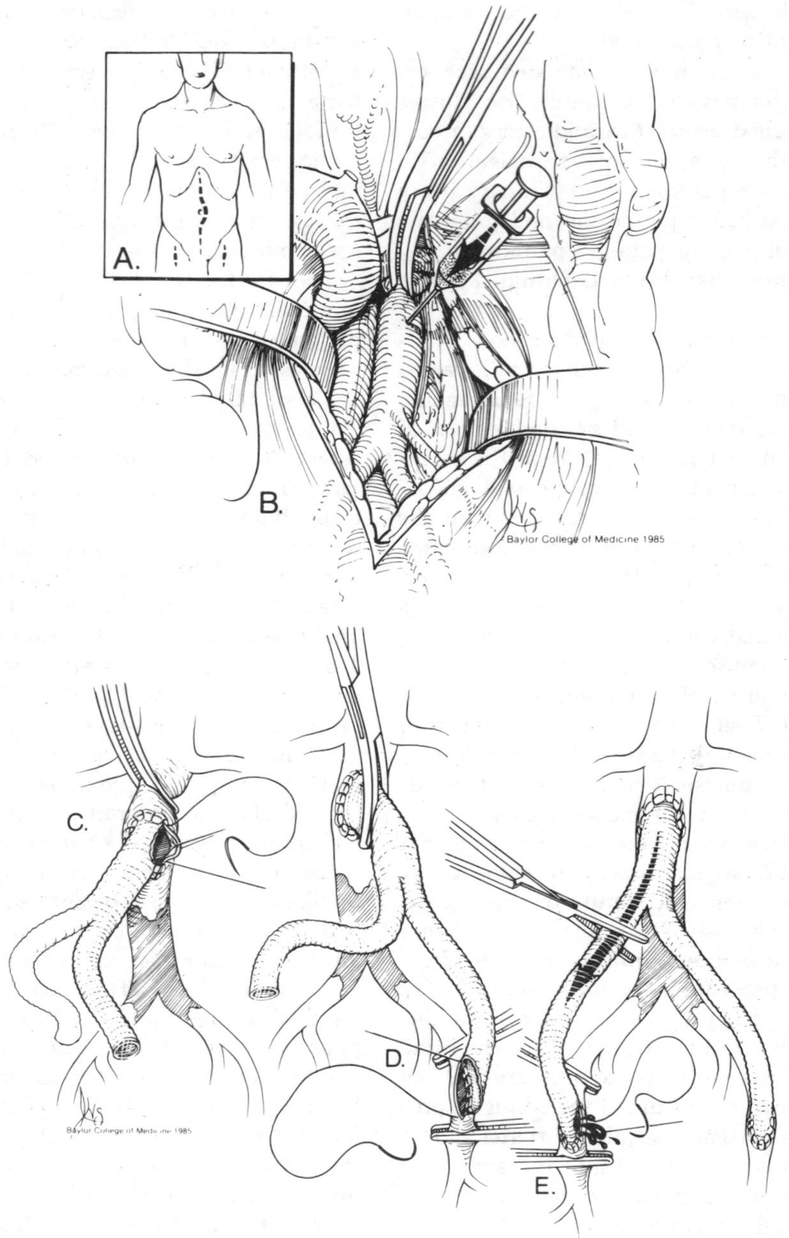

Figure 49.31. Technique for surgical correction of aortoiliac occlusive disease. *A*, Midline abdominal incision. *B*, Exposure of infrarenal abdominal aorta. Heparin injected into aorta as proximal vascular clamp applied. *C*, Proximal end-to-side aortic anastomosis. *D*, Completion of first distal anastomosis to left common femoral artery. *E*, Completion of last distal anastomosis.

femoral bypass. In our experience, under appropriate circumstances, these procedures have been useful for salvaging a limb and preventing amputation in the presence of threatening gangrene.

Our surgical results with these methods of treatment have been highly gratifying (Figure 49.32). The current operative mortality rate is 1% or less. Circulation may be restored and symptoms relieved in virtually all patients whose condition is surgically correctable. Long-term results are excellent, depending on the rate of progression of the disease. Patency rates exceeding 85% at five years should be expected. Our follow-up studies showed continued good function of the graft and circulation for as long as 20 years in some patients.

AORTITIS

A small group of systemic noninfected inflammatory diseases affect the aorta and its major branches. Their cause is not known, but they probably represent forms of autoimmune reactions. The condition is localized periaortitis, with inflammatory mononuclear infiltrates and giant cells, along with disruption and fragmentation of the elastic fibers of the arterial wall.[74] There are two major clinical patterns.

TAKAYASU'S ARTERITIS

This syndrome gets its name from M. Takayasu, a Japanese ophthalmologist, who in 1908 described a patient with changes in the retinal vessels, associated

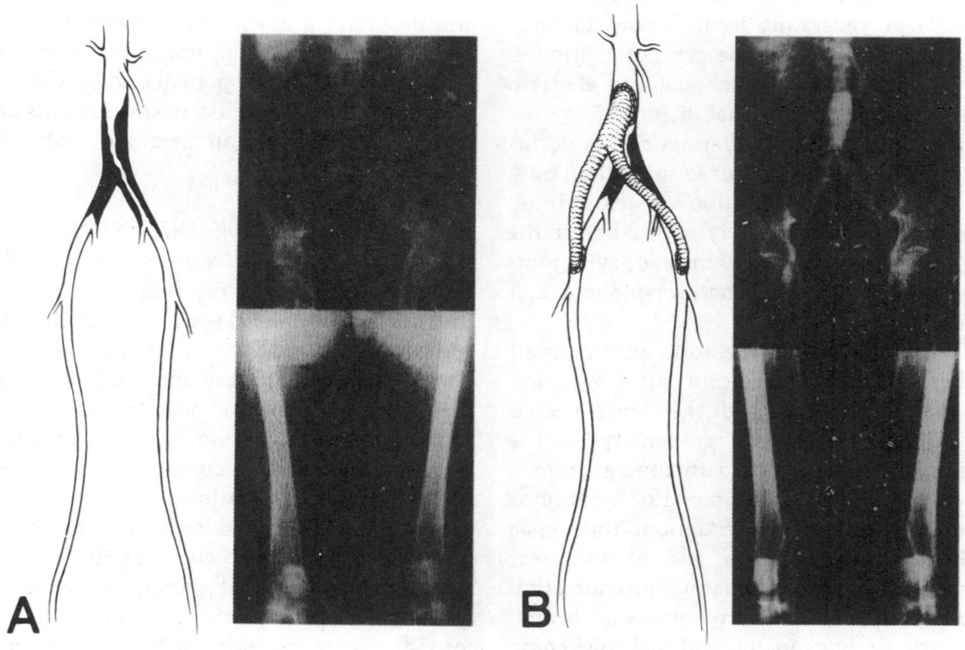

Figure 49.32. *A*, Drawing and aortogram in man with intermittent claudication of legs and impotence showing occlusion of distal abdominal aorta and patency of distal arteries below level of external iliac arteries. *B*, Drawing and aortogram illustrating surgical technique of inserting bypass graft from abdominal aorta to both external iliac arteries. Aortogram made 20 years later showing patent graft with restoration of circulation to legs. (From DeBakey ME: The current status of the Leriche syndrome. *Surgical Rounds* 1980; 3:20–30, with permission.)

with absence of pulses in the neck and arms.[49] It is also called pulseless disease, aortic arch syndrome, nonspecific aortoarteritis, giant-cell aortitis, and brachiocephalic arteritis. It was originally thought to be a disease of Orientals, but it is now known to affect all races throughout the world. It has a predilection for young females. It is a serious disease that can cause death from heart failure, myocardial infarction, stroke, hypertension, or rupture of the aneurysm.

The cause of this syndrome has not been elucidated. One observer noted a history of rheumatic fever in 9 of 28 of his patients.[75] Others noted a high incidence of tuberculosis and speculated that a hypersensitivity to tubercular infection occurs.[76] Most authors theorize that an autoimmune reaction is involved. Some have observed two phases of the disease, the "early systemic" or "prepulseless" phase and the "late occlusive" or "pulseless" phase. In the "early systemic phase," the patient has fever, articular pain, rash, splenomegaly, anemia, malaise, and elevation of the erythrocyte sedimentation rate. In the "pulseless" phase, the typical signs of end-stage occlusive vascular disease are noted.

The microscopic appearance is essentially that of panarteritis. The adventitia becomes thickened, secondary to fibrous tissue. If medial necrosis is a dominant feature, an aneurysm develops secondary to weakening of the wall. Indeed, Parulkar and Kelkar[77] reported aneurysms in 30% of their patients. The vasa vasorum shows a perivasal mononuclear infiltrate, but the intima is most severely affected. Intimal proliferation and fibrosis cause obstruction and thrombosis. Secondary atheromatous changes and calcification resemble those of atherosclerosis. The symptoms vary with the extent and site of the disease.

Certain patterns in the first group affect the aortic arch with the brachiocephalic vessels. This type produces symptoms resembling cerebrovascular insufficiency and ischemia of the arms. Surgical principles are similar to those described for correction of obstructive disease of the aortic arch vessels. Another type is limited to the descending thoracic, thoracoabdominal, or abdominal aorta. These patients resemble patients with abdominal coarctation. They often have renovascular hypertension or ischemia of the legs. Many will benefit from a bypass graft from the ascending aorta to the abdominal aorta if the descending thoracic or upper abdominal aorta is affected.[20(p270)] Still another group has mixed involvement or involvement primarily of the pulmonary artery. Patients with involvement of the pulmonary artery have elevated right ventricular pressure secondary to pulmonary artery stenosis. Unexplained pulmonary hypertension or heart failure may be the result of pulmonary artery involvement. Coronary artery lesions are rare but may produce aneurysms of the coronary arteries in young people. Surgical treatment includes the various techniques already described; the procedure selected will depend on the location of the occlusive or aneurysmal involvement.

GIANT-CELL ARTERITIS

Giant-cell arteritis, also known as temporal arteritis, cranial arteritis, and granulomatous arteritis, is a systemic vascular disease with chronic granulomatous inflammation of the medium-sized muscular and large elastic arteries including the aorta. It produces acute systemic manifestations of malaise, fever, headache, visual disturbances, myalgia, tenderness over the temporal arteries, claudication of the jaw, anorexia, anemia, and elevated erythrocyte sedimentation rate. Visual disturbances, secondary to ischemic optic or retrobulbar neuritis or occlusion of the central retinal artery, occur in more than 60% of the patients. Permanent loss of vision[78] develops in up to 42% of patients. The disease rarely occurs before the age of 50 years, and the average age of onset of symptoms in most patients is over 70 years. The preponderance of patients are white women.

Pathologic changes may affect the aorta and many of its major branches, including the carotid, subclavian, axillary, visceral, and femoral. Although the cranial vessels are not always affected, there is a propensity for the branches of the carotid artery. The pathologic picture is characterized by granulomatous inflammation with nonspecific inflammatory infiltrates throughout the vessel wall with both polymorphonuclear and mononuclear cells. In most patients, the granulomatous inflammation includes giant cells, but these cells are not always found. Additional histologic findings include intimal thickening and destruction of the media with infiltration of the inflammatory cells. These changes may produce arterial obstruction, which appears on arteriography as smooth, tapered narrowing of the medium-sized arteries. The medial destruction tends to be more diffuse in the aorta than in peripheral arteritis and may produce diffuse aneurysmal disease, aortic dissection, or obstruction.

The classic presentation is an elderly woman with headache, visual disturbances, and tenderness over the temporal artery. The diagnosis can be confirmed by biopsy of the temporal artery and an elevated erythrocyte sedimentation rate. The biopsy shows chronic inflammatory changes. Early diagnosis is important because prompt steroidal therapy will often reverse the inflammatory process with restoration of pulses and avoidance of blindness. Vascular reconstruction is contraindicated in the acute inflammatory stage. Arterial surgery should be delayed until a chronic, quiescent, or healed form of the inflammatory process is obtained with steroidal therapy. If the vascular complications of the arteritis are not resolved by steroidal therapy, vascular reconstruction should be performed.

INFECTIVE ANEURYSMS OF THE AORTA

SYPHILITIC ANEURYSMS

Syphilitic aneurysms are a complication of syphilitic aortitis, which is the tertiary form of syphilis. Syphilis used to be the most common cause of aneurysms of the thoracic aorta, but it is a rare occurrence in the United States today. The thoracic aorta, especially the ascending aorta and the aortic arch, is primarily infected with syphilis. Microscopically, chronic inflammatory changes develop in the adventitia and media. Focal destruction of the media causes loss of elastic and smooth-muscle fibers which are replaced by scar tissue. These irregularly shaped scars are characteristic of syphilitic aortitis. Medial destruction results in dilatation and aneurysmal formation.

Syphilitic aneurysms are usually sacciform but may be fusiform. Although these aneurysms usually develop in the proximal thoracic aorta, sacciform aneurysms have been observed on the posterior wall of the upper abdominal aorta.[20(p340)] Most patients with syphilitic aneurysms have a history of syphilis, positive results on the serologic test for syphilis, and an aneurysm in the typical site.

MYCOTIC ANEURYSMS/INFECTIONS OF THE AORTA

The term "mycotic" was originally used by Osler[79] to describe an aneurysm resulting from redundant bacterial invasion of the arterial wall. Because this term has caused confusion, newer classifications of arterial infections have been developed. Primary aortic infection may be due directly to bacteremia or indirectly to embolization of infected vegetation. Secondary aortic infection results from infection in adjacent contaminated tissues after aortic trauma or aortic operations.

Primary aortic infections are rare but do develop in the normal aorta, in atherosclerotic sites, in preexisting aneurysms, or in congenital anomalies. Patients usually have a history of primary infection in the urinary or gastrointestinal tract, lung, skin, or bone. A history of dental or genitourinary tract manipulation is common. The aortic wall becomes infected by pyrogenic organisms through the bloodstream, which produce abscess and destruction of the aortic wall. Because this aortic involvement leads to aneurysmal formation, the condition is called mycotic aneurysm. Many patients have a history of persistent fever, chills, and positive results of blood cultures. A pulsatile tender mass and pain may be present. Characteristically, these mycotic aneurysms are located on the lesser curvature of the aortic arch, in the region of the aortic isthmus, and on the posterior wall of the upper abdominal aorta.[20(p341)]

Primary treatment includes appropriate bacteriologic studies and administration of antibiotics. The infection can be completely eradicated by intensive antibiotic therapy and usually surgical excision of the infected aortic tissue; reestablishment of distal circulation is then necessary. Thus, surgical treatment includes wide local excision with proximal and distal occlusion, and extra-anatomic bypass in most patients. Rarely, local graft replacement is indicated.

Today, most aortic infections are secondary to infection in adjacent tissues or develop after vascular operations or other trauma. Although the reported incidence of infection after aortic surgery is low, this complication can be catastrophic. Infection of aortic grafts can occur in any artery, but the most common is the abdominal aorta affected by aortoiliac occlusive disease. The prosthetic graft may be directly contaminated at the original operation or bacteria may be hematogenously implanted on the graft surface. The more common and the most difficult to manage, however, is the infected abdominal aortic graft associated with an aortoenteric fistula. If the abdominal aortic graft comes in contact with the adjacent intestinal wall, usually duodenum or ileum, the intestinal wall erodes and permits bacteria from the intestines to contaminate the abdominal aortic graft. Eventually, the aortic anastomosis becomes infected, and anastomotic destruction leads to development of an infected false aneurysm.

When first seen, these patients may have a history of fever of unknown origin, septicemia, or a painful, pulsatile abdominal mass. More commonly, gastrointestinal hemorrhage may develop; initially, it may be occult. Leaking or rupture of the aneurysm into the gastrointestinal tract through the aortoenteric fistula can lead to sudden massive hemorrhage and death. The diagnosis should be suspected in a patient with a known aortic graft. If clinical manifestations of an infected aortic graft are present, bacteriologic studies, upper gastrointestinal endoscopy, upper gastrointestinal series, and computed tomographic scanning of the abdomen are all helpful in the diagnosis.

The best treatment is prevention. This complication can be avoided by interposition of adequate viable tissue between the aortic graft and the intestinal wall at the original operation. Once the complication occurs, debridement and removal of the graft become essential. The circulation to the limbs is restored with extraanatomic bypass procedures. Even after proper treatment of these problems, the infection may recur later, with or without aortic stump disruption, or an aneurysm may develop. Long-term suppressive antibiotic therapy is often indicated. Although these problems are difficult to treat and time-consuming, many satisfactory results have been achieved.

TRAUMA OF THE AORTA

Trauma of the aorta commonly results from battlefield injuries, but is not often seen in civilian practice. Because of the increasing incidence of violence and automobile accidents in our society, however, physicians must be aware of potential aortic injuries, their clinical manifestations, and their treatment.

Aortic injuries may be caused by penetrating or nonpenetrating objects. Gunshot and stab wounds account for most penetrating aortic injuries. When these patients are seen, they are in shock from loss of blood and require urgent surgical closure if they are to survive. Any part of the aorta may be involved.

The most common aortic injuries are nonpenetrating. Most of them are deceleration injuries, as in automobile or airplane accidents. As many as 16% of victims who die from automobile accidents have traumatic rupture of the thoracic aorta.[80] The severity of the aortic injury has been well documented. Among 275 patients with acute traumatic rupture of the aorta, only 14% were alive on arrival at the hospital.[81] Thus, most of these patients die immediately or soon after being injured. In almost two thirds of the patients in this same report, the site of aortic injury was the aortic isthmus or the descending thoracic aorta. All layers of the aorta were injured to a varying degree, but transverse tears were more common than longitudinal tears.

A high index of suspicion is mandatory, since delay in diagnosis is hazardous.[82] External evidence of trauma to the trunk is usually apparent. Many radiologic signs should alert the clinician to possible aortic injury, including a widened mediastinum, distortion of the aortic contour, obliteration of the medial aspect of the upper pulmonary field (apical capping), opacification of the space between the aorta and pulmonary artery, tracheal shift to the right, multiple rib fractures, depression of the main stem bronchus, or displacement of a nasogastric tube to the right. Aortography remains the most accurate diagnostic test and should be performed on any patient suspected of having an injury of the thoracic aorta[83] (Figure 49.33). Many of these patients have associated orthopedic and neurosurgical injuries.

In one reported series,[81] only two patients survived long enough after aortic injury for a chronic traumatic aneurysm to develop. Such an aneurysm is one that develops three or more months after a traumatic incident. In our report of 50 patients with traumatic thoracic aneurysms, the diagnosis was made three months to 32 years after the trauma occurred, the average interval being 11.9 years; these patients had successful surgical repair with a very low mortality rate.[84]

Once the diagnosis of acute trauma of the aorta is confirmed by aortography, prompt surgical intervention is mandatory. The approach to these injuries has previously been described. Injuries of the ascending and transverse arch are approached through a median sternotomy with use of cardiopulmonary bypass. Injuries of the descending thoracic aorta are generally approached through a left posterior lateral thoracotomy at the fourth intercostal space. Primary repair or resection with graft replacement is performed without adjuvant bypass or shunt techniques.

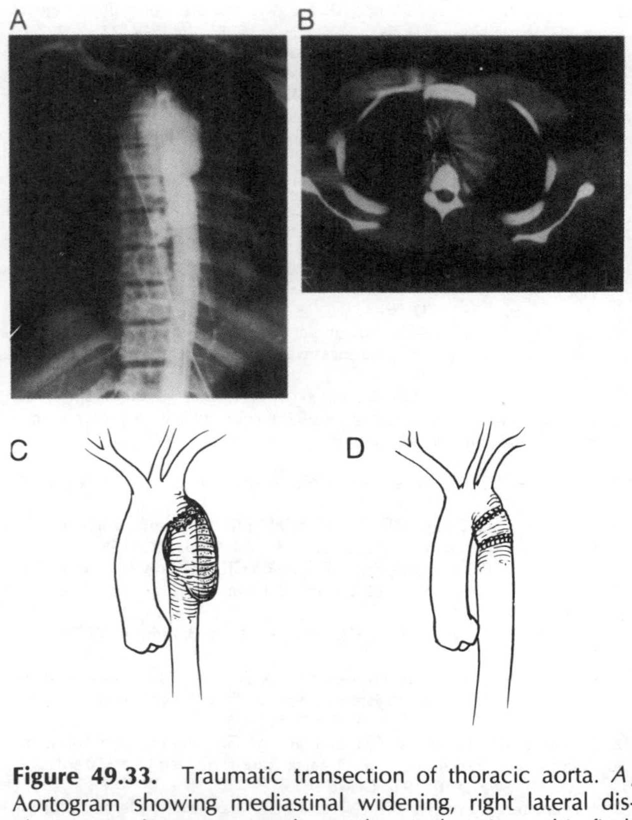

Figure 49.33. Traumatic transection of thoracic aorta. *A*, Aortogram showing mediastinal widening, right lateral displacement of nasogastric tube, and typical angiographic findings of aortic transection. *B*, Computed tomographic scan of chest showing nonhomogenous soft tissue density (hematoma) about thoracic aorta. *C*, Drawing showing transected aorta in proximal descending thoracic aorta with contained hematoma. *D*, Preoperative drawing showing resection of area of transected aorta with graft replacement. (Courtesy of Dr Rafael Espada.)

The incidence of spinal cord ischemia is higher in patients with acute aortic trauma than in those with chronic aneurysmal disease of the thoracic aorta. The acute trauma does not permit development of collateral circulation to the spinal cord. Whether distal perfusion provides any protection in acute trauma of the aorta is still controversial, but most agree that prolonged hypotension, with or without excessive cross-clamping, is a major factor in the development of posttraumatic ischemia of the spinal cord and paraplegia.

Traumatic aortic injuries are a serious problem. Only a few patients reach the hospital alive. Early index of suspicion and prompt aortography would yield an early diagnosis. Prompt surgical correction will help prevent subsequent rupture and death.

Acknowledgment: This work was supported in part by HEW Research Grant HL-17269, National Heart and Blood Vessel Research and Demonstration Center, Houston, Texas.

REFERENCES

1. Lindsay J Jr, DeBakey ME, Beall C Jr: Diseases of the aorta, in Hurst JW (ed): *The Heart: Arteries and Veins*, ed 6. New York, McGraw-Hill Book Co, 1986, pp 1321–1338.
2. Bahnson HT: Coarctation of the aorta and anomalies of the aortic arch. *Surg Clin North Am* 1952; 39:1313–1326.
3. Bayford D: An account of a singular case of obstructed deglutition. *Mem Med Soc London* 1794; 2:275–286.
4. Gross RE: Surgical relief for tracheal obstruction from a vascular ring. *N Engl J Med* 1945; 233:586–590.
5. DeBakey ME, Noon GP: Thoracic aorta and great vessels, in Effler DB (ed): *Blades' Surgical Diseases of the Chest*, ed 4. St Louis, The CV Mosby Co, 1978, pp 601–648.
6. Gross RE, Hubbard JP: Surgical ligation of a patent ductus arteriosus: report of first successful case. *JAMA* 1939; 112:729–731.
7. Lawrie GM, DeBakey ME, Morris GC Jr, Crawford ES, Wagner WF, Glaeser DH: Late repair of coarctation of the descending thoracic aorta in 190 patients: results up to 30 years after operation. *Arch Surg* 1981; 116:1557–1560.
8. Hope J: *A Treatise on the Diseases of the Heart and Great Vessels*, ed 3. London, John Churchill, 1839.
9. Lillehei CW, Stanley P, Varco RL: Surgical treatment of ruptured aneurysms of the sinus of Valsalva. *Ann Surg* 1957; 146:459–472.
10. DeBakey ME, Diethrich EB, Liddicoat JE, Kinard SA, Garrett HE: Abnormalities of the sinuses of Valsalva: experience with 35 patients. *J Thorac Cardiovasc Surg* 1967; 54:312–332.
11. Edwards JE, Burchell HB: The pathological anatomy of deficiencies between the aortic root and the heart, including aortic sinus aneurysms. *Thorax* 1957; 12:125–139.
12. Sakakibara S, Konno S: Congenital aneurysm of the sinus of Valsalva: anatomy and classification. *Am Heart J* 1962; 63:405–424.
13. Abbott ME: *Atlas of Congenital Cardiac Disease*. New York, American Heart Association, 1936, pp 18–21.
14. Sawyers JL, Adams JE, Scott HW Jr: Surgical treatment for aneurysms of the aortic sinuses with aorticoatrial fistula: experimental and clinical study. *Surgery* 1957; 41:26–42.
15. DeBakey ME, Lawrie GM: Aneurysm of sinus of Valsalva with coronary atherosclerosis: successful surgical correction. *Ann Surg* 1979; 189:303–305.
16. Dubost C, Allary M, Oeconomos N: Resection of an aneurysm of the abdominal aorta: reestablishment of the continuity by a preserved human arterial graft, with result after five months. *Arch Surg* 1952; 64:405–408.
17. DeBakey ME: The development of vascular surgery. *Am J Surg* 1979; 137:697–738.
18. Cooley DA, DeBakey ME: Resection of entire ascending aorta in fusiform aneurysm using cardiac bypass. *JAMA* 1956; 162:1158–1159.
19. Liddicoat JE, Bekassy SM, Rubio PA, Noon GP, DeBakey ME: Ascending aortic aneurysms: review of 100 consecutive cases. *Circulation* 1975; 52 (Suppl I): I-202–I-209.
20. Crawford ES, Crawford JL: *Diseases of the Aorta.* Baltimore, Williams & Wilkins, 1984.
21. DeBakey ME, Crawford ES, Cooley DA, Morris GC Jr: Successful resection of fusiform aneurysm of aortic arch with replacement by homograft. *Surg Gynecol Obstet* 1957; 105:657–664.
22. DeBakey ME, McCollum CH, Graham JM: Surgical treatment of aneurysms of the descending thoracic aorta: long-term results in 500 patients. *J Cardiovas Surg* 1978; 19:571–576.
23. McNamara JJ, Pressler VM: Natural history of arteriosclerotic thoracic aortic aneurysms. *Ann Thorac Surg* 1978; 26:468–473.
24. DeBakey ME, Cooley DA: Successful resection of aneurysm of thoracic aorta and replacement by graft. *JAMA* 1953; 152:673–676.
25. Valiathan MS, Weldon CS, Bender HW Jr, Topaz SR, Gott VL: Resection of aneurysms of the descending thoracic aorta using a GBH-coated shunt bypass. *J Surg Res* 1968; 8:197–205.
26. Crawford ES, Rubio PA: Reappraisal of adjuncts to avoid ischemia in the treatment of aneurysms of descending thoracic aorta. *J Thorac Cardiovasc Surg* 1973; 66:693–704.
27. Shennan T: *Dissecting Aneurysms*, Medical Research Council Special Report Series No. 193. London, His Majesty's Stationery Office, 1934.
28. Anagnostopoulos CE, Prabhakar MJS, Kittle CF: Aortic dissections and dissecting aneurysms. *Am J Cardiol* 1972; 30:263–273.
29. DeBakey ME, Cooley DA, Creech O Jr: Surgical considerations of dissecting aneurysm of the aorta. *Ann Surg* 1955; 142:586–612.
30. DeBakey ME, McCollum CH, Crawford ES, Morris GC Jr, Howell J, Graham JM: Dissecting aneurysms of the aorta, in Bergan JJ, Yao JST (eds): *Aneurysms: Diagnosis and Treatment*. New York, Grune & Stratton, 1982, pp. 97–103.
31. DeBakey ME, Henley WS, Cooley DA, Morris GC Jr, Crawford ES, Beall AC Jr: Surgical management of dissecting aneurysms of the aorta. *J Thorac Cardiovasc Surg* 1965; 49:130–148.
32. DeBakey ME, McCollum CH, Crawford ES, Morris GC Jr, Howell J, Noon GP, Lawrie G: Dissection and dissecting aneurysms of the aorta: twenty-year follow-up of five hundred twenty-seven patients treated surgically. *Surgery* 1982; 92:1118–1134.
33. Roberts WC: Aortic dissection: anatomy, consequences, and causes. *Am Heart J* 1981; 101:195–214.
34. DeBakey ME, Lawrie GM, Crawford ES, Morris GC Jr, Howell JF, Noon GP, McCollum CH: Surgical treatment of dissecting aortic aneurysms: 28 years' experience with 527 cases. *Contemporary Surg* 1984; 25:13–23.
35. DeBakey ME, Creech O Jr, Morris GC Jr: Aneurysm of thoracoabdominal aorta involving the celiac, superior mesenteric, and renal arteries. Report of four cases treated by resection and homograft replacement. *Ann Surg* 1956; 144:549–573.
36. DeBakey ME, Crawford ES, Garrett HE, Beall AC Jr, Howell JF: Surgical considerations in the treatment of aneurysms of the thoraco-abdominal aorta. *Ann Surg* 1965; 162:650–662.
37. Garrett HE, Crawford ES, Beall AC Jr, Howell JF, DeBakey ME: Surgical treatment of aneurysm of the thoracoabdominal aorta. *Surg Clin North Am* 1966; 46:913–918.
38. Estes JE Jr: Abdominal aortic aneurysm: study of one hundred and two cases. *Circulation* 1950; 2:258–264.
39. DeBakey ME, Cooley DA: Surgical treatment of aneurysm of abdominal aorta by resection and restoration of continuity with homograft. *Surg Gynecol Obstet* 1953; 97:257–266.
40. Carlsson J, Sternby NH: Aortic aneurysms. *Acta Chir Scandinav* 1964; 127: 466–473.
41. Rutherford RB: Infrarenal aortic aneurysms. *Vascular Surgery*, ed 2. Philadelphia, WB Saunders, 1984, pp 755–771.
42. Darling RC: Ruptured arteroisclerotic abdominal aortic aneurysms: a pathologic and clinical study. *Am J Surg* 1970; 119:397–401.
43. Bernstein EF, Dilley RB, Goldberger LE, Gosink BB, Leopold GR: Growth rates of small abdominal aortic aneurysms. *Surgery* 1976; 80:765–773.
44. Crawford ES, DeBakey ME, Morris GC Jr, Garrett HE, Howell JF: Aneurysm of the abdominal aorta. *Surg Clin North Am* 1966; 46:963–978.
45. McCollum CH, Garcia-Rinaldi R, Graham JM, DeBakey ME: Myocardial revascularization prior to subsequent major surgery in patients with coronary artery disease. *Surgery* 1977; 81:302–304.
46. Walker DI, Bloor K, Williams G, Gillie I: Inflammatory aneurysms of the abdominal aorta. *Br J Surg* 1972; 59:609–614.
47. Goldstone J, Malone JM, Moore WS: Inflammatory aneurysms of the abdominal aorta. *Surgery* 1978; 83:425–430.
48. Broadbent WH: Absence of pulsation in both radial arteries, the vessels being full of blood. *Trans Clin Soc London* 1875; 8:165–168.
49. Takayasu M: Case of unusual changes in central blood vessels of retina. *Acta Soc Ophthalmol Japan* 1908; 12:554.
50. Shimizu K, Sano K: Pulseless disease. *J Neuropathol Clin Neurol* 1951; 1: 37–47.
51. Porter JM, Taylor LM Jr, Baur GM: Nonatherosclerotic vascular disease, in Moore WS (ed): *Vascular Surgery: A Comprehensive Review.* New York, Grune & Stratton, 1983, pp 55–97.
52. Lupi-Herrera E, Sanchez-Torres G, Marcushamer J, Mispireta J, Horwitz S, Vela JE: Takayasu's arteritis. Clinical study of 107 cases. *Am Heart J* 1977; 93:94–103.
53. Crawford ES, DeBakey ME, Morris GC Jr, Howell JF: Surgical treatment

of occlusion of the innominate, common carotid, and subclavian arteries: a 10 year experience. *Surgery* 1969; 65:17–31.

54. DeBakey ME, Crawford ES: Surgical treatment of innominate, common carotid, and subclavian artery occlusion, in Gillespie JA (ed): *Extracranial Cerebrovascular Disease and Its Management.* London, Butterworths, 1969, pp 170–193.
55. Diethrich EB, Garrett HE, Ameriso J, Crawford ES, El-Bayar M, DeBakey ME: Occlusive disease of the common carotid and subclavian arteries treated by carotid-subclavian bypass: analysis of 125 cases. *Am J Surg* 1967; 114:800–808.
56. DeBakey ME, Morris GC Jr, Morgen RO, Crawford ES, Cooley DA: Lesions of the renal artery: surgical technic and results. *Am J Surg* 1964; 107:84–96.
57. DeBakey ME, Noon GP: Surgical treatment of chronic occlusive disease of the aorta and major arteries, in *Practice of Surgery*. Hagerstown, Harper & Row, Publishers, Inc, 1975, pp 1–44.
58. Dean RH: Renovascular hypertension, in Moore WS (ed): *Vascular Surgery: A Comprehensive Review*, New York, Grune & Stratton, 1983, chap 16.
59. Lawrie GM, Morris GC Jr, Soussou ID, Starr DS, Silvers A, Glaeser DH, DeBakey ME: Late results of reconstructive surgery for renovascular disease. *Ann Surg* 1980; 191:528–533.
60. Lawrie GM, Morris GC Jr, DeBakey ME: Long-term results of treatment of the totally occluded renal artery in forty patients with renovascular hypertension. *Surgery* 1980; 88:753–759.
61. Stanley JC, Fry WJ: Surgical treatment of renovascular hypertension. *Arch Surg* 1977; 112:1291–1297.
62. Dunphy JE: Abdominal pain of vascular origin. *Am J Med Sci* 1936; 192: 109–113.
63. Goodman EH: Angina abdominis. *Am J Med Sci* 1918; 155:524–528.
64. Shaw RS, Maynard EP III: Acute and chronic thrombosis of the mesenteric arteries associated with malabsorption. *N Engl J Med* 1958; 258: 874–878.
65. McCollum CH, Graham JM, DeBakey ME: Chronic mesenteric arterial insufficiency: results of revascularization in 33 cases. *South Med J* 1976; 69: 1266–1268.
66. Leriche R: Des oblitérations artérielles hautes (oblitération de la terminaison de l'aorte) comme causes des insuffisances circulatoires des membres inférieurs. *Bull Mém Soc Chir* 1923; 49:1404–1406.
67. Leriche R: De la résection du carrefour aortico-iliaque avec double sympathectomie lombaire pour thrombose artéritique de l'aorte: le syndrome de l'oblitération termino-aortique par artérite. *Presse Med* 1940; 48:601–604.
68. Leriche R, Morel A: The syndrome of thrombotic obliteration of the aortic bifurcation. *Ann Surg* 1948; 127:193–206.
69. Oudot J: La greffe vasculaire dans les thromboses du carrefour aortique. *Presse Med* 1951; 59:234–236.
70. dos Santos JC: sur la Désobstruction des thromboses artérielles anciennes. *Mem Acad Chir* 1947; 73:409–411.
71. Kunlin J: Le traitement de l'ischémie artéritique par la greffe veineuse longue. *Rev Chir* 1951; 70:206–235.
72. DeBakey ME, Crawford ES, Morris GC, Cooley DA: Patch graft angioplasty in vascular surgery. *J Cardiovasc Surg* 1962; 3:106–141.
73. Morris GC Jr, Edwards W, Cooley DA, Crawford ES, DeBakey ME: Surgical importance of profunda femoris artery: analysis of 102 cases with combined aortoiliac and femoropopliteal occlusive disease treated by revascularization of deep femoral artery. *Arch Surg* 1961; 82:32–37.
74. Titus J, Han-Seob K, Weilbaecher DG: Pathology of aortic aneurysm, in Saleh-Shenaq S (ed): *Anesthesia for Aortic Aneurysm Surgery*. California, Appleton & Davis, 1985, in press.
75. Ask-Upmark E: On the "pulseless disease" outside of Japan. *Acta Med Scandinav* 1954; 149:161–178.
76. Sen PK: *Non-specific Aorto-arteritis: A Monograph Based on a Study of 101 Cases*, Bombay, Tata McGraw-Hill Publishing Co, Ltd, 1973, p 8.
77. Parulkar GB, Kelkar MD: Nonspecific aortoarteritis, in Rutherford RB, (ed): *Vascular Surgery*, ed 2. Philadelphia, WB Saunders Co, 1984, pp 731–744.
78. Hollenhurst RW, Brown JR, Wagener HP, Shick RM: Neurologic aspects of temporal arteritis. *Neurology* 1960; 10:490–498.
79. Osler W: The Gulstonian Lectures on malignant endocarditis. *Br Med J* 1885; 1:467–470.
80. Greendyke RM: Traumatic rupture of aorta: special reference to automobile accidents. *JAMA* 1966; 195:527–530.
81. Parmley LF, Mattingly TW, Manion WC, Jahnke EJ Jr: Nonpenetrating traumatic injury of the aorta. *Circulation* 1958; 17:1086–1101.
82. Mattox KL: Invited commentary. *World J Surg* 1980; 4:551–552.
83. Pickard LR, Mattox KL, Espada R, Beall AC Jr, DeBakey ME: Transection of the descending thoracic aorta secondary to blunt trauma. *J Trauma* 1977; 17:749–753.
84. McCollum CH, Graham JM, Noon GP, DeBakey ME: Chronic traumatic aneurysms of the thoracic aorta: an analysis of 50 patients. *J Trauma* 1979; 19:248–252.

50 Nutritional Heart Disease

Suphachai Chaithiraphan, MD, Vichai Tanphaichitr, MD, PhD, and Tsung O. Cheng, MD, MS (Med)

Heart disease may result from undernutrition, malnutrition, or overnutrition. Among the entities to be discussed in this chapter are beriberi heart disease and the cardiovascular consequences of protein energy malnutrition, obesity, alcohol, dieting, anorexia nervosa, and bulimia.

BERIBERI

Beriberi is caused by a thiamin deficiency and can be classified into infantile and adult (childhood and adolescent are included) beriberi.[1,2] Two major systems, the cardiovascular and nervous systems, are involved.

INFANTILE BERIBERI

Infants may present with cardiac, aphonic, or pseudomeningitic forms or a combination of these.[1-3] Infants with cardiac beriberi usually have acute onset of symptoms including a loud piercing cry, cyanosis, dyspnea, vomiting, and tachycardia. Death may occur within a few hours after onset unless thiamin is administered.

ADOLESCENT OR ADULT BERIBERI

Patients may present with dry (paralytic or nervous), wet, cerebral, or subclinical forms.[1,2] The predominant features in dry beriberi are peripheral neuropathy of insidious onset and chronic course, tenderness of calf muscles, and difficulty in rising from a squatting position.[1,2,4,5]

In addition to peripheral neuropathy, common signs of beriberi include edema, tachycardia, wide pulse pressure, cardiomegaly, and congestive heart failure.[1,2,4,5] Some patients have abnormal electrocardiograms consisting of low or relatively low QRS complex voltages and nonspecific ST-T-wave abnormalities; these findings are most likely due to pericardial effusion.[2,6] Typical hemodynamic findings in wet beriberi include high cardiac output and low peripheral and pulmonary vascular resistance[2,7]; however, low cardiac output does not exclude the diagnosis of wet beriberi.

In some cases there is sudden onset of a cardiac manifestation known as acute fulminant or Shoshin beriberi (from the Japanese *sho* meaning acute damage and *shin* meaning heart).[7a] The predominant features are tachycardia, dyspnea, cyanosis, cardiac enlargement, and circulatory collapse.[2,7a]

CLINICAL DIAGNOSIS

Infants with beriberi are usually breast fed and have evidence of cardiac failure or aphonia, or both, whereas their nursing mothers often have a history of food restriction and numbness, of peripheral neuropathy, or both.[2,3]

Most cases of beriberi in occidental adults are confined to those with chronic alcoholism. Oriental patients usually have a history of excessive intake of carbohydrates derived mainly from milled rice and inadequate consumption of rich sources of thiamin, eg, pork, beef, and pulses. Some may consume foods containing antithiamin factors, eg, raw fermented fish. A sudden increase in thiamin requirements due to strenuous physical exertion or fever, or both, will precipitate the clinical manifestations of beriberi.[1,2,4,5]

In wet beriberi, improvement can be observed within 6 to 24 hours after thiamin administration[1-5] by less restlessness, the disappearance of cyanosis, a reduction in heart rate and respiratory rate, a decrease in pulse pressure, diuresis, a reduction in cardiac size, and clearing of pulmonary congestion. In dry beriberi, more time elapses before improvement is observed after thiamin administration. Other possible known causes of peripheral neuropathy must be carefully ruled out.

LABORATORY DIAGNOSIS

The biochemical diagnostic criteria for beriberi consist of low erythrocyte transketolase activity accompanied by a high thiamin pyrophosphate effect, which is usually greater than 15%.[1-5]

INCIDENCE

Although it was quoted in 1975 that beriberi had virtually disappeared from prosperous Asian countries,[8] there are still reports of beriberi in children, adolescents, and adults in Thailand[3-5,9] and Japan.[10,11]

TREATMENT

The current US recommended dietary allowance for thiamin is 0.5 mg/1,000 kcal.[12] However, patients with an acute condition usually receive a daily dosage of thiamin ranging from 50 to 100 mg intravenously or intramuscularly for 7 to 14 days, after which 10 mg/day are administered orally until the patient is fully recovered.[3-5] To prevent the recurrence of beriberi, patients should be advised to change their dietary habits.

PROTEIN-ENERGY MALNUTRITION

Although mass starvation in modern days has been greatly reduced, famine remains endemic and sometimes epidemic in developing nations.[13] In the Southeast Asian region, the major nutritional problem is protein-energy malnutrition (PEM). Bengoa[13] reported a median prevalence rate in Asia of 3.2% for severe PEM and 31.2% for moderate PEM. Although previously considered rare in the industrialized nations, PEM is now recognized and treated with increasing frequency.[14-16]

DEFINITION AND PATHOGENESIS

Severe PEM manifests in two forms: marasmus and kwashiorkor, which are often complicated by deficiency of other essential nutrients, including vitamins, minerals, and trace elements.[15,16] Marasmus is a consequence of inadequate intake of calories and protein due to inadequate breast-feeding complicated by frequent intercurrent infections. Kwashiorkor is primarily a protein deficiency accompanied by inadequate intake of calories, occurring in children who are weaned on starchy and sugary foods after prolonged breast-feeding. Adults with PEM usually have chronic debilitating diseases and often manifest with depletion of skeletal muscle and adipose tissue.

PATHOLOGY

The heart in PEM is usually small, flabby, and pale, epicardial fat is frequently absent, and pericardial effusion is often present in patients with generalized edema. The coronary arteries, valves, and endocardium are usually normal.[15-17] The microscopic features often include atrophy of myocardial fibers, which appear to be tightly packed and surrounded by an apparent increase in connective tissue. Other lesions include fragmentation of myofibrils, loss of striation, vacuolation, patchy necrosis of the fibers, and interstitial edema.

CARDIOVASCULAR ABNORMALITIES

In PEM, the loss of body weight is not accompanied by a proportional reduction in plasma volume. However, red cell volume declines at the same rate as lean body mass; thus, hematocrit decreases and anemia develops.[18] Cardiac chamber size and volume are usually normal or near normal per unit of body weight.[16] Hemodynamic studies reveal depression of stroke volume and cardiac output in starved subjects[16,19]; however, when cardiac output is adjusted for body weight, these parameters are not different from those of normal control subjects.[20] Gottdiener et al[21] reported normal systolic ventricular function in all emaciated men who were studied.

CLINICAL FEATURES

Undernourished subjects often experience fatigue, lethargy, and swelling of the extremities and abdomen; however, dyspnea, palpitations, and precordial pain are rarely noted.[15,16] Physical findings often reveal bradycardia, hypotension, cool extremities, and cyanotic nailbeds. Neck vein distension and gallop rhythm are rare unless cardiac failure is present. Heart sounds are muffled and the precordium is quiet. Systolic murmurs are mostly functional because most patients are anemic. Electrocardiographic abnormalities, which are common, include sinus tachycardia, right axis shift of QRS complex, diminished QRS amplitude, prolonged QT interval, and ST-segment depression with or without T-wave inversion.[22-24] Abnormal cardiac rhythms, which are occasionally present, include atrial fibrillation, junctional rhythm, premature ventricular beats, and exercise-induced ventricular tachycardia. Sudden death has been reported in advanced cases of PEM and was attributed to serious cardiac arrhythmias.

RECOVERY FROM PROTEIN-ENERGY MALNUTRITION

Although certain cardiac events such as heart failure or arrhythmia may emerge during recovery from PEM, changes in the cardiovascular state depend in part on the speed of recovery from PEM as well as the presence of underlying cardiac disease.[20] In cachectic men recovering gradually from prolonged starvation, cardiac abnormalities rarely develop. In most cases, abnormalities on the electrocardiograms resolved by the time body weight was restored. The reduced cardiac mass and the cardiac chamber size enlarge in proportion to the increase in body weight. Plasma volume remains unchanged, whereas red blood cell volume is restored at the same rate as lean body mass; therefore, the hematocrit level rises. A recent study using echocardiography revealed normal systolic left ventricular function in all patients recovering from anorexia nervosa.[21] In contrast, in undernourished subjects undergoing rapid recovery through enteral or parenteral hyperalimentation, cardiac failure may occur unpredictably under certain conditions, eg, a rapid rate of repletion, underlying heart disease, or excessive sodium in the diet. Rapid resolution usually followed diuretic therapy, a slower rate of hyperalimentation, and reduced dietary sodium. Children recovering from PEM are at greater risk of developing cardiac abnormalities.[16,20]

OBESITY

Obesity is an important problem in western countries because of its high prevalence[24a]; however, in Asia obesity plays a less significant role except in Singapore and Korea.[25] In general, there are two types of obesity: adult-onset and lifelong.[26] Adult-onset obesity is common in the developed countries in a major portion of the population between 20 and 40 years of age. The increased depot of adipose tissue in adult-onset obesity is due to hypertrophy of adipocytes only, whereas in lifelong obesity both the size and the number of adipocytes are increased.

PATHOLOGY

Although a previous study suggested that cardiac dysfunction in marked obesity was due to increased epicardial fat and fatty infiltration of the myocardium,[27] it is now recognized that these findings are nonspecific and of no functional significance because they are found in a variety of conditions other than obesity. Postmortem study revealed heart weight in marked obesity to be enormously greater than that predicted for ideal body weight. Severe left ventricular hypertrophy was found in virtually all cases and right ventricular hypertrophy in some.[28]

CARDIOVASCULAR ABNORMALITIES

Statistical data have shown that the increased morbidity and mortality in obesity are mostly related to cardiovascular abnormalities[29,30] including systemic hypertension, coronary heart disease, obesity heart disease, cardiac arrhythmias, sleep apnea, the obesity hypoventilation syndrome, and pulmonary hypertension.

Hypertension

Although it is frequently stated that indirect measurement of blood pressure by the standard cuff method tends to overestimate blood pressure, direct measurement of intraarterial pressure indicates that hypertension is not artifactual in obese men.[31] In a recent survey Stamler et al[32] found a nearly twofold increase in the prevalence of elevated diastolic pressure in men who were 15% above ideal weight versus those at or below ideal weight. Blood pressure can always be reduced with significant weight loss in obese men whether they are hypertensive or normotensive.

Coronary Heart Disease

The increased mortality associated with obesity has always been attributed to coronary heart disease.[29] Nonetheless, in a recent study when serum cholesterol and systolic blood pressure were excluded, the incidence of coronary heart disease was not different between the obese subjects and the control subjects.[30] Postmortem study in persons dying of accidental causes also failed to show any significant difference in the incidence and extent of coronary atherosclerosis in obese subjects when compared with men of ideal weight.[33] Conversely, obese diabetic women had a higher incidence of cardiac failure and increased mortality in the presence of acute myocardial infarction.[34] The increased incidence of these complications may be related to an increase in lipolysis of adipose tissue due to norepinephrine, with consequent high plasma free fatty acid levels leading to an increase in cardiac arrhythmias.

Obesity Heart Disease

It is now recognized that cardiac failure may occur in extremely obese subjects whether hypertension is present or not.[35] These patients often have cardiomegaly and clinical features of congestive heart failure indistinguishable from those due to other causes. Electrocardiograms frequently show left axis shift of the QRS complex, and atrial fibrillation may develop in the late stage.[36] Hemodynamic studies reveal a significant increase in blood volume and cardiac output in proportion to the excess body weight. Systemic and pulmonary hypertension is common and left ventricular filling pressure is often within upper normal limits but is elevated during exercise.[35]

Obesity Hypoventilation Syndrome (Pickwickian Syndrome)

This syndrome is characterized by hypoventilation, periodic respiration, cyanosis, twitching, polycythemia, and impaired consciousness.[37] The pathogenesis of this syndrome is thought to be depressed respiratory center activity and reduced expiratory reserve volume of the lungs, which result in hypoventilation, hypercapnea, and hypoxia. During periods of apnea during sleep, cardiac arrhythmias are common and include sinus arrest, asystole, heart block, and serious ventricular arrhythmias.[38]

Pulmonary Hypertension

The causes of pulmonary hypertension[35,37] in extreme obesity are multifactorial and include pulmonary vasoconstriction secondary to hypoxia and acidosis, increased pulmonary blood flow, and elevated left atrial pressure due to diminished compliance of the hypertrophic left ventricle.

MANAGEMENT

The effect of weight reduction on the prevention of coronary heart disease is difficult to assess. Improvement in angina pectoris may be anticipated after significant weight loss.[39] A low-calorie, low-sodium diet is often effective in achieving reduction in both weight and blood pressure.[35] Diuretic therapy may suffice in eliminating edema; however, digitalis may be needed in patients with heart failure due to myocardial insufficiency.

ALCOHOL AND THE HEART

Although cardiac failure, cardiac dilatation, and hypertrophy have been observed in chronic users of alcohol, these conditions were previously attributed to undernutritional states, especially thiamin deficiency.[40] A recent study, which specifically excluded subjects with evidence of malnutrition, demonstrated that excessive intake of alcohol can itself cause heart disease,[41] and thus the entity "alcoholic cardiomyopathy" was recently recognized.[42]

ACUTE ALCOHOLIC EFFECT

Acute alcohol ingestion may lead to alterations in either mechanical or electrophysiologic functions of the heart. In in vitro studies, alcohol reduces the contractile force of isolated cardiac tissue and electrophysiologically shortens the action potential.[43] Alcohol inhibits the ATPase activity of the cardiac plasma membrane and depresses the uptake of calcium by the sarcoplasmic reticulum.[44] These cellular effects of acute alcohol administration may inhibit the association of actin and myosin and lead to decreased contractility. Studies of the acute alcohol effect on mechanical function in nonalcoholic subjects without heart disease have produced variable results. An increase in cardiac output secondary to an increase in heart rate or stroke volume has been observed, whereas others report depressed myocardial function after alcohol ingestion in normal individuals.[43,44,44a] Conversely, studies in nonalcoholic patients with heart disease provide more consistent evidence of the myocardial depressant effect of alcohol. In patients with coronary artery disease, moderate alcohol consumption resulted in a decrease in blood pressure and cardiac output.[45] Furthermore, decreased exercise time to angina and increased ST-segment depression at the same workload were reported in patients after acute alcohol ingestion. Nonetheless, transient improvement in cardiac function was recently reported in patients with congestive heart failure after acute ingestion of alcohol. This was attributed to alcohol-induced peripheral vasodilation resulting in a reduction in afterload and preload.[46]

CHRONIC ALCOHOLIC ABUSE

Chronic alcohol consumption in man can lead to progressive cardiac dysfunction and ultimately congestive cardiomyopathy.[42,44] In animal studies, cardiac performance was generally impaired after long-term administration of a large quantity of alcohol comprising 35% to 40% of total calorie intake. A number of biochemical changes may lead to impaired contractile function of the chronic alcoholic heart. These include increased triglycerides in myofiber, decreased mitochondrial and sarcoplasmic reticulum calcium ion transport activity, decreased protein synthesis, and decreased density of β-adrenoceptor.[43,44] Most of these biochemical derangements, however, are not specific for the alcoholic heart because they are also reported in other myopathic hearts. Reversibility of alcohol-induced biochemical and physiologic dysfunction in animals has been reported after withdrawal of alcohol, which agrees with its clinical counterpart of improvement in patients with alcoholic cardiomyopathy following abstention from alcohol.[44]

CLINICAL ASPECTS

Alcoholic cardiomyopathy typically occurs in individuals 30 to 55 years of age who have a history of alcohol consumption in large quantity comprising 30% to 50% of daily calories over a 10- to 15-year period.[42] The cardiovascular presentations are usually variable and include cardiac failure, chest pain, palpitations, or syncope due to arrhythmias or thromboembolic phenomena. Physical signs of cardiac decompensation are indistinguishable from other causes of congestive cardiomyopathy.[43,44] Transient elevated diastolic pressure may be found during cardiac decompensation and may lead to a false diagnosis of hypertension. The elevated blood pressure usually returns to normal following response to therapy. Electrocardiograms often show sinus tachycardia and sometimes abnormal rhythm and conduction including atrial and ventricular ectopic depolarizations, atrial fibrillation or flutter, atrioventricular block, hemiblock, and bundle branch block.[47] Other electrocardiographic findings are abnormal P waves, slurred and notched QRS complexes, and ST-T segment abnormalities. Arrhythmias are also commonly reported in subjects without overt heart disease or cardiomegaly who indulge in heavy alcoholic intake on weekends or holidays ("holiday heart syndrome").[48] Typically this syndrome is characterized by acute rhythm disturbances associated with heavy ethanol consumption in a subject without heart disease and disappearing without residua on abstinence. Various atrial and ventricular arrhythmias including transient atrioventricular block were reported in holiday heart syndrome. The same arrhythmia may recur with subsequent episodes of alcohol intoxication.

CORONARY ATHEROSCLEROSIS AND MYOCARDIAL INFARCTION

An earlier postmortem study indicated less atherosclerotic disease of the coronary arteries in the cirrhotic than in the noncirrhotic alcoholic patient.[43] In a recent report relating alcohol intake to coronary arteriographic findings in patients with chest pain or previous myocardial infarction, less significant atherosclerotic occlusive disease was present in patients who had a history of heavy ethanol consumption.[49] The relation between alcohol consumption and myocardial infarction has recently received considerable attention. Habitual intake of a small quantity of alcohol may be associated with a decreased risk of nonfatal myocardial infarction and death from coronary artery disease.[43,44] Nevertheless, Regan et al[50] reported transmural myocardial infarction in ten alcoholic patients who had no traditional coronary risk factors and all had normal coronary arteries. There are also anecdotal reports of myocardial infarction in patients with normal coronary angiograms following acute ethanol intoxication.[51,52] In a recent study of myocardial infarction in young men, heavy ethanol intake was noted in 16%, suggesting a possible role of alcohol in the pathogenesis of acute myocardial infarction.[52] Alcohol has also been reported to induce coronary vasospasm and variant angina culminating in acute myocardial infarction.[43] However, increased total and MB creatine kinase (CK) isoenzyme values have been reported in patients with acute alcohol intoxication without infarction (67% and 8.3%, respectively, in one series[53]). Therefore, elevated MB-CK isoenzyme values per se should be used with extreme caution in the diagnosis of acute myocardial infarction in alcoholic patients.

The complex relation between alcohol and coronary heart disease was highlighted recently by some epidemiologic observational studies from New Zealand,[54] Puerto Rico,[55] Yugoslavia,[56] Honolulu (Japanese men),[57] Framingham,[58] and the Lipid Research Clinic Program Prevalence Study in North America,[59] all of which seemed to suggest a possible protective effect against coronary heart disease associated with moderate alcohol consumption. Clearly any potential protective effect against coronary heart disease cannot be used to justify alcoholic indulgence because of alcohol's effect on mortality from all causes such as dilated cardiomyopathy, cardiac arrhythmias, and coronary vasospasm, each of which may lead to sudden coronary death with or without acute myocardial infarction, as well as increased incidence of other alcohol-related problems.[60]

TREATMENT

Complete abstinence from alcohol is the key to management of alcoholic cardiomyopathy. Most patients who abstained from alcohol over a 3-year period had an improved or unchanged cardiac status.[61] Death occurred chiefly in those who did not abstain. Congestive heart failure should be treated with digitalis, diuretics, and peripheral vasodilators. Electrolyte abnormalities, when present, should be properly corrected. Cardiac arrhythmias may be treated with appropriate antiarrhythmic agents or direct-current countershock when indicated. Anticoagulant therapy may be needed to prevent thromboembolism in patients with severe heart failure, particularly when atrial fibrillation is present.

DIETING, ANOREXIA NERVOSA, AND BULIMIA

Although malnutrition is a disease of the underdeveloped countries of the world, it may seem paradoxical that it should also exist in the Western world. In the modern society of the Western world, where overeating and obesity are the rule rather than the exception, in certain sectors of the society, especially in the fashion and entertainment world where obesity becomes psychologically and cosmetically debilitating, there exists self-imposed starvation through the use of various weight reduction regimens. These include fasting, hypocaloric balanced diets, "fad" diets, total starvation, drugs, surgery, jaw wiring, and a combination of these methods. The extremes are exemplified by patients with anorexia nervosa and bulimia. In the mid 1970s, protein was added to a total fast to reduce the catabolism associated with total fasting. At about the same time, other diets such as very-low–calorie diets, protein-sparing modified fasts, and liquid protein diets were introduced and became very popular with the publication of the book *The Last Chance Diet* in 1976.[62]

CARDIAC ARRHYTHMIAS AND SUDDEN DEATH

Despite the high rate of success in achieving weight reduction in a small group of patients, these diets have been associated with potentially life-threatening cardiac arrhythmias[63–67] and in some cases sudden death.[68,69] Necropsy examination usually failed to establish an anatomic cause of death, and electrocardiograms recorded a short time before death showed various degrees of QT-interval prolongation and terminal ventricular tachyarrhythmias including torsades de pointes.[68–70] It is evident that sudden death in liquid-protein dieting, like sudden death in anorexia nervosa, results from ventricular tachyarrhythmias related to QT-interval prolongation.[70,71]

QT-INTERVAL PROLONGATION

Similar QT-interval prolongation has been reported after therapeutic starvation,[72] in anorexia nervosa,[23,70] in prisoners of war,[22] and in various malnutritional states.[73] Unlike the patient with anorexia nervosa who does not eat, patients with bulimia go through morbid food binging followed by purging. Because patients with bulimia do not lose a large amount of weight as do those with anorexia, their QT intervals might not be prolonged. However, one of the three patients reported on by Isner et al[70] exhibited elements of bulimia with cycles of gorging and purging as well as anorexia. Although the exact pathogenesis of QT-interval prolongation in all of these patients is unknown, it may be due to biochemical changes in the myocellular membrane, thereby altering potassium flux with prolongation or delay of electrical repolarization.[74] It is also possible that QT prolongation may result from a direct myocardial toxic effect of emetine secondary to abuse of ipecac in patients with major eating disorders.[75] Furthermore, severe weight loss and anorexia are associated with hypothalamic disturbances including impairment of thermoregulation and gonadotropin release[76,77]; almost all anorexic women are amenorrheic. It is therefore postulated that autonomic inflow to the heart might be deranged, particularly under conditions of stress, and an imbalance in the various components of the sympathetic innervation of the heart could contribute to QT-interval prolongation and malignant ventricular arrhythmias.[70,71,74] Hypokalemia resulting from diuretic abuse, cathartic abuse, and self-induced vomiting in these patients may also contribute to QT-interval prolongation.

LEFT VENTRICULAR DYSFUNCTION AND CONGESTIVE HEART FAILURE

In anorexia nervosa, as in malnutrition, the cardiac chamber size, left ventricular wall thickness, blood pressure, and cardiac output are all reported to be decreased.[20,21] However, left ventricular systolic function determined by echocardiography and radionuclide cineangiography both at rest and during exercise is unimpaired.[21]

Although most of the adverse cardiovascular effects of malnutrition and anorexia are reversible with nutritional rehabilitation,[20,21] caution is needed because too rapid replenishment of fluid or nutrients may precipitate heart failure.[78,79] It has been suggested that myocardial reserve recovers too slowly during refeeding in these patients to meet the demands imposed by improvement in the overall metabolic state.[20,78,79] Recommendations regarding the avoidance of "refeeding heart failure" include restriction of physical activity, use of low-salt regimens, serial monitoring of cardiac function, and treatment in a monitored unit equipped and staffed to handle cardiac emergencies until the patient's condition has been stabilized.[80,81]

REFERENCES

1. Tanphaichitr V, Wood B: Thiamin, in *Nutrition Reviews' Present Knowledge in Nutrition*, ed 5. Washington, DC, The Nutrition Foundation, Inc, 1984, pp 273–281.
2. Tanphaichitr V: *Clinical and Biochemical Studies in Beriberi*, thesis. Faculty of Graduate Studies, University of Medical Sciences, Bangkok, Thailand, 1968.
3. Cheunchit L, Tanphaichitr V: Infantile beriberi. *Supasitprasong Hospital Gazette* 1975; 1:97–101.
4. Tanphaichitr V, Vimokesant SL, Dhanamitta S, Valyasevi A: Clinical and biochemical studies of adult beriberi. *Am J Clin Nutr* 1970; 23:1017–1026.
5. Tanphaichitr V, Lerdvuthisopon N, Boongird P: Clinical and nutrition studies of adult beriberi. Abstracts of 4th Asian and Oceanian Congress of Neurology. Bangkok, Sompong Press, 1975, p 151.
6. Sukulmalchantra Y, Tanphaichitr V, Thongmitr V, Jumbala B: Electrocardiographic findings in adult beriberi: changes in the QRS voltage. *Mod Med Asia* 1975; 11:6–7.
7. Sukumalchantra Y, Thongmitr V, Tanphaichitr V, Jumbala B: Variability of cardiac output in beriberi heart disease. *Mod Med Asia* 1976; 12:7–10.

7a. Engbers G, Molhoek GP, Arntzenius AC: Shoshin beriberi: a rare diagnostic problem. *Br Heart J* 1984; 51:581–582.

8. Davidson S, Passmore R, Brock JF, Truswell AS: *Human Nutrition and Dietetics*, ed 6. Edinburgh, Churchill Livingstone, 1975, p 336.
9. Pattamakom V, Rattanasiri P, Roongpisuthipong C, Tanphaichitr V: Thiamin malnutrition in institutionalized subjects. *Thai J Intern Med* 1984; 4:1–4.
10. Kawai C, Wakabayashi A, Matsumara T, Yui Y: Reappearance of beriberi heart disease in Japan. A study of 23 cases. *Am J Med* 1980; 69:383–386.
11. Kuriyama M, Yokomine R, Arima H, Homada R, Igata A: Blood vitamin B_1 transketolase and thiamin pyrophosphate (TPP) effect in beriberi patients, with studies employing discriminant analysis. *Clin Chim Acta* 1980; 108:159–68.
12. Food and Nutrition Board, National Research Council: *Recommended Dietary Allowances,* ed 9. Washington, DC, National Academy of Science, 1980, pp 82–87.
13. Bengoa JM: The problem of malnutrition. *WHO Chron* 1974; 28:3–7.
14. Bistrian BR, Blackburn GL, Vitale J, Cochran D, Naylor J: Prevalence of malnutrition in general medical patients. *JAMA* 1976; 235:1567–1570.
15. Alleyne GAO, Hay RW, Picon DI, Stanfeld JP, Whitehead RG: *Protein-Energy Malnutrition*. London, Butler & Tanner Ltd, 1977, p 26.
16. Heymsfield SR, Nutter DO: The heart in protein-calorie undernutrition, in Hurst JW (ed): *The Heart-Update*. New York, McGraw-Hill Book Co, 1979, pp 191–209.
17. Chauhan S, Nayak NC, Ramalingaswami V: The heart and skeletal muscle in experimental protein malnutrition in Rhesus monkeys. *J Pathol Bacteriol* 1965; 90:301–309.
18. Alleyne GAO: Plasma and blood volumes in severely malnourished Jamaican children. *Arch Dis Child* 1960; 41:313–315.
19. Viart P: Hemodynamic findings in severe protein-calorie malnutrition. *Am J Clin Nutr* 1977; 30:334–348.
20. Heymsfield SB, Bethel RA, Ansley JD, Gibbs DM, Felner JM, Nutter DO: Cardiac abnormalities in cachectic patients before and during nutritional repletion. *Am Heart J* 1978; 95:584–594.
21. Gottdiener JS, Gross HA, Henry WL, Borer JS, Ebert MH: Effects of self-induced starvation on cardiac size and function in anorexia nervosa. *Circulation* 1978; 58:425–433.
22. Schnitker MA, Mattman PE, Bliss TL: A clinical study of malnutrition in Japanese prisoners of war. *Ann Intern Med* 1951; 35:69–96.
23. Thurston J, Marks P: Electrocardiographic abnormalities in patients with anorexia nervosa. *Br Heart J* 1974; 36:719–723.
24. Simonson E, Henschel A, Keys A: The electrocardiogram of man in semistarvation and subsequent rehabilitation. *Am Heart J* 1948; 35:584–602.

24a. National Institutes of Health: Health implications of obesity: National Institutes of Health Consensus Development Conference. *Ann Intern Med* 1985; 103:977–1077.

25. Wong HB, Jin SJ: Nutritional disorders in Southeast Asia. *Med Prog* 1984; 11(6):13–16.
26. Salans LB: Obesity and the adipose cell, in Bondy PK, Rosenberg LE (eds): *Metabolic Control and Diseases*, ed 9. Philadelphia, WB Saunders Co, 1980, p 150.
27. Balsaver AM, Morales AR, Whitehouse FW: Fat infiltration of myocardium as a cause of cardiac conduction defect. *Am J Cardiol* 1967; 19:261–265.
28. Amad KH, Brennan JC, Alexander JK: The cardiac pathology of chronic exogenous obesity. *Circulation* 1965; 32:740–745.
29. Lew EA, Garfinkel L: Variations in mortality by weight among 750,000 men and women. *J Chron Dis* 1979; 32:563–576.
30. Weinsier RL, Fuchs RJ, Kay TD, Triebwaser JH, Lancaster MC: Body fat: its relationship to coronary heart disease, blood pressure, lipids and other risk factors measured in a large male population. *Am J Med* 1976; 61:815–824.
31. Kvols LK, Rohlfing BM, Alexander JK: A comparison of intraarterial and cuff blood pressure measurements in very obese subjects. *Cardiovas Res Ctr Bull* 1969; 7:118–123.
32. Stamler R, Stamler J, Riedlinger WF, Algera G, Roberts RH: Weight and blood pressure. Findings in hypertension screen of one million Americans. *JAMA* 1978; 240:1607–1610.
33. Montenegro MR, Solberg LA: Obesity, body weight, body length and atherosclerosis. *Lab Invest* 1968; 18:594–603.
34. Tansey MJB, Opie LH, Kennelly BM: High mortality in obese women diabetics with acute myocardial infarction. *Br Med* 1977; 1:1624–1626.
35. Alexander JK: Obesity and the circulation. *Mod Concepts Cardiovasc Dis* 1963; 32:799–803.
36. Axelrod MA, Alexander JK: The electrocardiograms and cardiac anatomy in obesity. *Clin Res* 1965; 13:25.
37. Rochester DF, Enson Y: Current concepts in the pathogenesis of the obesity-hypoventilation syndrome. Mechanical and circulatory factors. *Am J Med* 1974; 57:402–420.
38. Shaw TRD, Coyyall RJM, Craib IA: Cardiac and respiratory standstill during sleep. *Br Heart J* 1978; 40:1055–1058.
39. Sharma B, Thadani U, Taylor SH: Cardiovascular effects of weight reduction in obese patients with angina pectoris. *Br Heart J* 1974; 36:854–858.
40. Weiss S: Occidental beriberi with cardiovascular manifestation. Its relation to thiamin deficiency. *JAMA* 1940; 115:832–839.
41. Regan TJ, Levinson GE, Oldewurtel HA, Frank MJ, Weisse AB, Moschos CB: Ventricular function in non-cardiacs with alcholic fatty liver: role of ethanol in the production of cardiomyopathy. *J Clin Invest* 1969; 48:397–407.
42. Burch GE, Giles TD: Alcholic cardiomyopathy: concept of the disease and its treatment. *Am J Med* 1971; 50:141–145.
43. Segal LD, Klausner SC, Gnadt JTH, Amsterdam EA: Alcohol and the heart. *Med Clin North Am* 1984; 68:147–161.
44. Regan TJ: Alcoholic cardiomyopathy. *Progr Cardiovasc Dis* 1984; 27:141–152.

44a. Lang RM, Borow KM, Neumann A, Feldman T: Adverse cardiac effects of acute alcoholic ingestion in young adults. *Ann Intern Med* 1985; 102:742–747.

45. Conway N: Hemodynamic effects of ethyl alcohol in patients with coronary heart disease. *Br Heart J* 1968; 30:638–644.
46. Greenberg BH, Schutz R, Grunkemeier GL, Griswold H: Acute effects of alcohol in patients with congestive heart failure. *Ann Intern Med* 1982; 97:171–175.
47. Bashour TT, Fahdul H, Cheng TO: Electrocardiographic abnormalities in alcoholic cardiomyopathy. A study of 65 patients. *Chest* 1975; 68:24–27.
48. Ettinger PO, Wu CF, de La Cruz C Jr, Weisse AB, Ahmed SS, Regan TJ: Arrhythmias and the "Holiday Heart": alcohol-associated cardiac rhythm disorders. *Am Heart J* 1978; 95:555–562.
49. Barboriak JJ, Rimm AA, Anderson AJ, Schmidhoffer M, Tristani FE: Coronary artery occlusion and alcohol intake. *Br Heart J* 1977; 39:289–293.
50. Regan TJ, Wu CF, Weisse AB, Moschos CB, Ahmed SS, Lyons MM: Acute myocardial infarction in toxic cardiomyopathy without coronary obstruction. *Circulation* 1975; 51:453–461.
51. Moreya AE, Kostis JB, Passannate AJ, Kuo PT: Acute myocardial infarction in patients with normal coronary arteries after acute ethanol intoxication. *Clin Cardiol* 1982; 5:425–430.

52. Chaithiraphan S, Ngam-U-Kos P, Watanachai K: Acute myocardial infarction at young age. A collaborative retrospective study of 55 cases from three medical centers in Thailand. *Intern Med* 1985; 1:1–6.
53. Siegel RJ, Kligerman M, Haywood LJ, Shell WE: Increased MB-creatine kinase isoenzymes in an alcoholic population. *J Nat Med Assoc* 1985; 77:459–464.
54. Alcohol and coronary heart disease, editorial. *N Zealand Med J* 1985: 98:896–898.
55. Kittner SJ, Garcia-Palmieri MR, Costas R Jr, Cruz-Vidal M, Abbott RD, Havlik RJ: Alcohol and coronary heart disease in Puerto Rico. *Am J Epidemiol* 1983; 117:538–550.
56. Kozarevic D, Demirovic J, Gordon T, Kaelber CT, McGee D, Zukel WJ: Drinking habits and coronary heart disease: the Yugoslavia cardiovascular disease study. *Am J Epidemiol* 1982; 116:748–758.
57. Blackwelder WC, Yano K, Rhoads GG, Kagan A, Gordon T, Palesch Y: Alcohol and mortality: the Honolulu heart study. *Am J Med* 1980; 68:164–169.
58. Gordon T, Kannel WB: Drinking habits and cardiovascular disease: the Framingham study. *Am Heart J* 1983; 105:667–673.
59. Little JA, Graves K, Suchindran CM, Milner J, McGuire V, Beaton G, Feather T, Christiansen D, Williams OD: Customary diet, anthropometry, and dyslipoproteinemia in selected North American populations. The Lipid Research Clinics Program Prevalence Study. *Circulation* 1986; 73(suppl I):I-80–I-90.
60. Wodak A: Australian alcohol consumption. *Med J Australia* 1986; 144:1–2.
61. Demarkis JG, Proskey A, Rahimtoola SH, Jamil M, Sutton GC, Rosen KM, Gunnar RM, Tobin JR: The natural course of alcoholic cardiomyopathy. *Ann Intern Med* 1973; 80:293–297.
62. Linn R, Stuart SL: *The Last Chance Diet.* Secaucus, NJ, Lyle Stuart, 1976.
63. Lantigua RA, Amatruda JM, Biddle TL, Forbes GB, Lockwood DH: Cardiac arrhythmias associated with a liquid protein diet for the treatment of obesity. *N Engl J Med* 1980; 303:735–738.
64. Siegel RJ, Cabeen WR Jr, Roberts WC: Prolonged QT interval-ventricular tachycardia syndrome from massive rapid weight loss utilizing the liquid-protein-modified-fast diet: sudden death with sinus node ganglionitis and neuritis. *Am Heart J* 1981; 102:121–123.
65. Lockwood DH, Amatruda JM: Very low calorie diets in the management of obesity. *Ann Rev Med* 1984; 35:373–381.
66. Felig P: Very low calorie protein diets. *N Engl J Med* 1984; 310:589–591.
67. Herzog DB, Copeland PM: Eating disorders. *N Engl J Med* 1985; 313:295–303.
68. Isner JM, Sours HE, Paris AL, Ferrans VJ, Roberts WC: Sudden, unexpected death in avid dieters using the liquid-protein-modified-fast diets: observations in 17 patients and the role of the prolonged QT interval. *Circulation* 1979; 60:1401–1412.
69. Sours HE, Frattali VP, Brand CD, Feldman RA, Forbes AL, Swanson RC, Paris AL: Sudden death associated with very low calorie weight reduction regimens. *Am J Clin Nutr* 1981; 34:453–461.
70. Isner JM, Roberts WC, Heymsfield SB, Yager J: Anorexia nervosa and sudden death. *Ann Intern Med* 1985; 102:49–52.
71. Editorial: Nutrition and the QT interval. *Lancet* 1985; 1:1431.
72. Pringle TH, Scobie IN, Murray RG, Kesson CM, Maccuish AC: Prolongation of the QT interval during therapeutic starvation: a substrate for malignant arrhythmias. *Int J Obesity* 1983; 7:253–261.
73. Ellis L: Electrocardiographic abnormalities in severe malnutrition. *Br Heart J* 1946; 8:53–61.
74. Moss AJ: Caution: very-low-calorie diets can be deadly. *Ann Intern Med* 1985; 102:121–123.
75. Palmer EP, Guay AT: Reversible myopathy secondary to abuse of ipecac in patients with major eating disorders. *N Engl J Med* 1985; 313:1457–1459.
76. Brown GM: Endocrine alterations in anorexia nervosa, in Darby PL, Garfinkel PE, Garner DM, Coscina DV (eds): *Anorexia Nervosa: Recent Developments in Research.* New York, Alan R Liss, 1983, pp 231–247.
77. Drossman DA: Anorexia nervosa: a comprehensive approach. *Adv Intern Med* 1983; 28:339–362.
78. Powers PS: Heart failure during treatment of anorexia nervosa. *Am J Psychiatry* 1982; 139:1167–1170.
79. Harris RT: Bulimarexia and related serious eating disorders with medical complications. *Ann Intern Med* 1983; 99:800–807.
80. Brotman AW, Stern TA: Case report of cardiovascular abnormalities in anorexia nervosa. *Am J Psychiatry* 1983; 140:1227–1228.
81. Arik TH, Desser KB, Benchimol A: Cardiac complications of intensive dieting and eating disorders. *Arizona Med* 1985; 42:72–74.

51 Iatrogenic Cardiovascular Disease

Hugh A. McAllister, Jr, MD, FACC and Robert J. Hall, MD, FACC

MORPHOLOGIC PATTERNS OF DRUG-INDUCED INJURY TO THE HEART AND BLOOD VESSELS

Although some drugs cause cardiac dysfunction by interfering with neural or biochemical mechanisms of conduction or contractility without structural alterations, many drugs induce patterns of injury that are morphologically similar. The major morphologic changes in the heart include hypersensitivity myocarditis, toxic myocarditis, cardiomyopathy, myocardial infarction, endocardial and valvular fibrosis, drug-associated infective endocarditis, pericarditis, and pericardial hemorrhage. The major morphologic changes in blood vessels include hypersensitivity vasculitis, toxic vasculitis, intimal proliferation, accelerated atherosclerosis, arterial calcification, thrombosis and thromboembolism, and drug-associated infective vasculitis.

Hypersensitivity myocarditis is characterized by an inflammatory cell infiltrate consisting of prominent numbers of eosinophils, lymphocytes, and plasma cells. Numerous foci of myocytolysis are common, but there is minimal, if any, muscle cell necrosis.[1] The inflammatory cell infiltrate is prominent in the interstitium and also is present in small intramural coronary arteries, arterioles, and venules, resulting in a bland appearing vasculitis that is similar to the hypersensitivity vasculitis associated with therapeutic drugs. Necrotizing vascular lesions such as those present in patients with Wegener's granulomatosis, systemic lupus erythematosus, and panarteritis nodosa are not a feature of hypersensitivity myocarditis.[2] The inflammatory cell infiltrates may also involve the pericardium, especially the visceral pericardium, but characteristically the cardiac valves are spared. The precise pathogenesis of hypersensitivity myocarditis remains unclear, but it appears to be immunologically mediated, perhaps as a delayed hypersensitivity reaction.[3] Other forms of myocarditis in which eosinophils are prominent, such as parasitic infections of the heart and Loeffler's endomyocardial fibrosis, usually can be distinguished from hypersensitivity myocarditis by the presence of focal myocardial necrosis and myocardial scarring.

The drugs that have been associated with hypersensitivity myocarditis in man are listed in Table 51.1. Many of these drugs have also been associated with hypersensitivity vasculitis. Early diagnosis of hypersensitivity myocarditis is important, as a majority of patients die suddenly.[1] Conduction disturbances from His bundle involvement may lead to heart block, and if ventricular tachycardia ensues it may become intractable.[3a] Obviously the first step in management is to stop the causal drug; early diagnosis therefore could be lifesaving.[3b]

In acute *toxic myocarditis* there is interstitial edema, necrosis of myocardial cells with contraction bands (myofibrillar damage leading to myocytolysis), and a mixed inflammatory cell infiltrate consisting of lymphocytes, plasma cells, and polymorphonuclear leukocytes. Prolonged therapy with a drug that is causing acute toxic myocarditis can allow progression to a chronic stage, with the gross and microscopic findings of dilated cardiomyopathy with scattered foci of myocytolysis and myocardial fibrosis, as well as focal endocardial thickening and mural thrombi. The progression of acute toxic myocarditis to cardiomyopathy can occur even after the drug has been discontinued (adriamycin and daunomycin). The increasing number of drugs that can cause acute as well as chronic toxic myocarditis are listed in Table 51.2.

Macroscopic *myocardial infarction* may occur when the extramural coronary arteries are involved by drug-induced arteritis (amphetamines), intimal proliferation (oral contraceptives), embolization from drug-associated endocarditis, or in patients with normal coronary arteries after exposure to toxic levels of carbon monoxide, nitrates, thyroid preparation, methysergide, or ergot deriv-

Table 51.1. Drugs Associated with Hypersensitivity Myocarditis*

Methyldopa	Penicillin
Hydrochlorothiazide	Phenindione
Sulfadiazine	Phenylbutazone
Sulfisoxazole	Oxyphenbutazone
Sulfonylureas	Tetracycline
Chloramphenicol	Diphenylhydantoin
Paramino-salicylic acid (PAS)	Acetazolamide
Amitriptyline	Ampicillin
Carbamazepine	Chlorthalidone
Indomethacin	Spironolactone
Streptomycin	

*From McAllister HA, Mullick FG: The cardiovascular system, in Riddell RH (ed): *Pathology of Drug Induced and Toxic Diseases*. New York, Churchill Livingstone, Inc, 1982. By permission of Churchill Livingstone, Inc.

atives.[4] Cardiac muscle cell damage secondary to capillary endothelial damage and microthrombosis with structural alterations similar to ischemic necrosis may also occur (cyclophosphamide, catecholamines, and selenium-vitamin E deficiency).[5] These areas are usually microscopic and patchy.

Endocardial fibrosis may occur adjacent to subendocardial areas of hypersensitivity or toxic myocarditis with or without mural thrombus. An identical form of endocardial thickening is commonly located adjacent to areas of myocardial ischemia and microscopically consists of collagen as well as elastic fibers, smooth muscle cells, and variable amounts of acid mucopolysaccharide. When the lesions are induced by drug hypersensitivity or toxicity alone, without antecedent valvular disease, the cardiac valves are seldom involved. In contrast, another form of drug-induced endocardial fibrosis commonly involves the cardiac valves. This latter form is most commonly associated with methysergide therapy, although ergotamine tartrate has also been implicated in the induction of these lesions.[6–8] The cardiac valves most commonly involved are the mitral and aortic; however, involvement of the tricuspid valve has also been reported.[6] The endocardium may contain similar lesions, with or without contiguity with the valvular lesions.

Infective endocarditis is one of several serious complications of parenteral narcotic abuse. Although the incidence of this infection in the addict population has not been precisely determined, an incidence of 1.5 to 2 cases per 1,000 at risk per year may be conservatively estimated. Because the number of daily narcotic users in the United States is believed to be between 400,000 and 600,000, almost 1,000 cases of narcotic-associated infective endocarditis can be anticipated annually.[9] Fungal endocarditis and endocarditis caused by gram-negative organisms are much more common in the addict population.

The fungus most commonly isolated in patients with this complication is Candida species. Also in contrast to the nonaddict population, the tricuspid valve is frequently involved in narcotic-associated infective endocarditis. Indeed, in one large study 50% of the patients with narcotic-associated infective endocarditis had primary tricuspid valve infection.[9]

Nonbacterial thrombotic endocarditis may affect the cardiac valves in patients with drug-induced disseminated intravascular coagulation. Nonbacterial thrombotic endocarditis differs morphologically from infective endocarditis in that no organisms are present in these lesions, and there is no significant destruction of the cardiac valve. The valves most commonly involved are the mitral and aortic.

Pericarditis, with or without effusion, has been reported in patients with drug-induced systemic lupus erythematosus. It is rare, however, for patients with drug-induced systemic lupus erythematosus to present with pericarditis as the major initial manifestation, and cardiac tamponade is the exception.[10] When the offending drug is discontinued, the signs and symptoms of pericarditis disappear but may recur promptly upon its readministration. There has been a steady accumulation of reports describing the induction of lupus-like syndromes by various drugs.[11] The list of drugs implicated in this manner continues to grow and is itemized in Table 51.3. In many of these reports the evidence linking drugs to disease is often highly circumstantial, and in some cases symptoms suggestive of systemic lupus erythematosus have antedated the use of the drug in question. The syndromes that have been most extensively investigated and most firmly established have been those that have followed the use of hydralazine and procainamide. Lupus-like syndromes with pericarditis usually occur only after prolonged treatment with large doses of the drug and then only affect a small group of patients exposed to the drug. As in spontaneously occurring systemic lupus erythematosus, women are affected more commonly than men.[11] Administration of procainamide, methysergide, or

Table 51.2. Drugs Associated With Toxic Myocarditis*

Adriamycin	Cyclophosphamide
Daunomycin	Arsenicals
Fluorouracil	Lithium carbonate
Emetine hydrochloride	Phenothiazines
Antimony compounds	Mitomycin C
Amphetamines	Catecholamines

*From McAllister HA, Mullick FG: The cardiovascular system, in Riddell RH (ed): *Pathology of Drug Induced and Toxic Diseases*. New York, Churchill Livingstone, Inc, 1982. By permission of Churchill Livingstone, Inc.

Table 51.3. Drugs That Induce Lupus-Like Syndrome*

Hydralazine	Sulfonamides
Procainamide	Tetracycline
Isoniazid	Propylthiouracil
Aminosalicylic acid	Methylthiouracil
Diphenylhydantoin	Alphamethyldopa
Methylphenylethylhydantoin	Barbiturates
Mephenytoin	Griseofulvin
Primidone	Streptomycin
Trimethadione	Quinidine
Ethosuximide	Phenylbutazone
Methsuximide	Chlorpromazine
Reserpine	Methotrimeprazine
Penicillin	Perphenazine
Penicillamine	Promazine

*From McAllister HA, Mullick FG: The cardiovascular system, in Riddell RH (ed): *Pathology of Drug Induced and Toxic Diseases*. New York, Churchill Livingstone, Inc, 1982. By permission of Churchill Livingstone, Inc.

practolol has been associated with the development of constrictive pericarditis.

Those drugs that cause hypersensitivity myocarditis or toxic myocarditis may also involve the contiguous pericardium, especially the visceral pericardium, resulting acutely in a fibrinous pericarditis with or without effusion. In toxic myocarditis, the pericardium is most commonly affected in patients receiving cyclophosphamide, anthracyclines, or arsenic.

Patients receiving immunosuppressive drugs may develop infective pericarditis with opportunistic organisms. Viral infections may result in fibrinous pericarditis, whereas bacteria and fungi commonly cause purulent pericarditis, which may occasionally be accompanied by myocardial abscess. Fibrinous or purulent pericarditis may result in cardiac tamponade or may evolve into chronic constrictive pericarditis. The rare occurrence of tuberculous pericarditis in these immunologically compromised patients must also be considered in the differential diagnosis. The organisms responsible for nontuberculous infective pericarditis have changed considerably since the introduction of antibiotics and immunosuppression.[12] In the preantibiotic and preimmunosuppressive era, gram-positive bacteria were responsible for most of these cases. Today, gram-negative bacteria and fungi are the most common etiologic agents. Although many different fungi have been implicated, the most common is *Candida* species in patients with leukemia receiving immunosuppressive drugs. Additionally, the types of gram-positive bacteria causing infective pericarditis have changed considerably. *Streptococcus* and *pneumococcus* were most common in the preantibiotic era, but these have been replaced by staphylococcus in the more recent antibiotic era.

Pericardial hemorrhage most commonly occurs in patients receiving anticoagulants and may exist as focal extravasations contained within the pericardium or may result in hemorrhage into the pericardial sac, occasionally resulting in cardiac tamponade. The latter is especially true in uremic patients receiving heparin in conjunction with hemodialysis.[10] If the pericardium is not damaged, the presence of blood within the pericardial sac leaves no residuum. However, in patients with pericarditis, hemorrhagic effusion frequently results in pericardial adhesions that initially are fibrinous. If these adhesions are extensive, chronic constrictive pericarditis may develop and can occur as early as 6 weeks and as late as 11 months after acute hemorrhagic pericarditis.

Hypersensitivity vasculitis related to therapeutic drugs most commonly involves arterioles, capillaries, and venules. Although small veins and occasionally small arteries may be affected, muscular and elastic arteries and large veins are spared. Although an inflammatory cell infiltrate is present in all three layers of the involved vessel walls, there is no evidence of necrotizing vascular lesions or fibrinoid necrosis.[13,14] Therefore, the media is not weakened, and in contrast to panarteritis nodosa, aneurysm formation is not a feature.

Drug hypersensitivity reactions are presumed to be the result of antigen–antibody interactions. However, numerous attempts to define the immunologic mechanisms of hypersensitivity angiitis have not been successful.[13] The interval between the first administration of the drug and the development of vasculitis is extremely variable. A history of drug-taking in a patient for months or years without side effects does not exclude it as a possible etiologic agent. Drug hypersensitivity is not dose- or time-dependent and may occur at any time while the drug is being administered; however, the temporal relation of drug administration to onset of symptoms is an important clinicopathologic correlation.[13] It is possible for lesions to occur one day to 1 week after medication has been discontinued. Therefore, in considering the diagnosis of drug-related vasculitis a complete drug history, including current medications as well as discontinued medications and the temporal relation of drug administration to the onset of symptoms, is imperative.

A continuing list of drugs that have been associated with hypersensitivity vasculitis is itemized in Table 51.4.

Toxic vasculitis is usually necrotizing, with morphologic similarities to panarteritis nodosa. The blood vessels involved most frequently are the medium-sized and small arteries; however, in contrast to classic panarteritis nodosa, capillaries, arterioles, and veins may also be affected by the inflammatory process. These lesions tend to be segmental, with a predilection for the bifurcations of arteries. An aneurysm may form in the weakened arterial wall. These lesions are usually present in varying stages of evolution and devolution, and the arterial lumen may be occluded by fresh thrombus or by formation of granulation tissue, fibrosis, and recanalization in varying combinations.

Patients who abuse drugs intravenously may also develop arterial lesions. Disseminated lesions morphologically identical to panarteritis nodosa are commonly seen in patients who inject amphetamines intravenously.[15] Although the cause of this necrotizing vasculitis in drug abusers is unclear, it has been speculated that it may be secondary to transmission of hepatitis B antigen from contaminated needles, resulting in antigen exposure and subsequent abnormal immunologic reactivity.[16] Indeed, the hepatitis B antigen has been demonstrated in the wall of an artery containing a lesion identical to panarteritis nodosa.[17] This association suggests the possibility that

Table 51.4. Drugs Associated With Hypersensitivity Vasculitis*

Allopurinol	Indocin
Ampicillin	Isoniazid
Bromide	Levamisole
Carbamazepine	Methylthiouracil
Chloramphenicol	Oxyphenbutazone
Chlorpropamide	Phenylbutazone
Chlortetracycline	Potassium iodide
Chromolyn sodium	Procainamide
Colchicine	Propylthiouracil
Dextran	Quinidine
Diazepam	Spironolactone
Diphenylhydantoin	Sulfonamides
Diphenhydramine	Tetracycline
Griseofulvin	Trimethadione

*From McAllister HA, Mullick FG: The cardiovascular system, in Riddell RH (ed): *Pathology of Drug Induced and Toxic Diseases*. New York, Churchill Livingstone, Inc, 1982. By permission of Churchill Livingstone, Inc.

immune complex deposition of viral antigen and antibodies may be a mechanism of vascular damage in some patients with necrotizing vasculitis. Drugs that have been associated with toxic vasculitis are listed in Table 51.5.

Intimal proliferation with and without associated thrombosis has been found in women taking oral contraceptives, in pregnant and postpartum women, and in a few men with severe liver disease.[18] These lesions may occur in any of the branches of the pulmonary, portal, or systemic arteries. Frequently, there is an occlusive thrombus that appears loosely attached to the intimal proliferative lesion without intimal ulceration or inflammation. Indeed, the presence of inflammatory cells in these lesions is rare, and there is no evidence of necrotizing arteritis or fibrinoid necrosis.[18–20]

The arterial lesions induced by ergotamine are those of intimal proliferation and hyalinization and medial hypertrophy resulting in compromise of the arterial lumen. Superimposed thrombosis frequently completes the occlusion, and gangrene results. The arteries most commonly involved are the tibial, radial, and ulnar arteries or small tributaries down to arterioles.[21–23] Methysergide malleate also may produce spasm and occlusive lesions in arteries.[24,25] The intimal proliferation may rarely be so extensive that distal ischemia persists after withdrawal of the drug.

The pulmonary arterioles may be occluded by intimal proliferation containing talc or magnesium silicate, fillers used in the manufacture of certain drugs, in those patients who inject these drugs intravenously.[26,27,27a] In patients with extensive intimal proliferation in pulmonary arterioles, pulmonary hypertension and cor pulmonale result. The drugs most commonly implicated in this pulmonary arteriopathy are methylphenidate, propoxyphene, and "blue velvet" (paragoric and tripelennamine).[27,27a]

Although scientific proof is lacking, epidemiologic studies have associated the chronic intake of certain drugs (oral contraceptives and oral hypoglycemic drugs) with *accelerated atherosclerosis*.[28] Oral contraceptives have also been associated with intimal proliferative lesions.[19] The proliferating cell in the arterial intima appears morphologically identical to the proliferating cell in early atherosclerosis by light and electron microscopy. Therefore, the chronic consumption of these drugs by patients with known atherogenic risk factors such as cigarette smoking, hypertension, or hyperlipidemia could possibly predispose to increased lipid accumulation in the thickened intima.

Table 51.5. Drugs Associated With Toxic Vasculitis*

Organic arsenicals
Gold salts
Mercurials
Bismuth
Amphetamine
Methamphetamine
DDT
Serum
Sulfonamides
Penicillin

*From McAllister HA, Mullick FG: The cardiovascular system, in Riddell RH (ed): *Pathology of Drug Induced and Toxic Diseases*. New York, Churchill Livingstone, Inc, 1982. By permission of Churchill Livingstone, Inc.

Epidemiologic studies have shown that plasma high density lipoprotein (HDL) concentration is negatively correlated with the risk of acquiring ischemic heart disease.[29,29a] Therefore, high density lipoprotein seems to retard the process of atherogenesis and protects against ischemic heart disease. Although women taking oral contraceptives containing more estrogen have higher levels of HDL, those taking contraceptives with mainly progestins have lower serum HDL.[30] Low plasma HDL has also been reported in patients taking oral hypoglycemic agents[31] and in patients being treated concurrently with hydrochlorothiazide and propranolol.[32,32a]

Drug-induced calcification of the arterial wall is a distinct process from atherosclerosis. Calcification of the internal elastic membrane and the adjacent media may occur in vitamin D intoxication or hypersensitivity.[10] The medial calcification in these disorders is similar to that seen in hyperparathyroidism, pseudoxanthoma elasticum, and juvenile intimal sclerosis (idiopathic arterial calcification of infancy) in that there is an associated fibromuscular hyperplasia of the intima resulting in significant luminal compromise. The calcification is not associated with any inflammatory reaction, and the adventitia is largely unaffected.

Thrombosis with or without subsequent *thromboembolism* may occur in both arteries and veins. Venous thrombosis may result from trauma caused by damage to the veins at injection site; toxic effects of the drug, diluent, or excipient; hypersensitivity to metals contained in the needle; or infection. Drugs that increase coagulation, damage endothelium, cause spasm, or stimulate intimal proliferation may result in localized or diffuse thrombosis.

Arterial thrombosis is less common, but usually more catastrophic than venous thrombosis. Arterial thrombosis may occur by inadvertent injection of drugs, resulting in an intimal flap, perivascular hematoma or perivascular injection, false aneurysm, infective arteritis with or without mycotic aneurysm, vasospasm, excipient injection with particulate embolism, or idiosyncratic reaction.

Other drugs administered by nonarterial routes may also result in arterial thrombosis. Most of these drugs are associated with intimal proliferation (oral contraceptives) or arterial spasm, acutely, and intimal proliferation, chronically (ergotamine and methysergide malleate). Arterial thrombosis has been associated with the conjunctive use of human chorionic gonadotropin and human menopausal gonadotropins (menotropins), although the precise mechanism of this reaction has not yet been defined.[33]

Drug-related infective vasculitis occurs almost exclusively in patients receiving intravenous drugs. The infection may remain localized to the injection site as phlebitis, or the organisms may become disseminated, resulting in infective endocarditis or infective arteritis. The inflammatory reaction to an infection of an artery depends on the infecting organism and the ability of the arterial wall to react to injury. Some organisms excite little or no inflammatory response, whereas others may completely destroy the arterial wall. A great variation is found in the inflammatory response, depending on the type of artery involved, the mode of involvement, and the stage of reaction. These lesions may be relatively diffuse or localized. In addition to routine histologic examination, cultures for bacteria and fungi, as well as serologic studies for viruses, frequently are necessary to identify the infective agent. The use of special histochemical strains for organisms and immunofluorescent techniques usually are helpful diagnostic aids.[34]

ANTIARRHYTHMICS

Many antiarrhythmic drugs can themselves be responsible for serious arrhythmias, the most notable example being digitalis. Quinidine, besides causing hypersensitivity vasculitis and inducing a lupus-like syndrome, as already mentioned, can also cause syncope due to polymorphic ventricular tachyarrhythmia, commonly of a specific variety called torsades de pointes.[34a] Furthermore, it can induce digitalis toxicity by increasing its serum level.[34b] Disopyramide can also cause torsades de pointes[34c] and heart block,[34d] besides its negative inotropic effect and anticholinergic side effects. Amiodarone, besides causing hypersensitivity pneumonitis,[34e] may cause life-threatening ventricular arrhythmias,[34f] symptomatic sinus bradycardia and sinus arrest requiring pacemaker implantation,[34g] and asystole.[34h] Flecainide may induce ventricular tachyarrhythmias, including ventricular fibrillation.[34i]

ANALGESICS

Most of the cardiovascular effects of aspirin are hoped to be beneficial in that aspirin is a potent inhibitor of platelet aggregation, which is instrumental in the progression of atherosclerosis. However, whether or not long-time ingestion of small amounts of aspirin will indeed inhibit atherogenesis in man has yet to be proved. There is preliminary evidence that large doses of aspirin may actually increase endothelial permeability, allowing the influx of lipids into the atherosclerotic plaque. Some patients with aspirin sensitivity may develop hemorrhagic vasculitis when exposed to the drug.[35] The precise mechanisms involved in aspirin sensitivity are unknown. An immunologic basis is suspected, but a specific allergic response has yet to be related to clinical sensitivity. Probably the most damaging effect of aspirin on the cardiovascular system is mediated by the effects of hypertension secondary to analgesic nephropathy. Analgesic nephropathy has been reported in patients who have consumed large amounts of aspirin and also in patients taking phenacetin.[35] Aspirin is teratogenic and embryotoxic in animals, and there is some evidence that it may cause congenital malformations in man, including congenital heart defects.[35]

Paracetamol (acetaminophen), when taken in overdosage, may result in myocardial damage with subendocardial hemorrhage and focal muscle necrosis.[36] Indomethacin has been associated with hypersensitivity vasculitis and experimentally reduces systemic blood pressure and myocardial blood flow when given intravenously to anesthetized cats, suggesting that indomethacin might aggravate angina pectoris and predispose toward myocardial infarction.[37] Phenylbutazone has been associated with both hypersensitivity myocarditis and the induction of a lupus-like syndrome.[37] Allopurinol and colchicine, drugs used in the treatment of gout, have been associated with hypersensitivity vasculitis, whereas gold, when used in the treatment of rheumatoid arthritis, has been associated with necrotizing vasculitis.[37]

Methysergide, and less frequently ergotamine, may induce cardiac valvular lesions microscopically identical to those present in the carcinoid syndrome. The endocardium may contain similar lesions with or without contiguity with the valvular lesions.[8] Ergotamine and methysergide are capable of inducing marked arterial spasm with resulting ischemia.[21,24] When the coronary arteries are involved, angina pectoris or myocardial infarction may be precipitated.[4] With prolonged administration of these drugs, intimal proliferation, hyalinization, and medial hypertrophy may occur, resulting in structural compromise of the arterial lumen. Arterial thrombosis may result either during the period of intense spasm or superimposed upon an intimal proliferative lesion. Tolazoline has been implicated as a precipitating factor in myocardial infarction and occasionally may produce hypertension.[38]

The cardiovascular complications of opiate dependence (generally heroin dependence) are usually of two types: (1) those directly related to the drug (overdose syndrome and acute pulmonary edema) and (2) infection associated with nonsterile techniques of injection by addicts. In addition, the pulmonary arterioles may be occluded by intimal proliferative lesions containing silicates or corn starch in patients who inject certain drugs intravenously.[27a] Usually granulomas containing foreign body giant cells are present in adjacent pulmonary parenchyma.[26,27]

Many of the mood-altering drugs are associated with adverse cardiovascular reactions, including hypersensitivity myocarditis (amitriptyline), hypersensitivity vasculitis (diazepam), toxic myocarditis (lithium carbonate, phenothiazines, and amphetamines) and toxic vasculitis (amphetamines).[39]

Malignant hyperthermia is an inherited disorder in which affected individuals may react adversely to certain anesthetic agents and other stressful stimuli. The condition is inherited as an autosomal dominant trait with variable penetrance and expressivity. In susceptible individuals, potent inhalation agents or skeletal muscle relaxants may cause fever, skeletal muscle rigidity, cardiac arrhythmias, and occasionally, sudden death. Those patients who are malignant hyperthermia susceptible may also develop myopathic disorders including cardiomyopathy. The heart in a patient dying during an episode of malignant hyperthermia usually contains extensive contraction band necrosis.[39] Recent studies indicated a defect of intracellular calcium channels; dantrolene, which staunches calcium outflow from the sarcoplasmic reticulum, has been effective in treating this disorder.[39a]

ANTICOAGULANTS

Hypersensitivity reactions to heparin are well known but fortunately are rare. The most dramatic cardiovascular effect of heparin hypersensitivity is a vasospastic reaction.[40] Vasospasm may develop independent of the route of heparin administration. These reactions usually occur six to ten days after initiation of injections of the drug and they last four to six hours. Women are affected more commonly than men. The affected limb is painful, ischemic, and cyanosed.[41] If heparin treatment is not discontinued, similar but progressively more severe reactions will occur after each injection. In addition, there may be signs of generalized vasospasm. These vasospastic reactions appear to be induced by heparin-protein complex, with heparin as a hapten inducing antibody production and an antigen–antibody reaction with histamine liberation.[42] Protamine sulfate treatment has no marked therapeutic effect. Generally, the prognosis is good, but ischemic necrosis has been reported.[43] Approximately 50% of patients with significant heparin immune-induced thrombocytopenia also have associated intravascular thrombosis. This problem occurs more frequently in the elderly and in patients with myeloproliferative disorders and is associated with high morbidity and mortality. With arteriography, isolated, broad-based, lobulated excrescences can be recognized that produce 30% to 95% narrowing of the arterial lumen proximal to the sites of arterial occlusion.[44] This "white-clot" syndrome is probably the result of heparin-dependent platelet membrane antibodies formed in predisposed patients. Disseminated intravascular coagulation, with or without cardiogenic shock, may rarely occur following heparin injection. In these patients, the disseminated intravascular coagulation may partly be due to antibodies against heparin.[40] There is evidence that neutralization of heparin with protamine in vivo induces a hypercoagulable state associated with an increased risk of thromboembolism. This might be caused by the activation of factor VII or factor XII or both by heparin–protamine, as evidenced by a marked shortening of the thrombotest in vitro.[45] Metastatic arterial calcification in patients with chronic renal failure undergoing hemodialysis may be enhanced by the action of heparin, because the intravenous injection of large doses of heparin induces mobilization of calcium and inorganic phosphate. The widespread use of intermittent hemodialysis in uremic patients appears to have increased the incidence of pericardial tamponade and fibrinohemorrhagic pericarditis, perhaps influenced by heparinization.[10] Heparin activates lipoprotein lipase, thereby inducing an increase in nonesterified fatty acids, an effect that may be associated with arrhythmias and death in patients with myocardial infarction.[46]

In patients receiving coumarin derivatives, skin necrosis may rarely develop secondary to vascular damage.[40] It has been suggested that coumarin conjugers exert a toxic effect at the site of the dermovascular loop near the junction of the capillary and precapillary arterioles, which may lead to hemorrhage into the skin, particularly in the presence of preexisting cutaneous lesions or after minor trauma.[47] Petechiae appear secondary to ruptured capillaries and often become confluent within 24 hours. During the next 24 hours, thrombotic occlusion of the veins causes infarction with necrosis of skin and subcutaneous fat. These lesions have a predilection for sites rich in adipose tissue, such as the breast, abdomen, buttocks, thighs, and calves; however, other sites of the body may occasionally be involved. Obese, elderly women account for the vast majority of the cases.[40] Hemorrhagic skin necrosis has been described as occurring with all coumarin derivatives and during combined therapy with heparin and phenindione; in the latter situation the necrosis may be unusually extensive.[48] Hemopericardium with or without cardiac rupture is distinctly more frequent in cardiac patients treated with anticoagulants as compared with patients not treated with these drugs.[49] Less commonly, cases of "spontaneous" hemopericardium in patients on long-term anticoagulant treatment have been reported.[50] Overdosage or virus infection has been suspected as a precipitating cause in some of these patients with spontaneous or idiopathic pericardial effusion.[51] The postmyocardial infarction syndrome and the postpericardiotomy syndrome may be intensified by anticoagulants. Although one study concluded that the frequency of hemorrhage into atherosclerotic plaques was no different in patients receiving anticoagulants as compared with untreated patients, additional investigation of this potential problem is needed.[52]

Although the indandione derivatives do not differ from coumarin derivatives with respect to their antivitamin K activity, bleeding complications, or liability to produce skin necrosis, their use, unlike that of the coumarins, involves the hazard of hypersensitivity, including hypersensitivity myocarditis.[53] It is conceivable that the benzene ring in the indandione molecule is significant in the pathogenesis of this hypersensitivity reaction.

Although the causal relation has not been proven, there is suggestive evidence that antifibrinolytic agents may be capable of inducing a thrombotic microangiopathy. In some patients with carcinomatosis, most probably associated with disseminated intravascular coagulation, acute heart failure[54] and renal failure due to glomerular capillary thrombosis[55] have occurred during treatment with epsilon-aminocaproic acid.

ANTIMICROBIALS

Most morphologic changes in the heart and blood vessels associated with antibiotic therapy are hypersensitivity myocarditis or hypersensitivity vasculitis, or both.[39,56] Those antibiotics that have been associated with hypersensitivity myocarditis in human subjects are included in Table 51.1. The antibiotics that have been associated with hypersensitivity vasculitis in human subjects are included in Table 51.3. Less commonly, antimicrobials may be associated with toxic myocarditis (emetine and antineoplastic antibiotics) or toxic vasculitis (penicillin and sulfonamides).[39]

Occlusion and thrombosis following penicillin injection into arteries are rare; however, the consequences of such complications may be catastrophic. Most often injection of depot-penicillin preparations into the gluteal area is involved, and the superior gluteal artery has been accidently entered.[57] Ischemic reactions followed by gangrene have been described not only after injection of depot-penicillin preparations, but also after injection of a water-soluble penicillin solution.[58] The high pressure used for injection of viscous fluids may produce a retrograde flow of the drug into the larger arteries, such as the common iliac, abdominal aorta, renal, and spinal cord arteries. Therefore, resulting ischemia not only may involve the region of the inferior branch of the superior gluteal artery, but also may result in intestinal and renal hemorrhage, necrosis of the entire lower extremity, or paraplegia from spinal cord damage.[57] Although benzathine penicillin crystals have been identified in an artery following arterial embolization, it is not certain whether the distal ischemia results from a direct vascular toxic effect of the drug on the endothelium, inducing thrombosis, or by the induction of arterial spasm resulting in secondary thrombosis.[59] In rare cases it is possible that a thrombotic vascular occlusion, with propagation of the thrombus or embolization, or both, may result from the trauma of arterial puncture alone. Accidental intravenous injection of penicillin compounds may also occur, resulting in venous thrombosis and occasionally pulmonary embolization.

The Jarish–Herxheimer reaction may occur in some patients with syphilis treated with penicillin, resulting in sudden aneurysmal dilation of the arch of the aorta,[60] or acute coronary occlusion resulting in myocardial infarction.[61] The Herxheimer reaction has also been documented in patients with typhoid fever or sepsis caused by *Salmonella*, *Escherichia coli*, or *Proteus* treated with chloramphenicol.

Isoniazid may produce a lupus-like syndrome with pericarditis. Antinuclear antibodies and lupus erythematosus cells can be uniformly demonstrated.[62] Discontinuance of this drug usually causes complete disappearance of the symptoms, but occasionally it may take many months for the lupus erythematosus cells and the antibodies to disappear. Spontaneous recurrences have been described.[62]

Although thrombophlebitis may be associated with the intravenous administration of any antimicrobial, it most commonly occurs with the intravenous administration of vancomycin or amphotericin B. Purpura-like vasculitis has been described rarely in patients receiving ethambutol.[62]

Other antimicrobials, especially the antihelminthic drugs, may be associated with electrocardiographic changes; however, the histologic changes in the heart have not been fully described. Because of the rapid onset of these electrocardiographic changes following administration of the drug and the usual disappearance of these changes following cessation of therapy, the mechanism of cardiac damage appears to be a toxic effect. Sinus tachycardia and nonspecific electrocardiographic changes have been described following injection of streptomycin.[63] Stibocaptate has been associated with myocardial enzyme changes together with T-wave changes on the electrocardiogram and chest pain.[64] Electrocardiographic changes, primarily T-wave inversion, which disappeared after the completion of treatment, have been described in patients receiving piperazine.[64] T-wave flattening and inversion have been observed in patients receiving hycanthone and niridazole.[64] The electrocardiographic changes associated with the administration of niridazole have been reversed with atropine.[64]

DIURETICS

Those diuretics associated with hypersensitivity myocarditis and hypersensitivity vasculitis are summarized in Tables 51.1 and 51.3. In addition, necrotizing vasculitis in the skin has been reported in patients taking benzothiazides or chlorthalidone.[65] Henoch–Schönlein purpura has been described in patients taking ethacrynic acid or chlorothiazide.[66,67] Carbonic anhydrase inhibitors (acetazolamide) may induce allergic reactions with cross antigenicity with sulfonamides.[68] Sudden death of presumed cardiac origin has occurred following the intravenous injection of furosemide and with the intravenous administration of mercurial diuretics.[68,69] Clorexolone, quinethazone, metolazone, and mefruside have metabolic effects similar to those of the benzothiazine diuretics, including hypokalemia, hyperuricemia, and hyperglycemia. Primarily because of their potassium-depleting effect, the incidence of adverse reactions to digitalis is two to three times as high if the patient is taking one of these diuretics.[68] There are no available data to indicate that the hyperglycemia and hyperuricemia caused by these drugs accelerate atherosclerosis in patients receiving them in the treatment of hypertension. Further investigation of this potential complication is necessary, however, in light of the recent report that concurrent treatment with hydrochlorothiazide and propranolol may decrease the HDL cholesterol.[32] In contrast to the hypokalemic effects of the diuretics just discussed, spironolactone, triamterene, or amiloride causes retention of potassium, which may result in the disturbances of cardiac rhythm attendant on hyperkalemia. Drugs often used in conjunction with diuretics in the treatment of hypertension may also cause hypersensitivity myocarditis. This is especially true of methyldopa.[14]

CORTICOSTEROIDS AND OTHER IMMUNOSUPPRESSANTS

Long-term treatment with corticosteroids may be accompanied by arteritis involving small and medium arteries. In most cases it is not clear whether the arteritis is caused by the underlying disease or causally related to the treatment with steroids. Most of the available evidence points to the first possibility.[70] Corticosteroids alter carbohydrate metabolism, inducing abnormal glucose tolerance, especially in patients with a family history indicating a predisposition to diabetes mellitus.[71] Treatment with steroids also predisposes to an increased incidence of thromboembolic complications in both adults and children.[70] Although the evidence is not conclusive, it has been suggested that corticosteroids may induce intimal proliferation in arteries and veins of susceptible individuals similar to that seen in patients receiving oral contraceptives. The combination of damage to the arterial wall with arteritis, an increased tendency to thrombosis, alteration of carbohydrate metabolism, and possible intimal proliferation suggests that the long-term administration of corticosteroids may accelerate atherosclerosis. Steroid-induced hypertension must also be considered an additional risk factor in accelerating atherogenesis.

Although focal myocardial necrosis has been induced in experimental animals receiving large doses of corticosteroids, the induction of these lesions in human subjects has not been documented.[72] Some patients who die while receiving large doses of corticosteroids will have cytoplasmic vacuoles in myocytes, similar to those seen in patients with Cushing's syndrome or hypokalemia. Patients with cardiac sarcoidosis treated with steroids have an increased incidence of ventricular aneurysm.[73] The immunosuppressive effect of corticosteroids predisposes the patient to infection of the heart and blood vessels by opportunistic organisms.

The immunosuppressants most commonly associated with cardiotoxicity are the anthracycline antibiotics (daunomycin and its analogs, especially adriamycin) and cyclophosphamide. Although the anthracycline antibiotics can produce acute and subacute cardiac toxicity, these agents are more notoriously known for the chronic congestive cardiomyopathy that they produce in human subjects and experimental animals. The cardiotoxic effects of adriamycin are dose-related, and the critical dose is 500 mg per square meter. An accumulative dose below 500 mg per square meter yields a low incidence of cardiomyopathy; whereas approximately 30% of the patients receiving a larger dose will develop cardiomyopathy.[74]

The pathogenesis of this complication remains uncertain; however, a number of possible mechanisms have been proposed, including damage to DNA in cardiac muscle cells and peroxidative damage to cell membranes, mitochondrial membranes, and membranes of sarcoplasmic reticulum.[5] Mural thrombi are frequently present in both ventricles. Microscopically, the lesions are both focal and disseminated. The earliest lesions are most common in the subendocardium. In these early lesions, single isolated myocytes with degenerative changes are often dispersed in an otherwise morphologically intact myocardium.[75]

The degeneration induced by anthracyclines is manifested microscopically by myofibrillar loss and cytoplasmic vacuolization.[76–78] The latter is a prominent but focal finding that involves individual cells rather than large, confluent areas of myocardium and is caused by massive dilatation of tubules of sarcoplasmic reticulum; some dilatation of T tubules also occurs. This vacuolar degeneration can occur with apparent preservation of the nucleus and mitochondria. The two types of degeneration may occur concomitantly in the same cell or in separate cells. There does not appear to be a relation between the two types of injury and the severity or course of the cardiotoxicity.[75]

These lesions eventually progress to the death of the myocyte, at which time the nuclei become pyknotic and disintegrate, and the mitochondria swell and develop myelin figures. When the myocardial cells die, they are replaced by fibrous tissue, resulting in patchy stellate scars throughout the myocardium. Although the microscopic and ultrastructural changes of anthracycline cardiotoxicity are characteristic, these changes are not specific and can be seen in cardiomyopathy due to other conditions. The severity of the cardiac morphologic changes induced by anthracyclines has been evaluated by myocardial biopsies, and these have been useful in determining whether or not patients suspected of developing anthracycline cardiomyopathy can receive additional amounts of the drug.[75] In addition to the myocardial degenerative lesions just described herein, which characteristically are not accompanied by an inflammatory cell infiltrate, patients receiving anthracycline antibiotics may develop acute myopericarditis, which is thought to be reversible.

Cyclophosphamide, an alkylating agent used in the treatment of cancer, also is associated with a high incidence of cardiac toxicity, especially when administered in high-dose combination chemotherapy.[79,80] Cyclophosphamide-induced cardiotoxicity usually has an acute onset within hours or days after the beginning of treatment. Morphologically, there may be numerous large foci of hemorrhagic necrosis in the myocardium associated with extensive capillary microthrombosis, erythrocytes, and fibrin in the interstitium and necrotic myocytes.[81] Subpericardial and subendocardial ecchymosis with an acute inflammatory infiltrate may also be present. Treatment with cyclophosphamide may result in acute myopericarditis with or without hemorrhagic necrosis of the myocardium.[75] Electron microscopic examination of the myocardial lesions reveals capillary endothelial damage and unraveling of nuclear chromatin in both myocytes and endothelial cell nuclei, producing prominent thick, thin, and intermediate filaments.[81]

Antineoplastic drugs may indirectly cause damage to the cardiovascular system by their immunosuppressive effect, resulting in infective vasculitis, endocarditis, myocarditis, or pericarditis by opportunistic organisms.

ORAL CONTRACEPTIVES

Some women receiving oral contraceptives have an increase in (1) superficial venous thrombosis, (2) thrombosis of deep veins, (3) pulmonary embolism, (4) cerebral ischemia and thrombosis, (5) hypertension, (6) intimal proliferation with or without associated thrombosis, and (7) accelerated atherosclerosis. Both retrospective and prospective studies indicate that the risk of deep vein thrombophlebitis and pulmonary embolism is fivefold, and that the risk of stroke is tenfold in women taking oral contraceptives as compared with age-matched control subjects.[82,83] The risk of thromboembolic disease is greatest in women under age 35 years and does not appear to correlate with smoking.[84] The duration of the use of oral contraceptives apparently does not affect the risk. The effect of contraceptive steroids on the clotting mechanism is complex. Platelet aggregation is increased, and the platelet count may decrease slightly.[85] There is an increase in platelet factor 3.[86] Some women demonstrate a slightly increased intravascular coagulation activity, and in some women blood viscosity is increased.[87] Soluble fibrin increases up to 97% in many patients.[88] Sequential therapy apparently causes more pronounced changes in clotting factors than the usual combined treatment.[89]

Retrospective epidemiologic studies have suggested an association between the use of oral contraceptives and myocardial infarction in premenopausal women.[84,90,90a] These studies indicate that the risk of myocardial infarction is increased fivefold in oral contraceptive users. This risk is greatest in women with preexisting medical conditions, especially diabetes mellitus, hypertension, or a history of ischemic heart disease. Intimal proliferation may be present in the extramural as well as intramural coronary arteries. Intimal proliferation may be extensive, resulting in marked luminal compromise, and occasionally there may be a superimposed occlusive thrombus.[19] Other women dying of myocardial infarction may have classic atherosclerotic lesions in the extramural coronary arteries. Oral contraceptives are associated with multiple risk factors known to accelerate atherosclerosis. These risk factors include the induction or exacerbation of hypertension in some patients, increased platelet aggregation and altered coagulation, increase in serum cholesterol, with an occasional decrease in the high density lipoprotein fraction, an increase in triglycerides as well as phospholipids and fatty acids, and altered carbohydrate metabolism with a decrease in glucose tolerance and increased plasma insulin levels. Additionally, women taking the contraceptive pill have significantly lower blood levels of vitamin B_6 than do other women.[91] Vitamin B_6 is necessary for the clearing of homocystine from the blood. Experimental studies in baboons indicate that homocystine is a potent inducer of atherosclerosis.[91] These alterations induced by the contraceptive pill, when combined with other risk factors such as cigarette smoking, may well accelerate atherogenesis.

Oral contraceptives may induce hypertension or exacerbate preexisting hypertension through alterations of the renin–angiotensin system.[92,93] Estrogen causes a marked elevation in plasma angiotensin (renin substrate). Renin acts on the substrate to produce angiotensin I, which is hydrolyzed to produce angiotensin II, an active pressor substance. Angiotensin II stimulates the adrenal cortex to produce aldosterone, which causes water and sodium retention. This, along with variables such as blood volume and increased arterial tone, may produce hypertension, especially if there is increased cardiac output and a compensatory failure of sodium and water excretion. The estrogen component of oral contraceptives appears to be the main agent responsible for the hypertension, but the progestin component has not been completely absolved.[94] It is not possible to explain the elevation of blood pressure on the renin–angiotensin system alone. Plasma renin substrate and plasma renin activity are increased in both hypertensive and normotensive patients taking oral contraceptives. When hypertension occurs, it is usually within the first 6 months. Both diastolic and systolic levels may be elevated. Usually the blood pressure returns to normal levels within 3 to 6 months after cessation of oral contraceptive therapy.[94] Although the hypertension is usually mild, there are reports of hypertensive crisis and renal failure in patients receiving contraceptive steroids.[95]

A rare but catastrophic complication associated with the use of oral contraceptives is hepatic vein thrombosis (Budd–Chiari syndrome).[96] Hereditary hemorrhagic telangiectasia is aggravated by oral contraceptives.[97]

RADIATION INJURY TO THE HEART

First reported by Seguy and Quenisset[98] in 1897, radiation-induced heart disease is now widely understood. The consequences of mediastinal radiation have been characterized by many investigators and involve the pericardium,[99–106] coronary arteries,[107–110] myocardium,[111–115] endocardium and cardiac valves,[116] and the conduction tissues[117–119] (Table 51.6).

Table 51.6. Spectrum of Radiation-Induced Cardiac Disease

I. Acute pericarditis
   - Early (during the course of irradiation)
   - Delayed

II. Chronic pericarditis
   - Pericardial effusion
   - Constrictive pericarditis

III. Myocardial involvement
   - Myocardial fibrosis
   - Myocardial necrosis secondary to radiation-induced coronary disease

IV. Endocardial fibrosis

V. Valvular dysfunction secondary to fibrosis and thickening

VI. Vascular: accelerated atherosclerosis with subintimal fibrosis of coronary artery and other vessels (aortic arch vessels, renal iliac, intestinal, etc)

VII. Conduction disturbances

Of the cardiac tissues, the pericardium is most commonly affected by radiation. Doses of radiation usually in excess of 4,000 rads produce acute pericarditis, usually after 1 to 6 or more months, in more than 30% of individuals so exposed. Pericarditis may occur acutely during the course of radiation or in some patients it may be considerably delayed. Chronic pericarditis may be manifested by pericardial effusion or chronic constriction, or both.[120]

Pericardial effusion is the most common manifestation of radiation injury,[121] and this may progress to tamponade[102] or chronic constrictive pericarditis.[100] Clinical features include pericarditic pain; elevated jugular venous pressure; an early diastolic filling sound (pericardial "knock"); and, to varying degrees, features of systemic venous hypertension, such as hepatic enlargement, ascites, and edema. There is enlargement of the cardiac silhouette on chest roentgenogram, and the electrocardiogram reveals evidence of changes compatible with pericarditis. Two-dimensional echocardiography is excellent for documenting pericardial effusion. Computed axial tomography aids in identifying both pericardial thickening and fluid, as well as malignant tumor involvement, which may coexist or mimic radiation involvement of the heart. Pericardiocentesis may be required to differentiate malignant from radiation pericarditis.[122] The differential diagnosis must also include myxedematous pericardial effusion, because hypofunction of the thyroid may follow mediastinal irradiation.[123] Treatment consists of salicylates and indomethacin.[121] The successful use of corticosteroid therapy also has been reported.[124,125] Pericardiocentesis may be required and aggressive surgical pericardiectomy has been recommended, even early in the course of effusive disease.[104,126] Constrictive pericarditis may occur many years after therapy,[127–130] and the patient may require surgical decortication, although differentiation from a restrictive myopathy may be difficult. In this regard computed axial tomography is particularly helpful in confirming major thickening of the pericardium.[131]

The genesis of postirradiation pericarditis has been the subject of some debate. A direct radiation effect is considered the most likely cause, but hypersensitivity reaction, radiation-induced vasculitis, and reaction to tumor-cell necrosis are possible factors.[121,129,132] Others have also considered radiation-induced obstruction of lymphatic vessels within the pericardium to be important in this process.[133]

Myocardial necrosis and hyalinization secondary to radiation were first described by Davis[134] in 1924; Stewart and Fajardo[105] noted pericarditis with neutrophilic infiltration within days of exposure of rabbits of 2,000 rads of radiation to the heart. A long period of time followed during which no changes were evident on light microscopy; however, during this period, electron microscopy disclosed abnormalities within the capillaries. After 8 to 10 weeks, a fibrotic reaction was visible on light-microscopic examination. These investigators postulate that the early capillary damage was responsible for the ultimate myocardial fibrosis, probably mediated by acute capillary endothelial injury and subsequent loss of capillaries, resulting in a chronic state of ischemia, late death of myocytes, and interstitial fibrosis.[112,113,135] These changes can ultimately result in clinical features of restrictive or congestive cardiomyopathy.[121,136,137] In some patients the right ventricle was involved more severely than the left, probably because of its anterior location. The consequent selective clinical features of right-sided heart failure may make the differential diagnosis of radiation-induced cardiomyopathy and constrictive pericarditis even more difficult.

Clinical abnormalities in the period following radiation may be of either myocardial or pericardial origin. Electrocardiographic changes usually consist of transitory ST–T-wave abnormalities. Cardiac enzymes may occasionally be elevated. Technetium-pyrophosphate uptake by the heart may also be noted after chest radiation,[110,138] and radiation-induced cardiomyopathy has been documented by gated radionuclide ventriculography.[139]

Additionally, the cancer chemotherapeutic agents may act synergistically with radiation in the genesis of a cardiomyopathic picture.

Coronary occlusion following mediastinal radiation therapy was first reported by Pearson[140] in 1957. Irradiation can cause coronary artery occlusive disease, either by coronary artery fibrosis or by accelerated atherosclerosis. Chest irradiation of experimental animals has produced coronary fibrosis and myocardial infarction.[110] These lesions were related to doses and demonstrated angiographically. Experimental animals, fed an atherogenic diet and exposed to cardiac irradiation, developed severe atherosclerotic coronary occlusive disease related in magnitude to the severity of the atherogenic diet and to the radiation dose.[110] The occurrence of coronary disease in patients more than 40 years of age who have received radiation therapy may be coincidental. Such does not appear to be the case, however, in younger subjects, many of whom lacked any other risk factors, who have developed postradiation angina, infarction, or sudden coronary death together with angiographically or anatomically demonstrable coronary occlusive disease.[110] These patients have anatomically demonstrated either fibrous changes or accelerated atherosclerosis in the coronary arteries.[107–109,115,141–144] An occasional patient with postradiation coronary artery occlusive disease has required aortocoronary saphenous vein bypass grafting as treatment for angina at a young age.[115,145]

Fajardo et al[112] in 1968 were the first to describe focal fibrosis endocardial changes. If severe, these changes may resemble congenital fibroelastosis. Valvular lesions, usually incompetence of the aortic or mitral valve, have been reported, and deformity and thickening of the valves have been described in postmortem findings.[104,129,136,146,147] Stenosis of cardiac valves is infrequent[116,148] but may lead to hemodynamic and clinical sequelae.

There have been several reported examples of complete heart block following radiation therapy.[117–119] Bundle branch block has also been reported.[144,146]

Radiation effects on the heart to varying degrees involve all of the cardiac tissues. Involvement is a function of the dose and the port of radiation exposure and, in lesser degrees, may be clinically inapparent yet evident on postmortem examination.[136] Furthermore, the length of time the patient is alive after exposure to radiation may be an important factor in the character and degree of the clinical expression of radiation injury.[116]

CARDIAC INJURY INVOLVING CATHETERS

Perforation of the right ventricle with a cardiac catheter is rare.[149] Perforation by a transvenous pacing electrode is more common,[150] although tamponade is uncommon. Perforation may also complicate endomyocardial biopsy.[151]

Complications during cardiac catheterization and coronary angiography additionally include acute myocardial infarction, cerebrovascular accidents, and arrhythmias, any of which may be fatal.[152–154] In a registry of over 53,000 patients studied, these complications were infrequent and mortality was 0.14%.[152]

Valve injury is rarely the consequence of trauma by an intracardiac catheter.[154a] Infective endocarditis may complicate placement of a permanent transvenous pacing catheter as well as thrombotic occlusion of the superior vena cava and recurrent thromboembolism of the pulmonary vascular bed.

Coronary angiographic catheter manipulation has resulted in both aortic dissection and coronary artery dissection, as well as coronary thrombotic occlusion.[155,156] Coronary air embolism may result from incomplete purging of air from catheter and syringe systems. Although this is usually of no consequence, ventricular fibrillation may ensue. Indeed, ventricular arrhythmias, including ventricular fibrillation, may complicate intracardiac catheterization, ventriculography, and coronary angiography.

Coronary balloon angioplasty may result in conversion of subtotal coronary occlusion into complete occlusion by thrombus formation or dissection of the coronary artery.[157,158] A pericarditis-like syndrome may occur early after coronary balloon angioplasty accompanied by ST- and T-wave changes and is probably the consequence of limited subepicardial ecchymosis resulting from minor coronary artery dissection.[159] A postpericardiotomy syndrome has not been recognized after this event, but it has occurred following recognized and apparent but unrecognized cardiac perforation with intracardiac catheters and biopsy devices. Coronary arterial damage and ultimate stenosis also have been reported following coronary artery cannulation at the time of aortic valve replacement.[160]

Balloon-tipped, flow-directed catheters (Swan–Ganz) currently are widely used for hemodynamic monitoring in intensive and critical care units. Complications following their use are rare, although right-sided infective endocarditis[161] and rupture of the pulmonary artery[162] have been reported recently.

Acknowledgment: We gratefully acknowledge the assistance of Debbie Charanza in the preparation of this manuscript.

REFERENCES

1. Fenoglio JJ, McAllister HA, Mullick FG: Drug related myocarditis. I. Hypersensitivity myocarditis. *Hum Pathol* 1981; 12:900–907.
2. McAllister HA: Collagen vascular disease and the cardiovascular system, in Silver MD (ed): *Cardiovascular Pathology.* New York, Churchill Livingstone, Inc, 1982, pp 1005–1033.
3. Kalikshtein DB, Odinokova VA, Paleev NR, Gurevich MA: Hypersensitivity of delayed type manifested during the development of allergic lesions of the myocardium. *Bull Exp Biol Med* 1975; 77:789-791.

3a. Taliercio CP, Olney BA, Lie JT: Myocarditis related to drug hypersensitivity. *Mayo Clin Proc* 1985; 60:463-468.

3b. Myocarditis related to drug hypersensitivity, editorial. *Lancet* 1985; 2:1165-1166.

4. Cheitlin MD, McAllister HA, DeCastro CM: Myocardial infarction without atherosclerosis. *JAMA* 1975; 231:951-959.
5. Ferrans VJ: Overview of morphologic reactions of the heart to toxic injury, in Balazs T (ed): *Cardiac Toxicology.* Boca Raton, Fl, CRC Press, 1981, pp 83–109.
6. Mason JW, Billingham ME, Friedman JP: Methysergide-induced heart disease. A case of multivalvular and myocardial fibrosis. *Circulation* 1977; 56:889-893.
7. Graham JR: Cardiac and pulmonary fibrosis during methysergide therapy for headache. *Am J Med Sci* 1967; 254:1-7.
8. Bana DS, McNeal PS, LeCompte PM, Shah Y, Graham JR: Cardiac murmurs and endocardial fibrosis associated with methysergide therapy. *Am Heart J* 1975; 88:640–647.
9. Simherkoff MS: Narcotic associated infective endocarditits, in Kaplan EL, Taranta AV (eds): *Infective Endocarditis: An American Heart Association Symposium.* American Heart Association Monograph, No. 42. Dallas, American Heart Association, Inc, 1977, p 46.
10. McAllister HA: Pathology of the cardiovascular system in chronic renal failure, in Lowenthal D, Pennock R, Likoff W, Onesti G (eds): *Management of Cardiovascular Disease in Renal Failure.* Philadelphia, FA Davis, 1981, pp 1–16.
11. Rodnan GP, McEwen C, Wallace SL (eds): Primer on the rheumatic diseases. *JAMA* 1973; 224 (suppl):662–812.
12. Lerner PI, Weinstein L: Infective endocarditis in the antibiotic era. *N Engl J Med* 1966; 274:199–201.
13. Mullick FG, McAllister HA Jr, Wagner BM, Fenoglio JJ: Drug related vasculitis: clinicopathologic correlation in 30 patients. *Hum Pathol* 1979; 10:313–325.
14. Mullick FG, McAllister HA: Myocarditis associated with methyldopa. *JAMA* 1977; 237:1699–1704.
15. Citron BP, Halpern M, McCarron M, Lundberg GD, McCormick R, Pincus IJ, Tatter D, Haverback BJ: Necrotizing angitis associated with drug abuse. *N Engl J Med* 1970; 283:1003–1005.
16. Gocke DJ, Hsu K, Morgan C, Hsu K, Bombardieri S, Christian CL: Association between polyarteritis and Australian antigen. *Lancet* 1970; 2:1149–1151.
17. Baker AL, Marshall MK, Wendy CB, Sidel JS, Wolfe HJ: Polyarteritis associated with Australian antigen-positive hepatitis. *Gastroenterology* 1972; 62:105–111.
18. Irey NS, Manion WC, Taylor HB: Vascular lesions in women taking oral contraceptives. *Arch Pathol* 1970; 89:1–6.
19. Irey NS, Norris HJ: Intimal vascular lesions associated with female reproductive steroids. *Arch Pathol* 1973; 96:227–234.
20. Irey NS, McAllister HA, Henry JM: Oral contraceptives and stroke in young women: a clinicopathologic correlation. *Neurology* 1978; 28:1216–1219.
21. Gould SE, Price AE, Ginsberg HI: Gangrene and death following ergotamine tartrate (Gynergen) therapy. *JAMA* 1936; 106:1631–1637.
22. Yater WM, Cahill JA: Bilateral gangrene of feet due to ergotamine tartrate used for pruritus and jaundice. *JAMA* 1936; 106:1625–1630.
23. Young JR, Humphries AW: Severe arteriospasm after use of ergotamine tartrate suppositories. *JAMA* 1961; 175:1141–1146.
24. Regan JF, Poletti BJ: Vascular adventitial fibrosis in a patient taking methysergide maleate. *JAMA* 1968; 203:1069–1074.
25. Schwarts DT: Relation of superior mesenteric artery obstruction to renal hypertension. *N Engl J Med* 1965; 272:1318–1321.
26. Siegel H: Human pulmonary pathology associated with narcotic and other addictive drugs. *Hum Pathol* 1972; 8:55–66.
27. Lewman LV: Fatal pulmonary hypertension from intravenous injection of methylphenidate (Ritalin) tablets. *Human Pathol* 1972; 3:67–70.

27a. Cheng TO: Cardiovascular complications, in Pradhan SN (ed): *Drug Abuse: Clinical and Basic Aspects.* St. Louis, CV Mosby, 1977, pp 388–399.

28. Kannel WB: Possible hazards of oral contraceptive use. *Circulation* 1979; 60:490–492.
29. HDL and CHD, editorial. *Lancet* 1976; 2:131–132.

29a. Rubenstein C, Romhilt D, Segal P, Heiss G, Chambless LE, Boyle KE, Ekelund L-G, Adolph R, Sheffield LT: Dyslipoproteinemias and manifestations of coronary heart disease. The Lipid Research Clinics Program Prevalence Study. *Circulation* 1986; 73(suppl I):I-91–I-99.

30. Bradley DD, Petitti DB, Wingerd J, Krauss RM, Ramcharan S: Serum high-density-lipoprotein cholesterol in women using oral contraceptives, estrogens and progestins. *N Engl J Med* 1978; 299:17–19.
31. Calvert GD, Mannik T, Graham JJ, Wise PH, Yeates RA: Effects of therapy on plasma-high-density-lipoprotein-cholesterol concentration in diabetes mellitus. *Lancet* 1978; 2:66–69.
32. Helgeland A, Hjermann I, Leren P: High-density-lipoprotein cholesterol and antihypertensive drugs. The Oslo study. *Br Med J* 1978; 2:403–412.

32a. LaRosa JC, Levy RI, Hazzard WR: Some clinical implications of the results of the Lipid Research Clinics Program Prevalence Study. *Circulation* 1986; 73(suppl I):I-126–I-133.

33. Humbert G, Delaunay P, Leroy J: Accident vasculaire cerebral an cours d'un traitment par les gonadotrophins. *Norv Presse Med* 1973; 2:28–36.
34. McAllister HA, Ferrans VJ: The heart and blood vessels, in Silverberg JS (ed): *Principles and Practice of Surgical Pathology.* New York, John Wiley & Sons, Inc, 1983, pp 615–652.

34a. Bauman JL, Bauernfeind RA, Hoff JV, Strasberg B, Swiryn S, Rosen KM: Torsade de pointes due to quinidine: observations in 31 patients. *Am Heart J* 1984; 107:425–430.

34b. Cheng TO: Digoxin–quinidine interaction. *J Am Geriatr Soc* 1982; 30:79.

34c. Azpitarte Almagro J, Casero A, Melgares R: Torsade de pointes induced by disopyramide: presentation of a case with fatal outcome. *Rev Esp Cardiol* 1984; 37:145–148.

34d. Timins BI, Gutman JA, Haft JI: Disopyramide-induced heart block. *Chest* 1981; 79:477–479.

34e. Akoun GM, Gauthier-Rahman S: Amiodarone pneumonitis: three further cases with a review of published reports. *Thorax* 1984; 39:800.

34f. Kumana CR, Tanser P, Eydt J: Life-threatening ventricular arrhythmias provoked by amiodarone treatment. *Hum Toxicol* 1985; 4:169–176.

34g. Raeder EA, Podrid PJ, Lown B: Side effects and complications of amiodarone therapy. *Am Heart J* 1985; 109:975–983.

34h. Kuo CS, Reddy CP, Paciotti MV: Asystole during treatment with amiodarone in a patient with persistent atrial tachycardia. *J Electrocardiol* 1985; 18:105–110.

34i. Ramhamadany E, MacKenzie S, Ramsdale DR: Dysarthria and visual hallucinations due to flecainide toxicity. *Postgraduate Med J* 1986; 62:61–62.

35. Vanecek J: Antipyretic analgesics, in Dukes MNG (ed): *Meyler's Side Effects of Drugs.* New York, American Elsevier, 1984, vol 10, pp 135–150.
36. Sanerkin NG: Acute myocardial necrosis in paracetamol poisoning. *Br Med J* 1971; 3:478–483.
37. Vrhovac B: Anti-inflammatory analgesics and drugs used in the treatment of rheumatoid arthritis and gout, in Dukes MNG (ed): *Meyler's Side Effects of Drugs,* New York, American Elsevier, 1984, vol 10, pp 151–182.
38. Huzulakova I, Dukes MNG: Drugs affecting autonomic functions, in Dukes MNG (ed): *Meyler's Side Effects of Drugs.* New York, American Elsevier, 1984, vol 10, pp 232–253.
39. McAllister HA, Mullick FG: The cardiovascular system, in Riddel R, (ed): *Pathology of Drug-Induced and Toxic Diseases.* New York, Churchill Livingstone, 1982, pp 201–228.

39a. Merz B: Malignant hyperthermia: nightmare for anesthesiologists and patients. Defect in intracellular calcium channels is culprit in malignant hyperthermia. *JAMA* 1986; 255:709–715.

40. Loeliger EA: Drug affecting blood clotting and fibrinolysis, in Dukes MNG (ed): *Meyler's Side Effects of Drugs.* New York, American Elsevier, 1984, vol 10, pp 648–693.

41. Turcotte JG, Kraft RO, Fry WJ: Heparin reactions in patients with vascular disease. *Arch Surg* 1965; 90:375–382.
42. Coon WW, Willis PW III: Some side-effects of heparin heparinoids and their antagonists. *Clin Pharmacol Ther* 1966; 7:379–384.
43. Gayer W: Seltene Blobachtungen von Heparin—Unvertaglichkeit. *Gynalcologia (Basel)* 1968; 166:25–32.
44. Lindsey SM, Maddison FE, Towne JB: Heparin-induced thromboembolism: angiographic features. *Radiology* 1979; 131:771–774.
45. Godal HC, Gjengedal G: Activation of coagulation by heparin-protamine complexes as demonstrated by thrombotest. *Scand J Haematol* 1971; 8:194–199.
46. Kurien VA, Yates PA, Oliver MF: Free fatty acids, heparin and arrhythmias during experimental myocardial infarction. *Lancet* 1969; 2: 185–188.
47. Nalbandian RM, Mader IJ, Barret JL, Pearce JF, Rupp EC: Petechiae ecchymoses and necrosis of skin induced by coumarin congeners. *JAMA* 1958; 192:603–607.
48. Desai SN: Extensive skin necrosis following anticoagulant therapy. *Br J Plast Surg* 1967; 20:325–331.
49. Aarseth S, Lange H: The influence of anticoagulant therapy on the occurrence of cardiac rupture and haemopericardium following heart infarction. *Am Heart J* 1958; 56:250–258.
50. Fell SC, Rubin IL, Enselberg, CD, Hurwitt ES: Anticoagulant-induced haemopericardium with tamponade; its occurrence in the absence of myocardial infarction or pericarditis. *N Engl J Med* 1965; 272:670–673.
51. Miller RL: Haemopericardium with use of oral anticoagulant therapy. *JAMA* 1969; 209:1362–1366.
52. Jorgensen L, Chandler AB, Borchgrevink CF: Acute lesions of coronary arteries in anticoagulant-treated and in untreated patients. *Atherosclerosis* 1971; 13:21–26.
53. Kerwin AJ: Fatal myocarditis due to sensitivity to phenindione. *Can Med Assoc J* 1964; 90:1418–1423.
54. Johansson S: Acute right heart failure during treatment with epsilon amino caproic acid (EACA). *Acta Med Scand* 1967; 182:331–337.
55. Charitan C, Purtilo D: Glomerular capillary thrombosis and acute renal failure after epsilon amino caproic acid. *N Engl J Med* 1969; 280:1102–1105.
56. Fighali F, Strickman NE, Hall RJ: Congestive cardiomyopathy presumably secondary to oxacillin. *Texas Heart Inst J* 1983; 10:421–423.
57. Hoigne R: Penicillins, cephalosporins and tetracyclines, in Dukes MNG (ed): *Meyler's Side Effects of Drugs.* New York, American Elsevier, 1975, vol 8, pp 551–593.
58. Hoigne R, Keller H, Sonntag R: Penicillins, cephalosporins and tetracyclines, in Dukes MNG (ed): *Meyler's Side Effects of Drugs.* New York, American Elsevier, New York, 1984, vol 10, pp 446–491.
59. Stiehl P, Weissbach G, Schroter K: Das nicolan-syndrom. Zur pathogenese and klinik arteriellembolischer penicillinzwischenfalle. *Schweiz Med Wchnschr* 1971; 101:377–378.
60. Diefenbach WCL: Fatal Jarish–Herxheimer reaction with sudden aneurysmal dilatation and complete bronchial occlusion following penicillin therapy. *N Engl J Med* 1949, 241:95–96.
61. Butterly JM, Fishman L: Jarish Herxheimer reaction following penicillin therapy in a case of syphilitic aortitis. *JAMA* 1952; 148:370–375.
62. Meyer H, Hoigne R: Drugs used in the treatment of tuberculosis and leprosy, in Dukes MNG (ed): *Meyler's Side Effects of Drugs.* New York, American Elsevier, 1984, vol 10, pp 572–590.
63. Martin PD: ECG change associated with streptomycin. *Chest* 1974; 65: 478–483.
64. Langman MJS: Anthelminthic drugs, in Dukes MNG (ed): *Meyler's Side Effects of Drugs.* New York, American Elsevier, 1984, vol 10, p 690.
65. Bjomberg A, Gisslen H: Thiazides: a cause of necrotizing vasculitis? *Lancet* 1965; 2:982–985.
66. Bar-On H, Eisenberg S, Eliakin M: Clinical experience with ethacrynic acid—with reference to a possible complication of the Schoenlein–Henoch type. *Israel J Med Sci* 1967; 3:113–117.
67. Reid JM, Stevenson JG, Orr M: Non-thrombocytopenic purpura due to chlorothiazide. *Scot Med J* 1969; 14:309–314.
68. Offerhaus L: Adverse reaction to diuretic drugs, in Dukes MNG (ed): *Meyler's Side Effects of Drugs.* New York, American Elsevier, 1984, vol 10, pp 369–385.
69. Machtely I: Sudden death after intramuscular furosemide. *Lancet* 1968; 2:1301–1303.
70. von Eickstedt KW: Corticotrophins and corticosteroids, in Dukes MNG (ed): *Meyler's Side Effects of Drugs.* New York, American Elsevier, 1984, vol 10, pp 727–743.
71. McKiddie MT, Jasani MK, Buchanan KD, Boyle JA, Buchanan WW: The relationship between glucose tolerance, plasma insulin and corticosteroid therapy in patients with rheumatoid arthritis. *Metabolism* 1968; 17:730–736.
72. Karstad L, Tabel H, Gordon D: Myocardial necrosis and mineralization in normal and Aleutian disease in mink fed dexamethasone. *Can J Comp Med* 1969; 33:253–257.
73. Roberts WC, McAllister HA, Ferrans VJ: Sarcoidosis of the heart: a clinicopathologic study of 35 necropsy patients (group I) and review of 78 previously described necropsy patients (group II). *Am J Med* 1977; 63:86–108.
74. Lefrak EA, Pitha J, Rosenheim S, Gottlieb JA: A clinicopathologic anatomy of adriamycin cardiotoxicity. *Cancer* 1973; 32:302–308.
75. Billingham ME: Some recent advances in cardiac pathology. *Human Pathol* 1979; 10:367–376.
76. Jaenke RS, Fajardo LF: Adriamycin-induced myocardial lesions; report of a workshop. *Am J Surg Pathol* 1977; 1:55–62.
77. Buja LM, Ferrans VJ, Mayer RJ, Roberts WC, Henderson ES: Cardiac ultrastructural changes induced by daunorubicin therapy. *Cancer* 1973; 32:771–779.
78. Billingham ME, Mason JW, Bistow MR, Daniels JR: Anthracycline cardiomyopathy monitored by morphologic changes. *Cancer Treat Rep* 1978; 62:865–872.
79. Buckner CD, Rudolf RH, Fefer A, Clift RA, Epstein RB, Funk DD, Weiman PE, Slichter SJ, Sturb R, Thomas ED: High dose cyclophosphamide therapy for malignant disease. *Cancer* 1972; 29:357–362.
80. Applebaum FR, Strauchen JA, Graw R, Savage DD, Kent KM, Ferrans VJ, Herzig GP: Acute lethal carditis caused by high dose combination chemotherapy. *Lancet* 1976; 1:58–61.
81. Buja LM, Ferrans VJ: Myocardial injury produced by antineoplastic drugs, in Fleckenstein A, Rona G (eds): *Recent Advances in Studies on Cardiac Structure and Metabolism.* Baltimore, University Park Press, 1975, vol 6, pp 487–509.
82. Sartwell PE, Masi AT, Arthes FG, Greene GR, Smith HE: Thromboembolism and oral contraceptives: an epidemiologic case-control study. *Am J Epidemiol* 1969; 90:365–372.
83. Kyser FA, Finsberg H, Gilbert NC: The effect of certain drugs upon the cardiotoxic lesions of digitalis in the dog. *Am Heart J* 1946; 31:451–459.
84. Jick H, Dinan B, Herman R, Rothman KJ: Myocardial infarction and other vascular diseases in young women: role of estrogen and other factors. *JAMA* 1978; 240:2548–2551.
85. Mettler Z, Selchow BM: Oral contraceptives and platelet function. *Thromb Diath Haemorrh* 1972; 28:213–221.
86. Renaud S, Gautheron P: Role of platelet factor 3 in the hypercoagulability induced by pregnancy and oral contraceptives. *Thromb Diath Haemorrh* 1973; 30:299–304.
87. Aronson HB, Magora F, Schewker JG: Effect of oral contraceptives on blood viscosity. *Am J Obstet Gynecol* 1971; 110:997–1004.
88. Pileram LO, Ellison J, Von Dern Bussche G: Oral contraceptives and increased formation of soluble fibrin. *Br Med J* 1974; 3:556–562.
89. Mink IB, Courey NG, Niswander KR, Moore RH, Lillie MA, Ambrus JL: Progestational agents and blood coagulation. V. Changes induced by sequential oral contraceptive therapy. *Am J Obstet Gynecol* 1974; 119: 401–408.
90. Mann JI, Inman WHW: Oral contraceptives and death from myocardial infarction. *Br Med J* 1975; 2:245–249.
90a. Stadel BV: Oral contraceptives and cardiovascular disease. *N Engl J Med* 1981; 305:612–618, 672–677.
91. Gruberg ER, Raymond SA: Beyond cholesterol: a new theory on arteriosclerosis. *Atlanta Mo* 1979; 59–61.
92. Beckerhoff R, Luetscher JA, Wilkinson R, Gonzalez C, Nokes JW: Plasma renin concentration, activity and substrate in hypertension induced by oral contraceptives. *J Clin Endocrinol Metab* 1972; 34:1067–1073.
93. Low J, Oparil S: Oral contraceptive pill hypertension. *J Reprod Med* 1975; 15:201–209.
94. Crane MG, Harris JJ: Plasma renin activity and aldosterone excretion rate in normal subjects. II. Effects of oral contraceptive agents. *J Clin Endocrinol Metab* 1969; 29:558–564.
95. Tobon H: Malignant hypertension, uremia and hemolytic anemia in a patient on oral contraceptives. *Obstet Gynecol* 1972; 40:681–686.
96. Dukes MNG: Hormonal contraceptives, in Dukes MNG (ed): *Meyler's Side Effects of Drugs.* New York, American Elsevier, 1984, vol 10, pp 744–763.
97. Rowley PT, Kurnick J, Cheville R: Hereditary haemorrhagic telangiectasia, aggravation by oral contraceptives. *Lancet* 1970; 1:474–477.
98. Seguy G, Quenisset F: Action des rayons X sur le coeur (abstr). *Comput Rendu Acad Sci* 1897; 124:790.
99. Maslund DS, Rotz CT, Harris JH: Postradiation pericarditis with chronic pericardial effusion. *Ann Intern Med* 1968; 69:97–102.
100. Muggia FM, Cassileth PA: Constrictive pericarditis following radiation therapy. *Am J Med* 1968; 44:116–123.
101. Blumenfeld H, Thomas SF: Chronic massive pericardial effusion following roentgen therapy for carcinoma of the breast. *Radiology* 1945; 44:335–340.
102. Hurst DW: Radiation fibrosis of pericardium with cardiac tamponade. *Can Med Assoc J* 1959; 81:377–380.
103. Teng CY, Nemickas R, Robin JR Jr, Szanto PB, Gunnar RM: Pericardial effusion following radiation to the chest: report of a case. *Dis Chest* 1967; 52:549–552.
104. Morton DL, Glancy DL, Joseph WL, Adkins PC: Management of pa-

tients with radiation induced pericarditis with effusion: a note in the development of aortic regurgitation in two of them. *Chest* 1973; 64: 291–297.
105. Stewart JR, Fajardo LF: Dose response in human and experimental radiation-induced heart disease. *Radiology* 1971; 99:403–408.
106. Byhardt R, Brace K, Ruckdeschel J, Chang P, Martin R, Wiernick P: Dose and treatment factors in radiation related pericardial effusion associated with the mantle technique for Hodgkin's disease. *Cancer* 1975; 35:795–802.
107. Dollinger MR, Lavine DM, Foye LV Jr: Myocardial infarction due to postirradiation fibrosis of the coronary arteries. *JAMA* 1966; 195:316–319.
108. Huff H, Saunders EM: Coronary artery occlusion after radiation. *N Engl J Med* 1972; 286:780.
109. McReynolds RA, Gold GL, Roberts WC: Coronary heart disease after mediastinal irradiation for Hodgkin's disease. *Am J Med* 1976; 60:39–45.
110. Kopelson G, Herwig KJ: The etiologies of coronary artery disease in cancer patients. *Int J Radiat Oncol Biol Phys* 1978; 4:895–906.
111. Bolti RE, Driscol TE, Pearson OH, Smith JC: Radiation myocardial fibrosis simulating constrictive pericarditis. *Cancer* 1968; 22:1254–1261.
112. Fajardo LF, Stewart JR, Cohn KE: Morphology of radiation-induced heart disease. *Arch Pathol* 1968; 86:512–519.
113. Fajardo LF, Stewart JR: Experimental radiation induced heart disease. *Am J Pathol* 1970; 59:299–316.
114. Rubin E, Camara J, Grayzel DM, Zak FG: Radiation-induced cardiac fibrosis. *Am J Med* 1963; 34:71–75.
115. Ali MK, Khalil KG, Fuller LM, Leachman RD, Sullivan MP, Loh KK, Gamble JF, Shullenberger CC: Radiation-related myocardial injury: management of two cases. *Cancer* 1976; 38:1941–1946.
116. Warda M, Khan A, Massumi A, Mathur V, Klima T, Hall RJ: Radiation-induced valvular dysfunction. *JACC* 1983; 2:180–185.
117. Cohen SI, Saroja B, Glass J, Lev M: Radiotherapy as a cause of complete atrioventricular block in Hodgkin's disease. *Arch Intern Med* 1981, 141: 676–679.
118. Tzivoni D, Ratzkowski E, Biran S, Brook JG, Stern S: Complete heart block following therapeutic irradiation of the left side of the chest. *Chest* 1977; 71:231–234.
119. Kremer DN, Laplace LB: Heart block following x-ray treatment for thyrotoxicosis. *Am Heart J* 1936; 11:227–232.
120. Wolf GL, Kumar PP: Radiation-induced pericarditis. *Pract Cardiol* 1980; 6(3):41–50.
121. Cohn KE, Stewart JR, Fajardo LF, Hancock EW: Heart disease following irradiation. *Medicine* 1967, 46:281–298.
122. Posner MR, Cohen GI, Skarin AT: Pericardial disease in patients with cancer. The differentiation of malignant from idiopathic and radiation-induced pericarditis. *Am J Med* 1981; 71:407–413.
123. Schimpff SC, Diggs CH, Salvatore PC, Wiernik PH: Radiation-related thyroid dysfunction: implications for treatment of Hodgkin's disease. *Ann Intern Med* 1980; 92:91–98.
124. Keelan MH Jr, Rudders RA: Successful treatment of radiation pericarditis with corticosteroids. *Arch Int Med* 1974; 134:145–147.
125. Biran S, Brufman G, Klein E, Hochman A: The management of pericardial effusion in cancer patients. *Chest* 1977; 71:182–186.
126. Morton DL, Kagan AR, Roberts WC, O'Brien KP, Holmes EC, Adkins PC: Pericardiectomy for radiation-induced pericarditis with effusion. *Ann Thorac Surg* 1969; 8:195–206.
127. Palmer HM, Colking JB, Emmanuel IG: Irradiation-induced constrictive pericarditis in intestinal lymphangiectasis. *Br Med J* 1970; 4:783–784.
128. MacLeod CA, Schwartz H, Linton OB: Constrictive pericarditis following irradiation therapy. *JAMA* 1969; 207:2281–2282.
129. Haas, JM: Symptomatic constrictive pericarditis developing 45 years after radiation therapy to the mediastinum: a review of radiation pericarditis. *Am Heart J* 1969; 77:89–95.
130. Applefeld MM, Cole JF, Pollack SH, Sutton FJ, Slawson RG, Singleton RT, Wiernik PH: The late appearance of chronic pericardial disease in patients treated by radiotherapy for Hodgkin's disease. *Ann Intern Med* 1981; 94:338–341.
131. Moncada R, Baker M, Salinas M, Demos CC, Churchill R, Love L, Reynes C, Hale D, Cardoso M, Pifarre R, Gunnar RM: Diagnostic role of computed tomography in pericardial heart disease: congenital defects, thickening, neoplasms, and effusions. *Am Heart J* 1982; 103:263–282.
132. Jones A, Wedgewood J: Effect of radiation on the heart. *Br J Radiol* 1960; 33:138–158.
133. Miller AJ, Jain S, Levin B: Radiographic visualization of lymphatic drainage of heart muscle and pericardial sac in the dog. *Chest* 1971; 59:271–275.
134. Davis KS: Intrathoracic changes following x-ray treatment: clinical and experimental study. *Radiology* 1924; 3:301–322.
135. Fajardo LF, Stewart JR: Pathogenesis of radiation-induced myocardial fibrosis. *Lab Invest* 1973; 29:244–257.
136. Brosius FC, Waller BF, Roberts WC: Radiation heart disease. *Am J Med* 1981; 70:519–530.
137. Burch GE, Sohal RS, Sun SC, Miller GC, Colcolough HL: Effects of radiation on the human heart. An electron microscopic study. *Arch Intern Med* 1968; 121:230–239.
138. Soin JS, Cox JD, Youker JE, Swartz HM: Cardiac localization of ^{99m}Tc-(Sn)-pyrophosphate following irradiation of the chest. *Radiology* 1977; 124:165–168.
139. Burns RJ, Bar-Shlomo B-Z, Druck MN, Herman JG, Gilbert BW, Perrault DJ, McLaughlin PR: Detection of radiation cardiomyopathy by gated radionuclide angiography. *Am J Med* 1983; 74:297–302.
140. Pearson HES: Coronary occlusion following thoracic radiotherapy, two cases. *Proc R Soc Med* 1957; 50:516.
141. Prentice RTW: Myocardial infarction following radiation. *Lancet* 1965; 2:388.
142. Ringrose TL: Radiation-"induced" coronary artery disease. *JAMA* 1974; 230:960–961.
143. Tracy GP, Brown DE, Johnson LW, Gottlieb AJ: Radiation-induced coronary artery disease. *JAMA* 1974; 228:1660–1662.
144. Totterman KJ, Pesonen E, Siltanen P: Radiation-related chronic heart disease. *Chest* 1983; 83(No. 6):875–878.
145. Iqbal SM, Hanson EL, Gensini GG: Bypass graft for coronary artery stenosis following radiation therapy. *Chest* 1977; 71:664–666.
146. Stewart JR, Cohn KE, Fajardo LE, Hancock W, Kaplan HS: Radiation-induced heart disease. *Radiology* 1967; 89:302–310.
147. Steinberg I: Effusive-constrictive radiation pericarditis: two cases illustrating value of angiocardiography in diagnosis. *Am J Cardiol* 1967; 19:434–449.
148. DeSanctis RW: Case records of the Massachusetts General Hospital. *N Engl J Med* 1978; 298:1184–1192.
149. Braunwald E, Swan HJC (eds): Cooperative study on cardiac catheterization. *Circulation* 1968; 37 (suppl III): III-1–III-113.
150. Escher DJW: Types of pacemakers and their complications. *Circulation* 1973; 47:1119–1131.
151. Caves P, Billingham MB, Coltart J, Rider A, Stinson E: Transvenous endomyocardial biopsy—application of a method for diagnosing heart disease. *Postgrad Med J* 1975; 51:286–290.
152. Kennedy JW: Complications associated with cardiac catheterization and angiography. *Cathet Cardiovasc Diagn* 1981; 8:5–11.
153. Davis K, Kennedy JW, Kemp HG Jr, Judkins MP, Gosselin AJ, Killip T: Complications of coronary arteriography from the collaborative study of coronary artery surgery (CASS). *Circulation* 1979; 59:1105–1112.
154. Abrams HL, Adams DF: The complications of coronary arteriography. *Circulation* 1975; 52(suppl 2):II-27.
154a. Travis WD, Balogh K, Wolf BC, Doos WG, Abraham JL: Silicone-induced endocarditis. A complication of transvenous cardiac pacing catheterization. *Arch Pathol Lab Med* 1986; 110:51–54.
155. Guss SB, Zir LM, Garrison HB, Daggett WM, Block PC, Dinsmore RE: Coronary occlusion during coronary angiography. *Circulation* 1975; 52:1063–1068.
156. Meller J, Friedman S, Dack S, Herman MV: Coronary artery dissection—a complication of cardiac catheterization without sequelae: case report and review of the literature. *Cathet Cardiovasc Diagn* 1976; 2:301–308.
157. Kent KM, Bentivoglio LG, Block PC, Cowley MJ, Dorros G, Gosselin AJ, Myler RK, Simpson J, Stertzer SH, Williams DO, Fisher L, Gillespie MJ, Detre K, Kelsey S, Mullin SM, Mock MB: Percutaneous transluminal coronary angioplasty: report from the Registry of the National Heart, Lung, and Blood Institute. *Am J Cardiol* 1982; 49:2011–2020.
158. Crowley MJ, Vetorovee GW, Wolfgang TC: Efficacy of percutaneous transluminal coronary angioplasty: technique, patient selection, laboratory results, limitations, and complications. *Am Heart J* 1981; 101:272–280.
159. Slack JD, Pinkerton CA, Nasser WK: Acute pericarditis after percutaneous transluminal coronary angioplasty. *Am J Cardiol* 1985; 55:843–844.
160. Sethi GK, Scott SM, Takaro T: Iatrogenic coronary artery stenosis following aortic valve replacement. *J Thorac Cardiovasc Surg* 1979; 77:760–767.
161. Rowley KM, Clubb KS, Smith GJW, Cabin HS: Right-sided infective endocarditis as a consequence of flow-directed pulmonary-artery catheterization. A clinicopathological study of 55 autopsied patients. *N Engl J Med* 1984; 311:1152–1156.
162. Klibaner MI, Hayes JA, Dobnick D, McCormick JR: Delayed fatal pulmonary hemorrhage complicating use of a balloon flotation catheter. *Angiology* 1985; 36:358–362.

52 Heart Diseases in the Tropics and Parasitic Heart Diseases

B.N. Datta, MD

INCIDENCE OF HEART DISEASE IN THE TROPICS

The cardiologist and the pathologist in tropical countries are likely to come across all the congenital and acquired heart diseases seen anywhere in the world, and in addition they will encounter conditions that may be exclusively or largely restricted to the tropics. The data presented in the succeeding pages is based on my own experience of nearly 2,000 cardiac autopsies performed in Chandigarh, a city in the northwest part of India,[1] and from a review of the published literature from India, Africa, and other tropical countries. The major emphasis is to highlight the different patterns of heart disease seen in the West and the tropics. No attempt will be made to provide detailed pathologic description of each disorder.

The epidemiology of cardiac disease in the underdeveloped countries is largely based on hospital statistics[1,1a] (Tables 52.1 and 52.2). In descending order of frequency, the pattern of heart disease may be stated as:

- Rheumatic heart disease in children and adolescents,
- Hypertensive heart disease in adults and the middle aged, and
- Cardiomyopathies/chronic cor pulmonale.

Atherosclerotic diseases—cardiac, peripheral, and intracranial—are far less frequent but are gradually mak- their presence felt in the urban populations in these countries.

THE CARDIOMYOPATHIES

Cardiomyopathy has been defined as myocardial disease of unknown or uncertain origin. The most recent internationally agreed upon classification is as follows[2-4]: (1) dilated cardiomyopathy (DCM); (2) restrictive cardiomyopathy (RCM); and (3) hypertrophic cardiomyopathy (HCM).

Of these three classes, the restrictive variety, in its classical form endomyocardial fibrosis, can be considered a truly tropical cardiac disease. Dilated cardiomyopathy has a worldwide prevalence. Perhaps it is more common in the tropics, whereas the hypertrophic variety is distinctly uncommon or rare.

An estimate of the autopsy incidence in India of the three classes can be seen in Table 52.3. At autopsy, in Africa, DCM in most reports and EMF in others contribute to 25% to 40% of cardiac diseases and HCM is still a subject of isolated case reports.

RESTRICTIVE CARDIOMYOPATHY

The fundamental cardiac problem, as the name implies, is the reduction in the capacity of one or both ventricles to fill because of endomyocardial disease. The presentation and pathophysiologic aspects are in many ways similar to those of constrictive pericarditis. Two main conditions are included in the group, endomyocardial fibrosis (EMF) and Loeffler's eosinophilic endocarditis fibroplastica or simply Loeffler's disease, the former prevalent in the tropics and the latter almost restricted to the temperate climates.[2,8] It is likely that the two conditions are a different spectrum of a common endomyocardial inflammatory disease in which the eosinophil leukocyte plays an immediate cardiotoxic role, but this hypothesis will be discussed later.[9-12]

Endomyocardial Fibrosis

Endomyocardial fibrosis is prevalent in the rain-drenched forests of Africa, India, and Sri Lanka on either side of the equator and South America. The two major

Table 52.1. Hospital Prevalence of Common Heart Diseases in India and Africa*

	Percentages of Total Cardiac Diseases				
Area	**Rheumatic**	**Hypertensive**	**Ischemic**	**Cardiomyopathy**	**Cor Pulmonale**
Africa	15–34 (21)	12–36 (22)	0–2 (1)	5–46 (20)	5–16 (8)
India	16–28 (28)	3–26 (16)	0–12 (8)	0–4 (2)	3–46 (9)

* Condensed from Datta[1] in 1983.

Note: A recent World Health Organization survey in Africa has attributed 23.8% of deaths to cardiovascular disease, with the prevalence per thousand population being 3 for rheumatic, 96 for hypertensive heart disease, and 9 for others.[1a]

habitats of the disease are East, Central Africa represented by Uganda and Nigeria and South India represented by Kerala. The two locations also have similar topography. Cases have been reported from almost all parts of India and Africa and rarely from Europe, the Middle East, and China also.[1,2,13–18,18a]

The clinical and pathologic knowledge of EMF has largely been built around the end stages of the disease. The onset, the early features, and their progression to cardiac failure are not exactly known.[19] Surveys of large numbers of autopsies even in endemic areas have rarely shown a case of "incidental" EMF.[16] The most common clinical onset suggests an infective/inflammatory illness; there is fever, malaise, at times itching, and urticaria soon followed by palpitations and effort dyspnea.[19,20] In tropical countries, such features can hardly be indicative of anything specific, with the prevalence of rampant parasitic and bacterial infection. In fact, even these nonspecific symptoms are infrequent in Kerala.[21–23] The patient in cardiac failure presents yet another problem, that of its differentiation from other equally or more common types of heart disease in the community, namely, rheumatic heart disease and, at times, DCM.

The cardiac features, both clinical and investigative, are an expression of the side of the heart predominantly involved in the fibrotic process. On this basis, EMF may be predominantly right ventricular (RV-EMF) or left ventricular (LV-EMF) or have a biventricular pattern (BiV-EMF). The RV pattern usually dominates the clinical picture, but the most common lesion is BiV-EMF, as investigations reveal even at that stage the involvement of the left ventricle.[16,18,22,24,25] Right ventricular endomyocardial fibrosis presents with high jugular venous pressure, ascites with little or no pedal edema, hepatomegaly, cyanosis, and clubbing of fingers. The patient is usually a child or adolescent with stunted growth and retarded sexual maturation.[19,20] Pericardial effusion is usual and may be massive and misleading.[16] In LV-EMF, the pulmonary circulation bears the brunt of the restrictive cardiac features. Dyspnea, cough with expectoration and hemoptysis, and signs of mitral regurgitation predominate. Pulmonary congestion and subsequent pulmonary hypertension supervene. In the BiV-EMF there is a mixture of features, with the right ventricular picture predominating.

Cardiomegaly may be detected on chest x-rays, with pericardial effusion. The electrocardiogram represents the underlying distribution of the EMF. Low voltage is usual, the QR pattern in leads V_{3R} and V_1 and inverted or flat T waves in leads V_1 to V_6 are found in most cases. Atrial fibrillation, P mitrale, P pulmonale, as well as a prolonged PR interval are reported in about 30% of the cases.[26] These features, with the clinical exclusion of myocardial infarction, cor pulmonale, and congenital heart disease, have been considered fairly diagnostic of EMF by the African workers but not so by Indians.[18,21,26] Echocardiography, especially two-dimensional and M-mode, has been helpful in the diagnosis and assessment of EMF. The thickened endocardium and the obliterated apices are easily picked up. Paradoxic motion and a crenelated appearance of the right ventricle with infundibular dilatation characterize RV-EMF.[14,18,24,27] Left ventricular endomyocardial fibrosis is recognised by a greater amplitude of septal motion and in most instances by the characteristic tethering of the posterior mitral leaflet.[28] Right heart angiography has been applied in many centers,[8,15,18,18a,19] to effectively demonstrate the obliteration of the apex and dilation of the infundibular chamber (Figure 52.1). Endomyocardial biopsy is a useful adjunct, although after the foregoing noninvasive techniques it may not be needed.

Table 52.2. Autopsy Incidence of Cardiac Diseases at Chandigarh, North India*

Disease	No.	% of Total	% of Cardiac Cases
Rheumatic	372	4.7	19.3
Hypertensive	336	4.3	17.4
Myocardial Infarction	272	3.6	13.2
Cor Pulmonale	177	2.3	9.2
Infective Endocarditis	139	1.8	7.2
Congenital	139	1.8	7.2
Isolated Aortic Valve Disease	94	1.2	4.8
Cardiomyopathies	65	0.3	3.4
Miscellaneous	144	1.9	7.6

* Total autopsies = 7670; cardiac cases = 1925; period = 1964–1982.

Table 52.3. Autopsy Incidence of Cardiomyopathies in India

Place	Total Cases	DCM	EMF	HCM
Chandigarh	68	52	12	4
Bombay[5]	34	20	12	2
Vellore[6]	38	25	9	2
New Delhi[7]	25	20	5	...

DCM = dilated cardiomyopathy; HCM = hypertrophic cardiomyopathy; EMF = endomyocardial fibrosis.

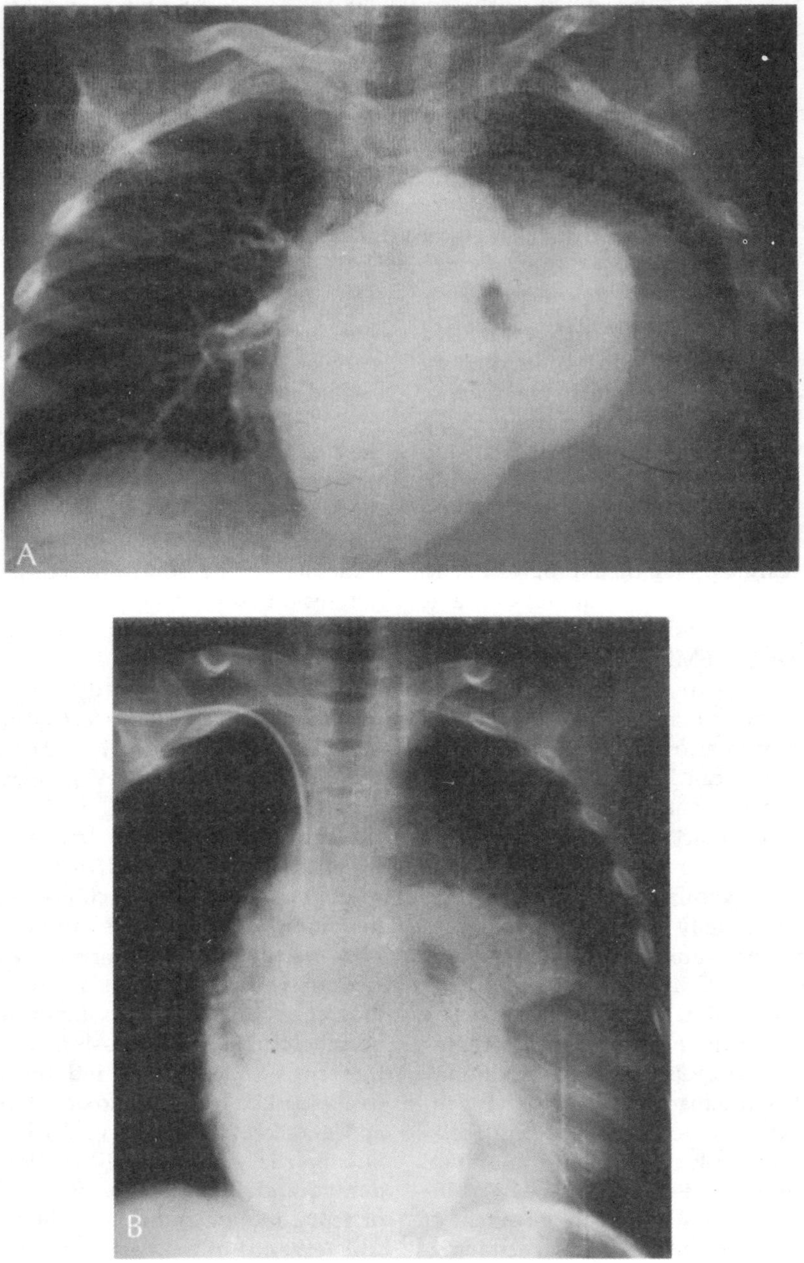

Figure 52.1. Angiograms of right atrium (*A*) and right ventricle (*B*) in two Chinese patients with endomyocardial fibrosis, showing marked atrial dilatation, obliteration of the right ventricular apex, and dilatation of the right ventricular outflow tract. (From Liu et al[18a] with permission.)

Pathology of Endomyocardial Fibrosis

In the routinely available, advanced, fully developed case the appearances are unmistakable. The heart may be normal in size or dilated. The dilatation is especially marked in cases of RV-EMF in which the obliteration of the apex produces a depressed notch outside and a markedly distended right atrium. The endocardial sclerosis in both ventricles is restricted to the inflow tracts and the apices; it may spread up the outflow tract for a few millimeters, but the subaortic endocardium and a major part of the septum on the left side remain unaffected. On the right side, the sclerosis does affect the outflow area a little more. The porcelain-white thick tissue overruns the papillary muscles, trabeculae carnae, and chordae tendineae and also the posterior mitral and septal leaflets of the tricuspid valves. This incarcerates and effectively immobilizes the valve apparatuses. The blood flow gradually undermines a ridge in the apical fibrosis towards the outflow tract (Figure 52.2). The endocardial fibrosis apparently begins as isolated patches that gradually coalesce, and five such patterns of endocardial plaques have been described.[29] Mural thrombi may be present in either ven-

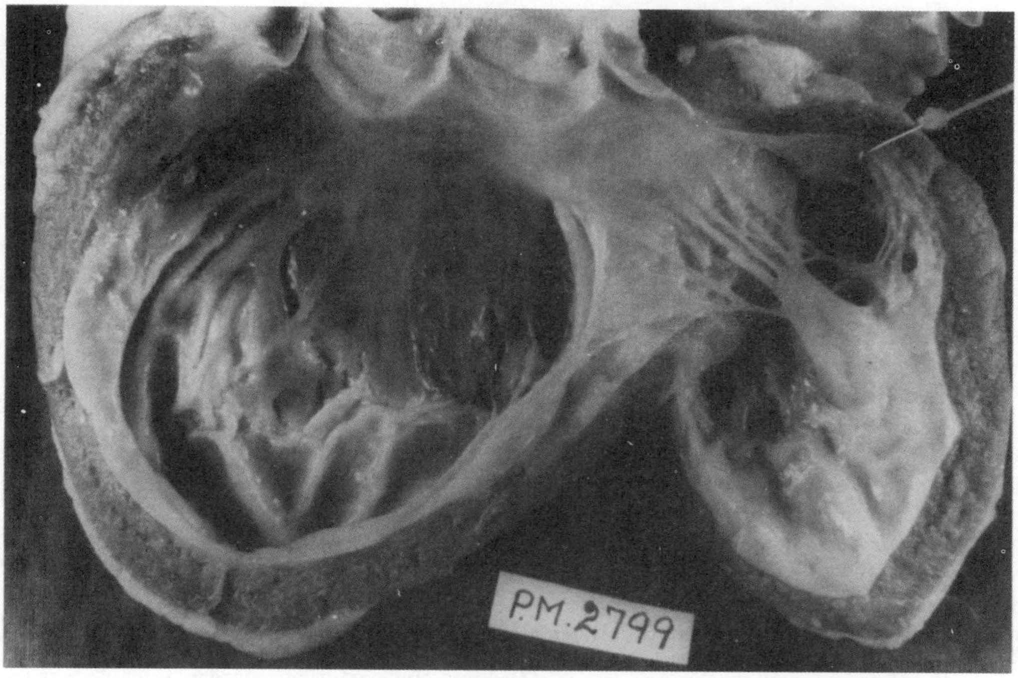

Figure 52.2. Endomyocardial fibrosis. Left ventricle opened up to show dense sclerosis in the inflow tract and apex forming a ridge towards the outflow tract. The chordae and papillary muscles are incarcerated and the subaortic endocardium is normal.

tricle. Histologically the endocardial sclerosis is composed of dense acellular collagen devoid of elastic tissue. It may be rather loose, cellular, and gelatinous in the "early" stages, and a layer of inflammatory granulation tissue of variable thickness separates the fibrosis from the underlying myocardium. This layer is composed of proliferating capillaries and dilated lymphatics and is infiltrated by lymphocytes, monocytes, plasma cells, and hemosiderin-laden histiocytes. Eosinophils may be rare or present in small numbers. The inflammation extends into the superficial myocardium for a variable degree. Ultrastructure of the lesion has no more than confirmed the histologic features.[30]

Etiology of Endomyocardial Fibrosis

A consideration of the etiology of EMF of necessity leans heavily upon the epidemiologic aspects of the disease; it is essential to tie the two together. Because of their geographic overlapping, a number of factors automatically become suspect, but so far other than a topographic association, no definite etiologic agent or agents have been recognized. Nor is it certain that the sporadic cases occurring outside the endemic zones really represent classic EMF. Among the dietary factors, bananas in Africa (because of the contribution to serotonin, a known endocardial sclerosing agent) and tapioca (cassava) in Kerala have been investigated in both man and experimental animals, but they have been exculpated.[31,32] Infective agents have received much attention. The tropical communities live almost in harmony with a variety of parasites and almost all such parasites have been implicated in the etiology of EMF. Filariasis has received maximum attention for its prevalence in both Africa and Kerala, and serologic evidence of filarial infection has been found more frequent in Africa than in Kerala,[21,23,33] but it has not been possible to go beyond the association. Malaria has been implicated in both Africa and South America.[14,34] A species of mice exposed experimentally to *Plasmodium berghei* infection was found to develop endocarditis followed by endocardial fibrosis (without the development of eosinophilia[35]). Toxoplasmosis, a well-known cause of myocarditis, was also investigated,[34] and trichinosis was reported to have caused mural endocarditis in association with eosinophilia.[36] However, none of the parasites has been considered to cause EMF as a direct manifestation of infection of the heart. Two mechanisms have been proposed to link the parasites to EMF; the two are not necessarily independent. One possibility is an immune-based cardiotoxicity; the other more recent and more popular is through the intervention of the eosinophil leukocyte.

Loeffler's Disease

The unity of Loeffler's endocardial disease and EMF has been built around the eosinophil.[37] Hypereosinophilic states, including eosinophilic leukemia, underlie Loeffler's disease, whereas some degree of eosinophilia is present in all cases of parasitic disease, and eosinophilia has been reported in many cases of EMF at some stage of the disease.[9,12,24,38,39] The degranulation of the eosinophils with release of the cardiotoxic cationic proteins in Loeffler's disease is presumably inherent in the eosinophils themselves, whereas in EMF an individual susceptibility possibly mediated through the parasite-related IgE has been postulated. The two conditions, Loeffler's disease and EMF, have been grouped under the common name, *endomyocardial disease*,[37] and three stages of the disease have been categorized on a clinicopathologic basis. The course is spread over about two and a half years, beginning as endomyocarditis and ending as endomyocardial fibrosis. At this end stage the two diseases are indistinguishable.[37] This unitarian hypothesis, however, has so far not found universal acceptance because of several facets in EMF. The entire unity lies in the morphologic end stage. Endocardial fibrosis is caused by a number of conditions including thrombi, infarcts, infections, and localized jet lesions in the chambers. Eosinophilia is not a consistent feature of EMF; in fact, it is usually not found towards the end stages. There is a wide disproportion between the population harboring parasites in the tropics and those in whom EMF actually develops; in fact, by comparison with the parasitic prevalence, EMF would be a rare disease. Moreover, there are clinical differences between EMF and Loeffler's disease.[37] Endomyocardial fibrosis occurs at a younger age, both sexes are affected equally, and there is a lack of multisystem involvement (cerebral, retinal, dermal, and lymph nodal involvement, which are features of Loeffler's disease), whereas orbital edema, hepatomegaly, and ascites are not found in Loeffler's disease. Endocardial eosinophilic infiltration and its degranulation, which is so readily discernible in Loeffler's disease is rarely seen in EMF.[38] A joint study of endomyocardial disease in the United Kingdom, Brazil, and Kerala[40] suggests that in temperate climates the eosinophil granule toxin produces a rapidly progressive form of disease, whereas in EMF in the tropics with less marked eosinophilia it takes much longer.

There is therefore no controversy in accepting that the eosinophil leukocyte is a potent cardiotoxic agent, but to accept it to the exclusion of all other possibilities for EMF is perhaps too premature and hasty.

Finally, immunologic aberrations have been postulated for EMF. In the Nigerian cases, IgE levels are elevated, but they are also elevated in cases of rheumatic heart disease and DCM.[41] The so-called "tropical immunologic syndrome" postulated by Shaper[42] for these diseases in Africa has little to support it in India where little, if any, immune disturbance has been found in EMF.[43] An overlap between EMF, DCM, and rheumatic heart disease both clinically and at autopsy, however, has been experienced by some.[34,44–46]

Surgical decortication of the thickened endocardium with replacement of the valves has been taken up in the last decade and offers good responses.[46a,46b,46c]

Endomyocardial fibrosis, therefore, remains a fascinating and enigmatic tropical cardiac disease.

DILATED CARDIOMYOPATHY

Congestive or dilated cardiomyopathy (DCM) or idiopathic cardiomegaly (ICM) is not restricted to the tropics although it is believed to be more common. It has been diagnosed as responsible for up to 36% of cardiac diseases in some parts of Africa.[47] The clinical profile of DCM in the African Black includes a consideration of local factors that possibly are not operative elsewhere.[47,48] These include thiamine deficiency or beriberi, alcoholism, chronic myocarditis due to Toxoplasma or coxsackie virus, pregnancy, and hypertension. Because proof of any one of these or additional conditions may not be available, the term DCM is possibly being used as a mixed bag. As Ikeme[49] wrote, "In the hands of the clinician, idiopathic cardiomegaly is an amorphous area in tropical cardiology." In the hands of a pathologist, DCM is best looked upon as end-stage heart failure.[1] This is one reason for the reportedly higher incidence of DCM in the tropics.

POSTPARTUM CARDIOMYOPATHY

Postpartum cardiomyopathy is a clinical syndrome[50] that satisfies all the clinical and morphologic criteria for the diagnosis of DCM except for its occurrence in relation to pregnancy or puerperium which gives it the special status. Appearing for the first time in the last trimester of pregnancy, the condition resolves in about two thirds of cases, but it may recur in the subsequent pregnancy. The disease is more common among Negro women all over the world, but it has its highest incidence of about 1% of childbirths in Zaria, Nigeria.[50,51] In this particular area the parturient woman is subjected to a ritual of a high salt diet while she is closeted in an artificially heated room. In this setting a number of factors in addition to pregnancy can overload the heart. These include malnutrition, vitamin deficiencies, viral myocarditis, endocrine influences, and genetic susceptibility. Hypertension in pregnancy looms large in the background. Salt overload, volume overload from pregnancy, splenomegaly, and anemia, which most of these women have, induce a state of high-output cardiac failure.[52] Prolapse of the mitral valve has also been documented in Nigerian women.[11] The Nigerian situation, however, does not exist elsewhere. The autopsy specimen of the heart is not distinguishable from that in DCM.

Hypertension, the most common cardiovascular disease in the tropics especially in the African Black, has been etiologically linked with DCM. That "DCM is hypertension in disguise" has been debated for some time.[53] In Nigeria, hypertension has been associated with 50% of cases of DCM in their course, and at autopsy in patients with hypertension, 50% of the heart specimens are dilated and flabby, similar to those with DCM.[47,48,54,55] Therefore, on account of modifying influences, including anemia and malnutrition, or unknown influences, the heart is unable to sustain the required high blood pressure and dilates and fails.[1] Among 50 autopsies in cases of DCM at Chandigarh, hypertensive renal arteriolar and arterial changes were found in 10% of patients under the age of 40 years. The best course, however, would be to exclude such cases from series of DCM.[11,47]

HYPERTROPHIC CARDIOMYOPATHY

Hypertrophic cardiomyopathy (HCM) is as yet uncommonly diagnosed in the underdeveloped countries,[56,57] because its recognition parellels the availability of echocardiographic facilities.[7,58] The clinical and morphologic features are no different from those described from the West.

RHEUMATIC HEART DISEASE

Rheumatic heart disease (RHD) has been identified as the most common cardiovascular disease of young persons in tropical countries.[59-67] In its natural history it differs from the pattern recorded in the West in certain aspects:

1. The initial attack of acute rheumatic fever occurs generally at a much younger age, by the fifth year of life.
2. The disease progresses much faster, leading to crippling valve deformities and death in the young (over 80% die before 30 years of age).
3. The incidence of pulmonary hypertension is much higher (60%) and severe grades of arterial changes are detected.
4. Organic tricuspid valve involvement occurs in a much higher proportion (about 35%) of cases at autopsy.

The epidemiologic and clinical aspects of the disease are covered in another chapter of this book. Some critical features of the valvular lesions will be touched upon here. Some areas of ignorance still exist in our understanding of the pathogenesis of rheumatic valvular lesions. The most common mitral valve dysfunction, based on surveys of schoolchildren and the general population, is stated to be mitral regurgitation in India, Pakistan, Africa, and Taiwan.[60,66-70] Statistics from hospitalized patients and from autopsies among adolescents and young adults, however, show mitral stenosis to be the most common and pure mitral regurgitation to be the rarest lesion.[59,63-65,69,71] The transition from the former to the latter has not been determined by adequate follow-up studies. The pathologic basis for the development of regurgitation in some cases and stenosis in others is not known. The morphologic lesions in both types are well documented.[69,72] It is hoped that with the availability of echocardiographic facilities it might be possible to study this aspect. Accelerated mitral stenosis has been shown to develop in early childhood if the initial acute rheumatic fever begins early, whereas delayed mitral stenosis develops when the initial disease begins in the adolescent.[73] No mention is made of mitral regurgitation in this recent study.

Organic tricuspid valve disease is reported in 34% to 46% of autopsy cases in India,[1] although severe degrees of tricuspid stenosis are much less frequent.[74,75]

Pulmonary arterial hypertension has been detected in 60% of hospitalized patients,[1] in many of them (up to 13%) at suprasystemic levels.[76] The existence and levels of pulmonary arterial hypertension have not shown any correlation with age, sex, duration of illness, mitral valve area, valve calcification, or atrial fibrillation.[77] Pathologists in India have come across more severe grades of arterial lesion in pulmonary arterial hypertension of rheumatic origin[78] including necrotizing arteriolar and plexiform lesions. Isolated aortic valve disease of rheumatic origin has been reported in 1% to 4% of autopsy cases in India.[66,71]

There is a paucity of studies on the basic immunopathologic studies on rheumatic heart disease in India and Africa. One such study compared lymphocytic infiltrates in mitral valve specimens in India with those in Mexico and found more cellular infiltrates in the calcified valves in Indian material. Residual streptococcal products were present in neither.[79]

INFECTIVE ENDOCARDITIS

Infective endocarditis, a common entity, again shows many differences from the picture seen in the West.[1,80] The vast majority of patients (73% to 89%) are under the age of 40; 40% to 55% at autopsy reveal no preexisting heart disease; 30% of cases occur over rheumatic valvular disease (Table 52.4). The category of "drug abusers" and postcardiac surgery cases is virtually nonexistent (as yet!), except in a report from Bombay.[82] Nonrheumatic acquired heart disease such as ischemic heart disease, atherosclerosis of valves, myxomatous degeneration of valves, syphilis, and cardiomyopathies is rarely encountered in the background of infective endocarditis.[81-87] Identification of the route of infection is uncommonly possible, but puerperal sepsis seems to be a common mode. Causative organisms have been isolated in about 50% of cases; the yield is higher (up to 80%) in tricuspid valve, right-sided endocarditis.[80,88] This valve presumably is just one more focus in a patient with septicemia and by itself would not cause significant mortality and morbidity. Staphylococci are the more common organisms; *Streptococcus viridans* has been identified in 20% of cases. Rare instances of fungal endocarditis, especially on prosthetic valves, have been identified.[80-82,88] The mitral valve is the frequent site of infection in cases of preexisting rheumatic heart disease and the aortic valve is more common in previously normal or congenitally deformed valves.[81]

MITRAL VALVE PROLAPSE SYNDROME

The detection of this condition, as that of hypertrophic cardiomyopathy, has been increasing because of the availability of echocardiographic setups in cardiology centers. Until about 1981, the condition was mentioned in isolated case reports from India and Africa,[1] but recent reports have shown mitral valve prolapse in 16% of healthy asymptomatic women[89] in one study, and 2.7% of asymptomatic and 18% of symptomatic women in another.[90]

ISCHEMIC HEART DISEASE

The underdeveloped countries on their way to westernized advancement and affluence are likely to catch up also with the high prevalence of ischemic heart disease in the West. The World Health Organization[91] has already taken note of the developing trends and has made a plea to avert the threat by applying appropriate measures. In India the death rate from ischemic heart disease in hospitals varies between 5% and 35% of cardiac diseases.[1] In population studies the figures are highly variable, from negligible in rural areas to 10 or 11 per 1,000 in urban areas, and one estimate of 2.5% above the age of 40 years.[92] In some old and recent reports the increasing incidence has been appreciated. In one state in India, the hospital incidence increased from 16.3% to 23.5% in five years[93]; in Fiji over a 20-year period from 1960 to 1979, it increased from 6.6 per 1,000 to 32 in hospitalized

Table 52.4. Infective Endocarditis in India and Africa

Location	No.	Source	Patients Under 40 Years (%)	Previous cardiac lesion (%)		
				Nil	VHD	CHD
India						
Chandigarh[81]	120	Autopsy	89	43	33	24
Bombay[82]	185	Autopsy	74	58	→42←	
New Delhi[88]	116	Clinical	77*	—	75	25
Africa						
Nigeria[85]	64	Autopsy	73	82		
		Clinical			→18←	
Ibadan[84]	90	Autopsy	85	35		
		Clinical			→65←	
Uganda[83]	102	Autopsy	65	39	53†	8
		Clinical				

CHD = congenital heart disease; VHD = valvular heart disease, mostly rheumatic. Figures between arrows indicate common number under previous cardiac lesions.

* All patients were under 30 years of age.

† Includes three cases of endomyocardial fibrosis.

cases[93a]; and in Hong Kong the increase was from 5.5% to 8.4% in the population in five years.[94]

Studies on the basic process of atherosclerosis of the aorta and coronary arteries in India and Africa were carried out in the late 50s and 60s.[1,95–97] Comparison with the West had established that the fatty streaks found in persons up to the third decade or so in tropical countries and in white persons in the United States occur to the same extent and severity, but in the subsequent development of fibrous plaques and calcific lesions the underdeveloped countries lag behind by two decades. Anatomic differences in the pattern of coronary arteries were also studied in considerable details by postmortem coronary arteriography.[1,95–98] These differences probably had no influence on the pattern of coronary atherosclerosis. In view of the current development of coronary artery surgery, attention has been focused on the angiographic patterns of coronary atherosclerosis. In some studies the Indian subjects had a lower incidence of single-vessel disease and a higher incidence of three-vessel disease than that found in the United States, the lesions beginning in the third decade and peaking in the seventh.[99–101]

Standard coronary risk factors were also recently evaluated and the usual difference was found between young patients (those under 40) and older patients with ischemic heart disease. The younger patients showed a lower profile of factors such as obesity, hypercholesterolemia, diabetes mellitus, and hypertension but a much higher prevalence of cigarette smoking.[102] The lipid status of patients in India is usually rated as normal in 54% to 80% of cases.[103,104] However, the pattern of elevated low density lipoprotein cholesterol, elevated very low density lipoprotein triglycerides, and depressed high density lipoprotein has also been confirmed in Indian subjects.[104] A higher component of manual laborers of poor socioeconomic class among patients with ischemic heart disease (up to 20%) was found in India.[105] Hypertension and diabetes mellitus have been recognized in 25% to 46% and 10% to 24% of cases, respectively.[93,105,106]

In Africa ischemic heart disease is among the rare diseases affecting the Black population, but the data need updating in view of recent changes in life-style and living standards. In Nigeria between 1961 and 1970, 26 hospital deaths were due to ischemic heart disease (1 in 20,000 patients)[107]; in the Congo area between 1975 and 1980, 25 cases of ischemic heart disease were detected in a total of 889 cases of heart disease[108]; and in the South African Black, 39 deaths were attributed to ischemic heart disease among 758 cases of sudden death.[109] A recent report from North Africa shows that ischemic heart disease contributed to 7.6% of all cardiac diseases; in 26.1% of these none of the coronary risk factors was identified, and in 16.2% three factors—hypertension, obesity, and hyperlipemia—were present.[110,110a] Hypertension occupies a unique position in Africa, being the most common cardiovascular disease; hypertension yet does not seem to have contributed towards ischemic heart disease.

The pathologic aspects of ischemic heart disease and myocardial infarction in Indian autopsy material in my experience have been no different from the usual textbook picture.[1]

NUTRITIONAL HEART DISEASE

Nutritional heart disease does not qualify as a single pathologic entity despite earlier descriptions.[111] The cardiac response to nutritional imbalance and deficiencies is highly variable. Other than beriberi, alcoholism, and possibly some trace metals, there are hardly any specific causes of nutritional heart disease. Even these examples produce a situation that is no different from that of DCM. However, malnutrition has a key role to play in the underdeveloped countries in determining the prevalence, age of onset, progression, morbidity, and mortality of most cardiac diseases.[1]

KWASHIORKOR

Kwashiorkor is among the best known nutritional disorders in children in the underdeveloped countries. Cardiac status in kwashiorkor varies. In the African famine of the mid-1960s,[112] 22.5% of children with kwashiorkor had atrophic hearts, whereas 43% with marasmus had cardiomegaly. In a recent study from Madras, India, microcardia (CT ratio under 0.40) was detected in a minority of cases of marasmic kwashiorkor, whereas cardiomegaly was more common in kwashiorkor. The cardiac size as well as the clinical features depend on the associated existence of the type of anemia and electrolyte imbalance. Electrocardiographic changes including sinus tachycardia, low voltage QRS complexes, ST-segment depression, flat T waves, and a prolonged QT interval appear to be expressions of metabolic acidosis and hypokalemia.[113] The autopsy appearance of the heart in kwashiorkor is nonspecific and includes atrophy of myofibers, fatty infiltration, patchy fibrosis, and stray lymphomononuclear infiltrates.

BERIBERI

Beriberi is a well-known deficiency disease, easily preventable and treatable. The thiamine deficiency may be dietary in origin or related to alcoholism; the former seems to be decreasing, whereas the latter is on the increase at least in the African Black.[114,115] Clinically, beriberi causes high-output cardiac failure, which can be distinguished from DCM only by red cell thiamine levels and therapeutic response to thiamine. Pathologic features of the heart are the same as those of DCM.

KESHAN DISEASE*

In some parts of China, notably along a broad belt running from northeast to southwest, dietary deficiency of selenium is believed to be responsible for producing Keshan disease, an endemic cardiomyopathy characterized by progressive cardiac failure, especially in children.[2] The disease, however, has been largely eradicated with selenium supplementation. The heart is dilated again as in DCM, although areas of necrosis and fibrosis on histologic study are more evident. It is of interest that a case was reported in Long Island, New York.[116] The patient was a 2-year-old child in progressive cardiac failure. She consumed no cereal products, no dairy products, and very little meat, all of which constitute the principal sources of dietary selenium in the United States. Low levels of zinc and selenium were found in her blood and she improved on selenium therapy.

PARASITIC DISEASES OF THE HEART

In their unique monograph, *Parasites of the Human Heart,* Kean and Breslau[117] in 1964 predicted that in years to come some obscure diseases of the heart (cardiopathies) were likely to be traced to a parasitic etiology. This expectation has so far not been realized, although advances in endomyocardial fibrosis point in that direction. In the last two or three decades great advances have been made in the science of parasitology and the host–parasite relation with parasites that cause heart disease has been elaborated. In the succeeding pages some parasitic diseases are described. For details on the biology and natural history of the parasites themselves, two recent books are recommended: *Manson's Tropical Diseases*[118] and *Tropical and Geographical Medicine.*[119]

Like all other organs of the body, the heart also may have a relationship with a parasite at four levels:

1. The cardiac parasite produces a major disease which is the dominant manifestation in the clinicopathologic picture. Chagas' disease, toxoplasmosis, and some cases of schistosomiasis are examples.
2. The cardiac involvement forms an important part of an otherwise systemic parasitic infestation. Conditions such as trichinosis, hydatid disease, cysticercosis, and amebic pericarditis belong in this category.
3. The cardiac involvement is just one incidental site of involvement by a systemic parasitic disease. All parasitic diseases of man, from malaria to guinea worm, may involve the heart with or without any cardiac manifestations.
4. The heart may indirectly have hematologic, hemodynamic, or immunopathologic aberrations caused by a systemic parasite. Pulmonary schistosomiasis, hookworm anemia, and possibly eosinophil-mediated cardiac damage in endomyocardial fibrosis may be examples of this group.

AMERICAN TRYPANOSOMIASIS: CHAGAS' DISEASE

American trypanosomiasis (Chagas' disease) is among the most important public health problems caused by an animal parasite in mankind. At risk are 35 million persons and 10-12 million actually have the disease in Latin America as per recent estimates of the World Health Organization.[120,121] The endemic areas include South and Central America, Texas, Argentina, as well as Trinidad and the Caribbean. Serologic tests indicating disease are positive in 40% to 50% of the population of Venezuela and 20% to 70% of that of Brazil.[122] The autopsy incidence of Chagas' disease is 6% in Brazil[123] and 1.16% in Trujillo.[124] In Curaçao 76.2% of cases diagnosed as cardiomyopathy at autopsy are due to Chagas' disease.[125] Isolated cases have recently been described from northern California[126] and Guyana.[127]

The parasite responsible for this devastation, *Trypanosoma cruzi,* is a hemoflagellate that alternates its life between an intermediate host, the winged reduviid bug, and a vertebrate host, man and animal, both wild and domestic. The animals form a vast reservoir of the disease. The *T cruzi* is passed with the insect's feces to the skin and mucous membranes of the victim and is rubbed into the tissues during itching or through wounds and abrasions (stercoral spread).[121,128] Infection also has been acquired across the placenta and through blood transfusions. Once in the tissues the parasite changes into its mastigote form and invades the cells. It multiplies by binary fission both inside and outside the cells, and distends the host cells into "pseudocysts" or packets of parasites. These rupture and produce parasitemia, so that the cycle is repeated. The cardiac and skeletal muscles are the favored sites for *T cruzi.*

Chagas' disease spreads over years, occasionally the life span of the human host. It sets in as an acute illness, lasting from one to three months, passes into a latent

* See also chapter 44.

phase over the next 10 to 20 years, to emerge as classic Chagas' cardiomyopathy, Chagas' heart disease, or chagasic cardiopathy. The acute phase often is subclinical,[128a] and the first presentation of the patient is in chronic Chagas' disease with failure. This aspect is of importance in countries such as the United States where immigrants from the endemic countries may present with confusing cardiac problems years after their entry into the United States. This has been well illustrated in a recent case report from New York where an Ecuadorian immigrant was diagnosed as having ischemic heart disease and only detailed investigations revealed Chagas' disease.[128b]

Clinical manifestations of acute Chagas' disease include fever, muscle pain, hepatomegaly, splenomegaly, and lymph node enlargement. Unilateral conjunctivitis with marked periorbital edema (Romana sign) and a local inflammatory reaction in the skin (chagoma) may indicate the portal of entry of the infection. Myocarditis and meningoencephalitis are important events and about 10% of patients die at this stage of the disease.[128]

Cardiac lesions dominate the acute as well as the chronic phase, and even during the clinically silent latent phase, electrophysiologic disturbances in cardiac function may be recorded.[129] In about 38% of acute cases of Chagas' disease there is acute diffuse granulomatous myocarditis accompanied by widespread or variable degrees of necrosis of small blood vessels. *T cruzi*, free as well in pseudocyst forms, are abundant; the cardiac conduction tissue does not show morphologic damage. An important, although inconsistent feature is the inflammatory destruction of nerve ends and ganglia, both sympathetic and parasympathetic, in the heart.

Chronic Chagas' disease emerges in about 90% of the patients, and about 70% die of cardiac failure. There is some variation in the "tissue tropism" of the *T cruzi*: whereas cardiac involvement is the principal lesion in Argentina and Venezuela, the gastrointestinal tract shows dominant lesions in cases in Brazil, producing the characteristic "megas" of Chagas' disease, that is, megaesophagus, megastomach, and megacolon.[129] The heart is enlarged, dilated, and flabby (Figure 52.3). Aneurysms, usually apical (47%) or retromitral (27%), are a characteristic feature and distinguish Chagas' heart disease from DCM.[130] The mitral and tricuspid valves, although morphologically normal, are functionally incompetent. Histologic study reveals myocardial atrophy, fibrosis, and inconspicuous inflammation. An occasional granuloma may be found, but parasites are rare. A characteristic feature is the destruction and fibrosis of the cardiac conduction tracts.[121,131] The right bundle branch and the anterior fascicular branch of the left bundle branch are preferentially involved. Atrophy of the cardiac ganglia is present. The similarity of the cardiac lesions to the piecemeal necrosis of viral hepatitis has been noted.[129] Arterioles show thickening and there is periarteriolar lymphocytic infiltration.

The electrocardiogram in the acute phase has no specific features.[121] Low voltage QRS complexes and some conduction abnormalities may be recorded. In the chronic stage, right bundle branch block, complete or incomplete, left anterior hemiblock, sinoatrial and atrioventricular nodal dysfunction, and QRS abnormalities are recorded in various combinations. Sick sinus syndrome requiring pacemaker implantation has been reported in 6% of cases.[132] Holter electrocardiographic monitoring is particularly useful in detecting subclinical damage in the latent phase. Two forms of Chagas' disease may be identified on the basis of electrophysiologic dysfunctions: a myogenic form affecting mainly the myocardium and a neurogenic form affecting the conduction tissue.[133]

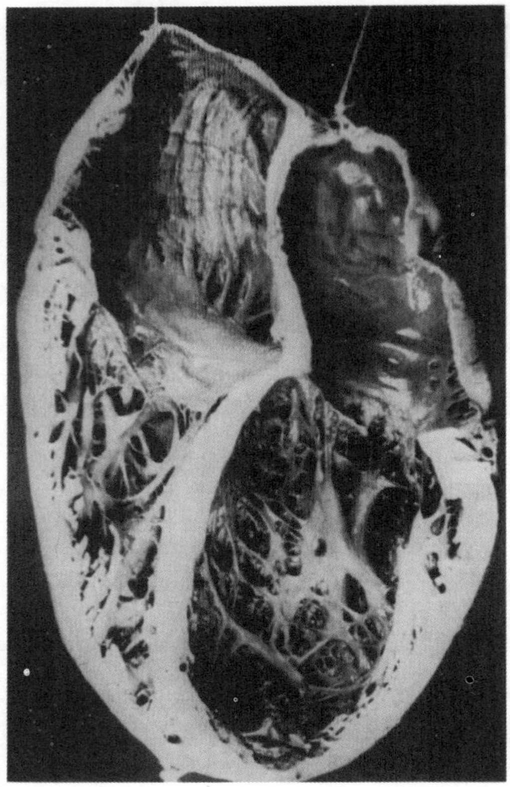

Figure 52.3. Chronic Chagas' disease of the heart. The chambers are thin walled and dilated; there is an apical aneurysm with thrombus. (Specimen provided by Dr J. Keystone of Toronto, Canada.) (From Silver MD [ed]: *Cardiovascular Pathology,* New York, Churchill Livingstone, 1983. Used with permission.)

Echocardiography, especially two-dimensional, is useful in demonstrating myocardial dysfunction, especially basic ventricular asynergy and aneurysms.[134] Angiocardiography supplements these findings by showing both systolic and diastolic dysfunction, namely, increased end-diastolic volume and decreased ejection fraction.[121] Aneurysms with or without thrombi are also visible. This investigation has been particularly useful in distinguishing Chagas' heart disease from dilated cardiomyopathy and endomyocardial fibrosis in Brazil.[122]

Pathogenesis of Chagas' Heart Disease

The host-parasite relation of a direct parasite-induced myocarditis is applicable only in the acute phase of the disease. The development of chronic "chagasic cardiopathy" appears to be a more complex issue. The prolonged latent phase in which the parasite has gone underground involves yet undefined interactions. Koberlé[135,136] described a state of "denervated heart" that emerges in chronic Chagas' disease as a result of destruction of the cardiac neuroganglia. Such a heart considered to be incapable of responding to neuroendocrine stimuli gradually dilates and fails. The parallel of neuroganglionic destruction in the gastrointestinal tract, with the development of the "megas," has a similar basis. This type of neuroganglionic destruction has also been induced in the rat[137] and in mice[138] and has been accompanied by a reduction in cardiac noradrenalin content.[137] The noradrenalin levels subsequently recover except when the rats are artificially made protein deficient. This part of the experimental observation lends further support to the human situation, because most patients with Chagas' disease belong to the poor malnourished groups.

The foregoing hypothesis is attractive, but it has three drawbacks. First, neuroganglionic destruction is not all that frequent in man and dog.[139] Second, controlled studies show similar atrophy of neurogangila in the rheumatic as well as hypertensive heart without the development of Chagas' type dilatation.[140] Third, the mechanism of neuroganglionic destruction is not clear; direct parasitic destruction is quite infrequent.

Immune reactivity to *T cruzi* initiated during the acute phase and nurtured during the latent phase has been put forward as an alternate hypothesis.[129,138] That there is considerable and consistent host immune reactivity to the parasite is well appreciated and forms the basis for the serologic detection of carriers and contacts at risk.[141] Such tests include indirect agglutination, complement fixation, indirect immunofluorescence, enzyme-linked immunosorbent assay (ELISA), and a recently added specific radioimmunoassay using biotin-^{3}H-avidin.[120,141-143] Another highly specific and sensitive serological test by competitive enzyme immunoassay (CEIA), using a *T cruzi*-specific monoclonal antibody, has been introduced recently and can differentiate Chagas' disease from other cross-reacting parasitic diseases in endemic areas where concomitant infections with leishmaniasis and *T rangeli* are suspected.[143a]

At tissue levels, immunoglobulin deposits have been detected on the plasma membrane of cardiac and other muscle cells. Antibodies to endocardium, vascular smooth muscle, and myocardial interstitium have been demonstrated and promise to become a useful diagnostic investigation using endomyocardial biopsies.[121,138] These observations in man have been partly supported and partly negated by experimental studies.[137,138,144,144a,145] In mice, for example,[138] the progressive loss of cardiac ganglia precedes the development of a demonstrable immune response against *T cruzi*, and the immune response may well be the result rather than the cause of cell destruction. On the other hand, more recent experiments with BALB/c mice indicate that the cardiac lesions seen in patients with Chagas' disease may be attributed to autoimmune reactions elicited by cross-reacting antigens (sarcoplasmic reticulum adenosine-triphosphatase [SRA]) shared by *T cruzi* and striated muscle.[145a]

Immune-mediated cardiac cell destruction and neuroganglionic changes, therefore, seem to hold greater promise in explaining Chagas' heart disease.

AFRICAN TRYPANOSOMIASIS: SLEEPING SICKNESS

Sleeping sickness caused by a subspecies of *Trypanosoma brucei* differs in many ways from *T cruzi*-induced Chagas' disease. The endemic areas include West, Central, and East Africa between the N20 and S20 parallels. Gambian sleeping sickness is rampant in West Africa, Zaire, the Southern Sudan, and along the Congo and Niger rivers and is caused by *T brucei gambiense.* The Rhodesian variety is caused by *T brucei rhodesiense* and occurs in Central and East Africa. The third subspecies, *T brucei brucei,* is nonpathogenic in man, affecting domestic animals only. Domestic cattle and pigs are the animal reservoirs for sleeping sickness and the tsetse fly (Glossina species), the insect vector. Unlike *T cruzi*, *T brucei* has the property of constantly changing its antigenic structure with each cycle in the animal host (variable antigenic type [VAT]).[146]

The bite of the fly leads to a local tissue reaction (trypanosomal chancre) and the parasite is spread through the salivary glands of the fly as is malaria (salivarian transmission). Cardiac involvement in the infection is uncommon but is quite varied. There may be only epicardial and endocardial hemorrhage, or full-fledged myocarditis develops with involvement of conduction tissue and the pericardium with effusion. In the mouse model of African trypanosomiasis,[147] pancarditis and valvulitis have been shown and appreciable damage to cardiac lymphatics occurs. Subsequently the heart shows atrophy, fibrosis, and dilatation. The possibility that the trypanosoma may be related to some cases of dilated cardiomyopathy and endomyocardial fibrosis in Africa has been debated.[148,149]

CARDIAC ECHINOCOCCOSIS: HYDATID DISEASE

Taenia echinococcus is a common parasite in most tropical and nontropical countries with large populations of sheep and dogs. Hardly any location in the human body has escaped infestation by the larval cyst. The heart is involved in 0.5% to 2% of cases and 41% present with complications arising out of rupture of one or more cysts[150] (anaphylaxis, pulmonary embolism, and systemic metastatic cysts) (Figure 52.4). Another 27% are incidentally found at autopsy.[150] The clinical features depend on the location of the cyst, and at autopsy at least five patterns have been described including a dead cyst with fibrosis, a living intact cyst, a cyst rupture into the pericardium, a pedunculated cyst in the cardiac chambers, or a cyst rupture into the cavity of the heart.[150] Most cysts (43% to 77%) are found in the left ventricle whereas rupture of the right ventricle is more frequent.[151-154] Pulmonary hydatid embolism has been reported in about 50 instances.[155] In recent years, clinical recognition of the cyst in the heart in known or suspected cases of hydatid disease elsewhere has been possible by echocardiography,[156-158] paving the way for successful surgical excision.[153,154,159]

CYSTICERCOSIS OF THE HEART

Infestation by the larva of the pig tape worm, *teania solium*, is a common problem in the South American and Indian subcontinents. Cardiac involvement is incidental and is rarely if ever diagnosed or suspected before death. A recent report from western India[160] lists six cases seen at autopsy, accounting for 1.3% of all autopsies and

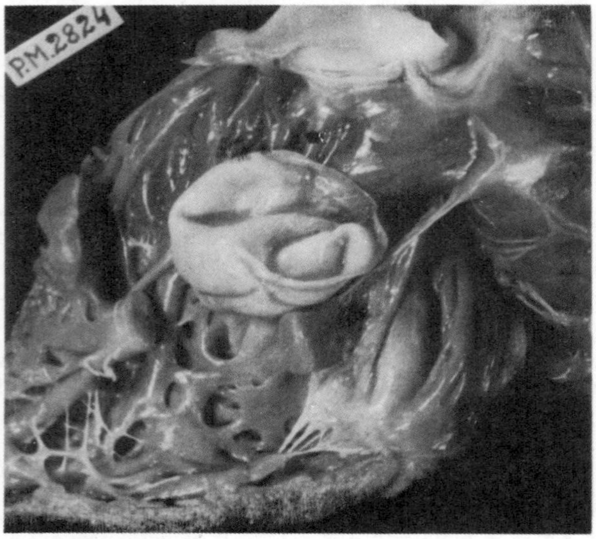

Figure 52.4. Hydatid cyst in the infracristal location of the right ventricle. The cyst had ruptured with hydatid embolization to the lungs. (From Silver MD [ed]: *Cardiovascular Pathology*. New York, Churchill Livingstone, 1983, with permission.)

46.1% of cases of generalized cysticercosis. In one case, pressure by the cyst led to coronary artery occlusion and death. Earlier reports included four instances of cysticercosis of the heart among 118 cases[161] and nine among 450 cases[162] (Figure 52.5).

SCHISTOSOMIASIS

Direct cardiac involvement by the circulating eggs of *Schistosoma hematobium* is rare and leads to myocarditis, pericarditis, and even coronary occlusion.[163] The common influence of schistosomiasis on the heart is exerted through pulmonary hypertension caused by widespread pulmonary schistosomiasis.[163,164] Other manifestations include anemia, myocarditis, even associated endomycardial fibrosis, and iatrogenic myocarditis.[164]

TRICHINOSIS: TRICHINELLOSIS

The nematode *Trichinella spiralis* invades the cardiac and skeletal muscles during its larval stage.[165] It is prevalent in Europe, the USSR, the United States, Canada, and Iceland. Larval cysts present in animal flesh, pork being the most common source of infection in man. The larva prefers to lodge in glycogen-poor muscle tissue.[166] Focal or widespread myocarditis results, which may rarely be fatal.[167] Transient electrocardiographic abnormalities,

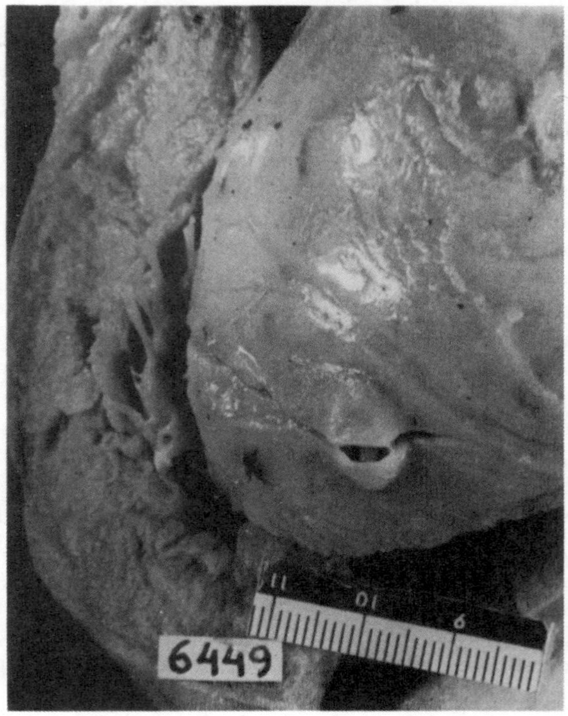

Figure 52.5. Cysticercus cellulosae cyst located in the epicardium. The larva can be seen in the cyst. Incidental autopsy finding.

including nonspecific T-wave changes, decreased QRS voltage, ventricular premature beats and conduction disturbances, occur in about one third of patients with trichinosis, often in the absence of cardiac symptoms; they parallel other evidence of myocarditis.[168] Trichinosis is another example of parasite-induced eosinophilia with associated endomyocardial fibrosis.[36]

OTHER PARASITES

Amebic pericarditis caused by rupture of an amebic liver abscess has occurred in up to 2.8% of the latter.[169] Similarly, filaria *Wuchereria bancrofti* produces chylous pericarditis.[1] Its possible role in endomyocardial fibrosis has already been discussed. The dog heart worm, *Dirofilaria immitis*, has sometimes been found in the human lung and skin and on rare occasions it has been detected incidentally in the heart.[170] Diethylcarbamazine and ivermectin are equally effective against *Wuchereria bancrofti* and *Dirofilaria immitis*.[171] Serologic tests such as enzyme-linked immunosorbent assay (ELISA) and indirect hemagglutination may be used to monitor antibody titers as an indicator of treatment efficacy.[172]

REFERENCES

1. Datta BN: Cardiovascular disease in tropics, in Silver MD (ed): *Cardiovascular Pathology*. New York, Churchill Livingstone, 1983, pp 1109–1152.

1a. Chukwuemeke AC, Pobee JOM, Larbi E, Kpodonu J, Ikeme IC, Pole D, William H, Chuwa ME: Are cardiovascular diseases important causes of mortality in Africa? Result of a WHO/UGMS follow-up study. *Trop Cardiol* 1982; 8:105–110.

2. World Health Organisation. *Cardiomyopathies*. WHO Tech Rep Ser 697, Geneva, 1984.

3. World Health Organisation and International Society and Federation of Cardiology: Report of the WHO/ISFC task force on definition and classification of cardiomyopathies. *Br Heart J* 1980; 44:672–673.

4. Davies MJ: The cardiomyopathies: a review of terminology, pathology and pathogenesis. *Histopathology* 1984; 8:363–393.

5. Kinare SG: Endomyocardial fibrosis in Bombay, in Sapru RP (ed): *Endomyocardial Fibrosis in India*. New Delhi, Indian Council of Medical Research, 1983, pp 155–162.

6. Bhaktaviziam A, Parameshwaran A: The pathology of endomyocardial fibrosis, in Sapru RP (ed): *Endomyocardial Fibrosis in India*. New Delhi, Indian Council of Medical Research, 1983, pp 143–154.

7. Bhatia ML, Reddy KS: Endomyocardial fibrosis: clinial, electrocardiographic and radiologic features, in Sapru RP (ed): *Endomyocardiol Fibrosis in India*. New Delhi, Indian Council of Medical Research, 1983, pp 14-21.

8. International Society and Federation of Cardiology Scientific Council on Cardiomyopathy: workshop on multicentric research project on endomyocardial disease, London, June 1982. *Postgrad Med J* 1983; 59:133–188.
9. Roberts WC, Buja LM, Ferrans VJ: Loffler's fibroblastic parietal endocarditis, eosinophilic leukaemia and Davies' endomyocardial fibrosis. The same disease in different stages. *Pathol et Microbiol* 1970; 35: 90-97.
10. Brockington IF, Olsen EGJ: Eosinophilia and endomyocardial fibrosis. *Postgrad Med J* 1972; 48:740–744.
11. Brockington IF: Heart disease in tropical Africa. The last ten years. *Acta Cardiol* 1980; 35:317-328.
12. Olsen EGJ: Pathological aspects of endomyocardial fibrosis. *Postgrad Med J* 1983; 59: 135–139.
13. Hutt MSR: Epidemiology aspects of endomyocardial fibrosis. *Postgrad Med J* 1983; 59:142–144.
14. Puigbo JJ, Combellas I, Acquatella H, Marsiglia I, Tortoledo F, Casal H, Suarez JA: Endomyocardial disease in South America: report on 23 cases in Venezuela. *Postgrad Med J* 1983; 59:162–168.
15. Indian Council of Medical Research: *Workshop on Endomyocardial Fibrosis in India, Trivandrum, 1981.* New Delhi, Indian Council of Medical Research, 1983.
16. Datta BN, Babu SK, Khattri HN, Bidwai PS, Wahi PL: Endomyocardial fibrosis in Chandigarh area, India. A study of nine autopsies. *Trop Geog Med* 1977; 29:346–352.
17. Datta BN, Aikat BK: Pathology of endomyocardial fibrosis: the Chandigarh experience, in Sapru RP (ed): *Endomyocardial fibrosis in India.* New Delhi, Indian Council of Medical Research, 1983, pp 163–167.
18. Fawzy ME, Ziady G, Halim M, Guindy R, Merces EN, Feteih N: Endomyocardial fibrosis: a report of eight cases. *J Am Coll Cardiol* 1985; 5:983–988.
18a. Liu YQ, Wang ZL, Wei EY: Radiological study of 4 cases of endomyocardial fibrosis. *Chin Med J* 1983; 96:569–574.
19. Falase AO: Endomyocardial fibrosis in Africa. *Postgrad Med J* 1983; 59:170–177.
20. Goodwin JF: Endomyocardial disease—clinical features. *Postgrad Med J* 1983; 59:154–155.
21. Sapru RP, Balakrishnan KG, Sasidharan K, Venkatachalam CG: Clinical profile of endomyocardial fibrosis, in Sapru RP (ed): *Endomyocardial Fibrosis in India.* New Delhi, Indian Council of Medical Research, 1983, pp 3–13.
22. Nair DV: Endomyocardial fibrosis in Kerala state. *Indian Heart J* 1982; 34:412–417.
23. Vijayaraghavan G, Sadanandan S: Immunological phenomena in tropical endomyocardial fibrosis. *Indian Heart J* 1984; 36:87–89.
24. Vijayaraghavan G: Endomyocardial fibrosis: clinical, electrocardiographic, and radiologic features, in Sapru RP (ed): *Endomyocardial Fibrosis in India.* New Delhi, Indian Council of Medical Research, 1983, pp 22–28.
25. Bijlsma F: The variety in endomyocardial fibrosis. A necropsy study. *Trop Geog Med* 1975; 28:199–205.
26. Jaiyesimi F: Scalar electrocardiogram in children with endomyocardial fibrosis. A useful diagnostic tool. *Trop Cardiol* 1981; 7:117–125.
27. Dienot B, Ekra A, Bertrand Ed: Echocardiographic signs in 45 cases of endomyocardial fibrosis. *Trop Cardiol* 1981; 7:107–114.
28. Davies J, Spry CJF, Sapsford R, Olsen EGJ, dePerez G, Oakley CM, Goodwin JF: Cardiovascular features of 11 patients with eosinophilic endomyocardial disease. *Q J Med* 1983; 52:23–39.
29. Shaper AG, Hutt MSR, Goles RM: Necropsy study of endomyocardial fibrosis and rheumatic heart disease in Uganda 1950-1965. *Br Heart J* 1968; 30:391–401.
30. Krishnaswamy H, Date A, Bhaktaviziam A, Krishnaswamy S, Cherian G: Electron microscopic changes in tropical endomyocardial fibrosis. *Trans Roy Soc Trop Med Hyg* 1984; 78:205–208.
31. Crawford MA: Endomyocardial fibrosis and carcinoidosis. A common denominator? *Am Heart J* 1963; 66:273–276.
32. Nair DV, Kurian S: Ecological study of endomyocardial fibrosis in Kerala; in Sapru RP (ed): *Endomyocardial Fibrosis in India.* New Delhi, Indian Council of Medical Research, 1983, pp 187–193.
33. Gerbaux A, Dubost Ch, Maurice P, Prigent C, Forman G, Baculard P, Valty J: Endomyocardite fibreuse observée au cours de la Filariose. A propos dún cas traité chirurgicalement. *Ann Med Interne* 1973; 124: 471–482.
34. Shaper AG, Hutt MSR, Fejfar Z (eds): *Cardiovascular Diseases in the Tropics.* London, British Medical Association, 1974.
35. Eling WMC, Jerusalem CR, Hermsen CC, Heinen-Borries UJ, Weiss ML, V. Run-V Breda CHJ: Endomyocardial lesion and endomyocardial fibrosis in experimental malaria (Plasmodium berghei) in mice. *Contr Microbiol Immunol* 1983; 7:218–229.
36. Andy JJ, O'Connell JP, Daddario RC, Roberts WC: Trichinosis causing extensive ventricular mural endocarditis with super-imposed thrombosis: evidence that severe eosinophilia damages endocardium. *Am J Med* 1971; 63:824–829,
37. Olsen EGJ, Spry CJF: Relation between eosinophilia and endomyocardial disease. *Prog Cardiovasc Dis* 1985; 27:241–254.
38. Olsen EGJ, Spry JFC: The pathogenesis of Loffler's endomyocardial disease and its relationship to endomyocardial fibrosis, in Yu PN, Goodwin JF (eds): *Progress in Cardiology*, Philadelphia, Lea & Febiger, 1979, pp 281–303.
39. Nambiar CA: Clinical features and etiology of endomyocardial fibrosis, in Sapru RP (ed): *Endomyocardial Fibrosis in India.* New Delhi, Indian Council of Medical Research, 1983, pp 42–48.
40. Davies J, Spry JFC, Vijayaraghavan G, DeSouza JA: A comparison of the clinical and cardiological features of endomyocardial disease in temperate and tropical regions. *Postgrad Med J* 1983; 59:179–183.
41. Jaiyesimi F, Salimonu LS, Antia AU: Serum immunoglobulins in children with cardiomyopathies. *Trans Roy Soc Trop Med Hyg* 1984; 78:127–131.
42. Shaper AG: Cardiovascular disease in tropics. II. Endomyocardial fibrosis. *Br Med J* 1972; 3:743–746.
43. Kartha CC, Mathai A, Balakrishnan KG, Valiathan MS: Immunological studies in endomyocardial fibrosis. *Indian Heart J* 1984; 36:90–91.
44. Edington GM, Jackson JG: The pathology of heart muscle disease and endomyocardial fibrosis in Nigeria. *J Path Bact* 1963; 86:333–344.
45. Datta BN, Aikat BK: Cardiomyopathy in N. India: an autopsy study of 30 cases. *Indian Heart J* 1974; 26:219–227.
46. Jaiyesimi F: From idiopathic cardiomegaly to endomyocardial fibrosis. *Trop Cardiol* 1981; 7:167–171.
46a. Metras D, Coulibaly AO, Ouattara K: The surgical treatment of endomyocardial fibrosis: results in 55 patients. *Circulation* 1985; 72(suppl II):II-274–II-279.
46b. Hess OM, Turina M, Egloff L, Jenni R, Krayenbühl HP: Clinical course of endomyocardial fibrosis following endocardial decortication. *Schweiz med Wchnschr* 1984; 114:1595–1598.
46c. Balakrishnan KG, Venkitachalam CG, Pillai VRK, Subramanian R, Valiathan MS: Postoperative evaluation of endomyocardial fibrosis. *Cardiology* 1986; 73:73–84.
47. Brockington IF, Edington GM, Olsen EGH: Nigerian "heart muscle disease." The late stages of untreated hypertensive heart failure? *Acta Cardiol* 1977; 32:245–267.
48. Falase AO, Fabiyi A, Ogunba EO: Heart muscle disease in Nigerian adults. A multifactorial disease. *Afr J Med Sci* 1977; 6:165–176.
49. Ikeme AC: Idiopathic cardiomegaly in Africa. *Bull WHO* 1976; 54: 455–461.
50. Julian DG, Szekely P: Peripartum cardiomyopathy. *Prog Cardiovasc Dis* 1985; 27:223–240.
51. Davidson N McD, Parry EHO: The etiology of peripartum cardiac failure. *Am Heart J* 1979; 97:535–536.
52. Sanderson JE, Adesanya CO, Anjorun FI, Parry EHO: Postpartum cardiac failure—heart failure due to volume overload? *Am Heart J* 1979; 97:613–621.
53. Dickinson J (ed): Debate: that congestive cardiomyopathy is really hypertensive heart disease in disguise. *Postgrad Med J* 1972; 48:777–789.
54. Falase AO: Cardiomegaly of unknown origin among Nigerian adults: role of hypertension in its etiology. *Br Heart J* 1977; 39:671–679.
55. Attah Ed'B, Falase AO: Large flabby hearts in hypertension. *Am Heart J* 1977; 94:189–195.
56. Beck W: Cardiomyopathies in South Africa—a brief survey of the problem and current therapeutic approaches. *Postgrad Med J* 1978; 54:469–474.
57. George BO, Okuwobi BO, Talabi AI, Jaiyeola BAO: Hypertrophic cardiomyopathy in Nigeria. *Trop Cardiol* 1981; 7:67–70.
58. Cherian G: Cardiomyopathy, in Ahuja MMS (ed): *Progress in Clinical Medicine*. New Delhi, Arnold Heinemann, 1976.
59. Bhatia ML: Juvenile rheumatic disease in India, in Ahuja MMS (ed): *Clinical Medicine*. New Delhi, Arnold Heinemann, 1976.
60. Padmavati S: The challenge of rheumatic fever and rheumatic heart disease in India. *Indian Heart J* 1982; 34:364–366.
61. World Health Organisation: Community control of rheumatic heart disease in developing countries. A major public health problem. *WHO Chron* 1980; 34:336–345.
62. Ferrans VJ, Roberts WC: Pathology of rheumatic heart disease, in Borman JB, Gotsman MS (eds): *Rheumatic Valvular Disease in Children.* New York, Springer Verlag, 1980, pp 28–58.
63. Lue Hung Chi, Tseng WP, Lin GJ, Hsieh KH, Hsieh RP, Chiou JF: Clinical and epidemiological features of rheumatic fever and rheumatic heart disease in Taiwan and the Far East. *Indian Heart J* 1983; 35:139–146.
64. Cole TO: Problems of rheumatic fever in Nigerians. *Trop Cardiol* 1980; 6:181–188.
65. Datta BN, Nograni B, Khattri HN, Sapru RP, Bidwai PS, Suri RK, Gujral JS, Wahi PL: Rheumatic heart disease at autopsy. An analysis of 260 cases at Chandigarh. *Indian Heart J* 1978; 30:39–48.
66. Datta BN: Cardiovascular disease in the tropics, in Silver MD (ed): *Cardiovascular Pathology*. New York, Churchill Livingstone, 1983, pp 1109–1152.
67. McLaren MJ, Hawkins DM, Koornhof HJ, Bloom KR, Bramwell-Jones DM, Cohen E, Gale GE, Kanarek K, Lachman AS, Lakier JB, Pocock WB, Barlow JB: Epidemiology of rheumatic heart disease in Black

school children of Soweto, Johannesburg. *Br Med J* 1975; 3:474–478.

68. Ilyas M, Peracha MA, Ahmed R, Khan N, Ali N, Janjua M: Prevalence and pattern of rheumatic heart disease in the frontier province of Pakistan. *J Pak Med Assoc* 1979; 29:165–168.
69. Lewis BS, Gotsman MS: Natural history of rheumatic heart disease in childhood, in Borman JB, Gotsman MS (eds): *Rheumatic Valvular Diseases in Children.* New York, Springer Verlag, 1980, pp 63–69.
70. Mathur KS, Wahal PK: Epidemiology of rheumatic heart disease. A study of 29,922 school children. *Indian Heart J* 1982; 34:367–371.
71. Kinare SG: Rheumatic heart disease in the young. Pathologic aspects. *Indian Heart J* 1983; 35:135–138.
72. Roberts WC: Morphologic features of the normal and abnormal mitral valve. *Am J Cardiol* 1983; 51:1005–1028.
73. Agarwal BL, Prasad S: Rheumatic mitral stenosis: accelerated and delayed types. *Indian Heart J* 1982; 34:286–287.
74. Uthaman B, Parameshwaram A, Bhaktaviziam A, Cherian G, Krishnaswamy S: Tricuspid valve involvement in rheumatic heart disease. A necropsy study. *Indian Heart J* 1978; 30:359–362.
75. Chopra P, Tandon HD: Pathology of chronic rheumatic heart disease with particular reference to tricuspid valve involvement. *Acta Cardiol* 1977; 32:423–434.
76. Moorthy JSSN, Reddy KN, Rajah S, Misra KP, Chitra M: Suprasystemic pulmonary hypertension in rheumatic mitral valve disease (abstr). *Indian Heart J* 1982; 34:297.
77. Mohan JC, Reddy KS, Karloopia BD, Venugopal P, Bhatia ML: Extreme pulmonary artery hypertension (PAH) in rheumatic heart disease in India—clinical, hemodynamic and surgical profile. *Indian Heart J* 1984; 36:313.
78. Tandon HD, Kasturi J: Pulmonary vascular changes associated with isolated mitral stenosis in India. *Br Heart J* 1975; 37:26–36.
79. Chopra P, Tandon HD, Raizada V, Gopinath N, Buttler C, William RC Jr: Comparative studies of mitral valves in rheumatic heart disease. *Arch Intern Med* 1983; 143:661–666.
80. Wahi PL, Kohli RS: Infective endocarditis, East and West. *Indian Heart J* 1982; 34:378–381.
81. Datta BN, Khattri HN, Bidwai PS, Suri RK, Gujral JS, Agarwal KC, Wahi PL: Infective endocarditis at autopsy in Northern India. A study of 120 cases. *Jpn Heart J* 1982; 23:330–336.
82. Mehta AP, Kalyani MD, Kinare SG: Infective endocarditis. *J Postgrad Med* 1978; 24:40–49.
83. Somers K, Patel AK, Steiner I, D'Arbela PG, Hutt MSR: Infective endocarditis—an African experience. *Br Heart J* 1972; 34:1107–1112.
84. Falase AO, Jaiyesimi F, Iyun AO, Attah EdB: Infective endocarditis: experience in Nigeria. *Trop Geog Med* 1976; 28:9–15.
85. Brockington IF, Edington GM: Adult heart disease in western Nigeria: a clinicopathologic synopsis. *Am Heart J* 1972; 83:27–40.
86. Steiner I, Patel AK, Hutt MSR, Somers K: Pathology of infective endocarditis: a postmortem evaluation. *Br Heart J* 1973; 35:159–164.
87. Datta BN, Misra NP: Infective endocarditis, in Misra NP (ed): *Progress in Cardiology.* New Delhi, Arnold Heinemann, 1981, pp 213–228.
88. Bhandari S, Kaul CL, Shrivastava S, Bhatia ML: Experience with infective endocarditis (abstr). *Indian Heart J* 1984; 36:330.
89. Nambiar U, Alurkar VM, Durairaj M, Saini P, Narayanan GR: Mitral valve prolapse in apparently healthy Indian women. *Indian Heart J* 1982; 34:285.
90. Antani J, Rao MS, Biradar NS, Nanjappa H, Thankur DS: Incidence and clinical profile of click-murmur syndrome in Indian female. *Indian Heart J* 1982; 34:285.
91. Dodu RAS: Coronary heart disease in developing countries: the threat can be averted. *WHO Chron* 1984; 38:3–7.
92. Banerjee JC: Some observation on the incidence of coronary atherosclerosis in India, in Datey KK, Pinto IJ, Bharucha PE (eds): *Proceedings of the International Seminar on Arteriosclerosis.* Bombay, Asia Publishing House, 1964, pp 12–18.
93. Naik CH: Incidence and epidemiology of coronary artery disease in Gujarat. *Indian Heart J* 1968; 20:3–7.

93a. Tuomilehto J, Ram P, Eseroma R, Taylor R, Zimmet P: Cardiovascular disease and diabetes mellitus in Fiji. *Bull WHO* 1984; 62:133–143.

94. Cheung FMF, Pang SW, Loke SL, Lan SH: Coronary atherosclerosis among Hong Kong Chinese. A histological and morphometric study using electronic digitizer. *Pathology* 1984; 16:381–386.
95. Chopra P, Sethi U, Gupta PK, Tandon HD: Coronary arterial stenosis. An autopsy study. *Acta Cardiol* 1983; 38:183–197.
96. Lee KT: Atherosclerosis in Africa. Studies of coronary arteries, blood lipids and coagulation profiles in Uganda. *Afr J Med Sci* 1971; 2:191–206.
97. Meyer BJ, Meyer AC, Pepler WJ: Chemical and structural aspects of atherosclerosis. *Afr J Med Sci* 1971; 2:283–299.
98. Langundoye SB, Edington GM, Ibeachun G, Cockshott NP: Postmortem coronary angiography in Nigerians: a radiologic view. *Afr J Med Sci* 1976; 5:9–17.
99. Krishnaswamy S, Satyamurthy I, Uthaman CB, Jaison TM, Kairnal NG, Sukumar IP: Angiographic pattern of coronary artery disease. *Indian Heart J* 1983; 35:200–203.
100. Krishnaswamy S, Satyamurthy I, Rao R, Padmakumar P: Age and coronary artery disease in Indians. *Indian Heart J* 1984; 36:152–154.
101. Wasir HS, Narula J, Mohan JC, Bhatia ML: Relationship of serum lipoproteins with angiographically defined coronary artery disease (abstr). *Indian Heart J* 1984; 36:329.
102. Bhandari S, Kaushik SK, Wasir HS, Bhatia ML: Critical evaluation of coronary risk factors profile in patients with myocardial infarction. *Indian Heart J* 1984; 36:297.
103. Kumar M, Chakravarti RN, Singh A, Wahi PL: Serum lipid profiles in patients of myocardial infarction in the Chandigarh area (North India). *Atherosclerosis* 1976; 24:355–361.
104. Taskar SP, Iyyer IR, Nerurkar SV, Sawant PN, Bhonsale DR, Kinare SG: Lipid profile in patients with myocardial infarction from the city of Bombay. *Indian Heart J* 1983; 35:169–171.
105. Banerjea JC, Mukherjea SK: Some observations on coronary heart disease. A study of 1000 cases. *Indian Heart J* 1970; 22:288–292.
106. Lal HB, Karoli RK, Sengupta D, Basumalik SN, Khan MA: Precocious myocardial infarction. *Indian Heart J* 1968; 20:11–15.
107. Falase AO, Cole TA, Osuntokun BO: Myocardial infarction in Nigerians. *Trop Geog Med* 1973; 25:147–150.
108. Bouramone C, Nkoua JL, Ekoba J: Les cardiopathies ischemiques en Republique Populaire du Congo. *Trop Cardiol* 1980; 6:17–29.
109. Van Staden DA, Kloppers PL, Fehrson JP: Ischemic heart disease in the South African Black. *S Afr Med J* 1980; 58:271–272.
110. Ben Ismail JL: Coronary heart disease in Africa. I. A multicentric prospective study. *Trop Cardiol* 1982; 8:93–97.

110a. Ben Ismail JL: Coronary heart disease in Africa. II. A multicentric prospective study. *Trop Cardiol* 1983; 9:105–112.

111. Higginson J, Gillanders AD, Murray JF: The heart in chronic malnutrition. *Br Heart J* 1952; 14:213–224.
112. Thomas J, Josserand C, Chastel C, Sagnet H, Lassale Y, LeVourch C: The cardiovascular manifestations of protein calorie malnutrition. *Med Trop* 1973; 32:505–509.
113. Lakshmikanthan C, Masilamani JA, Uthamalingam K, Thanikachalam S, Shetty V, Raju VB, Sreenivasan A: The heart in kwashiorkor. *Indian Heart J* 1982; 34:283.
114. Alexander CS: Nutritional heart disease in cardiomyopathy, in Burch GE (ed): *Cardiovascular Clinics 4.* Philadelphia, FA Davis, 1972.
115. Seftal HC, Metz J, Lakier JB: Cardiomyopathies in Johannesburg Bantu. Part I. Etiology and characteristics of beri-beri heart disease. *S Afr J Med* 1972; 46:1707–1713.
116. Collipp PJ, Chen SY: Cardiomyopathy and selenium deficiency in a two-year-old girl. *N Engl J Med* 1981; 304:1304–1305.
117. Kean BH, Breslau RC: *Parasites of the Human Heart.* New York, Grune & Stratton, 1964.
118. Manson-Bahr PEC, Apted FIC (eds): *Manson's Tropical Diseases,* ed 18. London, Bailliere Tindall, 1982.
119. Warren KS, Malsmond AEA (eds): *Tropical and Geographical Medicine.* New York, McGraw Hill, 1984.
120. World Health Organisation: Recent developments in the field of Chagas' disease. *Bull WHO* 1982; 60:463–473.
121. World Health Organisation. *Cardiomyopathies.* WHO Tech Report Ser 697, Geneva, 1984, pp 50–55.
122. Guimaraes AG, de Abreu NN, Santosfilho AA, Vinhaes LSA, Sousa JA de A: Haemodynamics in chronic Chagas' myocarditis and its differential diagnosis with endomyocardial fibrosis. *Trop Cardiol* 1977; 3:87–95.
123. Barbosa AJA, Pitella JEH, Tafuri WL: Incidence of chagasic cardiomyopathy in 15,000 necropsies. *Rev Soc Bras Med Trop* 1970; 4:219–223.
124. Leon A: Morphology of Chagas' myocarditis. *Kasmera* 1977; 3:299–341.
125. Suarez JA, Puigbo JJ, Rhode N, Valero JA, Gil Yepez: Cardiomyopathy in Venezuela. Morbid anatomy of 210 cases. *Acta Med Venez* 1968; 15:320–332.
126. Pearlman JD: Chagas' disease in Northern California. No longer an endemic diagnosis. *Am J Med* 1983; 75:1057–1061.
127. Rambajan I: The first autochthonous case of Chagas' disease with notes on possible vectors in Guyana. *Trop Geog Med* 1984; 36:73–76.
128. Puigbo JJ, Hirschault E, Boccalandro I, Aparicio JM, Valecillos R, Giordano H, Suarez C: Diagnosis of Chagas' cardiomyopathy. Non-invasive techniques. *Postgrad Med J* 1977; 53:527–532.

128a. Lima JAC, Szarfman A, Lima SD, Adams RJ, Russell RJ, Cheever A, Trischmann T, Weiss JL: Absence of left ventricular dysfunction during acute chagasic myocarditis in rhesus monkey. *Circulation* 1986; 73:172–179.

128b. Feit A, El-Sherif N, Korostoff S: Chagas' disease masquerading as coronary artery disease. *Arch Intern Med* 1983; 143:144–145.

129. Santos-Buch CA: American trypanosomiasis. *Intern Rev Exp Pathol* 1979; 19:63–100.
130. Suarez JA, Puigbo JJ, Valecillos R: Estudió clinicopatologico de la miocardiopatia cronica Chagasica de las miocardiopatias de etiologia dés conocida. *Acta Med Venez* 1970; 17:25–32.
131. Andrade ZA, Andrade SG, Oliviera GB, Alonso DR: Histopathology of the conducting tissue of the heart in Chagas' myocarditis. *Am Heart J* 1978; 95:316–324.

132. Palmero HA, Caeiro TF, Losa D: Prevalence of slow heart rates in chronic Chagas' disease. *Am J Trop Med Hyg* 1981; 30:1179–1182.
133. Pimenta J, Miranda M, Periera CB: Electrophysiologic findings in long-term asymptomatic chagasic individuals. *Am Heart J* 1983; 106:374–380.
134. Acquatella H, Schiller NB, Puigbo JJ, Giordano H, Suarez JA, Casal H, Arreaza N, Valecillos R, Hirschhaut E: M-mode and two-dimensional echocardiography in chronic Chagas' heart disease. A clinical and pathologic study. *Circulation* 1980; 62:787–799.
135. Koberlé F: Chagas' disease and Chagas' syndrome: the pathology of American trypanosomiasis. *Adv Parasitol* 1968; 6:63–110.
136. Koberlé F: Pathogenesis of Chagas' disease, in *Cardiomyopathies,* Ciba Foundation Symposia. No. 20. Amsterdam, North Holland, Elsevier/Excerpta Medica, 1974, pp 137–158.
137. Machado CRS, Moraes-Santos T, Machado ABM: Cardiac noradrenalin in relation to protein malnutrition in chronic experimental Chagas' disease in the rat. *Am J Trop Med Hyg* 1984; 33:835–838.
138. Ribeiro Dos Santos R, Hudson L: Denervation and the immune response in mice infected with Trypanosoma cruzi. *Clin Exp Immunol* 1981; 44:349–354.
139. Suarez JA: The intracardiac neurovegetative ganglia and the pathogenesis of Chagas' myocarditis. *Gaz Med Bahia* 1969; 69:73–104.
140. Lopez ER: Comparative study of intracardiac ganglia in rheumatic, hypertensive and Chagas' disease. *Rev Inst Med Trop S Paulo* 1970; 12:365–374.
141. Fife EH: Serodiagnosis of trypanosomiasis, in Cohen S, Saduri S (eds): *Immunology of Parasitic Infection.* Oxford, Blackwell Scientific, 1976, pp 77–93.
142. Camargo ME, Takeda GKF: Diagnostico de laboratorio, in Brener Z, Audrade Z (eds): *Trypanosoma cruzi e doenca de Chagas,* ed 1. Rio de Janeiro, Guanabara, 1979, pp 175–198.
143. Tarleton RL, Schulz CL, Grogl M, Kuhn RE: Diagnosis of Chagas' disease in humans using a Biotin-^{3}H-Avidin radioimmunoassay. *Am J Trop Med Hyg* 1984; 33:34–40.
143a. Lemesre JL, Afchain D, Orozco O, Loyens M, Breniere FS, Desjeux P, Carlier Y, Martin U, Nogueira-Queiroz JA, LeRay D, Capron A: Specific and sensitive immunological diagnosis of Chagas' disease by competitive enzyme immunoassay using a Trypanosoma cruzi-specific monoclonal antibody. *Am J Trop Med Hyg* 1986; 35:86–93.
144. Miles MA, Marsden PD, Petitt LE, Draper CC, Watson S, Seah SKK, Hutt MSR, Fowler JM: Experimental Trypanosoma cruzi infection in rhesus monkeys. III. ECG and histopathological findings. *Trans Roy Soc Trop Med Hyg* 1979; 73:528–532.
144a. Figueiredo F, Marin-Neto JA, Rossi MA: The evolution of experimental *Trypanosoma cruzi* cardiomyopathy in rabbits: further parasitiological, morphological and functional studies. *Int J Cardiol* 1986; 10:277–290.
145. Andrade ZA, Andrade SG, Sadigursky M, Maguire JH: Experimental Chagas disease in dogs. A pathologic and ECG study of the chronic indeterminate phase of infection. *Arch Path Lab Med* 1981; 105:460–464.
145a. Acosta AM, Santos-Buch CA: Autoimmune myocarditis induced by Trypanosoma cruzi. *Circulation* 1985; 71:1255–1261.
146. Vickerman K, Barry JD: in Cohen S, Warren KS (eds): *Immunology of Parasitic Infection.* Oxford, Blackwell Scientific, 1982, pp 204–260.
147. Poltera AA, Hochmann A, Lambert PH: A model for cardiopathy induced by Trypanosoma brucei brucei in mice. *Am J Pathol* 1980; 99:325–338.
148. Blackett K, Ngu JL: Immunological studies in congestive cardiomyopathy in Cameroon. *Br Heart J* 1976; 38:605–611.
149. Poltera AA, Cox JN: Pancarditis with valvulitis in endomyocardial fibrosis and in human African trypanosomiasis. *Virchows Arch [Pathol Anat]* 1977; 374:53–70.
150. Peters JM, Dexter L, Weiss S: Clinical and theoretical considerations of involvement of the left side of heart with echinococcal cysts. *Am Heart J:* 1945; 29:143–167.
151. Dighiero J, Canabal EJ, Aguitre CV, Hazan J, Horjales JO: Echinococcus disease of the heart. *Circulation* 1958; 17:127–132.
152. Di Bello R, Menendez H: Intracardiac rupture of hydatid cyst of the heart. A study based on three personal observations and 101 cases in the world literature. *Circulation* 1963; 27:366–374.
153. Heyat J, Mokhtari H, Hojaliloo J, Shakibi JG: Surgical treatment of echinococcal cysts of the heart. Report of a case and review of the world literature. *J Thorac Cardiovasc Surg* 1971; 61:755–764.
154. Saidi F: *Surgery of Hydatid Disease.* Philadelphia, WB Saunders, 1976, pp 302–321.
155. Palant A, Deutsch V, Kishon Y, Lieberman Y, Yahini JH, Neufeld HN: Pulmonary hydatid embolization. Report on 2 operated cases and review of published reports. *Br Heart J* 1976; 38:1086–1091.
156. Oliver JM, Benito LP, Ferrufino O, Sotillo JF, Nunez L: Cardiac hydatid cyst diagnosed by two-dimensional echocardiography. *Am Heart J* 1982; 104:164–165.
157. Ernst A, Čikes I, Radovanovič N: Two-dimensional echocardiographic study of a cardiac hydatid cyst. *Am J Cardiol* 1983; 52:1361–1363.
158. Malouf J, Saksouk FA, Alam S, Rizk GK, Dagher I: Hydatid cyst of the heart: diagnosis by two-dimensional echocardiography and computed tomography. *Am Heart J* 1985; 109:605–607.
159. Papo I, Ginsberg E, Albreht M, Martinovic N, Sokolic J: Surgical treatment of cardiac echinococcosis. Report of nine cases. *Texas Heart Inst J* 1982; 9:3–9.
160. Dutta SK, Banerjee AK, Pal A: Cysticercosis with involvement of the heart. Report of six cases. *Indian Heart J* 1982; 34:329.
161. Acha PN, Aguilar FJ: Studies on cysticercosis in Central America and Panama. *Am J Trop Med Hyg* 1964; 13:48–53.
162. Dixon HBF, Lipscomb FM: *Cysticercosis. An analysis and follow up of 450 cases.* MRC Special Rep Ser 299, 1961, pp 41–53.
163. Cheever AW, Kamel IA, Elwi AM, Mosimann JE, Danner R, Sipple JE: Schistosoma mansoni and schistosoma hematobium infection in Egypt. III. Extrahepatic pathology. *Am J Trop Med Hyg* 1978; 27:55–75.
164. Bertrand Ed, Charles D, Burdin CD, Ekra A, Girod FX, Lousdorfer J: Cardiac symptomatology in schistosomiasis. *Trop Cardiol* 1980; 6:167–179.
165. Spencer H: *Tropical Pathology.* Heidelberg, Springer-Verlag, 1973, pp 469–476.
166. Goldberg E: The glycolytic pathway in *Trichinella spiralis* larvae. *J Parasitol* 1958; 44:363–370.
167. Datta BN: Parasitic diseases of the heart, in Silver MD (ed): *Cardiovascular Pathology.* New York, Churchill Livingstone, 1983, pp 1153–1167.
168. Hurst JW: *The Heart,* ed 6. New York, McGraw Hill. 1986, p 1172.
169. Adeyemo AO, Aderoumu A: Intrathoracic complications of amoebic liver abscess. *J Roy Soc Trop Med Hyg* 1984; 77:17–21.
170. Takeuchi T, Asami K, Kobayashi S, Masuda M, Tanabe M, Miura S, Asakawa M, Murai T: Dirofilaria immitis infection in man. Report of a case of the infection in heart and inferior vena cava from Japan. *Am J Trop Med Hyg* 1981; 30:966–969.
171. Drugs for parasitic infections. *Medical Letter* 1986; 28:9–18.
172. Glickman LT, Grieve RB, Schantz PM: Serologic diagnosis of zoonotic pulmonary dirofilariasis *Am J Med* 1986; 80:161–164.

53 Diseases of the Peripheral Arteries

John A. Spittell, Jr., MD, FACP, FACC

Peripheral arterial disorders are common in both medical and surgical practice throughout the world. The ease with which the extremities can be examined and the characteristic symptoms, including pain, changes in skin color and temperature, and ulceration, make possible the bedside diagnosis of many peripheral arterial problems. At times a peripheral vascular abnormality is an early clue to an important, otherwise occult, process providing the alert clinician a significant diagnostic clue. Furthermore, even when asymptomatic, peripheral arterial disorders warrant proper management to lessen future morbidity and loss of limb.

GENERAL CONSIDERATIONS

Because atherosclerosis is the most common cause of both occlusive and aneurysmal arterial diseases, these diseases are common clinical problems.[1] In addition, the peripheral arteries can be involved by arterial spasm, inflammation, and trauma.

Intermittent claudication is the hallmark of symptomatic occlusive peripheral arterial disease. It is just as characteristic in its relation to walking and relief with standing still as angina pectoris is to exertion and rest. Many musculoskeletal and neurologic disorders causing symptoms in the extremities may mimic symptomatic peripheral occlusive arterial disease (Figure 53.1), but most are readily differentiated by careful history and physical examination. Perhaps the most difficult condition to differentiate is pseudoclaudication due to lumbar spinal stenosis; pseudoclaudication differs from true claudication in occurring with standing as well as walking, having a paresthetic quality, and requiring sitting or lying down for relief.[2]

When ischemia becomes severe, pain at rest, often disturbing sleep, develops; ischemic rest pain is severe and involves the foot or toes and is aggravated by a cool environment and elevation of the extremity.

The most common vasospastic disorder is Raynaud's phenomenon, but livedo reticularis and acrocyanosis deserve mention as well. Color change of the skin of the acral parts is the hallmark of these disorders because they are due to episodic constriction of the cutaneous and digital arterioles. Time taken to determine not only the time of onset but also the digits involved by the color change may provide the alert clinician with useful diagnostic information.

Because some commonly prescribed medications (beta blocking drugs and ergot preparations) may aggravate the symptoms of occlusive peripheral arterial disease or vasospastic disorders, their use should be included in the medical history. As a matter of fact, intermittent claudication in a patient on beta blocker therapy for angina pectoris may be the first presenting symptom of coexisting peripheral arterial disease. Occlusive peripheral arterial disease is common in persons with coronary artery disease and similarly coronary artery disease is often found in patients known to have peripheral artery disease.[2a] Such a patient with severe angina on exertion may not be able to walk a long distance as to develop intermittent claudication. On the other hand, patients with coexistent coronary artery disease and peripheral arterial disease may not experience much angina because of limited capacity to walk very much due to intermittent claudication. Very often satisfactory surgical relief of occlusive disease in one system will "worsen" the symptoms of occlusive disease in the other.

As noted, the extremities are easy to examine, but unless attention is paid to common symptoms and examination of the peripheral arterial system, including the brachial, radial, and ulnar pulses in the upper extremity

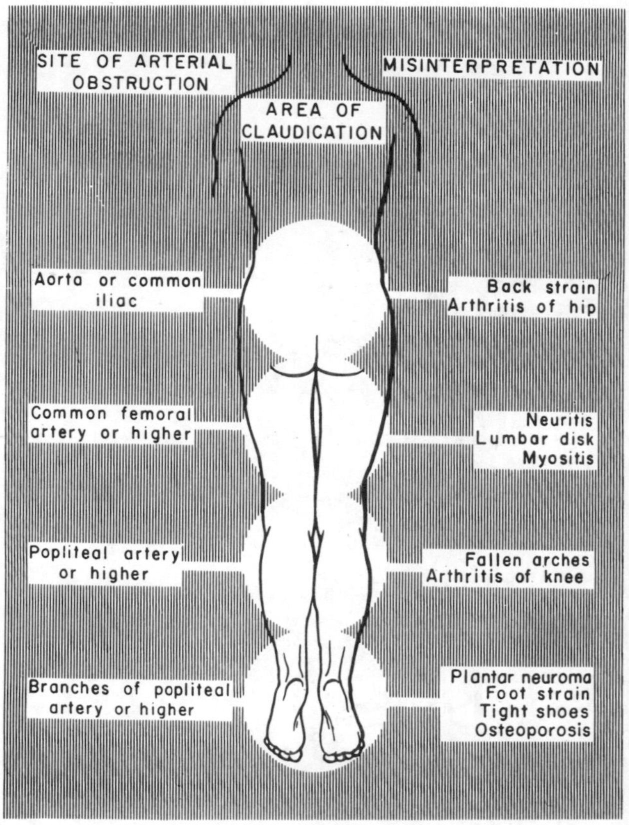

Figure 53.1. Common misinterpretations of claudication. Neurologic and musculoskeletal disorders are often incorrectly diagnosed as the cause of a patient's pain. Careful evaluation of mode of onset and relief will usually clarify distress as intermittent claudication. (Adapted from Gifford RW Jr, Hurst JW: A note on the location of intermittent claudication. *GP* 1957; 16:89, with permission of the American Academy of Family Physicians.)

and the femoral, popliteal, dorsal pedis, and posterior tibial pulses in the lower extremity, is complete, peripheral arterial disorders may be overlooked. Each arterial pulsation should be evaluated for its presence and character. Of interest in a recent study, an abnormal posterior tibial artery pulsation showed a sensitivity, specificity, and predictive value greater than any other historical or physical findings in the evaluation of occlusive peripheral arterial disease.[3] Auscultation for bruits over the larger arteries is an important finding in occlusive arterial disease, particularly after exercise.[4] A rough but reliable estimate of any ischemia of the extremity in the patient with occlusive arterial disease can be obtained by taking the few extra minutes required to perform the elevation and dependency tests (Tables 53.1 and 53.2).

In examination of the upper extremity, the Allen test (Figure 53.2) is useful to evaluate the patency not only of the arteries supplying the hand but also of the palmar arch and digital arteries.[5] When the principal symptoms or findings of arterial disease are confined to an upper extremity, the thoracic outlet compression syndrome must be a consideration and the appropriate maneuvers (Figures 53.3 to 53.5) included in the examination.[6]

Table 53.1. Grading of Elevation Pallor*†

Grade of Pallor	Duration of Elevation
0	No pallor in 60 seconds
1	Definite pallor in 60 seconds
2	Definite pallor in less than 60 seconds
3	Definite pallor in less than 30 seconds
4	Pallor on the level

* Elevation of extremity at an angle of 60 degrees above the level.

† From Spittell JA Jr: Recognition and management of chronic atherosclerotic occlusive peripheral arterial disease. *Mod Concepts Cardiovasc Dis* 1981; 50:19-23. (Tables 53.1, 53.2, and 53.4 are reproduced with permission of American Heart Association, Inc.)

The noninvasive diagnostic studies can both confirm objectively (Table 53.3) and provide a functional dimension to the diagnosis of occlusive peripheral arterial disease (Table 53.4). In aneurysms, ultrasound studies are excellent for diagnosis (Figure 53.6), but before any surgical treatment, contrast arteriography to evaluate both the proximal and distal circulation is necessary (Figure 53.7).

To confirm vasospasm in doubtful cases or to evaluate the effect of therapy on vasospasm we measure the skin temperature of the digits before and after 30 seconds of immersion in ice water[7]; in normal persons the digital skin temperatures return to normal in three to ten minutes, whereas in the patient with a vasospastic disorder more than ten minutes and often more than 20 minutes pass before preimmersion skin temperatures are reached. (If there is digital ulceration, gangrene, or a skin temperature of less than 22°C, we do not do ice water immersion studies for fear of inducing an injury.)

Although arteriography provides definitive information about occlusive peripheral arterial disease, it is usually necessary only when restoration of pulsatile flow is a consideration or when the origin of the occlusive arterial disease is uncertain. As noted earlier, when surgical treatment of peripheral arterial aneurysms is planned, contrast angiography is needed to assess the proximal and distal arterial circulation.

For every patient with occlusive peripheral arterial disease, whether involving the upper or lower extremities, or both, protection of the ischemic limb from trauma (mechanical, chemical, and thermal) and avoidance of vasoconstrictive influences, specifically tobacco, are basic therapeutic measures that may improve limb or digital survival. Time to explain these measures and their im-

Table 53.2. Color Return (CR) and Venous Filling Time (VFT)*

	Time for CR (s)	VFT (s)
Normal	10	15
Moderate ischemia	15–20	20–30
Severe ischemia	40+	40+

* From Spittell JA Jr: Recognition and management of chronic atherosclerotic occlusive peripheral arterial disease. *Mod Concepts Cardiovasc Dis* 1981; 50:19–23.

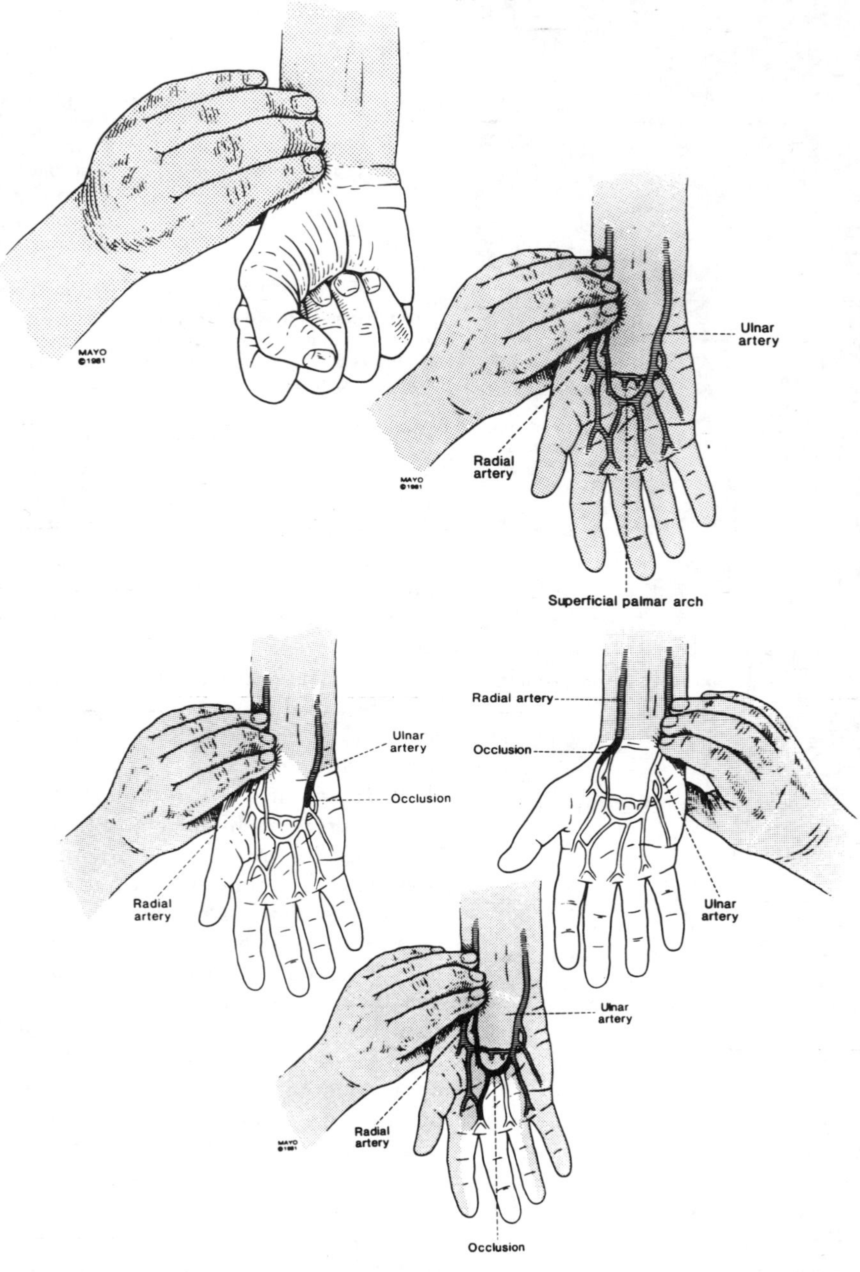

Figure 53.2. Allen test. *Top,* normal (negative) result, indicating patency of ulnar artery and superficial palmar arch. *Bottom,* abnormal (positive) results due to occlusion of ulnar artery (*left*), radial artery (*right*), and superficial palmar arch (*center*). (From Spittell JA Jr: Occlusive peripheral arterial disease: guidelines for office management. *Postgrad Med* 1982; 71:137–151. Reprinted with permission of McGraw-Hill Inc.)

portance to each patient is well worthwhile, whether other therapy is planned or not.

In the person with intermittent claudication a regular walking program, to the point of claudication, several times a day may significantly increase the walking distance.[8]

Chronic occlusive peripheral arterial disease is most often due to arteriosclerosis, but the less common types of occlusive peripheral arterial disease provide important therapeutic opportunities (Table 53.5).

CHRONIC OCCLUSIVE PERIPHERAL ARTERIAL DISEASE

ARTERIOSCLEROSIS OBLITERANS

In the nondiabetic person who has no symptoms or only intermittent claudication, restoration of pulsatile flow by either surgery or balloon angioplasty is an elective procedure (designed to relieve the claudication), because the outlook for limb survival is good, on the order of 95% over a five-year period, whereas their shortened life

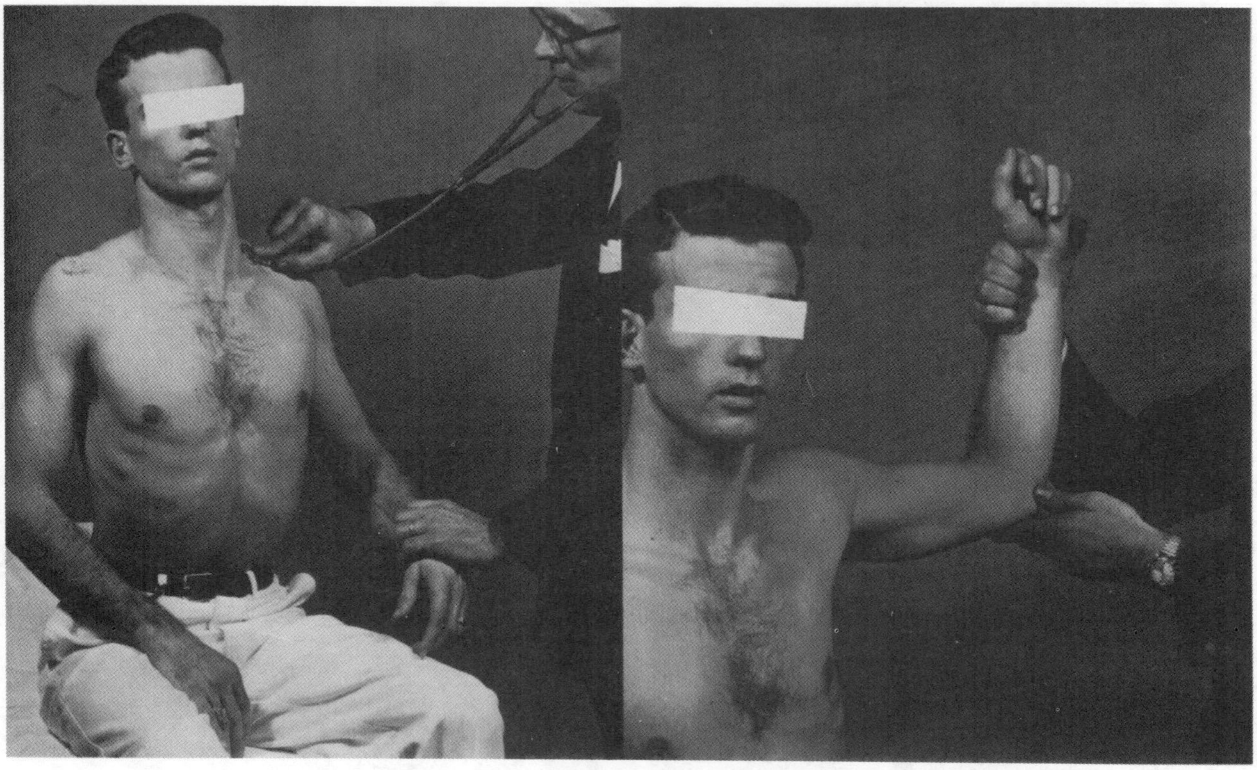

Figure 53.3. *Left,* costoclavicular maneuver, active. Auscultation over subclavian artery, above or below midportion of clavicle, may reveal systolic bruit as artery is compressed. Radial pulse and bruit over subclavian artery disappear when complete compression of subclavian artery occurs. *Right,* costoclavicular maneuver, passive. (From Fairbairn JF II, Campbell JK, Payne WS: Neurovascular compression syndrome of the thoracic outlet, in Juergens JL, Spittell JA Jr, Fairbairn JF II (eds): *Peripheral Vascular Diseases,* ed 5. Philadelphia, WB Saunders, 1980, pp 629–653. Figures 53.3–53.5, 53.9, 53.12 and 53.14 are reproduced with permission of the Mayo Foundation.)

expectancy is due to their associated atherosclerotic coronary and cerebrovascular disease.[9] However, when there is ischemic ulceration or ischemic rest pain, or both, the incidence of limb loss increases to the point that restoration of pulsatile flow is indicated. An even more aggressive approach to restoring pulsatile flow is justified by the poor prognosis of the diabetic person with occlusive peripheral arterial disease.[10]

Percutaneous transluminal balloon angioplasty provides a method of restoring pulsatile flow in selected cases with a lower morbidity, mortality, and cost than does arterial surgery. Although the indications are generally the same as those for arterial surgery, balloon angioplasty is best reserved for occlusions shorter than 10 cm in length in the iliac, femoral, or popliteal arteries. Reocclusion remains a problem, occurring in about one third of cases over three years, but it may improve as the technique evolves and postangioplasty antiplatelet therapy is better understood.[11]

With the excellent techniques of restoring pulsatile flow, the indications for sympathectomy are quite limited today. Because interrupting the sympathetic nerve supply to an extremity results mainly in increased blood flow in the skin, the principal indication of sympathectomy is ischemic ulceration when restoration of pulsatile flow to the extremity is not possible.

The oral vasodilators are not effective in the relief of intermittent claudication,[12] but they may be helpful in the patient with ischemic ulceration (just described for the use of sympathectomy) because they increase cutaneous blood flow.

A common finding in persons with atherosclerotic disease is an increased erythrocyte rigidity and increased blood viscosity.[13] Pentoxifylline, a methylated xanthine, has been used in Europe and recently introduced in the United States as a hemorrheologic agent for the treatment of intermittent claudication. In the dose of 400 mg three times daily it has been reported to increase the walking distance in some patients, presumably by improving the microcirculation as a result of increasing erythrocyte flexibility; however, it should be kept in mind that pentoxifylline has other actions that may contribute to any beneficial effect in intermittent claudication.[14,15,15a]

Clearly the person with atherosclerotic occlusive peripheral arterial disease who has associated hyperlipidemia, diabetes, or systemic hypertension warrants aggressive management of these risk factors in the hope of slowing the progression of the atherosclerotic process.[15b]

THROMBOANGIITIS OBLITERANS (BUERGER'S DISEASE)

That thromboangiitis is a distinct clinical entity has been well established by both clinical and pathologic

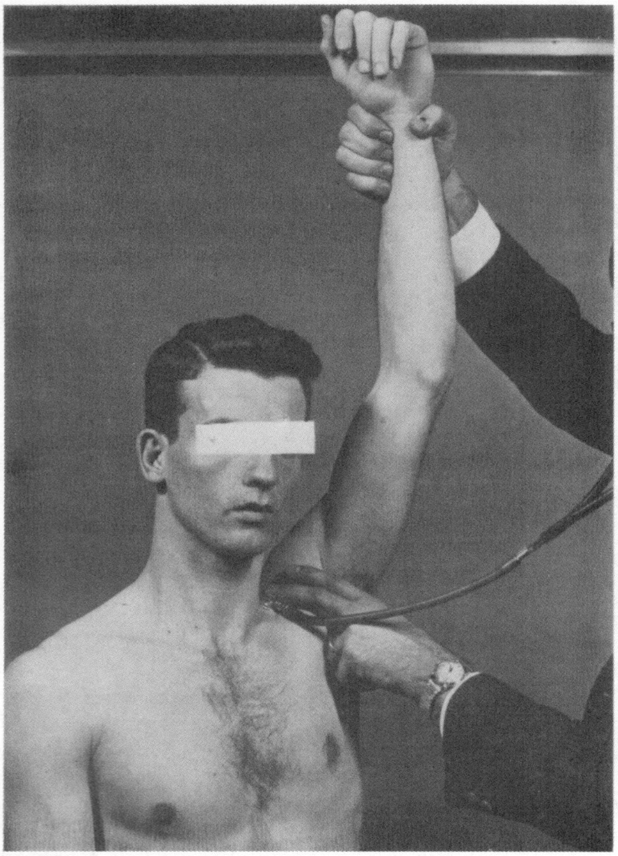

Figure 53.4. Hyperabduction maneuver. Axillary artery may be completely or incompletely compressed by maneuver. In the latter case, a bruit may be heard above or below the clavicle or on occasion deep in the axilla. (From Fairbairn JF II, Campbell JK, Payne WS: Neurovascular compression syndrome of the thoracic outlet, in Juergens JL, Spittell JA Jr, Fairbairn JF II (eds): *Peripheral Vascular Diseases,* ed 5. Philadelphia, WB Saunders, 1980, pp 629–653.)

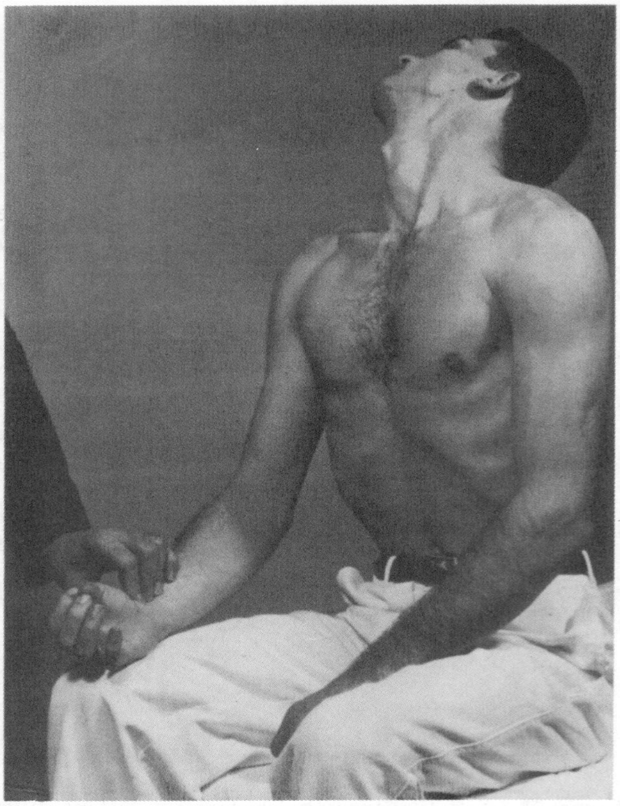

Figure 53.5. Scalene or Adson maneuver. This test is used in both cervical rib or anomalous first thoracic rib syndrome and scalenus anticus syndrome. Auscultation over subclavian artery being tested may reveal a bruit when artery is partially compressed. (From Fairbairn JF II, Campbell JK, Payne WS: Neurovascular compression syndrome of the thoracic outlet, in Juergens JL, Spittell JA Jr, Fairbairn JF II (eds): *Peripheral Vascular Diseases,* ed 5. Philadelphia, WB Saunders, 1980, pp 629–663.)

studies.[16,17] Its rather unique clinical features include its predilection for young males (usually less than 30 years and often less then 20 years of age), the involvement of small and medium-sized arteries of the wrist and hand with almost the same frequency as those of the leg and foot, the frequent association of superficial thrombophlebitis when the disease is active, and the association of the active disease with the use of tobacco. Although some have concluded that tobacco is an etiologic factor,[18] most believe it is contributory and perhaps related to the reaction of a specific phenotype to tobacco.[19] The recent report of a cell-mediated sensitivity to human collagen in persons with thromboangiitis obliterans raises the question of an immunologic basis.[20]

Regardless of etiology, the person with thromboangiitis obliterans can be advised with confidence that the activity of the disease will subside when the use of tobacco stops and will resume with the resumption of tobacco use. When ischemic ulceration is a problem, cutaneous vasodilation may be effected with one of the oral vasodilators or preferably by regional sympathectomy.

Table 53.3. Systolic Pressures and Indexes in Occlusive Arterial Disease*

	Supine Systolic Blood Pressure			
	Right		Left	
Level of Cuff	Pressure†	Index‡	Pressure†	Index‡
Arm	138/80	—	150/84	—
Thigh	62	0.41	144	0.96
Calf	54	0.36	138	0.92
Ankle	48	0.32	122	0.81

* From Spittell JA Jr: Peripheral arterial disease. Noninvasive diagnosis and management. *Resident & Staff Physician* 1982; 28:36s-45s. (Reproduced with permission of the Resident, Inc.)

† Pressure in millimeters of mercury.

‡ Index obtained by dividing the systolic ankle blood pressure by the systolic brachial blood pressure (normal, 0.95 or greater).

Table 53.4. Noninvasive Laboratory Assessment of Arterial Insufficiency of the Legs*

	Standard Exercise		Systolic Blood Pressure Index†	
Degree of Arterial Insufficiency	**Claudication**	**Duration (min)**	**Before Exercise**	**After Exercise**
Minimal	0	5	Normal to mildly	Abnormal
Mild	+	5	>0.8	>0.5
Moderate	+	<5	<0.8	<0.5
Severe‡	+	<3	<0.5	<0.15

* From Spittell JA Jr: Recognition and management of chronic atherosclerotic occlusive peripheral arterial disease. *Mod Concepts Cardiovasc Med* 1981; 50:19-23.

†Systolic pressure index is obtained by dividing the systolic ankle blood pressure by the systolic brachial blood pressure, both measured in the supine position (normal, 0.95 or greater).

‡Often the systolic ankle blood pressure is less than 50 mm Hg.

ARTERITIS

The arteritides that may involve arteries of the extremities are shown in Table 53.5. At times the occlusive peripheral arterial disease may dominate the clinical picture and on occasion may be the initial clinical manifestation.

Giant Cell Arteritis

Pathologically, cranial arteritis and Takayasu's disease are similar in that they present the picture of a focal granulomatous arteritis of the aorta and its branches. The difference in the two disorders is the age of the patient: cranial arteritis affects persons greater than 50 years of age and women slightly more often then men, whereas Takayasu's disease affects women four times more often than men and begins before age 40, often before the age of 20 years.

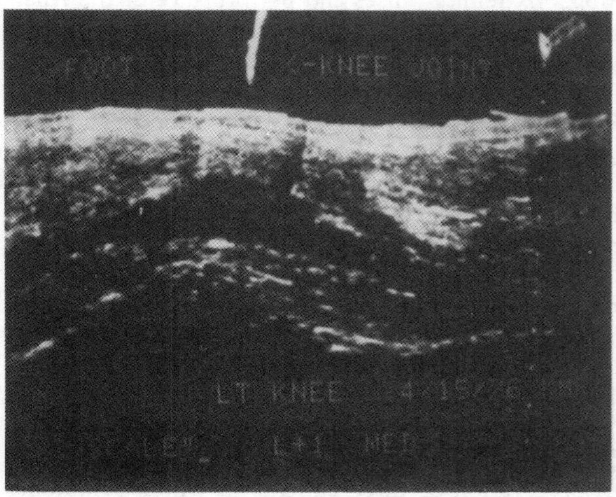

Figure 53.6. Longitudinal ultrasound scan of the left knee shows a popliteal aneurysm at about the level of the knee joint. (From Spittell JA Jr: Clinical aspects of aneurysmal disease. *Curr Probl Cardiol* 1980; 5:1–35. Figures 53.6 and 53.7 are reproduced with permission of Year Book Medical Publishers.)

Peripheral arterial involvement in both types of giant cell arteritis is fairly common and therefore the patient may complain of claudication of an extremity in addition to the systemic manifestations. In the person with peripheral arterial involvement, arteriography is useful in differentiating the arteritis from other types of occlusive arterial disease (Figures 53.8 and 53.9).

Giant cell arteritis is treated with adequate doses of corticosteroids. Decisions about arterial surgery or balloon angioplasty should be deferred until the activity of the arteritis has been suppressed[21,22] and, indeed, the peripheral arterial circulation at times will improve with corticosteroid therapy.[21,22a]

Connective Tissue Disorders

The arteritis seen with connective tissue disorders involves principally the digital arteries and the dermal arterioles. In the latter instance, rather typical painful ischemic ulceration of the skin of the lateral and posterior aspect of the legs occurs (Figure 53.10). When the digital arteries are involved, the clinical manifestations may be vasospasm (Raynaud's phenomenon), ischemic ulceration, gangrene, or a combination (Figure 53.11). The occlusive arterial problems described are seen most often in scleroderma, rheumatoid arthritis and systemic lupus erythematosus, and rarely in periarteritis nodosa. Management is directed at the systemic illness.

ARTERIAL TRAUMA

Acute arterial trauma can occur with penetrating or crush injuries, sudden deceleration, or fractures and dislocation of bones adjacent to arteries. The effects possible with acute arterial injury are illustrated in Figure 53.12. Establishing a cause and effect relation requires evidence that arterial disease was not present before the trauma, that the trauma was temporally and anatomically related to the arterial disease, and that the trauma was of the character to cause the arterial trauma.

Repetitive blunt or compressive trauma can cause arterial occlusive disease, particularly in the hand. Typically

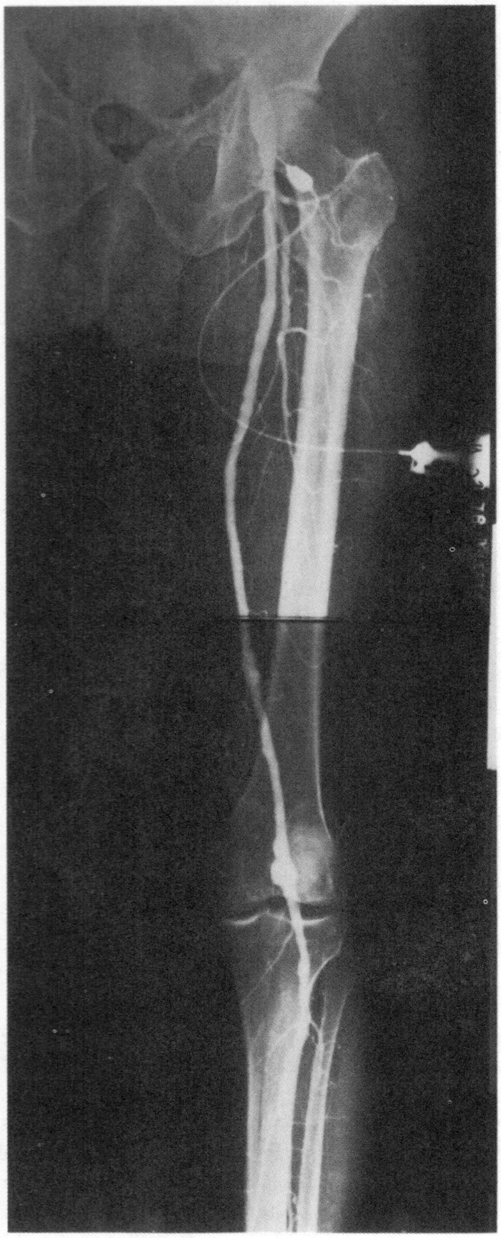

Figure 53.7. Left femoral arteriogram demonstrating popliteal aneurysm just above the level of the knee joint. Same patient as in Figure 53.6. (From Spittell JA Jr: Clinical aspects of aneurysmal disease. *Curr Probl Cardiol* 1980; 5:1–35.)

this occurs in the dominant hand and can be seen in a variety of occupations, as shown in Table 53.6. The symptoms vary from none or mild Raynaud's phenomenon to ischemic pain at rest and ischemic ulceration (Figure 53.13). The importance of making this diagnosis is to prevent continued trauma and progressive digital ischemia. The conservative measures already discussed and either pharmacologic agents (eg, prazosin or nifedipine) or regional sympathectomy to improve digital cutaneous circulation are indicated if there is significant digital ischemia or ischemic ulceration.

Table 53.5. Chronic Occlusive Peripheral Arterial Disease

A. Arteriosclerosis obliterans
B. Thromboangiitis obliterans (Buerger's disease)
C. Arteritis
  1. Giant cell arteritis
    a. Temporal (cranial) arteritis
    b. Idiopathic medial aortopathy (Takayasu's Disease)
  2. Connective tissue disorders
D. Trauma
  1. Blunt trauma
    a. Acute
    b. Chronic
  2. Arterial entrapment
    a. Thoracic outlet compression
    b. Superficial femoral artery
    c. Popliteal artery entrapment

ARTERIAL ENTRAPMENT

Arteries to the extremities may be chronically compressed at three principal locations: the thoracic outlet and the adductor canal outlet in the distal thigh and in the popliteal space. Each of these types of arterial compression can eventuate in arterial occlusion that can be limb threatening, and yet if diagnosed before such complications occur they are surgically remediable.

Thoracic Outlet Compression

The wall of the subclavian artery may be damaged by compression in the thoracic outlet, most often between the uppermost rib and the clavicle (Figure 53.14), resulting in thrombosis at the site of injury or embolization occluding more distal arteries in the arm or hand, or both. When the occlusive arterial complications of thoracic outlet compression occur, the symptoms vary from none or minor vasospastic phenomena to severe ischemia of the arm, hands, or fingers. In addition to careful examination of upper extremity pulses and performance of the Allen test (Figure 53.2), thoracic outlet maneuvers (Figures 53.3 to 53.5) should be performed. Arteriography is the best way to demonstrate any occlusive arterial process in the arm (Figure 53.15) and changes in the subclavian artery (Figure 53.16). In the patient with symptomatic or complicated thoracic outlet compression, resection of the uppermost rib is the most effective way to relieve the compression. Any needed surgery of the subclavian artery or sympathectomy to relieve ischemia of the affected hand can be performed at the same operation.[6]

Adductor Canal Outlet Compression of the Superficial Femoral Artery

Balaji and DeWeese[23] have proposed, on the basis of their observation of three patients in whom symptoms of occlusive disease of the femoral artery developed while skiing or jogging, that mechanical trauma to the artery is caused by the tendinous distal opening of Hunter's canal. Proper management consists of surgical release of the tendinous constriction and surgical restoration of pulsatile flow to the leg.

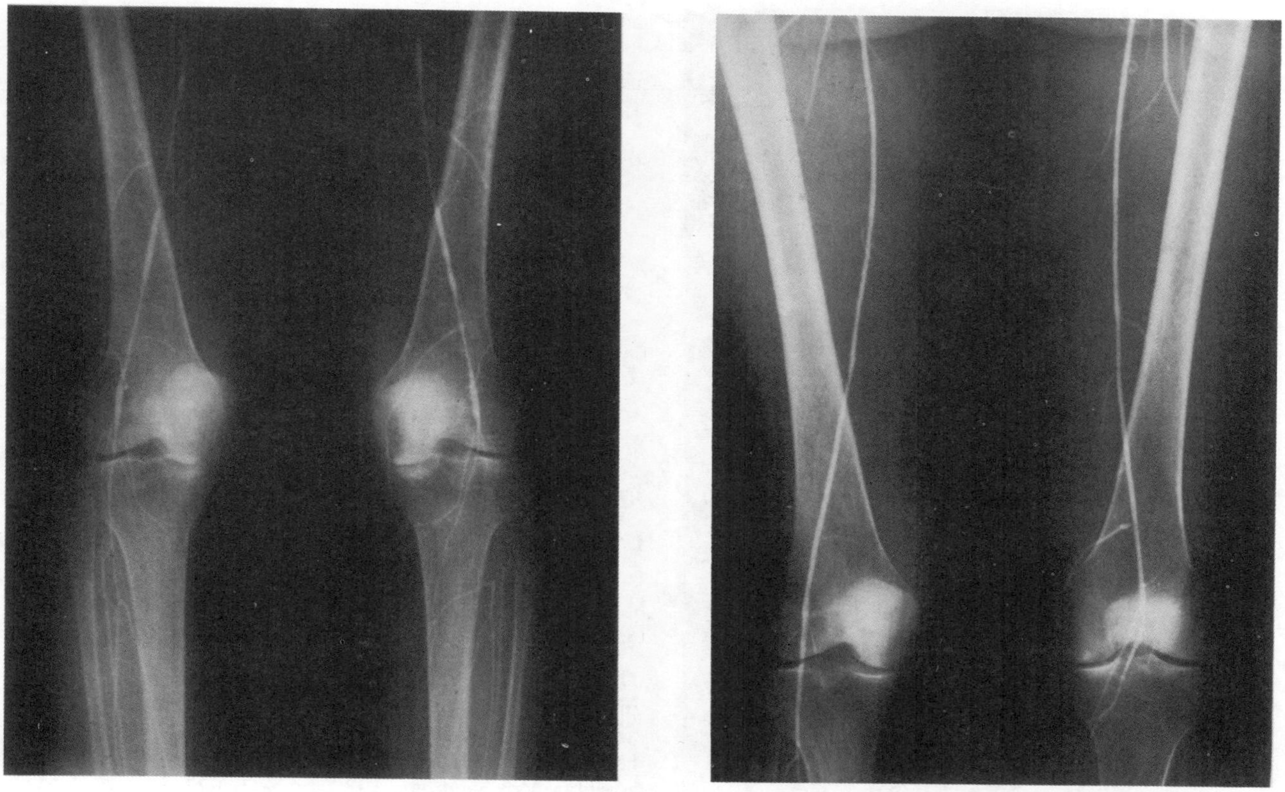

Figure 53.8. Angiogram demonstrating changes in lumina of arteries. *Left,* in polymyalgia rheumatica and intermittent claudication, segments are severely narrowed in both superficial femoral and both popliteal arteries; left popliteal artery is occluded. *Right,* same patient after six months of treatment with prednisone. Left popliteal artery remains occluded, but other zones of involvement have returned to almost normal appearance. (Modified from Hunder GG, Sheps SG: Intermittent claudication and polymyalgia rheumatica: association with panarteritis. *Arch Intern Med* 1967; 119:638–643, with permission of the Mayo Foundation.)

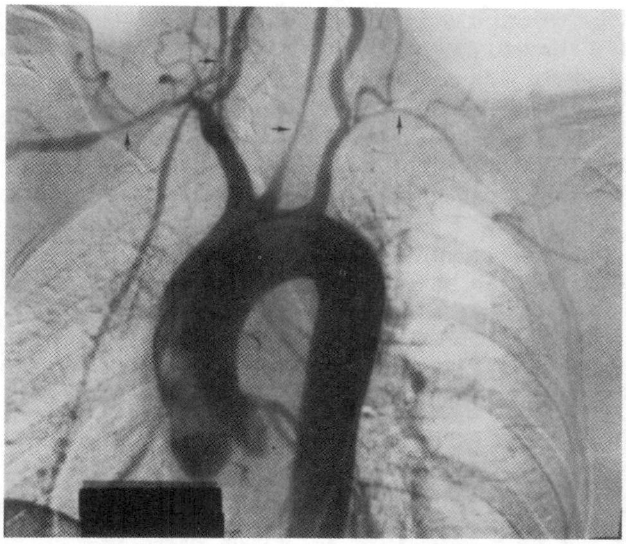

Figure 53.9. Arch aortogram in a 28-year-old woman with idiopathic medial aortopathy and arteriopathy (Takayasu's disease). Note severe narrowing of both common carotid arteries (*horizontal arrows*) and both subclavian arteries (*vertical arrows*). Left axillary artery is occluded in midcourse. (From Sheps SG, McDuffie FC: Vasculitis, in Juergens JA, Spittell JA Jr, Fairbairn JF II (eds): *Peripheral Vascular Diseases,* ed 5. Philadelphia, WB Saunders, 1980, pp 493–553.)

Popliteal Artery Entrapment

This unusual type of occlusive arterial disease occurs in young men. Typically they complain of calf or arch claudication with walking but not with running. If complete occlusion of the popliteal artery has not already occurred, the unusual observation of diminution of pedal pulses with sustained plantar flexion or passive dorsiflexion of the foot may be made.[24] The compression of the popliteal artery may be due to an anomalous insertion of one of the heads of the gastrocnemius muscle or the plantaris muscle or by the artery passing beneath rather than posterior to the popliteus muscle. The displacement or occlusion of the popliteal artery is demonstrated best by arteriography, and treatment is surgical release of the artery and reconstruction or resection of an occluded or aneurysmal popliteal artery to restore pulsatile flow to the leg and foot.

ACUTE ARTERIAL OCCLUSION

Acute peripheral arterial occlusion can result from the thrombotic or embolic occlusion of both diseased and normal arteries. The clinical picture varies according to the size and location of the artery occluded and the adequacy of the collateral circulation. One or all of the "5 P's" of acute arterial occlusion—pain, pallor, paresthesia, paralysis, and pulselessness—may be present when larger

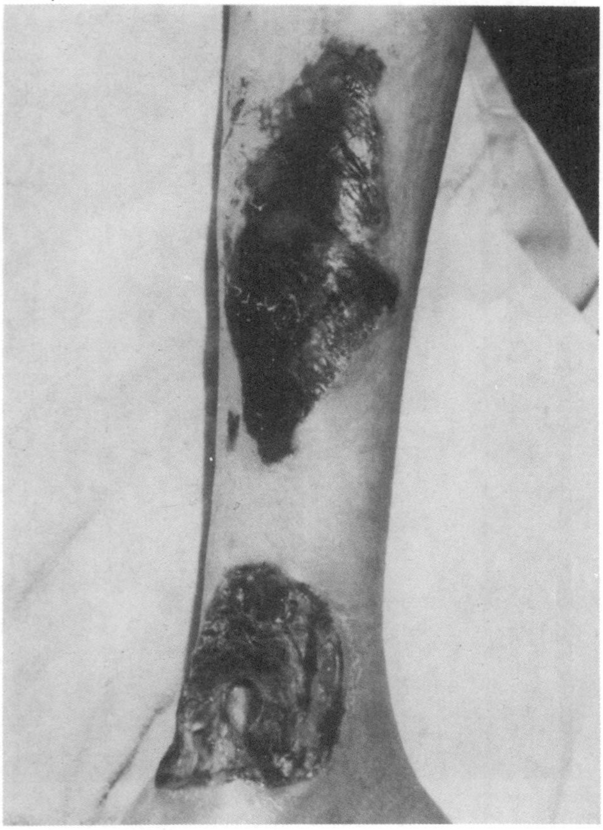

Figure 53.10. Arteriolar ischemic ulceration in a patient with rheumatoid arthritis. (From Spittell JA Jr: Diagnosis and management of leg ulcer. *Geriatrics* 1983; 38:57–65. Reproduced with permission of *Geriatrics*.)

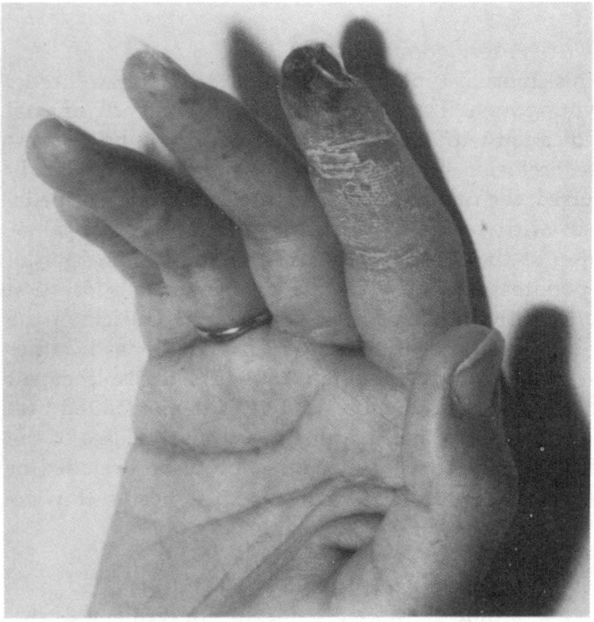

Figure 53.11. Gangrene of the tip of the index finger in a 29-year-old woman with scleroderma. Note the telangiectatic lesions of the skin of the digital phalanx of the adjacent finger. (From Spittell JA Jr: Occlusive arterial diseases in the upper extremities, in Spittell JA (ed): *Clinical Vascular Disease*. Philadelphia, FA Davis, 1983, pp 59–74. Figures 53.11 and 53.13 are reproduced with permission of FA Davis.)

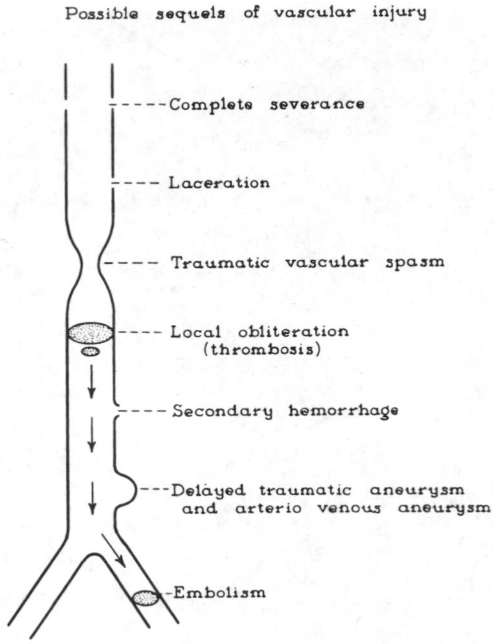

Figure 53.12. Diagrammatic representation of some effects of acute vascular injuries. (From Juergens JL, Pluth JR: Trauma and peripheral vascular disease, in Jeurgens JL, Spittell JA Jr, Fairbairn JF II (eds): *Peripheral Vascular Diseases,* ed 5. Philadelphia, WB Saunders, 1980, pp 607–627.)

extremity arteries are occluded, whereas occlusion of small arteries or arterioles may produce only a cold and painful digit or cutaneous infarction. Arteriography must be used to accurately localize the arterial occlusion, but a rough estimate can be made from noting the level of change in skin temperature (cold to normal) and sensation (anesthesia or hypesthesia to normal). In addition, in embolic arterial occlusion there often is tenderness over the site of arterial occlusion.

The many diverse types of acute arterial occlusion can be classified as shown in Table 53.7. The distinction between thrombotic and embolic arterial occlusion is an important one that is usually presumptive, based on clinical experience. Therefore, arterial occlusion is likely embolic in the patient with atrial fibrillation, a failing heart from any cause, recent acute myocardial infarction, or

Table 53.6. Occupations in Which Chronic (Traumatic) Occlusive Arterial Disease of the Hand Have Been Seen*

Farmer — tools and tractor steering wheel
Laborer — air hammer
Carpenter — hand tools
Mechanics — wrenches; "hammerhand"
Truck drivers — levers, valves, and steering wheel
Butcher — hand tools
Creamery worker — "hammerhand" on milk can lids
Forestry worker — chain saw
Packing house worker — "hammerhand"
Cash register operator — thenar "hammerhand"
Pharmacist — loosening bottle caps
Obstetrician — outlet forceps

* From Spittell JA Jr: Some uncommon types of occlusive peripheral arterial disease. *Curr Probl Cardiol* 1983; 8:1–35. (Reproduced with permission of Year Book Medical Publishers.)

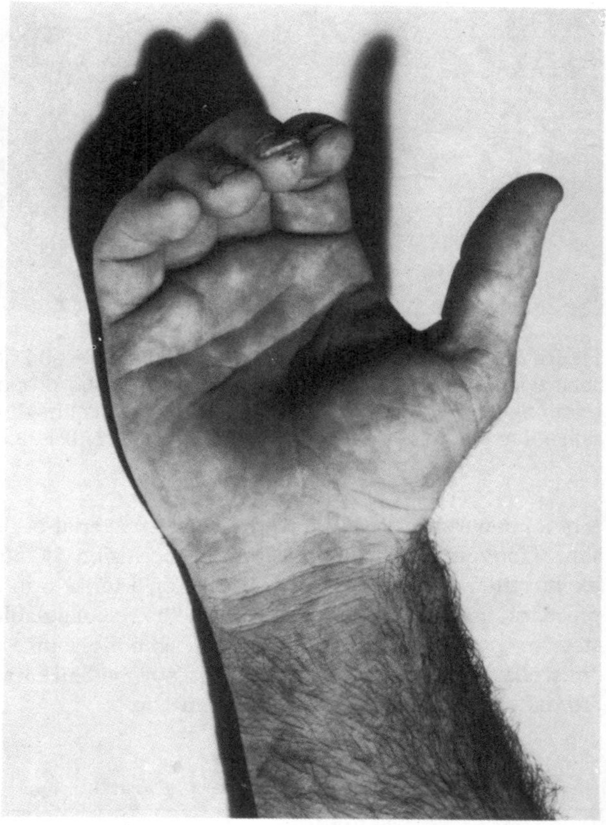

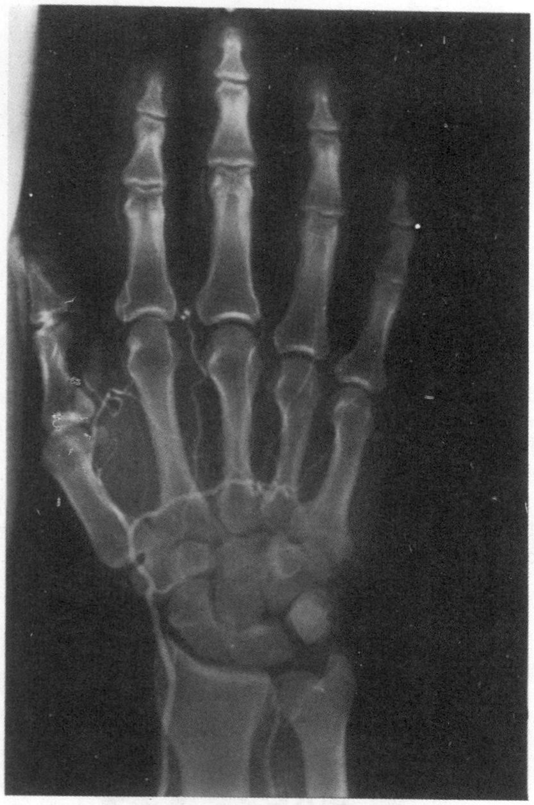

RIGHT	Sys B/P	PVR	Temp °C	LEFT	Sys B/P	PVR	Temp °C
Arm	138	22		Arm	124	31	
Forearm		17	27.9	Forearm		18	28.1
Radial	132 N		(wrist)	Radial	136 N		(wrist)
Ulnar	140 N			Ulnar	132 N		
Digits				Digits			
1st proximal	132	12		1st proximal	148	9	
distal		13	24.2	distal		7	24.3
2nd proximal	132	9		2nd proximal	142	7	
distal		4	23.5	distal		6	23.9
3rd proximal	90*	7		3rd proximal	132	7	
distal		4	23.2	distal		6	23.3
4th proximal	74*	4		4th proximal	140	4	
distal		1	22.7	distal		7	24.0
5th proximal	120*	5		5th proximal	132	6	
distal		3	23.3	distal		4	24.0

Figure 53.13. Occupational occlusive arterial disease in the hand. *Top Left,* ischemic ulcer of the tip of the right third finger of a man aged 27. He used the palm of his hand to "seat" a metal hook more than 300 times a day in his job. *Top Right,* arteriogram of the right hand shows occlusion of the ulnar artery, with the superficial palmar arch only partially filled via the radial artery. The digital arteries to the third and fourth fingers are occluded, as are the digital arteries to the ulnar side of the index finger and the radial side of the fifth finger. *Bottom,* laboratory findings indicate occlusive arterial disease in the third, fourth, and fifth fingers of the right hand. "N" means the arterial signal was normal. (From Spittell JA Jr: Occlusive arterial disease in the upper extremities, in Spittell JA (ed): *Clinical Vascular Disease.* Philadelphia, FA Davis, 1983, pp 59–74.)

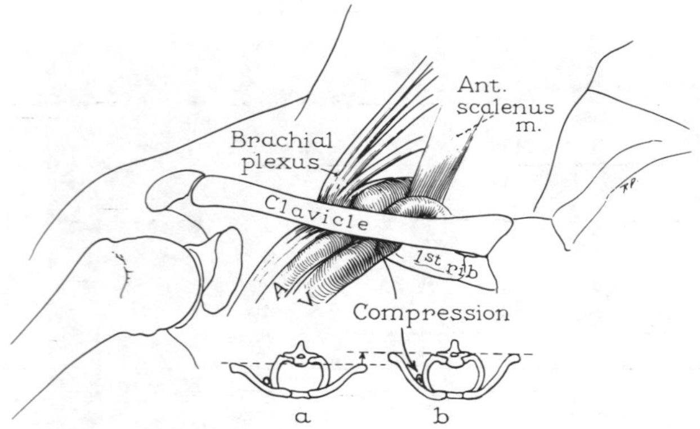

Figure 53.14. Costoclavicular syndrome. Compression of subclavian artery and brachial plexus occurs very commonly in the space between the clavicle and the first thoracic rib. (From Fairbairn JF II, Campbell JK, Payne WS: Neurovascular compression syndrome of the thoracic outlet, in Juergens JL, Spittell JA Jr, Fairbairn JF II (eds): *Peripheral Vascular Diseases,* ed 5. Philadelphia, WB Saunders, 1980, pp 629–653.)

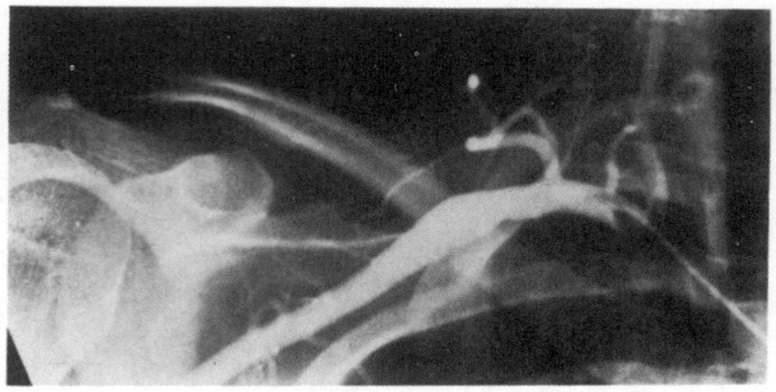

Figure 53.16. Arteriogram demonstrating compression of a subclavian artery by the first rib, with poststenotic dilation. (From Spittell JA Jr: Some uncommon types of occlusive peripheral arterial disease. *Curr Probl Cardiol* 1983; 8:1–35.)

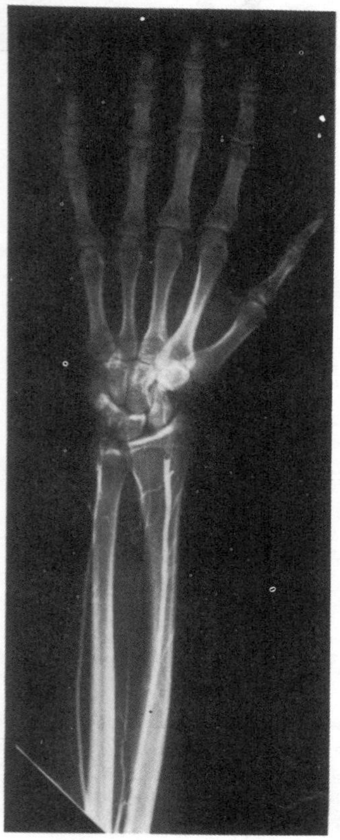

Figure 53.15. Arteriogram of the forearm and hand of the same patient in Figure 53.16 demonstrating embolic occlusion of the radial and ulnar arteries for the proximal thrombus in the dilated subclavian artery. (From Spittell JA Jr: Some uncommon types of occlusive peripheral arterial disease. *Curr Probl Cardiol* 1983; 8:1–35. Figures 53.15 and 53.16 are reproduced with permission of Year Book Medical Publishers.)

arterial aneurysm proximal to the level of arterial occlusion. Conversely, thrombotic arterial occlusion is more likely when occlusive arterial disease or arterial trauma precedes the acute occlusion or when a "hypercoagulable" state or arteritis is present. When an embolic source or "miscellaneous" cause (Table 53.7) is not evident, acute arterial occlusion is considered thrombotic.

Table 53.7. Acute Arterial Occlusion

- I. Thrombotic arterial occlusion secondary to:
  - A. Arteriosclerosis obliterans
  - B. Thromboangiitis obliterans (Buerger's Disease)
  - C. Arteritis
    - 1. Giant cell arteritis
    - 2. Connective tissue diseases
  - D. Hypercoagulable states
    - 1. Myeloproliferative diseases
      - a. Polycythemia vera
      - b. Thrombocytosis
    - 2. Neoplastic disease
    - 3. Ulcerative bowel disease
  - E. Arterial trauma from:
    - 1. Puncture and arteriotomy
    - 2. Fractures and dislocations
    - 3. Entrapment syndromes
- II. Embolic arterial occlusion (from thrombi of):
  - A. Cardiac origin
    - 1. Valvular heart disease
    - 2. Acute myocardial infarction
    - 3. Ventricular aneurysm
    - 4. Cardiomyopathy
    - 5. Atrial fibrillation
    - 6. Infective endocarditis
    - 7. Atrial myxoma
  - B. Proximal atherosclerotic plaques
  - C. Proximal arterial aneurysms
- III. Miscellaneous causes
  - A. Arterial spasm secondary to:
    - 1. Ergotism
    - 2. Intraarterial injection
    - 3. Penetrating trauma
  - B. Acute aortic dissection
  - C. Foreign bodies
    - 1. Guide wires and catheters
    - 2. Bullet embolism

The initial management of acute arterial occlusion should include relief of pain, protection of the ischemic limb, and intravenous heparin administration. After localization with arteriography, emboli can be removed with a Fogarty catheter. For thrombotic arterial occlusion there are several options, including thrombectomy, thrombolysis, arterial bypass, or anticoagulant therapy.

The mortality in patients with acute peripheral arterial occlusion (15% to 30%) is related in large measure to the age and cardiac status of the patients. With prompt and adequate treatment, limb salvage exceeds 85%.

ARTERIAL ANEURYSM

Aneurysms of peripheral arteries are most commonly atherosclerotic in origin, so they are common in men greater than 50 years of age; they are rare in women. They tend to occur at points where the artery is poorly supported by muscle or is subject to frequent bending, or both. The phenomenon of poststenotic dilatation plays a role in all likelihood when the artery is compressed, ie, the thoracic outlet, the outlet of the adductor canal, and the popliteal space.[25] Systemic hypertension contributes to aneurysm formation whether atherosclerotic or traumatic in origin.[26] Once formed, arterial aneurysms gradually enlarge and they commonly contain laminated thrombus, which may be both protective and a source of emboli.

Before the development of complications, aneurysms are asymptomatic and the only physical finding is an expansile pulsatile mass. Hence, care to evaluate not only the presence of pulsation but also the width of an arterial pulsation is essential. The complications of aneurysms include pressure on surrounding structures, rupture, thrombosis, distal embolization from contained thrombus, and rarely infection.

The most common peripheral arterial aneurysms occur in the femoral and popliteal arteries. Subclavian artery aneurysms are due to atherosclerosis or thoracic outlet compression, but are uncommon.

Although a soft tissue mass or calcification may be seen on roentgenograms, B mode ultrasound is the preferred diagnostic technique (Figure 53.6). Computed tomographic scan with contrast is an excellent but more expensive diagnostic method. Arteriography is the definitive diagnostic procedure and provides visualization of the proximal and distal arterial circulation (Figure 53.7).

The only effective method of treatment of a peripheral arterial aneurysm is resection and restoration of arterial circulation with a graft. Results are best when surgical treatment is performed before complications occur.

ARTERIOSPASTIC DISORDERS

RAYNAUD'S PHENOMENON AND RAYNAUD'S DISEASE

As noted earlier, color changes in the skin are the hallmark of vasospastic disorders, because the pathophysiologic aspect is intermittent constriction of the small arteries (digital) and arterioles (dermal); some believe that there is constriction of the venules as well in Raynaud's phenomenon. The arteriospastic disorders include Raynaud's phenomenon, livedo reticularis, and acrocyanosis. All are more common in women than in men. Typically, Raynaud's phenomenon consists of a triphasic color change; pallor or cyanosis occurs. During the pallor phase, arteriospasm prevents blood from entering the capillaries; during the cyanotic phase, blood flow is stagnant in the capillaries. Raynaud's phenomenon may be idiopathic (Raynaud's disease) or secondary to a variety of other disorders (secondary Raynaud's phenomenon) (Table 53.8).

Raynaud's disease is more common in women and may be diagnosed correctly about 95% of the time if the Allen–Brown criteria are adhered to.[27] These are: (1) Raynaud's phenomenon precipitated by exposure to cold or emotion; (2) bilateral, often symmetric, Raynaud's phenomenon; (3) lack of gangrene; (4) absence of an associated condition that may cause Raynaud's phenomenon; and (5) presence of Raynaud's phenomenon for at least two years. Secondary Raynaud's phenomenon should be suspected when the patient is a man, when Raynaud's phenomenon is asymmetric or unilateral, when there is significant digital ischemia or systemic symptoms, or a combination of these.

Patients with Raynaud's disease should protect themselves from cold, avoid tobacco and other vasoconstric-

Table 53.8. Classification of Raynaud's Phenomenon

I. Primary Raynaud's phenomenon (Raynaud's disease)
II. Secondary Raynaud's phenomenon, associated with:
  A. Occlusive arterial disease
    1. Arteriosclerosis obliterans
    2. Thromboangiitis obliterans
    3. Chronic occupational (traumatic) occlusive arterial disease in the hand
  B. Connective tissue diseases
    1. Rheumatoid arthritis
    2. Scleroderma
    3. Systemic lupus erythematosus
    4. Dermatomyositis
  C. Neurologic conditions
    1. Thoracic outlet compression
    2. Carpal tunnel syndrome
  D. Occupational
    1. Pneumatic hammer disease
    2. Arteriospasm of pianists and typists
    3. Occupational acro-osteolysis
  E. Drug induced
    1. Ergotism
    2. Beta blockers
    3. Clonidine
    4. Chemotherapy for testicular cancer
  F. Miscellaneous conditions
    1. Cold agglutinins
    2. Cryoglobulinemia
    3. Fabry's disease
    4. Hepatitis B antigenemia
    5. Myxedema
    6. Paroxysmal hemoglobinuria
    7. Pheochromocytoma
    8. Primary pulmonary hypertension

tors, and protect their fingers and toes from trauma. One of the following drugs may lessen the vasospastic episodes: (1) prazosin,[28] 1 mg one to three times a day, (2) phenoxybenzamine, 10 mg two to four times a day, (3) nifedipine,[29,29a] 10–20 mg three times a day, or (4) reserpine, 0.25 mg one to three times a day.

If the episodes of vasospasm are not controlled with one of the pharmacologic agents, two other modalities are available: (1) biofeedback[30] and (2) sympathectomy in the upper extremity. Moving to a warm climate often comes up for discussion; before making a permanent move, a trial period of several weeks to a month in the warmer climate is advisable to see if the benefit justifies the move.

In the patient with secondary Raynaud's phenomenon, in addition to the measures already noted, additional treatment may include: (1) treatment for the associated condition and (2) intraarterial reserpine (0.5 mg) to aid in healing ischemic digital ulceration resistant to healing with other measures.[31]

The prognosis for Raynaud's disease is excellent and the patient can be reassured that loss of digits is not to be expected. For the patient with secondary Raynaud's phenomenon the prognosis is that of the associated condition.

LIVEDO RETICULARIS

The bluish reticular pattern of livedo reticularis (Figure 53.17) is produced by spasm or occlusion of the dermal arterioles and associated capillary and venular dilatation. Livedo reticularis is persistent although more intense in the cold and therefore it should not be confused with cutis marmorata, a normal physiologic response to cold that clears with warming. Livedo reticularis is more common in women and, when idiopathic (Table 53.9), usually begins before the age of 20 years. In general, patients with livedo reticularis have no complaint other than discoloration of the skin; livedo reticularis of recent onset may be noted by an observant patient and is an important clinical clue to one of the causes of secondary livedo reticularis (Table 53.9).

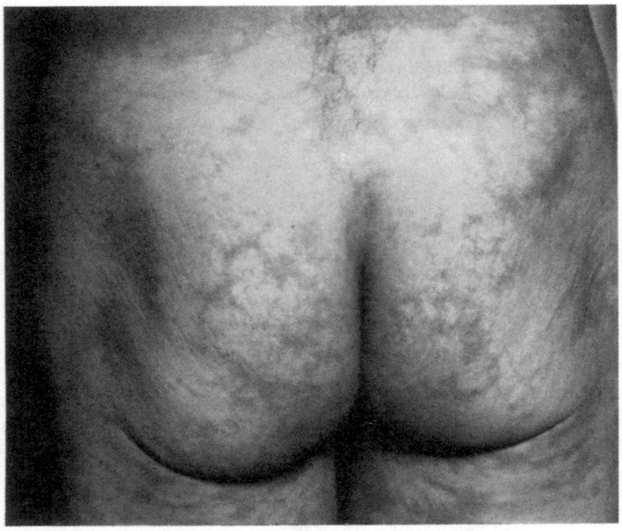

Figure 53.17. Livedo reticularis. (From Spittell JA Jr: Th vasospastic disorders. *Curr Probl Cardiol* 1984; 8:1–27. Fig ures 53.17 and 53.18b are reproduced with permission of Year Book Medical Publishers.)

Table 53.9. Classification of Livedo Reticularis*

Primary (idiopathic) livedo reticularis
Secondary livedo reticularis
Connective tissue diseases
Vasculitis
Myeloproliferative disorders
Dysproteinemias
Atheroembolism (cholesterol embolization)
After cold injury
Use of amantadine hydrochloride (Symmetrel)
Reflex sympathetic dystrophy

* From Spittell JA Jr: Vasospastic disorders. *Cardiovasc Clin* 1983; 13:75-88. (Reproduced with permission of FA Davis Co.)

ATHEROEMBOLISM (CHOLESTEROL EMBOLIZATION)

Atheroembolism (cholesterol embolization) is not a vasospastic disorder but is included because the atheromatous debris occludes dermal arterioles (Figure 53.18) producing a bluish purple mottling of the skin indistinguishable from that of true vasospastic livedo. Atheroembolism should be suspected in a person with recent onset of livedo after the age of 50 years. The atheromatous debris arises from atherosclerotic plaques of the aorta[32] or the laminated thrombus within an abdominal aortic aneurysm.[33] Because the atheromatous debris also occludes in the renal circulation, these patients have hypertension and renal insufficiency that are progressive unless the source of the atheromatous debris is surgically resected, the only effective therapy. Antithrombotic therapy, an attractive initial thought, is ineffective[33] and may actually precipitate atheroembolism[34]; discontinuing it may result in improvement.[35]

As noted in Table 53.9, amantadine hydrochloride prescribed for Parkinsonism may produce livedo reticularis in an occasional patient; this appears to be a benign side effect and will clear in two to four weeks if use of the drug is discontinued.

Because idiopathic livedo reticularis is generally asymptomatic except for its cosmetic effect, specific treatment is rarely indicated. If recurrent ulceration complicates it, a trial of prazosin or nifedipine would be appropriate.

ACROCYANOSIS

Acrocyanosis is an uncommon and benign vasospastic disorder that is caused by heightened digital arteriolar tone at usual environmental temperature.[36] The cyanosis and coolness of the fingers and toes are constant, simplifying the distinction from Raynaud's phenomenon. Cardiopulmonary causes of cyanosis should be excluded and then the patient, usually a young woman, can be reassured regarding the benign nature of acrocyanosis. If the patient desires relief of the cyanosis, a trial of prazosin or nifedipine would be in order.

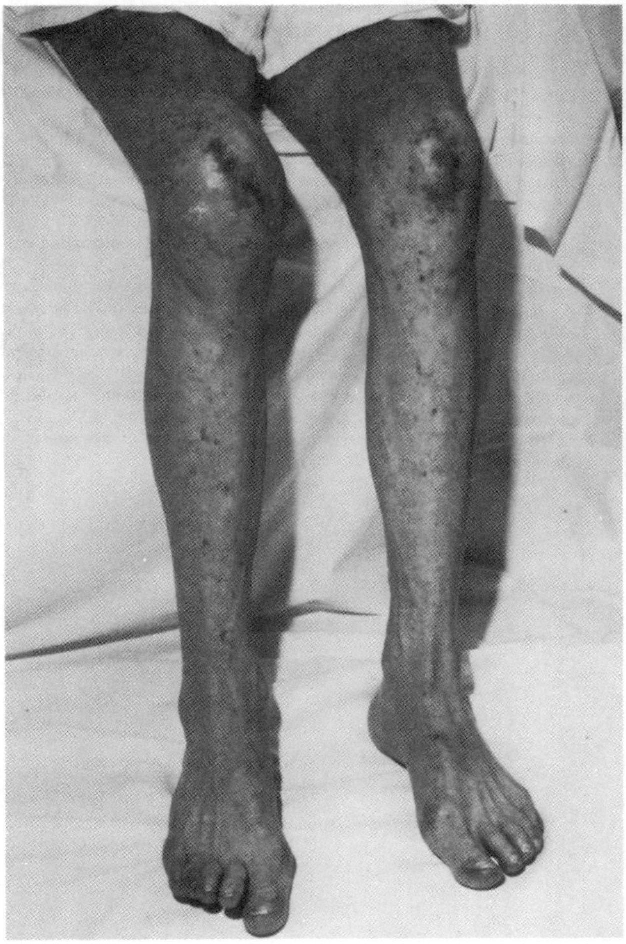

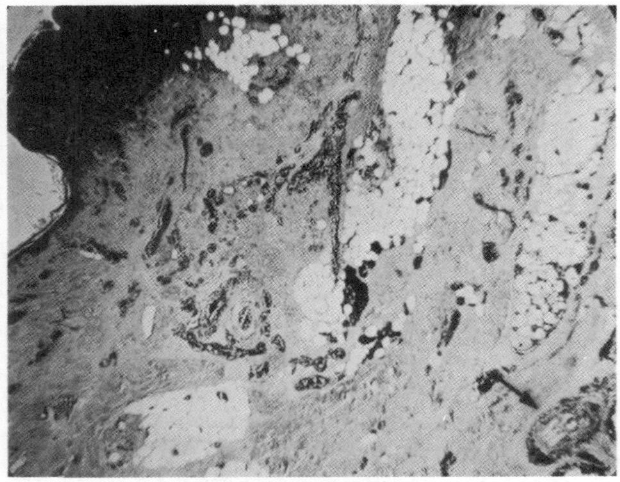

Figure 53.18. Atheroembolism (cholesterol embolization). *Left,* livedo reticularis and blue toes. (From Spittell JA Jr: Vasospastic disorders. *Cardiovasc Clin* 1983; 13:75–88. Reproduced with permission of FA Davis.) *Right,* skin biopsy specimen showing cholesterol clefts in dermal arteriole (*arrow*). (From Spittell JA Jr: The vasospastic disorders. *Curr Probl Cardiol* 1984; 8:1–27.)

REFERENCES

1. Criqui MH, Fronek A, Barret-Connor E, Klauber MR, Gabriel S, Goodman D: The prevalence of peripheral arterial disease in a defined population. *Circulation* 1985; 71:510–515.
2. Hall S, Bartelson JD, Onofrio BM, Baker HL Jr, Okazaki H, O'Duffy JD: Lumbar spinal stenosis: clinical features, diagnostic procedures and results of surgical treatment in 68 patients. *Ann Intern Med* 1985; 103:271–275.

2a. Spittell JA Jr: When CAD patients also have peripheral arterial disease. *J Crit Illness* 1986; 1:65–70.

3. Criqui MH, Fronek, A, Klauber MR, Barrett-Connor E, Gabriel S: The sensitivity, specificity, and predictive value of traditional clinical evaluation of peripheral arterial disease: results from noninvasive testing in a defined population. *Circulation* 1985; 71:516–522.
4. Carter SA: Arterial auscultation in peripheral vascular disease. *JAMA* 1981; 246:1682–1686.
5. Allen EV: Thromboangiitis obliterans: methods of diagnosis of chronic occlusive arterial lesions distal to the wrist with illustrative cases. *Am J Med Sci* 1929; 178:237–244.
6. Fairbairn JF II, Campbell K, Payne WS: Neurovascular compression syndromes of the thoracic outlet, in Juergens JL, Spittell JA Jr, Fairbairn JF II (eds): *Peripheral Vascular Diseases,* ed 5. Philadelphia, WB Saunders, 1980, pp 624–653.
7. Nielson SL, Nobin BA, Hirai M, Eklöf B: Raynaud's phenomenon in arterial obstructive disease of the hand demonstrated by locally provoked cooling. *Scand J Thorac Cardiovasc Surg* 1978; 12:105–109.
8. Jonason T, Jonzon B, Ringqvist I, Öman-Rydberg A: Effect of physical training of different categories of patients with intermittent claudication. *Acta Med Scand* 1979; 206:253–258.
9. Juergens JL, Barker NW, Hines EA Jr: Arteriosclerosis obliterans: review of 520 cases with special reference to pathogenic and prognostic factors. *Circulation* 1960; 21:188–195.
10. Schadt DC, Hines EA Jr, Juergens JL, Barker NW: Chronic atherosclerotic occlusion of the femoral artery. *JAMA* 1961; 175:937–940.
11. Hollier LH: Drugs as adjuncts to arterial surgery and balloon angioplasty, in Spittell JA Jr (ed): *Pharmacologic Approaches to Limb Ischemia.* Philadelphia, American College of Clinical Pharmacology, 1983, pp 143–151.
12. Coffman JD: Drug therapy: vasodilator drugs in peripheral vascular disease. *N Engl J Med* 1979; 300:713–717.
13. Reid HL, Dormandy JA, Barnes AJ, Lock PJ, Dormandy TL: Impaired red cell deformability in peripheral vascular disease. *Lancet* 1976; 1:666–667.
14. Porter JM, Cutler BS, Lee BY, Reich T, Reichle FA, Scogin JT, Strandness DE: Pentoxifylline efficacy in the treatment of intermittent claudication: multicenter controlled double-blind trial with objective assessment of chronic occlusive arterial disease patients. *Am Heart J* 1982; 104:66–72.
15. Spittell JA Jr: Pentoxifylline and intermittent claudication. *Ann Intern Med* 1985; 102:126–127.

15a. Strandness DE Jr: Intermittent claudication. Update on diagnosis and current therapy. *Consultant* 1986; 26(1):71–82.

15b. Pomrehn P, Duncan B, Weissfeld L, Wallace RB, Barnes R, Heiss G, Ekelund LG, Criqui MH, Johnson N, Chambless LE: The association of dyslipoproteinemia with symptoms and signs of peripheral arterial disease. The Lipid Research Clinics Program Prevalence Study. *Circulation* 1986; 73(suppl I):I-100–I-107.

16. McKusick VA, Harris WS, Otteson OE, Goodman RM, Shelly WM, Bloodwell RD: Buerger's disease: a distinct clinical and pathologic entity. *JAMA* 1982; 181:5–12.
17. Goodman RM, Elian B, Mozes M, Deutsch V: Buerger's disease in Israel. *Am J Med* 1965; 39:601–615.
18. Meyer W: Etiology of thromboangiitis obliterans (Buerger). *JAMA* 1918; 71:1268–1272.
19. McLoughlin GA, Helsby CR, Evans CC, Chapman DM: Association of HLA-A9 and HLA-B5 with Buerger's disease. *Br Med J* 1976; 2: 1165–1166.
20. Adar R, Papa MZ, Halpern Z, Mozes M, Shoshan S, Sofer B, Zinger H, Dayan M, Mozes E: Cellular sensitivity to collagen in thromboangiitis obliterans. *N Engl J Med* 1983; 308:1113–1116.
21. Klein RG, Hunder GG, Stanson AW, Sheps SG: Large artery involve-

ment in giant cell (temporal) arteritis. *Ann Intern Med* 1975; 83:806–812.

22. Hall S, Barr W, Lie JT, Stanson AW, Kazmier FJ, Hunder GG: Takayasu arteritis. A study of 32 North American patients. *Medicine* 1985; 64:89–99.

22a. Hayashi K, Fukushima T, Matsunaga N, Hombo Z: Takayasu's arteritis: decrease in aortic wall thickening following steroid therapy documented by CT. *Br J Radiol* 1986; 59:281–283.

23. Balaji MR, DeWeese JA: Adductor canal outlet syndrome. *JAMA* 1981; 245:167–170.

24. Darling RC, Buckley CJ, Abbott WM, Raines JK: Intermittent claudication in young athletes: popliteal artery entrapment syndrome. *J Trauma* 1974; 14:543–552.

25. Gedge SW, Spittell JA Jr, Ivins JC: Aneurysm of the distal popliteal artery and its relationship to the arcuate popliteal ligament. *Circulation* 1961; 24:270–273.

26. Spittell JA Jr: Hypertension and arterial aneurysm. *J Am Coll Cardiol* 1983; 1:533–540.

27. Allen EV, Brown GE: Raynaud's disease: a critical review of minimal requisites for diagnosis. *Am J Med Sci* 1932; 183:187–200.

28. Waldo R: Prazosin relieves Raynaud's vasospasm. *JAMA* 1979; 241:1037.

29. Rodeheffer R, Rommer J, Wigley F, Smith, CR: A randomized double-blind trial of nifedipine in the treatment of digital Raynaud's phenomenon (abstr). *Circulation* 1982; 66(Suppl II):II-381.

29a. White CJ, Phillips WA, Abraham LA, Watson TD, Singleton PT Jr: Objective benefit of nifedipine in the treatment of Raynaud's phenomenon. Double-blind controlled study. *Am J Med* 1986; 80:623–625.

30. National Institutes of Health: Biofeedback for patients with Raynaud's phenomenon. *JAMA* 1979; 242:509–510.

31. Spittell JA Jr: Raynaud's phenomenon and allied vasospastic disorders, in Juergens JL, Spittell JA Jr, Fairbairn JF II (eds): *Peripheral Vascular Diseases*, ed 5. Philadelphia, WB Saunders, 1980, pp 555–583.

32. Kempczinski RF: Lower extremity arterial emboli from ulcerating atherosclerotic plaques. *JAMA* 1979; 241:807–810.

33. Kazmier FJ, Sheps SG, Bernatz PE, Sayre GP: Livedo reticularis and digital infarcts: a syndrome due to cholesterol emboli arising from atheromatous abdominal aortic aneurysms. *Vasc Dis* 1966; 3:12–24.

34. Feder W, Auerbach R: "Purple toes": an uncommon sequela of oral coumarin drug therapy. *Ann Intern Med* 1961; 55:911–917.

35. Bruns FJ: Control of cholesterol embolization by discontinuation of anticoagulant therapy. *Am J Med Sci* 1978; 275:105–108.

36. Lewis T, Landis EM: Observations upon the vascular mechanism in acrocyanosis. *Am Heart J* 1930; 15:229–245.

54 Pulmonary Heart Disease (Cor Pulmonale)

Claude Lenfant, MD

"The lungs are connected to the skin and rule over the heart."
The Yellow Emperor's Classic of Internal Medicine.[1]

Although pulmonary heart disease has long been known as a clinical entity, it is only relatively recently that it has received the recognition and attention it deserves. Bhargava[2] cites no fewer than 11 definitions. The gist of these definitions is that pulmonary heart disease is an alteration of the right ventricle resulting from diseases affecting the structure and function of the lung, except when these pulmonary alterations are the result either of diseases that previously affected the left side of the heart or of congenital heart disease.

This definition was the one adapted in 1961 by the Expert Committee of the World Health Organization (WHO).[3] The only variance is the word *alteration*, chosen instead of *hypertrophy*, which is the hallmark of a chronic condition, whereas acute pulmonary heart disease is characterized by dilation produced by right heart strain or overload.[4]

The first description of cardiac hypertrophy shown to result from a preexisting lung condition seems to have been given by Laennec[5] in 1819. He described the case of a 41-year-old seamstress who appears to have had consumption later complicated by pulmonary emphysema. When Laennec first saw her, she displayed signs of right heart failure, such as peripheral edema, ascites, and crepitations in the lungs. According to Laennec, Jean-Nicholas Corvisant, his mentor, characterized the woman's illness as "an organic condition of the heart (resulting) from debility or original asthenia of the lung." Later in the same volume, Laennec stated that "all illnesses leading to severe and lasting dyspnea cause almost unavoidably hypertrophy (of the myocardium) or enlargement of the heart (right cavity)."

It is therefore not surprising that pulmonary heart disease remained popularly known as emphysema heart disease until White's[6] introduction of the term, cor pulmonale, in 1931. White wrote, "... (the term) emphysema heart ... is not actually satisfactory, for it is strictly limited to but one variety of pulmonary heart disease; . . . (it should be only) subsidiary to the designation pulmonary heart disease or cor pulmonale." Today, pulmonary heart disease and cor pulmonale are used synonymously.

ETIOLOGY

"The cause of pulmonary heart disease is increased resistance in the pulmonary circulation." With this statement White[6] clearly asserted that any event leading to pulmonary hypertension would, in effect, be a possible cause of pulmonary heart disease manifested by enlargement of the right heart cavity, myocardial hypertrophy, or both. More recently, Rubin[7] further emphasized the pluralistic etiology of pulmonary heart disease by pointing out that "right-sided failure is a late manifestation of pulmonary heart disease and need not to be present for the clinician to entertain the diagnosis of cor pulmonale." Implied in this statement is that elevation of pulmonary artery pressure is the earliest and most consistent feature of pulmonary heart disease.

In its Expert Committee Report[2] of 1967, WHO identified the diseases causing an increase in pulmonary artery pressure and therefore leading to cor pulmonale (Table 54.1). This list includes the causes of acute as well as chronic cor pulmonale. Among the former, thromboembolic disorders are foremost. As will be discussed in the next section, pulmonary embolism is extremely frequent, but it does not consistently cause an elevation in pulmonary artery pressure. Therefore, it is important to consider a high pulmonary artery pressure as the prepon-

Table 54.1. World Health Organization Classification of Chronic Cor Pulmonale According to Causative Diseases[2]

1. Diseases primarily affecting air passages of the lung and the alveoli
   - 1.1 Chronic bronchitis with generalized airways obstruction with or without emphysema
   - 1.2 Bronchial asthma
   - 1.3 Emphysema without bronchitis or asthma
   - 1.4 Pulmonary fibrosis, with or without emphysema, due to:
     - (a) Tuberculosis
     - (b) Pneumoconiosis
     - (c) Bronchiectasis
     - (d) Other pulmonary infections
     - (e) Radiation
     - (f) Mucoviscidosis
   - 1.5 Pulmonary granulomas and infiltrations
     - (a) Sarcoidosis
     - (b) Chronic diffuse interstitial fibrosis
     - (c) Berylliosis
     - (d) Eosinophilic granuloma or histiocytosis
     - (e) Malignant infiltration
     - (f) Scleroderma
     - (g) Disseminated lupus erythematosus
     - (h) Dermatomyositis
     - (i) Alveolar microlithiasis
   - 1.6 Pulmonary resection
   - 1.7 Congenital cystic disease of the lungs
   - 1.8 High-altitude hypoxia
2. Diseases primarily affecting the movements of the thoracic cage
   - 2.1 Kyphoscoliosis and other thoracic deformities
   - 2.2 Thoracoplasty
   - 2.3 Pleural fibrosis
   - 2.4 Chronic neuromuscular weakness, eg, poliomyelitis
   - 2.5 Obesity with alveolar hypoventilation
   - 2.6 Idiopathic alveolar hypoventilation
3. Diseases primarily affecting the pulmonary vasculature
   - 3.1 Primary affections of the arterial wall
     - (a) Primary pulmonary hypertension
     - (b) Polyarteritis nodosa
     - (c) Other arteritis
   - 3.2 Thrombotic disorders
     - (a) Primary pulmonary thrombosis
     - (b) Sickle cell anemia
   - 3.3 Embolism
     - (a) Embolism from thrombosis outside the lungs
     - (b) Schistosomiasis (bilharziasis)
     - (c) Malignancy embolism
     - (d) Other embolism
   - 3.4 Pressure on main pulmonary arteries and veins by mediastinal tumors, aneurysm, granuloma, or fibrosis

derant cause, if not the hallmark, of cor pulmonale, acute and chronic as well.

PREVALENCE AND INCIDENCE

Although some evidence seems to indicate that pulmonary heart disease is common, there is surprisingly little hard data to substantiate this belief. Yet, when considering the causative diseases listed in Table 54.1, it is clear that the prevalence and incidence of cor pulmonale must be high. Indeed, many of the listed diseases are extremely prevalent and even constitute major public health problems in certain countries or regions of the world.

The incidence, prevalence, mortality, and etiology of pulmonary heart disease and its subcategories, acute and chronic cor pulmonale, pulmonary embolism, and primary pulmonary hypertension, are described herein for various countries. The available statistics are incomplete and comparability among countries is poor. They are based on community studies, hospital statistics, and mortality statistics reported to WHO.

In the United States the annual incidence of pulmonary embolism is estimated to be 650,000, of which only 160,000 cases are diagnosed and treatment performed in hospitals.[8] An estimated 215,000 result in death, 65,000 within one hour, 137,000 because a diagnosis could not be made, and 13,000 (of the 160,000 hospitalizations) despite therapy. As many as 60% of patients who die of pulmonary embolism die before a diagnosis is made. These estimates cannot be verified because reporting of pulmonary embolism on hospital summary records and death certificates is incomplete.

At autopsy, chronic cor pulmonale is estimated to occur in 40% of cases of emphysema and chronic bronchitis.[9] The incidence of emphysema and chronic bronchitis, based on health interviews, is 2.1 million and 7.9 million persons, respectively[10]; in 1983 there were 60,000 hospitalizations for emphysema and 234,000 for chronic bronchitis as the "primary" diagnosis[11] and about 57,000 deaths from these diseases in 1982.[12]

In the Soviet Union chronic cor pulmonale is common, occupying the third or fourth place among cardiac diseases (personal communication with O.M. Eliseer, Soviet Union, December 17, 1984). It is also common in certain regions of China, among the Mongols, Kazaks, and Hans in Inner Mongolia and Xianjing.[13] Yet, it apparently does not occur in Ghana even though pulmonary tuberculosis and bronchial asthma are sizeable public health problems there: it occurred in only 4 of 776 cardiac cases in Accra from 1975 to 1979 (Personal communication, U.O.M. Pobee, Ghana, October 15, 1984). Although trend statistics are rarely available, the incidence of cor pulmonale appears to be increasing in the Soviet Union and Japan (personal communications, O.M. Eliseer, Soviet Union, December 17, 1984, and Y. Nimura, Japan, September 5, 1984).

In the late 1970s, WHO reported that in Europe the most common cause of chronic cor pulmonale was chronic pulmonary disease, including chronic bronchitis and emphysema.[14] This is also the case in the United States,[9] Nepal (personal communication, M.R. Pandey, Nepal, January 9, 1985), India (personal communication, S.K. Jindal, India, April 5, 1984), and China.[13] In the Soviet Union and Japan, however, most cases of cor pulmonale are attributed to pulmonary tuberculosis, although at a decreasing frequency in Japan. In recent years pulmonary tuberculosis has gained prominence as a cause of cor pulmonale in the Soviet Union, where 42.4% of patients who died of tuberculosis died of decompensated cor pulmonale. In regions of the world where many people live in highlands, the ratio of cor pulmonale to chronic bronchitis increases with altitude (personal communication, M.R. Pandey, Nepal, January 9, 1985).

Data on mortality from pulmonary heart disease in 15 countries reported to WHO[14a] are summarized in Figures 54.1 and 54.2. They show that the ranking of these countries is similar for two age groups (ie, 35 to 74 and 75 and over), but the rates are about ten times higher for the older age group. Death rates for all pulmonary heart diseases are higher in men than in women, particularly in the 35 to 74-year-old age group. This is especially the case in countries with the highest rates, with the exception of Ireland.

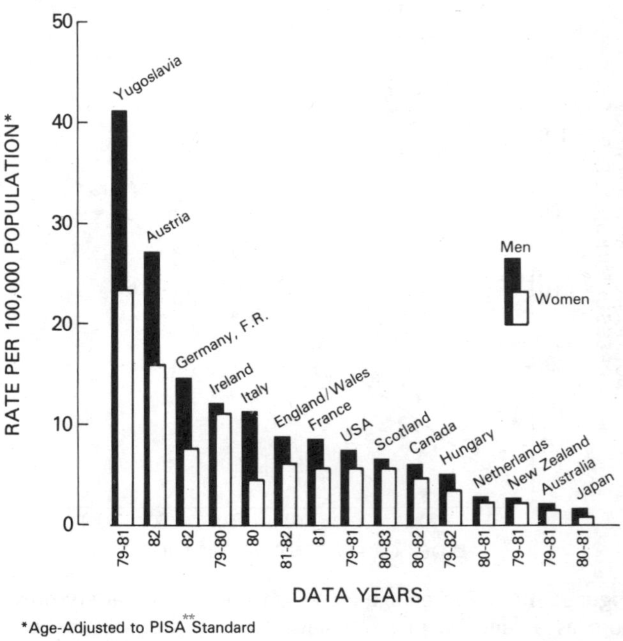

Figure 54.1. Annual death rate for pulmonary heart disease (ICD/9, codes 415 and 416). Ages 35 to 74 years by sex and country. Data collected from 1978 to 1983. (**Pisa and Yemura.[14a])

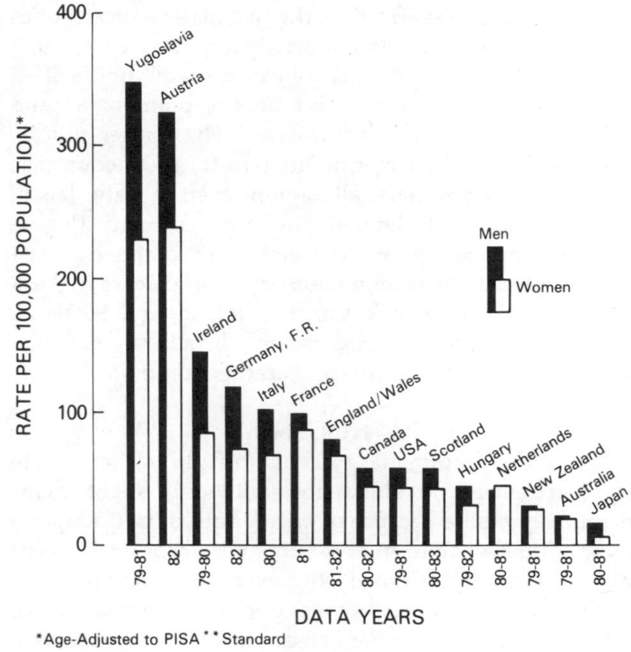

Figure 54.2. Annual death rate for pulmonary heart disease (ICD/9, codes 415 and 416). Ages 75 years and over by sex and country. Data collected from 1978 to 1983. (**Pisa and Yemura.[14a])

As a reported underlying cause of death in most countries, pulmonary heart disease accounts for no more than 2% of the mortality from all forms of heart disease combined (Table 54.2). The major exceptions are Yugoslavia, where death from pulmonary heart disease is 13.2% of all deaths from heart disease at ages 35 to 74 years and 8.4% of all deaths at age 75 and over, and Austria, with 7.1% and 8.6%, respectively, of deaths at these age groups.

Table 54.2. Percentage of Deaths from Heart Disease due to Pulmonary Heart Disease* by Age Group† (Men and Women Combined; 15 Countries)

Country	Percentage	
	Age 35-74	**Age 75+**
Yugoslavia	13.2	8.4
Austria	7.1	8.6
France	4.4	4.0
Germany, FR	3.6	2.3
Italy	3.4	1.9
Ireland	3.0	2.6
England/Wales	2.2	2.2
All others	< 2	< 2

* Nonrheumatic heart disease and hypertension (codes 26–28) in the World Health Organization's Statistics Annual for latest single year available.
† Average annual deaths from ICD/9 codes 415, 416 for latest data years (see Table 54.1).

In the WHO classification, the two major subcategories of pulmonary heart disease are "pulmonary embolism" (code 415.1) and "pulmonary heart disease" unspecified (416.9), which includes "chronic cor pulmonale" and "chronic cardiopulmonary disease." The former subcategory is by far the larger of the two for most countries; the latter is larger especially among men in Italy, Japan, Austria, and the Federal Republic of Germany (Figure 54.3). Deaths from pulmonary embolism comprise at least 85% of the deaths from pulmonary heart disease in Australia, the United States, Canada, Ireland, and Scotland. It is interesting that pulmonary embolism is rare in China where chronic cor pulmonale is rather common.[15]

PATHOGENESIS

The normal pulmonary circulation can accommodate large increments in blood flow with only slight increments in pressure because of one or both of two adaptive mechanisms, distension of existing vessels or recruitment of unused vessels. Conversely, severe constriction of existing vessels and extensive loss of cross-sectional surface of the pulmonary vascular bed can lead to a large increase in pulmonary artery pressure.

Of these two mechanisms, the loss of cross-sectional surface plays a relatively inconsistent role except in special situations. This role has been studied experimentally and clinically. Experiments in dogs[16] have established that the mechanical obstruction of the pulmonary artery to one segment, one lobe, or the entire right or left lung results in an increase in pressure in the unobstructed pulmonary artery (Figure 54.4). However, the percentage increase in blood flow in the parts of the lungs remaining open is much greater than the increase in pressure (Figure 54.5). This indicates a relative decrease in resistance which can be explained by opening of previously unused capillaries and dilation of vessels already open.

Unilateral occlusion of the pulmonary artery in patients undergoing diagnostic catheterization showed a twofold increase in blood flow in the nonoccluded lung, but an increase in pressure of only 30% in the main pulmonary artery.[17] Thus, in man too there appears to be a significant decrease in pulmonary vascular resistance which results from expansion of the pulmonary bed.

In patients who have had pneumonectomy, the development of pulmonary hypertension appears to be largely related to the preexisting condition of the lung, especially the presence of structural changes in the pulmonary capillaries, lung parenchyma, or both, which prevent compensatory mechanisms. This is probably why, following pneumonectomy, pulmonary hypertension rarely develops in children. However, pulmonary artery hypertension eventually develops in many patients who have had pneumonectomy[18] (Figure 54.6) and in time it leads to pulmonary heart disease. In summary, from experiments in dogs and in man, and from clinical observations, it is clear that a decrease in cross-sectional surface of the pulmonary vascular bed results in an increase in pulmonary artery pressure. This increase is present at rest in most cases, but it is consistently noted during exercise in which condition it is always much greater than that

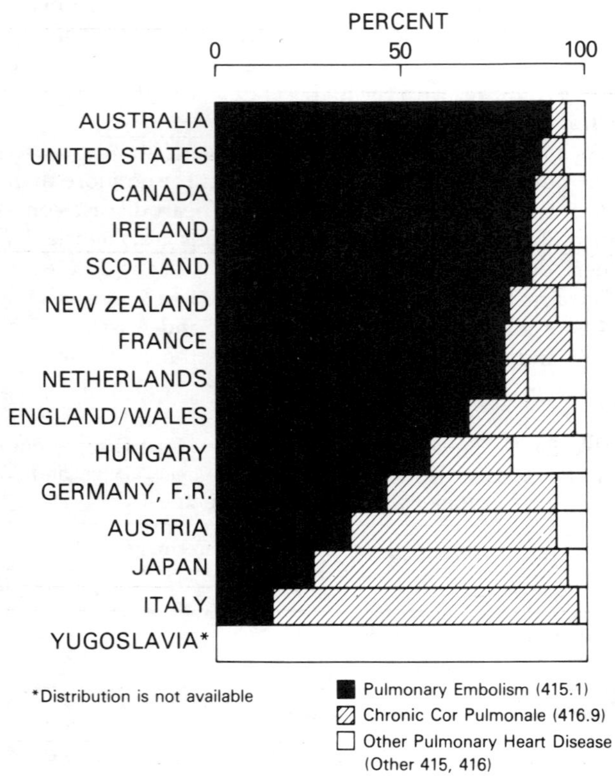

Figure 54.3. Proportion of deaths from pulmonary heart disease classified as due to pulmonary thromboembolism and to chronic cor pulmonale, in men aged 35 to 74 years. Fifteen countries. Data collected from 1978 to 1983. Classification based on ICD/9 codes.

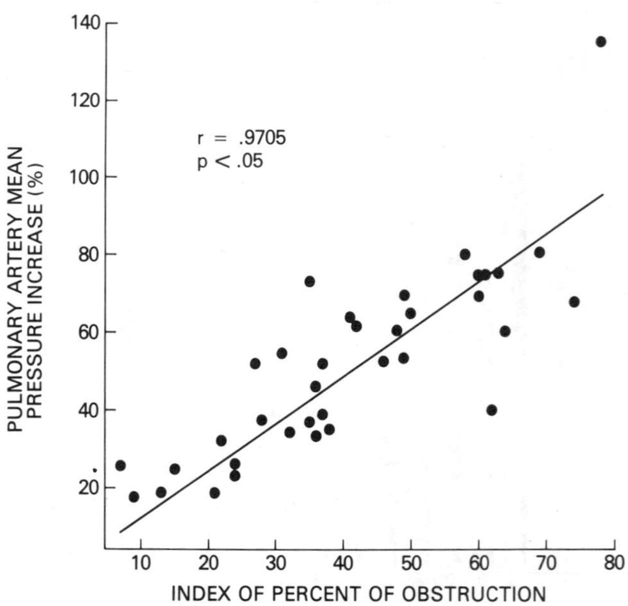

Figure 54.4. Percentage increase of pulmonary artery pressure as a function of percentage vascular bed obstruction. Pulmonary artery pressure increase was reported by the authors. The extent of vascular bed obstruction was derived from data on change in oxygen consumption in the right and left side of the lung after partial or total occlusion. (From Lategola,[16] with permission.)

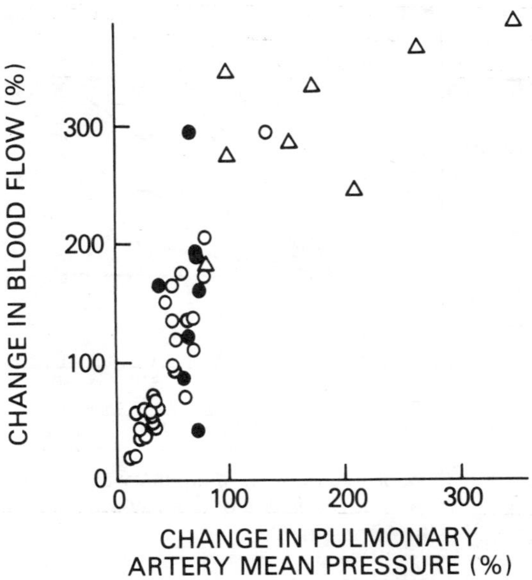

Figure 54.5. Percent change in blood flow in the nonoccluded parts of the lung as a function of percent change in pulmonary artery mean pressure after occlusion. (From Lategola,[16] with permission.)

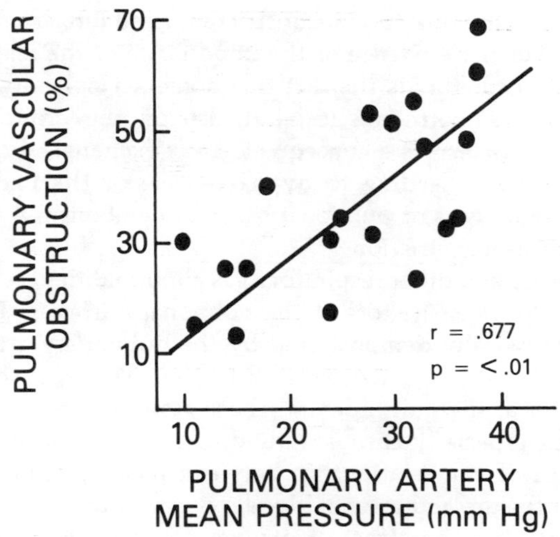

Figure 54.7. Relationship between pulmonary vascular bed obstruction as determined by angiography and pulmonary artery mean pressure. (From McIntyre and Sasahara,[19] with permission.)

observed when there is no reduction in cross-sectional surface of the pulmonary vascular bed.

That the loss of cross-sectional surface of the pulmonary vascular bed is a pathogenetic factor in acute and chronic cor pulmonale is certain. High pulmonary artery pressure is the hallmark of pulmonary thromboembolism and of the lung diseases associated with chronic cor pulmonale. However, although a linear relation between pulmonary vascular occlusion and pulmonary artery pressure has been found in patients with pulmonary thromboembolism[19] (Figure 54.7), it is also known that the clinical picture of acute cor pulmonale develops even when the obstruction is minimal. Moreover, nearly all pulmonary diseases leading to cor pulmonale are accompanied by a "restricted" vascular bed; yet, it is acknowledged that the degree of increase in pulmonary artery pressure in these patients exceeds that which can be accounted for by mechanical obstruction[20] (Figure 54.8).

Thus, it follows that mechanical obstruction alone cannot explain the entire magnitude of the pulmonary artery hypertension and that other pathogenetic factors, such as gas exchange abnormalities or release of neurohumoral mediators, or both, must intervene.

In pulmonary thromboembolism, blood clots traveling to the lung and obstructing some pulmonary vessels contain leukocytes and platelets that are rich in vasoactive mediators. As the blood clots settle in the capillaries, more platelet aggregation occurs and the release of humoral agents such as histamine, serotonin, catecholamines, prostaglandins, and thromboxane takes place. Although there may be some debate as to the relative importance of each of these mediators, that platelet aggregation and degran-

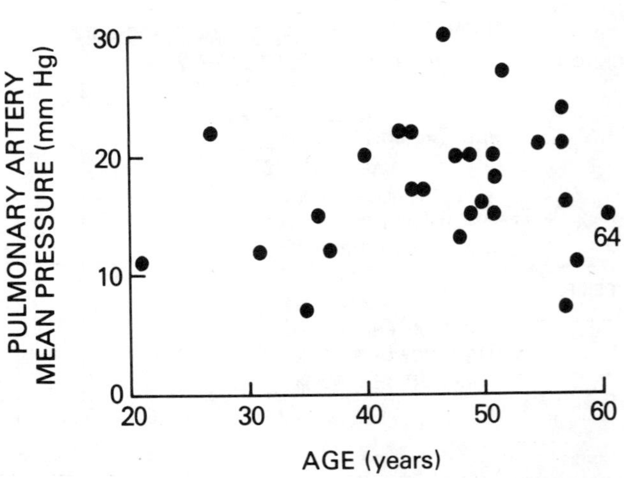

Figure 54.6. Relationship between age and pulmonary artery mean pressure after pneumonectomy. (From Denolin,[18] with permission.)

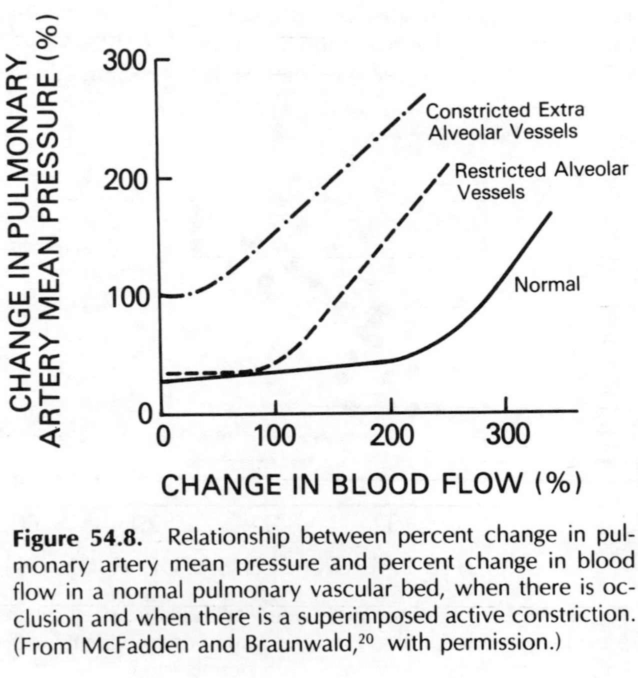

Figure 54.8. Relationship between percent change in pulmonary artery mean pressure and percent change in blood flow in a normal pulmonary vascular bed, when there is occlusion and when there is a superimposed active constriction. (From McFadden and Braunwald,[20] with permission.)

ulation are the link to vasoconstriction is no longer questioned. Further evidence of the importance of the release of these mediators is the fact that some act not only on the vessel smooth muscles, but also on the bronchial smooth muscles. As a consequence, gas exchange abnormalities occur, leading to hypoxia—one of the pathophysiologic signs of pulmonary thromboembolism—and further vasoconstriction.[21]

Hypoxia and other respiratory gas abnormalities are the most potent constrictors of the pulmonary arteries. This is unequivocally demonstrated by the pulmonary artery hypertension associated with all hypoxic states, such as residence at high altitude and those resulting from lung diseases, especially chronic lung diseases. There is ample evidence of the relationship between mean pulmonary artery pressure and arterial blood oxygen saturation (Figure 54.9), but the effect of oxygen depletion is significantly exacerbated by the synergistic effect of other abnormalities, such as hypercarbia and acidosis[22] (Figure 54.10).

In summary, the pathogenesis of acute and chronic cor pulmonale appears to be well understood. Cor pulmonale results from a "strain" of the right heart due to an increase in resistance in the pulmonary arteries. This increase in resistance may result from a mechanical obstruction, active vasoconstriction or, as it seems to be in nearly all cases, from both. The active vasoconstriction has one common denominator—hypoxia—but the effect of this factor is compounded and enhanced by the effect of other gas exchange abnormalities, as well as by the presence of potent mediators acting on the vascular and the bronchial smooth muscles.

CLINICAL MANIFESTATIONS

I. PULMONARY THROMBOEMBOLISM: ACUTE COR PULMONALE

Pulmonary thromboembolism occurs in a number of predisposing conditions, among which cardiovascular disease and chronic obstructive pulmonary disease are the most frequent (Personal communication, U.O.M. Pobee, Ghana, October 15, 1984) (Figure 54.11). The immediate

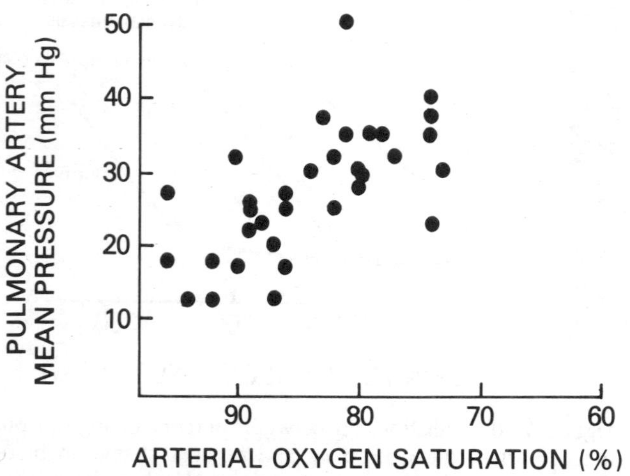

Figure 54.9. Relationship between pulmonary artery mean pressure and arterial blood oxygen saturation in patients with emphysema. (From Denolin,[18] with permission.)

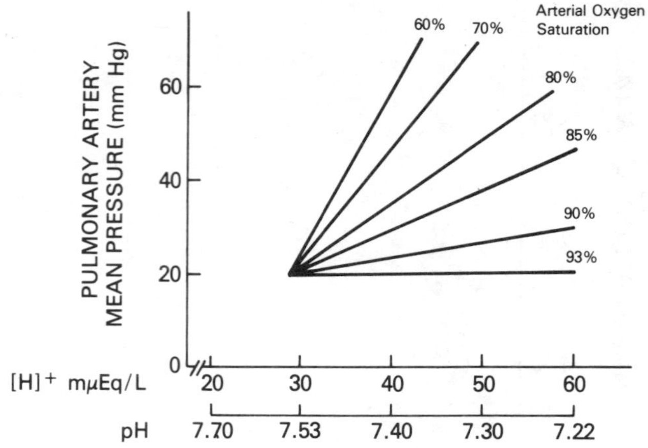

Figure 54.10. Relationship between pulmonary artery mean pressure, pH, [H]+, and arterial blood oxygen saturation. (From Ferrer,[22] with permission.)

and long-term clinical expression of pulmonary thromboembolism depends on its manifestation. A single massive episode is usually followed by complete resolution unless the event is so massive that death occurs, most frequently within a few hours. In contrast, recurrent embolism leads to chronic pulmonary artery hypertension followed by chronic cor pulmonale.

Fishman[23] describes four types of manifestations:

1. "Massive occlusion of the pulmonary arterial tree," which leads to a state of shock with all of its signs: the patient is pale, weak, if not unconscious and tachypneic. It is in this very desperate situation that the electrocardiogram (ECG) shows the features of acute cor pulmonale: rightward shift of the QRS axis in the frontal plane, $S_1Q_3T_3$ pattern with complete or incomplete right bundle branch block, P-pulmonale, deep T-wave inversion in V_1 to V_5, and clockwise rotation[24] (Figure 54.12).

2. "Embolism associated with infarction," an uncommon form expressed by characteristic pleural pain and breathlessness.

3. "Embolism without infarction," the most common form, but also the most difficult to detect. In contrast to

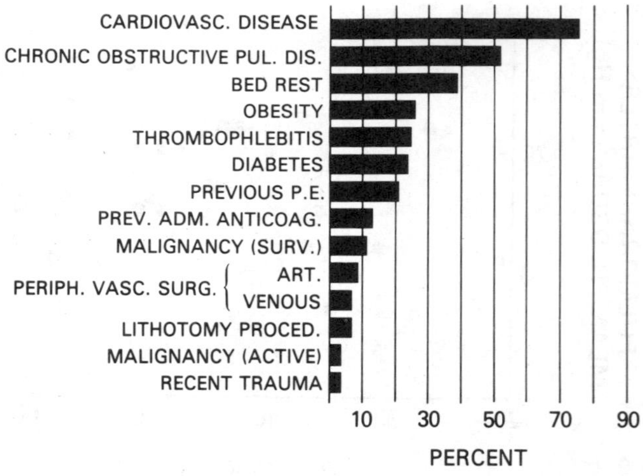

Figure 54.11. Percent frequency of risk factors in a series of 100 patients with angiographically proven pulmonary embolism (PE). (From McIntyre et al,[24] with permission. Copyright © 1972 by Year Book Medical Publishers, Inc, Chicago.)

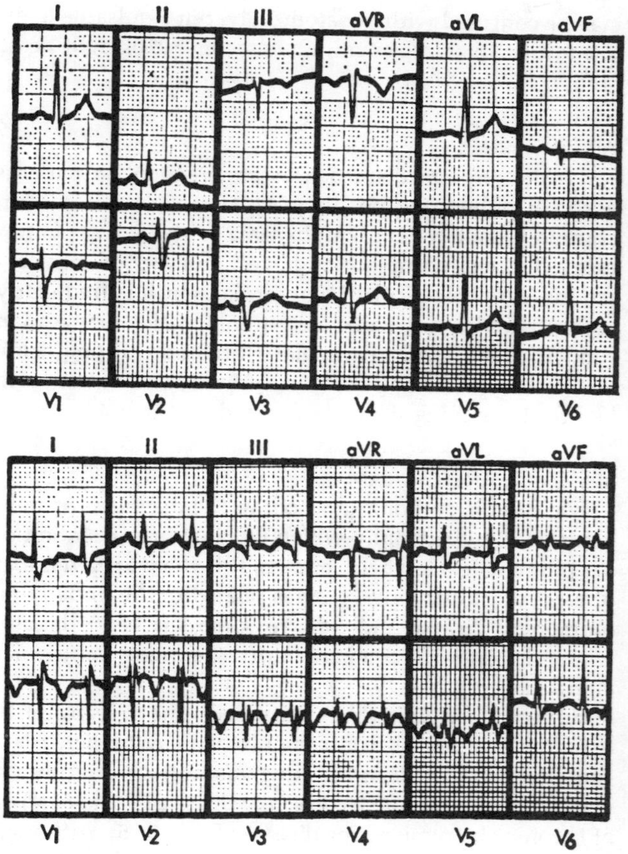

Figure 54.12. Electrocardiograms before (*upper tracings*) and after (*lower tracings*) massive pulmonary embolism in a 30-year-old patient with acute cor pulmonale. Changes include rightward shift of QRS axis in the frontal plane, $S_1Q_3T_3$ pattern, incomplete right bundle branch block, deep T-wave inversion in leads V_1 to V_5, and clockwise rotation. (From McIntyre et al,[24] with permission. Copyright © 1972 by Year Book Medical Publishers, Inc.)

massive occlusion, the pulmonary vessel obliteration is peripheral rather than central.

4. "Multiple pulmonary embolism," which may lead to widespread occlusion of the small and large pulmonary arteries followed by chronic pulmonary hypertension and cor pulmonale. It is often not diagnosed before irreversible consequences have occurred. However, from the large series of patients reported in the urokinase pulmonary embolism trial,[25] no single symptom or combination of symptoms appears as the hallmark of any of these forms. Therefore, chest pain, dyspnea, anxiety, cough, hemoptysis, and syncope can be observed with varying frequency. Examination can reveal tachypnea, tachycardia, rales, an increased pulmonic second sound, diaphoresis, murmur, and sometimes cyanosis.[8] Sometimes the combination of signs and symptoms resembles myocardial ischemia. Except in severe massive thromboembolism, electrocardiographic alterations are inconsistent and therefore nondiagnostic. The ECG must be recorded nonetheless to distinguish pulmonary thromboembolism from myocardial infarction.

The diagnosis of pulmonary thromboembolism is considerably aided by a number of measures, as follows:

Blood gas measurements: Gas exchange abnormalities, especially hypoxemia, are nearly always observed. They are caused by ventilation-perfusion ratio unevenness and sometimes also by a decrease in diffusing capacity due to a reduction in capillary blood volume.

Pulmonary scintigraphy: This is a very valuable diagnostic test of pulmonary thromboembolism. A normal perfusion scan nearly always rules out embolism, but conversely an abnormal scan does not necessarily reflect pulmonary thromboembolism because of a possible preexisting perfusion defect. A chest X-ray must be made to interpret accurately an abnormal perfusion scan. Ventilation scans are useful in assessing the degree of ventilation maldistribution.

Pulmonary angiography: The gold standard in the diagnosis of pulmonary thromboembolism is undoubtedly pulmonary angiography. Although not a technique readily available everywhere, it is a remarkably safe method in experienced hands. The urokinase pulmonary embolism trial[25] reported a mortality of 0.2% in 2,657 angiograms and a morbidity slightly less than 1% (mostly cardiac perforations and arrhythmias).

Chest X-ray: The chest X-ray usually has little diagnostic value per se, but it is useful to rule out other pulmonary disorders. There are, nonetheless, some features characteristic of pulmonary thromboembolism, such as elevated diaphragm and enlargement of the hilar arteries. Chest X-rays can be helpful in establishing the presence of lung infarction.

II. CHRONIC COR PULMONALE

Because chronic cor pulmonale is essentially a complication of severe chronic pulmonary disease, its clinical manifestations are largely influenced by the underlying disease. Table 54.1 shows all the diseases that may lead to cor pulmonale, but it is not possible to describe them all herein. As discussed in the section on pathogenesis, pulmonary hypertension always precedes cor pulmonale; in turn, pulmonary hypertension results from hypoxia (Figure 54.9).

In many patients with chronic pulmonary disease, the severity of pulmonary function alteration is often an indicator of the degree of pulmonary hypertension. Timsit et al[26] and Enson et al[27] evaluated patients with chronic obstructive or restrictive lung disease and found a correlation between the forced expired volume or the vital capacity and pulmonary artery pressure (Figure 54.13 and Table 54.3). In addition to hypoxia, other factors contribute to pulmonary artery hypertension. Most important is an increased blood viscosity owing to the polycythemia that occurs in patients with chronic hypoxia. Uncommonly, except during exercise, an increase in pulmonary blood flow can also be a cause of pulmonary artery hypertension. Finally, as mentioned earlier, loss of blood vessels or a decrease in the cross-sectional surface, or both, also contributes to an increase in pulmonary artery pressure.

SIGNS AND SYMPTOMS

Physical examination of the cardiovascular system of patients with chronic cor pulmonale may reveal a myriad of signs and symptoms that depend on the severity of the right heart involvement, if not failure. At auscultation, the pulmonic second sound is distinctly accentuated to

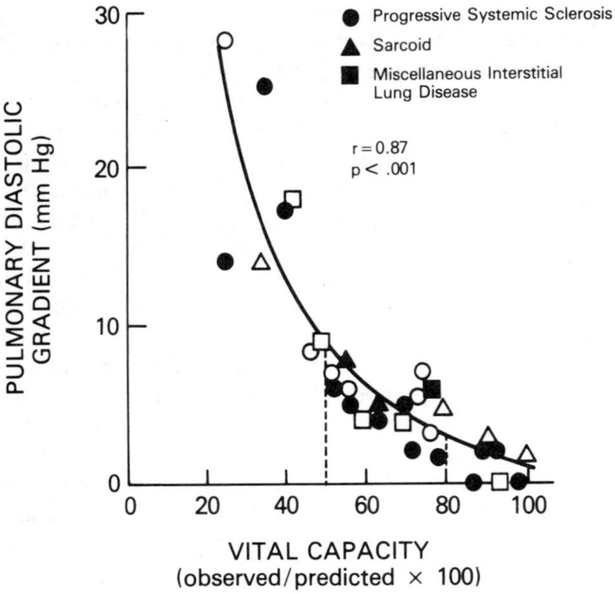

Figure 54.13. Relationship between pulmonary diastolic gradient and percent of predicted vital capacity in patients with chronic restrictive lung disease. The pulmonary diastolic gradient is the difference between the pulmonary artery diastolic pressure and the mean pulmonary capillary wedge pressure. (From Enson et al,[27] with permission.)

the point that it may become palpable. A precordial cardiac impulse is frequently noted in the xiphoid area. A left parasternal heave may be felt in conjunction with the presence of a pulmonary ejection click during systole. One of the most important signs is a right ventricular gallop which is subject to respiratory changes, ie, an increase with inspiration, if not heard only during inspiration.

Sometimes a right atrial gallop may also be heard, suggesting an increased filling pressure. One should also look for a tricuspid regurgitation murmur, which characterizes an acutely decompensated cor pulmonale. In severe forms of cor pulmonale, signs mimicking cardiac tamponade might be present such as diminished heart sounds, distended jugular veins, and a palpable liver. However, the latter two signs do not necessarily establish the presence of tamponade. Distension of the jugular veins during inspiration, with collapse during expiration, is a common occurrence in patients with chronic advanced lung disease; when heart failure is present, the distension is present throughout the respiratory cycle. Because of lung inflation (increased residual volume), lowering of the liver may be confused with hepatomegaly, but a pulsatile liver, in addition to enlargement, is characteristic of right heart failure.

ARRHYTHMIA

Cardiac rhythm disturbances are frequent in patients with cor pulmonale, but they are also often observed in chronic bronchitis and emphysema without cor pulmonale. The dysrhythmia may have a number of manifestations: supraventricular tachycardia, which is frequently asymptomatic; ventricular arrhythmia, which may lead to sudden death from ventricular fibrillation during acute respiratory failure; or bradyarrhythmia, which may also be life threatening if not recognized and treated.

ELECTROCARDIOGRAM

The ECG is an important tool in the diagnosis of right ventricular hypertrophy which is a late manifestation of cor pulmonale. However, prior to this there are a number of electrocardiographic changes related to the underlying pulmonary disease and even to some left heart disease, which is often a companion to the right ventricular alteration.

Holford[28] extensively described the electrocardiographic changes seen in cor pulmonale, whether it is a consequence of interstitial lung disease, chronic hypoventilation, or pulmonary vascular disease (Table 54.4) or of chronic obstructive lung disease (Table 54.5). Although the criteria listed in Table 54.4 are helpful, they depend on the interplay of factors such as hyperinflation of the lungs and displacement of, as well as structural changes in, the heart itself.

RIGHT VENTRICULAR FUNCTION

Alterations in right ventricular function depend essentially on the severity of the hypoxia and, in turn, of the pulmonary artery hypertension. Often, it is only with exercise that alterations can be detected in the form of excess increase in pulmonary artery pressure, increase in right ventricle stroke work, and decrease in the right ventricular ejection fraction.[29] The progressive changes in cardiovascular function with progressive cor pulmonale have been well depicted by Fishman[30] and are seen in Figure 54.14.

LEFT VENTRICULAR CHANGES

Autopsy studies in patients who died of chronic obstructive lung disease have shown frequent evidence of

Table 54.3. Relation of Spirographic Data to $\overline{PAP}$*

	FEV_1 (% pred)	VC (% pred)	FEV_1/VC (%)	$\overline{PAP}$ (mm Hg)
FEV_1 (% pred)	...	0.73†	0.65†	−0.43†
VC (% pred)	...	...	0.03	−0.58†
FEV_1/VC (%)	...	...	...	−0.10
PAP (mm Hg)	...	...	...	...

* From Timsit et al[26] with permission from S. Karger AG, Basel.

† The significance is marked, indicating that $0.001 < P < 0.05$.

FEV_1 = forced expiratory volume in the first second; $\overline{PAP}$ = mean pulmonary artery pressure; PRED = predicted; VC = vital capacity.

Table 54.4. Electrocardiographic Criteria for Cor Pulmonale without Obstructive Disease of the Airways*

1. Right axis deviation with a mean QRS axis to the right of +110†
2. R/S amplitude ratio in V_1 >1
3. R/S amplitude ratio in V_6 <1
4. Clockwise rotation of the electrical axis
5. P-pulmonale pattern
6. S_1Q_3 or $S_1S_2S_3$ pattern
7. Normal-voltage QRS

* From Holford,[28] Table 10-1; reproduced with permission.

† Any one of the first three criteria suffices to raise suspicion of right ventricular hypertrophy. The diagnosis becomes more certain if two or more of these findings are present. The last four criteria commonly occur in cor pulmonale secondary to primary alveolar hypoventilation, interstitial disease of the lung, or pulmonary vascular disease.

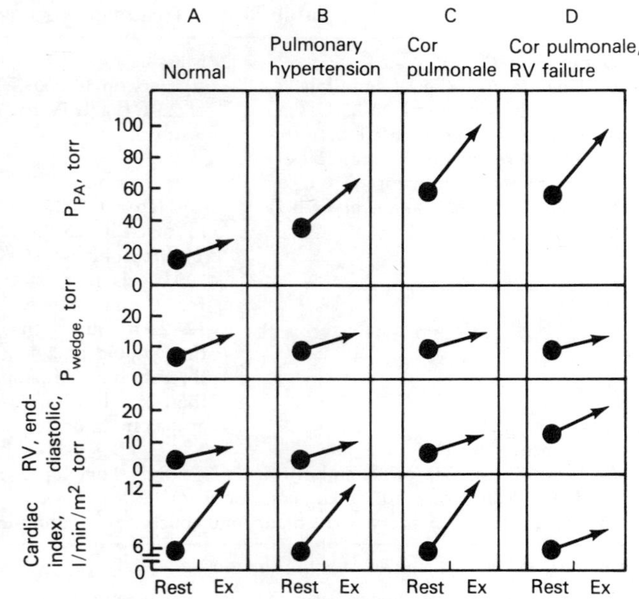

Figure 54.14. Schematic representation of the evolution of chronic cor pulmonale. Hemodynamic studies at rest and during exercise in a normal subject (A). The stage of pulmonary arterial hypertension (B) is succeeded by cor pulmonale (C) in which the right ventricle performs normally despite pulmonary arterial hypertension but is known to be enlarged because of radiographic and electrocardiographic findings. Once right ventricular failure supervenes (D), cardiac output fails to increase normally during exercise despite an increase in right ventricular filling pressure (end-diastolic) to abnormally high levels. Ex=exercise; RV=right ventricular. (From Fishman,[30] Figure 73-2, with permission.)

left ventricular hypertrophy. However, it is a subject of debate whether disease of the left ventricle is a consequence of cor pulmonale or the result of independent causes. The left ventricular dysfunction is manifested by electrocardiographic alterations, such as an important reduction in voltage of the precordial leads and prolonged QRS duration.

A number of mechanisms have been evoked to relate left ventricular changes to the right heart disease: (1) distorted configuration of the left ventricle due to right ventricular hypertrophy; this would impede the left ventricular ejection fraction, especially during exercise; (2) insufficient myocardial oxygen delivery owing to the chronic hypoxic state in patients with cor pulmonale; and (3) high-output cardiac failure in patients with carbon dioxide retention and increased bronchial circulation.

TREATMENT-PROGNOSIS

The most important treatment of cor pulmonale is treatment of the underlying disease.

I. PULMONARY THROMBOEMBOLISM: ACUTE COR PULMONALE

The hallmark in the treatment of pulmonary thromboembolism is anticoagulant therapy. Although most emboli resolve spontaneously in time, it is essential to speed up the process of resolution and to prevent recurrence. Bell and Simon[8] have provided a treatment based on the experience of the urokinase pulmonary embolism trial.[25]

Table 54.5. Electrocardiographic Changes in Chronic Cor Pulmonale with Obstructive Disease of the Airways*

1. Isoelectric P waves in lead I or right axis deviation of the P vector†
2. P-pulmonale pattern (an increase in P-wave amplitude in leads II, III, and aVF)
3. Tendency for right axis deviation of the QRS
4. R/S amplitude ratio in lead V_6<1
5. Low-voltage QRS
6. S_1Q_3 or $S_1S_2S_3$ pattern
7. Incomplete (and rarely complete) right bundle branch block
8. R/S amplitude ratio in lead V_1 >1
9. Marked clockwise rotation of the electrical axis
10. Occasional large Q waves or QS in the inferior or midprecordial leads, suggesting healed myocardial infarction

*From Holford,[28] Table 10-2; reproduced with permission.

† The first seven criteria are suggestive but nonspecific; the last three are more characteristic of cor pulmonale in obstructive disease of the airways.

As shown in Table 54.6, an approach is to prevent further thrombus formation with heparin and to enhance fibrinolysis with streptokinase. The drawback of such thrombolytic therapy is the risk of severe hemorrhage. However, the recent advent of recombinant DNA produced tissue-plasminogen-activator (tPA)[31] may soon provide a more effective and safer means of intervention.

The risk of massive recurrence in some instances makes it necessary to consider vena caval interruption (ligation). Fortunately this is needed less today than before because of better pharmacologic interventions, but also because morbidity and mortality of the intervention remain high. Moreover, a high mortality (more than 50%) is associated with pulmonary embolectomy, which is indicated only as a last resort in cases of massive embolism with a severe state of shock and heart failure.

By and large, the prognosis of patients with pulmonary thromboembolism has considerably improved during the last two decades. It nonetheless remains tied to the underlying disorder and to how well it is treated. The poorest prognosis is related to recurrence and, of course, to consequent pulmonary artery hypertension. Should it develop, all efforts must be made to limit its rise. The problem of controlling pulmonary hypertension is that except for oxygen, which acts selectively on the pulmonary arteries over the systemic arteries, all other vasodilators may produce systemic hypotension.[32] It is of interest, however, that recent work has demonstrated that some herbal

Table 54.6. Treatment Regimens in Pulmonary Embolism (PE)*

1. Submassive PE	2. Massive PE	3. Anticoagulants contraindicated
(a) Heparin 70 U/kg IV simultaneously with infusion of 20-25 U/kg/h IV regulated to keep APTT between 60 and 80 sec or Lee-White CT between 20 and 40 min for 7–10 d; or	(a) Heparin 10,000 U IV simultaneously with infusion of 25 U/kg/h IV for 7–10 d regulated by laboratory test; or	Vena caval ligation, umbrella or balloon, for life-threatening embolus; plication in other cause
(b) Heparin 55-70 U/kg every 4 h IV 7–10 d	(b) Heparin 7,000-10,000 U every 4 h IV for 24–48 h followed by 55-75 U/kg every 4 h for 7–9 d or	
	(c) Streptokinase 250,000 U IV for 30 min followed by 100,000 U/h for 24 h; or urokinase 4,400 CTA U/ kg for 10 min followed by 4,400 CTA U/kg/h for 12–24 h. During thrombolytic therapy, the thrombin time should be 2-7 × baseline. At completion of thrombolytic infusion when thrombin time is less than 2 × baseline (3–4 h later), start heparin therapy as in 2a or 2b	

Long-term therapy
(a) Warfarin to keep prothrombin 8%–25% activity, overlap 3–5 d with heparin and continue at least 12 wk; further therapy guided by status of predisposing conditions; or
(b) Heparin 5,000 U every 8–12 h subcutaneously for a minimum of 12 wk

* From Bell and Simon[8]; reproduced with permission.

APTT = activated partial thromboplastin time; CT = clotting time; CTA = Committee on Thrombolytic Agents.

drugs, eg, salviae miltiorrhizae, can decrease pulmonary hypertension due to chronic pulmonary thromboembolism without affecting the systemic circulation.[33]

II. CHRONIC COR PULMONALE

As chronic cor pulmonale is the consequence of pulmonary artery hypertension, the obvious treatment is to decrease the pulmonary artery pressure in order to limit the strain on the right side of the heart. To this end, and because of its selective action on the pulmonary circulation, supplemental oxygen is, and remains, the most important treatment of cor pulmonale secondary to advanced chronic pulmonary disease. In addition to relieving the pulmonary artery constriction caused by hypoxia, supplemental oxygen also corrects impaired tissue oxygen delivery. Two recent studies, one in England[34] and the other in the United States,[35] have convincingly demonstrated the value of supplemental oxygen. Figure 54.15, which shows the survival rate in several groups of patients, establishes that the longer supplemental oxygen is administered each day, the greater the survival. The American study also showed that the cost incurred by the use of oxygen 24 hours per day was, in the long run, compensated by a reduced number (as well as duration) of hospitalizations as compared to those of patients receiving oxygen for only 12 hours per day. It must be emphasized that in neither of these two studies did the pulmonary artery pressure of the patients receiving the most oxygen decrease significantly. Therefore, their longer survival could be accounted for by a limitation in further increase of the pulmonary artery pressure than would otherwise have occurred.

The effectiveness of supplemental oxygen is predicated upon efforts to improve lung function and to maintain

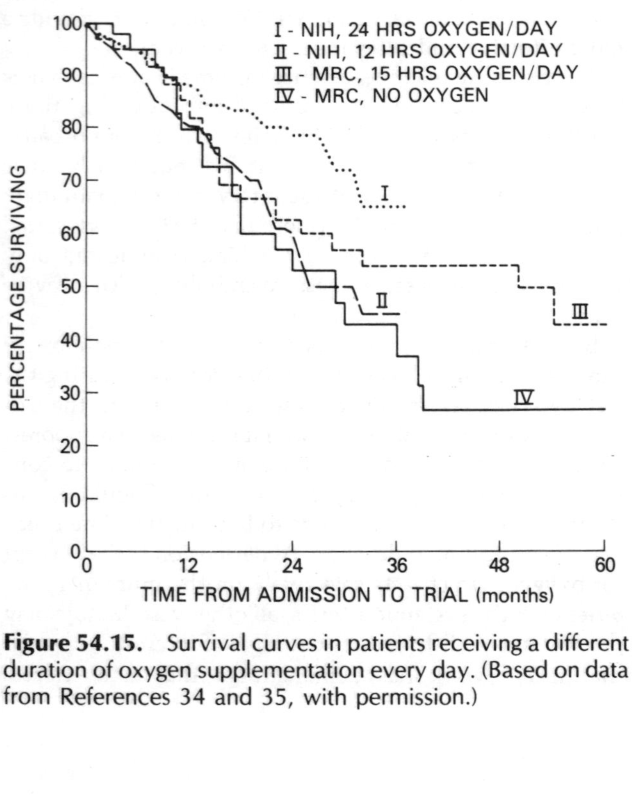

Figure 54.15. Survival curves in patients receiving a different duration of oxygen supplementation every day. (Based on data from References 34 and 35, with permission.)

Table 54.7. Vasodilator Agents of Possible Benefit in Primary Pulmonary Hypertension*

Alpha-adrenergic blocking agents	Direct smooth muscle relaxants
Tolazoline	Hydralazine†
Phentolamine†	Minoxidil†
Beta-adrenergic agonists	Prazosin†
Isoproterenol	Diazoxide
	Nitroprusside
	Nitrates†
Parasympathomimetics	Calcium channel blocking agents
Acetylcholine	Diltiazem†
	Nifedipine†
	Verapamil†
Vasodilator prostaglandins	Converting enzyme inhibitors
Prostacylin	Captopril

* From Rounds and Hill,[42] reproduced with permission.

† Indicates availability for oral administration.

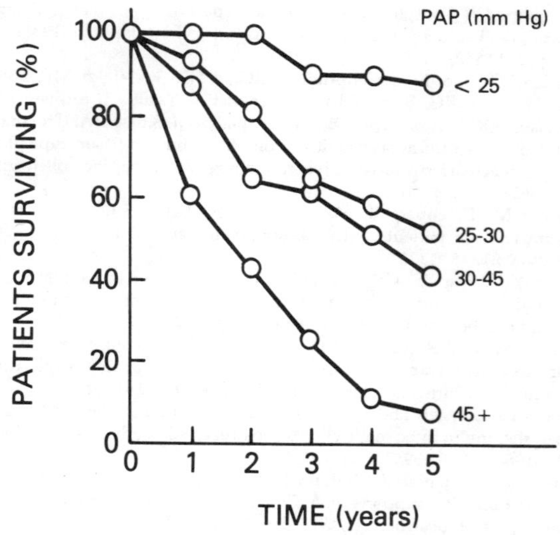

Figure 54.16. Survival of patients with chronic constrictive lung disease in relation to initial mean pulmonary artery pressure (PAP). (From Bishop,[43] with permission from S. Karger AG, Basel.)

bronchial hygiene, especially in patients whose underlying disease is characterized by excess secretions, such as cystic fibrosis. Therefore, smoking must be stopped, bronchodilators must be used when necessary, and recurring airway infections must be diligently treated. Although supplemental oxygen is the treatment of choice to reduce hypoxia, this may also be aided by pharmacologically improving the ventilation perfusion distribution; the drug almatrin[36] has been attributed to have such an effect, but clearly more studies are necessary before it becomes routinely used.

Although they have potential adverse effects, diuretics are important for the relief of edema and dyspnea. Possible complications are hypokalemia, metabolic alkalosis, and reduction in the right ventricular preload which in turn leads to a decrease in cardiac output.

Digitalis and other glycosides increase right ventricular function as well as act on the left ventricle.[37] They are also indicated in the management of supraventricular arrhythmia which occurs so often in advanced hypoxic pulmonary disease. Yet, glycoside toxicity has been reported in these patients, especially those with unsuspected hypokalemia. It is therefore prudent to carefully monitor patients receiving glycoside therapy.

more preponderant role in the treatment of pulmonary artery hypertension secondary to chronic pulmonary disease. The direct smooth muscle relaxant hydralazine has received considerable attention.[38,39] It improves right ventricular function. Other agents, such as beta-adrenergic agonists[40] and calcium channel blockers,[41] have been used with reported success, but again one must be vigilantly conscious that systemic hypotension and recurring hypoxia remain the adverse consequences of many of these drugs. In contrast, vasodilator agents are of great possible benefit in the treatment of primary pulmonary artery hypertension[42] (Table 54.7) or hypertension of iatrogenic origin. Prostaglandin E_1 offers a theoretical advantage over other vasodilators in that it has a high clearance in one passage through the lungs and thus may reduce pulmonary vascular resistance without producing systemic hypotension.[42a]

As shown by Bishop[43] (Figure 54.16), the prognosis of chronic pulmonary disease depends essentially on the severity of the pulmonary artery hypertension: "If pulmonary arterial pressure was initially normal, some 90% (of the patients) were still alive five years later, but with increasing levels of pressure, the mortality increased progressively." From this it can be concluded that the prognosis of chronic cor pulmonale is fearsome.

CONCLUSIONS

Cor pulmonale, acute or chronic, results from strain on the right side of the heart due to increased pulmonary artery pressure. Its severity and prognosis are directly related to the level of pulmonary artery pressure. Many underlying pulmonary disorders lead to an increase in pulmonary artery pressure, either because of a loss in cross-sectional surface or because of active constriction of the pulmonary vessels, or both.

The hallmark in the treatment of pulmonary artery hypertension is treatment of the underlying cause as well as pharmacologic dilation of the arteries. Despite considerable progress and the development of new and better drugs, there are possible adverse effects from all regimens. Therefore, each treatment must be individualized and closely monitored.

Acknowledgment: Mr. T. Thom assisted in the preparation and redaction of the section, "Prevalence and Incidence," and Dr. D. Williams in the analysis of the World Health Organization's data used in that section. Dr. A. Fishman critically reviewed the manuscript and Dr. D. Robinson provided assistance with the bibliographic search.

REFERENCES

1. Huang Ti Nei Ching Su Wen: *The Yellow Emperor's Classic of Internal Medicine,* Veith I, (trans). Baltimore, Williams & Wilkins, 1949.
2. Bhargava RK: *Cor pulmonale (Pulmonary Heart Disease)*. Mt Kisco, NY, Futura Publishing Co, 1973.
3. World Health Organization: Chronic cor pulmonale. Report of an expert committee. *Circulation* 1963; 27:594–615.
4. McGinn S, White PD: Acute cor pulmonale resulting from pulmonary embolism. *JAMA* 1935; 104:1473–1480.
5. Laennec RH: *Traité l'auscultatation médiate et des maladies des poumons et du coeur,* ed 4. Paris, Chaudé, 1837, vol 3 (first edition published 1819).
6. White PD: *Heart Disease*. New York, MacMillan Publishing Co Inc, 1931.
7. Rubin LJ: Pulmonary hypertension secondary to lung disease, in Weir EK, Reeves JT (eds): *Pulmonary Hypertension.* Mt Kisco, NY, Futura Publishing Co, 1984, pp 291–320.
8. Bell WR, Simon TL: Current status of pulmonary thromboembolic disease: pathophysiology, diagnosis, prevention, and treatment. *Am Heart J* 1982; 103:239–262.
9. *Respiratory Diseases.* Task Force Report on Problems, Research Approaches, Needs. Department of Health, Education, and Welfare publication No. (NIH) 73–432, National Heart and Lung Institute, 1972.
10. National Health Interview Survey, 1981. US Department of Health, Education, and Welfare. National Center for Health Statistics (unpublished data).
11. National Hospital Discharge Survey, 1983. US Department of Health and Human Services. National Center for Statistics (unpublished data).
12. Monthly Vital Statistics Report, Advance Report of Final Mortality Statistics, 1982. US Department of Health and Human Services. National Center for Health Statistics, 1984, vol 33, p 9.
13. Cheng TO: Prevalence of cardiovascular diseases among the national minorities of China. *Ann Intern Med* 1984; 101:562–563.

14. World Health Organization. *Chronic lung disease leading to cor pulmonale: report on a consultation in Florence* (December 6-7, 1976) 1977.

14a. Pisa Z, Yemura K: Trends of mortality from ischemic heart disease and other cardiovascular diseases in 27 countries, 1968–1977. *World Health Stat Q* 1982; 35:11–47.

15. Cheng TO: Medicine in modern China. *J Am Geriatr Soc* 1973; 21:289–313.

16. Lategola MT: Pressure-flow relationships in the dog lung during acute, subtotal pulmonary vascular occlusion. *Am J Physiol* 1958; 192:613–619.

17. Brofman BL, Charms BL, Kohn PM, Elder J, Newman R, Rizika M: Unilateral pulmonary artery occlusion in man. *J Thorac Surg* 1957; 34:206–227.

18. Denolin H: Contribution a l'etude de la circulation pulmonaire en clinique. *Acta Cardiol* (suppl X) 1961; 16:1–224.

19. McIntyre KM, Sasahara AA: The hemodynamic response to pulmonary embolism in patients without prior cardiopulmonary disease. *Am J Cardiol* 1975; 28:288–294.

20. McFadden ER, Braunwald E: Cor pulmonale and pulmonary embolism, in Braunwald E (ed). *Heart Disease; A Textbook of Cardiovascular Medicine,* ed 2. Philadelphia, WB Saunders Co, 1984, pp 1572–1604.

21. Wilson JE III, Pierce AK, Johnson RL Jr, Winga ER, Harrell WR, Curry GC, Mullins CB et al: Hypoxemia in pulmonary embolism, a clinical study. *J Clin Invest* 1971; 50:481–491.

22. Ferrer MI: Disturbances in the circulation in patients with cor pulmonale. *Bull NY Acad Med* 1965; 41:942–958.

23. Fishman AP: Pulmonary thromboembolism: pathophysiology and clinical features, in Fishman AP (ed): *Pulmonary Diseases and Disorders.* New York, McGraw-Hill Co, 1980, vol 1, pp 809–826.

24. McIntyre KM, Sasahara AA, Sharma GVRK: Pulmonary thromboembolism: current concepts. *Adv Intern Med* 1972; 18:199–218.

25. The Urokinase Pulmonary Embolism Trial: a national cooperative study. *Circulation* 1973; 47 (suppl II):II-1–II-108.

26. Timsit G, Neukirch F, du Perron MC, Verdier F, Drutel P, Legrand M, Botto MJ, Lesobre R: Statistical correlation between PAP spirographic data and arterial and mixed venous blood gases in 22 subjects with chronic obstructive lung disease. *Prog Resp Res* 1975; 9:105–111.

27. Enson Y, Thomas HM III, Bosken CH, Wood JA, Leroy EC, Blanc WA, Wigger HJ, Harvey RM: Pulmonary hypertension in interstitial lung disease: relation of vascular resistance to abnormal lung structure. *Trans Assoc Am Physicians* 1975; 88:248–255.

28. Holford FD: The electrocardiogram in lung disease, in Fishman AP (ed): *Pulmonary Diseases and Disorders*. New York, McGraw-Hill Co, 1980, vol 1, pp 139–145.

29. Burrows B, Kettel LJ, Niden AH, Rabinowitz M, Diener CF: Patterns of cardiovascular dysfunction in chronic obstructive lung disease. *N Engl J Med* 1972; 286:912–918.

30. Fishman AP: Cor pulmonale: general aspects, in Fishman AP (ed): *Pulmonary Diseases and Disorders*. New York, McGraw-Hill Co, 1980, vol 1, pp 853–862.

31. Collen D, Topol EJ, Tiffenbrunn AJ, Gold HK, Weisfeldt ML, Sobel BE, Leinbach RC, Brinker JA, Ludbrook PA, Yasuda I, Bulkley BH, Robison AK, Hutter AM Jr, Bell WK, Spadaro JJ, Khaw BA, Grossbard EB: Coronary thrombolysis with recombinant human tissue-type plasminogen activator: a prospective, randomized, placebo-controlled trial. *Circulation* 1984; 70:1012–1017.

32. Packer M, Greenberg B, Massie B, Dash H: Deleterious effects of hydralazine in patients with pulmonary hypertension. *N Engl J Med* 1982; 306:1326–1331.

33. Zhao Y, Cheng XS, Cai R: Effect of salviae miltiorrhizae compound on pulmonary artery hypertension caused by chronic pulmonary thromboembolism. *Chin Med J* 1984; 97:473–478.

34. British Medical Research Council Working Party: Long term domiciliary oxygen therapy in chronic hypoxic cor pulmonale complicating chronic bronchitis and emphysema. *Lancet* 1981; 1:681–685.

35. Nocturnal Oxygen Therapy Trial Group: Continuous or nocturnal oxygen therapy in hypoxemic chronic obstructive lung disease. *Ann Intern Med* 1980; 93:391:398.

36. Castaing Y, Manier A, Varene N, Guenard H: Almitrine orale et distribution des rapports VA/Q dans les bronchopneumopathies chroniques et obstructives. *Bull Eur Physiopathol Respir* 1981; 17:917–932.

37. Green LH, Smith TW: The use of digitalis in patients with pulmonary disease. *Ann Intern Med* 1977; 87:459–465.

38. Rubin LJ, Peter RH: Hemodynamics at rest and during exercise after oral hydralazine in patients with cor pulmonale. *Am J Cardiol* 1981; 47:116–122.

39. Rubin LJ, Handel F, Peter RH: The effects of oral hydralazine on right ventricular end-diastolic pressure in patients with right ventricular failure. *Circulation* 1981; 65:1369–1373.

40. Stockley RA, Finnegan P, Bishop JM: Effect of intravenous terbutaline on arterial blood gas tensions, ventilation, and pulmonary circulation in patients with chronic bronchitis and cor pulmonale. *Thorax* 1977; 32:601–605.

41. Simonneau G, Escourrou P, Duroux P, Lockhart A: Inhibition of hypoxic pulmonary vasoconstriction by nifedipine. *N Engl J Med* 1981; 304:1582–1585.

42. Rounds S, Hill NS: Pulmonary hypertensive diseases. *Chest* 1984; 85:397–405.

42a. Swan PK, Tibballs J, Duncan AW: Prostaglandin E_1 in primary pulmonary hypertension. *Critical Care Med* 1986; 14:72–73.

43. Bishop JM: Hypoxia and pulmonary hypertension in chronic bronchitis. *Prog Resp Res* 1975; 9:10–15.

55 The Heart and the Gastrointestinal System

Morris Traube, MD and Howard M. Spiro, MD

The gastrointestinal tract depends on the circulatory system to remain viable, but other more subtle relations exist between the gastrointestinal tract and the heart. Symptoms or signs that lead a patient to the cardiologist may ultimately prove to be of gastrointestinal origin. Diseases of the heart may bring substantial secondary gastrointestinal derangements, and some disorders primarily affecting the gut may bring secondary cardiac effects. Some systemic disorders affect both heart and gut. In this chapter, we will stress several of the more important issues faced by the practicing cardiologist.

CHEST PAIN OF ESOPHAGEAL ORIGIN

Patients with chest pain are usually first seen by the cardiologist because of the overriding concern about coronary artery disease. However, 10% to 30% of patients with typical or atypical angina pectoris have normal coronary arteries on arteriography.[1] One third of the patients hospitalized for acute anterior chest pain and suspected ischemic heart disease do not have that diagnosis confirmed.[2] Although such "noncardiac" chest pain may originate from disorders of the musculoskeletal, respiratory, or gastrointestinal system, the esophagus is implicated as a cause of chest pain more frequently than are other organs.

ANATOMY AND PHYSIOLOGY

The proximal esophagus contains only striated muscle, the middle esophagus has variable amounts of striated and smooth muscle, and the distal esophagus has only smooth muscle. Food is systematically propelled from mouth to stomach by primary peristalsis, the sequential propagation of contractions down the esophagus. The contractions are initiated by pharyngeal reflexes and require cholinergic input. Once initiated, however, the peristaltic wave traverses the esophagus without voluntary control.

In normal persons, 90% of all contractions after a swallow are peristaltic. Their amplitude increases as the contractions move toward the distal esophagus; 5 cm above the lower esophageal sphincter, waves usually have a pressure ranging from 50 to 150 mm Hg. A few waves are simultaneous, that is, they occur at the same time in different segments of the esophagus; orderly transit does not occur, and such waves are nonperistaltic.

The normal esophageal sphincter maintains high resting pressure, separating negative intraesophageal pressure from positive intragastric pressure, thus helping to prevent reflux of material from the high-pressure stomach into the low-pressure esophagus. The sphincter relaxes when food is swallowed, allowing food to enter the stomach, but it returns to its baseline level of 10 to 30 mm Hg when the peristaltic wave reaches the sphincter.

Physiologic mechanisms clear the esophagus of any acid that refluxes back into the esophagus, thereby minimizing damage to the esophageal mucosa. Acid clearance, as this process is called, depends on peristalsis and the presence of saliva. Most acid experimentally instilled into the esophagus is quickly emptied from the esophagus by one or two swallows; however, any residual acid maintains a low pH, which is independent of the volume of intraesophageal acid. Return of esophageal pH to normal occurs in a slow, stepwise manner as saliva is propelled down the esophagus to neutralize the acid.[3] For these reasons, any agent that inhibits peristalsis or salivary flow prolongs acid clearance time.

PATHOPHYSIOLOGY

Motility disorders of the esophagus or gastroesophageal reflux may lead to either chest pain or dysphagia. The best characterized motility disorders of greatest importance to the cardiologist are achalasia, diffuse esophageal spasm, and the high-amplitude peristaltic contractions known as "nutcracker esophagus." Current concepts of these motility disorders and of gastroesophageal reflux disease will be discussed.

Achalasia is characterized by complete loss of peristalsis in the body of the esophagus and failure of the lower esophageal sphincter to relax. Food empties only slowly from the esophagus because peristalsis in the esophageal body is absent and the sphincter is functionally obstructed. The pathogenesis of achalasia remains an enigma, studies suggesting a central nervous system or peripheral neurogenic mechanism.

Conversely, in diffuse esophageal spasm, an increased number of nonperistaltic or simultaneous contractions occur in the esophagus. Unlike normal waves, these nonperistaltic contractions often are repetitive, of high amplitude, or spontaneous, ie, not generated by swallowing. Nevertheless, such characteristics are of ancillary importance, the manometric diagnosis depending solely on demonstration of increased frequency of nonperistaltic waves.[4] The etiology of primary diffuse esophageal spasm is unknown, but spasm may sometimes occur as a consequence of long-standing reflux,[5] so-called secondary spasm. Acid reflux presumably damages the esophagus, leading to a disorder of peristalsis.

The abnormalities of nerve fibers seen in achalasia are not present in the esophagus of patients with spasm;[6] yet, a relation between the two disorders is suggested by several reports of patients with diffuse esophageal spasm in whom achalasia gradually developed.

Contractions in the distal esophagus in patients with nutcracker esophagus are, by definition, of high amplitude, but they also may be prolonged or repetitive. Peristalsis is normal, a characteristic that differentiates this disorder from classic diffuse esophageal spasm. An association with gastroesophageal reflux or psychiatric disturbance has been suggested,[7,8] but its pathogenesis remains unknown.

The pathogenesis of reflux esophagitis is complex and multifactorial. Reduced lower esophageal sphincteric pressure characterizes patients with reflux as compared with normal subjects. Much overlap exists, however, and sphincteric pressure in any one person is generally not diagnostic of the presence or absence of reflux. A significantly reduced pressure, perhaps 5 mm Hg, is generally suggestive of reflux. Patients with gastroesophageal reflux have more episodes of reflux than do normal subjects when monitored with pH probes; moreover, as in normal subjects, most episodes occur during transient unexplained relaxation of the sphincter.[9] Unlike in normal subjects, continuous low sphincteric pressure or transient increases in abdominal pressure are responsible for about one third of the episodes of reflux.[9] Acid clearance time may be prolonged in patients with reflux, resulting in prolonged exposure of the esophageal mucosa to noxious gastric contents. The delayed clearance of acid may result from abnormal peristalsis, which itself may be a consequence of reflux esophagitis, a vicious cycle of reflux-esophagitis-reflux. Delayed acid clearance has also been ascribed to hiatal hernia, a controversial matter not to be discussed herein. About half the patients with gastroesophageal reflux have delayed gastric emptying, indicating abnormal antral motility and suggesting that such gastric abnormalities contribute to the development of reflux.[10]

CLINICAL MANIFESTATIONS

Most patients with achalasia do not see a cardiologist, as their major complaint is dysphagia. Symptoms are insidious in onset, their history often dating back several years. Patients often change to soft food or chew their food longer than before, and only with progression of dysphagia do they seek medical attention. Weight loss or nocturnal cough from pulmonary aspiration of esophageal contents is not uncommon. Chest pain occurs in only 10% of patients, usually in those with "vigorous achalasia." In that disorder, esophageal contractions are nonperistaltic but remain normal in amplitude in contrast to the low amplitude contractions of classic achalasia. It is rare for a patient to complain of chest pain as the only symptom of achalasia.

In contrast to achalasia, chest pain and dysphagia are often striking features of diffuse esophageal spasm. Dysphagia is likely to be intermittent, and food stuck in the esophagus can be washed down by a glass of water. Chest pain lasting minutes to hours often accompanies an attack of dysphagia; however, many patients have chest pain without dysphagia. The pain may be located in the anterior chest, may be squeezing in nature, and may radiate down the left arm or to the jaw. In patients with such complaints, consideration of cardiac disease obviously is appropriate, so that such patients are often evaluated for esophageal disease only after having first been studied, and sometimes treated, for presumed cardiac disease. Patients with esophageal spasm sometimes also have heartburn, indicating acid sensitivity of the esophagus and suggesting the possibility of reflux-induced, or secondary, spasm.

Symptoms in patients with the high-amplitude peristaltic contractions of nutcracker esophagus are similar to those in patients with classic diffuse esophageal spasm. They may complain of intermittent dysphagia, which in retrospect has been occurring for years. They may have chest pain just like that of diffuse esophageal spasm. In some series,[7,11] evidence of reflux can be found in half the patients.

DIAGNOSTIC CONSIDERATIONS

The cardiologist aware of the esophagus as a source of perplexing chest pain should consider points in the history that suggest esophageal disease. Although his first emphasis will be placed on exclusion of more serious disorders such as coronary artery disease, the cardiologist should be familiar with tests that indicate the presence of an esophageal disorder and its causal relation to chest pain.

If chest pain accompanies or is initiated by dysphagia, there should be little difficulty in implicating the esophagus. The occurrence of both chest pain and dysphagia in the same patient, even at different times, should also lead to indictment of the esophagus as the cause of chest pain. Heartburn, suggesting esophageal reflux, should point to an esophageal origin of chest pain, from atypical reflux or secondary esophageal spasm.

In some series of patients with esophageal pain, the pain was described as "atypical" for angina pectoris, but complete characterization of its atypical nature was often lacking. Although some patients may have typical but short-lived squeezing pain like angina pectoris, other patients with esophageal dysmotility may have chest pain that lasts for hours.[12] Chest pain of esophageal origin is less likely to be related to exercise and more closely related to stress. Despite such clinical hints of an esophageal origin of chest pain, the history by itself can only lead to suspicion but not to a definite diagnosis, and it does not clearly exclude cardiac disease.[12]

Because of the difficulty in differentiating cardiac from esophageal pain, especially when dysphagia is absent, and the greater import of failing to recognize a cardiac disorder, most patients are evaluated for an esophageal disorder only after extensive cardiac testing. This approach is apparent from most reports of patients with esophageal chest pain. In two such series in which 18% to 31% of the patients were ultimately deemed to have chest pain of esophageal origin, all patients had previously undergone coronary arteriography with normal findings.[13,14] In another series in which gastroesophageal reflux was ultimately shown to be responsible for chest pain in nearly half the patients, all patients had earlier undergone coronary arteriography with ergonovine provocation with normal results.[15] In yet another series of patients with chest pain in whom there was a 20% incidence of esophageal disease, all had been hospitalized for evaluation of acute chest pain with a presumptive diagnosis of a cardiac disorder.[2]

Many patients with an ultimate diagnosis of chest pain of esophageal origin, however, do not undergo coronary arteriography as part of the initial workup. In recent reports of the nutcracker esophagus or spasm as a cause of chest pain, diagnostic studies for cardiac disease ranged from resting electrocardiography to coronary angiography, depending on clinical judgment.[7,16,17] In some reports, cardiac testing was not described.[11] Clearly, the level of investigation for cardiac disease is decided by the primary physician or cardiologist after considering individual and family risk factors, medical history, and physical findings, matters that will not concern us. For example, the 25-year-old otherwise healthy woman with dysphagia and chest pain may not need a cardiac workup, whereas the 60-year-old diabetic man with chest pain who has equivocal findings on a cardiac stress test will require coronary angiography to exclude ischemic disease.

When the esophagus is being considered as the cause of the patient's symptoms, certain diagnostic studies are appropriate. Even though an esophageal motility disorder is suspected, it is first necessary to exclude an anatomic disorder, especially in the patient with dysphagia. Barium studies of the esophagus are usually carried out first. The classic findings in achalasia are an atonic esophagus, dilatation of the esophagus, and a tight "beak-like" lower esophagus. In diffuse esophageal spasm, the esophagus may have a corkscrew appearance resulting from simultaneous contractions, but in many patients the esophagus remains normal in appearance. To a certain extent, simultaneous or tertiary contractions by themselves are not diagnostic of spasm as they may be found in normal subjects as well as in those with spasm. Findings in nutcracker esophagus are less dramatic than the corkscrew appearance of spasm, the esophagus usually remaining normal. Occasionally, some nonspecific tertiary contractions may be present.

Although the x-ray findings in achalasia or diffuse esophageal spasm may suggest a motility disorder, they are not diagnostic. Carcinoma of the gastric fundus can present an achalasia-like picture, and some physicians perform endoscopy to exclude a tumor, especially in elderly patients with new symptoms of rapid onset. Moreover, the diagnosis of achalasia[18] or diffuse esophageal spasm should be confirmed by manometric studies, which will display the findings already described. For the diagnosis of nutcracker esophagus, an esophageal manometric study is essential.

The presence of nonperistaltic or high-amplitude esophageal contractions, indicative of esophageal spasm or nutcracker esophagus, does not categorically prove that the pain originates in the esophagus, unless the patient has pain during the manometric study and the pain clears when the abnormalities disappear from the tracing. Such a situation occurs only rarely. In most patients, we can only presume that the identified manometric abnormalities are markers of underlying disorders that may in some as yet unknown way be connected with chest pain.

Despite the increasing awareness of esophageal motility disorders as a cause of chest pain, many patients referred for manometric studies have normal results because of the intermittent nature of the esophageal spasm. This has led to the use of provocative agents in an esophageal "stress test." In some patients with chest pain and a normal angiogram, ergonovine induced both the patient's typical chest pain and disordered esophageal motility.[19] The potentially serious cardiac side effects of ergonovine limit its routine use, perhaps only to those patients who have had normal coronary angiographic results on ergonovine stimulation. Recent interest in provocation of esophageal dysfunction centers on the use of the anticholinesterase edrophonium, because this drug has no effect on the coronary arteries. In 30% of patients with symptoms suspected to be of esophageal origin, edrophonium produced chest pain with manometric changes.[20] An agent that can induce both pain and objective findings with a high and accurate yield remains a goal of active current interest.

The diagnosis of gastroesophageal reflux disease is not

difficult in most patients. The available tests fall into three main categories: (1) those that indicate the potential for reflux, (2) those that show esophageal damage, and (3) those that indicate reflux.

Determining the presence of hiatal hernia or decreased lower esophageal sphincteric pressure may indicate potential for reflux, but the sensitivity and specificity of the findings are too low to be of diagnostic value.

The acid perfusion (Bernstein) test is performed by perfusing suitably dilute hydrochloric acid into the esophagus and asking the patient to report the development of heartburn or chest pain. A positive test result indicates esophageal damage or at least acid sensitivity of the esophagus, and it has an overall sensitivity and specificity of about 80%.[21] For the test result to be considered positive, pain should not occur during baseline perfusion with saline, it should appear during subsequent perfusion with acid, but it need not disappear immediately on termination of perfusion with acid or on restarting perfusion with saline.[22] Its ease makes this a valuable first-line test in the evaluation of patients with other than typical heartburn. Double-contrast barium techniques have improved the ability of the radiologist to recognize esophagitis, although many gastroenterologists believe that the sensitivity of x-ray studies is not as great as that of endoscopy, which also allows biopsy for histologic examination of the esophagus and greater precision in recognizing esophageal damage.

X-ray studies of the esophagus may show free reflux of barium, but its accuracy in predicting reflux disease is too low to be acceptable. The standard acid reflux test with monitoring of distal esophageal pH after various maneuvers is a highly specific (99%) but not too sensitive (40%) test for reflux.[21] Sensitivity is increased if acid is loaded into the stomach before the test, but specificity is then decreased. The most accurate indicator of reflux is 24-hour continuous pH monitoring of the esophagus, but until now this has generally required hospitalization. The recently introduced continuous ambulatory pH monitor (an "esophageal Holter") does away with hospitalization, but further assessment of its accuracy is needed. Monitoring pH for perhaps only 12 hours may have an accuracy approaching that of 24-hour pH monitoring, provided that both a postprandial period and nighttime supine period are included.[23]

The patient with typical heartburn who responds to simple measures needs no diagnostic workup, but the one with more severe, atypical, or refractory symptoms needs a definitive diagnosis. Barium studies of the esophagus, stomach, and duodenum are often performed primarily to exclude ulcer or stricture, and the acid perfusion test is carried out to determine whether acid elicits the patient's symptoms. If the results are consistent with reflux, appropriate therapy, as will be discussed, is instituted. Otherwise, testing that is more invasive and less readily available to the primary physician or cardiologist is in order. It includes standard acid reflux testing and endoscopy with biopsy. Negative or equivocal results may require the use of prolonged (24-hour) pH monitoring for determination of reflux status. However, as already discussed, introduction of the ambulatory pH probe may make pH monitoring a test of "earlier" resort.

We should reemphasize that finding gastroesophageal reflux does not categorically prove that reflux is the cause of the patient's chest pain unless evidence is strong. The acid perfusion test may induce chest pain, which closely mimics the patient's complaints. In a study of patients with chest pain and normal coronary arteriographic results, patients underwent 24-hour pH monitoring of the esophagus in conjunction with diary keeping. Those patients in whom chest pain occurred simultaneously with documented reflux episodes improved more after antireflux surgery than did patients in whom reflux and chest pain did not occur simultaneously, even if reflux was present.[15]

Several other studies give further evidence that identification of esophageal disorders does not clearly indict the esophagus as responsible for the patient's symptoms. In one report, patients with negative cardiac stress tests and normal coronary arteriograms underwent esophageal manometry, intraesophageal acid perfusion, and determination of coronary sinus lactate concentrations during maximal atrial pacing.[24] Eight patients had abnormal and 15 had normal lactate metabolism. Esophageal motor anomalies were observed in six of the eight with abnormal and in 9 of the 15 subjects with normal lactate metabolism. Thus, abnormal lactate metabolism was present in about one third of the patients, despite normal angiograms, indicating a possible cardiac cause for pain. Moreover, esophageal abnormalities were present without regard to abnormal lactate metabolism. Another report showed that patients with angiographic evidence of coronary artery disease in whom chest pain develops after intraesophageal acid perfusion have an increase in the heart rate–blood pressure product and may also have electrocardiographic ST-T wave changes.[25] Moreover, half the patients with coronary artery disease in whom pain developed during esophageal acid perfusion could not distinguish that pain from their usual angina.[25] Another study on 24 patients with angina-like chest pain—12 with normal coronary arteriograms and 12 with abnormal coronary arteriograms (stenoses more than 50% diameter)—used supine barium swallow and measurement of radionuclide and barium capsule transit times.[25a] Esophageal peristalsis on barium swallow was abnormal in 3 (25%) patients with normal coronary arteriograms and 6 (50%) patients with ischemic heart disease. There were no significant differences between the mean radionuclide or capsule transit times in the two groups. Such results indicate the difficulty in ascertaining precisely the source of chest pain, even if it suggests that some patients with documented coronary artery disease who fare poorly might benefit from investigations and appropriate therapy for gastroesophageal disease.

TREATMENT

Treatment of achalasia is designed to diminish obstruction of the nonrelaxing lower esophageal sphincter; no treatment can effect a substantial return of peristalsis. Either dilatation with a pneumatic bag or surgical myotomy will give adequate relief of symptoms in most patients.[26] It is reasonable to proceed with surgical myotomy only when pneumatic dilatation fails to give relief. Pharmacologic therapy has had a resurgence in the use of the calcium channel blockers to reduce sphincteric pressure and alleviate symptoms.[27-29] Although the manometric effect of decreasing sphincteric pressure is well established, the clinical experience in achalasia is still limited. Because the vasodilatory properties of the drugs cause hypotension and dizziness, many patients cannot tolerate doses that can otherwise substantially reduce sphincteric pressure.

Management of the patient with diffuse esophageal spasm should stress reassurance of the patient that the symptoms are not of cardiac origin. Antianxiety agents have been used for their nonspecific effects. Gastroesophageal reflux should be treated vigorously. More specific pharmacologic therapy includes anticholinergic agents, nitrates,[30-31] and hydralazine,[31] although controlled clinical trials of their efficacy are lacking. Most interest in pharmacologic therapy currently lies in the calcium channel blockers, but results of the limited reports are preliminary and contradictory.[32] Some reports indicate that nifedipine decreases the frequency of contractions but does not change the pattern of simultaneous contractions[33,34]; however, these reports differ on whether nifedipine decreased the amplitude of contractions. Another report describes the transient return of peristalsis after acute administration of nifedipine.[35] Chest pain in some patients was improved by nifedipine[34,35] but not in others.[36] When medication fails to relieve symptoms, measures such as bougienage or pneumatic dilatation should be performed, particularly in patients who have spasm associated with some dysfunction of the lower esophageal sphincter.[37] A long esophagomyotomy may be necessary in patients who do not respond to other treatment and who remain incapacitated by symptoms; however, this measure should be resorted to only rarely.

The approach to the patient with nutcracker esophagus remains uncertain because the disorder has been reported only in the past decade. It is appropriate to search for and to treat associated reflux as well as psychiatric disturbances. Pharmacologic intervention centers on the calcium channel blockers. Preliminary results with nifedipine and diltiazem suggest beneficial manometric and clinical effects,[29,38] but double-blind trials are lacking. Bougienage has no role in treatment in most patients[39] unless there is associated sphincter dysfunction.

Initial therapy for gastroesophageal reflux includes dietary modifications, elimination of smoking, and elevation of the head of the bed. It might be advantageous to avoid drugs that decrease lower esophageal sphincteric pressure such as theophylline and the calcium channel blockers. Initial therapy also has included antacids for relief of symptoms.

The H_2-histamine blockers cimetidine and ranitidine decrease gastric acid production and consistently improve symptoms. Histologic improvement of esophagitis has been more difficult to demonstrate probably because the drug trials were too short. Bethanechol, a cholinergic agent, has also been effective in treating reflux. Although it increases lower esophageal sphincteric pressure, its mechanism of action might also depend on its ability to stimulate saliva production and thereby improve acid clearance.[40] The dopamine antagonist, metoclopramide, which increases lower esophageal sphincteric pressure, is another drug effective in controlling symptoms of reflux. Because it also enhances gastric emptying rates, it is especially appropriate in patients with reflux with delayed gastric emptying.[41] The choice of drug generally remains a personal one, because there are insufficient data to attest to the superiority of one drug over another. It is, however, appropriate to consider concomitant medical conditions when selecting therapy. The patient with angina pectoris might best avoid bethanechol, as it could cause tachycardia. The patient taking warfarin might best avoid cimetidine because interactions between the two require retitration of the warfarin dose.

HEART FAILURE AND LIVER DYSFUNCTION

ANATOMY

The heart and liver lie close to each other, but that proximity is not as important as their interrelated vascular connections. Unlike other organs, the liver has a dual blood supply: (1) The hepatic artery supplies only one quarter of the blood flow to the liver, but that represents one half of the total oxygen supply to the liver. (2) The rest of the blood is supplied by way of the portal vein, which drains the splanchnic area. At the hilum of the liver, the portal vein divides into right and left branches, which accompany branches of the hepatic arteries and hepatic bile ducts. This pattern of portal vein, hepatic artery, and bile ducts carries on into the smallest network of the liver. The efferent blood supply of the liver is entirely by way of the hepatic veins, which drain into the inferior vena cava and thereby into the right atrium. Branches of the hepatic veins spread throughout the liver independent of the afferent blood supply and bile ducts. This separation of afferent and efferent blood supplies is responsible for the definition of the liver lobule as well as for specific abnormalities seen in the liver in various types of hepatic dysfunction, which are to be discussed.

PATHOPHYSIOLOGY

The lobule is commonly accepted as the basic unit of the liver. It is composed of a central efferent vein surrounded by parenchyma with numerous portal triads, each containing at the periphery a portal vein, hepatic artery, and bile duct. Definition of the lobule as the classic unit of the liver is arbitrary and results from its easy recognition at microscopy. The acinus, however, is the functional unit of the liver. It consists of the liver parenchyma supplied by blood from a single portal tract. Blood flows from the triads through sinusoids between the intervening liver cells in the surrounding parenchyma. Hepatocytes nearest the triad, in so-called zone 1, receive the highest concentration of oxygen and nutrients, and those farthest away, in zone 3, receive the least amount of nutrients. This is important because, as explained later, the location of hepatic changes seen in heart failure can be explained by this acinar distribution, although the changes are commonly described in terms of the classic lobule.

The effects of heart failure on the liver depend on whether cardiac failure is acute or chronic and primarily right-sided or left-sided. In acute congestive heart failure with right-sided dysfunction, the central hepatic veins become dilated and the sinusoids become engorged.[42–44] In severe heart failure, cells in the central part of the lobule, nearest the dilated efferent vein, may atrophy. Although necrosis in the mid-zone of the hepatic lobule usually is attributed to toxins such as those of yellow fever, hepatic necrosis in heart failure may be seen in the mid-zone as well as the centrilobular region.[45] Cell necrosis in heart failure is not associated with a substantial inflammatory infiltrate, which differentiates it from cell necrosis seen in viral hepatitis. With worsening congestive failure, hepatic necrosis spreads, leaving the only normal liver parenchyma in the periportal area. Fibrosis may even connect the central veins, the microscopic picture becoming that of a portal triad surrounded by fibrous strands connecting central veins, typical of cardiac cirrhosis. Previously found mainly in patients with long-standing rheumatic heart disease, cardiac cirrhosis currently is much less common but it may still be recognized in patients with constrictive pericarditis. Because of improved treatment in chronic, compensated congestive heart failure, the liver generally will not demonstrate much necrosis; signs of congestion or even fibrosis may be present.[43]

Perhaps the best known hepatic lesion of left-sided heart failure is "shock liver" or "ischemic hepatitis."[46,47] Although most patients with shock liver will have not only acute severe left-sided but also right-sided heart failure, centrilobular necrosis results primarily from decreased cardiac output and not from the passive congestion seen histologically. This explains the finding of centrilobular necrosis in some patients with isolated left-sided heart failure and no preceding hypotension.[48] Presumably the decreased delivery of nutrients to the acinar zone 3, or the centrilobular area, leads to localization of necrosis to this part of the lobule.

CLINICAL MANIFESTATIONS OF HEPATIC DYSFUNCTION IN HEART FAILURE

The manifestations of heart disease usually will dominate the picture of liver disease, so that the cardiologist will not be misled. The type of heart disease is unimportant in determining whether hepatic dysfunction occurs, but it will generally be known anyway. Occasionally, however, hepatic dysfunction appears in the absence of readily apparent cardiac disease. For example, left-sided heart failure may cause hepatic changes that present as acute hepatitis, with anorexia, fatigue, and right upper quadrant tenderness. Only after investigation is cardiac failure recognized as the source of hepatic dysfunction.[48] Likewise, hepatic dysfunction resulting from constrictive pericarditis, in the absence of left-sided heart failure, will not be attributed to a cardiac cause until the pericarditis is recognized.

Although symptoms of cardiac failure generally dominate the clinical picture, in some patients liver involvement will produce the major manifestations. In acute right-sided congestive failure, the swollen liver may cause pain and tenderness in the right upper quadrant; this finding is less frequent in chronic heart failure. Nausea, vomiting, and anorexia are nonspecific symptoms of either hepatic dysfunction or cardiac failure and its other complications of hypoxia and shock. Fulminant hepatic failure with hyperammonemia, encephalopathy, disseminated intravascular coagulation, and hypoglycemia is a rare complication of circulatory failure.[49–51] It may occur even after correction of circulatory failure and presents one to three days after acute cardiac injury.

As with the symptoms, the signs of heart failure are more apparent than those of liver involvement. Nevertheless, in right-sided heart failure, signs of hepatic involvement are almost always present. More than 95% of patients with acute or chronic right-sided failure will have hepatomegaly, the liver being palpable at least 5 cm below the right costal margin in half the patients.[43] Peripheral edema, which may occur in 75% of patients with right-sided heart failure, and ascites, which may occur in 15%, are primarily manifestations of heart failure and not of hepatic dysfunction.[44] However, splenomegaly has been noted in up to 25% of patients with right-sided heart failure and more frequently in the presence of cardiac cirrhosis.[44] Jaundice may be seen in 5% to 20% of patients, more frequently in acute than in chronic right-sided heart failure.[43,44] In acute left ventricular failure and "shock liver," cardiac failure and shock will obviously be overwhelming in the clinical picture. The development of hepatomegaly, liver tenderness, and edema may be influenced by the presence of right-sided heart failure, but they may also occur in its absence.[47]

Abnormalities in liver function tests are common in congestive heart failure without any clear relation between clinical findings and serum liver enzyme levels.[42] In 175 patients with acute or chronic right-sided congestive heart failure, the most common abnormality, seen in almost 80% of the patients, was in Bromsulphalein retention,[43] a test now infrequently used. Elevation of transaminase levels occurred in half the patients with acute failure but in only 5% of those with chronic failure. Most elevations were less than several times normal, but levels of serum glutamic oxalacetic transaminase (SGOT) greater than 1,000 U/ml were rare in patients with acute heart failure. Transaminase levels fell rapidly, reaching normal values within 1 week. Hyperbilirubinemia occurred in 31% of patients, more commonly in acute than in chronic heart failure; jaundice was visible in only 5% of patients. None of the patients in that series had a bilirubin level greater than 8 mg%. With improvement in heart failure, bilirubin levels decreased rapidly in all patients, usually returning to normal within a week. Serum alkaline phosphatase levels were increased in only 10% of patients and only to twice normal levels. Unlike bilirubin and transaminase levels, however, the decrease in alkaline phosphatase levels may be delayed longer than several weeks after the initial insult. A prolonged prothrombin time also occurred in about 80% of patients, correcting generally within 2 to 3 weeks. In acute left-sided heart failure without coexisting right-sided heart failure, dramatic increases in transaminase levels to greater than 3,000 U/ml, a prolonged prothrombin time, and hyperbilirubinemia up to 18 mg% have been reported.[47,48] Such elevated transaminase levels indicate centrilobular necrosis and do not occur in the presence of passive congestion alone.[43,47] As in right-sided heart failure, rapid reduction in serum enzyme and bilirubin levels takes place after correction of heart failure, unless hepatic failure has occurred.

DIAGNOSTIC CONSIDERATIONS

When cardiopulmonary symptoms of heart failure generally dominate the clinical picture, the physician should consider hepatic dysfunction a result of heart failure. Although a rapid increase and decrease in serum glutamic oxalacetic transaminase may also be seen when a stone transiently obstructs and then passes through the common bile duct, rapid return of liver function tests to normal in the setting of heart failure should reassure the physician enough to eliminate further workup.

If fever is associated with the aforementioned abnormalities, biliary tract disease should be suspected enough to require ultrasound examination. Although anorexia, nausea, and fatigue have led to considerations of chronic hepatitis in some patients, recognition of heart failure should delay any rush to biopsy the liver, and the rapid decrease in serum enzyme levels with treatment of heart failure will suggest the cause of hepatic abnormalities.

Drug-induced hepatitis must be considered in patients exposed to many cardiac drugs with known hepatotoxicity, such as methyldopa and procainamide. Acute deterioration in cardiac function usually makes liver dysfunction a likely result of cardiac disease, so that these drugs may be continued.

When heart and liver disease occur together, the physician should consider infiltrative diseases such as amyloidosis and hemochromatosis. Alcohol may lead to cirrhosis and to either alcoholic cardiomyopathy or beriberi heart disease. Patients with such abnormalities generally have evidence of chronic liver disease without rapid correction in hepatic dysfunction on appropriate cardiac therapy.

TREATMENT

Specific therapy for liver dysfunction in patients with heart failure is generally neither necessary nor effective. With cardiac therapy, liver abnormalities clear rapidly, with serum enzyme levels improving within days or occasionally weeks. Hypoprothrombinemia may last several weeks, and administration of vitamin K has little effect.

In the rare patient in whom hepatic failure develops, more specific measures are indicated. Correction of hypocoagulation may require blood products; hypoglycemia, the intravenous administration of glucose; and encephalopathy, treatment with lactulose or neomycin enemas to decrease serum ammonia levels, matters more appropriately discussed elsewhere.

During hypoperfusion and dysfunction of the liver, reduction in drug doses may be appropriate. This is especially true for lidocaine, whose serum concentrations can achieve toxic levels if the dosage is not reduced.

VASCULAR DISEASE OF THE INTESTINE

ANATOMY AND PATHOPHYSIOLOGY

The intestine receives a rich blood supply from the celiac, superior mesenteric, and inferior mesenteric arteries, with so many collateral connections that occlusion of one or more arteries does not necessarily lead to unfavorable consequences. The degree of obstruction, the rapidity of onset, and the status of the collateral circulation all interact to determine whether the intestine will remain normal or have pathophysiologic consequences.

Vascular disease of the gut may present as acute occlusion of a major artery, most often involving the superior mesenteric artery, regardless of its embolic or thrombotic origin.[52] Embolism may occur in patients with atrial fibrillation, mural thrombi after myocardial infarction, or cardiac vegetations after infectious endocarditis and in those who have recently undergone arterial manipulation during cardiac catheterization or surgery. Thrombosis occurs most often in patients with typical arteriosclerotic disease of the intestinal vasculature, but it also occurs with increased frequency in patients with clotting abnormalities such as polycythemia.

Mesenteric venous thrombosis is a less frequent cause of acute vascular injury to the gut. This disorder may be associated particularly with portal hypertension, intraabdominal sepsis, inflammatory bowel disease, hypercoagulable states such as those associated with oral contraceptives or deficiency of antithrombin III, or without known predisposing factors.[53]

Most intestinal infarctions occur, however, as a result of low-flow states without recognizable occlusion by emboli or thrombi. Hypoperfusion of intestinal vessels from shock of any origin or unusually low blood pressure, such as that after myocardial infarction or severe congestive heart failure, can lead to pathophysiologic consequences similar to those of occlusive disease. The potent splanchnic vasoconstrictive effect of digitalis has been deemed a contributory factor in some patients, but because evidence of a clinically important role for this effect is lacking, the drug should not be withdrawn if it is indicated for a cardiac condition.

The initial consequences of occlusion or hypoperfusion are ischemia of the mucosa and submucosa, with the development of edema, hemorrhage, and necrosis. Muscular atonia develops after initial spasm. With moderate injury, healing can occur with fibrosis and stricture formation. Extensive injury leads to infarction with acidosis and multisystem failure. It is not always easy for the pathologist to determine, even in the resected bowel, whether the initial injury is arterial, venous, or simply the result of a low-flow state.

Not all vascular insults lead to infarction of the bowel. Occlusion of a small branch of the mesenteric artery or hypoperfusion may lead only to transient ischemia of the colon, or ischemic colitis. This usually involves the splenic flexure or sigmoid colon, "watershed" areas that have the least reliable collateral circulation, but any segment of the intestine can be affected. In patients with so-called abdominal angina without colitis, symptoms are caused by occlusion of the intestinal blood vessels, but they may also follow the development of vasculitis, as in periarteritis nodosa or lupus erythematosus.

Angiodysplasia of the intestine, a lesion receiving much attention in recent years, will be discussed in a separate section.

CLINICAL MANIFESTATIONS

The manifestations of intestinal ischemia cover a broad spectrum, from abdominal angina to massive infarction with multisystem failure. However, the key symptoms of vascular disease of the intestine are abdominal pain or rectal bleeding.

Abdominal angina occurs about 30 minutes after eating; crampy or colicky, the pain centers around the umbilicus, often radiating to the back. It may last several hours and is usually so severe that the patient may decide to avoid pain by not eating. The resulting weight loss will lead both patient and physician to worry about malignancy. Curiously, however, abdominal angina, although often considered, is rare.

A more acute and certainly more common type of vascular disease of the gut is transient localized ischemia of the colon, or ischemic colitis. Symptoms may mimic those of inflammatory bowel disease, with the abrupt onset of lower abdominal pain followed by passage of bright red blood by rectum, or the major symptom may be rectal bleeding. The healing process after ischemic colitis is usually complete, resolving within a few weeks; however, it may lead to stricture, so that the disease is not always self-limited.

Patients with occlusion of major vessels are seen less frequently than are those with ischemic colitis. They ultimately will have dramatic findings; however, the initial manifestations may appear benign, with the patient restless and complaining of severe pain without abdominal tenderness or other objective signs. Once bowel infarction has occurred, however, vomiting, distention, abdominal tenderness, and fever will be evident.

DIAGNOSTIC CONSIDERATIONS

The rare patient with abdominal angina will have already undergone numerous imaging studies to exclude primary gastrointestinal disease. Only later is the possibility of vascular disease suspected, usually in someone with a disorder known to predispose to vascular disease of the gut. Often the decision to proceed with angiography is difficult, but recurrent and worsening symptoms will lead the physician in this direction. If no significant angiographic abnormalities (generally at least 50% stenosis of two major vessels) are present, the diagnosis is unlikely. However, the finding of considerable occlusive disease does not imply that the symptoms and vascular findings are related; in many elderly persons with no symptoms, considerable intestinal vascular disease can be detected on angiography or at autopsy.

The patient with localized ischemic colitis usually presents a picture that may mimic that of inflammatory bowel disease; therefore, considerations of inflammatory bowel disease in the elderly should include ischemic bowel disease.[54] "Thumbprinting," on abdominal films or barium study, which represents edema and submucosal hemorrhage, suggests ischemic or Crohn's disease; sigmoidoscopy will demonstrate submucosal hemorrhage or ulcerations, localized inflammation resembling that of Crohn's disease. Rapid resolution of the process suggests ischemic colitis. In some patients, however, stricture may lead to the incorrect diagnosis of colonic carcinoma.[55] The patient with a diagnosis of ischemic colitis on clinical, barium, and sigmoidoscopic findings should not undergo angiographic examination unless an accompanying disorder, such as atrial fibrillation, makes it necessary to exclude an embolism.

Diagnostic difficulties are more common in patients with major vessel disease leading to infarction. The task of the physician is to make the diagnosis before massive infarction occurs, with its high mortality, even with operative intervention. A plain film of the abdomen may show a gasless abdomen, further increasing the suspicion of vascular injury. Angiography may have an early role when embolism is strongly suspected, although some investigators urge an aggressive approach to angiography even when embolism is not suspected. Other diagnostic studies, such as barium enema or colonoscopy, occasionally may give clues, but they will not be carried out if events rapidly lead to full-blown infarction.

THERAPEUTIC CONSIDERATIONS

The rare patient with abdominal angina will learn on his own to decrease meal size. Nitrates should not be given for their vasodilatory effects because they may decrease systemic blood pressure and perfusion of the intestine. Vascular bypass is occasionally performed in the highly symptomatic patient with other diseases excluded and the "right" angiographic findings.

In the patient with acute ischemic colitis, watchful waiting is in order, with emphasis on maintaining systemic circulation. Some physicians administer steroids until Crohn's disease can definitely be excluded, a decision that will depend on clinical assessment of the possibilities.

When major vessel disease is suspected, improvement in the hemodynamic state is important. Shock must be treated first. However, if the diagnosis of infarction is likely, the only approach is operation, because medical measures alone will not prevent death. At laparotomy the surgeon will decide between embolectomy or resection of bowel. The availability of long-term parenteral nutritional support has made even massive intestinal resection a more valid maneuver, but such considerations are beyond the scope of this chapter.

INTESTINAL ANGIODYSPLASIA AND AORTIC STENOSIS

ANATOMY AND PATHOPHYSIOLOGY

Angiodysplasia of the intestinal tract is an important source of bleeding from the colon or upper gastrointestinal tract.[56,57] The apparent association between angiodysplasia and aortic stenosis makes it imperative that the cardiologist be familiar with this disorder, which is variously called angiodysplasia or vascular dysplasia. Vascular lesions of the intestinal tract may take the form of the sclerotic submucosal artery of Dieulafoy, the congenital hamartomatous hemangioma, or angiodysplasia. The latter, also called arteriovenous malformations or telangiectasia, consists of tortuous ectatic, thin-walled venous vessels that are usually submucosal but may also involve vessels of the lamina propria, muscularis propria, and serosa. Angiodysplasia may occur as (1) part of hereditary hemorrhagic telangiectasia, (2) a secondary disorder as from progressive systemic sclerosis with calcinosis, Raynaud's phenomenon, esophageal dysmotility, sclerodactyly, and telangiectasia (CREST syndrome), or (3) an isolated primary form. We will discuss primary angiodysplasia, especially as it relates to gastrointestinal bleeding in patients with aortic valve disease.

The pathogenesis of angiodysplasia remains unknown; the two main but unproven theories suggest either a vascular or a muscular origin. Proponents of the vascular theory have considered either ischemia from low-flow states or degeneration of vessel walls or connective tissue as important factors causing angiodysplasia.[58,59] They also have occasionally identified cholesterol emboli with adjacent ectatic blood vessels, suggesting the possibility that obstruction caused the ectasia.[60] The vascular theory has also been offered as an explanation for the apparent association between angiodysplasia and aortic stenosis. Nevertheless, the more attractive theory is that intestinal muscle hypertrophy leads to chronic, intermittent, low-grade obstruction of submucosal veins, with dilatation and tortuosity occurring initially in submucosal veins and subsequently in mucosal venules, capillaries, and arteries.[61]

A potential association between intestinal bleeding and aortic stenosis was first suggested in 1958,[62] and the combination was later explained by the presence of angiodysplasia.[63] In recent series of patients with angiodysplasia of the colon, 15% to 40% also had aortic stenosis, but that diagnosis was often based only on auscultatory findings, which might be misleading in the elderly.[59,61,64] Aortic stenosis also has been reported in 50% of patients with gastric angiodysplasia in one series,[58] and numerous case reports of angiodysplasia associated with aortic stenosis have appeared.[60,65,66] One series of gastroduodenal angiodysplasia, however, did not confirm an association with aortic stenosis, but it found one with uremia.[57] It is fair to conclude that an association between aortic stenosis and intestinal angiodysplasia has not clearly been shown; both lesions may be present in any person as part of the aging process.

CLINICAL MANIFESTATIONS

Gastrointestinal bleeding from angiodysplasia may take the form of acute hemorrhage or chronic, low-grade blood loss manifested as iron-deficiency anemia. Often, because the patients are elderly, concomitant colonic diverticula or polyps are blamed for persistent lower gastrointestinal tract bleeding. In the upper gut, bleeding might have been attributed to other lesions such as gastritis or ulcers. Repeated episodes of hemorrhage lead to further endoscopic or angiographic investigation and the diagnosis of angiodysplasia.

Angiodysplasia is increasingly being recognized at endoscopy as typical spider-like lesions most common in the ascending colon, but visible elsewhere. They also can be demonstrated at angiography. Barium studies are not helpful.

Some patients with severe aortic stenosis, angiodysplasia, and recurrent gastrointestinal bleeding have not had rebleeding after aortic valve replacement,[65,67] suggesting that bleeding from angiodysplasia should be considered a relative indication for aortic valve replacement.[67] Other reports, however, showed recurrent bleeding from angiodysplasia after valve surgery.[66] Therefore, unless surgery is necessary for hemodynamic reasons, we do not yet recommend valve replacement as acceptable treatment for bleeding colonic angiodysplasia.

Current therapy for bleeding angiodysplasia includes coagulation at endoscopy with various electrodes or lasers. Resection of the intestine is a last resort because it is more invasive and the recurrence rates for bleeding angiodysplasia in the remaining bowel are high.

Recurrent episodes of bleeding are frequent not only before the diagnosis of angiodysplasia is made, but also after treatment for angiodysplasia with either coagulation or surgery. In one series the incidence of rebleeding after intestinal resection was 38%.[59] Although others reported a lower rate, the long-term follow-up was too short for reliable conclusions to be drawn.[59]

STREPTOCOCCUS BOVIS ENDOCARDITIS AND COLONIC NEOPLASMS

Streptococcus bovis is a group D nonenterococcal organism found in the colon of both normal subjects and those with various intestinal disorders. Numerous reports show an association between *S bovis* endocarditis and bacteremia and intestinal disorders, so that the cardiologist seeing patients with *S bovis* endocarditis needs to be aware of this association.

Although this association has been known for more than a decade, it was only in 1979 that a prospective study of patients with *S bovis* bacteremia, most of whom probably had endocarditis, indicated a prevalence of greater than 50% for intestinal disease.[68] Although the patients did not have intestinal symptoms or occult blood in the stool, investigation showed that the majority had intestinal disorders. Most common were cancer or polyps of the colon, although cancer of the esophagus or stomach was also represented in this series of 30 patients with bacteremia. In a later retrospective series of 19 patients with *S bovis* bacteremia, 7 had cancer or adenomas of the intestinal tract, confirming the association between *S bovis* bacteremia and intestinal neoplasms.[69]

Recently, five patients who had had *S bovis* endocarditis several years previously underwent colonoscopy and two were found to have adenomatous polyps.[70] Carcinoma of the cecum developed more than 2 years after the occurrence of *S bovis* endocarditis in another patient.[71] Although these case reports by themselves are less convincing, they do suggest that endocarditis may precede the presentation of neoplasms by several years.

The physician caring for a patient with *S bovis* endocarditis (or bacteremia) should evaluate the colon, preferably by colonoscopy, for the presence of a neoplasm, even in the absence of intestinal symptoms or bleeding. If the results prove negative, it is appropriate to examine other portions of the gastrointestinal tract and keep the patient under close surveillance for colonic cancer.

REFERENCES

1. Ockene IS, Shay MJ, Alpert JS, Weiner B, Dalen JE: Unexplained chest pain in patients with normal coronary arteriograms: a follow-up study of functional status. *N Engl J Med* 1980; 303:1249–1252.
2. Alban Davies H, Jones DB, Rhodes J: Esophageal angina as the cause of chest pain. *JAMA* 1982; 248:2274–2278.
3. Helm JF, Dodds, WJ, Pek LR, Palmer DW, Hogan WJ, Teeter BC: Effect of esophageal emptying and saliva on clearance of acid from the esophagus. *N Engl J Med* 1984; 310:284–288.
4. Richter JE, Castell DO: Diffuse esophageal spasm: a reappraisal. *Ann Intern Med* 1984; 100:242–245.
5. Bennett JR, Hendrix T: Diffuse esophageal spasm: a disorder with more than one cause. *Gastroenterology* 1970; 59:273–279.
6. Freisen DL, Henderson RD, Hanna W: Ultrastructure of the esophageal muscle in achalasia and diffuse esophageal spasm. *Am J Clin Pathol* 1983; 79:319–325.
7. Traube M, Albibi R, McCallum RW: High-amplitude peristaltic esophageal contractions associated with chest pain. *JAMA* 1983; 250:2655–2659.
8. Clouse RE, Lustman PJ: Psychiatric illness and contraction abnormalities of the esophagus. *N Engl J Med* 1983; 309:1337–1342.
9. Dodds WJ, Dent J, Hogan WJ, Helm JF, Hauser R, Patel GK, Egide MS: Mechanisms of gastroesophageal reflux in patients with reflux esophagitis. *N Engl J Med* 1982; 307:1547–1552.
10. McCallum RW, Berkowitz D, Lerner E: Gastric emptying in patients with gastroesophageal reflux. *Gastroenterology* 1981; 80:285–291.
11. Orr WC, Robinson MG: Hypertensive peristalsis in the pathogenesis of chest pain: further exploration of the "nutcracker" esophagus. *Am J Gastroenterol* 1982; 77:604–607.
12. Cattau EL, Castell DO: Symptoms of esophageal dysfunction, in Castell DO, Johnson LF (eds): *Esophageal Function in Health and Disease*. New York, Elsevier Biomedical, 1983, pp 31–46.
13. Kline M, Chesne R, Sturdevant RAL, McCallum RW: Esophageal disease in patients with angina-like chest pain. *Am J Gastroenterol* 1981; 75:116–123.
14. Ferguson SC, Hodges K, Hersh T, Jinich H: Esophageal manometry in patients with chest pain and normal coronary arteriogram. *Am J Gastroenterol* 1981; 75:124–127.
15. DeMeester TR, O'Sullivan GC, Bermudez G, Midell AI, Cimochowsi GE, O'Drobiniak J: Esophageal function in patients with angina-type chest pain and normal coronary arteriograms. *Ann Surg* 1982; 196:488–498.
16. Benjamin SB, Gerhardt DC, Castell DO: High amplitude, peristaltic esophageal contractions associated with chest pain and/or dysphagia. *Gastroenterology* 1979; 77:478–483.
17. Patterson DR: Diffuse esophageal spasm in patients with undiagnosed chest pain. *J Clin Gastroenterol* 1982; 4:415–417.
18. Meshkinpour H, Glick ME, Sanchez P, Tarvin J: Esophageal manometry: a benefit and cost analysis. *Dig Dis Sci* 1982; 27:772–775.
19. Koch KL, Curry C, Feldman RL, Pepine CJ, Long A, Mathias JR: Ergonovine-induced esophageal spasm in patients with chest pain resembling angina pectoris. *Dig Dis Sci* 1982; 27:1073–1080.
20. Richter JE, Hackshaw BT, Wu WC, Castell DO: Edrophonium: a useful provocative test for esophageal chest pain. *Ann Intern Med* 1985; 103:14–21.
21. Richter JE, Castell DO: Gastroesophageal reflux: pathogenesis, diagnosis, and therapy. *Ann Intern Med* 1982; 97:93–103.
22. Winnan GR, Meyer CT, McCallum RW: Interpretation of the Bernstein test: a reappraisal of criteria. *Ann Intern Med* 1982; 96:320–322.
23. Fink S, McCallum RW: The role of prolonged esophageal pH monitoring in the diagnosis of gastroesophageal reflux. *JAMA* 1984; 252:1160–1164.
24. Ducrotte P, Berland J, Denis P, Galmiche JP, Cribier A, Letac B, Pasquis P: Coronary sinus lactate estimation and esophageal motor anomalies in angina with normal coronary angiogram. *Dig Dis Sci* 1984; 29:305–310.
25. Mellow MH, Simpson AG, Watt L, Schoolmeester L, Haye DL: Esophageal acid perfusion in coronary artery disease: induction of myocardial ischemia. *Gastroenterology* 1983; 85:306–312.

25a. Channer KS: Oesophageal abnormalities in patients with chest pain. *Lancet* 1986; 1:42–43.

26. Vantrappen G, Janssens J: To dilate or to operate: that is the question. *Gut* 1983; 24:1013–1019.
27. Bortolotti M, Labo G: Clinical and manometric effects of nifedipine in patients with esophageal achalasia. *Gastroenterology* 1981; 80:39–44.
28. Gelfond M, Rozen P, Gilat T: Isosorbide dinitrate and nifedipine treatment of achalasia: a clinical, manometric and radionuclide evaluation. *Gastroenterology* 1982; 83:963–969.
29. Traube M, Hongo M, Magyar L, McCallum RW: Effects of nifedipine in achalasia and in patients with high-amplitude peristaltic esophageal contractions. *JAMA* 1984; 252:1733–1736.
30. Swamy N: Esophageal spasm: clinical and manometric response to nitroglycerine and long acting nitrites. *Gastroenterology* 1977; 72:23–27.
31. Mellow MH: Effect of isosorbide and hydralazine in painful primary esophageal motility disorders. *Gastroenterology* 1982; 83:364–370.
32. Traube M, McCallum RW: Calcium-channel blockers and the gastrointestinal tract. *Am J Gastroenterol* 1984; 79:892–896.
33. Weiser HF, Lepsien G, Golenhofen K, Siewert R: Clinical and experimental studies on the effect of nifedipine on smooth muscle of the oesophagus and LES, in Duthie, HL (ed): *Gastrointestinal Motility in Health and Disease*. Lancaster, England, MTP Press, 1978, pp 565–572.
34. Blackwell JN, Holt S, Heading RC: Effect of nifedipine on oesophageal motility and gastric emptying. *Digestion* 1981; 21:50–56.
35. Nasrallah SM: Nifedipine in the treatment of diffuse esophageal spasm. *Lancet* 1982; 2:1285.
36. Alban Davies H, Lewis M, Rhodes J, Henderson A: Nifedipine for relief of esophageal chest pain? *N Engl J Med* 1982; 307:1274.
37. Ebert EC, Ouyang A, Wright SH, Cohen S, Lipshutz WH: Pneumatic dilatation in patients with symptomatic diffuse esophageal spasm and lower esophageal sphincter dysfunction. *Dig Dis Sci* 1983; 28:481–485.
38. Richter JE, Spurling TJ, Cordova CM, Castell DO: Effects of oral calcium blocker, diltiazem, on esophageal contractions: studies in volunteers and patients with nutcracker esophagus. *Dig Dis Sci* 1984; 29:649–656.
39. Winters C, Artnak EJ, Benjamin SB, Castell DO: Esophageal bougienage in symptomatic patients with nutcracker esophagus, a primary esophageal motility disorder. *JAMA* 1984; 252:363–366.
40. Helm JF, Dodds WJ, Riedel DR, Teeter BC, Hogan WJ, Arndorfer RC: Determinants of esophageal acid clearance in normal subjects. *Gastroenterology* 1983; 85:607–612.
41. McCallum RW, Fink SM, Lerner E, Berkowitz DM: Effects of metoclopramide and bethanechol on delayed gastric emptying in gastroesophageal reflux patients. *Gastroenterology* 1983; 84:1573–1577.
42. Sherlock S: The liver in heart failure: relation of anatomical, functional, and circulatory changes. *Br Heart J* 1951; 13:273–293.
43. Richman SM, Delman AJ, Grob D: Alteration in indices of liver function in congestive heart failure with particular reference to serum enzymes. *Am J Med* 1961; 30:211–225.
44. Dunn GD, Hayes P, Breen KJ, Schenker S: The liver in congestive heart failure: a review. *Am J Med Sci* 1973; 265:175–189.
45. de la Monte SM, Arcidi JM, Moore GW, Hutchins GM: Midzonal necrosis as a pattern of hepatocellular injury after shock. *Gastroenterology* 1984; 86:627–631.
46. Birgens HS, Henriksen J, Matzen P, Poulsen H: The shock liver. *Acta Med Scand* 1978; 204:417–421.
47. Bynum TE, Boitnott JK, Maddrey WC: Ischemic hepatitis. *Dig Dis Sci* 1978; 24:129–135.
48. Cohen JA, Kaplan MM: Left-sided heart failure presenting as hepatitis. *Gastroenterology* 1978; 74:583–587.
49. Kisloff B, Schaffer G: Fulminant hepatic failure secondary to congestive heart failure. *Am J Digest Dis* 1976; 21:895–900.
50. Kaymakcalan H, Dourdourekas D, Szanto PB, Steigmann F: Congestive heart failure as a cause of fulminant hepatic failure. *Am J Med* 1978; 65:384–388.
51. Nouel O, Henrion J, Bernuau J, Degott C, Rueff B, Benhamou J-P: Fulminant hepatic failure due to transient circulatory failure in patients with chronic heart disease. *Dig Dis Sci* 1980; 25:49–52.
52. Ottinger LW: Acute mesenteric ischemia. *N Engl J Med* 1982; 307:535–537.
53. Grendell JH, Ockner RK: Mesenteric venous thrombosis. *Gastroenterology* 1982; 82:358–372.
54. Brandt LJ, Boley SJ, Mitsudo S: Clinical characteristics and natural history of colitis in the elderly. *Am J Gastroenterol* 1982; 77:382–386.
55. Brandt LJ, Henry HJ, Wolf EL, Mitsudo S, Boley SJ: Simulation of colonic carcinoma by ischemia. *Gastroenterology* 1985; 88:1137–1142.
56. Richter JM, Hedberg SE, Athanasoulis CA, Schapiro RH: Angiodysplasia: clinical presentation and colonoscopic diagnosis. *Dig Dis Sci* 1984; 29:481–485.
57. Clouse RE, Costigan DJ, Mills BA, Zuckerman GR: Angiodysplasia as a cause of upper gastrointestinal bleeding. *Arch Intern Med* 1985; 145:458–461.

58. Weaver GA, Alpern HD, Davis JS, Ramsey WH, Reichelderfer M: Gastrointestinal angiodysplasia associated with aortic valve disease: part of a spectrum of angiodysplasia of the gut. *Gastroenterology* 1979; 77:1–11.
59. Meyer CT, Troncale FJ, Galloway S, Sheahan DG: Arteriovenous malformations of the bowel: an analysis of 22 cases and a review of the literature. *Medicine* 1981; 60:36–48.
60. Bank S, Aftalion B, Anfang C, Altman H, Wise L: Acquired angiodysplasia as a cause of gastric hemorrhage: a possible consequence of cholesterol embolization. *Am J Gastroenterol* 1983; 78:206–209.
61. Boley SJ, Sammartano R, Adams A, DiBiase A, Kleinhaus S, Sprayregen S: On the nature and etiology of vascular ectasias of the colon: degenerative lesions of aging. *Gastroenterology* 1977; 72:650–660.
62. Heyde EC: Gastrointestinal bleeding in aortic stenosis. *N Engl J Med* 1958; 259:196–200.
63. Galloway SJ, Casarella W, Shimkin P: Vascular malformation of the right colon as a cause of bleeding in patients with aortic stenosis. *Radiology* 1974; 113:11–15.
64. Howard OM, Buchanan JD, Hunt RH: Angiodysplasia of the colon: experience of 26 cases. *Lancet* 1982; 2:16–19.
65. Bourdette D, Greenberg B: Twelve-year history of gastrointestinal bleeding in a patient with calcific aortic stenosis and hemorrhagic telangiectasia. *Dig Dis Sci* 1979; 24:77–79.
66. Weaver GA, Arquin PL, Davis JS, Ramsey WH: More on aortic stenosis and gastrointestinal bleeding. *N Engl J Med* 1980; 303:584.
67. Love W: The syndrome of calcific aortic stenosis and gastrointestinal bleeding: resolution following aortic valve replacement. *J Thorac Cardiovasc Surg* 1982; 83:779–783.
68. Klein RS, Catalano MT, Edberg SC, Casey JI, Steigbeigel NH: *Streptococcus bovis* septicemia and carcinoma of the colon. *Ann Intern Med* 1979; 91:560–562.
69. Reynolds JG, Silva E, McCormack WM: Association of *Streptococcus bovis* bacteremia with bowel disease. *J Clin Microbiol* 1983; 17:696–697.
70. Friedrich IA, Wormser GP, Gottfried EB: The association of remote *Streptococcus bovis* bacteremia with colonic neoplasia. *Am J Gastroenterol* 1982; 77:82–83.
71. Robbins N, Klein RS: Carcinoma of the colon after endocarditis due to *Streptococcus bovis*. *Am J Gastroenterol* 1983; 78:162–163.

56 The Heart and Endocrine-Metabolic Disorders

T. S. Danowski, MD and James D. O'Toole, MD, FACC

Frequent endocrine–metabolic disorders, which in North America and Europe adversely affect the heart, include atherosclerosis, obesity, and diabetes mellitus in that order of frequency.[1–6] In fact, they are so frequent that they almost qualify as pandemics. Obesity carries with it the risk of the most common form of diabetes mellitus, viz, the adult onset type, and both obesity and diabetes increase the frequency and extent of atherosclerosis. Other endocrinopathies and metabolic disorders that predispose to myocardial or vascular disease are generally sporadic.

OBESITY

Excess body weight predisposes to diabetes mellitus and to atherosclerosis. A consensus panel of the National Institutes of Health in Bethesda has declared obesity a disease.[7] If the current more generous criteria of the Metropolitan Life Insurance Company based on mortality statistics, viz, a body weight increase greater than 20%, are applied, then 30% of North American women and 25% of the men are obese. However, the Framingham epidemiologic data indicate a significant correlation between disease states and a 5-pound increase in body weight in excess of the desirable range for age, height, and sex.[4,6,7]

Obesity present by itself has been recognized as a major health problem. In addition, it contributes to the morbidity and mortality attributable to atherosclerosis and to cancer. The other ailments that occur more frequently in obese persons in addition to diabetes mellitus and atherosclerosis include arthritis, cholelithiasis, gout, menstrual and reproductive problems, and cancer of the colon, rectum, and prostate in men and endometrial neoplasia in women.[5,6]

The hypertension and the atherosclerosis, myocardial infarctions, and strokes recorded in the Framingham population are statistically associated with increases in body weight and serum cholesterol and triglycerides, increased intake of saturated fat and carbohydrates, decreased physical exertion, and a host of other contributing factors such as cigarettes. In addition, certain multiplier variables accentuate the problem of obesity and atherosclerosis, viz, the early onset of obesity in children, the predisposition to lifelong obesity when it begins during childhood, the higher prevalence of obesity in black women, ie, 60% versus the 30% in white women, the higher cardiovascular death rates in black men, and the adverse atherosclerotic effects of hypertension, smoking, diabetes, and the like superimposed on obesity.

In America many citizens believe that a high intake of carbohydrate or of refined sugar, ie, sucrose, causes obesity. However, epidemiologic data indicate that obesity is more often due to excessive intake of fat.[8]

DIABETES MELLITUS

The data of the National Commission in 1976 indicate that diabetes mellitus is characterized by an increased incidence of myocardial infarction, gangrene, renal failure, and blindness.[1] More recent data compiled in 1984 by the National Diabetes Data Group indicate that coronary heart disease is present in 13% of adult diabetics, ischemic heart disease is involved in 50% to 60% of recorded deaths in adult diabetics and 15% of young diabetics, and the risk of death from ischemic heart disease in diabetics is twice that in nondiabetics.[1a]

However, the National Commission statistics do not distinguish among so-called mild chemical diabetes or impaired glucose tolerance, type II noninsulin-dependent maturity diabetes, or the far more severe insulin-dependent type I diabetes of juvenile and young adult onset. Each of these three types of diabetes may be associated with macroangiopathy (atherosclerosis and arteriolosclerosis), microangiopathy (thickening or damage to the capillary basement membrane, or both), and neuropathy.

In the Framingham study the prevalence of glycosuria and, hence, of diabetes mellitus increases sharply as relative body weight increases. Thus, the age-adjusted prevalence rate of diabetes mellitus is 16 per 1,000 in men below the 95th percentile for body weight compared with 75 per 1,000 in those with body weight 50% above the 95th percentile of the reference population.[4]

Does a high intake of carbohydrate or sugar exhaust the ability of the pancreas to produce insulin and result in diabetes? It is true that a high intake of sucrose can produce sucrogenic diabetes in animals, but support for this possibility in man is lacking.

More than 50 years ago Himsworth[8] presented epidemiologic data consonant with the hypothesis that the incidence of type II diabetes was highest in those nations that subsist on a high intake of fat, and West[9] has duplicated his findings. Yudkin[10] initially suggested that a high intake of sucrose accompanied the high fat diet, and hence sucrose was responsible for the diabetes. This hypothesis seemed to be supported by the increasing incidence of diabetes in Yemenites who began to consume a high sucrose diet on moving to Israel.[11] The issue of high sucrose versus high fat as a factor in obesity and diabetes was ultimately clarified by a prospective study of the intake of sucrose in 10,000 Israeli civil servants.[12] That study demonstrated that new cases of diabetes were related to a gain in weight and obesity rather than to a high sucrose intake. Indeed, the studies of Keen et al[13,14] indicated that the intake of sucrose was below average in those in whom diabetes developed, a finding in keeping with the older conclusion of Himsworth.[8]

Type II, ie, maturity-onset noninsulin-dependent diabetes, as well as milder chemical diabetes develops chiefly in older adults who become obese. Type II diabetes is almost always accompanied by overeating or underactivity, or both. Once the fasting blood glucose reaches about 115 mg/dl in obese and nonobese persons, there is a delay in insulin release. At that point, the patient meets the criteria for diabetes, namely, undue and prolonged fasting or postprandial hyperglycemia, or both, attributable to deficient insulin supplies, shortage of insulin receptors, or inadequate postreceptor responses. Also, in such persons neither the hyperglycemia nor the release of insulin in response to food produces the usual prompt suppression of hepatic glucose output. With time the hyperglycemia can result in damage to the beta cells of the pancreas even in the presence of early hyperinsulinemia in many obese diabetic persons. This accounts for the wide range of insulin titers in type II diabetes, ie, above normal, normal, or below normal. Moreover, insulin present in normal or excessive amounts does not exert its usual glucose-decreasing effect in the tissues, but it retains its usual lipogenic and antilipolytic actions.

The much less frequent insulin-dependent type I diabetes is unrelated to carbohydrate intake or to dietary customs in general. It is an autoimmune disorder in which the affected person is incapable of coping with viral infections that damage pancreatic islets. This susceptibility to islet damage by viruses is associated with several genetic patterns in loci A, B, C, and D of chromosome six.[15]

CARDIOVASCULAR RISKS OF DIABETES

In both nondiabetic and diabetic persons atherosclerosis begins with endothelial damage. Platelets aggregate and adhere to vessel walls, a process facilitated in the diabetic patient by increased levels of platelet-aggregating factors.[16] Also, in diabetes, atheromas are more common, hypertension is more frequent, the vessels are more permeable to protein, insulin antibodies bind to tissues, and so forth.

The erythrocytes of the incompletely controlled diabetic patient are rigid because of an increased burden of glycosylated hemoglobin A_{1c},[17] and they aggregate readily at sites where platelet collections have formed. Then too, cholesterol and triglycerides often present in excess in diabetes adhere to the plaque and/or break into intact cells at sites where high density lipoprotein (HDL) present at abnormally low levels in diabetic persons already had difficulty in removing excess cholesterol from the tissues. Finally, the fibrin that permeates the atheroma is less susceptible to dissolution, because fibrinolysis is relatively deficient in the diabetic patient. The result is a documented trend to earlier and more extensive atherosclerosis and to an increased frequency of circulatory insufficiency, myocardial infarction, stroke, and gangrene.

Similarly, the microangiopathy, ie, the thickening or damage to the basement membrane of capillaries, or both, the invasion and multiplication of smooth muscle cells in the subendothelium of the capillaries, and increased capillary permeability, the microaneurysms, the proteinuria, and the like, can proceed to vision-threatening retinopathy and glomerulosclerosis.

As indicated earlier, hyperglycemia can be divided into four subgroups: stress-related hyperglycemia and chemical, type II, and type I diabetes. All but the first of these carry the risk of vascular disease.

Stress-related hyperglycemia is usually transient. The adverse effect, if any, of such relatively brief increases in blood glucose on the cardiovascular system is not known.

Chemical diabetes, also known as impaired glucose tolerance, is characterized by normal blood glucose in the fasting state and undue and prolonged hyperglycemia following a carbohydrate load. Chemical diabetes predisposes to atherosclerosis and limited neuropathy, but it is not associated with capillary lesions of clinical significance. However, chemical diabetes can be a precursor of type II diabetes. The data of the United States Public

Health Service[18] indicate that in the course of a decade approximately one half the persons with persistent chemical diabetes progress to type II diabetes. This occurs most often in obese persons, and the combination of hyperglycemia progressing to type II diabetes, overweight, excessive dietary intake, decreased physical activity, and the passage of time increases the frequency of hypertension and atherosclerosis.

In type II adult onset diabetes hyperglycemia is present in the fasting state, and hence during the 24 hours of each day it increases further after food. As in chemical diabetes, type II diabetes is often associated with obesity, increased food intake, physical inactivity, and hyperlipidemia.[19] Untreated, this constant hyperglycemia and associated biochemical changes can result in atherosclerosis, capillary lesions with devastating effects on the eyes and kidneys, and neuropathy.

In type I diabetes of childhood or young adult onset the risks in the early years of the disease involve the capillaries of the eyes and kidneys, damage to the nervous system, and the so-called diabetic hand and foot changes in the connective tissues rather than the early atherosclerosis characteristic of type II diabetes. However, ultimately young and old type I diabetic adults are at increased risk with respect to myocardial infarction, stroke, and gangrene.

THE HYPERLIPIDEMIAS OF OBESITY, DIABETES, AND ATHEROSCLEROSIS

The earlier and more frequent onset of atherosclerosis and coronary heart disease and the higher incidence of myocardial infarction and stroke in patients with chemical, type I, or type II diabetes have been related to high levels of circulating cholesterol and perhaps triglycerides.[20]

The cholesterol and triglycerides in the circulation bound to apoproteins include: chylomicrons, very low density lipoproteins (VLDL), low density lipoproteins (LDL), intermediate density lipoproteins (IDL), and high density lipoproteins (HDL). The chylomicrons are of dietary origin and largely composed of triglycerides with some cholesterol and very little protein. Lipoprotein lipase normally disintegrates the chylomicrons and the liver removes the remnants. However, with a deficiency of lipoprotein lipase or its activator, chylomicrons accumulate in the plasma and can produce pancreatitis.[21]

The liver initially produces VLDL. This large, very low density molecule is then decreased in size to yield LDL, and the LDL in turn gives rise to HDL. The various apoproteins in VLDL, LDL, and HDL carry different amounts of triglycerides, cholesterol, and phospholipids. Thus, VLDL largely contains triglycerides, LDL is composed chiefly of cholesterol, and HDL predominantly carries phospholipids. However, each of these lipoprotein fractions also carries lesser amounts of other lipids. It has been suggested that apoprotein levels may surpass cholesterol and triglycerides as indexes predictive of the possible causal factors in coronary heart disease.[21a,21b]

Fredrickson et al[21] have identified chylomicron, VLDL, LDL, and HDL patterns in families with frequent and early myocardial infarction and stroke, which they grouped into categories that facilitate description of lipoprotein patterns (Table 56.1).

The Lipid Research Clinics Population Studies indicate that the normal 95th percentile values for cholesterol are 240 mg/dl in healthy young men and 270 in middle-aged men with lower values in women.[22]

NORMAL AND ABNORMAL LOW DENSITY LIPOPROTEIN CHOLESTEROL PATHWAYS

Excesses of LDL cholesterol are atherogenic. Normally, circulating LDL molecules attach to receptors on smooth muscle and other cells of arteries, enter the cell, and are separated into the carrier apoprotein and the free cholesterol which is then used to synthesize cell membranes.

The LDL receptors on cells have a high affinity for LDL and can satisfy the need for free cholesterol even when plasma cholesterol levels are low. At the same time the receptors also control the amount of free cholesterol that accumulates within the smooth muscle cell. Thus, when the free cholesterol within the cell reaches the requisite levels, the production of additional free cholesterol by the LDL mechanism ceases by reduction in the number or function of LDL receptors, or both. Thus, when such cells are in need of free cholesterol, the number of LDL receptors increases and vice versa. Any excesses of cholesterol can be converted to cholesterol esters.[23]

When circulating LDL cholesterol is abnormally high, it bypasses the physiologic LDL pathway and breaks into cells, damages the endothelium, and causes platelet aggregation. Several growth factors, including platelet-derived growth factor (PDGF), are also released and produce proliferation of smooth muscle cells which move into the subendothelial space and release collagen and mucopolysaccharides. Large amounts of cholesterol, triglycerides, platelets, macrophages, and protein accumulate and produce the atheromas.[23a]

Findings in the Framingham study have identified the importance of high HDL cholesterol levels as an anti-risk factor in atherosclerosis.[24] Thus, a high HDL cholesterol titer is protective, whereas low levels of HDL cholesterol predispose to atherosclerosis. Indeed, hyperalphalipoproteinemia, a familial trait, increases longevity. The apoproteins in HDL remove cholesterol from blood vessels and tissues and transport it to the liver where it is properly recycled or metabolized. Hence, the higher the level of HDL cholesterol, the more effective is the removal of cholesterol from blood vessels. The dividing line between high and low HDL cholesterol is between 35 and 45 mg/dl. The risk factor can be expressed as the ratio

Table 56.1. Categories of Lipoprotein Patterns

Type I	Chylomicron excesses
Type IIA	Increases in LDL and cholesterol
Type IIB	Increases in LDL, cholesterol, and triglycerides
Type III	"Broad-beta" band with LDL, remnants of cholesterol in VLDL, and cholesterol and triglycerides
Type IV	Excesses of VLDL and triglycerides
Type V	Excesses of VLDL, triglycerides, and chylomicrons

of total cholesterol to HDL cholesterol. Values less than 4.5 are considered favorable.

Women have higher levels of HDL than do men, and estrogen therapy increases HDL, whereas androgens lower it. Patients with low HDL have a higher incidence of coronary heart disease.[24a,24b] Factors associated with low HDL include diabetes, obesity, smoking, oral contraceptives, and high triglyceride levels. High density lipoproteins are increased by correction of diabetes, decreased obesity, long distance running, exercise,[24c] reasonable amounts of alcohol, and effective antihyperlipidemic drugs.[24d]

SIGNIFICANCE OF HYPERTRIGLYCERIDEMIA

The Lipid Research Clinics Population Prevalence Studies data indicate that the 95th percentile for triglycerides for healthy middle-aged men is over 300 mg/dl. Hypertriglyceridemia is more common than hypercholesterolemia in diabetes mellitus, but it is usually of limited degree, ie, less than 400 mg/dl, rather than massively elevated. One striking exception is the tremendous hypertriglyceridemia, up to 20,000 mg/dl, that on rare occasions develops in ketoacidosis and produces lipemia retinalis and the chronic hypertriglyceridemias above 500 mg/dl that can result in life-threatening pancreatitis. Limited hypertriglyceridemia is usually of metabolic origin and related to dietary intake and hyperglycemia, ie, so-called carbohydrate-induced hyperlipidemia, which occurs during high intake of carbohydrates. Diabetic persons overproduce VLDL, the chief carrier of triglycerides, and have difficulty in clearing IDL, a remnant of VLDL with a high cholesterol content. In type III hyperlipoproteinemia, remnant cholesterol in VLDL contributes to the broad beta pattern that is associated with a high atherosclerotic risk.

North American data indicate that high triglyceride levels accompany but may or may not cause increases in atherosclerosis and coronary heart disease. However, a sex difference is present in the cardiovascular risks associated with high serum triglycerides. Therefore, limited increases in triglyceride and VLDL levels (type IV hyperlipoproteinemias) are not a statistical risk factor in men in the Framingham study unless hypertension, glucose intolerance, or cigarette smoking is present alone or in combination. Conversely, type IV in women is a risk factor even in the absence of hypertension, diabetes, and smoking. Also, high VLDL and triglyceride levels are associated with low HDL.[24,25]

Population studies in Sweden indicate, however, that in that country hypertriglyceridemia exceeds hypercholesterolemia as a risk factor in coronary heart disease.[26,27] On the other hand, in a Japanese population study triglyceride level was less important than the total and HDL cholesterol levels as a risk factor in angiographically defined coronary artery disease.[27a] Then recent data from a British Regional Heart Study indicated that HDL cholesterol does not appear to be an important risk factor for ischemic heart disease in the present generation of middle-aged British men.[27b] It should also be noted that there are substantial interpopulation differences in cholesterol and triglycerides; for example, the recent report from the United States and Jerusalem Lipid Research Clinic population study showed clearly opposite trends in the levels of these lipids, ie, cholesterol higher in the United States and triglycerides higher in Jerusalem.[27c]

POSSIBLE CARDIAC RISKS OF SULFONYLUREAS IN DIABETES

In the view of the University Group Diabetes Program (UGDP) and the tenets of the US Food and Drug Administration, oral antidiabetic agents, viz, the tolbutamide and phenformin employed in the UDGP study, may increase cardiovascular mortality in diabetic patients.[28] These conclusions are by no means universally accepted in the United States and elsewhere. Hence, tolbutamide and other sulfonylureas and the second generation sulfonylureas, ie, glipizide and glyburide, are used in the treatment of adult onset diabetes although the package insert refers to the possibility of such cardiovascular risks. The phenformin used by the UGDP has been withdrawn by the Food and Drug Administration, because of the UDGP conclusions concerning cardiovascular mortality and because it may cause lactic acidosis.

ASYMPTOMATIC HEART DISEASE IN DIABETES MELLITUS

In managing diabetic patients it should be kept in mind that atypical symptoms without pain and indeed any new symptoms can indicate myocardial ischemia and silent infarctions. Thus, indigestion; any abnormal sensation in the upper half of the body; a sense of fullness with or without food; pain in the shoulders, neck, jaw, and teeth; a new cough; an earache; and the like can be indicators of myocardial ischemia.

Also, it is increasingly recognized that severe asymptomatic myocardial ischemia and electrocardiographic and echocardiographic evidence of myocardial infarction occur in diabetic patients who deny having any cardiac pain or other symptoms. In this regard the presence of cardiac neuropathy in diabetic persons, such as the delayed adjustments in heart rate on assuming the upright posture, raises the possibility that in diabetes pain fibers are also damaged, which accounts for the painless ischemia and the asymptomatic coronary occlusions and myocardial infarctions.

IDIOPATHIC CARDIOMYOPATHY IN DIABETES

The congestive heart failure and cardiac enlargement that occur in diabetic persons with normal blood pressure, patent coronary arteries, and intact cardiac indexes meet the criteria for idiopathic cardiomyopathy. Isolated instances of this combination and an undue frequency of congestive heart failure in diabetic persons without coronary artery disease in the Framingham study support the hypothesis that variables other than atherosclerosis and coronary sclerosis may contribute to the increased incidence of cardiac disease in persons with diabetes.

The origins of such idiopathic cardiomyopathy in the diabetic person are not clearly established, but there are suggestions that it is related to microangiopathy rather than macroangiopathy.[28a] Therefore, cardiac disease fulfilling the criteria of idiopathic cardiomyopathy has been noted with increased frequency in combination with proteinuria and presumed glomerulosclerotic microangiopathy.[29] Also, deteriorating left ventricular function and echocardiographic evidence of cardiac failure have been identified in diabetes with renal microangiopathy and found to be absent in those with intact kidneys. Finally, histopathologic assessment of heart muscle capillaries supports the view that they too are involved in basement membrane changes that represent microangiopathy. It has been suggested that the polyol pathway (glucose–sorbitol–fructose) may play a critical role in endothelial changes as the smooth muscle cells multiply and migrate from the endothelium to the subendothelial space. More recently a metabolic basis for cardiac dysfunction in diabetes—a slowing down of the Krebs cycle from the accumulation of ketone bodies—has been postulated.[29a]

PREVENTION OF OBESITY, DIABETES, AND CARDIOVASCULAR DISEASE

OBESITY

The logical method of coping with obesity is to avoid it entirely. In short, the most effective therapy for obesity is prevention.[30] The danger signal is a body weight just barely, ie, less than 5 pounds, above normal. At that point treatment should be most intense as the likelihood of success is then maximal.

The prevention of obesity is dependent on controlled intake of carbohydrate, fat, and protein, but especially of fat because of its high caloric density. Among people who are in caloric equilibrium, however, an increased intake of any one of the three foodstuffs will add weight in all but those individuals who may have a highly developed mechanism, perhaps akin to the brown fat of animals,[31] to dispose of some of the extra calories by increased conversion into heat. Similarly, weight reduction is possible by limiting either carbohydrate, fat, or protein, provided the intake of the other foodstuffs is not increased. However, the logical way to prevent or reduce excess weight is to eat all the usual foods, but in smaller quantities. Appetite suppressants of the amphetamine or methamphetamine type provide only transient support, ie, for only several weeks. It is of interest that one of the anorectic agents, fenfluramine, may ameliorate hyperglycemia. However, this drug shares the limitations of the other amphetamines and may have a marked depressive effect.

Exercise has effects other than the conversion of calories to heat. It reduces triglyceride levels, decreases cholesterol, increases HDL cholesterol, and has an insulin-like action on glucose. Although it is logical to attempt to lose weight by increasing caloric expenditure by physical labor, it is difficult to reverse obesity through exercise alone. The human body is remarkably efficient at converting food into work and even vigorous exercise may not take the place of restricted caloric intake.

DIABETES MELLITUS

As noted earlier, stress hyperglycemia is usually of short duration and intensity and is not a recognized diabetogenic hazard, but definite data are lacking.

Conversely, chemical diabetes does predispose to large vessel lesions and limited neuropathy, but it does not carry a significant risk, if any, of clinical microangiopathy. However, such chemical diabetes can be a precursor of overt diabetes. As noted earlier, the data of the United States Public Health Service indicate that in the course of a decade, approximately one half the patients with glucose tolerance tests of the chemical diabetes type progress to overt diabetes mellitus.[18] Jarett et al[32] have also documented this deterioration. The foregoing characteristics cited and the natural history of chemical diabetes indicate that one approach to prophylaxis of atherosclerotic, cardiac, and other complications of diabetes lies in the prevention and eradication of chemical diabetes. Identical measures can serve two purposes, that is, the prevention of chemical diabetes and the prevention of its progression to overt type II diabetes. These currently consist of avoidance of obesity, effective treatment of obesity, correction of any endocrinopathy, minimal exposure to agents such as diuretics and steroids which produce glucose intolerance, and reduction of the stresses and strains of daily living.

Weight loss is also strikingly effective in reducing the intensity of adult onset type II diabetes in persons who are obese and in minimizing macroangiopathy. In obese individuals even limited weight loss can produce a remission of diabetes. The decrease in weight reduces fasting hyperinsulinemia, accelerates insulin release, and increases the glucose disposal rate.[33]

ATHEROSCLEROSIS AND MICROANGIOPATHIES

The Multiple Risk Factor Intervention Trials,[34] the Oslo study,[35] and the Framingham study,[25] which epidemiologically relate hypercholesterolemia to atherosclerosis, provide evidence that low total cholesterol, high HDL cholesterol, and a favorable ratio between the two can reverse the risk of vascular catastrophes. It is not established, however, that these data apply equally to patients with diabetes.

Can we really speak of prevention of microangiopathies once diabetes has been diagnosed and appears to be permanently established? At one time it was suggested that thickening of the mesangium or glomerular basement, ie, glomerulosclerosis, may precede the advent of diabetes.[36] Subsequent data have established that thickening of the capillary basement membranes does not precede diabetes. Hence, prevention of the capillary lesions of diabetes is a realistic goal.

Most but not all authorities agree that control of the blood sugar level should be a constant goal in diabetes therapy in the hope of preventing coronary artery disease and the microangiopathies. Day-to-day individualized management of insulin-dependent diabetes with diet and insulin does avoid potential catastrophes such as the ketoacidotic, hypoglycemic, and hyperosmolar comas, but unfortunately it may not achieve consistent normoglycemia. Furthermore, at present we cannot clearly attribute microangiopathy to hyperglycemia per se, because disabling retinopathy and nephropathy in some patients increase in frequency with the passage of time, even when the glucose levels appear to be well controlled.

However, because we can do nothing about the effect of the duration of diabetes on the genesis of the microangiopathies, precise control of blood glucose levels presently offers the only hope of averting lesions of the small blood vessels. As indicated, such success can often be readily achieved in type II diabetes by reduction of excess weight. However, the limited success of current treatment programs in achieving normoglycemia in type I diabetes even with the open loop insulin pumps is generally acknowledged.[37] There is the hope, however, that implants of pancreatic islet cells or mechanical devices that release insulin in response to varying blood glucose levels (bionic pancreas) will be feasible in man. If one or the other of these research techniques becomes clinically available for long-term use, the precise role of hyperglycemia in causing the complications of diabetes may finally be clarified, and these complications may be prevented or even reversed. However, the complex origins of microangiopathy in diabetes mellitus is clearly evident in heterotransplants and homotransplants in type I diabetes. Such transplants, if they survive, will control hyperglycemia, but even the pancreatic islets of a transplant from a nondiabetic discordant identical twin ultimately acquire the histopathologic aspects and loss of insulin secretion characteristic of diabetes.[38]

HYPERLIPIDEMIA

The large blood vessel lesions of nondiabetic persons can be postponed or minimized by control of lipid levels. This may also be true in diabetes mellitus, but, as pointed out, it remains to be proved.

The hypercholesterolemias of diabetic persons are to be treated intensively by dietary measures designed to decrease excess body weight, reduce fat intake, decrease intake of saturated fats, increase intake of dietary polyunsaturated fats, increase physical activity, and control the hyperglycemia as precisely as possible. If hypercholesterolemia persists after these variables have been excluded or corrected, it is to be treated with a type IIA lipoprotein diet. If this diet does not return the elevated cholesterol level to normal, nicotinic acid in dosage of 3 to 6 gr per day, probucol (Lorelco®), or bile sequestrants such as cholestyramine or colestipol are administered. However, probucol also lowers HDL, and if the decrease in LDL is limited or the HDL alone decreases, probucol should be discontinued.

Hypertriglyceridemia that persists after decrease in body weight and control of hyperglycemia may be responsive to type IV or type V hyperlipoproteinemia diets. If need be, gemfibrozil or clofibrate may be added. The clofibrate may produce gallstones and gastrointestinal problems including a possibly increased risk of cancer.

Important clinical manifestations of incompletely treated hyperlipoproteinemia include xanthomatoses and pancreatitis. Xanthomas may provide a clue to an underlying lipid disorder. Therefore, the xanthomas on extensor surfaces indicate increased concentrations of chylomicrons (type I) due to lipoprotein lipase deficiency. Tendon xanthomas point to LDL cholesterol excesses (type IIA) of familial origin. The broad beta disease (type III with cholesterol remnants of VLDL in IDL) may be associated with tuberous or tuberoeruptive xanthomas.

Chylomicron excess, ie, the chylomicronemia syndrome, carries the risk of acute life-threatening pancreatitis, a particular hazard in type III broad beta disease identifiable by a VLDL cholesterol/total triglyceride ratio above 0.3. Regardless of cause, marked increases in serum triglyceride levels are associated with increased susceptibility to pancreatitis and require immediate therapy, ie, insulin in diabetes mellitus and clofibrate or gemfibrozil in nondiabetic persons.

CARDIOVASCULAR DISEASE IN OTHER ENDOCRINOPATHIES

ACROMEGALY

Hypertension is infrequent in acromegaly and, when present, is poorly tolerated. If cardiomegaly develops, it may be out of proportion to the general splanchnomegaly. Generalized weakness is an early sign of congestive heart failure and often precedes palpitations and dyspnea. In one report 18 of the 24 acromegalic patients had congestive heart failure and 6 died of this complication.[38a] Recent reports from China showed that even in the early stage of acromegaly, almost half the patients have abnormal left ventricular function, which is reversible after effective therapy.[38b]

HYPERTHYROIDISM

In any sizable series of thyrotoxic patients one or more evidences of cardiovascular abnormalities other than simple tachycardia will be found in some members of the group. These symptoms are quite similar to those present in other forms of heart disease, ie, angina, hypertension, cardiomegaly, and electrocardiographic changes. Also, age and its concomitant changes play a tremendously important role in determining the frequency of cardiovascular disease in hyperthyroidism. In those thyrotoxic patients who are 40 years of age or older, hypertension, cardiac enlargement, electrocardiographic abnormalities, and congestive heart failure occur three to six times as often as in the group below 40. If these figures are accepted at face value, it would appear that, at the most, only one third to one sixth the cases of cardiovascular disease can be attributed to thyrotoxicosis only, if such an entity as pure thyrotoxic heart disease does exist. However, one can argue the other way with even greater validity: the very fact that there are many instances of congestive heart failure in otherwise presumably normal hearts can be taken to indicate the hyperthyroidism can produce heart disease. It is logical that it would do so more often and to a greater degree in hearts already damaged by atherosclerosis.

Hyperthyroidism, conversely, may decrease the frequency of certain cardiopathies in view of the comparative rarity of myocardial infarction in patients with thyrotoxicosis. This could be related to the effect of thyroid overactivity on the net balance of calories available for storage as fat or to a hypolipemic effect exerted by thyroid hormone. However, the seeming nonsusceptibility of hyperthyroid patients to myocardial infarction has been questioned.

In any patient with congestive heart failure, atrial fibrillation, other disturbances of rhythm, angina, and the like, the possibility of occult thyrotoxicosis should be raised.

MYXEDEMA

With historical justification, we could refer to the cardiac changes encountered in some patients with myxedema as the "Zondek heart" in view of his clear description in 1918 of dilatation of the chambers, the low P and T waves on the electrocardiogram, and the changes in blood and pulse pressure.[38c] Reports since then have clarified the histologic aspects, the clinical manifestations, the occurrence of pericardial effusion, the electrocardiographic variants, and the danger that rapid thyroid replacement can produce an addisonian type of circulatory crisis. However, the fully developed picture of myxedema heart disease with congestive heart failure is relatively rare. It is so rare, as a matter of fact, that at one point the existence of this entity was questioned.

The patient with cardiac complications secondary to myxedema gives a history indistinguishable from that obtained in any other form of heart disease except that hypertension is usually absent. As in most types of heart disease, older patients are more apt to be affected. The heart is enlarged to the right and left, the pulse pressure is decreased by tamponade if pericardial effusion is present, and the sounds are distant. In early or less marked examples these findings are either incomplete or of lesser degree. Congestive heart failure need not be a feature even in advanced cases.

The globular or water bottle shape of the myxedematous heart stem from dilatation of the chambers and varying degrees of pericardial effusion. The infrequency of the latter is emphasized in some clinical reports,[38d] and yet in the experience of others pericardial effusion is a constant, early, and major factor in the cardiac syndrome of hypothyroidism.[38e] In some instances effusions are also found in the pleural and abdominal cavities, resembling those seen in other forms of congestive heart failure, and anasarca may be present.

Autopsy in patients with a myxedematous heart has revealed loss of myocardial striations, branching of muscle fibrils, irregularities of staining, and pyknosis of the nuclei; deposition of lipofuscin and basophilic substances has been reported.[38f] Although these changes are definite, they are neither specific nor diagnostic. Also, it has been suggested that even though increased generalized arteriosclerosis is present, the incidence of coronary atherosclerosis may be no greater than that in euthyroid individuals.

HYPERPARATHYROIDISM

Clinical findings in hyperparathyroidism may include fatigue, anorexia, nausea, vomiting, hypertension, congestive heart failure, peptic ulcer, loss of teeth, kidney calculi, renal failure, pathologic fractures, giant cell tumor, and the like. If diagnosis is delayed, death due to congestive heart failure, stroke, uremia, or bronchopneumonia may occur. Histologic examination has revealed calcium deposits and necrosis in various tissues including the kidneys, lungs, heart, salivary glands, pancreas, liver, dura mater, and arteries.

HYPOPARATHYROIDISM

In idiopathic hypoparathyroidism and hypocalcemia, physical and mental development may be retarded, dentition is poor, and the hair, skin, and nails are often brittle or atrophic. An immunologic association is suggested by the presence of moniliasis in the childhood form of idiopathic hypoparathyroidism. Also, it may be associated with Addison's disease.

Metabolic cataracts develop with continued tetany. Papilledema is rare in conjunction with convulsions and may become sufficiently marked to warrant the suspicion of brain tumor. Cardiac decompensation has been attributed to the hypocalcemia of idiopathic hypoparathyroidism.[39,39a] Calcification of basal ganglia may rarely occur in postoperative hypoparathyroidism[39b] (Figure 56.1).

CUSHING'S SYNDROME

Most untreated patients with hyperadrenocorticism of the Cushing type used to develop hypertension, cardiomegaly, congestive heart failure, nephrosclerosis, urolithiasis, and renal insufficiency. The ready availability of cortisol measurements now leads to diagnosis before these complications appear.

ALDOSTERONISM

Hypertension and edema formation are of limited degree in both primary and secondary aldosteronism.

In primary aldosteronism due to adenoma or bilateral nodular hyperplasia the potassium usually decreases, and serum aldosterone is increased and plasma renin activity is suppressed. The serum aldosterone is not decreased by a sodium load or by several days of treatment with desoxycorticosterone acetate. Also, administration of a diuretic, ie, furosemide, does not raise the aldosterone.

In secondary aldosteronism the plasma renin activity may or may not be increased, but it is not suppressed.

Follow-up studies of patients who had successful removal of an aldosterone-producing adenoma and the experience with other types of potassium depletion indicate that the hypertension and renal lesion can resolve completely. They may not do so, however, in patients with a prolonged history or superimposed pyelonephritis. If resolution occurs, disappearance of all of the serum, urinary, and body fluid solute changes can be anticipated.

Diabetes mellitus may persist following successful removal of an aldosterone tumor. The presumption is that in patients with persistent diabetes, irreversible beta-cell hyalinization has occurred.

ADDISON'S DISEASE

Melanin pigmentation and hypotension are the chief signs of established Addison's disease. The hypotension is systolic and diastolic, and an orthostatic component may be demonstrable. Part of the hypotension is pre-

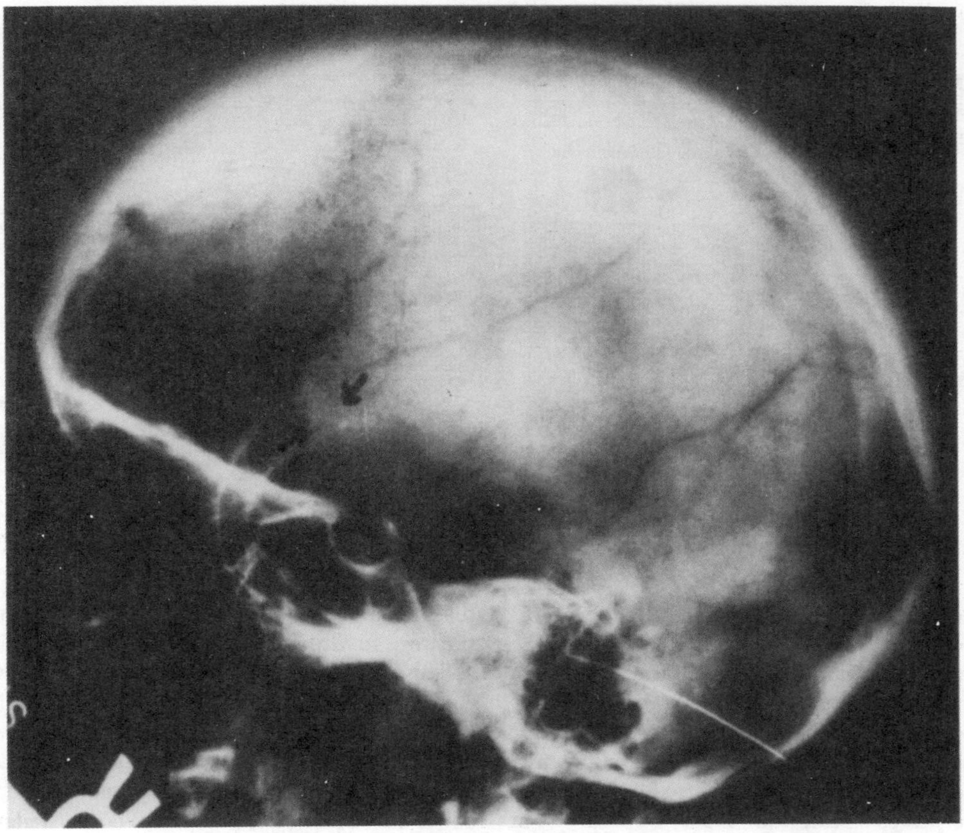

Figure 56.1. Calcification of basal ganglia in a patient with postthyroidectomy hypoparathyroidism. (From Danowski[39b] with permission).

sumably related to the decrease in plasma volume caused by depletion of sodium and extracellular fluid, but changes in vascular tone or incipient cardiac failure may play a role.

The routine chest film may reveal a small heart. The small heart presumably is a reflection of hypovolemia. However, overtreatment with adrenocortical-type steroids may produce cardiomegaly.

Electrocardiographic abnormalities not falling into any specific pattern will be encountered in approximately one half the patients. Hyperkalemia, if present, produces the characteristic peaking of T waves.

PHEOCHROMOCYTOMA

In addition to hypertension, patients with a pheochromocytoma may have headache, nervousness, anxiety, episodic abdominal or other pain, vomiting, convulsions, or a personality change. Also, polydipsia, polyuria, enuresis, and polyphagia are occasionally present. The patients are thin, and it has therefore been stated with some truth that pheochromocytoma and obesity are not often seen together. Pallor, generalized or limited to the extremities, can be present. The hands and lower part of the legs occasionally appear dusky or cyanotic. In either case they are cold. Hypertension may be sustained. Grade IV retinopathy, renal complications (proteinuria, abnormal sediment, decreased specific gravity, and azotemia), and cardiomyopathy (hypertrophy, angina, electrocardiographic abnormalities[40] (Figure 56.2), congestive heart failure, and diabetes mellitus) may be present. It is obvious, however, that such marked findings reflect delays in diagnosis and long-standing disease. With a higher index of suspicion, cases in which paroxysmal hypertension is the chief abnormality will be found.

Traditionally, the presence of nervousness, sweating, glucosuria, a high rate of oxygen consumption, and intermittent or persistent hypertension in a thin individual suggests the presence of a pheochromocytoma. Accurate measurement of urinary excretion of vanillylmandelic acid (VMA), total metanephrines, and fractionated catecholamines (norepinephrine and epinephrine) and of plasma catecholamines has greatly simplified the diagnosis. Abdominal computed tomography (CT), angiography, and [^{131}I] meta-iodobenzylguanidine scintigraphy[41] have further facilitated its localization.

With successful surgical removal of a pheochromocytoma, the prognosis for recovery from early vascular disease and freedom from permanent heart damage is usually good and diabetes mellitus can disappear.[42] In the remainder with permanent or only partially reversible changes, the hypertension and associated abnormalities persist. The most important elements in a successful outcome are proper preoperative preparation of the patient with an adrenolytic agent to avoid catastrophic hypertension as a result of anesthesia, surgery, or manipulation of the tumor and the administration of vasopressor agents once the tumor has been removed. Also in patients with bilateral pheochromocytoma of medullary origin, adre-

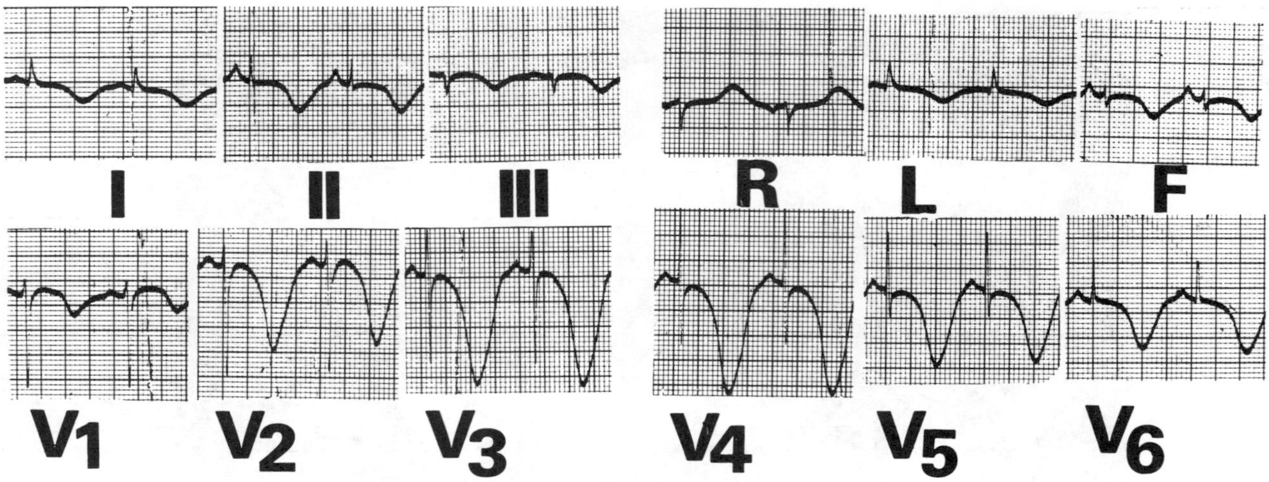

Figure 56.2. Symmetric giant T-wave inversion with marked prolongation of QT interval in a patient with pheochromocytoma. (From Cheng and Bashour[40] with permission).

nocortical replacement therapy is essential following bilateral adrenalectomy.

Cardiac pheochromocytomas, although rare, have been reported.[43,44] They should not be approached as ordinary posterior mediastinal tumors or, as they are in the abdomen, with the expectation that they will "shell away" from contiguous structures. Surgical treatment consists of either resection under cardiopulmonary bypass[43,44] or even cardiac explantation and autotransplantation.[45]

ARRHENOBLASTOMA

Hypertension may develop in patients with prolonged arrhenoblastoma or other androgen-secreting ovarian tumors. This is probably a reflection of the loss of the protective influence of estrogens or the hazards of androgens in this respect.

CARDIOVASCULAR COMPLICATIONS OF PAGET'S DISEASE OF BONE

Paget's disease, or osteitis deformans, is a common bone disease in the United Kingdom and in countries to which its inhabitants have migrated, including the United States, Canada, South Africa, Australia, and New Zealand.[46] The disease is also common in France, Germany, and Italy, but rare in China, Japan, India, and Scandinavia.[46]

The cardiovascular complications of Paget's disease derive from (1) increased vascularity of pagetic bones leading to a high cardiac output state, cardiomegaly, and occasionally heart failure[47,48]; (2) subendothelial calcification of cardiac valves, anulus, and endocardium, leading to aortic valve stenosis, mitral valve insufficiency, and conduction disturbances, respectively[48,49]; (3) atherosclerosis of both the coronary arteries and peripheral vascular systems, which may be coexistent or enhanced in Paget's disease.[49]

The pagetic basis of the cardiovascular abnormalities is sometimes very evident and sometimes subtle. Occasionally, cardiac insufficiency may be the initial clinical manifestation of Paget's disease.[50] The possibility of Paget's disease of the bones as a cause of an increased arterial pulse pressure must be considered in a middle-aged or older patient who has the three Bs (big head, bent back, and bowed legs). Fortunately, early diagnosis combined with effective therapy can reverse most of these complications.[51,52] Calcitonin therapy may decrease the elevated cardiac output.[47,51,52]

REFERENCES

1. Crofford OB: *Report of the National Commission on Diabetes, Vol 1: The Long-Range Plan to Combat Diabetes.* US Dept of Health, Education, and Welfare publication No. (NIH) 76-1010. Washington, DC, Public Health Service, National Institutes of Health, 1976.

1a. National Diabetes Data Group: *Diabetes in America. Diabetes Data Compiled 1984.* US Dept of Health and Human Services publication No. (NIH) 85-1468. Washington, DC, 1985, p I-4.

2. Danowski TS, Ohlsen PM, Sunder JH: Parameters of diabetes control, in Broff BN, Bleicher SJ (eds): *Diabetes Mellitus and Obesity.* Baltimore, Williams & Wilkins, 1982–83, chap 55.

3. Brody JE: Heart disease: big study produces new data. *New York Times,* January 8, 1985.

4. Kannell WB, Gordon T, Castelli WP: Obesity, lipids, and glucose intolerance: the Framingham study. *Am J Clin Nutr* 1979; 32:1238–1245.

5. Bray GA (ed): *Obesity in America.* Washington, DC, US Dept of Health, Education, and Welfare, National Institutes of Health, 1979.

6. Kolata G: Obesity declared a disease: a consensus panel says losing weight is not just a matter of vanity—it is a matter of health. *Science* 1985; 227:1019–1020.

7. National Institutes of Health: Health implications of obesity: National Institutes of Health Consensus Development Conference. *Ann Intern Med* 1985; 103:977–1077.

8. Himsworth HP: Diet and incidence of diabetes mellitus. *Clin Sci* 1935; 2:117–148.

9. West K: *Epidemiology of Diabetes and Its Vascular Lesions.* New York, Elsevier, 1978.

10. Yudkin J: Dietary fat and dietary sugar in relation to ischemic heart disease and diabetes. *Lancet* 1964; 2:4–5.

11. Cohen AM, Bayly S, Poznanski R: Change of diet of Yemenite Jews in relation to diabetes and ischemic heart disease. *Lancet* 1961; 2:1399–1401.

12. Kahn HA, Herman JB, Medalie JH, Neufeld HN, Riss E, Goldbourt U: Factors related to diabetes incidence: a multivariate analysis of two years' observation on 10,000 men. *J Chron Dis* 1971; 23:617–629.

13. Keen HA, Thomas BJ, Jarrett RJ, Fuller JH: Nutritional factors in diabetes mellitus, in Yudkin J (ed): *Diet of Man: Needs and Wants.* London, Applied Science Publishers, Ltd, 1978, p 89.

14. Keen H, Thomas BJ, Jarrett RJ, Fuller JH: Nutrient intake, adiposity and diabetes. *Br Med J* 1979; 1:655–658.

15. Illeni MT, Pellegris G, Del Guercio MJ, Tarantino A, Busetto F, DiPietro

C, Clerici E, Garotta G, Chiumello G: HLA antigens in diabetic children. *Diabetes* 1977; 26:870–873.

16. Danowski TS, Ohlsen P, Fisher ER, Sunder JH: Parameters of good control in diabetes mellitus. *Diabetes Care* 1980; 3:88–93.
17. Schmid-Schonbein H, Volger E: Red-cell aggregation and red-cell deformability in diabetes. *Diabetes* 1976; 25:897–902.
18. O'Sullivan JB, Mahan CM: Prospective study of 352 young patients with chemical diabetes. *N Engl J Med* 1968; 278:1038–1041.
19. Danowski TS: Classifications of diabetes mellitus, in Kryston LJ, Shaw RA (eds): *Endocrinology and Diabetes.* New York, Grune & Stratton, 1975, pp 321–328.
20. Danowski TS, Bahl VK, Fisher ER: Macrovascular and microvascular disease and their prevention, in Podolsky S (ed): *Clinical Diabetes: Modern Management.* New York, Appleton-Century-Crofts, 1980.
21. Fredrickson DS, Levy RI, Lees RS: Fat transport in lipoproteins—an integrated approach to mechanisms and disorders. *N Engl J Med* 1967; 276:34–44, 94–103, 148–156, 215–225, 273–281.

21a. Hoeg JM, Gregg RE, Brewer HB Jr: An approach to the management of hyperlipoproteinemia. *JAMA* 1986; 255:512–521.

21b. Franzen J, Fex G: Low serum apolipoprotein A-I in acute myocardial infarction survivors with normal HDL cholesterol. *Atherosclerosis* 1986; 59:37–42.

22. *Arteriosclerosis: A Report by the National Heart and Lung Institute Task Force on Arteriosclerosis. Vol 1.* US Dept of Health, Education and Welfare publication No. (NIH) 72–137. Washington, DC, National Institutes of Health, 1971.
23. Goldstein JL, Brown MS: The low-density lipoprotein pathway and its relation of atherosclerosis. *Ann Rev Biochem* 1977; 46:897–930.

23a. Ross R: The pathogenesis of atherosclerosis—an update. *N Engl J Med* 1986; 314:488–500.

24. Gordon T, Castelli WP, Hjortland MC, Kannel WB, Dawber TR: High density lipoprotein as a protective factor against coronary heart disease. The Framingham study. *Am J Med* 1977; 62:707–714.

24a. Rubenstein C, Romhilt D, Segal P, Heiss G, Chambless LE, Boyle KE, Ekelund L-G, Adolph R, Sheffield LT: Dyslipoproteinemias and manifestations of coronary heart disease. The Lipid Research Clinics Program Prevalence Study. *Circulation* 1986; 73(suppl I):I-91–I-99.

24b. Goldbourt U, Mandelzweig L, Neufeld HN: High density lipoprotein cholesterol: prognosis after myocardial infarction. *J Am Coll Cardiol* 1986; 7(suppl A):42A.

24c. Dufaux B, Order U, Muller R, Hollmann W: Delayed effects of prolonged exercise on serum lipoproteins. *Metabolism* 1986; 35:105–109.

24d. Krause BR, Newton RS: Gemfibrozil increases both apo A-I and apo E concentrations. Comparison to other lipid regulators in cholesterol-fed rats. *Atherosclerosis* 1986; 59:95–98.

25. Castelli WP: *Framingham Heart Disease Epidemiology Study.* Department of Health, Education and Welfare publication No. (NIH) 76–1083. Washington, DC, US Dept of Health, Education, and Welfare, 1976.
26. Pelkonen R, Nikkila EA, Koskinen S, Penttinen K, Sarna S: Association of serum lipids and obesity with cardiovascular mortality. *Br Med J* 1977; 2:1185–1187.
27. Carlson LA, Bottiger LE: Ischaemic heart-disease in relation to fasting values of plasma triglycerides and cholesterol. Stockholm prospective study. *Lancet* 1962; 1:865–868.

27a. Kanamori K, Nishijima H, Kojima S, Matsumura N, Sato I, Murakami R, Minami M, Yasuda H: Relationship between lipids and angiographically defined coronary artery disease in Japanese patients. *Am Heart J* 1984; 108:1207–1211.

27b. Pocock SJ, Shaper AG, Phillips AN, Walker M, Whitehead TP: High density lipoprotein cholesterol is not a major risk factor for ischemic heart disease in British men. *Br Med J* 1986; 292:515–519.

27c. Eisenberg S, Heiss G, Friedlander Y, Rifkind B, Segal P, Williams OD, Stein Y: Comparison of plasma lipids, lipoproteins and dyslipoproteinemia in Israel and the United States. The Lipid Research Clinics Program Prevalence Study. *Atherosclerosis* 1986; 59:63–74.

28. The University Group Diabetes Program: A study of the effects of hypoglycemic agents on vascular complications in patients with adult-onset diabetes. I. Design, methods and baseline results. *Diabetes* 1970; 70:747–783.

28a. Fein FS, Sonnenblick EH: Diabetic cardiomyopathy *Prog Cardiov Dis* 1985; 27:255–270.

29. Seneviratne BIB: Diabetic cardiomyopathy: the preclinical phase. *Br Med J* 1977; 1:1444–1446.

29a. Taegtmeyer H, Passmore JM: Defective energy metabolism of the heart in diabetes. *Lancet* 1985; 1:139–140.

30. Danowski TS: Five pounds, editorial. *Bull Allegheny County Med Soc* March 23, 1985; 73:215–217.
31. Rothwell NJ, Stock MJ: A role for brown adipose tissue in diet-induced thermogenesis. *Nature* 1979; 281:31–35.
32. Jarett RJ, Keen H, Fuller JH, McCartney M: Worsening to diabetes in men with impaired glucose tolerance ("borderline diabetes"). *Diabetologia* 1979; 16:25–30.
33. Ahmad U, Danowski TS, Nolan S, Stephan T, Sunder JH, Bahl VK: Remissions of diabetes mellitus after weight reduction by jejuno-ileal bypass. *Diabetes Care* 1978; 1:58–165.
34. Multiple Risk Factor Intervention Trial Research Group: Multiple Risk Factor Intervention Trial. Risk factor changes and mortality results. *JAMA* 1982; 248:1465–1477.
35. Hjermann I, Holme I, Byrek V, Leren P: Effect of diet and smoking intervention on the incidence of coronary heart disease. *Lancet* 1981; 2:1303–1313.
36. Siperstein MD, Norton W, Unger RH, Madison LL: Muscle capillary basement membrane width in normal, diabetic, and prediabetic patients. *Trans Assoc Am Phys* 1966; 79:330.
37. Danowski TS, Ohlsen P, Fisher ER: Diabetic complications and their prevention or reversal. *Diabetes Care* 1980; 3:178–183.
38. Sutherland DER, Goetz FC, Najarian JS: One hundred pancreas transplants at a single institution. *Ann Surg* 1984; 200:414–440.

38a. Courville C, Mason VR: The heart in acromegaly. *Arch Intern Med* 1938; 61:704–713.

38b. Hu G, Zhu B, Dan Y, Han Z, Dai X, Zhong X: The early effect of acromegaly on heart: clinical analysis of 28 cases. *Chin J Intern Med* 1985; 24:269–271.

38c. Zondek H: Das myxodemherz. *Munchen med Wchnschr* 1918; 65:1180–1182.

38d. Harrell GT, Johnson C: Pericardial effusion in myxedema. *Am Heart J* 1943; 25:505–511.

38e. Kern RA, Soloff LA, Snape WJ, Bello CT: Pericardial effusion: a constant, early and major factor in the cardiac syndrome of hypothyrodism (myxedema heart). *Am J Med Sci* 1949; 217:609–618.

38f. Zhao D: Myxedematous heart disease: report of 11 cases with 1 case of autopsy. *Chin J Intern Med* 1985; 24:77–79.

39. Bashour T, Basha HS, Cheng TO: Hypocalcemic cardiomyopathy. *Chest* 1980; 78:663–665.

39a. Levine SN, Rheams CN: Hypocalcemic heart failure. *Am J Med* 1985; 78:1033–1035.

39b. Danowski TS: *Clinical Endocrinology. III. Calcium, Phosphorus, Parathyroids, and Bone.* Baltimore, Williams & Wilkins Co, 1962, p 208.

40. Cheng TO, Bashour TT: Striking electrocardiographic change associated with pheochromocytoma, masquerading as ischemic heart disease. *Chest* 1976; 70:397–399.
41. Swensen SJ, Brown ML, Sheps SG, Sizemore GW, Gharib H, Grant CS, Van Heerden JA: Use of ^{131}I-MIBG scintigraphy in the evaluation of suspected pheochromocytoma. *Mayo Clin Proc* 1985; 60:299–304.
42. Stenstrom G, Holmberg S: Cardiomyopathy in phaeochromocytoma: report of a case with a 16-year follow-up after surgery and review of the literature. *Eur Heart J* 1985; 6:539–544.
43. Orringer MB, Sisson JC, Glazer G, Shapiro B, Francis I, Behrendt DM, Thompson NW, Lloyd RV: Surgical treatment of cardiac pheochromocytomas. *J Thorac Cardiovasc Surg* 1985; 89:753–757.
44. David TE, Lenkei SC, Marquez-Julio A, Goldberg JA, Meldrum DAN: Pheochromocytoma of the heart. *Ann Thorac Surg* 1986; 41:98–100.
45. Cooley DA, Reardon MJ, Frazier OH, Angelini P: Human cardiac explantation and autotransplantation: application in a patient with a large cardiac pheochromocytoma. *Texas Heart Inst J* 1985; 12:171–176.
46. Singer FR: Paget's disease of bone (osteitis deformans), in Wyngaarden JB, Smith LH Jr (eds): *Cecil Textbook of Medicine.* Philadelphia, WB Saunders, 1985, pp 1461–1463.
47. Fowler NO: High cardiac output states, in Hurst JW (ed): *The Heart.* New York, McGraw-Hill, 1986, pp 395–406.
48. Arnalich F, Plaza I, Sobrino JA, Oliver J, Barbado J, Pena JM, Vasquez JJ: Cardiac size and function in Paget's disease of bone. *Int J Cardiol* 1984; 5:491–505.
49. Wallach S: Neurological and cardiovascular complications of Paget's disease. *Geriatric Medicine Today* 1986; 5:38–49.
50. Pujadas Capmany R, Argimon Pallas J, Fernandez Monras F, Jane Pasquer J: Cardiac insufficiency as the initial clinical findings in Paget's disease. *Med Clin* (Barc) 1985; 84:337.
51. Zajac AJ, Phillips PE: Paget's disease of bone: clinical features and treatment. *Clin Exp Rheumatol* 1985; 3:75–88.
52. Ziegler R: Calcitonin as a therapeutic drug. *Ther Umsch* 1985; 42:358–365.

57 The Heart in Hematologic-Oncologic Disorders

Charles S. LaMonte, MD and Paul A. Marks, MD

With the simultaneous occurrence of both malignancy and heart disease in a patient, physicians may be uncertain of the priorities for treatment. In the past there was tendency to attach primacy to the malignant disorder, as more immediately life-threatening, and to relegate the cardiac disorder to secondary attention. However, treatment of hematologic and oncologic diseases is increasingly effective, cure rates are higher, and duration of remission is longer. Accompanying this increased efficacy of antineoplastic therapy has been the realization of the importance of the patient's other medical disorders. Among these, heart disease has been singular because of the many interactions of cancer or anticancer therapy with cardiovascular function and because of the rapidly expanding spectrum of physiologic insights and pharmacologic options for optimizing cardiac function.

Other chapters have considered heart disease independently of malignant disease. It should be emphasized that these independent cardiac conditions are concentrated in the same population at the highest risk for malignancy: those in the sixth decade or later. However, the purpose of this chapter is to summarize the cardiac disorders that arise *because of* the malignancy and hematologic disorders: that is, the neoplastic or hematopoietic disease itself, a humoral or paraneoplastic effect of the underlying tumor, or the antineoplastic treatment.

HEART DISEASE SECONDARY TO THE NEOPLASTIC DISEASE ITSELF

In addition to primary tumors of the heart or pericardium, there is increasing recognition during life of metastases or anatomic extension of noncardiac malignant lesions to these central cardiovascular structures. To a significant degree, this increased recognition reflects advances in technology: two-dimensional echocardiography, computed tomography of the chest, and, recently, magnetic resonance imaging of the heart and mediastinum. For example, there are several recent reports of serendipitous diagnosis of myocardial metastases of osteogenic sarcoma among patients who have undergone computed tomography of the chest as part of the preoperative workup for thoracotomy for pulmonary metastases.[1–4] Another factor contributing to the increased identification of cardiac metastases may be the altered course of many malignant diseases, because of more effective therapy and longer survival time, which permits the development of complications such as cardiac involvement.

From a partial review of the literature, it is difficult to ascertain the precise incidence of cardiac metastases from visceral malignancies. Most autopsy series from the United States, in the interval 1955 to 1977, suggest that the incidence of cardiac metastases among patients dying from solid tumors is between 17% and 21%.[5–7] The series by Lockwood et al[8] indicated an overall incidence of 14%, with more frequent cardiac metastases in the later interval between 1966 and 1977 than in the period 1952 to 1966. Two series published in 1980, from Italy and from Russia, indicated occurences of cardiac metastases of 6.4% and 5.1%, respectively, among patients autopsied after death from malignancy.[9,10] The Russian series reported from Moscow indicated an overall incidence of 5.1% (170 out of 3,327 patients in which death was caused by malignancies), with involvement of the pericardium in 55.9%, of both pericardium and myocardium in 33.5%, and of myocardium only in 10.6% of all cases.[10a]

These data raise several considerations. Clearly, the lack of contemporaneous occurrence of the different series is one factor in the varying reported incidences of cardiac metastases. The epidemiologic aspects of cancer among the different national and ethnic bases being considered, the different patterns of cancer treatment both by time and by nation, the different natural histories of solid tumors in different patient populations, and the recent longer duration of survival of cancer patients must also be considered. For discussion in this chapter, we have considered the analysis by McAllister and Fenoglio[7] to be reasonably representative. Finally, it should be noted that cardiac metastases are approximately equally divided between spread to the pericardium–epicardium and to the myocardium. Rarely is the endocardium the site of metastasis.

As shown in Table 57.1, virtually all types of malignant tumor can metastasize to the heart with the exception of primary nervous system tumors.[10b] Numerically, lung cancer involves the heart or pericardium more frequently than does any other; breast cancer, lymphoma, and malignant melanoma follow in that order. The lung and esophageal tumors usually involve cardiac structures by direct extension from the primary site. However, malignancies arising in anatomically distant sites almost always metastasize to the lungs or mediastinal lymph nodes as well as the pericardium and myocardium.

In addition to cardiac involvement with visceral neoplasms, a report by Commarosano and Lewis[11] indicates frequent cardiac involvement with manifestations of the acquired immune deficiency syndrome (AIDS). In their series of 41 autopsied patients four, or 10%, exhibited cardiac involvement by Kaposi's sarcoma. Other associated cardiac conditions included nonbacterial thrombotic endocarditis in 7%, fibrinous pericarditis without identifiable organisms in 7%, and cryptococcal myocarditis in 2%. In total, 24% of the patients exhibited significant disease-related pathology of the heart.[11]

Frequently, there are no signs or symptoms of the cardiac metastases. That most frequently observed is arrhythmia, usually supraventricular tachyarrhythmia, although ventricular ectopic beats are frequent, and occasionally conduction abnormalities and heart block have been described. Dyspnea, diminished energy, or other evidence of congestive heart failure may indicate pericardial effusion and early tamponade. Cardiac tamponade may sometimes be the first manifestation of cardiothoracic malignancy.[11a] They may also be the symptoms of intracardiac metastases with intermittent obstruction of a valve orifice or with progressive obstruction, such as that of the right ventricular outflow tract. On the electrocardiogram, nonspecific ST-segment depression and T-wave abnormalities, rare ST-segment elevations, and even less frequent Q waves or QS complexes characteristic of myocardial infarction may be observed. The critical diagnostic step, however, is to visualize the lesion. Two-dimensional echocardiography, which is internationally available, distinctly identifies almost all myocardial lesions and demonstrates pericardial effusion (Figure 57.1). In addition, however, computed

Table 57.1. Cardiac Metastases of Various Tumors*

Primary Tumor	Total Cases	Number of Cases with Cardiac Metastases	Percentage with Cardiac Metastases	Number with Parietal Pericardial Metastases Only	Number with Myocardial Metastases
Leukemia	99	46	46		
Melanoma	41	15	37	2	13
Carcinoma of thyroid	20	6	30	3	3
Carcinoma of lung	553	156	28	80	76
All sarcomas	69	18	26	8	10
Carcinoma of esophagus	107	25	23	6	19
Carcinoma of kidney	53	12	23	4	8
Lymphomas	245	55	22	13	42
Carcinoma of breast	492	104	21	61	43
Carcinoma of pancreas	96	14	15	6	8
Carcinoma of endometrium	69	8	12	3	5
Carcinoma of larynx	66	7	11	...	...
Carcinoma of renal collecting system	81	6	7	...	...
Carcinoma of cervix	187	13	7	...	...
Carcinoma of stomach	212	14	7	8	6
Oropharyngeal carcinoma	146	9	6	...	...
Carcinoma of liver and biliary tracts	75	4	5	...	...
Carcinoma of ovary	139	7	5	6	1
Myeloma	41	2	5	...	...
Colorectal carcinoma	273	13	5	...	...
Prostatic carcinoma	123	5	4	...	...
All others	61	7	12	...	...
Total	3248	546	17	200†	234†

* Adapted from McAllister and Fenoglio.[7]

† Sixteen patients with parietal pericardial metastases; 96 with myocardial metastases not enumerated in original article.

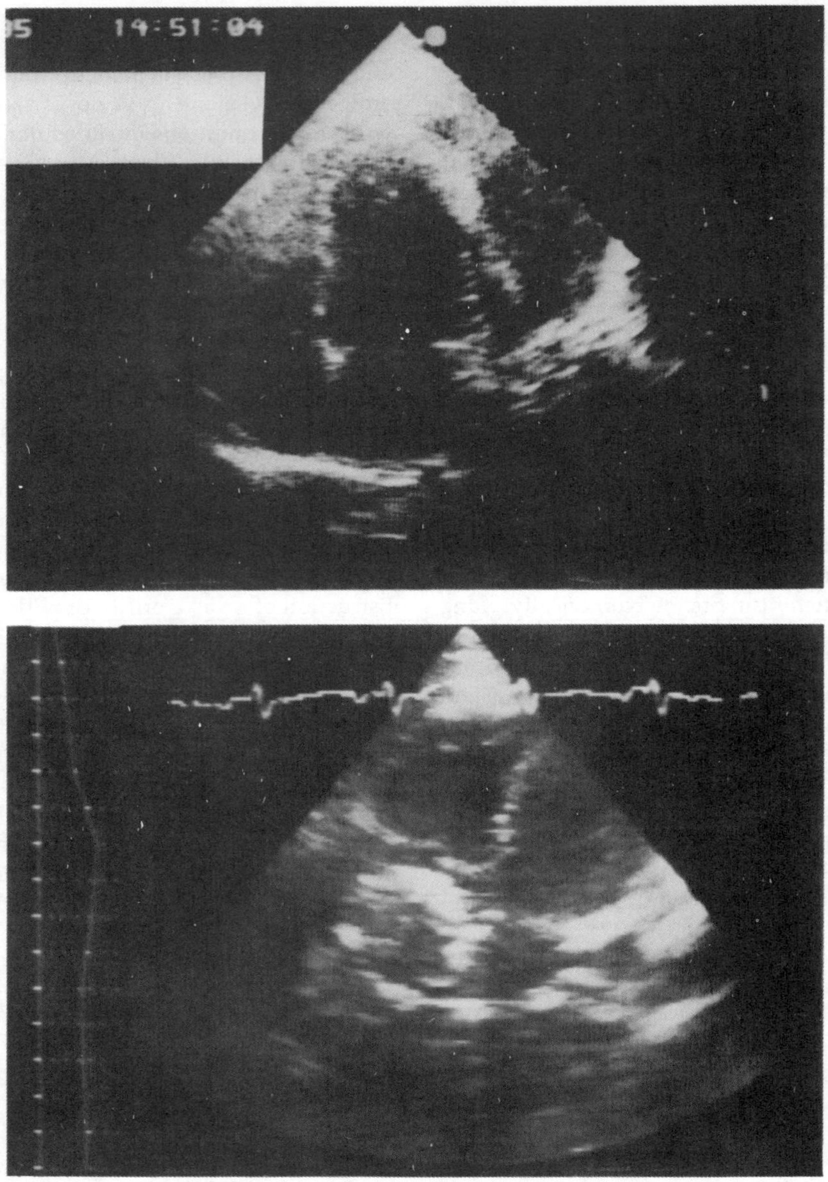

Figure 57.1. (*Top*) Echocardiograms showing cardiac involvement by tumor: Apical four-chamber view of a 20-year-old man with nodular sclerosing Hodgkin's disease, clinically suspected of pericardial effusion. Left ventricular cavity occupies center of field: free wall from 12 to 2:30 o'clock was akinetic with adjacent and adherent extracardiac mass. Computed axial tomography confirmed extension of mediastinal mass with probable epicardial and myocardial invasion. (*Bottom*) Apical four-chamber view of a 26-year-old woman with anaplastic carcinoma of right upper lobe, right paratracheal adenopathy. Right atrium, from 6 to 9 o'clock in lower left quadrant of scan, was completely occupied by mass. Superior vena cavogram showed mass occupying superior vena cava and right atrium.

tomography is sometimes required to demonstrate anatomic features such as the site of attachment or origin of an intracardiac mass, the extent of myocardial invasion, or possible valvular involvement. The characteristic nodular epicardial and parietal pericardial excrescences can be visualized by cross-sectional echocardiography, although such diagnostic elegance is rarely of clinical necessity.[12] It should be noted that M-mode echocardiography is usually insufficient to determine the anatomic or compositional features of myocardial or endocardial metastases, although it is definitive for pericardial effusion. In addition to echocardiography and computed tomography, recent reports have indicated a contribution of magnetic resonance imaging to the definition of metastatic disease of the pericardium or myocardium.[13,14] The value of this technology will be determined after further studies. Finally, there is a series of case reports and a small series in which cardiac scanning by means of ^{201}thallium and ^{99m}Tc pyrophosphate have furnished helpful information in the diagnosis and anatomic localization of cardiac metastases.[15,16] In at least one instance, endomyocardial biopsy established the histopathology of metastatic malignant melanoma in left ventricular endocardium.[17]

After localization of cardiac metastases, either by sector scanning or computed tomography, the cardiologist–oncologist team faces the decision of how or whether to treat. As mentioned, because myocardial metastases are usually asymptomatic, the decision in this situation is usually not urgent, and management of the cardiac lesion is incorporated into the management of the patient's usually widespread malignancy. Exceptions to this approach, however, include tumor that causes significant obstructive symptoms because of its location at a cardiac valve or at the right ventricular outflow tract, or osteogenic sarcoma that has been controlled except for one or two cardiac metastases. In these two situations, cardiac surgery with or without cardiopulmonary bypass should be considered and has been performed.

In contrast to myocardial metastases, pericardial tumor involvement, almost always with effusion, constantly poses the question of whether to intervene therapeutically. Frequently from physical examination and echocardiography alone, the cardiologist may be able to determine whether cardiac tamponade is present or imminent. On other occasions, right heart catheterization with or without fluid challenge may be necessary to determine whether the right atrial, right ventricular end-diastolic, and pulmonary capillary wedge pressures are elevated and equalized. If significant pulsus paradoxus or Kussmaul's sign is present, if there is diastolic collapse of the right ventricle on echocardiography, or if cardiac diastolic pressure is elevated and equalized, the patient may require urgent relief of the elevated intrapericardial pressure. Two techniques are presently employed: surgical creation of a pericardial window through a subcostal approach,[18] or pericardiocentesis, usually with an indwelling plastic catheter, and later instillation of a sclerosing agent such as tetracycline or thioTEPA.[19] Along with others, these authors favor the latter approach, using the fourth left intercostal space when possible, because it permits diagnostic study of the pericardial fluid before a commitment to therapy. Although analysis of the pericardial fluid, particularly cytologic examination, is helpful and indeed mandatory, the cardiologist should be cognizant that the cytologic study will be positive for malignant cells in most, but not necessarily all, pericardial effusions secondary to metastases; one report indicates 85% sensitivity.[20] In another series, adenocarcinoma is the most common cell type, with lung and breast, respectively, the most common sites of the primary tumor.[21] Conversely, the relatively simple surgical procedure of creation of a pericardial window with the patient under local anesthesia not only provides the needed treatment and symptomatic relief, but also furnishes a more reliable form of biopsy specimen for histopathologic analysis. The risk of surgical intervention without earlier diagnostic analysis of the pericardial fluid is that the pericardial effusion may prove to be due to a self-limited cause that would have resolved spontaneously, and that the patient may have been subjected needlessly to a procedure entailing a slightly greater morbidity.

In addition to decompression with or without instillation of a sclerosing agent, metastatic cancer to the pericardium should probably also be treated by radiation therapy.[11a] This treatment approach applies especially to patients whose malignant disease presents as constrictive pericarditis. Approximately 60% of such patients are eventually diagnosed to have bronchogenic carcinoma, with Hodgkin's or non-Hodgkin's lymphoma the second leading cause of cardiac tamponade as a presenting symptom.[22] In almost all series, the appearance of cardiac tamponade has been an ominous prognostic sign, with mean survival less than 30 weeks.

In addition to discrete metastases of visceral and epithelial tumors, two other types of cardiac involvement by malignancy deserve mention. First, causing symptoms of diminished cardiac output and less often of pulmonary or systemic venous congestion is cardiac infiltration by an acute leukemic process and occasionally by lymphoma. In a series of 420 autopsy cases reviewed from the National Cancer Institute, 69% of the patients demonstrated either leukemic infiltrates of the myocardium or pericardium, focal hemorrhage, or both.[23] Of the total 420 patients, 53% had infiltrates or hemorrhages within the myocardium and 38% had involvement of the pericardium. Of these patients, 13% had disease of the pericardium other than, or in addition to, petechiae or leukemic infiltrates, and 9% demonstrated significant pericardial effusion (greater than 25 ml in children and greater than 50 ml in adults). However, effusions greater than 300 ml were found in only four patients, and only one patient showed evidence of cardiac tamponade (Table 57.2). In such patients, management of cardiac involvement is the same as that of the underlying blood dyscrasia, often with the addition of cardiac radiation. The other cardiac involvement is extension of a benign or malignant tumor up the inferior vena cava into the chambers of the right heart. Examples include renal cell adenocarcinoma, Wilms' tumor, hepatocellular carcinoma, benign uterine leiomyomatosis, and leiomyosarcoma of the inferior vena cava or of pelvic organs. Such patients usually undergo resection of the intracardiac extension of the tumor, occasionally with cardiopulmonary bypass, at the same time

Table 57.2. Cardiac Involvement in Acute Leukemia; 420 Autopsied Cases*

	Cardiac Involvement	Pericardial Involvement
Infiltrates or petechiae	53.0%	38.0%
Valvular infiltrate	0.2%	—
Other pericardial disease (pericarditis, effusions)	—	13.0%
Significant effusions	—	9.0%
Greater than 300 ml	—	1.0%
Tamponade	—	0.2%
Normal heart (free of leukemic cells or extravasated erythrocytes)	31.0%	

*Adapted from Roberts et al.[23]

as laparotomy and resection of the primary abdominal, retroperitoneal, or pelvic tumor.

HUMORAL AND PARANEOPLASTIC EFFECTS OF TUMORS ON THE HEART

Aside from anatomic extension or metastasis of malignancy to the heart, selected tumors frequently cause pathognomonic changes within the heart. Cardiomyopathy secondary to pheochromocytoma will be discussed; carcinoid heart disease was reviewed in chapter 47 on Tumors of the Heart.

PHEOCHROMOCYTOMA

Myocarditis associated with pheochromocytoma and other conditions characterized by elevated blood levels of catecholamines, as in administration of levonorepinephrine to support blood pressure, has been described since the report of Szakacs and Cannon[24] in 1958. Although this myocarditis is morphologically nonspecific, the clinical setting and syndrome are characteristic. Review of this entity seems appropriate, because between 15% and 45% of pheochromocytomas are malignant.

Several investigators have described patchy areas with degeneration and necrosis of myocytes, with eosinophilic swollen myofibrils and interstitial edema or fibrosis. Focal areas have demonstrated infiltration with neutrophils, lymphocytes, histiocytes, and occasionally plasma cells. Other areas of the myocardium have demonstrated myocyte hypertrophy, whereas there were localized areas of hemorrhage elsewhere accompanied by endocardial proliferation, thickening, and edema. These lesions in the left ventricle are concentrated in the subendocardium and inner two thirds of the myocardium, especially in perivascular locations.[25,26]

The clinical presentation and management of uncomplicated pheochromocytoma has been presented in chapter 56 on endocrine–metabolic disorders. Pertinent to myocarditis, these patients frequently demonstrate abrupt deterioration of their physiologic state and may die suddenly of congestive heart failure.[27]

Hemodynamic measurements performed in patients with pheochromocytoma, but not correlated with the histopathologic condition of the heart, have revealed in hypertensive patients a normal cardiac output and elevated peripheral resistance. However, normotensive patients with pheochromocytoma have usually exhibited elevated cardiac output and normal peripheral resistance.[28]

The pathophysiologic mechanism of "pheochromocytoma myocarditis" is unclear. The existing literature on the subject implies that it represents an active inflammatory process. However, no specific explanation has been offered for a provocative agent. Furthermore, symptoms and signs of ischemia, even necrosis, have been associated in other organs or structures of the body with the paroxysmal discharge of functioning pheochromocytomas. The possibility of myocardial necrosis secondary to catechol-induced coronary arterial spasm should be considered.

Also associated with cardiac effects of pheochromocytoma is the echocardiographic finding of systolic anterior motion of the mitral valve. Such systolic anterior motion has been noted during hypertensive crisis, has been less prominent during the relatively quiescent periods of tumor activity, and has been eliminated by excision of the tumor.[29] No asymmetric septal hypertrophy has been noted on either echocardiographic or postmortem examination. Histopathologically, unlike those in patients with idiopathic hypertrophic subaortic stenosis, the myocytes of the interventricular septum have shown a normal orderly arrangement. Although an explanation for this phenomenon remains speculative, several investigators have likened it to the systolic anterior motion of the mitral valve in cases of intravascular volume depletion and have suggested that intermittently or consistently, during catechol-induced hypertension, the intraventricular blood volume may be diminished and that systolic anterior motion may develop.[30,31]

The complex treatment of this tumor, especially with reference to myocarditis and cardiomyopathy, has been indicated in chapter 56 on The Heart and Endocrine–Metabolic Disorders.

In summary, in some patients with pheochromocytoma there may be pathologic evidence of myocardial necrosis, termed pheochromocytoma myocarditis. This may cause intermittent or fixed myocardial dysfunction and left ventricular failure, which must be stabilized or corrected before surgical intervention. The echocardiographic finding of systolic anterior motion of the mitral valve may reflect decreased intravascular and intraventricular volume induced by this functioning tumor.

CARDIOTOXICITY FROM ANTINEOPLASTIC TREATMENT

Because nonsurgical anticancer treatment affects normal somatic cells in mitosis, the dominant organ systems also affected by anticancer treatment are the hematopoietic system, the gastrointestinal tract, the gonads, and dermal and mucosal tissue. Formerly the heart was considered resistant to both radiation and the early chemotherapeutic agents. However, with increasing experience, dosimetry, and patient survival, radiation therapy is now recognized to cause significant cardiac damage. Likewise with proliferation of the number of chemotherapeutic agents and with aggressive administration of these drugs, pharmacologic cardiac toxicity is a widely recognized fact.

RADIATION THERAPY

Until 1960, radiation was not recognized to have significant cardiac effects; the minor nonspecific ST-segment and T-wave abnormalities observed in some patients at varying intervals after external beam radiotherapy were thought to be "innocent."[32] Reports of cardiac dysfunction and of manifestations of coronary artery disease appeared in the 1960s, and cardiac radiation is now believed to cause different pathologic changes in pericardium, myocardium, endocardial structures, and epicardial and intramyocardial coronary arteries.[33]

Changes in the pericardium, occurring at varying intervals after radiotherapy, are the most frequently observed cardiac change, and are symptomatically and physiologically the most important. At varying intervals after delivery of relatively large doses of radiation, usually 3,500 rads or more, some patients may experience mid-precordial aching or the more typical sharp pleuritic type pain of acute pericarditis, may demonstrate ST-segment and T-wave abnormalities on the electrocardiogram, and may be found to have on echocardiography small to moderate pericardial effusions. More commonly, however, radiation-induced pericardial reaction is detected on a routine surveillance chest x-ray which discloses increased cardiac transverse diameter. Although pericardial reactions usually occur within the first year after radiotherapy, occasional radiation-induced pericardial changes are diagnosed 10 to 15 years after radiotherapy.[34]

The pathogenesis of the pericardial reactions and effusions is unclear, but it is generally considered to be inflammatory, possibly immunologically mediated. Accordingly, unless there is the threat of cardiac tamponade, this disorder is probably most appropriately treated with antiinflammatory agents in the expectation of spontaneous resolution. The late occurrence or recognition of the entity, however, is troubling. It may represent progressive insidious accumulation of pericardial fluid, which was not noted on the consecutive comparison of serial chest x-rays, it may reflect the recognition of cardiomegaly after a temporal gap in chest x-rays, or it may demonstrate the emergence of the inflammatory response after an interval of suppression by corticosteroids or other therapy incorporated in a cancer treatment protocol.

If pericardiocentesis is required for diagnosis or relief of cardiac tamponade, the fluid is usually straw-colored and clear. Usually there are mild to moderate mononuclear pleocytosis, an elevated protein level, and normal glucose and lactic dehydrogenase levels. Conversely, there may be occasionally little or no pericardial fluid, but the findings of pericardial thickening alone, occasionally with constrictive pericarditis. On inspection, the parietal pericardium is grossly thickened to as much as 1 to 2 cm, and in perhaps 25% of patients fibrous adhesions may be present. In another 25% of patients, in addition to the pericardial fluid, there may be fibrinous pericardial adhesions. The thickened pericardium itself is stiff and nondistensible. Histopathologically the pericardial membrane consists of a dense matrix of fibroblasts and collagen. In addition to the parietal pericardium, the epicardial surface of the heart also is affected and exhibits thickening by fibrous tissue.

In diagnosis, the physician may be alerted by the patient's symptoms of dyspnea and easy fatigability, and by the physical findings of distended neck veins, the inspiratory neck vein distention of Kussmaul's sign, narrow pulse pressure, or pulsus paradoxus. The electrocardiogram may display diffusely low QRS voltage, and the chest x-ray may or may not indicate cardiomegaly. Echocardiography usually identifies pericardial fluid, may arouse the cardiologist's suspicion of pericardial thickening, and in tamponade may exhibit diastolic collapse of the right ventricle. Computed tomography will confirm the findings of echocardiography, may resolve ambiguous features, and will demonstrate the absence of the epicardial and parietal pericardial nodularity that usually marks malignant pericardial disease. In some patients with only dyspnea as a symptom, cardiac catheterization with fluid challenge may be required to establish the diagnosis of occult constrictive pericarditis. This invasive procedure may also be necessary for confirmation of the diagnosis suggested by noninvasive evaluation or for management decisions.

The treatment options differ from those for malignant pericardial disease. The lack of specificity of cytologically negative malignant pericardial fluid examination has been noted, in the range of 15% false-negative results, and the cardinal feature of the thickened, noncompliant pericardial membrane in radiation-induced pericardial disease has received comment. Therefore, it is reasonable initially to perform diagnostic and therapeutic pericardiocentesis. However, instillation of a sclerosing agent seems imprudent and may lead to constrictive pericarditis, technically more complicated to manage in the future. Therefore, if pericardial fluid reaccumulates after the initial pericardiocentesis with normal fluid cytology, surgical creation of a pericardial window or partial pericardiectomy is indicated for long-range management of the process and to confirm histopathologically the absence of tumor.[35]

Rather than a progressive process like fibrosis of the pericardium, the myocardium exhibits two phases in its reaction to radiation therapy. In the acute stage, from a few hours to a few days after radiotherapy in experimental animals, diffuse polymorphonuclear infiltration is present. Accompanying this acute exudative reaction, as noted on electron microscopy, are diffuse changes in the myocardial microcirculation, especially evidence of widespread capillary endothelial cell injury demonstrated by disruption of the capillary basement membrane, endothelial cytoplasmic swelling, and often complete obstruction of the capillary lumen. Diffuse platelet aggregation at sites of basement membrane disruption and capillary endothelial cell proliferation reflect slightly later attempts at healing and reconstruction. After a latent interval, as long as two or three months, a diffuse fibrotic reaction is established throughout the myocardium.[35,36] Also of note in this late stage is a reduction in the number of capillaries proportional to myocytes. Fajardo and Stewart[36] hypothesize that this sequence of changes in the myocardium indicates primary damage to the microcirculation, resultant diffuse patchy ischemia, and resolution of the dynamic process in widespread interstitial myocardial fibrosis.

In itself, this myocardial reaction to radiotherapy is usually asymptomatic. In part, the nonspecific ST-segment and T-wave changes noted at intervals shortly after therapy may be the electrocardiographic manifestation. Despite the absence of overt signs and symptoms, subtle pathophysiologic abnormalities have been demonstrated by radionuclide cineangiography. Burns et al[37] demonstrated a significant decline in the right ventricular ejection fraction with exercise and a concomitant failure of the left ventricular ejection fraction to increase among 21 patients evaluated seven to 20 years after radiotherapy alone for Hodgkin's disease. Similarly, Gottdiener et al[38] and Gomez et al[39] independently documented subclinical cardiomyopathy in late follow-up after mediastinal irradiation. Being both asymptomatic and mild in severity on physiologic testing, these myocardial changes did not require treatment.

Although studied and reported less frequently than pericardial and myocardial changes, endocardial changes are common after radiation therapy. Brosius et al[40] reported necropsy findings among 16 patients who had received heavy mediastinal irradiation for lymphoma or carcinoid. In this series, 75% of the patients exhibited mural endocardial thickening: right atrium in 50%, right ventricle in 63%, left ventricle in 19%, and left atrium in none. In both the mural endocardium and the valve leaflets, this reaction consisted of proliferation of fibrous tissue with appreciable numbers of elastic fibers. The affected cardiac valves in 81% of the patients (mitral in 81%, aortic in 50%, tricuspid in 50%, and pulmonic in 13%) were considered to be so mildly abnormal as not to produce any hemodynamic abnormalities. However, there are several case reports of significant aortic insufficiency requiring valve replacement. One patient followed at Memorial Hospital has been treated not only for cardiomyopathy, but also with mitral valve replacement for severe valve thickening and regurgitation, with significant improvement.

In addition to changes in the pericardium, myocardium, and endocardium, radiotherapy has increasingly been recognized to cause narrowing and occlusion of epicardial coronary arteries and changes in the intramyocardial coronary vessels. In the study of 16 patients by Brosius et al,[40] 25% of the major epicardial coronaries exhibited greater than 75% reduction in cross-sectional area by intimal lesions composed of fibrous tissue with small amounts of lipid. In addition, there was fibrosis in the media and adventitia. Thirty-one percent of the patients showed focal medial, intimal, and adventitial fibrous thickening of the subepicardial intramyocardial coronary arteries in the right ventricular free wall. Although the reported symptoms of myocardial ischemia or infarction are not as common as the frequency of these reported anatomic lesions, there is a significant number of young women and men with angina pectoris and no risk factors other than mediastinal radiation. Some,[41] including a 28-year-old patient with Hodgkin's disease at Memorial, have required coronary artery bypass grafting. Other investigators have reported myocardial infarction among patients with a history of mediastinal irradiation and no other significant risk factors. The acute myocardial changes of endothelial cell swelling, platelet aggregation, and frequent vessel occlusion have been noted.

The reader should note that many of these physiologic and histopathologic studies were performed in patients who received radiotherapy delivery by outmoded techniques. Whether similar observations will be made in the future in patients who have been treated by present standards of radiation therapy is unknown.

The susceptibility of the other branches of the arterial system to these radiation-induced lesions must also be recalled including the carotid arteries, iliofemoral arteries, and axillary and brachial arteries after axillary irradiation.[42] When infection is superimposed on radiation and surgical changes, there may be insidious or catastrophic arterial rupture. Often these larger arterial stenoses, occlusions, and disruptions require appropriate surgical therapy. As well as for the epicardial coronary arteries, critical stenoses or occlusions of these major peripheral arteries may require bypass grafting. For disruption of arterial integrity, particularly of the carotids, ligation may be necessary. The reports of reconstructive surgery for these lesions are just beginning to accumulate.

ANTHRACYCLINE CARDIOMYOPATHY

In the late 1960s and early 1970s, the cytotoxic antibiotics daunorubicin and doxorubicin were shown to be highly effective against a wide variety of neoplasms: carcinoma of the breast, lung, and gonads: soft tissue sarcomas; leukemias; and lymphomas. Acute toxicity (namely, bone marrow suppression, alopecia, nausea, vomiting, and mucositis) has been reversible. However, cardiac toxicity resulting in severe and irreversible congestive heart failure has limited the cumulative dose of both drugs that could be administered to individual patients. This dose-dependent toxicity has required termination of chemotherapy often when the neoplasm has continued to exhibit gratifying response, and has stimulated a search for analogs without these deleterious side effects.

Acutely the anthracyclines also produce cardiac effects, although these are generally self-limited or reversible and convey no predictive information about the later development of cardiomyopathy. There are no significant symptoms of the acute changes, which consist of pericarditis, myocarditis, mild left ventricular failure, nonspecific ST-segment and T-wave abnormalities, and ventricular premature complexes.[43] To date there has been little methodical investigation of the acute cardiac response, although there are some anecdotal reports of mild dilatation of the left ventricle on echocardiogram shortly after administration of the anthracycline. This mild ventricular decompensation is asymptomatic, physiologically insignificant, and of little clinical concern. However, the arrhythmias occurring acutely after anthracycline administration have attracted attention. The ectopy, particularly the ventricular premature beats, are disturbing in view of at least two deaths recorded within 15 minutes of the administration of doxorubicin, presumably from lethal ventricular arrhythmia.[44]

Each cardiac effect of these agents is marked by cytopathologic changes. In the acute cardiac reaction in rabbit heart models, exposure to a perfusate for one to two hours, containing therapeutic concentrations of anthracycline, leads particularly to central clumping of nuclear chromatin with clear zones along the nuclear membrane, mitochondrial swelling and disruption, moderate disruption of sarcomeres, and small areas of cytoplasmic vacuolization.[45] The chronic changes from these drugs, documented on ultrastructural analysis of the heart of both experimental animals and human beings, consist of nuclear polymorphism, swollen cytoplasmic reticulum and mitochondria with prominent vacuolar coalescence, and disappearance of myofibrils.[46,47]

The cause or mechanism of this myocardial injury is unclear. Among hypotheses are direct nuclear alterations, inhibition of DNA-dependent RNA synthesis, peroxidation of the cell membrane lipids, inhibition of mitochondrial biosynthesis of coenzyme Q10, interference with the function of sodium-potassium ATPase, decrease in transport of calcium into the sarcoplasmic reticulum and concentration or retention of this ion within the cytoplasm, and/or response to histamine or catecholamines, or both. Concurrent with evidence for the roles for each of these mechanisms have been efforts to alter the biochemical reactions to prevent cardiac damage in experimental animals: entrapment of the anthracycline in electrically charged liposomes, concurrent administration of coenzyme Q10, parenteral treatment with free-radical scavenging N acetylcysteine, administration of vitamins A or E, and alteration of the drug structure or substitution of analog compounds. To date, none of these approaches has been successful, although the search for less cardiotoxic analogs seems promising.

The clinical manifestations of chronic anthracycline cardiotoxicity have aroused major concern and have stimulated research about its prevention, prediction, and early detection. Although the goal of this research has been to prevent the cardiopathic changes, the results to date have failed to identify reliable indicators to terminate chemotherapy before subtle physiologic deterioration. Therefore, investigators have sought reliable signs of this early cardiomyopathy, so that drug therapy could be terminated before the development of florid cardiac decompensation. An unresolved issue is whether noninvasive tests of cardiac function can appropriately satisfy this need or whether the invasive procedure of endomyocardial biopsy is required.

Historically, after clinical evaluation alone had been found inadequate, investigators reported the value of prolongation of the systolic time intervals (pre-ejection period/left ventricular ejection time) as determined from the simultaneously recorded electrocardiogram, carotid pulse and the phonocardiogram. A generalized decrease in QRS voltage was also associated with doxorubicin-induced cardiac changes. Changes in the ratio of pre-ejection period/left ventricular ejection time (greater than 0.43 or an increase of 0.10 over baseline) were noted to be sensitive but nonspecific and unreliable indicators of cardiomyopathy.[48] Similarly, a decrease in the electrocardiographic QRS voltage occurred late in the evolution of the toxicity and was nonspecific.

In the continuing search for both a specific and sensitive sign of early anthracycline cardiotoxicity, echocardiography and electrocardiogram-gated cardiac blood pool scans have offered more promise. Some investigators have found the percentage of shortening of myocardial fiber length to be reliable. Others, including ourselves, have noted dysfunction localized to the basal segments of the left ventricle to be an early sign of developing toxic cardiomyopathy, in contrast to the apical dysfunction characteristic of ischemic cardiac disease. The thickness of the intraventricular septum or the left ventricular free wall has been normal or slightly reduced.

Also among the noninvasive measures, radionuclide ventriculography is most frequently cited in the international literature for its sensitivity and specificity. However, there is no consensus on the protocol or precise criteria on which to base judgments about anthracycline dosing. Some investigators indicate that serial determination of resting left ventricular function suffices; others find greater sensitivity when both resting and exercise left ventricular ejection fraction are compared as increasing doses of anthracycline are administered.[49,50] In our institution we have relied on serial determinations of resting and exercise ejection fraction, provided the measurements are taken at least as frequently as dose increments of 100 mg/m^2 after an initial cumulative dose of 250 mg/m^2. Despite this protocol, the occasional sudden occurrence of symptomatic cardiac decompensation, documented by radionuclide study, has been disquieting. Although the quantitative documentation of left ventricular function has often indicated early cardiomyopathy and has dictated prompt discontinuation of anthracycline therapy, it occasionally lacks reliable predictive value.

Irrespective of the specific technique for serial evaluation of left ventricular function, the presence of risk factors for drug-induced cardiomyopathy lowers one's threshold for suspicion of drug-induced cardiac change and for vigilance in monitoring cardiac function as further chemotherapy is administered. The following conditions certainly place patients at higher risk for developing anthracycline cardiomyopathy: a cumulative doxorubicin dose exceeding 350 mg/m^2, patient age over 70 years, previous mediastinal radiation with a cardiac dose of over 2,000 rads, previous or concurrent therapy with cyclophosphamide, and an entity of "diminished cardiac reserve." This latter category may include specific diseases such as hypertension, coronary artery disease, and valvular heart disease, or may consist of patients with cardiomyopathy from other causes and a reduced number of viable myocytes. In addition, there are data suggesting that children younger than 18 months may have increased sensitivity to the cardiotoxic effects of anthracycline. If this interpretation of the risk factors is appropriate, then the proposed guidelines in Table 57.3 are suggested.[51]

From the reports of several investigators, however, such noninvasive documentation of cardiac function and left ventricular ejection fraction fails reliably to predict, and

Table 57.3. Guidelines from Radionuclide Ventriculograms for Continued Administration of Anthracycline*

Resting Ejection Fraction (%)	Increment with Exercise (%)	More Anthracycline?	
> 40	> 5	Yes	Without risk factors
> 40	< 5	With close monitoring	
<40	>5	With close monitoring	
< 40	< 5	No	
> 45	> 5	Yes	With risk factors
> 45	< 5	With close monitoring	
<45	> 5	With close monitoring	
< 45	< 5	No	

* Modified from Dresdale et al.[51]

therefore prevent, anthracycline cardiomyopathy among all patients receiving these drugs. Since the early 1980s, an increasing number of cardiologists have turned to the technique of right ventricular endomyocardial biopsy introduced by Konno and Sakakibara[51a] in 1963, and modified and applied extensively by Caves et al[52] at Stanford University in 1973. This procedure, performed percutaneously, provides several small specimens of myocardium. Bristow et al[53] analyzed a large number of such specimens, primarily by the electron microscope, and deduced a scoring system for anthracycline toxicity. When the histopathologic data are combined with results of right heart catheterization, the Stanford group[52] has been able to predict the risk of development of congestive heart failure with further anthracycline (Table 57.4). In addition, Bristow et al[53] reported a linear relation between biopsy score after a moderate cumulative dose of anthracycline (eg, 200 to 300 mg/m^2 of doxorubicin) and the dose at which the patient will experience cardiac decompensation. If this linear relation is consistent, then a single endomyocardial biopsy after such a moderate cumulative dose of anthracycline may permit prediction of the dose at which a given patient would develop clinical cardiomyopathy.

Table 57.4. Risk of Overt Cardiac Decompensation with 100 mg/m^2 Additional Doxorubicin*

Risk	Biopsy Score†	Catheterization§ Score	Number of Patients Developing Congestive Heart Failure Within 100 mg/m^2
No	≤ 1.5	< 1	0/42
Low (< 10%)	2	≤ 1	1/31
	≤ 1.5	2	
Moderate (10%–25%)	2	2	2/16
	2.5	≤ 1	
High (> 25%)	2.5	2	14/31
	3	—	
	≥ 1	3	

* Adapted from Bristow et al.[53]

† Biopsy scoring:

0 = normal myocardial ultrastructure
1 = < 5% myocytes with early distended cytoplasmic reticulum, myofibrillar loss
1.5 = 6%–15% myocytes with changes above, more marked
2 = 16%–25% with definite changes above
2.5 = 26%–35% with definite changes
3 = > 35% with marked change

§ Catheterization scoring:
0 = normal;
1 = any of following abnormalities:
(a) mild elevation right ventricular end-diastolic pressure (RVEDP), left ventricular end-diastolic pressure (LVEDP), mean right atrial pressure ($\overline{RA}$), mean pulmonary artery wedge pressure ($\overline{PW}$), A-VO_2 difference; mild reduction cardiac index (CI)
(b) exercise increase in pressures approximately 5 to 10 mm Hg;
$$\frac{\Delta \text{ cardiac output}}{\Delta\ O_2 \text{ consumption}} = 4-6$$
2 = Any of the following abnormalities:
(a) two or more of above,
(b) moderately elevated RVEDP, LVEDP, $\overline{RA}$, $\overline{PW}$, A-VO_2 difference; moderately reduced CI
(c) Exercise rise > 9 to 10 mm Hg in pressure, $\frac{\Delta \text{ cardiac output}}{\Delta\ O_2 \text{ consumption}} < 4$
3 = Any of the following:
(a) two or more of moderate abnormalities
(b) resting hemodynamics $\overline{PW}$ or LVEDP ≥ 20 mmHg, $\overline{RA}$ or RVEDP ≥ 16 and 18 mmHg, respectively, A-VO_2 difference > 5 vol% and CI < 1.8 L/min/m^2

The technique of endomyocardial biopsy also permits precise quantitative comparison of the cardiac toxicities of various anthracycline analogs: 4'-doxorubicin; aclacinomycin; rubidazone; mitoxantrone; demethoxydaunorubicin; N,L leucyldoxorubicin; and others. Additionally, the procedure permits evaluation of the efficacy of other maneuvers to reduce the cardiotoxicity of the anthracyclines presently used: for example, reducing the dose per treatment of doxorubicin and administering the doses more frequently or by continuous infusion.

Treatment of anthracycline-related cardiac congestive failure, by means of digitalis preparations and diuretics, occasionally results in apparent improvement in cardiac decompensation and reversal of the cardiomyopathy. More frequently, however, the physiologic changes are irreversible, and treatment requires long-term support of a failing heart. In addition to these standard drugs, reduction of left ventricular afterload with agents like hydralazine or of preload and afterload with captopril or prazosin may furnish satisfactory long-term improvement in hemodynamics.

In summary, the anthracycline antibiotics acutely cause mild myocyte injury and dysfunction and infrequent but potentially dangerous cardiac arrhythmias. These drugs chronically cause linearly dose-related myocyte injury with damage to nuclei, cytoplasmic organelles, and myofibrils, and, in more advanced stages, with marked loss of myocytes and ventricular decompensation. These ultrastructural abnormalities are more pronounced in biopsy specimens from the left ventricle, and light microscopy shows considerable fibrous thickening of the left ventricular endocardium, suggesting that chronic anthracycline cardiotoxicity is a restrictive endomyocardial disease.[53a] Measures of nonspecific cardiac function, particularly by radionuclide ventriculography, have permitted early detection of cardiomyopathy in most cases, but endomyocardial biopsy may be more reliable and probably does provide predictive information before the onset of physiologic dysfunction. Whereas the noninvasive tests are internationally widely available and require little specialized training of the supervising physician, the biopsy procedure requires a carefully organized and highly skilled team to assure patient safety and sophisticated, reliable data.

CYCLOPHOSPHAMIDE CARDIOMYOPATHY

Cyclophosphamide-induced cardiomyopathy has been reported in the treatment of solid tumors and in strategies for bone marrow ablation before engraftment of heterologous donor marrow. The first occurrence of this complication was reported by Santos et al[54] in 1970; the number of reports of clinical, physiologic, and pathologic analysis has accelerated within the last five years. In almost all instances, the cardiac complications of cyclophosphamide have been noted after large doses, generally exceeding 100 mg per kilogram within a one-week interval.[55,56]

In contrast to the progressive, chronic cardiomyopathy associated with anthracyclines, large doses of cyclophosphamide produce an acute deterioration of cardiac function one to three weeks after administration. The symptoms and signs are nonspecific but typical of left ventricular decompensation.

Pathologically, however, unlike anthracycline toxicity, evidence of drug-induced direct damage to myocytes is only mild to moderate. The early toxicity of cyclophosphamide observed in experimental animals is most striking in the intramyocardial coronary arterioles and capillaries, which exhibit endothelial cell swelling, intraluminal fibrin thrombi in capillaries, and lysis of the muscularis of larger vessels. In the myocardium itself of both human beings and experimental animals are hemorrhages, edema, fibrin deposition, and interstitial infiltrates of leukocytes. After the initial vascular damage and interstitial process, lesions appear in the myocytes primarily as vacuolization. This myocyte injury has been speculatively attributed to direct damage by a chemotherapeutic agent that has leaked into the interstitial space secondary to disruption of capillary integrity (Figure 57.2). As the interstitial leukocytic infiltration subsides and the cytoplasmic vacuolization resolves, early fibrosis and compensatory hypertrophy of the remaining undamaged myocytes are noted. Accompanying further recovery is evidence of more chronic scarring, focal calcification, and cartilaginous metaplasia.[56]

The clinical evidence of this process consists of the expected signs and symptoms of left ventricular decompensation and mild cardiac dilatation on chest x-ray. Particularly significant have been the echocardiographic findings: small to moderate pericardial effusion, a slight increase in the internal dimensions of the left ventricle, a reduction in the fractional shortening and in the computed left ventricular ejection fraction, and enlargement of the left atrium. However, the most significant finding is thickening of the interventricular septum and of the free wall of the left ventricle.[57] This is in contrast to the changes of anthracycline cardiomyopathy: more prominent chamber dilatation and thinning of the ventricular myocardium (Figure 57.3.)

Treatment of this iatrogenic complication has been supportive, using digitalis, techniques to reduce left ventricular preload and afterload, and especially diuretics.[58]

Other chemotherapeutic agents have been associated with cardiac complications in single case reports or small series: large doses of methotrexate with electrocardiographic changes, 5-fluorouracil with angina pectoris, busulfan with endocardial fibrosis, vincristine with myocardial infarction in a patient with known arteriosclerotic heart disease, cisplatinum with electrocardiographic changes, VP-16 with myocardial infarction after radiotherapy, amsacrine with ventricular arrhythmias and left ventricular dysfunction, and diethylstilbestrol with an increased frequency of coronary artery disease.[58a]

ENDOCARDITIS

Although no direct causal relation exists, features of endocarditis among patients with malignancy are unusual and deserve special comment. Usually, a complication of cancer or its treatment, a specifically reduced humoral or cellular immunity, or a coagulation disorder places the patient at increased risk for the cardiac process.

Infective endocarditis has been discussed in an earlier chapter (chapter 46). Although this complication occurs

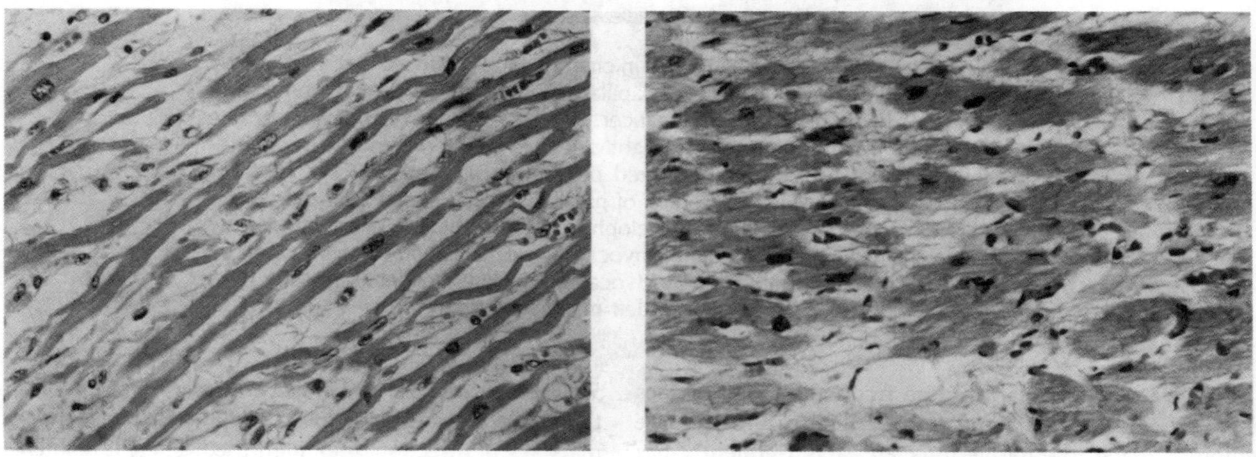

Figure 57.2. (*Left*) Acute myocardial changes after very high-dose cyclophosphamide therapy. Prominent interstitial edema with fibrin deposition, patchy hemorrhage, and leukocyte infiltration. Rare myocyte vacuolization; preservation of myofibrils and of nuclear chromatin. (Courtesy of Richard E. Slavin, MD). (*Right*) Anthracycline cardiotoxicity. Myocardium of 10-year-old boy with osteogenic sarcoma, after 675 mg/m^2 of daunorubicin. Heart weight 280 g (normal 150 g). Myocytes show cytoplasmic vacuolization with resulting disorganization of the myofibrils; virtually no inflammatory cell reaction (Courtesy of Stephen S. Sternberg, MD).

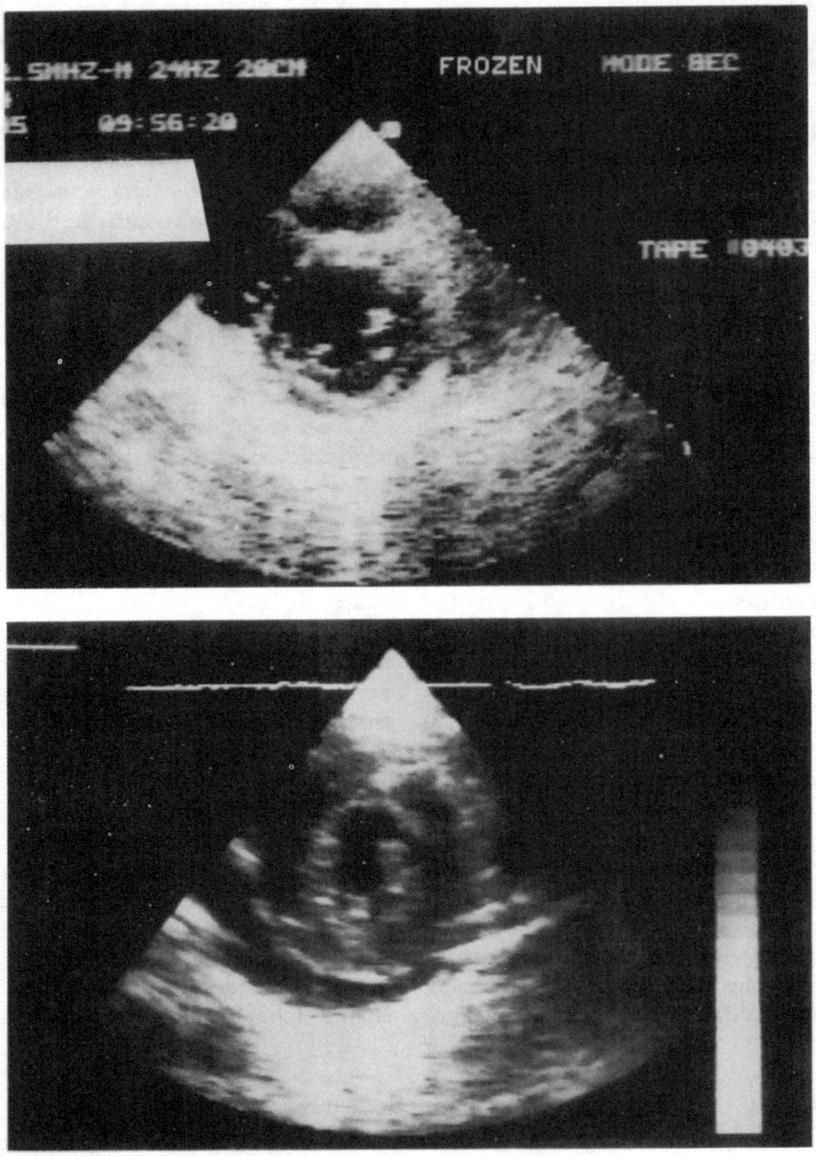

Figure 57.3. (*Top*) Echocardiograms in chemotherapy-induced cardiomyopathy. Parasternal short-axis view at level of papillary muscles in 53-year-old woman after 465 mg/m^2 doxorubicin for breast cancer. Dilated left ventricular cavity occupies center of frame with thinned, only slightly echogenic interventricular septum on the left. Posterior wall poorly visualized below the papillary muscles. (*Bottom*) Parasternal short-axis view at insertion of papillary muscles in 24-year-old woman with bone marrow transplant after cyclophosphamide ablation of native marrow. Prominent echogenic endocardium; myocardium of left ventricular free wall extending to echo-dense pericardium. Myocardial thickness of septum nearly twice as great, extending to faint echoes at left margin of sector.

among cancer patients no more frequently than it does in the general patient population, certain features deserve emphasis. First, the native infected valve frequently has been normal until the appearance of endocarditis (79% of cases[59]). Second, the valvular infection has frequently been associated with an indwelling venous catheter, and case reports are now indicating an association with Hickman–Broviac or other of the protected central venous access devices.[60,61] Third, among the infecting organisms, there is a disproportionate presence of staphylococci, both *Staphylococcus aureus* and *Staphylococcus epidermidis,* and also of the *candida* species. However, in many instances the primary site of infection is not identified. There is no increase in the frequency of opportunistic pathogens among the organisms.

Most significant among cancer patients is the occurrence of nonbacterial thrombotic endocarditis (NBTE). Although the appearance of new cardiac murmurs or a change in the existing ones may raise the suspicion of valvular vegetations, NBTE is usually first diagnosed because of evidence of systemic embolization. Most frequently such embolization is first noted in the cerebral circulation, with a sudden change of mental status or other neurologic sign, although peripheral systemic emboli are common, especially in the coronary circulation. Concerning diagnostic considerations, changes in preexisting murmurs are less frequent in patients with NBTE (17%) than among patients with infective endocarditis (50%). The nonbacterial process is frequently associated with coagulation abnormalities such as peripheral thrombophlebitis, an abrupt decline in platelet count, or other evidence of a consumptive coagulopathy. Whereas infective endocarditis is associated with a wide variety of malignant processes, without apparent predilection, NBTE is especially concentrated among patients with bronchogenic adenocarcinoma, bronchoalveolar adenocarcinoma, and less frequently pancreatic adenocarcinoma. Concerning incidence, among the two series from the same base of autopsied patients, Rosen and Armstrong[62] identified NBTE nearly three times as frequently as infective endocarditis. In addition, although NBTE is distinctly associated with malignancy, 58% of the cases occur among patients with no identified cancer.[63]

As would be expected, the treatment of infective endocarditis in patients with malignancy is the same as that among the unselected population of patients with this disorder: appropriate antibiotics and, in selected cases, cardiac valve replacement. Conversely, because of the usual association of NBTE with coagulopathies and the frequency of deaths in this disorder attributed to thromboembolic complications (85% in the Rosen and Armstrong series), heparinization is clearly indicated in patients with NBTE.

COR PULMONALE

Although right ventricular disease is similar in physical and physiologic characteristics in the cancer patient to that from other causes, the increased frequency of the disorder should be noted. Pulmonary arterial obstruction by neoplasm, vascular changes from mediastinal or pulmonary irradiation, progressive pulmonary interstitial disorders such as lymphangitic metastases, and pulmonary interstitial drug toxicity are among the causes. Cardiac dysfunction secondary to these pulmonary diseases has not been studied. However, unlike cor pulmonale secondary to chronic obstructive pulmonary disease, cor pulmonale in these disorders is not improved by oxygen administration. At this time, treatment is purely supportive.

SURGICAL MANAGEMENT OF SELECTED MALIGNANCIES

Cardiac evaluation and risk in noncardiac surgery is discussed in chapter 68. However, specific cardiac considerations in surgery for thoracic neoplasms deserves notation.

The management of thoracic neoplasms, especially esophageal and bronchogenic carcinoma, frequently entails radical surgery. In addition to the cardiac considerations outlined for general surgery, the specific threat of cardiac arrhythmias must be anticipated in the thorough perioperative management of patients undergoing surgery for these intrathoracic neoplasms. A modest literature documents the correlation of supraventricular arrhythmia with the increasing age of patients.[64,65] In addition, these arrhythmias are more likely in proportion to the volume of pulmonary parenchyma resected. A third risk factor, in addition to the patient's age and volume of pulmonary parenchyma excised, is the preexistence of cardiac disease. The literature on cardiac arrhythmias after esophageal surgery is only anecdotal, perhaps because of the compelling technical considerations and, until recently, the bleak prognosis of patients with this disease. However, in our institution, cardiac arrhythmias after radical mediastinal procedures have occurred in approximately 50% of patients. Most frequently on the second to fourth postoperative day, atrial fibrillation, atrial flutter, or atrial tachycardia may develop. In addition to experiencing discomfort and alarm, such patients are at risk for hypotension and thrombosis of cerebral, coronary, or other systemic arteries. To reduce the risk of these postoperative arrhythmias, several investigators[66,67] recommend preoperative prophylactic digitalization of patients undergoing thoracotomy, especially those 50 years of age or older. Among patients receiving digitalis prophylactically, the occurrence of supraventricular arrhythmias is 10% to 50% of that among untreated patients. It should be noted that there has been no recommendation for aggressive digitalization to avoid the risk of toxicity; a loading dose of 0.75 mg of digoxin is appropriate. Further, it should be noted that arrhythmias may occur despite prophylactic treatment, but they are generally asymptomatic, short-lived, self-limited, or responsive to the administration of additional small doses of digitalis, or some combination thereof.

HYPERCALCEMIA

Before concluding the portion of this chapter concerned with the interrelation between malignancy and the heart, the authors draw attention to the electrocardiographic changes observed in hypercalcemia, a common complicating or paraneoplastic effect of malignant disease. On the one hand, hypercalcemia is predictable in bony involvement with tumor: multiple myeloma, metastatic mammary carcinoma, disseminated prostatic carcinoma, metastatic lung carcinoma, and others. On the other, it is noted as a paraneoplastic complication of tumor not directly involving bone: pulmonary carcinoma, oropharyngeal carcinoma, and uroepithelial carcinoma.

Aside from the shortened QT interval traditionally associated with hypercalcemia, the electrocardiograms of such patients often exhibit low T waves and prominent U waves consistent with hypokalemia. However, the critical feature of the QT interval that is diagnostic of hypercalcemia remains unsettled. For example, Ellman et al[68] reviewed 48 electrocardiograms in patients with serum calcium exceeding 13 mg/dl, and estimated ionized calcium averaging 2.26 mmol/L, without noting a single abnormal $Q\text{-}T_c$ interval. In their analysis of components of the QT interval, Wortsman and Frank[69] did note shortened $Q\text{-}oT_c$ (beginning of QRS complex to onset of T wave), Q-aT_c (beginning of QRS complex to apex of T wave), and Q-eT_c (beginning of QRS complex to end of T wave) intervals in selected cases. In a carefully controlled series, Nierenberg and Ransil[70] established coefficients of correlation of −0.85 between Q-aT_c interval and serum calcium level, and of −0.59 between Q-oT_c and serum calcium.

We have found this suggested value of 0.29 second for the Q-aT_c interval a highly specific sign of hypercalcemia, but only moderately sensitive (Figure 57.4A). A combination of shortened Q-aT_c and shortened Q-oT_c intervals has increased the sensitivity of the electrocardiographic signs of hypercalcemia (Figure 57.4B). Because of the increased awareness of possible hypercalcemia among the patient population, cardiologists at Memorial Sloan-Kettering Cancer Center mention its possibility when they interpret electrocardiograms exhibiting either of these signs: the shortened or even absent Q-oT_c interval and the shortened Q-aT_c interval. Without this high index of suspicion, such electrocardiograms would erroneously be interpreted to indicate acute anteroseptal myocardial infarction.

NONMALIGNANT HEMATOLOGIC DISORDERS

HYPEREOSINOPHILIA

Since Loffler's description in 1936 of two patients with congestive heart failure and marked eosinophilia,[71] the occurrence of endomyocardial fibrosis has been associated with eosinophilia from diverse causes: parasitic infestations, especially among patients in West Africa, marked by larval migration (filariasis, trichinosis, ascariasis, hookworm disease, and schistosomiasis)[72]; myeloproliferative disorders; rare lymphomas[73,74]; idiopathic hypereosinophilic syndromes[75]; and various sustained hypersensitivity reactions. In all these conditions marked by chronic eosinophilia, the primary cardiac lesion is endocardial injury, then necrosis, followed by reparative platelet thrombus formation over the denuded endocardium. Subsequent steps include propagation of mural thrombus,

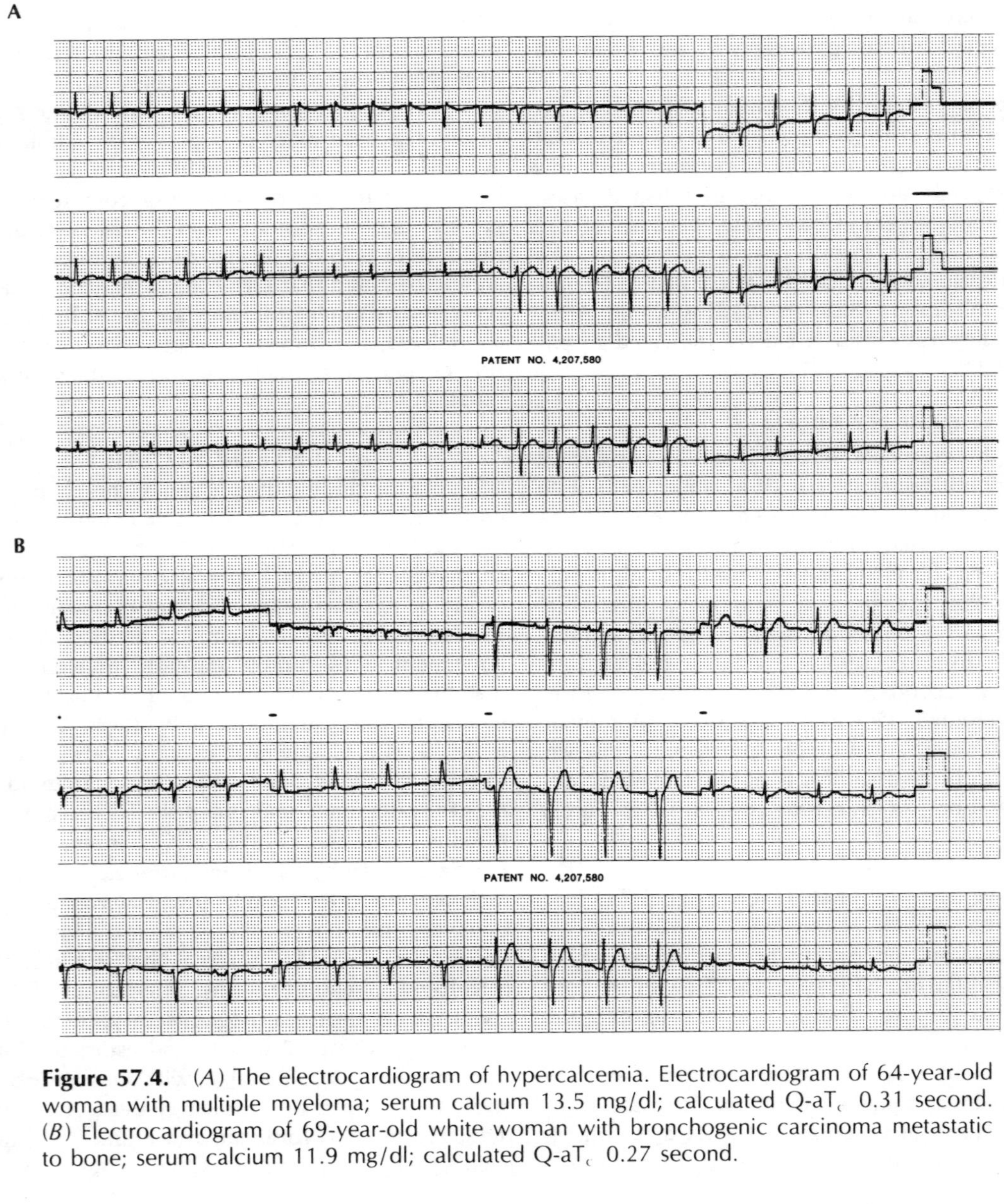

Figure 57.4. (*A*) The electrocardiogram of hypercalcemia. Electrocardiogram of 64-year-old woman with multiple myeloma; serum calcium 13.5 mg/dl; calculated Q-aT_c 0.31 second. (*B*) Electrocardiogram of 69-year-old white woman with bronchogenic carcinoma metastatic to bone; serum calcium 11.9 mg/dl; calculated Q-aT_c 0.27 second.

fibrosis, especially in the inflow tracts of the ventricles, and progression of the fibrosis to involve large portions or the entire ventricular endocardium and atrioventricular valves.[75] The latter may become bound down to the ventricular endocardium and may become grossly incompetent.[75] The fibrotic reaction may appear layered, contains collagen-rich connective tissue, may appear to penetrate the adjacent myocardium, and may contain granulation tissue and developing blood vessels in the deeper layers.[76] The superficial layers of this process appear to contain fibrin-like material, provide a nidus for mural thrombus formation, and are thought to cause the endocardial thickening by organization of these thrombi. Embolization may occur. This endocardial fibrosis persists, although circulating eosinophilia wanes or subsides.

Physiologically the manifestations of endomyocardial fibrosis, secondary to eosinophilia, consist of restrictive cardiomyopathy and atrioventricular valvular regurgitation. Supportive treatment by means of digitalis, diuretics, and trials of afterload reduction has been of limited success. Definitive treatment has been directed at reducing, during the active stage of disease, the hypereosinophilia that initiates and propagates the endocardial necrosis and fibrosis. When such active necrosis is diagnosed on endomyocardial biopsy or when there is documentation of progressive cardiac or neurologic deterioration, therapy is started with corticosteroids, 60 to 80 mg of prednisone daily or the equivalent. Chemotherapeutic agents are added in the myeloproliferative and idiopathic hypereosinophilic syndrome if the eosinophil count does not return to normal or if cardiac and neurologic function continues to deteriorate.[75] In the stable chronic condition of restrictive cardiomyopathy and congestive heart failure, best diagnosed by means of two-dimensional echocardiography,[77] cardiac surgery has been employed in several instances. Replacement of the mitral and occasionally of the tricuspid valve and even right ventricular endocardiectomy have been beneficial.[78,79]

IRON OVERLOAD: HEMOCHROMATOSIS AND THALASSEMIA

In both hemochromatosis and thalassemia, cardiomyopathy results from deposition or retention of iron particles within myocytes. Although congestive cardiomyopathy has frequently been described, there are occasional reports of restrictive cardiomyopathy.[80] Furthermore, although the ultimate pathophysiologic and pathologic mechanisms of hemochromatosis and thalassemia may be similar, the initiating pathogenic processes are sharply different.

Hemochromatosis is a genetically determined abnormality of iron metabolism. There is a close linkage between the loci of the histocompatibility human leukocyte antigen (HLA) and a gene for susceptibility to hemochromatosis. The frequency of occurrence of the hemochromatosis gene is about 0.05 in populations of Sweden, France, the United States, Canada, Australia, and Scotland; this figure implies a heterozygote frequency of about 1 person in 10 and a homozygote frequency of 2 or 3 persons per 1,000.[80a]

Hemochromatosis is marked by apparent loss of regulatory control of iron absorption from the small intestine. Although many features of this mechanism are not fully understood, there is probably absence or inefficiency of a negative feedback signal, so that the patient continues to absorb and retain excessive dietary iron in relation to total body stores. A second underlying pathogenic process is failure of the reticuloendothelial system to ingest, retain, and thereby physiologically inactivate this excess body iron.[81] As a consequence the iron is deposited in parenchymal cells of several organs: cardiac myocytes, hepatocytes rather than Kupffer cells, the genitalia, islets of Langerhans, anterior pituitary, and type B synovial cells. Within the heart, these iron deposits result in edema, fragmentation, necrosis and focal fibrosis, fatty infiltration, inflammatory infiltrate, and hemosiderin within myocytes. In both hemochromatosis and thalassemia, this intracardiac iron storage fails to elicit a diffuse fibrotic reaction, so that these abnormalities are potentially reversible. This intracellular iron may cause damage by stimulation of lipid membrane peroxidation or by intracellular lysosomal breakdown and cell damage.

Hemochromatosis becomes symptomatic and is usually diagnosed when the patient is in his forties or fifties. Although significant cardiac involvement is less frequent than hepatic or pancreatic involvement, between 35% and 50% of patients die of congestive heart failure. Since the 1960s, the clinical benefits of depleting this pathologically increased total body iron store have been recognized, and treatment has consisted of repeated phlebotomy to maintain a hemoglobin level of 10 g/dl or lower. Echocardiographic evaluation of these patients before treatment has revealed ventricular wall thickness at or near normal, occasional mild dilatation of the left ventricle with impaired systolic function, and an enlarged left atrium. On follow-up study after therapeutic phlebotomy, these functional abnormalities have shown improvement.[82,83]

The thalassemia syndromes constitute a spectrum of disorders of hemoglobin synthesis in which the homozygote expression of the abnormal gene is fatal at an early age, but the heterozygote expression confers an increased likelihood that the individual will survive infection with *Plasmodium falciparum.* Accordingly the original population distribution of this genetic variant was the Mediterranean region, Arabian peninsula, Indian subcontinent, Southeast Asia, and East Indies. In contrast to hemochromatosis, the signs and symptoms of this disease become severe in infancy and early childhood with dyspnea, tachycardia, and impaired growth and maturation. Hematologically the central abnormalities are defective hemoglobin synthesis, lack of erythrocyte maturation, red cell destruction within the marrow, and anemia. The hemolytic process floods the reticuloendothelial system with degraded red cells and iron-containing proteins; the severe anemia causes a state of high cardiac output. In addition, the small bowel is stimulated to physiologically normal, increased iron absorption. Even before transfusion therapy of the anemia there is overflow of the reticuloendothelial system and presentation of elemental iron to organ parenchyma, especially the heart.[84]

On the one hand, therefore, the heart of the patient with thalassemia must compensate for the demands of anemia by high cardiac output. On the other hand, cardiac function is impaired by the toxic effects of the intracellular iron. It is therefore not surprising that physiologic observations and measurements in these patients are varied. Tachycardia, variable cardiomegaly, normal systolic function on echocardiography, slight ventricular hypertrophy, and occasional slight abnormalities of ventricular filling have been commented.[85,86] Some thalassemic patients have pericarditis with possible causal relations to "iron-induced" pericardial siderosis and viral or mycoplasmal infection.[86a]

Treatment of this disorder by repeated transfusion to correct the anemia further adds to the total body stores of iron, although it does curtail gastrointestinal absorption of the element. Over the last 20 years, in the industrial nations, the chelating agent deferoxamine has been administered to reduce the accumulated tissue iron.[86b] Regrettably, this agent is prohibitively expensive to be widely available to the populations in which thalassemia syndromes are concentrated.[87] However, in follow-up echocardiographic studies there is evidence that deferoxamine has reduced the left ventricular diastolic dysfunction observed after treatment by transfusion alone.[88]

IRON DEFICIENCY

The hypochromic, microcytic anemia of iron deficiency places demands on the heart for increased cardiac output. As expected, such patients exhibit tachycardia and an insignificant change in cardiac diameter on chest x-ray. The echocardiogram in acute hemorrhagic anemia demonstrates a decrease in left ventricular end-systolic diameter and occasionally systolic apposition of the anterior mitral leaflet (SAM) to the interventricular septum.

The left ventricular changes of thickened, hypertrophied left ventricular walls in chronic iron deficiency are more complex than would be predicted from cardiac considerations alone. From the demands for increased cardiac output, in chronic iron deficiency, cardiac hypertrophy would be expected. Rossi and Carillo[89] demonstrated that in rats this hypertrophy can be prevented by adrenergic depletion by reserpine, and that on ultramicroscopic examination, in addition to myocyte hypertrophy in the untreated animals, areas of focal cellular degeneration and fibrosis suggest the role of norepinephrine. Furthermore, these investigators have documented decreased myocardial norepinephrine levels in the same experimental model.[90] In addition to the role of norepinephrine in the development of cardiac hypertrophy in chronic iron deficiency anemia, Florenjano et al[91] showed evidence of a noncatecholamine serum factor with positive inotropic effect.

Finally, not all the effects of iron deficiency are mediated through the anemia it causes. Among patients with chronic iron deficiency anemia being started on treatment, Mehta et al[92] showed correction of electrocardiographic abnormalities on treadmill stress testing, before improvement in the anemia. They postulate that this correction of the electrophysiologic abnormalities indicates an effect of iron at the tissue levels. In a detailed analysis of polycythemic patients who were maintained chronically iron deficient, but with a normal hematocrit level, Rector et al[93] reported normal exercise test results in six of their seven patients and normal neuromuscular and cardiovascular function, but they did observe the phenomenon of compulsive ice eating or pica.

From these data it appears that chronic iron deficiency alone has no direct deleterious effect on cardiac function.

MISCELLANEOUS BLOOD DYSCRASIAS AND HEMATOLOGIC DISORDERS

SICKLE CELL DISEASE

There has been a continuing controversy whether sickle cell anemia or trait is associated with a specific cardiomyopathy. Several investigators have concluded that parameters of left ventricular function are normal in sickle cell disease.[94] Others have noted a variable increase in left ventricular mass, dilatation of the left ventricle, and deterioration in left ventricular function among patients with sickle cell anemia, especially when echocardiographic measurements are corrected for volume overload.[95,95a] In a detailed study correcting for increased preload and decreased afterload, Denenberg et al[96] concluded that left ventricular systolic function is depressed in sickle cell anemia. Willems et al[97] believed that the appearance of left ventricular dysfunction required the addition of hypertension or other stress, as did the group at Johns Hopkins.[98,98a] A recent report by the National Cooperative Study of Sickle Cell Disease sponsored by the National Heart, Lung and Blood Institute, National Institutes of Health[98a] noted that a significant number of young patients with sickle cell anemia develop evidence of myocardial ischemia with exercise in the form of exercise-induced ST-segment depression and that the level of serum hemoglobin does not appear to play a major role in this occurrence.

Finally, Manno et al[99] performed rest and exercise testing of both right and left ventricular function among ten patients with sickle cell disease. Their finding of normal left ventricular function but of impaired right ventricular function was evaluated in conjunction with thallium-201 demonstration of increased right ventricular mass attributed to pressure/volume overload secondary to pulmonary vascular occlusion.

From these disparate data, it seems likely that in sickle cell disease there is right ventricular hypertrophy and dysfunction and that left ventricular function is variable. Although evidence fails to indicate a specific sickle cell left ventricular cardiomyopathy, it does suggest that the chronic high-output state reduces left ventricular reserve and that a nonspecific cardiomyopathy may be elicited by other coexisting diseases. On the other hand, the recent report from Saudi Arabia that patients with sickle cell anemia in association with α-thalassemia have a milder form of the disease, develop fewer complications, and receive fewer blood transfusions than the patients without α-thalassemia[99a] has important clinical implications in that these patients also may have fewer cardiovascular complications.

HEMOLYSIS FROM PROSTHETIC CARDIAC VALVES

Hemolytic reactions develop in 20% to 85% of patients after placement of prosthetic valves.[100] The frequency of hemolysis depends on the prosthetic device used; it is most frequent with ball valve prostheses, intermediate with tilting disk prostheses, and least common with tissue valves. Among patients with ball valves, wear and disruption of the cloth covering the valve ring and struts are a major factor in hemolysis.[101] Other factors contributing to hemolysis are the synthetic material of the valve; direct trauma to the red cells; and shearing forces created by gradients, high flow, and turbulence as may exist with perivalvular leaks or perforation or tear of bioprosthetic valve leaflets.[102,102a] In patients with the Lillehei–Kaster valves, Olesen et al[103] demonstrated that there is a modest increase in the frequency and severity of hemolysis with time. This complication has also been reported after prosthetic repair of septal defects, but it can be minimized by the use of biologic material such as pericardium. Iron replacement is indicated in patients in whom microcytic hypochromic red cell indices or overt anemia develops. Replacement of the defective prosthetic valve may be necessary if the hemolytic anemia is significant.[102,102a]

DIGOXIN METABOLISM IN ANEMIA

Pertinent to the subject of anemias is a report by Hamamoto et al[104] about abnormal features of digoxin metabolism in the setting of anemia. They noted reduced serum levels of the drug after its administration in anemic patients, increased urinary excretion in anemic experimental animals, and reduced myocardial binding of the glycoside.[104] Whether these observations carry clinical implications is unclear.

POLYCYTHEMIA AND ERYTHREMIA

Polycythemia vera contributes to cardiac dysfunction primarily through the increased blood viscosity and potential occlusion of vessels in the coronary microcirculation. Gemelli et al[105] demonstrated abnormal systolic time intervals among patients with polycythemia vera after the administration of amyl nitrite. A report by Ali et al[106] identifies another complication of polycythemia: massive intraventricular thrombus causing intractable congestive heart failure.

The same complications should be noted in the secondary polycythemias. For example, Yeager and Freed[107] described acute myocardial infarction in two patients with polycythemia secondary to cyanotic congenital heart disease.

REFERENCES

1. Dunnick NR, Seibert K, Cramer HR Jr: Cardiac metastases from osteosarcoma. *J Comput Assist Tomogr* 1981; 5:253–255.
2. Watts FB Jr, Zingas AP, Das L, Cushing BA: Computed tomographic diagnosis of an intracardiac metastasis from osteosarcoma. *CT* 1983; 7:271–272.
3. Das L, Farooki ZQ, Hakimi MN, Philippart AI, Watts FB Jr, Arciniegas E, Cushing B, Ryan J: Asymptomatic intracardiac metastases from osteosarcoma: a case report with literature review. *Med Pediatr Oncol* 1983; 11:164–166.
4. Daneman A, Martin DJ, Chan HS: Cardiac metastases from osteosarcoma. A report of two cases. *CT* 1983; 7:41–43.
5. Cohen GU, Perry TM, Evans JM: Neoplastic invasion of the heart and pericardium. *Ann Intern Med* 1955; 42:1238–1245.
6. Hanfling SM: Metastatic cancer to the heart. *Circulation* 1960; 22:474–483.
7. McAllister HA, Fenoglio JJ: *Tumors of the Cardiovascular System.* Washington, Armed Forces Institute of Pathology, 1978, pp 111–119.
8. Lockwood WB, Broghamer WL Jr: The changing prevalence of secondary cardiac neoplasms as related to cancer therapy. *Cancer* 1980; 45:2659–2662.
9. Ambrosio GB: Frequency of cardiac metastasis: review of 2222 autopsies and critical assessment. *Arch Sci Med (Torino)* 1980; 137:29–32.
10. Sokolova IN, Skhvatsabaja LV: Secondary tumors of the heart (based on autopsy materials in the Oncology Research Center of the Academy of Medical Sciences of the USSR...). *Arkh Patol* 1980; 42:38–41.
10a. Skhvatsabaja LV: Secondary malignant lesions of the heart and pericardium in neoplastic disease. *Oncology* 1986; 43:103–106.
10b. Lammers RJ, Bloor CM: Tumors of the heart and pericardium. *Med Concepts Cardiovasc Dis* 1986; 55:1–4.
11. Cammarosano C, Lewis W: Cardiac lesions in acquired immune deficiency syndrome (AIDS). *J Am Coll Cardiol* 1985; 5:703–706.
11a. El Allaf D, Burette R, Pierard L, Limet R: Cardiac tamponade as the first manifestation of cardiothoracic malignancy: a study of 10 cases. *Eur Heart J* 1986; 7:247–253.
12. Chandraratna PA, Aronow WS: Detection of pericardial metastases by cross-section echocardiography. *Circulation* 1981; 63:197–199.
13. Stark DD, Higgins CB, Lanzer P, Lipton MJ, Schiller N, Crooks LE, Botvinick EB, Kaufman L: Magnetic resonance imaging of the pericardium: normal and pathologic findings. *Radiology* 1984; 150:469–474.
14. Amparo EG, Higgins CB, Farmer D, Gamsu G, McNamara M: Gated MRI of cardiac and para-cardiac masses: initial experience. *Am J Radiol* 1984; 143:1151–1156.
15. Lubell DL, Goldfarb CR: Metastatic cardiac tumor demonstrated by ^{201} thallium scan. *Chest* 1980; 78:98–99.
16. Quaife MA, Boschult P, Baltaxe HA Jr, Dzindzio B: Myocardial accumulation of labeled phosphate in malignant pericardial effusion. *J Nucl Med* 1979; 20:392–396.
17. Hanley PC, Shub C, Seward JB, Wald LE: Intracavitary cardiac melanoma diagnosed by endomyocardial left ventricular biopsy. *Chest* 1983 84:195–198.
18. Prager RL, Wilson CH, Bender HW Jr: The subxiphoid approach to pericardial disease. *Am Thorac Surg* 1982; 34:6–9.
19. Davis S, Rambotti P, Grignani F: Intrapericardial tetracycline sclerosis in the treatment of malignant pericardial effusion: an analysis of thirty-three cases. *J Clin Oncol* 1984; 2:631–636.
20. Reyes CV, Strinden C, Banerji M: The role of cytology in neoplastic cardiac tamponade. *Acta Cytol* 1982; 26:299–302.
21. Yazdi HM, Hajdu SI, Melamed MR: Cytopathology of pericardial effusions. *Acta Cytol* 1980; 24:401–412.
22. Chen KT: Extracardiac malignancy presenting with cardiac tamponade. *J Surg Oncol* 1983; 3:167–168.
23. Roberts WC, Bodey GP, Westlake PT: The heart in acute leukemia. *Am J Cardiol* 1968; 21:388–412.
24. Szakacs JE, Cannon A: l-Norepinephrine myocarditis. *Am J Clin Pathol* 1958; 30:425–434.
25. Van Vliet PD, Burchell HB, Titus JL: Focal myocarditis associated with pheochromocytoma. *N Engl J Med* 1966; 274:1102–1108.
26. Kline IK: Myocardial alterations associated with pheochromocytomas. *Am J Pathol* 1961; 38:539–551.
27. Velasquez G, D'Souza VJ, Hackshaw BT, Glass TA, Formanek AG: Pheochromocytoma and cardiomyopathy. *Br Heart J* 1984; 57:89–92.
28. Levenson JA, Safar ME, London GM, Simon A Ch: Hemodynamics in patients with pheochromocytoma. *Clin Sci* 1980; 58:349–356.
29. Cueto L, Arriaga J, Zinser J: Echocardiographic changes in pheochromocytoma. *Chest* 1979; 76:600–601.
30. Bulkley BH, Fortuin NJ: Systolic anterior motion of the mitral valve without asymmetric septal hypertrophy. *Chest* 1976; 69:694–696.
31. Come PC, Bulkley BH, Goodman ZD, Hutchins GM, Pitt B, Fortuin NJ: Hypercontractile cardiac states simulating hypertrophic cardiomyopathy. *Circulation* 1977; 55:901–908.
32. Catterall M, Evans W: Myocardial injury from therapeutic irradiation. *Br Heart J* 1960; 22:168–174.
33. Selwyn AP: The cardiovascular system and radiation. *Lancet* 1983; II:152–154.
34. Cohn KE, Stewart JR, Fajardo LF, Hancock EW: Heart disease following radiation. *Medicine* 1967; 46:281–298.
35. Applefeld MM, Pollock SH: Cardiac disease in patients who have malignancies. *Curr Prob Cardiol* 1980; 4:1–37.

36. Fajardo LF, Stewart JR: Pathogenesis of radiation-induced myocardial fibrosis. *Lab Invest* 1973; 29:244–250.
37. Burns RJ, Bar-Shlomo B-Z, Druck MN, Herman JG, Gilbert BW, Perrault DJ, McLaughlin PR: Detection of radiation cardiomyopathy by gated radionuclide angiography. *Am J Med* 1983; 74:297–301.
38. Gottdiener JS, Katin MJ, Borer JS, Bacharach SL, Green MV: Late cardiac effects of therapeutic mediastinal irradiation: Assessment by echocardiography and radionuclide angiography. *N Engl J Med* 1983; 308:569–572.
39. Gomez GA, Park JJ, Panahan AM, Parthasarathy KL, Pearce J, Reese P, Bakshi S, Henderson ES: Heart size and function after radiation therapy to the mediastinum in patients with Hodgkin's disease. *Cancer Treat Rep* 1983; 12:1099–1103.
40. Brosius FC III, Waller BF, Roberts WC: Radiation heart disease. *Am J Med* 1981; 70:519–530.
41. Iqbal, SM, Hanson EL, Gensini GG: Bypass graft for coronary artery stenosis following radiation therapy. *Chest* 1977; 71:664–666.
42. McReady RA, Hyde GL, Bivins BA, Mattingly SS, Griffen WO: Radiation-induced arterial injuries. *Surgery* 1983; 93:306–312.
43. O'Bryan RM, Luce JK, Talley RW, Gottlieb JA, Baker LH, Bonadonna C: Phase II evaluation of adriamycin in human neoplasia. *Cancer* 1973; 32:1–8.
44. Wortman JE, Lucas VS, Schuster E, Thiele D, Logue GL: Sudden death during doxorubicin administration. *Cancer* 1979; 44:1588–1591.
45. Taylor AL, Applefeld MM, Wiernik PH, Grochaw LB, Mader LC, Bulkley BH: Acute anthracycline cardiotoxicity. *Cancer* 1984; 53:1660–1666.
46. Buja LM, Ferrans VJ, Mayer RJ, Roberts WC, Henderson ES: Cardiac ultrastructural changes induced by daunorubicin therapy. *Cancer* 1973; 32:771–788.
47. Lefrak EA, Pitha J, Rosenheim S, Gottlieb JA: A clinicopathologic analysis of adriamycin cardiotoxicity. *Cancer* 1973; 32:302–314.
48. Minow RA, Gottlieb JA: Adriamycin cardiotoxicity. *Ann Intern Med* 1975; 82:855–856.
49. Alexander J, Dainiak N, Berger HJ, Goldman L, Johnstone D, Reduto L, Duffy T, Schwartz P, Gottschalk A, Zaret BL: Serial assessment of doxorubicin cardiotoxicity with quantitative radionuclide angiocardiography. *N Engl J Med* 1979; 300:278–283.
50. Gottdiener JS, Mathisen DJ, Borer JS, Bonow RO, Myers CE, Barr LH, Schwartz DE, Bacharach SL, Green MV, Rosenberg SA. Doxorubicin cardiotoxicity: assessment of late left ventricular dysfunction by radionuclide cineangiography. *Ann Intern Med* 1981; 94:430–435.
51. Dresdale A, Bonow RO, Wesley R, Palmeri ST, Barr L, Mathison D, D'Angelo T, Rosenberg SA: Prospective evaluation of doxorubicin-induced cardiomyopathy resulting from postsurgical adjuvant treatment of patients with soft tissue sarcomas. *Cancer* 1983; 52:51–60.
51a. Konno S, Sakakibara S: Endo-myocardial biopsy. *Dis Chest* 1963; 44:345–350.
52. Caves PK, Stinson EB, Billingham ME, Shumway NE: Percutaneous transvenous endomyocardial biopsy in human heart recipients. Experience with a new technique. *Ann Thorac Surg* 1973; 16:325–336.
53. Bristow MR, Lopez MB, Mason JW, Billingham ME, Winchester MA: Efficacy and cost of cardiac monitoring in patients receiving doxorubicin. *Cancer* 1982; 50:32–41.
53a. Mortensen SA, Olsen HS, Baandrup U: Chronic anthracycline cardiotoxicity: haemodynamic and histopathological manifestations suggesting a restrictive endomyocardial disease. *Br Heart J* 1986; 55:274–282.
54. Santos GW, Sensenbrenner LL, Burke PJ, Colvin OM, Owens AH, Bias W, Slavin R: Marrow transplants in man utilizing cyclophosphamide: summary of Baltimore experience. *Exp Hematol* 1970; 20:78–81.
55. Slavin RE, Millan JC, Mullins GM: Pathology of high dose intermittent cyclophosphamide therapy. *Hum Pathol* 1975; 6:693–709.
56. Van Hoff DD, Rozencweig M, Piccart M: The cardiotoxicity of anticancer agents. *Semin Oncol* 1982; 9:23–33.
57. Hopkins HA, Betsill WL Jr, Hobson AS, Looney WB: Cyclophosphamide-induced cardiomyopathy in the rat. *Cancer Treat Rep* 1982; 66:1521–1527.
58. Steinherz LJ, Steinherz PJ, Mangiacasale D: Cardiac changes with cyclophosphamide. *Med Pediat Oncol* 1981; 9:417–422.
58a. Crawley IS: Effect of noncardiac drugs, radiation, electricity, and poisons on the heart, in Hurst JW (ed): *The Heart*, ed 6. New York, McGraw-Hill, 1986, pp 1479–1493.
59. Rosen P, Armstrong D: Infective endocarditis in patients treated for malignant neoplastic diseases. *Am J Clin Pathol* 1973; 59:241–250.
60. Press DW, Ramsey PG, Larson EB, Fefer A, Hickman RD: Hickman catheter infections in patients with malignancies. *Medicine* 1984; 63:189–200.
61. Liepman MK, Jones PG, Kauffman CA: Endocarditis as a complication of indwelling right atrial catheters in leukemic patients. *Cancer* 1984; 54:804–807.
62. Rosen P, Armstrong D: Nonbacterial thrombotic endocarditis in patients with malignant neoplastic diseases. *Am J Med* 1973; 54:23–29.
63. Biller J, Challa VR, Toole JF, Howard VJ: Nonbacterial thrombotic endocarditis. A neurologic perspective of clinicopathologic correlations of 99 patients. *Arch Neurol* 1982; 39:95–98.
64. Mowry F, Reynolds EF: Cardiac rhythm disturbances complicating resectional surgery of the lung. *Ann Intern Med* 1964; 61:688–694.
65. Kirsh MM, Rotman H, Behrendt DM, Orringer MB, Sloan H: Complications of pulmonary resection. *Ann Thorac Surg* 1975; 20:215–236.
66. Wheat MW, Burford TH: Digitalis in surgery: extension of classical indications. *J Thorac Cardiovasc Surg* 1961; 41:162–168.
67. Burman SO: The prophylactic use of digitalis before thoracotomy. *Ann Thorac Surg* 1972; 14:359–368.
68. Ellman H, Dembin H, Seriff N: The rarity of shortening of the Q-T interval in patients with hypercalcemia. *Crit Care Med* 1982; 10:320–322.
69. Wortsman J, Frank S: The QT interval in clinical hypercalcemia. *Clin Cardiol* 1936; 4:57–59.
70. Nierenberg DW, Ransil BJ: Q-aT, interval as a clinical indicator of hypercalcemia. *Am J Cardiol* 1979; 44:243–248.
71. Loffler W: Endocarditis parietalis Fibroplastica mit Bluteosinophilie. Ein eigenartiges Krankheitsbild. *Schwez Med Wochenschr* 1936; 66:817–820.
72. Andy JJ: Helminthiasis, the hypereosinophilic syndrome and endomyocardial fibrosis: some observations and an hypothesis. *Afr J Med Sci* 1983; 12:155–164.
73. Jacobs P, Dubovsky DW, King HS, Blumenthal I: Lymphocytic lymphoma, hypereosinophilia, and endomyocardial fibrosis (clinical conference). *S Afr Med J* 1982; 61:711–713.
74. Yakulis R, Bedetti CD: Loffler's endocarditis. Occurrence with malignant lymphoma with a high content of epithelioid histiocytes ("Lennert's lymphoma"). *Arch Pathol Lab Med* 1983; 107:531–534.
75. Fauci AS, Harley JB, Roberts WC, Ferrans VS, Gralnick HR, Bjornsan BH: The idiopathic hypereosinophilic syndrome. *Ann Intern Med* 1982; 97:78–92.
76. Sekiguchi M, Yu ZX, Take M, Hirae M, Hirosawa K, Shirai T, Ishide T, Takahashi T: Ultrastructural features of the endocardium in patients with eosinophilic heart disease. An endomyocardial biopsy study. *Jpn Circ J* 1984; 48:1375–1382.
77. Davies J, Spry CJ, Sapsford R, Olen EG, de Perez, G, Oakley CM, Goodwin JF: Cardiovascular features of 11 patients with eosinophilic endomyocardial disease. *Q J Med* 1983; 52:23–39.
78. Harley JB, McIntosh CL, Kirklin JJ, Maran BJ, Gottdiener J, Roberts WC, Fauci AS: Atrioventricular valve replacement in the hypereosinophilic syndrome. *Am J Med* 1982; 73:77–81.
79. Davies J, Sapsford R, Brooksby I, Olsen EG, Spry CJ, Oakley CM, Goodwin JF: Successful surgical treatment of two patients with eosinophilic endomyocardial disease. *Br Heart J* 1981; 46:438–445.
80. Cutler DJ, Isner JM, Bracey AW, Hufnagel CA, Conrad PW, Roberts WC, Kerwin DM, Weintraub AM: Hemochromatosis heart disease: an unemphasized cause of potentially reversible restrictive cardiomyopathy. *Am J Med* 1980; 69:923–928.
80a. Fairbanks VF, Baldus WP: Hemochromatosis: the neglected diagnosis. *Mayo Clin Proc* 1986; 61:296–298.
81. McLaren GD, Muir WA, Kellermeyer RW: Iron overload disorders: natural history, pathogenesis, diagnosis, and therapy. *CRC Crit Rev Clin Lab Sci* 1983-1984; 19:205–266.
82. Candell-Riera J, Lu L, Seres L, Gonzalez JB, Batlle J, Permanyer-Miralda G, Garcia-del-Castillo H, Soler-Soler J: Cardiac hemochromatosis: beneficial effects of iron removal therapy. *Am J Cardiol* 1983; 52:824–829.
83. Dabestani A, Child JS, Henze E, Perloff JK, Schan H, Figueroa WG, Schelbert HR, Thessamboon S: Primary hemochromatosis: anatomic and physiologic characteristics of the cardiac ventricles and their response to phlebotomy. *Am J Cardiol* 1984; 54:153–159.
84. Modell B, Berdaukas V: *The Clinical Approach to Thalassemia.* London, Grune & Stratton, 1984.
85. Lewis BS, Rachmilewitz EA, Amitai N, Halan DA, Gotsman MS: Left ventricular function in beta-thalassemia and the effect of multiple transfusions. *Am Heart J* 1978; 96:636–645.
86. Sapoznikov D, Lewis N, Rachmilewitz EA, Gotsman MS, Lewis BS: Left ventricular filling and emptying patterns in anemia due to beta-thalassemia. A computer-assisted electrocardiographic study. *Cardiology* 1982; 69:276–287.
86a. Giardina PJV, Hilgartner MW: Thalassemia: practical points. *Hosp Med* 1985; 21(6):162–205.
86b. Wolfe L, Olivieri N, Sallan D, Colan S, Rose V, Propper R, Freedman MH, Nathan DG: Prevention of cardiac disease by subcutaneous deferoxamine in patients with thalassemia major. *N Engl J Med* 1985; 312:1600–1603.
87. Yee H, Mra R, Nyunt KM: Cardiac abnormalities in the thalassemia syndromes. *Southeast Asian J Trop Med Pub Health* 1984; 15:414–421.
88. Freeman AP, Giles RW, Berdoukas VA, Walsh WF, Choy D, Murray PC: Early left ventricular dysfunction and chelation therapy in thalassemia major. *Ann Intern Med* 1983; 99:450–454.
89. Rossi MA, Carillo SV: Pathogenesis of cardiac hypertrophy in iron

deficiency anemia: the role of noradrenaline. *Br J Exp Pathol* 1982; 63:269–277.

90. Rossi MA, Carillo SV, Oliveira JS: The effect of iron deficiency anemia in the rat on catecholamine levels and heart morphology. *Cardiovasc Res* 1981; 15:313–319.
91. Florenjano F, Diaz G, Regonesi C, Escobar E: Left ventricular function in chronic anemia: evidence of noncatecholamine positive inotropic factor in the serum. *Am J Cardiol* 1984; 54:638–645.
92. Mehta BC, Panjwani DD, Jhala DA: Electrophysiologic abnormalities of heart in iron deficiency anemia. Effect of iron therapy. *Acta Haematol (Basel)* 1983; 70:189–193.
93. Rector WG Jr, Fortuin NJ, Conley CL: Non-hematologic effects of chronic iron deficiency. *Medicine* 1982; 61:382–389.
94. Falk RH, Hood WB: The heart in sickle cell anemia. *Arch Intern Med* 1982; 142:1680–1684.
95. Balfour IC, Covitz W, Davis H, Rao PS, Strong WB, Albert BS: Cardiac size and function in children with sickle cell anemia. *Am Heart J* 1984; 108:345–350.

95a. Arensman FW, Covitz W, Reyes LK, McKie V, McKie K, Davis HC: Digitized echocardiographic assessment of left ventricular wall motion in infants and adolescents with sickle cell anemia, in Doyle EF, Engle MA, Gersony WM, Rashkind WJ, Talner NS (eds): *Abstracts of Second World Congress of Pediatric Cardiology, June 2-6, 1985 New York*, New York, Springer-Verlag, 1985, p 119.

96. Denenberg BS, Criner G, Jones R, Spann JF: Cardiac function in sickle cell anemia. *Am J Cardiol* 1983; 51:1674–1678.
97. Willems HJ, Lawrence C, Frishman WH, Strom JA: The non-invasive comparison of left ventricular performance in sickle cell anemia and chronic aortic regurgitation. *Clin Cardiol* 1983; 6:542–548.
98. Gerry JL, Bulkley BH, Hutchins GM: Clinicopathologic analysis of cardiac dysfunction in 52 patients with sickle cell anemia. *Am J Cardiol* 1978; 42:211–216.

98a. Brown J, Geer M, Covitz W, Hellenbrand W, Leff S, Talner N, Robinson L: Electrocardiographic responses to exercise in sickle cell anemia, in Doyle EF, Engle MA, Gersony WM, Rashkind WJ, Talner NS (eds): *Pediatric Cardiology*, New York, Springer-Verlag, 1986, pp 1111–1116.

99. Manno BV, Burka ER, Hakki A-H, Manno CS, Iskandrian AS, Noone AM: Biventricular function in sickle-cell anemia: radionuclide angiographic and thallium-201 scintigraphic evaluation. *Am J Cardiol* 1983; 52:584–587.

99a. El-Hazmi MAF: Clinical manifestations and laboratory findings of sickle cell anemia in association with α-thalassemia in Saudi Arabia. *Acta Haemat* 1985; 74:155–160.

100. McClung JA, Stein JH, Ambrose JA, Herman MV, Reed GE: Prosthetic heart valves: a review. *Prog Cardiovasc Dis* 1983; 26:237–270.
101. Warnes CA, McIntosh CL, Roberts WC: Wear of the metallic studs on the composite seat of the 2320 Starr–Edwards aortic valve and its clinical consequences. *Am J Cardiol* 1983; 52:1062–1065.
102. Lader E, Kronzon I, Trehan N, Colvin S, Newman W, Roseff I: Severe hemolytic anemia in patients with a porcine aortic valve prosthesis. *J Am Coll Cardiol* 1983; 1:1174–1176.

102a. Schaer DH, Cheng TO, Aaron B: Hemolytic anemia and acute mitral regurgitation caused by a torn leaflet of a porcine mitral prosthetic valve. *Am Heart J*, in press.

103. Olesen KH, Andersen JK, Rygg I: Hemolysis and hyposideraemia in patients with Lillehei–Kaster prosthetic heart valves: a long-term follow-up. *Life Support Syst* 1983; 1:247–253.
104. Hamamoto H, Kitamura K, Takeda H, Bamba M, Takanashi T, Takino T: An altered distribution and elimination of digoxin in anemic patients and experimentally induced anemic rats. *Jpn Circ J* 1984; 48:1197–1202.
105. Gemelli A, Camericci S, Di Benedetto P, Di Nucci GD, Francescani M, Isacchi G: Study of left ventricular function using systolic time intervals in a group of patients with polycythemia vera (Vaquez–Osler disease). *Minerva Med* 1984; 75:2667–2672.
106. Ali M, Fayeni AD, Malcolm D, Braun EV: Intraventricular thrombosis in polycythemia vera: a cause of intractable cardiac failure. *Am Heart J* 1980; 100:520–522.
107. Yeager SB, Freed MD: Myocardial infarction as a manifestation of polycythemia in cyanotic heart disease. *Am J Cardiol* 1984; 53:952–953.

58 Heart in Connective Tissue Diseases

Douglas C. Conaway, MD and Allen R. Myers, MD

The systemic rheumatic diseases are often called collagen-vascular diseases or connective tissue diseases because these loosely linked disorders are typified by inflammatory reactions of connective tissue or blood vessels. Disordered immune responses seem to be important in all of these diseases, that is, an *autoimmune* attack by the body's cellular and humoral defenses on the basic structural components of tissues. However, the varying roles of external antigen triggers (viruses, drugs, and haptens) or primary abnormalities of immune regulation in initiating and perpetuating these disorders have not yet been well worked out. Furthermore, different clinical features of these diseases tend to obscure any pathogenetic similarities; the synovitis of rheumatoid arthritis and the fibrosing microvasculopathy of scleroderma may both be mediated by immunoregulatory abnormalities but with very differing results. Whatever the underlying mechanism of chronic inflammation, each of these rheumatic diseases shares the possibility of involving the heart or aorta in the pathologic process (Table 58.1).

RHEUMATOID ARTHRITIS

Rheumatoid arthritis (RA) is a chronic systemic disease of unknown origin usually dominated by a symmetrical inflammatory synovitis of the peripheral joints. Often, visceral organ involvement can be extremely important in ultimate prognosis and is not uncommon. Patients who have deforming arthritis, are rheumatoid factor positive (circulating antibodies to human IgG), and who have subcutaneous rheumatoid nodules or episcleritis are considered to have highly expressed RA and are much more likely to have significant extraarticular disease.

Cardiac disease associated with RA was initially not appreciated at autopsy; findings were thought to be due to rheumatic fever or nonspecific changes.[1] An evolution of understanding about cardiac involvement has occurred such that it is now understood that both specific granulomas and nonspecific inflammatory changes can occur as part of the basic rheumatoid pathologic process and can involve the entire heart, that is, the pericardium, myocardium, endocardium, and valves as well as the coronary arteries.[2]

PERICARDIAL INVOLVEMENT

Pericarditis is the most common manifestation of RA heart disease with an autopsy frequency of approximately 30% (sum of eight series).[3] This involvement is often inapparent, the clinical diagnosis of a pericardial abnormality being made in only about 2% of cases. A careful study of 100 patients admitted to a hospital and then followed prospectively indicated clinical evidence of pericarditis in only 10%.[3]

The autopsy findings in RA are most commonly nonspecific inflammatory changes and the pericardial abnormalities are no different. Whereas 75% of autopsied cases have a chronic fibrous and adherent pericarditis with gross thickening of the visceral and parietal pericardial surfaces, only 25% have acute fibrinous lesions. Only rarely are classic rheumatoid granulomas found.[3]

Typically, RA pericardial effusions are scanty exudates, yellow to bloody in appearance, with wide variations in white blood cell counts. Gamma globulin concentrations are increased and glucose concentrations are decreased as in rheumatoid pleuritis. Rheumatoid factor can be found,

Table 58.1. Clinical Involvement of the Heart by Connective Tissue Diseases

Type of Involvement	Disease Process					
	RA	SLE	PM/DM	SSc	AS	Vasculitis
Pericarditis	+[a]	+++	0	±	0	0
Myocarditis	±	+	++	++	0	0
Valvulitis	+	+[a]	0	0	±	+[b]
Coronary vasculitis	±		0	0	0	+++[c]
Aortitis	0	0	0	0	+[d]	+[b]

0 = rare or never; ± = unusual; + = occasionally seen; ++ = moderately common; +++ = common.

a = clinically unimportant involvement common at autopsy; b = occasionally seen in Takayasu's arteritis; c = common in polyarteritis nodosa and seen in Kawasaki disease; d = conduction disturbances common when this lesion present.

AS = ankylosing spondylitis; PM/DM = polymyositis/dermatomyositis; RA = rheumatoid arthritis; SSc = systemic sclerosis; SLE = systemic lupus erythematosus.

immune complexes are often present, and immunofluorescence studies have shown immunoglobulin and complement components deposited in pericardial vessels.[4] Thus, the deposition of immunoreactants in pericardial vessels may be the initiating event in an immune complex-mediated pericarditis. Cholesterol crystals or even a frank cholesterol pericarditis can be present as a reflection of the chronicity of the inflammation.[5]

Pericarditis, when active, usually becomes clinically detectable when the joint disease is active, but it can occur at any time in the disease or even precede arthritis.[3] Although clinically recognized cases are often asymptomatic, the diagnosis is usually made on the basis of nonspecific chest pains, electrocardiographic changes, or friction rubs.[3] Rheumatoid pleuritis often accompanies pericarditis (11 of 17 clinically diagnosed cases in one series)[6] and may obscure the interpretation of pain.

To some extent, echocardiography has resolved discrepancies between clinical and autopsy findings. Ultrasound series have shown pericardial thickening or effusion in about one third of the patients who were not selected for cardiac symptoms,[7] and these figures approximate the autopsy prevalence of pericardial inflammation.

Acute pericarditis symptoms are usually self-limited; if severe or prolonged, these symptoms may require the addition of salicylates or nonsteroidal antiinflammatory drugs if a patient is not on such treatment or even the brief use of corticosteroid treatment in modest doses. However, it is important to realize that drug treatment of these symptoms does not seem to alter the natural history of the inflammation or to hasten resolution of effusions.[8] In fact, rheumatoid pericarditis usually persists in a chronic, subclinical form that can smolder indefinitely.[3,9]

Pericardial tamponade or constriction can develop during the course of the pericarditis, but the appearance of these complications does not correlate with the duration of arthritis.[10] Tamponade is less common than constriction, and subacute effusive-constrictive pericarditis may occur.[8,11] This situation pertains when pericardial fluid accumulates in the presence of visceral and parietal pericardial thickening and the hemodynamic impairment that results is a combination of tamponade and constriction.

Any clinical evidence of right heart failure in a patient with RA should prompt investigation with echocardiography and consideration of hemodynamic monitoring. Because of the likelihood that a combination of constriction and tamponade will be present when either of these conditions is diagnosed, pericardiectomy is almost always required and is well tolerated.[12] Failure to treat surgically is associated with a high mortality.[10] Again, there is no evidence that corticosteroids are effective in treating these complications of rheumatoid pericarditis, but it is interesting that sudden discontinuation of corticosteroids has occasionally led to sudden tamponade.[13]

MYOCARDIAL INVOLVEMENT

Approximately 20% of patients with RA have nonspecific lymphocytic and plasma cell infiltrates in the cardiac interstitium at autopsy.[14] This type of infiltrate is a nonspecific inflammatory one, but it occurs more commonly and extensively in rheumatoid hearts than in controls.[14,15] Myocardial rheumatoid granulomas are even less common than nonspecific myocarditis (3% to 5%).[14] It is unusual for either of these processes to be so extensive that myocardial function is compromised, although occasional fatal cases of diffuse myocardial necrosis have been reported. As in other types of cardiac involvement, the presence and extent of myocarditis correlate roughly with the severity of the overall rheumatoid process. Rheumatoid vasculitis as well as pericardial and endocardial inflammation occur more frequently in patients with myocardial involvement.[14] Echocardiographic studies have not consistently shown left ventricular functional abnormalities in RA patients,[7] although some have revealed possible contractile abnormalities.[16]

Before concluding that RA myocarditis is contributing to cardiomegaly or impaired ventricular performance in an individual patient, the effects of hypertension, coronary artery disease (atherosclerotic or arteritic), rheumatoid lung disease, pericardial or valvular disease, or even cardiac amyloid infiltration (unusual in most autopsy series)[14,17] on right and left heart function must be considered. High dose corticosteroids might be useful in the rare case of overwhelming myocarditis, a diagnosis to be considered in systemically ill patients with evidence of vasculitis and sudden deterioration of myocardial function for no other apparent reason.

Conduction disturbances or arrhythmias are infrequent complications in RA that generally occur late in the course of highly expressed RA. Multiple types of pathologic lesions can interfere with conduction or impulse generation. First degree heart block is found at autopsy in cases of rheumatoid arthritis more often than in controls,[17] and the usual lesion responsible is a nonspecific inflammatory infiltrate or typical granuloma near the atrioventricular node or the bundle of His. These inflammatory lesions were found in cases of complete heart block in one RA series[18] and lesser degrees of block probably occur on the same basis. Transition from low to high grade block can occur suddenly, although gradual evolution through intermediate degrees of block is probably more common. Appropriate treatment for high grade block is permanent pacing, because the block is usually below the His bundle. Patients in one series had good results as long as generalized cardiac involvement was not present.[18]

Atrial arrhythmias occur with pericarditis because the superficial location of the sinoatrial node makes it vulnerable to extension of pericardial inflammation.[19] Vasculitic involvement of the sinoatrial or atrioventricular node nutrient arteries has been associated with arrhythmias in several cases.[14,19] Ventricular arrhythmias are unusual unless overwhelming myocardial involvement or coronary vasculitis is present.

VALVULAR INVOLVEMENT

Clinical valvular dysfunction in RA is uncommon, but autopsy evidence of nonspecific valvular inflammation or even rheumatoid granulomas is not rare.[14] The more common nonspecific inflammatory lesions are likely to be part of the rheumatoid process,[8,14] although not all authors agree that these lesions are related to RA.[15] Specific or not, the inflammatory lesions can lead to marked nodular or diffuse deformity of the valve cusp or they can cause minimal focal changes. Typically, they involve the central core of the cusp or valve ring and do not involve the endothelial surface.[8,20] This lack of endothelial involvement may account for the infrequent association of bacterial endocarditis with RA.[8]

Valvular involvement in RA classically occurs in highly expressed RA. The left-sided valves are more commonly affected than the right; mitral, aortic, tricuspid, and pulmonic involvement occurs in descending order of frequency.[8] Although abnormality of the mitral valve is most frequent at autopsy, dysfunction of the aortic valve is more common clinically.[21] Aortic insufficiency is more typically found than stenosis and the mitral valve lesion can be stenotic, incompetent, or both. It is not uncommon for both left-sided valves to have granulomas, and very rarely all four valves are involved.[22]

Valve dysfunction can be so severe that replacement is required, especially when the lesion is aortic insufficiency. Surgical results have been good when the patients are not moribund, although meticulous valve suturing is required to prevent later dehiscence from inflamed anular tissue.[21]

CORONARY ARTERY INVOLVEMENT

Atheromatous or arteritic involvement of coronary vessels in RA is common, and the vasculitic process can affect either small or large coronary arteries. Atherosclerotic lesions appear to be as frequent in RA subjects as in controls,[14,23] but the incidence of myocardial infarction in RA (11%) is significantly less than that in controls (34%) and remains significantly less on review of various autopsy series (8.6% as compared with 22% to 27%).[23] Perhaps concurrent treatment with platelet-inhibiting drugs (aspirin or nonsteroidal antiinflammatory agents) reduces the morbidity and mortality in the RA group.

The vasculitis found most often in autopsy series is a small-vessel, intramyocardial form with varying degrees of round cell infiltration, edema, intimal proliferation, and fibrosis.[14] This bland arteritis is usually clinically inapparent, but it can be associated with pericardial or endocardial abnormalities. Frank myocardial necrosis is uncommon with this lesion, and myocardial function is usually unimpaired.[24]

A rarer but more serious form of large epicardial vessel vasculitis with a polyarteritis nodosa pathologic appearance has been described occasionally in RA.[25] Angina, severe arrhythmias, and myocardial infarction in a patient with highly expressed RA and especially in the setting of active vasculitis elsewhere should suggest this large vessel arteritis. Otherwise, clinical cardiac abnormalities are much more commonly due to atherosclerosis.[8] Systemic corticosteroids or cytotoxic agents may be effective in active vasculitis, but the use of corticosteroids in myocardial infarction may impair healing and even lead to ventricular aneurysm formation.

SYSTEMIC LUPUS ERYTHEMATOSUS

Systemic lupus erythematosus (SLE) is a chronic immunologic disorder characterized by multisystem involvement and remissions and exacerbations. Circulating immune complexes and autoantibodies appear to cause tissue damage and hence organ dysfunction. The laboratory hallmark of the illness is the presence of serum antinuclear antibodies (ANA) in up to 95% of patients.

Early autopsy studies in SLE suggested almost universal cardiac involvement,[26,27] with approximately 50% of patients having clinical cardiac findings.[28] With the evolution of more sensitive laboratory parameters for diagnosis (ANA) and more uniform criteria for diagnosis (American Rheumatism Association criteria), milder cases of SLE are more commonly included in studies and less frequent clinical cardiac involvement is discovered (about 20%).[29,30] Furthermore, corticosteroid therapy in SLE may have affected the natural history of the cardiac lesions and added new drug-mediated detrimental cardiovascular effects.[31]

The basic pathologic process in the pericardial, myocardial, and endocardial lesions of SLE seems to be immune complex-mediated small-vessel injury leading to variable histologic inflammatory infiltration and consequent tissue damage.[27] In an immunofluorescence microscopy study of autopsied SLE subjects, diffuse granular deposits of immunoglobulin were seen in the walls of most myocardial or pericardial blood vessels and a more focal histologic inflammatory injury was noted in the same areas.[32] Similar deposits were seen in the inner zone vessels of endocardial vegetations, and a causal role for the deposits in the genesis of the vegetations was postulated.[33]

PERICARDIAL INVOLVEMENT

Pericarditis is the most common cardiac manifestation of SLE, occurring at autopsy in 43% to 74% of cases.[28,34] It is usually a serofibrinous reaction and occasionally has microscopic evidence of hematoxylin bodies,[35] the characteristic pathologic lesion of SLE. Fibrous change or adhesions predominate in healed forms, but this scarring is less widespread than that in RA. Present necropsy cases reflect the chronic adhesive form, probably because of corticosteroid effects on the inflammatory process.[31]

The pericardial fluid is commonly an exudate with white blood cells less than 10,000 per mm^3 and polymorphonuclear leukocyte predominance. Complement levels are frequently low to absent, and the presence of lupus erythematosus cells, rheumatoid factors, anti-N-DNA, and immune complexes has been recorded in such fluids.[30,36]

Clinically, pericarditis occurs less commonly than at autopsy (17% to 48%),[28,37,38] although some of the variation in incidence reflects differing criteria for diagnosis and disease severity between studies. Symptoms often occur acutely or recurrently in SLE, commonly reflecting the activity of the illness. Pleuritis commonly occurs in association with pericarditis[39]; therefore, either can be responsible for chest pain. Rubs are present in a minority of patients and may even be present in asymptomatic cases.

Using electrocardiography, nonspecific ST-T–wave changes rather than classic pericarditis patterns are usually found.[37] Echocardiography has demonstrated effusion in 6% of asymptomatic patients[40] and 66% of patients with clinically active pericarditis.[41] These findings suggest that pericardial effusions may be transient and that echocardiography is useful in following the activity of pericarditis.

Pericardial tamponade is a more common complication in SLE than in RA, just as clinical evidence of pericardial fluid is more common. Pericardial tamponade has been reported in up to 7% of cases of acute clinical pericarditis in SLE.[39] However, constrictive pericarditis seems to be rare in SLE.[42] Both of these complications have been reported as complications of drug-induced SLE[43,44] (especially procainamide-induced) as well as de novo SLE.

Acute pericarditis may respond to treatment with nonsteroidal antiinflammatory agents; otherwise, low-dose corticosteroid treatment may be required. Larger doses have been used in attempts to resolve large effusions before tamponade occurs, but definite evidence of the benefit of this approach is lacking. Tamponade may require pericardiocentesis, but this procedure should be performed only when tamponade exists or serious infection may be present. Laceration of epicardial coronary arteries or left ventricular punctures with resulting hemopericardium and death have been reported,[34] drastic complications in a situation in which resolution of effusion is the rule. Pericardiectomy is the usual treatment for constriction in SLE as in other causes of this condition.

MYOCARDIAL INVOLVEMENT

Myocardial inflammation rarely causes clinical cardiac failure in SLE and, when present, its severity correlates best with overall disease severity.[34] However, some noninvasive studies suggest that some degree of myocardial dysfunction is common in SLE.[45] Early studies[27,37] found myocardial interstitial lymphocyte and plasma cell infiltrates in about one third of autopsied subjects, but later studies[31] found focal myocarditis in only 8% with interstitial fibrotic lesions in others. Some investigators believe that these interstitial fibrotic lesions represent healed myocarditis and that corticosteroid treatment is responsible for the healing.[31] However, congestive heart failure is more frequent in steroid-treated than in nonsteroid-treated patients, despite healing of focal myocarditis. Presumably, atherosclerotic or hypertensive changes secondary to long-term corticosteroid therapy leads to congestive heart failure more often than does myocarditis.

Impaired myocardial contractility should not be treated any differently in an SLE patient than in a typical patient with congestive heart failure. However, sudden deterioration of myocardial function in the absence of acute large-vessel ischemia, severe hypertension, or other reversible causes of heart failure in a patient with active SLE is the appropriate clinical setting for severe acute myocarditis. A trial of large-dose corticosteroid therapy is warranted in this rare situation.

Serious arrhythmias and conduction disturbances are uncommon in SLE patients except in the preceding setting of generalized myocarditis. However, Ropes[46] found that 10% of 128 patients had first degree heart block, and atrial tachyarrhythmias can occur in acute pericarditis if the superficially located sinoatrial node is involved.[47] At autopsy in patients who had conduction or rhythm disturbances before death, nutrient sinoatrial and atrioventricular node artery inflammation is often present.[47]

ENDOCARDIAL INVOLVEMENT

Since Klemperer et al[27] extended Libman and Sacks' observations[48] on verrucous endocarditis by linking the lesion specifically to SLE, these endocardial and subvalvular excrescences have been repeatedly described in autopsy series, usually in about 50% of cases.[26,37] Active lesions contain lymphocyte and plasma cell infiltrates in areas of vascular degenerating valve tissue. More chronic lesions are fibrotic and thickened but still vascularized.[31] Early studies found these wart-like vegetations coalescing over ventricular endocardial surfaces, often in all four chambers, and especially on the undersurfaces of the mitral and tricuspid valves.[49] Modern autopsy studies have shown that most valve lesions are now left-sided, less frequent, and usually inactive or healed lesions, probably because of the effects of corticosteroid treatment.[31]

Most Libman–Sacks lesions are asymptomatic and rarely associated with murmurs (Figure 58.1). However, they can sometimes cause significant valvular deformity and dysfunction.[30] Mitral and aortic valve replacement has sometimes been required, usually because of regurgitant lesions.[50,51] Some believe that the healing process initiated by corticosteroids may cause retraction of valve tissue and adherence of valvular structures to underlying endocardium, thus causing a higher frequency of valve dysfunction than that in the presteroid era.[31]

Because verrucae often extend through the endothelial lining of the valve, fibrin thrombi can form on them and can therefore embolize[52] or provide a nidus for bacterial

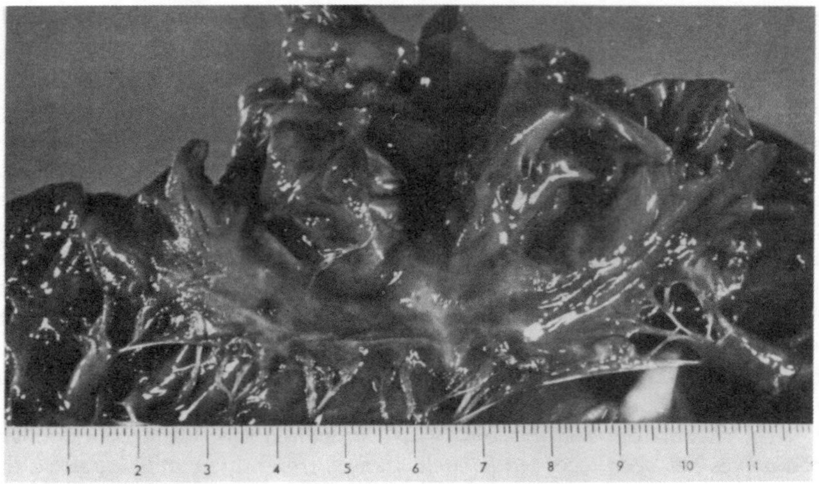

Figure 58.1. Libman–Sacks endocarditis verrucae on endothelial surface of mitral valve in patient with systemic lupus erythematosus.

growth. Therefore, the incidence of bacterial endocarditis is apparently higher than that in RA.[53] Echocardiography may demonstrate vegetations in patients with lupus erythematosus with infective endocarditis, but resolution of M-mode and two-dimensional machines is inadequate to visualize most noninfectious vegetations, which are usually smaller than 2 mm.[53]

CORONARY ARTERY INVOLVEMENT

Symptomatic coronary artery disease in SLE seems to be more frequent in the era of large-dose corticosteroid therapy. In the presteroid period, extramural coronary arteries were usually uninvolved, and occasionally small intramural coronary arteries had intimal proliferative lesions or fibrinoid necrosis.[31] In contrast, recent coronary pathologic specimens in steroid-treated patients show that 40% of the small intramural arteries are involved by endothelial proliferation and that significant extramural vascular atherosclerotic lesions are present in a similar percentage.[31] Although these lesions occurred only in patients treated with corticosteroids for longer than one year, another recent study[54] associated uncontrolled hypertension and cholesterol levels with the formation of lesions in steroid-treated patients. That these pathologic lesions are functionally important seems clear, and it has been shown that significant segmental perfusion abnormalities occurred in 38% of randomly selected patients with SLE studied by rest and exercise thallium scanning.[55]

Animal and human studies suggest that vasculitic involvement of coronary arteries can lead to the development of accelerated atherosclerotic plaques in the same areas. Rabbits subjected to immune complex-mediated vessel lesions quickly develop atherosclerotic plaques at the site of immunologic damage that cannot be distinguished from typical human atheromas.[56,57] Human autopsy studies have shown areas of atherosclerosis coexisting with areas of vasculitis,[46] and immunologic vessel injury has been found by immunofluorescence studies in intramural and extramural coronary arteries of patients with SLE.[32,58] Therefore, it is reasonable to hypothesize an immune complex-mediated vascular injury leading to intimal damage and initiation of atheromatous changes. Presumably, steroid-related alterations of blood pressure and lipids would facilitate the development and progression of the atheromatous lesion after injury.

Pure large vessel arteritic changes without atheromas have been described in case reports,[58,59] but these lesions are found most often in nonsteroid-treated patients who have active systemic disease and evidence of vasculitis elsewhere. These lesions have not been found in recent autopsy studies[31,54] of steroid-treated populations, suggesting that moderate-dose corticosteroids may have modified the injury.

It is apparent from the foregoing data that corticosteroids should be used cautiously in SLE and at the lowest possible dose to control manifestations of illness that can be treated in no less toxic way. Perhaps more importantly, hypertension and lipid disorders should be aggressively controlled. Oral contraceptive use and smoking should also be discouraged for their apparent contribution to accelerated atherogenesis. Clearly, coronary artery involvement is a serious complication of SLE with 20% of patients in a recent autopsy study dying of cardiac causes (myocardial infarction, congestive heart failure, and arrhythmia).[31]

Obvious large-vessel coronary arteritis should be aggressively treated with large-dose corticosteroids, but the clinical and perhaps arteriographic picture must be carefully evaluated before administering prednisone for coronary ischemia or infarction.

NEONATAL LUPUS SYNDROME

Infants with neonatal lupus syndrome can present with congenital heart block, typical lupus skin lesions, or both manifestations.[60] The pathophysiologic mechanism seems to be different from the diffuse immune complex-mediated small-vessel injury thought responsible for the cardiac lesions of adult SLE. In this syndrome, maternal IgG antibodies to *Ro* (a soluble tissue ribonucleoprotein) can be demonstrated in serum samples of mothers who give birth to infants with congenital heart block and transiently in the serum of the infants themselves.[61] Presumably, the anti-*Ro* antibodies cross the placenta, bind to fetal cardiac tissue, and are somehow associated with the immune injury. Immunofluorescence studies have confirmed diffuse immunoglobulin deposition in the cardiac tissue of an affected infant.[62]

Approximately 50% of the mothers giving birth to infants with neonatal lupus syndrome have clinical or serologic evidence of rheumatic disease, most commonly SLE or Sjögren's syndrome.[63] Mothers who have had one affected child seem to be at significant risk of having a second, but there is no evidence yet that treatment of the mother with corticosteroids protects against the development of the syndrome in the fetus.[60]

In most cases the conduction changes remain, and many children require permanent pacemaker implantation.[60] Despite the early onset of a serious conduction disorder, most affected children survive well into adulthood without clinical SLE, if they survive the neonatal period.[64]

POLYMYOSITIS/DERMATOMYOSITIS

Polymyositis/dermatomyositis (PM/DM) is an idiopathic inflammatory muscle disease associated with prominent proximal muscle weakness, muscle enzyme elevations, characteristic electromyographic myopathic patterns, and inflammatory infiltrates on skeletal muscle biopsy. Associated clinical features can include rash (dermatomyositis), arthritis, pulmonary interstitial disease, and cardiac involvement. Inflammatory myositis also occurs with other autoimmune diseases in "overlap" presentations (eg, scleroderma and SLE).

Cardiac involvement in PM/DM approaches 30%,[65,66] but autopsy studies select sicker patients with longer duration of disease. Findings include generalized interstitial and perivascular mononuclear cell infiltrates as well as fibrotic interstitial change, apparently early and late manifestations of the same inflammatory process. On occasion, abnormalities in skeletal and cardiac muscle are identical, but usually the skeletal muscle inflammation is more impressive. Also, intramyocardial small-vessel intimal proliferative change or medial hyperplasia is common, but resulting ischemic muscle necrosis is not.[66] Pericarditis or valvular involvement is unusual except in "overlap" syndromes. Cardiac findings appear to be more frequent in PM and less common in DM.[67] When symptomatic, patients present with cardiomyopathy, arrhythmias, and conduction disturbances.

Congestive heart failure occurred in about 7% of the series of Bohan et al,[67] but some of these patients may not have had cardiomyopathy. Myocardial cellular infiltrate and fibrosis are thought to be responsible for impaired myocardial contractility when generalized, and they apparently can lead to overt congestive failure if severe. A second form of cardiomyopathy has also been found in PM/DM: a hyperdynamic state. The prevalence of this form is unknown, but it has been described clinically[68] and echocardiographically[69] and it may be related to increased arteriovenous shunting of blood through diseased skeletal muscle. However, there is no definite proof that shunting occurs.

Atrial and ventricular arrhythmias occur commonly on routine electrocardiography,[69] and a high prevalence of abnormal Holter monitor abnormalities has been found in a population studied for probable myocardial involvement.[70] Conduction disturbances are not as frequent and high-grade blocks usually occur in patients with longstanding and generalized myocardial involvement.[71] Patients with PM/DM with complete heart block evaluated on electrophysiologic study generally have block distal to the atrioventricular node and have a poor prognosis unless treated by permanent pacemaker insertion.[71]

Recent noninvasive studies in PM/DM have helped to quantify subclinical cardiac involvement. An elevated MB fraction of creatine phosphokinase (CK) is thought to be a good indication of cardiac involvement, and serious abnormalities on one or more noninvasive tests (electrocardiography, echocardiography, Holter monitoring, exercise thallium-201 scanning, or radionuclide ventriculography) were found in all patients with elevated MB fractions studied.[70] Although other investigators point out that inflamed skeletal muscle may contain an MB band,[72] fractionation of CK may be a useful screening test for myocardial involvement. Holter monitoring picked up the greatest number of serious problems in one study[70] and appears to be a reasonable second step in evaluation, if the clinical situation warrants.

Although morbidity and mortality appear to be improved when corticosteroids are used to treat skeletal muscle disease,[67] treatment of cardiovascular manifestations with these agents or immunosuppressive drugs is less settled. Only random case reports[70] exist of the reversibility of cardiac abnormalities with large-dose corticosteroid treatment. Most commonly, the cardiac abnormalities are active when the skeletal muscle disease is active, and it is usually the skeletal muscle disease that prompts treatment. Echocardiography or radionuclide ventriculography may help to differentiate the hyperdynamic from the congestive forms of cardiomyopathy. Presumably, beta blockade is more useful for the high output state.[68]

SYSTEMIC SCLEROSIS (SCLERODERMA)

Systemic sclerosis (SSc) is characterized by widespread small-vessel obliterative disease and fibrotic changes involving the skin and multiple internal organs. A subtle disorder of immune regulation may be important in its pathogenesis, as suggested by abnormalities in cell-mediated immunity, the possible presence of a circulating factor toxic to endothelial cells, serologic evidence of autoantibody production, overlap syndromes with other rheumatic diseases, and a syndrome virtually identical to SSc developing in the graft-versus-host disease of bone marrow transplantation.[73]

The classic form of the disease presents as diffuse skin thickening involving not only fingers, face, and arms, but also trunk; this form is frequently associated with fibrotic involvement of the lungs, gastrointestinal tract, kidney, and heart. Myocardial and renal involvement are limited almost exclusively to this group of patients.[74] Raynaud's phenomenon is present in 95% of patients.

An apparently distinct form of SSc is the so-called CREST syndrome (subcutaneous Calcinosis, Raynaud's syndrome, Esophageal dysmotility, Sclerodactyly, and Telangiectasias). This distal, acrosclerotic form is usually more indolent, with finger skin thickening and Raynaud's syndrome dominating the early clinical picture. However, pulmonary vascular involvement can lead to pulmonary hypertension and death decades after the initial presentation.[75]

Cardiac involvement in SSc reflects the underlying obliterative microvascular abnormality characteristic of this disease. Patchy myocardial fibrosis is the predominant lesion, involving all layers of the heart and not related to extramural coronary artery flow distribution.[76] Another distinct pathologic lesion, contraction band necrosis, is often found as well, and may be a precursor of the fibrotic lesion.[77] This form of ischemic muscle death is different from coagulation necrosis, the lesion found with permanent coronary artery occlusion. Contraction band necrosis is a description of the peculiar segmentation of dying myocardial cell cytoplasm into transverse bands, and it was first recognized as a distinct entity in patients dying from coronary bypass surgery.[78] This type of myocardial death occurs when ischemia is followed by reperfusion. Therefore, in SSc, "reperfusion necrosis" might occur following prolonged myocardial vasospasm, especially if the vessels involved were the small intramural ones that often show medial hypertrophy and intimal proliferation. The necrotic-fibrotic lesion with its variable small-vessel involvement is found commonly at autopsy[77,79] and can involve the conduction system as well. Postmortem fibrous or fibrofibrinous pericarditis is also common, but valvular involvement is rare.[79,80] Atherosclerosis of epicardial vessels occurs with the same frequency as that in autopsy controls[79]; if SSc affects the large coronary arteries, it does so rarely.

PERICARDIAL INVOLVEMENT

Clinical pericardial involvement is much less common than autopsy evidence, which is seen in approximately one half of patients.[79,80] Only four of 210 patients in one large series[80] presented with symptoms or signs of acute pericarditis. Eleven other patients had chronic, moderately large effusions, and these clinically detectable effusions seemed to be associated with a high frequency of myocardial involvement, congestive heart failure, renal failure, and early mortality. Pericardial tamponade[81] and constriction,[79] two complications that are common in RA and SLE, are rare in SSc. Pericardial fluid from patients with scleroderma is usually an exudate, but it does not have the active immunologic characteristics of RA or SLE fluid.[82] Scleroderma is most often the only explanation for the pericarditis, although certainly congestive heart failure or uremia can be complicating factors. Echocardiographic studies suggest that pericardial involvement approaches autopsy figures.[83]

MYOCARDIAL INVOLVEMENT

In early studies, primary myocardial scleroderma has been confused with the secondary cardiac effects of systemic hypertension, atherosclerosis, and pulmonary hypertension.[84] However, more recent autopsy studies have clearly documented its importance in causing congestive heart failure, angina with normal coronary arteries, and arrhythmias or conduction disturbances.[77] Furthermore, noninvasive studies have matched functional impairments to the demonstrated pathologic changes and shown distinctions between the CREST and diffuse forms of SSc.[85]

Intractable congestive heart failure due to extensive myocardial fibrosis occurred in 8% of a large autopsy series,[77] a frequency approximated in other studies when secondary causes of congestive heart failure are eliminated. The typical presentation is a congestive cardiomyopathy, although a less common restrictive hemodynamic picture has also been described.[86]

Importantly, contrasting results in myocardial functional studies of CREST and diffuse scleroderma subsets have been demonstrated.[85,87] Using pulmonary function tests, radionuclide ventriculography, rest/exercise thallium-201 imaging, and cardiac catheterization, resting microvascular perfusion abnormalities were found in the diffuse group; these abnormalities worsened with exercise and were commonly associated with impaired left ventricular performance. Conversely, CREST patients had minor perfusion defects that did not increase with exercise and were not associated with left ventricular functional impairment. However, 36% of these patients did have abnormal right ventricular function, apparently due to isolated pulmonary vascular disease. Therefore, these different forms of SSc may have completely different forms of cardiac involvement, presumably with different prognoses.

Noncardiac chest pain is common in SSc, but angina with normal large coronary arteries can occur in as many as 25% of patients.[88] Ischemic electrocardiographic change or infarction has been noted in patients with normal coronary arteries, probably on the basis of vasospastic disease of the intramural coronary arteries.[89] Most of these patients died suddenly, apparently because of ischemia or arrhythmia. Obviously, the importance of this scleroderma anginal syndrome must not be minimized in a patient who has a normal coronary angiogram.

Arrhythmias and conduction disturbances occur in a high percentage of patients. A prospective study[90] with electrocardiography and Holter monitoring found resting electrocardiographic abnormalities in 32%, mostly first-degree heart block or left anterior hemiblock. Holter monitoring showed abnormalities in 62%, including 34% with atrial tachyarrhythmias and 40% with ventricular arrhythmias (10% with ventricular tachycardia). Electrophysiologic testing performed in some of these patients demonstrated that the sinoatrial node functional abnormalities were frequent and more common than atrioventricular node dysfunction and that His-Purkinje system abnormalities were unusual. These findings correlate well with anatomic studies showing frequent fibrosis of the sinoatrial node and proximal atrioventricular node but less common changes in the bundle branches.[91] Although it has been suggested that atrioventricular conduction disturbances correlate best with the extent of myocardial fibrotic damage,[77,92] other studies note that specific conduction system lesions are important and can occur before interference with myocardial function is manifest.[91,93] However, complex ventricular arrhythmias certainly seem to be more common when more extensive myocardial disease is present and are often responsible for sudden death.[89,90] Holter monitoring and exercise electrocardiography[94] are useful techniques for uncovering serious arrhythmias that require treatment.

Scleroderma is a disease with no satisfactory treatment, and symptomatic myocardial involvement is associated with short survival.[95] Separation of the subsets of diffuse scleroderma and CREST is useful for management and prognosis, because primary myocardial impairment occurs in the former and delayed pulmonary vascular changes in the latter. Case reports of reversal of myocardial abnormalities with D-penicillamine have been reported,[96,97] and preliminary conclusions from a large retrospective series[98] are that D-penicillamine treatment of patients with diffuse SSc is associated with a reduced rate of new visceral organ involvement and improved five-year survival rate. Clearly, prospective studies are needed, but these data are encouraging.

Finally, treatment of pulmonary hypertension due to fixed pulmonary arterial lesions or severe interstitial fibrosis has been discouraging. However, trials with traditional vasodilators (eg, nitroglycerine or hydralazine) or a calcium channel blocking agent (nifedipine) are warranted because patients without end-stage lesions may respond.[99]

SPONDYLOARTHROPATHIES

The spondyloarthropathies are enthesopathies, disorders associated with inflammatory changes where tendons and ligaments insert into bone.[100] Rheumatoid arthritis, in contrast, primarily involves inflammatory changes of the synovial lining of joints. Other important reasons for separating these disorders from RA are the presence of inflammatory changes of the sacroiliac joints and spine, association with histocompatibility antigen HLA-B27, typical absence of rheumatoid factor, and distinct extraarticular manifestations of disease including aortic and cardiac lesions.

Overlapping features of these syndromes often blur distinctions between them. Ankylosing spondylitis is the prototypical disease with a clinical course dominated by inflammation of axial joints and progressive spinal fusion and deformity. Usually less obvious and inconsistently present are anterior uveitis, asymmetric peripheral arthritis, and uncommonly apical pulmonary fibrosis. Reiter's syndrome usually has more prominent peripheral asymmetric arthropathy and less severe spondylitis, with variable urethritis, conjunctivitis, mucocutaneous lesions, and diarrhea. The arthropathy of psoriasis is categorized by its association with typical skin lesions, and the arthropathy of inflammatory bowel disease by its association with typical ulcerative colitis or granulomatous enteritis.

All of the spondyloarthropathies can be associated with typical cardiovascular lesions, but ankylosing spondylitis and Reiter's syndrome far more commonly than psoriatic or bowel-associated arthropathies.[101,102] In fact, recent investigations have popularized the concept of a proximal aortitis as an independent manifestation of an HLA-B27 associated disorder similar to anterior uveitis.[103] This hypothesis would explain occasional cases of severe aortic involvement and minimal joint disease or cases in which cardiac manifestations precede the joint changes by many years.[104]

The aortitis is primarily an adventitial process: scattered mononuclear cells, thick fibrous tissue proliferation, and vasa vasorum obliteration occur in the outer layer of the aorta, with secondary medial scarring and intimal fibrous proliferation. These pathologic changes are most prominent in the proximal aorta behind the sinuses of Valsalva and extending distally only a few centimeters. Proximally, the dense fibrous scarring involves the aortic valve cusps and the sinuses of Valsalva, and the lesion often extends as a thick band into the anterior mitral leaflet and interventricular septum.[104]

The areas of histologic abnormality predict the anatomic consequences. Aortic insufficiency results from thickening and shortening of aortic valve cusps, from displacement of the cusps into the ventricle by the fibrotic knob in the aorta, and from dilation of the aortic root. Mitral regurgitation occasionally occurs if the anterior mitral leaflet is thickened and distorted by the scar, and conduction disturbances can occur if the process extends into the interventricular septum to disrupt the atrioventricular node or proximal bundle branches. Myocardial fibrosis or perivascular lymphocytic infiltration is rarely seen and is not usually associated with hemodynamic compromise. Finally, pericarditis is very uncommon even at autopsy.[104]

Comparisons of relative frequency of aortic involvement between ankylosing spondylitis and Reiter's syndrome are difficult because self-limited Reiter's syndrome is common and some of the reported cases of ankylosing spondylitis with cardiac manifestations are probably Reiter's syndrome. In both, cardiac abnormalities increase with the duration of disease and the presence of other extraarticular manifestations such as anterior uveitis. Graham and Smythe's classic study[101] of ankylosing spondylitis suggests that 3.5% of patients with ankylosing spondylitis have aortic insufficiency after 15 years of disease, but that as many as 10% have this lesion after 30 years of illness. Prolongation of atrioventricular conduction also increases in frequency with time; 2.7% of patients at 15 years and 8.5% of those at 30 years of disease have an increased PR interval. The presence of these lesions is much more common when peripheral joint involvement accompanies spondylitis.

Clinical valvular involvement is much more commonly aortic insufficiency than mitral regurgitation, as would be expected from the pathologic findings.[104] The aortic lesion tends to become gradually more severe over time,[101] although precipitous functional deterioration can occur.[105] Cardiac involvement, once present, seems to stabilize and not require intervention,[106] but these findings may be a function of the indolent nature of the inflammation. Both aortic and mitral valve replacement surgery have been well tolerated in clinically severe lesions.[105] Two-dimensional echocardiography seems to be useful in screening for the presence of aortic root dilation as a manifestation of the inflammatory process.[107]

Conduction disturbances may occur early in the disease process as a result of acute inflammatory changes, but they generally occur as a late manifestation caused by fibrous involvement of the specialized conducting tissues. Electrophysiologic studies,[108] performed in several patients with late HLA-B27 associated conduction disturbances, demonstrated that all had proximal atrioventricular block with prolonged AH intervals and normal HV times. Fluctuating degrees of atrioventricular block are common, but the typical course is a gradually increasing impairment of conduction; however, if required, most of these patients tolerate permanent pacing well. Of interest is the report that patients with spondyloarthropathies made up 12.6% of a group of 223 men requiring permanent pacemaker insertion, thus highlighting the relative frequency of significant conduction disease in patients with these conditions.[109]

VASCULITIS

Although there is much disagreement about clinical and pathologic classifications of vasculitis, reasonably well-defined syndromes exist, which are characterized by necrosis and inflammation of blood vessel walls, some of which may be initiated by circulating immune complexes. Vasculitis can exist as a secondary manifestation of an infectious or rheumatic disease and can also be a primary feature of an idiopathic condition.

Clinical cardiac involvement in the vasculitides is generally a manifestation of large- or medium-sized vessel vasculitis.[110] Therefore, Takayasu's arteritis commonly affects the aorta or large systemic and pulmonary vessels with cardiac involvement only secondarily. Giant cell or temporal arteritis can affect the same vessels but much less commonly. Polyarteritis nodosa and mucocutaneous lymph node syndrome (Kawasaki disease) affect large coronary arteries and present as congestive failure, arrhythmias, or myocardial infarction. In contrast, Wegener's granulomatosus usually affects smaller vessels, and although cardiac involvement is not uncommon pathologically, it is rarely clinically manifest.

TAKAYASU'S ARTERITIS (PULSELESS DISEASE)

Takayasu's arteritis is predominantly a disease of young women and is more frequent in Orientals. Involvement of the aortic arch and its branches can lead to the characteristic presentation of "pulseless disease" because of the frequency with which large-vessel occlusion occurs. Pathologically, a granulomatous infiltration of mononuclear cells and occasionally multinucleated giant cells extends into all layers of the vessel, producing stenotic areas where endothelial proliferation occurs or aneurysms where the vessel structure has been weakened by the inflammatory process.[111]

Patients can present with a systemic prodrome such as polymyalgia rheumatica or with symptoms and signs of large-vessel occlusion, or both.[110] Aortic arch angiographic studies are usually required in the evaluation of these patients, because biopsy of the involved large arteries is difficult.[111] Either corticosteroid treatment or large-vessel reconstructive surgery may be needed, depending on the extent and reversibility of involvement at diagnosis.[110]

Cardiovascular manifestations are not uncommon in Takayasu's arteritis. Hypertension is present in more than 50% of patients, either from impaired vascular compliance due to large-vessel involvement or from ischemia due to renal artery involvement.[112] Blood pressure must be measured in the legs because of the common impairment of upper extremity blood flow by the disease. Right- or left-sided cardiac failure is present in about one third of patients, reflecting pulmonary artery involvement or systemic hypertension, respectively.[113]

Less common cardiovascular manifestations such as angina on the basis of narrowing of coronary artery ostia by the proximal aorta inflammatory process are also seen. These lesions have been successfully treated by coronary bypass grafting.[114] A peculiar lymphocytic and fibrotic process extending from the aortitis can occasionally involve cardiac valves (all four in one instance),[115] but significant hemodynamic compromise is unusual. This lesion may be responsible for the mild aortic insufficiency seen in 5% to 8% of cases.[116]

GIANT CELL ARTERITIS (TEMPORAL ARTERITIS)

Giant cell arteritis involves the same size of vessel as Takayasu's arteritis with a very similar pathologic process, although giant cells are more commonly found in biopsy specimens.[111] The clinical features of giant cell arteritis are typically much different, however. Giant cell arteritis usually occurs in older white patients and preferentially involves carotid artery branches. Consequently, vascular headache and ischemic ocular symptoms predominate over those of peripheral vessel occlusion. Polymyalgia rheumatica is present in up to 50% of cases, and systemic and ischemic symptoms seem more corticosteroid-responsive than do those in Takayasu's arteritis.[111]

Cardiac involvement can occur in the 10% to 15% of patients who have peripheral large-vessel involvement.[117] Aortitis has been reported to lead to aortic dissection,[118] rupture,[117] and aortic valvular insufficiency with congestive heart failure.[119] Giant cell arteritis can involve coronary arteries rarely and lead to myocardial infarction.[118]

POLYARTERITIS NODOSA

Small and medium-sized muscular arteries are the vessels most typically involved in classic polyarteritis nodosa; the gastrointestinal tract, kidney, peripheral nervous system, and the heart are the organ systems commonly affected.[110] Although some cases are associated with a history of hepatitis B infection or intravenous amphetamine abuse, many are idiopathic. Segmental panarteritic lesions of varying age are seen in pathologic specimens, and luminal obliteration, thrombosis, or aneurysm formation lead to clinical evidence of ischemic dysfunction.[111] Corticosteroids in large doses are used to treat acute manifestations,[120] and cytotoxic agents have been successfully employed in resistant cases.[111]

Cardiac lesions are extremely common[113] and usually present as congestive heart failure. As many as one half of patients have congestive heart failure primarily related to hypertension or coronary vasculitis.[121] A recent autopsy series[122] evaluated corticosteroid effects on cardiac lesions, and active vasculitis was much less common in steroid-treated patients, but congestive failure was just as common. Presumably, accelerated coronary atherosclerotic lesions led to myocardial infarction as often as vasculitis did, and hypertension was no better controlled in steroid-treated patients. Pericarditis can occur in 4% clinically[113] but up to 14% at autopsy[121] as part of the basic inflammatory process. Vasculitis of nutrient arteries to the sinoatrial node and occasionally atrioventricular node has been described,[123] and occasional cases of supraventricular tachycardia, atrial flutter, or atrial fibrillation may occur on the basis of this type of involvement.

MUCOCUTANEOUS LYMPH NODE SYNDROME (KAWASAKI DISEASE)

A puzzling and newly described syndrome referred to as the mucocutaneous lymph node syndrome can include coronary or systemic vasculitic involvement. Initially described in Japan by Kawasaki,[124] mucocutaneous lymph node syndrome is an acute febrile illness usually affecting young infants with prominent mucocutaneous lesions and lymphadenopathy. Although most cases are self limited, 1% to 2% of affected children die in the convalescent phase from complications of coronary vasculitis. This arteritis is pathologically identical to that previously recognized as infantile polyarteritis nodosa.[124] However, it appears to have more prominent adventitial inflammation than the late childhood or adult forms of polyarteritis nodosa and lacks fibrinoid necrosis.[125] Because of identical pathologic pictures, prominent coronary artery involvement, and potentially similar visceral vessel abnormalities, some have argued that fatal mucocutaneous lymph node syndrome and infantile polyarteritis nodosa are severe forms of a generally self-limited disease process.[125]

Using clinical parameters (electrocardiography, echocardiography, and chest x-ray), cardiac abnormalities can be found in as many as 70% of patients[126] and angiography shows coronary aneurysms in 15%.[127] However, early carditis does not predict later aneurysm formation,[128] although higher temperature and longer duration of fever do.[129] Two-dimensional echocardiography shows most aneurysms regressing spontaneously.[130,131] Left ventricular dysfunction may be present acutely and transiently in the absence of coronary aneurysm, but its duration is increased in the presence of coronary aneurysms.[132] Large doses of salicylates may facilitate regression of aneurysms or prevent thrombosis in an inflamed vessel.[133] The use of corticosteroids is controversial[134]; in one controlled study the incidence of coronary aneurysms was 65% in patients given steroids compared with 20% in those given no anti-inflammatory drugs and 11% in those given aspirin.[135] Treatment has not been clearly shown to affect either the course of coronary artery disease, including the development of myocardial infarction,[136] or the mortality; sudden death of patients who have apparently completely recovered is well recognized.[136,137]

More than two decades after its original description, Kawasaki disease remains a mystery. That it is not purely a Japanese disease is evidenced by the fact that outbreaks have recently occurred in Hawaii, the continental United States, Canada, Australia, and Finland, and sporadic cases have been reported among the Brazilian, British, Eskimo, French, German, Icelander, Italian, Spanish, Thai, and West Indian populations. The long-term outlook for patients who have had Kawasaki disease, even those who have not apparently had any cardiac involvement, is completely unknown at this time. Further research into all aspects of Kawasaki disease is therefore urgently needed.

REFERENCES

1. Baggenstoss A, Rosenberg F: Cardiac lesions associated with chronic infectious arthritis. *Arch Intern Med* 1941; 67:241–258.
2. Sokoloff L: The heart in rheumatoid arthritis. *Am Heart J* 1953; 45:635–643.
3. Kirk J, Cosh J: The pericarditis of rheumatoid arthritis. *Quart J Med* 1969; 38:397–423.
4. Butman S, Espinoza LR, Del Carpio J, Osterland CK: Rheumatoid pericarditis. Rapid deterioration with evidence of local vasculitis. *JAMA* 1977; 238:2394–2396.
5. Brawley R, Vasko J, Morrow A: Cholesterol pericarditis. Considerations of its pathogenesis and treatment. *Am J Med* 1966; 41:235–248.
6. Franco A, Levine H, Hall A: Rheumatoid pericarditis. Report of 17 cases diagnosed clinically. *Ann Intern Med* 1972; 77:837–844.
7. Mac Donald WJ, Crawford MH, Klippel JH, Zvaifler NJ, O'Rourke RA: Echocardiographic assessment of cardiac structure and function in patients with rheumatoid arthritis. *Am J Med* 1977; 63:890–896.
8. Iveson J, Pomerance A: Cardiac involvement in rheumatoid disease. *Clin Rheum Dis* 1977; 3:467–500.
9. Nomeir A, Turner R, Watts L: Cardiac involvement in rheumatoid arthritis. Follow-up study. *Arthritis Rheum* 1979; 22:561–564.
10. Thadani U, Iveson J, Wright V: Cardiac tamponade, constrictive pericarditis, and pericardial resection in rheumatoid arthritis. *Medicine* 1975; 54:261–270.
11. Hancock E: Subacute effusive–constrictive pericarditis. *Circulation* 1971; 43:183–192.
12. Burney D, Martin CH, Thomas CS, Fisher RD, Bender HW: Rheumatoid pericarditis. Clinical significance and operative management. *J Thorac Cardiovasc Surg* 1979; 77:511–515.
13. Matthew P: Pericardial tamponade secondary to sudden steroid withdrawal in chronic rheumatoid arthritis. *Chest* 1977; 72:532–534.
14. Lebowitz W: The heart in rheumatoid arthritis. A clinical and pathologic study of 62 cases. *Ann Intern Med* 1963; 58:102–123.
15. Bonfiglio T, Atwater E: Heart disease in patients with seropositive rheumatoid arthritis. A controlled autopsy study and review. *Arch Intern Med* 1969; 124:714–719.
16. Bacon PA, Gibson DG: Cardiac involvement in rheumatoid arthritis. An echocardiographic study. *Ann Rheum Dis* 1974; 33:20–24.
17. Cathcart E, Spodick D: Rheumatoid heart disease. A study of the incidence and nature of cardiac lesions in rheumatoid arthritis. *N Engl J Med* 1962; 266:959–964.
18. Ahern M, Lever JV, Cosh J: Complete heart block in rheumatoid arthritis. *Ann Rheum Dis* 1983; 42:389–397.
19. James TN: De subitaneis mortibus. Rheumatoid arthritis and ankylosing spondylitis. *Circulation* 1977; 55:669–677.
20. Roberts WC, Kehoe JA, Carpenter DF, Golden A: Cardiac valvular lesions in rheumatoid arthritis. *Arch Intern Med* 1968; 122:141–146.
21. Devlin A, Goldstraw P, Caves P: Aortic valve replacement in rheumatoid aortic incompetence. *Thorax* 1978; 33:612–615.
22. Carpenter DF, Golden A, Roberts WC: Quadrivalvular rheumatoid heart disease associated with left bundle branch block. *Am J Med*: 1967; 43:922–929.
23. Davis R, Engleman E: Incidence of myocardial infarction in patients with rheumatoid arthritis. *Arthritis Rheum* 1974; 17:527–533.
24. Sokoloff L, Bunim J: Vascular lesions in rheumatoid arthritis. *J Chronic Dis* 1957; 5:668–687.
25. Graef I, Hickey D, Altmann V, Rosenthal J: Cardiac lesions in rheumatoid arthritis. *Proc NY Path Soc* 1948; February 26:15–17.
26. Humphreys EN: The cardiac lesions of acute disseminated lupus erythematosus. *Ann Intern Med* 1948; 28:12–14.
27. Klemperer P, Pollack A, Baehr G: Pathology of disseminated lupus erythematosus. *Arch Pathol* 1941; 32:569–631.
28. Harvey AM, Shulman LE, Tumulty PA, Conley CL, Schoenrich EH: Systemic lupus erythematosus: review of the literature and clinical analysis of 138 cases. *Medicine* 1954; 33:291–437.

29. Grigor R, Edmonds J, Lewkonia R, Bresnihan B, Hughes GRV: Systemic lupus erythematosus: a prospective analysis. *Ann Rheum Dis* 1978; 37:121–128.
30. Chang RW: Cardiac manifestations of systemic lupus erythematosus. *Clin Rheum Dis* 1982; 8:197–206.
31. Bulkley BH, Roberts WC: The heart in systemic lupus erythematosus and the changes induced in it by corticosteroid therapy: a study of 36 necropsy patients. *Am J Med* 1975; 58:243–264.
32. Bidani A: Immunopathology of cardiac lesions in fatal systemic lupus erythematosus. *Am J Med* 1980; 69:849–858.
33. Shapiro RF, Gamble CN, Wiesner KB, Castles JJ, Wolf AW, Hurley EJ, Salel AF: Immunopathogenesis of Libman–Sack's endocarditis. Assessment by light and immunofluorescent microscopy in two patients. *Ann Rheum Dis* 1977; 36:508–516.
34. Kong TQ, Kellum RE, Haserik JR: Clinical diagnosis of cardiac involvement in systemic lupus erythematosus. *Circulation* 1962; 26:7–11.
35. Brigden W, Bywaters EGL, Lessof MH, Ross IP: The heart in systemic lupus erythematosus. *Br Heart J* 1960; 22:1–16.
36. Quismorio F: Immune complexes in the pericardial fluid in systemic lupus erythematosus. *Arch Intern Med* 1980; 140:112–114.
37. Hejtmancik MR, Wright JC, Quint R, Jennings FL: The cardiovascular manifestations of systemic lupus erythematosus. *Am Heart J* 1964; 68:119–130.
38. Shearn MA: The heart in systemic lupus erythematosus. *Am Heart J* 1959; 58:452–466.
39. Estes D, Christian C: The natural history of systemic lupus erythematosus by prospective analysis. *Medicine* 1971; 50:85–95.
40. Elkayam U, Weiss S, Laniado S: Pericardial effusion and mitral valve involvement in systemic lupus erythematosus: echocardiographic study. *Ann Rheum Dis* 1977; 36:349–353.
41. Davis P, Atkins B, Josse RG, Hughes GRV: Criteria for classification of systemic lupus erythematosus. *Br Med J* 1973; 111:88–89.
42. Jacobson E, Reza M: Constrictive pericarditis in systemic lupus erythematosus. Demonstration of immunoglobulins in the pericardium. *Arthritis Rheum* 1978; 21:972–974.
43. Ghose MK: Pericardial tamponade. A presenting manifestation of procainamide-induced lupus erythematosus. *Am J Med* 1975; 58:581–585.
44. Sunder S, Shah A: Constrictive pericarditis in procainamide-induced lupus erythematosus syndrome. *Am J Cardiol* 1975; 36:960–962.
45. del Rio A, Vazquez JJ, Sobrino JA, Gil A, Barbado J, Mate I, Ortiz-Vazquez J: Myocardial involvement in systemic lupus erythematosus. A non-invasive study of left ventricular function. *Chest* 1978; 74:414–417.
46. Ropes M: *Systemic Lupus Erythematosus*. Cambridge, Harvard University Press, 1976, pp 50–54.
47. James TN, Rupe CE, Monto RW: Pathology of cardiac conducting system in systemic lupus erythematosus. *Ann Intern Med* 1965; 63:402–410.
48. Libman E, Sacks B: A hitherto undescribed form of valvular and mural endocarditis. *Arch Intern Med* 1924; 33:701–732.
49. Gross L: The cardiac lesion in Libman–Sacks disease with a consideration of its relationship to acute diffuse lupus erythematosus. *Am J Pathol* 1940; 16:375–408.
50. Paget SA, Bulkley BH, Grauer LE, Seningen R: Mitral valve disease of systemic lupus erythematosus. A cause of severe congestive heart failure reversed by valve replacement. *Am J Med* 1975; 59:134–139.
51. Shulman HJ, Christian CL: Aortic insufficiency in systemic lupus erythematosus. *Arthritis Rheum* 1969; 12:138–146.
52. Fox IS, Spence AM, Wheelis RF, Healey LA: Cerebral emboli in Libman–Sacks endocarditis. *Neurology* 1980; 30:487–491.
53. Lehman TJA, Palmeri ST, Hastings C, Klippel JH, Plotz PH: Bacterial endocarditis complicating systemic lupus erythematosus. *J Rheum* 1983; 10:655–658.
54. Haider YS, Roberts WC: Coronary artery disease in systemic lupus erythematosus. Quantification of degree of narrowing in 22 necropsy patients aged 16 to 37 years. *Am J Med* 1981; 70:755–781.
55. Hosenspud JD, Montanaro A, Hart MV, Haines JE, Specht HD, Bennett RM, Kloster FE: Myocardial perfusion abnormalities in asymptomatic patients with systemic lupus erythematosus. *Am J Med* 1984; 77:286–292.
56. Hardin NJ, Minick CR, Murphy GE: Experimental induction of athero-arteriosclerosis by the synergy of allergic injury to arteries and lipid-rich diet. *Am J Pathol* 1973; 73:301–326.
57. Minick CR, Alonzo DR, Rankin L: Role of immunologic arterial injury in atherogenesis. *Thromb Haemost* 1978; 39:304–311.
58. Korbet S, Schwartz M, Lewis E: Immune complex deposition and coronary vasculitis in systemic lupus erythematosus. Report of two cases. *Am J Med* 1984; 77:141–146.
59. Homcy CJ, Liberthson RR, Fallon JT, Gross S, Miller LM: Ischemic heart disease in systemic lupus erythematosus in the young patient. Report of 6 cases. *Am J Cardiol* 1982; 49:478–484.
60. Lee L, Bias WB, Arnett FC, Huff JC, Norris DA, Harmon C, Provost TT, Weston WL: Immunogenetics of neonatal lupus syndrome. *Ann Intern Med* 1983; 99:592–596.
61. Reed BR, Lee LA, Harmon C, Wolfe R, Wiggins J, Peebles C, Weston WL: Autoantibodies to SS-A (Ro) in infants with congenital heart block. *J Pediatr* 1983; 103:889–891.
62. Litsey SE, Noonan JA, O'Connor WN, Cottrill CM, Mitchell B: Maternal connective tissue disease and congenital heart block. Demonstration of immunglobulin in cardiac tissue. *N Engl J Med* 1985; 312:98–100.
63. McCue CM, Mantakas MG, Tingelstad JB, Ruddy S: Congenital heart block in newborns of mothers in connective tissue disease. *Circulation* 1977; 56:82–90.
64. Michaëlson M, Engle MA: Congenital complete heart block. An international study of the natural history. *Cardiovascular Clin* 1972; 4(3):85–101.
65. Haupt H, Hutchins G: Heart and cardiac conduction system in polymyositis–dermatomyositis: a clinicopathologic study of 16 autopsied patients. *Am J Cardiol* 1982; 50:998–1006.
66. Denbow CE, Lie JT, Tancred RG, Bunch TW: Cardiac involvement in polymyositis. A clinicopathologic study of 20 patients. *Arthritis Rheum* 1979; 22:1088–1092.
67. Bohan A, Peter JB, Bowman RL, Pearson CM: A computer–assisted analysis of 153 patients with polymyositis and dermatomyositis. *Medicine* 1977; 56:255–286.
68. Babka J, Pepine C: Hyperkinetic cardiovascular state in polymyositis. *Chest* 1973; 64:243–246.
69. Gottdiener JS, Sherber HS, Hawley RJ, Engel WK: Cardiac manifestations in polymyositis. *Am J Cardiol* 1978; 41:1141–1148.
70. Askari A: Cardiac abnormalities. *Clin Rheum Dis* 1984; 10:131–149.
71. Kehoe RF, Bauerfeind R, Tommaso C, Wyndham C, Rosen KM: Cardiac conduction defects in polymyositis. Electrophysiologic studies in 4 patients. *Ann Intern Med* 1981; 94:41–43.
72. Larca L, Coppola J, Honig S: Creatine kinase MB isoenzyme in dermatomyositis. A noncardiac source. *Ann Intern Med* 1981; 94:341–343.
73. Jiminez S: Cellular immune dysfunction and the pathogenesis of scleroderma. *Semin Arthritis Rheum* 1983; 13:104–113.
74. Medsger TA: Progressive systemic sclerosis. *Clin Rheum Dis* 1983; 9:655–670.
75. Salneri R, Rodnan GP, Leon DF, Shaver JA: Pulmonary hypertension in the CREST syndrome variant of progressive systemic sclerosis (scleroderma). *Ann Intern Med* 1977; 86:394–399.
76. Weiss S, Stead EA, Warren JV, Bailey OT: Scleroderma heart disease with a consideration of certain other visceral manifestations of scleroderma. *Arch Intern Med* 1943; 71:749–776.
77. Bulkley BH, Ridolfi RL, Salyer WR, Hutchins GM: Myocardial lesions of progressive systemic sclerosis. A cause of cardiac dysfunction. *Circulation* 1976; 53:483–490.
78. Reichenbach D, Benditt E: Myofibrillar degeneration. A response of the myocardial cell to injury. *Arch Pathol* 1968; 85:189–199.
79. D'Angelo WA, Fries JF, Masi AT, Shulman LE: Pathologic observations in systemic sclerosis (scleroderma). *Am J Med* 1969; 46:428–440.
80. McWhorter J, LeRoy E: Pericardial disease in scleroderma (systemic sclerosis). *Am J Med* 1974; 57:566–575.
81. Uhl G, Koppes G: Pericardial tamponade in systemic sclerosis (scleroderma). *Br Heart J* 1979; 42:345–348.
82. Gladman DD, Gordon DA, Urowitz MB, Levy HL: Pericardial fluid analysis in scleroderma (systemic sclerosis). *Am J Med* 1976; 60:1064–1068.
83. Smith JW, Clements PJ, Levisman J, Furst D, Ross M: Echocardiographic features of progressive systemic sclerosis (PSS). Correlation with hemodynamic and post-mortem studies. *Am J Med* 1979; 66:28–33.
84. Sackner MA, Akgun N, Kimbel P, Lewis DH: The pathophysiology of scleroderma involving the heart and respiratory system. *Ann Intern Med* 1964; 60:611–630.
85. Follansbee WP, Curtiss EI, Medsger TA, Owens GR, Steen VD, Rodnan GP: Myocardial function and perfusion in the CREST syndrome variant of progressive systemic sclerosis. Exercise radionuclide evaluation and comparison with diffuse scleroderma. *Am J Med* 1984; 77:489–496.
86. Todesco S, Gatta A, Glorioso S, Chioin R, Pesarico A, Zuin R, Merkel C: Cardiac involvement in progressive systemic sclerosis. *Acta Cardiol (Brux)* 1979; 34:311–322.
87. Follansbee WP, Curtiss EI, Medsger TA Jr, Steen VD, Uretsky BF, Owens GR, Rodnan GP: Physiologic abnormalities of cardiac function in progressive systemic sclerosis with diffuse scleroderma. *N Engl J Med* 1984; 310:142–148.
88. Oram S, Stokes W: The heart in scleroderma. *Br Heart J* 1961; 23:243–259.
89. Bulkley B, Klacsmann P, Hutchins G: Angina pectoris, myocardial infarction, and sudden cardiac death with normal coronary arteries. A clinicopathologic study of 9 patients with progressive systemic sclerosis. *Am Heart J* 1978; 95:563–569.
90. Roberts NK, Cabeen W, Moss J, Clements PJ, Furst DE: The prevalence of conduction defects and cardiac arrhythmias in progressive systemic sclerosis. *Ann Intern Med* 1981; 94:38–40.

91. James TN: Coronary arteries and conduction system in scleroderma heart disease. *Circulation* 1974; 50:844–856.
92. Ridolphi R, Bulkley B, Hutchins G: The cardiac conduction system in progressive systemic sclerosis. *Am J Med* 1976; 61:361–366.
93. Clements PJ, Furst DE, Cabeen W, Tashkin D, Paulus HE, Roberts N: The relationship of arrhythmias and conduction disturbances to other manifestations of cardiopulmonary disease in progressive systemic sclerosis (PSS). *Am J Med* 1981; 71:38–46.
94. Blom-Bülow B, Jonson B, Bauer K: Factors limiting exercise performance in progressive systemic sclerosis. *Semin Arthritis Rheum* 1983; 13:174–181.
95. Medsger TA Jr, Masi AT, Rodnan GP, Benedek TG, Robinson H: Survival with systemic sclerosis (scleroderma). *Ann Intern Med* 1971; 75:369–376.
96. Muers M, Stokes W: Treatment of scleroderma heart disease by D-penicillamine. *Br Heart J* 1976; 38:864–867.
97. Kang B, Veres-Thorner C, Heredia R, Cha E, Bose S, Schwartz M: Successful treatment of far advanced scleroderma heart by D-penicillamine. *J Allergy Clin Immunol* 1982; 69:297–305.
98. Steen V, Medsger T, Rodnan G: D-penicillamine therapy in progressive systemic sclerosis (scleroderma). A retrospective analysis. *Ann Intern Med* 1982; 97:652–659.
99. McGoon M, Vlietstra R: Vasodilator therapy for primary pulmonary hypertension. *Mayo Clin Proc* 1984; 59:672–677.
100. Ball J: Enthesopathy of rheumatoid and ankylosing spondylitis. *Ann Rheum Dis* 1971; 30:213–223.
101. Graham D, Smythe H: The carditis and aortitis of ankylosing spondylitis. *Bull Rheum Dis* 1958; 9:171–174.
102. Bergfeldt L: HLA-B27 associated heart disease with severe cardiac bradyarrhythmias. Clinical features and prevalence in 223 men with permanent pacemakers. *Am J Med* 1983; 75:210–215.
103. Bergfeldt L, Edhag O, Rajs J: HLA-B27 associated heart disease. Clinicopathologic study of three cases. *Am J Med* 1984; 77:961–967.
104. Bulkley B, Roberts W: Ankylosing spondylitis and aortic insufficiency. Description of the characteristic cardiovascular lesion from study of eight necropsy patients. *Circulation* 1973; 48:1014–1026.
105. Stewart S, Robbins D, Castles J: Acute fulminant aortic and mitral insufficiency in ankylosing spondylitis. *N Engl J Med* 1978; 299:1448–1449.
106. Kinsella TD, Johnson LG, Sutherland RI: Cardiovascular manifestations of ankylosing spondylitis. *Can Med Assoc J* 1974; 111:1309–1311.
107. Tucker CT, Fowles RF, Calin A, Popp RL: Aortitis in ankylosing spondylitis: early detection of aortic root abnormalities with 2-dimensional echocardiography. *Am J Cardiol* 1982; 49:680–686.
108. Nitter-Haugh S, Otterstael J: Characteristics of atrioventricular conduction disturbances in ankylosing spondylitis. *Acta Med Scand* 1981; 210:197–200.
109. Bergfeldt L, Edhag O, Vedin L, Vallin H: Ankylosing spondylitis. An important cause of severe disturbance of the cardiac conducting system. *Am J Med* 1982; 73:181–187.
110. Parrillo J, Fauci A: Necrotizing vasculitis, coronary angiitis, and the cardiologist. *Am Heart J* 1980; 99:547–554.
111. Fauci A, Haynes B, Katz P: The spectrum of vasculitis. *Ann Intern Med* 1978; 89:660–676.
112. Ask-Upmark E: On the pathogenesis of the hypertension in Takayasu's syndrome. *Acta Med Scand* 1961; 169:467–477.
113. Cupps T, Fauci A: *The Vasculitides*. Philadelphia, WB Saunders, 1981, pp 107–115.
114. Cipriano PR, Silverman JF, Perlroth MG, Griepp RB, Wexler L: Coronary artery narrowing in Takayasu's aortitis. *Am J Cardiol* 1977; 39:744–750.
115. Roberts WC, Dangel JC, Bulkey BH: Nonrheumatic valvular cardiac disease: a clinicopathologic survey of 27 different conditions causing valvular dysfunction. *Cardiovasc Clin* 1973; 5(2):333–446.
116. Lupi-Herrera E, Sanchez TG, Marcushamer J, Mispireta J, Horowitz S, Vela JE: Takayasu's arteritis. Clinical study of 107 cases. *Am Heart J* 1977; 93:94–103.
117. Klein RG, Hunder GG, Stanson AW, Sheps SG: Large artery involvement in giant cell (temporal) arteritis. *Ann Intern Med* 1975; 83:806–812.
118. Huston K, Hunder G: Giant cell (cranial) arteritis: a clinical review. *Am Heart J* 1980; 100:99–107.
119. How J, Strachan R: Aortic regurgitation as a manifestation of giant cell arteritis. *Br Heart J* 1978; 40:1052–1054.
120. Frohnert P, Sheps S: Long-term follow-up study of periarteritis nodosa. *Am J Med* 1967; 43:8–14.
121. Holsinger D, Osmundson P, Edwards J: The heart in periarteritis nodosa. *Circulation* 1962; 25:610–618.
122. Schrader M, Bulkley B: The heart in polyarteritis nodosa: a clinicopathologic study of 36 patients. *Am J Cardiol* 1980; 45:395.
123. James TN, Birk RE: Pathology of the cardiac conduction system in polyarteritis nodosa. *Arch Intern Med* 1966; 117:561–567.
124. Kawasaki T, Kosaki F, Okawa S, Shigematsu I, Yanagawa H: A new infantile acute febrile mucocutaneous lymph node syndrome (MLNS) prevailing in Japan. *Pediatrics* 1974; 54:271–276.
125. Landing BH, Larson EJ: Are infantile periarteritis nodosa with coronary artery involvement and fatal mucocutaneous lymph node syndrome the same? Comparison of 20 patients from North America with patients from Hawaii and Japan. *Pediatrics* 1977; 59:651–662.
126. Fukushige J, Nihill MR, McNamara DG: Spectrum of cardiovascular lesions in mucocutaneous lymph node syndrome: analysis of eight cases. *Am J Cardiol* 1980; 45:98–106.
127. Kato H, Ichinose E, Yoshioka F, Takechi T, Matsunaga S, Suzuki K, Rikitake N: Fate of coronary aneurysms in Kawasaki disease: serial coronary angiography and long-term follow-up study. *Am J Cardiol* 1982; 49:1758–1766.
128. Hiraishi S, Yashiro K, Oguchi K, Kusano S, Ishii K, Nakazawa K: Clinical course of cardiovascular involvement in the mucocutaneous lymph node syndrome. Relation between clinical signs of carditis and development of coronary arterial aneurysm. *Am J Cardiol* 1981; 47:323–330.
129. Koren G, Lavi S, Rose V, Rowe R: Kawasaki disease: review of risk factors for coronary aneurysms. *J Pediatr* 1986; 108:388–392.
130. Yoshida H, Funabashi T, Nakaya S, Taniguchi N: Mucocutaneous lymph node syndrome. A cross-sectional echocardiographic diagnosis of coronary artery aneurysm. *Am J Dis Child* 1979; 133:1244–1247.
131. Kato H, Koike S, Tanaka C, Yokochi K, Yoshioka F, Takeuchi S, Matsunaga S, Yokoyama T: Coronary heart disease in children with Kawasaki disease. *Jpn Circ J* 1979; 43:469–475.
132. Stewart JM, Woolf PK, Burleson P, Gewitz MH: The relationship between myocardial dysfunction and coronary aneurysms in Kawasaki disease. *J Am Coll Cardiol* 1986; 7(suppl A):48A.
133. Koren G, Rose V, Lavi S, Rowe R: Probable efficacy of high-dose salicylates in reducing coronary involvement in Kawasaki disease. *JAMA* 1985; 254:767–769.
134. Price J: Kawasaki syndrome. *Br Med J* 1984; 288:262.
135. Kato H, Koike S, Yokoyama T: Kawasaki disease: effect of treatment on coronary artery involvement. *Pediatrics* 1979; 63:175–179.
136. Nakano H, Saito A, Ueda K, Nojima K: Clinical characteristics of myocardial infarction following Kawasaki disease: report of 11 cases. *J Pediatr* 1986; 108:198–203.
137. Kohr RM: Progressive asymptomatic coronary artery disease as a late fatal sequela of Kawasaki disease. *J Pediatr* 1986; 108:256–259.

59 Heart and Neuropsychiatric Disorders

Ewald W. Busse, MD and John I. Walker, MD

Cardiovascular disease exemplifies the interplay between emotional disturbances and medical disorders. Anxiety has been reported in 42% to 80% of patients with cardiovascular disease; depression in 23% to 58% of cases[1]; delirium following myocardial infarction in approximately 10% of patients over 65 years of age[2]; of 505 patients seen in a medical clinic complaining of chest discomfort, 25% received a psychiatric diagnosis.[3] Emotional conflicts contribute significantly to incapacitation in the 20% of individuals who become disabled from myocardial infarction each year.[1] Behavioral risk factors including smoking, lack of exercise, overeating, and improper diet increase cardiovascular morbidity and mortality.[4] This chapter will review the neuropsychiatric aspects of cardiovascular disease.

NEUROENDOCRINE AND CORTICONEURAL PATHWAYS

Pleasant or unpleasant emotions, ambiguous, unusual, or threatening environmental conditions; and significant life changes affect blood pressure, heart rate and rhythm, cardiac output, and blood flow through neuroendocrine and corticoneural pathways.[2] Lacey and Lacey,[5] for example, showed that cognitive work produces cardiac acceleration, whereas attention to environmental stimuli produces cardiac slowing. These changes probably reflect vagal effects. Taggart et al[6] studied 30 speakers before and after their performances. During their addresses all speakers developed tachycardia, whereas five speakers demonstrated multiple ectopic beats and three of seven speakers with coronary heart disease exhibited ischemic ST-segment depression. Free fatty acid and plasma noradrenaline levels were increased after the speaking engagement when compared with levels measured just before the performance. Beta blockers abolished these changes. Schiffer et al[7] demonstrated that heart rate and blood pressure significantly increased during a 12-minute intelligence test. Frankenhaeuser[8] found that individuals commuting to work on a train had higher catecholamine levels in their urine under crowded circumstances than under less crowded situations. Lynch[9] demonstrated the close relation between loss of love and premature death. These citations are only a few of the many studies that illustrate the highly complex reciprocal interactions between the mind and the cardiovascular system: they reflect the importance of emotional arousal on the etiology and prognosis of heart disease.[2]

ENVIRONMENTAL STRESSES AND BEHAVIORAL FACTORS IN CORONARY HEART DISEASE

SMOKING

Following an extensive review of the literature, Houpt et al[1] proposed that 8% to 10% of all health costs in the United States are directly related to smoking. Coronary heart disease (CHD) is the leading cause of excess mortality and morbidity among cigarette smokers, directly attributing to approximately 25% of coronary deaths. Coronary heart disease death rates dramatically improve after cessation of cigarette smoking.[10] Death rates are 50% lower for men who quit smoking than for men who continue to smoke, with almost two thirds of the excess risk disappearing within the first year after the person stops smoking.[1]

Blumenthal et al[10] found that approximately one half of patients who experience myocardial infarction will stop smoking on their own or on their physician's advice, although about one third of these patients can be expected to return to smoking. Antismoking advice of a physician is a particularly important factor in achieving cessation of smoking. In medical centers where the physician and medical team are committed to smoking control and where adequate rehabilitation and secondary prevention services are provided, 50% or more of patients have reported long-term cigarette smoking cessation following myocardial infarction.[11] Several psychologic and personal factors predict success in stopping smoking[1,10]: individuals with higher levels of education, married persons, and older persons are more likely to stop; encouragement, support, and cooperation from family and friends produce good results in cessation, whereas nagging and policing lead to poor results; poor self-image, lack of motivation, and anxiety adversely influence stopping.

Behavioral modification techniques can produce 6 months of abstinence in 30% to 76% of cigarette smokers.[1] Rapid smoking adversive conditions require that the individual inhale every 6 seconds until smoking becomes intolerable. This procedure is potentially hazardous, especially in post-myocardial infarction patients. Increased nicotine and carbon monoxide inhalation causes a significant increase in heart rate, blood pressure, and carboxyhemoglobin, and occasionally precipitates mild electrocardiographic abnormalities in healthy individuals.[1]

Alternatively, and more safely, normal paced adversive smoking requires that individuals smoke at the normal rate while concentrating on the disgusting qualities of smoking. Cognitive techniques to modify self-defeating beliefs, habits, and thoughts while reinforcing successful patterns of behavior can be effective in cessation of cigarette smoking. Behavioral nonsmoking skill training encourages behavior incompatible with smoking, such as exercise, yoga, and deep breathing. Training in relaxation techniques can help abstinent smokers relieve tension produced by not smoking.

OVEREATING AND SEDENTARY LIFE-STYLE

A diet high in saturated fat, cholesterol, salt, and calories and a sedentary life-style contribute to the risk of developing CHD.[1,10] Weight loss through exercise and reduction in salt intake, cholesterol, and total caloric consumption will lead to lower plasma cholesterol and triglyceride levels and contribute to the maintenance of normal blood pressure. Kannel and Gordon,[12] using data from the comprehensive Framingham study, estimate that the incidence of CHD, congestive heart failure, and stroke would be reduced by 35% if everyone maintained an ideal weight. A man whose serum cholesterol value falls below 194 mg/dl has a threefold reduction in the risk of CHD and stroke than one whose serum cholesterol value equals or exceeds 250 mg/dl.[13]

Physicians, pessimistic about the possibility of successful intervention, often fail to take an active role in proposing weight management and exercise programs.[1] A study of outpatient clinic charts in a major teaching hospital indicated that weight management programs were advised in only 24% of markedly obese patients and 4% of moderately obese patients.[14] Furthermore, most overweight persons who seek weight reduction drop out of treatment; those who remain in treatment lose fewer than 20 pounds; and most of those who lose weight regain it.[1] Only 10% to 20% of persons in nonbehavioral medical and self-help treatment programs achieve lasting weight loss.[1]

Diet

The American Heart Association[15] recommends a low salt diet containing 30% calories as fat, cholesterol limited to 300 mg/day, and saturated fat intake less than 10% of total calories. Saturated fats can be replaced by polyunsaturates and carbohydrates with carbohydrates consisting of 45% to 55% of total calories. Complex carbohydrates contained in vegetables, beans, cereals, and some fruits are recommended over simple sugars because they cause less risk of dental caries, prevent surges of hyperglycemia, and add more dietary roughage. Low salt intake helps control hypertension, whereas a low cholesterol diet will maintain plasma cholesterol at an ideal level of 130 to 190 mg/dl.

The best dietary plans change eating patterns, optimize individual choice through food exchanges, and encourage reasonable eating habits after weight loss. Most behavioral treatments employ the following procedures[1]: (1) educating the person on nutrition and exercise; (2) reducing the number of cues triggering inappropriate eating habits while increasing appropriate eating cues; (3) rewarding desired eating and exercise behaviors while discouraging unhealthy behaviors; (4) providing cognitive training to teach self-control skills; (5) teaching self-monitoring of eating and exercise patterns.

Nutrition counseling and emphasizing exercise instruction, food exchange strategy, and proper physical activity are essential for successful weight reduction treatments. Techniques to encourage caloric reduction include restricting times, places, and circumstances for eating; removing the availability and conspicuousness of high-calorie food; increasing access to healthful foods; restricting food portions; reducing the size of eating and serving dishes; posting signs near the refrigerator to deter overeating; and encouraging eating slowly while savoring each bite before taking another. Relaxation training can help reduce tension caused by restricting caloric intake. Positive social reinforcement from the physician, treatment team, family, and friends can enhance changes in eating and exercise habits. Teaching dieters to alter thoughts that stimulate eating can diminish urges to overeat, whereas training in stress management can help reduce anxiety and depression that contribute to overeating. Recording of eating and exercise behavior reinforces good health habits. Finally, setting reasonable short-term weight loss goals has beneficial effects by providing positive reinforcement when goals are accomplished.

Physical Exercise Training

Increased maximum oxygen uptake can be achieved primarily by improving maximum arteriovenous oxygen extraction following a program of regular exercise by coronary patients. Exercise may promote coronary collateral vascularization[16] and, in addition, exercise leads to a reduction in weight, triglycerides, cholesterol, and free fatty acids.[10] Higher pain threshold, increased work capacity, and enhanced self-esteem have been reported after several months of a cardiac rehabilitation program,[17] although evidence for prolongation of life remains equivocable.[10]

Although an estimated 25 million Americans run regularly,[17] behavior strategies designed to improve compliance with exercise have not been fully implemented internationally. The Duke University Preventive Approach to Cardiovascular Diseases (DUPAC), a model for cardiac rehabilitation programs, uses patient education, staff and peer support, personalized exercise plans, chart monitoring, regular assessment of cardiac status, and rewards for exercise improvement to encourage continued maintenance of exercise.

CORONARY-PRONE BEHAVIOR

During the past two decades, hundreds of studies have focused on the description and modification of coronary-prone behavior. The characteristics, known as type A behavior pattern (TABP), may be assessed using one of two methods: (1) a structured interview based on speech style and content of answers[18]; and (2) a self-rating questionnaire called the Jenkins Activity Survey.[19] The interview uses four principal sources of information[20]: (1) presence of characteristic speech and breathing patterns, gestures and movements, and facial expressions; (2) intensity of ambition and drive; (3) magnitude of competitive and aggressive strivings; and (4) severity of time urgency. Speech patterns have the greatest predictive value in classifying type A behavior.[4]

Type A behavior is marked by excessive competitive drive, aggressiveness, impatience, a sense of urgency, abruptness of speech and gesture, inability to relax without feeling guilty, preoccupation with quantity rather than quality, and hostility.[18] Type A behavior differs from stress and response to stress but rather reflects a behavior style to challenging situations.[20] There is a behavioral continuum with extreme type A behavior on the one hand, and on the other, extreme type B behavior (characterized by a lack of sense of urgency, freedom from hostility, ability to relax, no need to display achievements, and the ability to work without agitation). An individual with type A behavior need not have all the characteristics to be classified as coronary-prone, and several studies have begun to investigate which variables may be more predictive of CHD than others.[20] There is suggestive evidence that impatience, competitive drive, and hostility are pathogenic.[21]

Shekelle et al[22] recently found that higher hostility scores on the Minnesota Multiphasic Personality Inventory (MMPI) predicted increases in both CHD and mortality among more than 1,900 men in the Western Electric Study who were followed for 20 years after taking the test. These increases in both CHD and total mortality were independent of baseline smoking status, cholesterol, blood pressure, and alcohol use. Similarly, Barefoot et al[23] showed a correlation between CHD and high hostility scores on MMPI in a 25-year study of 225 physicians.

Type A behavior is clearly and independently associated with an increased risk of CHD. Middle-age type A men have over twice the risk of CHD of type B men, are more likely to have fatal myocardial infarction, and among survivors, to have reinfarction.[18] This risk appears to be of the same order of magnitude as the relative risk associated with hypertension, serum cholesterol, and smoking.[24] In comparing type A behavior with the severity of CHD using arteriographic findings, Blumenthal et al[25] found that types A and B were about equally represented in the group with mild vessel disease, whereas type A behavior was found in more than 90% of the group with severe CHD. Krantz et al[26] found angiographic evidence of disease progression in 75% of type A and 44% of type B persons. Type A behavior has also been associated with increased serum cholesterol, triglycerides, phospholipids, low-density lipoprotein lipids, decreased clotting time, and elevated levels during working hours of norepinephrine, epinephrine, 17-ketosteroids, 7-hydroxycorticosteroids, and 5-hydroxyindoles.[27]

In a study by Corse et al,[28] type A individuals showed higher systolic and diastolic pressure elevations while performing a series of frustrating cognitive tests than did type B subjects. Krantz et al[29] in studying 27 male patients before cardiac surgery found that type A behavior was related to systolic blood pressure increases during, but not before, surgery and that all 12 patients with surgical complications demonstrated type A behavior. Because blood pressure changes were demonstrated under general anesthesia, this study suggests that conscious mediation may not always be necessary to produce physiologic changes in type A individuals. Schwartz et al[30] examined blood pressure and heart rate following controlled imagery in 32 subjects while they rested and while they exercised. Exercising while imagining angry evoking scenes produced overwhelmingly higher cardiovascular changes than exercising in a normal or relaxed state. These findings suggest that the effects of running in type A individuals may be different from those in type B persons.

Behavioral Modification of Type A Behavior

Nineteen to 26% of coronary attacks present as sudden death; of those who survive, 10% die within the first few weeks following the attack; and the death rate is five times higher within the next 5 years compared with that in those with no history of CHD.[4] Clearly, primary prevention, reducing the frequency of first clinical episodes, represents the best protection against death from CHD. Brand et al,[31] based on the Western Collaborative Study findings, predicted that reduction in type A behavior would directly decrease the incidence of CHD by 31% with a standard error of 6.6%. This figure fails to take into account removal of all the risks associated with type A behavior (increased cholesterol, for example), which might produce a further reduction in morbidity.[4]

A behavior therapy program designed to teach stress management skills and methods for altering type A behavior demonstrated that modification of type A behavior results in major life-style changes and a significant decrease in serum cholesterol and triglyceride concentrations.[32] A controlled study[33] designed to reduce risk factors of cardiovascular disease indicated that mass media community health education may be effective in reducing the risk of cardiovascular disease, especially when reinforced by personal persuasion.

Although attempts to modify type A behavior are potentially beneficial,[10] the small amount of intervention research suffers from measurement ambiguity and subject selection.[21] Nevertheless, empirical evidence indicates that type A behavior can be altered by: (1) learning relaxation techniques; (2) modifying daily routines to reduce stress, eg, taking brief rest breaks during the day, scheduling regular exercise, and allowing time between meetings and appointments; (3) avoiding situations and persons who induce competitiveness and hostility in the individual; (4) cultivating relaxing hobbies and attitudes; and (5) diminishing the sense of time urgency. The major difficulty in altering type A behavior is convincing the individual that those behavior patterns are deleterious to health, happiness, and success.[10]

ENVIRONMENTAL STRESSORS

Since the studies of Holmes and Rahe[34] on the relation of life events and illness, the interplay between environmental stressors and cardiovascular disease has been extensively examined. Rahe and Romo[35] demonstrated that sudden death from CHD was preceded by a marked increase in life change events before death; the more dramatic the life changes, the sooner death occurred. According to trenchant statistics compiled by Lynch,[9] single, divorced, and widowed individuals have death rates from CHD two to three times higher than those of married men and women. Parkes et al[36] reported the death rate of 4,486 widowed men was 40% higher than expected during the first 6 months of bereavement; CHD was the cause in 75% of these cases.

Certain life change events seem to be related to CHD by influencing the major risk factors of coronary disease. Hinkle et al,[37] in a 5-year prospective study of 270,000 Bell System employees, found that men of white-collar family origin with college degrees who had been frequently transferred, had reached the higher managerial posts, and had been entrusted with the greatest responsibility had a 30% lower incidence of CHD than did men of blue-collar origin without college degrees who remained steadily employed at lower levels. Poorly educated, low income persons with little opportunity to improve their status may increase the probability of developing coronary disease secondary to excessive eating and smoking used to cope with their dull lives.[2] Holme et al[38] found that men of higher income and status had lower blood pressure, serum cholesterol, and rates of cigarette smoking than did men of lower socioeconomic status, reflecting perhaps that higher educated men attempt to avoid coronary risk factors more than do men with poor education.

Primary Prevention

Theorell,[39] in a review of environmental stress and CHD, recommended that life event information be used to prevent myocardial infarction following a significant crisis. Primary prevention would include providing social support and therapy for newly bereaved individuals and others suffering sudden emotional stress. Educating the public on the importance of life change events would encourage individuals to seek professional help if needed.

EMOTIONAL ASPECTS OF MYOCARDIAL INFARCTION AND ANGINA

As discussed in the section on CHD, life change events often precede myocardial infarction. Emotional states marked by increased autonomic arousal precipitate and exacerbate myocardial ischemia; chronically suppressed anger, anxiety, and elation may trigger anginal attacks.[2] Medalie and Goldbourt[40] found that a loving and supporting wife decreased the risk of angina even when high risk factors were present. Socioeconomic status and demographic indicators show weak or inconsistent associations with cardiac events.[21]

Postinfarction patients typically progress through certain stages of emotional adjustment.[41] Individuals may delay several hours before seeking medical attention, blaming their pain on gastrointestinal or respiratory difficulties. Following hospitalization, anxiety escalates, peaking on the first and second postinfarction days. On days 3 to 5, an increasing awareness of the lasting significance of the illness precipitates depression. Personality traits—hostility, dependency, and demanding behavior—become more evident on days 4 to 6. During the second week of convalescence, acceptance of the event allows the patient to cooperate more fully in the treatment program. Unfortunately, approximately one half the patients with myocardial infarction experience significant emotional distress that complicates recovery. Less educated individuals, blue-collar workers, and those with a previous history of emotional disorders have greater difficulty adjusting to myocardial infarction; mental stability and higher socioeconomic status are associated with better adjustment.[21]

ANXIETY

Symptoms of anxiety, ie, difficulty falling asleep, sweating, restlessness, tachycardia, and agitation, must be distinguished from the physical effects of myocardial infarction. Generally, anxious patients will require frequent reassurance, be obsessed with feelings of impending doom, complain of generalized aches and pains, and demonstrate sighing respirations more often than do patients experiencing cardiac distress.[42] Vigorous efforts to diminish the patient's anxiety reduces morbidity and mortality. Twenty-four–hour sedation with benzodiazepines is usually indicated. Those patients unresponsive to benzodiazepines can be given haloperidol (2 to 5 mg intramuscularly or orally) every hour as needed for agitation. Beta blockers can reduce excessive sympathetic nervous system activity.

Anxieties can be reduced by encouraging the patient to talk about his fears; for example, the patient may have difficulty falling asleep because of fantasies that his heart will stop or that he will not be watched closely enough when he is sleeping, or fears may escalate when the patient's regular physician is off duty.[42] The patient can be encouraged to talk about fears of death, dependency, separation, and nonproductivity. Explaining the usual course of the illness and medical procedures in nonmedical jargon can help relieve anxieties.

Environmental adjustments can also help decrease postcoronary anxiety. For example, some patients benefit from frequent staff or family visits, whereas others react adversely to excessive attention. Similarly, some patients may benefit by being moved from the coronary care unit as soon as possible, whereas others feel anxious with close monitoring for longer periods of time. Early mobilization helps relieve anxiety by reassuring the patient that his physical condition is improving. Biofeedback, hypnosis, or relaxation techniques can help relieve anxiety and hyperventilation.

DEPRESSION

Depression peaks on days 3 to 5 as the impact of the myocardial infarction is understood. Signs and symptoms suggesting depression include crying episodes and tearfulness; psychomotor agitation or retardation; early morning awakening; decreased appetite; feelings of helplessness or hopelessness; and suicidal thoughts. In addition, depressed patients may have excessive fears of dying and multiple somatic complaints.[42]

Helping the patient deal with the impact of myocardial infarction will in most cases relieve the symptoms. Allowing the patient to talk about how he feels the insult will interfere with his work and home life while maintaining a hopeful attitude will help the patient work through his grief. Active listening, reflecting back to the patient what he has said, and realistic optimism will be reassuring to the patient.

If the depressive symptoms persist longer than 6 weeks and are associated with the neurovegetative signs of depression, including terminal sleep disturbances, anorexia, and decreased libido, biomedical intervention is necessary. Desipramine or trazodone, because of their low anticholinergic side effects, may be the antidepressants of choice. Electroseizure therapy is safer, faster, and more effective than antidepressant medication for severe depression.

CHARACTER REACTIONS

The typical personality traits of the individual usually become manifest during post-myocardial infarction days 4 to 6. The aggressive patient will attempt to take charge of his care, whereas the dependent and clinging patient will become more demanding and helpless. Histrionic patients may overdramatize their symptoms. Paranoid personalities may become more suspicious and questioning, and so forth. The patient's character reactions may interfere with medical management and psychologic comfort. Intervention strategy for character disorders following myocardial infarction is beyond the breadth of this chapter.

DENIAL

From 25% to 40% of patients admitted for myocardial infarction unequivocably deny concern about their condition.[1] Denial in the acute phase has been associated with less anxiety and lower mortality.[21] Patients with persistent denial, however, will have a poorer prognosis because of interference with treatment recommendations.[1]

Because denial is an unconscious attempt to manage anxiety, depression, or threat to self-esteem, denial of the myocardial infarction will gradually remit when the physician helps the patient deal with these issues. Brief, frequent visits by the physician can help the patient gradually begin to discuss the impact of the illness on his life. Interventions can be empathetically educational and repetitive, but the physician would do best to avoid going into detail if the patient wants to change the subject. An honest, confident, and forthright approach encourages the patient to gradually discuss his reaction to the illness and the fear that is behind the denial: dependency, loss of control, inactivity, or death.

In addition, the physician can help the family deal with the patient's denial. The patient may feel a need to show no emotional distress to prevent the family from getting upset. Conversely, the family might be trying to guard the patient by minimizing the seriousness of the illness or failing to talk about their reactions to his myocardial infarction. By meeting together with the patient and family, the physician can help them deal appropriately with adjustments to the infarction by adapting realistic role changes.[21]

DELIRIUM

Delirium (also known as intensive care psychosis, acute confusional syndrome, coronary care psychosis, acute brain syndrome, cardiac psychosis, or toxic psychosis) has been reported in 3% to 10% of patients, usually begins on the third to fourth hospital day, and persists from two to five days.[2] The condition may be secondary to cerebral hypoxia, arrhythmias, cardiac drugs, and a metabolic or electrolyte disturbance that is exacerbated by psychosocial factors such as overstimulation or understimulation caused by the intensive care environment, lack of communication with familiar figures, and sleep deprivation.[21] Delirium fluctuates unpredictably with lucid intervals, being more common in the morning and confusion most marked at night ("sundowning"). The most prominent feature involves disattention, resulting in disordered thinking, incoherent speech, chaotic behavior, impaired memory and orientation, and a clouded sensorium ranging from drowsiness to stupor. Perceptual disturbances may produce illusions (misinterpretation of an actual event) or hallucinations (perception of something when nothing is there). Visual illusions predominate, although tactile sensations also occur and auditory hallucinations are sometimes present. The attention disorder can secondarily produce any type of emotional disturbance such as fear, sadness, anger, euphoria, or apathy. Tachycardia, dilated pupils, sweating, and tremor reflect an autonomic arousal.[43]

The most important aspect of treatment of delirium is correction of the underlying cause. Sensory deprivation can be alleviated by having a night light in the room with soft music playing over the radio. Staff should make certain to orient the patient when they enter the room, giving their name, the date, and the place. Signs in the room telling the patient where he is, the location of the bathroom, and other pertinent information are useful. A calendar should be prominently displayed. Because of its minimal anticholinergic effects, haloperidol 2 to 5 mg repeated every 30 minutes up to a total dose of 45 mg per day is recommended for treatment of the agitation that accompanies delirium. Sedatives and hypnotics, because they exacerbate the confusional state by depressing the level of consciousness, are contraindicated.[43]

IMPAIRED CONVALESCENCE

Most studies indicate that approximately 80% of individuals having myocardial infarction return to work, whereas 20% become disabled.[1] Several factors contribute to disability: poor physical condition, inconsistent premorbid work history; overcautionary advice from health professionals, and elevated anxiety and depression scores on the MMPI.[1]

Unwarranted emotional distress was found in 50% of male patients with ischemic heart disease at Work Assessment Centers in Australia.[1] Depression contributed to invalidism in 161 patients. Physicians had failed to recognize depression in 120 of these patients; antidepressants were required in 105 patients. Other effects contributing to disability included poor patient education, insufficient rehabilitation, and giving the patient a discouraging prognosis.

Family relations are altered by myocardial infarction: 20% of marriages deteriorate following myocardial infarction, whereas 25% improve[2]; 80% of the wives of postcoronary men report a sleep disturbance; 50% report a change in appetite; sexual activities are altered in as many as 75% of couples; 25% of wives are depressed and show poor adjustment 1 year following MI by their husbands.[1] A study of the sexual activity of 100 couples following a coronary attack in the husband revealed that 49 had decreased sexual activity; 24 failed to resume sexual activity; 22 maintained the premyocardial infarction frequency of sexual activity; and five couples increased sexual activity.[44] All of the wives reported concern that sexual activity would precipitate chest pain or another myocardial infarction.

PSYCHOLOGIC ASPECTS OF REHABILITATION

An analysis of 34 controlled studies demonstrated that patients who were given emotional support and provided with medical information concerning their condition did better than patients who were not informed, supported, or instructed in how to improve recovery.[45] Work or sexual inhibitions and physical complaints often can be diminished by patient education and a specific program of steadily increasing activities. For example, most patients are unaware how quickly bedrest can cause muscle atrophy and they often think that the damaged heart alone causes physical weakness. Patients can be reassured, and thus encouraged to become more active, by being told that simple bedrest alone can cause weakness. Treadmill testing performed before hospital discharge will help demonstrate to patients that they are capable of doing much more than they realized. Patients can be given specific exercise programs to follow, which will allow a steady increase in physical activity.

Families can be offered advice on how to encourage the patient to return to normal functioning. For example, because the strain on the heart during sexual intercourse is equivalent to climbing a flight of stairs, wives can be reassured that their husbands can be expected to return to normal sexual activity approximately 6 weeks after myocardial infarction. This sexual information combined with education about resumption of other routine activities can prevent an overprotective attitude from developing. Failure of the patient to resume normal activities should lead to prompt referral to a rehabilitation program and, if necessary, psychiatric consultation.[2]

OPEN HEART SURGERY

In an extensive review of the literature, Speidel et al[46] reported that psychic disturbances occur in approximately 40% of patients following heart operations; these disturbances were more severe following open heart surgery than closed heart surgery. There may be postoperative delirium without a lucid interval or delirium following a lucid interval of three to five days. Paranoid–hallucinatory conditions and episodes of depersonalization have also been reported and occur more commonly on the third postoperative day. Approximately 50% of the disturbances last one to two days, with almost 90% of the cases remitting within 1 week.

EMOTIONAL FACTORS IN CARDIAC ARRHYTHMIAS

Psychologic factors mediated through neural and hormonal influences contribute to cardiac arrhythmias[2]: in animal models, stimulation of the hypothalamus and midbrain reticular areas induces ectopic ventricular, atrial, and nodal arrhythmias attributed to sympathetic influences; stimulation of the medial temporal regions, cingulate gyri, and orbital cortex produces atrial flutter, sinus bradycardia, fibrillation, and cardiac arrest ascribed to parasympathetic overactivity; and amygdaloid complex stimulation produces both tachycardia and bradycardia. Patients with a variety of brain injuries have an increased incidence of cardiac arrhythmias. As Lipowski[2] points out, these findings suggest that psychologic responses may influence the electrophysiologic condition of the heart mediated by sympathetic and parasympathetic activity. Catecholamines that are increased by distressing or pleasant emotions may produce cardiac arrhythmias by their influence on the sinoatrial node. Compulsive, chronically anxious, and hostile individuals who are afraid to express anger demonstrated paroxysmal arrhythmias under conditions that produced emotional stress. Patients with an organic predisposition to arrhythmias, such as those individuals with the Wolff–Parkinson–White syndrome, are more prone to develop cardiac arrhythmias when subjected to sudden life changes.[2]

Management of patients with arrhythmias should consist of helping these patients understand the connection between emotional stress and cardiac symptoms. Educating the patient on how emotions influence heart action through neurologic and hormonal changes can help the patient be more willing to learn methods to reduce stress and resolve emotional conflicts. Patients can be taught more adaptive methods for coping with situations that precipitate arrhythmias and, in psychotherapy, can work through underlying guilts and resentments that contribute to emotional stress. Explaining the patient's fear of death can be investigated for its unconscious meaning, which usually involves guilt over unacceptable sexual and aggressive impulses. Psychotherapy, then, should be educative, supportive, and exploratory: the patient is educated on the cause of the arrhythmia, given reassurance that benign arrhythmias will not cause sudden death, and helped to understand the unconscious influences that contribute to the arrhythmia and fear.[2] Certain cardiac arrhythmias, especially premature ventricular contractions and sinus tachycardia, have been reduced by biofeedback.[10]

SUDDEN DEATH

Although myocardial infarction more commonly occurs in patients with chronic stress, sudden death from ventricular fibrillation more likely befalls individuals with a predisposition to myocardial instability who experience acute stress.[47,48] Myers and Dewar[49] found that emotional stress contributed significantly to sudden cardiac death in 100 men. Twenty-three of these men experienced severe stress within 30 minutes of their deaths; 40 men encountered intense stress in the preceding 24 hours. Depression may also contribute to sudden cardiac death in vulnerable individuals.[47] Rapid eye movement (REM) sleep may provoke sympathetic overactivity, producing electrical instability and malignant arrhythmias, whereas non-REM sleep decreases sympathetic outflow, stabilizing the myocardium.[47] Following an extensive review of the literature, De Silva[47] estimates that emotional stress may precede sudden death in 20% to 40% of cases.

CARDIOPULMONARY RESUSCITATION

Bedell et al[50] studied 294 patients who received cardiopulmonary resuscitation: in 166 patients resuscitation was successful; of the 128 patients in whom vital signs were restored, 31 patients died within 24 hours and another 56 patients died before hospital discharge. Therefore, only 42 patients (14%) of those having cardiopulmonary resuscitation left the hospital, and 8 of these survivors died within 6 months. In a study by Lemire and Johnson,[51] 230 of 1,204 resuscitated patients survived to discharge. Although most survivors are amnestic for the event, a few patients may report a pleasant "out of body" experience described by Moody.[52] Following successful resuscitation, transient anxiety, depression, and nightmares are common, but within 6 months most patients demonstrate good emotional adjustment. Post resuscitation fears can be allayed by allowing the patient to talk about his concerns and by frequent staff visits and 24-hour cardiac monitoring.[53]

EMOTIONAL ASPECTS OF CONGESTIVE HEART FAILURE

Emotional stress precedes hospitalization for congestive heart failure in approximately one half the patients. The most common stresses are separation from loved ones or interpersonal conflicts, producing increased heart rate, increased venous pressure, and decreased cardiac filling time presumably due to catecholamine release during emotional turmoil.[2] An awareness of the patient's current psychosocial conflicts can aid the physician in providing supportive and educational psychotherapy to help relieve the emotional stress that contributes to congestive heart failure.

Patients with chronic congestive heart failure have difficulty adjusting to their physical limitations and must be helped to find nonstrenuous outlets for normal aggressive drive. Insomnia, a chronic problem with congestive heart failure patients, may be accompanied by traumatic dreams, anxiety, and depression. Antidepressant medication may help relieve the dysphoric mood and sleep disturbance. Trazodone, a sedating serotonergic antidepressant with no anticholinergic side effects, may be the antidepressant of choice. It is prudent to keep the dose low, 50 to 100 mg at bedtime, unless the patient shows signs of a major depression, at which time therapeutic doses will be required (300 to 400 mg). Haloperidol, 2 to 5 mg at bedtime, can be used to control agitation and delirium which often accompany decompensating cardiac function.

ESSENTIAL HYPERTENSION

Since Alexander[54] first described hypertensive persons as individuals who had difficulty secondary to suppressed anger, numerous studies have shown correlations between psychosocial stress and elevated blood pressure: sympathetic overactivity, presumably due to unexpressed anger, has been found in some patients; anxiety and anticipation have been shown to increase renin secretion in a subset of patients; anger has been associated with increased diastolic pressure; patients who experience guilt over expressed aggression show elevated blood pressure; blacks living in high-stress urban areas have increased blood pressure hypothetically due to inhibited rage; in another study black men were thought to have increased blood pressure because of discontent and lack of control over their lives; increased diastolic blood pressure has been found in survivors of combat and natural disasters; air traffic controllers working in centers with congested airways have a higher incidence of hypertension; genetically predisposed mice exposed to approach-avoidance conflict showed persistent elevations of blood pressure. Essential hypertension most certainly develops from complex interactions involving constitutional, emotional, environmental, and dietary factors.[2]

NONCOMPLIANCE WITH MEDICAL TREATMENT

Although supportive psychotherapy and behavioral techniques including relaxation, transcendental meditation, and biofeedback may be helpful in reducing mild labile hypertension, these modalities should be considered adjuncts to pharmacotherapy.[2] The biggest problem in treating hypertension is dealing with noncompliance with medical treatment. Approximately 50% of hypertensive persons fail to keep follow-up appointments within the first year after they have been identified, and within 5 years, three fourths have dropped out of treatment.[1] A survey in the United States revealed that 34% of identified hypertensive persons were not taking their medications and 48% under age 35 were incorrectly following medication treatment recommendations.[1] The more behavior change required, the more likely is the patient to be noncompliant.[10] The hypertensive patient with multiple risk factors who is asked to stop smoking, decrease salt and caloric intake, begin exercise, and take medication is potentially at greater risk of noncompliance.

Compliance can be improved by education and reinforcement. Because most patients can remember only two thirds of what they are told after the first visit,[10] simple instructions need to be constantly repeated and the patient should understand the rationale for the medication and treatment plan. The following interventions can also increase compliance[1]: (1) frequent follow-up visits; (2) single daily dose drug administration; (3) returning to see the same physician each time; (4) short waiting times; (5) telephone calls and postcard reminders for missed appointments; (6) positive family support; and (7) guidance and encouragement from the physician.

THE HEART, THE MIND, AND MEDICATIONS

PSYCHIATRIC COMPLICATIONS OF ANTIHYPERTENSIVE DRUGS

Reserpine, clonidine, methyldopa, guanethidine, and beta-adrenergic blockers can cause depressive episodes. Reserpine depletes catecholamine stores and, in doses greater than 0.5 mg per day, produces major depression in 20% of patients. Methyldopa causes depression in 6% of patients. Although a rare complication, propranolol in doses as small as 80 mg per day has produced depression; paranoid reactions have also been reported with propranolol.[55] Hydralazine can cause psychosis, depression, and delirium from a lupus-like or lupus syndrome.[56] A hypertensive patient with mild depression can be treated with supportive psychotherapy and a diuretic for elevated blood pressure. For severe hypertension in a depressed patient, an antidepressant medication combined with a diuretic plus hydralazine can be used.[2]

PSYCHIATRIC COMPLICATIONS OF CARDIAC DRUGS

Digitalis intoxication causes arrhythmias and may produce delirium associated with visual hallucinations and paranoia. Disopyramide can also produce delirium. Psychiatric symptoms are more common in the elderly. Procainamide in moderate doses has been reported to cause dysphoria and fatigue, whereas larger doses have produced psychotic depression.[55]

CARDIAC EFFECTS OF PSYCHOTROPIC MEDICATIONS

Antidepressants

The tricyclic antidepressants produce orthostatic hypotension and block the antihypertensive effects of guanethidine, methyldopa, and clonidine.[56] In usual therapeutic doses the tricyclics may cause depressed ST segments, flattened T waves, prolonged QT intervals,[56a,56b] and tachycardia.[57] Because the tricyclics have quinidine-like effects, ventricular arrhythmias are likely to improve with TCA therapy.[58] Patients with preexisting bundle branch block have an increased risk of atrioventricular block at therapeutic levels; the tricyclics have little adverse effect on left ventricular function at usual dosages.[58] In large doses, atrial fibrillation, ventricular arrhythmias, and conduction blocks occur.[57] According to Boehnert and Lovejoy,[58a] in overdose situations QRS widening is a more sensitive measure of cardiotoxicity than are blood levels. Nontricyclic antidepressants such as trazodone and bupropion are reported to have a lower incidence of cardiovascular side effects.[56]

The monoamine oxidase inhibitors cause hypotension and must be used with caution in patients receiving antihypertensives.[56] Monoamine oxidase inhibitors can cause hypertensive crises if given simultaneously with guanethidine, reserpine, beta blockers, or sympathomimetics or with the ingestion of tyramine-containing foods.

Antipsychotics

Antipsychotic medications, especially the phenothiazines, can cause hypotension from alpha-adrenergic blockade. The antipsychotics may block the effects of clonidine, methyldopa, and guanethidine.[56] Haloperidol is the drug of choice in a cardiac patient with psychosis because of its low cardiovascular side effects.

Lithium

Because lithium and sodium compete for reabsorption at the proximal renal tubule, a decrease in sodium results in an increase in lithium reabsorption. Diminished body sodium from salt restriction, increased sweating, dehydration, or thiazide diuretics may lead to lithium toxicity.[56]

CARDIAC COMPLICATIONS OF ELECTROCONVULSIVE THERAPY

Electroconvulsive therapy (ECT), considered safer and more effective than drug therapy, is rarely associated with morbid cardiac complications. Myocardial failure or infarction, pulmonary edema, or vascular collapse rarely occurs in ECT modified by pretreatment atropine, short-acting intravenous barbiturate anesthesia, succinylcholine, and 100% positive pressure oxygenation.[59] Cardiac arrhythmias occurring in 8% to 75% of patients receiving ECT can be divided into vagal and extravagal categories.[60] Vagal arrhythmias marked by sinus bradycardia and premature ventricular contractions (PVCs) occurring postictally can be diminished by anticholinergic premedication. Extravagal arrhythmias occurring before, during, or after ECT are characterized by PVCs and can result from several conditions: increased cardiac sympathetic activity, hypoxia, succinylcholine-induced hypokalemia, and coronary artery insufficiency. Weiner et al[60] suggest that beta-adrenergic blocking agents may be useful in patients in whom PVCs develop secondary to increased sympathetic activity.

CARDIOVASCULAR MANIFESTATIONS OF PRIMARY NEUROLOGIC DISORDERS

Cardiac abnormalities are common in patients with cerebral embolism, hemorrhage, or infarction. Blood pressure is usually elevated in patients with cerebral infarction or hemorrhage; with cerebral embolism, blood pressure is usually normal. Cardiac enlargement and hypertension are commonly found in patients over 40 with primary subarachnoid hemorrhage. Over 90% of patients with cerebral embolism demonstrate cardiac enlargement or atrial fibrillation. Electrocardiographic changes, arrhythmias, conduction defects, and acute pulmonary edema can result from trauma to the cardioregulatory centers of the brain secondary to subarachnoid hemorrhage.[61] The postulated mechanism is increased levels of plasma catecholamines secondary to rapidly increasing intracranial pressure, irrespective of the cerebral pathology.[62]

Adult myotonic muscular dystrophy (Steinert's disease) is an autosomal dominant disorder that produces conduction abnormalities and arrhythmias involving the infranodal conduction system and the sinus node.[63,63a] Electrocardiographic evidence of conduction system disease is frequent, although the occurrence of clinically significant conduction block is rare.[63a,64] Dystrophy, but not myotonia, can be found in all four cardiac chambers, but involvement is usually insufficient to cause overt ventricular failure.[63]

Friedreich's ataxia is an autosomal recessive spinocerebellar neuromyelopathy in which cardiac involvement occurs in 50% to 100% of cases.[64a] In most cases hypertrophic cardiomyopathy has been noted,[64b] although dilated cardiomyopathy has also been reported.[64c,64d] Arrhythmias in Friedreich's ataxia usually consist of inappropriate sinus tachycardia, supraventricular and ventricular ectopic beats, paroxysmal atrial tachycardia, atrial fibrillation, and atrial flutter,[64a] although ventricular tachycardia has also been reported.[64c] Cardiac failure and persistent arrhythmias are rare and occur late in the evolution of the neurologic disease.[64d,64e]

NEUROLOGIC MANIFESTATIONS OF PRIMARY CARDIAC DISORDERS

Cerebral embolization is the most common neurologic manifestation of heart disease. Cerebral emboli, which are responsible for 15% to 20% of all cerebral infarctions,[64f] most commonly arise from the heart, major vessels, and thrombi from leg veins, via a patent foramen ovale.[65,65a] Atrial fibrillation and left atrial enlargement are two major risk factors for cerebral embolism.[65b] Embolization occurs suddenly in contrast to atheromatous thrombosis which is characterized by incremental neurologic deficits. Hemorrhage can result from hypertension, arteriovenous malformation, or congenital aneurysm.[65] In addition to causing localizing neurologic defects, primary cardiac disorders can cause delirium and dementia.

DELIRIUM

Myocardial infarction, microemboli of cardiac origin, arrhythmias, congestive heart failure, hypertensive encephalophathy, sensory deprivation, and cardiovascular drugs may produce delirium.[2] An interesting variety of delirium, transient global amnesia, involves a sudden episode of retrograde amnesia lasting a few hours and gradually clearing, but often leaving the victim without recollection of the episode. During the attack, anxiety may predominate. Whether the condition is vascular is unclear.[66] Brief episodes of delirium mandate an evaluation for cardiac arrhythmias. Sleep apnea should not be overlooked as a cause for arrhythmias.[66]

DEMENTIA

Multiple lacunar infarcts, almost exclusively related to hypertension, occur in approximately 10% of patients with dementia. Other cardiovascular causes for dementia include large vessel infarction, prolonged anoxia, and atherosclerosis.[67]

Dementia is marked by impaired memory, intellect, and judgment, in addition to lability and shallowness of affect. Recent events are forgotten more easily than remote events. The individual may attempt to conceal intellectual deficits, resulting in social withdrawal and confabulation. Dementia is irreversible.

PRIMARY PSYCHIATRIC DISORDERS

The variety of names used to describe the relation between the heart and psychiatric disorders, such as DaCosta's syndrome, anxiety neurosis, neurocirculatory asthenia, soldier's heart, nervous exhaustion, effort syndrome, and irritable heart, reflects the confusion that exists in the cardiologic and psychiatric literature regarding the impact of the psyche on the soma.[68] Some cardiologists believe that DaCosta's syndrome represents the mitral valve prolapse syndrome,[69] whereas psychiatrists contend that DaCosta's syndrome is psychogenic in origin.[68] During the American Civil War, DaCosta recognized a functional disorder of the heart, which he called irritable heart, that was marked by violent palpitations, constant dull pain, and physical exhaustion with the slightest exertion. DaCosta felt that the heart became irritable from frequent excitement and overaction. In the 1870s, symptoms of anxiety, depression, and exhaustion were labeled neurasthenia; in 1895, Freud coined the phrase "anxiety neurosis" because he felt the combination of heart spasms, sweating, and breathing difficulties centered on anxiety.[68] The Framingham heart study referred to this multinamed syndrome as neurocirculatory asthenia.[2] The third edition of the *Diagnostic and Statistical Manual of Mental Disorders*[70] has expanded and clarified psychiatric diagnostic categories, so that patients presenting with cardiac manifestations of anxiety could be classified under one of several syndromes depending on the clinical presentation.

ANXIETY DISORDERS

Patients with cardiac symptoms but without any organic evidence of heart disease could be classified under a variety of anxiety disorders: if the primary feature of the cardiac symptoms causes a persistent, irrational fear of leaving the home or other familiar setting unaccompanied, the condition would be classified as agoraphobia; if the main feature of the cardiac complaint consists of acute attacks of terrifying apprehension accompanied by dysphoria, palpitations, nausea, tremulousness, precordial discomfort, hyperventilation, dizziness, and weakness, the diagnosis of panic disorder would be made; if the condition consists of a persistent unprecipitated anxiety lasting for a least a month and accompanied by motor tension, autonomic hyperactivity, apprehensive expectation, edginess, impatience, distractability, poor sleep, and irritability, the disorder would be classified as generalized anxiety. Hyperventilation, a common symptom of anxiety disorders, may cause chest pain imitating angina or myocardial infarction.[2]

PSYCHOGENIC PAIN DISORDER

In psychogenic pain disorder, anxiety is converted into the physical symptom, pain. The conversion symptom prevents awareness of internal psychologic conflict (primary goal), while allowing the patient to avoid a noxious activity or gain a reward that would otherwise be unattainable (secondary gain). For example, after becoming enraged with his employer, an attack of chest pain prevents a man from confronting his boss (primary gain) and enables him to acquire a less tasking work assignment (secondary gain).

It may be difficult to distinguish myocardial ischemia from psychogenic pain disorder.[2] To be certain of the diagnosis of psychogenic pain disorder, physical findings must be absent and the psychologic factors must explain the cause of the pain. The angina symptoms may be atypical such as dull aches, fleeting stabs, or sticks of pain that cause dramatic grabbing of the chest and bending into a fetal position, or they may mimic exactly myocardial ischemia. The key depends on finding no organic disease after extensive diagnostic evaluation. Dyspnea at rest and frequent sighing respirations point toward psychogenic pain. A temporal relation between a psychologic conflict and the onset of pain seals the diagnosis. In some patients the pain has symbolic meaning, as in a man complaining of chest pain whose father died from myocardial infarction. Patients with psychogenic pain fail to obtain relief from medical reassurance, use analgesics excessively, assume a disabled role, and adamantly reject the role of psychologic factors in the pain.[70]

MANAGEMENT

Because these patients initially resist a psychologic interpretation of their illness, a special approach such as the Combined Medical Specialties Unit at Duke University Medical Center may offer the best prognosis. Patients are admitted to the unit under the care of a cardiologist. During extensive medical workup, psychiatric consultation is initiated and the patient begins biofeedback and stress management programs. As the diagnostic workup progresses, the patient is given a thorough, unambiguous explanation of how psychologic factors contribute to physical symptoms. Group therapy helps the patient understand the connection between soma and psyche: the short-term group is open ended, so that patients who are further along in therapy can help convince the newer members of the significance of emotional issues in causing physical symptoms. Individual psychotherapy aimed at uncovering unconscious psychologic conflicts is supplemented by educational and supportive psychotherapy from the nursing staff. Family therapy helps interrupt factors contributing to invalidism. Although the unit is too new to establish the long-term outcome of this approach, initial results are promising.

REFERENCES

1. Houpt JL, Orleans CS, George LK, Brodie HKH: *The Importance of Mental Health Services to General Health Care.* Cambridge, Mass, Ballinger Publishing Company, 1979.
2. Lipowski ZJ: Cardiovascular disorders, in Kaplan HI, Freedman AM, Sadock BJ (eds): *Comprehensive Textbook of Psychiatry/III,* ed 3. Baltimore, Williams & Wilkins, 1980, vol 2, pp 1891–1907.
3. Spaulding WB: The psychosomatic approach in the practice of medicine, in Lipowski ZJ, Lippsitt DR, Whybrow PC (eds): *Psychosomatic Medicine: Current Trends and Applications.* New York, Oxford University Press, 1977, pp 457–463.
4. Hartman LM: Behavioural prevention of ischemic heart disease. *Can Med Assoc J* 1978; 119:599–604.
5. Lacey BC, Lacey JI: Studies of heart rate and other bodily processes in sensorimotor behavior, in Obrist PA, Black AH, Brener J, di Cara LV (eds): *Cardiovascular Psychophysiology.* Chicago, Aldine Publishing Company, 1974, pp 538–564.
6. Taggart P, Carruthers M, Somerville W: Electrocardiogram, plasma catecholamines and lipids, and their modification by oxprenolol when speaking before an audience. *Lancet* 1973; 2:341–346.
7. Schiffer F, Hartley LH, Schulman CL, Abelmann WH: The quiz electrocardiogram: a new diagnostic and research technique for evaluating the relation between emotional stress and ischemic heart disease. *Am J Cardiol* 1976; 37:41–44.
8. Frankenhaeuser M: The role of peripheral catecholamines in adaptation to understimulation and overstimulation, in Serban G (ed): *Psychopathology of Human Adaptation.* New York, Plenum Press, 1976, pp 173–191.
9. Lynch JJ: *The Broken Heart.* New York, Basic Books, 1977.
10. Blumenthal JA, Calif R, Williams RS, Hindman N: Continuing medical education cardiac rehabilitation: a new frontier for behavioral medicine. *J Cardiac Rehab* 1983; 3:637–656.
11. Mulcahy R: Influence of cigarette smoking on morbidity and mortality after myocardial infarction. *Br Heart J* 1983; 49:410–415.
12. Kannel WB, Gordon T: Obesity and cardiovascular disease: the Framingham study, in Burland WL, Samuel PD, Yudkin J (eds): *Obesity Symposium.* New York, Churchill Livingstone, 1974, pp 24–51.
13. Ackerman AN: Factors influencing patient compliance in patients with ischemic heart disease, in Abbot EC, Becker MH, Biron P, Haynes RB, Laidlaw JC, Sackett DL, Taylor DW (eds): *A Workshop/Symposium on Compliance,* May 25–27, 1977. Hamilton, Ontario, Canada, McMaster University Medical Center, 1977, p 73.
14. Maddox GL, Anderson CF, Bogdonoff MD: Overweight as a problem of medical management in a public outpatient clinic. *Am J Med Sci* October 1966, pp 394–409.
15. Report of the American Heart Association Nutrition Committee: rationale of diet–heart statement of the American Heart Association. *Arteriosclerosis* 1982; 4:177–191.
16. Fergusun RJ, Pititclerc R, Choquette G, Chaniotis L, Gauthier P, Huot R, Allard C, Jankowski L, Campeau L: Effect of physical training on treadmill exercise capacity, collateral circulation and progression of coronary disease. *Am J Cardiol* 1974; 34:764–769.
17. Zoneraich S: Exercising testing and cardiac rehabilitation in patients with coronary artery disease. *Bull NY Acad Med* 1983; 59:635–659.

18. Rosenman RH, Friedman M, Straus R, Wurm M, Kositchek R, Hahn W, Werthessen NT: A predictive study of coronary heart disease: the Western Collaborative Group study. *JAMA* 1964; 189:15–22.
19. Jenkins CD, Rosenman RH, Friedman M: Development of an objective psychological test for the determination of the coronary-prone behavior pattern in employed men. *J Chron Dis* 1967; 20:371–379.
20. Blumenthal JA: Thoughts on the current status of investigations of personality patterns and coronary heart disease, in Reiffel J, de Bellis R, Mark LC, Kutscher AH, Patterson PR, Schoenbert B (eds): *Psychological Aspects of Cardiovascular Disease.* New York, Columbia University Press, 1980, pp 81–93.
21. Razin AN: Psychosocial intervention and coronary artery disease: a review. *Psychosom Med* 1982; 44:363–387.
22. Shekelle RB, Gale N, Ostfeld AM, Paul O: Hostility, risk of coronary heart disease, and mortality. *Psychosom Med* 1983; 45:109–114.
23. Barefoot JC, Dahlstrom G, Williams RB: Hostility, CHD incidence and total mortality: a 25-year followup study of 255 physicians. *Psychosom Med* 1983; 45:59–63.
24. The Review Panel on Coronary-Prone Behavior and Coronary Heart Disease: Coronary-prone behavior and coronary heart disease: a critical review. *Circulation* 1981; 63:1199–1215.
25. Blumenthal JA, Williams R, Kong Y, Schanberg SM, Thompson LW: Type A behavior and angiographically documented coronary disease. *Circulation* 1978; 58:634–637.
26. Krantz D, San Marco N, Selvester R, Matthews K: Psychological correlates of progression of atherosclerosis in men: a preliminary report. *Psychosom Med* 1979; 41:467–471.
27. Sheehan DV, Hackett TP: Psychosomatic disorders, in Nicholi AM Jr (ed): *The Harvard Guide to Modern Psychiatry.* Cambridge, Mass, The Belknap Press, Harvard University Press, 1978, pp 319–353.
28. Corse CD, Manuck SB, Kantwell JD: Coronary-prone behavior pattern and cardiovascular response in persons with and without coronary heart disease. *Psychosom Med* 1982; 44:449–459.
29. Krantz DS, Arabian JM, Davia JE: Type A behavior and coronary artery bypass surgery: intraoperative blood pressure and perioperative complications. *Psychosom Med* 1982; 44:273–284.
30. Schwartz GE, Weinberger GE, Singer JA: Cardiovascular differentiation of happiness, sadness, anger, and fear following imagery and exercise. *Psychosom Med* 1981; 43:343–364.
31. Brand RJ, Rosenman RH, Scholtz RI, Friedman M: Multivariate prediction of coronary heart disease in the Western Collaborative Group Study compared to the findings of the Framingham study. *Circulation* 1976; 53:348–355.
32. Suinn RM: Behavior therapy for cardiac patients. *Behav Ther* 1974; 5:569–577.
33. Farquahar JW, Maccoby N, Wood PD, Alexander JK, Breitrose H, Brown BW Jr, Haskell WL, McAlister AL, Meyer AJ, Nash JD, Stern MP: Community education for cardiovascular health. *Lancet* 1977; 1:1192–1195.
34. Holmes TH, Rahe RH: The social readjustment rating scale. *J Psychosom Res* 1967; 11:213–218.
35. Rahe RH, Romo N: Recent life changes and the onset of myocardial infarction and coronary death in Helsinki, in Gunderson EK, Rahe RH (eds): *Life Stress and Illness.* Springfield, Ill, Charles C Thomas, 1974.
36. Parkes CM, Benjamin B, Fitzgerald FG: Broken heart: a statistical study of increased mortality among widowers. *Br Med J* 1969; 1:740–743.
37. Hinkle LE, Whitney LH, Lehman EW, Dunn J, King BBR, Plakun A, Flehinger B: Occupation, education, and coronary heart disease. *Science* 1968; 161:238–246.
38. Holme I, Helgeland A, Hjermann I, Lund-Larsen PG, Leren P: Coronary risk factors and socio-economic status: the Oslo study. *Lancet* 1976; 2:1396–1398.
39. Theorell TG: Review of research on life events and cardiovascular illness. *Adv Cardiol* 1982; 29:140–147.
40. Medalie JH, Goldbourt U: Angina pectoris among 10,000 men. *Am J Med* 1976; 60:910–912.
41. Cassem NH, Hackett TP: Psychiatric consultation in a coronary care unit. *Ann Intern Med* 1971; 75:9–14.
42. Strain JJ, Grossman S: *Psychological Care of the Medically Ill: A Primer in Liaison Psychiatry.* New York, Appleton-Century-Crofts, 1975.
43. Walker JI: *Psychiatric Emergencies: Intervention and Resolution.* Philadelphia, JB Lippincott, 1983.
44. Papadopoulos C: How wives feel about coitus after husband's heart attack. *Med Aspects Human Sexuality* 1980; 14(8):57–66.
45. Mumford E, Schlesinger HJ, Glass GV: The effects of psychological intervention on recovery from surgery and heart attacks: an analysis of the literature. *Am J Public Health* 1982; 72:141–151.
46. Speidel H, Dahme B, Flemming B, Gotze P, Huse-Kleinstoll G, Meffert HJ, Rodewald G, Spehr W: Open-heart surgery unit. *Adv Psychosom Med* 1980; 10:30–56.
47. De Silva RA: Central nervous system risk factors for sudden cardiac death. *Ann NY Acad Sci* 1982; 382:143–161.
48. Lown B: Sudden cardiac death—1978. *Circulation* 1979; 60:1593–1599.
49. Myers A, Dewar HA: Circumstances attending 100 sudden deaths from coronary artery disease with coroners necropsies. *Br Heart J* 1975; 37:1133–1135.
50. Bedell SE, Delbanco TL, Cook EF, Epstein FH: Survival after cardiopulmonary resuscitation in a hospital. *N Eng J Med* 1983; 309:569–575.
51. Lemire JG, Johnson AL: Is cardiac resuscitation worthwhile? *N Engl J Med* 1972; 286:970–972.
52. Moody RA Jr: *Life after Life.* Atlanta, Mockingbird Books, 1975.
53. Cassem NH, Hackett TP: The setting of intensive care, in Hackett TP, Cassem NH (eds): *Massachusetts General Hospital Handbook of General Hospital Psychiatry.* St. Louis, CV Mosby, 1978, pp 319–341.
54. Alexander F: *Psychosomatic Medicine.* New York, WW Norton, 1950.
55. Ross DR, Walker JI, Covington T, Cools J: Psychiatric complications of nonpsychiatric drugs, in Sullivan JL, de Rimmer-Sullivan P (eds): *Biomedical Psychiatric Therapeutics.* Boston, Butterworth Publishers, 1984, pp 207–218.
56. Swift RM, Black HR: Essential hypertension: psychiatric aspects and use of psychotropics. *Psychosomatics* 1984; 25:737–742.
56a. Cheng TO: QRS duration in acute overdosage of tricyclic antidepressants. *N Engl J Med,* 1986; 314:989.
56b. Roberts DH: Cardiovascular effects of the tricyclic antidepressants. *IM* 1986; 7(2):52–61.
57. Davis JM: Antidepressant drugs, in Kaplan HI, Freedman AM, Sadock BJ (eds): *Comprehensive Textbook of Psychiatry/III,* ed 3. Baltimore, Williams & Wilkins, 1980, vol 3, pp 2290–2316.
58. Glassman AH: Cardiovascular effects of tricyclic antidepressants. *Ann Rev Med* 1984; 35:503–511.
58a. Boehnert MT, Lovejoy FH Jr: Value of the QRS duration versus the serum drug level in predicting seizures and ventricular arrhythmias after an acute overdose of tricyclic antidepressants. *N Engl J Med* 1985; 313:474–479.
59. Lewis WH, Richardson DJ, Gahagan LH: Cardiovascular disturbances and their management in modified electrotherapy for psychiatric illness. *N Engl J Med* 1955; 252:1016–1020.
60. Weiner RD, Henschen GM, Dellasega M, Baker JS: Propranolol treatment of and ECT-related ventricular arrhythmia. *Am J Psychiat* 1979; 136:1594–1595.
61. Toole JF: Vascular diseases of brain and spinal cord, in Merritt HH (ed): *A Textbook of Neurology,* ed 6. Philadelphia, Lea & Febriger, 1979, pp 149–211.
62. Kolin A, Norris JW: Myocardial damage from acute cerebral lesions. *Stroke* 1984; 15:990–993.
63. Perloff JK, Stevenson WG, Roberts NK, Caben W, Weiss J: Cardiac involvement in myotonic muscular dystrophy (Steinert's disease): a prospective study of 25 patients. *Am J Cardiol* 1984; 54:1074–1081.
63a. Hiromasa S, Ikeda T, Kubota K, Takata S, Hattori N, Nishimura M, Watanabe Y: A family with myotonic dystrophy associated with diffuse cardiac conduction disturbances as demonstrated by His bundle electrocardiography. *Am Heart J* 1986; 111:85–91.
64. Triffon DW, Ringel SP, Reiter MJ: Progression of electrocardiographic abnormalities in myotonic dystrophy. *Clin Res* 1985; 33:18A.
64a. Perloff JK: Neurological disorders and heart disease, in Braunwald E: *Heart Disease,* ed 2. Philadelphia, Saunders, 1984, pp 1711–1713.
64b. Gottdiener JS, Hawley RJ, Maron BJ, Bertorini TF, Engle WK: Characteristics of the cardiac hypertrophy in Friedreich's ataxia. *Am Heart J* 1982; 103:525–553.
64c. Zimmerman M, Gabathuler J, Adamec R, Pinget L: Unusual manifestations of heart involvement in Friedreich's ataxia. *Am Heart J* 1986; 111:184–187.
64d. Hawley RJ, Gottdiener JS: Five-year follow-up of Friedreich's ataxia cardiomyopathy. *Arch Intern Med* 1986; 146:483–488.
64e. Harding AE, Hewer RL: The heart disease of Freidreich's ataxia: clinical and electrocardiographic study of 115 patients with an analysis of serial electrocardiographic changes in 30 cases. *Quart J Med* 1983; 52:489–502.
64f. Kilgo GR, Toole JF, McGhee TB: Cerebrovascular disease and neurological manifestations of heart disease, in Hurst JW (ed): *The Heart,* ed 6. New York, McGraw-Hill, 1986, pp 1354–1363.
65. Preziosi TJ: Stroke syndromes and cerebrovascular disorders, in Harvey AM, Johns RJ, McKusick VA, Owens AH, Ross RH (eds): *The Principles and Practice of Medicine,* ed 20. New York, Appleton-Century-Crofts, 1980, pp 1278–1288.
65a. Cheng TO: Paradoxical embolism. A diagnostic challenge and its detection during life. *Circulation* 1976; 53:565–568.
65b. Caplan LR, D'Cruz I, Hier DB, Reddy H, Shah S: Atrial size, atrial fibrillation, and stroke. *Ann Neurol* 1986; 19:158–161.
66. Busse EW: Cardiovascular disease and psychopathology in the elderly. *Psychiatric Clin N Am* 1982; 5:159–169.
67. Sandok BA: Organic mental disorders associated with circulatory disturbances, in Kaplan HI, Freedman AM, Sadock BJ (eds): *Comprehensive*

Textbook of Psychiatry/III, ed 3. Baltimore, Williams & Wilkins, 1980, vol 2, pp 1392–1405.

68. Nemiah JC: Anxiety state (anxiety neurosis), in Kaplan HI, Freedman AM, Sadock BJ (eds): *Comprehensive Textbook of Psychiatry/III*, ed 3. Baltimore, Williams & Wilkins, 1980, vol 2, pp 1483–1493.
69. Wooley CF: From irritable heart to mitral valve prolapse: the Osler connection. *Am J Cardiol* 1984; 53:870–874.
70. American Psychiatric Association: *Diagnostic and Statistical Manual of Mental Disorders*, ed 3. Washington, DC, The American Psychiatric Association Press, 1980.

60 The Heart in Renal Disease

Henri A. Jahn, MD, Dominique C. Schohn, MD, and Renée L. Schmitt, MD

Disorders of the cardiovascular system are common in renal disease. They assume a prominent place when renal failure develops. These disorders exhibit a strong relation between cardiac function and volume regulation as well as electrolyte homeostasis. Cardiovascular impairment in renal disease demonstrates the important role of renal endocrine and metabolic regulations and comprises among others hypertension, which is a permanent threat to the heart, the whole arterial system, and the kidney.

Modern treatment of end-stage renal failure, such as long-term hemodialysis and transplantation, has been among the most important acquisitions of medicine. Treatment that corrects the humoral disorders of renal failure has allowed observations on the evolution of associated cardiovascular impairment. However, these techniques also display their own potential for deleterious effects on the cardiovascular system. Cardiovascular disturbances are the principal complications in the morbidity and mortality of renal failure.

CARDIOVASCULAR MORBIDITY AND MORTALITY IN END-STAGE RENAL FAILURE

Cardiovascular morbidity remains a limiting factor in the complete rehabilitation of patients with end-stage renal disease treated by either hemodialysis, peritoneal dialysis, or transplantation.[1] Cardiovascular complications represent the main cause of mortality in these patients.[2,3] The prevalence of cardiovascular disorders in patients with dialysis and transplantation is shown in the study of the registry of the EDTA-ERA[2] and the National Dialysis Registry of the United States.[4] The causes of mortality are of cardiovascular origin in nearly 50% of the patients, with only minor differences between the two registries. The mean age of cardiovascular-related mortality is 43.8 years in the United States, whereas it is 40 years in Europe. Both registries show that the mortality in male patients is higher than that in females (2/3 versus 1/3). Cardiac causes of death represent 35% of cases in the United States and 41% in Europe; cerebrovascular accidents, 7% in the United States and 10% in Europe. The respective role of pericarditis, hypertensive myocardiopathy, endocarditis, cardiac arrhythmias, and the like in mortality is analyzed in the European Registry (Table 60.1).[2] Hyperkalemia, hemorrhagic pericarditis, and hypertensive cardiac failure occur more often in younger patients. The origin of renal disease influences the distribution of causes of death[2] (Table 60.2). A high proportion of deaths are due to myocardial infarction, hy-

Table 60.1. Percentage of Cardiovascular Causes of Death in the EDTA-ERA Dialysis Registry*

Total Registry	Myocardial Infarction (%)	Hyperkalemia (%)	Hemorrhagic Pericarditis (%)	Other Causes of Cardiac Failure (%)	Cardiac Arrest (%)	Cerebrovascular Accidents (%)	Hypertensive Cardiac Failure (%)
Males							
30,470	12.5	3.4	2.2	8.4	9.0	10.3	5.2
Females							
20,369	7	3.4	2.3	9.3	9.3	12.2	4.8

*Adapted from Wing et al.[2]

pertensive cardiac failure, and cerebrovascular accidents in patients with renovascular disease, whereas there is a higher frequency of cerebrovascular accidents and a lower frequency of cardiac failure in patients with cystic disease of the kidney. Statistical evaluation is necessary to predict life expectancy in end-stage renal disease and to evaluate treatment costs.[5]

RISK FACTORS FOR CARDIOVASCULAR DISEASE

The clinician must be aware of all etiologic and potential risk factors in the cardiovascular system that may occur during the course of renal disease. Among the most important are:

- hypertension,
- fluid and sodium imbalances,
- electrolyte imbalances: dyskalemias and alterations in divalent ion metabolism,
- acidosis,
- anemia,
- uremic toxins (?),
- endocrine disorders (renin-angiotensin system, catecholamines, parathormone, and calcitriol),
- metabolic derangements:
    - lipid and hydrocarbon metabolism (atherosclerosis and diabetes mellitus)
    - oxalosis and hemochromatosis,
- nutritional deficiencies due to protein loss or to poor protein diet,
- infective episodes, and
- immunologic disorders.

Numerous important publications have been devoted to cardiovascular problems in renal disease.[6–12] In the course of chronic renal failure and in patients treated by renal replacement therapy, cardiac involvement may be disclosed by several clinical manifestations such as congestive heart failure, coronary heart disease, pericarditis, endocarditis, hypertension, or hypotension. These topics are treated elsewhere in this textbook, but because they have specific connotations in renal failure and its treatment modalities, their more specific aspects are disclosed in this chapter.

MYOCARDIAL PERFORMANCE IN CHRONIC RENAL FAILURE

Myocardial integrity is the main determinant of cardiac performance. Myocardial impairment appears to affect nearly 10% of dialysis patients and may be present before dialysis.[1,2]

In chronic renal failure, when myocardial evaluation is based on echocardiography, electrocardiography, and x-ray examination, an apparently normal myocardial status or, conversely, signs of electrocardiographic alterations and myocardial hypertrophy (eccentric or concentric) may be found. Cardiologic findings in these patients may be normal or they may display signs of congestive heart failure. These may be due to fluid overload (congested state[13]) with few signs of myocardial alteration as well as to small fluid overload in the case of significant impairment of myocardial performance. Hypertension has an additive effect in this latter situation. Nevertheless, its more specific effect is one of left ventricular failure.

CLINICAL MANIFESTATIONS

Different clinical stages can be delineated in patients with chronic renal failure and in those under replacement treament.

Early Signs of Cardiac Impairment

Patients with chronic renal failure (plasma creatinine levels up to 10 mg/dl), in the absence of hypertension, may appear to be without cardiac deterioration. Nevertheless, the response to exercise in these patients is impaired. They show limited exercise capacity and earlier fatigue in comparison with age-matched subjects without renal failure.[14–17] This exercise limitation may be due to uremia, anemia, volume overexpansion, or to a minor degree of myocardial impairment.[18]

Table 60.2. Percentage of Cardiovascular Causes of Death in Males, All Ages, According to the Primary Renal Disease. (Patients Treated by Hemodialysis—EDTA-ERA Registry 1983)*

Causes	Glomerulonephritis (%)	Hypertension (%)	Diabetes Mellitus (%)	Cystic Kidney Disease (%)	Other Kidney Diseases (%)
Myocardial infarction	12.4	17.5	16	18.2	13.3
Acute cardiac causes	17.3	15	17.8	13.8	16
Cardiac failure	17.2	15.9	12.2	9.1	15
Cerebrovascular accidents	10.6	14.9	12.2	13.6	10.7
All other causes	42.5	36.6	41.7	45.3	44.9

*Adapted from Wing et al.[1]

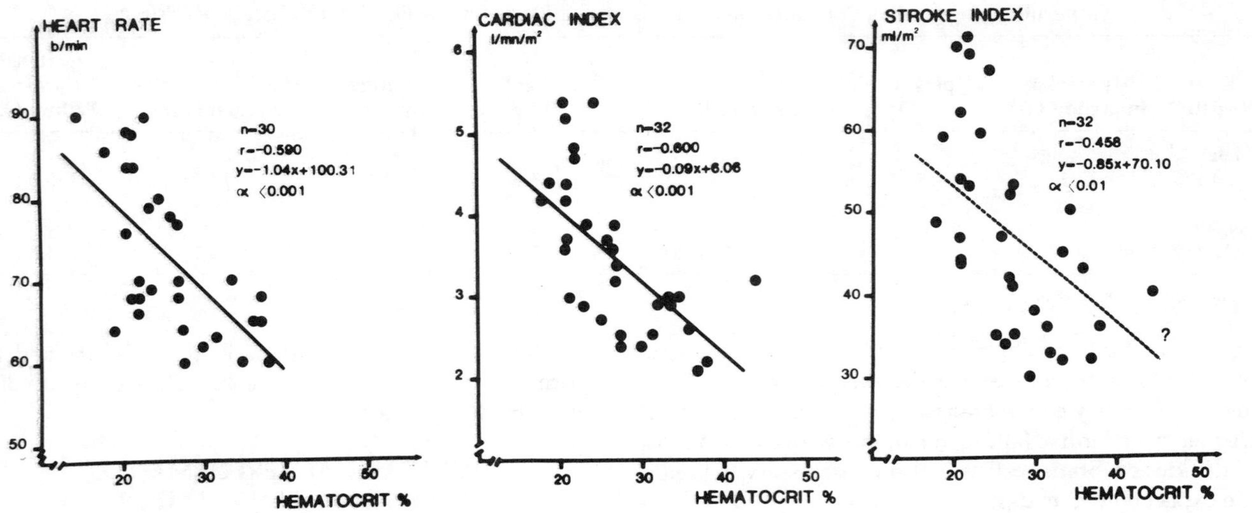

Figure 60.1. Heart rate, cardiac index, and stroke index as a function of hematocrit in patients with chronic renal failure. (From Jahn et al,[14] with permission.)

Assessment of Myocardial Function

The Sokolow index evaluated on the electrocardiogram and the cardiothoracic index measured on chest x-ray are not increased. Right atrial pressure and pulmonary wedge pressure are within the normal range,[14] whereas heart rate and cardiac index increase with the intensity of anemia and are inversely correlated with hematocrit (Figure 60.1). The study of diastolic properties of the myocardium as explored with cardiac function curves, following the Frank–Starling principle (cardiac output as a function of pulmonary wedge pressure) established after saline infusion,[19] shows on the average a reduced cardiac performance with high plasma creatinine levels[14–19] (Figure 60.2).

Investigation of the systolic properties of the myocardium explored by the left ventricular end-systolic pressure/volume ratio discloses slight left ventricular impairment. Left ventricular ejection fraction and circumferential fiber shortening determined by echocardiography correlate more or less with the preceding data. Cardiac performance is not perfect in most patients with chronic renal failure, and some degree of myocardial impairment can be speculated to exist when plasma creatinine levels are elevated above 6 mg/dl.[14,15] Most hemodialysis patients demonstrate an improvement in predialysis cardiac performance, but in some the cardiac performance remains altered.

Congestive Heart Failure

Signs of heart failure may appear in some patients with end-stage renal failure and also in patients on long-term hemodialysis.

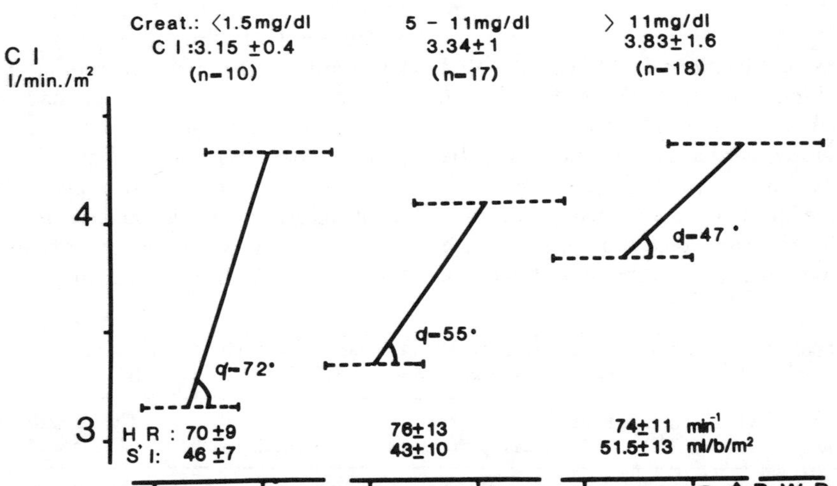

Figure 60.2. Heart function curves following Frank–Starling principles, showing flattening of the curve with increasing plasma creatinine levels. CI = cardiac index; HR = heart rate; PWP = pulmonary wedge pressure; SI = stroke index. (From Jahn et al,[14] with permission.)

Exertional Dyspnea. The patient is exercise intolerant, has shortness of breath after small efforts, and complains of fatigue. He has some ankle swelling, and pulmonary rales may exist. These symptoms may be related to volume overexpansion or myocardial impairment, or both.

Permanent Dyspnea. The patient presents with permanent dyspnea. Orthopnea may exist. He also presents with edema, pulmonary congestion, sometimes liver enlargement, and jugular vein distention. Cyanosis is rare because of the low hemoglobin levels associated with renal failure. On examination, the heart rate is increased, a gallop and a murmur of mitral regurgitation may be observed, and in some cases arrhythmia is also present. These patients often have elevated blood pressure. Large volume overexpansion, myocardial impairment, or both are responsible for this clinical stage.

Paroxysmal Pulmonary Edema. Paroxysmal pulmonary edema is rare in patients with apparently normal functional heart status. When it occurs, it is related to significant volume overload due to noncompliance of sodium and water dietary restriction. It is frequent when exertional dyspnea is present and coexists with hypertension. In hypertension, small volume overexpansion can be sufficient to initiate paroxysmal pulmonary edema because of the existing myocardial impairment. However, paroxysmal pulmonary edema is more specifically related to severe hypertension and to its effects on the left ventricle.

Assessment of Cardiac Function

In patients with signs of congestive heart failure, the Sokolow index and the cardiothoracic index are most often increased. The electrocardiogram may show signs of coexisting coronary heart disease or conduction disturbances, or both. Right atrial pressure and pulmonary artery wedge pressure are increased. Both high[20-22] and low[23] cardiac output states have been described.

Echocardiographic findings share many features with those found in cardiac patients without renal failure.[23-27] Left ventricular ejection fraction and circumferential fiber shortening are impaired. Moreover, echocardiography shows myocardial wall alterations. Echocardiographic findings allow several types of alterations to be distinguished, among which the following three are of particular interest in the management of fluid removal during dialysis[28]: (1) enlargement of cardiac chambers with normokinetic wall motion (Figure 60.3), (2) enlargement of cardiac chambers with hypokinetic wall motion (Figure 60.4), and (3) myocardial wall thickening with reduced chamber dimensions (Figure 60.5). Concentric hypertrophy usually is the consequence of severe hypertension, whereas eccentric hypertrophy may be the result of fluid overload.

The best evaluation of left ventricular contractility is the left ventricular end-systolic pressure/volume ratio. In these chronic renal failure patients it shows important alterations in left ventricular contractility.[14,29-31] This ratio, established before and after 500 ml of saline solution, demonstrates the incapacity of the left ventricle to adapt to volume overload. Suga et al[32] showed that these results permit a load-independent evaluation of left ventricular performance. Other noninvasive investigations, such as single-pass radionuclide ventriculography and equilibrium radionuclide ventriculography, may be of help in exploring myocardial function.[33]

It must be stressed that in patients with chronic renal failure, volume overexpansion induces signs of a congested state, which is sometimes difficult to distinguish

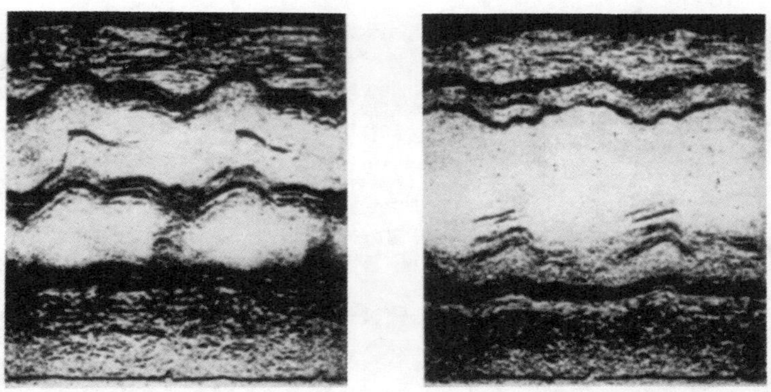

GRA... G..., 41 years, AP : 160/100 mm Hg

LA diastolic dimension : 3.2 cm

LV diastolic dimension : 6.2 cm — $\overline{\text{RAP}}$: 2 mm Hg

LV systolic dimension : 4.3 cm — $\overline{\text{PAP}}$: 12 mm Hg

LV posterior wall thickness : 0.8 cm — $\overline{\text{PWP}}$: 7 mm Hg

Interventricular septum thickness : 1 cm

Figure 60.3. M-mode echocardiograms showing dilation of left ventricle with normokinetic wall motion. (From Jahn et al,[28] with permission.)

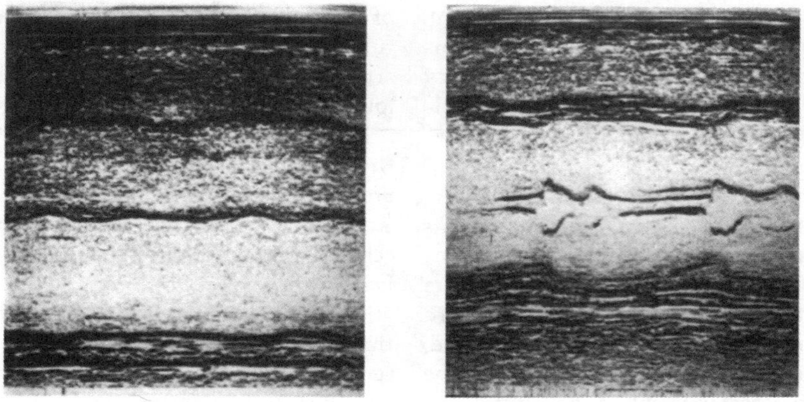

KEI... L..., 62 years, AP : 140/80 mm Hg

LA diastolic dimension : 4.8 cm

LV diastolic dimension : 7.3 cm, LV systolic dimension : 6.5 cm

LV posterior wall thickness : 0.5 cm

Interventricular septum thickness : 0.7 cm

Figure 60.4. M-mode echocardiograms showing dilatation of the left ventricle and the left atrium with hypokinetic wall motion. (From Jahn et al,[28] with permission.)

from true congestive heart failure. Frank–Starling curves provide a good pattern and means of distinguishing fluid overexpansion from myocardial impairment. The theoretic behavior of both left and right ventricles in Figures 60.6 and 60.7 demonstrates the effect of fluid overload producing increased cardiac output on the filling pressure when the left ventricle is normal (Figure 60.6) or impaired (Figure 60.7). In the latter case the pressure increment is tremendous with a small fluid overload. At the end of hemodialysis, retransfusion of extracorporeal blood gives a segment of the Frank–Starling curve that can be inserted in one of the curves in Figures 60.6 and 60.7. The steepness of this segment indicates the myocardial capacity to respond to a volume load. The steeper the segment, the better the myocardial performance.[6,14] This pressure/output relation gives information to differentiate volume overexpansion from myocardial failure.

The Frank–Starling curves also provide a scheme for managing uremic patients with right heart failure during hemodialysis. Too vigorous ultrafiltration decreases right ventricular filling pressure, which diminishes right cardiac output, endangers the pulmonary circulation and gas ex-

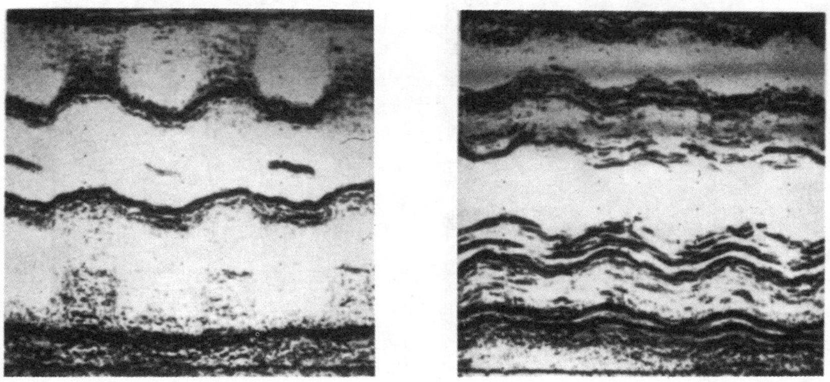

STR... J.C..., 35 years, AP : 170/110 mm Hg

LA diastolic dimension : 4.8 cm — $\overline{RAP}$: 14 mm Hg

LV diastolic dimension : 5.2 cm — $\overline{PAP}$: 46 mm Hg

LV systolic dimension : 3.1 cm — $\overline{PWP}$: 31 mm Hg

LV posterior wall thickness : 2.1 cm

Figure 60.5. M-mode echocardiograms showing wall and septum thickening (concentric hypertrophy). (From Jahn et al,[28] with permission.)

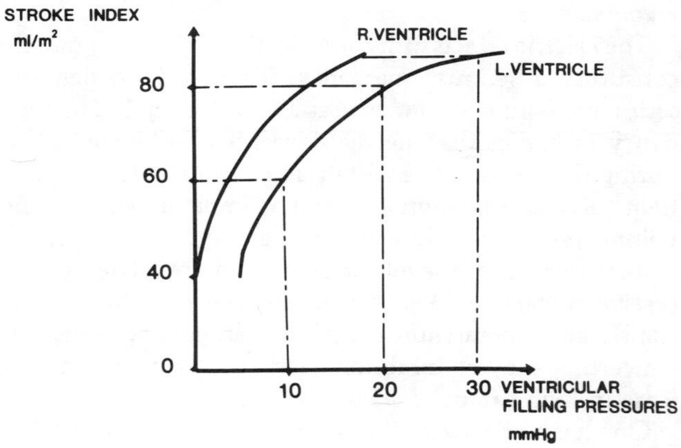

Figure 60.6. Pressure increment with increasing cardiac output, which can be correlated with fluid overload. With high stroke volume a dangerous pulmonary wedge pressure is reached, which can result in pulmonary edema.

changes in the lung, and leads to a dramatic decrease in left ventricular output.[28]

Uremic patients may show signs of myocardial impairment early in the course of renal failure, without important morphologic changes of the myocardium. In more advanced renal failure, serious impairment of myocardial performance appears associated with morphologic and electrocardiographic changes. At this stage of cardiac disorder, cardiomyopathy is multifactorial.

TREATMENT

The general treatment strategy becomes a matter of early prevention of increased myocardial work. The best hemodynamic conditions must be provided for the heart during renal failure and long-term dialysis treatment, maintaining a rigorous sodium and water balance, with overexpansion being a factor of increased preload and afterload.

Other factors that increase myocardial work or depress myocardial contractility must be suppressed or corrected as much as possible. There is much interest in the role of angiotensin converting enzyme inhibitors, nitrates, and other vasodilators to reduce afterload. The beta blockers tend to prevent or correct myocardial hypertrophy, but because of their negative inotropic effects, they must be given with caution. It is advisable to consult the specific treatment strategies that have to be applied in the different forms of hypertrophy.

The general trend in digitalis treatment currently is to limit its use to precise indications, such as congestive heart failure and certain arrhythmias, to administer rather small doses, and to take into account their pharmacokinetics and their interactions with other drugs.[34]

In patients with renal failure, these rules seem highly valuable. Nevertheless, before administering digitalis to patients in a congested state, a causal sodium and water retention that has to be managed by diuretics or fluid removal with dialysis techniques must be excluded. When digitalis is administered, it is necessary to control the kalemia and correct eventual hypokalemia in patients on diuretic or hemodialysis treatment. The practical impact of inhibition of Na^+-K^+-ATPase by uremic toxins or of an eventual circulating digitalis-like factor is not yet established.[35]

The digitalis glycosides most often used are digoxin and digitoxin. The choice between these two drugs is related to their respective properties. Digoxin is excreted in the urine and its excretion is directly proportional to the glomerular filtration rate,[36] with only minor modifications by tubular distal secretion.[37] Digoxin has a short half-life (1.5 days) in patients with normal kidney function and about 30% of the administered dose disappears per day.[34] During renal failure the dose has to be adapted to the renal excretion capacities. Control of its plasma levels is necessary to avoid signs of digitalis toxicity. During hemodialysis, only small quantities were dialyzed, the drug having an elevated protein-binding capacity. Dialysis treatment does not interfere much with the plasma levels of the drug.[38–40]

Digitoxin is advocated as the best drug in renal failure.[34] Its half-life (five to seven days) is longer than that of digoxin and it is not influenced by renal function. During dialysis the same behavior as for digoxin has to be observed. There are undesirable drug interactions with digitalis. Diuretics may produce hypokalemia. Antiarrhythmic drugs have negative inotropic effects and quinidine, procainamide, and beta blockers may favor the initiation of atrioventricular block. Calcium antagonists may increase the digitalis serum levels.

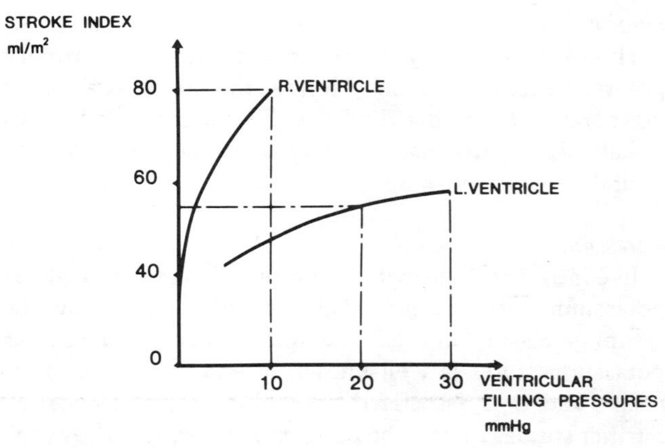

Figure 60.7. Graph showing that when left ventricular limitation exists, a small volume overload induces a dangerous pressure increment.

HUMORAL DISORDERS AND MYOCARDIAL FUNCTION

SODIUM

The disorders of sodium metabolism that are important for cardiovascular function in renal disease concern mainly the imbalances of this cation. Sodium balance is claimed to be maintained until glomerular filtration rates reach a low level, the adaptive mechanism being modifications of the tubular reabsorption of this ion. A natriuretic factor has been implied to inhibit sodium reabsorption in renal failure[41–43] and to enable adequate sodium excretion. This still hypothetical factor is claimed to inhibit Na^+-K^+-ATPase. There is now evidence for the existence of a natriuretic hormone of cardiac origin,[44] which has been isolated[45–47] and sequenced. The most common denominations are "cardionatrin" or "atrial natriuretic peptide." This hormone has important vasodilator potential and increases natriuresis through its effects on the glomerular filtration rate.[48,49] It is augmented in chronic renal failure,[50] but its exact effects in this condition are not yet established.

Positive Sodium Balance

Sodium retention occurs more frequently than expected in severe renal failure,[51] a difficult period of treatment in which sodium intake has to be well adapted to sodium excretion. In many cases, sodium and water retention is responsible for overexpansion of extracellular volume, hypertension, and congestive heart failure.[52]

Care must be taken to detect this overload and to interpret correctly its effects on hemodynamics. Treatment consists of dietary sodium and water restriction, large doses of furosemide, and in the absence of response to this treatment, hemodialysis to remove excess salt and fluid.

Negative Sodium Balance

A negative sodium balance is less frequent because of the increased urinary sodium loss. The consequences of negative sodium balance are hypovolemia and hypotension with an orthostatic syndrome. In such cases sodium administration has to be adapted to salt loss.

Both positive and negative sodium and fluid balances can occur during long-term hemodialysis treatment and have hemodynamic and cardiac consequences. Maintenance of an adequate salt and fluid balance is therefore important in the surveillance of patients with chronic hemodialysis. Hemofiltration is more efficient in achieving salt and water removal with fewer side effects.

METABOLIC ACIDOSIS

Metabolic acidosis may be detected in the early stages of renal failure when evaluated by plasma bicarbonate. It is due to renal incapacity to excrete H^+ ions and it increases in severity with the deterioration of renal function.[53] In end-stage renal disease, important decreases of pH associated with respiratory symptoms may occur.

Acidosis decreases myocardial performance and blunts the myocardial response to catecholamines.[54,55] Congestive heart failure may be initiated or, when it preexists, be severely aggravated.

Treatment. Treatment consists of the administration of bicarbonate. In mild acidosis oral compensation may be efficient; in severe cases infusion of bicarbonate is necessary. In end-stage renal failure, severe acidosis indicates that hemodialysis treatment, which corrects both acidosis and the associated electrolyte disorders, should be initiated.

POTASSIUM

The cardiologic effects of potassium metabolism in renal failure deserve major interest.

Hyperkalemia

The electric effects of hyperkalemia on the heart muscle constitute a serious emergency. They occur when the serum potassium level increases above 6 mEq/L. The tendency to higher than normal levels has to be controlled during the course of renal failure or in hemodialysis patients. Renal potassium excretion is impaired when urine volume decreases below 800 ml per day.

Increased plasma levels of potassium are related to excessive dietary intake, antialdosterone diuretics, blood transfusions, potassium-containing drugs, angiotensin II converting enzyme inhibitors, and cellular potassium release in high catabolic stages.

One has to be aware that hyperkalemia has no specific clinical symptoms. Weakness of skeletal muscles, dizziness, and nausea have been observed. Electrocardiographic signs are most important for diagnosis, but they do not always correlate with serum potassium levels. A tented T wave,[56] increased T amplitude, widening of the QRS, and a loss of atrial activity can be observed.[57,58] These signs may precede cardiac arrest.

Treatment. A suspicion of hyperkalemia indicates immediate treatment. Bicarbonate infusion can be initiated. Fifty to 100 mEq of sodium bicarbonate may be administered intravenously over a period of 30 minutes and repeated.[11] Like bicarbonate, infusion of glucose with insulin favors the entry of potassium into the cells. Intravenous calcium chloride may antagonize the electric effects of hyperkalemia (10 to 20 ml of 10% calcium chloride solution have been proposed).[6] Cation exchange resins such as sodium polystyrene sulfonate (Kayexalate®) act more slowly and exchange non-negligible amounts of sodium for potassium. They may be administered orally (15 g three times a day) or by enema in an emergency. During hemodialysis they may help to achieve the potassium balance.

In serious situations, which may also be encountered in long-term hemodialysis treatment, immediate dialysis will be more efficient. Nevertheless, the plasma levels of potassium must be decreased slowly. Hemodialysis also has the advantage in severe situations of correcting other electrolyte and acid-base disorders.

Hypokalemia

Hypokalemia rarely occurs from spontaneous urinary potassium loss, but it may follow the administration of nonpotassium-sparing diuretics. The occurrence of hypokalemia is particularly dangerous in patients receiving digitalis treatment.

Potassium Deficiency

In contrast to transient heart effects, there exist cellular potassium deficiencies[59] that are not reflected by the serum potassium levels. The role of decreased cellular potassium stores is well known in end-stage renal failure,[60] and it is associated with glucose intolerance.[60,61] Further studies have to be performed to explore the eventual effects of both potassium deficiency and glucose intolerance on the myofibrils.

Potassium deficiency may be due to fecal potassium

loss related to the aldosterone effect on intestinal potassium absorption. Aldosterone inhibition may explain the rapid hyperkalemias that follow antialdosterone therapy in end-stage renal failure.

CALCIUM

Calcium, through the plasma levels of ionized calcium, interferes with cardiovascular function. In renal failure, reduced intestinal calcium absorption is due to a lack of calcitriol, which is considered a renal hormone. The decrease in serum levels of ionized calcium implies two consequences on cardiovascular function: a decrease in myocardial contractility[62] and interference with norepinephrine release, which is directly related to serum calcium levels.[63,64] A direct relation seems to exist between contractility and ionized calcium plasma levels in chronic renal failure. There is a direct correlation between d*p*/d*t*/PD and the plasma ratio of Ca^{++}/K^{+} (Figure 60.8), arguing in favor of an effect of calcium on contractility.[14] In endocrine cardiology, an entity termed hypocalcemic cardiomyopathy may be isolated.[65] Heart failure has been observed in acute hypocalcemia, after parathyroidectomy, and after the administration of large amounts of citrates (transfusion), mithramycin, and intravenous phosphate.[62]

Alterations in calcium metabolism may also produce significant deleterious effects on the cardiovascular system by inducing metastatic phosphocalcic deposits. This phenomenon is frequent and occurs in relation to high plasma phosphate levels and hyperparathyroidism.[66] When the product of the plasma levels of calcium and phosphorus expressed in milligrams per deciliter is above 70, metastatic calcifications occur in soft tissues as in the media of arteries (mediacalcinosis).[66,67] Mitral anular locations have also been described.[68–71] In this context, one may speak of hypercalcemic cardiomyopathy.

Treatment. In hypocalcemia without hyperphosphatemia, oral calcium administration has some corrective effects,[72] but for adequate correction, calcitriol or other active metabolites of vitamin D are more efficient. They have been demonstrated to also improve left ventricular function.[73] Care must be taken to avoid hypercalcemia. When hyperphosphatemia exists, intestinal phosphate binders, either calcium carbonate or aluminum hydroxide, must be given.

NITROGEN WASTE PRODUCTS (UREMIC CARDIOMYOPATHY)

The degree of renal azotemic retention is best indicated by the glomerular filtration rate or serum creatinine levels, or both. Urea or blood urea nitrogen is less reliable in evaluating renal function because of its dependence on dietary management and cellular catabolism. Many waste products are classified as uremic toxins among which cyanate and guanidine compounds have been suspected to induce cardiovascular disturbances.[74–76] Uric acid and oxalic acid also undergo the renal retention process, but they depend more on endogenous metabolic alterations. Uric acid appears to be an important risk factor. Oxalic acid mainly in primary and secondary oxalosis, enhanced by retention, yields crystal deposits in the myocardium.

The term *uremic cardiomyopathy* has been coined. Both its existence and its etiology have become a matter of controversy. It has been difficult up to now to define a characteristic lesion or dysfunction of the myocardium, and it is also difficult to incriminate urea or a definite toxin in producing specific effects. Brass et al[77] introduced the broader term *urämische Herzkrankheit: UHK* (cardiomyopathy of uremia), which may imply other causes associated with azotemia such as myocardial calcium deposits[78] and carnitine deficiency.[79]

The problem appears still more entangled when the postulated effects of uremia on myocardial function are considered. Many reports stress the existence of myocardial depression,[6,7,10,11,74,76,80–83] and conversely, others present data showing enhanced myocardial perfor-

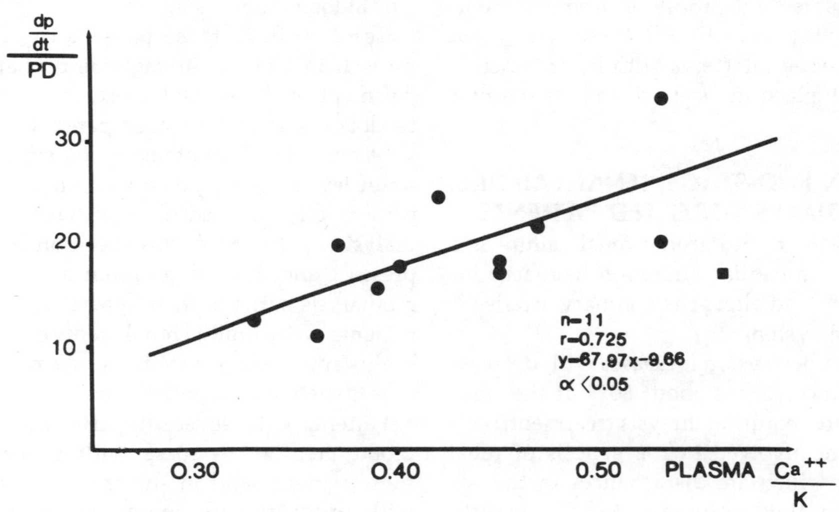

Figure 60.8. Correlation between d*p*/d*t*/PD and plasma ratio (Ca^{++}/K^{+}) in patients with chronic renal failure. d*p*/d*t* = instantaneous rate of rise of left ventricular pressure. PD = developed pressure (the total intraventricular pressure minus the end-diastolic pressure). (From Jahn et al,[14] with permission.)

mance[21,22,84–87] in renal failure. More experimental data must be gathered to elucidate this problem.

ANEMIA

Anemia is related to erythropoietin deficiency and to uremic toxins. Reduced hemoglobin levels and erythrocyte counts are associated with reduced oxygen-carrying capacity and reduced blood viscosity. Chronic anemia in man increases cardiac output when the hemoglobin level is below 7 g% and decreases systemic vascular resistance. Hyperkinetic states may be encountered.[88–90] In the preceding text, we showed the relation between hematocrit and heart rate and between hematocrit and cardiac output. We can speculate that both high cardiac output and reduced oxygen delivery may be etiologic factors in myocardial deterioration.[91] High cardiac output and decreased systemic vascular resistance may be corrected by blood transfusion.[92]

HYPERPARATHYROIDISM

Secondary hyperparathyroidism is common in chronic renal failure. Hyperparathyroidism has been claimed to depress cardiac function in uremia,[93] and a series of experimental studies by Massry[94] have shown that excess parathyroid hormone alters most of the energetic reactions at the cellular level, generating a specific heart muscle disease. Evidence indicates that parathormone inhibits in vitro oxygen uptake and phosphorylation by the heart mitochondria and reduces myocardial ATP and creatine phosphate in rat myofibrils.[95,96] Conversely, parathormone apparently inhibits the depressant effects of both l- and d-propranolol on the contractile force of the myofibrils,[97] and Katon et al[98] have demonstrated a positive inotropic effect of parathormone on the myocardium.

In clinical situations with high parathyroid hormone levels, investigation of myocardial performance using the Frank–Starling curves established before and after volume load discloses that the curves are shifted upward and to the left when compared with those of uremic patients without hyperparathyroidism.[14,99] All these data argue that parathyroid hormone interferes with heart function and has a prominent place in heart disease in chronic renal failure.

HYPERTENSION IN END-STAGE RENAL FAILURE AND IN HEMODIALYSIS-TREATED PATIENTS

Hypertension in patients in chronic renal failure is a most important factor in cardiac alteration in that it increases cardiac work[100] and alters the coronary arteries[101] and the entire arterial system.[102]

The prevalence of hypertension increases with decreasing kidney function and reaches about 80% at the stage of terminal renal failure requiring dialysis treatment.[103,104] Many mechanisms are involved in the genesis of renal hypertension, among which are disturbances in the sodium and extracellular fluid volume state,[51,105] disturbances in the renin–angiotensin[106] and sympathetic[107] pressor systems, disturbances in basal tone and in the cardiovascular reactivity to vasoactive stimuli,[107–109] and perhaps disturbances in the vasodepressor prostaglandin and kinin systems.[110] Disturbances in the sodium and extracellular fluid volume state are of primary importance and interfere with integrated hemodynamic autoregulation.[51,111]

Studies in patients with mild to moderate renal failure show a slightly elevated cardiac output and peripheral resistance when compared with those in normal subjects and patients with normal arterial pressure.[112] In end-stage renal failure, the major hemodynamic alterations maintaining high blood pressure are a commensurate and inappropriate increase in systemic vascular resistance coexisting with either a normal or high cardiac output.[113–117] Nevertheless, somewhat different hemodynamic patterns have also been reported.[15,114,118] Two main factors can be implied in the increase in cardiac output: anemia and extracellular fluid volume expansion. Structural as well as nonstructural and humoral mechanisms may contribute to these hemodynamic features.

Extracellular fluid volume and exchangeable body sodium are expanded in most patients with renal failure.[119–122] These alterations may also be found in patients on chronic hemodialysis.[107] Water and salt retention is a dominant factor in the hypertension accompanying renal failure[123,124] and also represents a factor in increased cardiac work. There exist close relations between blood pressure and exchangeable sodium and extracellular fluid volume in patients with terminal renal failure before the onset of hemodialysis.[121] These correlations were also found in patients on chronic hemodialysis.[107] The onset of hemodialysis and the removal of excess fluid and salt overload by vigorous ultrafiltration allow blood pressure control in approximately 80% to 90% of hypertensive patients on chronic hemodialysis.[52] This has led to the concept of volume-dependent hypertension in renal failure. In 10% to 20% of patients, blood pressure remains high, suggesting additional causes of blood pressure elevation.

With the progressive impairment of renal failure, many investigators described activation of the renin–angiotensin–aldosterone system.[106,119,121,125–127] The increased release of renin in these patients can be explained either by ischemia of the juxtaglomerular apparatus or by impairment of the juxtaglomerular perception of inhibitory feedback signals.[103,105] Compared with those in normal subjects and normotensive patients on hemodialysis, renin levels at any given sodium-volume state were approximately doubled in hypertensive patients on hemodialysis.[105,128,129–131] A close relation between mean blood pressure and the sodium renin product was found in hemodialysis patients with hypertension as in hypertensive patients with mild renal failure.[118,119] Therefore, the renin–angiotensin system also seems to contribute to volume-dependent hypertension.

Patients with severe hypertension have an important blood pressure decrease with saralazin infusion.[118] In these patients and in the chronic hemodialysis patients with uncontrollable hypertension, aggressive fluid and salt removal can lead to excessive activation of the renin–angiotensin system and so to aggravation of the high blood pressure.[130–131] In these patients the renin–angiotensin system plays a primary role.

Whether and to what extent the mechanisms of hypertension in chronic renal failure and in patients on chronic hemodialysis may also involve the sympathetic nervous system or disturbances in the cardiovascular responsiveness to various stimuli are still unclear.[108,109,132] The disturbances of this system in end-stage renal failure can be summarized as follows. Plasma norepinephrine concentrations are normal to high in end-stage renal failure; hemodialysis patients more often display high plasma concentrations.[133-137] These high plasma levels may be explained by a reduced neuronal re-uptake, reduced metabolism, and a lower plasma dopamine–beta-hydroxylase activity.[138] These normal to increased plasma levels coexist with decreased cardiovascular reactivity to infused norepinephrine.[118,136,139-141] The different evaluations of the autonomic nervous system, using tests of the integrity of the entire reflex arch and its limbs, favor altered function of the autonomic reflex arch.[108,132,142,143]

The definite participation of this system in the genesis of hypertension is suggested by pharmacologic autonomic blockade.[107,118,144,145] Selective norepinephrine inhibition with the sympathetic neurone blocker debrisoquine in hypertensive patients on chronic hemodialysis was followed by decreased arterial pressure and increased alpha- and beta-receptor sensitivity.[107] Injection of an alpha-adrenergic blocking agent in malignant hypertension accompanying end-stage renal failure leads to significant blood pressure decrease by a major decrease in systemic vascular resistance.[118] Such a decrease in blood pressure is also observed in mild to severe hypertension in patients on chronic hemodialysis.[145] All these arguments favor a norepinephrine-related mechanism, which participates as a sustaining factor in hypertension.

Finally, other pathogenic factors implied in the hypertension of renal failure could be impairment of the secretion of vasodepressor substances of renal origin (prostaglandins) or kinins.[146-149] The role of calcium is still unclear in the hypertension of renal failure.

Treatment. The management of hypertension in renal failure can be summarized as follows. Reduction in fluid and salt overload should be initiated by dietary restriction of salt intake. Diuretics can be useful for this. In patients on hemodialysis, removal of the excess weight and sodium may be achieved by hemodialysis and more efficiently by hemofiltration.[150] In hypertension resistant to hemodialysis, hemofiltration may normalize blood pressure within six months with normalization of the renin-angiotensin system and normalization of the disturbed hemodynamic features.[150]

Inhibition of the renin–angiotensin system can be achieved with beta-blocking agents[151] or angiotensin-converting enzyme inhibitors.[152,153] These latter drugs have allowed the control of blood pressure in drug resistant forms of hypertension and have been considered an alternative treatment to binephrectomy.

Inhibition or blockade of the autonomic nervous system (with guanethidine, debrisoquine, and alpha blockers)[107] is efficient but has significant side effects (including orthostatic hypotension). Normalization of the blood pressure is the keystone in the protection of the cardiovascular system. Calcium channel blockers have been proposed for the treatment; however, their effects still have to be explored.[154]

MYOCARDIAL PERFORMANCE IN GLOMERULONEPHRITIS

ACUTE GLOMERULONEPHRITIS

When a report on heart function, such as that of Derow,[155] was written in the 1950s, acute glomerulonephritis held a prominent place. Nowadays, acute glomerulonephritis occupies only a small space, whereas renal failure with its cardiovascular implications has assumed a primary place.[156] Nevertheless, there are some interesting features to underline.

Acute glomerulonephritis exhibits cardiac involvement in severe situations. Cardiac output appears to increase during the oliguric phase of the disease. High oxygen consumption has been noted. Systemic vascular resistance has been reported to be normal. We can conclude that acute glomerulonephritis induces a high cardiac output state, which reasonably has to be related to sodium and water overload. Pulmonary edema may be present and seems also to be a consequence of volume overexpansion. In such patients, the pulmonary wedge pressure appears to be very elevated. Eichna et al[157] coined the term *congested state* for this situation.[158-160] There is no definite proof of direct myocardial impairment, as suggested by cardiac enlargement and the presence of a gallop in some instances. The question remains as to whether these cardiac signs are related to salt and water retention.

Treatment. Overexpansion requires immediate institution of a severe salt- and water-restricted diet as long as the oliguric phase persists. Furosemide administration as well as hemodialysis may be of help in severe congestion.

CHRONIC GLOMERULONEPHRITIS

Several clinical features may be important in the course of chronic glomerulonephritis before renal failure occurs. Heavy proteinuria may induce nutritional deficiencies and is associated with reduced blood volume, reduced blood viscosity, and hypercholesterolemia with or without hypertriglyceridemia. Hypertension is often present.[155,156] These risks are still enhanced when chronic glomerulonephritis is secondary to lupus erythematosus[158] or other systemic diseases with severe immunologic disorders or to diabetes mellitus, which is very early complicated by hypertension and vascular degeneration. In these systemic diseases, characteristic heart alterations necessitate specific managements, which are described elsewhere in this textbook.

CORONARY HEART DISEASE

Atherosclerotic coronary artery disease is one of the most important factors of morbidity and mortality among the cardiovascular complications in patients treated by hemodialysis, peritoneal dialysis, or transplantation.[1-4]

In comparison with coronary heart disease in the general population, the risk factors (age, cigarette smoking, and hypertension) are more pronounced in patients with renal failure.[161] Moreover, the following factors also must be taken into account in patients with renal failure: (1) factors related to clinical features: existence or preexistence of the nephrotic syndrome with hypercholesterolemia; insulin resistance and glucose intolerance of renal failure; anemia; and the possibility of vascular metastatic calcifications; (2) factors related to replacement treatment: acceleration of preexisting atherosclerosis; high glucose delivery by the dialysate fluid in peritoneal dialysis; hypoxemia and vasodilatation occurring during acetate hemodialysis; biocompatibility phenomena with pulmonary leukostasis and complement activation causing hypoxemia when cuprophan membranes are used during hemodialysis; extracorporeal blood circulation during dialysis with the possibility of a "steal syndrome"; rapid changes in plasma potassium and calcium levels; and corticotherapy after renal transplantation.

CLINICAL MANIFESTATIONS

The clinical aspects of angina pectoris and myocardial infarction do not differ in renal failure patients from those of the general population.[162] However, the frequency of angina pectoris during the hemodialysis maneuvers must be mentioned. An evaluation of the exact coronary status must be performed with noninvasive methods,[163] with thallium scintigraphy,[164] and with coronary angiography.

TREATMENT

Elimination of known risk factors may be of primary importance including treatment of existing hypertension, correction of anemia (some patients present thoracic pain when hemoglobin falls under a certain level specific for each patient), suppression of smoking, correction of lipid disorders, and exercise training (cycling, walking and jogging).[164a]

The usual medications for coronary heart disease, among which nitrates have a prominent place, may be given to these patients. Medications with negative inotropic effects such as beta blockers and calcium antagonists[165] have to be monitored with care. Amiodarone administration has to be surveyed for its cumulative effects.

Concerning the treatment modalities of renal failure in patients with coronary heart disease, bicarbonate as a buffer in the dialysate can be tried instead of acetate to avoid hypotension. Polysulfone membranes and polyacrylonitrile membranes having better biocompatibility result in much less leukostasis in the lung and are to be preferred.

Coronary revascularization through aortocoronary bypass can be proposed to these patients, if necessary, to improve their comfort.[166,167]

ATHEROGENESIS AND LIPID DISORDERS IN RENAL DISEASE

The high incidence of coronary atherosclerosis in chronic renal failure patients can be related to accelerated atherogenesis consequent to lipid disorders.[168,169] Modifications of the plasma lipid fraction are frequent in chronic renal failure and are not improved by hemodialysis and transplantation.[170,171]

In non-nephrotic patients in chronic renal failure, the following types of hyperlipidemias may be encountered: (1) type IV: hypertriglycerideremia in 50% of the patients; (2) type IIa: hypercholesterolemia; (3) type IIb: hypercholesterolemia associated with hypertriglycerideremia.

Uremia seems to induce multiple disorders in lipid metabolism, which covers the domains of lipid production, transport, and catabolism.[6,12] The liver secretes molecular aggregates of triglycerides, cholesterol, and lipoproteins (very low-density lipoproteins [VLDL]). In chronic renal failure, there exists an abnormal production of VLDL due to the reduced activity of hepatic triglyceride lipase (HTGL)[172–175] and perhaps related to insulin resistance and glucose intolerance in these patients. Recent report that the affinity of LDL from uremic patients for the LDL receptor is decreased as compared to normal controls suggests that the dyslipoproteinemia in chronic renal failure may result also in part from alteration of lipoprotein binding and degradation at the cellular level.[175a]

Evidence exists that intestinal fat absorption is followed by the prolonged presence of chylomicrons in the serum. Now, lipoprotein lipase (LPL) activity is also impaired and there is no longer an increase in LPL activity after a meal as in normal subjects.[176] This impairment seems related to the presence of a nondialyzable uremic factor in the middle molecule range (600 to 3,400 daltons). The reduced activity of LPL may explain the absence of clearing of triglycerides. Moreover, lowered high-density lipoprotein (HDL) in uremic patients has been described, and a decreased transport capacity to the liver may therefore exist.[177,178] To these basic alterations must be added the altered function of apoproteins.

Apoproteins in the chylomicrons solubilize the lipid components of the chylomicrons and favor their transport. Rapaport et al[177] showed that the concentration of the apoproteins CII in the HDL molecules is decreased. This apoprotein is transferred from HDL in the plasma to VLDL, where it acts as an activator of LPL. Reduced triglyceride catabolism is common to all uremic patients. Finally, reduced carnitine in the muscle produces a disturbance in the intracellular transport of fatty acids to the mitochondria.[179]

Conflicting reports have been published as to the effects of hypercholesterolemia in the nephrotic syndrome. More recent studies confirm that the early existence of dyslipidemia may be a factor in subsequent atherogenesis.[180] Even if only a few signs of lipid disturbance are detectable in uremic patients, evidence exists that in the cascade of events in the blood, several processes may be responsible for endothelial lipid overload.[181,182]

TREATMENT

Plasma triglyceride levels can be reduced by limiting the dietary intake of carbohydrates and alcohol. A low cholesterol diet may lower HDL and LDL. Nevertheless, there is no proof that dietary management prevents atherogenesis. Clofibrate therapy lowers triglycerides plasma levels but may induce toxic effects such as myositis.[183]

When patients on long-term hemodialysis treatment

exhibit lipid disorders, bicarbonate dialysis and hemofiltration have been suggested as alternatives, but they are not universally agreed on.[182–186]

In transplantation, reduction in corticoid treatment has improved lipid metabolism.[187,188]

PERICARDIAL HEART DISEASE IN CHRONIC RENAL FAILURE

Pericardial disease is common in patients with end-stage renal failure. Since the introduction of hemodialysis treatment and with patients on replacement therapy before severe intoxication, the incidence of pericarditis has remarkably diminished. However, pericarditis continues to occur in patients maintained on hemodialysis, but this seems unrelated to uremic intoxication. This latter form is observed approximately in 15% of all dialyzed patients.[189,190] Both forms of pericarditis may display similar clinical signs and lead to similar complications.

The morphologic features of pericardial disease as observed at necropsy or surgery include acute pericarditis, subacute effusive-constrictive pericarditis, and chronic constrictive pericarditis.

In acute pericarditis there is a fibrinous reaction without (noneffusive type) or with (effusive type) serous effusion[191,192]; in hemodialysis patients, serosanguineous effusion is often present.

In subacute effusive-constrictive pericarditis, granulation tissue with capillary neoformation, serosanguineous effusion, adhesions, loculations, and thickening of pericardial membranes appear within the pericardial sac.[193–197] This form is seen in patients on chronic hemodialysis, and heparin administration can participate in its genesis.

In chronic constrictive pericarditis, there are either diffuse pericardial adhesions that obliterate the pericardial space or diffuse fibrosis and adherence of pericardial membranes with formation of a fibrous shell with no calcification.[198]

The initial fibrinous reaction may lead to any of the aforementioned abnormalities, but the evolution with serosanguineous exudate is most frequent in dialyzed patients. Hemopericardium may occur. The contact of blood with injured pericardial membranes causes the appearance of adhesions.[199,200]

CLINICAL MANIFESTATIONS

Today, the nephrologist may encounter "uremic pericarditis" in uremic patients when hemodialysis treatment is initiated too late and "dialysis-associated pericarditis" unrelated to uremic intoxication.[194,201–203]

Acute (Fibrinous) Pericarditis

The cardinal symptom of chest pain is not always present and the onset of pericarditis may be completely asymptomatic. A pericardial friction rub is an important clue in the diagnosis and must be searched for routinely in uremic patients and patients on hemodialysis. Echocardiographic examination is necessary to detect the presence of an effusion. A pericardial echo-free space may be found with effusions of no more than 20 ml.[204]

Effusive Pericarditis

Effusive pericarditis is most often the consequence of acute fibrinous pericarditis. Clinical symptoms are usually only present with large effusions. The occurrence of dyspnea should make one suspect the presence of effusion. A pericardial friction rub may persist despite effusion. Rapid enlargement of heart size without signs of pulmonary congestion is suggestive of the diagnosis. Echocardiography is the most reliable method to detect, locate, and estimate the volume of fluid.[204] On chest x-ray, the heart shadow may be enlarged when the volume of effusion exceeds 200 ml. Tamponade is an ever-impending threat; therefore, it is mandatory to carefully watch the patient for physical signs, eg, an increase in venous pressure, a decrease in blood pressure, a decrease of the systolo-diastolic amplitude of the arterial pressure, and the occurrence of paroxysmal tachyarrhythmia induced by hemodialysis.[205] When doubt exists as to the presence of tamponade, cardiac catheterization gives important information before the appearance of physical signs: an increase in right atrial pressure and right ventricular end-diastolic pressure is found, and occasionally a diastolic dip and plateau in the right ventricular pressure curve are observed.

Tamponade

Sudden development of cardiac tamponade may occur despite careful supervision. Patients complain of precordial oppressive chest pain and become anxious and dyspneic. The most important clinical signs are related to rising venous pressure and falling arterial pressure. The venous pressure increment causes jugular vein distention in the sitting position. Pulsus paradoxus is present in most cases. In emergency situations, therapeutic intervention cannot be delayed and the physician must rely on the aforementioned clinical signs to initiate lifesaving therapy. Thereafter, laboratory investigations may give valuable complementary information for patient management. Cardiac catheterization shows the following features: equilibration of the diastolic pressure of the right atrium, right ventricle, and pulmonary artery and pulmonary wedge pressure, the so-called "pressure plateau." Intrapericardial pressure equilibrates with the diastolic pressure of the cardiac chambers.[197,206] The difference between right atrial pressure and pulmonary wedge pressure must not exceed 5 mm Hg. This is important in differentiating tamponade from congestive heart failure.[204] A diastolic dip may also be present in cardiac tamponade and a W or M shape of the atrial pressure curve may be found. We would like to emphasize that hemodynamic investigations before and after a pericardial tap[196,197,206] may give valuable information in differentiating tamponade from constriction. Even a recording of the arterial pulse (finger transillumination pulsogram) can be helpful.[196]

Constrictive Pericarditis

The nephrologist may be confronted with the subacute effusive-constrictive form of pericarditis.[193,197,198] Its clinical features are usually a combination of tamponade and constriction. Progressive constrictive pericarditis is difficult to differentiate from congestive heart failure on the basis of clinical signs. As a rule, development is more insidious with dyspnea, edema, ascites, and hepatomegaly. Typical features are found on hemodynamic investigation.

ETIOLOGY

Uremic end-stage pericarditis seems related to uremic intoxication and there is evidence that uric acid may play a role in its genesis. The cause of hemodialysis pericarditis has not yet been detected, although poor dialysis, major phosphocalcic disturbances, and high uricemia have been suggested without definite proof. The possible infectious origin of pericarditis must be kept in mind; cytomegalovirus has been particularly incriminated. Circulating immune complexes have been suggested as a possible toxin responsible for uremic and hemodialysis pericarditis.[206a] This theory receives some support from a recent study which showed a much lower incidence of pericardial effusion in patients on continuous ambulatory peritoneal dialysis than on hemodialysis, the circulating immune complexes or other high molecular weight toxins being cleared more effectively through the peritoneum than by hemodialysis filters.[206b]

TREATMENT

Many modalities of treatment have been proposed in the management of uremic pericarditis and its accompanying complications.[196,207]

To avoid end-stage uremic pericarditis, hemodialysis must be initiated before plasma creatinine reaches high levels and severe biochemical disturbances occur. In asymptomatic pericardial effusion, it is generally agreed to intensify hemodialysis (four to seven times per week) with reduced anticoagulation by regional heparinization. When chest pain occurs, the administration of indomethacin is useful.

Pericardial tamponade indicates the need for emergency pericardiocentesis. In many cases the subsequent treatment with intensified dialysis is initiated or pursued with good results. Controversial opinions exist as to the choice of treatment when effusion appears resistant to conservative management. Some investigators use drainage techniques with instillation of nonabsorbable steroids or instillation of air associated with nonabsorbable steroids, and claim to have good results. Others prefer pericardiostomy.[208] Pericardiectomy is only indicated in severe constrictive pericarditis.

BACTERIAL ENDOCARDITIS IN END-STAGE RENAL FAILURE AND IN PATIENTS ON CHRONIC HEMODIALYSIS

The first description of bacterial endocarditis occurring in patients on hemodialysis was given by Brescia et al[209] in 1966. Many other cases were then reported. The frequency of this complication is 2.7% to 6.6%.[210–213] Endocarditis can be related to two main predisposing factors[214]: (1) the immunologic deficiency present in end-stage renal failure, and (2) the vascular access needed for hemodialysis treatment, that is, arteriovenous shunts, arteriovenous fistulas with synthetic materials or grafts, and venous cannulations.

The arteriovenous fistula could per se be a determinant or a predisposing factor for bacterial endocarditis through the highly increased work imposed on the heart. This fact was demonstrated in dogs[215] as in man with acquired arteriovenous fistula.[216,217] Infection occurs after septicemia or bacteremia.[218] The portal of entry of bacteria in hemodialysis patients is usually vascular,[219,220] but it can also be a dental infection[211,214] or kidney cyst infections.[221] Endocarditis is usually the first metastatic infectious localization preceding pulmonary[222] or bone localization.[223] Bacterial endocarditis can also occur during treatment with continuous ambulatory peritoneal dialysis, not necessarily following peritonitis episodes.

Mitral or aortic valves are the most commonly affected, but right heart bacterial endocarditis has also been described.[224] This latter type of endocarditis resembles the endocarditis found in heroin addicts.[225] The bacteriologic findings show *Staphylococcus aureus* (60% of all cases), *Streptococcus viridans* and gram-negative bacteria,[226] *Listeria,* and *Corynebacteria.*[211] A fungal or viral (cytomegalovirus) cause of endocarditis has also been described.[227]

Two-dimensional echocardiography is the main clue in the diagnosis of endocarditis. It allows definition of the lesions and their hemodynamic consequences.

TREATMENT

Bacterial endocarditis is treated with a combination of penicillinase-resistant antibiotics and aminoglycosides. Vancomycin[228] has been proposed as an alternative, its long half-life being useful in patients on chronic hemodialysis. Treatment most often provides a favorable clinical evolution, but death from sudden heart failure related to a major valvular injury can occur. Surgical valvular replacement can be proposed in hemodialysis patients when the valvular injury is severe.[229,230]

HEMODYNAMIC MODIFICATIONS RELATED TO HEMODIALYSIS

TECHNICAL ASPECTS

Artificial blood cleansing can be performed by conventional hemodialysis, hemofiltration, hemodiafiltration, or peritoneal dialysis. Whereas hemodialysis, hemofiltration, and hemodiafiltration need an extracorporeal blood circuit that may interfere with hemodynamics, peritoneal dialysis has only a few effects on cardiovascular function.[19,231]

In conventional dialysis the exchanges are realized between blood and the dialysate fluid, using both diffusion and convection as a means of exchange. Concentration gradients promote solute exchanges and induce ultrafiltration. Hemofiltration[232] is based only on convective transfer and ultrafiltration. A substitution fluid is administered to the patient to compensate for the excess fluid and solute loss. Hemodiafiltration is a combination of the two preceding techniques.[231]

Dialysate fluid and substitution fluid have an osmotic composition near to that of plasma and comprised the major electrolytes. The choice of buffer salt (acetate, bicarbonate, or lactate) induces several different hemodynamic modifications.[233–235]

Dialysators are manufactured with different types of membranes: cuprophane, cellulose acetate, polysulfone, polycarbonate, and polyacrylonitrile. These membranes may also interfere with the patient's hemodynamics.[236,237] For hemofiltration, only high porosity membranes can be used.

As will be mentioned, the onset of hemodialysis in patients in chronic renal failure improves heart function.[22,238] Nevertheless, there are some side effects that need to be analyzed.

HEMODYNAMICS DURING DIALYSIS

Low Pressure System (Pulmonary Circulation)

The low pressure system is influenced mainly by salt and water removal.[237–239] A relation exists between weight loss of the patient, ie, contraction of extracellular fluid volume, and the pressure decrements of the low pressure system (Figure 60.9) including the right atrial, mean pulmonary arterial, and pulmonary wedge pressure.[240,241]

The low pressure system may also be affected by the nature of the utilized membranes through biocompatibility phenomena.[236,237] Dialysis membranes, especially cuprophane, may induce pulmonary leukostasis and complement activation associated with hypoxemia (Figure 60.10). A slight increase in pulmonary pressure has been observed in these conditions.[236]

The nature of the buffer salt in the dialysate has only negligible effects on the low pressure system, but the sodium content of the dialysate may influence this pressure system. A high sodium concentration (greater than 145 mEq/L) in the dialysate allows fluid removal with lesser pressure decrement than does dialysate with a lower sodium content.[242]

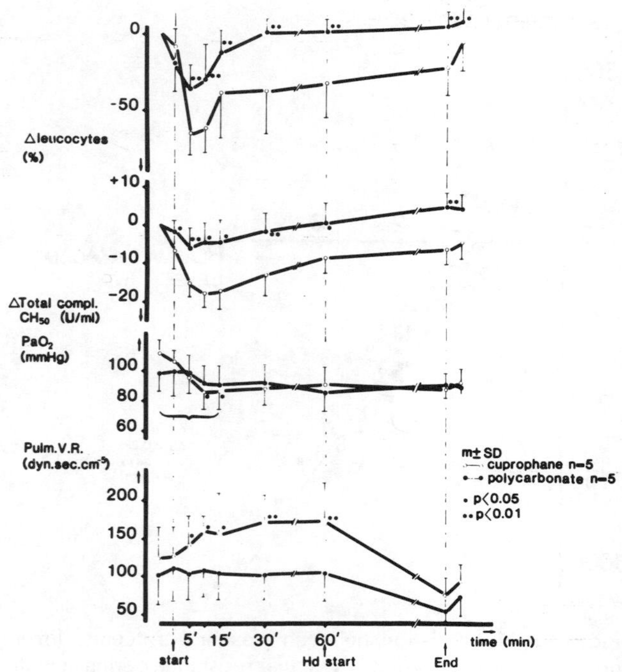

Figure 60.10. Evolution of the leukocyte count (expressed in percentage of variations), of total complement (CH 50) plasma level, of arterial blood partial O_2 tension, and of pulmonary vascular resistance (Pulm VR) during hemodialysis with two different membranes (polycarbonate versus cuprophane). (From Jahn et al,[241] with permission of S Karger AG, Basel.)

High Pressure System (Systemic Circulation)

Fluid and salt removal may decrease blood pressure.[19,243,244] Cardiac output and systemic vascular resistance are mainly influenced by technical modalities and the buffer salt in the fluid.[233,234,242,245] Pure ultrafiltration without any contact with dialysate fluid decreases cardiac

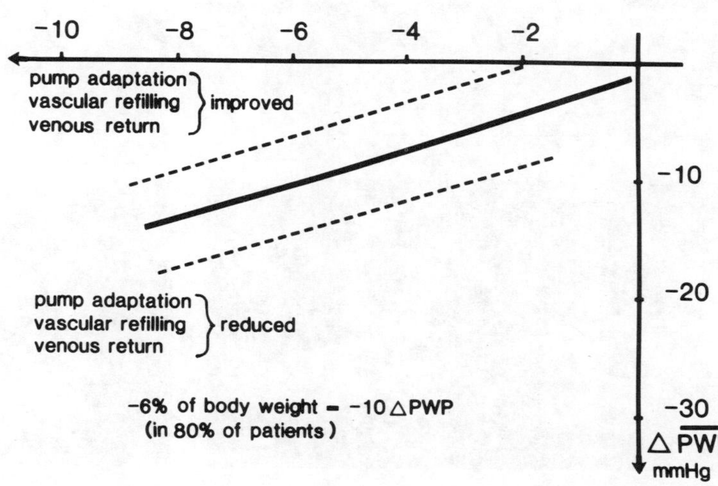

Figure 60.9. General relation between weight loss (expressed in percentage of body weight) and decrease in pulmonary wedge pressure during hemodialysis and related procedures. A shift to the X axis of this relation is observed during hemodialysis with high Na content in the dialysate. A shift to the Y axis is observed in patients with congestive heart failure.

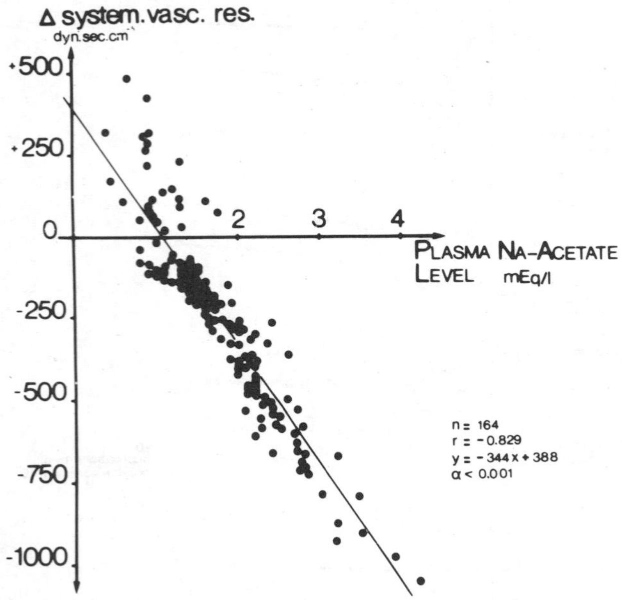

Figure 60.11. Relation between plasma Na acetate levels and the decrease in systemic vascular resistance during acetate hemodialysis. (From Schohn et al,[236] with permission of S Karger AG, Basel.)

output and increases systemic vascular resistance. Ultrafiltration during bicarbonate dialysis induces similar behavior,[234,246] whereas acetate dialysis increases cardiac output and decreases systemic vascular resistance.[235,239,247,248] There is a correlation as well between plasma acetate levels and stroke index, as between plasma acetate levels and decreased systemic vascular resistance (Figure 60.11). Acetate seems to promote vasodilatation and enhance cardiac contractility.[234,235,249–251] A greater intradialytic increase in serum ionized calcium concentration is associated with less fall in mean arterial pressure during dialysis.[251a]

FISTULAS AND SHUNTS

Vascular access is needed for dialysis treatment, and blood flows greater than 200 ml per minute are necessary to obtain satisfactory blood cleansing.[209] High blood flows must therefore be obtained with shunts and fistulas. There are usually only few impacts of these blood shuntings on heart function. Nevertheless, cardiac work may be increased, and increased cardiac output may occur.[252,253] In patients with congestive heart failure, the supplementary heart work imposed by a fistula may contribute to aggravation of the condition.

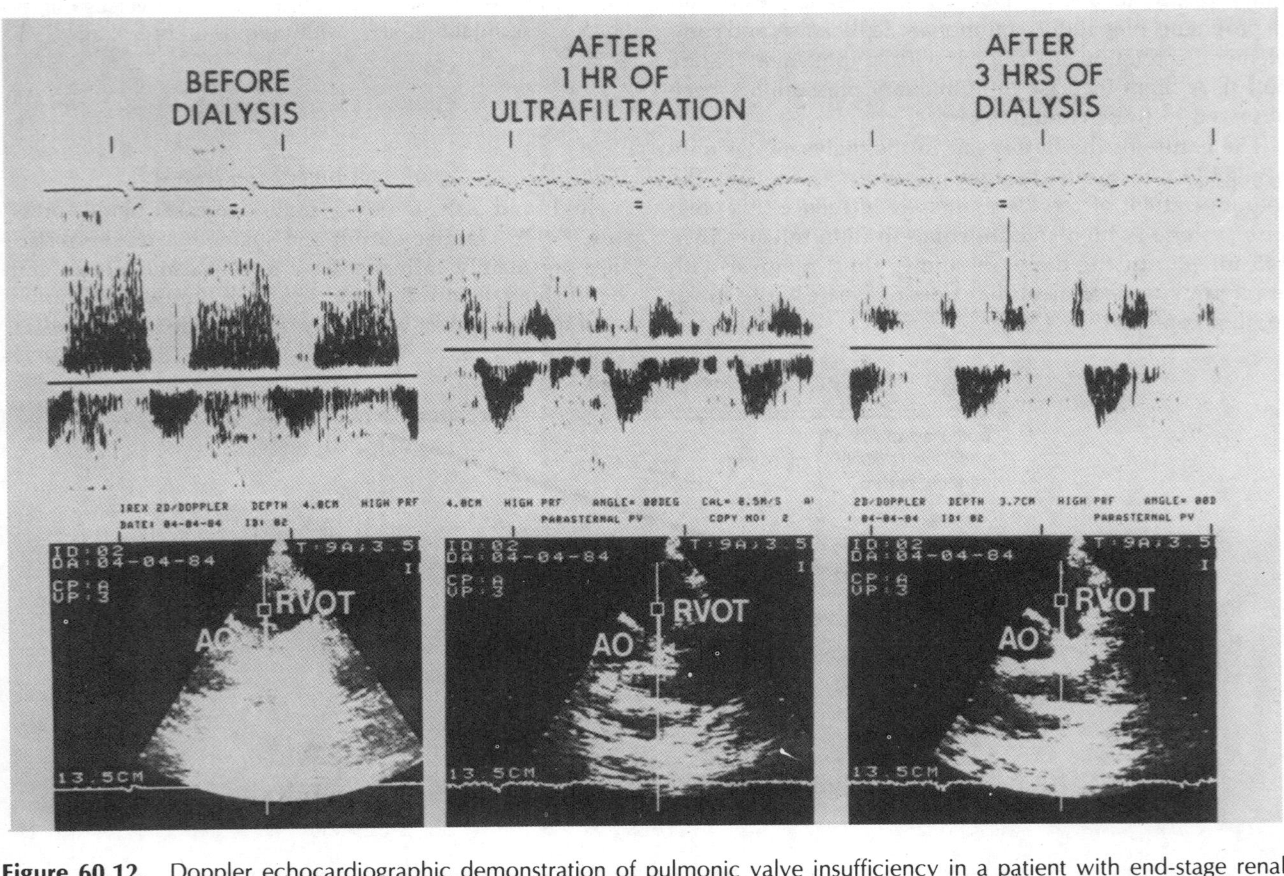

Figure 60.12. Doppler echocardiographic demonstration of pulmonic valve insufficiency in a patient with end-stage renal disease and a basal diastolic murmur before, after one hour of ultrafiltration, and after three subsequent hours of conventional hemodialysis. Pulmonic valve insufficiency, present before dialysis (*left panel*), is virtually abolished by extracellular fluid removal by ultrafiltration (*middle panel*), with little further modification of the Doppler recording after additional hemodialysis (*right panel*). AO = aorta; RVOT = right ventricular outflow tract. (From Perez et al,[262] with permission.)

DIASTOLIC MURMURS IN RENAL FAILURE

A transient early diastolic murmur may be heard in patients with renal failure.[254–259] Typically the murmur disappears after dialysis.[257,258] Although a pericardial origin has been suggested,[255,259] it has usually been attributed to functional aortic insufficiency.[255a,260,261] However, recent results from Doppler echocardiography[262] seem to suggest that pulmonic valve insufficiency may be a more frequent cause of diastolic murmur than aortic insufficiency in patients with renal failure. Fluid overload appears to be the principal pathophysiologic mechanism; the phenomenon is readily reversible by dialysis (Figures 60.12 and 60.13) and reflects correctable pulmonary hypertension.[262]

The early diastolic murmur of semilunar valve insufficiency in renal failure should not be confused with the early-to-mid-diastolic murmur associated with coronary artery stenosis,[263] a frequent complication of end-stage renal disease. The diastolic murmur in coronary artery stenosis, although high-pitched, is mid-diastolic in timing and may disappear following myocardial infarction.[263]

The early diastolic murmur in renal failure should not be confused with a cervical venous hum,[256] which sometimes may be quite loud in the presence of anemia.

Lastly, bacterial endocarditis must be excluded as a cause of early diastolic murmur in renal failure. This subject has been discussed earlier.

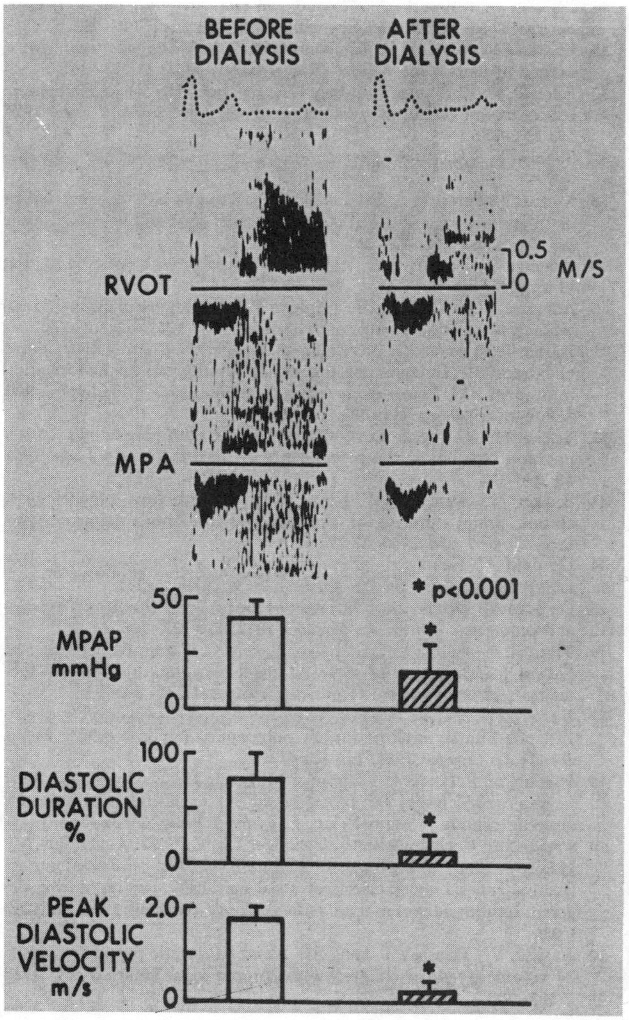

Figure 60.13. Comparison between Doppler echocardiograms and hemodynamic data obtained in patients with end-stage renal disease and pulmonic valve insufficiency before (*left panels*) and after hemodialysis (*right panel*). Reduction in pulmonic valve insufficiency with dialysis was associated with reduction in mean pulmonary artery pressure (MPAP). MPA = main pulmonary artery; RVOT = right ventricular outflow tract. (From Perez et al,[262] with permission.)

CARDIOVASCULAR FUNCTION AFTER KIDNEY TRANSPLANTATION

The altered cardiocirculatory function resulting from end-stage renal failure and hemodialysis would be expected to return to normal after successful kidney transplantation. In fact, however, after renal transplantation, cardiovascular problems continue to occupy an important place.[1,264] The main risk factors are hypertension, atherogenesis, and lipid abnormalities, perhaps related to steroid treatment.

Whereas hypertriglyceridemia is the predominant lipid abnormality in patients with chronic renal failure, hypercholesterolemia types IIa and IIb tend to predominate after renal transplantation, and in some transplanted patients hypertriglyceridemia persists.[170,178,265] These abnormalities are related in part to large doses of corticosteroids.[89,266,267] Alternate-day corticosteroid treatment was proposed to reduce the frequency of these lipid abnormalities. The introduction of new immunosuppressive drugs associated with small prednisone doses seems to reduce this cardiovascular risk factor.

The prevalence of hypertension remains high after allografting.[268–271] It occurs in approximately 50% of the recipients within one year after transplantation.[271a] Multiple etiologic factors are suspected: a daily dose of prednisone[272] not confirmed by all investigators,[271] age and sex of the patient,[271,273] origin of the graft,[271,274] body weight,[274,275] the role of the recipient's own kidneys,[273,276,277] the presence or absence of chronic or acute graft rejection,[271] and the presence or absence of a graft artery stenosis.[271,278–280] Among the etiologic factors, renin-induced hypertension remains the most accessible form to treatment that can be surgical by removing the recipient's own kidneys or by correcting the renal artery stenosis.[271] This correction can also be done by transluminal dilatation.[281] However, this form of hypertension can also respond to medical treatment by angiotensin II converting enzyme inhibitors[282,283] or vasodilatory drugs.[271]

Nevertheless, with transplantation, an improvement in heart performance may be expected as sodium and water balance is normally achieved.[284] Improvement in myocardial hypertrophy has been reported.[285]

Acknowledgment: We acknowledge the secretarial assistance of Pauline Wittemer, Chantal Schott, Gaby Milliere, Renée Leininger, and Sylvie Kopp, the technical assistance of Christian Klein, and the kind revision of the text by A. Pape.

REFERENCES

1. Wing AJ, Broyer M, Brunner FP, Brynger H, Challah S, Donckerwolcke RA, Gretz N, Jacobs C, Kramer P, Selwood NH: Combined report on regular dialysis and transplantation in Europe, *XIII, 1982. Proc Eur Dial Transplant Assoc-Eur Renal Assoc* 1983; 20:2–75.
2. Wing AJ, Brunner FP, Brynger H, Jacobs C, Kramer P, Selwood NH, Gretz N: Cardiovascular-related causes of death and the fate of patients with renovascular disease. *Contr Nephrol* (Karger Basel) 1984; 41:306–311.
3. Brunner FP, Brynger H, Chantler C, Donckerwolcke RA, Hathway RA, Jacobs C, Selwood NH, Wing AJ: Combined report on regular dialysis and transplantation in Europe. *IX, 1978. Proc Eur Dial Transplant Assoc* 1979; 16:4–73.
4. Bryan F: National dialysis registry. *Proceedings of the 6th Annual Contractor's Conference of the Artificial Kidney Program of the National Institute of Arthritis Metabolism and Digestive Diseases.* 1973, pp 201–202.
5. Stange PV, Sumner AT: Predicting treatment costs and life expectancy for end-stage renal disease. *N Eng J Med* 1978; 298:372–378.
6. Braunwald E, Gottlieb MN: Renal disorders and heart disease, in Braunwald E (ed): *Heart Disease,* ed 2. Philadelphia, WB Saunders, 1984, chap 52, pp 1748–1762.
7. Del Greco F: Cardiomyopathy and congestive heart failure, in Massry SG, Glassock RJ (eds): *Textbook of Nephrology.* Baltimore, Williams & Wilkins, 1983, pp 732–738.
8. Weidmann P: Hypertension, in Massry SG, Glassock RJ (eds): *Textbook of Nephrology.* Baltimore, Williams & Wilkins, 1983, pp 738–745.
9. Shapiro FL, Comty CM: Pericarditis, in Massry SG, Glassock RJ (eds): *Textbook of Nephrology.* Baltimore, Williams & Wilkins, 1983, pp 727–732.
10. Pabico RC, Freeman RB: Pericarditis and myocardiopathy, in Massry SG, Sellers AL (eds): *Clinical Aspects of Uremia and Dialysis.* Springfield, Ill, Charles C Thomas, 1976, pp 69–99.
11. Davidson RC, Schribner BH: Cardiovascular manifestations of renal failure, in Earley LE, Gottschalk CW (eds): *Strauss and Welt's Diseases of the Kidney,* ed 3. Boston, Little, Brown, 1979, Vol 1, pp 263–275.
12. Morrison G, Geheb MA, Earley LE: Chronic renal failure, in Seldin DA, Giebisch G (eds): *The Kidney: Physiology and Pathophysiology.* New York, Raven Press, 1985, pp 1901–1943.
13. Eichna LW: Circulatory congestion and heart failure. *Circulation* 1960; 22:864–886.
14. Jahn H, Schmitt R, Schohn D, Olier P: Aspects of the myocardial function in chronic renal failure. *Contr Nephrol* (S Karger AG, Basel) 1984; 41:240–250.
15. Pehrsson SK, Jonasson R, Lins LE: Cardiac performance in various stages of renal failure. *Br Heart J* 1984; 52:667–673.
16. Wizemann V, Kramer W, Thormann J, Kindler M, Schlepper M, Schütterle G: Rest and exercise response of left ventricular functions of patients on maintenance hemodialysis with and without coronary artery disease. *Contr Nephrol* (Karger Basel) 1984; 41:276–279.
17. Schäfer GE, Kober G, Schoeppe W: Veränderungen der Herz-Kreislauffunktion bei chronischer Niereninsuffizienz. *Nieren und Hochdruckkrankheiten* 1984; 13:S167–S174.
18. Heaton A, Amer H, Bellock RE, Ward MK, Hall RJC, Kerr DNS: Importance of impaired exercise tolerance in patients in renal replacement therapy. *Contr Nephrol* (Karger Basel) 1984; 41:272–275.
19. Jahn H, Schohn D, Schmitt R: Etudes hémodynamiques au cours de l'insuffisance rénale chronique terminale. Effets des techniques d'épuration extrarénale. *Néphrologie* 1981; 2:53–62.
20. Dongradi G, Kahn JC, Rocha P, Baron B, Moranne JB, Fendler JP: Courbes de fonction du ventricule gauche chez les patients hémodialysés chroniques: étude au cours d'un effort intense et au cours d'une perfusion de dextran. *Néphrologie* 1981; 2:73–76.
21. Rottembourg J, Rouby JJ, Durande JP, Guesde R, Guimont MC: Etudes hémodynamiques au cours de l'oedème pulmonaire chez 9 insuffisants rénaux chroniques (IRC) (abstr). *Néphrologie* 1981; 2:86.
22. Hung J, Harris PJ, Uren RF: Uremic cardiomyopathy: effect of hemodialysis on left ventricular function in end-stage renal failure. *N Engl J Med* 1980: 302:547–551.
23. Feigenbaum H: *Echocardiography,* ed 4. Philadelphia, Lea & Febiger, 1986, pp 127–187.
24. Cocchi A, Mori R, Carosella L, Iacono G, Greco A, Carbonin PU: Echocardiographic aspects of cardiac hypertrophy and dilatation in normo- and hypertensive hemodialyzed patients. *Contr Nephrol* (Karger Basel) 1984; 41:288–291.
25. Fea F, Bronzieri C, Ambroso GC, Casati S, Scalamogna A, Cantaluppi A, Grassi C, Mameli C, Planca E, Colombo G: Bimodal behavior of left ventricular function during hemodialysis. Echocardiographic study. *Contr Nephrol* (Karger Basel) 1984; 41:284–287.
26. Cohen MV, Diaz P, Scheuer J: Echocardiographic assessment of left ventricular function in patients with chronic uremia. *Clin Nephrol* 1979; 12:156–162.
27. Kasper W, Hoffmann T, Bechtold H, Treese N, Pop T, Meinertz T: Echocardiographic studies in cardiomyopathies, in Just H, Schuster HP (eds): *Myocarditis Cardiomyopathy* (International Boehringer Mannheim Symposia). New York, Springer Verlag, 1983, pp 213–223.
28. Jahn H, Schmitt R, Schohn D: Differentialdiagnose der myokardialen Herzinsuffizienz bei terminaler Niereninsuffizienz. *Nieren und Hochdruckkrankheiten* 1984; 13:374–380.
29. Grossmann W: Hemodynamic evaluation of congestive heart failure, in Braunwald E, Mock MB (eds): *Congestive Heart Failure: Current Research and Clinical Applications.* New York, Grune & Stratton, 1982, pp 167–178.
30. Grossmann W, Braunwald E, Mann T, McLaurin LP, Green LH: Contractile state of the left ventricle in man as evaluated from end-systolic pressure–volume relations. *Circulation* 1977; 56:845–852.
31. Merillon JP, Neukirch F, Motte G, Aumont MC, Curien ND, Prasquier R, Gourgon R: The left ventricular end-systolic pressure–volume ratio. Studies during changes in load and inotropism in the human. *Eur Heart J* 1981; 2:41–48.
32. Suga H, Sagawa K, Shoukas AA: Load independence of the instantaneous pressure–volume ratio of the canine left ventricle and effects of epinephrine and heart rate on the ratio. *Circ Res* 1973; 32:314–322.
33. Drüeke T, Zingraff J, Boudier L, Baubion N, Gambini D, Le Pailleur C: Non-invasive exploration of myocardial function in hemodialysis patients. *Contr Nephrol* (Karger Basel) 1984; 41:280–283.
34. Doherty JE: Modern use of digitalis, in Hurst JW (ed): *Clinical Essays on the Heart.* New York, McGraw-Hill, 1983, Vol 1, pp 145–171.
35. Kreusser W, Klooker P, Rambausek M, Ritz E: Digitalis treatment in uremic patients. *Contr Nephrol* (Karger Basel) 1984; 41:255–261.
36. Falch D: The influence of kidney function, body size and age on plasma concentration and urinary excretion of digoxin. *Acta Med Scand* 1973; 194:251–256.
37. Steiness E: Renal tubular secretion of digoxin. *Circulation* 1974: 50:103–107.
38. Marcus FI, Peterson A, Salel A, Scully J, Kapadia GG: The metabolism of tritiated digoxin in renal insufficiency in dogs and man. *J Pharmacol Exp Ther* 1966; 152:372–382.
39. Doherty JE, Perkins WH, Wilson MC: Studies with tritiated digoxin in renal failure. *Am J Med* 1964; 37:536–544.
40. Ackerman GL, Doherty JE, Flanigan WJ: Peritoneal dialysis and hemodialysis of tritiated digoxin. *Ann Intern Med* 1967; 67:718–723.
41. Seifter JL, Skorecki KL, Stivelman JC, Haupert G, Brenner BM: Control of extracellular fluid volume and pathophysiology of edema formation, in Brenner BM, Rector FC Jr (eds): *The Kidney,* ed 3, Philadelphia, WB Saunders, 1986, pp 343–384.
42. Bricker NS: The control of sodium excretion with normal and reduced nephron population: the preeminence of third factor. *Am J Med* 1967; 43:313–321.
43. Bricker NS, Morrin PAF, Kime SW: The pathologic physiology of chronic Bright's disease: an exposition of the "intact nephron hypothesis." *Am J Med* 1960; 28:77–98.
44. De Bold AJ: Heart atria granularity effects of changes in water-electrolyte balance. *Proc Soc Exp Biol Med* 1979; 161:508–511.
45. De Bold AJ: Atrial natriuretic factor of the rat heart. Studies on isolation and properties. *Proc Soc Exp Biol Med* 1982; 170:133–138.
46. Thibault G, Garcia R, Seidah NG, Lazure C, Cantin M, Chretien M, Genest J: Purification of three rat atrial natriuretic factors and their amino acid composition. *FEBS Letters* 1983; 164:286–290.
47. Kangawa K, Matsuo H: Purification and complete amino acid sequence of alpha-human atrial natriuretic polypeptide (alpha-h ANP). *Biochem Biophys Res Commun* 1984; 118:131–139.
48. Weidmann P, Hasler L, Gnädinger MP, Lang RE, Uehlinger DE, Shaw S, Rascher W, Reubi FC: Blood levels and renal effects of atrial natriuretic peptide in normal man. *J Clin Invest* 1986; 77:734–742.
49. Weidmann P, Hellmueller B, Uehlinger DE, Lang RE, Gnädinger MP, Hasler L, Shaw S, Bachman C: Plasma levels and cardiovascular endocrine and excretory effects of atrial natriuretic peptide during different sodium intakes in man. *J Clin Endocrinol and Metab* 1986; 62:1027–1036.
50. Rascher W, Tulassay T, Lang RE: Atrial natriuretic peptide in plasma of volume overload children with chronic renal failure. *Lancet* 1985; 2:303–305.
51. Davies DL, Schalekamp MA, Beevers DG, Brown JJ, Briggs JD, Lever AF, Medina AM, Morton JJ, Robertson JIS, Tree M: Abnormal relation between exchangeable sodium and the renin angiotensin system in malignant hypertension and in hypertension with chronic renal failure. *Lancet* 1973; 1:683–687.
52. Weidmann P, Maxwell MH: Hypertension, in Massry SG, Sellers AL (eds): *Clinical Aspects of Uremia and Dialysis.* Springfield, Ill, Charles C Thomas, 1976, pp 100–145.
53. Widmer B, Gerhard RE, Harrington JT, Cohen IJ: Serum electrolyte and acid base composition. The influence of graded degrees of chronic renal failure. *Arch Intern Med* 1979; 139:1099–1102.

54. Beierholm EA, Grantham RN, O'Keefe DD, Laver MB, Daggett WM: Effects of acid-base changes, hypoxia and catecholamines on ventricular performance. *Am J Physiol* 1975; 228:1555–1561.
55. Mitchell JH, Wildenthal K, Johnson RL Jr: The effects of acid base disturbances on cardiovascular and pulmonary function. *Kidney Int* 1972; 1:375–389.
56. Levine HD, Vazifdar JP, Lown B, Merril JP: "Tent-shaped" T waves of normal amplitude in potassium intoxication. *Am Heart J* 1952; 43:437–450.
57. Fisch C: Electrolytes and the heart, in Hurst JW (ed): *The Heart,* ed 6. New York, McGraw-Hill, 1986, pp 1466–1479.
58. Bashour TT, Cheng TO: Evidence for specialized atrioventricular conduction in hyperkalemia. *Electrocardiology* 1975; 8:65–68.
59. Hayes CP Jr, McLeod ME, Robinson PR: An extrarenal mechanism for the maintenance of potassium balance in severe chronic renal failure. *Trans Assoc Am Physicians* 1967; 80:207–216.
60. Bilbrey GL, Carter NW, White MG, Schilling JF, Knochel JP: Potassium deficiency in chronic renal failure. *Kidney Int* 1973; 4:423–430.
61. Spergel G, Bleicher JJ, Goldberg M, Adesman J, Goldner MG: The effect of potassium on the impaired glucose tolerance in chronic uremia. *Metabolism* 1967; 16:581–585.
62. Kleeman K, Singh BN: Serum electrolytes and the heart, in Maxwell MH, Kleeman CR (eds): *Clinical Disorders of Fluid and Electrolyte Metabolism,* ed 3. New York, McGraw-Hill, 1980, pp 145–180.
63. Axelrod J: The fate of noradrenaline in the sympathetic neurone, in *The Harvey Lectures, Series 67.* New York, Academic, 1971–1972, pp 175–197.
64. Manger WM: Catecholamines in normal and abnormal cardiac function. *Adv Cardiol* (Karger Basel) 1982; 30:1–145.
65. Bashour T, Basha HS, Cheng TO: Hypocalcemic cardiomyopathy. *Chest* 1980; 78:663–665.
66. Massry SG, Coburn JW: Divalent ion metabolism and renal osteodystrophy, in Massry SG, Sellers AL (eds): *Clinical Aspects of Uremia and Dialysis.* Springfield, Ill, Charles C Thomas, 1976, pp 304–387.
67. Friedman SA, Novack S, Thompson GE: Arterial calcification and gangrene in uremia. *N Engl J Med* 1969; 280:1392–1394.
68. Arora KK, Lacy JP, Schacht RA, Martin DG, Gutch CF: Calcific cardiomyopathy in advanced renal failure. *Arch Intern Med* 1975; 135:603–605.
69. Terman DS, Alfrey AC, Hammond WS, Donndelinger T, Ogden DA, Holmes JH: Cardiac calcification in uremia. A clinical, biochemical and pathologic study. *Am J Med* 1971; 50:744–755.
70. Depace NL, Rohrer AH, Kotler MN, Brezin JH, Parry WR: Rapidly progressing, massive mitral annular calcification. *Arch Intern Med* 1981; 141:1663–1665.
71. D'Cruz IA, Jain M, Fishman S, Abrahams C, Kathpalia S: Calcification in the mitral region in patients with chronic renal failure 2-D echocardiographic, hormonal and autopsy correlation. *J Am Coll Cardiol* (abstr). 1983; 1:625.
72. Eastwood JB, de Wardener HE: Renal osteodystrophy, in Jones NF (ed): *Recent Advances in Renal Disease.* Edinburgh, Churchill Livingstone, 1975, pp 177–209.
73. Coratelli P, Petrarulo F, Buongiorno E, Giannattasio M, Antonelli G, Amerio A: Improvement in left ventricular function during treatment of hemodialysis patients with 25-OHD_3. *Contr Nephrol* (Karger Basel) 1984; 41:433–437.
74. Giovanetti S, Biagini M, Cioni L: Evidence that methylguanidine is retained in chronic renal failure. *Experientia* 1968; 24:341–342.
75. Giovanetti S, Biagini M, Balestri PL, Navalesi R, Giagnoni P, De Matteis A, Ferro-Milone P, Perfetti C: Uremia-like syndrome in dogs chronically intoxicated with methylguanidine and creatinine. *Clin Sci* 1969; 36:445–452.
76. Scheuer J, Stezoski SW: The effects of uremic compounds on cardiac function and metabolism. *J Mol Cell Cardiol* 1973; 5:287–300.
77. Brass H, Krückels ED, Müller G, Heintz R: Pathomechanismen der Herzinsuffizienz bei Hämodialysepatienten. *Deutsche Medizinische Wochenschrift* 1971; 96:1319–1324.
78. Kraikitpanitch S, Lendeman RD, Yunice AA, Baxter DJ, Haygood CC, Blue MM: Effect of azotemia on the myocardial accumulation of calcium. *Min Elect Metab* 1978; 1:12–20.
79. Drueke T, Le Pailleur C: La cardiomyopathie urémique: aspects hémodynamiques et métaboliques. *Néphrologie* 1981; 2:63–66.
80. Prosser D, Parsons V: The case for a specific uraemic myocardiopathy. *Nephron* 1975; 15:4–7.
81. Drueke T, Le Pailleur C, Meilhac B, Koutoudis C, Zingraff J, DiMatteo J, Crosnier J: Congestive cardiomyopathy in uremic patients on long term hemodialysis. *Br Med J* 1977; 1:350–353.
82. Trznadel K, Luciak M, Wyszogrodzka M: The left ventricular systolic function after digoxin administration in patients with chronic renal failure. *Clin Nephrol* 1980; 13:231–234.
83. Penpargkul S, Bhan AK, Scheuer J: Studies of subcellular control factors in heart of uremic rats. *J Lab Clin Med* 1976; 88:563–570.
84. Scheuer J, Nivatpumin T, Yipintsoi T: Effects of moderate uremia on cardiac contractile responses. *Proc Soc Exper Biol Med* 1975; 150:471–474.
85. Mason MF, Resnik H Jr, Minot AS, Rainey J, Pilcher C, Harrison TR: Mechanism of experimental uremia. *Arch Intern Med* 1937; 60:312–336.
86. Kreusser W, Mann J, Rambausek M, Klooder P, Mehls O, Ritz E: Cardiac function in experimental uremia. *Kidney Int* 1983; 24 (suppl) 15:S83–S88.
87. Nivatpumin T, Yipintsoi T, Penpargkul S, Scheuer J: Increased cardiac contractility in acute uremia: interrelationship with hypertension. *Am J Physiol* 1975; 229:501–505.
88. Varat MA, Adolph RJ, Fowler NO: Cardiovascular effects of anemia. *Am Heart J* 1972; 83:415–426.
89. Duke M, Abelmann WH: The hemodynamic response to chronic anemia. *Circulation* 1969; 39:503–515.
90. Grossman W, Braunwald E: High cardiac output states, in Braunwald E (ed): *Heart Disease,* ed 2. Philadelphia, WB Saunders, 1984, pp 807–822.
91. Capelli JP, Kasparian H: Cardiac work demands and left ventricular function in end-stage renal disease. *Ann Intern Med* 1977; 86:261–267.
92. Kim KE, Onesti G, Schwartz AB: Hemodynamic alterations in hypertension of chronic end-stage renal disease, in Onesti G, Kim KE, Moyer JH (eds): *Hypertension—Mechanisms and Management.* New York, Grune & Stratton, 1973, pp 609–623.
93. Drueke T, Fleury I, Toure Y, De Vernejoul P, Fauchet M, Lesourd P, Le Pailleur C, Crosnier J: Effect of parathyroidectomy on left ventricular function in haemodialysis patients. *Lancet* 1980; 1:112–114.
94. Massry SG: Parathyroid hormone and uremic myocardiopathy. *Contr Nephrol* (Karger Basel) 1984; 41:231–239.
95. Bogin E, Massry SG, Harary I: Effect of parathyroid hormone on rat heart cells. *J Clin Invest* 1981; 67:1215–1227.
96. Bogin E, Levi J, Harary I, Massry SG: Effects of parathyroid hormone on oxidative phosphorylation of heart mitochondria. *Min Elec Metab* 1982; 7:151–156.
97. Lhoste F, Drüeke T, Larno S, Boissier JR: Cardiac interaction between parathyroid hormone, β-adrenoreceptor agents, and verapamil in the guinea pig in vitro. *Clin Exp Pharmacol Physiol* 1980; 7:119–127.
98. Katon Y, Klein KL, Kaplan RA, Sanborn WG, Kurokawa K: Parathyroid hormone has a positive inotropic action in the rat heart. *Endocrinology* 1981; 109:2252–2254.
99. Jahn H, Schohn D, Schmitt R: Plasma parathormone levels and heart function in end stage renal failure patients (abstr). IXth International Congress of Nephrology, Los Angeles, Calif, 1984, p 51 A.
100. Kennel WB, Danofer TR: Hypertension as an ingredient of cardiovascular risk profile. *Br J Hosp Med* 1974; 2:508–523.
101. Robert WC: The hypertensive diseases: evidence that systemic hypertension is a greater risk factor to the development of other cardiovascular disease than previously suspected. *Am J Med* 1975; 59:523–532.
102. Folkow B: The hemodynamic consequences of adaptive structural changes of the resistance vessels in hypertension. *Clin Sci* 1971; 41:1–12.
103. Weidmann P, Maxwell MH: The renin angiotensin aldosterone system in terminal renal failure. *Kidney Int* 1975; 8:S219–S234.
104. Lazarus JM, Hampers CL, Merrill JP: Hypertension in chronic renal failure. Treatment with hemodialysis and nephrectomy. *Arch Intern Med* 1974; 133:1059–1066.
105. Weidmann P, Beretta-Piccoli C, Steffen F, Blumberg A, Reubi FS: Hypertension in terminal renal failure. *Kidney Int* 1976; 9:294–301.
106. Weidmann P, Maxwell MH, Lupu AN, Lewin AJ, Massry SG: Plasma renin activity and blood pressure in terminal renal failure. *N Engl J Med* 1971; 285:757–762.
107. Schohn D, Weidmann P, Jahn H, Beretta-Piccoli C: Norepinephrine-related mechanism in hypertension accompanying renal failure. *Kidney Int* 1985; 28:814–822.
108. Campese VM, Iseki K, Massry SG: Plasma catecholamines and vascular reactivity in uremic and dialysis patients. *Contr Nephrol* (Karger Basel) 1984; 41:90–98.
109. McGrath BP: Autonomic component in hypertension accompanying renal failure. *Contr Nephrol* (Karger Basel) 1984; 41:83–89.
110. Weidmann P: Recent pathogenic aspects in essential hypertension and hypertension associated with diabetes mellitus. *Klin Wochenschr* 1980; 58:1071–1089.
111. Kim KE, Onesti G, Schwartz AB, Chinitz JL, Swartz C: Hemodynamics of hypertension in chronic end-stage renal disease. *Circulation* 1972; 46:456–464.
112. Brod J: Hypertension and renal parenchymal disease: mechanisms and management. *Cardiovasc Clin* 1978; 9(1):137–164.
113. Kim KE, Onesti G, Schwartz AB: The hemodynamic responses to salt and water loading in patients with end stage renal disease and anephric man. *Clin Sci Mol Med* 1976; 51 (Suppl 3):223S–225S.
114. Brod J, Fencl V, Ulrych M: General and regional hemodynamics in hypertension in chronic renal disease. *Clin Nephrol* 1975; 5:175–182.

115. Safar M: Etude hémodynamique, isotopique et biologique des variations tensionnelles chez les sujets en hémodialyse chronique après binéphrectomie et après transplantation rénale. *Actualités Néphrol Hôp Necker* 1969; 61–86.
116. Kim KE, Onesti G, Swartz CD: Hemodynamics of hypertension in uremia. *Kidney Int* 1975; 7 (Suppl 2):S155–S162.
117. Reubi FC, Tuckman J, Vorburger C, Weidmann P: Hypertension in chronic renal failure. *Verh Dtsch Ges Inn Med* 1974; 80:182–189.
118. Schohn D, Schmitt R, Jahn H: Malignant hypertension in end stage renal failure hemodynamic and hormonal status. *Contr Nephrol* (Karger Basel) 1985; 49:185–192.
119. Beretta-Piccoli C, Weidmann P, De Châtel R, Reubi F: Hypertension associated with early stage kidney disease. Complementary role of circulating renin, the body sodium/volume state and duration of hypertension. *Am J Med* 1976; 61:739–747.
120. Brennan BL, Yasamura SY, Letteri JM, Cohn SH: Total body electrolyte composition and distribution of body water in uremia. *Kidney Int* 1980; 17:364–371.
121. Dathan JRE, Johnson DB, Goodwin FJ: The relationship between body fluid compartment volumes, renin activity and blood pressure in chronic renal failure. *Clin Sci Mol Med* 1973; 45:77–88.
122. Tarazi RC, Dustan HP, Frohlich ED, Gifford RW, Hoffmann GC: Plasma volume and chronic hypertension. Relationship to arterial pressure levels in different hypertensive diseases. *Arch Intern Med* 1970; 125:835–842.
123. Guyton AC, Coleman TG, Cowley AW Jr, Scheel KW, Manning RD Jr, Norman RA Jr: Arterial pressure regulation. Overriding dominance of the kidneys in long term regulation and in hypertension. *Am J Med* 1972; 52:584–594.
124. Guyton AC, Coleman TG, Young DB, Lohmeier TE, DeClue JW: Salt balance and long term blood pressure control. *Ann Rev Med* 1980; 31:15–27.
125. Wilkinson R, Scott DF, Uldall PR, Kerr DNS, Swinney J: Plasma renin and exchangeable sodium in the hypertension of chronic renal failure. The effect of bilateral nephrectomy. *Q J Med* 1970; 39:377–394.
126. Kleinknecht D, Maxwell MH: Etude statistique des variations de l'activité rénine plasmatique dans les néphropathies bilatérales. Résultats préliminaires. *Act Nephrol Hôp Necker* (Flammarion Paris) 1970; 63–83.
127. Schalekamp MA, Beevers DG, Briggs JD, Brown JJ, Davies DK, Fraser R, Lebel M, Lever AF, Medina A, Morton JJ, Robertson JIS, Tree M: Hypertension in chronic renal failure. An abnormal relation between sodium and the renin angiotensin system. *Am J Med* 1973; 55:379–390.
128. Schohn D, Jahn H: Aggravation of hypertension by activation of the renin–angiotensin system in chronic hemodialysis patients by drastic ultrafiltration. (Unpublished observations.)
129. Laragh JH, Baer L, Brunner HR, Buhler FR, Sealey JE, Vaughan ED: Renin, angiotensin and aldosterone system in pathogenesis and management of hypertensive vascular disease. *Am J Med* 1972; 52:633–652.
130. Kahn T, Mohammad G, Bornia ME, Stein RM, Krakoff LR: Control of plasma renin activity in chronic stable renal disease. *J Lab Clin Med* 1975; 85:637–644.
131. Rosen SM, Robinson PJA: Interdependence of exchangeable sodium and plasma renin concentration in determining blood pressure in patients treated by maintenance dialysis. *Br Med J* 1973; 4:139–143.
132. Weidmann P: Pathogenesis of hypertension associated with chronic renal failure. *Contr Nephrol* (Karger Basel) 1984; 41:47–65.
133. Lilley JJ, Golden J, Stone RA: Adrenergic regulation of blood pressure in chronic renal failure. *J Clin Invest* 1976; 57:1190–1200.
134. Link L, Weidmann P, Beretta-Piccoli C, Boehringer K, Schiffl H, Reubi FC: Renal clearance of catecholamines in man. *Kidney Int* 1982; 21:902.
135. McGrath BP, Ledingham JGG, Benedict CR: Catecholamines in peripheral venous plasma in patients on chronic hemodialysis. *Clin Sci Mol Med* 1978; 55:89–96.
136. Campese VM, Romoff MS, Levitan D, Lane K, Massry SG: Mechanisms of autonomic nervous system dysfunction in uremia. *Kidney Int* 1981; 20:246–253.
137. Lake CR, Ziegler MG, Coleman MD, Kopin IJ: Plasma levels of norepinephrine and dopamine-β-hydroxylase in CRF patients treated with dialysis. *Cardiovasc Med* 1979; 4:1099–1111.
138. Spohr V, Ritz E, Kaden F: Plasma dopamine-β-hydroxylase activity in dialysed patients. *Klin Wschr* 1977; 55:1089–1093.
139. Brodde OE, Daul A: Alpha- and beta-adrenoreceptor changes in patients on maintenance hemodialysis. *Contr Nephrol* (Karger Basel) 1984; 41:99–107.
140. Lazarus JM, Hampers CL, Lowrie EG, Merrill JP: Baroreceptor activity in normotensive and hypertensive uremic patients. *Circulation* 1973; 47:1015–1021.
141. Rascher W, Schömig A, Kreye VA, Ritz E: Diminished vascular response to noradrenaline in experimental chronic uremia. *Kidney Int* 1982; 21:20–27.
142. Pickering TG, Gribbin B, Olivier DO: Baroreflex sensitivity in patients on long term hemodialysis. *Clin Sci Mol Med* 1972; 43:645–657.
143. Tomiyama O, Shiigai T, Ideura T, Tomita K, Mito Y, Shinohrae S, Takeuchi J: Baroreflex sensitivity in renal failure. *Clin Sci Mol Med* 1980; 58:21–27.
144. McGrath BP, Tiller DJ, Bune A, Chalmers JP, Korner PI, Uther JB: Autonomic blockade and the Valsalva maneuver in patients on maintenance hemodialysis: a hemodynamic study. *Kidney Int* 1977; 12:294–302.
145. Schohn DC, Jahn HA, Petitjean P: Acute hemodynamic effects of α and β adrenergic blockade in chronic hemodialysis patients. *Blood Purif* (abstr). 1983; 1:136.
146. Muirhead EE, Brown GB, Germain GS, Leach BE: The renal medulla as an antihypertensive organ. *J Lab Clin Med* 1970; 76:641–651.
147. Lee JB, Mookerjee BK: The renal prostaglandins as etiologic factors in human essential hypertension. Fact or fantasy? *Cardiovasc Med* 1976; 1:302–308.
148. Hornych A, Bedrossian J, Bariety J, Menard J, Corvol P, Safar M, Fontaliran F, Milliez P: Prostaglandins and hypertension in chronic renal disease. *Clin Nephrol* 1975; 4:144–151.
149. Russel GI, Taverner D, Jackson J, Bing RF, Swales JD, Thurston H: Role of the renal medulla in experimental hypertension. *Contr Nephrol* (Karger Basel) 1984; 41:163–166.
150. Jahn H, Schohn D, Gullberg C, Schmitt R: Hemodynamic long-term effects of hemofiltration on dialysis and drug resistant hypertension. *Contr Nephrol* (Karger Basel) 1982; 32:61–68.
151. Leski M, Phanh Tam N, Menard J: Traitement par le propranolol de l'hypertension artérielle de l'hémodialyse périodique. *J Urol Nephrol* 1973; 79:764–768.
152. Bauer JH: Role of angiotensin-converting enzyme inhibitor in essential and renal hypertension. *Am J Med* 1984; 77 (2A):43–51.
153. Delin K, Aurell M, Herlitz H: Captopril in the treatment of hypertension in predialytic end-stage renal disease. *Contr Nephrol* (Karger Basel) 1984; 41:299–303.
154. Jacobs C, Simon N, Patte R, Dupuy CA, Sari R: Control of blood pressure in patients treated by maintenance hemodialysis. *Contr Nephrol* (Karger Basel) 1984; 41:128–136.
155. Derow HA: The heart in renal disease. *Circulation* 1954; 10:114–128.
156. Fellner SK: The heart and chronic renal failure, in Hurst JW (ed): *The Heart*, ed 6. New York, McGraw-Hill, 1986, pp 1458–1465.
157. Eichna LW, Farber SJ, Berger AR, Rader B, Smith WW, Albert RE: Non-cardiac circulatory congestion simulating congestive heart failure. *Trans Assoc Am Phys* 1954; 67:72–85.
158. Binak K, Sirmaci N, Ucak D, Harmanci N: Circulatory changes in acute glomerulonephritis at rest and during exercise. *Br Heart J* 1975; 37:833–839.
159. McCrory WW: The heart in acute glomerulonephritis. *J Pediatrics* 1966; 69:1176–1178.
160. DeFazio V, Christensen RC, Regan TJ, Baer LJM, Morita Y, Hellems HK: Circulatory changes in acute glomerulonephritis. *Circulation* 1959; 20:190–200.
161. Haire H, Sherrard D, Scardapone D: Smoking, hypertension and mortality in a maintenance dialysis population. *Cardiovasc Med* 1978; 3:1163–1169.
162. Ibels LS, Stewart JH, Mahony JF, Neale FC, Sheil AGR: Occlusive arterial disease in uraemic and haemodialysis patients and renal transplant recipients. *Q J Med* 1977; 46:197–214.
163. Cheng TO: Non-invasive techniques in the evaluation of the patient with coronary heart disease. *Angiology* 1975; 26:820–836.
164. Boucek RJ, Morales AR, Romanelli R, Judkins MP: Clinical diagnosis of coronary stenosis, in *Coronary Artery Disease: Pathologic and Clinical Assessment.* Baltimore, Williams & Wilkins, 1984, pp 269–289.
164a. Goldberg AP, Geltman EM, Gavin JR III, Carney RM, Hagberg JM, Delmez JA, Naumovich A, Oldfield MH, Harter HR: Exercise training reduces coronary risk and effectively rehabilitates hemodialysis patients. *Nephron* 1986; 42:311–316.
165. Scheidt SS: The role of the calcium blockers in the treatment of chronic stable angina, in Flaim SF, Zelis R (eds): *Calcium Blockers: Mechanisms of Action and Clinical Applications.* Baltimore, Urban & Schwarzenberg, 1982, Vol 2, pp 231–244.
166. Crawford FA, Selby JH Jr, Bower JD, Lehan PH: Coronary revascularization in patients maintained on chronic hemodialysis. *Circulation* 1977; 56:684–687.
167. Lamberti JJ Jr, Cohn LH, Collins JJ Jr: Cardiac surgery in patients undergoing renal dialysis or transplantation. *Ann Thorac Surg* 1975; 19:135–141.
168. Kannel WB, Castelli WP, Gordon T, McNamara PM: Serum cholesterol, lipoproteins, and the risk of coronary heart disease. The Framingham study. *Ann Intern Med* 1971; 74:1–12.
169. Nicholls AJ, Catto GRD, Edward N, Engeset J, Macleod M: Accelerated atherosclerosis in long-term dialysis and renal transplantation patients: fact or fiction? *Lancet* 1980; 1:276–278.

170. Bagdade J, Casaretto A, Albers J: Effects of chronic uremia, hemodialysis and renal transplantation on plasma lipids and lipoproteins in man. *J Lab Clin Med* 1976; 87:37–48.
171. Brunzell JD, Albers JJ, Haas LB, Goldberg AP, Agadoa L, Sherrard DJ: Prevalence of serum lipid abnormalities in chronic hemodialysis. *Metabolism* 1977; 26:903–910.
172. Nestel PJ, Fidge NH, Tan MH: Increased lipoprotein-remnant formation in chronic renal failure. *N Engl J Med* 1982; 307:329–333.
173. Riesen WF, Mordasini R: Hyperlipidemia in renal failure: phenotypes and pathogenetic mechanisms. *Contr Nephrol* (Karger Basel) 1984; 41:312–320.
174. Mordasini R, Riesen W, Oster P, Walther A: Pathogenic aspects of hyperlipoproteinemia in chronic renal disorders, in Noseda G, Fragiacomo C, Fumagalli R, Paoletti R (eds): *Lipoproteins and Coronary Atherosclerosis.* Amsterdam, Elsevier, 1982, pp 317–327.
175. Mordasini R, Frey F, Flury F, Klose G, Greten H: Selective deficiency of hepatic triglyceride lipase in uremic patients. *N Engl J Med* 1977; 297:1362–1366.
175a. Shapiro RJ: Mechanism for hyperlipidemia in chronic renal failure. *Kidney Int* 1986; 29:326.
176. Murase T, Cattran DC, Rubenstein B, Steiner G: Inhibition of lipoprotein lipase by uremic plasma, a possible cause of hypertriglyceridemia. *Metabolism* 1975; 24:1279–1286.
177. Rapaport J, Aviram M, Chaimovitz C, Brook JG: Defective high density lipoprotein composition in patients on chronic hemodialysis. A possible mechanism for accelerated atherosclerosis. *N Engl J Med* 1978; 299:1326–1329.
178. Cattran DC, Fenton SSA, Wilson DR, Steiner G: Defective triglyceride removal in lipemia associated with peritoneal dialysis and haemodialysis. *Ann Intern Med* 1976; 85:29–33.
179. Maebashi M, Kawamura N, Sato M, Imamura A, Yoshinaga K: Lipid lowering effect of carnitine in patients with type IV hyperlipoproteinemia. *Lancet* 1978; 2:805–807.
180. Mallick NP, Short CD: The nephrotic syndrome and ischemic heart disease. *Nephron* 1981; 27:54–57.
181. Goldstein JL, Brown MS: Atherosclerosis. The low density lipoprotein receptor hypothesis. *Metabolism* 1977; 26:1257–1275.
182. Goldstein JL, Anderson RGN, Buja LM, Basu SK, Brown MS: Overloading human aortic smooth muscle cells with low density lipoprotein-cholesterol esters reproduces features of atherosclerosis in vitro. *J Clin Invest* 1977; 59:1196–1202.
183. Goldberg AP, Sherrard DJ, Haas LB, Brunzell JD: Control of clofibrate toxicity in uremic hypertriglyceridemia. *Clin Pharmacol Ther* 1977; 21:317–325.
184. Fuchs C, Armstrong VW, Cremer P, Henning HV, Wieland H, QuellHorst E, Seidel D: An investigation of the lipoprotein profiles of patients on hemofiltration as compared to those on hemodialysis and intermittent peritoneal dialysis. *Contr Nephrol* (Karger Basel) 1982; 32:92–96.
185. Kluge R, Heuck C, Ritz E: Lipidstoffwechsel unter Bikarbonatdialyse. *Nieren und Hochdruckkrankheiten* 1984; 13(4):143–151.
186. Kishimoto T, Ezaki K, Yamagami S, Maekawa M: Glucose tolerance and erythrocyte insulin receptors in undialyzed patients and patients on maintenance hemodialysis and hemofiltration. *Contr Nephrol* 1982; 32:97–110.
187. Morris PJ, Chan L, French ME, Ting A: Low dose oral prednisolone in renal transplantation. *Lancet* 1982; 1:525–527.
188. Curtis JJ, Galla JH, Woodford SY, Lucas BA, Luke RG: Effect of alternate-day prednisone on plasma lipids in renal transplant recipients. *Kidney Int* 1982; 22:42–47.
189. Comty CM, Shapiro FL: Cardiac complications of regular dialysis treatment, in Drukker W, Parsons F, Maher J (eds): *Replacement of Renal Function by Dialysis,* ed 2. Boston, Martinus Nijhoff, 1983, pp 595–610.
190. Degoulet P, Reach I, Aimé C, Berger C, Goupy F, Jacobs C, Rojas P, Legrain M: Epidémiologie des complications cardiaques. *Soc de Néphrologie* 1964; Commission Informatique IV.
191. Alfrey AC, Gross JE, Ogden DA, Vogel JHK, Holmes JH: Uremic hemopericardium. *Am J Med* 1968; 45:391–400.
192. Buja LM, Friedmann CA, Robert WC: Hemorrhagic pericarditis in uremia. Clinicopathologic studies in 6 patients. *Arch Path* 1970; 90:325–330.
193. Brogard JM, Brandt C, Kuntzmann F, Arnold P, Krivosic I, Fincker JL, Jahn H: Evolution des péricardites urémiques au cours de l'hémodialyse itérative. Etude hémodynamique à l'aide du cathétérisme cardiaque droit par sonde flottante. *Coeur Med Intern* 1969; 4:463–476.
194. Delahaye JP, Traeger S, Gonin A, Laurent J: Les péricardites urémiques. *Coeur Méd Intern* 1965; 4:3–13.
195. London G, Joly H, Valty J, Galey JJ, Man NK, Zingraff J, Vantelon J: Péricardites urémiques constrictives: deux nouvelles observations. *Presse Med* 1971; 79:341–344.
196. Reyman TA: Subacute constrictive uremic pericarditis. *Am J Med* 1969; 46:972–975.
197. Jahn H, Kieny R: Management of pericardial heart disease in uremia: tap, drainage, fenestration or pericardiectomy? *Contrib Nephrol* 1982; 33:197–209.
198. Comty CM, Wathen RL, Shapiro FL: Uremic pericarditis, in Spodick DH (ed): *Pericardial Diseases.* Philadelphia, FA Davis, 1976, pp 219–235.
199. Cliff WJ, Grobety J, Ryan GB: Postoperative pericardial adhesions. The role of mild serosal injury and spilled blood. *J Thorac Cardio Vasc Surg* 1973; 65:744–750.
200. Lindsay J Jr, Crawley IS, Callaway GM Jr: Chronic constrictive pericarditis following uremic hemopericardium. *Am Heart J* 1970; 79:390–395.
201. Meyrier A, Leroux-Robert C, Sraer JD, Marsac J, Richet G: Péricardites aiguës des insuffisants rénaux chroniques traités par hémodialyse itérative. *Ann Chir Thorac Cardiovasc* 1972; 11:201–206.
202. Pabico RC, Freeman RB: Pericarditis and myocardiopathy, in Massry SG, Sellers AL (eds): *Clinical Aspects of Uremia and Dialysis.* Springfield, Ill, Charles C Thomas, 1976, pp 69–99.
203. Renfrew R, Buselmeier TJ, Kjellstrand C: Pericarditis and renal failure. *Ann Rev Med* 1980; 31:345–360.
204. Lorell BH, Braunwald E: Pericardial disease, in Braunwald E (ed): *Heart Disease,* ed 2. Philadelphia, WB Saunders, 1984, pp 1470–1527.
205. Bashour TT, Guha A, Cheng TO, Parrish A, Kramer N: Paroxysmal atrial tachyarrhythmias induced by hemodialysis: an early sign of effusive pericarditis. *Clin Res* 1973; 21:403.
206. Hancock EW: On the elastic and rigid forms of constrictive pericarditis. *Am Heart J* 1980; 100:917–923.
206a. Twardowski ZJ, Alpert MA, Gupta RC, Nolph KD, Madsen BT: Circulating immune complexes: possible toxins responsible for serositis (pericarditis, pleuritis, and peritonitis) in renal failure. *Nephron* 1983; 35:190–195.
206b. Alpert MA, Van Stone J, Twardowski ZJ, Ruder MA, Whiting RB, Kelly DL, Madsen BR: Comparative cardiac effects of hemodialysis and continuous ambulatory peritoneal dialysis. *Clin Cardiol* 1986; 9:52–60.
207. Bashour TT, Kabbani SS, Jokhadar M, Hanna ES, Cheng TO: Constrictive pericarditis: Medical versus surgical treatment. *Cardiovasc Rev Reports* 1983; 4:1337–1340.
208. Jungers P, Zingraff J, Brefort G, Moynot A, Drueke T, Man NK, Crosnier J: Uremic pericarditis: beneficial effect of surgical pericardiostomy (abstr). *Kidney Int* 1978; 14:202.
209. Brescia MJ, Cimino JE, Appel K, Hurwich BJ: Chronic hemodialysis using venipuncture and a surgically created arteriovenous fistula. *N Engl J Med* 1966; 275:1089–1092.
210. Cross AS, Steigbigel RT: Infective endocarditis and access site infections in patients on hemodialysis. *Medicine* 1976; 55:453–466.
211. Leonard A, Raij L, Shapiro FL: Bacterial endocarditis in regularly dialysed patients. *Kidney Int* 1973; 4:407–422.
212. Vereerstraeten P: La survie du Brightique traité par hémodialyse. *J Sci Med Lille* 1970; 88:491–516.
213. Goodman JS, Crew HD, Ginn HE, Koenig MG: Bacterial endocarditis as a possible complication of chronic hemodialysis. *N Engl J Med* 1969; 280:876–877.
214. Ganeval D: Problèmes infectieux et immunologiques chez les hémodialysés, in Hamburger J, Crosnier J, Grünfeld PP (eds): *Nephrologie.* Paris, Flammarion, 1979, pp 1267–1268.
215. Lillehei CW, Bobb JRR, Visscher MB: Occurrence of endocarditis with valvular deformities in dogs with arteriovenous fistulas. *Ann Surg* 1950; 132:577–590.
216. Hook EW, Wainer HS, McGee TJ, Sellers TF: Acquired arteriovenous fistula with bacterial endarteritis and endocarditis. *JAMA* 1957; 164:1450–1454.
217. Fellner SK: Cardiovascular complications of chronic renal failure and dialysis, in Hurst JW (ed): *The Heart,* ed 3. New York, McGraw-Hill, 1974, pp 1119–1209.
218. Ribot S, Rothfeld D, Frankel HJ: Infectious endocarditis in maintenance hemodialysis patients. A report of four episodes among three patients. *Am J Med Sci* 1972; 264:183–188.
219. Ralston AJ, Harlow GR, Jones DM, Davis P: Infections of Scribner and Brescia arteriovenous shunts. *Br Med J* 1971; 3:408–409.
220. King LH Jr, Bradley KP, Shires DL Jr, Donohue JP, Glover JL: Bacterial endocarditis in chronic hemodialysis patients: a complication more common than previously suspected. *Surgery* 1971; 69:554–556.
221. Schohn DC, Jahn HA, Schmitt RL: Bacterial endocarditis following infected polycystic kidneys. (Unpublished observations.)
222. Schmidt P, Zazgornik J, Kopsa H, Kotzaurek R: Septicemia and pulmonary embolism complicating maintenance haemodialysis. *Lancet* 1972; 1:1129.
223. Wilson WEC, Kirkpatrick CH, Talmage DW: Suppression of immunological responsiveness in uremia. *Ann Intern Med* 1965; 62:1–14.
224. Laaban JP, Pasternac A: Endocarditis à staphylocoque. Nouvelles perspectives diagnostiques et therapeutiques. *Revue Médecine Intern* 1982; 3:155–162.
225. Roberts WC, Buchbinder NA: Right-sided valvular infective endocarditis. *Am J Med* 1972; 53:7–19.

226. Kurtz DM: Endocarditis after chronic hemodialysis. *N Engl J Med* 1969; 280:1302.
227. Leonard A, Raij L, Comty CM, Wathen R, Rattazzi T, Shapiro FL: Experience with endocarditis in a large disease program. *Trans Am Soc Artif Intern Organs* 1973; 19:298–301.
228. Saldanha LF, Goldman R, Adashek K, Mulder DG: Treatment of bacterial endocarditis: complicating hemodialysis. *Br Med J* 1972; 3:92–93.
229. Ribot S, Gilbert L, Rothfeld EL, Parsonnet V, Caobs MG: Bacterial endocarditis with pulmonary edema necessitating mitral valve replacement in a hemodialysis-dependent patient. *J Thor Cardiovasc Surg* 1971; 62:59–62.
230. Glabman S, Lukban S, Litwak R, Jurado R: Bacterial endocarditis leading to aortic valve destruction and open heart surgery in chronic dialysis patients (abstr). *V Int Congress of Nephrology,* Mexico, 1972, p 16.
231. Wizemann V, Kramer W, Knopp G, Siehla M, Schmidt H, Rawer P, Schutterle G: Cardiovascular function during hemodialysis, hemofiltration, hemodiafiltration, in *Proceedings Hemodiafiltration*. Friedberg, Giessen-Bindernagel, 1981, pp 89–104.
232. Schaefer K, Von Herrath D, Gullberg CA, Asmus G, Hufler M, Offermann G, Cremer H, Heuck CC, Ritz E: Chronic hemofiltration. A critical evaluation of a new method for the treatment of blood. *Artif Organs* 1978; 2:386–394.
233. Jahn H, Schohn D, Schmitt R, Moch S: Azetat und bikarbonat dialyse: hämodynamische wirkungen, in Seybold D, Schulz W, Pilgrim R (eds): *Nieren Insuffizienz, Aktuelle Klinische und Therapeutische Probleme.* Munich, Dustri-Verlag, 1983, pp 85–89.
234. Schohn D, Gessler W, Schmitt R, Jahn H: Einfluss der dialysatzusammensetzung auf die hämodynamik. *Nieren und Hochdruckkrankheiten* 1984; 13:S387–S395.
235. Schohn D, Klein S, Mitsuishi Y, Jahn H: Correlations between plasma sodium acetate concentration and systemic vascular resistances. *Proc XXVIII EDTA Meet* 1981; 18:160–168.
236. Schohn D, Jahn H, Eber M, Hauptmann G: Biocompatibility and hemodynamic studies during polycarbonate versus cuprophane membrane dialysis. *Blood Purif* 1986; 4:102–111.
237. Jahn HA, Bauler M, Schohn DC: Hemodynamic studies in chronic dialysis patients with a polysulfone dialyser. *Contr Nephrol* 1985; 46:151–161.
238. Nixon JV, Mitchell JH, McPhaul JJ Jr, Henrich WL: Effect of hemodialysis on left ventricular function. Dissociation of changes in filling volume and in contractile state. *J Clin Invest* 1983; 71:377–384.
239. Henry JP, Gauer OH, Sieker HO: The effect of moderate changes in blood volume on left and right atrial pressure. *Circ Res* 1956; 4:91–94.
240. Jahn H, Baubeau D, Fagalde A: Intérêt séméiologique du microcathétérisme cardiaque droit en hémodialyse. *J Urol Nephrol* 1973; 79:375–380.
241. Jahn H, Schohn D, Schmitt R: Hemodynamic modifications induced by fluid removal and treatment modalities in chronic hemodialysis patients. *Blood Purif* 1983; 1:80–89.
242. Brunois JP, Toupance O, Vistelle R, Choisy H, Chanard J: Sodium dependent transcellular water shift during dialysis. Change in extra cellular fluid volume. *Nephrol* 1984; 5:27–31.
243. Bergström J, Anaba H, Furst P: Dialysis ultrafiltration and blood pressure. *Proc EDTA Meet* 1976; 13:293–298.
244. Bergström J: Changes in blood pressure and hemodynamics during ultrafiltration and dialysis. *Dial Transplant* 1978; 7:1087–1092.
245. Kirkendol PL, Robie NW, Gonzalez, FM, Devia CJ: Cardiac and vascular effects of infused sodium acetate in dogs. *Trans Am Soc Artif Intern Organs* 1978; 24:714–718.
246. Sin Po Sit, Vatner SF: Integrated circulatory response to volume expansion, in Guyton AC (ed): *Cardiovascular Physiology.* Baltimore, University Park Press, 1982, pp 323–354.
247. Frohlich ED: Vascular effects of the Krebs intermediate metabolites. *Am J Physiol* 1965; 208:149–153.
248. Liang CS, Lowenstein JM: Metabolic control of the circulation. Effects of acetate and pyruvate. *J Clin Invest* 1978; 62:1029–1038.
249. Bauer W, Richards DW Jr: A vasodilatator action of acetates. *J Physiol* 1928; 66:371–378.
250. Schohn D, Jahn H, Doerflinger C, Hashimoto T: Increase of stroke index by acetate hemodialysis. *Contr Nephrol* 1984; 41:383–387.
251. Gessler W, Schohn D, Jahn H: Gefässreagibilität unter azetat bzw bikarbonat hämodialyse, in Seybold D, Schulz W, Pilgrim R (eds): *Niereninsuffizienz, Aktuelle Klinische und Therapeutische Probleme.* Munich, Dustri-Verlag, 1983, pp 100–106.
251a. Maynard JC, Cruz C, Kleerekoper M, Levin NW: Blood pressure response to changes in serum ionized calcium during hemodialysis. *Ann Intern Med* 1986; 104:358–361.
252. Conte J, Durand D, Ton That H, Guiraud R, Serres P: Etude du retentissement hémodynamique des fistules artério-veineuses chirurgicales chez les malades en hémodialyse périodique. *J Urol Nephrol* 1973; 79:351–354.
253. Anthony P, Chandraratna N: Determination of contribution of arteriovenous fistula to total cardiac output by Doppler computer. *Contr Nephrol* 1984; 41:251–254.
254. Salvesen HA: On a diastolic regurgitant murmur heard near and at the apical region of the heart in uremia with negative autopsy findings. *Acta Med Scand* 1938; 97:440–454.
255. Barratt LJ, Robinson MA, Whitford JA, Lawrence JR: The diastolic murmur of renal failure. *N Engl J Med* 1976; 295:121–124.
255a. Barratt LJ, Robinson MA: The evaluation of diastolic murmurs in renal failure. *Prac Cardiol* 1982; 8(12):143–148.
256. Editorial: Diastolic murmurs in renal failure. *Lancet* 1986; 1:482.
257. Adam WR, Dawborn JK, Rosenbaum M: Transient early diastolic murmurs in patients with renal failure. *Med J Aust* 1970; 2:1085–1086.
258. Alexander WD, Polak A: Early diastolic murmurs in end-stage renal failure. *Br Heart J* 1977; 39:900–902.
259. VandenBurg M, Foale R: Transient early diastolic murmur and end stage renal disease. *Br Heart J* 1980; 43:713.
260. Storstein O, Orjavik O: Aortic insufficiency in chronic renal failure. *Acta Med Scand* 1978; 203:175–180.
261. Matalon R, Moussalli ARJ, Nidus BD, Katz A, Eisinger RP: Functional aortic insufficiency—a feature of renal failure. *N Engl J Med* 1971; 285:1522–1523.
262. Perez JE, Smith CA, Meltzer VN: Pulmonic valve insufficiency: a common cause of transient diastolic murmurs in renal failure. *Ann Intern Med* 1985; 103:497–502.
263. Cheng TO: Diastolic murmur caused by coronary artery stenosis. *Ann Intern Med* 1970; 72:543–546.
264. Nerstrom B, Ladefoged J, Lund FL: Vascular complications in 155 consecutive kidney transplantations. *Scand J Urol Nephrol* 1972; 6(suppl 15):65–74.
265. Ibels LS, Alfrey AC, Weil R III: Hyperlipidemia in adult, pediatric and diabetic renal transplant recipients. *Am J Med* 1978; 64:634–642.
266. Ibels LS, Simons LA, King JO, Williams PF, Weale FC, Stewart JH: Studies on the nature and cause of hyperlipidemia in uremia, maintenance dialysis and transplantation. *Q J Med* 1975; 44:601–614.
267. Abbott LK, Elliot C, Aitken JM, Somer JB: Serum lipoprotein abnormalities in renal allograft recipients. *Atherosclerosis* 1978; 30:97–107.
268. Bachy C, Alexandre GJP, Van Ypersele de Strihou C: Hypertension after renal transplantation. *Br Med J* 1976; 2:1287–1289.
269. Ingelfinger JR, Grupe WE, Levey RH: Post-transplant hypertension in the absence of rejection or recurrent disease. *Clin Nephrol* 1981; 15:236–239.
270. Bewick M, Ogg CS, Parson V, Trafford AP, Goggin M, Rudge R: The arterial complications of 500 renal transplants, in Robinson BH, Vereenstraeten P, Hawkins JB (eds): *Dialysis, Transplantation, Nephrology.* London, Pitman Medical, 1976, pp 186–203.
271. Van Ypersele de Strihou C, Vereerstraeten P, Wauthier M, Toussaint C, Pirson Y, De Plaen JF, Vanherweghem JL, Dautrebande J, Kinnaert P, van Geertruden J, Dupont E, Alexandre GPJ: Prevalence, etiology, and treatment of late post-transplant hypertension. *Adv Nephrol* 1983; 12:41–60.
271a. Waltzer WC, Turner S, Frohnert P, Rapaport FT: Etiology and pathogenesis of hypertension following renal transplantation. *Nephron* 1986; 42:102–109.
272. Popovtzer MM, Pinnggera W, Kate FH, Corman JL, Robinette J, Lanois B, Halgrimson CG, Starzl TE: Variations in arterial blood after kidney transplantation: relation to renal function, plasma renin activity, and the dose of prednisone. *Circulation* 1973; 47:1297–1305.
273. Rao TKS, Gupta SK, Butt KMH, Kountz SL, Friedman EA: Relationship of renal transplantation to hypertension in end-stage renal failure. *Arch Intern Med* 1978; 138:1236–1241.
274. Jacquot C, Idatte JM, Debrossian J, Weiss Y, Safar M, Bariety J: Long term blood pressure changes in renal homotransplantation. *Arch Intern Med* 1978; 138:233–236.
275. Pollini J, Guttmann RD, Beaudoin JC, Morehouse DD, Klassen J, Knaack J: Late hypertension following renal allotransplantation. *Clin Nephrol* 1979; 11:202–212.
276. Cohen SL: Hypertension in renal transplant recipients. Role of bilateral nephrectomy. *Br Med J* 1973; 3:78–81.
277. Grünfeld JP, Kleinknecht D, Moreau JF, Kamoun P, Sabto J, Garcia-Torres R, Osorio M, Kreis H: Permanent hypertension after renal homotransplantation in man. *Clin Sci* 1975; 48:391–403.
278. Lacombe M: Arterial stenosis complicating renal allotransplantation in man: a study of 38 cases. *Ann Surg* 1975; 181:283–288.
279. Lindsey ES, Garbus SB, Golladay ES, McDonald JC: Hypertension due to renal artery stenosis in transplanted kidneys. *Ann Surg* 1975; 181:604–610.
280. Ricotta JJ, Schaff HV, Williams CM, Rolley RT, Whelton PK, Harrington DM: Renal artery stenosis following transplantation: etiology, diagnosis and prevention. *Surgery* 1978; 84:595–602.
281. Whiteside CI, Cardella CJ, Yeung H, De Veber GA, Cook GT: The role of percutaneous transluminal dilatation in the treatment of transplant renal artery stenosis. *Clin Nephrol* 1982; 17:55–59.
282. Gavras H, Biollaz J, Waeber B, Brunner HR, Gavras I, Davies RO:

Antihypertensive effect of the new oral angiotensin converting enzyme inhibitor "MK 421." *Lancet* 1981 2:543–546.

283. Seybold D, Lux E: Hypertonie nach Nierentransplantation, in Seybold D, Schulz W, Pilgrim R (eds): *Niereninsuffizienz, Aktuelle Klinische und Therapeutische Probleme.* Munich, Dustri-Verlag, 1983, pp 231–236.

284. Curtis JJ, Luke RG, Whelchel JD. Diethelm AG. Jones P, Dustan HP: Inhibition of angiotensin-converting enzyme in renal-transplant recipients with hypertension. *N Engl J Med* 1983; 308:377–381.

285. O'Regan S, Douste Blazy MY, Ducharme G, Fouron JC, Davignon A: Renal transplantation and cardiac function in pediatric patients. *Clin Nephrol* 1982; 17:237–240.

61 Cardiac Regulation of Renal Function

William C. Paganelli, MD, PhD, Mark A. Creager, MD,
and Victor J. Dzau, MD

Cardiovascular homeostasis is subserved by a series of neural and hormonal mechanisms that integrate cardiac and renal function. Blood pressure and plasma volume are kept within physiologic limits by mechanisms that regulate cardiac function, vascular tone, and renal excretion of sodium and water. The purpose of this chapter is to review the individual components of this regulatory system, which include cardiopulmonary and arterial baroreceptors, renal reflexes, the renin-angiotensin system, vasopressin, and atrial natriuretic factor (Figure 61.1). This chapter will discuss the interrelation between these components and examine how they are affected in certain disease states.

CARDIOPULMONARY BAROREFLEXES

Receptors are present in the heart which are capable of responding to changes in cardiac pressure or the chemical milieu of the heart. Alteration in receptor activity results in reflex responses that influence many aspects of renal and cardiovascular function.[1-3] Afferent fibers originating from receptors in the atria and ventricles travel through central nervous system relay centers through the vagi and spinal sympathetic nerves. These receptors are activated in response to blood volume expansion or mechanical stretch of the cardiac chambers.[4] As a result of this ability to sense volume and pressure changes in the central circulation, cardiac receptors may play a fundamental role in the control of blood pressure and sodium and water homeostasis.[5,6] Cardiac receptors initiate several reflex responses that influence renal function. These reflexes cause changes in renal sympathetic nerve activity, vasopressin secretion, and, indirectly, renal release of renin. Figure 61.2 illustrates the various relations between cardiac receptors and renal function.

CARDIAC DEPRESSOR REFLEX

Normally, cardiac receptors are tonically active and provide a constant input to central nervous system vasomotor centers that suppress sympathetic efferent activity and enhance vagal activity (Figure 61.2). For example, acute stimulation of cardiac ventricular receptors by injection of veratrum alkaloids results in bradycardia and hypotension.[7] The cardiac depressor reflex is interrupted by cooling or section of cardiac vagal afferent fibers. This results in augmentation of sympathetic efferent activity, especially to the kidney.[8] Hemorrhage or dehydration, situations that result in decreased cardiac filling pressures and unloading of the cardiopulmonary receptors, is associated with reflex renal vasoconstriction.[9] Therefore, cardiac receptors are able to modulate renal sympathetic nerve activity in response to physiologic changes in cardiac filling pressures. The cardiac depressor reflex is also pertinent in patients who have acute inferior or posterior myocardial infarction. In these patients significant bradycardia and hypotension often develop. Activation of vagal receptors in the posterior ventricular wall as a consequence of myocardial ischemia or infarction will result in a reflex decrease in sympathetic efferent activity and an increase in the vagal tone.[7]

CARDIAC PRESSOR REFLEXES

In addition to vasodepressor reflexes originating in the heart, several investigators have described cardiac pressor reflexes.[10,11] However, the physiologic significance of these reflexes is not clear. During experimental myocardial ischemia, a cardiac reflex mediated by sympathetic afferent and efferent nerves causes tachycardia and hypertension. This reflex may occur at the spinal level. In human subjects, anterior myocardial infarction has been

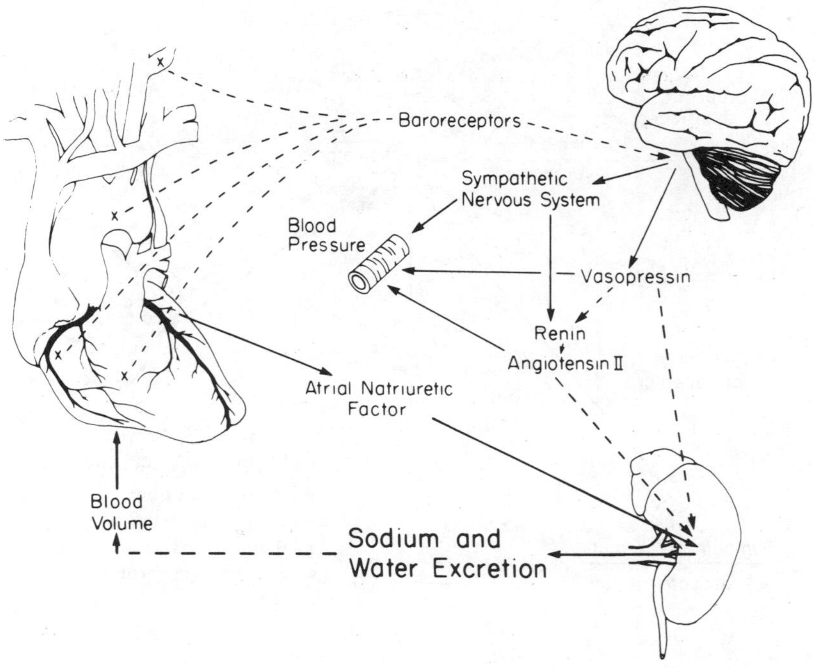

Figure 61.1. Overview of cardiovascular regulation of renal function. Inhibitory signals to each organ are indicated by *dashed lines* and stimulatory signals are indicated by *solid lines*. Increases in blood volume stimulate cardiopulmonary baroreceptors and secretion of atrial natriuretic factor. Increases in systemic arterial pressure stimulate arterial baroreceptors. Baroreceptor activation sends inhibitory signals to the central nervous system vasomotor center, resulting in suppression of sympathetic efferent activity and increased vagal efferent activity (not shown). Sympathetic efferent fibers carry stimulatory signals to the heart, blood vessels, and kidney and cause secretion of renin and reabsorption of sodium and water. Inhibition of sympathetic activity thereby favors sodium and water excretion. Baroreceptors also inhibit hypophyseal secretion of vasopressin, thereby promoting diuresis. Cardiac secretion of atrial natriuretic factor stimulates sodium and water excretion.

associated with hypertension. Therefore, the cardiac pressor reflex may be activated during myocardial ischemia. However, this reflex has not been shown to affect the circulation in normal individuals.

CARDIAC RECEPTORS AND VASOPRESSIN

Cardiac vagal afferent fibers are involved in regulating vasopressin release. Stimulation of atrial or ventricular receptors by stretch, volume expansion, or chemical agents results in reflex inhibition of vasopressin release. Conversely, decreased receptor activity due to decreases in atrial or ventricular pressure, or both, increases vasopressin secretion.[12,13] Figure 61.1 demonstrates these relations. Cardiac denervation eliminates all cardiac afferent nerves and markedly attenuates the increase in plasma vasopressin concentration that accompanies hemorrhage.[14] Thus, cardiac receptors contribute to volume homeostasis in part by stimulating or inhibiting vasopressin release. A further discussion of vasopressin's role in cardiovascular and renal function appears later in this chapter.

CARDIAC RECEPTORS AND RENIN RELEASE

Cardiac receptors contribute to the regulation of renal renin release indirectly through their effect on renal sympathetic nerve activity. Maneuvers that increase firing of cardiac receptors inhibit sympathetic efferent activity and suppress renin secretion, whereas decreases in receptor activity result in increased renin release. Thus, cardiac receptors can further contribute to salt and water homeostasis by their effect on the renin-angiotensin system.[15]

ARTERIAL BAROREFLEXES

The arterial baroreflexes comprise mechanoreceptors in the carotid sinus and the aortic arch. The afferent limb of the carotid sinus baroreflex travels in a branch of the glossopharyngeal nerve designated the carotid sinus nerve or nerve of Hering. The afferent limb of the aortic baroreflex is carried by a branch of the vagus nerve designated the depressor nerve. Afferent fibers from these receptors are predominantly myelinated. Stimulation of either nerve causes bradycardia and hypotension by augmenting parasympathetic activity and inhibiting peripheral sympathetic outflow (Figure 61.2). These receptors are excited by deformation of the vessel walls in which they reside. Thus, increases in transmural pressure, which increase the diameter of the carotid sinus or aortic arch, augment receptor firing. Decreases in carotid or aortic wall stretch diminish receptor activity.[16]

In animals, the threshold for carotid sinus stimulation

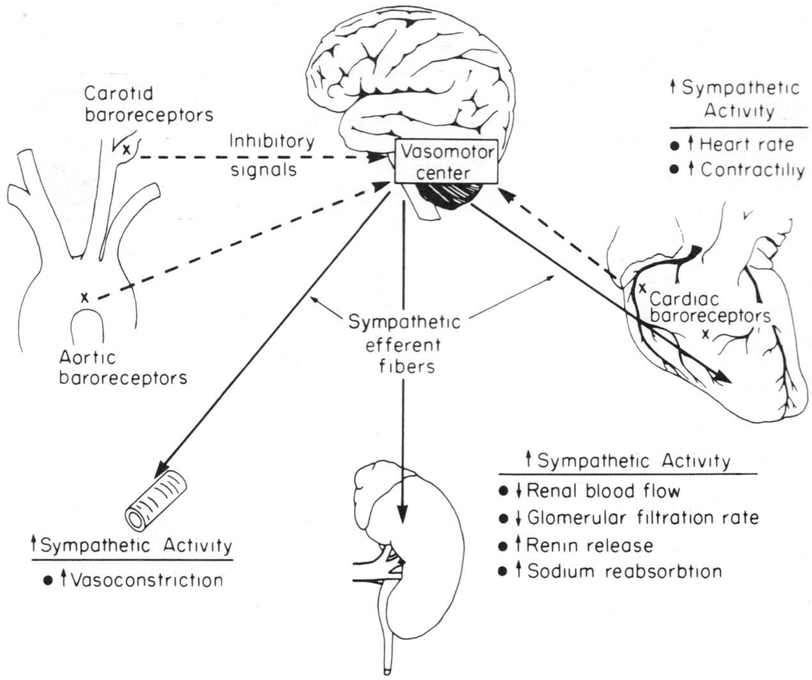

Figure 61.2. Integration of baroreflexes and renal function. Inhibitory signals from the cardiopulmonary and arterial baroreceptors are processed in the central vasomotor center. Sympathetic efferent activity causes vasoconstriction, increases heart rate and contractility, decreases renal blood flow and glomerular filtration rate, stimulates secretion of renin, and contributes to sodium reabsorption.

is approximately 60 mm Hg, with maximal effects occurring at approximately 200 mm Hg.[17] The threshold for stimulation of the aortic baroreflex is 90 to 100 mm Hg.[18] Both pulsatile and static pressures can stimulate the carotid sinus baroreflex, but the former augments the response.[19,20] The influence of pulsatility on the aortic baroreflex is controversial. The carotid sinus baroreceptor is tonically active; blockade of the carotid sinus nerve increases blood pressure and heart rate. Because the threshold of the aortic baroreflex approximates normal blood pressure, there is less tonic activity than that in the carotid sinus baroreflex. Blockade of the aortic depressor nerve causes only a small increase in blood pressure and heart rate. In human subjects neither electrical stimulation of afferent vagal fibers nor anesthetization of the vagi alters blood pressure.[9,21] These findings suggest that the aortic baroreflex does not exert a tonic influence on blood pressure in man.

BAROREFLEX REGULATION OF RENAL BLOOD FLOW

The cardiac and arterial baroreflexes can directly affect renal hemodynamics and sodium and water reabsorption by altering sympathetic nervous system activity. They can indirectly influence renal function by affecting secretion or activation of hormones such as vasopressin or angiotensin II (Figure 61.1). In animals, interruption of the cardiac baroreflex by vagal cold block or vagotomy constricts kidney resistance vessels. Stimulation of cardiac vagal afferents decreases renovascular resistance.[8]

Cardiac and arterial baroreflexes affect renal function directly by altering renal sympathetic efferent activity (Figure 61.2). Stimulation of renal sympathetic nerves results in an alpha-adrenoreceptor–mediated constriction of the renal afferent and efferent arterioles,[22,23] causing a reduction in total renal blood flow. Glomerular filtration rate decreases because glomerular capillary pressure falls. There is also a preferential shunting of blood away from the outer cortex, resulting in an increased juxtamedullary–cortical blood flow ratio.[24] Stimulation of beta-adrenergic receptors increases renin release and hence angiotensin II and aldosterone.[25] The net result is an increase in sodium reabsorption through the combination of a decrease in glomerular filtration rate, increase in tubular reabsorption, and redistribution of renal blood flow. In addition, neurally released norepinephrine directly increases sodium reabsorption by the proximal tubule.[26] Thus, changes in cardiac and arterial baroreceptor activity subserve reflex control of renal function through the sympathetic nervous system.

RENIN–ANGIOTENSIN SYSTEM

The renin-angiotensin system is a biochemical cascade system whose final product, angiotensin II, is intimately involved with sodium and volume homeostasis and blood pressure regulation (Figure 61.3). In this system, a proteolytic enzyme, renin, is secreted from the juxtaglomerular cells of the afferent arteriole in response to a variety of stimuli. Renin enzymatically cleaves a specific substrate, angiotensinogen, with resultant production of a decapeptide, angiotensin I. Angiotensin I, although essentially without physiologic effect, is the precursor to

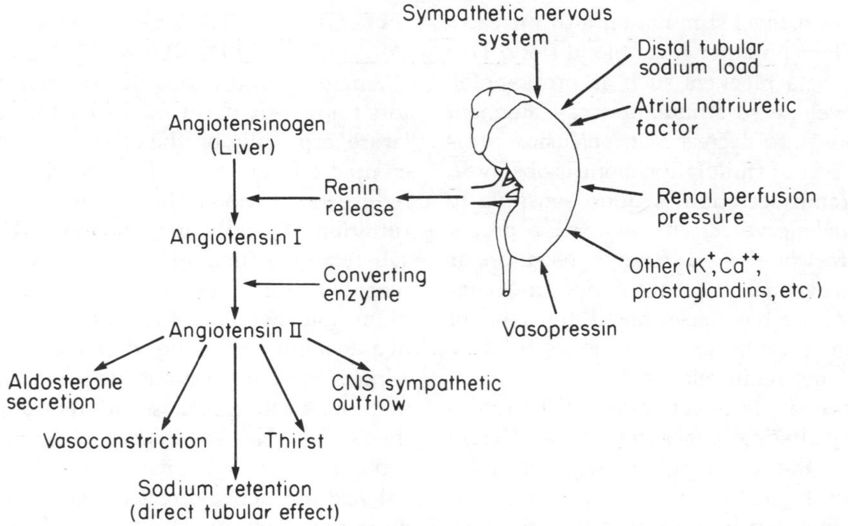

Figure 61.3. Overview of the renin–angiotensin system. Multiple signals affect renal release of renin (see text). Renin converts angiotensinogen to angiotensin I. This decapeptide is cleaved to angiotensin II by converting enzyme. Angiotensin II has multiple sites of action, including the blood vessels, adrenal glands, kidney, thirst center, and sympathetic nervous system.

angiotensin II. This next step in the pathway involves angiotensin converting enzyme, a dipeptidyl-peptidase that cleaves off the C-terminal dipeptide of angiotensin I to give the octapeptide angiotensin II.

Converting enzyme is located mainly on the endothelial membranes of the pulmonary capillaries. During a single pass through the pulmonary circulation, most of the circulating plasma angiotensin I is converted to angiotensin II. There are detectable amounts of converting enzyme present in the brain, kidney, and other vascular tissues that may subserve local renin-angiotensin effects on these tissues. Accordingly, angiotensin may serve not only as a circulating hormone affecting vascular tone, renal sodium reabsorption, aldosterone secretion, renal arteriolar resistance, and baroreflex pathways, but also as a local modulator of these functions.[27]

SIGNALS FOR RENIN RELEASE

The major determinants of renal renin release are: (1) renal perfusion pressure (as sensed by an intrarenal baroreceptor); (2) sodium delivery to the distal nephron (macula densa hypothesis); (3) beta-adrenergic stimuli resulting from release of catecholamines from intrarenal sympathetic nerve endings or circulating catecholamines; and (4) the effects of humoral agents such as prostaglandins, vasopressin, kinins, and possibly atrial natriuretic factor or factors (Figure 61.3). Each of these agents can individually affect renin secretion; there are also important interactions between the different stimuli which can enhance renin release in response to multiple inputs.[28,29]

Renal perfusion pressure can directly influence renin release. Increases in renal perfusion pressure will suppress renin release. Conversely, a decrease in perfusion pressure stimulates renin secretion from the juxtaglomerular cells. It is possible that Ca^{++} entry during pressure-mediated stretch of pressure-sensitive renal arterioles inhibits renin release, whereas increased Ca^{++} efflux accompanies decreases in perfusion pressure. Current evidence suggests that intracellular Ca^{++} levels may be important in determining renin secretion rates.[30,31] Of interest is the hypothesis that renin release seems to be inversely related to intracellular calcium, a finding different from that of other calcium-dependent hormone secretory systems.

The influence of sodium delivery to the distal tubules on renin secretion remains controversial. A decrease in dietary sodium intake results in increased synthesis, storage, and release of renin, both in the basal state and in response to other secretory stimuli.[32] These changes in intrarenal renin occur in the absence of renal innervation, so that at least part of the effect may be ascribed to intrarenal factors. High salt diet suppresses renin production and release in basal states and in response to other known stimuli. It has been argued that increased salt intake increases sodium delivery to the specialized cells of the distal tubule (the macula densa) which come into contact with the vascular pole of the glomerulus. These cells transduce this effect into a decrease in juxtaglomerular cell renin synthesis and release. Low salt diet depletes body sodium stores, decreases delivery of sodium to the macula densa, and increases renin secretion.

The juxtaglomerular cells are endowed with catecholaminergic receptors of both beta and dopaminergic type.[32] Stimulation of these receptors by endogenous agonists or exogenous pharmacologic probes results in increased renin release. Blockade of these receptors by specific antagonists inhibits renin secretion. These effects are seen in nonfiltering kidneys in which no direct effects of the agonists on tubular sodium transport occur, indicating a basic role of the receptors in mediating renin release.[33] Sympathetic nerve stimulation at high intensity augments renin secretion but also changes renal hemodynamics and sodium excretion. Lower level stimulation also increases renin release, but it does not alter renal blood flow. This effect is blocked by beta blockers such as propranolol. Finally, very low level nerve stimulation can augment renin release in response to decreases in perfusion pressure even when no effect of stimulation alone is observed. This suggests that renin secretion is quite sensitive to small changes in renal nerve activity under the proper conditions.[34] The effect of alpha-adrenergic receptors on renin release is controversial. Both inhibition and augmentation of renin release have been noted, but most of these experiments are complicated by changes in more than one factor affecting renin release.[33]

The baroreflexes contribute to activation of the renin-angiotensin system by altering renal sympathetic efferent activity. In animals, the cardiopulmonary baroreflex seems to be a primary regulatory mechanism for stimulation of the renin-angiotensin system, although some contribution is also provided by the arterial baroreflexes. Cardiac vagal afferents tonically inhibit renin release.[35] After vagotomy or during vagal cold block, plasma renin activity increases. Renin release also increases during nonhypotensive hemorrhage. Increased plasma renin activity has also been reported following carotid sinus hypotension in some studies but not in others.[36] In vagotomized, anesthetized dogs, carotid sinus hypotension increases renin release. In human subjects, there are few studies that have investigated baroreflex control of renin release, and the results are controversial. During water immersion, during which cardiac receptors are stimulated, plasma renin activity decreases.[37] Venous pooling caused by congestive thigh cuffs inhibits cardiac receptors and increases plasma renin activity in normal individuals.[38] In contrast, low levels of lower body negative pressure in which the cardiac baroreceptors are unloaded does not seem to increase plasma renin activity. High levels of lower body negative pressure and postural tilt maneuvers, during which both cardiopulmonary and arterial baroreceptors are unloaded, increase plasma renin activity.[39,40] Therefore, in human subjects the arterial baroreflex may be more pertinent to the regulation of the renin-angiotensin system.

Other humoral mediators of renin release include vasopressin, prostaglandins, and atrial natriuretic factor. Vasopressin can inhibit renin release acutely.[41] This effect is not seen when vasopressin is given as a chronic infusion during which total body fluid volume is closely regulated. The mechanism for this effect is unclear, although it may involve indirect effects on renal blood flow and vascular pressure. Prostaglandins PGE_2 and PGI_2 stimulate renin secretion, although acute prostaglandin blockade only inhibits renin release when some other stimulus of renin release is already active.[42] Prostaglandins may be intermediate modulators of renin release rather than direct mediators.[42a,42b] Atrial natriuretic factor appears to markedly inhibit renin secretion when infused intravenously.[43,44] No mechanism for this effect is certain, although there may be a direct effect of this peptide on the juxtaglomerular cells themselves or an indirect effect through alterations in tubular sodium load or renal hemodynamics.

EFFECTS OF THE RENIN–ANGIOTENSIN SYSTEM ON RENAL FUNCTION

Angiotensin II is one of the most potent vasoconstrictors known. It has a marked effect on the renal vasculature, especially on the efferent arteriole. Through preferential efferent arteriolar constriction angiotensin II can reduce renal blood flow while maintaining glomerular filtration at nearly normal levels. This may subserve a salt-retaining function while allowing for nearly normal renal excretory function. Of additional importance to sodium homeostasis is that angiotensin II mediates release of aldosterone from the adrenal cortex. Aldosterone is the adrenal hormone responsible for modulation of renal distal tubular sodium reabsorption through alteration in synthesis of the Na–K–ATPase transport system in the distal tubular cells. Angiotensin II also helps maintain sodium balance through a direct effect on proximal tubular sodium reabsorption. Through its dipsogenic effect on the brain's "thirst center," angiotensin II can further contribute to volume homeostasis by influencing drinking behavior. Central or peripheral angiotensin II may increase water intake in response to hypovolemic conditions such as hemorrhage or dehydration.[45]

Angiotensin II can also act as a central nervous system modulator/effector of cardiovascular function. Through effects on brain centers, such as the area postrema, angiotensin II can attenuate baroreflex sensitivity and increase regional vascular resistance.[46,47] These effects are thought to result from a facilitory effect of angiotensin II which stimulates central components of the sympathetic nervous system. There may also be an inhibitory effect on vagal vasomotor centers resulting in diminished vagal tone. Angiotensin II may thus be implicated in a positive feedback form of hypertension, because it increases pressure and attenuates baroreflex sensitivity.

VASOPRESSIN

Vasopressin or arginine vasopressin (AVP) or antidiuretic hormone (ADH) is a nonapeptide which is synthesized by the magnocellular neurons of the supraoptic and paraventricular nuclei and released from their axon terminals in the posterior pituitary (Figure 61.4). Stimuli for AVP release may be osmotic or nonosmotic.[48] Changes in plasma osmolality are sensed by brain osmoreceptors which are probably located in the hypothalamus. Stimulation of these osmoreceptors by increases in plasma tonicity increases AVP secretion.

The nonosmotic stimuli to AVP release include the cardiopulmonary baroreceptors and the arterial baroreceptors. Stimulation of cardiopulmonary baroreceptors decreases AVP secretion. Conversely, unloading of cardiopulmonary baroreceptors results in increased vasopressin release. Arterial baroreceptors also may be important in regulating AVP secretion. However, these usually function in concert with the cardiac baroreceptors. Thus, denervation of aortic baroreceptors does not increase plasma AVP if cardiac vagi are intact. However, carotid sinus denervation will increase plasma vasopressin if preceded by vagotomy and aortic nerve section.[49] The interaction between cardiopulmonary and

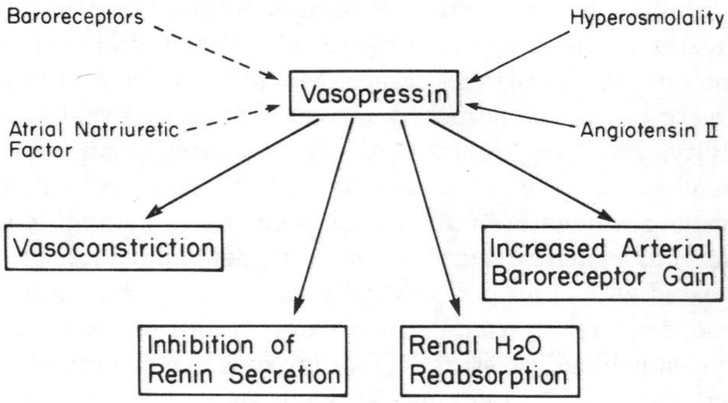

Figure 61.4. Vasopressin control mechanisms. Both osmotic and nonosmotic factors contribute to vasopressin release. Vasopressin secretion is inhibited by baroreceptor activation and by atrial natriuretic factor. Increased osmolality and angiotensin II stimulate vasopressin secretion. Vasopressin causes vasoconstriction and renal reabsorption of water and inhibits renal secretion of renin. Vasopressin also influences the sensitivity of arterial baroreceptors.

arterial baroreceptor-mediated control of AVP has been demonstrated in experimental animals and suggested by studies in human subjects.[50–54] Combined unloading of both receptor groups augments AVP release; simultaneous increase in receptor stimulation inhibits AVP release. The relative roles played by the two groups of baroreceptors may be different in animals and in man. Therefore, cardiopulmonary baroreceptors may be a dominant regulatory mechanism for AVP secretion in animals, whereas arterial baroreceptors may predominate in nonhuman primates and in man.

Vasopressin further interacts with baroreflex pathways by increasing baroreceptor sensitivity. Therefore, during exogenous administration of vasopressin, there is a greater reduction in sympathetic nervous system activity than during comparable pressor doses of other vasoconstrictive drugs. Similarly, the reduction in heart rate following AVP infusion is greater than that occurring secondary to phenylephrine.[55] Vasopressin sensitizes the arterial baroreflexes such that there is augmented reflex vasoconstrictive response to carotid hypotension. AVP also augments cardiopulmonary baroreflex-mediated peripheral vasoconstriction as demonstrated in humans during lower body negative pressure.[55a]

By stimulating or inhibiting release of AVP, the cardiovascular reflexes can further affect renal function and salt and water metabolism by several mechanisms. On a molar basis, AVP is a more potent vasoconstrictor than either norepinephrine or angiotensin II. Vasopressin may therefore decrease renal blood flow. In addition to its vascular effect, AVP directly increases renal tubular reabsorption of water. By activating cyclic AMP in the renal collecting tubules, AVP reduces diuresis and produces concentrated urine. Vasopressin also may suppress renal secretion of renin. This has been demonstrated in both anesthetized and conscious animals during intrarenal artery infusion of AVP. The mechanism for this effect is not known.

ATRIAL NATRIURETIC FACTOR

In addition to reflexes from the heart which are mediated through neural pathways, peptides with potent natriuretic and diuretic properties have been discovered in mammalian atria, raising the possibility that the heart may also serve an endocrine function.[56–58] De Bold et al[56] first showed that extracts of rat atrial tissue could produce large increases in urine flow and sodium excretion. Subsequent studies have shown that release of atrial natriuretic factor (ANF) in response to an increase in plasma volume may contribute to control of blood pressure as well as renal sodium and water conservation. Atrial natriuretic factor has also been referred to as atrial natriuretic peptide, cardionatrin, atriopeptin, and auriculin.[59] Depending on the laboratory, ANF contains 21 to 33 amino acid residues with a core sequence of 20 amino acids. There is evidence that the peptide is first synthesized as a high molecular weight precursor that is proteolytically cleaved into the shorter biologically active forms. Atrial natriuretic factor is stored in secretory storage granules within atrial myocytes. The quantity of atrial granules increases with sodium and water restriction and decreases with sodium and water loading.[60] This suggests that granular turnover and release of ANF depletes visible granular stores. Preliminary evidence has suggested that the right atrium contains greater quantities of ANF than does the left atrium. Increasing right atrial pressure in an isolated rat heart preparation[61] and the conscious dog[61a] increases release of ANF.[61] Removal of the rat right atrial appendage results in an attenuated natriuretic response to volume loading. A schema integrating circulatory and renal functions of ANF is presented in Figure 61.5.

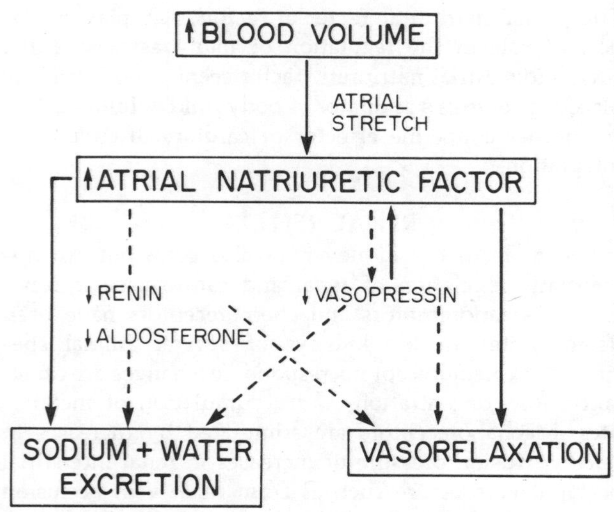

Figure 61.5. Contribution of atrial natriuretic factor to blood volume regulation. Inhibitory signals are indicated by *dashed lines* and stimulatory signals are indicated by *solid lines*. Increased blood volume stimulates the release of atrial natriuretic factor (ANF), which results in sodium and water excretion and vasorelaxation. Atrial natriuretic factor also affects blood pressure and sodium and water homeostasis by inhibiting the secretion of renin and vasopressin.

The mechanisms through which ANF promotes natriuresis are not yet well defined. Atrial natriuretic factor has been shown to increase glomerular filtration rate in some studies.[61b] In addition, ANF may act as a counter regulatory hormone to the renin-angiotensin system.[62] Atrial natriuretic factor suppresses renal release of renin through either a direct inhibitory effect on the juxtaglomerular apparatus or a feedback-induced suppression of juxtaglomerular cells which involves increased sodium delivery to the macula densa. Therefore, the angiotensin-mediated stimulation of aldosterone secretion is diminished[62a] and sodium reabsorption will thereby be decreased. Concomitantly, ANF may also directly inhibit release of aldosterone. Furthermore, it has been reported that ANF can decrease proximal reabsorption of sodium by an as yet unexplained mechanism. Atrial natriuretic factor does not seem to alter sodium transport in isolated epithelia and does not inhibit renal-sodium-potassium ATPase. It is therefore not established whether atrial natriuretic factor has any direct effect on renal tubular transport of sodium. Atrial natriuretic factor may indirectly affect renal excretion of water by inhibiting vasopressin release[63] or vasopressin action.[63a]

Atrial natriuretic factor may also reduce blood pressure by a mechanism other than its natriuretic effect. It has been shown to relax isolated strips of vascular smooth muscle precontracted by norepinephrine or angiotensin II.[64] Following intravenous injection, this agent has also been shown to decrease systemic blood pressure and cause transient renal vasodilation; however, with continuous infusion, renal blood flow returns to normal values despite the maintenance of a brisk natriuresis and diuresis. Atrial natriuretic factor conceivably may reduce blood pressure as a consequence of venous dilation, a decrease in cardiac output,[64a] or of direct arteriolar vasodilation.[64b] Thus, atrial natriuretic factor or factors may play an important role in the regulation of many aspects of the circulation. Atrial natriuretic factor seems to be critically placed to serve as a regulator of body fluid volumes acting as another endocrine effector of cardiorenal circulatory integration.[64c]

RENAL REFLEXES

Receptors in the kidney may also contribute to homeostatic regulation of renal and cardiovascular function. Mechanoreceptors and chemoreceptors have been demonstrated in the kidneys of several animal species.[65–68] Chemoreceptors respond to changes in osmolality, ion concentration, and accumulation of metabolites. Mechanoreceptors are stimulated by increases in renal perfusion pressure or increases in renal interstitial or capillary pressure such as from renal vein occlusion or ureteral obstruction. Stimulation of these receptors results in reflex inhibition of sympathetic activity to the contralateral kidney. A decline in renal sympathetic nervous activity may decrease renovascular resistance, increase renal blood flow, and also increase renal sodium and water excretion. Whether activation of renal mechanoreceptors alters sympathetic nervous system activity to the heart is controversial.

Unilateral renal hypoperfusion is accompanied by increases in mean blood pressure as well as hindlimb and mesenteric vascular resistance. Much of the pressure increase can be explained by increases in plasma renin activity. However, blood pressure responses occur independent of the renin-angiotensin system and these responses have been attributed to increased sympathetic nervous system activity. In sinoaortic denervated rats pretreated with captopril, unilateral renal hypoperfusion induced by renal arterial constriction results in increased systemic blood pressure.[69] This increase can be prevented by concomitant ganglionic blockade, suggesting that some of the pressure increase following renal artery hypoperfusion is a result of increased sympathetic vasoconstrictive tone. Therefore, just as the heart can send afferent signals to the brain and spinal cord, ultimately influencing renal function, so can the kidney act as an active sensory organ responding to its environment.

CARDIORENAL INTERACTION IN DISEASE STATES

In certain pathologic conditions, abnormalities in baroreceptor activity may adversely affect renal function and, consequently, sodium and water metabolism. This is particularly pertinent in patients with either hypertension or congestive heart failure in whom sodium retention is integral to the pathophysiologic and clinical manifestations of the disease.

HYPERTENSION

Studies in several animal models of hypertension and in patients with hypertension have suggested that cardiopulmonary and arterial baroreceptors are impaired. It is not clear whether abnormal baroreflexes are important in the pathogenesis of hypertension or occur as a secondary phenomenon in hypertensive states. Nonetheless, abnormalities in the baroreflexes are pertinent to the changes in renal function and sodium balance that occur in hypertension.

In experimental animal models of hypertension, the level of left atrial pressure required for cardiopulmonary baroreceptor stimulation is higher than that in normotensive animals.[70–72] Thus, renal sympathetic efferent activity is inhibited at higher left atrial pressure in hypertensive as compared with normotensive animals. Changes in baroreceptor structural properties or decreased cardiac compliance may explain the increased threshold. Furthermore, arterial baroreceptors are also reset to higher thresholds in hypertensive animals.[73–75] In fact, the carotid sinus pressure sufficient to discharge the baroreceptor is greater than 120 mm Hg compared with 60 mm Hg in normotensive animals. Furthermore, the sensitivity of these receptors is diminished. Compliance changes in the arterial wall may diminish deformation of the vessel and alter both the threshold and the sensitivity of the receptors.

Studies in human subjects with hypertension have also demonstrated baroreflex dysfunction. By measuring the heart rate response to vasoconstrictive or vasodilator drugs it has been suggested that arterial baroreflex sensitivity is reduced in hypertensive individuals.[76-78] Following phenylephrine infusion, the lengthening of the electrocardiographic RR interval is less in hypertensive than in normotensive subjects, and following nitroglycerin infusion, the shortening of the RR interval is less in hypertensive than in normotensive individuals. Using a neck chamber it has been possible to demonstrate that the carotid baroreceptor is reset to a higher threshold in hypertensive individuals.[79] Abnormalities in arterial baroreflex function cannot simply be attributed to the age of hypertensive patients, because decreased arterial baroreflex sensitivity is present in hypertensive patients compared with normotensive individuals when age-matched groups are studied.[77,78]

Not all studies have demonstrated decreased function of the cardiopulmonary baroreceptors in hypertension. In fact, several studies have suggested that impairment of the arterial baroreflexes may actually potentiate the inhibitory properties of the cardiopulmonary baroreflexes.[80,81] Abnormal arterial baroreceptor function and augmented cardiopulmonary baroreflex activity may therefore explain the increased plasma renin activity and catecholamine levels that have been observed during orthostasis in hypertensive patients.[82,83] Renal vasoconstriction during cardiopulmonary baroreflex inhibition could adversely alter intrarenal hemodynamics and contribute to renal sodium retention. In this regard, it might be postulated that abnormal cardiopulmonary baroreflex function can alter renal hemodynamics and subsequently contribute to sodium reabsorption.

Thus, in hypertension, baroreflex function is important in the regulation of renovascular resistance and, as such, indirectly affects sodium reabsorption and excretion. In addition, abnormalities in baroreceptor function may occasionally contribute to increased activity of the renin-angiotensin-aldosterone system, favoring both generalized vasoconstriction as well as renal sodium reabsorption.

CONGESTIVE HEART FAILURE

Abnormalities in cardiopulmonary and arterial baroreflex function may contribute to renal vasoconstriction and sodium reabsorption in congestive heart failure. In a dog model of congestive heart failure, atrial receptors with myelinated afferent vagal fibers have a decreased response to elevations of atrial pressure. Both the threshold of the receptor and the sensitivity to pressure changes are reduced.[84,85] The sensitivity of left atrial receptors, however, improves following reversal of experimental heart failure.[86] Altered cardiopulmonary baroreceptor function in heart failure may be secondary to decreased myocardial compliance or to structural changes within the baroreceptors. In addition, cardiac baroreceptor sensitivity may be diminished by decreased contractile states. In fact, digitalis compounds increase the sensitivity of ventricular receptors with vagal afferents either directly or indirectly by increasing contractility.[87,88] Arterial baroreflex sensitivity is also decreased in animal models of congestive heart failure. Reductions in baroreflex sensitivity or increases in threshold reduces baroreflex inhibition of sympathetic efferent activity. Thus, circulating levels of catecholamines, renin, and vasopressin may increase.[88a] As a result, activation of these neurohormonal systems may cause renal vasoconstriction and contribute to sodium and water reabsorption. A recent study in caval constricted dogs, however, demonstrated that cardiac baroreceptors did not contribute to sodium and water retention.[89]

Only a few studies have examined the cardiopulmonary and arterial baroreflexes in patients with heart failure.[88,90-92] The heart rate and systemic and regional vasoconstrictor responses to lower body negative pressure or postural tilt are reduced or absent in patients with heart failure.[92-95] Therefore, in contrast to that in normal individuals, renal vasoconstriction does not occur during upright posture in these patients. Furthermore, during postural tilt, the increases in plasma catecholamine concentrations, plasma renin activity, and plasma vasopressin concentrations that are usually observed in normal individuals are attenuated or absent in patients with heart failure. The arterial baroreflex control of heart rate is decreased in patients with Chagas' disease.[96] Following phenylephrine or nitroglycerin infusion, the heart rate response to changes in blood pressure is blunted in patients with heart failure.[97] Improvement in congestive heart failure by reducing cardiac filling pressures or by increasing contractility may restore cardiac baroreceptor sensitivity.

Baroreflex dysfunction in heart failure may contribute to activation of the sympathetic nervous system, the renin-angiotensin system, and possibly vasopressin, and may alter regional blood flow. Renal vasoconstriction occurs out of proportion to the vasoconstriction observed in most other regional circulations.[98] Therefore, renal blood flow may decrease from 20% to 10% of the total cardiac output. Not only is renal blood flow compromised, but glomerular filtration rate is also decreased. However, the reduction in glomerular filtration rate is not as great as the decrease in renal plasma flow. Thus, the ratio of glomerular filtration rate to renal plasma flow, the filtration fraction, actually increases in heart failure.[99,100] In both experimental and human heart failure, avid renal sodium retention is associated with a high filtration fraction and a presumed increase in peritubular oncotic pressure. Sodium reabsorption in the proximal tubule varies with the peritubular oncotic pressure. Consequently, an increase in filtration fraction would favor greater proximal sodium reabsorption. Increased levels of sympathetic nervous system and renin-angiotensin system activity could also directly influence tubular sodium transport mechanisms and favor sodium reabsorption. In addition, the stimulus of circulating angiotensin II on adrenal mineralocorticoid release would also favor sodium reabsorption.

Abnormal baroreflex function may also be responsible for the elevated plasma levels of vasopressin that have been reported in animal models of low output heart failure and in some patients with congestive heart failure.[101-106] Studies in man indicate that plasma vasopressin concentration is increased in approximately one third of patients with heart failure. Indeed, vasopressin may be increased even in the presence of hyponatremia. Abnormal baroreflex function could stimulate neurohypophyseal release of vasopressin. Elevated vasopressin levels would further increase renal reabsorption of water and contribute to hyponatremia.

Atrial natriuretic factor has not been studied in depth in either animal models of heart failure or in human subjects with congestive heart failure. In congestive heart failure, elevated atrial pressure could augment ANF release[107,108] and act as a compensatory mechanism to attenuate salt and water retention. Of interest is the observation that the atria of Syrian hamsters with congenital myopathic heart failure are deficient in ANF.[109] Symbiosis of normal hamsters with their myopathic kin prevents the development of fluid accumulation without altering the progression of cardiac degeneration, suggesting that a primary defect in ANF synthesis and release may contribute to increased renal sodium reabsorption in this animal model of heart failure. Further investigations should provide additional insight into the role of ANF in patients with, and therapy of, congestive heart failure.[110,111]

REFERENCES

1. Goetz KL, Bond GC, Bloxham DD: Atrial receptors and renal function. *Physiol Rev* 1975; 55:157–205.
2. Linden RJ: Function of cardiac receptors. *Circulation* 1973; 48:463–480.
3. Thames MD, Miller BD, Abboud FM: Baroreflex regulation of renal nerve activity during volume expansion. *Am J Physiol* 1982; 243:H810–H814.
4. Thoren PN, Donald DE, Shepherd JT: Role of heart and lung receptors with non-medullated vagal afferents in circulatory control. *Circ Res* 1976; 39(suppl II):2–9.
5. Quillen EW Jr, Skelton MM, Rubin J, Cowley AW Jr: Osmotic control of vasopressin with chronically altered volume states in anephric dogs. *Am J Physiol* 1984; 247:E355–E361.
6. Paintal AS: Vagal sensory receptors and their reflex effects. *Physiol Rev* 1973; 53:159–227.
7. Mark AL: The Bezold–Jarisch reflex revisited: clinical implications of inhibitory reflexes originating in the heart. *J Am Coll Cardiol* 1983; 1:90–102.
8. Thames MD: Acetylstrophanthidin-induced reflex inhibition of canine renal sympathetic nerve activity mediated by cardiac receptors with vagal afferents. *Circ Res* 1979; 44:8–15.
9. Pelletier CL, Shepherd JT: Circulatory reflexes from mechanoreceptors in the cardio-aortic area. *Circ Res* 1973; 33:131–138.
10. Peterson DF, Brown AM: Pressor reflexes produced by stimulation of afferent fibers in cardiac sympathetic nerves of the cat. *Circ Res* 1971; 28:609–610.
11. Malliani A, Lombardi F: Neural reflexes with myocardial ischemia, in Schwartz PJ, Brown AM, Malliani A, Zanchetti A (eds): *Neural Mechanisms in Cardiac Arrhythmias*. New York, Raven, 1978, pp 209–219.
12. Bishop VS, Thames MD, Schmid PG: Effects of bilateral vagal cold blood on vasopressin in conscious dogs. *Am J Physiol* 1984; 246:R566–R569.
13. Johnson JA, Moore WW, Segar WE: Small changes in left atrial pressure and plasma antidiuretic hormone titers in dogs. *Am J Physiol* 1969; 217:210–214.
14. Wang BC, Sundet WD, Hakamaki MO, Goetz KL: Vasopressin and renin responses to hemorrhage in conscious cardiac-denervated dogs. *Am J Physiol* 1983; 245:H399–H405.
15. Brennan LA Jr, Malvin RL, Jochin KE, Roberts DE: Influence of right and left atrial receptors on plasma concentrations of ADH and renin. *Am J Physiol* 1971; 221:273–278.
16. Kirchheim HR: Systemic arterial baroreceptor reflex. *Physiol Rev* 1976; 56:100–176.
17. Koshanpour E, Kelso DM: Partition of the carotid sinus baroreceptor response in dogs between the mechanical properties of the wall and receptor elements. *Circ Res* 1972; 31:831–845.
18. Pelletier CL, Clement DL, Shepherd JT: Comparison of afferent activity of canine aortic and sinus nerves. *Circ Res* 1972; 31:557–568.
19. Angell-James JE, de B Daly M: Comparison of the reflex vasomotor responses to separate and combined stimulation of the carotid sinus and aortic arch baroreceptors by pulsatile and non-pulsatile pressure in the dog. *J Physiol Lond* 1970; 209:247–293.
20. Schmidt RM, Kumeda M, Sagawa K: Cardiovascular responses to various pulsatile pressures in the carotid sinus. *Am J Physiol* 1972; 223:1–7.
21. Guz AM, Noble IM, Threnchard D, Cochrane HL, Makey AR: Studies on the vagus nerves in man: their role in respiratory and circulatory control. *Clin Sci* 1964; 27:293–304.
22. West JB: *Best and Taylor's Physiological Basis of Medical Practice*, ed II, Baltimore, Williams & Wilkins, 1985, p 466.
23. Block MA, Wakin KG, Mann FC: Renal function during stimulation of renal nerves. *Am J Physiol* 1952; 169:670–677.
24. Pomeranz B, Birtch AG, Barger AC: Neural control of intrarenal blood flow. *Am J Physiol* 1968; 215:1067–1081.
25. Vander AJ: Effect of catecholamines and the renal nerves on renin secretion in anesthesized dogs. *Am J Physiol* 1965; 209:659–662.
26. Slick GL, Aguilera AJ, Zambraski EJ, DiBona GF, Kaloyanides GJ: Renal neuroadrenergic transmission. *Am J Physiol* 1975; 229:60–65.
27. Hollenberg NK, Dzau VJ: The renin angiotensin system, in Narins RG, Maxwell MH, Kleeman CR (eds): *Clinical Disorders of Fluid and Electrolyte Metabolism*. New York, McGraw Hill, to be published.
28. Gibbons GH, Dzau VJ, Farhi ER, Barger AC: Interactions of signals influencing renin release. *Ann Rev Physiol* 1984; 46:291–308.
29. Farhi ER, Cant JR, Barger AC: Interactions between intrarenal epinephrine receptors and the renal baroreceptor in the control of PRA in conscious dogs. *Circ Res* 1982; 50:477–485.
30. Naftilan A, Oparil S: The role of calcium in the control of renin release. *Hypertension* 1982; 4:670–675.
31. Fray JCS: Stimulation of renin release in perfused kidney by low calcium and high magnesium. *Am J Physiol* 1977; 232:F377–F382.
32. Keeton TK, Campbell WB: The pharmacologic alteration of renin release. *Pharmacol Rev* 1980; 32:81–227.
33. Blaine EH, Davis JO, Prewitt RL: Evidence for a renal vascular receptor in control of renin secretion. *Am J Physiol* 1971; 220:1593–1597.
34. Thames MD, DiBona GF: Renal nerves modulate the secretion of renin mediated by non-neural mechanisms. *Circ Res* 1979; 44:645–659.
35. Stella A, Dampney RAL, Golis R, Zanchetti A: Afferent vagal control of renin release in the anesthetized cat. *Circ Res* 1978; 43(suppl I):I107–I111.
36. Rocchini AP, Barger AC: Renin release with carotid occlusion in the conscious dog: role of renal arterial pressure. *Am J Physiol* 1979; 236:H108–H111.
37. Epstein M: Renal effects of head-out water immersion in man: implications for an understanding of volume homeostasis. *Phys Rev* 1978; 58:529–578.
38. Kiowski W, Julius S: Renin response to stimulation of cardiopulmonary mechanoreceptors in man. *J Clin Invest* 1978; 62:656–663.
39. Mark AL, Abboud FM, Fitz AE: Influence of low- and high-pressure baroreceptors on plasma renin activity in humans. *Am J Physiol* 1978; 235:H29–H33.
40. Fasola AF, Martz BL: Peripheral venous renin activity during 70 degree tilt and lower body negative pressure in humans. *Am J Physiol* 1982; 243:H970–H973.
41. Gregory LC, Reid IA: Effect of renal denervation on the suppression of renin secretion by vasopressin in conscious dogs. *Am J Physiol* 1984; 247:F881–F887.
42. Gibbons G, Dzau VJ: Interaction of endogenous prostaglandin and angiotensin II in the regulation of renal baroreceptor-stimulated renin release in the conscious dog (abstr.). *Clin Res* 1984; 32:448A.

42a. Stoff JS: Prostaglandins and hypertension *Am J Med* 1986; 80(suppl 1A):56–61.

42b. Dzau VJ, Swartz SL, Creager MA: The role of prostaglandins in the pathophysiology of and therapy for congestive heart failure. *Heart Failure* 1986; 2:6–13.

43. Maack T, Marion DN, Camargo MJF, Kleinert HD, Laragh JH, Vaughn ED Jr, Atlas SA: Effects of auriculin (atrial natriuretic factor) on blood pressure, renal function, and renin-aldosterone system in dogs. *Am J Med* 1984; 77:1069–1075.
44. Seymour AA, Blaine EH, Mazack EK: Renal and systemic effects of synthetic atrial natriuretic factor. *Life Sci* 1985; 316:33–44.
45. Fitzsimmons JT: The effect on drinking of peptide precursors and of short chain peptide fragments of angiotensin II injected into the rat's diencephalon. *J Physiol* 1971; 214:295–303.
46. Lappe RW, Brody MJ: Mechanisms of the central pressor action of angiotensin II in conscious rats. *Am J Physiol* 1984; 246:R56–R62.
47. Stein RD, Stephenson RB, Weaver LC: Central actions of angioten-

sin II oppose baroreceptor-induced sympathoinhibition. *Am J Physiol* 1984; 246:R13–R19.
48. Schrier RW, Berl T, Anderson RJ: Osmotic and nonosmotic control of vasopressin release. *Am J Physiol* 1979; 236:F321–F332.
49. Share L, Levy MN: Cardiovascular receptors and blood titer of antidiuretic hormone. *Am J Physiol* 1962; 203:425–428.
50. Thames MD, Schmid PG: Interaction between carotid and cardiopulmonary baroreflexes in control of plasma ADH. *Am J Physiol* 1981; 241:H431–H434.
51. Gilmore JP, Zucker IH, Ellington MJ, Richards MA, Share L: Failure of acute intravascular volume expansion to alter plasma vasopressin in the nonhuman primate, *macaca fascicularis*. *Endocrinology* 1980; 106:979–982.
52. Epstein M, Preston S, Weitzman RE: Isoosmotic central volume expansion suppresses plasma arginine vasopressin in normal man. *J Clin Endocrinol Metab* 1981; 52:256–262.
53. Goldsmith SR, Francis GS, Cowley AW, Cohn JN: Response of vasopressin and norepinephrine to lower body negative pressure in humans. *Am J Physiol* 1984; 243:H970–H973.
54. Rogge JD, Moore WW: Influence of lower body negative pressure on peripheral venous ADH levels in man. *J Appl Physiol* 1968; 25:123–138.
55. Cowley AW Jr, Quillen EW Jr, Skelton MM: Role of vasopressin in cardiovascular regulation. *Fed Proc* 1983; 42:3170–3176.
55a. Ebert TJ, Cowley AW Jr, Skelton M: Vasopressin reduces cardiac function and augments cardiopulmonary baroreflex resistance in man. *J Clin Invest* 1986; 77:1136–1142.
56. De Bold AJ, Borenstein HB, Veress AT, Sonnenberg H: A rapid and potent natriuretic response to intravenous injection of atrial myocardial extract in rats. *Life Sci* 1981; 28:89–94.
57. Lang RE, Thölken H, Ganten D, Luft FC, Ruskoaho H, Unger T: Atrial natriuretic factor—a circulatory hormone stimulated by volume loading. *Nature* 1985; 314:264–266.
58. Garcia R, Thibault G, Gutkowska J, Hofky K, Hamet P, Cantin M, Genest J: Chronic infusion of low doses of atrial natriuretic factor (ANF Arg 101-Tyr 126) reduces blood pressure in conscious SHR without apparent changes in sodium excretion. *Proc Soc Exp Biol Med* 1985; 179:396–401.
59. Needleman P, Adams SP, Cole BR, Currie MG, Geller DM, Michener ML, Saper CB, Schwartz D, Standaert DG: Atriopeptins as cardiac hormones. *Hypertension* 1985; 7:469–482.
60. DeBold AJ: Heart atria granularity effects of changes in water-electrolyte balance. *Proc Soc Exp Biol Med* 1979; 1611:508–511.
61. Dietz JR: Release of natriuretic factor from rat heart–lung preparation by atrial distension. *Am J Physiol* 1984; 247:R1093–R1096.
61a. Paganelli WG, Pintal RR, Cotter RE, Kifor I, Cant JR, Dzau VJ: Influence of acute changes in atrial pressures on plasma atria natriuretic factor (ANF) in the conscious dog. *Clin Res* 1986; 34:605A.
61b. Weidmann P, Hasler L, Gnädinger MP, Lang RE, Uehlinger DE, Shaw S, Rascher W, Reubi FC: Blood levels and renal effects of atrial natriuretic peptide in normal man. *J Clin Invest* 1986; 77:734–742.
62. Borenstein HB, Cupples WA, Sonnenberg H, Veress T: The effect of a natriuretic atrial extraction on renal hemodynamics and urinary excretion in anaesthetized rats. *J Physiol* 1983; 334:133–140.
62a. Anderson IV, Struthers AD, Payne NN, Slater JDH, Bloom SR: Atrial natriuretic peptide inhibits the aldosterone response to angiotensin II in man. *Clin Sci* 1986; 70:507–512.
63. Samson WK: Atrial natriuretic factor inhibits dehydration and hemorrhage-induced vasopressin release. *Neuroendocrinology* 1985; 40:277–279.
63a. Dillingham MA, Anderson RJ: Inhibition of vasopressin action by atrial natriuretic factors. *Science* 1986; 231:1572–1573.
64. Huang CL, Lewicki J, Johnson LK, Cogan M: Renal mechanism of action of rat atrial natriuretic factor. *J Clin Invest* 1985; 75:769–773.
64a. Kleinert HD, Volpe M, Odell G, Marion D, Atlas SA, Camargo MJ, Laragh JH, Maack T: Cardiovascular effects of atrial natriuretic factor in anesthetized and conscious dogs. *Hypertension* 1986; 8:312–316.
64b. Needleman P, Greenwald JE: Atriopeptin: a cardiac hormone intimately involved in fluid, electrolyte, and blood-pressure homeostasis. *N Engl J Med* 1986; 314:828–834.
64c. Canton M, Genest J: The heart as an endocrine gland. *Scientific American* 1986; 254(2):76–81.
65. Recordati G, Genovesi S, Cerati D: Reno renal reflexes in the rat elicited upon stimulation of renal chemoreceptors. *J Auton Nerv Syst* 1982; 6:127–142.
66. Calaresu FR, Ciriello J: Renal afferent nerves affect discharge rate of medullary and hypothalamic single units in the cat. *J Auton Nerv Syst* 1981; 3:311–320.
67. Kostreva DR, Seagard JL, Castaner A, Kampine JP: Reflex effects of renal afferents on the heart and kidney. *Am J Physiol* 1981; 241:R286–R292.
68. Kopp UC, Olson LA, DiBona GF: Renorenal reflex response to mechano- and chemoreceptor stimulation in the dog and rat. *Am J Physiol* 1984; 246:F67–F77.
69. Katholi RE, Winternitz SR, Oparil S: Decrease in peripheral sympathetic nervous system activity following renal denervation or unclipping in the one-kidney, one clip Goldblatt hypertensive rat. *J Clin Invest* 1982; 69:55–62.
70. Thoren P, Noresson E, Ricksten SE: Resetting of cardiac C-fiber endings in the spontaneously hypertensive rat. *Acta Physiol Scand* 1979; 107:13–18.
71. Kezdi P: Cardiac reflexes conducted by vagal afferents in normotensive and renal hypertensive dogs. *Clin Sci* 1978; 51:353–355.
72. Ricksten SE, Noresson E, Thoren P: Inhibition of renal sympathetic nerve traffic from cardiac receptors in normotensive and spontaneously hypertensive rats. *Acta Physiol Scand* 1979; 106:17–22.
73. Ricksten SE, Thoren P: Reflex inhibition of sympathetic activity during volume load in awake normotensive and spontaneously hypertensive rats. *Acta Physiol Scand* 1980; 110:77–82.
74. Hallback-Nordlander M, Noresson E, Thoren P: Hemodynamic consequences of left ventricular hypertrophy in spontaneously hypertensive rats. *Am J Cardiol* 1979; 44:986–993.
75. Angell-James JE: Characteristics of single aortic and right subclavian baroreceptor fiber activity in rabbits with chronic renal hypertension. *Circ Res* 1973; 32:149–161.
76. Briston JD, Honour AJ, Pickering GW, Sleight P, Smyth HS: Diminished baroreflex sensitivity in high blood pressure. *Circulation* 1969; 39:48–54.
77. Gribbin B, Pickering TG, Sleight P, Peto R: Effect of age and high blood pressure on baroreflex sensitivity in man. *Circ Res* 1971; 29:424–431.
78. Korner PI, West MH, Shaw J, Uther JB: Steady-state properties of the baroreceptor—heart rate reflex in essential hypertension in man. *Clin Exp Pharmacol Physiol* 1974; 1:65–76.
79. Mancia G, Ludbrook J, Ferrari A, Gregormi L, Zanchetti A: Baroreceptor reflexes in human hypertension. *Circ Res* 1978; 43:170–177.
80. Chen HI: Interaction between the baroreceptor and Bezold–Jarisch reflexes. *Am J Physiol* 1979; 237:H655–H661.
81. Mancia G, Shepherd JT, Donald DE: Interplay among carotid sinus, cardiopulmonary and carotid body reflexes in dogs. *Am J Physiol* 1976; 230:19–24.
82. Esler MD, Nestel PJ: Sympathetic responsiveness to head-up tilt in essential hypertension. *Clin Sci* 1973; 44:213–226.
83. Kuchel O, Cuche J, Hamet P, Boucher R, Barbeau A, Genest J: The relationship between adrenergic nervous system and renin in labile hyperkinetic hypertension, in Genest J, Kolw E (eds): *Hypertension*. New York, Springer-Verlag, 1972, pp 118–125.
84. Higgins CB, Vatner SF, Eckberg DL, Braunwald E: Alteration in the baroreflex in conscious dogs with heart failure. *J Clin Invest* 1972; 51:715–724.
85. Greenberg TT, Richmond WH, Stocking RA, Gupta PD, Meehan JP, Henry JP: Impaired atrial receptor response in dogs with heart failure due to tricuspid insufficiency and pulmonary artery stenosis. *Circ Res* 1973; 32:424–433.
86. Zucker IH, Earle AM, Gilmore JP: Changes in sensitivity of left atrial receptors following reversal of heart failure. *Am J Physiol* 1979; 237:H555–H559.
87. Sleight P, Lall A, Meurs M: Reflex cardiovascular effects of epicardial stimulation by acetylstrephanthidin in dogs. *Circ Res* 1969; 25:705–711.
88. Ferguson DW, Abboud FM, Mark AL: Selective impairment of baroreflex-mediated vasoconstrictor responses in patients with ventricular dysfunction. *Circulation* 1984; 69:451–460.
88a. Creager MA: The role of vasopressin in congestive heart failure. *Heart Failure* 1986; 2:14–20.
89. Paganelli WC, Cant JR, Barger AC: Does cardiac denervation alter vasopressin and renin responses to chronic caval constriction in the conscious dog (abstr). *Fed Proc* 1985; 44:1727.
90. Brigden W, Sharpey-Schafer EP: Postural changes in peripheral blood flow in care with left heart failure. *Clin Sci* 1950; 9:93–100.
91. Kubo SH, Cody RJ: Circulatory autoregulation in chronic congestive heart failure: Responses to head-up tilt in 41 patients. *Am J Cardiol* 1983; 52:512–518.
92. Creager MA, Faxon DS, Rockwell SM, Gavras H, Coffman JD: The contribution of the renin–angiotensin system to limb vasoregulation in patients with heart failure: observations during orthostasis and alpha adrenergic blockade. *Clin Sci* 1985; 68:659–667.
93. Levine TB, Francis GS, Goldsmith SR, Cohn JN: The neurohormonal and hemodynamic responses to tilt in patients with congestive heart failure. *Circulation* 1983; 67:1070–1075.
94. Goldsmith SR, Francis GS, Levine TB, Cohn JN: Regional blood flow responses to orthostasis in patients with congestive heart failure. *J Am Coll Cardiol* 1983; 1:1391–1395.

95. Lilly LS, Dzau VJ, Williams GH, Rydstedt L, Hollenberg NK: Hyponatremia in congestive heart failure: implications for neurohormonal activation and responses to orthostasis. *J Clin Endocrinol Metab* 1984; 59:924–930.
96. Armorim DS, Godoy RF, Manco JC, Tanaka A, Gallo J: Effects of acute elevation in blood pressure and of atropine on heart rate in Chagas' disease. *Circulation* 1968; 38:289–294.
97. Eckberg DL, Drabinski M, Braunwald E: Defective parasympathetic control in patients with heart disease. *N Engl J Med* 1971; 285:877–883.
98. Zelis R, Flaim SF: Alteration in vasomotor tone in congestive heart failure. *Prog Cardiovasc Dis* 1982; 24:437–459.
99. Brenner BM, Falchuk KH, Keimowitz RI, Berliner RW: The relationship between peritubular capillary protein concentration and fluid reabsorption by the renal proximal tubule. *J Clin Invest* 1969; 48:1519–1531.
100. Brenner BM, Troy JL: Postglomerular vascular protein concentration: evidence for a causal role in governing fluid reabsorption and glomerulotubular balance by the renal proximal tubule. *J Clin Invest* 1971; 50:336–349.
101. Riegger GAJ, Liebau G: The renin–angiotensin–aldosterone system, antidiuretic hormone and sympathetic activity in an experimental model of congestive heart failure in the dog. *Clin Sci* 1982; 62:465–469.
102. Thrasher TN, Moore-Gillon M, Wade CW, Kiel LC, Ramsey DJ: Inappropriate drinking and secretion of vasopressin after caval constriction in dogs. *Am J Physiol* 1983; 244:R850–R856.
103. Yamane U: Plasma ADH level in patients with chronic congestive heart failure. *Jpn Circ J* 1968; 32:745–759.
104. Riegger GAJ, Liebau G, Kochsiek K: Antidiuretic hormone in congestive heart failure. *Am J Med* 1982; 72:49–52.
105. Szatalowicz VL, Arnold PE, Chaimovitz C, Bichet D, Berl T, Schrier RW: Radioimmunoassay of plasma arginine vasopressin in hyponatremic patients with congestive heart failure. *N Engl J Med* 1981; 305:253–266.
106. Goldsmith SR, Francis GS, Cowley AW Jr, Levine TB, Cohn JN: Increased plasma arginine vasopressin levels in patients with congestive heart failure. *J Am Coll Cardiol* 1983; 1:1385–1390.
107. Laragh JH: Atrial natriuretic hormone, the renin-aldosterone axis, and blood pressure-electrolyte homeostasis. *N Engl J Med* 1985; 313:1330–1340.
108. Hollenberg NK: The kidney in heart failure. *Hospital Practice* 1986; 21:81–100.
109. Chimoskey JE, Spielman WS, Brandt MA, Heidman SR: Cardiac atria of BIO 14.6 hamsters are deficient in natriuretic factor. *Science* 1984; 223:820–822.
110. Dzau VJ, Warren SE: Natriuretic hormones in heart failure. *Heart Failure* 1986; 2:33–39.
111. Dzau VJ, Creager MA: Neurohormonal mechanisms in congestive heart failure: are they beneficial or harmful? *Heart Failure* 1986; 2: 3–5.

62 Heart in Pregnancy

Chi-Sung Zee-Cheng, MD, Harry S. Jonas, MD, and Tommy N. Evans, MD

Cardiovascular disease, whether present before pregnancy or induced by the gravid state, can present a major health threat to both the mother and the fetus. Within the childbearing age group, the pattern of cardiovascular disorders will vary geographically and socioeconomically.[1-4] Worldwide, mitral stenosis due to rheumatic heart disease remains the major heart disease during pregnancy,[1,5,6] particularly in developing countries. In the last two to three decades, especially in industrialized nations, the incidence of mitral stenosis has decreased but still represents almost 70% of all cardiovascular disorders seen during pregnancy.[1-9] The decrease is probably due to antibiotics and a significant decrease in streptococcal infections and better living conditions. The increasing importance of congenital heart disease reflects advances in medical care and improved surgical techniques that have allowed these patients to reach childbearing age. Only a few decades ago the ratio of rheumatic to congenital heart disease was 20 to 1. Currently, the ratio is more like 3 to 1.[2,4] Other cardiovascular disorders, including peripartum cardiomyopathy, aortic dissection, and coronary artery disease, continue to contribute to maternal and fetal morbidity and mortality.

Risk assessment is important in evaluating the cardiac patient who is pregnant. Such an evaluation should take into consideration the age of the patient (risks increasing with age), the nature of the cardiac disease, and the functional classification of the cardiac status.

CARDIOVASCULAR CHANGES DURING PREGNANCY

The cardiovascular system undergoes a number of remarkable changes in response to the gravid state[10-23]: blood volume, cardiac output, and heart rate are increased, whereas systemic vascular resistance and systemic blood pressure are decreased. The adaptive changes, be they blood volume, cardiac output, or heart rate, can best be described in terms of the time of onset, the time of peak changes, and the magnitude of changes compared to the nonpregnant state. In general, the adaptive changes are associated with increased workload on the heart. These changes are well tolerated by the normal heart; however, they may adversely affect the mother and the fetus when maternal heart disease is present. A comprehensive understanding of these changes is important for the rational and logical management of the normal pregnant patient as well as the patient with a cardiovascular disorder.

Changes in blood volume constitute a major cardiovascular adaptation during pregnancy.[10,11,14-18,22] An increase in blood volume occurs as early as the 6th week of pregnancy, with a maximal increase during the 24th week; thereafter, the increase slows. The total change in blood volume varies considerably and ranges from 20% to nearly 100% with an average 50% increase from the nonpregnant state.[10,11,14-19,23] This increase in blood volume imposes great stress on the cardiovascular system and may overburden the diseased heart. Red blood cell volume also increases with pregnancy. However, there is a larger increase in plasma volume, resulting in a decreased hematocrit level and therefore a "physiological anemia of pregnancy."

A major change in the cardiovascular system during pregnancy is the alteration in the cardiac output.[10,12–14,16–21] An increase in cardiac output begins during the first trimester, generally around the 10th week of pregnancy. This rise is rapid, peaking by the 20th to 24th week. The maximum increase in cardiac output is usually 30% to 50% above the nonpregnant state.[10,12,13,17,21] Thereafter, the increase plateaus. There may be a decrease in cardiac output in the supine position, sometimes to nonpregnant levels, during the last few weeks of pregnancy as a result of inferior vena cava compression by the gravid uterus and decreased venous return.[24–26] The decreased cardiac output is abolished when the patient assumes a lateral recumbent position. Interestingly, when the fetal head becomes engaged in the pelvis, cardiac output is increased because of less caval compression.

During pregnancy the heart rate increases up to 20 beats per minute.[10,14,16,18,19] With twin pregnancy there is an even greater increase. The heart rate decreases somewhat from the sitting to the supine position and decreases more from the supine to the lateral position.[10,19,24,25] Significant decreases in systemic vascular resistance occur during pregnancy and may be related to hormonal changes.[10,14,16,18]

Most investigators have observed a decrease in blood pressure, mainly the diastolic component, beginning in the first trimester, reaching its nadir at mid-pregnancy, and returning to a nonpregnant level before term.[10,16,18,19,23,27] This change in blood pressure, resulting in widening of the pulse pressure, appears to be due mainly to the decrease in systemic vascular resistance. The magnitude of the decrease in blood pressure is variable, but increasing age and multiparity are associated with less of a decrease in both systolic and diastolic pressure.[23]

The adaptive cardiovascular changes seen during a normal pregnancy may be accompanied by symptoms, signs, and electrocardiographic, roentgenographic, and echocardiographic changes suggesting the presence of heart disease. These symptoms include dyspnea, easy fatigability, decreased exercise tolerance, lightheadedness, and syncope. Normally, a decrease in cardiac output in the supine position is not associated with a decrease in blood pressure.[10,12–14,17,19] However, a patient may occasionally experience lightheadedness, weakness, or even frank syncope when supine because of a decrease in blood pressure and heart rate. This so-called "supine hypotension syndrome of pregnancy" can be promptly relieved by assumption of a lateral position. Its cause may partly be inferior vena cava compression and partly a tendency toward a vasovagal response.[19,25] The signs are hyperventilation, peripheral edema, prominent neck veins, waterhammer pulse, brisk and laterally displaced left ventricular impulse, prominent right ventricular impulse, increased first heart sound, persistently split second heart sound with increased pulmonic component, third heart sound, midsystolic murmur over the pulmonic area, supraclavicular murmurs, continuous murmurs, and basilar pulmonary rales.

Hyperventilation may be present and basilar rales may be heard. Because of horizontal displacement of the heart due to the elevation of the diaphragm, the heart may appear enlarged on physical examination as lateral displacement of the point of maximal impulse occurs. A prominent left heart border on a chest roentgenogram may also suggest cardiomegaly.[28] There is generally a widened pulse pressure with a "collapsing" character simulating chronic aortic insufficiency. The neck veins may be distended, suggesting ventricular failure, and leg edema is frequently observed.

There is increased splitting of the first heart sound with accentuation of both components.[29] The second heart sound exhibits persistent expiratory splitting in the lateral position, especially during late pregnancy. There may be accentuation of the pulmonary component. The third heart sound, which is a frequent finding in children and young adults, may be noted in up to 90% of pregnant patients and is especially loud by the 30th week. It is diminished or disappears 1 week postpartum. The fourth heart sound normally is not present and should not occur during pregnancy. Because of hyperdynamic circulatory changes during pregnancy, the incidence of innocent systolic murmurs is extremely high (greater than 90%).[29] These murmurs are usually grade I/VI to grade III/VI in loudness, are usually early to midsystolic in timing, most often are located over the base of the heart and at the left sternal border, and are thought to be due to right or left ventricular ejection, or both. Diastolic murmurs are not normal before or during pregnancy. Continuous murmurs may be due to cervical hum, a frequent finding in the nonpregnant state, especially in the younger patient, and almost a universal finding during pregnancy.[29] Another cause of a continuous murmur is the mammary soufflé.[30] It is best appreciated during late pregnancy and the postpartum period; it is thought to be due to increased flow through mammary vessels.

It is important to realize that some murmurs due to structural heart diseases are accentuated during pregnancy.[29] They include the murmurs of pulmonary, mitral, and aortic stenosis. Other murmurs are attenuated or may disappear during gestation. The decrease in systemic vascular resistance during pregnancy may cause the murmur of aortic or mitral insufficiency to soften or disappear.[31] The increase in left ventricular volume during pregnancy may soften or abolish the murmur and click of mitral valve prolapse and the murmur of hypertrophic cardiomyopathy.[29,32]

With pregnancy, the QRS axis undergoes a leftward shift.[33] A small Q wave may accompany T-wave inversion in lead III, which is abolished with deep inspiration. There may be an occasional slight transient ST-segment depression and T-wave inversion in limb and precordial leads.[34]

During pregnancy there is a gradual increase in the left ventricular dimension during diastole in the lateral position but not in the supine position. The dimension during systole may also increase slightly or remain unchanged. Overall, the ejection fraction is either unchanged or increased slightly.[20,21]

Because a normal pregnancy may be accompanied by symptoms and signs suggestive of heart disease, obtaining a detailed history and performing a thorough physical examination are necessary. The electrocardiogram should be analyzed carefully. Because chest roentgenography may be associated with increased risk to the fetus, it may not always be advisable. However, with the advent of echocardiography, assessment of the patient's anatomic and physiologic status is simplified, although it does not necessarily contribute additional diagnostic information in the assessment of systolic murmurs in pregnancy in the absence of other clinical or electrocardiographic abnormalities.[34a] Echocardiography confirms the progressive increase in internal dimensions of the heart during pregnancy; the velocity of circumferential shortening and ejection fraction increase as pregnancy progresses.[20,21] If further data are needed, insertion of a Swan-Ganz catheter under pressure guidance may be performed to obtain hemodynamic parameters.[35,36] Because of possibly significant radiation exposure and the inability to do serial studies, cardiac catheterization with angiography is used only when absolutely necessary. Because of the availability of more effective noninvasive tests, the use of systolic time intervals has fallen out of vogue in some countries. Computed tomography may be employed to assess structural heart and aortic disease. Radionuclide scintigraphy may be employed in assessing right and left ventricular size and function as well as intracardiac shunt or valvular regurgitation. This modality is associated with a relatively low radiation risk to both the mother and fetus when compared with the risk of standard cardiac catheterization and angiography. Nevertheless, the stage of pregnancy still needs to be considered.

CARDIOVASCULAR CHANGES DURING LABOR, DELIVERY, AND THE POSTPARTUM PERIOD

The hemodynamic changes observed during labor and delivery are due to increased sympathetic activity secondary to pain and anxiety, uterine contractions, patient position, the analgesic and anesthetic used, blood loss, and the like.[10,11–13,15–18,37,40] In general, cardiac output during labor, particularly during uterine contractions, is increased. The change in heart rate is variable and in part dependent on the amount of sedation as well as the type of analgesics and anesthetics used.[37–40] Both systolic and diastolic blood pressures increase with uterine contractions and decrease to resting levels with uterine relaxation. Only a slight change occurs in systemic vascular resistance. Therefore, the increase in blood pressure is mainly due to the increase in cardiac output. These changes are less dramatic when the patient is in a lateral recumbent position than when supine.

Cardiac output increases 15% to 20% during labor as a result of uterine contractions.[10,12,13,16,18,38] During delivery there may be a further increase in cardiac output. In the first 2 weeks postpartum, there is a persistent increase in cardiac output of 10% to 20%,[10,12,13,15,16,18] mainly due to a blood shift from the emptied uterus to the systemic circulation and to a decrease in inferior vena cava compression. This is evidenced by an increase in the central venous pressure, a reflex decrease in the heart rate, with no change in blood pressure.

HEART DISEASE IN PREGNANCY

RHEUMATIC HEART DISEASE

The incidence of heart disease complicating pregnancy three or four decades ago was approximately 3.5%, with the vast majority of patients having rheumatic heart disease.[2,5] Today, the incidence is 0.5% to 1.5%.[2,5]

The clinical picture of acute rheumatic fever, which may be modified by pregnancy, should be considered when there is unexplained fever, arthralgia, arthritis, chest pain, or congestive failure.[41] Chorea can result in spontaneous abortion, preterm labor, intrauterine death, and maternal death. Myocarditis and heart failure are frequently fatal. The management of these patients should be similar to that of patients who are not pregnant. Steroids should be considered in those with severe myocarditis. Antibiotic prophylaxis against recurrent acute rheumatic fever should be instituted. Those with underlying chronic rheumatic heart disease should also receive acute rheumatic fever prophylaxis.[42]

Mitral stenosis continues to be the most common and most worrisome valvular lesion in pregnant women with rheumatic heart disease.[1,2,5,6–8,42,43] Because of the already impaired blood flow from the left atrium to the ventricle, the hemodynamic changes of pregnancy can precipitate congestive heart failure and pulmonary edema. Because of the time course of the hemodynamic changes, the time of maximum risk to the pregnant patient is late pregnancy, labor, and early puerperium. Patients in New York Heart Association functional classes III and IV have a maternal mortality of 4% to 5%.[1,2,5] If atrial fibrillation is present, the mortality increases to 14% to 17%.[1,2,5] Even if the patient has had mitral valve surgery before pregnancy, the maternal risk is still 2% to 3%.[1,2,5] Overall, the risk of death in all patients with mitral stenosis is 1%.[1,2,5] There is a general tendency toward an improved outcome because of the change in the natural course of the disease as well as improved medical management and cardiac surgery in selected cases.

Patients with rheumatic mitral valvular disease manifesting mitral regurgitation generally remain asymptomatic for years. It is rare for this lesion to produce problems during pregnancy. However, if regurgitation is severe and long-standing, heart failure and pulmonary congestion can eventually develop. These patients are at risk for developing atrial fibrillation with subsequent formation of atrial thrombi. Prophylaxis with digitalis is therefore recommended.[42]

Aortic stenosis is more common in males; therefore, it is only infrequently encountered during pregnancy. Patients with aortic stenosis, particularly a severe case, have a fixed cardiac output. Any decrease in systemic vascular resistance, as from pregnancy or anesthesia, and any decrease in blood pressure or venous return, as in compression of the inferior vena cava, blood loss during termination of pregnancy, vaginal delivery, or cesarean section, pose a great hazard to the mother and fetus.

If severe aortic stenosis is diagnosed before pregnancy, surgical intervention is recommended. Maintenance of adequate venous return is imperative. If conservative measures are unsuccessful, aortic valve surgery should be considered during pregnancy.

Aortic insufficiency due to rheumatic heart disease is more common than aortic stenosis in women of childbearing age. It is generally well tolerated during pregnancy and only rarely leads to hemodynamic embarrassment.

CONGENITAL HEART DISEASE

Cardiac disease is the most important nonobstetric cause of maternal death, being 18 times more common than any other nonobstetric cause.[1,2,5–8,43] Congenital heart disease is responsible for 3% to 10% of these deaths.[2,43–47]

The more common congenital lesions occurring during pregnancy are patent ductus arteriosus, atrial septal defect, ventricular septal defect, pulmonary stenosis, coarctation of the aorta, and tetralogy of Fallot.[2,44,46,47] Most patients with congenital heart disease generally can tolerate pregnancy. Most patients with acyanotic congenital heart disease will tolerate pregnancy without significant complications. In fact, overall mortality, with and without cardiac disease, is approximately the same, except in coarctation of the aorta, which is associated with an increased incidence of aortic dissection during pregnancy. Cyanotic congenital heart disease with or without pulmonary hypertension carries a significant increase in maternal and fetal morbidity and mortality.

Atrial septal defect is the most common maternal congenital defect. Most patients of childbearing age are asymptomatic and tolerate pregnancy, labor, and delivery well. The left-to-right shunt and the altered hemodynamics during pregnancy place an increased workload on the right ventricle. The increased pulmonary blood flow is well tolerated by the patient with an atrial septal defect. Pulmonary hypertension rarely occurs until the fourth decade. When present, it is associated with increased risks.

Ventricular septal defects can be an isolated finding or can be associated with other defects, such as transposition of the great arteries, coarctation of the aorta, pulmonic stenosis, or an endocardial cushion defect. In isolated ventricular septal defects, the clinical picture is determined by the size of the defect and the relation of pulmonary to systemic vascular resistance. A small defect is generally well tolerated during pregnancy, whereas the larger ones are associated with increased maternal risk. In those with persistent heart failure despite optimal medical management, the defect can be repaired during pregnancy, although this rarely is required.

Patent ductus arteriosus has become rare, as most cases are diagnosed and corrected in early childhood. Most patients with an uncorrected patent ductus arteriosus generally tolerate pregnancy without difficulty.

Coarctation of the aorta results in a narrowing of the aorta. In 95% of the cases this lesion is located just distal to the left subclavian artery. It can occur alone or in association with a bicuspid aortic valve (50%), cerebral aneurysms, and other congenital cardiovascular abnormalities. Mortality is 90% by age 50. The causes of death include heart failure, aortic rupture, aortic dissection, endarteritis, endocarditis, and intracranial hemorrhage. The incidence of dissection is increased during pregnancy.[48–50]

In uncomplicated cases, pregnancy is relatively safe for the mother, but fetal development may be impaired by the decreased blood flow to the distal aorta.[51–53] In complicated cases (those associated with other anomalies) the risk to the mother is increased as well, with a 3.5% maternal mortality.[51–53] Fetal mortality is 13% to 25%.[51–53]

It was previously thought that the stress of labor and vaginal delivery would produce aortic rupture; therefore, cesarean section was routinely performed. However, 80% of all ruptures occur before parturition.[51–53] Cesarean section is currently performed only for obstetric reasons. Surgical correction of coarctation of the aorta ideally should be performed before pregnancy. However, it may be carried out during pregnancy when aortic dissection, aortic rupture, uncontrolled severe hypertension, or persistent heart failure occurs.[51–53]

Most patients with pulmonic stenosis with or without sanative surgery will tolerate pregnancy well.[2,44,46,47] Right ventricular outflow obstruction is most commonly valvular but can be subvalvular or supravalvular. Valvulotomy may be performed in those in whom intractable heart failure develops during pregnancy. Most with uncorrected lesions, however, are asymptomatic, even with moderate stenosis.

Tetralogy of Fallot is currently the most common cyanotic congenital heart disease in children and adults and certainly the most common cyanotic congenital lesion found during pregnancy.[54–56] As definitive surgical repair of this anomaly continues to improve, more women with this lesion can be expected to reach childbearing age. Anatomically, tetralogy of Fallot is composed of pulmonic stenosis, ventricular septal defect, overriding aorta, and right ventricular hypertrophy. Physiologically, the two most important defects are pulmonic stenosis and ventricular septal defect. Right ventricular hypertrophy occurs secondary to pulmonic stenosis.

In most patients with tetralogy of Fallot, there is a gradual increase in the severity of pulmonic stenosis, with increasing symptoms and cyanosis. Most patients die by the fourth decade without surgery.[54–56] Pregnancy is well tolerated in those with definitive surgical repair.[56] However, in those without operative correction, pregnancy is associated with a perinatal mortality greater than 40%.[54–56] Patients who have a palliative procedure still have a relatively high maternal risk.[54–56] Pregnancy is poorly tolerated by those with tetralogy of Fallot because of a decrease in systemic vascular resistance, resulting in increased right-to-left shunting with increased hypoxemia. This right-to-left shunt may be further accentuated by a decrease in blood pressure during labor and delivery, worsening the hypoxemia even more.

Eisenmenger's syndrome is produced by pulmonary

vascular hypertension due to a high pulmonary vascular resistance with reversed or bidirectional shunting at the aortopulmonary, ventricular, or atrial level. A combination of a ventricular septal defect, an overriding aorta, and right ventricular hypertrophy is known as Eisenmenger's complex. Pregnancy is extremely poorly tolerated in patients with Eisenmenger's syndrome, with a 33% maternal mortality.[57–60] Cesarean section has generally been associated with a higher mortality than vaginal delivery[57–60]; however, this higher mortality may partly be due to patient selection. Most patients die during or within the first week of delivery. There is also a poor fetal outcome, with over 50% premature births and greater than 30% manifesting intrauterine growth retardation.[57–59] Eisenmenger's syndrome is considered by most authorities to be a contraindication to pregnancy.[57,59,60]

Mitral valve prolapse is a common congenital heart lesion[32] that is diagnosed frequently in women of childbearing age. The long-term prognosis of patients is generally good. Serious complications are rare and include severe mitral regurgitation, infective endocarditis, and sudden cardiac death. Patients with mitral valve prolapse generally tolerate pregnancy, labor, and delivery well.[32] The only exceptions are those with Marfan's syndrome in whom aortic dissection may lead to catastrophe.[50] Mitral valve prolapse has not been associated with an increased incidence of spontaneous abortion or preterm infants.

AORTIC DISSECTION

Aortic dissection is a rare but serious complication of pregnancy.[48–50] The aorta is primarily involved, but other arteries may be affected. Most patients with aortic dissection have no predisposing cardiovascular anomalies. In women under 40 years of age with dissection, about 50% were pregnant; therefore, pregnancy seems to predispose to dissection.[48–50] The highest incidence occurs from the third trimester to 1 month postpartum and most occur during rest. There is a low incidence of dissection during labor or delivery. Pathologically most of these patients exhibit medial necrosis. To date, the exact cause of dissection has not been clearly established. It may be due to hormonal changes associated with pregnancy. However, there is no evidence of an increased incidence in patients on hormonal drugs. Some investigators believe that nutritional deficiency may play a role in the pathogenesis. Certain cardiovascular malformations, such as coarctation or hypoplasia of the aorta, are predisposing factors. Patients with Marfan's syndrome, particularly those with a dilated aorta, are at an increased risk of dissection. It is recommended that those with an aortic root greater than 4 cm on echocardiography not undergo pregnancy.[50]

PRIMARY PULMONARY HYPERTENSION

Primary pulmonary hypertension is a progressive disease of unknown etiology occurring predominantly in young women.[61,62] It is generally associated with poor prognosis, with death occurring usually within 1 month to a few years after initial diagnosis. Early diagnosis may be hampered by symptoms attributed to pregnancy. However, women with primary pulmonary hypertension usually present during the second trimester with symptoms of fatigue, dyspnea, syncope, chest pain, or symptoms and signs of right ventricular failure. They typically become symptomatic during the second trimester because of the increased burden imposed on the cardiovascular system. Pregnancy is associated with a grave prognosis, with a 40% to 50% maternal mortality.[61,62] Most authorities strongly advise against pregnancy in patients with the disease. For those who become pregnant, early abortion is recommended.

CORONARY ARTERY DISEASE

Angina due to coronary artery disease is rare in women of childbearing age. In some, angina may be due to coronary artery spasm. Evidence exists of an increasing incidence of coronary artery disease in this group due to (1) postponement of pregnancy to later in life, (2) the increased use of birth control pills, and (3) increased smoking among women. Because of the increased burden imposed on the heart by the hemodynamic changes of pregnancy, angina can be precipitated or exacerbated. For those with angina refractory to maximal medical management during the first trimester, abortion is recommended. Those patients with refractory angina during the second or third trimester can be approached in the same manner as any nonpregnant patients with consideration of the risks of cardiac catheterization, intraaortic balloon pump counterpulsation, coronary angioplasty, and coronary bypass surgery.

Patients in whom uncomplicated myocardial infarction develops may be treated like other nonpregnant patients. Abortion is usually not necessary.[63,64] Those with myocardial rupture are considered as a medical emergency and treated aggressively as are nonpregnant patients. Induction of labor should be carried out when appropriate, with consideration of cesarean section.

HYPERTROPHIC CARDIOMYOPATHY

Hypertrophic cardiomyopathy is an idiopathic disease of the heart muscle with disorganized hypertrophy involving the interventricular septum and the muscles of the left ventricle. Pregnancy, labor, and delivery are frequently uneventful in these patients.[65–67] In the past, cesarean section was recommended in all patients with hypertrophic cardiomyopathy. However, vaginal delivery is well tolerated. Hence, cesarean section is now employed for obstetric reasons only.[65–67] In hypertrophic cardiomyopathy, left ventricular outflow tract obstruction is dynamic and depends on the location of hypertrophy as well as the size and contractility of the left ventricle. Measures that tend to decrease venous return (volume depletion and preload reducing drugs), increase contractility (digitalis), or decrease systemic blood pressure (epidural anesthesia) should be avoided. Beta blockers are preferable in those who demonstrate evidence of obstruction. These drugs may increase the incidence of small-for-date infants, cause low Apgar scores and neonatal hypoglycemia, and blunt a normal fetal stress response.[68,69]

PERIPARTUM CARDIOMYOPATHY

Peripartum cardiomyopathy is a primary dilated cardiomyopathy that develops during the last month of pregnancy or the first few months postpartum in the absence of another determinable cause.[70-72] Some limit the time period to the postpartum period to exclude the possibility that preexisting heart disease will be unmasked by the stress of pregnancy. Others exclude this diagnosis when toxemia or hypertension is present.

The exact origin remains unknown. Heart failure as well as cardiomegaly can resolve spontaneously only to recur during subsequent pregnancies.[70-72] This is unusual with idiopathic cardiomyopathy. Also, peripartum cardiomyopathy occurs most frequently in tropical climates, among blacks and those of lower socioeconomic status. A form of this disorder appears to be common in Africa, particularly in northern Nigeria where the incidence may be as high as 1% in women giving birth, with a seasonal peak in July.[72] This finding may be due in part to the puerperal customs of the Hausa people, which require the Hausa mother to lie for hours on a baked-mud bed over a fire and to ingest substantial quantities of "Kanwa," a dried lake-salt, to promote lactation.[72,72a,72b] Some investigators postulate an immunologic mechanism, viral infection, nutritional deficiency, or hypertension, or all, as etiologic factors. The incidence is about 1 in 1,300 to 4,000 pregnancies.[72a] There is a higher frequency in multiparous women. Toxemia is an associated complication in 15% to 30% with peripartum cardiomyopathy. The complications of this disorder are the same as with other types of dilated cardiomyopathy. Management of the patient in whom peripartum cardiomyopathy develops during pregnancy includes hospitalization with close observation, medical therapy for the cardiomyopathy, including consideration of anticoagulation and steroids, as some have a significant inflammatory response in the heart,[73] and hemodynamic monitoring. The route of delivery should be individualized. The long-term prognosis cannot be predicted on the basis of the initial presentation. The recurrence rate is high. Those with persistent heart failure and cardiomegaly may have significant cardiac deterioration with subsequent pregnancies. Therefore, further pregnancies are inadvisable and therapeutic sterilization should be considered.

INFECTIVE ENDOCARDITIS

Most of the general principles and therapeutic approaches to the nonpregnant patient with infective endocarditis apply to the pregnant patient as well.[74] Most commonly, infective endocarditis occurs in the pregnant patient with underlying heart disease. The etiologic organisms are the same as those in the nonpregnant patient. The clinical manifestations are similar to those of the nonpregnant state, but they may be more difficult to recognize because of the hemodynamic changes accompanying pregnancy. The confirmatory tests are also the same as those in nonpregnant patients. Antibiotics remain the mainstay of therapy, although the choice should be tailored to the possible adverse effects of these drugs on the fetus. Management of complications again is similar to that in the nonpregnant state, although drugs used must be assessed for their effects on both the mother and the fetus.

The role of antibiotic prophylaxis in the obstetric patient with heart disease remains controversial.[75-77] Factors to consider are the type of underlying heart disease, the probability of developing bacteremia, and the risk of developing infective endocarditis. In general, all patients with a prosthetic heart valve and those with rheumatic and congenital heart disease, with the exception of ostium secundum atrial septal defects, undergoing any obstetric procedure other than uncomplicated vaginal delivery should be given antibiotic prophylaxis.[75-77] The value of antibiotic prophylaxis in patients with mitral valve prolapse is debatable. (See chapter 31 on Mitral Valve Billowing and Prolapse.)

MEDICAL MANAGEMENT OF CARDIAC DISEASE IN PREGNANCY

Successful management of the pregnant patient with heart disease requires a multidisciplinary approach with cooperation among the obstetrician, a cardiologist knowledgeable of gestational hemodynamics, an anesthesiologist familiar with heart disease and its implication insofar as selection of anesthesia is concerned, and the patient. Medical management of the obstetric patient centers around the accurate diagnosis of heart disease and the treatment and prevention of congestive heart failure, hypertension, bacterial endocarditis, acute rheumatic fever, thromboembolism, and arrhythmia. It is imperative that the mother be given optimum treatment for the disease. However, no treatment should be administered to the mother without prior assessment of fetal risk. Essential therapeutic intervention for optimal maternal therapy may be employed even when some fetal jeopardy may be involved. Clearly any medical or surgical management of maternal disease during pregnancy often entails greater risk to the fetus than to the mother.

During pregnancy the demand placed on the cardiovascular system is profoundly increased; hence, it is desirable to eliminate unnecessary demands. Physical activity must be restricted when there are associated significant cardiopulmonary symptoms. Women with severe forms of heart disease may require as much bedrest as possible. Emotional stress should be avoided. A well-balanced high-protein diet during pregnancy complicated by heart disease is important. Excessive sodium must be avoided, while recognizing that excessive salt restriction may cause intravascular volume depletion detrimental to the fetus. Excessive weight gain places further demand on the heart and should be restricted in women with heart disease.

Only absolutely essential drugs are to be used. Those with the safest track record should be considered first. Diuretics and digitalis may be used to treat those with heart failure. A nondiuretic may be used to control systemic hypertension. A diuretic may be added when fluid retention occurs. Thromboembolism is common during pregnancy, especially in patients with heart disease and arrhythmias. Patients with previous episodes of thromboembolism or those with prosthetic cardiac valves are at the greatest risk. Infection should be avoided by appropriate immunization before pregnancy and the use of prophylactic antibiotics to decrease the risk of bacterial endocarditis. Women with a history of acute rheumatic fever and those with chronic rheumatic valvular heart disease should receive antibiotics for prophylaxis against recurrent acute rheumatic fever. When arrhythmia occurs, its severity should be assessed. Frequently, avoidance of cardiac stimulants and reassurance are all that is necessary. Antiarrhythmic agents are used only when absolutely necessary for termination, prevention, and rate control of an arrhythmia.

CARDIOVASCULAR DRUGS IN PREGNANCY

When administering cardiovascular or any drugs to a pregnant patient, certain principles need to be kept in mind. First, the pharmacologic and toxic effects of any drug on the fetus depend on the dose and disposition of the maternal-placental-fetal unit, stage of fetal development, and genetic susceptibility of the fetus. Second, with few exceptions, all drugs given to the mother pass to the fetus and may affect it either in utero or after birth. Third, during pregnancy, pharmacokinetics are modified. Fourth, during early embryogenesis, fetal tissues are highly susceptible to chemical and drug morphogenesis. Therefore, drug exposure may lead to abortion or malformations. To minimize these results, drugs should be avoided during the first trimester when possible. During the second and third trimesters, only drugs with a significant history of maternal and fetal safety should be considered.

TOCOLYTIC DRUGS

Cardiovascular changes secondary to medication used to treat complications of pregnancy must be carefully considered. Among the agents commonly used during pregnancy that can have a profound effect on the cardiovascular system are the tocolytic agents used to stop premature labor.[78,79] These include beta-adrenergic drugs, diazoxide, benzothiadiazine, magnesium sulfate, prostaglandin synthetase inhibitors, and alcohol. The primary use of tocolytic drugs is to prevent premature delivery. They may also be used to halt delivery temporarily while corticosteroids are being administered to accelerate fetal lung maturity.[80–82] On occasion, they are used for uterine relaxation to decrease fetal distress and for external cephalic version of breech presentation.

The beta-adrenergic drugs (terbutaline, ritodrine, and isoxysuprine hydrochloride) generally will increase the workload of the heart by increasing heart rate and contractility. These drugs are especially hazardous in patients with severe mitral and aortic stenosis because they precipitate pulmonary edema.[83,84] The hemodynamic effects of magnesium sulfate are similar to those of the beta-adrenergic drugs.[85] Diazoxide and benzothiadiazine may cause hypotension and reflex tachycardia.[86] The precise cardiovascular effects of prostaglandin synthetase inhibitors are unknown.[87] Large doses may impair contractility. Alcohol, especially in large doses, may impair left ventricular contractility.[88]

With tocolytic drugs, their effects on the mother and fetus as well as the length of use must be considered. Tocolytic drugs are contraindicated in a pregnant woman in New York Heart Association functional class III. Prostaglandin synthetase inhibitors may be considered, although a major concern is their potential for premature closure of the ductus arteriosus.[87] Because of their possible detrimental cardiovascular effects, beta-adrenergic agents, diazoxide, benzothiadiazine, and magnesium sulfate are contraindicated. Nifedipine, a calcium channel blocker, was recently shown to be an effective uterine relaxant.[88a] As a tocolytic agent, nifedipine is more effective and safer than ritodrine because of a lesser increase in the maternal heart rate.[88a] For short-term usage (24 to 48 hours) to delay delivery while corticosteroids are being administered to accelerate fetal lung maturity, intravenous ethyl alcohol is still the drug of choice,[88] although beta-adrenergic drugs may be considered. With ethyl alcohol, the fluid load must be carefully monitored to avoid precipitation of heart failure; the myocardial depressant effect of alcohol must also be considered. It should be kept in mind that the combined use of corticosteroids and tocolytic drugs may precipitate heart failure.

ANTIARRHYTHMIC AGENTS

Arrhythmias of any type may be noted during pregnancy. They frequently are benign and can be managed by reassurance and avoidance of cardiac stimulants. At times, the arrhythmia may cause hemodynamic compromise, leading to harm to the mother and fetus. Therapy should be directed toward all reversible causes, such as hypoxemia, electrolyte imbalance, acid/base disturbances, and underlying heart disease. Antiarrhythmic agents are used when necessary for termination of arrhythmia, prevention of recurrence, or rate control. In deciding to use an antiarrhythmic agent the nature and seriousness of the arrhythmia as well as the risks imposed on both mother and fetus must be considered. With regard to prophylaxis against an arrhythmia, one needs to consider the benefit/risk ratio. Antiarrhythmic agents generally are distributed to all tissues, including the placenta and fetus. They may act directly on the fetus, although studies of the effects of antiarrhythmic agents on the human fetus are scant. They may affect uteroplacental flow. Breast-fed neonates are also vulnerable, as a number of potentially harmful drugs are excreted in the milk. Digitalis, in longest use, is extremely safe in the pregnant patient for heart failure and as an antiarrhythmic agent.[89,90] Lidocaine is also safe for both mother and fetus. Its congeners, such as mexiletine and tocainide, are currently not recommended because data on their use in the pregnant patient are lacking. Quinidine may be used safely throughout pregnancy, although it does possess a minimal oxytocic effect and rarely causes premature labor. Toxic doses may lead to eighth cranial nerve damage in the fetus and to abortion. Procainamide is likewise relatively safe during pregnancy, but there is a high incidence of a lupus-like syndrome.[91] Dilantin® currently has limited use as an antiarrhythmic agent except in digitalis toxicity. When used during the first trimester, it can cause "fetal hydantoin syndrome"[92] with mental and growth retardation, craniofacial malformations, genital abnormalities in male infants, as well as cardiopulmonary disorders. Data on the use of disopyramide, diltiazem, and verapamil during pregnancy are insufficient.

Indications for, and maternal risks of, electrical cardioversion in terminating tachyarrhythmia are the same as in the nonpregnant patient. It has proved to be safe for the fetus, with only rare cases of transient fetal arrhythmia.[93]

ANTIHYPERTENSIVE AGENTS

All antihypertensive agents may decrease uteroplacental blood flow and may be detrimental to fetal growth. Whenever possible, decreased physical activity with bedrest should be instituted first, with the use of antihypertensive agents to decrease blood pressure gradually. Drugs that cause toxic effects to the fetus or neonates should be avoided.

For years, treatment of hypertension during pregnancy consisted of a low salt diet and diuretics. Better understanding of the pathophysiologic aspects of pregnancy-induced hypertension invalidates the role of dietary or drug-induced sodium depletion.[94–99] Nondiuretic antihypertensive agents have become the drug of choice in pregnancy-induced hypertension. Beta blockers currently are used as the first or second antihypertensive agent. They are used frequently for pregnancy-induced hypertension, but important maternal and fetal side effects have been reported with both cardioselective and noncardioselective agents. For example, they can increase the uterine tone and contractility and decrease umbilical blood flow.[68] Therefore, beta blockers should be used cautiously in the lowest possible dose, especially during the last phase of pregnancy, and should be discontinued before labor because of their effects on the uterus and to prevent neonatal complications. Abrupt discontinuation of beta blockers may cause rebound hypertension and exacerbate cardiac ischemia in patients with coronary artery disease. Recently a possible teratogenic effect of propranolol was also reported.[99a] Therefore, if the drug is not absolutely necessary for pregnant women, alternative therapy should be considered. The drugs that affect alpha receptors are methyldopa, clonidine, and prazosin. Methyldopa is generally safe for the mother and fetus. Insufficient data are available on clonidine and prazosin use during pregnancy. Hydralazine, a vasodilator, is effective and safe; however, a sudden decrease in blood pressure, especially when the drug is administered parenterally, can be deleterious to uteroplacental blood flow. There are insufficient data on the use of captopril during pregnancy. Most antihypertensive agents have been found to be present in the milk of nursing mothers. Breast feeding probably should be discontinued when antihypertensive agents are instituted.

Treatment of hypertensive emergencies during pregnancy represents a real challenge for the clinician. For the nonpregnant patient, a parenteral vasodilator is the drug of choice in most cases. The sudden decrease in blood pressure invariably leads to organ hypoperfusion and in the pregnant patient may decrease uterine perfusion, which is already severely compromised during vasoconstriction associated with hypertension. Hydralazine and diazoxide are both effective and relatively safe if used cautiously. Nitroprusside is not recommended, because accumulation of cyanide can occur in the fetus, possibly resulting in fetal death.

ANTICOAGULANTS DURING PREGNANCY

Anticoagulants are used during pregnancy in the treatment of, and prophylaxis against, thromboembolism, as in the patient with a nontissue prosthetic heart valve.[100–106] Their use during pregnancy poses difficult problems, requiring refined judgment and individualized care. The choice of anticoagulants in pregnancy requires consideration of toxicity in both mother and fetus. Heparin, a large molecule that does not cross the placenta, is considered the anticoagulant of choice during pregnancy. It still can induce fetal toxicity with prematurity and stillbirth. Coumadin, which does cross the placenta and does enter the mother's breast milk, may cause fetal mortality through fetal and placental hemorrhage, resulting in spontaneous abortion and stillbirth.[107] It has teratogenic effects, and when used during the 6th to 9th weeks of gestation, warfarin embryopathy can result, with nasal hypoplasia and stippled epiphyses.[108] Although coumadin is not approved by manufacturers for use during pregnancy, some consider it to be relatively safe if used judiciously during the second and third trimesters.[106] The patient on coumadin who becomes pregnant should be informed of the risks and termination of the pregnancy should be discussed. In patients who absolutely require anticoagulation during pregnancy, heparin is probably the safest to administer throughout pregnancy. Others have suggested using heparin during the first trimester and coumadin during the second and third trimesters.[106] Still others recommend using heparin during the first and third trimesters and coumadin during the second trimester.[106] In any case, although delivery can be performed with the patient fully anticoagulated, most suggest temporarily stopping the anticoagulant during labor and resuming it several hours after delivery. For proper timing, induction of labor may be preferable.

SURGICAL MANAGEMENT

Whenever possible, cardiac surgery should be performed before pregnancy. However, the obstetrician is still confronted with those who need surgical intervention even after pregnancy has been initiated. Cardiac surgery during pregnancy is necessary only infrequently and is considered if the disease is refractory to maximum medical management and if the operation can significantly improve the maternal hemodynamic status.[109] Cardiac surgery overall imparts a greater risk to the fetus than the mother, although the use of fetal monitoring has decreased the risk. Cardiac surgery has been performed at all stages of pregnancy; however, it is preferable to perform surgery during the 24th to 28th weeks of pregnancy, when organogenesis is complete.[109,110] Although cardiopulmonary bypass does not appear to expose the mother or fetus to undue risk, closed cardiac techniques generally offer a better result for the fetus than do open cardiac techniques.[111]

Cardiac surgery has been performed in pregnant patients with mitral stenosis and is considered when severe symptoms develop during the second trimester and are refractory to maximal medical therapy.[112] Even if the patient is doing well during the second trimester, hemodynamic changes that occur during labor and delivery can still precipitate pulmonary edema. When possible, it is best to use a porcine or tissue valve to avoid the need for anticoagulation.

Patients with acyanotic heart disease usually do well and do not require cardiac surgery during pregnancy. Surgery should be considered in those with cyanotic congenital heart disease when there is progressive shortness of breath, increasing hematocrit, enlarging cardiomegaly, and progressive arterial oxygen desaturation.

In infective endocarditis, indications for surgery are the same for pregnant as for nonpregnant women. Other indications for cardiac surgery during pregnancy include myxoma, severe constrictive pericarditis, and aortic dissection or rupture.

OBSTETRIC MANAGEMENT

Physiologic cardiovascular changes during pregnancy described previously have a major impact on obstetric management of heart disease during and after gestation. Average blood loss of approximately 600 ml with vaginal delivery and 1,100 ml with cesarean section results in significant reduction of blood volume within three days after delivery.

Obstetric management of heart disease ideally should begin before conception. When pregnancy occurs without prior evaluation, the cardiac patient must be carefully evaluated to determine whether pregnancy should continue and what risks are involved.

No treatment should be administered to a pregnant woman without prior assessment of the fetal risks. Both medical and surgical management of cardiovascular disease during pregnancy often entails greater risks to the fetus than the mother. Proper management of congestive heart failure in the mother may eliminate related symptoms and improve the placental circulation. However, rapid diuresis can have an unfavorable impact on the fetus by depleting the plasma volume.

Prophylactic antibiotics are important in any patient with valvular heart disease during parturition. A broad spectrum antibiotic is generally given approximately one hour before delivery and then additionally every eight hours.

Swan-Ganz catheterization is helpful in the management of pregnant women with heart disease. It should be used prophylactically during labor in women who have known cardiac disease and in whom symptoms develop at rest or with mild exercise.

With fetal monitoring, fetal tachycardia is being detected early with increasing frequency. Both digitalis and propranolol have been used successfully in the conversion of fetal tachycardia.

An accurate diagnosis of heart disease must be established before discussing its associated risks as well as the indicated medical management. It is imperative that the mother be given optimum treatment for the disease, while making every attempt to avoid, insofar as possible, any treatment that carries great fetal hazard.

A most important and often neglected aspect of management is the counselling of all women with heart disease. Ideally, this should be carried out before pregnancy, but frequently it is not. The risks of pregnancy to both the mother and the fetus should be assessed. If the mother has congenital heart disease, the risk of fetal development of a similar disorder should be considered.

Thromboembolic disease is more common in pregnancy, especially in those with heart disease associated with arrhythmia. Those who have had previous thromboembolic disease as well as those with valve prostheses are at the greatest risk. Probably all pregnant patients at high risk of developing thromboembolic disease when exposed to any surgical procedure should be treated with low dose prophylactic heparin (5,000 IU every 8 to 12 hours).

Anesthesia must be selected with care in the pregnant cardiac patient. Frequently, anesthetic agents used during parturition produce profound alteration in vascular tonus. Hemodynamic stability is important in the obstetric management of the parturient with heart disease.

The effects of cesarean section on the patient's hemodynamic status are variable. Although cesarean section alleviates the more marked hemodynamic alterations associated with vaginal delivery, the administration of anesthetics and the operative procedure are associated with significant deleterious hemodynamic changes.[37–40] Although the results of several studies are conflicting, spinal (subarachnoid) anesthesia in general may be associated with variable heart changes, a decrease in stroke volume with an overall decrease in blood pressure and cardiac output. Therefore, this method of administering anesthesia probably should not be employed in pregnant women with heart disease. The hemodynamic alterations are significantly less with balanced anesthesia (thiopental, nitrous oxide, and succinyl choline).[40] Hemodynamic stability is also seen with epidural anesthesia if used without epinephrine.[39]

Caution should be exercised in the use of the various diagnostic procedures commonly employed in nonpregnant patients with cardiovascular diseases. Ultrasonography has no confirmed risks when used in the pregnant woman. Characteristic changes with normal pregnancy also occur on the echocardiogram, which must be interpreted by someone familiar with normal gestational changes. X-ray procedures should be avoided as much as possible during pregnancy. When they are necessary, protective shielding must be used to diminish the chances of fetal damage, especially during the early organogenetic stages. Despite some degree of risk, termination of pregnancy is rarely indicated after conventional x-ray examinations.

During labor and delivery, patients with less severe heart disease usually do well. Women with severe heart disease may require hospitalization for close observation during the late phase of pregnancy. During labor and delivery, careful hemodynamic monitoring may be necessary. Prolonged labor, particularly the second stage, must be avoided in these patients with cardiac disease.

CONTRAINDICATIONS TO PREGNANCY

In assessing the advisability of pregnancy in a patient with heart disease, certain factors need to be considered.[4,42,43] These include (1) New York Heart Association functional class of the patient, (2) age of the patient (those greater than 35 years of age have an increased risk), (3) a history of congestive heart failure with pregnancy, (4) the quality of available medical care, and (5) the desire of the patient to become pregnant. Patients in functional classes I and II generally can be carried through pregnancy successfully. Those in functional class III should be followed carefully and be hospitalized with careful monitoring during the latter part of pregnancy. Those in functional class IV should not undergo pregnancy, except those whose functional class may be significantly improved by operative intervention.

With the establishment of sophisticated perinatal centers, abortions are rarely indicated for the pregnant woman with heart disease. In fact, it has been estimated that abortion is indicated in only 5% to 8% of all pregnant women with heart disease.[4,42,43] The reason is that patients with functional classes III and IV heart disease represent no more than 20% of all pregnant women with heart disease (but they represent 85% of all maternal deaths).[4,42,43] Therefore, the functional status of the pregnant woman with heart disease plays a large role in the decision making (Table 62.1).

Table 62.1. Mortality According to Functional Class*

New York Heart Association Functional Class	Mortality (%) Maternal	Fetal
I	0.4	0
II	0.4	—
III	6.8	—
IV	6.8	30

* From Braunwald E: *Heart Disease. A Textbook of Cardiovascular Medicine*, ed 2. Philadelphia, WB Saunders, 1984, p 1776, with permission.

In dealing with heart patients who should not become pregnant, counseling plays an important role. Methods of birth control must also be addressed. Because of the possibility of infective endocarditis, intrauterine devices are contraindicated in patients with valvular heart disease. Oral contraceptives, because of the increased incidence of the thromboembolic phenomenon, should be avoided in the patient with coronary artery disease, hypertension, and valvular heart disease, particularly mitral stenosis. Surgical sterilization is probably the safest and most reliable method of birth control in most heart patients. Because anesthesia may be associated with an inordinate risk to the woman, male sterilization is considered a preferable method for the couple.

REFERENCES

1. Szekely P, Turner R, Snaith L: Pregnancy and the changing pattern of rheumatic heart disease. *Bri Heart J* 1973; 35:1293–1303.
2. Szekely P, Snaith L: *Heart Disease and Pregnancy*. Edinburgh and London, Churchill Livingstone, 1974.
3. Krause RM: The influence of infection on the geography of heart disese. *Circulation* 1979; 60:972–976.
4. Conradsson T-B, Werko L: Management of heart disease in pregnancy. *Prog Cardiovasc Dis* 1974; 16:407–419.
5. Ueland K: Cardiovascular diseases complicating pregnancy. *Clin Obstet Gynecol* 1978; 21:429–443.
6. Wilson MG, Lim WN, Birch AM: The decline of rheumatic fever. Recurrence rates of rheumatic fever among 782 children for twenty-one consecutive calendar years (1936–1956). *J Chronic Dis* 1958; 7:183–197.
7. Etheridge MJ: Heart disease and pregnancy. *Med J Aust* 1968; 2:1172–1175.
8. Burch GE: Heart disease and pregnancy. *Am Heart J* 1977; 93:104–116.
9. Leman RB, Assey ME: Heart disease and pregnancy. *South Med J* 1981; 74:944–946.
10. Metcalfe J, Ueland K: Maternal cardiovascular adjustments to pregnancy. *Prog Cardiovasc Dis* 1974; 16:363–374.
11. Chesley LC: Plasma and red cell volumes during pregnancy. *Am J Obstet Gynecol* 1972; 112:440–450.
12. Lees MM, Taylor SH, Scott DB, Kerr MG: A study of cardiac output at rest throughout pregnancy. *J Obstet Gynaec Br Cwlth* 1967; 74:319–328.
13. Walters WAW, MacGregor WG, Hills M: Cardiac output at rest during pregnancy and the puerperium. *Clin Sci* 1966; 30:1–11.
14. Bader RA, Bader ME, Rose DJ, Braunwald E: Hemodynamics at rest and during exercise in normal pregnancy as studied by cardiac catheterization. *J Clin Invest* 1955; 34:1524–1536.
15. Pritchard JA: Changes in the blood volume during pregnancy and delivery. *Anesthesiology* 1965; 26:393–399.
16. Winner W, Romney SL: Cardiovascular responses to labor and delivery. *Am J Obstet Gynecol* 1966; 95:1104–1114.
17. Rovinsky JJ, Jaffin H: Cardiovascular hemodynamics in pregnancy. II. Cardiac output and left ventricular work in multiple pregnancy. *Am J Obstet Gynecol* 1966; 95:781–786.
18. Lees MM, Scott DB, Kerr MG: Hemodynamic changes associated with labour. *J Obstet Gynaec Br Cwlth* 1970; 77:29–36.
19. Ueland K, Novy MJ, Peterson EN, Metcalfe J: Maternal cardiovascular dynamics. IV. The influence of gestational age on the maternal cardiovascular response to posture and exercise. *Am J Obstet Gynecol* 1969; 104:856–864.
20. Lavid-Meeter K, Van de Ley G, Bom TH, Wladimiroff JW, Roelandt J: Cardiocirculatory adjustments during pregnancy: an echocardiographic study. *Clin Cardiol* 1979; 2:328.
21. Rubler S, Damani PM, Pinto ER: Cardiac size and performance during pregnancy estimated with echocardiography. *Am J Cardiol* 1977; 40:534–540.
22. Lund CJ, Donovan JC: Blood volume during pregnancy. Significance of plasma and red cell volume. *Am J Obstet Gynecol* 1967; 98:393–403.
23. Christianson RE: Studies on blood pressure during pregnancy. I. Influence of parity and age. *Am J Obstet Gynecol* 1976; 125:509–513.
24. Kerr MG: The mechanical effects of the gravid uterus in late pregnancy. *J Obstet Gynaec Br Cwlth* 1965; 72:513–529.
25. Bieniarz J, Crottogini JK, Curuchet E, Romero-Salinas G, Yoshida J, Poseiro JJ, Caldeyro-Barcia R: Aortocaval compression by the uterus in late human pregnancy. II. An arteriographic study. *Am J Obstet Gynecol* 1968; 100:203–217.
26. Abitbol MM: Inferior vena cava compression in the pregnant dog. *Am J Obstet Gynecol* 1978; 130:194–198.
27. Quilligan EJ, Tyler C: Postural effects on the cardiovascular status in pregnancy: a comparison of the lateral and supine postures. *Am J Obstet Gynecol* 1978; 130:194–198.
28. Turner AF: The chest radiograph in pregnancy. *Clin Obstet Gynecol* 1975; 18:65–74.
29. Cutforth R, MacDonald CB: Heart sounds and murmurs in pregnancy. *Am Heart J* 1966; 71:741–747.
30. Tabatznik B, Randall TW, Hersch C: The mammary souffle of pregnancy and lactation. *Circulation* 1960; 22:1069–1073.
31. Marcus FI, Ewy GA, O'Rourke RA, Walsh B, Bleich AC: The effect of pregnancy on the murmurs of mitral and aortic regurgitation. *Circulation* 1970; 41:795–805.
32. Rayburn WF, Fontana ME: Mitral valve prolapse and pregnancy. *Am J Obstet Gynecol* 1981; 141:9–11.
33. Carruth JE, Mirvis SB, Brogan DR, Wenger NK: The electrocardiogram in normal pregnancy. *Am Heart J* 1981; 102:1075–1078.
34. Boyle DM, Lloyd-Jones LL: The electrocardiographic ST segment in pregnancy. *J Obstet Gynaec Br Cwlth* 1966; 73:986–987.

34a. Northcote RJ, Knight PV, Ballantyne D: Systolic murmurs in pregnancy: value of echocardiographic assessment. *Clin Cardiol* 1985; 8:327–328.
35. Cotton DB, Benedetti TJ: Use of the Swan-Ganz catheter in obstetrics and gynecology. *Obstet Gynecol* 1980; 56:641–645.
36. Berkowitz RL, Rafferty TD: Invasive hemodynamic monitoring in critically ill pregnant patients: role of Swan-Ganz catheterization. *Am J Obstet Gynecol* 1980; 137:127–134.
37. Ueland K, Gills RE, Hansen JM: Maternal cardiovascular dynamics. I. Cesarean section under subarachnoid block anesthesia. *Am J Obstet Gynecol* 1968; 100:42–54.
38. Ueland K, Hansen JM: Maternal cardiovascular dynamics. III. Labor and delivery under local and caudal analgesia. *Am J Obstet Gynecol* 1969; 103:8–18.
39. Ueland K, Akamatsu TJ, Eng M, Bonica JJ, Hansen JM: Maternal cardiovascular dynamics. VI. Cesarean section under epidural anesthesia without epinephrine. *Am J Obstet Gynecol* 1972; 114:775–780.
40. Ueland K, Hansen J, Eng M, Kalappa R, Parer JT: Maternal cardiovascular dynamics. V. Cesarean section under thiopental, nitrous oxide, and succinyl choline anesthesia. *Am J Obstet Gynecol* 1970; 108:615–622.
41. Ueland K, Metcalfe J: Acute rheumatic fever in pregnancy. *Am J Obstet Gynecol* 1966; 95:586–587.
42. McAnulty JH, Metcalfe J, Ueland K: General guidelines in the management of cardiac disease. *Clin Obstet Gynecol* 1981; 24:773–788.
43. Hibbard LT: Maternal mortality due to cardiac disease. *Clin Obstet Gynecol* 1975; 18:27–36.
44. Schaefer G, Arditi LI, Solomon HA, Ringland JE: Congenital heart disease and pregnancy. *Clin Obstet Gynecol* 1968; 11:1048–1064.
45. Naeye RL, Hagstrom JWC, Talmadge BA: Postpartum death with maternal congenital heart disease. *Circulation* 1967; 36:304–312.
46. Neilson G, Galea EG, Blunt A: Congenital heart disease and pregnancy. *Med J Aust* 1970; 1:1086–1088.
47. Cannell DE, Vernon CP: Congenital heart disease and pregnancy. *Am J Obstet Gynecol* 1963; 85:744–753.
48. Cavanzo FJ, Taylor HB: Effect of pregnancy on the human aorta and its relationship to dissecting aneurysms. *Am J Obstet Gynecol* 1969; 104:567–568.
49. Konishi Y, Tatsuta N, Kumada K, Minami K, Matsuda K, Yamasato A, Usui N, Muraguchi T, Hikasa Y, Okamato E, Watanabe R: Dissecting aneurysm during pregnancy and the puerperium. *Jpn Circ J* 1980; 44:726–733.
50. Pyeritz RE: Risk of aortic complications in the Marfan syndrome during pregnancy (abstr). *Circulation* 1980; 62:III–304.
51. Deal K, Wooley CF: Coarctation of aorta and pregnancy. *Ann Intern Med* 1973; 78:706–710.
52. Barash PG, Hobbins JC, Hook R, Stansel HC, Whittmore R, Hehre FW: Management of coarctation of the aorta during pregnancy. *J Thorac Cardiovasc Surg* 1975; 69:781–784.
53. Mortensen JD, Joelsson I: Coarctation of the aorta in pregnancy. *JAMA* 1965; 191:596–598.
54. Meyer EC, Tursky AS, Sigmann P, Siber EN: Pregnancy in the presence of tetralogy of Fallot. *Am J Cardiol* 1964; 14:874–879.
55. Jacoby WJ: Pregnancy with tetralogy and pentalogy of Fallot. *Am J Cardiol* 1964; 14:866–873.
56. Ralstin JH, Dunn M: Pregnancies after surgical correction of tetralogy of Fallot. *JAMA* 1976; 235:2627–2628.
57. Loffer FD: Eisenmenger's complex and pregnancy. *Obstet Gynecol* 1967; 29:235–240.
58. Spinnato JA, Kraynack BJ, Cooper MW: Eisenmenger's syndrome in pregnancy: epidural anesthesia for elective cesarean section. *N Engl J Med* 1981; 304:1215–1217.
59. Devitt JH, Noble WH: Eisenmenger's syndrome and pregnancy. *N Engl J Med* 1980; 302:751.
60. Arias F: Maternal death in a patient with Eisenmenger's syndrome. *Obstet Gynecol* 1977; 50:76S.
61. McCaffrey RM, Dunn LJ: Primary pulmonary hypertension in pregnancy. *Obstet Gynecol Survey* 1964; 19:567–591.
62. Sleeper JC, Orgain ES, McIntosh HD: Primary pulmonary hypertension. Review of clinical features and pathologic physiology with a report of pulmonary hemodynamics derived from repeated catheterization. *Circulation* 1962; 26:1358–1369.
63. Sasse L, Wagner R, Murray FE: Transmural myocardial infarction during pregnancy. *Am J Cardiol* 1975; 35:448–451.
64. Brown A: Myocardial infarction associated with pregnancy. Report of two cases. *N Engl J Med* 1960; 262:1163–1166.
65. Turner GM, Oakley CM, Dixon HG: Management of pregnancy complicated by hypertrophic obstructive cardiomyopathy. *Br Med J* 1968; 4:281–284.
66. Kolibash AJ, Ruiz DE, Lewis RP: Idiopathic hypertrophic subaortic stenosis in pregnancy. *Ann Intern Med* 1975; 82:791–794.
67. Oakley GDG, McGarry K, Limb DG, Oakley CM: Management of pregnancy in patients with hypertrophic cardiomyopathy. *Br Med J* 1979; 1:1749–1750.
68. Pruyn CS, Phelan JP, Buchanan GC: Long-term propranolol therapy in pregnancy: maternal and fetal outcome. *Ann J Obstet Gynecol* 1979; 135:485–489.
69. Brinkman CR III, Woods JR Jr: Effects of cardiovascular drugs during pregnancy. *Cardiovasc Med* 1976; 1:231–251.
70. Demakis JG, Rahimtoola SH: Peripartum cardiomyopathy. *Circulation* 1971; 44:964–968.
71. Demakis JG, Rahimtoola SH, Sutton GC, Meadows WR, Szanto PB, Tobin JR, Gunnar RM: Natural course of peripartum cardiomyopathy. *Circulation* 1971; 44:1053–1061.
72. Davidson NM, Parry EHO: The etiology of peripartum cardiac failure. *Am Heart J* 1979; 97:535–536.
72a. Homan DC: Peripartum cardiomyopathy. *N Engl J Med* 1985; 312:1432–1437.
72b. Julian DG, Szekely P: Peripartum cardiomyopathy. *Prog Cardiovasc Dis* 1985; 27:223–240.
73. Faruque AA: Acute fulminating puerperal myocarditis. *Br Heart J* 1965; 27:139–143.
74. Crockett EJ, Batchelor TM, Corbeil J: Pregnancy and subacute bacterial endocarditis. *Obstet Gynecol* 1960; 16:93–95.
75. Shulman ST, Amren DP, Bisno AL, Dajani AS, Durack DT, Gerber MA, Kaplan EL, Millard HD, Sanders WE, Schwartz RH, Watanakunakorn C: Prevention of bacterial endocarditis. *Circulation* 1984; 70: 1123A–1127A.
76. Fleming HA: Antibiotic prophylaxis against infective endocarditis after delivery. *Lancet* 1977; 1:144–145.
77. Sugrue D, Blake S, Troy P, MacDonald D: Antibiotic prophylaxis against infective endocarditis after normal delivery: is it necessary? *Br Heart J* 1980; 44:499–502.
78. Fuchs F: Prevention of prematurity. *Am J Obstet Gynecol* 1976; 126:809–820.
79. Niebyl JR, Blake DA, Johnson JWC, King TM: The pharmacologic inhibition of premature labor. *Obstet Gynecol Survey* 1978; 33:507–515.
80. Liggins GC, Howie RN: A controlled trial antepartum glucocorticoid treatment for the prevention of respiratory distress syndrome in premature infants. *Pediatrics* 1972; 50:515–525.
81. Nochimson DJ, Petrie RH: Glucocorticoid therapy for the induction of pulmonary maturity in severely hypertensive gravid women. *Am J Obstet Gynecol* 1979; 133:449–451.
82. Ricke PS, Elliott JP, Freeman RK: Use of corticosteroids in pregnancy-induced hypertension. *Obstet Gynecol* 1980; 55:206–210.
83. Jacobs MM, Knight AB, Arias F: Maternal pulmonary edema resulting from betamimetic and glucocorticoid therapy. *Obstet Gynecol* 1980; 56:56–59.
84. Sackner MA: Changes in blood oxygen and in cardiac function following beta$_2$ and other bronchodilator drugs. *Chest* 1978; 73:985.
85. Elliott JP, O'Keeffe DF, Greenberg P, Freeman RK: Pulmonary edema associated with magnesium sulfate and betamethasone administration. *Am J Obstet Gynecol* 1979; 134:717–719.
86. Landesman R, deSouz JA, Coutinho EM, Wilson KH, deSousa MB: The inhibitory effect of diazoxide in normal term labor. *Am J Obstet Gynecol* 1969; 103:430–433.
87. Niebyl JR, Blake DA, White RD, Kumor KM, Dubin NH, Robinson JC, Egner PG: The inhibition of premature labor with indomethacin. *Am J Obstet Gynecol* 1980; 136:1014–1019.
88. Zlatnik F, Fuchs F: A controlled study of ethanol in threatened premature labor. *Am J Obstet Gynecol* 1972; 112:610–612.
88a. Golichowski AM, Hathaway DR, Fineberg N, Peleg D: Tocolytic and hemodyamic effects of nifedipine in the ewe. *Am J Obstet Gynecol* 1985; 151:1134–1140.
89. Szekely P, Desmond GJ: Heart disease and pregnancy. *Curr Probl Cardiol* 1979; 4:1–74.
90. Mendelson CL: *Cardiac Disease in Pregnancy*. Philadelphia, Davis, 1960.
91. Condemi JJ, Blomgren SE, Vaughn JH: The procainamide-induced lupus syndrome. *Bull Rheum Dis* 1970; 20:604–608.
92. Hanson JW, Myrianthopoulos NC, Harvey MAS: Risks of offspring of women treated with hydantoin anticonvulsant and emphasis on fetal hydantoin syndrome. *J Pediatr* 1978; 89:662–668.
93. Schroeder JS, Harrison DC: Repeated cardioversion during pregnancy. *Am J Cardiol* 1971: 27:445–446.
94. Lindheimer MD, Katz AI: Sodium and diuretics in pregnancy. *N Engl J Med* 1973; 288:891–894.
95. Lindberg BS: Salt, diuretics and pregnancy. *Gynecol Obstet Invest* 1979; 10:145–156.
96. Sarles HE, Hill SS, LeBlanc AL, Smith GH, Canales CO, Remmers AG: Sodium excretion patterns during and following intravenous sodium chloride loads in normal and hypertensive pregnancies. *Am J Obstet Gynecol* 1968; 102:1–7.
97. Symonds EM, Pipkin FB: Pregnancy hypertension, parity and the renin-angiotensin system. *Am J Obstet Gynecol* 1978; 132:473–479.
98. Soffronoff EC, Kaufmann BM, Connaughton JF: Intravascular volume determinations and fetal outcome in hypertensive diseases of pregnancy. *Am J Obstet Gynecol* 1978; 127:4–9.

99. Finnerty FA: Hypertension and pregnancy. *J Cardiovasc Med* 1980; 5:559–568.

99a. Campbell JW: A possible teratogenic effect of propranolol. *N Engl J Med* 1985; 313:518.

100. Taguchi K: Pregnancy in patients with a prosthetic heart valve. *Surg Gynecol Obstet* 1977; 145:206–208.

101. Tejani N: Anticoagulant therapy with cardiac valve prosthesis during pregnancy. *Obstet Gynecol* 1973; 42:785–793.

102. Limet R, Grondin CM: Cardiac valve prostheses, anticoagulation, and pregnancy. *Ann Thorac Surg* 1977; 23:337–341.

103. Ibarra-Perez C, Arevalo-Toledo N, Cadena OA, Noriega-Guerra L: The course of pregnancy in patients with artificial heart valves. *Am J Med* 1976; 61:504–512.

104. Hirsh J, Cade JK, Gallus AS: Anticoagulants in pregnancy: a review of indications and complications. *Am Heart J* 1972; 83:301–305.

105. Casanegra P, Aviles G, Maturana G, Dubernet J: Cardiovascular management of pregnant women with a heart valve prosthesis. *Am J Cardiol* 1975; 36:802–806.

106. Hall JG, Pauli RM, Wilson KM: Maternal and fetal sequelae of anticoagulation during pregnancy. *Am J Med* 1980; 68:122–140.

107. Palacios-Macedo X, Diaz-Devis C, Escudero J: Fetal risk with the use of coumarin anticoagulant agent in pregnant patients with intracardiac ball valve prosthesis. *Am J Cardiol* 1969; 24:853–856.

108. Pettifor JM, Benson R: Congenital malformations associated with the administration of oral anticoagulants during pregnancy. *J Pediatr* 1975; 86:459–462.

109. Selzer A: When is cardiac surgery necessary during pregnancy? *J Cardiovasc Med* 1982; 7:1332–1333.

110. Ueland K: Cardiac surgery and pregnancy. *Am J Obstet Gynecol* 1965; 92:148–162.

111. Levy DL, Warriner RA, Burgess GE III: Fetal response to cardiopulmonary bypass. *Obstet Gynecol* 1980; 56:112–115.

112. Sullivan JM, Ramanathan KB: Management of medical problems in pregnancy-severe cardiac disease. *N Engl J Med* 1985; 313:304–309.

63 Cardiovascular Pharmacology

Bramah N. Singh, MD, DPhil, FRCP, Nagammal Venkatesh, MD, and Gregory K. Feld, MD

Clinical cardiovascular pharmacology has grown rapidly into a major discipline within the specialty of cardiology over the last two or three decades. Numerous classes of agents have been developed and characterized for the treatment of major cardiocirculatory disorders such as ischemic myocardial syndromes, hypertension, cardiac arrhythmias, and cardiac failure with a host of lesser indications. The purpose of this chapter is to provide, within a relatively brief compass, the pharmacologic basis for the use of cardioactive drugs in the treatment of heart disease. The agents to be discussed include: (1) beta-adrenergic blocking drugs; (2) coronary dilators: nitrates and calcium channel blockers; (3) diuretics; (4) vasodilators; (5) cardiac stimulant drugs; and (6) antiarrhythmic agents.

The pharmacodynamics, pharmacokinetics, and clinical uses of vasodilators, cardiac stimulant drugs, and diuretics have been dealt with elsewhere in this volume in relation to the treatment of cardiac failure and hypertension and will be discussed here only briefly for completeness. The bulk of this chapter will therefore be devoted to the pharmacology of beta-antagonists, nitrates, calcium antagonists, and antiarrhythmic agents in relation to the salient features of the pathophysiology of diseases in which these drugs are of the greatest clinical utility.

BETA-ADRENERGIC BLOCKING DRUGS

Introduced in the early 1960s, this class of drugs has made major impact on the treatment of numerous cardiocirculatory disorders, especially myocardial ischemic syndromes, hypertension, certain cardiac arrhythmias, and obstructive cardiomyopathy. In recent years their role in reducing the incidence of sudden death and recurrent myocardial infarction in those surviving the acute episode has been clearly established.

PHARMACOLOGIC CONSIDERATIONS

Beta-adrenergic blocking drugs were developed by the modification of the basic isoproterenol molecule in relation to the observation that catecholamines exerted two distinct patterns of physiologic response due to differential receptor stimulation. The first was characterized by vasoconstriction in certain regional beds (mediated by alpha receptors) and the second by producing cardiac stimulation, vasodilatation, and bronchodilation (mediated by beta receptors). Beta-adrenergic blocking drugs are those that competitively antagonize beta receptor stimulation induced by endogenous or exogenous catecholamines. The bulk of the therapeutic effects of these drugs can be attributed to their propensity to produce beta receptor blockade. As a class, they tend to inhibit catecholamine-induced increases in cardiac contractility, heart rate, vasodilatation, atrioventricular nodal conduction, bronchodilation, renin release, lipolysis, and insulin release. An appreciation of these features with respect to individual agents of the class permits one to predict their therapeutic as well as their side effect profiles, especially when related to the pharmacokinetic features that are not related to the property of beta blockade.[1-3]

Certain beta receptors exhibit a greater predilection for blocking cardiac beta receptors (termed beta$_1$ receptors) than do the extracardiac ones (termed beta$_2$ adrenoceptors). The concept of *cardioselectivity* has therefore grown. However, it must be emphasized that cardioselectivity is relative rather than absolute, being apparent in small doses; in larger doses the differences between the so-called cardioselective and noncardioselective agents become indistinguishable. It has also been found that certain beta blockers have *intrinsic sympathomimetic activity* (ISA) in low concentrations and under resting conditions, stimulating beta receptors rather than blocking them. The clinical significance of this property still remains unclear, although there is evidence that beta antagonists that have ISA may be less depressant on the myocardium and atrioventricular nodal conduction, produce less resting bradycardia (or may even produce tachycardia), and do not elevate serum lipid levels during long-term administration. There is also tentative data to suggest that they may not exert similar cardioprotective effects in survivors of acute myocardial infarction when compared with those of agents lacking in ISA. Finally, it must be emphasized that certain beta antagonists have a *membrane stabilizing activity* (MSA) independent of their beta-blocking activity; therefore, they exert a depressant effect on the rate of depolarization in nerve and cardiac muscle. However, such an effect is only evident in extremely high concentrations and rarely may it be of clinical significance. Propranolol was the first beta blocker to be used widely in clinical therapeutics and continues to serve as the reference compound. The beta-blocking potencies of the commonly available beta antagonists and their associated properties of cardioselectivity, ISA, and MSA are summarized in Table 63.1. Labetalol is the only beta blocker that also exerts alpha receptor blocking property. Beta blockers differ significantly with respect to their metabolism, disposition in the body, lipid solubility, elimination half-lives, and other pharmacokinetic constants (Tables 63.2 and 63.3). It is known that lipophilic beta blockers generally have a high rate of hepatic metabolism, high brain penetration, and complex pharmacokinetic features. The converse occurs for those that are hydrophilic; they have a low hepatic metabolism and brain penetration and are excreted by the kidneys.[4]

HEMODYNAMIC AND ELECTROPHYSIOLOGIC EFFECTS

Beta-blocking agents exhibit a distinct pattern of hemodynamic and electrophysiologic actions. For example, when acutely administered, they reduce heart rate, systolic (but not diastolic) pressure, myocardial contractility, cardiac and stroke volume index, and stroke work index; elevate left ventricular filling pressure and dimensions; and prolong systolic ejection time at rest and after exercise. Following beta blockade, overall cardiac work and myocardial oxygen consumption are reduced coincident with a resultant decrease in coronary blood flow and coronary artery caliber. During acute administration there is an increase in peripheral resistance, but during chronic therapy, total systemic resistance decreases in hypertensive patients. Although the differences are not striking, agents such as pindolol may exert somewhat less depressant effect on the overall systemic hemodynamics. Sotalol appears to have a less depressant effect on cardiac contractility, an effect that may be related to prolongation of the action potential in cardiac muscle[5] which is unrelated to the drug's propensity to block beta receptors.

Beta blockers lengthen spontaneous sinus cycle and prolong sinus node recovery time and intranodal conduction time as well as the effective and functional refractory periods of the atrioventricular node.[6] Beta blockade has little or no effect on the effective refractory period in the atria, ventricles, His-Purkinje system, or accessory tracts of the heart.[7] Again, sotalol, because of its effects on the action potential duration in all cardiac tissues, differs from other agents. It lengthens the voltage-dependent refractoriness in all cardiac tissues, thus having a wide spectrum of electrophysiologic and antiarrhythmic effects.[8]

BETA BLOCKADE AND CLINICAL THERAPEUTICS

The major clinical uses of beta antagonists are summarized in Table 63.4.

Ischemic Myocardial Syndromes

Beta-blocking drugs have an established role in the treatment of *chronic stable angina.*[3] In this condition, they reduce the frequency of chest pain, prolong exercise capacity, and delay the onset of electrocardiographic evi-

Table 63.1. Pharmacodynamic Properties of Beta-Blocking Drugs

Drug	Beta$_1$-Blockade Potency Ratio	Relative Beta$_1$ Selectivity	Intrinsic Sympathomimetic Activity	Membrane Stabilizing Activity	Intravenous Dose (single doses; in mg)	Commonly Used Oral Dosage
Acebutolol	0.3	+	+	+	12.5–50.0	200–600 mg tid
Atenolol	1.0	+	0	0	5–15	25–200 mg/daily
Labetalol*	0.3	0	0	0	—	100–600 mg bid
Metoprolol	1.0	+	0	0	5–15	50–100 mg bid
Nadolol	1.0	0	0	0	—	40–240 mg/day
Oxprenolol	0.5	0	+	+	1–12	80–120 mg tid
Pindolol	6.0	0	++	+	0.4–2.0	2.5–7.5 mg tid
Propranolol	1.0 (reference agent)	0	0	++	1–10	20–160 mg tid
Timolol	6.0	0	0	0	0.4–1.0	10–30 mg bid
Sotalol	0.3	0	0	0	1–1.5 mg/kg	80–320 mg bid

* Also has alpha-adrenergic blocking properties.

Table 63.2. Elimination Characteristics of Orally Active Beta-Blocking Drugs

Drugs	Elimination Half-Life (h)	Total Body Clearance (ml/min)	Urinary Recovery of Unchanged Drug (% of dose)	Total Urinary Recovery (% of dose)	Predominant Route of Elimination	Active Metabolite	Drug Accumulation in Renal Disease
Acebutolol	3–4*	6–15	40	>90	HM†	Yes	Yes†
Atenolol	6–9	130	40	>95	RE	No	Yes
Labetalol	4–6	2,700	<1	>90	HM	No	No
Metoprolol	3–4	1,100	3	>95	HM	No	No
Nadolol	14–24	200	70	70	RE	No	Yes
Pindolol	3–4	400	40	>90	RE (40% unchanged), HM	No	No
Propranolol	3–4	1,000	<1	>90	HM	Yes	No
Propranolol LA (long-acting)	10	1,000	<1	>90	HM	Yes	No
Timolol	4–5	660	20	65	RE (~20% unchanged), HM	No	No
Sotalol	15–17	600	90	>90	RE	No	Yes

* $t_{1/2}$ of the pharmacologically active metabolite, diacetolol, is 12 to 15 hours.

† The predominant route of elimination of acebutolol is hepatic; however, its pharmacologically active metabolite, diacetolol, is excreted by the kidney and may accumulate in patients with renal dysfunction. HM = hepatic metabolism; RE = renal excretion.

Table 63.3. Pharmacokinetic Properties of Beta-Blocking Drugs

Drugs	Extent of Absorption (% of dose)	Extent of Bioavailability (% of dose)	Dose-Dependent Bioavailability (major first-pass hepatic metabolism)	Interpatient Variations in Plasma Levels	Beta-Blocking Plasma Concentrations	Protein Binding (%)	Lipid Solubility*
Acebutolol	70	50	No	7-fold	0.2–2.0 μg/ml	30–40	Weak
Atenolol	50	40	No	4-fold	0.2–5.0 μg/ml	< 5	Weak
Labetalol	> 90	25	Yes	10-fold	0.7–3.0 μg/ml	50	Weak
Metoprolol	> 90	50	No	7-fold	50–100 ng/ml	12	Moderate
Nadolol	30	30	No	7-fold	50–100 ng/ml	30	Weak
Pindolol	> 90	90	No	4-fold	5–15 ng/ml	57	Moderate
Propranolol	> 90	30	Yes	20-fold	50–100 ng/ml	93	High
Propranolol LA (Long-acting)	> 90	20	Yes	10–20-fold	20–100 ng/ml	93	High
Timolol	> 90	75	No	7-fold	5–10 ng/ml	10	Weak
Sotalol	> 90	> 60	No	10-fold	1,000–3,000 ng/ml	5	Weak

* Determined by the distribution ratio of octanol and water.

Note: The figures cited for all parameters are approximate.

dence of ischemia. Their salutary effect is mediated through the reduction in major determinants of myocardial oxygen consumption (at rest and with exercise), crudely assessed by heart rate and blood pressure product. Whether the known effect of these agents on the oxygen-dissociation curve or platelet adhesiveness contributes to their antiischemic actions is not certain. Over 60% of patients with chronic stable angina obtain symptomatic relief from beta blockade; the optimum response is judged from the degree of beta blockade attained rather than from arbitrarily defined dose regimens in the case of an individual agent. The effects of beta blockers may be complemented or supplemented by combination therapy with nitrates or, with certain precautions, with calcium antagonists. The role of beta blockers as single agents in the control of *Prinzmetal angina* or *unstable angina* is less clear. It is known, however, that in vasotonic angina with presumably normal coronary vessels, beta blockers may prolong the duration of ischemic episodes. Although spasm or abnormal vasoconstriction has been thought to be an important causative factor in the pathogenesis of unstable angina, there is no controlled data to suggest that beta blockers may aggravate ischemia in this syndrome. However, because beta blockers are almost invariably used in combination with nitrates in this setting, it is conceivable that any tendency for vasoconstriction induced by beta blockade is negated by the concomitant administration of nitrates.

Table 63.4. Clinical Applications of Beta-Adrenergic Blocking Agents

1. Ischemic myocardial syndromes
   a. Unstable angina
   b. Chronic stable angina
   c. Cardioprotective effect in survivors of acute myocardial infarction
   d. Reduction of infarct size (not established as a clinical indication)
2. Systemic hypertension
3. Cardiac arrhythmias
4. Cardiomyopathies
   a. Hypertrophic cardiomyopathy
   b. Dilated cardiomyopathy (role not fully established)
5. Thyrotoxicosis
6. Migraine
7. Glaucoma
8. Anxiety states
9. Alcohol withdrawal
10. Cyanotic spells in tetralogy of Fallot
11. Schizophrenia

The cardioprotective effects of beta blockers in the survivors of acute myocardial infarction have gained prominence in recent years.[9] When these drugs are given prophylactically, starting between 5 and 28 days after infarction, they reduce the incidence of sudden death and reinfarction by 25% to 35%[9] in the first year. It is not clear whether earlier administration may improve the mortality figures, nor is it clear whether the initiation of therapy remote from the time of infarction will also confer benefit. The mechanism of the salutary effect is also uncertain; it does not appear to be related to a primary antiarrhythmic action of these agents. There is some evidence that agents with ISA may be less effective, but other associated properties such as MSA or cardioselectivity do not appear to be relevant in this regard. Although beta blockers have been shown to reduce infarct size experimentally as well as in the clinical setting, there is little data at present to suggest that this can be translated into routine clinical practice, as the prognostic significance of infarct reduction in man remains to be defined.

Beta Blockade and Cardiac Arrhythmias

The spectrum of clinical effects here is predictable on the basis of the known action of these compounds in relation to involvement of the sympathetic nervous system in the genesis of cardiac arrhythmias. Their most consistent effect appears to be in tachyarrhythmias due to sympathetic excitation. The effects of these drugs on the atrioventricular node are consistent with the fact that these drugs may terminate reentrant paroxysmal supraventricular tachycardia and slow the ventricular response in atrial flutter and fibrillation. However, rarely do these agents convert atrial flutter-fibrillation to sinus rhythm except in those of recent onset. Either alone or in combination with other agents, beta blockers may be of value in preventing recurrent paroxysmal supraventricular tachycardia, both reentrant and ectopic. They are ineffective in arrhythmias complicating the Wolff-Parkinson-White syndrome in which the tachyarrhythmia is due to antegrade transmission over the bypass tract.

Beta blockers are not powerful suppressants of premature ventricular contractions except when sympathetically mediated, nor are these agents effective in controlling most forms of life-threatening ventricular tachycardias. They rarely suppress ventricular tachycardia inducible by programmed electrical stimulation of the heart. However, they are drugs of choice in the control of ventricular tachycardia/fibrillation complicating the hereditary long QT interval syndrome, which is due to "sympathetic imbalance" in the heart.[10] They are also effective in ventricular tachycardia induced by exercise. Except for sotalol, there is no evidence that different beta blockers have a differing spectrum of antiarrhythmic effects.

Control of Hypertension

Beta blockers are now used increasingly as first-line treatment of mild to moderate hypertension; however, the precise mechanism for their hypotensive effects is unclear. It may be multifactorial. They reduce cardiac output and plasma volume chronically and inhibit renin release. In experimental animals a central effect has been demonstrated. The hypotensive effects of beta blockers can be augmented in combination with diuretics, vasodilators, calcium antagonists, and other antihypertensive agents.

Miscellaneous Disorders

Beta blockers have been found to reduce the sympathetic manifestations of thyrotoxicosis and thyroid storm,[11] acute alcohol withdrawal, and attacks of migraine. In these conditions an agent without ISA is generally more effective. In hypertrophic cardiomyopathy, beta blockade has reduced provocative outflow tract gradient, ameliorated the diastolic abnormalities of the ventricle, increased exercise tolerance, and reduced symptoms of ischemia.[12] However, it appeared to have no effect on muscle hypertrophy, the incidence of sudden death, or ventricular arrhythmias. Chronic therapy may lead to cardiac failure. Recent studies have suggested that carefully administered doses of a beta-blocking agent may be effective in improving hemodynamic function and exercise tolerance in patients with dilated cardiomyopathy.[13]

Contraindications and Side Effects

These are predictable on the basis of the known pharmacodynamics of beta blockers. When given acutely, these agents may produce excessive bradycardia, sinus arrest, atrioventricular block, asystole, and hypotension, which may be reversed by the use of sympathomimetic amines or glucagon. Acute bronchospasm or acute pulmonary edema has also been known to occur following single intravenous doses of beta-blocking compounds. These agents are therefore contraindicated in patients with conduction system disease, impaired ventricular function, and bronchospastic disease. They also aggravate depression and vasospastic disorders such as Raynaud's phenomenon. In insulin-dependent diabetes, they may interfere with control of diabetes. Often the most striking unwanted reactions are fatigue, central nervous system depression, and impotence. It has been suggested that cardioselective agents have a lower propensity to produce fatigue and that agents that are hydrophilic lead to less central nervous system disturbances than do those that are lipophilic. It should be emphasized that the major therapeutic effects as well as the adverse reactions of beta blockers are related to their ability to block beta receptors. Therefore, clinically, the net effects of different agents are similar and the potential differences of direct clinical relevance slight. However, familiarity with these nuances is sometimes of value in an individual patient requiring beta blockade. The recent introduction of esmolol, a short-acting beta-blocker with rapid onset of action, short half-life (9 minutes), and rapid reversal of effects upon discontinuation, may provide an increased margin of safety, particularly in the perioperative setting for control of tachyarrhythmias[13a] and hypertension[13b] and in acutely ischemic patients.[13c]

CORONARY DILATORS: NITRATES AND CALCIUM CHANNEL BLOCKING DRUGS

These two groups of agents, one old and the other relatively new, have gained prominence recently because of the increasing appreciation of the dynamic nature of coronary arterial obstruction in the pathogenesis of myocardial ischemia in patients with coronary artery disease.[14] This has provided an additional impetus for the development of calcium antagonists because of the demonstration of the ubiquitous role of calcium in many physiologic processes, the abnormalities of which appear to underlie numerous cardiocirculatory disorders. The spectrum of therapeutic utility of calcium antagonists appears to be at least as wide as that of beta-adrenergic blocking agents.

NITRATES

Although nitroglycerin was introduced in cardiovascular therapeutics over a century ago for the relief of angina pectoris, its precise mechanism of action is still debated.[15] However, it is known that this three-carbon organic nitrate acts primarily to relax vascular smooth muscle, so that the overall hemodynamic effects of the compound reflect a balance between its coronary vasodilator actions and those due to peripheral venodilator and arteriolar dilator actions with the attendant reflex effects on heart rate and cardiac contractility. In the periphery, the strongest effect appears to be exerted on the venous capacitance vessels. It is thought that the drug exerts fundamental actions to relax smooth muscle by combining with the sulphydryl groups of nitrate receptors on the smooth muscle membrane. It is possible that nitrates may also act by augmenting cyclic 3′,5′-guanosine monophosphate (GMP) formation and by inducing release of prostacyclin from vessel walls. Nitrates may relax smooth muscle in nonvascular tissue such as the esophagus.

Hemodynamic Effects

Nitrates, regardless of the route of administration, reduce preload and afterload and produce reflex increases in heart rate and contractility. The cardiac output may decrease if the filling pressure is normal, because the reduction in preload exceeds that in afterload. In patients with elevated ventricular filling pressure, cardiac output may increase as nitrates may reduce the increased filling pressures into the optimal range. The overall effect may also be altered in the presence of myocardial ischemia.

It must be stressed that rarely the reflex sympathetic drive may lead to worsening of myocardial ischemia in patients with fixed atherosclerotic coronary artery disease, although in most patients the reduction in myocardial ischemia leads to an amelioration of ischemia. The beneficial effects in ischemia may also be mediated through dilatation of coronary stenosis at sites in which the narrowing is due to an eccentrically placed plaque.[14] In fact, lesion dilatation is now thought to be an important mechanism of the antiischemic action of nitrates,[15] an action that may be additive to that mediated through a reduction in myocardial oxygen consumption due to reduced afterload and reduced ventricular wall tension following a decrease in preload. Finally, the antiischemic effects of nitrates may also result from relief of focal coronary artery spasm.

Nitrate Formulations

Sublingually administered nitrates have been used for relief of individual episodes of angina for over 100 years. Little doubt exists about their efficacy. In recent years numerous preparations have been developed to prolong the action of nitrates for prophylactic use in the treatment of angina and heart failure.

By altering the molecular structure, a number of synthetic nitrate esters with longer elimination half-lives than nitroglycerin (eg, isosorbide dinitrate, erythritol tetranitrate, and pentaerythritol tetranitrate) for oral and topical use has been introduced. The use of various delivery systems has also led to the formulation of long-acting nitroglycerin. Therefore, in addition to intravenous and sublingual nitroglycerin, long-acting topical, transmucosal, and transdermal nitroglycerin preparations are now available for prophylactic therapy in myocardial ischemic syndromes, heart failure, and possibly hypertension.

The salient features of the currently available nitrate preparations are summarized in Table 63.5. Although the bioequivalence of these newer preparations has been deemed satisfactory, their efficacy remains to be established by stringently controlled clinical trials. There is evidence that tolerance to these agents may develop especially during the use of the longer acting formulations; neither the precise nature of the tachyphylaxis nor its magnitude is certain at present, and further studies are needed to define the regimens that might be effective in various clinical indications.[16]

Clinical Uses of Nitrates in Cardiac Disorders

Ischemic myocardial syndromes remain the major indication for the use of intravenous, sublingual, oral, transmucosal, or transdermal preparation of nitrates. There is substantive evidence that nitrates relieve anginal attacks, prolong exercise capacity, minimize electrocardiographic evidence of myocardial ischemia, and reduce the frequency and duration of silent ischemic myocardial episodes documented by Holter recordings in patients with coronary artery disease. Nitrates are effective in Prinzmetal angina, unstable angina, and chronic stable angina. An unequivocal superiority of nitrates over calcium channel blockers in unstable or Prinzmetal angina has not been demonstrated. However, there is a clear rationale for combining nitrates with beta blockers or calcium antagonists in the treatment of angina in relation to the hemodynamic properties of these agents.

Numerous studies have also indicated that in patients with congestive heart failure or pulmonary edema nitrates may acutely reduce mean pulmonary wedge pressure and increase cardiac output. These agents may also be used

Table 63.5. Dosage Kinetics of Nitroglycerin and Long-Acting Nitrates

Medication	Usual Dosage (mg)	Onset of Action (min)	Duration of Action
Sublingual NTG	0.3–0.6	2–5	10–30 min
Intravenous NTG	0.6–12.0 mg/h	. . .	During infusion and 30 seconds post infusion
Sublingual and chewable ISDN	2.5–10	3–15	1–2 h
Sublingual and chewable ET	5–15, 10	3–15	2 h
Oral NTG (SR)	2.5–9	30–45	2–8 h*
Oral ISDN	5–30	15–30	3–6 h*
Oral ISDN (SR)	20–40	30–40	6–10 h
Intravenous ISDN	1.25–5.0 mg/h	Minutes	During infusion
Oral ET	10	30	Variable
Oral PET	10–40	30	3–6 h
Oral PET (SR)	30–80	Slow	6–10 h
NTG ointment (2%)	1/2–2 inches	20–60	3–8 h
Transdermal NTG (Ciba-Geigy)	5–10	30–60	Up to 24 h
Nitrodur® (Key)	10–20 cm^2	30	Up to 24 h
Nitrodisc® (Searle)	5–10	30–60	Up to 24 h

*Duration increases with increasing dosage.

ET = erythritol tetranitrate; ISDN = isosorbide dinitrate; NTG = nitroglycerin; PET = pentaerythritol tetranitate; SR = sustained released.

in the chronic treatment of congestive heart failure especially in conjunction with vasodilators such as hydralazine. Whether long-term administration of nitrates in congestive cardiac failure leads to the development of tolerance is uncertain.

Intravenous Nitrates in Cardiovascular Therapy

The development of intravenous formulations of nitroglycerin has led to its use in a variety of cardiovascular disorders. Infusions may be used in dilutions ranging from 25 to 400 μg/ml, with the concentration based on the patient's fluid requirements. The initial dosage is usually 5 μg per minute with increases of about 4 μg per minute every three to five minutes until the desired response is obtained. Higher infusion rates and more rapid increases in the dosage regimen may be permissible in individual patients in relation to the predetermined level of hemodynamic function. Intravenous nitroglycerin infusions have been used in complicated myocardial infarction, unstable angina, coronary vasospasm, pulmonary edema, and hypertension during coronary bypass surgery or neurosurgical procedures. At high concentrations, nitroglycerin is a potent arteriolar dilator while being a powerful venodilator.

Side Effects and Contraindications

The main contraindication to nitrate therapy is marked hypotension. The side effects of various nitrate preparations are predictable: headaches, postural hypotension, syncope, and, less commonly, palpitations. Rarely, a marked decrease in blood pressure may impair coronary perfusion with aggravation of ischemia and angina. Very uncommonly, nausea and paradoxically bradycardia have been reported. The phenomenon of nitrate withdrawal may develop after the abrupt cessation of therapy.[17]

CALCIUM CHANNEL BLOCKING DRUGS

It is over 20 years since the prototype of calcium antagonists, verapamil, was first introduced. Rapid advances in our understanding of the pharmacodynamics of these agents and their clinical applications followed only after the important conceptual framework was provided by Fleckenstein in the early 1970s.[18] These drugs were found to block the slow channel in the heart while they blocked calcium fluxes in vascular smooth muscle; thus, they were all peripheral and coronary vasodilators.[19-22]

Classification of Calcium Antagonists

Fleckenstein[18] suggested that calcium antagonists may be classified into two categories. He placed agents such as verapamil, diltiazem, and nifedipine with its derivatives, which have a marked selectivity for inhibiting the slow channel versus the fast sodium channel in the heart, into one group (group A) and those such as prenylamine, terodiline, fendiline, and perhexiline, which also inhibit the slow channel but have a broad array of other electrophysiologic actions, into another group (group B). However, the expanding knowledge of the electropharmacologic aspects of these and newer agents suggests a need for an alternative classification. The one proposed in Table 63.6[22] appears to have clinical relevance.

Table 63.6. Clinical Classification of Calcium Antagonists

Type I. *Calcium antagonists with in vivo myocardial, electrophysiologic, and vascular effects:*		
	Verapamil	Diltiazem
	Gallopamil (D-600)	Tiapamil
Type II. *Calcium antagonists with predominant vascular effects in vivo:*		
	Nifedipine	Nicardipine
	Nitrendipine	Niludipine
	Nisoldipine	Felodipine
	Nimodipine	
Type III. *Calcium antagonists with selective vascular effects:*		
	Cinnarizine	
	Flunarizine	
Type IV. *Calcium antagonists with complex pharmacologic profile:*		
	Bepridil	Perhexilene
	Lidoflazine	

Type I: Calcium Antagonists with in vivo Myocardial Effects. Except for diltiazem, there are structural similarities among the other three compounds. All four are moderately potent peripheral and coronary vasodilators and are effective in mild to moderate hypertension. Their predominant electrophysiologic actions are to lengthen conduction time and to prolong refractoriness in the atrioventricular node, properties that account for their known antiarrhythmic effects especially in supraventricular tachyarrhythmias.

Type II: The Dihydropyridine Subgroup of Calcium Antagonists. Numerous dihydropyridine derivatives are currently under investigation for the control of a variety of cardiocirculatory disorders, depending on each drug's presumed specific pharmacologic properties. Of the newer compounds, these are the most closely related structurally. As a group, the potency of the dihydropyridines is much greater in relation to smooth muscle compared with cardiac muscle; these agents in vivo are nearly or completely devoid of clinically significant electrophysiologic properties, their overall hemodynamic effects being dominated by striking peripheral vasodilatation. From a therapeutic standpoint this may prove of particular value in the control of hypertensive emergencies as well as in the long-term management of essential hypertension either as single agents or in combination with diuretics, beta-adrenergic blocking drugs, or other hypotensive agents. It is also emphasized that because all of these agents produce marked reflex increases in heart rate and contractility, angina may be aggravated in some patients with coronary artery disease if concomitant sympatholytic agents are not used. The dihydropyridines may exert tissue selectivity.[23] For example, nimodipine appears to have selectivity of action in the cerebral vasculature.[23]

Type III: The Piperazine Derivatives: Flunarizine and Cinnarizine. The properties of the compounds in this type of calcium antagonist drug, namely, cinnarizine and its difluro derivative, flunarizine, are highly selective for calcium channels in vascular smooth muscle relative to cardiac muscle.[24]

The properties and therapeutic uses of flunarizine have recently been reviewed by Holmes et al.[24] Flunarizine has a much longer plasma elimination half-life than does cinnarizine. Most therapeutic trials with flunarizine have been in the prophylaxis of migraine, occlusive peripheral vascular disease, and vertigo of central and peripheral origin.

Type IV: Calcium Antagonists with Complex Pharmacologic Profile. Another group of pharmacologic agents that have a selectivity of action either for vascular tissues (eg, lidoflazine) or, in the case of perhexiline[25] and bepridil,[26,27,27a] for both cardiac as well as smooth muscle while also having the propensity to block the fast-sodium channel in the heart to a variable degree may be categorized as calcium antagonists. Some of these agents have yet other electrophysiologic properties. Therefore, not only are these agents heterogeneous chemically but also, by virtue of their overall complex pharmacologic properties, they may exert a somewhat different spectrum of therapeutic effects. This pertains particularly to their cardiac electrophysiologic actions and to the control of cardiac arrhythmias; bepridil is the most important in this regard, having a long elimination half-life (almost 40 hours).

Pharmacodynamic and Pharmacokinetic Properties

The bulk of available data pertain to the properties of verapamil, diltiazem, and nifedipine. Their structural features are shown in Figure 63.1 in relation to those of tiapamil and gallopamil (which are similar to verapamil).

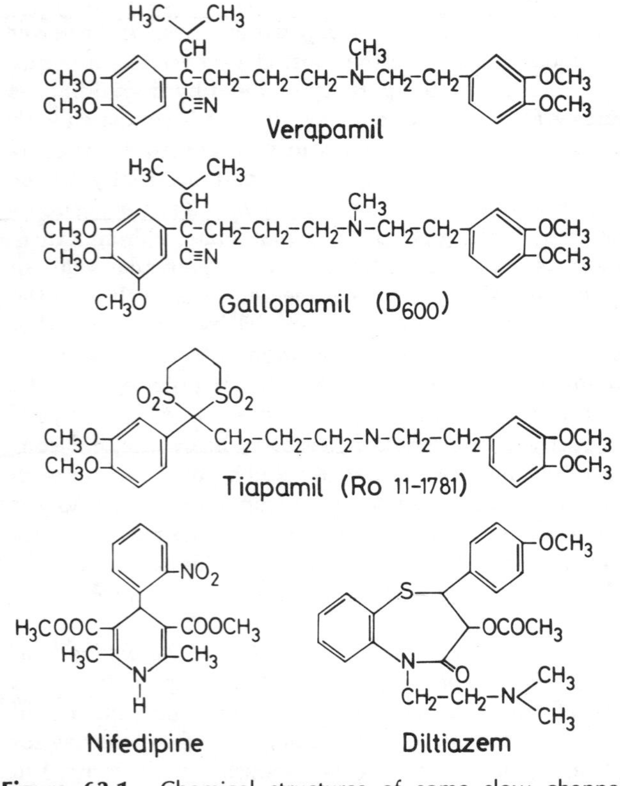

Figure 63.1. Chemical structures of some slow channel blocking drugs. Despite the structural heterogeneity, these compounds block the myocardial slow channel and calcium fluxes in the vascular smooth muscle. They are peripheral and coronary vasodilators.

Their in vitro and in vivo characteristics are summarized in Table 63.7. In isolated cardiac muscle, verapamil, gallopamil, diltiazem, and nifedipine block the slow inward current without much effect on the fast sodium channel. However, nifedipine in vivo has little effect on the electrophysiologic properties of the atrioventricular node.[27] Whether this is due to the fact that the marked peripheral vasodilator effects of the drug inducing reflex sympathetic effect nullifies or reverses the intrinsic negative dromotropic effects of the compound on the atrioventricular node and the negative chronotropic effects on the sinus node is not certain.[21] Other factors may contribute to the differences between the in vitro and in vivo effects of nifedipine and other dihydropyridines on the senoatrial and atrioventricular nodes. These effects of the various compounds are concordant with their observed clinical electrophysiologic actions. The clinical effects are dominated by the inhibition of intranodal conduction and prolongation of the effective and functional refractory period of the atrioventricular node in the case of type I calcium antagonists, with little or no effect on the refractory periods in the atria, ventricles, or accessory tracts of the heart.[27] The lack of effect on these tissues is consistent with the fact that neither type I or II nor type III calcium antagonists exert significant effects on the depolarization or repolarization phases of the fast-channel dependent cardiac action potentials.[21] These overall findings provide the basis for delineation of the effects of various types of calcium antagonists in different cardiac arrhythmias.

The hemodynamic effects of calcium antagonists are characterized by a complex interplay of simultaneous changes in the preload, afterload, heart rate, contractility, and coronary blood flow.[21] The net effect may be determined by the level of ventricular function, the presence or absence of myocardial ischemia, the state of the autonomic tone, and the properties of the individual compound. For example, diltiazem and verapamil have a noncompetitive sympatholytic effect that may attenuate the sympathetic stimulation that may follow in the wake of their albeit weak peripheral vasodilator action. For these reasons, verapamil has a variable effect on heart rate and diltiazem generally a depressant one, whereas nifedipine and other dihydropyridines almost invariably produce tachycardia because they do not exhibit sympatholytic actions. In patients with reduced ventricular function, verapamil may aggravate cardiac decompensation; this is less common with diltiazem and least common with the dihydropyridines such as nifedipine. The effects of calcium antagonists on the coronary circulation are similar. They are all weak epicardial dilators, but they dilate both the resistance as well as the capacitance vessels; they do not produce "coronary steal." They all have the propensity to dilate coronary artery lesions,[14] with a tendency to augment coronary sinus flow.

The pharmacokinetic features and dosage schemes for the three commonly used calcium antagonists are outlined in Table 63.8. The significant interaction between digoxin and verapamil should be emphasized; this interaction is either minimal or absent in the case of diltiazem and nifedipine. However, diltiazem is known to interact markedly with cimetidine.

Table 63.7. Comparative Experimental and Clinical Electrophysiologic Effects of Calcium Channel Blockers

	Verapamil	Nifedipine	Diltiazem
1. Inhibitory effects of cardiac slow-channel (in vitro)	+++	++++	+++
2. Relaxation of smooth muscle			
(in vitro)	+++	++++	
(in vivo)	+++	++++	+++
3. Nonspecific sympathetic antagonism	+	0	+
4. Effect on heart rate			
Isolated atria	↑+++	↓++++	↓+++
Intact organism and man	↑↓	↑	↓
5. Effect on atrioventricular conduction			
In isolated heart	↓+++	↓++++	↓+++
In intact organism and man	↓++++	0 to ↑	↓+++
6. Clinical electrophysiologic properties			
RR interval	↓↑	↓	↑↓
QRS	0	0	0
Q-Tc	0	0	0
PR	↑	0	↑
AH	↑	0	↑
HV	0	0	0
Atrial ERP	0	0	0
AV node ERP	↑↑	±	↑
AV node FRP	↑↑	±	↑
Ventricular ERP	0	0	0
His-Purkinje ERP	0	0	0
Bypass tract ERP	±	0	?
Sinus node recovery time	0*	0	0*
Ventricular automaticity	0	0	0

* Prolonged in sick sinus syndrome.

↓ = decrease, ↑ = increase; ↑↓ = variable effect; + → ++++ = indicates graded intensity of effect; ERP = effect refractory period; RFP = functional refractory period.

Therapeutic Applications of Calcium Antagonists

The clinical indications are summarized in Table 63.9. The major ones are for certain cardiac arrhythmias, ischemic myocardial syndromes, hypertension, and hypertrophic cardiomyopathy.

Supraventricular Arrhythmias. When these agents are given intravenously, paroxysmal reentrant supraventricular tachycardia is promptly terminated in most cases, especially after verapamil; the ventricular rate is slowed in atrial flutter and fibrillation, with rare cases converting

Table 63.8. Pharmacokinetics and Side Effect Profiles of Three Major Calcium Channel Blockers

	Verapamil	Nifedipine	Diltiazem
Absorption	90%	90%	90%
Bioavailability	10–20%	45–65%	24–90%
Protein binding	85–95%	90–98%	75–80%
Therapeutic plasma concentration	80–100 ng/ml	25–100 ng/ml	40–80 ng/ml
Oral dose (tid or qid)	80–120 mg	10–40 mg	30–90 mg
Metabolism	Extensive demethylation in liver (85% first-pass effect) but saturable	Metabolized to inactive acid or lactone by liver	Deacetylated glucuronidated in liver (50% first-pass but saturable)
Active metabolite	Norverapamil	...	Deacetyldiltiazem
Elimination half-life	3–7 h (increases with time)	1.5–6 h	2–6 h
Recovered in urine	70%	80%	30–40%
Recovered in feces	15%	15%	60%
Major interactions	Digoxin	...	Cimetidine
Overall side effects*	9–15%	9–39%	1–5%
Hypotension	+	+++	+
Headaches	+	+++	+
Peripheral edema	++	+++	++
Constipation	±	+	++
CHF	+	+	++
AV Block	++	±	++
Hepatotoxicity	+	?	?

* These are crude estimates rather than from controlled studies.

AV = atrioventricular; CHF = congestive heart failure.

Table 63.9. Therapeutic Applications of Calcium Antagonists

A. Established clinical indications
1. Ischemic myocardial syndromes
   a. Prinzmetal angina
   b. Unstable angina
   c. Chronic stable angina
2. Cardiac arrhythmias
3. Hypertension and hypertensive emergencies
4. Hypertrophic cardiomyopathy

B. Potential indications
1. Cardioprotection
2. Pulmonary hypertension and afterload reduction
3. Migraine and cluster headaches
4. Cerebral insufficiency
5. Raynaud's phenomenon
6. Disorders of gastrointestinal motility
7. Exercise-induced bronchospasm
8. Prevention of atherosclerosis

to sinus rhythm. Verapamil is generally given at a dose of 0.145 mg/kg intravenously over 30 to 120 seconds, diltiazem at 0.15 to 0.25 mg/kg intravenously over 1–2 minutes. The role of the oral drugs in the prophylaxis of recurrent arrhythmias is less certain. Type I calcium antagonists are highly effective in reducing the ventricular response in atrial flutter and fibrillation at rest as well as during exercise. They are effective alternatives to beta blockers and digoxin in this setting. The effect of calcium antagonists in multifocal atrial tachycardia is generally poor, although they may occasionally be effective. Their role in ectopic atrial tachycardia is poorly defined.[28]

Ventricular Arrhythmias. Calcium antagonists have a limited role in the control of ventricular tachyarrhythmias except in cases in which ventricular tachycardia or fibrillation is due to coronary artery spasm. They are weak suppressants of premature ventricular contractions in either normal subjects or those with organic cardiac disease; they rarely suppress ventricular tachycardia inducible by programmed electrical stimulation. The effects of bepridil, perhexiline, and lidoflazine, which do increase ventricular and atrial refractoriness, are not defined. Calcium antagonists are effective in controlling ventricular tachycardia induced by exercise in patients with coronary artery disease; they appear to be effective also in young patients without organic heart disease but with ventricular tachycardia with the right bundle branch block morphologic characteristics associated with left axis deviation, an arrhythmia that may be due to triggered automaticity.

Myocardial Ischemic Syndromes. Calcium antagonists are potent coronary vasodilators and may antagonize a vasoconstrictive tendency in various anginal syndromes. It has also been shown that these drugs reverse or negate the vasoconstrictive effects of ergonovine on the coronary arteries, and they prevent the sympathetically mediated vasoconstriction induced by handgrip or other physiologic interventions.[14] Therefore, unlike the effects of beta blockers, a significant action of calcium antagonists in ischemic syndromes may be mediated by their effects on coronary vessels over and above those on myocardial oxygen consumption.

Variant or Prinzmetal Angina. The advent of calcium antagonists has constituted a major advance in the control of variant angina. All the available agents (eg, verapamil, diltiazem, or nifedipine and those currently under investigation) have been found to reverse coronary artery spasm and reduce the frequency of ischemic episodes as judged by symptoms as well as ST-segment deviation documented on Holter recordings.[29,30] Clinical studies have shown no significant differences among various calcium antagonists with respect to their effects on coronary hemodynamics in man.[21] Neither has there been evidence of a striking difference in the potency of individual types of various calcium antagonists (types I, II, and III) in the control of Prinzmetal variant angina.[29] The overall clinical impression is that over 80% of patients with Prinzmetal angina respond to calcium antagonists.[30]

Unstable Angina. Nearly all cases of unstable angina occur in the setting of advanced coronary artery disease and, as already indicated, there may be a significant incidence of abnormal coronary vasomobility in these patients. Numerous studies have established the effectiveness of calcium channel blockers in relieving symptoms of unstable angina and reducing the electrocardiographic abnormalities that accompany symptomatic ischemia. The efficacy of intravenous calcium antagonists in unstable angina remains to be established, nor is it established that these agents prolong survival or avert infarction in unstable angina.

Chronic Stable Angina. Verapamil and its congeners, nifedipine and diltiazem, have been shown to reduce the frequency of angina and the number of sublingual nitroglycerin tablets consumed while they increase exercise capacity during treadmill testing and delay the onset of ischemia as judged by electrocardiographic parameters.[30] These drugs also elevate the anginal threshold and attenuate the ischemic manifestations during rapid atrial pacing in patients with coronary artery disease undergoing cardiac catheterization.[31] They also reduce the extent of decrease in left ventricular ejection caused by ischemia induced by either exercise or rapid atrial pacing.[32]

It is in the setting of chronic stable angina that a significant difference in the overall effects of type I and II calcium antagonists becomes clearly evident. For example, type I calcium antagonists tend to have a heart rate-lowering effect, whereas the dihydropyridines (eg, nifedipine) may induce significant tachycardia. In a proportion of such patients this may lead to an increase in oxygen demand and aggravation of ischemia, and rarely myocardial infarction may be precipitated. Therefore, the dihydropyridines are best used in combination with beta blockers in patients with chronic stable angina.

Hypertension. Although the vasodilator properties of calcium antagonists have been recognized for many years, it is only recently that these agents have begun to be used in the control of hypertensive emergencies and in the control of mild to moderate essential hypertension. In the chronic treatment of essential hypertension, the response is dependent on the initial level of arterial pressure, but it is independent of the renin status of the patient. There is some evidence that the older patient may be more responsive.

When calcium antagonists are given orally or intravenously in patients with hypertension, they reduce systemic vascular resistance, increase cardiac output, and increase stroke volume index. These properties have been used in the treatment of hypertensive emergencies with or without encephalopathy. Numerous studies have indicated that verapamil, nifedipine, and diltiazem are as potent as beta blockers or diuretics in the control of mild to moderate systemic hypertension.[33,34] As might be expected, there does not appear to be a significant difference in efficacy among the different agents. However, in hypertensive emergencies, the strikingly rapid onset of action and the potent vasodilator properties of the dihydropyridines are clearly different from the activity of the other calcium antagonists.

Hypertrophic Cardiomyopathy. Because hypertrophic cardiomyopathy is characterized by augmented systolic ventricular performance and impaired diastolic function, calcium antagonists might be expected to be effective in normalizing the hemodynamic abnormalities of the disease and in ameliorating symptoms. The data with verapamil suggest that intravenously and orally administered drugs produce an improvement in the diastolic function in patients with hypertrophic cardiomyopathy; the overall effect is similar to that found with propranolol.[35] However, as with propranolol and other beta blockers, there is no evidence that verapamil alters the incidence of serious ventricular arrhythmias and sudden death or halts the progression of ventricular hypertrophy. The effects of other type I calcium antagonists are likely to be similar, but because the dihydropyridines are much more potent vasodilators, they are likely to be less effective.

Calcium Antagonism and Other Miscellaneous Disorders

Numerous studies in a wide variety of cardiovascular and noncardiovascular conditions suggest that the overall spectrum of therapeutic utility of calcium antagonists is exceedingly wide. Calcium antagonists may be effective in the control of migraine and cluster headaches[36]; they may prevent or minimize cerebral damage in cases of developing strokes by reversing cerebral vasoconstriction.[23] Certain calcium antagonists (eg, verapamil) reduce platelet aggregability, but the clinical relevance of this property has not been established. Similarly, although the cardioprotective effect of calcium antagonists in experimental animals has been clearly demonstrated, the clinical utility of this finding in the survivors of acute myocardial infarction or during cardioplegia at open heart surgery remains to be determined.

Contraindications and Side Effects

The contraindications to the use of calcium antagonists vary somewhat in relation to the individual agent. For example, in the case of type I agents, especially in the presence of conduction system disease, sinus arrest, atrioventricular block, and even asystole may develop, especially in a beta-blocked patient and when these agents are administered intravenously. These effects may be reversed by the administration of intravenous calcium, isoproterenol, or glucagon. Pacing may be required in some patients. Atrioventricular block may also develop during chronic therapy especially with the use of verapamil and to a lesser extent with diltiazem; rarely may it follow the use of nifedipine especially if there is autonomic dysfunction. Cardiac failure may develop after verapamil and diltiazem and sometimes after nifedipine. The side effects attributed to nifedipine are generally related to marked peripheral vasodilator actions, the commonest being leg edema and dizziness or syncope. The most common side effect caused by verapamil is constipation, but derangement of liver function tests and rarely hepatitis have been reported.

DIURETICS

The synthesis and characterization of diuretics, agents that inhibit the renal tubular reabsorption of sodium and chloride resulting in the excretion of a greater fraction of the glomerular filtrate into the urine, have been major advances in the development of drugs in the treatment of cardiac failure and other disorders accompanied by edema. These agents have also played a major role in the treatment of mild to moderate hypertension. The clinical utility and the mode of action of various diuretics in these conditions have been dealt with elsewhere in this book. Therefore, only a few salient features will be discussed herein.

The main classes of diuretics and their clinical pharmacologic characteristics are presented in Table 63.10.[37] Each class of agent often has distinctive chemical features and affects ion transport in different segments of the nephron. However, little is known about the precise biochemical or molecular basis of action of different diuretic agents.

CARBONIC ANHYDRASE INHIBITORS

These were the first orally active diuretics. They act by inhibiting the enzyme carbonic anhydrase in the proximal and distal tubules as well as in the collecting ducts. These agents have little effect on the glomerular filtration rate. The diuretic effect of carbonic anhydrase inhibitors is generally self-limited because of the metabolic acidosis that results from their action. Their overall potency is low, but they can be effective natriuretic compounds in patients with elevated levels of sodium bicarbonate. They are also of value in the treatment of glaucoma.

ORGANOMERCURIALS

Of the three agents, organomercurials, ethacrynic acid and furosemide, all of which exert their effects by inhibiting chloride transport in the thick ascending limb of Henle's loop, the organomercurials are the oldest agents. Their diuretic effects are ineffective after oral administration and are now rarely used.

ETHACRYNIC ACID

This compound can be administered orally or intravenously. In man it has little or no effect on renal blood flow or the glomerular filtration rate. It is likely that ethacrynic acid is converted to ethacrynic-cysteine, which is the active compound. During the action of the diuretic,

Table 63.10. Various Classes of Diuretics and Their Clinical Pharmacologic Features*

Generic Names (Brand names)	Usual Dosage	Onset (h)	Peak (h)	Duration (h)
A. Carbonic anhydrase inhibitor				
Acetazolamide (Diamox)	250–1,000 mg/day	1	2–4	8
B. Thiazides and related agents				
Chlorothiazide (Diuril)	500–2,000 mg/day	1	4	6–12
Hydrochlorothiazide (Esidrix)	25–100 mg/day	2	4	>12
Chlorthalidone (Hygroton)	100 mg/day	2	6	>24
Trichlormethiazide (Metahydrin, Naqua)	4–8 mg/day	2	6	24
Metolazone (Zaroxolyn)	5–10 mg/day	1	2–4	24–28
C. Mercurials				
Meralluride (Mercuhydrin)	0.5–2.0 ml IM	2	6–9	12–24
Mercaptomerin (Thiomerin)	0.25–2.0 ml IM	2	6–9	12–24
D. Loop diuretics				
Ethacrynic acid (Edecrin)	50–200 mg/day	Oral, 30 min IV, 15 min	Oral, 1–2 IV, 30–45 min	Oral, 6–8 IV, 2–3
Furosemide (Lasix)	40–120 mg/day	Oral, 1 IV, 10–15 min	Oral, 1–2 IV, 30–45 min	Oral, 6–8 IV, 2–3
E. Potassium-sparing diuretics				
Spironolactone (Aldactone)	25–200 mg/day	Gradual	1–3 days	2–3 days after administration
Triamterene (Dyrenium)	100–300 mg/day	2	6–8	12–16
Amiloride	5–10 mg/day	2	5–8	24

* Adapted from Cannon.[37]

20% to 25% of sodium chloride filtered may be delivered into the urine. By its action on the thick ascending limb of the nephron, urinary dilution is reduced and the urinary concentrating power is impaired. There is increased excretion of potassium and hydrogen in the increased volume of bicarbonate-free and chloride-rich urine, resulting in hypochloremic metabolic alkalosis. However, unlike the situation with the organomercurials, the diuretic effect of ethacrynic acid is maintained despite the electrolyte derangement.

FUROSEMIDE

The diuretic action of furosemide is similar to that of ethacrynic acid despite a marked difference in chemical structure. Furosemide can also be given intravenously or orally. In the usual therapeutic doses, furosemide does not depress renal function or the glomerular filtration rate. At large doses, furosemide inhibits carbonic anhydrase. Furosemide impairs urinary dilution to a lesser extent than does ethacrynic acid. *Bumetanide* also exerts its major action in the loop of Henle; like ethacrynic acid or furosemide, it can be used orally or intravenously.[37a]

THIAZIDE AND RELATED AGENTS

These agents, generally sulfonamide derivatives, exert their predominant action in the cortical diluting segment of the nephron. The major effect is to augment urinary chloride excretion, and they are now widely used as safe, effective, and orally active agents of moderate potency. At peak diuresis action, they facilitate the removal of 5% to 8% of the filtered load of sodium chloride. The thiazides depress glomerular filtration rate and renal blood flow. The individual agents differ with respect to their duration of action, maximal dosage for optimal diuresis, and potency for inhibiting carbonic anhydrase. During diuresis with these compounds, there is an increase in urinary potassium, titratable acid, and ammonium. The thiazides differ from the loop diuretics in not promoting urinary calcium excretion; therefore, in certain patients hypercalcemia may result. *Metolazone* is a quinethazone derivative, but its action is similar to that of the thiazides, although it does not depress renal blood flow or the glomerular filtration rate. Its action can be combined with that of the thiazides.

POTASSIUM-SPARING DIURETICS

These are agents that increase sodium excretion but retard the loss of potassium in the distal tubule. There are two types of these agents. The first, spironolactone, is the competitive inhibitor of aldosterone; the second, as exemplified by amiloride and triamterene, directly blocks distal potassium secretion. All three agents have a modest effect in producing natriuresis, removing 2% to 3% of the filtered sodium chloride load from the nephron during their peak actions. *Spironolactone* does not affect glomerular filtration or renal blood flow; it acts essentially in the distal convoluted tubules and the collecting ducts, its full effect being delayed for several days. Its overall effect is characterized by a weak natriuresis but inhibition of the potassium and hydrogen ion excretion induced by other diuretics. Because the compound is a competitive inhibitor of aldosterone, it is most effective in situations in which the circulating level of the hormone is high (ie, right heart failure and cirrhosis of the liver). In contrast, *triamterene* and *amiloride,* while producing a pattern of changes in the urine similar to that induced by spironolactone, have a completely different mode of action, which is incompletely understood. However, they do antagonize aldosterone action but not by competitive inhibition. Triamterene and amiloride may also depress renal blood flow and glomerular filtration rate. The potassium-sparing diuretics are best used in conjunction with diuretics that lead to potassium depletion; dangerous hyperkalemia may result when they are used alone, especially in patients with impaired renal function in whom they may also induce renal acidosis.

CLINICAL USES OF DIURETICS

These agents are used essentially for the control of edema due to cardiac, renal, and hepatic disease. The use of diuretics in the control of cardiac failure and essential hypertension has been dealt with elsewhere in this book. In the treatment of acute pulmonary edema, intravenous ethacrynic acid and furosemide have both been reported to be effective. The salutary effect is related to the onset of diuresis, although in the case of furosemide it was initially thought that the venodilator actions of the diuretic led to a decrease in the filling pressure of the left ventricle, with apparent clinical improvement before the onset of diuresis. The most recent data do not support earlier observations.

ADVERSE REACTIONS

These occur as a result of either the pharmacologic actions of the various classes of diuretics or the toxic or idiosyncratic reactions peculiar to individual compounds. Electrolyte and acid-base derangements during diuretic therapy may lead to hypovolemia and azotemia, hyponatremia, dilutional hypoosmolality, metabolic alkalosis, or acidosis. Hyperkalemia is most common with the potassium-sparing diuretics especially in patients with renal insufficiency. In the case of most diuretics the occurrence of hypokalemia is most significant in cardiac patients because it may aggravate cardiac arrhythmias especially in the setting of digitalis therapy. Both hyperuricemia and hypouricemia may occur.

Toxic manifestations include skin rashes after thiazides, abdominal pain after ethacrynic acid, hyperglycemia after thiazides or furosemide, and gynecomastia, impotence, and loss of libido in males and menstrual disturbances in females following the use of spironolactone. Ototoxicity following large intravenous doses of ethacrynic acid or furosemide has been reported. In recent years, following prolonged therapy in hypertension, it has been suggested that diuretics may be a risk factor in the acceleration of coronary artery disease.

VASODILATORS AND CARDIAC STIMULANT DRUGS

The treatment of cardiac failure by a reduction of impedance to ventricular ejection has been one striking example of pharmacologic therapy based on an understanding of the pathophysiologic aspects of disease.[38] The enthusiasm for this mode of therapy has not, however, detracted from the development of newer agents that improve pump performance by their direct inotropic actions. Vasodilator compounds are now also used widely in the treatment of hypertension and hypertensive emergencies. The clinical applications of vasodilators and cardiac stimulant drugs have been discussed at length in other sections of this book. Their pharmacology is briefly summarized in this chapter.

VASODILATORS

These agents have their major utility in the treatment of systemic (rarely pulmonary) hypertension and for impedance reduction in the the control of cardiac failure. The major classes of vasodilators are indicated in Table 63.11.

Arteriolar Dilators

As just indicated, *nitrates* relax venous smooth muscle with a lesser effect on systemic arterioles. Therefore, they reduce preload, but for adequate reduction of impedance they are usually combined with more potent arteriolar dilators such as *hydralazine* or *minoxidil.* These have little or no venodilator actions. *Hydralazine* has been used widely in the acute and chronic treatment of resistant cardiac failure. It increases cardiac output[39] which is most evident in patients with large left ventricular chamber size. Reflex tachycardia occurs in a proportion of patients undoubtedly accompanied by a positive inotropic effect. The vasodilator actions of hydralazine accompanied by relief of symptoms and improved hemodynamics are sustained over months of therapy in doses of 25 to 150 mg four times a day, but larger doses are sometimes necessary.[39] The metabolism of hydralazine occurs in the liver; the compound is acetylated and toxicity is greater in patients in whom acetylation is slow and who are particularly prone to develop the syndrome of systemic lupus erythematosus. This develops as a function of dose as well as duration of therapy in 10% to 20% of patients, especially those with hypertension. The syndrome, however, is reversible. The elimination half-life of the compound is short, but the duration of action is much longer, presumably because of the formation of its active metabolite. Barring the development of systemic lupus erythematosus, other side effects are minor but include nausea, fluid retention, pyridoxine-responsive peripheral neuropathy, and if not administered with a sympatholytic agent, reflex increases in heart rate and contractility; in

Table 63.11. Vasodilator Agents for Afterload Reduction

Compound	Site of Action	Dosage Regimens
Parenteral		
Sodium Nitroprusside	Arterial and venous	10–500 μg/min IV
Nitroglycerin	Venous >> arterial	10–60 μg/min or higher IV
Oral		
Isosorbide dinitrate	Venous >> arterial	10–60 mg, 4–6 hourly
2% nitroglycerin ointment	Venous >> arterial	0.5–2 inches, 4–6 hourly
Prazosin	Arterial and venous	1–6 mg, 8 hourly
Hydralazine	Arterial	25–100 mg, 6–8 hourly
Captopril	Arterial and probably venous	12.5–100 mg, 8 hourly
Trimazosin	Arterial and venous	50–300 mg, 8 hourly

a patient with atherosclerotic coronary disease, this may lead to increased angina or even myocardial infarction.

Minoxidil is available in the treatment of systemic hypertension and cardiac failure. Its hemodynamic effects in patients with cardiac failure resemble those of hydralazine.[40] Minoxidil is metabolized 90% in the liver; its elimination half-life is about 4 hours, but its therapeutic effect is manifest for about 24 hours. The role of minoxidil currently is unclear and limited to refractory cases because of the high incidence of fluid retention and often serious hypertrichosis.

Mixed Venous and Arteriolar Dilators

Included in this group are nitroprusside and alpha-adrenergic blocking drugs. *Nitroprusside*[41] produces a balanced relaxing effect on resistance as well as capacitance vessels, thus reducing preload as well as afterload but having inotropic properties. This increases cardiac output in patients with elevated ventricular filling pressure; if these are normal, cardiac output may decrease, the maximum beneficial effect occurring when the left ventricular end-diastolic pressure is maintained between 15 and 18 mm Hg. Following intravenous nitroprusside the effect is almost immediate, and because of its extremely short elimination half-life, it needs to be given by continuous infusion, the hypotensive effect dissipating within a few minutes of cessation of therapy. There is variability of response among patients, necessitating an individualized approach to dosage although the average dose is about 75 μg per minute. The infusion rate is determined by decrements in arterial or pulmonary artery wedge pressure. Nitroprusside is metabolized in the liver to thiocyanate, which may accumulate over a period of days with symptomatic, potentially lethal toxicity. In the treatment of cardiac failure, nitroprusside may be combined with cardiac stimulant drugs such as dopamine or dobutamine, as will be discussed. Rebound changes in both hypertension and cardiac failure can occur during abrupt withdrawal of nitroprusside infusion.

The underlying principle that accounts for the clinical utility of the alpha-adrenergic blocking drugs in the treatment of cardiac failure is that such agents block adrenergically mediated vasoconstriction in arterioles and venules. The oldest alpha-blocking drugs, *phentolamine* and *phenoxybenzamine*, inhibit both $alpha_1$ and $alpha_2$ receptors; in contrast, *prazosin* has a greater blocking effect on the $alpha_1$ receptors, with less effect on norepinephrine release. For this reason, prazosin produces less reflex tachycardia.

Prazosin has been widely used in hypertension and has been extensively studied in the control of cardiac failure.[42] Its effects on systemic hemodynamics resemble closely those of intravenous nitroprusside; like nitroprusside, it does not exert a positive inotropic effect. After single doses the effect of the drug may last six hours, but tolerance may develop, the underlying mechanism of which remains unclear. The "first-dose" phenomenon with prazosin is often striking, with the development of severe and abrupt hypotension. The metabolism of prazosin occurs essentially in the liver, with less than 10% being excreted unchanged in the urine. The half-life of prazosin, normally 2.5 hours, may be increased to four to six hours, but the kinetics of the drug are not altered by renal insufficiency. Beneficial effects with prazosin may be evident with doses of 3 mg daily (in three divided doses), but larger doses (16 to 24 mg per day) are often required for sustained effect in hypertension and cardiac failure. However, in the latter case, the development of tolerance may constitute a significant problem. The side effect profile of prazosin is essentially benign. It is characterized by fluid retention, orthostatic hypotension, headache, weakness, nausea, and rarely priapism.

Phentolamine and *phenoxybenzamine* are now rarely used in therapeutics. Both are vasodilators, with arteriolar dilatation predominating. Phentolamine is used intravenously for constant infusion, but the kinetics of long-term drug infusion are not known. Although oral doses of phenoxybenzamine may produce long-lasting alpha-adrenergic blockade, its clinical use has been limited. Little is known about its metabolism and disposition. Nasal congestion, orthostatic hypotension, and inhibition of ejaculation may be seen following alpha-adrenergic blockade with phentolamine and phenoxybenzamine.

Angiotensin-Converting Enzyme Inhibitors

Both congestive cardiac failure and hypertension are characterized by increases in systemic vascular resistance in the resting state. In many such patients, there is an increase in the level of angiotensin II, inhibition of the formation of which leads to a reduction in systemic vascular resistance and ventricular afterload and an increase in cardiac output with improvement in ventricular performance. The synthesis and characterization of the orally active angiotensin-converting enzyme inhibitors, *captopril*[43] and *enalapril*,[44] have provided a new approach to the treatment not only of hypertension but also of cardiac failure resistant to nonspecific vasodilators.

Sustained symptomatic and hemodynamic improvement has been reported with chronic therapy of cardiac failure with *captopril*. The drug has been found to reduce preload as well as afterload. The beneficial effect of the drug does not always correlate with the renin status of the patient, suggesting that other pharmacologic effects of the drug may be involved. Captopril is usually given in doses of 25 to 150 mg, every eight hours; 75% of the drug is absorbed. The drug is metabolized by oxidation to mixed disulfides, its elimination half-life being about four hours. Captopril is well tolerated but it may induce rashes, serum sickness with fever and rash, metallic taste in the mouth, and rarely agranulocytosis. Of particular importance is the development of proteinuria or the nephrotic syndrome in patients receiving long-term treatment with the drug. *Enalapril* is a nonsulphydryl angiotensin-converting enzyme inhibitor which, in doses of 10 to 40 mg/day orally, is effective in decreasing blood pressure in patients with essential hypertension and in improving the signs and symptoms of congestive cardiac failure. Unlike captopril, enalapril does not produce agranulocytosis, taste loss, rash, or proteinuria. Enalapril is well absorbed after oral administration; it is hydrolyzed to the active molecule, enalaprilat,[45] predominantly in the liver without further metabolism. Excretion is essentially renal. The elimination half-life of the compound is long, approximately 11 hours. The most common side effects of the drug include dizziness, headaches, and asthenia. More experience is needed with the compound to precisely define its role in cardiovascular therapeutics.

CARDIAC STIMULANT DRUGS

These include sympathomimetic amines, cardiac glycosides, and agents such as amrinone which exert direct positive inotropic effects on the heart.

Sympathomimetic Amines

The net hemodynamic effects of the *sympathomimetic amines* are a balance between their positive inotropic effects on the myocardium and their peripheral vascular actions with consequent reflex actions in relation to dose. Their beneficial as well as their deleterious effects may vary in relation to the clinical setting in which they are used and with the dosage regimens. For example, in patients with coronary artery disease, the tachycardia and increased contractility they produce may aggravate ischemia, and in the case of evolving infarction, infarct size may be increased and arrhythmias may be precipitated. For the increase in cardiac performance the commonly used agents are now *dopamine* and *dobutamine.* Norepinephrine is rarely used. When used in small doses (eg, less than 5 μg/kg per minute, *dopamine* increases renal blood flow and cardiac output with little effect on systemic resistance or heart rate. At larger doses, because of alpha-receptor augmentation, increases in systemic resistance occur followed by tachycardia and possibly arrhythmias. The usual initial doses of dopamine are 1 to 3 μg/kg per minute.

Dobutamine produces less tachycardia and fewer arrhythmias in doses in which it augments contractility. However, it lacks the beneficial effects on renal vasculature and produces less vasoconstriction than dopamine. Furthermore, dobutamine has the additional effect of decreasing the left ventricular filling pressure. The usual doses of dobutamine are 2.5 to 10 μg/kg per minute. Other sympathomimetic amines that may also be used include terbutaline, salbutamol, pirbuterol, and prenolterol.

Cardiac Glycosides

The role of *cardiac glycosides* in the therapy of cardiac failure is undergoing change. *Digoxin* is the most commonly used compound both parenterally as well as orally, digitoxin being rarely used now. The pharmacology of the drug has been described elsewhere in this book. It is now well established that digoxin exerts a positive inotropic effect on the normal and the failing heart, but only in the latter is the effect on contractility translated into an increase in cardiac output. There is evidence that the effect on contractility is most beneficial in patients with marked cardiomegaly and is maintained over several months. However, there is no evidence that cardiac glycosides exert a salutary effect on mortality in patients with cardiac decompensation. The available data do not support the use of these drugs in patients with mild cardiac failure, because they have serious or potentially serious side effects. The use of cardiac glycosides in severe cardiac failure is now also questioned in view of the increasing availability of newer vasodilators and nonglycoside-positive inotropic agents.

The role of digoxin is also undergoing change in the treatment of supraventricular tachyarrhythmias. The major action of the drug relevant to its use here is its ability to prolong intranodal atrioventricular conduction and refractoriness, essentially by its vagomimetic action. Whereas the compound has been, for many decades, the agent of choice for acute and chronic therapy in the control of the ventricular response in patients with atrial flutter and fibrillation, beta blockers and certain calcium antagonists (eg, verapamil and diltiazem) are now being used increasingly for this purpose. Similarly, for the termination and prophylaxis of recurrent paroxysmal supraventricular tachycardia, the use of digoxin is being increasingly superseded by newer modalities of pharmacologic treatment.

Amrinone

Amrinone and related compounds represent a new departure in the development of new compounds that exert a positive inotropic effect.[46,46a] The augmentation in contractility is effected by an increase in transcellular influx of calcium independently of alterations in adrenergic receptors, adenyl cyclase, or Na-K ATPase. The precise mechanism of the positive inotropic effect of amrinone is not understood; it is possible that it may act through the cyclic nucleotide system, but its action is not blocked by beta blockade. The drug is active intravenously as well as orally. It increases cardiac output and decreases systemic resistance and left ventricular filling pressure, changes that are not accompanied by major alterations in heart rate or blood pressure. The overall magnitude of the effect is comparable to that of dobutamine, and despite the decrease in coronary blood flow and increase in contractility, ischemia does not appear to be aggravated in patients with coronary artery disease. However, amrinone has been shown to increase experimentally induced myocardial ischemia, and therefore, the potential for the drug to worsen clinical ischemia exists. Much experience with the drug has been gained during acute intravenous treatment; the long-term effect on hemodynamics, symptoms, and mortality remains unclear. During acute infusion, premature ventricular contractions and nausea may be encountered, and during chronic oral therapy thrombocytopenia and nephrogenic diabetes insipidus have been reported. *Milrinone* and a number of similar compounds are currently under investigation.[46a]

ANTIARRHYTHMIC AGENTS

Since the introduction of quinidine into therapeutics in 1918, a great deal has been learned about the cellular and clinical electrophysiology of the heart, the genesis of cardiac arrhythmias, and the way in which antiarrhythmic drugs exert their salutary effects[7,47] in controlling disorders of impulse formation and impulse generation. The beneficial effects of antiarrhythmic compounds may be derived from their direct or indirect effects. The direct effect is usually mediated through a lengthening of the effective refractory period in the relevant cardiac tissue. For instance, the conversion of atrial flutter or fibrillation to sinus rhythm by the intravenous injection of sotalol is an example of the direct effect of the drug insofar as it lengthens the effective refractory period by prolonging the action potential duration. In contrast, the conversion by verapamil of ventricular tachycardia due to coronary artery spasm is an example of an indirect effect of an antiarrhythmic agent, because verapamil has little or no effect on the ventricular effective refractory period, but it is active in this setting by ameliorating ischemia by reversing spasm.[48] In discussing the antiarrhythmic properties of various compounds, it is essential to delineate the extent to which direct electrophysiologic effects of the compounds are modified by their indirect pharmacologic effects.[49]

The direct antiarrhythmic effects are best elucidated by studying the effects of these compounds on the gross parameters of the cardiac action potential, with particular attention to the changes effected by these drugs on depolarization, automaticity, excitability threshold, and particularly the time and voltage-dependent refractory period in various cardiac tissues in vitro (eg, atria, ventricles, Purkinje fibers, and nodal tissues) and in vivo in animals and man (eg, sinoatrial and atrioventricular nodes, atria, ventricles, His-Purkinje system, and bypass tracts). When this is done, the overall mechanism of action of antiarrhythmic agents falls reasonably discretely into four categories.[25,49,50] In the first category (class I) are compounds that inhibit the fast depolarizing current in cardiac muscle and influence variably the kinetics of the sodium channel. In the second category (class II) are compounds that essentially are inhibitors of sympathetic stimulation (especially beta blockers) and that do not normally influence the gross parameters of the normal cardiac action potential in fast-channel dependent myocardial fibers. Class III compounds are those that selectively or somewhat selectively lengthen the repolarization phase of the action potential with little or no effect on depolarization, and hence lengthen the voltage-dependent effective refractory period. Finally, class IV antiarrhythmic agents are compounds that selectively block the so-called slow channel in the myocardium, thus having the propensity to abort arrhythmias that arise on the basis of slow conduction due to abnormally generated slow responses in the heart. This framework continues to provide the basis for interpreting the actions of currently available as well as investigational antiarrhythmic compounds (Table 63.12). The salient pharmacokinetic and clinical pharmacologic features of various antiarrhythmic agents are summarized in Table 63.13.

FAST SODIUM CHANNEL BLOCKERS OR CLASS I ANTIARRHYTHMIC AGENTS

These agents are potent local anesthetic agents on nerves with a depressant action on cardiac fibers in lower concentrations. The dominant action of these agents is to depress the maximal rate of increase (hence conduction velocity) of the action potential, shifting the membrane-

Table 63.12. Electrophysiologic Classification of Antiarrhythmic Drugs*

	Depression of Fast Response	Inhibition of Sympathetic Activity	Homogeneous Prolongation of the Action Potential Duration	Depression of the Slow Response
Class Ia	Quinidine Procainamide Disopyramide	...	...	...
Class Ib	Lidocaine Mexiletine Tocainide Aprindine Diphenylhydantoin Ethmozin	...	...	...
Class Ic	Encainide Lorcainide Flecainide Cibenzoline Propafenone Encainide Indecainide Recainam	...	...	...
Class II	...	Propranolol and other β-antagonists	...	...
Class III	...	...	Amiodarone Bretylium Sotalol NAPA	...
Class IV	...	...	...	Verapamil D-600 Nifedipine Diltiazem Tiapamil Bepridil

*See text for details.

Table 63.13. Clinical Pharmacologic Properties of Antiarrhythmic Compounds

Drug	Usual Dosage (mg/day)	Dosing Intervals (h)	"Therapeutic" Serum (μg/ml)	Elimination Half-life (h)	Major Route of Elimination	Active Metabolite
*Quinidine	1,200–1,800	6–8	2–5	4–9	Renal, hepatic	?
*Procainamide	2,000–6,000	3–4	4–10	3–4	Renal, hepatic	Yes
*Disopyramide	300–900	6–8	2–5	5–8	Renal, hepatic	...
Tocainide	1,200–2,400	6–12	3–10	8–15	Renal	Yes
Lidocaine	1–4 μg/min	Constant infusion	1.5–6	1½	Hepatic	Yes
Phenytoin	300–400	8	10–25	20–26	Hepatic	...
Mexiletine	300–1,200	6–12	0.5–2	8–15	Hepatic	...
Encainide	50–200	6–12	0.01–0.1	2–4	Hepatic	Yes
Indecainide	100–200	8–12	?	4–6	Hepatic	?
Flecainide	200–400	8–12	0.3–1	12–24	Renal	?
Amiodarone	200–600	Once daily	1–2.5	15–150 days	Hepatic	Yes
Bretylium	5–10 mg/kg IV	8	0.5–1	7	...	...
NAPA	3,500 ± 900	8	20–35	7	Renal	...
Sotalol	320–640	9–12	1.5–3.0	12	Renal	...

* Long-acting preparations are available. The pharmacologic features of beta blockers and calcium antagonists are indicated elsewhere in this chapter.

responsiveness curve to the right and increasing the effective refractory period without a major effect on repolarization. They have little effect on membrane resting potential, but they depress phase 4 depolarization. They have little or no effect on the slow response fibers. These agents share certain common properties: their effects are more pronounced in partially depolarized fibers (eg, in ischemia), in hyperkalemia (converse in hypokalemia), and during fast-stimulation frequencies (so-called use-dependent effects). In man these agents widen the QRS interval, lengthen the HV interval, and prolong the effective refractory period in atria, ventricles, His-Purkinje system, and bypass tracts, ie, tissues in which the main depolarizing current is carried by sodium ions. As a group, these agents exhibit a wide spectrum of antiarrhythmic activity being effective in arrhythmias due to enhanced automaticity and to reentry, but they do not appear to be effective in those arrhythmias due to triggered automaticity. One other feature that has emerged from recent observations is that in ventricular arrhythmias in man, when these agents acutely prevent the arrhythmia inducible by programmed electrical stimulation of the heart (which they do in about 10% to 30% of cases), this effect correlates reasonably well with their long-term beneficial prophylactic effect.

Another feature that has emerged from experimental studies is the necessity to further classify the so-called class I agents into subcategories. This has followed in the wake of the understanding that these agents as a class do not behave in an identical manner either experimentally or clinically. The first attempt to do this was made by Singh and Hauswirth,[49] and recently the concept was further refined on the basis of either the changes in repolarization[51] that may accompany the major effects of these drugs on depolarization or the effects of the compounds on the kinetics of recovery from inactivation of the sodium channel[52] in relation to the receptor-modulated hypothesis.[53] The details of the subclassification of class I agents are presented in Table 63.12.

Class Ia Compounds

In addition to blocking the fast sodium channel, these agents variably lengthen the action potential duration in all cardiac tissues. This latter property appears to confer on these agents additional properties such as the propensity to convert atrial flutter and fibrillation to sinus rhythm. They slow the atrial rate in flutter and may accelerate the ventricular response in these conditions. Because these agents decrease conduction and increase the effective refractory period of the bypass tract, they are effective in slowing the ventricular response in atrial flutter and fibrillation complicating the Wolff-Parkinson-White syndrome. While being effective in most types of ventricular arrhythmias, they are contraindicated in torsades de pointes. They are not effective in exercise-induced tachycardia. The most significant agents in class Ia category are quinidine, procainamide, and disopyramide.

Quinidine. This is the oldest antiarrhythmic agent and continues to be used widely for the prophylactic control of supraventricular and ventricular arrhythmias. It is metabolized by hydroxylation in the liver, with a small amount being excreted in the kidney. Therefore, in heart failure and cirrhosis of the liver, metabolism is retarded and blood levels may increase disproportionately to the dose. The dose of the drug should be regulated by plasma level determinations. The longer-acting preparations (quinidine gluconate or polygalacturonate) are available. Intravenous formulations are available but are rarely used because of hypotension, although the intramuscular regimen may be used for acute drug testing during electrophysiologic studies. The use of quinidine for chemical conversion has largely been superseded by electrical cardioversion, but the drug continues to be used for maintaining stability of sinus rhythm following conversion of atrial fibrillation.

The overall electrical effects of quinidine in the atria and atrioventricular node may be modified by its anticholinergic effects and in all tissues by its alpha- and beta-adrenergic antagonistic actions. The major effects are however exerted on the QRS and QT_c intervals. Prolongation of these intervals should be monitored carefully, because depression of conduction and lengthening of repolarization may lead to torsades de pointes, the cause of the so-called quinidine syncope, which may be irreversible. The drug, as with all class Ia agents, is contraindicated in ventricular arrhythmias because of the long QT syndromes. Quinidine does not depress sinus frequency or atrioventricular nodal conduction except in patients with conduction system disease.

Recently, it was shown that quinidine increases the steady-state levels of digoxin, and dosage adjustment of these drugs is essential during combination therapy. The steady-state levels of quinidine are also increased by the concomitant administration of amiodarone, but the nature of this interaction is not well understood.

Not all the side effects of quinidine are related to the dose of the drug; idiosyncratic reactions (which includes torsades) are recognized. Following intravenous drug injection, sudden cardiovascular collapse can occur. Following oral therapy, the common side effects are diarrhea, headache, nausea, dizziness, cinchonism, visual disturbances, disturbed hearing, thrombocytopenic purpura, and agranulocytosis. Toxicity resulting from excess quinidine ingestion may result not only in torsades but also in severe bradycardia and atrioventricular block. Therapy to reverse the changes includes stopping the drug, decreasing potassium if elevated, acidification of the urine, and the administration of molar lactate to increase the serum concentration of sodium. Transvenous pacing and intravenous infusion of isoproterenol may also be helpful as in the case of toxicity with all class Ia agents.

Procainamide. The electrophysiologic properties of procainamide in isolated cardiac muscle and in intact animals and man closely resemble those of quinidine. However, unlike quinidine, procainamide has vasodilator actions and weaker anticholinergic actions. It produces less hypotension following intravenous injections and is therefore preferred to quinidine for acute parenteral administration.

When the drug is given intravenously, it is usually given at a dose of 100 mg every one to two minutes with blood pressure and electrocardiographic control to a total dose of about 1 g in the first hour; subsequently intravenous infusions may be used at a rate of 1 to 4 mg per minute. Orally the drug is given every three to four hours (preceded by a loading regimen), although with the slow release preparations (ie, Procan-SR ®), a much longer dosing interval is possible.[53a] The actual dosing regimen used in an individual patient is determined by the response, side effects, and plasma drug concentrations.

In man the action of procainamide is complicated by its metabolism (by slow or fast acetylation) in the liver to n-acetylprocainamide, which differs from the parent compound not only in its electrophysiologic prcperties but also in its pharmacokinetic properties (as will be described). In renal failure, the concentration of n-acetylprocainamide may increase significantly and not only may contribute to the antiarrhythmic effects of the parent compound but also may lead to arrhythmogenicity.

The clinical indications for procainamide closely resemble those of quinidine, but the side effect profile of the two drugs differs. Procainamide as a function of dose and duration of therapy, especially in those with slow acetylation, may produce immunologically mediated side effects including the production of high titers of antinuclear antibody resulting in the development of systemic lupus erythematosus in about 30% of patients treated for over six months. Other side effects include gastrointestinal disturbances, fever, joint pains, arthralgias and arthritis, pericarditis, and skin rashes. The drug may also increase the ventricular response in atrial fibrillation and flutter and occasionally produce heart block in cases of preexisting conduction system disease. The drug is contraindicated in shock, severe heart failure, myasthenia gravis, unstable heart block (unless pacemaker is in situ), and severe renal failure. Toxicity developing as a result of excess dosage may be treated in the same manner as that found during quinidine intoxication.

Disopyramide. The electrophysiologic properties and the spectrum of antiarrhythmic activity in supraventricular and ventricular arrhythmias of disopyramide are similar to those of quinidine, although the compound has more potent anticholinergic and negative inotropic effects.[54] These properties influence the drug's overall side effect profile. Disopyramide is available as the free base as well as the phosphate salt; the bioavailability of both formulations is similar. On oral ingestion, about 50% of the drug undergoes metabolism by N-dealkylation, the remainder being excreted unchanged in the urine. Therefore, the dose of the drug should be reduced in renal failure. One of the metabolites of disopyramide has a strong anticholinergic effect.

Oral disopyramide is generally given in a loading dose of about 400 mg, followed by a maintenance dose of approximately 600 mg per day in three divided doses. Long-acting slow release formulation of the drug is now available, permitting twice daily dosing.

As in the case of all class I agents the effects of disopyramide are affected greatly by serum potassium levels and, as in the case of quinidine, depression of conduction and prolongation of the QT interval may lead to torsades de pointes in a proportion of patients. The drug is not effective in digitalis-induced tachyarrhythmias. The drug is contraindicated in patients with depressed ventricular ejection fraction, especially those with a history of previous cardiac failure.[55] Disopyramide may also induce a negative inotropic effect in patients with beta blockade and in combination with certain calcium antagonists such as diltiazem and verapamil which have an intrinsic potential to depress cardiac contractility. There is no significant interaction between digitalis or lidocaine and disopyramide.

The side effects of disopyramide relate to its electrophysiologic effects, eg, in patients with the sick sinus disease the drug may induce sinus arrest either by itself or in combination with digoxin or other agents that exert a depressant effect on cardiac conduction. The development of torsades de pointes has also been documented in a proportion of patients given oral disopyramide. The anticholinergic effects include dryness of mouth, nausea, abdominal pain, visual disturbances, and urinary retention.

Class Ib Agents

These agents (Table 63.12) share certain common properties. First, although they are all fast channel blockers, they exert a relatively modest effect on conduction and refractoriness in healthy hearts; their effects are augmented in depolarized (diseased) or ischemic cardiac fibers. Second, these agents either have no influence on cardiac repolarization (eg, ethmozin) or they shorten it (eg, lidocaine, mexiletine, tocainide, phenytoin sodium, and aprindine). As a group, their use is associated with a low incidence of torsades de pointes. Aprindine and phenytoin have additional electrophysiologic properties that allow their use in the control of certain supraventricular arrhythmias. The major use of this class of compounds is to control ventricular arrhythmias.

Lidocaine and Its Oral Congeners. Lidocaine is most commonly used for the acute therapy of ventricular arrhythmias, especially those complicating acute myocardial ischemia or cardiac surgery.[56] The effects of the drug are exaggerated by hyperkalemia and reduced by hypokalemia. The exact electrophysiologic actions of lidocaine are still controversial.

Lidocaine is rapidly deethylated in the liver microsomes. Therefore, the levels of the drug in the plasma are greatly dependent on hepatic blood flow and on factors or concomitant drugs that influence hepatic microsomal activity. There is a marked effect requiring dosage reduction during cimetidine administration. The side effects of the drug include those related to central nervous system toxicity: drowsiness, numbness, speech disturbances, and dizziness. At higher plasma drug concentrations sudden respiratory arrest or convulsions may develop. Alternatively, the patient may lapse gradually or relatively suddenly into coma; the incidence of toxicity rises with age. Rarely does lidocaine induce ventricular fibrillation, but a sudden large bolus injection may produce complete atrioventricular block or asystole.

The use of lidocaine in the prophylactic treatment of ventricular arrhythmias complicating acute infarction is undergoing change. Although it has been shown to reduce the incidence of primary ventricular fibrillation in the setting of acute infarction, the relatively low incidence of the disorder in patients with transmural infarction, the lack of a relation between the so-called warning arrhythmias and the onset of ventricular fibrillation, and the high incidence of side effects with the effective dose regimen of the drug indicate that the routine use of lidocaine in this setting may not be warranted. Similarly, there is little evidence to indicate that the drug should be given routinely to patients admitted to the coronary care unit with unstable angina for the exclusion of acute myocardial infarction.

It has been postulated that if the patients with ventricular arrhythmias respond to the acute administration of lidocaine, its congeners, *mexiletine*[57] and *tocainide*[58] will be effective in the chronic prophylaxis of the same arrhythmia. This premise has not been completely substantiated. However, both mexiletine and tocainide are effective in the suppression of symptomatic and asymptomatic premature ventricular contractions, but their role in the prevention of sudden arrhythmic deaths has not been established. Uncontrolled studies indicate that in a relatively small number of patients these drugs prevent recurrence of symptomatic ventricular tachycardia. Their efficacy may be limited by the inability to use the optimal suppressant dose, because troublesome gastrointestinal (nausea, vomiting, and metallic taste) and central nervous system symptoms (ataxia, tremors, nystagmus, and disorientation) develop in a significant number of patients as the dose is escalated. In the case of tocainide, pulmonary fibrosis and agranulocytosis may also develop. There are some uncontrolled data to suggest that mexiletine and tocainide may be combined with other antiarrhythmic agents in doses at which side effects are less common.

Phenytoin Sodium (Dilantin®). The electrophysiologic effects of dilantin are well defined in experimental and clinical studies. Dilantin does not have a major depressant effect on cardiac conduction and may facilitate conduction and shorten the refractory period at the atrioventricular node. This effect is probably due to the anticholinergic effect of the agent. It mildly shortens the QT interval. The major use of the drug is in the treatment of digitalis-induced tachyarrhythmias and perhaps torsades de pointes. It was ineffective in reducing mortality in survivors of acute myocardial infarction. During chronic therapy the drug exerts a wide variety of side effects, among which are gingival hypertrophy, pulmonary infiltrates, megaloblastic anemia, and cerebellar toxicity, but they are all reversible. There is a pharmacokinetic interaction with amiodarone.

Aprindine. This is a powerful antiarrhythmic agent[59] which, apart from exerting effects on the fast channel, appears to have some slow-channel blocking propensity. Thus, it delays conduction at the atrioventricular node. It is effective in certain supraventricular tachycardias including those complicating the Wolff-Parkinson-White syndrome and has been effective in a proportion of patients with ventricular tachycardias resistant to the antiarrhythmic compounds. The clinical use of the drug is limited by its side effects, because it can produce severe agranulocytosis, hepatic toxicity, and central nervous system disturbances.

Ethmozin. This compound, developed in the USSR,[60] is a phenothiazine derivative. Its major action is mediated through inhibition of the fast sodium channel; therefore, its major use is in the treatment of ventricular arrhythmias. Its side effects include headache, dizziness, nausea, and vomiting. Its role in the treatment of various cardiac arrhythmias needs further delineation.

Class Ic Compounds

These agents, which are structurally heterogeneous, share numerous common electrophysiologic properties but differ in their overall effects because of differences in their kinetic as well as associated properties. The feature that distinguishes them from other class I agents is their propensity to markedly delay conduction with a lesser effect on refractoriness. Their effects on the reactivation kinetics of V_{max} are similar. They also have a differential effect on repolarization in the Purkinje fibers and ventricular muscle,[51] shortening it in the former and either having no effect or lengthening it in the latter (Figure 63.2).

The best known are *flecainide, encainide,* and *propafenone.* Also under investigation are *lorcainide, indecainide,* and *recainam.* These compounds are potent suppressants of premature ventricular contractions, some of them producing complete or near complete suppression in a significant numbers of patients but in concentrations at which there is often a striking lengthening of the QRS duration. The major drawback of these compounds is their propensity to aggravate ventricular arrhythmias, especially serious ones, often in patients with reduced ventricular ejection fraction.[61–65]

Flecainide. Flecainide is more potent in suppressing premature ventricular contractions than quinidine, suppressing them markedly after intravenous, short-term, or long-term oral therapies.[61,62] However, the effects of flecainide on recurrent symptomatic sustained ventricular tachycardia are less clear; the drug does not prevent reinduction in many patients, and although the premature ventricular contractions in this setting are eliminated, exercise-induced tachycardia may develop with use of the drug. At large doses, flecainide exerts some slow channel blocking actions and depresses the ventricular ejection fraction, producing cardiac failure in a small number of patients with reduced ventricular performance.

Encainide. The properties and clinical effects of encainide are similar to those of flecainide, but the electrophysiologic effects of encainide may not be immediately apparent. Its net effects during chronic therapy may be mediated by the formation of at least two active metabolites which have longer elimination half-lives. Encainide lengthens the PR interval, the nature of which is not understood. Preliminary studies have shown that the drug may be effective in terminating a variety of supraventricular arrhythmias with or without Wolff-Parkinson-

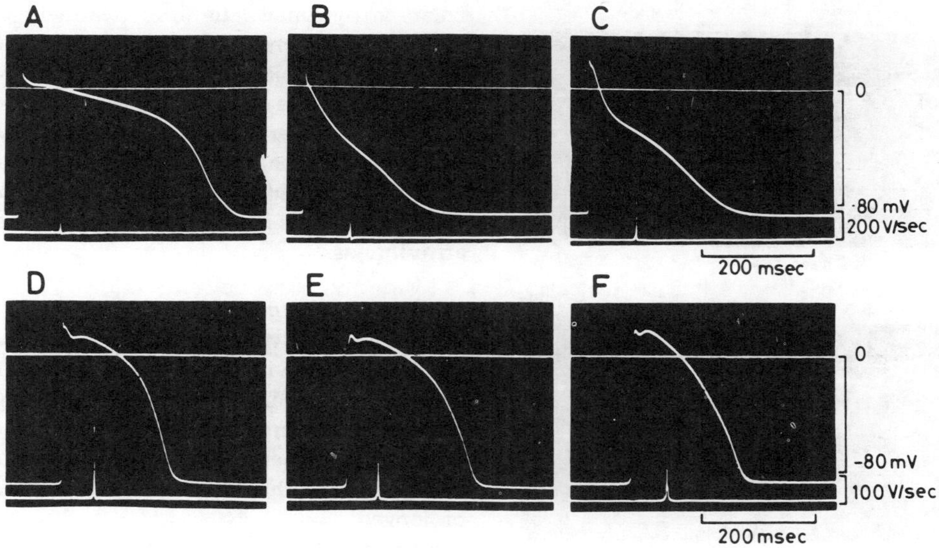

Figure 63.2. Differential effects of flecainide on the action potential duration in Purkinje fibers (*upper panel*) and in ventricular muscle (*lower panel*). *A,* Control in Purkinje fibers; *B,* after 10 μg/ml of flecainide; *C,* after elevation of extracellular calcium concentration. *D,* control in ventricular muscle; *E,* after 10 μg/ml of flecainide; *F,* on elevation of extracellular calcium. This differential effect is characteristic of class Ic sodium channel blockers including encainide and its metabolites, flecainide, indecainde, recainam, and propafenone.

White syndrome. The major use of the drug is in the suppression of symptomatic and asymptomatic premature ventricular contractions, but, as in the case of other class Ic agents, the role of encainide in ventricular tachycardia/fibrillation is not established, there being a major concern regarding its arrhythmogenic potential, especially in patients with reduced ventricular ejection fraction.

Propafenone. This agent differs from other class Ic agents on a number of counts.[66] It exhibits modest beta-blocking and calcium channel blocking properties while not depressing conduction to the same extent as is the case with flecainide or encainide. It produces a dose- and concentration-dependent increase in the AH interval with a lesser effect on QRS duration. Perhaps because it is less potent in depressing conduction, its arrhythmogenic potential also appears lower than that of encainide and flecainide. During short-term as well as long-term administration, the drug produces marked suppression of premature ventricular contractions in patients with and without heart disease.[66a] In a small number of patients the drug prevents the reinduction of ventricular tachycardia by programmed stimulation of the heart, but failure to do this does not, as in the case of amiodarone, preclude a favorable clinical outcome in patients with life-threatening ventricular arrhythmias. However, the effect of the drug on survival in this subset of patients remains to be defined. Because of the known pharmacodynamics of the drug, a wide spectrum of antiarrhythmic effects might be expected; the preliminary data are in line with these predictions.[66] The major side effects of the drug relate to central nervous system and gastrointestinal disturbances, but heart failure may be aggravated in patients with severely depressed ventricular function.

CLASS II ANTIARRHYTHMIC AGENTS

The most important agents in this class are beta blockers. Their electrophysiologic and pharmacokinetic properties and their use in arrhythmias have already been dealt with herein. It is emphasized that their role in the treatment of arrhythmias stems essentially from their ability to block beta-receptors. It should also be appreciated that many other antiarrhythmic agents may exhibit sympatholytic actions (a class II effect), which may be competitive receptor antagonism (eg, propafenone), adrenergic neurone-blocking action (eg, bretylium and bethanidine), or noncompetitive antagonism (eg, amiodarone, verapamil, diltiazem, and bepridil). However, such actions, in the case of these agents, are subsidiary ones but may contribute to their dominant antiarrhythmic effects achieved by other electrophysiologic mechanisms.

CLASS III ANTIARRHYTHMIC AGENTS

As just indicated, the concept of lengthening the action potential duration and hence the voltage-dependent refractoriness in cardiac muscle is a significant approach to the control of cardiac arrhythmias. Agents that do this in a selective manner do not appear to exert a depressant effect on cardiac function, have a lower incidence of arrhythmogenicity when compared with class I agents, and exert an antifibrillatory action. This effect may be of particular importance in the control of life-threatening ventricular arrhythmias. The concept of class III antiarrhythmic action has burgeoned with recent experience with the use of amiodarone in a variety of cardiac arrhythmias. The major compounds are bretylium, N-acetylprocainamide, (Figure 63.3), and amiodarone. Their pharmacokinetic and dosing schedules are summarized in Table 63.13.

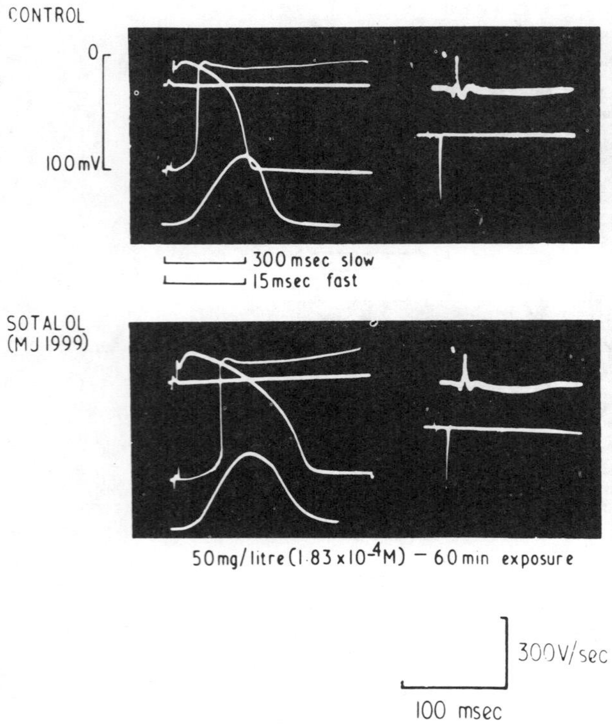

Figure 63.3. Effect of sotalol (in J1999) on the transmembrane action potentials recorded from cat papillary muscle. The horizontal line on the left at the top panel represents zero potential; the middle tracing represents the action potential at slow and fast sweep speeds. The bottom tracing represents isometric tension. The upper tracing on the right represents surface potential and the lower tracing, the differential signal for the maximal rate of increase of the action potential. Note that sotalol has little or no effect on the upstroke velocity (maximal rate of increase) of phase 0 or on isometric contraction. Its dominant effect is the lengthening of the action potential duration and hence, by inference, the effective refractory period (a class III action).

Bretylium

The factors responsible for the overall beneficial effects of bretylium are not fully defined.[67] The drug exerts a neurone-blocking action, but its administration is followed by the release of catecholamines which tend to increase heart rate by augmenting phase 4 depolarization. Subsequently, the effect on sympathetic excitation is blunted. The acute electrophysiologic effect is characterized by a lengthening of the action potential duration in ventricular tissues and Purkinje fibers but not in the atria. The effects of the drug on the atrioventricular node and the bypass tracts have not been established. The effect on ischemic myocardium is such that the drug tends to normalize the disparate changes in repolarization and refractoriness between ischemic and normal tissues, a feature that may be of importance in its well known beneficial actions in arrhythmias complicating acute myocardial infarction. Whether the drug is effective in controlling ventricular arrhythmias from causes other than myocardial infarction has not been convincingly established. There are no experimental or clinical data to indicate that bretylium might be effective in supraventricular arrhythmias. In the treatment of ventricular arrhythmias, there is a finite delay in the onset of action of the drug despite intravenous administration.

The major side effect of the drug is hypotension when it is used intravenously; when used orally, postural hypotension may be troublesome even if the drug is insufficiently absorbed. It is doubtful whether the drug has an important role in prophylactic oral treatment of cardiac arrhythmias.

N-acetylprocainamide (NAPA)

This is the active metabolite of procainamide produced by N-acetylation in the liver. This process results in three clinically significant differences when compared to those of the parent compound. The metabolite has no effect on conduction, it does not produce systemic lupus syndrome during chronic therapy, and the elimination half-life is prolonged.

Systemic studies have shown that the major electrophysiologic actions of NAPA are dominated by isolated lengthening of the action potential duration and the effective refractory period in the atria, ventricles, and the His-Purkinje system, without effecting sinus node automaticity or the atrioventricular node.[68] Although not well studied, the drug is likely to lengthen the refractory period of the bypass tracts. These clinical data are consistent with the effects of the drug in isolated cardiac muscle.[69] The drug has no significant effect on myocardial function and is devoid of major interaction with the autonomic nervous system.

NAPA has linear pharmacokinetics, being excreted essentially by the kidney. Preliminary data have suggested that the drug suppresses premature ventricular contractions and prevents reinduction of ventricular tachycardia by programmed electrical stimulation of the heart. Electrophysiologic properties suggest that NAPA is likely to be effective in the conversion of atrial flutter and fibrillation to sinus rhythm, but it is unlikely to be effective in terminating paroxysmal supraventricular tachycardia.

The major side effects of NAPA are gastrointestinal and central nervous system disturbances. Occasional cases of Coomb's positive hemolytic anemia, agranulocytosis, and allergic vasculitis have been reported; torsades de pointes may also develop in situations in which the concentrations of the drug rise to high levels. The clinical role of NAPA is under study.

Sotalol (MJ1999)

Although a beta-blocking agent, sotalol has recently drawn considerable attention as a class III antiarrhythmic compound established many years ago.[5] Both intravenously and orally, sotalol has properties that represent a composite of its beta-blocking actions and its propensity to lengthen the action potential duration and refractoriness in all myocardial fibers.[8,70] Thus, it slows the heart by decreasing sinus node frequency and it delays the conduction and lengthens the functional and effective refractory periods across the atrioventricular node. It prolongs sinus node recovery time, and lengthens the effective refractory period in the atria, ventricles, His-Purkinje system, and over the bypass tracts. It has no effect on

QRS duration, but it lengthens the QT and AH intervals without affecting the HV interval.

The elimination half-life of sotalol is long, permitting twice daily dosing schedules. It is excreted primarily by the kidneys. Given orally, it has a lower propensity to depress hemodynamic function in man than do other beta blockers. It is well tolerated during cardiac failure in most patients.

As an antiarrhythmic agent, sotalol has broad spectrum activity, being effective in supraventricular as well as ventricular arrhythmias. Acutely administered, it may convert atrial flutter and fibrillation to sinus rhythm; if conversion does not occur, the ventricular response is slowed. In a proportion of cases, intravenous drug administration terminates paroxysmal supraventricular tachycardia as do other beta blockers. The drug also slows or abolishes incessant ventricular tachycardia. When administered orally, sotalol is of value in the prophylaxis of recurrent atrial flutter/fibrillation and paroxysmal supraventricular tachycardia. When compared with other beta blockers, sotalol not only can suppress premature ventricular contractions, but also can prevent the reinduction of ventricular tachycardia in a high percentage of patients subject to recurrent ventricular tachyarrhythmias. It is also of prophylactic value in this setting. The currently available data suggest that the drug is a major advance in the treatment of cardiac arrhythmias.

The side effects of sotalol are those related to beta blockade and to the development of torsades de pointes, which is uncommon except with large doses or abnormal electrolyte disturbances, especially hypokalemia. It might be possible to minimize the beta-blocking adverse reactions by using the dextroisomer of the compound which has the same electrophysiologic properties as the levoisomer or the racemate[71] (Figure 63.4).

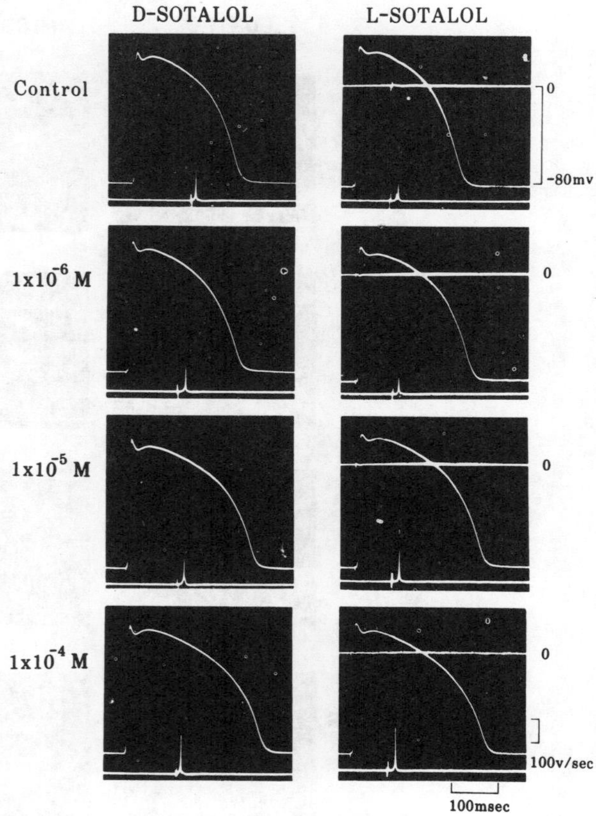

Figure 63.4. The effects of d- (*left panel*) and 1-sotalol (*right panel*) on the action potentials recorded from isolated rabbit ventricular muscle. Both agents produce a concentration-dependent increase in the action potential duration, although the 1-sotalol has 50 times the beta-blocking potency of the d-isomer (Kato R, Singh BN, unpublished observations). Thus, lengthening of the action potential is a property independent of beta-adrenergic blockade.

Amiodarone

Introduced as an antianginal agent about 20 years ago, amiodarone has recently emerged as an extremely potent broad spectrum antiarrhythmic compound,[72–74] with a complex pharmacologic profile (Table 63.14). Electrophysiologically, its action differs somewhat when injected intravenously and given orally. This is in accord with the acute in vitro studies indicating that even with extremely high concentrations in the superfusate, the lengthening of the action potential duration is minimal. In contrast, when given chronically, the drug produces a stepwise increase in action potential duration as a function of time on a constant dose of the drug in the rabbit (Figure 63.5). In man, when the drug is given intravenously, there is little change in the QT interval or in the refractory period of the atria or ventricles. However, there is an increase in the AH interval and the effective refractory period of the atrioventricular node. These effects are due to the calcium antagonistic as well as sympatholytic action of the drug when given acutely. Such effects are accentuated in chronic drug administration during which there is lengthening of the effective refractory period also of the atria, ventricles, His-Purkinje system, as well of those of the bypass tracts. Under resting conditions, amiodarone does not affect conduction, but at fast stimulation frequencies it exhibits a fast-channel inhibitory effect, a "use-dependent" property characteristic of sodium channel blockers.[75]

Amiodarone is a systemic and coronary vasodilator which produces bradycardia during chronic therapy. The drug is an iodinated molecule that has a complex inter-

Table 63.14. Pharmacologic Profile of Amiodarone

1. Electrophysiologic effects
   A. Lengthening of action potential duration in all cardiac tissues (chronic)
   B. Depression of phase 4 depolarization (acute/chronic)
   C. Fast channel blockade at high stimulation frequencies ("use-dependency")
2. Coronary arterial dilatation
3. Systemic vasodilation
4. Noncompetitive alpha and beta catecholamine receptor antagonism
5. Probably little or no vagomimetic action
6. Probably little or no intrinsic negative inotropic propensity
7. Complex interrelationship with thyroid hormone metabolism
8. Complex pharmacokinetics with long and variable elimination half-life
9. Complex interactions with numerous cardioactive compounds

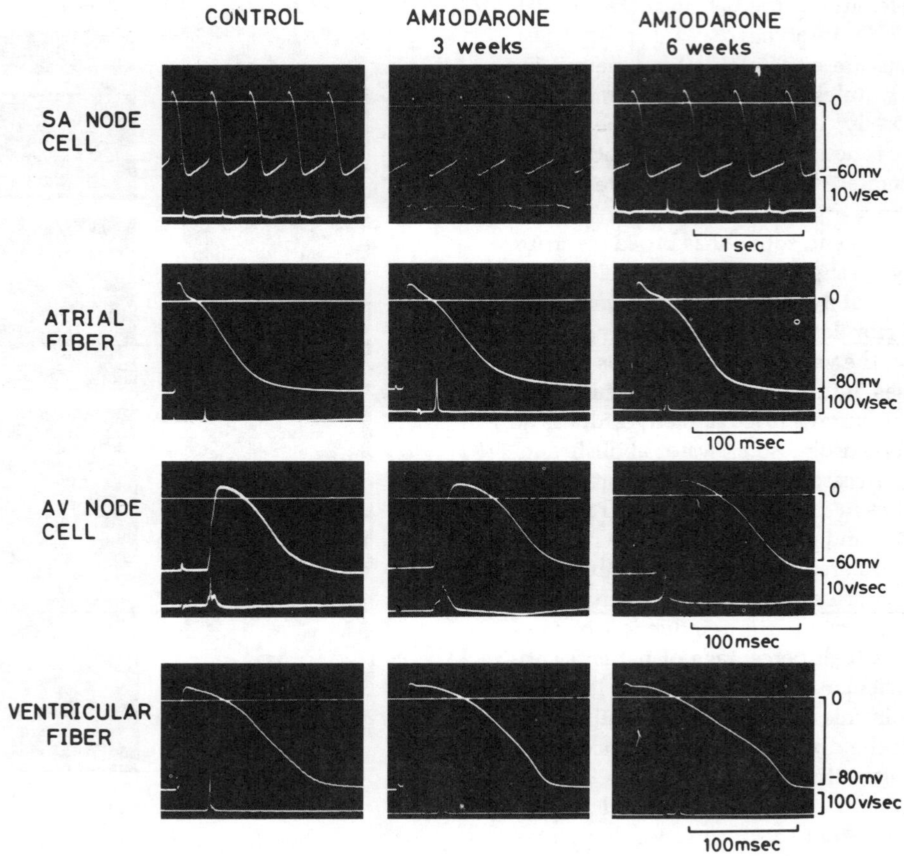

Figure 63.5. The effects of chronic treatment of amiodarone on the action potential characteristics of various types of myocardial fibers. Note that the main effect is the lengthening of the action potential duration. Note the time-dependent increase in repolarization at a constant daily dose of amiodarone.

relationship with thyroid hormone metabolism[76,77] (Figure 63.6). Its electrophysiologic actions closely resemble those of hypothyroidism and they are attenuated or prevented from developing by the concomitant administration of thyroid hormone. Intravenous injection of the drug

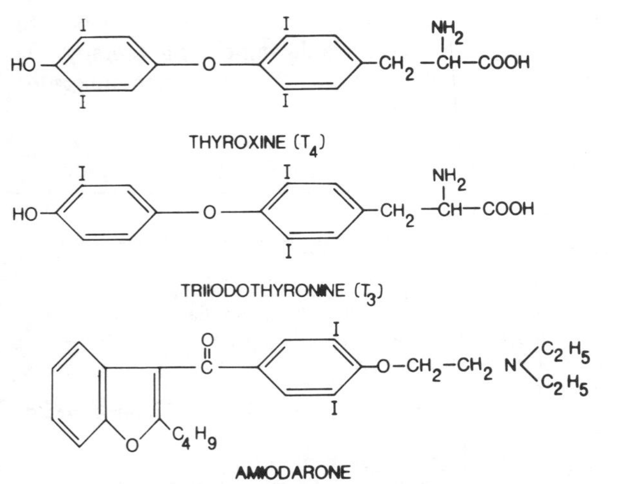

Figure 63.6. Chemical structures of amiodarone and of thyroid hormones. The structural similarities are evident and raise the possibility of a relationship between amiodarone action and that of hypothyroidism.

suspended in the commercial diluent produces peripheral vasodilatation, but transient increases in the left ventricular filling pressures may occur, suggesting a mild negative inotropic effect. However, during chronic oral therapy with amiodarone, the left ventricular ejection fraction does not decrease even with patients with severely depressed ventricular function. This is consistent with the observation that amiodarone rarely aggravates cardiac failure.

The pharmacokinetics of amiodarone are complex. It is well absorbed, with a bioavailability between 35% and 55%. It is highly protein bound; it is metabolized in the liver to a number of metabolites, the most prominent being desethylamiodarone, which is pharmacologically active. The elimination half-life of amiodarone varies between 15 and 150 days, that of the metabolite being even longer. The serum levels of the drug tend to be higher during acute intravenous administration despite the fact that the actions of the drug during chronic therapy are much more pronounced with lower tissue and serum levels of the drug. This suggests that tissue-receptor interaction requiring a finite period of time for the drug to exert its pharmacologic effects may mediate the chronic pharmacologic actions of the drug.

When the drug is given intravenously, the major effect is on the atrioventricular node. Therefore, the ventricular response in atrial flutter and fibrillation is slowed, but conversion to sinus rhythm is uncommon. Similarly, a fraction of cases of reentrant paroxysmal supraventricular tachycardia using antegrade atrioventricular nodal conduction during tachycardia are terminated by the drug. However, ventricular tachycardia is rarely terminated or inducible ventricular tachycardia/ventricular fibrillation suppressed. Occasionally, the ventricular tachycardia cycle length is somewhat prolonged. In contrast, after an adequate period of chronic oral dosing (amiodaronization) there is sinus bradycardia; slowing of the ventricular response in atrial flutter and fibrillation with attenuation of the exercise-induced increases also occurs, with a high conversion rate to sinus rhythm with maintenance of a stable sinus mechanism. Amiodarone is effective in paroxysmal atrial fibrillation and flutter as well as in paroxysmal supraventricular tachycardia in patients with and without accessory tracts in the heart. The demonstrated efficacy of amiodarone in atrial flutter and fibrillation complicating the Wolff-Parkinson-White syndrome has reduced the necessity for surgery in a significant number of such patients.

Orally administered amiodarone is extremely effective in suppressing premature ventricular contractions in patients with structural heart disease, suppressing complex premature ventricular contractions in smaller drug doses than those necessary to suppress total premature ventricular contractions. However, amiodarone is of particular value in suppressing life-threatening sustained ventricular arrhythmias and in preventing recurrent cardiac arrest in survivors of sudden cardiac death. Uncontrolled data indicate that the drug may prolong survival in these subsets of patients. The long-term outcome may be predictable on the basis of the suppression of complex premature ventricular contractions in such patients but not by the suppression of inducible ventricular tachycardia/ventricular fibrillation by programmed electrical stimulation of the heart. It is now appreciated that failure of the drug to prevent inducible ventricular tachycardia/ventricular fibrillation does not preclude a salutary long-term outcome with prophylactic use of amiodarone in malignant ventricular tachyarrhythmias.

The role of amiodarone in certain arrhythmias such as parasystole, torsades de pointes, and exercise-induced ventricular tachycardia has not been defined.

In view of the slow onset of drug action, various loading regimens have been used, including intravenous as well as oral regimens, which have reduced the latency of onset of drug action but not abolished it. Intravenously, the drug may be given initially at a dose of 5 mg/kg over ten minutes followed by about 1,000 to 1,200 mg/24 hours by constant infusion. The oral loading doses have been up to 2,000 mg daily (in two divided doses) for one to two weeks, the dose being reduced if there are side effects (usually of gastrointestinal or central nervous system origin). Subsequently, the dose is reduced in a stepwise fashion over six to eight weeks to about 200 to 400 mg per day for supraventricular arrhythmias and somewhat higher maintenance doses for ventricular arrhythmias. The dose adjustments may be made in relation to the clinical response and the changes in reverse T_3 levels and in levels of amiodarone and especially its metabolite, desethylamiodarone. The role of combination therapy with other antiarrhythmic agents is not defined. However, it must be emphasized that amiodarone exerts a pharmacokinetic interaction with a number of cardioactive agents: digoxin, coumadin, quinidine, phenytoin, procainamide, NAPA, and disopyramide among others. Electrophysiologic and hemodynamic interactions may also occur with other antiarrhythmic agents, beta blockers and calcium antagonists, necessitating timely dose adjustments.

Although the potency and efficacy of amiodarone in a wide variety of arrhythmias are no longer in doubt, the widespread use of the compound in recent years has indicated its proclivity to induce a complex and varied array of adverse reactions. These may be considered as those that occur early during the loading phase and those that occur as a function of dose and duration of therapy with the drug. The early side effects are of central nervous sytem origin and those referable to the gastrointestinal tract (headaches, insomnia, ataxia, tremors, memory impairment, nausea, vomiting, weakness, and malaise). During chronic therapy, corneal microdeposits occur in most adult patients, but rarely do they interfere with vision. However, haloes may develop in a small number of patients, but they are reversible. Photosensitivity is common, although other skin lesions may also develop in some patients. A slate-grey or bluish skin pigmentation develops as a function of duration of therapy in over 10% of patients and may regress slowly over many months. In some patients there is elevation of the serum levels of hepatic enzymes, and rarely toxic hepatitis has been reported. Because amiodarone is an iodinated compound, both hypothyroidism as well as hyperthyroidism may develop in predisposed patients. The incidence is about 1% to 5% in relation to the geographic area.

The most serious side effects of the drug relate to the development of pulmonary infiltrates, the nature of which is not understood. The exact incidence of the complication is debated, but it is unlikely to be more than 5% if a timely reduction of dose is carried out. However, some cases appear to be unrelated to dose, but they generally occur in relation to marked increases in reverse T_3 levels and are not systematically related to serum levels of the drug or its metabolite. Other side effects include sinus arrest, atrioventricular block, aggravation of heart failure, peripheral neuropathy, aggravation of arrhythmia (probably in less than 5% of the patients), epididymitis, and generalized lipidosis. When drug usage is monitored meticulously, less than 10% of patients require discontinuation of therapy. Clearly, with such a potent drug an appropriate perspective needs to be developed with regard to its role in the control of cardiac arrhythmias. Such a perspective should recognize that the drug is effective in over 75% of patients after other drugs have failed, but a large number of side effects may develop, most of which are reversible but a few of which may be potentially lethal. Clearly, a detailed knowledge of the fundamental action of amiodarone may lead to better understanding of the nature of cardiac arrhythmias and to the development of potent and safer antiarrhythmic compounds in the future.

CALCIUM CHANNEL BLOCKERS (CLASS IV AGENTS) AS ANTIARRHYTHMIC AGENTS

The role of these agents in cardiovascular therapeutics has been discussed herein. They have indirect as well as direct antiarrhythmic actions. The newer agents may have a broad pharmacologic profile.

CONCLUSIONS

In this chapter, we have attempted to review the pharmacology of a number of classes of cardioactive agents used in the treatment of ischemic myocardial syndromes, hypertension, and cardiac failure and in the acute and chronic management of cardiac arrhythmias. Focus has been placed on the salient features of the underlying mechanisms that lead to the salutary effects in clinical disorders in which an individual agent might be of value. A knowledge of the fundamental action of drugs is essential in predicting their clinical effects, adverse reactions, and potential for pharmacokinetic, hemodynamic, or electrophysiologic interaction. However, our knowledge of these various facets of drug action is essentially incomplete, but it is growing. Some of the newer developments are indicated in order that an appropriate focus may eventually evolve so that cardiovascular therapy may assume an increasingly rational approach. This is likely to occur with greater understanding of the mode of action of cardioactive agents in relation to the pathophysiologic aspects of various cardiocirculatory disorders in which they are used for a particular clinical effect.

Acknowledgment: This work was supported by the Medical Research Service of the Veterans Administration and the American Heart Association, The Greater Los Angeles Affiliate, Los Angeles, California.

REFERENCES

1. Conolly ME, Kersting F, Dollery CT: The clinical pharmacology of beta-adrenoceptor-blocking drugs. *Prog Cardiovasc Dis* 1976; 19:203–234.
2. Frishman WH: Beta-adrenoceptor antagonists: new drugs and new indications. *N Engl J Med* 1981; 305:500–506.
3. Frishman WH: Beta-adrenergic blockade in the treatment of coronary artery disease, in Hurst JW (ed): *Clinical Essays on The Heart.* New York, McGraw-Hill, 1984, vol 2, pp 25–63.
4. Cruickshank JM: The clinical importance of cardioselectivity and lipophilicity in beta blockers. *Am Heart J* 1980; 100:160–178.
5. Singh BN, Vaughan Williams EM: A third class of antiarrhythmic action. Effects on atrial and ventricular intracellular potentials, and other pharmacological actions on cardiac muscle, of MJ 1999 and AH 3474. *Br J Pharmacol* 1970; 39:675–687.
6. Singh BN, Jewitt DE: Beta-adrenergic receptor blocking drugs in cardiac arrhythmias. *Drugs* 1974; 7:426–461.
7. Singh BN, Collett JT, Chew CYC: New perspectives in the pharmacologic therapy of cardiac arrhythmias. *Prog Cardiovasc Dis* 1980; 22:243–301.
8. Nademanee K, Feld G, Hendrickson JA, Singh PN, Singh BN: Electrophysiologic and antiarrhythmic effects of sotalol in patients with life-threatening ventricular tachyarrhythmias. *Circulation* 1985; 72:555–564.
9. Singh BN, Venkatesh N: Prevention of myocardial reinfarction and of sudden death in survivors of acute myocardial infarction: role of prophylactic β-adrenoceptor blockade. *Am Heart J* 1984; 107:189–200.
10. Schwartz PJ: Idiopathic long QT syndrome: progress and questions. *Am Heart J* 1985; 109:399–411.
11. Zonszein J, Santangelo RP, Macklin JF, Lee TC, Coffey RJ, Canary JJ: Propranolol therapy in thyrotoxicosis. A review of 84 patients undergoing surgery. *Am J Med* 1979; 66:411–416.
12. Frank MJ, Abdulla AM, Canedo MI, Saylors RE: Long-term medical management of hypertrophic obstructive cardiomyopathy. *Am J Cardiol* 1978; 42:993–1001.
13. Engelmeier RS, O'Connell JB, Walsh R, Rad N, Scanlon J, Gunnar RM: Improvement in symptoms and exercise tolerance by metoprolol in patients with dilated cardiomyopathy: a double-blind, randomized, placebo-controlled trial. *Circulation* 1985; 72:536–546.

13a. The Esmolol vs Placebo Multicenter Study Group: Anderson S, Blanski L, Byrd RC, Das G, Engler R, Laddu A, Lee R, Rajfer S, Schroeder J, Steck JD, Sung R, Turlapaty P, Williams D, Wilner G, Zoble R: Comparison of the efficacy and safety of esmolol, a short-acting beta blocker with placebo in the treatment of supraventricular tachyarrhythmias. *Am Heart J* 1986; 111:42–48.

13b. Gray RJ, Bateman TM, Czer LSC, Conklin CM, Matloff JM: Esmolol for hypertension early after cardiac surgery. *J Am Coll Cardiol* 1986; 7:178A.

13c. Sung RJ, Blanski L, Kirshenbaum J, MacCospe P, Turlapaty P, Laddu AR, Esmolol Research Group: Clinical experience with esmolol, a short-acting beta-adrenergic blocker in cardiac arrhythmias and myocardial ischemia. *J Clin Pharmacol* 1986; 26(suppl A):A-15–A-26.

14. Brown BG, Bolson EL, Dodge HT: Dyanmic mechanisms in human coronary stenosis. *Circulation* 1984; 70:917–922.
15. Brown BG, Bolson EL, Petersen RB, Pierce CD, Dodge HT: The mechanisms of nitroglycerin action: stenosis vasodilatation as a major component of the drug response. *Circulation* 1981; 64:1088–1097.
16. Abrams J: Nitrate tolerance and dependence. *Am Heart J* 1980; 99:113–123.
17. Franciosa JA, Nordstrom LA, Cohn JN: Nitrate therapy for congestive heart failure. *JAMA* 1978; 240:443–446.
18. Fleckenstein A: History of calcium antagonists. *Circ Res* 1983; 52 (suppl I):I-3–I-16.
19. Epstein SE, Rosing DR, Conti CR: Calcium-channel blockers: present status and future directions. *Am J Cardiol* 1985; 55:1B-221B.
20. Singh BN, Ellrodt G, Nademanee K: Calcium antagonists: cardiocirculatory effects and therapeutic applications, in Hurst JW (ed): *Clinical Essays on the Heart.* New York, McGraw-Hill, 1984, vol 2, pp 65–97.
21. Singh BN, Hecht HS, Nademanee K, Chew CYC: Electrophysiologic and hemodynamic effects of slow-channel blocking drugs. *Prog Cardiovasc Dis* 1982; 25:103–132.
22. Singh BN, Baky S, Nademanee K: Second-generation calcium antagonists: search for greater selectivity and versatility. *Am J Cardiol* 1985; 55:214B–221B.
23. Allen GS, Ahn HS, Preziosi TJ, Battle R, Boone SC, Chou SN, Kelly DL, Weir BK, Crabbe RA, Lavik PJ, Rosenbloom SB, Dorsey FC, Ingram CR, Mellits DE, Bertsch LA, Biosvert DPJ, Hundley MB, Johnson RK, Strom JA, Transou CR: Cerebral arterial spasm—a controlled trial of nimodipine in patients with subarachnoid hemorrhage. *N Engl J Med* 1983; 308:619–624.
24. Holmes B, Brogden RN, Heel RC, Speight TM, Avery GS. Flunarizine: a review of its pharmacodynamic and pharmacokinetic properties and therapeutic use. *Drugs* 1984; 27:6–44.
25. Vaughan Williams EM: *Antiarrhythmic Action and the Puzzle of Perhexiline.* London, Academic Press, 1980, pp 1–135.
26. Bianco R, Albert J, Katz RJ, Spann J, Chesler E, Ferri DP, Larca LJ, Costello RB, Gore JM, Eisenman MJ: Bepridil for chronic stable angina pectoris: results of a prospective multicenter, placebo-controlled, dose-ranging study in 77 patients. *Am J Cardiol* 1984; 53:35–41.
27. Singh BN, Nademanee K, Feld G, Piontek M, Schwab M: Comparative electrophysiologic profiles of calcium antagonists with particular reference to bepridil. *Am J Cardiol* 1985; 55:14C–19C.

27a. Kato R, Singh BN: Effects of bepridil on the electrophysiologic properties of isolated canine and rabbit myocardial fibers. *Am Heart J* 1986; 111:271–279.

28. Singh BN, Nademanee K, Baky S: Calcium antagonists. Clinical use in the treatment of arrhythmias. *Drugs* 1983; 25:125–153.
29. Johnson SM, Mauritson DR, Willerson JT, Hillis LD: A controlled trial of verapamil in Prinzmetal's variant angina. *N Engl J Med* 1981; 304:862–866.
30. McCall D, Walsh RA, Frohlich ED, O'Rourke RA: Calcium entry blocking drugs: experimental studies and clinical uses. *Curr Probl Cardiol* 1985; 10:1–80.
31. Hecht HS, Chew CYC, Burnam MH, Hopkins J, Schnugg S, Singh BN: Verapamil in chronic stable angina: amelioration of pacing-induced abnormalities of left ventricular ejection fraction, regional wall motion, lactate metabolism and hemodynamics. *Am J Cardiol* 1981; 48:536–544.
32. Josephson MA, Hecht HS, Hopkins J, Guerrero J, Singh BN: Comparative effects of oral verapamil and propranolol on exercise-induced myocardial ischemia and energetics in patients with coronary artery disease: single-blind placebo crossover evaluation using radionuclide ventriculography. *Am Heart J* 1982; 103:978–985.
33. Bühler FR, Hulthén L: Calcium channel blockers: a pathophysiologically based antihypertensive treatment concept for the future? *Eur J Clin Invest* 1982; 12:1–3.

34. Frohlich EA: Calcium channel blockers: a new dimension in antihypertensive therapy. *Am J Med* 1984; 77:1–45.
35. Rosing DR, Idänpään-Heikkilä U, Maron BJ, Bonow RO, Epstein SE: Use of calcium-channel blocking drugs in hypertrophic cardiomyopathy. *Am J Cardiol* 1985; 55:185B–195B.
36. Gelmer JH: Nimodipine, a new calcium antagonist in the prophylactic treatment of migraine. *Headache* 1983; 23:106–109.
37. Cannon PJ: The pharmacology of diuretics, in Rosen MR, Hoffman BF (eds): *Cardiac Therapy*. Boston, Martinus Nijhoff, 1983, pp 413–434.
37a. Whelton A: A symposium: current trends in diuretic therapy. *Am J Cardiol* 1986; 57:1A–53A.
38. Mason DT: Afterload reduction and cardiac performance. Physiologic basis of systemic vasodilators as a new approach in treatment of congestive heart failure. *Am J Med* 1978; 65:106–125.
39. Chatterjee K, Parmley WW, Massie B, Greenberg B, Werner J, Klausner S, Norman A: Oral hydralazine therapy for chronic refractory heart failure. *Circulation* 1976; 54:879–883.
40. Linas SL, Nies AS: Minoxidil. *Ann Intern Med* 1981; 94:61–65.
41. Cohn JN, Burke LP: Nitroprusside. *Ann Intern Med* 1979; 91:752–757.
42. Graham RM, Pettinger WA: Prazosin. *N Engl J Med* 1979; 300:232–236.
43. Captopril Multicenter Research Group: A placebo-controlled trial of captopril in refractory chronic congestive heart failure. *J Am Coll Cardiol* 1983; 2:755–763.
44. Webster MWI, Fitzpatrick MA, Hamilton EJ, Nicholls MG, Ikram H, Espiner EA, Wells JE: Effects of enalapril on clinical status, biochemistry, exercise performance and haemodynamics in heart failure. *Drugs* 1985; 30(suppl 1):74–81.
45. Maskin CS, Ocken S, Chadwick B, LeJemtel TH: Comparative systemic and renal effects of dopamine and angiotensin-converting enzyme inhibition with enalaprilat in patients with heart failure. *Circulation* 1985; 72:846–852.
46. Benotti JR, Grossman W, Braunwald E, Carabello BA: Effects of amrinone on myocardial energy metabolism and hemodynamics in patients with severe congestive heart failure due to coronary artery disease. *Circulation* 1980; 62:28–34.
46a. Braunwald E: Newer positive inotropic agents. *Circulation* 1986; 73(Supp III):III-1–III-239.
47. Zipes DP, Troup PJ: New antiarrhythmic agents. Amiodarone, aprindine, disopyramide, ethmozin, mexiletine, tocainide, verapamil. *Am J Cardiol* 1978; 41:1005–1024.
48. Ellrodt G, Chew CYC, Singh BN: Therapeutic implications of slow-channel blockade in cardiocirculatory disorders. *Circulation* 1980; 62:669–679.
49. Singh BN, Hauswirth O: Comparative mechanisms of action of antiarrhythmic drugs. *Am Heart J* 1974; 87:367–382.
50. Singh BN, Vaughan Williams EM: A fourth class of antidysrhythmic action? Effect of verapamil on ouabain toxicity, on atrial and ventricular intracellular potentials, and on other features of cardiac function. *Cardiovasc Res* 1972; 6:109–119.
51. Singh BN, Ikeda N, Nademanee K, Hauswirth O: Cellular electrophysiology of the heart: basis for elucidating the origin of cardiac arrhythmias and the action of antiarrhythmic agents, in Levy S, Scheinmann MM (eds): *Cardiac Arrhythmias*. Mt Kisco, NY, Futura, 1984, pp 1–36.
52. Harrison DC: Antiarrhythmic drug classification: new science and practical applications. *Am J Cardiol* 1985; 56:185–187.
53. Hondeghem L, Katzung BG: Test of a model of antiarrhythmic drug action: effects of quinidine and lidocaine on myocardial conduction. *Circulation* 1980; 61:1217–1224.
53a. Feld GK, Singh BN: Clinical experience with sustained-release procainamide. *Arrhythmia Clinic* 1986; 3:13–19.
54. Heel RC, Brogden RN, Speight TM, Avery GS: Disopyramide: a review of its pharmacological properties and therapeutic use in treating cardiac arrhythmias. *Drugs* 1978; 15:331–368.
55. Podrid P, Schoeneberger A, Lown B: Congestive heart failure caused by oral disopyramide. *N Engl J Med* 1980; 302:614–617.
56. Pfeifer HJ, Greenblatt DJ, Koch-Weser J: Clinical use and toxicity of intravenous lidocaine. A report from the Boston Collaborative Drug Surveillance Program. *Am Heart J* 1976; 92:168–173.
57. Chew CYC, Collett J, Singh BN: Mexiletine: a review of its pharmacological properties and therapeutic efficacy in arrhythmias. *Drugs* 1979; 17:161–181.
58. Winkle RA, Meffin PJ, Harrison DC: Longterm tocainide therapy for ventricular arrhythmias. *Circulation* 1979; 57:1008–1016.
59. Danilo, P Jr: Aprindine. *Am Heart J* 1979; 97:119–124.
60. Podrid PJ, Lyakishev A, Lown B, Mazur N: Ethmozin, a new antiarrhythmic drug for suppressing ventricular premature complexes. *Circulation* 1980; 61:450–457.
61. Holmes B, Heel RC: Flecainide. A preliminary review of its pharmacodynamic properties and therapeutic efficacy. *Drugs* 1985; 29:1–33.
62. The Flecainide-Quinidine Research Group: Flecainide versus quinidine for treatment of chronic ventricular arrhythmias. A multicenter clinical trial. *Circulation* 1983; 67:1117–1123.
63. Roden DM, Reale SB, Higgins SB, Mayol RF, Gammans RE, Oates JA, Woosley RL: Total suppression of ventricular arrhythmias by encainide. *N Engl J Med* 1980; 302:877–882.
64. Winkle RA, Mason JW, Griffin JC, Ross D: Malignant ventricular tachyarrhythmias associated with the use of encainide. *Am Heart J* 1981; 102:857–864.
65. Morganroth J, Horowitz LN: Flecainide: its proarrhythmic effect and expected changes on the surface electrocardiogram. *Am J Cardiol* 1984; 53:89B–94B.
66. Zipes DP: Recent advances in antiarrhythmic therapy: symposium on propafenone. *Am J Cardiol* 1984; 54:1D–73D.
66a. Hammill SC, Sorenson PB, Wood DL, Sugrue DD, Osborn MJ, Gersh BJ, Holmes DR: Propafenone for the treatment of refractory complex ventricular ectopic activity. *Mayo Clin Proc* 1986; 61:48–103.
67. Anderson JL, Patterson E, Wagner JG, Stewart JR, Behm HL, Lucchesi BR: Oral and intravenous bretylium disposition. *Clin Pharmacol Ther* 1980; 28:468–478.
68. Dangman KH, Hoffman BF: In vivo and in vitro antiarrhythmic and arrhythmogenic effects of N-acetyl procainamide. *J Pharmacol Exp Ther* 1981; 217:851–862.
69. Sung RJ, Juma Z, Saksena S: Electrophysiologic properties and antiarrhythmic mechanisms of intravenous N-acetylprocainamide in patients with ventricular dysrhythmias. *Am Heart J* 1983; 105:811–819.
70. Senges J, Lengfelder W, Jauernig R, Czygan E, Brachmann J, Rizos I, Cobbe S, Kübler W: Electrophysiologic testing in assessment of therapy with sotalol for sustained ventricular tachycardia. *Circulation* 1984; 69:577–584.
71. Kato R, Ikeda N, Yabek SM, Kannan R, Singh BN: Electrophysiologic effects of sotalol in isolated cardiac muscle and their in vivo pharmacokinetics. *J Am Coll Cardiol* 1986; 7:116–125.
72. Singh BN, Vaughan Williams EM: The effect of amiodarone, a new antianginal drug, on cardiac muscle. *Br J Pharmacol* 1970; 39:657–667.
73. Singh BN, Zipes DP: Amiodarone: basic concepts and clinical application. *Am Heart J* 1983; 106:787–964.
74. Podrid P, Lown B: Amiodarone therapy in symptomatic, sustained refractory atrial and ventricular tachyarrhythmias. *Am Heart J* 1981; 101:374–379.
75. Yabek SM, Kato R, Singh BN: Effects of amiodarone and its metabolite, desethylamiodarone, on the electrophysiologic properties of isolated cardiac muscle. *J Cardiovasc Pharmacol* 1986; 8:197–207.
76. Martino E, Safran M, Aghini-Lombardi F, Rajatanavin R, Lenziardi M, Fay M, Pacchiarotti A, Aronin N, Macchia E, Haffajee C, Odoguardi L, Love J, Bigalli A, Baschieri L, Pinchera A, Braverman L: Environmental iodine intake and thyroid dysfunction during chronic amiodarone therapy. *Ann Intern Med* 1984; 101:28–34.
77. Monteiro E, Galvao-teles A, Santos ML, Mourao L, Correia MJ, Lopo Tuna J, Ribeiro C: Antithyroid antibodies as an early marker for thyroid disease induced by amiodarone. *Br Med J* 1986; 292:227–228.

64 Herbal Pharmacology in Cardiovascular Therapeutics

Ming-xin Huang, MD, DSc, Shu-xia Chen, MD, and Tsung O. Cheng, MD, MS (Med)

The usefulness of certain herbal medicines in cardiovascular therapy has been known for thousands of years. Many of today's cardiac drugs are derived from ancient remedies, such as digitalis, ephedrine, quinidine, and atropine. Chinese medical scientists have made remarkable advances in the field of traditional herbal medicine during the past 30 years. In the field of cardiovascular diseases, three drugs, higenamine, hyoscine drugs, and danshen, are most important not only because of their promising results in clinical application but also because they have been the subject of numerous animal experiments and clinical trials; therefore, their use is based more on sound scientific principles than on mere empiric experiences in the category of folk medicine.

HIGENAMINE

Radix Aconiti Praeparata, a commonly used Chinese medicinal herb, is the main drug in the application of the "warming" method. Classified as an "inferior" drug, it was considered a substance for producing "great heat" in Shen Nong's herbal classic (神農本草). It possesses multiple pharmacologic actions. Zhang Zhong-jing (張仲景) 2,187 to 2,205 years ago in his "Shang Han Lun" used aconite in "reviving the Yang for resuscitation" (回陽救逆) in the treatment of the symptom complexes of "Deficiency of Yang" and "Depletion of Yang." The manifestations of both symptom complexes are generally cold intolerance, cold extremities, fatigue, and sleepiness, with a forceless pulse, possibly indicating cardiac insufficiency, circulatory disturbance, and slowing of metabolism. Reviving the Yang for resuscitation may possibly enhance cardiac contraction, improve circulation, and promote metabolism.

PHARMACOLOGY

In 1975, The Institute of Pharmacology, Chinese Academy of Medical Sciences, synthesized higenamine (aconite No. 1) with the structural formula shown in Figure 64.1. From 1975 through 1977 Chou et al,[1] in investigations of the effect of higenamine on the cardiovascular system, proved that higenamine had strong physiologic activities, its action closely resembling that of isoprenaline, both of which could be blocked by propranolol, a beta-blocker.

To test whether aconite also possesses effects similar to those of higenamine, Huang et al[2] in 1978 compared the pharmacologic action of aconite injection (supplied by the No. 9 Shanghai Pharmaceutical Factory) and higenamine. The results indicated that aconite possessed the effect of vasodilatation, similar to that of higenamine.

Aconite can increase cardiac output, cardiac index, and myocardial oxygen consumption in the anesthetized dog. After intravenous injection of extract equivalent to 2 g/kg of herbal aconite in the unanesthetized dog, heart rate was accelerated, blood pressure elevated, and heart sounds accentuated. Moreover, herbal aconite extract injection (0.15 to 0.3 g) increased contraction and output of the isolated heart of the frog. These results demonstrated that aconite also acts as a cardiac stimulant similar to higenamine (Tables 64.1 and 64.2).

The aforementioned results indicate that aconite injection acts as both a cardiac stimulant and a vasodilator, although much weaker than higenamine. The effect of 5 μg of higenamine is stronger than that of 2 g of the raw drug of aconite.

From 1979 through 1980 Li et al[3] proved that higenamine could activate the beta-receptor of cultured myo-

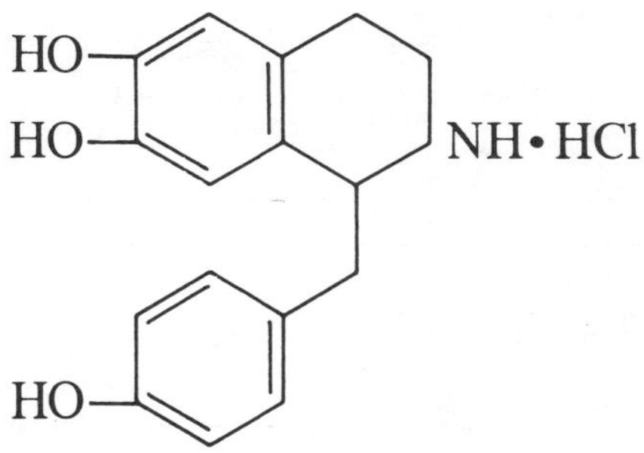

Figure 64.1. Structural formula of higenamine.

cardial cells of rats, increasing markedly the pulsating frequency and amplitude of contraction of the myocardial cells. Because higenamine accelerates cardiac rate, it might result in an increase in oxygen consumption.

From 1975 through 1977 Chou et al[1] applied the principle of the specific affinity of injured myocardium to radioisotope ^{169}Yb. They found that higenamine had an injurious effect on myocardial tissue. However, this injurious effect induced by higenamine was less than one tenth of the therapeutic dose of isoprenaline (Table 64.3).

CLINICAL APPLICATION

From 1978 through 1980, altogether 147 patients treated with aconite No. 1 and 59 patients treated with isoprenaline as the control were observed clinically. Those with complete data were selected and are reported on as follows:

Bao et al[4] administered higenamine injections (supplied by the Shanghai No. 9 Pharmaceutical Works, 2.5 mg/amp) of 5 mg in 250 ml of 10% glucose solution intravenously at a rate of approximately 20 drops per minute per day for two weeks in the treatment of 14 patients with bradyarrhythmia from coronary heart disease, myocarditis, atrioventricular (AV) block, sick sinus syndrome, and so forth. A markedly effective rate of 23% and an overall effective rate of 77% suggested that higenamine was able to ameliorate both sinoatrial (SA) node and AV node bradyarrhythmias, to promote conduction, to accelerate the heart rate rapidly, and to ameliorate pathologic disturbances in AV conduction. These results confirmed the therapeutic effects of higenamine reported in 33 other cases of clinical bradyarrhythmia.[5,6]

Another study[7] was conducted in 1981 on a total of 68 cases of bradyarrhythmia treated by higenamine: sinus bradycardia in 39 cases; AV block in 20 cases (II° AV block in ten cases, in three of which the QRS was ≥0.12 second and in seven it was <0.12 second; III° AV block in ten cases, in six of which the QRS was ≥0.12 second and in four it was <0.12 second); nodal rhythm in three cases; and SA block in six cases. Higenamine 2.5 mg was dissolved in 100 to 150 ml of 5% to 10% glucose for an IV drip at a rate of 15 to 25 μg/min and 30 to 60 μg/min to observe changes in heart rhythm, heart rate, blood pressure, pulse, heart sound, etc, before and after administration. The results were as follows:

(1) Heart rhythm and rate: There was improvement in conduction in most cases and an increase in heart rate in all cases after IV drip of higenamine (Table 64.4).

(2) Blood pressure: In most cases, either systolic BP was elevated or diastolic BP was lowered within 10 to 20 mm Hg after IV higenamine. An individual case might show elevation in systolic pressure of as high as 30 mm Hg or a decrease in diastolic pressure of 10 to 20 mm Hg, values essentially similar to those in the control group of isoprenaline.

(3) Time of action of the drug and its elimination: The shortest time of action of the drug was two minutes after IV drip of higenamine; generally it acted within ten minutes and lasted five to ten minutes after cessation of administration and occasionally as long as two to eight hours.

(4) Changes in signs and symptoms: After IV higenamine, most patients showed less chest distress, fewer palpitations, and a subjective sensation of forceful heartbeat with an increase in heart rate, warmth in the extremities, accentuation of heart sounds, and flushing of the face.

(5) Side reactions: In some cases IV higenamine caused dryness of the mouth, numbness of the lips, dizziness, headache, and ventricular extrasystoles.

In 1980 at the Fu Wai Hospital and Cardiovascular Institute, Chinese Academy of Medical Sciences,[8] a nuclear stethoscope was used to measure left ventricular ejection fraction (LVEF) in 15 patients treated with IV drip of higenamine and in six treated with isoprenaline. All except one demonstrated improvement in LVEF ($P < 0.01$) (Figure 64.2).

Higenamine, therefore, can increase heart rate, ameliorate SA block, and improve AV conduction in bradyarrhythmia. Furthermore, according to the measurement by ^{113}In with the nuclear stethoscope, this drug can improve LVEF, enhance cardiac stroke volume, and ameliorate cardiac contractile abnormality. It also decreases peripheral vascular resistance and causes a decrease in diastolic blood pressure as manifested by flushing of the face and warmth of the extremities. Therefore, aconite indeed has the function of "warming the Yang" and "re-

Table 64.1. Effect of Higenamine on the Isolated Heart of the Frog

Drug Concentration (g/ml)	Increase of Amplitude of Contraction	Increase of Cardiac Output (%)
1×10^{-8}	22 ± 9	15 ± 7
1×10^{-7}	33 ± 5	20 ± 10
1×10^{-6}	74 ± 27	35 ± 7
5×10^{-6}	98 ± 27	80 ± 37

Table 64.2. Effect of Intravenous Drip of Higenamine on Organ Blood Flow and Vascular Resistance in Four Anesthetized Dogs

	Coronary Artery			Internal Carotid Artery			Femoral Artery		
Dog No.	Before Medication	After Medication	Difference	Before Medication	After Medication	Difference	Before Medication	After Medication	Difference
				Mean Blood Flow (ml/100 g/min)					
Higenamine									
1	70	87	17*	67	65	−2	37	33	−4
2	76	109	33	83	86	3	38	35	−3
4†	84	120	36*	82	95	13	36	42	6
Isoprenaline									
1	67	107	40*	73	74	1	35	38	3
				Mean Vascular Resistance (mm Hg/ml/min)					
Higenamine									
1	1.9	1.1	−0.8*	2.2	1.5	−0.7	3.5	3.1	−0.4
2	1.5	0.8	−0.7*	1.4	1.1	−0.3	3.1	2.5	−0.6‡
4†	1.3	0.6	−0.7‡	1.3	0.8	−0.5	2.9	1.9	−1.0
Isoprenaline									
1	1.2	0.5	−0.7‡	1.2	1.0	−0.2	2.3	1.6	−0.7‡

* Significant.
† Mean value of four dogs.
‡ Very significant.

Table 64.3. Effect of Intraperitoneal Injection of Higenamine and Isoprenaline on Rat Myocardial Absorption of ^{169}Yb

Group	Dosage	Animals (No.)	Deaths (No.)	Absorption Rate (%)
Control	Saline	5	0	0.21 ± 0.02
Higenamine	20	5	0	0.32 ± 0.21
	40	5	0	0.43 ± 0.12*
	80	5	0	0.53 ± 0.11†
	160	6	0	0.48 ± 0.09†
	320	6	5	1.50‡
Isoprenaline	2	5	0	0.37 ± 0.05
	4	5	1	0.62 ± 0.29*
	8	5	1	0.80 ± 0.15‡
	16	6	2	1.37 ± 0.07‡
	32	7	3	1.85 ± 0.36‡

* $P < 0.05$.
† $P < 0.01$.
‡ $P < 0.001$.

viving the Yang for resuscitation" according to traditional Chinese medical practices. The clinical impression that higenamine seems to possess a beta-receptor stimulating effect similar to that of isoprenaline is verified by experimental results. The intensity of drug action is about 1/20 to 1/25 that of isoprenaline. The incidence of ventricular extrasystoles after IV drip of higenamine is lower than that of isoprenaline, with total disappearance after decreasing the drip rate. Although there is transient numbness of the lips and dizziness, continued use of the drug is not contraindicated. The drug is useful in emergency, life-threatening situations because of its immediate effect after IV drip and the rapid disappearance of its action after its discontinuation.

ELECTROPHYSIOLOGIC STUDY

To further investigate the mechanism of higenamine's action on the heart, Bao et al[4] in 1979 made observations by means of His bundle electrography. Results of animal experiments showed that the drug acted by shortening the AH interval, thus ameliorating AV conduction disturbances.

In 1983, 1982, and 1985, Qiao et al,[9] Wang et al,[10] and Yu et al,[11,11a] successively applied glass microelectrode technology in investigating the effect of isoprenaline and higenamine on action potentials of isolated Purkinje and ventricular myocardial cells in dogs and pigs. Their results showed that isoprenaline could significantly shorten the effective refractory period of action potentials of Purkinje cells; therefore, it could induce the side reaction of severe cardiac arrhythmia. Conversely, higenamine occasionally could induce cardiac arrhythmia, such as ventricular extrasystole, only at a comparatively higher concentration. Moreover, our experiment[11a] proved that higenamine could relatively prolong the refractory period of Purkinje cells at a comparatively lower concentration (10^{-7} g/ml): $\Delta APD/\Delta ERP < 1$. Accordingly, higenamine is much safer than isoprenaline in the treatment of cardiac arrhythmia.

Table 64.4. Comparison of Cardiac Rate and Rhythm Before and After Treatment With Higenamine

Type of Cardiac Arrhythmia	Cases (No.)	AR		VR		Increase in:		Change of Conduction Block
		Before	After	Before	After	AR	VR	
Sinus brady-cardia; I° AV block	39	49.8	74.4	49.8	74.4	24.6	24.6	1 case of I° AV block; PR restored to normal
Sinoatrial block	6	54.0	72.5	54.0	72.5	18.5	18.5	Normal; disappearance of sinoatrial block
Nodal rhythm	3	...	...	61.0	127.0	...	66.0	1 case of rapid atrial fibrillation with VR 130/min
II° AV block	10	73.8	80.3	49.5	80.3	6.5	30.8	4 cases of block improved, QRS < 0.12 s;
		79.0	96.8	43.0	56.3	17.8	13.3	6 cases of block with no change: QRS ≥ 0.12 s and QRS < 0.12 s, 3 cases each, respectively
III° AV	10	94.0	115.0	47.0	83.0	21.0	36.0	1 case of block with improvement, QRS = 0.12 s;
		76.7	111.0	37.3	48.0	34.3	10.7	9 cases without change: QRS ≥ 0.12 s, 5 cases; QRS < 0.12 s, 4 cases

AR = atrial rate; AV = atrioventricular; VR = ventricular rate.

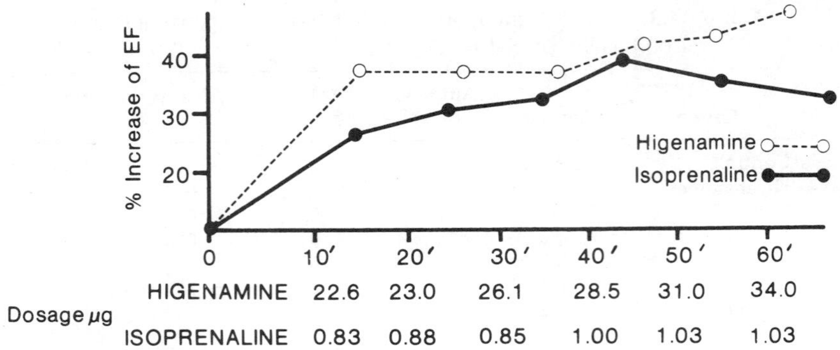

Figure 64.2. Change in left ventricular ejection fraction (EF) after intravenous infusion of higenamine and isoprenaline. Data derived from nuclear stethoscope measurement and ^{113m}In.

We[10] also demonstrated that higenamine could ameliorate the conduction block elicited by hyperkalemia.

Significant improvement was seen in the abnormal corrected sinus node recovery time and SA interval on the His bundle electrogram after injection of higenamine.[12] Experimental studies indicated that higenamine exerted an overall effect on SA node function and AV node conduction of the canine heart (Table 64.5).

Both SA and AV node cells are slow reaction cells and are mainly calcium dependent.[11] Their velocity of depolarization depends on activation of the calcium channel. When calcium electroconductivity increases along with acceleration of influx, the depolarization slope of diastole becomes steep as the frequency of the impulse initiated by the SA node accelerates. As a result, heart rate increases. With acceleration of depolarization velocity of O phase, there is also acceleration of intra-SA node conduction. A close relation therefore exists between higenamine and the inward current of calcium ions.

CALCIUM CHANNEL AND BETA BLOCKERS

To determine whether the action of higenamine could influence the calcium channel, verapamil, a typical calcium channel blocker, was used in our experiments. We found that higenamine exerted a distinct action against verapamil (Table 64.6). It therefore confirmed that higenamine can reactivate the inactivated calcium channel and render the transferring process of calcium ions back toward normal, thereby restoring SA and AV node function to normal.

To find out whether the action of higenamine on the calcium channel is direct or indirect, propranolol, a beta-receptor blocker, was used. Observation revealed that once propranolol showed its effect by combining with beta-receptors on myocardial cells, higenamine lost its original effect of accelerating the heart rate as well as shortening the AH interval (Table 64.7). It was therefore concluded that higenamine exerts its effect only after it has combined with the beta-receptors of the myocardium. It does not act directly on the calcium channel, but it activates the calcium channel indirectly by combining first with beta-receptors. In the experiment, isoprenaline, a beta-receptor stimulant, also was used as a control. The actions of higenamine and isoprenaline on SA node and AV conduction of the heart were similar. We therefore concluded that higenamine is an activator of cardiac beta-adrenergic receptor.[12]

HYOSCINE DRUGS

The use of the herbal drug Yang Jin Hua (洋金花), belonging to class Solanaceae plant, suborder Datura metel linn sicca, dates back 2,200 years as recorded in Shen Nong's herbal classic (神农本草). This herbal drug, in terms of Western medicine, possesses hyoscine-like action. Through close integration of traditional and Western medicine, Chinese medical scholars found that hyoscine drugs inhibit not only acetylcholine, but also the catecholamines. Therefore, it seems advisable to call this group of drugs hyoscine or hyoscine-like drugs rather than anticholinergic drugs.

Table 64.5. Effect of Higenamine on Cardiac Rate, Corrected Sinus Node Recovery Time, Sinoatrial (SA) Interval, and AH Interval

Comparison Between Injection	Atrial Rate (times/min)	Corrected Sinus Node Recovery Time (ms)	SA Interval (ms)	AH Interval (ms)
Before injection	148 ± 13	137 ± 23	21 ± 1	44 ± 2
After injection				
1 min	209 ± 21*		17 ± 1*	30 ± 2*
5 min	186 ± 20*	78 ± 23*	17 ± 1*	33 ± 2*
15 min	174 ± 16*		17 ± 2†	38 ± 3
30 min	166 ± 18†	140 ± 24	18 ± 3	40 ± 2

* Very significant difference $P < 0.01$.
† Significant difference $P < 0.05$. Absence of an asterisk indicates no difference.

Table 64.6. Antagonistic Effect of Higenamine on the Slowing of Cardiac Rate and Prolongation of AH Interval Caused by Verapamil

Comparison	Cardiac Rate (times/min)	AH Interval (ms)
Before injection	167 ± 12	47 ± 7
After injection of verapamil		
1 min	71 ± 17	111 ± 9
5 min	68 ± 9	152 ± 10
After injection of higenamine		
1 min	117 ± 15*	51 ± 14*
5 min	128 ± 15*	51 ± 14*
15 min	127 ± 12*	61 ± 8*

* Very significant difference $P < 0.01$.

HISTORY

In 1955 Huang et al[13–15] first applied massive doses of atropine, averaging 2 to 5 mg of atropine intravenously followed immediately by 5 to 10 mg in 500 ml of a 10% to 15% glucose solution administered by intravenous drip, for the most dreaded complication of Adams-Stokes syndrome caused by intravenous injection of antimony and potassium tartrate. This antimonial drug was used for more than 15 years as the sole agent during a nationwide antischistosomiasis campaign in which more than 10 million patients were treated. Tens of millions of these tartar emetic ampuls were consumed. The Adams-Stokes syndrome averaged about 1% of cases. Initially (1949 to 1954), the mortality rate was about 50% to 70%; none of the routine sympathomimetic agents seemed to have any therapeutic effect, if indeed they did not hasten death. After massive doses of atropine, mortality was reduced to an average of 0.03%. Thereafter, in 1959 atropine in large dosage was used in infectious shock of toxic dysentery[16] and in 1966 anisodamine, another hyoscine drug, was used in shock of epidemic meningitis and in various severe shocks.[17–19] All of these reports revealed a significant decrease in the mortality rate.

PHARMACOLOGY

Through the efforts of Chinese pharmacologists and medical scholars, an attempt was made to study the hyoscine drugs. From the raw herbal plants Atropa belladonna linn and Datura stramonium linn, atropine was isolated and chemically synthesized. Atropine was then named dl-hyoscyamine. From Anisodus tanguticus (茄科植物唐古特山莨菪), Chinese pharmacologists first isolated anisodamine (山莨菪碱), also known by the number "654" indicating its date of clinical introduction (April 1965), which subsequently was proven to have outstanding effects in the treatment of various shock states.[17–19] From Datura metel linn and Hyoscyamus niger linn, scopolamine was isolated. The structural formulas are shown in Figure 64.3.

Chinese pharmacologists found that the oxygen bridge and the –OH group, both located at the far left of the structural formula, exert just the opposite action on the hyoscine drugs. The oxygen bridge enhances the therapeutic action, whereas the –OH radical weakens it. Scopolamine possesses the oxygen bridge, so it exerts the strongest action on the central nervous system. Atropine possesses neither oxygen bridge nor –OH group and ranks second in potency. Anisodamine possesses an –OH group only and is therefore the weakest in action among the hyoscine drugs.[20] Another hyoscine drug, anisodine, possessing both –OH group and oxygen bridge, ranks third in potency, that is, between atropine and anisodamine. The weakening effect of the –OH group apparently overrides the enhancing effect of the oxygen bridge. The order of decreasing intensity of the central action of hyoscine drugs is therefore as follows: scopolamine → atropine → anisodine → anisodamine. Hence, scopolamine clinically has the best anticonvulsive action. Regarding pupil dilation, anisodamine is five times weaker than anisodine. Atropine followed by anisodine and anisodamine is the

Table 64.7. Lack of Antagonistic Effect of Higenamine on the Slowing of Cardiac Rate and Prolongation of AH Interval Caused by Propranolol

Comparison	Cardiac Rate (times/min)	AH Interval (ms)
Before injection	152 ± 16	46 ± 2
After injection of propranolol		
1 min	115 ± 16	74 ± 6
5 min	111 ± 14	83 ± 5
After injection of higenamine		
1 min	117 ± 14	85 ± 4
5 min	113 ± 15	85 ± 5
15 min	106 ± 14	84 ± 5

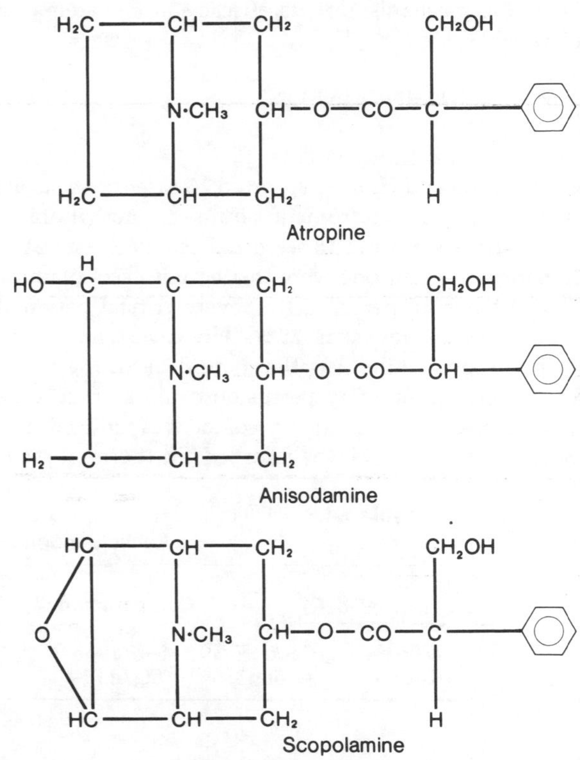

Figure 64.3. Chemical formulas of atropine (dl-hyocyamine), anisodamine, and scopolamine.

strongest in the inhibition of saliva secretion. Scopolamine and anisodine are stronger than anisodamine with respect to antitoxic action against organic phosphorus poisoning.

The main therapeutic action of hyoscine-like drugs is the antispasmodic, antitremor, and analgesic function against blood vessel or smooth muscle spasm. Therefore, good therapeutic effect can be obtained in all diseases with small blood vessel or smooth muscle spasm, or both, eg, infectious shock, bronchospasm, hemorrhagic enteritis, and the like. Some untoward side reactions, such as thirst, tachycardia, and urinary retention, may appear. With large dosage, mental disturbance and high fever may occur. The occurrence of the toxic side reaction and its intensity is greatly influenced by the functional state of the human body. Generally speaking, the younger the patient, the more severe are the side reactions. However, young patients have great tolerance. Sometimes such patients can tolerate a dose much greater than the toxic dosage.

INFECTIOUS SHOCK

In the treatment of infectious shock, as reported in the Third National Microcirculation and Hyoscine-like Drugs Research Seminar held in 1981, 42 cases of infectious shock were treated with anisodamine hydrochloride. The mortality rate was reduced to 4.5%. This favorable result was attributed to improvement in the microcirculation of the shock patients.[19] Xiu et al[21] found anisodamine to be a modest inhibitor of granulocyte aggregation and a powerful inhibitor of platelet aggregation; thromboxane synthesis was inhibited in anisodamine-treated platelets, further suggesting that inhibition of prostaglandin synthesis is a possible mechanism of its efficacy in bacteremic or other types of shock.

OTHER CLINICAL INDICATIONS

Diseases of Respiratory System

In 1980 Yang and Hong[20] reported 20 cases of the acute respiratory distress syndrome in adults, among whom 17 were in a shock state and 18 were assisted by a respirator; all 20 patients except one were treated with scopolamine (0.01 to 0.1 mg/kg per dose for severe critical patients) and the mortality rate was 25%. The investigators felt that when scopolamine was the main drug in the treatment of shock, pulmonary perfusion could markedly be improved, interstitial pulmonary edema was reduced, and pulmonary alveolar fluid was resorbed. Furthermore, scopolamine possesses certain therapeutic efficacy in stimulating respiration while sedating the cerebral cortex.[22]

Datura metel linn was the major drug employed in the treatment of 122 cases of cor pulmonale during the quiescent stage.[22] About one third of the patients received small doses of antibiotics in addition. Follow-up study demonstrated that this therapeutic regimen alleviated the symptoms and signs in most patients, improved the general mental and physical condition, and decreased the incidence of acute exacerbation of cold. Objectively, results of x-ray film of the chest, electrocardiogram, and blood gas analysis all improved. Simple and easy to administer, low in price, and effective in outcome, this herbal medicine is well received by all.

Diseases of the Cardiovascular System

In 20 cases of ischemic coronary heart disease treated by extract of hyoscine tablets with the addition of propranolol 10 to 20 mg three times a day continuing for one and a half to two months, the overall effective rate was 80% with improvement in the ST-T wave abnormality.[22] In two patients with intractable angina in whom many combinations of Chinese and Western medicines were used without improvement, the addition of hyoscine extract tablets controlled symptoms with improvement in the electrocardiogram. A patient with severe variant angina pectoris was relieved of attacks on the use of extract of hyoscine drugs.[22]

In recent years, further investigations were carried out on the mechanism of hyoscine drugs in the treatment of shock. It was found that 654-2, the synthetic anisodamine, possessed protective action against endotoxic shock and myocardial ischemic shock by relieving the vascular spasm induced by noradrenaline, improving the microcirculation, significantly reducing blood plasma content of fibrinogen, elevating the activity of fibrinolytic enzymes, liberating histamine, activating histaminic acid carboxylase activity, and thus reducing blood 5-HT, tryptophan, and noradrenaline contents.

Effect on the Reticuloendothelial System

A study carried out on the phagocytic function of the reticuloendothelial system of the rat revealed a definite enhancing effect of phagocytosis (Table 64.8).

Hematologic Diseases

Eight patients with shock following disseminated intravascular coagulopathy were treated with 654-2 or scopolamine. Four of them were given dibenzyline and one

Table 64.8. Effect of Hyoscine-Scopolamine on the Function of Phagocytosis of the Reticuloendothelial System in the Rat

Category		Concentration of Medication (ng/ml)	Time of Medication (days)	K Value (Index of Phagocytosis)		
Medicine Group	Control Group			Medication Group	Control Group	*P* Value
8	7	0.05	3	0.0023 ± 0.00056	0.0009 ± 0.00046	$P < 0.1$
10	10	0.1	14	0.0022 ± 0.0003	0.0009 ± 0.0004	$P < 0.05$

a hyoscine drug. All eight patients were cured completely.[22,23] The investigators attributed the successful outcome to the relief of blood vessel spasm by hyoscine drugs.

Effect on Renal Function

The superior effect of scopolamine on renal function in patients in shock during surgical anesthesia is illustrated in Table 64.9.

Effect on Platelets

Xu et al[23a] studied the effects of anisodamine (654-2) on platelet aggregation rate and release and morphologic changes by scanning electron microscope in endotoxemic rabbits (Figure 64.4). They suggested that the 654-2 protective action may be due to stabilizing of the lysosome membrane or other ways of inhibiting beta-glucuronidase release, which may also be its antishock mechanism.[23a]

DANSHEN (RADIX SALVIAE MILTIORRHIZAE)

The traditional Chinese herbal medicine, danshen (丹参) (Salvia miltiorrhizae Bge), has long been judged highly effective in "activating circulation and dispersing stasis or sludging of blood."[24–26] Among the classic teachings of traditional Chinese medicine, it is stated that, "When blockage is opened, pain is relieved"(通则不痛.不通则痛). Those trained in Western medicine, especially Chinese cardiologists, who at the same time are interested in traditional Chinese medicine, naturally tend to select some herbal drugs, such as danshen, as a subject for investigation. They are the vanguards, attempting to integrate the two completely different systems of medicine, traditional Chinese and modern Western, into a new school which has for the first time become a major endeavor in China.

HISTORY

In 1971, Yu from the Shanghai Second Medical College, Shanghai, China, began the earliest study of danshen. He found that oral administration of crude powder or concoction was effective in the treatment of angina pectoris. Ampuls of danshen injected into animals produced similar favorable results without untoward reactions. Finally, Yu himself received the intravenous injection of the danshen concoction, the first instance of intravenous administration of Chinese herbal medicine in man. The second intravenous injection was given to a house staff member, who had frequent attacks of precordial distress and occasional attacks of angina pectoris. The electrocardiogram showed inverted T waves. Immediately after injection, symptoms improved and the inverted T waves became isoelectric for more than eight hours. Subsequently, 11 cases of ischemic coronary heart disease were treated by intravenous injection of the drug at the Shanghai Third People's Hospital (which in October 1984 resumed the former name of Ren Ji Hospital). All of them noted improvement of symptoms within one day associated with T-wave changes from inversion to upright or isoelectric levels for two or three days. The authorities of Shanghai Public Health Bureau paid great attention to this remarkable event and called for further investigation of this drug. The Shanghai Cooperative Group for Study of Danshen was organized in 1971,[27,28] and the supply of ampuls of danshen concoction for parenteral use was taken over by the 9th Pharmaceutical Factory of Shanghai.[29]

From 1972 to 1974, 311 patients with ischemic coronary heart disease were treated with danshen; 80% demonstrated symptomatic and objective improvement and 50% electrocardiographic improvement.[25] These favorable results with danshen aroused great interest among Chinese cardiologists and led to extensive study of its action. Jin[24] presented a general comprehensive review of danshen's pharmacologic actions in 1978, but unfortunately by the end of his article no reference was given.

PHARMACOLOGY

Microcirculation was observed in the nail fold of 22 coronary patients.[24] In 70%, blood flow velocity increased after 22 weeks of danshen concoction injection; 50% showed persistent and definite improvement, which coincided with symptomatic and electrocardiographic T-wave improvement.

Blood rheology study showed significant improvement, as demonstrated by reduced blood viscosity in 75% of the patients, and reduced red blood cell electrophoresis in 92.9%.[24] Another coincidental finding during observation of blood rheologic change was the significant increases in the number and size of new capillary networks.[24] Results of the patients' vascular fragility tests became normal.[24]

The tolerance to anoxia was much greater in danshen-treated mice than in untreated ones; therefore, danshen was used in shock, epidemic hemorrhagic fever, throm-

Table 64.9. Comparison of Changes in Urinary Amount and Routine Urinalysis

Category	Cases (No.)	Changes in Urinary Amount (ml/h)				Amount of Urine During BP <60 MM Hg	Rate (%) of Improvement on Routine Urinalysis	
		>100	>50	50-30	>30		Intraoperatively	Postoperatively
Scopolamine group	76	23	41	10	2	Yes	70	100
Ether anesthesia group	20	1	8	7	4	No	47.2	96
Acupuncture anesthesia group	25	3	9	8	5	No	46	95

BP = blood pressure.

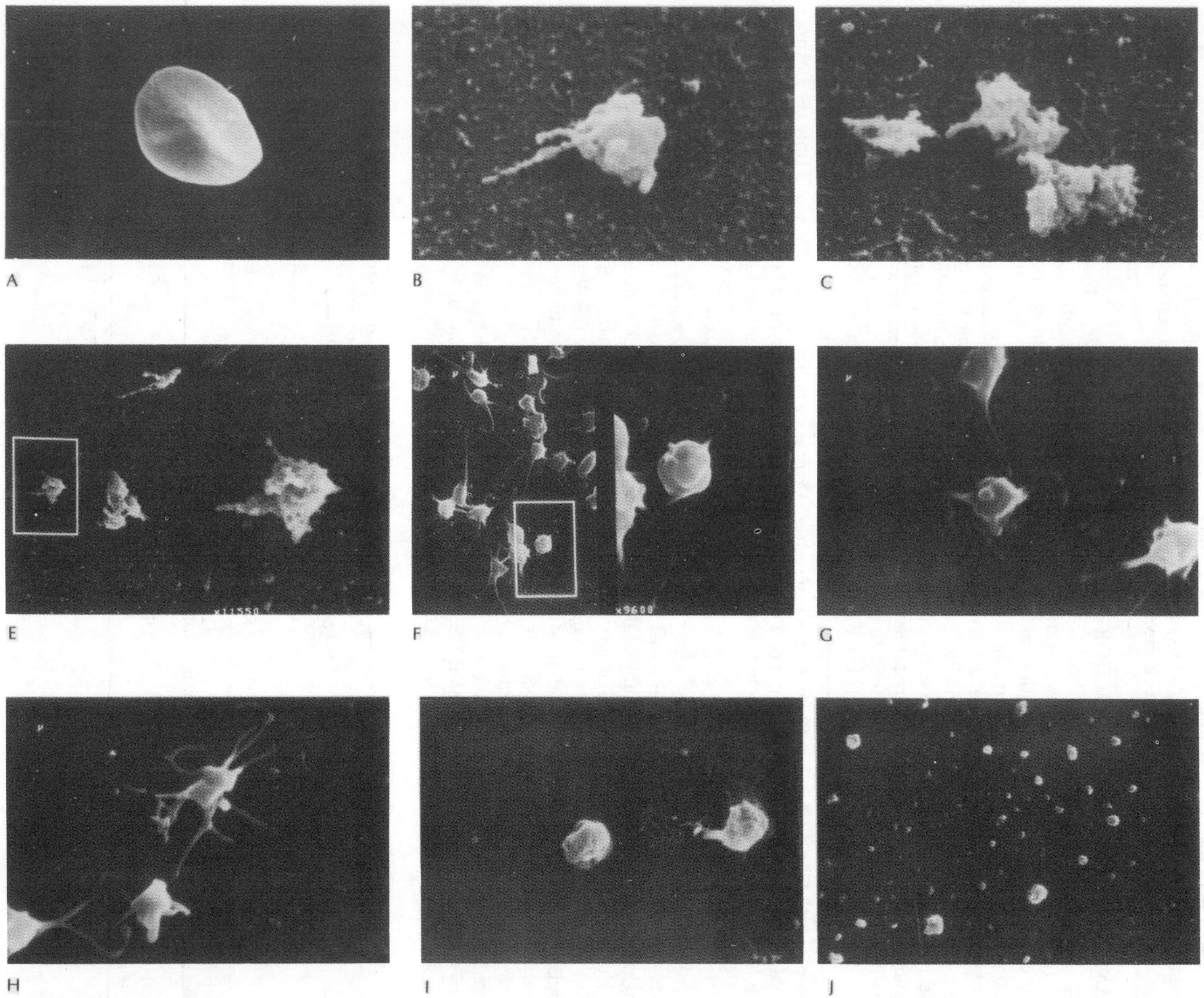

Figure 64.4. *A*, Rabbit platelet (PRP) before endotoxin injection; most of these platelets are disk shaped with smooth surfaces. *B and C*, PRP after endotoxin injection; platelet aggregation and long bifurcated pseudopods are present. Platelet surfaces have roughened, the shapes are irregular, and their density is decreased. *D and E*, PRP after 654-2 injection, platelet aggregation is partially dispersed, and the pseudopods are shortened and thickened. *F and G*, Washed platelets incubated with normal saline; platelets are spherechinocytes with smooth surfaces; some have a few long filopods or several bubbles on the surface. *H*, Washed platelets incubated with endotoxin; long bifurcated pseudopods are generally found. Rough surfaces, irregular shapes, and transparent hole-like areas have formed. *I*, Washed platelets incubated with 654-2; most of the platelets are spherechinocytes, pseudopods are shortened and thickened, and secretory granules may be found. *J*, Washed platelets incubated with both endotoxin and 654-2; platelets are mostly spherechinocytes, and pseudopods are rare. (From Xu et al,[23a] with permission.)

bolic vasculitis, and as an important adjuvant in antibiotic treatment.[24,30]

Danshen also possesses the action of coronary artery dilatation by temporarily increasing coronary blood flow which effectively improves cardiac function without increasing oxygen consumption.[24,31]

At the Shanghai Institute of Pharmacology, Academia Sinica, many active constituents were found to exist in the alcohol- and water-soluble extracts of danshen.[24,28] The alcohol-soluble constituents, after being subjected to aluminum oxide (Al_2O_3) chromatography and recrystallization from methanol, yielded tanshinone I, tanshinone IIA, and other tanshinone derivatives. The water-soluble constituents consisted chiefly of sodium-tanshinone IIA sulfonate, the structural formula of which, prepared from the Shanghai Institute of Pharmacology, is $C_{19}H_{17}O_6SNa$ with a molecular weight of 396.391 (Figure 64.5).

CLINICAL APPLICATION

Cardiologists from six hospitals in Shanghai recently organized the Shanghai Sodium Tanshinone IIA Sulfonate Cooperative Group[28] and carried out a double-blind study. Forty-six patients with proven coronary heart disease, ranging in age from 41 to 75 years (average 57), were given sodium tanshinone IIA sulfonate 160 mg in 250 ml of 5% glucose for intravenous infusion. Results showed that the effective rate was 73.1% ($\chi^2 = 19.05$; $P < 0.001$); electrocardiographic changes showed improvement in 59.7%, with a significant drug and placebo difference ($\chi^2 = 14.215$; $P < 0.001$).

Blood rheologic changes from sodium tanshinone IIA sulfonate, including blood viscosity, plasma viscosity, and blood fibrinogen content, showed insignificant changes or minor improvement only. This finding further emphasized that danshen concoction is more effective than sodium tanshinone IIA sulfonate. The findings of this double-blind study were fully in accord with Wang's results in animal experiments,[32] ie, the extent of acute myocardial infarction was reduced after sodium tanshinone IIA sulfonate treatment.

This double-blind study also verified previous reports that the capillary nail bed showed an increase in blood flow three to five minutes after intravenous injection of the drug. An increase in blood flow also was demonstrated in the mesenteric capillaries of the dog. However, this action of sodium tanshinone IIA sulfonate was shorter in duration than that of total extract of S miltiorrhizae.[28,33] We believe that the discrepancy in effectiveness is due to the difference between crude extract and sodium tanshinone IIA sulfonate.[28]

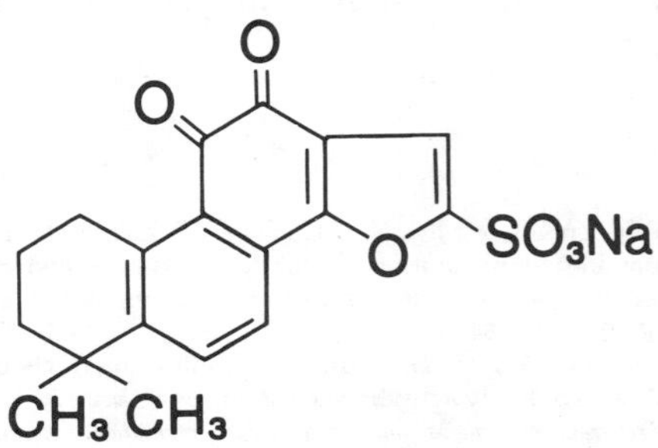

Figure 64.5. Structural formula of Danshen.

By Doppler's effect of laser light, the speed of blood flow in canine mesenteric microvasculature of a diameter of 14 to 40 μm was studied.[34] In 19 dogs, before and 5, 10, 15, and 20 minutes after intravenous injection of S miltiorrhizae, blood velocity was 0.426 ± 0.02, 0.49 ± 0.025 ($P < 0.001$), 0.553 ± 0.025 ($P < 0.001$), 0.526 ± 0.04 ($P < 0.005$), and 0.508 ± 0.04 mm/s ($P < 0.05$), respectively. The investigators concluded that the beneficial effect of S miltiorrhizae in angina pectoris probably was due to the increased microcirculatory blood velocity, which improved the perfusion of the ischemic myocardium.[34] The drug apparently improves tissue perfusion by increasing the oxygen supply. The absence of change in blood pressure and heart rate with no significant change in the caliber of the microvessels suggested that the danshen concoction might increase 2,3 diphosphoglyceride (2,3-DPG) of red blood cells, thus allowing red blood cells to change their shape readily during passage through microvessels whose caliber was smaller than the diameter of the red blood cell.

Danshen can also increase right ventricular myocardial contractility and reduce the afterload of the right ventricle. Using the method of systolic time intervals, Zhou et al[35] studied 26 patients with chronic cor pulmonale before and after intravenous injection of danshen. Right ventricular function and blood rheology improved significantly as follows: PEP time was reduced from 0.133 ± 0.018 second to 0.118 ± 0.017 second; RVET time increased from 0.292 ± 0.019 second to 0.324 ± 0.020 second; and PEP/RVET ratio decreased from 0.460 ± 0.083 to 0.395 ± 0.084. Whole blood viscosity and red blood corpuscle electrophoresis were also significantly improved ($P < 0.05$). The investigators concluded that a positive correlation exists between PEP, whole blood viscosity, and red corpuscle electrophoresis, that the increase in whole blood viscosity and hematocrit may increase the pulmonary arterial pressure, and that danshen by favorably influencing the PEP time, whole blood viscosity, and red cell electrophoresis reduces the afterload of the right ventricle, thus improving right ventricular contraction. It is interesting that danshen recently was incorporated into some Chinese cigarettes (Figure 64.6).

PROTECTION AGAINST MYOCARDIAL ISCHEMIA

Recently, the protective effect of danshen on ischemia of heart muscle during stoppage of cardiac pulsation was observed during extracorporeal circulation in 15 dogs.[36] "Protective infusion solution" with glucose, KCl, $MgCl_2{\cdot}6H_2O$, NaCl, and $CaCl_2{\cdot}H_2O$ was given, immediately followed by ice packages placed directly on the surface of the heart for rapid cardiac standstill, maintaining the temperature at 15° to 17°C. The ascending aorta was cross-clamped, and an infusion tube was inserted at the root of the aorta. Dogs that had danshen concoction in the infusion showed no increase in serum glutamic

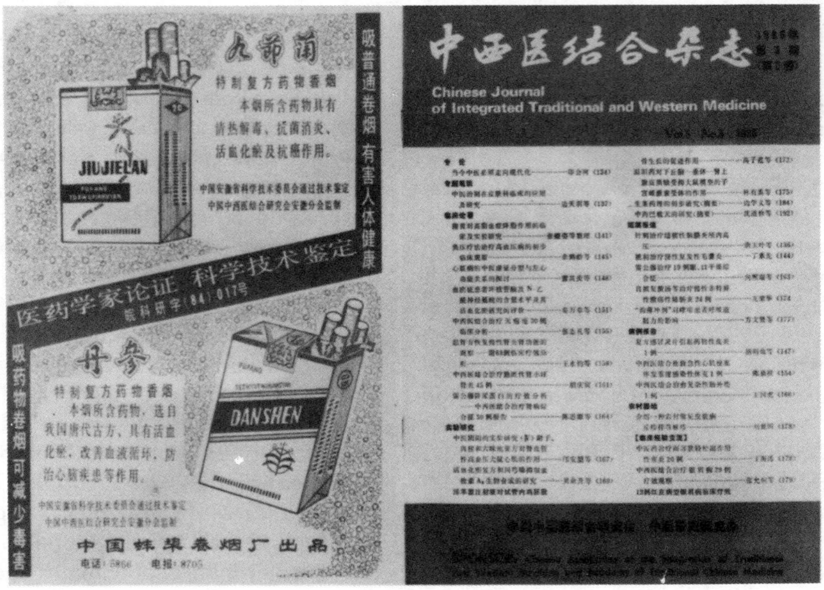

Figure 64.6. Danshen cigarettes advertised in a recent issue of the *Chinese Journal of Integrated Traditional and Western Medicine*.

oxalacetic transaminase content, denoting that permeability of the myocardial cellular membrane was fortified. Ultramicroscopic examination of specimens taken four hours after ligation of the coronary arteries revealed that mitochondrial damage in danshen-infused dogs was much less than that of dogs not receiving the infusion.[36]

In a group of three dogs that received $CaC1_2 \cdot 2H_2O$ 11.60 mMol/L in the protective solution without danshen, the nucleus, mitochondria, and capillaries were severely damaged. However, one group of four dogs with danshen and a similar concentration of $CaC1_2 \cdot 2H_2O$ in the infusion solution revealed only mild ultrastructural damage. Similar mild damage was observed in dogs receiving $CaC1_2 \cdot 2H_2O$ at only 2.04 mMol/L with danshen concoction added into the infusion solution. From the degree of damage observed, Zhu et al[36] concluded that danshen exerted a protective action on cardiac muscle cells by blocking the influx of calcium ions and combining the calcium into a nonionizing state at pH 7.15 in the intracellular milieu. In the extracellular fluid compartment, where acidic metabolites accumulated during extracorporeal circulation, calcium in a combined state was dissociated and changed back into calcium ions. This mechanism, in fact, protects the body from hypocalcemia. Danshen is therefore a calcium antagonist. Its usefulness in treating angina pectoris might well be partly attributed to this calcium antagonist action.[36–38]

THROMBOXANE SUPPRESSION

In 1984 a study of danshen on the effect of release of the vascular constricting factor of platelet was reported.[39] Injection of a watery extract of danshen (10 mg/100 g of body weight) led to suppression of the release of the vasoconstricting factor in rats. Before injection of danshen, 1 ml of the rat's platelet-rich plasma and 0.1 mg/ml of ADP were dropped into the incubation fluid, and a fresh rabbit aorta strip was placed in the solution equivalent to 1×10^{-9} of noradrenaline (NA). Contraction of $107 \pm 26\%$ occurred at 1×10^{-7} NA for one and a half hours. After danshen injection the rat's platelet-rich plasma induced a contraction of $38 \pm 22\%$ at 1×10^{-7} NA for less than one hour. Comparing the two tests the P value was highly significant, being less than 0.01. On the basis of these findings, the investigators concluded that danshen suppressed both the formation and the release of thromboxane A_2.[39] These effects of danshen, like those of persantin and aspirin, in inhibiting prostaglandin synthesis and platelet adhesion and aggregation have also recently been demonstrated in patients with diabetes mellitus.[40]

REFERENCES

1. Chou YP, Fen LL, Chang LY, Zheng GY: Studies on pharmacologic action of aconite. 1. Cardiovascular effect of higenamine. *Nat Med J China* 1978; 58:664–669.
2. Huang NH, Chou YP, Liu WL, Fen LL, Zheng GY: Cardiovascular comparison of effects of aconite root and higenamine in dogs. *Acta Pharmacol Sinica* 1980; 1:34–38.
3. Li LD, Xu CH, Zhang JM, Gao FH, Tu XY, Liu JX, Zhang J: The effect of higenamine on the pulsation of myocardial cells in vitro. *Chin J Cardiol* 1980; 8:141.
4. Bao YX, Yu GR, Xu JM, Xu YQ, Bian YT, Zheng DS: Effect of acute higenamine administration on bradyarrhythmias and His bundle. A clinical study of 14 cases and an animal experiment on dogs. *Chin Med J* 1982; 95:781–784.
5. Guo SK, Li JM, Zhao SH, Guo XZ: Studies on effects of higenamine on 33 cases of bradyarrhythmias. *Compilation of Data of Research on Prevention and Treatment of Cardiovascular Diseases by Combination of Chinese and Western Medicine* 1979; 6:49–51.
6. Jiang WQ, Tao SQ, Li JM, Fan AP, Chen KJ, Zhang WQ, Guo SK,

Qian ZW, Xu XH, Zhu QY, Sheng KH, Gu FS, Zheng GY: Effect of higenamine on bradyarrhythmias. A preliminary clinical observation. *Chin J Cardiol* 1980; 8:95–97.

7. Cardiovascular Institute and Fu Wai Hospital, Chinese Academy of Medical Sciences, Academy of Traditional Chinese Medicine, Friendship Hospital and Institute of Pharmacology, Chinese Academy of Medical Sciences. Unpublished data.
8. Liu XJ, Hu QW, Wang YQ, Wang SH, Chen ZJ, Wagner HN: Evaluation of left ventricular function by using nuclear stethoscope and ^{113m}Indium. *Chin J Cardiol* 1980; 8:90–93.
9. Qiao SY, Huang MX, Yu GR, Zheng DS, Bian YT, Chen SX: Effects of higenamine on action potentials of Purkinje and ventricular myocardial cells in dogs. *Chin J Cardiol* 1983; 11:260–264.
10. Wang BY, Huang MX, Yu GR, Zheng DS, Gu PK: Effect of higenamine on electrophysiological characteristics of myocardial cell. *Acta Pharmacol Sin* 1982; 3:112–115.
11. Yu GR, Wang BY, Zheng DS, Huang MX, Gu BK, Chen YL, Shang M, Jin ZJ, Cheng TO: Effect of higenamine on action potential of ventricular myocardial cells. *J Electrocardiol* 1985; 18:97–104.

11a. Yu GR, Chia SY, Zheng DS, Huang MX, Bien YT, Cheng TO: Effect of higenamine on action potential of Purkinje and ventricular myocardial cells. *Acta Cardiologica* 1985; 40:409–420.

12. Tong JS, Li HP, Yang MY, Yu DD, Zhang HD: Influence and mechanism of rehmania-root No. 1 on electrogram of sinus and bundle of His and corrected sinus recovery time. *Acta Acad Med Secondae Shanghai* 1984; 2:123–129.
13. Huang MX, Jiang SJ, Yu GR: Preliminary report of treatment of atropine in the treatment of cardiac arrhythmia and tartar emetic induced Adams-Stokes syndrome. Symposium of data in research on schistosomiasis. Published by the Hubei Provincial Anti-Schistosomiasis Commission, Hubei, China, Vol 2, 1957, p 102.
14. Huang MX, Jiang SJ, Pan RS, Yu GR, Lu ZW, Xu JY, Gao WS: Mechanism and treatment of cardiac arrhythmias in tartar emetic intoxication with special reference to atropine therapy. *Chin Med J* 1958; 76:103–115.
15. Huang MX, Jiang SJ, Yu GR, Lu ZW, Xu JY: The severe arrhythmias induced by tartar emetic poisoning. Collected works of the study on protecting and treating schistosomiasis. Shangai, Shanghai Science and Technique Publishing House, 1958, p 191.
16. Qian C, Xu XL, Wang ZC, Cai TZ, Wu PT, Cao MD: The effect of using atropine as the major drug in the comprehensive treatment of toxic bacterial dysentery. *Chin J Intern Med* 1961; 47:163–166.
17. Qian C: Mechanism and therapeutic effect of atropine in the treatment of toxic dysentery. *Chin J Pediat* 1964; 13:363–366.
18. Zhu SH: Experience in the emergency treatment of acute epidemic meningitis. *Chin J Pediat* 1966; 15:5–9.
19. Zhou SH, Liang WF, Zhou TL: Clinical experiences of 42 cases of infectious shock treated with anisodamine-HCL. *Chin J Emerg Med* 1982; 2:30–32.
20. Yang GD, Hong ZL: Clinical application of hyoscine-like drugs in medicine. *Chin J Intern Med* 1980; 19:303–305.
21. Xiu RJ, Hammerschmidt DE, Coppo PA, Jacobs HS: Anisodamine inhibits thromboxane synthesis, granulocyte aggregation, and platelet aggregation. A possible mechanism for its efficacy in bacteremic shock. *JAMA* 1982; 247:1458–1460.
22. Third National Research Symposium on Microcirculation and Hyoscine-like Drugs. Zhangzhou, China, December 14–22, 1981.
23. Yang GD, Wei SG: Some advances on the research of mechanism of hyoscine-like drugs in the treatment of shock. *Chin J Emerg Med* 1982; 2:50–52.

23a. Xu SH, Wu QX, Chen HC: Anisodamine effects on functional and morphologic changes of platelets in endotoxinemic rabbits. *Chin Med J* 1985; 98:106–110.

24. Jin HM: Clinical application of Salvia miltiorrhizae and the investigation of its mechanism for activating the blood circulation to eliminate blood stasis. *Nat Med J China* 1978; 58:180–183.
25. Cooperative Group for Study of Salvia Miltiorrhizae: Clinical observation of therapeutic effect of Salvia miltiorrhizae in patients of coronary heart disease. *Chin J Cardiovasc Dis* 1974; 2:143–150.
26. Shanghai First Medical College, Physiological Teaching Research Department, Pathological Teaching Research Department, Biological-Physics Teaching Research Department, Shanghai 9th Pharmaceutic Factory, Zhong Shan Hospital, Shanghai Cardiovascular Institute: A preliminary investigation of Salvia miltiorrhizae intravenous infusion in patients with coronary heart disease. *Chin J Intern Med* 1977; 2:203–206.
27. Shanghai Cooperative Group for Study of Tanshinone IIA: Therapeutic effect of sodium tanshinone IIA sulfonate intravenous infusion on 108 cases of coronary heart disease. *J Chin Herbal Inf* 1978; 1:37–40.
28. Shanghai Cooperative Group for the Study of Tanshinone IIA: Therapeutic effect of sodium tanshinone IIA sulfonate in patients with coronary heart disease: a double blind study. *J Trad Chin Med* 1984; 4:20–24.
29. Shanghai 9th Pharmaceutic Factory: An investigation of salvia miltiorrhizae and its infusion. *Medical Industry* 1973; 1:14–17.
30. Yu GR, Tang XM, Zheng DS, Huang MX, Han YS: Change of ischemic myocardium and ultrastructure in mice after Salvia miltiorrhizae infusion. *Chin J Integrated Trad West Med* 1981; 1:30–31.
31. Cardiovascular Department, Second Hospital, Chekiang Medical University: Clinical and laboratory investigation of coronary heart disease. *Compilation of Data of Research on Prevention and Treatment of Cardiovascular Disease by Integrating Traditional Medicine and Western Medicine*, 1978; 5:50.
32. Shanghai First Medical College, Zhong Shan Hospital, Shanghai Cardiovascular Institute, Bio-physics Teaching Department, Shanghai First Medical College, Shanghai 9th Pharmaceutic Factory: Therapeutic effect of experimental myocardial infarction after intravenous Danshen compound infusion. *Chin J Cardiovasc Dis* 1975; 3:197–199.
33. Shen WL, Yu GR, Zheng DS: Nail bed microcirculation in patients with coronary heart disease after Danshen injection. Proceedings of Symposium in Commemoration of the 30th Anniversary of Shanghai Second Medical College, Shanghai, China, October 1982, pp 9.54–9.55.
34. Yu GR, Zheng SH, Xie XL, Xin LL, Shou PY, Shi XF, Xu SC, Mao YF, Zheng SX: Effect of Salvia miltiorrhizae on dog's mesenteric microcirculatory blood flow measured by Doppler's effect of laser light. *Chin J Integrated Traditional and Western Med* 1984; 4:546–547.
35. Zhou HK, Hong ZL, Liu MS, Zhand SL, Wang ZL, Zheng FH: The effect of danshen on right ventricular function and blood rheology in chronic cor pulmonale. *Chin J Integrated Trad West Med* 1984: 4:220–221.
36. Zhu HS, Jiang TF, Wang YS, Feng ZR, Fan QR, Lu RX: An investigation of effect of Salvia miltiorrhizae on the protection of myocardium during ischemic cardiac arrest. *Acta Acad Med Secondae Shanghai* 1984; 3:177–179.
37. Patmore L, Whiting RL: Calcium entry blocking properties of tanshinone II-A sulphonate, an active principal of the antianginal extract Dan Shen. *Br J Pharmacol* 1982; 75:149P.
38. Huang WM, Digerness SB, Chen DGF, Tracy WG, Andrews NF: Increased protection against ischemic damage with the Chinese drug Danshen. In preparation.
39. Li CZ, Lin JB, Yang SC, Zhao FD, Zhang JC: Effect of Salvia miltiorrhizae on the release of vasoconstrictor substance of platelets. *Chin J Integrated Trad West Med* 1984; 4:565.
40. Zhu XX, Wang ZQ, Chen SH, Jin WM, Yan YZ, Zhu ZR: Effect of danshen and persantin on the alteration of platelet aggregation and microcirculation in diabetics. *Chin J Intern Med* 1985; 24:197–199.

65 Antibodies in Cardiology

Edgar Haber, MD

Progress in both medical diagnosis and therapy can often be identified with the discovery of a more selective reagent or drug. The antibiotic revolution is a most cogent example. The first antibiotic to be used, penicillin, is still the prototypical example of this principle. It kills bacteria at concentrations many orders of magnitude below those that harm mammalian cells and thereby it is exceptionally selective for its intended target. Antibodies have proven their value as diagnostic agents of even greater selectivity. An immunoassay may bind a single component present in low concentration in an incredibly complex biologic fluid that may contain hundreds of different substances. It is time now to examine whether antibody specificity may be harnessed beyond its well-accepted application in measurement, to in vivo detection and therapy.

The property that makes antibodies so attractive is their incredible diversity. There are at least 10 billion different antibody specificities.[1,2] With so many different binding sites to choose from, selective recognition of any structure within the human body should be possible.

We are in the midst of a period of explosive growth in our ability to make and utilize antibodies. Although antibodies have been recognized as serum components since the early 1900s, it was never possible to obtain sufficient quantities for any purpose other than a diagnostic assay. Antiserum samples always contain many more than one antibody, often hundreds characterized by differing affinities and specificities. Each animal produces a different mixture, which may vary from time to time even in the same individual. Standardization was therefore impossible. Antibodies could not be considered single chemical components.

These problems have now been solved by the discovery of the means to amplify a single antibody-producing clone.[3] These uniform cultures secrete a single antibody that may be considered a pure chemical. Recently, methods have been devised that allow large-scale production of antibodies in this manner in industrial fermenters.[4] It is already possible to transfect lymphoid cells with immunoglobulin genes, which results in the secretion of new proteins.[5,6]

The application of recombinant DNA methods has now permitted the production of antibodies in yeast.[7] We are not far from the point where antibodies will be produced in fermenters as cheaply as antibiotics.

Today, limitations in the use of antibodies in clinical medicine as in vivo diagnostic and therapeutic agents relate to their immunogenicity as foreign proteins, their long persistence in the circulation, and their propensity to form damaging immune complexes. A partial solution is already at hand, and the longer-term remedy is in sight.

Two clinical studies have already employed an antigen-binding fragment (Fab), a smaller fragment of the immunoglobulin molecule.[8,9] Immunoglobulin molecules and the immune complexes that may be formed, comprising simply a single antigen molecule with several Fabs attached, are smaller than those that cause nephrotoxicity.

Although smaller antibody fragments reduce the risk of immunogenicity, they are not likely to eliminate it entirely. Human immunoglobulins may now be produced by cell fusion techniques in vitro.[10,11] An even more promising potential development is in the application of molecular genetics techniques. Immunoglobulin genes are now routinely cloned for study.[1,2,12] It is reasonable to envision their manipulation and expression as antibody fragments that carry the minimal structure necessary to effect antigen binding. Recombinant DNA methods permit the introduction of human immunoglobulin framework sequences, so that tolerance to intrinsic proteins can prevent the mounting of an immune response.

Applications of antibodies that I would like to discuss include the treatment of digitalis intoxication, the evaluation of myocardial infarct size, the visualization and dissolution of thrombi in vivo, inhibition of the action of renin, and the selective blockade of adrenergic receptors. Two of these applications have reached the point of clinical investigation.

ANTIBODIES TO THE BETA-ADRENERGIC RECEPTOR

Pharmacologic agonists are often either peptides of modest size or organic compounds, both of which can be readily synthesized. For some receptors, a variety of antagonists has been created in the organic chemist's laboratory. Could an antibody for the receptor be obtained by using the ligand (agonist or antagonist) as a template? The vast diversity of antibody combining sites, as suggested herein, provides the potential for creating a complementary fit to almost any shape. If a figurative plaster mold could be cast on the surface of the ligand that would bind it to the receptor, then a second mold made from the first one should fit the receptor perfectly. The well-known immunologic principle of raising antibodies specific to another antibody's combining site (antiidiotypical antibodies) may be used to mold the desired shape.

This principle is effected by selecting antibodies that recognize common structures on all beta-adrenergic agonists and antagonists. These antibodies are nearly perfect mimics of the receptor, in that they bind all the compounds that would interact with the beta-adrenergic receptor, but they do not interact with similar compounds that are neither beta-specific agonists nor beta-specific antagonists. A second generation of antibodies (antiidiotypical antibodies) is then raised by using the first antibodies as immunogens. The antiidiotypical antibodies are selective beta receptor blockers, as is shown by their abilities to compete with beta-blocking drugs for the receptor and to inhibit the generation of adenylate cyclase when stimulated by isoproterenol[13] (Figure 65.1). Some potential uses of such receptor-specific antibodies are the recognition of structural differences among subsets of beta-adrenergic receptors; more rigorous examination of their respective physiologic roles using reagents of greater resolution; the isolation of receptors by antibody affinity chromatography; and the ultimate application of antibody fragments as highly selective drugs.

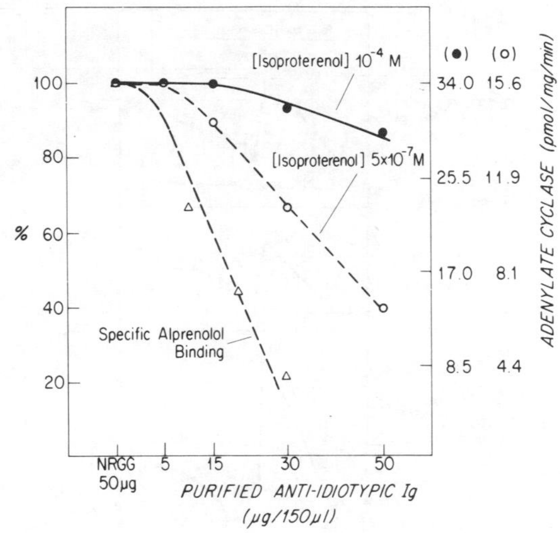

Figure 65.1. The effects of DEAE-purified Ig fraction on the percentage of (^{3}H)alprenolol (2 nmol) binding to turkey erythrocyte membranes and on isoproterenol-mediated adenylate cyclase stimulation. The ability of the anti-idiotypic Ig fraction to inhibit adenylate cyclase stimulation in turkey erythrocyte membrane was tested at isoproterenol concentrations of 0.5 μmol and 0.1 mmol in the presence of 0.1 mmol guanisine triphosphate. In contrast to the effects seen at the nonsaturating isoproterenol concentration of 0.5 μmol, only a slight amount of inhibition is seen at the highest Ig concentrations in the presence of 0.1 mmol of isoproterenol. NRGG = normal rabbit gamma globulin. (From Homcy et al,[13] with permission of the American Society for Clinical Investigation.)

RENIN-SPECIFIC ANTIBODIES

Although renin has been known to play a role in circulatory control since the classic work of Goldblatt et al[14] in the 1930s, its precise importance in a number of specific circumstances has been in doubt. Much has been learned from the application of inhibitors directed at several of the steps in the sequence leading to angiotensin II, the final product of renin. However, most of the inhibitors used lack specificity. The competitive inhibitors of angiotensin II's action on receptors, such as saralysin, are partial agonists.[15] The angiotensin-converting enzyme is identical to the enzyme that deactivates bradykinin; therefore, its inhibitors also affect the kinin system.[16] In addition, compounds such as captopril have been shown to stimulate prostaglandin synthesis.[17] Because both the kinin and the prostaglandin systems affect vasoregulation, it is difficult to define renin's specific role when interpreting experiments in which these inhibitors are used.

A specific antibody for renin should be a highly selective antagonist. Indeed, polyclonal renin-specific antibodies and their Fabs were shown to be effective renin-blocking agents in experimental hypertension[18,19] (Figure 65.2). Salt-depleted animals show a significant decrease in blood pressure when the antibodies are infused intravenously; in animals with renovascular hypertension, blood pressure is normalized. Monoclonal antibodies to human renin are now available and may provide the potential for using a highly selective renin blocker[20] to examine the role of renin in human essential hypertension, a question that is still largely unsettled.

DIGOXIN-SPECIFIC ANTIBODY IN THE CLINICAL REVERSAL OF TOXICITY

Digitalis intoxication is one of the most frequently reported adverse drug reactions. There is no specific antidote, and the cardiac arrhythmias that are a feature of digitalis intoxication are commonly fatal. We reasoned that if an antibody specific to the digitalis glycosides had a higher affinity for the drug than did the physiologic receptor, it should be possible to simply transfer the ligand from the receptor to the antibody. If Fab rather than intact antibody were used, the antibody-drug complex would be rapidly excreted in the urine.

After demonstrating safety and effectiveness in animal

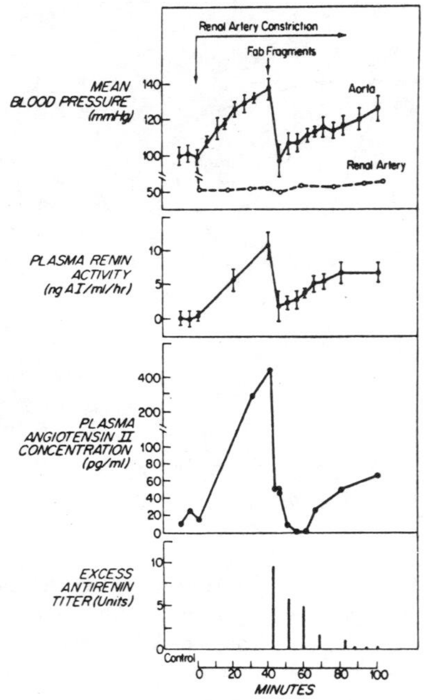

Figure 65.2. Immediate reduction by renin-specific Fab of systemic blood pressure, plasma renin activity, and angiotensin II levels to normal in acute renovascular hypertension. Duration of action was short-lived (30 to 60 minutes). (From Dzau et al,[19] with permission.)

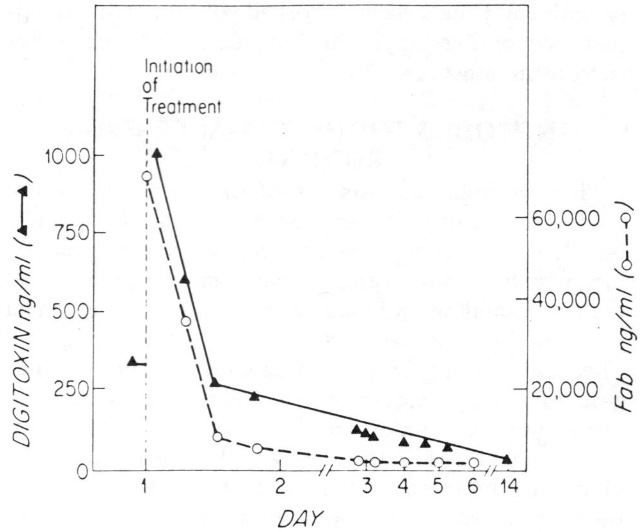

Figure 65.3. Blood levels of digitoxin and Fab fragments after intravenous administration of antibody Fab in a 34-year-old woman with a series of life-threatening arrhythmias as a result of a massive overdose (20 mg) of digitoxin. Within one hour of intravenous administration of antibody Fab, atrioventricular conduction had returned. (From Aeberhard et al,[23] with permission.)

studies, clinical studies were initiated. Results in 26 patients with life-threatening digitalis intoxication were reported in 1982 as the result of a multicenter national trial.[8] Twenty geographically dispersed university-based centers participated. Patients were chosen for the trial if they presented a life-threatening rhythm disturbance or hyperkalemia and were resistant to conventional therapeutic approaches. The patients ranged in age from 19 months to 35 years, and overdoses occurred either during the course of therapy or as a result of accidental or suicidal overdose. In each case a dramatic reversal of the presenting cardiac arrhythmia occurred. Five of the 26 patients died, one because inadequate quantities of Fab were available in the participating hospital and the rest because treatment was initiated after irreversible brain or cardiac damage had already occurred. In a more recent report of 63 patients so treated, results were remarkably similar to those in the earlier study.[21] An instructive example is that of a young woman who took 20 mg of digitoxin with suicidal intent.[22] She progressed through a series of dysrhythmias that included complete atrioventricular block with a very slow ventricular response, ventricular tachycardia, and ventricular fibrillation. She became hyperkalemic and was in cardiovascular shock. Within one hour after the intravenous administration of antibody Fab, atrioventricular conduction returned, and she was soon in normal sinus rhythm. No further dysrhythmias occurred. The patient was discharged from the hospital without sequelae several days later. Figure 65.3 demonstrates the initial marked increase in serum digitoxin concentration in this patient as tissue-bound drug equilibrated with the antibody (antibody-bound drug is pharmacologically inactive), followed by the rapid clearance of both drug and Fab.[23] It should be noted that the half-life of digitoxin in man is normally seven days, with hepatic metabolism of the drug being the major source of removal. It is apparent that excretion has been markedly accelerated by the antibody Fab, and the half-life is seemingly reduced to about 12 hours. Figure 65.4 shows

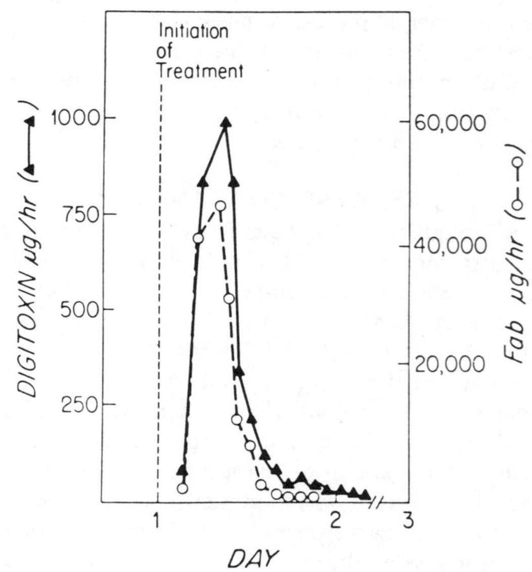

Figure 65.4. Urinary excretion of digitoxin and Fab fragments following intravenous administration of antibody Fab in a 34-year-old woman with digitalis intoxication (20 mg). (From Aeberhard et al,[23] with permission.)

that both antibody and Fab appear in the urine largely within the first day after Fab administration.

This approach to the neutralization of a toxic substance could be applied to many other substances. The accelerated excretion of a substance that is normally metabolized slowly is of particular interest. Digitoxin has a half-life of seven days and is metabolized by the liver. When bound to Fab, it has a biologic half-life of less than one day (Figure 65.3) and is excreted by the kidney (Figure 65.4).

IMAGING OF MYOCARDIAL INFARCTS

The diagnosis of myocardial infarction does not often present a significant challenge to the clinician. Symptoms may be pathognomonic and the so-called objective findings unequivocal. Quite often, however, when it is most important to identify myocardial infarction, associated injury or disease masks symptoms and distorts the results of laboratory tests, none of which is entirely specific. Beyond the question of diagnosis is quantification. Many attempts have been made to investigate methods for arresting the progress of infarction, thereby salvaging as much tissue as possible. It is difficult to evaluate the efficacy of these interventions without an objective in vivo measurement of the extent of cardiac tissue necrosis. To the present time, quantification of infarct size has only been possible in retrospect.

The hallmark of cell death is the loss of membrane integrity; when there is no longer a physical separation between inside and outside, the cell ceases to exist. This principle is commonly employed in clinical practice to diagnose tissue infarction. Intracellular enzymes are lost to extracellular fluid, and their increased concentration in the blood may be used as a measure of tissue necrosis. An alternative approach is to measure the inward diffusion of a marker that is normally excluded from cells. We have selected myocardial infarction as a model, and radioactively labeled myosin-specific antibody as a marker.[24] Myosin is the principal protein of the cardiac cell. Its covalent structure is unique to the heart, allowing the development of antibodies that differentiate cardiac myosin from skeletal and smooth-muscle myosins. In the intact organism, cardiac myosin is protected from extracellular fluid by the cell's plasma membrane. When cell death occurs and the membrane breaks down, myosin is exposed to extracellular fluid. It is then available to react with labeled antibodies or antibody fragments.

In the first clinical study, Fab fragments of antimyosin antibodies labeled with technetium-99m by means of a bifunctional chelating agent, diethylene triamine pentaacetic acid, were used in the scintigraphic examination of 32 patients with myocardial infarction and unstable angina pectoris.[9] The results were compared with regional wall motion studies by ventriculography or gated blood pool scanning at 10 to 14 days after the onset of symptoms. Figure 65.5 shows a typical antimyosin scintigram of an anterior infarct and a tracing of the late ventriculogram.[25] Concordance in the apparent region of injury defined by these different methods is excellent. Initial clinical studies in over 50 patients show substantial promise that a highly selective method may be developed for imaging and sizing myocardial infarcts. This approach will be of particular value in assessing methods of evaluating reperfusion therapy following coronary thrombosis.

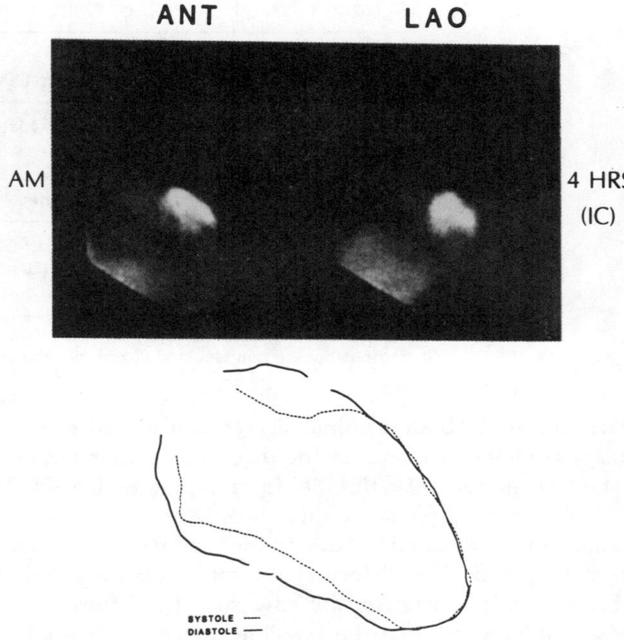

Figure 65.5. Antimyosin images in the anterior position (*top left panel*) and left anterior oblique position (*top right panel*) of a patient with acute anterior infarction. Antimyosin was administered by the intracoronary (IC) route 4 hours prior to imaging. There is antimyosin concentration in the anterolateral wall and upper septum. *Bottom panel* shows end-diastolic (*solid lines*) and end-systolic (*dotted lines*) outlines of the contrast ventriculogram performed at ten days. Akinesia of the anterolateral wall of the left ventricle corresponds to the zone of antimyosin uptake. (From Haber,[25] with permission.)

DETECTING THROMBI IN VIVO

It would be highly desirable to have an antibody specific for fibrin that did not react with fibrinogen. Immunization with fibrin usually results in antibodies to epitopes common to both fibrin and fibrinogen, that cannot differentiate between the two molecules. An alternate approach is to synthesize an immunogen that duplicates the unique structural features of fibrin. Fibrinogen is converted to fibrin in three steps. Thrombin, a proteolytic enzyme, cleaves the alpha and then the beta chain of fibrinogen, revealing two new amino termini. Factor XIII effects amide bond cross-links between the gamma and alpha chains. Potential candidate epitopes include all of these structures. We synthesized peptides of the sequence of the amino termini of the alpha and beta chains of fibrin and showed that both polyclonal and monoclonal antibodies could be identified that bound fibrin uniquely, even in the presence of physiologic concentrations of fibrinogen.[26,27] One of the monoclonal antibodies, 64C5, has been shown to bind to human fibrin precipitated on a filter paper disk when injected intravenously in an ex vivo circulatory model in the chicken[27,28] (Table 65.1). With this encouragement, we have labeled the antibody with indium-111, a radionuclide suitable for scintigraphy.

Table 65.1. Detection of Human Fibrin: Chicken Ex Vivo Circulatory Model

Experiment	Paper Disk	Circulation Ex Vivo (min)	Counts per Minute†
Ex vivo detection of fibrin disks by intravenous antibody 64C5*	Fibrin-coated	0	1,935 ± 250
	Fibrin-coated	10	13,116 ± 450
	Fibrin-coated	60	15,396 ± 600
	Uncoated	60	442 ± 60

* Two disks containing 30 to 35 μg of human fibrin were placed in a cylindrical plastic chamber and exposed to intravenously administered 64C5 (50 μg) for the indicated time before in vitro treatment with the second antibody.

† Mean radioactivity associated with ^{125}I-labeled antibody to mouse Fab, used to detect monoclonal antibody 64C5 bound to human fibrin-coated disks. Data are means ± standard deviations for two separate determinations. (From Hui et al,[27] with permission. Copyright 1983 by AAAS.)

Early results in both a pulmonary embolism and a coronary thrombosis model in the dog suggest that localization of intravascular thrombi in vivo may be feasible.

The exciting promise of this work is not only in the delineation of thrombi in both arteries and veins, but also in the potential for detecting ulcerated atherosclerotic plaques that characteristically have superficial fibrin deposits. It may one day be possible to map potentially troublesome arterial lesions before occlusive thrombosis occurs.

ANTIBODY-DIRECTED FIBRINOLYSIS

Selective fibrinolysis of thrombi has long been an attractive concept. Fibrinolytic agents, such as streptokinase, urokinase, or tissue-type plasminogen activator exert their effect by activating plasminogen to plasmin, which in turn degrades fibrin. Plasmin is a proteolytic enzyme that is not selective for fibrin and therefore readily degrades fibrinogen. Of the three plasminogen activators used in clinical therapy, tissue-type plasminogen activator has the greatest affinity for fibrin and is therefore the most selective. However, all three result in fibrinogenolysis as well as fibrinolysis, which leads to bleeding as a complication of therapy.

We sought to use a fibrin-specific antibody that binds to fibrin specifically with very high affinity, to direct a plasminogen activator to a single substrate. By increasing the concentration of the plasminogen activator solely in the vicinity of fibrin, plasminogen would be locally activated to effect fibrinolysis, but it would be inactivated by circulating antiplasmin before attacking circulating fibrinogen.

Reduced urokinase was coupled to fibrin-specific monoclonal antibody 64C5 by means of its intrinsic sulfhydryl using N-succinimidyl 3-(2-pyridyldithio) propionate (SPDP) as a cross-linking agent.[29] Unconjugated urokinase and its component subunits were separated from the urokinase-antibody conjugate (^{125}I-UK)-SS-(64C5) by gel filtration on Sephacryl® S-200. Two radioactive fractions were clearly resolved; the first contained the antibody-urokinase conjugate and was free of unconjugated urokinase. The molecular weight of this fraction was greater than 150 kilodaltons (KD) as assessed by sodium dodecylsulphate polyacrylamide gel electrophoresis and it proved to be radioactive on subsequent autoradiography. Because radioactivity was initially associated with the 30 KD subunit of urokinase, this observation demonstrated the covalent linkage of urokinase to antibody. Further evidence of the association of urokinase activity with antibody was obtained by affinity chromatography of the antibody-urokinase conjugate on a column constructed by coupling a synthetic amino terminal beta chain fibrin peptide (Gly-His-Arg-Pro-Leu-Asp-Lys-Cys, beta peptide)[28] to maleimidobenzoyl lysine-Sepharose® Cl-4B.[30] The eluate of this column (0.2 M glycine hydrochloride, pH 2.8) was radioactive and fibrinolytic, both properties of urokinase, in the assay to be described. The same methods were used to synthesize and purify a conjugate of urokinase and a monoclonal antibody of irrelevant specificity, (^{125}I-UK)-SS-(3H3).[31]

A quantitative fibrinolytic assay was devised by linking fibrin monomer to Sepharose. Fibrinogen was purified of plasmin contaminates by passage over lysine-Sepharose and then mixed with trace labeled ^{125}I-fibrinogen. It was then coupled to cyanogen bromide activated Sepharose Cl-4B. The immobilized fibrinogen was converted to fibrin by the addition of human thrombin in the presence of 100 mM $CaCl_2$.

To assess their relative fibrinolytic activity, increasing amounts of (^{125}I-UK)-SS-(64C5) and unconjugated urokinase were incubated with ^{125}I-fibrin-Sepharose for four hours. Thereafter, the resin was incubated with purified plasminogen. After intervals of 2.5 and 15 hours, the mixture was centrifuged and the radioactivity of the supernatant was determined. This procedure was repeated with the control conjugate, (^{125}I-UK)-SS-(3H3).

To obtain kinetic information, (^{125}I-UK)-SS-(3H3) and (^{125}I-UK)-SS-(64C5), each in a plasminogen-containing solution, were continuously circulated over a column of ^{125}I-fibrin-Sepharose. At set intervals, samples were collected and their radioactivity was determined.

Figure 65.6 indicates that the concentration of (^{125}I-UK)-SS-(64C5) required to release labeled peptides from fibrin-Sepharose was 1/100 that of unconjugated urokinase.[32] The myosin antibody conjugate, (^{125}I-UK)-SS-(3H3), did not differ significantly from unconjugated urokinase. Figure 65.7 shows that (^{125}I-UK)-SS-(64C5) markedly enhances the rate of release of peptides from fibrin-Sepharose and that this effect is unimpaired by fibrinogen at a physiologic concentration.[32] Beta-peptide inhibits fibrinolysis of (^{125}I-UK)-SS-(64C5), whereas it has no effect on the fibrinolytic rate of unconjugated urokinase or (^{125}I-UK)-SS-(3H3).

A monoclonal antibody specific for fibrin is thus able

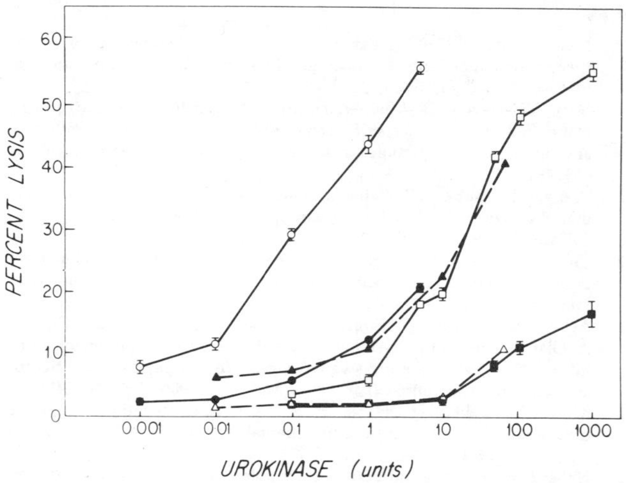

Figure 65.6. Release of labeled peptides from fibrin-Sepharose by a conjugate of urokinase and fibrin-specific antibody (urokinase antifibrin conjugate) (black circles, 2.5 hours; white circles,15 hours), urokinase control conjugate (white triangle, 2.5 hours; black triangles, 15 hours) and unconjugated urokinase (black squares, 2.5 hours; white squares, 15 hours). The two conjugates and the unconjugated urokinase (100 μl containing the indicated amount of urokinase) were each incubated for four hours with 100 μl of ^{125}I-fibrin-Sepharose, washed once with 3 ml 0.1 M Tris, 0.1 M NaCl, 0.5% bovine serum albumin, 0.5% Triton X-100, and three times with 3 ml tris-buffered saline azide and incubated for 2.5 and 15 hours with purified plasminogen (120 mg/liter). Lysis is expressed as the quotient of released radioactivity and total radioactivity. Each point represents the mean ± standard deviation of three independent determinations. (From Bode et al,[32] with permission. Copyright 1985 by AAAS.)

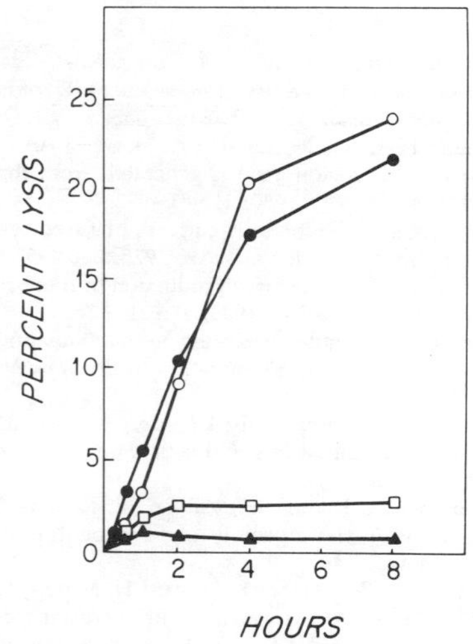

Figure 65.7. Release of ^{125}I-labeled peptides from fibrin-Sepharose during continuous circulation of a solution containing plasminogen (0.12 mg/ml) and urokinase antifibrin conjugate in the presence (*white circles*) and absence (*black circles*) of 3.5 mg/ml of fibrinogen. The experiment is repeated with control conjugate in the presence (*black triangles*) and absence (*white squares*) of fibrinogen. In each instance the circulating fluid contained 0.25 units of urokinase per milliliter coupled to either of the antibodies. Each point represents the mean of three determinations with a standard deviation of less than 1.6%. (From Bode et al,[32] with permission. Copyright 1985 by the AAAS.)

to target the plasminogen activator urokinase to fibrin and, by virtue of enhanced local concentration, to increase the efficiency of plasmin lysis 100-fold. The antibody is sufficiently fibrin-specific so that physiologic concentrations of fibrinogen do not interfere with enhanced fibrinolysis. Fibrinolytic effectiveness is not enhanced by the coupling of urokinase to a monoclonal antibody of irrelevant specificity, and it is significantly diminished by a peptide representing the epitope recognized by the fibrin-specific antibody. If these effects can be demonstrated in vivo, the dose of urokinase required for effective lysis of a thrombus would result in only minimal fibrinogenolysis, the major impediment to the widespread application of this form of therapy.

WHAT ARE THE NEXT STEPS?

Selection of hybridomas among the many candidates that present is a rather powerful method for finding antibodies suitable to any given application. This approach may certainly be enhanced by selecting epitopes for immunization, as already detailed in the fibrin antibody discussion. A further refinement that may be necessary if these steps do not yield an antibody of either appropriate selectivity or affinity may be the manipulation of the amino acid sequence of the antigen combining site by recombinant DNA methods, such as site-directed mutagenesis. Before this can be applied, we need to know much more about the relation between antibody structure and antigen binding specificity.

To diminish immunogenicity, it would be most desirable to use antibodies that contain constant and perhaps even variable region sequences homologous with human immunoglobulins. Hybrid molecules that contain mouse variable regions and human constant regions have already been constructed.[33,34] As noted earlier, widespread practical application will require large-scale production, most economically by either bacterial or yeast fermentation.[35]

I have only scratched the surface of what I believe to be a vast potential for tapping the specificity and selectivity of antibodies as both diagnostic and therapeutic agents in medicine.[36] Wherever there is a unique structure, be it tissue determinant or circulating hormone or drug, an antibody should be able to recognize it. Once recognized, it can be located, blocked, or deactivated. I believe that we are on the brink of a new pharmacology based on the unique resolution of the antibody combining site.

Acknowledgment: This work was supported in part by Grants HL 26215 and HL 19259 from the National Institutes of Health, Bethesda, Maryland.

REFERENCES

1. Sakano H, Kurosawa Y, Weigert M, Tonegawa S: Identification and nucleotide sequence of a diversity DNA segment (D) of immunoglobulin heavy-chain genes. *Nature* 1981; 290:562–565.
2. Early P, Huang H, Davis M, Calame K, Hood L: An immunoglobulin heavy chain variable region gene is generated from three segments of DNA: VH, D, and JH. *Cell* 1980; 19:981–992.
3. Köhler G, Milstein C: Continuous cultures of fused cells secreting antibody of predefined specificity. *Nature* 1975; 256:495–497.
4. Fazekas de St Groth S: Automated production of monoclonal antibodies in a cytostat. *J Immunol Methods* 1983; 57:121–136.
5. Rice D, Baltimore D: Regulated expression of an immunoglobulin kappa gene introduced into a mouse lymphoid cell line. *Proc Natl Acad Sci USA* 1982; 79:7862–7865.
6. Oi VT, Morrison SL, Herzenberg LA, Berg P: Immunoglobulin gene expression in transformed lymphoid cells. *Proc Natl Acad Sci USA* 1983; 80:825–829.
7. Wood CR, Boss MA, Kenten JH, Calvert JE, Roberts NA, Emtage JS: The synthesis and *in vivo* assembly of functional antibodies in yeast. *Nature* 1985; 314:446–449.
8. Smith TW, Butler VP Jr, Haber E, Fozzard H, Marcus FI, Bremner WF, Schulman IC, Phillips A: Treatment of life-threatening digitalis intoxication with digoxin-specific Fab antibody fragments: experience in 26 cases. *N Engl J Med* 1982; 307:1357–1362.
9. Khaw BA, Gold HK, Yasuda T, Leinbach RC, Strauss HW, Fallon JT, Cahill SL, Haber E: Acute myocardial infarct imaging with technetium-99m-DPTA-antimyosin Fab (abstr). *Circulation* 1982; 66:272.
10. Olsson L, Kaplan HS: Human-human hybridomas producing monoclonal antibodies of predefined antigenic specificity. *Proc Natl Acad Sci USA* 1980; 77:5429–5431.
11. Croce CM, Linnenbach A, Hall W, Steplewski Z, Koprowski H: Production of human hybridomas secreting antibodies to measles virus. *Nature* 1980; 288:488–489.
12. Seidman JG, Leder A, Nau M, Norman B, Leder P: Antibody diversity. The structure of cloned immunoglobin genes suggests a mechanism for generating new sequences. *Science* 1978; 202:11–17.
13. Homcy CJ, Rockson SG, Haber E: An antiidiotypic antibody that recognizes the beta-adrenergic receptor. *J Clin Invest* 1982; 69:1147–1154.
14. Goldblatt H, Lynch J, Hanzal RF, Ramon F, Summerville WW: Studies on experimental hypertension. 1. The production of persistent elevation of systolic blood pressure by means of renal ischemia. *J Exp Med* 1934; 59:347–379.
15. Hollenberg NK, Williams GH, Burger B, Ishikawa I, Adams DF: Blockade and stimulation of renal, adrenal, and vascular angiotensin II receptors with 1-Sar, 8-Ala angiotensin II in normal man. *J Clin Invest* 1979; 57:39–46.
16. Swartz SL, Williams GH, Hollenberg NK, Moore TJ, Dluhy RG: Converting enzyme inhibition in essential hypertension: the hypotensive response does not reflect only reduced angiotensin II formation. *Hypertension* 1979; 1:106–111.
17. Goldstone R, Martin K, Zipser R, Horton R: Evidence for a dual action of converting enzyme inhibitor on blood pressure in normal man. *Prostaglandins* 1981; 22:587–598.
18. Dzau VJ, Kopelman RI, Barger AC, Haber E: Renin-specific antibody for study of cardiovascular homeostasis. *Science* 1980; 207:1091–1093.
19. Dzau VJ, Kopelman RI, Barger AC, Haber E: Comparison of renin-specific IgG and antibody fragments in studies of blood pressure regulation. *Am J Physiol* 1984; 246:H404–H409.
20. Dzau VJ, Devine D, Mudgett-Hunter M, Kopelman RI, Barger AC, Haber E: Antibodies as specific renin inhibitors: studies with polyclonal and monoclonal antibodies and Fab fragments. *Clin Exper Hypertens* [A]1983; 5:1207–1220.
21. Wenger TL, Butler VP, Haber E, Smith TW: Treatment of 63 severely digitalis toxic patients with digoxin-specific antibody fragments. *J Am Coll Cardiol* 1985; 5:118A–123A.
22. Bismuth C, Gaultier M, Conso F, Efthymiou ML: Hyperkalemia in acute digitalis poisoning: prognostic significance and therapeutic implications. *Clin Toxicol* 1973; 6:153–162.
23. Aeberhard P, Butler VP, Smith TW, Haber E, Eng DT, Brau J, Chalom A, Glatt B, Thébaut JF, Delangenhagen B, Morin B: Le traitement d'une intoxication digitalique massive (20 mg de digitoxine) par les anticorps anti-digoxine fractionnés (Fab). *Arch Mal Coeur* 1980; 73:1471–1478.
24. Khaw BA, Beller GA, Haber E, Smith TW: Localization of cardiac myosin-specific antibody in experimental myocardial infarction. *J Clin Invest* 1976; 58:439–446.
25. Haber E: Monoclonal antibodies: their potential as *in-vivo* diagnostic and therapeutic agents, in Bizollon CA (ed): *Monoclonal Antibodies and New Trends in Immunoassays.* Amsterdam, Elsevier Science Publishers BV, 1984, pp 81–90.
26. Matsueda GR, Hui KY, Pacella BL Jr, Young JD, Haber E: Synthetic fibrin-like peptides used as antigens yield fibrin-specific antibodies, in Hruby VJ, Rich DH (eds): *Peptides: Structure and Function.* Proceedings of the Eighth American Peptide Symposium, Tucson, Arizona. Rockford, Ill, Pierce Chemical Co, 1984, pp 873–876.
27. Hui KY, Haber E, Matsueda GR: Monoclonal antibodies to a synthetic fibrin-like peptide bind to human fibrin but not to fibrinogen. *Science* 1983; 222:1129–1131.
28. Hui KY, Haber E, Matsueda GR: Immunodetection of human fibrin using monoclonal antibody-64C5 in an extracorporeal chicken model. *Thromb Haemost* 1985; 54:524–527.
29. Carlsson J, Drevin H, Axen R: Protein thiolation and reversible protein-protein conjugation. N-Succinimidyl 3-(2-pyridyldithio)propionate, a new heterobifunctional reagent. *Biochem J* 1978; 173:723–737.
30. Kitagawa T, Aikawa T: Enzyme coupled immunoassay of insulin using a novel coupling reagent. *J Biochem (Tokyo)* 1976; 79:233–236.
31. Khaw BA, Mattis JA, Melincoff G, Strauss HW, Gold HK, Haber E: Monoclonal antibody to cardiac myosin: imaging of experimental myocardial infarction. *Hybridoma* 1984; 3:11–23.
32. Bode C, Matsueda GR, Hui KY, Haber E: Antibody-directed urokinase: A specific fibrinolytic agent. *Science* 1985; 229:765–767.
33. Morrison SL, Johnson MJ, Herzenberg LA, Oi VT: Chimeric human antibody molecules: mouse antigen-binding domains with human constant region domains. *Proc Natl Acad Sci USA* 1984; 81:6851–6855.
34. Boulianne GL, Hozumi N, Shulman MJ: Production of functional chimaeric mouse/human antibody. *Nature* 1984; 312:643–646.
35. Haber E: Antibodies in cardiovascular diagnosis and therapy. *Hospital Practice* 1986; 21(2):147–172.
36. Haber E: In vivo diagnostic and therapeutic uses of monoclonal antibodies in cardiology. *Annu Rev Med* 1986; 37:249–261.

66 Cardiac Rehabilitation: A Strategy for the 1990s and Beyond

Robert F. DeBusk, MD

CARDIAC REHABILITATION: A PARADOX IN CLINICAL MEDICINE

Cardiac rehabilitation is the process by which patients with cardiac disease, especially ischemic heart disease, are brought to their highest level of function after *acute clinical events* such as myocardial infarction (MI) or *interventions* such as coronary artery bypass graft (CABG) surgery. Cardiac rehabilitation represents a paradox in clinical medicine: it is highly regarded by most patients and disparaged by most physicians. That patients prize cardiac rehabilitation is hardly surprising: it emphasizes the personalized side of medicine—information, encouragement, and support—which patients and their families consider lacking in the increasingly technology-intensive care of patients with ischemic heart disease. Cardiac rehabilitation is an example of what John Naisbitt, author of the best-selling book, *Megatrends*, calls "high touch," which complements the "high tech" approach to the management of ischemic heart disease with sophisticated imaging techniques, invasive studies, and surgery.[1]

The medical profession's low regard for cardiac rehabilitation results primarily from the fact that this discipline is not considered "main line." The most tangible success of cardiac rehabilitation is the enhancement of functional capacity, which is perceived by most physicians to be of secondary importance. Cardiac rehabilitation has not convincingly improved prognosis (a criticism that can be leveled at most medical and surgical interventions!), which is regarded as the paramount objective of medical care. Second, cardiac rehabilitative services are provided in facilities, such as gymnasia, which are unfamiliar to physicians who spend their time in hospitals, offices, and clinics. Third, although physicians perceive their own efforts to provide comprehensive services, such as risk factor modification, to be inadequate, they are generally reluctant to relinquish this role to others, fearing that their authority may be undermined: at the least there is the potential for misunderstanding and at worst a loss of control over patient care.

To understand why cardiac rehabilitation as a discipline has not thrived within the American medical care system, it is instructive to compare cardiac rehabilitation and CABG surgery. The point of this comparison is differences in structure and function rather than efficacy of these two interventions. Coronary artery bypass graft surgery is preceded not only by coronary arteriography but also often by a variety of noninvasive tests. The testing that precedes the surgery and tests performed subsequently benefit the cardiologists and pathologists who interpret these tests and those who operate the laboratories in which the tests are performed. A busy surgical service helps to assure the fiscal health of the hospital on which all physicians depend. Both the referring physician and the surgeon share the gratitude of the patient for the favorable effects of surgery, which are observed in the great majority of cases. The referring physician is confident that the surgeon will promptly return the patient to his or her care. Moreover, the surgeon often refers patients for medical care to the same physicians who refer their patients for surgical care. Importantly, the entire process of surgical care occurs within a few days, in a physical environment with which the referring physician is familiar. Finally, the entire transaction does not take place without prearranged payment to all the parties just noted.

Contrast this neat scenario with that of cardiac rehabilitation after acute MI, which occurs over a span of many weeks to months, in an environment with which the referring physician is generally unfamiliar, with no benefits to health care providers or laboratories other than those operating the cardiac rehabilitation program. Exercise training, risk factor modification, and other elements of cardiac rehabilitation are provided by a variety of professionals whose advice may differ from that of the referring physician. Reimbursement for these services is marginal and no professional benefit, such as the referral of patients from the cardiac rehabilitation program, accrues to physicians who refer patients to these programs.

Pressures to limit medical expenditures during the next decade are likely to force many American cardiac rehabilitation programs out of existence and to limit the scope of those that manage to survive. In part this reflects the fact that cardiac rehabilitation programs are currently not structurally or functionally integrated into the traditional medical care system. This chapter presents a strategy for accomplishing this.

CURRENT OBJECTIVES OF CARDIAC REHABILITATION PROGRAMS IN THE MANAGEMENT OF ISCHEMIC HEART DISEASE

TO IMPROVE PROGNOSIS

Conclusive proof that the prognosis of patients with ischemic heart disease can be improved through cardiac rehabilitation is lacking, although a favorable trend has been found in most studies of heart attack survivors.[2] There are several reasons for this:

1. Patients who are medically eligible for exercise training, which is the centerpiece of cardiac rehabilitation, are generally at low risk; patients at high risk due to severe angina and heart failure are not considered eligible for such programs. Moreover, the low risk patients who have entered these programs after MI have generally done so after three months, at which time the mortality rate has fallen sharply.[3] It is difficult to demonstrate the benefit of any treatment on prognosis in low risk patients.

2. Formidable logistical constraints have limited the number of patients participating in trials of cardiac rehabilitation. Supervised group exercise training programs are costly to operate and regular attendance at these programs over a period of many months is inconvenient for patients; participation in such programs at 6 months after MI rarely exceeds 50%.[4]

3. Evaluation of the efficacy of cardiac rehabilitation is confounded by dropouts from exercise training and by "drop-ins," ie, individuals in the "control" group who undertake regular physical activity. Moreover, prognosis is also influenced by alteration of risk factors such as smoking, which are not directly related to the primary intervention of exercise training. Finally, patients participating in randomized trials receive a variety of medications that may influence prognosis apart from the primary intervention of exercise training. Consequently, it has been impossible to demonstrate that cardiac rehabilitation programs emphasizing exercise training demonstrably improve prognosis in patients with ischemic heart disease.

In the one study that demonstrated a clear-cut improvement in prognosis, the contribution of exercise training was not well established, for functional capacity was no higher in patients receiving intervention than in control subjects.[5] Although multifactorial programs combining physical exercise training and risk factor modification are more likely to succeed than those featuring only exercise training, the cost of the exercise training component vastly exceeds that of other components such as risk factor modification, which in any event, can be offered in a non-group setting.

It is instructive to compare the effects of cardiac rehabilitation and beta-blocking drugs on the prognosis of patients after MI. Whereas fewer than 4,000 patients have participated in randomized trials of cardiac rehabilitation, more than 10,000 have participated in drug trials.[2] Beta blockers can be safely administered to the vast majority of post-MI patients, commencing within hours or days after the acute event. The inclusion of clinically high risk patients in drug studies helps to insure that significant differences between treated and untreated patients will be found. It is vastly more convenient to take medication than to attend a group rehabilitation program over an extended period. This eliminates one major logistical limitation of rehabilitation programs, ie, declining participation in regimens of exercise training and the possibility of "drop-in" to treatment by patients assigned to the control group. These considerations largely explain why beta blockers have been shown to lower mortality in post-MI patients, whereas cardiac rehabilitation has not.

The claim that cardiac rehabilitation can improve prognosis is not convincing to most physicians. Even if cardiac rehabilitation and beta blockers were equally effective, simple economic and logistical considerations would favor the latter in practice.

TO ENHANCE FUNCTIONAL CAPACITY

The restoration of physical vigor following acute coronary events and interventions has been the centerpiece of cardiac rehabilitation. Exercise training alleviates cardiac symptoms and leads to an enhanced sense of well-being. However, recent studies indicate a substantial degree of *spontaneous* improvement in functional capacity following acute MI.[6,7] The *independent* contribution of exercise training to a restoration of functional capacity has until recently been poorly defined. Early ambulation after acute MI and CABG surgery has tended to limit the degree of deconditioning which in years past was the major contributor to physical disability following these events. Physicians generally do not perceive an increase in functional capacity as an important therapeutic objective. Moreover, exercise training has not been shown to improve functional status, eg, the resumption of occupational work. Enhancement of functional capacity apart from relief of angina pectoris has a relatively narrow appeal. Alleviation of angina pectoris is as effectively accomplished by drug therapy as by exercise training. Moreover, the former is much more widely available!

TO IMPROVE PSYCHOLOGIC WELL-BEING

Patients often report an enhanced sense of well-being resulting from their participation in cardiac rehabilitation programs. The support provided by the professional staff and by peers also contributes. Cardiac rehabilitation programs provide information, support, and encouragement that are often otherwise lacking. These services tend to alleviate the mild to moderate anxiety and depression that are almost universal following acute MI. These psychologic states tend to regress spontaneously, however. Most patients with MI who are incapacitated by anxiety or depression usually have a history of psychologic dysfunction before MI. Patients with severe anxiety or depression, or both, are generally referred to psychologists and psychiatrists for specific therapy. Although the identification of these patients is often facilitated by the staffs of the cardiac rehabilitation programs, it is difficult to demonstrate that participation in cardiac rehabilitation programs diminishes these psychologic sequelae of acute MI.

TO MODIFY RISK FACTORS

An important element of cardiac rehabilitation programs is the assistance provided to patients in altering coronary risk factors, especially smoking and hypercholesterolemia. Participants in cardiac rehabilitation programs often *do* adopt a healthier life-style including nonsmoking and less fat in the diet. However, assistance in modifying these and other risk factors is available outside cardiac rehabilitation programs.

STRUCTURE AND FUNCTION OF CARDIAC REHABILITATION PROGRAMS

The services provided by cardiac rehabilitation programs are multidisciplinary in scope and therefore tend to be provided by groups of professionals that may include physicians, nurses, vocational rehabilitation specialists, physical therapists, dietitians, psychologists, and psychiatrists. The chief requirement of such programs is a facility large enough to accommodate groups of patients undergoing exercise training. The facility also provides space for individual or group counseling of patients and for housing the professional and administrative staff of the program. Facilities large enough for all these activities are expensive. Because few cardiac rehabilitation programs have a sufficiently large patient population to warrant full-time use, they often share the costs of the multiuse facility with other organizations such as the YMCAs.

The structure and function of cardiac rehabilitation programs reflect the need to assure the safety of, and adherence to, relatively intensive regimens of exercise training. Because intensive exercise in patients with ischemic heart disease occasionally results in cardiac arrest, it has until recently been considered axiomatic that such training occur in a supervised group setting. A substantial proportion of the costs of participation in many cardiac rehabilitation programs, especially for-profit ones, is devoted to continuous electrocardiographic "hard-wire" monitoring. Whether such monitoring contributes to the safety of exercise training has not been established. Third party reimbursement for participation in medically supervised cardiac rehabilitation programs that use hard-wire monitoring is under close scrutiny and is likely to be substantially reduced.

A multidisciplinary group approach to rehabilitation, which emphasizes intensive exercise training, involves large capital and personnel expenses. These factors have considerably increased the costs and limited the availability of such rehabilitative services to as few as 15% to 20% of post-MI patients. Because such programs are popular with patients, they are likely to continue to operate; however, it seems increasingly clear that they may have to do so outside the traditional system of third party reimbursement.

NEW STRATEGY FOR CARDIAC REHABILITATION IN THE 1990s AND BEYOND

The goal of decreasing mortality through cardiac rehabilitation has remained elusive, and the elaborate structure of cardiac rehabilitation programs that has evolved during the last three decades now threatens to collapse under its own weight. Cardiac rehabilitation as a scientific discipline has now come of age: the early research models that were important in developing the individual components of rehabilitation have brought this discipline to the threshold of widespread clinical application.

The centerpiece of the new rehabilitation strategy is the development of effective techniques for the *assessment of prognosis* soon after important clinical events such as acute MI.[8–10] In patients with a good prognosis, *functional capacity* is generally maintained; customary activities, including occupational work, can generally be resumed soon after the acute event.[11,12] *Counseling* of low risk patients regarding prognosis and functional capacity, including provision for the resumption of customary activities, usually eliminates medically unwarranted fears, enabling these patients to make a more rapid and complete recovery.[13,14] Finally, long-term *risk factor modification* can be accomplished through medically directed self-care: patients who engage in regular physical activity[15,16] can also learn to become or remain nonsmokers and modify their diet at home with the assistance of periodic telephone and other contact with nurses and other health care professionals.

This strategy for rehabilitation employs a stepwise approach to the evaluation of prognosis to separate low risk patients, who comprise the majority, from high risk patients, who comprise the minority. There is no consensus regarding the management of the latter: these patients will likely continue to receive relatively more intensive diagnosis and therapy. However, the rehabilitation strategy described herein enables a more cost-effective evaluation of the prognosis in high risk patients after acute MI. This strategy results in a lesser use of diagnosis and therapy in low risk patients and the reduction of disability through the earlier return to work of these individuals.

IMPROVED METHODS FOR THE ASSESSMENT OF PROGNOSIS

The unpredictable course of ischemic heart disease sets it apart from other serious medical conditions such as head and spinal cord injury in which sudden unexpected clinical deterioration is relatively rare. Although uncertainty about the long-term outcome remains a feature of ischemic heart disease, this uncertainty has been dramatically reduced in recent years by systematic follow-up studies which have examined patients recovering from myocardial infarction and other acute ischemic heart syndromes.

A wide variety of historical and clinical characteristics and specialized tests have been used to distinguish high risk and low risk patients soon after the acute event. For example, a combination of historical and clinical characteristics and symptom-limited exercise testing 3 weeks after acute MI has enabled the identification of nearly three quarters of patients who had recurrent MI and death in the 6 months following the evaluation (Figure 66.1). Other studies have also indicated that very low risk patient subsets, comprising 30% to 60% of the entire post-MI population, can be identified by a combination of history and clinical characteristics and specialized tests including radionuclide ventriculography, thallium perfusion scintigraphy, and ambulatory electrocardiography.[17–19] It is important to define these very low risk patient subsets, for they are least likely to benefit from currently available medical or surgical therapies. Further diagnostic testing will predictively increase the cost of care for these patients without improving their outcome.

In general, the prognosis of patients with ischemic heart disease reflects the *extent of infarcted myocardium* and the *extent of myocardial ischemia*. The extent of infarcted myocardium is reflected in clinically evident left ventricular failure, ie, the presence of one or more of the following: pulmonary rales, cardiac gallops, radiographic evidence of pulmonary congestion, cardiomegaly, extensive Q waves on the electrocardiogram including a QRS score greater than 10, and substantial elevation of cardiac enzymes, eg, peak CPK-MB greater than 500 U/L.[20] Patients with clinically evident left ventricular failure have a poor prognosis. No further diagnostic testing is required to establish this fact. However, severe left dysfunction, which is not clinically evident, can be detected by exercise testing performed 7 to 14 days after MI. Such testing has its greatest independent value in patients without clinically severe left ventricular dysfunction. A low peak treadmill exercise workload, especially in the absence of angina pectoris, and failure to increase the systolic pressure or a decrease in systolic pressure generally reflect significant left ventricular dysfunction. Patients with these exercise-induced abnormalities have an annual mortality several times greater than that of patients without such abnormalities.

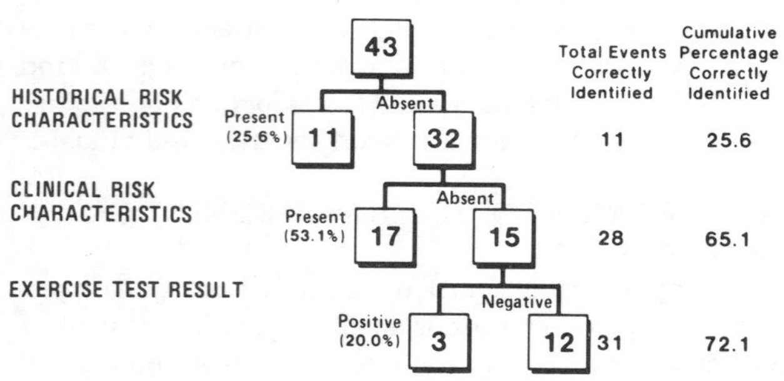

Figure 66.1. Stepwise risk stratification procedure: hard medical events within 6 months (6.4% of patients). (From DeBusk et al[8] with permission.)

The other major determinant of prognosis in post-MI patients is the extent of ischemic myocardium. Patients with recurrence of ischemic chest pain 24 to 48 hours after acute MI have a substantially increased mortality rate compared with that in those without recurrent pain.[21] Specialized testing is not required to establish the presence of myocardial ischemia in such individuals, although coronary arteriography is often a necessary prelude to the treatment of such syndromes with percutaneous transluminal coronary angioplasty (PTCA) or CABG surgery. However, patients without ischemic chest pain at rest may manifest evidence of ischemia during exercise testing performed 7 to 14 days after MI. Predischarge exercise testing limited to 5 METs (multiples of resting energy expenditure) or 70% of predicted maximum for age often discloses severe exercise-induced myocardial ischemia manifested by ST-segment depression equal to or greater than 0.2 mV. The sensitivity of submaximal predischarge exercise testing for the prediction of subsequent death and reinfarction is enhanced by exercise thallium perfusion scintigraphy[22] and radionuclide ventriculography.[23]

Thus, from a practical standpoint the evaluation of prognosis after MI is a stepwise process: patients at the very highest risk for subsequent cardiac events are those with historical characteristics including prior infarction, angina before infarction, and angina after infarction.[8] Many of these clinically high risk patients also demonstrate significant clinical abnormalities, eg, clinically evident myocardial ischemia and left ventricular dysfunction (Figure 66.2). Exercise testing 14 to 21 days after MI is relatively hazardous and may contribute little to the evaluation of prognosis in these individuals. Patients with clinically evident myocardial ischemia and left ventricular dysfunction who lack the high risk historical triad have an intermediate risk. Exercise testing is also relatively

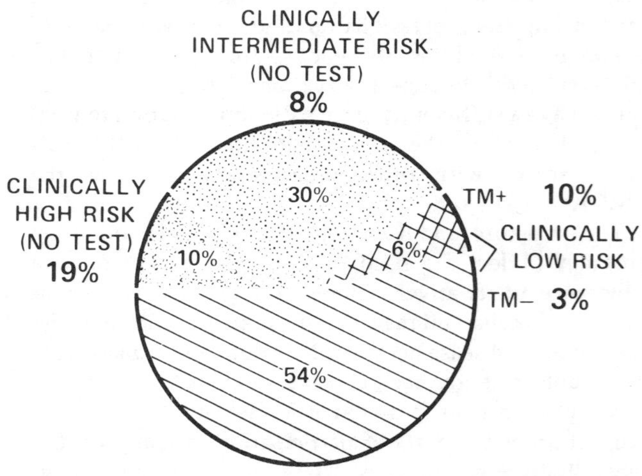

Figure 66.2. Prognosis in 722 male survivors of acute myocardial infarction. Rate of medical events (death and reinfarction) within 6 months. TM+ = treadmill test positive (ST-segment depression ≥0.2 mV at a heart rate ≤135 beats per minute); TM− = treadmill test negative (ST-segment depression <0.2 mV or occurring at a heart rate >135 beats per minute).

hazardous in such patients. Patients without clinically evident ischemia or left ventricular dysfunction comprise a clinically low risk group. Within this group, symptom-limited exercise testing is effective in distinguishing the few patients at high risk (TM+) from those at low risk (TM−) (Figure 66.2). Importantly, the same exercise test that is used to evaluate prognosis can be used to provide individualized guidelines for physical activity in patients after MI.

IMPROVED METHODS FOR EVALUATING AND ENHANCING FUNCTIONAL CAPACITY

The classic autopsy study of Mallory et al[24] in 1939 concerning patients who had died within 6 weeks after MI was an important milestone in the management of this clinical syndrome.[24] If 6 weeks were required for complete tissue healing, it seemed logical that 6 weeks of absolute bedrest would be required to facilitate and assure this healing. However, experience has shown that patients can be safely mobilized at a much earlier point. Recent physiologic studies have indicated that the influence of acute MI on left ventricular dysfunction has largely stabilized within 1 week after the acute event.[25]

Recognition that bedrest, even in normal individuals, has deleterious effects gradually led to the adoption of early ambulation, but the notion persisted that formal exercise training would be required to restore functional capacity to preinfarction levels. This belief was furthered by another classic study, that by Saltin et al[26] of five normal college men who underwent 21 days of bedrest. This study was designed to elucidate the mechanisms by which functional capacity was restored after bedrest, rather than to assess the need for exercise training to accomplish this purpose.

A more recent study of normal middle-aged men undergoing ten days of bedrest indicates that the major cause of the bedrest-induced decline in functional capacity was simple hypovolemia,[27] which can be eliminated by four hours or more per day of sitting quietly in a chair. Spontaneous restoration of bedrest-induced volume deficits occurs relatively quickly, ie, within days. Restoration of functional capacity after ten days of bedrest was not facilitated by a program of vigorous exercise training commencing on the day after bedrest and extending over the next 2 months.[28] This calls into question the need for formal inhospital rehabilitation programs of structured physical activity to increase functional capacity in patients after MI.

Identification of low risk patients has important implications for the provision of physical activity following acute cardiac events such as MI. In general, functional capacity is well maintained in the absence of critical left ventricular dysfunction and unstable angina pectoris. Moreover, even in the absence of formal exercise training, large spontaneous increases in functional capacity occur in the 3 to 6 months following acute MI. This appears to reflect an increase in the peak exercise heart rate, rather than a substantial improvement in myocardial perfusion or in exercise left ventricular function (Figures 66.3 and 66.4).

The ability to define clinically very low risk patient

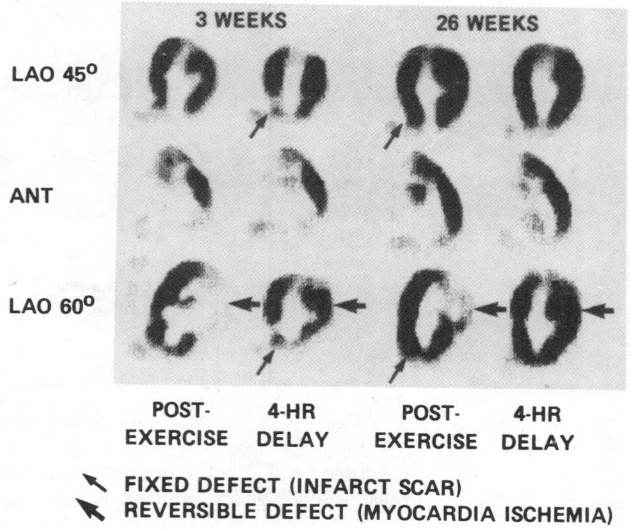

Figure 66.3. Thallium perfusion scintigrams from a patient with inferior Q waves. A fixed inferoapical defect (infarct zone) and a reversible thallium defect posterolaterally (periinfarctional) appear 3 weeks after infarction. At 26 weeks after infarction, the "fixed" inferoapical defect has undergone substantial regression, but the "reversible" posterolateral ischemic defect persists. This patient had treadmill-induced angina pectoris and ischemic ST-segment depression at 3 and 26 weeks. ANT = anterior; LAO = left anterior oblique. (From Hung J, Gordon EP, Houston N, Haskell WL, Goris ML, DeBusk RF: Changes in rest and exercise myocardial perfusion and left ventricular function 3 to 26 weeks after clinically uncomplicated acute myocardial infarction: effects of exercise training. *Am J Cardiol* 1984; 54:943–950. Reprinted with permission.)

subsets has enabled a reevaluation of the rationale and methodology for exercise training following acute MI. In a randomized trial of clinically low risk post-MI patients, at-home exercise training was as effective as group exercise training in increasing functional capacity[15] (Figure 66.5). From a baseline capacity of approximately 7 METs at 3 weeks after MI, functional capacity increased to an average of 8 METs at 11 weeks and 9 METs at 26 weeks. "No-training" patients underwent symptom-limited exercise testing at 3 weeks but received no formal instruction in exercise training. Patients in the control group had no exercise testing until 26 weeks and received no formal instruction in exercise training. Patients of this study represented 60% of men aged 70 or less, and 80% of patients remained in the study without cardiac events during the first 6 months after infarction.

No training-related cardiac events were noted. Adherence to both the home and gymnasium regimens of physical exercise exceeded 90% through the 11th week and 75% through the 26th week after infarction.[15] Contributors to the safety and efficacy of home training included individualized activity guidelines based on the 3-week exercise test, the use of heart rate monitors to assist patients to remain within prescribed limits of intensity during exercise, and systematic brief surveillance of patients during exercise training sessions by means of a transtelephonic electrocardiogram-transmitting device. Nurses called patients during two of their five training sessions

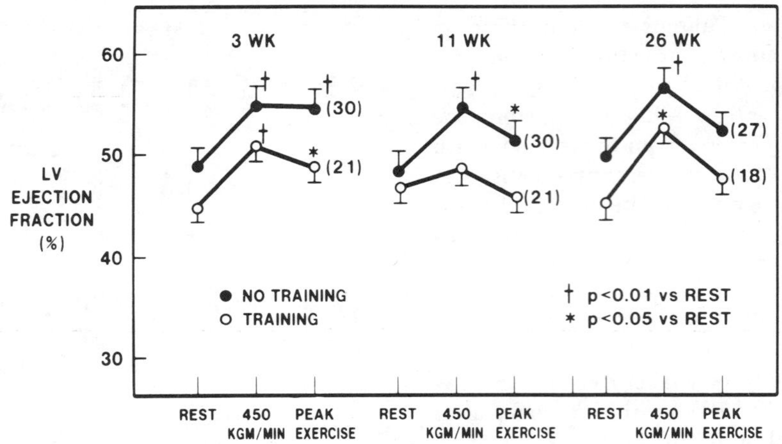

Figure 66.4. Left ventricular (LV) function 3 to 26 weeks after infarction. KGM/MIN = kilogram · meter/minute. (From Hung J, Gordon EP, Houston N, Haskell WL, Goris ML, DeBusk RF: Changes in rest and exercise myocardial perfusion and left ventricular function 3 to 26 weeks after clinically uncomplicated acute myocardial infarction: effects of exercise training. *Am J Cardiol* 1984; 54:943–950. Reprinted with permission.)

each week to record the electrocardiogram for one minute during peak exercise and the first minute of recovery. No patient was dropped from the home training program on the basis of ischemic ST-segment depression or ventricular arrhythmias recorded on these brief electrocardiographic transmissions. Of the patients with worsening angina who were referred for coronary arteriography, most underwent CABG surgery. Thus, the nurse-initiated systematic telephone surveillance not only provided important reassurance and information to patients regarding the general course of their recovery, but also helped to facilitate the appropriate evaluation and management of patients whose clinical course deteriorated during the study.[16]

"No-training" patients stated that they were quite physically active during the first 6 months: the self-reported extent of vigorous nonprescribed exercise performed by these patients rivaled that of patients participating in prescribed home or gymnasium training.

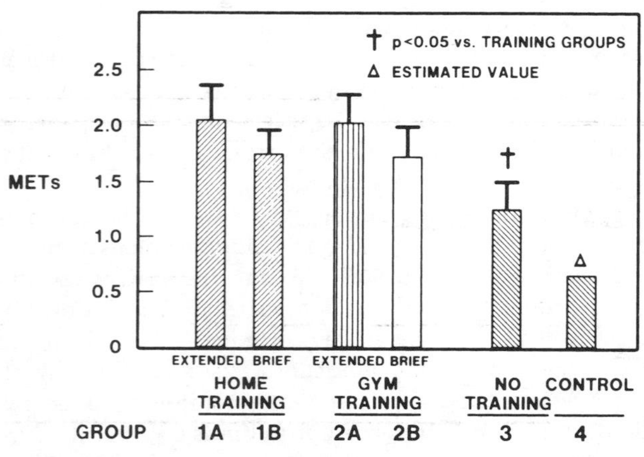

Figure 66.5. Change in functional capacity occurring between 3 and 26 weeks after infarction, expressed in METs or multiples of resting energy expenditure. Extended = 23 weeks of training; brief = 8 weeks of training.

Therefore, it appears that symptom-limited exercise testing soon after acute MI provides substantial reassurance to clinically low risk patients and may provide guidelines for a simple program of physical exercise that does not require stationary cycles or transtelephonic transmitting devices.

The overall importance of this study is *not* the fact that functional capacity increased to a greater extent in those who underwent training than in those who did not. Two findings were of special clinical importance[16]:

1. Symptom-limited exercise testing at 3 weeks identified nearly half of the patients who experienced a cardiac event in the following 6 months: of the five patients with profound myocardial ischemia who were not randomized, three experienced a subsequent cardiac event, as did seven of ten randomized patients (70%) who demonstrated prognostically important ischemic ST-segment depression equal to or greater than 0.2 mV at a heart rate of 135 beats per minute or less. The high incidence of subsequent cardiac events in these patients justifies the performance of coronary arteriography and consideration for CABG surgery or PTCA as early as 3 weeks after acute MI.

2. Patients appreciated the continuity of care provided by systematic telephone contact with a nurse. Patients realized that the nurse was working under the direction of the physician and that significant changes in clinical course would immediately be reported to the physician so that appropriate responses could be initiated promptly. Patients also appreciated the information and support provided by the nurse: their high level of adherence to the prescribed exercise training regimen reflected this.

Occupational Work Evaluation in Ischemic Heart Disease

In clinically low risk post-MI patients, symptom-limited exercise testing at 3 weeks not only serves to define prognosis and to provide the basis for individualized physical activity guidelines, but also provides a measure of occupational work potential.[12] Automation has dramatically reduced the physical requirements of occupational work in the United States during the past 30 years. Most heavy occupational work is performed by younger individuals. For these reasons, neither exercise conditioning nor job retraining is required to restore the physical work capacity of the great majority of patients recovering from acute MI and CABG surgery. Patients whose exercise tests reveal a good prognosis and well-preserved functional capacity are quite capable of performing even relatively vigorous physical effort soon after the acute event.

As early as the 1940s, Levine[29] observed that the time at which physicians recommended to patients that they could return to work after a heart attack coincided with the point at which mortality from this condition had declined. Despite the fact that modern techniques have enabled a relatively accurate assessment of prognosis and functional capacity by techniques just described herein, these developments have had little impact on physicians' recommendations to patients regarding the time at which they can return to work after a heart attack.

Recent research indicates that low risk "white collar" workers can return to work earlier than the customary 6 to 8 weeks and low risk "blue collar" workers can return much earlier than 8 to 12 weeks after MI. Even if their jobs require relatively heavy physical effort, most clinically low risk patients can safely return to work 3 to 4 weeks after MI. Such patients are free of significant myocardial ischemia during symptom-limited exercise testing performed 3 weeks or more after MI.

Patients who do not demonstrate significant myocardial ischemia on symptom-limited treadmill exercise tests are also unlikely to do so during tests in which symptom-limited treadmill or bicycle effort is combined with a variety of other stimuli such as static effort, the postprandial state, and exposure to cold[30] (Figures 66.6 and 66.7). In other words, the absence of significant ischemic and arrhythmic abnormalities on a symptom-limited exercise test provides a generic measure of the robustness of the heart and the ability of patients to resume their occupational activities. The common practice of deferring

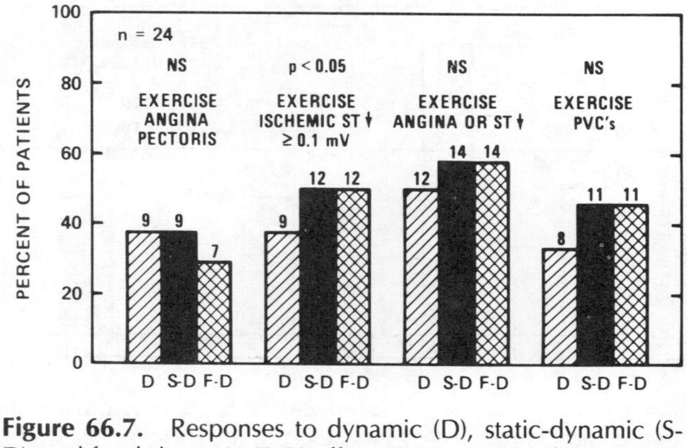

Figure 66.7. Responses to dynamic (D), static-dynamic (S-D), and food-dynamic (F-D) effort. NS = not significant; PVCs = premature ventricular contractions; ST↓ = ST segment depression.

occupational work evaluation, ie, exercise testing, until 6 weeks after MI is self-fulfilling: patients are not likely to return to work before this time, even though most are medically capable of doing so. Once public and private disability insurers and self-insuring employers understand the potential of early exercise testing to reduce the duration of disability, they are more likely to support the costs of such testing.

Exercise Training of High Risk Coronary Patients

Close medical surveillance of patients who are moderately symptomatic from congestive heart failure or angina pectoris is a potentially important application of cardiac rehabilitation. Prolonged observation of these patients in a group exercise training program over a period of weeks or months often facilitates clinical decision-making. Titration of drug regimens to obtain optimal control of symptoms is an important objective for such patients. In those whose symptoms improve, coronary arteriography may be eliminated or deferred; in those whose symptoms deteriorate, coronary arteriography can be recommended with confidence. This method of surveillance and close follow-up of more symptomatic patients affords an opportunity to determine whether "op-

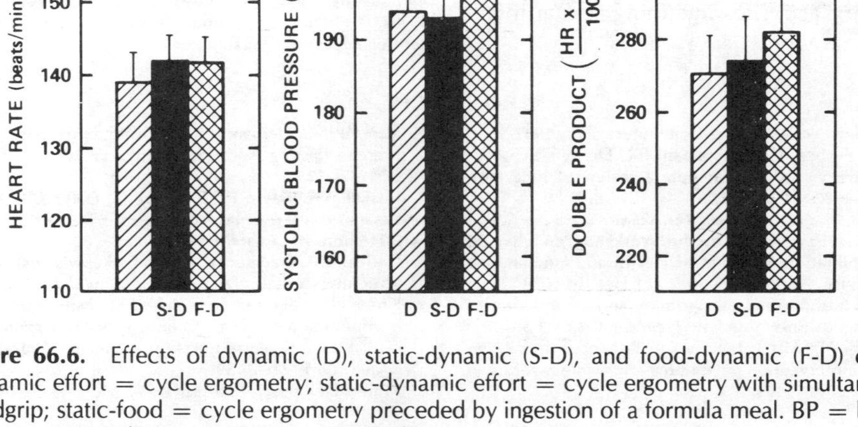

Figure 66.6. Effects of dynamic (D), static-dynamic (S-D), and food-dynamic (F-D) effort. Dynamic effort = cycle ergometry; static-dynamic effort = cycle ergometry with simultaneous handgrip; static-food = cycle ergometry preceded by ingestion of a formula meal. BP = blood pressure; HR = heart rate; NS = not significant.

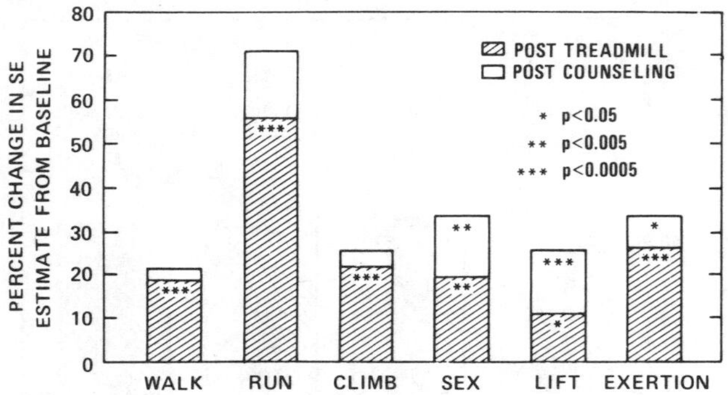

Figure 66.8. Increases in self-efficacy (SE) after treadmill and counseling. Changes in self-efficacy (confidence) are measured after treadmill exercise and counseling, respectively. (From Ewart et al,[13] with permission.)

timal" medical treatment has been achieved before the selection of CABG surgery or PTCA. In this respect, the modified exercise program serves as an outpatient analog of the coronary care unit: the same close observation and monitoring that are the principal rationale for acute in-hospital coronary care are extended to the outpatient setting.

IMPROVED METHODS FOR REDUCING PSYCHOLOGIC DISTRESS AFTER MYOCARDIAL INFARCTION

Much anxiety following acute MI results from patients' uncertainty about their ability to resume their customary activities, including gainful employment. Many post-MI patients develop a phobic reaction to physical activity, fearing that any excess exertion may precipitate a cardiovascular catastrophe. The uncertainty of such individuals is heightened by the lack of explicit, forceful guidelines from their physicians regarding the kinds of activities they can carry out with safety. Physicians' counseling regarding the safety of resuming customary activities, especially those that are dissimilar from those of exercise testing, is often of enormous benefit to patients and spouses (Figure 66.8). Patients' confidence or self-efficacy is usually increased by exercise testing: most clinically low risk patients report that they performed much more treadmill exercise than they had expected to. Successful completion of a treadmill exercise test affords substantial reassurance to patients regarding their ability to resume their customary activities including sexual intercourse and occupational work.

IMPROVED METHODS FOR RISK FACTOR REDUCTION AFTER ACUTE MYOCARDIAL INFARCTION

Acute MI provides strong motivation for patients tc alter habits that they believe may have contributed to their initial cardiac event or might contribute to future events. Despite this motivation, however, a change in long-standing health-related habits is difficult. As many as one half of the patients who were smoking at the time of acute MI have resumed this habit within 1 year after the acute event.[31,32] However, this recidivism rate reflects in large part the absence of effective behavioral strategies to alter health-related behavior.

The medically directed at-home program of physical exercise training described above provides a useful structure for a broad-based program of risk factor modification. The same nurse who assists patients to undergo individualized exercise training also assists them to become or remain nonsmokers. The strategy is this: (1) the physician indicates to patients that it is important to modify the smoking habit, (2) the physician expresses his or her confidence that the patient can modify the habit, (3) the physician and nurse provide explicit guidelines for relapse prevention including the prior identification of circumstances in which relapse is most likely to occur, (4) patients contact the nurse in case of an actual or a threatened relapse, and (5) the nurse provides ongoing support and encouragement for patients attempting to remain nonsmokers. Further experience with this model has indicated that the nurse's telephone contact with the patient need not be so frequent and that other informational materials such as videocassettes and printed materials may help patients to adopt healthy habits.

This behavioral strategy for risk factor modification may enable some patients to adopt and maintain healthful habits permanently with little or no ongoing support or instruction from health care professionals. This prospect, that patients can learn to alter behavior permanently without the continued support of the medical profession, has heretofore received little serious attention. The present high level of health awareness among the public affords an ideal opportunity to explore this approach.

Acknowledgment: This work was supported by Grant HL18907 from the National Heart, Lung, and Blood Institute, Bethesda, Maryland, and Grant G008435049 from the National Institute of Handicapped Research, Department of Education, Washington, DC.

REFERENCES

1. Naisbitt J: *Megatrends*. New York, Warner Communications, 1982.
2. May GS, Eberlein KA, Furberg CD, Passamani ER, DeMets DL: Secondary prevention after myocardial infarction: a review of long-term trials. *Prog Cardiovasc Dis* 1982; 24:331–352.
3. Naughton J: *Exercise and Myocardial Infarction: The National Exercise and Heart Disease Project: An Overview*. Proceedings of the Workshop on Physical Conditioning and Rehabilitation. US Dept of Health and Human Services, Public Health Service, National Institutes of Health, 1979.
4. Oldridge NB: Compliance and exercise in primary and secondary prevention of coronary heart disease: a review. *Prev Med* 1982; 11:56–70.
5. Kallio V, Hamalainen H, Hakkila J, Luurila OJ: Reduction in sudden deaths by a multifactoral intervention programme after acute myocardial infarction. *Lancet* 1979; 2:1091–1094.
6. Haskell WL, DeBusk R: Cardiovascular responses to repeated treadmill exercise testing soon after myocardial infarction. *Circulation* 1979; 60:1247–1251.
7. Haskell WL, Savin W, Oldridge N, DeBusk R: Factors influencing estimated oxygen uptake during exercise testing soon after myocardial infarction. *Am J Cardiol* 1982; 50:299–304.
8. DeBusk RF, Kraemer HC, Nash E: Stepwise risk stratification soon after acute myocardial infarction. *Am J Cardiol* 1983; 52:1161–1166.
9. Krone RJ, Gillespie JA, Weld FM, Miller JP, Moss AJ, Multicenter Postinfarction Research Group: Low-level exercise testing after myocardial infarction: usefulness in enhancing clinical risk stratification. *Circulation* 1985; 71:80–89.
10. Waters DD, Bosch X, Bouchard A, Moise A, Roy D, Pelletier G, Theroux

P: Comparison of clinical variables and variables derived from a limited predischarge exercise test as predictors of early and late mortality after myocardial infarction. *J Am Coll Cardiol* 1985; 5:1–8.
11. DeBusk RF, Houston N, Haskell W, Fry G, Parker M: Exercise training soon after myocardial infarction. *Am J Cardiol* 1979; 44:1223–1229.
12. DeBusk RF, Dennis CA: Occupational work evaluation of patients with cardiac disease: a guide for physicians. *West J Med* 1982; 137:515–520.
13. Ewart CK, Taylor CB, Reese LB, DeBusk RF: Effects of early postmyocardial infarction exercise testing on self-perception and subsequent physical activity. *Am J Cardiol* 1983; 51:1076–1080.
14. Taylor, C, Bandura A, Ewart CK, Miller NH, DeBusk RF: Exercise testing to enhance wives' confidence in their husbands' capability soon after clinically uncomplicated myocardial infarction. *Am J Cardiol* 1985; 55:635–638.
15. Miller NH, Haskell WL, Berra K, DeBusk RF: Home versus group exercise training for increasing functional capacity after myocardial infarction. *Circulation* 1984; 70:645–649.
16. DeBusk RF, Haskell WL, Miller NH, Berra K, Taylor CB: Medically directed at-home rehabilitation soon after clinically uncomplicated myocardial infarction: a new model for patient care. *Am J Cardiol* 1985; 55:251–257.
17. Weld FM, Chu KL, Bigger JT Jr, Rolnitzky LM: Risk stratification with low-level exercise testing 2 weeks after acute myocardial infarction. *Circulation* 1981; 64:306–314.
18. Theroux P, Waters DD, Halphen C, Debaisieux JC, Mizgala HF: Prognostic value of exercise testing soon after myocardial infarction. *N Engl J Med* 1979; 301:341–345.
19. Starling MR, Crawford MH, Kennedy GT, O'Rourke RA: Exercise testing early after myocardial infarction: predictive value for subsequent unstable angina and death. *Am J Cardiol* 1980; 46:909–914.
20. Palmeri ST, Harrison DG, Cobb FR, Morris KG, Harrell FE, Ideker RE, Selvester RH, Wagner GS: A QRS scoring system for assessing left ventricular function after myocardial infarction. *N Engl J Med* 1982; 306:4–9.
21. Henning H, Gilpin EA, Covell JW, Swan EA, O'Rourke RA, Ross J Jr: Prognosis after acute myocardial infarction: a multivariate analysis of mortality and survival. *Circulation* 1979; 59:1124–1136.
22. Gibson RS, Watson DD, Craddock GB, Crampton RS, Kaiser DL, Denny MJ, Beller GA: Prediction of cardiac events after uncomplicated myocardial infarction: a prospective study comparing predischarge exercise thallium-201 scintigraphy and coronary angiography. *Circulation* 1983; 68:321–336.
23. Corbett JR, Dehmer GJ, Lewis SE, Woodward W, Henderson E, Parkey RW, Blomqvist CG, Willerson JT: The prognostic value of submaximal exercise testing with radionuclide ventriculography before hospital discharge in patients with recent myocardial infarction. *Circulation* 1981; 64:535–544.
24. Mallory GK, White PD, Salcedo-Salgar J: The speed of healing of myocardial infarction. A study of the pathologic anatomy of seventy-two cases. *Am Heart J* 1939; 18:647–671.
25. Borer JS, Rosing DR, Miller RH, Stark RM, Kent KM, Bacharach SL, Green MV, Lake CR, Cohen H, Holmes D, Donohue D, Baker W, Epstein SE: Natural history of left ventricular function during 1 year after acute myocardial infarction: comparison with clinical, electrocardiographic and biochemical determinations. *Am J Cardiol* 1980; 46:1–12.
26. Saltin B, Blomqvist G, Mitchell JH, Johnson RL, Wildenthal K, Chapman CB: Response to exercise after bedrest and after training. *Circulation* 1968; 38 (suppl VII): VII-1–VII-55.
27. Convertino V, Hung J, Goldwater D, DeBusk RF: Cardiovascular responses to exercise in middle-aged men after 10 days of bedrest. *Circulation* 1982; 65:134–140.
28. DeBusk RF, Convertino VA, Hung J, Goldwater D: Exercise conditioning in middle-aged men after ten days of bedrest. *Circulation* 1983; 68:245–250.
29. Levine SA: Physician's fear: a deterrent to rehabilitation among cardiacs. *Geriatrics* 1960; 15:534–536.
30. Hung J, McKillop J, Savin W, Magder S, Kraus R, Houston N, Goris M, Haskell W, DeBusk R: Comparison of cardiovascular response to combined static-dynamic effort, postprandial dynamic effort and dynamic effort alone in patients with chronic ischemic heart disease. *Circulation* 1982; 65:1411–1419.
31. Salonen JT: Stopping smoking and long-term mortality after acute myocardial infarction. *Br Heart J* 1980; 43:463–469.
32. Wilhelmsson C, Vedin JA, Elmfeldt D, Tibblin G, Wilhelmsen L: Smoking and myocardial infarction. *Lancet* 1975; 1:415–420.

67 Cardiopulmonary Limitations in Exercise

Karlman Wasserman, MD, PhD

To achieve the increased energy required by the contracting muscles during exercise, O_2 delivery to and CO_2 removal from the muscle cells are necessarily accelerated. The cardiovascular and pulmonary systems provide the means by which the increased cellular respiration can be accommodated. Normally, these systems behave as though they are functionally coupled to the rate of cell respiration. Abnormalities in function affect the gas exchange coupling between internal respiration (gas exchange within the tissues) and external respiration (gas exchange with the environment). The description of abnormal patterns of gas exchange caused by specific defects in this cardiopulmonary coupling provides valuable insight into the degree of impairment and it may define the underlying pathophysiologic mechanism. The aim of this chapter is to describe the more common cardiovascular and pulmonary disorders limiting exercise performance and the gas exchange abnormalities that may be found with each. First, however, the mechanisms involved in the normal cardiopulmonary coupling of external to cellular respiration are reviewed.

COUPLING OF EXTERNAL TO CELL RESPIRATION

OVERVIEW OF THE METABOLIC–CARDIOVASCULAR–VENTILATORY COUPLING MECHANISMS

The large increase in muscle O_2 requirement during exercise demands that O_2 flow to the muscle be increased if muscular contractions are to be sustained. Simultaneously, the large quantity of CO_2 produced in the cell must be removed to avoid severe tissue acidosis with its adverse effects on cell function. Thus, exercise poses a gas transport problem. To accomplish the increased gas exchange needed for exercise, a close coupling of physiologic mechanisms involved in gas transport involving the lungs, pulmonary circulation, heart, and peripheral circulation is required (Figure 67.1). These subsystems must efficiently accommodate the increased metabolic rate to maintain tissue O_2 supply and CO_2 elimination as well as to achieve arterial blood gas homeostasis.

When exercise is initiated, the relatively large quantity of energy stores in the form of creatine phosphate in the muscles allows contraction to begin immediately. Within seconds, however, mitochondrial PO_2 must decrease in the metabolically active muscles since O_2 utilization increases. To allow this increased O_2 utilization by the muscles, the blood vessels perfusing the exercising muscles dilate. The initial dilation is neurogenic, whereas subsequent dilation is under local humoral control, enabling blood flow to increase to the muscle units with the highest metabolic activity.

Cardiac output is increased at the start of exercise by an increase in stroke volume and heart rate. Stroke volume appears to increase approximately to its maximum as soon as exercise begins. This is accomplished by increased cardiac inotropy and increased venous return secondary to compression of veins as muscles contract. As exercise progresses, further increases in cardiac output are accomplished almost exclusively by increasing heart rate.

In response to the increase in right ventricular output, the pulmonary vascular bed dilates, primarily by perfusing lung units that were unperfused or underperfused at rest. This dilation is essential for the normal exercise response of the left ventricle; without it, the weakly muscled right ventricle could not readily pump the increased venous return through the lungs to the left atrium to effect a normal increase in cardiac output.

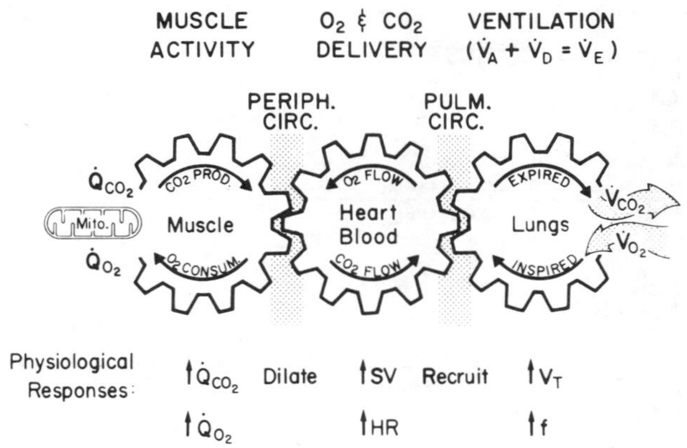

Figure 67.1. Schematic drawing of physiologic mechanisms coupling external (V) to internal (Q) respiration. Gears are used to illustrate that the physiologic responses are linked to metabolism. New O_2 is brought to the muscle as it is consumed by the mitochondria (mito) of cells, and CO_2 is simultaneously washed out of the tissues by the increase in muscle blood flow. The initial increase in cardiac output is largely dependent on the increase in stroke volume (SV), whereas subsequent changes are accounted for by an increase in heart rate (HR). In response to the increase in venous return (right ventricular output), the pulmonary vascular resistance decreases, largely by recruitment of poorly perfused or nonperfused pulmonary blood vessels. Arterial chemoreceptors are stimulated to increase ventilation to prevent respiratory acidosis in response to the increase in pulmonary blood flow and CO_2 and H^+ in the venous return. At work rates below the anaerobic threshold, the increase in ventilation is achieved primarily by an increase in tidal volume (V_T), and at higher work rates it is largely increased by breathing frequency (f). Oxygen uptake ($\dot{V}O_2$) and CO_2 output ($\dot{V}CO_2$) of the lungs equals the oxygen consumption ($\dot{Q}O_2$) and CO_2 production ($\dot{Q}CO_2$) by the cells except for circulatory delays. Because cardiac output does not increase in a one-to-one proportion with $\dot{Q}O_2$ or $\dot{V}O_2$, the O_2 content of venous blood decreases and the arterial-mixed venous difference widens as work rate is incremented. In contrast, alveolar ventilation does increase in a one-to-one relation with CO_2 delivered to the lungs in excess of rest, and arterial $PaCO_2$ is regulated at resting levels through moderate work rates. At higher work rates, ventilation accelerates to reduce $PaCO_2$ for respiratory compensation of the metabolic acidosis. (Figures 67.1, 67.5, and 67.7 are from Wasserman K, Hansen JE, Sue DY, Whipp BJ: *Principles of Exercise Testing and Interpretation*. Philadelphia, Lea & Febiger, in press. Copyright 1986 by Lea & Febiger. Reprinted with permission.)

Minute ventilation ($\dot{V}E$) increases at a rate required to remove the CO_2 added to the blood by the tissues. The increase in $\dot{V}E$ is so precise that arterial isocapnia and isohydria are generally maintained through moderate levels of exercise despite a manifold increase in the metabolic rate. Simultaneously, the pulmonary capillary blood is reoxygenated. At work rates above the anaerobic threshold, metabolic acidosis occurs that further increases ventilation.[1] The increase in ventilation is accomplished at low and moderate work rates primarily by increasing tidal volume and, to a lesser degree, breathing frequency; the latter increases more significantly at work rates above the anaerobic threshold.

Oxygen Requirement

Oxygen uptake increases as soon as exercise begins, reflecting the immediate increase in cardiac output and the rapid use of O_2 by the exercising muscles. The amount of O_2 stored in the tissues is small. The use of the creatine phosphate stores stimulates mitochondrial activity (Figure 67.2) to replenish the high energy phosphate.[2] Figure 67.3 shows the time course of O_2 uptake for different cycle ergometer work rates. Oxygen uptake reaches a plateau by three minutes at moderate work intensities. At heavy work intensities, $\dot{V}O_2$ continues to increase slowly. This slow drift in $\dot{V}O_2$ beyond three minutes for heavy work intensities appears to be related to mechanisms that involve increased lactate production, because it occurs at work rates only above the anaerobic threshold.

Oxygen Cost of Work

When $\dot{V}O_2$ reaches a steady-state, all of the energy required for exercise is generated from atmospheric O_2. To determine the O_2 cost of work, the steady-state $\dot{V}O_2$ can be related to the amount of external work performed. The normal relation for moderate work rate cycle ergometry is shown in Figure 67.4. The slope is uniform from one subject to another and it is unaffected by training, age, and sex. However, the curve is displaced upward because of obesity, the magnitude of the displacement depending on the degree to which the subject is overweight.[3] The slope of the relation is approximately 10 ml per watt. When numerator and denominator are converted to caloric equivalents, work efficiency for cycle ergometer work can be calculated and is found to be approximately 30%.[1]

Oxygen Supply

The increased O_2 supply to the mitochondria of exercising muscles depends on: (1) increased muscle blood flow, (2) oxygen content of the arterial blood, and (3) degree of O_2 extraction by the exercising muscles.

Blood Flow. The increase in blood flow to the muscles at the start of exercise seems to be primarily due to neurogenic vasodilatation as evidenced by a decrement in arterial pressure during the first 15 seconds of exercise. However, as exercise proceeds, blood flow apparently comes under local control, allowing it to increase to the tissues in greatest need of oxygen. The precise mechanisms are not clear, but locally produced humoral factors appear to provide the control needed for optimal blood flow distribution.[4] The increase in cardiac output combined with altered resistances in regional capillary beds allows marked increases in O_2 flow to the exercising muscles.

Arterial Oxygen Content. The O_2 in arterial blood depends on the hemoglobin concentration and the partial pressure of O_2 in the alveoli. Anemias that reduce the hemoglobin concentration in the blood or lung diseases, because of ventilation/perfusion mismatching or diffusion impairment (reduction in the alveolar or pulmonary capillary partial pressure of O_2), cause reductions in O_2

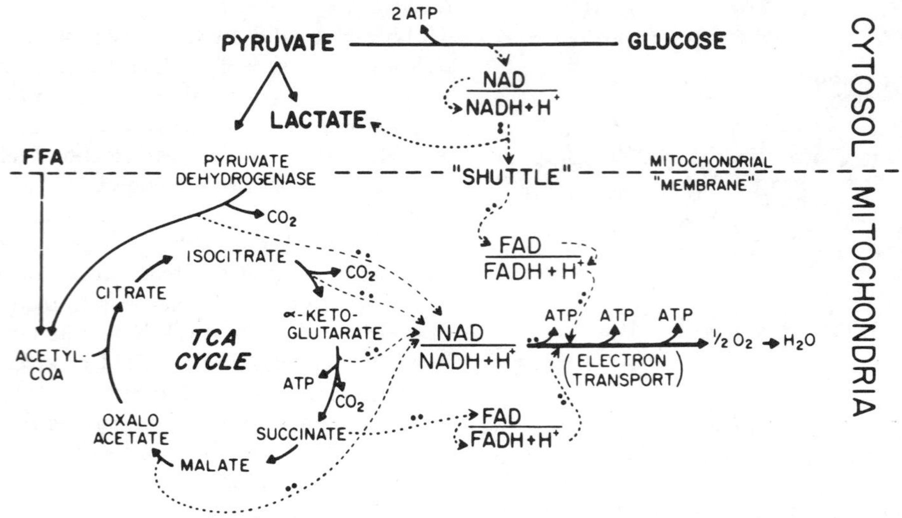

Figure 67.2. A skeletal version of the biochemical pathways for adenosine triphosphate (ATP) production. The ability of the "shuttle" mechanisms to reoxidize cytoplasmic NAD (nicotinamide adenine dinucleotide) is the key step in determining lactate production. See text for further details. ACETYL-COA = acetyl coenzyme A; FFA = free fatty acid; FAD = flavin adenine dinucleotide; FADH = reduced FAD; NADH = reduced NAD; TCA cycle = tricarboxylic acid (Krebs) cycle. (From Wasserman et al.[1])

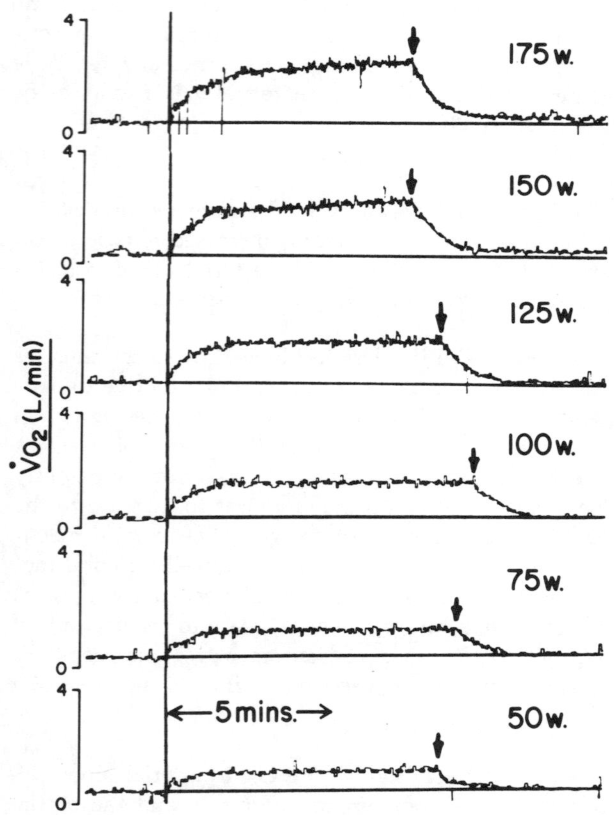

Figure 67.3. Oxygen uptake kinetics as related to work rate. (From Whipp BJ, Wasserman K: Oxygen uptake kinetics for various intensities of constant-load work. *J Appl Physiol* 1972; 33:351-356. Copyright 1972 by the American Physiological Society. Reprinted with permission.)

content of pulmonary capillary blood and impair peripheral oxygen delivery.

Arterial-mixed Venous Oxygen Difference (Oxygen Extraction). The extent to which the venous O_2 content can increase in the blood perfusing an exercising muscle depends on the minimum partial pressure gradient needed to allow O_2 to diffuse from the capillary to the mitochondria. The PO_2 decreases in the capillary as oxygen is extracted. The critical PO_2 in the capillary below which diffusion of O_2 might be impaired depends on the rate of O_2 consumption.

A rightward shift of the oxyhemoglobin dissociation curve, as induced by a decrease in pH and heat, will allow more O_2 to be extracted at a given capillary PO_2. Increased carbon monoxide in the blood, as found in heavy cigarette smokers, will cause a leftward shift in the oxyhemoglobin dissociation curve and slow the release of O_2 from hemoglobin. Thus, the position of the oxyhemoglobin dissociation curve, as described by its P_{50}, determines the extent to which O_2 will unload from hemoglobin and the venous O_2 content for a given PO_2. The arterial-venous O_2 difference depends on blood flow and O_2 consumption.

Carbon Dioxide Production

Like O_2 consumption, CO_2 production increases during exercise because of the increased metabolic activity of the exercising muscles. The amount of CO_2 generated from this process is related to O_2 consumption by the metabolic respiratory quotient (RQ). The RQ can range between 0.7 and 1.0 depending on the mix of fatty acids and carbohydrates used for energy. Ordinarily, the RQ is between 0.8 and 0.9 for moderate exercise.

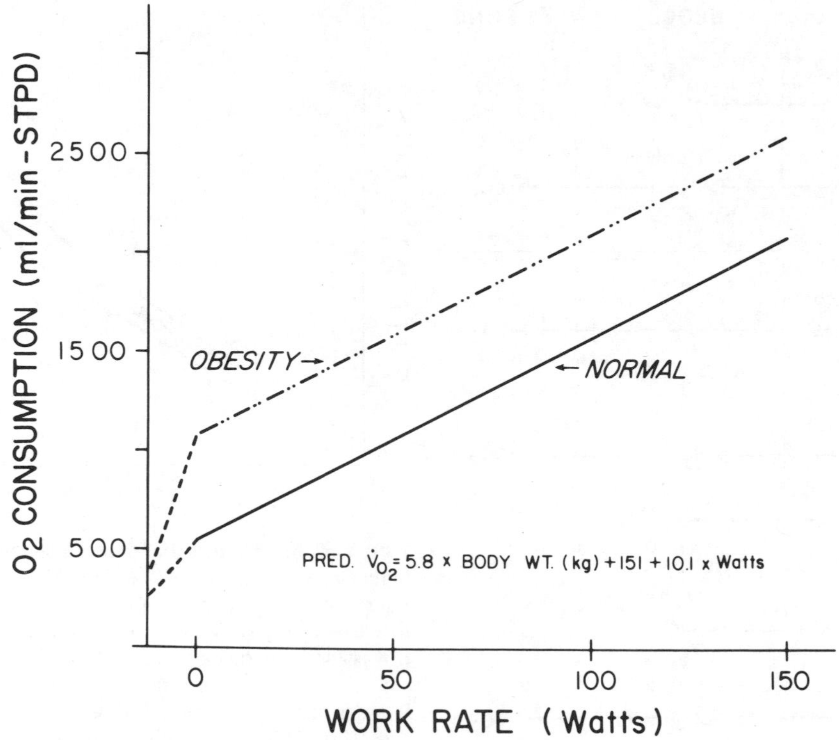

Figure 67.4. Oxygen (O_2) cost ($\dot{V}O_2$) of performing cycle ergometer work. Slope of work rate – $\dot{V}O_2$ relation is the same for all persons and unaffected by training, age, or gender. However, the relation is replaced upward by increasing weight. Predicted (pred) $\dot{V}O_2$ = 5.8 × body weight (kg) + 151 + 10.1 × watts. STPD indicates standard temperature and pressure, dry. (From Wasserman K: Dyspnea or exertion. Is it the heart or lungs? *JAMA* 1982; 248:2039–2043.)

At work rates high enough to cause an increase in blood lactate, additional CO_2 is derived from the buffering of this acid by bicarbonate. The only way CO_2 can be eliminated from the body in significant quantity is by its delivery to the lungs in the venous return. In contrast to tissue O_2 supply, CO_2 elimination is not critically dependent on cardiac output. It is the ventilation rate that determines arterial P_{CO_2} (Pa_{CO_2}). The tissue P_{CO_2}, in turn, is defined by Pa_{CO_2}, blood flow, and metabolic activity.

Lactic Acid Production

The only acid-base disturbance that develops during exercise in man is metabolic acidosis. It occurs only at work rates above which lactate concentration increases. Although at low work rates, lactate may increase by a few tenths of a milliequivalent per liter due to accelerated glycolysis, the lactate/pyruvate ratio does not increase.[5] Lactate increases significantly at a threshold of work rate at which the mitochondrial membrane proton shuttle (Figure 67.2) cannot reoxidize the cytosolic NADH + H^+, generated by glycolysis, fast enough to maintain the redox state of the cytosol.[6] Because this threshold appears to be due to an imbalance between the O_2 supply and O_2 requirement of the metabolically active muscles, it is referred to as the anaerobic threshold.[7] The magnitude of the metabolic acidosis that develops during exercise depends on the degree to which the work rate performed is above the anaerobic threshold.

Under conditions in which the total energy can be derived aerobically, there are no increases in lactate of any significance (Figure 67.5A). However, when some of the energy required for muscle contraction is generated from anaerobic glycolysis with a consequent increase in lactate in the muscle, the hydrogen ion that accompanies the production of lactate will be buffered immediately as it is produced (Figure 67.5B), because lactic acid is virtually completely dissociated at the pH of cell water (approximately 7.0). This is accomplished primarily by the bicarbonate buffer system. Therefore, as lactate is increased in the cell, CO_2 efflux from the cell increases above that derived from aerobic metabolism (22 ml of CO_2 for each milliequivalent of lactic acid buffered by bicarbonate). This CO_2 will be reflected quickly at the level of the lungs and measured as an increase in CO_2 output relative to O_2 uptake. This increase in CO_2 output will occur only during the period of a rising lactate level, ie, during a period of a decreasing bicarbonate level. As lactate increases and bicarbonate decreases in the cell water, an electrochemical potential is generated and lactate diffuses out of and HCO_3^- diffuses into the cell. Therefore, there is an anion exchange between the cell water and the extracellular water when lactate increases during exercise.

Conditions that limit O_2 flow to the tissues, such as those associated with low cardiac output states (heart

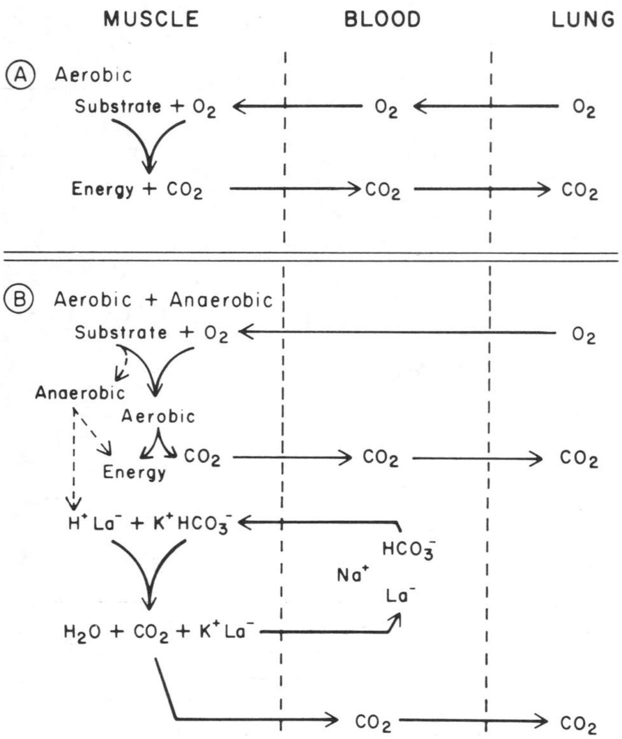

Figure 67.5. Gas exchange when energy generation is totally aerobic (*A*) and when aerobic energy generation is supplemented by anaerobic mechanisms (*B*). The acid-base consequence of the latter is an increase in cell lactic acid production. The buffering of the newly formed lactic acid takes place in the cell at the site of formation and almost wholly by bicarbonate buffer. The latter mechanism will increase CO_2 production of the cell by approximately 22 ml per milliequivalent of lactate formed. The increase in cell lactate and the decrease in cell bicarbonate will result in chemical concentration gradients causing lactate to diffuse out of a bicarbonate to diffuse into the cell. HCO_3^-=bicarbonate; La^- = lactate; H^+ La^- = lactic acid.

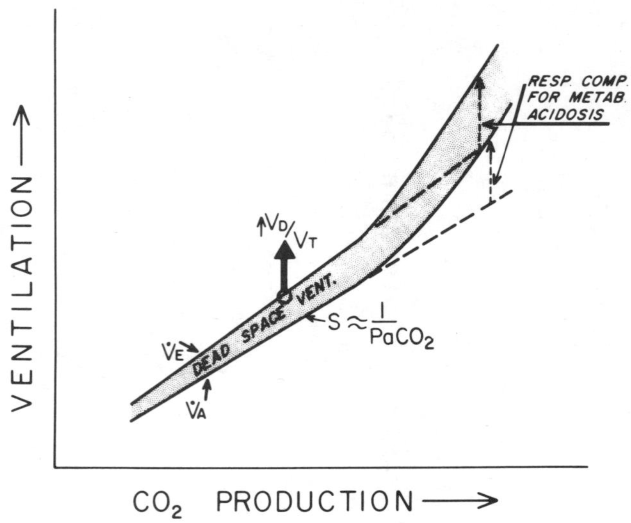

Figure 67.6. Factors that determine alveolar and minute ventilation during exercise ($\dot{V}A$ and $\dot{V}E$, respectively). S = 1/ Pa_{CO_2} means that the slope of the line is inversely related to the arterial P_{CO_2}. VD/VT is the fraction of the breath that is physiologic dead space. RESP COMP FOR METAB ACIDOSIS = respiratory compensation for metabolic acidosis. (From Wasserman K: Breathing during exercise. *N Engl J Med* 1978; 298:780–785. Used with permission.)

disease and disorders of the pulmonary circulation), peripheral vascular diseases (peripheral atherosclerosis and microvascular disease, eg, diabetes), or reduced arterial O_2 content (lung disease or anemia) can cause an increase in lactate and a consequent metabolic acidosis at relatively low work rates.[7]

Determinants of the Ventilatory Response to Exercise

Figure 67.6 describes the various factors that affect the ventilatory response to exercise. Because of regulation of arterial CO_2 and pH at work levels below the anaerobic threshold, ventilation increases linearly with CO_2 production. However, the slope of this relation is inversely related to the arterial CO_2 tension and directly to the fraction of tidal volume that is not involved in gas exchange, ie, the physiologic dead space/tidal volume ratio (VD/VT). At work rates performed above the anaerobic threshold, minute ventilation increases more steeply because: (1) there is an increase in CO_2 production from the buffering of lactic acid, and (2) respiratory chemoreceptors (carotid bodies) are stimulated by the increased hydrogen ion. This stimulation increases the ventilatory response, causing arterial CO_2 tension to decrease as partial compensation for the metabolic acidosis. This hyperventilation (reduction in Pa_{CO_2}) functions to constrain the magnitude of the decrease in arterial pH.

Thus, cardiopulmonary disorders accompanied by: (1) an increase in metabolic rate for the amount of external work performed, eg, obesity, (2) ventilation/perfusion mismatching in which VD/VT is increased, eg, lung and pulmonary vascular diseases, (3) a reduction in Pa_{CO_2}, eg, chronic metabolic acidosis, and (4) an increase in lactate at a relatively low work rate (low anaerobic threshold), eg, heart disease, all cause an abnormally increased ventilatory response to exercise.

DETECTING CARDIOPULMONARY DYSFUNCTION FROM GAS EXCHANGE MEASUREMENTS DURING EXERCISE

CARDIOVASCULAR AND OXYGEN FLOW LIMITATIONS TO EXERCISE

Maximal $\dot{V}O_2$ ($\dot{V}O_2$max) and Maximum $\dot{V}O_2$

The maximal O_2 uptake or the maximal aerobic power ($\dot{V}O_2$max) is a measure of the greatest capacity of the circulation to deliver O_2 to the tissues under conditions of supramaximal work. Usually, however, a symptom-limited maximum $\dot{V}O_2$ is obtained during incremental exercise testing and this can be interpreted in the same way as the $\dot{V}O_2$max, for clinical purposes.

The maximum $\dot{V}O_2$ becomes reduced in any condition in which O_2 flow to or O_2 use by the tissues is impaired, eg, cardiovascular diseases, lung diseases, or anemias. Note that the maximum $\dot{V}O_2$ does not describe all of the energy expended by the subject, because it does not account for the anaerobic (lactic acid generating) contribution to energy production, an important energy source at high work rates.[8] The maximum $\dot{V}O_2$ establishes whether the patient's physiologic responses allow normal maximal aerobic function. Other measurements are needed to differentiate the cause of a reduced maximum $\dot{V}O_2$.

$\dot{V}O_2$-Work Rate Relation

Although the O_2 uptake measurements are made at the mouth, they reflect the O_2 utilization by the cells. Because $\dot{V}O_2$ equals cardiac output multiplied by the arterial-mixed venous O_2 difference (Fick equation), this measurement depends on cardiovascular performance. In disorders that limit the rate of increase in O_2 flow to the tissues, the $\dot{V}O_2$ might increase at a slower rate than normal.

Anaerobic Threshold

The best way to determine the work level at which O_2 flow to the exercising muscle becomes inadequate for its need is to progressively increase the work rate and measure the $\dot{V}O_2$ at which lactate starts to rise rapidly. Alternatively, the gas exchange effects of buffering lactic acid might be used to detect the anaerobic threshold. Figure 67.7 is an example showing a progressively increasing work rate test in which O_2 uptake rises relatively linearly, but CO_2 output increases more steeply above the work rate identified as the anaerobic threshold. Because $\dot{V}CO_2$ is significantly increased relative to $\dot{V}O_2$ only during the period of buffering of the rising lactate concentration and not after it is already buffered, a progressive work rate test is needed to detect the anaerobic threshold using gas exchange measurements. Gas exchange methods to detect the anaerobic threshold are described elsewhere.[7] The anaerobic threshold is an extremely important measurement because it demarcates the work rate above which: (1) cellular and extracellular metabolic acidosis occurs, (2) the steady state in O_2 uptake is delayed, and (3) cardiorespiratory endurance is reduced. Also, the threshold denotes the work rate where ventilation is stimulated beyond that needed to keep pace with metabolism.

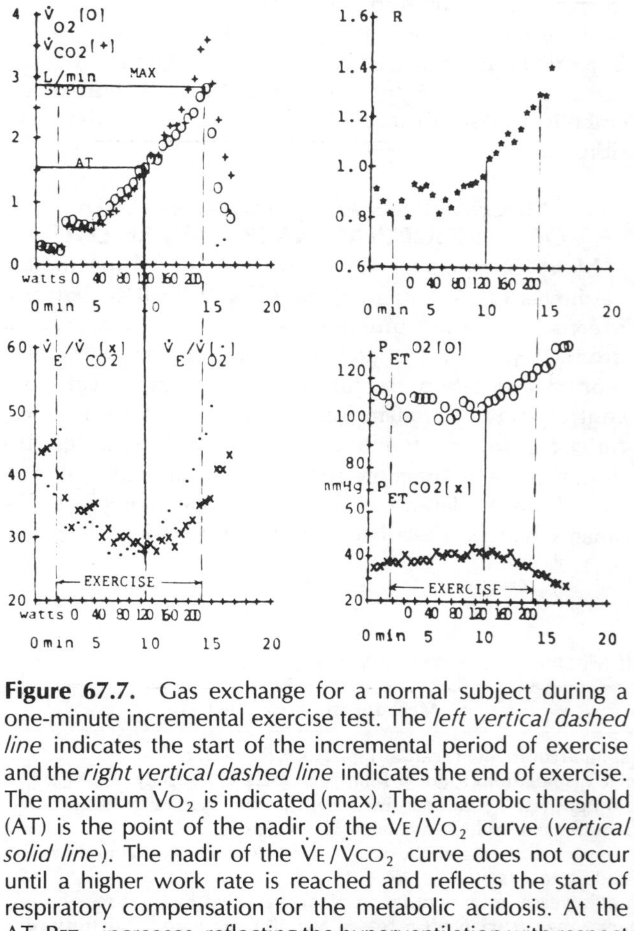

Figure 67.7. Gas exchange for a normal subject during a one-minute incremental exercise test. The *left vertical dashed line* indicates the start of the incremental period of exercise and the *right vertical dashed line* indicates the end of exercise. The maximum $\dot{V}O_2$ is indicated (max). The anaerobic threshold (AT) is the point of the nadir of the $\dot{V}E/\dot{V}O_2$ curve (*vertical solid line*). The nadir of the $\dot{V}E/\dot{V}CO_2$ curve does not occur until a higher work rate is reached and reflects the start of respiratory compensation for the metabolic acidosis. At the AT, PET_{O_2} increases, reflecting the hyperventilation with respect to $\dot{V}O_2$, whereas there is no change in PET_{CO2} until approximately two minutes later. At the AT, R increases strikingly, reflecting the increase in $\dot{V}CO_2$ relative to $\dot{V}O_2$. PET_{CO_2} = end-end-tidal CO_2 tension; PET_{O_2} = end-tidal O_2 tension.

Any of the cardiorespiratory disorders that impair O_2 flow to the tissues will cause the anaerobic threshold to be reduced. These are notably (1) heart disease, (2) disorders of the pulmonary circulation (increased pulmonary vascular resistance), (3) failure to provide a normal increase in muscle blood flow as a consequence of peripheral vascular disease, (4) marked reductions in arterial PO_2, and (5) anemias.

Heart Rate-$\dot{V}O_2$ Relation and Heart Rate Reserve

Heart rate normally increases linearly with $\dot{V}O_2$ during exercise. In cardiac and pulmonary vascular disorders, the heart rate increase is relatively steep for the increase in $\dot{V}O_2$ because the stroke volume is low. As the patient with heart disease approaches his maximum work rate, $\dot{V}O_2$ commonly slows its rate of increase while the heart rate continues to increase. Therefore, the heart rate increases even more steeply relative to $\dot{V}O_2$. Although this phenomenon is not always seen in patients with cardiovascular disease, it is a diagnostically useful observation.

The heart rate reserve expresses the fraction of predicted heart rate increase that remains at the end of maximum exercise:

$$\frac{\text{heart rate predicted max} - \text{max exercise heart rate}}{\text{heart rate predicted max}}$$

In normal subjects, the heart rate reserve is relatively small (less than 0.1). It is usually also small in patients with myocardial dysfunction and in patients with disorders of the pulmonary circulation. However, patients with peripheral vascular disease or coronary artery disease may discontinue exercise because of pain before the maximal heart rate is reached. Other patients in whom heart rate reserve is high are: (1) those taking beta-adrenergic blocking drugs, (2) those limited in exercise because of primary lung disease, (3) patients limited by musculoskeletal dysfunction, and (4) patients who make a poor effort.

Oxygen-Pulse ($\dot{V}O_2$/HR)

The oxygen-pulse is calculated by dividing the $\dot{V}O_2$ by heart rate. It is the volume of O_2 extracted by the tissues per heart beat and is equal to the product of stroke volume

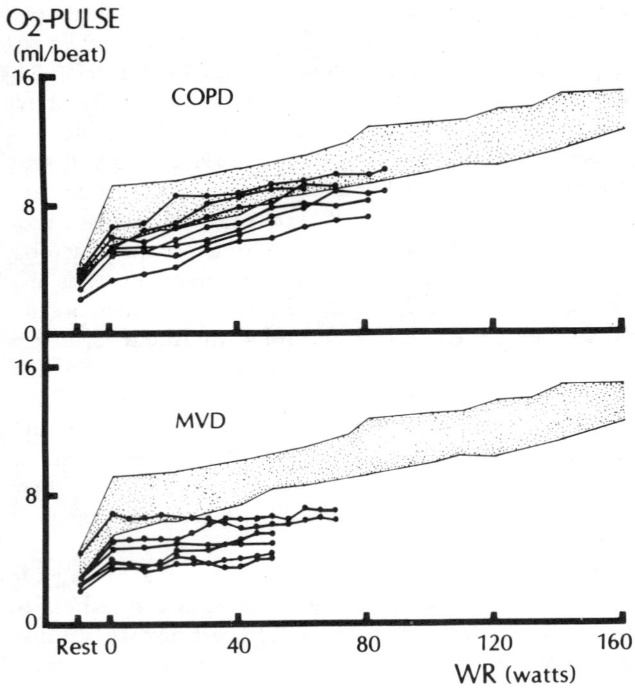

Figure 67.8. Oxygen-pulse ($\dot{V}O_2$/HR) response to incremental exercise in patients with chronic obstructive pulmonary disease (COPD) (*upper panel*) and those with mitral valve disease (MVD) (*lower panel*) compared with range of values of a matched control group (*stippled area*). WR = work rate. (From Nery et al[9] with permission.)

and the arterial-mixed venous O_2 difference. The initial increase in O_2-pulse is due to the increase in stroke volume. As work rate is increased, the further increase in O_2-pulse is primarily due to the increasing arterial-mixed venous O_2 difference. When the stroke volume is reduced, the arterial-mixed venous O_2 difference and therefore the O_2-pulse reach maximal values at a relatively low work rate (Figure 67.8).

VENTILATORY LIMITATION TO EXERCISE

Except when performing exercise at high altitude, most normal individuals are not ventilatory limited in the performance of exercise. At altitudes near sea level, normal subjects exercise to their predicted maximum heart rate, leaving a ventilatory reserve (computed as the difference between the maximum voluntary ventilation and the maximum exercise minute ventilation). However, in patients with lung diseases, the maximum ability to breathe is reduced. Consequently, they generally have no or a very small breathing reserve. Because of the ventilatory limitation, the heart rate commonly does not reach its predicted value, ie, cardiac reserve at maximum work rate is increased.

GAS EXCHANGE EFFICIENCY AND PHYSIOLOGIC DEAD SPACE/TIDAL VOLUME RATIO (VD/VT)

When there is uneven ventilation relative to perfusion, some lung units are relatively hyperventilated, whereas other lung units are hypoventilated. The hypoventilated areas of lung affect minute ventilation ($\dot{V}E$) very little but cause arterial hypoxemia and CO_2 retention; in contrast, the hyperventilated lung units cause a relatively large ventilatory change to unload the newly produced CO_2 arriving at the lungs. The net effect is a much greater increase in minute ventilation than that achieved if the ventilation/perfusion relations in the lungs were uniform. Because $\dot{V}E$ is higher than normal when there is ventilation/perfusion mismatching, the calculated VD/VT will be increased. The greater $\dot{V}E$ needed to eliminate CO_2 at the rate it is produced by metabolism reflects inefficiency in the gas exchange system. Disorders in which VD/VT is particularly increased are those associated with disturbances in the pulmonary circulation, eg, pulmonary embolic disease, obstructive lung disease, and pulmonary fibrosis.

MECHANISMS AND MEASUREMENTS OF CARDIOPULMONARY IMPAIRMENT

Many disorders interfere with the normal metabolic–cardiovascular–ventilatory coupling needed to perform exercise, including primary disorders of red blood cell production, the peripheral circulation, the heart, the pulmonary circulation, the lungs, the chest wall, respiratory control, and metabolism. Limiting symptoms are dyspnea, fatigue, pain, or a combination of these. A brief description of some of the more common disorders contributing to exercise intolerance and their pathophysiologic mechanisms will be described and are summarized in Table 67.1.

Table 67.1. Cardiorespiratory Disorders and Mechanisms Impairing Work Tolerance

Disorder	Mechanism
1. Obesity	Increases metabolic requirement; cardiorespiratory restriction
2. Peripheral vascular disease	Prevents normal vasodilation, thereby limiting muscle O_2 supply
3. Heart disease	Limits cardiac output (stroke volume) increase, thereby creating imbalance between O_2 requirement and O_2 available for exercising muscle
4. Anemia (or carboxyhemoglobinemia)	Limits muscle oxygenation; metabolic acidosis at low work rates stimulates breathing, leading to dyspnea
5. Pulmonary vascular occlusion	Prevents normal increase in $\dot{Q}$; ventilation of nonperfused lung causes decreased gas exchange efficiency (increased VD/VT) and high ventilatory response to exercise; causes hypoxemia with exercise
6. Lung disease	Reduces maximum ability to breathe; decreases efficiency of gas exchange (increased VD/VT); exercise induces hypoxemia
7. Chest wall disease	Reduces maximum ability to breathe

HEART DISEASE

The major and most immediate role of the heart is to pump blood to provide O_2 to the tissues to support their metabolic requirements. During exercise, the heart is under particular stress. Primary disorders of the heart limit blood and O_2 flow to the exercising muscles. Therefore, exercise testing provides a measure of the functional capacity of the heart.

Coronary Artery Disease

Coronary artery disease can best be detected under conditions that increase cardiac work. When blood flow perfusing the myocardium is inadequate to provide the O_2 required to support the bioenergetics needed for generation of adenosine triphosphate for cardiac contraction, repolarization of the myocardium is slow. This usually results in abnormal electrocardiographic complexes during exercise performance, such as ST-segment and T-wave changes. Also, ventricular arrhythmias developing during exercise should be regarded as evidence of myocardial ischemia. Evidence that myocardial ischemia is affecting myocardial function becomes evident from a failure of $\dot{V}O_2$ to increase linearly with work rate and of the O_2-pulse to reach a maximum at a relatively low work rate. Also, the anaerobic threshold is likely to be reduced.

Valvular Heart Disease

The heart may be unable to eject a normal stroke volume because of dysfunction of one of the heart valves as a result of either stenosis or incompetence. This limits the increase in cardiac output that can be generated during exercise, and O_2 transport to the exercising muscles can become inadequate. Therefore, the maximum $\dot{V}O_2$ and anaerobic threshold will be reduced, the heart rate increase with respect to $\dot{V}O_2$ will be steep, and the O_2-pulse will be low and will fail to increase normally with work rate[9] (Figure 67.8).

Cardiomyopathy

A disorder of the myocardium caused by either metabolic dysfunction, hypertrophy, dilatation, or fibrosis replacing muscle will cause stroke volume to be reduced and will limit cardiac output increase. The physiologic measurements that will be abnormal during exercise are similar to those described for valvular heart disease; however, the heart rate reserve may be abnormally high in patients in whom abnormalities in the conduction system prevent the normal increase in heart rate.

Congenital Heart Disease

Most varieties of congenital heart disease result in limited exercise tolerance because of failure to develop a normal cardiac output in response to exercise. In patients with cyanotic congenital heart disease, the problem is compounded because of the increased O_2 desaturation that occurs during exercise, as a larger fraction of the cardiac output bypasses the lungs. The gas exchange abnormalities during exercise testing are similar to those in valvular heart disease. In addition, ventilatory requirements are strikingly increased when a right-to-left shunt is present or develops during exercise because, to achieve CO_2 regulation, the fraction of the cardiac output going through the lungs must be hyperventilated to make up for the high P_{CO_2} in the shunted blood.

Arrhythmias

Heart block, failure to increase heart rate appropriately consequent to sinoatrial node dysfunction, or the development of an inappropriate tachycardia in which cardiac ejection is inefficient can reduce exercise tolerance.

PERIPHERAL VASCULAR DISEASE

The increase in peripheral blood flow essential for increasing the availability of O_2 to the working muscles is problematic in patients with peripheral vascular disease. Consequently, the exercising muscles may become ischemic and produce lactic acid locally. The circulation may be unable to efficiently remove the acid and the patient may experience claudication. Although the number of mitochondria in the ischemic muscle is increased, presumably a compensatory mechanism, it is inadequate to make up for the deficiency in O_2 flow.[10]

The maximum $\dot{V}O_2$ and the anaerobic threshold are reduced, although the latter can be so low that it may not be measurable by gas exchange measurements. Because of reduced muscle perfusion, lactate may not readily enter the central circulation and evidence of systemic lactic acidosis may be minimal. The slope of the $\dot{V}O_2$/work rate relation may be more shallow than normal, reflecting diminished O_2 utilization and increased anaerobic energy production.

Blood pressure measurements are important in these patients because exercise can induce arterial hypertension in those with peripheral vascular occlusive disorders.

LUNG DISEASE

The pathophysiologic aspects of exertional dyspnea in patients with chronic obstructive airway disease (eg, asthma, bronchitis, and emphysema) are shown in Figure 67.9. Two basic defects exist, both limiting the maximum metabolic rate that these patients can achieve: (1) because of limited ability to breathe, the maximum ventilation that the patient can develop is reduced; (2) the ventilation required by the patient to perform exercise is increased because gas exchange is inefficient as a result of mismatching of ventilation relative to perfusion (increased $\dot{V}D/\dot{V}T$).

The maximum $\dot{V}O_2$ is reduced in patients with obstructive lung disease, but the $\dot{V}O_2$-work rate relation does not approach a plateau as it commonly does in patients with cardiovascular disorders. Generally, the anaerobic threshold, if it can be determined, is on the low side of normal, consistent with that of a typically sedentary subject. Because patients with obstruction are ventilatory limited, the heart rate at their maximum work rate is generally low (high heart rate reserve). However, it will increase if the maximum work rate can be improved

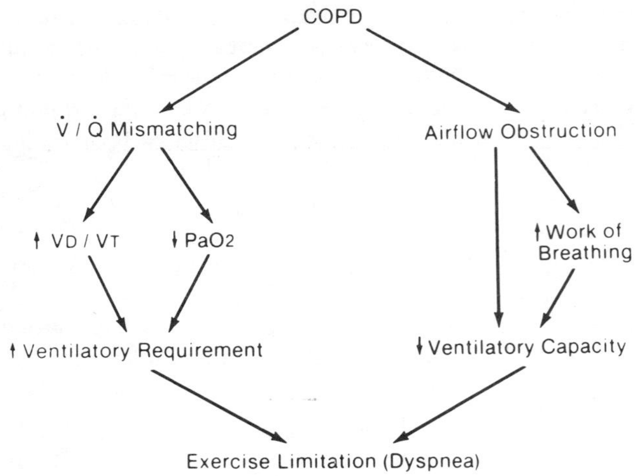

Figure 67.9. Pathophysiology of exercise limitation in patients with chronic obstructive pulmonary disease (COPD). $\dot{V}_D/\dot{V}_T$ indicates physiologic dead space/tidal volume ratio; $\dot{V}/\dot{Q}$ is the ratio of ventilation to perfusion in lung gas exchange units. (From Brown HV, Wasserman K: Exercise performance in chronic obstructive pulmonary diseases. *Med Clin North Am* 1981; 65:525-547. Copyright 1981 by WB Saunders Co. Reprinted with permission.)

(eg, O_2 therapy, bronchodilators, and discontinuance of smoking). Because of the mismatching of ventilation relative to perfusion, patients with primary lung disease have a high $\dot{V}_D/\dot{V}_T$. Therefore, the ventilatory response is elevated for the exercise metabolic rate and level at which Pa_{CO_2} is regulated. Arterial hypoxemia usually develops during exercise because of ventilation–perfusion mismatching, although Pa_{CO_2} may be normal. This provides a further stimulus to breathe and adds to the symptom of dyspnea.

The ventilatory response of patients with pulmonary fibrosis is steep because of both hyperventilation (reduced Pa_{CO_2}) and high $\dot{V}_D/\dot{V}_T$. Arterial hypoxemia, which systematically increases with work rate, is common. Because of associated pulmonary vascular disease and hypoxemia, these patients may appear to be O_2-flow limited.

PULMONARY VASCULAR DISEASE

Diseases of the pulmonary circulation characteristically result in reduced perfusion of ventilated alveoli. Because these alveoli are so poorly perfused, a large ventilatory component is wasted (alveolar dead space). Likewise, alveoli that are perfused must be ventilated to a greater degree than normal to remove the metabolic CO_2 and maintain Pa_{CO_2} at a normal level. Because minute ventilation is the sum of alveolar ventilation and physiologic dead space ventilation, it is increased relative to the metabolic rate.

Hemodynamically, pulmonary vascular occlusive diseases represent stenosis in the central circulation, making it difficult for the right ventricle to deliver blood to the left atrium at a rate sufficient to meet the increased cardiac output needed for exercise. The cardiac output increase in patients with pulmonary vascular disease can be limited, and reductions in maximum $\dot{V}_{O_2}$, anaerobic threshold, and O_2-pulse are usually observed to be similar to those found in patients with primary heart disease.

OBESITY

Despite some increase in the resting metabolic rate ($\dot{V}_{O_2}$) relative to lean body mass, the increase in $\dot{V}_{O_2}$ is even more marked during dynamic exercise in obese subjects because of the additional energy needed to move their large body segments. Consequently, for the obese individual to do any form of physical work, the cardiovascular and respiratory stress is greater than normal.[11]

In obese patients, the resting metabolic rate and therefore the cardiac output and minute ventilation per kilogram of lean body weight are already high because of the large body mass that must be provided with O_2. Because of fat deposition in the chest wall and abdomen, however, a constraint is imposed on the maximal performance of the cardiovascular and respiratory systems by obesity. Therefore, the degree to which ventilation and cardiac output can be further increased during exercise is limited.

Because of the reduced alveolar volume at end expiration consequent to the pressure imposed on the chest by obesity, peripheral lung units spontaneously become atelectatic. This causes a resting hypoxemia that usually disappears during exercise, presumably because of the deep breathing and the re-aeration of atelectatic alveoli.

The increased O_2 demand for obese subjects to perform cycle ergometer work is predictable and well worked out.[3,12] The $\dot{V}_{O_2}$-work rate relation is displaced upward without a discernible change in slope as compared to normal. The extent of displacement depends on the degree of obesity (Figure 67.4).

The maximum V_{O_2} and anaerobic threshold are low when related to actual body weight in obese individuals, but they are normal when related to height[12] or lean body mass.[13] Ventilation–perfusion relations are usually normal during exercise in these patients. Also, the O_2-pulse is normal or high when related to predicted values determined from normal body weight.

ANEMIA AND ABNORMAL HEMOGLOBINS

Anemic states (blood with reduced O_2 content) compromise delivery of O_2 to the mitochondria because the blood P_{O_2} falls more rapidly than normal as the red cells travel through capillaries of exercising muscle. Because of the reduced capillary blood P_{O_2}, the diffusion gradient for O_2 from the blood to the mitochondria might reach critically low levels, causing anaerobic energy generation at relatively low work rates.

Similarly, the presence of abnormal hemoglobins that have a leftward shift in the O_2 dissociation curve (reduced P_{50}) results in a decrease in capillary blood P_{O_2} at a given O_2 consumption. Because at high rates of O_2 consumption the O_2 partial pressure difference between the capillary blood and mitochondrion may not provide adequate O_2 flow, the mitochondrial membrane proton shuttle would not get reoxidized rapidly enough to maintain the cytosol redox state.[6] Therefore, lactic acidosis occurs at reduced work rates.[14]

Breathlessness during exercise in subjects with anemia

is well recognized. The increased ventilatory drive (mediated by the carotid body stimulation) is presumably due to the metabolic acidosis that accompanies the low anaerobic threshold.

Patients with reduced O_2-carrying capacity have a relatively high cardiac output, with a higher than expected heart rate for a given submaximal work rate, ie, relative tachycardia. In contrast to patients with cardiac diseases and disorders of the pulmonary circulation in which the stroke volume is reduced, the stroke volume is normal or even increased in this disorder. However, because the arterial and venous O_2 content is low at rest, the potential increase in the arterial-venous O_2 difference is limited. Therefore, the O_2-pulse increases to a maximum and reaches a plateau value at a relatively low work rate.

SUMMARY

Cardiovascular and respiratory disorders limit exercise by interfering with the normal coupling of the physiologic responses that allow the gas exchange needs of the cells to be met. Each type of disorder manifests unique pathophysiologic aspects in the gas exchange responses to exercise. Therefore, measurement of gas exchange in response to a known exercise stimulus can provide valuable insight into not only the degree of impairment, but also the site of the defect in the normal coupling of external to cell respiration.

Acknowledgment: This work was supported in part by PHS Grant HL-11907, National Institutes of Health, Bethesda, Maryland.

REFERENCES

1. Wasserman K, Whipp BJ, Davis JA: Respiration in exercise, in Widdicombe JG (ed): *International Review of Physiology, Respiration Physiology*. Baltimore, University Park Press, 1981, Vol 3, pp 149–211.
2. Chance B, Eleff S, Leigh JS Jr, Sokolow D, Sapega A: Mitochondrial regulation of phosphocreatine/inorganic phosphate ratios in exercising human muscle: A gated ^{31}P NMR study. *Proc Natl Acad Sci* 1981; 78:6714–6718.
3. Wasserman K, Whipp BJ: Exercise physiology in health and disease. *Am Rev Resp Dis* 1975; 112:219–249.
4. Sparks HV Jr, Belloni FL: The peripheral circulation: local regulation. *Ann Rev Physiol* 1978; 40:67–92.
5. Wasserman K, Beaver WL, Davis JA, Pu J-Z, Heber D, Whipp BJ: Lactate, pyruvate and lactate-to-pyruvate ratio during exercise and recovery. *J Appl Physiol* 1985; 59:935–940.
6. McGilvery R: *Biochemistry: A Functional Approach,* ed 3. Philadelphia, WB Saunders Co, 1983, pp 469–470.
7. Wasserman K: The anaerobic threshold measurement to evaluate exercise performance. *Am Rev Resp Dis* 1984; 129(Suppl):S35–S40.
8. DiPrampero, PE: Energetics of muscular exercise. *Rev Physiol Biochem Pharmacol* 1981; 89:143–222.
9. Nery LE, Wasserman K, French W, Oren A, Davis JA: Contrasting cardiovascular and respiratory responses to exercise in mitral valve and chronic obstructive pulmonary diseases. *Chest* 1983; 83:446–453.
10. Bylund-Fellenius AC, Walker PM, Elander A, Scherstén T: Peripheral vascular disease. *Am Rev Resp Dis* 1984; 129(Suppl):S65–S67.
11. Alexander JK, Amad KH, Cole VW: Observations on some clinical features of extreme obesity, with particular reference to circulatory effect. *Am J Med* 1962; 32:512–524.
12. Hansen JE, Sue DY, Wasserman K: Predicted values for clinical exercise testing. *Am Rev Resp Dis* 1984; 129(Suppl):S49–S55.
13. Buskirk E, Taylor HL: Maximal oxygen intake and its relation to body composition, with special reference to chronic physical activity and obesity. *J Appl Physiol* 1957; 11:72–78.
14. Butler WM, Spratling L, Kark JA, Schoomaker EB: Hemoglobin Osler: Report of a new family with exercise studies before and after phlebotomy. *Am J Hemat* 1982; 13:293–301.

68 Noncardiac Surgery in Cardiac Patients

Lee Goldman, MD

The evaluation and management of the cardiac patient for noncardiac surgery requires cooperation among the surgeon, anesthesiologist, and medical consultant. Each must be prepared to provide expertise, but at the same time to appreciate the unique contributions that may be made by the other participants, so that their efforts are synergistic and not contradictory or antagonistic.

Some issues in the management of the cardiac patient for noncardiac surgery refer to the particular type of cardiac disease that is evident on preoperative evaluation. Other principles are pertinent to all types of patients, regardless of their cardiac condition.

CARDIAC ISSUES

CORONARY ARTERY DISEASE

It has long been recognized that patients with coronary artery disease are at increased risk of cardiac complications with major noncardiac surgical procedures. Several studies from the 1960s and 1970s[1–6] emphasize that a recent preoperative myocardial infarction is a major risk factor for reinfarction or cardiac death. In most of these studies, risk appeared to return to plateau by about 6 months after infarction.

In pooled data from the 1960s and 1970s, the risk of reinfarction or cardiac death was reported to be about 30% in patients operated on within 3 months after preoperative myocardial infarction and about 15% in those operated on between 3 and 6 months after infarction.[1,4,5] However, recent data suggest that this risk may be declining. For example, in 1973 to 1976, Rao et al[7] reported reinfarction rates of 36% and 26% in patients who were less than 3 and 3 to 6 months after myocardial infarction, respectively, but then they reported that these rates decreased to 6% and 2%, respectively, between 1977 and 1982. The principal explanation for this decline in complication rates was the application of cardiovascular anesthetic techniques in cardiac patients undergoing major noncardiac surgery. Patients were monitored aggressively with pulmonary artery catheters whenever the operation was expected to last more than 30 minutes, pressures were not allowed to fluctuate more than 20% from the preinduction values for more than five minutes, blood gases and electrolytes were closely monitored, and the hematocrit was not allowed to decrease below 30%. The benefits of aggressive monitoring appeared to apply to virtually all groups of patients, with special benefits in those undergoing emergency surgery. Similarly optimistic results were reported recently by Wells and Kaplan,[8] who also used analogous management techniques.

Consistent with substantial data from the cardiologic literature,[9,10] the risk in patients with recent preoperative subendocardial infarction seems to be similar to the risk in patients with preoperative transmural infarction. These data do not imply that every postinfarction patient has the same surgical risk. For example, left ventricular function[11,12] and ventricular arrhythmias[12] are important prognostic factors in the postinfarction patient, and it is not surprising that they are also important correlates of risk when such patients undergo noncardiac surgery.[5]

Despite the apparently lower risk in patients with preoperative infarction in the 1980s, it still would be appropriate to delay non-urgent surgery for the 4 to 6 weeks or so required for full pathologic healing and hopefully until the patient has returned to the preinfarction exercise level. Nevertheless, when such delay is impossible, the data suggest that the risks of operation in the current era of cardiovascular anesthesia will be lower than those often quoted. For the patient with a semiurgent condition, such as carcinoma potentially requiring resection, a 6- to 12-week delay is often practical, but earlier surgery may be appropriate in patients whose overall cardiac status is favorable. (See section on Multifactorial Assessment of Cardiac Risk.)

ANGINA

In patients with chronic anginal symptoms, the risk of major cardiac complications is increased about fourfold.[5,13] Furthermore, in patients with peripheral vascular disease, asymptomatic coronary disease is a frequent concern, especially if the patient's exercise capacity is sufficiently reduced by the peripheral vascular condition so that angina may not be induced by activity. Therefore, several investigators[14–18] have proposed routine preoperative exercise tests, coronary arteriography, or pulmonary artery catheterization in patients with suspected or known coronary artery disease or in elderly patients undergoing major surgery. Unfortunately, controlled data to support these aggressive preoperative approaches are limited, and one study[19] reported that pulmonary artery hemodynamic measurements at rest and during exercise did not supplement clinical data alone for the prediction of major cardiac complications in noncardiac surgery.

The appropriate preoperative approach to the patient with known or suspected coronary artery disease is currently controversial. Exercise tests have known limitations as screening tests for the detection of asymptomatic coronary artery disease,[20,21] but they are better at assessing the severity of disease in patients with known coronary artery disease.[22,23] Furthermore, in the most difficult clinical situation, as in patients with orthopedic or peripheral vascular disease that renders treadmill exercise impractical, other tests would be needed.

In terms of the benefits of potential intervention, we must ask whether prophylactic medical therapy or coronary artery bypass surgery to precede the noncardiac surgery would reduce overall risk. Again, no randomized controlled data are available, but several studies indicate that patients who survive bypass surgery can have subsequent noncardiac surgery with rather low risks.[16,24–27] Data from the cardiac surgery literature suggest that bypass surgery will prolong life in patients who have left main coronary artery disease[28] and probably in patients who have stable angina with more than mild symptoms and triple-vessel disease, especially if they also have left ventricular dysfunction.[29,30] In patients who have class I or II stable angina or who are asymptomatic after myocardial infarction, the Coronary Artery Surgery Study[31] showed no overall benefit from surgery, although patients with triple-vessel disease and left ventricular dysfunction benefited.

Therefore, there seem to be two principal issues: which patients require preoperative evaluation because their symptom level is unclear, and what to do in patients in whom the symptomatic status is clear.

In most patients, symptomatic status can be evaluated on the basis of a good history to determine whether they have mild angina[32] or are asymptomatic after myocardial infarction, as were patients in the Coronary Artery Surgery Study, or have more symptomatic, although technically stable, coronary artery disease, as did patients in the Veterans Administration Cooperative Study and the European Study. In patients in whom such a determination cannot be made by the history, preoperative exercise testing is a reasonable alternative. It is difficult to be precise about the types of exercise test abnormalities that should then lead to a consideration of preoperative coronary artery catheterization. For example, Podrid et al[33] demonstrated an excellent prognosis in mildly symptomatic patients with 2 mm or more ST-segment depression on exercise testing. Nevertheless, if 2 mm or more ST-segment depression occurs in a patient who cannot exercise more than three minutes of a standard Bruce protocol, the patient should be considered to have class III disease and cardiac catheterization commonly would be appropriate before major noncardiac surgery. If angina cannot be assessed by history or by exercise testing because of noncardiac limitations from conditions such as orthopedic or peripheral vascular disease, options for determining the physiologic severity of any underlying coronary artery disease are limited. One option, although still experimental, is dipyridamole thallium testing,[34] in which imaging after dipyridamole-induced vasodilatation may mimic the response that would be expected in exercise thallium testing. A second option is thallium imaging during cardiac catheterization with right atrial pacing to simulate the physiologic responses to exercise.[35] In patients who have precipitation of typical anginal pain at low-paced heart rates or who have major changes in left ventricular hemodynamics, the observed anatomic lesions must be considered physiologically important and coronary artery bypass surgery before major noncardiac surgery will often be appropriate. The issue of coronary artery bypass surgery in patients with significant coronary artery disease prior to their major noncardiac surgery has been further explored by the Coronary Artery Surgery Study (CASS) registry experience. Patients with significant coronary artery disease undergoing noncardiac operation without prior coronary artery bypass grafting had a general surgical mortality of 2.4%, as compared to an operative mortality of 0.9% in those who had survived prior coronary artery bypass grafting.[35a] This study is limited in that all-cause mortality was considered, so that specific cardiac mortality, as well as nonfatal cardiac events, were not included. Furthermore, in the CASS study, the mortality associated with elective coronary artery bypass grafting was 1.4%. Thus the sequence of elective coronary bypass grafting followed by noncardiac surgery would yield a total mortality of 2.3% (1.4% + 0.9%), as compared to 2.4% in patients undergoing noncardiac surgery without prior coronary artery bypass grafting. While coronary artery bypass grafting should undoubtedly benefit certain subgroups of patients, data from the CASS study cannot be used to support a policy of routine coronary artery bypass grafting in all patients with significant coronary artery disease who are about to undergo major noncardiac surgery.

In general, the risks of catheterization and surgery in patients with truly stable class II angina or less probably outweigh the prophylactic benefits of such surgery before nearly all noncardiac surgical procedures. Another approach would be to say that if a patient does not meet these usual criteria for catheterization and coronary artery surgery and can be evaluated on the basis of history, then neither catheterization nor surgery need be performed prophylactically before noncardiac surgery except in the unusual situation in which the stress of surgery is greater than the stresses associated with the patient's daily activities.

Despite earlier concerns about the safety of beta-adrenergic antagonists,[36] patients who are taking such medications preoperatively should continue them until surgery.[37-41] The medication can be given with a small sip of water the morning of surgery. Postoperatively, several options are reasonable. One is to begin propranolol, 1 mg intravenously, up to a total loading dose of 10 mg followed by 1 mg every 20 to 60 minutes. An alternative regimen is a loading dose of 5 to 10 mg over 60 minutes followed by an infusion of 0.01 to 0.05 mg per minute[42] or 3 mg per hour.[43] Alternatively, propranolol can be begun orally at its usual interval postoperatively, by crushing the medication, inserting it through a nasogastric tube, then clamping the tube for about 60 minutes to obtain reasonable absorption; if this fails, one of the preceding intravenous regimens can be used.

It may be hazardous to wait for signs or symptoms before reinstituting beta-adrenergic antagonists postoperatively. If a patient has required beta blockade to control important anginal symptoms, then propranolol should be continued either orally (if successful) or intravenously. In some situations, other medications, such as sublingual calcium channel antagonists or topical nitrates, may be used to reduce the dependence on beta-adrenergic medications. If patients are being treated for mild hypertension, they often will not require medication postoperatively. If patients are being treated for more severe hypertension, propranolol can be continued with one of the foregoing regimens or adequate antihypertensive therapy can be attempted with alpha methyldopa or nitroprusside.

The peak risk for perioperative myocardial infarction is not during anesthesia but rather about three to five days after the surgical procedure.[1,7,13,44] Therefore, patients with ischemic heart disease must be observed carefully for several days postoperatively, and it has been suggested that if a pulmonary artery catheter was an important part of the management, as in patients with recent preoperative myocardial infarction, it should be continued for three to four days postoperatively.[7]

CONGESTIVE HEART FAILURE

All available data clearly indicate that congestive heart failure is a major risk factor in noncardiac surgery.[13,45] This is not surprising because a diminished ejection fraction is perhaps the worst prognostic factor in survivors of myocardial infarction,[11] and congestive heart failure carries nearly a 50% five-year mortality rate.[46]

There are no controlled data to indicate the precise benefit to be gained by the preoperative control of congestive heart failure. Nevertheless, the aggressive preoperative control of heart failure is an important part of the management of a cardiac patient for noncardiac surgery. Although diuresis must be appropriately aggressive and successful, care must be taken to avoid dehydration. Dehydration can cause major surgical problems, because the early hemodynamic response to both general anesthesia and spinal or epidural anesthesia is peripheral vasodilatation and potential hypotension. Operating on dehydrated patients will worsen this complication, which can be especially dangerous in patients with underlying ischemic heart disease. Virtually every study that has investigated the issue has shown that intraoperative hypotension is a major correlate of perioperative myocardial infarction.[7,13,47,48] Perioperative hemodynamic monitoring, including a pulmonary artery catheter, is appropriate in patients with advanced class III or IV congestive heart failure who undergo noncardiac surgery.

Many general anesthetic agents cause direct myocardial depression; nevertheless, congestive heart failure is not a contraindication to standard general anesthetic techniques. Decisions regarding anesthetic agents and techniques should be made by qualified, experienced anesthesiologists. However, in patients with far-advanced (eg, class IV) heart failure, spinal or epidural anesthesia may occasionally be preferable to general anesthesia.[13]

The two periods of peak risk for perioperative pulmonary edema are soon after the cessation of positive pressure ventilation and again about 48 hours after surgery when fluid that was "third-spaced" during the procedure returns to the intravascular space. Patients in whom postoperative pulmonary edema develops usually have a history of preoperative congestive heart failure, or are elderly and have undergone major surgical procedures. In at least half the cases, postoperative pulmonary edema may be directly attributable to the fluids that were given intraoperatively.[49] When pulmonary edema or worsening congestive heart failure occurs in the early postoperative period, intravenous furosemide is the treatment of choice, and it should be accompanied by appropriate fluid restriction. However, fluid-induced postoperative congestive heart failure is not always an indication for the chronic use of diuretic therapy. Unlike patients with ischemic heart disease, whose risks actually increase during the first three or more postoperative days, patients whose indication was congestive heart failure can usually have the pulmonary artery catheter discontinued 24 to 48 hours after surgery.

VALVULAR HEART DISEASE

In most series, about 20% of patients with important valvular heart disease have new or worsening heart failure in the perioperative period.[13,44] Patients with valvular heart disease, especially those with subcritical aortic or mitral stenosis, tend to tolerate fluid overload poorly and may be at especially high risk for major noncardiac surgery. In general, patients with valvular heart disease who do not require surgery on the basis of their symptoms also do not require prophylactic surgery preoperatively. The principal exception would be patients whose usual exercise level is so limited that the expected stress of a major procedure, such as repair of an abdominal aortic aneurysm, may be greater than that associated with the patient's usual activity.

If a patient is suspected of having aortic stenosis as the cause for controllable or uncontrollable cardiac symptoms, aggressive preoperative evaluation is mandatory. If a noninvasive evaluation cannot exclude severe aortic stenosis as the cause of angina, congestive heart failure, or syncope, cardiac catheterization is required.

It is recommended that patients with valvular heart disease, including mitral valve prolapse in the presence of a murmur,[50] should receive prophylactic antibiotic therapy if the procedure is likely to be associated with bacteremia. For both native valvular heart disease and prosthetic valves, the American Heart Association recommends antibiotic prophylaxis for incision and drainage of an infection, all dental procedures likely to induce gingival bleeding, tonsillectomy or adenoidectomy, surgical procedures or biopsy of respiratory mucosa, and bronchoscopy (especially with a rigid bronchoscope), and for the following gastrointestinal and genitourinary procedures: cystoscopy, prostatic surgery, indwelling urethral catheterization or brief catheterization in the presence of bacteriuria, urinary tract surgery, vaginal hysterectomy, gallbladder surgery, colonic surgery, esophageal dilatation, sclerotherapy of esophageal varices, colonoscopy, and upper gastrointestinal endoscopy with biopsy or proctosigmoidoscopic biopsy.[50] The official American Heart Association recommendations[50] do not suggest prophylactic antibiotics in patients with native valvular heart disease who have vaginal delivery, cesarean section, dilatation and curettage of the uterus, therapeutic abortion, pelvic examination, upper gastrointestinal endoscopy or sigmoidoscopy without biopsy, barium enema, percutaneous liver biopsy, or uncomplicated insertion or removal of an intrauterine device in the absence of pelvic infection.[50] For all of the aforementioned procedures, however, prophylaxis is suggested as prudent in patients with prosthetic heart valves.[50]

The chosen prophylactic regimen must be appropriate to cover the type of bacteremia that is expected given the surgical site. For oral or respiratory tract procedures in patients with native valvular disease, the recommendations[50] suggest penicillin V, 2 g one hour before and then 1 g six hours later. Alternative regimens include: for the patient who cannot take oral medication, penicillin G (intravenously or intramuscularly) 2 million units 30 to 60 minutes before and 1 million units six hours after a procedure; for penicillin-allergic patients, erythromycin 1 g one hour before and then 500 mg six hours later; for penicillin-allergic patients who cannot tolerate oral medication, one dose of vancomycin, 1 g intravenously given slowly during the hour before the procedure.[50] For patients with prosthetic valves who are having more than routine maintenance dental procedures in the context of a high level of oral health, the American Heart Association[50] recommends ampicillin 1 to 2 g (intramuscularly or intravenously) and gentamicin 1.5 mg/kg (intramuscularly or intravenously) 30 minutes before the procedure and then either 1 g of oral penicillin V six hours later or a repeat of the parenteral regimen eight hours later. For genitourinary or gastrointestinal procedures, the standard recommendations are for ampicillin 2 g (intramuscularly or intravenously) and gentamicin 1.5 mg/kg (intramuscularly or intravenously) 30 to 60 minutes before the procedure and then commonly repeated eight hours later. If the patient is penicillin-allergic, vancomycin (as just described) should be substituted for ampicillin. For minor or repetitive procedures, amoxicillin alone (3 g orally one hour before the procedure and 1.5 g six hours later) may be sufficient.

Patients with prosthetic valves, and many patients with underlying valvular heart disease with or without atrial fibrillation, are often receiving anticoagulants. For patients whose reason for anticoagulation is a left ventricular aneurysm or atrial fibrillation from native valvular heart disease, anticoagulation should usually be discontinued about three or four days preoperatively and a normal or near-normal coagulation profile should be documented preoperatively. Regardless of whether low-dose prophylactic heparinization is used perioperatively, full-dose anticoagulation can be restarted orally with warfarin about three to five days postoperatively or with heparin at a slightly later date. In general, the actuarial daily risk of embolization in patients with these conditions is so small that discontinuation of anticoagulation for about ten days to 2 weeks does not pose a substantial risk. In patients with prosthetic nontissue valves, however, the actuarial daily risk of embolization is substantially higher. For such patients, two probably equally effective regimens have been proposed. In one, oral warfarin is discontinued about two days preoperatively and then resumed one to three days after surgery.[51] The hemorrhagic complication rate was reported to be about 13%. A second alternative is to discontinue oral warfarin about three to five days before surgery and to begin heparin treatment at that time. The heparin is then discontinued about six hours before surgery and resumed 12 to 24 hours after surgery. Warfarin is reinstituted when the patient is able to take oral medication.[52] Either of these options has about the same complication rate, but the latter more aggressive approach is preferable in patients with highly thrombogenic caged disk valves.

ARRHYTHMIAS

Patients with frequent premature ventricular contractions or rhythms other than normal sinus rhythm have an increased risk of cardiac complications in noncardiac surgery,[5,13,44] principally because these arrhythmias are markers of more severe heart disease.[12,53,54] There is no evidence that alterations from the usual ambulatory management of arrhythmias need be undertaken preoperatively to reduce risk, and special prophylactic perioperative therapy is rarely required. The one exception is in patients who have a history of truly symptomatic ventricular arrhythmias, in whom prophylactic lidocaine is commonly appropriate, because the usual oral medications may not have adequate durations of action to cover the perioperative period when the patient will not be able to take medications by mouth. Therapeutic, as opposed to prophylactic, lidocaine should be used in patients in whom perioperative arrhythmias develop that cause hemodynamic compromise or who have runs of ventricular tachycardia. The approach to perioperative arrhythmias generally is similar to that used in ill medical patients, with reliance on intravenous medication because of the difficulties in obtaining rapid or reliable levels with oral or intramuscular therapy.

When postoperative arrhythmias develop, the arrhythmias are commonly precipitated by noncardiac problems such as fluid overload, pain, hypoxia, infection, or electrolyte abnormalities.[55] The cornerstone of therapy is the detection and appropriate therapy of these noncardiac problems, in addition to any therapy that may be appropriate for the arrhythmia itself. The mortality rate in patients with postoperative supraventricular tachycardias is as high as 40% to 50%,[55] principally because of these underlying medical conditions. Cardioversion is rarely required for postoperative supraventricular tachycardias, and most patients will respond to continuation of their usual medications or the addition of digitalis or intravenous verapamil. Often, new medications begun to treat the perioperative arrhythmia can be discontinued after the patient's condition has been stabilized.

Digitalis may be appropriate for patients who have a high risk of perioperative supraventricular tachycardia, such as elderly patients undergoing pulmonary surgery or patients with a history of paroxysmal tachycardia or subcritical valvular heart disease.[55,56] However, the availability of intravenous verapamil has reduced the need for prophylactic digitalis except in these occasional subgroups of patients.[57]

Ample data[13,44,58] indicate that even in patients with bifascicular or trifascicular block, the risk of perioperative complete heart block is not high enough to warrant prophylactic pacemaker therapy. Patients with sick sinus syndrome will rarely require pacemakers for surgery if they do not require chronic pacing. If a patient who requires a new pacemaker is expected to have bacteremia with the planned surgery, it is appropriate to insert a temporary pacemaker preoperatively and then to insert the permanent pacemaker after the risk of bacteremia has passed.

HYPERTENSION

Although patients with hypertension have an increased risk of cardiac complications with noncardiac surgery,[5,59] most of their increased risk is a function of their already manifest heart disease. Patients with stable diastolic blood pressure below 110 mm Hg generally do not need to have their operation postponed to achieve hypertension control, providing that excellent anesthetic care is available.[59,60] Antihypertensive medication commonly should be continued at least until the day before surgery, and concerns about hypotensive responses in patients on antihypertensive medication seem to be largely unfounded.[61–64]

Perioperative hypertension most commonly occurs during intubation, during periods of inadequate anesthesia, or soon after cessation of anesthesia. Much like postoperative arrhythmias, the most common causes of postoperative hypertension include pain, hypoxia, and fluid overload. Postoperative hypertension will occur in about 25% of patients with a history of hypertension, regardless of the adequacy of preoperative therapy, and also occurs in about 30% of patients having major vascular surgery.[59,65] The initial approach should emphasize oxygen, sedation, and adequate analgesia. Because fluid overload is a common precipitant of postoperative hypertension, intravenous furosemide is an important therapeutic maneuver. Nitroprusside generally is the best drug to control severe postoperative hypertension, with guidelines similar to those used in hypertensive crises. Intravenous alpha methyldopa has a delayed onset of action and will not be helpful initially, although it may be helpful in controlling hypertension four to six hours later. Intravenous hydralazine therapy is often used, but caution must be used by starting with small doses, such as 2 to 5 mg intravenously, because of its potential for precipitating postoperative supraventricular tachycardia. If postoperative hypertension is adequately controlled, it rarely causes other major cardiac sequelae.[59,66]

GENERAL MEDICAL AND SURGICAL ISSUES

Regardless of the type and severity of the underlying heart disease, the stress of surgery and the general health of the patient are important correlates of perioperative cardiac complications. Cardiac risks are increased in the elderly,[5,13,44] with a marked increase in cardiac risk in patients over the age of 70. Cardiac complications are more common after major intraabdominal or intrathoracic procedures[5,7] even in the modern era. Risk is especially high with abdominal aortic aneurysm surgery.[67] The length of surgery generally does not correlate with cardiac risk after controlling for the type of surgery.[3,13,44] Cardiac complications are significantly more common after emergency operations.[5,7,13,44] In addition, in patients whose general medical condition is poor because of noncardiac disease or laboratory abnormalities, cardiac risk is clearly increased.[5]

ANESTHETIC TECHNIQUE

There is little evidence that the choice among general anesthetic agents or between general versus spinal anesthesia is a major determinant of risk for patients with ischemic heart disease. Spinal anesthesia causes peripheral vascular dilatation and is at least as likely to cause un-

Table 68.1. Computation of the Cardiac Risk Index for the Estimation of Cardiac Risk in Noncardiac Surgery

Criteria	Points
1. History:	
(a) Age > 70 yr	5
(b) MI in previous 6 mo	10
2. Physical examination:	
(a) S_3 gallop or JVD	11
(b) Important VAS	3
3. Electrocardiogram:	
(a) Rhythm other than sinus or PACs on last preoperative ECG	7
(b) >5 PVCs/min documented at any time before operation	7
4. General status:	
Po_2 <60 or Pco_2 >50 mm Hg, K <3.0 or HCO_3 <20 mEq/L, BUN >50 or Cr >3.0 mg/dl, abnormal SGOT, signs of chronic liver disease, or patient bedridden from noncardiac causes	3
5. Operation:	
(a) Intraperitoneal, intrathoracic, or aortic operation	3
(b) Emergency operation	4
Total possible	53

BUN = blood urea nitrogen; Cr = creatinine; ECG = electrocardiogram; HCO_3 = bicarbonate; JVD = jugular vein distension; K = potassium; MI = myocardial infarction; PACs = premature atrial contractions; Pco_2 = partial pressure of carbon dioxide; Po_2 = partial pressure of oxygen; PVCs = premature ventricular contractions; SGOT = serum glutamic oxalacetic transaminase; VAS = valvular aortic stenosis. (Adapted from Goldman et al,[5] with permission of the *New England Journal of Medicine.*)

Table 68.2. Performance of the Cardiac Risk Index

No. of Points	Class	Life-Threatening Complications (%)*		Cardiac Death (%)	
		Goldman et al†	Zeldin‡	Goldman et al†	Zeldin‡
0–5	I	0.7	0.5	0.2	0.2
6–12	II	5	2	2	1
13–25	III	12	11	2	4
≥26	IV	22	4	56	26

* Recognized nonfatal myocardial infarction, pulmonary edema, or ventricular tachycardia.
† Based on 1,001 general surgical patients over age 40 on whom the index was derived in 1975 to 1976.[5]
‡ Based on 1,140 general surgical patients over age 40 on whom the index was prospectively evaluated at four hospitals, not including the one from which it was derived, in 1978 to 1982.[71]

planned intraoperative hypotension as is general anesthesia.[13] For patients with ischemic heart disease, well-balanced general anesthesia is preferable to potentially inadequate local or spinal anesthesia. Spinal anesthesia may be less likely to cause an exacerbation of congestive heart failure because, unlike many general anesthetic agents, it is not a direct myocardial depressant. Therefore, it may occasionally be preferable to use spinal anesthesia or agents that are not major myocardial depressants, such as droperidol, fentanyl, or intravenous narcotics,[68] in patients with severe heart failure. Generally, however, the medical consultant should not join in the debate about anesthetic agents and technique, but should leave this responsibility to the anesthesiologist, with advice from the surgeon and the consent of the patient.[69]

MULTIFACTORIAL ASSESSMENT OF CARDIAC RISK

One way to assess overall cardiac risk is to use the multifactorial cardiac risk index (Tables 68.1 and 68.2). It is not clear whether the routine availability of newer diagnostic techniques, such as exercise thallium scans, exercise left ventricular function studies, or dipyridamole thallium scanning will improve risk assessment beyond what is available with the history and physical examination. Recent data, however, suggest that dipyridamole thallium scanning can be very helpful in patients undergoing vascular surgery[34] and that exercise testing may be helpful in assessing the risk of major surgery in the elderly.[70] This index, which was originally derived from patients seen in the mid-1970s, has performed well in prospective testing at several other institutions during the subsequent years.[24,71,72] It should be emphasized, however, that more recent data[7,8,71] suggest that patients with recent preoperative myocardial infarction and class IV patients may have a better outcome in the 1980s because of the application of cardiovascular anesthetic techniques to sick cardiac patients undergoing noncardiac surgery. Data also suggest that the multifactorial cardiac risk index underestimates the risk of patients undergoing abdominal aortic aneurysm surgery, because it does not take into account that their risk is higher than that among patients undergoing other abdominal and thoracic procedures.[67] In one large series, the risk of major cardiac complications from abdominal aortic aneurysm surgery was 7%, 11%, and 38%, respectively, in patients who were in class I, II, and III in the cardiac risk index.[67] These latter figures, rather than those in Table 68.2, should be used to estimate risk in aortic aneurysm surgery. Furthermore, there are some situations, such as unstable angina, that were too infrequent to be analyzed by the original cardiac risk index[5] but that likely carry a high enough risk to warrant special attention and management strategies similar to those used for other high risk patients.

Generally the application of cardiovascular anesthetic techniques, including arterial and pulmonary artery catheterization, is appropriate in patients who are class IV on the index, are class III on the index and undergoing major surgery, have late class III or class IV heart failure, or have had recent preoperative myocardial infarction. Some have suggested the use of the same routine in all patients over age 65 who have major noncardiac surgery,[17,18] but it is not clear that such a strategy is warranted in patients who are otherwise at low risk except for their age. It should also be emphasized that the interplay between general medical status and cardiac complications mandates careful consideration of noncardiac maneuvers to improve the patient's general condition. Because complications of surgery often do not appear until three to five days after surgery,[7,13] it is imperative that postoperative cardiac follow-up continue until the patient has regained an ambulatory status and recovered from the surgical procedure.

REFERENCES

1. Tarhan S, Moffitt EA, Taylor WF, Guiliani ER: Myocardial infarction after general anesthesia. *JAMA* 1972; 220:1451–1454.
2. Arkins R, Smessaert AA, Hicks RG: Mortality and morbidity in surgical patients with coronary artery disease. *JAMA* 1964; 190:485–488.
3. Topkins MJ, Artusio JF: Myocardial infarction and surgery: a five year study. *Anesth Analg* 1964; 43:716–720.
4. Steen PA, Tinker JH, Tarhan S: Myocardial reinfarction after anesthesia and surgery. *JAMA* 1978; 239:2566–2570.
5. Goldman L, Caldera DL, Nussbaum SR, Southwick FS, Krogstad D, Murray B, Burke DS, O'Malley TA, Goroll AH, Caplan CH, Nolan J, Carabello B, Slater EE: Multifactorial index of cardiac risk in noncardiac surgical procedures. *N Engl J Med* 1977; 297:845–850.
6. Fraser JG, Ramachandran PR, Davis HS: Anesthesia and recent myocardial infarction. *JAMA* 1967; 199:318–320.
7. Rao TLK, Jacobs KH, El-Etr AA: Reinfarction following anesthesia in patients with myocardial infarction. *Anesthesiology* 1983; 59:499–505.
8. Wells PH, Kaplan JA: Optimal management of patients with ischemic heart disease for noncardiac surgery by complementary anesthesiologist and cardiologist interaction. *Am Heart J* 1981; 102:1029–1037.
9. Cannom DS, Levy W, Cohen LS: The short- and long-term prognosis

of patients with transmural and nontransmural myocardial infarction. *Am J Med* 1976; 61:452–458.

10. Scheinman MM, Abbott JA: Clinical significance of transmural versus nontransmural electrocardiographic changes in patients with acute myocardial infarction. *Am J Med* 1973; 55:602–607.
11. Sanz G, Castaner A, Betriu A, Magrina J, Roig E, Coll S, Pare JC, Navarro-Lopez F: Determinants of prognosis in survivors of myocardial infarction. A prospective clinical angiographic study. *N Engl J Med* 1982; 306:1065–1070.
12. The Multicenter Postinfarction Research Group: Risk stratification and survival after myocardial infarction. *N Engl J Med* 1983; 309:331–336.
13. Goldman L, Caldera DL, Southwick FS, Nussbaum SR, Krogstad D, Murray B, Burke DS, O'Malley TA, Goroll AH, Caplan CH, Nolan J, Carabello B, Slater EE: Cardiac risk factors and complications in noncardiac surgery. *Medicine* 1978; 57:357–370.
14. Gage AA, Bhayana JN, Balu V, Hook N: Assessment of cardiac risk in surgical patients. *Arch Surg* 1977; 112:1488–1492.
15. Fudge TL, McKinnon WMP, Schoettle GP, Ochsner JL, Mills NL: Improved operative risk after myocardial revascularization. *South Med J* 1981; 74:799–801.
16. Hertzer NR, Young JR, Kramer JR, Phillips DF, deWolfe VG, Ruschhaupt WF III, Beven EG: Routine coronary angiography prior to elective aortic reconstruction: results of selective myocardial revascularization in patients with peripheral vascular disease. *Arch Surg* 1979; 114:1336–1344.
17. Del Guercio LRM, Cohn JD: Monitoring operative risk in the elderly. *JAMA* 1980; 243:1350–1355.
18. Babu SC, Sharma PVP, Raciti A, Mayr CH Jr, Elrabie NA, Clauss RH, Stahl WM, Del Guercio LRM: Monitor-guided responses: operability with safety is increased in patients with peripheral vascular diseases. *Arch Surg* 1980; 115:1384–1386.
19. Bille-Brahe NE, Eickhoff JH: Measurement of central haemodynamic parameters during preoperative exercise testing in patients suspected of arteriosclerotic heart disease: value in predicting postoperative cardiac complications. *Acta Chir Scand* 1980; 502:38–45.
20. Goldman L, Cook EF, Mitchell N, Flatley M, Sherman H, Rosati R, Harrell F, Lee K, Cohn PF: Incremental value of the exercise test for diagnosing the presence or absence of coronary artery disease. *Circulation* 1982; 66:945–953.
21. Rifkin RD, Hood WB Jr: Bayesian analysis of electrocardiographic exercise stress testing. *N Engl J Med* 1977; 297:681–686.
22. DeBusk RF, Kraemer HC, Nash E, Berger WE, Lew H: Stepwise risk stratification soon after acute myocardial infarction. *Am J Cardiol* 1983; 52:1161–1166.
23. De Feyter PJ, van Eenige MJ, Dighton DH, Visser FC, de Jong J, Roos JP: Prognostic value of exercise testing, coronary angiography and left ventriculography 6–8 weeks after myocardial infarction. *Circulation* 1982; 66:527–536.
24. Kaplan JA, Dunbar RW: Anesthesia for noncardiac surgery in patients with cardiac disease, in Kaplan JA (ed): *Cardiac Anesthesia*. New York, Grune & Stratton, Inc, 1979, pp 377–389.
25. Bernhard VM, Johnson WD, Peterson JJ: Carotid artery stenosis—association with surgery for coronary artery disease. *Arch Surg* 1972; 105:837–840.
26. Mahar LJ, Steen PA, Tinker JH, Vlietstra RE, Smith HC, Pluth JR: Perioperative myocardial infarction in patients with coronary artery disease with and without aorta-coronary bypass grafts. *J Thorac Cardiovasc Surg* 1978; 76:533–537.
27. Crawford ES, Morris GC, Howell JF, Flynn WF, Moorhead DT: Operative risk in patients with previous coronary artery bypass. *Ann Thorac Surg* 1978; 26:215–221.
28. Takaro T, Hultgren HN, Lipton MJ, Detre KM, Participants in the VA Cooperative Study Group: VA Cooperative Randomized Study of Surgery for Coronary Arterial Occlusive Disease. II. Subgroup with significant left main lesions. *Circulation* 1976; 54(suppl 3):III-107–III-117.
29. European Coronary Surgery Study Group: Long-term results of a prospective randomised study of coronary artery bypass surgery in stable angina pectoris. *Lancet* 1982; 2:1173–1180.
30. The Veterans Administration Coronary Artery Bypass Surgery Cooperative Study Group: Eleven-year survival in the Veterans Administration randomized trial of coronary bypass surgery for stable angina. *N Engl J Med* 1984; 311:1333–1339.
31. CASS Principal Investigators and Their Associates: Myocardial infarction and mortality in the Coronary Artery Surgery Study (CASS) randomized trial. *N Engl J Med* 1984; 310:750–758.
32. Goldman L, Hashimoto B, Cook EF, Loscalzo A: Comparative reproducibility and validity of systems for assessing cardiovascular functional class: advantages of a new Specific Activity Scale. *Circulation* 1981; 64:1227–1234.
33. Podrid PJ, Graboys TB, Lown B: Prognosis of medically treated patients with coronary artery disease with profound ST-segment depression during exercise testing. *N Engl J Med* 1981; 305:1111–1116.
34. Boucher CA, Brewster DC, Darling RC, Okada RD, Strauss HW, Pohost GM: Determination of cardiac risk by dipyridamole-thallium imaging before peripheral vascular surgery. *N Engl J Med* 1985; 312:389–394.
35. Heller GV, Aroesty JM, Parker JA, McKay RG, Silverman KJ, Als AV, Come PC, Kolodny GM, Grossman W: The pacing stress test: thallium-201 myocardial imaging after atrial pacing: diagnostic value in detecting coronary artery disease compared with exercise testing. *J Am Coll Cardiol* 1984; 3:1197–1204.

35a. Foster ED, Davis KB, Carpenter JA, Abele S, Fray D: Risk of noncardiac operation in patients with defined coronary disease: the Coronary Artery Surgery Study (CASS) registry experience. *Ann Thorac Surg* 1986; 41:42–50.

36. Viljoen JF, Estafanous FG, Kellner GA: Propranolol and cardiac surgery. *J Thorac Cardiovasc Surg* 1972; 64:826–830.
37. Nattel S, Rangno RE, Van Loon G: Mechanism of propranolol withdrawal phenomena. *Circulation* 1979; 59:1158–1164.
38. Goldman L: Noncardiac surgery in patients receiving propranolol: case reports and a recommended approach. *Arch Intern Med* 1981; 141:193–196.
39. Moran JM, Mulet J, Caralps JM, Pifarre R: Coronary revascularization in patients receiving propranolol. *Circulation* 1974; 50(suppl 2):II-116–II-121.
40. Kaplan JA, Dunbar RW, Bland JW Jr, Sumpter R, Jones EL: Propranolol and cardiac surgery: a problem for the anesthesiologist? *Anesth Analg* 1975; 54:571–572.
41. Kopriva CJ, Brown ACD, Pappas G: Hemodynamics during general anesthesia in patients receiving propranolol. *Anesthesiology* 1978; 48:28–33.
42. Woolsey RL, Shand DG: Pharmacokinetics of antiarrhythmic drugs. *Am J Cardiol* 1978; 41:986–995.
43. Smulyan H, Weinberg SE, Howanitz PJ: Continuous propranolol infusion following abdominal surgery. *JAMA* 1982; 247:2539–2542.
44. Salem DN, Homans DC, Isner JM: Management of cardiac disease in the general surgical patient. *Curr Probl Cardiol* 1980; 5:1–41.
45. Skinner JF, Pearce ML: Surgical risk in the cardiac patient. *J Chronic Dis* 1964; 17:57–72.
46. McKee PA, Castelli WP, McNamara PM, Kannel WB: The natural history of congestive heart failure: The Framingham Study. *N Engl J Med* 1971; 285:1441–1446.
47. Mauney FM, Ebert PA, Sabiston DC Jr: Postoperative myocardial infarction: a study of predisposing factors, diagnosis and mortality in a high risk group of surgical patients. *Ann Surg* 1970; 172:497–503.
48. Von Knorring J: Postoperative myocardial infarction: a prospective study in a risk group of surgical patients. *Surgery* 1981; 90:55–60.
49. Cooperman LH, Price HL: Pulmonary edema in the operative and postoperative period: a review of 40 cases. *Ann Surg* 1970; 172:883–891.
50. Shulman ST, Amren DP, Bisno A, Dajani AS, Durack DT, Gerber MA, Kaplan EL, Millard HD, Sanders WE, Schwartz RH, Watanakunakorn C: Prevention of bacterial endocarditis. *Circulation* 1984; 70:1123A–1127A.
51. Tinker JH, Tarhan S: Discontinuing anticoagulant therapy in surgical patients with cardiac valve prostheses: observations in 180 operations. *JAMA* 1978; 239:738–739.
52. Katholi RE, Nolan SP, McGuire LB: The management of antiocoagulation during noncardiac operations in patients with prosthetic heart valves: a prospective study. *Am Heart J* 1978; 96:163–165.
53. Schulze RA Jr, Rouleau J, Rigo P, Bowers S, Strauss HW, Pitt B: Ventricular arrhythmias in the late hospital phase of acute myocardial infarction: relation to left ventricular function detected by gated cardiac blood pool scanning. *Circulation* 1975; 52:1006–1011.
54. Schulze RA Jr, Strauss HW, Pitt B: Sudden death in the year following myocardial infarction: relation to ventricular premature contractions in the late hospital phase and left ventricular ejection fraction. *Am J Med* 1977; 62:192–199.
55. Goldman L: Supraventricular tachyarrhythmias in hospitalized adults after surgery: clinical correlates in patients over 40 years of age after major noncardiac surgery. *Chest* 1978; 73:450–454.
56. Selzer A, Walter RM: Adequacy of preoperative digitalis therapy in controlling ventricular rate in postoperative atrial fibrillation. *Circulation* 1966; 34:119–122.
57. Singh BN, Ellrodt G, Peter CT: Verapamil: a review of its pharmacological properties and therapeutic use. *Drugs* 1978; 15:169–197.
58. Pastore JO, Yurchak PM, Janis KM, Murphy JD, Zir LM: The risk of advanced heart block in surgical patients with right bundle branch block and left axis deviation. *Circulation* 1978; 57:677–680.
59. Goldman L, Caldera DL: Risks of general anesthesia and elective operation in the hypertensive patient. *Anesthesiology* 1979; 50:285–292.
60. Prys-Roberts C: Hypertension and anesthesia—fifty years on (editorial). *Anesthesiology* 1979; 50:281–284.
61. Katz RL, Weintraub HD, Papper EM: Anesthesia, surgery and rauwolfia. *Anesthesiology* 1964; 25:142–147.
62. Prys-Roberts C, Meloche R, Foex P: Studies of anesthesia in relation

to hypertension. I. Cardiovascular responses of treated and untreated patients. *Br J Anaesth* 1971; 43:122–137.

63. Prys-Roberts C, Foex P, Greene LT, Waterhouse TD: Studies of anaesthesia in relation to hypertension. IV. The effects of artificial ventilation on the circulation and pulmonary gas exchanges. *Br J Anaesth* 1972; 44:335–349.
64. Foex P, Prys-Roberts C: Anaesthesia and the hypertensive patient. *Br J Anaesth* 1974; 46:575–588.
65. Lehv MS, Salzman EW, Silen W: Hypertension complicating carotid endarterectomy. *Stroke* 1970; 1:307–313.
66. Gal TJ, Cooperman LH: Hypertension in the immediate postoperative period. *Br J Anaesth* 1975; 47:70–74.
67. Jeffrey CC, Kunsman J, Cullen DJ, Brewster DC: A prospective evaluation of cardiac risk index. *Anesthesiology* 1983; 58:462–464.
68. Bille-Brahe NE, Sorensen MB, Mondorf T, Engel HC: Central hemodynamics during induction of neurolept anaesthesia in patients with arteriosclerotic heart disease. *Acta Anaesth Scand Suppl* 1978; 67:47–54.
69. Goldman L: When the cardiac patient has noncardiac surgery. *Hospital Physician* 1985; 26:32A–40A.
70. Gerson MC, Hurst JM, Hertzberg VS, Doogan PA, Cochran MB, Lim SP, McCall N, Adolph RJ: Cardiac prognosis in noncardiac geriatric surgery. *Ann Intern Med* 1985; 103:832–837.
71. Zeldin RA: Assessing cardiac risk in patients who undergo noncardiac surgical procedures. *Can J Surg* 1984; 27:402–404.
72. Weathers LW, Paine R: The risk of surgery in cardiac patients. *Intern Med* 1981; 2:57–64.

69 Anesthesia for Cardiac Surgery

Edward Lowenstein, MD and E. Greg Koski, MD, PhD

Cardiac anesthesia has evolved with, and contributed to, the rapid growth of cardiac surgery, and it is now a recognized subspecialty of anesthesiology. Conceptually, there are two divisions of this field, the first being anesthesia for the patient undergoing cardiac surgery and the second being management of the patient with heart disease undergoing noncardiac surgery. This discussion is limited to the former, as the latter has been covered in chapter 68. We believe it is crucial that the lessons learned from patients undergoing open heart surgery, who are routinely monitored intensively and who undergo routine perioperative intensive care, be disseminated to all anesthetists. Such dissemination has occurred, and the esoteric practices in the cardiac surgical operating room of only a few years ago are now standard for patients with cardiac disease undergoing other types of surgery, as well as all critically ill patients, whether undergoing surgery or receiving intensive care.

This chapter will present only a limited perspective of the field, highlighting information we perceive to be of interest to physicians other than anesthesiologists, and reflecting methods and philosophies developed by the Cardiac Anesthesia Group of the Department of Anesthesia of the Massachusetts General Hospital.

Nowhere in medical practice is success more dependent on interdisciplinary cooperation and understanding. For the anesthetist, this can best be achieved by participating in the total care of the patient. The anesthetist must have an understanding of the physiologic aspects of the particular lesion, the surgical procedure, the physiologic aspects of cardiopulmonary bypass, and the normal and pathologic circulatory, respiratory, and renal physiology to effectively care for the cardiac surgical patient.

Priorities of anesthetic practice include, in order of importance, (1) preservation of cardiovascular and respiratory integrity, (2) provision of suitable operating conditions, and (3) patient comfort. When dealing with patients as seriously ill as are many candidates for cardiac surgery, it is imperative not to sacrifice the first two priorities for utmost patient comfort. Although it is usually possible to provide all three, it is frequently necessary to impose temporary discomfort on a patient to preserve life. Most patients are willing to accept this if it is properly clarified at the time of the preoperative visit.

PREOPERATIVE CARE

MANAGEMENT OF CARDIAC MEDICATIONS

An important aim of cardiac anesthesia practice is to maintain physiologic normalcy as much as possible during the entire perioperative period. In patients who are receiving "cardiac medications" (digitalis, beta blockers, calcium channel blockers, and antihypertensive drugs) for valid indications, this implies that unless an adverse interaction between anesthetic drugs or perioperative surgical maneuvers is anticipated, the drug should be continued through the perioperative period. Over the past generation, the perioperative management of each of the aforementioned classes of compounds has undergone a cycle of (1) fear of adverse drug interactions, (2) discontinuation of the drug preoperatively, (3) recognition of the adverse consequences of an inadequate drug level, and (4) a more liberal policy of either routine continuation or a modified regimen of continuation of smaller doses for specific indications.

A review of the initial drug category that went through this cycle is illuminating. A study indicated that severe hypotension on induction of anesthesia was more common in treated hypertensive patients than in nontreated normotensive patients.[1] The conclusion was drawn that antihypertensive therapy should be discontinued preoperatively. Years later, hypertension per se was recognized as the responsible factor, rather than the antihypertensive medication. A study in which hypertensive patients whose medication was continued were compared with hypertensive patients whose medication was discontinued indicated that the incidence of hypotension was similar but the morbidity was greater in patients whose medication had been withdrawn.[2] Additional studies then indicated that the incidence of myocardial ischemia in hypertensive patients prophylactically receiving the beta-adrenergic blocker practolol was reduced by 90% from 38% to 4%.[3] Thus, the philosophy arose that initiation of treatment in untreated patients with this condition was actually advantageous.

It is interesting to speculate why this cycle has been repeated so many times. We believe it reflects the generalization of anecdotal data, in essence a certain anti-intellectualism and sloppiness of thought. As noted herein, however, even small well-conducted studies were successful in disabusing the physician population of misleading ideas. It is reassuring that this cycle has been shorter and less profound with the latest group of compounds, the calcium channel blockers, than with any of the previous groups.

Digitalis Preparations

The interaction of digitalis with hypokalemia to increase ventricular automaticity is well established. Furthermore, shifts in serum potassium are common during all types of surgery, but virtually the rule in patients undergoing cardiac surgery with cardiopulmonary bypass. The frequency of hyperventilation with respiratory alkalosis leading to hypokalemia is great both intraoperatively and postoperatively, whenever mechanical ventilation without continuous carbon dioxide monitoring is employed. The potassium-wasting effect of many diuretics is well established. The inotropic effect of digitalis preparations may be effectively substituted by infusion of inotropic drugs. For all these reasons, there has been a consensus for many years to discontinue digitalis preparations several days preoperatively.

By and large, this practice holds. It is common also to discontinue diuretics 24 to 48 hours before operation so that the patient may be slightly hypervolemic rather than hypovolemic, because this is thought to decrease the incidence of hypotension attendant on the venodilation invariably associated with induction of anesthesia. This practice was initiated in the early days of cardiac surgery before the ability to rapidly measure serum potassium. The universally available ability to measure serum potassium levels rapidly and repeatedly has decreased the necessity for rigidly applying this practice.

Our present approach is as follows[4]: (1) Acute digitalization is warranted in the patient who has preoperative heart failure. (2) Prophylactic preoperative digitalization is not employed if it is intended solely to counteract the cardiac depressant effect of anesthetic drugs or other perioperative physiologic alterations. (3) Digitalis therapy is continued in patients with chronic atrial fibrillation if the ventricular rate is in excess of 80 beats per minute, unless digitalis intoxication is suspected or confirmed.

The influence of preoperative digitalization on the frequency of postoperative supraventricular tachyarrhythmias in patients subjected to open heart surgery is unclear. Numerous studies have examined the incidence of supraventricular arrhythmias, conversion to atrial fibrillation, rate of ventricular response, and serum digoxin levels.[5–7] There is little consistency among the studies. In one, the incidence of atrial fibrillation postoperatively was actually twice as great after prophylactic digitalization.[8]

Because of the equivocal nature of the evidence and the hazards associated with digitalis intoxication, we do not employ prophylactic digitalization to reduce the incidence and hemodynamic consequences of supraventricular arrhythmias in patients undergoing coronary artery or other cardiac surgical procedures. The utility of both beta-adrenergic blockers and calcium channel blockers for treatment of supraventricular tachyarrhythmias, if they occur, has reinforced our decision.

Beta-Adrenergic Blockers

Continuation of beta-adrenergic blockers until the cardiac operation is now universally accepted, because both ischemic episodes and morbidity are reduced.[9] Discontinuation over four days was associated with a higher incidence of arrhythmias, angina pectoris, and electrocardiographic signs of myocardial ischemia in patients with coronary artery disease scheduled to undergo noncardiac surgery.[10]

Interactions of beta-adrenergic blockers with anesthetics have been established but primarily with those anesthetics (diethyl ether, cyclopropane, trichloroethylene) that depend on liberation of catecholamines for maintaining circulatory stability. Such anesthetics are now obsolete in virtually all countries and no longer used during cardiac surgery anywhere.

Many studies attest to the safety of modern anesthetics (halothane, enflurane, isoflurane, and narcotics) in beta-blocked animals or man. For instance, the circulatory response to halothane in the normovolemic or hypovolemic animal is similar at several levels of halothane anesthesia, whether or not the animal has received a beta-adrenergic blocker.[11] Kopriva et al[12] reported the response of two groups of patients with ischemic heart disease, one of which received an average of 140 mg of propranolol per day, to a standard anesthetic regimen. The only preoperative difference observed was a lower heart rate in the group treated with propranolol. No differences in mean arterial pressure, cardiac output, stroke volume, or systemic vascular resistance were present in response to anesthesia or endotracheal intubation. Ventricular filling pressures were not measured in this study. Slogoff et al[13] compared the response to isoproterenol of propranolol-blocked dogs receiving either halothane or morphine anesthesia. No increased sensitivity to any measured effect of propranolol, expressed as the slope of the log dose-response curve, was observed, indicating a lack of potentiation by morphine or halothane of the effects of propranolol.

Deep (3%) enflurane anesthesia leads to circulatory decompensation or collapse in beta-blocked dogs that are made hypovolemic by withdrawal of 20% of the estimated blood volume.[14] However, there is no clinical evidence of such circulatory interaction. Perhaps this disparity is due to the fact that such high concentrations are seldom achieved in man. In contrast, no differences in cardiac output, systemic arterial blood pressure, systemic vascular resistance, heart rate, or left ventricular filling pressure were associated with the administration of 0.5 mg/kg of propranolol in dogs lightly or deeply anesthetized with isoflurane.[15]

In the aggregate, these studies indicate that myocardial depression observed with anesthesia in the presence of beta blockers is additive rather than synergistic. The fear that surgical stimulation would increase afterload to such a degree that the anesthetically depressed, beta-blocked myocardium would be unable to pump effectively has not been realized in clinical practice.

Two recent pieces of information modify, to a minor degree, the recommendation to continue the use of beta blockers. Wechsler,[16] in a double-blind, controlled study, reported that patients receiving large doses (320 to 480 mg per day) of propranolol had an increased need for postoperative inotropic support. Interestingly, cardiac morbidity was not increased in patients who required such support (Figure 69.1). Wechsler recommended reducing the preoperative dose of propranolol accordingly. The only substantive question concerning the validity of the conclusions is whether the patients who required such large doses of beta blockers constituted a group at higher risk for requiring postoperative support.

The Johns Hopkins Cardiac Surgical Unit noted a higher incidence of postoperative hypertension in patients receiving preoperative beta blockers[17] and a linear ($P = 0.7$, $P < .001$) correlation between postoperative serum propranolol levels and the nitroprusside dose required to maintain mean blood pressure between 80 and 90 mm Hg.[18] To achieve a sufficiently high concentration to establish this, however, required the administration of supplemental propranolol postoperatively. This indicates that this is an unusual problem with the current practice of not administering beta blockers during operation. This phenomenon appears to be due to beta$_2$ receptor blockade and emphasizes the desirability of absolute specificity of receptor blockade.

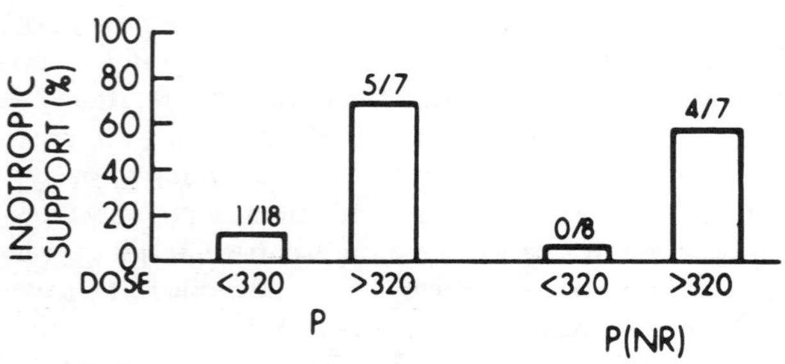

Figure 69.1. Requirement for inotropic support to terminate bypass or postoperatively as a function of propranolol dosage in patients undergoing myocardial revascularization. The results were similar in randomized (P) and nonrandomized (P[NR]) groups. (From Wechsler,[16] with permission of Little, Brown.)

Calcium Channel Blockers

Discontinuation practices are still in flux, and little definitive information exists concerning the administration of anesthesia in patients receiving calcium channel blockers. One report indicated that hypotension was more common on induction of anesthesia with fentanyl in patients receiving nifedipine, but this has not been confirmed.[19] We have a clinical impression that systemic vascular resistance is lower during and following termination of cardiopulmonary bypass in patients receiving large doses of nifedipine and diltiazem, and that such patients more often require alpha-adrenergic agonist infusions.

Beta-adrenergic antagonists and calcium channel blockers are frequently given in combination, making it difficult to determine whether calcium channel blockers by themselves are responsible for any difficulties encountered. Furthermore, we believe patients are coming to operation later in the course of the disease, because this combination of drugs is so effective in reducing symptoms. This makes it even more difficult to judge with certainty whether an adverse drug interaction has occurred.

PREANESTHETIC MEDICATION

The topic of preanesthetic medication appears initially to be mundane and unimportant. This is untrue in patients with severe cardiac disease who are scheduled for cardiac surgery, a most anxiety-provoking situation. We have found that such patients are among the most motivated and suggestible patients encountered. Thus, we have applied the lessons learned by Egbert et al,[20] who documented the profound benefits of a compassionate, unhurried, and informative preanesthetic visit (Figure 69.2).

Specifically, we apprise the patient of the procedures to which he will be subjected, starting with the mild annoyance of having food and water withheld through the administration of sedatives, transportation to the operating room, the insertion of monitoring cannulas, and the breathing of oxygen before anesthesia induction. We also discuss the postoperative course, including the discomfort of prolonged endotracheal intubation, endotracheal suction, chest physical therapy, inability to speak, weakness, and the various discomforts and noisy atmosphere of the intensive care unit. Lastly, we discuss in a nonthreatening way the possibility of dreams or recall, stressing that they are unusual but do occur occasionally and that such recall does not imply either fault in anesthetic administration or a psychologic disturbance in the patient. This is done because of the rare occurrence of the so-called traumatic psychosis after cardiac surgery due to recall of parts of the procedure.[21] The condition is promptly relieved by a thorough explanation to the patient.

The backbone of pharmacologic premedication has remained the combination of morphine and scopolamine, despite the synthesis of myriad sedatives and anxiolytic

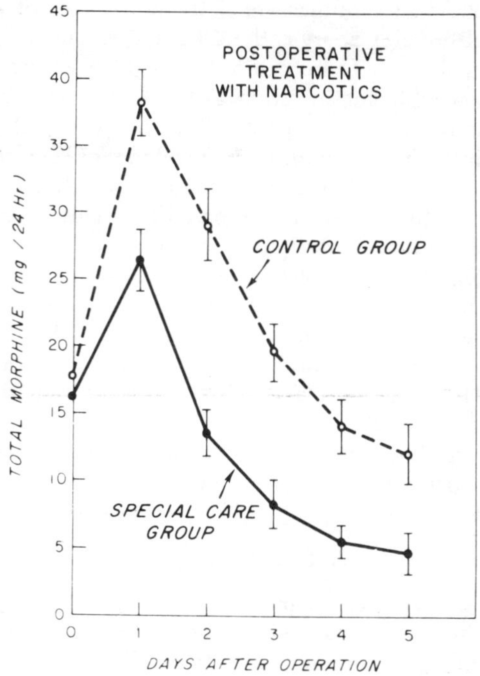

Figure 69.2. Effect of a supportive preoperative and periodic postoperative visit by an anesthetist on postoperative narcotic requirement in general surgical patients. Patients in the "special care" group left the hospital an average of two days earlier. (From Egbert et al,[20] with permission of The American Medical Association.)

compounds. Morphine by itself produces dysphoria. Scopolamine alone may well produce excitement. The combination, however, is associated with no change in heart rate or blood pressure and provides sedation more predictably than does any other combination tested.[22] Preoperative nausea or vomiting is astonishingly rare.

The basic dose employed is 0.1 mg/kg of morphine plus 0.4 mg of scopolamine intramuscularly in all adults. In patients with cardiac cachexia the dose of morphine is reduced by as much as one half. In robust patients, particularly those with ischemic heart disease and normal ventricular contractility, the dose may be increased, although we employ a maximum of 12 mg of morphine. Supplementary sedation and amnesia are frequently provided by a benzodiazepine, either diazepam or lorazepam, administered orally the night before surgery and the day of surgery at least one half hour before the intramuscular medications. It is important to monitor the patient for signs of hypertension, tachycardia, or excitement during insertion of the monitoring cannulas, so that supplementary sedation may be given promptly and myocardial ischemia or cardiac failure prevented.

The respiratory consequences of this preanesthetic regimen are present, although minimal (Table 69.1). Of 100 patients, randomly assigned to receive either morphine, scopolamine, the combination, or a placebo, those given morphine sustained an average decrease of 7 mm Hg of Pa_{O_2}.[22] Interestingly, the only patient in this series who became severely hypoxemic was one in the placebo group with severe mitral stenosis who became tachycardiac and had an episode of pulmonary edema. This case emphasizes the importance of adequate sedation.

The Pa_{CO_2} was increased approximately 3.5 mm Hg by morphine, an equivalent amount by scopolamine, and 7 mm Hg by the combination.[23] Patients who became most sedated retained the most carbon dioxide.

Patients with chronic mitral valve disease are most likely to become hypoxemic, and we recommend that they be transported to the operating room in a semi-Fowler position and with either mask or nasal oxygen. The same is true for any patient with a history of recent congestive heart failure.

MONITORING

The goal of all monitoring practices is to detect with safety the early signs of organ dysfunction to allow initiation of therapy before irreversible tissue damage. The ability to monitor cardiac surgical patients now exceeds the wildest dreams of even the physiologist of a decade or two ago. Modalities formerly available only in advanced research laboratories are now used routinely. Several points are worth emphasizing, however. We advocate and practice continuous recording of as many variables as possible, marking on the strip chart the clinical events as they take place. Review of such records has led to recognition of many phenomena, which have then become understood and often avoidable. (Tape or disk storage, permitting subsequent review at different speeds to allow waveform analysis and trend recording, is desirable

Table 69.1. Effect of Premedication on Pa_{O_2} and Pa_{CO_2}*†

	Placebo	Morphine	Scopolamine	Morphine and Scopolamine
Pa_{O_2}				
Control	80.7 ± 10.4	79.3 ± 11.7	82.0 ± 12.0	81.3 ± 12.1
Medicated	82.8 ± 12.8	73.1 ± 12.9	79.2 ± 13.9	73.2 ± 12.1
Mean change	+2.1	−6.2‡	−2.8	−8.1‡
Pa_{CO_2}				
Control	37.8 ± 4.7	37.5 ± 5.1	36.7 ± 5.5	35.0 ± 5.1
Medicated	38.9 ± 4.3	41.0 ± 4.6	40.0 ± 4.2	42.4 ± 5.4
Mean change	0.9	3.5‡	3.3‡	7.4†

*Data from four groups of 25 cardiac surgical patients each. Morphine+scopolamine premedication provides excellent sedation at an acceptable cost to blood gas exchange.

†After Katz et al.[22]

‡$P < 0.05$.

and now within the scope of current technology.) The hypotensive–vasodilatory effect of 5% plasma protein fraction solution[24] and pulmonary vasoconstriction associated with protamine reversal of heparin are two examples[25] (Figure 69.3). That hypertension and tachycardia occurred predictably with laryngoscopy and tracheal intubation was widely accepted only after routine vascular cannulation and continuous strip chart recording were practiced.

We advocate routine "aggressive" monitoring, because we continue to be impressed that many patients experience events that would be unrecognized without it, and that early institution of therapy often avoids serious problems. We institute monitoring before induction of anesthesia, rather than after induction and endotracheal intubation, because this is one of the most hazardous times during the procedure. We and others have demonstrated that vascular cannulation can be performed safely in the properly sedated patient.[26,27] We generally measure arterial, pulmonary artery, and right atrial pressure continuously, and pulmonary capillary wedge pressure and cardiac output intermittently. Left atrial pressure is recorded after cardiac repair. One inferior and one precordial electrocardiographic lead is displayed throughout anesthesia. Arterial blood is sampled at regular intervals for blood gases, pH, Na^+, K^+, Ca^{++}, hematocrit, total protein, osmolarity, and blood glucose analysis.

Although many complications of monitoring have been documented, perhaps the most insidious and distressing is bacteremia. Particularly in the presence of distorted natural or prosthetic heart valves, it causes bacterial endocarditis, which may in turn cause significant morbidity and mortality.

All vascular cannulas are potential sources of bacteremia, although urinary catheters may present the greater problem overall. Therefore, strict sterile procedures must be followed during insertion. All catheters must be handled with appropriate precautions and changed at frequent intervals to minimize the incidence of bacteremia.[28]

More recent monitoring techniques, which are still research methods, include esophageal two-dimensional echocardiography (ejection fraction, regional ventricular function, and air embolization), sonomicrometry (regional ventricular function), cardiokymography (anterior left ventricular wall ischemic dysfunction), processed electroencephalogram (compare hemispheric activity, not useful during hypothermia), and spinal evoked potentials (thoracic aneurysms). It remains to be determined which of these techniques will provide sufficient data beneficial to patient care to justify routine use in cardiac surgical patients.

DRUGS FOR ANESTHESIA

The goal of this chapter is clearly not to instruct the reader how to administer an anesthetic. Reference textbooks of up to three volumes in length are available for this purpose, including over a half dozen on cardiac anesthesia alone. As in the rest of medical practice, most of the drugs commonly employed have become available in the past two decades, ie, after initiation of the young field of cardiac surgery. Generally the trend has been toward anesthetics that reduce myocardial work and muscle relaxants that release less histamine.

We are including tables that present cardiovascular properties of the major anesthetic drugs, so the diversity of their hemodynamic effects can be appreciated, and the

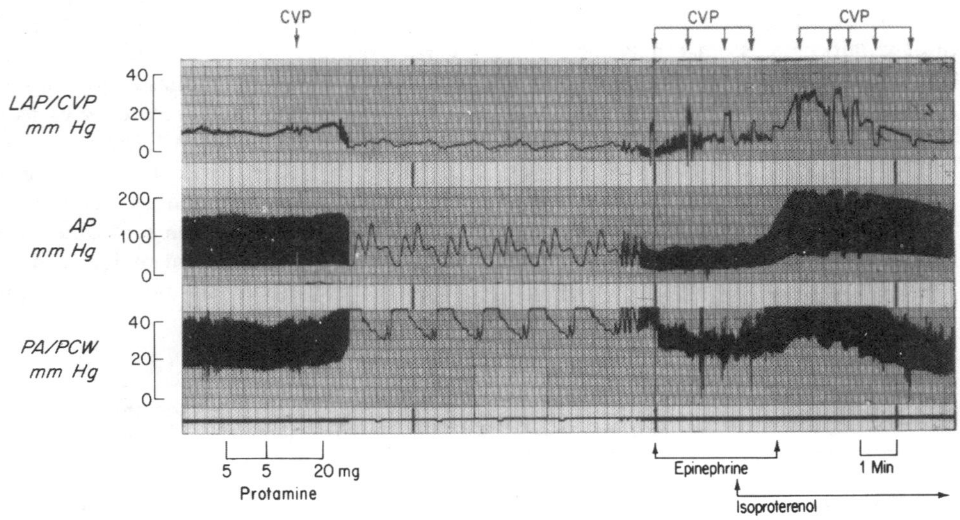

Figure 69.3. Continuous recording permits review and subsequent understanding of events occurring during operation. This strip chart documents acute pulmonary vasoconstriction and right ventricular failure associated with protamine reversal of heparin, as evidenced by pulmonary hypertension, left atrial and systemic hypotension, and right atrial hypertension. Reversal of the episode and normalization of pressure occur subsequent to epinephrine and isoproterenol administration. AP = arterial pressure; CVP = central venous pressure; LAP = left atrial pressure; PA = pulmonary arterial pressure; PCW = pulmonary capillary wedge pressure. (From Lowenstein et al[25] with permission of JB Lippincott.)

Table 69.2. Cardiovascular Effects of Major Drugs Used for Anesthesia and Neuromuscular Blockade

			Vascular					
	Contractility	CBF	Resistance	Capacitance	Heart Rate	Rhythm	Automaticity	Other
Opioids								
Morphine	– or ↑	–	– or ↓	↑↑↑	– –	–	–	Histamine release prominent; slow onset
Fentanyl	–	–	– or ↓	?↑	↓↓	–	–	1,000 times as potent as morphine
Sufentanil	–	–	– or ↓	?↑	↓↓↓	–	–	5 to 10 times as potent as fentanyl; more rapid in onset of action than fentanyl
Volatile Anesthetics								
Halothane	↓	↓	–	↑	–	Junctional Frequent	Sensitized to catecholamines	Decreases size of myocardial infarction
Enflurane	↓	↑	↓	↑	↑	–	Sensitized to catecholamines	
Isoflurane	↓	↑↑↑	↓↓	↑	↑↑	–	Not sensitized	Coronary steal prominent in severe CAD
Induction Drugs								
Thiopental	↓↓	↑	↑Initially	–	↑Initially	–	–	Must be used sparingly in presence of valvular heart disease
Etomidate	↓	–	– or ↓	– or ↑	– or ↑	–	–	Inhibits adrenal steroidogenesis
Ketamine	↓↓ direct	– or ↑	↓ Indirect	↓	↑ Indirect	–	↓↓	Induces release of catecholamines
Diazepam	–	↑	↓ (with fentanyl)	–	–	–	–	Induces anesthesia in large doses 0.3 to 0.5 mg/kg; excellent amnesiac
Muscle Relaxants								
Succinyl choline	–	–	– or ↑	↓	↑	–	↑	Bradycardia in children and with repeated doses/infusion
D-Tubocurarine	– or ↓	–	↓↓↓	↑↑↑	↑	–	–	Vasodilation due principally to histamine release
Metocurine	–	–	↓↓	↑↑	–	–	–	Less histamine release than d-tubocurarine
Pancuronium	– or ↑	–	↑	–	↑↑	Junctional prominent	– or ↑	Some sympathomimetic activity, heart rate acceleration unpredictable
Vecuronium	–	–	–	–	–	–	–	Short duration of action; fewest cardiovascular effects
Gallamine	↑	–	– or ↑	–	↑↑↑	–	↑	Predictable increase in heart rate
Atracurium	–	–	– or ↓	↑	– or ↑	–	–	Histamine release unusual; Hoffman degradation

CAD = coronary artery disease; CBF = coronary blood flow.

portion of this chapter devoted to a presentation of these properties as they pertain to specific situations can be minimized (Table. 69.2). We believe the cardiologist is well advised to leave to the anesthetist the decision of which drug to employ in each clinical setting.

No single pharmacologic approach is suitable in all cardiac surgical patients. Virtually all drugs used in anesthesia affect the cardiovascular system to some degree, particularly at the upper end of the dose range. Furthermore, hemodynamically significant interactions occur when some of these drugs are used in combination, as exemplified by the vasodilation induced by fentanyl when administered following diazepam.[29] Therefore, the anesthetist must judiciously select a combination of agents that will provide the essential elements of anesthesia, namely, analgesia, amnesia, and muscle relaxation plus hemodynamic stability. Thus, drugs are frequently selected according to their hemodynamic "side effects."

Just as aggressive monitoring permits early recognition of adverse hemodynamic trends, appropriately aggressive pharmacologic intervention will favorably alter their course. The agents chosen in specific situations will depend largely on the anesthetist's interpretation of hemodynamic data, the physiologic aspects of the cardiovascular system, and the cardiovascular effects of the available drugs. For instance, succinylcholine may be chosen to provide neuromuscular blockade in a patient with severe mitral stenosis and a poorly controlled ventricular response, specifically to decrease the heart rate. In contrast, a small dose of gallamine may be administered to increase heart rate in a patient with coronary artery disease who has received a high dose of a synthetic narcotic that has caused the blood pressure to decline secondary to severe bradycardia. In the latter instance, gallamine is given for its circulatory effect despite lack of a need for further neuromuscular blockade at that time.

ANESTHESIA IN CORONARY ARTERY DISEASE

The mandate of the anesthetist in coronary artery disease is to prevent episodes of ischemia whenever possible, to detect them promptly, and to relieve them when present. An episode of ischemia before bypass, whether before or after induction of anesthesia, is associated with a tripling of perioperative myocardial infarction.[30] *Res ipsa loquitur.*

Patients with coronary artery disease may be placed in three major categories: (1) patients with normal myocardium but limited coronary blood flow due to stenoses of coronary vessels; (2) patients with permanent myocardial damage or complications of infarction (such as decreased ejection fraction, regional wall motion abnormalities, papillary muscle dysfunction or rupture, ventricular septal defect); and (3) patients with primary valvular disease but coexisting coronary artery disease. Each category requires a somewhat different strategy.

Patients with normal myocardium must be protected from an increase in myocardial oxygen demand. Tachycardia is particularly important, perhaps partly because diastolic filling time is reduced, but hypertension and ventricular distension are also associated with increases in demand. Many different anesthetic regimens have been used successfully, and myocardial depressants have been recommended.[31] No single pharmacologic regimen can reliably prevent such an occurrence. Therefore, combinations of anesthetics are employed, varying administration according to the degree of stimulation and response. For instance, an oxygen-narcotic technique may be supplemented by an inhalation anesthetic when hypertension or tachycardia occurs with sternotomy or aortic cannulation. Importantly, it often appears prudent to block the effector systems rather than to attempt to control the hemodynamics solely by anesthetic drugs. For example, a vasodilator such as nitroprusside or nitroglycerine might be used to normalize blood pressure, or a beta-adrenergic blocker or verapamil to reduce an elevated heart rate, rather than depending on an inhalation anesthetic or further narcotic.

The myocardial oxygen supply may be jeopardized by decreased blood flow secondary to a pressure gradient across a stenosis, despite a systemic pressure compatible with normal blood flow and regional function in myocardium supplied by a normal coronary artery[32] (Figure 69.4). If the region supplied by the narrowed artery is less than 40%, this decrease may occur without global evidence of ischemia and may set the stage for perioperative myocardial infarction.[33] Recognition of this phenomenon has led to great interest in intraoperative measurement of regional function by echocardiography and cardiokymography.[34] The role of coronary spasm as an anesthetic-mediated event is controversial, as is its incidence. However, ischemia with minimal change in global hemodynamics has been repeatedly demonstrated during anesthesia.[35] Profound coronary spasm following cardiopulmonary bypass is a devastating event, often leading to circulatory collapse. Its cause is not well understood, although neurogenic mechanisms, prostaglandins, or leukotrienes may play a role. Patients with preinfarction angina who have been on high (>100 $\mu g/min$) doses of nitroglycerine appear to present a higher risk of coronary vascular spasm. Although intracoronary nitroglycerin in doses of up to 37 mg has been effective in relieving this condition, systemic nitroglycerin has been less so. Calcium channel antagonists offer promise for this purpose. Intravenous preparations are anxiously awaited, although verapamil has been used effectively on occasion.

Patients with impaired myocardial function are relatively intolerant of myocardial depressant anesthetics, and high-dose narcotic anesthetics are often preferred, because narcotics do not impair myocardial performance. The development of potent synthetic narcotics (fentanyl, sufentanil) which release little or no histamine has permitted administration of narcotizing doses one to two orders of magnitude greater than of morphine. Such doses, combined with a muscle relaxant, are sufficient for induction of anesthesia with little circulatory deterioration in most such patients.[36] Preoperative initiation of intraaortic balloon counter-pulsation may allow stabilization and less emergent operation in conditions such as acute papillary muscle rupture and ventricular septal defect. Balancing the need for decreased work and oxygen demand, and sufficiently high blood pressure to prevent further ischemia or infarction is a challenge that demands continuous attention and flexibility.

Coronary disease may be incidental and noncontrib-

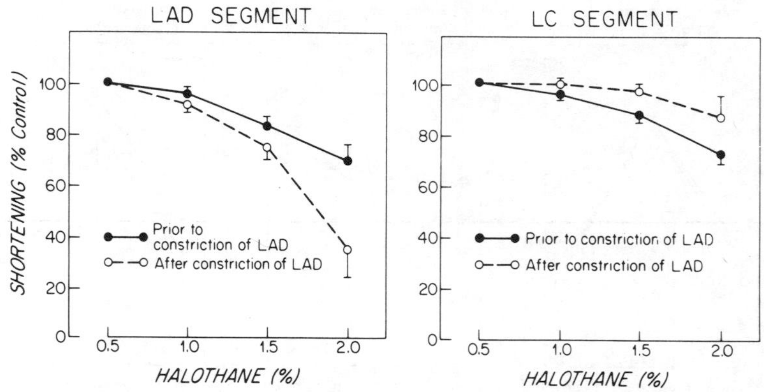

Figure 69.4. Effect of increasing concentrations of halothane anesthesia on myocardial function in a region supplied by a narrowed (LAD) or normal (LC) canine coronary artery. Flow across the stenosis is decreased as concentration is increased and blood pressure declines. Regional function is preserved by coronary autoregulation in the normal area. Regional function is more sensitive than other monitors for detection of ischemia. (From Lowenstein et al,[32] with permission of JB Lippincott.)

utory in the presence of valvular heart disease, or may be the primary disease. For example, the patient with exercise-induced angina and a 30 mm Hg aortic valve gradient stands a good chance of having primarily coronary artery disease. There is no substitute for a careful examination of the patient, his catheterization data, and coronary angiography when deciding upon management strategies. Communication between surgeon, cardiologist, and anesthetist becomes of utmost importance in such cases.

SPECIFIC DRUG STRATEGIES IN CORONARY ARTERY DISEASE

Calculations have been performed to indicate that a low oxygen demand, low arterial pressure anesthetic regimen is less likely to lead to ischemia in an area supplied by a coronary stenosis than is a high pressure, high demand anesthetic. Such calculations are based on many assumptions. In any individual patient, in whom the state of the coronary circulation is never precisely known (despite coronary angiography), monitoring of ischemia is still the most crucial maneuver.[37]

A recent double-blind study in patients with stable angina and normal ventricular function indicated that when muscle relaxation for intubation is provided by pancuronium, it is associated with higher heart rates, marginally higher blood pressure, and significantly more ischemia than when metocurine alone or a combination of smaller doses of pancuronium and metocurine are employed.[38] This clearly demonstrates that each aspect of management must be considered as a potential cause of ischemia.

Isoflurane, a volatile anesthetic that causes marked vasodilation when used to control hypertension associated with surgical stimulation, produces normalization of CI, PCWP, and SVR. The PCWP and SVR remain elevated, and stroke volume and CI decrease when halothane is used for this purpose[39] (Figure 69.5). On the other hand, isoflurane anesthesia has been documented to impair coronary autoregulation and to cause a coronary steal in patients with severe coronary artery disease.[40,40a,41] This occurs despite returning blood pressure and left ventricular filling pressure to control and maintaining heart rate constant at control levels. Ischemic episodes were not observed in similar studies when a halothane anesthetic was employed.[42] Preliminary experiments in dogs with a narrowed right coronary artery and RV dysfunction have shown that substitution of halothane for isoflurane, keeping blood pressure constant, results in decreased *left* coronary blood flow and improved RV function, probably from relieving the coronary steal (H. Priebe, personal communication, 1985).

Nitrous oxide, long considered innocuous and previously even administered to provide analgesia for patients with myocardial infarction, has been shown to cause postsystolic shortening in an area of myocardium supplied by a narrowed coronary artery, despite unchanged hemodynamics and coronary blood flow, in dogs anesthetized with fentanyl or sufentanil.[43] This raises the possibility of ischemia due to intramyocardial redistribution of blood flow, but metabolic data are not yet available to support this conclusion.

ANESTHESIA FOR PATIENTS WITH VALVULAR HEART DISEASE

The pathophysiology of valvular heart disease has been discussed fully elsewhere in this book (see chapters 30–32). The basic clinical features characterizing various stages of valvular lesions are summarized in Table 69.3. The information in this section is limited to factors affecting the anesthetic management of these patients. Specific management goals are based on the pathophysiology of the patient's specific cardiac lesion or lesions. A knowledge of the natural history of those lesions and the physiologic adaptations that accompany their progression often enables the anesthetist to predict the patient's response to administration of specific anesthetic agents and to anticipate the need for pharmacologic cardiovascular support. Frequently, a patient will present with a combination of valvular lesions. The lesion that presents the

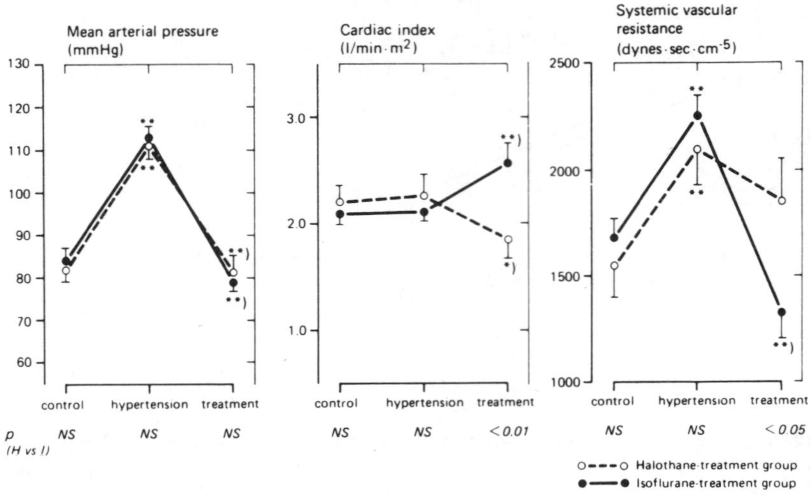

Figure 69.5. Comparison of halothane and isoflurane in the treatment of intraoperative hypertension. Both anesthetics reduce blood pressure and heart rate effectively. However, halothane is associated with a decline in cardiac output and unaltered systemic vascular resistance and left ventricular filling pressure, whereas isoflurane is associated with a decreased systemic vascular resistance and pulmonary capillary wedge pressure and elevated cardiac output. Response in individual patients is best gauged by hemodynamic measurement. (From Hess et al,[39] with permission of Elsevier.)

most important impediment to the pumping function of the heart should be identified, if possible. Failure to appropriately deal with the principal lesion may lead to rapid decompensation or cardiovascular collapse.

As previously outlined,[44] the anesthesiologist's "sphere of influence" is limited to the cardiovascular variables over which some measure of control can be exerted. Advances in recent years have enlarged this "sphere of influence." These include the availability of new muscle relaxants and anesthetic agents with fewer, or more predictable, cardiovascular side effects and the ability to easily and reliably pace either the atria or ventricles, or both, with electrodes on a pulmonary artery catheter inserted prior to induction.[45]

HEMODYNAMIC CONSIDERATIONS IN VALVULAR DISEASE

In the early stages of most chronic valvular abnormalities, ventricular function is well preserved. Regurgitant lesions are characterized by volume overload of the ventricle leading to dilatation. Acute insufficiency of either the mitral or aortic valve is poorly tolerated, but chronic regurgitation stimulates the serial growth of new myofibrils,[46] so that ventricular function and systemic

Table 69.3. Essential Features of Valvular Heart Disease

	Aortic Valve		Mitral Valve	
	Stenosis	Regurgitation	Stenosis	Regurgitation
Principal hemodynamic features	↑ impedance to LV ejection ↑ LV systolic pressure LV pressure overload	Regurgitation into left ventricle ↑ LV diastolic pressure LV volume overload	↑ impedance to LV filling ↑ LA pressure with ↓LV volume	Regurgitation into left atrium ↑ LA pressure with ↑ LV volume
Pathologic change	LV hypertrophy and ↓ compliance	LV dilation and ↑ compliance	LA distension with pulmonary vascular congestion	LA and LV dilation and ↑ compliance
Management goals	Maintain coronary perfusion pressure Prevent bradycardia or tachycardia	Minimize LV afterload Prevent bradycardia	Maintain LV filling time Prevent tachycardia	Minimize LV afterload Prevent bradycardia
Support measures	(1) Vasopressors (2) Inotropes (3) Avoid hypovolemia	(1) Vasodilators (2) Inotropes	(1) Avoid hypovolemia (2) Inotropes	(1) Vasodilators (2) Inotropes (3) IABP (acute MR)

IABP = intraaortic ballon pumping; LA = left atrial; LV = left ventricular; MR = mitral regurgitation.

cardiac output are maintained despite increased end-diastolic volume. This condition may persist for years before signs of ventricular dysfunction begin to appear. Once dysfunction is apparent, however, its progression is rapid and largely irreversible. Even with replacement of the affected valve or valves, ventricular function is unlikely to return to normal, particularly after long-standing periods of elevated end-diastolic pressure that may be accompanied by fibrosis and loss of ventricular compliance.[47] In the presence of stenotic lesions, ventricular function may also be maintained for long periods before symptoms appear. With aortic stenosis, ventricular hypertrophy due to parallel growth of new sarcomeres in response to increased pressure work leads to a thickened, noncompliant ventricle.[46] The onset of symptoms, including angina, heart failure, and syncope, is an ominous sign heralding a rapidly progressive functional deterioration or sudden death. Only in mitral stenosis is the left ventricle relatively spared from the pathological effects of volume or pressure overload, but even then, the ventricle is abnormal late in the course of the disease.[48]

Heart rate and rhythm are very important variables in perioperative management of patients with valvular heart disease. Tachycardia is poorly tolerated in patients with mitral stenosis because of limited time for left-ventricular filling. Bradycardia is particularly detrimental in patients with aortic insufficiency because it increases regurgitation, which leads to ventricular distension and reduced forward cardiac output. In patients with aortic stenosis, stroke volume is effectively limited and myocardial perfusion is compromised by ventricular hypertrophy and reduced coronary perfusion pressure. Consequently, either tachycardia or bradycardia may cause decompensation. There is a high incidence of dysrhythmias in patients with valvular lesions, including atrial fibrillation and conduction disturbances accompanying high intracavitary volumes and pressures and coexisting coronary artery disease. Acute loss of the atrial contribution during anesthesia often produces rapidly progressive decompensation. In the management of these patients our goal is to control rate and rhythm in such a way as to optimize cardiac output and provide adequate myocardial nutrition.

Aggressive control of systemic and pulmonary vascular resistances is critical in the perioperative management of patients with valvular lesions. Appropriate use of vasodilators can dramatically improve cardiac output in patients with regurgitant lesions.[49] Patients with aortic stenosis require a high myocardial perfusion pressure and usually benefit from pharmacological support of their systemic vascular resistance. Finally, the pulmonary vascular resistance may be markedly elevated and reactive in patients with mitral disease or end-stage aortic disease. Failure to properly control pulmonary vascular resistance can lead to ineffective transfer of blood through the pulmonary vasculature, right ventricular volume overload and failure, functional tricuspid insufficiency, and decreased cardiac output and hypotension due to left ventricular hypovolemia. The right ventricular overload may further compromise left ventricular filling by leftward shift of the septum and decreased left ventricular compliance. In this instance, the left atrial pressure may not adequately reflect the volume status of the left ventricle.

SPECIFIC DRUG STRATEGIES

In the anesthetic management of these patients, we take advantage of the direct pharmacologic and indirect, reflex-mediated effects of the drugs used for anesthesia and neuromuscular blockade; these have been summarized in Table 69.2. Frequently, we resort to electrical pacing through electrodes in a pulmonary artery catheter or, after sternotomy, applied directly to the heart. In general, patients with cardiac cachexia are extremely sensitive to depressant medications of all types. Consequently, anesthetic agents that depress the myocardium should generally be avoided in patients with advanced valvular disease. We prefer high-dose narcotic anesthetic techniques for these patients, either morphine (1 to 3 mg/kg) or the synthetic opioids, fentanyl (50 to 100 mg/kg) or sufentanil (8 to 20 μg/kg).

Fentanyl and sufentanil, which are sympatholytic and vagotonic, generally slow the heart, sometimes to a profound bradycardia, particularly in the presence of beta receptor blockade. These effects can be partially or completely reversed by the sympathomimetic, chronotropic effects of the neuromuscular blocking agents pancuronium or gallamine. We frequently administer gallamine in doses of 10 to 20 mg instead of atropine because the increase in heart rate is more predictable and less dramatic. Large doses of either relaxant occasionally induce junctional rhythm. The combination of pancuronium with halothane is particularly likely to lead to junctional rhythm.[50] Atrial pacing is almost invariably successful in converting this to a sinus mechanism. In the case of bradycardia refractory to these drugs, atropine, or intravenous infusions of small doses of beta-adrenergic agonists (isoproterenol, dopamine, and epinephrine) may be necessary if pacing is not possible.

Metocurine, curare, and to a lesser extent atracurium, may indirectly or reflexly increase heart rate due to histamine and epinephrine liberation and systemic vasodilation, but such changes are not always predictable. Sodium nitroprusside and other direct acting vasodilators are more likely to increase heart rate through this mechanism. In contrast to the neuromuscular blocking drugs just mentioned, vecuronium is essentially free of cardiovascular side effects[51] and may be particularly useful in critically ill patients who are judged to have little or no tolerance for changes in heart rate or blood pressure.

Of the commonly used inhalational anesthetics, isoflurane, enflurane and, to a lesser extent, nitrous oxide are more prone to increase heart rate than is halothane, probably largely because of their vasodilating (enflurane and isoflurane) or sympathomimetic (nitrous oxide) effects. Because of their myocardial depressant effects, we seldom rely on them as primary anesthetics for critically ill patients with valvular heart disease, but use them to supplement a narcotic-based anesthetic technique.

Both fentanyl and sufentanil usually provide hemodynamic stability. However, patients with end-stage valvular lesions frequently depend on a high level of sympathetic tone for hemodynamic compensation. The rapid administration of these drugs can reduce sympathetic tone by a central mechanism so quickly as to produce hypotension. Morphine has a less rapid onset of action because it crosses the blood brain barrier more slowly and it may be better tolerated. Morphine causes vasodilation by histamine release when delivered rapidly. The latter effect, which may be beneficial in patients with regurgitant lesions, can be blocked effectively by pretreatment with histamine-receptor (H_1 and H_2) blocking drugs.[52]

The ventricular rate response to the drugs described earlier is not always predictable in patients with atrial fibrillation. Patients with severe mitral stenosis suffer most commonly from increases in the ventricular response rate, and patients with severe aortic insufficiency are least likely to tolerate bradycardia. In the former case, we generally continue to administer digitalis until surgery if the ventricular response rate is greater than 80 beats per minute and, if necessary, we may judiciously use propranolol or verapamil to control the rate perioperatively. In the latter patients, particularly when conduction disturbances accompany severe aortic insufficiency, placement of a pulmonary artery catheter with pacing electrodes preoperatively has been useful (Figure 69.6). Electrical pacing of the heart during the institution of cardiopulmonary bypass allows a longer period of ejection before ventricular fibrillation and aortic cross-clamping, which in turn allows more effective cooling of the myocardium before arrest and administration of the cardioplegic solution.

The vasodilating properties of the neuromuscular blocking agents curare, metocurine, and, to a small extent, atracurium argue against their use in patients with aortic stenosis. Phenothiazines and butyrophenones, notably droperidol and Thorazine®, also produce vasodilation, partially through alpha receptor blockade, and must also be used carefully. When direct systemic arterial vasodilation is desired, sodium nitroprusside provides potent, short-lived effects that are ideally suited to perioperative management of these patients.[53] For hypotension in the presence of aortic stenosis, we prefer norepinephrine to phenylephrine because of its inotropic action, unless lowered systemic vascular resistance is documented.

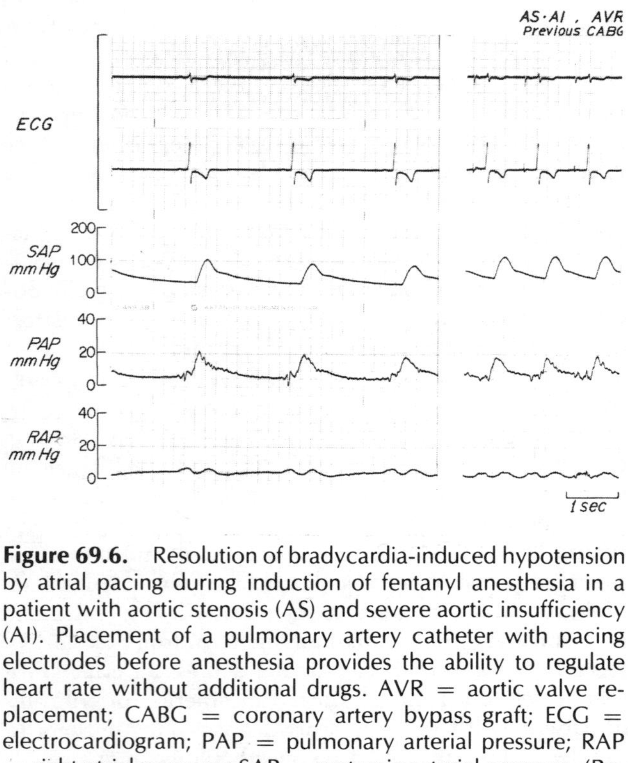

Figure 69.6. Resolution of bradycardia-induced hypotension by atrial pacing during induction of fentanyl anesthesia in a patient with aortic stenosis (AS) and severe aortic insufficiency (AI). Placement of a pulmonary artery catheter with pacing electrodes before anesthesia provides the ability to regulate heart rate without additional drugs. AVR = aortic valve replacement; CABG = coronary artery bypass graft; ECG = electrocardiogram; PAP = pulmonary arterial pressure; RAP = right atrial pressure; SAP = systemic arterial pressure. (Reproduced by courtesy of Dr Demetrios Lappas.)

The pulmonary vasculature is not as well understood as the systemic vasculature, but the effects of a given drug will generally be qualitatively the same on both. However, this is less than ideal, because in many instances specific and selective dilation of the pulmonary circuit is desired. Of the drugs presently available, nitroglycerin and isoproterenol probably come closest to this ideal, but both also dilate the systemic vasculature in a dose-dependent fashion in the absence of fixed obstructive disease. Recently, D'Ambra et al[54] reported that patients with refractory right heart failure and pulmonary vasoconstriction and hypertension after mitral valve replacement benefit from infusion of prostaglandin E_1 into the pulmonary circulation, while systemic vascular resistance is maintained by infusion of norepinephrine into the left atrium (Figure 69.7). The strategy of infusing vasoconstrictors in the left-sided circulation to minimize pulmonary vascular effects is one we have employed frequently with apparent benefit. The development of new agents for specific control of pulmonary vascular resistance without affecting systemic vascular tone remains a challenging goal for biochemical pharmacologists.

Most valvular heart diseases are chronic and are accompanied by profound compensatory changes in the heart and blood vessels. Acute lesions due to papillary muscle rupture, chordal disruption, or bacterial endocarditis are poorly tolerated. The right ventricle is suddenly faced with the necessity of overcoming retrogradely transmitted left ventricular pressure. If prompt intervention, pharmacologic, mechanical, or surgical, is not forthcoming, right ventricular distension may limit survival despite insertion of a competent mitral or aortic valve and a functioning left ventricle.

Just as a normal circulation tolerates poorly an acute valvular lesion, a well-compensated abnormal circulation may not tolerate valve replacement. Even though prosthetic valves are functioning normally, patients often require intense support during the immediate postoperative period, sometimes for several days. Ventricular function may be severely impaired. For instance, the massively dilated left ventricle in a patient with profound mitral regurgitation may be unable to accommodate the dramatic increase in afterload following corrective surgery. A period of afterload reduction through systemic vasodilation allows the ventricle to compensate to this. The use of sodium nitroprusside for this purpose has been particularly gratifying and is largely responsible for the decrease in surgical mortality from mitral insufficiency.

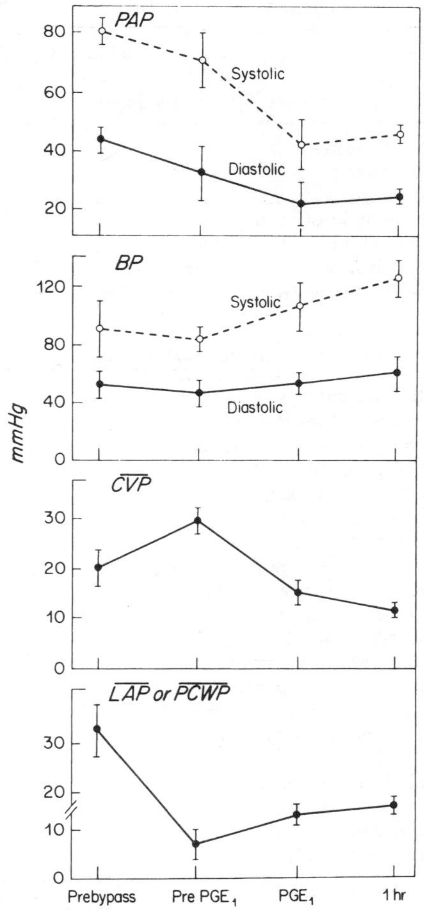

Figure 69.7. Effect of prostaglandin E_1 infusion in the treatment of right heart failure in five patients after mitral valve replacement. PGE_1 dilates the pulmonary vascular bed, reduces impedance to right ventricular ejection, and permits transfer of blood to the left side of the heart. See text for details. BP = blood pressure; $\overline{CVP}$ = mean central venous pressure; $\overline{LAP}$ = mean left atrial pressure; PAP = pulmonary artery pressure; $\overline{PCWP}$ = mean pulmonary capillary wedge pressure. (From D'Ambra et al,[54] with permission of CV Mosby Company.)

ANESTHESIA FOR CARDIAC SURGERY IN INFANTS AND CHILDREN

Congenital heart disease has been discussed in detail elsewhere in this textbook (chapters 26 and 27). For this discussion, it is sufficient to note that congenital heart defects are generally classified as either cyanotic or noncyanotic according to the degree of oxygen saturation of the systemic arterial blood (see Table 69.4). Obviously, an infant with a "noncyanotic" lesion, such as a ventricular septal defect, can present with systemic desaturation in the presence of severe congestive failure or intrinsic pulmonary vascular disease, but in most cases hypoxemia will improve with the administration of oxygen. Any infant with an adequate cardiac output who fails to show a significant improvement in arterial oxygenation after effective administration of oxygen, or who remains cyanotic for more than a few hours after birth should be considered to have a cyanotic congenital heart lesion until proven otherwise and therefore needs a full evaluation to define his/her cardiovascular anatomy.

Infants with congenital heart disease are often critically ill when presenting for anesthesia and surgery, either with severe congestive heart failure or with hypoxemia and acidosis, despite optimal medical management. Providing perioperative life support for these infants, in addition to providing satisfactory analgesia and amnesia during the surgical procedure, requires specific knowledge of the normal and pathologic physiology of the neonatal cardiorespiratory system as well as an understanding of the special metabolic requirements and anatomic features of this age group.

HEMODYNAMIC CONSIDERATIONS IN CONGENITAL HEART DISEASE

Congenital cardiac lesions characterized by severe hypoxemia that is unresponsive to oxygen administration may be divided into three groups according to the magnitude of pulmonary blood flow and the nature of the anomalous connections between the pulmonary and systemic circulations. Frequently, congenital heart defects will be complex, including features of both "cyanotic" and "noncyanotic" lesions, and the condition of the affected infants may be extremely unstable. Although certain lesions are fixed anatomically, the cardiovascular system in infants is remarkably reactive to a number of variables, including sympathetic tone, humoral mediators, metabolic status, and patterns of ventilation. In patients with abnormal cardiovascular communications, the relative pressures within the chambers of the heart and the relative resistance to flow in the pulmonic and systemic circuits determine the direction and amount of blood flow. This fact governs the basic principles underlying the perioperative management of these patients.

PHYSIOLOGIC AND METABOLIC CONSIDERATIONS IN INFANTS

The cardiorespiratory physiology of the neonate differs markedly from that of the adult. Because of its small size and large surface area, an infant rapidly loses heat by radiation and convection, resulting in dramatic increases in oxygen consumption as metabolic activity increases during thermogenesis.[55] Accompanying peripheral vasoconstriction further increases the workload on the already strained heart and reduces the delivery of oxygen to the tissues. A resulting metabolic acidosis may rapidly lead to cardiovascular collapse. Fever can be equally detrimental in infants unable to deliver adequate amounts of oxygen to the tissues. The need for maintaining a neutral thermal environment and euthermia cannot be overstated.

Adequate delivery of oxygen to the tissues depends on cardiac output more in infants than in adults because of the higher resting oxygen requirements and the decreased ability of fetal red blood cells to unload oxygen at the tissue level.[56] In infants, the arteriovenous difference of oxygen content may be only one third that of adults, so that three times more relative blood flow may be required to ensure adequate oxygen delivery. This problem is obviously magnified in patients with hypoxemia due to cy-

Table 69.4. Classification of Congenital Heart Disease

Cyanotic Lesions
Right-to-Left Shunting

Increased Pulmonary Flow	Decreased Pulmonary Flow
Transposition of great arteries (TGA)	Tetralogy of Fallot
Double-outlet right ventricle (DORV)	Pulmonary atresia
Common ventricle	Tricuspid atresia
Single ventricle	Ebstein's anomaly of tricuspid valve
Truncus arteriosus	Single common or double outlet right ventricle with pulmonary stenosis
Total anomalous pulmonary venous return (TAPVR)	Truncus arteriosus with pulmonary stenosis

Noncyanotic Lesions

Left-to-Right Shunting	Valvular and Vascular Lesions
Atrial septal defect	Left ventricular outflow tract anomalies
Ventricular septal defect	Hypoplastic left heart syndrome
Patent ductus arteriosus	Idiopathic hypertrophic subaortic stenosis (IHSS)
Partial anomalous pulmonary venous return	Valvular aortic stenosis
Endocardial cushion defect	Supravalvular aortic stenosis
Aortopulmonary window	Interrupted aortic arch
	Coarctation of aorta
	Right ventricular outflow tract anomalies
	Hypoplastic right heart syndrome
	Infundibular hypertrophic stenosis
	Valvular pulmonic stenosis
	Peripheral pulmonary artery stenosis
	Pulmonary artery hypoplasia
	Absent pulmonic valve syndrome
	Mitral valve and left atrial anomalies
	Cleft mitral valve
	Congenital mitral stenosis
	Mitral valve prolapse
	Cor triatriatum
	Parachute mitral valve

anotic congenital heart lesions. To achieve this high level of flow, the infant heart must beat more frequently, because it has a limited ability to increase stroke volume in response to increased end-diastolic volume. An adequate hematocrit is also essential for maintaining oxygen delivery to the tissues. The development of metabolic acidosis due to either inadequate cardiac output or hypoxemia is a grave sign that signals the need for urgent therapy, usually surgical intervention.

SPECIFIC ANESTHETIC CONSIDERATIONS

Many approaches to management of the pediatric patient undergoing correction of a congenital heart defect appear to yield equally satisfactory results, provided the general hemodynamic and physiologic considerations discussed herein are kept in mind. Selection of specific drugs is therefore best left to the judgment and experience of the individual anesthetist. However, we will address some specific management considerations directly.

Surgical intervention in neonates and infants with congenital heart disease is often urgent, as deterioration often continues despite optimal medical management. Delaying an operation because a child is "too sick" may only worsen the situation. Only in infants for whom specific lifesaving nonsurgical treatment is available can surgery safely be delayed. For instance, prostaglandin E_1 may maintain ductal patency in infants with lesions where the ductus arteriosus provides the only pathway for pulmonary or systemic blood flow.[57] In these cases, the beneficial effects of prostaglandin infusion may justify a period of stabilization before surgery.

Inadequacy of pulmonary blood flow is obviously incompatible with life. When a fixed anatomic limitation to pulmonary blood flow is present, all blood leaving the lungs is virtually fully saturated, so increasing the inspired concentration of oxygen will not increase systemic oxygenation importantly. Furthermore, in ductus-dependent lesions, saturated pulmonary blood flow may promote closure of the ductus arteriosus and cause further deterioration. Conversely, if high pulmonary vascular resistance alone is responsible for decreased pulmonary flow, as in persistent fetal circulation, a decline in resistance in response to higher inspired oxygen tensions with relief of hypoxic vasoconstriction, improved ventilation, and correction of systemic acidosis may effect dramatic improvement.

A remarkable difference between infants under 6 months of age and older patients is the sensitivity of the pulmonary vasculature to various stimuli that mediate vasoconstriction.[58] Pulmonary vascular resistance remains relatively high for several weeks after birth, gradually diminishing to adult levels by about 3 months of age in normal infants. However, the reactivity of the vessels remains high, particularly in infants with congenital heart defects. Because of the small caliber of the neonatal pulmonary vessels, small changes in diameter can cause large changes in resistance. This becomes very important during anesthetic management of these patients. Even infants with noncyanotic lesions characterized by large systemic-to-pulmonary shunts can experience shunt reversal in the presence of systemic vasodilation or pulmonary vasoconstriction, or both.

Although pulmonary vascular resistance is determined in part by the intrinsic tone of the pulmonary vessels, it is also importantly influenced by lung volume.[59] Resistance is lowest at functional residual capacity. Above this level, compression of the vessels increases the impedance to pulmonary blood flow. The increasing resistance at lower lung volumes is probably related to compression of vessels in areas of atelectasis and hypoxic pulmonary vasoconstriction.[60] As already mentioned, the pulmonary vasculature of neonates is particularly sensitive to hypercarbia or acidosis as well.

On the basis of these considerations, hyperventilation at relatively low lung volumes can be predicted to provide optimal conditions for maintaining pulmonary blood flow in such critically ill infants. In fact, rapid ventilatory rates (120 per minute) with short inspiratory times are optimal. The expiratory time must be sufficient to permit deflation of the lungs and to prevent elevated lung volumes and pulmonary vascular resistance. Ventilation by hand with a high gas flow T-piece system *with minimal dead space* is most effective. Mechanical ventilation, even when efforts are made to duplicate the pattern of ventilation, often leads to elevated pulmonary vascular resistance.

This pattern of ventilation also effectively assists the pumping function of the heart during periods of inadequacy, as during separation from cardiopulmonary bypass or resuscitation. The role of phasic increases in intrathoracic pressure in augmentation of cardiac output, as applied in cardiopulmonary resuscitation,[61] can easily be demonstrated in a fully monitored infant by observing the improvement in arterial pressure when positive pressure ventilation is provided as just described at a rate approximating that of the infant's heart. Because of the sensitivity of the infant's cardiovascular system to the pattern of ventilation, we avoid mechanical ventilation of infants during critical periods, including transfer from the operating room to the intensive care unit. We recommend ventilation by hand until the child's condition is fully monitored and stabilized.

The foremost goal in the anesthetic management of patients with congenital heart disease is maintenance of adequate cardiac output. This goal is probably best achieved by maintaining heart rate, limiting direct depression of the myocardium by either metabolites or drugs, preventing sympathetic reflexes that can produce intense vasoconstriction, and adjusting intravascular volume to provide optimal filling pressures without either distending the heart or producing ventricular hypovolemia.

Optimal systemic blood pressure in neonates with congenital heart disease is not well established. Given evidence of adequate systemic perfusion, such as appropriate urine output and absence of metabolic acidosis, we do not aggressively support systemic arterial pressure because of the potentially adverse effects of vasoconstrictive drugs on the pulmonary circulation. Continuous measurement of systemic arterial oxygen saturation by pulse oximetry[62] appears to be a sensitive, reliable monitor of overall cardiopulmonary integrity in infants, and we have found such measurements to be useful during the entire perioperative period.

It is important that patients are brought to the operating room adequately sedated to avoid struggling and to permit smooth induction of anesthesia. At our institution, infants less than 3 months of age and those critically ill are not routinely premedicated. For elective procedures, most infants receive a single intramuscular injection containing chlorpromazine (0.6 mg/kg), promethazine (1.0 mg/kg), meperidine (3 mg/kg), and atropine (0.02 mg/kg) approximately one hour before surgery. Even in infants with significant right-to-left shunts in whom avoidance of systemic vasodilation, as may occur with the administration of phenothiazines, is desired, this combination has usually been well tolerated. The occasional infant who is inadequately premedicated with this drug combination may be given a supplemental dose of ketamine (1 to 4 mg/kg intramuscularly) or methohexital (15 to 20 mg/kg rectally) in the preinduction area with the parents present to calm and soothe the child. Fears that ketamine might increase pulmonary vascular resistance and reduce pulmonary blood flow in cyanotic patients or compromise right ventricular function in patients with large volume overload appear to be unjustified. Ketamine can be used safely in these patients, provided hypoventilation is avoided[63] (Figure 69.8). Once adequately sedated, a quiet,

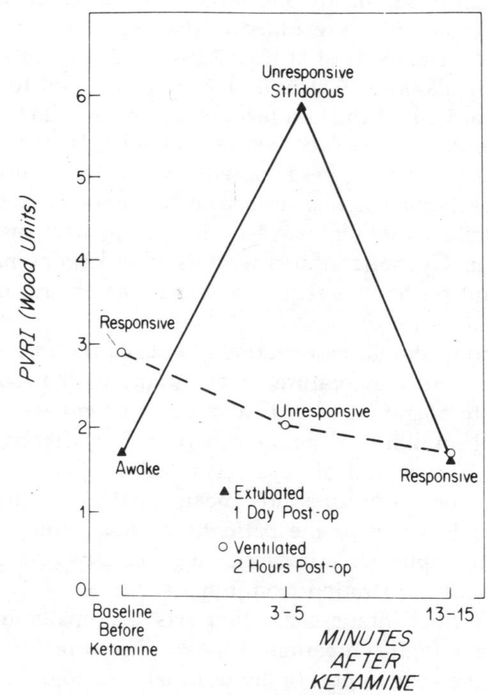

Figure 69.8. Response of pulmonary vasculature to ketamine in one child on two occasions. When the trachea was intubated, pulmonary vascular resistance (PVR) declined. When not intubated, the patient experienced partial upper airway obstruction and PVR became substantially elevated. Thus, the pulmonary vasoconstriction reported in association with ketamine is not a pharmacologic effect. PVRI = pulmonary vascular resistance index. (From Hickey et al,[63] with permission of JB Lippincott.)

cooperative patient can safely be taken from the parents without a struggle. In most infants, invasive monitoring is instituted and intravenous access is established to permit administration of fluids and additional drugs only after induction of anesthesia.

Early control of the airway is important, with endotracheal intubation a high priority. Our preferred anesthetic technique includes halothane by mask until an intravenous line is available, followed by the administration of pancuronium (0.1 to 0.15 μg/kg) for muscle relaxation and fentanyl (50 to 100 mg/kg), a potent synthetic narcotic that does not release histamine, for anesthesia. We administer pancuronium, a neuromuscular blocking agent with vagolytic effects, before fentanyl to avoid or minimize the bradycardia associated with administration of this narcotic. Halothane or ketamine is used to supplement the anesthetic as required. This technique accomplishes most of the goals previously set forth in that heart rate and cardiac output are preserved and adverse reflexes are blocked. Infants tolerate manipulation of the great vessels poorly and may require pharmacologic support during and after cannulation until cardiopulmonary bypass is begun. Infusion of dopamine (5 μg/kg per minute) or isoproterenol (0.1 μg/kg per minute) is usually effective.

After surgical repair, before separation from cardiopulmonary bypass, the patient's hematocrit and metabolic status, including the level of ionized calcium and acid-base balance, should be optimized. Packed red cells and sodium bicarbonate are added to the bypass reservoir to achieve a hematocrit of at least 28% to 30% and a slight metabolic alkalosis. Calcium gluconate is added to raise the serum ionized calcium level to 1.2 to 1.3 mEq/L; this level should be measured before separation from cardiopulmonary bypass. These maneuvers usually ensure adequate systemic vascular resistance and myocardial function, while avoiding increases in pulmonary vascular resistance. Cyanotic infants who have undergone palliative shunt procedures require a higher hematocrit, in the 45% to 55% range.

The body should be rewarmed to normothermia. Usually, the core temperature of an infant with nasopharyngeal temperature of 38°C and a rectal temperature of 35°C will equilibrate to a normothermic state after bypass. An adequate period of reperfusion of the heart with a *satisfactory* perfusion pressure (mean arterial pressure approximately equal to the patient's normal value) is essential to replenish myocardial high-energy phosphate stores before separation from bypass.

The normal infant heart contracts maximally in the presence of high sympathetic tone.[56] Therefore, inotropic drugs have little impact on myocardial function. Any increases in cardiac output depend on an increasing heart rate. In contrast, inotropic support appears to improve performance in the depressed heart of an infant after cardiac surgery. Inotropic and chronotropic support with dopamine or isoproterenol often permits discontinuation of bypass at lower filling pressures,[64] thereby avoiding distension of the heart. These drugs alone do not always elicit a response, perhaps because coupling of the beta receptors and their effector system is altered. Calcium gluconate or phosphodiesterase inhibitors (amrinone and theophylline), or both, have proven to be useful adjuncts when beta-adrenergic agonists alone are not sufficient. It is our clinical impression that calcium is the most effective agent for short-term inotropic support in infants. Failure to respond to calcium administration is a very grave sign.

Once bypass is discontinued, we administer warmed, *fresh* whole blood exclusively for maintenance of intravascular volume, together with sufficient calcium gluconate to overcome chelation by a citrate anticoagulant. This requires approximately 100 mg of calcium gluconate for every 100 ml of whole blood administered. Frequent determinations of the serum ionized calcium level are indicated, because total serum calcium levels do not reflect the functionally significant pool of calcium ions in the presence of large amounts of citrate.[65] Reversal of heparinization is accomplished by the administration of protamine, 4 to 6 mg/kg, usually over five to ten minutes. Adverse hemodynamic consequences appear rare in children. Our goal is to establish normal coagulation and metabolic balance as quickly as possible in the postbypass period to minimize the need for transfusion of large amounts of bank blood with its attendant problems.[66]

The postoperative period after a palliative or corrective procedure in a child with congenital heart disease is crucial for survival. Despite normal postoperative anatomy, the cardiovascular system remains labile and has little compensatory reserve. Usually no attempt is made to reverse the effects of narcotics, sedatives, and muscle relaxants and awaken these patients from anesthesia. Maintaining profound sedation, analgesia, and pharmacologic neuromuscular paralysis for several hours, if not days, is beneficial. It allows the heart a period of optimal oxygenation and circulation and minimal work requirement to more fully recover from the adverse effects of cardioplegia and surgical trauma, and to allow the entire cardiovascular system to accommodate to the new hemodynamic state. The sickest of these patients may require weeks or even months of intensive care before they are able to survive without intensive cardiopulmonary support.

MANAGEMENT OF PATIENTS AFTER CARDIOPULMONARY BYPASS

Separation from cardiopulmonary bypass and the early postbypass period are critical times when communication among anesthesiologist, surgeon, and perfusionist is absolutely essential. All systems should be checked before attempting to terminate bypass, including transducers, pacers, ventilator, and the like. The anesthetist should position himself or herself in an area where he or she can see the heart, the monitors, the anesthetic machine, and the cardiopulmonary bypass machine to have maximum possible information on which to make informed decisions.

Strategies for terminating bypass vary greatly. In general, they involve an iterative process whereby myocardial function is assessed. For instance, ventricular function may be assessed during bypass by providing deep inspiration. Blood is thereby transferred from the pulmonary veins to the left heart, allowing estimation of the ability of the left ventricle to generate pressure and eject blood into the aorta. If excessively high (greater than 15 mm Hg) filling pressures are required for ejection, the need for inotropic support can be anticipated. Appropriate interventions are then made on a moment-to-moment basis, while the level of extracorporeal perfusion is progressively reduced.

Myocardial function during separation from bypass can best be assessed by observing the heart and monitoring right and left ventricular filling pressures. Direct comparison of these pressures permits rapid diagnosis of right or left ventricular dysfunction.[67] Concomitant measurements of systemic and pulmonary artery pressures and cardiac output permit calculations of vascular resistances on which to base the choice of pharmacologic support. The proper atrial–ventricular contraction sequence is extremely useful in the depressed, impaired, or incompliant heart. We attempt to convert to sinus rhythm whenever possible and are not hesitant to initiate atrioventricular (AV) sequential pacing for a prolonged AV interval as well as for complete heart block.[68]

Within this general framework, a few points deserve emphasis. First, recovery of myocardial function after cardioplegia or nonpulsatile perfusion requires adequate reperfusion. This necessitates sufficient perfusion pressure to open myocardial capillary beds and time for replenishment of high-energy phosphates. Thickened hypertrophic ventricles and those with severe distal coronary artery disease require especially high pressure, both during reperfusion and immediately after bypass, to sustain myocardial perfusion. It is most impressive to observe a distended, dusky, poorly contracting ventricle abruptly begin to contract vigorously with only an increase in perfusion pressure, despite an increase in the work demand of the myocardium.

Patients may be profoundly vasodilated because of systemic rewarming, mediator liberation, or other unknown factors. Furthermore, hyperthermia per se is a severe myocardial depressant.[69] Therefore, it is important to ensure that blood temperature not exceed 38°C and that systemic vascular resistance is optimized before discontinuation of bypass.

In contrast, poorly functioning, noncompliant ventricles, like those found in patients with end-stage aortic regurgitation, may fail if afterload is excessive. In this instance, inotropic rather than vasopressor support is indicated in the immediate postbypass period, although the need for adequate reperfusion before separation from bypass is no less important.

In some patients, particularly those with severe pulmonary hypertension, right ventricular failure or inability to transfer blood across the pulmonary vasculature may prevent successful termination of cardiopulmonary bypass. In these patients, inotropic agents and pulmonary vasodilators (isoproterenol, dobutamine, phentolamine, amrinone, sodium nitroprusside, and prostaglandin E_1) can be infused through the venous system into the pulmonary circulation while systemic vascular resistance is maintained by the administration of norepinephrine, epinephrine, or calcium chloride through a surgically placed, left atrial line[54] (Figure 69.9). This approach diminishes

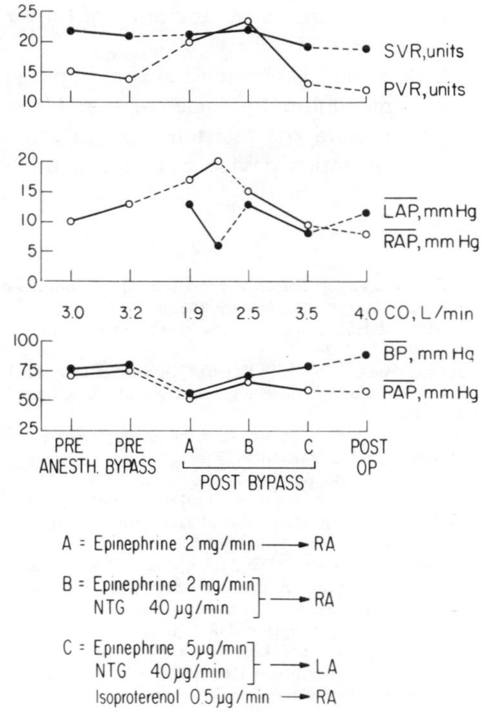

Figure 69.9. Reversal of pulmonary vasoconstriction and circulatory decompensation in a patient with mitral lung disease. Initial attempts to terminate cardiopulmonary bypass while administering epinephrine into the venous circulation were associated with right ventricular failure. Note the reversal of the right (RA) and left atrial (LA) pressure. By infusing isoproterenol into the venous system and a vasoconstrictive and inotropic dose of epinephrine into the left atrium, pulmonary vasoconstriction and right ventricular failure were relieved, blood was transferred across the pulmonary vasculature, and circulatory integrity was restored. $\overline{BP}$ = mean blood pressure; CO = cardiac output; $\overline{LAP}$ = mean left atrial pressure; NTG = nitroglycerin; PVR = pulmonary vascular resistance; $\overline{RAP}$ = mean right atrial pressure; SVR = systemic vascular resistance.

direct and alpha receptor-mediated pulmonary vasoconstriction, and has been employed frequently at our institution for over a decade. In this case, the left atrial medication line is connected by sterile intravenous tubing in the sterile field to an intravenous bottle. Strict "bubble precautions" are required. We have not recognized systemic embolic complications from this practice.

Air embolization is a well-recognized complication of open heart surgery, but its occurrence during coronary artery bypass surgery is also relatively common. Air may be entrapped within the aortic root or a vein graft or it can enter the left ventricle through a vent cannula. Although cerebral embolization can occur, more commonly air enters the coronary circulation through the right coronary ostium or a proximal vein graft anastomosis, because they are superior in the aorta. Such embolization is manifested by acute elevation of ST segments of the electrocardiogram, visual deterioration of heart function, abrupt increases in filling pressure, and sometimes hypotension or cardiovascular collapse. Elevation of perfusion pressure and coronary vasodilation with nitroglycerin frequently causes distal migration of the air with recovery of function.

Patients who cannot be weaned from cardiopulmonary bypass despite maximum pharmacologic and electrical pacing support require the assistance of an intraaortic balloon counter-pulsation device. Survival in this group of patients is high, and in many centers this is the leading indication for counterpulsation.

Acknowledgment: This work was supported in part by USPHS SCOR Grant NHLBI 23591 and Center Grant GM15904-17, National Institutes of Health, Bethesda, Maryland.

REFERENCES

1. Munson WM, Jenicek JA: Effect of anesthetic agents on patients receiving reserpine therapy. *Anesthesiology* 1962; 23:741–746.
2. Katz RL, Weintraub HD, Papper EM: Anesthesia, surgery and Rauwolfia. *Anesthesiology* 1964; 25:142–147.
3. Prys-Roberts C, Foex P, Biro GP, Roberts JG: Studies of anaesthesia in relation to hypertension. V. Adrenergic beta-receptor blockade. *Br J Anaesth* 1983; 45:671–680.
4. Laver MB, Lowenstein E: Anesthesia and the patient with heart disease, in Johnson RA, Haber E, Austen WG (eds): *Clinical Cardiology*. Boston, Little, Brown & Co, 1980, pp 1090–1109.
5. Johnson LW, Dickstein RA, Fruehan CT, Kane P, Potts JL, Smulyan H, Webb WR, Eich RH: Prophylactic digitalization for coronary artery bypass surgery. *Circulation* 1976; 53:819–822.
6. Rose MR, Glassman E, Spencer FC: Arrhythmias following cardiac surgery: relation to serum digoxin levels. *Am Heart J* 1975; 89:288–294.
7. Smith R, Grossman W, Johnson L, Segal H, Collins J, Dalen J: Arrhythmias following cardiac valve replacement. *Circulation* 1972; 45:1018–1023.
8. Tyras DH, Stothert JC Jr, Kaiser GC, Barner HB, Codd JE, Willman VL: Supraventricular tachyarrhythmias after myocardial revascularization: a randomized trial of prophylactic digitalization. *J Thorac Cardiovasc Surg* 1979; 77:310–314.
9. Oka Y, Frishman W, Becker RM, Kadish A, Strom J, Matsumoto M, Orkin L, Frater R: Clinical pharmacology of the new beta-adrenergic blocking drugs. Part 10. Beta-adrenoceptor blockade and coronary artery surgery. *Am Heart J* 1980; 99:255–269.
10. Ponten J, Biber B, Bjuro T, Henriksson BA, Hjalmarson A: Beta-receptor blocker withdrawal. A preoperative problem in general surgery? *Acta Anaesth Scand* 1982; 76(suppl):32–37.
11. Roberts JG, Foex P, Clarke TNS, Bennett MJ: Haemodynamic interactions of high-dose propranolol pretreatment and anaesthesia in the dog. I. Halothane dose-response studies. *Br J Anaesth* 1976; 48:315–325.
12. Kopriva CJ, Brown ACD, Pappas G: Hemodynamics during general anesthesia in patients receiving propranolol. *Anesthesiology* 1978; 48:28–33.
13. Slogoff S, Keats AS, Hibbs CW, Edmonds CH, Bragg DA: Failure of general anesthesia to potentiate propranolol activity. *Anesthesiology* 1977; 47:504–508.
14. Horan BF, Prys-Roberts C, Hamilton WK, Roberts JG: Haemodynamic responses to enflurane anesthesia and hypovolemia in the dog, and their modification by propranolol. *Br J Anaesth* 1977; 49:1189–1197.
15. Philbin DM, Lowenstein E: Lack of beta-adrenergic activity of isoflurane in the dog: a comparison of circulatory effects of halothane and isoflurane after propranolol administration. *Br J Anaesth* 1976; 48:1165–1170.
16. Wechsler AS: Assessment of prospectively randomized patients receiving propranolol therapy before coronary bypass operation. *Ann Thorac Surg* 1980; 30:128–136.
17. Whelton PK, Flaherty JT, MacAllister NP, Watkins L, Potter A, Johnson D, Russell RP, Walker WG: Hypertension following coronary artery bypass surgery. Role of preoperative propranolol therapy. *Hypertension* 1980; 2:291–298.
18. Bolling SF, Flaherty JT, Potter AM, Gardner TJ: Propranolol-induced postoperative hypertension following coronary artery bypass grafting. *J Thorac Cardiovasc Surg* 1984; 87:112–119.
19. Fries ES, Lappas DG: Chronic administration of calcium entry blockers and the cardiovascular responses to high doses of fentanyl in man. *Anesthesiology* 1982; 57:A295.
20. Egbert LD, Battit GE, Turndorf H, Beecher HK: The value of the preoperative visit by an anesthetist. *JAMA* 1963; 185:553–555.
21. Blacher RS: On awakening paralyzed during surgery. A syndrome of traumatic neurosis. *JAMA* 1975; 234:67–68.
22. Katz AM, Lappas DG, Lowenstein E: Cardio-respiratory effects of morphine and scopolamine premedication in adult cardiac surgical patients (abstr). *J Anesth* 1974; 41:225–226.
23. Lipton B, Litwak RS, Gadboys HL, Rendell-Baker L: Preanesthetic medication in cardiac disease. Effect on oxygenation of arterial blood and use in predicting need for postoperative ventilatory assistance. *NY State J Med* 1969; 69:1161–1168.
24. Bland JHL, Laver MB, Lowenstein E: Vasodilator effect of commercial 5% plasma protein fraction solutions. *JAMA* 1973; 224:1721–1724.
25. Lowenstein E, Johnston WE, Lappas DG, D'Ambra MN, Schneider RC, Daggett WM, Akins CW, Philbin DM: Catastrophic pulmonary vasoconstriction associated with protamine reversal of heparin. *Anesthesiology* 1983; 59:470–473.
26. Thomson IR, Dalton BC, Lappas DG, Lowenstein E: Right bundle-branch block and complete heart block caused by the Swan-Ganz catheter. *Anesthesiology* 1979; 51:359–362.
27. Waller JL, Zaidan JR, Kaplan JA, Bauman DI: Hemodynamic responses to preoperative vascular cannulation in patients with coronary artery disease. *Anesthesiology* 1982; 56:219–221.
28. Anon: Monitoring devices and septicaemia. *Br Med J* 1979; 1:1747–1748.
29. Tomichek RC, Rosow CE, Schneider RC, Moss J, Philbin DM: Cardiovascular effects of diazepam–fentanyl anesthesia in patients with coronary artery disease. *Anesth Analg* 1982; 61:217–218.
30. Slogoff S, Keats AS: Does perioperative myocardial ischemia lead to postoperative myocardial infarction? *Anesthesiology* 1985; 62:107–114.
31. Hamilton WK: Do let the blood pressure drop and do use myocardial depressants! *Anesthesiology* 1976; 45:273–274.
32. Lowenstein E, Foex P, Francis CM, Davies WL, Yusuf S, Ryder WA: Regional ischemic ventricular dysfunction in myocardium supplied by a narrowed coronary artery with increasing halothane concentration in the dog. *Anesthesiology* 1981; 55:349–359.
33. Francis CM, Foex P, Lowenstein E, Glazebrook CW, Davies WL, Ryder WA, Jones LA: Interaction between regional myocardial ischaemia and left ventricular performance under halothane anesthesia. *Br J Anaesth* 1982; 54:965–980.
34. Bellows W, Bode RH Jr, Levy JH, Foex P, Lowenstein E: Noninvasive detection of periinduction ischemic ventricular dysfunction by cardiokymography in humans: preliminary experience. *Anesthesiology* 1984; 60:155–158.
35. Lowenstein E: Perianesthetic ischemic episodes cause myocardial infarction in humans: a hypothesis confirmed. *Anesthesiology* 1985; 62:103–106.
36. Lowenstein E, Philbin DM: Narcotic "anesthesia" in the eighties. *Anesthesiology* 1981; 55:195–197.
37. Lowenstein E, Hill RD, Rajagopalan B, Schneider RC: Winnie the Pooh revisited, or, the more recent adventures of piglet. *Anesthesiology* 1982; 56:81–83.
38. Thomson IR, Putnins CL: Adverse effects of pancuronium during high-dose fentanyl anesthesia for coronary artery bypass grafting. *Anesthesiology* 1985; 62:708–713.
39. Hess W, Arnold B, Schulte-Sasse U, Tarnow J. Comparison of isoflurane and halothane when used to control intraoperative hypertension in patients undergoing coronary artery bypass surgery. *Anesth Analg* 1983; 62:15–20.
40. Reiz S, Balfors E, Sorenson MB, Ariola S, Friedman A, Truedsson H: Isoflurane: a powerful coronary vasodilator in patients with coronary artery disease. *Anesthesiology* 1983; 59:91–97.

40a. Moffitt EA, Barket RA, Glen JJ, Imrie DD, DelCampo C, Landymore RW, Kinley E, Murphy DA: Myocardial metabolism and hemodynamic responses with isoflurane anesthesia for coronary arterial surgery. *Anesth Analg* 1986; 65:53–61.

41. Merin RG, Lowenstein E, Gelman S: Is anesthesia beneficial for the ischemic heart? III. *Anesthesiology* 1986; 64:137–140.
42. Reiz S, Balfors E, Gustavsson B, Haggmark S, Nath S, Rydvall A, Truedsson H: Effects of halothane on coronary haemodynamics and myocardial metabolism in patients with ischemic heart disease and heart failure. *Acta Anaesth Scand* 1982; 26:133–138.
43. Philbin DM, Foex P, Drummond G, Lowenstein E, Ryder WA, Jones LA: Postsystolic shortening of canine left ventricle supplied by a stenotic artery when nitrous oxide is added in the presence of narcotics. *Anesthesiology* 1985; 62:166–174.
44. Thomas SJ, Lowenstein E: Anesthetic management of the patient with valvular heart disease. *Int Anesth Clin* 1976; 17:67–96.
45. Zaidan JR, Freniere S: Use of a pacing pulmonary artery catheter during cardiac surgery. *Ann Thorac Surg* 1983; 35:633–636.
46. Grossman W, Jones D, McLauren LP: Wall stress and patterns of hypertrophy in the human left ventricle. *J Clin Invest* 1975; 56:56–64.
47. Clark DG, McAnulty JH, Rahimtoola SH: Valve replacement in aortic insufficiency with left ventricular dysfunction. *Circulation* 1980; 61:411–421.
48. Rappaport E: Natural history of aortic and mitral valve disease. *Am J Cardiol* 1975; 35:221–227.

49. Stone JG, Hoar PF, Faltas AN, Johnson LL, Edie RN, Bowman FO Jr, Malm JR: Comparison of intraoperative nitroprusside unloading in mitral and aortic regurgitation. *J Thorac Cardiovasc Surg* 1979; 78:103–109.
50. Miller RD, Eger EI II, Stevens WC, Gibbons R: Pancuronium-induced tachycardia in relation to alveolar halothane, dose of pancuronium, and prior atropine. *Anesthesiology* 1975; 42:352–355.
51. Morris RB, Cahalan MK, Miller RD, Wilkinson PL, Quasha AL, Robinson SL: The cardiovascular effects of vecuronium (ORG NC45) and pancuronium in patients undergoing coronary artery bypass grafting. *Anesthesiology* 1983; 58:438–440.
52. Philbin DM, Moss J, Rosow CE, Akins CW, Rosenberger JL: Histamine release with intravenous narcotics: protective effects of H_1- and H_2-receptor antagonists. *Klin Wochenschr* 1982; 60:1056–1059.
53. Stone JG, Faltas AN, Hoar PF: Sodium nitroprusside therapy for cardiac failure in anesthetized patients with valvular insufficiency. *Anesthesiology* 1978; 49:414–418.
54. D'Ambra MN, LaRaia PJ, Philbin DM, Watkins WD, Hilgenberg AD, Buckley MJ: Prostaglandin E_1. A new therapy for refractory right heart failure and pulmonary hypertension after mitral valve replacement. *J Thorac Cardiovasc Surg* 1985; 89:567–572.
55. Stern L, Lees MH, Leduc J: Environmental temperature, oxygen consumption, and catecholamine excretion in newborn infants. *Pediatrics* 1965; 36:367–373.
56. Klopfenstein HS, Rudolph AM: Postnatal changes in the circulation and responses to volume loading in sheep. *Circ Res* 1978; 42:839–845.
57. Olley PM, Coceani F, Bodach E: E-type prostaglandins: a new emergency therapy for certain cyanotic congenital heart malformations. *Circulation* 1976; 53:728–731.
58. Rudolf AM, Yuan S: Response of the pulmonary vasculature to hypoxia and H^+ ion concentration changes. *J Clin Invest* 1966; 45:399–411.
59. Simmons DH, Linde LM, Miller JH, O'Reilly RJ: Relation between lung volume and pulmonary vascular resistance. *Circ Res* 1961; 9:465–471.
60. Benumof JL: Mechanism of decreased blood flow to atelectatic lung. *J Applied Physiol* 1978; 46:1047–1048.
61. Criley JM, Blaufuss AH, Kessel GL: Cough-induced cardiac compression. Self-administered form of cardiopulmonary resuscitation. *JAMA* 1976; 236:1246–1250.
62. Yelderman M, New W Jr: Evaluation of pulse oximetry. *Anesthesiology* 1983; 59:349–352.
63. Hickey PR, Hansen DD, Cramolini GM, Vincent RN, Lang P: Pulmonary and systemic hemodynamic responses to ketamine in infants with normal and elevated pulmonary vascular resistance. *Anesthesiology* 1985; 62:287–293.
64. Lang P, Williams RG, Norwood WI, Castaneda AR: Hemodynamic effects of dopamine in infants after cardiac surgery. *Circulation* 1978; 58 (suppl 2):II-149.
65. Drop LJ, Scheidegger D: Plasma ionized calcium concentration. Important determinant of the hemodynamic response to calcium infusion. *J Thorac Cardiovasc Surg* 1980; 79:425–431.
66. Miller RD: Complications of massive blood transfusions. *Anesthesiology* 1973; 39:82–93.
67. Sarin CL, Yalav E, Clement AJ, Braimbridge MV: The necessity for measurement of left atrial pressure after cardiac valve surgery. *Thorax* 1970; 25:185–189.
68. Daggett WM, Bianco JA, Powell WJ Jr, Austen WG: Relative contributions of the atrial systole–ventricular systole interval and of patterns of ventricular activation to ventricular function during electrical pacing of the dog heart. *Circ Res* 1970; 27:69–79.
69. D'Ambra MN, Margrassi P, Derkac WM, Lowenstein E, Kyo S, Austen WG, Buckley MJ, LaRaia PJ: Regional myocardial hyperthemia/hypothermia: effects on segmental cardiac function, coronary blood flow, and metabolism. *Fed Proc* 1983; 42:1109.

70 Physiologic and Neurochemical Basis of Acupuncture Analgesia

Ji-Sheng Han, MD

From the historical record of *Huangdi Neijin* (*The Yellow Emperor's Classic*), acupuncture has been used in China as a therapeutic measure for at least 2,000 years. However, only in the recent 10 to 20 years has acupuncture become popularly known to the whole world.

In the 1970s two events seemed to play a role in accelerating the popularity of acupuncture. One was the clinical application of "acupuncture anesthesia," which gained access to the whole world after the US President's first visit to China in 1974. The other was the discovery of endogenous opioids in 1975 and the great expectation of their possible role in the basic mechanisms of acupuncture analgesia.

A decade has passed since these events. It appears worthwhile to make a scientific evaluation of what acupuncture can do as an analgesic measure and what the basic mechanisms are underlying this millennium-old medical treatment.

THE BASIC PHENOMENA OF ACUPUNCTURE ANALGESIA

ACUPUNCTURE ANALGESIA IN HUMANS

Acupuncture traditionally has been used to ameliorate the already existing painful syndromes such as frozen shoulder and sciatica. Only in recent decades was it also used to prevent the pain elicited by surgical trauma. After wide application in millions of patients during the 1960s and 1970s in a variety of surgical operations, it has generally been accepted in the Chinese medical field that (1) acupuncture or electroacupuncture can be used to reduce or even prevent the pain of surgical trauma in completely awake patients; (2) analgesia is more satisfactory in operations involving the head, neck, and chest regions (craniotomy in the anterior cranial fossa, tooth extraction, thyroidectomy, operations on cervical vertebrae through an anterior approach, pneumonectomy, and cardiac surgery) as compared with abdominal and pelvic operations, of which only cesarean section was claimed to be the most successful operation performed under acupuncture analgesia; (3) individual variation in the response to acupuncture stimulation and insufficient analgesia in certain patients (nonresponders to acupuncture analgesia) constituted the major problems in large scale application of acupuncture analgesia as a standard anesthetic procedure in surgical operations; (4) besides its analgesic effect, acupuncture can stabilize the vital parameters during surgical intervention, lessening the postoperative pain and accelerating the postoperative recovery probably because of its activation of the immunologic system; (5) a proper combination of acupuncture analgesia and an adequate amount of sedatives and analgesics which were supposed to be synergistic or additive to acupuncture analgesia is strongly suggested; (6) a deeper understanding of the basic mechanisms of acupuncture analgesia will probably increase the efficacy of acupuncture analgesia and change nonresponders into responders.

The complexity of the pathologic conditions encountered in various diseases with the symptom of pain makes it difficult to pick up the "pure" analgesic component elicited by acupuncture. Thus, a decrease in epigastric pain in patients with duodenal ulcer by acupuncture treatment may well be the result of a suppression of gastric acid secretion. Immediate relief of frozen shoulder could be the outcome of muscle relaxation by acupuncture treatment to break the vicious cycle.

An alternative to exploring the basic characteristics of acupuncture analgesia is to measure the pain threshold or pain tolerance change during and after the acupuncture stimulation. This was the first study we made when we first came across this field in 1965. A series of experiments were performed in human subjects using a potassium iontophoresis method for assessing the pain threshold in eight representative areas distributed over the head, neck, chest, abdomen, and extremities. Control experiments in 22 subjects with pain threshold assessed every ten minutes showed a reasonably stable level in a period of 100 minutes. In 66 subjects undergoing acupuncture stimulation in "hegu" point (large intestine 4) located on the dorsal surface of the thenar eminence of the hand, a significant increase in pain threshold was seen, which was slow in onset, reaching a plateau in about 20 to 30 minutes, remained at the high level during the 50-minute stimulation period, and declined exponentially after removal of the needle with a half-life of 15 to 17 minutes. The characteristic time course which was found not only in hegu point, but also in seven other points, together with the generalized spatial distribution of the analgesic effect, pointed to the possible participation of chemical factors as the underlying mechanism, rather than simple distraction or suggestion. That this analgesic effect was abolished by local infiltration of procaine deep into the needling site and was absent when acupuncture was applied to the afflicted extremities of paraplegic or hemiplegic patients further indicated an intact afferent neuronal pathway as the prerequisite for mediation of acupuncture analgesia. The aforementioned basic observation was reported at the First All-China Acupuncture Conference held in Shanghai in 1966, and was published in 1973.[1] In the same year Andersson et al[2] reported the effect of acupuncture on the pain threshold experimentally induced by tooth pulp stimulation in healthy volunteers. These studies were then verified by an explosion of reports in the late 1970s, showing that acupuncture was capable of suppressing the pain that originated not only from the skin and tooth pulp, but also from deep structures as elicited by intramuscular injection of hypersaline or by tourniquet ischemia.[3] Moreover, the suppression of pain resulted not only from the central biasing effect expected by the profound psychologic influence supposedly exerted by the acupuncturist, but also from a biologic component as depicted by procedures based on the signal detection theory.[4,5]

ACUPUNCTURE ANALGESIA IN EXPERIMENTAL ANIMALS

The phenomenon of acupuncture analgesia has amply been demonstrated in varieties of animals ranging from mouse to monkey, using different kinds of noxious stimuli (thermal, electrical, mechanical, and chemical) and different physiologic parameters as the end point for nociceptive response ranging from single neuron discharge, tail flick, and vocalization, up to complicated instrumental avoidance response.[6] That acupuncture is capable of inducing an analgesic effect can therefore be regarded as a general phenomenon existing at least in mammals. It might be advantageous to describe some of the animal models in detail, so that the advantages and limitations in methodology can be evaluated.

In rabbit experiments, radiant heat emanating from a projection bulb was applied on the shaved nostrils or on the shaved tail as noxious stimulus and the latency of head jerk or tail flick was recorded as a nociceptive threshold. Acupuncture was given to the animal by inserting a stainless steel needle (0.15 mm in diameter) into the "zusanli" point, located 8 mm lateral to the anterior tubercle of the tibia, and manipulating it for ten minutes. In about 80% of the animals there was an increase in the escape response latency. A cutoff level of 200% increase in latency was set to avoid burning of the skin. For electroacupuncture, another needle was inserted into the "sanyinjiao" point, located in front of the Achilles tendon, 5 mm above the level of the medial malleolus, and electric stimulation generated from a 57-6D electronic stimulator was applied through these two needles. The parameters of the electric impulses were: biphasic square waves 0.3 ms in width, a constant output of 1 V from the baseline (2 V peak-to-peak), and a frequency automatically changed from 2 to 15 Hz, 12 cycles per minute, unless otherwise stated. In some experiments mechanical pressing of the point was used instead of needling. Escape response latencies were measured before and every ten minutes after the administration of acupuncture for a total of 60 minutes. Details of the method are described elsewhere.[7] Because of the ease in handling a number of animals at a time and the lesser degree of stress to the animal, electroacupuncture has been used more frequently than manual needling.

The method of electroacupuncture in rats was similar to that in rabbits except for two modifications, ie, the intensity of electroacupuncture stimulation was increased stepwise from 1 V to 3 V within 30 minutes, and electroacupuncture was applied to both hind legs bilaterally. Nociceptive threshold was measured by tail flick latency[8] or by the squeak threshold induced by electric stimulation applied to the tail through hypodermic needles.

PAIN PATHWAYS

Nociceptors that sense noxious stimulation are distributed over the skin and mucosa as well as in some deep structures. They are free nerve terminals of some A_δ and C afferent fibers, the central end of which terminates mainly in the first and fifth laminae of the dorsal horn or the spinal tract nucleus of the trigeminal nerve. There are at least six neuronal pathways carrying nociceptive information from spinal cord to brain stem. They have been categorized into two groups: the fast conducting lateral group ending in the lateral thalamus and the multineuronal slow conducting system ending in the medial thalamus.[9] About 10% of the total neuronal population in the nucleus parafascicularis and nucleus centrolateralis of the medial thalamus react to noxious stimuli with a specific pattern of discharge, therefore regarded as nociceptive units.[10] Neurons with similar discharge patterns were also found in the reticular formation of the lower brain stem, although the incidence might have been lower as in the nucleus parafascicularis and nucleus centrolateralis. Recent findings show that noxious information can be transmitted further upward to the cerebral cortex, presumably by multisynaptic neuronal pathways[11] (Figure 70.1).

From the brief account just given, it is evident that the dorsal horn neurons and the medial thalamic nuclei are the two strategic links in mediating nociceptive information. The measures intervening in the transmission through these two links will be anticipated to produce an analgesic effect.

TRANSMISSION OF ACUPUNCTURE INFORMATION

In classic acupuncture treatment, a needle is inserted into the skin, passing through subcutaneous tissue to the deep structures including muscle, tendon, fascia, ligament, and even periosteum. When the needle is mechanically twisted (manual needling) or connected to an electronic stimulator (electroacupuncture), it is bound to stimulate the surrounding tissues, including certain receptors, nerve terminals, nerve fibers, and muscle fibers. To evaluate the role of peripheral structures sensing acupuncture stimulation, procaine was injected subcutaneously or intramuscularly into the point "hegu" of ten healthy volunteers followed by conventional manual needling. The characteristic needling sensation, the so-called "deqi" (soreness, heaviness, numbness, and sense of swelling) as well as the analgesic effect induced by manual needling was almost totally abolished by local administration of procaine deep into the muscle but not by its subcutaneous infiltration, suggesting that afferent impulses arise mainly from the deep structures rather than the skin and subcutaneous ones.[1]

Another study in human subjects was performed to further localize the categories of deep structures implicated in the needling sensation. An injection needle connected with a syringe was inserted into a certain acu-point of the affected limb immediately before its amputation. The needle was inserted downward along with a twisting movement until a characteristic needling sensation was obtained, and a minute amount of dye was delivered into the point. Serial histologic examination of the relevant tissue obtained from the amputated limb revealed divergent structures including bundles of nerve fibers, nerve terminals, muscle spindles, and some afferent structures along with the blood vessels.[12] There was a consensus from at least two different sources that various components of the complex needling sensation may arise from stimulation of different structures: the sense

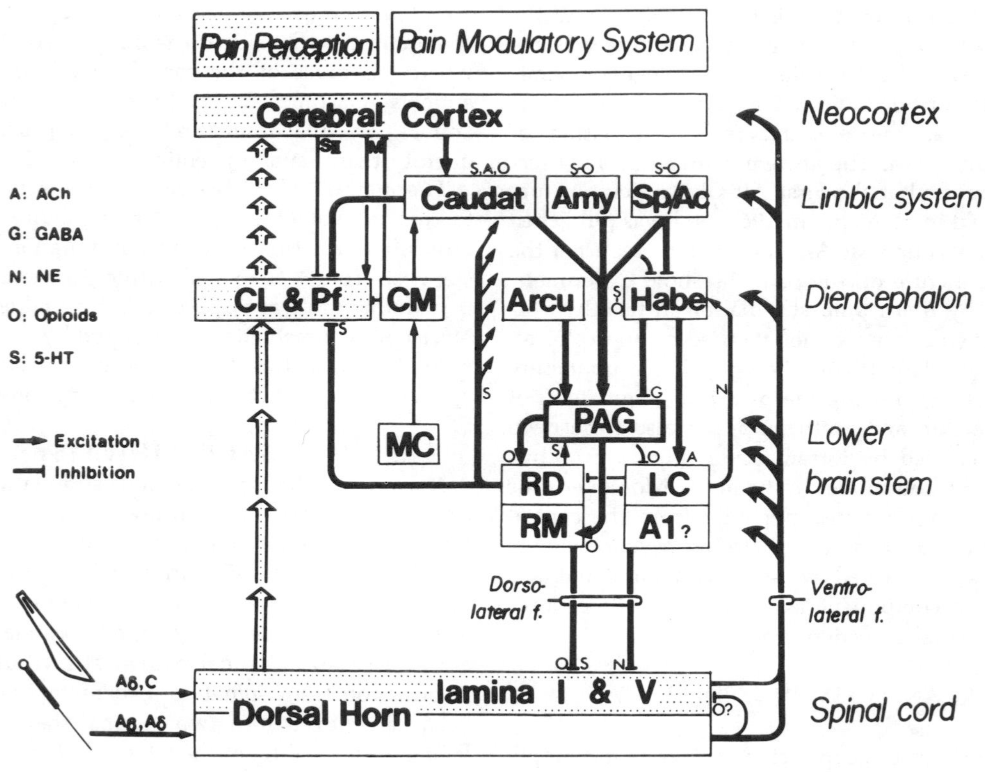

Figure 70.1. Diagram showing the possible mechanisms of acupuncture analgesia. For details, see text. A_1? = perikarya of noradrenergic neurons with descending fibers to the spinal cord (Whether it is group A_1 or A_{5-7} remains to be identified); Ac = nucleus accumbens; Amy = nucleus amygdala; Arcu = nucleus arcuatus hypothalami; Caudat = nucleus caudatus; CL = nucleus centrolateralis hypothalami; CM = nucleus centromedianus hypothalami; Habe = nucleus habenula; LC = locus ceruleus; MC = nucleus megalocellularis; PAG = periaqueductal grey; Pf = nucleus parafascicularis; RD = nucleus raphe dorsalis; RM = nucleus raphe magnus; Sp = septum.

of swelling and heaviness from the muscles, soreness from tendons and periosteum, and numbness and a sense of electric shock from stimulation of the nerve trunk.[10,13]

The afferent nerve fibers pertinent to acupuncture analgesia have been composed mainly of medium-sized fibers (groups II and III).[10,14] In addition, some thin fibers (group IV) arising from muscle spindles[15] or heavy pressure receptors located in muscles and tendons[16] have also been shown to take part in transmitting acupuncture signals. In fact, the types of nerve fibers implicated in electroacupuncture analgesia depend on the frequency and intensity of the electroacupuncture stimulation being used. While more and more thin fibers will be recruited in low-frequency high-intensity electroacupuncture stimulation, high-frequency low-intensity stimulation is apt to be transmitted by thicker fibers because of their low threshold and short refractory period. Evidence obtained from focal destruction of the spinal cord[17] indicates that the signals coded with acupuncture stimulation are transmitted along the ventrolateral column of the spinal cord. Evoked neuronal activities coincident with electroacupuncture stimulation have been picked up from all levels of the central nervous system, starting from the reticular formation of the lower brain stem to the cerebral cortex.[10,11] These form the structural and physiologic basis for multilevel interaction between acupuncture signals and those arising from noxious stimulation (Figure 70.1).

INTERACTION BETWEEN ACUPUNCTURE AND NOXIOUS INFORMATION AT THE SPINAL LEVEL

The gate control theory of Melzack and Wall[18] suggests that the ascending transmission of nociceptive information carried by thin (A_δ and C) afferent fibers could be gated at the spinal level by afferent signals carried by thick fibers emanating from the same dermatome. This mechanism may play a role in acupuncture given to a point in the vicinity of the wounded area. In surgical operations performed under "acupuncture anesthesia," a good analgesic effect was obtained when high-frequency (100 Hz or more) electroacupuncture was administered along both sides of the line of incision. Theoretically, the neuronal circuitry mediating the gate control effect should be completed in the spinal cord per se; therefore, it should exist in spinalized animals. Woolf et al[19] reported that electric stimulation at the root of the tail was capable of prolonging the latency of tail flick response in the spinalized rat in which both the conditioning stimulus (electric stimulation) and the noxious stimulus (hot water immersion) were given to the tail.[19] However, when electric stimulation was given at the zusanli point located near the knee joint and tail flick response was elicited by radiant heat applied on the tip of the tail, no increase in tail flick latency was noted in the rat with transection of the third thoracic vertebra as was clearly demonstrated in the intact animal.[20] The results indicate that when electroacupuncture is given at a point remote from the site of noxious stimulation, the analgesic effect of electroacupuncture could be completed only when the spinal cord is under the control of the suprasegmental structures. In other words, the electroacupuncture signal should be transmitted upward to the brain to activate the pain modulatory system, which then sends a descending signal downward to the spinal cord to produce an analgesic effect.

Recent studies reveal that some monoamines and endogenous opioids in the spinal cord exhibit an important antinociceptive effect. Marked analgesia was found after the administration of 5-hydroxytryptamine (5-HT),[21] norepinephrine (NE),[22] [Met^5]enkephalin,[23] β-endorphin,[24] dynorphin A,[25] and dynorphin B[26] into the subarachnoid space of the spinal cord. To evaluate whether these neurochemical substrates play a role in acupuncture analgesia, various pharmacologic tools have been used to manipulate the effects of the endogenously released neurotransmitters to determine their effects on acupuncture analgesia. Results in rats clearly show that the analgesic effect of electroacupuncture is markedly potentiated by intrathecal injection of 5-hydroxytryptophan[27] and dihydroxyphenylserin,[22] the direct precursors of 5-HT and NE, respectively, and is dramatically reduced by cinanserin[27] and phentolamine,[22] the blockers of 5-HT and NE receptors, respectively, indicating that both 5-HT and NE are important mediators in acupuncture analgesia at the spinal level.

As for endogenous opioids, 20 or more individual opioid peptides have been found in the central nervous system, and they can be grouped into three families: enkephalins, endorphins, and dynorphins.[28] The multiplicity of opioid peptides has added some difficulties to opioid study, at least from the methodologic point of view. Because all of these opioid peptides act on opiate receptors to produce an analgesic effect, blockade of the acupuncture effect by the opiate receptor blocking agent naloxone can hardly differentiate which of the opioid families is actually involved. Another paradoxic finding is that intrathecal injection of β-endorphin produced marked analgesia,[24] although this peptide did not naturally exist in the spinal cord. We have therefore chosen another approach, ie, to inject intrathecally antibodies recognizing specific opioid peptide, thus preventing the released peptide from receptor activation. Using this antibody microinjection technique we found that the effect of electroacupuncture analgesia can be significantly reduced by intrathecal injection of antibodies (IgG) directed to [Met^5]enkephalin, dynorphin A, and dynorphin B, but not by IgG-recognizing [Leu^5]enkephalin or β-endorphin,[29,30] indicating that in the spinal cord it is [Met^5] enkephalin, dynorphin A, and dynorphin B that are relevant in mediating the effect of acupuncture analgesia.

LOWER BRAIN STEM

THE RAPHE NUCLEI

The raphe nuclei stretch along the midline of the lower brain stem, where serotonergic neuronal somas aggregate and send ascending fibers to the forebrain and descending fibers to the spinal cord. The descending 5-HT fibers emanate mainly from the nucleus raphe magnus of the medulla oblongata, traveling downward along the dorsolateral funiculus to the spinal cord. Electric stimulation of the nucleus raphe magnus or microinjection of morphine into the nucleus produced behavioral analgesia and inhibition of the dorsal horn cells receiving noxious input.[31,32] From the nucleus raphe dorsalis located in the midbrain, ascending 5-HT fibers are sent to the medial thalamus, especially to the nucleus parafascicularis, the strategic nucleus for nociception, to suppress its activities.[33] At the same time, ascending 5-HT fibers are sent to forebrain structures to activate the pain-modulating system, including the periaqueductal grey, habenula, amygdala, septum, and nucleus accumbens. Administration of cinanserin, the 5-HT blocking agent, into these nuclei resulted in marked suppression of the effect of acupuncture analgesia without a dramatic change in the basal pain threshold. The results suggest that 5-HT released in these nuclei during acupuncture stimulation is essential for acupuncture analgesia.[34-36]

NORADRENERGIC NEURONAL STRUCTURES

The perikarya of the noradrenergic neurons in the brain aggregate in six pairs of small nuclei (A_{1-2}, A_{4-7}) in the pons/medulla, from where noradrenergic fibers radiate to the forebrain structures and also downward to the spinal cord. The descending norepinephrine fibers reach the spinal cord through the dorsolateral funiculus[37] to release norepinephrine which exerts an inhibitory effect on dorsal horn cells through alpha receptors.[22] Ascending norepinephrine fibers emanate largely from the locus ceruleus and are distributed extensively to the forebrain structures. That the efficacy of acupuncture analgesia was facilitated by destruction of the locus ceruleus and suppressed by electrical stimulation of the nucleus[38] seems to indicate that the overall effect of the locus ceruleus in acupuncture analgesia was an antagonistic one. However, more elaborate studies have shown that the influence on acupuncture analgesia of the ascending norepinephrine fibers depends on the target sites being innervated. Although the effect of acupuncture analgesia was markedly potentiated by a noradrenergic blocking agent microinjected into the periaqueductal grey or habenula[39] of the rabbit, the reverse was true when the blocking agent was injected into the hypothalamus of the rat.[40]

From these results it becomes evident that the functional roles played by central monoamines in mediating acupuncture analgesia are unique for 5-HT in the whole central nervous system and are site specific for norepinephrine. Moreover, a reciprocal inhibitory relation was reported to exist between the raphe nuclei and the locus ceruleus (Figure 70.1).

PERIAQUEDUCTAL GREY

Early in 1964 Tsou and Jang[41] reported that the periaqueductal grey and periventricular grey matter of the rabbit are the central sites of action for morphine analgesia. In 1969 Reynolds[42] claimed significant analgesia following electrical stimulation of the periaqueductal grey of the rat. This stimulation-produced analgesia was later abolished by naloxone, suggesting the involvement of endogenous opioids in this reaction. Using an antibody microinjection technique we demonstrated that [Met^5] enkephalin,[29] [Met^5]enkephalin-Arg^6-Phe^7,[43] and β-endorphin,[29] but not dynorphin,[44] were important mediators of acupuncture analgesia in the periaqueductal grey of the midbrain. Substance P in the periaqueductal grey releases enkephalins,[45] thus enhancing the effect of acupuncture analgesia, which is opposing the effect of substance P in the spinal cord where it acts as a neurotransmitter for the nociceptive afferents.

As seen in Figure 70.1, the periaqueductal grey receives afferent input from peripheral tissue as well as the descending influence from higher centers. Efferent impulses from the periaqueductal grey are capable of activating both ascending 5-HT pathways from the nucleus raphe dorsalis and descending pathways from the nucleus raphe magnus. For these reasons the periaqueductal grey is regarded as one of the most important structures in the neuronal circuitry mediating acupuncture analgesia. It will be discussed in some detail later in this chapter.

DIENCEPHALON

HABENULA

The habenula is an important relay station between the forebrain structures and the lower brain stem. Because destruction of the habenula led to a potentiation of acupuncture analgesia and stimulation of the habenula brought about a suppression of acupuncture analgesia, it was suggested that the habenula might play an antagonistic role against acupuncture analgesia. Efferents from the habenula were shown to activate the locus ceruleus through a cholinergic mechanism[46] and inhibit raphe nuclei through a GABAergic mechanism.[47] Considering the importance of the raphe in mediating acupuncture analgesia, and the antagonistic role of the locus ceruleus against it, it would be rational to assume that suppression of the raphe and activation of the locus ceruleus would lead to deterioration of the acupuncture effect.

ARCUATE NUCLEUS OF THE HYPOTHALAMUS

Immunohistochemical studies have shown that within the arcuate nucleus of the hypothalamus there are aggregates of the somas of β-endorphinergic neurons[48] together with some enkephalinergic neurons. Radioimmunoassay reveals that in rats with prominent analgesic effect after electroacupuncture stimulation (good responders) there was a marked increase in the β-endorphin content in the hypothalamus, whereas in nonresponders no significant changes in β-endorphin content were encountered.[49] Efferents from the arcuate nucleus course along limbic structures to end in the periaqueductal grey and locus ceruleus.[48] The importance of β-endorphin in the periaqueductal grey for electroacupuncture analgesia has been discussed in the preceding paragraph. In the meantime, a strong suppressive effect of β-endorphin on the locus ceruleus is also beneficial in the mediation of acupuncture analgesia.[50]

CENTROMEDIAN NUCLEUS OF THE HYPOTHALAMUS

The centromedian nucleus is part of the intralaminar nuclei of the hypothalamus. This nucleus is anatomically close to, but functionally different from, another intralaminar nucleus, the parafascicularis nucleus. According to Chang[10,51] the parafascicularis is an integral part of the nociceptive pathways and is constantly under the inhibitory influence of the centromedian nucleus. Low-frequency (4 to 6 Hz) electroacupuncture stimulation, but not that of higher frequency (60 Hz), was very effective in activating the centromedian nucleus which then exerted an inhibitory modulation on the parafascicularis nucleus through three routes: (1) removal of the tonic excitatory influence from the cortex to the parafascicularis,[51] (2) strengthening of the inhibitory influence from caudate to the parafascicularis,[10] and (3) a direct inhibitory influence from the centromedian nucleus to the parafascicularis.[51]

LIMBIC SYSTEM AND BASAL GANGLIA

SEPTUM AND NUCLEUS ACCUMBENS

The nucleus accumbens is part of the limbic system, lying ventrolateral to the septum. Involvement of the nucleus accumbens in acupuncture analgesia was evidenced by the finding that the efficacy of acupuncture analgesia was dramatically decreased by the destruction of the bilateral accumbens.[52] Further studies revealed that 5-HT and endogenous opioids were the major neurochemical substrates mediating acupuncture analgesia, because 5-HT or morphine microinjected into the nucleus accumbens produced marked analgesia, whereas antagonists of 5-HT (cinanserin) or opioids (naloxone) microinjected into the same nuclei attenuated electroacupuncture analgesia.[35,53] Given the supposition that both 5-HT and opioids play a role in acupuncture analgesia, what then would be the possible interrelation between them? Because the analgesic effect of 5-HT microinjected into the nucleus accumbens could be abolished by naloxone administered into the same site, whereas the analgesic effect of morphine could not be reversed by the 5-HT blocker cinanserin, it would be rational to propose that serotonergic terminals are connecting in series with opioidergic interneurons.[54]

The serotonergic fibers innervating the nucleus accumbens are derived from the nucleus raphe dorsalis located in the periaqueductal grey area. It would therefore be interesting to evaluate the interconnection between the periaqueductal grey and the accumbens. The analgesic effect produced by microinjection of morphine into the periaqueductal grey was found to be dose-dependently attenuated by cinanserin or [Met[5]]enkephalin antibodies[55] microinjected into bilateral nuclei accumbens, indicating that the ascending serotonergic fibers emanating from the nucleus raphe dorsalis were capable of activating the antinociceptive mechanisms in the nucleus accumbens. Conversely, electrical stimulation of the nucleus accumbens was reported to activate the nucleus raphe magnus in the medulla oblongata, and this effect was readily blocked by naloxone administered into the periaqueductal grey.[56] It implies that a descending pathway from the nucleus accumbens to the periaqueductal grey might exist which uses endogenous opioids as its final linkage.

From the aforementioned material there seems to be a neuronal circuitry connecting the periaqueductal grey, the nucleus raphe dorsalis, and the nucleus accumbens into a loop tentatively termed the mesolimbic loop of analgesia. The neurotransmitters used in this loop have been clarified to some extent (eg, a 5-HT/enkephalin link within the nucleus accumbens and an opioid link in the periaqueductal grey), but not yet completely resolved. If such a neuronal loop is proved to function, it might be helpful to explain why the effect of acupuncture analgesia could be blocked by and large when naloxone was injected only into one nucleus such as the periaqueductal grey or nucleus accumbens.[53]

The role played by the septum in acupuncture analgesia seems to be similar to that of the nucleus accumbens. Microinjection of naloxone into the septum was capable of blocking the effect of acupuncture analgesia to a moderate extent.[57] Electric stimulation of the septum resulted in activation of the periaqueductal grey as well as inhibition of the habenula.[58] Because the habenula has an inhibitory influence on the periaqueductal grey,[47] removal of this inhibitory influence might contribute to activation of the periaqueductal grey.

AMYGDALA

The amygdala is known to be related to emotion. Only recently has its involvement in pain control been evaluated. The importance of the amygdala in mediating acupuncture analgesia was suggested by the notion that stimulation of the amygdala increased the pain threshold of the rabbit and that destruction of the amygdala resulted in attenuation of electroacupuncture analgesia.[59]

The amygdala is innervated by serotonergic fibers from the nucleus raphe dorsalis. Within the nucleus are a number of enkephalinergic neurons condensed especially in the central nucleus of the amygdala. Microinjection studies have shown that the effect of electroacupuncture analgesia can be blocked by the 5-HT antagonist cinanserin or narcotic antagonist naloxone, and the effective sites of these two blockers overlap almost completely.[60] These results indicate that the serotonergic fibers terminating in the amygdala form a synapse with short-axon enkephalinergic interneurons which release enkephalin to act on opiate receptors. In fact, direct administration of morphine into the amygdala produced marked analgesia.[60] The possible connections between the amygdala and the periaqueductal grey are currently under study.

CAUDATE NUCLEUS

The caudate nucleus, which is part of the extrapyramidal system related to complicated locomotor function, recently was found to play a role in pain control. Intolerable pain could be ameliorated by electrical stimulation of the caudate nucleus in human subjects,[61] and the effectiveness of electroacupuncture analgesia was decreased by destruction of the head of the caudate nucleus in the rabbit.[62]

Among the multiple neurotransmitters contained in the caudate nucleus, acetylcholine and dopamine are the two most thoroughly studied in relation to behavior control. The turnover rate of acetylcholine was significantly accelerated during electroacupuncture stimulation.[63] This was in line with the finding that the effect of acupuncture analgesia was decreased when the synthesis of acetylcholine was blocked by microinjection of hemicholine-3 and augmented when the degradation of acetylcholine was retarded by the acetylcholine esterase inhibitor eserine administered into the caudate nucleus of the rabbit.[64] The effect of dopamine seemed to oppose that of acetylcholine. Therefore the effect of acupuncture analgesia was augmented by l-dopa, the precursor of dopamine, and attenuated by haloperidol, the blocker of dopamine, when these chemicals were microinjected into the caudate nucleus.[65]

There were also findings favoring an enkephalinergic mechanism in the caudate nucleus for mediation of acupuncture analgesia: the steady state content[66] and release[67] of enkephalins were significantly increased during electroacupuncture stimulation; the effect of electroacupuncture analgesia in the rat bore a positive correlation with the content of [Met^5]enkephalin but not with that of [Leu^5]enkephalin[66]; the effect of acupuncture analgesia was significantly potentiated when the degradation of enkephalin was hindered by bestatin and thiorphan, leading to an increase in the content of enkephalins in the caudate nucleus.[68]

The caudate nucleus receives a lot of afferent fibers from the cerebral cortex. Among the efferent connections from the caudate nucleus, there are at least three pathways related to pain and analgesia: (1) an inhibitory influence on the thalamus to suppress nociception,[69] (2) an inhibitory influence on the habenula, resulting in disinhibition of the periaqueductal grey,[58] and (3) modulation of periaqueductal grey activity through opioid mechanisms.[70] All these connections seem to favor the mediation of electroacupuncture analgesia (Figure 70.1).

CEREBRAL CORTEX

The suppression of nociceptive somatosensory evoked potential by acupuncture stimulation has been taken as evidence for the possible involvement of the cerebral cortex in mediating the effect of acupuncture,[11] although this suppression of evoked potential might well be the result of a blockade of ascending nociceptive pathways at the brain stem level.[71] Detailed studies reveal that the role of the cerebral cortex in pain and analgesia is a complex modulatory action rather than a simple inhibition or excitation. Therefore, the effect of electric stimulation of the somatosensory I area (S_I) on the pain threshold of the monkey could be facilitatory or inhibitory,[72] although stimulation of the S_{II} area resulted predominantly in a suppressive effect.[73] The influence of cortical stimulation on the activities of the parafascicularis nucleus was also site dependent: a suppressive influence from the S_I area[74] and a facilitatory influence from the motor area.[51] What is even more complicated is that while the functional activities of the parafascicularis and centromedian nuclei were opposing each other, both were tonically excited by the motor cortex. When the acupuncture signals reached the centromedian nucleus and proceeded further to remove the tonic excitatory influence from the cortex to the parafascicularis nucleus, it also weakened the tonic excitation from the cortex to the centromedian nucleus.[51] The existence of these complicated feedback controls probably made it impossible for the intensity of acupuncture analgesia to reach a level of complete analgesia.

CONCLUSIONS

The mechanism of acupuncture analgesia is to activate the body's pain modulatory system, thereby suppressing the transmission and perception of noxious information at various levels of the central nervous system. A variety of manipulations can be used to activate the pain modulatory system or the endogenous analgesia system, eg, electric stimulation of specific sites in the central nervous system (brain stimulation produced analgesia),[42] strong stressors (stress analgesia),[75] strong noxious stimulus (diffuse noxious inhibitory control, DNIC),[76] transcutaneous electric nerve stimulation (TENS), and the like. Even the analgesia induced by morphine was due, at least in part, to activation of this system.[31,54,55,77] However, acupuncture or electroacupuncture stimulation applied on certain points of the body can be regarded as a more powerful and less stressful means to activate the analgesia system.

Despite the use of acupuncture for thousands of years, much still needs to be done to use this technique to its full extent. In this context, a combination of traditional medical experience with modern scientific technique would be profitable not only for clarification of its mechanisms of action, but also for selection of optimal parameters and sites of stimulation for various therapeutic purposes. In a recent study we found that electroacupuncture of different frequencies was able to activate different opioid systems in the spinal cord of the rat: low frequency (2 Hz) for [Met^5]enkephalin release and high frequency (100 Hz) for dynorphin A release.[78] An optimal combination of electroacupuncture parameters is now under study for maximal release of endogenous opioids in the central nervous system.

The diagram in Figure 70.1 summarizes our current knowledge of the mechanisms of acupuncture analgesia. It can be seen, for example, that the periaqueductal grey of the midbrain is located in the central part of the neuronal circuitry. The influence from higher centers is funneled down directly or through the relay of the habenula to the periaqueductal grey which is the cardinal link of a neuronal loop (mesolimbic loop of analgesia), giving rise to constant control of the pain perception pathways from the spinal cord up to the cerebral cortex.

Although useful in describing a general principle, this kind of sketch has the innate drawback of oversimplification. Division of the pain perception system and pain modulatory system is more ideologic than anatomic, because one and the same nucleus could perform both functions. Thus, the centromedian nucleus, periaqueductal grey, and the nucleus raphe magnus have been implicated as integral parts of the pain modulatory system, yet they contain neurons with typical nociceptive characteristics and could therefore be regarded as part of the pain perception system. Moreover, the mark that indicated excitation could actually be a manifestation of disinhibition. With these limitations in mind, this diagram is presented in the hope that it may stimulate a deeper interest into the complicated mechanisms of acupuncture analgesia and thereby lead to a better understanding of pain and analgesia as a whole.

REFERENCES

1. Research Group of Acupuncture Anesthesia, Peking Medical College: Effect of acupuncture on pain threshold of human skin. *Chin Med J* 1973; 3:151–157.
2. Andersson SA, Ericson T, Holmgren E, Lindqvist G: Electroacupuncture: effect on pain threshold measured with electrical stimulation of teeth. *Brain Res* 1973; 63:393–396.
3. Han JS, Terenius L: Neurochemical basis of acupuncture analgesia. *Ann Rev Pharmacol Toxicol* 1982; 22:193–220.
4. Chapman CR, Gehrig JD, Wilson ME: Acupuncture compared with 33% nitrous oxide for dental analgesia. *Anesthesiology* 1975; 42:532–537.
5. Jiang ZY, Ye Q, Shen YT, Zhu FX, Tang SQ, Liang NJ, Zeng XC: Effects of naloxone on experimental acupuncture analgesia evaluated by sensory decision theory. *Acta Zool Sin* 1978; 24:1–8.
6. Ren MF: Experimental studies of acupuncture analgesia, in Ji Z-P (ed): *Progress in Acupuncture Research.* Beijing, People's Medical Press, 1981, pp 133–141.
7. Han JS, Zhou ZF, Xuan YT: Acupuncture has an analgesic effect in rabbits. *Pain* 1983; 15:83–91.
8. Ren MF, Han JS: Rat tail flick acupuncture analgesia model. *Chin Med J* 1979; 92:576–582.
9. Dennis SG, Melzack R: Comparison of phasic and tonic pain in animals. *Adv Pain Res Ther* 1979; 3:747–760.
10. Chang HT: Neurophysiological basis of acupuncture analgesia. *Sci Sin* 1978; 21:829–846.
11. Wan YZ, Xu W: The role of the cerebral cortex in acupuncture analgesia: a review. *Acup Res* 1981; 6:1–7.
12. Joint Research Group from Xian Medical College, Shangdong Medical College and Anhuei Traditional Medical College: Morphological studies on the structures under acu-point related with needling sensation. *Acupunct Anesth* 1979; 2:59–64.
13. Lin WZ, Xu MH, Wang ZY, Dai JD, Chen GM, Shen JY: Some observations on structures in certain acupuncture points and their afferent pathways subserving "needling sensations" in humans. National Symposia of Acupuncture and Moxibustion and Acupuncture Anesthesia, Beijing, 1979, pp 417–418.
14. Lu GW: Characteristics of afferent fiber innervation on acupuncture point zusanli. *Am J Physiol* 1983; 245:R606–R612.
15. Chen LS, Tang JS, Yan JQ: Analysis of afferent fibers for acupuncture analgesia. *Kexue Tongbao* 1981; 26:564–569.
16. Wei JY, Feng CC, Chu TS, Chang SC: Observations on discharge of certain deep receptors during acupuncture on the hind leg of cat. *Kexue Tongbao* 1973; 18:184–186.
17. Chiang CY, Liu JY, Chu TH, Pai YH, Chang SC: Studies on spinal ascending pathway for effect of acupuncture analgesia in rabbits. *Sci Sin* 1975; 18:651–658.
18. Melzack R, Wall PD: Pain mechanisms: a new theory. *Science* 1965; 150:971–979.
19. Woolf CJ, Mitchell D, Barrett GD: Antinociceptive effect of peripheral segmental electric stimulation in the rat. *Pain* 1980; 8:237–252.
20. Han JS, Zhang M, Ren MF: The effect of spinal transection on electroacupuncture analgesia and morphine analgesia in the rat. *Kexue Tongbao* 1985; 30:1446–1449.
21. Schmanss C, Hammond DL, Ochi JW, Yaksh TL: Pharmacological antagonism of the antinociceptive effects of serotonin in the rat spinal cord. *Eur J Pharmacol* 1983; 90:349–357.
22. Xie CW, Tang J, Han JS: Central norepinephrine in acupuncture analgesia: differential effects in brain and spinal cord. *Acta Physiol Sin* 1983; 35:186–192.
23. Yaksh TL, Huang SP, Rudy TA, Frederickson RCA: The direct and specific opiate-like effect of met[5]-enkephalin and analogues on the spinal cord. *Neuroscience* 1977; 2:593–596.
24. Yaksh TL, Henry JL: Antinociceptive effect of intrathecally administered human β-endorphin in the rat and cat. *Can J Physiol Pharmacol* 1978; 56:754–759.
25. Han JS, Xie CW: Dynorphin: potent analgesic effect in spinal cord of the rat. *Life Sci* 1982; 31:1781–1783.
26. Han JS, Xie GX, Goldstein A: Analgesia induced by intrathecal injection of dynorphin B in the rat. *Life Sci* 1984; 34:1573–1579.
27. Tang J, Li SJ, Han JS: The role of central 5-hydroxytryptamine in acupuncture analgesia and acupuncture tolerance, in Takagi H, Simon EJ (eds): *Advances in Endogenous and Exogenous Opioids.* Tokyo, Kodansha, 1981, pp 300–302.
28. Höllt V: Multiple endogenous opioid peptides. *Trends Neurosci* 1983; 6:24–26.
29. Han JS, Xie GX, Zhou ZF, Folkesson R, Terenius L: Acupuncture mechanisms in rabbits studied with microinjection of antibodies against β-endorphin, enkephalin and substance P. *Neuropharmacology* 1984; 23:1–5.
30. Han JS: Antibody microinjection technique as a tool to clarify the role of opioid peptides in acupuncture analgesia. *Pain* 1984; 2(suppl):667.
31. Rivot JP, Weil-Fugazza J, Godefroy F, Bineau-Thurotte M, Ory-Lavollee L, Besson JM: Involvement of serotonin in both morphine and stimulation-produced analgesia: electrochemical and biochemical approaches. *Adv Pain Res Ther* 1984; 6:135–150.
32. Du HJ, Kitahata LM, Thalhammer JG, Zimmermann M: Inhibition of nociceptive neuronal response in the cat's spinal dorsal horn by electrical stimulation and morphine microinjection in nucleus raphe magnus. *Pain* 1984; 19:249–258.
33. Chang KL, Wei CP, Lin YM, Chou LP, Chou LH, Lo CL, Chang TC: Effect of stimulation of midbrain raphe nuclei on the discharge of pain sensitive cells in nucleus parafascicularis of thalamus and its significance in acupuncture analgesia. *Acta Physiol Sin* 1979; 31:209–218.
34. Kang BE, Zhou ZF, Han JS: The involvement of serotonergic transmission in periaqueductal grey for electroacupuncture analgesia and morphine analgesia in rabbits. *Kexue Tongbao* 1984; 29:116–122.
35. Xuan YT, Zhou ZF, Wu WY, Han JS: Antagonism of acupuncture analgesia and morphine analgesia by cinanserin injected into nucleus accumbens and habenula in the rabbit. *J Beijing Med Coll* 1982; 14: 23–26.
36. Xu DY, Zhou ZF, Han JS: Amygdaloid serotonin and endogenous opioid substances are important for mediating electroacupuncture analgesia and morphine analgesia. *Acta Physiol Sin* 1985; 37:162–171.
37. Westlund KN, Bowker RM, Ziegler MG, Coulter JD: Noradrenergic projections to the spinal cord of the rat. *Brain Res* 1983; 263:15–31.
38. Du HJ, Chao YF: Effect of destruction or stimulation of locus coeruleus on inhibition of viscero-somatic reflex activities. *Acta Physiol Sin* 1979; 31:153–161.
39. Zhou ZF, Du MY, Wu WY, Han JS: Effect of intracerebral injection of clonidine or phentolamine on acupuncture analgesia in rabbits. *Acta Physiol Sin* 1981; 33:1–7.
40. Pan JC, Jin GZ, Hong GX: Receptors involved in potentiation of electroacupuncture analgesia by microinjection of noradrenaline into hypothalamus in rats. *Acta Physiol Sin* 1982; 34:179–184.
41. Tsou K, Jang CS: Studies on the site of analgesic action of morphine by intracerebral microinjection. *Sci Sin* 1964; 13:1099–1109.
42. Reynolds DV: Surgery in the rat during electrical analgesia induced by focal brain stimulation. *Science* 1969; 164:444–445.
43. Han JS, Fei H, Zhou ZF: Met-enkephalin-Arg[6]-Phe[7]-like immunoreactive substances mediate electroacupuncture analgesia in the periaqueductal grey of the rabbit. *Brain Res* 1984; 322:289–296.
44. Han JS, Xie GX: Dynorphin: important mediator for electroacupuncture analgesia in the spinal cord of the rabbit. *Pain* 1984; 18:367–376.
45. Zhou ZF, Xie GX, Han JS: Substance P produces analgesia by releasing enkephalins in periaqueductal grey of the rabbit. *Kexue Tongbao* 1983; 28:1716.
46. Wang S, Xie L: The facilitatory effect of habenular nucleus on locus coeruleus. *Acta Physiol Sin* 1981; 33:66–73.
47. Wang S, Jian Y, Xiao JS, Liu MZ, Liu SP: Spontaneous discharge of habenula and its inhibitory action on nucleus raphe magnus. *Kexue Tongbao* 1980; 25:36–39.
48. Bloom F, Battenberg E, Rossier J, Ling N, Guillemin R: Neurons containing β-endorphin in rat brain exist separately from those containing enkephalin: immunocytochemical studies. *Proc Natl Acad Sci USA* 1978; 75:1591–1595.
49. Cheng QS, Xie CW, Tang J, Han JS: Effect of electroacupuncture on the β-endorphin content in different brain areas of the rat. *Kexue Tongbao* 1983; 28:312–315.
50. Gao YS, Ku YH: Mechanism underlying the inhibitory effect of rat nucleus arcuatus hypothalami on unit discharge of locus coeruleus with reference to electroacupuncture. *Acta Physiol Sin* 1983; 35:163–171.
51. Chang HT: Pain related neuronal discharges and their modification by activity of centrum medianum. *Jpn J EEG EMG* 1981; Suppl:133–136.
52. Zhang DX, Gu XG, Shan HY: Effects of lesions in the nucleus accumbens on acupuncture analgesia in rats. *Acta Physiol Sin* 1978; 30:95–97.
53. Zhou ZF, Du MY, Wu WY, Jian Y, Han JS: Effect of intracerebral microinjection of naloxone on acupuncture and morphine analgesia in the rabbit. *Sci Sin* 1981; 24:1166–1178.
54. Xuan YT, Shi YS, Zhou ZF, Han JS: A serial connection of serotonergic and enkephalinergic mechanism on nucleus accumbens. *Kexue Tongbao* 1985; 30:304–307.
55. Han JS, Xuan YT: Serotonergic pathway from periaqueductal grey to nucleus accumbens. *Kexue Tongbao* 1985; 30:1352–1354.
56. Liu X: The role of nucleus raphe magnus in acupuncture analgesia and its control by some higher analgesic structures. *Acupunct Res* 1984; 9:91–100.
57. Mo WY, Chou YF, Wang GN: Analgesia by injection of morphine and antagonism of electroacupuncture analgesia by injection of naloxone into septal area of rabbits. *Acta Pharmacol Sin* 1982; 3:150–154.
58. Fu JY, Fu QG, Wang S: Inhibitory effect of caudate nucleus region on nociceptive discharges of lateral habenular nucleus in rats. *Acta Physiol Sin* 1982; 34:400–405.
59. Zhai XZ, Chen GB, Mo WY, Jiang CC, Li SC, Xu MF: Role of amygdala in acupuncture analgesia. Experimental report in animals. *Acupunct Res* 1981; 6:215–220.
60. Zhou ZF, Xuan YT, Han JS: Analgesic effect of morphine injected into habenula, nucleus accumbens or amygdala of rabbits. *Acta Pharmacol Sin* 1984; 5:150–153.

61. Chen GB, Jiang CC, Li SC: The role of the human caudate nucleus in acupuncture analgesia. *Acupunct Electrother Res* 1982; 7:255–265.
62. Research Group of Acupuncture Anesthesia, Shanghai Institute of Physiology: The possible role of caudate nucleus in acupuncture analgesia. *Chin Med J* 1975; 5:340–342.
63. Guan XM, Wang CY, Zhang YW, Zeng YY, Liu XH: Studies on the acetylcholine turnover in the brain of rat during acupuncture analgesia. *Acupunct Res* 1982; 7:137–144.
64. Lu WX, Zeng DY, Xu SF: Effect of cholinergic activity in caudate nucleus on acupuncture analgesia. *Acupunct Res* 1983; 8:109–113.
65. Zhou GZ, Wang DL, Xu SF: The role of dopamine system in caudate nucleus on acupuncture analgesia in rabbit. *Kexue Tongbao* 1981; 26:951–953.
66. Xie CW, Zhang WG, Hong XJ, Han JS: Relation between the content of central met- and leu-enkephalin and the analgesic effect of electroacupuncture in rats. *Acta Physiol Sin* 1984; 36:192–197.
67. Lu RL, Pan XP: The relationship between acupuncture analgesia and opioid peptides or inorganic ions in rabbit caudate nucleus. *Acupunct Res* 1984; 9:65–71.
68. Yuan H, Han JS: Electroacupuncture accelerates the biogenesis of central enkephalins in the rat. *Acta Physiol Sin* 1985; 37:265–273.
69. Rogers DK, McKenzie JS: Regional difference within the caudate nucleus for suppression of extralemniscal thalamic units. *Brain Res* 1973; 56:345–349.
70. Dong WC, He LF: Effect of microiontophoretic opiates and caudate stimulation on neurons in periaqueductal grey (PAG). *Acta Physiol Sin* 1982; 34:63–70.
71. Shen E, Ma WH, Lan C: Involvement of descending inhibition in the effect of acupuncture on the splanchnically evoked potential in the orbital cortex of cat. *Sci Sin* 1978; 21:677–685.
72. Han XW, Huang ZZ, Lu YY: Influence of intracortical stimulation or cryogenic blockade of somatosensory area I upon the operant conditioning and acupuncture analgesia in monkeys. *Acta Physiol Sin* 1982; 34:165–171.
73. Huang ZZ, Han XW, Xie HM, Zeng YC: Influence of intracortical microstimulation of somatosensory area II upon operant avoidance conditioning and acupuncture analgesia in Rhesus monkeys. *Acta Physiol Sin* 1983; 35:286–294.
74. Hong YG, Dai TL, Zang QZ, Lu ZZ: Effect of somatosensory cortex on nociceptive discharges of parafascicular neurons in rabbit's thalamus. *Acta Physiol Sin* 1983; 35:156–162.
75. Lewis JW, Terman GW, Shavit Y, Nelson LR, Liebeskind JC: Neural, neurochemical and hormonal bases of stress-induced analgesia. *Adv Pain Res Ther* 1984; 6:277–288.
76. Le Bars D, Dickenson AH, Besson JM: Diffuse noxious inhibitory controls (DNIC) I. Effects on dorsal horn convergent neurons in the rat. *Pain* 1979; 6:283–304.
77. Xie GX, Xu H, Han JS: Involvement of spinal met-enkephalin and dynorphin in descending morphine analgesia. *Acta Physiol Sin* 1984; 36:457–463.
78. Han JS, Xie GX, Ding XZ, Fan SG: High and low frequency electroacupuncture analgesia are mediated by different opioid peptides. *Pain* 1984; 2(suppl):543.

71 Cardiac Surgery Under Acupuncture Anesthesia

Yi-shan Wang, MD and Chun-xiu Ye, MD

The history of acupuncture for relieving pain in Chinese ancient traditional medicine can be traced back to the Warring State period (战国) more than 2,000 years ago.[1] However, not until the late 1950s was acupuncture accepted as a method of anesthesia. The first type of operation successfully performed under acupuncture anesthesia was tonsillectomy.[2] Since then, acupuncture anesthesia had been widely employed in various operations, including thoracic operations such as lobectomy and mitral commissurotomy.

CLOSED MITRAL COMMISSUROTOMY UNDER ACUPUNCTURE ANESTHESIA

Over the past 25 years, acupuncture anesthesia has been applied in a series of selected cases of mitral stenosis undergoing closed mitral commissurotomy in Ren-Ji Hospital, Shanghai, China. The results were comparable to those of conventional general anesthesia with fewer cardiac arrhythmias during the operation and fewer respiratory complications postoperatively. However, it is advisable not to use acupuncture anesthesia for those who are emotionally unstable or have severe cardiac lesions.

PREOPERATIVE PREPARATIONS

One to two weeks of preoperative preparation, including a thorough interview with the patient explaining all the details of the disease, are usually necessary. It is important to inform the patient of the main operative procedures and to instruct him carefully in how to react during specific surgical maneuvers. For instance, he should wink or open his eyes if he is asked. Also, the physicians should answer all of the patient's questions no matter how unusual. In general, patients must have complete confidence in the physicians and the hospital and also be kept stable and quiet preoperatively. This can only be achieved by an intimate and sincere interview between the physician and patient.

Of utmost importance is an abdominal breathing exercise which should be practiced right after admission. The patient is instructed to take a deep breath ten times a minute for 30 minutes each time with a sandbag weighing 5 to 10 kg on his chest. This exercise is repeated several times a day until the patient is well accustomed to it and can breathe quietly depending largely on his diaphragmatic motion. This is important because the patient can be instructed to shift chest respiration immediately into abdominal breathing when the chest is opened during the operation, so that the sense of oppression due to unilateral open pneumothorax can be lessened greatly.

Premedication is more or less the same as that in conventional general anesthesia except for the minimized dosage. Intramuscular sodium phenobarbital is usually given in a dose of 2 mg/kg of body weight, or diazepam, 0.2 mg/kg, given two hours before operation. Pethidine is given intramuscularly, 0.5 to 1.0 mg/kg 15 minutes before operation. Scopolamine is used to reduce saliva secretion with better results if used together with pethidine or diazepam; the usual dose is 0.3 to 0.4 mg/kg intramuscularly one hour before operation. Cortisone, 25 to 50 mg intramuscularly, should be given the night before and two hours before the operation in those who are in a state of adrenocortical deficiency or have had cortisone therapy for a prolonged period. Sometimes, droperidol, 50 to 100 mg/kg, should be given before the incision in nervous patients; however, its hypotensive effects should always be kept in mind.

PRESCRIPTION OF NEEDLING POINTS

The prescription of the needling points follows the ancient theory of channels and collaterals. It was taught by an ancient acupuncturist that, "wherever the Channels and Collaterals pass, the keynote of treatment lies." The prescription depends largely on experiences of the acupuncturists after extensive clinical trials. Two sets of points of equal efficiency were chosen for closed mitral commissurotomy by the Department of Anesthesiology of Ren-Ji Hospital (Table 71.1).

It is customary to use the patient's own finger as a measuring unit to localize an acupuncture point. One Cun (unit) represents the distance between the ends of the creases of the two interphalangeal joints at the side of the middle finger (Figure 71.1). The location of the different points for closed mitral commissurotomy is shown in Figure 71.2.

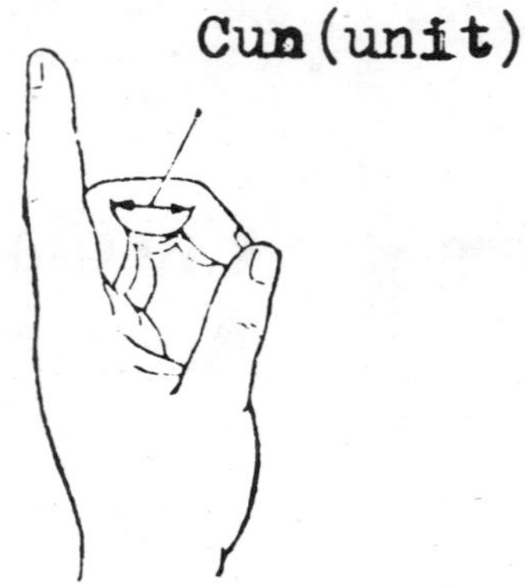

Figure 71.1. Measurement of Cun (unit).

STIMULATION

The usual method of needling is manual twirling of needles together with up-and-down motion. The needles should puncture the skin swiftly over the selected points vertically at first, then tilted and deepened gradually toward the direction of the points. However, because the points prescribed for closed mitral commissurotomy are in close vicinity of the surgical field, electrical stimulation is thus preferable. Either a type G6805 or type BT-701 electrical stimulator can be used; it produces biphasic triangular or square waves with a wave width of 0.5 to 2.0 ms. The frequency is set at 120 to 180 per minute. The extent of stimulation depends on the patient's tolerance and is individualized. Too strong stimulations probably would place more strain on the patient and not infrequently induce tachycardia. If strong stimulation is necessary, the frequency should be reduced. The usual induction time is 20 minutes.

MEDICATION DURING OPERATION

Various auxiliary drugs should be given according to the patient's reaction during different stages of the operation. Usually a few milliliters of 1% lidocaine is used to block the intercostal nerves if the patient complains of pain on retraction of the ribs. Three to 4 ml of 1% lidocaine should be instilled into the pericardial cavity before its incision to reduce the irritability of the heart. Endotracheal tubes should routinely be kept at hand if signs of early respiratory distress are noted; however, this seldom occurs. The anesthetist should never hesitate to intubate the patient and the artificial respirator can be installed within a minute. If the operation lasts more than two hours, it is reasonable to give an additional dose of pethidine (50% of the previous preoperative dose).

Table 71.1. Acupuncture Points for Closed Mitral Commissurotomy

Set	Major Point	Adjunct Points
1	Neiguan	Hegu, Lieque, Zhigou, or Sanyanglou (bilateral)
2	Neiguan	Hegu, Binao

MONITORING

Acupuncture itself seldom or never induces any physiologic disturbances in closed mitral commissurotomy. However, monitoring is always necessary in any cardiac operation; routine, simple, and noninvasive measures such as electrocardiography, blood pressure measurements, and central venous pressure monitoring through the internal jugular veins are used in every case.

THE OPERATION

The operation should strictly follow the most fundamental principle of surgery, that is, minimal trauma to tissue. It should always be borne in mind that the keys to the success of this operation are speed and gentleness. It should be performed preferably by experienced surgeons or young surgeons under the guidance of experienced hands. Subcutaneous bleeding can be minimized by local infiltration of 20 ml of saline with 1 to 2 drops of 1:1000 adrenaline over the incisional line. No electrocautery should be used. The incision down into the muscular layer is made within a second. Hot pads are used to control oozing. No unnecessary blunt dissections and only a sharp cut are allowed. A pinpoint hole is made on the intercostal pleura and immediately covered with the fingertip. The patient is then instructed to do the abdominal breathing exercise. The fingertip is removed for 2 to 3 seconds to expose the hole and then covered again. This maneuver is repeated several times, so that open pneumothorax takes place gradually until the patient is accustomed to it. The ribs are gently retracted; if there is any complaint of pain or discomfort, intercostal nerve block, as already mentioned, is performed. Retraction of the ribs should be carried out gradually in a stepwise fashion. The operating field should be wide enough to admit the surgeon's hands and no more than that. The left lung is gently retracted by hand to expose the heart. After instillation of lidocaine into the pericardial cavity, the pericardium is incised and the commissurotomy is carried out as usual with definite steadiness, swiftness, and gentleness (Figure 71.3). There is nothing of particular

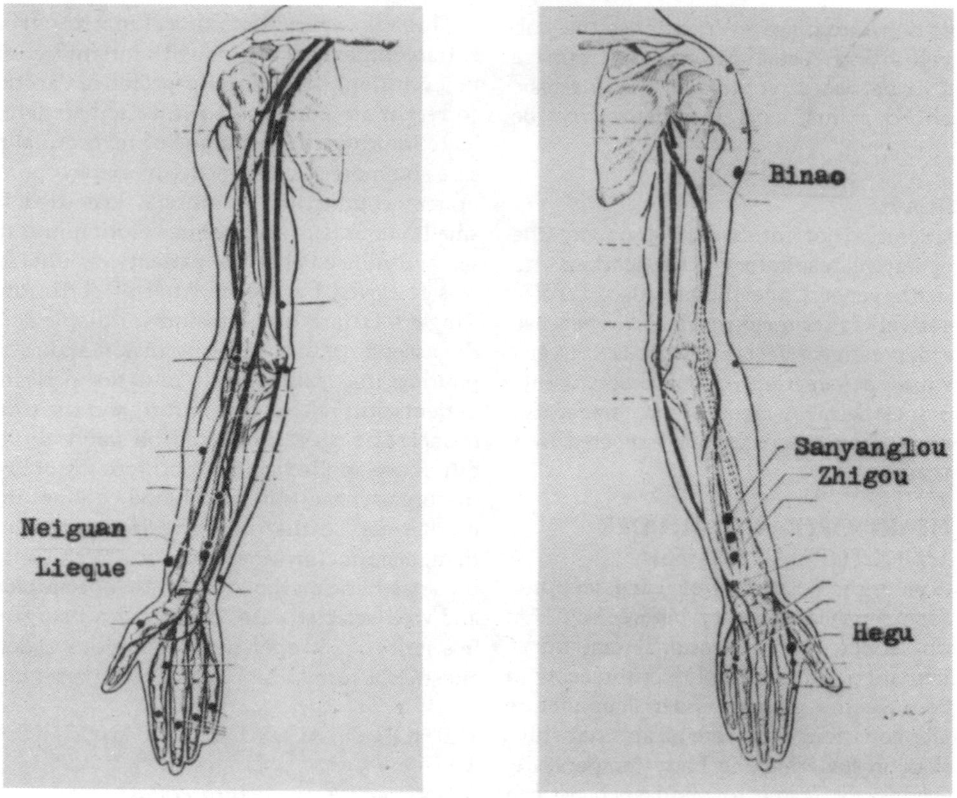

Figure 71.2. Anterior (*left*) and posterior (*right*) surfaces of the forearm showing the various points. *Neiguan:* Located at the anterior surface of the lower forearm, 2 Cun above the wrist, between the tendons of the palmaris longus and flexor carpi radialis. *Hegu:* Located at the posterior aspect of the hand between the first and second metacarpi (the anatomic snuff box), near the radial aspect of the middle point of the second metacarpus. *Lieque:* 1.5 Cun above the transverse crease of the wrist, external to the radial artery just above the radial styloid. *Zhigou:* Located at the posterior aspect of the forearm, 3 Cun above the wrist, between the ulnar and radius bones. *Sanyanglou:* 1 Cun above the Zhigou point. *Binao:* 7 Cun above the elbow, posterior to the apex of the deltoid muscle.

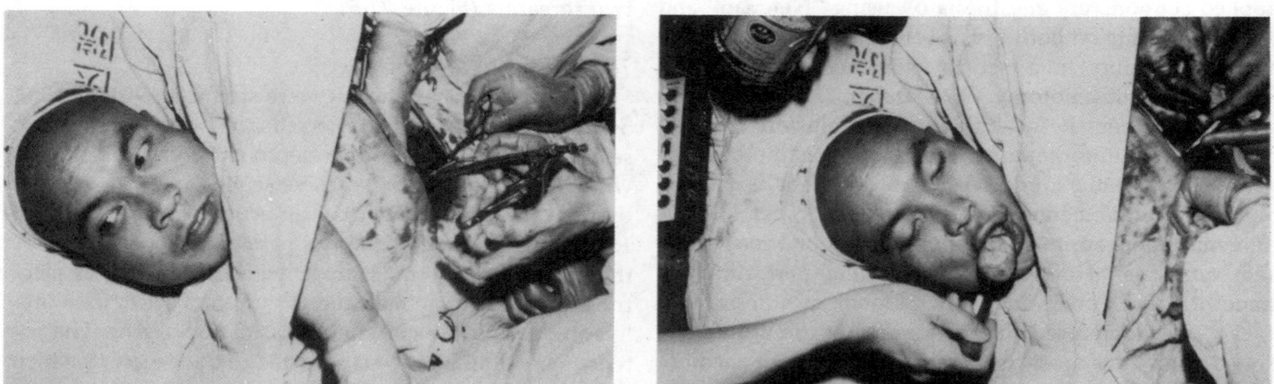

Figure 71.3. Closed mitral commissurotomy under acupuncture anesthesia: *left*, during transventricular dilation; *right*, during oral feeding in the middle of the operation. (From Cheng TO: Cardiology in the People's Republic of China, in Russek HI (ed): *New Horizons in Cardiovascular Practice.* Baltimore, University Park Press, 1975, pp 1–27. Reproduced with permission.)

note in closure of the wound; however, because the stab wound over the eighth intercostal space for the drainage tube is supposed to be out of control of the analgesic area of the prescribed points, local anesthetics may be necessary.

POSTOPERATIVE CARE

Because the patient is not intubated, obviously the chances of postoperative respiratory complications are less than those with general anesthesia. Also, cardiac function postoperatively is resumed much faster because the usual cardiac depressive effects of various conventional anesthetics are not experienced by those patients with acupuncture anesthesia. A smooth and uneventful postoperative course could reasonably be expected in a great majority of cases.

OPEN HEART OPERATION UNDER ACUPUNCTURE ANESTHESIA

We began to explore the possibility of using acupuncture anesthesia for open heart surgery before 1970. On our cardiothoracic service the conventional method of extracorporeal circulation was routinely combined with blood cooling. Because the patient under acupuncture anesthesia is totally conscious, we were afraid that shivering could develop on lowering the body temperature. Many other questions also came to mind such as: can patients tolerate intracardiac manipulations or electric defibrillation? Can respiration be maintained without embarrassment when the mediastinum or pleural cavity is accidentally entered? Fortunately, we were handicapped by these problems not long before solutions were found. We recalled that under acupuncture anesthesia patients felt nothing while intracardiac manipulation was applied during commissurotomy for mitral stenosis. Moreover, we reviewed the history of a female patient with sudden cardiac arrest postoperatively. She was kept conscious by efficient cardiac massage, and she could even converse with physicians resuscitating her heart. Sinus rhythm resumed after several electrical shocks for defibrillation, and the patient recovered uneventfully. Then, to determine whether the patient could tolerate mediastinotomy, we applied acupuncture anesthesia by using "Neiguan" and "Lieque" points on both wrists for resection of thymoma and thymectomy in a patient with myasthenia gravis through a mediastinotomy. On March 8, 1972, we applied acupuncture anesthesia with inflow occlusion of caval blood under normothermia through a mediastinotomy for valvulotomy under direct vision in a patient with pulmonary valvular stenosis with complete success. Dissection and taping around superior and inferior venae cavae and subsequent inflow occlusion were performed as smoothly as if done under conventional anesthesia.

We were therefore fully convinced by the aforementioned facts that open heart operation through mediastinotomy under normothermia could be performed under acupuncture anesthesia to correct intracardiac defects. Therefore, after adequate preoperative preparation, the first patient, a girl of 15 years with trilogy of Fallot, was successfully operated on with extracorporeal circulation under normothermia and acupuncture anesthesia on April 19, 1972.

Through a period of clinical practice of normothermic extracorporeal circulation with intermittent ischemic aortic occlusion, the desire for prolonged aortic occlusion to correct more complicated intracardiac defects prompted us to improve the technique of myocardial protection for safe and more secure practice of extracorporeal circulation under acupuncture anesthesia. We tried instillation of small amounts of iced saline solution into the pericardial sac and noticed that the patient was unaware of it. This was followed by another trial of perfusion of 0° to 4°C Ringer's lactate or potassium cardioplegic solution into the ascending aorta after occlusion and at the same time pouring iced saline slush into the pericardial sac. The patients still felt no discomfort, and the time allowed for intracardiac operation could be safely prolonged. In addition, we applied mild hypothermia (not lower than 33°C [nasopharyngeal] by mild blood cooling) instead of normothermia, so that no shivering was noted. Ever since then, acupuncture anesthesia has been considered one of the anesthetic methods that might be employed in simple and well-selected cases of open heart surgery. Experience in a series of 250 open heart operations under acupuncture anesthesia forms the basis of this presentation.

METHOD OF ACUPUNCTURE ANESTHESIA

Selection of Acupuncture Points

Many points on both upper and lower extremities in the course of the proper meridian leading to the chest had been chosen for acupuncture to control chest pain. Many points on the ears reflect the anatomic distribution of the viscera and organs of the human body (Figure 71.4). Therefore, selection of ear points was based on the theory of "Zang-Shiang" (藏象). In our practice most point groups chosen for operation were prescribed with combinations of points on both ears and extremities. Ten groups of various combinations of points had been applied in our hospital. In the order of sequence, the sixth group of points was the most effectual one,[3] and it was chosen in most cases. It is comprised of the "thorax," "neck," "kidney," and "lung" points on the left ear lobe (Figure 71.5) and "Neiguan" and "Lieque" points on the two forearms (Figure 71.6).

Technique of Needling

The fields of acupuncture were sterilized with alcohol. Stainless steel needles of selected sizes were inserted into selected points to the proper depth and twirled manually with a rapid up-and-down traverse motion of the needles by the thumb and fingers of an acupuncturist for about 15 minutes for the induction period. The needles were then connected by small clips on electric wires to an electrical stimulator, a small direct current battery unit delivering a pulsatile current at 150 to 200 c/min. The intensity of stimulation was adjusted to the degree to which the patient could adapt (Figure 71.7).

PREOPERATIVE PREPARATION

It was most important after admission to instruct the patient to practice the abdominal breathing exercise. A sandbag weighing 5 to 10 kg was placed on the front of the chest. With the patient in the supine position, slow

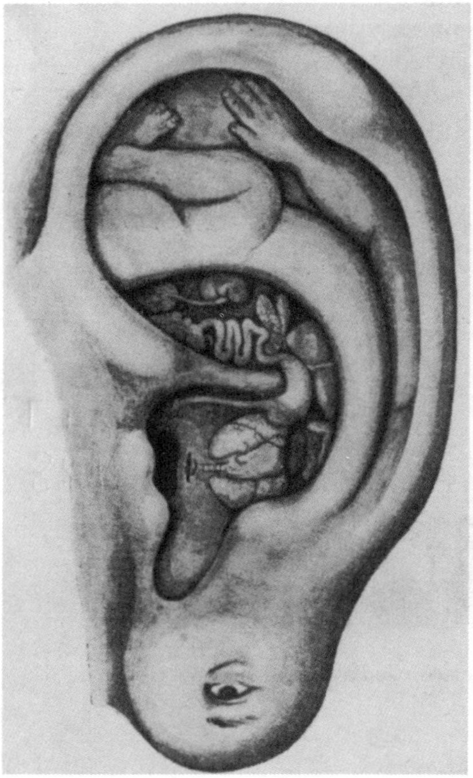

Figure 71.4. Distribution of body organs at specific sites on the auricle.

breathing with the abdomen at a frequency of ten times per minute was practiced to accommodate the oppressive sensation that usually occurs after splitting of the sternum. Thus, the patient actually breathed by a diaphragmatic motion. The patient was then interviewed, acupuncture anesthesia was described, and the operative procedure generally discussed in order to relieve the patient's anxiety and to secure his or her cooperation. A preoperative needling trial applied to the patient was an important step in helping the patient adapt to acupuncture stimulation.

Other preparative measures were similar to those carried out in ordinary open heart anesthesia.

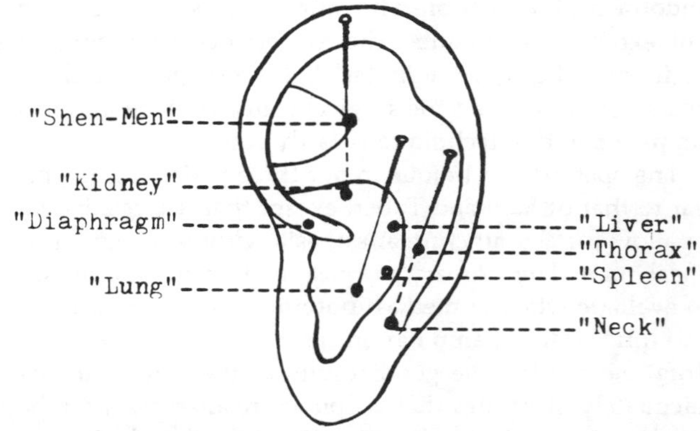

Figure 71.5. Bilateral ear points used: "Shen-Men" through "Kidney," "Lung," "Thorax" through "Neck."

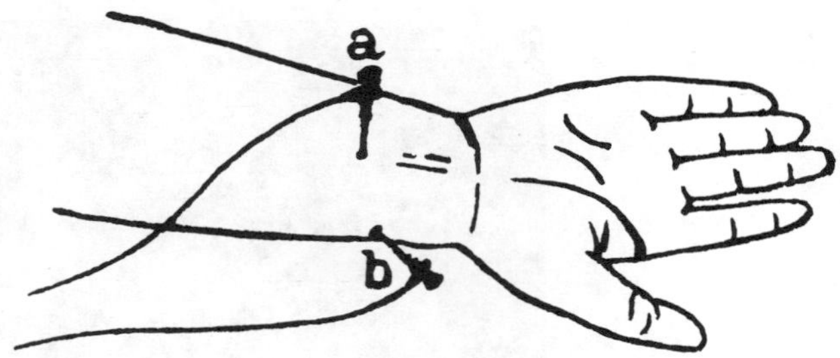

Figure 71.6. Acupuncture points on forearm: (a) "Neiguan" point; (b) "Lieque" point.

SUPPLEMENTARY MEDICATION

Sodium phenobarbital 2 mg/kg was given intramuscularly two hours before operation, and pethidine 1 mg/kg, not exceeding 50 mg, was administered intravenously 15 minutes before skin incision. An additional dose of pethidine 20 to 30 mg or fentanyl 0.1 to 0.2 mg may be necessary before splitting the sternum or closing the wound.

Local infiltration of 1:200,000 adrenaline-saline solution at the incision line was employed to reduce bleeding so that electrocauterization of the skin and subcutaneous tissue might be reduced. Early in this series 0.25% to 0.5% lidocaine solution in a small dose was used to infiltrate the incision line to relieve pain. As the technique of acupuncture anesthesia improved, its application was nearly abandoned.

DIRECT VISION PULMONARY VALVULOTOMY UNDER NORMOTHERMIA AND ACUPUNCTURE ANESTHESIA

Needling Points Selected

Bilateral ear points included "Shen-Men" through "Kidney," "Lung," and "Thorax" through "Neck" (Figure 71.5). Bilateral body points were the "Futu" points (Figure 71.8).

Technique of Operation

The patient was placed in the supine position with the upper half of the body elevated 20° and the left side of the body 15° higher. After skin sterilization, the third through the sixth intercostal nerves at both midclavicular lines were infiltrated with 1% lidocaine solution, 2 ml to each space; a similar dose was infiltrated into the suprasternal notch and infraxiphoid process area. A mediastinotomy was made with an electric motor saw, electric cauterization was avoided as much as possible, longitudinally incised pericardial flaps were gently pulled up and sewed to the presternal tissue, and sternal parts were gradually spread. Superior and inferior venae cavae were dissected carefully and gently and tapes were wound around them. The anterior wall of the dilated main pulmonary artery trunk was partially clamped, four traction stitches were placed, and a 2 cm incision was made between these stitches. Superior and inferior vena caval blood inflow was occluded in sequence by tightening the tapes, which usually took 10 s. After another 10 s, the pulmonary artery occlusion clamp was removed, and the

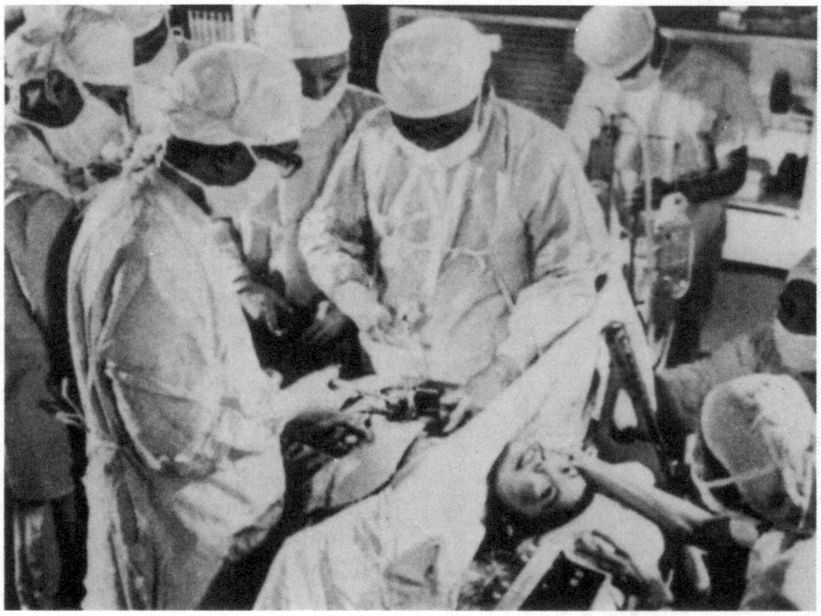

Figure 71.7. Open heart surgery in progress; acupuncture needles on wrist connected by electric wires to an electrical stimulator.

incised edges of the pulmonary arterial wall were gently retracted apart. The assistant grasped the stenosed valve edge and pulled it up into direct vision, and the operator incised the stenosed valve at its commissures. Blood gushing out of the right ventricle was sucked continuously into a sterile bottle containing citrate solution and transfused back into the patient through a venous route. Thereafter, an assistant removed the superior vena caval occlusion, the first assistant gently pulled superior and inferior traction stitches, while the surgeon occluded the pulmonary artery incision using curved nontraumatic clamps as the blood gushed out, so that air was expelled from the right ventricle. The inferior vena caval occlusion was gradually relieved, usually one minute after relief of the superior vena caval occlusion. The anesthetist should have a mask on hand for assisted ventilation, because after this intracardiac procedure the patient's respiration can become shallow and slow. After careful hemostasis the pericardium was loosely brought together by a few stitches, the sternal spreader was gently and slowly removed, and the sternum was approximated with stainless steel wires. Finally, the skin incision was sewed.

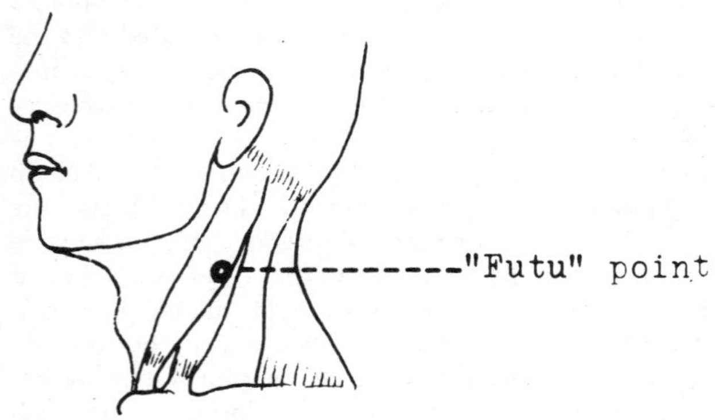

Figure 71.8. "Futu" point located at the middle of the posterior border of the sternocleidomastoid muscle.

Clinical Material

Three patients, two female and one male, aged 14, 15, and 22, were operated on with this technique between March 8, 1972 and July 11, 1972. The diagnosis, pathology, inflow occlusion time, and perioperative status are given in Table 71.2. The effect of acupuncture anesthesia in these three patients was graded as excellent, good, and good, respectively. All recovered quite well and were discharged uneventfully in about 10 to 14 days.

Comments

Lam and Taber[4] in 1959 reported on a simple technique for direct vision pulmonary valvulotomy which was carried out under general anesthesia with normothermia and endotracheal intubation. The inflow occlusion time could not exceed two minutes, the longest occlusion time in their series being 1.5 minutes. If the preoperative diagnosis is accurate, and the surgical team is competent, this simple operative technique is fairly safe.

The operative technique in our three patients was similar to that of Lam and Taber, except that it was adapted to allow for acupuncture anesthesia without an endotracheal tube. The primary purpose of this technique was to evaluate whether mediastinotomy and intrapericardial and intracardiac manipulation can be carried out without drug anesthesia. The good results in the three patients adequately illustrates that acupuncture anesthesia can be employed in such a major operative procedure instead of conventional anesthesia.

Table 71.2. Clinical Data in Three Patients With Pulmonary Stenosis Operated on Under Acupuncture Anesthesia

Case	Diagnosis	Size of Stenosed Orifice of PV (cm^2)	Size After Valvulotomy (cm^2)	Occlusion Time of SVC Flow	Time (minutes) of Assisted Ventilation	Consciousness	Immediate Response	Postoperative Appetite	Effect of Acupuncture Anesthesia
1	Trilogy of Fallot	0.4	1.5	1′10″	5	Temporary loss; 20 min later, fully recovered	Pupils contracted; temporary apnea	Liquids day of operation	Excellent
2	Simple pulmonary stenosis	0.5	1.8	1′25″	9	Conscious throughout	Pupils contracted; temporary apnea	Liquids day of operation, semiliquid diet 2nd day	Good
3	Simple pulmonary stenosis	1.2	2.5	1′20″	12	Conscious throughout	Temporary apnea	Liquids day of operation semiliquid diet 3rd day	Good

PV = pulmonary valve; SVC = superior vena cava.

OPEN HEART OPERATIONS WITH EXTRACORPOREAL CIRCULATION

Needling Points Selected

Left ear points included the "Thorax," "Neck," "Kidney," and "Lung" (Figure 71.5). Bilateral body points were "Neiguan" and "Lieque" (Figure 71.6).

Technique of Operation

The surgical procedure was basically the same as that in standardized open heart operations. However, under acupuncture anesthesia the patient is conscious, so that handling of tissue and operative manipulation of bone, heart, or great vessels should be done with extreme care and gentleness. The general principle is that all maneuvers should be steady, accurate, gentle, and speedy. Rough handling is strictly forbidden. Electrocauterization might be avoided if bleeding from skin and subcutaneous tissue can be prevented by infiltration of adrenaline-saline solution. Suprasternal and subxiphoid spaces are sensitive to blunt separation, so sharp dissection is preferred. Spreading and retraction on sternal parts or removal of retractor should be gradual and very gentle. Manipulation of the inferior vena cava and elevation of cardiac apex should not be prolonged; otherwise, low cardiac output may ensue, causing a decrease in blood pressure and loss of consciousness. After the first vena caval tube is inserted, extracorporeal circulation should be started with initially a low but later a gradually increasing perfusion rate. The priming saline solution was pumped into the patient's arterial system at speed slow enough to allow the body to accommodate itself to the effect produced by acute hemodilution; otherwise, blood pressure tended to decrease. The patient could be kept fully conscious only when mean blood pressure was maintained over 50 mm Hg.[5] On many occasions, by closely monitoring blood pressure, we noted that consciousness changed quickly in response to blood pressure fluctuations. The perfusion rate was gradually increased to the calculated level, while the surgeons continued to insert another tube into the other vena cava. The left ventricular venting tube, which is inserted after caval intubation, should be opened only after aortic clamping. Then, 1° to 4°C cardioplegic solution is perfused into the root of the aorta, which was then cross-clamped. Meanwhile, saline ice slush was poured into the pericardial sac. After the intracardiac procedure was completed, the heart was resuscitated. The left ventricle vent was removed before termination of extracorporeal circulation.

The endotracheal tube was inserted in only three patients. Oxygen was administered by nasal tube. As soon as perfusion was stopped, spontaneous respiration usually resumed. Assisted respiration with a mask was applied for a brief interval only in some patients (Figure 71.9).

Perfusion Technique

A Shanghai type II or III heart-lung machine was primed mainly with normal saline balanced solution. Blood was added if necessary. Hemodilution was controlled with a hematocrit in the range of 20% to 25%. The perfusion rate was 60 to 80 ml/kg per minute. Body hypothermia should not be lowered to less than 33°C; otherwise, chilliness and shivering would disturb the patient. If body temperature tends to decrease further, rewarming must begin with the blood heat exchanger.

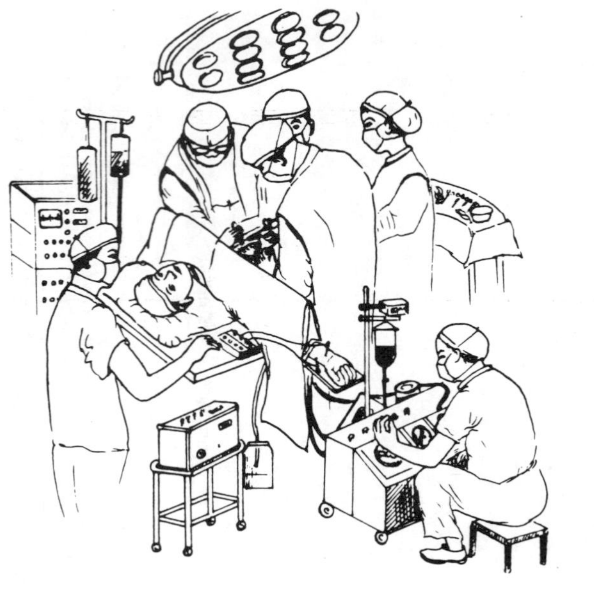

Figure 71.9. Endotracheal tube was not inserted, and oxygen was administered by a nasal tube. The patient was conscious during the open heart procedure.

Clinical Data

A series of 250 patients, 135 male and 115 female, aged 10 to 48 years (average 21.4) were operated on. There were 237 cases of congenital heart disease, most of which were ventricular septal defects. Cyanotic heart disease was mainly tetralogy of Fallot; all of the patients were subjected to total correction. There were 16 patients with ruptured aneurysm of the sinus of Valsalva; among these, ten had coexisting ventricular septal defects, all of which were corrected at one operation. All patients with acquired lesions had rheumatic heart disease with mitral stenosis and atrial fibrillation with heart function graded III to IV; all had a history of thromboembolism. Commissurotomy together with removal of thrombus from the atrium was performed. One patient with mitral stenosis and mild insufficiency was subjected to mitral valvular replacement (Table 71.3).

Time of Perfusion and Occlusion of the Ascending Aorta

Perfusion time lasted 9 to 132 minutes, being greater than 60 minutes in 76 cases and over 100 minutes in 16 cases. In all cases except nine, the ascending aorta was occluded for 6 to 85 minutes, the average occlusion time being 31.8 minutes.

Electroencephalograms

Tracing records in 30 patients during the entire course of perfusion showed predominance of α-waves with sporadic β-waves. During perfusion in some cases there was sporadic or transient θ or δ rhythms. Whenever slowing

Table 71.3. Diagnosis and Surgical Procedure in 250 Cases of Open Heart Operation Under Acupuncture Anesthesia

Diagnosis	Surgical Procedure	Cases (No.)
Ventricular septal defect	Closure by suture or patch	114
Atrial septal defect (ostium secundum)	Closure by suture or patch	45
Atrial septal defect (ostium primum, partial cushion defect)	Closure with patch and suturing of mitral valve cleft	8
Trilogy of Fallot	Pulmonary valvulotomy	
Cyanotic		6
Acyanotic		5
Tetralogy of Fallot	Intracardiac repair	
Cyanotic		14
Acyanotic		19
Pulmonary valvular stenosis	Valvulotomy	8
Right ventricular infundibular stenosis	Infundibulotomy	2
Rupture of aneurysm of sinus of Valsalva	Repair of defect	
With VSD		10
Without VSD		6
Rheumatic mitral stenosis, atrial fibrillation	Open mitral commissurotomy	12
Mitral stenosis and insufficiency	Mitral valve replacement	1

VSD = ventricular septal defect.

of the electroencephalogram wave appeared, a number of patients were found asleep; yet, soon after termination of cardiopulmonary bypass, the patients regained consciousness, and the electroencephalographic pattern gradually returned to normal.[6]

Electrocardiogram

Electrocardiograms of 39 patients during operation were analyzed. There was usually no arrhythmia from the beginning of acupuncture to insertion of the caval tubes. Only a few patients had atrial and ventricular premature beats; otherwise, the ECG was essentially normal. After termination of cardiopulmonary bypass, there was generally sinus rhythm, except in occasional cases in which ventricular extrasystole was the only abnormal rhythm.

Monitoring of Respiratory Wave and Measurements of Ventilatory Volume

Respiratory wave pattern was continuously monitored throughout the course of cardiopulmonary bypass in 40 cases. Respiration wave ceased as soon as bypass was initiated in 24 cases, and reduction in frequency and amplitude of the wave with lengthening of the intervals was observed in 16 cases. Respiratory waves always returned spontaneously and resumed normal patterns within one to two minutes after termination of cardiopulmonary bypass. Ventilatory volumes in terms of total expiratory volume per minute in 35 adult cases were measured at various periods in the operation. The average volumes before operation, during the induction period, after skin incision, during mediastinotomy, after cardiopulmonary bypass, and after operation were 5.24, 5.39, 6.50, 5.50, 5.20, and 5.50 L/min, respectively. These figures illustrate that the ventilatory volumes at various stages of operation without endotracheal intubation or assisted respiration showed no significant changes, even when the chest was opened.

Blood Gas Analysis

Arterial blood samples were collected in 20 cases before, during, and at the termination of bypass and also three hours after operation. Values of pH, buffer base, standard bicarbonate, pO_2, pCO_2, and the like were determined. The mean values ± standard error of these parameters were all within the normal range (Figure 71.10). During

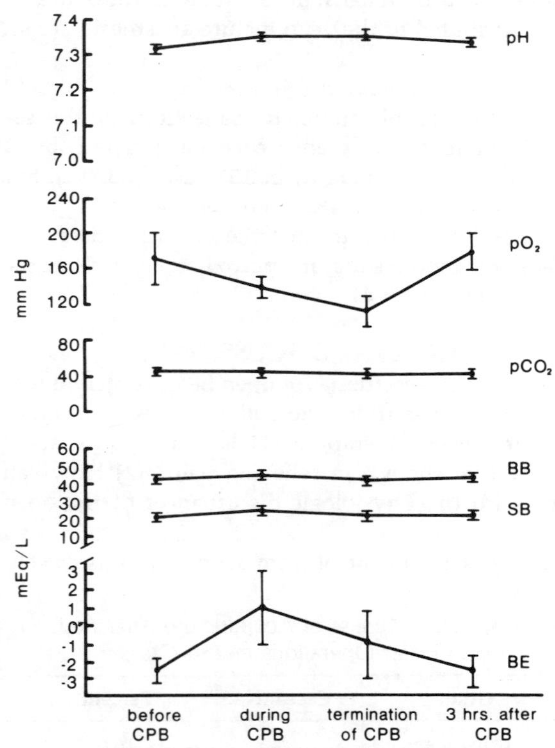

Figure 71.10. Mean values (± standard error) in blood gas analysis in 20 patients before, during, and after cardiopulmonary bypass (CPB). BB = buffer base; SB = standard bicarbonate; BE = base excess.

mediastinotomy, unilateral perforation of the pleura occurred in 41 cases, bilateral perforation in two. Immediate repair by simple suture and covering with reflected pericardial flaps or insertion of an intercostal tube connected to an underwater drainage bottle with suction, or both, was carried out. Mean arterial blood pO_2 in 14 patients with ruptured pleura before institution of cardiopulmonary bypass was 108 mm Hg, arterial blood O_2 saturation was 94%, and mean pH and pCO_2 were 7.3 and 49 mm Hg, respectively; however, latter values returned to normal during bypass or postoperatively. These measurements showed that even with rupture of pleurae during mediastinotomy, there were no untoward effects.

Postoperative Deaths

There were 12 early postoperative deaths, an operative mortality rate of 4.8%. Among these were four patients with ventricular septal defects. One of them died of extradural hematoma, two died of acute renal failure, and one with pulmonary hypertension died of respiratory failure. Four patients with tetralogy of Fallot died of low cardiac output syndrome. Three patients with rheumatic heart disease died postoperatively; one of them with mitral stenosis complicated by cerebral thrombosis died of heart failure. Another patient with heavy calcific mitral stenosis, poor cardiac function, and a history of hemiplegia preoperatively died of low cardiac output syndrome in the immediate postoperative period. The third patient with mitral insufficiency subjected to valve replacement died of disseminated intravascular coagulopathy. One patient with a ruptured aneurysm of the sinus of Valsalva died of renal failure. None of these deaths could be attributed to the acupuncture anesthesia per se.

Effectiveness of Acupuncture Anesthesia

The effectiveness of acupuncture anesthesia in this series of 250 patients was graded excellent (grade I) in 42 cases (16.4%), good (grade II) in 133 cases (53.2%), fair (grade III) in 56 cases (22.4%), and poor (grade IV) in 19 cases (7.6%). Acupuncture anesthesia was satisfactory (excellent and good results) in approximately 70% of the entire series (Table 71.4).

GENERAL DISCUSSION

In acupuncture anesthesia for open heart surgery under extracorporeal circulation, the following two questions are of primary consideration: (1) Is acupuncture anesthesia effective enough in relieving pain? (2) How can we cope with the physiologic disturbances of the open chest?

The effect of pain control from acupuncture is closely related to the choice of acupuncture points, technique of needling, and skill of operative maneuver by the surgeon. In this series we used "Neiguan" and "Lieque" points more frequently and they proved to be most effective. According to the channels and collaterals theory of Chinese traditional medicine and its modern interpretation, the "Neiguan" point is closely related to regulation of the circulatory organs in terms of heart rate and blood pressure. The "Lieque" point is related to pain elimination in the chest wall. The combined needle stimulation of these two points would inhibit thoracic wall pain as well as regulate the physiologic disturbance of the cardiovascular system.

Physiologic disturbance of respiration in the open chest without respiratory control is a major problem in acupuncture anesthesia. However, it is easier for patients when they are in the supine position and a mediastinotomy is used. If the pleura is not opened, negative intrathoracic pressure is maintained. Fixation of pericardial flaps by stitches to the presternal tissue will stabilize the paradoxical motion of the mediastinum. If the preoperative breathing exercise is practiced sufficiently, there should be no significant respiratory disturbance.

Blood gas analysis was performed in 20 patients undergoing open heart operation under acupuncture anesthesia. The PaO_2 was in the normal range, $PaCO_2$ was slightly elevated, and pH was slightly low, but normal values were restored soon after cardiopulmonary bypass was established. No significant change in ventilatory volume was observed pre-, intra-, or postoperatively. Even in cases of pleural perforation, arterial blood PaO_2 and oxygen saturation were within the normal range, although the pH value of central venous blood was low and the PCo_2 high; yet, both became normal soon after the establishment of cardiopulmonary bypass and during the postoperative period.

Acupuncture anesthesia for open heart operations under extracorporeal circulation has definite advantages. It is indicated in patients who are poor risks for general anesthesia because of either a bad reaction to anesthetic drugs or depression of myocardial function. Theoretically, acupuncture may regulate cardiac function and prevent arrhythmias. Moreover, with acupuncture anesthesia we have observed fewer rhythmic problems during open heart operations. Blood pressure and heart rate during operation were more stable. We compared reactions in 191 patients with open heart operations under acupuncture anesthesia with the findings in 100 patients treated under general anesthesia. A decrease in blood pressure requiring vasopressors was observed in 30 patients (30%) in the general anesthesia group before perfusion and 52 patients (52%) after perfusion. In the acupuncture group this need occurred in only 17 patients (8.9%) before perfusion and in 49 (25.6%) after perfusion ($P < 0.01$).

The rate of respiratory complications in these two groups was also compared. In the general anesthesia group there were 23 patients (23%) with respiratory complications including pneumonia, pleuritis, atelectasis, hoarseness of the voice, and the like. There were only six patients (3%) ($P < 0.01$) with such complications in the

Table 71.4. Effectiveness of Acupuncture Anesthesia in Open Heart Operations in 250 Cases

Grade	Cases (No.)	Percent
I. Excellent	42	16.8
II. Good	133	53.2
III. Fair	56	22.4
IV. Poor	19	7.6

acupuncture anesthesia group. The reduction in respiratory complications in the acupuncture anesthesia group was evidently due to elimination of endotracheal intubation. Patients are usually free from cough and expectoration in the postoperative period; therefore, cough-induced pain along the incision is also eliminated.

Gastrointestinal function is less affected by acupuncture anesthesia, which also hastens the patient's recovery.

Although acupuncture anesthesia in open heart surgery is feasible and may be advantageous in carefully selected cases, there are many limitations. It is not practical in young children and highly nervous patients because they do not cooperate well during the operation. This type of anesthesia obviously should not be considered in complicated and prolonged operations. As to perfection of pain elimination, we believe there is room for improvement by better conduction of acupuncture stimulation and the use of supplementary medication.

It is suggested that further research be continued in acupuncture anesthesia. It will remain one type of anesthesia for carefully selected patients requiring thoracic and cardiac surgery and may be conducted with greater success only by a well-organized and trained team of anesthetists and surgeons in the future. We are gratified to note that equally successful results have been reported on non-Chinese patients undergoing cardiac surgery, including coronary bypass operations, in other parts of the world.[7-10]

REFERENCES

1. "Ling Shu Jing"(灵枢經) of "Huang Di Nei Jing"(黄帝内經).
2. Department of ENT and Acupuncture Clinic of the First People's Hospital of Shanghai: Preliminary observation on acupuncture anesthesia applied clinically as a local anesthesia. *Shanghai Chin Trad Med Drug J* 1959; 1:25–27.
3. Ren-Ji Hospital (the Third People's Hospital) of Shanghai Second Medical University: Intracardiac operations with extracorporeal circulation under acupuncture anesthesia. *Sci Sin* 1975; 18:271–280.
4. Lam CR, Taber RE: Simplified technique for direct vision pulmonary valvotomy. *J Thorac Surg* 1959; 38:309–316.
5. Ren-Ji Hospital (the Third People's Hospital) of Shanghai Second Medical University: Open heart operations with extracorporeal circulation under acupuncture anesthesia. *Chin J Surg* 1978; 16:197–199.
6. Ren-Ji Hospital (the Third People's Hospital) of Shanghai Second Medical University: Acupuncture anesthesia for open heart operation under extracorporeal circulation. *Chin Med J* 1976; 2:51–58.
7. Hollinger I, Richter JA, Pongratz W, Baum M: Acupuncture anesthesia for open heart surgery: a report of 800 cases. *An J Chin Med* 1979; 7:77–90.
8. Caracausi SR: Electroacupuncture in thoracic and cardiovascular surgery. *Minerva Med* 1979; 70:3859–3860.
9. Boros M, Matko I, Kovac G, Tanosh T, Tarnoky K: The use of electroacupuncture during operations on the heart. *Anesteziol Reanimatol* 1980; 6:33–35.
10. Kuzmenko VM, Datsenko NYa, Govenko AV: First experiences with acupuncture in cardiosurgical patients. *Klin Khir* 1983; 7:62–63.

72 Circulatory Assist

David Bregman, MD and Peter S. Kaskel

The objective of a circulatory assist device is to provide support under conditions in which the natural circulation is unable to meet the presenting metabolic requirements. Circumstances that can produce a need for circulatory assistance include circulatory shunting, septic shock, and ventricular pump failure secondary to valvular dysfunction or myocardial ischemia. The earliest circulatory assist techniques used powerful pharmacologic agents including inotropic agents (cardiac glycosides and digitalis preparations), diuretic agents (both purine and mercurial), antihypertensive agents, and vasodilators. In addition, antiarrhythmic agents and pacemakers were developed to control abnormal cardiac rhythms. Circulatory assist devices currently refer exclusively to a mechanical technology that augments a compromised circulatory flow. We include in our list the intraaortic balloon pump (IABP), the left ventricular assist device (LVAD), the right ventricular assist device (RVAD), pulmonary artery balloon pumping (PABP), the pulsatile assist device (PAD), and the total artificial heart (TAH). All of these devices come in a myriad of forms, and all require invasive implantation with some associated risks. These devices are only employed in situations in which the foreseen benefits greatly outweigh the risks involved.

INTRAAORTIC BALLOON PUMPING

The intraaortic balloon pump (IABP) currently is the most widely used temporary circulatory assist device. Since its inception in 1962 by Moulopoulos et al,[1] intraaortic balloon pumping has represented a simple and atraumatic approach to support the failing circulation. The principles of counterpulsation come from the pioneering work of Harken,[2] Kantrowitz and Kantrowitz,[3] and Kantrowitz and Mckinnon[4] who, through their efforts, demonstrated that the failing left ventricle indexes could be positively influenced by augmenting the diastolic pressure. Counterpulsation, as employed by the IABP, is accomplished when the balloon is positioned in the descending aorta; the balloon is rapidly inflated in diastole concurrent with closure of the aortic valve, augmenting coronary perfusion pressure seen at the aortic root (Figure 72.1). With the onset of systole, the balloon is rapidly deflated, allowing the forthcoming ventricular ejection to pass unhindered. When the IABP is properly synchronized with the electrocardiogram, the balloon is rapidly deflated during systole and creates a "vacuum" effect, helping the contracting ventricle to expel its volume. Therefore, the mechanism of the balloon pump is twofold: (1) by augmenting diastolic pressure (Figure 72.2), coronary blood flow and myocardial oxygen supply can be increased, which can improve myocardial contractility in ischemic regions; (2) rapid deflation of the balloon in systole reduces impedance in the left ventricle, aiding its contraction and reducing its myocardial oxygen requirements.[5]

After 7 years of experimental research, Kantrowitz et al[6] in 1969 introduced the IABP to the clinical setting for patients in cardiogenic shock. Careful follow-up of such patients showed that mortality rates remained largely unaltered.[7] However, the findings that counterpulsation decreases the extent and severity of ischemic injury[8–11] and opens dormant coronary vessels[12] suggested that counterpulsation ought to be considered in patients with uncomplicated myocardial infarction. This procedure then could minimize the quantity of myocardium that ultimately becomes necrotic.[13] Recently, application of IABP has been expanded to prophylactic management of patients with mild to moderate hemodynamic decompen-

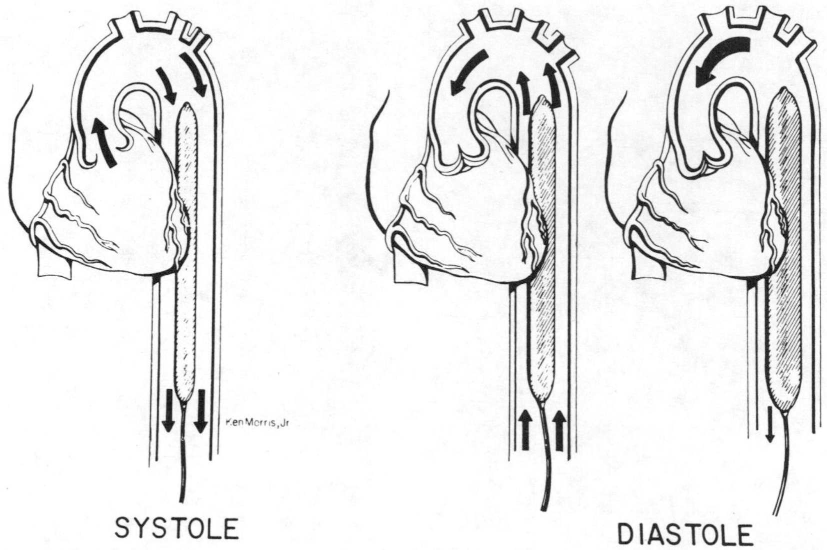

Figure 72.1. Mechanism of action of the percutaneous intraaortic balloon. In systole the balloon is collapsed, causing ventricular unloading; in diastole the balloon inflates, displacing blood toward the coronary tree, thereby improving the balance between myocardial oxygen supply and demand.

sation. At the present time, IABP is widely used for circulatory support in patients with postoperative left ventricular failure, unstable angina refractory to medical treatment, and recurrent myocardial ischemia following acute myocardial infarction.

In 1979 a single-chambered 40-cc percutaneous intraaortic balloon (Figure 72.3) was constructed around a central wire.[14–17] The intraaortic balloon (IAB) was wrapped manually about the wire, which then allowed for percutaneous insertion into the femoral artery. A 12F sheath-dilator assembly was previously inserted into the artery, using a modified Seldinger technique[18] (Figure 72.4). Percutaneous balloon insertion requires approximately five to ten minutes and has been successfully performed in the cardiac catheterization laboratory, coronary care unit, and operating suite. Fluoroscopy during percutaneous IAB insertion is not necessary—many insertions having been performed without it—but it can be of great help, and during a difficult insertion it is indispensable. Difficulties with percutaneous insertion were sometimes encountered in the following circumstances: (1) tortuous vessels preventing IAB insertion; (2) small femoral pulse, making it difficult to find the vessel; (3) balloons failing to unfurl due to overwrapping; and (4) dislodging of atherosclerotic plaques or thrombus. The clinical experience gained through the use of the first percutaneous balloon[16] allowed identification of these problem areas and resulted in a new series of percutaneous balloons.

In 1981, the second generation of percutaneous IABs was introduced, featuring a dual-lumen IAB (Percor DL-II®).[19] The dual-lumen IAB has a flexible inner lumen

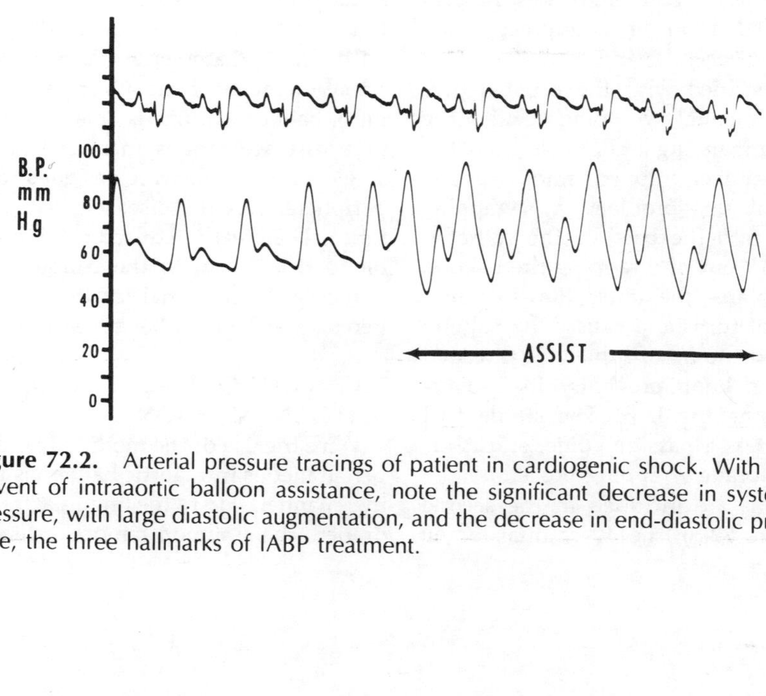

Figure 72.2. Arterial pressure tracings of patient in cardiogenic shock. With the advent of intraaortic balloon assistance, note the significant decrease in systolic pressure, with large diastolic augmentation, and the decrease in end-diastolic pressure, the three hallmarks of IABP treatment.

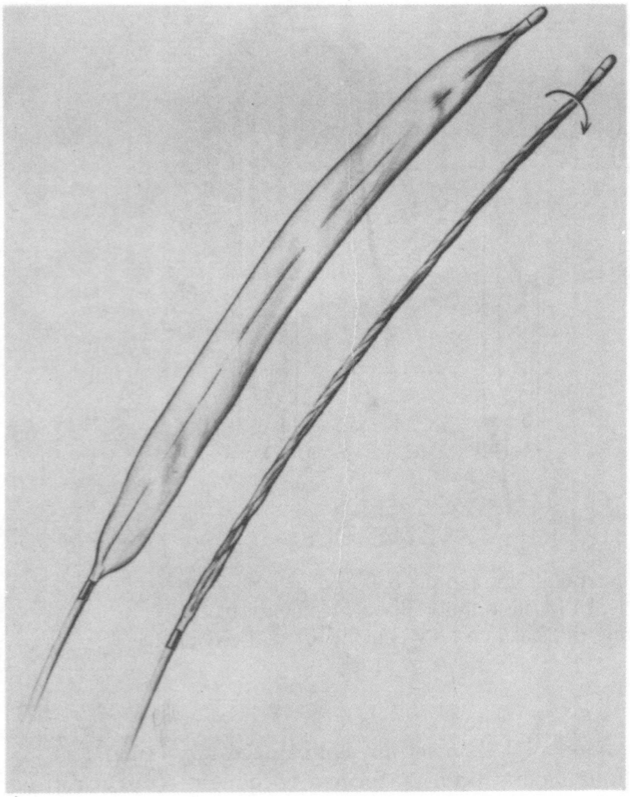

Figure 72.3. Manual wrapping of original Percor balloon proceeded from proximal to distal end.

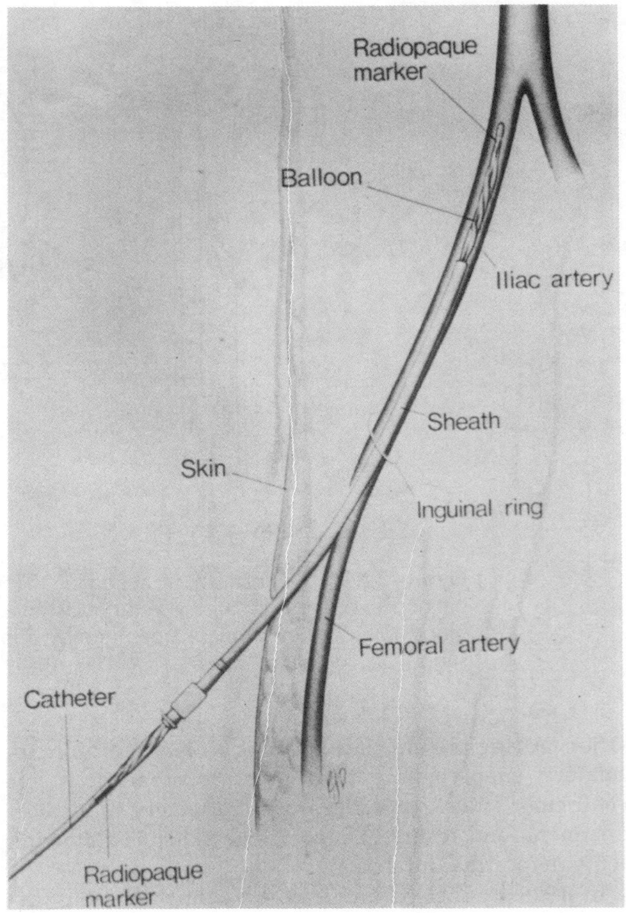

Figure 72.4. Schematic representation of percutaneous intraaortic balloon within sheath in common femoral artery.

incorporated inside the catheter that allows the balloon to be advanced over the 0.038-inch J-tip guidewire, the guidewire already having been advanced into the descending thoracic aorta. Access to this central lumen is achieved by removing the central stylet that is attached to the "wrapping-knob" assembly. After the balloon is advanced over the 0.038-inch J-tip guidewire, the wire is removed and the central lumen can either be closed with a male Luer-Lok cap or be used to monitor aortic arch pressure.[19] The ability to quickly establish an arterial line, along with rapid insertion of the balloon, makes the percutaneous dual-lumen IAB a powerful adjunct in an emergency situation.

One early problem identified with the original percutaneous IAB involved manual wrapping. Under the tense circumstances accompanying IABP insertion, too often the balloon was either overwrapped or not wrapped uniformly. To circumvent this problem, a "wrapping knob" was incorporated into the base of the catheter, taking all of the guesswork out of wrapping the balloon membrane. This knob rotates the inner lumen a mechanically fixed number of turns and causes the balloon membrane to wrap around the inner lumen. A threaded screw assembly inside the knob prevents either overwrapping or underwrapping the IAB. The sterile IAB package is designed to act as a passive guide, and it facilitates this balloon membrane wrapping procedure.

Four new adult balloons are included in the second generation of IABs (Figure 72.5): the 40-cc dual-lumen IAB available on a 10.5F catheter; the 50-cc dual-lumen IAB also available on a 10.5F catheter; a 9.5F 40-cc single-lumen balloon that can use either carbon dioxide or helium; and finally a narrow 8.5F 40-cc single-lumen balloon that can only be operated with helium as the shuttle gas. All four balloons incorporate the wrapping-knob assembly into the base of the catheter. The 50-cc dual-lumen balloon was specially developed for the patient with a large diameter aorta. By increasing the cross-sectional diameter of the 40-cc balloon (an increase of 1.25 mm), balloon volume is enlarged to 50 cc and blood volume displacement is increased 25%. The two-catheter single-lumen IABs were designed for patients with severe peripheral vascular disease or small tortuous femoral arteries. The greatly reduced catheter diameters allow more blood flow distal to the balloon insertion site, thereby reducing the potential for limb ischemia. A prewrapped Percor-Stat balloon has recently been introduced.

TECHNIQUE OF PERCUTANEOUS INTRAAORTIC BALLOON INSERTION

With the use of the modified Seldinger technique,[18] the percutaneous intraaortic balloon is inserted in the following manner. First, the inguinal region is prepared and draped, the common femoral artery is punctured with a

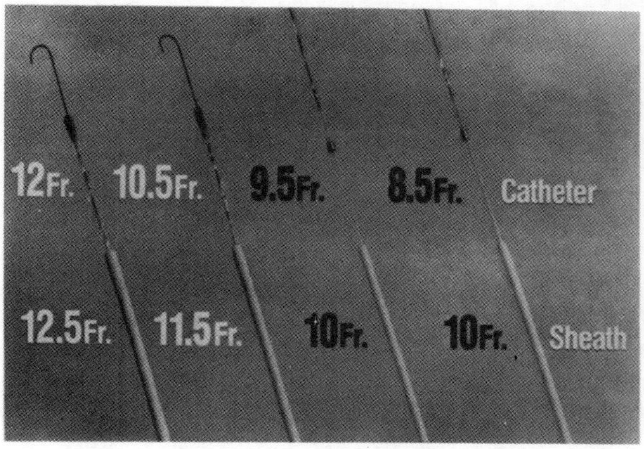

Figure 72.5. Current family of percutaneous intraaortic balloon pumps. The most widely employed is the 10.5F dual-lumen balloon, which is inserted through an 11.5F sheath. In smaller patients the 8.5F balloon is used through a 10F sheath, but measurement of intraaortic pressure is not possible through this single-lumen balloon.

standard 18-gauge arterial needle, and an 0.030-inch (0.097-cm) J-tip guidewire is introduced through the needle (Figure 72.6). The needle is removed, and an 8F dilator is passed over the guidewire to pre-dilate the subcutaneous tissues and the arterial puncture site (Figure 72.7). The 10F sheath-dilator combination is then advanced over the guidewire into the puncture site (Figure 72.8). One inch of sheath is left exposed to control hemorrhage.

The percutaneous balloon is prepared in the following manner. The sterile package is opened and the balloon and inner package are removed as a single unit. While the package is held firmly, the wrapping knob is rotated clockwise in a smooth motion. The wrapping knob will stop turning when the balloon is completely wrapped (Figure 72.9). The balloon membrane is inspected to determine if the membrane is evenly wrapped over the entire length. If incomplete wrapping is observed, the knob is rotated a few turns counterclockwise to unfurl the membrane, and the balloon is rewrapped. Next, the one-way valve is connected to the IAB Luer connector and a

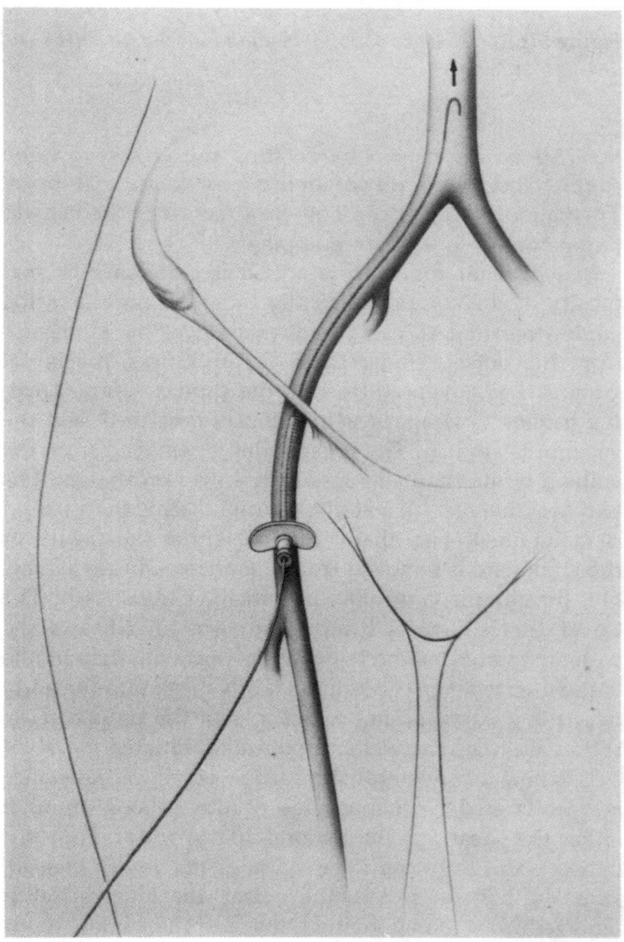

Figure 72.6. Modified Seldinger technique for insertion of percutaneous intraaortic balloon. An 18-gauge needle punctures the common femoral artery and a 0.035 J-tip guidewire is inserted through a needle in the common femoral artery into the aorta.

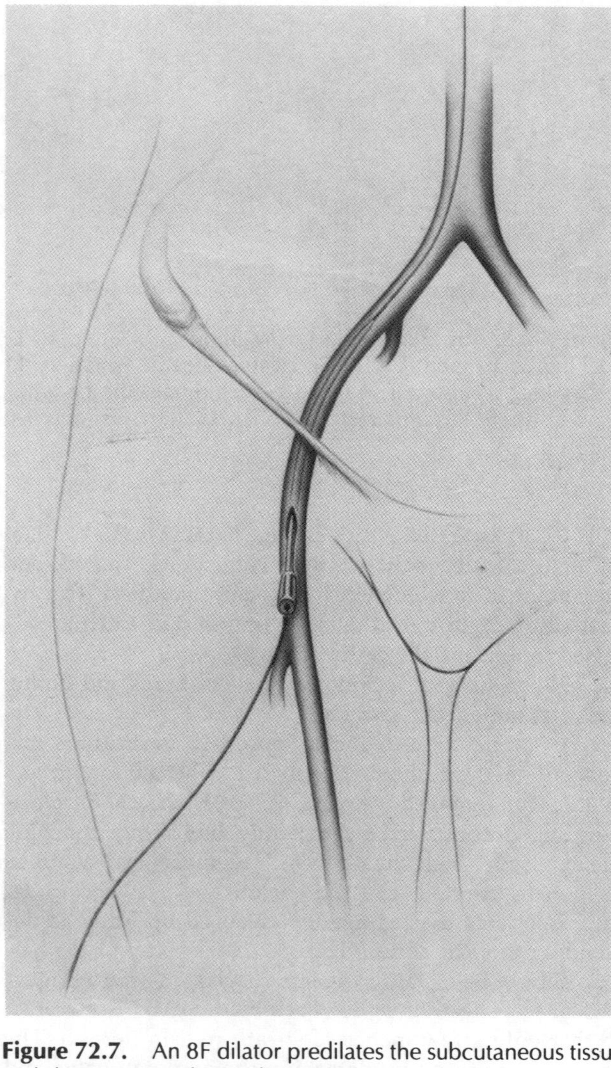

Figure 72.7. An 8F dilator predilates the subcutaneous tissue and the common femoral artery.

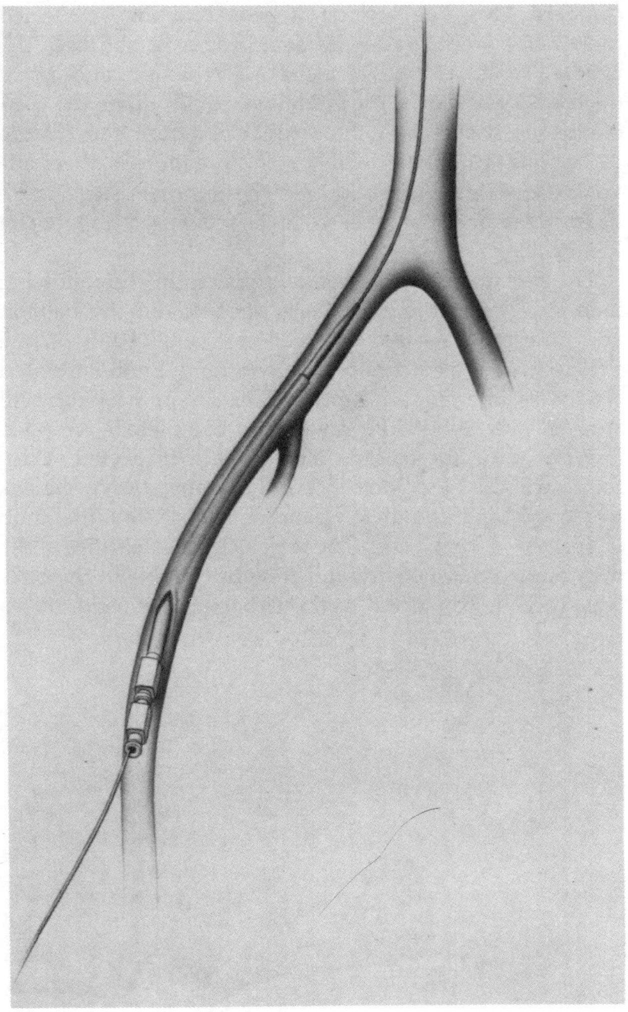

Figure 72.8. In preparation for insertion of a 40-cc 10.5F dual-lumen balloon, an 11.5F dilator sheath, which is 11 inches long, is inserted over the guidewire into the common femoral artery. Approximately 1 inch of the sheath is left exposed.

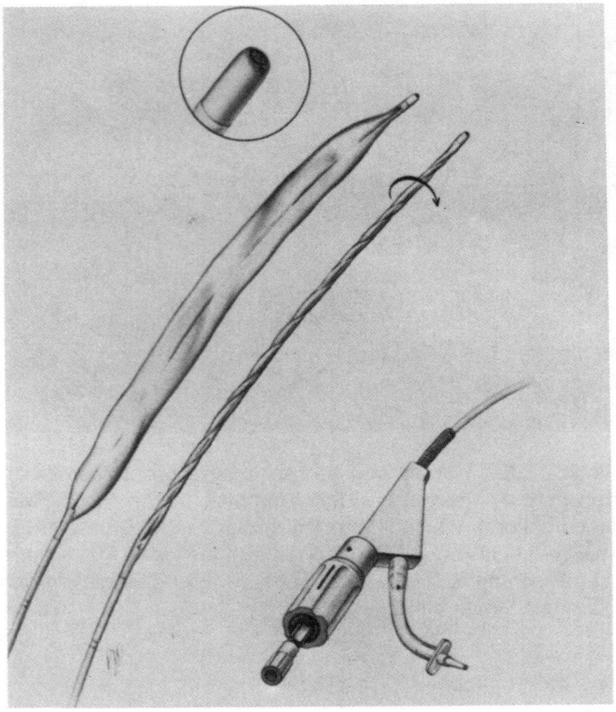

Figure 72.9. A 10.5F balloon is automatically wrapped and vacuum applied.

full 50 cc is aspirated with a syringe to remove the residual air in the furled balloon. In a large bowl, the balloon membrane is moistened in sterile saline solution. The appropriate length of catheter to be inserted can be estimated by placing the catheter on the patient's chest with the balloon tip 1 cm below the angle of Louis and noting the marking on the catheter.

After preparation of the balloon, IAB insertion is carried out in the following sequence. The guidewire and dilator are removed, leaving the 10F sheath in place. Bleeding is controlled by carefully but firmly pinching the exposed 1-inch sheath stem. The moistened wrapped balloon is inserted into the sheath and watched under fluoroscopy as the catheter is advanced up into the descending thoracic aorta (Figure 72.10). The tip of the balloon should be distal to the left subclavian artery (Figure 72.11). The sheath is pulled back before IABP is initiated, so that only a few inches of sheath remain in vivo. The vacuum is released by detaching the one-way valve and the IAB is unwrapped by rotating the wrapping knob counterclockwise until rotation is mechanically stopped. The balloon catheter can now be attached to the balloon pump console to initiate pumping.

If a difficult insertion is anticipated because of tortuosity of the aorta or difficulty in advancing the initial guidewire, the IAB can be advanced over the guidewire from the outset. Under these circumstances, the initial guidewire is advanced up into the thoracic aorta. Next, the balloon is wrapped as previously described, and the vacuum is applied. The inner stylet is removed from the balloon while the balloon is held with both hands. The IAB is submerged in a sterile solution, while the vacuum is maintained. The dilator but not either the sheath or the guidewire is removed from the dilator-sheath assembly. Bleeding is controlled by pinching the sheath. The tip of the balloon is inserted into the sheath and the balloon rotated counterclockwise; this will tighten the balloon wrapping. The balloon is advanced into the aorta over the guidewire, and when it is in the proper place, the vacuum is removed and pumping initiated.

If during a conventional insertion sequence, resistance is encountered in the passage of the balloon through either the sheath or the femoral artery, force is not imparted, so as to prevent dissection of the vessel. Instead, with the balloon still in the vessel, the inner stylet is removed from the wrapping knob, and the guidewire inserted through the inner lumen. The dual-lumen balloon is flexible and will follow the tortuous path of the guidewire. Sometimes, as the balloon is advanced, the tip may be felt against the aortic arch. Should this occur, the catheter is withdrawn 1 inch, so the tip will lie immediately

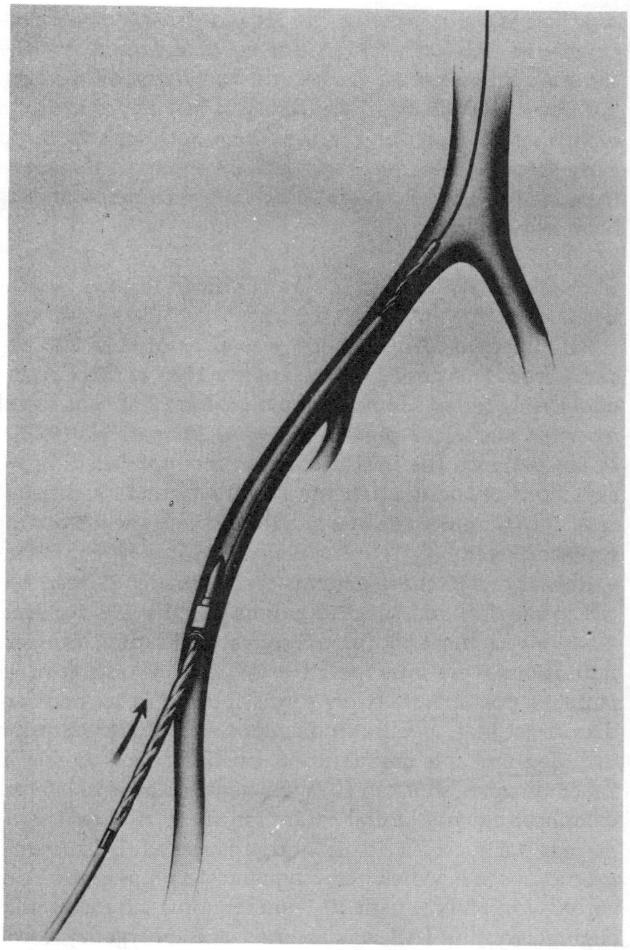

Figure 72.10. The balloon is inserted over the guidewire, after the dilator is removed, into the descending thoracic aorta.

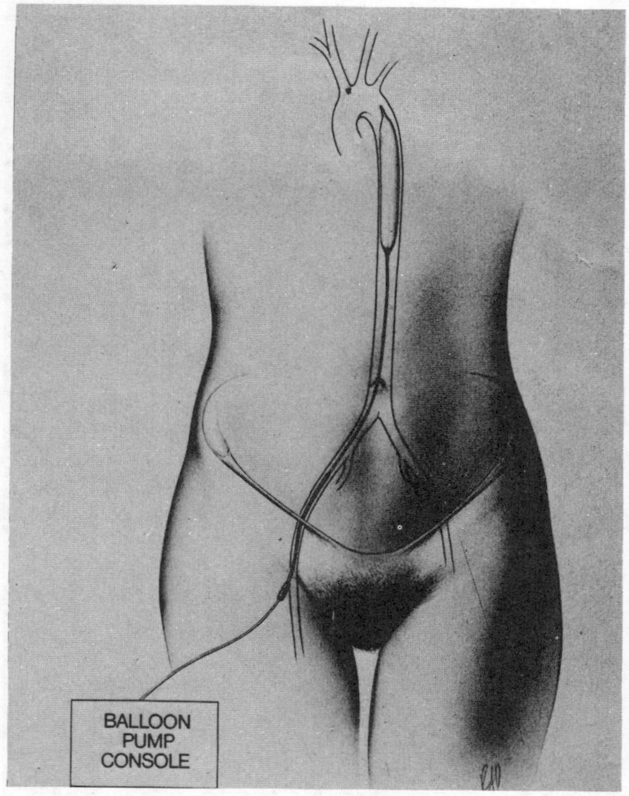

Figure 72.11. Final position of the percutaneous intraaortic balloon just distal to left subclavian artery. The distal end of the balloon is attached to the balloon pump console.

below the left subclavian artery. Correct inflation and deflation of the balloon may be confirmed with fluoroscopic visualization. The sheath seal prevents bleeding from the sheath catheter junction, and a sterile dressing is applied to the insertion site. The sheath seal is sutured to the skin to secure the catheter position.

MANAGEMENT OF THE PATIENT WITH A PERCUTANEOUS INTRAAORTIC BALLOON

It has been demonstrated that the functioning of the percutaneous IAB is identical to that of its predecessor, the surgically inserted dual-chambered IAB. In studies designed to compare both balloons, all parameters of left ventricular work were diminished identically.[20] The management and weaning of patients during intraaortic balloon pumping have been described previously.[21] A new computerized balloon pump, the Datascope System 90 (Figure 72.12), has just been introduced clinically.

REMOVAL OF THE PERCUTANEOUS INTRAAORTIC BALLOON

Before removal of the balloon catheter, the balloon is completely collapsed by aspiration with a 50-cc syringe and a stopcock. The balloon is pulled down to (but not into) the sheath. The femoral artery is compressed distal to the insertion site, and the balloon and sheath are removed as a single unit. Blood is allowed to spurt from the artery for a few seconds, so that any thrombus material will be removed. Compression of the femoral artery is shifted over the puncture site for 30 minutes. Distal pulses are monitored with a Doppler apparatus and manual compression is adjusted so that an audible pulse is registered. A compression dressing is applied to the puncture site for 24 hours.

RECENT OBSERVATIONS ON PERCUTANEOUS INTRAAORTIC BALLOON PUMPING

During our first 4 years of clinical experience with the percutaneous balloon pump catheter at Columbia–Presbyterian Medical Center, certain observations were made which can reduce the "hazards" associated with this technique[22]:

1. The percutaneous IAB must be inserted by a physician skilled in the Seldinger technique of cardiac catheterization. Those institutions adhering to this suggestion have a reduced morbidity associated with this procedure.
2. Ideally, the insertion procedure should be carried out under fluoroscopic control.
3. The use of a longer dilator-sheath assembly has significantly increased the success of insertion.[23]
4. In critically ill patients undergoing cardiac catheterization who have poor ventricular function, study of the aorto-iliac system is highly desirable as a guide for subsequent balloon insertion.

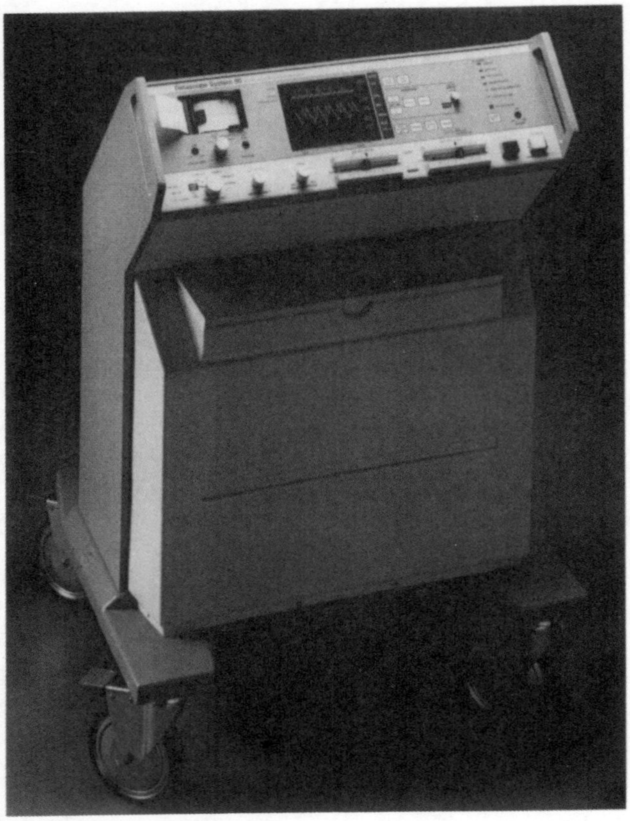

Figure 72.12. Datascope System 90 balloon pump.

5. In high-risk cardiac patients undergoing open heart surgery in whom an IABP was not inserted before induction of anesthesia, we recommend preparing for potential IABP insertion. With an arterial needle, femoral artery access is obtained and the guidewire inserted. Should IABP be required for separation from cardiopulmonary bypass, arterial access is then already established for IABP insertion.

6. The development of the second generation of percutaneous IAB catheters, including dual-lumen, narrow catheter single-lumen IABs, and prewrapped balloons, has given the clinician flexibility when approaching a difficult IAB insertion (Figure 72.5). Although it is too early to tell, these new catheters are expected to reduce the vascular complications associated with percutaneous balloon pumping.

CLINICAL EXPERIENCES WITH PERCUTANEOUS BALLOON PUMPING

Percutaneous IAB insertion was attempted in 202 patients from February 1979 to January 1985 at the Columbia–Presbyterian Medical Center (Table 72.1). Successful insertion was accomplished in 196 of 202 patients (97%). In ten patients, the initial insertion attempt failed; however, four of the ten patients eventually underwent successful IAB implantation when the 11-inch sheath-dilator was employed.

Indications in these patients were broadly divided between medical and surgical groups. Of the 196 patients, 91 received the IAB for a surgical indication. Surgical indications were intraoperative low cardiac output in 71 patients, postoperative low cardiac output in 16, and cardiac arrest in 4. Medical indications for counterpulsation included unstable angina in 36, postinfarction angina in 21, cardiogenic shock in 13, acute ventricular septal defect complicating myocardial infarction in 4, recurrent ventricular tachycardia in 1, and unsuccessful Gruentzig procedures in 6. When hemodynamic decompensation occurred in six patients undergoing transluminal angioplasty, the IAB was inserted and emergency coronary revascularization carried out. Four patients subsequently were discharged from the hospital. Only one patient received the IAB prophylactically for unstable angina before a general surgical procedure. This patient survived and the balloon was removed in the immediate postoperative period.

The location of the balloon insertion procedure varied.

Table 72.1. Percutaneous Intraaortic Balloon Insertions from February 1979 to January 1985 at Columbia–Presbyterian Medical Center.

	SUCCESSFUL INSERTIONS	CCU	Cath Lab
Preop	Unstable angina with general surgery	1	—
	Unstable angina with cardiac surgery	18 (3)	13 (2)
	Unstable angina—treated with medication	4 (1)	1
	Postinfarction angina—treated with medication	4 (2)	4 (1)
	Postinfarction angina with surgery	10 (1)	3
	Cardiogenic shock—treated with medication	2	4 (3)
	Cardiogenic shock with surgery	2	5 (2)
	Cardiac arrest	4 (3)	1
	Recurrent ventricular tachycardia—medication	1	—
	Failed Gruntzig Procedure with emergency surgery	—	6 (2)
	Acute VSD with surgery	1	2 (1)
	Acute VSD without surgery	—	1 (1)
	Anesthesia support for open heart surgery	6 (1)	12 (1)
Periop	Low output—OR	71 (44)	
Postop	Low output	16 (9)	
	Cardiac arrest	4 (3)	
	*Parentheses indicate number of deaths		
	Total Number Assisted	196	
	Total Number Discharged	116 (60%)	

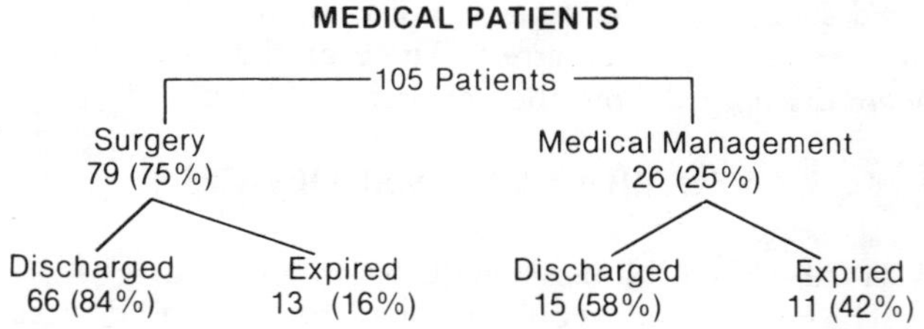

Figure 72.13. Successful percutaneous intraaortic balloon insertions at Columbia–Presbyterian Medical Center (1979–1985).

Seventy-one patients had the balloon implanted in the operating room, 20 in the open heart recovery room, 52 in the cardiac catheterization laboratory, and 53 in the cardiac intensive care unit.

Of the 105 patients in whom the IAB was successfully inserted for a medical indication (Figure 72.13), 79 (75%) eventually underwent cardiac surgery, whereas 26 (25%) were treated medically. Only 13 of the 79 patients (16%) receiving preoperative IAB support combined with definitive surgical procedures died. In contrast, 56 of the 91 patients (61%) requiring intraoperative or postoperative IAB died. We reviewed the first 113 consecutive patients undergoing percutaneous IAB insertion. Complications of percutaneous IAB insertion, which occurred in 11 of the 113 patients, included one guidewire perforation of the aorta. Complications related to the maintenance and removal of the IAB included femoral thrombi requiring embolectomy in four patients, asymptomatic iliac occlusion in one, and weak dorsalis pedis pulses in one. There were no false aneurysms, aortic dissections, or septic complications resulting from the percutaneous balloon in our series. However, it should be noted that extensive necropsy examinations were not performed.

Four patients in whom percutaneous IAB insertion by a conventional approach was unsuccessful underwent successful balloon implantation by the long inserter technique.[23] There were no insertion-related complications in these four patients. Another noteworthy case concerned a patient with an improperly positioned IAB which intermittently occluded the origin of the superior mesenteric artery. The resulting abdominal pain was relieved when the balloon was advanced to its correct position.[24]

PULMONARY ARTERY BALLOON PUMPING

There has always been a great need to mechanically support the right side of the heart in both right and biventricular failure. In 1969 Kralios et al[25] experimentally placed a balloon pump in the main pulmonary artery and in one of its branches. By timing the balloon to inflate during diastole, improved hemodynamic indexes were recorded. Opravil et al[26] reported marked improvement in experimentally induced right ventricular failure, including reduced right ventricular preload, reduced right ventricular afterload, and increased cardiac output, when using pulmonary artery balloon counterpulsation. Other laboratories have also reproduced these positive results.[27,28] Recently, pulmonary artery balloon pumping (PABP) was clinically applied for profound right ventricular failure.[29] In the surgical setting, a Dacron® side graft was attached to the main pulmonary artery, just beyond the pulmonic valve, and an intraaortic balloon was placed within this graft. The graft was then ligated distally. The Dacron graft serves as a reservoir, so that the balloon can counterpulsate a greater volume of blood; the amount of blood within the pulmonary artery is often too small for counterpulsation to effectively unload the right ventricle. With this technique, the patient was successfully weaned from the cardiopulmonary bypass circuit. Moran et al[30] reported on two patients with biventricular failure in whom they implanted an intraaortic balloon and a pulmonary artery balloon. Hemodynamically the intraaortic balloon was not sufficient to separate the patient from the heart-lung machine; the combination of both balloons counterpulsating synchronously with the existing myocardium produced a physiologic output, and separation was achieved.

PULSATILE ASSIST DEVICE

The pulsatile assist device (PAD) is the first clinical inline device (Figure 72.14) to produce atraumatic synchronized pulsatile cardiopulmonary bypass (CPB) and also to function as an arterial counterpulsator.[31] The PAD is a disposable plastic unit designed to be easily inserted into the arterial line of the cardiopulmonary bypass circuit (Figure 72.15). When not in use, the PAD will not interfere with cardiopulmonary bypass; rather, it becomes a passive tube. It is constructed of a valveless polyurethane tube that can be squeezed rhythmically by the application of pneumatic pressure between the outer plastic housing and the inner flexible tubular membrane. Before cardiopulmonary bypass is instituted, a tubing clamp is applied between the PAD and the roller pump. Synchronized to the electrocardiogram, the PAD can act as an arterioarterial counterpulsator through the arterial cannula.[32] The effectiveness of the PAD as a counterpulsator stems from its proximity to the aortic root and its ability to rapidly withdraw and return 35 cc of blood. At the start of cardiopulmonary bypass, the tubing clamp is removed and the PAD either can be used to pulsate synchronously with the heart or can be left as a passive tube. When the heart has a regular rhythm, the PAD will be triggered to produce diastolic augmentation and thus acts as a more effective IABP. When the heart is either cross-clamped or in ventricular fibrillation, the PAD is switched to an internal trigger of 80 beats/min to produce a pulsatile cardiopulmonary bypass. At the end of cardiopulmonary bypass, when the patient is to be weaned from the pump, the PAD can once again be switched to the

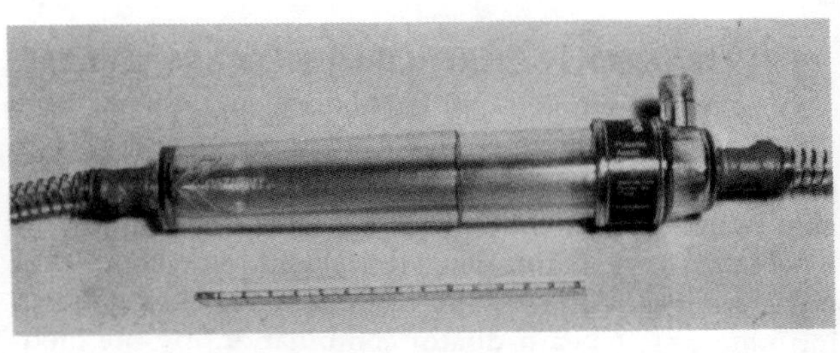

Figure 72.14. Pulsatile assist device (PAD) for creation of pulsatile cardiopulmonary bypass.

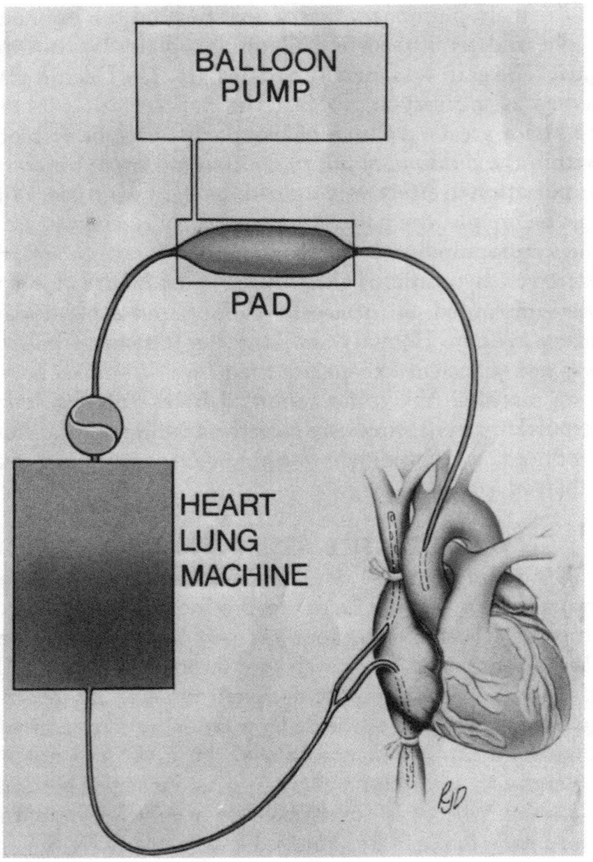

Figure 72.15. Schematic representation of pulsatile assist device in circuitry of the heart-lung machine.

counterpulsation mode. Counterpulsation may be continued until protamine is administered.

Clinically, the PAD has been routinely employed at the Columbia–Presbyterian Medical Center since 1975. Over this period, we had the opportunity to study 200 consecutive patients who underwent elective open heart surgery.[33] During bypass, urinary output in the PAD patients was compared with that in the control group. The PAD patients had more than double the urinary output as compared with the control group (9.18 $\pm$0.68 cc/min versus 3.90 $\pm$ 0.35 cc/min). In addition, intraoperative coronary graft flow measurements revealed a 21.4% increase in coronary blood flow with pulsatile cardiopulmonary bypass, when compared with that in the control group. Therefore, we believe that the PAD is a simple inline device that can be used routinely during open heart surgery to create either pulsatile flow or counterpulsation.

PERCUTANEOUS CARDIOPULMONARY BYPASS

A novel system of rapid circulatory support has been developed by Phillips et al.[34] Utilizing advances in percutaneous introducer technology, they constructed a portable bypass circuit consisting of a centrifugal pump and a pediatric oxygenator. One arterial and two venous cannulas are inserted femorally through a 12F percutaneous introducer set (sheath-dilator combination) by the modified Seldinger technique.[18] Circulatory assistance can be initiated within five minutes. This procedure has been used successfully to support and resuscitate five people who were in cardiac arrest. Three of the five patients were discharged from the hospital.

VENTRICULAR ASSIST DEVICES

LITWAK LEFT ATRIAL–AORTIC BYPASS

The need for more powerful circulatory support devices stems from the diminishing effectiveness of the IABP as the severity of left ventricular failure increases. To fill this need, investigators have proposed an assortment of mechanical pumps, some of which have been successful despite limited clinical exposure. One example of the ingenuity generated by this problem is the left atrial–aortic bypass system designed by Litwak et al.[35] This system utilizes two permanently implanted obturator occluding cannula assemblies (Figure 72.16). These silicone elastomer cannulas are sutured to the left atrium and ascending aorta and positioned subcutaneously in the abdominal wall. During diminished cardiac output, the cannulas are exposed, the obturators are removed, and a nonocclusive roller pump is connected to maintain adequate circulation. Bypass flows up to 5 L/minute can be produced. Once the heart has recovered and can carry a full load, the obturators are reinserted into the cannulas and the entire assembly is covered by abdominal wall tissue. Of the 18

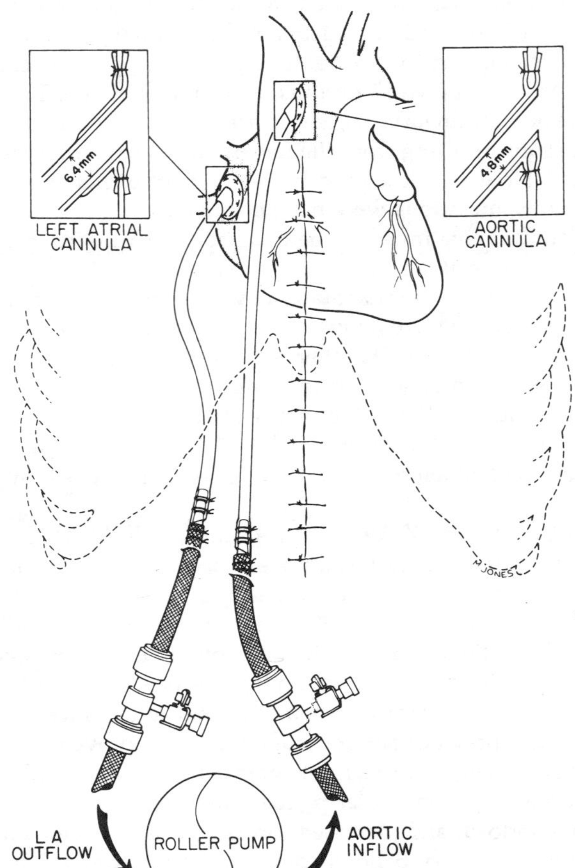

Figure 72.16. Litwak left heart bypass setup with permanent silicone cannulas.

patients who could not be weaned from cardiopulmonary bypass and who had implantation, 6 were discharged from the hospital and 4 are considered late survivors.[36]

ABDOMINAL LEFT VENTRICULAR ASSIST DEVICE

To achieve even greater circulatory support in left ventricular power failure, larger capacity pumps had to be developed. However, as the scale of circulatory support increases, so do the dimensions of the devices. Schemes using bypass circuits with long lengths of tubing are too fragile for long-term support. One alternative solution, the abdominal left ventricular assist device (ALVAD), was developed in the 1970s at the Texas Heart Institute in Houston.[37] The ALVAD is a compact pneumatic bladder pump with a one-way valve at both inlet and outlet ports (Figure 72.17). The ALVAD is inserted at the apex of the left ventricle and delivers blood to the abdominal aorta. To date, the ALVAD has been implanted in 22 patients for periods ranging from one day to 1 week.[37] In three cases, the pump was removed after left ventricular recovery, and in one patient, a cardiac allograft replaced an evolving ALVAD dependency.

HERSHEY LEFT VENTRICULAR ASSIST DEVICE

A completely different philosophy is embodied in the approach taken by Pennock et al[38] at the Pennsylvania State University at Hershey. Here, an extracorporeally placed pneumatic pump containing a smooth polyurethane oblate spheroid sac is used to withdraw blood through a cannula in the left atrial appendage. The return flow is sent to the ascending aorta through a woven Dacron prosthesis. At both the inlet and outlet ports, a Björk-Shiley tilting disk valve is used to maintain unidirectional flow. The inflow and outflow cannulas exit the chest wall below the costal margin, and the pump rests on the anterior abdominal wall. This paracorporeal ventricular assist pump has been in use since 1976. However, it was not until the 1980s that the device's true potential became apparent. Of the 12 patients requiring circulatory assistance, 9 have been weaned from the Hershey pump, and 6 of these (50%) have survived. One patient who received the pump for right ventricular assistance is among the survivors, and three patients who required biventricular assistance using two separate pumps did not survive.[38] Pennington[38a] at St. Louis reported 21 patients, 10 of whom were weaned from the ventricular assist device, with 7 being discharged from the hospital.

It seems clear now that temporary ventricular assistance has a definite role in those patients who cannot be successfully weaned from cardiopulmonary bypass despite inotropic support and IABP. Pierce, Norman, Litwak, Pennington, Loop, Spencer, and others[35–40] have all reported positive clinical results using ventricular assist devices. Although survival of these patients is at best 50%, this figure should improve as our experience with these devices grows.[41,41a]

CIRCULATORY SUPPORT FOR CARDIAC TRANSPLANTATION

Patients with end-stage heart disease who fulfill the Stanford University heart recipient criteria are prime candidates for receiving a donor allograft.[42] The process of locating a suitable donor organ can take several weeks. Too often during this waiting period the transplant candidate can slide into rapid circulatory failure. It is now feasible to consider temporary mechanical support for these unstable transplantation candidates. At the Columbia–Presbyterian Medical Center, we have begun to consider such patients for cardiac transplantation.[43] In five patients the IABP was used to support the circulation for an average of 7.8 days, until a donor heart became available. Orthotopic cardiac transplantation was performed in all instances, and the IABP was discontinued immediately following transplantation. All five patients were discharged from the hospital. Disler et al[44] recently maintained a cardiac transplantation candidate on the IABP for 30 days until a suitable donor was located. Even more remarkable was that while on IABP support, the patient was transported 1,400 km by airplane. At Stanford University, two patients received cardiac transplants following IABP circulatory assistance.[45] Both patients are alive and well 14 and 28 months later. Norman et al[46] reported on a patient supported for 122 hours by the ALVAD before cardiac transplantation. The patient died 15 days after transplantation. Cooley[47] supported a patient using the ALVAD for 39 hours before allografting. This patient died of renal failure 14 days after transplantation. In an-

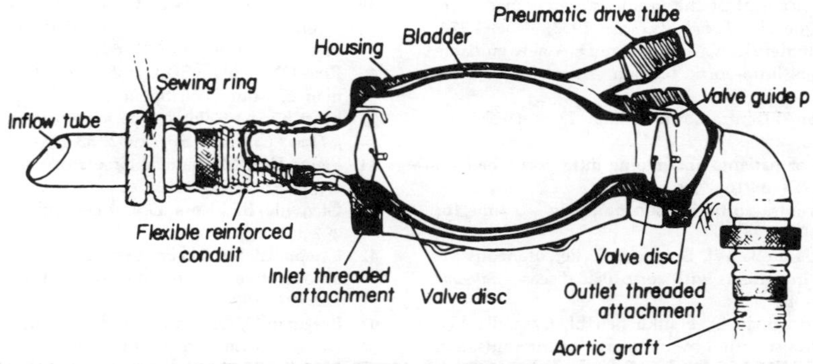

Figure 72.17. Clinical abdominal left ventricular assist device developed at the Texas Heart Institute.

other two patients, Cooley performed two-stage cardiac transplantation, first using a total artificial heart and then implanting a donor heart. The two patients were supported for 64 hours and five days, respectively, by the total artificial heart. The allograft then supported the circulation for 7.5 and 20 days.[48] Other more recent successful examples of use of a prosthetic ventricle as a bridge to cardiac transplantation have been performed at Stanford University, St. Louis University Hospital, Hershey Medical Center, Jewish Hospital at Louisville, Kentucky, University of Arizona at Tucson, University of Pittsburgh, Minneapolis Heart Institute, and Pacific Presbyterian Medical Center at San Francisco.[49] The temporary use of the available models of mechanical circulatory support in patients awaiting cardiac transplantation seems to receive a great deal of support.[50]

REFERENCES

1. Moulopoulos SD, Topaz S, Kolff WJ: Diastolic balloon pumping (with carbon dioxide) in the aorta — a mechanical assistance to the failing circulation. *Am Heart J* 1962; 63:669–675.
2. Harken DE: Presentation at the International College of Cardiology Meeting, Brussels, Belguim, 1958.
3. Kantrowitz A, Kantrowitz A: Experimental augmentation of coronary flow by retardation of the arterial pressure pulse. *Surgery* 1953; 34:678–687.
4. Kantrowitz A, Mckinnon WMP: The experimental use of the diaphragm as an auxiliary myocardium. *Surg Forum* 1958; 9:266–268.
5. Maroko PN, Bernstein EF, Lippy P, DeLaria GA, Covell JW, Ross J, Braunwald E: Effects of intra-aortic balloon counterpulsation on the severity of myocardial ischemic injury following acute coronary occlusion. Counterpulsation and myocardial injury. *Circulation* 1972; 45:1150–1159.
6. Kantrowitz A, Tjonneland S, Freed PS, Phillips SJ, Butner AN, Sherman JL Jr: Initial clinical experience with intra-aortic balloon pumping in cardiogenic shock. *JAMA* 1968; 203:113–118.
7. Bregman D, Bailin M, Bowman FO, Parodi EN, Haubert SM, Edie RN, Spotnitz HM, Reemtsma K, Malm JR: A pulsatile assist device (PAD) for use during cardiopulmonary bypass. *Ann Thorac Surg* 1977; 24:574–580.
8. Nachlas MM, Siedband MP: The influence of diastolic augmentation on infarct size following coronary artery ligation. *J Thorac Cardiovasc Surg* 1967; 53:698–706.
9. Feola M, Limet RR, Glick G: Direct and reflex peripheral vascular effects of intra-aortic balloon counterpulsation (IABC) in dogs at four levels of aortic pressure. *Clin Res* 1971; 19:313.
10. Haddy FJ: Pathophysiology and therapy of the shock of myocardial infarction. *Ann Intern Med* 1970; 73:809–827.
11. Johnson SA, Scanlon PJ, Loeb HS, Moran JM, Pifarre R, Gunnar RM: Treatment of cardiogenic shock in myocardial infarction by intra-aortic balloon counterpulsation and surgery. *Am J Med* 1977; 62:687–692.
12. Gold HK, Leinbach RC, Buckley MJ, Mundth ED, Daggett WM, Austen WG: Refractory angina pectoris: follow-up after intra-aortic balloon pumping and surgery. *Circulation* 1976; 54(suppl 3): III-41–III-46.
13. Levine FH, Gold HK, Leinbach RC, Daggett WM, Austen WG, Buckley MJ: Safe early revascularization for continuing ischemia after acute myocardial infarction. *Circulation* 1979; 60(suppl 1):I5–I9.
14. Bregman D, Casarella WJ: Percutaneous intra-aortic balloon pumping: initial clinical experience. *Ann Thorac Surg* 1980; 29:153–155.
15. Bregman D: Intra-aortic Balloon Counterpulsation. Circulatory Assistance and the Artificial Heart, in Pierce WS (ed): *USA–USSR Joint Symposium, Tbilisi, USSR, September 20–22, 1979.* US Dept of Health and Human Services, PHS, NIH, 1980, pp 155–165.
16. Bregman D, Cohen SR: Mechanical techniques of circulatory support: a percutaneous intra-aortic balloon device. *Artif Organs* 1983; 7:38–48.
17. Bregman D, Nichols AB, Weiss MB, Powers ER, Martin EC, Casarella WF: Percutaneous intra-aortic balloon insertion. *Am J Cardiol* 1980; 46:261–264.
18. Seldinger SI: Catheter replacement of the needle in percutaneous arteriography: a new technique. *Acta Radiol (Stockholm)* 1953; 39:368–374.
19. Merav AD, Solomon N, Montefusco CM, Bregman D: A new guidable double lumen percutaneous intra-aortic balloon. *Trans Am Soc Intern Organs* 1981; 27:593–594.
20. Bregman D: A new percutaneous intra-aortic balloon. *Trans Am Soc Artif Intern Organs* 1980; 26:8–10.
21. Bregman D: Management of patients undergoing intra-aortic balloon pumping. *Heart and Lung* 1974; 3:916–928.
22. Bregman D: Percutaneous intra-aortic balloon pumping—a time for reflection. *Chest* 1982; 82:397–398.
23. Nichols AB, Weiss MB, Casarella WJ, Bregman D: Percutaneous intraaortic balloon insertion in patients with aorto-iliac disease. *Cath and Cardiovasc Diag* 1981; 7:443–449.
24. Karlson KB, Martin EC, Bregman D, Frankuchen EI, Casarella WJ: Superior mesenteric artery obstruction by intraaortic counterpulsation balloon simulating embolism: a case report. *Cardiovasc Intervent Radiol* 1981; 4:236–238.
25. Kralios AC, Zwart HHJ, Moulopoulos SD, Collan R, Kwan-Gett CS, Kolff WJ: Intrapulmonary artery balloon pumping. Assistance of the right ventricle. *J Thorac Cardiovasc Surg* 1970; 60:215-232.
26. Opravil M, Gorman AJ, Krejcie TC, Michaelis LL, Moran JM: Pulmonary artery balloon counterpulsation for right ventricular failure. I. Experimental results. *Ann Thorac Surg* 1984; 38:242–253.
27. Jett GK, Siwek LG, Picone AL, Applebaum RE, Jones M: Pulmonary artery balloon counterpulsation for right ventricular failure. An experimental evaluation. *J Thorac Cardiovasc Surg* 1983; 86:364–372.
28. Gaines WE, Pierce WS, Prophet GA, Holtzman K: Pulmonary circulatory support. A quantitative comparison of four methods. *J Thorac Cardiovasc Surg* 1984; 88:958–964.
29. Miller DC, Moreno-Cabral RJ, Stinson EB, Shinn JA, Shumway NE: Pulmonary artery balloon counterpulsation for acute right ventricular failure. *J Thorac Cardiovasc Surg* 1980; 80:760–763.
30. Moran JM, Opravil M, Gorman AJ, Rastegar H, Meyers SN, Michaelis LL: Pulmonary artery balloon counterpulsation for right ventricular failure. II. Clinical experience. *Ann Thorac Surg* 1984; 38:254–259.
31. Habal SM, Parodi EN, Hanson B, Wolvek S, Bregman D: A new pulsatile assist device (PAD) for use in cardiac surgery. *Am Soc Artif Intern Organs* 1976; 5:32.
32. Habal SM, Weiss MB, Spotnitz HM, Parodi EN, Wolff M, Cannon PJ, Hoffman BF, Malm JR: Effects of pulsatile and nonpulsatile coronary perfusion on performance of the canine left ventricle. *J Thorac Cardiovasc Surg* 1976; 72:742–755.
33. Bregman D, Parodi EN, Haubert SM, Szarnicki R, Edie RN, Spotnitz HM, Bowman FO Jr, Reemtsma K, Malm JR: Counterpulsation with a new pulsatile assist device (PAD) in open heart surgery. *Med Instrum.* 1976; 10:232–238.
34. Phillips SJ, Ballentine B, Slonine D, Hall J, Vandehaar J, Kongtahworn C, Zeff RH, Skinner JR, Reckmo K, Gray D: Percutaneous initiation of cardiopulmonary bypass. *Ann Thorac Surg* 1983; 36:223–225.
35. Litwak RS, Koffsky RM, Jurado RA, Lukban SB, Ortiz AF, Fischer AP, Sherman JJ, Silvay G, Lajam FA: Use of a left heart assist device after intracardiac surgery: technique and clinical experience. *Ann Thorac Surg* 1976; 21:191–202.
36. Litwak RS, Koffsky RM, Jurado RA, Lukban SB, Ortiz AF, Grana V, Fischer A, Sherman JJ, Silvay G, Lajam FA, deAsla RA, Fitzkee HL: Management of low cardiac output after open intracardiac operation with a left heart assist device, in Bregman D (ed): *Mechanical Support of the Failing Heart.* New York, Appleton-Century-Crofts, 1977, pp 47–59.
37. Norman JC, Duncan MJ, Frazier OH, Hallman GL, Ott DA, Reul GJ, Cooley DA: Intracorporeal (abdominal) left ventricular assist devices or partial artificial heart: a five-year clinical experience. *Arch Surg* 1981; 116:1441–1445.
38. Pennock JL, Pierce WS, Wisman CH, Bull AP, Waldhausen JA: Survival and complications following ventricular assist pumping for cardiogenic shock. *Ann Surg* 1983; 198:469–478.
38a. Pennington DG: Unilateral and bilateral bypass, in Glenville BE, Ross DN (eds): *Update in Circulatory Support and Artificial Heart—Third International Symposium on Cardiac Bioprostheses,* London, AMI Health Care Ltd, 1986, pp 11–15.
39. Golding LR, Jacobs G, Groves LK, Gill CC, Nose Y, Loop F: Clinical results of mechanical support of the failing left ventricle. *J Thorac Cardiovasc Surg* 1982; 83:597–601.
40. Rose DM, Colvin SB, Culliford AT, Cunningham JN, Adams PX, Glassman E, Isom OW, Spencer FC: Long-term survival with partial left heart bypass following perioperative myocardial infarction and shock. *J Thorac Cardiovasc Surg* 1982; 83:483–492.
41. Pierce WS: Mechanical circulatory assistance — current state of the art. *Heart Transpl* 1983; 3:6–7.
41a. Glenville BE, Ross DN: Ventricular assist devices. *Br Med J* 1986; 292:361–362.
42. Griepp RB, Stinson EB, Dong E, Clark DA, Shumway NE: Determinants of operative risk in human heart transplantation. *Am J Surg* 1971; 122:192–197.
43. Bregman D, Drusin R, Lamb J, Reemstma K, Rose E: Heart transplantation in patients requiring mechanical circulatory support. *Heart Transpl* 1982; 1:154–156.
44. Disler PB, Scott Millar RN, Obel IWP: Prolonged circulatory support with the intra-aortic balloon pump after myocardial infarction. *Thorax* 1978; 33:504–507.
45. Pennock JL, Wisman CB, Pierce WS: Mechanical support of the cir-

culation prior to transplantation. *Heart Transpl* 1982; 1:299–301.

46. Norman JC, Brook MI, Cooley DA, Klima T, Khan BD, Frazier OH, Keats AS, Hacker J, Massin EK, Duncan JM, Solis RT, Dacso CC, Luper WE, Winston DS, Reul GJ: Total support of the circulation of a patient with post-cardiotomy stone heart syndrome by a partial artificial heart (ALVAD) for 5 days followed by heart and kidney transplantation. *Lancet* 1978; 1:1125–1127.
47. Cooley DA: Staged cardiac transplantation: report of three cases. *Heart Transpl* 1982; 1:145–153.
48. Cooley DA, Akutsu T, Norman JC, Serrato MA, Frazier OH: Total artificial heart in two-staged cardiac transplantation. *Bull Texas Heart Instit* 1981; 8:305–319.
49. Hill JD, Farrar DJ, Hershon JJ, Compton PG, Avery GJ II, Levin BS, Brent BN: Use of a prosthetic ventricle as a bridge to cardiac transplantation for postinfarction cardiogenic shock. *N Engl J Med* 1986; 314:626–628.
50. Relman AS: Artificial hearts—permanent and temporary. *N Engl J Med* 1986; 314:644–645.

73 Cardiac and Cardiopulmonary Transplantation

John C. Baldwin, MD, Edward B. Stinson, MD, Philip E. Oyer, MD, PhD, Stuart W. Jamieson, FRCS, and Norman E. Shumway, MD, PhD

The idea of cardiac replacement is an old one, but its realization as a clinical alternative has occurred as a result of laboratory and clinical investigation over the last 80 years. Surgical technique, graft preservation, maintenance of recipient circulation during surgery, and diagnosis and treatment of rejection were formidable obstacles, and the solution to all of these problems has depended on continuing experimentation and innovation. Investigative efforts continue on a broad front, but cardiac transplantation has emerged during the past few years as a realistic therapeutic method with excellent outlook for survival and rehabilitation in patients who would otherwise face certain death. With improved results in cardiac transplantation, increasing knowledge in lung preservation, and the advent of newer forms of immunosuppression, clinical cardiopulmonary transplantation is being introduced with some success. Significant problems related to donor availability and management, optimum graft preservation, postoperative pulmonary management, and long-term airway disease do exist, and all of them are being aggressively addressed in continuing laboratory and clinical efforts.

HISTORY

On December 30, 1905, the first report of cardiac transplantation appeared in the literature. Carrel and Guthrie[1] reported the results of several experiments, which represented a continuation of their work on the surgery of blood vessels. Cervical heterotopic transplantation was carried out in a dog, and effective ventricular contraction was achieved. The heart beat for approximately two hours. Nearly 30 years later, Mann et al[2] reported on further work, refining the technical aspects of heterotopic transplantation. During the 1950s, Demikhov[3] carried out experiments in which heterotopic cardiac transplantation was carried out within the thorax in the canine model. In addition, he demonstrated the ability of the donor heart to sustain the animal's circulation independently.

Lower and Shumway[4] in 1960 reported the first series of successful orthotopic cardiac transplantations. This pioneering work, characterized by the use of safe and reliable cardiopulmonary bypass, topical hypothermia for preservation of the cardiac graft, and surgical excision and reimplantation of the heart at the mid-atrial level, was the touchstone for subsequent investigative work in cardiac transplantation, and the methods employed constitute the paradigm for clinical cardiac transplantation as it is currently practiced.

Because the loss of graft function in orthotopic cardiac transplantation is immediately fatal, the ability to diagnose and treat rejection was essential to the further development of the technique. When loss of QRS voltage on the electrocardiogram was found to correlate with tissue rejection, this indication became the standard noninvasive method for establishing the diagnosis.[5] The pharmacologic means for the prevention and treatment of rejection in the laboratory model were based on experience with immunosuppressive agents used in cancer chemotherapy and renal transplantation.[6] The immunologic aspects of cardiac transplantation and the selection of immunosuppressive regimens subsequently became areas of independent and intensive investigation, and tremendous advancement has occurred, with concomitant improved survival in both laboratory and clinical populations.

The first human heart transplant was carried out by Hardy et al.[7] in 1964, when they unsuccessfully transplanted a chimpanzee heart into a patient dying of left ventricular failure. This effort focused considerable attention on the evolving laboratory experience and on the possibility of clinical implementation. Barnard[8] in 1967 performed the first human orthotopic cardiac allograft transplantation at the Groote-Schuur Hospital in Cape Town. Although the patient did not achieve long-term survival, this operation did usher in a period of intense interest and widespread clinical activity in cardiac transplantation. During the first year following the operation in South Africa, more than 100 cardiac transplants were performed, with generally poor results. Disillusionment based on these poor results culminated in a precipitous decline in clinical interest (Figure 73.1).

On the basis of a long laboratory experience, clinical orthotopic cardiac transplantation was begun at Stanford University Medical Center in January 1968. The program at Stanford, both in the laboratory and in the clinical sphere, has continued without interruption since its inception, and the clinical volume has steadily increased (Figure 73.1). This continual increase in clinical activity was based upon gradual but steady improvement in survival (Table 73.1).

Table 73.1. Stanford Cardiac Transplantation: One-Year Survival by Program by Year

Year	Percent
First	22
Fifth	54
Tenth	58
Fifteenth	83

SELECTION OF RECIPIENTS

Appropriate candidates for cardiac transplantation are patients who have end-stage congestive heart failure, placing them in New York Heart Association class IV for symptoms. These are patients for whom no other conventional medical or surgical therapy is applicable; life expectancy is measured in weeks or months without transplantation. There is currently no lower age limit for cardiac transplantation, and certain congenital anomalies, such as the hypoplastic left heart, may ultimately be best treated by cardiac transplantation; however, this area remains investigative. The current upper age limit is 60 years; experience with patients over 50 years of age is still limited, but recent reports suggest that transplantation is a satisfactory method in this group.[9]

There are several contraindications to cardiac transplantation. The first of these is the presence of another major systemic disease, such as a malignancy or collagen vascular disease. Insulin-requiring diabetes mellitus is a contraindication because of the expected exacerbation with postoperative steroid immunosuppression. Moderate prerenal azotemia and passive hepatic congestion are common in the cardiac transplant recipient group, but irreversible degrees of renal or hepatic dysfunction do constitute contraindications to transplantation. Recent pulmonary infarction generally precludes transplantation because of the risk of bleeding with heparinization and the possibility of related pulmonary infection.

Fixed elevation of pulmonary vascular resistance above 6 to 8 Wood units generally makes orthotopic cardiac transplantation unfeasible because of the inability of the normal donor right ventricle to sustain function against high pulmonary pressure. Decisions regarding the influence of pulmonary vascular resistance on transplantation require considerable judgmental input, and factors to be considered include reversibility with vasodilator agents, availability of an on-site donor, the use of a donor with a larger body mass than the recipient's, the use of special operative and pharmacologic techniques for augmentation of right ventricular function, heterotopic transplantation techniques, and possibly the use of temporary right ventricular assistance devices.

The importance of a thorough and accurate preoperative psychologic evaluation cannot be overstressed. It is essential to ascertain, inasmuch as possible, that the potential recipient will be able to cope successfully with the stress of operation and the requirements of postoperative medication compliance and clinical follow-up.

DONOR SELECTION

Cardiac allograft donors are chosen from persons who have sustained brain death, usually due to cerebral trauma

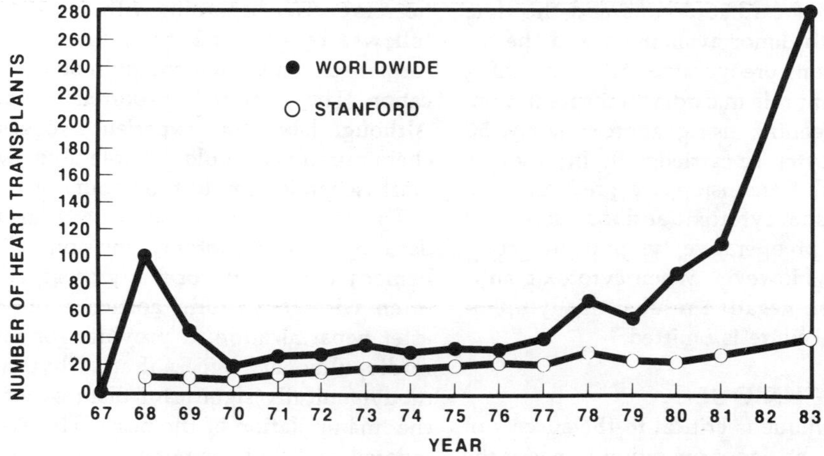

Figure 73.1. Number of cardiac transplants performed by year from 1967 to 1983.

or acute cerebrovascular accident, but who have continued stable cardiopulmonary function. To avoid unrecognized coronary artery disease and other acquired conditions, donors should be less than 35 years of age. They should have no history of cardiac disease and no evidence of active infection. Frequently, brain-dead organ donors maintained on mechanical ventilation will have purulent tracheobronchial secretions, but this finding does not represent a contraindication, and appropriate antibiotic coverage should be employed. It should be ascertained that no chest trauma likely to have resulted in direct cardiac contusion has occurred; serial electrocardiograms and isoenzyme determinations will assist in this judgment. Prolonged efforts at cardiopulmonary resuscitation preclude the use of the heart in transplantation. In addition, with appropriate fluid management and the treatment of diabetes insipidus, the condition of the donor should remain hemodynamically stable with little or no vasopressor support. When larger dose pressor support is required on a continuing basis despite adequate volume replacement, the donor heart should not be transplanted.

MATCHING OF DONOR AND RECIPIENT

When a donor heart that is appropriate for transplantation becomes available, the organ is matched with an appropriate recipient. Given the exigencies of cardiac transplantation and donor availability, clinical immunologic matching in the preoperative period is rudimentary. Recipients are considered on the basis of ABO blood group compatibility with the donor. Within this constraint, donors and recipients are matched for body mass, with the general stipulation that the donor's body mass be not more than 20% smaller than the recipient's. When the recipient's pulmonary vascular resistance is elevated, it is helpful to choose donors of at least equal if not greater body mass.

A limited retrospective analysis of HLA incompatibility in cardiac transplantation has shown no discernible correlation between the degree of HLA incompatibility and the severity or frequency of rejection.[10] Early analysis suggested that the incidence of coronary artery disease was greater when mismatching occurred at the HLA-A2 locus between donor and recipient. However, recent retrospective analysis does not support this relation. Therefore, given the scarcity of cardiac donors and the time pressure in terms of both donor availability and the recipient's clinical condition, preoperative HLA matching does not play an important role in cardiac transplantation. Cytotoxic antibody screening using approximately 50 random donor lymphocytes is carried out. In cases of previous surgery, blood transfusion, or pregnancy, in which the results of random cytotoxic antibody screening tests may be positive, preoperative lymphocyte cross-matching is carried out. However, when cytotoxic antibody screening has given negative results, this lymphocyte cross-matching procedure is omitted.

TECHNIQUE

Optimal surgical technique is critical to the success of cardiac transplantation. The donor operation provides the final opportunity for accurate donor assessment and requires meticulous attention to physiologic graft preservation. The recipient operation requires continued focus on preservation of the graft and exemplifies all of the basic principles of open heart surgery, with special emphasis on exclusion of air from the heart and appropriate resuscitative measures.

Since 1977, most of our cardiac transplant operations have been carried out using distant organ procurement. Several advantages obtain when distant procurement of cardiac allografts is used. The available donor pool is greatly expanded, and the very real personal needs of families and physicians who prefer that the bodies of organ donors not be moved are fulfilled. Furthermore, this technique has facilitated cooperation between cardiac transplantation groups and other organ transplantation groups. Given the continuing shortage of organs for transplantation, the importance of this aspect cannot be overemphasized. Special circumstances exist in which distant organ procurement may be inappropriate. In particular, recipients with pulmonary vascular resistance in the borderline elevated range are best served when an on-site donor with minimal graft ischemic time can be used.

The donor operation is carried out without cardiopulmonary bypass. A standard median sternotomy incision is employed, and the heart and great vessels are carefully inspected particularly for unrecognized trauma, coronary artery disease, valvular disease, or other congenital anomalies. The heart and great vessels are dissected out in the usual fashion and the superior and inferior venae cavae are isolated. The donor is given 30,000 units of intravenous heparin via the superior vena cava. Inflow occlusion is achieved through ligation of the superior vena cava and clamping of the inferior vena cava. The heart is allowed to beat for four or five cycles to empty, and the aortic cross-clamp is then applied. Cold crystalloid potassium cardioplegic solution is administered through the aortic root. The superior vena cava and right superior pulmonary vein are immediately incised to eliminate the possibility of distension of either the right or the left side of the heart. Topical cooling with normal saline (4°C) is carried out during administration of the cardioplegic solution. Graft dysfunction related to procurement most often results from distension or inadequate cooling, and attention to the details of the donor operation is mandatory. The heart is excised beginning with division of the venae cavae followed by the aorta, the pulmonary veins at the pericardial reflection, and the pulmonary artery at its bifurcation. The graft is transported in normal saline (4°C). Although laboratory experience suggests that longer ischemic periods would be tolerable, we currently limit graft ischemic time to four hours or less.

The recipient operation is performed through a standard median sternotomy incision. Given the tenuous hemodynamic status of many prospective recipients, it is often wise to perform aortic cannulation immediately after heparinization. It provides for rapid institution of cardiopulmonary bypass if an arrhythmia or another hemodynamically significant disturbance occurs after further manipulation of the heart. The aorta should be cannulated as distally as possible, usually at the base of the innominate artery. Cannulation of the venae cavae is performed using a lateral approach to the right atrium with uncrossed cannulas. Snares are placed around the superior and inferior cavae to exclude air from the circuit.

After institution of cardiopulmonary bypass, the caval snares are tightened and the aortic cross-clamp is applied. The aorta should be clamped before manipulation of the heart to avoid dislodgement of thrombi. The heart is excised, beginning in the right atrium, just lateral to the right atrial appendage. The incision is carried caudally along the atrioventricular groove so as to maximize the available right atrial cuff. This portion of the incision is carried down through the coronary sinus and the atrial septum into the left atrium, emptying the blood from the left side of the heart. The aorta and pulmonary artery are then transected at the immediate supravalvular level. Excision of the heart is completed by continuation of the incision through the atrial septum superiorly and posterior to the left atrial appendage. Electrocautery is used to control bleeding from small vessels in the atrial cuffs.

The donor heart is brought into the field, and the aorta and pulmonary artery are separated. The transverse sinus is dissected out, and the pulmonary artery is fashioned with an appropriate circumference for the recipient. The pulmonary veins are interconnected to form a uniform left atrial circumference.

Implantation of the graft is begun with the left atrial anastomosis, beginning at the recipient left superior pulmonary vein and the donor left atrial appendage (Figure 73.2). This anastomosis is made using a continuous polypropylene suture technique. On completion of the posterior portion of the left atrial anastomosis, topical cooling with normal saline is recommenced. When the left atrial anastomosis is completed in the midportion of the atrial septum, a second catheter containing cold saline is introduced. This so-called bubble-free line is introduced into the left atrium through a small incision in the tip of the left atrial appendage. Infusion of cold saline through this line further enhances endomyocardial cooling and excludes air from the left side of the graft during the remainder of the operation.

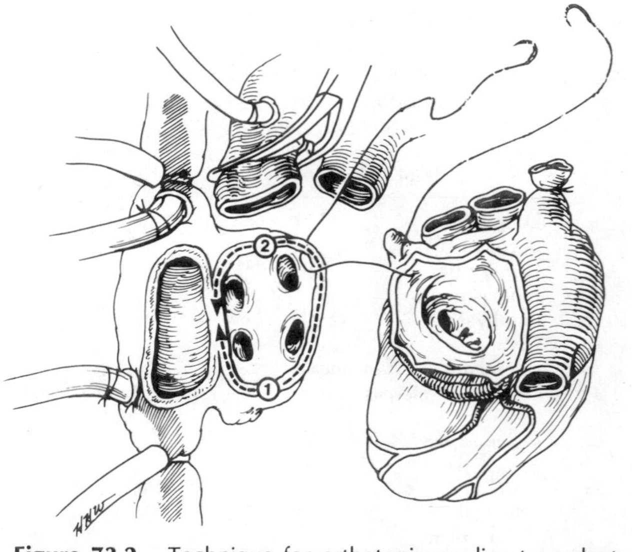

Figure 73.2. Technique for orthotopic cardiac transplantation.

The right atrium is then incised, beginning at the inferior vena cava and proceeding in a curvilinear direction toward the atrioventricular groove to avoid injury to the sinus node.[11] The length of this incision is made to correlate with the size of the recipient right atrial cuff. Anastomosis is then begun in the midportion of the atrial septum and is carried out using the same running polypropylene technique.

Systemic cooling to 28°C is used during cardiopulmonary bypass, and systemic warming is begun on commencement of the aortic anastomosis. This end-to-end anastomosis is carried out again using polypropylene. With careful attention to evacuation of air, the aortic cross-clamp is removed and resuscitation is actively pursued. If distension intervenes, rhythm should quickly be established through cardioversion or epicardial pacing or both, but spontaneous defibrillation usually occurs.

The pulmonary arterial anastomosis is carried out with the aortic cross-clamp removed and in a similar manner to that described for the aorta. This maneuver is not technically difficult and serves to minimize graft ischemic time.

Gradual warming and resuscitation are accomplished, and pressor support, usually with isoproterenol, is instituted. Atrial and ventricular epicardial pacing wires are usually placed, along with appropriate drainage catheters.

POSTOPERATIVE MANAGEMENT

The early postoperative respiratory and hemodynamic management of cardiac transplant recipients is similar to that of patients undergoing other cardiac operations. Early ventilator weaning and extubation and early ambulation are of considerable importance. Patients are usually maintained on low-dose isoproterenol support for four to five days because graft dysfunction has been observed in patients who are weaned earlier. Arrhythmias occurring in the early postoperative period are treated with digoxin, quinidine, and procainamide or with electrical cardioversion when appropriate. Beta-blocking agents are generally best avoided. Prophylactic postoperative antibiotic coverage with cephalosporin is continued for five days.

The progressive improvement in survival for clinical cardiac transplantation correlates with advances in immunosuppressant techniques. Cyclosporine is currently the mainstay of immunosuppression. However, because of many observed adverse effects possibly related to cyclosporine, the recent trend is toward lower dosages.

Current immunosuppression protocols in our institution are indicated in Table 73.2. This two-armed regimen includes cyclosporine with a target level of 200 to 300 ng/ml during the first six weeks after transplantation. After an initial loading dose of 18 mg/kg orally, patients are maintained on doses of 10 to 12 mg/kg/day depending on renal and hepatic function. Lower serum levels are targeted after the early postoperative period, when the frequency and seriousness of rejection are greatest. With the lower dosage of cyclosporine, azathioprine is employed, with modulation of dosage according to the WBC count. All patients receive an early prophylactic course of intravenous equine antithymocyte globulin and intravenous perioperative steroid coverage. As noted in the

Table 73.2. Immunosuppression Protocols Using "Low-Dose" Cyclosporine

Protocol 1

1. *Cyclosporine:* 18 mg/kg orally as preoperative loading dose; 10 mg/kg/day orally postoperatively, with target level of 200 to 300 ng/ml for first six weeks
2. *Azathioprine:* 4 mg/kg intravenously (IV) as preoperative loading dose; 2 mg/kg/day (according to WBC count) as postoperative maintenance
3. *Equine antithymocyte globulin:* 10 mg/kg/day IV (dose adjusted according to rosette count) for seven days.
4. *Steriods:* methylprednisolone 500 mg IV at discontinuation of cardiopulmonary bypass, 125 mg IV every eight hours for three doses; prednisone 0.2 mg/kg/day as maintenance

Protocol 2

Same as Protocol 1, without maintenance prednisone

Table 73.3. Cause of Death after Cardiac Transplantation (N=307; 177 Deaths)

Cause of Death	No.
Infection	93
Rejection	30
Graft atherosclerosis	18
Malignancy	12
Pulmonary hypertension	7
Cerebrovascular accident	3
Pulmonary embolism	2
Cerebral edema	1
Myopathy	1
Suicide	1
Acute graft failure	2
Hepatic failure	1
Sudden death, unknown cause	6

table, one arm of the protocol includes maintenance prednisone coverage, whereas the other does not.

Endomyocardial biopsy is ordinarily carried out on the seventh postoperative day. Rejection occurring earlier than this is extremely rare, but when clinical conditions mandate, earlier biopsy should be contemplated. Cardiac biopsy is performed under local anesthesia using a percutaneous Seldinger technique for introduction of the bioptome through the right internal jugular vein. Under fluoroscopic guidance, the bioptome is advanced into the right ventricle and apposed against the interventricular septum. Because cardiac rejection in the cyclosporine-treated group may be heterogeneous in its distribution, it is important to obtain multiple (four or five) biopsy specimens.

Rejection with myocyte necrosis is initially treated with steroid boluses. Patients are given methylprednisolone 1,000 mg intravenously every day for three days. Histologic resolution normally occurs within four days, and endomyocardial biopsy is repeated at that time. If histologic rejection has not resolved, the three-day course of intravenous methylprednisolone is repeated. If rejection persists on a third consecutive biopsy, intravenous methylprednisolone therapy is combined with intramuscular rabbit antithymocyte globulin therapy. Occasionally, rejection may be so fulminating or recalcitrant to therapy that retransplantation must be contemplated. Six patients in our experience have required emergency retransplantation for rejection.

When complications do not intervene, patients are discharged approximately three weeks after operation. The frequency of clinic visits and outpatient endomyocardial biopsies is based on the individual patient's clinical history.

COMPLICATIONS

The range of complications involved in cardiac transplantation is suggested by the causes of death depicted in Table 73.3. Clearly, infection and rejection constitute the greatest threat to the cardiac transplant recipient. The sites of infection and the wide distribution of organisms that may be involved in the immunosuppressed host underscore the great importance of clinical vigilance (Table 73.4). Antimicrobial therapy must be applied promptly and aggressively, but it does not differ qualitatively from that used in other patients. In the era of cyclosporine immunosuppression, the importance of identifying a minimal effective level of immunosuppression still pertains, and the incidence of infection has not declined significantly compared with that in conventional immunosuppression. However, the severity of clinical illness for a given infection is less among cyclosporine-treated patients and the response of patients on cyclosporine therapy to appropriate antimicrobial therapy is generally better than that of patients taking conventional drugs.

Rejection remains a major source of morbidity and mortality in cardiac transplant recipients. The introduction of cyclosporine immunosuppression has statistically reduced the frequency of rejection significantly. As noted in Figure 73.3, approximately half the recipients will have experienced an episode of rejection by one month postoperatively. However, as with infection, the introduction of cyclosporine has been associated with a reduction in the clinical severity of illness when rejection does occur. Severe acute rejection is seen in the cyclosporine-treated group, but the general trend has been toward less severe rejection episodes, making possible the outpatient treat-

Table 73.4. Site of and Organisms Involved in Infection After Cardiac Transplantation with Cyclosporine Immunosuppression (12/80–9/83; N=80 patients)

Site of Infection	No.
Lung	30
Bacteremia	16
Urinary tract	6
Mediastinum	7
Emphysema	1
CNS	1
Cutaneous, Herpes simplex	24
Cutaneous, Herpes zoster	7
Organisms Involved	
Bacterial	77
Viral	56
Fungal	16
Protozoan	2
Nocardia	3

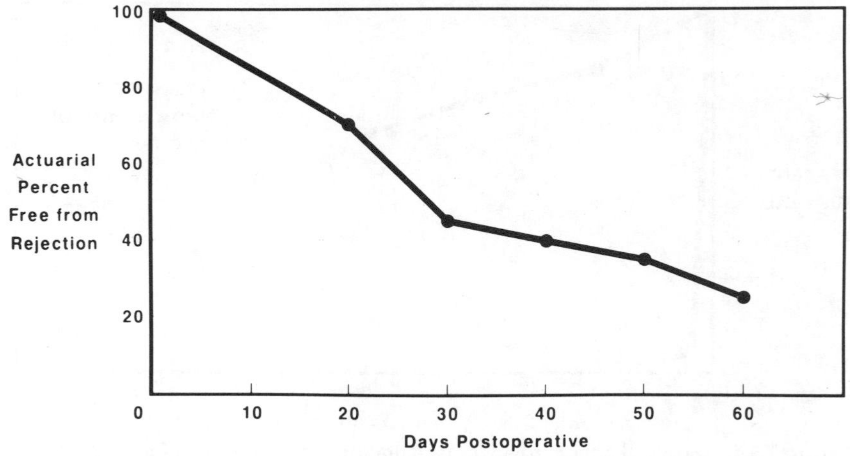

Figure 73.3. Frequency of rejection after cardiac transplantation (cyclosporine patients), as indicated by actuarial percent free from rejection.

ment of some episodes with modulation of oral steroid therapy.

Graft atherosclerosis is a persistent and disturbing cause of mortality among cardiac transplant recipients. Because of the denervated state of the transplanted heart, the occurrence of coronary artery disease is insidious, manifested only by the gradual onset of congestive heart failure or by sudden death. The occurrence of this phenomenon is the basis for our practice of yearly angiographic follow-up. It is surprising that the incidence of graft atherosclerosis among recipients who underwent cardiac transplantation for coronary artery disease is similar to that among patients who received transplants for cardiomyopathy. The basis for this affliction is incompletely understood, but it is presumed to be a chronic, immunologically mediated rejection process resulting in intimal injury, platelet adherence, and atherogenesis. Typically, this form of atherosclerosis is particularly aggressive and diffuse, involving the distal coronary vasculature in a way that precludes consideration of coronary artery bypass grafting. When severe, graft atherosclerosis may require consideration of retransplantation, and this problem has been the most frequent reason for retransplantation in our series.

Malignancy is many times more common in organ transplant recipients than in the general population. Lymphoma, in particular, has been a frequent complication after cardiac transplantation and is characterized by large cell immunoblastic (diffuse histiocytic) histopathology, by early occurrence after transplantation (within four months), and by frequent central nervous system involvement. In approximately 160 transplants at our institution since the introduction of cyclosporine immunosuppression in December 1980, there have been six lymphomas. Retrospective analysis of the quantitative degree of immunosuppression in these patients suggests that the overall degree of immunosuppression correlates with the risk of lymphoma, with high mean cyclosporine levels and high cyclosporine levels during periods of T-cell suppression from antithymocyte globulin therapy best differentiating the lymphoma from the nonlymphoma group.[12] No specific role for the Epstein-Barr virus could be demonstrated, although the concurrence of high cyclosporine levels and Epstein-Barr virus antibody titer conversion did appear to predict a high risk of lymphoma. Optimal therapy for these neoplasms remains speculative, although conventional radiation and chemotherapy as well as acyclovir therapy for presumed virologic etiologies have been employed. Other patients have been treated with reduction of immunosuppression on the assumption that the lymphoma is due to the overall level of immunosuppression. Analysis of our data substantiates this assumption, and the importance of identifying the lowest effective level of immunosuppression is again pointed out.[12]

RESULTS

Since the inception of the clinical program at Stanford University Medical Center in January 1968, some 400 cardiac transplants have been performed in more than 360 patients. There has been steady improvement in survival results, and current one-year survival exceeds 80%. Actuarial survival statistics, comparing the results of cardiac transplantation since the introduction of cyclosporine in 1980 with survival among prospective recipients for whom no donor is found, show the dramatically improved outlook for survival that it provides (Figure 73.4). Because cardiac transplantation is performed in relatively young patients with disease limited to the cardiac axis and its direct ramifications, these results translate into an excellent rehabilitation outlook, with 84% of one-year survivors being able to return to work or to school.

CARDIOPULMONARY TRANSPLANTATION

The great difficulties encountered in the treatment of patients with end-stage pulmonary vascular disease have generated considerable laboratory interest in the possibility of combined heart and lung transplantation. During the late 1950s and early 1960s, several laboratory experiences with cardiopulmonary transplantation in animals were reported.[13,14] However, success in the laboratory was complicated by the tremendous problems related to postoperative pulmonary insufficiency. These problems reflected the complex interrelation between postoperative

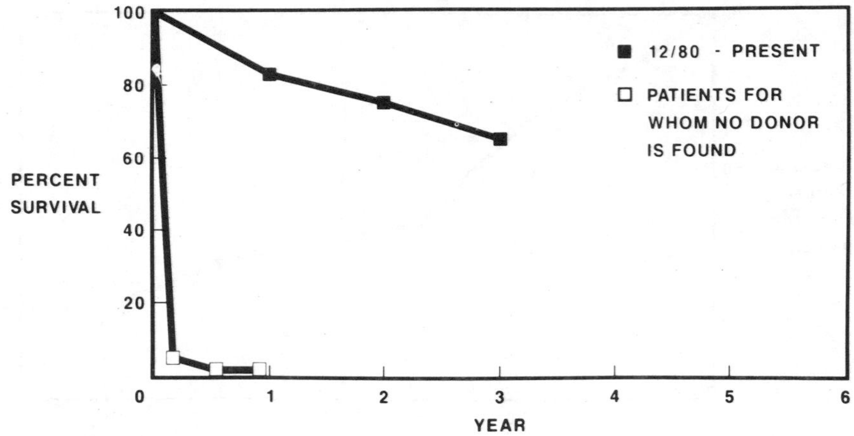

Figure 73.4. Survival after cardiac transplantation in the Stanford University Medical Center program.

atelectasis, infection, surgical denervation, and interruption of lymphatic drainage, pulmonary edema, "reimplantation," and rejection. However, efforts in the laboratory continued, and with favorable results in primates in our laboratory and evident improvement in cardiac transplantation results with the use of cyclosporine, a clinical cardiopulmonary transplantation program was begun at our institution in 1981.[15,16]

The range of potential indications for combined heart and lung transplantation is great. The many patients with end-stage left ventricular failure due to atherosclerotic, valvular, or congenital heart disease associated with left ventricular failure and elevated pulmonary vascular resistance are particularly evident in this regard, because they are frequently disqualified from consideration for orthotopic cardiac transplantation. In addition, patients with primary pulmonary hypertension, cystic fibrosis, and end-stage pulmonary disease associated with cor pulmonale could all be considered as potential candidates for this therapy. Thus far, we have limited our clinical application to patients with primary pulmonary hypertension and Eisenmenger's syndrome, who are less than 45 years of age and who have no other systemic illnesses. The contraindications to cardiac transplantation, with the exception of elevated pulmonary vascular resistance, pertain in this group. Early clinical experience has suggested that because of formidable problems with postoperative bleeding, patients with prior thoracotomy do represent a substantially higher risk group.

Basic criteria for donor selection are the same as those for cardiac transplantation. Donor availability is the salient and rate-limiting aspect of clinical cardiopulmonary transplantation and is affected primarily by the great difficulty in maintenance of adequate pulmonary toilet and function in the brain-dead patient. This fact underscores the importance of early identification of the brain-dead person as a potential organ donor, so that the organ can be procured before pulmonary deterioration occurs. In addition to the criteria already mentioned for potential cardiac donors, donors for cardiopulmonary transplantation should exhibit a pO_2 greater than 100 on 40% inspired oxygen, peak inspiratory pressures less than 30 to 35 mm Hg, and clear chest radiographs. The management of potential cardiopulmonary donors may be somewhat more difficult than that of potential heart donors because of the importance of meticulous pulmonary toilet and the avoidance of neurogenic pulmonary edema. Fluid restriction is of greater importance, and manipulation of peripheral vascular resistance with alpha agents and aggressive treatment of diabetes insipidus with intramuscular vasopressin minimize the requisite fluid replacement for the donor.

The recipient operation has been described in detail[17] and is diagrammed in Figure 73.5. Safe removal of recipient organs is paramount, and the technique emphasizes the avoidance of injury to the phrenic nerves, vagi, and recurrent laryngeal nerve. Furthermore, particularly in patients with Eisenmenger's syndrome, meticulous attention to hemostasis of the bronchial circulation is essential, because this portion of the surgical dissection is subjected to systemic pressure after discontinuation of cardiopulmonary bypass and is inaccessible after implantation of the heart/lung graft. Implantation of the graft

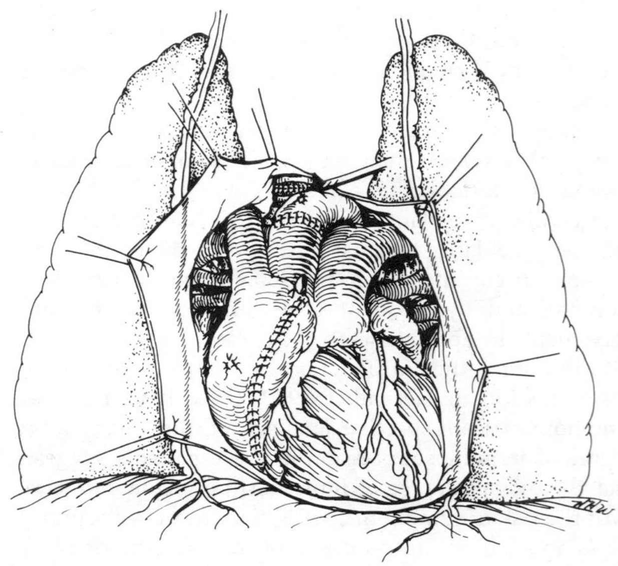

Figure 73.5. Technique for combined heart and lung transplantation.

is begun with tracheal anastomosis using end-to-end running polypropylene sutures. The right atrial and aortic anastomoses are then performed sequentially.[18]

Postoperative management of combined heart and lung transplant recipients is similar to that of heart transplant recipients. However, in cardiopulmonary transplantation with surgical interruption of lymphatic drainage, rigorous fluid restriction and meticulous pulmonary toilet are extremely important. Postoperative immunosuppression includes cyclosporine, azathioprine, and rabbit antithymocyte globulin. Steroid therapy is avoided for the first two weeks after transplantation, to enhance the conditions for tracheal healing.

Surveillance for rejection is carried out in the same manner as for cardiac transplantation. However, recent evidence suggests that isolated pulmonary rejection may occur, and when clinical and radiologic evidence of pulmonary dysfunction occurs in the absence of evidence of infection, the possibility of pulmonary rejection must be contemplated.[19]

Thirty combined heart and lung transplant operations have been performed in 29 patients at our institution. These patients have been nearly evenly divided between the categories of primary pulmonary hypertension and Eisenmenger's syndrome. Fourteen patients are currently surviving at intervals of 8 to 49 months. Early mortality was due to postoperative hemorrhage, principally related to intrathoracic adhesion from previous surgery, and multisystem failure in sepsis. One late death 18 months after cardiopulmonary transplantation was due to graft atherosclerosis and myocardial infarction. Obstructive airway disease of varying severity developed in 7 of 17 long-term survivors; one patient required retransplantation for this problem.

CONCLUSION

Evolving from laboratory experience near the turn of the century to clinical implementation over the past 17 years, cardiac transplantation has emerged as a standard mode of clinical therapy for end-stage congestive heart failure. It currently provides an excellent outlook for relatively long-term survival and rehabilitation. Cardiopulmonary transplantation is emerging as a clinical alternative in certain patients with end-stage pulmonary vascular disease. Further clinical application will depend upon increased availability of suitable donors, improved understanding of postoperative respiratory failure and the interrelation of pulmonary rejection and infection, and better understanding of long-term obstructive pulmonary changes.

Ongoing investigation in cardiac and cardiopulmonary transplantation focuses on improved control of the immune response, noninvasive diagnosis of rejection, improved techniques of graft preservation, the possibility of xenograft transplantation, and the interrelation between the fields of mechanical heart replacement and cardiac transplantation.

REFERENCES

1. Carrel A, Guthrie CC: The transplantation of veins and organs. *Am Med* 1905; 10:1101–1102.
2. Mann FC, Priestley JT, Markowitz J, Yates WM: Transplantation of the intact mammalian heart. *Arch Surg* 1933; 26:219–224.
3. Demikhov VP: *Experimental Transplantation of Vital Organs,* Basil Haigh (trans). New York, Consultants Bureau, 1962, p 126.
4. Lower RR, Shumway NE: Studies on orthotopic transplantation of the canine heart. *Surg Forum* 1960; 11:18-19
5. Lower RR, Dong E Jr, Glazener FS: Electrocardiograms of dogs with heart homografts. *Circulation* 1966; 33:455–460.
6. Reemtsma K, Williamson WE Jr, Iglesias F, Pena E, Sayegh SF, Creech O Jr: Studies in homologous canine heart transplantation: prolongation of survival with a folic acid antagonist. *Surgery* 1962; 52:127–133.
7. Hardy JD, Chavez CM, Kurrus FD, Neely WA, Eraslan S, Turner MD, Fabian LW, Labecki TD: Heart transplantation in man: developmental studies and report of a case. *JAMA* 1964; 188:1132–1140.
8. Barnard CN: The operation. A human cardiac transplant: an interim report of a successful operation performed at Groote-Schuur Hospital, Cape Town. S *Afr Med J* 1967; 41:1271–1274.
9. Emery RW, Levinson MM, Copeland JG: Cardiac transplantation in patients over 50 years of age, abstracted. *J Am Coll Cardiol* 1985; 5:534.
10. Stinson EB, Payne R, Griepp RB, Dong E Jr, Shumway NE: Correlation of histocompatibility matching with graft rejection and survival after cardiac transplantation in man. *Lancet* 1971; 2:459–462.
11. Barnard CN: What we have learned about heart transplants. *J Thorac Cardiovasc Surg* 1968; 56:457–468.
12. Brumbaugh J, Baldwin JC, Stinson EB, Oyer PE, Jamieson SW, Bieber CP, Henley W, Shumway NE: Quantitative analysis of immunosuppression in cyclosporine treated patients with lymphoma. *Heart Transplant* 1985; 4:307–311.
13. Webb WR, Howard HS: Cardiopulmonary transplantation. *Surg Forum* 1957; 8:313–317.
14. Lower RR, Stofer RC, Hurley EJ, Shumway NE: Complete homograft replacement of the heart and both lungs. *Surgery* 1961; 50:842–845.
15. Reitz BA, Burton NA, Jamieson SW, Bieber CP, Pennock JL, Stinson EB, Shumway NE: Heart and lung transplantation: auto-transplantation and allo-transplantation in primates with extended survival. *J Thorac Cardiovasc Surg* 1980; 80:360–372.
16. Oyer PE, Stinson EB, Jamieson SW, Hunt SA, Reitz BA, Bieber CP, Schroeder JS: One year experience with cyclosporin A in clinical heart transplantation. *Heart Transplant* 1982; 1:285–290.
17. Jamieson SW, Stinson EB, Oyer PE, Baldwin JC, Shumway NE: Operative technique for heart-lung transplantation. *J Thorac Cardiovasc Surg* 1984; 87:930–935.
18. Baldwin JC, Jamieson SW, Stinson EB, Oyer PE, Shumway NE: Cardiopulmonary transplantation. *Cardiovasc Rev Rep* 1984; 5:148–154.
19. McGregor CGA, Baldwin JC, Jamieson SW, Yousem SM, Burke CM, Oyer PE, Stinson EB, Shumway NE: Isolated pulmonary rejection after combined heart/lung transplantation. *J Thorac Cardiovasc Surg* 1985; 90: 623–625.

74 The Artificial Heart

Domingo Liotta, MD, José A. Navia, MD, Jorge Jordana, Pedro del Rio, MD, Miguel del Rio, MD, Omar Lima Quintana, MD, Robert Leachman, MD, Denton A. Cooley, MD and O.H. Frazier, MD

THE DEONTOLOGIC PRINCIPLE

Is life possible with a mechanical heart? Furthermore, is it reasonable to maintain life with a mechanical heart? These fundamental questions, which depend on the profound importance of religious feelings, philosophical attitudes, and logical concepts of modern science, have been answered affirmatively only in recent years.

Since the earliest times, the heart has been considered the organ of life. Life, pureness of feelings, ethical behavior toward others, goodness in human acts, and commiseration for the weak have, in all the history of mankind, been symbolized by the heart. The Egyptians believed their hearts were weighed before being admitted to the presence of the god Osiris, the balancing weights being a statue of the truth or an ostrich feather. If the equilibrium did not incline on the side of the heart, this was thrown to the tenebrae.* Homer had considered the heart in seventh century BC the dwelling place of feelings and passions. Biblical passages and the Judeo-Christian tradition are rich in metaphors, among which the heart is the symbol of the purity of love among human beings. The custom of separating the hearts of princes and distinguished dead extended over centuries. The heart of young Napoleon II, King of Rome, is found in the Loreto chapel in San Agustin Church in Vienna, whereas the body lies in *Les Invalides* in Paris.

In the philological study of ancient languages the heart always symbolizes life. In Sanskrit for the Indo-European languages and in Tibeto-Burman for the Chinese language, the word heart means life. In Sanskrit the word heart (*hrid, Krid*) also means jump, the observation of the concrete fact of an organ bounding in the chest. If this movement stopped, life was no longer possible. The terms *cord* in Latin, *Kardia* in Greek, *crudize* in Leton, *Ssird* in Armenian, and *hertz, heart, hearte,* and *hairt* in Germanic languages, all derived from the Sanskrit *Hrid, Krid*, the bouncer in the chest, the movement always meaning life.

The study of the Chinese language proves useful for these investigations. The graphic representation of the phonemes appears like photographs of the ideas (ideogram). The study of the Chinese phonemes in which the word *heart* is incorporated shows a strong spiritualistic connotation. In our investigation we were able to identify 18 hieroglyphs† (Figures 74.1, 74.2, and 74.3).

Modern scientific thinking has resulted in a fantastic reevaluation of concepts, a change in the comprehension and appreciation of the traditional intact being. Modern science now considers the heart as an object being. Science is not interested in the symbol of the everyday experience; its main concern is an a priori determination of the verifiable concepts of the nature of the heart entity, a separate organ, dissected, scrutinized with precision instruments, and finally having its function defined by mathematic calculations and numeric symbols. More than

* The Egyptian papyrus representing the symbol of the weight, together with the Chinese hieroglyphs of Yin-Zhou (XVI–XI BC) (Figure 74.1), is probably the oldest graphic document referring to the heart. Egyptian papyrus of the Royal Museums of Art and History of Brussels, Belgium. (From Boyadjian N (ed): *The Heart*. Antwerpen, Esco, 1980, p 16.)

† These linguistic works were initiated in China in 1973, 1975, and 1978 by one of us (DL). Recently (1981–1982), Mr Zhang Zhiya, second secretary of the Embassy of the People's Republic of China in Buenos Aires, and Dr Wang Yi-Shan, Professor of Cardiac Surgery, Shanghai Second Medical University, have greatly contributed to these investigations.

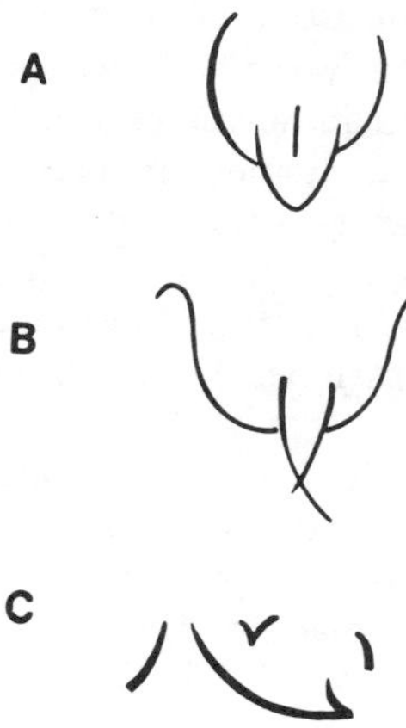

Figure 74.1. The original hieroglyph of the word *heart* in Chinese; note the shape of the natural heart in the ideogram. *A*, Jin Wen (ancient inscription in the brass vessels of the Yin-Zhou epoch of XVI to XI BC). *B*, Xiao Zhuan (a type of writing from the Qin dynasty of the twentieth century BC). *C*, The present writing.

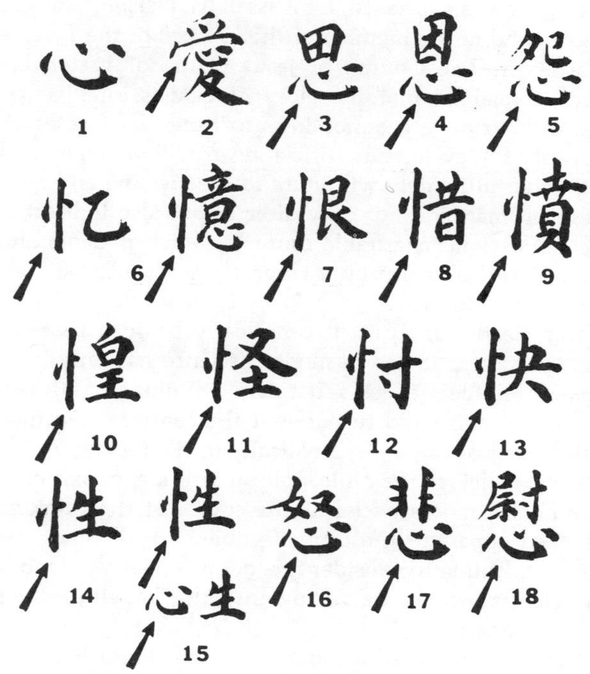

Figure 74.3. Many phonemes in the Chinese language have strong spiritualistic connotations. Their graphic representation incorporates the word *heart* (phonemes 1 to 18). *Arrows* indicate the position of the word *heart* in the phonemes. The pronunciation (in italics) and the meaning are as follows: 1, *xin*, heart, feel, center; 2, *ai*, love; 3, *si*, think, recall; 4, *en*, favor, kindness; 5, *yuan*, rancor, hate; 6, *yi*, remember, the left being a simplified version of the right; 7, *hen*, hate; 8, *xi*, hurt, regret, pity; 9, *fen*, irritate, resent, angry; 10, *huang*, alarmed; 11, *guai*, blame, strange; 12, *cun*, reflect, consider; 13, *kuai*, happy, rapid, sharp; 14, *xing*, sex, characteristics; 15, *xing*, heart + birth, heart + life; 16, *nu*, anger; 17, *bei*, sad; 18, *wei*, comfort. Numbers 14 and 15 are highly interesting; note how the ideas of sex and characteristics (*xing*) are integrated into birth and life (*sheng*), the right radical in number 15. (Chinese calligraphy is presented through the courtesy of the Honorable Han Xu, Ambassador of the People's Republic of China to the United States.)

a philosophic symbol, the heart entity in modern science is determined by natural laws, previously established by the scientific community to describe structure and function by a quantitative mathematic structure.

The description of the mechanical function, the hemodynamics of the heart, appears as one of the milestones of modern cardiology. Therefore, heart replacement becomes a mechanical problem rather than a physiologic, philosophic, or deontologic one.

In 1959, when we started work on mechanical circulation, we were aware only of the physiologic problems to be solved. We were all seduced, in those early days, by the magic of body cellular preservation achieved by means of extracorporeal circulation. The idea that naturally arose was how to provide long-term artificial circulation with a mechanical heart instead of extracorporeal pumping. This happened at least to us in the European spring of 1959 while working in the experimental laboratory of Lyon University in France.

The same thought had perhaps struck Pierre Salisbury when he presented his idea of a mechanical heart during one of the early meetings of the American Society of Artificial Internal Organs (ASAIO) in 1957. Soon, the challenging idea was carried out by Willem J. Kolff in the laboratories of Cleveland Clinic.

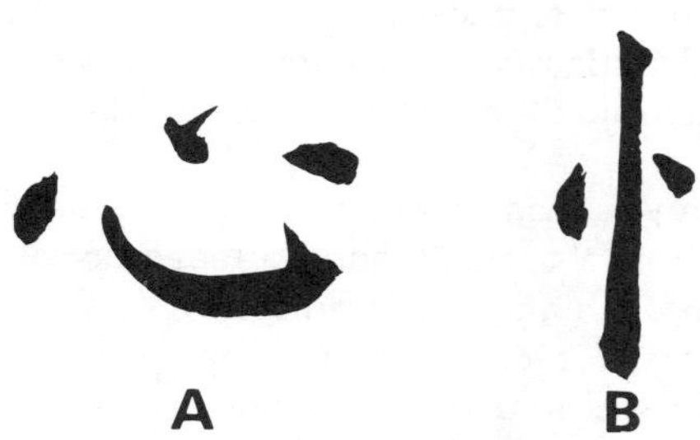

Figure 74.2. Two ways of representing the ideogram of the word *heart* in the modern Chinese language; *B* is usually a left radical of another Chinese character. (Chinese calligraphy is presented through the courtesy of the Honorable Han Xu, Ambassador of the People's Republic of China to the United States.)

After a decade of uncertainties in the search for a mechanical heart, our own hearts found spiritual encouragement in the words of Pope Paul VI in the European summer of 1969. In April of that year, together with Dr Cooley, we had implanted the first artificial heart in the history of medicine. During a personal interview with one of us (DAC), the Pope prudently declared: "In the advancement of man's science, the defense of life, *in an act of sincere love*, is the doctrine of Christianity itself. If the function of the natural organ reaches the extreme point where it can no longer maintain life, and if science has progressed to the extent that replacing the organ will maintain life, science must act."

From another scholar and church leader, a similar supporting view is expressed. Dr Russell M. Nelson,* cardiac surgeon and now a member of the Council of the Twelve Apostles in The Church of Jesus Christ of Latter-day Saints, explained that the glory of God is intelligence. Light and truth are ennobling attributes. The research necessary to develop an artificial heart will unveil eternal truths that ultimately will inure to the blessing and benefit of all mankind not only directly but also indirectly. The selfless and charitable cause to which patients and medical staff all contribute embraces service to our fellowman and to God.

From deeper analysis, it can clearly be seen that the change of heart image in modern science has only been apparent. In fact, it seems that man's thinking has drawn a complete circle and throughout the centuries returned to the point of origin. Symbolically in the feeling, in the religious belief, in the philosophical attitude, or as a concrete fact in modern science, the course of the thinking has been apparent: the ultimate object of all times has been life. Failing to consider this point of view, the modern scientist would be falling into the haughtiness of pseudoscience.

Man's intuition, reason, and belief reveal him as a spiritual being with a more or less lucid vocation to avoid perishing in time. The last call, the primary one, is that of existence. Defending existence is the radical vocation, the most honorable, with the condition that it is not exercised with deceit; a "sincere act of love to a fellow being."

The ethical principles that underlie all human behavior must be preserved in this difficult stage of medical research on a mechanical heart.

MECHANICAL CIRCULATION: EVOLUTION OF SYSTEMS

The development of mechanical systems for permanent circulatory support is the cardiologic challenge of the present and the future.

THE CRUCIAL 1960

Our own studies on the mechanical heart were begun in Lyon, France, in 1959, but it was in 1960 that we, together with a remarkable bioengineer, Tomas Taliani, and a group of co-workers, developed three models of the artificial heart. Oddly enough, the initial device was not constructed according to arrant principles, because of our obvious lack of understanding of the problems.

The first model, a pusher-plate type pump, incorporated a direct current electric motor. It was implanted orthotopically in a dog on May 8, 1960, after ablation of the natural heart (Figure 74.4). This animal maintained acceptable blood pressure levels and vital reflexes for three hours, 30 minutes. When the chest was closed, only the skin could be approximated because of the excessive size of the unit.[1–5]

The second model consisted of a continuous flow pump, a subocclusive roller type, with two separate chambers for each ventricle. It had no valves, and three rollers with a 120° separation maintained unidirectional blood flow (Figure 74.5). Energy was transmitted to the roller system by means of a percutaneous flexible shaft from an extracorporeal electrical motor. The model was implanted in a dog on September 15, 1960, and the dog survived eight hours.[2–5]

Finally, the third, a predecessor of the present models, used a pneumatic system. It was made of Plexiglas® and the two ventricles had valves of trileaflet (aortic) design, each valvular cusp being made of thin Dacron® tissue fabric (Figures 74.6, 74.7, 74.8). The blood pump diaphragm was made from thin latex rubber. The external power source was a pneumatic, piston type, with variable systolic volume. The elasticity of the latex regulated the diastolic negative pressure. This cardiac prosthesis was orthotopically implanted on November 6, 1960, in a dog which survived 13 hours.[3–5]

Looking back, it seems almost impossible to us that in only 1 year we were able to develop such diverse systems that reflected the subsequent course of experimentation and development of the artificial heart (Figure 74.9). Because of ignorance of the problems in the first model, we considered the hemodynamic and energy aspects together as one question. It was then realized that these two fundamental aspects must be separated; therefore, the second and third models were of a different and progressive design. Animal implantation of the three models was carried out in the Universidad Nacional de Cordoba and in the Hospital Provincial Nuestra Señora del Valle. The construction and in vitro circulation tests were performed in the factory and private laboratories of Tomas Taliani, who in 1960 was 77 years old.

In September 1961, experiments at the School of Medicine of Baylor University in Houston were started. The concept of an intracorporeal artificial left ventricle was presented for the first time. Various models were studied in in vitro circulation and in animal experimentation[6–15] (Figures 74.10, 74.11, 74.12). In 1963, together with Dr Stanley Crawford, we had the opportunity to implant in a patient the left ventricular assist device (LVAD) prosthesis represented in Figure 74.11.[8,8a] The patient, who had considerable left ventricular hypertrophy, was in postcardiotomy shock after undergoing replacement of a severely calcified aortic valve. The pump inlet was situated in the left atrium and the outlet in the descending thoracic aorta.

Implantation was made through a left thoracotomy at the fourth intercostal space 30 hours after aortic valvular replacement through a median sternotomy.†

During 1964 and 1965, the search for a better blood pump interface was initiated. A pseudoendocardium or neoendocardium, consisting of a fibrin substratum and blood cells, was produced by lining the blood chamber

*Russell M. Nelson, MD, PhD, DSc (Hon), was a member of the team of Dr Clarence Dennis developing a heart-lung machine used for the first time in a human being in March 1951 in Minneapolis, Minnesota. After a lifetime of service as a cardiac surgeon, he was called to render full-time service to The Church of Jesus Christ of Latter-day Saints as a member of the Council of the Twelve Apostles in April 1984.

†This clinical experience represents the first implantation of a mechanical circulatory system in the history of medicine. The original artificial ventricular pump used in this patient is permanently exhibited at the Smithsonian Institution in Washington, DC.

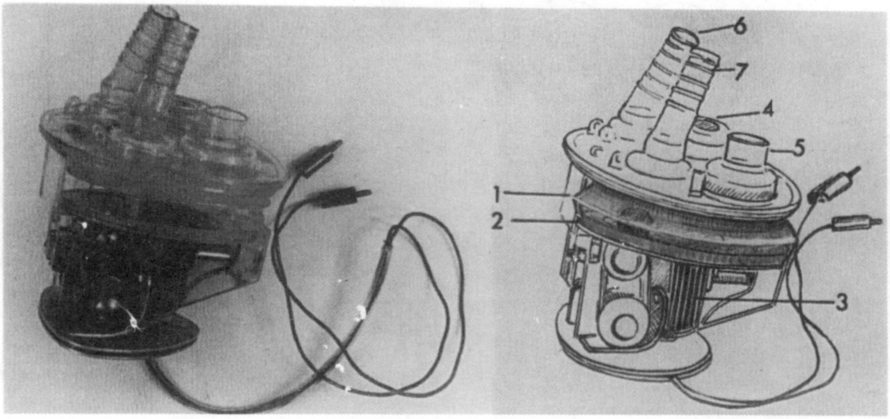

Figure 74.4. Photograph (*left*) and drawing (*right*) of the electric motor-driven orthotopic total artificial heart (implanted in May 1960). 1,2, pusher-plate type blood pump; 3, DC, brushless electric motor; 4,5, inlet connectors with Plexiglas ball valves; 6,7, outlet connectors with Plexiglas ball valves.

with velour type Dacron tissue fabric.[15-19] These investigations and those of others subsequently led to the design of a vascular prosthesis lined with velour type fabric.[20,21]

Near the end of 1965, the concept of a circulatory pump in a paracorporeal position was advanced, with blood pump connectors passing through the chest wall.[22] This system can be eliminated or disconnected without a new thoracotomy by closing and leaving the intrathoracic portions of the atrial and aortic conduits. The paracorporeal position seems ideal in patients with cardiogenic shock in the operating room, eg, perioperative myocardial infarction.

In 1966, after extensive animal studies, the clinical value of the left ventricular assist device (LVAD) in paracorporeal pumps was assessed at the Methodist Hospital of Houston.[23] The valves were Silastic® ball type, and the blood chamber was completely lined by velour Dacron fabric. The neoendocardial interface noted in clinical studies was surprising because of its uniform thickness and absence of irregular deposits in the fibrin layer. In calves, irregular excessive fibrin was frequently seen in selective areas of the ventricular chamber.

Conclusions from the clinical experience at the Methodist Hospital were difficult to reach and uncertain. Complications not related to the prosthesis under evaluation often occurred. However, the experience was valuable in the individual analysis of each patient. A patient in shock after double valve replacement was assisted over 14 days by a paracorporeal LVAD. This patient died 6 years later in a car accident.

In 1966, we studied the possibility that sepsis was caused by sinus tract formation around the percutaneous tubes to the external power source of the circulatory me-

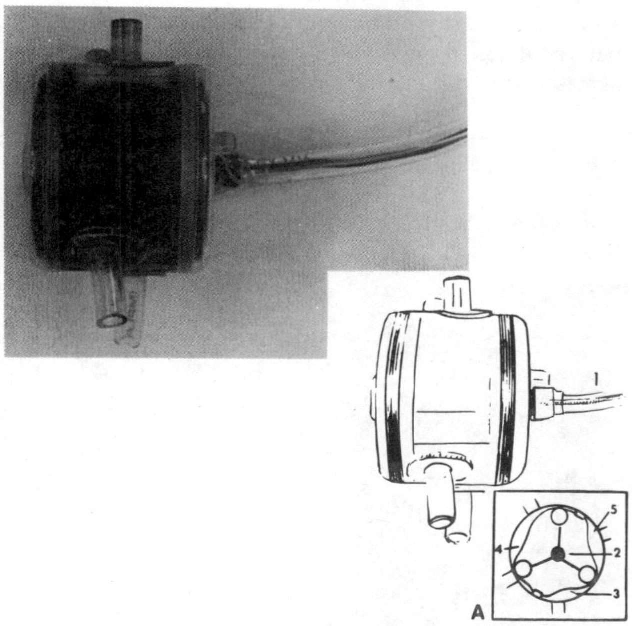

Figure 74.5. Photograph (*left*) and drawing (*right*) of the roller type, valveless, continuous flow orthotopic total artificial heart with external (paracorporeal) electric motor (implanted in September 1960). 1, flexible shaft for external electric motor; 2, central axis of blood pump; 3, membrane of blood chamber; 4, right ventricular blood chamber; 5, left ventricular blood chamber.

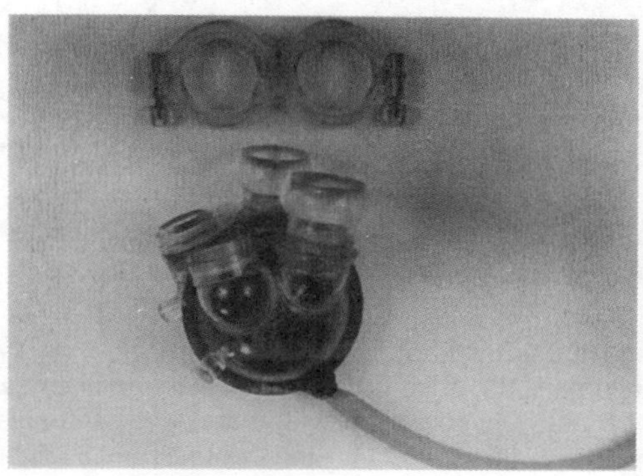

Figure 74.6. Photograph (lateral view) of the pneumatically driven orthotopic total artificial heart (implanted in November 1960).

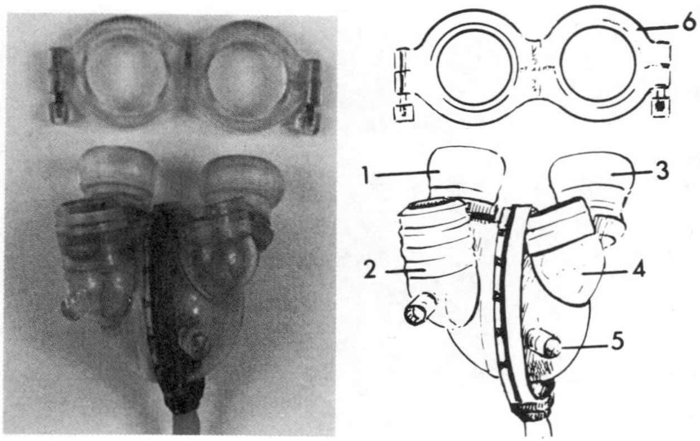

Figure 74.7. Photograph (*left*) and drawing (*right*) of the pneumatically driven orthotopic total artificial heart (frontal view) in Figure 74.6. 1, right ventricular inlet connector; 2, right ventricular outlet connector; 3, left ventricular inlet connector; 4, left ventricular outlet connector; 5, left ventricular air removal system; 6, right and left atrial quick connector system.

chanical system.[24-26] By sealing the percutaneous ducts with a subcutaneous velour Dacron fabric, the formation of sinus tracts was blocked by the growth of subepidermic tissue inside the Dacron tissue fabric. These works provoked investigations by others.[27]

On April 4, 1969, at the Texas Heart Institute in Houston, we implanted a biventricular heart in the orthotopic position in a patient with terminal ischemic myocardiopathy.* The pneumatic biventricular heart was implanted as part of a staged procedure at the height of initial enthusiasm for cardiac transplantation.[28,29] The four valves were of monocuspid hingeless design. The

* This clinical experience is the first implantation of an artificial heart in man in the history of medicine. The original cardiac prosthesis used in the patient is pemanently exhibited at the Smithsonian Institution in Washington, DC.

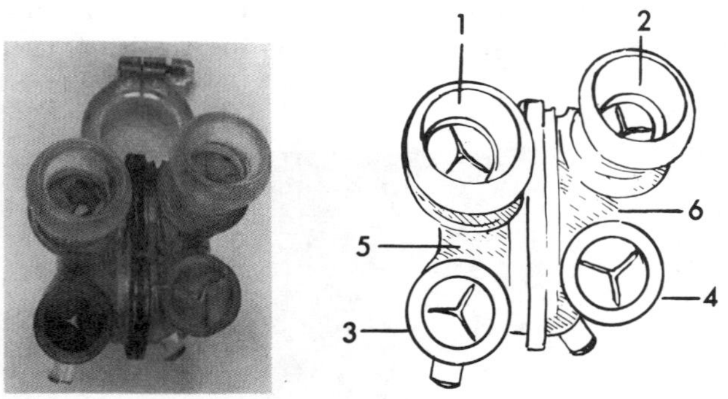

Figure 74.8. Photograph (*left*) and drawing (*right*) of the pneumatically driven orthotopic total artificial heart in Figures 74.6 and 74.7 (cephalic view). 1, right ventricular inlet connector; 2, left ventricular inlet connector; 3, right ventricular outlet connector; 4, left ventricular outlet connector; 5, right ventricular blood pump; 6, left ventricular blood pump. The four valves of a trileaflet (aortic) design; each valvular cusp is made of thin Dacron tissue fabric.

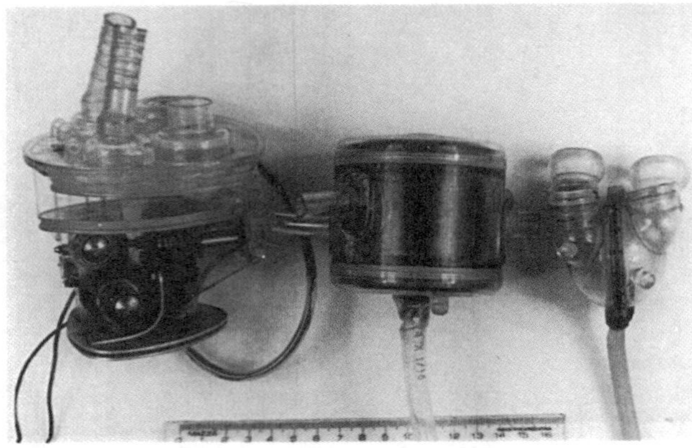

Figure 74.9. Photograph showing the comparative size in centimeters of the three models of the total artificial heart studied in vitro and in vivo in dogs in 1960.

blood pump chambers were lined with a velour Dacron fabric. For 64 hours the biventricular prosthesis worked acceptably, although its output remained lower than was necessary for the patient. The regurgitation present in the Wada-Cutter prosthesis substantially contributed to the marginal pump output.

The level of plasma hemoglobin unexpectedly increased in the early hours after implantation, but later stabilized. This effect had not been observed in the clinical implantation of the paracorporeal LVAD in 1966. It was thought secondary to the increased surface area within the blood chambers of the biventricular prosthesis. This observation later encouraged us to use polymers, such as polyurethane and Silastic, to create a smooth glossy interface in contact with blood. It was also of great interest that reduction of peripheral resistance with Arfonad® increased the volume output of the pump without any

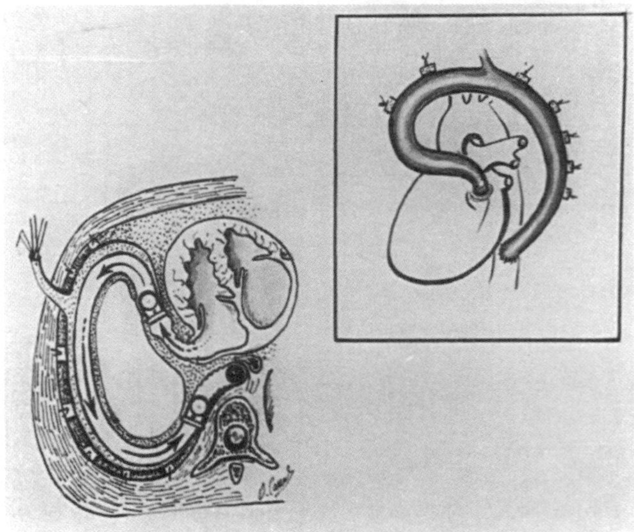

Figure 74.10. Model of an intrathoracic pneumatically driven LVAD positioned between the left atrium and descending thoracic aorta. The blood chamber made of Silastic had two Silastic ball valves studied in vitro and in vivo in calves in 1961 to 1962.

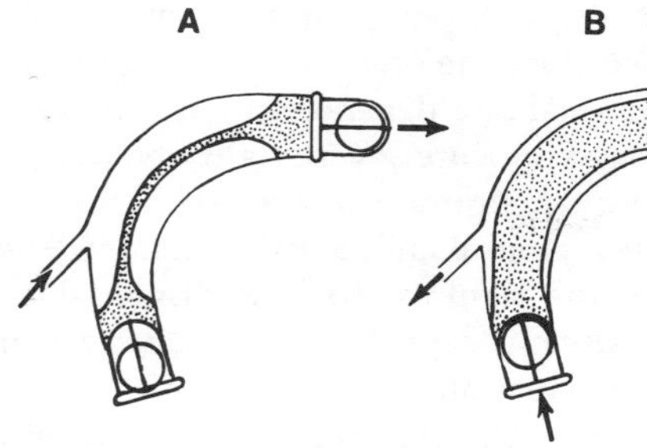

Figure 74.11. Model of an intrathoracic pneumatically driven LVAD positioned between the left atrium and descending thoracic aorta. The blood chamber made of Silastic had two Silastic ball valves. This model corresponds to the first intracorporeal auxiliary left ventricle implanted in man in 1963.[8,8a] *A*, Pump systole; *B*, pump diastole.

change in rate and pressure settings, an early example of afterload reduction.

In April 1969, the Baylor-Rice University program of total artificial heart research was discontinued.[30,31]

THE UNIVENTRICULAR TOTAL ARTIFICIAL HEART

On May 1, 1983, The International Council for Clinical Research on Mechanical Circulation, The International Council of Cardiac Surgeons was formed. There are currently 45 cardiac surgery services around the world willing to offer mutual aid for research on the mechanical circulation of blood.

The orthotopic univentricular artificial heart project was given priority by the council.[32-36] The possibility of excluding the right ventricular pump is a significant step in total artificial heart research. This new concept decreases the incidence of problems seen in biventricular hearts such as unbalanced output of the two ventricles, two valvular prostheses, the volume of blood pump, hemolysis, thromboembolism, sepsis, bleeding due to a disturbance of the hemostatic system (platelet dysfunction), and mechanical failure of the system. Because the energy required is reduced, the orthotopic univentricular artificial heart can be powered by a fully implantable battery-powered system. Pulmonary circulation is achieved with a direct right atrium–pulmonary artery shunt (Figure 74.13).

The rationale for this project is based on the good late results observed after the Fontan-Kreutzer operation for the treatment of tricuspid atresia. The pneumatically actuated, polyurethane-lined, single-chambered diaphragm type blood pump is positioned between the left atrium and aorta. The device displaces a thoracic volume of 210 cc, weighs 110 g, and provides a stroke volume of 90 cc (Figure 74.14). After acute experiments on right atrium–pulmonary artery shunts, we found that the most important factor in maintaining an adequate cardiac output was the volume of venous blood returned to the right atrium. To maintain this central volume, an abdominal compressor or splanchnic venous system assistance may be required for 24 to 48 hours (Table 74.1). Mean aortic pressure (AoP), right atrial pressure (RAP), and left atrial pressure (LAP) increased with abdominal compression. Pump minute output ($\dot{Q}$p) increased 78%.

Pierce et al[37,38] reported experiments in dogs using a single intrathoracic blood pump for a total artificial heart. Takano and Taenaka[39] reported their observations of paracorporeal left ventricular and right atrium–pulmonary artery shunts in goats.

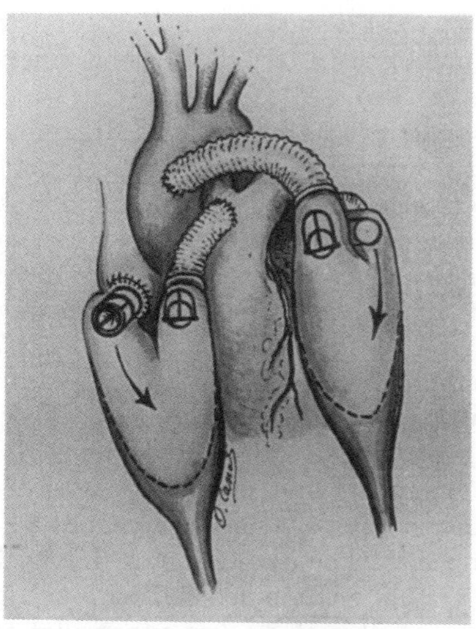

Figure 74.12. Model of an intrathoracic pneumatically driven auxiliary biventricular artificial heart. The two blood chambers made of Silastic have four Silastic ball valves studied in vitro and in vivo in calves in 1963 and 1964.

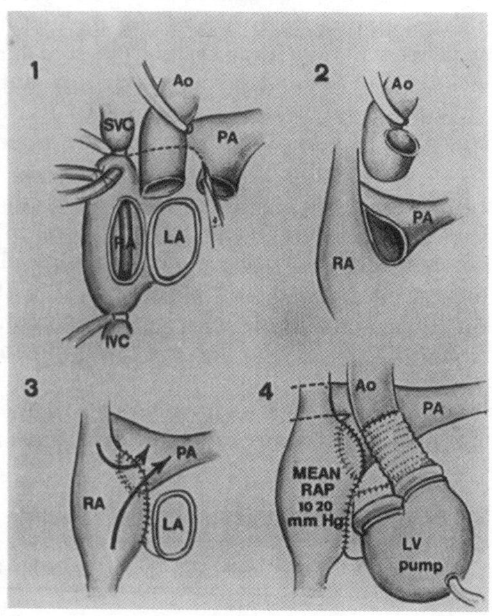

Figure 74.13. The orthotopic univentricular artificial heart surgical procedure: 1, removal of right ventricle and left ventricle; 2, longitudinal opening of pulmonary artery (PA) for right atrium (RA)–pulmonary artery shunt; 3, RA-PA shunt has been performed; 4, the orthotopic left ventricular pump positioned between the left atrium (LA) and aorta (Ao). IVC = inferior vena cava; SVC = superior vena cava.

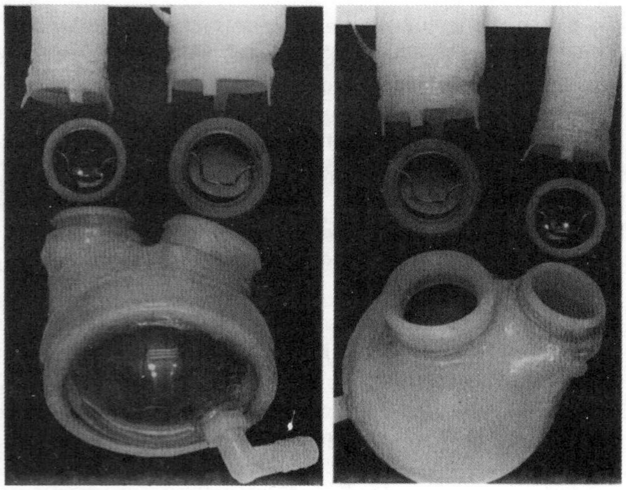

Figure 74.14. *Left*, Photograph (superior view) of pneumatically actuated single-chambered diaphragm type polyurethane (avcothane) blood pump for orthotopic univentricular artificial heart. Quick connection system for left atrium and aorta with two Björk-Shiley valve prostheses (Bioimplant Canada, Inc. Laboratory). *Right*, Photograph (inferior view) of blood pump.

PHYSIOLOGIC BASIS OF THE UNIVENTRICULAR ARTIFICIAL HEART

The anatomy and physiology indicate that the right ventricle is a volume pump rather than a pressure pump. At rest and during exercise, the right ventricle develops volumes per minute similar to those of the left ventricle, although with lower pressure. Right ventricular end-diastolic pressure (RVEDP) is lower than 5 mm Hg even during maximum effort. Mean pulmonary artery pressure (PAP) increases approximately 1 to 3 mm for each liter per minute increase in flow. Peak systolic pressure during exercise exceeds 30 to 40 mm Hg. Right ventricular output is determined, as is left ventricular output, by its characteristics as a blood pump: cardiac frequency, preload, afterload, and contractility. Furthermore, because the right ventricle is a volume pump, venous return is crucial. Pulmonary artery pressure is interrelated with intra-alveolar pressure, and pulmonary venous pressure plays a major role in the regional distribution of blood flow through the lung. The pulsatile character of pulmonary flow also contributes to the inciease in pulmonary circulation.

Both ventricles are functionally interrelated, sharing pericardium, myocardial structure (ventricular anatomic interdependence), and pump function of the right ventricle that conditions the preload of the left ventricle (circulatory functional interdependence). It is almost impossible to conceive of acute severe right ventricular failure without severe compromise of the left ventricle or vice versa. However, clinical and experimental evidence demonstrates that the right ventricle is dispensable, ie, the left ventricle alone is capable of maintaining pulmonary and systemic circulation.

The Fontan-Kreutzer procedure for tricuspid atresia has proven to be an adequate clinical model to study the physiologic consequences of acute and chronic exclusion of the right ventricle. Hemodynamic studies during late follow-up show that cardiac output is lower than that of the normal population, both at rest and during exercise. However, cardiac frequency, pulmonary resistance, and LVEDP are normal. High central venous pressure (CVP) is constant, 15 ± 4 mm Hg at rest and 25 ± 3.6 mm Hg during exercise. Arterial oxygen saturation is normal and most patients are in New York Heart Association class I functional capacity.[40,41]

In summary, after a right atrium–pulmonary artery shunt, right atrial pressure is sufficient to maintain adequate forward pulmonary flow. Indirect clinical evidence indicates that forward flow is enhanced by atrial systole.[41] Studies by Doppler technique demonstrate that flow is biphasic and antegrade even during left ventricular systole. Peak flow is to be expected during diastole, because it is the moment of higher gradient between the right atrium and left atrium. The absence of a functional right ventricle in the chronic state after a right atrium–pulmonary artery shunt probably affects left ventricular function by the mechanical and circulatory ventricular interdependence mentioned previously. If this is the case, the univentricular artificial heart should be spared this problem.

Venous return is another mechanism to be considered. In the direct right atrium–pulmonary artery derivation, the high central venous pressure contributes to preload in the left ventricle. However, it may limit venous return. Despite the apparent hemodynamic limitations after the right atrium-pulmonary artery shunt, good functional capacity can be reached.

Another excellent clinical model is acute right ventricular myocardial infarction. Acute right ventricular ischemia has two effects: low cardiac output and high central venous pressure. Although acute right ventricular infarction as a clinical model approximates the univentricular artificial heart model, mechanical and circulatory interdependence has a negative effect on left ventricular function. In acute right ventricular infarction, the right atrium and right ventricle become a single functional cavity. The diastolic and mean pressures tend to equalize in the right atrium, right ventricle, and pulmonary artery. Loss of right ventricular pump function is evidenced by the fact that increasing diastolic volume is not followed by increases in the systolic work index. Furthermore, right ventricular failure rapidly affects left ventricular function. Improvement in cardiac output with massive blood transfusion indirectly demonstrates this phenomenon.

A fundamental aspect of right ventricular function con-

Table 74.1. Effect of Abdominal Compression

	AbC OFF	AbC ON	Change (%)
AoP	113	153	+ 35
RAP	17	29	+ 71
LAP	3	10	+233
SV	42	75	+ 79
Qp	3.95	7.05	+ 78

AbC = abdominal compression; AoP = aortic pressure; LAP = left atrial pressure; Qp = pump output/min; RAP = right atrial pressure; SV = stroke volume.

cerns the regulation of venous return.[42] The principal element contributing to venous return is the pressure gradient between the mean circulatory filling pressure and the mean right atrial pressure. The natural resistance of the venous ductal system and gravitational forces are opposing venous flow return. Then, venous return flow ($\dot{Q}$) is equal to the following formula:

$$\dot{Q} = \frac{MCFP-RAP}{R}$$

The mean pressure of the circulatory system (Pms), which was originally reported by Guyton,[43] is the mean pressure of the cardiovascular system when the circulation is arrested; ie, a condition of non-flow.[44] The factors determining Pms are intravascular volume, capacity of the system, and system compliance,[45] where

$$Pms = \frac{V-Vo}{C} .$$

Vo is the volume necessary to fill the system without generating pressure (system capacity), V is the total intravascular volume (Vo + added volume), and C is the system compliance (Δ v/Δ p). The role of the entire venous bed is essential in the central venous pressure determination, because its compliance is 20 to 40 times greater than arterial compliance. Figure 74.15 shows the relation between right atrial pressure and venous return. Venous return is zero when the right atrial pressure is equal to the Pms. It is maximum when the gradient between the Pms and right atrial pressure is also maximum. Pms may be increased by a reduction in system capacity (Vo), an increase in total intravascular volume (V), and a reduction in system compliance (C).

Expansion of intravascular volume in clinical situations such as right ventricular infarction precisely seeks to increase venous return and thereby increase left ventricular preload. This approach is useful but may be transitory. The high Pms is transmitted backwards, 60% to 70%, to the splanchnic microvascular bed because arteriolar sphincters regulate hydrostatic pressure more than do the venous sphincters in the splanchnic microvascular bed. The increase in hydrostatic pressure favors edema formation in the small bowel, liver, pancreas, and the resulting ascites. The buildup of a large third space requires expansion of the intravascular volume with only transitory hemodynamic improvements. Another way of increasing Pms, when the intravascular volume is kept constant, is by reducing system capacity or system compliance.

Heck and Doty[46] used external phasic compression of the splanchnic circuit and lower limbs with pneumatic antishock trousers for circulatory assistance after the Fontan procedure. The immediate response is that right and left atrial pressure and cardiac output increased. Hemodynamic stability with less intravascular expansion required is the consequence.

We have used phasic abdominal compression in seven calves that underwent univentricular artificial heart implantation.[36] The results are shown in Table 74.1. One of the most important findings was the response of mean circulatory filling pressure (MCFP) with and without abdominal compression. Figure 74.16 shows the MCFP to be 15 mm Hg without abdominal compression and 25 mm Hg with compression, an increase of 70%. Calculation of resistance to venous return flow is as follows: without abdominal compression:

$$\frac{15 \text{ mm Hg (MCFP)} - 17 \text{ mm Hg (RAP)}}{3.95\ (\dot{Q})} = 0.50 \text{ (resistance)};$$

with abdominal compression:

$$\frac{25 \text{ mm Hg (MCFP)} - 29 \text{ mm Hg (RAP)}}{7.05\ (\dot{Q})} = 0.57 \text{ (resistance)}.$$

The gradients between MCFP and RAP, with or without abdominal compression, were not significantly different. What really has increased is flow ($\dot{Q}$). It seems

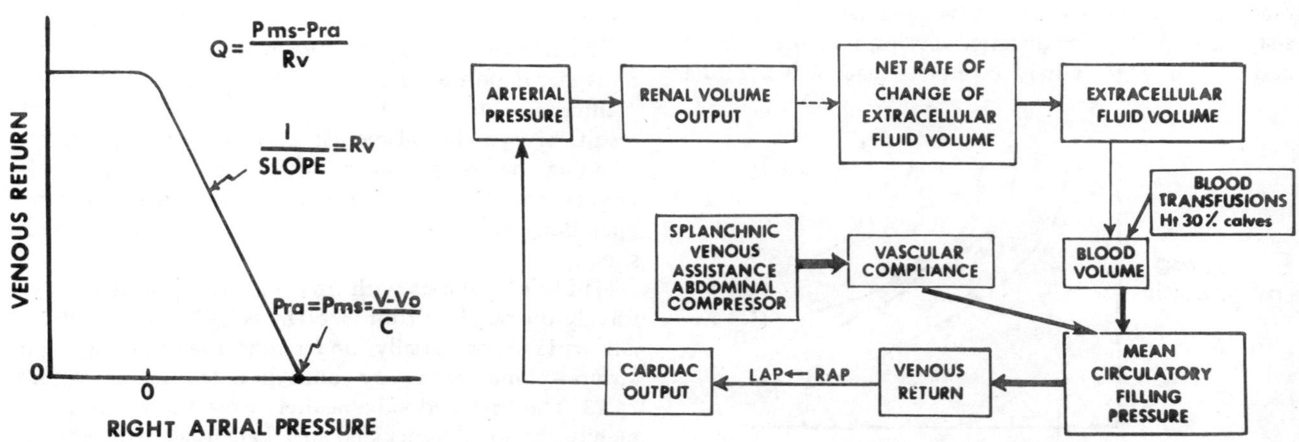

Figure 74.15. *Left*, Effect on the venous return curve of progressive increase in the mean systemic pressure (Pms) measured as the mean circulatory filling pressure (MCFP). *Right*, Orthotopic univentricular artificial heart regulation of blood volume and mean circulatory filling pressure. C = system compliance; Pra = right atrial pressure; Q = venous return flow; Rv = resistance to venous return; V = total intravascular volume; Vo = system capacity.

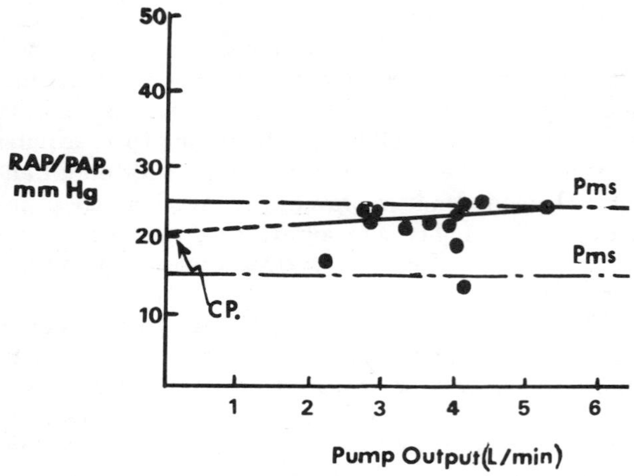

Figure 74.16. Determination of capillary closing pressure (CP) in pulmonary circulation. Behavior with and without abdominal compression. (See text.) PAP = pulmonary artery pressure; RAP = right atrial pressure.

that absolute pressure values may be more important than pressure gradients per se.

Furthermore, Figure 74.15 illustrates that when right atrial pressure is similar to MCFP, venous return is zero. This consideration is valid either with or without abdominal compression, because venous resistance is similar in both cases. Then it is necessary to discuss when the compression improves cardiac output. It is well recognized that with low cardiac output, pulmonary resistance is greatly influenced by the closing pressure of the pulmonary vasculature,[47] the critical closing pressure (CCP). Total pulmonary resistance (TPR) is calculated as follows:

$$TPR = \frac{RAP - CCP}{\dot{Q}} .$$

Critical closing pressure is obtained by extrapolating $\dot{Q} = O$ to the RAP/PAP ratio (Figure 74.16). In our animal studies this value was 20 mm Hg. At this intravascular pressure, blood flow is null because of closure or collapse of the pulmonary venous circulation. In Figure 74.17, cardiac output isopleths were drawn against pulmonary resistance (RAP/Q) for different closing pressures (10, 20, and 30 mm Hg). It may be noted that with a cardiac

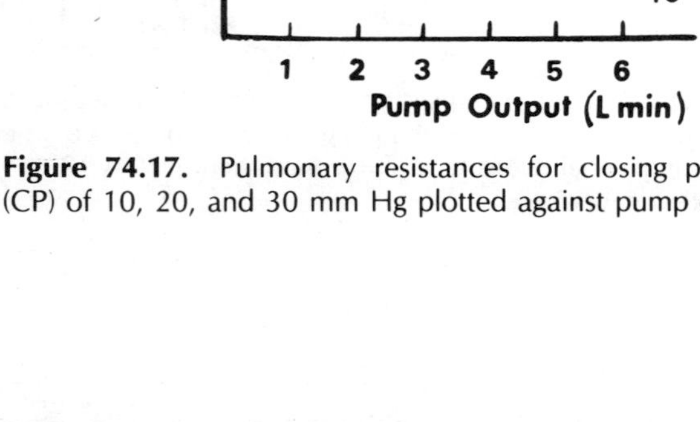

Figure 74.17. Pulmonary resistances for closing pressure (CP) of 10, 20, and 30 mm Hg plotted against pump output.

output of less than 4 liters (calves), pulmonary resistance increases exponentially. Conversely, normal values are observed with high cardiac output. These considerations demonstrate the influence of cardiac output on pulmonary resistance. It should be noted that during low cardiac output with high pulmonary resistance, right atrial pressure was lower than critical closing pressure. Right atrial pressure exceeded critical closing pressure only when abdominal compression was added. Right atrial pressure exceeding critical closing pressure probably improves cardiac output.

During abdominal cyclic compression (20 to 30 minutes), right atrial pressure was nonpulsatile, indicating that the change in the natural right atrial flow had no effect on the results observed.

The concept of a dispensable right ventricle may be misleading.[48–50] As seen in the late follow-up of patients in whom the pulmonary circulation is maintained through a right atrium–pulmonary artery shunt, the right ventricle has never functioned significantly and is dispensable. Conversely, after acute right ventricular infarction, serious hemodynamic disturbances may occur: (1) venous return may be impaired; and (2) the right ventricular–left ventricular anatomic and functional unit becomes affected.

After univentricular artificial heart implantation, mean circulatory filling pressure and consequently venous return are the most important determinants of forward flow. In the acute postoperative period, massive blood transfusion is detrimental. It is well recognized that a 50% increase in blood volume causes an increase in mean circulatory filling pressure from approximately 7 to 20 mm Hg. After two hours, however, the blood volume is still 35% above normal, whereas mean circulatory filling pressure returns to normal (7 mm Hg). This phenomenon of vascular stress relation[51] is due to an increase in vascular compliance. The assistance of the splanchnic venous circulation with a cyclic abdominal compressor (already pointed out by Guyton et al[52] in 1952) decreases the compliance of the vascular system. The mean circulatory filling pressure increases to 15 to 20 mm Hg, causing an increase in venous return and consequently in cardiac output.

The long-term compensatory mechanisms of the venous circulation after univentricular artificial heart implantation have not yet been studied. However, the late results of two clinical models may be useful for understanding the compensatory chronic mechanisms of venous return: (1) tricuspid atresia after the Fontan-Kreutzer operation; and (2) acute right ventricular infarction with shock.

(1) Eleven patients with tricuspid atresia were consecutively operated on from September 1979 to July 1985.* All patients essentially underwent the type of right atrium–pulmonary artery connection described in Figure 74.13. The tricuspid valve leaflets were sutured to completely occlude the tricuspid area. Late follow-up (August

*Neirotti R and Alvarez J, Division of Pediatric Cardiac Surgery, Italian Hospital, Buenos Aires, September 1985.

1985, two years average) revealed that one patient died immediately after surgery, and ten patients survived and are totally asymptomatic in New York Heart Association functional class 1 with normal ergometric tests.

(2) The angiograms of the patient in Figures 74.18, 19, and 20 were taken 6 months after acute right ventricular infarction with shock. The contractility of the right ventricle is null. However, 6 months after the acute episode, the patient is asymptomatic in New York Heart Association class 1 functional capacity.

OTHER RESEARCH

Willem J. Kolff, who in 1943 had already initiated clinical experience with the artificial kidney, had early evaluated his own and others' experience with mechanical circulation. The number of theoretic works and laboratory findings is so great that it is impossible to present it herein concisely, and we shall refer to systems potentially valid clinically.

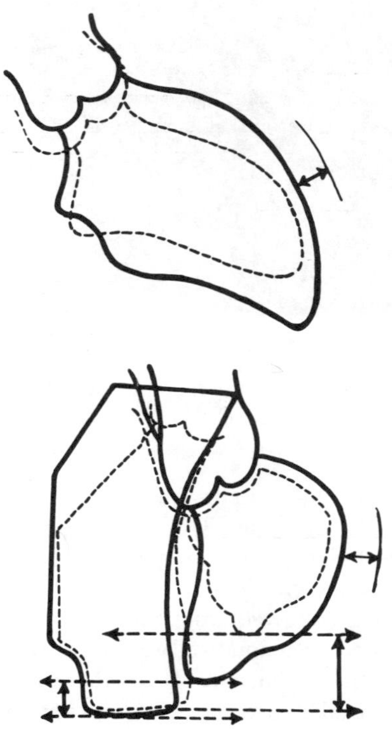

Figure 74.18. Schematic drawing of 30° right anterior oblique (RAO) (*top*) ventriculogram and simultaneous 60° left anterior oblique (LAO) (*bottom*) under the effects of nitrite and of postextrasystolic beat, respectively. A patient, a 40-year-old man, was catheterized (study No. 24606) 6 months after acute myocardial infarction, with severe compromise of right ventricular function during the acute episode. At present, he is in functional class I, reaching 11 METs during ergometric test. Coronary angiography shows occlusion at the origin of the right coronary artery and proximal occlusions of the left anterior descending coronary artery and first diagonal branch. The circumflex artery has 70% to 80% proximal stenosis. The distal bed of occluded coronary vessels is suitable for revascularization. *Top*, The left ventricle shows good motility (*continuous line*, end of diastole; *discontinuous line*, end of systole). *Bottom*, simultaneous 60° LAO biventriculogram. The left ventricle shows good contractility. However, the right ventricle demonstrates akinesia in most visualized regions. The right ventricle has a horizontal bottom level clearly descended compared with the left ventricle (extensive chronic right ventricular infarction).

Stroke volume (80 to 100 cc) may be activated by three different types of blood pumps: (1) diaphragm, (2) sac, and (3) pusher-plate. The primitive model in Figures 74.6 to 74.8 is a diaphragm-type system, whereas the model in Figure 74.4 is a pusher-plate type pump with an implantable motor. During recent years the diaphragm design has prevailed and has been used clinically. Pusher-plate systems have been evaluated with data presented in numerous publications.

The biocompatible material used for blood pump chambers belongs to the group of polyurethanes (Avcothane 51®, Biomer,® Pellethane®).[53] The valves incorporated are low-profile pyrolytic carbon disk types (Björk-Shiley, Medtronic-Hall). Static surfaces (pressure connectors and enlargements of atrial chambers) may be covered by Silastic.[54]

In any of the three designs mentioned (diaphragm, sac, or pusher-plate), the prosthetic blood chamber must be activated by a transmission system with an externally fixed power module. These power supplies have been used clinically (Figures 74.21 and 74.22). Portable pneumatic systems to allow mobility of the patient are also available.[55,56] Hydraulic transmission and pusher-plate types in general can be powered by implantable electric systems (motor solenoid). LVAD devices with implantable electrical power supplies have been extensively investigated.[57,58] A totally artificial heart with implantable electric energy source will be ready in the near future for clinical use.[59]

The systems with potential for clinical use must have precise requirements related to duration of the material, total volume occupied in the chest, acceptable weight, simplicity of implantation, and compact energizing system. The prosthetic heart with a frequency of 72 beats per minute must perform 40 million cycles per year. To be clinically acceptable the intracorporeal components should last at least 5 years, an average of 200 million cycles. The energy needed to activate the ventricular prosthesis must change according to the demand of the activity. For mean pressure, aortic 100 mm Hg and pulmonary 15 mm Hg with a cardiac prosthesis of 60% efficiency, the estimated requirements are as follows[60]:

for men,	3.23 w	(energy)	= 7.6	L/min (cardiac output)
	4.9 w		=11.5	L/min; for
women,	2.9 w	(energy)	= 6.9	L/min (cardiac output)
	3.9 w		= 9.3	L/min.

In 1968 at the University of Utah, Clifford S. Kwan-Gett designed 7- and 8-cm models from which the later Jarvik type prostheses were derived. The design of the Kwan-Gett prosthesis with a flexible nondistensible diaphragm permitted partial regulation of the prosthesis output by the atrial filling pressure.[61]

This automatic regulation approximates Frank-Starling's law of the natural heart. However, the hemody-

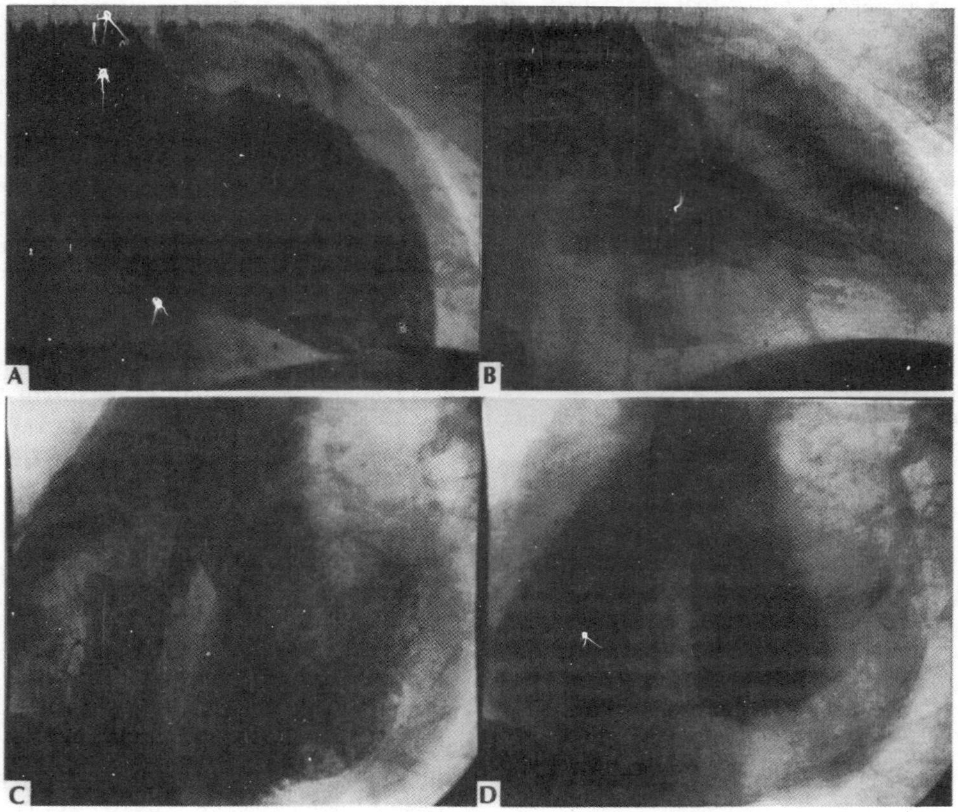

Figure 74.19. Photographs of ventriculogram in Figure 74.18, top. *A*, 30° RAO left ventriculogram (diastole); *B*, 30° RAO left ventriculogram (systole); *C*, 60° LAO simultaneous biventriculogram (diastole); *D*, 60° LAO biventriculogram (systole).

namic principle of Frank-Starling's law loses its effectiveness in the prosthetic heart. The atrial contraction that normally increases the cardiac output 30% to 40% is also compromised.* Depending on the elasticity of the materials employed, an increase in intraventricular pressure of 15 mm Hg may be observed during the maximum filling period. This 15-mm Hg pressure and the kinetic energy of filling may cause premature closure of the mitral and tricuspid valves. The increase in pulmonary resistance, which may lead to failure of the right blood pump, may be related to a low minute volume. (See section on Univentricular Artificial Heart.) In the biventricular replacement, other factors related to the right ventricular prosthesis may cause an increase in lung resistance.

The obvious disconnection of the artificial heart from the central nervous system may cause relaxation of the peripheral vasculature, with pooling of a considerable volume of blood in the splanchnic venous circuit. The use of abdominal and inferior limb compression in a cyclical way, 20 to 30 cycles per minute, may help to increase atrial pressure and cardiac output. (See section on Univentricular Artificial Heart with concomitant abdominal compression.)

In 1957 Kolff began the theoretic work on the artificial heart at the Cleveland Clinic and it was only after 17 years that he achieved survival in calves (3 months) at the University of Utah. The indefatigable tenacity of Kolff permitted the beginning of the clinical work by William DeVries on December 2, 1982.[62] New clinical experience has followed from that historic date.

DeVries used a pneumatically activated diaphragm type cardiac prosthesis (Jarvik 7®) made of polyurethane (Biomer®), similar in its general conception to the mechanical circulatory system implanted in a patient in 1969 at the Texas Heart Institute and also to the device used in animal experimentation in 1960.

On April 7, 1985, Bjarne K.H. Semb implanted a Jarvik 7 total artificial heart at the Karolinska Institute, Stockholm. Although the patient had to be returned to surgery to have the left ventricular pump replaced because of a dislodged left atrial pressure catheter impacted in the mitral valve, he was doing remarkably well in the early postoperative months. Although Semb was prepared to remove the total artificial heart and proceed with cardiac transplantation when a proper donor became available, the patient died 228 days later after suffering a massive cerebral stroke.[62a] Even so, the two-staged procedure (carried out in Tucson, St. Louis, Louisville, Pittsburgh, Hershey, Stanford, San Francisco, and Minneapolis),[62b] supporting our point of view in 1969, will permit rapid progress in the field.[62c]

At first sight, these mechanical systems seem to the clinician to be rather primitive devices. Nevertheless, the

* On June 23, 1985, Kolff in his laboratory at the University of Utah showed one of us (DL) the in vitro function of the vacuum-molded TAH. In general, the output of these pumps seems to respond to a sort of Starling's law.

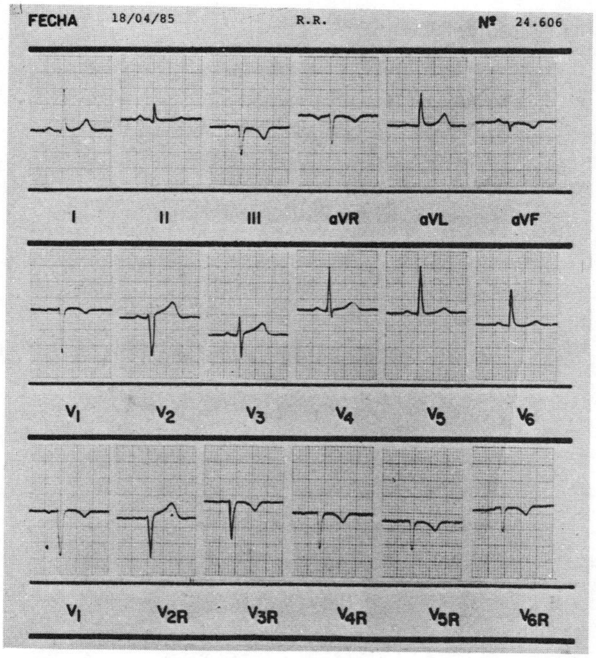

Figure 74.20. Electrocardiogram of the patient in Figures 74.18 and 74.19. Pathologic Q waves with repolarization disorders in the anteroseptal (leads V_{1-2}) and diaphragmatic regions (III and aVF) can be observed *simulating* a left ventricular infarction of the anterolateral, apical, and inferior diaphragmatic regions. However, the compromised right ventricle may be identified by means of the right precordial leads (V_{2R} to V_{4R}).

demonstration of life maintenance, as mentioned in the first paragraph of this chapter, is the main concern in this decisive stage of clinical application. Mechanical perfection will, no doubt, soon follow.

Kolff's basic understanding of clinical experiences with the total artificial heart follows the same concept. On July 14, 1969, he was quoted in the *Hospital Tribune* as follows: "The implantation of an artificial heart in Houston, Texas, on April 4th, was a step forward in the history of medicine. Dr. Cooley, Dr. Liotta, and others kept a patient alive during 64 hours with a mechanical heart before a natural heart was transplanted. Although the patient died due to complications subsequent to the second operation, the significant fact is that the Houston physicians demonstrated that an artificial heart can really substitute for a man's natural heart."

CRITERIA FOR SELECTING PATIENTS WITH INTRACTABLE HEART FAILURE FOR MECHANICAL CIRCULATORY SUPPORT

Three groups of patients may be considered for mechanical circulatory assistance (Table 74.2): group 1 includes patients in cardiac surgery who cannot be weaned from extracorporeal circulation. It is estimated that 1,800 patients per year die in the United States[63] who could benefit from mechanical assistance. Two basic etiologies of this perioperative acute myocardial failure are recognized: (1) acute myocardial infarction and (2) stunned

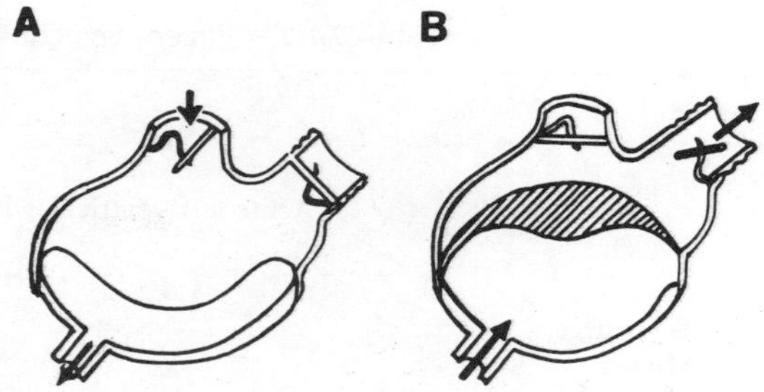

Figure 74.21. A pneumatically actuated diaphragm type polyurethane blood pump for either biventricular or univentricular total artificial heart with Medtronic-Hall valve prostheses. *A*, Pump diastole; *B*, pump systole.

myocardium (ie, temporary cardiac dysfunction that may be relieved with support).[64] Recognition in surgery of stunned heart permits a selective indication for short-term assistance (24 to 48 hours). In this situation the choice is prolonged partial left ventricular bypass with closed chest. When right ventricular function is also severely compromised (biventricular failure), the choice is prolonged partial extracorporeal circulation with membrane oxygenator and closed chest or biventricular jump support. The use of extracorporeal circulation exceeding 96 hours may produce disorders in coagulation factors and severe organic dysfunction, both of which are usually irreversible situations. Postcardiotomy shock due to extensive acute myocardial infarction would prolong the requirement of mechanical assistance over a 48-hour period. In this case, the choice is LVAD with paracorporeal blood pump[65–68] (Figures 74.14 and 74.23).

Group 2 includes patients with intractable chronic heart failure. It is estimated that 10,000 to 15,000 patients die every year in the United States in this category.[63] A pre-

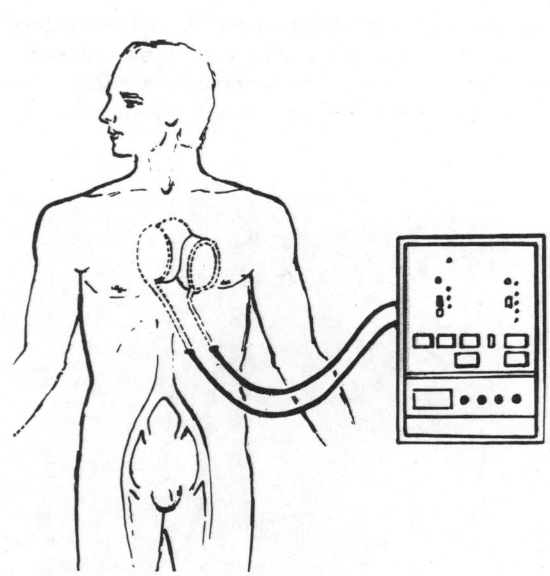

Figure 74.22. A pneumatically driven orthotopic biventricular total artificial heart with extracorporeal pneumatic source of energy.

Table 74.2. Patient Selection for Mechanical Circulatory Assistance

Group	Condition	Option
1 PTS in surgery (TMA)	Acute left ventricular failure	—Prolonged partial LV bypass (closed chest); short-term assistance (hours)
		—LVAD with paracorporeal blood pump; long-term assistance (days/weeks)
	Acute biventricular failure	—Prolonged partial ECC with MO (closed chest); few hours' assistance
		—Paracorporeal biventricular blood pumps; long-term assistance
2 Intractable Congestive Cardiac Failure (PMA)		—Intracorporeal LVAD
		—Orthotopic Univentricular AH
		—Orthotopic Biventricular AH
3 AMI with shock (PMA)		—Intracorporeal LVAD
		—Orthotopic Univentricular AH
		—Orthotopic Biventricular AH

AH = artificial heart; ECC = extracorporeal circulation; MO = membrane oxygenator; PMA = permanent mechanical assistance; TMA = temporary mechanical assistance.

operative right ventricular function study is indispensable to elaborate the clinical strategy of employing permanent mechanical assistance. A simultaneous biventriculogram in the left anterior oblique position is used to evaluate comparatively the contractility of both ventricles[69–79] (Figures 74.24 and 74.18,19). The absence of a contractile deficit of the right ventricle, even with a moderate increase in pulmonary pressure, should indicate implantation of an intracorporeal LVAD (in either the chest or abdomen).

Use of an orthotopic artificial heart is a more advanced decision, with two alternatives: (1) orthotopic univentricular artificial heart and (2) orthotopic biventricular artificial heart. A sine qua non requirement for the orthotopic univentricular artificial heart procedure is the finding of normal pulmonary pressure. Conversely, the biventricular artificial heart is not contraindicated, even with moderately high pulmonary pressure and mildly elevated pulmonary resistance.

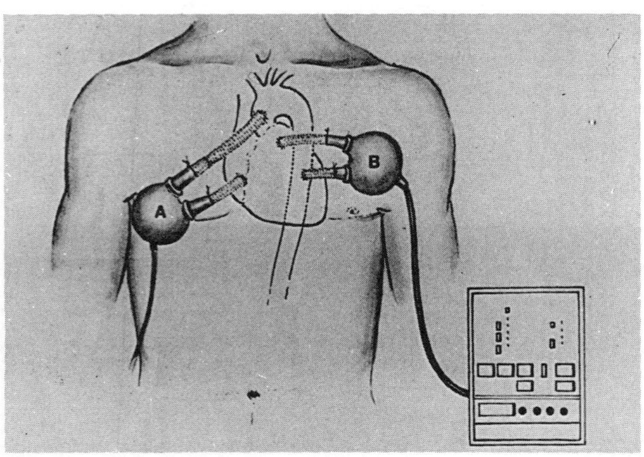

Figure 74.23. Paracorporeal left ventricular assist device (A and B).

Group 3 are patients in cardiogenic shock after acute myocardial infarction. Patients dying in the hospital following acute myocardial infarction exceed 150,000 a year in the United States. Arrhythmias are the primary cause in most patients, followed by cardiogenic shock due to 30% to 40% destruction of myocardial muscle. The three options mentioned for group 2 are also valid for this group of patients. In these patients without previous illness, pulmonary pressure and resistance are normal. The choice should be an orthotopic univentricular artificial heart.

In summary, for patients in group 1 (postcardiotomy shock in the operating room), prolonged partial left ventricular bypass with the chest closed should be done. Cardiac recovery should be observed within a few hours of assistance (stunned heart). If the cause is extensive acute myocardial infarction requiring prolonged assistance, the logical indication is a paracorporeal LVAD. Certainly, stone heart requires either a biventricular or a univentricular artificial heart, if the previous study of pulmonary circulation renders it possible.

Group 2 requires careful preoperative recognition of biventricular function and the pulmonary circulation.

Group 3 is most challenging from both the medical and the social point of view. These are young patients with the remainder of their vital organs functioning normally. In this group lies the challenge for simplified mechanical circulatory systems, including the orthotopic univentricular artificial heart.

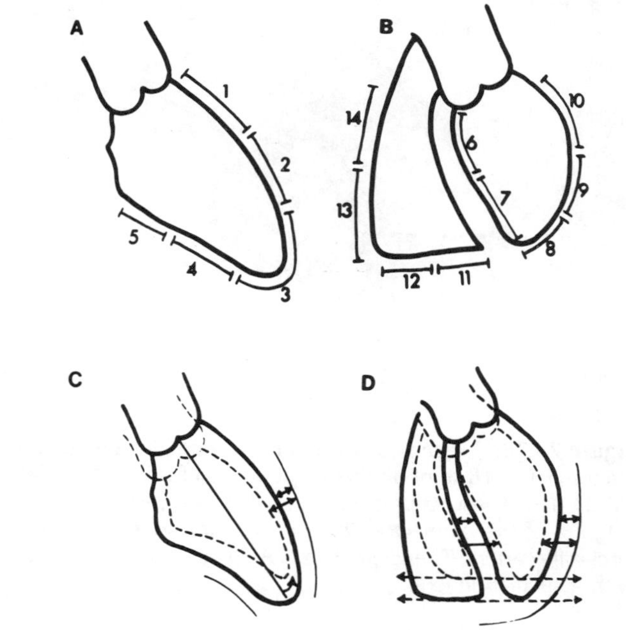

Figure 74.24. Schematic drawing of left ventricular (LV) angiogram in 30° right anterior oblique position (*A and C*) and of simultaneous biventriculogram in 60° left anterior oblique position (*B and D*). *A and B*, The regions of the LV are determined according to the American Heart Association classification: 1, anterobasal; 2, anterolateral; 3, apical; 4, inferodiaphragmatic; 5, inferobasal; 6, septobasal; 7, septoapical; 8, inferobasal; 9, posterobasal; 10, superolateral. For the right ventricle the following original classification has been adopted: 11, medial diaphragmatic; 12, lateral diaphragmatic; 13, inferolateral; 14, superolateral. *C and D*, The thick continuous line corresponds to the end of diastole and the discontinuous line to the end of systole. The continuous thin line indicates the cardiac silhouette. It serves as the reference to measure the thickness of the LV wall at the end of diastole (*short arrow*) and at the end of systole (*long arrow*). The thickness of the interventricular septum (*short and long arrows*) can also be measured. During systole the apex elevates (*curved arrow*) and the motion must be considered to measure parietal motility. In *D*, the horizontal lines in systole and diastole indicate the same level, respectively, for the normal two ventricles.

SURGICAL TECHNIQUES

TEMPORARY ASSISTANCE

Left Ventricular Bypass with Prolonged Extracorporeal Circulation and a Closed Chest

The Litwak cannula[80] or simply a No. 28 Bardic cannula is advanced into the left atrial cavity through either the left atrial appendage or behind the interatrial groove (Figure 74.25). The left atrium is sutured to a Teflon felt band securely attached 3 to 4 cm from the distal end of the Bardic cannula. An untied purse-string suture around the cannula (No. 2–0 polyester) is left for controlling hemostasis when at the second thoracotomy the extracorporeal circulatory system is removed. A 6- to 8-mm low-porosity woven Dacron graft is sutured to either the ascending or descending aorta or the femoral artery. A

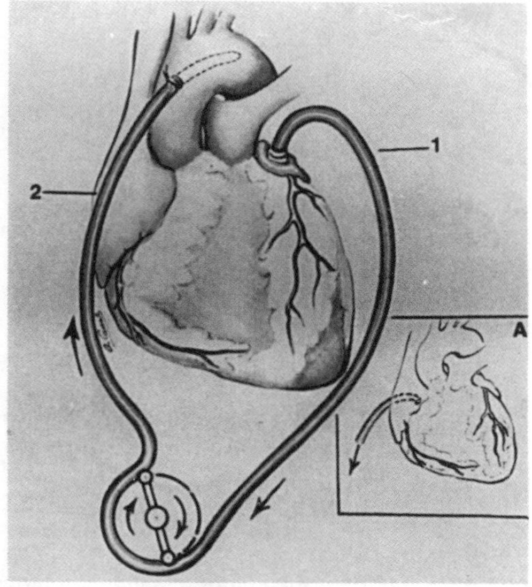

Figure 74.25. Surgical technique of left ventricular bypass with prolonged extracorporeal circulation and closed chest using a standard roller pump: 1 = cannula in the left atrial cavity through the atrial appendage; 2 = cannula in the ascending aorta through which a 6- to 8-mm Dacron graft is advanced into the proximal descending thoracic aorta to prevent central nervous system embolism. Inset *A* shows cannula reaching left atrial cavity behind the interatrial groove.

No. 18 Bardic cannula is secured in the lumen of the graft. Usually 1.5 to 2.5 liters per minute of flow through the roller pump is needed in patients with stunned myocardium (Figure 74.25). We recently treated two patients (January 20, 1984 and April 18, 1985).* In both patients the roller pump flow ranged from 1.5 to 2.0 liters per minute. Both patients were assisted in the recovery room for six hours. At late follow-up (16 months), the first patient who had undergone aortocoronary bypass oper-

* Service of Cardiovascular Surgery, Italian Hospital, Buenos Aires, Argentina.

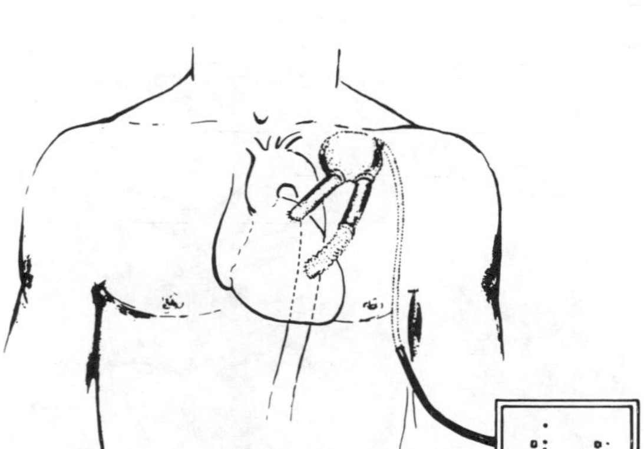

Figure 74.26. Intracorporeal (left chest) left ventricular assist device. Pump inlet: in the left atrium via the atrial appendage. Pump outlet: sutured to the descending thoracic aorta.

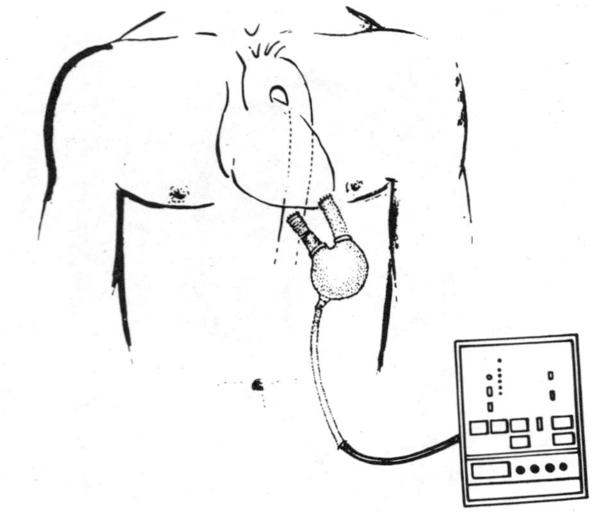

Figure 74.27. Intracorporeal (abdominal) left ventricular assist device. Pump inlet is in the left ventricular cavity. Pump outlet is sutured to the descending thoracic aorta.

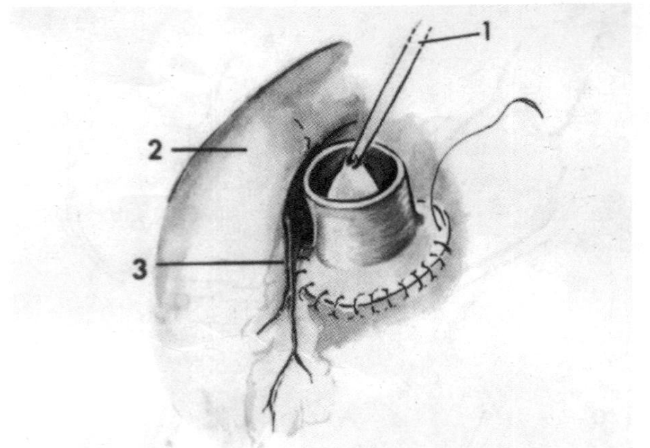

Figure 74.28. Technique of suturing a large inlet pump connector (16 to 18 mm) on the left atrial wall for intracorporeal LVAD. 1 = The forceps is pulling up the LA appendage during suturing of the connector; 2 = Pulmonary artery; 3 = Left circumflex artery. The LA wall and LA appendage are removed with a special punch.

ation is completely asymptomatic and in New York Heart Association functional class 1. The second patient underwent replacement of the ascending aorta for acute dissecting aneurysm. He left the hospital after 20 days in good condition.

Continuous blood flow through the pump prevents the activation of clotting mechanisms.[82] The circulating systemic heparin must be counteracted with protamine. The activated partial thromboplastin time is maintained 1.5 to 2.0 times normal; otherwise, uncontrollable loss of blood may occur with the chest closed. The extracorporeal circulatory system is removed after 24 to 48 hours and requires a second thoracotomy. Often the pericardial sac is under tension, full of clots. Once extracorporeal circulation is discontinued, even for a short time, it cannot be resumed. Clots are always found distally in the atrial cannula. A balloon catheter (counterpulsation catheter) inflated at the end of the atrial cannula may prevent clot formation. If the patient's condition requires reinitiation of cardiac assistance, the left atrial cannula must be aspirated and all extracorporeal tubes replaced.

A centrifugal pump has advantages for temporary cardiac assistance. Unger et al[81] recently reported data on nonpulsatile blood pumps.

LVAD with Paracorporeal Blood Pumps

The pneumatically activated blood pump is the choice for this temporary assistance. The specially designed atrial and aortic connectors are exteriorized through the chest wall and connected to the blood pump (Figure 74.23). The paracorporeal LVAD may work for a prolonged period of time (weeks to months).[14–19,22,23]

If synchronized with extracorporeal circulation, a diastolic counterpulsation effect is achieved. Coagulation

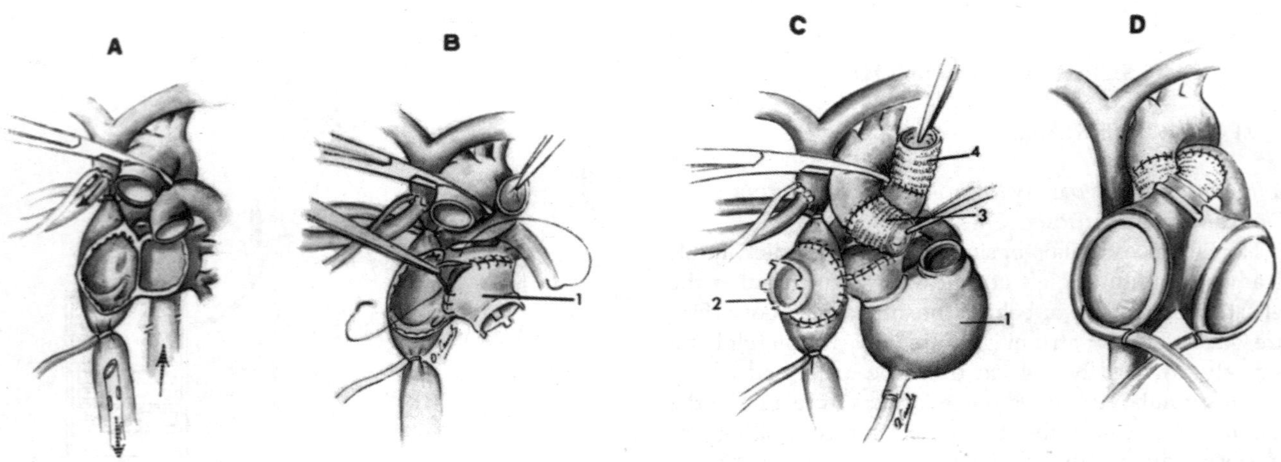

Figure 74.29. Implantation of the total artificial heart. *A*, right and left ventricles are excised; *B*, suturing of left atrial quick connector (1); *C*, (1) left ventricular blood pump; (2) right atrial quick connector; (3) graft and quick connector of ascending aorta; (4) graft and quick connector of pulmonary artery. *D*, operation completed.

time remains normal, and coumadin therapy may be started after 36 hours.

The paracorporeal pump is removed using local anesthesia around the left atrial and aortic connectors. Dissection is advanced until the external intercostal muscles are exposed. With gentle tension the connectors are occluded and then sutured. The intrathoracic segments of both connectors are left in place.

PERMANENT CIRCULATORY DEVICES

LVAD with Intracorporeal Pump

Some models implanted in calves in 1961 to 1963 are shown in Figures 74.10–74.12.[6–13] The inlet connector may be placed in the left atrium or left ventricle (Figures 74.26 and 27). A technique for an ample diameter left atrium inlet connector (16 to 18 mm) is illustrated in Figure 74.28.[6–10] The left ventricular apex connector may essentially be inserted with the technique described by Cooley et al[83] in 1965 for the valved apicoaortic conduit.

Orthotopic Univentricular Artificial Heart

The right atrium–pulmonary artery shunt technique is illustrated in Figure 74.13.[84,85] When the right atrium–pulmonary artery connection is placed anterior to the aortic graft, the anterior aspect of the shunt must be closed with a pericardial or Dacron woven patch graft. In the univentricular artificial heart model, sinoatrial node function is important; it should not be disturbed with surgical maneuvers. Left ventricular orthotopic implantation does not differ from the described biventricular technique (Figure 74.29).

Orthotopic Biventricular Artificial Heart

The technique used for implantation of an orthotopic total artificial heart in 1969[28,29] is similar to that used today. Important technical progress has been made in the use of left atrial, right atrial, pulmonary artery, and aortic quick connectors sutured separately from the blood pumps[62] (Figure 74.29). The two pneumatic conduits, after an intraparietal course, are exteriorized in the left side of the abdominal region (Figure 74.22).

Table 74.3. Summary of Clinical Pneumatic Artificial Heart Patient Implantations*

No.	Patient	Investigator	Age	Implant Date	Device	Period on TAH	Transplant	Outcome
1	Karp	Cooley	47	4/4/69	Liotta	64 hr	Yes	Died
2	Meuffels	Cooley	36	7/23/81	Akutsu	54 hr	Yes	Died
3	Clark	DeVries	61	12/2/82	JARVIK-7	112 days	No	Died
4	Shroeder	DeVries	52	11/24/84	JARVIK-7	Ongoing	--	Alive
5	Haydon	DeVries	58	2/17/85	JARVIK-7	Ongoing	--	Alive
6	Stenberg	Semb	53	4/7/85	JARVIK-7	227 days	No	Died
7	Burcham	DeVries	62	4/14/85	JARVIK-7	10 days	No	Died
8	Creighton	Copeland	33	3/6/85	Phoenix	11 hr	Yes	Died
9	Drummond	Copeland	25	8/29/85	JARVIK-7	9 days	Yes	Alive
10	Mandia	Pierce	44	10/18/85	Penn State	10 days	Yes	Died
11	Gaidosh	Griffiths	47	10/24/85	JARVIK-7	4 days	Yes	Alive
12	Lund (female)	Joyce	40	12/18/85	JARVIK-7-70	45 days	• Yes	Alive
13	Chayrez (female)	Copeland	40	2/3/86	JARVIK-7-70	4 days	Yes	Rejected, reimpl.
14	Burello	Griffiths	39	2/3/86	JARVIK-7	12 days	Yes	Alive
15	Kent	Frazier Cooley	41	2/3/86	JARVIK-7	31 days	Yes	Alive
16	Chayrez (female)	Copeland	40	2/9/86 (reimp.)	JARVIK-7-70	Ongoing	No	Alive
17	(male)	Unger	26	3/6/86	Unger	~1 day	Yes	Alive
18	Holzwig	Bucherl	39	3/7/86	Berlin	4 days	Yes	Died
19	Cresswell	Pierce	48	3/17/86	Penn State	Ongoing	--	Alive
20	Blake	Griffiths	43	3/23/86	JARVIK-7	17 days	No	Died
21	(male)	Cabrol	26	4/11/86	JARVIK-7-70	Ongoing	--	Alive

* This information was compiled by Don B. Olsen, DVM, Director, Institute For Biomedical Engineering, University of Utah, Salt Lake City, Utah, USA.

ADDENDUM

Clinical experience in the field of mechanical circulation is moving rapidly. In the area of left ventricular assistance, the etiology of perioperative ventricular failure is not well understood. Myocardial ischemia, acute myocardial infarction, and prolonged cardiopulmonary bypass all result in myocardial edema and decreased ventricular compliance. It is not possible to foresee the required duration of cardiac assistance necessary to reverse this state and regain adequate function. Today, LVAD pumps are available for clinical use. Short-term cardiac assistance with left ventricular bypass using extracorporeal circulation should be avoided.

The OUAH research is currently being investigated at the University of Utah under the direction of Drs Willem J. Kolff, Donald Olsen, Jerome B. Riebman and George Pantalos. A small ASD (4 mm diameter) has been incorporated into the surgical technique. This right-to-left shunt helps maintain an adequate cardiac output during the crucial hours following surgery.

The TAH as a bridging procedure for cardiac transplantation has gained world-wide acceptance. Patients awaiting transplantation as a treatment for rapidly progressing intractable left ventricular failure (due to acute viral and other cardiomyopathies, valvular or ischemic heart disease) may now be offered a period of total mechanical circulatory support for recovery of depressed organ function and an improvement in overall metabolic condition, permitting these patients to become more ideal transplantation candidates. To this date, fifteen bridging implantations have been performed internationally by pioneering cardiac surgeons: Dr Denton Cooley, Dr John G. Copeland, Dr William Pierce, Dr Bartley Griffith, Dr O. Howard Frazier, Dr Felix Unger, Dr E. Bucherl, and Dr C. Cabrol (Table 74.3). The continuing efforts of these and other bold surgeons and their brave patients will move us rapidly into an exciting era of practical clinical application of mechanical cardiac replacement.

Acknowledgment: This work was supported by an Alberto Juan Lacroze Grant from the Alfredo Fortabat and Amalia Lacroze de Fortabat Foundation, Buenos Aires, Argentina. Dr Jerome B. Riebman wrote the Addendum section.

REFERENCES

1. Liotta D, Taliani T: Replacement of the heart by means of intrathoracic prosthesis. *Bol Ministerio Salud Pública Córdoba,* May 8, 1960, pp 2–3.
2. Liotta D, Taliani T: Artificial heart of roller type implanted inside the chest. *Bol Ministerio Salud Pública Córdoba,* Sept 15, 1960, pp 1–2.
3. Liotta D, Taliani T, Giffoniello AH, Sarria Deheza F, Liotta S, Lizarraga R, Tolocka L, Pagano J: Total maintenance of the pulmonary and systemic blood circulation by mechanical means. Artificial heart inside the chest. *Bol Ministerio Salud Pública Córdoba,* November 6, 1960, pp 5–6.
4. Liotta D, Taliani T, Giffoniello AH, Sarria Deheza F, Liotta S, Lizarraga R, Tolocka L, Pagano J, Bianciotti E: Artificial heart in the chest: preliminary report. *Trans Am Soc Artif Intern Organs* 1961; 7:318–319.
5. Liotta D, Taliani T, Giffoniello A, Liotta S, Lizarraga R, Tolocka L, Pagano J: Ablation experimentale et replacement du coeur par un coeur artificiel intra-thoracique. *Lyon Chir* 1961; 57:704–714.
6. Liotta D, Crawford ES, Cooley DA, De Bakey ME, Urquia M, Feldman L: Prolonged partial left ventricular bypass by means of an intrathoracic pump implanted in the left chest. *Trans Am Soc Artif Intern Organs* 1962; 8:90–99.
7. Liotta D, Hall CW, Henly WS, Beall AC, Cooley DA, De Bakey ME: Prolonged assisted circulation during and after heart or aortic surgery. I. Prolonged partial left ventricular bypass by means of an intrathoracic circulatory pump. II. Diastolic pulsation of the descending thoracic aorta. *Trans Am Soc Artif Intern Organs* 1963; 9:182–185.
8. Liotta D, Hall CW, Henly WS, Cooley DA, Crawford ES, DeBakey ME: Prolonged assisted circulation during and after cardiac or aortic surgery. Prolonged partial left ventricular bypass by means of intracorporeal circulation. *Am J Cardiol* 1963; 12:399–405.

8a. DeBakey ME, Liotta D, Hall CW: Left-heart bypass using an implantable blood pump, in Eiseman B (ed): *Mechanical Devices to Assist The Failing Heart.* Publication 1283. National Academy of Sciences–National Research Council, Washington, DC 1966, pp 223–239.

9. Liotta D, Descotes JP, Cooley DA, Crawford ES, Morris GC, Henly WS, DeBakey ME: L'assistance circulatoire prolongee par pompe intrathoracique réalizant un bypass partiel du ventricule gauche, étude expérimentale. *Ann Chir Thorac Cardiovasc* 1963; 2:108–114.
10. Liotta D, Hall CW, Cooley DA, DeBakey ME: Prolonged ventricular bypass with intrathoracic pumps. *Trans Am Soc Artif Intern Organs* 1964; 10:154–156.
11. Hall CW, Liotta D, Henly WS, Crawford ES, DeBakey ME: Development of artificial intrathoracic circulatory pumps. *Am J Surg* 1964; 108:685–692.
12. Liotta D, Hall CW, Maness JH, DeBakey ME: The implantable intrathoracic circulatory pump: surgical technique. *Cardiovasc Res Cent Bull* 1964; 3:54–61.
13. Hall CW, Akers WW, O'Bannon W, Liotta D, DeBakey ME: Intraventricular artificial heart. *Trans Am Soc Artif Intern Organs* 1965;11:263–264.
14. Liotta D, Maness J, Bourland H, Rodwell D, Hall CW, DeBakey ME: Recent modifications in the implantable left ventricular bypass. *Trans Am Soc Artif Intern Organs* 1965; 11:284–288.
15. Liotta D, Hall CW, Villanueva A, O'Neal RM, DeBakey ME: A permanent autologous lining for implantable blood pumps: a pseudoendocardium. *Cardiovasc Res Cent Bull* 1966; 4:69–80.
16. Liotta D, Hall CW, Akers WW, Villanueva A, O'Neal RM, DeBakey ME: A pseudoendocardium for implantable blood pumps. *Trans Am Soc Artif Intern Organs* 1966; 12:129–134.
17. Ghidoni J, Liotta D, Villanueva A, Adams D: Rapid organization of fibrinous pseudointimas within impermeable arterial prostheses following implantation of autologous tissue fragments (abstr). *Fed Proc* 1967; 26:360.
18. Ghidoni J, Liotta D, Adams JG, O'Neal RM, Hall CW: Implantation of autologous tissue fragments in velour fabric used to line cardiovascular prosthesis: an in vivo culture system to produce cellular blood-prosthesis interfaces. *J Biomed Mater Res* 1968; 2:201–208.
19. Ghidoni JJ, Liotta D, Adams JG, Hall CW, O'Neal RM: Culture of autologous tissue fragments in paracorporeal left ventricular bypass pumps. *Arch Path* 1968; 86:308–311.
20. Hall CW, Liotta D, Ghidoni JJ, DeBakey ME: Velour fabrics applied to medicine. *J Biomed Mater Res* 1967; 1:179–196.
21. Bernhard WF, LaFarge CG, Robinson T, Yun I, Shirahige K, Kitrilakis S: An improved blood-pump interface for left-ventricular bypass. *Ann Surg* 1968; 168:750–764.
22. Akers WW, O'Bannon E, Hall CW, Liotta D: Design and operation of a paracorporeal bypass pump. *Trans Am Soc Artif Intern Organs* 1966; 12:86–93.
23. DeBakey ME: Left ventricular bypass pump for cardiac assistance: clinical experience. *Am J Cardiol* 1971; 27:3–11.
24. Hall CW, Liotta D, DeBakey ME: Artificial skin. *Trans Am Soc Artif Intern Organs* 1966; 12:340–343.
25. Hall CW, Eppright RH, Engen T, Liotta D: A permanently attached artificial limb. *Trans Am Soc Artif Intern Organs* 1967; 13:329–331.
26. Hall CW, Liotta D, DeBakey ME: Biologic interfacing with synthetic fabrics. *J Soc Plast Eng* 1968; 24:94–98.
27. Kessler TR, Foote JL, Andrade JD, Kolff WJ: Methods to construct artificial organs. *Trans Am Soc Artif Intern Organs* 1971; 17:36–41.
28. Cooley DA, Liotta D, Hallman GL, Bloodwell RD, Leachman RD, Milam JD: First human implantation of cardiac prosthesis for staged total replacement of the heart. *Trans Am Soc Artif Intern Organs* 1969; 15:252–263.
29. Cooley DA, Liotta D, Hallman GL, Bloodwell RD, Leachman RD, Milam JD: Orthotopic cardiac prosthesis for two-staged cardiac replacement. *Am J Cardiol* 1969; 24:723–730.
30. Curran WJ: The first mechanical heart transplant: informed consent and experimentation. *N Engl J Med* 1974; 291:1015–1016.
31. Strauss MJ: Special report: The political history of the artificial heart. *N Engl J Med* 1984; 310:332–336.
32. Liotta D: Orthotopic univentricular artificial heart. Japanese Artificial

Organs Society, Atami Congress, February 1984.

33. Liotta D: Orthotopic univentricular artificial heart. *Recent Adv Cardiovasc Surg* 1984; 1(6):6–17.
34. Liotta D, Cooley DA, Navia JA, Frazier H: Orthotopic univentricular artificial heart. Proceedings of 2nd Symposium on the Artificial Heart, Berlin, 1984. In press.
35. Frazier OH, Cooley DA, Liotta D, Navia JA, Jordana J: A univentricular artificial heart: in-vivo results with concomitant abdominal compression (abst). *Artificial Organs* 1985; 9A:32.
36. Liotta D, Cooley DA, Navia JA, Frazier OH, Jordana J, del Río P, Lima Quintana O: Orthotopic univentricular artificial heart (abstr). Submitted to the ESAO, September 1985.
37. Pierce WS, Morris L, Gardiner BN, Burney RG, Leppik I, Malmud L, Danielson GK: Experimental use of a single mechanical ventricle to replace the dog's heart. *Trans Am Soc Artif Intern Organs* 1965; 11:271–276.
38. Pierce WS, Gardiner BN, Livingston M, Burney RG, Leppik IE, Danielson GK: Total heart replacement by a single intrathoracic blood pump. *J Surg Res* 1965; 5:387–394.
39. Takano H, Taenaka Y, Nakatani T, Umezu M, Matsuda T, Iwata H, Tanaka T, Noda H, Hayashi K, Takatani S, Nakamura T, Seki J, Akutsu T, Manabe H: Circulatory maintenance with a single artificial heart. *Trans Am Soc Artif Intern Organs* 1984; 30:550–552.
40. Shachar GB, Fuhrman BP, Wang Y, Lucas RV, Lock JE: Rest and exercise hemodynamics after the Fontan procedure. *Circulation* 1982; 65:1043–1048.
41. Laks H, Milliken JC, Perloff JK, Hellenbrand WE, George BL, Chin A, Di Sessa TG, Williams RG: Experience with the Fontan procedure. *J Thorac Cardiovasc Surg* 1984; 88:939–951.
42. Funey SA, III, Zieske HA, Levy MN: The essential function of the right ventricle. *Am Heart J* 1984; 107:404–410.
43. Guyton AC, Polizo D, Armstrong GG: Mean circulatory filling pressure measured immediately after cessation of heart pumping. *Am J Physiol* 1954; 179:261–267.
44. Guyton AC: *Circulatory Physiology: Cardiac Output and its Regulation.* Philadelphia, WB Saunders, 1983.
45. Guyton AC: Venous return, in Hamilton WF, Dow P (eds): *Handbook of Physiology.* Washington, DC, American Physiological Society, sect 2, vol 2, 1963, pp 1099–1133.
46. Heck HAJ, Doty DB: Assisted circulation by phasic external lower body compression. *Circulation* 1981; 64:II-118–II-122.
47. McGregor M, Sniderman A: On pulmonary vascular resistance: the need for more precise definition. *Am J Cardiol* 1985; 55:217–221.
48. Bakos ACP: The question of the function of the right ventricular myocardium: an experimental study. *Circulation* 1950; 1:724–732.
49. Haller JA Jr, Adkins JC, Worthington M, Rauenhorst J: Experimental studies on permanent bypass of the right heart. *Surgery* 1966; 59:1128–1132.
50. Sade RM, Castaneda AR: The dispensable right ventricle. *Surgery* 1975; 77:624–631.
51. Manning RD Jr, Guyton AC: Control of blood volume. *Rev Physiol Biochem Pharmacol* 1982; 93:69–114.
52. Guyton AC, Satterfield JH, Harris JW: Dynamics of central venous resistance with observations on static blood pressure. *Am J Physiol* 1952; 169:691–699.
53. Lemm W, Pirling L, Bucherl ES: Biodegradation of some biomaterials. *ESAO Proceedings* 1980; 3:86–90.
54. Zartnack F, Dunkel W, Affeld K, Bücherl ES: Fatigue problems in artificial blood pumps. *Trans Am Soc Artif Intern Organs* 1978; 24:600–605.
55. Affeld K, Frank J, Baer P, Mohnhaupt A, Bücherl ES: A new portable driving unit for implantable blood pumps. *Trans Am Soc Artif Intern Organs* 1978; 24:6–10.
56. Thoma H: Drive and management of circulation support systems, in Unger F (ed): *Assisted Circulation 2.* New York, Springer Verlag, 1984, pp 340–366.
57. Portner PM, Oyer JS, Jassawalla H, Chen PJ, Miller DH, La Forge DH, Green GF, Shumway NE: A totally implantable ventricular assist device for end-stage heart disease, in Unger F (ed): *Assisted Circulation 2.* New York, Springer-Verlag, 1984, pp 115–141.
58. Igo SR, Fuqua JM, McGee MG, Creager GJ, Pool GE, Krudewig TW, Frazier OH: An implantable ventricular assist system: chronic in vivo performance. *Trans Am Soc Artif Intern Organs* 1984; 30:81–85.
59. Rosenber G, Snyder AJ, Landis DL, Geselowitz DB, Donachy JH, Pierce WS: An electric motor-driven total artificial heart: seven months survival in the calf. *Trans Am Soc Artif Intern Organs* 1984; 30:69–74.
60. Donovan FM, Kolff WJ: Power requirement of the artificial heart. Meeting of the Fed of Am Soc of Exp Biol and US Government Report (C002155-4), Atlantic City, 1972.
61. Kwan-Gett C, Backman DK, Donovan FM Jr, Eastwood N, Foote JL, Kawai J, Kessler TR, Kralios AC, Peters JL, Van Kampen KR, Wong HK, Zwart HHJ, Kolff WJ: Artificial heart with hemispherical ventricles II and disseminated intravascular coagulation. *Tr Am Soc Artif Intern Organs* 1971; 17:474–481.
62. DeVries WC, Anderson JL, Lyle LD, Anderson FL, Hammond EH, Jarvik RK, Kolff WJ: Clinical use of the total artificial heart. *N Engl J Med* 1984; 310:273–278.

62a. Marwick C: Pondering past, future of implantable heart. *JAMA* 1985; 254:3288–3292.

62b. Hill JD, Farrar DJ, Hershon JJ, Compton PG, Avery GJII, Levin BS, Brent BN: Use of a prosthetic ventricle as a bridge to cardiac transplantation for post-infarction cardiogenic shock. *N Engl J Med* 1986; 314:626–628.

62c. Relman AS: Artificial hearts—permanent and temporary. *N Engl J Med* 1986; 314:644–645.

63. DeVries WC: Total artificial heart, in Sabiston DC, Spencer FC (eds): *Gibbon's Surgery of the Chest,* ed 4. Philadelphia, WB Saunders, 1983, pp 1629–1636.
64. Braunwald E, Kloner RA: The stunned myocardium: prolonged, postischemic ventricular dysfunction. *Circulation* 1982; 66:1146–1149.
65. Pierce WS, Parr GVS, Myers JL, Pae WE Jr, Bull AP, Waldhausen JA: Ventricular-assist pumping in patients with cardiogenic shock after cardiac operations. *N Engl J Med* 1981; 305:1606–1610.
66. Bernhard WF, Berger RL, Stetz JP, Carr JG, Colo NA, McCormick JR, Fishbein MC: Temporary left ventricular bypass: factors affecting patient survival. *Circulation* 1979; 60:I-131–I-141.
67. Pennington DG, Merjavy JP, Codd JE, Swartz MT, Willman VL: Temporary mechanical support of patients with profound ventricular failure, in Unger F (ed): *Assisted Circulation 2.* Springer-Verlag, 1984, pp 85-99.
68. Bernhard FJ, Schoen FJ, Poirier V, Carr J: A temporary ventricular assist device for patients exhibiting intractable postcardiotomy shock, in Unger F (ed): *Assisted Circulation 2.* Springer-Verlag, 1984, pp 49-69.
69. AHA Committee Report: A reporting system on patients evaluated for coronary artery disease. *Circulation* 1975; 51:5–40.
70. Dodge HT, Sandler H, Baxley WA, Hawley RR: Usefulness and limitations of radiographic methods for determining left ventricular volume. *Am J Cardiol* 1966; 18:10–24.
71. Sandler H, Dodge HT: The use of single plane angiocardiograms for the calculation of left ventricular volume in man. *Am Heart J* 1968; 75:325–334.
72. Rackley CE, Dodge HT, Coble YD Jr, Hay RE: A method for determining left ventricular mass in man. *Circulation* 1964; 29:666–671.
73. Lichtlen P, Huhmann W: Right ventricular angiograms in patients with coronary artery disease, in Lichtlen PR (ed): *Coronary Angiography and Angina Pectoris.* Symposium of the European Society of Cardiology (1975). Hanover, Publishing Sciences Group, 1976, pp 168–176.
74. Fisher EA, Dubrow IW, Hastreiter AR: Right ventricular volume in congenital heart disease. *Am J Cardiol* 1975; 36:67–75.
75. Redwood DR, Scherer JL, Epstein SE: Biventricular cineangiography in the evaluation of patients with asymmetric septal hypertrophy. *Circulation* 1974; 49:1116–1121.
76. Helfant RH, Pine R, Meister SG, Feldman MS, Trout RG, Banka VS: Nitroglycerin to unmask reversible asynergy. Correlations with post coronary bypass ventriculography. *Circulation* 1974; 50:108–113.
77. Dyke SH, Cohn PF, Gorlin R, Sonnenblick EH: Detection of residual myocardial function in coronary artery disease using post-extrasystolic potentiation. *Circulation* 1974; 50:694–699.
78. Popio KA, Gorlin R, Bechtel D, Levine JA: Postextrasystolic potentiation as a predictor of potential myocardial viability: preoperative analyses compared with studies after coronary bypass surgery. *Am J Cardiol* 1977; 39:944–953.
79. Report of the Inter-Society Commission for Heart Disease Resources: Optimal resources for examination of the chest and cardiovascular system. *Circulation* 1976; 53:A1–A37.
80. Litwak RS, Koffsky RM, Jurado RA, Lukban SB, Ortiz AF, Fisher AP, Sherman JJ, Silvay E, Lajam FA: Use of a left heart assist device after intracardiac surgery: technique and clinical experience. *Ann Thorac Surg* 1976; 21:191–202.
81. Unger F, Genelin A, Hager J, Kemkes BM, Koller I, Schistek R: Functional heart replacement with nonpulsatile assist devices, in Unger F (ed): *Assisted Circulation 2.* Springer-Verlag, 1984, chap 2, pp 163–174.
82. Rose DM, Colvin SB, Culliford AT, Cunningham JN, Adams PX, Glassman E, Isom OW, Spencer FC: Long-term survival with partial left heart bypass following perioperative myocardial infarction and shock. *J Thorac Cardiovasc Surg* 1982; 83:483–492.
83. Cooley DA, Norman JC: Apical left ventricular-abdominal aortic composite conduits for left ventricular outflow obstructions. *Cardiovasc Dis Bull Texas Heart Institute* 1978; 5:112–127.
84. Kreutzer G, Galindez E, Bono H, de Palma C, Laura JP: An operation for correction of tricuspid atresia. *J Thorac Cardiovasc Surg* 1973; 66:613–621.
85. Kreutzer GO, Vargas FJ, Schlichter AJ, Laura JP, Suarez JC, Coronel AR, Kreutzer EA: Atriopulmonary anastomosis. *J Thorac Cardiovasc Surg* 1982; 83:427–436.

75 International Practices of Cardiovascular Surgery

Charles Hahn, MD

During a reunion organized by the World Health Organization in 1977 in The Hague, the main aim of which was to study the long-term effects of coronary bypass, certain norms were defined in relation to the needs in cardiac surgery in the West. The resultant conclusion was that approximately 400 patients out of 1 million inhabitants would possibly benefit from cardiac intervention. Assuming that all conditions or prerequisites for efficient screening of cardiovascular lesions are realized, that the diagnosis is correct, that judgment is logical, the need for cardiac surgery on a world scale would be 2 million cardiac operations per year, estimating the world population to be 5 billion. This number, which appears either impressive or nearly insignificant, depending upon how it is viewed, has not yet been reached. To calculate the number of cardiac operations performed in the world, computer statistics, mainly from the United States, have been studied. Despite detailed research, no overall conclusion has been reached. Such information cannot be obtained from international organizations. Such a study has never been attempted, and the establishment of a world cardiovascular register would require several years of research at least. Even if a maximum number of figures are obtained, their accuracy, in terms of common definitions applicable to all, must be ascertained. This is far from evident. For this reason, we have had to limit ourselves, within the context of this chapter, to a number of examples that reflect an overall picture of cardiovascular surgery as practiced on the five continents, and from this experience a given number of conclusions can be drawn. The enormous discrepancy that exists between the needs in cardiac surgery and the ability to fulfill them is due to several causes:

The first is to be found in the great clinical traditions our generation experienced, which directed all medical effort toward diagnosis. Thus, for example, it was traditional for our generation to learn all details that allowed clinical observation, from inspection to percussion, to auscultation, with a thoracic x-ray and an electrocardiographic study as the only complementary tests. This practice resulted in endless discussions, usually useless in terms of therapeutic approach. The means of therapy were so limited that it was known in advance, whether a correct or an incorrect diagnosis, that ultimately all would result in the administration of an herbal infusion, digitalis, or diuretics. However, since the advent of drugs containing more or less active components, the current situation has become totally different.

In the context of medicine in general, it must be admitted that it was in the field of cardiovascular surgery that all records were broken in the underestimation of needs and requirements. Yet, it was 5,000 years ago (estimated date of the papyrus of Edwin Smith) that discoveries succeeded one another and finally had to result in surgical solutions. As an improved understanding of anatomy, physiology, and pathology was evolving, surgical solutions to the treatment of vascular lesions, from simple wounds to aneurysms, were reached. The spread of knowledge and of such therapy followed the evolution of human civilization: those in which importance was given to culture reached peaks of development. One could speak of an international practice of vascular surgery from the time of antiquity, but not of cardiac surgery.

The development of cardiac surgery in particular, which will be discussed subsequently, played a role in stimulating a conservative approach to the treatment of cardiopathy, or arteriopathy, because of the increasing interest that knowledge of the cardiovascular system and its lesions produced. The search for medical solutions did not limit itself to cardiac insufficiency, but it was directed toward many forms of complications related to cardiopathology in general, and it rapidly progressed on an international scale through the development of an impressive pharmaceutical industry, especially in developed countries. This effort, on a surgical as well as medical scale, widely affected the interest of the medical profession in the preservation of life and its quality, especially in the cardiovascular domain.

TREATMENT VERSUS PREVENTION

If the treatment of cardiovascular lesions found justification in a better understanding of the underlying pathology and its frequency, then the prevention of cardiovascular disease apparently was even more important. On the whole, medical prevention has always been a specific preoccupation of therapists, whether physicians, priests, or witch doctors. From the instant at which knowledge and identification of infectious diseases improved (the Committee of Hygiene of the League of Nations in Geneva, which existed in 1945 and was a predecessor of the World Health Organization, placed much effort in the study of infectious diseases to better understand, avoid, and eradicate them from the surface of the earth), it became possible to modify the life-style of people toward better protection, even before the discovery of antibiotics. However, it is to the latter that we attribute the complete upheaval in the profile of infectious diseases, one of which is acute rheumatic fever, responsible for much damage to the cardiac valves. It is perfectly logical to have an international policy for the prevention of acute rheumatic fever, or to combat it from the moment of diagnosis with the use of antibiotics, even at long term. This system can be applied in any country without seriously compromising a health budget, even in the presence of a weak economy.

The efficiency of such a medical approach cannot be doubted, just as the efficiency of the means widely used in the past to prevent other infectious diseases such as smallpox, tuberculosis, and poliomyelitis cannot be denied. The danger lies in posing prevention against more aggressive therapy, which is what occurred in many places. Discussions on a government level with countries from Africa, South America, or Asia Minor often demonstrated that the financial effort was entirely devoted to preventive measures, and that no means were available for direct therapy despite the fact that in many such countries where preventive measures were emphasized, the number of patients with valvular pathology, usually children, constituted an absolute scourge, so malignant was the disease process. It was in fact a passive genocide produced by an unacceptable apportionment of the budget because of an inability to recognize existing problems and possible solutions. This was so despite a complete change in prognosis established after the introduction of closed heart surgery followed by open heart surgery for valvulopathy, usually mitral.

Before discussing the current situation in cardiovascular surgery in the world, let us return to the subject of prevention. One of the banes of human civilization, which up to a few years ago was limited to the western world but which is spreading further into other countries, whether this relates to South America or Asia, is arteriosclerosis. This degenerative process, which is poorly understood on a scientific level, is misleading in both its geographic as well as its individual distribution. The identification of risk factors, although useful, tended to produce dogmatic attitudes rather than statistical certitudes. An artillery of preventive measures is at the origin of an already international distribution of regulations; however, these are insufficient, and the systematic cult of exercise is not necessarily an effective prophylaxis to sudden death. Preventive concepts in congenital heart malformations are passing through profound changes in human philosophy. Birth control should be encouraged not only in areas with a high birth rate, but also in developed countries whose healthier economy allows for procedures permitting intrauterine diagnosis of severe congenital heart malformations, and hence the taking of necessary measures to interrupt pregnancy when the pathology is irreversible.

From the moment of conception, the problem arises of avoiding all factors that could affect the later development of the embryo (eg, the intake of a toxic drug by the mother at a vulnerable period in the embryo's development). The placental "barrier" is well known to be a myth in most cases. It is perfectly feasible that with the further development of genetics, we may be able to predict cardiac malformations or at least reduce their frequency or gravity. Let us not forget that inheritance is a consequence (through successive stages in the evolution of the cardiovascular system parallel to those in animal life) of the incomplete growth of certain elements, particularly the septa, as well as the persistence of structures that should disappear but that remain in the form of lesions whose physiopathologic significance can be important.

Thus, if in the international practice of cardiovascular surgery, prevention is a chapter of capital importance, its therapeutic application faces a whole series of limitations. Its value, although indisputable in the case of infectious disease with cardiac complications (valvular, myocardial, or pericardial), takes on a more symbolic aspect in the case of arteriosclerotic lesions, the real "disease" of civilization.

HISTORY OF CARDIAC SURGERY

The history of cardiac surgery contains many lessons in surgical techniques for the correction of cardiac lesions, as well as in the spread of such methods on a world scale. It is widely known that cardiac surgery developed in the 19th century in the same manner as vascular surgery, ie, in the repair of direct traumatic lesions of the heart. The first operation for cardiac trauma with suture of the damaged myocardium is generally attributed to Rehn in Frankfurt. However, Daniel Hale Williams of Chicago in 1893 had already performed exploration of the heart for a myocardial wound that had stopped bleeding after slight tamponade. Surgical procedures succeeded each other but at a discreet pace. Thus, in 1902, Hill in Louisiana operated on a patient with tamponade secondary to a myocardial lesion which he sutured with catgut. Pericardial drainage has also been known since the end of the last century. The idea of an intracardiac procedure such as mitral commissurotomy was due to Brentano and Samways. It was performed on autopsy specimens by Sir Brunton, and in the same country, Souttar from London then proceeded to perform the operation in May 1925. It was not until 1938 that closed heart surgery began to develop after the successful closure of a patent ductus arteriosus by Gross. Once again, this operation had previously been performed by Munro in 1907. Let us recall the first successful resection for coarctation of the aorta followed by reestablishment of aortic continuity in October 1944 by Crafoord in Stockholm, and ten days later, the operation of Blalock for cyanotic lesions associated with pulmonary stenosis.

A review of these various stages in heart surgery reflects the extent of the difficulties encountered and explains its slow development. This is not without interest as at this time, when so many centers wish to begin cardiac surgery, the importance of the difficulties encountered should not be underestimated, even if the means developed to overcome them are different. That certain works destined to obtain results in a given domain may result in unexpected applications should not be forgotten. The operation of Blalock, for instance, has been applied in situations of low pulmonary blood flow, although it was originally invented ten years previously to create under experimental conditions a pulmonary arterial hypertension, without success.

The topic of congenital pulmonary valvular stenosis also contains many lessons. The development of a safe and efficient surgical procedure took many years. It is to Doyen in Paris that we attribute the first operation for pulmonary valvulopathy in 1913, a failure due to an error in diagnosis. This form of intervention, however, was reinstated 35 years later by Brock and Holmes Sellors, and has since become a routine procedure. Many historical examples can be given relating to the development of the surgery of valves and aneurysms. The only point of interest in this summary, however, is the manner in which it demonstrates that cardiac surgery, like vascular surgery, was at the start the product of the imagination and ability of surgeons living in different countries and even different continents. In another manner it indicates the international nature of surgery, which is also true of medicine. This was even more marked in the cardiovascular domain because of its very rapid progression since the end of the World War II.

In effect, closed heart surgery showed that contrary to the assertions of reputable physicians and surgeons, the heart was accessible, that instruments could be slipped in without provoking cardiac arrest, and that if the latter occurred, cardiac massage was possible, as demonstrated by Niehans in 1909, thus successfully restoring the circulation.

Other restrictions were definitely removed when, after 20 years of work, Gibbon of Philadelphia successfully performed open heart surgery using an artificial heart-lung model. Three weeks later the Hammersmith Hospital team was also successful with its first open heart operation. In the same year Lillehei, lacking a team for the circulation of oxygenated blood, used the principle of cross circulation in 45 cases during the following year.

DeWall developed a system of bubble oxygenation during this period. At the time, American, British, Danish (Rygg), Swedish, and French teams were ready for the systematic application of open heart surgery in the correction of more complex intracardiac lesions.

Other solutions presented themselves between the apparatus of Gibbon, which was used by Kirklin at the Mayo Clinic, and the bubble oxygenator of DeWall, particularly the plastic disposable bubble oxygenator of Rygg, developed in 1956 and mounted on a very simple apparatus. To remain as close as possible to normal physiologic conditions, Kolff and Cloves in 1956 were developing a membrane oxygenator with the aim of avoiding direct contact between the blood and oxygen or carbon dioxide. Thus, in 1956, American and European groups, followed rapidly by Japanese teams, had at their disposal a wide range of material from which to choose depending upon their work and economic conditions.

DEVELOPMENT OF CARDIAC SURGERY

The generalization of cardiac surgery in all five continents, however, was subject to a number of conditions.

For example, the need for open heart surgery in various countries had to be recognized. At the time, approximately 30 years ago, the demand for cardiac surgery was estimated to be very low, the number of teams trained in the latter field was to be limited, and the argument of cost was put forward each time a center wished to apply such new techniques and methods. Soon after, it was shown that the cost of open heart surgery was not much greater than that of any other major surgical procedure, especially in cases of severe illness or even of fractures necessitating prolonged hospitalization and often repeated operations. For a long time, the risk associated with open heart intervention was used as a reason against its systematic application in developing as well as developed countries. As cardiovascular surgery developed, the surgical risk diminished with increasing experience, thus allowing the definition of conditions related to the number of patients to be operated on. It is currently known that a group that operates on less than 250 patients per year cannot guarantee good results, particularly in complicated lesions. Moreover, once the number of patients is too great, the adaptation of the components of the total structure must be strict, otherwise the quality will certainly diminish.

TRAINING OF CARDIAC SURGEONS

The training of a cardiosurgical team is of primordial importance. During the early years of cardiac surgery, many general surgeons wished to practice such interventions because of interest and novelty. Such an attitude led to many poor results; this result should be taken into account when assisting in the development of a center in a country where surgical expertise is not sufficiently developed.

There are three different methods of training a cardiosurgical team:

(1) One consists of accepting inside a well-trained department the basic members of a future surgical center in order to pass on the knowledge required for their improvement. In such an elaborate specialty as cardiac sur-

gery, training applies not only to surgeons, but also to anesthesiologists, cardiologists, technicians, and even engineers. Nurses play a main part in postoperative care as well as in cardiosurgical instrumentation. The surgeon undergoes the longest training to be able to overcome any difficulty and to adapt himself to the many different situations in the field of congenital and acquired cardiopathies.

(2) Training can be taken abroad to a hospital, providing it offers the strictly necessary basic conditions for major operations. This method of conveying medical knowledge has been widely used. Pioneers in cardiac surgery were often asked to teach in foreign centers; for instance, Blalock demonstrated his procedure abroad as did entire surgical teams, such as that of the Hammersmith Hospital[1] which introduced cardiac surgery in the USSR, Finland, and other countries ranging across the Middle and Far East. We believe in this second method of training, although we combine it as often as possible with the first. Its advantage is that we then can find in the autochthonous team abroad a number of already trained members.

(3) The third form of internationalization of cardiovascular surgery consists mainly of the exportation of patients. There are two main reasons behind this form of exportation:

(a) Because cardiology is well developed in certain countries that also have a good medical organization, allowing correct detection of all surgical diseases and precise diagnosis, the number of patients is continuously increasing. The introduction of coronary artery surgery in 1967–1968 has resulted in an explosive increase in cardiosurgical centers in the United States as well as in Europe. In some cases, the increased number of patients rapidly surpassed the latter framework's ability to absorb them all, creating waiting lists, which are particularly harmful in difficult cases. Therefore, such countries had a moral obligation to send their worst cases to foreign centers whose surgical capacity had not been fully utilized.

(b) In countries where cardiac surgery is either nonexistent or only starting, those aware of the possibilities of being operated on abroad to improve their condition of life have taken the chance and travelled to foreign centers well known for their good operative results.

INTERNATIONAL PRACTICES OF CARDIAC SURGERY

A consequence of these two phenomena, although their origins were poles apart, was a deep change in cardiovascular surgery which in many places has lost its regional or national complexion. This may be one reason why it is impossible most of the time to quantify the real needs in cardiac surgery in different countries in the world.

Where there is a good economy and a well-developed medical technology, figures mentioned at the start of the chapter, ie, 400 open heart surgery cases per 1 million inhabitants, are nearly satisfied or even surpassed.

Less privileged countries, those whose social systems are sometimes more restrictive, can operate on one half, more often only on one fourth of this figure, which has been taken as a reference.

Because it has been impossible to obtain global figures despite an in-depth search, we shall successively analyze those to be found in the literature from different countries in the world.

EUROPE

We shall start with Europe and consider a number of overall figures. In *France*, a working group headed by Dubost[2] showed in 1980 that 41 teams had performed 15,621 cardiac operations, of which 13,241 were open. In 1982, 51 centers had performed 17,292 open heart interventions. These figures compared with those of the United States, which will subsequently be discussed, led to the conclusion that a good relation exists between the needs of the population and the number of centers, which in turn are well spread out over the French territory to meet these needs. The working group concludes with another argument, that prospectively the number of open heart operations will not diminish during the following years. There is one center (Institut Arnault Tzanck in Nice, headed by Professor Vincent Dor) where 800 to 1,000 open heart operations are currently being performed each year, 85% without the use of blood. The total number of operations from 1973 to 1985 is approximately 6,000.

Open heart surgery in certain countries is quantitatively limited. In *Portugal*, with a population of 10 million inhabitants, five centers are performing 160 open heart interventions per 1 million inhabitants. This figure represents approximately one third of that proposed as a reference in terms of requirements in open heart surgery by the World Health Organization.

In *Greece*, where the population is 9.5 million, the estimated number of patients who would be candidates for surgery is about 3,000 per year; only one third of this number are being operated on.

In *Norway*, a country of 4 million inhabitants, four centers are performing between 1,250 and 1,400 operations a year because of the increase in coronary artery disease. These figures are considered sufficient for the needs of the country. If we relate them to the average previously defined, then approximately 350 patients per million inhabitants are operated on in Norway. This constitutes a tremendous effort if we consider that Norway geographically is a huge country more than 2,000 km in length with many fjords and mountains. In conclusion, detection, investigation, and transportation of patients is very well organized and can act as an example for other countries in the northern hemisphere in a similar situation.

In *Sweden*, a country of 8 million inhabitants where, as in Finland, arteriosclerosis is extremely common, Ekeström et al[3] studied the number of cardiac interventions during the years 1970 to 1979. In 1970, only a few patients were operated on, approximately 15 in the main hospital in Stockholm; this number increased to 200 in 1979. Some three other centers are also performing open heart procedures; altogether, however, it is estimated that only one third of the hypothetical needs are being met.

Higher figures have been shown for Germany, the Netherlands, and the United Kingdom.

In *Germany*, in 1983, a study performed by 22 units with data received from 21 centers was published on the situation of cardiac surgery in the Federal Republic.[4] It included all the figures on cardiac surgery performed in 1982 with or without extracorporeal circulation and showed the respective numbers of valvular, coronary, and congenital heart procedures (Table 75.1). For a total population of nearly 62 million inhabitants, 15,476 operations were performed in 1982. All the centers recorded more than 100 interventions for 1982, 21 showed more than 200, 19 more than 300, 1 more than 400, 15 more than 500, 11 more than 600, 8 more than 700, 2 more than 800, 2 more than 900, and none of the centers more than 1,000 interventions (Table 75.2).

Germany as well as the Netherlands provides a very good example of the destabilization created by the tremendous increase in ischemic heart disease and the resultant increasing need for operations which could not be met by the surgical structures in place when the rush occurred. This is mainly due to an excellent cardiologic background, good investigative techniques, and a medical body that rapidly understood that revascularization of the myocardium could tremendously improve the quality of life and, a little later, the life expectancy. Conversely, Germany and the Netherlands were wise enough to avoid limiting their activities to patients with coronary artery disease. As shown in Table 75.1, they kept a correct distribution in their treatment of different forms of cardiac disease. Of interest is the relatively new philosophy of operating on young children with congenital heart disease, as shown in Table 75.3. The 21 centers that replied to the register indicated that 721 infants under 1 year of age were operated on without extracorporeal circulation and 273 with a heart-lung machine. In the group over 1 year of age, 666 had closed heart interventions (less than the number in the group under 1 year of age) and 1,642 underwent procedures with extracorporeal circulation (almost six times more than the infants). The surgical mortality with a closed procedure was less than 1% in the group over 1 year of age against 10% in the infant group. In open heart cases, however, the surgical risk amounts to 4.2% in children and 14.7% in infants.

These findings could argue for a reassessment of the position relative to intervention in young infants, either closed or open methods, when there is not an absolute need for surgical correction. It is probably preferable for such operations in infants, who also represent a higher risk category of patients, to be limited to highly specialized centers.

Great Britain is particularly well organized and is carefully formulating a very good cardiac surgical register. This is mainly the result of work undertaken by very active surgeons including English et al.[5]

Table 75.4 shows the activity in the United Kingdom. The number of cases of valvular heart disease did not change significantly, nor did the surgical risk which oscillated between 7% and 9%. The same was applicable for congenital heart disease, which remained constant, as well as for the surgical risk, which did not change (around 10% for the past six years). From 1977 until 1982, the number of coronary operations more than doubled. It is interesting to compare what occurred in Australia and in the United Kingdom in 1982 (see following section).

Again, it is interesting to look at the development of cardiac surgery in infants (Table 75.5). The number of patients operated on during the six years decreased slightly without any change in the surgical risk which remained, altogether, 7% to 8%. The number of patients operated on, over 1 year of age, almost doubled between 1977 and 1982, but the surgical risk remained extremely high. This higher surgical risk indicates that the waiting period is too long, a well-known occurrence in severe congenital heart disease, and may explain such a high risk.

Interesting too is the number of operations for revascularization of the myocardium (Table 75.6). The number of coronary patients has almost tripled during the six years and the surgical risk has been cut by half.

The United Kingdom is very different from one area to another. There are, for example, 14 health regions varying between 1.9 million inhabitants (in East Anglia) and 5.2 million (in the West Midlands).

With Figures 75.1 and 75.2, we have tried to relate the number of cases of ischemic, valvular, and congenital heart disease in different parts of the country in terms of the number of operations performed (in Figure 75.1, fewer than 400 per 1 million inhabitants; in Figure 75.2, more than 400 per 1 million inhabitants per annum). A great discrepancy can be seen between the different regions in terms of the number of operations. Thus, most calculations based on regional populations are probably not as significant as one may think, because many centers are draining patients from other areas or from abroad. This is one reason why this chapter should be considered as giving estimations rather than precise data. The 1983 statistics from the United Kingdom go further and point out the number of different procedures performed with extracorporeal circulation: Of a total of 16,874 procedures, 4,683 were performed for valvular disease, 9,617 for coronary artery disease, 2,166 for congenital defects, and 408

Table 75.1. Summary of Cardiac Surgery Performed in West Germany in 1982

	Disease				
	Valvular	Coronary	Congenital	Miscellaneous	Total
With ECC	3,788	7,287	2,126	470	13,671
Without ECC	87	1	1,498	219	1,805
Total	3,875	7,288	3,624	689	15,476

ECC = extracorporeal circulation.
From Rodenwald and Polonius,[4] with permission.

Table 75.2. Number of Procedures Per Unit

Number of ECC	1978	1979	1980	1981	1982
0–99	0	0	0	0	0
100–199	4	1	1	1	1
200–299	3	1	3	1	2
300–399	5	9	4	4	3
400–499	3	2	4	3	1
500–599	2	3	2	3	4
600–699	2	2	2	1	2
700–799	1	2	2	3	3
800–899	1	1	3	3	2
900–1,000	0	0	0	2	2
Over 1,000	0	0	0	0	2

ECC = extracorporeal circulation.
From Rodewald and Polonius,[4] with permission.

for miscellaneous lesions. The surgical risk was, respectively, 7.7%, 4.8%, 12.8%, and 20%. In closed operations, the total number was 1,810, 128 for valvular disease with a surgical risk of 1.6%, 1,553 for congenital defects, the risk being 7%, and 19 for miscellaneous lesions with the surgical risk a little less than 15%. Altogether, 18,684 patients were operated on during 1983, which means about 332 patients per million inhabitants, an almost ideal calculated figure.

In the United Kingdom cardiac surgery register, some figures are particularly interesting as they reflect some of the choices made in valvular surgery. The importance of this is that a great number of cardiac surgeons in the world were trained in Great Britain, even after the independence of the British colonies. A comparison of the material used in the mitral and aortic positions in 2,001 patients who underwent single valve replacement during 1983 shows almost similar figures for mechanical prostheses and bioprostheses. As expected, the number of patients who had conservative surgery was ten times greater in the mitral than in the aortic position. One interesting fact should be retained for the future: the low surgical risk of mitral valvuloplasty compared with the risk of mitral or aortic replacement.

Many double valve interventions were performed, 538 involving the mitral and aortic valves, 132 the mitral and

Table 75.3. Operations for Congenital Heart Disease in 1982 in West Germany

Age	Number	Deaths	%
Without ECC			
Over 1 yr	666	5	0.8
Under 1 yr	721	73	10.1
Total	1,387	78	5.6
With ECC			
Over 1 yr	1,642	69	4.2
Under 1 yr	273	40	14.7
Total	1,915	109	5.7
Total of both procedures	3,302	187	5.7

ECC = extracorporeal circulation.
From Rodewald and Polonius,[4] with permission.

tricuspid, and 6 the aortic and tricuspid, with a surgical risk of 10% for mitral and aortic procedures and about 20% for mitral and tricuspid procedures. In triple valve operations the mortality rate was 27% in 44 patients.

Revascularization of the myocardium (Table 75.7) quantitatively shows the type of revascularization procedure in 8,332 patients. The surgical risk is studied in terms of the number of revascularized vessels. Apart from these 8,332 patients, 1,111 had an additional surgical procedure (left ventricular aneurysmectomy, mitral or aortic valve replacement or repair, or closure of a ventricular septal defect) with an average surgical risk of 11%.

Once again, with reference to cardiac surgery in infants, without entering into details, 1,749 infants over 1 year of age were operated on with a mortality rate of 8.7%, and 417 infants under 1 year of age, with a mortality of 29.7%. These findings agree with what was previously mentioned, that the surgical risk in open procedures is about three times greater in infants under 1 year of age. For closed procedures, 1,553 patients were operated on; 768 were over 1 year of age, whereas 785 were under 1 year of age, the younger group having a surgical risk six times greater than the older group.

In *Holland*, information was obtained from the Department of Thoracic Surgery of Professor Hans Huysmans in Leiden. With a population of 14.5 million, ten centers performed 8,260 open heart procedures in 1983; 6,225 were coronary, 1,235 valvular, 602 congenital, and 189 miscellaneous procedures.

In 1984, the total number of open heart operations was 8,750 with an additional 450 closed cardiac procedures. Government calculations indicate that the current need, which is probably an underestimation, is 12,000 open heart operations per year, approximately double the needs estimated by the World Health Organization. Again, it reflects the good organization in cardiology in Holland. The discrepancy between the needs of patients and the availability of surgery is still very high; 25% of the cardiac patients in the Netherlands are still waiting. Again, the constant number of patients requiring surgery for valvular and congenital disease is not going to decrease.

In *Yugoslavia*, a country of 22 million inhabitants, with which we have rather privileged relations, the number of open heart operations recorded in three centers was between 200 and 300 from 1958 to 1963. This number progressively increased, from 1974 to 1983, to 400 to 500 interventions in seven centers. In 1984, 1,800 open heart operations were performed. From 1958 to mid-1985, a total of 20,000 Yugoslav patients were operated on with extracorporeal circulation.

In *Switzerland*, approximately 4,000 open heart operations are performed each year. Because the population is estimated at 6,330,000 inhabitants, then about 650 open heart operations are performed per 1 million inhabitants every year. This is a typical example of a totally incorrect figure as two thirds of the patients operated on in this country come from abroad. Contrary also to what this figure appears to demonstrate, the need for open heart surgery in different parts of Switzerland is not satisfied as there are many areas where a very conservative approach to cardiac disease is practiced.

Table 75.4. Summary of All Cardiac Operations from 1977 to 1982 in the United Kingdom*

	Disease				
	Valvular	Ischemic	Congenital	Miscellaneous†	Total
1977	4,832	3,040	3,344	386	11,602
1978	4,873	3,345	3,385	340	11,943
1979	4,791	3,688	3,275	402	12,156
1980	4,814	5,011	3,472	442	13,739
1981	4,762	6,123	3,501	401	14,787
1982	4,652	7,403	3,392	443	15,890
Total	28,724	28,610	20,369	2,414	80,117

* From English et al,[5] with permission.

† Miscellaneous acquired heart disease in adults.

AUSTRALIA

In *Australia*, the National Heart Foundation of Australia in April 1984 published the cardiac surgical register for 1982.[6] In that year, 16 cardiac units performed 9,005 cardiac operations compared with 8,151 in 1981 and 6,865 in 1980. Also in 1982, 1,299 operations for congenital heart disease were recorded; this figure is very similar to those obtained in the past years. An important progressive increase in the number of coronary artery bypasses has been recorded since 1979: 6,244 patients underwent intervention for coronary artery disease compared with 5,517 in 1981, 4,224 in 1980, and 3,233 in 1979. The report shows a tendency toward stabilization in the number of myocardial revascularizations: a 13% difference between 1981 and 1982 compared with an average annual increase of 40% for the past nine years.

An analysis of valve surgery between 1972 and 1982 shows the number of operations on individual valves: 6,927 mitral, 7,270 aortic, 510 tricuspid, and 563 pulmonary. Moreover, there were many double and triple valve procedures, either repair or replacement. The number of valve repairs was very stable at about 260 over this period of 11 years. Mechanical prosthetic valve replacements increased from approximately 650 to nearly 1,000 per year. Homograft replacements decreased altogether, as have autografts, which have been nearly totally replaced by heterografts since 1976. Thus, heterografts increased tremendously over the past seven years and were used in 569 cases in 1982. With regard to cardiac surgery in infants and children, 970 operations were recorded in 1982 for children over 6 months of age (663 open and 307 closed procedures). There was no difference in mortality between the group of children older than 6 months and the 137 patients between 1 and 6 months of age, the mortality being 26% in both groups, whereas the group of 192 newborns (less than 1 month of age) had a mortality rate of 23%. The number of operations for congenital heart diseases showed a slight and regular increase between 1971 (961 interventions) and 1982 (1,299 cases). In summary, this perfectly well-formulated cardiac register, which can be used as an example, in addition to those from the United Kingdom and Germany, shows that Australia is well organized and able to face its requirements in cardiac surgery. In 1982, 600 cardiac operations per 1 million inhabitants were performed.

THE UNITED STATES

Data from the National Center for Health Statistics and other sources cited by Rimm[7] include global figures on coronary artery bypass surgery as well as the total number of open heart operations performed in the United States from 1970 to 1984.

Figure 75.3 shows a total of about 250,000 open heart operations for 1982, of which 170,000 were coronary artery bypass procedures, as compared with the number performed between 1970 and 1982.

Details and figures given by Kennedy et al[8,9] reveal that in 1973, 15 patients with coronary artery disease were operated on in Olmsted County, Minnesota (100,000 inhabitants); in other words, 150 per 1 million inhabitants. Four years later in 1977, 40 patients underwent coronary artery surgery, ie, 400 per 1 million inhabitants. The re-

Table 75.5. Operations for Congenital Heart Disease in Patients Over and Under One Year of Age in the United Kingdom*

Year	Patients Over 1 Year	Patients Under 1 Year	Total No. of Operations
1977	1,830	275	2,105
1978	1,820	333	2,153
1979	1,638	377	2,015
1980	1,619	390	2,009
1981	1,620	426	2,046
1982	1,637	570	2,207

* From English et al,[5] with permission.

Table 75.6. Number of Operations for Ischemic Heart Disease in the United Kingdom*

	Coronary Bypass Grafts		
Year	Alone	With Other Procedures	Procedures Without Graft
1977	2,297	584	159
1978	2,653	537	155
1979	2,918	620	150
1980	4,057	802	152
1981	5,130	839	154
1982	6,008	1,224	171

* From English et al,[5] with permission.

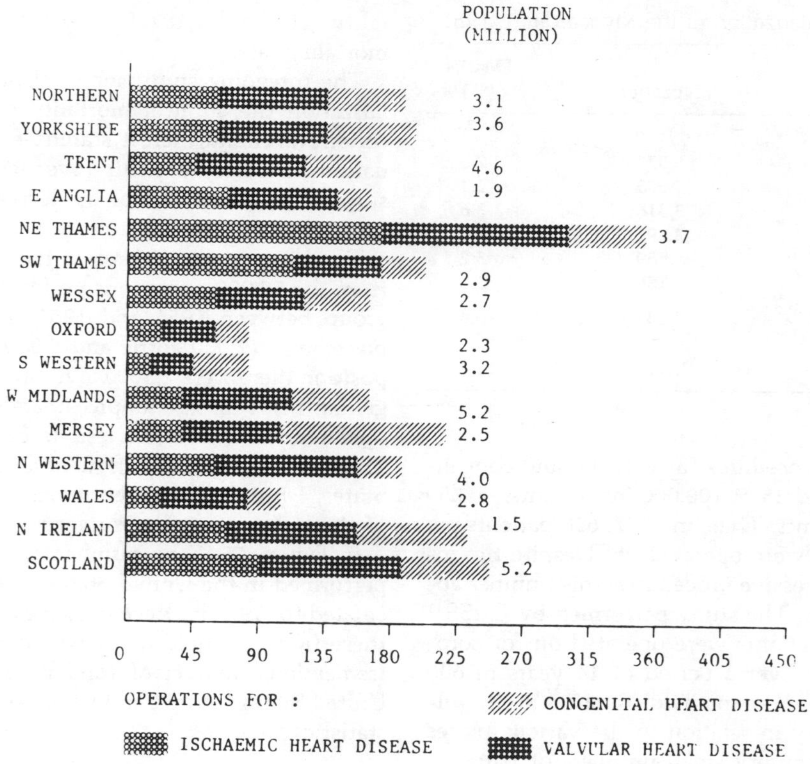

Figure 75.1. The number of cardiac operations per 1 million inhabitants per year in the United Kingdom (1977 to 1982). (From English et al,[5] with permission.)

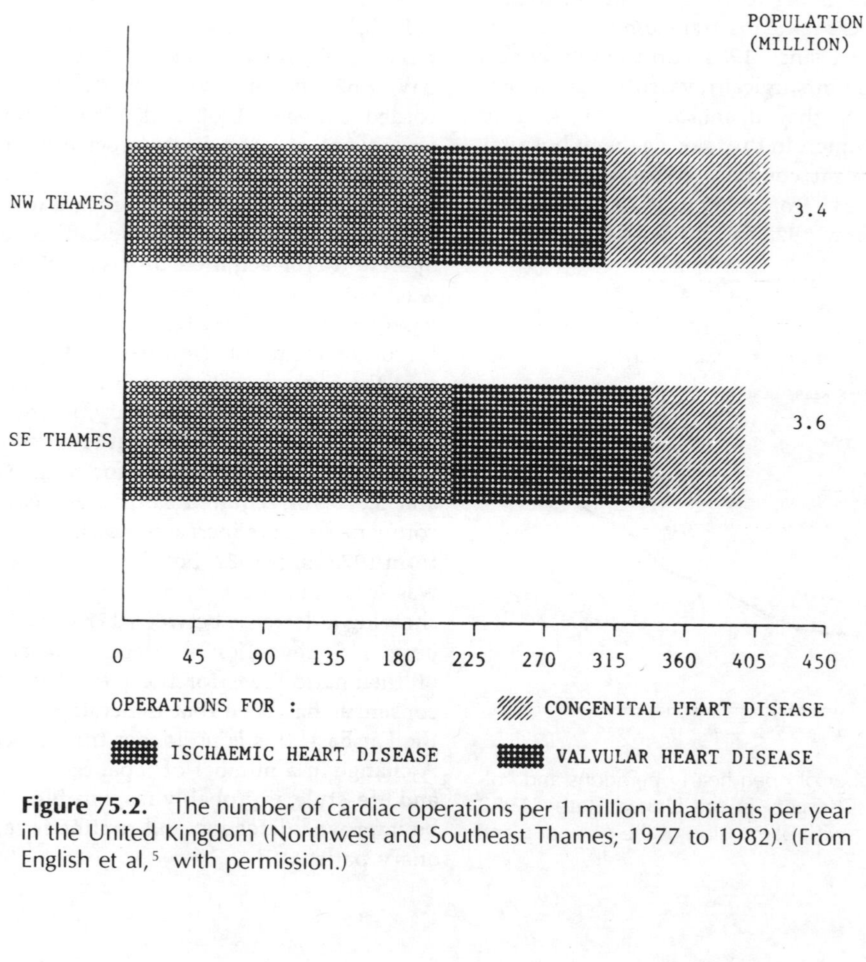

Figure 75.2. The number of cardiac operations per 1 million inhabitants per year in the United Kingdom (Northwest and Southeast Thames; 1977 to 1982). (From English et al,[5] with permission.)

Table 75.7. Revascularization of the Myocardium: 1983

Operation	Number	Deaths (%)
Isolated bypass grafts		
Single	533	2.8
Double	1,675	2.4
Triple	3,316	3.6
Quadruple	2,191	3.6
Quintuple	459	5.2
Others	158	3.8
Total	8,332	3.4
Grafts and other procedures	1,111	11.3

maining open heart procedures for valvular and congenital disease represented 25 of 100,000 inhabitants, ie, 250 per 1 million inhabitants. Thus, in 1977, 650 patients per 1 million inhabitants were operated on. Despite the introduction of less aggressive procedures, this number appears to remain stable. The study performed by CASS[10] shows that 500,000 patients were operated on for coronary revascularization over a period of 14 years in 600 different hospitals. There are many differences in the volume of cardiac surgery in relation to the various places considered. Some have very small numbers of patients; others, such as the Texas Heart Institute under the direction of Denton Cooley, have a tremendous turnover in patients undergoing open heart intervention.[11] In the so-called late period shown in Figure 75.4, a tremendous increase can be seen since 1970, because of coronary bypass surgery. It is interesting to note on this histogram that the number of percutaneous transluminal coronary angioplasties performed since 1981 corresponds almost exactly to the decrease in surgical revascularization procedures. If compared to that at another center, such as that of Dr George Schimert in Buffalo, a general hospital, 5,466 patients underwent coronary bypass surgery between 1969 and 1984: 218 from 1969 to 1973 with a 3.7% mortality rate, 1,051 from 1973 to 1977 with a 1.8% mortality rate, and 4,167 from 1977 to 1983 with a 1.6% mortality rate.

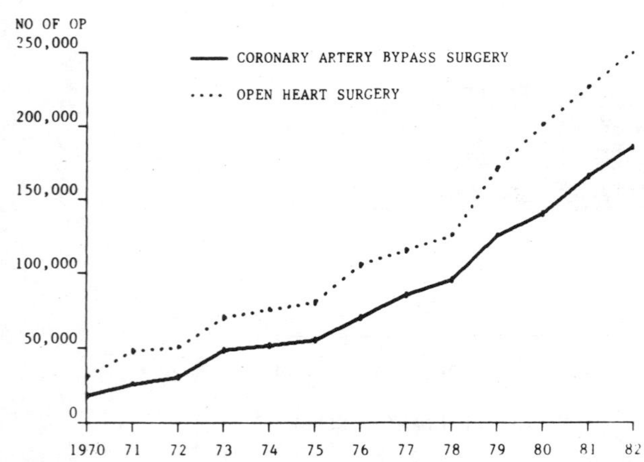

Figure 75.3. The number of open heart operations and volume of coronary bypass surgery in the United States (1970 to 1982). (From Rimm,[7] with permission of the *New England Journal of Medicine*.)

The foregoing study shows that in coronary revascularization the surgical mortality can be improved to a certain level and then it stabilizes. This is the exact situation in elderly patients (over 65 years of age) where surgical mortality cannot be decreased further than approximately 5% in most centers, American or European.

To return to the figures at the Texas Heart Institute, from the 50,000 operations performed by Cooley and his group between 1956 and 1983, 12,000 were valve replacements (7,000 aortic and 5,000 mitral). In the mitral position there were 2,500 valvuloplasties. In terms of congenital heart disease, approximately 6,000 patients were operated on for different lesions, cyanotic or noncyanotic. There are many other figures available for the United States,[12] but the ones mentioned give an excellent picture of the status of cardiac surgery in the country.

In Figure 75.3, the number of open heart operations performed in the United States in 1982 is twice that calculated for 1977 by the World Health Organization. Also, these figures should be viewed critically because of the tremendous number of foreign patients referred to the United States for operation and who appear in American statistics.

ASIA

In considering the *Asian continent*, a choice had to be selectively made; thus, figures were obtained for India, Japan, the Philippines, South Korea, and Indonesia. The situation in China will be described in the following chapter.

In *India*, valve surgery was a main concern in the different cardiovascular centers. In the KEM hospital, Bombay, 7,626 patients with mitral valve disease were recorded between 1962 and 1984. From this total 1,261 underwent an open heart procedure and 237 had valve replacement.

In *Japan*, the situation with regard to open heart surgery in 1982 was indicated by Wada.[13] The total number of operations for acquired disease (valvular and coronary) was 5,875. Of these patients 65% were operated on for valvular disease, 29% for ischemic heart disease, and 6% for other forms of acquired cardiopathy. During these past three years, patients with all types of disease, valvular, congenital, and coronary, increased in number. In 1982, the total number of patients recorded was 12,421; from this: 6,546 procedures for congenital heart disease, and 5,875 for acquired cardiac diseases. The number of coronary patients increased constantly and progressively from 1975 until 1982, but the increase in valvular patients was less dramatic between 1955 and 1979, whilst even showing a decrease between 1979 and 1982. This reflects improved prevention of infectious diseases and treatment of rheumatic fever for the past few years. The general consensus has been that ischemic heart disease is rare in the Far East; this is no longer true, especially from 1975. A change in a number of Japanese habits, mainly in diet and life-style, is probably responsible. Other reasons may be improved detection and routine investigations of coronary patients.[14]

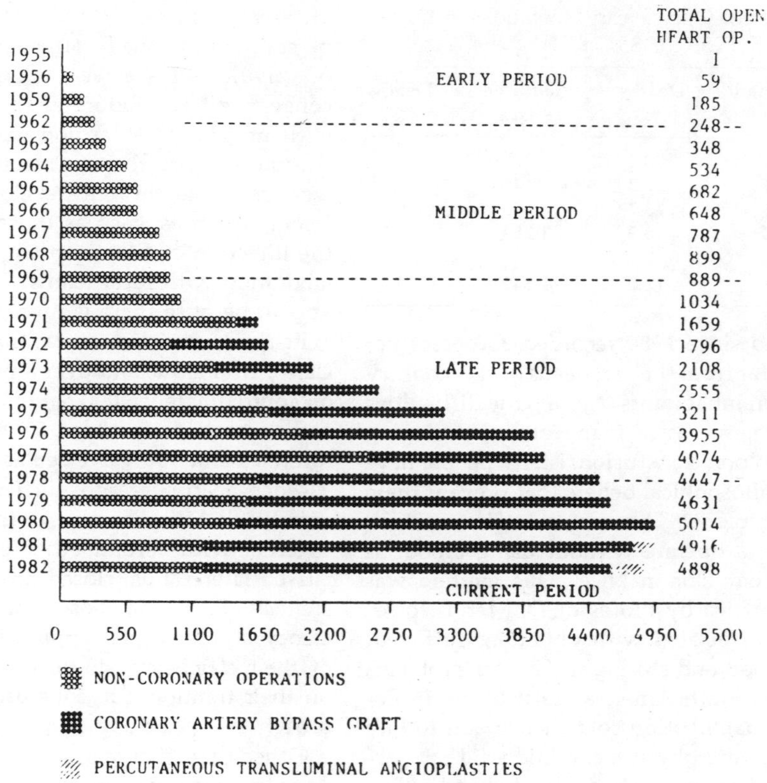

Figure 75.4. Open heart operations per year at the Texas Heart Institute. (From Keats,[11] with permission.)

It is a general rule that most countries that claim a low incidence of arteriosclerosis, regardless of the type or location, are underestimating this problem. The same situation was applicable to Europe prior to the development of the correct means of making a precise diagnosis, even in congenital disease.

The population of Japan consists of 116 million inhabitants. The total number of operations for acquired heart disease was 5,875 in 1982, which represents 51 patients per 1 million inhabitants, and 107 operations per 1 million inhabitants for all forms of cardiac surgery.

For *South Korea*, we have figures concerning the entire country and other more specific ones from the Seoul University Hospital by Lee.[15] As in most countries in the Far East and the Pacific area, the number of babies born with congenital cardiovascular lesions is extremely high. In Korea, which has 37.5 million inhabitants, 870,000 births were registered in 1980; of these infants, 5,000 to 7,000 had congenital anomalies. Rheumatic fever is still so widespread that many children are developing valvular disease. As previously mentioned, the number of coronary patients is still small; Figure 75.5 shows that an open heart procedure was performed in 1959 in one patient who died. There was a slight increase in numbers until 1971; then from 1977 to 1982 a relatively important and systematic rise was noted. The different types of congenital or acquired diseases treated surgically between 1969 and 1983 are summarized in Table 75.8. This table indicates that the number of open heart operations for congenital malformations is increasing at a much more rapid pace than that for acquired diseases, probably because coronary revascularization is not performed as a routine procedure.

In the *Philippines*, at the Heart Center for Asia, 10,000 patients underwent cardiac surgery over a period of ten years; 2,151 operations were for valvular heart disease. The problem arising from American type institutions created in underdeveloped countries is always the same: at a certain point, the cost of cardiac surgery will overload the financial budget of the country. This is applicable not only in the developing countries of Asia but also in those of Africa and South America.

In *Indonesia*, the two centers at which cardiac operations

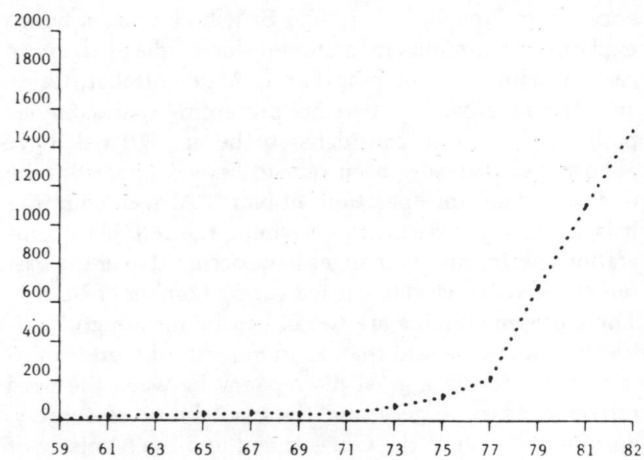

Figure 75.5. Open heart surgery in Korea (1959 to 1982).

Table 75.8. Number of Open Heart Operations in Korea (1959–1983)

Years	Congenital Cases	Deaths (%)	Acquired Cases	Deaths (%)
1959	1	100.0	...	...
1961–1969	114	27.2	40	37.5
1970–1979	1,316	13.7	555	15.1
1980–1983	2,760	8.9	1,254	6.5
Total	4,191	11.0	1,849	9.8

have been performed since 1980 recorded 350 cases per year in 1983. This is far from the real needs of this country which has 160 million inhabitants. Among the difficulties encountered in Indonesia, as in many other developing countries, is that of blood transfusion. Many people have either religious or philosophical beliefs that prevent them from donating their blood. The best solution for such countries would be to operate without using blood, as does Professor Vincent Dor in Nice. This method was employed in Black Africa by Professor D. Metras to resolve the problems associated with obtaining sufficient amounts of clean blood and storing it. Greater problems were encountered in South America, particularly in Ecuador: donors with malnutrition sold their blood to buy food. However, their poor physical condition did not permit the withdrawal of amounts normally obtained in Europe or America, as many collapsed after the removal of 100 cc of blood. This caused many problems for cardiosurgical teams, because the bags prepared for open heart procedures contained almost no blood if the usual amount of citrate had been placed in them. Conversely, operating without blood for transfusion requires tremendous experience and an enormous discipline from the different members of a team; therefore, this method cannot be adopted without having previously solved many basic prerequisites.

AFRICA

Africa can be divided into three parts, each of which has developed independently of the others because of differences in their historical past.

In *North Africa*, which consists of Tunisia, Algeria, Morocco, Egypt, and Libya, there were strong cultural influences from French, Italian, and British colonizers which explains the attempts made to develop cardiac surgery in certain main cities such as Tunis, Algiers, Rabat, Cairo, and Tripoli. However, patients presenting with complex pathology or those considered to be at high risk have almost systematically been sent to France, Great Britain, or Switzerland for operation. In North African countries it is extremely difficult to determine the number of operations performed as changes have occurred over the past ten years with regard to the increasing number of centers. Thus, present figures are too old to be meaningful. Altogether it can be said that, as in most third world countries, there is still a great discrepancy between the need for open heart surgery and the availability of surgery, despite the wish of the Government and the Ministry of Public Health to develop this type of surgery. Generally speaking, valvular diseases are the most malignant in the different countries of North Africa. Rheumatic fever can be severe and usually affects children. Prior to the time of valvular replacement, many children died of chronic congestive heart failure at the ages of 11 and 15 years, with unbelievable cardiomegaly and severe progressive shortness of breath. As a result, most surgical procedures were performed in well-developed centers within the different countries, such as those in Tunis or Egypt, under the direction of European surgeons who worked in collaboration with local teams. The precise figures are unknown because there is no register.

In *Egypt*, statistics are available from Dr El Sayed in Cairo, who alone and over a period of 20 years, operated on approximately 6,000 patients with rheumatic heart disease; operations included 5,000 closed mitral commissurotomies and 950 valve replacements.

Open heart surgery is difficult in North Africa as well as in Black Africa, because of the cost of such a procedure, together with certain other problems that will be discussed later. Thus, closed procedures, mainly for mitral stenosis, including those associated with slight insufficiency, still have great application in North Africa because of their efficiency, simplicity, and low cost. Depending on their training, surgeons use either a left thoracic approach or a right one as described by Bailey.

Other than rheumatic heart disease, many congenital disorders are found in North Africans. The less difficult anomalies, such as atrial and ventricular septal defects and certain degrees of tetralogy of Fallot, and those requiring closed procedures, such as patent ductus arteriosus and coarctation of aorta, are treated within the country.

The most difficult cases, those requiring a higher degree of technology, are mostly sent to Europe. There is a special Swiss organization, Terre des Hommes, that supports sick children whose families have no means. This is to indicate that open heart surgery for third world countries is not reserved only for wealthy patients, but it can be offered by countries in a better economic situation without any charge or with limited fees to the former. We subsequently shall return to such social problems.

In *Black Africa*, apart from those of Nigeria and the Ivory Coast, the number of cardiac procedures performed is totally unknown because most patients are sent to European countries that had previously colonized these different places, as in the case of North Africa.

In *Nigeria*, Adebonojo et al[16] reported the following statistics. From January 1975 to December 1980, 1,450 thoracic surgical procedures were performed at the Uni-

Table 75.9. Number of Cardiovascular Operations at the University College Hospital, Ibadan, from 1975 to 1980

Disease	No.	%
Thoracic surgical disease (total cases)	1,450	100
Cardiovascular disease	227	16.0
Acquired heart disease	100	7.0
Congenital heart disease	94	6.5
Vascular disease	33	2.0

From Adebonojo et al,[16] with permission.

Table 75.10. Analysis of 100 Patients With Acquired Heart Disease

Disease	Total No. of Patients	No. of Operations
Rheumatic heart disease		
Mitral stenosis	16	15
Mitral incompetence	5	0
Aortic valve disease	4	0
Multiple valve disease	2	0
Pyopericarditis	32	31
Complete heart block	17	10
Constrictive pericarditis	12	12
Endomyocardial fibrosis	12	10
Total	100	78

From Adebonojo et al,[16] with permission.

versity College Hospital of Ibadan (Table 75.9). Of this number, 227 were performed for cardiovascular diseases, of which 194 were cardiac (100 were acquired diseases and 94 congenital anomalies). Among the 100 patients who underwent operation for acquired heart disease, the distribution is surprising (Table 75.10) as almost one half had pericardial lesions (pyopericarditis or constrictive pericarditis) and only 27 had rheumatic fever; 15 of the 27 had closed commissurotomy. Table 75.11 shows the number of operations for congenital heart disease recorded as of July 1982; there were only five open heart procedures, the rest being closed.

This feature is typical of different Black African countries, that is, the number of patients operated on is very low, and experience with difficult cases is almost nonexistent. The explanation for the lack of development in such an important field always lies in the tremendous scarcity of diagnostic facilities, the poor equipment for open heart surgery both during and after the operation, and a total absence of well-trained personnel. This is true for most countries of Black Africa as they are "young" countries, having had independence for a short time only

Table 75.12. Analysis of 300 Open Heart Operations Performed in Abidjan

Cardiopathy	No. of Patients	No. of Deaths
Congenital cardiopathy	100	18
Endomyocardial fibrosis	40 (+2)*	9
Mitral valvulopathy		
Insufficiency	57	2
Stenosis	42	2
Mitral insufficiency + left ventricular aneurysm	2	1
Aortic valvulopathy		
Insufficiency	14	1
Stenosis	6	1
Insufficiency + aneurysm of ascending aorta	3	2
Polyvalvulopathy	30 (+2)*	3
Aortic arch aneurysm	2	2
Total	300	41 (13.3%)

* Reoperation for endocarditis of a bioprosthesis.
From Metras et al,[17] with permission of Masson SA, Editeur—Paris.

and facing huge economic and political problems. The worst enemies to the development of cardiovascular surgery are a poor economy and political or tribal problems leading to military solutions, creating new problems instead of solving them. As soon as good seed can be planted in the fertile soil of Africa the situation can change totally.

It is what occurred in Abidjan, and in the Ivory Coast where, owing to the medical background and understanding of the chief of state, a French team[17] has taken care of the Institute of Cardiology in Abidjan since 1977. Up to the present time, this institution is the only one of its kind. For more than six years, because of the tremendous involvement of the cardiovascular team, more than 800 thoracic and cardiovascular operations have been performed in patients coming from all parts of tropical West Africa. Table 75.12 analyzes the 300 open heart operations performed; a third of these operations involved congenital heart disease and 154 valvular disease. It is interesting to

Table 75.11. Analysis of 94 Patients Operated on for Congenital Heart Disease at the University College Hospital, Ibadan, 1975 to 1980

Disease	Total No.	No. of Operations	Operation Procedure: Operation	Operation Procedure: No.
Patent ductus arteriosus	39	38	Double ligation	22
			Division and closure	16
			No operation	1
Tetralogy of Fallot	38	35	Palliative shunt	34
			No operation	3
			Total correction	1*
Transposition of great arteries	5	3	Blalock-Hanlon	
Coarctation of aorta	3	3	Coarctectomy	
Atrial septal defect	2	2*	Closure	
Pulmonary stenosis	2	2*	Pulmonary valvotomy	
Tricuspid atresia	2	2	Palliative shunt	
Congenital vascular anomalies	2	0	None	
Ectopia cordis	1	0	None	
Total	94	85		

* Open heart procedure (total 5).
From Adebonojo et al,[16] with permission.

note the huge number of cases of endomyocardial fibrosis (more than 40) which is a typical feature of certain African countries. Particular diseases can be found in limited geographic areas such as Chagas disease in South and Central America and certain severe, very malignant cardiomyopathies in Zaire and Senegal. These are only some examples in the distribution of acquired diseases. There are similar differences in other countries. In Guayaquil, Ecuador, where we built a center, a case of atypical septation of the atria was found only because of our good background in embryology. When performing surgery in other countries, we must be aware that one may not necessarily find the same diseases faced at home. Lack of information or insufficient preparation can explain certain disasters that might be encountered. The results in the 300 patients with open heart surgery (46 of whom were operated on without the use of blood) are very good, the surgical risk being 13%. Of this group, three patients died of hepatitis after blood transfusion and four from endocarditis of a bioprosthesis; these deaths are mainly due to local problems.

The third part of Africa is *South Africa*, and particularly the experience of the Groote Schuur group in Cape Town. This country differs completely from the rest of the African continent. It permits a number of surgical procedures similar to those used in Western Europe or the United States. Statistical work performed in 1982 and reported in 1983[18] shows 6,161 cardiac operations between 1971 and 1981, of which 4,618 (75%) were for acquired heart disease and 1,543 (25%) for congenital heart disease. There are other centers in South Africa where closed and open procedures are performed, but their exact figures are not known. As in many other countries, coronary patients who were almost never submitted to surgery in the past are taking on a greater importance. In the acquired heart disease group there were close to 20% in 1976. Figure 75.6 illustrates the increase in the number of open heart procedures despite a decrease in the progression in 1980, particularly in valvular and congenital

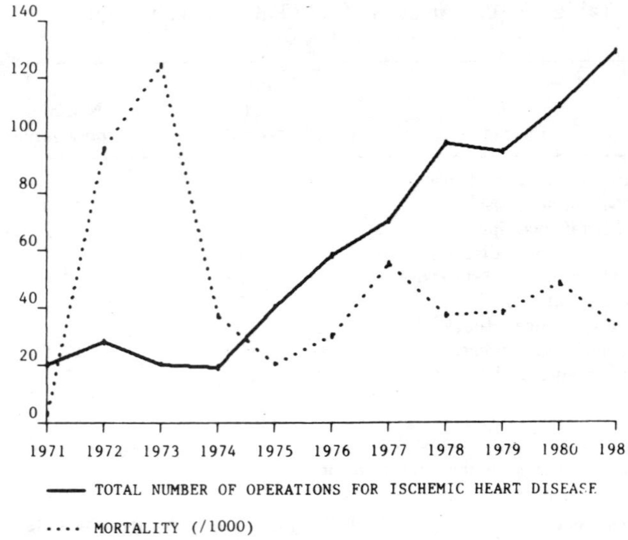

Figure 75.7. The number of operations for ischemic heart disease in Cape Town, South Africa. (From Parry et al,[18] with permission.)

heart surgery. Myocardial revascularization by aortocoronary bypass remained at a low level up to 1975 and then increased slowly up to 1981. The total amount of valvular surgical procedures almost doubled between 1971 and 1978 and then subsequently decreased. Rheumatic valvular disease is still an important problem in the lower socioeconomic classes of South Africa. Many bioprostheses were considered the ideal material, as in most countries where good anticoagulation cannot safely be maintained. However, many such patients had malfunction of the valve, requiring mechanical valve replacement.

Figure 75.7 indicates the number of operations for ischemic heart disease between 1977 and 1981 as well as the evolution in surgical risk. This small number can be explained by ethnic differences among the three groups of patients: white, colored, and black. During these five

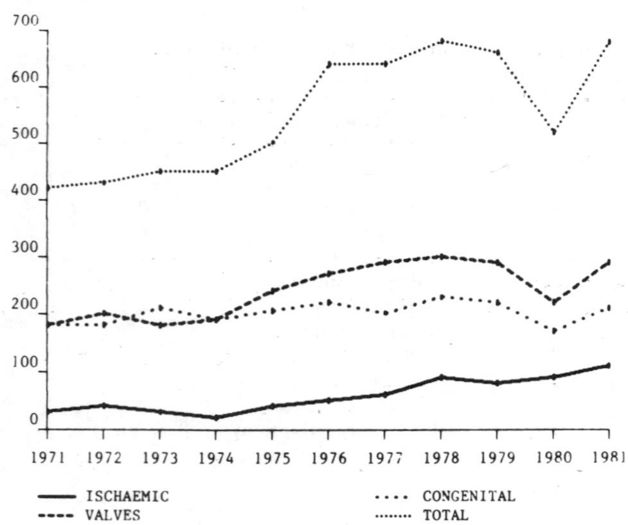

Figure 75.6. The number of cardiac operations performed in Cape Town, South Africa. (From Parry et al,[18] with permission.)

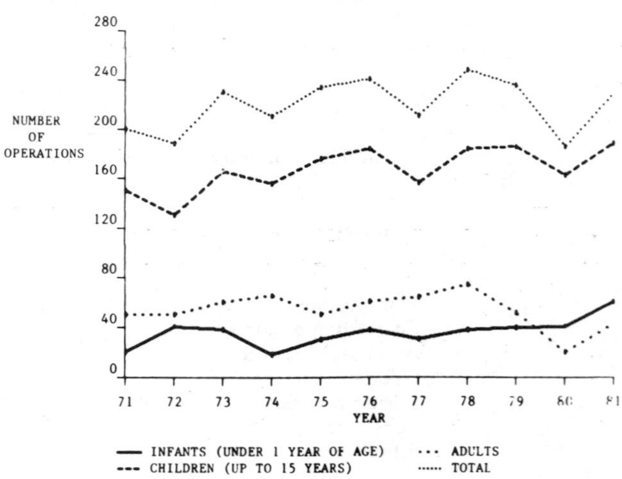

Figure 75.8. The number of operations performed for congenital heart disease; Cape Town's Statistic. (From Parry et al,[18] with permission.)

years no black patient received coronary artery bypass. Among the colored people, the number of surgical patients increased from 14 in 1977 to 28 in 1981. During the same period, the number of white patients increased from 56 in 1977 to 101 in 1981. The number of females, which was extremely low in 1977 (2), went up to 14 in 1981. The data presented cannot give a satisfactory explanation for these differences. For congenital heart disease (Figure 75.8) treated surgically throughout this 10-year period, the number of adults, infants, and children under 15 years of age is almost stable. The mortality is very high, approximately 26%, and it appears to be related to the greater number of children coming from the country probably in very poor condition.

LATIN AMERICA

The only figures obtained for Latin America are those from *Brazil* where 120 to 150 open heart operations are performed per 1 million inhabitants, and this figure is less in *Argentina*. Despite the excellent centers that exist in South America, figures are unknown; no doubt they are far from what the population would actually require. This discrepancy is mainly due to economic reasons and a lack of efficient manpower.

CARDIAC TRANSPLANTATION

There exists another problem common in Africa, South America, and a number of Far Eastern countries: certain patients with valvular or congenital disease are referred to the small number of existing centers when they are almost in an end-stage condition. The same situation still exists in patients with ischemic heart disease in more developed countries. Patients still come to surgery when all the risk factors of the operation are met: one or several infarctions in the past, diffuse coronary lesions, or age over 65. This explains the increase in the indications for cardiac replacement, which will probably change the profile of open heart surgery in the future. In an attempt to understand the future prospectives of cardiovascular surgery, the needs in cardiac replacement in Europe and the United States were studied. The 1984 figures for the United States were obtained from the National Heart Transplantation Study. Patients who met the conditions for cardiac transplantation (mainly age under 55 years) were estimated at 335,000 per year. The same study gave a figure for donors: those who met the criteria allowing use of their heart for transplantation, assuming none are lost, were estimated at 17,000 per year. In January 1984, the statistics from eight centers to which 1,269 patients were referred for heart transplantation were studied; 23% of these patients obtained a heart whereas 20% on the waiting list died. Some are still on the list, but 55% were rejected because of contraindications. If we look at more homogeneous statistics, those of Shumway[19] for instance, orthotopic heart transplantation definitely appears to be the method of choice for cardiac replacement. In Shumway's group, 325 patients were operated on up to January 1985. The current surgical curves are extremely good with an 80% survival rate, particularly after the introduction of cyclosporine. Of these 325 patients, 85 are living normally after one year. There are many other figures that also demonstrate the degree of perfection attained by excellent centers in human heart transplantation.

However, there will always be a chronic lack in donors, thus requiring the development of other means of replacing heart function or the chronic support of the latter by mechanical means. These future prospectives in cardiac surgery raise the question as to the conditions necessary for the establishment of an institute of cardiology and cardiac surgery.

THE FUTURE

Experience indicates that unless certain rules are respected, success in building active and efficient centers in developing countries will not be achieved.

Among the various conditions that determine success or failure are the procedures used, the type of material for valves such as homografts, xenografts, or mechanical valves, as well as the material or technical procedure used to repair difficult congenital heart abnormalities. Our experience indicates that many surgeons would like to have some open heart surgery performed in their centers for different reasons, usually nothing to do with scientific achievement. Those responsible for spreading knowledge over the world must remember that the work currently being done in the best centers cannot be implemented everywhere. All the steps that had to be taken must also be cleared by the new teams, although they can proceed more rapidly because of technologic progress. For example, it is of no use to start with the most complicated open heart procedures if simple closed operations cannot be performed. The latter do not require sophisticated measures, and they can succeed and instill confidence in the medical personnel as well as in the patients and their families. Then, teams must be trained in the proper manner, according to norms that have been established in terms of the number and quality of different components of this team. Thereafter, in perhaps the most important step, these different specialists must really become a team through correct training in an experimental laboratory. Coordination within a group that performs open heart surgery and that takes the responsibility for patients in an intensive care unit is essential. The team must work as a body and have the proper equipment to perform such work.

The attitude in most countries around the world, where the economic or political situation does not favor the treatment of cardiovascular disease, must be changed, and those responsible must be made to understand that open heart surgery is not a luxury but a necessity. Few would accept the lack of treatment in cancer of the esophagus or in many of the traumatic or degenerative lesions of the bones or articulations. If the cost of open heart surgery is actually compared rather than just claiming that it is prohibitive, the conclusion is easily reached that the cost of medicine generally is not within the means of our societies in their current organization. We believe that it is the responsibility of government or private institutions to organize the financial aspect of medicine in a more rational way. Many patients are still paying in terms of the quality of life or life expectancy, mainly because of a lack of responsibility in terms of medical care. In other words, we must direct our thoughts to a more social attitude in the treatment of patients, even if the term *social* has nothing to do with political involvement. Liberal medicine as well as socialized medicine must follow parallel pathways to solve the problems of cardiovascular disease. A real international practice of cardiovascular surgery must be instituted, which is far from the present situation. The lack of information faced when writing this chapter is direct proof. However, the data we found demonstrate or at least give an indication of the distribution of the different types of cardiac lesions in different continents. The need to develop methods to prevent infection, arteriosclerosis, or severe congenital heart disease exists and should be considered on a worldwide level. The same is also true for less aggressive forms of treatment like those currently being used in the treatment of arteriosclerotic stenosis in different locations, particularly the coronary arteries. Much development is required with new procedures, such as the laser in the treatment of arteriosclerosis as well as certain arrhythmias. Much work must continue in the field of cardiac replacement which has just opened. However, all these new procedures must be developed in a small number of centers that have all the appropriate facilities, before they can be spread all over the world. It is up to the developed countries and to international organizations to train the teams necessary for the care of patients in their own countries.

CONCLUSIONS

In summary, this study shows that in the cardiovascular field, particularly in its surgical aspect, there is an enormous difference in the application of surgical procedures in different countries of the world. Those with a strong economy or an incentive to give priority to their health services are close to, or even higher than, the ideal number of cardiac operations estimated by an international group of experts chosen by the World Health Organization. Most cardiac diseases, particularly in countries with lower socioeconomic conditions, are very severe and can be considered as malignant as cancer. Hence, it is unacceptable that a tremendous number of patients should be invalid or dying because of a lack of organization in their own countries. The cost of open heart surgery cannot continue to be a "screen" to explain why proper treatment is not instituted. It is becoming more frequent to speak of crimes against humanity, and yet the situation in cardiovascular disease is nothing less than a passive method of allowing people to die without the required care. This has been true for the last 30 years. Unfortunately, however, there is a great risk that it will continue to be true in the future if we do not take the correct measures to apply our scientific and human knowledge in the treatment of those in need.

Acknowledgment: I thank Miss Z. Kadry, MD, and Mrs C. Joran for taking part in the preparation of this chapter.

REFERENCES

1. Cleland WP: The evolution of cardiac surgery in the United Kingdom. *Thorax* 1983; 38:887–896.
2. Dubost C: Données sur l'état actuel et l'avenir de la chirurgie cardiaque en France. Presented at the Académie Nationale de Médecine, Paris, March 6, 1984.
3. Ekeström S, Westrom L, Ramstrom LM, Otto U, Scholander T: Hjärtkirurgi i arktisk miljö och i kyligt svenskt klimat. *Lakartidningen* 1980; 77:1289–1290.
4. Rodewald G, Polonius MJ: Cardiac surgery in the Federal Republic of Germany during 1982. A report by the German Society for Thoracic and Cardiovascular Surgery. *Thorac Cardiovasc Surg* 1983; 31:188–190.
5. English TAH, Bailey AR, Dark JF, Williams WG: The UK Cardiac Surgical Register 1977–82. *Br Med J* 1984; 289:1205–1208.
6. Cardiac Surgery 1982: A report by the National Heart Foundation of Australia. April 1984, National Heart Foundation of Australia, Woden; Act 2606.
7. Rimm AA: Trends in cardiac surgery in the U.S.A. *N Engl J Med* 1985; 312:119.
8. Kennedy RH, Kennedy MA, Frye RL, Giuliani ER, McGoon DC, Pluth JR, Smith HC, Ritter DG, Nobrega FT, Kurland LT: Cardiac-catheterization and cardiac-surgical facilities: use, trends, and future requirements. *N Engl J Med* 1982; 307:986–993.
9. Kennedy RH, Kennedy MA, McGoon DC, Pluth JR, Nobrega FT: Trends in cardiac surgery: five-year study of a defined population. *J Thorac Cardivasc Surg* 1980; 80:702–707.
10. CASS Principal Investigators and their associates: Coronary artery surgery study: a randomized trial of coronary artery bypass surgery. Survival data. *Circulation* 1983; 68:939–950.
11. Keats AS: The Rovenstine lecture 1983: cardiovascular anesthesia: perceptions and perspectives. *Anesthesiology* 1984; 60:467–474.
12. Mills NL: Valvular heart surgery-1984. *J La State Med Soc* 1984; 136:43–46.
13. Wada J: Cardiovascular operations in Japan in 1982. *Rinsho Kyobu Geka* 1983; 3:641–642.
14. Nakamura Y: Medical management of ischemic heart disease. Proceedings of the VIII Asia-Pacific Congress on Diseases of the Chest, July 11-15, 1983, Tokyo, Japan. Edited by Records Committee, 1984, p 137.
15. Lee YK: Open heart surgery in Korea. Proceedings of the VIII Asia-Pacific Congress on Diseases of the Chest, July 11-15, 1983, Tokyo, Japan. Edited by Records Committee, 1984, pp 24–26.
16. Adebonojo SA, Grillo IA, Osinowo O, Adebo OA: The spectrum of thoracic and cardiovascular surgery in Nigeria. *East Afr Med J* 1982; 59:451–464.
17. Metras D, Ouezzin-Coulibaly A, Ouattara K, Chauvet J, Longechaud A, Millet P: Chirurgie à coeur ouvert en Afrique tropicale. *Presse Méd* 1983; 12:621–624.
18. Parry MMW, Cooper DKC, Barnard CN: Trends in cardiac surgery at the University of Cape Town, 1971-1981. *S Afr Med J* 1983; 63:189–193.
19. Shumway N: Heart transplantation 1985, in *Congress on Heart Surgery 1985 International Symposium on Cardiac Surgery,* in press.

76 Cardiac Surgery in China: History and Present Status

Xi-ch'un Lan, MD, Zhuo-rong Feng, MD, and Tsung O. Cheng, MD

Cardiac surgery in China started in the mid-1940s. Wu et al[1,2] first performed ligation of patent ductus arteriosus in 1944 and successful pericardiectomy for constrictive pericarditis in 1948. Anastomosis between the subclavian and pulmonary arteries for tetralogy of Fallot was performed in the early 1950s.[3]

In February 1954, Lan et al[4] first successfully performed closed mitral commissurotomy for mitral stenosis. This was the beginning of intracardiac surgery in China.

In January 1957, Liang et al[5] were the first to perform pulmonary valvulotomy with circulatory arrest under hypothermia, marking the beginning of open cardiac surgery in China. In June 1958, Su et al[6] repaired a ventricular septal defect using cardiopulmonary bypass. Subsequently, with the availability of Chinese-made heart-lung machines and progress in perfusion techniques, an increasing number and variety of congenital and acquired heart diseases, such as atrial septal defect, trilogy of Fallot, tetralogy of Fallot, ruptured aneurysm of the sinus of Valsalva, ventricular aneurysm, and atrial myxoma, were treated with direct-vision intracardiac operations. In June 1965, Cai et al[7] first implanted a Shanghai-made caged-ball mitral valve prosthesis in a woman with advanced mitral valve disease. She is currently living and well 21 years after the operation (Figure 76.1).

In November 1974, Guo et al[8] were the first to perform aortocoronary bypass. In May 1976, Guo et al[9] used self-made bovine pericardial cardiac prostheses and porcine aortic valves for valve replacement, which has since become a popular procedure. In April 1978, Zhang et al[10] performed the first orthotopic cardiac transplantation, and the patient survived 109 days. In May of the same year, the surgical treatment of the Wolff-Parkinson-White syndrome was carried out successfully by Zhang et al.[11] In December 1978, Cai et al[12] employed a Shanghai-made low-profile tilting-disk prosthesis for valve replacement.

New types of heart-lung machines have recently been manufactured and counterpulsation devices installed into the cardiopulmonary bypass system. Also, infant cardiac surgery has been developed, and more complicated congenital heart diseases are being treated surgically.

PRESENT STATUS

A general survey of cardiac operations performed between 1978 and 1982, conducted through questionnaires sent in early 1983,[13] shows that open heart operations are undertaken in 28 of the 29 provinces, autonomous regions, and municipalities (Taiwan not being included in the survey), the only exception being the autonomous region of Tibet where only closed mitral commissurotomy is practiced. Thirty-eight cardiac centers responded to our questionnaire. For the five-year period 1978 to 1982 inclusive, a total of 24,442 cardiac operations were performed. There was a yearly increase in the number of open heart procedures, averaging about 17%. The percentages of operations for congenital and acquired heart disease were 59.5% and 40.5%, respectively (Figure 76.2). The percentages of closed and open heart operations were 45% and 55% respectively (Figure 76.3). The number of cardiac valve replacements was only 88 as of September 1977; however, it rapidly increased to 2,085 within a five-year period, a jump of 23.7 times.

The present status of cardiac surgery in China will be presented under the following subheadings: (1) basic techniques for open heart surgery, (2) surgery for congenital heart disease, (3) valvular heart surgery, and (4) coronary artery surgery.

OPEN HEART SURGERY: BASIC TECHNIQUES

With the ever-increasing perfection of the techniques of cardiopulmonary bypass, open heart operations in most institutions are carried out with the aid of heart-lung machines. For complicated direct-vision intracardiac op-

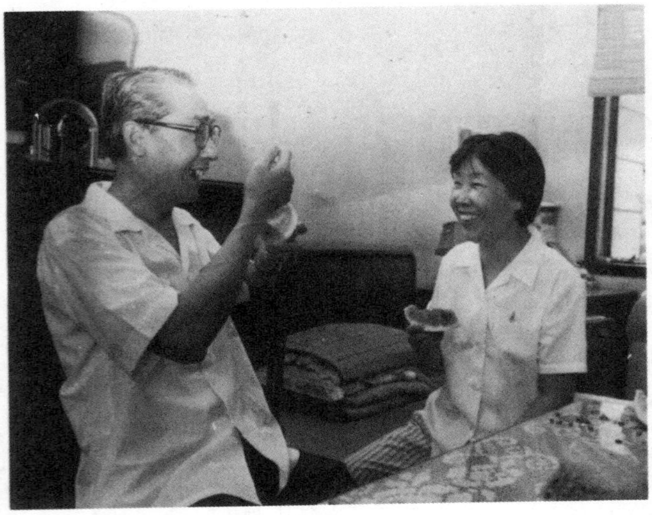

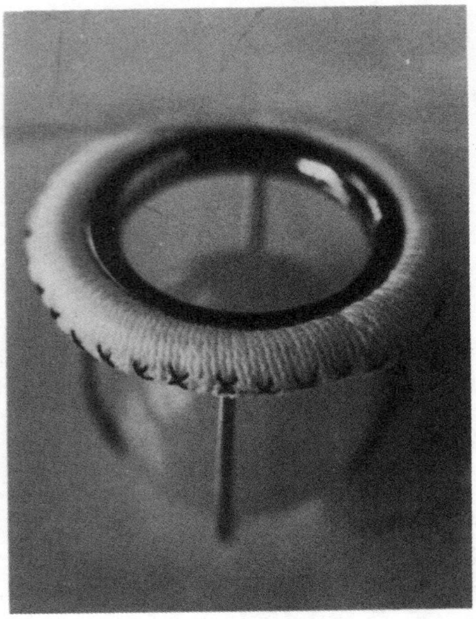

Figure 76.1. China's first and world's longest surviving patient 21 years after mitral valve replacement by Dr. Y. Z. Cai (*left*) with a Shanghai-made caged-ball prosthesis (*right*).

erations in infants, the use of selective profound hypothermia and limited cardiopulmonary bypass has also been adopted. It is only in a few institutions that pulmonary valvular commissurotomy and repair of secundum atrial septal defects are still undertaken under hypothermia with circulatory arrest. In our recent survey of 13,440 open heart operations, 20 (0.2%) were performed at normal temperature, 1,200 (8.9%) under hypothermia, and 12,220 (90.9%) during cardiopulmonary bypass.

In a few institutions a counterpulsation device is added to the extracorporeal circulation unit to change the blood flow into a pulsatile one, which is more physiologic and provides more adequate tissue perfusion. Such a technique is especially beneficial during cardiopulmonary bypass of longer than three hours. As for the oxygenator, the rotating disk type Shanghai heart-lung machine (models II and III) is gradually being replaced by a disposable bubble machine such as the bent tube type made in Shanghai and Guangdong and the plastic bag type from Tianjin and Changchun. The hollow fiber membranous type has also been developed in 1984 and in use since.

To decrease blood cell destruction and coagulation disturbances as well as to promote microcirculation and renal excretion, the hemodilution technique has been used extensively during extracorporeal circulation in many institutions. Electrolyte solution, mainly Ringer's, is used for priming the heart-lung machine. Hemodilution is usually 40 to 50 ml/kg of body weight; the deficit is made up by banked blood so as to keep the hematocrit above 20 vol%. In some institutions, good results were reported with extreme hemodilution, ie, a hematocrit of 10 to 15 vol% without replacement of any blood.

Myocardial preservation during open heart operations has been used widely in recent years. The common method is to induce rapid complete standstill of myocardial electromechanical activity and to attain cardiac arrest by topical deep hypothermia in combination with a decrease in myocardial temperature to 15° to 17°C or

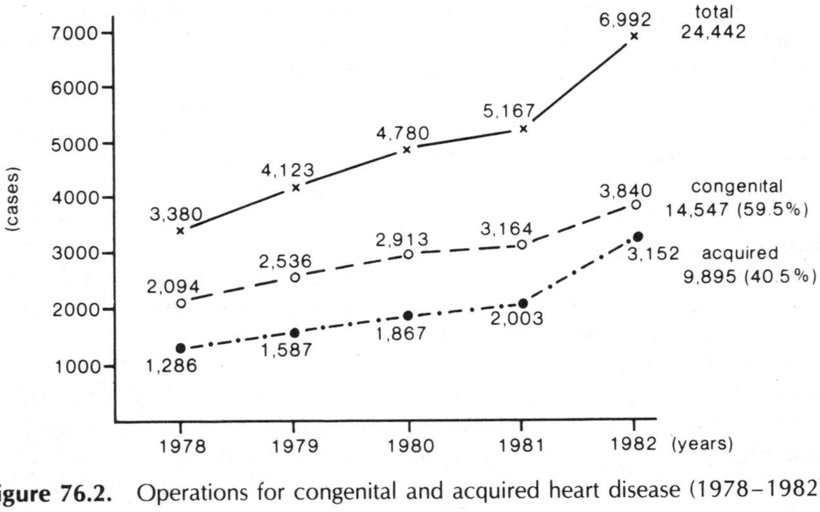

Figure 76.2. Operations for congenital and acquired heart disease (1978–1982).

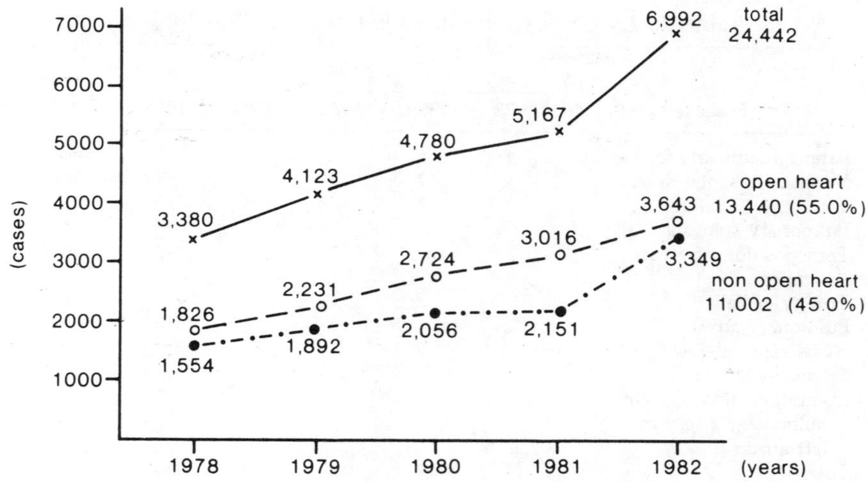

Figure 76.3. Open heart and non-open heart operations (1978–1982).

below by perfusion of 0° to 4°C cardioplegic solution, which is to be repeated every 30 to 45 minutes. Although the components of the cardioplegic solutions differ somewhat in different institutions, the main element is potassium, and in about two-thirds of the institutions magnesium ions together with glucose, procaine, energy ingredients, steroids, or mannitol is included in the prescription. In some institutions herb medicine such as Radix astragali (黄芪) or Radix salviae miltiorrhizae (丹参) is added to the solution. Shang[14] reported a 63.0% rate of spontaneous resumption of heartbeat when Radix astragali was added to the cardioplegic solution. Recently, Su reported a rate of 80.6% simply by keeping the myocardial temperature below 15°C (personal communication).

SURGERY FOR CONGENITAL HEART DISEASE

Most of the 14,547 operations for congenital heart disease (Table 76.1) were for the more common types. The operative mortality rate averaged 4.0%.

(1) Repair of ventricular septal defect (VSD) heads the list of all cardiac operations for congenital heart disease (27.3%). Recently, its scope has been extended, and closure of VSDs in infants (the youngest being 8 months old) associated with pulmonary hypertension or cardiac failure has been undertaken with satisfactory results in some centers with pediatric cardiac surgical programs. The statistics from 36 institutions indicate that 65.0% of 3,261 VSDs were closed by simple suture and 35.0% were repaired with patches.

Table 76.1. Operations for Common Congenital Heart Disease

Disease	No. of Cases	Operative Mortality	
		No.	%
Ventricular septal defect	3,969	135	3.4
Patent ductus arteriosus	3,937	21	0.5
Atrial septal defect	2,816	49	1.7
Tetralogy of Fallot	1,890	291	15.4
Pulmonary stenosis	876	16	1.8
Trilogy of Fallot	401	32	8.0
Ruptured aneurysm of sinus of Valsalva	170	15	8.8
Total	14,059*	559	4.0

* The 488 miscellaneous cases are not included.

There is a high incidence of the supracristal type of VSD in China. Operative findings in 3,113 cases collected from 32 institutions reveal that 19.6% represented this type. In a series of 1,187 operations for VSD reported by Guo et al[15] the incidence of supracristal VSD was as high as 31.8%. Long-term follow-up study of their 572 cases (203 of which were associated with pulmonary hypertension) showed good results in 84.3%, fair results in 11.3%, and poor results in 4.4%.

(2) Operations for patent ductus arteriosus were second in frequency (27.1%) in our survey. The youngest patient operated upon was 33 days old. In most centers, ligation of the ductus under induced hypotension was the method of choice and was especially suitable for children. Among the 3,937 operations for patent ductus arteriosus, ligation was used in 3,199 cases (81.3%), staplers were used to obliterate the ductus in 498 cases (12.6%), and division and suturing were carried out in 240 cases (6.1%). A 0.6% postoperative recanalization rate of the ductus was reported by Xiao et al[16] in their series of 1,016 cases.

(3) Repair of atrial septal defect was performed in 2,313 patients in 37 institutions; 2,159 (93.3%) of these defects were the ostium secundum type and 154 (6.7%) the ostium primum type.

Most of the ostium secundum defects (1,820 cases or 84.3%) were repaired during cardiopulmonary bypass. In a few institutions they (339 cases or 15.7%) were repaired under hypothermic conditions. All of the 154 ostium primum defects were repaired with patches and suturing of the clefts in the mitral valves during cardiopulmonary bypass. Liu et al,[17] in their long-term follow-up study of 35 patients over 35 years of age, reported good results in 25, fair results in seven (efficacy rate 91%), and poor results in three.

(4) Operation for tetralogy of Fallot is mainly one-stage total correction, except for shunting or closed enlargement of the outflow tract in severely cyanotic children. Of the 1,890 cases of tetralogy of Fallot in the survey, only 80

Table 76.2. Cardiac Operations in Infants (1978–1982)

Disease	Year 1978	1979	1980	1981	1982	Total
Patent ductus arteriosus	4	16	5	18	15	58
Ventricular septal defect	4	9	7	7	7	34
Tetralogy of Fallot	3	2	2	3	1	11
Pulmonary stenosis	...	...	2	1	2	5
Transposition of great arteries	...	...	1	...	3	4
Trilogy of Fallot	...	...	...	1	...	1
Pulmonary atresia	...	...	...	...	3	3
Atrial septal defect	...	...	...	...	1	1
Tricuspid atresia	...	...	...	...	1	1
Communication of right pulmonary artery to left atrium	...	...	...	...	1	1
Total	11	27	17	30	34	119

patients (4.2%) had a palliative operation, and 1,810 patients (95.8%), the youngest of whom was 15 months old, had total correction.

The operative mortality for total correction was 15.4%. With the recent accumulation of surgical experience, it has gradually been decreasing. Wang et al[18] had the lowest operative mortality rate, it being 4.5% in a series of 605 cases. The operative mortality rate in 20 children in a series by Ding et al[19] was 5%. Their primary method is to enlarge and reconstruct the outflow tract of the right ventricle. Wang's indications for patch grafting to enlarge the outflow tract are: (1) multiple pulmonary stenoses including infundibular, pulmonary valve and ring, and/or trunk and branch orifice stenoses, (2) small third ventricles, actually high infundibular stenoses, especially in adults, in whom, after the infundibular muscle is partially resected, the residue may still obstruct the pulmonary valvular orifice, and (3) subpulmonary ventricular septal defect.[20]

(5) *Repair of ruptured aneurysm of the aortic sinus of Valsalva*, which has a comparatively high incidence in China,[21] was performed in 170 cases (1.2%) in our survey. In most of them (153 cases or 90.0%), the aneurysm had ruptured into the right ventricle, whereas in only 17 cases it had ruptured into the right atrium. In the former group, 94.0% of the aneurysms were excised and repaired through right ventriculotomy and 6.0% through incisions in the root of the aorta. The associated lesions discovered at operation were ventricular septal defects (37.1%) and aortic insufficiency (10.5%), or both. Lan and Feng[13] followed up 155 cases and found that the results were good in 69.7%, fair in 23.2%, and poor in 7.1%. The less satisfactory results are due to the complexity of the lesions as well as the lack of experience in the early development of surgical treatment.

In addition, surgical treatment of less common congenital cardiac anomalies such as double outlet right ventricle,[22] Ebstein's anomaly,[23,24] total anomalous pulmonary venous connection,[25] tricuspid atresia, aortopulmonary window, transposition of the great arteries, single ventricle,[26] cor triatriatum,[27] and congenital aortic stenosis has also been reported in small series.

Cardiac surgery in infants developed in China only in recent years. In this five-year survey, 119 cardiac operations in infants had been undertaken in eight institutions. These operations were mostly for patent ductus arteriosus and ventricular septal defects (77.3%) (Table 76.2).

VALVULAR HEART SURGERY

Following the wide application of antibiotics, the incidence of rheumatic heart disease has been reduced remarkably in the last 30 years, and it has dropped from first place to second place[28] (Zheng DS et al, personal

Table 76.3. Changing Incidence of Cardiac Disease in the Shanghai Area During a 30-Year Interval

	Chen and Dong's Series (1982)[28]			Series of Zheng et al (1985) *	
Cardiac Disease	1948–1958: % of 5,031 Cases	1959–1971: % of 13,414 Cases	1972–1979: % of 7,152 Cases	1951–1963: % of 13,943 Cases	1964–1980: % of 25,831 Cases
Coronary	6	18	29.11	8.5	31.7
Rheumatic	50	40	26.41	43.7	26.8
Congenital	4	9	14.64	16.9	6.6
Pulmonary	8	11	6.45	7.2	14.4
Hypertensive	16	12	4.64	11.0	3.5
Other	16	10	18.75	12.7	17.0
Total			25,597		39,774

* Data collected from the four affiliated hospitals of Shanghai Second Medical University and two other institutions, namely, Shanghai First People's Hospital and Shanghai Sixth People's Hospital. (Zheng, DS et al, personal communication)

Table 76.4. Types of Prostheses Used for Valve Replacement

Type of Prosthesis	Mitral Valve	Aortic Valve	Tricuspid Valve	Multiple Valves	Total	
Mechanical valve						
Caged-ball valve	9	2	0	0	11	444
Tilting disk valve	325	68	1	39	433	(20.7%)
Bioprosthetic valve						
Porcine aortic valve	803	25	9	112	949	
Bovine pericardial valve	443	76	10	138	667	1,702
Dura mater valve	45	18	0	23	86	(79.3%)
Total	1,625	189	20	312	2,146	

communication) (Table 76.3). However, it currently is still the most common cardiac lesion requiring surgical intervention in adults, mitral stenosis being the most frequent. From the data submitted by 36 institutions, there were 6,667 patients with mitral stenosis who underwent operation, 27.3% of all cardiac operations.

For the surgical treatment of mitral stenosis, closed mitral commissurotomy is a simple but effective operation that has been practiced for many years in China with comparatively satisfactory long-term results. In a ten-year follow-up study, 73.9% of the patients operated upon had good or improved results.[29] Therefore, it currently is still the method of choice in well-selected cases. Of the total 6,667 patients requiring mitral valve surgery, 6,314 or 94.7% were treated by closed commissurotomy, 5,380 procedures (85.2%) being performed through a left approach, whereas 934 associated with atrial fibrillation or small left auricular appendages were operated upon through a right approach. The operative mortality rate was 1.8%, and the main cause of death was cardiac failure.

Open mitral commissurotomy or valve replacement, however, is indicated in (1) cases associated with a history of atrial fibrillation and embolism, (2) cases accompanied by mitral insufficiency (concomitant or post-commissurotomy), and (3) reoperated cases with severely calcified valvular lesions. Of the 6,667 cases, 353 or 5.3% were treated by direct-vision intracardiac surgery.

Since valve replacement has become an accepted procedure, the scope of valvular heart surgery has been extended to mitral stenosis or insufficiency, or both; aortic stenosis or insufficiency, or both; multivalvular disease; and Ebstein's anomaly. Operations for valve replacement have increased yearly. From 1978 to 1982 there were 133, 310, 472, 548, and 620 procedures in each consecutive year for a total of 2,083; there was an increase of 4.7 times in 1982 as compared with 1978. There were 275 operative deaths, a mortality rate of 13.2%.

Analysis of 1,988 cases with complete data collected from 35 institutions shows that there were 1,834 single valve replacements (92.3%), most often the mitral valve (1,625 cases), next the aortic valve, and least of all the tricuspid valve, usually for Ebstein's anomaly (Table 76.4). Of the 154 multiple valve replacements, a total of 312 valves were replaced, with combined mitral and aortic valve replacement in 144 cases, combined mitral and tricuspid replacement in 6 cases, and combined mitral, aortic and tricuspid valves in 4 cases. The operative mortality was lowest (11.8%) in single mitral valve replacement and highest (26%) in multiple valve replacement (Table 76.5).

Late in 1983 at the Tianjin convention of the Chinese Surgical Society and the Shanghai Cardiovascular Surgical Meeting, Cai et al[30] reported a series of 124 consecutive cases in which Shanghai-made tilting disk valves were used without any operative mortality, and 86.6% of the patients followed up longer than one year resumed work. Zheng et al[31] in 1984 reported an operative mortality of 6.8% in 74 patients undergoing mitral valve replacement with porcine heterografts and functional improvement in 100% in a follow-up study averaging 24 months. Ren et al[32] in 1983 reported a mortality rate of 18.6% in 59 cases of multiple valve replacement, which had been reduced to 12% since 1980 with improvement in surgical technique.

In the 547 patients who had valve replacement followed up longer than 6 months, the efficacy rate was 92.1% in 277 porcine aortic valves, 94.4% in 124 bovine pericardial valves, and 80.1% in 146 tilting disk valves (Table 76.6). In comparison, results with the bioprosthetic valve are better than those with the mechanical valves.

CORONARY ARTERY SURGERY

In the last 30 years there has been a remarkable change in the epidemiologic characteristics of coronary arteriosclerotic heart disease in China; its incidence has jumped from less than 10% of all cardiac diseases in the 1950s

Table 76.5. Operative Mortality in Valve Replacement

	Mitral Valve	Aortic Valve	Tricuspid Valve	Multiple Valves	Total
Operations (no.)	1,625	189	20	154	1,988
Deaths (no.)	192	29	3	40	264
Mortality rate (%)	11.8	15.3	15.0	26.0	13.3

Table 76.6. Long-Term Results With Different Types of Valve Prostheses

Results	Porcine Aortic Valve (4)*		Bovine Pericardial Valve (3)*		Tilting Disk Valve (1)*	
	No.	%	No.	%	No.	%
Good	192	69.3	89	71.8	77	52.7
Fair	63	22.8	28	22.6	40	27.4
Poor	10	3.6	6	4.8	29	19.9
Late fatality	12	4.3	1	0.8	0	0
Total	227	100.0	124	100	146	100

* Number of institutions.

to about 30% in the 1970s (Table 76.3). Combined Chinese traditional and Western medicines currently remain the main method of treatment, and coronary bypass surgery is rather uncommon. Through 1983, using incomplete statistical materials, about 30 ventricular aneurysms complicating coronary heart disease had been resected. Thus, in China coronary surgery is still at an early stage of development.

Congenital coronary arterial fistula is not uncommon in China. The data from 11 institutions indicate that there were 23 operative cases, and all of these patients survived with satisfactory late results. The fistula involved the right coronary artery in 18 patients, the left coronary artery in four, and both coronary arteries in one.

CONCLUSIONS

In China, cardiac surgery, especially valvular surgery, has grown rapidly in recent years. However, coronary artery surgery and cardiac surgery in infants, especially surgery for correction of complicated cardiac anomalies, still require enormous efforts to promote their development.

Acknowledgment: Statistical data in this report on the present status of cardiac surgery in China were provided by Affiliated Children's Hospital of Shanghai Medical University, Affiliated Renji Hospital, Ruijin Hospital and Xinhua Hospital of Shanghai No. 2 Medical University, Affiliated Zhongshan Hospital of Shanghai Medical University, Beijing Children Hospital, Beijing Friendship Hospital, Peking Union Medical College Hospital of Chinese Academy of Medical Sciences, Chongqing Municipal Surgical Hospital, First Affiliated Hospital of Chongqing Medical College, First Affiliated Hospital of Fourth Military Medical University, First and Second Affiliated Hospitals of Harbin Medical University, First Affiliated Hospital of Nanjing Medical College, First Affiliated Hospital of Hubei Medical College, First Affiliated Hospital of Second Military Medical University, First Affiliated Hospital of Suzhou Medical College, First Affiliated Hospital of Third Military Medical University, First Affiliated Hospital of Wuhan Medical College, First Affiliated Hospital of Xian Medical College, First and Second Affiliated Hospitals of Zhejiang Medical University, First Affiliated Hospital of Zhongshan Medical College, Fujian Provincial Hospital, General Hospital of Chinese People's Liberation Army, Nanjing Gulou Hospital, Henan Medical College Hospital, Quangdong Provincial People's Hospital, Second Affiliated Hospital of Hebei Medical College, Second Affiliated Hospital of Hunan Medical College, Second Affiliated Hospital of Jiangxi Medical College, Shandong Medical College Hospital, Shandong Provincial People's Hospital, Shanghai Municipal Chest Hospital, Shenyang Army General Hospital, Szechuan Medical College Hospital, Tianjin Heping Hospital and Xinjiang Medical College Hospital.

REFERENCES

1. Wu YK: Ligation of patent ductus arteriosus. *Chin Med J* 1947; 65:71–76.
2. Wu YK, Huang KC: Surgical treatment of constrictive pericarditis. *Chin Med J* 1953; 71:274–284.
3. Lan XC, Fu PB, Dong FZ: *Cardiac Surgery.* Beijing, People's Health Publ, 1964, pp 3–7.
4. Lan XC, Feng ZR, Huang MX, YU KJ: Surgical treatment of mitral stenosis. *Chin Med J* 1955; 73:278–292.
5. Liang QS, Wang YS, Sung XM, Ye CX: Transpulmonary valvulotomy under direct vision for the correction of pulmonic stenosis. *Chin Med J* 1959; 78:559–561.
6. Su HX, Lin CJ, Mou SC, Li Q, Liu WY, Zhang WL, Shi HL, Wang PL: Direct vision repair of ventricular septal defect under extracorporeal circulation. *Chin J Surg* 1959; 7:557–565.
7. Shi MX, Guo JQ, Qiu JH: Summary report of symposium of valvular heart surgery, in *Proceedings of National Conference of Cardiovascular Surgery*, Changchun, September 1977.
8. Guo JQ, Zhu XD, Le XH, Xue GX, Cao JX: Aorto-coronary bypass operation: a report of 15 cases. *Chin J Surg* 1983; 21:686–689.
9. Guo JQ, Zhu XD, Zhi QH, Tang YF, Zhou QW, Yue XH, Chen BT, Gong DF, Tang CJ, Liu HJ: Preliminary clinical experience with Chinese bioprosthetic heart valves. *Chin Med J* 1981; 94:441–448.
10 Zhang SZ, Zhou SB, Fang LD, Wang XC, Lu LJ, Weng SW, Chen ZY, Zhu MH, Zheng KY, Hong HQ, Gong LS, Yang Q, He GX, Ding HY: Heart transplantation: a case report. *Chin J Surg* 1980; 18:204–207.
11. Zhang QF, MA CZ: Surgical treatment of Wolff-Parkinson-White syndrome. *Chin Med J* 1983; 96:695–697.
12. Cai YZ, Zhang BR, Long GC, Geng ZJ, Chen RK, Zhu JL, Hao JH, Sun DH: Research study and clinical application of Shanghai-made low profile tilting disc mitral valve. *Shanghai Med J* 1980; 3:1–4.
13. Lan XC, Feng ZR: The advances of cardiac surgery during recent five years in China. *Acta Acad Med Secondae Shanghai* 1983; 3:1–4.
14. Shang DY: Myocardial protection in cardiac surgery, in *Proceedings of Beijing Symposium on Cardiothoracic Surgery.* Beijing, China Academic Publisher, 1982, p 227.
15. Guo JQ, Xue GX, Zhu XD, Yue XH, Hu BZ, Zhi QH, Xu QZ, Fan DJ, Chen YC, Zhou QW, Shen ZL, Cao JX, He MX, Xiao MD: Surgical treatment of congenital ventricular septal defect. A 21-year experience of 1,187 patients. *Chin Med J* 1983; 96:323–329.
16. Xiao MD, Quo JQ: The operative indications and results of patent ductus arteriosus in children. *Annual Report of Fu Wai Hospital,* Cardiovascular Institute, Chinese Academy of Medical Sciences, Beijing, 1980.
17. Liu JF, Li SM, Zuo CG, Zhi XZ, Pan Z: Surgical treatment of atrial septal defect over 35 years old. *Chin J Surg* 1984; 22:169–170.
18. Wang ZW, Fei CG, Zhang RF, Xu FX, Qian WY: Corrective surgery of tetralogy of Fallot in childhood, in Doyle EF, Engle MA, Gersony WM, Rashkind WJ, Talner NS (eds). *Pediatric Cardiology,* New York, Springer-Verlag, 1986, pp 493–497.
19. Ding WX,Cai DF, Su ZK: An experience of total correction of tetralogy of Fallot in children below 5 years old. *Chin J Cardiol* 1983; 11:172–175.
20. Wang ZW: Corrective surgery of tetralogy of Fallot. *Chin Med J* 1983; 96:21–26.
21. Zhu M, Zhou SZ, Jia WC: Diagnosis of the ruptured sinus of Valsalva. *Chin J Cardiol* 1984; 12:106–107.
22. Guo DW, Lin ML, Gu ZQ,Cheng TO: Double outlet right ventricle. A clinical-roentgenologic-pathologic study of 28 consecutive patients. *Chest* 1984; 85:526–532.
23. Zhang ST, Ning SB, Ren CY: Tricuspid valve replacement in Ebstein's anomaly in children, in Doyle EF, Engle MA, Gersony WM, Rashkind WJ, Talner NS (eds). *Abstracts of Second World Congress of Pediatric Cardiology,* June 2–6, 1985, New York City. New York, Springer-Verlag, 1985, p 165.
24. Wang ZW, Fei CJ, Zhang RF, Xu FX, Sun LZ, Zhu HY, Wang WX, Gong HD, Qian WY: Surgical management of Ebstein's anomaly of the heart. *Chin J Thorac Cardiovas Surg* 1985; 1:26–28.
25. Ruan XM, Luo ZX: Surgical treatment of total anomalous pulmonary venous drainage. *Chin J Cardiol* 1984; 12:104–105.
26. Wang ZW, Fei CJ, Zhang RF, Xu FX, Qian WY, Sun LZ, Zhu HY, Wang

WX, Gong HD: Modified Fontan operation for univentricular heart. *Chin J Surg* 1984; 22:365–367.
27. Liu WY, Yang JX, Zhang WL, Tian ZZ, Liu ZH: Diagnosis and surgical treatment of cor triatriatum. *Chin J Surg* 1983; 21:351–353.
28. Chen HZ, Dong CL: Cardiac diseases, in *Encyclopedia of Chinese Medicine, cardiology section*. Shanghai, Shanghai Scientific & Technological Publ, 1982, p 3.
29. Third People's Hospital, Rui-jin Hospital, Xin-hua Hospital, Ninth People's Hospital of Shanghai Second Medical College: Retrospect of cardiac surgery in the past thirty years. *Acta Acad Med Secondae Shanghai* 1982; 2(4):40–44.
30. Cai YZ, Zhang BR, Chen RK, Chu JL, Hao JH, Gen ZJ: Elective mitral valve replacement with Shanghai made tilting disc mechanical valves: no early mortality in 124 consecutive cases. *Acta Acad Med* Secondae Militaris 1983; 42:247–251.
31. Zhang XL, Qian XX, Li LS, Jia GL: Mitral valve replacement with porcine heterograft. A follow up study of 74 cases. *Chin Med J* 1984; 97:495–499.
32. Ren CY, Shi MX, Wang MS, Jiang ZW, Mao LY, Zhang TY, Zhao QF: Multiple valve replacement: experiences in 59 cases. *Chin J Cardiol* 1985; 13:84–86.

77 Geriatric Cardiology

Neil D. Berman, MD

In 1950, 8% of the population of the United States consisted of people aged 65 and older.[1] By 1969, this figure had risen to 9.6% and by 1980 to over 11%.[2] Similar increases in the relative size of the elderly population have been noted in all developed countries (Table 77.1). The same trend has been noted in China.[2a] Moreover, not only is the elderly segment of the population increasing in size, but it is also increasing in age, as attested to by the fact that the percentage of this population greater than 75 years of age is steadily increasing. Heart disease is a major cause of morbidity and mortality in the aged. Although representing only about 10% of the population of the United States in 1976, the elderly accounted for 75% of all deaths from ischemic heart disease (Table 77.1). Heart disease was responsible for approximately two thirds of all deaths in this age group and the majority were classified as ischemic in origin. It is of interest that although the relative size of the elderly population continues to increase, the contribution of this population to the total deaths from heart disease appears to be leveling off in some countries. It is premature to interpret this as a definite trend, but it does coincide temporally with the emergence of interest in the problem of geriatric cardiology.

Although morbidity data are less well documented, heart disease affects at least one quarter of the elderly population and is a major source of disability in this age group[3-6] (Table 77.2). In 1974, circulatory diseases accounted for 39% of total hospital care days for Canadians 65 years of age and older.[7] This amount was approximately three times that of the next highest disease group. However, acute hospital care is a relatively small, although readily quantitated, aspect of morbidity. It is extremely difficult to ascertain the extent to which heart disease results in major disability in this age group, but it is certainly less important in this regard than disorders of the central nervous or musculoskeletal system.

With this large and ever-increasing population at risk, it is not surprising that more attention is being focused on the problem of heart disease in the elderly. Reviewing the cardiology literature is complicated by the fact that no clearly defined line of demarcation exists between the elderly population and the population as a whole. Various investigators have used ages ranging from 50 to 80 depending on the disease or therapy being discussed and the time at which the paper was written.[8-13] Furthermore, many of these reports contain insufficient data on population distribution to allow data on a specific age group to be extracted. Finally, both medical and surgical therapy have been subject to dramatic changes over the past decade, and much of the information published just 5 years ago is of questionable validity today. Increased interest in the problem of geriatric cardiology has led to many recent studies of cardiac problems as they relate to the aged population, but the long-term results of these studies will not be available for years.

The major overriding concern in dealing with heart disease in elderly patients is the discrepancy between chronologic and physiologic age. This area is the one in which the art of medicine takes precedence. It is the clinician's estimation of the physiologic age of the patient that guides his therapeutic approach. Although it is the most important factor in determining optimal therapy and long-term outcome, there are, unfortunately, no rec-

Table 77.1. Cardiac Mortality in the Elderly: Data for Two European and Two North American Countries

Country	Year	Elderly Population (% of Total Population)	Cardiac Deaths in the Elderly (% of Total Cardiac Deaths)
Canada	1950	7.8	69.0
	1970	7.8	73.6
	1975	8.6	74.4
	1980	9.5	75.2
USA	1950	8.2	64.9
	1969	9.6	73.1
	1976	10.7	75.6
	1980	11.2	74.1
UK	1950	10.9	78.2
	1970	13.0	76.1
	1977	14.6	78.2
	1981	15.3	77.9
Sweden	1950	10.3	79.6
	1970	13.7	83.6
	1977	16.2	85.4
	1981	16.5	86.8

Note: Data are based on references 1 and 2. The elderly are persons 65 years and older. Cardiac deaths include those from ischemic, hypertensive, and chronic rheumatic heart disease.

ognized markers for physiologic age. It is not subject to definition nor can it even readily be dissected into its component parts. It represents a fusion of a host of small clues gleaned from both history and physical examination.

A detailed discussion of all that the term *geriatric cardiology* encompasses is clearly beyond the scope of this chapter. The purpose here is to survey the field, emphasizing those aspects in which the elderly population differs from the population at large, and detailing the work that has appeared in the press since I reviewed this area in 1982.[14]

AGING AND THE HEART

Theories of aging can be divided into two basic schools of thought: programmed (genetic) or random.[15] For each of these possibilities, a variety of mechanisms has been proposed to explain aging. There is some experimental support for all of these theories, and therefore the issue remains unresolved. Nevertheless, the various postulated mechanisms all lead to a common endpoint: cellular dysfunction and ultimately cell death because of either a lack of an adequate amount of a vital component or an accumulation of a deleterious component.[16–18] In either case, it is clear that tissues comprised largely of postmitotic cells, which lack the capacity to replace malfunctioning or dead cells, are more likely to feel the brunt of "cellular aging." Therefore, it is not surprising that the heart is one of the organs most apparently affected by aging.

Table 77.2. Incidence of Heart Disease in the Aged*†

Heart Disease	Percent Men	Percent Women
Ischemic	20	12
Hypertensive	10	14
Combined (ischemic and hypertensive)	3	7
Valvular	2	6
Pulmonary	3	1
Other	9	6
Total definite heart disease	47	46

* Persons over 65 years of age.
† From Wei JY: Heart disease in the elderly. *Cardiovasc Med* 1984; 9:971–982. Reproduced with permission.

The frequent occurrence of heart disease in the elderly has made it difficult to define the pathologic processes that are specific to aging. At the molecular level, the most important changes are related to collagen. Although the amount of collagen in the heart increases with advancing age,[19,20] of greater importance is the qualitative change by which collagen becomes increasingly insoluble, chemically stable, and increasingly stiff.[21,22] Because collagen is interspersed between all myocardial cells, changes in its physical properties can affect both contractile and distensile properties of the heart. Collagen is also a major component of all arteries. These alterations in the amount and nature of collagen affect the functioning of arteries throughout the body, but the consequences are clinically most apparent in the aorta. Decreased aortic distensibility (increased stiffness) reduces the extent of amplification of the pressure wave while increasing the velocity of the pulse wave in the major arteries.[23] Of greater importance, for a given stroke volume, the increase in aortic pressure is greater in older persons because of the reduced distensibility.[24] To some extent, the dilatation of the aorta commonly seen with aging, by increasing aortic volume, compensates for the decrease in distensibility and reduces the amount of cardiac work required to maintain cardiac output. Nevertheless, increased impedance to ventricular ejection is a major factor in the altered cardiac performance of the elderly.[25]

Lipofuscin is thought to originate in the breakdown products of intracellular organelles.[26] Its deposition in aggregates of granules near the poles of the nuclei is a specific, age-related change.[27] The accumulation of lipofuscin appears to have no effect on myocardial function, nor is it related to the presence of any other cardiac disease.

Although amyloid deposition can be demonstrated in a number of tissues with advancing age, senile cardiac amyloid appears to be a specific form of amyloidosis.[28,29] It is found in up to 50% of senescent hearts and extracardiac involvement is uncommon.[28–30] Although its incidence increases with advancing age,[28] its presence is not universal, suggesting that it likely represents a pathologic process.

With aging, the fibrous stroma of the valves show a decrease in the number of nuclei.[30,31] At the sites of maximum cusp movement there is collagen degeneration, lipid accumulation, and calcification. Microscopically identifiable calcification will be found in at least one valve in about one third of the patients over 70 years of age.[30] These changes are found more commonly in the aortic than the mitral valve. Nodular thickening on the atrial surface of the mitral leaflets appears to be an age-related alteration, whereas the incidence of nodules on the aortic cusps does not increase after middle age, suggesting this is not an age-dependent change. Tricuspid and pulmonary valves are rarely involved. Mucoid degeneration of the mitral leaflets is pathologically identical to the myxomatous change described in younger patients and may produce the clinical syndrome of mitral valve prolapse. It is unclear whether this represents a true, age-associated abnormality or a clinically unimportant abnormality that has been present from a younger age. Myxomatous change has been attributed to a variety of etiologies and age-associated degeneration may be one cause of this abnormality. Calcification of the mitral anulus, although not universally present in the elderly, is found with increasing frequency with age and is generally considered an exaggeration of normal aging changes. In about 10% of autopsies in patients over 50 years of age, some calcification of the mitral anulus will be found, varying from small spicules to solid calcification of the entire ring.[30]

These age-associated changes in heart valves may progress to hemodynamically important valve lesions. Calcific degeneration of the aortic valve is the most common cause of aortic stenosis in the elderly.[30] Heavily calcified mitral rings have been associated with obstruction, incompetence, heart block, and endocarditis.

The conduction system is the focus of important changes.[32] In the sinoatrial node, the number of pacemaker cells decreases with age to the point where often less than 10% of the normal complement remain after age 75. Beginning at age 60, there is a detectable loss of fibers from the fascicles of the left bundle branch. Commonly less than half the original number remain, the others having been replaced by fibrous tissue. Microcalcification is often found in this region, but it is uncertain as to whether this represents an age-associated change or a pathologic process. There is also some fibrous tissue replacement of conduction fibers in the distal conduction system, whereas no age-related changes have been documented in the atrioventricular node or common His bundle. Although fibrosis and hyalinization occur in the media of the blood vessels supplying the conduction tissue, they do not appear to be causally related to the cellular depletion and fibrosis noted in the conduction system itself.[33,34]

Resting cardiac output decreases with age, primarily because of reduced stroke volume.[35] Cardiac output increases linearly with workload as in younger persons, but because resting output is lower, the output at any given workload will also be lower.[35,36] Furthermore, because peak heart rate decreases with age, maximum cardiac output is markedly decreased in the elderly.[36] Some of these changes in cardiac performance may reflect the decline in cardiac conditioning that results from the sedentary life-style of most elderly and might be amenable to a conditioning program.[36] However, although a training effect could be demonstrated in 24 apparently normal older persons subjected to a 12-week physical conditioning program, this was not reflected in improved left ventricular performance as assessed by exercise radionuclide angiography.[37]

Four factors have been identified as possibly being responsible for these age-related changes.[38] With aging, the function of the *autonomic nervous system* is altered, resulting in decreased responsiveness of the homeostatic mechanisms.[39–44] Decreased sympathetic responsiveness, in particular, has been well documented and attributed at least in part to alterations related to the adrenergic receptors.[38,45] Whether this represents a decrease in the number of receptors or a decrease in their affinity has not yet been determined. These alterations may partly be responsible for the altered cardiac response to exercise; however, because resting autonomic tone does not appear to change with age, functional changes in the resting heart cannot be attributed to these alterations.

With aging, there is a *prolongation of the time course of contraction and relaxation*.[46] The relaxation phase in particular is prolonged 20% to 35%.[38,47] This has been attributed to age-related alterations in the function of the sarcoplasmic reticulum or contractile proteins or both. Prolongation of systole reduces the relative duration of diastole at any given heart rate, thus shortening the period that is most important for myocardial perfusion.

Alterations in the myocardial collagen, just noted, result in *decreased compliance* (increased passive stiffness) of the myocardium. Although not having a significant effect on resting hemodynamics, in the absence of other disease any increase in left ventricular diastolic volume would lead to a disproportionally greater increase in pressure in a ventricle with reduced compliance.

The increase in *vascular impedance* increases the work of the myocardium and its oxygen requirements for any level of cardiac output. Although the increase in work at rest is minimized by aortic dilatation and mild ventricular hypertrophy, with exercise there is an excessively steep increase in impedance, resulting in a marked increase in ventricular work.

PHARMACOLOGIC CONSIDERATIONS

Adverse drug effects are frequently encountered in elderly patients for a variety of reasons. The elderly are more likely to be taking multiple drugs.[48,49] They are often confused as to which drug is intended for which problem and medication errors are frequent. Medications are often prescribed for specific problems and continued even when the need for them is no longer active. This is best illustrated in the case of digoxin. Recent studies have shown that as many as 15% of elderly patients may be receiving digoxin.[50] In the absence of any evidence of congestive heart failure, digoxin can be withdrawn in up to 85% of patients with sinus rhythm without any apparent adverse consequences.[50,51] Digoxin is more likely to be successfully discontinued if serum levels are subtherapeutic.[51] Therefore, when dealing with an elderly patient, it is imperative to take a careful, detailed drug history; to attempt to clarify, as much as possible, the indication for the prescription of any of these drugs; and to ascertain whether there is any current need for the various medications to be maintained. Care must be observed when taking a drug history to include any over-the-counter medications that the patient may also be using. Furthermore, when prescribing medication for the elderly, extra effort must be made to clarify for the patient the purposes of the various drugs, the dosage schedule, and the appearance of the various drugs. This situation may be one in which drugs are better ordered by specific trade names, and substitutions should be discouraged. These considerations are important with all patients but even more so with the elderly.

Factors other than medication errors play a role in the increased incidence of adverse drug effects in the elderly. With many drugs, altered responsiveness can be demonstrated in elderly patients. Many potential mechanisms may account for this variation. Differences in drug absorption from the gastrointestinal tract may occur, but they have not yet been demonstrated with cardioactive drugs in human subjects.[52] With aging, total body water decreases.[52,53] A decrease in body muscle mass is often counterbalanced by an increase in body fat, so that body weight itself may be unaltered. Serum albumin also tends to decrease with advancing age.[54] These three factors significantly alter the volume of distribution of many drugs. Renal function decreases with advancing age, thereby altering the decay curves of drugs that depend largely on renal excretion for their elimination.[55,56] Drug metabolism may also be altered, but again this has not been conclusively demonstrated with cardioactive drugs in human subjects.[52]

In addition to all these factors that may affect drug concentration, there are situations in which altered drug responsiveness appears attributable to a change in drug receptors. It is unclear whether this change represents an alteration in the number or kinetics of the receptors. Many of these adverse effects can be attributed to deficiencies in homeostatic mechanisms that in younger patients are capable of preventing or minimizing an adverse drug effect. Furthermore, the frequent presence of other diseases, either directly or by virtue of medications being given for their treatment, may alter the response to a newly prescribed drug.

In view of the foregoing considerations, prescribing for the elderly may be summarized as follows: the fewest possible drugs, in the smallest possible doses, for the shortest possible duration.

CARDIAC ASSESSMENT IN THE ELDERLY

HISTORY

Generally, history in the elderly patient is taken in the same manner as in the younger patient. In the elderly patient with a long history of numerous diseases, the chronology may be more difficult to clarify. The importance of the drug history, as already mentioned, cannot be overemphasized. Specific cardiovascular symptoms often will be absent or overshadowed by nonspecific complaints or symptoms related to other systems. In addition to assessing the symptoms attributable to the cardiovascular system, it is especially important in elderly patients to determine the general health and overall functional capacity and the extent to which the cardiovascular illness affects these two. These considerations form the basis of many therapeutic decisions made in regard to the cardiac disease. The presence of other illnesses is of importance in terms of their interaction with the cardiovascular system. Other diseases may aggravate the cardiac illness and vice versa. Also, cardiac therapy may interact with the other illness or its therapy and vice versa.

PHYSICAL EXAMINATION

The approach to physical examination is the same as that with younger patients and includes the effects of postural changes and other maneuvers in most elderly patients. The general physical examination is extremely important because of the frequent occurrence of other diseases that may interact with the cardiac problem. Care must be taken, when determining blood pressure, not to underestimate the systolic pressure because of the presence of an auscultatory gap or localized obstruction in the subclavian, axillary, or brachial artery. Therefore, pressure in both arms should be determined by inflating the cuff until the radial pulse is no longer palpable. The effects of altered distensibility on the characteristics of the pulses were alluded to earlier. The rigidity and tortuosity of the peripheral arteries have no clinical significance, but they may produce bruits not related to functionally important abnormalities[31,57] or prominent neck pulsations due not to aneurysms but to buckling of the great vessels.[57a]

The loss of subcutaneous fat may make the jugular venous pulse easier to see, but kinking of the external jugular veins at the junction with the subclavian makes these veins unreliable in assessing venous pressure. Furthermore, compression of the central veins by the unfolded aortic arch may falsely elevate the pressure in the internal jugular vein. Therefore, when determining venous pressure, care must be exercised to be certain that pulsations are visible. Deep inspiration will usually reduce the compression, allowing the column of blood to drop to the appropriate level.[58] The characteristics of the wave form have the same implications as they do in younger patients. Ankle edema does not necessarily imply heart failure and local causes must be excluded.

Skeletal deformities make localization of the apical impulse more difficult and less meaningful, but the quality of the impulse, when felt, carries the same diagnostic weight as in younger patients. Heart sounds are generally less intense, but the significance of their intensity relative to one another remains the same. Splitting of the second heart sound is usually narrower in the elderly.[59] Abnormalities of splitting have the same diagnostic implications. Fourth heart sounds may be normal in the elderly, whereas third heart sounds are always abnormal, the opposite of the situation in young adults.[60] Systolic murmurs can be detected in up to 60% of elderly patients.[61] The majority have ejection murmurs not associated with significant valvular disease and attributed to aortic sclerosis.[61,62] The valvular abnormalities underlying murmurs, other than the ejection murmur, are the same as in younger patients.

INVESTIGATIONS

All the investigations that are applied to younger patients are applicable to the elderly, but it must be recognized that the range of normal variation may be different. Particularly in noninvasive cardiologic investigations, normal values for the elderly have not been well defined. Much of this deficit derives from the difficulties in defining an elderly population known to be free of heart disease. Electrocardiographic changes are common in the elderly,[63,64] but this is not to imply that these changes should be accepted as normal variants.[2a] Even nonspecific T-wave changes have been associated with an increased mortality.[57] About 10% of the aged will have electrocardiograms that would be considered entirely normal by criteria applicable to younger patients.[2a,63,65] With aging, the PR interval shows a gradual lengthening and 0.22 second has been suggested as the upper limit of normal in the elderly.[66-68] The QRS axis gradually moves leftward,[69-71] but values less than −45° are definitely abnormal although not necessarily indicative of underlying heart disease.[63,71] Limb lead voltages decrease with advancing age,[69] precordial voltages are less consistent, and increases may not necessarily indicate hypertrophy.[72] The initial 20-ms vector decreases with increasing age, producing the "poor R-wave progression" pattern that is not indicative of anterior infarction in the elderly.[67]

Some degree of left ventricular hypertrophy is a normal concomitant of aging and is reflected in increased echocardiographic left ventricular wall thickness,[73-75] but changes in other echocardiographic parameters are less well defined. Although there have been attempts to determine normal echocardiographic values in elderly patients,[75] these have not yet been generally accepted. However, the qualitative features of the echocardiogram are as reliable as in younger patients,[76] and grossly abnormal dimensions are quite clearly abnormal.

Stress testing with or without thallium imaging appears to be as valuable as in younger patients, provided an adequate level of stress can be achieved.[77] Protocols that include lower levels of stress appear to be the most useful.[78] Initially, it was thought that the response to exercise radionuclide angiography was significantly different in normal elderly patients in that the ejection fraction often decreased with exercise and the development of regional wall abnormalities was common.[37,79] However, a more recent study in patients whose coronary anatomy had been angiographically documented found that both ejection fraction response and regional wall motion were determined by the extent of coronary disease and not the patient's age.[80] This study suggests that the same criteria for interpreting radionuclide angiography are applicable regardless of age.

CONGESTIVE HEART FAILURE

Before discussing specific cardiac conditions, it is reasonable to consider the problem of congestive heart failure in the elderly as it may occur as a consequence of any form of cardiac disorder. The most common causes of heart failure in the elderly are ischemic and hypertensive heart disease. These two are commonly combined. Valvular disease is less common. Although arrhythmias may provoke heart failure, in the elderly this usually occurs in conjunction with organic heart disease.

The pathogenesis of congestive heart failure in the general population (see chapter 16 on Congestive Heart Failure) is equally applicable to the elderly and the resultant signs and symptoms are similar. However, in the elderly, the diagnosis of congestive heart failure is more likely to be complicated by the presence of other diseases. The coexistence of chronic pulmonary disease makes assessment of effort dyspnea, the dominant symptom of congestive failure, extremely difficult. The presence of ankle edema does not necessarily imply the presence of congestive heart failure. There are many other causes for ankle edema. It should not be attributed to congestive heart failure in the absence of other signs of failure, such as a gallop, elevated jugular venous pressure, or hepatomegaly.

Therapy is directed at the four determinants of cardiac performance: heart rate, myocardial contractility, venous filling, and impedance to ventricular ejection.

Restriction of physical activity continues to have a role in the treatment of congestive heart failure, but it must be applied judiciously in the elderly. Similarly, the extent to which sodium intake is restricted must be tempered by the possibility of further impairing the nutritional status of an older patient whose diet may already be less than adequate.

Although recently a matter of controversy, digitalis remains the mainstay of therapy for congestive heart failure, particularly in the presence of atrial fibrillation. Skeletal muscle is the major body reservoir of digoxin. With aging, the proportion of lean muscle mass to body fat decreases.[52] This is a major reason for the reduced maintenance dose requirement seen in the elderly. Another is the decrease in glomerular filtration rate that accompanies aging even in the absence of renal disease.[81-83] Generally, there is no indication for rapid digitalization. Daily administration of the maintenance dose will result in steady state blood levels within 1 week. Prevention of toxic effects can best be achieved by carefully tailoring the dose for each patient, maintaining an awareness of interactions with other drugs, and assessing the patient frequently, particularly early in the course of therapy. Such assessment should include specific questioning about possible symptoms and monitoring of the electrocardiogram, electrolytes, renal function, and serum digoxin levels.

Because the symptoms of digitalis intoxication are often deceptive in the elderly, the possibility should be considered in the presence of any unusual symptom. Intoxication may be manifest as weakness, fatigue, confusion, or hallucinations. Gastrointestinal disturbances are often absent.[84] An arrhythmia may be the sole manifestation. Atrioventricular block combined with atrial tachycardia or ventricular irritability are the most specific arrhythmias; however, virtually any arrhythmia can occur.

The potential dangers of over-diuresis must always be considered in treating elderly patients. Loop diuretics should not be used when thiazides will suffice.[52] Altered central nervous system function may be related to fluid or electrolyte depletion and often can be improved with appropriate therapy.[85] Slight fluid retention generally is preferable to slight dehydration.

Vasodilator therapy has been recognized as a useful adjunct in the treatment of congestive heart failure and has been used for this purpose in elderly patients.[86] Particular care must be taken to avoid hypotension. There are few published data regarding the relative benefits and risks of this form of therapy in the elderly. Almost any vasodilator can be used in this situation. Long-acting nitrates appear to be of particular use because of the important role of underlying coronary artery disease in the etiology of congestive heart failure in the elderly. They also increase venous capacitance, thereby reducing ventricular filling pressure as well as reducing afterload. The use of hydralazine in congestive heart failure is often counterproductive because of its tendency to cause reflex tachycardia. In older patients, this reflex is often blunted, and hydralazine may therefore prove to be more useful in this age group.

ARRHYTHMIAS

Arrhythmias are common in the elderly. The reported frequencies vary depending on the population studied and the technique employed for their detection. Electrocardiograms of elderly patients, not being specifically investigated for cardiac disease, demonstrated atrial premature beats in about 10%, ventricular premature beats in 6% to 11%, and atrial fibrillation in 5% to 8%.[63,64,68] Twenty-four hour ambulatory monitoring of healthy elderly persons provides additional insight into the frequency of arrhythmias in this age group.[87–90] Unfortunately, differences in patient selection and in classification of the results of ambulatory monitoring make it difficult to compare these studies. The results of two studies are compared in Table 77.3. Camm et al[87] studied a population of active elderly subjects of whom 8% had mild but clinically recognized heart disease and presumably more had latent heart disease. Fleg and Kennedy[89] used maximal treadmill exercise testing to define a normal population for their study. This may account in part for the significant differences in the frequencies of supraventricular arrhythmias detected. What is more noteworthy is the similarity in detection frequency of ventricular arrhythmias. Atrial fibrillation and flutter were surprisingly uncommon, compared with data derived from standard electrocardiographic studies. This is likely a consequence of differences in population selection.

Table 77.3. Ambulatory Monitoring in the Elderly

Study	Camm et al[87]	Fleg and Kennedy[89]
Subjects (No.)	106	98
Age range (yr)	75–95	60–85
Supraventricular arrhythmias	40*	86
Premature beats	25	86
Atrial fibrillation	11	0
Atrial flutter	0	1
Other tachycardias	3	13
Ventricular arrhythmias	73	78
Isolated premature beats	45	76
Frequent premature beats†	13	7
Complex premature beats‡	27	45
Ventricular tachycardia	4	4

* Number of subjects.
† Frequent: Camm et al[87] > 100/h; Fleg and Kennedy[89] > 60/h.
‡ Includes multiform and couplets.

In acute myocardial infarction, arrhythmias were no more frequent in the elderly; in fact, ventricular premature beats were seen less commonly in patients 70 years of age and older.[91] Age is not a factor in determining the success of resuscitation from cardiac arrest,[91–95] although it may be a predictor of 6-month survival.[94]

In general, there is nothing unique about the presentation, diagnosis, and treatment of arrhythmias in the elderly. Arrhythmia may occur in an otherwise normal heart but with increasing age, associated cardiac disease becomes more likely.[63] Atrial flutter, to some extent an exception, has been considered an arrhythmia of the aged.[96] In younger patients, its presence is almost always indicative of a serious cardiac disorder, most commonly mitral valve disease, but with advancing years its implications are much less ominous. Digoxin remains the basis of therapy, but, as in younger patients, atrial flutter is often very resistant and large doses will be required. Intravenous verapamil has become the drug of choice in controlling the ventricular rate during the digitalization period,[97] thus eliminating the need for rapid digitalization or cardioversion.

Sick sinus syndrome also merits specific comment as it is seen with increasing frequency with advancing age.[98,99] The term includes a variety of disorders thought to originate in abnormalities of the sinoatrial node, its neurogenic control, or the perisinus tissue.[100] Its presentation varies from sinus bradycardia (or inappropriately normal sinus rate in situations in which tachycardia would be anticipated) to a bradycardia-tachycardia syndrome. The treatment of sick sinus syndrome is pacemaker therapy and it should be reserved for symptomatic patients as even moderate bradycardia may be associated with normal rest and exercise hemodynamics in the elderly.[101] Because of the frequency of associated disease elsewhere in the conducting system, single-chamber atrial pacing should be avoided. Advanced age is not a contraindication to pacemaker therapy.[13,102] In the bradycardia-tachycardia syndrome, antitachycardia drug therapy may also be required, but often pacing alone will control both aspects of the arrhythmia.[102a,102b]

HYPERTENSION

The systematic study of hypertension in the elderly is a relatively recent topic of investigation and long-term results are not yet available.[103] Although the prevalence of hypertension after age 65 has been estimated as high as 50%,[104] a 1978 review of major hypertension studies disclosed that only about 10% of the patients included in these studies were older than 60 years of age.[105] Information derived from the older subgroups of patients in these studies indicates that hypertension is a significant risk factor in both coronary heart disease and cerebrovascular disease.[106–108] For example, half the hypertension-associated morbidity detected in the Veterans Administration Study occurred in patients aged 60 or older.[106] Furthermore, systolic hypertension is at least as important a risk factor as diastolic pressure.[109] In elderly patients with normal diastolic blood pressure, systolic pressure greater than 160 mm Hg was associated with a sevenfold increase in cardiovascular mortality.[110]

In the very old, hypertension may lose its prognostic significance.[111] One study of people aged 85 and older actually demonstrated an inverse relation between blood pressure and 2-year mortality.[112] The interpretation of these data is complicated by the actions of competitive risk factors.[113,114] Moreover, blood pressure may have been decreased by the presence of disease that may ultimately have been responsible for the higher mortality.[115,116]

Arterial compliance decreases with aging,[24,109] resulting in an increase in systolic and a decrease in diastolic pressure. Therefore, the presence of systolic hypertension associated with normal or only mildly elevated diastolic pressure suggests the coexistence of essential hypertension.[117] The pathophysiologic process responsible for essential hypertension in elderly patients is almost always an increase in peripheral vascular resistance.[109,117,118] This process should affect both systolic and diastolic pressure proportionately; however, the decrease in aortic compliance leads to a disproportionate elevation in systolic pressure. The extent by which systolic pressure exceeds two times (diastolic pressure − 15) is thought to represent the contribution of aortic rigidity.[119] This factor is important in therapeutic considerations, because antihypertensive therapy reduces both systolic and diastolic pressure. In the patient with a disproportionate elevation of systolic blood pressure, attempts to decrease the systolic pressure to normal may result in diastolic pressures that are below normal. Particularly in view of the frequency of atherosclerotic disease in the elderly, sustained reduction of diastolic pressure might compromise vital organ function. However, antihypertensive medication reduces systolic pressure to a greater extent than it does diastolic pressure; therefore, even isolated hypertension is amenable to therapy.[109,120]

Based on these considerations, treatment can readily be recommended in all elderly hypertensive patients with evidence of complications of high blood pressure and patients with symptoms that may be aggravated by hypertension, eg, angina. All patients with systolic pressure greater than 160 mm Hg or diastolic pressure greater than 120 mm Hg, or both, should receive therapy. The merits of treating elderly hypertensive patients whose pressures are below these levels have not yet been demonstrated and the decision must be individualized.

Treatment of the elderly hypertensive patient is complicated by the inadequacy of homeostatic reflexes. Orthostatic hypotension of significant degree is common in the otherwise healthy elderly person and will be aggravated by antihypertensive medication. General measures such as weight reduction and decreased salt intake maintain their importance, although they are particularly difficult to institute.

The drug of choice for initiating antihypertensive therapy in elderly patients is currently a subject of much debate. Although beta blockers have been recommended by some, the high incidence of adverse effects to beta blockers in elderly patients makes them a poor choice in my mind. Thiazides have established themselves as being relatively safe and effective in elderly patients.[109,120,121] Furthermore, because hypertension in the elderly is characterized by low plasma renin activity, thiazides appear to be more effective than beta blockers.[119,122] The likelihood of electrolyte imbalance is significantly reduced by the currently recommended small doses. However, monitoring of electrolytes early in the course of therapy remains important. Calcium antagonists may play a role in the initial therapy of elderly hypertensive patients, but this remains to be determined. The selection of a second drug, if required, is even more controversial than the initial therapy. Beta blockers, calcium antagonists, methyldopa, and hydralazine have all been suggested. If more potent antihypertensive medication is required, almost any of the antihypertensive drugs currently in use may be added. These drugs must be administered with caution and close supervision.

ISCHEMIC HEART DISEASE

Ischemic heart disease is the most common cause of cardiac disease in the elderly. It may be manifest in all the forms seen in younger patients. However, some aspects of ischemic heart disease are peculiar to the aged population, and these will be the focus of the discussion that follows.

Hypertension is the most significant risk factor in the elderly, although, as discussed earlier, it may not be true in the very old. Similarly, smoking and family history are no longer relevant risk factors after age 65.[114,123] Glucose intolerance[123] and lipid disorders appear to retain their prognostic importance, but these factors have not been widely studied. Aside from control of hypertension, risk factor modification is unlikely to be practical or beneficial in the elderly.

ANGINA PECTORIS

Stable angina pectoris tends to be associated with less frequent and less severe pain in elderly patients.[31] Although unstable patterns such as crescendo angina do occur, they are less frequent than would be the case in a middle-aged population. Furthermore, the description of the discomfort is often somewhat atypical and the angina may be manifest as dyspnea or dizziness rather than pain.

Control of symptoms is the major therapeutic objective, the precision of the diagnosis being less important than that in a younger patient. Therefore, a therapeutic trial of antianginal therapy, if successful, may be sufficient for a presumptive diagnosis and the resulting freedom from symptoms constitutes a therapeutic success. Failure to readily control symptoms by simple antianginal regimens will require a more definitive diagnosis. Stress testing can be applied to many elderly patients as readily as to younger ones. The electrocardiographic changes seen with stress carry the same weight as they do in younger populations.[77] Unfortunately, the frequent coexistence of resting electrocardiographic abnormalities may make interpretation of the stress test difficult. To this end, thallium imaging in conjunction with stress testing can often help to clarify the stress response. The sensitivity and specificity of thallium stress testing have not been well defined in the elderly population. Stress radionuclide angiography has also been applied to elderly patients. Initial reports suggested that normal elderly subjects may demonstrate wall motion abnormalities under stress,[79] but more recent studies indicate that these abnormalities are of the same significance in elderly (ie, suggestive of disease) as in younger patients.[80] More work is obviously required to clarify the use of nuclear-assisted stress tests in the elderly.

Coronary angiography generally should be reserved for patients for whom surgery is being considered, essentially patients refractory to medical therapy.

Therapy consists of nitrates, beta blockers, and calcium antagonists, used essentially as they would be in younger patients. Because of the increased likelihood of borderline conduction and contractility and of chronic pulmonary disease, beta blockers must be used with extra caution. Similarly, the propensity of calcium antagonists, particularly verapamil, to aggravate underlying atrioventricular node disease must be borne in mind.

Complete relief of symptoms is not always necessary. The patient is often prepared to accept the occasional mild episode of angina, and the physician should be prepared to accept this as well, providing it does not constrain the patient's life-style too much.

Other causes of chest pain become increasingly important in the differential diagnosis in elderly patients. Musculoskeletal disorders, particularly as they affect the cervical vertebrae, as well as mediastinal and aortic diseases, must be considered. When manifest as dyspnea on exertion, the differentiation between cardiac and chronic pulmonary disease is extremely important, although at times very difficult.

MYOCARDIAL INFARCTION

The major feature of myocardial infarction that distinguishes the elderly population is the wide variety of atypical presentations. Typical chest pain is less frequent and nonspecific symptoms are more common (Table 77.4). The importance of painless infarction appears to have been overstated in the past.[95] Pathy[124] reported a typical presentation of myocardial infarction in less than 20% of elderly patients. Over 60% of the patients of MacDonald et al[95] presented with chest pain. Whether or not this pain was typical of infarction is not defined. Moreover, this presenting symptom was significantly less common than in the younger patients (77%). Even with these diagnostic difficulties, acute myocardial infarction remains a most frequent cause of emergency hospital admission and inhospital death in the elderly.

Although chest pain may be less common in older patients, syncope tends to be significantly more common.[95] In addition to differences in the manifestation of acute myocardial infarction in the elderly, the cardiac enzyme profile may also be altered with advanced age. In acute infarction, the phenomenon of an elevated myocardial fraction of creatine kinase (CK-MB isoenzyme) with a normal total CK level tends to occur twice as often in patients aged 70 years and over than in younger patients.[124a] It is not known whether a lower total CK level represents smaller infarcts, decreased numbers of myocytes or myofibers in the myocardium, an altered isoenzyme distribution (increased MB fraction), or other changes in the older heart.

Complications of myocardial infarction are somewhat more frequent in the elderly population; congestive heart failure, in particular, is the most common complication in this population.[91,95] Ventricular arrhythmias are no more frequent; in fact, ventricular fibrillation is less common.[91,95] Resuscitation in a coronary unit is as successful with elderly as with younger patients.[91-95] Thus, the elderly patient benefits as much from coronary care unit care as does the younger patient.[91,95,125] Treatment of the complications is the same. The elderly require extra effort to minimize the possibility of thromboembolic disease by encouragement of in-bed exercise, mobilization as early

Table 77.4. Presentation of Acute Myocardial Infarction in the Elderly

Study	MacDonald et al[95]	Pathy[124]
Patients (No.)	317	387
Minimum age (yr)	70	60
Presenting symptom		
Pain	61*	19
Dyspnea	18	20
Syncope	12	15†
Other	9	56

* Percentage of patients.
† Includes syncope and sudden death.

as possible, and subcutaneous heparin if bedrest is prolonged or congestive heart failure is present. The elderly also will often require more assistance during the rehabilitation period to return to their former level of activity.

CORONARY ARTERY SURGERY

If surgery is considered feasible, elderly patients whose angina, stable or unstable, cannot be controlled medically should be subjected to coronary angiography, a procedure that carries a risk only slightly higher than that in younger patients.[14 (pp 36–38)] Whether this is also the best approach for uncontrolled pain in the course of myocardial infarction is currently not clear.

The results of bypass surgery in the elderly have been the subject of numerous publications.[126–128] These data must be interpreted in light of the results in younger patients in the same institution during the same period. Improved overall surgical results have made the older publications obsolete. For example, Elayda et al[126] report an early mortality of 13.9% in elderly patients (70 and older) operated on in the early 1970s and 4.7% in the late 1970s. This compares to a reduction in mortality from 4.6% to 2.1% in patients under 70 years of age. Other recent studies also suggest that early mortality in the elderly is about twice that in younger patients.[126a,127,128] All complications are significantly more frequent in the elderly.[126–128]

Little information is available concerning the long-term results of surgery in the aged. Faro et al[128] report 94% survival after a follow-up period of 20 days to 78 months. The patients of Knapp et al[127] experienced a 95% 36-month survival, with more than 95% pain-free or improved at that time. These figures were identical to those for their younger patients. Both Elayda et al[126] and Loop et al[126a] found an 80.6% 5-year survival rate, with 50% and 74%, respectively, being asymptomatic. The Coronary Artery Surgery Study (CASS) also suggested that coronary bypass surgery appeared to improve survival at least in some subsets of elderly patients.[128a]

Percutaneous transluminal coronary angioplasty is a relatively recent alternative to bypass surgery in some patients.[129] Initial results in elderly patients were less successful than those in younger patients[130]; both fatal and nonfatal complications and major clinical events in the first year of follow-up were more frequent in the elderly. However, recent results are more encouraging.[130a] The criteria for patient selection for angioplasty as opposed to surgery are still under development, especially those for older patients. The higher morbidity and mortality of surgery in the aged make angioplasty an attractive alternative in the opinion of some,[130,130a] whereas others believe it has its greatest applicability in the young.[131]

These figures all suggest that angioplasty and surgery can be performed in the elderly with an acceptable level of morbidity and mortality and with a reasonable expectation of sustained symptomatic relief. However, each clinician must remain aware of the current experience in his own institution, specifically that with elderly patients, as this rather than figures culled from the literature will form the basis for his decision-making.

VALVULAR HEART DISEASE

Heart murmurs are common in the elderly population, being found in up to 60% of patients.[61] This finding does not negate their importance.[62] A murmur in an elderly patient must be assessed in light of the potential benefits of medical versus surgical therapy for some valve lesions. Patients with symptomatic aortic stenosis, in particular, have a poor prognosis with medical therapy and such a good prognosis with surgical therapy that the approach to the elderly patient with a systolic murmur might be considered a search for and correction of those patients with hemodynamically significant, symptomatic aortic stenosis. Overall, calcification of a congenitally bicuspid valve is the most common cause of aortic stenosis, but the frequency of this pathologic finding decreases with advancing age. Isolated aortic stenosis after age 75 is almost always a result of degenerative calcification of a normal valve.[30,132] In about one half of elderly patients with aortic stenosis, associated aortic incompetence can be demonstrated.[31] Aortic stenosis combined with mitral valve disease is usually rheumatic in origin.

The major clinical manifestations of aortic stenosis remain angina, congestive heart failure, and syncope. Systolic ejection murmurs are frequently found in elderly patients. The distinction between aortic sclerosis and aortic stenosis often cannot be made on clinical grounds. In fact, it can be argued that the two processes are basically the same and that the only true distinction between them is the presence or absence of a gradient across the aortic valve. The decrease in arterial elasticity that accompanies aging will mask the otherwise slow upstroke of the pulse wave in aortic stenosis. The heart sounds are generally reduced in intensity in elderly patients; therefore, the reduction and intensity of the aortic component that accompanies aortic stenosis may be difficult to appreciate. The murmur of hemodynamically significant aortic stenosis is generally louder and longer than that in the absence of a gradient and tends to peak later in systole,[133,134] but these criteria are too indefinite to be helpful clinically. Although physical findings indicative of left ventricular hypertrophy may not be demonstrable in the presence of significant aortic stenosis, electrocardiographic and echocardiographic evidence of hypertrophy will usually be present. As other causes of hypertrophy can coexist with aortic sclerosis, this finding is of limited usefulness. Echocardiography can demonstrate thickening of the aortic cusps, but attempts to determine the orifice area have been hampered by the amount of calcification usually present. The absence of any evidence of left ventricular hypertrophy makes hemodynamically significant stenosis unlikely. The extent of calcification as seen on chest x-ray films is thought to correlate with the severity of the stenosis.[135]

The poor prognosis for patients with symptomatic aortic stenosis treated medically compared with the low risk and potential benefits of surgery (discussed subsequently in detail) emphasizes the importance of not overlooking this diagnosis. Even though the elderly patient with severe aortic stenosis represents a relatively high risk for cardiac catheterization,[136] this procedure must be offered to any suitable patient in whom the diagnosis cannot be otherwise excluded. Although the need for cardiac catheterization before aortic valve replacement remains somewhat controversial,[137,138] current noninvasive tests cannot be relied on to determine the severity of stenosis in the elderly patient with valvular calcification. Doppler ultrasound may overcome many of these problems and allow a definitive diagnosis to be established. Although patients who do not complain of angina are statistically unlikely to have associated obstructive coronary disease, only coronary angiography can determine this with certainty. In our experience as in that of others, failure to correct significant coronary disease compromises the long-term results of aortic valve replacement, even in elderly patients.[139,140] Furthermore, in our laboratory, the complications of cardiac catheterization have been related primarily to left ventricular angiography. Therefore, unless we suspect the presence of associated mitral insufficiency, we do not perform contrast angiography at the time of catheterization, but we do perform radionuclide angiography separately.

The most common valve lesion found in the elderly is aortic incompetence.[31] It occurs as an isolated lesion in about 1% of patients, but is associated in over 50% of patients with aortic stenosis and in about 40% of patients with rheumatic mitral disease. Degenerative dilatation of the aortic root, calcific degeneration of the aortic valve, and rheumatic heart disease are the most common causes. Syphilitic aortitis, once an important cause, is still seen in the elderly population but with decreasing frequency. All the recognized causes of aortic incompetence in younger patients may be seen in older patients, but most are relatively rare.

Aortic incompetence in the elderly is similar in its presentation and clinical features to aortic incompetence in the young. The clinical diagnosis poses no particular problems in the aged. Its presence can often be confirmed by noninvasive means, which may also provide evidence for its etiology. Except when sudden in onset, aortic incompetence is well tolerated hemodynamically, and surgery in elderly patients should therefore be considered only in patients whose symptoms cannot be controlled medically.

Mitral incompetence may be secondary to left ventricular enlargement of any cause. Papillary muscle dysfunction[140a] and mitral valve prolapse[141] are also recognized causes of mitral insufficiency in the elderly population. Rheumatic mitral valve disease has an estimated prevalence of 2% to 3% in the elderly population.[31] Stenosis dominates in one third of these patients; incompetence dominates in the remainder. Calcification of the mitral anulus occasionally presents as mitral stenosis as does the rare, left atrial myxoma.[142] The clinical presentation of mitral valve disease in elderly patients is generally similar to that in younger patients. Angina is more common, occurring in about 10% of patients.[31] In most of these cases, coronary artery disease is also present. The features of the physical examination carry the same implications as in younger patients. Because of the extent of valvular calcification, the increased intensity of the first heart sound and the opening snap may both be absent. In the elderly patient with mitral stenosis, the electrocardiographic features of right ventricular hypertrophy are uncommon, but the characteristics of left atrial enlargement may be seen if sinus rhythm is still present. Electrocardiographic evidence of left ventricular hypertrophy will be seen in the presence of moderate mitral incompetence. Echocardiography has proven itself to be reliable, not only in the diagnosis of mitral stenosis, but often in the assessment of its severity. It is also a useful technique in the diagnosis of mitral valve prolapse, but it is of limited usefulness in other cases of mitral incompetence. The extent of mitral valve calcification as seen on chest x-ray films correlates with the gradient in mitral stenosis.[143]

Mitral valve disease not associated with atrial fibrillation or congestive failure appears to have no significant effect on the life expectancy of elderly patients.[134] Because mitral valve replacement generally has been considered a less satisfactory operation than aortic valve replacement, surgery is usually reserved for patients whose symptoms cannot be controlled by medical means including attempts to maintain sinus rhythm, control ventricular response rate in atrial fibrillation; and treat congestive heart failure. However, as a result of these considerations, mitral valve surgery is often delayed longer than aortic valve surgery, perhaps accounting for some of the lack of benefit from mitral valve replacement.

Many reports have appeared concerning the results of valve replacement surgery in the elderly.[8–12,139] As in coronary bypass surgery, current results are far superior to earlier experience, particularly in older patients.[143a,143b] For isolated aortic valve replacement with or without coronary bypass grafting, operative mortality is almost negligible, 3-year survival is 90%, and greater than 80% of patients are functionally improved. Isolated mitral valve replacement still carries a 4% to 10% mortality and a 3-year survival of only 66%; however, 90% of survivors are clinically improved. More complex procedures continue to be associated with a high operative mortality that is usually not clinically justifiable. The results of valve surgery in our hospital from 1979 to 1983 in patients aged 75 and older are presented in Table 77.5.

MISCELLANEOUS CONDITIONS

THYROID DISORDERS

Many endocrine disorders may play a role in cardiac disease, but disorders of thyroid function are by far the most important in the elderly patient. Hypothyroidism in particular is relatively common in the elderly, and its associated symptoms including slowing of mental and physical functioning, dry skin, hair loss, constipation, and cold intolerance are frequently attributed to aging. Moreover, an elderly patient commonly presents with cardiac abnormalities in the absence of other definitive evidence of hypothyroidism. These presentations include congestive cardiomyopathy with cardiomegaly and pleural and pericardial effusion. Bradycardia, which may or may not be symptomatic, is a consistent feature of hypothyroidism. Physical examination may suggest the diagnosis. The deep tendon reflex response is often typical, if one remembers to assess it, but the diagnosis really depends on

Table 77.5. Results of Valve Surgery in Patients Aged 75 and Older (1979–1983)*

Procedure	Patients (No.)	Age (yr)		Patients With Coronary Bypass	Deaths		Follow-up (yr)	
		Mean	Range		Early	Late	Mean	Range
Single Valve Replacement								
Aortic valve replacement	10	76.5	75–83	4	0	1	2.6	1–4
Mitral valve replacement	7	75.7	75–77	2	0	0	3.7	1–5
Complex Procedures								
Double valve replacement	4	76.8	75–79	. . .	1	0	2.0	1–3
Aortic valve + aortic root replacement	2	75.5	75–76	. . .	0	0	2.0	1–3

* Berman ND and David TE, unpublished data.

consideration of the possibility and ordering of the appropriate blood tests, which are usually definitive.

The diagnosis of hyperthyroidism is often equally difficult. Apathetic hyperthyroidism, a common presentation in the elderly, is usually associated with cardiomegaly, congestive heart failure, and atrial fibrillation.[144] The latter may be the only demonstrable abnormality in older patients with hyperthyroidism,[145] and the rate may prove difficult to control. The diagnosis should be considered in any patient with atrial fibrillation whose ventricular response and rate appear unusually resistant to the negative chronotropic effect of digoxin. The development of angina or congestive heart failure in a patient with hyperthyroidism usually suggests an associated underlying primary cardiac condition.

INFECTIVE ENDOCARDITIS

Infective endocarditis is commonly overlooked in the elderly because of the misconception that it is usually a disease of young and middle-aged patients. In fact, the clinical spectrum has shifted toward older age groups, and most patients in more recent series have been 60 years of age and older.[146] The typical symptoms of malaise, weakness, anorexia, and weight loss occur in less than one third of the patients and even these tend to be modified in the aged. Psychiatric disturbances, persistent back pain, or embolic episodes are common presenting symptoms.[147–149] The disease may also present as progressive renal insufficiency[150] or metastatic abscess. The presence of other pathologic processes further obscures the diagnosis.

As in younger patients, one third have no underlying heart disease. Although rheumatic valvular disease remains an important cause,[151] nonrheumatic cardiac abnormalities, particularly those involving the aortic valve, are increasingly important in the elderly.[31,152,153]

The combination of fever and heart murmur is the most obvious clue to the diagnosis, but both may be absent. High fevers are uncommon and low-grade fevers are apt to be overlooked because basal body temperature is generally lower in the elderly.[154] Murmurs are usually soft and not readily distinguishable from those commonly found in healthy older patients. Atrial fibrillation is not uncommon and does not militate against the diagnosis.[148] The classic peripheral manifestations are rare.

Echocardiography has proven useful in the diagnosis and monitoring of patients with endocarditis.[155,156] Blood culture remains the basis of diagnosis and treatment. Treatment is essentially the same as in younger patients and consists of a minimum of 4 weeks of intravenous antibiotic therapy based on blood culture results. Infective endocarditis in the elderly is associated with a 30% mortality, approximately twice that in younger patients.[148] The delay in diagnosis does not account for all of this excess mortality. Surgical intervention is indicated for medically refractory failure or persistent infection despite adequate antibiotic therapy. Although surgery is associated with an extremely high risk, medically refractory congestive heart failure is associated with a 90% mortality, and persistent infection is universally fatal.[157]

Antibiotic prophylaxis is warranted in elderly patients with known hemodynamically significant valvular disease. However, murmurs are common in elderly patients and have no hemodynamic significance in most situations. The use of prophylaxis in these patients is controversial. The consequences of endocarditis generally are so devastating that prophylactic therapy should probably be given when a structural abnormality underlying the murmur is suspected.

MYOCARDITIS AND PERICARDITIS

Myocarditis is rarely diagnosed in elderly patients because the presentation of chest discomfort associated with transient electrocardiographic changes is almost always attributed to coronary artery disease. The diagnosis is more commonly considered in the course of a systemic illness in which myocardial involvement is common. Postmortem evidence of myocardial inflammation is significantly more common than is the clinical diagnosis of myocarditis.[158] Although the distinction may not be important in its effect on therapy of the acute illness, the importance in both the short and long term of labeling a patient as having coronary artery disease rather than a self-limiting viral infection cannot be overemphasized. Unfortunately, there is no ready way of making this diagnosis clinically. In the absence of solid evidence of coronary artery disease, the possibility of myocarditis should be considered.

Similar considerations apply to the diagnosis of pericarditis in the elderly. Idiopathic pericarditis is uncommon in the elderly. The typical electrocardiographic progression is rarely seen, especially in the secondary forms.[159] The ST-segment and T-wave changes, the presence of supraventricular arrhythmias, and even the reduced voltages of the QRS complexes do not specifically point to this diagnosis. A pericardial friction rub, the pathognomonic feature of pericarditis, may occur in ischemic heart disease. Echocardiography, by demonstrating the presence of pericardial effusion, may lend weight to the diagnosis, although neither the presence nor the absence of effusion can be considered specific for either diagnosis.[160]

Pericarditis in the elderly is usually a complication of some other disease, most commonly uremia, malignancy, postmyocardial infarction, or a collagen vascular disease. Purulent pericarditis has become relatively rare, but when it does occur, it is usually in older patients who have some other intrathoracic focus of infection.[161]

The typical pain is sharper, more localized than ischemic pain, and aggravated by respiration and by lying supine. Radiation to the arms is uncommon and rarely extends distal to the elbows. In the elderly, these features are rarely well defined and pain is commonly mild or absent, particularly in patients whose pericarditis is secondary to some other disease process.

Both the acute complication of pericarditis, cardiac tamponade, and the chronic complication, constrictive pericarditis, may occur in elderly patients. The clinical presentation and treatment of these complications do not differ from those in younger patients.

CARDIOMYOPATHIES

Although cardiomyopathies of any form may be seen in the elderly, only congestive cardiomyopathies are seen with any frequency. The presence of cardiomyopathy is a diagnosis of exclusion. Noninvasive tests have not been reliable in ruling out the possibility of ischemic heart disease in this setting, and coronary angiography is usually not warranted in elderly patients with this clinical presentation. However, the inability to make this distinction does not alter therapy, which is basically that of congestive heart failure. Moreover, the prognosis depends on the severity of congestive heart failure rather than its etiology.

The variety of disease processes recognized to cause congestive cardiomyopathies in younger patients are equally applicable in the elderly but are uncommon. In the absence of preexisting ischemic or hypertensive heart disease, these possibilities should be considered as they are readily amenable to therapy. The systemic manifestations may be subtle and specific laboratory tests are readily available to aid in most of these diagnoses.

Restrictive cardiomyopathies are extremely rare in the elderly and almost always secondary to a myocardial infiltrative process such as amyloid. Conduction disturbances often occur at an early stage in these disorders and pacemaker implantation should be considered. Congestive heart failure often becomes resistant to the usual therapeutic modalities, but the rate of progression of this complication is extremely variable, depending on the primary process.

Hypertrophic cardiomyopathy is more common in the elderly than is generally considered.[162–164] In one series one third of such patients were over 60 years of age, and in two thirds of these older patients the diagnosis had not been considered clinically.[162] Echocardiography is useful in confirming the diagnosis of hypertrophic cardiomyopathy and its widespread use has resulted in an increased frequency of clinical recognition of this condition in the elderly. The importance of making this diagnosis in the elderly cannot be overemphasized as treatment is specific and often contrary to the usual treatment employed in a patient thought to have coronary artery or valvular heart disease. Surgery can be performed in the appropriate elderly patient with this disorder. The risks and benefits in the aged are comparable to those in younger patients,[165] but the role of surgery in this condition is generally a matter of controversy. Medical therapy is indicated in most symptomatic elderly patients. The best approach for asymptomatic patients remains to be defined.

COR PULMONALE

Although chronic obstructive pulmonary disease is common in elderly patients, true cor pulmonale is not.[166,167] Chronic obstructive pulmonary disease severe enough to lead to right ventricular hypertrophy and failure is not compatible with survival into the elderly age group.[167,168] Furthermore, the emphysematous aspect of chronic pulmonary disease dominates in the elderly[166] and the risk of developing cor pulmonale relates to the severity of the bronchitic component.[169] Although right ventricular failure is common in elderly patients with chronic obstructive pulmonary disease, it is almost always secondary to left ventricular failure. Three problems commonly interact in this situation: congestive failure, exacerbation of chronic pulmonary disease (with or without infection), and arrhythmias. Each may contribute to the development and increased severity of the other two. Each factor also increases the resistance of the others to treatment. Therefore, therapy must be directed at all three components simultaneously.

CONGENITAL HEART DISEASE

Congenital heart disease is occasionally encountered in the elderly and almost every conceivable defect has been reported.[170–176] Even anomalies not associated with lengthy survival may be seen either in a mild form or in a complex of deformities that somehow result in hemodynamic balance. The superimposition of ischemic or hypertensive heart disease or the development of arrhythmias often will precipitate symptoms in later life. This is particularly true of atrial septal defect, probably the most common congenital defect to become manifest and require intervention in the aged. Surgical correction of many congenital abnormalities is feasible in the elderly if symptoms cannot otherwise be controlled. Most congenital defects are now surgically corrected in childhood with the objective of prolonging survival. We can expect survival of increasing numbers of these patients into the geriatric age group. It will be of interest to see what specific problems these patients will pose for the geriatric cardiologist.

PSYCHOSOCIAL CONSIDERATIONS

The psychologic and social implications of cardiac illness are important at any age, but their significance is magnified in the elderly. Although a detailed discussion of psychosocial factors pertinent to geriatric cardiology is clearly beyond the scope of this chapter, it would be impossible to leave this topic without reviewing some of its most pertinent aspects, where the disciplines of geriatrics and cardiology blend.

The elderly are more likely to decompensate emotionally when hospitalized for an acute illness, particularly in the intensive care unit setting. Unfortunately, psychotropic drugs have a higher incidence of adverse effects in the elderly. Moreover, the elimination of these drugs is generally prolonged. Central nervous system reactions to nonpsychotropic drugs are also more common in the aged. It is of interest that reported cases of intoxication due to the ethanol diluent of intravenous nitroglycerin have, to date, been confined to patients over 70 years of age.[177,178] An awareness of these factors may reduce the problems associated with these drugs and allow for earlier recognition and correction of the adverse effects.

The dislocation produced by the acute illness tends to be less readily reversible in the aged. Complete recovery to premorbid functional level is less likely, and as a result the patient may be unable to return to his previous environment. Instead, a higher level of supervised environment may be required such as independent domicile to a child's home or supervised apartments. This change in life-style will require detailed planning with patients and relatives. Moreover, this change further aggravates the psychologic effects of the illness. Early involvement of family, community agencies, and psychiatric and social work departments are important in smoothing this transition.

A prominent feature of the increasing size of the elderly segment of the population has been an increased utilization of hospital beds for longer periods. Part of the response to this phenomenon must be the increased development of a variety of community- and hospital-based alternative forms of care. These alternatives must be fully integrated so that many or all of them can serve the same patient at different phases in his illness and the transition from one to the other can be made smoothly and quickly when required. Different societies have succeeded to different extents in the development of these interrelated facilities.

Many limitations of the traditional outpatient department have been addressed by the concept of a day hospital. Not only does it provide a more acceptable environment in which to follow up the elderly patient, but it also provides an opportunity to readily assess and aid the patient in routine activities. Furthermore, the day hospital is associated with a communal atmosphere that plays a vital role in the social rehabilitation of the patient.

Home treatment is an important modality that has largely been forgotten in many developed societies. The elderly fear even "temporary" institutionalization. They recognize that it is all too uncommon for the older patient to be returned to his pre-morbid environment following such admission. It is in the best interest of the patient, the family, and the community to rely to a greater extent on home treatment, where more of the elderly patient's requirements for care can be met, than is the current practice in many societies. However, this requires a high level of organization of support resources including information, personnel, and special equipment. Of fundamental importance is the confidence that if a crisis develops with either the patient or those responsible for his care, relief will be readily available. Such a program requires the integration of acute care, chronic care, and outpatient facilities as well as community service agencies. In addition, periodic relief must be provided for those responsible for the patient's care and may consist of involvement of additional family members, visiting nurses, attendance at day programs, or possibly even some form of "holiday admissions."

REFERENCES

1. World Health Organization: *Annual Epidemiological and Vital Statistics, Part I. Vital Statistics and Causes of Death.* Geneva, 1960 (and previous publications under similar title).
2. World Health Organization: *World Health Statistics Annual.* Geneva, 1982 (and previous publications under similar title).

2a. Cheng TO: Medicine and health care along the Silk Road in China. *Am J Med* 1985; 78:3–8.

3. Kraus AS, Spasoff RA, Beattie EJ, Holden EW, Lawson JS, Rodenburg M, Woodcock GM: Elderly applicants to long-term care institutions: I. Their characteristics, health problems and state of mind. *J Am Geriat Soc* 1976; 24:117–125.
4. Shanas E: *The Health of Older People.* Cambridge, Harvard, 1962, p 8.
5. Caird FI, Kennedy, RD: Epidemiology of heart disease in old age, in Caird FI, Dall JLC, Kennedy RD (eds): *Cardiology in Old Age.* New York, Plenum Press, 1976, pp 1–10.
6. Kennedy RD, Andrews GR, Caird FI: Ischemic heart disease in the elderly. *Br Heart J* 1977; 39:1121–1127.
7. Statistics Canada, Hospital Morbidity 1974, Ottawa, June 1977.
8. Calson RG, Shafer RB, Eliot RS, Sellers RD, Lillehel CW: Results of cardiac surgery in 273 older patients. *Geriatrics* 1967; 22:173–183.
9. Ahmad A, Starr A: Valve replacement in geriatric patients. *Br Heart J* 1969; 31:322–236.
10. Oh W, Hickman R, Emanuel R, McDonald L, Sommerville J, Ross D, Ross K, Gonzalez-Lavin L: Heart valve surgery in 114 patients over the age of 60. *Br Heart J* 1973; 35:174–180.
11. Barnhorst DA, Giugliani ER, Pluth JR, Danielson GK, Wallace RB, McGoon DC: Open heart surgery in patients more than 65 years old. *Ann Thorac Surg* 1974; 18:81–90.
12. Stephenson LW, MacVaugh H III, Edmunds LH Jr: Surgery using cardiopulmonary bypass in the elderly. *Circulation* 1978; 58:250–254.
13. Strauss HD, Berman ND: Permanent pacing in the elderly. *PACE* 1978; 1:458–464.
14. Berman ND: *Geriatric Cardiology.* Toronto, Collamore Press, 1982.
15. Davies I: Biology of aging—theories of aging, in Brocklehurst JC (ed): *Textbook of Geriatric Medicine and Gerontology*, ed 3. New York, Churchill Livingstone, 1985, pp 62–81.
16. Guthrie RD: Senescence as an adaptive trait. *Perspect Biol Med* 1969; 12:313–324.
17. Norwood TH, Pendergrass WR, Sprague CA, Martin GM: Dominance of the senescent phenotype in heterokaryons between replicative and post-replicative human fibroblast-like cells. *Proc Natl Acad Sci USA* 1974; 71:2231–2235.
18. Hart RW, Setlo RB: Correlation between deoxyribonucleic acid excision repair and lifespan in a number of mammalian species. *Proc Natl Acad Sci USA* 1974; 71:2169–2173.
19. Lenkiewicz JE, Davies MJ, Rosen D: Collagen in human myocardium as a function of age. *Cardiovasc Res* 1972; 6:549–555.
20. Kohn RR: Heart and cardiovascular system, in Finch CE, Hayflick L (eds): *Handbook of the Biology of Aging.* Toronto, Van Nostrand Reinhold, 1977, pp 281–317.
21. Kohn RR, Rollerson E: Age changes in swelling properties of human myocardium. *Proc Soc Exp Biol Med* 1959; 100:253–256.
22. Bailey AJ, Robins SP, Balian G: Biological significance of the intermolecular crosslinks of collagen. *Nature* 1974; 251:105–109.
23. Yin FCP: The aging vasculature and its effects on the heart, in Weisfeldt

ML (ed): *The Aging Heart: Its Function and Response to Stress.* New York, Raven Press, 1980, pp 137–213.
24. Hallock P, Benson IC: Studies on the elastic properties of human isolated aorta. *J Clin Invest* 1937; 16:595–602.
25. Weisfeldt ML: Aging of the cardiovascular system. *N Engl J Med* 1980; 303:1172–1173.
26. Limas CJ: Aging of the myocardium. *Acta Cardiol* 1971; 26:249–259.
27. Strehler BI, Mark DD, Mildvan AS, Gee MV: Rate and magnitude of age pigment accumulation in the human myocardium. *J Gerontol* 1959; 14:430–439.
28. Cornwell GG III, Westermark P: Senile amyloidosis: a protean manifestation of the aging process. *J Clin Pathol* 1980; 33:1146–1152.
29. Cornwell GG III, Murdoch WL, Kyle RA, Westermark P, Pitkanen P: Frequency and distribution of senile cardiovascular amyloid: A clinicopathologic correlation. *Am J Med* 1983; 75:618–623.
30. Pomerance A: Pathology of the myocardium and valves, in Caird FI, Dall JLC, Kennedy RD (eds): *Cardiology in Old Age.* New York, Plenum, 1976, pp 11–55.
31. Caird FI, Dall JLC, Williams BO: The cardiovascular system, in Brocklehurst JC (ed): *Textbook of Geriatric Medicine and Gerontology*, ed 3. New York, Churchill Livingstone, 1985, pp 230–267.
32. Davies MJ: Pathology of the conducting system, in Caird FI, Dall JLC, Kennedy RD (eds): *Cardiology in Old Age*. New York, Plenum Press, 1976, pp 57–80.
33. Sims BA: Pathogenesis of atrial arrhythmias. *Br Heart J* 1972; 34:336–340.
34. Kennel AJ, Titus JL, McCallister BD, Pruitt RD: The vasculature of the atrioventricular conducting system in heart block. *Am Heart J* 1973; 85:593–600.
35. Strandell T: Cardiac output in old age, in Caird FI, Dall JLC, Kennedy RD (eds): *Cardiology in Old Age.* New York, Plenum Press, 1976, pp 81–100.
36. Raven PB, Mitchell JH: Effect of aging on the cardiovascular response to dynamic and static exercise, in Weisfeldt ML (ed): *The Aging Heart: Its Function and Response to Stress.* New York, Raven Press, 1980, pp 269–296.
37. Schocken DD, Blumenthal JA, Port S, Hindle P, Coleman RE: Physical conditioning and left ventricular performance in the elderly: assessment by radionuclide angiocardiography. *Am J Cardiol* 1983: 52:359–364.
38. Weisfeldt ML: Left ventricular function, in Weisfeldt ML (ed): *The Aging Heart: Its Function and Response to Stress.* New York, Raven Press, 1980, pp 297–316.
39. Frolkis UV, Bezrukov VV, Shevchuk VG: Hemodynamics and its regulation in old age. *Exp Gerontol* 1975; 10:251–271.
39a. Weisfeldt ML: The aging heart. *Hosp Prac* 1985; 20:115–130.
40. Gribbin B, Pickering TG, Sleight P, Peto R: Effect of age and high blood pressure on baroreflex sensitivity in man. *Circ Res* 1971; 29:424–431.
41. Rothbaum DA, Shaw DJ, Angell CS, Shock NW: Cardiac performance in the unanesthetized senescent male rat. *J Gerontol* 1973; 28:287–292.
42. Kalbfleisch JH, Stowe DF, Smith JJ: Evaluation of the heart rate response to the Valsalva maneuver. *Am Heart J* 1978; 95:707–715.
43. Gooden BA, Holdstock G, Hampton JR: The magnitude of the bradycardia induced by face immersion in patients convalescing from myocardial infarction. *Cardiovasc Res* 1978; 12:239–242.
44. Finch CE: Neuroendocrine and autonomic aspects of aging, in Finch CE, Hayflick L (eds): *Handbook of the Biology of Aging.* Toronto, Van Nostrand Reinhold, 1977, pp 262–280.
45. Vestal RE, Wood AJJ, Shand DG: Reduced β-adrenoceptor sensitivity in the elderly. *Clin Pharmacol Ther* 1979; 26:181–186.
46. Willems JL, Roelandt J, De Geest H, Kesteloot H, Joossens JV: The left ventricular ejection time in elderly subjects. *Circulation* 1970; 42:37–42.
47. Harrison TR, Dixon K, Russell RO Jr, Bidwai PS, Coleman HN: The relation of age to the duration of contraction, ejection, and relaxation of the normal human heart. *Am Heart J* 1964; 67:189–199.
48. Schwartz D, Wang M, Zeitz L, Goss MEW: Medication errors made by elderly, chronically ill patients. *Am J Public Health* 1962; 52:2018–2029.
49. Kennedy RD: Drug therapy for cardiovascular disease in the aged. *J Am Geriatr Soc* 1975; 23:113–120.
50. Krakauer R, Petersen B: The effects of discontinuing maintenance digoxin therapy. A study of elderly cardiac patients in sinus rhythm. *Dan Med Bull* 1979; 26:10–13.
51. Johnston GD, McDevitt DG: Is maintenance digoxin necessary in patients with sinus rhythm? *Lancet* 1979; 1:567–570.
52. O'Malley K, Judge TG, Crooks J: Geriatric clinical pharmacology and therapeutics, in Avery G (ed): *Drug Treatment, Principles and Practice of Clinical Pharmacology and Therapeutics.* ed 2. Sydney, ADIS Press, 1980, pp 158–181.
53. Lamy PP: Therapeutics and the elderly. *Addict Res* 1978; 3:311–335.
54. Triggs EJ, Nation RL: Pharmaco-kinetics in the aged: a review. *J Pharmacokinet Biopharm* 1975; 3:387–418.
55. Davies DF, Shock NW: Age changes in glomerular filtration rate, effective renal plasma flow, and tubular excretory capacity in adult males. *J Clin Invest* 1950; 29:496–507.
56. Friedman SA, Raizner AE, Rosen H, Solomon NA, Sy W: Functional defects in the aging kidney. *Ann Intern Med* 1972; 76:41–45.
57. Caird FI: Clinical examination and investigation of the heart, in Caird FI, Dall JLC, Kennedy RD (eds): *Cardiology in Old Age.* New York, Plenum Press, 1976, pp 127–142.
57a. Hsu I, Kistin AD: Buckling of the great vessels. A clinical and angiographic study. *Arch Intern Med* 1956; 98:712–719.
58. Sleight P: Unilateral elevation of the internal jugular pulse. *Br Heart J* 1962; 24:726–730.
59. Gerstenblith G: Non-invasive assessment of cardiac function in the elderly, in Weisfeldt ML (ed): *The Aging Heart*. New York, Raven Press, 1980, pp 247–267.
60. Spodick DH, Quarry-Pigott VM: Fourth heart sound as a normal finding in older persons. *N Engl J Med* 1973; 288:140–141.
61. Bethel CS, Crow EW: Heart sounds in the aged. *Am J Cardiol* 1963; 11:763–767.
62. Blumgart HL: The systolic murmur: innocent or guilty? *N Engl J Med* 1968; 279:268–269.
63. Bowers D: Electrocardiogram of nonagenerians. *Geriatrics* 1969; 24:89–92.
64. Fisch C: Electrocardiogram in the aged: an independent marker of heart disease? *Am J Med* 1981; 70:4–6.
65. May SH, Avila V, Margoulaff D: Hearts in the tenth decade. A study of one hundred nonagenerians. *Arch Intern Med* 1968; 121:141–144.
66. Rodstein M, Brown M, Wolloch L: First-degree atrioventricular heart block in the aged. *Geriatrics* 1968; 23:159–165.
67. Simonson E: The effect of age on the electrocardiogram. *Am J Cardiol* 1972; 29:64–73.
68. Mihalik MJ, Fisch C: Electrocardiographic findings in the aged. *Am Heart J* 1974; 87:117–128.
69. Simonson E: *Differentiation Between Normal and Abnormal in Electrocardiography.* St. Louis, CV Mosby, 1961, pp 82–99.
70. Ostrander LD, Brandt RL, Kjelsberg MO, Epstein FH: Electrocardiographic findings among the adult population of a total natural community, Tecumseh, Michigan. *Circulation* 1965; 31:888–898.
71. Blackburn H, Vasquez CI, Keys A: The aging electrocardiogram: a common aging process or latent coronary artery disease? *Am J Cardiol* 1967; 20:618–627.
72. Michie I: Electrocardiographic changes in the elderly. *Gerontol Clin* 1970; 12:193–202.
73. Sjogren AL: Left ventricular wall thickness determined by ultrasound in 100 subjects without heart disease. *Chest* 1971; 60:341–346.
74. Gerstenblith G, Frederiksen J, Yin FCP, Fortuin NJ, Lakatta EG, Weisfeldt ML: Echocardiographic assessment of a normal adult aging population. *Circulation* 1977; 56:273–278.
75. Gardin JM, Henry WL, Savage DD, Ware JH, Burn C, Borer JS: Echocardiographic measurements in normal subjects: evaluation of an adult population without clinically apparent heart disease. *J Clin Ultrasound* 1979; 7:439–447.
76. D'Cruz IA, Wallner H: Echocardiography in elderly patients. *Med Instrum* 1982; 16:12–14.
77. Lester FM, Sheffield LT, Reeves TJ: Electrocardiographic changes in clinically normal older men following near-maximal and maximal exercise. *Circulation* 1967; 36:5–14.
78. Sheffield LT: Exercise stress testing, in Braunwald E (ed): *Heart Disease: A Textbook of Cardiovascular Medicine.* Toronto, Saunders, 1980, vol 1, pp 253–277.
79. Port S, Cobb FR, Coleman RE, Jones RH: Effect of age on the response of the left ventricular ejection fraction to exercise. *N Engl J Med* 1980; 303:1133–1137.
80. Hakki A, DePace NL, Iskandrian AS: Effect of age on left ventricular function during exercise in patients with coronary artery disease. *J Am Coll Cardiol* 1983; 2:645–651.
81. Ewy GA, Kapadia GG, Yao L, Lullin M, Marcus FI: Digoxin metabolism in the elderly. *Circulation* 1969; 39:449–453.
82. Caird FI: Metabolism of digoxin in relation to therapy in the elderly. *Gerontol Clin* 1972; 16:68–74.
83. Cusack B, Kelly J, O'Malley K, Noel J, Lavan J, Horgan J: Digoxin in the elderly. Pharmacokinetic consequences of old age. *Clin Pharmacol Ther* 1979; 25:772–776.
84. Goldberg PB, Roberts J: Pharmacology, in Weisfeldt ML (ed): *The Aging Heart. Its Function and Response to Stress.* New York, Raven Press, 1980, pp 215–246.
85. Leaf A: Dehydration in the elderly. *N Engl J Med* 1984; 311:791–792.
86. Satinsky JD: Chronic heart failure in the elderly: vasodilator therapy. *Angiology* 1983; 34:509–516.
87. Camm AJ, Evans KE, Ward DE, Martin A: The rhythm of the heart in active elderly subjects. *Am Heart J* 1980; 99:598–603.
88. Abdon NJ: Frequency and distribution of long-term ECG-reduced car-

diac arrhythmias in an elderly population. *Acta Med Scand* 1981; 209:175–183.

89. Fleg JL, Kennedy HL: Cardiac arrhythmias in a healthy elderly population: detection by 24-hour ambulatory electrocardiography. *Chest* 1982; 8:302–307.
90. Taylor IC, Stout RW: Is ambulatory electrocardiography a useful investigation in elderly people with "funny turns"? *Age Ageing* 1983; 12:211–216.
91. Berman ND: The elderly patient in the coronary care unit. I. Acute myocardial infarction. *J Am Geriatr Soc* 1979; 27:145–151.
92. Linn BS, Yurt RW: Cardiac arrest among geriatric patients. *Br Med J* 1970; 2:25–27.
93. Gulati RS, Bhan GL, Horan MA: Cardiopulmonary resuscitation of old people. *Lancet* 1983; 2:267–269.
94. Suljaga-Petchel K, Skovron ML, Goldberg E: Cardiopulmonary resuscitation of old people. *Lancet* 1983; 2:685.
95. MacDonald JB, Baillie J, Williams BO, Ballantyne D: Coronary care in the elderly. *Age Ageing* 1983; 12:17–20.
96. Schamroth L: *The Disorders of Cardiac Rhythm.* Oxford, Blackwell, 1975, p 54.
97. Waxman HL, Myerberg RJ, Appel R, Sung RJ: Verapamil for control of ventricular rate in paroxysmal supraventricular tachycardia and atrial fibrillation or flutter: a double-blind randomized cross-over study. *Ann Intern Med* 1981; 94:1–6.
98. Rubenstein JJ, Schulman CL, Yurchak PM, DeSanctis RW: Clinical spectrum of the sick sinus syndrome. *Circulation* 1972; 46:5–13.
99. Berman ND, Mitchell JM, Dickson SE: Pacemaker therapy in the seventies: interaction of patient age, time of implant, and indications for pacing. *PACE* 1983; 6:247–252.
100. Ferrer MI: The sick sinus syndrome. *Circulation* 1973; 47:635–641.
101. Agruss NS, Rosin EY, Adolph RJ, Fowler NO: Significance of chronic sinus bradycardia in elderly people. *Circulation* 1972; 46:924–930.
102. Siddons H: Management of heart block, in Caird FI, Dall JLC, Kennedy RD (eds): *Cardiology in Old Age.* New York, Plenum Press, 1976, pp 347–367.
102a. Cheng TO: Transvenous ventricular pacing in the treatment of paroxysmal atrial tachyarrhythmias alternating with sinus bradycardia and standstill. *Am J Cardiol* 1968; 22:874–879.
102b. Berman ND: Antiarrhythmic therapy in the elderly: pacemakers and drugs. *Geriatrics* 1986; 41(2):61–72.
103. Amery A, Berthaux P, Birkenhager W, Bulpitt C, Clement D, De Schaepdryver A, Dollery C, Ernould H, Fagard R, Forette F, Hellermans J, Kho T, Lund-Johansen P, Meurice J, Pierguin L: Antihypertensive therapy in elderly patients. Pilot trial of the European Working Party on High Blood Pressure in the Elderly. *Gerontology* 1977; 23:426–437.
104. Ostfeld AM: Elderly hypertensive patient: epidemiologic review. *NY State J Med* 1978; 78:1125–1129.
105. Koch-Weser J: Arterial hypertension in old age. *Herz* 1978; 3:235–244.
106. Veterans Administration Co-operative Study Group on Antihypertensive Agents: Effects of treatment on morbidity in hypertension. II. Results in patients with diastolic blood pressure averaging 90 through 114 mm Hg. *JAMA* 1970; 213:1143–1152.
107. Kannel WB, Castelli WP, McNamara PM, McKee PA, Feinleib M: Role of blood pressure in the development of congestive heart failure: The Framingham study. *N Engl J Med* 1972; 287:781–787.
108. Kannel WB, Gordon T: Evaluation of cardiovascular risk in the elderly: The Framingham study. *Bull NY Acad Med* 1978; 54:573–591.
109. Rowe JW: Systolic hypertension in the elderly. *N Engl J Med* 1983; 309:1246–1247.
110. Colandrea MA, Friedman GD, Nichaman MZ, Lynd CN: Systolic hypertension in the elderly: an epidemiologic assessment. *Circulation* 1970; 41:239–245.
111. Lindholm L, Schersten B, Thulin T: Letters to the editor; *Lancet* 1983; 2:745–746.
112. Rajala S, Haavisto M, Heikinheimo R, Mattila K: Blood pressure and mortality in the very old. *Lancet* 1983; 2:520–521.
113. Burch PRJ: Blood pressure and mortality in the very old. *Lancet* 1983; 2:852–853.
114. Burch PRJ: Ischemic heart disease: epidemiology, risk factors and cause. *Cardiovasc Res* 1980; 14:307–338.
115. MacLennan WJ: Letter to the editor; *Lancet* 1983; 2:746.
116. Coope JR: Letter to the editor; *Lancet* 1983; 2:746.
117. Koch-Weser J: The therapeutic challenge of systolic hypertension. *N Engl J Med* 1973; 289:481–483.
118. Simon AC, Safar MA, Levenson JA, Kheder AM, Levy BI: Systolic hypertension: hemodynamic mechanism and choice of antihypertensive treatment. *Am J Cardiol* 1979; 44:505–511.
119. Koch-Weser J: Correlation of pathophysiology and pharmacotherapy in primary hypertension. *Am J Cardiol* 1973; 32:499–510.
120. Vardan S, Mookherjee S, Warner R, Smulyan H: Systolic hypertension in the elderly: hemodynamic response to long-term thiazide diuretic therapy and its side effects. *JAMA* 1983; 250:2807–2813.
121. Chobanian AV: Pathophysiologic considerations in the treatment of the elderly hypertensive patient. *Am J Cardiol* 1983; 52:49D–53D.
122. Messerli FH, Sundgaard-Riise K, Ventura HO, Dunn FG, Glade LB, Frohlich ED: Essential hypertension in the elderly: hemodynamics, intravascular volume, plasma renin activity and circulating catecholamine levels. *Lancet* 1983; 2:983–985.
123. Hammond EC: Coronary heart disease, stroke and aortic aneurysm. *Arch Eviron Health* 1969; 19:167–182.
124. Pathy MS: Clinical presentation of myocardial infarction in the elderly. *Br Heart J* 1967; 29:190–199.
124a. Heller GV, Blaustein AS, Wei JY: Implications of elevated myocardial isoenzymes in the presence of normal serum creatinine kinase activity. *Am J Cardiol* 1983; 51:24–27.
125. Chaturved NC, Walsh MJ, Shivalingappa G, Scaria K, Shanks B, Lynas P, Mckay A, Courtney D, Cumming K, Barber JM, Boyle DM: Myocardial infarction in the elderly. *Lancet* 1972; 1:280–281.
126. Elayda MA, Hall RJ, Gray AG, Mathur VS, Cooley DA: Coronary revascularization in the elderly patient. *J Am Coll Cardiol* 1984; 3:1398–1402.
126a. Loop FD, Golding LR, Cosgrove DM, Lytle BW, Estafanous FG: Coronary bypass surgery in the elderly. *Geriatr Med Today* 1985; 4:55–67.
127. Knapp WS, Douglas JS Jr, Craver JM, Jones EL, King SB, Bone DK, Bradford JM, Hatcher CR: Efficacy of coronary artery bypass grafting in elderly patients with coronary artery disease. *Am J Cardiol* 1981; 47:923–930.
128. Faro RS, Golden MD, Javid H, Serry C, DeLaria GA, Monson D, Weinberg M, Hunter JA, Najafi H: Coronary revascularization in septuagenarians. *J Thorac Cardiovasc Surg* 1983; 86:616–620.
128a. Gersh BJ, Kronmal RA, Schaff HV, Frye RL, Ryan TJ, Mock MB, Myers WO, Athearn MW, Gosselin AJ, Kaiser GC, Bourassa MG, Killip T: Comparison of coronary artery bypass surgery and medical therapy in patients 65 years of age or older: a nonrandomized study from the Coronary Artery Surgery Study (CASS) Registry. *N Engl J Med* 1985; 313:217–224.
129. Gruentzig A: Transluminal dilatation of coronary-artery stenosis. *Lancet* 1978; 1:263.
130. Mock MB, Holmes DR Jr, Vlietstra RE, Gersh BJ, Detre KM, Kelsey SF, Orszulak TA, Schaff HV, Piehier JM, VanRaden MJ, Passamani ER, Kent KM, Gruentzig AR: Percutaneous transluminal coronary angioplasty (PTCA) in the elderly patient: experience in the National Heart, Lung and Blood Institute PTCA Registry. *Am J Cardiol* 1984; 53:89C-91C.
130a. Raizner AE, Hust RG, Lewis JM, Winters WL Jr, Batty JW, Roberts R: Transluminal coronary angioplasty in the elderly. *Am J Cardiol* 1986; 57:29–32.
131. Jones EL, Craver JM, Guyton RA, Bone DK, Hatcher CR Jr: Trends in the treatment of coronary disease today: selective use of PTCA and bypass surgery. *Ann Surg* 1983; 197:728–736.
132. Pomerance A: Pathogenesis of aortic stenosis and its relation to age. *Br Heart J* 1972; 34:569–574.
133. Devision TE, Friedman SA, Significance of systolic murmurs in the aged. *N Engl J Med* 1968; 279:225–230.
134. Caird FI: Valvular heart disease, in Caird FI, Dall JLC, Kennedy RD (eds): *Cardiology in Old Age.* New York, Plenum Press, 1976, pp 231–247.
135. Glancy DL, Freed TA, O'Brien KP, Epstein SE: Calcium in the aortic valve: roentgenologic and hemodynamic correlations in 148 patients. *Ann Intern Med* 1969; 71:245–250.
136. Davis MA, Taylor JL: The risk of catheterization in elderly patients. *Clin Res* 1981; 29:810A.
137. St. John Sutton MG, St. John Sutton M, Oldershaw P, Sacchetti R, Paneth M, Lennox SC, Gibson RV, Gibson DG: Valve replacement without preoperative cardiac catheterization. *N Engl J Med* 1981; 305:1233–1238.
138. Parisi AF, Folland ED: Are non-invasive tests sufficient for preoperative evaluation of aortic stenosis? *J Am Coll Cardiol* 1984; 3:1092–1095.
139. Berman ND, David TE, Lipton IH, Lenkei SC: Surgical procedures involving cardiopulmonary bypass in patients aged 70 or older. *J Am Geriatr Soc* 1980; 28:29–32.
140. Jamieson WRE, Thompson DM, Munro AI: Cardiac valve replacement in elderly patients. *Can Med Assoc J* 1980; 123:628–632.
140a. Cheng TO: Some new observations on the syndrome of papillary muscle dysfunction. *Am J Med* 1969; 47:924–945.
141. Kolibash AJ, Bush CA, Fontana MB, Ryan JM, Kilman J, Wooley CF: Mitral valve prolapse: analysis of 62 patients aged 60 years and older. *Am J Cardiol* 1983; 52:534–539.
142. Guillet P, Baconnet C, Labrousee A, Aigueparse I, Andre A, Grosgogeat Y, Laurenceau JL, Temkine J, Vanetti A: Left atrial myxoma in the elderly: diagnosis by M-mode and bidimensional echocardiography. *J Am Geriatr Soc* 1981; 29:453–459.
143. Lachman AS, Roberts WC: Calcific deposits in stenotic mitral valves: extent and relation to age, sex, degree of stenosis, cardiac rhythm,

previous commissurotomy and left atrial body thrombus from study of 164 operatively-excised valves. *Circulation* 1978; 57:808–815.

143a. Wei QM, Kusagawa M: Heart valve surgery in geriatric patients. *Natl Med J China* 1985; 65:87–90.

143b. Rich MW, Sandza JG, Kleiger RE, Connors JP: Cardiac operations in patients over 80 years of age. *J Thorac Cardiovasc Surg* 1985; 90:56–60.

144. Thomas FB, Mazzaferri EL, Skillman TG: Apathetic thyrotoxicosis: a distinctive clinical and laboratory entity. *Ann Intern Med* 1970; 72:679–685.

145. Forfar JC, Miller HC, Toft AD: Occult thyrotoxicosis: a correctable cause of 'idiopathic' atrial fibrillation. *Am J Cardiol* 1979; 44:9–12.

146. Von Reyn CF, Levy BS, Arbeit RD, Friedland G, Crumpacker CS: Infective endocarditis. An analysis based on strict case definition. *Ann Intern Med* 1981; 94:505–518.

147. Weinstein L, Rubin RH: Infective endocarditis—1973. *Prog Cardiovasc Dis* 1973; 16:239–274.

148. Wedgwood J: Remediable heart disease, in Caird FI, Dall JCL, Kennedy RD (eds): *Cardiology in Old Age.* New York, Plenum Press, 1976, pp 249–265.

149. Churchill MA, Geraci JE, Hunder GG: Musculoskeletal manifestations of bacterial endocarditis. *Ann Intern Med* 1977; 87:754–759.

150. Zeman FD: Subacute bacterial endocarditis. *Am Heart J* 1945; 29:661–684.

151. Gleckler WJ: Diagnostic aspects of subacute bacterial endocarditis in the elderly. *Arch Intern Med* 1958; 102:761–765.

152. Wallach JB, Glass M, Lukash L, Angrist AA: Bacterial endocarditis in the aged. *Ann Intern Med* 1955; 42:1206–1223.

153. Thell R, Martin FH, Edwards JE: Bacterial endocarditis in subjects 60 years of age and older. *Circulation* 1975; 51:174–182.

154. Weinstein L: Infective endocarditis, in Braunwald E (ed): *Heart Disease: A Textbook of Cardiovascular Medicine*, ed 2. Toronto, Saunders, 1984, pp 1136–1182.

155. Melvin ET, Berger M, Lutzker LG, Goldberg E, Mildvan D: Noninvasive methods for detection of valve vegetations in infective endocarditis. *Am J Cardiol* 1981; 47:271–278.

156. Stewart JA, Silimperi D, Harris P, Wise NK, Fraker TD, Kisslo JA: Echocardiographic documentation of vegetative lesions in infective endocarditis: clinical implications. *Circulation* 1980; 61:374–380.

157. Parrott JCW, Hill JD, Kerth WJ, Gerbode F: The surgical management of bacterial endocarditis: a review. *Ann Surg* 1976; 183:289–292.

158. Saphir O: Nonrheumatic inflammatory diseases of the heart. C Myocarditis, in Gould SE (ed): *Pathology of the Heart.* Springfield, Charles C Thomas, 1953, pp 784–835.

159. Surawicz B, Lasseter KC: Electrocardiogram in pericarditis. *Am J Cardiol* 1970; 26:471–474.

160. Connolly DC, Burchell HB: Pericarditis: a ten year survey. *Am J Cardiol* 1961; 7:7–14.

161. Klacsmann PG, Bulkley BH, Hutchins GM: The changed spectrum of purulent pericarditis: an 86 year autopsy experience in 200 patients. *Am J Med* 1977; 63:666–673.

162. Whiting RD, Powell WJ Jr, Dinsmore RE, Sanders CA: Idiopathic hypertrophic subaortic stenosis in the elderly. *N Engl J Med* 1971; 285:196–200.

163. Hamby RI, Aintablian A: Hypertrophic subaortic stenosis is not rare in the eighth decade. *Geriatrics* 1976; 31:71–74.

164. Krasnow N, Stein RA; Hypertrophic cardiomyopathy in the aged. *Am Heart J* 1978; 96:326–336.

165. Koch JP, Maron BJ, Epstein SE, Morrow AG: Results of operation for obstructive hypertrophic cardiomyopathy in the elderly: septal myotomy and myectomy in 20 patients 65 years of age or older. *Am J Cardiol* 1980; 46:963–966.

166. Burrows B, Niden AH, Barclay WR, Kasik JE: Chronic obstructive lung disease. 1. Clinical and physiologic findings in 175 patients and their relationship to age and sex. *Am Rev Resp Dis* 1965; 91:521–540.

167. Hanley T: Pulmonary heart disease, in Caird FI, Dall JLC, Kennedy RD (eds): *Cardiology in Old Age.* New York, Plenum Press, 1976, pp 209–230.

168. Burrows B, Earle RH: Course and prognosis of chronic obstructive lung disease: a prospective study of 200 patients. *N Engl J Med* 1969; 208:397–404.

169. Fishman AP: Chronic cor pulmonale. *Am Rev Resp Dis* 1976; 114:775–794.

170. Loeffler E: Unusual malformation of left atrium: pulmonary sinus. *Arch Pathol* 1949; 48:371–376.

171. Coulshed N, Littler TR: Atrial septal defect in the aged. *Br Med J* 1957; 1:76–80.

172. Pouget JM, Kelly CE, Pilz CG: Congenital absence of the pulmonic valve: report of a case in a 73 year old man. *Am J Cardiol* 1967; 19:732–734.

173. Perloff JK, Lindgren KM: Adult survival in congenital heart disease. Part I. Common defects with expected adult survival. *Geriatrics* 1974; 29:94–104.

174. Perloff JK, Lindgren KM: Adult survival in congenital heart disease. Part 2. Uncommon defects with expected adult survival. *Geriatrics* 1974; 29:99–109.

175. Perloff JK, Lindgren KM: Adult survival in congenital heart disease. Part 3. Common and uncommon defects with exceptional adult survival. *Geriatrics* 1974; 29:93–102.

176. Haldane JH: Coarctation of the aorta in an elderly man. *Can Med Assoc J* 1983; 128:1298–1299.

177. Shook TL, Kirshenbaum JM, Hundley RF, Shorey JM, Lamas GA: Ethanol intoxication complicating intravenous nitroglycerine therapy. *Ann Intern Med* 1984; 101:498–499.

178. Shorey J, Bhardwaj N, Loscalzo J: Acute Wernicke's encephalopathy after intravenous infusion of high-dose nitroglycerine. *Ann Intern Med* 1984; 101:500.

78 Environmental Factors Affecting the Heart

Wilbert S. Aronow, MD, FACC

TOBACCO SMOKING

Numerous studies have documented that cigarette smoking is a risk factor contributing to the pathogenesis of coronary heart disease (CHD). Cigarette smoking is associated with an increased mortality from CHD (Table 78.1) and with a higher incidence of myocardial infarction (MI) (Table 78.2).[1-9] Men and women cigarette smokers also have an increased incidence of sudden death from CHD as compared with nonsmokers.[10-12] In addition, cigarette smokers who stop smoking have a lower incidence of MI and death from CHD than do those who continue smoking.[2,5,9,10,13,14] Furthermore, autopsy studies have demonstrated an association between cigarette smoking and coronary atherosclerosis, even in men without a history of clinical CHD.[15,16] Cigarette smokers also have a higher risk of developing peripheral vascular disease than of developing CHD.[17]

Increased exposure to cigarette smoke from smoking more cigarettes daily, for a greater number of years, with an increased depth of inhalation, and from an earlier age of beginning smoking increases the risk of developing CHD.[3,14] Cigarette smoking acts synergistically with other coronary risk factors, especially hypercholesterolemia and hypertension, to greatly increase the risk of developing CHD.[17a] The greater the tobacco consumption and the number and severity of other coronary risk factors, including hyperlipidemia, hypertension, diabetes mellitus, marked obesity, and sedentary living, the greater the risk of developing CHD. The risk of nonfatal MI among women of childbearing age is increased approximately two times by the use of estrogen-containing contraceptives. Cigarette smoking in women who use estrogen-containing contraceptives increases the incidence of nonfatal MI approximately ten times.[18,19] Cigarette smoking is associated with decreased serum high-density lipoprotein cholesterol in men and women.[20,20a]

Cigar and pipe smokers have a smaller increase in risk of CHD than do cigarette smokers. However, in one large study, the risk of developing CHD was 1.82 times greater in male cigar and pipe smokers than in nonsmokers and 2.14 times greater in male cigarette smokers than in nonsmokers.[9] Wald et al[21] found that the relative risk of developing CHD or intermittent claudication was 21.2 times greater in persons with carboxyhemoglobin levels of 5% or greater than in persons with carboxyhemoglobin levels below 3%. The magnitude of risk was not significantly different for different types of tobacco. Gyntelberg et al[22] found that the relative risk of developing MI was 4.2 in Danish cheroot smokers compared with 2.1 in cigarette smokers. Because they tend to inhale less smoke, pipe and cigar smokers may have a smaller increase in risk of CHD than do cigarette smokers. The tendency of some smokers who have switched from cigarettes to cigars and pipes to continue to inhale the smoke may eliminate the decrease in risk of CHD that might be expected after switching to cigars and pipes from cigarettes.

An association between cigarette smoking and the incidence of angina pectoris has been demonstrated in some studies.[9,23-25] Cigarette smoking also aggravates angina.[26-30] Patients with angina who stop smoking experience fewer anginal attacks and can perform more exercise before developing angina. Smoking high-nicotine cigarettes aggravates exercise-induced angina more than does smoking low-nicotine cigarettes.[26,27] Smoking low-nicotine cigarettes aggravates exercise-induced angina more than does smoking nonnicotine cigarettes.[27,31] Patients develop angina sooner after exercise following cigarette smoking for at least three reasons: (1)

Table 78.1. Coronary Heart Disease Mortality Ratios Related to Cigarette Smoking

Study	Cigarettes Smoked Daily	Mortality Ratio	Follow-up (Yr)	Comments
Hammond,[1] 1964	None	1.00	3	Men aged 40–59 yr
	1–9	1.95		
	10–19	2.42		
	20–39	2.65		
	40 +	3.00		
Doyle et al,[2] 1964	None	1.00	10	Men aged 40–49 yr
	All smokers	2.40		
	> 20	3.50		
Doll and Peto,[3] 1976	None	1.00	20	British male physicians
	1–14	1.47		
	15–24	1.58		
	25 +	1.92		
Pooling Project,[4] 1978	None	1.00	8.6	Men aged 40–59 yr
	20	1.70		
	> 20	3.00		
Friedman et al,[5] 1979	None	1.00	11	Women and men aged 35–54 yr
	All smokers (men)	4.85		
	All smokers (women)	5.42		
Doll et al,[6] 1980	None	1.00	22	British female physicians
	1–14	0.97		
	15–24	2.20		
	25 +	2.12		

nicotine causes an increase in myocardial oxygen demand,[26,27,29,32–34] (2) carboxyhemoglobin causes a decrease in oxygen delivery to the myocardium,[28–30,35–37] and (3) tobacco components other than nicotine or carbon monoxide cause a small reduction in oxygen delivery to the myocardium.[30]

NICOTINE

Smoking high-nicotine cigarettes increases resting systolic and diastolic blood pressure and resting heart rate but does not change systolic ejection period, thereby increasing the myocardial oxygen demand.[26,27,29,32–34] This increase in resting systolic and diastolic blood pressure and in resting heart rate does not occur after smoking nonnicotine cigarettes[28,30,31] and is greater after smoking high-nicotine cigarettes than after smoking low-nicotine cigarettes.[32]

Nicotine increases heart rate and systolic and diastolic arterial pressure by releasing norepinephrine locally from adrenergic axon terminals within the cardiovascular system[38] and by increasing catecholamine discharge from the adrenal medulla and from chromaffin tissue in the heart. Nicotine also acts on chemoreceptors in the carotid and aortic bodies, reflexly causing increases in arterial pressure and heart rate. In addition, nicotine acts directly on the myocardium, inducing positive inotropic and chronotropic effects.

Nicotine may induce ventricular arrhythmias in smokers. In canine papillary and trabecular muscle, nicotine causes simultaneous enhancement of ectopic pacemaker activity and slowed conduction in both Purkinje and ventricular fibers, predisposing to ventricular arrhythmia.[39] Inhalation of cigarette smoke caused a 30% to 40% reduction in ventricular fibrillation threshold in dogs with acute MI and in normal dogs.[40] Nicotine also increases platelet stickiness and aggregation, thereby increasing a thrombotic tendency.[41] In animal experiments, nicotine in amounts much higher than the nicotine uptake by a smoker does not cause coronary atherosclerosis.[42]

Both nicotine and carbon monoxide contribute to the

Table 78.2. Coronary Heart Disease Morbidity Ratios Related to Cigarette Smoking

Study	Cigarettes Smoked Daily	Morbidity Ratio	Follow-up (Yr)	Comments
Doyle et al,[2] 1964	None	1.00	10	Men aged 40–49 yr
	All smokers	2.36		
	> 20	3.04		
Jenkins et al,[7] 1968	None	1.00	4.5	Men aged 39–59 yr
	> 16	3.06		
Stamler et al,[8] 1966	None	1.00	4	Men aged 40–49 yr
	> 20	3.83		
Shapiro et al,[9] 1969	None	1.00	3	Men and women aged 35–64 yr
	All smokers (men)	2.14		
	All smokers (women)	2.00		
	> 20 (men)	2.33		
	> 20 (women)	1.77		
Pooling Project,[4] 1978	None	1.00	8.6	Men aged 40–59 yr
	10	1.79		
	20	2.07		
	> 20	3.16		

increase in nonfatal and fatal MI and sudden death in cigarette smokers. Nicotine may do so by (1) increasing the myocardial oxygen demand but not the myocardial oxygen supply during an episode of myocardial ischemia, (2) increasing platelet adhesiveness, and (3) decreasing the threshold for ventricular fibrillation during an episode of myocardial ischemia.

CARBON MONOXIDE

Smoking high-nicotine, low-nicotine, or nonnicotine cigarettes raises the carboxyhemoglobin level, decreasing the amount of oxygen available to the myocardium.[28-30,32,34] The increase in carboxyhemoglobin in the smoker is a result of incomplete combustion of any organic material in the cigarette. The carbon contained therein is oxidized to carbon monoxide and inhaled in the gaseous phase along with the other volatile products of smoking. As cigarette smoke exposes the pulmonary capillary blood to at least 400 ppm of carbon monoxide, smokers who inhale develop high carboxyhemoglobin levels.

As the affinity of hemoglobin for carbon monoxide is approximately 245 times greater than its affinity for oxygen, carbon monoxide displaces oxygen from hemoglobin, reducing the amount of oxygen available to the myocardium. Acute elevation of the venous carboxyhemoglobin level from 0.98% to 8.96% in patients with heart disease caused a 20% average decrease in mixed venous oxygen tension.[43,44] This greater decrease in mixed venous oxygen tension relative to the increase in venous carboxyhemoglobin level resulted from a leftward shift of the oxyhemoglobin dissociation curve. Tighter binding of oxygen to hemoglobin in the presence of carboxyhemoglobin further decreased the availability of oxygen to the myocardium. The increased carboxyhemoglobin level caused an increase in coronary blood flow in their patients with noncoronary heart disease but not in their patients with CHD.[43,44] The increased carboxyhemoglobin level also caused a reduction in myocardial oxygen extraction and myocardial oxygen, lactate, and pyruvate extraction ratios in their patients with CHD and with noncoronary heart disease, but the myocardial lactate extraction ratio changed to lactate production only in their patients with CHD.[43,44]

Carbon monoxide also combines with myoglobin and can impair the facilitated diffusion of oxygen to mitochondria.[45] In addition, carbon monoxide combines directly with cytochrome oxidase (a_3), slowing oxidation of reduced nicotinamide-adenine-dinucleotide.[46]

Increased carboxyhemoglobin levels after smoking in patients with angina cause a decrease in the product of systolic blood pressure (SBP) times heart rate (HR) at the onset of angina, an indirect index of myocardial oxygen delivery.[28-30] Increased carboxyhemoglobin levels after smoking cause exercise-induced ischemic ST-segment depression to develop earlier in patients with angina, after less exercise and at a lower SBP × HR at the onset of angina.[28-30] Because patients with angina due to CHD cannot have an adequate increase in coronary blood flow with exercise, and because an increased carboxyhemoglobin level makes less oxygen available for delivery to the myocardium, the patients' myocardial oxygen demand exceeds their myocardial oxygen supply, inducing angina earlier and after less myocardial work.

The hemodynamic effects of breathing tobacco smoke or carbon monoxide in patients with angina were studied during cardiac catheterization.[34] Three standard-brand nonfilter cigarettes containing 1.8 mg of nicotine were smoked within 50 minutes. One week later, the patients breathed carbon monoxide 150 ppm to produce an increase in coronary sinus carboxyhemoglobin level similar to that observed after smoking three cigarettes. The results indicated an increase in systolic and diastolic arterial pressure and heart rate after smoking attributable to nicotine, and a decrease in stroke index and an increase in left ventricular end-diastolic pressure caused by carbon monoxide.

Carbon monoxide increases platelet adhesiveness, thereby increasing a thrombotic tendency.[47] Carbon monoxide also reduces the ventricular fibrillation threshold, predisposing patients with CHD to sudden death.[48-50] Inhalation of carbon monoxide to increase the arterial carboxyhemoglobin level to 10.2% enhanced ventricular fibrillation in monkeys with acute MI.[48] Inhalation of carbon monoxide to increase arterial carboxyhemoglobin level to 6.5% caused a reduction in ventricular fibrillation threshold in dogs with acute MI and in normal dogs.[49,50] Carbon monoxide may contribute to the increase in nonfatal and fatal MI and sudden death in cigarette smokers (1) by interfering with myocardial oxygen delivery, aggravating an episode of myocardial ischemia,[51] (2) by its negative inotropic effect, (3) by increasing platelet adhesiveness, and (4) by reducing the threshold for ventricular fibrillation during an episode of myocardial ischemia.

Animal experiments on atherogenesis and carbon monoxide have provided conflicting data. Lipid synthesis and cholesterol uptake in vitro were measured in perfused human coronary arteries obtained at autopsy.[52] Nicotine failed to influence cholesterol uptake or lipid synthesis, and carbon monoxide did not influence lipid synthesis in the arterial wall. However, carbon monoxide led to a marked increase in cholesterol uptake in perfused human coronary arteries, regardless of the concentration of carbon monoxide in the perfused fluid.

Carboxyhemoglobin levels in tobacco smokers correlate better than the smoking history with the development of MI, angina, and intermittent claudication.[21] However, the higher levels of carboxyhemoglobin may also reflect the absorption of other constituents of tobacco smoke in addition to carbon monoxide. Nonsmoking foundry workers exposed to carbon monoxide have a high prevalence of CHD.[53] The prevalence of angina in foundry workers showed a clear dose response relation with regard to carbon monoxide exposure from either smoking, occupation, or both.

OTHER TOBACCO COMPONENTS

Tobacco smoke contains more than 4,000 components. In addition to nicotine and carbon monoxide, other components including carbon disulfide, hydrogen cyanide, oxides of nitrogen, and cadmium may contribute to CHD. Carbon disulfide has been suggested as the risk factor responsible for the increased incidence of CHD in viscose rayon factory workers.[54]

A greater reduction in exercise duration until the onset of angina was demonstrated after smoking nonnicotine cigarettes (−45%) than after breathing carbon monoxide (−35%).[30] A greater decrease in SBP × HR at the onset of angina was also observed after smoking nonnicotine cigarettes (−23%) than after breathing carbon monoxide (−18%). These data indicate that tobacco components other than nicotine or carbon monoxide cause a small decrease in exercise duration until angina and a small probable decrease in oxygen supply to the myocardium. Further research is needed to investigate the cardiovascular effects of concentrations of hydrogen cyanide, oxides of nitrogen, carbon disulfide, cadmium, and other components inhaled in tobacco smoke. Coronary vascular reserve is less in chronic tobacco smokers than in nonsmokers.[55] Cigarette smoking also acutely increases coronary resistance in patients with CHD.[56] Further research is needed to determine the mechanism of these adverse effects on coronary circulation induced by smoking.

NO SAFE CIGARETTE

Smokers of filter cigarettes do not have a lower incidence of CHD than do smokers of nonfilter cigarettes.[57] Young men who smoke cigarettes with decreased amounts of nicotine and carbon monoxide do not have a lower risk of MI than do those smoking cigarettes with increased amounts of nicotine and carbon monoxide.[58] Smokers of low-nicotine cigarettes usually inhale more deeply, increasing exposure to the various harmful components of smoke.[59] There is no safe level of smoking. Both nicotine and carbon monoxide cause harmful effects on the cardiovascular system, and these effects may be critical in patients with cardiovascular disease.[60] Because there is no known safe level of either nicotine or carbon monoxide in the cardiovascular system, the best advice for those with cardiovascular disease is to stop smoking tobacco[60] completely, not only cigarettes,[60a] but also pipes and cigars.[60b]

PASSIVE SMOKING AND ANGINA PECTORIS

Passive smoking in patients with angina increases resting systolic and diastolic blood pressure, heart rate, and venous carboxyhemoglobin; decreases SBP × HR at the onset of angina; and reduces exercise duration until the onset of angina.[61] These changes were greater in an unventilated room than in a well-ventilated room. In some patients, premature ventricular complexes developed after exercise following exposure to passive smoking in an unventilated room. A prospective study has also demonstrated that passive smoking causes an increase in mortality from ischemic heart disease.[61a] Passive smoking causes increased venous carboxyhemoglobin levels,[61] increased blood[62] and urinary nicotine[62,63] levels, and increased urinary cotinine levels[63,64] in nonsmokers.

MARIJUANA SMOKING

The long-term effects of smoking marijuana on the risks of developing cardiovascular disease are unknown. However, smoking marijuana increases the resting SBP × HR and venous carboxyhemoglobin, decreases the SBP × HR at the onset of angina, and reduces the exercise time until the onset of angina.[29,65] Smoking one marijuana cigarette decreases the exercise time until the onset of angina more (−50%) than does smoking one high-nicotine cigarette (−23%).[29] Smoking marijuana also causes a decrease in stroke index and in left ventricular ejection fraction in patients with CHD.[66]

AIR POLLUTION

CARBON MONOXIDE

Heavy atmospheric carbon monoxide pollution increases carboxyhemoglobin levels. A major source of carbon monoxide in the urban atmosphere is automobile exhaust in which carbon monoxide emission is highest during idling and deceleration. Peak atmospheric carbon monoxide exposures have been reported as high as 147 ppm in Los Angeles freeway traffic, 141 ppm in New York expressway traffic, 135 ppm at traffic intersections in Dayton, Ohio, and 217 ppm for one hour in a tollbooth at the Queens midtown tunnel in New York. Exposure to heavy freeway traffic increases carboxyhemoglobin levels and causes patients with angina to have a reduction in exercise time until the onset of anginal pain associated with a decrease in SBP × HR at the onset of angina.[35]

Three double-blind, randomized studies have demonstrated that exposure to carbon monoxide in concentrations found during heavy atmospheric carbon monoxide pollution aggravates exercise-induced angina.[36,37,67] Double-blind, randomized studies have also shown that exposure to carbon monoxide in concentrations found during heavy atmospheric carbon monoxide pollution shortens exercise time until the onset of intermittent claudication in patients with intermittent claudication of the calf or thigh due to iliofemoral occlusive arterial disease,[68] reduces exercise time until the onset of marked dyspnea in patients with chronic obstructive pulmonary disease,[69] and decreases exercise time until the onset of marked fatigue in patients with chronic anemia.[70] Hypoxia induced by high altitude would increase adverse health effects due to carbon monoxide exposure in susceptible patients.

An association between community carbon monoxide concentrations and mortality was observed in Los Angeles County.[71] An association between atmospheric carbon monoxide pollution and case fatality rates for acute MI was demonstrated in patients admitted to 35 Los Angeles hospitals.[72] A higher death rate from acute MI occurred in hospitals in more polluted areas when the ambient carbon monoxide levels were above 7.7 ppm. Reductions in mortality from cardiovascular disease occurred in San Francisco County and Alameda County during the fuel crisis of 1974.[73] The ambient level of carbon monoxide in Denver was also shown to have a low level association with the frequency of acute cardiorespiratory complaints in a hospital emergency room.[74] Excessive numbers of cardiorespiratory complaints were seen above a carbon monoxide level of 5 ppm for the 24-hour mean and 11 ppm for the 1-hour mean maximum ambient carbon monoxide. These findings lead to the conclusion that carbon monoxide in the macroenvironment must be considered a risk factor for cardiopulmonary disease. Carbon monoxide exposure from heavy smoking or heavy atmospheric carbon monoxide pollution depresses the pump performance of the heart muscle in patients with CHD, aggravates angina, aggravates intermittent claudication of the calf or thigh, increases myocardial ischemia in patients with clinical and subclinical CHD, and contributes to an increased incidence of nonfatal and fatal MI and sudden death from CHD.

OTHER AIR POLLUTANTS

Acute episodes of heavy air pollution with increased concentrations of sulfur dioxide and particulates have caused mortality, especially in patients with cardiovascular or respiratory disease, in the Meuse Valley of Belgium in 1930, in Donora, Pennsylvania in 1948, in London in 1952,[75] in New York in 1953,[76] in London in 1962, and in Chicago in 1966.[77] Sulfur dioxide ambient levels measured in upper Manhattan during 1962 to 1966 correlated with the residual daily mortality in the New York metropolitan area.[78] Patients with cardiovascular disease should avoid exposure to heavy atmospheric pollution. Research is needed to determine the effects of low levels of atmospheric pollutants including oxidants, especially ozone,[79] oxides of sulfur, and oxides of nitrogen on cardiovascular performance in patients with CHD.

TRACE METALS, HEAT, AND COLD

Data relating a deficiency or an excessive intake of trace metals to the pathogenesis of CHD and to sudden death are conflicting. At this time, altering the hardness or trace metal content of drinking water in an attempt to reduce the incidence of CHD or sudden death cannot be recommended.

Performing exercise in a hot environment is stressful for the cardiovascular system. Heart rate is increased for the same workload, the ability to constrict peripheral cutaneous veins is decreased, the redistribution of blood volume to working muscles is impaired, central blood volume is diminished, stroke volume is reduced, and peak cardiac output, maximal oxygen consumption, and working capacity are decreased.[80] A hot, humid environment may precipitate congestive heart failure in patients with cardiovascular disease and compensated congestive heart failure. Patients with cardiovascular disease should avoid excessive exertion in a hot, humid environment.

A cold environment is well known to precipitate angina in patients with CHD. A cold environment or emotional stress may precipitate myocardial ischemia in patients with angina by adrenergic stimulation. Exposure of patients with CHD to cold at rest and during mild exercise caused an increased systemic vascular resistance, mean arterial blood pressure, and SBP $\times$ HR, indicating an increased myocardial oxygen demand in the presence of a restricted coronary reserve.[81] Exposure to cold also causes a reflex increase in coronary vascular resistance in patients with CHD.[82] Therefore, patients with angina should avoid excessive exertion in a cold environment and may need to take sublingual nitroglycerin before stepping out in a cold environment and an increased amount of antianginal drugs during cold weather.

NONCORONARY HEART DISEASE

SMOKING AND ETHANOL

Smoking is associated with diffuse hypokinesis independent of coronary artery disease in men younger than 55 years old, suggesting that smoking causes cardiomyopathy.[83] Ethanol aggravates exercise-induced angina pectoris,[84] may induce variant angina pectoris,[85] and causes in heavy drinkers a higher mortality from CHD and all cardiovascular diseases.[86] Ethanol also causes alcoholic cardiomyopathy with congestive heart failure and arrhythmias.[87] The effect of ethanol on the cardiovascular system is discussed in detail in chapter 50 on Nutritional Heart Disease.

PULMONARY HEART DISEASE

The most frequent cause of chronic cor pulmonale is chronic obstructive pulmonary emphysema. Cigarette smoking is the most important cause of chronic obstructive pulmonary emphysema. Passive smoking also causes adverse effects in small airways function in both children[88] and adults.[89] Tobacco smoking may have a cumulative or synergistic action with air pollution exposure in causing chronic obstructive pulmonary emphysema.[90] Exposure to asbestos fibers, silica dust, coal dust, granite dust, beryllium, cotton fibers, other dusts, or toxic chemicals in the form of gases and vapors affecting the lungs causes an increased incidence of chronic pulmonary disease which may lead to pulmonary hypertension and chronic cor pulmonale. This risk is increased further by cigarette smoking.

CHANGES IN ALTITUDE AND IONIZING RADIATION

Noncardiogenic pulmonary edema may develop in unacclimatized persons who ascend to altitudes in excess of 9,000 feet.[91] Physical exertion and cold weather exacerbate high altitude pulmonary edema, which is more common in persons under 21 years of age and in males. Some persons remaining at high altitudes lose their acclimatization and develop alveolar hypoventilation with chronic cor pulmonale.[92] Decompression sickness with intracardiac nitrogen bubbles may lead to syncope, hypotension, and shock from circulatory obstruction.

Therapeutic chest irradiation may induce heart damage with fibrosis of the pericardium, myocardium, and endocardium.[93] Occasionally, acute pericarditis may develop. Months or years after exposure to radiation therapy, chronic pericardial effusion or pericardial constriction may occur. Patients with radiation-induced myocardial fibrosis may develop refractory congestive heart failure. Therapeutic chest irradiation may also induce CHD.[94]

TOXIC OCCUPATIONAL EXPOSURES

Nonsmoking foundry workers exposed to carbon monoxide[53] and viscose rayon factory workers exposed to carbon disulfide[54] have an increased incidence of CHD. Firefighters may develop myocardial damage following marked exertion during heavy carbon monoxide exposure.[95] Organic phosphorus insecticides, many other chemical agents, and many drugs may cause cardiovascular toxicity by the mechanisms of cholinesterase inhibition, a direct toxic effect on the myocardium, interference with the oxygen-carrying capacity of the blood, or by causing hypersensitivity myocarditis. Occupational exposure to toxic gases or fumes may cause noncardiogenic pulmonary edema.

Munitions workers constantly exposed to nitroglycerin become nitrate dependent. Symptomatic nonatherosclerotic ischemic heart disease developed in 9 of 200 munitions workers when they were withdrawn from nitroglycerin exposure.[96] Other investigators have also demonstrated withdrawal syndromes with chest pain, acute myocardial infarction, and sudden death in workers chronically exposed to nitrate powder and vapor.

Fatalities have been reported from the abuse of consumer aerosol products[97] and misuse of aerosol bronchodilators through the mechanism of cardiac arrhythmia or arrest.[98] Fortunately, several years ago the use of fluorocarbons in consumer aerosol products was banned.

REFERENCES

1. Hammond EC: Smoking in relation to mortality and morbidity. Findings in first thirty-four months of follow-up in prospective study started in 1959. *J Natl Cancer Inst* 1964; 32:1161–1188.
2. Doyle JT, Dawber TR, Kannel WB, Kinch SH, Kahn HA: The relationship of cigarette smoking to coronary heart disease: the second report of the combined experience of Albany, NY, and Framingham, Mass. studies. *JAMA* 1964; 190:886–890.
3. Doll R, Peto R: Mortality in relation to smoking: 20 years' observations on male British doctors. *Br Med J* 1976; 2:1525–1536.
4. Pooling Project Research Group: Relationship of blood pressure, serum cholesterol, smoking habit, relative weight and ECG abnormalities to incidence of major coronary events: final report of the Pooling Project. *J Chron Dis* 1978; 31:201–306.
5. Friedman GD, Dales LG, Ury HK: Mortality in middle-aged smokers and nonsmokers. *N Engl J Med* 1979; 300:213–217.
6. Doll R, Gray R, Hafner B, Peto R: Mortality in relation to smoking: 22 years' observations on female British doctors. *Br Med J* 1980; 1:967–971.
7. Jenkins CD, Rosenman RH, Zyzanski SJ: Cigarette smoking: its relationship to coronary heart disease and related risk factors in the Western collaborative group study. *Circulation* 1968; 38:1140–1155.
8. Stamler J, Berkson DM, Levinson M, Lindberg HA, Majonnier L, Miller WA, Hall Y, Andelman SL: Coronary artery disease. Status of preventive efforts. *Arch Environ Health* 1966; 13:322–335.
9. Shapiro S, Weinblatt E, Frank CW, Sager RV: Incidence of coronary heart disease in a population insured for medical care (HIP): myocardial infarction, angina pectoris, and possible myocardial infarction. *Am J Public Health* 1969; 59(suppl): 1–101.
10. Inter-Society Commission for Heart Disease Resources. Atherosclerosis Study Group and Epidemiology Study Group: Primary prevention of the atherosclerotic diseases. *Circulation* 1970; 42:A54–A95.
11. Spain DM, Siegel H, Bradess VA: Women smokers and sudden death. The relationship of cigarette smoking to coronary disease. *JAMA* 1973; 224:1005–1007.
12. Doyle JT, Kannel WB, McNamara PM, Quickenton P, Gordon T: Factors related to suddenness of death from coronary disease: combined Albany-Framingham studies. *Am J Cardiol* 1976; 37:1073–1078.
13. Aberg A, Bergstrand R, Johansson S, Ulvenstam G, Vedin A, Wedel H, Wilhelmsson C, Wilhelmsen L: Cessation of smoking after myocardial infarction. Effects on mortality after 10 years. *Br Heart J* 1983; 44:416–422.
14. Hammond EC, Garfinkel L: I. Coronary heart disease, stroke, and aortic aneurysm. Factors in the etiology. *Arch Environ Health* 1969; 19:167–182.
15. Auerbach O, Carter HW, Garfinkel L, Hammond EC: Cigarette smoking and coronary artery disease: a macroscopic and microscopic study. *Chest* 1976; 70:697–705.
16. Strong JP, Richards ML: Cigarette smoking and atherosclerosis in autopsied men. *Atherosclerosis* 1976; 23:451–476.
17. Gordon T, Kannel WB: Predisposition to atherosclerosis in the head, heart, and legs. The Framingham study. *JAMA* 1972; 221:661–666.

17a. Ramsdale DR, Faragher EB, Bray CL, Bennett DH, Ward C, Beton DC: Smoking and coronary artery disease assessed by routine coronary arteriography. *Br Med J* 1985; 290:197–200.

18. Mann JI, Vessey MP, Thorogood M, Doll R: Myocardial infarction in young women with special reference to oral contraceptive practice. *Br Med J* 1975; 2:241–245.
19. Ory HW: Association between oral contraceptives and myocardial infarction. A review. *JAMA* 1977; 237:2619–2622.
20. Kannel WB: Update on the role of cigarette smoking in coronary artery disease. *Am Heart J* 1981; 101:319–328.

20a. Criqui MH, Cowan LD, Heiss G, Haskell WL, Laskarzewski PM, Chambless LE: Frequency and clustering of nonlipid coronary risk factors in dyslipoproteinemia. The Lipid Research Clinics Program Prevalence Study. *Circulation* 1986; 73:140–150.

21. Wald NJ, Howard S, Smith PG, Kjeldsen K: Association between atherosclerotic diseases and carboxyhemoglobin levels in tobacco smokers. *Br Med J* 1973; 1:761–765.
22. Gyntelberg F, Lauridsen L, Pedersen PB, Schubell K: Smoking and risk of myocardial infarction in Copenhagen men aged 40 to 59 with special reference to cheroot smoking. *Lancet* 1981; 1:987–989.
23. Mulcahy R, Hickey N: Cigarette smoking habits of patients with coronary heart disease. *Br Heart J* 1966; 28:404–408.
24. Reid DD, Hamilton PJS, McCartney P, Rose G, Jarrett RJ, Keen H: Smoking and other risk factors for coronary heart disease in British civil servants. *Lancet* 1976; 2:979–984.
25. Dawber TR: *The Framingham Study: The Epidemiology of Atherosclerotic Disease*. Cambridge, Harvard University Press, 1980, pp 1–267.
26. Aronow WS, Kaplan MA, Jacob D: Tobacco: a precipitating factor in angina pectoris. *Ann Intern Med* 1968; 69:529–536.
27. Aronow WS, Swanson AJ: The effect of low-nicotine cigarettes on angina pectoris. *Ann Intern Med* 1969; 71:599–609.
28. Aronow WS, Rokaw SN: Carboxyhemoglobin caused by smoking nonnicotine cigarettes: effects in angina pectoris. *Circulation* 1971; 44:782–788.
29. Aronow WS, Cassidy J: Effect of smoking marihuana versus a high-nicotine cigarette on angina pectoris. *Clin Pharmacol Ther* 1975; 17:549–554.
30. Aronow WS: Effect of non-nicotine cigarettes and carbon monoxide on angina. *Circulation* 1980; 61:262–265.
31. Aronow WS, Swanson AJ: Non-nicotinized cigarettes and angina pectoris. *Ann Intern Med* 1969; 70:1227.
32. Aronow WS, Dendinger J, Rokaw SN: Heart rate and carbon monoxide level after smoking high-, low-, and non-nicotine cigarettes: a study in male patients with angina pectoris. *Ann Intern Med* 1971; 74:697–702.
33. Aronow WS, Goldsmith JR, Kern JC, Cassidy J, Nelson WH, Johnson LL, Adams W: Effect of smoking cigarettes on cardiovascular hemodynamics. *Arch Environ Health* 1974; 28:330–332.
34. Aronow WS, Cassidy J, Vangrow JS, March H, Kern JC, Goldsmith JR, Khemka M, Pagano J, Vawter M: Effect of cigarette smoking and breathing carbon monoxide on cardiovascular hemodynamics in anginal patients. *Circulation* 1974; 50:340–347.
35. Aronow WS, Harris CN, Isbell MW, Rokaw SN, Imparato B: Effect of freeway travel on angina pectoris. *Ann Intern Med* 1972; 77:669–676.
36. Aronow WS, Isbell MW: Carbon monoxide effect on exercise-induced angina pectoris. *Ann Intern Med* 1973; 79:392–395.
37. Aronow WS: Aggravation of angina pectoris by two percent carboxyhemoglobin. *Am Heart J* 1981; 101:154–157.
38. Cryer PE, Haymond MW, Santiago JV, Shah SD: Norepinephrine and epinephrine release and adrenergic mediation of smoking: associated hemodynamic and metabolic events. *N Engl J Med* 1976; 295:573–577.
39. Greenspan K, Edmands RE, Knoebel SB, Fisch C: Some effects of nicotine on cardiac automaticity, conduction, and inotropy. *Arch Intern Med* 1969; 123:707–712.
40. Bellet S, Deguzman NT, Kostis JB, Roman L, Fleischmann D: The effect of inhalation of cigarette smoke on ventricular fibrillation threshold in normal dogs and dogs with acute myocardial infarction. *Am Heart J* 1972; 83:67–76.
41. Levine PH: An acute effect of cigarette smoking on platelet function: a possible link between smoking and arterial thrombosis. *Circulation* 1973; 48:619–623.
42. Schievelbein H, Londong V, Londong W, Grumbach H, Remplik V, Schauer A, Immich H: Nicotine and arteriosclerosis. *Z Klin Chem* 1970; 8:190–196.
43. Ayres SM, Mueller HS, Gregory JJ, Giannelli S Jr, Penny JL: Systemic and myocardial hemodynamic responses to relatively small concentrations of carboxyhemoglobin (COHB). *Arch Environ Health* 1969; 18:699–709.
44. Ayres SM, Giannelli S Jr, Mueller HS: Effect of low concentrations of carbon monoxide: myocardial and systemic responses to carboxyhemoglobin. *Ann NY Acad Sci* 1970; 174:268–293.
45. Wittenberg JB: The molecular mechanism of hemoglobin-facilitated oxygen diffusion. *J Biol Chem* 1966; 241:104–114.
46. Whereat AF: Is atherosclerosis a disorder of intramitochondrial respiration? *Ann Intern Med* 1970; 73:125–127.

47. Birnstingl MA, Brinson K, Chakrabarti BK: The effect of short-term exposure to carbon monoxide on platelet stickiness. *Br J Surg* 1971; 58:837–839.
48. DeBias DA, Banerjee CM, Birkhead NC, Greene CH, Scott D, Harrer WV: Effects of carbon monoxide inhalation on ventricular fibrillation. *Arch Environ Health* 1976; 31:38–42.
49. Aronow WS, Stemmer EA, Wood B, Zweig S, Tsao KP, Raggio L: Carbon monoxide and ventricular fibrillation threshold in dogs with acute myocardial injury. *Am Heart J* 1978; 95:754–756.
50. Aronow WS, Stemmer EA, Zweig S: Carbon monoxide and ventricular fibrillation threshold in normal dogs. *Arch Environ Health* 1979; 34:184–186.
51. DeBias DA, Banerjee CM, Birkhead NC, Harrer WV, Kazal LA: Carbon monoxide inhalation effects following myocardial infarction in monkeys. *Arch Environ Health* 1973; 27:161–167.
52. Tillmans H, Sarma ISM, Seeler K, Bing RI: Lipid metabolism in perfused human coronary arteries and saphenous veins, in Schettler G, Weizel A (eds): *Atherosclerosis*. New York, Springer-Verlag, 1974, vol 3, pp 118–125.
53. Hernberg S, Käräva R, Koskela R, Luoma K: Angina pectoris, ECG findings and blood pressure of foundry workers in relation to carbon monoxide exposure. *Scand J Work Environ Health* 1976; 2(suppl 1):54–63.
54. Davidson M, Feinleib M: Carbon disulfide poisoning: a review. *Am Heart J* 1972; 83:100–114.
55. Klein LW, Pichard AD, Holt J, Smith H, Gorlin R, Teichholz LE: Effects of chronic tobacco smoking on the coronary circulation. *J Am Coll Cardiol* 1983; 1:421–426.
56. Klein LW, Ambrose J, Pichard A, Holt J, Gorlin R, Teichholz LE: Acute coronary hemodynamic response to cigarette smoking in patients with coronary artery disease. *J Am Coll Cardiol* 1984; 3:879–886.
57. Castelli WP, Dawber TR, Feinleib M, Garrison RJ, McNamara PM, Kannel WB: The filter cigarette and coronary heart disease. The Framingham study. *Lancet* 1981; 2:109–113.
58. Kaufman DW, Helmrich SP, Rosenberg L, Miettinen OS, Shapiro S: Nicotine and carbon monoxide content of cigarette smoke and the risk of myocardial infarction in young men. *N Engl J Med* 1983; 308:409–413.
59. Herning RI, Jones RT, Bachman J, Mines AH: Puff volume increases when low-nicotine cigarettes are smoked. *Br Med J* 1981; 283:187–189.
60. McMillan GC, Aronow WS: Recommendations: sub-section B: Relation of smoke components to cardiovascular disease, in Wynder EL, Hoffman D, Gori GB (eds): *Smoking and Health. I. Modifying the Risk for the Smoker. Proceedings Third World Conference on Smoking and Health.* US Government Printing Office, 1976, pp 548–549.
60a. Oliver MF: Prevention of coronary heart disease—propaganda, promises, problems, and prospects. *Circulation* 1986; 73:1–9.
60b. Ockene JK, Goldberg RJ, Dalen JE: Pipes, cigars and cardiovascular health. *Cardiovasc Med* 1985; 10:53–55.
61. Aronow WS: Effect of passive smoking on angina pectoris. *N Engl J Med* 1978; 299:21–24.
61a. Garland C, Barrett-Connor E, Suarez L, Criqui MC, Wingard DL: Effects of passive smoking on ischemic heart disease mortality of nonsmokers. A prospective study. *Am J Epidemiol* 1985; 121:645–650.
62. Russell MAH, Feyerabend C: Blood and urinary nicotine in non-smokers. *Lancet* 1975; 1:179–181.
63. Greenberg RA, Haley NJ, Etzel RA, Loda FA: Measuring the exposure of infants to tobacco smoke. Nicotine and cotinine in urine and saliva. *N Engl J Med* 1984; 310:1075–1078.
64. Matsukura S, Taminato T, Kitano N, Seino T, Hamada H, Uchihashi M, Nakajima H, Hirata Y: Effects of environmental tobacco smoke on urinary cotinine excretion in nonsmokers. Evidence for passive smoking. *N Engl J Med* 1984; 311:828–832.
65. Aronow WS, Cassidy J: Effect of marihuana smoking on angina pectoris. *N Engl J Med* 1974; 291:65–67.
66. Prakash R, Aronow WS, Warren M, Laverty W, Gottschalk LA: Effects of marihuana and placebo marihuana smoking on hemodynamics in coronary disease. *Clin Pharmacol Therap* 1975; 18:90–95.
67. Anderson EW, Andelman RJ, Strauch J, Fortuin NJ, Knelson JH: Effect of low-level carbon monoxide exposure on onset and duration of angina pectoris. A study in ten patients with ischemic heart disease. *Ann Intern Med* 1973; 79:46–50.
68. Aronow WS, Stemmer EA, Isbell MW: Effect of carbon monoxide exposure on intermittent claudication. *Circulation* 1974; 49:415–417.
69. Aronow WS, Ferlinz J, Glauser F: Effect of carbon monoxide on exercise performance in chronic obstructive pulmonary disease. *Am J Med* 1977; 63:904–908.
70. Aronow WS, Schlueter WJ, Williams MA, Petratis M, Sketch MH: Aggravation of exercise performance in patients with anemia by 3% carboxyhemoglobin. *Environ Res* 1984; 35:394–398.
71. Hexter AC, Goldsmith JR: Carbon monoxide: association of community air pollution with mortality. *Science* 1971; 172:265–267.
72. Cohen SI, Deane M, Goldsmith JR: Carbon monoxide and survival from myocardial infarction. *Arch Environ Health* 1969; 19:510–517.
73. Brown SM, Marmot MG, Sacks ST, Kwok LW: Effect on mortality of the 1974 fuel crisis. *Nature* 1975; 257:306–307.
74. Kurt TL, Mogielnicki RP, Chandler JE, Hirst K: Ambient carbon monoxide levels and acute cardiorespiratory complaints. An exploratory study. *Am J Public Health* 1979; 69:360–363.
75. Logan WPD: Mortality in the London fog incident. *Lancet* 1953; 264:336–338.
76. Greenburg L, Jacobs MB, Drolette BM, Field F, Braverman MM: Report of an air pollution incident in New York City, November, 1953. *Public Health Rep* 1963; 78:1061–1064.
77. Carnow BW: Fossil fuel pollutants: current thinking and future needs. *Calif Air Environ*, Winter 1974; 4:6–7.
78. Buechley RW, Riggan WB, Hasselblad V, VanBruggen JB: SO_2 levels and perturbations in mortality. A study in the New York-New Jersey metropolis. *Arch Environ Health* 1973; 27:134–137.
79. Superko HR, Adams WC, Daly PW: Effects of ozone inhalation during exercise in selected patients with heart disease. *Am J Med* 1984; 77:463–470.
80. Rowell LB: Human cardiovascular adjustments to exercise and thermal stress. *Physiol Rev* 1974; 54:75–159.
81. Epstein SE, Stampfer M, Beiser GD, Goldstein RE, Braunwald E: Effects of a reduction in environmental temperature on the circulatory response to exercise in man. *N Engl J Med* 1969; 280:7–11.
82. Mudge GH Jr, Grossman W, Mills RM Jr, Lesch M, Braunwald E: Reflex increase in coronary vascular resistance in patients with ischemic heart disease. *N Engl J Med* 1976; 295:1333–1337.
83. Hartz AJ, Anderson AJ, Brooks HL, Manley JC, Parent GT, Barboriak JJ: The association of smoking with cardiomyopathy. *N Engl J Med* 1984; 311:1201–1206.
84. Orlando J, Aronow WS, Cassidy J, Prakash R: Effect of ethanol on angina pectoris. *Ann Intern Med* 1976; 84:652–655.
85. Takizawa A, Yasue H, Omote S, Nagao M, Hyon H, Nishida S, Horie M: Variant angina induced by alcohol ingestion. *Am Heart J* 1984; 107:25–27.
86. Dyer AR, Stamler J, Paul O, Berkson DM, Shekelle RB, Lepper MH, Mckean H, Lindberg HA, Garside D, Tokich T: Alcohol, cardiovascular risk factors and mortality: The Chicago experience. *Circulation* 1981; 64(suppl III):III-20–III-31.
87. Regan TJ, Haider B: Ethanol abuse and heart disease. *Circulation* 1981; 64(suppl III):III-14–III-19.
88. Tager IB, Weiss ST, Rosner B, Speizer FE: Effect of parental cigarette smoking on the pulmonary function of children. *Am J Epidemiol* 1979; 110:15–26.
89. White J, Froeb HF: Small-airways dysfunction in nonsmokers chronically exposed to tobacco smoke. *N Engl J Med* 1980; 302:720–723.
90. Wyatt JP: Environmental factors in chronic lung disease, in Lee DHK (ed): *Environmental Factors on Respiratory Disease. Fogarty International Center Proceedings No. 11.* New York, Academic Press, 1972, pp 119–137.
91. Hultgren HN: High altitude pulmonary edema. *Adv Cardiol* 1970; 5:24–31.
92. Penaloza D, Sime F: Chronic cor pulmonale due to loss of altitude acclimatization (chronic mountain sickness). *Am J Med* 1971; 50:728–743.
93. Stewart JR, Fajardo CF: Radiation-induced heart disease. Clinical and experimental aspects. *Radiol Clin North Am* 1971; 9:511–531.
94. McReynolds RA, Gold GL, Roberts WC: Coronary heart disease after mediastinal irradiation for Hodgkin's disease. *Am J Med* 1976; 60:39–45.
95. Sammons JH, Coleman RL: Firefighters' occupational exposure to carbon monoxide. *J Occupational Med* 1974; 16:543–546.
96. Lange RL, Reid MS, Tresch DD, Keelan MH, Bernhard VM, Coolidge G: Nonatheromatous ischemic heart disease following withdrawal from chronic industrial nitroglycerin exposure. *Circulation* 1972; 46:666–678.
97. Reinhardt CF, Azar A, Maxfield ME, Smith PE Jr, Mullin LS: Cardiac arrhythmias and aerosol "sniffing." *Arch Environ Health* 1971; 22:265–279.
98. Aviado DM: Toxicity of aerosols. *J Clin Pharmacol* 1975; 15:86–104.

79 Computers and Cardiovascular Practice: Old Dreams and Current Realities

Eugene A. Stead, Jr, MD

Computers and microprocessors are now built into many instruments used in medicine and cardiology. Computerized axial tomography (CAT) scans, computerized echocardiography, and various digital techniques for enlarging the gray scale of x-ray films are in daily use.

Computers have not modified the collection of data and the keeping of records to any great extent. The entry of computers into the office practice of cardiology has been slow because of the same factors that have prevented computers from having a great effect on other medical specialties.[1] This chapter summarizes those factors that have inhibited wider use of computers and offers suggestions for the future.

Computers have a certain fascination for persons who have spent their careers developing young minds to explore uncharted waters. Men exposed naked to the world have too little force to make a major impact on their environment, but armed with instruments of their own creation, they have tremendous power to perturb and even destroy large parts of the world. With the development of speech, writing, and printing, information could be saved and transferred. Man could begin with stored information and ascend to new plateaus.

Books, charts, and journals were passive aids. Each brain had to assimilate and process available information before it could advance knowledge. Now computers allow information to be stored and manipulated in ways previously restricted to the brain. For the first time, man is extending not only the power of arms and legs, but also the power of the brain.

DNA contributed by egg and sperm dictates the structure of the brain, but after the first cell division, feedback from the environment becomes important. The result is a biologic machine programmed to carry out many functions before the infant leaves the womb. The combination of continued DNA programming and environmental factors leads to the adult brain.

The computer is a tool created and controlled by man. We all agree that there are no computers on the horizon with the flexibility and reprogramming ability of the brain. The combination of multiple sensory inputs, rich association pathways, and many motor outlets gives the brain a large lead. Early dreams of reviewing lifetime medical records and applying the wisdom of several specialists to an individual patient's care remain unfulfilled.

The future is less certain. In the last 50 years, computers have repeatedly increased their range of function. The brain has developed over millions of years. Major mutations increasing the power of the brain occur slowly, one at a time, so diffusion through the world's population is very slow. It is doubtful that major improvements will occur in the next thousand years. However, millions of individuals can share in constructing computers. Over time they may develop a nonbiologic system as complex and functional as the human brain, making our dreams come true.

EVOLUTION OF COMPUTERS IN MEDICINE: A MIXTURE OF SUCCESS AND FAILURE

Twenty years ago the National Institutes of Health and the National Aeronautics and Space Administration (NASA) recognized that introducing computers into bioscience laboratories might open up many new areas of investigation. Computers at that time were large, bulky instruments guarded by computer scientists, programmers, and technicians. They were housed in specially air-conditioned laboratories. They were too remote to be integrated into day-to-day research. A way was needed to unleash the creativity of the biomedical researcher. The way became a standardized laboratory computer small enough to be a working laboratory instrument and easy for non-computer–trained researchers to program. Fred Stone, director of the Institute of General Medical Sciences, and Bruce Waxman, executive secretary of the

Computer Science Study Section, arranged for financing. The Institute of General Medical Sciences supplied $3,200,000, the Institute of Mental Health $300,000, and NASA transferred $600,000 to General Medical Sciences for the venture. Wesley Clark, William Paoian, Charles Molnar, and others of the Massachusetts Institute of Technology (MIT) faculty created the LINC computer. Scientists were able to acquire 1 of 16 LINCS by submitting a research protocol and agreeing to spend 2 months at MIT learning to assemble and service a computer to be located in the laboratory. When the bioscientists departed with their new tool, the minicomputer and personal computer were on their way. Putting computers directly into scientists' hands produced many creative new uses for the technology.

The ability of the computer to create three-dimensional images and to manipulate the arrangements of atoms in space has helped theoretical and experimental chemists to design a variety of new compounds. Several computer banks have brains containing the sequences of nucleotides found in DNA, RNA, and the amino acid sequences of proteins.

The National Library of Medicine recognized that information was exploding and that old methods of cataloging sources and searching scientific literature were no longer adequate. They created Medline, sparked by Martin Cummings. This computerized system supplied a complete set of references for any topic. Today the system is very sophisticated. Subgroups can be specified much more definitely and most of the irrelevant titles eliminated. The group at Beth Israel Hospital in Boston has made its library more user-friendly with a program called Paper Chase. The terminals in a modern medical library are in constant use. The librarian's ability to identify sources of interest from only a modicum of information is constantly amazing. We no longer need to focus our efforts on finding facts; we can spend our time synthesizing them.

In clinical areas, physicians' great expectations were not realized. Instead, computers entered large clinics and hospitals as tools of the accounting office. Even here, change was slow because the computer was used only to speed up standard accounting methods. For example, accountants used the computer to generate a batch report identifying records missing a diagnosis rather than using it interactively to prevent creation of a record without specifying a diagnosis. New approaches based on the capabilities of the new tools appeared slowly. With on-line computing, orders can be entered and a charge made when the order is filled, eliminating the need for an audit trail. Much of the paperwork and the paper can be eliminated, but old-line accountants are slow to change.

Accounting personnel had no incentive to experiment with clinical uses of computers. In areas where physicians have developed medical information systems, there has been little cross talk between the business office and the clinic. One group rarely knows what hardware and software are in other parts of the institution and future purchases are planned by one group without regard for other users. Therefore, they have not achieved cost-savings by eliminating redundant special purpose hardware such as graphics or laser printers, nor have they increased reliability through shared backup facilities or increased function through networking. In the last 30 years, eager beavers have created a large variety of databases for teaching, care, and guiding diagnosis. Most of these are rarely used. Medical schools do not recognize computer science as an important component of the curriculum. Medical schools and hospitals do not support computerized information systems in their budgets. Database creators have largely been entrepreneurs supported by noninstitutional funds. Operating outside the traditional medical practice, they have usually failed to engage physicians in using their systems routinely. When the entrepreneur leaves, the computer program disappears.

Another problem has been the seduction of some physicians by computers. As a result, few persons writing medical information systems have continued to practice medicine. They have created a great variety of interesting material that is useless in practice. The average physician overestimates the accuracy and usefulness of written information in traditional medical charts. When asked what information should be stored in the computer, the reply is "I need everything." When that advice is followed, the computer record becomes as overloaded and unworkable as its manual counterpart. We need teams of practicing physicians who are knowledgeable about software and engineers who are comfortable as colleagues.

Most physicians have been slow to lay hands on the computer. They have not entered information directly into the system or extracted needed data from the computer. Because they have employed interface personnel for these functions, a system has had to bear this overhead. However, the overhead for this isolation is greater than just salaries. The support personnel ask the computer to do what they think the physician wants. Because the physician does not understand the computer's capabilities and the support personnel do not understand the physician's needs, the effort is often wasted.

Computer software for practice has usually had narrowly focused purposes such as billing, checking for drug–drug interactions, interpreting electrocardiograms, calculating values for pulmonary function testing, or interpreting blood gas and electrolyte data in renal failure. Most of the practice continues without using the computer. For this reason the physician is not involved in developing a new mode for his practice, and the computer is underused. To give a specific example, while the computer prints prescriptions, it could silently check for drug–drug interactions. This type of cross talk is rarely built into the system because the physician is peripheral to the venture.

Physicians think of computerization when facing an administrative problem such as processing insurance forms on time or rescheduling a day's appointments. Each practice's day-to-day routine is a patchwork of procedures evolved to solve past problems. The first thought is to use a computer to speed existing processes. This instinct overlooks the fact that taking advantage of a computer requires that old processes be replaced. One way to schedule appointments is to divide the day into units, each of which is the size of the shortest appointment, and to let the secretary flip pages of a book until she sees the right number of units for each patient. Such a system is flexible but depends on a person's visual ability to level the workload. The physician may have one day with six new patients and the next with 40 returning patients. Using a computer to keep a book that is visually managed is more tedious than using a paper book. If a physician accepts the discipline imposed by the computer and gives up the flexibility of personally establishing time schedules of different types and lengths, he or she can use the computer to match patients to resources and have a more efficient practice.

Customizing a program to fit a physician's habits is expensive in time. In today's programs, sophisticated data dictionaries allow nonprogrammers to tailor a system to their needs, but developing and maintaining the dictionaries can require months of the physician's time. Each procedure performed by a practice must be defined. Coding data requires listing all the items usually scribbled under "others" in a paper system. Defining the system and then encoding the data are hard work, but once you have them in the computer, you can arrange the data in many ways and get a variety of useful outputs.

The physician is a better diagnostician than the computer. Initially, all diagnoses are possible for a patient. The physician quickly narrows the range until only a few possibilities remain. At this stage, the computer could in many areas be used to determine the most likely diagnosis. However, the physician faces one of two situations: He is an expert in evaluating the data because the practice has many patients with this set of problems. If so, computer evaluation is unnecessary. Or, he sees very few patients with this set of problems. If so, no computer program is easily available to cover the issues at hand. It is much simpler to refer the patient to the appropriate specialist. Interacting with a computer consultation program is not as rewarding as consulting with a specialist. The primary physician can ask another physician exactly what he or she wants to know, skipping over known and understood facts. A computer program straightforward enough to be used by a novice will likely force a more experienced user through a tedious dialogue. The specialist provides a dual function of caring for the patient and educating the primary physician. The primary physician in turn educates the specialist by providing follow-up data about the patient. Although the computer program may educate the physician, it learns nothing from the interchange.

Diagnostic programs go out of date rapidly. Because no one is really using them, their format is rigid and not easily modified. Because they are not widely used, no one knows how many modifications are needed to help the physicians who did not have a hand in writing the program. There are no methods to keep programs up-to-date and user-friendly. Artificial intelligence techniques attempt to solve this problem by placing medical information in a database that can be changed by nonprogramming physicians, but the experimental systems have not been complete enough to achieve general use.

The initial hope that on-line interactive computers would have a major impact on medical education has not been realized. We doubt that this will change until specialty boards incorporate computers more completely into the examination process. Faculty believe that the curriculum is an important determinant of students' activities. The practical student focuses on passing examinations. The present examination system places a premium on memorized facts. A student receives no credit for knowing where information is stored and how to extract it from a computerized data bank.

Given this somewhat discouraging picture, can we realistically predict a brighter future for information systems?

WHAT COMPUTERS CAN DO FOR MEDICAL PRACTICE IN THE NEAR FUTURE

Inexpensive personal computers, which can fit into any office, put the practicing physician in a position similar to that of the basic laboratory scientist given a LINC computer 20 years ago. However, innovative uses of this tool in medical practice are developing at a slower pace than they did in the laboratory. The sources of support for the basic scientist are more limited than those for medical practice, and this makes the competition keener. The scientists' jobs are creating, recording, analyzing, and publishing data leading to progress in the field of bioscience. They are involved personally in handling and manipulating data and are willing to get involved with the computer. The physician in practice does many things and relegates tasks to technical staff. There is no need to analyze and change activities each day. This creature of habit tries to speed up or ease customary procedures. Other people put data into the computer and extract information from it. These physicians miss the fact that material entered can be rearranged and that the output can be of many kinds only loosely linked to input. The computer offers them a chance to develop new strategies and to change financial and medical records. When practicing physicians devote personal time and energy to use the computer in new ways, they can see real benefits.

A computer can produce many different outputs if the data have been collected with more than one type of report in mind. If business office procedure codes for established hypertension, a limited physical examination, and serum electrolytes are stored, a computer can generate a bill for the visit and create utilization statistics for practice management, but the program can provide no medical data except that the patient has hypertension. If, however, the computer keeps a date of onset along with the diagnosis of hypertension, the actual results of the vital signs, funduscopic and cardiac examination, and values for each electrolyte, a program can interpret the data to produce a variety of administrative or medical reports. After the initial entries are made, the computer can be updated rapidly by entering values for items that change. Unchanged parameters can be carried forward automatically. The computer can summarize data or expand a report, depending on its purpose. Even if only abnormal physical findings have been recorded, the computer can generate a detailed executive physical examination, supplying pertinent negatives from a dictionary containing those parts of the examination the physician always performs.

Physicians have routines they follow when a medical

problem has been defined. In an encounter with acute illness, the computer can remind the physician of the way in which he intends to handle the problem and can note deviations from the routine. The computer can record the therapy and remind the physician of a potential drug incompatibility. It can remind the physician of the date of the next visit and generate instructions to prepare the patient for the visit.

A large part of any practice involves fairly standard prescriptions. These may be for single drugs on a short-term basis or complex prescriptions for chemotherapy, dialysis, or nutrition schedules. The computer can decrease the time needed to initiate these schedules by physically printing the necessary mathematics, such as adjusting an antibiotic dose for renal insufficiency.

In chronic illness the computer can create flow sheets to record needed information and remind the physician that it is time to collect new information. As data are recorded, the computer can tell whether there have been changes since the last entry, using the patient's own data as a control rather than the normal limits from a larger population.

Moreover, in chronic illness the computer can tell the physician the findings at the first visit, the treatment undertaken, and the patient's current state. It allows the physician to stratify patients with the same diagnosis into a set of subgroups. Outcome data can help determine the effectiveness of treatment. By gradually increasing the intervals between visits and tests in one portion of the practice, the physician can determine optimal timing. The computer is like a timelapse camera. It compresses time and allows the physician to examine quickly the data from many patients over years of time.

The computer can inform the physician of the sensitivity and specificity of procedures and tests. It can tell how often a CAT scan of the brain alters the outcome of patients with the clinical picture of Alzheimer's disease or how often an asymptomatic patient profits from determining the serum uric acid level. Given data from history, physical examination, chest plate, and electrocardiogram, the computer can tell whether an exercise stress test will change the patient's probabilities of having coronary artery disease enough to change the physician's management.

The computer can make life easier by managing appointments and scheduling. As diagnostic protocols are entered into the computer, scheduling algorithms optimize the use of all scarce resources, such as procedure rooms, and not just the physician's time.

The computer can enhance business management in a practice. Charge capture and management of accounts receivable can be automated, reducing lost charges and speeding up payments. Electronic links to third party payers allow analysis of reasons for under-reimbursement. Utilization statistics permit planning for growth of the practice.

The computer offers the physician entering practice the opportunity to establish a practice profile. Using demographic data, inactive and active problems, and treatments, the physician can test new drugs and procedures. He can use this database in a business designed to sustain his own intellectual growth.

These uses of the computer are more mundane than the grander schemes we once dreamed about. The notion of placing every person's medical record on a centrally located computer with a terminal in each physician's office is certainly appealing. The trouble is that most of us rarely need all medical information. We want what relates to our own area of activity. This information can be carried much more cheaply in flip charts, bulletin boards, or paperback books. Actually, all medical information needed for emergency services can be entered on a 3 by 5 inch card and kept in one's pocket book.

It is intriguing to consider placing all medical knowledge into computers. In so doing, we can build an excellent reference library, but the physician will be a better clinician than the computer until we build a computer that is more like the human brain in its ability to synthesize information, recognize patterns, and learn from its mistakes.

Computers are here; they are storing usable medical information and medical practice is slowly changing. As in most cases, the tortoise will outdistance the hare. Those of us who are hares will have to develop patience.

REFERENCE

1. Stead EA Jr, Stead WW: Computers and medical practice: old dreams and current realities. *MD Computing* 1985; 2(6):26–31.

80 Preventive Cardiology

Jeremiah Stamler, MD

CENTRAL ROLE OF PRIMARY PREVENTION

TWO LEVELS (STAGES) OF PREVENTIVE CARDIOLOGY

Preventive cardiology involves two stages: primary and secondary prevention. Primary prevention encompasses all measures to prevent the development of clinical disease in persons currently free of evidence of disease, ie, it aims to reduce or eliminate risk of onset of disease and thereby decrease or end its incidence in the population. Secondary prevention focuses on persons who already have manifest disease; it involves all efforts to limit and control disease in such persons, to cure disease when possible, to avoid or postpone acute recurrent episodes, and to delay or halt disease progression and thereby improve prognosis. Thus, secondary prevention merges with clinical treatment and rehabilitation.

Irreversible damage to the heart characterizes the main forms of cardiac disease currently afflicting mankind: first and foremost, hypertensive and atherosclerotic heart disease, also pulmonary heart disease, rheumatic heart disease, Chagas' disease, alcoholic heart muscle disease, the cardiomyopathies of unknown causes, and congenital heart disease. This is manifest in its most dramatic, forceful, and extreme form in the high incidence of premature sudden death as the first manifestation of coronary heart disease (CHD) in the industrialized countries where CHD is epidemic. It is also significantly expressed in the fact that for most living persons with heart disease, a complete cure is not attainable. Therefore, the goals of secondary prevention and clinical care are necessarily limited. In this sense, the old adage, "prevention is better than cure," is deceptive and misleading in regard to most cases of heart disease, because there is no cure.

must be the primary prevention of the heart diseases. Only long-term strategy giving prominence to primary prevention can accomplish the effective abatement and control of the common cardiovascular diseases.[1-12] Hence, the focus of this chapter is on the primary prevention of the principal present-day heart diseases.

POSSIBILITIES FOR PRIMARY PREVENTION

The last 100 years have been epoch-making in demonstrating that epidemic onslaughts of disease can be brought under control and ended, first and foremost, by the application of strategies of primary prevention. In the industrialized countries and in some of the economically developing countries, broadly based socioeconomic advances and population-wide applications of specific public health and medical care measures for primary prevention have long since ended the era when infectious and undernutritional diseases (pestilence and famine) were the main killers.[1] As a result chiefly of these spectacular achievements, more years have been added to life expectancy in the 20th century than in the preceding two millennia. For US newborns, for example, life expectancy in 1900 was 47.3 years; in 1983, 74.7 years (for whites, 47.6 and 75.2 years at the two time points; for blacks, 33.0 and 71.3 years), and the US achievement is not the greatest among the industrialized nations.[13-15]

These advances have had their cardiovascular components, eg, beriberi, diphtheritic, luetic, and rheumatic heart diseases have all become very low incidence events in industrialized countries. These transformations unequivocally demonstrate two fundamental points: (1) heart diseases are preventable; (2) primary prevention is the key strategy for achieving control of mass diseases, including those of the cardiovascular system. The marked and sustained downturn in mortality rates from coronary heart disease during the last 15 to 20 years, most notable in the United States and Australia, is an important confirmation that the contemporary epidemic forms of heart disease can also be controlled and prevented, and that primary prevention is of key importance also in relation to this latest achievement (see below).[3,5,8–12,16]

GENERAL METHODOLOGY OF PRIMARY PREVENTION

The general strategy of prevention is to break links in the chain of causation; the particular strategy of primary prevention is to break early links in this chain, ie, from early childhood on to block exposures to etiologic factors leading to disease. This is accomplished by a combined effort of public health and medical care. The former is concerned with large population groups, whereas the latter focuses on individuals and families. The two complement and enhance each other. Both use a two-pronged approach, ie, preventive efforts for the whole population, plus special pinpointed and intense efforts for higher risk individuals and groups (including those who already manifest disease).

As to sources of disease causation, for diseases occurring at high rates in the population, Virchow[17] over a century ago formulated a basic scientific generalization (law) that is key to breaking links in the chain of their causation. Mass diseases, Virchow concluded, are due to " . . . disturbances of human culture." Rectification and elimination of these disturbances are of decisive importance in controlling epidemics.

This concept has stood the test of time, as dramatically attested to for the cardiovascular diseases by the patterns of progress, ranging from spectacular to nonexistent, in different countries against rheumatic fever and rheumatic heart disease.[18] Virchow's concept is particularly seminal in regard to the main forms of cardiac disease in the world today, ie, hypertensive and atherosclerotic disease.

PRIMARY PREVENTION OF HYPERTENSIVE AND ATHEROSCLEROTIC DISEASE, PARTICULARLY CORONARY HEART DISEASE

HYPERTENSIVE DISEASE

The concept, essential hypertension: Most cases of hypertensive disease are still labeled essential hypertension, ie, high blood pressure (HBP) of unknown etiology. If causes are indeed unknown, how is it possible to undertake breaking links in the chain of causation? In my judgment, the current state of knowledge concerning risk factors for HBP, particularly risk factors amenable to prevention and control, warrants, even requires, a fresh evaluation of the concept of essential hypertension. Many data sets of widely varied type, such as animal experimental, clinical, and epidemiologic, as illustrated in Figure 80.1 and Tables 80.1 to 80.3 are now available and demonstrate a significant association between at least three aspects of life-style and mass occurrence of HBP: caloric imbalance with consequent obesity, high salt intake, and heavy alcohol consumption.[1,12,19–42] *

The research findings fulfill criteria for assessing these associations as etiologically significant, at a high level of probability. A sizable proportion of the total risk of HBP in the United States and similar populations is attributable to the three cited traits. It follows that prevention and control of obesity, high salt intake, and heavy drinking should contribute importantly to the prevention and control of HBP.

Other aspects of life-style have been implicated in the etiology of HBP, eg, low intake of potassium, calcium, magnesium, polyunsaturated fats, and fiber; high intake of total fats, saturated fats, and animal proteins; low level of habitual physical activity, with consequent poor cardiopulmonary fitness; high psychosocial stress; also, such life-style–related metabolic traits as hyperuricemia, hyperglycemia, and hypercholesterolemia.[30,33–37,39–42] At the present stage of knowledge in my judgment, these other factors remain to be established as causes of HBP, ie, as etiologically significant links in the chain of pathogenesis.

If it is indeed reasonable to conclude that the relations between obesity, high salt intake, heavy alcohol consumption, and HBP are etiologically significant, then persistence of the view that HBP is of unknown cause is ipso facto an anachronistic distortion that should be abandoned. Instead of continuing to use the term essential hypertension, it would seem wise to drop it from the medical lexicon, and speak instead of primary hypertension, ie, HBP without a demonstrable pathologic basis (renal, adrenal, aortic, and the like).

Empirical evidence, most of it in the area of secondary prevention thus far, is available to support the foregoing conclusion. Thus, there are many reports, in both the older and the more recent literature, showing that weight loss decreases blood pressure in obese hypertensive persons. Years ago it was shown that marked reduction in sodium intake to low levels controlled HBP in many patients with severe hypertension. Several, but not all, recent trials have found that a moderate decrease in sodium intake decreases blood pressure in persons with moderate hypertension. Cessation of alcohol consumption by problem drinkers with HBP resulted in normotension in a high proportion of cases.[30,35–37,39,41,42]

A four-year multifactorial randomized controlled trial of ability to control HBP by nutritional means was recently completed in Chicago and Minneapolis.[30,43,44] This Hypertension Control Program dealt with middle-aged men and women with established moderate HBP, in most cases a mean diastolic pressure of 90 to 104 mm Hg, previously well controlled by stepped care drug treatment. One half the participants were counseled on nutritional measures to decrease overweight, high sodium intake, and heavy alcohol consumption (when present), and antihypertensive medication was stopped. A control group was taken off drugs without dietary recommen-

*In view of new data emerging from current research in the People's Republic of China on the relation of level of habitual sodium intake to mean blood pressure and prevalence of hypertension (eg, Tables 80.2A and 2B),[23,24] the generalization in the oldest Chinese medical book (circa 2698 to 2598 BC) is intriguing: "hence if too much salt is used for food, the pulse hardens..."[25]

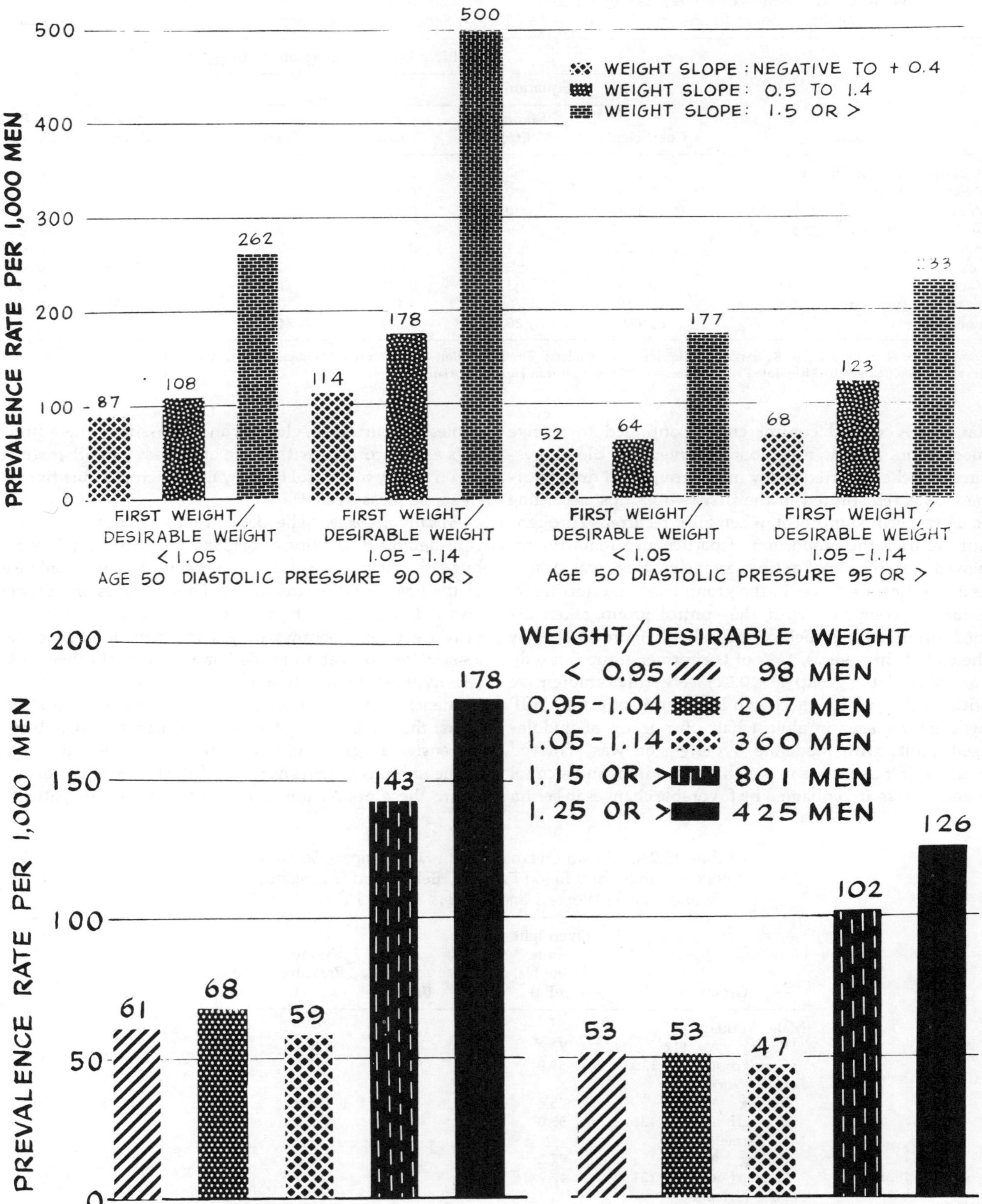

Figure 80.1. Peoples Gas Company Study; relation between initial weight as a young adult, slope of the weight curve over the next 20 years, and development of hypertensive disease in middle age, 20-year follow-up data on 746 men aged 40–59 in 1958–59 (*top*), and relation between the ratio of observed weight to desirable weight and prevalence of various blood pressure levels on initial examination, men aged 40–59 in 1958; all prevalence rates are age-corrected by five-year age groups to the United States male population, 1950 (*bottom*). (From Stamler J.[1] Reprinted with permission of Grune & Stratton, Inc.)

Table 80.1. Mean Seven-Day 24-Hour Sodium Excretion, Other Variables, and Systolic Blood Pressure: Multiple Linear Regression Analyses—73 Chicago School Children Aged 11 to 14, Study A

	Multiple Linear Regression Analyses					
	Equation 1			Equation 2		
Variable	Coefficient	Standard Error	P Value	Coefficient	Standard Error	P Value
$\bar{X}$ 24-hour sodium (mEq)	0.059	±0.029	0.045	0.085	±0.029	0.005
Height (inches)	0.308	±0.327	0.350	...	...	...
Weight (lb)	0.159	±0.061	0.011	...	...	...
Body mass index ($\frac{wt(kg)}{height(m^2)}$)	...	...	...	0.614	±0.323	0.062
Age (years)	-1.527	±1.816	0.403	-0.903	±1.917	0.639
Sex	-1.239	±2.476	0.618	-0.573	±2.616	0.827
Race	0.670	±3.416	0.845	1.869	±3.595	0.605
Heart rate (per min)	0.101	±0.124	0.418	0.055	±0.131	0.676
Constant	61.425	±26.526	0.024	74.969	±24.563	0.003

From Cooper R, Soltero T, Liu K, Berkson D, Levinson S, Stamler J: The association between urinary sodium excretion and blood pressure in children. *Circulation* 1980; 62:97–104. Reprinted with permission of the American Heart Association, Inc.

dations. A second control group continued to receive medication, with no nutritional intervention. Blood pressure was checked frequently in all groups and drug treatment was reinstituted in the first two groups, according to a prespecified protocol, when HBP recurred. Throughout the trial, the proportion of participants requiring renewed prescription of antihypertensive drugs was sizably and significantly lower in the group receiving nutritional guidance, compared with the control group taken off medication without dietary counseling (Figure 80.2).[43] By the end of three years, 44% of the former group but only 16% of the latter group ($P < 0.01$) were still normotensive without drugs. This success in long-term control of HBP by dietary means in almost half of a group of middle-aged adults with moderate hypertension was achieved with modest decreases in weight and sodium and alcohol intake. It was accompanied by favorable changes in serum cholesterol, uric acid, glucose, and potassium. These findings are concordant with those of at least two other studies on ability to control HBP by multifactorial nutritional-hygienic measures.[45,46]

Primary prevention: The data just cited show that in a considerable proportion of persons with HBP, nutritional-hygienic means can control hypertension, with avoidance of the need for drug treatment. These studies and others also indicate that such measures are useful adjuvants to drug treatment, because they serve both to reduce the amount of medication needed and to control other traits (eg, hyperlipidemia, hyperglycemia, and hyperuricemia) influencing the long-term prognosis of people with HBP. Thus, the skillful use of these measures and of antihypertensive drugs is highly important in the effective care of the millions of persons with HBP. However, important as are these opportunities nowadays to benefit patients

Table 80.2A. Mean Overnight Eight-Hour Urinary Sodium, Other Variables, and Blood Pressure, Beijing and Guangzhou: Male and Female Workers and Farmers Aged 35 to 54 Years*

Group	Overnight 8-hour Urine Na (mEq)	Age (yrs)	Body Mass (Index △)	Systolic Pressure (mm Hg)	Diastolic Pressure (mm Hg)
Male Workers					
Beijing $N=113$	73.8	46.8	23.6	123.1	81.7
Guangzhou $N=125$	59.9	44.1	21.1	115.2	74.9
Female Workers					
Beijing $N=102$	75.8	45.0	24.7	116.6	75.8
Guangzhou $N=136$	58.0	44.4	21.9	113.0	74.3
Male Farmers					
Beijing $N=109$	97.2	46.7	21.9	123.5	79.1
Guangzhou $N=131$	47.7	44.7	19.9	115.0	75.4
Female Farmers					
Beijing $N=113$	86.4	43.0	22.8	115.3	73.6
Guangzhou $N=119$	48.5	42.8	19.9	108.1	70.2
All Beijing[△△] $N=437$	83.3	45.4	23.2	119.6	77.5
All Guangzhou[△△] $N=511$	53.5	44.0	20.7	112.8	73.7

*From Tao et al.[24]

[△]Weight (kg)/Height (m²)

[△△]Unweighted means

Table 80.2B. Multiple Regression of Three-Day Average Blood Pressure on Mean Three-Day Eight-Hour Overnight Electrolyte Excretion Controlling for Age, Body Mass Index (BMI), and Pulse, by Sex

	Systolic Blood Pressure				Diastolic Blood Pressure			
Variable	Electrolyte	Age	BMI	Pulse	Electrolyte	Age	BMI	Pulse
Men (N = 40)								
Sodium	0.081	0.531	0.536	0.373	0.065*	0.158	0.228	0.150
Potassium	−0.602	0.656	0.715	0.490†	−0.292	0.245	0.333	0.234*
Sodium/potassium	2.092‡	0.378	0.930	0.292	1.520§	0.053	0.518	0.098
Sodium/creatinine	39.277‡	0.541	0.703	0.378*	25.741‡	0.177	0.346	0.166
Potassium/creatinine	501.868	0.618	0.561	0.408*	324.804	0.228	0.253	0.186
Women (N = 50)								
Sodium	0.037	0.446	0.833†	−0.145	−0.012	0.171	0.625†	0.031
Potassium	−0.384	0.360	0.919†	−0.096	−0.777†	0.112	0.656†	0.088
Sodium/potassium	0.649*	0.422	0.826†	−0.063	0.585†	0.209	0.544*	0.083
Sodium/creatinine	27.013*	0.416	0.833†	−0.100	8.490	0.193	0.586†	0.034
Potassium/creatinine	−7.838	0.397	0.893†	−0.127	−151.902	0.182	0.582†	0.037

From Hsiao et al.[23] Reprinted with permission.

*$P \le 0.10$, 1-tailed;

†$P \le 0.05$, 1-tailed;

‡$P \le 0.01$, 1-tailed;

§$P \le 0.001$, 1 tailed

Table 80.3. Percent with High Blood Pressure among Problem Drinkers and Nonproblem Drinkers: Chicago Peoples Gas Company (1,233 White Men Aged 40 to 59 in 1958)

Variable	Problem Drinkers (N = 38)	Nonproblem Drinkers (N = 1,195)	t	Adjusted* t
SBP ≥ 140	55.3	33.1	2.85	2.92
SBP ≥ 160	18.4	10.7	1.50	1.68
DBP ≥ 90	34.2	20.4	2.06	2.66
DBP ≥ 95	15.8	9.1	1.39	1.95

Chicago Western Electric Company (1,899 White Men Aged 40 to 55 in 1957)

Variable	Heavy Drinkers (N = 117)	Non-Heavy Drinkers (N = 1,782)	t	Adjusted* t
SBP ≥ 140	59.0	36.9	4.75	4.30
SBP ≥ 160	28.2	11.7	5.18	4.66
DBP ≥ 90	64.1	42.1	4.65	4.27
DBP ≥ 95	40.2	20.4	5.02	4.75

* Adjusted by analysis of covariance for age, serum cholesterol, pulse, relative weight, and cigarettes/day.

Tables 80.3, 80.7A, and 80.7B are from Stamler J: Improved life styles: their potential for the primary prevention of atherosclerosis and hypertension in childhood, in Lauer RM, Shekelle RB (eds): *Childhood Prevention of Atherosclerosis and Hypertension,* New York, Raven Press, 1980, pp 3–36. Reprinted with permission.

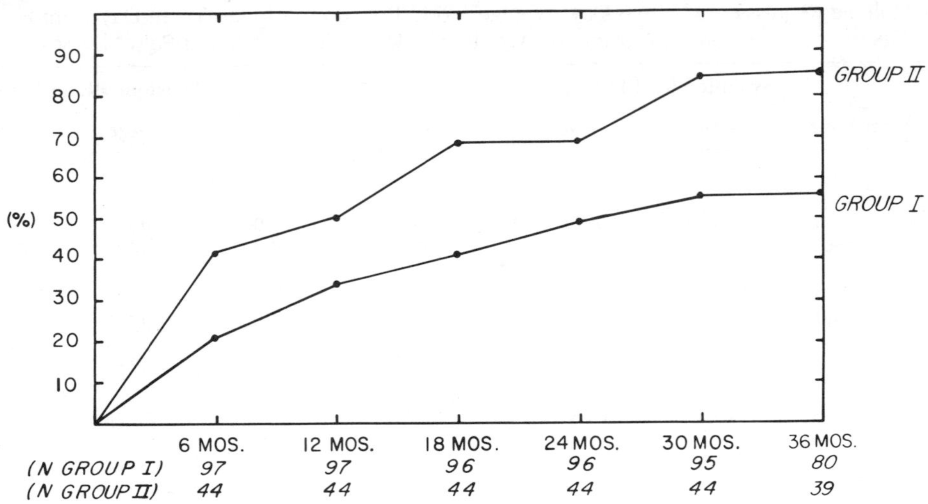

Figure 80.2. Hypertension Control Program; percentage of participants returned to antihypertensive medication by group (Group I off drugs with nutritional counseling, Group II off drugs, no counseling). (From Stamler R, et al.[44] Reprinted with permission of Gower Medical Publishing.)

with HBP, they must be recognized as limited interim approaches to this epidemic problem. The ultimate, and only full, solution of the hypertension problem is its primary prevention. This requires a whole new emphasis over and above that of treating HBP once it has developed; it means putting high on the contemporary agenda the task of preventing HBP from developing in the first place. A broad foundation of knowledge exists, anthropologic, epidemiologic, animal-experimental, and clinical, as a basis for practical efforts along these lines.[1,6,9,12,19–24,26–38,40,42,45,47,48] It includes the following: Among preliterate isolated populations consuming little salt, blood pressure does not increase with age and HBP is rare. The addition of salt to food is a relatively recent practice for the human species, dating back no more than 10,000 years, since the invention of agriculture and animal husbandry. Supplemental salt feeding produces HBP in several animal species, and low sodium intake inhibits the development of experimental hypertension. The sodium ion is pivotally involved in the pathophysiologic aspects of HBP. In populations of "western" industrialized countries habitually ingesting a high salt diet, a high proportion of cases of hypertension is attributable to the further effects of obesity or a heavy alcohol intake, or both. In these circumstances, rapid heart rate, due often to sedentary habits and low cardiopulmonary fitness, is also a risk factor for HBP (Table 80.4).[32–34] Persons with high-normal blood pressure, eg, diastolic levels averaging 80 to 89 mm Hg, are particularly prone to HBP, especially when they manifest one or more of the foregoing risk factors for hypertension.

These facts indicate the strategic thrusts appropriate for safe and reasonable efforts for the primary prevention of hypertension: (1) moderate salt intake, eg, under 4 g of sodium chloride per day (equivalent to less than 1.6 g of sodium or less than 50 mEq); (2) regular frequent moderate rhythmic (isotonic) exercise to maintain high cardiopulmonary fitness and to aid, together with improved eating habits, in preventing obesity; (3) for those who choose to use alcohol, a moderate intake (under 40 g per day).

General nutritional recommendations for prevention of the major adult cardiovascular diseases also include: (1) moderation in total fat intake (no more than 30% of total calories); (2) low cholesterol intake (under 100 mg per 1,000 calories); (3) low saturated fat intake (under 10% of calories); (4) moderate polyunsaturated fat intake from vegetable and fish sources (up to 10% of calories); (5) ingestion of food of low caloric and high nutrient density (including low fat dairy products, egg whites, lean poultry, fish, seafood, meat, vegetables, legumes, whole grain products, and fruits) to assure high intake of all essential nutrients (potassium, calcium, magnesium, and other minerals, vitamins, amino acids, and essential fatty acids) and of fiber, without excess calories; (6) no more than modest ingestion of refined and processed sugars and of visible fats low in saturates and cholesterol, including spreads, salad dressings, and cooking fats.

In essence, these nutritional recommendations entail enjoying the pleasures of Mediterranean (Greek and southern Italian) and Far Eastern (Chinese and Japanese) cooking styles, but with moderation in salt intake. Encouraging these improved life-style patterns is best initiated early, after weaning, because hypertensive disease, as well as the atherosclerotic diseases, has its roots in childhood, and in any case it is easier to form good habits than to change habits in youth or adulthood. The guidelines for primary prevention are applicable for the population as a whole and especially for individuals and families at higher risk of hypertension (and the atherosclerotic diseases). With current life-styles, most Americans experience a steady more-or-less marked nonphysiologic increase in blood pressure from youth into middle age. By middle age, only a minority, no more than 20%, have optimal blood pressure levels, ie, systolic and diastolic levels less than 120 and 80 mm Hg, respectively.[1,32,49–52]

Table 80.4A. Relation Between 1958 Levels, 1958 to 1966 Changes in Levels for Several Variables and 1966 Blood Pressure, Subcohort of 549 White Men Originally Aged 40 to 55, Free of Evidence of Organic Disease at Baseline, not on Drug Treatment for Hypertension, with 1958 Blood Pressure <135/<85 mm Hg, Western Electric Co. Study, 1958-1966

Variable, Statistic	Systolic Blood Pressure (SBP), 1966	Diastolic Blood Pressure (DBP), 1966	Systolic Blood Pressure, 1966	Diastolic Blood Pressure, 1966
Relative weight, 1958	.2113*†	.1339†	.1887†	.1074†
Change in relative weight, 1958-1966	.5647†	.2914†	.5614†	.2951†
Pulse, 1958	.2661‡	.1493‡	.2404‡	.1137§
Change in pulse, 1958-1966	.2224‡	.1429‡	.2147‡	.1231†
Age, 1958	.6125†	.1070	.5977†	.1101
Blood pressure, 1958‖	---¶	---¶	.4359†	.4056†
Constant	55.0551†	48.6650†	8.1564	22.7946‡
Multiple R	.3252	.2774	.4014	.3485
R^2	.1058	.0770	.1611	.1215
F for significance	12.8444†	9.0550†	17.3513†	12.4911†

*Coefficient for the multiple linear regression equation.

†$P \leq 0.001$.

‡$P \leq 0.01$.

§$P \leq 0.05$.

‖In analyses with 1966 SBP as the dependent variable, 1958 SBP was used as the independent variable; with 1966 DBP as the dependent variable, 1958 DBP was used as the independent variable.

¶Blood pressure not included as an independent variable in the analysis.

Table 80.4B. Relation between Several Variables and Incidence of Hypertension—Expected Incidence Based on Multiple Logistic Analysis and Observed Incidence, Subcohort of 549 White Men Originally Aged 40 to 55, Free of Evidence of Organic Disease at Baseline, not on Drug Treatment for Hypertension, with 1958 Blood Pressure <135/<85 mm Hg, Western Electric Co. Study, 1958–1966

Quintile, Expected Incidence of Elevated Pressure, 1958-1966	Incidence Rate per 1,000 of Elevated Pressure, 1958-66: Diastolic Blood Pressure (DBP) ≥ 90 mm Hg, 5-Factor Analysis		6-Factor Analysis		DBP ≥ 95 mm Hg, 5-Factor Analysis		6-Factor Analysis	
	E	O	E	O	E	O	E	O
1	99.3	100.9	87.1	82.6	32.0	18.3	25.4	18.3
2	151.5	146.8	142.8	119.3	51.8	45.9	47.3	27.5
3	194.2	156.0	194.6	238.5	72.1	82.6	69.9	64.2
4	246.2	302.8	258.3	284.4	98.2	128.4	98.9	119.3
5	390.7	380.5	399.1	362.8	182.4	159.3	192.0	203.5
All	217.6	218.6	217.7	218.6	88.0	87.4	87.5	87.4
Ratio: 5/1	4.1	3.9	4.8	4.6	5.9	9.0	7.8	11.5
% of All with Elevated DBP in 5	36.9%	35.8%	37.7%	34.2%	42.7%	37.5%	45.2%	47.9%

E is expected; O is observed.

The five variables are: 1958 relative weight, 1958 pulse, 1958 age, 1958-1966 change in weight, 1958-1966 change in pulse.

The six variables are the foregoing five, plus 1958 DBP.

Tables 80.4A and 80.4B are from Stamler J,[34] and are reprinted with permission of Health Learning Systems, Inc.

A high proportion have definite HBP or high-normal pressures (diastolic levels in the 80 to 89 mm Hg range) and are on a collision course for premature cardiovascular sickness, disability, and death. Therefore, a two-pronged strategy, including recommendations for improved life-styles for the whole population and special focused counseling for higher risk individuals and families, is necessary for substantial progress in the primary prevention of HBP.

To date, findings are sparse from research studies designed to test ability to achieve primary prevention of HBP by the foregoing means. One double-blind controlled trial has been done involving 476 newborn infants in The Netherlands, 245 randomized to a usual sodium diet and 231 to a low sodium diet for the first six months of life.[53] Sodium intake of the latter group was one third that of the former. Mean systolic pressure of the two groups differed progressively in monthly readings. At 25 weeks, it was 2.1 mm Hg lower in the low sodium group than in the usual sodium group.

A recently reported Australian trial of the effects of bicycle ergometric exercise involved 12 sedentary normotensive adults randomly assigned, according to a Latin square design, to four different levels of physical activity: (1) two weeks at less than their usual activities, followed by two weeks in the hospital; (2) four weeks of their usual sedentary activities; (3) four weeks of bicycle ergometric exercise, three times weekly for 45 minutes at 60% to 70% of maximum work capacity; and (4) four weeks of similar exercise daily.[47] Mean resting blood pressure, 126/63 mm Hg at the end of the sedentary period, decreased 6/4 mm Hg after a month of three-times weekly exercise, and 10/5 mm Hg after daily exercise (both *P*s <0.05). Peripheral resistance decreased with exercise, as did overall sympathetic tone, plasma noradrenaline, and total body spillover into plasma of noradrenaline.

Our group has accrued experience in two trials of multifactorial nutritional-hygienic intervention involving adults with high-normal pressure. In the Coronary Prevention Evaluation Program carried out in Chicago from 1957 to 1973, one subgroup among coronary-prone men aged 40 to 59 years at entry had baseline diastolic blood pressure in the 80 to 89 mm Hg range.[45] This pilot trial included recommendations to reduce intake of total fat, saturated fat, cholesterol, and refined and processed carbohydrate; to increase moderately intake of polyunsaturated fat; to eat more low calorie vegetable products; to control calories to reduce excess body weight; to undertake regular, frequent, moderate rhythmic (isotonic) exercise; to avoid high sodium intake; and to abstain from smoking. With sustained moderate weight loss and slowing of resting heart rate, reduction in systolic blood pressure and diastolic pressure was achieved for almost a decade, instead of the usual increase over these years of age for such American men. Both weight loss and slowing of pulse were significantly and independently related to decrease in blood pressure.

During the last years, our group has been engaged in a systematic randomized controlled trial on ability to influence blood pressure and prevent high blood pressure by nutritional and hygienic means. Employed men and women aged 30 to 44 years were evaluated for susceptibility to HBP and invited to join the study if they had diastolic pressure 85 to 89 mm Hg, or 80 to 84 with overweight or rapid pulse or both and were found to be generally healthy. More than 200 persons were recruited and are participating in this ongoing trial. For the active intervention group, recommendations are multifactorial: a calorie-controlled, fat-modified diet to reduce weight; decreased sodium intake; cessation of heavy drinking and smoking (if present at baseline); and regular, frequent, moderate rhythmic exercise. Over the first three years, for those in the intervention group in the upper 50% of weight loss (with a mean loss of 16 pounds) and in the upper 50% of decrease in sodium intake (with a mean daily reduction of 2.1 g), diastolic pressure was reduced by 5 mm Hg. This was greater than the diastolic change in those with weight loss or sodium decrease, or both, less than the median amount, and it was greater than the blood pressure change in the control group.[48] Also, in 19% of those in the active intervention group an increase in diastolic blood pressure developed to hypertensive levels, whereas this occurred in 27% of the control group. This trial is continuing.

These data are encouraging with regard to ability to influence blood pressure favorably by safe nutritional and hygienic means. Given the safety of these measures, they merit extensive use in efforts to achieve primary prevention of HBP both in further research and in general medical practice.

ATHEROSCLEROTIC DISEASES, PARTICULARLY CORONARY HEART DISEASE

The vast array of congruent data on the relations between life-styles, life-style–related risk factors, and premature CHD is the foundation for the mounting efforts for the primary prevention of CHD and the other atherosclerotic diseases. This data base is derived from all major research methodologies—clinical, pathologic, animal-experimental, and epidemiologic.[1–12,16,19,30,54–61] It affords a profound rationale for societal, public health, and medical care efforts to have an impact on the etiologic and pathogenetic mechanisms producing severe atherosclerosis and its clinical manifestations, first and foremost to break *early* links in the chain of causation, for the purpose of primary prevention. The modern "disturbances of human culture" causing the epidemic of premature CHD in "western" industrialized countries are first and foremost "rich" diet and cigarette smoking, aided and abetted in all probability by sedentary life-style and also probably by contemporary psychosocial stresses-tensions and incongruent behavior patterns. Mass consumption of "rich" diet, a unique 20th century development, so far still involving only a minority of mankind, is of central importance as a primary and essential etiologic factor. This is a habitual diet high in total fat, cholesterol, saturated fat, refined and processed sugars, calories (for level of energy expenditure), salt, and (for many persons) alcohol as well. Such a diet leads to a high prevalence in the population of hypercholesterolemia-hyperbetalipoproteinemia and hypertension, two of the established major risk factors for CHD and the other atherosclerotic diseases. "Rich" diet and resultant mass hypercholesterolemia are sine qua non for the mass occurrence of premature severe atherosclerosis. Also, rich diet, along with sedentary habits, promotes severe obesity and type II diabetes, risk factors for both hypertensive and atherosclerotic diseases. All these aspects of modern life-style, producing the epidemic of premature CHD, have emerged willy-nilly as consequences of economic development in the maturity of "western" industrial society, in marked contrast to the different "disturbances in human culture" of its infancy and childhood, producing the epidemics of infectious and undernutritional diseases of yesteryear.

Among the findings that have contributed to quantification of the impact on man of these causes of mass CHD, data from long-term prospective epidemiologic studies have made a preeminent contribution. It is now almost 30 years since the first such data became available, from investigations of three US population samples.[62] Over these decades, more than a score of such investigations in many different populations in different countries have accumulated extensive results.[1–12,16,19,49–52,54–62] Three life-style–dependent traits, including elevated serum cholesterol, high blood pressure, and use of cigarettes, have demonstrated a relation to the risk of premature CHD that is strong, graded, consistent, independent (one from the other, and also independent of age, sex, ethnicity, and the like), temporally appropriate (ie, demonstrable prospectively), predictive (from one population to another), and coherent (in regard to findings of other research methodologies and to pathogenetic mechanisms). That is, these three traits meet established criteria for judging epidemiologic associations to be etiologically significant.[3–5,7] They have therefore been appropriately characterized as established major risk factors for CHD.[2] The designation, major, serves to emphasize not only that the impact of each of these is strong, but also that each is widely prevalent in the population of the United States and of other "western" industrialized countries and, unlike age and sex, is amenable to prevention and control, first and foremost by safe nutritional-hygienic means. These cardinal facts about the established major risk factors create a firm basis for mass approaches to prevention, including early (primordial) prevention, ie, prevention of the major risk factors themselves from emerging, in populations in both industrialized and economically developing countries.[4]

Until recently, the prospective epidemiologic studies producing the foregoing data and conclusions dealt with population samples numbering in the hundreds, thousands, or in a few instances tens of thousands. In the last year or two, findings from a much larger investigation have become available, ie, prospective data on the 361,662 men age 35 to 57 years screened in 18 US cities in 1973 to 1975 by the Multiple Risk Factor Intervention Trial (MRFIT) Research Group.[63–65,65a] Of these men, 356,222 were free at baseline of a history of hospitalization for myocardial infarction. With such an unprecedentedly large cohort, characterized at baseline in standardized fashion, there is an extraordinary ability to make quantitative assessments of the relation to long-term prognosis of each of the established major risk factors, each considered singly and in various combinations with the other two. Table 80.5 gives such data for 20 subgroups based on division of the cohort into nonsmokers and smokers, with and without HBP, and by quintile of serum cholesterol at baseline. There was one measurement of these risk factors per man. The mean duration of follow-up was six years; the end point was the age-adjusted CHD mortality rate per 1,000. The range of risk across the 20 cells was more than 13-fold, from a low of 1.6 per 1,000 per six years to a high of 21.4. Only 10% of these men were in the lowest risk subgroup, ie, the increase in risk was spread broadly throughout the cohort. The increase in relative risk was substantial in all 19 other subgroups, compared with the 10% at lowest risk, eg, a 56% increase in risk for the next subgroup (nonsmoking normotensive men in the second serum cholesterol quintile, 182 to 202 mg/dl).

At any level of serum cholesterol in men with and without HBP, the age-adjusted CHD mortality rate was much higher in cigarette smokers than in nonsmokers, at least 1.7 and as much as 3.2 times greater and 2.4 times greater in all cigarette smokers, making up 37% of the cohort (Table 80.5).[64]

At any level of serum cholesterol in both nonsmokers and smokers, the age-adjusted CHD mortality rate was much higher in men with HBP than in men without HBP, at least 1.2 and as much as 2.3 times greater and 1.8 times greater in all men with HBP, constituting 28% of the cohort (Table 80.5).[64]

For both nonsmokers and smokers with and without HBP, the age-adjusted six-year CHD death rate increased progressively over the entire range of serum cholesterol, from the second through the fifth quintile (Table 80.5).[64] With the large number of men and the consequent substantial number of CHD deaths in each of the 20 subgroups, this unique cohort permitted a definitive assessment of the question: Is the relation between serum cholesterol and CHD risk a continuous graded one or a threshold one, as some investigators have implied in recent years? The MRFIT data unequivocally confirm that in nonsmokers and smokers with and without HBP aged 35 to 39, 40 to 44, 45 to 49, and 50 to 54 at baseline, the relation is continuously graded (not threshold); it is nonlinear, ie, the risk increases curvilinearly. Overall, for the second quintile of the MRFIT cohort (182 to 202/mg/dl), the risk of premature CHD death was increased by 31%; for the third quintile (203 to 220 mg/dl), by 70%; for the fourth quintile (221 to 244 mg/dl), it was 2.15 times higher, compared with the first quintile; for the fifth quintile (245 mg/dl or greater), it was increased 3.4 times. Within the fifth quintile, the levels for the two highest deciles were 246 to 263 mg/dl and 264 mg/dl or greater, respectively; for these two subgroups the risk of premature CHD death was increased more than threefold and almost fivefold, respectively (data not shown).

The impact of combinations of these three established major risk factors merits emphasis, because it has profound implications, both practical and theoretic. For example, compared with the 10% of men in the lowest risk group of the MRFIT primary screenee cohort (serum cholesterol less than 182 mg/dl, nonhypertensive, nonsmok-

Table 80.5. Baseline Serum Cholesterol, Diastolic Blood Pressure, Smoking Status and Six-Year Age-Adjusted Coronary Heart Disease Death Rate per 1,000: 356,222 Men Aged 35 to 57 and Free at Baseline of a History of Hospitalization for Myocardial Infarction

	Serum Cholesterol Quintile (mg/dl)	Diastolic Pressure < 90 mm Hg			Diastolic Pressure ≥ 90 mm Hg			All		
		No. of Deaths	No. of Men	Rate per 1,000	No. of Deaths	No. of Men	Rate per 1,000	No. of Deaths	No. of Men	Rate per 1,000
Nonsmokers										
1	<182	47	35,741	1.6	36	9,612	3.7	83	45,353	2.1
2	182-202	82	34,553	2.5	51	11,599	4.0	133	46,152	2.9
3	203-220	87	31,939	2.7	80	12,839	5.6	167	44,778	3.5
4	221-244	126	30,431	3.8	94	14,500	5.6	220	44,931	4.4
5	≥245	188	26,996	6.4	200	16,930	10.7	388	43,926	8.0
All		530	159,660	3.3	461	65,480	6.4	991	225,140	4.3
Smokers										
1	<182	82	20,017	5.2	31	5,002	6.3	113	25,019	5.4
2	182-202	95	19,675	5.5	60	5,977	10.0	155	25,652	6.7
3	203-220	128	18,812	7.3	100	6,397	15.5	228	25,209	9.5
4	221-244	186	19,119	10.2	127	7,533	16.6	313	26,652	12.1
5	≥245	250	18,907	13.3	208	9,643	21.4	458	28,550	16.0
All		741	96,530	8.4	526	34,552	15.1	1,267	131,082	10.3
All										
1	<182	129	55,758	2.8	67	14,614	4.6	196	70,372	3.2
2	182-202	177	54,228	3.5	111	17,576	6.0	288	71,804	4.2
3	203-220	215	50,751	4.3	180	19,236	8.8	395	69,987	5.6
4	221-244	312	49,550	6.2	221	22,033	9.2	533	71,583	7.1
5	≥245	438	45,903	9.1	408	26,573	14.4	846	72,476	11.1
All		1,271	256,190	5.2	987	100,032	9.3	2,258	356,222	6.3

ers; six-year CHD mortality rate of 1.6 per 1,000), men in serum cholesterol quintile 4 ("moderate" hypercholesterolemia, levels of "only" 221 to 244 mg/dl) had the following increases in relative risk of CHD death, depending on their status in regard to HBP and cigarette use: diastolic blood pressure less than 90 mm Hg, a nonsmoker, "only" a 2.4-times increase in risk (3.8:1.6); diastolic blood pressure 90 mm Hg or greater, nonsmoker, a 3.5-times increase; diastolic blood pressure less than 90 mm Hg, a smoker, a 6.4-times increase; diastolic blood pressure 90 mm Hg or greater, a smoker, a 10.4-times increase (Table 80.5).[64] Absolute excess risk, ie, the difference in risk for a given subgroup compared with the subgroup at lowest risk, also increased progressively and steeply with various combinations of these three traits, eg, for the four aforementioned strata, from 2.2 (3.8 minus 1.6), to 4.0, to 8.6, to 15.0 per 1,000 in the six years from an average age of about 45 to 51 years.

These in-depth findings from the MRFIT screenee cohort exquisitely confirm for the 1970s and 1980s the conclusions reached on the basis of data from earlier prospective epidemiologic studies begun in the late 1940s, 1950s, and 1960s, eg, those of the national cooperative Pooling Project.[2,66] The Pooling Project life-table analyses add a further dimension to our understanding and comprehension of the combined impact of the three major risk factors, because they give data on long-term cumulative risk from age 40 through age 64, ie, a 25-year span of middle age (Table 80.6).[66] In these data, the full scope of the modern CHD epidemic is laid bare: for the entire cohort, the overall risk of a first major coronary event (nonfatal myocardial infarction or CHD death) before age 65 was almost one in four (221 per 1,000). For the 20% of men in the lowest quintile of risk, based on joint assessment of the three established major risk factors, the probability of a first major coronary event was about one in 17 (58 per 1,000). For American men, this is a relatively low risk, but it is hardly a miniscule risk absolutely. Moreover, it is a good deal higher than that in all Japanese and Chinese men over this age span, reflecting first and foremost the contrasting patterns of diet and serum cholesterol. Whereas the men in the Pooling Project in the lowest quintile of risk had a mean serum

Table 80.6. Three Major Risk Factors and Risk of a First Major Coronary Event Between Ages 40 and 64: 8,162 White Men, Pool 5, Pooling Project, Final Report

Quintile of Level	Number of Events	Risk of an Event Per 1,000	Relative Risk	Absolute Excess Risk Per 1,000	Percent of all Excess
I	23	57.9	1.00	---	---
II	66	118.3	2.04	60.4	8.7%
III	107	168.0	2.90	110.1	15.9%
IV	167	241.1	4.16	183.2	26.5%
V	271	395.7	6.83	337.8	48.9%
All	634	221.0	---	---	---

$$\frac{\text{QII–V Excess Events, 4,000 Men}}{\text{All Events, 5,000 Men}} = \frac{691.5}{981.0} = 70.5\%$$

of all events are excess events, attributable to the three major risk factors.

From Pooling Project Research Group.[66] Reprinted with permission.

cholesterol of 206 mg/dl (Table 80.7),[6,66] representative groups of middle-aged men in Japan and China have repeatedly shown overall mean levels no greater than 180 mg/dl and as low as 158 mg/dl.[58,60,67] Thus, the status of men in quintile I of the Pooling Project cohort may be viewed as a first, but by no means an optimal and final, goal in American men, as is evident from the rates of hypercholesterolemia, hypertension, and cigarette smoking prevalent even in this quintile (Table 80.7).

As to the men of the US Pooling Project in the highest 20% of risk (quintile V), based on their high levels of the three major risk factors (Table 80.7), their risk of a first major coronary event by age 65 was well over one in three (396 per 1,000), almost seven times greater than that of the lowest quintile (Table 80.6).[66] Excess risk was widely spread throughout the cohort, twice as great for the second quintile as for the first, three times greater for the third quintile, and four times greater for the fourth quintile. More than half (51%) the total excess risk was in quintiles II to IV; the remaining 49%, in quintile V. These findings, along with the MRFIT and multiple other data sets on the ubiquity of excess risk in the US population, document the essentiality of a two-pronged strategy for the prevention and control of epidemic premature CHD, ie, the need for population-wide improvements in life-styles to shift the distributions of the major risk factors to the left for the whole population, plus special pinpointed efforts for the higher risk strata. The potential for major shifts in risk factor distributions is illustrated, for serum cholesterol and blood pressure, respectively, in Figure 80.3.[68,69] Actual achievements by the US population in the last decade or two are summarized below. Because people with clinically manifest CHD are at especially high risk of acute events and death, and because their prognosis is significantly and sizably influenced by their status in regard to the major risk factors, they must be included among the higher risk strata deserving special attention as part of this two-pronged strategy.

The data in Table 80.6 also permit an estimate of the proportion of all first major coronary events that were excess events, attributable to the presence of hypercholesterolemia, hypertension, or cigarette smoking, or a combination of these, to a degree greater than that in quintile I. The excess risk of an event before age 65, over and above the risk for quintile I (57.9 per 1,000 men), was 60.4, 110.1, 183.2, and 337.8 per 1,000 men for quintiles II, III, IV, and V, respectively, with an average excess risk for these four quintiles of 172.9 per 1,000 men. These excess risks summate to 691.5 excess events per 4,000 men in quintiles II to V. Total or absolute risk per 5,000 men in quintiles I to V is the sum of the age-adjusted rates per 1,000 persons, ie, 981.0 per 5,000 men (57.9 + 118.3 + 168.0 + 241.1 + 395.7, Table 80.6). Therefore, the proportion of all events that were excess events is 691.5 per 981.0, ie, 70.5%.

This calculation is also an estimate of the potential that existed for prevention of premature CHD among middle-aged American men in the 1950s and 1960s. With shifts of the distributions of the established major risk factors to the left, eg, as a first goal, to levels for the whole middle-aged population like those prevailing for the low-

Table 80.7A. Prevalence of Major Risk Factors at Entry, Quintiles of Expected Risk, Three-Factor Logistic Analysis: Final Report, Pooling Project

	Serum Cholesterol		Systolic Pressure		Diastolic Pressure		Cigarettes	
Quintile	≥ 220 (%)	≥ 240 (%)	≥ 140 (%)	≥ 160 (%)	≥ 90 (%)	≥ 95 (%)	½+ Pks/Day (%)	1+ Pks/Day (%)
I	33.8	17.6	16.9	2.1	13.2	3.1	33.2	17.1
II	52.6	30.8	29.0	5.9	28.3	11.9	57.0	41.1
III	63.6	42.7	38.6	10.0	37.1	14.6	69.6	56.7
IV	73.2	53.8	47.8	15.2	46.6	23.8	80.9	71.9
V	83.9	68.6	68.4	34.2	69.2	47.1	90.5	84.3
All	61.4	42.7	40.1	13.5	38.9	20.1	66.2	54.2

est quintile of risk, it may be projected that about 70% of all first major coronary events before age 65 could have been prevented. Over the last two decades, the distributions of the three major risk factors have indeed been moving to the left, with sizable declines in mean levels of serum cholesterol and in prevalence rates of hypercholesterolemia, hypertension, and cigarette smoking for the adult population (see subsequently). Concomitantly, death rates from premature CHD have decreased steadily and substantially from the late 1960s to the early 1980s by about 30% overall (see subsequently). These data support the central thesis of this chapter, set forth at its beginning, that the contemporary mass forms of heart disease, like earlier forms of epidemic disease, are preventable.

A key reason for the great success of cardiovascular epidemiologic factors in identifying and quantitating the role of the three established major risk factors for CHD was the fact that a single measurement, readily made with high-level accuracy, was sufficient to characterize individuals within a population and validly distinguish them one from another with little misclassification. This is the case despite measurement error, short-term physiologic fluctuations, and possible long-term changes in serum cholesterol and blood pressure, and the fact that during the years of these studies many cigarette smokers became exsmokers. The reason behind this ability of one measurement of these three variables to characterize persons satisfactorily for research classification is that for each of them the ratio of intraindividual to interindividual variation is well below 1.0, eg, for serum cholesterol and blood pressure, about 0.3.[70] That is, for these traits, people vary much more from each other than they do over time from themselves. This is not the situation, however, in regard to other life-style–related traits of concern in regard to the etiology of epidemic premature CHD, eg, intake of dietary lipids, level of physical activity at work and leisure, psychosocial stresses–tensions, and incongruent behavior patterns. For these latter variables, compared with the three established major risk factors, the problems of achieving validity in measurement and classification of individuals within a population are much greater. Thus, when systematic studies were made of the ratios of intraindividual to interindividual variability for these latter variables, as were done for dietary lipids and physical activity, ratios are well above unity.[71–74] Under this circumstance, a single measurement, such as the oft-used 24-hour recall of food eaten on the previous day, is generally inadequate to classify individuals satisfactorily. Day-to-day variation in eating practices is too great; people differ much more from themselves day-to-day than from each other. The failure until recently to appreciate this key problem, together with other methodologic difficulties, accounts in a major way for negative results reported by some studies on the relation of dietary lipids to serum cholesterol and long-term CHD risk of individuals within a population.[71,75,76]

To overcome the methodologic difficulties, either or

Table 80.7B. Mean Levels of Major Risk Factors at Entry, Quintiles of Expected Risk, Three-Factor Logistic Analysis: Final Report, Pooling Project

Quintile	Mean Serum Cholesterol (mg/dl)	Mean Systolic Pressure (mm Hg)	Mean Diastolic Pressure (mm Hg)	Mean Cigarettes Packs/Day (All)	Mean Cigarettes Packs/Day (Smokers Only)
I	206.0 ± 36.2*	124.7 ± 13.6	78.5 ± 8.1	0.36 ± 0.65	1.08 ± 0.71
II	221.9 ± 37.1	131.1 ± 15.1	83.1 ± 9.1	0.85 ± 0.93	1.48 ± 0.77
III	234.3 ± 41.0	134.6 ± 17.0	85.1 ± 9.7	1.20 ± 1.04	1.73 ± 0.81
IV	246.5 ± 43.3	138.8 ± 18.6	87.9 ± 10.5	1.63 ± 1.06	2.02 ± 0.79
V	269.1 ± 53.9	151.1 ± 23.8	95.8 ± 13.7	2.05 ± 0.97	2.27 ± 0.74
All	235.6 ± 47.8	136.1 ± 20.0	86.1 ± 11.9	1.22 ± 1.11	1.84 ± 0.85

* Standard deviation.

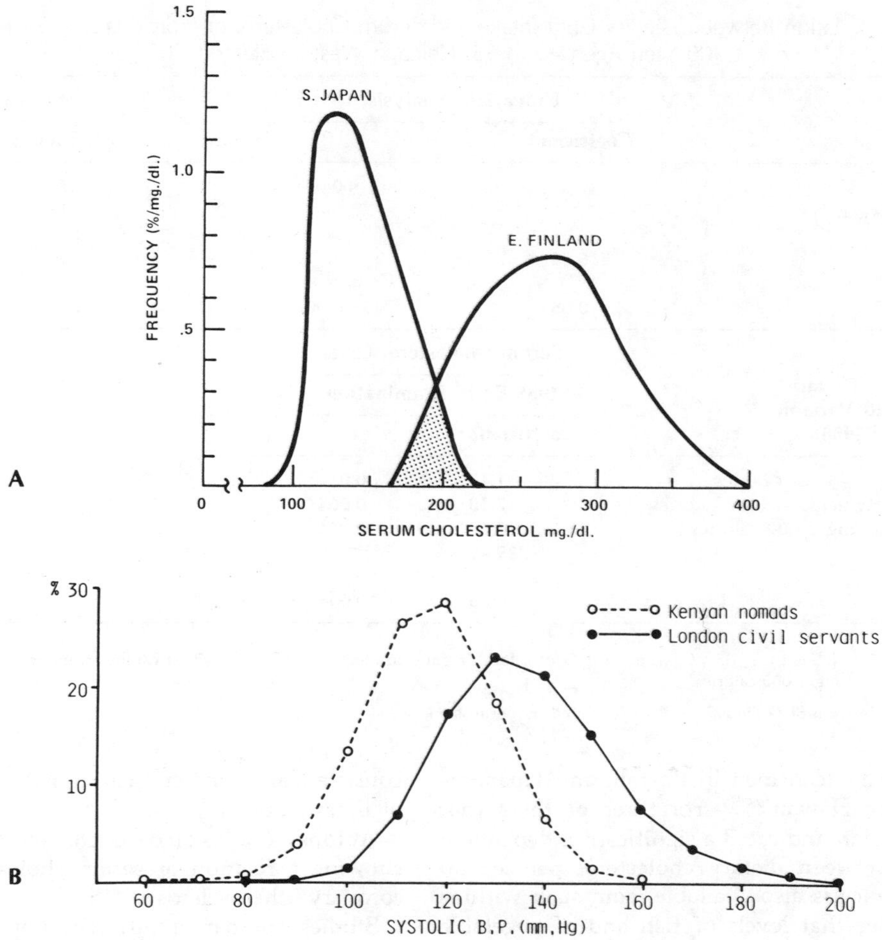

Figure 80.3. Distributions of serum cholesterol in samples of men from southern Japan and east Finland (*A*), and distributions of systolic blood pressure in men aged 40 to 59 years in Kenyan nomads and in London civil servants (*B*). (Figure 80.3A is from Blackburn H: Diet and mass hyperlipidemia: a public health view, in Levy RI, Rifkind BM, Dennis BH, Ernst ED (eds): *Nutrition, Lipids, and Coronary Heart Disease—A Global View*. New York, Raven Press, 1979, pp 309–347. Reprinted with permission. Figure 80.3B is from Rose G.[69] Reprinted with permission of Springer-Verlag.)

both of two alternative approaches must be used for proper nutritional assessment of individuals within a population: multiple 24-hour recalls (eg, 3 to 11 per person depending on empiric assessment of the ratio of intraindividual to interindividual variation and precision of individual classification desired), or a standardized in-depth interview to assess individual habitual eating pattern (eg, that during the previous 30 days). To account for possible confounding of the data, pains must also be taken to ascertain whether individuals have changed their eating habits recently, particularly in response to information about their risk factor status (eg, altered dietary lipid intake because of hypercholesterolemia, decreased salt intake due to hypertension, and reduction in calories and weight in response to one or the other or both of these). Failure to take this aspect into account can lead to spurious findings.[76]

When dietary methods are satisfactory, clearcut significant relations are demonstrable at three levels: (1) the level and composition of dietary lipids (and also of relative body weight) of individuals are related to their level of serum cholesterol (Table 80.8)[75,77]; (2) change in the level and composition of dietary lipids (and weight) by individuals over time is related to change in serum cholesterol (Table 80.9)[75,77]; (3) most important of all, baseline lipid intake, particularly dietary cholesterol intake, is significantly related to long-term risk of death from CHD and all causes (Table 80.10).[75–77] These relations are independent of the significant relations of serum cholesterol, blood pressure, cigarette use, and age to risk of death.

Until 1984–1985, these findings from the Chicago Western Electric Study on the significant independent relation of dietary lipid to long-term risk of CHD in individuals within a population stood virtually alone. However, confirmatory data were published in 1984 and 1985 for four other populations studied long-term: California Seventh Day Adventists, Dutch men in Zutphen, Irish

Table 80.8. Relation Between Dietary Lipid Intake and Serum Cholesterol of Individuals, 1958 Entry Examination, 1,900 Men Aged 40 to 55, Chicago Western Electric Co. Study

	Univariate Analysis		Trivariate Analysis	
Regressor	Coefficient	*P*	Coefficient	*P*
Dietary lipid score	0.51	<0.001	0.54	<0.001
Body mass index (kg/m²)	···	···	1.15	0.003
Age (yrs)	···	···	0.38	0.171
Constant	216.89		167.90	
R	0.08	<0.001	0.11	<0.001

Entry Dietary Lipid Variable (1958)	Serum Cholesterol Level 1958 Entry Examination Coefficient	*P*
Saturated fatty acids—% of calories	1.10	0.014
Polyunsaturated fatty acids—% of calories	-2.10	0.064
Dietary cholesterol—mg/1,000 calories	0.03	0.044
Constant	229.41	
R	0.08	0.006

Dietary lipid score = 1.26 (2S − P) + 1.5 $\sqrt{C}$, where S is % of calories from saturated fatty acids, P is % of calories from polyunsaturated fatty acids, and C is dietary cholesterol in mg/1,000 calories.

Tables 80.8 and 80.9 are from Shekelle RB, et al.[75] Reprinted by permission.

men and Irish-American men in Boston, and Japanese-American men in Hawaii.[78-83] For three of these four populations, the data indicated a significant independent direct relation between dietary cholesterol per se and CHD risk. Evidence is also available from such within-population studies that levels of fish and of vegetable products high in fiber have a significant independent inverse relation to CHD risk.[78-84] These findings from within-population prospective epidemiologic research are consistent and coherent with those from many other types of investigations:

Autopsy studies on decedents within such populations, showing a relation of serum cholesterol to severity of coronary atherosclerosis[85-88];

Studies comparing different populations around the world, eg, the autopsy data of the International Atherosclerosis Project, the results of the Seven Countries Study and the Ni-Hon-San Study, the multiple analyses

Table 80.9. Relations Between Change in Dietary Lipid Intake and Change in Serum Cholesterol of Individuals, Entry to Year 1, 1,900 Men Aged 40 to 55 at Entry, Chicago Western Electric Co. Study, 1958–1959

	Univariate Analysis		Trivariate Analysis	
Regressor	Coefficient	*P*	Coefficient	*P*
Change in Dietary Lipid Score	0.64	<0.001	0.62	<0.001
Change in Body Mass Index—kg/m²	···	···	5.53	<0.001
Age (yr)	···	···	0.10	0.627
Constant	-10.31		-16.37	
R	0.12	<0.001	0.18	<0.001

Variable: Change, 1958→1959	Change in Serum Cholesterol, 1958→1959: Three Variable Analysis Coefficient	*P*	Four Variable Analysis Coefficient	*P*
Change in Dietary Sat. Fatty Acids—% of Calories	1.68	<0.001	1.58	<0.001
Change in Dietary Poly. Fatty Acids—% of Calories	-0.02	0.492	-0.38	0.334
Change in Dietary Cholesterol—mg/ 1,000 Calories	0.03	0.041	0.03	0.029
Change in Body Mass Index—kg/m²	···	···	5.47	<0.001
Constant	-10.31		-11.37	
R	0.13	<0.001	0.18	<0.001

Dietary lipid score = 1.26 (2S − P) + 1.5 $\sqrt{C}$.

Table 80.10. Relation Between Dietary Lipid Intake and 19-Year Mortality From Coronary Heart Disease and All Causes: 1,884 Men Aged 40 to 55 At Entry, Chicago Western Electric Co. Study

	Coronary Heart Disease (213 Deaths)		All Causes (448 Deaths)	
Baseline Variable	Multiple Logistic Coefficient	*P*	Multiple Logistic Coefficient	*P*
Dietary lipid score	0.0264	0.015	0.0161	0.048
Serum cholesterol (mg/dl)	0.0056	<0.001	0.0030	0.018
Systolic pressure (mm Hg)	0.0242	<0.001	0.0220	<0.001
Cigarettes (no./day)	0.0379	<0.001	0.0376	<0.001
Age (yr)	0.1026	<0.001	0.1104	<0.001
Saturated fatty acids (% of cal.)	0.0320	0.398	0.0154	0.589
Polyunsaturated fatty acids (% of cal.)	−0.2352	0.025	0.0993	0.182
Dietary cholesterol (mg/1,000 cal.)	0.0032	0.015	0.0023	0.026
Serum cholesterol (mg/dl)	0.0056	<0.001	0.0031	0.014
Systolic pressure (mm Hg)	0.0234	<0.001	0.0212	<0.001
Cigarettes (no./day)	0.0384	<0.001	0.0382	<0.001
Age (yr)	0.0945	<0.001	0.1057	<0.001

Also included in analyses, but not significantly related to either end point: BMI, alcohol intake, ethnic background.

From Stamler J.[77] Reprinted with permission.

correlating overall data on national food patterns and CHD mortality rates for sets of countries[1–12,16,54–61,89];

Clinical angiographic studies on the relation of serum cholesterol, its subfractions, and other major risk factors to severity of coronary atherosclerosis[5,90];

Animal-experimental research, from the first decade of this century on, repeatedly demonstrating, in virtually all species worked with in the laboratory, including nonhuman primates, the crucial role of dietary cholesterol in the development of significant atherosclerosis, and the ability to stop atherogenesis and achieve regression of lesions with cessation of administration of a cholesterol supplement to the diet[1–12,54,57,61,91];

Recent clinical trials and community demonstration projects showing ability to achieve primary and secondary prevention of CHD and other atherosclerotic diseases, eg, the significant positive results from the Oslo Primary Prevention Trial involving severely hypercholesterolemic cigarette-smoking nonhypertensive men and the similar findings from the MRFIT Oslo-like cohort; the positive data from the Belgian factory trial and the Lipid Research Clinics Coronary Primary Prevention Trial; the repeated angiographic demonstration in people with severe clinical atherosclerotic disease, coronary and peripheral, of ability to slow and stop progression of atherogenesis by treatment with diet and drugs to lower serum cholesterol, the data on declining CHD rates in relation to development and demonstration projects in Finland, Norway, and elsewhere.[3–5,12,16,30,92–107]

In fact, the multiple sets of impressive new data on the role of the major risk factors and on ability to prevent CHD by improving life-styles and life-style–related risk factors are essentially profound confirmations of findings available for many years.[1,2,7,8,26,45,54–57,62,66,91] Correspondingly it is now many years, about a quarter of a century, since the first statements on the possibilities of CHD prevention were formulated by expert groups, for dissemination to physicians, other health professionals, policy makers, and the general public.[5,8] Over the ensuing years, these recommendations for Americans were reiterated, elaborated, and reinforced from several influential and prestigious sources (professional, voluntary health, quasi-governmental, governmental), particularly in the periodic statements of the American Heart Association (AHA); the periodic Reports of the Joint National Committee advising the National High Blood Pressure Education Program; the Reports to the Surgeon General on Smoking and Health; the 1970 and 1984 Reports of the Inter-Society Commission for Heart Disease Resources; the 1971 and 1981 Reports on Arteriosclerosis to the National Heart, Lung, and Blood Institute (NHLBI); the Proceedings of the Bethesda Conference on the Prevention of Coronary Heart Disease, under the leadership of the American College of Cardiology, and cosponsored by AHA and NHLBI; the Dietary Goals set forth by the US Senate Select Committee on Nutrition and Human Needs; the Dietary Guidelines jointly developed by the US Departments of Agriculture and of Health and Human Services; and most recently, in 1984 and 1985, the NIH Consensus Development Conference on Lowering Blood Cholesterol to Prevent Heart Disease.[2,3,5,7,8,39,57,61]

These recommendations have been widely disseminated. The message has evidently registered. One consequence is that the proportion of people in whom high blood pressure is detected, treated, and controlled (only 10% to 15% in the late 1960s and early 1970s) now represents a majority of hypertensive persons from all socioeconomic and ethnic groups.[3,5,8,12,108]

In regard to life-styles, surveys by the US Department of Agriculture show that by 1979 almost two thirds of all Americans had changed eating patterns for reasons of health.[109,110] Correspondingly, intakes of foods high in cholesterol and saturated fats, eg, eggs, fat-containing dairy products, and lard, have declined steadily and substantially.[5,8,12,111] Adults in the CHD-prone age groups have also reduced their intake of beef and meat and have curtailed their consumption of visible fats.[5,8,12,112] Mean serum cholesterol levels in the population are down, as expected given the diet trends, eg, among middle-aged men, the level has declined from 235 to 245 mg/dl in the late 1940s, 1950s, and early 1960s to 210 to 215 in the late 1970s and early 1980s.[5,8,12,55,56] These changes may be especially important, given the extensive evidence that a "rich" diet and diet-related hypercholesterolemia play a primary and pivotal part in the etiology of severe atherosclerosis.

Over the same period, the proportion of cigarette smokers in the adult population has also decreased steadily.[5,8,12,113] A majority of men smoked at the time of the *Report to the Surgeon General* in 1964; now only about a third do. In addition, as part of the emergence of a new mass health consciousness, tens of millions of American adults have taken up leisure-time exercise.

For all these life-style changes in eating, smoking, and exercise habits, there is evidence of a socioeconomic connection: the more educated have changed more than the less educated.[5,8,12,55,56,114]

Concomitantly, since the late 1960s, US death rates from coronary heart disease have fallen steadily and markedly (Figure 80.4).[115] This decline has involved all sectors of the adult population.[5] For persons aged 35 to 74 years, the rate of mortality from CHD has fallen by over 30%, resulting in more than 800,000 lives saved since 1968. Death rates from stroke have declined even more precipitously. Therefore, death rates for the broad generic group, the major cardiovascular diseases (made up largely of CHD and stroke), are also down markedly, as are death rates from all causes—the "bottom line" item. Without doubt, these declines are real; there is absolutely no reason to believe they are spurious or artifactual.

The decline in CHD mortality can be a result of two trends: decreasing incidence of the disease or a lower case fatality rate (this latter, in turn, due possibly to a tendency for the disease to become more mild and/or better medical care for those developing CHD), or both. No national data are available on these matters, for the US population as a whole or for random samples, and the valid collection of representative data on these trends is a complex and difficult task. In recent years, a few reports have appeared on selected populations in different parts of the country, eg, subscribers to the Kaiser-Permanente Health Plan in California; residents of Olmsted County, Minnesota,

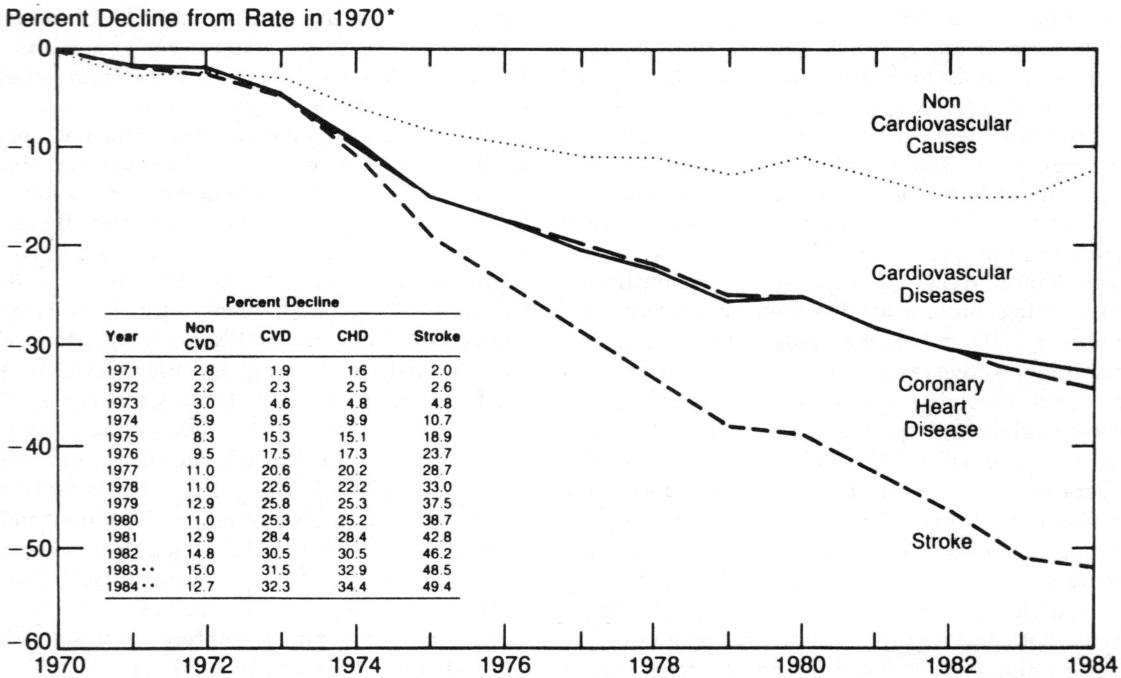

Percent Decline

Year	Non CVD	CVD	CHD	Stroke
1971	2.8	1.9	1.6	2.0
1972	2.2	2.3	2.5	2.6
1973	3.0	4.6	4.8	4.8
1974	5.9	9.5	9.9	10.7
1975	8.3	15.3	15.1	18.9
1976	9.5	17.5	17.3	23.7
1977	11.0	20.6	20.2	28.7
1978	11.0	22.6	22.2	33.0
1979	12.9	25.8	25.3	37.5
1980	11.0	25.3	25.2	38.7
1981	12.9	28.4	28.4	42.8
1982	14.8	30.5	30.5	46.2
1983**	15.0	31.5	32.9	48.5
1984**	12.7	32.3	34.4	49.4

*Based on Age-Adjusted Death Rates.
**Estimated
Source: Vital Statistics of the U.S., NCHS.

Figure 80.4. Trends in mortality for cardiovascular disease and noncardiovascular causes of death. Percentage decline in age-adjusted death rates, United States, 1970 to 1984. (From National Heart, Lung, and Blood Institute.[115])

served by the Mayo Clinic; the population of the State of Minnesota; and employees of the DuPont Company.[116–120] Most of these studies indicate that the decline in CHD mortality reflects in a major way a decline in overall incidence of major coronary events; the DuPont data are illustrative (Table 80.11).[120] Correspondingly, data from serial autopsy studies in New Orleans indicate that for young adult men, the prevalence of severe coronary atherosclerosis at autopsy was lower in the 1970s than in the 1960s, particularly for white men.[121] Thus, the limited information available supports the inference that decreases in the underlying disease and its clinical manifestations have contributed importantly to the decreases in CHD mortality rates.

The decline in mortality from coronary heart disease is all the more remarkable because it occurred after a sustained period of rising death rates from this cause,[5] going back to at least 1940. The recent decline in the United States is also striking in that it is larger than that observed in any other country (Figure 80.5).[5] In the late 1960s, the death rate in the United States from premature CHD was the second highest in the world; only Finland was doing worse. By the late 1970s, the US rate ranked eighth among rates in 27 economically developed countries. The decline in the United States has continued into the early 1980s. Only Australia has approached the US rate of decline in mortality from CHD. Several European countries have registered little or no change in rates or rising rates. Thus, the decrease in coronary heart disease rates is not universal, not a contemporary "cohort effect" for the human species overall. It is a reasonable inference, in light of all the other supporting data, that the improvements in life-style and the resultant lower rates in the US population of life-style–related major risk factors have contributed importantly to the decline in CHD mortality rates (Table 80.12).[16] Several analyses support this conclusion. They include data showing good quantitative correspondence between the observed decreases in CHD death rates and expected decreases, as estimated from the earlier experience of US prospective epidemiologic studies and from the recorded population changes in major risk factors.[89,116,122] Perhaps the most impressive, and practically significant, data on this matter relate to an important aspect of the improvement in life-styles and the related shift downward in prevalence rates of life-style–related risk factors: In regard to the key area of eating habits and diet-dependent serum cholesterol levels, cigarette smoking, and leisure-time exercise, the higher the level of education-affluence, the greater has been the favorable change. This set of facts leads to an important inference: If improvements in life-style and life-style–related risk factors have contributed sizably to the decline in CHD death rates, should not the more educated-affluent have experienced a greater decline than the less educated-affluent? Three data sets are now extant testing this inference; all of them are consistent with it. One of these is the recent report of the long-term follow-up of almost 100,000 employees of the DuPont Company. The CHD incidence rate among salaried employees fell twice as steeply as that of wage workers, 38% and 18%, respectively.[120] A second data set is available from the Metropolitan Life Insurance Company. Its male policy holders, as compared with age–race-matched men in the general US population, had a steeper decline in recent years in CHD mortality rates.[123] The third data set, comparing California physicians and age–race-matched men in the general US population, particularly merits attention in a modern textbook of cardiology: During 1950 to 1954, the rate of death from CHD for white male physicians in California was 15% higher than that for all age-matched white men in the United States (Table 80.13).[124] By the period 1975 to 1979, the rate was 31% lower, ie, the decline in the rate for physicians exceeded that for all white men by 40%. In the period 1950 to 1954, a majority of male physicians, like men in the general population, were cigarette smokers. Over the next decades, the proportion who became exsmokers was much higher among physicians than among men overall. By the period

Table 80.11. Trend of Age-Adjusted Incidence Rates of Myocardial Infarction, 1957–1983: Male Employees of the DuPont Co. in the USA

	All Male Employees			Wage Workers			Salaried Employees		
Period	No. of Events	Rate per 1,000 per Yr	Decline (%)	No. of Events	Rate per 1,000 per Yr	Decline (%)	No. of Events	Rate per 1,000 per Yr	Decline (%)
1957–1959	641	3.19	...	384	3.13	...	257	3.30	...
1960–1962	704	3.12	2.2	△	△	△	△	△	△
1963–1965	733	2.92	8.5	△	△	△	△	△	△
1966–1968	819	2.98	6.6	△	△	△	△	△	△
1969–1971	758	2.70	15.4	△	△	△	△	△	△
1972–1974	710	2.57	19.4	△	△	△	△	△	△
1975–1977	739	2.70	15.4	△	△	△	△	△	△
1978–1980	644	2.33	27.0	△	△	△	△	△	△
1981–1983	538	2.29	28.2	272	2.56	18.2	266	2.06	37.6

During these years, DuPont Co. male employees in the USA numbered 75,000 to 94,000; 55 to 60% were production workers receiving hourly wages; the remainder were salaried employees in managerial, supervisory, professional, technical, and clerical occupations.

△Data not available.

From Pell S, Fayerweather WE.[120] Reprinted with permission.

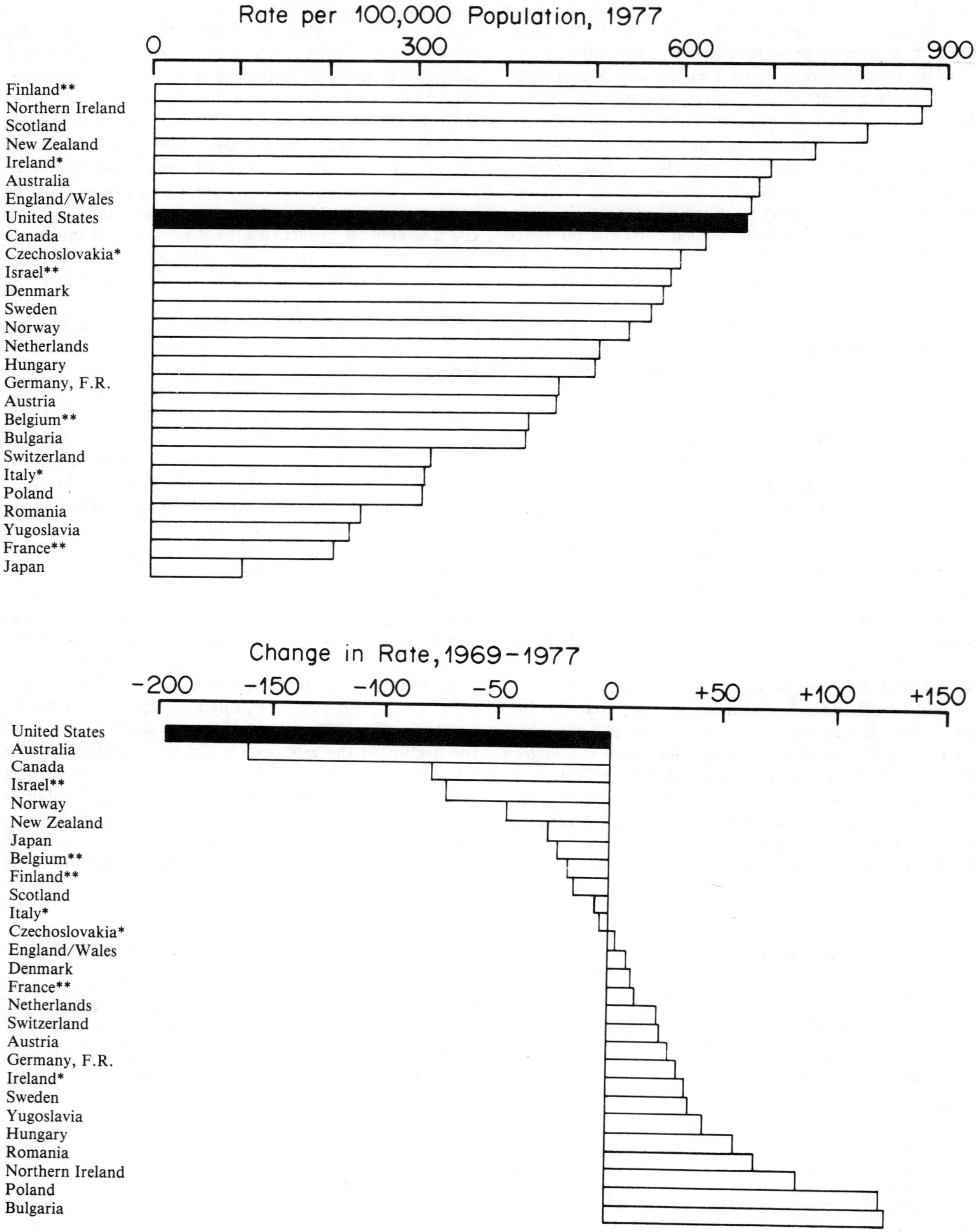

*1975 Data
**1976 Data
Source: Prepared by NHLBI; data from the World Health Organization.

Figure 80.5a. Death rates in 1977 for coronary heart disease by country for men, 35 to 74 years of age, and changes in rates, 1969 to 1977. (From Working Group on Arteriosclerosis of the National Heart, Lung, and Blood Institute.[5])

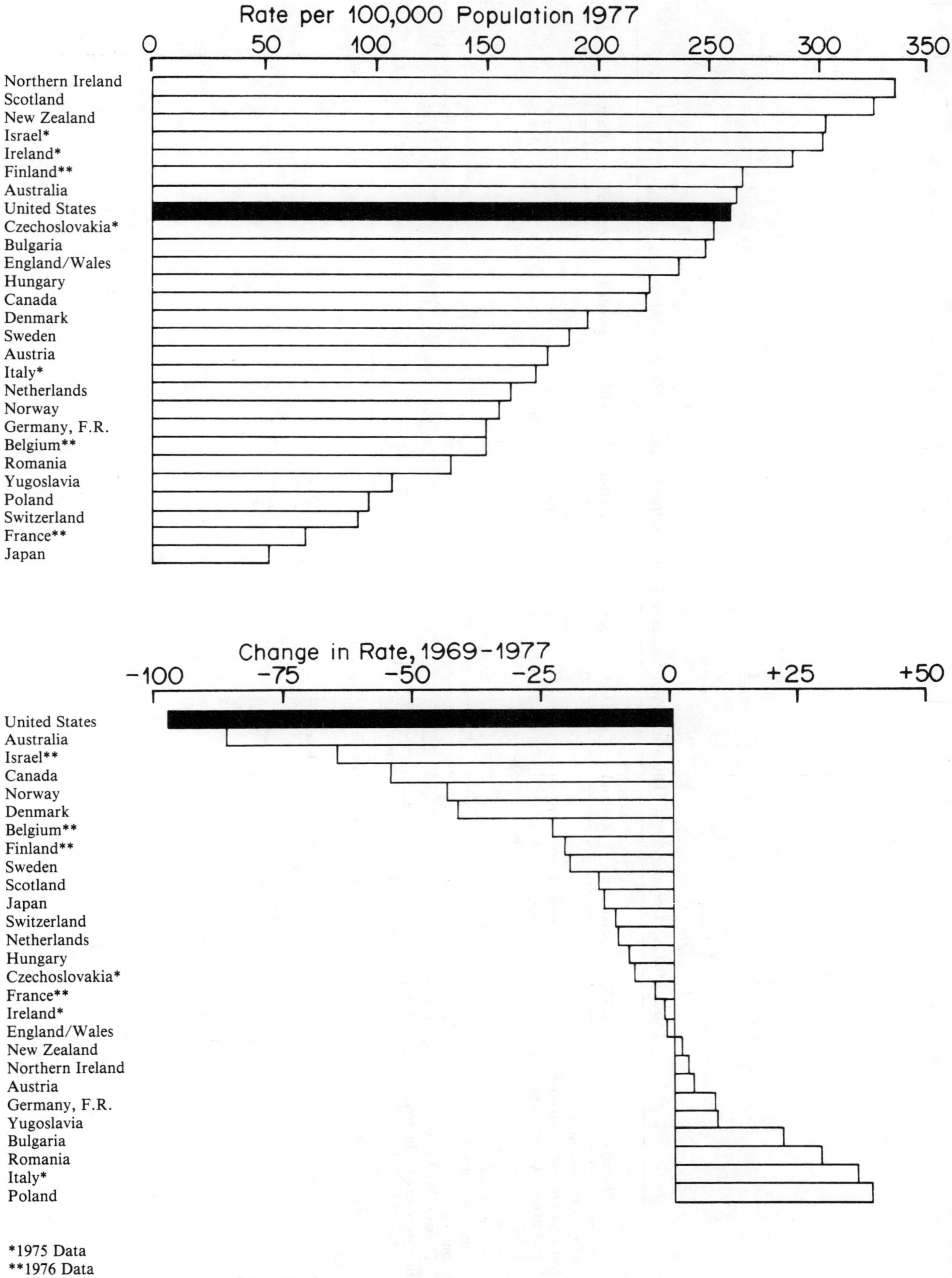

*1975 Data
**1976 Data
Source: Prepared by NHLBI; data from the World Health Organization.

Figure 80.5b. Death rates in 1977 for coronary heart disease by country for women, 35 to 74 years of age, and changes in rates, 1969 to 1977. (From Working Group on Arteriosclerosis of the National Heart, Lung, and Blood Institute.[5])

Table 80.12. Coronary Heart Disease (CHD) Mortality Trends in the 1970s: Contributory Influences

Trends	USA	Australia	New Zealand	Finland	Norway	Belgium	Israel	Sweden	Poland	Italy	Spain
CHD mortality trends[1]	↓	↓	↓	↓	↓	↓	↓	↑	↑	↑	↑
National preventive efforts[2]	++	++	+	++	++	++	0	+	0	+	0
Trend toward better dietary habits[2]	++	++	+	+	+	++	0	0	0	0	0
Risk factors[1]											
Serum cholesterol	↓	?	(↓)	↓	↓	↓	ø	ø	(↑)	(↑)	(↑)
Blood pressure	↓	(↓)	↓	↓	↓	(↓)	↓	(↓)	(↓)	(↓)	(↓)
Smoking	↓	↓	↓	↓	↓	↓	ø	↓	?	(↑)	(↑)
Physical inactivity	↓	?	↓	↓	↓	?	?	(↓)	?	(↓)	?
Improvement in the treatment of CHD[2]	++	++	+	+	+	++	++	+	+	+	+

[1] ? = no data: ↓ = decline; ø = no change; ↑ = increase; ( ) = possible change.

[2] Scale of 0 to ++.

From Pyörälä, et al.[16] Reprinted with permission of the author and S Karger AG, Basel.

Table 80.13. Standardized Mortality Ratios, Five-Year Periods: California Male Physicians Compared with Age-Matched US White Men

Years	Cause of Death		
	Coronary Heart Disease	Lung Cancer	All Causes
1950–4	115	51	89
1955–9	97	70	80
1960–4	86	52	79
1965–9	80	57	78
1970–4	74	29	67
1975–9	69	30	67
% Change: 1950–1954→1975–1979	−40.0%	−41.2%	−24.7%
% Change: 1965–1969→1975–1979	−13.7%	−47.4%	−14.1%

From Enstom JE.[124] Reprinted with permission.

1975 to 1979, no more than 10% of physicians were still smoking cigarettes, as compared to about 40% of white men generally. Physicians in the United States have also paced the rest of the population in regard to changes in eating and exercise habits.[125]

These data lend strong support to the conclusion that improvements in life-style and in life-style–related risk factors have contributed substantially to the decline in the rates of coronary heart disease.[126]

As indicated, over the last quarter of a century, with statesman-like leadership from American cardiology, sound public policy has been developed and disseminated on the prevention, first and foremost the primary prevention, of coronary heart disease. Wide-ranging activities have been set in motion at many levels, in public health and medical care, in the general channels of popular communication, in the food industry, and the like, to implement the sound two-pronged strategy of general recommendations for the whole population and special ones for the many persons at higher risk (including those who already have clinical coronary heart disease). Critical mass has been achieved in the effort to influence the disturbances of human culture that produced the epidemic, ie, the changes in life-styles and life-style–related risk factors are detectable in routine statistics for the US population as a whole and its various strata. Links in the chain of the causation have been broken for many people, and the tide of the epidemic has been turned. However, rates of morbidity, disability, and premature death from coronary heart disease remain very high in the United States. All the efforts in primary prevention, and in secondary prevention as well, need to be extended and intensified, as noted in recent reports on prevention for the United States.[127,128] A sound goal is to sustain a 3% annual decline in the rate of death from coronary heart disease for the remainder of the century, with special efforts to realize this goal for all socioeconomic strata of our population, not only the more educated and affluent.

PRIMARY PREVENTION OF OTHER HEART DISEASES

As indicated in the introductory paragraphs of this chapter, the other heart diseases afflicting mankind in a major way today are: pulmonary heart disease, alcoholic heart muscle disease, congenital heart disease, which have a significant incidence in both industrialized and economically developing countries of the world, and rheumatic heart disease, Chagas' disease, and the cardiomyopathies of unknown causes, which are large-scale problems particularly in developing countries.

In one way or another, insofar as one or another of these diseases has a mass incidence in different populations, each of these challenges to modern preventive cardiology reflects the soundness of Virchow's concept that mass disease is due to disturbances of human culture. Thus, at least in the industrialized countries, pulmonary heart disease is first and foremost related to mass use of cigarettes;[1] the disturbance of human culture producing a high incidence of alcoholic heart muscle disease is self-evident. In the economically developing countries, the combined effects of such mass disturbances of human culture as gross overcrowding and chronic undernutrition, plus inadequacies in preventive and primary health care, combine to make rheumatic heart disease an unsolved persistent epidemic problem.[1,9,18,129] The relation of mass Chagas' disease to inadequate housing is well known. Although much remains to be learned about the etiology and pathogenesis of the cardiomyopathies of unknown causes,[130] it is a reasonable inference, both from what is currently known about their epidemiologic patterns of incidence and from general experience with other common diseases, that in due course research will uncover the environmental factors causing their high incidence in certain populations in the developing countries. The specifics of their primary prevention will then emerge more forcefully as a challenge. In the interim, it is also reasonable to anticipate that general socioeconomic progress, if it can be accomplished with improvements in the living standards for the masses of the populations afflicted by these diseases, will lead to declines in their incidence, as well as in the incidence of the other heart diseases afflicting these deprived sectors of mankind. Even for congenital heart disease, or, more correctly, in terms of etiology and pathogenesis, as well as pathology and pathophysiology, the congenital heart diseases, where much still remains obscure in terms of causes, mounting knowledge, and experience, eg, in regard to rubella, illustrate the potentials, present and future, for prevention through dealing with known and probable environmental causes, even before any future era of prophylactic genetic engineering.[1,9,131,132]

Other chapters in this book and publications by this writer, dealing with each of the foregoing problems, and recent expert reports present specifics of modern knowledge concerning the primary prevention of these forms of heart disease.[1,9,132–134]

Acknowledgments: It is a pleasure to acknowledge the fine contributions over many years of the author's colleagues involved in the research work of our group reported here, including: Ruth Anderson, MPH, David M. Berkson,

MD, Robert Byington, PhD, Jean Civinelli, Richard Cooper, MD, Alan R. Dyer, PhD, Eduardo Farinaro, MD, Joan Fishman, MS, RD, Dan Garside, BS, Flora Gosch, MD, Dante Giumetti, MD, Yolanda Hall, MS, Ron Hoeksema, ZG Hong, MD, Emanuel Larbi, MD, Sophie Levinson, MD, Kiang Liu, PhD, Howard Lindberg, MD, John Marquardt, MD, Arline McDonald, PhD, Jeffrey McKeever, MD, Patricia McKeever, MS, Dorothy Moss, MS, Peter Rhomberg, MD, Richard B. Shekelle, PhD, Ivan Soltero, MD, Rose Stamler, MA, Elizabeth Stevens, RN, Maurizio Trevisan, MD, Ton Tokich, Yi Tsong, PhD, and Linda Van Horn, PhD, RD.

Appreciation is also expressed to the several groups of colleagues from other institutions, involved with our group in cooperative research efforts, including those of the Hypertension Control Program, especially Reuben Berman, MD, Patricia Elmer, RD, Richard Grimm, MD, Nancy Van Heel, RD; the Multiple Risk Factor Intervention Trial, especially James Neaton, PhD and Deborah Wentworth, MPH; the Cardiovascular Institute, Chinese Academy of Medical Sciences, People's Republic of China, especially CK Hsiao, MD, ZD Huang, MD, LS Liu, MD, and SC Tao, MD; the principal investigators of the prospective studies of Albany civil servants, Chicago Western Electric Company employees, Framingham community residents, Los Angeles civil servants, Minneapolis–St. Paul business and professional men, Northwest Railroad workers, Tecumseh community residents, and to the coordinators of the National Cooperative Pooling Project. It is a pleasure to acknowledge the cooperation and aid of our colleagues in this endeavor, Drs Henry Blackburn, John M Chapman, Thomas R Dawber, Joseph T Doyle, Frederick H Epstein, William B Kannel, Ancel Keys, Felix J Moore, Oglesby Paul, and Henry L Taylor; the Western Electric Company study, especially Drs Mark Lepper, Harlley McKean, Oglesby Paul, and Anne M Shryock.

The author is pleased to express gratitude to the following colleagues whose data were cited: Drs Henry Blackburn, James Enstrom, Frederick H Epstein, Marcel Kornitzer, Li-sheng Liu, Sidney Pell, Kalevi Pyörälä, Geoffrey Rose, SC Tao, and the above-colleagues of the Pooling Project.

The author's research reported here has been supported by the American Heart Association; Chicago Heart Association; National Heart, Lung, and Blood Institute; also by CIBA-GEIGY; CPC International (Best Foods); Nabisco Brands; and the Marsteller Company (Flora Information Service).

REFERENCES

1. Stamler J: *Lectures on Preventive Cardiology*. New York, Grune & Stratton, 1967.
2. Inter-Society Commission for Heart Disease Resources. Atherosclerosis Study Group and Epidemiology Study Group: Primary prevention of the atherosclerotic diseases, in Wright IS, Fredrickson DT (eds): *Cardiovascular Diseases—Guidelines for Prevention and Care,* Washington DC, US Government Printing Office, 1974, pp 15–58.
3. Inter-Society Commission for Heart Disease Resources. Atherosclerosis Study Group: Optimal resources for primary prevention of atherosclerotic diseases. *Circulation* 1984; 70:153A–205A.
4. WHO Expert Committee on the Prevention of Coronary Heart Disease: *Prevention of Coronary Heart Disease,* World Health Organization Technical Report Series No 678, World Health Organization, Geneva, Switzerland, 1982.
5. Working Group on Arteriosclerosis of the National Heart, Lung, and Blood Institute: *Report of the Working Group on Arteriosclerosis of the National Heart, Lung, and Blood Institute*, vols 1 and 2. US Department of Health and Human Services, Public Health Service, National Institutes of Health, NIH Publication Nos 81-2034 and 81-2035, Bethesda MD, June and September, 1981.
6. Stamler J: Improved life styles: their potential for the primary prevention of atherosclerosis and hypertension in childhood, in Lauer RM, Shekelle RB (eds): *Childhood Prevention of Atherosclerosis and Hypertension*. New York, Raven Press, 1980, pp 3–36.
7. American Heart Association Committee Report: Risk factors and coronary disease: a statement for physicians. *Circulation* 1980; 62:449A–455A.
8. Stamler J, Abelmann WH (eds): Bethesda Conference Report—Eleventh Bethesda Conference: prevention of coronary heart disease. *Am J Cardiol* 1981; 47:713–776.
9. Stamler J: Disease of the cardiovascular system, in Clark DW, MacMahon B (eds): *Preventive and Community Medicine*. Boston, Little, Brown & Co, 1981, pp 193–217.
10. Stamler J: Primary prevention of epidemic premature atherosclerotic coronary heart disease, in Yu PN, Goodwin JF (eds). *Progress in Cardiology* vol 10. Philadelphia, Lea & Febiger, 1981, pp 63–100.
11. Stamler J: The prevention and control of epidemic coronary heart disease: scientific foundations and strategic approaches. *Int J Cardiol* 1983; 4:207–215.
12. Kaplan NM, Stamler J (eds): *Prevention of Coronary Heart Disease—Practical Management of the Risk Factors*. Philadelphia, WB Saunders, 1983.
13. US Bureau of the Census: *Historical Statistics of the United States, Colonial Times to 1970*, Bicentennial edition, Part 1. Washington DC, 1975, p 55.
14. US Bureau of the Census: *Statistical Abstract of the United States:* 1985, ed 105. Washington DC, 1984, p 69.
15. World Health Organization: *World Health Statistics Annual, 1983.* Geneva, Switzerland, 1983, pp 20–21.
16. Pyörälä K, Epstein FH, Kornitzer M (eds): Changing trends in coronary heart disease mortality—possible explanations. *Cardiology* 1985; 72:4–104.
17. Ackerknecht EH: *Rudolf Virchow—Doctor, Statesman, Anthropologist.* Madison, University of Wisconsin Press, 1953.
18. Agarwal BL: Rheumatic heart disease unabated in developing countries. *Lancet* 1981; 2:910–911.
19. Stamler J: Overweight, hypertension, hypercholesterolemia and coronary heart disease, in Mancini M, Lewis B, Contaldo F (eds): *Medical Complications of Obesity*. London, Academic Press, 1980, pp 191–216.
20. Dyer AR, Stamler J, Shekelle RB, Schoenberger JA, Stamler R, Shekelle S, Berkson DM, Paul O, Lepper MH, Lindberg HA: Relative weight and blood pressure in four Chicago epidemiologic studies. *J Chronic Dis* 1982; 35:897–908.
21. Cooper R, Soltero I, Liu K, Berkson D, Levinson S, Stamler J: The association between urinary sodium excretion and blood pressure in children. *Circulation* 1980; 62:97–104.
22. Cooper R, Liu K, Trevisan M, Miller W, Stamler J: Urinary sodium excretion and blood pressure in children: absence of a reproducible association. *Hypertension* 1983; 5:135–139.
23. Hsiao CK, Wang SY, Hong ZG, Liu K, Cheng TY, Stamler J, Tao SC: Timed overnight sodium and potassium excretion and blood pressure in steel workers in North China. *J Hypertension,* 1986; in press.
24. Tao SC, Huang ZD, Stamler J: Timed overnight Na, K, Na/K and blood pressure in middle-aged men and women in urban and rural populations in North and South China. Council on Epidemiology, American Heart Association, 25th Annual Conference on Cardiovascular Disease Epidemiology, Tucson, AZ, March 1985.
25. From the "Nei Ching," cited by Ruskin A: Introduction, in *Classics in Arterial Hypertension*. Springfield, IL, Charles C Thomas, 1956, p xi.
26. Stamler J, Katz LN, Pick R, Rodbard S: Dietary and hormonal factors in experimental atherogenesis and blood pressure regulation, in Pincus G (ed): *Recent Progress in Hormone Research*. New York, Academic Press, 1955, vol 11, pp 401–452.
27. Denton D: *The Hunger for Salt: An Anthropological. Physiological and Medical Analysis*. Berlin/Heidelberg/New York, Springer-Verlag, 1982.
28. Fregly MJ, Kare MR (eds): *The Role of Salt in Cardiovascular Hypertension*. New York, Academic Press, 1982.
29. World Health Organization: *Primary Prevention of Essential Hypertension.* Report of a WHO Scientific Group. World Health Organization Technical Report Series 686, Geneva, Switzerland, 1983.
30. Stamler J, Stamler R: Intervention for the prevention and control of hypertension and atherosclerotic diseases: United States and international experience. *Am J Med* 1984; 76 (suppl 2A):13–36.
31. Larbi EB, Cooper RS, Stamler J: Alcohol and hypertension. *Arch Intern Med* 1983; 143:28–29.
32. Stamler J, Nadler HL, Davis AT, Christoffel KK, Berkson D, Levinson S, Whipple IT: Blood pressure in children. Scientific Exhibit. CIBA-GEIGY Corporation, Summit, NJ, 1980.
33. Stamler J, Berkson DM, Dyer A, Lepper MH, Lindberg HA, Paul O, McKean H, Rhomberg P, Schoenberger JA, Shekelle RB, Stamler R: Relationship of multiple variables to blood pressure: Findings from four Chicago epidemiologic studies, in Paul O (ed): *Epidemiology and Control of Hypertension*. Miami, FL, Symposia Specialists, 1975, pp 663–672.
34. Stamler J: Aspects of risk, in Hunt JC, Cooper T, Frohlich ED, Gifford RW Jr, Kaplan NM, Laragh JH, Maxwell MH, Strong CG (eds): *Hypertension Update: Cardiovascular Risk Factors and Consequences of Hypertension*. Bloomfield NJ, Health Learning Systems, Inc, 1979, pp 22–37.
35. Gutzwiller F, Epstein FH, Rickenbach M (eds): Proceedings of the Symposium on Epidemiology and Prevention of Hypertension and its Cardiovascular Complications, Saanen-Gstaad, Switzerland, June 17–21, 1984. *Prev Med* 1985; 14:395–552.
36. Horan MJ, Blaustein M, Dunbar JB, Kachadorian W, Kaplan NM, Simopoulos AP (eds): NIH Workshop on Nutrition and Hypertension. Proceedings from a Symposium, Bethesda, Maryland, March 12–14, 1984. New York, Biomedical Information Corporation, 1985.
37. Tuomilehto J, Wolf E (eds): Proceedings of the Symposium on Diet and Primary Prevention of Hypertension, June 25–27, 1984, Kuopio, Finland. *Ann Clin Res* 1984; 16 (suppl 43):1–183.
38. Blair D, Habicht J-P, Sims EA, Sylwester D, Abraham S: Evidence for an increased risk for hypertension with centrally located body fat and the effect of race and sex on this risk. *Am J Epidemiol* 1984; 119:526–540.
39. Joint National Committee on Detection, Evaluation, and Treatment of

High Blood Pressure: The 1984 Report of the Joint National Committee on Detection, Evaluation, and Treatment of High Blood Pressure. *Arch Intern Med* 1984; 144:1045–1057.

40. Rouse IL, Beilin LJ: Vegetarian diet and blood pressure. *J Hypertension* 1984; 2:231–240.
41. Kaplan NM: Non-drug treatment of hypertension. *Ann Intern Med* 1985; 102:359–373.
42. Epstein FH, Strazzullo P (eds): Proceedings, International Symposium on Nutritional and Metabolic Aspects of Arterial Hypertension, Anacapri, Italy, June 3–4, 1985, to be published.
43. Stamler R, Stamler J, Grimm R, Dyer A, Gosch FC, Berman R, Elmer P, Fishman J, Van Heel N, Civinelli J, Hoeksema R: Nonpharmacological control of hypertension. *Prev Med* 1985; 14:336–345.
44. Stamler R, Stamler J, Grimm R, Gosch F, Dyer A, Berman R, Civinelli J, Elmer P, Fishman J, Van Heel N, McDonald A, McKeever P: Trial on control of hypertension by nutritional means: three-year results. *J Hypertension* 1984; 2 (suppl 3):167–170.
45. Stamler J, Farinaro E, Mojonnier LM, Hall Y, Moss D, Stamler R: Prevention and control of hypertension by nutritional-hygienic means: long-term experience of the Chicago Coronary Prevention Evaluation Program. *JAMA* 1980; 243:1819–1823.
46. Langford HG, Blaufox D, Oberman A, Hawkins M, Curb JD, Cutter GR, Wassertheil-Smoller S, Pressel S, Babcock C, Abernethy JD, Hotchkiss J, Tyler M: Dietary therapy slows the return of hypertension after stopping prolonged medication. *JAMA* 1985; 253:657–664.
47. Jennings G, Nelson L, Nestel P, Esler M, Korner P, Burton D, Bazelmans J: Effects of changes in physical activity on major cardiovascular risk factors, hemodynamics, sympathetic function, and glucose utilization in man: a controlled study of four levels of activity. *Circulation* 1986; 73:30–40.
48. Stamler R, Stamler J, Gosch FC, McDonald AM: Primary prevention of hypertension: a randomized controlled trial. *Ann Clin Res* 1984; 16 (suppl 43):136–142.
49. Stamler J: Population patterns of blood pressure and the problem of high blood pressure: their nature, impact, correlates, and estimated effects of its control. World Health Organization, WHO Expert Committee on Prevention of Coronary Heart Disease. Geneva, November 30–December 8, 1981. World Health Organization, Geneva, Switzerland, 1981, CVD/CHD/EC/81.23.
50. Stamler J, Stamler R, Liu K: High blood pressure: role in coronary heart disease, and implications for prevention and control. Position paper prepared at the request of the Non-Communicable Disease Division, and the Cardiovascular Section, World Health Organization. Geneva, Switzerland, WHO/CVD/83.5, August 1983.
51. Giumetti D, Liu K, Stamler R, Schoenberger JA, Shekelle RB, Stamler J: Need to prevent and control high-normal and high blood pressure, particularly so-called "mild" hypertension: epidemiological and clinical data. *Prev Med* 1985; 14:396–412.
52. Stamler J: The risks of hypertension. Proceedings of the Symposium on Control of Arterial Hypertension in the Prevention of Cardiovascular Disease, Höhenreid, Federal Republic of Germany, April 1984.
53. Hofman A, Hazebroek A, Valkenburg HA: A randomized trial of sodium intake and blood pressure in newborn infants. *JAMA* 1983; 250:370–373.
54. Katz LN, Stamler J, Pick R: *Nutrition and Atherosclerosis*. Philadelphia, Lea & Febiger, 1958.
55. Stamler J: Population studies, in Levy RI, Rifkind BM, Dennis BH, Ernst ND (eds): *Nutrition, Lipids, and Coronary Heart Disease: A Global View.* New York, Raven Press, 1979, pp 25–88.
56. Stamler J: Nutrition-related risk factors for the atherosclerotic diseases: present status. *Prog Biochem Pharmacol* 1983; 19:245–308.
57. Grundy SM, Bilheimer D, Blackburn H, Brown WV, Kwiterovich PO Jr, Mattson F, Schonfeld G, Weidman WH: Rationale of the diet heart statement of the American Heart Association. *Circulation* 1982; 65:839A–854A.
58. Keys A (ed): *Seven Countries: a Multivariate Analysis of Death and Coronary Heart Disease.* Cambridge, MA, Harvard University Press, 1980.
59. Keys A, Menotti A, Aravanis C, Blackburn H, Djordevic BS, Buzina R, Dontas AS, Fidanza F, Karvonen MJ, Kimura N, Mohaček I, Nedeljkovic S, Puddu V, Punsar S, Taylor HT, Conti S, Kromhout D, Toshima H: The seven countries study: 2,289 deaths in 15 years. *Prev Med* 1984; 13:141–154.
60. Stamler R, Stamler J (eds): Asymptomatic hyperglycemia and coronary heart disease: a series of papers by the International Collaborative Group, based on studies in fifteen populations. *J Chronic Dis* 1979; 32:683–837.
61. NIH Consensus Development Conference: Lowering blood cholesterol to prevent heart disease. *JAMA* 1985; 253:2080–2086.
62. Measuring the risk of coronary heart disease in adult population groups. *Am J Public Health* 1957; 47 (suppl):1–63.
63. Neaton JD, Kuller LH, Wentworth D, Borhani NO: Total and cardiovascular mortality in relation to cigarette smoking, serum cholesterol concentration, and diastolic blood pressure among black and white males followed for five years. *Am Heart J* 1984; 108:759–769.
64. Stamler J, Wentworth DN, for the MRFIT Research Group: Baseline serum cholesterol and 6-year mortality from coronary heart disease (CHD) in 356,222 men screened by the Multiple Risk Factor Intervention Trial (MRFIT) (abstr). *Circulation* 1985; 72(suppl III):III-185.
65. Kannel WB, Neaton JD, Wentworth D, Thomas HE, Stamler J: Overall and coronary heart disease (CHD) mortality in relation to major risk factors in MRFIT screenees, unpublished data.

65a. Stamler J, Wentworth D, Neaton JD, for the MRFIT Research Group: Prevalence and prognostic significance of hypercholesterolemia in men with hypertension. Prospective data on the primary screenees of the Multiple Risk Factor Intervention Trial. *Am J Med* 1986; 80 (Suppl 2A):33–39.

66. Pooling Project Research Group: Relationship of blood pressure, serum cholesterol, smoking habit, relative weight and ECG abnormalities to incidence of major coronary events: final report of the Pooling Project. *J Chronic Dis* 1978; 31:201–306.
67. Tao SC, Huang ZD, Stamler J: Serum lipids in middle-aged men and women in urban and rural populations in North and South China. International Conference on Preventive Cardiology, Moscow, June 23–26, 1985, Abstracts. Moscow, USSR, 1985, p 42.
68. Blackburn H: Diet and mass hyperlipidemia: a public health view, in Levy RI, Rifkind BM, Dennis BH, Ernst ND (eds): *Nutrition, Lipids, and Coronary Heart Disease—A Global View.* New York, Raven Press, 1979, pp 309–347.
69. Rose G: Social class and coronary heart disease, in Hofmann H (ed): *Primary and Secondary Prevention of Coronary Heart Disease—Results of New Trials*. Berlin/Heidelberg/New York/Tokyo, Springer-Verlag, 1985, pp 44–49.
70. Liu K, Stamler J, Stamler R, Cooper R, Shekelle RB, Schoenberger JA, Berkson DM, Lindberg HA, Marquardt J, Stevens E, Tokich T: Methodological problems in characterizing an individual's plasma glucose level. *J Chronic Dis* 1982; 35:475–485.
71. Liu K, Stamler J, Dyer A, McKeever J, McKeever P: Statistical methods to assess and minimize the role of intra-individual variability in obscuring the relationship between dietary lipids and serum cholesterol. *J Chronic Dis* 1978; 31:399–418.
72. Liu K, Cooper R, McKeever J, McKeever P, Byington R, Soltero I, Stamler R, Gosch F, Stevens E, Stamler J: Assessment of the association between habitual salt intake and high blood pressure: methodological problems. *Am J Epidemiol* 1979; 110:219–226.
73. Liu K, Dyer AR, Cooper RS, Stamler R, Stamler J: Can overnight urine replace 24-hour urine collection to assess salt intake? *Hypertension* 1979; 1:529–536.
74. Anderson RM: *Assessment of Individual Physical Activity Level: Intra-Individual versus Inter-Individual Variability.* MPH Thesis, Department of Community Health and Preventive Medicine, Northwestern University Medical School, Chicago, IL, 1981.
75. Shekelle RB, Shryock AM, Paul O, Lepper M, Stamler J, Liu S, Raynor WJ Jr: Diet, serum cholesterol, and death from coronary heart disease: The Western Electric study. *N Engl J Med* 1981; 304:65–70.
76. Shekelle RB, Stamler J, Paul O, Shryock AM, Liu S, Lepper M: Dietary lipids and serum cholesterol level: change in diet confounds the cross-sectional association. *Am J Epidemiol* 1982; 115:506–514.
77. Stamler J: Does cholesterol change alter coronary artery disease risk? Epidemiological evidence. *Proceedings of a Symposium on the Decline in Coronary Heart Disease Mortality: The Role of Cholesterol Change.* New York, Science and Medicine, 1983, pp 27–45.
78. Yano K, Reed DM, McGee DL: Ten-year incidence of coronary heart disease in the Honolulu Heart Program: Relationship to biologic and lifestyle characteristics. *Am J Epidemiol* 1984; 119:653–666.
79. McGee DL, Reed DM, Yano K, Kagan A, Tillotson J: Ten-year incidence of coronary heart disease in the Honolulu Heart Program: relationship to nutrient intake. *Am J Epidemiol* 1984; 119:667–676.
80. Kromhout D, Coulander C: Diet, prevalence and 10-year mortality from coronary heart disease in 871 middle-aged men: The Zutphen study. *Am J Epidemiol* 1984; 119:733–741.
81. Kromhout D, Bosschieter EB, Coulander C: The inverse relation between fish consumption and 20-year mortality from coronary heart disease. *N Engl J Med* 1985; 312:1205–1209.
82. Kahn HA, Phillips RL, Snowdon DA, Choi W: Association between reported diet and all-cause mortality: twenty-one-year follow-up on 27,530 adult Seventh-Day Adventists. *Am J Epidemiol* 1984; 119:775–787.
83. Kushi LH, Lew RA, Stare FJ, Ellison CR, Lozy M, Bourke G, Daly L, Graham I, Hickey N, Mulcahy R, Kevaney J: Diet and 20-year mortality from coronary heart disease: The Ireland-Boston Diet-Heart Study. *N Engl J Med* 1983; 312:811–818.
84. Shekelle RB, Paul O, Shryock AM, Stamler J: Fish consumption and mortality from coronary heart disease. *N Engl J Med* 1985; 313:820.
85. Feinleib M, Kannel WB, Tedeschi CG, Landau TK, Garrison RJ: The

relation of antemortem characteristics to cardiovascular findings at necropsy. The Framingham Study. *Atherosclerosis* 1979; 34:145–157.

86. Rhoads GG, Blackwelder WC, Stemmermann GN, Hayashi T, Kagan A: Coronary risk factors and autopsy findings in Japanese-American men. *Lab Invest* 1978; 38:304–311.
87. McGill HC Jr (ed): *Geographic Pathology of Atherosclerosis.* Baltimore, Williams & Wilkins, 1968.
88. Hubbard JD, Inkeles S, Barnard RJ: Nathan Pritikin's heart. *N Engl J Med* 1985; 313:52.
89. Byington R, Dyer AR, Garside D, Liu K, Moss D, Stamler J, Tsong Y: Recent trends of major coronary risk factors and CHD mortality in the United States and other industrialized countries, in Havlik RJ, Feinleib M (eds): *Proceedings of the Conference on the Decline in Coronary Heart Disease Mortality.* US Department of Health, Education, and Welfare, Public Health Service, National Institutes of Health, NIH Publication No 79-1610, Washington, DC, May 1979, pp 340–379.
90. Pearson TA: Coronary arteriography in the study of the epidemiology of coronary artery disease. *Epidemiologic Rev* 1984; 6:140–166.
91. Katz LN, Stamler J: *Experimental Atherosclerosis.* Springfield IL, Charles C Thomas, 1953.
92. Hjerrman I, Holme I, Velve KB, Leren P: Effect of diet and smoking intervention on the incidence of coronary heart disease. Report from the Oslo Study Group of a randomised trial in healthy men. *Lancet* 1981; 2:1303–1310.
93. Holme I, Hjermann I, Helgeland A, Leren P: The Oslo Study: diet and antismoking advice: additional results from a 5-year primary preventive trial in middle-aged men. *Prev Med* 1985; 14:279–292.
94. Cutler JA, Neaton JD, Hulley SB, Kuller L, Paul O, Stamler J: Coronary heart disease and all-cause mortality in the Multiple Risk Factor Intervention Trial: subgroup findings and comparisons with other trials. *Prev Med* 1985; 14:292–311.
95. Kornitzer M, Rose G: WHO European Collaborative Trial of Multifactorial Prevention of Coronary Heart Disease. *Prev Med* 1985; 14:272–278.

95a. World Health Organisation European Collaborative Group: European collaborative trial of multifactorial prevention of coronary heart disease: final report on the 6-year results. *Lancet* 1986; 1:869–872.

96. Kornitzer M, de Backer G, Dramaix M, Kittel F, Thilly C, Graffar M, Vuylsteek K: Belgian Heart Disease Prevention Project: incidence and mortality results. *Lancet* 1983; 1:1066–1070.
97. Lipid Research Clinics Program: The Lipid Research Clinics Coronary Primary Prevention Trial results. I. Reduction in incidence of coronary heart disease. *JAMA* 1984; 251:351–364.
98. Lipid Research Clinics Program: The Lipid Research Clinics Coronary Primary Prevention Trial results. II. The relationship of reduction in incidence of coronary heart disease to cholesterol lowering. *JAMA* 1984;251:365–374.
99. Barndt R Jr, Blankenhorn DH, Crawford DW, Brooks SH: Regression and progression of early femoral atherosclerosis in treated hyperlipoproteinemic patients. *Ann Intern Med* 1977; 86:139–146.
100. Duffield RGM, Lewis B, Miller NE, Jamieson CW, Brunt JNH, Colchester ACF: Treatment of hyperlipidaemia retards progression of symptomatic femoral atherosclerosis: a randomised controlled trial. *Lancet* 1983; 2:639–642.
101. Brensike JF, Levy RI, Kelsey SF, Passamani ER, Richardson JM, Loh IK, Stone NJ, Aldrich RF, Battaglini JW, Moriarty DJ, Fisher MR, Friedman L, Friedewald W, Detre KM, Epstein SE: Effects of therapy with cholestyramine on progression of coronary arteriosclerosis: results of the NHLBI Type II Coronary Intervention Study. *Circulation* 1984; 69:313–324.
102. Levy RI, Brensike JF, Epstein SE, Kelsey SF, Passamani ER, Richardson JM, Loh IK, Stone NJ, Aldrich RF, Battaglini JW, Moriarty DJ, Fisher ML, Friedman L, Friedewald W, Detre KM: The influence of changes in lipid values induced by cholestyramine and diet on progression of coronary artery disease: results of the NHLBI Type II Coronary Intervention Study. *Circulation* 1984; 69:325–337.
103. Nikkila E, Viikinikoski P, Valle M, Frick MH: Prevention of progression of coronary atherosclerosis by treatment of hyperlipidaemia: a seven year prospective angiographic study. *Br Med J* 1984; 289:220–223.
104. Arntzenius AC, Kromhout D, Barth JD, Reiber JHC, Bruschke AVG, Buis B, van Gent CM, Kempen-Voogd N, Strikwerda S, van der Velde EA: Diet, lipoproteins, and the progression of coronary atherosclerosis: The Leiden Intervention Trial. *N Engl J Med* 1985; 312:805–811.
105. Salonen JT, Puska R, Kottke TE, Tuomilehto J, Nissinen A: Decline in mortality from coronary heart disease in Finland from 1969 to 1979. *Br Med J* 1983; 286:1857–1860.

105a. Tremoli E, Petroni A, Socini A, Maderna P, Colli S, Paoletti R, Galli C, Ferro-Luzzi A, Strazzullo P, Mancini M, Puska P, Iacono J, Dougherty R: Dietary interventions in North Karelia, Finland and South Italy. Modification of thromboxans B_2 formation in platelets of male subjects only. *Atherosclerosis* 1986; 59:101–111.

106. Bjartveit K: The effect of intervention on coronary heart disease risk factors in some Norwegian counties. *Am J Med* 1986; 80(supp 2A): 12–17.
107. International Conference on Preventive Cardiology, Moscow, June 23–26, 1985. Abstracts, Moscow, 1985.
108. Lenfant C: Longterm high blood pressure control programmes: achievements and challenges, abstracted. International Conference on Preventive Cardiology, Moscow, June 23–26, 1985.
109. Jones J, Weimer J: A survey of health-related food choices. *National Food Review,* NFR-12, US Department of Agriculture, Washington DC, 1980, pp 16–18.
110. Jones JL, Weimer J: Health-related food choices. *Family Economics Rev* 1981, pp 16–19.
111. US Bureau of the Census: *Statistical Abstract of the United States: 1985,* ed 105. Washington DC, 1984, p 121.
112. US Department of Agriculture: *Dietary Levels: Households in the United States, Spring 1965 and Spring 1977, Nationwide Food Consumption Surveys, 1965–66 and 1977–78.* Washington, DC, 1968 and 1982.
113. US Bureau of the Census: *Statistical Abstract of the United States: 1985,* ed 105. Washington DC, 1984, p 766.
114. Stamler J: The marked decline in coronary heart disease mortality rates in the United States, 1968–1981: summary of findings and possible explanations. *Cardiology* 1985; 72:11–22.
115. National Heart, Lung, and Blood Institute: *Vital Statistics of the United States.* National Center for Health Statistics, Rockville, Maryland, 1986.
116. Havlik RJ, Feinleib M (eds): *Proceedings of the Conference on the Decline in Coronary Heart Disease Mortality.* US Department of Health, Education, and Welfare, Public Health Service, National Institutes of Health, NIH Publication No 79–1610, US Government Printing Office, Washington DC, 1979.
117. Friedman GD: Decline in hospitalizations for coronary heart disease and stroke: the Kaiser-Permanente experience in northern California 1971–1977, in Havlik RJ, Feinleib M (eds): *Proceedings of the Conference on the Decline in Coronary Heart Disease Mortality.* US Department of Health, Education, and Welfare, Public Health Service, National Institutes of Health, NIH Publication No 79–1610, US Government Printing Office, Washington, DC, 1979, pp 109–114.
118. Elveback LR, Connolly DC, Kurland LT: Coronary heart disease in residents of Rochester, Minnesota. II. Mortality, incidence and survivorship, 1950–1975. *Mayo Clin Proc* 1981; 56:665–672.
119. Gillum RF, Hannan PJ, Prineas RJ, Jacobs DR Jr, Gomez-Marin O, Luepker RV, Baxter J, Kottke TE, Blackburn H: Coronary heart disease mortality trends in Minnesota, 1960–80: The Minnesota Heart Survey. *Am J Public Health* 1984; 74:360–362.
120. Pell S, Fayerweather WE: Trends in the incidence of myocardial infarction and in associated mortality and morbidity in a large employed population, 1957–1983. *N Engl J Med* 1985; 312:1005–1011.
121. Strong JP, Guzman MA: Decrease in coronary atherosclerosis in New Orleans. *Lab Invest* 1980; 43:297–301.
122. Beaglehole R, LaRosa JC, Heiss GE, Davis CE, Rifkind BM, Muesing RM, Williams OD: Secular changes in blood cholesterol and their contribution to the decline in coronary mortality, in Havlik RJ, Feinleib M (eds): *Proceedings of the Conference on the Decline in Coronary Heart Disease Mortality.* US Department of Health, Education, and Welfare, Public Health Service, National Institutes of Health, Public Health Service, NIH Publication No 79–1610, US Government Printing Office, Washington, DC, 1979, pp 282–295.
123. Recent trends in mortality from cardiovascular diseases. *Stat Bull Metropol Life Ins Co* 1979; 60:3–8.
124. Enstrom JE: Trends in mortality among California physicians after giving up smoking: 1950–79. *Br Med J* 1983; 286:1101–1105.
125. Wyshak G, Lamb GA, Lawrence RS, Curran WJ: A profile of the health-promoting behaviors of physicians and lawyers. *N Engl J Med* 1980; 303:104–107.
126. Stamler J: Coronary heart disease: doing the "right things." *N Engl J Med* 1985; 312:1053–1055.
127. US Department of Health and Human Services: *Health United States, 1983.* US Department of Health and Human Services, Public Health Service, Office of Health Research, Statistics, and Technology, DHHS Publication No (PHS) 84–1232, Hyattsville, MD, 1984.
128. Prepared for the Investigator Group by Klimt CR, Knatterud GL, Stamler J, Meier P: Persantine–Aspirin Reinfarction Study. Part II. Secondary coronary prevention with persantine and aspirin. *J Am Coll Cardiol* 1986; 7:251–269.
129. Zabriskie JB: Rheumatic fever: the interplay between host, genetics, and microbe. Lewis A. Conner Memorial Lecture. *Circulation* 1985; 71: 1077–1086.
130. World Health Organization: *Cardiomyopathies.* Report of a WHO Expert Committee, Technical Report Series 697, WHO, Geneva, Switzerland, 1984.
131. Kalter H, Warkany J: Congenital malformations: etiologic factors and their role in prevention. *N Engl J Med* 1983; 308:424–431, 491–497.

132. Rabo E, Taranger J: Scandinavian model for eliminating measles, mumps, and rubella. *Br Med J* 1984; 289:1402–1404.

133. Schulman ST, Amren DP, Bisno AL, Dajani AS, Durack DT, Gerber MA, Kaplan EL, Millard D, Sanders E, Schwartz RJ, Watanakunakorn C: Prevention of rheumatic fever: a statement for health professionals by the Committee on Rheumatic Fever and Infective Endocarditis of the Council on Cardiovascular Disease in the Young. *Circulation* 1984; 70:1118A–1122A.

134. Schulman ST, Amren DP, Bisno AL, Dajani AS, Durack DT, Gerber MA, Kaplan EL, Millard D, Sanders E, Schwartz RJ, Wantanakunakorn C: Prevention of bacterial endocarditis: a statement for health professionals by the Committee on Rheumatic Fever and Infective Endocarditis of the Council on Cardiovascular Disease in the Young. *Circulation* 1984; 70:1123A–1127A.

81 Cardiovascular Nursing

Grace E. Brown, RN, MA, FAAN

The practice of cardiovascular nursing is embedded in the care needs of individuals with cardiovascular disease regardless of age. As scientific discovery has uncovered the reasons for cardiovascular disease, not only has the care of individuals become more precise and targeted, but also a decrease in heart disease is evident. Historically, nursing care of individuals with cardiovascular disease has generally evolved from physician practices. However, current day cardiovascular nursing care has become discrete and refined. Standards for nursing care activities have evolved, providing a data base from which nurses can predict that specific regimens of care will provide cardiovascular wellness to the individual.

The care of individuals with cardiovascular disease is not profession-specific. Collaboration with colleagues in all disciplines is necessary for the health of persons with cardiovascular disease. Nursing care and reinforcement of prescriptive care are essential if the individual is to maintain as optimum a degree of health as possible.

Consideration of cardiovascular nursing internationally necessitates an overview of priorities of the different countries. Because nursing is a service-oriented discipline, and one in which nurses must work with the cultural and socioeconomic heritage of patients, it is important to realize that different countries have different priorities. In developing countries, infant deaths, literacy, life-styles and beliefs, sanitation, and socioeconomic problems are interlocked with health problems. In addition, the physician and nurse are often confronted not only with cardiovascular problems but also with other major problems such as poor nutrition, tuberculosis, schistosomiasis, and other parasitic diseases as well as literacy and cultural gaps that often need to be bridged for some degree of health to be maintained.[1] A great difference exists between the needs of developed countries and those of developing countries, and it is often the cardiovascular nurse who is required to bridge that gap through understanding, knowledge, and creativity. It is with this thought that the present chapter is presented.

ESSENCE OF CARDIOVASCULAR NURSING PRACTICE

Cardiovascular nursing care represents a practice that is consistent throughout the world. It answers the question of what it is that nurses do to help cardiovascular patients maintain or regain health. The outcome of the practice does not change across cultures; however, the processes by which the nurse accomplishes the objective will change as they will be based on approaches that will be successful considering the individual's sociocultural background, the cardiac problem, and the environment in which the patient is to maintain health. Nursing care of cardiac patients is more standardized than that of care in some specialties primarily because of early research that was performed in coronary care that directed not only the development of coronary care units but also the development of training curriculum for nurses. The curriculum has currently evolved with the practice and nurses have become highly sophisticated in the care of cardiovascular patients.

Nursing care is generally provided in three types of settings: the intensive cardiac care unit where the acutely ill patient is managed, the general care unit which is an admission and discharge unit, or primary care in the community. The acute care management of patients has changed rapidly and nurses have had to maintain a fast pace to be current in knowledge and skills. A primary responsibility of cardiovascular nursing is to monitor the patient's response to the disease as well as the patient's response to therapy. Table 81.1 defines those steps in monitoring. To perform accurate assessment and monitoring, in-depth understanding of cardiovascular pathophysiology is necessary. The nurse will build on theory to give understanding to nursing actions. Discrete clinical judgment is dependent on theory plus practice as the following equation demonstrates:

Knowledge + Clinical Practice = Clinical Judgment
& Theory

Table 81.1. Steps in Constant Monitoring

Observation and awareness of the implications of what is observed.
Collecting data and then synthesizing it to discover trends or patterns.
Relating information and knowledge so that certain combinations of data have meaning.
Initiating nursing activity as a result of observation and monitoring.

Clinical judgment is critical to a nurse's practice as continual assessment is based on astute observation of the patient and evaluation of clinical data. Prevention is a major objective in the care of cardiac patients and is a primary responsibility of the nurse who will be monitoring patient response to therapy to initiate preventive measures. Regardless of the presenting disease and its management, the prevention of further cardiac problems should be the goal.

Nursing assessment of the cardiac patient requires evaluation of several parameters. The patient's health history establishes the baseline from which changes can be measured. Assessment factors included in a cardiac health history are found in Table 81.2.[2] The health history obtained from the patient is updated on a regular basis. It provides the data for defining patient care problems and for developing the plan of care that will give specificity and priority to nursing care to achieve problem resolution. Nursing care is based on a process that provides for a systematic approach to a cardiac patient's care. The parts of the care process are to assess, plan, implement, and evaluate. The process is inherent in nursing action and gives orderliness to nursing care that is provided.[3]

Clinical assessments of cardiovascular function are another important part of the nurse's evaluation of the patient. Table 81.3 defines specific assessment parameters relevant to all cardiovascular patients. Cardiovascular diseases prevalent in one country may not be prevalent in another. Rheumatic fever and rheumatic heart disease are well controlled in North America; however, they have a high prevalence in South America. Stroke is a major cardiovascular problem in Japan and a primary population for which nurses will provide care. Clinical assessment of cardiovascular function transcends the general nature of the disease and gives it its definition. Viewed as cardiovascular-specific, the assessments can be used across settings and populations. It is the results of the assessment and their interpretation in conjunction with the health history that give definition to the cardiovascular problem. For example, in a coronary care unit, a patient who has had myocardial infarction may develop rales or rhonchi. An immediate postoperative patient who has had a coronary artery bypass graft may also develop rales or rhonchi as may a stroke patient who is stable and recovering. The assessment is significant to each of these cardiovascular populations; however, the reasons for and the nursing activity to solve the problem may be different. In one instance the nurse may need to suction the cardiac surgical patient's endotracheal tube, but yet in another the nurse's

Table 81.2. Cardiac Health History*

1. *Perceptions, expectations and adherence to previously prescribed or self-initiated therapy*
2. *Description of current cardiac symptoms*
   - Onset
   - Duration
   - Quality
   - Location
   - Radiation
   - Associated symptoms
   - Precipitating factors
   - Symptom relief factors
3. *Risk factor profile*
   - Family history of cardiovascular disease
   - Serum lipid levels (hypercholesterolemia/hypertriglyceridemia)
   - Smoking
   - Hypertension
   - Obesity
   - Sedentary living
   - Diabetes
   - Alcohol intake
   - Oral contraceptives
   - Psychosocial factors
4. *Previous health status*
   - Hospitalizations
   - Operations
   - Injuries
   - Infectious diseases
5. *Personal and social factors*
   - Caffeine intake
   - Meals
   - Sleep
   - Occupation
   - Activities
   - Living arrangements
   - Environment
   - Economic situation
   - Cultural values and beliefs
   - Psychosocial considerations
   - Spiritual beliefs/practices
   - Education
6. *Systems review*
   - Skin
   - Head, eye, ear, nose, throat
   - Respiratory
   - Cardiovascular
   - Gastrointestinal—food preferences, appetite, etc
   - Genitourinary
   - Metabolic—weight changes
   - Neuropsychiatric—memory changes, vertigo, etc
   - Fatigue
   - Emotional changes
7. *Current medical diagnosis and therapy*

*Adapted from American Nurses' Association.[2]

function may be to report to the physician the development of the rales and rhonchi as those may be the first symptoms of pulmonary edema and cardiac failure. It is important to view the assessment in the context of each patient and in conjunction with all clinical data that might be helpful in problem identification and resolution.

An individual may seek health care on the basis of an actual problem he is experiencing or because of a potential problem. If an individual has a family history of hypertension, he may seek health care monitoring in order that

Table 81.3. Clinical Assessment of Cardiovascular Functions*

1. *Cardiac*
   Chest wall size, configuration, and movements
   Point of maximal intensity, thrills, heaves, pulsations
   Heart sounds and murmurs
   Pericardial friction rub
   Apical/radial pulses; rate, quality, rhythm
   Korotkoff sounds
2. *Pulmonary*
   Respiratory rate, quality, pattern
   Chest expansion
   Intercostal retractions/bulging
   Trachea position
   Diaphragm excursion
   Tactile fremitus
   Breath sounds
   Rales, rhonchi, wheezes, pleural friction rub
   "E" to "A" changes, whispered pectoriloquy, bronchophony
   Clubbing
3. *Vascular*
   Skin color, moisture, temperature
   Petechiae
   Nailbed, mucous membrane color
   Peripheral pulses
   Homans' sign
   Blood pressure
   Pulsus alternans
   Pulsus paradoxus
   Bruits, carotid, renal artery
   Eye grounds
4. *Circulatory*
   Jugular venous distention
   Jugular venous pulsations
   Hepatojugular reflux
   Kussmaul's sign
   Edema
   Ascites
   Liver engorgement and enlargement
   Skin turgor
5. *Effects on the neurological system*
   Visual acuity
   Level of consciousness
   Restlessness
   Confusion
   Syncope
   Pupil response
6. *Related data*
   Body temperature
   Xanthelasma
   Arcus senilis
7. *Laboratory results*
   Electrocardiogram
   Chest x-ray
   Exercise testing
   Complete blood count
   Serum electrolytes
   Fasting blood sugar
   Uric acid
   Blood coagulation studies
   Serum creatinine and blood urea nitrogen
   Serum lipids
   Serum enzymes
   Arterial blood gases
   Urine studies

*Adapted from American Nurses' Association.[2]

he can maintain optimal health for as long as possible. A plan of management such as weight control, regular blood pressure measurement, and cessation of smoking are all strategies to assist this individual in maintaining health. The potential for developing high blood pressure is present, but prevention is the intent of management. Actual cardiovascular problems are easier to define than potential problems, because the problem exists now. Potential problems may occur if strategies are not implemented, such as salt control in the patient with cardiac failure. For the past several years, nursing has identified patient care needs as problems. Care plans have been developed around patient problems and nursing interventions for those problems. Patient problems currently are being defined as nursing diagnoses.[4,5] A nursing diagnosis is a statement of the individual's problem, either actual or potential, and is based on evaluation of the data derived from the cardiovascular nursing assessment. A nursing diagnosis is a patient problem in which the nurse has primary responsibility for implementing nursing intervention or activity in solving the problem.[6] Whether a nursing diagnosis or nursing problem approach is used on the plan of care is not the important issue. The important issues are that there is consistency to the care plan and that the goals are derived from the problem or diagnosis. Broad goals of cardiovascular nursing for individuals with cardiovascular problems are: (1) prevention of complications, (2) restoration, maintenance, and promotion of optimum cardiac function, and (3) acceptable quality of life. Within each of these goals, specific outcomes can be defined for the individual with cardiovascular disease. The outcomes are based on the known cardiovascular health status of the patient which was derived from the initial and on-going health assessment. The following example demonstrates how patient outcomes can be written:

The individual maintains a pharmacologic regimen that is compatible with therapeutic and personal goals (outcome statement).

The individual will: (1) explain the rationale for the specific drug regimen prescribed, (2) state specific action and side effects of prescribed medication, (3) assist in determining the schedule for taking medication, and (4) plan a method to assist with drug compliance in the home.

The foregoing patient behaviors deal with a patient's cardiac medications, and if each of the behaviors is achieved before the individual's discharge, it is anticipated that the drug regimen the patient maintains will be the one he learns before discharge. Goals for cardiovascular patients generally fall into the areas of diet (salt and fluid control), activity/exercise, medications, adjustments to a changed life-style, coping mechanisms, and iatrogenic infections. If the individual is in the acute phase of a cardiovascular illness, physician and nurse collaboration is frequent and often the goals of both are identical and take precedence as they represent lifesaving activities. Nursing problems such as skin care, mouth care, and body position remain important and should be part of the plan of care. Developing a plan of care for the individual provides for an organized systematic process in which nursing problems are defined and strategies for resolution are stated through goals and outcomes. The plan is also collaborative as it provides for the implementation of physician orders.

The nursing care of cardiovascular patients is complex because of the discrete nature of the therapy. With the introduction of calcium channel and beta blockers, thrombolytic therapy, percutaneous transluminal coronary angioplasty as well as better differential diagnostic techniques, cardiovascular nurses often have had to monitor and care for patients without the advantage of experience in knowing what patient responses should be.[7] Assessment factors become critical background data from which the nurse can extract, so that presenting symptoms have some meaning.[8,9] It is important that nurses create standards, protocols, and flow sheets so that responses by staff are consistent and quality care is provided. Cardiovascular care units are highly sophisticated because of telemetry systems that provide computer arrhythmia diagnosis, monitoring equipment that has data management components, and additional technology that has increased the necessity for nurses to be able to interpret data rapidly and thus respond to patient needs. Establishing nursing care plans, cardiac arrest guidelines of accountability, medication regimens, and emergency dilution standards for drugs all provide support to the nurse in a rapidly changing environment. In addition, evolving practice requires evolving skill and knowledge. Nurses working in cardiovascular settings must keep up to date with medical therapy and thus be able to define nursing therapy as the practice evolves. Creating an organized, skilled environment for the patient whether it is a rehabilitation unit, a pediatric cardiac unit, or a medical floor on which cardiac patients receive care assures that responses to the needs of individuals with cardiovascular disease will be focused, rapid, and of quality. As mentioned earlier, prevention is primary; the person with cardiovascular disease regains optimal health if the team works together toward that end.

PATIENT TEACHING

Cardiovascular patient teaching is based on the principles of adult learning, and content is patient specific. Cardiovascular patient teaching takes into consideration the disease process of the individual and the prescribed regimens. Individuals with cardiovascular disease may be in one of several phases of illness: high risk but not yet ill, experiencing an acute event, recovering from an acute episode, or in a compensated state of chronic illness. Part of the nurse's responsibility is to help the patient at each stage of illness to attain and then maintain the highest degree of health for that individual. This is accomplished not only through physical care of the patient but also through an assessment of the learning needs of the person, then providing the appropriate teaching at the most opportune time. Patient teaching occurs at two levels (American Heart Association Council on Cardiovascular Nursing, unpublished data, December 1980). The first level can occur on a formal or informal basis and focuses on a general cardiovascular related content that any patient needs to know. It may be to help the person to recognize a need for care if he is at high risk. It may also be orientation to diagnostic procedures, and to cardiovascular care settings, risk factor information, or review of the patient's plan of care with him. The second level generally occurs on a more formal basis and derives from the patient's specific needs. Teaching and information are directed toward assisting the patient to recognize risk factors and to modify them in relation to his life-style, to clarify and reinforce the physician's orders, and to prevent the complications as well as the recurrence of additional cardiac problems. Teaching may include information about the patient's disease, related anatomy and physiology, medication, diet and activity, specific treatment modalities, and recognition of specific symptoms (ie, shortness of breath or chest pain) that require medical intervention and steps the person can take to receive that care. The nurse through teaching helps the patient and family to make the adjustment from acute illness to wellness and to accept specific limitations imposed by cardiovascular disease and its treatment. A goal of teaching is to assist the individual with cardiovascular disease to modify his life-style, thereby reducing his risk factors and the potential of the disease to occur or extend.

The teaching role of the nurse is well utilized in primary intervention in such areas as rheumatic fever and hypertension. To change life-styles the individual needs to understand the presence and nature of the risk to him. Health teaching is crucial in defining life-style behavior change for the individual at risk but currently without cardiac disease. Once cardiovascular disease is present (ie, coronary artery disease, high blood pressure, and rheumatic fever), the nurse will coordinate the patient teaching with the medical plan of care. Teaching should focus on adaptation of the patient to his current cardiovascular health status. Counseling will focus on making the individual aware of feelings and attitudes that influence his behavior. Teaching provides the information necessary to regain personal health and is inherent in almost all cardiovascular patient-related activities. In the hospital patient, teaching ranges from risk factor identification to modification, and pre-test, preoperative, postoperative, and discharge teaching. Within each of these areas standards have been developed based on medical therapy and patient specific needs. A standard teaching plan is useful as it can be adapted to each patient. Table 81.4 illustrates a basic teaching plan. Following this basic plan assists the nurse to develop with the patient a specific cardiovascular teaching plan. If anticoagulant therapy is being taught, the content format will evolve around anticoagulants. If pacemaker teaching is occurring, the content format will relate to the patient's learning needs concerning the pacemaker.[10]

To effectively teach patients the nurse and patient must have a relationship that will allow both patient and nurse access to necessary information. Teaching requires a flexible, clear and well-organized understanding of content that is partially based on information drawn from the patient. Teaching should be developed from specific objectives that are behaviors the patient or learner will demonstrate as outcomes of the teaching process. Before

Table 81.4. Teaching Plan

1. *Goal*
   Statement of why the learner needs the content
2. *Specify behavioral objectives*
   Describe what it is the learner should do with the information
   Written behavioral objectives contain measurable verbs as well as one verb for each objective
3. *Content outline*
   List assessment factors related to the content
   Describe nursing interventions, which may consist of integration of nursing and medical management
   State outcomes for the individual; what are the results expected from the interventions
4. *Summary*
5. *Evaluation of the plan*
   The plan should achieve the health goal in a systematic process
   The plan should be evaluated in terms of patient outcomes
   The process is based on the behavioral objectives

teaching takes place the desired outcomes must be known. What one hopes to attain through teaching is defined in the outcome statement. To direct learning and achieve outcomes, the nurse can do many things to assist patients such as: (1) provide for imitation through the use of models, (2) give facts succinctly, demonstrate the skill, and allow the patient to practice what is taught, (3) express understanding and insight that will in turn help the individual to perform the desired behavior, and (4) match the patient's behavior with goals or expected outcomes and evaluate his progress.

In directing the learning process the nurse should keep in mind the domains of learning that are motor skills, verbal information, intellectual skills, and cognitive strategies and attitudes. It is not often that all of the learning domains become operational at once, but rather particular ones are drawn upon depending on the learning needs. If taking a pulse is the behavior to be learned, motor skills are important. If the patient is learning alternate doses of cardiotonic medications, intellectual skills will be used. To know the domain of learning necessary for the behavior directs the nurse to help the patient develop that skill.

Although teaching is universal and should be a primary responsibility of all nurses, it is important to recognize that approaches to teaching must be compatible with the culture, life-style, and belief system of the individual. Often it is not only the patient but also the family members who are being taught. Understanding age-specific needs allows the nurse to use appropriate methods (visual aids, terminology, and language) that the individual will understand and comprehend. Understanding the culture in which the teaching is provided and its impact on the individual allows the nurse to create a learning environment and develop behavioral outcomes that the patient can accept and become an active participant in achieving outcomes he has agreed he can meet. Equally important is family acceptance and adherence, which will enhance patient compliance.

NURSING EDUCATION FOR CARDIOVASCULAR PRACTICE

Although education and training for cardiovascular nursing care continue to be primarily an apprenticeship in many countries, a systematic approach to gaining knowledge and skills generally occurs. Mason[11] has identified three interrelated patterns of nursing education that have influenced the development of nursing education systems throughout the world. They are the English, the French, and the American. The French curriculum, at one extreme, is medically oriented with lectures on nursing skills and medical pathology, although most learning is achieved through apprenticeship. The English pattern is a hospital-based apprenticeship with greater definition to the nursing role and activities. As we know, the American pattern is based on academia. These patterns influence what is taught and how it is taught. In the United States generic nursing education contains some cardiovascular content, but on the whole most of what the nurse learns occurs in short-term courses in a hospital setting after which an apprenticeship is completed in the area to which the nurse has been assigned. If the nurse is interested in primary intervention, small short-term courses must be found in order to learn the basic skills and knowledge.

Historically, physicians have played a large part in evolving the curriculum for nurses as they have been the educators of nurses and still are in many countries.

Education for cardiovascular nursing practice is comprised of technical skill and theory underlying heart disease. A typical basic cardiac care course should include most of the content areas listed in Table 81.5. This list is not all inclusive as learning needs will be based on patient groups and their care requirements. Breadth and depth of content will depend on the patient population for which the nurses will be caring. In those countries in which rheumatic fever is prevalent, epidemiology and primary intervention of the disease will be essential content to learn. Coronary artery disease is significant in the

Table 81.5. Curriculum Content for Cardiac Care

Cardiac anatomy
Cardiac physiology—pulmonary physiology
Neurophysiology of the heart
Coronary artery disease
Angina
Myocardial infarction
Electrophysiology and arrhythmia interpretation
Nursing history—physical assessment of the heart and lungs
Diagnostic studies
Respiratory management
Technology—computers, hemodynamic monitors, patient data management systems, respirators, etc
Valvular heart disease
Blood studies and component therapy
Cardiotonics, calcium channel and beta blockers
Basic cardiac life support (often advanced cardiac life support)
High blood pressure
Stroke
Shock
Cardiac assist devices (intraaortic balloon pumping, pacemakers)

United States and Canada, but Japanese nurses would focus on stroke prevention and care. In almost all countries congenital heart disease care is taught; however, the focus may be on primary intervention and maintenance, not surgical correction.

In underdeveloped countries, a nurse needs to learn not only cardiovascular nursing, but also basic health care principles relevant to patient life-styles and environment. If an individual's heart disease is successfully treated, but yet the patient returns to an environment that creates risks to his newly gained health, the nurse must be able to assist the patient in adapting to his environment, again without compromising his recently gained health.

Apprenticeship-type learning is necessary in fields in which skill practice is essential. Beginning learners need to practice their knowledge and skills in a supervised environment. Repetition of skills increases efficiency and accuracy which are necessary to achieve rapid response to acute events. The application of theory and knowledge makes nursing care an intellectual process and not a rote, habitual action. The most skilled nurses are those who can assess cardiovascular patient data, give meaning to the data, and initiate action. Prevention is built on this premise. Too often, however, data are not assessed as a whole pattern or reviewed for trends that give subtle cues to what is occurring.

Several countries have begun to use the concept of preceptoring. A preceptor is a clinical teacher. Most programs will teach nurses how to be teachers. Once again, adult learning principles are used. The nurse preceptor should be a very skilled nurse in cardiovascular care who accepts the responsibility for teaching and guiding the learning process of a new cardiovascular nurse. The preceptor will work side by side with the new nurse, teaching cardiovascular regimens to the new person as well as providing a support system in an often tense environment. Standards of cardiovascular care concerning all activities are followed, so that the new nurse learns correct behavior and can adapt and adjust as more experience is gained. Although not a new idea, preceptoring has become an important teaching/learning model in high technology areas.[12] By using this model it is hoped that staff retention will occur and that an experienced staff will feel a responsibility for their new colleagues.

Understanding normal anatomy and physiology provides the basis for understanding cardiovascular pathophysiology. This in turn leads to accurate and appropriate cardiovascular patient health assessments which, when utilized with appropriate behavioral skills, can only enhance patient care.

CARDIOVASCULAR NURSING RESEARCH

Research by nurses has been a significant part of the literature for many years. Nurses have participated in cardiovascular research studies in universities, laboratories, and clinical units; however, cardiovascular nursing research by prepared nurses has evolved primarily in the last 20 years in the United States[13] (S.B. Foster, RN, unpublished data, 1974). European nurse researchers, conversely, convened their first conference in the Netherlands in 1978.[14] The conference hoped to obtain a profile on the state of nursing research in participating countries. Twelve European countries did report on the development of nursing research in their countries. In 1984 the fifth European research conference was held in London in collaboration with the Research Society of the Royal College of Nursing. Approximately 600 nurse researchers attended, representing most of the countries of Europe.[15] In Canberra, Australia, in 1982 the nursing and health services branch of the Commonwealth Department of Health of Australia published the second edition of the *Directory of Nursing Research in Australia*.[16] Then in 1983 the International Council of Nurses surveyed the known nursing research units of all countries except the United States. Although several findings resulted from this survey, the two most significant were that: (1) the greatest number of research units reported that they were associated with a university and (2) research in the practice of nursing was the most frequently cited focus for their research.

Currently in the United States as well as in other countries, cardiovascular nursing research is combined into the broad program of nursing research. In the United States, Canada, the Netherlands, and a few other European countries, cardiovascular research by nurses has begun to be defined by clinical specialty and patient data rather than by role or what a nurse does. In addition, prepared nurses are defining their areas of special interest for research, which will enhance national and international replication and collaboration studies.

Cardiovascular nursing is an applied science, the practice of which requires the nurse to use new knowledge and evaluate clinical manifestations of the response of individuals (human response) to cardiovascular problems and to new and changing modes of therapy. Cardiovascular nursing research can not only enrich the patient's quality of life but also benefit the individual's ability to deal with cardiovascular problems. It generates reasons through a systematic process for the nursing therapy provided. Instead of intuitive, repetitive practice, cardiovascular nursing care becomes an intellectual process toward which specific objectives are directed.

Research in cardiovascular nursing care has a wide range. Initial studies attempted to define the nurse's role, which is evident in the coronary care and high blood pressure literature.[17] However, in the past ten years, studies have begun to focus on clinical nursing interventions such as patient teaching, compliance to regimens, cardiovascular nursing practice problems, physical as well as psychosocial responses, and laboratory research. Breadth in research studies is needed to develop a cardiovascular nursing knowledge base; however, too much breadth without replication of studies does not allow verification of findings in different populations and settings under varying conditions. As cardiovascular nursing research matures and the results of studies become the essence of practice, it is hoped that an international network can occur wherein nurses throughout the world can do parallel and collaborative studies that will enhance nursing practice and provide standards of care for cardiovascular patients.

As cardiovascular nurses provide a scientific base for

their practice, problems can occur as cultures are crossed. Communication depends on the ability of nurses to speak a common language, which at this point in time is often not the case. Publications must be in a common language, so that international use will result. Once that link is in place, collaboration and exchange will occur as a routine.

The roots of good research have been planted; it is now the responsibility of cardiovascular nurses on behalf of their patients to feed and nourish this beginning into an expectation for continued growth.

REFERENCES

1. Ohlson VM: Issues in professional nursing practice. 6. *An International Perspective on Nursing Practice*. Kansas City, MO, American Nurses' Association, 1985, pp 1–7.
2. American Nurses' Association, Division on Medical-Surgical Nursing Practice and American Heart Association, Council on Cardiovascular Nursing: *Standards of Cardiovascular Nursing Practice.* American Nurses' Association, Kansas City, MO, 1981, pp 1–14.
3. Yura H, Walsh MB: *The Nursing Process,* ed. 4. Connecticut, Appleton-Century-Crofts, 1983, p 330.
4. Dossey B, Guzzetta CE: Nursing diagnosis. *Nursing* 1981; 11:34–38.
5. Carpenito LJ: *Handbook of Nursing Diagnosis*. Philadelphia, JB Lippincott, 1985, pp 1–226.
6. Carpenito LJ: Is the problem a nursing diagnosis? *Am J Nurs* 1984; 84:1418–1419.
7. Frishman WH, Furberg CD, Friedewald WT: Beta adrenergic blockade for survivors of acute myocardial infarction. *New Engl J Med* 1984; 310:830–837.
8. Taylor JW: Nursing management of stroke: acute care — part I. *Cardiovasc Nur* 1985; 21:1–5.
9. Taylor JW: Nursing management of stroke: acute care — part II. *Cardiovasc Nur* 1985; 21:7–12.
10. Sadler D: *Nursing for Cardiovascular Health*. Connecticut, Appleton-Century-Crofts, 1984, pp 7–9, 136–137.
11. Mason V: International collaboration in nursing education: the people to people approach. *J Nur Ed* 1980; 19:48–54.
12. Yee BH, Zoyb SL: *Cardiac Critical Care Nursing*. Boston, Little, Brown & Co, 1986, p 13.
13. Kinney MR: Trends in cardiovascular nursing research, 1972–1983. *Cardiovasc Nur* 1985; 21:25–30.
14. National Hospital Institute: *Collaborative Research and Its Implementation in Nursing: First Conference*. Utrecht, The Netherlands, The Institute, 1979.
15. International nursing research—Does it make a difference? *Intern Nurs Rev* 1984; 31:127.
16. Australian Government Publishing Service: *Directory of Nursing Research in Australia,* ed. 2. Canberra, the Service, 1982.
17. McCauley CA, Anderson AD: The nurse as primary therapist in the management of the patient with stroke. *Circulation* 1972; 45 (suppl II):II-242.

82 The Cardiologist and the Pharmaceutical Industry

Lars Werkö, MD

The rapid development of cardiovascular medicine since the Second World War has had many reasons. The war effort stimulated the use of new invasive methods for hemodynamic research, which led to a wealth of new information regarding cardiovascular diseases and especially their pathophysiologic aspects. At first, interest was focused mainly on valvular diseases, both acquired and congenital, but later studies included hypertension, coronary artery disease, and cardiomyopathies. Coupled with these advances in our understanding of heart disease was the vast expansion in therapeutic possibilities. The surgical treatment of cardiovascular disease has been a continuous story of success ranging from the first operation for coarctation of the aorta to heart transplantation. Similarly, the medical treatment of cardiovascular diseases has progressed since the middle of the 20th century. The advances in surgical intervention in heart disease have also depended on advances in anesthesia and preoperative and postoperative care.

It is in this latter context that the pharmaceutical and health care industries have constituted strong forces aimed at improved therapy for patients with cardiovascular disorders. These industries have by no means concentrated their resources on cardiology, but through the successive increase in knowledge in cardiovascular physiology, biochemistry, and pharmacology, not to speak of marked advances in all aspects of clinical cardiology, a background has been created that has stimulated research in cardiovascular pharmacology both in medical schools and in the pharmaceutical industry.

The development of new therapies constitutes a combined effort of various kinds of preclinical and clinical scientists and the pharmaceutical industry. To be able to institute a new and improved therapy, both a thorough knowledge of physiologic and pathophysiologic mechanisms and some special tool to influence these mechanisms are needed. The biochemists of the industry may be successful in defining such a tool in the form of a new medicine. Through the interaction between knowledgeable clinicians and the industry many such new medicines have been designed, adequately tested, and become used as the basis of a new therapy in clinical practice all over the world. The constant interaction between scientists working in industry and their clinical counterparts working in medical schools or in other clinical facilities has ensured both high efficacy and marked safety with these new medicines when used in clinical practice.

The invention and further development of new medicines has become an exercise that is almost totally confined to the scientific laboratories of the pharmaceutical industry. Various estimates have shown that whereas at the turn of the century a single scientist might have invented a new medicine as a basis for improved therapy, currently the vast resources of a dedicated industrial laboratory are necessary for the creation of any new medicine. This is due not only to the need for in-depth studies of the metabolic and pharmacologic actions of the new chemical entity (NCE), but also to the requirement that its possible mutagenic, oncogenic, and toxic effects be described in a continuously increasing, sophisticated battery of animal and other tests. It has been calculated that the vast resources used in the industry for research aimed at new medicines, to an increasing extent, are employed in such safety assessment studies, from 5% to 10% in 1960 to 25% to 35% in 1980. If this trend continues, fewer and fewer resources will be available for real innovative efforts.

THE PHARMACEUTICAL INDUSTRY

It is not always realized that the modern pharmaceutical industry is a fairly recent development. Some new chemical entities were recommended as medicines at the turn of the century, but it was not until the Second World War that a determined, concentrated effort was made to produce new effective medicines on an industrial scale. The invention of sulfa drugs by Domagk just before the war and the development of the penicillins by Fleming, Florey, and Chain during the war demonstrated that it was possible to create new, lifesaving therapies through concentrated efforts in industrial laboratories in cooperation with outside scientists, especially when stimulated by governmental interest. The American and, to a certain extent, the Swiss industry led the rapid development of this new industrial venture. British and German companies damaged by war efforts later joined the race for new drugs.

The most important research-based pharmaceutical companies of today either have their origin in the successful chemical industry, especially the dye-stuff developers such as Ciba-Geigy, Sandoz, Merck, Hoechst, Bayer, and Imperial Chemical Industries—or were developed from old druggists such as Eli Lilly, Astra, and the Japanese companies. Some, like Syntex, have been able to start de novo based on hormonal biochemistry. The distinction may be important as those companies that originated in the chemical industry have been influenced by the chemical philosophy prevalent in that industry, whereas the companies that developed out of old drug sellers have been able to keep a more biologic outlook on their activities. Some of the early "misbehavior" of the pharmaceutical industry may have been due to the fact that it grew out of chemical enterprises and had little input from the medical and hospital world in their top management. It is of interest that still the two largest companies in the world, Hoechst and Bayer, only have 17.5% and 16.6%, respectively, from their pharmaceutical divisions in 1983 to 1984, whereas most of the top 15 companies have half their activities in divisions unrelated to medicine or medical-related needs. This means that the top management may use value scales other than those related to sickness and human suffering.

The growth of the pharmaceutical industry can be described as passing through many phases. The first was the optimistic, mainly antibiotic-based, rapid growth phase of the 1940s and 1950s—the golden age. The second started with the thalidomide disaster of the early 1960s, with increasing criticism from government and the public. This phase was characterized by negative publicity and many investigations into the conduct of the industry in toto or some specific companies. The output of new medicines slowed down. At the same time many of the most important new medicines in the treatment of cardiovascular disorders, such as antihypertensives, were created in the 1960s.

The third phase, from the early 1970s to the present, is characterized by continuing public criticism of the industry, some disturbing series of adverse reactions to drugs that had been adequately tested in preclinical, toxicologic, and clinical studies before marketing, but also a new optimism due to rapid expansion of biologic knowledge. The first targeted medicines, developed through the use of specific actions on receptors or enzymes, appeared and became great successes such as the specific H_2-blocker cimetidine and beta-adrenergic agonists and antagonists.

We now are probably entering a fourth phase based on the development of what is diffusely called the new biotechnology, in which the use of recombinant DNA, hybridoma, and cloning techniques is going to permit the creation of completely new medicines and also completely new, and hopefully better, ways of production. It is within the companies belonging to this group that biologically inclined scientists, and especially those with a clinical background, can contribute to the creation of new and improved therapies for the next century.

PARTICIPATION WITH INDUSTRY

There are many ways that a physician can contribute to the development of new medicines in a pharmaceutical company: (1) as an outside consultant; (2) as a clinical trialist; (3) as a part-time employee; and (4) as a full-time employee.

AS AN OUTSIDE CONSULTANT

An outside consultant may work with the medical department, the research laboratories, or the marketing department of the pharmaceutical company. In all these instances, what the company needs is a balanced view of the outside medical world, the prevailing philosophy regarding current therapies, and the need for new ones. It is also necessary to transfer the attitude of the medical community towards the pharmaceutical industry as such and the specific company in particular.

Suggestions for ways of improving the therapeutic armamentarium within the specialty in question are welcome. Constructive criticism both on the research philosophy of the company and the means the company is using to promote its product to the medical profession should always be part of the knowledge represented. The position of an outside consultant may be sensitive as the researchers in the company may be extremely negative to any criticism, especially that from someone they regard as an outsider. Similarly, the marketing personnel may also believe that they know best how to handle the medical information to the profession, based, as their efforts are, on what they believe to be outstanding marketing research. To make the best impact and to contribute to the development of the company the outside consultant must have (1) a firm position in his daily medical occupation, (2) a good connection with various outside medical societies, both in his specialty and, if possible, in general societies, (3) a keen interest in therapeutic problems, and (4) solid personal integrity.

It is also important that he has a written contract with the company, explicitly spelling out his responsibilities toward different levels in the company (the person or persons to whom he is reporting, what special advice is wanted, and whether he is supposed to represent the company in his local medical circles). The contract should also contain some statement about the amount of work that is envisaged and the remuneration for that work. Last but not least it has to contain how long he is going to stay with the company and how (and possibly on what grounds) he can be released from the terms of the contract.

Such a document may seem unnecessarily bureaucratic, but it is needed if the consultant is to influence the medical work in the company, an influence that both he and the leadership of the company wanted when he was hired.

Up to now it has not been used to a large extent and most written papers between outside consultants and pharmaceutical companies usually contain only some economic terms coupled with a time limit. Nevertheless, with the increasing interest of the public and the media regarding the relation or relations between the medical profession and the pharmaceutical industry, I believe that some formal agreement is needed to save both the company and the physician later trouble.

AS A CLINICAL TRIALIST

The clinical trialist can be looked upon as a special form of consultant with more specified responsibilities. To conduct a clinical trial with a new chemical entity constitutes a great responsibility, both toward the company that has developed the new medicine and toward the patients taking part in the study. Different companies have different routines, but most will appoint a person within the medical department as a monitor who is required to work closely with the clinical investigator. This monitor may be medically qualified but is usually not. In that case he or she frequently has some basic science degree and special education and training within the company. A protocol for the intended trial has to be formulated and agreed upon. Sometimes the company has a master protocol for the medicine in question, but it is important that the investigator who wants to take part in the trial scrutinizes any suggestions, makes his own comments, and suggests details in the protocol that may suit his own scientific interest better or that conform better with his type of patient and medical routine. Any sensible company will accept changes in a suggested protocol as long as they are medically relevant and the study can still be incorporated in the file that has to be submitted to the authorities in different countries.

It is the responsibility of the investigator to secure approval for the study by both the authorities and the institutional review board or its equivalent (in Europe, usually some kind of scientific ethics committee) before the study starts. It is also the responsibility of the investigator that informed consent for the study be obtained in writing from each patient participating in the study. When obtaining such consent, the investigator must explain (1) the nature of the study drugs, (2) the nature and purpose of the study, (3) the procedure that the subject should follow, (4) the benefits or risks, or both, associated with participation in the study, (5) alternative treatments available, and (6) the assurance that the subject may withdraw from the study at any time without prejudice. In some cases, when emergency medicines are tried out, the consent may be given by some relative to the patient after he or she has been properly informed.

It is important that the investigator perform the study with the highest scientific standard possible and that he follow the protocol agreed upon regarding the registration of effects of the new medicine, both positive (therapeutic) and negative (adverse reactions). Before the start of the study, agreement must be reached concerning statistical analysis of the data produced. It is also important that the investigator and representatives of the company agree beforehand how the results should be presented, both in the internal reports of the company (that may be used for regulatory purposes) and in scientific publications. The way the company will keep track of the trial (eg, through visits by the monitor) and how the investigator should be remunerated should also be clearly stated before the start of the investigation.

For the patients, the investigator, and the company it is of great importance that clinical trials of new medicines be regarded as a high-class scientific activity comparable to any other clinical research. Only then will the investigator get the necessary satisfaction out of taking part in this phase of the development of a new medicine.

The importance of outside clinical contacts in the development of new therapies can be illustrated with many examples. I have chosen two examples within the cardiovascular field that illustrate how the outside clinical consultant may alter the whole emphasis of the use of a new medicine. His or her observations and thorough knowledge of clinical medicine may lead to the opening up of a completely new field of therapy. A solid clinical background coupled with a keen interest in treating patients enables the well-trained cardiologist to relate his observations on a new medicine to the present frontiers of therapeutic research and thus judge its possibilities in relation to present therapy.

The following examples illustrate this.

When Karl Beyer and his team at Merck Sharpe & Dohme developed the first oral thiazide, the aim was to improve the treatment of edema in congestive heart failure. It was an immediate success, but it was two clinicians, Ed Freis and Robert Wilkins, who both observed that treatment of congestive heart failure in hypertension with the new agent not only cleared the edema but also decreased the blood pressure in these patients. This observation was the start of the very successful use of thiazide and similarly the use of diuretics in the treatment of high blood pressure.

Similarly, when Sir James Black at Imperial Chemical Industries developed propranolol as the first adrenergic beta-blocking agent, the aim was to shield the heart and hopefully to diminish symptoms in anginal pain and certain arrhythmias. It was when Pritchard studied patients with angina and high blood pressure that he noted that the new medicine also affected the blood pressure. He suggested that propranolol should be used as an antihypertensive agent, but lacking any animal studies demonstrating on antihypertensive effect and without any scientific explanation to the mode of action, he was not believed. It is sobering, at least for scientists working in the industry, to see that it took several years and much effort on the part of Pritchard and his followers before both of the companies that had developed propranolol and other beta-blocking drugs accepted the fact that this was indeed a most valuable tool in the treatment of hypertension. Similarly, clinical scientists in many countries were slow to accept the new treatment approach, to a large extent on the basis of theoretic considerations.

These two examples illustrate that the development of new therapies requires not only an efficient industrial research organization with highly skilled and motivated scientists but also astute clinicians who use their power of clinical observation to look for unexpected results of any intervention. They should also be so certain of their clinical knowledge that they are willing to fight for their opinion, even against their preclinical colleagues in the industry (and in academies also for that matter).

I stress this point as I believe that not enough credit is given to the power of clinical observation during the development of new medicines. It is unfortunately possible that new important ways for the treatment of disease are never opened because evidence from the clinical use of new compounds has not been analyzed with the necessary open mind, or the responsible clinician has not been certain enough in his conduct of the initial trials of the new medicines. The message to the cardiologist is: use your clinical judgment, observe any and all effects when using new medicines, believe your own observations in sick patients, and avoid being overruled in this matter by preclinical studies in healthy animals, the result of which may be totally irrelevant to the clinical setting. It seems to be a safe bet that also in the future new therapies will originate from clinical research, especially if this can be conducted in close collaboration with biochemical, physiologic, and pharmacologic research in industry.

AS A PART-TIME OR FULL-TIME EMPLOYEE

To move from the status of outside consultant to become an employee of a pharmaceutical company is a drastic step. Even if it encompasses only part-time employment, the relations with both clinical colleagues, patients, and civil servants in the government are changing. This may be due partly to preconceived ideas about the industry and the way it will express its hold over the new employee; partly it reflects a real change in status. As an employee in a private, profit-oriented enterprise, its rules of conduct have to be followed which may be quite different from those relevant for a government employee (in hospital or outside) or for a physician deriving most of his income, if not all, from private practice.

The larger the companies, the more bureaucratic are the rules they have created to keep the increasing organization performing smoothly. Many physicians, especially those in countries with nationalized health services such as the United Kingdom and Sweden, believe that work in private business would mean fewer rules and more flexibility in their daily chores than in the public service. How wrong they are! On the contrary, private business with its orientation toward profit-generating work calculates on getting as much as possible out of the newly acquired specialist. Conversely, the manager of the private company has an important carrot to offer the new co-worker coming from academia or a hospital service: he can offer a salary that is commensurate with actual capability. However, as in all profit-oriented activities, the employer does not want to pay more than the value of what he gets, which means stricter control of activities, responsibilities, and general conduct in private industry compared with the public sector.

When it comes to the requirement for part-time or full-time employment in a pharmaceutical company, it is more difficult to give detailed advice. Different companies have different policies; some want to give a fair amount of internal education, whereas others are satisfied with university, academic, or other special outside education.

Frequently, what has started as an outside consultancy may end in more formal employment. The personal and scientific requirements are therefore similar to what has been described herein. One main difference may be that the status of an employee in a company further strengthens the requisite for absolute loyalty to the company and its more or less clearly defined goals. To be an employee in a pharmaceutical company may therefore encompass a greater risk for conflict between loyalty to the medical profession and loyalty to the commercial or other goals of a business organization. Such conflicts can always be easily handled by the adequately equipped, scientifically educated person. However, they may nevertheless put some strain on the person and probably also on his personal relations with other people inside and outside the enterprise. It is therefore necessary to give some thought to solving such conflicts before entering into an employer-employee relation with a member of the pharmaceutical industry. The better prepared one is, the better the long-term results will be for all parties involved.

CONTINUING MEDICAL EDUCATION

There is one activity in which the relation between a physician and the pharmaceutical industry has been rather extensively discussed and that is continuing medical education (CME). During the last years, more and more states and specialty organizations have required that a physician practicing as a specialist upgrade his knowledge within his specialty through special courses, symposia, and similar learning activities, ie, active participation in CME. At the same time, universities and medical schools have had few, if any, resources in their budgets for CME. To a large extent the increasing amount of CME that has appeared in the United States has been organized by specialty organizations such as the American College of Cardiology and the American College of Physicians, organizations with limited funds for such activities. A similar situation prevails in other countries. When public funds are lacking, it has seemed natural to ask the large pharmaceutical firms to help fund such activities in CME that might be of interest to them. There has been no difficulty in raising money this way, but the ethical question then arises: does the society or the physician "sell" his prescribing to the company that supports its CME or can he receive this monetary support without being caught in an ambiguous situation? This is an important question not at all typical only for the United States and not only for CME activity. It has therefore been discussed at length in many societies. The result of this discussion has not surprisingly been dependent upon who started the discussion and with what background it was entered.

One special feature of this CME is the funding of large international congresses. The International and Continental Congresses of Cardiology, now taking place every fourth year, have become very big enterprises with more than 10,000 active participants, lavish social programs, and meeting places often in countries with some tourist attraction. The scientific program, always of a high caliber, tends to become repetitive and the news value in these congresses for scientists working in the field is probably nil.

The value for continuing education may be greater, especially for those participants coming from scientifically less developed countries. Discussion is now going on in many quarters as to whether the resources—time and money—spent on this endeavor are properly used. However, both the medical profession and many other parties (not least of which are the travel and tourist industries) still seem to want to continue these meetings as long as they can be funded. This is where the pharmaceutical industry has to make up its mind. The main source of financial support, both for the congress as such (exhibitions, symposia, and round tables) and for the participant (travel support and sometimes fees for participation), comes from the different companies working with new therapies within the specific field. With the keen competition among the large research-oriented companies in the cardiovascular field, there has been no difficulty for the congress host to find sponsors willing to pay even millions of dollars. It is not absolutely clear, however, that this source of money will continue.[1] One reason is generally rising costs; another is the increasing criticism from different public media. The consumer organizations, now organized in Health Action International, specifically created to scrutinize the marketing methods of the pharmaceutical industry, especially its relation to physicians and their organizations, are increasing their scrutiny. Others are also critical. In a testimony before a senate subcommittee in the United States, Dr Richard Crout, then director of the Food and Drug Administration Bureau of Drugs, stated that "the growing influence of the pharmaceutical industry in medical education is a long-term threat to the integrity of the medical profession."[2] This probably still reflects the view of many regulators, even though the statement was made long ago (and Dr. Crout now has joined the industry). Rules that may curtail the possibility of funding large congresses may occur in governmental decrees, within medical professional organizations, or from the industry itself.

It is therefore important that the cardiologist plan to fund his own CME in the future. As long as the present arrangements continue with heavy subsidies from the pharmaceutical industry to many or all forms of CME, it is wise of the cardiologist always to contemplate what the American College of Physicians has stated in its Ethics Manual.

"The physician should avoid any business arrangement that might, because of personal gain, influence his decisions in patient care. Activities of physicians relating to the business aspects of his own or his group's practice should be guided by the principle that such activities be intended for the reasonable support of that practice and for the effective provision of quality care for patients. Similarly, activities relating to the provision and maintenance of research and education endeavours of his group or institution should be guided by the same principle."[3]

As I have tried to outline in this presentation, the research-oriented international pharmaceutical industry needs the cooperation of well-trained, clinically oriented physicians. It also offers interesting, meaningful, and challenging tasks for the therapeutically interested cardiologist. Work in or with the industry can therefore be recommended as long as the physician always remembers his responsibility to the patient as first spelled out in the Hippocratic oath.[4]

REFERENCES

1. Kaplan NM: The support of continuing medical education by pharmaceutical companies. *N Engl J Med* 1979; 300:194–196.
2. Hearings before the US Senate, Select Committee on Small Business, Subcommittee on Monopoly, April 28, May 10, and May 24, 1976. 94th Cong, 2nd sess (statement of JR Crout, Director, Food and Drug Administration, Bureau of Drugs).
3. Ad Hoc Committee on Medical Ethics of the American College of Physicians: American College of Physicians Ethics Manual. Part I. History of medical ethics, the physician and the patient, the physician's relationship to other physicians, the physicians and society. *Ann Intern Med* 1984; 101:129–137.
4. Relman AS: The new medical–industrial complex. *N Engl J Med* 1980; 303:963–970.

83 Medical Communications in Cardiology

Arthur M. Sackler, MD and Richard S. Gubner, MD, FACP

Communication in cardiology, as in all medicine, occurs at different levels, initially between cardiovascular researchers and cardiologists, then between cardiologists and primary care physicians, and ultimately between the medical profession, its patients, and the public. Each level involves a different mix in media and each tends to relate to the interests and needs of the target audience.

RANGE OF MEDICAL COMMUNICATIONS

Since the development of print from movable type, the medical journal (periodical in print) has been the medium of record in this as in other branches of science. In point of time, this was preceded by personal interchanges between teachers and scholars in the groves of academia. Regional, national, and international meetings are extensions of the traditional manner in which the earliest teachers of medicine in the Mediterranean Basin and on the Asiatic mainland communicated with scholars. Today, teaching lectures continue as a critical and basic form of communication of medical knowledge from physicians' first days in medical school, through their exposure to clinical medicine on ward rounds and to their mentor in the research laboratories, through their postgraduate and continuing medical education. With the development of electronic media, preceptors and scholars have entered what is now an expanding technology. Today, the marvels of the computer, fiber optics, and the satellite era promise to outstrip the most advanced audiovisual exchanges ever dreamed possible by the most imaginative of minds.

At medical meetings, the constraints of time and the volume of reports have led to the extension of collateral activities beyond plenary sessions and sections, beyond seminars and symposia, into scientific exhibits and poster sessions, which have become integral to most major meetings over the past four to five decades.

THE NEED FOR MORE AND BETTER MEDIA OF COMMUNICATIONS

The exponential growth of new clinical technologies, diagnostic modalities, pharmacotherapy, and cardiovascular surgery has forced a collateral development of specialty journals for interchanges between researchers, between cardiovascular clinicians and surgeons, and between them and specialists in other areas such as internal medicine and pediatrics. It has further led to a significant increase in cardiovascular reports appearing in major general medical as well as specialty medical journals. Thus far, most of the expansion of communication has occurred through traditional media, such as print and meetings (symposia, seminars, colloquia, congresses, etc). Although audiovisual and electronic media have begun to make their appearance, the major development of this field lies ahead.

MEDICAL COMMUNICATIONS BETWEEN PHYSICIANS AND PATIENTS

For cardiologic prophylaxis, diagnosis, and therapeutics, the patient and physician must be in communication. Living patterns and habits must be improved to prevent cardiovascular disease; early diagnosis is essential to assure the greatest potentials for beneficent intervention. For adjustments in life-style and physical status to be successful; dietaries to be changed; abuse of smoking, alcohol, and excess salt intake to be controlled; and compliance with medicinal regimens assured, patient education is essential.

For millennia, disease constituted a mystery. Empiric medicine developed at different rates in different societies, to a high level in China and the Middle East and to a lesser level on other continents. The medicine man and the doctor were authorities in societies that were authoritarian. With the development of the printing press, literacy began to spread throughout the world and with it the recognition of causality and interest in natural processes on the part of an increasingly educated public. By the 1930s the appetite for information on health subjects began to increase, as reflected in the growing frequency of articles on health and science in lay publications. The explosive interest in different aspects of disease is now reflected in a public that manifests as great an interest in exercise and physical activity and perhaps an even greater interest in the details of nutrition than do many in the medical professions. It is the rare magazine or newspaper that does not carry in each issue some story on health, medicine, diet, and exercise. The growing dominance of electronic media has markedly amplified the channels of communication in these areas. The public, which previously was exposed to its medical information either solely through the profession or in the schoolroom, is now immersed in an environment in which problems of health and disease are addressed with infinite repetition editorially, in advertising, and in public service messages in all media of communication— print, radio, and television— and the speed of communication is such that the patient may frequently hear of a new development at the same time his/her physician does. The physician/patient relationship, which from the earliest days of the medicine man through to the present remained critical to most diagnosis and therapeutics and to the maintenance of a healthy life-style, is now placing incredible demands on both the physician and the patient.

Relevant to the importance of physician/patient communication is a recent book whose title expresses the problem, *The Silent World of Doctor and Patient,* by Katz.[1] As stated by Hellerstein[2] in his review in *The Sciences,* "The problem in medicine may indeed be a failure to communicate. . . . Medicine is filled with unnecessary mystery and mystification. Patients are enjoined to speak up for their rights, to ask questions, to challenge the doctor's advice. Doctors are told to explain procedures, to detail the side effects of drugs, to quantify the risk of operations . . . [contrasting with] the tradition of unquestioning compliance, and the patient's acquiescence in the physician's decision. . . ." Informed consent involving explicit communication between physician and patient expressing benefits, risks, and uncertainties is becoming an obligatory aspect of the physician/patient relationship.

INTERNATIONALIZATION OF THE MEDICAL PRESS

The internationalization of the medical press is a rather recent event. Only 25 years ago the development of a physician's newspaper format made the greatest breakthrough in truly internationalizing medical news. The establishment of *Medical Tribune,* which first took place in the United States, led to its companion publications in Germany and France as well as England. A world network of correspondents was developed, followed by the establishment of a medical news syndicated network. Today, with offices in eight countries, a newspaper for physicians, *Medical Tribune,* appears in seven languages, reaching physicians in over 20 countries. It is truly international in coverage as well as in language. The staffs of physicians, editors, writers, and other specialists are indigenous to their countries. In China, Japan, and Korea in the Far East; in German-speaking countries in Europe (Germany, Austria, and Switzerland); as well as in Italy, France, England, and the United States, national and regional offices process medical news from abroad for their countries and in return report medical events in *their* country to their fellow publications abroad. Such internationalization has not occurred in comparable measure in more highly specialized journals. It is, however, reflected through satellite transmission and wire news services in presenting news of medicine to the lay public.

MEDICAL COMMUNICATIONS AND MODERN CARDIOLOGY

"A Brief Outline of the 350 Years Prelude to an Explosive Growth" is the subtitle of the *History of Cardiology.*[3] Such "explosive growth," which is aptly stated, may be considered to have begun in the immediate post–World War II period. Medical communication and growth in cardiology have been synergistically interrelated, each reflecting and fostering the development of the other.

During the 1930s, the *American Heart Journal* appeared every second month, sufficing for clinical studies, which comprised the greater number of papers published, largely from those presented at the modestly attended annual meeting of the American Heart Association. A rapidly burgeoning succession of publications followed soon after the war. The *American Heart Journal* became a monthly publication and has continued vigorously until the present, although the American Heart Association left its publisher and began *Circulation* as its official monthly organ. This too proved inadequate for the steadily increasing stream of new reports. In addition to its briefer publications, *Modern Concepts of Cardiovascular Diseases* and the *Heart Bulletin, Circulation Research, Hypertension,* and *Stroke* all followed as major journals under the aegis of the American Heart Association. Additionally, the several Councils of the American Heart Association undertook to publish sizable newsletters, such as the Councils on Epidemiology and on Thrombosis. An overt expression of how the American Heart Association has grown to its present gigantic size is reflected in the annual October supplement of *Circulation* containing the abstracts of nearly 2,000 papers presented at the November meeting. The development of the American College of Cardiology is equally illustrative of the growth of cardiology.

When Hitler and his Nazis brutally throttled the arts and sciences, first in Germany and then in Austria in the 1938 Anschluss, there was mass emigration of those in the arts, sciences, and academia who foresaw their work and themselves threatened with suppression and extinction. The United States was the principal haven for these refugees. In New York, the New School for Social Research became literally a university in exile where distinguished scholars in all fields assembled and taught, many then moving on to other academic posts in their new country. This exodus and resettlement have recently been described in a book, *The Muses Flee Hitler.*[4]

Equally so in cardiology, eminent physicians sought

refuge in the United States, particularly in New York. New York State was hospitable in granting licensure to practice medicine, but universities and well-established cardiologists were less cordial initially. In measure, this was responsible for the formation of a society of predominantly Viennese and German cardiologists, joining with the New York Cardiologic Society. Spearheaded by Franz Maximilian Groedel of Bad Nauheim, a spa renowned then as now for its focus on cardiovascular disease, this group comprised such European luminaries as David Scherf, Wilhelm Dressler, Bruno Kisch, Professors Loewi and Pick, with a few such as Hugo Roesler and Wilhelm Raab finding their way to new posts in Philadelphia and Vermont, respectively. All of these had made and continued to make important research contributions. This was the nidus of the American College of Cardiology, soon complemented after the war by well-known American cardiologists such as Ashton Graybiel, Simon Dack, and others. *The American Journal of Cardiology,* under Simon Dack's editorship, soon followed, and the membership and readership had an explosive growth. Eventually, the American College of Cardiology parted ways from its publisher, as had the American Heart Association, and began its own monthly journal, the *Journal of the American College of Cardiology. The American Journal of Cardiology,* meanwhile, has continued as an independent vigorous monthly journal with a new editorial board.

A host of publications, either society organs, such as *Angiology* (American College of Angiology), *The Journal of Heart Transplantation* (International Society of Heart Transplantation), *Chest* (American College of Chest Physicians), or numerous independent journals and newsletters followed. Today, the practicing cardiologist is literally overwhelmed with cardiovascular literature, to which may be added the very substantial proportion of articles on cardiovascular topics in all the journals and newsletters he receives, together with an endless profusion of books, all reflecting the enormous growth of cardiovascular medicine and surgery.

Even more important in magnitude than the volume of cardiologic literature is the overwhelming size of the annual conventions of the American Heart Association in November and the American College of Cardiology in March, limiting consideration to these two organizations alone, although there are hosts of other meetings in the United States and abroad. Both these giant organizations each attract some 15,000 participants at their annual meetings, greater in number than any other medical meetings of whatever specialty.

Manifestly, it is impossible for any single physician to attend more than a few of the many concurrent sessions at the American Heart Association, American College of Cardiology, or World Congress of Cardiology. A welcome expansion in the format of these conventions, and indeed in all large medical meetings today, has been the advent of poster sessions. In these, each author has a poster space exhibiting his/her abstract for a limited period where he can be sought out and queried by those attending, whereas this is impossible in a 10- or 15-minute presentation, or longer, in large assembly halls where "plenary sessions" are attended by hundreds or more.

A tacit indication of how the enormous volume of medical literature has changed the method of presentation not only in cardiologic literature but in all fields of medicine is the now universal custom of placing summaries, often in heavy type, heading up the article rather than at its end. It has become akin to window-shopping. If the exterior appears of interest, one enters to browse or look seriously; otherwise, it is passed by.

Another change in medical literature, still the primary vehicle of communication, is the number of authors participating in a report. In former years, a single author-researcher was the rule rather than the exception, occasionally with one or two coauthors. Currently, multiple authorship is the rule.* Individual creative research, responsible for so many medical advances, hopefully will continue, but evidently today research is a multi-scientist effort requiring expensive technology and cooperative specialized expertise.

A further trend in medical research and communication is indicated by an analysis, not only of authorship, but also of sources of the studies, such as those in the May 1985 issue of *The American Journal of Cardiology.* Among the 51 articles, it is of interest that 18 derive from fully 12 countries other than the United States. It might appear from this that medical communication is truly international. Unfortunately, such is not the case, as is shown by review of the bibliographic references of both American and foreign articles in this issue. Provincialism, if not outright xenophobia, is most conspicuous among American contributors. Excepting short articles and case reports, which average six references, the major articles by United States and foreign authors range from 7 to 54 references, averaging 20. Only 8 of the 33 articles deriving from United States institutions have any references to foreign sources (excepting British and Canadian journals). All foreign sources quoted are in English, except a single reference to a 1929 study by the eminent French cardiologist, Gallavardin. The very few foreign references are principally to journals whose articles are published in English, such as the *European Heart Journal* and the *Japanese Heart Journal.*†

INTERNATIONALIZATION OF CARDIOPHARMACOLOGY; PROVINCIALISM OTHERWISE

Pharmacologic developments are more internationalized than are developments in other fields of cardiology because so many new drugs are often first developed and tested in countries around the world before being sanctioned by the Food and Drug Administration for mar-

* In the May 1985 issue of the *American Journal of Cardiology,* now an independent nonsociety-related publication, there are 51 articles. None has a single author, and joint authorships range from 2 to 11, the most frequent number being 4 and 5 joint coauthors.

† It is of interest that among the 18 articles from outside the United States published in the May 1985 issue of *The American Journal of Cardiology,* there is also a great preponderance of references to the American (and British) medical literature. The very few exceptions, from whatever country, are also to articles in English in the *European Heart Journal, International Journal of Cardiology,* and *Japanese Heart Journal,* with a few references to pharmacologic journals in countries other than the United States.

keting in the United States. Accordingly, this is a particularly important area of international communication in cardiology.

One is left with the conclusion that English is the predominant language of communication in recent cardiologic literature, as judged not only by the overwhelming preponderance of bibliographic references to United States and British sources and not only by American but foreign investigators as well. However, what is equally evident is the provincialism of American authors in their almost exclusive references to American (and British) literature, allowing no alternative explanation other than that literature search of foreign research is not carried out despite ready availability through the *Index Medicus* and other literature search sources.

An overt illustration of the practice of authors to refer in their bibliographic references to their countrymen's literature (as well as to their own previous reports) is illustrated in a two-part chapter in *Progress in Cardiology* (edited by Paul N. Yu of Rochester, NY and John F. Goodwin of London, England, vol 10, Lea & Febiger, 1981). Part I of the chapter on Future Trends in Cardiovascular Surgery is by Charles Dubost, Professor and Chief of Cardiovascular Surgery at Hopital Broussals, Université Curie, Paris, France, and part II by David C. Sabiston, Jr, Professor and Chairman of Surgery at Duke University, Durham, North Carolina. Dubost's 22-page contribution has 14 references, of which 12 are to French authors, including seven of his own studies, and 2 to American authors writing in the American journal *Surgery*. Sabiston's part II of this chapter, which is of equal length, has 73 references, 2 German, 2 French, and 1 to Barnard's pioneer report on cardiac transplantation in the *South African Medical Journal* in 1967. The remaining references, 68 in number, are to American sources.

A different and far greater international perspective in communication is offered by the journal *Clinical Cardiology*, published in English, but with a distinguished editorial board comprising cardiologists from 22 countries. The May 1985 issue contains four articles from the United States, two from Italy, and also some from Norway and New Zealand. The preceding issue (April 1985) contains nine articles, with three contributions from the United States, three from Japan, and one each from West Germany, Australia, and England.

It is worthy of note that represented on the editorial board of *Clinical Cardiology* are E. I. Chazov of Moscow (who has contributed a chapter to this volume) and Z. Fejfar of Prague. Both are widely known to cardiologists of western Europe and the United States. Recently there was published (1984) a massive two-volume text, *Cardiology: An International Perspective.*[5] It is hoped that this will help bridge the gap between East and West. A notable opening of dialogue between American cardiologists and Professor Chazov and others in the USSR was made by Dr Bernard Lown of Harvard. Such meetings as the International Conference on Preventive Cardiology in Moscow in 1985, immediately following the Interamerican Congress of Cardiology in Vancouver, BC, Canada, reflect an internationalism in cardiologic communication, and it would be salutary to have their proceedings widely disseminated to foster international awareness and cooperation. Also worthy of note is the X World Congress of Cardiology in 1986 in Washington, DC.

Dr Fejfar of Prague was exemplary in promoting international communication in cardiology during his tenure in charge of cardiovascular disease at the World Health Organization. The writers, who participated, recall his very effective chairing of an international conference on preventive cardiology in the 1970s, which was held in Madrid under the auspices of the World Health Organization, sponsored by the International Medical Tribune.

INTERNATIONAL EPIDEMIOLOGIC CARDIOVASCULAR STUDIES

Thus far, such communication as has developed in cardiology internationally has been principally in the area of epidemiology, such as the seven-country study headed by Keys,[6] demonstrating that differences in diet, with accompanying differences in serum cholesterol, have important bearing on coronary heart disease morbidity and mortality. Among those participating with Keys and his associate, Henry Blackburn of the University of Minnesota, were such figures as Paul Dudley White of the United States, Kimura of Japan, Karvonen of Finland, Puddu of Italy, and others of similar eminence in their countries.

Two valuable epidemiologic studies from China may be cited. One from the Beijing Heart, Lung and Blood Vessel Medical Center by Wu et al[7] emphasizes that cardiovascular disease has recently become a major health problem in China, with doubling of the mortality rate in the brief period 1958 to 1979. The authors stress that, "Further development of international exchange and collaboration in cardiovascular epidemiology will be emphasized in the coming years." In another study from the Shanghai Sixth People's Hospital, by Tung et al,[8] it was similarly noted that in a study of over 25,000 patients with heart disease admitted to three general hospitals in Shanghai in the years 1948 to 1979, analysis showed a remarkable near fivefold rise in the relative proportions of ischemic heart disease from the first period (1948 to 1958) to the third period (1972 to 1979). The increase is attributed to the same factors that have been implicated in the western world, ie, an increase in cigarette smoking and in the consumption of saturated fat in pork and other meats, and of eggs, with a significant rise in serum cholesterol and other lipids.

Other international studies recently reported in the *New England Journal of Medicine* by Kromhout et al[9] of Leiden, Netherlands, as well as two further studies[10,11] and an editorial[12] in the same issue emphasize the importance of diet in coronary heart disease mortality. Significantly lower mortality is found in populations with high fish consumption, the fish oil eicosapentanoic acid possessing the salutary property of decreasing platelet aggregation involved in the initial phase of thrombosis. These observations confirm those originally made on Greenland Eskimos, who have a very low occurrence of ischemic heart disease. The important conclusion is drawn by Kromhout et al[9] that consumption of as little as one or two fish dishes per week may confer some protection against coronary heart disease. Two other studies and an accompanying editorial in the *New England Journal of Medicine* further stress the significance of blood lipids in coronary disease. One is that of Arntzenius et al,[13] also of Leiden, Netherlands. The other, by Kushi et al,[14] is the Ireland-Boston Diet Heart Study representing a joint undertaking by the Department of Nutrition, Harvard School of Public Health, and the Department of Preventive Cardiology and Department of Community Medicine and Epidemiology, Trinity College, Dublin. The foregoing all reflect a broad international approach in cardiovascular research.

DEPARTMENTALIZED SPECIALTIES IN CARDIOLOGY

When cardiology began its explosive growth immediately after World War II, referred to earlier, there were no or very few such departmental disciplines as cardiovascular epidemiology, nutrition, and community medicine and certainly no preventive cardiology. It is evident that apart from the great strides made possible by newer technology, including surgery, in the conquest of cardiovascular disease (creating numerous subspecialties in cardiovascular disease), cooperative international studies have made major contributions to the control and prevention of heart disease. Communication is the lifeline of such progress, and it is to be hoped that increasing international efforts and communication in cardiology will further promote health, understanding, and amity among nations. A macabre but useful example of international communication is the recently published volume, *The Cold and the Dark: The World After Nuclear War.*[15] This derived from a congress of some 100 physical and biologic scientists, followed by a conference, jointly sponsored by 31 scientific organizations held in Washington, DC. A two-way live satellite link with Soviet scientists in Moscow, following the Washington Conference, resulted in a general consensus and in the establishment of a new educational center on nuclear war. Medicine, which has no aims but peaceful ones, can and should take examples from such international communication.*

CONTINUITY IN MEDICAL COMMUNICATIONS

The continuity of man's probing the mysteries of disease is reflected in the manner in which different societies have addressed the problems of its control. The magnum opus of Joseph Needham, *Science and Civilization in China,*[16] provides a great panoramic view of the subject even as the publications of Vesalius and Malpighi, Harvey and Hunter, Helmholtz and Virchow, and Claude Bernard and Pasteur presented the classic communications of pioneers in medical research. Cardiology as an essential part of medicine, and medicine as an essential part of science, society, and life, must reflect in its communications within countries and beyond the boundaries of countries and continents the ultimate role of the physician. The goal of that role is probably most succinctly expressed by the immortal Pasteur who, at the inauguration of his Institute in 1888, used the occasion to communicate his conviction as to the unique mission of science:

> *"Two opposing laws seem to me now in contest. The one, a law of blood and death, opening out each day new modes of destruction, forces nations to be always ready for the battle. The other, a law of peace, work and health, whose only aim is to deliver man from the calamities which beset him. The one seeks violent conquests, the other the relief of mankind. The one places a single life above all victories, the other sacrifices hundreds of thousands of lives to the ambition of a single individual. . . . Science, in obeying the law of humanity, will always labour to enlarge the frontiers of life."*[17]

* The organization called International Physicians for the Prevention of Nuclear War, of which Lown and Chazov were cofounders, received the 1985 Nobel Peace Prize.

REFERENCES

1. Katz J: *The Silent World of Doctor and Patient.* New York, The Free Press, 1984.
2. Hellerstein D: Bedside manners. *The Sciences* 1984; 24:53–54.
3. Snellen HA: *History of Cardiology: A Brief Outline of the 350 Years Prelude to an Explosive Growth.* Rotterdam, Douker Publications, 1984.
4. Jackman JC, Borden CM (eds): *The Muses Flee Hitler.* Washington, DC, Smithsonian Institution Press, 1983.
5. Chazov EJ, Smirnov VN (eds): *Cardiology: An International Perspective.* New York, Plenum Press, 1984.
6. Keys A, Menotti A, Aravanis C, Blackburn H, Djordevic BS, Buzina R, Dontas AS, Fidanza F, Karvonen MJ, Kimura N: The seven countries study: 2289 deaths in 15 years. *Prev Med* 1984; 96:141–154.
7. Wu YK, Wu ZS, Yao CH: Epidemiologic studies of cardiovascular diseases in China. *Chin Med J* 1983; 96:201–205.
8. Tung CL, Chen WC, Liang SP, Pan SR, Xue W: A reappraisal of the changing proportion of the various types of heart diseases in Shanghai and its relationship to serum cholesterol levels. *Chin Med J* 1984; 97: 171–174.
9. Kromhout D, Bosschieter EB, Coulander CL: The inverse relation between fish consumption and 20-year mortality from coronary heart disease. *N Engl J Med* 1985; 312:1205–1209.
10. Phillipson BE, Rothrock DW, Connor WE, Harris WS, Illingworth DR: Reduction of plasma lipids, lipoproteins, and apoproteins by dietary fish oils in patients with hypertriglyceridemia. *N Engl J Med* 1985; 312:1210–1216.
11. Lee TH, Hoover RL, Williams JD, Sperling RI, Ravalese J, Spur BW, Robinson DR, Corey EJ, Lewis RA, Austen KF: Effect of dietary enrichment with eicosapentaenoic and docosahexaenoic acids on in vitro neutrophil and monocyte leukotriene generation and neutrophil function. *N Engl J Med* 1985; 312:1217–1224.
12. Glomset JA: Fish, fatty acids, and human health. *N Engl J Med* 1985; 312: 1253–1254.
13. Arntzenius AC, Kromhout D, Barth JD, Reiber JHC, Bruschke AVG, Buis B, van Gent CM, Kempen-Voogd N, Strikwerda S, van der Velde EA: Diet, lipoproteins, and the progression of coronary atherosclerosis: the Leiden intervention trial. *N Engl J Med* 1985; 312:805–811.
14. Kushi LH, Lew RA, Stare FJ, Ellison CR, el Lozy M, Bourke G, Daly L, Graham I, Hickey N, Mulcahy R, Kevaney J: Diet and 20-year mortality from coronary heart disease: the Ireland–Boston diet heart study. *N Engl J Med* 1985; 312:811–818.
15. Ehrlich P, Sagan C, Kennedy D, Roberts WR, Thomas L: *The Cold and the Dark: The World After Nuclear War.* New York, WW Norton, 1984.
16. Needham J: *Science and Civilization in China.* London, New York, Cambridge University Press, 1954–1984, vols I–VI.
17. Pasteur L (entry): *Encyclopedia Britannica.* Chicago, Encyclopedia Britannica, Inc, 1956, vol 17, p 359.

Index

Note: Page numbers preceded by *f* or *t* indicate figures or tables.

About the Editor

Tsung O. Cheng, M.D., M.S. (Med) is a Professor of Medicine at The George Washington University School of Medicine and Health Sciences, Washington, D.C. Born in Shanghai, China where he was graduated from the University of Pennsylvania School of Medicine at the St. John's University, Dr. Cheng came to the United States and completed his graduate training at the University of Pennsylvania, Northwestern University, Harvard Medical School, and Johns Hopkins University. Before moving to Washington, D.C., he was on the faculty of the State University of New York Downstate Medical Center, Brooklyn, New York. He was a student of Drs. Paul D. White, Isadore Snapper and William Dock.

He is board certified in both internal medicine and cardiovascular disease, and a Fellow of the American College of Physicians, American College of Cardiology, American College of Chest Physicians, American College of Angiology, International College of Angiology, and Society for Cardiac Angiography. His special interests, in addition to cardiac catheterization, coronary artery spasm and mitral valve prolapse, include geographic cardiology and international medicine.

Dr. Cheng was the first Chinese-American physician to visit China in 1972 following renewal of friendly relations between the United States and the People's Republic of China. Since then he has been a guest lecturer of the Chinese Medical Association, Chinese Ministry of Health, making numerous return visits to China for exchange of medical and cardiological information. In 1983 he received the honor of being appointed the Visiting Professor at the Shanghai Second Medical University, Shanghai, China.

Dr. Cheng, in addition to his close to 300 publications on cardiovascular disease and international medicine including contributions to three books, is a senior editor of *Vascular Medicine*, an associate editor of *Angiology*, and a peer reviewer for such journals as *American Heart Journal*, *American Journal of Cardiology*, *Angiology*, *Annals of Internal Medicine*, *Catheterization and Cardiovascular Diagnosis*, *Chest*, *Circulation*, *Investigative Radiology*, *Journal of the American Medical Association*, and the *New England Journal of Medicine*. He is listed in *Who's Who in America*, *Who's Who in the World*, *American Men and Women of Science*, and *Dictionary of International Biography*.